OXFORD MEDICAL PUBLICATIONS

Oxford Textbook of Medicine

 KT-229-166

Oxford
Textbook of
Medicine

Edited by

D. J. Weatherall
Nuffield Professor of Clinical Medicine, University of Oxford

J. G. G. Ledingham
May Reader in Medicine, Nuffield Department of Clinical Medicine, University of Oxford

D. A. Warrell
*Director, Wellcome–Mahidol University, Oxford Tropical Medicine Programme,
Faculty of Tropical Medicine, Bangkok, Thailand
Wellcome Reader in Tropical Medicine, Nuffield Department of Clinical Medicine,
University of Oxford*

VOLUME 1
Sections 1–12

Oxford New York Toronto
OXFORD UNIVERSITY PRESS
1983

Oxford University Press, Walton Street, Oxford OX2 6DP

London Glasgow New York Toronto
Delhi Bombay Calcutta Madras Karachi
Kuala Lumpur Singapore Hong Kong Tokyo
Nairobi Dar es Salaam Cape Town
Melbourne Auckland
and associates in
Beirut Berlin Ibadan Mexico City Nicosia

Oxford is a trade mark of Oxford University Press

© D. J. Weatherall, J. G. G. Ledingham, and D. A. Warrell 1983

Published in the United States by
Oxford University Press Inc., New York

All rights reserved. No part of this publication may be reproduced,
stored in a retrieval system, or transmitted, in any form or by any means,
electronic, mechanical, photocopying, recording, or otherwise, without
the prior permission of Oxford University Press

This book is sold subject to the condition that it shall not, by way
of trade or otherwise, be lent, re-sold, hired out or otherwise circulated
without the publisher's prior consent in any form of binding or cover
other than that in which it is published and without a similar condition
including this condition being imposed on the subsequent purchaser

British Library Cataloguing in Publication Data
Oxford textbook of medicine.—(Oxford medical
publications)
1. Pathology   2. Medicine
I. Weatherall, D. J.   II. Ledingham, J. G. G.
III. Warrell, D. A.
616   RB111
ISBN 0-19-261159-3

Set by Western Printing Services Ltd
Printed in the United States of America

Preface

The *Oxford Textbook of Medicine* is the reincarnation of 'Price' which, after 60 years as the major British postgraduate textbook of medicine, has been laid to rest by the Oxford University Press. The first edition of a *Textbook of the Practice of Medicine (including Sections on Diseases of the Skin and Psychological Medicine)* edited by Frederick Price was published in 1922. There were 26 contributors, all from London teaching hospitals. The book was updated roughly every four years up to the ninth edition (1957); for the tenth edition (1966) Sir Ronald Bodley Scott took over as editor. The last (twelfth) edition was published in 1978. Sir Ronald did much to modernize and expand the book during his time as editor and it is sad to record that his tragic death in an accident in 1982 prevented his seeing its successor.

When Sir Ronald Bodley Scott retired as editor of 'Price' in 1978, Oxford University Press approached us with the idea of producing a completely new textbook to replace it. This was a daunting proposal. There were several excellent American postgraduate textbooks of medicine already available and the undergraduate was well served on both sides of the Atlantic. Furthermore, although many of the reviewers of the twelfth edition of 'Price' were quite complimentary, others raised doubts about whether there was a place in the 1980s for a general textbook of medicine of its size and scope. Among the most critical reviews was a characteristically acerbic piece by J. R. A. Mitchell. After weighing the book he reminded us that dinosaurs became extinct because of their sheer bulk. 'Price' would suffer the same fate; it could not be lifted and therefore it could not be read! In addition, Professor Mitchell and other reviewers voiced the often-heard criticism that big textbooks are out of date before they are published, and suggested that smaller paperback textbooks, together with occasional forays into specialist monographs, provide the most economical and accessible guidance for students and general practitioners, while postgraduates are best served by specialist monographs and up-to-date review journals.

After considering these arguments very carefully we came to the conclusion that there is still an important role for a larger textbook of medicine. Certainly, the basic and clinical sciences are moving so fast that no textbook of medicine can hope to be absolutely up to date. However, relatively few of the advances in these fields lead to major changes in patient-care, and those that do require several years of critical evaluation before they become an integral part of routine clinical practice. Although we agree that the specialist monograph is often the best source of information in any particular area of medicine, the very breadth of the subject and the tendency to overspecialization means that few students and practitioners have immediate access to monographs on every branch of the subject, and even when they are available they are not always written by clinicians who are used to evaluating their patients in a general medical setting. Another reason for retaining at least a few broadly based textbooks of medicine is that medical practice varies very much in different parts of the world. Although it is important for students and practitioners to appreciate these differences as part of their general education, there is a more pragmatic reason for stressing this aspect of modern medicine. With increasing international travel and massive movement of refugee populations no practitioner can be sure that he will not be expected to deal with diseases with which he is unfamiliar and which may present in a variety of unexpected ways. The steadily rising number of deaths from malaria in the United Kingdom in the last few years is just one example of this new phenomenon.

Thus we believe that the rapid expansion of knowledge, increasing specialization, and the blossoming of narrow specialist monographs have, if anything, strengthened the case for the general reference book. Therefore we have attempted to produce a reference book of internal medicine which we hope will reflect current British practice, but which also includes the views of an international group of authors. We have also tried to present some of the problems of clinical practice in the developing countries and to describe how the pattern of disease varies in different parts of the world. We have included some background chapters describing how some of the important basic clinical sciences such as microbiology, genetics, immunology, epidemiology, and oncology are contributing to an understanding of the pathogenesis of the diseases which are described in the book. With Professor Mitchell's criticisms of 'Price' in mind, we have remembered the frail and divided the book into two volumes.

For whom is this book intended? The short answer is anyone who is studying or practising clinical medicine. Our overall aim has been to provide a bird's eye view of the subject; the book is designed primarily for general practitioners and specialists as a first reference source. In addition, we hope that it will provide medical students and postgraduates with an adequate guide to the more important clinical disorders and point them in the right direction when looking up the rarities. It is an impossible task to produce a balanced reference book of general medicine first time round and we are only too aware of the shortcomings of our first effort. However, we hope that we have laid a basis on which future editions can develop a more mature and balanced view of this increasingly complicated field.

We cannot acknowledge everyone who has helped us in this enterprise. Several of the major sections were planned with a sub-editor. These are: Nutrition: Dr Roger Smith; Reproductive medicine: Dr C. W. G. Redman; Gastroenterology: Dr D. P. Jewell; Cardiology: Dr D. G. Gibson; Respiratory disease: Dr D. J. Lane; Neurology: Professor W. B. Matthews; Psychiatry: Professor M. G. Gelder. We were cajoled into this impossible task by Richard Charkin of Oxford University Press. His colleagues at the Press, particularly Alison Langton, Nicholas Dunton, and Christopher Riches have managed to see it to a conclusion despite innumerable difficulties caused by errant authors and a typesetting process which, in the best traditions of an ancient University, persisted in producing sections of the book in ancient Greek. On a more personal note we take particular pleasure in acknowledging the help of our secretaries, Janet Watt, Jenny Stephens, Jeanne Packer, Sheila Hatton, Judith Last, Jacqueline Teodorczyx, Eunice Berry, and Patchari Prakongpan. Finally, we are happy to record that the marriages of the three editors have survived the production of this book; the forbearance of our wives during its difficult gestation is the major reason for its ever seeing the light of day.

Oxford, August 1982

D. J. WEATHERALL
J. G. G. LEDINGHAM
D. A. WARRELL

While every effort has been made to check drug dosages in this book, it is still possible that errors have been missed. Furthermore, dosage schedules are being continually revised and new side-effects recognized. For these reasons the reader is strongly urged to consult the drug companies' printed instructions before administering any of the drugs recommended in this book.

Contents

List of contributors   xiii

Section 1. On textbooks and medicine *A. M. Cooke*   1.3

Section 2. Health and sickness in the community
M. J. Goldacre and *M. P. Vessey*   2.3

Section 3. Medicine in an unjust world *M. H. King*   3.3

Section 4. Genetics, immunology, and neoplasia
Genetic factors in disease *D. A. Price Evans*   4.1
Molecular genetics in clinical medicine
   D. J. Weatherall   4.20
Immune mechanisms in health and sickness
   E. J. Holborow   4.28
Neoplasia   4.46
   General characteristics of neoplasia *H. Harris*   4.46
   Epidemiology of cancer *R. Doll* and *R. Peto*   4.51
   Medical aspects of neoplasia *D. A. G. Galton*   4.79
     The causation of neoplasia: medical aspects   4.79
     Metabolic effects of neoplasms (paraneoplastic
     syndromes)   4.82
     Chemotherapy of malignant disease   4.87

Section 5. Infections
The host response to infection *B. M. Greenwood*   5.3
Epidemiology and public health *A. B. Christie*   5.12
Physiological changes in infected patients
   P. A. Murphy   5.19
Principles of antimicrobial therapy *A. Percival*   5.23
Practical aspects of antimicrobial chemotherapy
   Mary P. E. Slack   5.30
Specific infectious agents   5.44
   Viruses   5.44
     Respiratory viruses *J. Nagington* and
     D. Rubenstein   5.44
     The herpesviruses *B. E. Juel-Jensen*   5.49
     Varicella–zoster virus infections: chickenpox and
     zoster *B. E. Juel-Jensen*   5.57
     Infectious mononucleosis: Epstein–Barr virus
     disease *B. E. Juel-Jensen*   5.61
     Infections caused by simian herpesviruses
     B. E. Juel-Jensen   5.64
     Cytomegalovirus infection *J. O'H. Tobin*   5.65
     Poxviruses *K. R. Dumbell*   5.68
     Paramyxoviruses
      Mumps: epidemic parotitis *A. B. Christie*   5.73
      Measles *W. C. Marshall*   5.76
      Rubella *J. O'H. Tobin*   5.80
     Enteroviruses *N. R. Grist*   5.82
     Stool viruses *C. R. Madeley*   5.90
     Rhabdoviruses: rabies and rabies-related viruses
     D. A. Warrell   5.93
     Alphaviruses *D. I. H. Simpson*   5.99
     Flaviviruses *D. I. H. Simpson*   5.101
     Bunyaviridae *J. S. Porterfield*   5.105

     Arenaviruses *D. I. H. Simpson* and
     E. T. W. Bowen   5.112
     Hepatitis viruses *A. J. Zuckerman*   5.116
     Tumour viruses *R. A. Weiss*   5.123
     Marburg and Ebola fevers *E. T. W. Bowen* and
     D. I. H. Simpson   5.127
     Slow virus encephalopathies *W. B. Matthews*   5.130
     Papovaviruses *S. D. Gardner*   5.131
   Bacteria   5.133
     Diphtheria *A. B. Christie*   5.133
     Pathogenic streptococci *M. T. Parker*   5.137
     Pneumococcal infection *B. M. Greenwood*   5.149
     Staphylococci *I. Phillips* and *S. J. Eykyn*   5.158
     Meningococcal infection *B. M. Greenwood*   5.165
     Enterobacteria and miscellaneous entero-
     pathogenic and food-poisoning bacteria
     M. B. Skirrow   5.174
     Typhoid and paratyphoid fevers *E. B. Adams*   5.183
     Anaerobic bacteria *S. J. Eykyn* and *I. Phillips*   5.189
     Cholera *C. C. J. Carpenter*   5.195
     Haemophilus *D. C. Turk*   5.198
     Bordetella *C. C. Linnemann, Jr.*   5.203
     Plague *A. B. Christie*   5.205
     Tularaemia, glanders, and melioidosis
     R. G. Mitchell   5.210
     Yersiniosis *N. S. Mair*   5.213
     Anthrax *A. B. Christie*   5.217
     Brucellosis *E. Williams*   5.221
     Tetanus *E. B. Adams*   5.226
     Botulism, gas gangrene, and clostridium
     gastrointestinal infections *H. E. Larson*   5.230
     Tuberculosis *K. M. Citron* and *D. J. Girling*   5.237
     Particular problems of tuberculosis in
     developing countries *M. Aquinas* and
     D. Todd   5.262
     Leprosy *M. F. R. Waters*   5.266
     Mycobacterium ulcerans infection
     M. F. R. Waters   5.273
     Actinomycosis *R. G. Mitchell*   5.274
     Nocardiasis *R. G. Mitchell*   5.276
     Spirochaetes   5.277
      Syphilis *G. W. Csonka*   5.277
      Rat bite fevers *D. A. Warrell*   5.293
      Borrelia infections *D. A. Warrell*   5.293
      Leptospirosis *V. Sitprija*   5.297
      Non-venereal treponemes: yaws, endemic
      syphilis, and pinta *P. L. Perine*   5.301
     Granuloma inguinale *P. L. Perine*   5.303
     Chancroid *P. L. Perine*   5.305
     Lymphogranuloma venereum *P. L. Perine*   5.307
     Gonorrhoea *G. W. Csonka*   5.309
     Genital candidiasis *G. W. Csonka*   5.314
     Clinical approach to non-gonococcal urethritis
     (NGU) *G. W. Csonka*   5.315
     Clinical approach to pelvic inflammatory disease
     (PID) *G. W. Csonka*   5.319

Contents

Venereologist's approach to Reiter's disease
G. W. Csonka — 5.321

Venereologist's approach to herpes simplex
infections G. W. Csonka — 5.327

Listeria Rosalind Hurley — 5.329

Legionnaires' disease J. O'H. Tobin — 5.331

Rickettsial diseases T. E. Woodward — 5.334

Chlamydial infections S. Darougar,
M. A. Monnickendam, and J. D. Treharne — 5.346

Mycoplasmas D. Taylor-Robinson — 5.355

Bartonellosis D. A. Warrell — 5.361

'Newer' and lesser known organisms causing
infection in man R. G. Mitchell — 5.362

Fungal infections (mycoses) R. J. Hay and
D. W. R. Mackenzie — 5.369

Protozoa — 5.384

Amoebic infections R. Knight — 5.384

Malaria L. H. Miller — 5.393

Pneumocystis carinii W. T. Hughes — 5.399

Toxoplasmosis W. Kwantes — 5.400

Giardiasis, balantidiasis, sacrocystosis, and
isosporiasis S. G. Wright — 5.404

African trypanosomiasis B. M. Greenwood — 5.406

American trypanosomiasis: Chagas' disease
P. D. Marsden — 5.410

Leishmaniasis P. E. C. Manson-Bahr — 5.412

Trichomoniasis G. W. Csonka — 5.417

Babesia T. K. Ruebush II — 5.419

Nematodes —

Filarial infections and diseases B. O. L. Duke — 5.420

Guinea worm disease (dracunculiasis,
dracontiasis) B. O. L. Duke — 5.427

Hookworm and strongyloides P. A. J. Ball — 5.428

Pathogenic, free-living nematodes P. A. J. Ball — 5.432

Other gut nematodes V. Zaman — 5.432

Toxocara and visceral larva migrans D. R. Bell
and M. J. Clarkson — 5.437

Angiostrongyliasis S. Punyagupta — 5.438

Gnathostomiasis P. Suntharasamai — 5.440

Cestodes — 5.442

Hydatid disease A. J. Radford — 5.442

Gut cestodes V. Zaman — 5.444

Diphyllobothriasis and sparganosis S. Y. Cho — 5.448

Trematodes — 5.449

Schistosomiasis K. S. Warren — 5.449

Liver fluke diseases of man N. Bhamarapravati,
W. Thamavit, and A. Limsuwan — 5.455

Other liver flukes D. A. Warrell — 5.457

Other hermaphrodite flukes parasitic in man
D. A. Warrell — 5.458

Non-venomous arthropods A. J. Radford — 5.462

Pentastomiasis (porocephalosis) D. A. Warrell — 5.468

Infectious disease syndromes — 5.469

Pyrexia of uncertain origin P. B. Beeson — 5.469

Septicaemia P. A. Murphy — 5.472

Infection in the compromised host C. Bunch — 5.478

Infection in pregnancy Rosalind Hurley — 5.484

Possibly infectious diseases — 5.490

Sarcoidosis J. G. Scadding — 5.490

Whipple's disease H. J. F. Hodgson — 5.501

Cat scratch fever C. M. P. Bradstreet — 5.502

Benign myalgic encephalomyelitis
W. B. Matthews — 5.504

Section 6. Chemical and physical injuries. Climatic and occupational diseases

Poisoning with chemical substances G. N. Volans,
B. Widdop, R. Goulding, T. J. Meredith, and
J. A. Vale — 6.3

Venoms and toxins of animals and plants
D. A. Warrell and L. G. Goodwin — 6.35

Environmental extremes W. R. Keatinge and
D. Rennie — 6.52

Aviation medicine F. S. Preston and D. M. Denison — 6.64

Diving medicine D. M. Denison — 6.76

Electric shock and lightning B. A. Pruitt, Jr and
A. D. Mason, Jr — 6.83

Radiation R. J. Berry — 6.86

Noise D. H. Glaister — 6.90

Air pollution P. J. Lawther — 6.93

Non-filarial endemic elephantiasis of the lower legs
E. W. Price — 6.97

Occupational diseases G. Kazantzis and R. T. Booth — 6.99

Section 7. Principles of clinical pharmacology and therapeutics A. Breckenridge and M. L' E. Orme

— 7.3

Section 8. Nutrition

Introduction R. Smith and W. P. T. James — 8.3

Biochemical background R. Smith and
D. H. Williamson — 8.4

Undernutrition — 8.12

Protein energy malnutrition A. A. Jackson and
M. H. N. Golden — 8.12

Vitamins and trace elements D. S. McLaren — 8.21

Obesity W. P. T. James — 8.26

Special nutritional problems R. Smith — 8.43

Anorexia nervosa G. F. M. Russell — 8.51

Diseases of overnourished societies and the need for
dietary change J. I. Mann — 8.55

Section 9. Metabolic disorders

The inborn errors of metabolism: general aspects
R. W. E. Watts — 9.3

Diabetes mellitus K. G. M. M. Alberti and
T. D. R. Hockaday — 9.5

Hypoglycaemia R. C. Turner — 9.49

Inborn errors of carbohydrate metabolism
R. W. E. Watts — 9.52

Inborn errors of fructose metabolism H. F. Woods — 9.56

Disorders of lipid transport B. Lewis — 9.58

Disorders of purine metabolism G. Nuki — 9.70

Porphyrin metabolism and the porphyrias
A. Goldberg, M. R. Moore, K. E. L. McColl, and
M. J. Brodie — 9.81

Inborn errors of amino acid and organic acid
metabolism R. W. E. Watts — 9.89

Amino acid transport defects R. W. E. Watts — 9.101

Lysosomal storage diseases R. W. E. Watts — 9.105

Wilson's disease A. G. Bearn — 9.114

Disturbances of acid–base homeostasis R. D. Cohen
and H. F. Woods — 9.116

Section 10. Endocrine disorders

Introduction to endocrinology Pamela C. B. MacKinnon — 10.3

Pituitary and hypothalamic disorders R. Hall — 10.7

Thyroid disorders R. Hoffenberg — 10.24

Disorders of calcium metabolism J. A. Kanis — 10.41

Adrenocortical diseases C. W. Burke — 10.58

Disorders of the reproductive systems
D. R. London — 10.69

Disorders of the breast D. R. London — 10.91

Corticosteroid and corticotrophin treatment in
non-endocrine disease R. I. S. Bayliss — 10.93

Section 11. Reproductive medicine

Benefits and risks of oral contraceptives
M. P. Vessey — 11.3

Contents

ix

Hypertension in pregnancy *C. W. G. Redman* — 11.6
Renal disease in pregnancy *C. W. G. Redman* and *J. G. G. Ledingham* — 11.10
Heart disease in pregnancy *C. W. G. Redman* and *P. Sleight* — 11.11
Thyroid disease in pregnancy *C. W. G. Redman* — 11.13
Systemic lupus erythematosus and related disorders in pregnancy *C. W. G. Redman* — 11.14
Diabetes in pregnancy *C. W. G. Redman* and *T. D. R. Hockaday* — 11.16
Blood disorders in pregnancy *C. W. G. Redman* and *D. J. Weatherall* — 11.21

Section 12. Gastroenterology
Methods for investigation of gastrointestinal and related diseases — 12.3
　Endoscopy *D. P. Jewell* — 12.3
　Radiological investigation of the digestive system *D. J. Nolan* and *E. W. L. Fletcher* — 12.4
　Computerized tomography *R. Dick* — 12.9
　Liver biopsy *J. M. Trowell* — 12.11
Symptomatology of gastrointestinal disease *D. P. Jewell* — 12.11
The mouth and salivary glands *T. Lehner* — 12.17
The tonsils and pharynx *R. F. McNab Jones* — 12.30
Disorders of motility *D. L. Wingate* — 12.33
Hormones and the gastrointestinal tract *R. G. Long*, *Julia M. Polak*, and *S. R. Bloom* — 12.47
Peptic ulcer *J. J. Misiewicz* and *R. E. Pounder* — 12.57
Gastritis *K. B. Taylor* — 12.70
Immune disorders *A. D. B. Webster* — 12.80
Malabsorption *M. S. Losowsky* — 12.84
Crohn's disease *D. P. Jewell* — 12.102
Ulcerative colitis *S. C. Truelove* — 12.107
Tumours of the gastrointestinal tract *M. L. Clark*, *A. B. Price*, and *C. B. Williams* — 12.112
Vascular and collagen disorders *G. Neale* — 12.124
Infections of the gastrointestinal tract *A. M. Tomkins* — 12.129
Congenital abnormalities of the gastrointestinal tract *J. A. Walker-Smith* and *V. Wright* — 12.140
The appendix, the peritoneum and omentum *E. G. Lee* — 12.148
Miscellaneous disorders of the gastrointestinal tract *D. J. Weatherall* and *D. P. Jewell* — 12.152
Diseases of the pancreas *K. G. Wormsley* — 12.156
Diseases of the gall bladder and biliary tree *J. A. Summerfield* — 12.168
Jaundice *E. Elias* — 12.175
Cirrhosis of the liver *Sheila Sherlock* — 12.182
Disorders of the hepatic veins and arteries *D. J. Weatherall* — 12.192
Acute hepatitis and fulminant hepatic failure *A. L. W. F. Eddleston* — 12.195
Chronic hepatitis *H. C. Thomas* — 12.203
Alcohol and the liver *P. W. Brunt* — 12.209
Drugs and liver damage *J. M. Trowell* — 12.213
Liver tumours *I. M. Murray-Lyon* — 12.215
Infections of the liver *S. G. Wright* — 12.218
Metabolic, genetic, and congenital disorders of the liver and biliary tract *A. P. Mowat* — 12.221

Section 13. Cardiovascular disorders
Introduction to cardiovascular disorders *Sir John McMichael* — 13.3
Clinical physiology — 13.3
　Biochemistry and cellular physiology of heart muscle and membranes *P. A. Poole-Wilson* — 13.3
　Clinical physiology of the normal heart *D. E. L. Wilcken* — 13.10

Ventricular disease ('heart failure') *D. G. Gibson* — 13.16
Clinical assessment of cardiovascular function — 13.29
　The chest X-ray in heart disease *R. S. O. Rees* — 13.29
　Echocardiography *D. G. Gibson* — 13.34
　Nuclear techniques *D. J. Rowlands* — 13.41
　Cardiac catheterization *G. A. H. Miller* — 13.46
　The electrocardiogram *D. J. Rowlands* — 13.48
Principles of drug treatment — 13.58
　Digitalis *D. A. Chamberlain* — 13.58
　Diuretics *J. G. G. Ledingham* — 13.61
　Beta-adrenoceptor blocking drugs *B. N. C. Prichard* — 13.63
　Vasodilators *K. Chatterjee* — 13.66
　Anti-arrhythmic agents *D. H. Bennett* — 13.71
　Catecholamines and their derivatives *P. Foëx* and *A. Fisher* — 13.74
Cardiac arrhythmias *D. H. Bennett* — 13.78
Pacemakers *R. Sutton* — 13.92
Congenital heart disease — 13.94
　The anatomy of congenital heart disease *R. H. Anderson* and *E. A. Shinebourne* — 13.94
　Congenital heart disease in adults *Jane Somerville* — 13.108
Valvular disease *D. G. Gibson* — 13.130
　Rheumatic fever *K. G. Nair* — 13.148
Ischaemic heart disease — 13.151
　Epidemiology of ischaemic heart disease *J. I. Mann* and *M. G. Marmot* — 13.151
　Pathology *M. J. Davies* — 13.161
　Detection of ischaemic heart disease *R. Balcon* — 13.163
　Myocardial infarction *B. L. Pentecost* — 13.174
　Cardiac transplantation *S. W. Jamieson* — 13.188
　Angina with normal coronary arteries *W. Somerville* — 13.190
　Da Costa's syndrome *W. Somerville* — 13.194
Cardiomyopathies — 13.195
　Cardiomyopathies and specific heart muscle disorders *Celia M. Oakley* — 13.195
　Specific heart muscle diseases *Celia M. Oakley* — 13.212
Infective endocarditis *B. Gribbin* — 13.221
Cardiovascular syphilis *B. Gribbin* — 13.231
Left atrial myxoma *T. A. Traill* — 13.233
Pericardial disease *D. G. Gibson* — 13.234
Disorders of the pulmonary circulation — 13.241
　Pulmonary hypertension *M. Honey* — 13.241
　Cor pulmonale *J. S. Prichard* — 13.248
　Pulmonary embolism *G. A. H. Miller* — 13.252
Hypertension — 13.258
　Essential hypertension *P. Sleight* — 13.260
　Secondary hypertension *J. G. G. Ledingham* — 13.278
Peripheral arterial disease *P. J. Morris* — 13.288

Section 14. Intensive care *R. D. Bradley*
Major acute derangements of the circulation — 14.3
Positive-pressure ventilation — 14.14
Haemodialysis in the presence of circulatory disorder — 14.17

Section 15. Respiratory disorders
The structure of the lung and its investigation — 15.3
　Pulmonary anatomy *M. S. Dunnill* — 15.3
　Diagnostic bronchoscopy and tissue biopsy *M. F. Muers* — 15.6
　Radiology *F. W. Wright* — 15.8
The functions of the lung and its investigation *N. B. Pride* — 15.21
The responses of the lung to inhaled particles *Margaret E. H. Turner-Warwick* — 15.30
The clinical presentation of chest diseases *D. J. Lane* — 15.39

Structural disorders of the thoracic cage and lungs
  C. Ogilvie   15.52
Diseases of the airways M. K. Benson   15.60
Parenchymal lung diseases   15.71
  Infection of the respiratory tract J. E. Stark   15.71
    Pneumonia   15.72
  Pneumoconioses A. Seaton   15.83
  Alveolitis I. W. B. Grant   15.89
Drug-induced pulmonary disease G. J. Gibson   15.101
Tumours of the lung, mediastinum, and pleura
  N. W. Horne   15.103
End-stage lung disease   15.115
  Adult respiratory distress syndrome A. Fisher and
  P. Foëx   15.115
  Respiratory failure J. B. L. Howell   15.119
  The respiratory cripple D. J. Lane   15.122

Section 16. Joints and connective tissues
Immunopathology of rheumatoid arthritis
  G. S. Panayi   16.3
Clinical features of rheumatoid arthritis
  M. I. V. Jayson and D. M. Grennan   16.5
Seronegative arthritides P. Hickling and V. Wright   16.13
Osteoarthritis and related disorders P. Dieppe   16.22
The connective tissue diseases M. A. Byron and
  G. R. V. Hughes   16.28
Other inflammatory arthritides B. L. Hazleman   16.40
Non-inflammatory arthropathies and soft tissue
  rheumatism I. Haslock   16.47
The management of inflammatory joint disease
  A. G. Mowat   16.51

Section 17. Disorders of the skeleton R. Smith
Physiology of bone   17.3
The diagnosis of bone disease   17.7
Osteoporosis   17.10
Osteomalacia and rickets   17.15
Paget's disease of bone   17.19
Parathyroids and bone disease   17.22
Osteogenesis imperfecta. The brittle bone syndrome   17.25
The Marfan syndrome, homocystinuria, the
  Ehlers–Danlos syndrome, and alkaptonuria   17.27
The mucopolysaccharidoses   17.29
The osteopetroses   17.29
Disorders of alkaline phosphatase   17.31
Fibrous dysplasia   17.32
Skeletal dysplasias   17.33
Assorted bone disorders   17.34
Ectopic mineralization   17.35

Section 18. Nephrology
Clinical physiology of the kidney: tests of renal
  function and structure R. B. I. Morrison,
  J. M. Davison, and D. N. S. Kerr   18.3
Water and electrolyte disturbances   18.19
  Water and sodium homeostasis
  J. G. G. Ledingham   18.19
  Disorders of potassium metabolism
  J. G. G. Ledingham   18.28
Glomerulonephritis and renal manifestations of
  systemic disease D. Gwyn Williams and
  D. K. Peters   18.33
Proteinuria and the nephrotic syndrome
  J. S. Cameron   18.52
Interstitial nephritis and urinary tract infections
  A. W. Asscher   18.63
Familial renal disease C. Chantler   18.75
Renal calculi R. W. E. Watts   18.81

Urinary stone disease (urolithiasis)
  R. W. E. Watts   18.81
  Idiopathic hypercalciuria R. W. E. Watts   18.86
  Primary hyperoxaluria R. W. E. Watts   18.87
Metabolic disorders of the kidney R. W. E. Watts   18.88
Urinary tract obstruction L. R. I. Baker   18.93
Toxic nephropathies F. P. Marsh   18.100
Drugs and the kidney F. P. Marsh   18.107
Acute renal failure J. G. G. Ledingham   18.111
Chronic renal failure, dialysis, and transplantation
  D. O. Oliver   18.118
Renal bone disease J. A. Kanis   18.135
Cystic and congenital abnormalities of the kidneys
  D. B. Evans   18.143
Genito-urinary tuberculosis J. C. Smith   18.149

Section 19. Diseases of the blood
Introduction D. J. Weatherall   19.1
Erythropoiesis, the red cell, and anaemia
  A. J. Bellingham and D. J. Weatherall   19.8
  The anaemia of chronic disorders Sheila Callender   19.15
Iron metabolism; deficiency and overload
  A. Jacobs   19.17
Megaloblastic anaemia A. V. Hoffbrand   19.28
Other anaemias resulting from defective red cell
  maturation D. J. Weatherall   19.40
Haemolytic anaemia D. J. Weatherall   19.54
  Acquired haemolytic anaemias
  E. C. Gordon-Smith and D. J. Weatherall   19.66
Other metabolic disorders of the red cell:
  methaemoglobinaemia, carboxy-
  haemoglobinaemia, and sulphaemo-
  globinaemia D. J. Weatherall   19.76
Polycythaemia D. J. Weatherall   19.78
The white cell   19.84
  Leucocytes in health and disease C. Bunch   19.84
  The leukaemias Sheila Callender   19.89
Haemostasis and thrombosis J. A. Davies and
  G. P. McNicol   19.111
Disorders of all cell lines   19.137
  The myeloproliferative disorders D. J. Weatherall   19.137
  Aplastic anaemia and other causes of bone
  marrow failure E. C. Gordon-Smith   19.141
Disorders of the spleen S. M. Lewis   19.150
The lymphomas Sheila Callender and
  R. I. Vanhegan   19.160
Histiocytosis X Sheila Callender   19.174
Paraproteinaemia Sheila Callender and D. Y. Mason   19.175
Blood transfusion H. H. Gunson   19.187
Bone marrow transplantation C. Bunch   19.193
Haematological manifestations of systemic disease
  D. J. Weatherall   19.197

Section 20. Skin diseases T. J. Ryan
Introduction   20.3
Factors determining or modifying skin disease   20.12
Dermatitis   20.29
Pruritus   20.37
Psoriasis   20.38
Lichen planus and lichenoid eruptions   20.43
Acne vulgaris   20.45
Pigmentation   20.47
Diseases of nails, hair, and sweat glands   20.52
Skin disorders affecting the genitalia   20.59
Urticaria   20.61
Cutaneous vasculitis   20.63
Vesico-blistering diseases   20.69
Abnormal vascularity of the skin, angioma, and
  telangiectasia   20.74

Disorders of collagen and elastic tissue 20.78
Atrophy 20.80
Malignant disease 20.82
Viral warts 20.86
Granulomata and other infiltrations of the skin 20.87
Management of skin disease 20.92

Section 21. Neurology
Introduction W. B. Matthews 21.3
Investigations used in neurological disease 21.3
  Electroencephalography W. B. Matthews 21.3
  Principles of neuroradiology I. Isherwood 21.4
  The cerebrospinal fluid W. B. Matthews 21.9
  Electrophysiological investigation of the peripheral
    nervous system W. B. Matthews 21.9
Disturbance of higher cerebral function
  J. M. Oxbury 21.11
Stupor, coma, and brain death W. B. Matthews 21.17
The motor and sensory systems and effects of
  subcortical brain lesions W. B. Matthews 21.19
The autonomic nervous system W. B. Matthews 21.22
Lesions of the cranial nerves 21.23
  The olfactory nerve W. B. Matthews 21.23
  The optic nerve and visual pathways
    J. M. Oxbury 21.24
  Other cranial nerves P. K. Thomas 21.26
Peripheral neuropathy P. K. Thomas 21.31
Lesions of the spinal roots W. B. Matthews 21.43
Spinal cord disease W. B. Matthews 21.44
Bacterial meningitis J. B. Foster 21.50
Neurosyphilis J. B. Foster 21.55
Virus infections of the nervous system R. S. Kocen 21.58
  Other viral infections or disorders in which viruses
    may play a role in the pathogenesis of
    neurological disease R. S. Kocen and
    W. B. Matthews 21.61
Tetanus: clinical aspects J. M. K. Spalding 21.63
Cerebrovascular disease C. P. Warlow 21.65
Intracranial tumours A. A. Jefferson 21.75
Intracranial abscess A. A. Jefferson 21.79
Benign intracranial hypertension A. A. Jefferson 21.81
Head injury A. A. Jefferson 21.81
  Chronic traumatic encephalopathy
    W. B. Matthews 21.84
Developmental abnormalities W. B. Matthews 21.84
Inherited disorders P. K. Thomas 21.88
Degenerative disease and dementia W. B. Matthews 21.92
Demyelinating disease W. B. Matthews 21.95
Movement disorders C. D. Marsden 21.100
Central nervous system involvement in systemic
  disease W. B. Matthews 21.121
Metabolic disorders of the nervous system
  C. D. Marsden 21.123
Neurological disorders due to physical agents
  C. D. Marsden 21.126
Alcohol and the central nervous system
  W. B. Matthews 21.127
Epilepsy A. Hopkins 21.128
Narcolepsy and related sleep disorders
  C. D. Marsden 21.142
Syncope, dizziness, and vertigo W. B. Matthews 21.143
Headache W. B. Matthews 21.145
Neurology in developing countries 21.149
  Neurological disorders in India N. H. Wadia 21.149
  Neurological disorders in Africa D. A. Warrell
    and D. J. Weatherall 21.153

Neurological disorders in Southeast Asia
  A. Vejjajiva 21.156

Section 22. Diseases of voluntary muscle
The muscular dystrophies J. N. Walton 22.8
Myotonic disorders J. N. Walton 22.11
Inflammatory diseases of muscle J. N. Walton 22.13
Myasthenia gravis J. N. Walton 22.14
The myasthenic–myopathic syndrome J. N. Walton 22.16
Metabolic myopathies J. N. Walton 22.17
Periodic paralysis syndromes J. N. Walton 22.19
Some miscellaneous muscular disorders J. N. Walton 22.21
Tropical pyomyositis (tropical myositis)
  D. A. Warrell 22.23

Section 23. Disorders of uncertain aetiology
Recurrent polyserositis (familial Mediterranean
  fever, periodic disease) M. Eliakim and
  M. Rachmilewitz 23.3
Fibrosing syndromes (multicentric fibrosclerosis)
  P. B. Beeson 23.5
Eosinophilia and the hypereosinophilic syndromes
  P. B. Beeson 23.6
Laurence–Moon–Biedl syndrome
  J. G. G. Ledingham 23.8
Acatalasia D. J. Weatherall 23.8
Adenoma sebaceum, tuberose sclerosis, renal, lung,
  and other hamartomata, and the 'formes frustes'
  F. W. Wright 23.9
Werner's syndrome J. G. G. Ledingham 23.11
Unclassified granulomatous diseases J. O'D. McGee 23.11
Behçet's disease D. J. Weatherall 23.12

Section 24. Psychiatry and medicine
Introduction M. G. Gelder 24.3
Psychological and psychiatric disorders secondary to
  medical illness 24.3
  Abnormal emotional reactions to physical illness
    D. H. Gath 24.3
  Organic mental states G. Stores 24.11
  Specific conditions giving rise to mental disorders
    W. A. Lishman 24.16
  Sexual problems associated with physical illness
    K. Hawton 24.23
Psychiatric disorders presenting as physical disease
  M. G. Gelder 24.26
Psychological factors and the course of illness
  R. A. Mayou 24.31
Important practical problems 24.34
  The alcoholic patient D. H. Gath 24.34
  The patient who has attempted suicide
    H. G. Morgan 24.38
  Psychiatric emergencies H. G. Morgan 24.40
  Drug addiction M. Mitcheson 24.43
Psychiatry and medicine in developing countries
  J. H. Orley and M. T. Tsuang 24.47

Section 25. Medicine in old age F. I. Caird 25.3

Section 26. Terminal care Cicely M. Saunders 26.3

Appendix. Normal or reference values for biochemical
  data Angela M. Giles and B. D. Ross 27.3

Index follows page 27.8

Colour plates appear between pages 5.238 and 5.239

List of contributors

E. B. Adams, Emeritus Professor of Medicine, University of Natal, South Africa.

K. G. M. M. Alberti, Professor of Clinical Biochemistry, University of Newcastle upon Tyne, Royal Victoria Infirmary, Newcastle upon Tyne, U.K.

R. H. Anderson, Joseph Levy Professor of Paediatric Cardiac Morphology, Department of Paediatrics, Cardiothoracic Institute, University of London, Brompton Hospital, London.

M. Aquinas O.B.E., Honorary Clinical Lecturer in Medicine (Tuberculosis), University of Hong Kong.

A. W. Asscher, Professor of Medicine and Honorary Director, The Kidney Research Unit Foundation, Institute of Renal Disease, Welsh National School of Medicine, Royal Infirmary, Cardiff, U.K.

L. R. I. Baker, Consultant Physician and Nephrologist, St. Bartholomew's Hospital, London.

R. Balcon, Consultant Cardiologist, The London Chest Hospital, London.

P. A. J. Ball, Consultant Physician, Middlesex Hospital, London.

Sir Richard Bayliss, K.C.V.O., Honorary Consultant Physician and Endocrinologist, Westminster Hospital, London; Consulting Physician, King Edward VII's Hospital for Officers, London.

A. G. Bearn, Senior Vice President, Medical and Scientific Affairs, Merck Sharp and Dohme International; Professor of Medicine, Cornell University Medical College; Attending Physician, The New York Hospital, New York, U.S.A.

P. B. Beeson, Distinguished Physician, United States Veterans Administration; Professor of Medicine, University of Washington, U.S.A.

D. R. Bell, Senior Lecturer in Tropical Medicine, Liverpool School of Tropical Medicine, Liverpool, U.K.

A. J. Bellingham, Professor of Haematology, University of Liverpool, U.K.

D. H. Bennett, Consultant Cardiologist, Wythenshawe Hospital, University of Manchester School of Medicine, Manchester, U.K.

M. K. Benson, Consultant Physician, Chest Clinic, Churchill Hospital, Oxford, U.K.

R. J. Berry, Professor of Oncology, Middlesex Hospital Medical School, London.

S. R. Bloom, Professor of Endocrinology and Honorary Consultant Physician, Royal Postgraduate Medical School, Hammersmith Hospital, London.

R. T. Booth, Professor of Occupational Health and Safety, University of Aston in Birmingham, U.K.

E. T. W. Bowen, Deputy Director, the PHLS Centre for Applied Microbiology and Research, Special Pathogens Reference Library, Porton Down, Salisbury, U.K.

R. D. Bradley, Consultant Physician, Intensive Therapy Unit, St. Thomas's Hospital, London.

C. M. P. Bradstreet, Formerly Director, Standards Laboratory for Serological Reagents, Central Public Health Laboratory, London.

N. Bhamarapravati, Professor of Pathology, Faculty of Medicine, Ramathibodi Hospital, Bangkok, Thailand.

A. M. Breckenridge, Professor of Clinical Pharmacology, University of Liverpool, Department of Pharmacology and Therapeutics, Royal Liverpool Hospital, Liverpool, U.K.

M. J. Brodie, Lecturer, Department of Clinical Pharmacology, Royal Postgraduate Medical School, Hammersmith Hospital, London.

P. W. Brunt, Consultant Physician (Gastroenterology), Aberdeen Royal Infirmary, Aberdeen, U.K.

C. Bunch, Clinical Reader and Honorary Consultant Physician, Nuffield Department of Clinical Medicine, University of Oxford, John Radcliffe Hospital, Oxford, U.K.

C. W. Burke, Consultant Physician, Department of Endocrinology, Radcliffe Infirmary, Oxford, U.K.

Margaret A. Byron, Senior Registrar, Department of Rheumatology, Nuffield Orthopaedic Centre, Oxford, U.K.

F. I. Caird, David Cargill Professor of Geriatric Medicine, University of Glasgow, Southern General Hospital, Glasgow, U.K.

Sheila T. E. Callender, Formerly Clinical Reader and Honorary Consultant Physician, Nuffield Department of Clinical Medicine, University of Oxford, John Radcliffe Hospital, Oxford, U.K.

J. S. Cameron, Professor of Renal Medicine, Guy's Hospital Medical School, London.

C. C. J. Carpenter, Chairman, Department of Medicine, Case Western Reserve University, Cleveland, Ohio, U.S.A.

D. A. Chamberlain, Consultant Physician, Royal Sussex County Hospital, Brighton, U.K.

C. Chantler, Professor, Evelina Department of Paediatrics, Guy's Hospital Medical School, London.

K. Chatterjee, Professor of Medicine, Associate Chief, Cardiovascular Division, Director of Coronary Care Unit, University of California, School of Medicine, San Francisco, California, U.S.A.

S.-Y. Cho, Associate Professor of Parasitology, College of Medicine, Chung-Ang University, Korea.

A. B. Christie, Honorary Consultant, Fazakerly Hospital, Liverpool, U.K.

K. M. Citron, Consultant Physician, Wandsworth and Battersea Chest Clinic, St. John's Hospital, London.

M. L. Clark, Consultant Physician, St. Mark's Hospital, London.

M. J. Clarkson, Professor of Veterinary Preventive Medicine, University of Liverpool, Field Station 'Leahurst', Neston, Wirral, U.K.

R. D. Cohen, Professor of Medicine, London Hospital Medical College, London.

A. M. Cooke, Honarary Consulting Physician to the United Oxford Hospitals; Emeritus Fellow of Merton College, Oxford, U.K.

G. W. Csonka, Consultant Venereologist, The Praed Street Clinic, St. Mary's Hospital, London.

S. Darougar, Professor of Public Health Ophthalmology, Head of Sub-Department of Virology, Institute of Ophthalmology, London; Honorary Consultant, Moorfields Eye Hospital, London.

J. A. Davies, Lecturer in Medicine, University of Leeds, General Infirmary, Leeds, U.K.

M. J. Davies, Professor of Cardiovascular Pathology, St. George's Hospital Medical School, London.

J. M. Davison, Member of Scientific Staff, MRC Human Reproduction Group, Princess Mary Maternity Hospital, Newcastle upon Tyne, U.K.

D. M. Denison, Professor of Clinical Physiology, Cardiothoracic Institute, University of London.

R. Dick, Consultant in Diagnostic Radiology, Royal Free Hospital, London.

P. Dieppe, Senior Lecturer in Rheumatology, University of Bristol, Bristol Royal Infirmary, Bristol, U.K.

Sir Richard Doll, Emeritus Regius Professor of Medicine, University of Oxford, Green College, Oxford, U.K.

B. O. L. Duke, Chief, Filarial Infections Parasitic Disease Programme, World Health Organization, Geneva, Switzerland.

K. R. Dumbell, Professor of Virology, St. Mary's Hospital Medical School, London.

M. S. Dunnill, Consultant Pathologist, Histopathology Department, John Radcliffe Hospital, Oxford, U.K.

A. L. W. F. Eddleston, Professor of Liver Immunology and Honorary Consultant Physician, Liver Unit, King's College Hospital, London.

M. Eliakim, Professor of Medicine, Hebrew University, Hadassah Medical School; Chairman, Department of Medicine A, Hadassah University Hospital, Jerusalem, Israel.

E. Elias, Consultant Physician, Queen Elizabeth Hospital, Birmingham, U.K.

D. A. Price-Evans, Professor and Chairman, Department of Medicine, University of Liverpool, Royal Liverpool Hospital, Liverpool, U.K.

D. B. Evans, Consultant Physician and Nephrologist, Addenbrookes Hospital, Cambridge, U.K.

S. J. Eykyn, Senior Lecturer, Department of Bacteriology, St. Thomas's Hospital, London.

A. Fisher, Consultant Anaesthetist, Clinical Lecturer, Intensive Care Unit, John Radcliffe Hospital, Oxford, U.K.

E. W. L. Fletcher, Consultant Radiologist, John Radcliffe Hospital, Oxford, U.K.

P. Foëx, Clinical Reader and Honorary Consultant, Nuffield Department of Anaesthetics, University of Oxford, Radcliffe Infirmary, Oxford, U.K.

J. B. Foster, Honorary Reader in Neurology, University of Newcastle upon Tyne, U.K.

D. A. G. Galton, Professor of Haematology, University of London; Honorary Director, MRC Leukaemia Unit, Royal Postgraduate Medical School, Hammersmith Hospital, London.

S. D. Gardner, Consultant Virologist, Virus Reference Laboratory, Central Public Health Laboratory, London.

D. H. Gath, Clinical Reader in Psychiatry and Honorary Consultant, University Department of Psychiatry, Warneford Hospital, Oxford, U.K.

M. G. Gelder, Professor of Psychiatry, University of Oxford, Warneford Hospital, Oxford, U.K.

D. G. Gibson, Consultant Cardiologist, National Heart and Chest Hospitals and The Brompton Hospital, London.

G. J. Gibson, Consultant Physician; Clinical Lecturer, Freeman Hospital, Newcastle upon Tyne, U.K.

Angela Giles, Chief Medical Laboratory Scientific Officer, Department of Clinical Biochemistry, John Radcliffe Hospital, Oxford, U.K.

D. J. Girling, Member of Scientific Staff, MRC Tuberculosis and Chest Diseases Unit, Brompton Hospital, London.

D. H. Glaister, Head, Biodynamics Division, RAF Institute of Aviation Medicine, Farnborough, U.K.

M. J. Goldacre, Lecturer, Department of Community Medicine and General Practice, University of Oxford, Radcliffe Infirmary, Oxford, U.K.

A. Goldberg, Regius Professor of the Practice of Medicine, University of Glasgow, Department of Medicine, Gardiner Institute, Western Infirmary, Glasgow, U.K.

M. H. N. Golden, Wellcome Senior Research Fellow, Department of Nutrition, London School of Hygiene and Tropical Medicine. On secondment to Tropical Research Unit, U.W.I., Jamaica, West Indies.

L. G. Goodwin, Formerly Director of Science, The Zoological Society of London.

E. C. Gordon-Smith, Senior Lecturer and Honorary Consultant, Royal Postgraduate Medical School, Hammersmith Hospital, London.

R. Goulding, Formerly, Director, Poisons Unit, Guy's Hospital, London.

I. W. B. Grant, Consultant Physician, Respiratory Unit, Northern General Hospital, Edinburgh, U.K.

B. M. Greenwood, Director, M. R. C. Laboratories, Fajara, Banjul, The Gambia, West Africa.

D. M. Grennan, Consultant Physician, Hope Hospital, Salford; Senior Lecturer, Department of Rheumatology, University of Manchester, U.K.

B. Gribbin, Consultant Cardiologist, John Radcliffe Hospital, Oxford, U.K.

N. R. Grist, Professor of Infectious Diseases, University of Glasgow, Glasgow, U.K.

H. H. Gunson, Reader in Haematology, University of Manchester, U.K.

R. Hall, Professor of Medicine, Welsh National School of Medicine, Cardiff, U.K.

H. Harris, Regius Professor of Medicine and Head of Department, William Dunn School of Pathology, University of Oxford, U.K.

I. Haslock, Consultant Rheumatologist, Middlesborough General Hospital, Middlesborough, U.K.

K. Hawton, Clinical Lecturer, University of Oxford, Department of Psychiatry, Warneford Hospital, Oxford, U.K.

R. J. Hay, Consultant Dermatologist, St. John's Hospital for Diseases of the Skin, London.

B. L. Hazleman, Consultant Rheumatologist, Addenbrooke's Hospital, Cambridge, U.K.

P. Hickling, Professor of Rheumatology, University of Leeds, Rheumatism Research Unit, University Department of Medicine, General Infirmary, Leeds, U.K.

T. D. R. Hockaday, Consultant Physician, Radcliffe Infirmary, Oxford, U.K.

H. J. F. Hodgson, Senior Lecturer and Consultant Physician, Department of Medicine, Royal Postgraduate Medical School, Hammersmith Hospital, London.

A. V. Hoffbrand, Professor of Haematology, Royal Free Hospital School of Medicine, London.

R. Hoffenberg, William Withering Professor of Medicine, University of Birmingham, Queen Elizabeth Hospital, Birmingham, U.K.

E. J. Holborow, Professor of Immunopathology, Bone and Joint Research Unit, The London Hospital Medical College, London.

M. Honey, Consultant Cardiologist, Brompton Hospital, London.

A. Hopkins, Physician-in-charge, Department of Neurological Sciences, St. Bartholomew's Hospital, London.

N. W. Horne, Consultant Chest Physician, City Hospital, Edinburgh, U.K.

J. B. L. Howell, Dean and Professor of Medicine, University of Southampton, Southampton General Hospital, Southampton, U.K.

G. R. V. Hughes, Senior Lecturer in Medicine, Royal Postgraduate Medical School, Hammersmith Hospital, London.

W. T. Hughes, Eudowood Professor of Pediatric Infectious Diseases, Director, Division of Infectious Diseases, The Johns Hopkins University School of Medicine, Baltimore, U.S.A.

Rosalind Hurley, Professor of Microbiology, Institute of Obstetrics and Gynaecology, University of London, Queen Charlotte's Maternity Hospital, London.

I. Isherwood, Professor of Diagnostic Radiology, University of Manchester, U.K.

A. A. Jackson, Senior Lecturer, AG Director, Tropical Metabolism Unit, University of West Indies, Mona, Kingston, Jamaica, West Indies.

A. Jacobs, Professor of Haematology, Welsh National School of Medicine, University Hospital of Wales, Cardiff, U.K.

W. P. T. James, Assistant Director, MRC, Dunn Clinical Nutrition Center, Palto Alto, California, U.S.A.

S. W. Jamieson, Assistant Professor, Cardiovascular Surgery, Co-Director, Heart Transplantation Program, Stanford University Hospital, Stanford, Staff Surgeon and Co-Director of Cardiac Surgical Services, Veterans Administration Medical Center, Palo Alto, California, U.S.A.

M. I. V. Jayson, Professor of Rheumatology, University of Manchester, Rheumatic Diseases Centre, Hope Hospital, Salford, U.K.

A. A. Jefferson, Consultant Neurosurgeon, Hallamshire Hospital, Sheffield, U.K.

D. P. Jewell, Consultant Physician, John Radcliffe Hospital, Oxford, U.K.

B. E. Juel-Jensen, Consultant Physician (Communicable Diseases), Radcliffe Infirmary, Oxford, U.K.

J. A. Kanis, Reader in Human Metabolism, Department of Human Metabolism and Clinical Biochemistry, University of Sheffield Medical School, Sheffield, U.K.

G. Kazantzis, Senior Lecturer in Occupational Medicine, London School of Hygiene and Tropical Medicine; Honorary Consultant Physician, The Middlesex Hospital, London.

W. R. Keating, Professor of Physiology, London Hospital Medical College, London.

D. N. S. Kerr, Professor of Medicine, University of Newcastle upon Tyne, Royal Victoria Infirmary, Newcastle upon Tyne, U.K.

M. H. King, Staff Member, Kenyan/German Project for Hospital Technology, Nyeri, Kenya.

R. Knight, Senior Lecturer, Liverpool School of Tropical Medicine, Liverpool, U.K.

R. S. Kocen, Consultant Physician, National Hospital for Nervous Diseases, Queen Square, London.

W. Kwantes, Director, Public Health Laboratory, Swansea, U.K.

D. J. Lane, Consultant Chest Physician, Churchill Hospital, Oxford, U.K.

H. E. Larson, Member, MRC Scientific Staff, Division of Communicable Diseases, Clinical Research Centre, Harrow, Middlesex, U.K.

P. J. Lawther, Professor of Environmental and Preventive Medicine, St. Bartholomew's and London Hospital Medical Colleges, London.

J. G. G. Ledingham, Formerly Director of Clinical Studies, May Reader in Medicine, Nuffield Department of Clinical Medicine, University of Oxford; Honorary Consultant Physician, John Radcliffe Hospital, Oxford, U.K.

E. G. Lee, Consultant Surgeon, Department of Surgery, Radcliffe Infirmary, Oxford, U.K.

T. Lehner, Professor of Oral Immunology, Guy's Hospital Dental School, London.

B. Lewis, Professor of Chemical Pathology, St. Thomas's Hospital Medical School, London.

S. M. Lewis, Reader in Haematology, Royal Postgraduate Medical School, Hammersmith Hospital, London.

A. Limsuwan, Professor of Medicine, Ramathibodi Hospital, Bangkok, Thailand.

C. C. Linnemann, Jr, Associate Professor of Medicine, Division of Infectious Diseases, University of Cincinnati, Ohio, U.S.A.

W. A. Lishman, Professor of Neuropsychiatry, Institute of Psychiatry, University of London.

D. R. London, Consultant Physician, Queen Elizabeth Hospital, Birmingham, U.K.

R. G. Long, Senior Registrar, St. Thomas's Hospital, London.

M. S. Losowsky, Professor of Medicine, University of Leeds, St. James's Hospital, Leeds, U.K.

K. E. L. McColl, Lecturer in Medicine, University of Glasgow, Gardiner Institute, Western Infirmary, Glasgow, U.K.

J. O'D McGee, Professor of Morbid Anatomy, University of Oxford, Department of Pathology, John Radcliffe Hospital, Oxford, U.K.

D. W. R. MacKenzie, Director, Mycological Reference Laboratory, London School of Hygiene and Tropical Medicine, London.

Pamela C. B. MacKinnon, Lecturer, Department of Human Anatomy, University of Oxford, U.K.

D. S. McLaren, Reader in Clinical Nutrition, University Department of Medicine, The Royal Infirmary, Edinburgh, U.K.

Sir John McMichael, Emeritus Professor of Medicine, University of London.

R. F. McNab Jones, Consultant Surgeon-in-charge, ENT Department, St. Bartholomew's Hospital, London.

G. P. McNichol, Principal and Vice-Chancellor, Aberdeen University; Formerly, Professor of Medicine, University of Leeds, Honorary Consultant Physician, General Infirmary, Leeds, U.K.

C. R. Madeley, Professor of Clinical Virology, University of Newcastle upon Tyne, Royal Victoria Infirmary, Newcastle upon Tyne, U.K.

N. S. Mair, Honorary Reader in Microbiology, School of Medicine and School of Biological Sciences, University of Leicester, U.K.

J. I. Mann, University Lecturer and Honorary Consultant in Social and Community Medicine, Department of Social and Community Medicine, University of Oxford, Radcliffe Infirmary, Oxford, U.K.

P. E. C. Manson-Bahr, Consultant Physician, Ministry of Overseas Development and Commonwealth Development Corporation, London.

M. G. Marmot, Senior Lecturer, Department of Medical Statistics and Epidemiology, London School of Hygiene and Tropical Medicine, London.

C. D. Marsden, Professor of Clinical Neurology, King's College Hospital Medical School, London.

P. D. Marsden, Professor of Tropical Medicine, University of Brasilia, Brasilia, Brazil.

F. P. Marsh, Consultant Nephrologist, The London Hospital, London.

W. C. Marshall, Senior Lecturer, Department of Microbiology, Institute of Child Health, University of London.

A. D. Mason, Jr, Chief Laboratory Division, U.S. Army Institute of Surgical Research, Brooke Army Medical Center, Fort Sam, Houston, Texas, U.S.A.

D. Y. Mason, University Lecturer and Honorary Consultant, Department of Haematology, John Radcliffe Hospital, Oxford, U.K.

W. B. Matthews, Professor of Clinical Neurology, University of Oxford, Radcliffe Infirmary, Oxford, U.K.

R. A. Mayou, Honorary Consultant Psychiatrist, University Department of Psychiatry, Warneford Hospital, Oxford, U.K.

T. J. Meredith, Research Fellow, Department of Gastroenterology, Guy's Hospital, London.

G. A. H. Miller, Director, Cardiac Laboratories, Brompton Hospital, London.

L. H. Miller, Head, Malaria Section, Laboratory of Parasitic Diseases, National Institute of Allergy and Infectious Diseases, Bethesda, Maryland, U.S.A.

R. G. Mitchell, Consultant Microbiologist, Department of Medical Microbiology, John Radcliffe Hospital, Oxford, U.K.

J. J. Misiewicz, Consultant Physician, Department of Gastroenterology, Central Middlesex Hospital, London.

M. Mitcheson, Consultant Psychiatrist, Drug Dependance Clinic, University College Hospital, London.

M. A. Monnickendam, Lecturer, Sub-Department of Virology, Institute of Ophthalmology, London.

M. R. Moore, Lecturer in Medicine, University of Glasgow, Gardiner Institute, Western Infirmary, Glasgow, U.K.

H. G. Morgan, Professor of Mental Health, University of Bristol, U.K.

P. J. Morris, Nuffield Professor of Surgery, Nuffield Department of Surgery, University of Oxford, John Radcliffe Hospital, Oxford, U.K.

R. B. I. Morrison, Consultant Physician, Renal Unit, Wellington Hospital, Wellington, New Zealand.

A. G. Mowat, Clinical Lecturer in Rheumatology, University of Oxford; Consultant Rheumatologist, Department of Rheumatology, Nuffield Orthopaedic Centre, Oxford, U.K.

A. P. Mowat, Consultant Paediatrician, Department of Child Health, King's College Hospital Medical School, London.

M. F. Muers, Consultant Physician and Honorary Clinical Lecturer, St. James's University Hospital, Leeds, U.K.

I. M. Murray-Lyon, Consultant Physician and Gastroenterologist, Charing Cross Hospital, London.

P. A. Murphy, Associate Professor of Medicine, Department of Microbiology, The Johns Hopkins University School of Medicine, Baltimore, Maryland, U.S.A.

J. Nagington, Consultant Virologist, Addenbrooke's Hospital, Cambridge, U.K.

K. G. Nair, Honorary Cardiologist, Jaslock Hospital, Bombay, India.

G. Neale, Consultant Physician, Addenbrooke's Hospital, Cambridge, U.K.

D. J. Nolan, Consultant Radiologist, John Radcliffe Hospital, Oxford, U.K.

G. Nuki, Professor of Rheumatology, University of Edinburgh; Consultant Rheumatologist, Rheumatic Diseases Unit, Northern General Hospital, Edinburgh, U.K.

Celia M. Oakley, Consultant Cardiologist, Royal Postgraduate Medical School, Hammersmith Hospital, London.

C. Ogilvie, Consultant Physician, Royal Liverpool Hospital, Liverpool Cardiothoracic Centre, and The King Edward VIIth Hospital, Midhurst, U.K.

D. O. Oliver, Consultant Nephrologist, The Renal Unit, Churchill Hospital, Oxford, U.K.

J. H. Orley, Lecturer, University Department of Psychiatry, Warneford Hospital, Oxford, U.K.

M. L'E. Orme, Reader in Clinical Pharmacology, Department of Pharmacology and Therapeutics, University of Liverpool, U.K.

J. M. Oxbury, Consultant Neurologist, Department of Neurology, Radcliffe Infirmary, Oxford, U.K.

G. S. Panayi, Arthritis and Rheumatism Research Council Professor of Rheumatology, Guy's Hospital and Medical School, London.

M. T. Parker, Formerly Director, Cross Infection Reference Laboratory, Colindale, Manchester, U.K.

B. L. Pentecost, Consultant Physician, United Birmingham Hospitals; Senior Clinical Lecturer, University of Birmingham, U.K.

A. Percival, Professor of Clinical Bacteriology, Department of Bacteriology and Virology, University of Manchester, U.K.

P. L. Perine, Associate Professor, Department of Epidemiology, School of Public Health and Community Medicine, University of Washington, Seattle, U.S.A.

D. K. Peters, Professor of Medicine, Royal Postgraduate Medical School, Hammersmith Hospital, London.

R. Peto, Imperial Cancer Research Fund Reader in Cancer Studies, Nuffield Department of Clinical Medicine, University of Oxford, Radcliffe Infirmary, Oxford, U.K.

I. Phillips, Professor of Microbiology, St. Thomas's Hospital Medical School, London.

Julia M. Polak, Senior Lecturer in Histochemistry, Department of Medicine and Histochemistry, Royal Postgraduate Medical School, Hammersmith Hospital, London.

P. A. Poole-Wilson, Reader in Cardiology, Department of Cardiac Medicine, The Cardiothoracic Institute; Honorary Consultant Physician, National Heart Hospital, London.

J. S. Porterfield, Reader in Bacteriology, Sir William Dunn School of Pathology, Oxford, U.K.

R. E. Pounder, Senior Lecturer in Medicine, Royal Free Hospital Medical School; Honorary Consultant Physician and Gastro-enterologist, Royal Free Hospital, London.

F. S. Preston, Deputy Director of Medical Services, British Airways Medical Service, London (Heathrow) Airport, Middlesex, U.K.

A. B. Price, Consultant Histopathologist, Northwick Park Hospital, Harrow, Middlesex, U.K.

E. W. Price, Honorary Research Fellow, Department of Clinical Tropical Medicine, London School of Hygiene and Tropical Medicine, London.

B. N. C. Prichard, Professor of Medicine, University College Hospital Medical School, London.

J. S. Prichard, Senior Lecturer in Medicine, Trinity College, Dublin, Consultant Physician, St. James's Hospital, Dublin, Eire.

N. B. Pride, Consultant Physician, Hammersmith and Ealing Hospitals; Honorary Senior Lecturer in Medicine, Royal Postgraduate Medical School, Hammersmith Hospital, London.

B. Pruitt, Jr, Commander and Director, U.S. Army Institute of Surgical Research, Brooke Army Medical Center, Fort Sam, Houston, Texas, U.S.A.

S. Punyagupta, Medical Director, Vischaiyut Clinic, Bangkok, Thailand.

M. Rachmilewitz, Professor Emeritus, Hebrew University; Hadassah Medical School, Jerusalem, Israel.

A. J. Radford, Professor of Primary Care and Community Medicine, Flinders Medical Centre, The Flinders University of South Australia, South Australia.

C. W. G. Redman, Lecturer in Obstetric Medicine, Nuffield Department of Obstetrics and Gynaecology, University of Oxford, John Radcliffe Hospital, Oxford, U.K.

R. S. O. Rees, Consultant Radiologist, St. Bartholomew's Hospital and National Heart Hospital, London.

D. Rennie, Associate Professor of Medicine, Harvard University; Senior Associate in Medicine, The Brigham and Women's Hospital, Boston, Massachusetts, U.S.A.

B. D. Ross, Honorary Consultant Physician, Nuffield Department of Clinical Medicine, John Radcliffe Hospital, Oxford, U.K.

D. J. Rowlands, Consultant Cardiologist, Manchester Area Health Authority; Lecturer in Cardiology, University of Manchester, U.K.

D. Rubenstein, Physician, Addenbrooke's Hospital, Cambridge; Associate Lecturer, University of Cambridge, U.K.

T. K. Ruebush II, Bureau of Tropical Diseases, Center for Disease Control, Public Health Service, U.S. Department of Health and Human Services, Atlanta, Georgia, U.S.A.

G. F. M. Russell, Professor of Psychiatry, Institute of Psychiatry, University of London, Bethlem Royal and Maudsley Hospitals, London.

T. J. Ryan, Consultant Dermatologist, The Slade Hospital, Oxford, U.K.

Dame Cicely Saunders, C.B.E., Medical Director, St. Christopher's Hospice, London.

J. G. Scadding, Emeritus Professor of Medicine, University of London.

A. Seaton, Director, Institute of Occupational Medicine, Edinburgh, U.K.

Dame Sheila Sherlock, D.B.E., Professor of Medicine, Royal Free Hospital School of Medicine, London.

E. A. Shinebourne, Consultant Paediatric Cardiologist, Brompton Hospital, London.

D. I. H. Simpson, Director, Special Pathogens Reference Laboratory, Centre for Applied Microbiology and Research, Porton Down, Salisbury, U.K.

V. Sitprija, Professor of Medicine and Associate Dean, Division of Nephrology, Department of Medicine, Chulalongkorn Hospital, Bangkok, Thailand.

M. B. Skirrow, Consultant Microbiologist, Department of Pathology (Microbiology), Worcester Royal Infirmary, Worcester, U.K.

Mary E. P. Slack, University Lecturer in Bacteriology, University of Oxford; Honorary Consultant Microbiologist, John Radcliffe Hospital, Oxford, U.K.

P. Sleight, Field Marshal Alexander Professor of Cardiovascular Medicine, University of Oxford, Department of Cardiology, John Radcliffe Hospital, Oxford, U.K.

J. C. Smith, Consultant Urological Surgeon, Radcliffe Infirmary, Oxford, U.K.

R. Smith, Consultant Physician and Consultant in Metabolic Medicine, John Radcliffe Hospital, Oxford, U.K.

J. Somerville, Consultant Physician in Congenital Heart Disease, National Heart Hospital, London.

W. Somerville, C.B.E., Consultant Physician, Department of Cardiology, The Middlesex Hospital, London.

J. M. K. Spalding, Formerly Consultant Neurologist, Oxford; Senior Research Fellow, St. Peter's College, Oxford, U.K.

J. E. Stark, Consultant Chest Physician, Department of Respiratory Medicine, Addenbrooke's Hospital, Cambridge, U.K.

G. Stores, Consultant Neuropsychiatrist, The Park Hospital for Children, Oxford, U.K.

Jane A. Summerfield, Lecturer, Department of Medicine, Royal Free Hospital School of Medicine, London.

P. Suntharasamai, Associate Professor, Faculty of Tropical Medicine, Mahidol University, Bangkok, Thailand.

R. Sutton, Consultant Cardiologist, Westminster Hospital, London.

K. B. Taylor, The Barnet Professor of Medicine, Stanford University School of Medicine, California, U.S.A.

D. Taylor-Robinson, Head, Division of Communicable Diseases, Transmitted Diseases Research Group, Clinical Research Centre, Harrow, Middlesex, U.K.

W. Thamavit, Associate Professor, Department of Pathobiology, Faculty of Science, Mahidol University, Bangkok, Thailand.

H. C. Thomas, Senior Wellcome Fellow, Honorary Senior Lecturer, Honorary Consultant Physician, Royal Free Hospital, London.

P. K. Thomas, Professor of Neurology, Royal Free Hospital School of Medicine, London.

J. O'H. Tobin, Demonstrator in Pathology, Sir William Dunn School of Pathology, University of Oxford, U.K.

D. Todd, Professor of Medicine, University of Hong Kong, Queen Mary Hospital, Hong Kong.

A. M. Tomkins, Medical Research Council Laboratories, Fajara, Banjul, The Gambia, West Africa; Department of Human Nutrition, London School of Hygiene and Tropical Medicine, London.

T. A. Traill, Assistant Professor of Medicine, The Johns Hopkins Hospital, Baltimore, Maryland, U.S.A.

J. D. Treharne, Senior Lecturer in Virology, Sub-Department of Virology, Institute of Ophthalmology, London.

Joan M. Trowell, Oxford Regional Health Authority Research Fellow and Honorary Consultant Physician, Radcliffe Infirmary, Oxford, U.K.

S. C. Truelove, Formerly, Reader in Clinical Medicine, University of Oxford; Nuffield Department of Clinical Medicine, University of Oxford, John Radcliffe Hospital, Oxford. Consultant Physician, John Radcliffe Hospital, Oxford, U.K.

M. T. Tsuang, Professor and Vice-Chairman, Section of Psychiatry and Human Behavior, Brown University, Butler Hospital, Providence, U.S.A.

D. C. Turk, Consultant Microbiologist, Public Health Laboratory, Northern General Hospital, Sheffield, U.K.

R. C. Turner, Clinical Reader and Honorary Consultant Physician, Nuffield Department of Clinical Medicine, Radcliffe Infirmary, Oxford, U.K.

Margaret E. H. Turner-Warwick, Professor of Medicine (Thoracic Medicine), Department of Medicine, Cardiothoracic Institute, London.

J. A. Vale, Director, West Midlands Poisons Unit, Birmingham, U.K.

R. I Vanhegan, Consultant Pathologist, Princess Margaret Hospital, Swindon, U.K.

A. Vejjajiva, Professor of Neurology, Division of Neurology, Department of Medicine, Rama Thibodi Hospital, Mahidol University, Bangkok, Thailand.

M. P. Vessey, Professor of Social and Community Medicine, Department of Community Medicine and General Practice, University of Oxford, U.K.

G. N. Volans, The Director, Poisons Unit, Newcross Hospital, London.

N. H. Wadia, Honorary Professor of Neurology, Grant Medical College; Director of Neurology, Jaslok Hospital and Research Centre; Consultant Neurologist, The B.D. Petit Parsee General Hospital, Bombay, India.

J. A. Walker-Smith, Consultant Paediatrician, St. Bartholomew's Hospital, London.

Sir John Walton, Professor of Neurology, University of Newcastle upon Tyne; Consultant Neurologist, Newcastle Area Hospitals, Regional Neurological Centre, General Hospital, Newcastle upon Tyne, U.K.

C. P. Warlow, Clinical Reader, Department of Neurology, University of Oxford, Radcliffe Infirmary, Oxford, U.K.

D. A. Warrell, Director, Wellcome-Mahidol University, Oxford Tropical Medicine Programme, Faculty of Tropical Medicine, Bangkok, Thailand.

K. S. Warren, Director, Health Sciences Division, The Rockefeller Foundation, New York, U.S.A.

M. F. R. Waters, O.B.E., Consultant Leprologist, Hospital for Tropical Diseases, London.

R. W. E. Watts, Head, Division of Inherited Metabolic Diseases, Medical Research Council Clinical Research Centre, Harrow, Middlesex, U.K.

D. J. Weatherall, Nuffield Professor of Clinical Medicine, University of Oxford, Nuffield Department of Clinical Medicine, John Radcliffe Hospital, Oxford, U.K.

A. B. D. Webster, Consultant Physician, Northwick Park Hospital, Harrow, Middlesex, U.K.

R. A. Weiss, Director, Institute of Cancer Research, Royal Cancer Hospital, Chester Beatty Research Institute, London.

B. Widdop, Consultant Biochemist, Poisons Unit, Guy's Hospital, London.

D. E. L. Wilcken, Associate Professor of Medicine, University of New South Wales, The Prince Henry Hospital, Sydney, New South Wales, Australia.

C. B. Williams, Consultant Physician, Endoscopy Unit, St. Mark's Hospital, London.

E. Williams, Consultant Physician, Withybush General Hospital, Haverfordwest, Dyfed, U.K.

D. Gwyn Williams, Consultant Physician in Renal Medicine, Clinical Science Laboratories, Guy's Hospital, London.

D. H. Williamson, Member of Medical Research Council External Staff, Metabolic Research Laboratories, Radcliffe Infirmary, Oxford, U.K.

D. L. Wingate, Senior Lecturer in Gastroenterology, and Honorary Consultant Physician, The London Hospital, London.

H. F. Woods, Professor of Therapeutics, University of Sheffield, The Royal Hallamshire Hospital, Sheffield, U.K.

T. E. Woodward, Professor and Chairman, Department of Medicine, University of Maryland School of Medicine and Hospital, Baltimore, Maryland, U.S.A.

K. G. Wormsley, Consultant Physician, Ninewells Hospital, Ninewells, Dundee, U.K.

F. W. Wright, Consultant Radiologist, Clinical Lecturer in Radiology, Department of Radiology, Churchill Hospital, Oxford, U.K.

S. G. Wright, Senior Lecturer, Department of Clinical Tropical Medicine, London School of Hygiene and Tropical Medicine; Honorary Consultant Physician, Hospital for Tropical Diseases, London.

V. Wright, Professor of Rheumatology, Rheumatism Research Unit, Leeds, U.K.

V. Wright, Consultant Surgeon, Queen Elizabeth Hospital for Children, London.

V. Zaman, Professor of Parasitology, Faculty of Medicine, University of Singapore.

A. J. Zuckerman, Professor of Microbiology, Director of the Department of Medical Microbiology and WHO Collaborating Centre for Reference and Research on Viral Hepatitis, London School of Hygiene and Tropical Medicine, University of London.

Section 1
On textbooks and medicine

On textbooks and medicine

A. M. Cooke

'Of making many books there is no end; and much study is a weariness of the flesh.' Nevertheless, physicians have been writing textbooks of medicine for at least 5000 years. The first Oxford text, the *Rosa Medicinae*, was written about 1314.

What is expected of a modern textbook? It can never be fully comprehensive nor completely up-to-date. It should aim to give an overall view of the commoner diseases (that is, the important ones), avoiding undue detail and extreme views. It should not be merely descriptive, but should deal with the factors behind disease, genetic and environmental, with the mind as well as the body, and with the pathophysiology of disease processes. Doctors are given to quasi-philosophical discussions on whether or not diseases exist, and if they do, how they are to be defined. It is true that Armand Trousseau said '*Il n'y a pas de maladies, seulement des malades*', but most of us, medical and lay, have little difficulty in understanding what is meant by 'a disease', and the concept is a convenient one.

In effect, a textbook of medicine maps out the terrain where the physician will face and try to solve the problems of diagnosis and treatment. Beginners will find that a textbook tends to make diagnosis appear to be easier than it is, because every symptom and every sign are recorded, but in real life the patient may show only a few of the known symptoms and signs, and these may not be typical. Richard Cabot pointed out that in any serious or complicated illness there is always at least one symptom or sign that does not fit in or make sense.

Important as textbooks are for the student, and indeed for the experienced physician, they form only a small part of medicine. It has been said that the physician who practises medicine without a textbook is like a sailor who goes to sea without a chart, while the physician who studies books rather than patients is like a sailor who does not go to sea at all. Thomas Sydenham put it more forcibly when he said to the young Hans Sloane '. . . you must go to the bedside, it is there alone that you can learn disease'. Books or no books, medicine is essentially a practical art. At the bedside, whatever the difficulties in diagnosis, decisions *must* be made and action taken.

Textbooks outline the treatment of the diseases described, but physicians do not treat diseases, they treat human beings, all of whom differ from each other, with individual likes and dislikes, fears and prejudices, a unique set of genes, and widely differing environmental backgrounds. A patient is not merely an example of some disease described in the textbook, but is a fellow creature and emphatically not 'a case'. Used in this sense the word 'case' should be expunged from the medical vocabulary.

Physicians should not need to be reminded that all their patients have minds as well as bodies. A study made by a physician and a hospital chaplain has drawn much-needed attention to the many fears and worries that can afflict patients in hospital. This is so important an aspect of medicine that with the kind permission of the authors the results of their survey are given in full.

Feeling of strangeness and helplessness. While many patients experience a feeling of great relief at being admitted to hospital, there are others who, especially in the first few days, find difficulty in adapting themselves to the new environment. The following are the main matters that we have found to be a cause of concern to the patient at this time.

Away from home, perhaps for the first time.

Confined to bed; strange high bed; surrounded by patients in other beds.

Clothes are taken away; given strange backward gown to wear.

Cannot come and go as one pleases.

Cannot select own food; food is different and strange; do not like this food, but don't like to say so.

Cannot take own bath; must be bathed by a stranger when and how ordered. Sense of shame at being bathed by a nurse.

Cannot go to WC; must use urinal and bedpan; great difficulty in performing exhausting task of using bedpan.

Not in control of situation; must submit to nurses, doctors, students, etc.

No privacy; must submit to examination by any and all who desire.

Can't sleep for the noise of nurses working in the early hours of the morning.

The doctor in direct charge is too young, and the older ones are too busy to listen to my long story.

Can't tell the doctor all the facts, as it would embarrass me too much.

Life is made a misery by medical students using me as a guinea-pig for practising taking off blood, etc.

I'm not a person. I'm just another case.

Worry about relatives and dependants. It is surprising how frequently the hospital patient worries a great deal about his family, often unnecessarily, without confiding this fact to the doctors or nursing staff. This is most commonly the case when the mother of a young family is hospitalized, and it is evident that such a patient must undergo severe emotional stress if she is apprehensive about the way in which her children are being cared for in her absence.

How will (wife, husband) get on without me?

Who will take care of the children?

Who will take my place in the family circle of activities?

How can I keep the family from worrying about me?

I am so lonely in this strange place!

Worry about job, examinations, etc. In many diseases, mental rest is perhaps the most important part of the treatment. The duodenal ulcer of the business executive is not likely to heal while he lies in bed fretting about the way in which his office is being run in his absence.

I am indispensable. The work cannot go on without me.

Supposing they find they *can* get on without me!

I cannot be idle like this, I must get out tomorrow.

I'm missing so many classes that I'll fail my examinations. I might even miss the examinations.

Supposing I have a deformity, or some weakness, and have to change occupations.

It's all very well to tell me to take an open-air job, but what can I do?

Financial worries. It is fortunate that in the United Kingdom the person who has the bad luck to fall ill does not have the further worry of how he is going to pay for his illness. Nevertheless, the patient may be very disturbed about financial matters in relation to himself or his family.

How will my family be supported while I'm in hospital?

Supposing I become an invalid for life?

While I'm here my business will be ruined, and so will I.

It's all very well to say to take a light job, but how can we live on the pay?

Concern about the illness itself. It is natural that the patient should be apprehensive about the nature and results of his illness. This is often made worse by injudicious reading of home medical books or newspaper medical articles, and the patient may develop a state of extreme anxiety through misunderstanding such matter, or from overhearing injudicious remarks made near his bedside.

What is the nature, duration of this illness? How long will I be in hospital?

Will I have to have an operation?

Will they tell me the truth? Will they operate without warning me? What are they hiding?

Will it hurt? How much? Can I stand it? Will I make a fool of myself?

What about the anaesthetic? I might say things I should not say.

Can I trust the doctor, the surgeon, the nurse?

Why do they keep asking these foolish questions?

Why do they keep taking my blood pressure, blood tests etc.?

Mrs Brown says her sister died of something just like I've got.

I saw my chart lying on the table. I've got a fatal disease.

I overheard the professor (doctor, sister, nurse, student, visiting doctor), saying I have cancer (six months to live, a hopeless outlook, came to hospital too late).

Is it hereditary? Is it infectious?

Fear about the diagnosis. Many patients have a fear of cancer, and many of those are afraid even to mention this to the doctor in case their fear should be realised.

Perhaps I have cancer (leukaemia, tuberculosis, syphilis), and they are hiding it from me.

I don't believe their diagnosis.

The doctor can find nothing organically wrong, and says it is imagination. But I still have the pain.

I don't want to see the psychiatrist. I'm not mad. Think of the disgrace.

I am a diagnostic problem. Nobody can find out what is wrong with me.

I can't tell them about the lump I feel in case it's cancer.

It's just like my father had, and he died of cancer.

Fear of pain. It is surprising how much pain many patients can endure without complaint, but there is considerable individual variation in this respect.

Will it hurt? Will I be able to stand it?

I'd rather die than have another sternal puncture.

If only that other doctor would do it. He realises it can hurt, and does his best to make it painless.

Will I make a fool of myself, and show that I'm a coward?

Will I become a dope addict with all those drugs?

Will they give me something to make me sleep tonight?

Fear of the operation. Possibility of dying on the operating table.

Fear of the anaesthetic; fear of talking, and revealing inner thoughts.

Fear of not getting sufficient anaesthetic, or of the operation being started too soon.

Difficulty of surrendering life into the hands of the surgeon and of God.

Is this operation necessary?

Fear of pain after the operation, evidence of this from seeing other patients after operation.

Modesty about being exposed during the operation.

Fear of physical handicap or deformity. Will my handicap or deformity spoil my appearance? Will people stare, pity?

Will my activities, job, sports be curtailed?

Will I become less attractive sexually? Incapable of sexual relations?

Will I lose my job? Have to change my occupation?

Will I be distasteful aesthetically? Repulsive to others?

Will I always have to have this colostomy?

Sense of guilt. A sense of guilt is not uncommon in association with illness, and may be revealed more readily to the chaplain than to the doctor or nurse.

Why did this happen to me?

Am I being punished for some sin that I have committed?

Is it my fault? I did not take care of myself. I have waited too long.

Is it someone else's fault—my family, my doctor, my employer, my heredity?

Will they find out that I had VD? Think of the disgrace if my family find out.

I can't tell them how much alcohol I drink.

It must be because . . . (review of all past sins, wickedness, disobediences, warnings, old wives' tales).

Fear of getting well. This short summary is not intended to be an exhaustive treatise on the psychology or psychiatry of the hospital patient, but every physician is faced with the patient who prefers to be in hospital.

Welcome haven and protection of hospital care.

Afraid of unpleasant environment of home, job, school, etc.

Love of attention received in hospital.

Compensation neurosis.

Need of an excuse for not succeeding in work, life, etc.

Fear of death. This matter is one that the patient usually discusses more readily with the chaplain.

Am I going to die? How long have I got to live?

Are they telling me the truth?

Am I ready to die? Why have I not led a better life?

What will happen if I die? To my family? To myself?

Will it be a long, lingering, painful death?

If I am to die, would it be wrong to take my own life to avoid misery?

Won't they give me something to put an end to it?

Can't they keep me going just a little longer in case some new cure is discovered?

I read in the Sunday newspaper about a cure for cancer. Why don't they get it for me?

Most of these fears may seem obvious, specially when they are pointed out. They occur not only in hospital but also in the out-patient clinic and the doctor's consulting room. There can be very few patients who have not experienced some of them. How seldom in hospital does a patient say openly 'What is the matter with me?' It is certain that nearly all wish to know. These aspects of illness are of course related to the important question of communication. The complaint of laymen that there is an iron curtain between doctor and patient is unfortunately often true. It is essential for the physician to explain and discuss the patient's illness with him, and preferably not in front of a large ward round. In a perfect world no one would qualify as a doctor, or nurse, without having been ill, experienced bewilderment and fear, or faced the rigours of modern investigation and treatment.

Technology. Once the physician has introduced diagnostic apparatus into medicine—the tape-measure, thermometer, watch, or stethoscope—it is logical to use any and every device that can assist diagnosis. As well as departments of pathology, radiology, and biochemistry, no up-to-date hospital is now without electric typewriters, electronic devices for measuring and recording, a department for radioactive isotopes, X-ray scanners, ultrasound, and the like. These aids are good servants, but bad masters. One danger of too much technology is that the physician may become so dependent on laboratory and mechanical help, that without them he is at a loss. Moreover, there is a tendency to use new and expensive apparatus simply because it is available.

There is a strong case for keeping alive purely clinical medicine, that is diagnosis by the history and the five senses (of which common sense is still the most important). It is not only a fascinating intellectual exercise, but in some circumstances indispensable. In a disaster such as earthquake, tidal wave, tornado or flood, in war, or in the middle of a desert, there may be no laboratory aids of any kind, but doctors will still be required to diagnose and treat patients.

Experimentation. There can be no progress in medicine without the trial of new methods and new remedies. Somebody had to give the first anaesthetic, the first antibiotic, had to do the first valvotomy, replace the first hip. These turned out to be successes, but it has to be confessed that there have been experiments on patients which were badly planned, unnecessary, useless, painful, or even dangerous. It is well for enthusiastic experimenters to ask—would I like this done to myself, my wife, or my child? They should remember the dictum of Chevalier Jackson, a noted endoscopist—practise your method first on a rubber tube, then on a cadaver, then on an animal, then on a man, and lastly on a child. Many hospitals have a committee to study the ethical aspects of experiments on patients, and so to exercise some control over what is done.

Research. Ideally, every doctor should try to add to medical knowledge, but there are two practical difficulties. First, only a small proportion of doctors have the special gifts required for doing research of value, and secondly, there are not enough important discoveries to go round. Every young doctor should be encouraged to try his hand at research, partly for its educational value, and partly to see if he or she has the particular mental equipment and outlook essential for successful research. The deplorable doctrine of 'publish or perish' is responsible for many repetitive, second-rate and third-rate publications. There can be no question about the importance of supporting the gifted researcher, but there is the problem of what to do with the large number of keen but undistinguished or inadequate workers. As world medical literature now requires at least one mile of shelf space every two years, adding to this torrent is a serious matter. Important papers may be buried in a mass of uninspired writing, and so be overlooked, as Mendel's classic paper on heredity was for 34 years. The problem of what to do with unsuccessful researchers is unsolved, but their keenness and energy could surely be diverted to useful channels.

Specialization. The ever increasing range and complexity of medicine has inevitably led to more and more specialization, and to the fragmentation of medicine. Will the process ever stop? Who is to direct the patient to the right doctor in the correct subdivision of the appropriate specialty? There is still a case for the general physician, specially in non-teaching hospitals where the more esoteric specialties are not represented. Also, junior students are best taught the principles of medicine by those with general interests, and not by those obsessed by some small specialty. There is a natural law in medicine that the smaller the specialty the more demands it makes for increased funds, premises, and staff. There is also the danger that those who shout loudest get most.

Medical students. The selection and training of medical students determine the quality of the next generation of doctors. Selection is now mainly on academic record, but general education, personality, and motivation are equally important. As John Stuart Mill said over a century ago 'Men are men before they are lawyers, physicians or manufacturers, and if you make them capable and sensible men, they will make themselves capable and sensible lawyers and physicians.' Although students must of necessity learn an enormous number of facts, more important is the training to develop the attitude of mind which questions, reasons, can weigh evidence, and acts logically when faced by some entirely new situation—above all a mind which has not been stifled by cramming.

Medicine abounds in many other problems. As well as the immediate and day-to-day problems of diagnosis and treatment, there are important wider issues that concern not only doctors, but the public and the state. It is an axiom that no hospital or department has all the money that it considers necessary for its work. How then are limited resources to be allocated—for the aged? for backward children? for organ transplants? for mental disease? for academic research? In a major disaster, who should be treated and who left to expire? Many of these problems are at present insoluble and of such complexity that they cannot be solved by any one person, or indeed by the medical profession alone. The solutions, if found, will be reached by co-operative studies by doctors, laymen, administrators, and even by government.

Art and science. Medicine is an art based on science, and is slowly moving away from art and towards science. The process is slow and can never be complete. Despite astonishing advances in technology in recent years, the crude death rate for England and Wales was exactly the same in 1977 as it was in 1955. The future of medicine is bound to involve more and more technology, but it is to be hoped technology curbed by common sense and tempered by humanity. Whatever technological empires are built, the most *important* person in the hospital will still be the patient.

Reference

Girdwood, R. H. and Ballinger, M. B. (1949). The factors that commonly worry the patient in hospital. *Edin. med. J.* **56**, 347–52.

Section 2
Health and sickness in the community

Section 2
Health and sickness in the community

Health and sickness in the community

M. J. Goldacre and M. P. Vessey

The World Health Organization has defined health as a state of 'complete physical, mental and social well-being and not merely the absence of disease and infirmity'. This definition emphasizes that our attitude towards health should be a positive one but, for practical purposes, heavy reliance is placed on negative indices—mortality, morbidity, and disability—in measuring the health status of communities.

Mortality in the United Kingdom. Mortality statistics have been collected and analysed routinely in the United Kingdom since 1838. They occupy a special place in the measurement of disease because of their ready availability both for geographical and historical comparison. Tables 1 and 2 show annual death rates, expressed per 1000 individuals within each age-group, for England and Wales at

Table 1 Annual death rates per 1000 people within each age-group for selected years, England and Wales: males

Age (years)	1871–5	1901–5	1931–5	1951–5	1961–5	1971–5	1978
Less than 1*	167	151	70	30	23	19	15
1–4	NA	NA	6.9	1.2	0.9	0.8	0.6
5–9	7.1	3.7	2.3	0.6	0.5	0.4	0.3
10–14	4.0	2.1	1.4	0.5	0.4	0.4	0.3
15–19	5.7	3.2	2.5	0.9	1.0	0.9	0.9
20–24	8.1	4.4	3.2	1.2	1.1	1.0	1.0
25–34	10	5.9	3.3	1.4	1.1	1.0	1.0
35–44	14	9.7	5.4	2.7	2.5	2.2	2.0
45–54	20	17	11	7.9	7.4	7.2	6.8
55–64	35	32	24	23	22	20	19
65–74	70	65	57	55	54	51	49
75–84	150	138	135	127	121	116	112
85 and over	323	275	279	266	253	241	234
All ages	23.3	17.1	12.7	12.5	12.4	12.4	12.4
SMR†	314	234	127	98	95	89	85

* Deaths under one year of age per 1000 live births
† Standardized mortality ratio (base years, 1950–2 = 100), see page 2.7
NA = not available
Source: Office of Population Censuses and Surveys *Mortality Statistics*

Table 2 Annual death rates per 1000 people within each age-group for selected years, England and Wales: females

Age (years)	1871–5	1901–5	1931–5	1951–5	1961–5	1971–5	1978
Less than 1	138	124	54	23	18	15	12
1–4	NA	NA	6.2	1.0	0.8	0.6	0.5
5–9	6.6	3.8	2.1	0.4	0.3	0.3	0.2
10–14	4.0	2.2	1.4	0.3	0.3	0.2	0.2
15–19	5.9	3.0	2.2	0.5	0.4	0.4	0.4
20–24	7.4	3.7	2.8	0.7	0.5	0.4	0.4
25–34	9.2	5.0	3.1	1.1	0.7	0.6	0.6
35–44	12	8.1	4.3	2.1	1.8	1.6	1.4
45–54	16	13	8.0	4.9	4.4	4.4	4.2
55–64	29	25	17	12	11	10	9.8
65–74	61	55	43	33	30	27	25
75–84	135	120	109	92	84	75	70
85 and over	294	249	245	222	207	194	191
All ages	20.7	15.0	11.4	10.9	11.2	11.4	11.5
SMR	371	264	141	95	87	81	77

See footnote to Table 1

various times during the past century. Mortality rates have declined substantially at all ages during the period although the changes are more impressive in those under 45 years of age than in older people. Analysis of mortality rates by cause leaves no doubt that numerically the most important factor in the decline has been the fall in deaths from infectious diseases. The reasons for this fall are to some extent a matter of speculation although it is clear that for many diseases the greater part of the reduction occurred prior to the introduction of specific medical intervention, such as the use of immunization or antimicrobial chemotherapy, directed to the care of the individual patient (Fig. 1). McKeown has suggested that the main reasons for the downward trend in mortality have been, in order of importance, rising standards of living (of which possibly the most significant factor was improvement in diet), developments

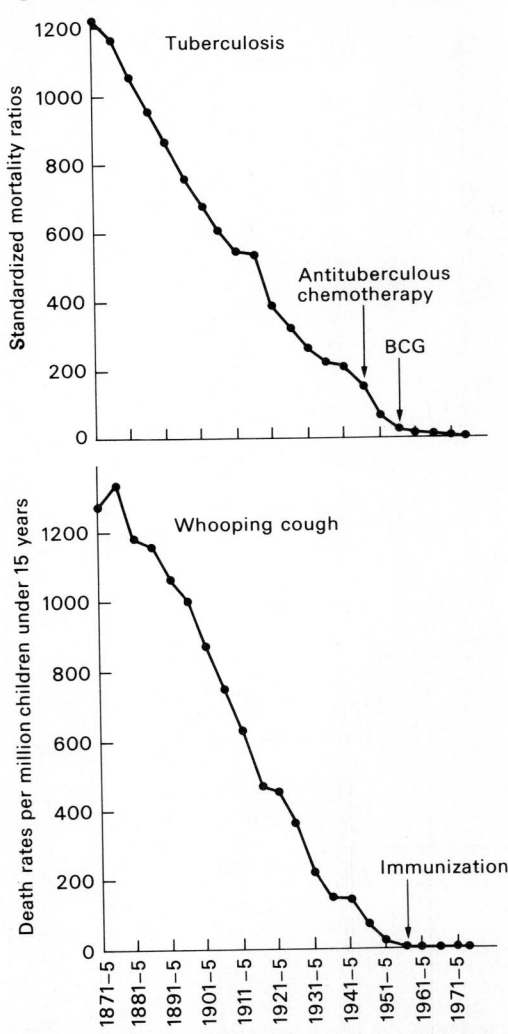

Fig. 1 Deaths from (a) tuberculosis expressed as standardized mortality ratios and (b) whooping cough expressed as annual death rates per million children under 15 years of age. (Source: Office of Population Censuses and Surveys *Mortality Statistics*)

in hygiene and the control of the physical environment, limitation of population growth, and the introduction of preventive and therapeutic medical measures.

The infant mortality rate (i.e. deaths under one year of age per 1000 live births) has declined dramatically in the United Kingdom during this century (Fig. 2). Nonetheless, death rates are still higher in the first year of life than in any other single year below the age of 55 in males or 60 in females. The main causes of death in the neonatal period (the first four weeks of life) are now those associated with low birth weight, complications of pregnancy and childbirth, and congenital malformations. The main causes of death in the post-neonatal period (from the end of the fourth week to the end of the first year of life) are respiratory and other infective diseases, congenital malformations, the sudden infant death syndome, and accidents.

Death rates in children aged 1–14 years have shown about a ten-fold decline since the turn of the century, mainly due to the reduction in deaths from infectious diseases, and now stand at very low levels. Accidents presently account for about one-third of all deaths in this age-group and neoplasms for one-fifth. Other numer-

ically important causes of death include congenital malformations and respiratory infections.

For adolescents and young adults, mortality has fallen more steeply in females than in males (see, for example, Fig. 3). The importance of accidents as a cause of death in these age groups (especially in males) is shown in Table 3.

Table 3   Death rates in people aged 15–24 and 25–34 years of age per million people of each sex in each age-group: England and Wales, 1978 (percentage of all deaths in each age-group in parentheses)

Causes	Males		Females	
	15–24	25–34	15–24	25–34
Neoplasms	92 (9.7)	178 (18.8)	64 (16.3)	184 (31.3)
Circulatory diseases	36 (3.8)	132 (14.0)	28 (7.1)	82 (13.9)
Respiratory diseases	35 (3.7)	49 (5.2)	25 (6.4)	35 (6.0)
Accidents	662 (69.9)	455 (48.1)	191 (48.6)	156 (26.5)
All other causes	122 (12.9)	131 (13.9)	85 (21.6)	131 (22.3)
Total	947 (100.0)	945 (100.0)	393 (100.0)	588 (100.0)

In older age-groups, neoplasms and circulatory diseases are now the dominant causes of death (Table 4). Mortality rates among men in middle- and late middle-age showed a marked improvement during the early part of the present century (Fig. 4), but began to level off in the 1920s and have shown only modest changes from then up to the present day. Interestingly, mortality rates among women have continued to decline steadily throughout the century. The past 50 years have seen the emergence of two conditions in

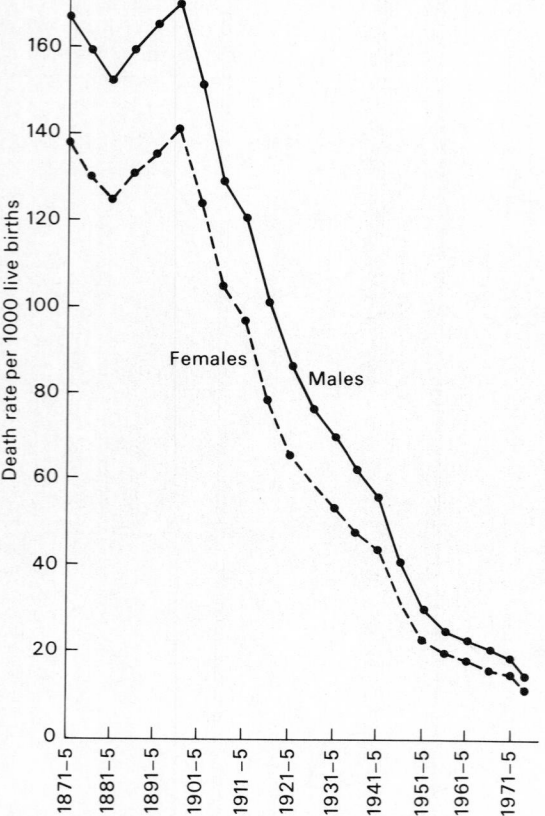

Fig. 2   Infant mortality rates for males and females.

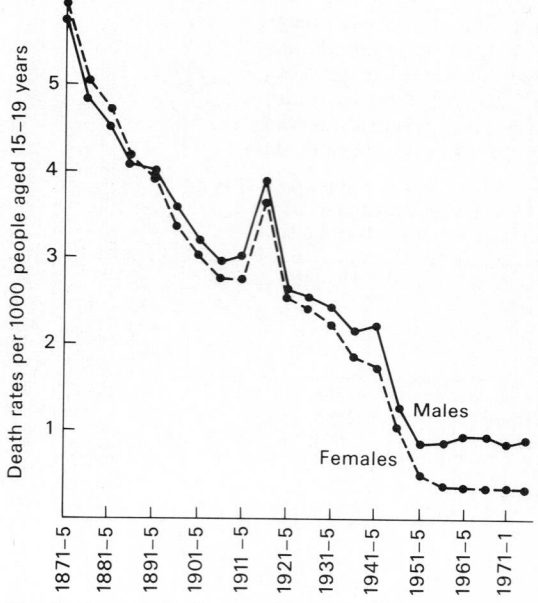

Fig. 3   Annual death rates in people aged 15–19 years.

Table 4   Death rates in people aged 35–74 years per million people in each age-group for selected causes of death: England and Wales, 1977 (percentage of all deaths within each age-sex group in parentheses)

Causes	35–44 years		45–54 years		55–64 years		65–74 years	
	Males	Females	Males	Females	Males	Females	Males	Females
Malignant neoplasm of lung	95 (4.7)	44 (3.1)	701 (10.3)	249 (6.0)	2507 (13.3)	702 (7.1)	5712 (11.6)	1066 (4.2)
Malignant neoplasm of breast		253 (17.6)		669 (16.1)		928 (9.4)		1219 (4.8)
All other neoplasms	351 (17.2)	350 (24.3)	1161 (17.0)	1121 (27.0)	3140 (16.7)	2394 (24.3)	7623 (15.5)	4510 (17.8)
Acute myocardial infarction	470 (23.0)	76 (5.3)	2129 (31.3)	388 (9.3)	5522 (29.3)	1522 (15.5)	12172 (24.8)	4974 (19.7)
Cerebrovascular disease	101 (4.9)	110 (7.7)	355 (5.2)	314 (7.6)	1213 (6.4)	907 (9.2)	4764 (9.7)	3556 (14.1)
Other circulatory diseases	254 (12.4)	119 (8.3)	1052 (15.4)	433 (10.4)	3080 (16.3)	1340 (13.6)	8605 (17.5)	4592 (18.2)
Accidents	423 (20.7)	208 (14.5)	491 (7.2)	262 (6.3)	559 (3.0)	343 (3.5)	767 (1.6)	572 (2.3)
All other causes	347 (17.0)	276 (19.2)	921 (13.5)	720 (17.3)	2831 (15.0)	1699 (17.3)	9447 (19.2)	4778 (18.9)
All causes	2041 (100.0)	1436 (100.0)	6810 (100.0)	4156 (100.0)	18852 (100.0)	9835 (100.0)	49090 (100.0)	25267 (100.0)

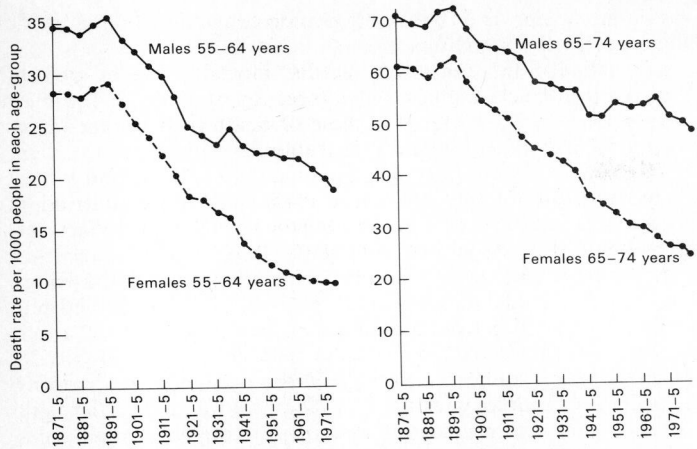

Fig. 4 Annual death rates in people aged 55–74 years.

particular, ischaemic heart disease (notably acute myocardial infarction) and lung cancer, which have increased substantially as causes of death and which, at present, are both commoner among men than women. Death rates for men aged 55–64 and 65–74 years are now almost double those for women of the same age.

Morbidity in the United Kingdom: the hospital perspective. Most routinely available information on morbidity in the population comes from statistics about the contact of people with health services. Hospital inpatient statistics have been collected nationally since 1949. Figures for episodes of hospitalized illness (conventionally counted as discharges from and deaths in hospital) show a predominance of patients under the care of acute medical, acute surgical, and maternity services (Table 5). A census measure shows that patients cared for by the specialties of mental illness, mental handicap, and geriatrics account for over half of all patients in hospital at any one time (Table 5).

Table 5 Annual number of hospital episodes (discharges from and deaths in hospital) and beds occupied daily: England, 1977. (Figures in thousands of patients and thousands of beds)

Specialty	Hospital episodes		Hospital beds occupied daily	
	No.	%	No.	%
Acute medical	1350.7	25.3	42.1	13.8
Acute surgical	2595.1	48.6	58.3	19.0
Maternity	694.7	13.0	12.9	4.2
Geriatrics	226.0	4.2	51.8	16.9
Mental illness	177.8	3.3	80.8	26.4
Mental handicap	19.6	0.4	47.9	15.6
Other	281.1	5.2	12.6	4.1
Total	5345.0	100.0	306.4	100.0

Some of the commonest causes of death are, of course, also among the commonest reasons for hospital admission—notably, acute myocardial infarction, other manifestations of ischaemic heart disease, cerebrovascular disease, and cancers (Table 6). But other conditions are also prominent: these include head injuries, adverse effects of medicinal agents (mainly self-poisoning), diabetes mellitus, pneumonia, bronchitis, and a number of surgical and gynaecological conditions.

Outpatient attendances exceed inpatient episodes in the acute specialties by an overall ratio of about six to one. Detailed information on the use made of outpatient services in the United Kingdom is not routinely collected but a general comparison of outpatient and inpatient workload in the acute specialties is show in Table 7.

Morbidity in the United Kingdom: the general practitioner's perspective. Hospital patients constitute a small proportion of all doc-

Table 6 Some common reasons for hospital admission: number of episodes, England and Wales, 1977 (percentage of all admissions for each sex in parentheses)

Disease	Number of episodes			
	Males		Females	
Malignant neoplasm of lung	38 310	(1.8)	10 370	(0.4)
Malignant neoplasm of breast	560	(<0.1)	36 510	(1.6)
Other malignant neoplasms	113 560	(5.5)	105 660	(4.6)
Diabetes mellitus	22 940	(1.1)	25 960	(1.1)
Cataract	16 090	(0.8)	24 210	(1.0)
Acute myocardial infarction	61 020	(2.9)	29 070	(1.3)
Other ischaemic heart disease	31 360	(1.5)	19 990	(0.9)
Cerebrovascular disease	46 940	(2.3)	58 280	(2.5)
Pneumonia	31 390	(1.5)	28 130	(1.2)
Bronchitis and emphysema	29 410	(1.4)	13 420	(0.6)
Hypertrophy of tonsils and adenoids	40 240	(1.9)	43 640	(1.9)
Appendicitis	36 090	(1.7)	36 830	(1.6)
Hernia	80 220	(3.9)	21 750	(0.9)
Cholelithiasis, cholecystitis	18 380	(0.9)	43 510	(1.9)
Hyperplasia of prostate	32 840	(1.6)		
Disorders of menstruation			94 770	(4.1)
Abortion			102 400	(4.4)
Arthritis	23 780	(1.1)	47 980	(2.1)
Fractures, dislocations, sprains	102 300	(4.9)	88 480	(3.8)
Intracranial injury	75 940	(3.7)	43 030	(1.9)
Adverse effects of drugs	39 640	(1.9)	67 070	(2.9)
All causes	2 071 500	(100.0)	2 315 560	(100.0)

Source: *Hospital Inpatient Enquiry*

Table 7 Comparison of number of inpatient episodes and number of outpatient attendances: medical and surgical specialties, England, 1977 (percentage of total in parentheses)

Specialty	Inpatient episodes		Outpatient attendances	
General medicine*	954.8	(24.2)	5121.0	(21.2)
Paediatrics	343.8	(8.7)	1100.4	(4.6)
Dermatology	20.6	(0.5)	1457.4	(6.1)
Sexually transmitted diseases	0.3	(<0.1)	1174.8	(4.9)
Rheumatology, physical medicine	31.3	(0.8)	830.4	(3.4)
General surgery	1084.4	(27.5)	3584.5	(14.9)
Trauma and orthopaedic surgery	446.3	(11.3)	4346.1	(18.0)
Ophthalmology	125.9	(3.2)	2562.2	(10.6)
ENT surgery	254.7	(6.5)	1904.9	(7.9)
Gynaecology	497.8	(12.6)	1596.4	(6.6)
Other surgical†	186.0	(4.7)	428.6	(1.8)
Total	3945.8	(100.0)	24 106.7	(100.0)

Notes: Figures in thousands of patients
Specialty given is the designated specialty of the consultant responsible for the case
* Includes infectious diseases, diseases of chest, cardiology, neurology
† Includes neurosurgery, plastic surgery, thoracic surgery

tor–patient contacts. An estimated 98 per cent of all episodes of illness which result in medical consultation are managed wholly within general practice. In addition, the majority of patients who are seen in hospital are referred from general practice. Table 8 shows, by broad classification, the illnesses managed in a year by the general practice with an average list-size of 2500 patients. Some of the commonest, and some of the serious but less common, diseases seen annually in an average general practice are shown in Table 9.

Morbidity in the United Kingdom: the individual's perspective. Data on illnesses which do not result in contact with the health service are relatively sparse but some information on self-reported illness is available from the General Household Survey in which samples of the population are interviewed about various matters

Table 8   Number of consultations per year in general practice per 2500 patients on practice list for selected broad disease groupings

Condition	No. of consultations
Diseases of respiratory system	1475
Mental disorders	813
Diseases of circulatory system	671
Diseases of musculoskeletal system	529
Diseases of skin	488
Diseases of digestive system	456
Diseases of eye and ear	441
Accidents	413
Diseases of genito-urinary system	404
Neoplasms	108

Source: *Morbidity Statistics from General Practice*

Table 9   Number of individual patients seen per year in general practice per 2500 patients on practice list for selected diseases

Disease	No. of patients
Acute nasopharyngitis, pharyngitis, tonsillitis	461
Anxiety neurosis, depressive neurosis	181
Acute bronchitis, bronchiolitis	148
Otitis media	73
Hypertension	50
Cerebrovascular disease	12
Acute myocardial infarction	9
Acute appendicitis	5
Neoplasm of lung	2
Leukaemia	0.2

including health. In the most recent survey short-term health problems experienced during the 14 days prior to interview were reported by just over half the population. Just under half the population reported taking some kind of medication in the same period; and medication prescribed by doctors was taken by 13 per cent of all males and 18 per cent of all females. Diseases of the upper respiratory tract comprised the largest single group of disorders resulting in self-reported, short-term health problems, followed by injuries, bronchitis, and digestive disorders.

Chronic health problems were reported by 56 per cent of males and 70 per cent of females and, as might be expected, the percentage of respondents with self-reported illness rose with advancing age. Conditions which accounted for self-reported, long-standing illness are shown in Table 10.

Sources of information about disease in the community. Sample surveys are undertaken from time to time by research workers to

Table 10   Self-reported long-standing illness: rate per 1000 individuals within each age-group according to condition

Condition	Age group (years)		
	15–44	45–64	65 or over
Mental disorders	9.0	18.7	18.2
Diseases of the nervous system	7.6	14.2	14.0
Diseases of the eye and ear	7.6	16.5	56.2
Heart disease and hypertension	4.9	43.5	96.9
Other diseases of circulatory system	2.5	17.1	43.6
Bronchitis	5.4	27.5	56.0
Other diseases of respiratory tract	9.3	19.5	14.5
Diseases of the digestive system	5.3	18.7	38.5
Arthritis and rheumatism	5.8	41.8	123.3
Other diseases of the musculoskeletal system	6.6	18.3	16.1
Injuries	11.4	27.6	37.2

Source: *General Household Survey*

determine the occurrence of particular diseases in the community. However, most systematic information comes from routinely collected statistics and these are usually worth consulting before embarking on special studies. In addition to the sources of information referred to so far, there are some diseases which are recorded in systems of notification and registration. Notification of certain infectious diseases was introduced gradually in England and Wales around the turn of the 20th century as a means of controlling individual outbreaks and of monitoring the occurrence of infectious disease. Statistics are published regularly. Registration of cancers is undertaken in a number of countries including the United Kingdom. International data from cancer registries are now pooled and the latest publication from the International Association of Cancer Registries provides data on cancers from 78 populations in 28 countries. Many studies which make inter-population comparisons in cancer epidemiology use this source of information. There are also registration or notification systems for congenital malformations, some industrial diseases, and certain forms of handicap.

Diseases in the community: the epidemiological approach

The physician engaged in clinical practice is concerned with the diagnosis, treatment, and care of his patients as individuals. There are, however, circumstances where it is important to relate the illness of individuals to the populations from which they are drawn. Epidemiology is the study of disease and its distribution in defined populations. The hallmark of epidemiology is that it is concerned with identifying both the individuals who have the disease under study and with enumerating those who do not. In this way it is possible to calculate rates of occurrence of disease and to estimate whether the disease is commoner in people with particular characteristics than in others, whether it is commoner in one place than another, and whether its occurrence has changed over time. The term 'population' means more to the epidemiologist than simply a geographically defined group of people: it includes, for example, groups of people defined by their age, sex, or occupation, or who share particular social, behavioural, or environmental characteristics.

Measurement in epidemiology. Several general measures are commonly used in epidemiology. The *incidence* of a disease is the number of new cases occurring during a specified period of time. The incidence rate is this number per specified unit of population. A conventional expression of an incidence rate would be the number of new cases of the disease which occurred per year per thousand (or million) population. The *prevalence* of a disease is the total number of cases of the disease existing in the population at a specified time; and the prevalence rate is this number expressed per unit of population, say, per thousand individuals. There is an obvious numerical relationship between the measures of incidence and prevalence: the prevalence of a disease varies according to the product of its incidence and duration. In circumstances where the incidence of a disease and its duration—the length of time from onset to recovery or death—remain constant over time, the prevalence of the disease equals the product of its incidence and duration.

As we have already shown, the occurrence of most diseases and death varies considerably with age. It is therefore usually more appropriate to calculate age-specific mortality, incidence, or prevalence rates than 'all-ages' rates. Indeed, a comparison of, say, mortality rates between populations of different age-compositions which does not take account of age-specific rates can be very misleading. For example, whilst mortality rates have declined in every single age-group over the past 50 years, the all-ages mortality rate has shown virtually no change (Tables 1 and 2). The reason for this seeming paradox is that the percentage of elderly people in the population has increased over the years; and that, because the risk of dying is much higher in the elderly than in the young, the population has contained a much greater percentage of people at 'high risk' of dying by virtue of their age in recent than earlier years.

In practice a comparison between populations across a whole range of age-specific rates is usually rather cumbersome. Statistical methods have therefore been developed to summarize the disease experience of populations in a single figure which is standardized for differences in the age structure of the populations. One statistic which is commonly used for this purpose is the *standardized mortality ratio* (SMR). This is the ratio of the number of deaths actually observed in a study population to the number of deaths which would have occurred in the population if it had experienced the age-specific death rates of a standard population. The SMRs in Table 1 indicate that the age-standardized death rate for males in 1931–5 was 27 per cent higher, and that in 1978 was 15 per cent lower, than that in 1950–52. The methods of standardization can be applied to the study of morbidity as well as mortality rates, can be used to take account of differences between the sexes as well as differences in age, and can be used to compare populations defined by any number of characteristics.

Epidemiology in the study of causes and risks. The main application of epidemiology has been to study the determinants of the distribution and spread of disease in populations. The aim of this approach to disease—aetiological epidemiology—is to identify factors which are causally associated with the occurrence of disease and which may be manipulated in order to prevent the disease.

A classic example is the demonstration by John Snow in mid-19th century London that mortality from cholera was higher in areas which received their water supply from a particular company which obtained its water from a part of the river Thames heavily polluted with sewage. Snow recognized that factors other than differences in water supply might have correlated with the geographical differences in mortality from cholera. He took account of this possibility in the design of his studies which, indeed, finally implicated contaminated water as an important means by which cholera had spread. More recent examples of aetiological epidemiology include (among many others) the studies of the association between smoking and lung cancer; the use of oral contraceptives and the risk of cardiovascular disease; X-irradiation and leukaemia; maternal rubella and congenital malformations; work in the dye and rubber industry and cancer; and dietary factors, exercise, and ischaemic heart disease.

The concept of a causal association is one of profound importance in epidemiology. First, an observed association may be causal (factor A causes disease B) either directly or indirectly such that a change in the factor will result in a change in the frequency of the disease. Secondly, the possibility must sometimes be considered that the disease has caused the factor associated with it, rather than vice versa, as when the occurrence of the disease itself leads to a change in (say) the dietary, behavioural, or physiological variable under study. Thirdly, an observed association may be non-causal. For example, if factor A influences both factor B and disease C, factor B and disease C will be associated statistically. The association between B and C will, however, be non-causal and there would be no hope of producing a change in disease C by manipulating factor B. Awareness of the possibility of obtaining spurious associations, through 'confounding' variables, is a central feature in the design, analysis, and interpretation of epidemiological studies.

Descriptive studies. Descriptive epidemiological studies are undertaken to determine whether a disease varies in frequency from place to place, has changed in frequency over time, and whether particular characteristics of populations with a high frequency of the disease distinguish them from populations in which the frequency of the disease is low. Examples of *geographical variation* in disease frequency are legion—see for instance, pages 4.51 *et seq.* and page 13.151 in relation to cancers and heart disease—and, indeed, all countries exhibit their own patterns of disease.

Studies of variation in disease frequency over *time* may be concerned with long-term trends (for example, the increase in the

frequency of lung cancer or coronary heart disease over decades), with the cyclical changes characteristic of an infectious aetiology, or with short-term fluctuations in association with other environmental factors (e.g. atmospheric pollution).

Some data on the type of person affected by particular diseases are often available from routine health statistics and, in assembling epidemiological information about a disease, these usually receive early consideration both because of their ready availability and because of the clues they may give to aetiology. They include such factors as patients' age, sex, socio-economic status, occupation, and marital status. For example, the facts that death rates from cancer of the lung and myocardial infarction are strikingly higher among men than women (see Table 4) indicate that aetiological factors exist which predispose males to, or protect females from, these diseases.

Descriptive studies are useful for generating or testing the plausibility of aetiological hypotheses and may occasionally go far towards implicating a particular exposure. However, the investigator will usually wish to proceed to analytical studies (Fig. 5) to test whether the observations made on populations as a whole can be confirmed in groups of people defined according to whether they, as individuals, manifest the disease and have experienced the aetiological factor under study.

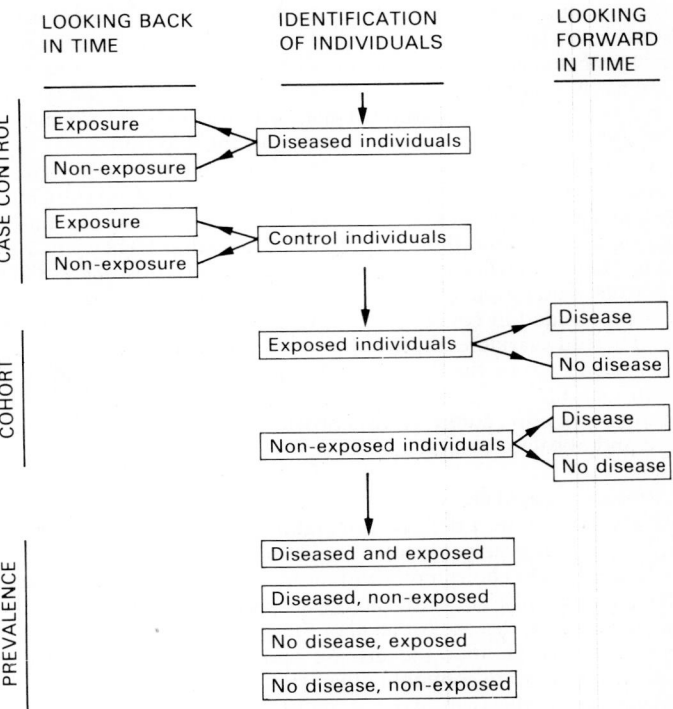

Fig. 5   Comparison of methods of case-control, cohort, and prevalence studies.

Case-control and cohort studies. The starting point for the *case-control study* is the identification of a group of individuals who have the illness under study and of an appropriate 'control' group of individuals who do not. Information about prior exposure to the suspected cause is then sought. The exposure of each group to the suspected cause is compared to determine whether it is any commoner among the cases than the controls. In a case-control study the diagnostic criteria for the inclusion of cases must be carefully defined; and the control subjects should be chosen such that they are comparable with the cases in all relevant respects except that they do not manifest the disease under consideration. Information about exposure to the suspected cause should be obtained in the same way for both cases and controls. Case-control studies are commonly used to investigate a specific hypothesis—for example, that there is a relationship between thrombo-embolic disease in young women and the use of oral contraceptives. Sometimes, however, if a specific hypothesis is not apparent, case-control studies may be used to explore a wide range of possible aetiological variables.

In a *cohort study* groups of people are identified according to whether or not they have been exposed to a factor (or possess a characteristic) which is thought to be related to the subsequent development of a disease. People in the non-exposed cohort are chosen such that they are comparable with the exposed cohort in all relevant respects except that they have not been exposed to the factor under study. These groups of people are then observed over a period of time to determine and compare the frequency of disease among the exposed and non-exposed groups.

Case-control and cohort studies each have advantages and disadvantages. Case-control studies involve many fewer patients than cohort studies; they are usually fairly quick, cheap, relatively easy to undertake, and they are the only feasible way to study rare diseases. Cohort studies usually need observations on large numbers of individuals and may require a period of follow-up over many years. They are therefore usually slow, expensive, and relatively difficult to undertake, and are only practicable for fairly common diseases. The smaller numbers in a case-control study will often permit study of individual cases in depth whilst the large numbers in a cohort study usually preclude collection of very detailed information on each subject. A case-control study is usually concerned with only a single disease but many possible aetiological factors may be sought. A cohort study is usually concerned with only one type of exposure but allows the study of many different diseases which may subsequently develop in association with the exposure.

Case-control studies are dependent on obtaining information about events which occurred at a time in the past and are subject to deficiencies and biases in patients' recall of past events and/or deficiencies of recording in old medical records. They are also sometimes subject to problems of bias in the selection of cases and controls. The problems of recall and some of the problems of bias can be avoided in cohort studies. Case-control studies cannot be used to study variables (such as physiological measurements) which may be altered by the disease while such factors can be studied in cohort studies. Case-control studies usually provide an estimate of relative risk only; cohort studies provide information on both relative and absolute risk (see below).

Prevalence studies. In a *prevalence study* the investigator studies individuals within a defined population to discover those with a disease (or with various levels of a quantitative attribute, e.g. blood pressure, serum cholesterol) and, at the same time, also measures the presence or absence of factors suspected to be related to the existence of the disease (or level of the attribute). The investigator then assesses whether the disease and the suspected causative factor coexist more commonly than would be expected by chance. Prevalence studies can avoid some of the biases inherent in the selection of cases in a case-control study, or in the identification of exposed individuals in a cohort study, because the whole population is sampled. Uniform criteria can be used readily in both the measurement of disease and of factors associated with it because both are studied simultaneously. As with cohort studies, prevalence studies usually require large numbers of individuals and are only appropriate for common conditions with a chronic course; but, unlike cohort studies, information on the occurrence of disease in relation to the factors associated with it does not need to await the passage of years. A common problem with prevalence studies, however, is that of distinguishing whether the disease preceeded the factor associated with it or vice versa. A prevalence study may be indispensable when no means exists through available records of identifying cases of the disease or of individuals with a particular exposure. In these circumstances a prevalence survey may be the essential first step in identifying cases for a case-control study or cohorts of individuals for further follow-up.

Interpretation of observational studies. The results of the methods of observational study described so far must be interpreted with due regard to the validity of the observations made and to the possibilities of bias and confounding. For example, the investigator who uses routine sources of data such as death certificates must consider the likely accuracy of certification of the cause of death. Interpretation of studies based on patients' recall must include the possibility that diseased individuals may be more likely than others to recall past events which they believe could be associated with their current disease. Bias in the identification of cases must also be considered as when, for example, subjects exposed to a suspected cause of illness are under more intensive medical surveillance than controls because of their exposure. The possibility that an association between a disease and a factor has arisen through the influence of a confounding variable related to both must be considered.

If an association does not seem to be attributable either to chance or to methodological problems in the design of the study, a causal interpretation can be considered. The likelihood that an observed association is causal is strengthened by (*a*) an appropriate temporal relationship in which the exposure clearly preceded the onset of the disease; (*b*) a high relative risk; (*c*) a dose response and/or duration response such that the risk of disease is associated with the degree of exposure; (*d*) consistency with findings from other epidemiological studies, with the results of laboratory research, and with other known facts about the disease.

Intervention studies. An *intervention study*, if practicable and ethical, is the definitive experimental way of testing an aetiological hypothesis. The effect of the removal of a factor thought to be related to the development of a disease, or the addition of a factor thought to confer protection, is tested (preferably in a randomized, controlled trial) to see whether the expected changes in disease frequency occur.

Risk. The *risk* of acquiring a disease can be expressed in several ways (Table 11). The *absolute risk* of developing a disease per year is given by the annual rate at which the disease occurs. The absolute risk over a period of years can be estimated simply by accumulating the successive annual incidence rates for the period required. The *relative risk* of acquiring a disease in association with an exposure is given by the incidence rate of the disease in the exposed group divided by the incidence rate in the non-exposed group. The *attributable risk* is given by subtracting the incidence rate in the non-exposed group from the incidence rate in the exposed group.

Table 11 Annual death rates, relative and attributable risks: death from lung cancer and ischaemic heart disease in non-smokers and heavy smokers

Disease	Death rate among non-smokers per 100 000 men	Death rate among heavy smokers per 100 000 men	Relative risk	Attributable death rate per 100 000 men
Cancer of lung	10	251	25.1	241
Ischaemic heart disease	413	792	1.9	379

Based on figures reported by Doll and Peto (1976)

Uses of epidemiology to complete the clinical picture. The experience of disease gained in clinical practice, and notably in hospital practice, is often incomplete for a number of reasons. Patients with an illness who are seen in one hospital or locality may not necessarily be representative of all patients with the illness. Selective factors, such as a hospital's special interests and reputation, may influence whether a patient is admitted to a particular hospital. Selective factors, such as the severity of the illness, whether its presentation is typical, the readiness and confidence with which a diagnosis can be reached and the patient treated outside hospital, may influence whether a patient is admitted to hospital at all.

Patients vary in the extent to which they seek medical services for symptoms: some patients with symptoms do not seek medical help. Information about disease in the community as a whole, as well as from particular medical institutions, may greatly aid understanding of the natural history of disease as the following examples illustrate.

1. Community-based studies of fatal acute myocardial infarction show that the majority of deaths occur outside hospital and that 40 to 50 per cent of deaths occur within one hour of the onset of the acute attack. These findings indicate that the outcome of heart attacks is considerably worse than would be apparent from observations made only on patients admitted to hospital. Furthermore, it cannot be assumed that hospital patients, who constitute only a selected proportion of all patients with the disease, are necessarily typical of all patients in respect of, say, factors which precipitated their attack. The findings also have implications for the organization of coronary care services; and, since a proportion of patients with coronaries are always likely to die before the arrival of care, they underline the importance of seeking means to prevent the disease.

2. The search for methods of early detection of presymptomatic disease, in order to screen for and prevent the development of disease, by definition requires the study of individuals in the community rather than of patients with manifest illness.

3. With some attributes (e.g. blood pressure, serum cholesterol) the distinction between disease and normality cannot be made from the study of clinical populations alone. The definition of levels of low intermediate, and high risk of developing disease depend on observations made on normal individuals as well as those made on patients with the disease.

Epidemiology in planning health services. The clinical management of a patient requires a clinical diagnosis. Management of medical resources to meet the medical needs of the community requires knowledge of the occurrence and distribution of disease in the community. The epidemiological approach can be used to monitor the health of the community, to show changing patterns of disease in the community, to identify groups of people who are at special risk, to assess local health problems and to quantify needs for local health services. In these ways epidemiological knowledge can be applied to the organization and planning of health services.

References

Doll, R. and Peto, R. (1976). Mortality in relation to smoking: 20 years' observations on male British doctors. *Br. med. J.* **ii**, 1525.

International Agency for Research on Cancer (1976). *Cancer incidence in five continents*, vol. 3 (eds. J. Waterhouse, C. Muir, P. Correa, and J. Powell). International Agency for Research on Cancer, Lyon.

McKeown, T. (1976). *The role of medicine.* Rock Carling Series, Nuffield Provincial Hospitals Trust.

Office of Population Censuses and Surveys. *Mortality Statistics.* HMSO, London, annual. (Prior to 1974: Registrar-General's *Statistical Review of England and Wales, Medical Tables*)

— *Hospital In-patient Enquiry.* HMSO, London.

— *General household survey.* HMSO, London.

— *Statistics of infectious diseases.* HMSO, London.

Royal College of General Practitioners. (1979). *Morbidity statistics from general practice, 1971–2: second national study.* HMSO, London.

Section 3
Medicine in an unjust world

Medicine in an unjust world

M. H. King

Four and a half billion patients in the practice

As the doctors of today we have four and a half billion people in our care. The practice has doubled in the past thirty years, and it will double again even faster, unless there is some colossal famine or disaster. Of the nearly two billion more people to be cared for by the end of the century, about 1.5 billion will be citizens of the developing world. The poorest 30 per cent of the practice are the low income countries whose per capita gross national product amounts to $300 or less. They are mostly in Asia and Africa, and include India, Bangladesh, Pakistan, Zaire, and Tanzania. Next come the middle income countries with a little less than half the world's population and a per capita GNP of between $300 and $3000. They include China, Nigeria, and most of Latin America. The richest countries, with a per capita GNP of over $3000, form about a quarter of the world's population. They include the industrial countries belonging to the OECD (USA, Japan, Scandinavia, and most of the countries of Europe), the centrally planned economies, such as the USSR, and the capital surplus oil exporters of the Middle East.

Places in the GNP league are changing. The newly developing countries such as Taiwan, South Korea, and Singapore, for example, are rapidly lifting themselves out of poverty. Some, such as Britain, whose place has fallen to 24th in the league, and whose GNP is presently declining, are rapidly becoming the post industrial 'new poor'.

The injustice of the world is such that three-quarters of the world's patients live on only a fifth of its income. About 800 million people are desperately poor, and, as Fig. 1 shows, most of them are

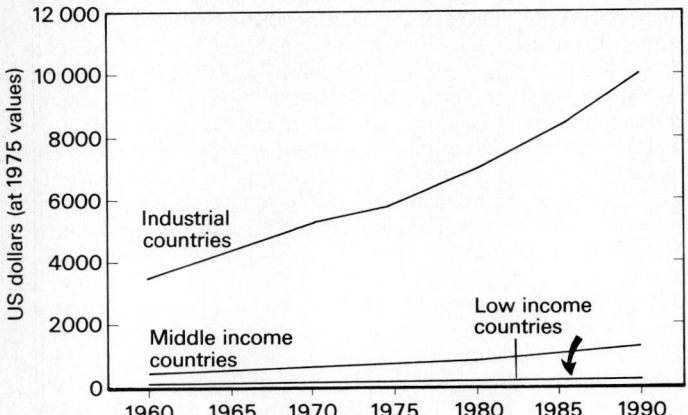

Fig. 1 Projected trends in per capita GNP. (From Fig. 4, *World Development Report* (1979). World Bank, Washington.)

likely to remain so. A recent World Bank report concluded that, even if optimistic rates of economic growth are achieved in the developing world, there will still be 600 million people trapped in absolute poverty in the year 2000. This, the Bank defines, as a condition of life so characterized by malnutrition, illiteracy, disease, high infant mortality, and low life expectancy as to be beneath any reasonable definition of human decency. Somehow these 600 million patients have to be cared for.

Despite the enormous inequalities between nations, the survival

of the world economy, with all that this means for the health of mankind, depends absolutely on the recognition of our dependence upon one another. Yet development is everywhere checked by political and economic uncertainties, and over us all hangs the ultimate cataclysm, that the escalation of tension among the superpowers, or even some malfunction of their military computer systems, will produce a scenario of unimaginable desolation, disease, and death.

The purpose of this section is to consider some of the challenges before us in our care of the world's sick, and to look widely at some of the adaptations that must take place in our own minds, if medicine is to do all that it might for mankind in the latter years of this century, and particularly for the sick poor of this planet. If it is mostly concerned with the developing world, this is because most of the world's patients live here. If it is disturbing, this is because the present state of the world can hardly be anything else. If it is unpopular, this may be because what needs saying and doing, often has been so.

Half the practice are villagers. Picture the village of Tubuan in the Philippines whose 550 people live in 95 houses hidden in a coconut grove and surrounded by paddy fields. At present, more than a billion people live in villages like this, and if you include China it is almost 2 billion, or nearly half the people in the world. But the picture is changing. The cities of the developing countries are now growing even faster than their total populations, with the result that the biggest of them are likely to exceed 30 million people by the end of this century. Providing these gigantic urban slums with health care promises to be hardly less difficult than caring for the villagers.

At present, in most developing countries three-quarters of the people still live in villages. Yet, despite this, three-quarters of the health expenditure is usually in towns. In the Indian state of Maharashtra, for example, although $1.60 per person per year is spent on health, only 2 cents are spent on the villagers, and 80 per cent of the total sum is spent in only three cities. As the result of such patterns of expenditure, over half of the people in villages and urban slums have no access to organized health services, nor are they likely to get them in the near future. Yet, despite the poor conditions of the present urban slums, the people who live in them are usually better off than the villagers, their infant mortality is lower, they are richer, they have cleaner water and better sanitation, they are more likely to go to school, and they have more personal health services. The situation is thus the reverse of that in England during the industrial revolution, when health was better in the villages.

Trade, aid, arms, and energy. The health of the absolute poor can only be improved by relieving their poverty. This requires much more international trade for the benefit of everyone, the investment of more private capital in the developing world, and better domestic development strategies designed specially to reduce absolute poverty. Although just what these strategies should be, under particular circumstances, is far from being fully understood, much can be done, and much more must be done.

As evidence of our priorities, there can be no greater indictment of our generation than to compare the resources we devote to arms with those we spend on helping the poor. Global defence expenditures have now grown so large that it is difficult to grasp their full dimensions. The overall total is now $450 billion each year, or about a million dollars a minute. The world's military expenditure of only half a day could finance WHO's entire malaria eradication programme. A modern tank costing about $1 million could provide 1000 classrooms for 30 000 children. A jet fighter for $20 million is the equivalent of 40 000 village pharmacies. Public expenditure on weapons research approaches $30 billion a year and occupies half a million scientists and engineers throughout the world. This is a greater research effort than on anything else on earth, and is more than that on the problems of energy, health, education, and food combined. Only about $20 billion is spent annually on development aid, and even this declined as a percentage of the combined GNP of the donors from 0.52 per cent in 1960 to 0.31 per cent in 1977. Of the $75 billion spent every year on health care in the developing world, only about 0.5 per cent comes as aid from the richer countries.

Few things are going to have a greater influence on what can or cannot be done for the sick than their access to energy. Every time the price of oil rises by $1 per barrel, the non-oil producing developing countries have to find an extra $2 billion a year to pay for their oil imports. Part of this section was written in Tanzania, 40 per cent of whose foreign exchange is now required to buy its meagre supply of oil. Where there is no foreign exchange left for health care, there are no drugs, no X-ray films, no surgical sutures, and no spares. For lack of fuel, supplies cannot reach distant hospitals and dispensaries, electricity cannot be generated, nor can water be pumped to enable a surgeon to wash his hands. Mostly for the lack of fuel to cook with, the forests of the developing world are being cleared at the rate of 50 acres a minute, with the result that it will be as tree-bare as the Middle East in two generations, with all the ecological implications that this will have for health. Land which could grow food is increasingly being used to produce motor fuel. No single factor so starkly outlines the wealth or poverty of nations as their access to energy. Most westerners use more energy in a year than the average Asian does in his liftime. Even in the industrial world, a 30-fold rise in the price of oil in 15 years has accelerated inflation, reduced industrial growth, and increased unemployment to such an extent that we may well see political instability added to economic stagnation and disorder, with all the consequences that this will have for health.

The health of the world

Despite what has just been said about the present prevalence of absolute poverty and the slow pace of development, both the health and the wealth of mankind is better than it was. Even in the developing world, the health conditions of many communities have improved considerably in recent decades. Since this has usually been accompanied by economic progress, there is now a marked association between the per capita income of a developing country and the state of its health. The best measure of this is life expectancy at selected ages. For the developing countries as a whole, life expectancy at birth increased from about 32 years before the Second World War, to about 49 years in the 1960s, compared with about 70 years for the industrial world. Unfortunately, the rate of improvement in the developing world is declining. These are moreover averages, and disguise the much lower expectations of the poor within a country.

Figure 2 shows the overall differences in patterns of disease between a typical developing country with a life expectancy at birth of only 40 years, and a young population, nearly half of whom are under 15; and an industrial country with an older population, nearly half of whom are over 40. A developing country has about four times as many deaths from infectious parasitic and respiratory diseases, only a quarter as many deaths from cancer, and only about half as many from cardiovascular disease or trauma.

The burden of preventable disease. In the world as a whole, the mere numbers of the sick with preventable diseases soon overwhelm us by their magnitude. Later editions of this Textbook will probably have much more to say about exercise, diet, fat and fibre,

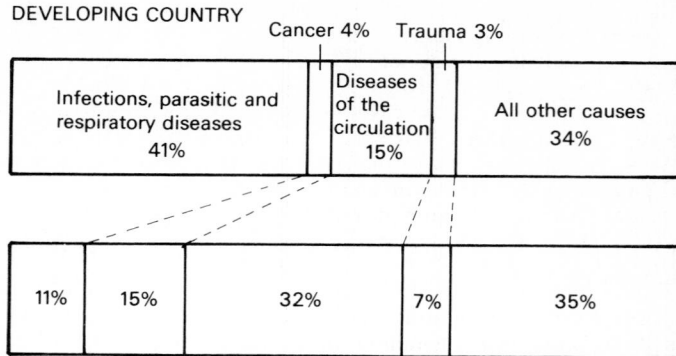

Fig. 2   Causes of death in a model developing country and a model industrial country. (From Table 3, *Health Sector Policy Paper* (1975). World Bank, Washington.)

and indeed about altering much of the western way of life in order to prevent the diseases it causes, particularly those of the cardiovascular system. Since these factors are complex and still controversial, this brief survey will confine itself to some factors which are less so.

Fifty million people were living in England and Wales in 1975 and 600 000 of them died. Half of them did so from diseases of the cardiovascular system, with cancer and respiratory diseases killing most of the rest. Of these deaths, over 10 per cent, and perhaps as many as 100 000 were due to smoking. In spite of this, nearly half the population of Britain, including one doctor in five, still smokes. If only it were possible to control tobacco, 40–50 per cent of all cancer deaths in males would be prevented. Although the tobacco companies are doing their utmost to promote the sale of cigarettes in the developing world, their major effect on mortality here has yet to come.

In spite of the 'green revolution' more people are hungry, even starving, than at any time in the past. A billion people are said to be malnourished, and 400 million on the brink of starvation. The mortality rate of children between one and five, which is perhaps the best indicator of nutrition, is 10 to 40 times higher in parts of Asia, Africa, and Latin America, than it is in Europe or the United States. In Africa alone, 30 per cent of children are estimated to be clinically underweight for their age, and 4 per cent of them seriously so, with either kwashiorkor or marasmus. Nevertheless, the population continues to increase, often at 3 per cent or more, in countries least able to increase food production, with the result that food aid can no longer be considered a transitional phenomenon, at least until the end of the century, the suppliers being always the industrial west, and the recipients the 29 least developed countries.

Human faeces transmit some of the most important diseases of the developing world, particularly the diarrhoeas of childhood, but also poliomyelitis, typhoid, cholera, and the worms of the gut. These and the airborne respiratory infections are the main cause of death in poor communities. Both the prevalence and severity of most of them are increased by malnutrition. In the developed world economic progress has fortunately controlled them by providing enough food, clean water, safe sanitation, and decent houses.

In 1975 there were about 500 million episodes of diarrhoea in the children of Asia, Africa, and Latin America, causing 5–18 million deaths, a situation comparable to that in the industrial world at the end of the last century. It is fortunate, therefore, that one of the great recent advances has been the use of rehydration fluids by simply trained workers to reduce the case mortality of even severe cases of dehydrating diarrhoea to less than 1 per cent. A major task now is to see that all the world's children benefit from it.

About a billion people have worms. Studies in Sri Lanka, Bangladesh, and Venezuela found that over 90 per cent of six-year-old children were infected. About 700 million people are said to have hookworm and probably even more have *Ascaris*.

The airborne infections include pneumonia, bronchitis, whooping cough, measles, influenza, diphtheria, meningitis, and tuberculosis. One study in Latin America found that, between them, these diseases accounted for between 20 and 30 per cent of all deaths. There are at least 7 million cases of infectious tuberculosis in the world, more than three-quarters of them in the developing countries. Although diagnosis is usually easy, and the drugs both effective and cheap, there are more than 3.5 million new infectious cases each year, and more than half a million people die.

At a conservative estimate there are 10 million leprosy patients in the world.

In sub-Saharan Africa alone, about 270 million people remain exposed to malaria without any organized protection, with the result that it kills nearly a million children each year. Over the past five years the total number of cases in the world has doubled, and in some countries it has increased forty times. As the result of air travel, there is now more malaria in Europe than there was when the global eradication programme began.

Although the other vector-borne diseases are less prominent than malaria in statistics of morbidity and mortality, they are important in certain areas. Two hundred million people have schistosomiasis, and another 200 million filariasis. Trypanosomiasis, and particularly Chagas' disease, are also serious problems.

One per cent of mankind cannot see, three-quarters of the blind live in the developing countries, and half of them suffer from such preventable and curable diseases as xerophthalmia, trachoma, and onchocerciasis.

Once a community has overcome malnutrition and the infectious diseases, the 'backward child' is one of its next urgent problems. There are at least 80–100 million mentally handicapped people in the world, most of whom could lead happy and socially useful lives, if only they received adequate care, support, and education, particularly during childhood. Much of this handicap is preventable by better perinatal care, and even such an eminently preventable disease as iodine embryopathy is still endemic in some areas.

Although as doctors we do not usually consider teeth our business, they cause much pain and suffering. This is quite unnecessary, since dental caries and periodontal disease are among the most widespread and preventable of all diseases.

This catalogue of organic diseases must not end without mention of the fact that perhaps 40 per cent of all the patients who seek help from the dispensaries, health centres, and outpatient departments of the developing world have no obvious organic complaint. Patients here seek help for all the major and minor ailments of body and mind, just as they do everywhere else.

Resources for the care of the sick

If these then are some of the diseases to be prevented and treated, what resources are available for such a gigantic task, both in absolute terms, and as a percentage of GNP? How does the money available differ in different parts of the world, and what trends are there in health expenditure? Finally, what might the global health bill look like, and how is it distributed?

Since the distribution of health manpower tends to follow that of money, it will merely be observed that in 1976 the doctor to population ratio ranged from 1:84 000 in Ethiopia to 1:410 in Israel. For the low income countries overall it is 1:10 300, and for the industrial ones 1:630. For nursing staff the ratios are even less favourable. Thus the low income countries have 16 times fewer doctors per head than the industrial ones, but 46 times fewer 'nursing persons' with all that this means for the sick. The inequality with which health staff are distributed within developing countries is no less serious. Thus about three-quarters of the doctors are in the cities where only a quarter of the people live.

The poorer third of the world. Improving health is a popular priority in the developing countries. Such data as there are suggest that in the public and private sectors combined, between 6 and 10 per cent of GNP is spent on health, in addition to what is spent on family planning, water, sanitation, and nutrition. For the poorest countries with a per capita GNP of only $100 this amounts to between $6 and $10. For those with a per capita GNP of $300 it is between $18 and $30. Of this, the government often spends less than half, $1 to $8 being the figure given by the World Bank for government health expenditure in the developing world, the remainder being spent by the patients themselves on private doctors and hospitals, on traditional practitioners, and on drugs from pharmacies.

Most government money is spent on expensive, well-equipped hospitals in towns, and on highly trained staff, with the result that most villagers and indeed many slum dwellers cannot reach it. Since it is modelled after care in the industrial world, it is heavily biased towards the cure of inpatients, and away from preventive medicine. Since it is politically impracticable to reduce such expenditure in order to make health care more equitable, the most that can usually be done is to try to curtail it.

The richer quarter of the world. Much better data are available for health expenditure in the industrial world. In the 1950s the countries of Europe spent about 4 per cent of their GNP on health, but by 1978 this had doubled, the Netherlands, for example, was spending 8 per cent, and Sweden 8.6 per cent. Even more serious, as Fig. 3 shows, the rate of increase has recently been rising, particularly since 1965. Thus in Europe in the decade of the 1950s, it typically increased by 1 per cent, in the 1960s by 1.5 per cent, and for the 1970s the figure is likely nearly 2 per cent. In 1971 it was estimated that the 10 per cent level would be reached by the end of the century, but if the present trend continues many countries will have reached it long before that. The USA is said to have got there already. The result is that, in per capita terms, a typical industrial country already spends more on health alone than the entire income of many developing ones.

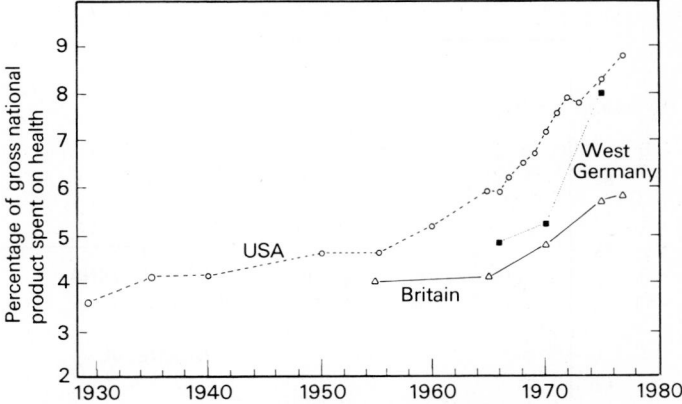

Fig. 3 The rising percentage of the GNP spent on health. (From Knowles, J. H. (1980) *Doing better and feeling worse*, Appendix Table A. Rockefeller Foundation and NCHSR (1980) *Research proceedings series*, Table 1. DHEW publications, PHS 79–3256.)

These figures are, however, all percentages of GNP. In terms of money spent, even at constant prices, the increases in health expenditure have been much greater, since the GNPs of all industrial countries have been increasing. That of North America for example increased by 4 per cent annually between 1970 and 1978. In current dollars total health expenditure in the USA rose nearly five times between 1960 and 1978.

In Europe and elsewhere the rising cost of medicine is causing much public concern. Although this is often focused on the high salaries of doctors, these are less important than the urge for every clinic to have and use every possible form of prestigious equipment. This trend cannot continue, since no country can afford to provide everyone with every possible form of technology, nor would this necessarily be good for the patient, or for society. Ways must be found to prevent the health industry from consuming an unjust proportion of the community's resources, to the detriment of education, industry, the environment, or any other legitimate human endeavour.

USA leads the way, but where to? The high and rapidly increasing cost of modern medicine is seen at its most extreme in the USA. In 1968 a week's stay in a hospital there cost $469, in 1978 it cost $1543. In 1983 it is expected to cost $2872. Even a normal antenatal patient can be asked to pay $900 on booking in, and $1000 later in pregnancy. Falling ill in America can be financially ruinous, and no less than half the private bankruptcies there are said to be caused by medical costs. Medicine has often failed to reach the very poor, but this is the first time that it has been able to bankrupt the middle classes in significant numbers.

When so much money is spent on health, it is important to know how and when it is spent. Much of it is spent when no reasonable expectation of useful life is possible. For example, one study showed that no less than $35 billion, or about 17 per cent of all health expenditure in the United States, was spent on the care of the terminally ill.

There can hardly be a more terrible reflection on the futility and indulgence of modern medicine than this. Of our roles as physicians to struggle so pointlessly, so cleverly, and so expensively to keep people alive, and of our roles as patients to refuse to accept that ultimately we too must die. In our determination to grasp even a few more days or even hours of life, we use resources that are badly needed elsewhere in the community and the world. We have long had placebo medicines, we now have an enormously more expensive placebo technology. If ever there was need for a change in the direction of modern medicine, it is this. Away from the emphasis on coronary bypass surgery and silastic aortas towards the prevention of preventable disease and the saner and more equitable use of the world's resources.

The global health bill. The per capita health expenditure of a country is the product of two factors, its per capita GNP, and the percentage of this that it spends on health. Of these, per capita GNP has much the greatest influence, since it varies a hundredfold, from about $100 to $10 000, whereas the percentage spent on health varies only about two-fold, from about 6 to 10 per cent. This means that Fig. 4, which shows the cumulative global GNP of the world's people arranged in order of their increasing wealth, is also a close indication of their per capita health expenditure.

Assuming that 10 per cent of the gross global product of about $8 trillion is spent on health, the high estimate for the world's total health bill is $800 billion, a figure which is likely to be closer to the true one than the low estimate of $480 billion. Of the high figure, $200 billion, or a quarter of the global sum is spent in the USA on only about 5 per cent of the world's people. If the estimate of the rest of the world's health expenditure proves to be high, the USA's share may well be nearer a third. Only 3 per cent of the world's health expenditure is spent on the poorest third of its people, and the poorest half of the world have only 10 per cent spent on them. The richest quarter of the world is responsible for 80 per cent of its entire health expenditure.

Figure 4 also plots the cumulative infant mortality. Half of all the world's children who die before their first birthday do so in the 30 per cent of the world who make up the low income countries. Of the 11.6 million infants who die each year 2.7 million do so in India alone. At the other end of the scale, only 4 per cent of infant deaths take place in the richest 25 per cent of the world.

A just share of the manpower pool. Besides consuming an ever increasing share of a country's wealth, the health industry also consumes such a high proportion of its available manpower, particularly the most talented members of the community, that this too may be impairing economic development. This is particularly true for the United Kingdom. Thus a recent circular from Britain's Royal College of Physicians remarked that 'Whatever the political influence of the United Kingdom in the world, its prestige in world

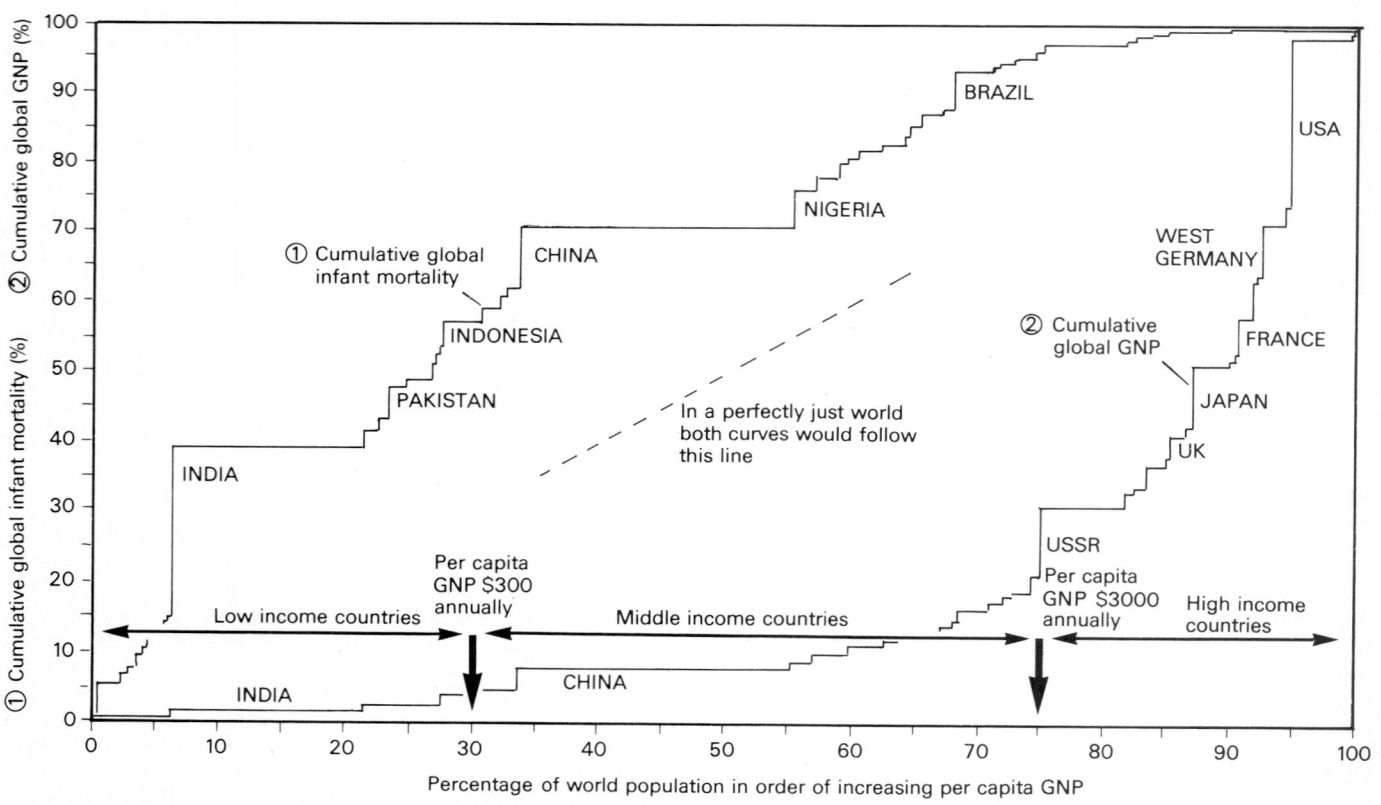

Fig. 4 Cumulative global infant mortality and cumulative global GNP. (Data from the World Population Data Sheet 1979.)

medicine has never been higher.' Unfortunately, political influence depends on economic strength and the College failed to observe that its two observations might possibly be connected. The unquestioned tradition that medicine should recruit a higher proportion of the ablest school-leavers than engineering for example, and subsequently accord them higher status and pay them more, must, over several generations, so seriously impair the creation of wealth as to diminish the share of it that can be devoted to health care. This same tradition has been exported to much of the developing world. It is typical of many and perhaps most developing countries, that medicine requires some of the highest entrance qualifications of any university course.

Modern medical technology

How effective and at what cost? Although some of the miracles of modern medicine, such as penicillin, now cost less than the bottle they are put in, the price of others is enormous. At the time of writing, interferon, for example, costs upwards of $30 000 a course, or more than $20 billion a kilo, if indeed such a quantity existed. Modern technologies have become so expensive because of the huge number of man-hours they now demand, not only in directly investigating and caring for the patient, but also in developing and manufacturing new drugs and equipment by the industries that have arisen to serve modern medicine. These man-hours have ultimately to be paid for, and account for most of the cost of the new medical care. It was formerly impossible to spend nearly $400 000 on a single piece of equipment, which is what a 16-channel auto-analyzer costs today.

Since to spend resources on one thing makes it impossible to spend them on another, we must also ask what the opportunity costs are. Of this there can be no more extreme case than that of the Prime Minister of one developing country who asked that the entire allocation of WHO funds for his country be used to buy one sophisticated scanner. For the same money he could have immunized all the children in his country against measles for several years, and have saved half a million lives.

Something for everyone, or more for the fortunate few? Technologies do not exist in isolation, and if a patient has access to a technology of a particular degree of cost and sophistication, he probably has access to other technologies of a similar kind, and to any that are simpler. For example, if he can reach a health centre, he has access to all the simple things it can do. If a mother can get a Caesarean section at a district hospital, she can get a Pott's fracture set, or a chest X-ray, or any of the other services which such a hospital offers. If a patient is so fortunate as to be able to get a kidney transplant, he certainly has access to almost anything that modern medicine can provide. It is thus possible to make a scale of technologies of increasing sophistication and cost, such that a patient having access to those at one particular point on the scale can expect to get any of those beneath it, should he need them. This scale can also show the technologies that can be provided by a community health worker, a health centre, a district hospital, and a regional or national one.

Figure 5 uses this scale as one axis of a graph, the other axis of which is the percentage of a population having access to health care at a particular technological level. A hypothetical developing country and an industrial country are shown on it. In a developing country, the fortunate urban elite have access to almost any highly sophisticated technology, either in the capital city or abroad, while many of the rural poor have no modern health care whatever. In an industrial country, not only is the average technological level of care much higher, but it is also distributed much more equitably.

It is also possible to insert a level in Fig. 5 to represent a 'basic human right' in health care, or the essential technologies that might constitute the primary health care described later. Caesarean section, for example, and anything simpler, should surely now be one of the rights of all the world's mothers?

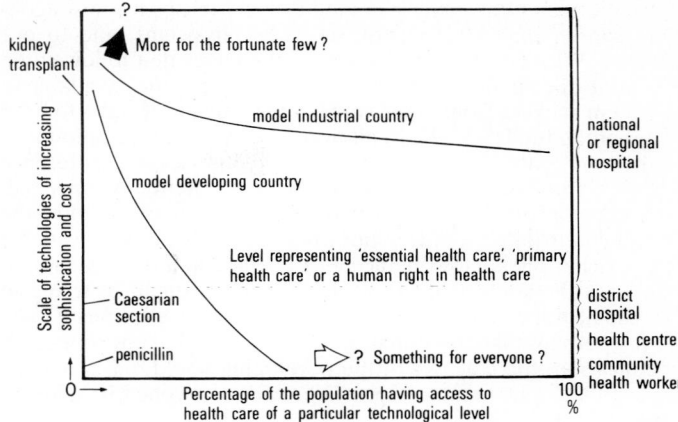

Fig. 5 Percentage of the population having access to health care at a particular technological level in a model industrial country and a model developing one. The black and white arrows represent policy choices in the deployment of resources.

The two arrows in Fig. 5 represent one of the major dilemmas in modern medicine. Are limited resources to be spent in the direction of the white arrow or the black one? To increase the quantity and the sophistication of medical care at the top end of the scale, or to see that everyone has at least something at the bottom end? Which is of the greater benefit, when resources are scarce? To transplant kidneys, or to see that every mother has surgical help when her labour obstructs?

If the arrows were to be coloured red and blue, they would give a better representation of the political tensions within a society, of which equity or inequity in health care is only one of many expressions. Since the pattern of health care in a society is such an integral part of it, some would argue that as individual doctors we can do nothing about it. We do however have a complete responsibility for one small part of it, what we ourselves choose to do.

Prestigous and capable, but only potentially universal. This Textbook of Medicine describes what physicians can now do. It defines the scope, the sophistication, the technical magnificence, and even the beauty of scientific medicine as it now is in 1982. Here, in three million words is the global technology of medicine. However, its very prestige, capability, and universality, each has serious consequences.

The present prestige of high technology medicine is such that it dominates the ambition of our profession. As the site of between a quarter and a third of the health expenditure of the entire world, the USA has become medicine's global pace-setter. Consciously, or unconsciously, not to follow the North American lead may be to be labelled, or to feel, technically inadequate, or socially deviant or both. To go against such a powerful trend may require considerable courage. Nowhere is courage more badly needed than in some of the medical schools of the developing world, torn between the technological sophistry of North America, and the dire need of the villages and slums. Paradoxically, to fail to resolve this dilemma may be to lose simultaneously, both the major opportunity to be of service to the sick, and the prestige that wider recognition might bring. It is surely no accident that one of the most famous and original medical books of the decade, *Where there is no doctor*, by David Werner, a biologist, required such an imaginative leap in the medical care of the disadvantaged, that no doctor could write it.

The capability of high technology medicine often leads its patients, and indeed sometimes their doctors, to expect it to do more than it can. Much of the pressure to provide it comes from a public who have a false idea of what medicine can do. We must tell our patients when we do not have an answer to a problem, and when doing something would be at least as dangerous, and certainly very much more expensive than not doing it.

The potential universality of medicine is perhaps its most agonizing consequence, both to ourselves as physicians, and to our patients. Whereas the technologies in the pages that follow could potentially be applied to anyone anywhere, the money available to buy them ranging from a few cents in the villages of India to $750 and more in the USA. When allowance is made for the amount of health care a dollar will buy in different countries, the difference narrows. But even so, although medicine is potentially universal, the money available to buy it varies at least a hundred fold—the poorer countries have only about 1 per cent of the money available to the richer ones. How medicine can be adapted to such circumstances is the subject of the next few pages. But, if in trying to provide health care for everyone, we think we have a difficult task, we can perhaps take some comfort from the fact that our colleagues in education, the teachers of the developing world, have an even more difficult one in their efforts to provide everyone with a meaningful education.

Seven axioms

Although medicine is inevitably different when there is so little money to spend, it can offer us great professional satisfaction but only provided that it is actively adapted to reality. If the attempt is made to follow North America blindly, with only 1 per cent of its money, then most, if not all, is lost. Should we allow ourselves to be seduced by the irresistable technological imperative, the seductive *non sequitur*, that because some expensive and sophisticated procedure is done in Detroit or San Diego, it must also be done in Dacca, Delhi, or Dar-es-Salaam, or even in Dover, then not only is frustration likely to follow, but there will be less money to spend in Tubuan and the millions of villages like it, all over the developing world.

Here are seven linked axioms, which although they are particularly relevant to the medicine of poverty, are in reality universal. They are followed by the most promising lead so far, in medicine in the latter years of this century—WHO's programme for Primary Health Care, which attempts to implement them as a programme.

1. Care for all men. Jack Bryant has put this in another way—for whom are we responsible? Only for those who seek our help, or for those outside, who do not? The sick in the greatest need of care, both globally and near us, either cannot afford it, or cannot reach it, or would not want it, even if they could. Are we responsible for them too, and if so, how? This is perhaps the central question in medicine, not only in the developing world, and is no less escapable for being a moral rather than a medical one. The answer will depend on who we are. For each of us there is a 'more' and a 'less', a narrow limited view, and a wider, more embracing one.

Often we do not realize that we have this choice, and by not realizing it, we make it by default. We take it for granted that the responsibility of a hospital extends only to those who present themselves as sick. This failure to realize even that there is such a choice is being increasingly criticized. Are we to provide care, perhaps of superb technical sophistication, for the fortunate few? Or should we see that the limited resources at our disposal are used in the most cost-effective way possible to reduce the mass of human suffering and improve the quality of life?

2. Create. This Textbook of Medicine describes the cure of diseases. It assumes that a health service machine exists for turning this knowledge into actions which will heal the sick. Unfortunately, such a health delivery system may not exist, or if it does exist, it may be ineffective, disorganized, remote, expensive, extravagant, inequitable, unacceptable, or even downright dangerous. So the social structures for a health service delivery system may have to be created, improved, or, one hopes, even perfected. The care of all men may thus require the raising of money, the hiring and firing of staff, the improvement of morale, the ordering of stores, the mending or making of equipment, attending committees, and even the writing and reading of huge books, as well as continually teaching and delegating, supervising, congratulating, and inspiring. Such acts of health service creation are no less a part of medicine than laying a hand on the epigastrium, making a burr hole, or managing isovalericacidaemia, or the blue diaper syndrome. Indeed, they are often the necessary vehicle for such acts.

3. Teach. Personal health care is essentially a skilled service that one human being does for another. Motivation, compassion, skill, and knowledge are usually the limiting factors in providing it, rather than staff, drugs, or equipment. The increase of all these critical attributes by every possible means is thus one of the great imperatives in medicine. It requires an appreciation of the fact that 'doctor' originally meant teacher, and often should do so still. It means teaching on every possible occasion—individual teaching on the job, group teaching, and the provision of teaching materials. It means retraining even more than initial training, and a careful study of what one particularly effective doctor-teacher so aptly termed 'the epidemiology of continuing ignorance'.

4. Delegate. Caring for everyone requires that the ordinary tasks of medicine be done on a huge scale. Besides teaching people how to do them, this requires that each task should be delegated to the humblest and cheapest member of the health team capable of doing it effectively. Since a useful level of personal health care can be provided widely and cheaply by such auxiliaries as medical assistants and rural medical aides, the key to providing at least some health care for everyone is to train these workers on a wide scale, to delegate tasks to them, and then to supervise them carefully. The most recent trend is to continue the process still further, and to delegate the simplest forms of health care to workers from the community itself. They are a doctor's extra hands and the best hope that the world's two billion villagers have of getting some health care close to their homes. Managing the provision of such care is now one of the most critical and necessary tasks in medicine. It was said by one sometime professor, who had started his career teaching post-graduates, continued it teaching graduates, and ended it teaching auxiliaries, that he found the last task much the most difficult, the most valuable, and the most rewarding.

5. Apply the most cost-effective technologies. The task here is no less than a systematic shopping expedition through the whole hypermarket of modern medicine for just those procedures which might give the maximum benefit in terms of death prevented, and suffering and disability relieved. It is a hunt for what medicine might so readily do, even when money is so scarce. There can be no better example than the freeze-dried smallpox vaccine applied with a bifurcated needle which enabled WHO to eradicate smallpox globally. So cost-effective was this programme that it is reported to have saved the developed world alone about a billion dollars a year in vaccination and supervision costs.

Smallpox was, however, a unique case. The same process of selection, relentless development and application must now continue for the whole of personal health care. Once selected, the chosen technologies must be carefully described and printed in the languages of all the world's workers. This must be followed by providing the necessary equipment, devising the appropriate evaluation procedures and management targets, and producing the necessary teaching aids. The attempt to do this 'health microplanning' systematically from a ministry of health has hardly begun, nor indeed do most ministries consider it their business. The result is that highly cost-effective technologies are not applied nearly as widely as they should be. District hospital surgery, for example, particularly needs such an approach, and the writer is presently engaged in doing just this.

Drugs are the main technology in the hands of the physician, and since they now account for a rising percentage of the cost of health care in almost every country, economy in their use is critical. In a developing country they may consume up to 40 per cent of the health budget. The major choice to be made is between generic drugs, and proprietary ones, between diazepam, for example, and 'Valium'. Since the difference in cost between the two may exceed 100 per cent, the routine prescription of only generic drugs must thus be considered one of the essential attributes of the good physician, and one of his main opportunities for containing the rising costs of health care.

6. Go widely rather than deeply. If lack of facilities to investigate our patient prevents us going deeply into some minute corner of medicine, we should at least not be constrained by the historically arbitrary and increasingly impenetrable barriers between specialties, and be prepared to go widely instead. Is the broadly skilled doctor who can read an ECG, put up a scalp vein drip, repair a hernia, set a Pott's fracture well, pass an endotracheal tube, do a barium swallow, identify *Entamoeba histolytica*, teach medical assistants competently, and do a tolerable post mortem, more or less to be admired than his colleague who specializes in the diseases of one organ in one age group, or does only one operation, or looks down only one orifice with one kind of endoscope? Since the best definition of a surgeon is that he is merely a physician who can operate, even this great division in our profession should surely not be absolute. The reader should not, therefore, be tempted to let the confines of even these two huge volumes set the limits to his practice. The opportunity to be 'a very general practitioner' with such broadly based skills is, alas, now only possible in the developing world, and is surely one of its major advantages. Fortunately, there are signs that the tide may be turning and that the high water mark of hyperspecialization may be passing. No less a person than Mrs Indira Gandhi has been exhorting her doctors not to become too specialized.

Lack of facilities for investigation also means that much greater reliance has to be placed on a patient's physical signs, hence the great importance given to them in this text. As with other technologies, those for special investigations have to be carefully selected for their cost-effectiveness. Many, which could be available much more widely, blood culture, for example, are not, partly because too little trouble has been taken to choose and implement what could reasonably be done. The reader may indeed have to create facilities for the easier, and often the most useful methods of investigation, first by learning how to do them himself, and then by teaching someone else. Although it may be frustrating to have mastered the metabolic minutiae responsible for mental handicap, and to be unable to get the special investigations done, they may not be the priority in a children's ward. It may be much more important to teach the laboratory assistants to examine cerebrospinal fluid properly, so that at least the children with meningitis are diagnosed and treated as they should be.

7. Make the community master. The best interests of the individual sick patient in his bed have always been the ultimate objective of the best medical care. The ultimate authority, economy, and convenience of the patients collectively, rather than that of ourselves, their physicians, has however had less attention. Hence the increasing dissatisfaction of many communities, both rich and poor, with the services they get, and the importance of making these services acutely sensitive to communal need. Communities must, wherever possible, be given a bigger say, and indeed the ultimate responsibility for the services they get. Listening for this still small voice, obeying it, and encouraging it to speak up, decide, and take charge, must in future become an integral part of medicine. It is also one of the major inspirations of the section which follows.

Health for all by the year 2000

Comprehensive primary health care. What can we do to prevent disease, disability, and untimely death in two-thirds of the world's

people, especially those locked into absolute poverty? The most hopeful solution is comprehensive primary health care, as this was defined at the international conference held by WHO and UNICEF at Alma Ata in Soviet Asia in 1978. The Declaration of Alma Ata which followed this meeting has as its aim:

The attainment by all the people of the world by the year 2000, of a level of health that will permit them to lead a socially and economically productive life. Primary health care includes, at least, education concerning the prevailing health problems and the methods of preventing and controlling them, the promotion of an adequate food supply and proper nutrition together with a sufficient supply of safe water and basic sanitation. It also includes maternal and child health, family planning, and immunization against the major infectious diseases, as well as the prevention and control of locally endemic diseases, the appropriate treatment of the common diseases and injuries, and the provision of essential drugs.

Some other features of primary health care are brought out in the definition that Alma Ata provided.

Primary health care is essential health care, made universally accessible to individuals and families in the community by means acceptable to them, through their full participation and at a cost the community and the country can afford. It forms an integral part, both of the country's health system, of which it forms the nucleus, and of the overall social and economic development of the country.

The definition of primary health care is not a rigid one, and wisely so. In the words of Dr Halfdan Mahler, Director General of WHO, it is more a goal, a purpose, or a direction which medicine should take. The principles behind it are equity, universality, cost-effectiveness, and most especially the involvement of the community in its own health. It is held to be equally valid for all countries, from the most to the least developed, although the form it takes will vary in each of them. For the developing countries it is a burning necessity. It seeks to narrow the gap between the 'haves' and the 'have-nots', both between nations and within them. It is at once both the means and the expression of social and economic development, besides being at least part of their purpose. Primary health care also has a potentially dangerous political objective, in that it may be a way of awakening and encouraging a demoralized and inert community to care for itself and seek its own destiny. The treatment of common diseases and injuries comes almost last in the Declaration, after enough food, clean water, and a sanitary environment, since these are likely to have a greater effect in improving health and reducing infant mortality than personal health care, as they did in the last century in industrial Europe. It has indeed been estimated that improved water and sanitation would prevent 80 per cent of the deaths in the developing world.

Although it is easy to say that the Declaration of Alma Ata is full of pious and impractical hopes, that it did not define its terms in sufficient detail, and indeed that it seeks an impossible utopia, the

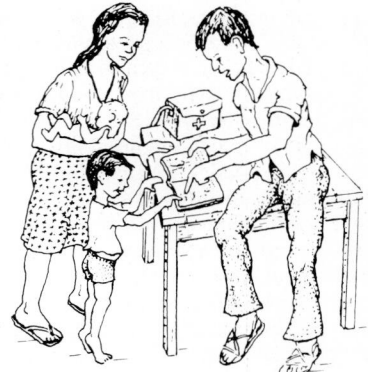

The village health worker lives and works at the level of his people. His first job is to share his knowledge

Fig. 6   An illustration from *Where there is no doctor* (Werner 1977).

Declaration can also be considered the most inspiring lead that the WHO has yet provided. Many of the aims of primary health care could be achieved in many countries within 20 years, if they were promoted with the same energy and devotion that eradicated small-pox and sent men to the moon. Perhaps the greatest criticism that can be levelled against it is that it has yet to define detailed strategies and targets.

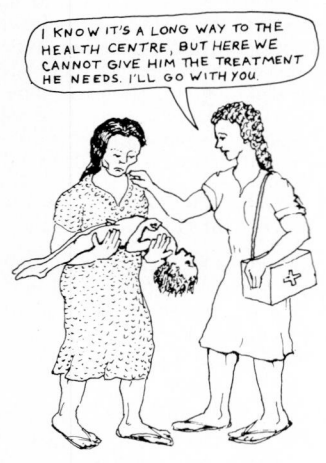

Know your limits

Fig. 7   Another illustration from *Where there is no doctor*.

Needless to say, primary health care means different things to different people, and can be used in two equally valid ways. It sometimes means only the care given by village-based community health workers (CHWs). At other times it is used to mean all cost-effective health care, from the district hospital downwards, including that given by CHWs. As such it resembles the older term 'basic health services'. Primary health care is however much wider, in that it includes the concepts of community participation, integration in the rest of the development process, and a greater emphasis on appropriate technology.

Unfortunately, if it is to be comprehensive, even primary health care with its minimal emphasis on curative medicine and hospital services, will cost more than the aid funds that are likely to be available. For example, the World Bank estimated that to provide community water supplies and sanitation to all those in need by the year 2000 would cost $260 billion. Although this may seem a huge sum, it is only half a single year's global arms expenditure.

Community Health Workers (CHWs). Much highly cost-effective health care can be given by workers with only a few months training, and who may even be illiterate. CHWs can treat respiratory infections, dehydrating diarrhoea, malaria, worms, and minor injuries. They can immunize children and advise mothers on family planning. Although such care may seem trivial in the context of this textbook. CHWs can satisfy a high proportion of a villager's needs and considerably reduce disease and death, particularly in children. Such simply trained CHWs have one great advantage, they live in the community, where the need is, and can thus be the spearhead of primary health care in disadvantaged societies. Although CHWs may be the most important means of delivering such care on a global scale, they are not the only ones, and Britain's general practitioners, for example, or the medical assistants and rural medical aides of East and Central Africa all have a similar role.

Since villagers do not have the knowledge to train their own CHWs, or to supervise them technically, this has to be done by someone else, either working for a voluntary agency, or for government. In this lies one of the main difficulties with these programmes, particularly on a national scale, since CHWs are neither better nor worse than those who teach and supervise them. The technical leadership of such workers and particularly monitoring

and improving the quality of the care they give, is thus one of the major opportunities for the reader who is interested in maximizing his own role in the care of the sick.

At the present time the Alma Ata declaration is hardly more than three years old, and most CHW programmes are still run on a small scale under the devoted leadership of their charismatic founders. How well they will succeed on a national scale as part of a government health service remains to be seen, since national programmes for the provision of primary health care by CHWs have only just begun. The Iranian programme is the oldest, largest, and best documented. In that programme, using community health workers, trained for only a few months, the infant mortality rate was reduced from 130 to 80 per thousand, the crude birth rate from 40 to 27 per thousand, and the crude population growth rate from 2.5 per cent to 1.8 per cent. Under some circumstances these workers can therefore be very effective.

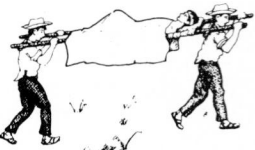

Fig. 8   A further illustration from *Where there is no doctor*.

For many of the sick of the world, especially its sick children, the future of primary health care in the hands of CHWs is going to be one of the most critical issues in medicine during the lifetime of this book. Are they going to be a passing hope which is soon forgotten? Or, are they going to be one of the main means of providing at least a little health care for everyone? Tragically, and as so often in development strategy, the people in most dire need, such as the villagers in the Sahel, are less likely to get it than communities which are not quite so disadvantaged. Alas, governments like those of the Sahel are least able to provide the support, supervision, and transport which CHWs must have.

WHO expanded programme of immunization (EPI). Since immunization is one of the most cost-effective ways of preventing disease, it is tragic that 90 per cent of the 80 million children born each year in the developing world are never immunized. Five diseases: diphtheria, pertussis, tetanus, measles, and poliomyelitis, which have almost disappeared from the industrial world, kill 5 million children each year. And for every child who dies, another is crippled, blinded or otherwise disabled by diseases that immunization could prevent. It had been hoped that the ravages of tuberculosis in the developing world might be controlled by immunization, but unfortunately the results of the recent BCG trial in India, although incomplete, are negative. In the developing countries, where BCG is most wanted, its value has never been proved. Despite this setback, WHO has launched its expanded programme of immunization in order to make use of such vaccines as there are, and in the hope that more will be developed. The aim of the programme, which is one aspect of the global programme for primary care, is to immunize all the world's children by 1990. Unlike the smallpox programme, the new one hopes to control diseases rather than eradicate them. Instead of being a once-and-for-all programme, it is to be an integrated part of primary health care, and particularly of the care of mothers and children.

Primary health care and population. Improvements in health usually reduce mortality and accelerate the growth of the population. Since this is such a problem in so many developing countries, there is a narrow view which holds that the improving health must in the end be futile and self-defeating. It is, however, essential in the longer term, since only when people perceive that their children are not going to die, will they want smaller families. Unfortunately, they take some time to perceive this. Nevertheless, the spectre of massive global overpopulation is slightly less desperate than it was. Although rapid population growth is still an acute problem in Africa, between 1960 and 1977 falls in the crude birth rate of over 30 per cent have occurred in China, Korea, Chile, Colombia, Tunisia, and Turkey. There have also been smaller, but significant decreases in India, Indonesia, and elsewhere. But even if fertility does decline significantly during the 1980s and 1990s, it will not make a big difference to total numbers by the year 2000. It will, however, be decisive in determining what happens after that. Depending on whether the decline in fertility accelerates or slows down, the world population could possibly stabilize or turn down at levels anywhere between 8 and 15 billion during the next century. Even if it is assumed that fertility will decline, the population of most developing countries are likely to double. Nigeria and Bangladesh will each have as many people as the United States has today, and India will have at least 1.2 billion citizens.

The danger is that, if the improvements that better primary care might bring are not accompanied by other measures to promote socio-economic progress, faster population growth will reduce the stimulus to economic development that better health might bring. In the industrial world socio-economic progress was accompanied by falls in both mortality and fertility, and the hope is that this will happen again in the developing world. Health programmes, particularly those for primary health care, must therefore be part of broad programmes of social and economic development, which will reduce both mortality and fertility simultaneously.

Conclusion

No man shall want for what medicine might readily do. Historically, so many of the real problems are opportunities in medicine that have not at the time seemed obvious, and were certainly not popular. Today is unlikely to be an exception. The major problem now, both in rich countries and in poor ones, is to provide effective and economical primary care. Others are the absence, in many parts of the world, of any sort of equity in health care, and the tragedy that drugs, including alcohol and cigarettes, now kill more people than did all the epidemics of earlier centuries. No profession is likely to welcome the fact that effective mechanisms to limit its expenditure are an urgent need. If, in Britain, one of the major problems of medicine is the increasing estrangement between one group of health workers and another which causes each to strike to the detriment of all, then might not one of the ways of healing the lack of communication between them be that they should meet and dine together daily instead of segregating themselves, each to his own faction? However abhorrent to English traditions of class, this would merely be following the long-established practice of much of Europe and of all Scandinavia.

The real problems before the medicine of now are thus moral, political, social, and administrative, rather than purely technical. For the most part we have the knowledge and the technologies, but the sick still want for what medicine might so readily do. What we ourselves might do will depend on who and where we are. Enthuse unity, purpose, hope, and economy into a divided, demoralized and wasteful National Health Service? Make sure that the villages have at least some care? In 1900 medicine was awaiting the discovery of antibiotics, and the advances in organic chemistry that could isolate and purify them. As it approaches the year 2000, it waits for leadership of another kind, and the vision and determination on which these are founded. It waits also for the zeal and enthusiasm which money cannot buy, and without which nothing is achieved.

From the edge of the abyss. The major need for zeal, enthusiasm, and indeed courage, now, if many of us and our patients are going to see the year 2000, is to disarm the nuclear arsenals of the world, unilaterally if necessary. There are now said to be three tons of TNT equivalent waiting for every man, woman, and child in the world. Taking a long-term historical view, a strong case can be argued for a period of disciplined solidarity and oppression under conditions like those of Poland, being far preferable to a nuclear holocaust, in which 50 million people might die in a few hours in the United Kingdom alone. It is this, just this, and the benefit that the massive turning of swords into ploughshares might bring to the deprived of the world that is the ultimate challenge to all of us now. An unjust world it may be, but, as the doctors of tomorrow, we shall not justly be able to complain of its injustice, those of us who might survive, if we do not now do all we can now to prevent this nuclear madness, this ultimate expression of mankind's most insidious disease, the arms race.

References

Bryant, J. (1969). *Health and the developing world*. Cornell University Press, Ithaca.
Caldicott, Helen (1979). *Nuclear madness*. Wildwood House, London.
Knowles, J. H. (1977). *Doing better and feeling worse*. Norton, New York.
McNamara, R. (1979). *Development and the arms race*. World Bank, Washington.
Morley, D. (1973). *Paediatric priorities in the developing world*. Butterworth, London.
Mushkin, S. J. (1979). Economic issues in terminal illness. *Mimeo.*
King, M. H. (1966). *Medical care in developing countries*. Oxford University Press, Nairobi.
—, King, F. M. A., and Martodipoero, S. (1979). *Primary child care*, Vols. 1 and 2. Oxford University Press, Oxford.
Sampson, A. (ed.) (1980). *North-South: a programme for survival. The report of the Brandt Commission*. Pan Books, London.
Werner, D. (1977). *Where there is no doctor*. TALC, Institute of Child Health, London.
World Bank (1979). *World Development Report*. World Bank, Washington.
World Health Organization, Alexandria (1980). *An Iranian Experiment in Primary Care*. Oxford University Press, Oxford.
World Health Organization and UNICEF (1978). *Primary Health Care*. WHO, Geneva.

Section 4
Genetics, immunology, and neoplasia

Genetic factors in disease

D. A. Price-Evans

The science of genetics is of increasing importance in medicine, partly because more is now known about the basic facts of inheritance, and partly because with the control of infections, genetic disorders are relatively more frequent than they were. It is also being increasingly realized that genetic factors are important in common clinical problems.

Before proceeding further it may be useful to define the main genetic terms used in this section. Further information on terminology can be obtained from Rieger *et al.* (1968) and King (1974); the former provides information about the date of introduction of terms into usage, e.g. 'gene' was first used by Johannsen in 1909.

Definition of terms

Acrocentric. Chromosomes where the centromere is very close to one end, so that there is one long arm and one very short arm.

Allelomorph (allele). One of two or more alternative forms of a gene occupying the same locus on a particular chromosome.

Ascertainment. The finding or selection of individuals or families for inclusion in a genetic study.

Autosome. Any chromosome other than the sex chromosomes. In humans there are 22 pairs of autosomes.

Centromere. The region of each chromosome with which the spindle fibres become associated during mitosis and meiosis.

Character (synonym: trait). Any observable phenotypic feature of the individual.

Concordance. When both members of a pair of twins exhibit the same trait, they are said to be concordant.

Crossing-over. The event leading to genetic recombination by exchange of genes between homologous chromosomes. This occurs at meiosis and at mitosis. Meiotic crossing-over allows genes to be arranged in new combinations (recombinants) in the next generation.

Deletion. Loss of a section of chromosome with the genes contained therein. Sometimes also used on a molecular scale to denote loss of a piece of DNA molecule.

Discordance. When only one twin has the trait they are said to be discordant.

Dominant inheritance. This is said to be present when a genetic character is expressed by the heterozygote so that it is similar to a homozygote. It is a property of the phenotype and not of the genes themselves *per se*. In measured characters different degrees of dominance are possible increasing from the position where the properties of the heterozygote are mid-way between those of the two homozygotes (in a two-allele system) to complete dominance where the heterozygote is identical with a homozygote. The concept of dominance no longer applies when individual gene products can be recognized, e.g. haemoglobin A and S (sickle cell haemoglobin).

Expressivity. The degree to which the effect of a gene is expressed. If the gene is controlling a disease, some of those inheriting it will be more severely affected than others, e.g. in neurofibromatosis some individuals will have skin tumours, pigmentation, and bone changes whereas others will have pigmentation only.

Gene pool. The total genetic information encoded in the sum total of the genes in a breeding population at a given time. The gametes of all breeding individuals in a population furnish a pool of genes from which the genes of the next generation are chosen. The concept is frequently restricted to consideration of alleles at one locus, but of course alleles at different loci may interact.

Genetic marker. Any genetically controlled phenotypic difference used in genetic analysis. For example, ABO blood groups have been used in studies of both genetic linkage and of associations with specific disorders.

Genetics. The science of heredity and variation.

Genetic variability. Variability due to differences of genetic constitution in contrast to environmentally induced differences which cause non-heritable changes of the phenotype.

Genotype. Strictly means the total of the genetic information in an individual. In practice it is often used to refer to the genetic constitution of an individual at one or a few loci, e.g. a blood group A individual may be of genotype AA or AO.

Heterozygous. Possessing two different alleles at the two corresponding loci on a pair of homologous chromosomes.

Homozygous. Possessing two identical alleles at the two corresponding loci on a pair of homologous chromosomes.

Isochromosome. A type of chromosomal aberration in which one of the arms of a particular chromosome is duplicated because the centromere has divided transversely and not longitudinally during cell division. There is a corresponding loss of the genes in the other arm. The two arms of an isochromosome are, therefore, of equal length and contain the same genes (Fig. 1).

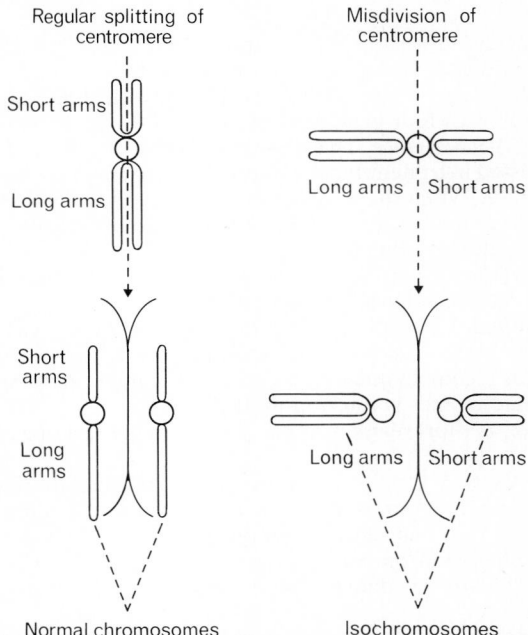

Fig. 1 Isochromosomes (from Harnden (1962) in *Chromosomes in medicine*. Heinemann, London).

Metacentric. Chromosomes where the centomere is localized roughly half-way along the length.

Meiosis. The type of nuclear division which occurs during gametogenesis and involves two divisions of the nucleus, resulting in halving the somatic number of chromosomes so that each gamete is haploid.

Mitosis. The type of nuclear division which produces daughter nuclei which contain identical numbers of chromosomes and all the genes present in the parent cell.

Monosomy. Lack of one chromosome of a homologous pair, hence in man the individual has only 45 chromosomes.

Non-disjunction. Abnormal distribution of chromosomal material occurring at either meiosis or mitosis. In meiosis homologous pairs of chromosomes may fail to separate and so gametes may receive two or none instead of one.

Penetrance. An allelic gene is said to have full penetrance when the dominant character which controls is always evident in an individual possessing one such allele. An allelic gene controlling a recessive character is said to be fully penetrant if the character is always evident in individuals possessing two such alleles.

Phenocopy. A condition in an individual which is due to environmental factors but resembles one which is genetic.

Phenotype. The properties observable in a single individual. These properties are due to effects of both genes and environment, but where penetrance is high, e.g. in ABO blood groups, the influence of environment and of genes at other loci may have little effect. Examination of the pedigree as well as the individual may reveal information concerning the individual's genotype which cannot be deduced from his phenotype, e.g. a phenotype blood group A may be found to be due to genotype AA or AO.

Pleiotropy (synonym: pleiotropism). The effects of an allele being shown in different parts of the body, e.g. (*a*) in Marfan's syndrome anatomical abnormalities may occur in eyes, heart, and skeleton; (*b*) tylosis is one of many forms of dyskeratosis. The most conspicuous feature is great thickening of the skin of palms and soles and hyperidrosis is also often present. Rarely tylosis is confined to the soles. It is usually inherited as an autosomal dominant, but the same morphologic features can be due to different genes. One genetic variety exhibits pleiotropism in that persons with the skin abnormality are prone to develop oesophageal carcinoma.

Polyploidy. Possession of the entire basic set of chromosomes more than the normal twice. Hence every chromosome is represented three or more times (e.g. triploidy with three basic sets; tetraploidy with four basic sets, etc.).

Recessive inheritance. This is said to be present when the character expressed in a phenotype is associated with alleles in the homozygous state. When these alleles occur singly they are masked by the effect of an allele controlling the dominant character. Recessivity is a feature of the phenotype and not of the genes and so it is inappropriate to refer to 'the recessive gene' (and likewise it is inappropriate to refer to 'the dominant gene').

Recombinant. Any of the individuals or cells arising as a result of interchromosomal genetic recombination by crossing-over. The number of recombinants in relation to the number of offspring in appropriate crosses is referred to as the 'recombinant fraction'.

Satellite. A short segment constricted from the rest of a chromosome.

Sex-linkage. A gene is said to be sex-linked when it is on either the X or the Y chromosome. If it is situated on the non-pairing part of the Y, it can never cross on to the X and will therefore always be handed from father to son. If a gene is on the X, a man will pass it on to his daughter and a woman to either her son or daughter.

Submetacentric. When the centromere is away from the centre of the chromosome so that the chromosome appears J-shaped at anaphase.

Translocation. This happens when either a piece of one chromosome is transferred to another, or two pieces of chromosome (not necessarily of the same size) are broken off from two non-homologous chromosomes and their positions exchanged (reciprocal translocation).

Trisomy. Where one chromosome is represented by three homologues as opposed to the normal two. Hence the individual has 47 chromosomes.

Patterns of pedigrees

The behaviour of genes in families will now be discussed and methods described of how the various types of inheritance are recognized.

Single gene inheritance. The single-gene Mendelian type of pedigree in which affected and unaffected individuals segregate in well-defined ratios is the corner-stone of classical medical genetics. Much more often, however, illness is caused by a subtle interaction between genetic and environmental factors. When this is so it is usually not one gene but many, each with a small and additive effect, which are responsible for the inherited component (see Multifactorial variability below).

Autosomal dominant inheritance. Figures 2 and 3 show two situations. In Fig. 2 we are dealing with a rare gene, e.g. that responsible for Huntington's chorea. This will originally have arisen as a mutation, and since it controls a dominant character will have manifested itself from the beginning. Homozygotes are not likely to occur, and if they did would certainly not be viable. Therefore, the chance of any given offspring having the disease if one parent be affected and the other normal is one in two, and the risk is similar for subsequent siblings (chance has no memory). In Fig. 3 is shown a common and innocuous trait in which an individual heterozygous for blood group A (and therefore genotypically AO) has married someone of the same blood type. Because A is dominant to O, the offspring are, on average, three group A to one group O, but the As are of two genotypes AO and AA.

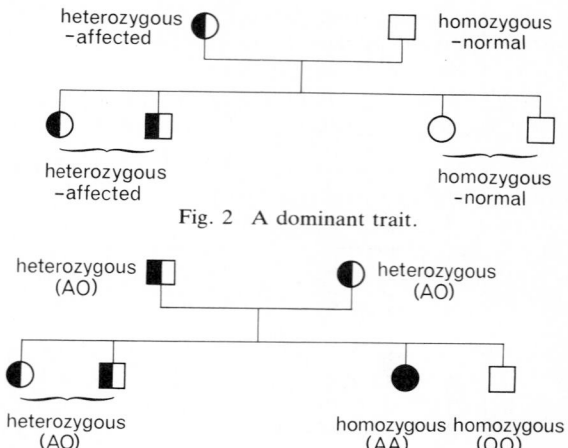

Fig. 2   A dominant trait.

Fig. 3   Mating between two individuals heterozygous for a common dominant trait, e.g. blood group AO (typing as AO because A is dominant to O).

In general, diseases which are dominant characters and therefore manifesting in the heterozygotes are less damaging than recessives. This may be partly due to the fact that the abnormal gene is present only in single dose, but additionally, if a dominant character is disadvantageous enough in the heterozygous condition to prevent reproduction, it will be selected against and the responsible allele will rapidly disappear. A recessive, on the other hand, however lethal it may be in the homozygote will (since the heterozygous carriers are normal) have ample opportunity to spread through the population. This is even more likely to happen than might be expected since carriers of some deleterious recessives probably have increased fertility.

Another peculiarity of dominant inheritance is that characters inherited in this manner are of varying seriousness in different individuals, the degree of severity being known as the expressivity of the gene. When the effect is so reduced that the individual carrying the gene appears quite normal, the trait is said to be 'non-penetrant'. This can cause a good deal of uncertainty when families are being studied as the gene seems to 'skip' a generation (which in fact it does not do). Part of this variability in expression is dependent on the normal allele which has been received from the unaffected parent and which accompanies the abnormal gene in the heterozygotes. That this is so can be proved because it can be demonstrated that sibling–sibling correlations for the expressivity of a given disease are stronger than the parent–sibling ones. This is because the affected siblings will each have one of the two normal alleles from their unaffected parent and these may well be different from that possessed by their affected parent.

Autosomal recessive inheritance. These characters also usually occur equally often in males and females, and the parents of patients are as a general rule normal, though both must be heterozygous carriers of the gene concerned. Since related individuals are more likely to be carrying the same gene, affected children are not infrequently the offspring of cousin marriages, and it is also a fact that the rarer the recessive trait the higher the proportion of consanguineous parental matings in the families of affected individuals.

Figure 4 shows the general situation. If a child is born with an autosomal recessive trait (e.g. albinism, fibrocystic disease, phenylketonuria) the risk of each subsequent offspring being affected is one in four. Phenylketonuria, however, requires further comment. With treatment, affected girls may survive, marry genotypically normal men, and produce children who, being heterozygous, would all be expected to be phenotypically normal. However, phenylalanine from the affected mother (who often relaxes the strictness of her diet in pregnancy) can cross the placental barrier and render all the children mentally defective. This is a loose example of a 'phenocopy' (see page 4.2).

If an affected individual marries a homozygous normal person, none of the children will be affected but all will be carriers. It is

unlikely that an affected individual will marry a heterozygote unless there is inbreeding or the gene is common, but when they do, half the children will be affected so here the pedigree might resemble one containing a dominant character. If two affected (and therefore homozygous) people marry, one would expect all their children to be affected, but this is not invariably so because, though the phenotypes of the two parents are the same, the genes controlling them can be at different loci. The same phenotype can, therefore, be produced by different genotypes, and furthermore an environmental cause can produce the same phenotype as a genetic one, e.g. the congenital deafness caused by rubella is indistinguishable from the purely inherited type (see phenocopy, page 4.2).

Intermediate inheritance. The terms 'dominant' and 'recessive' are often incorrectly used and indeed are sometimes almost interchangeable. For instance, if the heterozygote in a 'recessive' condition can be detected by a sensitive test, it is not completely recessive. Also, if a 'dominant' condition is clearly recognizable in the heterozygote and yet the homozygote for this gene is affected in a different way, it is inaccurate to call the character a dominant one, and it would be better to refer to such genes as being 'intermediate' in effect; this is illustrated in Fig. 5.

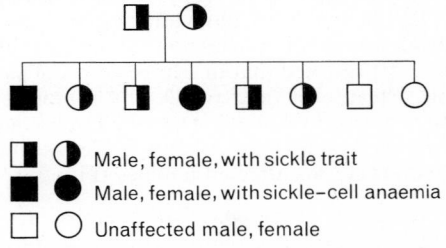

◧ ◖	Male, female, with sickle trait
◼ ●	Male, female, with sickle–cell anaemia
☐ ○	Unaffected male, female

Fig. 5   Pedigree pattern of an autosomal intermediate trait as illustrated by sickle state. The anomaly in the heterozygote can be revealed if the oxygen tension of a drop of blood is lowered (from McKusick (1962) in *Principles of internal medicine*. McGraw-Hill, New York).

The term 'co-dominant' is used to describe allelic characters which are both expressed when they come together in the heterozygote—such as the blood group antigens A and B; in an individual of blood group AB both manifest equally.

Sex (X)-linked recessive inheritance. X-linked genes can control dominant or recessive characters in just the same way as autosomal genes. In a male, however, a large portion of the X chromosome is unpaired, and so genes on this portion will be manifest, whether they control a dominant or recessive character in the female. A father will usually hand on all his X-linked genes to all of his daughters and to none of his sons. (There is a small chance of crossing-over between the small paired portion of the X and Y chromosomes.) Figure 6 illustrates the pattern of the sex-linked

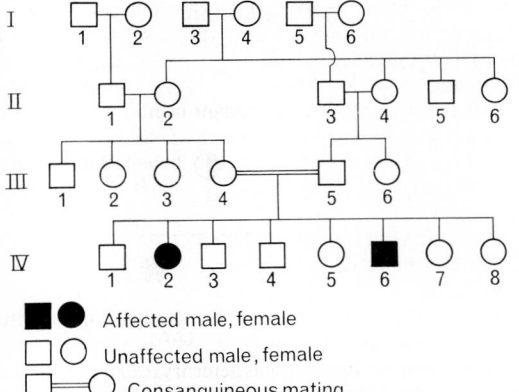

◼ ●	Affected male, female
☐ ○	Unaffected male, female
☐—○	Consanguineous mating

Fig. 4   Pedigree pattern of an autosomal recessive trait (from McKusick (1962) in *Principles of internal medicine*. McGraw-Hill, New York).

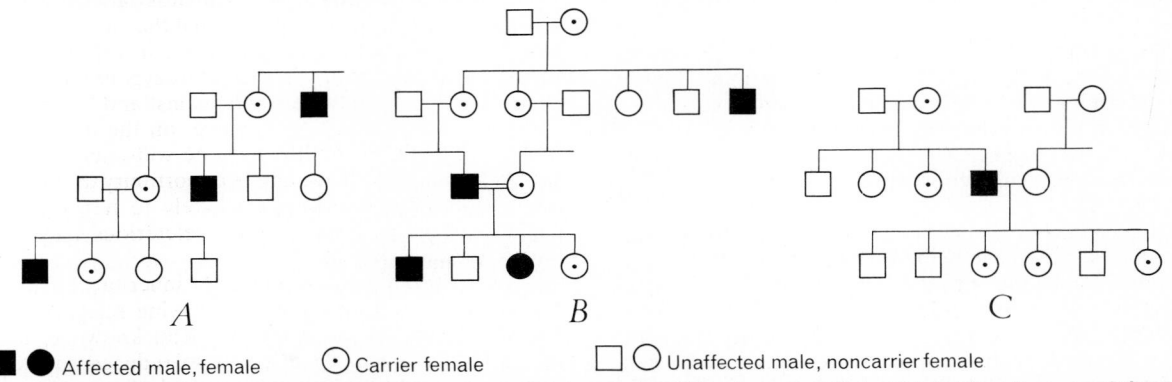

◼ ● Affected male, female	⊙ Carrier female	☐ ○ Unaffected male, noncarrier female

Fig. 6   Pedigree patterns of a sex-linked recessive trait, e.g. haemophilia. (a) Note the 'oblique' pattern. (b) An affected female can result from the mating of an affected male and a carrier female, as in the case of consanguineous marriage shown here. (c) An affected male mating with a normal non-carrier female has all normal sons, all carrier daughters (from McKusick (1962) in *Principles of internal medicine*, McGraw-Hill, New York).

recessive character, haemophilia, which is due to a gene carried on the X chromosome. It will be seen that the daughters of a carrier female are half carriers and half normal, and that the same pattern (though not the same result) applies to her sons—they are half affected and half normal. A haemophiliac man cannot transmit the disease to any of his sons so that, provided his spouse is not a carrier, the sons can be sure of being normal. Generally speaking, women are only very rarely affected by the disease of haemophilia. The rare female patient can arise in two ways; first, the female homozygous for the deleterious allele (a potential adverse effect of specialized counselling and treatment clinics); and secondly, because of an effect of 'Lyonization' (q.v.) which, as it is a random process, produces a spectrum of individuals (phenotypes) from amongst heterozygous genotypes. Some heterozygous women can have that X chromosome on which is sited the normally functioning allele inactivated, and furthermore this process can occasionally occur in a sufficient proportion of the factor-VIII synthesizing cells to produce a significantly low level of the factor in the plasma. Such individuals are termed 'manifesting heterozygotes'.

Sex (X)-linked dominant inheritance. Sex-linked gene-controlled dominant characters are rare, vitamin D-resistant rickets being the best example of a disease and the Xg blood group of a trait inherited in this way. Half the daughters of an affected woman will have the condition and all the daughters (but none of the sons) of an affected man. It will be appreciated that in a large series of cases, females with the trait (because of their two X chromosomes) will occur twice as often as males. In the case of vitamin D-resistant rickets the hemizygous affected males tend to have the disease more severely than do the heterozygous affected females (Fig. 7).

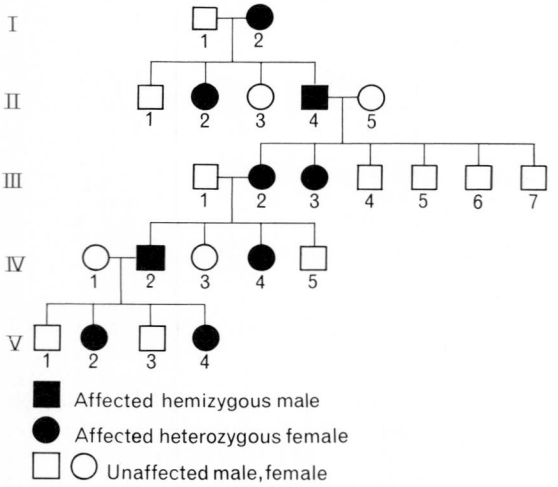

Fig. 7   Pedigree pattern of a sex-linked dominant trait (from McKusick (1962) in *Principles of internal medicine*, McGraw-Hill, New York).

Y-linkage. The chromosome carries a locus regulating the histocompatibility antigen H-Y. This may well determine heterogametic sex determination. The existence of factors controlling spermatogenesis on the non-fluorescent part of the long arm of Y (distal part of Yq ll) was suggested by the finding of six men with the deletion of this segment with azoospermia.

Sex-limited inheritance. Some phenotypes are modified by sex without being sex-linked—the gene being carried on an autosome but manifesting only in one sex. Frontal baldness appears to be an autosomal dominant in men, but in women it behaves like a recessive, a woman needing to have the gene in double dose. Haematochromatosis in the reproductive period is sex-limited to the male because menstruation and parturition are safety valves in the female.

The inheritance of testicular feminization is an interesting gen-

netic problem, for the affected male does not reproduce. The normal females are carriers and therefore the pattern of inheritance could be that of a sex-linked recessive. It could equally well be a sex-limited autosomal dominant, but since the males are sterile there is no easy means of testing which theory is correct. However, recent studies in mice (in which a similar syndrome occurs) indicates that the allele concerned is on the X chromosome. Since many X-carried genes seem common to all mammals, it is quite probable that the testicular feminization gene is sex-linked in humans.

Diagnostic aid. A directory of published single-gene disorders which is most useful for diagnostic purposes has been compiled and updated by McKusick (1979).

The Hardy–Weinberg equilibrium

Many experiments performed by geneticists in the years following the rediscovery of Mendel's paper utilized pure lines of plants. Then researchers wondered what would be the outcome of random mating in wild populations. The answer was found independently in 1908 by Hardy, a Cambridge mathematician, and Weinberg, a Stuttgart physician, and can be simply stated thus: 'In the absence of mutation, non-random mating, selection, and genetic drift, the genetic constitution of the population remains the same from one generation to the next.' The mathematical proof of this statement is based upon a simple application of the binomial theorem.

This genetic principle has clinical importance. In order to illustrate this it is necessary to introduce the concept of a 'gene pool'. Consider a population of, say, 10 000 men and women with regard to the locus whereat the allele for fibrocystic disease of the pancreas is situated. For the purpose of this discussion, it will be assumed there is one allele which in the homozygote confers the disease, representable by a green bead, and that there is one 'normal' allele representable by a white bead. Each individual person in the population is the bearer of two alleles, so there are three different genotypes. All 20 000 alleles could be represented by 20 000 beads in a bottle. Some would be white and some would be green. The contents of the bottle represent the 'gene pool' of the population under consideration. Let the proportion of white beads be p and the proportion of green beads q, so that $p + q = 1$. The genotypes can then be represented by pairs of beads drawn randomly from the bottle. Some pairs will be two white beads, some pairs will consist of one green and one white bead, and some pairs will be of two green beads. The frequencies of these three types of pairs can be represented by p^2, $2pq$, and q^2 respectively. Note that $(p + q)^2 = p^2 + 2pq + q^2 = 1$. One obvious application of this idea is that it can be used to compute the frequency of heterozygous carriers.

In fibrocystic disease the homozygous affected individual occurs about once in 2000 live births in the British population. So $q^2 = 1/2000 = 0.0005$, and $q = 0.02248$. Hence $p = (1 − q) = 0.9775$, and therefore $2pq = 0.0439$. That is to say one out of every 23 persons (1/0.0439) is a heterozygous carrier.

Viewing this in terms of the 20 000 beads in the bottle, 19 550 would be white ('normal alleles') and 450 would be green ('fibrocystic alleles').

Multifactorial variability

Biological measurements vary between individuals within populations. The variability can be expressed as a frequency distribution histogram or curve. For most biological variables this curve is unimodal and is (or can be transformed into) a symmetrical 'normal' (or 'Gauss') curve with well-known mathematical properties. The normal distribution curve can be described in terms of its mean and of its variance (or standard deviation which is the square root of the variance). A typical example is height in human populations.

The variability between individuals portrayed by such a curve is due to both genetic and environmental factors. In the case of the genetic component of variance it is thought that a number of alleles at a number of loci are involved giving rise to additive effects. Hence the use of the term 'polygenic' in this context. Since this branch of genetics deals mainly with measured variables it is often called quantitative or biometical genetics. The alleles and loci involved cannot be individually identified. (If they were identifiable, the events they controlled could be described by means of single-gene terminology.)

Formerly it was thought that a large number of loci and alleles might be involved in the genetic component of multifactorial variability. It turns out, however, in certain examples such as the control of red cell acid phosphatase activity, that three alleles at one locus can account for a large proportion of the variability.

Because most human genes have not been individually defined, the heritable component of many important physiological, morphological, and biochemical events can be described only in terms of quantitative genetics.

The relative sizes of the genetic and environmental components of the phenotypic variance may be estimated in human populations by using data obtained from families and from twins (Falconer 1960).

There has been a relative lack of application of quantitative genetics to medical problems, but despite this some notable examples exist, e.g. the analysis of variability of arterial blood pressure. In this example, symptoms and pathological signs arise when physiological mechanisms fail. It appears likely that in other instances a physiological process may show multifactorial variability, and symptoms arise above a certain threshold. An individual may possess such a constitution (which is largely genetically determined) so that relatively minor environmental or ageing processes may cause him to cross the threshold. This type of model is obviously applicable to diabetes mellitus and may form the basis for a clearer understanding of other common disorders such as duodenal ulcer, coronary artery disease, and emphysema.

Sometimes a different type of approach reveals the production of a pathological process by the action of a number of genes. Consequently, phenomena which cannot easily be measured can sometimes be examined for polygenic control. An example is congenital hypertrophic pyloric stenosis, the underlying biochemical basis of which is unknown. This disease is much commoner in boys than in girls. Carter (1965) showed that if a girl has the disease, she has more affected relatives than does a boy with the disease. This is interpreted as meaning that a higher concentration of the relevant genes is required to produce the disease in girls than in boys.

Yet another way of showing that alleles at several loci are important in the aetiology of a particular disorder is provided by studying 'associations' (see page 4.11).

Genetic counselling

Counselling is usually sought because of a positive family history—commonly by parents who have already produced one or more abnormal offspring. According to Fraser Roberts (1970), about 1 pregnancy in 30 will produce a serious developmental abnormality which appears early in life; whereas Emery (1974) states that roughly 1 in 20 children admitted to hospital have a disorder which is almost entirely genetic in origin—either a single-gene disorder or chromosomal abnormality, and these disorders account for about 1 in 10 of childhood deaths in hospital. Multifactorial disorders in which a genetic element is prominent account for about 15 per cent of paediatric inpatients and 11 per cent of adult inpatients.

Only a minority of families afflicted with a disorder which is largely or partly genetic in origin seek expert counselling.

Precise information can be given only (a) in instances of single-gene Mendelian disorders with high penetrance and expressivity, and (b) in chromosomal disorders. It is essential to have karyotyping facilities in order to provide proper counselling. Very often, particularly in common disorders, the genetic component can be assessed only empirically and Table 1 gives some examples.

Heterozygous carriers may be detected particularly in X-linked

Table 1 Empirical risks for some common disorders (in percentages)

Disorder	Incidence	Sex ratio M:F	Normal parents having a second affected child	Affected parent having an affected child	Affected parent having a second affected child
Anencephaly	0.20	1:2	5*	—	—
Cleft palate only	0.04	2:3	2	7	15
Cleft lip ± cleft palate	0.10	3:2	4	4	10
Club foot	0.10	2:1	3	3	10
Congenital heart disease (all types)	0.50	—	1–4	1–4	—
Diabetes mellitus (early onset)	0.20	1:1	8	8	10
Dislocation of hip	0.07	1:6	4	4	10
Epilepsy ('idiopathic')	0.50	1:1	5	5	10
Hirschsprung's disease	0.02	4:1			
male index			2	—	—
female index			8	—	—
Hypospadias (in males)	0.20	—	10	—	—
Manic-depressive psychoses	0.40	2:3	—	10–15	—
Mental retardation ('idiopathic')	0.30	1:1	3–5	—	—
Profound childhood deafness	0.10	1:1	10	8	—
Pyloris stenosis	0.30	5:—			
male index			2	4	13
female index			10	17	38
Renal agenesis (bilateral)	0.01	3:1			
male index			3	—	—
female index			7	—	—
Schizophrenia	1–2	1:1	—	16	—
Scoliosis (idiopathic, adolescent)	0.22	1:6	7	5	—
Spina bifida	0.30	2:3	5*	3*	—

* Anencephaly *or* spina bifida
From Emery, A. E. H. (1979). *Elements of medical genetics*, 5th edn. Churchill Livingstone, Edinburgh, by courtesy of the author

disorders, and this information can have counselling value. The proportion detected varies with the condition, e.g. about two-thirds in haemophilia A, about one quarter in haemophilia B (Christmas disease), and all in the Lesch–Nyhan syndrome (see Table 2).

It is for the patients to make the decision. The physician counsellor should explain the risk of a further offspring being affected in terms of probability, and the opportunity should also be taken to discuss the prognosis and availability of treatment since parents are so often influenced as much by the 'burden' of a disease as they are by the chances of producing a further abnormal offspring. Sound family-planning advice must be readily available if a decision is made by parents not to produce more children (see Bonaitti-Pellie and Smith 1974; Bundey 1975; Emery 1974).

Antenatal diagnosis. Antenatal diagnosis is advantageous for a variety of conditions:

1. Chromosome abnormalities in which the diagnosis is based on cytogenetic techniques.

2. X-linked disorders in which specific diagnosis is not yet possible but where the determination of the sex of the fetus is the guide for action.

3. Metabolic disorders, the so-called 'inborn errors of metabolism' in which the diagnosis depends on assay of a specific enzyme or possibly some other biochemical characteristic.

4. Malformations, such as anencephaly and spina bifida, where the concentration of alpha-fetoprotein in the amniotic liquid is often elevated. Here suspicions would be generated by: (a) a high maternal serum alpha-fetoprotein concentration found on routine screening after twins had been excluded by ultrasound examination

Table 2 Carrier detection in X-linked disorders

Disorder	Abnormality
Haemophilia A	factor VIII reduced*
Haemophilia B	factor IX reduced
G6PD deficiency	erythrocyte G6PD reduced
Lesch–Nyhan syndrome	hypoxanthine-guanine phosphoribosyl transferase in skin fibroblasts reduced. Two populations of cells
Hunter's syndrome	iduronosulphate sulphatase reduced in skin fibroblasts. Two populations of cells
Ocular albinism	patchy depigmentation of retina and iris
Vitamin D resistant rickets (hypophosphataemia)	serum phosphorous reduced
Duchenne muscular dystrophy	serum creatine kinase raised
Becker muscular dystrophy	serum creatine kinase raised
Diabetes insipidus (nephrogenic)	urine concentration diminished
Fabry's disease (angiokeratoma)	α-galactosidase in skin fibroblasts reduced. Two populations of cells
Chronic granulomatous disease (one type)	leucocyte phagocytosis and nitro blue tetrazolium test abnormal
Retinitis pigmentosa	tapetal reflex
Anhidrotic ectodermal dysplasia	sweat pore counts reduced
Lowe's syndrome	lenticular opacities

* More precisely a reduction in the ratio of factor VIII activity to inactive antigen
From Emery, A. E. H. (1979). *Elements of medical genetics*, 5th edn. Churchill Livingstone, Edinburgh, by courtesy of the author

and time after conception checked; (b) by a history that the woman concerned had produced a previous offspring with neural tube defect; and (c) when investigating a suspected abnormality finding an alpha-fetoprotein level inappropriate for stated duration of pregnancy.

5. In later pregnancy the fetus may be ill as a result of environmental illnesses. Accurate diagnosis is required to decide about premature delivery.

6. Intra-uterine treatment, e.g. blood transfusion, is a new technical advance whose implementation depends on accurate diagnosis.

This section focuses on the first four conditions listed above. The main aim is to decide whether the fetus should be aborted. Consequently the information to make the decision should be available before about 20 weeks.

Some 15 ml of amniotic liquid are withdrawn with a needle, ideally at about 15 weeks gestation when the total volume is about 130 ml. The cells in the amniotic liquid removed are grown for two to three weeks to make a diagnosis of chromosomal abnormality and for four to six weeks for biochemical tests. All specimens of amniotic liquid removed for prenatal diagnosis should have the alpha-fetoprotein determined.

There is evidence that the procedure of amniocentesis carries risks. Early fetal death and abortion may occur, sometimes several weeks later. Each attempt at amniocentesis carries a 1 per cent risk of abortion. There is also an increase in neonatal respiratory disease, death from hyaline membrane disease, and an association with fetal pressure deformities, especially talipes equinovarus.

The commonest indication for amniocentesis is suspicion of chromosomal abnormality, and in fact mongolism is the commonest condition diagnosed by amniocentesis. The most common indicators are maternal age over, say, 40 years or the birth of a previous trisomic Down's offspring.

With regard to X-linked disorders, tests are available which may indicate heterozygosity for haemophilia and X-linked Duchenne-type muscular dystrophy in the mother. If such is the case and the embryo is karyotyped XY, then if the mother wishes, she can forgo the one in two risk of the affected son. For Fabry's disease,

the Lesch–Nyhan syndrome, and Hunter's syndrome a direct diagnosis of the abnormality can be made by enzymic or metabolic studies in amniotic cells grown in tissue culture. So for these X-linked disorders a decision can be made knowing the fetus is definitely abnormal.

There are about 37 fairly rare conditions in which metabolic abnormalities can be detected in cells grown after amniocentesis. Many of these are autosomal recessive disorders and the information would be of value in conceptions of matings which had already produced one abnormal child. However, there are some notable exceptions. Phenylketonuria, for example, cannot be diagnosed in this way because the fibroblasts grown from the amniotic liquid do not contain phenylalanine hydroxylase.

If heterozygous adult carriers could be detected by population screening, then it might not be necessary for a mating of heterozygotes to have produced one abnormal offspring to institute amniocentesis studies. The best example where such a technique is available is for Tay–Sachs disease in communities of Ashkenazi Jews. Estimations of N-acetyl hexaminidase-A in serum and white cells of adults can identify adult heterozygotes. The enzyme is detectable in normal fibroblasts grown from amniotic fluid, but is absent if the embryo is an abnormal homozygote.

The phenomenon of linkage (see page 4.7) can be used in prenatal diagnosis. Supposing a disease is due to alleles occupying a locus which is very close to another locus occupied by alleles which control a genetic marker, e.g. a polymorphism, then the marker can be studied in the amniotic cells or fluid and a deduction made about the genotype at the 'disease' locus. It has been suggested that this approach can be utilized in myotonic dystrophy which is due to alleles closely linked to the 'secretor' locus. Another possible example is haemophilia A due to a locus on the X chromosome very near that for G6PD.

A total of 2428 amniocenteses were performed in the United Kingdom in 1976 and a follow-up of more than 90 per cent revealed only four wrong diagnoses.

Quite recently the technique of fetal blood sampling has been applied to the prenatal diagnosis of some genetic disorders. It has particular application to the prenatal identification of fetuses homozygous for different forms of thalassaemia and sickle cell anaemia, haemophilia, and rare haematological disorders such as chronic granulomatous disease. Another recent development in this field is the application of the techniques of human gene mapping (see page 4.21) to antenatal diagnosis using DNA obtained from amniotic fluid cells. At the present time this technology is only applicable to he abnormal haemoglobin disorders, in particular those which result from gene deletion (see page 4.26). It is now believed that human DNA is extremely polymorphic and that there will be many restriction enzyme sites which may be linked to specific gene loci responsible for human disease (see page 4.27). It is hoped to utilize this new information for the prenatal diagnosis of disorders such as cystic fibrosis and Huntington's chorea even though the precise molecular defects in these conditions remain to be determined (see page 4.2).

Antenatal diagnosis programmes require adequate laboratory facilities and genetic counselling services.

The effects of selective abortion of deleterious genotypes can, if vigorously prosecuted, affect the genetic structure of the population. The effect would be small as far as alleles controlling recessive characters are concerned. However, a significant reduction could be effected in a few generations in the frequency of alleles responsible for dominant conditions such as Huntington's chorea.

Twinning

A study of twins is a commonly used technique in genetic research but there has recently been a growing awareness of its limitations. Some of these are as follows:

1. Bias in the collection of twin data. Concordance is much more likely to be reported in monozygotic twins than discordance (an

editor is unlikely, for instance, to accept a report of appendicitis occurring in only one of a pair of monozygotic twins). Concordance should, however, be computed on randomly ascertained twinships.

2. There is a multiplicity of twin types. The monozygous and dizygous forms are well known, but in addition two sperm may fertilize an ovum at the same time so that, although the maternal genes are similar, the paternal ones differ. Furthermore, monozygous twins are not always both of the same sex and 'identical' twins have even been reported in which one of the pair was normal and the other a mongol. Non-disjunction can occur after fertilization. Consider two examples: first, a fertilized egg with karyotype (XY + 44) can undergo non-disjunction in the sex chromosomes at its first division. Two cells, one (XO + 44) and the other (XYY + 44) can result each developing into an individual. Secondly, a fertilized egg with karyotype (XY + 44) can divide to give two cells with the same karyotype. Both of these then are destined to develop into an individual. In the case of one cell, disjunction does not occur and a normal individual is produced. In the case of the other cell, non-disjunction occurs in the autosomes (e.g. number 21) at the very next division giving (XY + 45) and (XY + 43), the latter probably being eliminated), so in this instance a normal individual and a mongol are produced from what started out to be a monozygous twinship. (Explanations of the chromosome descriptive terms are given below.)

3. Twinning may affect pathology. For example, cerebral palsy is more frequent in twins than in single births, and there is possibly an increase in cancer in twins compared with the single born.

4. Very often, monozygous ('identical') twinships are compared with dizygous ('non-identical') twinships on the assumption that the intra-twinship environment variance is the same in both types. This is an unwarranted assumption since common observation reveals that the environment is often less disparate between monozygous twins than between dizygous twins.

Despite these limitations it may be very rewarding to study discordant monozygotic twins for this may point to the environmental factor in the disease.

An example of this approach is the study of concordance of diabetes mellitus in monozygous twinships in an attempt to delineate the environmental factors. Another aspect of twin research which may be useful is the study of the frequency of a condition in twins compared with that in the single born, such as in cancer mentioned above.

Linkage and genetic mapping

Genes are said to be linked when the loci they occupy are situated on the same chromosome. If they are sufficiently near together, then the alleles which occupy the loci will only infrequently be separated by the process of 'crossing over'. Consequently the phenomenon can be observed by pedigree analysis. Even though it is an infrequent event, crossing-over does occasionally occur between closely linked loci, so linkage between different alleles at the two loci can be observed in different pedigrees.

An allied field of genetics is genetic 'mapping' by which is meant the localization of genes on individual chromosomes. The information enabling the construction of such a map in man has been derived mainly from studies of traits in families and studies of traits and chromosomes in somatic cell hybrids; also, in certain instances from *in situ* DNA–RNA annealing ('hybridization'), deductions from the amino acid sequence of proteins, and deletion mapping and gene dosage effects (see below for further explanation).

Sex (X)-linkage and mapping the X chromosome. Due to the peculiar disposition within families of characters controlled by genes situated on the X chromosome, 116 confirmed and 118 suspected genetic loci have been ascribed to it. Two clusters of close linkages are known (see Fig. 8).

Autosomal linkages and mapping. A growing number of autosomal linkages have been recognized. A total of 50 000 loci for structural

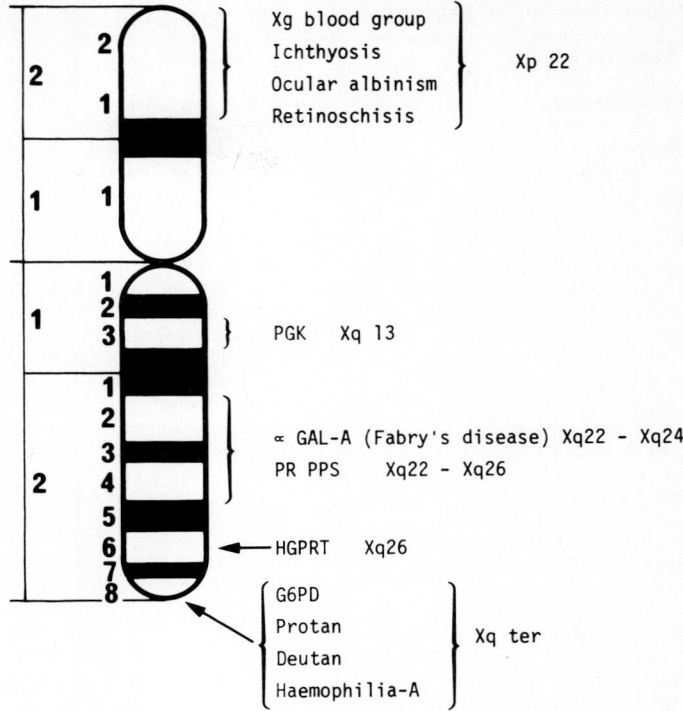

Abbreviations:-

PGK	Phosphoglycerate kinase
∝ GAL-A	Alphagalactosidase-A
PRPPS	Phosphoribosyl-pyrophosphate synthetase
HGPRT	Hypoxanthine-guanine phosphoribosyl transferase
G6PD	Glucose-6-phosphate dehydrogenase

Note:- Ichthyosis = steroid sulphatase deficiency

Fig. 8 Map of the human X chromosome. 116 loci have been mapped to this chromosome and a selection are shown in this diagram. There are two linkage clusters, one containing the Xg blood group and the other containing G6PD.
(The author wishes to acknowledge the help of Dr Ruth Sanger and *The Human Gene Map Newsletter* distributed 26 October 1981, by Professor V. A. McKusick, Johns Hopkins Hospital, Baltimore, Maryland, USA in preparing this diagram).

genes are thought to exist in man. About 3500 gene loci have been confidently identified by pedigree analysis techniques. Some mapping information is available concerning at least 10 per cent of these loci.

A considerable number of loci have been located on autosomes 1, 2, and 6 (Table 3). Gene loci are now being mapped on some of the smaller chromosomes, e.g. alleles controlling the structures of haemoglobin chains β, γ, and δ are on chromosome 11, whereas the alleles controlling the structure of haemoglobin chain α is on chromosome 16. Chromosome 9 carries the closely linked genes governing ABO blood groups, nail–patella syndrome, adenylate kinase, and arginosuccinate synthetase. Chromosome 21 carries genes governing superoxide dismutase-l (soluble) and phosphofructokinase (liver type). Chromosome 22 carries genes controlling β-galactosidase 2 and α-galactosidase B (N-acetyl α-D-galactosaminidase).

Some close linkages are known which have, as yet, not been ascribed to any particular chromosome (Table 4).

An addressing system and measuring distances on chromosomes. In order to be able to state where a gene locus is sited on a chromosome a system exists based upon the morphologic 'banding' staining characteristics of the chromosome (see section on Chromosomes

Table 3 Some loci on specific autosomes

Chromosome 1	Chromosome 6
6-phosphogluconate dehydrogenase	Major histocompatibility complex (HLA)
Elliptocytosis-1	Properidin factor B
Rhesus blood group	Complement 4, including
Alpha-L-fucosidase	Chido blood group
Adenylate kinase-2	Rodgers blood group
Phosphoglucomutase-1	Haemochromatosis
Retinitis pigmentosa 1	21-hydroxylase deficiency
Elliptocytosis-2	1-Glyoxylase-1
Amylase-1 (salivary)	Phosphoglucomutase-3
Amylase-2 (pancreatic)	Hypercholesterolaemia
Cataract zonular pulverulent	B cell receptor for monkey red cells
Duffy blood group	Superoxide dismutase-2 (mitochondrial)
Charcot Marie Tooth disease, slow nerve conduction type	
Uridyl diphosphate glucose	
Pyrophosphorylase	
Classical phenylketonuria	
Antithrombin III	
Succinate dehydrogenase	

below). First, for an autosome the chromosome number is given (or X or Y for a sex chromosome), then either p or q, the former signifying the short arm (conventionally drawn pointing upwards) and the latter the long arm (pointing downwards). It is to be noted that this usage of p and q has nothing to do with the Hardy–Weinberg equilibrium (see page 4.4). Within each arm, prominent bands are constantly found using quinacrine or Giemsa staining. These bands define regions and within these regions are sub-regions numbered from the centromere in relation to minor bands (see Fig. 8).

Finer detail in addressing is derived from non-morphologic information. Recombination frequency is information derived from examination of characters in progeny (see Definitions on page 4.1). The map unit (cross-over unit: Morgan unit) is the unit of map distance between linked genes. It is used to measure chromosome length and equals the total cross-over frequency between the genes con-

Table 4 Linkages of autosomal loci for which assignment to a specific chromosome has not yet been achieved

Phenylthiocarbamide tasting
Kell blood group

Ii blood group
Congenital cataract

Epidermolysis bullosa progressiva
Hypoacusis (a recessive partial deafness)

Cerebellar ataxia, a recessive form
Tyrosinase-negative albinism

cerned (corrected for the effect of double cross-over and chromosome interference) and is expressed as a percentage. A corrected cross-over frequency of 1 per cent equals 1 map unit. On a molecular scale it is now possible to express gene length in terms of kilobases. For example, in the study of haemoglobins it is possible to proceed in the following way: (*a*) RNA from reticulocytes can be prepared and matching DNA synthesized using reverse transcriptase; (*b*) this DNA can be cut up into pieces using various restriction endonucleases; (*c*) the sizes of the pieces of the DNA can be determined and correlated with the phenotype of the donor (see page 4.21). Information obtained in this way shows that the two linked genes for the α-chains of haemoglobin are contained in a fragment of DNA of 14.5 kilobase in length on chromosome 16 (haemoglobin β is at address 11 p 12).

The nail–patella syndrome and the ABO blood group locus. One of the autosomal linkages discovered by means of the study of traits in families will be discussed in more detail.

The nail–patella syndrome, inherited as an autosomal dominant with full penetrance, is characterized by absent or hypoplastic patellae, nail dystrophy, abnormalities of the elbow joints, the presence of iliac horns, and the gradual development of glomerular pathology. Fig. 9 illustrates part of a family with the condition.

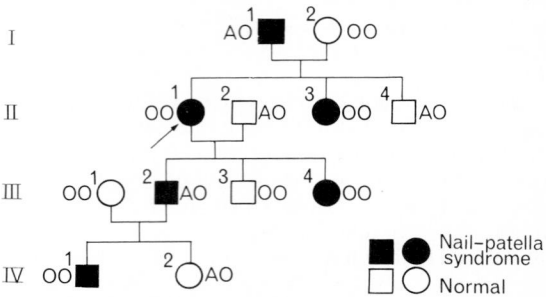

Fig. 9 Nail–patella syndrome. (From Clarke (1964) *Genetics for the clinician*. Blackwell, Oxford).

At first sign there might not appear to be linkage at all, as in generation I the nail–patella syndrome appears in an A individual (I.1), in the next in two O people (II.1, the proposita, indicated by an arrow, and II.3), in the next in an A and an O (III.2 and 4), and in the next in O (IV.1). In fact, however, the linkage is only masked by the dominance of group A. The proposita (II.1) has received the nail–patella gene with her group O and she has handed them on together to her son, III.2. As, however, the mother of III.2 was group O, he must have received O from her and A from his father. He types as an A individual because A is dominant to O and the linkage of the syndrome with O is masked by this dominance of A. In generation IV it will be seen that III.2 has handed on the condition with O again. The situation is not due to crossing-over—if it were, IV.1 would have recieved the nail–patella deformity with A.

Figure 10 shows what happens when crossing-over does take place. Here the nail–patella syndrome is linked with group A₁, as in

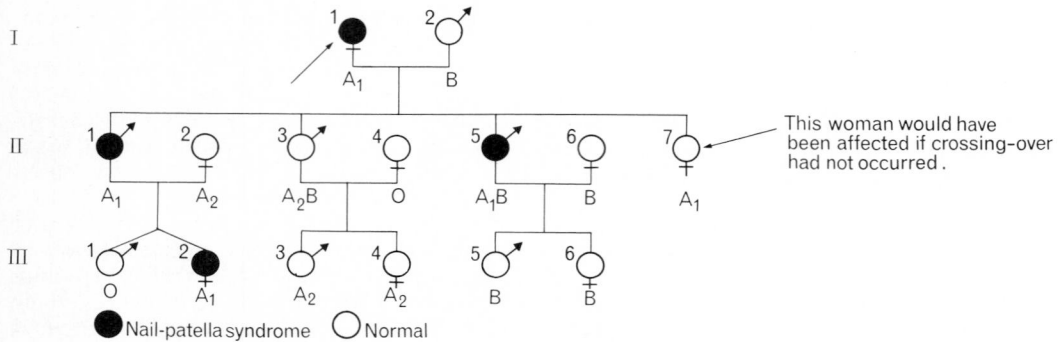

Fig. 10 Nail–patella syndrome. (From Clarke (1964) *Genetics for the Clinician*, Blackwell, Oxford)

I.1, II.1, II.5 and III.2. Crossing-over has occurred at gamete formation with I.1, after the birth of II.5, and before the birth of II.7, who is, as will be seen, blood group A_1 and yet is *not* affected. It will be noticed that the other A individuals in this family who are unaffected are A_2 and not A_1 (A_1 and A_2 are alleles and are distinguishable).

The cross-over value of about 12 per cent agrees with that found in many other families. It is calculated by looking at those individuals where the linkage can clearly be seen, i.e. II.1, II.3, II.5, II.7, III.1, III.2, III.5, and III.6. In one case out of the 8 (12 per cent) where the linkage could be detected, a *new* combination is seen instead of the previous one, and this is quite close linkage. If the cross-over value reaches 50 per cent, it will be clear that there is an equal likelihood of the characters occurring separately as there is of them occurring together, and therefore there is no linkage at all, but 'free recombination'.

It is of great interest that Renwick, on analysing the linkage data from 27 pedigrees of the nail–patella syndrome, found that crossing-over occurred twice as often in women as in men, and in men less frequently as they grew older. If this is characteristic of many loci, it would mean that there would be less recombination, i.e. shuffling, of the paternal than the maternal genes.

Other methods of mapping genetic loci. As stated above, methods other than studying characters in family pedigrees can be used to map loci on individual chromosomes. One example of these methods is described below.

A new way of mapping chromosomes is by means of mixed cell cultures. The procedure is to mix animal cells from two species, each set of cells having particular genetic markers, and to grow a hybrid cell line for many generations in culture. When this was done with cells from Chinese hamsters and men it was found after about 50 generations *in vitro*, that there were two populations of cells, the first with a human chromosome 1 containing a break deleting a portion of the short-arm, whereas the second contained a normal chromosome 1. Biochemical analysis showed that the products of alleles at the phosphoglucomutase-1 and 6-phosphogluconate dehydrogenase loci were absent from the first cell population thus enabling them to be 'mapped' on a specific region of the short arm of chromosome 1. A refinement of this method is provided by breaking up the human chromosomes with ionizing radiations prior to cell infusion. It is then possible to see in suitable cells whether loci have been separated or have stayed together.

The recently developed techniques of DNA analysis and their application to linkage analysis are considered in the next section.

Computational aspects. The basic idea of linkage, i.e. the closeness together of two loci on a chromosome, is very simple. However, to provide a mathematically precise estimate of the closeness is rather more complicated. It involves computation of the odds of the two loci becoming separated in the process of crossing-over. The tedium of these lengthy computations has now been annulled by the availability of tried and tested programmes for large digital computers.

Practical usefulness of linkage and gene mapping. Hitherto little of immediate practical value has emerged from these exciting new developments in the knowledge of the genes of man. It has long been known that the clinical picture of elliptocytosis due to a locus linked to Rhesus, differs from that of elliptocytosis due to another locus not linked to Rhesus which gives a much more serious haemolytic anaemia. So it can be seen that linkage could be used for more precise diagnosis.

Another important practical application can be envisaged in the management of Huntington's chorea families. Here the problem is that a dominant is not manifest until middle age, by which time progeny may already exist perpetuating the abnormal gene in the population. In the present stage of knowledge the heterozygote cannot be identified before clinical manifestations arise. If it could

be shown that a genetic marker locus was closely linked to the Huntington's chorea locus, then it might enable the 'carrier' to be detected early in life (see also Antenatal diagnosis, page 4.27).

Genetic polymorphism

General considerations. Genetic polymorphism is a type of variation in which individuals with clearly distinct qualities exist together in a freely inter-breeding single population. Ford (1940) defined the condition as 'the occurrence together in the same habitat of two or more discontinuous forms or "phases" of a species in such proportions that the rarest of them cannot be maintained merely by recurrent mutation'. This definition excludes several very familiar types of variation. For example, the white, Mongolian, and Negroid races of man do not constitute a polymorphism since, when inter-breeding occurs, the hybrid populations are intermediate and variable. Again, continuous variation, as in human height or blood pressure, is not an example of polymorphism. In these examples, genes at a number of loci are at work and the variation is brought about by the cumulative effects of segregation taking place at more than one locus, and not by 'switch' genes giving rise to distinct alternative forms.

Furthermore, segregation in human populations into normal and phenylketonurics, or normal and achondroplastics are not examples of polymorphism.

What do fall into the definition are many enzyme and blood group systems, certain of the haemoglobinopathies and, perhaps most important from the practical point of view, polymorphisms of drug metabolism and pharmocological responses. In each case the biological problem is to find out the selective advantages and disadvantages which keep the various 'morphs' in balance.

A classical example of this is provided in the work on the peppered moth *Biston betularia*. A melanic form of this moth is found in polluted industrial areas and it is dominant to the peppered form. Both forms are eaten by birds. The peppered form is well camouflaged on lichen-covered tree trunks in the unpolluted countryside, where the melanic is most conspicuous. On a soot-coated tree trunk the reverse applies. Clarke and Sheppard immobilized numbers of peppered and melanic moths on both backgrounds and observed that birds selectively removed the uncamouflaged form. Thus is clearly shown the manner of operation of Darwinian selection. The camouflaged form in both environments survives selectively to propagate the species. In non-human work it can often be demonstrated that heterozygous advantage is the mechanism, but in man there is only one certain example of this, that of the individual who, heterozygous for normal and sickle cell haemoglobin (HbA/HbS), is at an advantage over the normal because he is protected against malaria and clearly better off than the homozygous sickler who dies young. Malaria is also probably responsible for the high incidence of glucose 6-phosphate dehydrogenase (G6PD) deficiency in some malarious areas. More often we simply do not know whether or not heterozygous advantage exists, and in one troublesome polymorphism, that of the Rhesus blood group system, the baby who develops Rh haemolytic disease is always a heterozygote.

Pharmacogenetic polymorphisms. Pharmacogenetic polymorphisms are of practical importance. They can be sub-divided into polymorphisms of drug metabolism and polymorphisms of drug effect (see World Health Organization Technical Report Series 1973, no. 524, *Pharmacogenetics* for much detailed information).

A polymorphism of drug 'metabolism' is shown in the acetylation by *N*-acetyl transferase of eight commonly used compounds. A simple *in vivo* test using either sulphadimidine (synonym: sulphamethazine) or isoniazid reveals two phenotypes—rapid and slow acetylators. The latter phenotype constitutes about 55 per cent of European populations. The effect of the polymorphism in treatments employing five drugs is summarized in Table 5. The increased incidence of isoniazid hepatitis reported in rapid acetyla-

Table 5 Acetylator phenotypes in practical therapeutics

Drug (i.e. environmental factor)	Genetic phenotype	Effect observed in the phenotype noted
Isoniazid	slow	more prone to develop peripheral neuropathy on therapy with conventional doses
	slow	more prone to phenytoin adverse effects when simultaneously being treated for tuberculosis with INH
	slow	more prone to hepatotoxicity when being treated for tuberculosis with rifampicin and INH
	rapid	less favourable results of treating open pulmonary tuberculosis with a once-weekly isoniazid dosage regimen
	rapid	more prone to develop isoniazid-hepatitis
Hydralazine	slow	develop antinuclear antibodies and systemic lupus erythematosus-like syndrome
	rapid	require higher doses to control hypertension
Salicyl-azo-sulphapyridine	slow	increased incidence of various adverse reactions in healthy subjects and when drug used to treat ulcerative and Crohn's colitis
Dapsone	rapid	higher doses needed to control dermatitis herpetiformis (disputed)
	slow	more haematological adverse effects

Genetic polymorphism of acetylation has been described for sulphadimidine, sulphapyridine, and the amine metabolite of nitrazepam produced in the body as a result of reduction, and for these drugs no firm association of a clinical event with either phenotype has been defined. Procaine amide has been shown to be polymorphically acetylated; and the correlation of clinical effects with plasma concentration makes it likely that the acetylator phenotype is relevant in clinical practice

tors is interesting since it may be due to the toxic effect of acetyl isoniazid which is present in large amounts in this phenotype.

The fact that patients developing the hydralazine-induced SLE-like syndrome are almost invariably slow acetylators has prompted different groups of researchers to investigate patients with spontaneous SLE. Their reports conflict, some groups find a high incidence of slow acetylators amongst these patients and others do not.

A natural substrate for the polymorphic N-acetyl transferase is unknown but its ecological importance is suggested by the fact that the polymorphism is 'set' differently in various ethnic groups, e.g. Japanese are 90 per cent and Eskimos almost 100 per cent rapid acetylators.

When the muscular relaxant drug suxamethonium (succinylcholine) was introduced into clinical practice, it was found to have an unusually potent effect on some 1 in 2000 otherwise healthy persons which was clinically apparent as prolonged apnoea. The drug is hydrolysed in the plasma by the enzyme pseudocholinesterase, and the activity of this enzyme was found to be low in susceptible subjects. However, it was the introduction of enzyme inhibition studies which resulted in the recognition of discrete phenotypes. The percentage inhibition of the enzyme by the local anaesthetic dibucaine is called the 'dibucaine number' (DN). Most normal persons have a DN of about 80. A small number of persons have a DN of about 60 and they are heterozygous. The very few persons prone to prolonged apnoea have a DN of about 15 and they are homozygous for an autosomal gene. Further work on this system has defined four alleles at this autosomal locus. It is of practical relevance as well as of theoretical interest that these alleles have widely different frequencies in different ethnic groups. Again no natural substrates are known for this enzyme and its ecological significance is a mystery.

The insecticide, parathion, is converted in the body of man and other mammals to paraxon by means of microsomal oxidation. Paroxon is a powerful anticholinesterase and has in the past been used in eye drops. Paroxon is hydrolysed by an enzyme present in human plasma. The activity of this enzyme exhibits a clear genetic polymorphism. There are considerable inter-ethnic differences in the polymorphism. No clinical association or significance has yet been discovered.

Two rare families have been described in each of which there is a genetically determined distinct abnormality of drug metabolism. The first concerns diphenylhydantoin, which occasionally in the usual clinical doses causes ataxia and nystagmus, and this has been shown in the propositus to be due to an inability to hydroxylate the drug; the same defect has been disclosed in siblings of the affected person. The second relates to methaemoglobinaemia caused by phenacetin because of the patient's relative inability to de-ethylate the drug to paracetamol. In these circumstances, phenacetin is metabolized to a much greater extent than usual along minor pathways to hydroxyphenetidin and to hydroxyphenacetin, both of these being potent causes of methaemoglobinaemia. The same defect was shown to be present in a sister of the patient.

Most drugs are metabolized in the liver by the endoplasmic reticulum. Biotransformation is in many cases firstly by means of oxidation, and the rate at which this process can be carried out has long been known to vary greatly between individuals.

Recently polymorphisms have been described for the oxidation of debrisoquine and sparteine, there being two phenotypes in each polymorphism. Family studies have disclosed that 'poor metabolizers' of debrisoquine are Mendelian recessive characters (Evans et al. 1980) and they are much more prone to hypotension when given modest doses of the drug than are 'extensive metabolizers'.

The metabolism of each of the two compounds is controlled by two alleles at an autosomal locus. About 95 per cent of persons in the population are well able to metabolize both compounds. Most individuals who are poor at metabolizing one compound are also poor at metabolizing the other compound. Rare individuals, however, have the ability to metabolize one compound extensively, but metabolize the other compound poorly. This is interpreted as indicating that the two loci are closely linked and that there is 'linkage disequilibrium' (i.e. some combinations of alleles on a chromosome—'haplotypes'—do not occur at their expected frequencies, possibly because of selection).

The most important genetic polymorphism of drug response concerns G6PD deficiency. This X-linked character has an incidence of 25 per cent on males in some areas and predisposes these subjects to haemolysis in response to a large variety of drugs. They are also prone to haemolysis on eating the bean Vicia faba, giving the syndrome of favism, and to haemolytic disease of the newborn (see Section 19).

A polymorphism of response to the oral anticoagulants has been described in both humans and in rats. In both species the anticoagulant resistant phenotype is a rare autosomal dominant. In a number of areas a population of resistant rats has developed due to selective advantage in the presence of warfarin rodenticide.

Resistance in both humans and rats is exhibited to all the commonly used oral anticoagulants, but not to heparin.

The biochemical basis of the unusual phenotype in man is unknown, but its effect appears as an increased affinity of the appropriate receptor for vitamin K and so much larger amounts than usual of warfarin are required to counteract its action. Doses of 75–80 mg warfarin sodium daily are required in the resistant patient to maintain satisfactory therapeutic prothrombin complex activity in the rate 20–40 per cent. No natural substrate is known for this polymorphism.

A genetic polymorphism has been described for the manner in which intra-ocular pressure responds to topical corticosteroids. Two alleles P^H and P^L at one autosomal locus have been postulated giving rise to the three genotypes $P^L P^L$, $P^L P^H$, and $P^H P^H$. The allele P^H governs the ability to respond with a high-pressure increase to steroids, whereas the allele P^L confers a low-pressure response. The original account of the existence of this polymorphism has been confirmed and also refuted by subsequent independent groups of researchers, and so an element of doubt remains. Ophthalmologists, who have described the polymorphism, have described an increased incidence of glaucoma associated with possession of the P^H allele, so that the P^HP^H genotype is at the greatest risk of developing this disorder with advancing age.

Malignant hyperpyrexia is a rare but often fatal complication of general anaesthesia. The main manifestations of the syndrome are a rapid rise in body temperature, generalized muscular rigidity, and a severe metabolic acidosis. It occurs in persons who inherit, as a Mendelian dominant, a phenotype characterized by mild myopathy—often subclinical—and a raised serum creatine phosphokinase. Halothane and succinylcholine have been used in many of the fatal cases, but other major anaesthetics have also precipitated malignant hyperpyrexia. Moulds and Denborough showed that muscle strips taken from survivors of malignant pyrexia exhibited pronounced contractures *in vitro* when exposed either to halothane or succinylcholine. This contracture was inhibited by procaine. It is suggested that the basic defect is an increased release of calcium ions from the calcium-storing membranes in the muscle cell.

The practical importance of this information is that close attention must be given to any patient who gives a family history of 'anaesthetic deaths'. Causes other than malignant hyperpyrexia may be responsible. However, a careful clinical examination for minor myopathic signs and a serum creatine phosphokinase estimation should be carried out, and, if indicated, a pharmacological test *in vitro* of a small piece of muscle. Patients with a rised creatine phosphokinase from other causes are not at risk during general anaesthesia.

Some diabetics who are being treated with chlorpropamide experience marked flushing after ethanol ingestion. Recent investigations suggest this is a Mendelian autosomal dominant character which is significantly associated with non-insulin-dependent diabetes (but not with insulin-dependent diabetes). Recent studies suggest that non-insulin-dependent diabetics who develop retinopathy and large vessel disease are likely to be persons who do not flush in response to ethanol and chlorpropamide.

Human lymphocyte antigens polymorphism

Human lymphocyte antigens (HLA) (see also page 4.31) first came into prominence in connection with organ transplantation, and now important associations have been found between certain genotypes and various medical disorders (see below).

The A, B, and C antigens can be recognized by using, as sources of antibody, sera either from parous women or from patients having received transfusions or from immunized volunteers. The antibodies can detect minor differences in the chemical structure of glycoproteins present on virtually all cell membranes.

In the testing procedure, lymphocytes are separated from peripheral blood and are incubated with a range of antibodies of known specificity in the presence of complement. The results are determined by assessing the viability of the lymphocytes, e.g. by showing their ability to exclude trypan blue. If the antibody does not react with the antigen, the lymphocyte remains alive and excludes the dye. If the antibody 'recognizes' the antigen and binds to it (with complement) the cell membrane is damaged and the trypan blue enters the cell.

D antigens are recognized by the mixed lymphocyte culture (MLC) technique. A 'standard' lymphocyte thought to be homozygous for a defined antigen is treated with mitomycin to prevent it responding with a proliferative reaction. When an unknown lymphocyte is cultured with this standard cell, it will not undergo a proliferative reaction (measured by the incorporation of radioactive thymidine) if it possesses the same D antigen as the standard cell, but will show proliferation if it lacks this antigen (in this case it recognizes the standard cell as 'foreign'). So if there is available a panel of different homozygous standard typing cells, an unknown lymphocyte can be typed.

The DR antigens are thought to be very closely related to the D antigens and are detected (on B lymphocytes only) by a cytotoxic antibody test as for the A, B, and C antigens, using appropriate antisera.

The important loci for this discussion are those for the first segregant series HLA–A and the second segregant series HLA–B. There are over 20 different antigens produced by different alleles at HLA–A and over 30 different antigens produced by different alleles at HLA–B. These antigens have different frequencies in a given population, some being very frequent, e.g. HLA–A2 (about 45 per cent) and HLA–B7 (about 29 per cent) in a British white population. Some of the antigens however are rare. It might be expected that the distribution of the alleles of the two loci in different individuals of the population might be entirely at random. However, this is not so. There is a pronounced 'linkage disequilibrium' so that some combinations of alleles appear in the population more frequently than random. For example, HLA–A1 at locus A is often accompanied by HLA–B8 at locus B. This combination is called a haplotype. Presumably the phenomenon of linkage disequilibrium indicates that some haplotypes possess a biological advantage, but there is no clear understanding of how this operates.

HLA antigens show wide inter-ethnic variability. For example, HLA antigens giving haplotype A1–B8 are predominantly Caucasoid, whereas antigen B13 is most frequent in Orientals.

Other polymorphisms. Polymorphisms of haemoglobins and blood groups are described in Section 19.

Association between genetic markers and disorders

An association is essentially a statistical finding—for example, it is well known that populations of hospitalized duodenal ulcer patients possess a higher frequency of blood group O individuals than do the general populations from which they are derived. Usually an association is between a particular phenotype in a genetic polymorphism and some reasonably well-defined clinical disorder.

In comparison with genetic linkage which, as explained above, is a precise concept, statistical associations are findings which can be due to a variety of phenomena.

First, an association can arise because of the admixture of two populations possessing different properties. A classical example of this arose in a study of ABO blood groups and hair colour conducted in the Netherlands. A strong association was found between dark hair and blood group B. On closer examination of the data it was revealed that the result had been produced because of the inclusion of Indonesian students (who had a high incidence of blood group B and, of course, dark hair) in the population studies. This phenomenon is called 'stratification' and produces essentially an artefactual association. Although association is basically different from genetic linkage, where only a limited number of individuals is available for examination, it may be difficult or impossible to distinguish between the two. For example, tylosis and carcinoma of the oesophagus sometimes occur together in families. This could be due either to an association or to two linked genes, one for tylosis and one for the carcinoma. However, with linkage, if sufficient individuals in sufficient different families were examined, then crossing-over would sometimes occur and then in a particular family some members would have the cancer without the tylosis. Pleiotropism is another possible explanation.

Sometimes a strong statistical association indicates that the biochemical or physiological products of the genetic marker play some part in the production of the disorder. Examples where knowledge is in this stage of development are Rhesus haemolytic disease and various pharmacogenetic polymorphisms (see above).

In the mid-1950s there was considerable interest in associations and many of the methodological difficulties were overcome. For example, the demonstration of an association between blood group O and duodenal ulcer within sibships ruled out stratification as the explanation.

Consequently some firm statistical associations came to be recognized, including the following:

Blood group O and bleeding duodenal ulcer
Salivary ABH non-secretion and duodenal ulcer
Blood group and thrombosis
PTC taster phenotypes and various thyroid disorders

Important associations are those between the HLA antigens and certain disorders. The most startling association is between antigen B27 and ankylosing spondylitis (AS). Furthermore, the possession of antigen B27 predisposes to the development of arthropathy with psoriasis and with the recognizable environmental infectious agents chlamydia (in urethritis), *S. typhi, yersinia enterocolitica*, and *campylobacter*.

Other associations have been discovered (Table 6). Most associations are with antigens controlled by alleles at the B locus.

Table 6 Associations between clinical disorders and HLA antigens

Clinical disorder	A	C	B	DR
Ankylosing spondylitis			27	
Reiter's syndrome			27	
*'Reactive' arthritis			27	
Psoriatic arthritis			27	
Acute anterior uveitis			27	
Coeliac disease			8	
Dermatitis herpetiformis			8	
Thyrotoxicosis: Caucasian			8	DRw3
Thyrotoxicosis: Chinese			(w46)	
Chronic active hepatitis (Hb-Ag negative)			8	
Addison's disease			8	
Myasthenia gravis (young, no thymoma)			8	
Sicca syndrome			8	
Psoriasis		w6†	13	
			17	
Behçet's disease			5	
Insulin-dependent diabetes			8	DRw3
			15	DRw4
			18	
Haemochromatosis	3		14	
Nasopharyngeal carcinoma: Chinese			w46	
Multiple sclerosis			7	DRw2
Rheumatoid arthritis				DRw4
Idiopathic membranous nephropathy				DRw3

* Arthritis following gastrointestinal infections due to certain Gram-negative bacteria
† The letter 'w' in this context stands for 'workshop' and indicates a provisional antigenic specificity not as yet completely established as being determined by a separate allele
This Table was kindly compiled and supplied by Professor J. C. Woodrow

An example of another possibly more informative way of viewing these associations is provided by the study of HLA types in families containing diabetics. It has been found that insulin-dependent diabetes is associated in populations with HLA–B8, Bw15, and B18, but, of course, the disease can occur with other phenotypes. In a family in which more than one sibling with insulin-dependent diabetes is present, the affected members share either one or two identical chromosomes no. 6 (as far as their HLA region is concerned) to a degree far in excess of that expected by chance. This is interpreted as showing that there is a major 'diabetogenic' gene locus closely linked to the HLA chromosomal region.

Three hypotheses have been advanced to explain HLA and disease associations: (a) that there are 'immune response genes' situated on chromosome 6 very near to the HLA genes so that the latter act as a 'flag' or indicator for the former, (b) that the HLA antigen concerned may be responsible possibly because it is structurally very similar to an antigen produced by a micro-organism. Consequently the body fails to mount a reaction to the latter; (c)

that a particular HLA antigen is a receptor site on a cell surface for a particular virus or hormone.

In a totally different category are two other associations: (a) the locus for 21 hydroxylase deficiency has been shown to be linked to HLA; and (b) likewise, the disorder of complement C2 deficiency is associated with A25, B18, and DRw 2, and the structural gene is thought to be in the HLA region (Fig. 11).

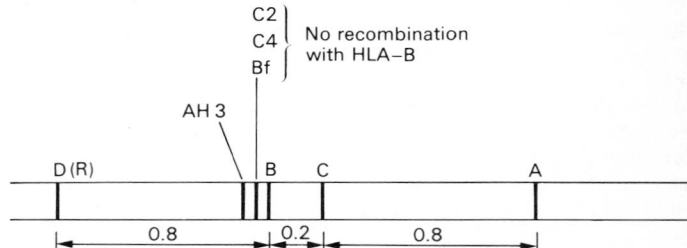

Approximate recombination fractions
AH3 = adrenal hyperplasia – 21 hydroxylase deficiency
C2 = complement component 2   C4 = complement component 4
Bf = properidin factor

Fig. 11 The HLA region on chromosome 6.
The loci for alleles controlling HLA antigens of the A,B,C, and D (R) series are shown.

Various disorders having an 'immunologic' basis have long been known to 'run in families' and in some instances polygenic inheritance has been unequivocally demonstrated. It appears now that genes carried in the vicinity of the HLA loci on chromosome 6 are important in determining the constitution prone to such disorders. Preliminary evidence indicates that the clinical picture produced in a leprosy patient is determined by his HLA-linked genes.

A practical application of HLA typing occurs in the management of hyperthyroidism. When a patient with Graves' disease has been successfully treated with an antithyroid drug such as carbimazole, the clinician has to decide what to do next. The severity of the initial disease and the size of the thyroid gland may give an indication whether the patient will relapse or not if the carbimazole is stopped. Often, however, it is difficult to tell what will happen. Now it is clear that patients possessing antigen DRw3 relapse much more readily than patients who lack this antigen. So HLA phenotyping may be an aid in this clinical situation.

As mentioned previously, HLA antigens show inter-ethnic variability. The HLA–A1, B8–DRw3 haplotype is known to be characteristic of north European populations and also to be associated with coeliac disease. This may be the reason why coeliac disease seems to have a particularly high incidence in this ethnic group.

HLA and adverse reactions to drugs. The most common adverse reactions to drugs are clinical phenomena such as rashes, proteinuria, and haematological changes, which appear to have a basis of hypersensitivity. A convincing immunologic mechanism has, however, been demonstrated in very few instances (e.g. 'Sedormid' and quinine purpuras).

New light has now been shed on this area in that in a few instances associations have been found between HLA antigen and adverse reactions.

Patients with systemic lupus erythematosus induced by hydralazine have been known for some time to be largely slow acetylators. It has now been found by Batchelor et al. (1980) that three-quarters of these hydralazine-SLE subjects had antigen HLA–DRw4 which was possessed by only about one quarter of the two control groups, (a) slow acetylators treated with hydralazine but who did not develop hydralazine-SLE, and (b) idiopathic SLE patients.

One of the most toxic of medications is sodium aurothiomalate given for rheumatoid arthritis. Wooley et al. (1980) have found that out of 15 rheumatoid patients developing proteinuria on aurothiomalate, 14 possessed antigens B8 and DRw3. About 30 per cent of rheumatoid patients possess antigen DRw3—a proportion similar to that of the general population. Latts *et al.* (1980), however, report that a mixed bunch of adverse reactions to gold therapy for rheumatoid arthritis is more prone to occur in B12-positive patients (especially women) than in those patients who are B12-negative. Obviously this topic merits closer scrutiny.

Leucopenia and agranulocytosis during levamisole therapy for rheumatoid arthritis has been noted particularly in B27-positive individuals. B27-positive patients account for about 6 per cent of the rheumatoid population—a figure resembling that in the general population (Veys *et al.* 1978).

The way in which the possession of these HLA alleles confers increased susceptibility to the adverse reactions is at present unknown. This lack of understanding need not, however, prevent attempts at the practical application of the knowledge to identify patients with above average risks.

Chromosomes

DNA. Chromosomes contain deoxyribonucleic acid (DNA), a molecule of which consists of two chains, each made up of a deoxyribose phosphate backbone and a series of purine and pyrimidine bases which pair with those of the opposite chain (Watson and Crick 1953) (see also page 4.22). The molecule is constructed like a double spiral staircase of which the deoxyribose phosphate backbones form the 'bannisters' and the nitrogenous bases the 'steps'. The pyrimidine bases are thymine and cytosine and the purines, adenine and guanine. Thymine normally always pairs with adenine, whereas guanine pairs with cytosine (see Figs. 12 and 13). A single molecule of DNA may have as many as 10 000 purine–pyrimidine pairs and its molecular weight is about 6 000 000.

The two chains reproduce themselves by unwinding and separating and the bases then pick up new partners—guanine plus its deoxyribose phosphate if cytosine is needing one, and adenine plus its sugar and phosphate if thymine needs one, and so on. Each new double chain consists therefore of one old and one new chain (the semiconservative mode of replication).

Goulian, Kornberger, and Sinsheimer (1967) made the great advance of synthesizing DNA *in vitro*. They put the tritium-labelled DNA of a virus in a test-tube with the bases adenine, guanine, and (instead of thymine) bromouracil, and added the enzyme DNA polymerase. This caused artificial DNA to be formed around the natural DNA and the two could be separated because bromouracil is heavier than thymine. This artificial DNA was found to be capable of reproducing itself, and, if this were the case in man, it might be possible in the future to attach a needed gene to harmless viral DNA and use this as a vehicle for delivering it to the cells of a patient with an hereditary defect (a form of 'genetic engineering') (see page 4.27).

The vital importance of DNA is that it can initiate the transmission of information to the cytoplasm, so that amino acids can be formed into polypeptide chains containing the correct sequences and hence form the appropriate proteins. For example:

$$G—C$$
$$C—G$$
$$A—T$$

would carry a different message from that of:

$$A—T$$
$$G—C$$
$$T—A$$

A gene is, therefore, that portion of DNA responsible for coding a single polypeptide sequence and this functional unit is also known as a cistron. It is, of course, vastly smaller than a DNA molecule.

Although the genetic information arises in the DNA of the nucleus, the proteins are manufactured in the cytoplasm on small particles called ribosomes. Messenger ribonucleic acid (mRNA) is similar to DNA but has only one strand and thymine is replaced with uracil, and transmits the correct order of the bases and hence

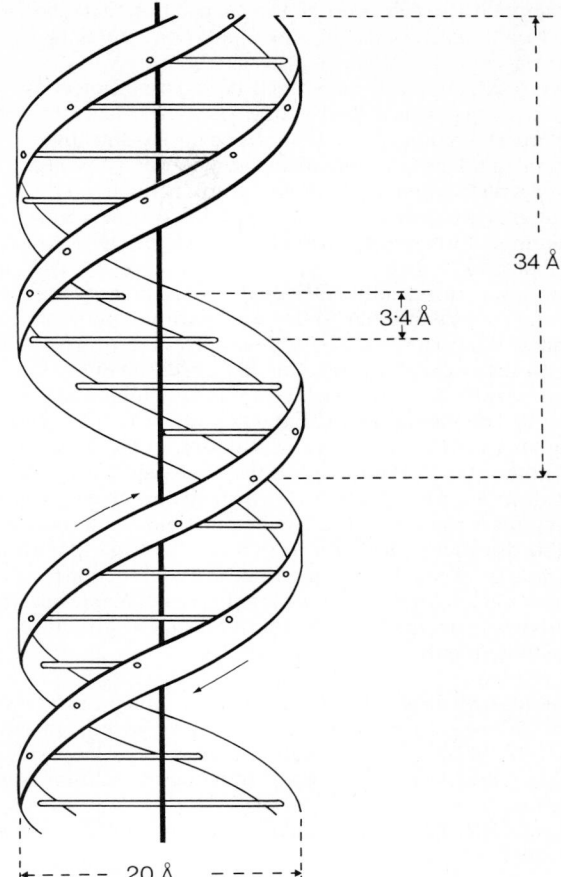

Fig. 12 Diagram representing the double spiral 'staircase' of the DNA molecule, giving dimensions in Angstrom (10^{-10}) units. The outer bands represent the phosphate-sugar chains and the horizontal rods the paths of the bases holding the chains together. The arrows indicate that the sequence of bases goes one way in one chain and the opposite way in the other. The vertical line represents the axis of the molecule. (From Clarke (1964) *Genetics for the clinician*. Blackwell, Oxford).

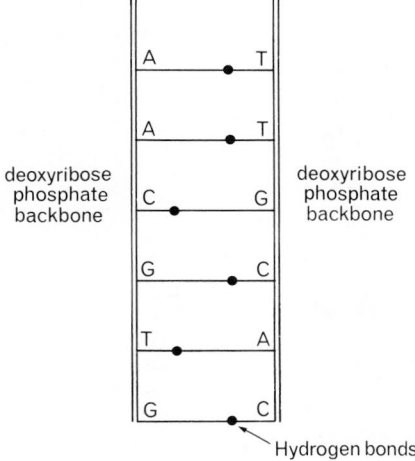

Fig. 13 Diagram showing the way in which the nitrogenous bases of DNA are paired, facing inwards from the phosphate-sugar chain and joined together by hydrogen bonds. (From Clarke (1964). *Genetics for the clinician*. Blackwell, Oxford).

of the amino acids. Transfer RNA (tRNA) picks up the necessary amino acids from the cytoplasm and positions them on a ribosome for chain synthesis.

It has been shown in the bacteriophage T_4 that:

1. Three of the four bases form a 'word' which codes for an amino acid. If four bases formed the 'word', this would produce only 16 combinations—4×4—and there are 20 amino acids so this was unlikely. Selecting any 3 bases out of a given 4 will make 64

combinations (4 × 4 × 4), i.e. too many; but there are several triplet 'words' which code for the same amino acid, e.g. GGC, GGA, and GGG all code for glycine.

2. The code is 'read' in one direction. If a mutation consisting of the addition of a purine or pyrimidine base takes place, the coding is altered after the addition. If, however, a base is shortly afterwards deleted in the DNA of the phage, the order goes back to the original correct sequence. The same result is obtained if, after the first addition, two further bases are added. It will be seen that either of these procedures will restore the subsequent DNA sequence to its original form.

Another way in which the DNA can be altered is by the substitution of one base for another. If this occurs within one triplet, it only alters one amino acid—the one coded for by that triplet. It does not alter the amino acids controlled by the 'words' on either side of the mutated 'word'. In man, in sickle-cell haemoglobin the single substitution of the amino acid valine for glutamic acid is enough to change HbA to HbS, this being a mutation in the sense of alteration. Another type of mutation in the base sequence of the DNA can result in no given protein (for instance an enzyme), and this may account for many of the biochemical blocks in the inherited metabolic disorders. Other forms of mutation and other aspects of human molecular genetics are described in a later section (page 4.25).

What has been discussed above is at the molecular level, whereas what follows concerns whole chromosomes, i.e. structures which can be studied under the microscope.

Techniques of chromosome identification. Much of the information and the figures on chromosome studies have been obtained from Dr S. Walker, Cytogenetics Laboratory, Department of Genetics, University of Liverpool, to whom the author is greatly indebted.

Chromosomes can be seen only in actively dividing cells and so

marrow cells, peripheral blood lymphocytes stimulated with phytohaemagglutinin (PHA), or skin cells in tissue culture are usually those investigated.

Bone marrow cells are most often looked at in leukaemia and other blood disorders and are examined without culture so as to reveal the real *in vivo* picture. For most other investigations, peripheral blood lymphocytes are taken and incubated in a medium containing amino acids, PHA, and either AB or pooled human serum. There is an interval of two or three days before chromosome preparations can be made. In the case of skin it is at least one and sometimes several weeks before results are obtainable.

In cultures, colchicine is added after the requisite incubation time. This markedly retards cell division at the metaphase (i.e. the middle of mitosis) which then lasts several hours. At this phase the chromatids remain attached at the centromere and so this is an advantageous time to count and study the forms of the chromosomes. The cells are next caused to swell by exposure to an hypotonic solution, the preparation is fixed, then spread on a slide, and finally stained. Now the chromosomes are clearly visible microscopically. A chromosome is described and classified by four criteria: (*a*) its length; (*b*) the position of the centromere; (*c*) distinguishing features such as the presence of a satellite; and (*d*) by characteristic banding patterns obtained by the techniques of fluorescence and Giemsa (or Leishman) staining. Each chromosome shows a characteristic banding pattern which allows it to be individually identified. Variations of the banding technique bring out particular features of individual chromosomes, e.g. staining at pH 11 reveals a dark blob near the centromere of chromosome 9. Quite a number of these morphological features revealed by banding techniques exhibit genetic polymorphism (e.g. the size of the dark blob on chromosome 9 which may be used to see from which parent an offspring has derived this autosome).

In Fig. 14 is shown how by convention the 22 pairs of autosomes

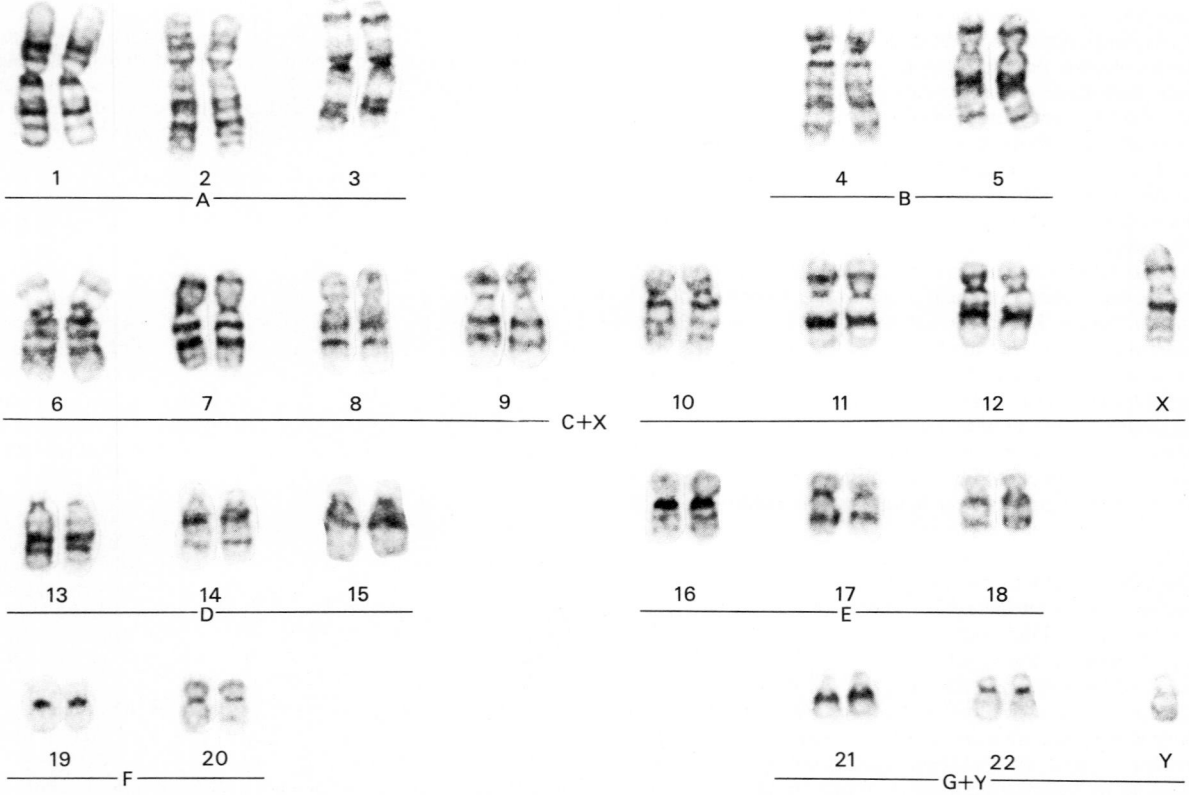

Fig. 14 Normal male karyotype, prepared from cultured lymphocytes treated with trypsin and Leishman stained. This gives typical G-banding, so called because it was originally discovered using Giemsa stain. The chromosomes are arranged in the order as determined at the Paris Conference 1971. Letter grouping as per Patau's classification (London Conference 1963). In terms of absolute size, the length of chromosome 1 at this stage of division is approximately 7 μm. Chromosomes 21 and 22 are about 1–1.5 μm long. (Photograph kindly supplied by Dr Stanley Walker).

are arranged and numbered in decreasing order of size (except that 21 is smaller than 22). The order in which the chromosomes are numbered is according to the Paris Conference of 1971. The X and Y chromosomes are not numbered.

Chromosomal abnormalities

Non-disjunction. Non-disjunction is an abnormality of nuclear division. It can occur in meiosis or mitosis. In meiosis there may be a failure of chromosomes to separate at the first division. A failure of chromatids to separate can occur at the second division of meiosis or in mitosis.

Non-disjunction can occur with the autosomes or with X and Y, and in the case of the autosomes the individuals who have received the extra chromosome are known as trisomic for that chromosome. However, in the case of the sex chromosomes the constitution XXY, for example, is not strictly speaking trisomic because there are not three homologous chromosomes.

Non-disjunction in the autosomes. Mongolism (Down's syndrome) is caused by trisomy 21, and the much rarer Edwards and Patau syndromes (both characterized by mental retardation and various congenital physical defects) by trisomy 18 and 13 respectively. It is probable that the mental deficiency of these three disorders is due to the increase in chromatin and that it is not specific for trisomy of any particular chromosome.

Translocation in the autosomes. Although the majority of cases of mongolism are due to non-disjunction, in about 5 per cent of cases and especially in those produced by younger mothers no additional chromosome is present, but simply extra chromatin resulting from an exchange of parts from one chromosome with another non-homologous chromosome. This process is termed a translocation. Translocations are usually reciprocal, implying exchange of chromatin between two non-homologous chromosomes. A special type of reciprocal translocation is known as 'Robertsonian' where two acrocentric chromosomes give rise to one meta- or submeta-centric chromosome with loss of the two short arms. In other reciprocal translocations all the exchange products are retained.

The most common Robertsonian translocation in the general population is 13/14 which occurs in about 1 in 1000 persons (but this figure includes some familial aggregation). The Patau syndrome, which is a possible clinical outcome in the offspring of carriers of this translocation, occurs far less commonly than it theoretically should (i.e. 1 in 4). The reason for this is unknown but possibly it is due to a selection process at nuclear division or fertilization.

The most frequent Robertsonian translocation giving rise to Down's syndrome is a 14/21 translocation (Fig. 15). Other Robertsonian translocations such as 15/21, 21/21, and 21/22 may also be responsible for transmission of mongolism in families. Satisfactory counselling depends on knowing the exact mechanism occurring in the family being counselled. For example, a 21/21 translocation carrier mated to a normal person can produce only offspring which are effectively 21 trisomic or 21 monosomic, and there is no chance of producing a normal offspring.

In 14/21 translocation trisomy the theoretical chance of a subsequent offspring being a mongol is 1 in 4. However, in practice the risk is less than this—somewhere between 1 in 5 and 1 in 10 if the mother is a carrier, and between 1 in 10 and 1 in 20 if the father is a carrier. This is possibly due to either selection during separation of chromosomes at meiosis, or selection against unbalanced sperm.

From the point of view of genetic advice, it is very important to known whether mongolism is caused by a translocation or by a non-disjunction in a parent. In the former, one parent (more often the mother) may be the carrier, and some of her children are likely to be mongols. Consequently of course the risk of recurrence is high. The occurrence risks for non-disjunction cases (by far the commonest) are shown in Table 7. The recurrence risk for non-disjunction type trisomy-21 is not accurately known, but recent amniocentesis

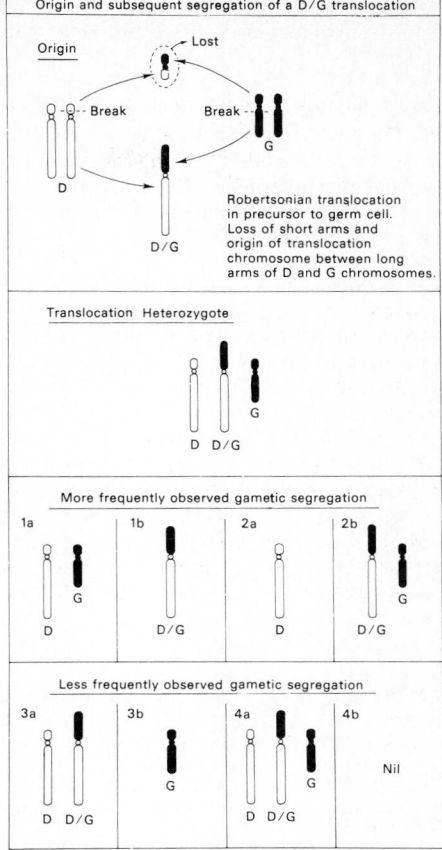

Fig. 15 Mongolism. Robertsonian translocation involving a D group chromosome (e.g. 14) and a G group chromosome (e.g. 21). The chromosomes produced and shown in the lower half of the picture will eventually be paired with normal chromosomes from the gametes of the other parent.

data suggests that it may be about 1 in 100 irrespective of material age. This is a substantial contribution to the occurrence figure of total mongolism at a young maternal age, but only a small contribution in mothers aged 40 years (personal communication, Dr C. O. Carter).

Mongol mosaicism. The non-disjunction in the autosomes described above occurs during meiosis and so all the cells in the resulting individual are abnormal. Sometimes, however, non-disjunction occurs shortly after the two gametes have united; in which case it occurs during mitosis with the result that two or more cell lines may be established. This is known as chromosomal mosaicism. Mongol mosaics may sometimes be normal mentally but have some of the physical stigmata of mongolism such as the facies or abnormal palm-print patterns.

Mosaicism in a parent may also explain the occurrence of more than one mongol in a family when this is not due to translocation. It

Table 7 Relationship of maternal age to trisomy 21

Maternal age	Risk of occurrence (live births)
20–29	1:1000
30–34	1: 600
35–39	1: 200
40–45	1: 60
45 upwards	1: 30

Data kindly supplied by Dr C. O. Carter (1980) and reproduced here with his permission is then possible that some of the gametes, either maternal or paternal, have 24 chromosomes, the extra one being a second chromosome 21.

Deletion. A disorder due to deletion of part of the short arm of chromosome 5 is the *cri-du-chat* syndrome. Deletions are also referred to in the section on the mapping of chromosomes. These deletions are visible microscopically, whereas other deletions occur at the molecular level, the classical example of which is one form of thalassaemia (see page 4.26).

Non-disjunction in the sex chromosomes. Because men and women are respectively XY and XX with regard to the sex chromosomes, the consequences of non-disjunction are different in the two sexes, and Figs. 16 and 17 show the production of possible gametes.

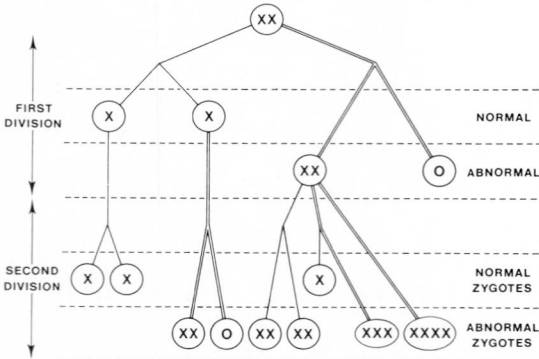

Fig. 16 Possible results of normal meiosis and of non-disjunction during meiosis in a female. Pathways involving non-disjunction are denoted =).

Furthermore, by various combinations of gametes 18 potentially viable sex chromosomal constitutions can arise, the most exotic theoretically being XXXXXXYY. Some theoretically possible combinations, not including an X, e.g. YO and YYO, are not viable. The situation can be further complicated by mitotic non-disjunction early in embryogenesis giving rise to a mosaic.

Despite this complexity, the important clinical syndromes are relatively few and the discussion here will be restricted to them (see Table 9).

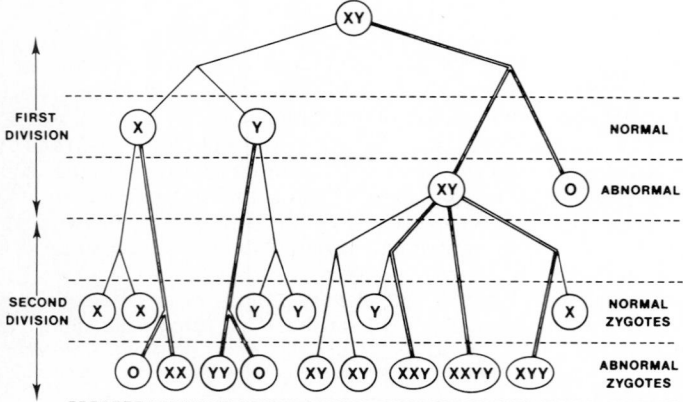

Fig. 17 Possible results of normal meiosis and of non-disjunction during meiosis in a male. Pathways involving non-disjunction are denoted =).

Turner's syndrome. The clinical features of Turner's syndrome are well known and most cases have 45 chromosomes, particularly those with webbing of the neck. The genotype of the sex chromosomes is usually XO and the patients are chromatin negative (see Nuclear sexing below). However, about one-fifth of patients are chromatin positive and the explanation for this may be that they are: (*a*) mosaics, e.g XO/XX; (*b*) possessors of a normal X and an

isochromosome of the long arms of the X (see definitions of terms and Fig. 1); (*c*) carriers of a normal X and part of a second X (a 'deleted' X); or (*d*) in a minority of cases, the syndrome may be due to loss of a piece of both arms and the chromosome forming a ring; (*e*) finally, the Turner's syndrome may be confused with Noonan's syndrome in which the sex chromosomes are normal and additional features, e.g. mental impairment and pulmonary stenosis, are present.

The shortness of stature and the other somatic abnormalities frequently associated with an XO sex chromosome complement are not present in females who have a normal X and an isochromosome of the short arm of the X; they are present, however, when the isochromosome is formed of the the two long arms. It appears, therefore, that the genes influencing height and the other somatic characters, which are abnormal in XO females, are situated on the short arm of the X chromosome and that for normal development of these characters in the female the short arms of two X chromosomes should be present. It would seem that genes present on the long and short arms of both X chromosomes are necessary for the development of a functioning ovary.

It is important to recognize Turner's syndrome in the female since at some stage after the age of 12 years, oestrogens can be administered to bring about spurious menstruation and secondary sex development, which is helpful for psychological reasons. Furthermore, a definite diagnosis also enables a prognosis of permanent infertility to be given with almost complete certainty.

Klinefelter's syndrome. The clinical features of Klinefelter's syndrome include elongated limbs and trunk, small testes, and gynaecomastia. Most men with the syndrome have 47 chromosomes and are chromosomally XXY. They are chromatin positive on nuclear sexing. As might be expected because of the presence of two X chromosomes, the incidence of colour-blindness is comparable to that found in normal women. The IQ may be low. Some cases are mosaics, e.g. XY/XXY, but those of this genotype who have been described are not phenotypically different from patients whose cells are all XXY. XXXYY and XXXXY are well described variants. A few patients for unknown reasons are chromatin negative and have the normal complement of 46 chromosomes with an XY sex pair.

The psychiatric features of Turner's and Klinefelter's syndromes are discussed in Section 25.

Parental source of the X chromosome. Though clinically immaterial it is of interest to know in which parent non-disjunction has occurred. This point can sometimes be decided either by colour vision studies, or more efficiently by means of the sex-linked blood group system Xg. Because the responsible alleles are on the X chromosome, normal males can only be either Xg^a or Xg. Normal women however, can be Xg^{a}Xg^a (homozygous positive), XgXg (homozygous negative), or Xg^{a}Xg (heterozygous). Since the frequency of the heterozygote is as high as 36 per cent in Europe, many families will segregate for Xg^a and Xg. Using this blood group it has been shown that in Turner's syndrome the non-disjunction is more usually paternal (74 per cent of cases) whereas in Klinefelter's syndrome it is more usually maternal (60 per cent of cases).

The XYY syndrome. This karyotype occurs in 1 in 700 live male births, so many persons possessing it are normal members of the population. Some subjects with this karyotype are very tall. Probably the idea that there was an association between this genotype and behavioural disturbances and criminal tendencies is artefactual due to a bias of ascertainment. However, it does seem that larger numbers than random of XYY persons have difficulty in social adaptation and delayed speech and language development (as in many other chromosomal abnormalities).

The XXX syndrome. The triple X female with 47 chromosomes shows very little physical abnormality, is often fertile, but may have a low IQ. It is possible that only one X is working in any cell at a given time and so an extra non-working X may not constitute much of a handicap (see Lyon hypothesis below). It could be expected that they might produce chromosomally abnormal offspring—on average half their sons should be XXY and half their daughters XXX, but 90 per cent of their offspring who have been investigated have in fact normal sex chromosome karyotypes.

Anomalous sex chromosome karotype. The outward phenotypic appearance of a person may be at variance with the sex chromosome karyotype.

XX males are rare and due to a type of translocation since the H–Y antigen is usually present.

XY females are common and are usually due to gonadal agenesis or gonadal dysgenesis or to testicular feminization.

Shorthand description of chromosomal abnormalities. An addressing system based upon the microscopic morphologic banding pattern of chromosomes has been described above. The same system can be used to describe chromosomal abnormalities. In this system the short arm is identified as 'p' and the long arm as 'q'. A gain or loss of a whole chromosome is indicated by '+' or '−' before the chromosome number (e.g. 47, XY + 21 = male mongol). A translocation is indicated by the letter 't', followed by the chromosomes involved in parentheses. An illustrative example is that described by Bass and Sparkes (1979) where two balanced translocations are described in a pedigree as follows:

t (7;10) (q 11; q 22)   and
t (14;21) (14 q ter→cen→21 q ter)

The first expression infers a reciprocal translocation between chromosomes 7 and 10. The break in chromomosome 7 has taken place in the long arm region 1 band 1 (q 11). The break in chromosome 10 has occurred in the long arm region 2 band 2 (q 22).

The second expression infers a Robertsonian translocation between chromosome 14 and 21. Here the long arm of chromosome 14 from its end (ter = terminal) to the centromere has fused with the long arm of chromosome 21. It may be of interest to point out that is latter translocation is the one commonly found in carriers for translocation Down's syndrome.

Nuclear sexing. In a high proportion of somatic cells of the normal female, lying closely adjacent to the nuclear membrane, can be seen a small stainable body (Barr body) which is rarely seen in males. Sexing from the buccal mucosa has therefore become a routine procedure. The absence of a Barr body (synonym: chromatin negative), however, does not necessarily mean that the individual is a male, but merely that there are not two X chromosomes. This is of some importance when a patient presents with some male and some female sex characters.

It is thought that the Barr body is the inactive X, and tritium labelling shows that this X synthesizes DNA very late. The fact that it is tightly coiled (hence the deep staining) may prevent the production and release of messenger RNA which transmits the chemical instructions from the genes.

The Y chromosome can now be detected in interphase using fluorescent dyes (either mepacrine hypochloride or mepacrine mustard). This is known as Y chromatin and fluoresces brightest of all the chromosomes present.

The Lyon hypothesis. Mosaicism was referred to on page 4.15 and in the examples given the indiviuals were always abnormal, but the Lyon hypothesis suggests that all women are mosaics with regard to their two X chromosomes. This is an important concept and well worth serious study.

Lyon (1961) postulated that at about the twelfth day after fertilization one of the X chromosomes in every cell of the female fetus becomes inactive. Which of the two Xs does so is decided at random for every cell but once it is decided, all the descendants of that cell follow the same pattern. The result is that about half the somatic cells of the female will have an inactive maternal X chromosome and the paternal one will be 'working', whereas the opposite will be the case in the remaining half. In men the single X will always be

working in all the cells. Lyon showed that this was certainly the case in mice, as female animals which occur carrying both an allele controlling a dominant coat colour on their maternal X and an allele controlling a recessive colour on their paternal X show patchiness of coat colour—just what would be expected if in one piece of skin one allele was in action and at other places the alternative allele was active.

The hypothesis explains why too much or too little chromatin does not greatly upset the mental or physical development of individuals where an X chromosome is concerned, but trisomy or monosomy for any of the autosomes is highly damaging. The hypothesis also explains why women are in many ways so little different from men; if both their X chromosomes were active they would have twice as many active X-linked genes as males, which they do not. This can actually be tested when a dosage effect might be expected, for example in glucose 6-phosphate dehydrogenase production, it is found that normal women do not make twice as much of the enzyme as do normal men.

Chromosomes and abortions. In about quarter of all spontaneous abortions the chromosomes are abnormal (60 per cent in first trimester) whereas in legalized abortuses the figure is around 2 per cent.

Table 8 gives the distribution of different types of chromosomal abnormality in 120 spontaneous abortions in which the chromosomes were not normal.

Table 8 Distribution of chromosomal abnormalities in unselected spontaneous abortions

	Abnormality	Number of abortuses	Total	Percentage
Monosomy	XO	57	60	20.48
	autosomal	3		
Trisomy	A (1–3)	6		
	B (4–5)	6		
	C (6–12)	10		
	D (13–15)	27	132	45.05
	E (16–18)	47		
	F (19–20)	6		
	G (21–22)	25		
	double trisomy	5		
Triploidy	69, XXX	25		
	69, XXY	42	71	24.23
	69, XYY	4		
Tetraploidy	92, XXXX	8	14	4.78
	92, XXYY	6		
Others	mosaics, translocations, etc.	16	16	5.46
Totals		293	293	100

Adapted by Dr S. Walker (1976) from data supplied by D. H. Carr (1971)

The very high incidence of autosomal trisomy (53.3 per cent) represents about 13 per cent of all recognized spontaneous abortions and probably about 1.3 per cent of all conceptions, and this contrasts markedly with the figure of 0.2 per cent for autosomal trisomy in live births, suggesting that such abnormality usually ends in abortion.

Monosomy, mainly XO, has a high incidence but surprisingly few abortuses are recognized with autosomal deficiencies, probably because they are lethal at such an early age that they have not been detected. The high frequency of XO abortions is somewhat unexpected since individuals with Turner's syndrome can lead a reasonably normal though sterile life. The data in fact suggest that the XO condition at conception may be as high as 0.7 per cent and that approximately 98 per cent of the resulting fetuses are aborted.

Synoptic view of chromosomal abnormalities. The most common chromosomal abnormalities in living humans and the phenotypic features which are associated with them are listed in Table 9. The phenotypes associated with abnormal chromosomal constitution include the following clinical abnormalities at high frequency: abortion; amenorrhoea; infertility (both sexes); mental retardation; and multiple congenital malformations of skeleton and organs. Consequently these conditions are indications for karyotyping the patient and possibly the parents and siblings. The following example illustrates the value of this approach.

A family doctor sent along a girl aged 20 years who was perfectly healthy, with the following question: 'Though her parents are normal, the fact that she has three brothers who are high grade mental defectives makes her ask for genetic counselling in view of her impending marriage'. Chromosome studies revealed that the three affected boys each had some cells in which their X chromosome exhibited readiness to break very near to the end of its long arm. This is recognized as *'Fragile-X' mental retardation* and inherited in an X-linked recessive manner with a high risk to sons of mothers who also carry the Fragile-X but are themselves not affected (as they also carry one normal X). A low percentage of cells showing one Fragile-X chromosome was found in the sister of these three brothers and accordingly she was counselled, indicating that she was most probably at a high risk of having similarly affected sons (Evans and Walker, unpublished material).

Chromosomes and neoplasia. (See also page 4.47). A high proportion of tumours have abnormal chromosomes. There is disagreement on the significance of this observation. Two extreme viewpoints are: (a) that the chromosomal changes are epiphenomena

with little or no relevance to the development of neoplasia; and (b) that the changes are a fundamental and integral part of the neoplastic process.

In favour of the first viewpoint, the following facts are adduced. Some tumours have normal chromosomes. In a single neoplasm the chromosomal aberrations may be much more marked in a metastasis than in the primary.

Support for the second viewpoint rests mainly on the following considerations:

1. Ionizing radiations are responsible for clones of cells with abnormal chromosomes seen in lymphocytes of thorotrast-treated patients, bone marrow of patients with polycythaemia treated with ^{32}P and lymphocytes of patients treated with radiation for ankylosing spondylitis. It is however, not clear whether the malignancies which arise in such patients originate from these abnormal cells. The 'Philadelphia' (Ph[1]) chromosome (see below) is an abnormality of the type that can be produced by radiation and is seen in chronic myeloid leukaemia arising after irradiation.

2. Patients subjected to vigorous cytotoxic therapy show chromosomal aberrations and have a high risk of developing a second primary neoplasm. Likewise, environmental chemicals, such as benzene and vinyl chloride, produce both chromosome aberrations and malignancy.

3. Many viruses cause chromosome damage. RNA viruses (such as the humble measles) cause chromosome fragmentation without rearrangement. DNA viruses cause chromosome gaps, breaks, and rearrangements. Some viral infections (notably the Epstein–Barr virus) are followed by neoplasia, and the chromosomal effects of

Table 9   Reference guide to more common chromosomal abnormalities

Descriptive title	Chromosomal complement	Phenotypic features
Sex chromosomal abnormalities		
Turner's syndrome	45, XO 46, XXqi (isochromosome for long arm of X)	female, ovarian dysgenesis, short stature, cubitus valgus, webbed neck, wide-spaced nipples, coarctation of aorta; normal IQ range
Triple-X syndrome	47, XXX	female, no distinctive somatic features, some with mental retardation, occasional behavioural disturbances, mostly fertile
Klinefelter's syndrome	47, XXY	male, eunuchoid habitus, testicular atrophy, sterile, gynaecomastia, feminine distribution of hair, some with mental retardation
Double-Y syndrome	47, XYY	male, usually tall (> 180 cm) and fertile. Some with mental retardation. Some have antisocial behaviour leading to incarceration; hence a higher incidence in tall prisoners
Mosaics	46, XX/45, XO 46, XY/45, XO 46, XX/46, XY	low grade mosaicism; may not affect the phenotype. If mosaicism affects a higher proportion of cells, intersex states or hermaphroditism may be present. A high proportion of 45, XO cells usually gives features of Turner's syndrome
Autosomal abnormalities		
Down's syndrome	47, + 21	mental retardation, brachycephaly with flattened occiput, epicanthic folds, short metacarpals and phalanges, simian crease, hypotonia, male genitalia infantile
Edwards' syndrome	47, + 18	mental retardation, hypertonicity, failure to thrive, micrognathia, low-set malformed ears, clenched hands, short sternum, rocker-bottom feet, congenital heart disease (CHD)
Patau's syndrome	47, + 13	severe mental retardation, deafness, holoprosencephaly, microphthalmia, coloboma, cleft lip/palate, polydactyly, abnormal male genitalia, haemangiomata, scalp defects, narrow hyperconvex finger-nails, CHD
Cat eye syndrome	47, + 22	mental and growth retardation, microcephaly, micrognathia, pre-auricular skin tags, low-set malformed ears, cleft palate, males with small penis and undescended testes, CHD
Mosaic trisomy-8	46/47, + 8	mental retardation, craniofacial dysmorphia, prominent and bulging forehead, hypertelorism, micrognathia, high-arched palate, hypertonia, camptodactyly, bone dysplasia
Cri-du-chat syndrome	45, 5p −	low birth weight, slow growth, cat-like cry, mental retardation, hypotonia, microcephaly, hypertelorism, epicanthic folds, simian crease

References for less common chromosomal abnormalities: Smith (1977), Yunis (1977), and Therman (1980)
The author acknowledges the help of Dr S. Walker in constructing this Table

viruses invites the hypothesis that chromosome damage is the mechanism. However, most viral-induced chromosomal damage is repaired.

4. The rare Mendelian autosomal recessive disorders of ataxia telangectasia, Fanconi anaemia, Bloom syndrome, and xeroderma pigmentosum (XP) shows a predisposition to malignancy (see page 4.48). The first two have a high frequency of spontaneous chromosome abnormalities and a DNA repair defect. There is a defect of DNA replication in Bloom syndrome and spontaneous chromosome breakage. XP has a DNA repair defect and, whilst the cells in this condition do not show spontaneous chromosome breaks, they are susceptible to do so after exposure to ultraviolet light. The patients with the first three conditions show various internal malignancy whereas XP shows skin malignancies only. Hence the suggestion that the induced chromosomal abnormalities are important in generating potentially malignant clones.

Specific chromosomal abnormalities in particular neoplasms. The Ph^1 chromosome (mentioned above) is the typical marker chromosome found in the majority of patients with chronic granulocytic (myeloid) leukaemia (and occasionally in other forms of leukaemia) and results from a reciprocal translocation of the long arm of 22, with, in the majority of cases, the long arm of 9, so the Ph^1 is a small fragment of 22 with possibly a tiny piece of 9. It can be found both in the marrow cells and in peripheral blood cultures in the acute phases, but during the haematological remissions, either natural or following chemotherapy or radiotherapy, the Ph^1 cell line disappears from the blood though it persists in the marrow. It has been detected only in the immature granulocytes, erythroblasts, and megakaryocytes suggesting a possible common stem cell origin for these since other tissues do not show the abnormality.

In children under 15 years of age, chronic myeloid leukaemia appears in two forms, a juvenile and an 'adult' type, and the presence or absence of the Ph^1 chromosome provides the most certain method of distinguishing them though they also differ in their haematological and clinical features. The juvenile form is Ph^1 negative, with thrombocytopenia usually present and the total white cell count not as high (rarely over 100×10^9/l) as in the 'adult' form which is Ph^1 positive. Another striking difference is the increased level of Hb-F (from 15 to 55 per cent) in the juvenile form whereas this is not the case of Ph^1 positive cases even when the disease occurs in infancy. The juvenile type has a poorer response to chemotherapy than the adult form and the mean survival time after diagnosis is much reduced (see also Section 19).

Other neoplasms also possess characteristic chromosomal abnormalities which are repeatedly found in different patients with the same clinical and histological diagnosis.

In Burkitt's lymphoma a band from 8 q is reciprocally translocated to the distal end of 14 q (14 q +). Human meningiomas lose chromosome 22(−22).

In many cases of retinoblastoma band 13 q 14 is absent (13 q −)

Specific chromosomal abnormalities have also been described in mixed salivary gland tumour and cancers of the breast and ovary.

It is clear that the future holds interesting possibilities for the study of chromosomes in neoplastic conditions, for example to elucidate causative mechanisms, as a method of classification and as 'markers' to assist in assessments of therapy. (For review of this topic see Harden and Taylor 1979, and Therman 1980.)

References

Bass, H. N. and Sparkes, R. S. (1979). Two balanced translocations in three generations of a pedigree: t (7; 10), (q 11; q 22) and t (14;21) (14 q ter→cen→21 q ter). *J. med. Genet.* **16(3)**, 215.

Batchelor, J. R., Welsh, K. I., Tinoco, R. M., Dollery, C. T., Hughes, C. R. V., Bernstein, R., Ryan, P., Naish, P. F., Aber, G. M., Bing, R. F., and Russell, G. I. (1980). Hydralazine-induced systemic lupus erythematosus: influence of HLA-DR and sex on susceptibility. *Lancet* i, 1107.

Bonaiti-Pellie, C. and Smith, C. (1974). Risk tables for genetic counselling in some common congenital malformations. *J. med. Genet.* **11**, 374.

Bundey, S. (1975). Genetic counselling. *Br. J. hosp. Med.* **13**, 466–3.

Carr, D. H. (1971). Chromosomes and abortions. In *Advances in human genetics* (eds. H. Harris and K. Hirschhorn), vol. 2, 201. Plenum Press, New York.

Carter, C. O. (1965). The inheritance of common congenital malformations. In *Progress in medical genetics* (eds. A. G. Steinberg and A. G. Bearn), vol. 4, 59. Grune and Stratton, New York.

— (1975). Personal communication.

Clarke, C. A. (1964). *Genetics for the clinician*, 2nd edn. Blackwell Scientific Publications, Oxford.

— and Sheppard, P. M. (1966). A local survey of the distribution of industrial melanic forms in the moth *Biston betularia* and estimates of the selective values of these in an industrial environment. *Proc. R. Soc. B.* **165**, 424.

Emery, A. E. H. (1974). Genetic counselling—or what can we tell parents? *Practitioner* **231**, 641.

— (1979). *Elements of medical genetics*, 5th edn. Churchill Livingstone, Edinburgh.

Evans, D. A. P., Mahgoub, A., Sloan, T. P., Idle, J. R., and Smith, R. L. (1980). A family and population study of the genetic polymorphism of debrisoquine oxidation in a white British population. *J. med. Genet.* **17**, 102.

Falconer, D. S. (1960). *An introduction to quantitive genetics* (reprinted with amendments 1964). Oliver and Boyd, Edinburgh.

Ford, E. B. (1940). Polymorphism and taxonomy, p. 493. In *The New Systematics* (ed. J. Huxley). Clarendon Press, Oxford (quoted in E. B. Ford 1965).

Goulian, M., Kornberger, A., and Sinsheimer, R. L. (1967). Enzymatic synthesis of DNA, XXIV Synthesis of infectious phage phi- X174 DNA. *Proc. nat. Acad. Sci.* **58**, 2321.

Harnden, D. G. (1965). In *Chromosomes in medicine* (ed. J. L. Hammerton). Heinemann, London.

— and Taylor, A. M. R. (1979). Chromosomes and neoplasia. In *Advances in human genetics* (eds. H. Harris and K. Hirschhorn), vol 9, p. 1. Plenum Press, New York.

Johannsen, W. (1909) *Elemente der exackten erblichkeitslehre*. Fisher, Jena. (quoted by Rieger *et al.* 1968).

King, R. C. (1974) *A Dictionary of genetics*, 2nd edn. New York.

Lyon, M. F. (1961). Gene action in the X chromosome of the mouse (*Mus musculus* L), *Nature, Lond.* **190**, 372.

London Conference (1963). The normal human karyotype. *Ann. hum. Genet.* **27**, 295.

McKusick, V. A. (1979). *Mendelian inheritance in man*, 5th edn. Johns Hopkins University Press, Baltimore.

— (1962). In *Principles of internal medicine* (ed. T. R. Harrison). McGraw-Hill, New York.

Moulds, R. F. W., and Denborough, M. (1974). Identification of susceptibility to malignant hyperpyrexia. *Br. med. J.* ii, 245.

Paris Conference (1971). Standardization in human cytogenetics, *Birth defects: original article series* (1972) **8**, no. 7. National Foundation, New York.

Penrose, L. S. and Smith, G. F. (1966). *Down's anomaly*, Churchill, London.

Renwick, J. H. (1963). Male and female recombination functions in man. *Genetics today*. Proceedings of the eleventh International Congress of Genetics, vol. 1, Abstract 15.30. The Hague, Netherlands.

Rieger, R., Michaelis, A., and Green, M. M. (1968). *A glossary of genetics and cytogenetics*, 3rd edn. Allen and Unwin, London.

Roberts, J. A. Fraser and Pembrey, M. (1978). *An introduction to medical genetics*, 7th edn. Oxford University Press.

Smith, D. W. (1977). *Recognizable patterns of human malformation*, 2nd edn. W. B. Saunders, Philadelphia.

Therman, E. (1980). *Human chromosomes*. Springer-Verlag, New York.

Veys, E. M., Mielants, H., and Verbruggen, G. (1978). Levamisole-induced adverse reactions in HLA-B27 positive rheumatoid arthritis. *Lancet* i, 148.

Watson, J. D. and Crick, F. H. C. (1953). The structure of DNA. *Cold Spr. Harb. Symp. quant. Biol.* **18**, 123.

World Health Organization (1973). Pharmacogenetics. Report of a WHO Scientific Group, *Wld Hlth Org. techn. Rep. Ser.* no. 524.

Wooley, P. H., Griffin, J., Panayi, G. S., Batchelor, J. R., Welsh, K. I., and Gibson, T. J. (1980). HLA-DR antigens and toxicity to sodium auro thiomalate and D-penicillamine in rheumatoid arthritis. *New Engl. J. Med.* **303**, 300.

Yunis, J. J. (Ed.) (1977). *New chromosomal syndromes*. Academic Press, New York.

Molecular genetics in clinical medicine

D. J. Weatherall

As pointed out by Francis Crick, the term molecular biology is unsatisfactory because it has two meanings. In the broad sense, it encompasses an explanation for any biological phenomenon in terms of atoms and molecules. However, as currently used it describes the study of interactions of proteins and nucleic acids, especially gene structure, replication, and expression including protein synthesis and structure. Crick claims that he was forced to call himself a molecular biologist because it was more convenient to do so when asked what he did by enquiring clergymen, rather than to explain that it is a mixture of crystallographer, biophysicist, biochemist, and geneticist!

During the last few years there have been some remarkable developments in molecular biology. In particular, it has become possible to analyse the fine structure of mammalian genes and to start to gain some insight into the way that they are regulated. Although these extraordinary achievements have yet to make a major impact on clinical practice, the signs are that this will not be the case for long. Indeed, in the last two years the newer techniques for molecular genetics have started to find medical applications in areas ranging from the pharmaceutical industry to the antenatal diagnosis of genetic disorders.

In this short section the techniques which are available for analysing human genes, what is known about their structure and regulation, some of the molecular mechanisms which underlie genetic diseases, and some potential practical applications of this new information will be described. It is only possible to give the briefest outline of the topic here and the reader is advised to consult the more extensive reviews which are cited at the end of this section for a more detailed discussion of each of these subjects.

Methods for analysing the fine structure of the human genome

Until recently the only approach to the analysis of the molecular basis of genetic disorders was to attempt to isolate and purify gene products, i.e. enzymes or proteins, and to try to determine whether the condition resulted from a structural change or from a reduced rate of production of the protein. From information gained in this way it was only possible to speculate about what might be happening at the DNA level. However, during the last few years the application of the new approaches of gene mapping and recombinant DNA technology has revolutionized the study of human molecular genetics, and it is now possible to analyse human genes and their messenger RNAs in great detail and to define precisely the causes of at least some genetic disorders at the molecular level.

Molecular hybridization. The general structure of DNA was described in the previous section. In the early 1960s it was shown that two strands of native DNA can be dissociated and reassociated *in vitro* by heating and subsequent cooling. In addition, it was found that hybrid DNA molecules could be made from the DNAs of different viruses or bacteria and, furthermore, that it was possible to form double-stranded DNA/RNA molecules using this approach. These annealing reactions are highly specific and, under suitable conditions, only occur between DNA or RNA strands which have identical or almost identical base sequences.

In 1970, an enzyme was isolated from certain RNA tumour viruses which is capable of synthesizing a DNA molecule from an RNA template. This enzyme, RNA-dependent DNA polymerase, or reverse transcriptase, can be used to synthesize a DNA copy (cDNA or complementary DNA) from any messenger RNA

(mRNA) that can be isolated from mammalian cells. Furthermore, if radioactive bases are added to the reaction the synthesized DNA can be made radioactive and hence used as a hybridization probe to look for complementary sequences in either genomic DNA or in cellular RNA. A schematic representation of the synthesis of cDNA using reverse transcriptase is shown in Fig. 1.

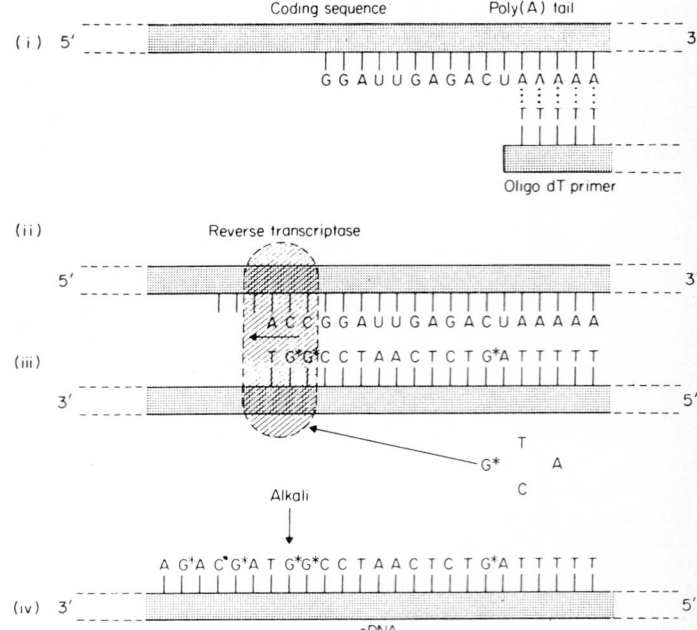

Fig. 1 The synthesis of cDNA using reverse transcriptase. A complementary DNA copy is synthesized on an mRNA template (i) primed with oligo (dT) (ii) which binds to the poly-A tail of the mRNA, using reverse transcriptase and labelled* deoxyribonucleotides, (iii). The double stranded mRNA/dDNA hybrid is then treated with alkali, which destroys the mRNA leaving the cDNA (iv). (From Weatherall and Clegg, 1981)

Under the right conditions cDNAs hybridize in a highly specific manner to appropriate DNAs or RNAs. Hence it is possible not only to test for the presence of complementary RNA or DNA sequences, but actually to quantify them. An example of this type of experiment is illustrated in Fig. 2 which shows the steps in determining the ratios of human α and β globin mRNAs in cellular RNA. A similar approach can be used to quantify the number of genes for a particular protein in the total genome. All that is needed is a source of DNA and a purified mRNA to act as a template for producing radioactive cDNA.

The development of these techniques was of great value in human genetics. They enabled questions to be asked about the relative amounts of mRNAs for differnt protein subunits that might be present in reduced quantities in inherited diseases. Thus it was possible to determine whether a defect in protein synthesis is due to a reduced rate of production of normal mRNA or to the synthesis of normal amounts of a defective mRNA. Even more important, one was now able to ask whether a genetic disorder in which no gene product is produced is due to the absence of a particular structural gene or to a more subtle abnormality later in the complicated pathway of protein synthesis. It was the application of the techniques of cDNA/DNA hybridization which led, in 1974, to the first

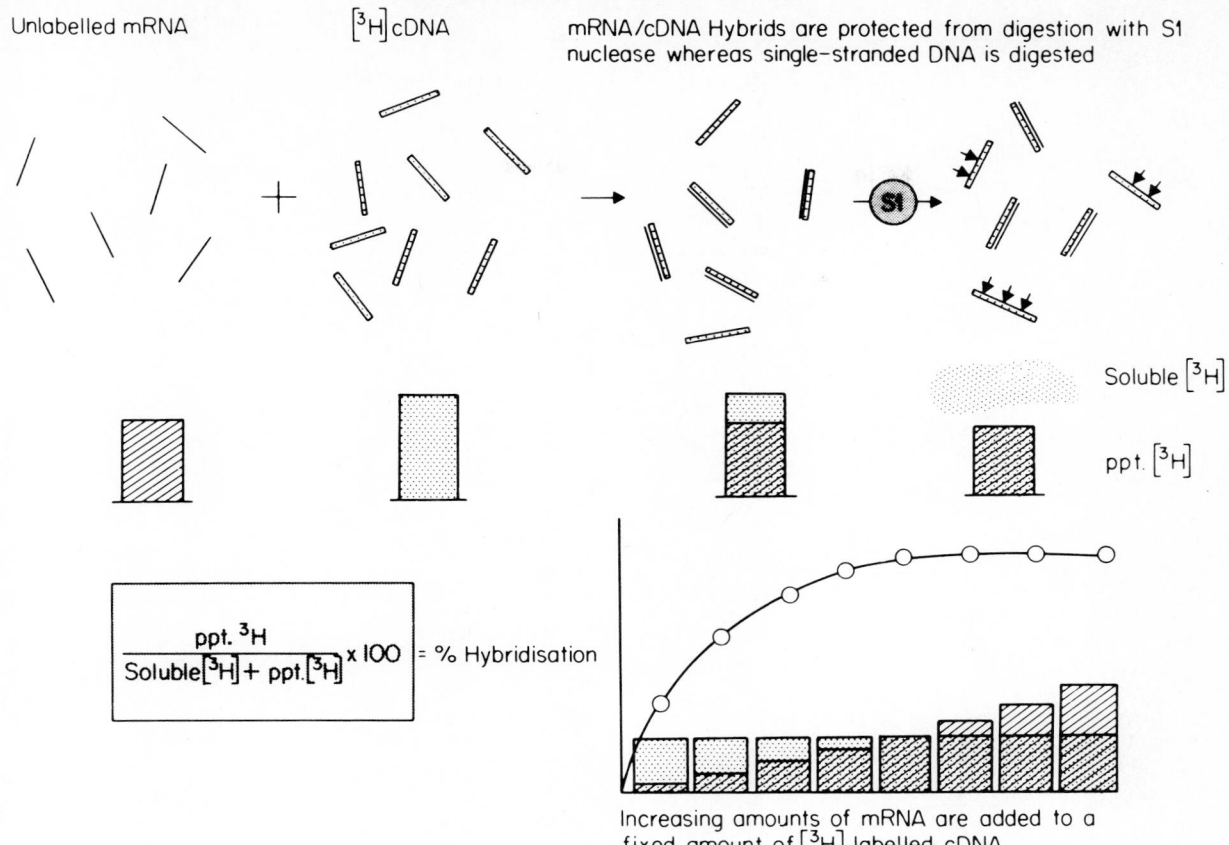

Fig. 2 cDNA/RNA hybridization to measure the relative amounts of cytoplasmic mRNA. Labelled cDNA is mixed with total cellular RNA containing the mRNA to be quantified. After hybridization the reaction mixture is treated with a nuclease which degrades single stranded nucleic acid. Hence, any unhybridized cDNA is digested and the remaining hybrids can be precipitated and counted. By carrying out a number of reactions with an increasing amount of RNA hybridized to a fixed amount of cDNA, the concentration of the unknown mRNA can be calculated from the kinetics of the hybridization curve. (From Weatherall and Clegg, 1981)

demonstration of a gene deletion in man, i.e. the molecular basis for one form of thalassaemia (see Section 19).

However, these techniques only allowed an approximate estimation of the amount of mRNA or the number of genes. They told us nothing about the structure of the DNA and how it might be altered in genetic disease. To answer this type of question new techniques were needed.

Gene mapping. The techniques described above rely on hybridization reactions that take place in solution. Experiments of this type give quantitiative information about the relative number of gene sequences present in DNA, or about relative levels of cytoplasmic mRNA, but provide no information about the physical arrangements of the genes on the chromosome. Over the last few years it has become possible to approach this problem, largely because of the development of methods for fractionating DNA. The major advance in this field came from the discovery of a family of bacterial enzymes called restriction endonucleases. These enzymes cleave DNA in a small number of reproducible sites, typically of the order of one cleavage per few thousand base pairs. After treatment of the DNA with a particular enzyme the mixture of fragments is subjected to electrophoresis on agarose gel. After separation of the DNA fragments according to their size, the DNA in the gel is denatured by alkali treatment and the separated fragments are then transferred to a nitrocellulose filter by a process called Southern blotting. The filter is then exposed to a radioactively labelled cDNA probe under conditions which favour the reformation of hybrid molecules. The position of the gene-containing fragment(s) is then determined by radioautography. By using a series of different enzymes which cleave the DNA either within or outside the gene or

genes under study, and by orientating some of the fragments defined in this way, it is possible to build up what are called restriction enzyme maps of appropriate areas of the genome.

The technique of restriction enzyme mapping is extremely powerful and requires relatively little DNA. For example, maps of the human globin genes can be obtained from the DNA contained in the white cells of approximately 5 ml of peripheral blood, and gene mapping can also be carried out on DNA obtained from 10 to 20 ml of amniotic fluid.

Recombinant DNA technology. In the last few years the advent of recombinant DNA technology has made things even simpler, since it is now possible to clone (i.e. selectively purify and amplify) a chosen DNA or cDNA sequence. This approach is shown in Fig. 3. The principle is to insert foreign DNA into a bacterial plasmid or phage. Plasmids are extremely simple organisms which live and replicate in the cytoplasm of bacteria. They are probably best known for their ability to transfer antibiotic resistance between bacterial species. They consist essentially of a circular ring of DNA. In recombinant DNA technology plasmids are cleaved by a specific restriction endonuclease to produce a linear structure. The DNA to be inserted is fragmented by the same endonuclease and the plasmid and DNA fragments are mixed and joined by a ligase. Some plasmids rejoin to form the original circular DNA, but others, recombinants, incorporate the foreign DNA. Suitable bacteria are then transformed by the reformed plasmids, i.e. plasmids and bacteria are mixed and a small proportion of the former enter the bacterial cytoplasm. The frequency of transformation is low enough so that on average each bacteria contains only one plasmid. Those containing recombinants can be selected by various

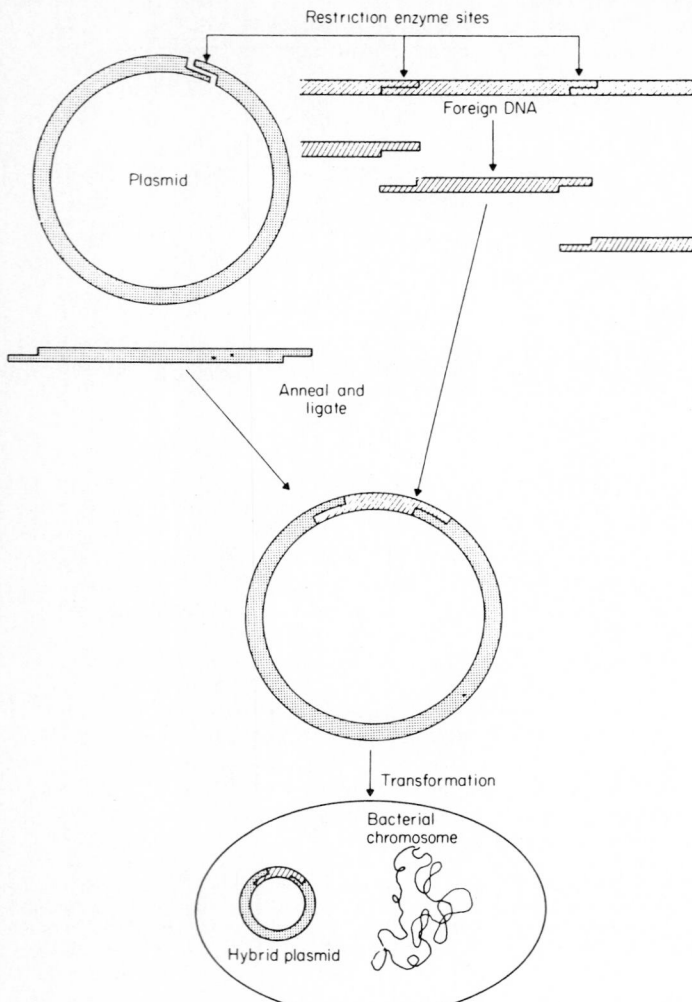

Fig. 3   The construction of a bacterial plasmid containing a foreign DNA insert (for details see text). (From Weatherall and Clegg, 1981)

microbiological tricks such as allowing the plasmid to confer anti-biotic resistance to the growth of the bacteria in selective media. Bacterial colonies can be screened by hybridization for the presence of various foreign DNA inserts, and when a positive clone is obtained it can be grown in large quantities to produce the particular DNA which is required.

Recombinant DNA technology has become extraordinarily sophisticated, and now whole libraries of cloned DNA fragments representing the entire human genome are available for study. Thus, it is possible to isolate individual genes for sequencing or to make probes for gene mapping. Furthermore, this technology has many wider applications which will be considered at the end of this chapter.

The genetic control of protein structure and synthesis

The organization of the genetic control of protein synthesis is summarized in Fig. 4. The amino acid sequence of any particular protein is determined by the order of bases of the DNA which forms its structural gene. The cytoplasmic determinant for protein synthesis is a form of RNA called messenger RNA (mRNA) which carries the genetic information derived from the DNA of the gene from the cell nucleus to the cytoplasm where it acts as a template for protein synthesis. The latter takes place on polysomes, groups of ribosomes which have become attached to mRNA and carry the growing peptide chains. Amino acids do not bind directly to mRNA, but first become covalently attached by their carboxyl

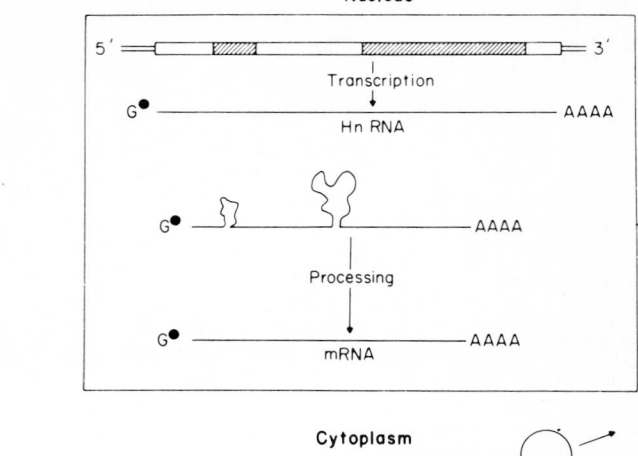

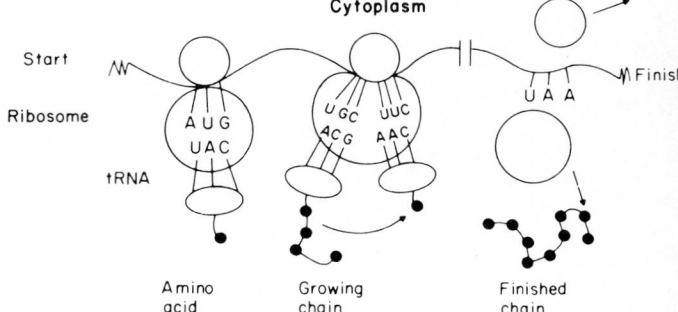

Fig. 4   The general organization of the genetic control of protein synthesis. (From Weatherall and Clegg, 1981)

groups to another type of RNA, transfer RNA (tRNA). Each tRNA molecule is specific for both a particular amino acid and for a group of three mRNA nucleotides (i.e. a codon). Suitably modified tRNA molecules bind to the appropriate codons of the mRNA by hydrogen bonding with their anti-codons, groups of three nucleotides with complementary sequences to the mRNA codon.

Ribosomes act as pulleys which move along the mRNA as it is translated, and hold growing peptide chains in position. They have two binding sites for tRNA, the peptide site which binds the pep-tide-tRNA complex, and the amino site which binds the next incoming tRNA molecule. Protein synthesis results from the movement of ribosomes along the mRNA strand, so exposing successive codons to tRNA anticodons. As the ribosome moves from one codon to the next, the tRNA in the amino site moves to the peptide site, and the peptide chain is transferred to it from the tRNA previously in the peptide site, thus being lengthened by one amino acid residue.

Hence, in examining the genetic control of protein synthesis we have to consider the organization of DNA, the way in which mRNA is transcribed from DNA and is processed and transported into the cell cytoplasm, and the mechanisms whereby peptide chains are synthesized on the mRNA template and combine to form definitive proteins. Clearly, a genetic disorder of protein synthesis could result from a defect at any of these stages.

The organization of DNA.   The general organization of the structure of DNA was described in the previous section. The monomers, the letters of the DNA code, consist of four different nucleotides each attached to a 2-deoxyribose sugar and held together in a polymeric structure by phosphodiester bonds between the dexoyribose moieties. In the Watson–Crick model of DNA the double-stranded molecule consists of chains of nucleotides held together by hydrogen bonds between the purine and pyrimidine bases. The pairing between purine and pyrimidine nucleotides on opposite strands is highly specific and dependent on the hydrogen bonding of adenosine (A) with thymidine (T), and guanosine (G) with cytidine (C)

(Fig. 13, page 4.18). The genetic information which determines the sequence of amino acids in any particular protein resides in the order of nucleotides on one strand of DNA called the sense strand; the opposite or antisense strand is complementary to the sense strand.

It seems likely that the majority of proteins or enzymes which are of particular interest in medical genetics are coded for by only one or two copies of DNA in a total genome which contains enough DNA to code for, perhaps, several million proteins. These genes are called unique sequences and account for approximately 60 per cent of the total DNA. Ten per cent of the DNA exists as highly repetitive, non-transcribed sequences repeated many thousands of times. Finally, about 30 per cent of the DNA is present as moderately repetitive sequences which are repeated several hundred times. These sequences are spaced throughout the genome, alternating with unique sequences, and may have some regulatory function.

The genes in mammalian cells are present, not as simple strands of DNA, but complexed with histones and other proteins in chromatin. This means that the transcriptional activity of the total DNA can be quite limited, so that in erythroid cells, for example, only a few per cent of the total DNA sequences are transcribed. Some of this selectivity is achieved by gross alterations in chromatin structure. Chromatin is composed of repeating subunits called nucleosomes which consist of eight histone molecules, two each of a specific type associated with about 200 base pairs of DNA. It is currently believed that one of the major factors which regulate gene activity is chromatin structure. It seems probable that superimposed on this is a hierarchy of more subtle regulators, probably involving the interaction of accessible DNA regions with non-histone proteins, and possibly with RNA.

Until recently it was thought that the structural genes consist simply of lengths of DNA which contain sufficient nucleotide triplets to code for the appropriate number of amino acids in the polypeptide chains of a particular protein. One of the great surprises arising from recent work in molecular biology has been that this notion is a gross oversimplification. In fact, nearly all the mammaliam genes that have been analysed to date have coding sequences which are interrupted by so-called intervening sequences (introns) at various positions along their length. For example, the human globin genes each contain two such 'inserts' of approximately 120 and 900 nucleotide base pairs. Thus mammalian structural genes contain alternating regions of non-coding introns and coding sequences or exons. As well as having specific triplets for regulating initiation and termination of protein synthesis at their left-hand (5′) and right-hand (3′) ends, they also contain sequences of varying length at both ends which code for non-translated regions of mRNA. Furthermore, it appears that many mammalian genes have coding sequences in their 5′ flanking regions which are very similar to those found in micro-organisms or Drosophilia. The first of these is AT rich, a sequence originally found in the histone gene cluster of Drosophilia and called the Hogness box. The second region is called the CCAAT box and is found about 70 base pairs upstream (5′) from the various structural genes. These regions may be involved in transcription initiation or RNA processing, or both.

A typical mammalian gene is illustrated in Fig. 5. It consists of various regulatory regions, an area coding for the 5′ non-translated portion of messenger RNA, an initiation codon, a coding region interspersed with various introns, a terminating codon, and an area which codes for the 3′ non-translated part of the messenger RNA.

Transcription. The initial step leading to protein synthesis is the production of an RNA transcript of the DNA coding sequence. This requires the action of a family of enzymes called RNA polymerases. Three types of RNA polymerase have been identified in mammalian cells, two of which are involved in the transcription of the genes for various cytoplasmic RNAs such as ribosomal RNA, and one which transcribes the unique sequence of DNAs for

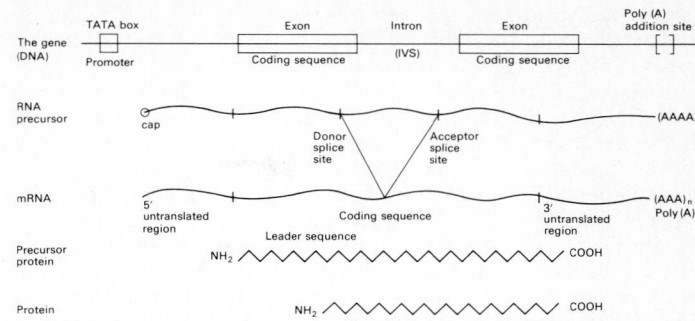

Fig. 5   A schematic model of a typical mammalian gene showing the processing of the large mRNA precursor and the various steps which take place down to the production of a definitive protein. (By permission of the Editor of *Science*)

specific proteins. All these enzymes are complex multimeric molecules which require co-factors for their correct functioning. While the latter have been isolated and characterized from bacterial cells, very little is known about their mammalian equivalents. Nevertheless, it seems very likely that mammalian RNA synthesis follows essentially the same pattern as that seen in micro-organisms.

Processing of the primary transcript. As mentioned above, genes coding for mammalian peptide chains are interrupted by a number of non-coding sequences or introns. The first step in the production of mRNA is the transcription of the entire unit, coding and non-coding sequences included, in the form of a large RNA precursor molecule which may be two to three times the length of the definitive mRNA molecule which finally moves into the cell cytoplasm. This huge precursor molecule is called heterogeneous nuclear RNA (HnRNA). It is first chemically modified at its 5′ end by establishing a complex structure containing methylated nucleotides (CAP) and by having a string of adenylic acid residues (poly-A) attached to the other (3′) end. The non-coding introns are then removed by a successive series of excision and ligation reactions to form the mature mRNA. It seems likely that during their time in the nucleus, and for much of their time in the cytoplasm, HnRNA and mRNA are associated with various protein molecules which may serve to stabilize and protect them from nuclease attack.

Messenger RNA. Most of what is known about the structure of human mRNAs has been derived from the study of the globin mRNAs. They all contain the modified 5′ end CAP structure and the 3′ poly-A tail (Fig. 5). In addition, there are non-coding sequences at the 5′ and 3′ ends. Thus there are a variable number of nucleotides after the CAP structure before the AUG initiation codon and between the UAA termination codon and the poly-A tail (Fig. 5). It seems likely that the CAP structure is involved in the initiation of mRNA translation, but the function of the non-coding sequences at the ends of the mRNA is not yet understood; these regions may play a role in determining the stability of the mRNAs in the cell cytoplasm. Certainly, there are highly conserved sequences in the 5′ non-coding region suggesting some important function.

Peptide chain synthesis. Peptide chain synthesis results from a complex series of interactions between tRNA, ribosomes, and mRNA. The initial step involves the formation of a complex between an initiation factor and an initiation transfer RNA which binds to one of the ribosomal subunits. With the help of other initiation factors, mRNA and the large ribosomal subunits are added to this complex so that in its final configuration the mRNA is aligned with the ribosomes with the AUG initiation codon opposite the UAC anticodon of the initiation transfer RNA. Protein synthesis then proceeds by stepwise addition of amino acids from the N-terminal end to form the growing peptide chain. This cycle involves at least three distinct stages. The first is a codon-directed binding of transfer RNA to the ribosome site next to that occupied by the initiator transfer RNA. With two amino acids now in place a peptide bond is formed and the tRNA containing the dipeptide and the mRNA are both shifted from the acceptor to the donor site on the ribosome. In this way the acceptor site is freed and the process can be repeated over and over again with the formation of a growing peptide chain. In fact, most mRNAs are long enough to support a number of ribosomes active in synthesis along their length. Once a ribosome has moved away from the initiation site another ribosome can bind and start the whole process all over again, so forming a polyribosome complex. Finally, peptide chain synthesis stops when the ribosome reaches a chain termination codon (UAA, UAG, or UGA) in the mRNA. At this point the peptide chain is split from the tRNA to be released into the cell cytoplasm, where it combines with similar chains to produce either a definitive protein or subunits of a protein which combine in turn with their fellows to form a complete molecule.

A variety of different mechanisms are involved in the later stages of protein synthesis. For example, haemoglobin consists of two different pairs of peptide chains called α and β chains. These are synthesized independently and combine with haem after release from the ribosomes to form $\alpha\beta$ subunits which then combine with each other to form the definitive haemoglobin molecules. Some proteins are synthesized in the form of large precursor molecules. For example, insulin is synthesized as a single chain precursor called proinsulin. However, the immediate translation product of proinsulin mRNA is a larger peptide containing 23 additional amino acid residues at the N-terminal end. This molecule, which is called preproinsulin, is rapidly cleaved to proinsulin by proteases. Interestingly, the peptide extension in preproinsulin is similar in size and amino acid composition to the additional sequences found in *in vitro* translational products of mRNA for a variety of hormones such as proparathyroid and growth hormone as well as non-hormonal proteins such as immunoglobulin light chains. Preproinsulin is cleaved to proinsulin in the rough endoplasmic reticulin, and proinsulin is then transferred to the Golgi apparatus and to the secretory granules where it is cleaved into equimolar amounts of insulin and C-peptide.

Even more complex post-synthetic processing must occur during the synthesis of some of the other peptide hormones. For example, recent evidence suggests that both ACTH, β-lipoprotein, and β-endorphin are synthesized in the pituitary as segments of a single large prohormone (pro-ACTH).

Regulation. As we have seen in the preceeding sections, the processes of gene transcription and the translation of genetic information from DNA into protein are now understood in some detail. What is not known, however, is how this complex mechanism is regulated. This is a question of fundamental importance in human genetics. How does a fertilized egg with 10^9 nucleotide pairs of DNA make a human being? How is it that although every cell in the body contains the genetic information to make every protein, only a limited number of genes are transcribed in any particular tissue or organ? How are genes or batteries of genes turned on and off at different stages during development? How are genes which determine the structure of the different subunits which make up a single protein regulated so that neither subunit is produced in excess? How are the genes turned on and off during the lifespan of a cell and co-ordinated with the activity of other genes for enzymes with similar metabolic functions?

It is becoming apparent that most regulation must take place in the nucleus of the cell by determining the relative amounts of various mRNAs which find their way into the cytoplasm. Unfortunately, virtually nothing is known about how this is achieved despite endless speculation about the regulation of transcription and mRNA processing and transport. Numerous models have been derived, based on mechanisms pirated from microbial genetics, and applied to both normal and abnormal gene regulation in human

beings. However, so far there is no evidence that any human disease results from a regulatory gene mutation.

A little more information is available about cytoplasmic protein synthesis and its regulation. It appears that chain initiation is the rate-limiting step in some forms of protein synthesis and that some fine tuning of the amounts of peptide chains which are synthesized occurs at the translational level. There is evidence that small molecules such as haem, for example, may play a role in regulating peptide chain synthesis, probably by their action on chain initiation, although the overall importance of these cytoplasmic mechanisms in the regulation of protein synthesis is probably small as compared with translational control of mRNA levels.

Some clue as to how external agents such as hormones might be involved in the regulation of gene expression has come from an analysis of the mechanism of action of certain steroid hormones. The latter have specific receptor proteins which are found in the cell cytoplasm rather than on the cell surface as is the case for polypeptide hormones. The steroid hormones traverse the plasma membrane and are bound with great affinity to the receptors. This interaction appears to alter the receptor in some way (possibly by changing its allosteric form) so that it can now enter the cell nucleus and interact with chromatin of appropriate genes. By a mechanism which is still not worked out, the active steroid receptor complex induces gene transcription and new mRNA formation, and hence the synthesis of specific peptides and proteins. Some of these are enzymes, whilst others are receptors for other hormones, e.g. oestrogen induces the synthesis of progesterone receptors. Yet other products may be involved with the regulation of cell replication.

Complex genetic systems. The previous sections have attempted to summarize what is known about the structure and regulation of the genes which code for single proteins or parts of a protein. Clearly, there must be much more complex genetic systems involved in the regulation of such processes as human development or antibody production. Although virtually nothing is known about human developmental genetics, some remarkable information has come to light recently regarding the genetic regulation of the immune system. It seems likely that this is going to have major implications in clinical medicine over the next few years.

How might something as complex and diverse as the immune system be genetically regulated? This fascinating question has led to intense speculation over the years. For example, one theory suggested that the entire antibody population is encoded in a vast array of germ-line genes. However, many workers guessed that this is much too complicated and favoured the notion that there might be somatic generation of variation on the basis of a limited number of germ-line genes. How this might be mediated was far from clear, however. In the last two years, following the advent of recombinant DNA technology, some quite extraordinary information has been obtained about the organization of the immunoglobulin genes and how they function (see also page 4.31).

During lymphocyte ontogeny single antigen binding sites are associated successively with various effector sites to produce first immunoglobulin M (IgM), then IgD, and later IgG, IgA, or IgE. Each of these different immunoglobulins are expressed first as a membrane-bound receptor molecule, and later, after terminal differentiation of the lymphocyte, as a secreted protein which is identical to the receptor except for a few residues at its CO terminal end. Both the immunoglobulin class and its membrane-bound or secreted status depend on the structure of the constant region of its heavy chains (Fig. 6). Each heavy chain has a variable (V_H) region which is associated with a constant (C_H) region coding for μ, δ, and γ, α or ε chains which correspond to IgM, IgD, IgG, IgA, and IgE. During development of the B cell there is a remarkable series of alterations in the position and structure of the genes which regulate the variable and constant regions of the immunoglobulin chains. Thus the class switch from IgM to IgG, IgA, or IgE is mediated by translocation of the variable region DNA with a deletion of the C_H

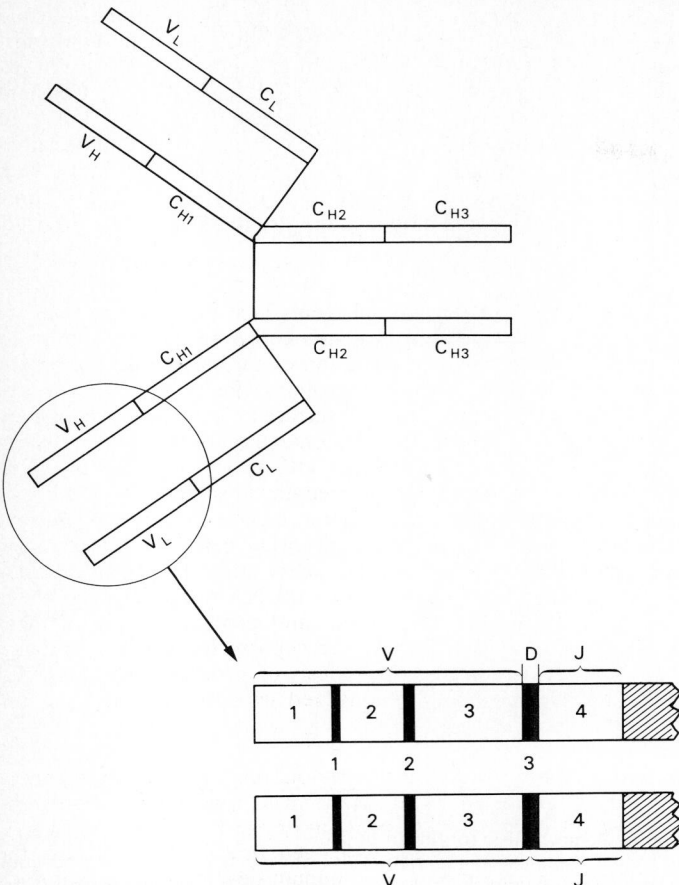

Fig. 6 A schematic representation of the genetic control of the immuno-globulin molecule. Each molecule consists of four chains; one pair of heavy chains and one pair of light chains. Each chain is divided functionally into two regions; the variable (V) region which mediates antigen recognition, and the constant (C) region which in the case of the heavy chain mediates the effector function of the molecule. The constant regions are further divided into a series of domains i.e. C_{H1}, C_{H2}, C_L, etc. The variable region is further subdivided into four zones which vary slightly from one antibody molecule to another and are known as the framework regions (numbered 1 to 4) and these are separated from each other by three hypervariable regions which are very much more variable and in the definitive protein form the actual antigen binding sites. Each light chain is coded by three separate genes; the C gene coding for the constant region, a J gene coding for the fourth framework region and part of the third hypervariable region, and a V gene coding for the first three framework regions. Each heavy chain is coded for by four separate genes: a C gene coding for the constant region, a J gene coding for the fourth framework region, a D gene coding for the third hypervariable region and a V gene coding for the first three framework regions including hypervariable regions 1 and 2 (modified from Robertson 1981).

region DNA upstream to the one that is expressed. The IgM to IgD switch is even more complicated and involves the excision of a series of introns together with complex splicing of the remaining DNA.

In addition to explaining some of the developmental changes in the immune system, recent work has gone some way to providing a molecular basis for the remarkable diversity of antibodies. First, there appear to be quite a large number of germ-line genes for the variable region subgroups. Secondly, during the translocation of the V_H region DNA during B cell lymphocyte maturation, the V genes for the light chains undergo translocation and join up with a cluster of genes called J genes which control part of the so-called hypervariable region of the light chain (Fig. 6). Since these joins are random, this process generates considerable diversity. This diversity is even greater in the case of the heavy chain genes in which the

V_H genes combine with a D gene which comprises a hypervariable region which in turn recombines with one of a cluster of J genes (Fig. 6). Recently, the whole of these areas of the genome have been sequenced and a highly complex and elegant scheme of rearrangements has been proposed which is believed to provide a basis for V–J and V–D–J joining in light and heavy chain variable region genes. Further variation occurs by the association of different light chains with the heavy chains, and possibly by changes of the rearranged immunoglobulin genes by somatic mutations in the course of B cell ontogeny.

Thus, from these remarkably complex and sophisticated series of gene rearrangements, excisions, translocations, and mutations it is possible to begin to envisage a system with the diversity and functional adaptability required of the immune system.

The molecular pathology of human disease

Because of the difficulties inherent to obtaining pure mRNA for many human proteins or enzymes, the techniques outlined in earlier sections have so far had relatively limited application to human gentic disease. This new technology has transformed the human haemoglobin field, however, and much of what we know about the molecular mechanisms for human genetic disease has been gleaned from the study of the inherited disorders of haemoglobin synthesis (see Section 19). However, from evidence which is accumulating from studies of other systems such as red cell enzymes and the insulin mutants, it seems unlikely that the molecular mechanisms which underlie other human diseases will be very different, and hence I shall describe a few of the molecular defects which have been defined for the haemoglobin disorders.

Single base mutations. Because of the degeneracy of the genetic code, i.e. the ability of several different nucleotide triplets to code for the same amino acid, only about four-fifths of the possible mutations in the structural genes will result in amino-acid changes. Furthermore, of those changes which can result in amino-acid substitutions, only about a third will be expected to lead to an alteration in the charge of the molecule so that the variant can be identified electrophoretically.

Over 300 structural haemoglobin variants have been defined during the last 25 years. The majority of these have single amino-acid substitutions which have been detected because they alter the electrophoretic mobility of haemoglobin. Undoubtedly there are many other amino-acid substitutions which do not alter the charge of the molecule and therefore have usually remained undetected. Indeed, it has been estimated that about 1 in 800 individuals carries an electrophoretic haemoglobin variant; perhaps one in 300 have variants of any sort. It is likely that other human proteins will show similar variability.

If the various amino-acid substitutions in human haemoglobin are examined within the framework of the genetic code as derived from micro-organisms, it is clear that, without exception, the variants are explicable on the basis of single base changes in the coding DNA of the structural genes. This remarkable observation provides good evidence that the genetic code is universal throughout the animal kingdom.

Whether or not an amino-acid substitution in a protein produces a clinical disorder will depend on whether the substitution occurs at a critical part of the molecule, the active site of an enzyme for example, or whether it changes the stability of the molecule leading to its premature destruction. Some substitutions have no effect on the function or stability of proteins and hence are completely harmless. Others, the substitution which produces the sickle cell haemoglobin and the other haemoglobinopathies for example, can result in profound functional abnormalities and hence lead to crippling diseases.

Examples of single amino-acid substitutions as a basis for other genetic diseases are starting to accumulate. For example, the common form of glucose 6-phosphate dehydrogenase deficiency in

Negroes (see Section 19) results from the production of an enzyme variant with a single amino-acid difference from its normal counterpart. Several human insulin variants have been described. One form of diabetes results from a single amino-acid substitution which prevents the normal cleavage of proinsulin to insulin. Considerable progress is being made in sorting out various structural variations of collagen in some of the inherited disorders of connective tissue. As judged by the various techniques of enzyme chemistry, many genetic disorders which are caused by defined enzyme deficiencies result from the production of structural enzyme variants, although, with the exception of the red cell enzymes, the precise structural changes remain to be determined.

Frameshift mutations Genetic lesions that result in the deletion or insertion of bases other than in groups of three produce variants in which the amino-acid sequence beyond the site of the mutation is completely changed owing to an alteration of the reading frame of the genetic code. Several examples of frameshift mutations have been discovered as the basis for abnormal human haemoglobins. As would be predicted, these haemoglobin variants have globin chains which are completely normal in their sequence up to a particular point, after which there is a complete change of sequence because of the 'frame shift' in reading the genetic code.

Deletions and insertions. It is possible to synthesize proteins which have lost or gained one or more amino acids along their sequence. It seems likely that these variants result from non-homologous crossing over at meiosis with loss or gain of groups of three DNA bases. Larger deletions involving part or all of a structural gene have been found to be the cause of some forms of thalassaemia or growth hormone deficiency.

Fusion genes. If there is chromosomal misalignment with mispaired synapsis, it is possible for linked genes to become fused with each other during crossing over with the production of abnormal fusion genes. An example of this derived from the abnormal haemoglobin field is shown in Fig. 7. Other examples of this mechanism have been demonstrated as the basis for the production of abnormal glycoproteins which form part of the red cell membrane.

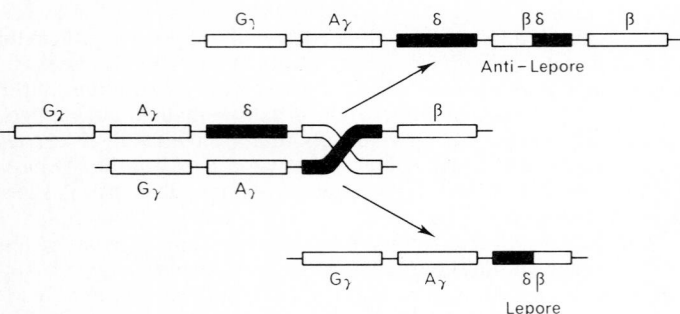

Fig. 7 Abnormal genetic crossing over between the δ and β globin genes for human haemoglobin. Normally the δ and β globin genes responsible for the direction of the synthesis of the δ and β globin chains of the adult haemoglobins lie linked together on chromosome 11. Because of mispaired synapsis of the two genes at meiosis, unequal crossing over has occured with the production of a δβ fusion gene on one chromosome (the Lepore gene) and its opposite number, a βδ fusion or anti-Lepore gene on the other. Unequal crossing over of this type is responsible for many different haemoglobin variants. Because the Lepore globin chains are synthesized inefficiently, this genetic event produces a form of thalaassaemia (see Section 19). Lepore was the family name of the first patient to be found with this disorder.

Chain termination mutants. Normal chain termination occurs when the ribosomes on the mRNA reach a chain termination codon, UAA, UAG, or UGA. A family of human haemoglobin variants have been found which result from a single base change in the chain termination codon which, instead of reading 'stop', allows the

insertion of an amino acid. Hence, translation continues beyond the normal chain termination point on what is usually non-translated mRNA until another termination codon is reached. For example, the human haemoglobin variant, haemoglobin Constant Spring, results from a change in the termination codon, UAA, to CAA which is the code word for glutamine. This variant has an α-chain with an elongated 'tail' of amino acids which starts with glutamine and goes on for 30 more residues (Fig. 8). For some reason these elongated globin chains are inefficiently synthesized.

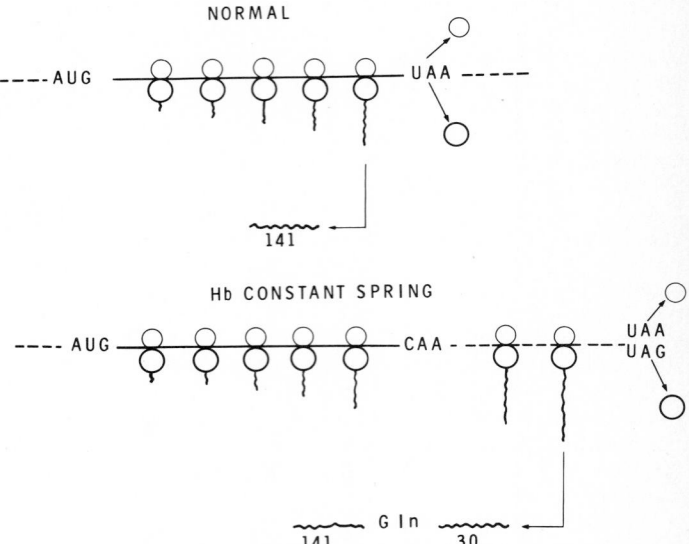

Fig. 8 A mechanism for the production of an elongated protein chain due to a chain termination mutation. This is the mechanism for the production of the human haemoglobin variant, haemoglobin Constant Spring. (Constant Spring is a suburb of Kingston, Jamica where the condition was first identified.) It results from a single base mutation in the chain termination codon for the α chain (UAA). The substitution of cytosine (C) for uracil (U) produces a codon CAA which is the code word for glutamine. Thus, instead of terminating, the ribosomes move along and glutamine is inserted into the growing peptide chain at the position where it would normally stop. Further elongation of the chain continues along messenger RNA (shown by the dotted line) which is not normally translated until another in-phase termination codon appears. Thus the globin chain is elongated by 30 amino acid residues.

Premature termination mutations. If a single base change in a codon which normally codes for an amino acid in a peptide chain produces a chain termination codon, then chain synthesis will cease at this site and a shortened polypeptide chain will be synthesized. For example, there is a form of β thalassaemia (see Section 19) in which there is a change in the AAG codon for lysine at the seventeenth position in the β-chain of haemoglobin to the chain termination codon UAG. This causes premature chain termination with the production of a short fragment of the β-chain which is rapidly destroyed. Hence no adult haemoglobin molecules can be synthesized.

Gene inversions. Although inversions of sections of the genome have been recognized in Drosophilia for many years, it is only in the last year that this type of molecular abnormality has been found as the basis for a human disease. One form of thalassaemia (see Section 19) results from an inversion of a large piece of DNA between two groups of globin genes. How can part of the human genome become orientated back to front? One tends to think of genes as existing in long strings of sausage-like structures set out in a linear fashion. Of course, nothing could be further from the truth. DNA and the chromosomes have a great deal of secondary and tertiary structure and are probably coiled in an extremely complex fashion. It seems likely that a major gene inversion has arisen by deletions and rearrangements occurring on a single chromosome strand.

Splice mutations. As mentioned earlier, the primary transcript is a long RNA molecule which has to be processed before a definitive mRNA molecule can be produced to act as a cytoplasmic template for protein synthesis. The various introns in the structural genes have to be removed and the exons spliced together. These splice reactions are highly specific, and in the last year it has become apparent that mutations at critical splicing sites may interfere with the processing of the large nuclear mRNA precursors. Several forms of thalassaemia seem to result from this type of mutation.

Summary of human molecular pathology. Although there is a long way to go, we are gaining some remarkable insights into abnormal gene action in human disease. It is interesting to reflect that until a few years ago it was only possible to define human genetic diseases that are due to structural protein variants, and those disorders which result from a decreased rate of synthesis or absence of a particular protein or protein subunit were thought to arise from mutations of putative 'operator' or 'regulator' genes, perhaps based on the hope that the evolutionary jump from *Escherichia coli* to man might not be reflected in any fundamental difference in the methods of gene regulation! With the advent of recombinant DNA technology and gene mapping, the whole picture has changed. It is now evident that many genetic diseases result from relatively straightforward molecular lesions and that much of the earlier speculation about regulatory gene mutations was incorrect.

We have seen how single base mutations, deletions and insertions, nonsense mutations, fusion genes, chain termination mutations, inversions, splice junction defects, and so on form the basis for some of the human haemoglobin disorders. As these mechanisms are worked out it is becoming apparent that all of them result from structural changes involving specific genetic determinants for the globin genes, and that all these molecular lesions act primarily in *cis*, i.e. on the same chromosome. Although they may give rise to secondary effects on loci 'up or downstream' from the defective loci, and may have other secondary effects in *trans*, i.e. on the opposite pair of homologous chromosomes, the primary defect in all these conditions is related to the structural gene or its flanking regions.

This new information raises the fascinating question as to whether genuine regulatory gene mutations occur as a basis for human disease. As mentioned earlier, nothing is known about the regulation of genes during different phases of human development. Presumably some kind of regulatory genes must exist which control and co-ordinate whole batteries of structural genes. Whether mutations of genes of this type would be compatible with survival is uncertain. This would almost certainly not be the case for mutations involving genes which regulate such fundamental biological systems as the Krebs' cycle or oxidative phosphorylation pathways, histone structure, nucleic acid polymerases, or major contractile proteins. It is possible that some forms of multiple congenital anomalies result from lesions at loci of this type. However, it seems likely that the majority of human genetic disorders have underlying molecular mechanisms which are very similar to those which have been unravelled recently in the human haemoglobin genome. This emerging pattern of relatively simple molecular pathology is extremely encouraging for medical geneticists in their further attempts to determine the basis for other human diseases.

The future

What might we hope to gain from some of the extraordinary advances in recombinant DNA technology which have occurred over the last year or two? There are many possible applications; I shall mention just three.

The pharmaceutical industry. The pharmaceutical industry has not been slow to appreciate the possibilities of recombinant DNA technology, and many 'gene companies' have appeared almost overnight! The commercial exploitation of the recent advances in molecular genetics has been encouraged by several 'tours de force' For example, it has been possible to clone human insulin genes, interferon genes, and genes for several small peptide hormones. The pharmacological properties of the products of these cloned genes are still being evaluated but it seems likely that at least some of them will be of considerable value. This technology has immense possibilities for the production of a whole variety of products including diagnostic agents, hormones, and vaccines.

Antenatal diagnosis. The major goal in medical genetics is the development of techniques for preventing genetic disease. In practice, antenatal diagnosis may well be the most efficient way of achieving this end. Many disorders can be diagnosed by enzyme analysis of amniotic fibroblasts grown in cell culture, though this is a difficult and time-consuming technique. Other genetic disorders can be diagnosed by fetal blood sampling. Again, this is technically difficult and still carries a significant and often unacceptable fetal mortality and maternal morbidity. For this reason there is considerable interest in the possibility of antenatal diagnosis using analysis of DNA obtained from amniotic fluid cells. This approach has already been used in the human haemoglobin disorders in which it is possible to map the globin genes in amniotic fluid DNA and identify fetuses at risk for various gene deletions which give rise to thalassaemia. Unfortunately, many human haemoglobin disorders are not associated with definable changes in the structure of the globin genes. Furthermore, the biochemical basis for some of the commonest and most serious genetic conditions such as cystic fibrosis and Huntington's chorea is not known. It is in the antenatal diagnosis of latter disorders that recombinant DNA technology promises some of the most exciting prospects in medical genetics.

It is becoming apparent that human DNA is highly polymorphic with regard to the action of bacterial restriction enzymes. In other words, there are base changes scattered throughout the human genome which create different cleavage sites for the same restriction enzyme, and therefore there is considerable inherited variation between different people in the size of the fragments produced when their DNA is digested by a particular enzyme. For example, there is a restriction enzyme which produces a DNA fragment of about 7.6 kilobases long (a kilobase =1000 bases) containing the human β globin gene. In some people, because of a polymorphism near but not involving the β globin gene, the enzyme produces a larger fragment containing the gene. It happens that many individuals with the sickle cell mutation at their β globin loci have this particular polymorphism, i.e. their β globin genes are on this larger restriction fragment. Hence, it is possible to carry out antenatal diagnosis for sickle cell anaemia using a restriction enzyme polymorphism which is easily demonstrable in amniotic fluid DNA.

Many laboratories are looking for further restriction enzyme polymorphisms in the human genome, not necessarily related to any particular structural genes. As these are found it will be possible to carry out detailed family studies to see whether any of them are linked to genetic determinants for such serious genetic disorders as cystic fibrosis or Huntington's chorea. Although the search for linkage relationships of this type will take time and a considerable amount of good luck, there seems little doubt that such linkages will be found and that ultimately it may be possible to produce maps of the whole human genome which relate serious genetic defects to particular restriction enzyme polymorphisms. Once this is achieved, the antenatal diagnosis of most common human genetic disorders should be feasible. The beauty of this approach is that it does not matter whether the molecular or cellular basis for these conditions is worked out; their genetic determinants can be defined by linked restriction enzyme polymorphisms even though nothing is known about the basic defects at their respective loci. This approach should be facilitated by the recent observation that there are a series of highly variable (polymorphic) regions scattered through the human genome.

Gene replacement therapy. With the possibility of obtaining 'pure' human genes in relatively large amounts by recombinant DNA technology, it is not surprising that thoughts are turning towards gene replacement therapy. However, the fact that one has a gene in a test-tube does not mean that it is going to be easy to insert it into human cells and encourage it to synthesize normal amounts of a particular product. A gene would have to be inserted in the appropriate orientation and with its regulatory regions intact. Presumably, it would have to be put into the correct cell and it should not express itself in other cell populations. For example, it seems unlikely that it would be beneficial to insert globin genes into haemopoietic stem cells such that their progeny produce white cells or platelets which synthesize haemoglobin! These genes would have to come under the same regulation as normal genes and be expressed at an appropriate time during cellular maturation. These are formidable problems, and although experiments which have attempted to replace missing globin genes have already been carried out in man, they seem to be rather premature and much has to be learnt about the transfer of genes into mammalian cells before this new technology can be applied to the treatment of human genetic diseases. So much has happened in the field of human molecular genetics in the last few years, however, that gene therapy may not be long in coming.

Ethical problems. I hope that in this short section I have managed to provide some insights into the remarkable developments in molecular biology over the last few years and of the extremely powerful technology that is moving rapidly into the hands of medical geneticists. Progress has been so fast that clinicians may not have had time to appreciate some of the ethical problems which the existence of these new techniques will pose in the near future. What appears to be high technology at the moment is rapidly becoming commonplace—any science student can now master most of the techniques of recombinant DNA methodology (and is expected to!). Furthermore, when compared with much of modern medicine, they are not expensive. Undoubtedly antenatal recognition of genetic disease will become easier and more widely applied. As it does, we are going to have to think very carefully about the whole question of the indications for antenatal diagnosis; which genetic defects are society and individual families willing to accept, and when is therapeutic abortion indicated on grounds of potential genetic disabilities. Gene transfer between individuals will undoubtedly become feasible; this will raise even more fundamental moral dilemmas. Already there are worrying signs that, given the increasing ease of antenatal diagnosis, individual families and communities may wish for the termination of pregnancies which are at risk for a disorder which may be moderately incapacitating, rather than lethal or incompatible with any form of decent life. This is a dangerous road, and the whole question of how much genetic imperfection is acceptable needs very careful thought. The molecular biologists are not going to wait for the doctors to make these decisions before perfecting these new techniques and, judging by progress over the last few years, they will be with us all too soon.

References

Abelson, J. (1980). A revolution in biology. *Science* **209**, 1319.

Lewin, R. (1981). Jumping genes help trace inherited diseases. *Science* **211**, 690.

Little, P. F. R., Annison, G., Darling, S., Williamson, R., Camba, L., and Modell, B. (1980). Model for antenatal diagnosis of β thalassaemia and other monogenic disorders by molecular analysis of linked DNA polymorphisms. *Nature, Lond.* **285**, 144.

Maniatis, T. (1980). In *Cell biology, a comprehensive treatise* (eds. M. Goldstein and D. M. Prescott), vol, 3, 564. Academic Press, New York.

Martin, D. W. (1981). In *Pathophysiology. The biological principles of disease* (eds. L. N. Smith and S. O. Their), 57. W. B. Saunders, Philadelphia.

Porter, R. and O'Connor, M. (1979). *Human genetics: possibilities and realities*. Ciba Foundation Symposium 66. Excerpta Medica, Amsterdam.

Robertson, M. (1981). Genes of lymphocytes I: Diverse moves to antibody diversity. *Nature, Lond.* **290**, 625.

— and Hubert, M. (1981). Antibodies, introns and biosynthetic versatility. *Nature, Lond.* **290**, 543.

Watson, J. D. (1977). *Molecular biology of the gene*, 3rd edn. W. A. Benjamin, San Francisco.

Weatherall, D. J. (1979). Mapping human genes. *Br. med. J* **ii**, 353.

— and Clegg, J. B. (1979). Recent developments in the molecular genetics of human hemoglobin. *Cell* **16**, 467.

— and — (1981). *The thalassaemia syndromes*, 3rd edn. Blackwell Scientific Publications, Oxford.

Williamson, R. (1976). The direct measurement of the number of globin genes. *Br. med. Bull.* **32**, 246.

— (1977). DNA insertions and gene structure. *Nature, Lond.* **270**, 295.

— (1981). *Genetic engineering*, vols. 1 and 2. Academic Press. London.

Immune mechanisms in health and sickness

E. J. Holborow

The immune character of specific hypersensitivity was demonstrated when Richet in 1902 elicited anaphylactic shock in dogs with the second of two spaced injections of sea-anemone extract. In the investigation of immune phenomena in general much confusion at first arose from the puzzling contrast between, on the one hand, the beneficial immunity—that is, enhanced specific resistance to infection—conferred by, say, antitoxic antibodies against tetanus or diphtheria, and, on the other, the deleterious effects such as anaphylaxis that were equally clearly attributable to antibody. The explanation of this paradox began to appear when von Pirquet a few years later pointed out that, looked at from the biological rather than the clinical point of view, both effects evidently reflect aspects of the same *altered reactivity* that develops in the individual as a result of initial exposure to antigen. This altered reactivity, however mediated and expressed, von Pirquet called 'allergy'.

Initial lodgement in the tissues of alien biological material may more or less immediately induce local inflammation to the extent that the material is particulate or of a chemical nature capable of activating directly mechanisms of non-specific or natural immunity such as complement and phagocytic cells. *Adaptive immunity* is the specific amplifying contribution that the immune system makes to non-specific mechanisms of tissue defence. Conditions of foreign antigenic challenge stimulate the immune system through its highly developed ability to recognize particular arrays of the accessible, relatively small chemical groupings—antigenic determinants or *epitopes*—which characterize the molecular configurations of different antigenic macromolecules and distinguish each of them specifically from the vast range of other configurations subsumed in the myriad of potential antigens, natural or artificial, in the environment. Through their participation in this process of specific recognition, lymphocytes, which constitute the predominant cell population of the immune system, are triggered to produce the humoral and cellular effector components of adaptive immunity, that is to say antibody and sensitized cells, together with the non-antibody active products of the latter. These in turn exercise their biological functions by recruiting humoral and cellular non-specific defence mechanisms, bringing them to bear in selective fashion on the specific antigenic material in question wherever they encounter it in the body. Furthermore, *recognition* of a given foreign antigen in this way by the immune system leads to expansion of the initially small fraction of its lymphocyte population which is genetically endowed with the matching specific recognition equipment. This has the double effect of augmenting the scope of cellular and humoral attack against the antigenic material in question, and generating the cellular basis of specific immunological memory for it, which confers one of the principle advantages of adaptive immunity, *acquired specific resistance*.

The terms 'allergy', 'hypersensitivity', and 'immunity' at an early stage acquired restricted usage according to the recognizable clinical outcome of such contact with antigen, a development which for long obscured the fact that the same range of normal immune mechanisms underlies all three responses. To overcome the challenge presented by invading micro-organisms, parasitic infestation, virally infected cells, or non-replicating foreign antigenic material, the destructive humoral and cellular manifestations of the adaptive response need not necessarily exceed the microscopic level—the level at which clinically we recognize 'immunity'. Where the degree, extent, nature, or effect of an immune response are such as to amount to a clinical disability, we recognize 'hypersensitivity' and 'allergy'.

Immunopathology seeks (*a*) to identify the underlying immune effector mechanisms common to immunity, hypersensitivity, and allergy; (*b*) to elucidate the disorders of control and organization in the immune system which result in failures of response (immune deficiencies) or in loss of ability to distinguish self from non-self antigens (autoimmunity); and (*c*) to map genetic factors which influence the range and degree of responsiveness of the immune system.

Immunobiological knowledge, especially of the complex genetic and micro-environmental factors which determine the co-operative interactions between the cells of the immune system which are necessary to develop, and equally important, to regulate immune responses, has increased abundantly in the last two decades, and the rate of progress shows no sign of slackening. The discovery and elucidation of underlying immune mechanisms or disorders in a continually increasing number of human diseases has engendered in medicine the rapidly expanding and many-faceted speciality of clinical immunology, each facet reflecting a partnership between immunopathologists and practitioners of a given medical or surgical speciality.

A brief account of the developmental genetics of the immune system is given on page 4.24.

The cells of the immune system

The immune functions of the body have two aspects, afferent and efferent. The afferent side deals with recognition of antigen, its processing, and other events leading up to induction of the immune response, while on the efferent side are the specific effector mechanisms, cellular or humoral, activated by contact or re-encounter with antigen to put immune responses into practical effect. This dual function requires, for its smooth performance, a high degree of collaboration, mainly through cell surface receptors and soluble mediators, between lymphocytes themselves, and between lymphocytes and other cells which share the same haemopoietic stem cell ancestry in the bone marrow. On the afferent, antigen recognition side, the chief of these auxiliary cells is the macrophage. On the efferent side, both macrophages and phagocytic cells of the granulocyte series (polymorphs, eosinophils, and basophils) play a variety of executive roles in the range of effector mechanisms, antibody-mediated or otherwise, which lymphocytes may generate in response to antigenic stimulation.

Lymphoid organs. As we have seen, a major part of the cell population of the lymphoid tissues of the body consists of small lymphocytes. The lymphoid organs comprise the thymus, the spleen, the lymph nodes, and the mucosa-associated lymphoid tissue (MALT). The latter consists of the collections of lymphoid cells in the gut (in Peyer's patches and the lamina propria), in the pharynx (tonsils, adenoids, and submucosal lymphoid tissue, together constituting Waldeyer's ring), in the bronchial mucosa, and in the breasts, the lacrimal and salivary glands, and the genito-urinary system.

The thymus and T cells. On leaving the bone marrow, some of the progeny of lymphoid stem cells migrate to the thymus, where they constitute the densely packed population of thymocytes. The thymus reaches its largest size in early life, undergoing slow atrophy subsequently. Thymocytes migrate from the thymic cortex to the medulla, undergoing at the same time both frequent mitoses and an intensive process of weeding-out, which is probably strongly influenced by the presence of the thymic epithelial cells which are particularly prominent in the medulla.

The lymphocytes that finally emerge from the thymus into the circulation are mature cells which have acquired *immunological competence*, that is to say they are qualified to respond to antigenic stimuli and to undertake the various effector roles discussed below. Because of the thymus-dependent nature of their competence, the lymphocytes of this subpopulation are known as T cells. This essential role of the thymus as a primary lymphoid organ is testified by the gross immune deficiencies seen in babies with rare congenital absence or hypoplasia of the thymus (diGeorge and Nezelof syndromes).

Cells leaving the thymus join the mobile population of lymphocytes in the blood and lymph *en route* to the spleen, lymph nodes, and MALT. In thoracic duct lymph, T cells are the principal cell type, while of the blood lymphocytes 75–80 per cent are T cells.

These mobile lymphocytes recirculate from the lymph nodes via the lymphatics and thoracic duct to the blood, through the white pulp of the spleen, and, leaving the blood stream again through the post-capillary venules in the lymph nodes, rejoin the lymphatic flow into the thoracic duct. The cells of this recirculating pool are antigen-sensitive, responding to antigenic stimuli by transforming into large pyroninophilic 'blast' cells and undergoing mitosis. Proliferation of pyroninophilic cells following antigenic stimulation occurs in the paracortical region in lymph nodes and in the peri-arteriolar lymphocytic sheaths in the white pulp of the spleen, both traffic areas of the recirculating lymphocyte pool. When white cells from the blood are cultured *in vitro*, addition of antigen causes a similar transformation of a small proportion of lymphocytes, especially from an individual previously immunized to the same antigen. Antigen-induced proliferation of cells in response to a given antigenic stimulus implants the immunological memory of the same antigen referred to above.

The plant lectins concanavalin A and phytohaemagglutinin (PHA) are also activators of T cells which induce markedly polyclonal blast transformation with DNA synthesis, and this effect is used as a broad *in vitro* test of T cell function. T cells also have the property of binding sheep erythrocytes to their surface, a phenomenon known as E-rosetting, and may be enumerated in this way among lymphocytes separated from blood samples.

B-cells. T cells do not themselves differentiate into antibody-forming cells. This is a function of small lymphocytes belonging to another subpopulation, which are not subject to thymic conditioning, and which, for their functional equivalence to the lymphocytes produced in the avian bursa of Fabricius as precursors of antibody-forming cells, are known as B cells.

The B cells of man, as of other mammals, originate from the same stem cells in the bone marrow as T cells, and migrate via the blood stream to the lymphoid organs, contributing plentifully to the sessile lymphocyte population of all lymphoid tissues except the thymus.

B cells in lymphoid tissue respond to appropriate antigenic

stimulation by proliferating and differentiating into plasma cells. These are short-lived end cells whose sole function is to synthesize and secrete antibody molecules into the lymph and blood.

The maturation of B cells is independent of the thymus, and they form a second functionally distinct population of lymphocytes, readily distinguishable from T cells by the surface immunoglobulin (sIg) which provides them with the cell membrane receptors by means of which they recognize and respond to specific antigens. The immunoglobulin (Ig) molecules which plasma cells elaborate are identical in antigen-combining specificity with the sIg of their B cell precursors. The Ig of both types of cell may be visualized under the microscope by its reactivity with fluorescein-labelled anti-Ig antibodies. The use of this and other techniques involving anti-Ig reagents shows that 10–20 per cent of blood lymphocytes belong to the B cell subpopulation.

Clonal selection. The clonal selection theory of antibody production put forward by Burnet in 1956, together with the concept of immunological tolerance (see below) forms the basis upon which modern immunology has developed. It proposes that antigen plays no direct part in shaping the combining specificity of antibody molecules, but instead selects for stimulation only lymphocytes whose antigen receptors (sIg) are already genetically encoded to provide the best available fit. Immunogenetic observations are in close accord with this hypothesis. The sIg membrane receptors on B cells are immunoglobulin proteins coded for by three gene families, for the κ and λ light chains, and for the various types of heavy chain respectively (see below). Joining and recombination of gene sets within these families encode the antigen receptor sIg protein in the cell membrane of B cells as they undergo maturation in such a way as to confer different antibody combining specificities on each cell, the population as a whole thus covering reactivity with the widest possible range of potential antigens (see also page 4.24). Stimulation by a given antigen leads to expansion by proliferation of cell clones arising only from B cells with suitably specific sIg antibody, as predicted by Burnet's theory.

T cells do not carry sIg but have an individual surface receptor with specificity for antigen less well understood but as good as, or even better, than that of B cells. Although the nature of the surface antigen receptor of T cells is still controversial, it appears likely that some of the genes implicated in immunoglobulin encoding are also involved here, possibly V genes.

Since antigens are usually macromolecules bearing several different antigenic determinants, and since a restricted range of lymphocytes may carry receptors capable of binding a given antigenic determinant with more or less affinity, antibody responses are mostly polyclonal in character. Many forms of malignant disease arising in the lymphoid system (myelomas, lymphomas, and leukaemias) are clearly monoclonal, in contrast, and presumably originate in a single aberrant cell.

Functional subsets of lymphocytes. We have seen that although lymphocytes share a common morphology as small mononuclear cells, their maturation pathways and surface properties differentiate them into two major subpopulations, T and B cells. Both of these display further important, functionally distinct subdivisions.

T cell subsets. The crucial observation that while T cells and B cells together can produce an antibody response to most antigens, alone neither is capable of doing so, revealed the essential interdependence of lymphocytes in mounting immune responses.

Helper and suppressor T cells. Antigenic macromolecules are polyvalent with regard to the number and specificities of their antigenic determinants (epitopes). The epitopes of most antigens, especially proteins, may be considered as those binding to appropriately specific B cell sIg, and those binding to T cell antigen receptors. In accordance with the classical hapten-carrier concept of immunogenicity, carrier epitopes of a given antigen activate T cells with appropriately specific antigen receptors, and these T cells

in turn stimulate into antibody production B cells which are at the same time ready to undergo proliferation as a result of specifically binding the haptenic epitopes of the same antigen. T cells which promote antibody responses in this way belong to the T-'helper' (T_H) subset, and have proved to be of a phenotype identifiable serologically by possession of their own characteristic surface antigens which differ from those of other functionally distinct T cells.

The latter include cells of another subset, T-suppressor (T_S) cells. These exert an immunoregulatory effect which limits the promotion by T_H cells of antibody production by B cells. T_S cells are likewise separately identifiable phenotypically by their possession of distinctive surface antigens.

Cytotoxic T cells. An important, perhaps the paramount, immune effector function of T cells is to recognize and destroy cells infected with virus. Viruses replicate in a variety of host cells, and in a variety of ways, ranging from a productive cycle with release from the damaged cell of fresh infectious virus particles to incomplete, non-productive or latent infections with only partial expression of viral function in the form of protein synthesis. Neutralizing antibodies have access to released virus, but cells carrying incompletely replicating virus are accessible to immune attack only through viral antigens expressed on their surface. Cytotoxic T cells act by lysing such cells with exquisitely selective specificity by cell-to-cell contact, independently of antibody. Such T-cell-induced lysis is the result of a process of specific binding, alteration in membrane permeability of the target cell, osmotic swelling, and finally membrane disruption.

Allograft rejection is another clinically important cell-mediated immune reaction, and here again cytotoxic T cells play a central role. In both antiviral and anti-allograft responses, however, optimal development of T cell cytotoxicity depends upon the collaborative effect of T_H cells proliferating in response to the foreign antigen. T_H cells thus deploy their powers not only in the T–B cell interactions necessary to antibody production, but also in the T–T collaboration required to activate cell-mediated immunity.

Another form of cell-mediated immunity originally thought of as a typically bacterial allergy is *delayed hypersensitivity*. The classical example is the tuberculin reaction, and contact hypersensitivity to chemicals and drugs has identical features. Both reactions are the result of mononuclear cell infiltration at the site of activation of T cells by antigen. Activated T cells respond by releasing soluble non-antibody mediators, known as *lymphokines*, which attract or activate other cells, including macrophages. Lymphokines are 20–100K molecules to which various biological activities have been assigned, viz. macrophage migration inhibitory factor (MIF), macrophage activating factor (MAF), lymphocyte activating factor (LAF), and others. Since these factors act as communicating signals between leucocytes, they have been termed *interleukins*. Another form of lymphokine is interferon, which stimulates cells to produce a protein which blocks viral protein synthesis, and enhances the cytotoxicity of T cells, natural killer (NK), and killer (K) cells, and the phagocytic activity of macrophages.

Of the T lymphocytes in the blood, 55–65 per cent are helper cells, and 20–30 per cent suppressor cells. Although four different T cell subgroups are distinguishable functionally—helper, suppressor, cytotoxic, and delayed hypersensitivity— it appears that cells of the suppressor subset mediate cytotoxic effects, while helper cells produce the lymphokines that mediate delayed hypersensitivity.

B cell subsets. As stated above, B cells can make antibody to most antigens only with T cell help. The B cells co-operate with T cells in this way by intercellular signals involving products of the immune response (Ir) region of the major histocompatibility gene complex (see below). These products, termed 'immune associated' (Ia) antigens, have been most studied in the mouse, but in man the HLA-D and HLA-DR antigens (see below) appear equivalent, and phenotypically characterize the B1 cell subset which produces antibody to such T dependent antigens. B1 cells also carry receptors for IgG-Fc determinants and complement.

A minority of antigens, especially those carrying numerous identical epitopes such as macromolecular polysaccharides, are T-independent, being capable of stimulating directly a second subset of B cells (B2 cells) which probably lack both HLA-D and complement receptors.

Null cells. A small proportion of circulating lymphoid cells originating in the bone marrow do not carry the phenotype markers of either T or B cells. Some of these appear to be 'killer' (K) cells with cytotoxic properties against target cells coated with antibody. Others may be 'natural killer' (NK) cells to which a lytic role against certain tumour cells has been ascribed. The *in vivo* significance of both types of killer activity is at present uncertain.

Clinical relevance of lymphocyte phenotypes. During their ontogeny from bone marrow stem cells, lymphocytes of the different subpopulations and subsets acquire new characteristic phenotypic surface antigens and lose others. The programming of specific cell function appears to be linked to expression of particular cell-surface phenotypes, and has already occurred before cell activation. As methods of recognizing such markers become routinely available, leukaemias, lymphomas, and other malignancies of the lymphoid tissues are becoming more precisely classifiable according to the stage of maturation arrest which they represent. Since immunological functions are acquired only at the end stages of lymphocyte ontogeny, congenital or acquired immunodeficiencies may likewise be more precisely analysed with regard to the stages of T or B cell maturation at which aberration has occurred. Furthermore, phenotypic identification and enumeration of lymphocyte subsets has begun to elucidate the nature of defects of immune regulation which result in auto-immune diseases. Finally, the recent development of monoclonal antibodies against defined lymphocyte phenotypic determinants is bringing immunotherapy by selective T-cell subset manipulation within the bounds of probability.

The genetics of the immune response

Patients receiving multiple blood transfusions, and pregnant women, may develop antibodies against the transfused leucocytes, or against leucocytes of the fetus which have crossed the placenta. These allo-antibodies, which are analogous to blood group isoantibodies, define by their different specific reactivities a complex range of genetically related leucocyte surface antigens which constitute the HLA (human leucocyte) antigen system. The fact that kidney grafts from HLA-identical sibling donors survive almost perfectly, unlike dissimilar donor grafts, established HLA as the major histocompatibility system.

HLA gene products form five separate segregant allelic series of antigens. The five HLA gene loci are closely linked in the major histocompatibility complex (MHC) on chromosome 6, and designated HLA-A, HLA-B, HLA-C, HLA-D and HLA-DR, each with its own set of alleles, distinguished numerically.

The gene products of three of the HLA loci, A, B, and C, were the first to be identified and were distinguished serologically as described above. These are 45K molecules which are associated with a common protein, β microglobulin, and are grouped together as MHC class I antigens. The HLA-D locus was identified in a different way, by the mixed lymphocyte culture (MLC) test. In this, the blood lymphocytes of two individuals are grown together in mixed culture. The cells of one are first rendered unresponsive by treatment with mitomycin or X-rays. The untreated (responder) cells of the other react in culture to HLA-D antigen differences in the treated (stimulator) cells, and undergo blast transformation measurable by new DNA synthesis.

The biological significance of the MHC, however, goes far beyond transplantation. Gene products of the MHC play a critical directing role in most forms of immune response. Much of our present understanding of what the MHC is for has come from studies of inbred mouse strains, in which 'immune response' (Ir) genes controlling major differences in magnitude of antibody responses to defined antigenic epitopes have been identified and located in the equivalent murine MHC. The molecules which are the products of these Ir genes are distinct 'immune-associated' (Ia) antigens and are present on the surfaces of B cells and macrophages. In man, attempts to use pregnancy sera instead of MLC techniques to detect D-locus specificities led to the discovery of another distinct allelic series of antigens which also are present on B lymphocytes, but not on most T cells. It is not possible in outbred humans to demonstrate directly the existence of Ir genes, but it is nevertheless likely that the B cell allo-antigens in question are the human analogues of immune Ia antigens. These appear to be the products of a single locus in the human MHC which is very closely linked to, but probably distinct from HLA-D, and is hence designated HLA-DR (D-related). HLA-D antigens are 28–32K molecules and are grouped together as class II determinants.

The stage of the immune response at which Ir genes operate is T_H cell recognition of macrophage-bound antigen. At the beginning of this section it was pointed out that immune responses are in essence devices to amplify non-specific defence mechanisms, and in the latter macrophages play a leading part. It is not surprising, therefore, to find that macrophage-bound antigen is many thousand times more immunogenic than free soluble antigen, and that T_H cells recognize and respond to antigen far better when it is associated with macrophages.

The recognition process itself is not simply a matter of fitting antigenic epitopes to lymphocyte receptors, but involves additional apparently complex molecular interactions which are increasingly becoming recognized as immunoregulatory in function. Experiments on the cellular interactions involved in antibody production in mice have shown that T_H cells co-operate only with B cells that share Ia antigens with the T cell donor, and furthermore that the macrophages presenting a given antigen to T_H cells must also share the same Ia antigens if antibody production is to result. Relevant to such conclusions is the fact that human anti-B cell sera defining the analogous HLA-DR alleles react also, and with the same specificity, with human monocytes and macrophages. Many other cell types lack this Ia-like antigens.

It thus appears that recognition of antigen by T_H cells involves parallel recognition of Ia-like (HLA-DR) surface molecules on the macrophage presenting the antigen, while stimulation of B cells to produce the relevant antibody requires similar recognition by T_H cells of Ia-like molecules on the B cell surface.

The animal experiments mentioned established the further important corollary that the macrophage Ia-molecules involved in priming T_H cells with a given antigen in this fashion determine the Ia specificity required to promote a successful secondary challenge with the same antigen. Regarded in the context of *in vivo* events, this means that foreign antigen is recognized by T_H cells in association with 'self' Ia (or HLA-DR). Since Ia (HLA-DR) molecules are the products of Ir genes, an Ir allele governing a good antibody response to a given antigen presumably codes for Ia molecules interacting with the antigen in question. Lack of the same allele would mean that the corresponding gene product was lacking on both macrophages and B cells, with resultant failure of the relevant foreign antigen to present itself in immunogenic association with a complementary Ia molecule. To express this idea in another way, T_H cells recognize 'antigen plus "self" Ia'.

This type of genetic restriction of the immune response is also evident with cytotoxic T lymphocytes (CTL). As we have seen, the natural function of CTL seems to be to eliminate virus infected cells. Tests with human lymphocytes show that CTL lyse cells from the same donor which have been infected with virus – and in the case of influenza virus, for example, with the expected specificity for virus type A or B. However, virus-infected cells from a different donor are not lysed. The genetic restriction here is that HLA-A and/or HLA-B antigens must be shared between target cell and T effector.

It seems likely that these genetic restrictions imposed on T cell function are controlled by the thymus. It is postulated, again from the result of animal experiments, that immature thymocytes in their passage through the thymus are repeatedly exposed to HLA antigens expressed on the surfaces of thymic epithelial cells. This results in the proliferation and consequent elimination within the thymus of thymocytes with receptors for 'self' HLA molecules, while those with receptors for non-self molecules (including non-self HLA) pass through to become mature immunocompetent T cells. It is thought that the interaction between virus and HLA antigens necessary to induce CTL (here any cell type might be the target according to the virus implicated, and most cell types carry HLA-A or HLA-B antigens), or between foreign antigen and Ia antigen necessary for the activation of T_H cells, leads to an alteration of the HLA molecular configuration ('altered-self') so that together the latter and the foreign antigen form a dual complex for which recognition receptors on T cells exist. A pendant to this concept of MHC function is that different virus antigens may interact in this way better with one HLA molecule type than with another to engender an effective dually immunogenic product. If this were the case, it would account for the marked polymorphism which the HLA system has developed in evolution.

In summary of the foregoing, then, it may be said that the main function of MHC molecules is to govern the activities of T cell subsets in such a way to promote immune responses appropriate to infectious agents as different as bacteria (antibody), viruses (T cytotoxicity), and intracellular parasites (macrophage activation), at the same time ensuring through their 'altered self' property that the normal cells of the body do not undeservedly become the subject of their own T cells' attention.

Immunoglobulins

Antibodies belong to the immunoglobulin fraction of the serum proteins and as we have seen are synthesized and secreted by plasma cells maturing from B lymphocyte precursors present in all lymphoid tissue except the thymus. Although conforming to a common molecular structure in which two pairs of polypeptide chains [light (L) and heavy (H)] are covalently linked through cysteine residues by disulphide bonds to form the single or repeating unit of the finished molecule (Fig. 1), immunoglobulin molecules display a remarkable inner heterogeneity that reflects the highly complex genetic patterns directing synthesis of their constituent peptide chains, and determining both their combining specificities for antigen and their biological properties as immune effectors.

Domains and effector functions of antibody molecules.

The unit of structure of the immunoglobulin molecule is the domain, a polypeptide homology unit comprising a sequence of about 110 amino acid residues. The typical H chain is made up of four linked domains, the L chain two. Each domain fulfils a particular biological function of the Ig molecule. The two domains at the N-terminal ends of each pair of H and L chains together form the antigen-combining site. The sequences of amino acid residues in these two N-terminal domains are highly variable, and for this reason they are termed the V_H and V_L domains respectively. It is a genetically coded hypervariability within the V_H and V_L domains that confers different antibody combining specificities on each lymphocyte at an early stage of maturation, thus providing the wide spectrum of antigen-recognizing receptors which is the basis of the clonal selection mechanism of antibody production.

The other three domains of the H chain, and the remaining L chain domain have constant sequences of amino acids. In the H chain these differ only between the five different classes (isotypes) of Igs and their subclasses (Fig. 2) which are present in all normal individuals. The H chain constant domains are numbered consecutively from the N-terminal region CH1, CH2, CH3, and, for IgM and IgE, which each have an extra H chain domain, CH4. The H chains of the different Ig isotypes take the Greek letter equivalents

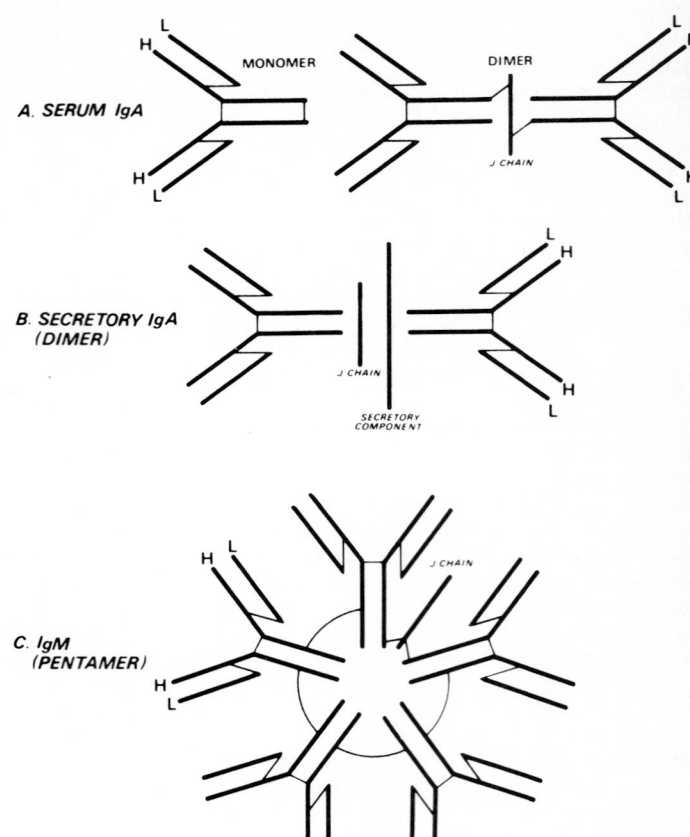

Fig. 1 Highly schematic illustration of polymeric human immunoglobulins. Polypeptide chains are represented by thick lines; disulphide bonds linking different polypeptide chains are represented by thin lines. (From Goodman, J. W. and Wang, A. C. (1980). In *Basic and clinical immunology*, ed. H. H. Fudenberg *et al.*, 32. Lange, Los Altos, by permission)

of their class, i.e. γ, μ, α, ε, and δ, so that the CH2 region of the H chain of IgG, for example, is designated Cγ2.

The L chain constant domains fall into two types, κ and λ, any given Ig molecule having either κ or λ, but not both. Urinary Bence Jones protein, long recognized as a characteristic feature of multiple myeloma, results from passage through the kidney of free L chains, their dimers, or their fragments. Since this condition is one of the monoclonal gammopathies, a given myeloma patient excretes Bence Jones protein of κ or λ type, but not both. In addition to these C domain differences within individuals, Ig molecules express certain minor genetic polymorphisms which define differences between individuals (allotypes). The best-known of these structurally variant products of allelic genes are the Gm series of γ-chain markers and the InV series of κ chain markers.

The section of H chain between the CH1 and CH2 domains contains cysteine residues that provide disulphide bonds which link H chains in their characteristic pairs. This region (the hinge region) is also rich in proline residues, which confer a marked degree of flexibility on the Ig molecule at this point, a feature which, on binding of the antigen-combining sites with their specific epitopes, appears to favour activation of the effector functions of the different C_H domains in the rest of the antibody molecule.

The apportionment of effector functions to different parts of the Ig molecule has been demonstrated by study of the properties of Ig molecule fragments produced by enzymic digestion (Figs. 2 and 3). The proline residues in the hinge region are particularly vulnerable to digestion by papain, the action of which cleaves the IgG molecule into (*a*) antigen binding (Fab) fragments, comprising the two L chain domains (VL and CL) linked to the complementary H chain

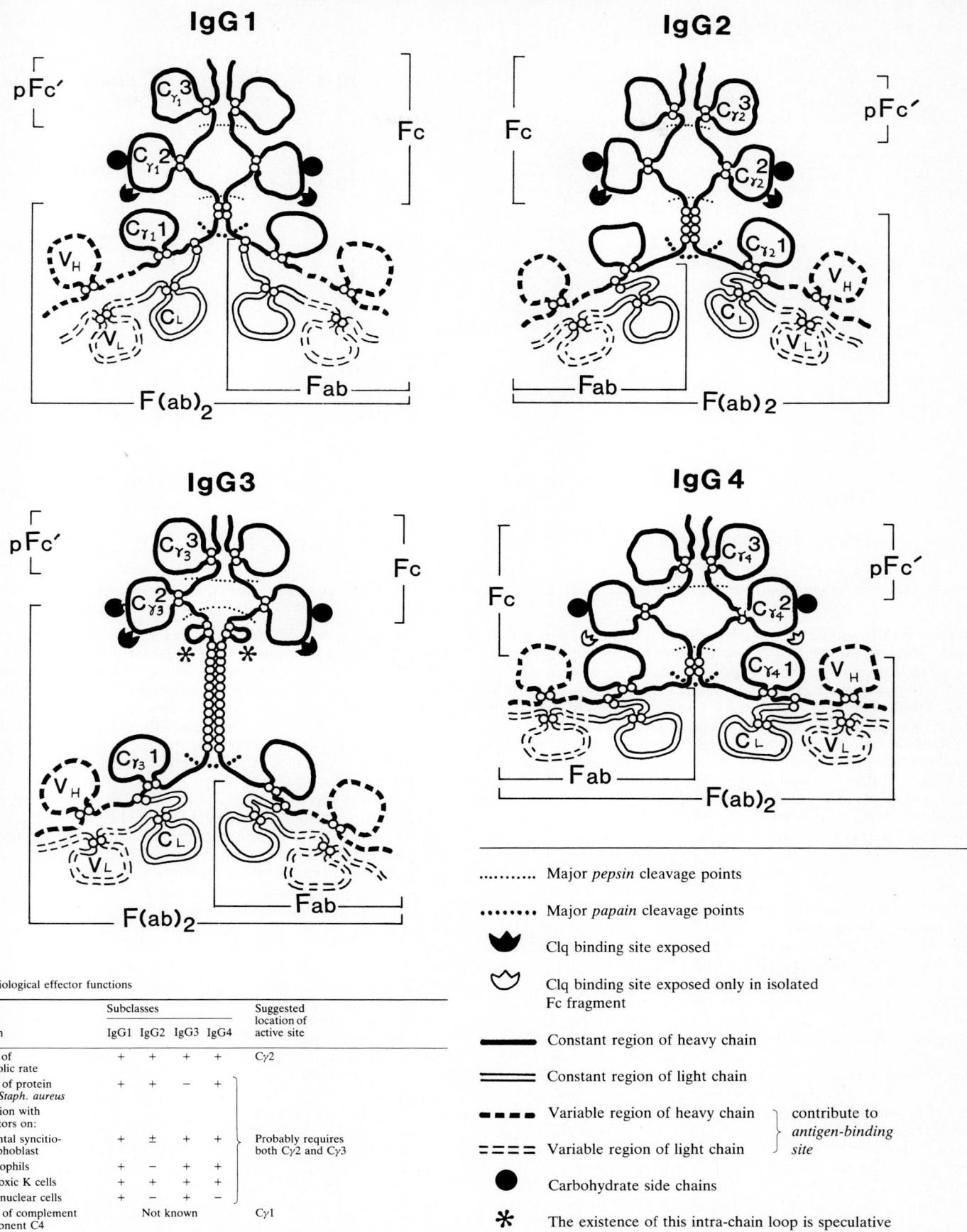

Other biological effector functions

Function	Subclasses				Suggested location of active site
	IgG1	IgG2	IgG3	IgG4	
Control of catabolic rate	+	+	+	+	Cγ2
Binding of protein A of *Staph. aureus*	+	+	−	+	
Interaction with receptors on:					
Placental syncitio-trophoblast	+	±	+	+	Probably requires both Cγ2 and Cγ3
Neutrophils	+	−	+	+	
Cytotoxic K cells	+	+	+	+	
Mononuclear cells	+	−	+	−	
Binding of complement component C4		Not known			Cγ1

.... Major *pepsin* cleavage points

.... Major *papain* cleavage points

Clq binding site exposed

Clq binding site exposed only in isolated Fc fragment

Constant region of heavy chain

Constant region of light chain

Variable region of heavy chain ⎫ contribute to

Variable region of light chain ⎭ *antigen-binding site*

Carbohydrate side chains

* The existence of this intra-chain loop is speculative

Fig. 2   The domain structure of the subclasses of human immunoglobulin G. (From *Immunology Today*, (1980), **1**, by permission)

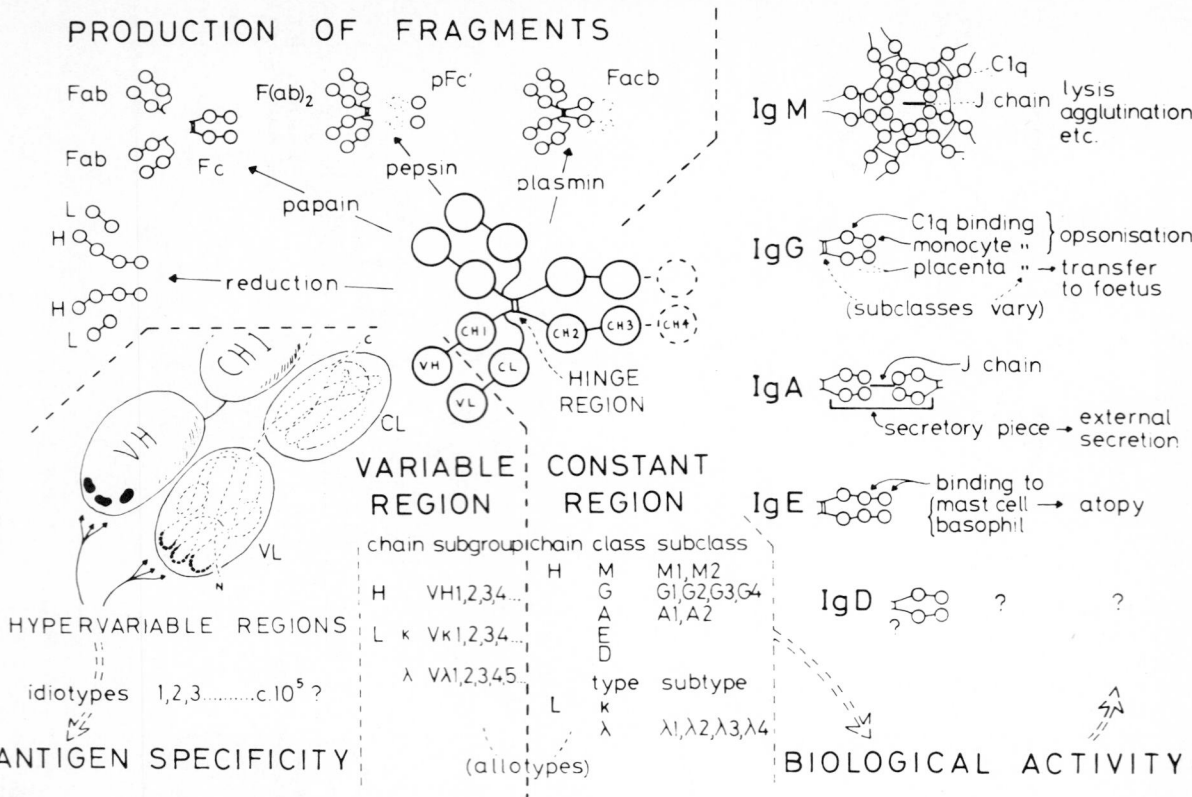

Fig. 3   Antibody structure and function. (From Playfair, J. H. L., 1979. *Immunology at a glance.* Blackwell Scientific Publications, Oxford, by permission)

fragment (VH and CH1) by cysteine residues, and (*b*) paired CH2 and CH3 domains similarly linked to form a fragment designated Fc (c stands for crystallizable). Pepsin cleaves the Ig molecule differently, digesting the CH2 domain and leaving the two Fab portions still linked together as the F(ab)$_2$ fragment. Plasmin digests the CH3 domain, leaving the CH2 domains linked to F(ab)$_2$.

Antibody may exert its useful effect simply by neutralizing toxin or virus by combining with and masking active sites through its V domains. Bordet showed early in the present century, however, that, although mixing live cholera vibrios with specific antiserum which had been heated at 56 °C produced clumping of the organisms, this did not kill them, the agglutinated bacteria retaining the ability to grow on in culture. If fresh antiserum was used, however, or with added fresh normal serum, the antibody-coated vibrios were killed, an outcome due to the lytic action of complement. Studies with enzymically or chemically derived fragments of H chains have shown that the complement-activating site of IgM and IgG antibody molecules is in the CH2 domain. It likewise proved to be the case that phagocytic cells induce adherence of antigen–antibody complexes to their surfaces by means of their membrane receptors for Fc determinants located in the CH3 domains of Ig molecules. Through such precise interactions with complement on the one hand and surface receptors on different functional types of phagocytic and mononuclear cells on the other, antigen-bound antibody molecules promote a range of inflammatory effects (discussed more fully below) and stimulate disposal or destruction of antigenic material. As well as these effects, antibodies exert a regulatory influence on the activities of the cells of the immune system themselves, which, through receptors for IgM or IgG, receive positive or negative feedback signals, according to local conditions of isotype concentration and reactivity with antigen. Table 1 shows some properties of antibody molecules of different classes.

Immunoglobulin classes and their functions. Analysis by electrophoresis and ultracentrifugation shows a wide range of molecular size and charge among immunoglobulin molecules (Table 1). Immunological analysis shows their heterogeneity in much greater detail. Here separated immunoglobulins, or their constituent fragments or polypeptides are treated as antigenic proteins and antisera raised against them in a different species. The ability of such antiglobulin antisera to discriminate different types and classes of immunoglobulins is based on their specific reaction with different antigenic determinants in the different domains of the L or H chains.

As free proteins in the body, immunoglobulins show very wide differences in distribution and behaviour. In healthy adults the total free IgG is distributed equally between the blood and the interstitial tissues, about a quarter passing across capillary walls each day and the same amount returning via the thoracic duct. IgM, on the other hand, being a macromolecular pentamer, is mostly intravascular. In man only IgG among the immunoglobulin classes passes the placenta and reaches the fetal circulation, and this is not due to simple filtration, but to active transport across the cells of the trophoblast layer. In the major immunoglobulin class, IgG, four subclasses differing in biological behaviour are distinguished Table 1 and Fig. 2).

Thus, although antibodies in the shape of immunoglobulin molecules are initially secreted into the lymph, blood, or tissue fluids in the immediate environment of the plasma cells that produce them, their subsequent distribution in the body is largely determined by the physicochemical and biological properties of the immunoglobulin class to which they belong.

The heterogeneity of antibodies with regard to immunoglobulin class and subclass is an evolutionary development which reflects the diverse range of protective functions they are called upon to fulfil at many different possible sites of encounter with antigen in the body. The relationship between structure and function of Ig molecules is well exemplified by the manner in which IgA antibodies provide protection against infection at the mucous membranes (Fig. 4). IgA is a relatively minor component of the blood immunoglobulins, but

Table 1 Some properties of human immunoglobulins

	IgG	IgA	IgM	IgD	IgE
Molecular weight	160 000	170 000	900 000	184 000	188 000
Sedimentation coefficient	7S	7S (monomer)	19S	7S	8S
Mean serum level (g/l) normal range in parentheses	9.4 (5.0–14.0)	1.8 (0.5–3.0)	1.1 (0.5–1.9)	3 mg	5 μg

	Subclasses								
	1	2	3	4	1	2			
Complement fixation							IgM	IgD	IgE
Classical (C1q binding)	++	±	+++	−	−	−	+++	−	−
Alternative pathway	+	+	+	?	+	+	+	−	+
Placental transfer	+	+	+	+	−	−	−	−	−
Binding to mononuclear cells and polymorphs	+	−	+	−	−	−	−	−	?
Binding to mast cells and basophils	−	−	−	−	−	−	−	−	++

From Turner, M. W. (1977). *Immunology in medicine* (eds. E. J. Holborow, and W. G. Reeves), p. 108. Academic Press, London

an important constituent of the secretions. Secretory IgA (s-IgA) has a molecular weight more than twice that of the predominantly monomeric serum IgA. It is a major product of the plasma cell population in the lamina propria of the gut, the IgA-synthesizing members of which secrete IgA in dimeric form, the two pairs of Hα chains being linked by a joining polypeptide, J chain.

As s-IgA passes to the adjoining gut epithelium, it unites with membrane receptors (secretory-component, SC) on the gut epithelial cell, and the whole complex of dimeric IgA with J chain and SC is transported through the epithelium in endocytic vesicles to reach the luminal surface. Monomeric IgA cannot unite with SC and so does not appear in secretions.

Pathogenic bacteria and viruses in the gut gain their initial invasive foothold by adhering to epithelial cell surfaces. A function of the SC element of secreted IgA appears to be to anchor the molecule in the mucous layer overlying the epithelium, thus providing a barrier of specific antibody against micro-organisms prone to adhere.

Some of the s-IgA produced in the lamina propria finds its way not into the gut but into the mesenteric lymph, and thence by the blood to the liver. In many animals, and, it is thought, in man also, liver cells, like gut epithelium, carry SC receptors for s-IgA. These, by a similar mechanism, capture s-IgA reaching the blood and return it to the lumen of the gut via the bile. Other secretions, such as saliva and colostrum, probably also acquire from the blood by the same means at least some of the s-IgA they contain. This efficient clearance mechanism keeps the level of s-IgA in the blood low by comparison with that of monomeric IgA, the function of which is still not clearly understood. An additional biological advantage of the system described is that immune complexes formed by s-IgA antibodies encountering dietary or microbial antigens which have penetrated the tissues of the lamina propria are likewise rapidly cleared into the bile by this liver mechanism. It will thus be seen that s-IgG performs its protective function in the gut and secretions without recourse to the inflammatory sequelae of complement activation, upon which much of the biological effectiveness of IgM and IgG depends. It is also evident that measurement of the largely monomeric serum IgA level alone is not enough to define the functional depletion of s-IgA in the secretions, or lack of its production by the plasma cells of the lamina propria, which characterize selective IgA deficiency disease.

As we have seen, antibody molecules which have combined with antigen exert their biological functions in the body through reactions initiated by determinants in their CH domains. Both IgM and IgG molecules carry Fc determinants which are capable of binding to Fc receptors present on cells of several different types, viz.

polymorphonuclear leucocytes, macrophages, and other mononuclear cells including some T lymphocytes which play immunoregulatory roles. Other IgM and IgG Fc determinants activate complement by specifically binding the C1q recognition unit of the first complement component, C1. IgE has yet another type of Fc determinant, specific receptors for which on the membranes of basophils and tissue mast cells bind it so efficiently that the bulk of IgE in the body is cell-bound (homocytotropic) and the normal level of free IgE in the plasma is consequently very low.

Interactions of antibody with cells having Fc receptors. 'Professional' phagocytes such as polymorphs and macrophages are characterized by possessing Fc receptors with special affinity for sequences on the Fc regions of IgG molecules of subclasses IgG1 and IgG3. These antibodies, belonging to the group of immunologically reactive serum components classically designated 'opsonins', facilitate ingestion of antigenic particles they have combined with by attaching them closely to the phagocyte cell membrane and thus initiating immune phagocytosis. Immune precipitates and soluble immune complexes of sufficient size are disposed of likewise. Antibodies of these two subclasses are also independently cytophilic (although this has much less effect in depleting their serum levels than the marked cytotropism of IgE), so that they may become bound in the first instance to the Fc receptors of neutrophils or macrophages, 'arming' these cells with powers of specific binding and ingestion towards subsequently encountered antigenic material of matching epitope specificity.

A somewhat different outcome of opsonization is seen when cells coated with antibody (examples are virus-infected cells, and protozoal and metazoal parasites) become the target of attack of 'killer' cells carrying Fc receptors. Such K cells are typically non-phagocytic and lymphocyte-like, although lacking B or T cell markers (polymorphs, eosinophils, and macrophages may in some circumstances behave similarly). The antibody-coated target cell is killed as a result of direct contact with the K cell. This process, which is independent of complement, is termed antibody-dependent cellular cytotoxicity (ADCC), and requires only a very low density of antibody molecules of any IgG class on the target cell surface to initiate killing. The Fc receptors on K cells bind free cytophilic antibody molecules poorly and in practice bind only to arrays of Fc determinants of antibodies already complexed with the target cell. Conversely, the F(ab) sites of homocytotropic IgE molecules bound to the receptors of mast cells and basophils have to be crosslinked by reacting with di- or polyvalent antigen before preformed histamine and other pharmacological mediators of inflammation are released from these cells as a result of antigen–antibody interaction.

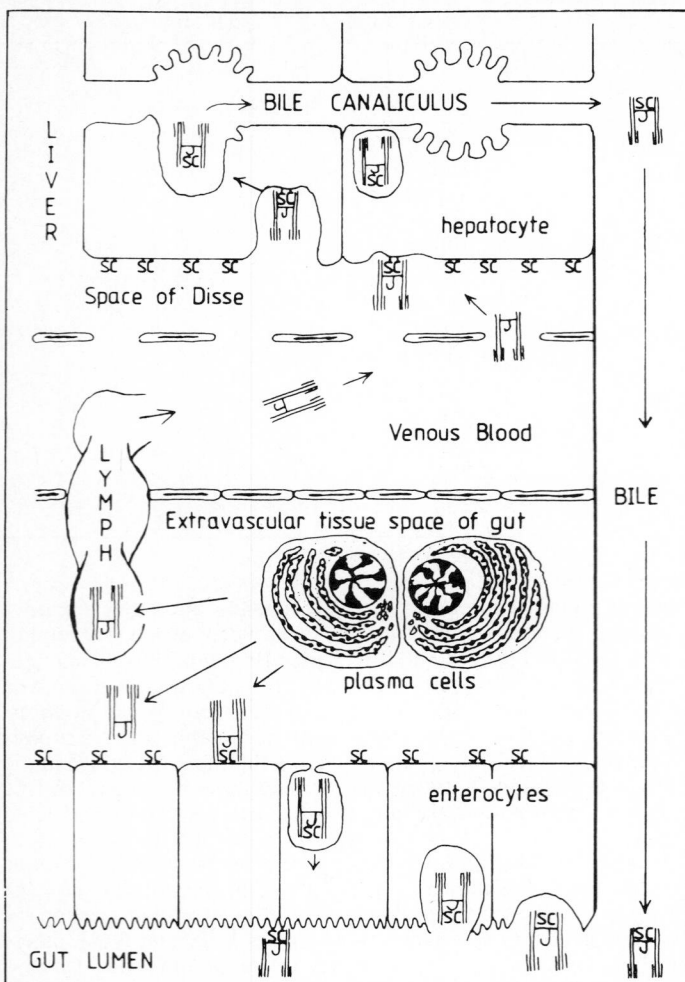

Fig. 4 Diagram of the pathways by which IgA reaches the gut. The submucosal plasma cells secrete IgA, dimerized by J chain, into the extravascular tissue space of the gut. Some of this dimeric IgA unites immediately with secretory component (SC) on the basal aspect of the enterocytes; the IgA-SC complex is transported across the cytoplasm in endocytic vasicles and discharged into the lumen of the gut. The remaining IgA is collected into the lymphatic lacteals and conveyed, via the intestinal and thoracic ducts, to the great veins.

The IgA then circulates in the blood until it reaches the portal vein where it quickly passes through the fenestrated endothelium of the portal sinusoids and unites with SC on the hepatocyte membrane. Endocytic vesicles carry the IgA-SC complex across the hepatocyte cytoplasm and discharge it into the biliary system which conveys it to the duodenum. (From Hall, J. G. and Andrew, E. (1980). *Immunology Today*, **1**, 100, by permission)

Interactions of complement with cells. Complement is a multimolecular activation system of plasma proteins dependent in part on the sequential activation of a series of proteolytic zymogens which promote phagocytosis, inflammation, and, when activation is at or near the surface of a target cell, membrane damage leading to cell lysis.

The predominant component of the complement cascade both quantitatively and functionally is the third component, C3. Initiation of complement activation leads by different pathways to cleavage of C3 into a larger fragment (C3b) and a smaller fragment (C3a), both of which have important biological properties. In C3b two functional sites are revealed, a hydrophobic site for attachment to cell membranes, or to the initiating antigen–antibody complex, and an enzymatic site for the next component in the sequence.

Antigen–antibody complexes initiate the *classical pathway* of C3 activation by generating a protease, C3 convertase, from the early-

acting complement components. When the first component of complement, C1, is bound to IgG or IgM antibody complexed with antigen, it becomes an active protease, $\overline{C1}$, which catalyses activation of C4 and C2. Together, as $\overline{C42}$, these form C3 convertase. $\overline{C42}$, as well as cleaving C3 into its two active fragments, combines with one of them, C3b, to form $\overline{C423}$, another protease, which in turn activates C5 by cleavage. This is the last enzymatic step in the complement activation sequence, the final event being the formation of a C5b6789 complex (the 'attack' mechanism) which inserts as a macromolecular protein into cell membranes, causing 'holes' (visible on electron microscopy) through which electrolytes escape from and water enters into the cell, leading to lysis.

The C1 component of complement is a complex of three subcomponents, C1q, C1r, and C1s, held together by calcium ions. C1q is a unique protein, of molecular weight 400 000, formed of 18 very similar peptide chains formed into three-stranded fibrils, and having collagen-like sequences near their N-terminal ends. These collagen-like tails associate to give the whole C1q molecule a hexameric structure of six fibrils with six radiating globular heads. It is with these heads that C1q binds to CH2 domains of antibody complexed to antigen, an event that in turn activates the other two C1 sub-components, C1r and C1s, as esterases. Binding of a C1q molecule to even a single molecule of antigen-bound IgM antibody leads to activation of C1 esterase in this way, but at least two adjoining molecules of IgG antibody are required to produce the same effect. If antigen sites binding IgG antibody on a target cell membrane are sparse, the bound antibody may fail to initiate C1 activation. In mediating complement lysis of, say, red cells, IgM antibodies are thus much more efficient than IgG antibodies. For example, rhesus immunization in pregnancy usually produces IgG antibodies which are 'non-complement fixing' because the relevant Rh determinants on the red cell surface are widely spaced. In the classical pathway, in short, C1 esterase activation follows interaction of C1 with IgM or aggregated IgG antibody.

Next, $\overline{C1}$ activates C4 and C2 by splitting both proteins into a and b fragments. C4b, the major fragment of C4, has an attachment site for cell membranes, so that some C4b molecules attach directly to cell membranes in the vicinity of bound $\overline{C1}$, generating C3 convertase there also.

C2 is highly labile, however, and this modulates production of C3 convertase. Another controlling factor is the presence in normal plasma of $\overline{C1}$INH, an inhibitor of C1 esterase activity (and also of kallikrein and Hageman factor). $\overline{C1}$INH is absent, or, if present, non-functional, in hereditary angioedema, an episodic disorder due to an autosomal dominant gene. As a result serum levels of C4 and C2 (but not C3) are chronically reduced in this condition, and even more so during attacks.

C3 convertase splits the main complement component, C3, into C3a and C3b, fragments which both undertake important interactions with cells. C3a is released into the fluid phase, where on reaching mast cells and basophils in the vicinity it stimulates histamine release. This is a property it shares with C5a, as noted below, and for this functional resemblance to IgE, these two fragments are designated anaphylotoxins.

The largest fragment, C3b, plays a central part in immunological inflammation, subserving several different roles (Fig. 5). Cell surface receptors for C3b are present on polymorphs and on macro-

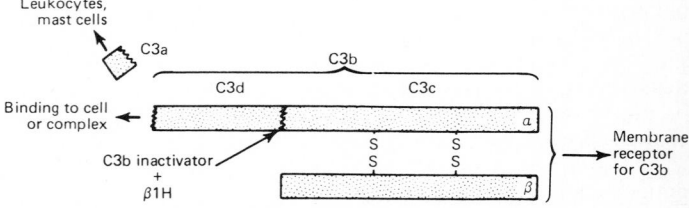

Fig. 5 Schematic model of the C3 molecule. (From Cooper, N. R., 1980. In *Basic and clinical immunology*, ed. H. H. Fudenberg, et al., 86. Lange, Los Altos, by permission)

phages, so that complement activation on antibody-coated particles (bacteria, red cells, and immune complexes), with deposition of C3b promotes efficient *adherence* of such particles to these phagocytic cells. With IgM class antibody alone, adherence produced in this fashion by complement does not itself facilitate subsequent ingestion, but if IgG antibody is also involved, ingestion is strongly expedited through collaboration with Fc receptors on the same cells. Fixed C3b thus plays a highly important role in defence as an opsonin.

As well as this, however, C3b is also an *initiator of cell function*. Macrophages exposed even to isolated C3b become activated, acquiring an increased tendency to spread on surfaces and increased pinocytotic activity, together with an ability to secrete proteases and, now, to ingest particles coated only with IgM antibody and complement.

B lymphocytes, too, have C3b receptors, which are thought to play a part in triggering antibody synthesis, and, in addition, to be involved in the complement-dependent trapping of circulating soluble antigen–antibody complexes in germinal centres in lymphoid organs. Such localization of complexes in germinal centres is part of the mechanism for generating B cell memory to T-dependent antigens.

C3b receptors are also present on primate erythrocytes, where their function is at present unknown. Their presence explains the immune-adherence reaction, long recognized as occurring between human red cells and complement-fixing immune complexes. Finally, it must be mentioned that C3b receptors are found on human renal glomeruli, which may well account at least in part for the localization of certain circulating immune complexes in the kidney.

The various activities of the C3b fragment are restricted by the presence of another proteolytic enzyme, C3b inactivator, which acts together with a second protein termed β1H, and possibly also with serum plasmin, to cleave C3b into inactive fragments, C3c and C3d. C3c diffuses away in the fluid phase, but if the C3b has been bound to a membrane or particle, C3d remains firmly bound at the site. Macrophages carry a special receptor for C3d, so that phagocytosis of IgG coated particles on which bound C3b has been inactivated is still assured. Likewise, to ensure elicitation of a positive direct Coomb's test with complement-coated erythrocytes, antisera with unequivocal anti-C3d specificity are to be preferred.

Because of its small molecular weight (30 000), C3d diffuses rapidly into the plasma from extravascular sites of fluid phase activation of complement. For this reason, and its relative stability, determination of plasma C3d levels are a useful index of complement activation in systemic disease.

Of the C3b activated by membrane-bound $\overline{C42}$, a portion combines with the latter, as noted above, to form a new $\overline{C423}$ protease which cleaves C5, again into a and b fragments. C5a is released into the fluid phase where, as we have seen, it has an anaphylotoxic activity similar to that of C3a. C5a also serves as a potent chemotaxin, attracting directed migration of polymorphs and macrophages to the site of its formation. At the same time it increases the adhesiveness of polymorphs, thus favouring their margination in the local blood vessels.

C5b joins with C6 and then with C7 to form a trimolecular complex which is inserted into the lipid of the cell membrane. On addition of C8, channels are opened in the membrane, initiating lysis, and this is accelerated by the presence of the last component, C9.

Although cell lysis by the classical pathway C1–C9 is triggered by the combination of C1q with antibody aggregates (with or without antigen), other substances which bind C1q may also initiate this pathway. These include DNA, heparin, and dextran sulphate (all polyanions), and also C-reactive protein, one of the *acute phase reactants* that are part of the rapid non-specific inflammatory response to tissue damage. On binding its substrate, phosphatyl choline, which is a ubiquitous component of mammalian cell membrane phospholipid, C-reactive protein also acquires the ability to bind C1q, and in this way activates the classical pathway as efficiently as antibody.

C3 convertase, however, may equally be generated by a different route, independent of both the early complement components and antibody. Activation of this *alternative pathway* involves two steps —initiation and amplification. Initiation requires cleavage of C3 in the fluid phase, with deposition of the resulting C3b on particle or membrane sites which are protected from the action of C3b inactivator and β1H. The initial cleavage mechanism is not clearly understood, but it is suggested that spontaneous conformational change allows C3 to bind to a plasma zymogen termed factor B. A second zymogen, factor D, activates the C3B complex to generate the first C3 convertase of this pathway, $\overline{C3Bb}$. The proteolytic action of this enzyme on native C3 then generates metastable C3b which is capable of binding to membrane or particle sites. Among particles active in this respect are solid polysaccharides such as zymosan and inulin, aggregated IgA, certain bacteria, viruses, virus-infected cells, and parasites. Amplification begins with the binding of factor B to the newly generated C3b molecule and its subsequent cleavage into Ba and Bb by factor D. The resulting surface-bound complex $\overline{C3bBb}$ is capable of cleaving C3, and thus generating more C3b which on binding repeats the process, and so on, providing positive feedback (Fig. 6). Thus the product (C3b) of the substrate (C3) of the activating enzyme ($\overline{C3bBb}$) becomes a subunit of that enzyme. Furthermore, addition of another C3b molecule to the activating enzyme forms a protease which activated C5. This C5 convertase is very labile, and the protein properdin plays its part in the alternative pathway by stabilizing it. Control of the whole amplification stage of alternative pathway activation of C3 is exercised by β1H protein, which blocks the factor B binding site on C3b, the resulting complex being rapidly inactivated by C3b INA. In some patients with mesangiocapillary glomerulonephritis the very low levels of plasma C3 found are due to the effect of an auto-antibody (C3 NeF) against $\overline{C3bBb}$ protecting it against inactivation by C3b INA. This is an example of persistent activation of the alternative pathway in human disease.

It has been suggested that the alternative pathway of complement activation, being independent of antibody, is phylogenetically older as a defence against micro-organisms. In many biological contexts it produces the same effects as the classical pathway, but is less efficient on dilution and acts more slowly. The C3b-dependent positive feedback mechanism, however, markedly augments the antibody-mediated classical activation pathway.

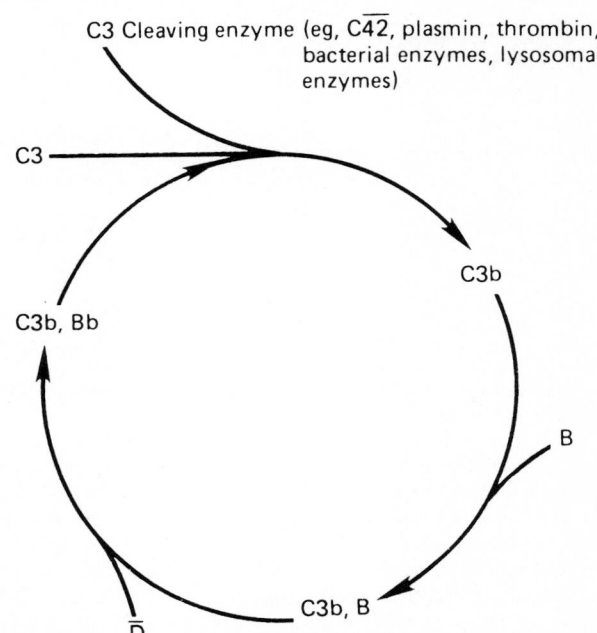

Fig. 6 The C3b-dependent positive feedback mechanism. (From Cooper, N. R., 1980. In *Basic and clinical immunology*, ed. H. H. Fudenberg *et al.*, 88. Lange, Los Altos, by permission)

Types of allergic tissue damage

Immune reactions which trigger the non-specific tissue mechanisms of inflammation discussed above can be amplified to a level which is recognizable clinically as immunologically mediated disease.

The most useful classification of tissue-damaging hypersensitivity reactions at present available is based on initiating mechanisms—that is, the circumstances of the initial reaction with antigen. Three types of initiating mechanism involving humoral antibody may be distinguished under the general heading of immediate hypersensitivity.

Antibody-mediated tissue damage

Reaginic damage. The signs and symptoms of generalized anaphylaxis that may follow within minutes the parenteral injection of foreign serum, protein, or drugs, or sometimes even insect bites or stings in a sensitized individual, include a marked fall in blood pressure with profound and possibly fatal shock, intense dyspnoea, and urticaria. They occur because combination of antigen with cell-bound IgE antibody activates enzymes in mast cells and basophils and causes the release of vaso-active agents—histamine, serotonin, slow-reacting substance, and kinins—which increase capillary permeability, alter vascular tone, and stimulate contraction of smooth muscle (Fig. 7). General anaphylaxis is rare in man, however; in the 10 per cent or so of the population who becomes sensitized by ordinary everyday exposure to antigens like pollen or house-dust mites, the antigen–antibody interaction takes place not systemically, but locally. At a mucosal surface of such atopic individuals—the eye, nose, or bronchus—local activation and release of these same agents produces immediate conjunctivitis, rhinorrhoea, or bronchospasm.

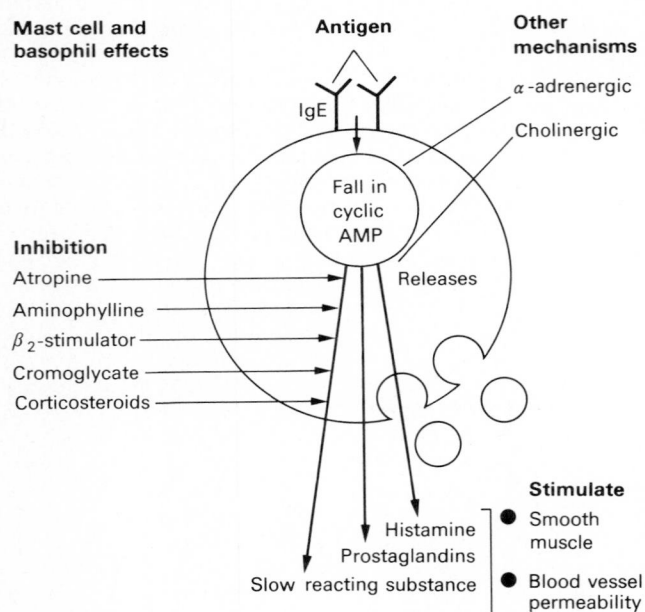

Fig. 7   Mast cell and basophil effects. (From *Medicine International* (1981), **1**, no. 5., by permission)

The cytotropic property of IgE is demonstrated in the classical Prausnitz–Kustner (P–K) test which makes use of another manifestation of local anaphylaxis, the wheal response to a skin prick with test antigen. This was initially shown by injecting a small quantity of serum from an atopic individual into the skin of a non-atopic person, a reaction at the injection site being elicited by a subsequent challenge with the same antigen. What is relevant here is that the challenge could be withheld for several days after the initial passive sensitization; yet when the challenge was eventually made, it elicited an immediate unequivocal specific reaction. The

essential feature of such cytotropic antibodies, known as reagins, is this ability to become absorbed to Fc receptors on the surfaces of basophil (mast) cells that produce histamine and other pharmacologically active agents. In effect, such cells become 'allergized' with respect to antigen; and it is only when cell-bound in this way that reaginic antibody is able to produce an anaphylactic response as a result of encounter with specific antigen.

In man, reaginic antibodies of IgE class are the chief mediators of human atopic hypersensitivity of immediate type. The term atopy describes a familial tendency to develop abnormal hypersensitivity to common antigens, and the atopic trait may be defined as the spontaneous tendency in an individual to produce high levels of IgE antibody against one or more common antigens, in association with antigen-provoked disorders in which reaginic mechanisms can be identified. Examples of atopic disorders are extrinsic allergic asthma, allergic rhinitis and hay fever, vernal keratoconjunctivitis, and cow's milk hypersensitivity in infants. Apart from familial factors, immunoglobulin deficiencies, especially of IgA production in the MALT system, and immunoregulatory defects of T cell function, appear to predispose to atopy. The efficacy of antigen avoidance in infancy in circumventing such predisposition is seen in the advantage conferred by breast-feeding as against bottle-feeding. In the commonest clinical manifestations of atopy, such as extrinsic asthma and allergic rhinitis, serum IgE levels are usually normal, but raised antigen-specific IgE antibody levels are demonstrable by the radio-allergosorbent test (RAST), the results of which mostly parallel those obtained by prick tests in the patient's skin, although the RAST is rather less sensitive. In atopic eczema and bronchopulmonary aspergillosis IgE levels may reach several times normal values and are often raised in some parasitic, especially helminthic, diseases particularly in tropical countries, where vigorous IgE responses are seen in parasitic infection of the bowel. IgE-mediated expulsive reactions play a large part in host immunity against worm infections of the gut, and IgE also mediates the mast cell and eosinophil responses to schistosomula tissue infestation in schistosomiasis. A lesser incidence is claimed for atopic conditions in the tropics where parasitic infestation is rife, and it may well be that the emergence of clinical forms of atopy in developed countries is a result of a reduction in parasitic load.

Membrane-reactive damage. We have next to consider tissue damage arising from the interaction of free circulating antibody with antigen already forming part of a cell surface or a tissue membrane. Such antigen may be a normal integral component, or may have been initially separate and have become bound by surface adsorption. In either case one result of an encounter with specific antibody is damage to the membrane carrying the antigen, and if this is a cell membrane, lysis and death of the cell.

A familiar illustration of the cytotoxic action of antibody through cell membrane damage is immune haemolysis following incompatible blood transfusion. To reproduce such haemolysis in the test-tube, complement must be added to the mixture of incompatible red cells and serum, and it is characteristic of most cytotoxic antibodies that they achieve their effect by directing the cytotoxic action of serum complement toward a specific target cell in this way. In complement activation, as we have seen, at several points short of final lytic activity intermediate compounds are produced which themselves have important biological effects. These are: (*a*) anaphylatoxins, which are histamine releasers and hence the means by which formation of complement-fixing IgM and IgG antigen–antibody reactions in the tissues can lead to altered vascular permeability and smooth muscle contraction; (*b*) leucocyte chemotactic factors; and (*c*) opsonizing factors which promote phagocytosis locally by causing immune complexes to adhere to the surfaces of red cells, leucocytes, or platelets (immune adherence) and indeed to the surfaces of phagocytic cells themselves, in this way considerably enhancing the function of the latter.

Cytotoxic antibodies are not invariably complement-fixing. In haemolytic disease of the newborn where placental bleeds of

Rhesus-positive red cells have provided an antigenic stimulus for production of anti-Rh iso-antibodies by a Rhesus-negative mother, the destruction of fetal red cells is due to IgG 'incomplete' antibody passively acquired across the placenta. Complement is not involved here, since the Rhesus epitopes involved are too widely spaced to permit C1q molecules to bind to more than one IgG antibody molecule, and there is little intravascular haemolysis. The cytotoxic action of the anti-red-cell antibody is due rather to its opsonizing effect, the red cells being cleared from the circulation and destroyed later by the phagocytic cells of the spleen. Immune haemolytic anaemia may also arise following administration of drugs which form a stable haptenic bond with circulating red cells. Penicillin and cephalosporin act in this manner, their active metabolites binding to both plasma proteins and membrane-associated proteins of the red cell. In this way is provided both the immunogenic stimulus to production of anti-drug antibodies (which, in the case of penicillin, are present in the IgM class in more than 90 per cent of normal people), and the potential target for their action. Immune haemolytic anaemia due to penicillin, however, occurs only in patients receiving very large doses, whose red cells become heavily coated, and even then in only a small percentage of cases. In the latter, the antibody is usually of the IgG class, so that red cell destruction is non-lytic and effected by splenic sequestration. The comparative rarity of these drug-induced immune blood dyscrasias presumably reflects the instability of most drug-cell complexes and their resulting very poor immunogenicity.

It is not surprising that examples of antibody-mediated cell damage are most easily found among blood dyscrasias, where cells can readily be tested for antibody and complement. The immunopathology of each condition, however, whether affecting red cells, platelets, or leucocytes, has its own characteristic features, so that in the auto-immune haemolytic anaemias, for example, the breadth of the clinical spectrum of disease due to shortened red cell survival reflects the wide variety of red cell auto-antibodies of different isotypes, specificities, affinities, thermal optima, and complement fixing ability that have been distinguished. The effects produced by auto-antibodies against membrane components of other tissue cells depend upon the functions of the membrane antigens involved, and cover a clinical spectrum ranging from thyrotoxicosis, where antibody against thyrotrophin receptors on thyroid epithelial cells stimulates the latter to pathological activity, to myasthenia gravis, where antibody to the acetyl-choline receptor of muscle end plates impairs transmission at the neuromuscular junction. Damage brought about by the action of specific antibody against basement membrane is seen rarely in the kidney, where it affects not individual cell surfaces but the integrity of the glomerular basement membrane itself. In man, immunofluorescent studies show that in about 1 per cent of cases of chronic glomerulonephritis immunoglobulin is bound in linear fashion to the injured basement membrane together with complement. In Goodpasture's syndrome anti-basement membrane antibody is deposited on the alveolar basement membrane in the lung as well as in the glomeruli, and free antibody is often present in the blood also.

Immune complexes. So far, we have considered the effects of immune reactions on local tissues when the participating antibody or antigen is bound, for one reason or another, at the surfaces of cells or membranes. When both participants in the antigen-antibody encounter are free, the immune complexes that result are no less able to provoke tissue responses, especially when complement is activated in the reaction; but the distribution of tissue damage is now independent of localizing effects due to antigen or antibody separately, and is determined instead by the site of deposition of the immune complexes formed. This in turn is influenced by their solubility.

A high degree of lattice formation between interacting antigen and antibody molecules leads to formation of large complexes which eventually become insoluble, precipitate, and, partly through complement activation, induce Arthus reactions in which

the granulocytes play a prominent phagocytic role in their disposal. Lesser degrees of lattice formation produce complexes which remain soluble. This occurs under conditions of antigen excess, or when there is a low density of determinants on antigen molecules, or when the affinity of the antibody involved is low. Complement also plays an important role in stabilizing complex deposits, as discussed below.

The immunopathogenetic potential of soluble immune complexes is inversely related to their rate of clearance from the circulation. This depends both upon their composition and upon their ability to activate the phagocytic cells of the reticulo-endothelial system. Phagocytic human macrophages have surface receptors for the Fc portions of IgG subgroups 1 and 3, and bind complexes containing these immunoglobulins. Here again the degree of lattice formation is an important factor in their removal, small complexes with mono- or bivalent antigen persisting in the circulation, but the role of antibody of other immunoglobulin classes is less clearly identified. It seems that specific receptors on macrophages can become saturated under conditions of persistent antigen and immune complex formation, resulting in the continued circulation of complexes which would otherwise have been cleared.

Soluble complexes in the circulation eventually become deposited in capillary endothelium. The factors governing the site of deposition of circulating immune complexes are imperfectly understood, but they presumably operate by increasing vascular permeability locally, or through properties of the antigen itself. It appears, for example, that DNA has an affinity for renal basement membrane, so that the immune complex deposits demonstrable in the glomeruli in the glomerulonephritis of systemic lupus erythematosus, which contain DNA as antigen and anti-DNA as antibody, may localize in the kidney as a result of this property of DNA. Alternatively, IgE antibodies interacting with antigen locally may induce the vascular permeability which determines localization of immune complexes containing antibodies of other classes. A third possibility is primary vascular damage due to viral infection. Most of the resulting damage seems to follow from the deposition and activation of complement at the site, and the accompanying activation of the enzymic systems of coagulation, fibrinolysis, and kinin formation compound the tissue injury.

The Arthus reaction, and serum sickness, are respectively effects due to insoluble and soluble complexes. In the experimental animal, the Arthus reaction is a localized acute necrotizing vasculitis, initially appearing about four hours after injection of soluble antigen locally in the presence of circulating precipitating IgG antibody. Essential to its development is the coexistence of a high serum concentration of antibody and a high extravascular concentration of soluble antigen; the resulting contrary diffusion gradients lead to antigen–antibody interactions under conditions favouring formation of precipitates, which are deposited in considerable amounts in the local vessel walls. Fixation of complement follows, with production of the biologically active intermediates already noted, increased vascular permeability, and—characteristic of the Arthus reaction—attraction of leucocytes, especially polymorphs, which engulf and digest the immune precipitates. In doing so they contribute significantly to local tissue damage through the high concentration of acid hydrolytic enzymes released from their activated lysosomes.

In man Arthus reactions of this type occur when antigen is introduced extravascularly in the presence of high titre intravascular precipitins. These conditions used to occur in patients receiving repeated therapeutic serum injections, and are seen in patients receiving heterologous antilymphocyte antibodies as an immunosuppressant. In pulmonary disease due to certain inhaled organic antigens, such as thermophilic actinomyces (farmer's lung) and *Aspergillus fumigatus* (bronchopulmonary aspergillosis), serum precipitins against these fungal antigens commonly develop, and an Arthus type of reaction is elicited by skin-testing these patients with the appropriate antigen. Challenge (carefully monitored) by the endobronchial route causes an Arthus reaction clinically manifested by severe symptoms, systemic as well as local, and character-istic of the disease itself.

The serum sickness that in man and animals follows a single large injected dose of foreign serum, is, in contrast, a generalized con-dition, with onset after about 10 days. The signs and symptoms arise when antibodies to the foreign protein begin to appear at a time when the latter is still present in the body in considerable amount. Some of them—bronchospasm, vomiting, diarrhoea, urticaria, and shock—are immediate anaphylactic responses due to IgE anti-body binding to mast cells and involving mucous membrane, skin, and smooth muscle in its interaction with antigen. More prolonged effects on the joints, heart, and especially the kidney are brought about by immune complexes formed in the circulation by combi-nation of IgG antibody with persisting antigen. Figure 8 shows the temporal relationship between the latter events. After an initial drop due to equilibration between intra- and extravascular fluids serum levels of antigen fall slowly; but after a week or so the rate of loss from the serum increases sharply, and soon free antigen is replaced by free antibody. The phase of rapid antigen loss rep-resents elimination due to interaction with newly formed antibody. Antigen–antibody complexes begin to form in a milieu at first of gross, and later of moderate antigen excess. As in the classical quantitative precipitin curve, immune complexes formed in antigen excess are soluble. It is during this phase, when soluble complexes are circulating in the blood, that acute inflammatory lesions begin to occur in the joints, heart, and kidney. When formed under appropriate conditions of moderate antigen excess, complexes at-tain a critical macromolecular size which favours their trapping by basement membranes or by the internal elastic laminae of blood vessels. Once trapped on membranes, their complement-fixing prop-erty is enhanced, and the inflammatory changes ensue. Immuno-fluorescence shows that in the kidney of experimental serum sick-ness immune complexes are deposited on the glomerular base-ment membrane in a pattern that is characteristically granular and irregular, and contrasts with the smoothly linear attachment of specific antibasement-membrane antibody described above. Elec-tron microscopy of affected glomeruli shows electron-dense aggre-gates deposited on the epithelial side of the basement membrane.

In 'one-shot' serum sickness the scattered lesions are transient, since with increasing antibody production soluble complexes are no longer formed, and recovery occurs. Acute post-streptococcal glomerulonephritis is a parallel condition, for here too, although renal biopsies taken during the attack have shown immunoglobu-lin, complement and streptococcal antigen bound to the glomeru-lus, complete recovery is the rule. Immune complexes probably play a part in this way in many acute infections. Another example is meningococcal meningitis, where following penicillin treatment there may be a second phase of fever, skin rash, and arthritis due to formation of immune complexes between newly formed antibody and bacterial polysaccharide disseminated in the tissues. Since this occurs in only about 10 per cent of such patients, other host factors affecting antigen disposal or antibody production are presumably operating as well. Thus (to take a further example) the acute haemorrhage shock seen in a small minority of children developing dengue fever is attributable to previous sensitization with a cross-reacting strain of the arbovirus responsible. Some drug-induced haemolytic anaemias and thrombocytopenic purpuras are likewise the result of immune complex formation. Binding of the drug to serum protein may produce an immunogenic compound, and when this happens immune complexes with antibody result, which in turn bind to red cells by immune adherence involving complement. Cell destruction is brought about by opsonization or by lysis.

Chronic progressive disease can develop when conditions are such that soluble complexes are constantly renewed in the blood. When rabbits are repeatedly injected intravenously with soluble antigen, some of them develop proteinuria, rising blood urea, and renal failure, and their kidneys show glomerular deposits of Ig, C3, and antigen on immunofluorescent examination. The amount of antigen given at each injection is critical, chronic glomerulonephri-tis developing only if periods of antigen excess are induced, with resulting chronic formation of circulating soluble immune com-plexes. This experimental regimen mimics events in several chronic infectious diseases in which immune complex deposition rather than direct infection appears to be responsible for complications which frequently include glomerulonephritis, arthritis, skin lesions such as erythema nodosum, and vasculitic lesions. Well docu-mented examples of such chronic infections are subacute bacterial endocarditis, viral hepatitis (especially when a chronic carrier state for HBsAg supervenes), leprosy, and quartan malaria. In malarial nephrosis in African children, the parasite (*Plasmodium malariae*) has been constantly present in the blood from infancy, but when antibody begins to be formed during early childhood under condi-tions as yet unexplained, formation of soluble complexes with malarial antigen occurs (Fig. 9), nephrosis develops, and renal biopsy shows the characteristic deposits of immunoglobulin, com-plement, and *P. malariae* antigen. The worst prognosis is in cases where the fixed IgG is not complement-fixing, which may parallel the situation in immune complex nephritis complicating comple-ment deficiencies (see below).

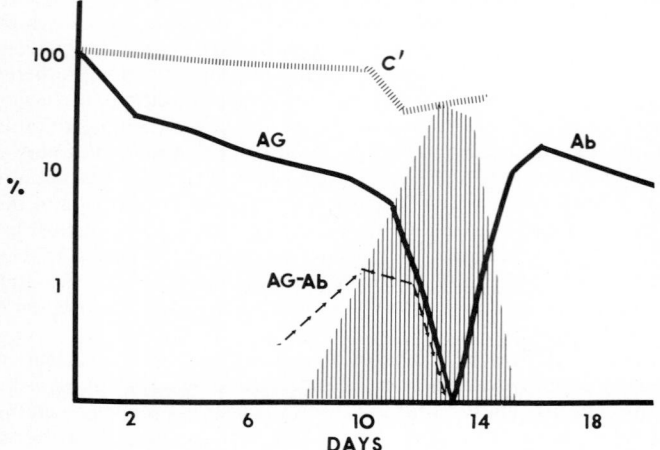

Fig. 8 'One-shot' serum sickness in the rabbit. 250 mg isotope-labelled bovine serum albumin injected intravenously at day 0. With the appearance of antigen-antibody complexes (AG–Ab) there is a fall in serum com-plement (C) and the appearance of lesions in heart, blood vessels, joints, and kidneys (shaded area). With elimination of complexes free antibody (Ab) appears in the serum, and the inflammatory lesions subside. (Redrawn from Cochrane, C. G. and Dixon, F. J., (1969). In *Immunopathology*, vol. 1. Grune and Stratton. New York, by permission)

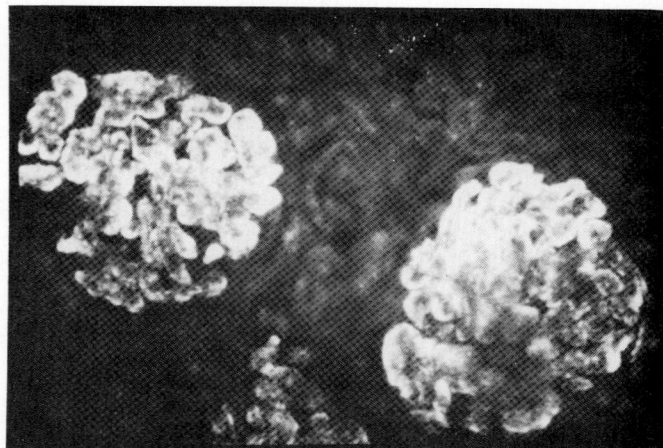

Fig. 9 Cryostat section of renal biopsy from an African child with malarial nephrosis, treated with fluorescein-labelled antihuman IgG antibody and viewed on a fluorescence microscope. Staining of the IgG component shows the immune complexes deposited in granular fashion on the glomerular basement membrane. (Courtesy of Dr V. Houba)

Another source of persistent antigen in the body is tissue constituents which have acquired auto-immune status. In rheumatoid arthritis the major antigen contributing to immune complex formation is the IgG molecule. In patients with this condition immune complexes result predominantly from self-association of IgG molecules that themselves have rheumatoid factor (anti-IgG) activity, as well as from additional or alternative association with IgM rheumatoid factor as auto-antibody. A main site of rheumatoid factor synthesis in rheumatoid disease is in the inflamed synovial membrane of the affected joints. The immune complexes thus generated in the rheumatoid joint are complement-activating and have an inflammatory effect, so that rheumatoid arthritis, so far as the joints are concerned, may be regarded as an extravascular form of immune complex disease. Similar complexes circulating in the blood appear to account for the systemic vasculitic lesions which are seen in a minority of cases of rheumatoid disease, but in most rheumatoid arthritis patients, even when systemic lesions are absent or trivial, complexes in which IgG is a major component are detectable in the blood, circulating apparently harmlessly.

In another disease of connective tissue, systemic lupus erythematosus, auto-antibodies to several different autologous tissue antigens are present, of which anti-DNA, giving rise to DNA–anti-DNA complex deposits in the renal and skin lesions, is most clearly incriminated in the immune complex pathology. As noted above, however, the circulating immune complexes frequently present in the blood of SLE patients probably mainly involve tissue antigens other than DNA.

The relationship between circulating immune complexes and clinical features of diseases, or disease activity, is thus not a simple one. Many methods are in use to detect soluble immune complexes, based on physiochemical separation techniques, or on the ability of complexes to interact with humoral or cellular receptors either for the determinants of antibody molecules, or for complement components bound to the complexes. Most available methods therefore do not detect or identify the antigen component. A given test, moreover, may detect only a restricted population of complexes which carry appropriate determinants. The question arises, therefore, what is the value to the clinician of measurement of immune complexes, especially as immune complexes are to be found, for example, even in the sera of apparently healthy people after meals? We have seen above, furthermore, that IgA immune complexes participate in normal clearance mechanisms, and this presumably holds also for complexes containing antibodies of other isotypes.

At present, detection of circulating immune complexes provides no diagnostic aid to the clinician. The pathogenetic potential of immune complexes relates to their ability to saturate or otherwise avoid the normal clearance mechanisms of complement and the mononuclear phagocytic system, or to functional disturbance of the latter.

The size, range, and the concentration of complexes determine their fate and hence their pathogenicity. The usefulness of immune complex determinations on serum specimens in monitoring disease activity, or the effects of treatment, thus depends as much upon qualitative as quantitative assessment. In biopsy specimens, however, the separate identification of antibody classes and complement components in immune deposits in the kidney or in the skin, for example, may have important diagnostic implications.

Cell-mediated tissue damage. In individuals sensitized by exposure, application of some chemicals to the skin produces a local dermatitis that takes 24 hours or so to develop. The substances that produce this contact hypersensitivity have in common the property of reacting with skin proteins to form hapten–protein conjugates of potent antigenicity in the individual concerned. Skin hypersensitivity arising in this way is a common cause of acute or chronic allergic contact dermatitis associated with exposure of the skin to metals, solvents, resins, some simple reactive chemicals like picryl chloride or dinitrochlorobenzine, cosmetics, antibiotics, and other drugs.

Contact hypersensitivity resembles in kind delayed hypersensitivity—formerly known as bacterial allergy, and represented by the tuberculin reaction; this is another relatively slowly developing hypersensitivity reaction elicited by injecting a protein or hapten—protein conjugate into the skin of an appropriately sensitized subject. Contact hypersensitivity and delayed hypersensitivity reactions are highly specific and share the characteristic feature that for the eliciting antigen specificity resides as much in the protein-carrier as in the hapten carried. This is unlike antibody-mediated (immediate or anaphylactic) hypersensitivity, where the response is hapten-specific. Landsteiner and Chase showed that contact hypersensitivity induced in guinea-pigs to the simple chemical picryl chloride could be transmitted to normal guinea-pigs by injecting them with living peritoneal exudate cells from hypersensitive animals, but not by antiserum, however potent, and this introduced the notion that lymphoid cells themselves can effect immune responses directly, without antibody as intermediary.

The essential histological change in delayed hypersensitivity reactions in the skin is local tissue damage in the neighbourhood of an infiltrate of mononuclear cells made up of lymphocytes and monocytes, and both of these cell types contribute to producing the lesion. The lymphocytes are drawn from the recirculating pool of immunologically competent, and in this case, immunologically active cells, already sensitized and thus arrested at the site of local concentration of antigen by specific interaction with it. This interaction liberates lymphokines which attract and activate blood monocytes, cells that have originated from rapidly proliferating precursors in the bone marrow, and eventually contribute 80–90 per cent of the inflammatory cells in the delayed hypersensitivity lesion. It is these activated monocytes which are evidently the nonspecific (in the immunological sense) effectors of actual tissue damage, for in the Chase type of transfer experiment recipients deprived by irradiation of these bone marrow precursors cannot mount delayed reactions. Activated macrophages produce damage to target cells by direct membrane action or by secretion of damaging hydrolytic enzymes. That the interaction of sensitized lymphocytes with antigen produces a biological effect is demonstrated in vitro by the inhibition of macrophage migratory activity brought about by adding antigen to tissue cultures containing both normal macrophages and lymphocytes from specifically sensitized donors. This provides a useful method of studying delayed hypersensitivity in vitro. Other effects of lymphokines are to recruit lymphocytes, and to act as interferons.

A similar histological picture of lymphocyte and macrophage infiltration is seen in homografts undergoing rejection. Medawar's classical experiments on induction of acquired immunological tolerance of skin homografts in mice, and more particularly the demonstration that tolerance could be terminated by adoptive immunization using transferred lymphoid cells, though not immune serum alone, established that cell-mediated rather than humoral immunity provides a major effector mechanism of homograft rejection. Furthermore, guinea-pigs that had rejected skin homografts gave delayed hypersensitivity reactions to intradermal injection of killed cells, or cell-free extracts, from the same skin donor; while their own lymphocytes excited a typical delayed hypersensitivity when injected intradermally into the same donor. To elicit the latter, however, the lymphocytes had to be living, thus reproducing essentially the conditions of the Chase passive transfer system, except that now sensitized lymphocytes were being injected locally into skin in which transplantation antigens were naturally present.

Thus contact hypersensitivity, delayed hypersensitivity, and the homograft reaction are examples of tissue damage brought about by cell-mediated immunity. As well as producing inflammatory changes through the agency of macrophages and monocytes, sensitized lymphocytes are apparently capable of direct cytotoxic effects on cells carrying histocompatibility antigens, viral antigens, passively acquired antigens, and tumour antigens. The specifically sensitized lymphocytes are T cells, probably belonging to the cytotoxic subpopulation mentioned above. As mobile cells, they bring themselves into close surface-to-surface apposition with one or more target cells and the effect of this close contact between cell membranes is to produce local damage to the target cell which progresses to osmotic cell death.

Another type of cell-mediated cytotoxicity is antibody-dependent. Mononuclear cells present in human blood which have no readily demonstrable surface Ig but possess receptors for IgG Fc regions act against target cells which have been sensitized by coating with specific antibody, the killer (K) cells in question not being specifically sensitized themselves. Their cytotoxic activity towards cells sensitized with histocompatibility antibodies, certain tumour antibodies, and viral antibodies is demonstrable *in vitro*, and it seems likely that they form a significant proportion of the cells in mononuclear cell infiltrates in tissues or organs which are the site of chronic immunologically mediated inflammatory damage.

Auto-immunity and self-tolerance

The specificity of the acquired immunological tolerance experimentally inducible in animals by inoculation of, say, newborn mice of one strain with tissue cells from a mouse of another strain is expressed in the identical strain-selective nature of the ability of the recipient subsequently to accept homografts. This was strong support for Burnet's clonal selection hypothesis of antibody production (and of cell-mediated immunity).

An intrinsic feature of adaptive immunity is self-tolerance, that is, the ability to adjust immune responsiveness to discriminate between self and foreign antigens. A healthy person is continually making immune responses to a multiplicity of foreign antigens gaining access to his tissues. Nevertheless, he remains immunologically unresponsive towards his own tissues' constituent macromolecules, although they are immunogenic when injected or grafted into another individual of genetically different make-up (e.g. blood groups or transplantation antigens).

Ideas about self-tolerance have developed in parallel with ideas about how the immune system regulates its own activity. These in turn take their origin from experiments on acquired tolerance (or unresponsiveness) induced to foreign antigens, and from elucidation of the role of the MHC in controlling lymphocyte function.

Potentially immunogenic self-components obviously vary widely in biochemical composition, molecular structure, manner of access, and presentation to the immune system, and in the time during fetal or post-natal life at which they appear. The marked biological diversity of self-antigens, together with the complexity of the cellular organization of the immune system, and the damaging potential of immune reactivity towards self, are likely to have imposed strong evolutionary pressures favouring development of multiple mechanisms for monitoring self-tolerance.

Possible mechanisms of self-tolerance. *Functional deletion of antigen-reactive lymphocytes.* Burnet's clonal selection theory of antibody production carried the corollary that self-reactive lymphocyte clones, generated as a result of rapid somatic mutation during fetal development, are eliminated ('forbidden clones') by contact with the corresponding auto-antigens during this initial period of development. Thus clonal deletion during fetal life was postulated to explain self-tolerance. Since normal individuals were later shown to possess B cells capable of specifically binding a range of auto-antigens such as thyroglobulin and DNA, this could not be retained as a general explanation. However, lymphocytes undoubtedly pass through a stage of ontogeny during which they are particularly susceptible to induction of tolerance. In the case of B lymphocytes, specific reactivity with antigen depends upon the presence of surface antigen receptor in the form of sIg. In the B cell lineage, the first detectable Ig is intracytoplasmic IgM in 'pre-B cells'. Before these cells emerge from their site of origin from haemopoietic stem cells in the fetal liver or bone marrow, Ig appears on their surface. At this stage 'baby B cells' are exquisitely sensitive to cross-linking of surface Ig receptors by antigen, and, when this occurs it aborts further maturation, possibly because it leads to internali-

zation and subsequent failure of re-expression of the receptors in question.

The efficiency of this mechanism of *clonal abortion*, acting at the stage of B cell differentiation, probably depends upon two factors inter-relating surface Ig receptors and antigen, viz. binding affinity and epitope density. Although direct proof is difficult to obtain, clonal abortion probably accounts for the elimination of most self-reactive lymphocytes. Immature B cells that escape this weeding out of autoreactivity probably do so because the concentration of auto-antigen is too low, or its binding affinity too weak. It may be that the postulated elimination within the thymus of thymocytes with receptors for 'self' HLA molecules also represents a species of clonal abortion of T cells.

Receptor blockade. Exposure of mature B cells to high concentrations of specific antigen leads to saturation of their antigen receptors, and this blocks further stimulation. The relevant clones are not eliminated, however, since blockade is reversed *in vitro* by incubation in antigen free medium, or by enzymic degradation of the blocking antigen. Soluble antigens are usually more 'tolerogenic' than aggregated or particulate ones, since they escape phagocytosis and the accompanying macrophage processing, and are thus likely to blockade lymphocyte receptors if presented in sufficient concentration.

Suppressor T cells. A normal consequence of the immune response to foreign antigen is the generation of suppressor T cells which play an essential part in modulating both antibody production and cell-mediated activity. Helper T cells and suppressor T cells are activated by two closely related subsets of 'inducer' T cells (Fig. 10) which control cell interactions at T–T, T–B, and T–macrophage levels. The interactions of these T cell subsets constitute a feedback circuit weighted in favour of suppression to ensure that the effect of antigen is ultimately to dampen the immune response initially engendered. Although suppressor cell activity has been demonstrated experimentally in many instances of induced tolerance to foreign antigen in adult animals, it has also been unequivocally shown that such tolerance can be efficiently established in the

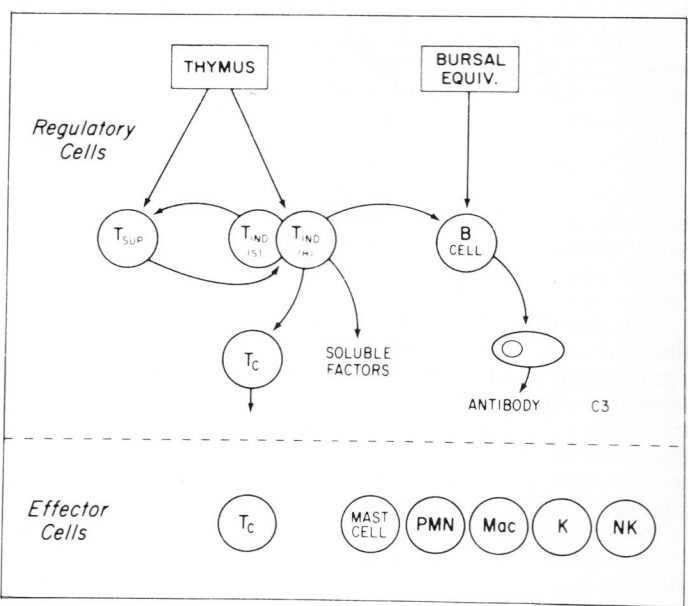

Fig. 10 The human T cell circuit. Cellular and humoral responses are regulated by inducer (T_{IND}) and suppressor (T_{SUP}) T lymphocytes. One subpopulation of cells ($T_{IND(S)}$) induces suppressor cell activation while a second subpopulation of cells ($T_{IND(H)}$) induces help for cytotoxic T cell (T_C) effector function, B cell differentiation, and immunoglobulin production. Many of the effector cells illustrated above including NK, K, mast cells, polymorphonuclear leucocytes (PMN), and macrophages (Mac) are under the influence of these regulatory cells and their products. (From Reinherz, E. L. and Schlossman, S. F. (1981). *Immunology Today*, **2**, 69, by permission)

absence of antigen specific suppressor cells. It seems *a priori* unlikely that suppressor T cells are less susceptible to developing tolerance to antigen than helper or inducer cells, which would appear to be a necessary condition for suppressor cells to play an active part in the maintenance of tolerance to self antigens. At all events, direct evidence of the existence of autosuppressor cells is still fragmentary.

Idiotypes. The heterogeneity which is such a characteristic feature of immunoglobulin molecules arises from the differences in constant domain sequences which distinguish isotypes, the intraspecies differences due to genetic polymorphism which distinguish allotypes, and the myriad differences of sequence in the hypervariable region of Ig V domains which confer antibody diversity. These latter differences themselves have antigenic specificity, and for this reason antibody molecules can be immunogenic in genetically identical individuals, and indeed in the individual in whom the antibody is produced. The antigenic determinants in question are in the V_H and V_L domains, and are termed idiotypes, while antibodies against them are anti-idiotypic.

The network theory (Jerne) of regulation of the immune system proposes that an antigen-specific response results in an antibody response to the idiotypes of the antibody molecules produced by the lymphocyte clones which first respond. The anti-idiotype antibodies produced themselves have idiotype specificity, and hence induce an anti-anti-idiotype response, and so on. The effects of anti-idiotype antibodies appear to be variable, some suppressing and some stimulating cells with surface receptors bearing the complementary idiotype pattern or idiotype. It thus appears that auto-immune responses based on idiotypy may play a fundamental immuno-regulatory role, antibody molecules and B cells forming a network of interactions tending towards a stable condition. The hypervariability of antibody molecules in their V_H and V_L domains makes it inevitable that some of them can recognize self antigens, as Burnet's clonal theory postulates. If idiotypes are immunogenic, this means that the repertoire of self antigens that can be recognized (which includes idiotypes) is vast, and at least co-extensive with the repertoire of antibody idiotypes. This in turn implies that the repertoire of specific responses to foreign antigenic determinants that a given individual can make reflects the extent of the idiotype network his own immune system comprises. The stability of this network, the theory postulates, normally militates against uncontrolled auto-immune responses.

Possible mechanisms of auto-immunity. The 'forbidden clone' theory postulated that somatic mutation could replace clones that had been eliminated during the developmental stage. The ability of experimenters to induce selectively in animals auto-immune conditions such as thyroiditis by injection of thyroglobulin together with appropriate adjuvants, put this interpretation in doubt, and abundant evidence has since been adduced that auto-antigen binding cells, and indeed low titre auto-antigen binding cells, are frequently present in normal subjects. The ability of normal B cells to produce auto-antibodies has been further demonstrated by the use of certain mitogenic substances which behave as B cell activators independently of antigen. Polyclonal B cell mitogens such as pokeweed mitogen, Nocardia antigen, and Epstein–Barr (EB) virus stimulate lymphocytes in culture to produce a heterogeneous range of IgM molecules, some of them with autoreactivity. EB virus is a herpesvirus with a narrow tropism for human B cells, and patients with infectious mononucleosis due to EB virus show the same effect of polyclonal B cell activation, producing transient raised serum levels of IgM auto-antibodies including rheumatoid factors, antinuclear antibodies, and antibodies to cytoskeletal structures. Unlike antibodies produced by antigenic stimulation, the antibodies resulting from polyclonal B cell activation are of relatively low average affinity, since no selection of cells by antigen-binding affinity is involved.

While high concentrations of soluble antigen are required to induce B cell tolerance, T cells are rendered tolerant by exposure to much lower antigen doses. Since most antigens are T-dependent, this means that tolerance produced by low doses of soluble antigen depends upon the unresponsiveness of T cells only, potentially responsive B cells being held in check only because they are deprived of the requisite helper T-cell collaboration. T-dependent antigens behave as if they are composed of two antigenic moieties, a carrier portion with epitopes matching appropriate T cell receptors, and a haptenic portion with high binding affinity for appropriate B cell sIg. It follows that in an individual made tolerant to a T-dependent antigen by low-dose exposure, B cells potentially responsive to the haptenic epitopes in question can be provided with the necessary T-cell help by stimulation with another T-cell dependent antigen of a different specificity but sharing some epitopes with the original tolerogen. By this manoeuvre low-dose tolerance induced experimentally in animals may be broken, and antibody reactive with the shared epitopes of the original tolerogen induced. This T-cell by-pass is illustrated in Fig. 11, which shows the mechanism at work experimentally for inducing auto-antibodies to thyroglobulin and to mouse red cells respectively. A similar mechanism is seen in some forms of human autoimmunity where self-antigens share determinants with micro-organisms gaining access to the tissues. Thus antibodies to Group A haemolytic streptococcal cell wall constituents cross-react with heart muscle antigens, and antibodies to *Escherichia coli* and other intestinal bacteria cross-react with the cells of the colonic mucosa. Such tissue reactive auto-antibodies are found in rheumatic fever and in ulcerative colitis.

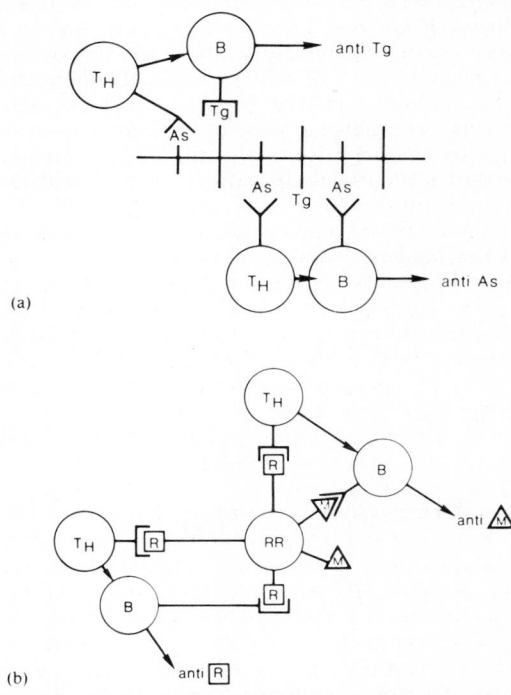

Fig. 11 The proposed bypass mechanism which allows the stimulation of helper T-cells (T_H) and, hence, auto-antibody production. This is compared with the induction of antibody to foreign determinants, where specific T-help is normally provided. (*a*) Tg: determinant on autologous native thyroglobulin. As: foreign group linked to the native thyroglobulin. (*b*) RR: rat red cell. R: determinant unique to rat cells. M: determinant common to both mouse and rat cells. (From Russell, A. S., (1981). In *Clins. Immunol. Allergy* **1**, 57, by permission)

By a somewhat similar mechanism, cells acquiring new surface antigens through infecting virus may by this means recruit and activate T cells which are capable of co-operating with self-reactive B cells to allow auto-antibody production. This T-cell by-pass mechanism is effective only when the shared and the newly introduced determinants are physically linked in the same molecule or on the same cell.

Auto-immune disease. Whether tissue damage or alteration of function results from the interaction of auto-antibody and auto-antigen depends, as with the hetero-immune reactions in the body discussed above, upon the circumstances of the encounter and upon the properties of the effector antibody or cell.

Auto-antibodies reactive with cell surface constituents are manifest clinically in the auto-immune haemolytic anaemias—where the precise red cell surface antigens are in many cases identifiable—and also in idiopathic thrombocytopenic purpura. The effects of the lymphocytotoxic auto-antibodies seen in systemic lupus erythematosus are less easily recognized, since, despite the lymphopenia in this disease, there is also a loss of suppressor T cells and an accompanying increase in activated helper cells and of B cells secreting Ig in the circulating blood. In thyrotoxicosis, a thyroid-stimulating auto-antibody has been identified which interacts with the thyrotrophin receptor on thyroid epithelial cells, and is the agent responsible for producing the hyperthyroidism. In other endocrine glands, auto-immunity against different components and secretions of the parenchymal cells may produce damage by any combination of the above mechanisms, and may interfere with normal physiological function by combining with active secretions, e.g. intrinsic factor in pernicious anaemia.

Immune complex formation is especially favoured in some forms of auto-immunity. Deposition of soluble complexes is an important immunopathogenetic event in the glomerulonephritis of systemic lupus erythematosus, where anti-nuclear, especially anti-DNA antibodies are involved, and in rheumatoid arthritis were anti-globulin antibodies (rheumatoid factors) play a significant part in inducing and maintaining inflammatory changes in the synovial membrane. In rheumatoid arthritis the presence of lymphokines in the synovial fluid or in the synovial membrane suggests that lymphocyte cytotoxicity is producing some of the joint damage, although much of the latter is more certainly attributable to immune complexes formed intra-articularly between rheumatoid factor and IgG.

The different types of immune effector mechanisms which may be at work in producing tissue changes in auto-immune disease, and their relative importance, are often difficult to disentangle. Furthermore, some antibodies are clearly auto-immune in nature and occur exclusively, principally or prominently in certain well-defined conditions—reticulin antibodies in coeliac disease and dermatitis herpetiformis, and smooth muscle antibodies in some forms of chronic active hepatitis, are examples—but whether they contribute to the pathology or are merely markers accompanying disease is not clear.

HLA associations of auto-immune disease. An increased frequency of HLA-B8 has been noted in a number of diseases with auto-immune features, and with the introduction of the serological method of detecting HLA-D and D-related antigens, it has emerged that in some of these conditions it is the B8/DR3 haplotype frequency that is increased. Conditions for which this has been shown include myasthenia gravis, thryrotoxicosis, primary Addison's disease, Sjögren's syndrome, chronic active hepatitis, and systemic lupus erythematosus. In rheumatoid arthritis it is the frequency of HLA-DR4 that is increased, and in the case of insulin-dependent diabetes mellitus both HLA-DR3 and HLA-DR4 frequencies are raised. Since the relative risk factors for the conditions mentioned are of the order 5–10, it is likely that in each case other susceptibility factors are also involved, but it is noteworthy that possession of the DR3 antigen is related to high immune responsiveness. Patients positive for DR3 not only have higher titres of auto-antibodies of various specificities, but also higher titre antibodies against viruses and other antigens. Patients with DR2 have lower titre auto-antibodies, and the risk for insulin-dependent diabetes or myasthenia gravis, for example, is also less in HLA-DR2 subjects. It has been suggested that DR3-positive individuals are better able to resist microbial pathogens at the cost of a greater risk of developing auto-immune disease, while for HLA-DR2

individuals the reverse is the case. The raised frequency of DR2 found in multiple sclerosis might, if this argument held, imply decreased resistance of DR2 subjects to a postulated virus.

Immunodeficiency

T cells, B cells, phagocytes, and complement work together in the body to combine natural and adaptive immunity mechanisms to provide a versatile and durable defence in depth against numerous microbial and other incidental biological invaders. Thus defects of more than a trivial nature in one or more components of this intricate organization commonly manifest themselves through chronic or unduly recurrent infections, infections with unusual agents, incomplete recovery from infection, or unsatisfactory response to treatment. Disturbances of immune regulation, which might also be classed as deficiencies, may lead to immunopathology by routes other than infection, e.g. auto-immunity.

Immunodeficiency may be primary, due to genetic defects, or secondary, due to malignancy, auto-immune disease, protein-losing states, and other disorders including certain congenital or chronic infections. Primary immunodeficiencies are increasingly classifiable on a logical basis as the lineages of the cells of the immune system which develop from stem cells in the fetal liver and the bone marrow are brought to light, largely from phenotypic studies of leukaemias, lymphomas, and lymphoproliferative diseases (see Section 19).

Defects of antibody production (see also Section 12, page 12.80)
Transient hypogammaglobulinaemia of infancy. Infants are born with IgG derived by placental transfer from the mother, and their IgG levels are thus at birth those of normal adults (see Table 1). By four to six months their serum IgG has fallen to about 3 g/l, rising thereafter as the baby's own IgG synthesis takes over, together with IgM and later IgA. Occasionally, IgG levels remain dangerously low (1 g/l or less) for several months, and recurrent infections, especially of the respiratory tract, may occur until IgG synthesis picks up. Premature babies are at similar risk, and injected gamma-globulin is protective in both conditions.

Selective IgA deficiency is the most common immunodeficiency, serum levels less than 50 mg/l occurring with an incidence of between 1 in 400 and 1 in 2500 in both children and adults. Such individuals often have otherwise normal antibody responses and normal numbers of IgA B cells, and while some appear healthy, others suffer repeated mild respiratory tract infections. Affected children may in addition have asthma, and in babies with IgA deficiency, atopic eczema may develop. The benefits of breast feeding in avoiding the infantile food allergy are well-established, and the association of the latter with IgA deficiency may reflect increased absorption of intact food proteins. Patients with gluten-sensitive enteropathy show an additional increase in incidence of IgA deficiency, and both conditions are associated with HLA-B8. Several auto-immune diseases are described in IgA deficiency, as well as the occurrence of a variety of auto-antibodies without accompanying disease. More than half the patients have serum antiglobulin antibodies directed against IgA, and these may produce anaphylactic reactions on attempted treatment with gamma-globulin, which may contain IgA.

The presumed defect in IgA deficiency is a failure of terminal differentiation of B cells, and IgA plasma cells are markedly lacking in the lamina propria of the gut, while the frequency of IgM plasma cells is increased. The latter is a feature also of gluten enteropathy, irrespective of serum IgA level.

Selective deficiencies of IgG, its different subclasses, IgM, and IgE are rare.

X-linked infantile hypogammaglobulinaemia (Bruton type) is characterized by the early onset in males (five to six months of age) of recurrent pyogenic infections. The serum IgG level is less than 2 g/l and IgM, IgA, IgE, and IgD are absent. There is usually an absence also of circulating B cells, and of plasma cells in the lamina propria and in stimulated lymph nodes. Without treatment, death from infection during the first decade is usual. The estimated incidence in the United Kingdom is 1 in 100 000 and the family history clearly shows X-linked recessive inheritance. Occasional children have normal numbers of circulating B cells and raised IgM levels. T cell numbers and functional behaviour, and delayed hypersensitivity skin reactions are normal. The infections are readily controlled with gamma-globulin injections and antibiotics.

Patients with this condition have a defect in the B cell lineage which appears to be impairing differentiation at the transition from 'pre-B cells' to B cells. Their blood lymphocytes stimulated with antigen in culture produce as much antibody as normal lymphocytes. It is not yet clear whether this differentiation block is attributable to excessive suppressor T cell activity.

'Variable' (acquired) hypogammaglobulinaemia. This term is used to describe the condition of patients of either sex who develop recurrent pyogenic infections with onset at any age, and do not have affected relatives. In these patients total serum immunoglobulins are less than 3 g/l, (except in a few cases with raised IgM) and IgG levels less than 2.5 g/l. Their circulating B cell numbers are normal. There is a lack of normal antibody response (e.g. positive Schick test after a booster injection of diphtheria antigen), and isohaemagglutinins are of low titre (1:10) or absent.

Cell-mediated immunity is usually normal, but a minority give negative delayed hypersensitivity skin tests, and show depressed responses to phytohaemagglutinin stimulation. The patients have a high incidence of gastrointestinal and haematological disorders, and a rheumatoid arthritis-like condition, systemic lupus erythematosus, and other auto-immune diseases have also been noted. The causes of variable (acquired) hypogammaglobulinaemia are unknown. The serum IgG molecules show restricted electrophoretic mobility, abnormal proportions of IgG subclasses, and abnormal κ/λ chain ratios. The B cells of some patients appear to have a defect of immunoglobulin secretion and/or synthesis, suggesting an intrinsic B cell defect. An effect due to suppressor T cells has also been demonstrated, but not consistently.

Other rare forms of hypogammaglobulinaemia occur in association with thymoma, in a small proportion of infants with the rubella syndrome, and following post-natal infection with Epstein–Barr virus. In Down's syndrome, despite raised IgG levels, there is a defect in antibody production affecting both primary and secondary responses.

Hypogammaglobulinaemia associated with lymphoma and haematological disorders is considered in Section 19.

Defects of cell-mediated immunity. Isolated severe defects of cell-mediated immunity are very rare, and probably only associated with congenital partial or complete absence of the thymus. In the *diGeorge syndrome* there is a failure of development of the third and fourth pharyngeal pouches during embryonic life, with resulting absence of thymus and parathyroid glands. T cells are low or absent, delayed hypersensitivity skin reactions absent, and PHA responses are usually grossly depressed. There is often a relative expansion of the B cell population and Ig levels in the serum are normal. A fetal thymus graft can result in permanent reconstitution of T cell immunity. If thymus tissue from a less than 14 week fetus is used, this reduces the likelihood of a subsequent graft-versus-host reaction. Some success has also been achieved by treatment with the thymus humoral factor, thymosin. The accompanying lack of parathormone in diGeorge's syndrome requires treatment with calcium in conjunction with vitamin D or parathormone.

Nezelof's syndrome, in which the thymus is hypoplastic but the parathyroids normal, presents a similar picture of T cell deficiency, but with accompanying abnormalities of immunoglobulin levels and antibody responses. Gamma-globulin injections and antibiotics are used to combat the chronic infections seen in Nezelof patients. Bone marrow or thymus transplants have both had some success in treatment, and transfer factor has also been used.

A group of clinical syndromes characterized by *chronic muco-*

cutaneous candidiasis appears to be due to a defect of T cell function restricted to an inability to mount a protective immune response to *Candida albicans* and some related yeast-like fungi.

Chronic candida infection of mucous membranes, skin, and nails develops with the formation of granulomatous lesions. In some patients there is an accompanying endocrinopathy, most often hypoparathyroidism or Addison's disease. The delayed hypersensivity skin test to candida antigen is negative, and there may be impaired ability of the patient's lymphocytes to proliferate or to produce lymphokine migration inhibition factor (MIF) in response to candida antigen. The numbers of T and B cells in the blood and immunoglobulin levels and antibody responses are normal. There is evidently a specific T cell defect, but whether due to a genetic factor or to an induced tolerance is not known. In cases with endocrinopathy a more widespread disturbance, possibly of suppressor cell function, seems likely.

Defects of both antibody production and cell-mediated immunity
Severe combined immune deficiency (SCID) of infancy is apparent within the first three months of life, and most affected infants die before two years of age. Circulating T lymphocytes are severely depleted. While B cells may be present, and some patients have raised serum immunoglobulin levels, the immunoglobulins produced appear to be non-functional as antibodies. Delayed hypersensitivity skin tests, leucocyte inhibition factor, and PHA responses are all severely depressed or absent.

SCID is heterogeneous both clinically and in aetiology. It may occur spontaneously, or show a sex-linked recessive or autosomal recessive mode of inheritance, the former accounting for the male predominance.

A proportion of cases occur in association with other diseases, including short-limbed dwarfism and cartilage-hair hypoplasia. About half the cases with the autosomal recessive form are caused by a deficiency of the purine enzyme, adenosine deaminase (ADA), which catalyses the conversion of adenosine to inosine in the purine metabolism pathway. This leads to raised levels of adenosine and deoxyadenosine in the blood and tissue fluids. This affects lymphocytes preferentially, apparently because they have specific kinases which convert deoxyadenosine to deoxyadenosine triphosphate (dATP). The lymphocytes in ADA deficiency contain high concentrations of dATP, which is a potent inhibitor of ribonucleotide reductase and so reduces the synthesis of deoxynucleotide triphosphates. In these ADA deficient patients T cell function, it is suggested, is more impaired than B-cell function. Another rarer deficiency is due to lack of the enzyme purine nucleoside phosphorylase (PNP). These patients are not as severely ill as those with SCID. The reported cases are children with recurrent respiratory tract infections, who have also had severe infections with common viruses. PNP deficiency leads to high concentrations of circulating guanosine and deoxyguanosine, and this leads to accumulation of deoxyguanosine triphosphate (dGTP). This appears to affect T cell function selectively, since PNP deficient patients have normal serum immunoglobulin levels and, if anything, exaggerated antibody responses. It is noteworthy that transfusions of blood benefit both ADA and PNP deficient patients, an effect due to the presence of both these enzymes in red cells.

Bone marrow grafts are the best curative treatment at present available in SCID, and with well-matched grafts are relatively uneventful procedures. However, graft-versus-host reactions of varying and even fatal degree occur.

Monoclonal antibodies with specificity for different immature and mature T cell subsets are being increasingly used to investigate congenital and acquired immunodeficiences, and results underline the heterogeneity of the cell defects responsible in different cases. These reagents are also being used to isolate lymphocyte precursers required for treatment, and to deplete cells obtained for transplant of subsets likely to mediate graft-versus-host reactions.

Immunodeficiency with ataxia-telangiectasia. This is a multi system disease characterized by oculocutaneous telangiectasia, cerebellar ataxia, immunodeficiency and autosomal recessive inheritance. Onset is in early childhood, with ataxia becoming obvious as the child starts to walk. Patients usually die in the second decade from chronic lung infections. Varying degrees of T and B cell defects are found. E-rosetting cells (T cells) are reduced and delayed skin test responses depressed to varying extents in different patients. IgA deficiency, with or without IgE deficiency, is a frequent feature, the former, at least, representing a defect in terminal B cell differentiation, since IgA B cell numbers are normal. As with selective IgA deficiency, circulating auto-antibodies of various tissue specificities are often present.

The underlying defect has not been defined. Patients have an increased sensitivity (severe tissue necrosis) to ionizing radiation, and spontaneous and radiation-induced chromosome breaks are found with increased incidence. These observations suggest a DNA repair defect. Another suggestion is that interactions between primordial germ-line tissues during embryogenesis is defective. The thymus resembles that of a three month fetus, while the liver is not fully differentiated and the alpha-fetoprotein levels are high, and patients may produce collagen of immature type.

Wiskott–Aldrich syndrome. A sex-linked recessive condition in males characterized by thrombocytopenia, eczema, and immunodeficiency. A bleeding tendency is present from birth, and recurrent infections begin after six months, especially with pneumococcus, meningococcus, and *Haemophilus influenzae*. Decreased IgM levels, and low or absent isoagglutinins are often found with raised IgA and IgE. Immunoglobulins are catabolized at two or three times the usual metabolic turnover rate. Cellular immunity is abnormal, with anergy to the range of skin test antigens, but T cell numbers and PHA responsiveness normal. A major cause of mortality is the development of a lymphoma, often in the brain.

The underlying defect has not been defined.

Complement deficiencies. The commonest inherited complement deficiency is of C2, homozygotes constituting approximately 1 in 10 000 blood donors and heterozygotes (with half normal C2 levels) about 1 per cent of random individuals. C1 and C4 deficiencies are much rarer, but it has been noted that homozygous C1, C4, or C2 deficient patients have a disproportionate incidence of systemic lupus erythematosus-like illness, or other systemic rheumatic disorders.

As discussed above, the role of the classical pathway C3 convertase, $C\overline{4b2a}$, is to cleave C3, thus generating C3b, a process which takes place on antibody-coated particles, including deposits of immune complexes. C3b molecules generated in this way by the classical pathway accumulate on the lattice of antigen-antibody complexes, where they serve as seeds to initiate assembly of the alternative pathway properdin-stabilized C3 convertase, $C\overline{3bBb}$. This participation of both pathways leads to intercalation of C3b and C4b in the lattice, solubilizing the deposited complexes and thus favouring their dispersal and subsequent up-

take and degradation by phagocytic cells with C3b and C4b receptors. It might be expected, therefore, that in the absence of early complement components solubilization of immune complex deposits would be defective, and this hypothesis has been advanced to explain the incidence of auto-immune disease resembling systemic lupus erythematosus in complement deficiency states. While homozygous C2 deficient relatives of propositi have been shown to have a lower incidence of auto-immune disease, this does not rule out the hypothesis, since it is known that the structural genes for C4 and C2 and factor B are located within the human major histocompatibility complex, and hence may be in linkage disequilibrium with immune response genes at the HLA-D or DR loci. It may also be noted that the depletion of C3 levels in patients with C3NeF and mesangio-capillary glomerulonephritis occurs before detectable involvement of the kidney.

Despite the role of complement in opsonization, phagocytosis, and killing of micro-organisms, the inherited complement component deficiencies are not characterized by undue frequency of infection, except in the case of lack of C3, another rare deficiency. Children with this defect present with recurrent bacterial infections, clinically resembling patients with hypogammaglobulinaemia.

The interfering effect of auto-antibody to C3bBb (C3NeF) on its disposal by C3B inactivator (C3b INA) has been mentioned above. A few cases are known of inherited C3b INA deficiency, some of which, though not all, having histories of repeated severe infections.

Deficiency of C1 inhibitor has also been referred to above, and its association with hereditary angioedema (see Section 20). The oedema appears to be caused by a polypeptide kinin which increases vascular permeability and is released from plasmin by a fragment split from C2 by C1.

C1 INA is normally synthesized in the liver, and in subjects lacking even non-functional C1 INA, the liver cells do not contain demonstrable amounts. Treatment with the anabolic steroid danazol induces synthesis and release of normal C1 INA into the plasma of affected individuals, and clinical remissions have been obtained in this way (see Section 20).

References

Fudenberg, H. H., Stites, D. P., Caldwell, J. L., and Wells, J. V. (eds.) (1980). *Basic and clinical immunology*, 3rd edn. Lange, Los Altos.

Holborow, E. J. (ed.) (1981). *Clinics in immunology and allergy: autoimmunity* W. B. Saunders, London.

— and Reeves, W. G. (eds.) (1982). *Immunology in medicine*, 2nd edn. Academic Press, London.

Lachmann, P. J. and Peters, D. K. (eds.) (1982) *Clinical aspects of immunology*, 4th edn. Blackwell Scientific Publications, Oxford.

Parker, C. W. (ed.) (1980). *Clinical immunology*. W. B. Saunders, Philadelphia.

Playfair, J. H. L. (1982). *Immunology at a glance*, 2nd edn. Blackwell Scientific Publications, Oxford.

Neoplasia

GENERAL CHARACTERISTICS OF NEOPLASIA

H. Harris

The control of cell multiplication. A tumour is produced by the growth of cells that have become in some measure insensitive to normal growth control mechanisms. Some consideration of these mechanisms is thus a prerequisite of any informed discussion of the

cancer problem. The fundamental principles were first elucidated by the analysis of regeneration in epidermis and especially, for an interesting biological reason, the epidermis of insects. In insects, once the cuticle has been laid down, the epidermis is composed of a single layer of contiguous epithelial cells which do not undergo further multiplication during the life of the insect unless the epidermis is wounded. This tissue thus provides an initially static two-dimensional system that lends itself to more precise analysis than is normally possible in the heterogeneous three-dimensional arrays of which most animal tissues are composed. In a classical study, Wigglesworth showed that, when insect epidermis is wounded, a wave of mitoses is induced in the cells near the wound and that this mitotic activity is controlled in a quite specific way. The initial response is a migration of epithelial cells to the edge of the wound. This redistribution of the cell population occurs well before any multiplication of cells begins, with the result that the cell density immediately adjacent to the wound is increased, whereas, further away, a zone is produced in which the cell density is reduced. When, later, the cells begin to multiply, the mitoses are observed, not in the region of high cell density adjacent to the wound, but in the region of reduced cell density further away. The cells continue to multiply until the cell density is restored to normal and then cease. Throughout the whole process of repair, the epidermal cells remain in contact with one another through cytoplasmic bridges. The multiplication of the cells is therefore initiated not by diffusible factors generated at the edge of the wound, nor by the disruption of cell contact, but by some mechanism associated with a reduction in the normal cell density. Similar experiments on young insects in which the volume of the body is reduced by starvation provide strong support for this interpretation. The reduction in body volume produces a greatly increased density of cells in the epidermis. In this crowded epidermis, the migration of cells to the edge of a wound does not generate an outer zone in which cell density is reduced below normal; and the healing of the wound is achieved without the intervention of a wave of cell multiplication.

These simple experiments delineate a cardinal property of metazoan cells: their ability to register and respond to cell density. It will be obvious that the acquisition of this property during evolution must have been essential for the development of metazoan life. If cells within a tissue were not able to sense changes in cell density and respond to them by increasing or decreasing the rate of cell multiplication, it is difficult to see how organized metazoan forms could ever have evolved. We are therefore dealing here with a very primitive cell response. The process of differentiation, of course, imposes on the basic density-sensing mechanism specializations and refinements appropriate to the tissue architecture in which particular cells find themselves; but the long evolutionary history of this mechanism makes it reasonable to suppose that certain elements in it might well be common to all metazoan cells. Cells in which the density-sensing mechanism is intact maintain a density appropriate to the tissue in which they function; they do this by limiting their rate of multiplication to what is necessary to replace, and no more than replace, the cells that are lost. Thus, in tissues such as the intestine or bone marrow, where the rate of cell loss under physiological conditions is high, the basal rate of cell multiplication is also high; where the physiological rate of cell loss is low, as, for example, in the adult liver, the basal rate of cell multiplication is also low. Non-physiological destruction of cells in any tissue, provided that the cells in that tissue remain capable of mitosis, initiates a wave of cell multiplication, and this ceases when normal cell density is restored. The whole process is a paradigm of balanced feedback control.

Impairment of the density-sensing mechanism. Disease processes may impair the density-sensing mechanism in various ways. Cells may fail to respond, or may respond inadequately, to a reduction in cell density or a disruption of tissue architecture. In this case, a wound may fail to heal or may heal imperfectly. Cells may respond in the appropriate way, but they may fail to stop multiplying when normal cell density has been restored. Exuberant masses of superfluous tissue may then be produced. Or cells may be induced to multiply even though cell density and tissue architecture remain normal. Some viruses, for example, may initiate a wave of mitotic activity in certain cells without first perturbing their topological interrelationships. In some way the virus renders the cell insensitive to the normal restraints on its multiplication. The gratuitous cell multiplication induced by viruses is usually limited: the cells either recover their sensitivity to growth controls or they die. Under

certain conditions, however, cells may undergo a more stable change. Not only do they become insensitive to normal growth controls, but this insensitivity becomes heritable. Cells so affected beget daughter cells that are also insensitive and hence continue to multiply without responding to changes in cell density, and without respect for the integrity of tissue architecture. This kind of rogue growth is called a tumour. The cardinal biological characteristic of a tumour cell is thus the presence of a heritable lesion that determines insensitivity to the normal restraints governing cell multiplication.

The nature of the heritable lesion. These days, when one talks about heritable lesions, one thinks naturally of alterations in the nucleotide sequences of DNA or RNA; and the simplest explanation of the heritable cellular aberration that produces a tumour is that it is caused by a mutational event or series of events in the genetic material of the cell. This idea, which is sometimes called the 'somatic mutation' theory of cancer, is so consonant with our present understanding of cell biology, and with our knowledge of the behaviour of tumours, that it is perhaps difficult to see why other kinds of explanation should be entertained. There are two essential reasons: first, the argument, based on histological appearances, that tumours do not arise from a single cell, as would be expected for a mutational event, but by the large scale transformation of a 'field' of cells; and secondly, the observation that the tumour cell phenotype can, under certain conditions, apparently be restored to normal. These considerations have led some authors to propose that the heritable lesions that determine the tumour cell phenotype are not genetic in the classical sense, but epigenetic, that is, akin to the cellular changes that determine stable forms of differentiation. A tumour is then envisaged as an aberration of the normal process of differentiation.

With respect to the 'field' theory of carcinogenesis, it seems surprising that it is still necessary to say that histological methods cannot, in principle, resolve questions of this kind. A single cell, provided it retains the ability to undergo appropriate forms of differentiation, may generate a population of cells that can organize itself into an easily recognizable tract of differentiated tissue. This has been formally demonstrated *in vitro*, where clonal populations of cells have been grown for long periods of time without losing the ability to form, under appropriate conditions, specialized tissues such as muscle, cartilage, or lens. There is no way of telling, simply by looking at the histology of the tumour, whether it arose from a single cell or by the wholesale transformation of a 'field' of normal tissue. But it is clearly of cardinal importance to determine whether tumours do indeed arise from single cells or from large numbers of contiguous cells, for, if the latter were the case, a somatic mutation model for carcinogenesis would be difficult to sustain. Mutations are rare and, to a first approximation, random events, which could not reasonably be held to explain a co-ordinate change occurring more or less simultaneously in a large group of cells. The best available evidence indicates, however, that in the great majority of cases, tumours, whether they form recognizable tissues or not, are clones that arise from the proliferation of a single cell.

Evidence for the clonal origin of human tumours. Three main lines of evidence support the conclusion that tumours are usually clonal growths.

The presence of marker chromosomes. It often happens that all, or almost all, of the cells in a tumour carry the same specific marker chromosome. Morphologically recognizable marker chromosomes are generated by chromosomal rearrangements, such as breaks and translocations, which are comparatively rare events. It is hardly conceivable that within a tumour the same rearrangement could occur independently but simultaneously in a high proportion of the cells. When one finds such a situation, the only plausible explanation is that all the cells bearing the specific marker are the progeny of a single cell in which that particular chromosomal rearrangement initially occurred. Cells carrying a diagnostic chromosome marker may, of course, generate subpopulations that have lost it, so that the presence in the tumour of cells not carrying the marker is no argument against a clonal origin. Nor is the fact that there are tumours that do not show consistent chromosomal abnormalities; for one would not expect that every cell capable of giving rise to a tumour would necessarily show a chromosomal abnormality that could be recognized in cytological preparations. It is, however, notable that as the resolution of cytogenetic techniques improves, marker chromosomes are discovered in tumours with increased frequency. The cytogenetic evidence does not exclude the possibility that initially more than one cell might have escaped growth control, but it does indicate that during the growth of the tumour the progeny of one such cell has an overwhelming selective advantage.

Tumours that form single antibodies. It is now well established that once a cell is committed to antibody production, it can produce only one kind of antibody; and its descendants form a clone in which all the cells produce the same antibody. The heterogeneity of antibody molecules seen in the natural immune response of an animal to an antigen is due to contributions from a number of different antibody-forming clones. Myelomas, which are tumours derived from antibody-forming cells, often synthesize and secrete antibodies. It has, however, been shown that each myeloma produces an antibody that is chemically homogeneous and distinct from the antibody produced by any other myeloma. The homogeneity of the antibody has been formally established by the analysis of amino-acid sequence. This provides compelling evidence for the conclusion that myelomas are clones derived from single antibody-forming cells.

Tumours arising in mosaic tissues. In placental mammals, such as man, the cells of the female normally contain two X chromosomes, but one of these is rendered inactive at an early stage of embryological development. Inactivation affects the paternal and the maternal X chromosome in a random fashion, so that the tissues of the adult female are an intiminately mixed mosaic of two populations of cells, one containing an inactive maternal X, the other an inactive paternal X. This mosaicism may be revealed where X-linked enzymes show polymorphisms that permit the paternal form of the enzyme to be distinguished, usually by its electrophoretic mobility, from the maternal form. The tissues of the adult female, and even the smallest fragments of them that can be analysed, will then show both the paternal and the maternal forms of the enzyme. If a tumour arose by conversion of a substantial number of cells in such a tissue, then one would expect that the tumour would also show the mosaicism of the tissue of origin. But if the tumour arose from a single cell (or from a very few, depending on how intimately mixed the two cell populations were in the tissue), then one would expect the cells of the tumour to contain only one form of the enzyme, either the paternal or the maternal. The X-linked enzyme most extensively used for this sort of analysis is glucose 6-phosphate dehydrogenase which shows an easily demonstrable polymorphism in man. A very wide range of human tumours of different kinds taken from individuals whose tissues contain a mixture of two electrophoretic variants of glucose 6-phosphate dehydrogenase have now been examined. The majority of these tumours have been found to contain only one form of the enzyme. This again argues strongly for the view that most tumours arise from single cells, or, at the very least, from the selective overgrowth of a very small number of cells.

The cumulative weight of all this evidence effectively eliminates the idea that tumours are produced by the wholesale conversion of large 'fields' of cells. An animal may be exposed to ionizing radiation at a dose sufficient to ensure that every cell in it is subjected to multiple ionizing events; a chemical carcinogen may be administered at a concentration that ensures that every cell in the target tissue receives many thousands of molecules; a tumorigenic virus may be injected in an inoculum large enough to ensure that every accessible cell is infected with many viral particles. But, in each case, only an occasional cell among the huge numbers of like cells at risk gives rise to a tumour. The heritable change that renders a cell insensitive to normal growth control is thus a rare and, at least superficially, a random event. In this respect it clearly resembles a mutation rather than a form of differentiation. For differentiation is not a clonal event. It is, on the contrary, the process par excellence in which an induced change affects a 'field' of cells, not a single cell; and there is nothing random about the character of the transformation.

Evidence from hereditary abnormalities of DNA metabolism. There is a group of hereditary diseases that are produced by defects in the enzymes involved in the replication or repair of DNA. These diseases are associated with an extremely high incidence of malignant tumours, and, in some cases, these tumours arise inevitably if the patient lives long enough. The best studied condition of this kind is *Xeroderma pigmentosum* in which the inherited defect involves one of the enzymes responsible for the repair of damage produced in DNA by ultraviolet light. Those parts of the body that are exposed to ultraviolet light become progressively disfigured by chronic inflammatory processes, and eventually generate multiple carcinomas. Malignant tumours are not notably more common than usual in those parts of the body that are not exposed to ultraviolet light. In the case of *Ataxia telangiectasia* and Bloom's syndrome, the enzymatic basis of the defect in DNA metabolism has not been delineated as precisely as in *Xeroderma pigmentosum*, but here again aberrant DNA synthesis or repair leads to a very high incidence of malignant disease, especially leukaemia. These observations make it very difficult to escape the conclusion that the generation of a tumour must involve some alteration in the structure of the DNA (see also pages 4.19 and 4.81).

The correlation between carcinogenicity and mutagenicity. Earlier studies which, on the whole, had failed to establish a good correlation between carcinogenicity and mutagenicity have now been undermined by the discovery that many carcinogens require metabolic activation before they are effective. If metabolic activation systems that convert inert carcinogens to more reactive intermediates are incorporated in the test procedure, then an astonishingly good correlation between carcinogenicity and mutagenicity emerges. The most extensively used test is that devised by Ames, which measures reversion in auxotrophic histidine mutants of *Salmonella typhimurium*. A liver homogenate is added to the bacterial culture to achieve metabolic activation of the compound being tested. Several hundred carcinogens have now been screened by this procedure, and some 90 per cent of them have been found to be highly mutagenic. Animal cells growing *in vitro* can also be used as screens for mutagens. Although the data so far obtained with animal cells is not very extensive, the correlation between carcinogenicity and mutagenicity holds. The importance of the small proportion of cases in which the correlation breaks down should not be overestimated. It is always possible that the metabolic activation system incorporated in the test is not the appropriate one for any particular carcinogen, or that other special conditions operating in the whole animal are not mimicked in the *in vitro* tests. What is impressive is that the results of simple *in vitro* tests for mutagenicity should correlate so well with a phenomenon as complex as the generation of a tumour *in vivo*. This striking correlation further strengthens the argument that tumours are produced by cellular events that involve structural alterations in DNA.

The problem of reversibility. The main support for the idea that tumorigenicity might be determined by epigenetic events comes from experiments in which the insensitivity to growth control is suppressed or reversed by the processs of differentiation: cells known to be tumorigenic cease to be so when they undergo certain specialized changes. In a sense, this is a very old piece of information. The whole of tumour histopathology is based on the fact that tumour cells may undergo recognizable forms of differentiation, and, in many tumours, differentiation generates cells that are no longer capable of continued multiplication. In extreme cases, for example, keratinization of skin tumours or the generation of enucleated erythrocytes by erythroid tumour cells, differentiation actually results in cell death. There is, therefore, no problem about accepting the fact that differentiation can override whatever it is that produces the unphysiological growth of tumour cells; but this fact does not in itself constitute evidence for the view that tumorigenicity is determined by epigenetic mechanisms. Some recent experiments provide an illuminating analysis of the problem.

In both plants and animals it has now been demonstrated that the progeny of certain kinds of tumour cells can contribute to many, if not all, of the specialized tissues of the developing organism. The experiments that have been done with plant cells are more dramatic than those with animal cells. Single cells isolated from crown gall tumours of *Nicotiana tabacum* are capable of generating apparently normal, and fertile, tobacco plants. This striking observation clearly demonstrates that the malignant phenotype can be suppressed in every one of the cells that go to form the mature plant. But this fact is not a decisive argument for the view that tumorigenicity is determined by epigenetic mechanisms. Further investigation of the cells that form the regenerated plants shows that they are not normal cells: when these are re-explanted *in vitro*, these cells are found to have retained the biochemical and cultural abnormalities characteristic of crown gall tumour cells. In fact the whole problem has been transformed by experiments of another kind. It has been shown that the production of a crown gall tumour involves the incorporation into the plant cell of a plasmid normally carried by the tumorigenic bacterium *Agrobacterium tumefaciens*; and there is strong genetic and biochemical evidence that specific DNA sequences in the plasmid are responsible for certain critical steps in the generation of the neoplastic state. Moreover, the plasmid DNA is still present in the somatic cells of the phenotypically normal plants generated from the crown gall tumour cells. We must therefore conclude either that the process of differentiation can override the expression of the plasmid DNA sequences that contribute to the production of the malignant phenotype, or that the process of plant growth selects for cells in which the plasmid DNA sequences are in some way defective. In any case, it is now difficult to avoid the conclusion that the formation of the crown gall tumour does involve genetic changes in the classical sense, that is, changes in DNA nucleotide sequence.

We cannot yet generate a phenotypically normal adult individual from a single somatic animal cell, but the experiments that have been done on the reversibility of the malignant phenotype during animal development, and the interpretations that have been given to them, are very reminiscent of the work with crown gall tumour cells. It has been shown that embryonal teratocarcinoma cells injected into mouse blastocysts may generate progeny that contribute to the apparently normal development of many different tissues. As in the case of the crown gall tumour, this observation has been used as an argument for the view that tumorigenicity is determined by epigenetic mechanisms, but, once again, these experiments merely show that the insensitivity to growth control can be suppressed by the process of differentiation. It is altogether possible that if the cells derived from the injected embryonal carcinoma cells were re-isolated from the chimaeric tissues and grown again *in vitro*, they might, as in the comparable case of the crown gall tumour, retain or regain elements of the tumour cell phenotype. In this connection, it is of interest that, under certain conditions, many of the animals derived from blastocysts that have received embryonal carcinoma cells eventually develop embryonal carcinomas and other tumours at various sites.

Compared with the massive circumstantial evidence supporting genetic mechanisms for the generation of tumours (the fact that tumours arise as rare and essentially random events, the correlation between the carcinogenicity of chemical agents and their mutagenicity, the inordinately high incidence of tumours in patients with inherited defects of DNA metabolism), the case for epigenetic mechanisms is very weak.

Genetic analysis of the cellular lesions determining tumour growth. The introduction of cell fusion techniques has made it possible to apply genetic methods to the analysis of somatic cells. This new approach involves the construction of hybrid cells in which the genomes of two different parent cells are initially combined, and in which different genes are subsequently segregated by chromosome loss and rearrangement. Consistent co-segregation of a particular marker with a particular chromosome usually permits the assignation of the gene specifying the marker to that chromosome. A very large number of human genes have now been mapped in this way. Regional mapping within a chromosome, which establishes the order of genes and the distances between them, can be achieved by techniques that combine cell fusion with radiation-induced chromosome rearrangement. A beginning has been made in the application of these new genetic techniques to the problem of tumour growth, and some interesting findings have emerged.

When a variety of different highly malignant transplantable mouse tumour cells were fused with normal diploid cells, it was found that the resulting hybrids, so long as they retained something close to the sum of the two parental chromosome sets, were unable to grow progressively in immuno-suppressed genetically compatible hosts. On continued cultivation *in vitro*, however, these hybrid cells, like all others, underwent chromosome losses and rearrangements; and, with a variable frequency, they generated sub-sets of cells which regained the ability to grow progressively *in vivo*. Interpreted in simple Mendelian terms, these findings suggest that, if they are mutational events, the lesions determining escape from growth control behave as if they were recessives. This conclusion is in line with a good deal of circumstantial evidence derived from the incidence of tumours in human populations. Since dominant mutations occurring in one of two homologous genes would be expressed in diploid cells, it is difficult to see how any of us could ever reach adult life without developing a tumour if tumours were determined by dominant mutations occurring at a frequency within the normal range. If only one or two dominant mutations were required, we would rarely, if ever, survive fetal life. The literature does contain some experiments in which tumorigenicity appears not to have been suppressed when tumour cells were fused with diploid cells; but these experiments have not yet been analysed in enough detail to provide convincing evidence for the view that, in these cases, the genetic determinants of tumorigenicity are transmitted in a dominant fashion. The reappearance of tumorigenicity in hybrids in which it was initially suppressed is sometimes associated with the loss of identifiable chromosomes derived from the diploid parent cell. This chromosome loss forms the basis of attempts to map the genetic determinants of the tumour phenotype. This has proved to be a more difficult task than might have been anticipated, but it has none the less been shown that certain specific genetic loci are indeed commonly involved even in different kinds of tumour. This conclusion is supported by two additional pieces of evidence derived from hybrid cells. The first of these is based on complementation tests in which different tumour cells are fused with each other. These tests also indicate that many different kinds of tumour may have lesions at the same genetic locus. The second is based on the analysis of hybrids in which parent cells of different morphological types are fused together. If, for example, a lymphoma is fused with a normal fibroblast, the sub-sets of tumorigenic cells that arise in the hybrid cell population may produce either lymphomas or sarcomas when injected into the animal. This indicates that the same genetic lesions may determine tumorigenicity in both lymphoid cells and cells of fibroblastic type. Similar observations have been made with other parental combinations in hybrid cells.

Cell fusion experiments have also thrown some light on the mode of action of oncogenic verses. Tumorigenicity may also be suppressed in hybrids produced by the fusion of virus-induced tumour cells with normal diploid cells. Such hybrid cells may be unable to grow progressively *in vivo* even though they can be shown to carry the oncogenic virus, and even though the normal parent cell is known to be susceptible to the virus. This finding indicates that at least some oncogenic viruses must act indirectly by inhibiting or modifying certain cellular genes whose defective function is made good in the hybrid by the activity of homologous genes contributed by the normal parent cell.

The natural history of a tumour. Once a cell has undergone the heritable change that confers insensitivity to growth control, it generates within the tissues of the affected animal a subpopulation of cells whose subsequent evolution is governed by principles that are very familiar to population geneticists. A population of this kind is subjected to extreme selection pressure which continually favours the emergence of cells with increased growth potential. Thus, any cellular change, mutational or other, which results in an increased rate of multiplication confers a selective advantage: the progeny of a cell that has undergone such a change will progressively increase its representation in the growing tumour. A cell may undergo a change affecting substrate utilization; this may endow it with the ability to survive under conditions that inhibit the growth of other cells. A cell may lose the ability to maintain normal coaptation with its neighbours. It might then move away from the primary tumour mass, where conditions are crowded, and thus gain for itself an increased nutrient supply. A detached cell, or group of cells, may be translocated by lymph or the blood stream to other sites in the body. If these new sites provide a favourable milieu for cell multiplication, a secondary growth or metastasis is produced. Thus, the tumour cell population, like any other growing population, continually generates variants, and the tissues of the body select those variants that are best fitted for growth at the particular site where they find themselves. It is this Darwinian process that determines the histopathology of a tumour and ultimately its clinical course.

Tumour histopathology rests on the fact that, in general, tumour cells retain enough of the morphological characteristics of differentiation to permit their tissue of origin to be recognized. Thus, for example, tumours arising from muscle cells or cartilage cells are usually composed of tissue that unmistakably resembles muscle or cartilage. The histological appearances of very early tumours suggest that the event that determines initial escape from growth control does not, in general, produce a gross alteration in the morphology of the cell affected. Some tumours never lose the specific morphological characteristics of their tissue of origin; but others, at some stage of their development, do. This loss is often called 'dedifferentiation', which is a rather misleading term as it implies reversal of the process of differentiation, that is, a wholesale conversion of a population of cells from one phenotype to another. There is, in fact, every reason to believe that 'dedifferentiation' is simply the selective overgrowth within the tumour of cells that have lost a particular morphological marker or group of markers that permits the differentiated state of the tissue of origin to be recognized. If the loss of any particular marker of differentiation results in an increased rate of cell multiplication, then cells lacking the marker will eventually come to dominate the tumour. Since expression of most differentiated states involves the synthesis of molecules that are not essential to cell survival, it will be obvious that changes that determine the loss of differentiated markers will very commonly confer a growth advantage. It is for this reason that a broad correlation is found between the degree of 'dedifferentiation' of a tumour and its rate of growth.

From the clinical point of view, the most important property of a tumour cell population is whether it has the ability to generate secondary deposits elsewhere in the body. Cancer would be a trivial disease if tumour cells did not sometimes have this ability. There is very little information about either the biochemical or the genetic basis of metastasis. Cell fusion experiments have demonstrated that the heritable determinants of metastasis are different from those that determine progressive growth: hybrids between the cells of

tumours that metastasize and normal diploid cells generate subsets of tumorigenic cells that do metastasize and others that do not. Attempts are being made to use genetic methods to delineate the biochemical basis of metastasis, but these are at a very preliminary stage, more preliminary, indeed, than the comparable analysis of progressive growth.

Is cancer one disease or many? There is a trivial sense in which cancer is, of course, many diseases. Since cancers arise at different sites, grow at different rates, may be either benign or lethal, it is clear that, in terms of symptomatology, clinical course, and prognosis, the term cancer covers a very wide spectrum of disease entities. This is, however, also true of tuberculosis or syphilis, and should not blind one to the very real possibility that an essential unity of biochemical malfunction might none the less exist. Despite an apparent multiplicity of causative agents and a multiplicity of clinical syndromes, it remains true that all tumour cells show the same fundamental aberration in their response to the physiological mechanisms that govern cell multiplication. It is also true that, as far as they have gone, genetic and biochemical studies make it much more probable that many different kinds of tumour have the same, or very similar, heritable defects. To work on this assumption is, in any case, a more intelligent approach to the cancer problem at the present time, than to suppose that every different tumour is a law unto itself.

References

Ames, B. N., Durston, W. E., Yamasaki, E., and Lee, F. D. (1973). Carcinogens are mutagens: a simple test system combining liver homogenates for activation and bacteria for detection. *Proc. natn. Acad. Sci. U.S.A.* **70**, 2281.
Bramwell, M. E. and Harris, H. (1978). An abnormal membrane glycoprotein associated with malignancy in a wide range of different tumours. *Proc. R. Soc.* **B201**, 87.
Braun, A. C. and Wood, H. N. (1976). Suppression of the neoplastic state with the acquisition of specialized functions in cells, tissues, and organs of crown gall teratomas of tobacco. *Proc. natn. Acad. Sci. U.S.A.* **73**, 496.
Cleaver, J. E. (1968). Defective repair replication of DNA in *Xeroderma pigmentosum*. *Nature, Lond.* **218**, 652.
Fialkow, P. J. (1976). Clonal origin of human tumours. *Biochim. biophys. Acta. Reviews on Cancer* **3**, 283.
Harris, H. (1971). Cell fusion and the analysis of malignancy. The Croonian Lecture. *Proc. R. Soc.* **B179**, 1.
—— (1979). Some recent progress in the analysis of malignancy by cell fusion. In *Human genetics: possibilities and realities*, 311. Ciba Foundation Series 66.
Huberman, E. and Sachs, L. (1976). Mutability of different genetic loci in mammalian cells by metabolically activated carcinogenic hydrocarbons. *Proc. natn. Acad. Sci. U.S.A.* **73**, 188.
Illmensee, K. and Mintz, B. (1976). Totipotency and normal differentiation of single teratocarcinoma cells cloned by injection into blastocysts. *Proc. natn. Acad. Sci. U.S.A.* **73**, 549.
Jonasson, J., Povey, S., and Harris, H. (1977). The analysis of malignancy by cell fusion. VII. Cytogenetic analysis of hybrids between malignant and diploid cells and of tumours derived from them. *J. Cell Sci.* **24**, 217.
Knudson, A. G., Strong, L. C., and Anderson, D. E. (1973). Heredity and cancer in man. *Prog. med. Genet.* **9**, 113.
McCann, J., Choi, E., Yamasaki, E., and Ames, B. N. (1975). Detection of carcinogens as mutagens in the *Salmonella*/microsome test: assay of 300 chemicals. *Proc. natn. Acad. Sci. U.S.A.* **72**, 5135.
Marshall, C. J. (1980). Suppression of the transformed phenotype with retention of the viral 'src' gene in cell hybrids between Rous sarcoma virus transformed rat cells and untransformed mouse cells. *Expl. cell Res.* **127**, 373.
Meyer, G., Berebbi, M., and Klein, G. (1974). Expression of polyoma-induced antigens in low malignant hybrids derived from fusion of a polyoma-induced tumour with a fibroblast line. *Nature, Lond.* **249**, 47.
Mintz, B. (1978). Gene expression in neoplasia and differentiation. *Harvey Lect.* **71**, 193.
Nowell, P. C. (1976). The clonal evolution of tumour cell populations. *Science, N.Y.* **194**, 23.
Papaioannou, V. E., Gardner, R. L., McBurney, M. W., Babinet, C., and

Evans, M. J. (1978). Participation of cultured teratocarcinoma cells in mouse embryogenesis. *J. Embryol. exp. Morph.* **44**, 93.

Papaioannou, V. E., McBurney, M. W., Gardner, R. L., and Evans, M. J. (1975). Fate of teratocarcinoma cells injected into early mouse embryos. *Nature, Lond.* **258**, 70.

Schell, J., Van Montagu, M., de Beuckeleer, M., de Block, M., Depicker, A., de Wilde, M., Engler, G., Genetello, C., Hernalsteens, J. P., Holsters, M., Seurinck, J., Silva, B., van Vliet, F., and Villarroel, R. (1979). Interactions and DNA transfer between *Agrobacterium tumefaciens*, the Ti-plasmid and the plant host. *Proc. R. Soc.* **B204**, 251.

Stoker, M. G. P. (1972). Tumour viruses and the sociology of fibroblasts. *Proc. R. Soc.* **B181**, 1.

Turgeon, R., Wood, H. N., and Braun, A. C. (1976). Studies on the recovery of crown gall tumour cells. *Proc. natn. Acad. Sci. U.S.A.* **73**, 3562.

Wiener, F., Cochran, A., Klein, G., and Harris, H. (1972). Genetic determinants of morphological differentiation studied in hybrid tumours. *J. natn. Cancer Inst.* **48**, 465.

—, Klein, G., and Harris, H. (1971). The analysis of malignancy by cell fusion. III. Hybrids between diploid fibroblasts and other tumour cells. *J. Cell Sci.* **8**, 681.

—, —, and — (1974). The analysis of malignancy by cell fusion. V. Further evidence of the ability of normal diploid cells to suppress malignancy. *J. Cell Sci.* **15**, 177.

—, —, and — (1974). The analysis of malignancy by cell fusion. VI. Hybrids between different tumour cells. *J. Cell Sci.* **16**, 189.

Wigglesworth, V. B. (1937). Wound healing in an insect (*Rhodnius prolixus* Hemiptera). *J. exp. Biol.* **14**, 364.

EPIDEMIOLOGY OF CANCER

R. Doll and R. Peto

Note: readers of this chapter may, on first examination, wish to pass over the central part (pages 4.55–71) which lists separately the epidemiological features of each separate type of cancer, as the preceding and subsequent parts may be read without much reference to it.

The epidemiology of cancer, by which is meant the study of the incidence of the disease in man under different conditions of life, has a history dating back nearly 300 years to Ramazzini's observation that cancer of the breast occurred more often in nuns than in other women and to Pott's observation, some 75 years later, that scrotal cancer in young men occurred characteristically in chimney sweeps. Both observations have been confirmed many times since, but whereas the reason for the first is still incompletely understood (except insofar as it is attributable to the avoidance of pregnancy), the second led to the realization that the combustion products of coal could cause cancer on any part of the skin with which they came into repeated contact, and became the foundation stone on which our knowledge of chemical carcinogenesis was built.

These observations and a few other similar ones that were made before the First World War on, for example, lung cancer in miners of Schneeberg and Jachymov (who it was subsequently realized were heavily exposed to radon), skin cancer in radiologists and radiographers exposed to X-rays and in farmers and seamen exposed to ultraviolet light, bladder cancer in aniline dye workers, and buccal cancer in betal chewers, depended for the most part on the acumen of individual physicians, surgeons, and pathologists who were struck by seeing a cluster of cases of a particular type of cancer in patients with a similar occupational or cultural background, and they provided almost all that was known at the time about the causes of cancer. Later on, between the wars, when Stocks and others began to apply to the study of cancer the formal techniques that had been evolved for the epidemiological study of infectious disease, little attention was paid to their results. By then, Yamagiwa and Ishikawa had produced cancer on a rabbit's ear by painting it with tar and the potential of laboratory experiment had captured the imagination of the scientific world. Epidemiological data, by contrast, were observational in origin and required an element of subjective interpretation. They were, therefore, commonly ignored on the grounds that the conclusions drawn from them were liable to be misleading. They carried little weight in comparison with those obtained by experiment and there appeared to be little point in worrying about them, as it was confidently believed that the mechanisms by which all cancers were produced, and hence the factors that caused them, would be discovered within a few years.

After the Second World War, this attitude changed dramatically and interest in the use of epidemiological observations as a means of investigating the causes of cancer was reawakened. The results have been so successful that it is now generally realized that epidemiological data can both suggest hypotheses for testing in the laboratory and identify causes in the field with sufficient certainty to justify preventive action. It may be, too, that they can help to define the mechanisms by which the disease is commonly produced in man.

Methods of epidemiology. The epidemiological methods that are applied to the study of cancer are the same as those that are used for the study of any other disease and are described in textbooks of the subject (for example, Barker and Rose 1979, and Lilienfeld 1976). The simplest method is to compare the incidence of, or the mortality from, cancer in different phases of life, in different countries or communities, in different occupations or social groups, and at different dates, in the hope that it may be possible to correlate the rates with factors in the environment or patterns of behaviour that might be suspected of causing the disease. Another method is to compare the personal characteristics and past experience of people with and without some preselected type of cancer (case-control studies). A third is to record some preselected characteristic of each member of a group of people and to follow them up prospectively to observe the incidence of cancer in each subgroup defined by these recorded characteristics (cohort studies). Finally, hypotheses may be tested in practice by monitoring the effect of any changes in exposure or behaviour that may take place as a result of the suspicions aroused by other investigations.

Biological factors

Each type of cancer, defined by the type of cell from which it originates and the organ in which it occurs, has a characteristic relationship to age and sex, and these relationships provide some useful clues to the causes of the disease. For some of these relationships the general shape is invariant, being, so far as is known, the same everywhere and at all times. Retinoblastoma of the eye, for example, always occurs about equally in both sexes with its maximum incidence in the second year of life, while carcinoma of the stomach is always more preponderant in men (being about 1½ or 2 times as common as in women), and increases in incidence progressively from adolescence. For others, the patterns vary in different communities or at different times. Carcinoma of the female breast, for example, increases in incidence from adolescence to the menopause in all countries, but the incidence may then decline (as in Japan), or decline for a year or two before increasing again more slowly (as in western Europe, North America, and Australasia); while carcinoma of the lung in men has shown a different relationship to age at different times in one country after another, a peak incidence at around 60 years of age earlier this century gradually moving to older ages.

Another important characteristic is the long 'latent period' that occurs between the first exposure to the carcinogenic agent and the appearance of the clinical disease.

Age. Cancers occur at all ages and the different types show a variety of patterns that defy precise classification. By far the commonest general pattern, which is shown by carcinomas of the skin and the gastrointestinal and urinary tracts, and by a few cancers of non-epithelial cells, such as myelomatosis and chronic lymphatic leukaemia, is a progressive increase in incidence from near zero in late adolescence to a high incidence in extreme old age. The rate of increase is rapid, being typically proportional to the fourth, fifth, or sixth power of the age, so that cancers that affect only 1 or 2 persons per 1 000 000 each year at around 20 years of age may affect 1 or 2 per 1000 each year at age 80. With most of these cancers, the recorded rate of increase diminishes after about 75 years of age and the recorded incidence may stabilize, or even decrease, in the oldest age groups; but this is partly or wholly an artefact due to incomplete investigation of the terminal illnesses of old people. With the continuing development of medical services, the increasingly intensive investigation of the old, and the collection of progressively more complete data, the cancer incidence rates that are recorded in old age may be expected to increase still more, even if there is no secular change in the risk of developing the disease at a given age. This pattern of a rapidly increasing incidence with age is observed for skin carcinoma due to exposure to ultraviolet light and for bronchial carcinoma both in non-smokers and in men who regularly smoke a constant number of cigarettes a day, and is observed in the laboratory in skin-painting experiments on mice. It is probable (Peto 1977) that it reflects lifelong exposure to small amounts of a carcinogen, starting at or within a decade or two of birth.

Two much less common patterns are a peak incidence early in life followed by a decline virtually to zero, or a slow rise to a second peak in old age. For example, retinoblastoma and nephroblastoma occur only in childhood, teratomas and seminomas of the testis have peak incidence rates respectively at about 20 and 30 years of age and later almost cease to occur, and osteogenic sarcoma has a peak incidence in adolescence and then shows a slow increase from a lower rate in young adult life.

The remaining cancers show a bewildering variety of patterns. For example, carcinoma of the cervix uteri begins to appear in adolescence, becomes rapidly more common up to the menopause, and then shows a constant or declining incidence, like carcinoma of the breast in most parts of Africa and Asia. In contrast, Hodgkin's disease appears in childhood and then continues to occur more or less evenly throughout life with minor peaks in young adult life and in old age, while connective tissue sarcomas become progressively more common from childhood on, but with a much slower rate of increase than is shown by the common carcinomas. All these various patterns provide information, either about the period of activity of the stem cells from which the cancers derive, or about the times when exposure to the causative agents occurs and the length of time the exposure lasts. Some of it has already helped to explain the causes of cancer, as has been the case with the shift in the peak incidence of bronchial carcinoma; but much of it still awaits elucidation.

Sex. Cancer used to be more common in women than in men in nearly all countries due to the great frequency half a century ago of carcinoma of the cervix uteri and the rarity of bronchial carcinoma, and it still is in populations for which these conditions hold, as in much of Latin America. Elsewhere, cancer is now more common in men. This overall male preponderance hides, however, a wide range of relative rates for cancer of different organs. If the sites of cancer which are peculiar (or almost peculiar) to one sex are ignored, the ratio of the rates varies in Britain from a male excess of about 14 to 1 for carcinoma of the lip and 7 to 1 for carcinoma of the larynx, through many types of cancer with a small male preponderance, to carcinomas of the right side of the colon, thyroid, and gallbladder, which may be up to twice as common in women.

For many types of cancer the sex ratio is much the same in different countries and at different times. For some, however, and particularly for cancers of the mouth, oesophagus, larynx, and bronchus, the sex ratio may be extremely variable—not only between different countries and at different times, but sometimes also between different ages at the same time and in the same country. The most marked variation is shown by cancer of the oesophagus,

which may affect both sexes equally or be 20 times more common in men than in women. As with the various patterns of incidence with age, these different sex ratios and the variation between countries and times can provide useful clues to the causation of the various types of cancer, only few of which have yet been successfully followed up.

Latent period. One reason why it has been difficult to recognize causes of cancer in man is the long delay that characteristically occurs between the start of exposure to a carcinogen and the appearance of the clinical disease. This 'latent period', as it is commonly but not very helpfully called, usually lasts for 20 to 40 years, although it may be as short as one or as long as 60. The exact relationship between the date of exposure and the date of the appearance of human cancer is still uncertain, partly because the interval is subject to random factors, partly because few cancers are induced by a single brief exposure, and partly because there are still very few sets of quantitative data in which we have detailed information about the dates when exposure began and ended.

When cancer is induced by short but intensive exposure to ionizing radiation, as in Hiroshima and Nagasaki following the explosions of the atomic bombs or in patients treated by radiotherapy, the excess incidence of solid tumours rises for at least 15 to 20 years and then may level off or decline. In the case of leukaemia, however, a peak in the incidence occurs earlier (about five years after exposure) and few cases appear after more than 20 years.

Short intensive exposure to a carcinogen is, however, exceptional. The more usual situation is for exposure to a carcinogen to be prolonged for years—perhaps a decade or two in the case of occupational exposure, several decades in the case of tobacco smoking, and a lifetime in the case of ultraviolet sunlight. In this situation the incidence of cancer increases progressively with the length of exposure. In the last two cases cited, the incidence appears to vary approximately in proportion to the fourth power of the duration of exposure so that the effect after (say) 40 years is about 10–20 times as great as that after 20 years and two or three hundredfold as great as that after 10 years. Whether the same holds for occupational exposure is not known; but it has been shown to hold in skin-painting experiments on mice and it may well prove to be a general biological rule for many types of tumour and many (but definitely not all) carcinogens.

There is still less quantitative information about what usually happens when exposure ceases; but in the case of cigarette smoking the excess annual risk appears to stabilize and to remain at approximately the same level for one or two decades thereafter. The ex-smoker, therefore, avoids the enormous progressive increase in risk suffered by the continuing smoker. Such substantial benefits will, however, be conferred only by agents that affect at least one of the *later* stages of the process that culminates in clinical cancer and cannot always be anticipated, particularly if the carcinogen persists in the body (as happens following exposure to asbestos). For initiating agents that affect only an *early* stage in the process it may be safer to assume that the risk continues to increase, though not at the same rate.

It is not clear how these findings accord with current knowledge of the mechanisms of carcinogenesis; but they would certainly fit in better with the idea that the appearance of clinical cancer was the end-result of a multi-stage process in which different effects were exerted by initiating and promoting agents than with the idea that it was the immediate effect of a single specific change in cellular DNA. From the point of view of the clinician the important conclusions are that cancer is more likely to occur after prolonged exposure to a carcinogen than after short exposure, that it is seldom likely to appear within five years after first exposure (except in the case of leukaemia and the specific cancers of childhood), that it commonly occurs several decades after first exposure, and that it may continue to occur for many years after exposure has stopped. The exact relationship may differ for different carcinogens and different types of tumour. Bladder tumours, for example, began to appear within five years of intensive exposure to 2-naphthylamine in the dye industry, while mesotheliomas of the pleura seldom, if ever, appear within 10 years of exposure to asbestos, but continue to increase in incidence for up to 50 years after first exposure, even if the exposure was relatively brief.

Preventability of cancer

Perhaps the most important result of epidemiological observation has been the realization that the common cancers occur, in large part, as a result of the way people behave and the nature of the environment in which they live and are, therefore, in principle preventable. This does not mean that we can envisage a society in which any of the common cancers are completely eliminated (although this may prove to be possible when we understand more clearly the mechanisms by which the disease is produced); but that it is reasonable to envisage a society in which the risk of developing cancer by any particular age is greatly diminished.

The evidence that much human cancer is preventable can be summarized under four heads: differences in the incidence of a particular type of cancer between different settled communities, differences between migrants from a community and those who remained behind, variation with time within particular communities, and the actual identification of a large number of specific and controllable causes.

Differences in incidence between communities. Evidence of variation between communities has not been easy to establish because of differences in the provision and utilization of medical resources and changes in terminology and methods of diagnosis. Detailed clinical and pathological comparisons backed up by surveys of limited populations have, however, shown that the sort of differences now reported by good cancer registries throughout the world are for the most part real, particularly if comparisons are restricted to the limited range of ages between 35 and 64 years, which excludes the youngest ages, at which cancer is rare, and the oldest ages, at which the records of the diagnosis are least reliable.

Table 1 shows for selected types of cancer the range of variation recorded by cancer registries that have produced data sufficiently reliable for the purpose of international comparison. Types of cancer have been included if they are common enough somewhere to have a cumulative incidence among men or women of at least 1 per cent by 75 years of age. The ranges of variation shown are for incidence rates between 35 and 64 years, because these are the ages at which cancer is reasonably common and reliably recorded. The range of variation is never less than sixfold and is sometimes more than a hundredfold. Despite the selection of reliable registries, some of this tabulated variation may still be artefactual, due to different standards of medical service, case registration, and population enumeration; but in many cases the true ranges will be greater. First, there are still large gaps in the cancer map of the world so that some extreme figures may have been omitted, since no accurate surveys have been practicable in the least developed areas and it is just these areas that are likely to provide the biggest contrasts (both high and low) with western society. Secondly, the figures cited refer to cancers of whole organs and do not distinguish between different histological types or different locations within the organ. This does not matter for cancer of the oesophagus because this is nearly always squamous and the various causes thus far discovered all produce cancer in the same part of the organ (the lower two-thirds), but it does matter for many other types of cancer. It is, for example, not satisfactory to compare the aggregate of non-melanomatous skin cancers with each other, for these include such unrelated diseases as basal cell carcinomas of the face, which affect more than half the fair-skinned population of Queensland by 75 years of age, scar epitheliomas of the leg, which develop on the site of old ulcers in Africa and account for 10–20 per cent of all cancers seen in some hospitals in Malawi and Rwanda Burundi, 'dhoti' cancers of the groin in India, and occupational cancers

Table 1 Range of incidence rates of common cancers (men, unless specified otherwise)

Site of origin of cancer	High incidence area	Cumulative incidence (%) in high incidence area*	Low incidence area	Ratio of rates in high and low incidence areas†
Skin	Australia (Queensland)	> 20	India (Bombay)	> 200
Oesophagus	Iran, N. E.	20	Nigeria	300
Lung	England	11	Nigeria	35
Stomach	Japan	11	Uganda	25
Cervix uteri††	Columbia	10	Israel (Jewish)	15
Prostate	USA (blacks)	9	Japan	40
Liver	Mozambique	8	England	100
Breast††	Canada (British Columbia)	7	Israel (non-Jewish)	7
Colon	USA (Connecticut)	3	Nigeria	10
Corpus uteri††	USA (California)	3	Japan	30
Buccal cavity	India (Bombay)	2	Denmark	25
Rectum	Denmark	2	Nigeria	20
Bladder	USA (Connecticut)	2	Japan	6
Ovary††	Denmark	2	Japan	6
Nasopharynx	Singapore (Chinese)	2	England	40
Pancreas	New Zealand (Maori)	2	India (Bombay)	8
Larynx	Brazil (Sao Paulo)	2	Japan	10
Pharynx	India (Bombay)	2	Denmark	20
Penis	Parts of Uganda	1	Israel (Jewish)	300

* By age 75 years, in the absence of other causes of death
† At ages 35–64 years, standardized for age
†† Women

on the forearm due to exposure to tar and oil in industrialized countries.

The variation in incidence that is shown in Table 1 is not limited to the common cancers, but is also shown by many others. Burkitt's lymphoma, for example, never affects more than 1 in 1000 of the population, but it is at least 100 times as common among children in parts of Uganda as it is in Europe and North America; while Kaposi's sarcoma, which is extremely rare in most of the world, is so common in children and young adults in parts of Central Africa that it accounted for 16 per cent of all tumours seen in one of the African hospitals surveyed by Cook and Burkitt (1971). Some few cancers, such as the nephroblastoma of childhood, may perhaps occur with approximately the same frequency in all communities; but, if any do, they will certainly not be common anywhere.

The figures that have been cited so far all refer to the incidence of cancer in different communities defined by the area in which they live. Communities can, however, be defined in other ways and no matter what method is used, including categorization by ethnic origin, religion, or socio-economic status, similar differences may be found. Jewesses, for example, have a low incidence of cervical cancer irrespective of the country in which they live, and the Mormons of Utah and the Seventh Day Adventists of California suffer fewer cancers of the respiratory, gastrointestinal, and genital systems than members of other religious groups living in the same American States.

It does not seem likely that the large differences observed between communities can be explained by genetic factors (apart from cancer of the skin, the risk of which is much greater for whites than blacks, and possibly also chronic lymphocytic leukaemia, which rarely affects people of Chinese or Japanese descent, and cancer of the nasopharynx, which is much more common in Chinese from south China than in any other group). Genetic factors certainly cannot explain the differences observed on migration or with the passage of time, discussed below, nor can they explain the correlations that are often observed between the national rates for particular types of cancer and some measures of the lifestyle of the different countries.

Changes in incidence in migrant groups. That changes in the incidence of cancer occur on migration is beyond reasonable doubt. Many groups have been studied, including Indians who went to Fiji and South Africa, Britons who went to Fiji and Australia, and Central Europeans who went to North America. Among the most reliable data are those for the black Africans who went to America and the Japanese who went to Hawaii. The former experience cancer incidence rates that are generally much more like those of white Americans than like those of the black population in West Africa from which they were chiefly taken, while the latter have experienced rates that are much more like those of the Caucasian residents in Hawaii than like those of the Japanese in Japan (Table 2). The ancestors of black Americans and Hawaiian Japanese will have come from many different parts of West Africa and Japan, some of which are likely to have cancer rates somewhat different from those that have been cited in Table 2. Nevertheless, the contrasts are so great that there can be little doubt that new factors were introduced with migration.

Table 2   Comparison of cancer incidence rates in migrants and residents in homelands and adopted countries (men, unless otherwise specified)

Primary site of cancer	Annual incidence per million persons*					
	Japan†	Hawaii		Nigeria	USA	
		Japanese	Caucasians	(Ibadan)	Blacks†	Whites†
Oesophagus	131	46	75			
Stomach	1311	397	217			
Colon	83	371	368	34	351	315
Rectum	93	297	204	34	204	225
Liver				272	77	36
Pancreas				55	225	124
Larynx				37	193	141
Lung	268	379	962	27	1532	981
Prostate	14	154	343	134	651	275
Breast††	315	1221	1869	337	1187	1650
Cervix uteri††	364	149	243	559	569	276
Corpus uteri††	26	407	714	42	222	568
Ovary††	53	160	274			
Non-Hodgkin's lymphoma				133	8	4

*Rates are standardized for age among people aged 35–64 years. Data are provided only for those types of cancer where there are marked differences in incidence between residents of countries of origin and of destination.
†Average of rates in two regions
††Women

Changes in incidence over time. Changes in incidence with time provide still more conclusive evidence of the existence of preventable factors. Such changes are, however, difficult to be sure about, chiefly because it is difficult to compare the efficiency of case finding at different periods and partly because few incidence data have been collected for long enough, so that we have to compare mortality rates and these may be influenced by changes in treatment as well as changes in incidence. There are no simple rules for deciding which of the many changes in recorded cancer incidence and mortality rates are reliable indicators of real changes in incidence. Each set of data has to be assessed individually. It is relatively easy to be sure about changes in the incidence of cancer of the oesophagus as the disease can be diagnosed without complex investigations and its occurrence is nearly always recorded, at least in middle age, because it is nearly always fatal. It is much more difficult to be sure

about changes in the incidence of many other types. The common basal cell carcinomas of the skin, for example, are also easy to diagnose, but they seldom cause death and can be treated effectively outside hospital, so that they often escape registration. What appears to be a change in incidence may, therefore, be a change only in the completeness of registration. Cancers of the pancreas and liver and myelomatosis, in contrast, are usually fatal, but may be overlooked or diagnosed as cancer of another type, so that an increased incidence or mortality rate may be wholly or partly due to improvements in diagnosis, in the availability of the medical services, or in the readiness of physicians to inform cancer registries of the cancers they find. Such changes are particularly likely to affect the rates recorded for people over 65 years of age, as many old people who are terminally ill used not to be intensively investigated. Despite these difficulties some changes have been so gross that there can be no doubt about their reality. These include the increase in oesophageal cancer in the black population of South Africa, the continued increase in lung cancer throughout most of the world, the increase in mesothelioma of the pleura in males in industrialized countries, the decrease in cancer of the tongue in Britain, and the decrease in cancers of the cervix uteri and stomach throughout western Europe, North America, and Australasia.

Identification of causes. Finally, it has been possible to obtain evidence of the preventability of cancer by defining agents or circumstances that are a cause of the disease and are capable of control. The most straightforward evidence would be the demonstration by scientific experiment that an alteration led to an alteration in the incidence of the disease. Such evidence is, however, extremely difficult to obtain and we often have to be content with the type of strong circumstantial evidence that would be sufficient to secure a conviction in a court of law. Action, based on such evidence, has in practice often been followed by the desired result—for example, a reduction in the incidence of bladder cancer in the chemical industry on stopping the manufacture and use of 2-naphthylamine and the avoidance on stopping smoking of the progressive increase in the risk of developing lung cancer that would otherwise have occurred with increasing age. Cancer research workers throughout the world have, therefore, accepted that the type of human evidence that has been obtained, often, but not invariably, combined with laboratory evidence that the suspected agents are carcinogenic in animals, is strong enough to conclude that a cause of human cancer has been identified and that, as a corollary, the disease can be prevented by controlling the conditions under which it is produced. Such causes, which amount altogether to about 40, are listed in Tables 4 (page 4.71), 5 (page 4.72), and 7 (page 4.76), or are described under the specific types of cancer they are known to produce.

Epidemiology of cancer by site of origin

In all the preceding discussion, cancers in different anatomic sites have been treated as if they were diseases as different from each other as the different infectious diseases. They have certain obvious pathological and clinical characteristics in common, but they are in many ways aetiologically distinct, or the causes that can be eliminated are different, and there is scant evidence that the prevention of any one type of cancer need necessarily augment the age-specific risk of any other. It is, therefore, impossible to review the epidemiology of cancer as a whole. One must rather examine separately the epidemiology of each type and such an examination now follows. There are a few exceptions to be dealt with subsequently when one agent does or may cause cancer at all or most sites (e.g. ionizing radiations or overnutrition or deficiency of certain micronutrients) but, in general, the agents responsible for the production of human cancer vary with the site of origin of the tumour. In the examination that follows 'cancer' includes both carcinoma and sarcoma (although the causes are likely to be different), and the incidence and mortality figures refer to Britain.

The description of each type of cancer is preceded by notes showing its importance. One figure gives the proportion of all cancers arising in the site, as indicated by the data for the seven British cancer registries around 1970 collected by the International Agency for Research on Cancer (1976), and another gives the proportion of all cancer deaths allocated to the site in the national mortality statistics for 1979 (Registrar General 1980). A third gives the ratio of the age-standardized incidence rates for each sex obtained from the same seven registries. The way in which the incidence of the disease varies with age in each sex is shown in a graph. For this purpose the age-specific incidence rates recorded for the Birmingham and South Metropolitan Cancer Registries during the years 1969–73 and 1968–72 respectively have been averaged (International Agency for Research on Cancer 1976). Major differences between Britain and other countries are commented on in the text and are described more fully in the report on *Cancer Risks by Site* Published by the International Union Against Cancer (1980) and in the publications of the International Agency for Research on Cancer (1970 and 1976).

Lip

0.4 per cent of all cancers and 0.04 per cent of cancer deaths. Sex ratio of rates 13.6 to 1 (Fig. 1).

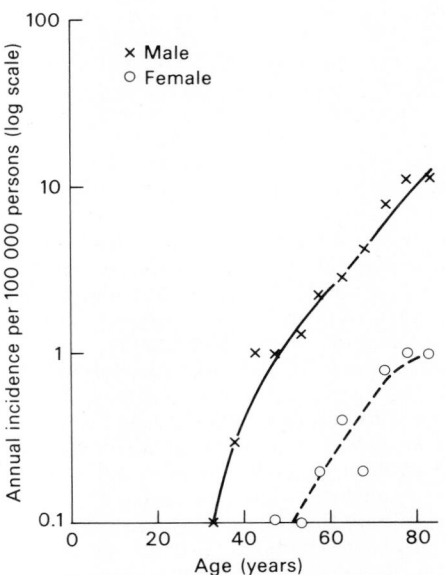

Fig. 1   Annual incidence of cancer of the lip

Carcinoma of the lip was one of the first types of cancer to be related to an extrinsic cause when, more than 200 years ago, it was noted to occur characteristically in pipe smokers. Many years later it was realized that the disease could also be produced by smoking tobacco in other ways so that it must be produced by the chemicals in smoke rather than by a non-specific effect of local heat. It is also much more common in outdoor workers than in indoor workers and is evidently induced by ultraviolet light in the same way as other cancers of the exposed skin. Ultraviolet light and tobacco account, between them, for the great majority of all cases in Britain; but whether they act independently or synergistically (to multiply each other's effects) is unknown. The disease is now much less common than it used to be, due presumably to the decrease in pipe smoking and in outdoor work.

Buccal cavity and pharynx (excluding nasopharynx)

1.2 per cent of all cancers and 1.0 per cent of cancer deaths. Sex ratio of rates 2.2 to 1 (Fig. 2).

Cancers of the tongue, mouth, and pharynx (other than nasopharynx) can be classed together as all are related to smoking (of

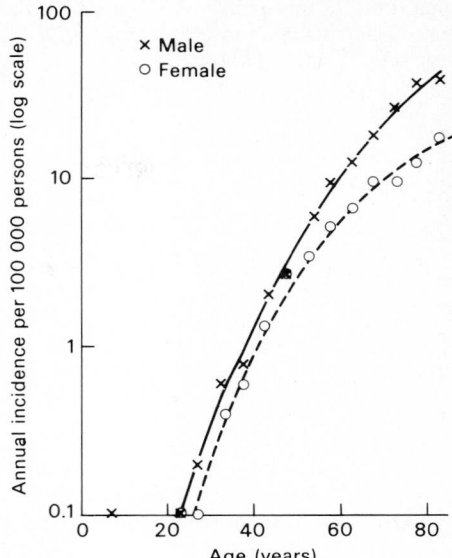

Fig. 2   Annual incidence of cancer of the buccal cavity and pharynx (excluding nasopharynx)

pipes, cigars, and cigarettes) and to the consumption of alcohol. The two factors act synergistically and cancers in these sites are extremely rare in non-smokers who do not drink alcohol. When cases occur in people who neither smoke nor drink alcohol, a disproportionate number (according to one American study) occur in habitual users of commercial mouthwashes that are 20–24 per cent alcohol. Some evidence suggests that textile workers may have an occupational hazard of developing them; but there is no obvious reason why such a hazard should exist and the limited data need confirmation.

Cancer of the tongue is much less common now in Britain than it was early this century, but the reason for the sharp decline in incidence is unknown. One possible explanation could be the decrease in syphilis, which was commonly believed to be a predisposing factor because of the clinical association between cancer and leucoplakia.

Cancers that occur low in the hypopharynx are distinguished by a tendency to affect women who have suffered from iron deficiency anaemia and dysphagia.

Outside Britain, cancers of the buccal cavity and pharynx (excluding nasopharynx) are particularly common in Southeast and Central Asia where tobacco smoking is largely replaced by chewing of tobacco, betel nut or leaf, and lime (calcium hydroxide). A close association with chewing has been established by case-control studies which have demonstrated that the cancers tend to originate in that part of the mouth in which the quid is usually held—a characteristic that varies both between individuals and between areas. The materials chewed differ in different places and although the disease is commonly described as 'betel chewers' cancer', betel is not invariably a component of the quid and the most characteristic constituent seems to be a small amount of lime. In some parts of Asia the disease is so common that it accounts for 20 per cent of all cancers and the abandonment of chewing would be the single most effective means of reducing the total incidence of cancer—so long as the habit was not replaced by smoking. One other preventive measure that might be of value would be to improve nutrition, as several studies have suggested that the disease tends to be associated in Southern Asia with vitamin A deficiency.

In parts of India where women tend to smoke the local small cigars and cigarettes with the burning end inside the mouth to prevent them going out, this habit is associated with cancer of the palate, a type of cancer that is extremely rare everywhere else.

Salivary glands

0.4 per cent of all cancers and 0.1 per cent of cancer deaths. Sex ratio of rates 1.0 to 1 (Fig. 3).

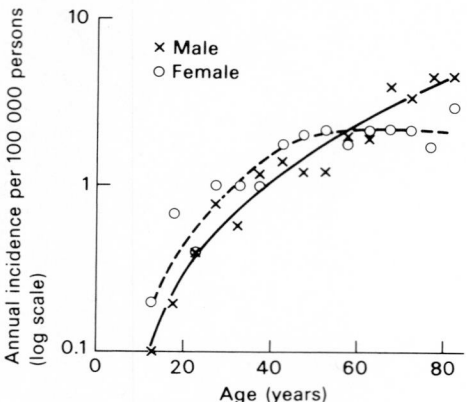

Fig. 3   Annual incidence of cancer of the salivary glands

The salivary glands are not common sites for cancer anywhere. They are, however, relatively more common in the Asiatic populations of Hawaii and in Canadian Indians than elsewhere. A small proportion of cases occur specifically in families which also have a high incidence of breast cancer. No causative factors are known and no notable changes in incidence have occurred over time.

Nasopharynx

0.1 per cent of all cancers and 0.1 per cent of cancer deaths. Sex ratio of rates 1.9 to 1 (Fig. 4).

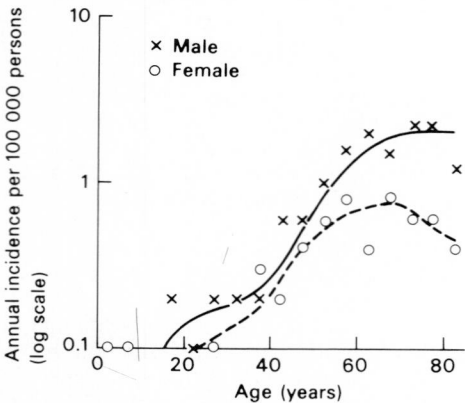

Fig. 4   Annual incidence of cancer of the nasopharynx

Cancers of the nasopharynx, unlike those in other parts of the pharynx, are not related to tobacco or alcohol. They are rare throughout most of the world, but are common in populations that originated from southern China, where the disease is the most common type of cancer. Moderately high rates have also been observed in Alaskan Eskimos and American Indians, and intermediate rates are observed in Malaysia, Kenya, and North Africa. A relationship with HLA type has been reported from Singapore, and it is widely believed that the southern Chinese have some specific genetic susceptibility to the disease. Incidence rates appear, however, to have been decreasing among Chinese Americans and the existence of a specific genetic predisposition remains to be proved. DNA characteristic of the Epstein–Barr (EB) virus has been detected in the nuclei of nasopharyngeal cancer cells and patients with the disease tend to have unusually high antibodies against EB virus-related antigens. Infection with the EB virus is, however, almost universal and if the virus is an aetiological agent, as seems likely, it can be only one of several that act in combination to produce the disease. Some reports have suggested that certain Chinese herbal medicines may be a cause of some cases of the disease.

Oesophagus

1.8 per cent of all cancers and 2.8 per cent of cancer deaths. Sex ratio of rates 1.9 to 1 (Fig. 5).

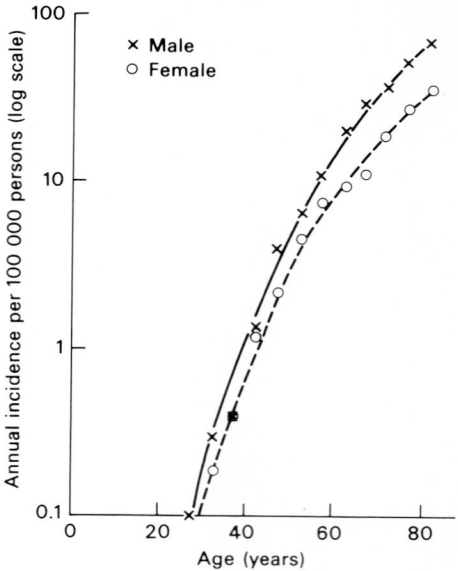

Fig. 5   Annual incidence of cancer of the oesophagus

Cancer of the oesophagus, like other cancers of the upper respiratory and digestive tracts, is closely related to smoking and to the consumption of alcohol. All types of smoking have comparable effects and, so it appears, do all alcoholic drinks, although in producing cancer spirits may be slightly more effective per gram of ethyl alcohol than other types of drink. Alcohol and tobacco act synergistically and, in the absence of either, the incidence is reduced by approximately three-quarters. In France, where the consumption of alcohol is greater than in Britain, it is reduced even more. A few cases originate from the scars produced by poisoning with corrosive substances and a very few in conjunction with a particular hereditary form of tylosis (presenting with keratoses of the palms and soles). The relatively small excess in men probably reflects the existence of other unknown causes in women, possibly nutritional in origin and similar to those responsible for cancers of the hypopharynx. Mortality (which, because of the high fatality rate, is almost identical with incidence) fell progressively in the first half of the century *pari passu* with the fall in the consumption of alcohol, and has risen again in young and middle aged men since 1950 when the trend in the consumption of alcohol reversed. Since pipe smoking affects oesophageal cancer risks at least as strongly as cigarette smoking does, no large effects on male oesophageal cancer trends can be predicted from the male switch from pipes to cigarettes, although the switch by females from nothing to cigarettes should, other things being equal, produce a large upward trend. It appears, however, that other things are not equal and some other, possibly nutritional, cause of oesophageal cancer seems to have decreased, for any upward trends in oesophageal cancer in Britain are surprisingly moderate.

In Africa and Asia the epidemiological features are different and present some of the most striking unsolved problems in the whole field of cancer epidemiology. In parts of China (particularly in north Honan but also elsewhere) and on the east coast of the Caspian Sea in Turkmenistan and Iran, oesophageal cancer is the commonest type of cancer, with incidence rates in both sexes that are equal to the highest rates observed for lung cancer in men in

European cities. In parts of Africa, particularly in the Transkei region of South Africa and on the east coast of Lake Victoria in Kenya, extremely high rates are also observed, sometimes equally in both sexes and sometimes only in men. In these and several other areas, the high incidence zones are strictly localized and the incidence falls off rapidly over distances of only 200 or 300 miles. When tobacco and alcohol are used, they increase the hazard but they are not the principal agents and in some areas, particularly in Iran and China, they are hardly used at all. Many causes have been proposed, including mineral deficiency in the soil (resulting in a deficiency of the plant enzyme nitrate reductase and a build-up of nitrosamines), contamination of food and pickled vegetables by fungi (particularly by species of *Fusaria*) with the production of carcinogenic metabolites, an agent associated with the production of beer from maize, and the residues left behind in pipes from smoking opium (which are commonly swallowed). None, however, are supported by any impressive epidemiological data. The high incidence area in Iran, which has been intensively investigated, is characterized by extreme poverty and a restricted diet consisting chiefly of home-made bread and tea, with some sheep's milk and milk products, and very little meat, vegetables, or fruit. In this area the disease has been common for centuries. In Southern Africa, however, it seems to have become common only since the First World War.

Stomach

7.4 per cent of all cancers and 8.8 per cent of cancer deaths. Sex ratio of rates 2.2 to 1 (Fig. 6).

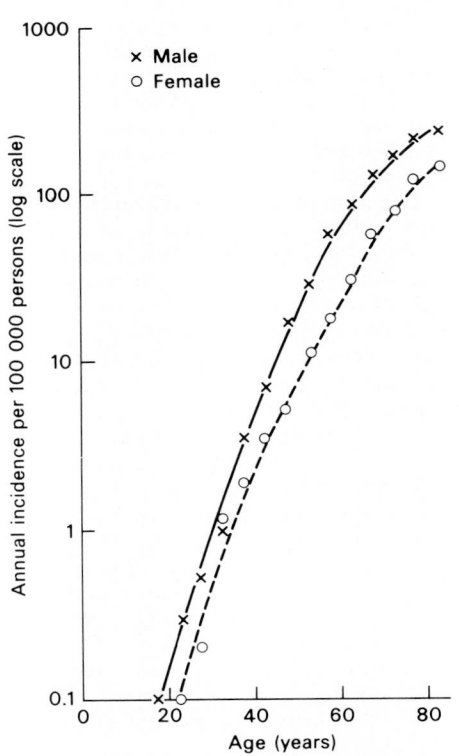

Fig. 6   Annual incidence of cancer of the stomach

Cancer of the stomach was, and possibly still is, responsible for more deaths from malignant disease throughout the world than any other type. Over the last 50 years, however, the incidence has declined rapidly in western Europe, North America, and Australasia and is still continuing to do so. More recently it has begun to decline also in South America and Japan. High rates are now confined to China, Japan, the USSR, and Central and South America, while the lowest rates are, perhaps surprisingly, found equally in North America, Australasia, and some of the least developed

parts of Africa. In nearly all areas the sex ratio is between 1.5 and 3 to 1, irrespective of whether the incidence is high or low.

Within Britain cancer of the stomach is most common in North Wales and becomes progressively less common from north to south and from west to east. Over the last 60 years it has been consistently some five times more common in unskilled labourers than in members of the major professions and this gradient with socio-economic class has been one of the most marked for any disease. Relatively high rates are consistently observed in coal miners and have also been recorded in some chemical workers; but no specific hazards have been identified in these groups and the excess in coal miners is paralleled by a similar excess in their wives. An occupational hazard has been associated with exposure to asbestos in the USA, but not apparently in Britain.

Despite these clues, there is no firm evidence about the nature of the causes. Genetic factors play some part, the incidence being 20 per cent greater in people belonging to blood group A than in people belonging to the other groups, irrespective of whether they live in high or low incidence areas. Pathologically, stomach cancer tends to be preceded by atrophic gastritis or intestinal metaplasia of the gastric mucosa, and patients who have developed pernicious anaemia run three times the normal risk of developing the disease. Innumerable writers have suggested an origin in chronic gastric ulcers, but given an accurate initial diagnosis it is doubtful if this occurs more often than would be expected from the socio-economic status of the patient. The risk may, however, be raised slightly after gastroenterostomy.

Diet is almost certainly important and a number of ways in which it could contribute to the production of the disease (or to its prevention) are discussed later (see page 4.73). Smoking and cooking food in ways that produce polycyclic hydrocarbons or other carcinogenic or mutagenic substances do not seem to be important and modern methods of preservation, particularly by refrigeration, seem more likely to have reduced the hazard than the reverse.

Large bowel

12.1 per cent of all cancers and 12.9 per cent of cancer deaths. Sex ratio of rates 1.3 to 1 (Fig. 7).

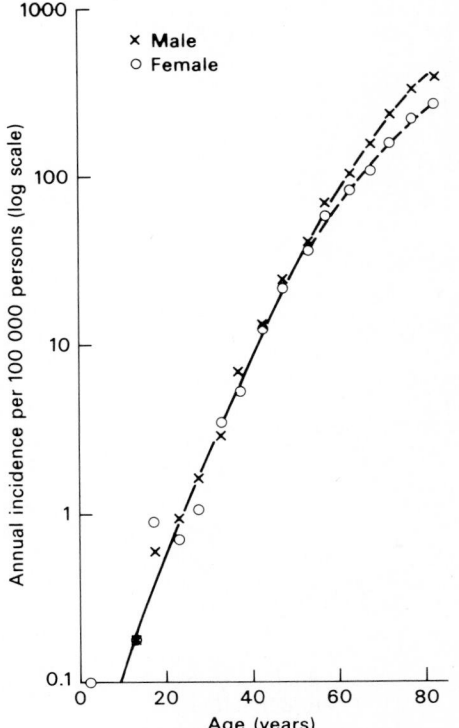

Fig. 7   Annual incidence of cancer of the large bowel

Cancers of the colon and rectum ought to be considered separately, as their causes are not identical. Cancer of the colon, for example, tends to occur more often in women than in men, particularly when it occurs on the right side, while cancer of the rectum is nearly twice as common in men. The geographical distribution also differs slightly, the former varying in incidence more than the latter. Unfortunately, cancers occur commonly at the rectosigmoid junction and the site of origin of these cases is not always recorded consistently. Moreover, there is a growing tendency to describe both diseases merely as 'cancers of the large bowel' which, according to the internationally agreed rules, are classed with cancers of the colon. The two diseases will, therefore, be considered together.

Incidence rates have been approximately static for many years, apart from a possible slight decrease in some countries in the immediate post-war period. Close examination, however, suggests a gentle decline in mortality, especially among women. The disease is still uncommon in most parts of Africa, Asia, and Eastern Europe, but has become common in Japanese migrants to Hawaii.

International variations in incidence are generally thought to be due to differences in diet. Incidence rates in different countries correlate closely with the per caput consumption of fat and meat and crudely with the consumption of processed foods from which the natural fibre has been removed. Ways in which these and several other dietary constituents might influence the development of the disease are discussed later (see page 4.73).

Within Britain there is no clear relationship to socio-economic status and no occupational hazards have been detected. An association with exposure to asbestos has, however, been reported in the USA. Unlike other carcinomas, some cases occur in childhood or early adult life when they are a complication of polyposis coli or (more rarely) Gardner's syndrome. These conditions are determined by dominant genes which so increase the susceptibility to the disease that it almost invariably develops before middle age. Many other cases develop from adenomatous polyps and a few occur as a complication of long-standing ulcerative colitis. Anal intercourse may predispose to anal carcinoma.

Liver
0.3 per cent of all cancers and 0.7 per cent of cancer deaths. Sex ratio of rates 2.1 to 1 (Fig. 8).

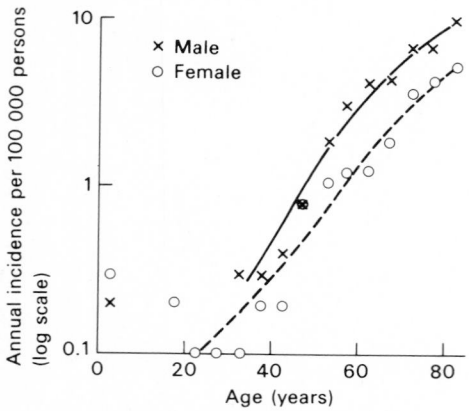

Fig. 8   Annual incidence of cancer of the liver

Incidence rates tend to be overestimated even in developed countries because the primary condition is often confused with metastases to the liver from cancer in various other organs, particularly over 65 years of age when carcinomas of the gastrointestinal and respiratory tracts are common. Changing standards of medical services make reliable estimation of trends difficult, but there is no reason to suppose that there are at present any appreciable increases or decreases in liver cancer rates either in the United States or in Britain, where current rates are among the lowest

anywhere. Compared with Britain and America, liver cancer is much more common in Southeast Asia, including parts of China, and in large parts of tropical Africa it is the most common type of cancer in men.

Most cases derive from the main cells of the organ (hepatocellular carcinomas) and are probably due to the combined effect of exposure to aflatoxin (a toxin secreted by the fungus, *Aspergillus flavus*, which may contaminate stored food) and infection with the hepatitis B virus. This double aetiology illustrates the point that just because one agent is an avoidable cause of one particular case of cancer, this does not mean that the same case does not also have other avoidable causes.

In developed countries such as Britain it is uncertain whether the minute amounts of aflatoxin that are consumed could account for many of the few cases of liver cancer that occur. A more important cause of hepatocellular carcinoma is cirrhosis, irrespective of whether it is due to hepatitis, chronic alcoholism, or haemochromatosis. Occasionally liver cancer is produced by drugs. A few cases have occurred in young men who have taken androgenic-anabolic steroids to increase their muscular strength and it seems probable that it may rarely complicate the development of the benign adenomas of the liver which are themselves rare complications of the use of steroid contraceptives.

A second histological type (cholangiosarcoma) arises from the intrahepatic bile ducts, tends to occur at a somewhat later age than hepatocellular carcinoma, and, although generally less common than hepatocellular carcinoma, nevertheless accounts for an appreciable proportion of cases. In China it can be produced by chronic infection with liver flukes (clonorchiasis). Elsewhere a few cases may appear as a complication of the sort of intensive immunosuppression that is required to prevent rejection of organ transplants, but the data are sparse.

A third histological type that is extremely uncommon everywhere has been variously described as reticulo-endothelioma or angiosarcoma. It was first recognized as a complication of the use of thorotrast as a contrast agent in neuroradiology, a practice which led to chronic retention of insoluble radionuclides in the marrow, spleen, and liver. In 1973 it was found to be an occupational hazard for men exposed to vinyl chloride. Fewer than 100 cases have occurred throughout the world in men who were heavily exposed in the manufacture of vinyl chloride polymer, and it seems improbable that the minute amounts that have leached out of plastic consumer products can have caused more than one or two cases altogether, if indeed they have produced any. A third, and ever rarer, cause is prolonged exposure to inorganic arsenic, as used to result from the medical prescription of Fowler's solution. Despite these multiple causes only one or two cases occur each year in Britain, which is why the recognition of new causes has been so easy. The frequency does not appear to be increasing and the majority of the cases that do occur are of unknown cause.

Cancer of the liver is almost uniformly fatal and it is fortunate that it should be so rare in developed countries. The fact of its rarity is intriguing, since most of the animal carcinogens thus far discovered induce, perhaps *inter alia*, tumours of the liver, so the lack of any high or increasing liver cancer rate in Britain and America suggests that, on average, people have not been importantly exposed to the sort of chemical carcinogen that is currently recognized (see, however, Clemmesen 1981).

Gallbladder and extrahepatic bile ducts
0.7 per cent of all cancers and 0.8 per cent of cancer deaths. Sex ratio of rates 0.9 to 1 (Fig. 9).

Cancers of the gallbladder and extrahepatic ducts are nearly always classed together, which is unfortunate as the causes are certainly different. The former is more than twice as common in women as in men, is strongly associated with obesity, and is nearly always accompanied or preceded by cholelithiasis. The latter is slightly more common in men and is increased in incidence by clonorchiasis and perhaps also by long-standing ulcerative colitis.

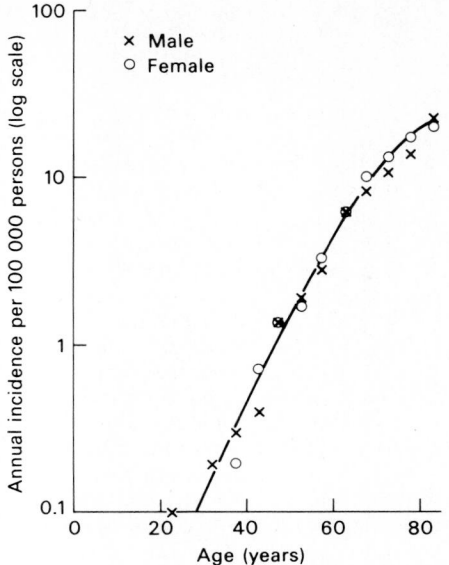

Fig. 9 Annual incidence of cancer of the gallbladder and extrahepatic bile ducts

Both types are rather rare, and their aggregate varies only slightly from one population to another. Relatively high rates are recorded among Jewesses in Israel, especially among those born in Europe and America.

The incidence of cancer of the gallbladder has fallen sharply in the USA in the last 15 years, which might be due to the decreased consumption of animal fat or, perhaps more likely, to an increase in the rate of cholecystectomy among people who, having gallstones, should be at greatest risk of cancer of the gallbladder.

Pancreas
2.8 per cent of all cancers and 4.7 per cent of cancer deaths. Sex ratio of rates 1.7 to 1 (Fig. 10).

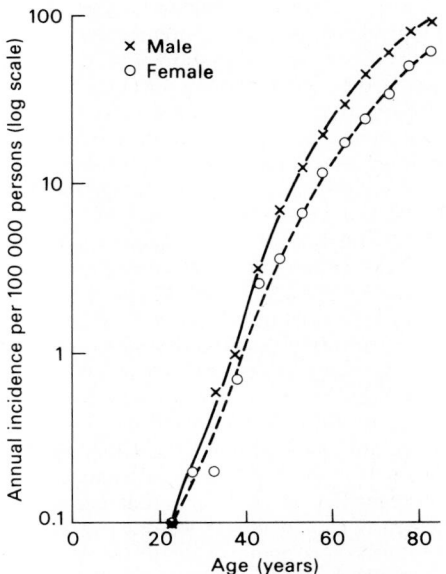

Fig. 10 Annual incidence of cancer of the pancreas

Cancer of the pancreas is two to three times more common in regular cigarette smokers than in lifelong non-smokers. Cigarette smoke contains many hundreds of chemicals including minute amounts of volatile nitrosamines and it is possible that a pancreatic carcinogen is absorbed from the alveoli and carried to the pancreas

in the bloodstream, although, since no particular such agent is known, other mechanisms may be more important. The incidence of the disease is correlated with a high standard of living and is twice as common in diabetics as in the population as a whole. It should not, therefore, be surprising that the highest rate recorded is among New Zealand Maoris, a population that smokes heavily and is prone to obesity, hypertension, myocardial infarction, and diabetes. An association has been reported with the consumption of coffee, but the reality of the relationship has yet to be proved.

Cancer of the pancreas is generally regarded as a disease of the developed world, but the diagnosis is difficult in the absence of a well-developed medical service and some of the relatively small geographical and temporal variations may be artefacts. Mortality rates in Britain and the USA have begun to decrease under 65 years of age and this is more likely to reflect a real reduction in incidence (due perhaps to changes in diet and smoking habits) than to improvement in treatment, as the five-year survival rate remains well under 10 per cent.

Nose and nasal sinuses
0.3 per cent of all cancers and 0.2 per cent of cancer deaths. Sex ratio of rates 2.0 to 1 (Fig. 11).

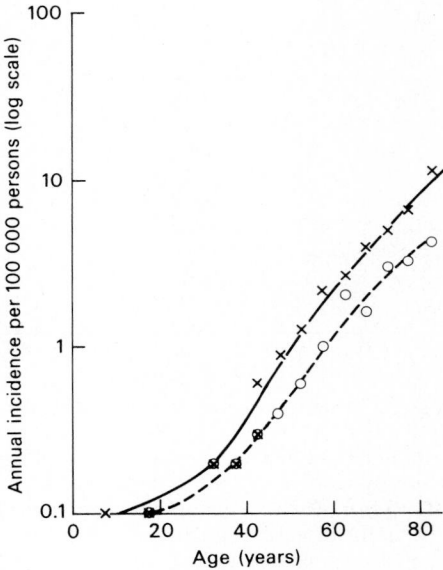

Fig. 11 Annual incidence of cancer of the nose and nasal sinuses

Cancers of the nasal cavity itself are extremely rare and most of the cancers in this group arise from the paranasal sinuses. Several occupational hazards have been recognized including the refining of nickel, the manufacture of isopropyl alcohol and hardwood furniture, and some aspect of the manufacture of leather goods. This should not, however, be taken to mean that all contact with nickel, hardwood dust, etc. creates a hazard. The hazards have been observed in special situations in which exposure has been intensive and probably also in which specific physical and chemical conditions have occurred. The nickel hazard was first observed in a refinery in south Wales where the nickel carbonyl process was used, but similar hazards have since been observed with other processes in Canada, Norway, and the USSR. Despite the continued use of the process in Wales no hazard of nasal sinus cancer has been observed among men first employed since 1930. The hazard in furniture workers was first observed in High Wycombe and appears to have followed the introduction of high-speed wood working machinery early in the century. It certainly affects some other groups but should not be assumed to affect furniture workers in general.

Most occupational and other cancers in this group are squamous carcinomas, but the hazard from hardwood dust characteristically produced adenocarcinomas. In some of the exposed groups as many as 5 per cent of the men developed the disease; but it is normally so rare that this meant that the risks were increased up to 1500 times (in the case of the woodworkers' adenocarcinoma) and were, in consequence, easy to confirm once suspicion had been aroused.

Chromate workers are sometimes said to experience a hazard of nasal cancer, but this is perhaps an error due to confusion with the characteristic 'chrome ulcer' of the nasal septum. These ulcers have not been shown to become malignant.

Larynx

1.0 per cent of all cancers and 0.6 per cent of cancer deaths. Sex ratio of rates 6.9 to 1 (Fig. 12).

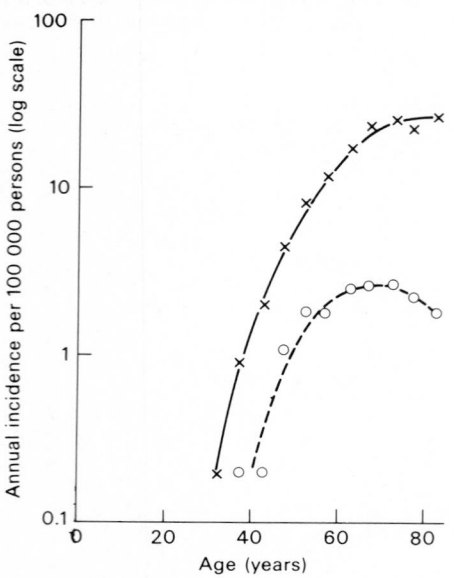

Fig. 12 Annual incidence of cancer of the larynx

Cancers of the larynx, like cancers of the oesophagus and buccal cavity, are closely associated with tobacco smoking and the consumption of alcohol. The two agents act synergistically and in the absence of either the disease would be extremely rare, more than 90 per cent of cases being due to one or other factor or both in combination. Cancers of the glottis are (like cancers of the lung) associated particularly closely with cigarette smoking, while all types of tobacco smoking may equally cause cancers of the extrinsic larynx.

In Scandinavia the incidence has increased *pari passu* with the increase in cancer of the lung. A similar increase has not, however, been seen in Britain and it seems probable that some other aetiological factor has become less prevalent. That other causal factors exist is evident from the relatively high incidence rates in parts of India, Turkey, North Africa, and Brazil.

The disease has occurred as an occupational hazard of the manufacture of mustard gas and possibly also from exposure to asbestos.

Lung

18.6 per cent of all cancers and 27.0 per cent of cancer deaths. Sex ratio of rates: see below (Fig. 13).

Nearly all lung cancers are bronchial carcinomas and should be so described. The term 'lung cancer' is, however, in such common use that it will be used here as synonymous with bronchial carcinoma, although it actually includes a very small proportion of alveolar cell carcinomas with different characteristics.

Until the 1920s, lung cancer was uniformly rare. In the next two decades German and then British pathologists began to comment on an apparent increase, but this tended to be dismissed as an

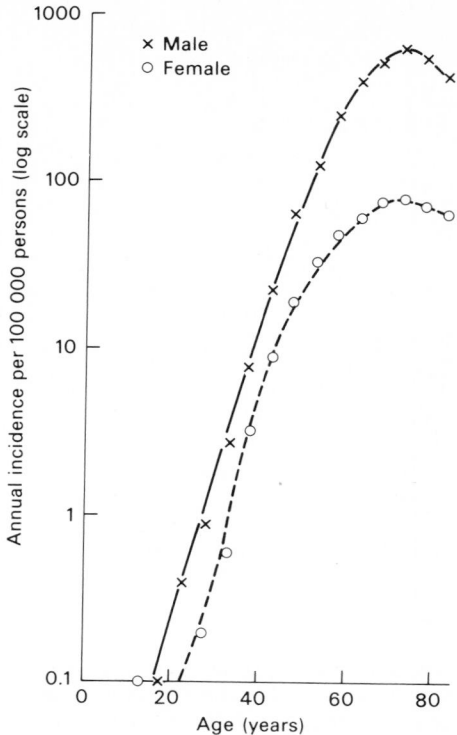

Fig. 13 Annual incidence of cancer of the lung

artefact of improving methods of diagnosis combined with the establishment of special centres for thoracic disease based on the university centres, and undoubtedly most of the increase among females and some of the (larger) increase among males was indeed artefactual. Gradually, however, the increase became so pronounced, and the change in the sex ratio so marked, that it could no longer be wholly dismissed in this way, and by the late 1940s, when in Britain the age-standardized mortality rate in men had increased 20 times, it was clear that the developed world had begun to see an epidemic of lung cancer that was comparable in severity to, though with a longer time scale than, the epidemics of infectious diseases in the past. Up to the 1940s, the increase among women can be regarded as being largely a diagnostic artefact, and so it provides a useful indication of the quantitative extent to which diagnostic artefacts may have affected the male rates prior to 1950. Since 1950, however, diagnostic standards have changed very little, the increase in British men has eventually slowed down and begun to reverse itself, and the increase in women has gathered speed. As a result, the sex ratio (male rate divided by female rate), which rose from 2.0 after the First World War to 6.7 in 1959, fell to 3.6 in 1979. The male excess in the first quarter of the century may have existed partly because of the effects of pipe smoking (an almost exclusively male habit in the nineteenth century) and partly because, even among non-smokers, male lung cancer rates are about 50 per cent greater than female rates.

Changes in treatment have had little effect on the fatality rate, which remains extremely high, and real changes in mortality can therefore be regarded as reflecting real changes in incidence. These, in their turn, can be almost entirely explained by the effects of smoking tobacco, particularly in the form of cigarettes, and tobacco now (c 1980) causes about 91 per cent of all British lung cancer (94 per cent male, 81 per cent female). Evidence of the effect of smoking was first obtained by comparing the smoking histories of patients with different diseases. It was found that the proportion of patients who had never smoked was much smaller if they had lung cancer than if they had some other disease, and the proportion who had smoked heavily was correspondingly greater. Further evidence was obtained by asking large numbers of apparently healthy men and women what they smoked, and then following them all up to determine the causes of death of those that had died. Typical findings of one such study, in which British doctors were first approached in 1951 and then followed for between 20 and 22 years (with later changes in their smoking habits also being recorded periodically) are shown in Table 3. Similar results, all of which show a progressive increase in risk with the amount smoked without any indication of a safe amount of tobacco below which no effect is produced, have been observed in many other countries. Particularly large and impressive studies have been carried out in the United States (by the American Cancer Society and the National Cancer Institute), in Japan (by Hirayama), and in Sweden, and all point to the conclusion that, in countries in which many cigarette smokers have been smoking regularly since early adult life, lung cancer is some 10 to 15 times commoner in regular cigarette smokers than in lifelong non-smokers and up to 40 times commoner in very heavy smokers. The differences are in general less marked in women than in men, not only because women still smoke less but also because most female smokers who are now old enough to have a high risk of cancer either did not begin smoking heavily in *early* adult life or smoke (or have smoked) less intensively (being, for example, less inclined to inhale).

Table 3 Mortality from lung cancer in British doctors by amount smoked (cigarette smokers only) and sex

| Sex | Death rate per 100 000 persons per year* | | | | |
| | Lifelong non smokers | Ex-cigarette smokers | Continuing regular cigarette smokers No. of cigarettes smoked per day | | |
			1–14	15–24	25 or more
M	10	44	78	127	251
F	7	23	9	45	208

* Standardized for age on age distribution of man-years at risk of male doctors.
After Doll and Peto, (1976); Doll, Gray, Hafner, and Peto, (1980)

These observations that smokers were at far greater risk of lung cancer than non-smokers did not, in themselves, prove that smoke caused the disease, although it was difficult to think of any other way in which such a close quantitative relationship could have been produced; but other observations effectively exclude any alternative. These include the fact that the relative risk of lung cancer increased with decreasing age of starting to smoke and decreased with the number of years that smoking had been stopped; that the increase in incidence appeared at an appropriate time after the increase in cigarette sales (after due allowance is made for a spurious increase due to improved diagnosis) and with an appropriate lag in time between the increase among men (who started to smoke cigarettes early this century) and that among women (who started about a quarter of a century later); and that there is a general parallelism between the incidence of the disease in different countries and social and religious groups and the corresponding figures for the consumption of cigarettes. (Furthermore, it was found that when extracts of cigarette smoke were applied repeatedly to the skins of laboratory mice many tumours developed.) Finally, and most encouragingly, the trend in mortality at young ages has now reversed following the change to a type of cigarette that delivers substantially less tar. By 1979 the mortality from lung cancer among men in their thirties, many of whom had smoked low tar cigarettes for the greater part of their smoking lives, was only about half that of men in their thirties a quarter of a century earlier in Britain, the smokers among whom had always smoked high-tar cigarettes. At older ages the decreases are less striking, but they are seen at all ages up to 75 in British men, and up to 50 in British women.

Several other causes of lung cancer have been discovered as a result of observations in industry. Many thousands of men and women have experienced significant hazards from exposure to asbestos or to polycyclic hydrocarbons (in the combustion products of fossil fuel). The former has given rise to hazards in asbestos mines, asbestos textile works, and in a wide variety of occupations in the shipbuilding and construction industries, particularly in insulation work. The latter gave rise to specific hazards in the manufacture of coal-gas, in coking ovens in steel works, in aluminium foundries, and wherever else tar fumes were released into the working environment. Much smaller numbers of men have experienced substantial hazards from radon in the air of mines (not only when mining radioactive materials but also when mining haematite and fluorspar under conditions in which radon seeped into the mine air from streams and the surrounding rock), from the manufacture of chromates and chrome pigments, from the refining of nickel, from arsenic (in the manufacture of arsenical pesticides and in the refining of copper, which is always contaminated with arsenic), and probably from the manufacture of mustard gas. In one extreme situation, the absolute risk of contracting lung cancer due to the occupational hazard was so large that more than half the workers contracted the disease (in the cobalt mines of Schneeberg and Jachymov in Central Europe, which were subsequently mined for radium and uranium). In several other situations with heavy exposure to asbestos or the early stages of nickel refining the occupational hazard has affected as many as 20–30 per cent of the exposed men.

Some of the materials responsible for these occupational hazards —particularly the combustion products of fossil fuels—are or have been widely distributed in the air of towns and it is still a matter for debate how far they, in this way, contributed to the production of the disease in the general population. That lung cancer is more common in big towns — and in particular in capital cities—than in smaller towns and rural areas is certain, but this holds as strongly for Oslo and Helsinki, two relatively unpolluted cities, as for London, Birmingham, Manchester, Chicago, Los Angeles, and Pittsburgh. Differences between the largest towns and the least populated ares are seldom more than threefold and it is difficult to estimate how far these present-day differences can be accounted for by present-day or, perhaps more importantly, past differences in cigarette smoking, a habit which has tended to spread outwards from the major cities. Attempts to 'allow for' cigarette smoking are probably inadequate, as it is impossible to take full account of such factors as the age of starting to smoke cigarettes, the amount smoked daily at different periods, and the method of smoking (number of puffs, depth of inhaling, etc.). The results of the large study carried out by the American Cancer society showed some small differences between residents of the different areas after standardizing for current cigarette smoking to the best of the authors' ability, but they concluded that their data offer 'little or no support to the hypothesis that urban air pollution has an important effect on lung cancer' (Hammond and Garfinkel 1980). One thing is certain, that in the absence of cigarette smoking any effect of urban pollution is relatively so small that it has been impossible to measure it reliably. Some synergism between smoking and urban air pollution, however, is possible and estimates based on extrapolation from the effects observed in heavily polluted factories suggest that previous levels of atmospheric pollution may have contributed to as much as 10 per cent of all lung cancers in certain big cities. In Britain, present levels of air pollution by benzypyrene and various other components of smoke are, however, much lower than the levels of a quarter of a century ago, and their effects on future lung cancer rates are, therefore, likely to be substantially less than this.

The development of the male lung cancer epidemic and the early signs of its departure have been most prominent in Britain and Finland, since the switch of young men to cigarettes was largely complete in these countries by the 1920s. In the United States, where cigarette consumption doubled during the Second World War, the resultant increases in lung cancer among older men (older than 55) are still in progress, and only among younger men (younger than 50) are the benefits of reduced smoking and a switch to low tar cigarettes causing decreases in lung cancer mortality. In some other developed countries the development of the epidemic is still further behind and it is only just beginning to appear in many undeveloped countries. Two populations show unusually high mortality rates in women. One is the Maori population in New Zealand, whose women began to smoke regularly at the turn of the century, well before any other national group. The other is the Chinese, whose women, both in China and abroad, have an unusually high mortality on non-smokers, perhaps from their special mode of cookery.

The different histological types of bronchial carcinoma have different relationships to the various causative factors. Squamous carcinoma is most closely related to smoking and adenocarcinoma least. The same criteria have, unfortunately, not always been used for the diagnosis of adenocarcinoma—reports of an increase in the proportion of cancers of this type among bronchial carcinomas may be evidence merely for changes in the source of materials and an increasingly intensive search for small mucus-secreting structures in poorly differentiated neoplasms rather than for any material increase in causes of lung cancer other than tobacco. 'Oat cell' carcinoma (a term that describes only the histological appearance of the neoplastic cells, since the nature of their precursors is uncertain) has an intermediate position in relation to smoking, but is particularly easily induced by ionizing radiations and bischloromethyl ether.

Pleura and peritoneum
0.2 per cent of fatal cancers.
Sex ratio of rates (from mortality data) 3.4 to 1.

The existence of a specific type of tumour arising from the pleura or peritoneum was debated by pathologists until 1960 when Wagner and his colleagues reported that six African patients with a similar type of 'peripheral lung cancer' had all lived in villages that were heavily polluted with dust produced by the mining of blue asbestos (i.e. crocidolite). Since then many cases have been reported throughout the world, the great majority, but not all, of which have been specifically associated with exposure to asbestos at work. A few cases arise from secondary contamination by asbestos (e.g. from household contact with asbestos workers); but some 20 or 30 per cent are probably due to spontaneous biological accident or other causes, including the large number of cases that have occurred in two Turkish villages due probably to natural exposure to mineral fibres that are physically similar to, but chemically different from, asbestos. Most mesotheliomas arise from the pleura, but some originate from the peritoneum. It is still uncertain whether they are peculiarly likely to occur after exposure to crocidolite or whether they are produced equally by exposure to white asbestos (chrysotile) and other types.

Mesothelioma seldom occurs less than 15 years after first exposure to asbestos, commonly occurs 25 to 30 years afterwards, and may be delayed for 50 years or more. Almost all cases are fatal, so that the mortality would reflect incidence, if all cases were correctly diagnosed. Due to the rarity of the disease and the possiblity of confusion with lung or other types of cancer, it is still uncertain how many cases occur each year; but the recorded rate, which rose rapidly during the 1960s, appears to have stabilized at around 250 cases a year and there is reason to hope that, at least in Britain, the increases have abated. Pleural mesothelioma is not related to cigarette smoking and the occupational hazard affects cigarette smokers and non-smokers alike.

Bone
0.3 per cent of all cancers and of all cancer deaths.
Sex ratio of rates 1.7 to 1 (Fig. 14).

Tumours can affect any bone, but characteristically affect the long bones in adolescence. After 45 years of age they occur most commonly in bones affected by Paget's disease (osteitis deformans). This predisposes to bone tumours so strongly that as many as 1 per cent of all affected people eventually develop one.

Many different histological variaties occur, some of which appear

to have different causes. Osteogenic sarcomas and chondrosarcomas are the most common, the former accounting for nearly all the adolescent peak. One rare type (Ewing's tumour) occurs only in childhood and adolescence and is almost unknown in black people, irrespective of the society in which they live.

Ionizing radiations are the only known extrinsic cause. Cases have been produced after intensive radiotherapy or the medicinal use of thorium (a bone-seeking radionuclide). In industry they have occurred in luminizers who have ingested radium, possibly as a result of pointing the luminous paint brushes in their mouths.

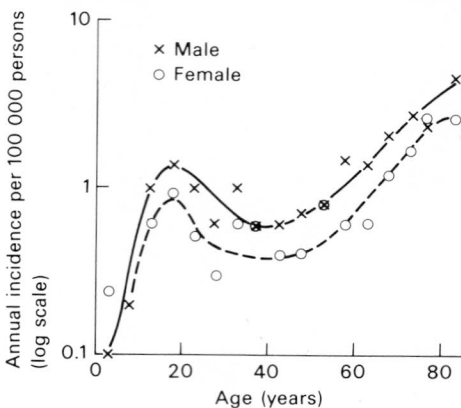

Fig. 14   Annual incidence of cancer of the bone

National statistics record a reduction in mortality over the last 40 years, but are unreliable indicators of incidence as many deaths attributed to tumours of bone are in reality due to cancers that have spread from other sites. The recorded decrease in mortality in adult life is, therefore, an artefact due to improved diagnosis (and contributed to in recent years by higher survival rates in childhood) and the true incidence may have remained roughly constant.

Connective tissues
0.4 per cent of all cancers and 0.2 per cent of cancer deaths.
Sex ratio of rates 1.3 to 1 (Fig 15).

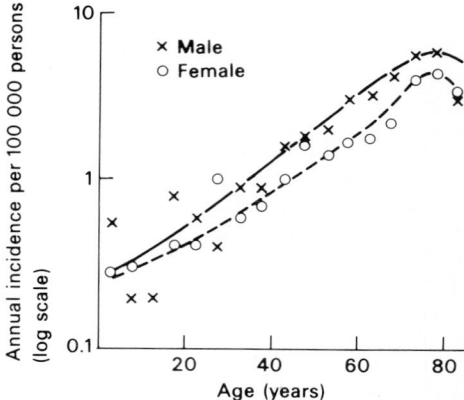

Fig. 15   Annual incidence of cancer of the connective tissues

Sarcomas of the soft tissues include a wide variety of different disease, all of which are rare throughout the world, with the sole exception of Kaposi's sarcoma which is one of the commonest types of cancers in parts of Central Africa. A few cases are due to ionizing radiations and to the phenoxy acids and chlorophenols used as herbicides, while some may be caused by intensive immunosuppression; but the causes of the majority of cases are unknown.

Skin (melanoma)
0.8 per cent of all cancers and 0.6 per cent of cancer deaths.
Sex ratio of rates 0.6 to 1 (Fig. 16).

The incidence of the disease varies inversely with the amount of skin pigmentation. In white people the tumour occurs most commonly on the legs (in women) and the trunk, head, and neck (in men). It is extremely rare in blacks in the USA, but is more common in Africa where it occurs at the junction of the pigmented and unpigmented skin on the sole of the foot, particularly if the junction is irregular, as it tends to be in some tribes. Like basal cell and squamous carcinoma of the skin, it is particularly common in sufferers from xeroderma pigmentosum.

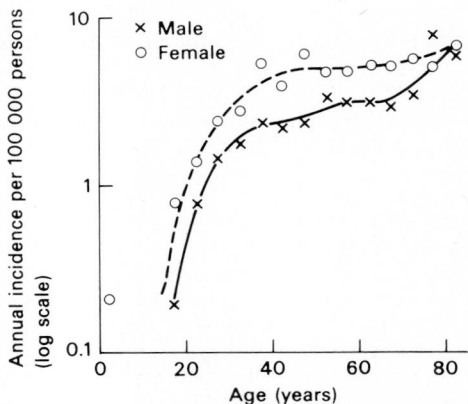

Fig. 16   Annual incidence of cancer of the skin (melanoma)

Incidence rates in white people vary roughly in proportion to the flux of ultraviolet light in the countries in which they live. It is not, in general, more common in outdoor than indoor workers (rather the reverse, in fact, perhaps due to the protective effects of a semi-permanent sun-tan), but it may be associated with periodic bouts of sunbathing. Incidence and mortality rates have been increasing in Britain, the USA, and many other countries with mainly white populations. The increase began in cohorts born early this century, who exposed their skin more readily to the sun than their predecessors had, and it appears to have slowed or stopped in more recent cohorts. The totality of the evidence suggests that ultraviolet light is the principal cause, but there are some discrepant observations and other factors (possibly hormonal) may also be important.

Skin (non-melanoma)

11 per cent of all cancers (or more, since few registries collect reliable data), but only 0.3 per cent of cancer deaths.

Sex ratio of rates 1.7 to 1. (Fig. 17).

Non-melanomatous skin cancers are of two main types, basal cell and squamous carcinomas. The former, which are also known as rodent ulcers, are produced by ultraviolet light. They occur mainly on parts of the body that are regularly exposed to the sun and, in particular, on the face, head, and neck. They are more common in outdoor workers, such as seamen and farmers, than in indoor workers, more common in fair-skinned than in dark-skinned people, and are almost unknown in blacks unless they suffer from albinism. Some few cases have been produced by exposure to X-rays, but the risk is very small unless the dose is very large and they seldom occur after normal courses of radiotherapy. People who are unfortunate enough to suffer from xeroderma pigmentosum, a hereditary condition in which there is a defect in the enzyme responsible for the repair of the principal form of ultraviolet damage to DNA, invariably develop large numbers of skin tumours at an early age in response to even quite mild exposure to diffuse sunlight (see pages 4.19, 4.48, and 4.81).

Squamous carcinoma is also produced by ultraviolet light, but less easily, so that it accounts for only about 20 per cent of cancers on the exposed skin. It is, however, the principal type of skin cancer produced by various carcinogenic chemicals, and particularly by polycyclic hydrocarbons in the combustion products of coal. These chemicals have been responsible for the scrotal cancers of chimney sweeps, who accumulated soot in the folds of the scrotal skin, of mule-spinners, whose clothes were saturated with carcinogenic oils, and of various other groups of workers whose clothes were contaminated with tar. They have caused (and still do cause) cancers of the forearm in industrial workers whose arms are regularly splashed with tar or carcinogenic oils, cancers of the groin in India, localized by the continued friction of the dhoti cloth, and cancers of the abdomen in Kashmir that are associated with the habit of carrying a kangri, or small stove, inside the clothes in winter to keep warm. Occasionally they have been caused on the legs or other parts of the body when prolonged courses of coal tar ointment were prescribed for the treatment of chronic skin diseases.

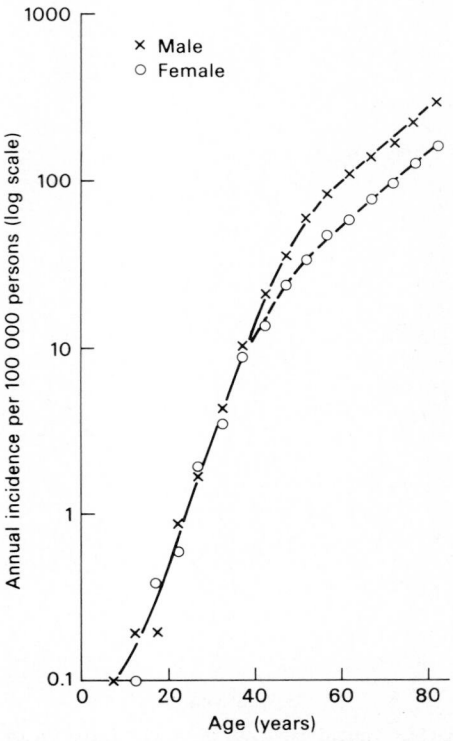

Fig. 17   Annual incidence of cancer of the skin (non-melanoma)

Squamous carcinomas of the skin may also be due to prolonged exposure to arsenic, which is excreted by the skin, although arsenic has not been shown to cause any type of cancer in any experimental animal thus far studied. Pigmentation and, less often, cancer of the skin sometimes occur after prolonged medical treatment with arsenic, which was prescribed for a variety of chronic diseases, and both conditions have occurred in arsenic-exposed smelters of copper and cobalt and in arsenical pesticide manufacturers, many of whom have been exposed chronically to as much as 100 µg of arsenic per cubic metre of air.

One iatrogenic cause of squamous carcinoma of the skin that is difficult to eliminate is the intensive immunosuppression that is required to ensure the survival of organ transplants. Whether immunosuppression of this type, prolonged over many years, will eventually lead to an increased risk of cancer in all organs is still a matter of speculation. On present evidence it certainly produces a gross increase in the risk of non-Hodgkin's lymphoma (see page 4.69) and a material increase in the risk of squamous, but not basal cell, carcinoma of the skin. Why these two cancers should be selectively affected is unclear; but, in the latter case, it may be related to the fact that squamous carcinomas of the skin are among the most strongly antigenic of all human cancers.

Breast

10.8 per cent of all cancers and 9.5 per cent of cancer deaths. Sex ratio of rates 0.01 to 1 (Fig. 18).

Cancer of the breast is the commonest fatal cancer in women throughout most of the developed world, where it is responsible for approximately 20 per cent of all female cancer deaths. It is less common in eastern Europe and much less common in Asia and in black African populations south of the Sahara. Incidence rates have tended to rise slowly in many countries but the changes are relatively small and decreases have been recorded in some age groups. The geographical differences are unlikely to be chiefly due to genetic factors as black women in the USA and Japanese women in Hawaii have rates that are similar to those in their white American compatriots but much greater than those in their country of origin.

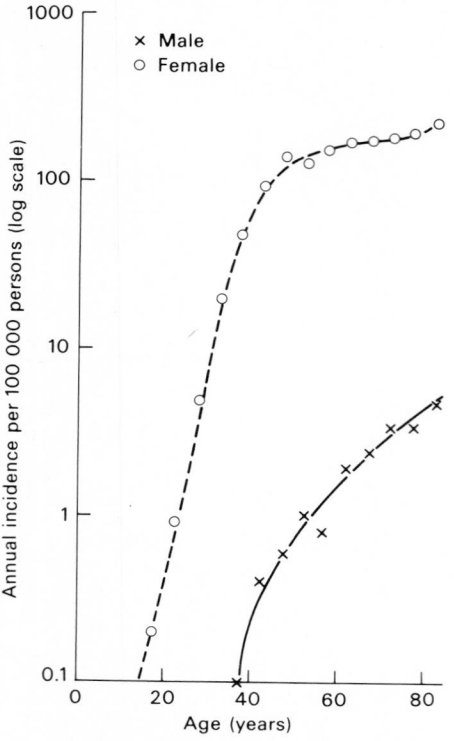

Fig. 18   Annual incidence of cancer of the breast

Hormonal factors are important in the production of the disease, but it has not been possible to define them precisely. The duration of ovarian activity appears to be relevant as the disease is particularly common in women who have an early menarche and a late menopause. The incidence in later life increases progressively with a woman's age at the time of her first full-term pregnancy, being about three times greater when the first birth occurs after 35 years of age than when it occurs before 18 years. Pregnancies after the first have little or no further effect and neither do abortions before the first full-term birth. It is probable, therefore, that the effect depends on the age at which lactation is first stimulated. The duration of lactation, however, is of little importance. The widespread belief that breast feeding protects against the development of the disease is, unfortunately, not generally true. The inverse correlation that has been reported between the duration of breast feeding in different countries and the incidence of the disease in those countries is a secondary effect of the age at which the first child is born, and does not hold up when comparisons are made between women who have their first child at the same age.

Parity differences are insufficient to account for the large variations in the incidence of the disease in different countries, which seem to be correlated with a 'high' standard of living: that is, with life in a developed country. Internationally, incidence rates corre-

late closely with the consumption of fat (and somewhat less closely with the consumption of meat), and within countries there is some evidence that the risk of developing the disease increases with the degree of obesity. Although this relationship is not as strong as the correlations with national fat consumption might lead one to expect, it is nevertheless important, at least for extremely obese women. It may be due to the fact that after the menopause the only natural source of oestrogen is from adrenal hormones which are converted to oestrone in adipose tissue. Whether oestrogens prescribed medically increase the risk of the disease is uncertain, but what little evidence there is suggests that they may. Oestrogens combined with progestogens, as in the contraceptive pill, do not appear to affect the risk; but the evidence is conflicting, and it is, in any case, too early to be sure what the effect of prolonged use of oral contraceptives (for, say, 10 years or more) may be, particularly if they are used before the birth of the first child.

Choriocarcinoma

0.01 per cent of all cancers and 0.005 per cent of cancer deaths. Occurs only in women.

Choriocarcinomas are malignant tumours of the trophoblastic (placental) tissue. Most cases occur as a result of malignant degeneration of remnants of a hydatidiform mole left behind after a miscarriage, but a few cases occur after completion of apparently uncomplicated pregnancies. The condition is extremely rare in developed countries but somewhat less rare in Maoris, Hawaiians, Malays, and American Indians and in parts of China. Within developed countries there is no evidence of a relationship with socio-economic status and no causes are known.

Cervix uteri

2.6 per cent of all cancers and 1.6 per cent of cancer deaths. Occurs only in women (Fig. 19).

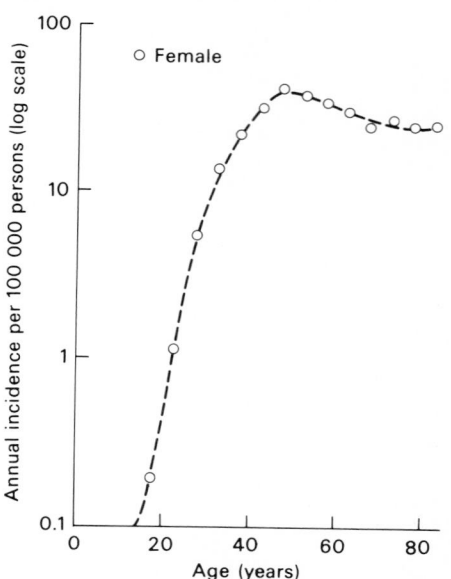

Fig. 19   Annual incidence of cancer of the cervix uteri

Carcinoma of the cervix is the commonest type of cancer throughout much of Africa, Asia, and Latin America, and it used also to be common in Europe and North America. It has always been rare in Jewesses and has tended to be less common in Muslim women than in women of other faiths living in the same country (as, for example, in Christian women in Yugoslavia and in Hindu women in India).

Changes in incidence have been difficult to assess, partly because mortality data did not distinguish between deaths due to cancer of the cervix and those due to cancer of the corpus uteri (or endometrium), partly because the introduction of screening programmes has made it possible to diagnose and treat premalignant lesions (see below), and partly because hysterectomy well prior to the onset of the disease has been performed progressively more often with a corresponding reduction in the number of uteri in which the disease could occur. Despite these complications there can be no doubt that the disease has become substantially less common in Europe and North America than it used to be before the Second World War. Unfortunately, however, mortality rates under 35 years of age have begun to increase again in Britain in the last 10 years despite the introduction of screening and, if this reflects an increase in incidence (as it presumably does), the increase must be expected to spread to older ages with the passage of time.

The rarity of the disease in Jewesses and its relative rarity in Muslim women suggests that male circumcision might materially reduce the risk of its development, but this is unlikely to be true as the state of circumcision of her husband has no substantial effect on the risk a woman runs of developing the disease in religious communities in which only some men are circumcized. Cleanliness is likely to be an important factor, as the disease is relatively uncommon in communities that practise ritual ablution before and after intercourse and, within each community, it becomes less common with rising socio-economic status.

Squamous carcinoma, which constitutes the vast majority of all cases, is the type that is intimately connected with sexual activity. It almost never occurs in virgins, and is common in prostitutes. Moreover, the risk of developing it increases with the number of children and with the number of marriages and inversely with the age at which intercourse first occurs. All of these observations can largely be explained by a single variable: that is, the number of sexual partners. Moreover, for those women who report only one partner, the risk increases with the number of partners that that partner has had. Finally, among women who use contraceptives, the disease is less common among those who use occlusive contraceptives than among those who use an intrauterine device or an oral contraceptive. It may be hypothesized (see page 4.72) that the excess risk among pill users is in part due to some special effect of the pill, but it is difficult to avoid the general conclusion that the disease is chiefly venereal in origin—and perhaps, therefore, due to a virus. A strong correlation with cigarette smoking has been consistently found, but this is probably largely or wholly because of an association between cigarette smoking and behaviour conducive to venereal infection. Infection with the herpes simplex type 2 virus and (to a lesser extent) the condyloma virus have both been associated with it, but no part of their genomes has been recovered from the DNA of the malignant cells and the nature of the causative infection(s) is still uncertain.

If cervical cancer is due to a virus, the same virus is probably also responsible for the much more common lesions of dysplasia and carcinoma-in-situ, as they both have the same epidemiological features as cervical cancer, save only that they occur at younger ages. Progression may not occur at all and dysplasia (and even, occasionally, carcinoma-in-situ) may regress and disappear. Why this should be so, and what the factors are that determine regression or progression, is unknown. The presence of dysplasia and carcinoma-in-situ can be recognized simply in cervical smears and screening for these lesions, followed by cone biopsy (or amputation of the affected cervix), provides a simple means of preventing the development of clinical malignancy. Protection is not, however, complete as the presence of abnormal cells may in practice be overlooked and a few cases seem to appear and develop so rapidly that it would be difficult to detect them in the premalignant stage unless screening was repeated at impracticably short intervals.

Nothing is known about the epidemiology of adenocarcinoma of the cervix, except that it is uniformly rare and has little or nothing in common with that of squamous carcinoma of the cervix.

Endometrium (corpus uteri)
1.9 per cent of all cancers and 0.9 per cent of cancer deaths. Occurs only in women (Fig. 20).

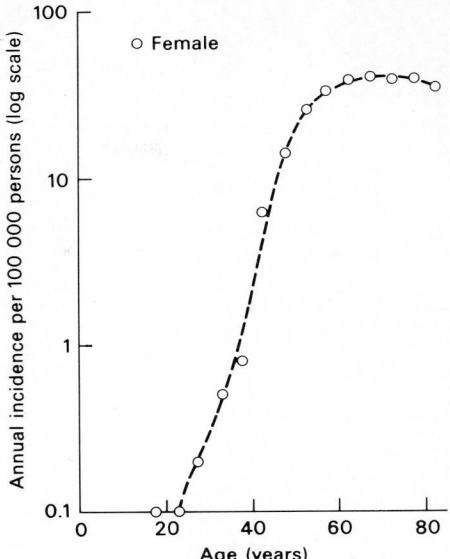

Fig. 20 Annual incidence of cancer of the endometrium

The epidemiological features of endometrial cancer are in many respects the opposite of those of cervical cancer. Histologically, it is nearly always an adenocarcinoma. It is common in developed countries, rare in poor countries, and is, if anything, becoming more common with the passage of time. It is inversely related to parity, the risk of developing the disease being greatest in nulliparae, but is not otherwise related to coitus and is unaffected by the number of sexual partners. Like cancer of the breast, it is positively associated with early menarche and a late menopause.

The one factor that is known to produce the disease is regular exposure to oestrogen, unopposed by progestogen. This leads first to endometrial hyperplasia and eventually, in some cases, to cancer. Known causes include oestrogen-secreting tumours of the ovary, the use of oral contraceptives in which oestrogens and progestogens are prescribed sequentially (which have now been abandoned), the use of 'natural' conjugated oestrogens to relieve menopausal and post-menopausal symptoms, and adiposity. That the last should cause the disease is not surprising, when it is borne in mind that the only oestrogens to be produced in the body after the menopause are produced in adipose tissue from the adrenal hormone, androstenedione.

It is improbable, however, that oestrogens are initiating agents. They are not mutagens in vitro and the changes that took place in the incidence of the disease in the USA following the increase and the subsequent reduction in the use of premarin (a conjugated oestrogen) for the treatment of menopausal symptoms occurred so quickly that they make sense only if oestrogens act on some late stage(s) of the carcinogenic process.

Whether the consumption of fat has a specific effect apart from its contribution to the total of energy producing foods is uncertain. That it may do is suggested by the very close correlation between the incidence of the disease and the per caput consumption of fat in different countries, which is closer than for any other item of food or indicator of a high standard of living. An excess consumption of fat, moreover, seems to have a specific effect in producing maturity onset diabetes and hypertension, both of which tend to be clinically associated with endometrial cancer.

Ovary
2.3 per cent of all cancers and 2.9 per cent of cancer deaths. Occurs only in women (Fig. 21).

Cancer of the ovary is not one disease but many, each of which is defined by its histological appearance. Most types are too rare to have been considered separately in epidemiological studies and the

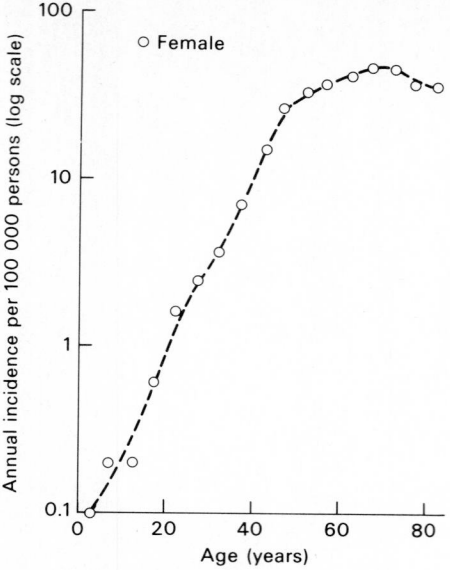

Fig. 21 Annual incidence of cancer of the ovary

few characteristics that have been recognized may refer only to adenocarcinoma, which is the most common type. These characteristics resemble those of endometrial cancer, in that the risk of developing the disease is greatest in countries with a high standard of living, increases with the length of time from menarche to menopause, and decreases progressively with increasing numbers of children. They differ in that ovarian cancer is not produced by oestrogens. The incidence of the disease appears to be diminished by the use of oral contraceptives, and its development may prove to depend on the cyclic activity of the ovary.

Prostate
4.6 per cent of all cancers and 3.8 per cent of cancer deaths. Occurs only in men (Fig. 22).

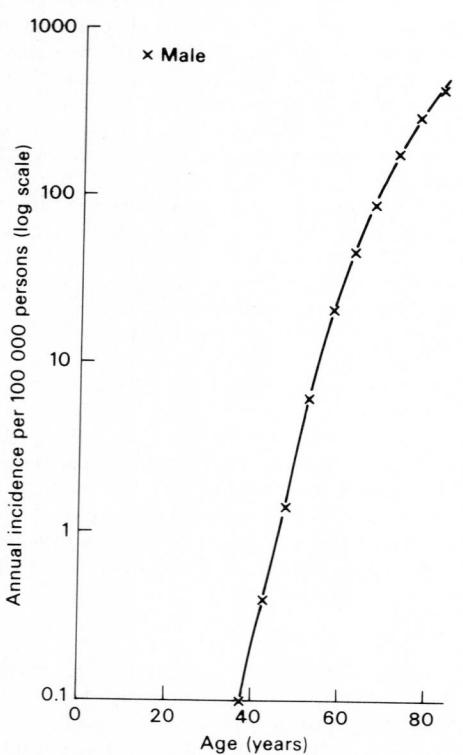

Fig. 22 Annual incidence of cancer of the prostate

Cancer of the prostate is more characteristically a disease of old age than any other cancer, so that it has of necessity come to play a much larger part in clinical experience as the proportion of old people in the population has increased. It is also unusual in that foci of cells resembling prostatic cancer can be found in a high proportion of clinically normal prostates, so that the recorded incidence rate can be increased dramatically by increasing the number of prostatic biopsies. Death rates at each age have remained fairly constant in Britain and North America and the weight of evidence suggests that the disease is due to factors that have affected society for many years. What these factors are remains obscure. Associations have been reported with both increased and decreased sexual activity. On general grounds it seems likely that the disease is dependent on hormonal imbalance, but the nature of the imbalance is unknown.

Two epidemiological observations stand out: the high incidence in black populations throughout the world, and the low incidence in Japanese. Both may be partly due to genetic factors, but they are not wholly so, as both Japanese and blacks have higher rates in the USA than in Japan and Africa. Some cases may be due to cadmium, as increased mortality rates have been observed in several studies of men who have worked with the metal. This is not, however, a major factor, as the occupation is uncommon, the exposures have been heavy, and the increased mortality small.

Testis
0.4 per cent of all cancers and 0.2 per cent of cancer deaths. Occurs only in men (Fig. 23).

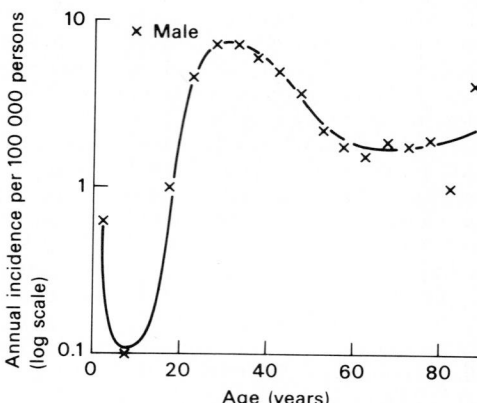

Fig. 23 Annual incidence of cancer of the testis

Testicular cancers are of two main types which differ epidemiologically in that one tends to occur at slightly younger ages than the other. Seminomas, which are the more common, have a peak incidence at about 30 years, but some continue to occur in old age. Teratomas, which are more often called embryomal carcinomas in the USA, have a peak incidence about 10 years earlier and very rarely occur after 50. Both genetic and environmental factors are important. On the one hand, the disease is uniformly rare in black populations, whether in Africa or in the USA. On the other, it has increased in incidence. In Britain, the increase began in the 1920s and affected first the higher socio-economic groups. The increase trebled the mortality at 15 to 34 years of age, producing a sharp peak in young adult life that had not previously been present, and was compensated for, to a small extent, by a decrease at ages over 55. The disease is much more likely to occur in an undescended than in a normal testis, but otherwise its causes are unknown.

Penis
0.2 per cent of all cancers and 0.1 per cent of cancer deaths. Occurs only in men (Fig. 24).

The most striking fact about the epidemiology of cancer of the penis is that circumcision protects against its development. Carried

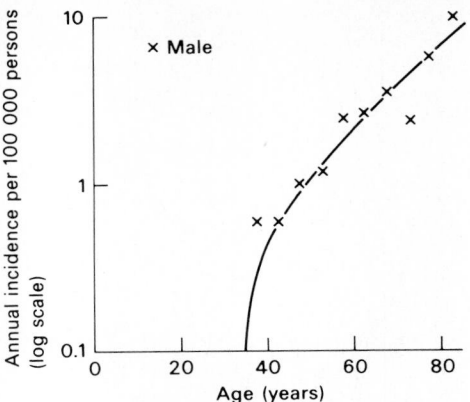

Fig. 24 Annual incidence of cancer of the penis

out within a week or two of birth, the protection is almost complete; carried out later in boyhood, the effect is obvious, but less marked. Circumcision is not the only way of preventing the disease, as marked variations in incidence occur among tribal groups in Africa who are alike in not practising circumcision, but otherwise have different social customs. In some the disease accounts for as much as 10 per cent of all cancers in males; in others it is only slightly more common than in developed countries. Personal cleanliness may be an important factor, as it is in relation to some forms of cancer of the skin, and it seems that as long as the glans, coronary sulcus, and foreskin are kept clean, the risk of developing the disease is remote.

An observation that suggests the possibility of a venereal (and hence perhaps a viral) origin is an association between cancers of the penis and cervix uteri in marital pairs. The association is not strong, but it has been observed in several countries and cannot be accounted for simply by confounding with socio-economic class.

Bladder
4.7 per cent of all cancers and 3.3 per cent of cancer deaths. Sex ratio of rates 4.2 to 1 (Fig. 25).

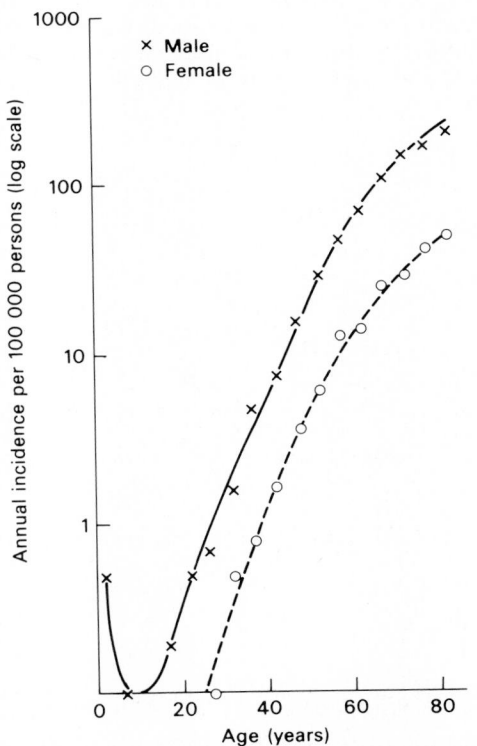

Fig. 25 Annual incidence of cancer of the bladder

Cancer of the bladder is known to be produced by cigarette smoking, occupational exposure to a group of chemicals classed together as aromatic amines, infestation of the bladder with *Schistosoma haematobium*, and the medical prescription of chlornaphazine (N,N'-bis(2-chloroethyl)-2-naphthylamine) and cyclophosphamide. It has also been suspected of being due to the consumption of coffee, saccharin, and cyclamates, but these claims are not confirmed. It is not surprising that the bladder should be affected by so many chemicals, as any noxious small molecules in the blood will tend to be found at greatly increased concentration in the urinary tract. For example, cigarette smoke contains various mutagenic chemicals that enter the bloodstream and thence the bladder, so that, when tested on bacterial DNA, the urine of cigarette smokers is found to be mutagenic, while that of non-smokers is barely active.

Smoking. Of all these causes, the most important numerically is cigarette smoking, which probably accounts for about half the total number of cases in Britain and North America. 2-naphthylamine is present in cigarette smoke; but although it is a very powerful bladder carcinogen (see below), the amount present is probably too small to account either for the cacinogenic effect or for the mutagenicity of smokers' urine.

Occupation. An occupational cause was first suspected in 1898 in Germany, when Rehn commented on a cluster of cases in men using aniline for the manufacture of dyes. Aniline, however, is not carcinogenic in experimental animals, more recent studies have failed to incriminate it epidemiologically, and it seems likely that other carcinogenic chemicals were present as impurities. Four aromatic amines that are carcinogenic in experimental animals have been shown to cause bladder cancer in man: 2-naphthylamine, benzidine, 3,3'-dichlorobenzidine, and 4-amino-biphenyl. The first of these is one of the most powerful human carcinogens so far discovered and was responsible for the development of bladder cancer in all the 19 men who were at one time employed in distilling it in a British factory. Its manufacture was stopped in Britain in 1949, but small quantities continued to be imported until the 1960s. Other aromatic amines that may cause bladder cancer include auramine, magenta, and, perhaps, l-naphthylamine. The last is only dubiously carcinogenic in experimental animals and it seems probable that the many cases associated with its use have been due to the few per cent of 2-naphthylamine that was present as an impurity in the commercial material. These substances were used in the manufacture of dyes, in the rubber industry as antioxidants (1-naphthylamine and 4-amino-biphenyl) and hardeners (benzidine), and in laboratories as a reagent (benzidine). 2-naphthylamine is also found in the combustion products of coal and was presumably chiefly responsible for the hazard of bladder cancer in men who made coal-gas. The proportion of cases attributable to occupational causes has varied from place to place and time to time. In recent years a reasonable estimate for Britain and North America would be between 5 and 10 per cent.

Medicines. The two medicinal causes have, by contrast, been responsible for only a handful of cases. Chlornaphazine was used briefly for the treatment of myelomatosis, but it was rapidly found to produce bladder cancer, which was hardly surprising as it was metabolized into 2-naphthylamine. Cyclophosphamide is used primarily for the treatment of malignant disease but also as an immunosuppressant. In large doses it may cause sloughing and, occasionally, cancer of the bladder mucosa.

Parasitic infestation. The association between schistosomiasis and cancer of the bladder is particularly marked in Egypt and Tanzania. The schistosomes should not be thought of as carcinogenic in themselves, but probably as the start of a chain of events that may lead to cancer through chronic bacterial infection and, perhaps, the formation of nitrites and nitrosamines. Cancer associated with schistosomiasis is characteristically squamous in appearance and this type of carcinoma is predominant in countries where schistoso-miasis of a type (*S. haematobium*) that affects the bladder is common. Elsewhere the predominant type is a transitional cell carcinoma.

Diet. The evidence linking bladder cancer to diet is weak. Several case-control studies have suggested a positive relationship with the consumption of coffee, but the results are inconsistent and it is difficult to exclude the effect of confounding with the stronger relationship with cigarette smoking. Artificial sweeteners have come under suspicion because of the results of animal experiments in which first mixtures of cyclamates and saccharin and then sac-charin alone were shown to cause bladder cancer in rats. The human use of cyclamates was banned before saccharin came under suspicion, but it now appears that the 'positive' results of animal experiments with cyclamates alone were due to impurities. Saccharin has been shown to cause cancer of the bladder in rats in straightforward feeding experiments, especially when given over two generations and when given after a single instillation into the bladder of a powerful carcinogen. In both instances the quantities that had to be given were large, constituting a few per cent of the feed. The human evidence consists of an analysis of time trends in consumption and cancer mortality, of observations on diabetics (who consume more saccharin and experience less bladder cancer than average), and large case-control studies which show relative risks of developing bladder cancer in users and non-users that range neatly on either side of one. In summary, it could hardly be more negative (although it is still possible that *lifelong* use of saccharin will produce a measurable risk of bladder cancer).

Variations in incidence. Existing knowledge of the causes of the disease accounts for most of the geographical variations in inci-dence, but temporal variations are more difficult to interpret, due to the changing attitudes to the classification of papillomas of the bladder. It is possible that there is an increasing tendency to de-scribe what would previously have been called 'papillomas' as 'carcinomas' of the bladder, in which case this will produce artefac-tual upward trends in the recorded incidence rates. Consequently, as curative treatment has not improved greatly over the past quar-ter of a century, the trends in the true onset rate of the disease are probably best estimated from a study of the trends in mortality from the disease. Surprisingly, in view of the presumably increasing effect of tobacco on the disease, mortality rates are if anything decreasing rather than increasing. The reasons for this are not clear, and reduction of occupational exposure to aromatic amines is unlikely to account for much of the decrease that is being observed.

Kidney
1.4 per cent of all cancers and 1.8 per cent of cancer deaths. Sex ratio of rates 2.2 to 1 (Fig. 26).

Cancers of the kidney are of three main types: nephroblastomas (or Wilm's tumours), adenocarcinomas (or hypernephromas), and transitional and squamous cell carcinomas of the renal pelvis. The first are limited to childhood, occur with almost equal frequency everywhere, and are of unknown aetiology. The second constitute by far the majority of all cases, are more common in Western Europe and North America than in Africa and Asia, and have been slowly increasing in incidence. Cigarette smoking may account for a quarter of the cases but the association is weak and the conclusion that it is causal would not be regarded as probable were it not for the mutagenicity of the urine of cigarette smokers and the much stronger association of smoking with cancer of the bladder. This, however, is less conclusive than might appear as there is no firm evidence that hypernephromas are also produced by any of the occupational exposures that have given rise to substantial risks of bladder cancer.

The third type of renal cancer (carcinoma of the pelvis) consti-tutes some 10 per cent of all cases. Two established causes are occupational exposure (as for cancer of the bladder) and the con-

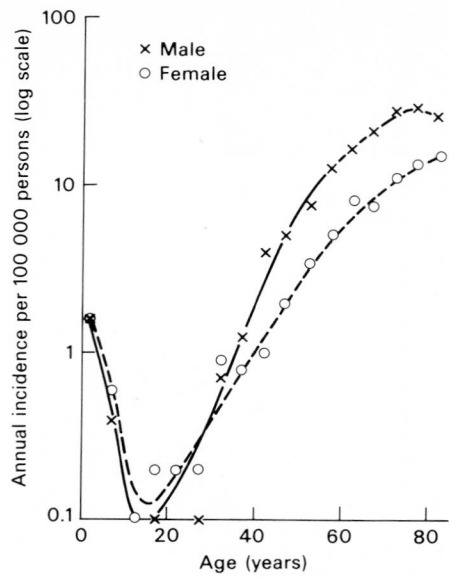

Fig. 26   Annual incidence of cancer of the kidney

sumption of amounts of phenacetin large enough to produce anal-gesic nephropathy. In both cases the hazards are small.

Brain and nervous system
1.8 per cent of all cancers and 2.3 per cent of cancer deaths. Sex ratio of rates 1.5 to 1 (Fig. 27).

Tumours of the brain and nervous system are of many different histological types and many of them fall into a category that histolo-gists find extremely difficult to decide whether to call malignant or benign. Some occur characteristically in childhood (medulloblasto-mas), others in adult life (glioblastomas), and others at all ages (astrocytomas). Despite the overall male excess, some types (men-ingiomas) are more common in females. No environmental causes have been established, but some occupations in the chemical indus-try are under suspicion. A small excess of brain tumours was re-ported in children whose mothers were vaccinated against polio-myelitis while the children were *in utero*. The vaccine was an early preparation that was contaminated with SV 40 virus from

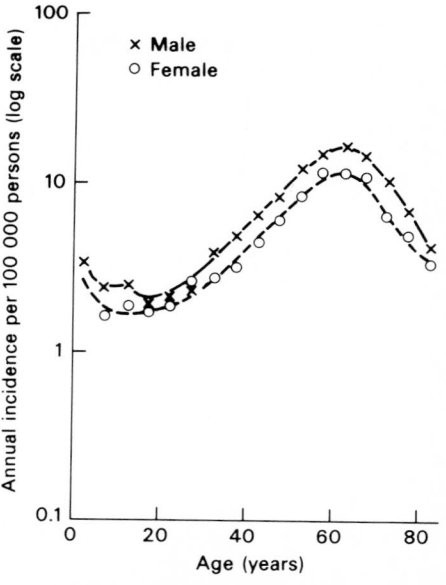

Fig. 27   Annual incidence of cancer of the brain and nervous system

monkey kidney cells that were used as a culture medium. It is unlikely that a similar situation will ever arise again and it is impossible to tell now whether the excess was a chance event or not.

Cerebral reticulosarcomas are described under non-Hodgkin's lymphoma (see below).

Thyroid
0.4 per cent of all cancers and 0.3 of cancer deaths.
Sex ratio of rates 0.5 to 1 (Fig. 28).

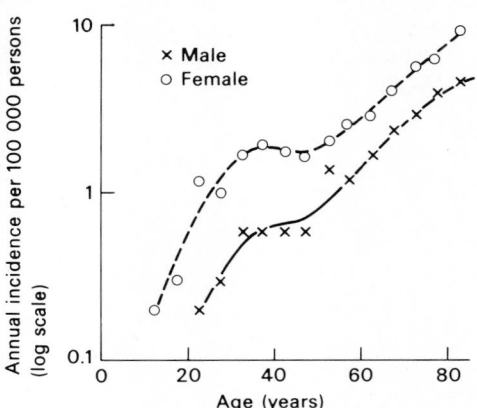

Fig. 28   Annual incidence of cancer of the thyroid

The thyroid is particularly sensitive to ionizing radiations in childhood. Substantial numbers of cases have occurred among the survivors of the atomic explosions in Hiroshima and Nagasaki and in young people whose necks were irradiated in infancy for the treatment of an enlarged thymus. This condition, which is now considered to be perfectly normal, was at one time thought to be a cause of sudden death. Fortunately, the thyroid tumours produced in this way have nearly all been of the papillary and follicular types which respond well to treatment. No causes are known of the medullary and anaplastic types, which occur only in adult life and have a high fatality.

The disease is several times more common in Iceland, Hawaii, Fiji, and Israel than in other countries, and in these countries it affects all racial groups.

Hodgkin's disease
0.9 per cent of all cancers and 0.5 per cent of cancer deaths.
Sex ratio of rates 1.8 to 1 (Fig. 29).

Hodgkin's disease is, perhaps, best thought of as at least two diseases, one affecting primarily youths and young adults, the other primarily the middle-aged and elderly. This division is suggested partly by the existence of two peaks in the age-specific incidence rates, partly by the histological appearances (younger patients

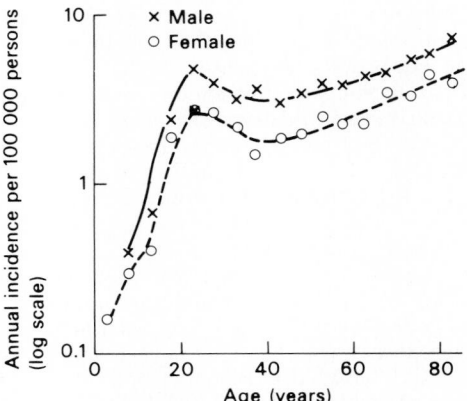

Fig. 29   Annual incidence of Hodgkin's disease

tending to have the nodular sclerotic form of the disease and older patients the mixed cellular form), and partly by the clinical distinction that young patients show mediastinal involvement in more than 50 per cent of cases and infradiaphragmatic involvement in less than 5 per cent, while the reverse tends to be true in the elderly.

No specific causes are known, but there are several reasons for thinking that the type developed by young people may be at least partly infective in origin. A report of a large cluster of cases in which the patients had been in personal contact with each other, either directly or through an intermediary, has not been substantiated by controlled studies elsewhere; nor is there any convincing evidence that the disease occurs in epidemic form in schools. It is notable, however, that it occurs in childhood in undeveloped countries and that as the standard of living rises, the childhood cases disappear and are replaced by a larger number in young adults. This changing pattern is reminiscent of what happened to poliomyelitis in the first half of the century and suggests that the disease may be due to a ubiquitous infective agent that becomes less widespread as hygiene improves. One agent that may play some part is the Epstein–Barr virus that causes infectious mononucleosis, a disease which is followed between 5 and 20 years later by a slightly increased incidence of Hodgkin's disease. The virus, however, cannot be recovered from the lymphomatous cells nor can any part of it be identified in the malignant DNA. If it exerts any effect at all, it may, therefore, do so simply by stimulating division of the relevant stem cells.

Non-Hodgkin's lymphoma
1.4 per cent of all cancers and 1.7 per cent of cancer deaths.
Sex ratio of rates 1.6 to 1 (Fig. 30).

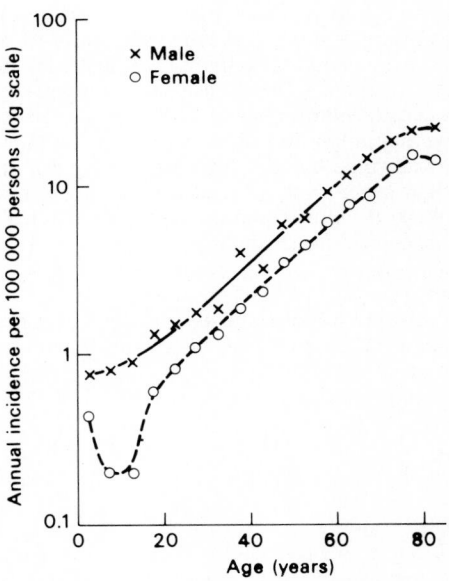

Fig. 30   Annual incidence of non-Hodgkin's lymphoma

Non-Hodgkin's lymphoma is a non-specific term that embraces several diseases with different histological appearances. The histological classification has, however, varied from place to place and from time to time, so that it has been difficult to collect epidemiological information about the individual conditions.

One that has been clearly distinguished epidemiologically, and that can be distinguished histologically by experts, is Burkitt's lymphoma. This affects children throughout the world but is rare everywhere, except for a few places in which malarial infection is both heavy and widespread. In these areas (for example, parts of Uganda, Tanzania, and Nigeria) the disease is 100 times more common than in Europe and North America. The Epstein–Barr (EB) virus can nearly always be recovered from the lymphomatous cells and part of its genome is identifiable in the cells' DNA.

Infection with the EB virus is, however, not necessary for the development of the disease, as some cases occur in its absence; nor is it sufficient, as infection is almost universal and occurs at a very young age in high incidence areas. It seems, therefore, that the EB virus is one cause and that its carcinogenic effect is precipitated by the gross stimulation of the reticulo-endothelial system that is characteristic of heavy and chronic malarial infection.

Other forms of non-Hodgkin's lymphoma, taken altogether, have become more common since the end of the Second World War as registered causes of death; but the increase in the last decade has chiefly been limited to people over 65 years of age. This could be explained either as an effect of improving diagnosis or, perhaps more likely, as a cohort effect reflecting an increase in the prevalence of the causes of the disease some time in the past. One new factor that is responsible for a few cases each year (but insufficient to be reflected in the national statistics) is the introduction of immunosuppressive drugs. When given in the large doses required to prevent rejection following a renal transplant (for example, daily doses of 100–150 mg azathioprine plus 15–30 mg prednisone) they lead to the development of reticulosarcomas in about 1 per cent of treated patients within 5 years, which is approximately 60 times the normal incidence of all types of non-Hodgkin's lymphoma in other circumstances. There is also a lower, but still substantially increased, incidence when these drugs are given for the medical treatment of patients with arthritis, Crohn's disease, and variety of other medical conditions.

The lymphomas following immunosuppression are remarkable in two respects: firstly, they commonly arise in the brain, which is otherwise very seldom the site of origin of a lymphoma, and secondly, they begin to occur within six months of the start of treatment and continue to occur at much the same rate for at least several years. These last features are never seen with other chemical carcinogens and weigh heavily in favour of some idiosyncratic mechanism (for example, the release of a carcinogenic virus previously controlled by immune reactions). That the disease is related to the immunosuppression, rather than to any mutagenic effect of the drug, is confirmed by the grossly increased risk of developing the disease that occurs with a variety of rare hereditary disorders, such as the Wiskott–Aldrich syndrome, which are characterized by major immunological impairment.

Myelomatosis
0.7 per cent of all cancers and 1.2 per cent of cancer deaths. Sex ratio of rates 1.3 to 1 (Fig. 31).

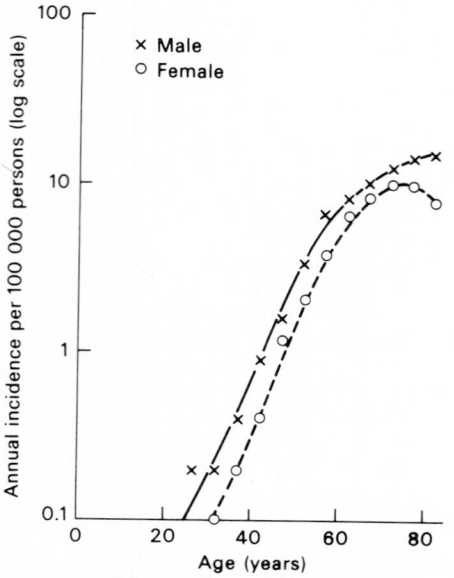

Fig. 31   Annual incidence of myelomatosis

Myelomatosis has been much easier to diagnose since marrow puncture and then serum electrophoresis became standard diagnostic tools and since the managment of renal failure (as which it often presents) has improved. As a result it is difficult to be sure whether the increase that has been recorded in both incidence and mortality rates, and which has now slowed down or stopped at young ages, is due solely to improved diagnosis, or whether it also reflects the introduction of major new causes into Europe and North America between the two World Wars.

The disease is uncommon in undeveloped areas, but is almost certainly underdiagnosed. Genetic factors could be important, as it is twice as common in blacks in the United States as in whites and is rare in Japanese irrespective of where they live.

Leukaemia
2 per cent of all cancers and 2.6 per cent of cancer deaths. Sex ratio of rates 1.5 to 1 (Fig. 32).

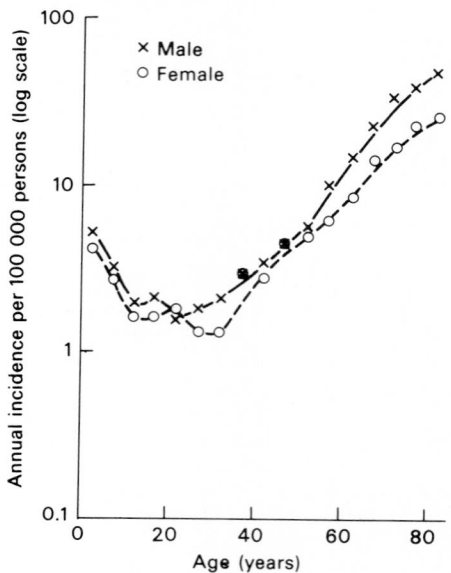

Fig. 32   Annual incidence of leukaemia

Leukaemia may be subdivided reasonably consistently into chronic lymphatic leukaemia (CLL), chronic myeloid leukaemia (CML), acute myeloid leukaemia (AML), and acute lymphatic leukaemia (ALL). Each of these is probably in turn an amalgam of two or more importantly different types, perhaps with different causes, a different age distribution, and a different prognosis, but the distinction between them is still undergoing rapid evolution, so that epidemiological descriptions of each separate sub-type are not possible (see Section 19).

The first of these increases progressively with age in the same way as myelomatosis and most of the common epithelial cancers. It is extremely rare in Chinese, Japanese, and Indians, which is presumably due to genetic differences in susceptibility as it continues to be rare in these racial groups even when they migrate to other countries. Unlike nearly every other type of cancer CLL does not appear to be induced by ionizing radiations. This may be because the induction period is so long that no study of irradiated subjects has been continued for long enough to observe the increased risk. Alternatively, the relevant stem cells may be so sensitive that they are killed by relatively small doses.

In contrast to CLL, the other three main types are induced by ionizing radiations more easily than are most other types of cancer (except possibly thyroid cancer) and they constitute a major part of the risk of fatal cancer attributable to a particular dose to the whole of the body. One of these (ALL) accounts for most of the childhood cases. Whether its incidence varies much between different countries is debatable as affected children are very susceptible to infection and may die quickly in the absence of good medical services, so the rates recorded in underdeveloped countries are undoubtedly too low.

AML occurs at all ages. It becomes slowly but progressively more common from childhood on and is the most common type in young adult life. In this age group, its incidence is probably less variable throughout the world than that of any other reasonably common type of cancer. CML, by contrast, is very rare in youth, but becomes more common than AML in later middle age. The few cases that occur in childhood should perhaps be regarded as constituting a separate disease, as they lack the Philadelphia chromosome that normally characterizes the CML of adult life.

Causes of leukaemia, other than ionizing radiations, include several chemicals and genetically determined diseases. The most important such chemical is benzene, which is used widely in industry and in large amounts has caused a substantial number of cases of erythroleukaemia, other types of acute myeloid leukaemia and, less commonly, acute lymphatic leukaemia. Erythroleukaemia, which is a variant of myeloid leukaemia, is normally so rare that its occurrence acts as a pointer to a possible benzene hazard. Many cases are preceded by periods of aplastic anaemia and, as benzene is not a mutagen, there is still some doubt whether doses insufficient to cause anaemia are capable of causing leukaemia.

Two other chemicals, melphalan and busulphan, are used in the treatment of cancer and the small risk of AML that follows their use is unimportant in relation to the benefit obtained if they are used intelligently. Melphalan is an alkylating agent and so presumably mutagenic. Busulphan, however, has been observed to produce leukaemia only after producing aplastic anaemia. Phenylbutazone may, perhaps, act in the same way, but whether it produces leukaemia or not is unsettled.

Of the hereditary causes, Down's disease is the most common and, for this reason, is probably responsible for the greatest number of cases, although the relative risk in some of the other syndromes may be greater than the 20-fold increase in childhood leukaemia that occurs with Down's disease. Ataxia telangiectasia and Bloom's syndrome predispose to ALL, while Fanconi's anaemia predisposes to AML.

Quantitative apportionment of risk

In this review of cancers of different organs it has not been possible to examine in detail the evidence relating to pervasive causes that affect many different types of cancer. Some of these are, therefore, examined separately in the following sections before an estimate is made of the proportion of cancers attributable to each category of cause.

Ionizing radiations. Ionizing radiations, of whatever sort, share the characteristic of being able to penetrate animal tissues and damage DNA. It is not surprising, therefore, that they have been found to increase the incidence of cancer in practically every organ. It has not been possible to detect by direct observation the effect of the small amounts of radiation that adults receive as a result of exposure to (for example) radiological examination, atmospheric pollution, and natural background; but it has been possible to make an estimate of their effect by extrapolating from the observed effects of the much larger doses received by the survivors of the atomic explosions at Hiroshima and Nagasaki, patients given radiotherapy for a variety of benign conditions, patients who were screened radiologically on many occasions in the days when pulmonary tuberculosis was treated by the induction of an artificial pneumothorax, and men who were exposed to high concentrations of radon in the air of mines. Theoretical considerations and the observed effects of these relatively large doses both indicate that there is unlikely to be any threshold dose below which no effect is produced. This conclusion is reinforced by the discovery that children who received doses of only one or two rad *in utero* (because their mothers were irradiated for diagnostic purposes whilst they

were pregnant) were subject to an added risk of developing cancer in childhood of approximately 1 in 2000. At low doses it seems probable that the carcinogenic effect is likely to be proportional to the dose, but it is not yet clear whether the effect should be regarded as proportional to the dose or to the square of the dose at the higher levels at which most of the observations have been made. It is unlikely, however, that we should be far out in our estimate if we accepted the conclusions of the United Nations Scientific Committee on the Effects of Atomic Radiation (1977) and assumed that the lifetime risk of developing a fatal cancer is approximately 250 per million for each rem of radiation to the whole body, with corresponding reductions if only part of the body is exposed. It should be noted, however, that for many, though not all, of the people who are irradiated in medical practice the risks per rem will be smaller, either because they already have a shortened life expectancy because of disease or old age, and so will not live long enough to develop a radiation-induced cancer, or because the doses given for the treatment of cancer are so large that most of the cells that might be made cancerous are actually destroyed.

According to Pochin (1976), who estimated the whole body doses of radiation received by typical people from different sources, the average was about 101 mrem/year from naturally occurring sources (cosmic radiation, soil, air, and body tissues), plus about 46 mrem/year from medicines and medical procedures (diagnostic X-rays, radiotherapy, and radioisotopes), plus about 6 mrem/year from fallout from past bomb tests, plus about 1 mrem/year from all other sources (nuclear power industry, other occupations, and miscellaneous). Taken altogether, these would produce just under 2000 fatal cancers a year in a population of 55 million, or a few hundred less if allowance is made for the diminished effects of some medical irradiation, which is about 1.5 per cent of all fatal cancers.

Medical drugs. Apart from ionizing radiations there are 12 agents which have been used therapeutically that are known to cause cancer in man. These are listed in Table 4. Other cytotoxic agents that are used medically (particularly in the treatment of cancer) may well be added before long and several other drugs in common use are suspected of being liable to cause cancer, but have not been proved to do so. That so many carcinogenic agents should have been prescribed medically is not surprising when it is borne in mind that treatment often requires modification of cellular metabolism and is sometimes intended to interfere with the DNA itself. The hazard of cancer, however, need not necessarily be a bar to the use of a drug if the risk of loss of life due to iatrogenic cancer is materially less than the chance of saving life that is brought about by treatment—as may commonly be the case with busulphan, immunosuppressive drugs, and radiotherapy.

Table 4 Carcinogenic agents used in medical practice (other than ionizing radiations)

Agent	Site of cancer
Alkylating agents:	
cyclophosphamide	bladder, ?other sites
melphalan	marrow
Arsenic	skin, liver (angiosarcoma), lung
Busulphan	marrow
Chlornaphazine	bladder
Immunosuppressive drugs	reticulo-endothelial system
Oestrogens:	
(unopposed)	endometrium
(transplacental)	vagina (adenocarcinoma)
Phenacetin	kidney (pelvis)
Polycylic hydrocarbons	skin
(coal-tar ointment)	
Steroids:	
oxymetholone	liver (hepatoma)
contraceptives	liver (adenoma,? hepatoma)
Ultraviolet light	skin

Some of the agents listed in the Table were soon abandoned, while others continue to be used for the treatment of uncommon conditions, and the sum of the cancers they produce cannot amount to more than a hundred or so a year. Two, however, are used extensively: oestrogens and steroid contraceptives. The former were used almost routinely for the treatment of post-menopausal symptoms and the prevention of osteoporosis in some parts of the USA. This led to an 'epidemic' of endometrial cancer which, at one time, may have doubled the normal incidence. Endometrial cancer, however, has a relatively good prognosis, and those cases associated with the use of oestrogen a particularly good one, so that the total increase in the number of deaths from this cause was relatively small. Unfortunately, there is some evidence to suggest that their prolonged use may also cause cancer of the breast, and if this is confirmed, the position may be very different. They are certainly not responsible for more than a small proportion of cases, but breast cancer is so common and the fatality still so high (breast cancer accounting for a total of 20 per cent of all cancer deaths in women) that the production of an excess risk of as little as 10 per cent among users would be important although it would be extremely difficult to detect.

Oestrogens produce cancer of the endometrium when given unopposed by a progestogen and a similar effect was observed with the use of the sequential type of contraceptive pill in which an oestrogen was given for 21 days followed by a progestogen for 7 days. The current pills, which combine both types of drug, not only do not cause endometrial cancer, but according to the results of several case-control studies may actually diminish the risk of endometrial cancer and possibly of ovarian cancer as well. Unfortunately, this does not conclude the tale and there is some reason to think that the combined pills could produce some other types of the disease. Firstly, they can produce benign tumours of the liver. These 'adenomas' have become more common in recent years and, although still extremely rare—probably not affecting more than 1 in 50 000 pill users per year—they are many times more common in women who use the pill than in women who do not. Such tumours often recede when the pill is stopped, but otherwise they may rupture and lead to internal haemorrhage, or, very rarely, they may become malignant.

Secondly, it is still uncertain whether oral contraceptives can produce cancers of the breast and cervix uteri. In one sense the use of the pill must lead to an increase of breast cancer, since early pregnancy reduces the risk of cancer of the breast at all subsequent ages and any effective form of contraception (male or female) if practised early in reproductive life will delay pregnancy. But whether, other things being equal, the combined steroid pill actually increases the risk of cancer of either breast or cervix is uncertain. A review of the evidence available up to 1977, undertaken by an expert committee of the World Health Organization (WHO 1978), did not permit any definite conclusion and the evidence available four years later is still conflicting.

Taken altogether it seems unlikely that medically prescribed drugs can be responsible for more than 1 per cent of all today's fatal cancers.

Occupation. In the years that followed Pott's observation that chimney sweeps tended to develop cancer of the scrotum, many other groups of workers have been found to suffer from specific hazards of cancer and more substances that are known to be carcinogenic to man have been unearthed by the search for occupational hazards than by any other means. These hazards, many of which were described in the sections referring to individual types of cancer, are listed in Table 5 together with the agents responsible for them. The hazards that have been recognized were substantial, or at least relatively very large, and it may well be that other occupational hazards exist that have not yet been detected, either because the added risk is small in comparison with that due to other causes, or because only a few men have been exposed, or simply because a hazard has not been suspected and so not looked for. It must also be

Table 5 Occupational causes of cancer

Agent	Site of cancer	Occupation*
Aromatic amines: 4-amino-diphenyl benzidine 2-naphthylamine	Bladder	Dye manufacturers Rubber workers Coal gas manufacturers Some chemical workers
Arsenic	Skin, lung	Copper and cobalt smelters Pesticide manufacturers Some gold miners
Asbestos	Lung, pleura, peritoneum (and maybe stomach, large bowel, oesophagus)	Asbestos miners Asbestos textile manufacturers Insulation workers Shipyard workers
Benzene	Marrow, especially erythroleukaemia	Workers with glues and varnishes
Bischloromethyl ether	Lung	Makers of ion-exchange resins
Cadmium	Prostate	Cadmium workers
Chromium	Lung	Manufacturers of chromates from chrome ore; pigment manufacturers
Ionizing radiations	Lung	Uranium and some other miners
	Bone	Luminizers
	Marrow, all sites	Radiologists, radiographers
Isopropyl oil	Nasal sinuses	Isopropyl alcohol manufacturers
Mustard gas	Larynx, lung	Poison gas manufacturers
Nickel	Nasal sinuses, lung	Nickel refiners
Phenoxy acids and/or chlorophenols	Connective and lymphoid tissues	Herbicide users
Polycyclic hydrocarbons in soot, tar, oil	Skin, scrotum, lung	Coal gas manufacturers, roofers, asphalters, aluminium refiners, and many groups exposed to tars and selected oils
Ultraviolet light	Skin	Farmers, seamen
Vinyl chloride	Liver (angiosarcoma)	PVC manufacturers
?	Nasal sinuses	Hardwood furniture manufacturers
?	Nasal sinuses	Leather workers

* Typical occupations with proven hazards

borne in mind that cancer in man seldom develops until one or more decades after exposure to the carcinogen first occurs and it is, therefore, too soon to be sure whether agents that have been introduced into industry only during the last 20 years are carcinogenic or not.

Many groups of workers other than those listed in Table 5 have been suspected of having a special risk of cancer, but it has not yet been possible to decide whether the risk is real and attributable to their work. Such groups include beryllium workers (lung cancer), lead workers and coal miners (gastric cancer), and professional chemists and agricultural workers in various countries (lymphoma). Some of the excess mortality rates that have been described may be due to chance. Many types of cancer have been examined in each occupational group and, in these circumstances, some differences that are traditionally 'statistically significant' (that is to say, likely to turn up by chance less than once in 20 times) are bound to be observed and they should be regarded as pointing to the presence of a hazard only if highly significant ($P < 0.001$), or if excess rates are confirmed in other studies, or if a risk of the specific type of cancer was predicted from the nature of the agent to which they were exposed.

Other excess rates may be due to confounding; that is, they may be produced by social factors that are associated with the occupation in question rather than by the occupation itself. The potential importance of such confounding was illustrated by Fox and Adelstein's (1978) analysis of the occupational mortality statistics for England and Wales over the period 1970–72. They aggregated the occupations of men aged 15–64 years into 25 major categories and found that the lung cancer rates in these categories differed up to two-fold, a spread that was far too wide to be attributed to chance alone. However, data obtained from random samples of the general population showed that the proportions of men who smoked in each of these 25 large occupational categories varied from about 65 per cent of the national average to about 130 per cent, and that these proportions correlated closely with the 25 mortality rates from lung cancer and could account for nearly all the variation among them.

Given sufficient details and the ability to repeat the observations, it is usually possibly to obtain a fairly clear idea of whether or not an excess incidence in an occupational group does or does not reflect an occupational hazard by (for example) seeing whether the effect is related to the length of employment (or the time after first exposure) and to any specific type of work within the industry. Unfortunately these details are not always available and so the reasons for many of the moderate excesses of cancer incidence or mortality that have been reported in certain industries are still uncertain.

Although occupational hazards may not account for a large proportion of the total number of cancers in the nation as a whole, such hazards may be of great importance to the groups of individuals concerned. Even in the absence of conclusive proof, it is often advisable to err on the side of safety by restricting exposure if any strong suspicion of a hazard has been aroused, particularly if the occupation results in exposure to an agent that can be shown by animal or other laboratory tests to be potentially carcinogenic. The closure of an industry may, however, have serious social implications which also have to be taken into account and it is no help to government, the employers, or the employees at risk if medical research workers allow themselves to express judgements about the existence of a hazard on anything other than strict objective scientific criteria.

On present evidence it seems likely that occupational hazards account for about 4 per cent of all fatal cancers in the USA and perhaps slightly fewer in Britain. The three principal causes of today's occupational cancers are probably previous exposure to asbestos dust (lung and pleural cancer), to the combustion products of fossil fuels (skin and lung cancer), and to a group of aromatic amines (bladder cancer). The evidence is, however, incomplete and this estimate could be out by a factor of two in either direction.

Pollution. The idea that pollution might be an important cause of cancer has been in the forefront of the minds of cancer research workers since it was realized that the incidence of lung cancer tended to be higher in towns than in the countryside and that the combustion products of coal, which used to produce a pall of smoke over all large British cities, contained substantial amounts of carcinogenic hydrocarbons. More recently, with the rapid expansion of the chemical industry and the discovery that some of its products are mutagenic *in vitro* and carcinogenic in laboratory animals, anxiety has increased about the possible effects of distributing such products ubiquitously in the air we breathe, the water we drink, and the food we eat.

The effects of pollution of this sort are, however, peculiarly difficult to assess directly by epidemiological methods since many pollutants are likely to be present in each area, the absolute risks from each are likely to be low, and there may be little difference in the extent to which individuals are exposed over a wide area. Reliance is, therefore, often placed on two indirect methods: extrapolation downwards from the effects of chronic exposure to much larger amounts of some pollutants in an occupational setting, and prediction of the effects in man from laboratory tests. Both have their difficulties (see page 4.77) and it is essential, whenever

the situation permits, to check the results obtained against the actual experience of people living in the polluted areas.

So far as atmospheric pollution is concerned the epidemiological picture is complicated by the personal pollution produced by tobacco smoke and the social distribution of smoking habits, but despite this complication, the various methods that have been discussed under lung cancer (see page 4.61) all lead to the conclusion that the pollution of the past may have contributed to the production of a few per cent of all current lung cancers (and thus perhaps 1 per cent of all cancers); but that current levels of pollution from the combustion of fossil fuels (and from asbestos, arsenic, and various other materials) are unlikely to be responsible for more than a fraction of 1 per cent of future cancers—although there may be exceptions awaiting discovery in the neighbourhood of particular factories.

No other air pollutant seems likely to produce more cancer than these agents except perhaps for the chlorofluorocarbons that have been used extensively as refrigerants and air propellants. These persist in the atmosphere and, it is thought, will eventually reach the stratosphere where they will react with ozone, reduce its concentration, and hence permit more ultraviolet light to reach the surface of the earth. If this happens, the incidence of skin cancer, including the relatively fatal melanoma, must be expected to rise. Some arguments, which are complex and based on a number of unproved assumptions, lead to the conclusion that the mortality from skin cancer might eventually be increased by as much as 20 per cent (i.e. that total cancer mortality rates might be increased by 0.2 per cent); but the present excess produced by these agents, if indeed there is any at all, should be at least one order of magnitude less.

The effect of polluted drinking water and food is even more obscure. Until recently no serious consideration had been given to the possibility that either might be important, except for the possible effect of the contamination of food with smoke from urban air. Now, however, analytical techniques permit the detection of chemicals at concentrations of less than 1 p.p.b. in both food and water and many have been detected, in consequence, that are arguably carcinogenic, including pesticide residues and a variety of halogenated organic materials produced by the chlorination of water supplies. Relationships have been reported between the concentrations of some of these compounds in water and the mortality from cancers of the bladder and, possibly, the large intestine, in different localities; but it is extremely difficult to know what these relationships mean as there are so many potentially confounding factors.

Mortality rates from cancers of the liver and gastrointestinal and urinary tracts are, for the most part, stable or decreasing in middle age, when the effects of new agents might be expected to show themselves first, and, in the absence of more specific evidence, it seems unlikely that chemical pollution of water and food could have a greater effect than the small effect already estimated for pollution of the air. It is important, however, to monitor the situation and, in particular, to seek an explanation for any irregularities in the geographical distribution of any type of cancer that may be observed.

Diet. For many years now there has been suggestive evidence that most of the cancers that are currently common could be made less so by modification of the national diet; but, with few exceptions, there is still little reliable evidence as to what modifications would be of major importance. If we define diet to include all materials that occur in natural foods, are produced during the normal processes of storage, cooking, and digestion, or are added as preservatives or to give food colour, flavour, and consistency, the ways in which diet could influence the development of cancer are legion.

Ingestion of preformed carcinogens. The most obvious is the ingestion of small quantities of powerful carcinogens or precarcinogens. Several have been identified in foodstuffs but only one has been related at all clearly to the production of cancer in man: that is aflatoxin, a metabolic product of *Aspergillus flavus*, which contaminates stored carbohydrates in many countries, and is a major cause of liver cancer in the tropics (see page 4.58). Another possible source is bracken fern, an extract of which is carcinogenic in animals. It is eaten extensively in Japan and has been linked with the development of oesophageal cancer. The polycyclic hydrocarbons and other mutagens that are produced in food by grilling or smoking have often been suspected of playing a role, but intensive investigation has failed to define one. It seems, therefore, that if diet does affect the incidence of cancer in the western world in any material way, it is likely to do so by some more indirect means.

Indirect mechanisms. Some of the indirect ways in which diet could influence the incidence of cancer are summarized in Table 6. Only the effect of overnutrition has been established with certainty; but the evidence to suggest that others are important is mounting. Two examples, fibre, and retinoids and carotenoids, illustrate the strengths and the weaknesses of the available evidence.

Table 6 Some ways in which diet may influence the incidence of cancer indirectly

Possible ways	Example
Affecting the formation of carcinogens in the body	Providing substrates for the formation of carcinogens (e.g. nitrites, nitrates, secondary amines) Inhibiting formation of carcinogens (e.g. vitamin C in the stomach) Altering intake or excretion of cholesterol and bile acids and hence the production of carcinogenic metabolites in the bowel Altering the bacterial flora and hence the capacity to produce carcinogenic metabolites.
Affecting contact of carcinogens with stem cells	Altering transport of carcinogens (e.g. alcohol, fibre) Altering concentration of carcinogens (e.g. effect of fibre on faecal mass)
Affecting activation or deactivation of carcinogens	Induction or inhibition of enzymes that effect metabolism of carcinogens (e.g. indoles in *Brassica*) Deactivation or prevention of formation of short-lived intracellular species (e.g. by selenium and vitamin A, by otherwise trapping free radicals, by quenching singlet oxygen with betacarotene, or by antioxidants used as preservatives)
Affecting 'promotion' of cells that are already initiated	Serum retinol levels (e.g. vitamin A deficiency) or other factors affecting blood retinol binding protein Otherwise affecting stem cell differentiation (e.g. possible effect of beta-carotene, or of determinants of lipid 'profiles')
Overnutrition	Bringing forward age at menarche Formation of adipose-tissue-derived oestrogens

Overnutrition. That overnutrition could affect the incidence of cancer was first suggested by Tannenbaum's experiments on mice during the Second World War. These showed that the incidence of spontaneous tumours of the lung and breast and of a variety of tumours produced experimentally by known carcinogens could be halved by restricting the intake of food without modifying the proportions of the individual constituents. This protective effect has been demonstrated repeatedly since, sometimes with considerably more striking results, but until recently it has attracted surprisingly little attention (perhaps because reports of such results emphasized the benefits of restriction rather than the harm of overeating). It is now clear, however, that obesity is also associated with an increased incidence of certain types of human cancer; but the effect

is marked and progressive only for cancer of the endometrium (see page 4.65) and cancer of the gallbladder in women. For several other types (that is, for cancers of the cervix uteri, breast, and kidney in women and for cancer of the colon in men) the American Cancer Society's massive follow-up study of a million Americans (Lew and Garfinkel 1979) shows that the mortality rates in people who are 40 per cent or more above the standard weight for their height are approximately double those in people who are more than 20 per cent below the standard weight. These results are not easy to interpret, however, partly because obesity may delay diagnosis (and hence lead to an increased fatality) and partly because obesity is associated with a variety of socio-economic factors that may affect the incidence of cancer for other reasons.

Fibre. That fibre may play a part was suggested by Burkitt's observation that several intestinal diseases, including cancer of the colon, were common in countries in which cereals were processed to remove the fibre and rare in rural Africa and Asia where they are not. Fibre, defined as the remnants of the cell wall that are not hydrolysed by the alimentary enzymes of man, consists of a variety of concatenated sugar molecules, some of which pass through the gut unchanged, while some are partially (15 per cent) and others are almost wholly (85 per cent) degraded by the gut flora, and each of which has its own characteristic physiological effects. The types of fibre that seem most likely to exert a protective effect are those in which pentose sugars are abundant, as the amount of these in the diet has been found to correlate closely and inversely with the incidence of colon cancer in different parts of Britain, Finland, and Denmark. These polymers, which are particularly abundant in unrefined cereals and are present in most vegetables other than potatoes, help to produce soft bulky stools, by increasing the number of faecal bacteria. The evidence that they exert a protective effect is far from complete, but, if they do, it may be by changing the make-up of the bacterial flora in the gut, or, more simply, by increasing the faecal bulk and hence diluting any carcinogens present or reducing the length of time they are in contact with the mucosa.

Retinoids and carotenoids. Experiments on animals and on cell cultures *in vitro* have suggested that vitamin A (retinol) and its esters and analogues (retinoids) may, in appropriate circumstances, reduce the risk of cancer by reducing the probability that partially transformed cells become fully transformed and successfully proliferate into a clinically detectable tumour, although in other circumstances they appear to have opposite effects. Now, however, it appears in two of four small cohort studies of apparently healthy people that the incidence of human cancer varies inversely with the level of serum retinol. In view of the experimental data, these results suggest (but do not prove) that circulating retinol protects against the development of the disease. Consequently, if the dietary or other factors that determine the level of serum retinol were known, they might offer a means of cancer prophylaxis. Unfortunately, the simple expedient of adding more vitamin A (retinol) or provitamin A (β- carotene or other carotenoids) to the diet has little effect on the blood retinol level, except in poor countries in which clinical vitamin A deficiency is common, as retinol is normally stored in the liver and released from it at a rate that is approximately independent of the amount that is stored. This makes it unlikely that, in developed countries, supplementing the normal diet with vitamin A or provitamin A could protect against cancer by affecting blood retinol levels. Despite this, however, people who give a history of an intake of less than average amounts of 'vitamin A' have been reported to have an increased risk of cancers of the larynx, lung, oesophagus, stomach, large bowel, bladder, and prostate. If this does reflect a cause-and-effect relationship then the explanation may, perhaps, be that the measures of 'vitamin A' that have been used include amounts estimated from the dietary content of the pro-vitamin (β-carotene), much of which is absorbed from the gut unchanged, circulates in the blood and reaches and is stored in peripheral tissues. In principle, β-carotene could be protective in two main ways, either by being converted into some molecule with retinol-like effects in the peripheral tissues, or directly by, for example, scavenging some reactive excited molecules that might otherwise damage the cell. (For review, see Peto *et al.* 1981.)

Conclusion. Many other components of the diet, including the indoles in cabbages and sprouts, vitamins C and E, and selenium have also been proposed as protective agents; while meat, nitrates, nitrites, secondary amines, and fat have been proposed as liable to increase the hazard. (For a review, see Doll and Peto 1981.) The evidence is, as yet, too weak to justify any firm conclusions, but the current interest in the subject should lead to a much clearer understanding within the next decade. The outcome may well be that some dietary factors will be shown to be important determinants of cancers of the stomach and large bowel, as well as of the endometrium, gallbladder, and (in tropical countries) the liver. They may also prove to have a material effect on the incidence of cancers of the breast and pancreas and, perhaps through some antipromoting or anti-oxidant effects, on the incidence of epithelial tumours in many other tissues. It would not be surprising if, in total, dietary factors were found to provide a means for reducing cancer death rates by a third; but the range of uncertainty about this figure is large.

Interaction of agents. The attribution of the risk of cancer to different causes is complicated by the fact that some agents interact with others to produce effects that are much greater than the sum of the separate effects of each on its own. An example is provided by smoking and asbestos which multiply each other's effects so that the incidence of cancer of the lung among a group of insulation workers in the USA who did not smoke was increased sixfold (above that among non-smokers in the country in general), that among cigarette smokers in general who do not work with asbestos is increased 10-fold or 20-fold, but that among asbestos insulation workers who also smoked cigarettes regularly was increased nearly 90-fold (Hammond, Selikoff, and Seidman 1979). Others are provided by smoking and radon, which interact similarly to produce cancer of the lung and by smoking and alcohol, which interact to produce cancer of the oesophagus. Evidence is now beginning to accumulate that some dietary factors may act similarly by modifying the risk of cancer in several different organs in response to a variety of other causes.

Such interactions may come about through some analogue of the dual mechanism of initiation and promotion that was suggested many years ago by the experiments of Rous and Kidd and Berenblum and Shubik, that has since been extended to include the concept of 'antipromotion'. They could, however, also be produced in many other ways, some of which are discussed in the section on diet (see above). From a statistical point of view they complicate the attribution of risk, since we may find ourselves appearing to claim that we can prevent more cancer than actually occurs by attributing, say, 80 per cent of lung cancers in men heavily exposed to asbestos to their occupational exposure and 90 per cent of the same cancers to cigarette smoking. But they greatly facilitate the task of the specialist in preventive medicine, since they provide a choice between two methods of prevention, one of which may be simpler or more acceptable than the other or, perhaps, quicker acting if, as seems likely, some act as promoting or anti-promoting agents in a late stage of the development of the disease.

Role of genetic susceptibility. (See also pages 4.18 and 47.) The factors that determine whether a person of a given age will develop cancer in the course of the year are of three types: 'nature', 'nurture', and 'luck', or the play of chance. The first describes a person's genetic make-up at conception and affects the liability to react to a given environment by developing a specific type of cancer. The second is the sum of the effects of everything that people do or have done to them in the womb, in childhood, and in adult life, and has been the main topic of this chapter. The third is commonly ignored. It is,

however, the reason why two animals of identical genetic constitution that have been treated in the same way do not develop cancer in the same place at the same age. It reflects the element of chance that determines whether a particular series of events all occur in the appropriate relationship to each other in the same cell and may be as important in determining who next develops cancer as it is in determining who is next involved in a traffic accident. For any one individual the role of good or bad luck may be enormous, but in a population of a million it has only a trivial effect and only nature and nurture are important.

The existence of genetic differences in susceptibility may, in principle, be recognized in two ways: by laboratory demonstration of biochemical or other characteristics of human cells, or by epidemiological observation that particular types of cancer tend to cluster in families or to be associated with genetically determined factors like blood groups. In practice, laboratory evidence has been hard to obtain and is only now becoming available for a few conditions, such as xeroderma pigmentosum, that have already been recognized as hereditary because they cluster in families. The epidemiological evidence, for its part, has been relatively simple. It has consisted mainly of two sorts, (*a*) the recognition of clusters that are so marked that no statistical analysis is needed to show the reality of their existence, and (*b*) the demonstration that if one member of a family develops a specific type of cancer, other members are somewhat more likely to develop that particular type of cancer than would be expected from the experience of some control series.

The first has shown that several rare genes have such a gross effect on susceptibility that bearers of one such gene (in the case of dominance) or two (if the genes are recessive) almost invariably develop a particular type of cancer. Examples include the dominant genes for polyposis coli and Gardner's syndrome, leading to cancer of the large bowel, and for a rare type of tylosis leading to carcinoma of the oesophagus, and the recessive genes for xeroderma pigmentosum leading to squamous carcinoma and melanoma of the skin and for factors that confer a high probability of developing retinoblastoma. The same sort of evidence has also shown that other genetic syndromes frequently, but not invariably, lead to the development of cancer, including von Recklinghausen's neurofibromatosis leading to fibrosarcoma, the Peutz–Jegher syndrome leading to carcinoma of the small bowel, the Wiskott–Aldrich syndrome leading to non-Hodgkin's lymphoma, ataxia-telangiectasia, Bloom's syndrome, and Fanconi's anaemia leading to leukaemia, and many others. The recognition of these syndromes is important to the individual, as it may provide an opportunity for prophylactic surgery, or enable the diagnosis of malignancy to be made at an early stage when treatment is likely to be effective, or (rarely) enable precautions to be taken to prevent exposure to the relevant carcinogens, as in the case of sufferers from xeroderma pigmentosum and albinism who can be protected against sunlight.

The proportion of all cancers that occur in people who are highly susceptible to cancer in this way is very small and the important question is, therefore, whether the risk of developing various common types of cancer in the absence of the stigma of one or other of the specific syndromes that have been described is related to the possession of specific genes that do not produce any gross abnormalities that can be recognized clinically, but yet substantially increase the risk of developing the disease.

The second sort of epidemiological evidence has shown that there is no material tendency for cancer as such to cluster in families and confirms that there are no genes that materially increase the risk of developing cancer as a whole—or, if there are, that they are extremely rare. It has also shown, however, that the common types of cancer do tend to cluster in families to a small extent, in that a sibling of an affected patient has about twice the normal risk of developing a cancer in the *same* site. Differences of this sort do not, of course, necessarily imply that the familial clusters are genetic in origin; they could be due to familial habits of behaviour, which, for example, encourage the development of similar habits of smoking, drinking, and eating. Nor, however, do they necessarily imply that any genetic difference in susceptibility that may exist is necessarily small. Calculations show that they are compatible with fifty- to a hundred-fold differences in genetic susceptibility if the genes for high susceptibility have the appropriate prevalence in the population. That such genes exist is demonstrated by the grossly increased risk of developing basal cell and squamous carcinomas of the exposed skin in fair-skinned populations, and there is no reason why there should not be other genes associated with localized groups which, for example, increase the risk of nasopharyngeal carcinoma in the southern Chinese, or diminish the risk of chronic lymphatic leukaemia and myelomatosis in Chinese, Japanese, and Indians. It is clear also that some genes do exist that influence, or correlate with, the risk of developing other types of cancer, but only to a minor extent. An example is the gene for blood group A, the possession of which increases the risk of gastric cancer by about 20 per cent over that of people belonging to blood groups O or B.

Discovery of genetic factors that affect particular types of cancer is unlikely to explain much of the differences in the social and geographical distribution of cancer that have been described previously (see page 4.53); but it might help to elucidate mechanisms, and perhaps to focus health education and costly methods of early diagnosis on the sections of the population that are most at risk.

Conclusion. Estimates of the proportions of fatal cancers that can be attributed to each of the known causes of cancer are given in Table 7. For this purpose many individual causes (such as the various carcinogenic drugs and occupational hazards) have been grouped together in 13 main categories. The evidence on which these estimates are based is summarized in previous sections of this chapter and is available in greater detail elsewhere in a review of the avoidable risks of cancer in the USA (Doll and Peto 1981).

Table 7 Proportion of cancer deaths attributable to different environmental factors

Factor or class of factors	Best estimate of proportion (%)	Range of acceptable estimates (%)
Ionizing radiations		
background	1	
medical procedures	0.5	} 1 to 2
industry	< 0.1	
Ultraviolet light	0.5	< 0.2 to 1
Occupation	4	2 to 8
Industrial products	< 1	1 to 2
Pollution		
atmospheric	1	} < 1 to 5
water	< 1	
Medical drugs	< 1	< 1 to 2
Diet	30	10 to 70
Food additives	< 1	−5 to 2
Tobacco	30	25 to 35
Alcohol	3	2 to 4
Reproductive and sexual behaviour	7	1 to 13
Infection	(10)	?
Other and unknown	?	?

The sum of the estimates in Table 7, it will be noted, amounts to less than 100 per cent, despite the fact that some of the listed agents interact with one another to augment each other's effect (see page 4.75) and that some fatal cancers are counted twice. The total would be somewhat more than 100 per cent, however, if the true proportions attributable to some of the categories turn out to be nearer the upper end of the acceptable estimates and it would be a great deal more than 100 per cent if it had been possible to characterize the factors that have been classified as 'other and unknown'.

Two categories (tobacco and diet) stand out as contributing by far the largest effects. Both are estimated to cause about 30 per cent of cancer deaths; but whereas the effect of smoking can be calculated with precision, that of diet is speculative and could prove to be either much more or much less; moreover, it is not known which dietary factors are of chief importance. On present knowledge, the diminution of smoking and, to a lesser extent, the substitution of low for medium or high tar cigarettes, constitute the most effective methods for reducing the incidence of cancer in developed countries. It may eventually be possible to produce as great or greater benefits by various dietary changes; but it is possible now to advise, with confidence, only the avoidance of obesity and, less confidently, to suggest that beneficial effects may perhaps be produced by decreasing the consumption of animal and dairy products and increasing the consumption of cereal fibre and of various green or yellow vegetables.

The only other categories that seem at all likely to cause as much as 10 per cent of cancers are infection and reproductive and sexual behaviour. Viral infection certainly plays some part in the production of liver cancer (though perhaps not as an initiating agent), almost certainly does so in the production of cervical cancer, and may well do so in the production of several other types; while bacterial infection may play a part in the production of many cancers by helping to produce chemical carcinogens in vivo. The figure cited for reproductive and sexual factors allows for the known effect of promiscuity on the risk of cervical cancer and for the possibility that in the future socially acceptable ways will be found for mimicking the favourable effects of pregnancy on the risks of endometrial, ovarian, and breast cancer in women; but it is not impossible that some aspects of sexual behaviour also affect the risks of prostatic and testicular cancer in men by, for example, modifying hormonal secretions. It cannot be expected that sexual behaviour or reproduction will be much influenced by knowledge that they are likely to affect the incidence of cancer some decades later, but it may prove possible to diminish the risks associated with them by preventing infection or simulating or modifying the effects of hormonal secretion, when more is known about the ways in which hormonal factors affect the genesis of cancer.

Occupational hazards do not seem likely to account for a large proportion of all cancers, but they may give rise to substantial risks for small groups. Once recognized, they can usually be reduced or eliminated by immediately practicable methods, so that their identification is particularly valuable.

With a few outstanding exceptions (affecting particularly cancer of the stomach), the main determinants of avoidable cancer are much the same in all developed countries. Elsewhere priorities are different and major opportunities for prevention exist in Southeast Asia to prevent buccal cancer by the diminution of chewing and, in the tropics, to prevent liver cancer by the development of practicable techniques for immunization against hepatitis and the storage of food in such a way as to avoid fungal contamination.

For the practical purpose of preventing death from cancer in Britain and the USA the data in Table 7 are unsatisfactory as they treat equally future knowledge and aetiological factors that are sufficiently understood to enable specific action to be taken with a guarantee of success. Table 8, which has been constructed to show the potential effect of such practicable strategies for the prevention of fatal cancer, looks very different. The paucity of reliable, useful information in it is disturbing, especially when it is noted that, when effects on causes of death other than cancer are also taken into account, even the direction of the net effect of alcohol avoidance on total mortality becomes uncertain (since, in small amounts, alcohol may help to prevent vascular disease), leaving as certain and substantial only the net effects of tobacco.

Consequently, a doctor who is asked by a non-smoking patient what actions will substantially reduce the risk of death from cancer can describe only certain general dietary changes (Table 8) which, although probably important, lack detail and lack conclusive proof of benefit. For a patient who smokes cigarettes the picture is different because not only dietary modification but also avoidance

Table 8   Reliably established practicable ways of avoiding fatal cancer*

Method	Percentage of all cancer deaths known to be thus avoidable
Avoidance of tobacco smoke	30%†
Avoidance of alcoholic drinks and mouthwashes	3%††
Regular cervical screening and genital hygiene	1%
Avoidance of inessential medical use of hormones or radiology	< 1%
Avoidance of unusual exposure to sunlight	< 1%
Avoidance of current industrial levels of exposure to currently known§ occupational carcinogens	< 1%
Avoidance of current levels of pollution of food, water, or urban air by known§ environmental carcinogens	< 1%
Avoidance of obesity§§	2%

* Excluding ways such as undergoing prophylactic prostatectomy, mastectomy, hysterectomy, oophorectomy, artificial menopause or pregnancy

† About 50 per cent of the cancer deaths among smokers, but less than 1 per cent among non-smokers. Avoidance of tobacco smoke also decreases the risk of tobacco-induced vascular or respiratory disease causing disability or death (and, among smokers, the excess risk of death from these probably exceeds that of death from tobacco-induced cancer). The net effects of avoidance of tobacco on the aggregate of all causes of death other than cancer are also therefore substantial

†† Avoidance of alcohol also reduces the risk of death from cirrhosis, violence or accident, perhaps by an absolute amount comparable with the reduction in risk of death from cancer, but, in view of the (inconclusive) evidence that moderate alcohol consumption decreases the risk of death from vascular disease, the direction of the net effect of avoidance of alcohol on total mortality cannot be predicted with confidence except for heavy drinkers

§ Including only agents for which there is good epidemiological evidence of human hazard

§§ Other dietary information is not yet reliable, but a general reduction of animal products and increase of plant products might well reduce risks substantially

of tobacco can be prescribed, and the quantitative effects of the latter are large and known with reasonable certainty. Until dietary, infective, and hormonal factors are much better understood, the epidemiology of cancer will therefore remain in a frustratingly unsatisfactory state.

Relative roles of laboratory tests and epidemiology

Until some years ago all the known causes of human cancer, or the circumstances that gave rise to them, had been discovered by clinical, pathological, or epidemiological observation, and the specific agents responsible had been identified (if indeed they have yet been identified at all) by subsequent laboratory investigation. More recently a variety of laboratory methods have been developed for predicting which chemicals would be likely to cause cancer in humans, if men and women were exposed to them acutely in one or a few high doses or chronically in repeated low doses.

Laboratory tests. Many methods of testing have been proposed and the most favoured ones are reviewed by the International Agency for Research on Cancer (1980). These include not only 'long-term' tests involving repeated application of the test chemical to living animals but also a variety of 'short-term' tests that are both quicker and cheaper to perform. In a long-term test, a few dozen small laboratory animals are fed or otherwise repeatedly exposed to the test chemical, usually in very high doses throughout a substantial part of their lives, to see if they develop an excess of tumours of any particular type. In most short-term tests, the chemicals are applied to isolated cultures of bacterial or mammalian cells to see whether the cellular DNA can be made to suffer a permanent change that can be detected by allowing selective proliferation of the changed cells, by causing certain cellular side-effects, or by

'transforming' some of the cells so that they appear cancerous and have a selective advantage over their unaltered neighbours. Alternatively, the test chemicals may be given to animals that are killed a few hours later, to see if the DNA extracted from any particular organ shows signs of recent damage (see page 4.48).

The use of these tests has led to the discovery of a few agents that have subsequently been shown to be carcinogenic to man, together with hundreds of other substances that are carcinogenic to one or more animal species. Many of these have, as a result, not been manufactured for general use. Others, however, are already in deliberate use or are found as unintended pollutants of air, water, food, or industrial products, and the question arises how far efforts should be made to remove them from the environment.

Unfortunately, it is not yet possible to answer this question in a sensible way as knowledge of the mechanisms of carcinogenesis is too incomplete. Alteration of a normal cell into the seed of a growing clone of cancerous cells seems to require at least two qualitatively different types of change and the chief causes of one may not be important causes of the other, and vice versa. Agents that increase the risk of cancer may, therefore, do so in a variety of ways: by, for example, facilitating early changes, by conferring a selective advantage on partially altered cells relative to their normal neighbours, by facilitating the later changes, or by interfering with any hypothetical host defence factors that may exist to restrain fully cancerous cells from proliferating. There are, moreover, important differences between man and the small short-lived animals that laboratory workers must necessarily study, not only in the ways in which particular chemicals are metabolized and detoxified (which differ somewhat haphazardly in different species) but also in the ways that humans have evolved to allow most of us to remain free of cancer despite having a far larger body size and a far longer lifespan than that of laboratory animals.

Direct evidence that the short- and long-term tests are both moderately reliable is provided by the qualitative observation that most chemicals that have been found to be carcinogenic in both rats and mice also damage DNA in one or more short-term tests for mutagenicity; whereas most chemicals that have been found not to cause any excess of cancer in either species are inactive in all such tests. It is not surprising, however, in view of the difficulties that have been discussed, that it has not yet been possible to demonstrate reliably any quantitative relationship between the results of short- or long-term laboratory tests and the risk of human cancer over the whole range of conditions that are known to cause human cancer. Nor, according to the International Agency for Research on Cancer (1980), are we yet even at the point where useful quantitative estimates of animal risk in long-term feeding studies can be derived from the findings in the various short-term tests.

So many thousands of chemicals are active in one or other laboratory test that it is hardly practicable to promulgate regulations that are based solely on these qualitative results. A more sensible procedure might be to multiply the potency of each chemical in certain such tests by whatever crude estimate of total human exposure is available to yield some sort of index of human hazard. When this has been done for a variety of tests, including long-term animal tests, it is likely that a few chemicals will, for each separate type of test, stand out head and shoulders above the rest and efforts could reasonably be made to reduce exposure to those few chemicals without necessarily requiring direct evidence of human harm. Before priorities for action could be set in this way, however, it would be necessary to seek out as many important sources as possible (including formation *in vivo* and externally in complex materials such as smoke) of human exposure to agents that are active in the particular test being considered. In the absence of any way of calibrating the relevance to humans of each test, a policy of concentrating regulatory efforts against the few principal exposures may confer benefits nearly as great as those that would be conferred by a much more expensive policy of broad action against all apparently active chemicals, and it would certainly be less socially disruptive. The chief exception to this approach might be that heavy chronic exposure to a highly active agent in industry should, if possible, be prevented, even if the product of laboratory potency and total human exposure was not outstandingly large, because the number of individuals exposed was small.

Epidemiological observation. Epidemiological observation, for its part, may be displaced almost entirely by laboratory investigation in the course of time, if the mechanisms by which cancer is produced ever come to be completely understood. Meanwhile it has many advantages.

Firstly, observations of the vagaries of human behaviour may suggest ideas that might never occur to a laboratory investigator. Historically they provided the starting point for a large part of all cancer research by pinpointing many specific risks (see page 4.71), and they are continuing to provide new ideas by, for example, pointing to the possible role of various dietary fibres and vegetables and to the role of pregnancy, menarche, and the menopause.

Secondly, study of national trends in age-specific mortality from particular diseases draws attention to types of cancer likely to be due to newly introduced factors (as happened in the 1940s with cancer of the lung and is happening now with melanoma of the skin). Similarly, study of the recent trends in incidence among occupational or other groups in which an excess of cancer had previously been shown to be present for reasons that were incompletely understood provides a monitoring system to check whether any measures that have been instituted have effectively reduced exposure to the actual cause of the disease.

Thirdly, positive epidemiological observations provide quantitative data relating directly to the species whose cancers we are trying to prevent, and to some of the doses to which humans are actually exposed (for example, from ionizing radiations). By so doing they avoid or reduce the pitfalls in extrapolating from one species to another and from one dose level to an extremely different one and so provide estimates of human risk that are reliable enough for a rational comparison of risks and benefits. Moreover, such large numbers of people can be studied that direct evidence of the effect of very small doses can sometimes be obtained. Humans feed and house themselves and arrange their own medical care at no cost to the epidemiologist, so that observations can be made on hundreds of thousands of individuals, while comparable-sized studies on experimental animals would be prohibitively expensive.

Fourthly, apparently negative epidemiological observations (that is, ones that are consistent with the absence of risk) may provide a useful upper limit to the effect that certain agents, which have been shown to be carcinogenic in the laboratory, can be expected to have in a human population. Epidemiology cannot prove that an effect could never occur; but it may be able to provide data for so many people who have been exposed for such a long time that it is possible to conclude that the effect is small enough to be neglected (as with limited use of isoniazid and phenobarbitone).

Trustworthy epidemiological evidence nearly always requires the demonstration that a relationship holds for individuals (or at least for small groups) within a population, as well as between large population groups as a whole. Correlations between the incidence of cancer in whole towns or whole countries and, say, air or water pollution on the consumption in those areas of certain items of food are unlikely to provide reliable evidence, although they may provide hypotheses for testing by other means. In such 'ecological' studies attempts to separate the role of causative and confounding factors by statistical analysis are often made, but the information obtained in this way is, at best, of only marginal value.

In practice the danger of reaching wrong conclusions is slight when observations are made on individuals rather than on whole populations and when the risk of the disease is increased many times by exposure to the agent under suspicion. In these circumstances risks have been detected that are quite small in absolute terms (affecting perhaps one 1 in 1000 exposed people) and some have been detected after only a handful of cases of a rare type of cancer have occurred. The situation is very different, however, when the induced disease is as common as cancer of the lung or

cancer of the breast. In these circumstances risks that will ultimately kill as many as 1 per cent or more of the exposed population may easily be overlooked or attributed to chance, unless the population studied is very large. In these circumstances, too, when cancer rates are only a moderate multiple of those among the unexposed (that is, when the relative risk lies between 1 and 2, as it does for kidney cancer in smokers), problems of interpretation become acute and it may be extremely difficult to disentangle the various contributions of biased information, confounding with other factors, and cause and effect. There is, moreover, a special difficulty in the study of cancer, because the disease is seldom induced within five years of starting exposure and may not be induced to any great extent until exposure has continued for two or three decades. In short, unless epidemiologists have studied reasonably large, well-defined groups of people who have been heavily exposed to a particular substance for a long time, they can offer no guarantee that continued exposure to moderate or low levels will be without material risk.

Conclusion

Epidemiology and laboratory investigation complement each other and both are needed to understand the important causes of cancer and learn how to prevent it. The latter is essential if risks of cancer are to be predicted before they occur and so avoided; and it must be expected that laboratory investigation will gradually replace epidemiology as we come to learn more about the mechanism by which cancer is produced. The former, meanwhile, has the advantage that it starts not with the 10 000 trace chemicals that may be found in one or other organ of the body or in the environment of a particular city, but with the 10 000 deaths that occur each year in that city. Epidemiology is more likely to overlook many small effects of a variety of chemicals than is laboratory investigation; but it is much less likely to overlook the main determinants of cancer rates and trends, especially if these are not simple industrial products or environmental pollutants.

References

Barker, D. J. P. and Rose, G. (1979). *Epidemiology in medical practice.* Churchill Livingstone, Edinburgh.

Clemmesen, J. (1981a). Increase in liver cancer. *J. nat. Cancer Inst.* **67**, 3.

— (1981b). Uses of a cancer register in carcinogenesis. *J. nat. Cancer Inst.* **67**, 5.

Cook, P. J. and Burkitt, D. P. (1971). Cancer in Africa. *Br. med. Bull.* **27**, 14.

Doll, R., Gray, R., Hafner, B., and Peto, R. (1980). Mortality in relation to smoking: 22 years' observations on female British doctors. *Br. med. J.* **280**, 967.

— and Peto, R. (1976). Mortality in relation to smoking: 20 years' observations on male British doctors. *Br. med. J.* **ii**, 1525.

— and — (1981). The causes of cancer: quantitative estimates of avoidable risks of cancer in the United States today, *J. Nat. Cancer Inst.* **66**, 1191. (Also reprinted as an Oxford University Press paperback, published in 1981.)

Fox, A. J. and Adelstein, A. M. (1978). Occupational mortality: work or way of life? *J. Epidemiol. Community Hlth* **32**, 73.

Hammond, E. C. and Garfinkel, L. (1980). General air pollution and cancer in the United States. *Prev. Med.* **9**, 206.

—, Selikoff, I. J., and Seidman, H. (1979). Asbestos exposure, cigarette smoking, and death rates. *Ann. N. Y. Acad. Sci.* **330**, 473.

International Agency for Research on Cancer (1976). *Cancer incidence in five continents, vol. 3* (eds. J. Waterhouse, C. Muir, P. Correa, and J. Powell). International Agency for Research on Cancer, Lyon.

— (1980). Molecular and cellular aspects of carcinogen screening tests. *IARC Scientific Publications no. 27.* International Agency for Research on Cancer, Lyon.

International Union Against Cancer (1970) *Cancer incidence in five continents, vol. 2* (eds. R. Doll, C. S. Muir, and J. A. H. Waterhouse). International Union Against Cancer, Geneva.

— (1980). *Cancer risk by site* (eds. T. Hirayama, J. A. H. Waterhouse, and J. F. Fraumeni, Jr). International Union Against Cancer, Geneva.

Lew, E. A., and Garfinkel, L. (1979). Variation in mortality by weight among 750 000 men and women. *J. Chron. Dis.* **32**, 563.

Lilienfield, A. M. (1980). *Foundations of epidemiology*, 2nd edn. Oxford University Press, New York.

Peto, R. (1977). Cancer epidemiology and multistage models. In *Origins of human cancer* (ed. H. H. Hiatt, J. D. Watson, and J. A. Winsten), 1403. Cold Spring Harbor Publications, New York.

Pochin, E. E. (1976). *Estimated population exposure from nuclear power production and other radiation sources*. OECD, Paris.

Registrar General (1980). *Mortality statistics: Cause*. Office of Population Censuses and Surveys, HMSO, London.

United Nations Scientific Committee on the Effects of Atomic Radiation (1977). *Sources and effects of ionizing radiation*. United Nations, New York.

World Health Organization (1978). Steroid contraception and the risk of neoplasia. *Technical Report Series no. 619*, World Health Organization, Geneva.

MEDICAL ASPECTS OF NEOPLASIA

D. A. G. Galton

THE CAUSATION OF NEOPLASIA: MEDICAL ASPECTS

From the preceding chapter, it is apparent that a high proportion of human malignant disease is likely to arise from contact with environmental carcinogens, which include ionizing radiation, specific chemical carcinogens, and possibly viruses.

The role of genetic factors is difficult to assess. Thus the lower incidence of and lower mortality rates of breast cancer were once correlated with the different pattern of oestrogen metabolism in Japanese women who, in comparison with white Americans, excrete relatively more of the anticarcinogen oestriol and less of the carcinogenic oestrone and oestradiol. Differences in diet rather than genetic factors could account for this difference. On the other hand, the possible role of genetic factors is suggested by the higher incidence of breast cancer in Japanese American women with the genetic marker of wet cerumen than in those with dry cerumen. The incidence of several neoplasms has been examined in relation to other genetic markers, especially to the ABO blood groups and the HLA histocompatibility antigens. The positive correlations so far found are of a low order of magnitude and do not suggest any major role in carcinogenesis. In general genetic factors appear to play only a small part in the effect of environmental carcinogens. However certain families are on record in which breast cancer or leukaemia and lymphoproliferative disease have recurred at high frequency through several generations, indicating an inherited predisposition to cancers for which a genetic factor is not generally implicated. There are also many inherited disorders in which the risk of malignant disease is high, and some of these are referred to below.

Tests of carcinogenicity. Ionizing radiation, the carcinogenic hydrocarbons, and the naphthylamines are carcinogenic for small laboratory animals, as well as for man, and it would appear logical to use these animals to test suspected substances for carcinogenicity. The use of Butter Yellow, at one time added to margarine as a colouring agent, was prohibited when it was found to cause liver cancer in laboratory rodents. Since then many governments have introduced legislation whereby all types of food additives, whether intended as colouring agents, flavouring agents, or preservatives, must be submitted to tests of carcinogenicity, and some governments require similar tests for pharmaceutical products, cosmetics, and chemicals used in industry and agriculture.

The interpretation of the results of carcinogenicity tests is fraught with difficulty. Different animal species vary greatly in their susceptibility to carcinogens, and in any one species the effect of a given agent varies according to the dose, frequency, and route of administration, and the sex and age of the animals. A compound may be carcinogenic for one species only because it is metabolized in a unique manner, one of the products being the active carcinogen. Arsenic is an established carcinogen for man but not for any laboratory animal. Negative results are sometimes obtained when known carcinogens are administered to specific-pathogen-free animals. In some cases supposed 'carcinogens' are thought to activate latent oncogenic viruses. In others carcinogenicity can be demonstrated only when the test substance is administered by a non-physiological route in massive doses for long periods. The significance of such results is very uncertain in assessing the possible hazards to man. Rapid screening tests for mutagenicity in bacteria, such as the Ames test (see page 4.77), or for the capacity to transform the growth pattern of cells in tissue culture, are increasingly used, but are not, by themselves, adequate for disclosing carcinogenicity. This subject is considered on page 4.77.

Oncogenic viruses. Many neoplasms in laboratory animals and wild animals are of viral origin, and an increasing number of animal neoplasms are suspected to be of viral origin. No human neoplasm is yet known to be caused by a virus, but there is circumstantial evidence that some tumours will prove so to be, the most likely being acute myeloid leukaemia in which, as in all avian and mammalian leukaemias of established viral aetiology, evidence for the involvement of a C-type RNA virus is rapidly accumulating. The use of chromosome markers has shown that the cells of 'recurrent' lymphoblastic leukaemia in two children who received marrow grafts from sibs after destruction of the leukaemia by whole-body irradiation were donor cells which had been transformed to leukaemic cells perhaps by the action of a virus. Even in the animal tumours of viral origin, the relationship between the presence of an oncogenic virus and the initiation and subsequent growth of the neoplasm is highly complex, and much influenced by genetic, endocrine, and immunological factors. Wild mice carrying the polyoma virus are tolerant to it and do not develop tumours. In laboratory conditions the polyoma virus will induce multiple neoplasms in different tissues. The leukaemogenic properties of the Gross leukaemia virus could be demonstrated only when inoculated into newborn mice belonging to a strain not carrying it. Gross leukaemia also illustrates the importance of the target organ; mice heavily infected with the virus do not develop leukaemia if the thymus is removed soon after birth, but leukaemia develops if the animals are provided with a thymus from a normal animal. Some radiation-induced murine leukaemias are now known to be of viral origin. The virus is tolerated in the intact animal, but when the thymic lymphoid tissue regenerates rapidly after having been depleted by radiation, the thymic cells become susceptible to infection and become leukaemic. Similarly, the mouse mammary carcinoma virus is not oncogenic unless the mammary gland is activated by the appropriate hormonal environment. Thus, in viral neoplasia, although the cells of many tissues become infected with virus, only the cells of the target tissue undergo neoplastic transformation, and then only in special circumstances. The nature of the event, or events, that effect the transformation is unknown. In some cases, transformation is likely to be an excessively rare event, because the resulting tumour can be shown to be monoclonal. Biochemical genetic markers have indicated the monoclonal nature of Burkitt's lymphoma, of suspected though not established viral aetiology. Moreover, the finding of different markers in late 'recurrences' in apparently cured cases suggests the reinduction of a second neoplasm rather than recurrence. In contrast, biochemical genetic markers have established the polyclonal nature of condyloma acuminatum which may be considered as a benign neoplasm, and is caused by papovavirus. Here, a high proportion of the infected cells undergo neoplastic, though not malignant, transformation.

Oncogenic viruses are not a specific taxonomic group. Some, like the leukaemogenic viruses, are RNA viruses, others like the polyoma virus are DNA viruses. Oncogenic viruses, unlike the viruses that cause acute infection, do not proliferate within and kill the cells they invade. Infective virus cannot always be recovered from the cells but the presence of the viral genome incorporated in the host genome can be detected because of the presence of viral-coded neoantigens within the cell or its membranes. In the case of oncogenic RNA viruses ('oncorna viruses'), the RNA genome is transcribed as a DNA homologue by a viral DNA polymerase ('reverse transcriptase'). Oncornaviruses are therefore also described as 'retraviruses'. The presence of the viral polymerase in human leukaemia cells has been interpreted as evidence of oncornavirus infection.

The herpesviruses are becoming increasingly suspect as potential oncogenic agents. They are known to be causal agents in several naturally occurring animal tumours including the Lucké renal carcinoma of the leopard frog, Marek's disease of chickens, as well as in the malignant lymphomas in owl monkeys and marmosets experimentally induced by the Saimiri herpes virus of squirrel monkeys. DNA-free Marek virus vaccines confer 94 per cent protection on chickens challenged with virulent virus, and similar protection against *Herpes virus saimiri* has been conferred on marmosets by the use of a heat-inactivated vaccine. A herpes-like virus (EBV) was isolated from cultures of Burkitt's lymphoma by Epstein and Barr, but has not been isolated from tumours obtained directly from the patients. The disease occurs predominantly in certain areas of tropical Africa and New Guinea where malaria is holoendemic. All patients have been found to contain antibodies against EBV in their serum, and in a prospective epidemiological study in East Africa, every child who subsequently developed Burkitt's lymphoma had undergone seroconversion from negative to positive. Antibodies are present in the sera of a high proportion of normal adults, and the proportion of positive reactors increases during childhood and adolescence, but the antibody titres are not as high as those of 'Burkitt' sera except in persons who have recently had infectious mononucleosis (IM), a disease known to occur only in persons whose sera do not contain anti-EBV antibodies. The highest titres are found in the sera of patients whose Burkitt lymphoma has been successfully treated by chemotherapy. The sera of patients with Burkitt's lymphoma also react with suspensions of Burkitt's lymphoma cells, and the reaction is thought to indicate the presence of specific neoantigens on the cell surface. Apparently identical neo-antigens are present in cultured lymphocytes from patients suffering from IM. Remarkably, almost all established cultures of human transformed B lymphocyte cell lines are known to be infected with EBV, and few clones proliferate indefinitely in culture unless they are infected with EBV.

The relationship between EBV, Burkitt's lymphoma, and IM is unknown, but it is suggested that infection with EBV is common in man and usually tolerated, that a minority who escape infection and reach adolescence without acquiring antibodies are likely to succumb to IM when they are infected, and that a much smaller minority, predisposed by unknown factors, possibly holoendemic malaria in tropical Africa and New Guinea, react by developing Burkitt's lymphoma. Though speculative, this hypothesis is consistent with what is known of the circumstances in which viruses induce neoplasms in animals.

Burkitt-type lymphoma occurs sporadically throughout the world and is frequently not associated with the presence of anti-EBV antibodies; but the same chromosome abnormality, a translocation involving chromosomes 8 and 14, is found in about one half of the cases of both the endemic African and the sporadic forms, a finding reminiscent of bovine leucosis where the enzootic form but not the sporadic form is associated with a C-type retravirus. Besides African Burkitt's lymphoma the only other condition in which the serum consistently contains high-titre anti-EBV antibodies is the nasopharyngeal carcinoma found in East Africa and China. Here again, the possibility of a single virus causing more than one type of neoplasm is consistent with the facts of animal oncology.

Carcinoma of the uterine cervix has a greatly differing incidence in different social groups. The strong association with sexual activity and with promiscuity have raised the suspicion of a transmissible aetiology. *Herpesvirus hominis* type II has been isolated from the genital tract of a higher proportion of patients than control subjects, but the significance of the finding is not yet clear.

Iatrogenic carcinogenesis. Several of the agents used for treating malignant disease are themselves carcinogenic, especially ionizing radiation and the biological alkylating agents. Acute myeloid leukaemia is being encountered more frequently now that larger numbers of patients treated intensively with radiotherapy, alkylating agents, or both, for Hodgkin's disease, myelomatosis, breast cancer, and ovarian cancer are surviving long enough for the induced leukaemia to become manifest. The average latent period is four to five years, but the incidence rises from about one year from treatment and persists for more than ten years. It is accepted that the risk is higher for patients who have received both radiotherapy and alkylating agents. It is possible that the risk is higher for some conditions than others, the majority of reports so far having been for myelomatosis and Hodgkin's disease, in which the risk for patients who survive beyond five years is about 10 per cent for myelomatosis, about 800 times the expected risk, and between 5 and 10 per cent for Hodgkin's disease. It is also possible that the alkylating agents differ in their leukaemogenecity; in the Medical Research Council's therapeutic trials in lung cancer and in myelomatosis, busulphan and melphalan were more leukaemogenic than cyclophosphamide. The risk of inducing leukaemia is at present acceptable in the treatment of malignant disease by radiotherapy and alkylating agents, but the use of these agents in the treatment of non-malignant conditions, such as the nephrotic syndrome or rheumatoid arthritis, requires careful consideration.

Organ transplantation is another situation in which the recipients are exposed to a risk of developing malignant disease. Malignant lymphomas are the most frequently reported conditions arising in recipients of kidney, heart, or liver allografts. The incidence is about ten times greater than expected, and the latent period is much shorter than for acute myeloid leukaemia following radiotherapy and treatment with alkylating agents, being on average two years, but sometimes only a few months. A high proportion of the tumours arise in and are often confined to the central nervous system which is otherwise a rare site for lymphoreticular tumours. The neoplasia is thought to result from the long-term immunosuppressive treatment given to the recipients, usually involving corticosteroids, azathioprine, cyclophosphamide, antilymphocyte globulin, and more recently the cyclic polypeptide cyclosporin A. On the other hand the recipient's lymphoid tissue is under constant stimulation by foreign antigens from the graft and this may generate clones of immunoreactive cells with an increased risk of becoming transformed. Kaposi's sarcoma, a very rare tumour in the general population, is about five times more common in transplant recipients.

Inherited disorders and malignant disease. Many inherited disorders carry an increased risk of malignant disease. Examples are:

1. Epidermodysplasia verruciformis is a multisystem hereditary disorder inherited as an autosomal recessive. Warty lesions appear in childhood, become increasingly numerous, and several types of epidermoid carcinoma develop, including intra-epidermal carcinoma *in situ* (Bowen's disease), basal-cell and squamous-cell carcinoma. Wart virus, though widespread in the warty skin lesions cannot be demonstrated in the cells of the malignant lesions. This is reminiscent of the Shope papilloma-virus lesions in rabbits in which the virus can be recovered from the warty lesions but not from the malignant epidermoid carcinomata that develop from them.

2. Polyposis coli is inherited as an autosomal dominant, and there is a high risk of malignant change developing in affected persons, though the malignant change occurs in only a small proportion of the numerous polyps. Chromosomal abnormalities that vary from case to case have been described and are considered to be secondary.

3. Several hereditary conditions with cytogenetic abnormalities carry an increased risk of leukaemia, but the risk is far less than in the diseases just described. In Down's syndrome and D-trisomy one member of a particular pair of chromosomes is duplicated, but in Fanconi's syndrome the chromosome abnormalities are inconstant and variable. In Fanconi's anaemia, there is also an increased

risk of skin cancers, and hepatoma has been reported in patients who have not received androgens.

4. Several hereditary immunological deficiency syndromes carry a high risk of malignant lymphoma. The Wiskott–Aldrich syndrome is inherited as an X-linked recessive, and is characterized by thrombocytopenia and eczema as well as by gross immunological deficiency. The ataxia–telangiectasia syndrome (Louis–Bar) is inherited as an autosomal recessive, and other similarly inherited cases, less well characterized, are associated with amyloidosis. It is not known whether the increased risk of neoplasia in these conditions is related to the genetic disturbance, or to the immunological defects caused by them. The incidence of malignant disease is higher than in the inherited conditions not associated with immunological deficiency. In ataxia–telangiectasia, variable chromosome breaks and an almost constant involvement of chromosome 14 are found.

5. Nephroblastoma (Wilms' tumour). This is an embryonal tumour with a high incidence in children with multiple congenital anomalies, including cases of hemihypertrophy, aniridia, and hypospadias. Chromosomal defects have been described.

6. Retinoblastoma is an embryonal tumour with a high risk of developing in both eyes. There is a strong familial tendency, with a high incidence in the sibs of affected children, and there is an increased risk of other malignant diseases, including rhabdomyosarcoma, lymphoblastic leukaemia, and melanoma.

7. Cancer of the oesophagus and tylosis. Rare families exist in which there is a close association between tylosis, a skin disease inherited as an autosomal dominant character, and cancer of the lower oesophagus. In tylosis, there is marked hyperkeratosis of the palms and soles. Affected members of the family are at high risk of developing oesophageal cancer, but unaffected members are no more susceptible than the general population and no case of cancer has yet occurred in one. It is therefore not known whether the gene for tylosis renders the oesophageal epithelium exceptionally vulnerable to neoplastic transformation, or whether two separate genes are involved, so closely linked that the chances of segregation by crossing over are remote.

A further example illustrates how complex the problem of carcinogenesis in a clinical setting can be. In adult coeliac disease there is an increased risk of malignant histiocytosis; the disease is frequently multifocal, and is another instance of multifocal malignancy arising in already abnormal tissue. In addition, there is an increased risk of other digestive tract malignancies, including cancer of the tongue, oesophagus, stomach, duodenum, colon, rectum, and anus. The frequency of both the lymphomas and the cancers is reported to be lower in patients treated with a gluten-free diet. However, an increased incidence of cancer but not of lymphomas has been reported in the relatives of patients suffering from coeliac disease.

Malignant-cell phenotypes and target cells. Tumour-cell populations vary greatly in the characteristics of the cells of which they are composed. Thus some are essentially monomorphic, almost all the cells having the same overall characteristics. In 'common' acute lymphoblastic leukaemia all the cells appear to be undifferentiated blast cells, in Burkitt's lymphoma they are early B-lymphoid cells, while in myelomatosis the cells have both differentiated into the B-cell lineage and have also undergone complete maturation to immunoglobulin-producing plasma cells. In contrast a malignant teratoma may contain apparently undifferentiated cells and mixtures of cells that have differentiated to such types as bone, cartilage, muscle, nerve, and gut cells, each type showing, in varying degree, maturation to the appropriate end cell. In colloid carcinomas of the bowel, a substantial part of the tumour mass may consist of mucin secreted by goblet cells that are clearly end cells: they and the mature cells of each lineage in the teratoma are the products of malignant cells but are not themselves capable of perpetuating the growth of the tumour. Tumour-cell populations are clones derived by common descent from a single transformed normal cell, the

target of the carcinogenic process. It is the capacity for self renewal of the target cell, or of a proportion of its descendants, that perpetuates the tumour. These clonogenic cells may or may not resemble the original target cell; they may, for example, have become committed to a line of differentiation and yet retained their clonogenicity. The extent to which their descendants undergo maturation, and in doing so lose their clonogenicity, determines the overall heterogeneity of the tumour-cell population. As discussed earlier see page 4.47), the clonogenic cells are unable to respond to the environmental signals that lead their normal counterparts to undergo further differentiation and maturation. The absolute number of clonogenic cells is, however, often large enough to permit the characterization of the clone by a large number of ascertainable features. The resulting phenotype may at first appear to differ from that of cells from the tissue of origin. Only a few years ago such phenotypes were thought to be 'tumour-specific'. New methods of characterization have shown that tumour-cell clones are often derived by the expansion of a very small population of normal cells previously undetected, because they are heavily outnumbered by their differentiated and maturing descendants. As suggested above, however, the stage in differentiation along a particular lineage at which further development is blocked varies from one tumour to another, and therefore the predominant cell type of a malignant clone may be more differentiated than the original transformed target cell whose numbers remain too small to permit accurate characterization.

The original demonstration by Greaves of a unique surface membrane antigen of the leukaemia cells of the common type of acute lymphoblastic leukaemia (c-ALL) was thought to have revealed a leukaemia-specific determinant. These cells were further characterized by the possession of the Ia-like antigen, coded by the DR locus of the HLA gene complex, and of the nuclear enzyme terminal deoxynucleotidyl transferase (TdT). Recently it has become possible to identify these substances in individual cells in a large population by means of specific antisera labelled with suitable fluorochromes. In this way, it has been shown that in certain states of bone-marrow regeneration, small numbers of cells having the same phenotype as c-ALL cells are present in non-leukaemic or normal persons. The phenotype of these cells is now thought to be present during a short period only in the normal differentiation of early haemopoietic stem-cell precursors, and was unmasked only as a result of its preservation and amplification in the expanded clone of c-ALL cells. It now seems probable that most 'tumour-specific' antigens are differentiation antigens like the c-ALL antigen. Some, however, are coded by viruses incorporated in the cell genome, and others in experimentally induced tumours are coded by DNA altered by the chemical carcinogen used or by one of its metabolites. They are called tumour-associated antigens.

Some malignant tumours are composed of cells for which a normal counterpart has not been identified, while in others, the phenotype is not identical with that of any recognized normal cell. The 'hairy cell' of hairy-cell leukaemia, and the large nucleolated lymphocyte of prolymphocytic leukaemia have no known normal counterparts. In thymic acute lymphoblastic leukaemia (thy-ALL), the cell phenotype is identical with that of early cortical thymic cells except that thy-ALL cells have the HLA-A, -B, and -C core antigen strongly represented on their surface membrane; this antigen is absent in cortical thymic cells. It has been suggested that the difference is not related to the malignancy of thy-ALL cells, but arises because these cells, when in the bone marrow and peripheral blood, are released from the environmental influence of thymic epithelium which suppresses the expression of the antigen in cortical thymocytes. The analysis of tumour-cell phenotypes by refined methods is at an early stage, and will be greatly extended by the use of monoclonal antibodies against a large number of cellular antigenic determinants.

Philadelphia-chromosome (Ph[1])-positive chronic granulocytic leukaemia (CGL) illustrates the relationship between tumour-cell populations and the target cells from which they are derived. CGL is characterized by an enormous clonal expansion of myeloid tissue, in particular of the granulocytic series. However, the red-cell, megakaryocytic, and monocytic lines belong to the clone which is perpetuated during the chronic phase by a clonogenic myeloid stem cell. This cell often undergoes transformation to a cell of enhanced malignancy, with restriction of its capacity for differentiation, usually to the granulocytic line, less often to one of the other lines, and of the capacity of its differentiated descendants for maturation. The new clone gives rise to the clinical events of 'myeloid' blast-cell transformation which occurs in about 80 per cent of all cases of CGL. In the remainder, however, the malignant phase of the disease results from the proliferation of a clone of 'lymphoid' blast cells which carry a phenotype identical with that of the c-ALL cell which is thought to be an early precursor of the B-lymphocyte lineage. This suggests that the clonogenic myeloid stem cell responsible for maintaining the chronic-phase erythrocytic, granulocytic, megakaryocytic, and monocytic cell populations is a derivative of a still earlier haemopoietic stem-cell target which may become transformed to a malignant clonogenic blast cell with the c-ALL phenotype. The Ph^1-positive target cell of CGL would thus appear to be a pre-myeloid, pre-lymphoid, haemopoietic cell precursor. It is thus not surprising that occasionally this target cell first manifests its presence as Ph^1-positive acute lymphoblastic leukaemia, and subsequently as CGL, the lymphoblastic leukaemia having been controlled by appropriate treatment. The target cell may not produce any myeloid-committed descendants, thus accounting for Ph^1-positive ALL which is not at any stage followed or accompanied by CGL.

METABOLIC EFFECTS OF NEOPLASMS (PARANEOPLASTIC SYNDROMES)

Most of the harmful effects of malignant tumours are caused by their local effects on neighbouring structures. They are locally destructive to the tissues they invade, and although they advance along paths offering the least resistance, they infiltrate and destroy the walls of lymphatics, capillaries, venules, veins, arterioles or larger arteries, nerve sheaths, and bone; they invade, encircle, and obstruct the tubular structures of the respiratory, gastro-intestinal, and genito-urinary tracts and their associated glands and ducts, and they ulcerate mucous membranes and skin, while their plaque-like deposits on serous membranes exude fluid, often in large quantities.

The clinical consequences of these local effects are essentially fortuitous and depend on the anatomical position of the tumour. At certain sites, tumours or their metastases may produce profound systemic disturbances as a result of the damage they cause to vital tissues or organs. The symptoms resulting from this damage may be the first of which the patient has complained, and may not at first raise a suspicion of underlying malignant disease. In some instances the diagnosis is easily made from the history and physical examination, while in others sophisticated investigations may fail to reveal the underlying cause. Examples are the following:

1. Uraemia resulting from bilateral ureteric obstruction due to a pelvic tumour. Pelvic examination will usually suffice to detect its presence.

2. Partial or complete bone marrow failure resulting from widespread skeletal deposits of metastatic carcinoma (usually secondary to mammary, prostatic, bronchial, renal, or thyroid carcinoma, malignant melanoma, or neuroblastoma). The patients may have had a primary tumour excised years before, or the primary tumour may remain small and undetected at the time of presentation. The presentation is with anaemia, neutropenia, or thrombocytopenia in varying combinations and occasionally eosinophilia. Paradoxically, an abnormally high platelet count is occasionally found in association with malignant disease with or without metastatic deposits in the bone marrow: increased numbers of megakaryocytes are found in the marrow (see Section 19).

Myelomatosis may also present with bone marrow failure, the patient having at no time experienced bone pain. The finding of leucoerythroblastic anaemia suggests a diagnosis of secondary carcinoma, melanoma, or neuroblastoma, and rouleaux formation and background protein in the blood films suggest a diagnosis of mylomatosis, in which leucoerythroblastic anaemia is less common. Bone marrow examination permits the recognition of myelomatosis, secondary melanoma, and neuroblastoma, and when carcinoma cells are found, a positive L-tartrate-sensitive acid-phosphatase reaction suggests a prostatic origin. The radiological appearance of the bones may give some indication of the nature of the disease. Metastases from prostatic carcinoma are usually osteoplastic, those from mammary carcinoma only occasionally are.

3. Acute hypercalcaemia resulting from widespread skeletal deposits of metastatic carcinoma [see (2) for the common primary sites] or from myelomatosis. The loss of bone calcium is due to a local effect of the malignant cells on the surrounding bone, mediated by the action of osteoclasts. Myeloma cells in culture have been shown to release an osteoclast-activating substance. Hypercalcaemia may also result from the release of hormone-like substances from extraskeletal tumours in the absence of skeletal metastases, but skeletal metastases must be carefully sought before concluding that they are not present. Widespread but diffuse infiltration of bone may not give rise to pain and may not be detected radiologically until considerable demineralization has occurred. Recent active discrete deposits may cause pain but may not be visible on plain X-rays. However, they are sometimes surrounded by a hyperaemic zone in which reactive new-bone formation is taking place. Tracer doses of a bone-seeking radionuclide such as radiofluoride are concentrated in these areas, and permit their early detection. The presence of leucoerythroblastic anaemia provides supporting evidence of skeletal involvement and the presumptive diagnosis is clinced by finding malignant cells in a bone marrow aspirate or trephine specimen perferably taken from a site of suspected involvement. In rare cases, usually of metastatic disease from a primary mammary cancer, the spleen and liver are enlarged as a result of myeloid metaplasia, but these patients are usually thrombocytopenic, and it is not safe to attempt a needle biopsy of the liver. Skeletal X-rays may show at least some demineralization even though discrete metastases or irregularities in the bone pattern are not visible (see Section 17).

4. Diabetes insipidus resulting from deposits of tumours (other than those arising primarily in the hypophysis) in the neighbourhood of the hypothalamus and hypophysis. The nature of the tumours may be suggested by their radiological appearances, and a full skeletal survey is desirable to reveal other deposits. Eosinophilic granuloma and Hand–Schüller–Christian disease may present in this way.

5. Hypoadrenalism resulting from replacement of both adrenals by metastatic carcinoma. Bronchial carcinoma is the commonest source of this.

6. Hepatorenal encephalopathy resulting from extensive replacement of the liver or kidneys by secondary carcinoma. This is a terminal condition usually readily recognized by physical examination, and the search for a primary tumour is academic and rarely undertaken.

The above examples refer to the distant effects of tumours growing in specific organs or tissues. Certain profound general effects associated with tumours, usually but not necessarily disseminated, may cause clinical disability before the onset of any symptoms resulting from the local effects of the tumour, but cannot be related to the involvement of any particular organs or tissues. Neuromuscular disorders and disturbances of coagulation are discussed below.

7. Neuromuscular disorders of several types are associated with

carcinoma arising from the bronchus, breast, stomach, rectum, ovary, and other organs, and with malignant lymphoma. Minor usually asymptomatic proximal muscle weakness and wasting associated with diminution or loss of tendon reflexes are found in a small proportion of cases of carcinoma on routine examination. Occasionally there is severe disability months or years before the discovery of the neoplasm. The neurological disturbances are occasionally associated with small localized tumours and disappear when the tumour is excised. Dermatomyositis, in which the rash may be inconspicuous and transient, is more often associated with breast cancer than with other neoplasms.

The commonest disorder is of the neuromyopathic type described above, but predominantly sensory neuropathies occur, as well as mixed types. In some cases the disorder is essentially myopathic with myasthenic features, or simulates those of motor neurone disease. Cerebellar dysfunction has been associated with ovarian adenocarcinoma, and occasionally with carcinoma of the breast and lung, but carcinoma of the lung accounts for the majority of cases of all types of neurological disturbances. The cause of the carcinomatous neuromyopathies remains unknown, but they are not due to the physical presence in or near nervous tissue of the tumours or their metastases. Local infiltration of nervous structures must always be exluded by appropriate investigation. A rapidly progressive and lethal leucoencephalopathy due to widespread multifocal demyelinating lesions throughout the white matter of the central nervous system occurs rarely in cases of disseminated malignant disease with immunodeficiency, most often of malignant lymphoma and Hodgkin's disease. It is caused by papovagroup viruses (see page 4.79).

8. Disturbances of blood coagulation may cause the presenting symptoms in cases of unsuspected though often widely disseminated malignant disease, almost always of mucin-secreting adenocarcinoma arising in pancreas, stomach, bronchus, prostate, or colon. Migratory thrombophlebitis has been associated with cancer for a century, but the existence of disseminated intravascular coagulation and microangiopathic haemolytic anaemia has been recognized only recently; malignant disease is one of the causes of the latter (see Section 19).

Successive thrombotic episodes in superficial veins, or in the veins draining muscles and viscera, result from a hypercoagulable state of the blood, believed to be initiated by the thromboplastic activity of substances released from mucin-secreting carcinoma cells. In some cases, sometimes associated with eosinophilia, nonbacterial thrombotic endocarditis is found, usually involving the mitral valve; secondary arterial embolic disease affecting arteries in the brain, limbs, heart, kidneys, or other viscera may supervene.

Hypergranular promyelocytic leukaemia accounts for 7 per cent of the acute myeloid leukaemias, and is more frequent in children and young adults. The heavily granulated leukaemia cells release tissue thromboplastin that precipitates intravascular coagulation which is rapidly lethal unless emergency supportive treatment with heparin and massive platelet transfusions are administered.

Malignant cachexia and the metabolism of bulky tumours. Tumours also affect the host by their own metabolic activities. When the total mass of tumour tissue is very large in relation to the body weight, some effect on the general metabolism would be expected either as a result of the diversion of essential nutrients from the tissues of the host to the tumour, or as a result of intoxication by metabolites liberated by the tumour. 'Malignant cachexia' has been attributed to these effects without definite evidence. Patients with widespread deposits of metastatic malignant disease often remain well nourished until secondary phenomena lead to cachexia. They include ulceration of skin with supervening infection, compression of tubular structures with subsequent infection resulting from poor drainage, and anorexia resulting from obstructive dysphagia, persistent vomiting, or from the prolonged use of opiates administered to relieve pain. Some have attributed malignant cachexia entirely to

secondary effects. However, cachexia not secondary to local effects has been associated with small tumours, and has disappeared following their excision. Malignant cachexia in man requires detailed investigation, for its explanation remains unknown.

Few instances of gross interference with metabolism result from the activities of massive tumours. Chronic myeloid leukaemia patients lose weight because their basal metabolic rate is raised, due to the metabolic activity of the greatly increased total mass of granulocytic tissue. Raised serum urate levels are associated with deposits of cellular tumours whose nuclei account for a substantial fraction of the total nucleic acid content of the body. The raised levels reflect the enlarged total body pool of nucleic acids. Clinical gout occurs in myeloproliferative disorders associated with raised serum urate levels, but not in lymphoproliferative disorders and myelomatosis in which equally high levels are found. In lymphosarcomatosis and lymphoblastic leukaemia when cell turnover is excessively rapid, the metabolic breakdown of the purines of the nucleic acids leads to the production of urate at a rate beyond the excretory capacity of the kidneys. The urate concentration exceeds the maximum solubility and microcrystals of urate precipitate in the renal tubules, pelves, and ureters. The microcrystals confer a consistency of mud on the urine, and obstructive oliguric nephropathy results. This is rare in untreated disease, but not uncommon when massive breakdown of tumour cells occurs rapidly during cytotoxic therapy. Administration of the xanthine oxidase inhibitor, allopurinol, reduces the concentration of urate by causing part of the total metabolites of the purines to be excreted as xanthine and hypoxanthine; the solubility of the three metabolites is independent, the concentration of any one of them does not reach saturation, and crystallization does not take place.

Anaemia is rarely attributable to a specific metabolic effect of tumours. When iron deficiency resulting from chronic blood loss or malabsorption are excluded, there remain cases in which defective iron transport results from hypotransferrinaemia or from an inability to mobilize storage iron; this is found in many wasting diseases and chronic infections and is not specific for malignant disease. Rarely, patients later found to have acute leukaemia or malignant lymphoma present with megaloblastic anaemia resulting from folate deficiency. The malignant disease becomes overt only when folate therapy is begun, and it is inferred that the malignant tissue functions as a folate trap.

Anaemia resulting from a selective aplasia of the erythropoietic cells in the bone marrow is sometimes associated with a thymic tumour, usually of benign encapsulated spindle-cell or lymphocytic type though occasionally infiltrating or metastasizing to the pleura. The anaemia may remit after the tumour has been removed, but the same type of anaemia has occurred following the removal of similar tumours when the patients were not anaemic. The patients are usually elderly women, and some have myasthenia gravis.

Fever in malignant disease is usually accounted for by infection, haemorrhage, or necrosis, but these do not explain the fever of Hodgkin's disease, chronic myeloid leukaemia, or renal cortical carcinoma. Dying neutrophil leucocytes release pyrogen that is believed to cause the fever accompanying infections; in chronic myeloid leukaemia, the fever subsides when the leucocyte count is lowered by treatment and is likely to be due to leucocyte pyrogen. The cause of the fever of Hodgkin's disease and renal cortical carcinoma is not known.

Pruritus, a common symptom of Hodgkin's disease, rarely of other lymphomas, may precede the appearance of any lesions detectable by physical examination by many months. When persistent unexplained pruritus is accompanied by fever, sweats, weight loss, a raised erythrocyte sedimentation rate, and a raised alkaline phosphatase content of the neutrophil leucocytes, Hodgkin's disease should be suspected and deep-seated involvement sought by lymphangiography, CT scanning, and laparotomy. The spleen may contain deposits of Hodgkin's disease even when not enlarged, and should be removed.

The hyperviscosity syndrome is a feature of those cases of Waldenström's macroglobulinaemia and myelomatosis in which the concentration of paraprotein in the serum is high enough to increase its viscosity sufficiently to impede the microcirculation in the tissues. The effect of immunoglobin molecules on the viscosity of the serum depends on their size, shape, and extent of polymerization as well as on their concentration. IgM increases viscosity at lower serum concentration that IgG, and within a narrow range, small increases in the concentration lead to great increase in the viscosity. The subclass IgG_3 behaves more like IgM. Whole-blood viscosity is markedly increased in polycythaemia rubra vera by the high redcell count, and cerebral blood flow is reduced; when the packed-cell volume is reduced by appropriate treatment the rate of flow returns to normal.

Increased serum viscosity causes weakness and exhaustion, headache, drowsiness, haemorrhages from the nose, gums, gastrointestinal or genital tract, visual disturbance, isolated neuropathies, congestive cardiac failure, and coma. The sequence of symptoms varies from patient to patient, but in any one case the sequence is usually the same whenever the serum concentration of the paraprotein reaches the critical level for that patient. The symptoms are often preceded by a regular sequence of changes in the fundi that provide a warning of their impending onset. The fundal veins become first dilated, then tortuous, and later their calibre becomes irregular; finally constrictions alternate with dilated segments, giving a beaded or 'string of sausages' appearance, and papilloedema, exudates, and haemorrhages appear. The symptoms and signs may be rapidly relieved by removing blood, separating, and discarding the plasma, and returning the red cells to the patient. The removal of as little as 1 l of blood may suffice in some cases. Plasmapheresis is most easily performed with a continuous flow blood-cell separator.

Cryoglobulins are immunoglobulins that precipitate when cooled. They occur in some cases of myelomatosis and Waldenström's macroglobulinaemia as well as in non-malignant conditions in which the cryoprotein may consist of IgG/IgM complexes.

They precipitate in the superficial capillaries and sub-papillary venules or outside the vessels in the coldest parts of the skin where they produce purpura or micro-infarcts. The affected areas are painful, and at first show livid purplish discoloration within which dark brown or blackish necrotic patches appear. The lesions occur on the coldest parts of the skin, usually on the extensor aspects of the limbs and are more numerous distally. Perforation of the anterior parts of the nasal septum is often found.

Amyloidosis is found in some 3 per cent of cases of myelomatosis and Waldenström's macroglobulinaemia and in some cases of longstanding Hodgkin's disease. The main clinical consequences result from involvement of ligaments, fasciae, tendons, synovial membranes, nerves, the liver, the tongue, the larynx, the myocardium, and renal cortex. The carpal tunnel syndrome, focal amyloid deposits in joints and overlying the limb and trunk musculature, macroglossia, hoarseness due to laryngeal involvement, firm enlargement of the liver, and cardiomyopathy are the commoner manifestations. In rare cases coarse purpuric spots appear in clusters over the cheeks, neck, and upper chest. Biopsy of the rectal mucosa offers the best chance of establishing the diagnosis. The amyloid material has been identified as containing amino-acid sequences of the variable portion of the light immunoglobulin chain.

Nephrotic syndrome is occasionally associated with, and may even be the presenting feature of, bronchial, gastric, colonic and other cancers, Hodgkin's disease, other lymphomas and chronic lymphocytic leukaemia. It may disappear following resection of the tumour and its reappearance may be the first indication of the presence of metastases. Renal biopsy usually shows a membranous glomerulopathy, and occasionally antibody reacting with the cancer cells has been eluted from the deposits, or immune complexes containing tumour-associated antigens including carcinoembryonic antigen have been found. Amyloid is sometimes found.

Nicotinamide deficiency and *hypoproteinaemia* occur in a small proportion of patients with the carcinoid syndrome who have massive tumour deposits in the liver. The tumour acts as a tryptophan trap, diverting its metabolism to the synthesis of 5–hydroxytryptamine, and away from its major pathways to protein synthesis and the synthesis of nicotinamide. Affected patients develop pellagra-like skin lesions, and become hypoproteinaemic.

Metabolic effects of small tumours. The effects described above are brought about by the metabolic activities of large masses of tumour tissue and are not usually a feature of the early stages of the same diseases, although they may be responsible for the first symptoms.

Profound metabolic disturbances, however, are associated with the activities of quite small tumours which would otherwise remain undetected until they are large enough to cause local manifestations. The association in some instances is so frequent that the appearance of the characteristic syndrome should immediately arouse the suspicion of the presence of a neoplasm, whereas in others, the systemic disturbance, though characteristic, is only rarely associated with a particular neoplasm and is more commonly due to other causes. An example of the former type is phaeochromocytoma, the functional tumour of chromaffin tissue, which releases catecholamines, especially noradrenalin. These cause attacks of paroxysmal hypertension and a variety of vasomotor phenomena. All the functional tumours of the endocrine organs are of this type. An example of the latter type is the association of *acute haemolytic anaemia* with *ovarian tumours* usually *teratomas*, including *dermoid cysts*, occasionally *pseudomucinous cystadenocarcinoma*. Marked spherocytosis is usually present, and splenectomy fails to relieve the anaemia. Subsequently, removal of the ovarian tumour is followed by relief of the anaemia. The pathogenesis of the anaemia remains unknown, but is thought to involve autoimmunization. Between these two extremes are a wide variety of manifestations, most of which are poorly understood. Attempts to classify them are necessarily arbitrary and provisional, and the basis of the attempts depends on the standpoint adopted.

From the medical standpoint, metabolic disturbances caused by small tumours are important because they are clinically harmful, and because they provide information that prompts the search for a tumour the presence of which would otherwise remain unsuspected; in some cases the symptoms may be relieved by removing the tumour. In an increasing number of cases, some at least of the metabolic disturbances can now be attributed to the production by the tumour of substances with powerful hormonal or pharmacological activity often closely resembling or even identical with normally occurring substances. In many cases, however, including the ovarian tumours causing haemolytic anaemia, the relation between the tumour and the metabolic disturbance remains obscure.

From the biological standpoint, the release by tumours of substances with powerful hormonal or pharmacological activity should be regarded as a special case of the disturbed metabolism of the tumour cells. Some identifiable products of tumour cells cause no metabolic disturbances but are clinically useful indicators of the presence of a tumour, especially when almost every tumour of a specific type releases the substance: in some instances changes in the serum concentrations of the substances reflect the activity of the tumour. Examples of such substances are alpha-fetoprotein associated with hepatocellular carcinoma, L-tartrate-sensitive acid phosphatase with prostatic adenocarcinoma, leucineaminopeptidase with pancreatic carcinoma, chorionic gonadotrophin with trophoblastic tumours, and lysozyme with monocytic leukaemia. Some of the substances produced by the tumour cells are also produced by their normal counterparts, but others are not normally associated with the tissues of origin. An isoenzyme of alkaline phosphatase resembling placental alkaline phosphatase biochemically and immunologically has been found in the serum and in the tumour in some cases of carcinoma of the lung, breast, uterus, ovary, colon, and of malignant lymphoma and myelomatosis. Other isoenzymes of alkaline phosphatase have been found in association with malignant tumours arising in the lung, gastrointestinal tract, pancreas, and liver. The clinical importance of these isoenzymes is that the raised serum levels do not indicate the presence of metastases in the bones or the liver. The anomalous synthesis of alkaline phosphatase by tumours is unexplained, but presumably involves the utilization of part of the facultative genome that is normally inactive, and it has been suggested that this synthesis is mediated by the activity of a virus incorporated into the genome. Alternatively, and perhaps more likely, the substance may be the product of the target cell or an immature descendant which is normally present in such low numbers that its product is undetectable. Its production in large quantities when the target cell proliferates as a malignant clone with limited maturation then appears anomalous.

Thus, metabolically active products that have been identified in tumours and sometimes in the serum are of two main types, namely those characteristically produced by the tissue from which the tumour arose, and those not known to be produced by the tissue of origin. The former type includes all the hormones and substances with hormonal activity produced by the classical functional endocrine tumours and by those more recently described, which arise in normal anatomical structures appropriate to the endocrine tissue concerned, or in ectopic sites often associated with that tissue in embryological development. Characteristically, the production of the hormones is unphysiological and not subject to the homeostatic control that regulates their secretion by the normal endocrine glands. To a large extent the resulting syndromes are explicable in terms of the overproduction of hormones of known activity, and when two or more hormones are produced by the same tumour, the variations in the clinical manifestations may be explained by the differing proportions in which the several hormones are represented. However, persistent and striking symptoms that disappear when the tumour is removed often remain unaccounted for by any known hormone or pharmacologically active agent. Occasionally a characteristic syndrome associated with the persistent overproduction of a single hormone is explicable in terms of secondary as well as primary effects of the hormone. Thus, in the glucagonoma syndrome produced by pancreatic islet *a-2* cells, and characterized by an apparently specific rash ('necrolytic migratory erythema'), stomatitis, anaemia, weight loss, and diabetes, all but the last feature are considered secondary to the catabolic action of glucagon. From the biological standpoint, the production of specific hormones by the functional endocrine tumours is analogous to the production of the identifiable but apparently functionally inert substances by specific tumours.

The functional endocrine tumours are considered elsewhere in this volume (see Section 10) as are the *carcinoid tumours* (see Section 12) that release several pharmacologically active substances including 5-hydroxytryptamine and other tryptophan metabolities, histamine, and the proteolytic enzyme kallikrein, as well as other peptides such as substance P, motilin, kinins, and also prostaglandins. It should be noted that, in contrast to the functional endocrine tumours, only a minority of carcinoid tumours produce pharmacologically active substances, and of those that do, only a small proportion cause the carcinoid syndrome, because the active products of those tumours whose venous blood drains into the tributaries of the portal vein are inactivated in the liver. When metastases of those tumours grow in the liver, however, the active products are released into the systemic circulation.

The carcinoid tumours illustrate the difficulty in deciding whether the metabolic products of tumours are appropriate to the presumptive tissue of origin. Most carcinoid tumours arise from the epithelium of those parts of the gastrointestinal tract and its derivatives that contain argentaffin cells and the tumour cells are thought to arise from these cells. Similar argentaffin-cell tumours, occasionally responsible for the carcinoid syndrome, arise from ectopic gastrointestinal epithelium within ovarian or testicular teratomas. However, some tumours responsible for the carcinoid syndrome do not resemble the classical argentaffin-cell tumours in any respect and arise from bronchial epithelium, the pancreas, the thyroid and elsewhere. Some apparently monomorphic pancreatic islet-cell tumours have been responsible for the carcinoid syndrome, and have also released gastrin, with the production of peptic ulceration (Zollinger–Ellison syndrome), and insulin. Whatever the embryological derivation of the tumour cells they appear to be capable of synthesizing and releasing a greater variety of specific products than is the case with any commonly represented normal cell in post-natal life, but their activities, unlike those of normal cells, are not integrated with the physiological requirements of the host.

The APUD-cell series illustrates how a widely distributed system of specialized cells of common developmental origin may undergo divergent differentiation according to the tissue in which the cells settle (see Section 12). The APUD cells (characterized by their capacity for *a*mine *p*recursor *u*ptake and for the *d*ecarboxylation of amino acids) arise in the neural crest and migrate to the anterior pituitary, thyroid, pancreatic islets, stomach, small bowel, carotid body, adrenal medulla, and lung. The cells, at different sites, produce one of the biogenic amines 5-hydroxytryptamine, or one of the catecholamines, or one of the polypeptide hormones described below. In the neoplastic state, however, the cells readily synthesize amines or polypeptides normally synthesized only by APUD cells in other locations, and they may synthesize products not normally associated with APUD cells.

Like the carcinoid tumours the even less common non-argentaffin tumours of the APUD system may present with symptoms and signs caused by the biological effects of the substances they synthesize and release rather than with those caused by the presence of a tumour mass. The substances concerned are peptides identical with, or similar to those produced by the normal cells of the diffuse endocrine system, and not all have yet been fully characterized. They are identified in the serum by radio-immunoassay, and specific peptides with characteristic biological actions have been located to specific cell types in the pancreatic islets, in the gastrointestinal tract, and other tissues by immunocytochemical methods involving light- and electron-microscopy. Some normal cells produce more than one peptide, and this is true of some tumours also, though one product usually predominates. Methods for characterizing the peptides and their biological properties, and the cells producing them have been only recently developed, and are still being applied to the analysis of the variable clinical syndromes.

The best characterized syndromes are those resulting from tumours of the specific cells that secrete insulin, gastrin, glucagon, somatostatin, and vasoactive intestinal polypeptide. Insulinomas cause spontaneous hypoglycaemic attacks that are relieved by the administration of glucose; gastrinomas cause hyperchlorhydria and consequent intractable peptic ulceration, and diarrhoea; glucagonomas cause diabetes often associated with a characteristic painful necrolytic migratory erythema and diarrhoea; somatostatinomas are somatostatin-producing pancreatic apudomas associated with raised serum concentrations of somatostatin and give rise to diarrhoea, flushing, hypochlorhydria, and abnormal glucose tolerance. Watery diarrhoea in apudomas is often associated with raised plasma concentrations of vaso-active intestinal polypeptide. When persistent and copious, it leads to hypokalaemia and achlorhydria (Verner–Morrison syndrome) (see also Section 12).

Aberrant hormone production by non-endocrine tumours. Hormonally active substances are produced by tumours arising from many tissues that do not secrete them. It is likely that the tumours arise from the target cells normally present only in very small numbers in the tissue concerned: these target cells are of different origin from the major components of the tissue, having migrated there in embryonic life, for example from the neural crest. The hormone they produce in appreciable quantities when neoplastic transformation has led to clonal expansion is a reflection of the phenotype of the target cell. It is 'ectopic' only in the sense that recognizable, and physiological amounts of the hormone are not produced by the few target cells present in the normal adult tissue, and 'inappropriate' only in the sense that the transformed tumour cells are not producing the hormone in response to physiological demand. Substances so far identified in association with non-endocrine tumours include those with the activity of vasopressin, antidiuretic-hormone, renin, adrenocorticotrophic hormone, melanophore-stimulating hormone, follicle-stimulating hormone, thyroid-stimulating hormone, parathormone, calcitonin, prostaglandins, glucagon, and insulin. As in the case of carcinoid tumours, the hormone-like substances are produced by only a minority of the tumours of each type, although the incidence of clinical syndromes resulting from their activity is higher than was formerly believed. The metabolic disturbance may precede the onset of any symptoms caused by the local effects of the tumour, whereas in other cases in which the primary tumour has been treated, it results from the development of recurrence or of metastases. The commoner syndromes are now summarized:

The adrenocorticotrophin syndrome (ectopic-ACTH syndrome) is especially associated with oat-cell and undifferentiated carcinoma of the lung, but has also been described in association with thymoma and with carcinoma of the stomach, pancreas (islet-cell), neuroblastoma, thyroid, including medullary carcinoma, parotid, ovary, testis, breast, colon, stomach, and with thymic tumours. It may also be associated with carcinoid tumours, including bronchial carcinoids. It should be emphasized that although the ectopic-ACTH syndrome is most frequent in small-cell bronchial carcinoma, the cells of which contain the neurosecretory granules indicating their origin from neural crest, the syndrome occurs in only a minority of the cases.

The clinical features resemble those following the administration of ACTH and are attributable to a substance having adrenocorticotrophic properties. This has been found in large amounts in the tumours. The adrenocorticotrophic activity of the serum is greatly elevated, but in contrast to the findings in Cushing's syndrome due to other causes is not suppressed by the administration of adrenal corticosteroids, indicating that the pituitary is not the source. When the secretory activity of the tumour is relatively low and the tumour only slowly progressive, the symptoms closely resemble those of Cushing's syndrome, but they are often atypical. More rapidly growing tumours may secrete large amounts of ACTH-like substance over a short period, and the adrenal cortex is under maximal stimulation. The patients complain of severe muscle weakness, they have a cushingoid facies and may become diabetic. The adrenal output of cortisol is very high and this leads to excessive loss of potassium of the urine. The administration of ACTH does not lead to any increase in the serum cortisol level, or in the urinary excretion of its metabolites.

The patients sometimes become deeply pigmented, and this results either from the similarity of structure of the peptide produced by the tumour to adrenocorticotrophin which has melanocyte-stimulating activity, or from the production of another slightly different peptide resembling the melanocyte-stimulating hormone more closely.

Hypercalcaemia has been described already as resulting from massive skeletal involvement by malignant tumours. It may also result from the secretion by small tumours of a substance having parathormone activity, and may subside when the tumour is resected only to reappear with the growth of metastases. The parathyroid glands are not involved. A parathormone-like substance has been isolated from the tumours. It occurs most commonly in association

with carcinoma of the bronchus, breast, renal cortex, and ovary, and the clinical manifestations depend partly on the duration of the exposure to the parathormone-like substance, and partly on the intensity of the stimulation. In the slowly developing syndrome, calcific corneal deposits and metastatic calcification with nephrocalcinosis may occur, but more commonly the syndrome appears too rapidly for their development. In breast cancers a substance resembling 7-dehydrocholesterol has been demonstrated, but it is not known whether it is released or whether it affects calcium metabolism.

The hyponatraemic syndrome may result from hypocorticism due to adrenal replacement by metastatic tumour. Bronchial carcinoma is a more common source of bilateral adrenal metastases than other primary tumours. The symptoms are those of hypocorticism with extreme lethargy, mental confusion, and drowsiness. In these cases the serum potassium concentration is normal. In rare cases of oat-cell carcinoma of the bronchus hyponatraemia may occur in association with a raised plasma volume. The haemoglobin concentration, the packed-cell volume, and the blood urea concentration are low, while the osmolality of the urine is high. In these cases the adrenals are not infiltrated by growth and the hyponatraemic state is thought to arise from the effects of a vasopressin-like peptide with antidiuretic activity that has been identified in the tumours. The urinary sodium loss is increased by the reduced secretion of aldosterone which follows the haemodilution.

The carcinoid syndrome has been mentioned in connection with bronchial adenoma and other non-argentaffin-cell tumours. It also occurs rarely in association with oat-cell and undifferentiated bronchial carcinoma.

Hypertrophic pulmonary osteoarthropathy (HPOA) is especially associated with peripheral lung carcinoma and pleural mesothelioma, but, like all the other conditions discussed, it occurs in only a minority of patients. The patients complain of severe pain in the wrists, ankles, and sometimes knees, and the joints are hot and swollen. There is almost always marked clubbing of the fingers and toes, though this sign is much more common in the absence of HPOA, and some patients have gynaecomastia, which may also occur in the absence of HPOA. HPOA is much more specifically associated with lung cancer than is clubbing, and may precede the onset of chest symptoms by several years. The pain may disappear instantly when the lung is resected, though the physical signs and radiological changes resolve only slowly. In one such case, the histology of the resected tumour showed Hodgkin's disease. The cause of HPOA remains unknown. In some cases with gynaecomastia, high levels of urinary oestrogens are found. In some of these, the high levels persist after the tumour has been resected, but in one case, the levels of serum follicle-stimulating hormone activity were higher in the venous effluent from the tumour than in the arterial blood, and the resected tumour contained large amounts of both follicle-stimulating and luteinizing hormone.

Hypoglycaemia, though usually associated with insulin-secreting β-cell islet tumours of the pancreas, also occurs occasionally in association with other tumours, especially retroperitoneal fibrosarcoma, spindle-cell sarcoma, pseudomyxoma, haemangiopericytoma, and even less commonly with bronchial and gastric carcinoma and malignant lymphoma. Histochemical examination of all tumours is essential to make sure that they do not contain the granules characteristic of pancreatic islet β-cells, indicating an origin in ectopic islet tissue. The symptoms occur especially in the early mornings, when fasting, or after exercise, and are relieved by food. During attacks the blood sugar level may fall to 2.5 mmol/l (45 mg/dl). In some cases substances with insulin-like activity have been isolated from the tumours, but the plasma insulin levels have not been raised. Tolbutamide administered intravenously does not raise the plasma-insulin concentration as it does in insulin-secreting islet-cell tumours (see also Section 9).

Hyperthyroidism, usually not clinically significant, is commoner in association with some tumours than would be expected by chance, notably in gastrointestinal and ovarian tumours. In some trophoblastic tumours the symptoms disappear after successful cytotoxic therapy, and in some cases there is evidence of the production by the tumour of a substance with thyroid-stimulating properties.

CHEMOTHERAPY OF MALIGNANT DISEASE

Chemotherapy specific for malignant disease would exploit some property of malignant cells not shared with normal cells. No such property is yet known and chemotherapy still involves the use of agents known as cytotoxic drugs that damage growing cells. The great majority of these drugs interfere with one or more of the cellular processes concerned in the preparation for cell division, or with the mechanical process of mitosis when the newly formed chromosomes of the two daughter cells move apart. Because the process of cell division is common to normal and malignant growing cells, cytotoxic drugs are entirely non-specific in their effect on malignant disease, and cannot destroy malignant cells without also destroying normal growing cells. However, normal growing cells from different tissues vary in their susceptibility to cytotoxic drugs, though the reasons for this variation are largely unknown, and malignant growths also vary in their sensitivity to these drugs. In a few instances the malignant cells are just sensitive enough in relation to the sensitivity of the most vulnerable normal growing cells for worthwhile effects to be obtained by treatment. In addition, following destruction by cytotoxic drugs, the homeostatic responsiveness of surviving malignant cells is usually far less efficient than that of surviving normal cells, so that populations of the latter recover or even overshoot before the malignant-cell population has regrown to its former size. Without these two sources of selectivity chemotherapy would not be possible at all. Practical chemotherapy is a compromise in which the attempt to destroy the greatest possible number of tumour cells has to be balanced against the inevitability of causing damage to the normal proliferating cells that are essential to life.

The mitotic cycle includes the following phases after the preceding cell division. (a) The 'first gap' (G$_1$) of variable duration in which active synthetic processes have not been shown to occur. (b) The phase of deoxyribonucleic acid (DNA) synthesis (S) in which the cell synthesizes from simple organic molecules the purine and pyrimidine bases adenine, guanine, cytosine, and thymine, combines them with deoxyribose to form the corresponding deoxyribosides, and with phosphate to form the deoxyribotides adenylic acid, guanylic acid, cytidylic acid, and thymidylic acid. These deoxyribotides are assembled in an order determined by that present in the parent chain into the double helix of the new DNA chain. At the end of the S phase the total amount of DNA in the cell is exactly double the amount present at the beginning. The whole process requires a rapid uptake of the simple molecules from which the DNA is synthesized, an assembly of enzymes that control each step in the process, and a source of energy. (c) The 'second gap' (G$_2$) of variable duration before the final phase (d) of mitosis itself in which the DNA threads shorten by spiralization and become condensed into the two sets of compact daughter chromosomes that move apart along the mitotic spindle to form the nuclei of the two daughter cells, each of which receives an identical set of chromosomes. A population of cells continuously engaged in the process of division is said to be 'in cycle'.

Classes of cytotoxic drugs

The biological alkylating agents. These are synthetic compounds of great chemical diversity that have in common the ability to add alkyl groups to a wide range of electronegative groups under mild aqueous conditions that prevail in the living cell. The cytotoxic alkylating agents have two or more active groups, and it is thought that they destroy growing cells by cross-linking the adjacent guanine molecules on a strand of DNA or the molecules on adjacent strands, thus mechanically preventing the uncoiling of the strands and so halting the replication of the DNA. Although the alkylation of DNA may be the basic mechanism by which the cells are killed, there are many differences in the pharmacological properties of the alkylating agents in different chemical classes and in those of the members of each class. Some alkylating agents cause conspicuous breaks in chromosomes, while others at equivalent doses cause no visible chromosome damage but prevent cell division and lead to the production of polyploid giant cells.

The chloroethylamines mustine, chlorambucil, and melphalan dissociate electron transport and energy transformation processes at the inner mitochondrial membrane, thus uncoupling oxidative phosphorylation and leading to a rapid loss of ADP and ATP, and accumulation of AMP. Chlorambucil has been shown to cross link and so to polymerize transfer RNA thus reducing the efficiency of translation of messager RNA in protein synthesis.

In any one alkylating agent the alkylating groups become active as a result of hydrolysis, and the rate of hydrolysis, which depends on the structure of the whole molecule, determines a large part of the biological reactivity. In some, such as chlorambucil and melphalan, the rate of hydrolysis is entirely dependent on the properties of the molecule itself, while in others, such as busulphan, the rate is dependent on the availability of suitable groups that can be alkylated. Cyclophosphamide is an inactive compound from which alkylating compounds are liberated only by enzymic breakdown mainly in the liver.

Alkylating agents differ greatly in their physicochemical properties, and consequently in their biological effects. Highly reactive compounds like mustine hydrocholride are vesicants and can be administered only intravenously, intra-arterially, or into serous cavities. Because of its high reactivity, mustine is particularly valuable clinically when it is important to obtain a rapid response, for example to relieve toxaemia in generalized Hodgkin's disease, or superior vena cava obstruction from bronchial carcinoma. It is less useful for maintenance therapy. Milder agents like cyclophosphamide may also be administered intramuscularly or orally, while highly insoluble compounds like busulphan are suitable only for oral administration. They may be used in maintenance therapy for months or years and their dosage adjusted in relation to the response and to the side-effects.

The clinical usefulness of the alkylating agents is determined by their efficacy, their convenience in administration, their immediate and delayed toxicity, and by their side-effects. All are mutagenic in experimental animals but the risks in man are not well understood; they are also teratogenic and are to be avoided during the first 16 weeks of pregnancy. They are carcinogenic in experimental animals and probably in man also. Already long-term treatment of myelomatosis, breast and ovarian cancer with melphalan, cyclophosphamide, or chlorambucil is thought to have led to the development of acute myeloid leukaemia in about 3 per cent of patients. All are myelosuppressive, and in practice this property is the chief limiting factor in treatment because bone marrow aplasia resulting from overdosage is often irreversible. The effect on haemopoietic cells relative to that on other growing cells whether normal or malignant varies; it is so great in the case of busulphan, that the usefulness of this drug is practically limited to haemopoietic neoplasms; cyclophosphamide has relatively less effect on the platelet counts than other alkylating agents.

Because the antitumour effect of the alkylating agents is in most diseases small in relation to their myelosuppressive effect, it is usually necessary in order to obtain worthwhile benefit, to administer these drugs at an order of dosage close to the limits of bone marrow tolerance. Meticulous and continuous supervision is therefore essential if these drugs are to be used to the greatest advantage and with safety.

Alkylating agents damage lymphocytes, and unlike other cells, non-dividing small lymphocytes as well as those in the mitotic cycle are vulnerable. Alkylating agents are therefore immunosuppressive, especially when administered continuously for long periods.

Anorexia, nausea, and vomiting are common side-effects of alkylating agents that limit their acceptability to some patients. Most patients vomit within two hours of receiving mustine hydrochloride, but not before six hours of receiving cyclophosphamide or melphalan intravenously. Orally administered cyclophosphamide often causes anorexia, sometimes nausea, and less often vomiting. These effects are less often caused by melphalan and chlorambucil, but a patient intolerant to one of these three drugs may accept one of the other two without difficulty. At high dosage, melphalan and cyclophosphamide, administered intravenously, and cyclophosphamide but not melphalan, administered orally at low daily dosage for several months cause alopecia in women and sometimes in men. All alkylating agents administered for long periods cause amenorrhoea and hot flushes in women of child-bearing age. Busulphan often causes skin pigmentation not usually in the distribution characteristic of Addison's disease, but a minority of patients, treated continuously for several years, rarely for less than one year, develop a wasting syndrome resembling Addison's disease but lacking evidence of adrenal cortical hypofunction. There is evidence, however, of defective but reversible pituitary responsiveness as shown by the metyrapone test. Busulphan also causes the appearance of giant hyperchromatic polyploid cells in many tissues, and very rarely damages the pulmonary alveolar cells with consequent exudation of fibrin and subsequent intra-alveolar fibrosis. Cyclophosphamide has also caused the wasting syndrome and pulmonary fibrosis. Cyclophosphamide is activated in the liver, and some of its metabolites are excreted in the urine. One metabolite, acrolein, causes hyperaemia of the urothelium, microscopic haematuria, occasionally dysuria, frequency, and episodes of gross haematuria persisting long after treatment has been discontinued, associated with chronic inflammation, trabeculation, and contraction of the bladder lining. The toxic effect of acrolein on the urothelium can be prevented by the administration, at the same time as the cyclophosphamide, of mercaptoethanosulphonic acid.

After varying periods of time, malignant cells, but not normal cells become resistant to alkylating agents. Further treatment with the same or with any other alkylating agent still causes bone marrow depression and other toxic effects but no longer influences the tumour. It is believed that resistant cells acquire the property of excising cross-linked parts of the DNA chain and restoring functional continuity.

Melphalan enters cells by active transport requiring leucine and alanine as carriers. Entry into the cell can be prevented by specific inhibitors of these transport systems, and in some experimental models, resistance is a consequence of decrease in the rate of entry of the drug into the cells.

Some tumours such as ovarian adenocarcinoma, Hodgkin's disease, other lymphomas, and lymphoblastic leukaemia remain sensitive to other types of cytotoxic drugs when they have become resistant to alkylating agents, but when chronic myeloid leukaemia becomes resistant to busulphan, the most commonly used alkylating agent, treatment with other drugs of any class is only partially effective.

Occasional patients develop allergic reactions to alkylating agents, usually in the form of irritating generalized blotchy maculopapular rashes that become confluent and later desquamate. These reactions are specific for the drug concerned and treatment may be safely continued with another alkylating agent.

Highly reactive alkylating agents like mustine are taken out of the circulation within a few minutes of injection and are fixed by alkylation to the tissues. More slowly reacting compounds and those with a slower spontaneous hydrolysis rate are eliminated through the kidneys before they have exerted their maximum possible effect. Thus in uraemia, the toxic effect of agents like chlorambucil, cyclophosphamide, or melphalan is greatly increased.

Clinical uses. Alkylating agents, alone or in combination with other drugs or radiotherapy, are now indispensable in the treatment of Hodgkin's diesease, lymphocytic lymphoma (including Burkitt's lymphoma, chronic lymphocytic leukaemia, follicular lymphoma, Waldenström's macroglobulinaemia), plasma-cell tumours (myelomatosis and extramedullary plasmacytoma), chronic myeloid leukaemia and lymphoblastic leukaemia. They are less useful but have a place in the management of immunoblastic and lymphoblastic lymphoma, testicular seminoma, ovarian adenocarcinoma, mammary carcinoma, neuroblastoma, nephroblastoma, and embryonal sarcoma. Their value in bronchial carcinoma (other than oat-cell) and gastrointestinal carcinoma is doubtful. However, with the exception of Burkitt's lymphoma, in the early stage of which alkylating agents may effect a cure, and perhaps chronic myeloid leukaemia, in the treatment-responsive stage of which alkylating agents alone, especially busulphan, provide the best method of controlling the disease, the other conditions are best treated by a carefully prepared programme of management in which alkylating agents have a place alongside other methods of treatment. Examples illustrating the circumstances in which they are used are Hodgkin's disease and chronic lymphocytic leukaemia (see Section 19).

The antimetabolites. The antimetabolites are synthetically prepared structural analogues of naturally occurring substances that play essential parts in the metabolism of proliferating cells. The antimetabolites differ structurally from their normal counterparts only very slightly and compete with them by a variety of mechanisms, to interfere with their specific functions in the synthesis of the pyrimidine and purine bases, their assembly into nucleotides, or their incorporation into the DNA chain. These processes are blocked at different stages in the S phase of the cell cycle by different antimetabolites, and the affected cells fail to divide and often die, though it is not understood how this happens.

Antimetabolites like all other cytotoxic drugs affect normal as well as malignant poliferating cells, and the margin of safety is therefore narrow. This greatly limits their usefulness in practice. The three main types of antimetabolite are analogues of folic acid, of the purines, and of the pyrimidines. Tumour cells, but not normal proliferating cells eventually become resistant to antimetabolites, but because the several types of agent act by different mechanisms there is no cross-resistance between them. A tumour that has become resistant to a folic acid antagonist may still respond to a purine antagonist, or to a pyrimidine antagonist.

Folic-acid antagonists. Folic acid, which cannot be synthesized by mammalian cells, plays an essential part in the biosynthesis of the nucleic acids, and of several amino acids, and in amino acid metabolism. To become metabolically active it has to be reduced in two steps to tetrahydrofolic acid (FH_4) by a specific enzyme, dihydrofolate reductase (DFR). FH_4 transfers single carbon groups from suitable donors such as serine to the precursor molecules for the purine skeleton. Two transfers for the carbon atoms at positions 2 and 8 are required. FH_4 also donates a methyl group to deoxyuridylic acid (UMP, the deoxyribotide of uracil) thus converting it to deoxythymidilic acid (TMP, the deoxyribotide of thymine), while itself becoming oxidized to dihydrofolate (FH_2). To continue its metabolic activity FH_4 must be regenerated from FH_2 by the action of DFR. The conversion of UMP to TMP is the rate-determining step of DNA synthesis, and if it is blocked, DNA synthesis cannot proceed. Thymidine also reverses the block in the methylation of UMP to TMP but does not affect the block in purine biosynthesis. It can therefore be used to examine the relative importance of the two main effects of methotrexate (MTX) in inhibiting tumour growth and in causing toxicity to normal tissues. Thus, in experimental mice continuously infused with MTX, the conversion of UMP to TMP is blocked at plasma levels of about 10^{-8} mol/l, but levels of 10^{-7} mol/l are required to inhibit purine synthesis. However, it is the latter that appears to control the proliferation of the transplanted lymphoma L1210, because the survival of the mice can be prolonged by reversing the block to thymidine synthesis with thymidine infusions. As is so often the case, it is not known whether this mechanism is of general relevance or applies only to the specific circumstances of the experiments. Another factor that greatly influences the effects of MTX is the extent to which it forms polyglutamates. MTX polyglutamates accumulate in the liver and are slowly released over many months; MTX-5-glutamate is a powerful inhibitor of thymidylate synthetase.

MTX is the 4-amino-N^{10}-methyl-subsituted analogue of folic acid. It blocks the conversion of folic acid to FH$_4$ because it binds DFR irreversibly; its affinity for DFR is much greater than that of folic acid itself so that the blocking action of MTX cannot be reversed by treatment with folic acid at high dosage. It can, however, be bypassed by folinic acid (CF) which is 5-formyl FH$_4$, already fully reduced.

Experimental and human tumours originally sensitive to MTX may acquire resistance rapidly, but the normal proliferating tissues retain their original sensitivity. In some laboratory situations resistance to MTX has been shown to be due to the increased capacity of the tumour cells to synthesize DFR, as a result of gene reduplication, while in others resistance has been shown to be due to reduction in the permeability of the cells to MTX. Thus tumour cells become resistant in different ways and attempts to overcome resistance would require knowledge of the underlying mechanism in each case.

MTX is readily absorbed from the gut, and may be administered intravenously, intramuscularly, and intra-arterially. It does not pass the blood-brain barrier, except at high plasma concentrations and must be administered intrathecally in the treatment of meningeal leukaemia or lymphoma. Although it enters cells readily, it is also rapidly excreted unchanged by the kidneys, so that the effect of a given dose administered by intravenous injection is much less than that of the same dose administered by prolonged intravenous infusion. In uraemic subjects, however, an intravenous dose is cleared slowly from the blood stream and the toxicity greatly increased. The killing power of a single dose administered by injection against proliferating normal or malignant cells is limited not only by the excretion rate but also by the proportion of cells in the S phase in the population at risk. The enhancement of activity by prolonging the duration of an infusion is due to the trapping of an increasing number of cells in the population at risk, as they enter the sensitive phase of the cell cycle. Up to 48 hours the homeostatic triggering of the non-dividing (and therefore MTX-insensitive) bone-marrow stem cells seems not to occur, so that folinic acid administered for several days from the end of an infusion protects haemopoietic cells leaving the pool and entering mitosis. These cells are destroyed when infusions are prolonged beyond 48 hours and folinic acid cannot then reverse the damage.

The major immediate toxic effects of MTX are seen in the buccal mucosa, the gastrointestinal tract, and the bone marrow. Buccal ulceration is an early sign, and if administration is continued after the appearance of an ulcer, extensive confluent and extremely painful ulceration ensues. If the platelet count is falling rapidly the ulcers may be haemorrhagic. Intestinal ulceration may cause abdominal pain and diarrhoea. MTX causes megaloblastic change in the bone marrow, neutropenia and thrombocytopenia, and the blood films show macrocytosis and hypersegmentation of the neutrophils. These changes are seen also in the films of patients on long-term MTX therapy whose blood counts are substantially normal. Severe toxic effects include transient alopecia and confluent maculo-erythematous rashes mainly on the face and neck, and in the flexures, and the perineum; the rashes become purpuric before the adjacent normal skin if the platelet count falls.

Patients receiving continuous MTX therapy either on a daily or twice-weekly basis succumb more often than normal subjects to upper respiratory and pulmonary infections which tend to run a prolonged course; herpetic lesions on the lips may not heal until the MTX is withheld. Increase in the serum levels of alkaline phospha-

tase and transaminases sometimes occurs during prolonged intra-arterial infusions of methotrexate. Rarely, hepatic fibrosis has been recorded during long-term oral or intramuscular MTX therapy, and more rarely still fibrinous exudation into the pulmonary alveoli which has resolved when the administration was stopped. Fetal abnormalities and abortion were recorded when aminopterin, and anologue of MTX, was administered during early pregnancy, and are likely to be caused by MTX also.

Clinical uses. MTX, alone or in combination with other drugs is now indispensable in the treatment of lymphoblastic leukaemia, choriocarcinoma in women, Burkitt's lymphoma, and other lymphoma. It is sometimes effective when admininstered by prolonged intra-arterial infusion in the treatment of epidermoid carcinoma of the skin and mucosae of the head and neck. Its value is more difficult to assess in the treatment of mammary cancer and of soft tissue sarcomata because there is no way of predicting the small proportion of patients likely to respond well. An even smaller proportion of patients suffering from other forms of malignant disease have responded to MTX, and no general recommendations of practical value can be made. The use of methotrexate is illustrated in the treatment of lymphoblastic leukaemia (see Section 19) and choriocarcinoma.

Choriocarcinoma is so rare and its manifestations, complications, and response to treatment are so varied that useful experience in its management can be accumulated only in special centres, where cure rates exceeding 70 per cent are obtained. The two features that contribute to this high rate are, first, the relative sensitivity of the tumour cells to MTX and other cytotoxic drugs in relation to that of the normal proliferating cells, and secondly, the fact that choriocarcinoma cells secrete human chronionic gonadotrophin (HCG) the β-subunit of which can be detected in the serum and urine by radio-immunoassay: levels just above the background level of luteinizing hormone from which HCG cannot be distinguished, indicate the presence of about 10^6 tumour cells, far fewer than could be detected by any other method. A test of comparable sensitivity is not yet available for any other human tumour; for example, in myelomatosis, paraprotein at the lowest detectable concentration in the serum or urine represents between 10^9 and 10^{10} myeloma cells. The existence of the assay for HCG makes it possible to set the end point for treatment in choriocarcinoma far more accurately than is possible for other tumours where the duration of treatment is decided arbitrarily and empirically. In choriocarcinoma the rate of fall in the concentration of HCG can be plotted during treatment, the curve extrapolated beyond the level equivalent to 10^6 residual tumour cells, and the treatment continued for a period beyond the time when the curve suggests that there are no surviving tumour cells. The HCG assays are continued at regular intervals; rising concentrations indicate relapse long before the presence of tumour could be detected in any other way, and treatment can be resumed without delay.

Purine analogues. 6-Mercaptopurine (MP), and 2-amino-6-mercaptopurine (thioguanine) (TG) are the best known purine analogues. MP is inactive until it has been converted within the cell to its ribonucleotide by the enzyme hypoxanthine guanine ribosyl transferase (HGRT). This competes with the normal ribonucleotide, inosinic acid, by blocking its conversion to adenylosuccinic acid and to xanthylic acid which are precursors of adenine and guanine deoxyribotides. The excess inosinic acid, and perhaps MP itself, suppress the de novo synthesis of inosinic acid at an early stage by feed-back inhibition. MP also interferes with the synthesis of the hydrogen acceptor nicotine–adenine dinucleotide (NAD). There is some doubt as to which of these and other effects of MP and TG are important in their anti-tumour action, or even how affected cells die.

The final effect of MP is to suppress DNA synthesis. In vivo MP is powerfully myelosuppressive, and clinically this is its main toxic property. Damage to the gastrointestinal epithelium usually occurs only at higher dosage but hepatotoxicity may occur. Like the alkylating agents and MTX, mercaptopurine is teratogenic and immunosuppressive.

MP is usually administered orally and is well tolerated, only occasionally causing nausea and diarrhoea, and hardly ever mouth ulcers. It is metabolized to thiouric acid by the enzyme xanthine oxidase, and its activity is therefore prolonged if it is administered in combination with the xanthine-oxidase inhibitor allopurinol. Allowance should be made for this effect when allopurinol is administered to reduce the load of purine metabolites derived from breaking down tumour cells excreted as uric acid. MP occasionally causes jaundice with evidence of liver cell damage.

MP is an indispensable drug in the treatment of lymphoblastic leukaemia and the acute myeloid leukaemias, and it is also of some value in busulphan-resistant chronic myeloid leukaemia. Because of the danger of overdosage with MP if allopurinol is not administered simultaneously, it has become customary to replace MP by the much more expensive TG in the treatment of the acute and chronic myeloid leukaemias, although there is no good evidence that TG is more effective: in the treatment of lymphoblastic leukaemia MP is still the most widely used antipurine. Tumour cells acquire resistance to the thiopurines in various ways, involving the enzyme HGRT, or an increase in membrane-bound alkaline phosphatase derivatives.

Pyrimidine analogues. 5-Fluorouracil (FU) and cytosine arabinoside (Ara-C) are the best known pyrimidine analogues. FU is uracil in which the hydrogen atom at position 5 has been replaced by a fluorine atom. Like uracil it is converted within the cell to its deoxyribotide. The false deoxyribotide competes with the naturally occurring deoxyribotide for the enzyme thymidylate synthetase which converts the normal substrate to deoxythymidylic acid by transferring a methyl group from methylenetetrahydrofolate to position 5 of the uracil moiety. Methylation of the fluoro-substituted deoxyribotide does not occur. The inhibition of deoxythymidilic acid synthesis results in the failure of DNA synthesis and so in the death of proliferating cells. FU is thus specially toxic to the mucosa of the buccal cavity and of the gastrointestinal tract, to the bone marrow, to embryonic tissues, and it is also immunosuppressive. In clinical practice the pattern of toxicity differs from that resulting from methotrexate administration. Diarrhoea is usually the first sign of toxicity, followed by evidence of bone marrow depression with megaloblastosis, and by ulceration of the tongue more often than of the mucosa of the lips, palate, and cheeks characteristic of MTX toxicity.

FU is administered intravenously by injection or infusion, the latter being less toxic but also less effective. It is well tolerated. The margin between toxic damage and therapeutic efficacy is too narrow for FU, used alone, to be a useful drug in practice, but it is occasionally effective in mammary, urothelial, gastric and colorectal carcinoma and ovarian adenocarcinoma. It is more useful when administered in combination with drugs of other classes.

Cytosine arabinoside (Ara-C) is an analogue of cytidine in which the ribose moiety is replaced by its stereo-isomer D-arabinose. It is phosphorylated within the cell by the enzyme deoxycytidine kinase, and the triphosphate blocks DNA synthesis by inhibiting the DNA polymerases I and II. However its cytotoxic effect is attributed to its entry into RNA. *In vivo* it is powerfully myelosuppressive, causing severe megaloblastosis and marrow hypoplasia.

Ara-C may be administered intravenously by injection or by infusion, intramuscularly, subcutaneously, and intrathecally. It causes anorexia, nausea, and vomiting which, during the continuous infusions now often used in the treatment of acute myeloid leukaemia and kept going for as long as ten days, can lead to rapid weight loss and protein energy malnutrition: the symptoms subside two to three days after the end of the infusion. Resistance to Ara-C can occur by a variety of mechanisms, some involving the enzyme deoxycitidine kinase, the reduced activity of which diminishes the supply of the active Ara-C triphosphate, or an increase in the activity of the enzyme cytosine deaminase which inactivates the drug.

Ara-C is one of several drugs used, usually in combination, in the treatment of acute myeloid leukaemia, lymphoblastic leukaemia, and malignant lymphoma.

Cytotoxic antibiotics. In the course of testing bacterial filtrates for antibiotic activity, several were found to be powerfully cytotoxic and therefore unsuitable as antibiotics. However, some were found to cause the regression of transplanted tumours in laboratory animals, and the less toxic agents were submitted for clinical trial. The clinically useful antibiotics dactinomycin, mitomycin C, mithramycin, daunorubicin, and doxorubicin were isolated from filtrates of bacteria in the genus *Streptomyces*. These antibiotics are structurally varied and they differ in the mechanism whereby they inhibit mitosis, though the effect of all is to inhibit the synthesis of ribonucleic acid, and hence to block protein synthesis. Most are myelosuppressive and immunosuppressive.

Dactinomycin is the most active of a large group of actinomycins. It combines with DNA and blocks its template activity in directing the synthesis of messenger RNA. The cross-linking of adjacent strands of DNA interferes with their separation.

Dactinomycin is active when administered intravenously, but not when administered by mouth. Extravasation causes severe necrotizing effects. At therapeutic doses it is usually well tolerated, but may cause anorexia, nausea, vomiting, and diarrhoea. Overdosage causes profound bone marrow damage, destruction of mature lymphocytes, erythema, thinning and ulceration of the buccal mucosa and gastrointestinal tract, and intense erythema of the skin with exfoliation, thinning, and ulceration. Even at therapeutic dosage, previously irradiated areas of the skin become erythematous. In experimental systems dactinomycin is immunosuppressive, damages germinal epithelium, and is teratogenic and carcinogenic.

It is now an essential drug in the treatment of nephroblastoma (Wilms' tumour) in children, and is occasionally effective in other embryonal tumours and in testicular teratoma. Dactinomycin causes regression of metastatic deposits in recurrent nephroblastoma, but it is used to greatest advantage in conjunction with surgery and radiotherapy in the management of the localized primary disease. Injections are given before the affected kidney is excised, and for 18 months further courses are administered after the completion of a radical course of postoperative radiotherapy. The recurrence rate is much lower in patients so treated than when chemotherapy is omitted.

Daunorubicin and doxorubicin are the best known of the family of anthracycline antibiotics. Several recently isolated analogues said to be more effective and less toxic are undergoing preliminary trials. Three mechanisms of action are known: the flat molecules enter the cell nucleus and bind to the DNA but at different sites to those bound by dactinomycin; the molecules impair the activity of DNA polymerase, and so affect the elongation of the newly formed DNA chain. RNA synthesis is also impaired as a result of damage to the DNA template. The anthracyclines also interact with cell enzymes to generate free radicals which react with molecular oxygen to produce the superoxide radical which damages membrane lipids. Lastly, the anthracyclines bind directly to the cytoskeletal protein spectrin and to cardiolipin with resulting disturbance of ion transport.

The anthracyclines are toxic to the bone marrow, but higher doses damage the gastrointestinal mucosa, and cause lymphoid atrophy and alopecia. Long-term administration causes irreversible myocardial toxicity which imposes an upper limit to the total dosage. Daunorubicin and doxorubicin are too myelotoxic for use as single agents, but both are useful in combination with other drugs in the treatment of the acute leukaemias, and doxorubicin is active in the malignant lymphomas, embryonal sarcomas, and many 'solid' tumours. Extravasation is painful and causes severe tissue necrosis. There is no cross-resistance between daunorubicin and any of the other antileukaemic agents, and its inclusion with other agents in treatment programmes would be expected to reduce further the likelihood of resistance emerging. Regimens of treatment suitable for routine use are still being developed (see Section 19).

Doxorubicin and daunorubicin illustrate how minor molecular changes can have profound biological effects. Doxorubicin differs from daunorubicin only in the substitution of a hydrogen atom in a methyl component of a side chain by a hydroxy group, yet it has activity against a far wider range of tumours than daunorubicin. The minor chemical change is associated with a major change in the steric configuration of the molecule. The common form of resistance to the anthracyclines is associated with increased efflux of the drugs, an energy-dependent process, from the cells.

Bleomycin is a glycopeptide which inhibits DNA synthesis. It causes drying, thickening, and discoloration of the skin over the extensor surfaces of joints; it also causes diffuse lung damage, but is not myelotoxic. It has some activity in Hodgkin's disease and in squamous-cell carcinoma of the skin, but is mainly used in combination with other drugs.

The plant alkaloids. The vinca alkaloids vinblastine (VLB), vincristine (VR), and the recently introduced vindesine, extracted from the plant *Catharanthus roseus*, have a variety of toxic effects other than those on dividing cells. In spite of their close structural similarity VLB and VCR differ strikingly in their toxic properties. VCR damages the microtubular fibrils in the axons of peripheral nerves, first manifest in the longest fibres with resulting depression and loss of the ankle reflexes, paraesthesiae in the toes, and later weakness of the dorsiflexors and evertors of the foot. These effects occur with VLB only after prolonged treatment or when high doses are used. VCR almost always causes some degree of neuropathy at commonly used doses that do not depress the bone marrow. VCR, but not VLB, frequently causes severe constipation and occasionally prolonged ileus, thought to result from an effect on the autonomic plexuses. The neurological effects of the vinca alkaloids as well as their effects on mitosis depend on their high affinity for tubulin. The binding sites are not the same as those occupied by colchicine.

VCR, but not VLB, occasionally causes pain in the jaw, teeth, and gums, which begins one to two days after an injection and passes off within three days. Both VLB and VCR cause tissue necrosis if leakage outside a vein occurs. Both are immunosuppressive.

Vinblastine is used, usually in combination with other drugs, in the management of generalized Hodgkin's disease.

Vincristine is used in the treatment of Hodgkin's disease, lymphoblastic leukaemia, and the non-Hodgkin's lymphomas. It is also most effective when administered in combination with other drugs.

Miscellaneous drugs

Dibromomannitol (DBM) is one of a series of halogenated sugars with cytotoxic properties. It is thought to act as an alkylating agent. It is administered orally but often causes anorexia, nausea, and vomiting. It is a powerful myelotoxic agent, and is effective in the treatment of chronic myeloid leukaemia, sometimes in busulphan-resistant patients.

Hydroxyurea, structurally the simplest cytotoxic drug, inhibits the reduction of the ribonucleotides to the corresponding deoxyribonucleotides and so interferes with DNA synthesis. Its effect, though powerful, is short-lived. It is myelotoxic and useful in the management of the chronic myeloid leukaemias. The leucocyte count often rises steeply when administration is stopped.

Procarbazine, a methylhydrazine derivative, whose mode of action is unknown, is an indispensable drug in the management of generalized Hodgkin's disease. It is effective in patients who have become resistant to alkylating agents and the vinca alkaloids. It is a powerful myelotoxic drug, and frequently causes anorexia, nausea, and vomiting. Procarbazine is administered in short courses in combination with vincristine or vinblastine, chlorambucil, cyclophosphamide or mustine, and prednisolone.

L-Asparaginase represents an entirely different class of chemotherapeutic agent from all others. The L-asparaginases are proteins with enzyme activity, splitting an amino group from the amino acid L-asparagine which becomes converted to aspartic acid. The enzymes are produced by several birds, one order of mammals (*Caviidae*), and by several genera of bacteria. The detailed structures of the enzymes vary according to their source, and some of those of bacterial origin have glutaminase activity, believed to reside in the asparaginase molecule itself. The preparations in clinical use are derived from *Escherichia coli*, and from a strain of *Erwinia caratovora*, a plant pathogen. The antitumour activity of L-asparaginase, first demonstrated in murine leukaemia, was attributed to the destruction of the body pool of asparagine required by the tumour cells and which they were unable to synthesize. The lack of toxicity was explained by the capacity of all the normal cells to synthesize asparagine: thus they were independent of an external supply.

L-Asparaginase will induce temporary remissions in lymphoblastic leukaemia but continuous treatment fails to maintain remission. It is now regarded as an important component of remission-induction therapy, being administered in conjunction with vincristine and prednisolone.

Asparaginase preparations, being proteins, are antigenic, and allergic reactions can be troublesome. Other side-effects are fever, anorexia, and nausea. The synthesis of at least two serum proteins, fibrinogen and albumin, is impaired during therapy. Serum fibrinogen levels may fall by 90 per cent during the first week of treatment, but the level subsequently returns to normal although the treatment is continued; the liver cells normally obtain part of their asparagine from an external source and require time to repace the loss by increasing their own synthetic activity. The serum albumin levels usually fall by less than 50 per cent. The haemoglobin concentration of anaemic patients who remit during asparaginase therapy often rises less rapidly than would be expected, and this may indicate that erythroblasts depend in part on externally derived asparagine for haemoglobin synthesis. Asparaginase is immunosuppressive and it prevents the regeneration of neutrophils when administered in combination with myelotoxic drugs.

Interferons. These are a group of glycoproteins with molecular weights of the order of 20 000 dalton. Type I interferons are produced by B lymphocytes in response to viral infections: *in vitro*, stimulation by *Corynebacterium parvum*, *Brucella* species, bacterial lipopolysaccharides, and tilorone also induces interferon production. Type II interferons, which bind to different receptors on the cell membrane, are produced by T lymphocytes in response to stimulation by mitogens such as phytohaemagglutinin, concanavalin A, by antigens such as BCG or its PPD, by anti-lymphocyte serum, and by allogeneic lymphocytes in the mixed-lymphocyte reaction. The interferons induce changes in cells that render them less susceptible to viral infection, and they also retard the growth of certain animal tumours and several cell lines established from human tumours. Type II interferons appear to be more active against tumours than type I interferons. The action of interferons is largely species specific, and clinical trials so far have been confined to type I interferons obtained from human blood donor leucocytes, fibroblasts, or a lymphoblastoid-cell line derived from a Burkitt lymphoma. The extraction and processing are complex, the yields small and the supplies limited; little information is available yet on the clinical value of the very impure preparations of interferon so far used in human malignant disease. The recent development of methods for obtaining interferons by recombitent DNA technology may overcome some of these problems.

The interferons arrest cell division in sensitive cells but the mechanism is unknown and may be independent of the antiviral effect. Preliminary reports suggest that some beneficial effects have been observed in osteogenic sarcoma, myelomatosis, Hodgkin's disease, non-Hodgkin's lymphoma, malignant melanoma, breast cancer, and lymphoblastic leukaemia, but the extent and frequency of the benefit and the place of interferon in the management of these conditions remain to be worked out.

Deoxycoformycin is a specific antagonist of the enzyme cytosine deaminase. In some cases of thymic acute lymphoblastic leukaemia, the leukaemia cells have a high content of cytosine deaminase. Preliminary trials in relapsed thy-ALL resistant to other agents have shown dramatic, though shortlived, responses to deoxycoformycin when the leukaemia-cell content of cytosine deaminase was high. Deoxycoformycin may, after further study, be incorporated into the standard early treatment for thy-ALL in the same way as L-asparaginase is now used in the initial treatment of common-ALL.

cis-Diamminodichloroplatinum (cis-platinum), is the best known of a series of platinum complexes with growth inhibitory properties. It binds to DNA and appears to act as an alkylating agent with unusual properties. Its limiting toxicity is renal, and special precautions are necessary to reduce this. It also causes nausea and vomiting, tinnitus, and loss of hearing as well as other toxic effects. In spite of these disadvantages, it has an established place, in combination with other drugs, in the management of testicular teratoma and ovarian cancer, and its possible value in the treatment of cancer of the bladder, prostate, and of 'head-and-neck' cancers is being assessed.

Hexamethylmelamine is structurally but not functionally similar to the triazine alkylating agents: its mechanism of action is not known. It has some effect in cancer of the lung, ovary, cervix, breast, and colon, but its role in the management of these conditions remains to be established.

Principles of chemotherapy

From the previous section, it will be appreciated that the majority of cytotoxic drugs are effective only in a limited range of conditions, that their antitumour activity depends on the same properties that render them harmful to normal growing cells, and that any selectivity they possess against malignant tissues depends on the same type of variation in growth characteristics that is found in normal growing tissues. Therapeutic efficacy is almost always obtained only at the cost of considerable toxicity, and because of this it is never justified to begin chemotherapy without careful consideration of the maximum benefit likely to be obtained in relation to the toxic effects certain to be produced. The aims of treatment, and therefore its strategy, vary according to the disease. The prospect of eradicating the tumour, or at least of inducing prolonged remissions, justifies the production of toxic effects, even when the treatment has to continue for long periods (see below) during most of which the patient feels well. However, in conditions for which chemotherapy is merely palliative, it is not justified to incur a burden of toxic effects out of proportion to the benefits conferred. On the other hand chemotherapy must be administered at doses likely to be effective. There is no justification for using cytotoxic drugs at low doses as placebos as is done all too frequently. This type of treatment may cause cumulative toxicity and yet be totally ineffective in its antitumour activity.

The strategy of clinical chemotherapy is based on the necessity for achieving a balance between maximal destruction of the tumour cells and an acceptable burden of toxic effects. Two assumptions, based on experimental work and not fully established in human malignant disease, underlie the practice of chemotherapy. The first is that tumour-cell growth, being largely independent of the homeostatic control that regulates the growth of normal cells, proceeds exponentially, and the second is that at a given dose, some chemotherapeutic agents destroy the same proportion of cells whatever the size of the population at risk. Thus the same dose that

reduces a population of 10 million cells to 1 million cells would be required to reduce a population of 10 cells to 1 cell.

At the present time the practice of chemotherapy is undergoing rapid expansion, and attempts at radical therapy are being made in many conditions which would, only a few years ago, have been considered incurable. It is already clear that a high proportion of patients suffering from choriocarcinoma and Burkitt's lymphoma can be cured by intensive chemotherapy alone. It is possible that cure is being achieved in some cases of state IV Hodgkin's disease and of lymphoblastic leukaemia. Because chemotherapy is thought to have the best chance of eradicating a tumour when the total mass of tumour cells is small, intensive therapy is now being added to surgery and radiotherapy in several tumours of childhood in which no detectable metastases are present following the excision of an apparently localized tumour and the irradiation of its bed. The presence of disseminated micrometastases at the time of operation is inferred because of the high rate of early generalized recurrence following excision and radiotherapy alone, and this justifies the policy of adding to the treatment programmes intensive chemotherapy already known to cause regressions in overt disease. For a few years long recurrence-free intervals were being recorded for nephroblastoma, embryonal rhabdomysarcoma, Ewing's tumour, and osteogenic sarcoma. Courses of vincristine, dactinomycin, doxorubicin, methotrexate, and cyclophosphamide in varying combinations for periods for up to 18 months were used. The same principle was extended to some of the commoner cancers of adults, especially breast cancer in which the long-term survival rate is very low when spread to the axillary nodes has already occurred. At present, the practice of chemotherapy is in a state of transition, in respect to its aims, the range of conditions for which a radical approach is envisaged, and the tactics of combining different drugs in ways likely to be as effective and innocuous as possible. In the circumstances a list of agents and the conditions for which they were formerly used individually is not considered to be helpful and is omitted from this edition of this Textbook.

All the drug combinations used in the conditions mentioned, as well as in others, were arrived at empirically, with little possibility of assessing precisely the complex interactions between the drugs in respect of additive, synergistic, or antagonistic effects on the tumour and the toxic effect on different normal tissues. The general tendency has been to increase the overall intensity of therapy both by increasing the dosage of individual drugs and by adding more drugs. There is, however, always the danger that any increase in antitumour effect may be offset by unacceptable toxicity. It has, for example, been found that the addition of two more drugs to the basic mercaptopurine/methotrexate combination used in the long-term management of acute lymphoblastic leukaemia in children added nothing to the proportion of long-term survivors because of the increased death rate resulting from the increased toxicity of the more intensive treatment while, in addition, the relapse rate after treatment was ended was higher. For the same reason, the recent enthusiasm for intensive adjuvant chemotherapy for osteogenic sarcoma is now waning. On the other hand, the importance of adequate chemotherapy in the initial treatment of acute lymphoblastic leukaemia was formerly underestimated, and it is now thought that the long-term prospects are influenced by the character of the initial treatment: it is usual now to administer a third agent, L-asparaginase or an anthracycline in conjunction with the well-established combination of vincristine and prednisolone; the remission rate is no higher, but the percentage of cures may be.

In some circumstances tumour cells almost certainly do grow exponentially, and are more likely to do so when they grow in a free-living state in optimal conditions for the inflow of oxygen and nutrients and the removal of metabolites. Such conditions apply more closely to undifferentiated leukaemic cells growing in the bone marrow than to a 'solid' tumour, where the vascularization is precarious, and overcrowding leads to massive necrosis. Even in undifferentiated leukaemic-cell populations, however, there is evidence that only a proportion of the cells are 'in cycle' and growing exponentially. Even if the exponentially growing cells are considered as a separate sub-population, the total increase in that sub-population will proceed exponentially only if all the daughter cells in each generation live to divide again. There is evidence that a variable proportion of the actively proliferating cells in each generation die, so that the doubling time of the sub-population is longer than the generation time of its cells. The doubling time of the whole population (that is the sum of the exponentially dividing sub-population and the resting cells) is longer still. In undifferentiated free-living tumour-cell populations therefore, the doubling time is determined by the relative proportions of resting cells and dividing cells, the death-rate in the dividing-cell population, by the generation time of the dividing cells, and by the survival curve of the resting-cell population.

Measurements in experimental and human tumours (notably myelomatosis) have shown that the retardation of the exponential growth-rate increases as the tumour-cell population increases, and the extent of the retardation can be expressed by the mathematical formula of Gompertz. In solid tumours with cell maturation the relatively simple condition just described is complicated by the following features: first, the stromal and vascular components account for a variable and often substantial proportion of the tumour mass; secondly, some of the component cells undergo maturation to cells with a long life span during which they may elaborate a specific product, for example keratin or mucin, that adds materially to the bulk of the tumour. Regional necrosis resulting from vascular insufficiency adds to the non-proliferating part of the tumour. Thus a large tumour may increase in size from factors other than cell division, and the proportion of clonogenic cells proliferating exponentially may be relatively small. The doubling time of the tumour mass will be very long in relation to the generation time of the proliferating tumour cells. Nevertheless, the whole tumour may increase in size exponentially, as shown for example in serial radiological measurements of discrete cannonball metastases in lung parenchyma.

The hypothesis of the exponential cell-killing effect of cytotoxic drugs is important because, in theory, it points to the possibility of killing every cell in a given population. Thus, if a course of treatment destroys 90 per cent of tumour cells, then with an initial population of 10^9 cells, a series of nine similar courses would reduce the population to a single cell, and there would be a 90 per cent chance that a tenth course would destroy that cell. The hypothesis has been successfully applied to several experimental tumours, and its success led to attempts to eradicate human lymphoblastic leukaemia by repeated courses of intensive chemotherapy. It seems likely, however, that for some drugs, the survival curves for tumour-cell population are hyperbolic rather than exponential; the percentage of cells killed by a given dose of drug falls increasingly rapidly as the cell population declines.

In spite of the qualifications just summarized, the exponential growth of tumours and the exponential cell-killing effect of cytotoxic drugs are probably the most accurate available descriptions on which to plan clinical chemotherapy, and are accepted in the following account.

It should be emphasized that the lack of a differential killing effect on the tumour cells and their normal counterparts does not preclude the possibility of selective total-cell kill of the tumour-cell population provided that the normal cells and the tumour cells differ in their capacity to respond to the physiological homeostatic influences that lead residual cells to proliferate when their population has been largely depleted. If normal cells respond briskly, while tumour cells respond sluggishly, it should be possible by the appropriate spacing of courses of treatment to secure progressive diminution in the tumour-cell population while ensuring the survival of the normal cells. In practice, the limiting toxicity of cytotoxic chemotherapy is often for a tissue other than the one from which the tumour has arisen. Thus the destruction of certain 'solid' tumours may require treatment at a higher dosage than the bone marrow could tolerate; in this circumstance it may be possible to administer the required treatment by first removing enough bone marrow to ensure subsequent regeneration, the marrow being returned to the patient after an interval following the treatment long enough for the concentration of active drug remaining in the body to have declined below levels that would damage the returned haemopoietic cells. This approach is not possible if the marrow is known to contain, or is suspected of containing, metastatic tumour cells, though in the future methods may be developed for 'sterilizing' the marrow before it is returned to the patient.

Extent of control of tumour growth achieved by different methods of using cytotoxic drugs

Figures 1 and 2 illustrate the effect on the growth of a population of tumour cells of chemotherapy administered by two methods in various clinical circumstances, at different time intervals. The first (Fig. 1, curves 2 and 4; Fig. 2, curves 1, 2, and 3) represents courses of treatment with one drug, or several drugs in combination, at sufficiently high dosage to destroy a substantial fraction of the tumour, assumed to be the same fraction in every course of treatment; the second (Fig. 1, curves 1a and 1b) represents continuous chemotherapy with one drug or several drugs in combination, at low dosage designed for maintenance therapy. In Fig. 1, curves 1 and 1a, the dosage is such that the number of tumour cells destroyed is exactly balanced by the number of new cells produced, resulting in a steady state, whereas in curve 1b, the dosage is the same, but some of the tumour cells have become resistant to the treatment and are increasing in number more rapidly than the sensitive cells which are still being destroyed at the same rate as they are produced; thus the continuous treatment previously effective in maintaining a steady state is no longer effective.

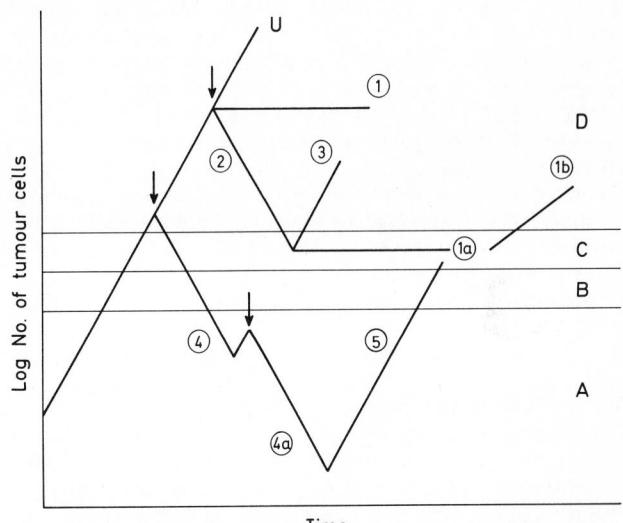

Fig. 1   The effect of chemotherapy on the size of a tumour-cell population. The clinical condition is shown in relation to the number of tumour cells.

Sections A, B, and C: the patient has no symptoms; A, no evidence of the presence of tumour; B, the presence of tumour is shown by special laboratory tests only; C, there is radiological or clinical evidence of disease. Section D: the patient has symptoms. The tumour growth is assumed to be exponential (U). Three courses of chemotherapy (2, 4, 4a) at the same dosage destroy the same proportion of tumour cells whatever the total number of cells when the treatment is begun (indicated by arrows). In 2, the symptoms are relieved, but clinical or radiological evidence of disease persists; in 4, symptoms are relieved, all clinical and laboratory evidence of the presence of tumour disappears; in 4a, the treatment is given to an apparently healthy patient. After the effect of the treatment has worn off, the tumour grows at the same rate as before; in 3, symptoms return rapidly; after 4, the further growth is arrested by course 4a; and in 5, the return of symptoms is delayed. Maintenance therapy at low dosage that sustains a steady state does not relieve symptoms in 1, and does not cause any tumour regression in 1a; maintenance therapy is continued in 1b, but the tumour has become resistant to the treatment.

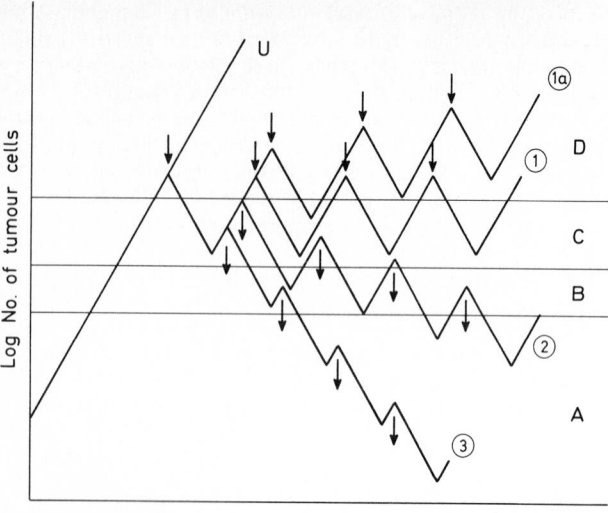

Fig. 2   The effect of varying the interval between courses of treatment at the same dosage on the size of a tumour-cell population. Letter symbols as in Fig. 1. In 1, the interval between courses permits the return of symptoms, but is short enough to maintain an essentially steady state. In 1a, the intervals are rather longer, and after the second course the treatment fails to relieve symptoms. In 2, the second course is begun before the return of symptoms, and the fifth is begun when there are no clinical or radiological signs of the disease, although the presence of tumour is revealed by special tests. In 3, the intervals between courses are short enough to permit considerable reduction in the size of the tumour-cell population.

Both Figs. 1 and 2 are divided into 4 sections, A, B, C, and D, which relate the clinical effects of the tumour to the total number of cells. Thus in section A the number of tumour cells is too small to be detected by any known means; in section B their presence can be detected by laboratory methods (for example, human chorionic gonadotrophin assay in choriocarcinoma, serum acid phosphatase assay in prostatic carcinoma, paraprotein assay in myelomatosis) but not by clinical or radiological means; in section C, the tumour is large enough to give rise to physical signs or radiological abnormalities, but the patient has no symptoms; in section D, the patient has symptoms.

This subdivision is admittedly artificial and the extent to which it can be applied to different forms of malignant disease varies greatly, but it is useful to illustrate the principles of chemotherapy.

Maintenance therapy. Figure 1 (curve 1a) shows that continuous therapy at low dosage that prevents the tumour from growing but does not reduce its size, provides excellent symptomatic control when applied to a tumour that has been already reduced by more aggressive treatment (curve 2) below the size at which it causes symptoms. However, the same treatment is useless if administered when the tumour has advanced into section D and is giving rise to symptoms (curve 1). No matter how long the treatment is continued, the total number of tumour cells will not decrease and the symptoms will persist. At best, the treatment will prevent the situation deteriorating. The use of busulphan at low daily dosage for maintenance in chronic granulocytic leukaemia after an initial course at higher dosage illustrates the practical application of curves 2 and 1a, while the onset of busulphan-resistance is illustrated by curve 1b.

Maintenance therapy is only practicable in conditions that respond to drugs which can be safely administered for long periods without incurring insupportable side-effects, and which do not rapidly engender resistance.

Single-course therapy. A single course of treatment at high dosage given to a patient in an advanced state of relapse with symptoms may completely relieve the symptoms (Fig. 1, curve 2) but at

the end of the course, if maintenance therapy is not given, the tumour will resume its growth at the same rate (U) as before, and in a short time the symptoms will return (curve 3). The same course of treatment administered at an earlier stage of relapse will produce a better effect in that all evidence of active disease will disappear (curve 4) and the time before symptoms return will be much longer than in situation 2. The length of remission will be still further increased if a second similar course is administered as soon as possible after the first (curve 4a), but the possibility of doing so will depend on the toxic effects brought about and the speed of recovery. It will be noted that treatment 4a is given to a patient who has no evidence of active disease and who considers himself to be well. Until recently physicians have been reluctant to administer further treatment in these circumstances, because they were unwilling to inflict distressing and potentially dangerous toxic injury to fit patients whom they knew they could not cure, or were most unlikely to cure. However, attitudes have changed since it has been demonstrated beyond doubt that carefully planned intensive therapy was to the patients' long-term advantage in particular forms of malignant disease.

Once the desirability of attempting more than relief of symptoms is accepted, the logical inference is to continue treatment as far beyond the limit shown in Fig. 1, curve 4a, as the patient will tolerate. In current practice the possibility of doing so is severely limited by the toxicity of the available drugs, which limits the amounts that can be administered and determines the intervals at which courses of treatment can be repeated. Figure 2 illustrates the consequences of varying the interval between courses of treatment.

Curve 1 illustrates the outcome when four courses of treatment are administered, each course being started when the patient complained of symptoms. The symptoms are successfully relieved by each course, but clinical or radiological evidence of disease persists throughout, and the condition of the patient at the end of the period is substantially the same as at the beginning. If the same series of four courses were begun when the disease was at a less advanced stage (for example, in section C of Fig. 2), and the intervals between the courses were the same, the disease would be controlled to the extent that the patient would be free of symptoms throughout the period, but as before his overall condition would not have improved.

If a series of courses designed to relieve symptoms on the lines of curve 1 is planned, but symptoms recur before the patient has fully recovered from the toxic effects of the first course there will be no possibility of controlling the disease with this form of treatment, because only two alternatives are available. Either treatment must be deferred until the patient has recovered from the toxic effects (curve 1a), or the dosage used in each course must be reduced. The effect will be the same, in that the disease will continue to advance and the treatment will no longer relieve the symptoms. On the other hand, courses of treatment that can be repeated at frequent intervals without incurring insupportable toxicity will lead to progressive reduction in the total number of tumour cells (Fig. 2, curves 2 and 3) and so will lengthen the duration of remission. Curve 3 shows that the most satisfactory result follows when successive courses are administered at very short intervals. The symptoms are relieved after the first course, all clinical and radiological evidence of disease disappears after the second, while after the third evidence of activity is not obtainable at all. In choriocarcinoma, the line dividing section A from section B could be drawn lower in the figure, because the assay of HCG in the urine permits the recognition of a smaller number of tumour cells in the body (about 10^6) than can yet be achieved with any other tumour, and this assay is used to determine the end-point of treatment. No comparable assay of minimal tumour activity is available for any other human malignant disease and the end-point has to be determined empirically by clinical trials. In lymphoblastic leukaemia, for example, the frequency of long-term remission is higher when treatment is ended only after $2\frac{1}{2}$–3 years than when it is discontinued earlier.

Advantages of multiple-drug therapy. The use of several drugs in sequence or in various combinations is now common practice and is justified by the following considerations: first, the need to reduce the likelihood of the development of resistance; secondly, the need to reduce the severity of toxic effects; thirdly, the hope of increasing the therapeutic effect by synergism, or by the use of drugs acting independently by different mechanisms and affecting tumour cells at different stages in the cell cycle.

Sequential therapy was an inevitable result of the introduction of new drugs. For ethical reasons, new drugs were first given only to patients who had become resistant to the drugs already available, and as more new drugs were found to be effective, patients were treated by using each drug in turn, usually in the order in which they were introduced, the change from one to another being determined by the onset of resistance, or poor tolerance.

The acquisition of resistance, though highly characteristic of malignant cells, is not confined to them. Thus patients with idiopathic cold haemagglutinin disease become resistant to chlorambucil, and those with systemic lupus erythematosus become resistant to immunosuppressive drugs. The nature of resistance of cytotoxic drugs by cells that were formerly sensitive is unknown and is unlikely to be the same in all cases. In some cases resistance may result from a change in the growth characteristics of the tumour-cell population and not from a specific biochemical change. There are experimental systems in which resistance may be shown to arise by a genetic change akin to mutation in a very small number of tumour cells in a large population. The change is stable, heritable, and confers a selective advantage on the cells bearing it, enabling them to replace the original population. The initial change is considered to arise by chance and to be a rare event. If the population were exposed to two drugs simultaneously, a mutant cell resistant to one drug would be as likely to be killed by the other as sensitive cells, and the same reasoning would apply to a mutant cell resistant to the second drug. Since mutation is always a rare event the chance of a single cell bearing two independent mutations conferring resistance to both drugs would be infinitesimally small: it would be the reciprocal of the product of the frequency of each mutation. The frequency of resistant mutants arising would be correspondingly lower if more than two drugs were administered simultaneously.

The toxic effects that accompany an effective course of treatment with any particular drug may be insupportable. If two drugs of equal efficacy, but acting independently and having different limiting toxic effects, are each administered at one half of the dosage necessary to obtain the desired effect, their therapeutic actions will summate, but their specific toxic effects will be one half of those resulting from the full dose, if the ratio of the toxic effect and the therapeutic action is the same at all dose levels. A further reduction in toxicity would result if more drugs were added.

Synergism would be expected if two drugs having a comparable antitumour effect acted by unrelated mechanisms. Thus a drug acting only on cells actively synthesizing DNA (S-phase cells) would affect the proliferating cells in a tumour only if its administration were continued long enough to permit all those cells to enter the S phase, but those tumour cells that were out of cycle during the period of exposure would not be affected at all. If a second drug, active also against resting cells, were administered simultaneously, the proportion of susceptible cells in the tumour would be correspondingly greater than if an equivalent dose of the S-phase-active drug had been administered instead. Unfortunately, little is known about the basic mechanisms of action of most of the available drugs, and the combinations that have proved useful in practice have largely been chosen empirically and the basis of selection has depended more on the desire to minimize toxicity than on an established rationale of differential mechanism of action.

The possibility must be considered also that certain drug combinations deemed suitable from the standpoint of tolerance, might be antagonistic. Thus a drug that reduced the proportion of cells entering the S phase would limit the efficacy of a drug that acts only on cells in the S phase. Without doubt, improvements in multiple drug therapy will depend on a better understanding of the mechanisms of action of the drugs. Attempts, so far unsuccessful, at deliberately altering the growth characteristics of tumour populations so as to render them more susceptible to cytotoxic drugs have been made. Thus drugs that inhibit entry into the S phase might be expected to lead to an accumulation of cells ready to synthesize DNA when the effect wore off. S-phase-active drugs could then be expected to destroy a higher proportion of cells than in an unsynchronized population.

Pharmacokinetics. The aim of cytotoxic chemotherapy is to ensure that every cell of a tumour-cell population is exposed to the lethal drug at a concentration sufficient to kill it if the duration of exposure is adequate. Until recently it has not been possible to determine accurately by conventional pharmacological methods even the basic facts concerning the fate in the body of cytotoxic drugs administered by different routes, at different doses and frequencies. In the absence of this information chemotherapy schedules have been devised empirically, and it is probable that many drugs are not being used in the best possible way to secure effective anti-tumour action and minimal toxicity. For example a rapidly metabolized or excreted drug that acts on cells only during the DNA-synthetic phase (S) of the cell cycle would be expected to act optimally if administered by continuous infusion, because there is probably a continuing entry of small numbers of cells into S phase: continuous exposure to the drug at the optimal concentration would ensure that each cell is affected as it enters S phase, whereas a high proportion would pass through S unscathed and so complete their mitosis if the drug were administered intermittently. Another S-phase-active drug with slightly different pharmacological properties would be equally effective administered intermittently if the doses and intervals between doses were adjusted to ensure that every cell entering S phase would be exposed to damaging concentrations of the drug. Sensitive methods, mostly involving radioimmunoassay, are now being developed for assaying the concentrations of the most commonly used cytotoxic drugs and their metabolites in body fluids and urine, and this will permit a critical review of currently used drug schedules. It is already known, for example, that constant blood levels of the S-phase-active drug cytosine arabinoside can be maintained by continuous intravenous infusion but not by 12-hourly subcutaneous injection as frequently used. The efficiency of absorption of orally administered drugs is often variable: it has now been shown that a proportion of children taking methotrexate by mouth each week absorb the drug much more slowly than the remainder, and that the relapse rate in the slow absorbers is higher. These examples suffice to illustrate the potential importance of accurate pharmacokinetic investigations in accounting for some at least of the variability in response to apparently identical treatments, and in improving the efficiency of existing drug schedules.

Clinical trials. The experience of the past two decades at the major cancer-treatment centres has shown that for each type of malignant disease, the treatment policy must be carefully planned on a long-term basis and in the greatest detail, incorporating appropriate contributions from surgery, radiotherapy, chemotherapy, and endocrine therapy. In spite of considerable improvements in the results in some conditions, the overall results, especially in the most common forms of cancer, are poor. The incentive for the closest integrative effort internationally, and between the therapists in the several disciplines concerned, is therefore very strong, and the machinery now exists for carrying out and evaluating clinical trials in such a way that encouraging results can be readily acted upon in subsequent trials. In malignant disease the prospects for survival depend on many factors, including the histological or cytological features, sex and age of the patient, and the stage of advancement of the disease. In well-organized trials these features, and others appropriate to particular conditions are carefully recorded for each patient, and every detail of the highly complex treatment programmes, which may continue for several years, is specified. Potential improvements suggested by small-scale trials are tested by the method of random allocation, whereby a series of patients are allocated at random to receive either the standard regiment of treatment considered at the time to be the best available, or the potentially superior treatment. Powerful methods of statistical analysis are now available which permit the detection of significant variations between the treatments and of the effect of different characteristics of the patients and the features of their disease on the outcome. It is possible, too, to ask several different questions in a single trial, each involving a separate process of randomization. For example, in the current (eighth) Medical Research Council trial in acute myeloid leukaemia, three questions are asked: first, whether patients who enter remission fare better if they receive intensive 'consolidation' therapy for a short (two courses) or long (six courses) period; secondly, whether further intensive therapy after maintenance therapy for one year is beneficial; and thirdly, whether 'prophylactic' intrathecal chemotherapy is beneficial. The exact procedure at every stage of the treatment in this and all similar trials is specified. It has become clear that the discipline required in the conduct of these trials has had a remarkable effect in raising the standards of diagnosis, investigative procedure, and management in all forms of malignant disease; it has already improved the general standard of care, and provides an effective framework within which future improvements can be developed.

Chemotherapy records. The expectation of life in several forms of advanced malignant disease has been increased by cytotoxic - chemotherapy. On the other hand chemotherapy is inevitably hazardous and potentially lethal because of the toxic effects of the drugs, and thus imposes a grave responsibility on the clinician. A patient may receive repeated courses of treatment with ten or more different cytotoxic drugs during as many years, and it is clearly essential that the records of the treatment, of the response to it, and of the toxic effects produced, be kept in such a way that at all stages it must be possible to survey every detail of the previous course of the disease, to discovery exactly which drugs had been administered, by which routes, and in which doses and combinations, and to review the indications for which each course of treatment had been administered, and the criteria by which its efficacy had been assessed. It is important to be able to find out rapidly whether the response to recent courses of treatment was as satisfactory and as long lasting as the response to earlier courses, and whether the severity of the toxic effects was greater than before. This information makes it possible to plan the future treatment rationally. Hospital records are not adapted for retrieving the information in a form that permits the exacting assessment essential for the most efficient management of patients receiving chemotherapy with cytotoxic drugs. Long experience has shown that the simplest way of recording the essential information is by the use of a chart with a linear time scale on which the details of all drugs administered are entered by a system of bars indicating the doses and the dates on which the treatment was begun and ended. Most cytotoxic drugs are myelotoxic, and the trends in the haemoglobin concentration, platelet, total leucocyte, and neutrophil counts provide the best index of bone marrow depression. The chart should include a section with a logarithmic scale for plotting the platelet and leucocyte counts. The details of treatment and the blood counts are entered at every visit and other clinical, radiological, or biochemical details relevant to the particular case are entered also. Potentially dangerous trends resulting from the treatment are much more easily appreciated by the inspection of the chart than is possible from hospital records or from numerical data in tabular form. The intervals between courses of treatment indicate the duration of remissions, and the extent to which control of the disease is being maintained or lost can be appreciated at a glance. The charts are as

indispensable in the practice of chemotherapy as are conventional ward temperature charts in the management of febrile illnesses.

Endocrine therapy

Prostatic, mammary, and endometrial carcinoma have some of the characteristics of the conditional neoplasms (Foulds) of experimental oncology. Conditional neoplasms grow in certain specific environmental conditions; when the conditions are altered the neoplasms regress but do not die. They persist in a non-proliferating state of residual neoplasia and resume active growth when their specific requirements are restored. At any time some or all of the cells in a conditional neoplasm change their character by acquiring the capacity to grow in the absence of the specific conditions that were previously essential. Alteration of the specific conditions will now lead to regression of that part of the neoplasm that has retained its conditional character, but not of the part that has lost its former dependence on those conditions. Conditional neoplasia in hormone-dependent tissues may be regarded as an expression of differentiation. The growth of these tissues is determined by their hormonal environment, and in the absence of the appropriate stimuli the tissues remain dormant. When such a tissue becomes neoplastic its capacity for growth may remain wholly or partly dependent on hormonal stimuli for some time. Thus *prostatic carcinoma* and its metastases, like normal prostatic epithelium, may regress and remain dormant following orchidectomy, but unlike the normal epithelium, some or all of the deposits of the carcinoma will at some stage acquire the capacity to grow in the absence of testicular control. Treatment with oestrogens is as effective as orchidectomy, and is thought to suppress testicular activity by inhibiting the production of pituitary gonadotrophins. However, oestogens may have a direct inhibitory effect on the carcinoma, because regression may be occasionally observed in orchidectomized patients in relapse.

Normal adult prostatic epithelial cells secrete acid phosphatase, but lose their capacity for doing so after orchidectomy. Prostatic carcinoma cells often secrete acid phosphatase, and the trend in the serum concentration provides an index of the activity of the disease. Following orchidectomy or oestrogen treatment, the serum acid-phosphatase level falls to the normal range. In relapse, however, the tumour cells may secrete acid phosphatase although they are no longer under the influence of androgens, and no longer respond to oestrogen therapy. On the other hand, the tumour cells responsible for the relapse may no longer secrete the enzyme, and in this circumstance serial estimations of the serum acid phosphatase do not provide a warning of impending relapse.

In practice, it has been found that the quality of response to orchidectomy or oestrogen therapy is superior when the cancer cells possess a cytoplasmic androgen receptor. The treatment for metastatic disease, introduced by Huggins as a result of physiological experimentation on the dependence of normal prostatic epithelium on its hormonal environment, is highly effective in relieving symptoms, and was the first instance in modern times of dramatic benefit in human malignant disease conferred by altering the endocrine environment. However, it has not been proved to prolong life, and oestrogen therapy was shown to have increased the incidence of fatal cardiovascular disease, a dose-related effect. Symptomatic relief occurs, on average, sooner after orchidectomy than after the start of oestrogen therapy. Orchidectomy is preferable except in slowly progressive disease causing relatively minor symptoms which are usually controlled by oestrogen therapy at low daily dosage.

The conditional nature of murine mammary cancers with respect to oestrogen dependence has been long known. More recently their dependence on prolactin has been established. The incidence of mammary cancer after exposure to carcinogens (chemical, viral, or radiation) was enormously increased in animals with high secretion rates of prolactin and growth hormone from oestrogen-induced pituitary tumours. Short-term cultures of biopsy specimens from human *breast cancers* have shown enhancement of specific hormone-dependent metabolic pathways in about one half of the cases with respect to human growth hormone as well as prolactin and oestrogen.

Although it has been known for many years that alteration of the hormonal status of the patient may lead to favourable effects, sometimes dramatic and of long duration, in recurrent breast cancer, the endocrine manipulations used in practice have been - worked out empirically. The major factor influencing responsiveness is whether the patient is premenopausal or postmenopausal. In addition, patients whose cancer cells possess cytoplasmic receptors for oestrogen respond better than those whose cells lack them, and the proportion of receptor-positive patients who respond is higher in premenopausal women. In contrast, responsiveness to cytotoxic chemotherapy is not related to the presence of receptors. Although postmenopausal patients may respond to oophorectomy, the proportion is much higher in premenopausal patients, more than 50 per cent in oestrogen-receptor-positive cases. Postmenopausal patients are usually treated with the anti-oestrogen tamoxifen; about 50 per cent of oestrogen receptor-positive patients respond. The duration of response to oophorectomy in premenopausal, and to tamoxifen in postmenopausal cases, is of the order of one year, though some patients remain well for several years. Oophorectomized patients who relapse may respond to tamoxifen, and following a subsequent relapse they may still respond to adrenalectomy or hypophysectomy; the latter is less often performed nowadays, and 'chemical' instead of surgical adrenalectomy is often accomplished by the administration of aminoglutethimide which blocks an early stage in adrenal steroid synthesis by inhibiting the enzyme that converts cholesterol to pregnenolone. Unless prednisolone is given as well, the suppression of adrenal steroid synthesis leads to increased corticotrophin secretion by the anterior pituitary; the resulting stimulation of the adrenal cortex eventually overcomes the effect of aminoglutethimide. The administration of prednisolone concurrently with aminoglutethimide prevents the rebound increase in corticotrophin production. A favourable response to this endocrine ablation therapy may last for one to two years, but in the event of relapse, cytotoxic chemotherapy offers a chance of further response. Before abandoning endocrine therapy, the use of progestational agents, of bromocriptine, an inhibitor of prolactin secretion, or of androgens may be considered, though the severe virilizing effects of androgens in premenopausal women limits their value. Oestrogens are often effective in postmenopausal patients. At all ages, the benefits of endocrine therapy are greatest and long lasting in those patients who have relapsed after a long interval after the treatment of the primary disease, that is to say, patients whose cancer is inherently slowly growing. When rapid growth rate leads to early relapse, it is likely that the duration of response to the first attempt at endocrine therapy, oophorectomy in premenopausal, or tamoxifen in postmenopausal patients, will be short: subsequent endocrine therapy is not likely to be more effective, and cytotoxic chemotherapy should not be unduly postponed. Patients who relapse within five years after the menopause rarely respond well to endocrine therapy.

About one-third of patients suffering from disseminated *endometrial carcinoma* respond to treatment with progestational agents, administered continuously for months or years until one or more of the metastases lose their sensitivity. Patients whose disease has recurred following a previous hysterectomy respond as well and as frequently as those who present with disseminated disease. Even numerous large pulmonary deposits may regress during progestogen therapy. Regression is usually evident within three months of starting the treatment, and when no significant change has occurred after three months, the patient is unlikely to benefit by continuing the treatment.

References

Bodley Scott, R. B. (1979). *Cancer—the facts.* Oxford University Press, Oxford. p. 208.

Buchanan, K. D. (1980). Gut hormones and gut endocrine tumour syndromes. *Br. J. hosp. Med.* **24**, 190.

Burchenal, J. H. (1977). The historical development of cancer chemotherapy. *Semin. Oncol.* **4**, 135.

Cairns, J. (1978). *Cancer, science and society.* W. H. Freeman. San Francisco.

Chabner, B. A., Myers, C. E., and Oliverio, V. T. (1977). Clinical pharmacology of anticancer drugs. *Semin. Oncol.* **4**, 165.

Cline, M. J. and Haskell, C. M. (1980). *Cancer chemotherapy*, 3rd edn. W. B. Saunders, London.

Hughes, R. O. (ed.) (1979). *Surfaces of normal and malignant cells.* Wiley, Chichester.

Montesano, R., Bartsch, H., and Tornatis, L. (eds.) (1980). *Molecular and cellular aspects of carcinogen screening tests.* WHO–IARC. Lyons.

Valeriote, F. A. and Edelstein, M. B. (1977). The role of cell kinetics in cancer chemotherapy. *Semin. Oncol.* **4**, 217.

Waldenström, J. (1979). *Paraneoplasia: biological signals in the diagnosis of cancer.* Wiley, Chichester.

Section 5
Infections

Section 5
Infections

THE HOST RESPONSE TO INFECTION

B. M. Greenwood

Introduction. Many factors determine what happens when a potentially harmful organism reaches a new host. The characteristics of an organism that determine its virulence are considered in the individual sections. In this section the immune response of the host to infection is reviewed briefly and some of the genetic and environmental factors that can influence this response are discussed. The physiological response of man to infection is considered on page 5.19.

Protection against infection

Introduction. A complex system of surface defences, non-specific, and specific immune mechanisms allows man to survive in a hostile microbiological environment (Fig. 1). Damage to any one of these protective mechanisms increases the risk of serious infection. In the following paragraphs the nature of these defences is reviewed briefly. Further details of the way in which complement, antibody, polymorphonuclear neutrophil leucocytes (PMN) and lymphocytes aid in protection against infection are given in Section 4.

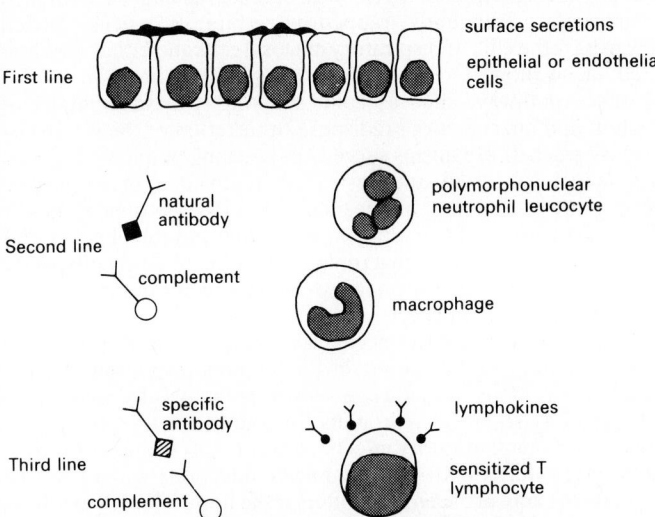

Fig. 1 Three lines of defence against infection.

Surface barriers. Skin and mucosa provide an important mechanical barrier to invasion by many pathogenic organisms. Secretion of bactericidal substances, such as free fatty acids and lysozyme, on to the surface of the skin increases its protective properties. The mechanical barrier to infection provided by the gastric epithelium is aided by the acid pH of the contents of the stomach. Subjects with achlorhydria, a common consequence of malnutrition, have an increased susceptibility to infection with organisms such as *Vibrio cholerae* and *Giardia lamblia*.

Phagocytic cells

Polymorphonuclear neutrophil leucocytes. Polymorphonuclear neutrophil leucocytes (PMN) are usually the first cells to be brought into action against an invading micro-organism. They are attracted to sites of invasion by chemotactic factors produced either directly by the organism or as a result of complement activation. The way in which PMN ingest and destroy micro-organisms has been described in Section 4. Polymorphonuclear neutrophil leucocytes can phagocytose some organisms unaided but many virulent bacteria can be phagocytosed only if they have been trapped against a mechanical barrier, such as a pulmonary alveolar membrane, or if they have been coated with antibody or complement. Patients with neutropenia or with PMN which are functionally defective show an increased susceptibility to infection with many bacteria, including infection with species that are not usually pathogenic. Defective PMN function may result from a hereditary defect, such as chronic granulomatous disease, or it may result from environmental factors such as an overwhelming infection or diabetes.

Macrophages. Organisms which are not destroyed by PMN may be taken up by fixed, tissue macrophages or by phagocytic cells derived from blood monocytes. Such cells are attracted to sites of infection by organisms, such as *Mycobacterium tuberculosus*, which produce monocyte chemotactic factors. Phagocytosis and killing of micro-organisms by macrophages follows similar lines to those described for PMN except that the myeloperoxidase enzyme system is not as well developed in macrophages as it is in PMN. Some micro-organisms, for example *M. leprae* and *Toxoplasma gondii* can survive unharmed in macrophage phagosomes, thus escaping the harmful effects of antibody, unless the macrophages have been activated by lymphokines produced as a consequence of a specific cell-mediated immune reaction.

The macrophages of the spleen play an important part in protection against pneumococcal infection, malaria, and babesiosis. Patients without a spleen or with a non-functioning spleen, as may occur in sickle cell disease, have an increased susceptibility to these infections. It is likely that the unusual vascular anatomy of the spleen provides an environment in which circulating micro-organisms can be brought into close proximity with tissue macrophages which can then ingest and destroy them.

Antibodies. Some individuals possess antibodies which act against organisms to which they have not been exposed previously. Such 'natural' antibodies, which belong mainly to the IgM class, are probably formed as a result of exposure to a cross-reacting antigen. Thus, infection with the harmless bacterium *Neisseria lactamica* can induce the formation of antibodies which are bactericidal for the meningococcus and some strains of *Escherichia coli* induce the formation of antibodies which cross react with capsular surface antigens of *Haemophilus influenzae* type b, an important pathogen in young children. It has been suggested that deliberate infection of children with *E. coli* type O 75:K 100:H 5 might be a more effective method of immunizing against *H. influenzae* infection than vaccination with purified capsular polysaccharide antigen, for the latter is poorly immunogenic in the very young.

Recovery from some infections can be achieved only with the aid of specific antibody. Formation of such antibody takes seven to ten days unless the immune system of the host has been primed by previous infection with the organism or by previous vaccination. During this time lag death or irreparable tissue damage may occur. Antibody can aid recovery from infection, or prevent reinfection, by a number of mechanisms. These are summarized in Table 1.

Patients with a primary or with an acquired defect in antibody production show an increased susceptibility to infection with many species of bacteria, including some which are not usually pathogenic.

Table 1 Methods by which specific antibody can protect against infection

Mechanism	Examples
Prevention of attachment of a Micro-organism to a cell membrane	many bacterial and viral gastro-intestinal and respiratory tract infections
Prevention of spread of a micro-Organism from cell to cell	malaria many viral infections
Enhancement of opsonization	most coccal infections
Immune lysis	*E. coli* infections neisserial infections
Neutralization of a toxin	diphtheria tetanus

The synergistic action of antibody and PMN in the destruction of bacteria has long been recognized. More recently it has been shown that other types of cell can co-operate with antibody in killing micro-organisms. Killing of some species of protozoa and bacteria and of virally infected cells by a subpopulation of lymphocytes (K cells) acting in conjunction with antibody has been demonstrated *in vitro*, but it is still uncertain how important a protective mechanism this is in life. Eosinophils, with the aid of antibody, can kill schistosomula of *Schistosoma mansoni* and larvae of *Trichinella spiralis*. Eosinophils obtained from patients with schistosomiasis are more effective killers than eosinophils obtained from controls.

Complement. The complement pathway is described in detail in Section 5. Complement activation commonly accompanies systemic infections as a result of activation of the classical complement pathway by immune complexes, as a result of activation of the alternative complement pathway by microbial products such as pneumococcal polysaccharides or endotoxin, or as a result of direct digestion of complement components by bacterial proteases. Activation of complement by any of these pathways can aid in protection against infection in three main ways. These are summarized in Fig. 2.

Patients with C3 deficiency suffer from recurrent pyogenic infections. Patients with deficiency of late complement components show an increased susceptibility to infection with neisseria.

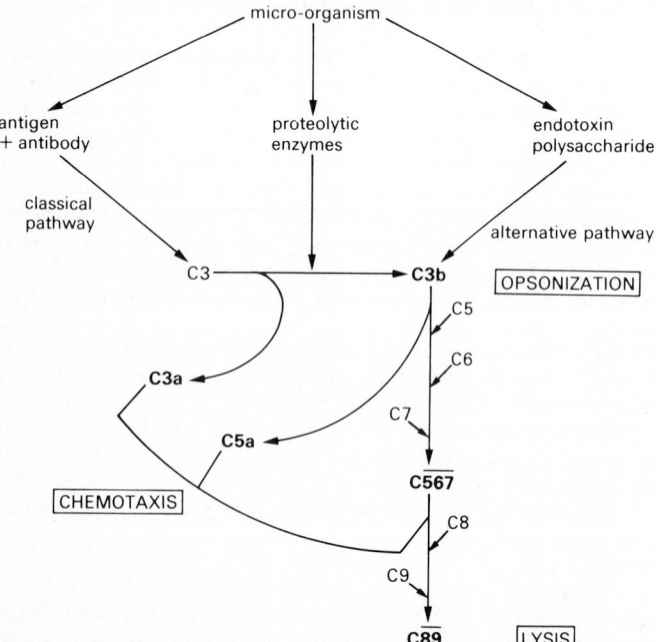

Fig. 2 Complement activation as a result of infection and the protective role of activated complement components.

Specific cellular immunity. Parasites within a cell are safe from the harmful effects of antibody. Recovery from infection with many intracellular organisms is thus dependent upon specific cell-mediated immune mechanisms mediated by thymus-dependent (T) lymphocytes. Sensitized T lymphocytes can destroy a micro-organism or, more usually, an infected host cell by a direct cytolytic action. How this is achieved is not completely understood. Direct contact between the T lymphocyte and the target cell is required and the effector cell must be metabolically active. Neither antibody nor complement are required. In most systems killing is only achieved when the effector cell and the target cell share the same histocompatibility (HLA) antigens.

Sensitized lymphocytes can also protect against infection through their influence on macrophages. Macrophages activated by lymphokines produced as a result of contact between sensitized T lymphocytes and the appropriate antigen are able to destroy organisms against which they were previously impotent. Such activated macrophages show enhanced activity against organisms other than the one which induced the cell-mediated immune reaction that lead to their formation.

Patients with deficient cell-mediated immunity have an increased susceptibility to infection with many viruses, some intracellular bacteria, and protozoa, and they are susceptible to infection with fungi and yeasts.

Protective mechanisms acting at mucosal surfaces. As many pathogenic organisms invade through either the alimentary tract or through the respiratory tract, protective mechanisms acting at these sites play an especially important part in determining susceptibility to infection.

Organisms that invade through the respiratory tract must be able to overcome a number of mechanical defence mechanisms. Inhaled organisms are frequently trapped by respiratory mucus, carried upwards by the cilia of respiratory mucosal cells and either expectorated or swallowed. Factors which impair the function of this clearance pathway, such as cold, smoking, excessive intake of alcohol, and anaesthetics predispose to infection of the lower respiratory tract. If organisms succeed in reaching pulmonary alveoli they may be ingested and destroyed by alveolar macrophages. Respiratory secretions contain small amounts of antibody, mainly of the IgA class, and complement which may aid the phagocytosis of organisms by alveolar macrophages. Large amounts of specific antibody are required for phagocytosis of virulent organisms such as capsulated pneumococci.

Damage to the defence mechanisms of the respiratory tract by adverse climatic factors is one of the features responsible for the seasonal variations in incidence shown by many infections which are spread by respiratory droplets. In countries with a temperate climate, serious respiratory infections occur most frequently during the winter whilst in tropical countries infections spread by the respiratory route are seen most often at the hottest and driest times of the year (Fig. 3). Atmospheric absolute humidity is low under both these sets of climatic conditions, and a low absolute humidity may predispose to respiratory infection by impairing the secretion of respiratory mucus and antibody and by impairing the function of ciliated respiratory tract epithelial cells. Other factors, such as changes in social activities, also contribute to seasonal variations in the pattern of individual infectious diseases.

The role of the acid contents of the stomach in protection against infection of the gastrointestinal tract has been mentioned already. Organisms which manage to pass this barrier and thus to reach the small bowel are susceptible to attack by IgA antibodies produced by plasma cells in the lamina propria of the small gut. These cells produce secretory IgA antibodies (two IgA molecules linked by a polypeptide secretory piece) which are resistant to digestion by small bowel enzymes. The epithelium of the gut is capable of mounting a specific cell-mediated immune reaction but the possible role of cell-mediated immunity in protection against gastrointestinal infections has been little studied. The resident gut flora protect against colonization of the bowel by pathogenic organisms. Susceptibility to gastrointestinal infection is increased when the normal flora is disturbed, for instance by the administration of antibiotics.

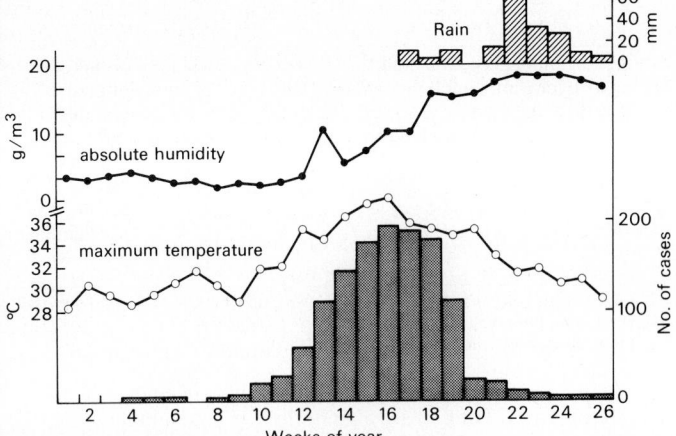

Fig. 3   The relationship between atmospheric humidity and an epidemic of meningococcal disease in northern Nigeria. (From Greenwood *et al.* (1979). *Trans. R. Soc. Trop. Med. Hyg.* **73**, 557.)

Breast milk protects an infant from gastrointestinal infection in several ways. It provides a relatively sterile source of food and it contains IgA antibodies, lysozyme, and other less clearly defined substances which have an adverse effect on the growth of many bacteria and viruses. Bottle-fed babies experience gastrointestinal infections more frequently than breast-fed babies, especially in developing countries where preparation of uncontaminated bottle feeds is difficult.

Genetic factors and susceptibility to infection

Introduction. It is widely believed that genetic factors influence susceptibility to infectious diseases and their clinical outcome, but it has proved difficult to document this assertion in man. Clustering of patients with an infection may suggest that genetic factors play a part in its pathogenesis but such clusters can equally well result from environmental factors, such as exposure of several members of a family to a common source of infection. Racial differences in the pattern of individual infectious disease, for example, the tendency of Indian patients with tuberculosis to show bone involvement, and the severity of yellow fever in Europeans, suggest that genetic factors may have an influence on the clinical course of an infection but, in such situations, it is once again difficult to differentiate between the likely roles of genetic and environmental factors. The firmest clinical evidence supporting the role of genetic factors in determining susceptibility to infection comes from studies of identical twins, which have shown that the twin of a patient with tuberculosis or leprosy has a higher risk of contracting the infection than a control, even when the twin is brought up in a different environment from his sibling.

Delineation of the HLA (histocompatibility) antigen system has provided a valuable new tool for investigating the possible role of genetic factors in determining susceptibility to infection.

HLA and infection. Genes situated at four loci on the sixth chromosome determine the structure of cell surface antigens (histocompatibility locus antigens) which play a major part in transplantation reactions (see Section 4). Studies undertaken during the past few years have shown that susceptibility to a variety of diseases, most of which are associated with some kind of immunological abnormality, is linked to the possession of specific HLA haplotypes. Surprisingly, only a few such studies have been carried out in patients with infectious diseases. The possible relationship between

the HLA system and susceptibility to infection has been investigated in three main ways. At a population level it has been shown that the distribution of certain HLA haplotypes is related to the geographical distribution of widespread infections such as malaria. At the individual level it has been demonstrated that patients with certain infections possess specific HLA haplotypes significantly more frequently than carefully matched controls. Thus, in two studies, HLA-B8 and Bw15 were found more frequently in patients with tuberculosis than in controls. An alternative approach to the use of direct case control studies has been employed to investigate the possible role of genetic factors in determining susceptibility to leprosy. Study of families with more than one case of the infection has shown that affected siblings carry the same haplotype as the index cases significantly more frequently than non-affected siblings, although the haplotype involved varies from family to family. Thus, genetic factors are probably important in determining susceptibility to leprosy. A similar study carried out in families of patients with meningococcal disease showed no such relationship indicating that, in this infection, clustering of cases is probably due to environmental rather than to genetic factors.

Histocompatibility related factors may influence the clinical outcome of an infection as well as its incidence. Thus, the likelihood that hepatitis B infection will progress to chronic liver disease is HLA-related.

How possession of certain HLA haplotypes influences susceptibility to infection is still not certain. Linkage of HLA haplotypes to immune response genes situated on an adjacent area of the same chromosome is one possibility. Such a system has been convincingly established in experimental animals. The fact that the immune response to influenza, tetanus, and smallpox vaccines is influenced by the HLA haplotype of the recipient supports this view. An alternative explanation for the association between certain infections and specific HLA haplotypes is that some organisms possess antigens which cross-react with HLA antigens and that possession of such antigens confers upon them a degree of protection from the host's immune response. Some evidence to support this hypothesis has been obtained from study of patients with ankylosing spondylitis for some strains of Klebsiella isolated from patients with this disease possess an antigen which cross-reacts with the HLA-B27 antigen found on the lymphocytes of many patients with this condition.

Other genetic markers and susceptibility to infection. Immune responsiveness is related to the possession of certain genetically determined allotypes of immunoglobulin molecules. In man immune responsiveness to meningococcal and *H. influenzae* polysaccharides is related to the presence of a specific Km allotype of IgG and responsiveness to flagellin is influenced by Gm allotype, perhaps because the genes controlling these alleles are in linkage disequilibrium with an immune response gene. It is likely that susceptibility to some bacterial infections is influenced by possession of specific immunoglobulin allotypes but this has yet to be shown.

Possession of specific blood group antigens is related to susceptibility to some infections. Severe schistosomiasis mansoni and giardiasis are encountered more frequently in blood group A individuals than in controls, the latter association perhaps being due to the fact that hypochlorhydria is found more frequently in group A subjects than in individuals with other ABO blood groups. The relationship between Duffy blood group antigens and *Plasmodium vivax* is discussed below.

Mechanisms by which genetic factors increase susceptibility to infection. Genetic factors can influence susceptibility to infection in at least three ways.

(a) Influence on surface receptors. Invasion of a host cell by an intracellular parasite initially involves attachment of the microorganism to the surface of its new target. This attachment is often achieved by binding to a specific surface membrane receptor. The presence or absence of a suitable membrane receptor may be under

genetic control. This situation has been demonstrated most clearly in man in connection with *P. vivax* infection. Red cells can be infected with this malaria parasite only if they possess a surface receptor closely related to a Duffy red cell antigen. Most blacks lack Duffy antigens, thus offering a possible explanation for the infrequent occurrence of *P. vivax* malaria in West Africa. It is likely that genetic factors influence susceptibility to other infections by a similar mechanism.

(b) Influence on host cell constituents. An intracellular parasite is dependent for its nutrition upon the constituents of the host cell that it has invaded. The nature of these constituents may be under the influence of genetic factors. Malaria offers an example of this phenomenon also. Red cells which contain a high concentration of fetal haemoglobin (HbF), a situation found in patients with various forms of haemoglobinopathy, do not support the growth of *P. falciparum* as well as red cells containing haemoglobin A (Fig. 4).

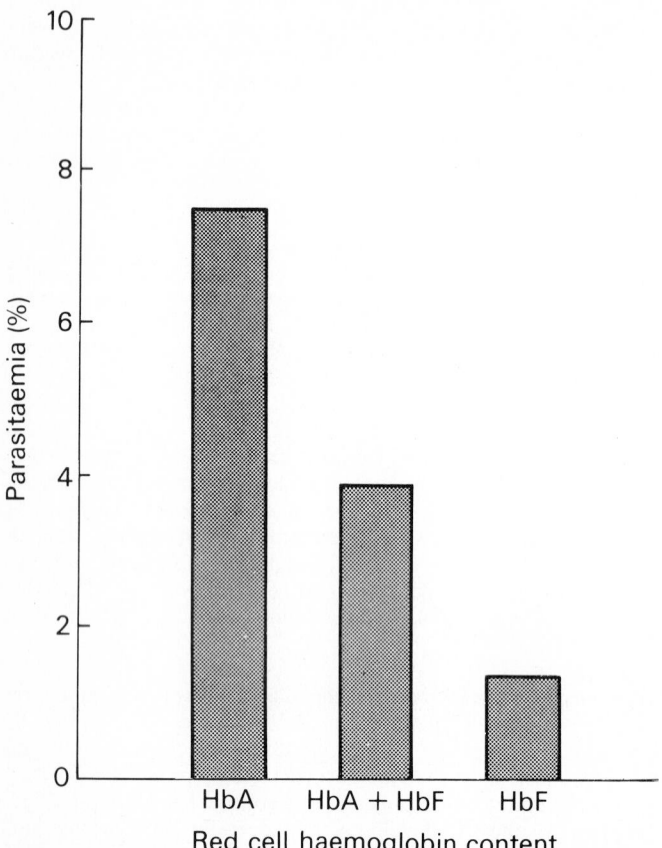

Fig. 4   The distribution of parasites observed in red cells containing different types of haemoglobin observed in 13 infants infected with *P. falciparum*. (From Wilson *et al.* (1977). *Bull. Wld Hlth Org.* **55**, 179.)

The mechanism of the protection against severe *P. falciparum* malaria observed in subjects with the haemoglobin genotype AS is still not certain. Red cells containing haemoglobin AS support the growth of *P. falciparum* normally under standard tissue culture conditions, although not under conditions of low oxygen tension. Possibly malaria parasites can use sufficient oxygen to cause an AS red cell to sickle, with consequent removal of both red cell and parasite from the circulation.

(c) Influence on the specific immune response. A number of clearly defined primary immunodeficiency syndromes have been described which are associated with an increased susceptibility to infection. Most of these conditions are genetically determined. Lymphocytes, immunoglobulins, complement, and PMN may all be involved. Table 2 lists some of the most important forms of specific primary immune deficiency and their usual mode of inheritance. The inherited complement deficiencies which are associated

Table 2   Some well characterized primary defects of specific immunity and their usual mode of inheritance

Condition	Defect		Inheritance
	Antibody	Cell-mediated	
X-linked agammaglobulinaemia	+		X-linked
Transient hypogammaglobulinaemia	+		unknown*
Selective IgA deficiency	+		variable
Severe combined immunodeficiency	+	+	AR†
Thymic hypoplasia	+	+	not familial
Ataxia telangiectasia	+	+	AR
Wiskott–Aldrich syndrome	+	+	X-linked
Variable immunodeficiency	+	+	not familial or unknown

* Found with an increased frequency in the families of patients with severe combined immunodeficiency
† AR = autosomal recessive

with an increased susceptibility to infection (deficiency of C3, C3b inactivator, C6, C7 or C8) are all inherited as autosomal recessives. Chronic granulomatous disease, one of the most important primary defects of PMN, is usually inherited in an X-linked manner but the condition can occasionally affect girls when it is presumed to be inherited as an autosomal recessive.

These well characterized primary immune deficiencies are responsible for only a tiny fraction of all severe infections. It is possible that more subtle defects of the immune system, some of which may be genetically determined, contribute to the pathogenesis of a much larger proportion of cases of infectious disease. Such defects may be highly specific, for example the recently described defect in a patient with fatal Epstein–Barr virus (EBV) infection whose lymphocytes were unable to produce interferon or immune challenge. Highly specific defects have been described also in patients with severe mucocutaneous candidiasis. As immunological techniques for probing the integrity of the immune system become more sophisticated it is likely that more such defects will come to light.

Constitutional factors and susceptibility to infection

Introduction. Environmental, as well as genetic, factors play an important role in determining susceptibility to infection and in determining its severity. Some of the most important of these constitutional factors are now considered.

Age. Many infectious diseases show a characteristic age distribution. Age exerts an influence on susceptibility to infection in various ways. Infections with ubiquitous organisms are seen first in young infants shortly after they have lost the maternal antibody transferred to them across the placenta. The peak incidence of infections such as measles, mumps, and whooping cough, is thus in early childhood. Older children are resistant to these common infections because they have experienced a sub-clinical attack of the infection or because they have been immunized. As immunity declines in the very old, susceptibility to infection increases once again.

The age distribution of many infectious diseases is determined by age-dependent occupational or social activities. Venereal infections are an obvious example of this phenomenon. Other examples can be cited which depend upon more subtle changes in social behaviour. Thus, in endemic areas, the clinical features of schistosomiasis are seen most frequently in young boys and they are only rarely encountered in adults. Gradual acquisition of protective immunity may play some part in reducing the severity of this infection in adults but the fact that small boys, unlike adults, bathe frequently in infected water is likely to be an equally important factor.

Age influences not only susceptibility to infection but also its clinical severity. Thus, in endemic areas, malaria is a milder infection in adults than in children because adults have acquired some protective immunity as a result of numerous previous infections. The converse situation applies to many viral infections. Poliomyelitis, yellow fever, infectious hepatitis, EBV infection, and mumps are all milder infections in children than in adults. Why this should be the case has never been satisfactorily explained. It is possible that, because of maturation of the immune system, immunopathological reactions are more marked when infection occurs in adult life than when infection occurs during childhood but this is unlikely to be the only explanation for this phenomenon.

Sex and hormonal factors. Variation in the sex distribution of infectious diseases may be brought about by both social and hormonal factors. Some infections are commoner in men than in women because men come into close contact with the source of the infection more frequently than women as a result of their occupation. However, for reasons that are not obvious young women are more susceptible to tuberculosis than young men. Certain infections, for example hepatitis, pneumococcal infection, amoebiasis, and malaria, are more severe when they occur during pregnancy than when they occur at other times. An enhanced susceptibility to infection during pregnancy is probably a reflection of the generalized impairment of immunity that occurs at this time.

An excess of glucocorticosteroids, resulting from adrenal hyperplasia, an adrenal tumour, or steroid therapy, increases susceptibility to many infections and increases their severity. Herpes simplex and herpes zoster can cause severe, and sometimes fatal, infections in patients receiving large doses of corticosteroids. Tuberculosis, amoebiasis, and strongyloidiasis can all be activated by corticosteroids; strongyloidiasis may be especially severe when it occurs in such circumstances. Corticosteroids probably exert their effect by their action on the immune response. In large doses they cause depletion of T lymphocytes, impairment of cell-mediated immunity, and impairment of some functions of PMN.

Patients with diabetes, especially when the condition is poorly controlled, show an increased susceptibility to several infections. Boils, abscesses, and urinary tract infections are common. Tuberculosis may be activated, and pulmonary infection with yeasts or fungi may occur. A high tissue concentration of glucose favours the growth of some bacteria. Cell-mediated immune reactions and chemotaxis by PMN are impaired in patients with diabetes and these defects may contribute to the increased susceptibility to infection shown by patients with this condition.

Trauma. Trauma predisposes to infection in several ways. Damage to the surface defences, for example by a severe burn, opens the way to systemic invasion by organisms which are normally confined to the body's surface. Severe burns have a depressive effect on the immune system also. Tissue destruction as a result of mechanical trauma or vascular damage can create an environment in which anaerobic organisms such as *Clostridium tetani* and *C. welchii* can thrive. In such an area, the normal immune defence mechanism cannot be brought into play. Thus, pulmonary infarcts and bone infarcts may become infected by organisms which have difficulty in establishing themselves in normal tissue. Such a process is likely to be one of the reasons for the high incidence of salmonella osteomyelitis observed in patients with sickle cell disease. Tonsillectomy and intramuscular injections predispose to paralytic poliomyelitis but the mechanism of this association is uncertain.

Malnutrition. Numerous studies in experimental animals have shown that dietary deficiency of protein, of individual vitamins, and of trace elements increases susceptibility to infection with a wide variety of organisms. Likewise in man clinical studies have shown that certain infections are more frequent or more severe in malnourished subjects than in healthy controls (Table 3). In developing countries, most attention has been paid to children with severe protein energy malnutrition, for such children frequently die from infection. The response to infection of children with marasmus or

Table 3 Some common infections seen more frequently, or with increased severity, in the malnourished

Protozoa	Bacteria	Viruses	Yeasts
Amoebiasis	Cholera	Herpes simplex	Candidiasis
Giardiasis	Gram-negative sepsis	Infection	
Pneumocystis	Infectious diarrhoea	Infectious hepatitis	
	Tuberculosis	Measles	

with milder degree of protein energy malnutrition has been little investigated. In industrialized countries, severe malnutrition is encountered as a complication of conditions such as disseminated cancer or cirrhosis more frequently than as a result of pure dietary deficiency. It is likely that associated malnutrition contributes to the increased susceptibility to infection shown by patients with these conditions.

The pathogenesis of the enhanced susceptibility to infection shown by subjects with protein energy malnutrition is complex, for this form of malnutrition adversely affects nearly all host defence mechanisms (Table 4).

Table 4 The harmful effects of protein energy malnutrition on defences against infection

Surface defences	damage to the skin and other epithelial surfaces achlorhydria
Non-specific immunity	impaired microbial killing by PMN depression of serum complement levels
Specific immunity Cellular	diminished cutaneous delayed hypersensitivity depletion of T lymphocytes diminished proliferative response of lymphocytes *in vitro* diminished lymphokine production inhibitory serum factors
Humoral	impaired antibody production to some antigens

In man, severe isolated deficiencies of metals and vitamins are rarely encountered, but it has been shown that iron deficiency increases susceptibility to certain bacterial infections, and that deficiency of vitamin A predisposes to infection at epithelial surfaces, such as the cornea.

Although, in general, malnutrition enhances susceptibility to infection, it is possible that under certain circumstances the reverse situation applies. Studies in severely malnourished refugees have shown that refeeding is associated with an increased incidence of tuberculosis, brucellosis, amoebiasis, malaria, and herpes. These observations suggest that famine adversely affects the nutrition of some pathogenic organisms as well as adversely affecting the nutrition of their host.

Infection. The fact that one infection frequently follows hard upon the heels of another is well known. Some examples of this phenomenon are given in Table 5. The mechanisms underlying these associations vary from infection to infection and they are, in some instances, very complex. A large parasite can act as a nidus for infection by a smaller one. Thus, salmonellae can colonize the cuticle of adult schistosomes, and, from this protected site in the portal vein, they can cause recurrent episodes of septicaemia. Tissues damaged by one organism may provide a favourable environment for invasion by another. *Clostridium tetani* can colonize infected wounds that are the site of a pyogenic infection, and old tuberculous cavities may be colonized by moulds such as *aspergillus*. Damage to the epithelium of the respiratory tract by viruses may predispose to subsequent pulmonary infection with bacteria. However, the most important mechanism by which one infection predisposes to another is by depressing the immune response of the host.

Table 5 Examples of situations in which one infection predisposes to another

Primary infection	Secondary infection	Likely mechanism
Bartonellosis	salmonella septicaemia	? ↑ serum iron
Influenza	bacterial pneumonia	damage to epithelium ↓ PMN function
Malaria	salmonella septicaemia	↓ humoral immunity ? ↑ serum iron
Measles	bacterial pneumonia gastroenteritis herpes simplex tuberculosis	severe impairment of cellular and humoral immunity
Meningococcal disease	herpes simplex	↓ cell mediated immunity
Pneumococcal disease	herpes simplex	↓ cell mediated immunity
Schistosomiasis	salmonella septicaemia	adult worm acts as focus
Septic abortion	tetanus gas gangrene	tissue damage
Tuberculosis	aspergillosis	tissue damage
Trypanosomiasis	pneumococcal pneumonia	↓ humoral immunity

Some degree of immunosuppression accompanies most infections; it is the rule rather than the exception. In some cases immunodepression produced in this way is of interest to the immunologist but is of little importance to the patient. However, in a few instances, suppression of the immune response of the host regularly leads to a secondary infection which has a major influence on the outcome of the patient's illness. Measles is an important example of this phenomenon. Children with this infection frequently develop secondary bacterial infections, such as pneumonia and severe gastro-enteritis. Tuberculosis may be activated and activation of herpes simplex may result in severe ulceration of the mucosa of the mouth and of the cornea, or, occasionally, in an overwhelming viraemia.

The pathogenesis of the immunosuppression that accompanies infection is complex and varies considerably from infection to infection. In some instances the immune defect is very specific, for example, patients with lepromatous leprosy have a specific cellular immune defect to products of *M. leprae*, but they are able to respond normally to other antigens. In contrast many components of the immune response are impaired in patients with measles. In general, cellular immune reactions are depressed more frequently by infections than humoral immune mechanisms, but both these components of the immune response, as well as PMN and macrophages, may be adversely affected. The complex interactions that may arise between infection, nutrition, and immunity are well illustrated by measles (Fig. 5).

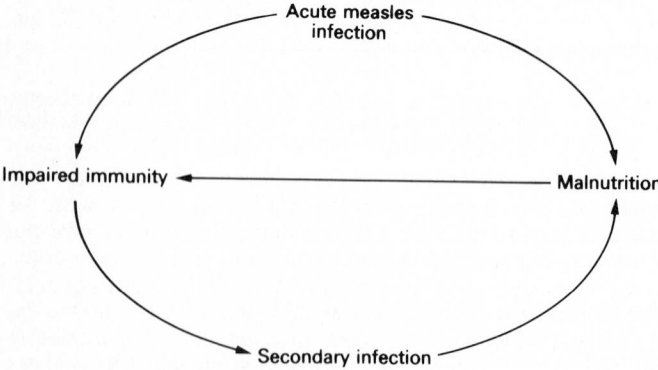

Fig. 5 The complex interaction between infection, nutrition, and impaired immunity seen in measles.

Drugs. The problem of infection in patients receiving cytotoxic or immunosuppressive drugs is considered on pages 5.478–84. Alcohol in excess increases susceptibility to many infections, especially when cirrhosis of the liver has supervened. Septicaemia is a common terminal event in hard-line drug addicts who neglect simple hygienic precautions when administering their intravenous injections. Smoking, by damaging the epithelium of the respiratory tract, predisposes to respiratory infections.

Malignant disease. Immune responsiveness is impaired in patients with widespread malignant disease, and such patients have an increased risk of infection, sometimes with organisms of low virulence. The risk of such infections may be increased further by extensive radiotherapy or by treatment with cytotoxic drugs.

Conclusion. In this section some of the numerous environmental factors that can influence susceptibility to infection have been considered. This list must be born in mind whenever a patient with a serious infection is seen. In such a situation the first task of the physician is to identify correctly the causative organism and to start an appropriate form of treatment. However, he must also try to establish why the patient was infected by this particular organism at this particular time. Does the patient belong to a population group at special risk from this infection or could he have some underlying predisposing condition? In the vast majority of patients, a negative answer will be obtained to both these questions, but failure to ask them may lead occasionally to failure to diagnose an underlying systemic illness and to consequent failure of the patient to respond satisfactorily to treatment with an appropriate course of chemotherapy.

Tissue damage and the host response to infection

Introduction. The value of the immune response in achieving recovery from infection and in preventing re-infection is illustrated clearly by the serious consequences that ensue when the integrity of the immune system is damaged by one of the genetic or environmental factors considered in the previous section. However, there is often a price to be paid for elimination of micro-organisms by the immune system. Destruction of an intracellular parasite can be achieved only at the cost of destruction of the host cell within which the parasite resides. At sites such as the liver, where cell regeneration is rapid, damaged cells are easily replaced. However, immunologically mediated recovery from infections of the nervous system can often be achieved only at the expense of irreversible tissue damage.

The factors that determine why immunopathological complications are associated with some infections but not with others are poorly understood. Thus, immune complex-mediated arthritis and vasculitis are well recognized complications of meningococcal infection, but are rarely, if ever, seen as a complication of pneumococcal infection. Perhaps meningococcal capsular polysaccharides possess some special characteristics, not shared by pneumococcal polysaccharides, which predispose to the formation of harmful immune complexes. Alternatively, vascular damage by endotoxin, produced by meningococci but not by pneumococci, might predispose to immune complex-mediated tissue damage. Further uncertainties surround the question of why only a small proportion of patients with an infectious disease develop immunopathological complications. Thus, immune complex-mediated glomerulonephritis complicates only a small proportion of group A β-haemolytic streptococcal infections and progressive glomerulonephritis is an even rarer complication of *P. malariae* malaria. Both microbial and host factors are likely to be involved. Thus, certain antigenic types of group A β-haemolytic streptococci are more likely to produce renal disease than others, and genetic factors influence the host's immune response to streptococcal antigens.

Types of immunologically mediated tissue damage. In 1963 Gell and Coombs introduced a new classification of allergic reactions which delineated four main categories of immunopathological response. Application of this classification to the immunopathology of infectious diseases has introduced some order into an area which was previously very confused. All four types of immunopathological reaction can complicate infections. Further details of the immunological mechanisms involved in the pathogenesis of these reactions are given in Section 4.

Type 1 (immediate hypersensitivity) allergic reactions. Type 1 mediated allergic reactions result from the release of histamine and other vasoactive amines from basophils and mast cells which have been sensitized with IgE antibody, and which have then been exposed to the relevant antigen. Such reactions often complicate helminth infections which are associated with enhanced synthesis of IgE antibody. Some examples of type 1 reactions complicating an infection are shown in Table 6. The clinical features of type 1 allergic reactions, which are largely those of histamine poisoning, vary in severity from a mild skin lesion to peripheral circulatory collapse and death.

Table 6 Some examples of type 1 allergic reactions complicating infections and their different clinical manifestations

Peripheral circulatory collapse	Pulmonary infiltration or asthma	Rashes
Onchocerciasis (treatment reaction)	Aspergillosis	Animal hookworm larvae (cutaneous larva migrans)
Ruptured hydatid cyst	Migrating round worm larvae	Animal schistosome cercariae
	Migrating schistosomula	Hookworm larvae (ground itch)
	Tropical eosinophilia	Onchocerciasis (treatment reaction)
		Trypanosomiasis

Eosinophilia is a frequent accompaniment of many infections which are complicated by type 1 allergic reactions. Eosinophils can inactivate histamine and other vasoactive compounds, such as slow-reacting substance, released by mast cells. Thus, in patients with a helminth infection, eosinophilia may, in part, be a protective response aimed at modulating some of the harmful effects of an immunopathological reaction.

Type 2 (antibody-mediated) allergic reactions. Sensitization of host cells with microbial antigens may render such cells susceptible to immune attack. Such a process probably plays a part in the pathogenesis of the haemolytic anaemia associated with *Mycoplasma pneumoniae* and with some viral infections. The anaemia of malaria has a complex aetiology, for non-parasitized cells, as well as parasitized cells, are destroyed more rapidly than normal during this infection. It is probable that binding of malaria antigen, followed by antibody and complement, on to the surface of non-infected red cells renders them susceptible to elimination by phagocytic cells. Tissue damage by antibody may occur during the course of other infections. Antibodies which react with myocardial cells and with Schwann cells are often found in sera obtained from patients with South American trypanosomiasis but it is uncertain whether these antibodies play any part in bringing about the cardiac and neurological damage characteristic of this infection. Sera from some patients with chronic hepatitis B infection contain an antibody which, with the help of mononuclear cells (K cells), can damage healthy hepatocytes. This antibody may play a part in the pathogenesis of chronic active hepatitis.

Type 3 (immune complex-mediated) allergic reactions. Tissue damage as a result of immune complex deposition is one of the most frequently encountered immunopathological complications of infection. It is likely that immune complex-mediated tissue damage can be produced in two ways. Immune complexes are formed within the circulation during the course of recovery from many systemic infections. In some instances, for example, in patients with streptococcal infection, acute hepatitis, or dengue fever, such complexes are trapped in the kidneys, skin, or synovium where, as a result of complement activation, they induce an acute inflammatory reaction. Deposition in the kidney is favoured by the organ's high blood flow and by the presence of C3b receptors on the basement membrane of renal capillaries. During the course of other infections, for example, lepromatous leprosy, large amounts of antigen accumulate in the peripheral tissues; such aggregates may be the site of local immune complex formation (an Arthus reaction). Such a process is the likely cause of erythema nodosum leprosum and the arthritis associated with meningococcal disease. Immune complexes can cause a variety of clinical syndromes, dependent upon the site at which they are formed, ranging in severity from a mild rash to peripheral circulatory collapse and associated disseminated intravascular coagulation. Table 7 lists some of the most frequently encountered clinical manifestations of immune complex disease and the infections with which these features may be associated.

Table 7 Some examples of immune complex-mediated tissue damage arising as a complication of an infection.

Shock syndrome	Acute glomerulno-	Chronic glomerulonephritis	Rashes and/or arthritis
Dengue	Bacterial endocarditis	*P. malariae* infection	Hepatitis B infection
	Dengue	Streptococcal infection	Meningococcal infection*
	Hepatitis B infection		Leprosy*
	Leprosy		Syphilis
	P. falciparum malaria		
	Pneumococcal infection		
	Schistosomiasis mansoni		
	Streptococcal infection		
	Syphilis		
	Typhoid		

* Due to local information of immune complexes

Type 4 (delayed hypersensitivity) allergic reactions. Damage to host cells is inevitable whenever a cell-mediated immune attack is mounted against an intracellular parasite. For some infections tissue damage produced in this way is more important than that produced directly by the causative micro-organism. Thus, in experimental animals, the outcome of some viral meningo-encephalitides is less serious in immunodeficient animals than in animals with an intact immune system, even though the virus is not eliminated by the animals with defective immunity.

Cell-mediated immune damage plays an important role in the pathogenesis of the clinical features of tuberculoid leprosy. Patients with this form of leprosy are able to contain, and eventually to eradicate, *M. leprae* but this may be achieved only at the expense of severe and irreversible damage to peripheral nerves. A sudden deterioration in the clinical features of patients with borderline leprosy may follow an increase in the patient's ability to mount a cellular immune response following the start of treatment or as a consequence of other less clearly defined factors.

Conclusion. Although it is convenient to ascribe the immunopathological complications of an infection to one or other of the Gell and Coombs categories of immunopathological reaction, it is important to remember that these types of reaction are not mutually exclusive and that two or even more types of reaction may take place concurrently. Thus type 1, type 3, and type 4 reactions probably all contribute to the pathology of pulmonary aspergillosis.

Stimulation of the immune response to infection

Introduction. A physician often wishes to increase the resistance of a patient, or of a community, to an infection. There are several ways in which this can be achieved. It may be possible to eliminate predisposing factors to the infection in either an individual or in a community by general health measures. Alternatively, it may be possible to achieve protection by passive or by active immunoprophylaxis. Protection through chemoprophylaxis is considered on page 5.39.

Correction of predisposing factors. Improvement in general living standards is sometimes as important a factor in controlling an infectious disease as specific immunoprophylaxis. This point is clearly illustrated by study of the incidence of major infectious diseases in industrialized countries throughout the twentieth century. In many cases, for example, whooping cough, the incidence of the infection, and the mortality that it caused, fell considerably before the discovery of antibiotics or before the introduction of vaccination (Fig. 6). This decline probably resulted from improvements in housing, nutrition, and sanitation.

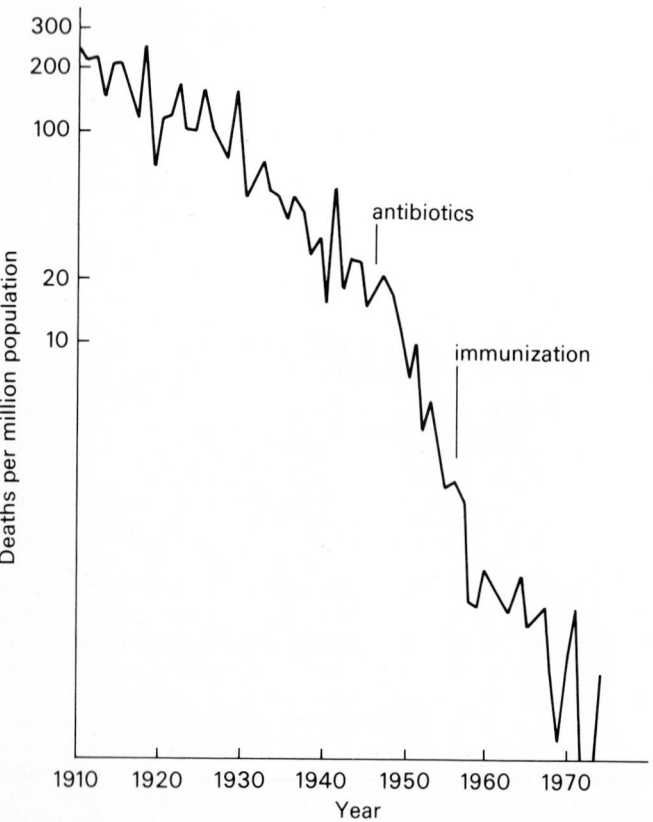

Fig. 6   Whooping cough deaths per million population in England and Wales in relation to the introduction of antibiotics and whooping cough immunization. (Modified from Dick (1978) in *New trends and developments in vaccines* (eds. A. Voller and H. Friedman) 29. MTP Press, Lancaster.)

For some groups of patients with an enhanced susceptibility to infection, for example, patients with diabetes or malnutrition, it is possible to cure or control their underlying illness, thus restoring their resistance to infection to normal. However, for others, for example, patients with sickle cell disease, cure of the underlying condition is not possible and vaccination, or prophylactic antibiotic administration, are needed to protect patients with such conditions against infection.

Passive protection
Serum and gammaglobulin. Serum and gammaglobulin can confer short-lived protection against a number of infections. Immune serum may either prevent an infection or it may reduce its clinical severity. Gammaglobulin is of proven value in preventing infection in patients with agammaglobulinaemia or hypogammaglobulinaemia; it is of less certain value in patients with poorly defined reasons for an increased susceptibility to infection. Antiserum has been used widely to prevent tetanus in patients with dirty wounds. There is convincing evidence that, in developing countries, antiserum is a more effective prophylactic than tetanus toxoid and an antibiotic. Antiserum given together with vaccine is more effective than vaccine alone in preventing rabies in patients at high risk, such as those bitten by a rabid wolf. Gammaglobulin is partially effective in preventing hepatitis A and hepatitis B infection.

Antiserum or gammaglobulin prepared in animals can cause severe anaphylaxis in man. This risk is greatly reduced if human antiserum or gammaglobulin is used. Such preparations can now be prepared by plasmaphersis of immunized volunteers.

Polymorphonuclear neutrophil leucocytes. Granulocyte transfusion can help to prevent septicaemia in patients with severe leucopenia resulting from cytotoxic drug therapy, malignant disease, or infection. However, a cell separator and large number of leucocytes are required, and granulocyte transfusion is thus a very expensive form of therapy.

Lymphocytes and their products. Patients with chronic infections caused by leishmania, *M. leprae* and *C. albicans* have a specific defect in cell-mediated immunity to antigens derived from the causative organism. This immunological abnormality probably contributes to their inability to overcome the infection. Thus, attempts have been made to overcome this defect by the administration of immune lymphocytes or by the administration of lymphocyte-derived transfer factor. Transfer factor, unlike lymphocyte suspensions, does not transmit hepatitis. Claims have been made that transfer factor enhances recovery from borderline leprosy, cutaneous leishmaniasis, systemic candidiasis, systemic mycoses, hepatitis, and other infections. Most of these claims have been based upon uncontrolled studies. However, recently carefully conducted controlled trials have shown that transfer factor is effective in hastening the recovery of patients with cutaneous leishmaniasis and in preventing varicella–zoster infections in immunocompromised patients. Therapy with transfer factor may, therefore, find an accepted place in the management of a limited number of clinical situations.

Interferon is produced by lymphocytes and other cells such as fibroblasts. Using cell lines, it has only been possible to produce sufficient interferon to undertake a limited number of clinical trials. However, interferon produced by genetically programmed *E. coli* may soon become more widely available. Controlled trials have shown that interferon increases the resistance of immunodepressed patients to herpes and cytomegalovirus infections. Interferon diminishes the rate of viral replication in patients with chronic hepatitis B infection, but it has little or no effect on the clinical course of the infection. Many further controlled trials will be required before the place of interferon in the management of infectious diseases has been defined.

Active immunoprophylaxis
Problems with existing vaccines. A number of controversies still surround the use of well-established vaccines. Changing environmental circumstances raise new problems for old vaccines. Difficulties may arise when a successful vaccination campaign leads to the virtual disappearance of an infection. Under such circumstances it may be difficult to achieve adequate coverage with a vaccine and, if this is achieved, the risks of serious illness resulting from vaccination may excede the risks of the infection. This situation arose in many countries during the course of the highly successful smallpox campaign, and, in some developed countries, it now applies to poliomyelitis. In such circumstances, the unfortunate victim of a

vaccine accident pays the price of protection of the community at large, a situation which raises difficult social and ethical problems.

The past few years have seen a lively controversy over the use of whooping cough vaccine in the United Kingdom. Reports of occasional serious neurological side-effects following administration of this vaccine, taken in conjunction with some doubts over its efficacy, led to the suggestion that vaccination against whooping cough might no longer be appropriate in the United Kingdom. As a result of this controversy, a fall in the number of babies immunized with triple vaccine (whooping cough, tetanus, and diphtheria) was observed. This fall in vaccine coverage was accompanied by an increase in the number of reported cases of whooping cough. As whooping cough can still be a severe disease in young children in industrialized countries, and because effective whooping cough vaccines can be made, it would seem premature to abandon whooping cough vaccine unless new surveys reveal a high incidence of serious vaccine associated side-effects. In developing countries, where whooping cough is still a major cause of morbidity and mortality, very strong evidence of harmful vaccine side-effects would be required before routine immunization against whooping cough was abandoned.

In Holland and in parts of Scandinavia, killed vaccine is used for routine prophylaxis against poliomyelitis but in the rest of the world oral polio vaccine, which is much cheaper than killed vaccine, is widely used. Studies undertaken in many developing countries have shown poor rates of seroconversion following immunization with oral polio vaccine, perhaps because of the inhibitory effects of breast feeding or because of prior infection with enteroviruses. Therefore, it has been suggested that, despite its high cost, killed polio vaccine should be used instead of oral vaccine in developing countries. However, it is possible that too much attention has been paid to the serum antibody response to oral polio vaccine as opposed to its clinical effect. Studies in several developing countries have shown that oral polio vaccine can control outbreaks of poliomyelitis very effectively. Perhaps it can produce good gut immunity without inducing seroconversion.

In the United Kingdom vaccination with bacillus Calmette–Guérin (BCG) is believed to be an effective means of preventing tuberculosis, a view based on the results of carefully conducted clinical trials. In the United States, enthusiasm for BCG has always been less marked than in the United Kingdom, and serious doubts have been raised about the efficacy of this vaccine in developing countries. These doubts have recently been reinforced by the results of a large study carried out in India, which showed that BCG immunization of children had no protective effect against tuberculosis. The results of this study are very disquieting, for many developing countries devote a significant proportion of their very limited health resources to vaccinating infants with BCG as soon as possible after birth.

New vaccines. The past decade has seen the introduction into clinical practice of several new vaccines (Table 8). The development

Table 8   Vaccines introduced into clinical practice during the 1970s

Bacterial	Viral
Clostridium welchii type C (pig bel)	Hepatitis B
Haemophilus influenzae	Rabies (human cell line)
Meningococcal A + C	
Pneumococcal (polyvalent)	
Pseudomonas	

of effective group A and group C meningococcal polysaccharide vaccines is a major advance, for previous attempts at vaccination against meningococcal disease using whole cell vaccines met with very limited success. Purified polysaccharide vaccines effective against *H. influenzae* and the pneumococcus have also been developed. These polysaccharide vaccines have certain interesting

properties in common which are not shown by more familiar protein vaccines. They act as T lymphocyte independent antigens and they are poor at inducing immunological memory. Thus, it is difficult to achieve an enhanced antibody response by booster immunization. The vaccines are poorly immunogenic in the very young in whom they produce only a weak and transitory antibody response. Formulation of a rational vaccination policy must take into account the unusual properties of these polysaccharide vaccines.

Protective levels of group A and group C meningococcal antibody can be achieved throughout childhood by administration of three carefully spaced doses of vaccine. Such a regimen is likely to be beyond the resources of many of the countries of sub-Saharan Africa where meningococcal disease is still a major clinical problem. In such areas, restriction of vaccination to the control of epidemics may be a more rational policy. Studies are in progress in several countries to determine the most cost-effective way in which pneumococcal polysaccharide vaccines can be used. At present most authorities advocate vaccination only for high risk groups, such as patients with sickle cell disease, the nephrotic syndrome, or cirrhosis, and for those who are over the age of 60 years.

Rabies vaccines produced in infected human cell lines are safer and much more effective than vaccines produced in duck eggs or prepared from brain tissue. Unfortunately these new vaccines are very expensive, thus precluding their widespread use in developing countries where they are most needed.

Preparation of a vaccine from infected human serum is an unconventional approach to immunization but this technique has now been used successfully to obtain protection against hepatitis B infection. Vaccines prepared by partial purification of HB$_s$Ag positive serum produce raised antibody levels in a high proportion of vaccinated subjects. The results of the first large scale trials of hepatitis B vaccines are now becoming available. Vaccination with two doses of vaccine gave American homosexuals over 90 per cent protection against hepatitis B infection and a similar success rate has been achieved in infants immunized with hepatitis B vaccine in Senegal.

Prospects for further new vaccines. The next decade will probably see the introduction of at least as many new vaccines as the last. In the field of bacterial diseases, more effective typhoid and cholera vaccines are likely to be introduced, and some progress is being made towards the development of a vaccine active against toxin producing strains of *E. coli*. Leprosy bacilli grown in the armadillo are providing material for a leprosy vaccine which, it is hoped, will be more effective in preventing this infection than BCG.

Vaccines effective against animal herpes infections have been developed and it should be possible to produce vaccines which will protect against infection with herpes simplex virus, Epstein–Barr virus, and cytomegalovirus. Whether the use of such vaccines would be cost-effective will have to be established. Now that rotavirus can be propagated *in vitro*, it should be possible to develop an attenuated rotavirus vaccine. Such a vaccine might be of considerable value in developing countries where diarrhoea is a major cause of morbidity and mortality among young children.

Progress in the field of parasite vaccines has been slow, and is likely to remain so, because of the complexity of the host's immune response to infection with protozoa and helminths. Furthermore, many of these parasites have evolved highly effective means of outwitting the host's immune response. The optimism of a few years ago that envisaged a malaria vaccine just over the horizon has now waned, and attention has once again been turned to investigation of the basic mechanisms involved in protective immunity to malaria and related infections. The monoclonal antibody technique provides a new tool for carrying out such investigations. By application of this technique it is becoming possible to identify which antigens and antibodies are involved in protective immunity against malaria and other parasites. If the antigens responsible for producing protective antibody can be identified, it should be possible to isolate them in a pure form with the aid of monoclonal antibodies. Such material might provide the source for an effective vaccine.

Non-specific immunostimulants. Resistance to infection can be stimulated actively by immunopotentiators as well as by vaccines. In experimental animals, BCG enhances resistance to malaria and schistosomiasis as well as to tuberculosis. In man, BCG is used to stimulate immunity to tumours and it gives some protection against infection with *M. leprae* and *M. ulcerans*, the cause of Buruli ulcer, as well as tuberculosis.

Levamisole, initially developed as an anti-helminthic, provides an easier means of stimulating immunity non-specifically than BCG. Levamisole enhances the function of PMN and of T lymphocytes. It is more effective in subjects with impaired immunity than in subjects with a normal immune response. Levamisole has been tried in the treatment or prevention of a wide variety of infectious diseases and many claims as to its efficacy have been made. However, few controlled trials have been undertaken and the potential of levamisole in enhancing resistance to infection has yet to be clearly established.

Suppression of the immune response to infection. When an immunopathological response dominates the clinical features of an infection, it may be necessary to depress the immune response of the host, even if this carries the risk of allowing enhanced growth of the causative organism. Such severe reactions are prone to occur at the time at which chemotherapy is started, for this may result in the release of large amounts of antigen from dead or dying microorganisms. The drug used most frequently to prevent or control immunopathological complications of infections are cortiscosteroids. Some examples of the use of corticosteroids to diminish an immunopathological complications of infections are corticoster-

Table 9   Some examples of the use of corticosteroids to diminish the immunopathological response to an infection

Condition	Comments
Acute rheumatic carditis	short-term beneficial effect no protection against valve damage
Chronic hepatitis B infection (chronic active hepatitis)	corticosteroids given with azathioprine increase survival
Mumps orchitis	symptomatic relief; no protection against sterility
Onchocerciasis	diminish reaction to treatment with diethylcarbamazine
P. malariae nephritis	ineffective in most patients
Acute schistosomiasis (Katayama fever)	reported to be effective
Tuberculous meningitis	probably reduces late sequelae

References

Bodmer, W. F. (1980). The HLA system. *Br. med. Bull.* **34**, 213.
Chandra, R. K. (1979). Nutritional deficiency and susceptibility to infection. *Bull. Wld Hlth Org.* **57**, 167.
Fearon, D. J. and Austen, K. F. (1980). The alternative pathway of complement—a system for host resistance to microbial infection. *New Engl. J. Med.* **303**, 259.
Greenwood, B. M. and Whittle, H. C. (1981). *Immunology of medicine in the tropics.* Arnold, London.
Kirkpatrick, C. H. (1980). Therapeutic potential of transfer factor. *New Engl. J. Med.* **303**, 390.
Scott, G. M. and Tyrrell, D. A. J. (1980). Interferon: therapeutic fact or fiction for the 80's. *Br. med. J.* **i**, 1558.
Voller, A. and Friedman, H. (1978). *New trends and developments in vaccines.* MTP Press, Lancaster.
Weller, P. F. and Goetzl, E. J. (1979). The regulatory and effector roles of eosinophils. *Adv. Immun.* **27**, 339.

World Health Organization (1978). Immunodeficiency. *Tech. Rep. Ser. Wld Hlth Org.* **630**.
— (1979). Intestinal immunity and vaccine development: a WHO memorandum. *Bull. Wld Hlth Org.* **57**, 719.

EPIDEMIOLOGY AND PUBLIC HEALTH

A. B. Christie

An infected world. It is an infected world in which we have to live, along with the hordes of other legitimate inhabitants, for example, protozoa, bacteria, and viruses and their phages. To regard these other inhabitants as illegitimate and expendable is to adopt an instinctive, yet highly biased, human attitude. We are in competition but we have no exclusive territorial rights. When we look at other, and larger inhabitants, the mammals, birds, worms, and insects, our rights are even more in question. We have more obviously to share living space with them and the fruits of the earth. Our attitude towards them is more liberal, but the competition is still keen. There has to be some kind of balance. If the viruses and the bacteria became too dominant, man would be dislodged from his high eminence or even cease to exist. Vast pandemics in the past, of plague or influenza, for example, have shown how intense can be the competition from these other teeming inhabitants of our world—but it is their world just as much as ours. To maintain our place we have to study how to meet, or better how to forestall these threats to our well-being or our existence. That study is known as epidemiology, the study of things that can happen to man.

The epidemiological outlook. The outlook must be both detailed and wide. An investigation might at one and the same time include wide geographical cover of a whole country and detailed examination of one local factory; the health of hundreds of travellers over several weeks and the conditions for a few hours on a ship or plane; or the study might extend over many years and look at season, temperature, housing, and movement; flocks, rainfall, and transport; race, religion and politics. The habits of a people are obviously important: smoking, alcohol, occupation and leisure pursuits; family size, breast-feeding, age, sex, heredity, and social position; medical history, operations, drugs, accidents, and deaths from all causes. The natural resources of a country are important: its ability to feed man, or to supply him with fuel to heat his house or drive his machinery; its vegetation and forests, its place above or below sea level, the cover it offers to its animal population, and the delicate microclimate it provides for the survival of overwintering ticks or fleas. All these, and many more, influence the health of man and the spread of disease. Any or all of them may be important in the epidemiology of an infectious disease.

The agent and the disease

Ultimately, the agent and host must come together. The agent is a microbe, helminth, or other pathogen, the host, man. But mere coming together need not mean infection. An organism may live on the skin of man and cause no inconvenience whatever so long as the skin remains intact and healthy. It is a parasite but not a pathogen. Another organism may grow and multiply in man's intestine, still, from the embryological point of view, outside his body. It causes no reaction nor any symptom. This is colonization, but still not infection. In the third instance the body reacts to the presence of the parasite, perhaps by producing antibody against it. There are still no symptoms, but this is infection; subclinical, inapparent, asymptomatic. This infection may be fleeting and the parasite be destroyed, or it may persist, and the host becomes a carrier. In the final instance, symptomatic infection, the parasite forestalls or breaks through the body's defences. The host now suffers from an infectious disease. These are all close encounters between host and parasite: just how they operate may best be studied by examples from different parts of the epidemiological field.

Intestinal infections

Cholera and *E.coli* infections. Many different organisms cause intestinal infections but they do not all act in the same way. *Vibrio cholerae* (see page 5.195) is highly sensitive to gastric acidity, and unless the number of organisms swallowed is very high or the gastric acidity low, very few will get through to the duodenum, and there will be no disease. There are two facts of epidemiological importance here. The water or food swallowed must be heavily contaminated due to bad hygiene or bad sanitation; and if the person swallowing the contaminated food or drink has hypochlorhydria or achlorhydria, he is more likely to suffer from cholera than a person with normal gastric acidity. This association with low gastric acidity, sometimes with previous gastrectomy, has in some outbreaks been very clear. The one factor concerns the external environment, the other concerns an internal host abnormality, but the two are related in an epidemiological sense.

With *E. coli* gastroenteritis of infancy (see page 5.179), there is a similar link between external and internal factors. Human breast milk has a poorer buffering capacity than cow's milk, and the intestinal contents of the breast-fed baby are therefore more acid than those of the bottle-fed baby. *E. coli*, like *V. cholerae*, is sensitive to acid, and *E. coli* gastroenteritis is certainly more common in bottle-fed babies. The lower acidity of their intestinal contents may have something to do with this though it is not the whole explanation. This association is an example of how a cultural or social factor may affect the epidemiological reaction between host and parasite.

When *V. cholerae* does get through the stomach it finds the duodenal environment more alkaline and can multiply freely there. This is colonization only, not infection. Unless the vibrios can first adhere and then bind to the epithelium of the mucosa, they simply pass down the intestinal tract and are excreted in the faeces, causing no symptoms in the host. Antibiotics can at this stage attack and destroy *V. cholerae*. Adherence and binding can be prevented by antibody, adherence by O antibody, binding by antibody against the light toxin (LT) of the vibrio. Disease is caused by the heavy toxin (HT) of the vibrio, which activates adenyl cyclase, but it cannot act until the LT causes binding. The binding is a biological state and cannot be undone by antibiotics. These facts emerge only from study of the internal environment of the host, by aspiration, biopsy, and other means: it is a study just as epidemiological in nature as any study of the external environment. Its immediate aim is an understanding of the encounter between parasite and host; its ultimate aim is to discover some method of treatment or prevention.

Giardiasis. *Giardia lamblia* (see page 5.404) is a protozoon and very much larger than *V. cholerae* or *E. coli*. It is, in fact, its size that is mainly responsible for its pathogenicity. It too dislikes acid but flourishes in the more alkaline duodenal environment where it adheres by a suction disc on its flat surface to the intestinal mucosa. On light microscopy of a biopsy specimen, it can be seen to cover three epithelial cells, and it produces its effects by simply smothering the absorptive epithelial surfaces. However, the attachment is only mechanical rather than biological and can be undone. A drug such as metronidazole which can kill and dislodge the adhering giardiae can therefore lead to clinical cure, whereas, in cholera, a bactericidal drug can affect only those vibrios which are not yet bound to the epithelium and which are therefore not yet causing symptoms. Once again a study of the internal environment reveals the vital elements in a host–parasite conflict.

Rotavirus enteritis. A virus must, of course, invade a cell in order to replicate and survive. Rotavirus (see page 5.91) penetrates the epithelial cells of duodenum and jejunum. As it does so, it loses its outer coat, possibly as a result of interaction between a polysaccharide on the viral cell wall and the enzyme lactase which is secreted on the epithelial surfaces. Intestinal lactase is very high in the infant, especially at the suckling stage, and this may explain why

rotavirus so easily penetrates the epithelial cells of infants. More and more of the infant's lactase-producing sites are used up in the interaction, and there is less and less lactase available to convert the disaccharide lactose in the milk feed into easily absorbable monosaccharides. This leads to an increase in osmotic pressure in the fluid intestinal contents: as a result, more fluid is drawn into the lumen, and this increased fluid load with its high lactose content passes down into the colon. Here the lactose is split by bacteria into various acids which raise still higher the osmotic pressure. The symptom is diarrhoea, as in cholera or giardiasis. The interactions between host and parasites, albeit in the same environment, are very different in all three.

Other forms of intestinal infections. Although *S. typhi* (see page 5.183) enters the body in contaminated food or drink as in these other infections, its behaviour in the intestinal tract is very different. It passes rapidly from the tract through the epithelium and into the host's bloodstream to cause a septicaemic, febrile type of illness. It is not in fact primarily an intestinal pathogen: any effect on the intestinal epithelium is a late one and entirely secondary. Shigellae are also conveyed to man in contaminated food or drink, but they cause diarrhoea mainly by invading and inflaming the intestinal mucous membrane. With campylobacter infection (see page 5.181) diarrhoea is common, but the mechanism of the reaction between parasite and host is not yet understood. There is, however, one epidemiological difference between campylobacter and these other infections. Campylobacters are common parasites of many other parasites, cattle, voles, sea-birds, rats, dogs, sheep, turkeys, and chickens. Not all the campylobacters which infect animals also infect man, but some do, and campylobacter enteritis may come to be regarded as one of the zoonoses, infections which move over very wide and varied epidemiological fields.

The competition between man and parasite does not stop after the latter has entered the human body: it goes on. The pursuit may pass from the epidemiologist to the microbiologist or histologist, and it may be classed as pathogenesis rather than epidemiology, but the study is still essentially an epidemiological one. The aim is to scrutinize every stage of the conflict, now at close quarters, in the hope of finding some way of intervening. Such intervention may eventually take the form of a vaccine to build up the host's defences against the parasite, or a drug to attack it if it breaks through. It is the host, man, that must finally defeat the parasite: the vaccine or the drug helps him to that end.

Zoonoses

Salmonellosis, anthrax, and Q fever. With the campylobacters we reach the zoonoses, and epidemiological enquiry must now cover the needs and habits not only of man, but also of animals, and how, through vector, reservoir host, or otherwise, infection in an animal passes to man. Sometimes the passage is direct and crude, as when man eats animal flesh contaminated with salmonellae (see page 5.175) and so becomes infected. Though the method of transfer in this case is crude, tracing the infection to its origin, back through the abattoir, sale ring, farm, field, and feed, and then overseas to a factory which supplied the feed can be an exacting epidemiological task. A goatherd or shepherd may get his anthrax (see page 5.217) by direct contract with animals in his flock dying under his care, but another worker thousands of miles away may be infected in a factory where the animal's contaminated bones are rendered down for glue. Q fever (see page 5.345) may strike the slaughterer in an Australian abattoir where infected animals are killed. However, the infection may also be spread in contaminated milk, or by aerosol, from animals at pasture, or from straw contaminated by them when under cover. Measures which might remove the danger to man of salmonellosis from contaminated meat would have no effect on the spread of anthrax in a glue factory or of Q fever on a farm.

Plague. The study of the zoonoses is wide, in many senses of the word. It may be wide in the geographical sense as in the case of anthrax just mentioned, or in the epidemic spread of plague across seas and continents. It is wide, too, in the fields of study covered. In plague a mammalogist is required to study in detail the habits of several hundred rodents and other animals that may harbour *Y. pestis* (see page 5.205) or die from the infection. An entomologist is needed to study the many fleas that may act as vectors; their life-style, their feeding habits, which animals they infest, their breeding pattern, and how they overwinter. A microbiologist must study the yersiniae in a plague focus; which variety of *Y. pestis* is around, or perhaps what titre of anti-plague antibody is present in the rodent population.

Rabies. The field is less wide in the case of rabies (see page 5.94), but no less difficult to explore. There are no insect vectors so that spread from animal to man is more direct than in plague, but the variety of animal life and certainly the diversity of animal life-style is scarcely less varied. The fox is the most obvious source of man's infection, but there are resident foxes and itinerant foxes, and it is no easy matter to find out how a fox lives and how it spends its time. Computers and radiotelemetry have been used to study fox ecology, but the findings are not clear. Yet without a precise knowledge of the animal's foraging habits and breeding rites, it is not possible to evolve a reliable method of fox control.

Bats are usually gregarious animals: vampire, insectivorous, and fruit-eating bats roost together in caves, and, though the vampire bats are mainly concerned in the spread of rabies to cattle, the infection can be passed to these other bats, and from them to man. There are 40 known species of bats in North America and 25 have been found to be infected with rabies. Even non-colonial bats may be infected and their infection may be linked, geographically at least, with rabies in foxes in the same area. So the epidemiology is complex. But rabies is not an infection of foxes and bats only: it is found in many other animals, from cattle to mongooses. Man is not a natural host for the rabies virus, for he dies with his infection and the virus dies with him.

Other zoonoses. Rabies, plague, and anthrax are obviously animal-borne diseases or zoonoses, but there is an equally varied picture in the epidemiology of the leptospiroses, the arbovirus diseases, helminth infections, the rickettsioses, and others. The diagnosis of a human infection in any of them merely marks the end, or the beginning, of a long chain of infection through wild life to man. Treatment and control depend on accurate study of all the links in that chain.

Other modes of infection

Airborne infections. In the zoonoses and in the intestinal diseases infectious agents enter the body by fairly obvious and direct routes: they are rubbed into the skin on close contact, injected into the tissues in a sting or bite, or swallowed in our food or drink. In theory, control and prevention are likewise straightforward; prevent bites and stings and swallow only wholesome food and drink and most of these diseases would disappear.

The air, however, may appear to be no other than 'a foul and pestilent congregation of vapours', and while Hamlet was no epidemiologist his view of the atmosphere we may have to live and breathe in is not inapt. The source of airborne infection is always some infected person or animal but whether the agent coughed or breathed out infects some other person depends on many factors more insubstantial than bites, stings, and foul water. Distance is one factor, and temperature and humidity have an influence on the survival of the agent over distance. So clearly crowding and density of exposed people, confinement, ventilation, the everyday manner of life, work, and recreation all affect the spread of the agent from one person to another.

The climate, the weather, and the season of the year all influence spread, but it is no easy matter determining how these act. Cold weather may seem to favour the spread of respiratory diseases, but

the cold may have no more specific effect than causing people to stay indoors and heat their homes. Moreover it has been shown in well-controlled experiments that chilling the body does not increase susceptibility to the viruses of the common cold, and it is now well-established that respiratory infections are no less common in the tropics than in temperate climates. Indeed workers in Arctic and Antarctic stations have often remained remarkably free from colds and other respiratory infections until relief ships in the spring bring visitors and their viruses from countries with much milder climates.

Rheumatic fever. The incidence of rheumatic fever (see page 5.142) was at one time thought to be influenced by damp and cold, but the disease has almost disappeared from damp, cold Britain but remains a common and severe disease of childhood in some hot, dry climates. Why the streptococcus has lost its grip in Britain but not in the Middle East or West Indies, for example, is far from clear. What element is responsible in the climate, in the mode of life, or in the state of nutrition? There seem to be no strains of streptococci which especially lead to rheumatism, although there are strains which appear to be highly nephritogenic. So the epidemiologist has to look for evidence of higher susceptibility or lower resistance in one population than in another, without any clear idea of how such differences might have come about. His investigation must cover age and sex incidence, the rate of infection in siblings and neighbours, the seroconversion state of the population, the frequency of relapses, the response to specific treatment and prophylaxis, and the relation of all these to factors outside the host such as housing, rainfall, and social structure. In this and other diseases there are many variables.

Periodicity of infections. Diseases come and go. In some, like measles, this periodicity seems to depend almost mathematically on the number of susceptibles in the childhood population. It is so highly infectious that few susceptible children escape. The virus does not change, and it cannot spread until the number of susceptibles rises again as new children are born into the population. So unless this natural rise and fall is altered by immunization, the disease will tend to occur in epidemics every few years, the interval varying according to the size and structure of the population. The same kind of periodicity can be seen in other common infections such as rubella and mumps, although in both these examples the disease is not so infectious, asymptomatic infections are common and the time pattern as a result is less obvious.

Influenza. With influenza (see page 5.46) a very different factor affects the epidemiology and periodicity of the disease, namely the changing antigenic pattern of the virus itself. The virus is not stable, like the measles virus, but highly protean. Haemagglutinin (H) and neuramidase (N) are antigens on the surface of the virus and over the years they keep changing. The change may be a minor one in the H or N antigen. Thus the A/England/42/72 and the A/Port Chalmers/1/73 are both still Hong Kong viruses with H_3N_2 surface antigens. These antigens, though basically the same, may differ slightly in their amino-acid sequences, and it may be that, as antibody builds up in the human population against one virus, a minor mutation, or antigenic drift, takes place in the virus and that this new variant can then circulate in the population in spite of its antibody. When virus is grown in the laboratory in the presence of specific antibody such variants do emerge, as they also do when the influenza virus is passaged in immunized mice. This might affect any attempt at mass immunization of man, although sometimes antibody against one variant still gives protection against a closely related one, and antigenic drift does not usually give rise to massive human epidemics by the new variant.

In antigenic shift, by contrast, there is a dramatic change from one H or N antigen, or from both, to completely new and unrelated antigens. H_1 becomes H_2, or H_2 becomes H_3, or H_1N_2 becomes H_2N_3. Here there is no possibility of antibody against one antigen, say H₁, having any effect on another antigen, say H₂, and severe epidemics or a pandemic in human populations may be the result. The mechanism which underlies these major changes is obscure. It is unlikely that the genetic apparatus of the virus could code for all the necessary proteins: nor could the multiple changes in the base sequences of the RNA coding for an antigen take place as rapidly as occurs in the sudden change in the epidemic field, more especially when both H and N antigens change. There is no evidence of any 'bridging' strains linking one antigenic subtype with a succeeding one. It is conceivable that there are several fixed types of influenza virus, a 1918 virus, a 1957 virus, a 1968 virus, and so on, and that one virus takes over as the population with antibody against it dies out leaving a younger population susceptible. There is certainly evidence, serological and virological, that one antigenic type may cause outbreaks separated by many years, though there is little known about where it may be in the interval: perhaps in some animal other than man, perhaps in some human parasite or in a human cell protected in some way from the immune system until recycled into activity by some unknown influence. Perhaps a human influenza virus combines with an animal one to produce a variant with new epidemic thrust. Much is conjecture, but epidemiological and virological research can turn conjecture into fact.

Summary. In this infected world, to take account of the human condition, of the animal creation, and of the micro-organisms and other parasites that plague both, requires an outlook on the part of the epidemiologist as wide and detailed as in any other field of scientific enquiry. The rewards can be great, for the control, treatment, prevention, or even eradication of a disease depends on understanding what causes the disease and how the disease spreads.

The control of infection

Incidence and prevalence To control an infection one must know how it is spreading in a population; its incidence and its prevalence. Incidence measures the number of new cases which occur in a population throughout a given time; the number of cases of typhoid fever, for example, per 100 000 of a city population in one year. Prevalence measures the number of new and old cases per 100 000 at any time during the year; how many cases of typhoid fever there are per 100 000 of the city population on 1 October 1980, for example.

Notification. To obtain these figures there must be some form of notification or ascertainment. Notification may be statutory, that is required by law. In Britain there is a list of diseases which must be notified under Act of Parliament to the health authority: the officer concerned is usually the medical officer for environmental health (MOEH). The person who must notify the MOEH is either the head of the house, or another relative present, or the doctor in attendance: in practice the doctor notifies. The list of diseases comprises the common and also some very uncommon diseases. The purpose of notification is to enable the MOEH or other officer to take any immediate action which may be necessary to control the spread of the disease. It also helps to provide reliable statistics of prevalence and incidence on which wider methods of control, such as immunization or improved sanitation, may be based.

The value of a notification scheme depends on how well it is carried out. This depends somewhat on the importance of the disease: a doctor in Britain might overlook notification of cases of measles during a busy period but would at once notify a case of typhoid fever. Elsewhere because of immense distances, the absence of effective central control, the bureaucracy, or simply because many of the patients who suffer or die from an infection are never seen by a doctor, diseases may be grossly undernotified, and any calculation of incidence or prevalence be highly misleading.

Laboratory ascertainment. A good laboratory service can provide additional information. In Britain and America, for example, weekly statements are published on microbial types isolated throughout the country: these add to the information given by statutory notification and also cover many diseases that are not notifiable. In Britain enterovirus infections are not notifiable, but there are few weeks when such infections do not occur: the laboratory reports reveal these. Illness or deformity caused by cytomegalovirus may not at the time of clinical diagnosis be recognized as an infection and it is not notifiable, but if a laboratory grows the virus the information eventually appears in one of the reports issued by the central public health laboratory service. The same applies to such conditions as herpes simplex encephalitis, psittacosis, salmonellosis, brucellosis, bacteraemia of various types, some animal diseases, and any others that from time to time occur.

A further advantage of such laboratory reports is that whereas infections notified by individual doctors may appear on paper to be unconnected, laboratory reports from different parts of the country may show that they are. This may be most obvious in salmonella infections. One type, say *S. hadar*, may be isolated in widely separated areas of the country: notification to a local health authority would lead to action by the local MOEH, but he might not know that the local outbreak was part of a wide national outbreak of food poisoning. Results coming in from many laboratories would make this clear and might lead to the discovery of one item of food distributed all over the country.

The tracing of a salmonella infection across a country illustrates in a dramatic fashion the value of good reporting and good collaboration. Other studies proceed in a quieter manner but are no less important. The incidence and follow-up of cases of congenital infection, for example, or of deafness or deformity caused by rubella and other congenital or perinatal infections are important examples.

Hospital infection. Infection in hospital is not an 'infectious disease' in the common sense of the term, but hospital infection is an important and possibly an increasing public health hazard. A hospital is a community. There is a fairly stable hospital staff of nurses, doctors, porters, administrative staff, and so on, but hospital patients make up a population highly unstable in the epidemiological sense. They come from all sorts of backgrounds, they are already ill, and during their stay in the hospital community, which may be long or short, many unusual things happen to them, from an injection to a major operation.

The staff and the patients are not the only inhabitants of the hospital. There are many micro-organisms as well. They may already be in or on the patient's body, the endogenous organisms; or they may be in the environment of the hospital, or in or on another person, staff or patient, the exogenous organisms. These organisms can move around in the hospital: operations and other procedures assist their movement.

Venepuncture. Taking a sample of blood is a simple and very common operation. It should be a sterile procedure but organisms from the patient's or the doctor's skin can easily get into the vein. Moreover, if glass syringes are used and not properly sterilized, infection can be transferred from one patient to another. In the old days jaundice in syphilitic patients on treatment was usually regarded as due to the arsenic in the arsphenamine injections—it came on after the first course of ten weekly injections, an incubation period that fitted exactly with that of hepatitis B infection which we now know was the true cause of the jaundice. Disposable syringes have removed this kind of danger, but they must still be used with aseptic care to prevent the entry of chance organisms.

When fluids are injected into a vein, the danger of infection is increased and few doctors have not seen infection follow a badly handled infusion. Even with careful screening, transfused blood can still convey infection, perhaps hepatitis other than A or B. These are simple everyday hospital precedures: when faulty, they take infection straight into the patient's circulation.

Urethral Catheters. The passage of a urethral catheter is a minor procedure to the nurse or the doctor. To the patient, it is a common cause of infection. An indwelling catheter almost always causes infection unless technique and management are perfect. Infection may be regarded as almost a normal complication of catheterization, yet it is an induced infection, an injury for which the hospital is responsible.

Hospital environment. The atmosphere in which a patient is nursed is peopled with micro-organisms. They may come to him in breath from a member of the staff or from a patient in a nearby bed. From the infected wound of another patient they may fall on his bedding and then on to his skin or into his throat. He may have to use a bed-pan or other utensil that has not been properly sterilized. The food or drink he is offered may come from a not-too-hygienic kitchen. Perhaps the unwashed hands of a nurse or doctor are more dangerous to him than anything else in the hospital.

Surgery. Surgery adds a new hazard to the hospital patient. He is wheeled into a new environment, the hospital theatre: and it can be dangerously contaminated with micro-organisms. His tissues are cut and manipulated by the surgeon: peritoneal, pleural, and other internal cavities are laid open and micro-organisms, endogenous and exogenous alike, have a new chance to spread and multiply in his body. Even anaesthesia is not completely safe. The complicated apparatus may not be sterile, and organisms can then be blown into the patient's lungs; or the unconscious patient may aspirate micro-organisms from his gastrointestinal tract during or after the operation. These are hazards unrelated to the condition for which the operation is required, and are examples of hospital infection. After the operation the danger is not over: germs may contaminate the wound, from his own body, from the hospital environment, or carried to him on hands or through the air from some other patient. Mild wound infection may be regarded as almost unavoidable, but it is a hospital infection, a hazard to which the patient is unknowingly exposed.

The high-risk patient. Every normal patient is exposed to hospital infection. Some patients are not 'normal' and are especially prone to infection. These are patients with some immune defect, patients with leukaemia, or on immunosuppressive treatment for some other condition, transplant patients, patients on dialysis or intensive care, or patients undergoing cardiac surgery. These patients may have to undergo complicated surgical manipulations which carry high risks of infection, but these patients are less able than 'normal' patients to withstand such infection, and the intense drug treatment which is part of the programme may itself undermine their resistance. So hospital infection is to them a very special hazard: to those who have to care for them, the doctors and nurses, the risks add greatly to their task. In spite of all the difficulties they must regard them as avoidable.

An unavoidable hazard is age, the very old and the very young. Hospital infection is especially dangerous in geriatric and neonatal wards.

A common hazard. Hospital infection is not a hazard which occurs only after complicated procedures; after cardiac catheterization, intra-arterial cannulation, gastric endoscopy, heart valve replacement, and the like. Nor is it a hazard which occurs only in poor, badly staffed, unsanitary institutions. It is a hazard even in the most sophisticated, modern hospital. It can ruin the best-planned operation, lead to longer stays in hospital, to legal difficulties, and to higher hospital costs. It is not an unusual, unfamiliar occurrence. It is very common in ordinary hospital wards, conveyed most often on hands during simple patient care. Something can be done about hands.

Improving the environment

In its epidemiological sense, the environment covers everything outside a person which may in any way affect him. This includes the air which he breathes and which may carry infective matter towards him; clothing and bedding; all household, school, workshop, and ward equipment; water, sanitary equipment, and plumbing; tools for preparing food, and cooking and storage apparatus in kitchens; heating, ventilating, and air-conditioning appliances. Any of these improperly controlled can lead to infection.

Food hygiene. In some circumstances control is straightforward, if rules are followed. Frozen food should be thoroughly thawed, heat must penetrate to the centre of food during cooking, cooked food must be kept separate from raw food, and if not to be eaten at once it must be quickly cooled. Hands must at all times be carefully washed. Good food hygiene can be achieved by simple measures: but the foodhandlers must be informed, intelligent, and willing.

Water and sanitation. In the developed world, safe water can be had from the tap: it has been processed and rendered free of pathogens at the waterworks. In the underdeveloped world, well or surface water can be far from safe, although something can be done by chlorine baskets in wells if used with care: but often only boiled water is safe. To provide safe water for everyone to drink is one of the heaviest public health tasks of the twentieth century and it may be at least the end of the century before it is achieved.

What goes for water goes also for sanitation. In the developed world it is taken for granted, although it involves immense public works. In the underdeveloped world, sanitation is usually non-existent. One must try to teach latrine or earth closet hygiene, realizing that in this matter one is dealing with aspects and habits of life that are deep in tradition and culture, however unscientific they may be as regards health. It is useless installing modern equipment, even if that were possible, unless life habits also change.

Sterilization. Sterilization means the destruction of all microbial life so that none can reproduce. This is required for instruments used in surgical operations, for dressings, for intravenous fluids, and other medicaments. Disinfection means the destruction of pathogens, germs that might cause disease, and as many other organisms as possible. The skin can be disinfected but never made sterile. Pasteurization of milk is a form of disinfection: pathogens in the milk, such as typhoid or tubercle bacilli, are killed, but thermophilic organisms survive and eventually multiply and turn the pasteurized milk sour. Sterilization can be achieved only by heat: chemicals can be used as disinfectants.

Wet heat is the most effective form of sterilization. An autoclave is an apparatus in which articles are exposed to steam at high pressure. Materials must be placed carefully in the autoclave so that steam can penetrate them. All the air must be evacuated from the autoclave so that only saturated steam is inside, and the pressure must then be raised to ensure penetration and to raise temperature. If all the air is evacuated, the steam turned on and a pressure of 100 kPa (15 lb/in^2) applied, the temperature rises to 121 °C. Twenty minutes at this temperature and pressure kills all bacteria, spores, fungi, and viruses. The steam is then turned off, and the materials inside are dried by vacuum pump. Filtered air is introduced, pressure returns to atmospheric, the autoclave is opened and the sterile contents removed. This is the process still in most common use, but high pressure vacuum autoclaves can produce much higher temperatures and pressures, which cut the operation time to only a few minutes.

Figures on temperature and pressure gauges may not reflect exactly what is going on inside an autoclave; whether, for example, these temperatures and pressures are reaching the centre of materials wrapped in packs. Tests must be carried out routinely with cultures of highly resistant organisms placed in such packs. A culture or spore strip of *Bacillus stearothermophilus* is commonly used: at a temperature of 121 °C it requires 12 minutes to kill 100 000 of these spores.

Some materials cannot withstand steam sterilization; for example, powders, oils and greases, and cutting instruments which may lose their sharp edge. These can be sterilized by dry heat but this takes much longer. Dry heat at 160 °C can take from one to three hours to sterilize some materials, and in a large drying oven there must be a fan to make sure the hot air circulates. Higher temperatures, up to 190 °C, can sterilize in a few minutes but it may not be easy to produce such dry heat.

Ethylene oxide is a gas which mixes completely with air at low pressures: it is an effective sterilizing agent and acts at much lower temperatures than is required in autoclaves or hot air ovens. It acts by denaturing bacterial proteins. It is especially useful for materials which cannot withstand heat sterilization, such as plastics, rubber, and much electronic equipment. The gas is absorbed into many plastics and it must be allowed to diffuse out after sterilization, a process known as aeration, to avoid the local irritant effect. This aeration can take many hours, from 24 to 48 hours, unless a special aeration cabinet is fitted. Ethylene oxide sterilization is highly effective, but it is an explosive gas, the equipment is expensive, and it requires very expert handling.

Sterilization by gamma and other forms of radiation is effective but costly. It is used in very large-scale operations for the supply of disposable syringes, catheters, and surgical dressing packs.

Disinfection. Many chemicals are available as disinfectants but it must be emphasized that none can guarantee sterility, and some give only poor disinfection. Coal-tar disinfectants, such as Lysol, and various phenols, such as Dettol, are useful as 'sanitizers', that is they reduce the level of bacteria over a floor or similar area. They act in the presence of organic material, they have an immediate and a residual effect, especially phenols mixed with neutral detergents (not soaps), but they do not destroy spores and have little action against some Gram-negative organisms: some of these can grow in solutions of phenolic disinfectants. Their main use is in mopping and cleaning storerooms, lavatories, and the like. They often have a strong 'disinfectant smell', but this is not closely related to their disinfectant efficacy.

Formalin is a 37 per cent solution of formaldehyde in water. A 20 per cent solution in ethanol or isopropanol kills bacteria, spores, fungi, and many viruses although it may take many hours to do so. A 1 in 8 solution in water in combination with potassium permanganate is useful for the disinfection of ambulances used for dangerous infections and for the terminal disinfection of rooms. Its disadvantages are that the mixture is explosive and that a highly irritant gas is liberated in the process. The room or vehicle must be sealed for 24 hours, and protective clothing and breathing masks worn by operators.

Glutaraldehyde is chemically distinct from formaldehyde. A 2 per cent alkaline solution in water kills vegetative bacilli and some fungi within five minutes, tubercle bacilli and enteroviruses in ten minutes, and some spores within three hours. The solution must be stored carefully at room temperature, but not for more than a week or two, as otherwise it polymerizes and loses activity. Glutaraldehyde can be used for metal instruments and glass lenses provided they are clean: it is not active in the presence of organic matter.

Ethyl alcohol in a 70 per cent solution in water kills non-sporing organisms within seconds, but not in the presence of blood or pus: it is useful for rapid hand cleansing but does lead to roughening of the skin if used too often. Ethyl alcohol or isopropyl alcohol can be added to other disinfectant agents such as iodine and quaternary ammonium compounds and this greatly increases their speed of action and efficacy.

Iodine in alcohol is a very useful skin disinfectant, though not highly active against spores. Its disadvantages are staining and irritant action: these can to some extent be reduced by combining iodine with anionic detergent surfactants to form iodophors, but these still depend on the release of sufficient free iodine.

Chlorinated lime depends for its action on the release of free chlorine: it acts quickly on vegetative bacteria and some viruses but not so well against spores. Its action is brief because the free chlorine is rapidly lost to the air. It is inactivated by organic matter

and is useful mainly for disinfecting clean utensils. At 1 part per million concentration of free chlorine, it is used for disinfecting drinking water and swimming pools, but the concentration must be kept constant by continuous inflow of chlorine. A chlorinated soda surgical solution is sometimes used in cleaning superficial wounds.

Quaternary ammonium compounds are cationic detergents. They must not be mixed with anionic detergents or soaps. They are active against some Gram-positive bacteria but inactive against many Gram-negative organisms, including pseudomonas, some klebsiellas species, and enterobacters, and have no action against tubercle bacilli, spores, fungi, or viruses. They are good cleansing agents but not reliable disinfectants.

Chlorhexidine and hexachlorophane are often used as skin disinfectants. Care must be taken, especially with hexachlorophane, not to use it over large areas of skin, especially in babies, for there may be danger of toxic absorption. Used with care, either will remove most pathogens which are not normally resident in or on the skin.

Isolation of patients

In many diseases the patient is highly infectious before the typical signs of the disease appear. This is true, for example, of measles and of hepatitis A: in both the organism is passing from the patient before the infection is diagnosed, and in both the patient becomes non-infectious very soon after the typical signs of his illness appear. As far as prevention of spread to contacts or in the community is concerned there is little point in sending such a patient to an isolation hospital. In other diseases, such as typhoid fever, the patient may excrete the organism for weeks after the onset of his illness so that isolation is necessary for the protection of others. Such isolation could be provided in an intelligent, modern home, but the disease can be severe and requires expert nursing and medical care, so that most patients must go to hospital—if there is a hospital to which they can go. In some remote areas of third world countries the patient is isolated in another sense: isolated from all nursing and medical care. Infection is only one of the many health problems in such areas of the world.

The isolation unit. The main duties of the staff of an isolation or infectious diseases unit is to investigate and treat patients suffering from infectious disease. They must try to do this in such a way that infection does not spread to other patients. Sterilization and disinfection, as already discussed, help towards this end, but efforts must also be made to prevent organisms leaving the patient's bedside. This is the essence of isolation. The patient should ideally be structurally separated from other patients, and staff must employ, as far as possible, aseptic techniques in handling the patient, his clothing, bedding, and other equipment.

A completely separate room for each patient is the ideal. There should be an air-lock between the room and the outside corridor. Each room should be separately ventilated and the ventilation system must be constantly supervised to avoid air cross-contamination: legionnaires' disease seems to be related to air-conditioning apparatus.

The aim of structural separation is to prevent micro-organisms being conveyed through the air from one patient to another. Staff are responsible for seeing that organisms do not pass in any other way; for example, on their own hands, on laundry, on soiled instruments and dressings, or on any other fomites. When there is no structural division between patients, prevention of spread of infection depends entirely on staff techniques. This is known as barrier nursing, but the real barrier is staff discipline: it can be surprisingly effective, but not against airborne infection.

Negative-pressure isolators. For the most dangerous infections, especially when no form of immunization is available for staff, it may be desirable to nurse the patient in a sealed negative-pressure plastic isolator. This provides a self-contained microbiologically controlled environment around the patient, and full medical and nursing procedures can be carried out from outside the isolator. The isolator can be set up in a large room and no structural alterations are required other than inlet and outlet for filtered air. The apparatus for filtering the air passing into and out of the isolator must be expertly maintained. The isolator looks cumbersome, but with trained staff there are no great medical or nursing difficulties. The isolator does, however, take up hospital space, it requires constant maintenance, and months or years may pass without its being required at all.

Improving resistance

The standard of life. Micro-organisms can flourish only when they have a good standard of life. One of the two main aims of public health measures must be to reduce that standard by all the methods already discussed. The other must be to improve the standards for the other competitors for environmental space, the human population. Good housing with less overcrowding must lessen the direct spread of infection from person to person, as also must decrease in actual numbers, through family planning: both immense tasks. Most children in the world are undernourished and the state of nutrition is probably linked with infection. Undernutrition may itself interfere with resistance, and certainly after infection an undernourished child does less well than a strong, healthy one. So making sure that everyone is properly fed is another immense public health task in the struggle against infection.

Outside the home there are other dangers: insect vectors of malaria, yellow fever, and other diseases, rodents and the plague, foxes, wolves, and dog bites and rabies, and poor sanitation leading to unsafe food and water and so to typhoid, dysentery, cholera, hepatitis, and poliomyelitis. It is an infected world, unsafe for man in many areas. To improve the standard of life in such areas and so improve resistance to infection is a severe challenge to the public health.

Immunization for travellers. Immunization has probably eradicated one disease, smallpox. Others, such as diphtheria, poliomyelitis, and tetanus, have almost been defeated in the developed world. Elsewhere immunization campaigns are not so easy to manage and with rapid travel there is a two-way danger of spread of infection for travellers to and from the underdeveloped world. They should take precautions.

Smallpox vaccination is no longer required. Yellow fever vaccine is a live vaccine containing an attenuated strain of the virus: only one injection is required and immunity lasts for ten years. Cholera vaccine contains killed strains of the two main serotypes and sometimes El Tor strains as well: two injections are required separated by at least one week but preferably four weeks. Immunity is not very dependable and lasts not more than six months. It need be given only to travellers going to an endemic or epidemic area, but, once there, they must still be careful what they eat or drink. Against the enteric fevers travellers may be given either TAB or monovalent typhoid vaccine. Two doses are required, either 0.5 ml followed by 1.0 ml subcutaneously, or 0.1 ml twice intradermally. The interval should be at least four weeks. Immunity is only partial and will not protect against massive doses of the organism in contaminated food, but may protect against the smaller doses present in drinking water: this immunity may last for three years. Against hepatitis A travellers to areas of poor sanitation should be given one dose of immunoglobulin; this gives protection for several months, possibly not against infection but against symptomatic disease. They may acquire active immunity under cover of passive immunity, and frequent travellers should have their blood tested for hepatitis A antibody: if positive they have become immune. Plague and typhus vaccines are available but should be given only to travellers at very high risk from these infections.

Poliomyelitis is still very much an endemic disease in many parts of the world, and travellers should be given poliomyelitis vaccine, killed or live, either as a booster dose or as the full course of three

doses if not previously immunized. Depending on the traveller's occupation abroad, tetanus can be a greater danger than at home and tetanus vaccine should be given, combined if desired with typhoid vaccine. If children are travelling abroad they should be fully immunized, if not already immune, against measles, diphtheria, whooping cough, tetanus, and poliomyelitis, to all of which they may be exposed in the new country.

For travellers going frequently abroad to tropical countries, the following schedule may be used:

Week	Vaccine	
1	Yellow fever	
3	TAB and tetanus	(1)
	oral polio vaccine	(1)
7	TAB and tetanus	(2)
	oral polio vaccine	(2)
11	oral polio vaccine	(3)
33	tetanus	(3)

Reinforcing doses will be required after the schedule as follows: yellow fever and tetanus vaccines every 10 years, TAB every year, if at special risk, otherwise every three years. Only yellow fever vaccination and cholera vaccination are now required by International Sanitary Regulations, the yellow fever vaccination for travellers to defined areas, and the cholera vaccination only for travellers to infected areas.

Travellers must sometimes travel at short notice, and for them a shorter schedule may be used as follows:

Day	Vaccine
1	yellow fever, TABT (1), and oral polio vaccine (1)
14	TAB (2) and cholera (1) given as TABC
28	tetanus (2), cholera (2), and oral polio vaccine (2)

The third dose of polio vaccine must be given one month later, probably abroad, and the third dose of tetanus vaccine six months later.

Travellers to countries where malaria is a risk, even if they spend only an hour or two in a port or airport there, should have correct advice about prophylaxis, which differs according to the drug resistance of the prevailing malaria parasite. Daily proguanil or weekly pyrimethamine were once effective, but there remain few areas where the parasites are sensitive to these drugs. For resistant strains, a combination of pyrimethamine and dapsone (Maloprim) or pyrimethamine and sulfadoxine (Fansidar) may be effective. Chloroquine is best reserved for treatment. The drugs should be taken immediately before or on entry and continued for at least one month after leaving the area. Expert up-to-date advice should always be obtained.

Immunization in epidemics. Routine immunization against the common infectious diseases is dealt with elsewhere. Is immunization of any avail during outbreaks or epidemics? In smallpox outbreaks in Britain in the past, vaccination certainly prevented the spread of the disease, but it was vaccination of contacts or exposed persons, ring vaccination, not mass vaccination. It was this policy of ring vaccination that eventually led to success in the world eradication programme. When cases of poliomyelitis begin to appear in a population which is normally free of it, the feeding of live oral polio vaccine on a wide scale can bring the threatened outbreak to an end: the attenuated vaccine virus colonizes the intestinal tracts of the population, and the wild virus cannot then circulate. Influenza vaccine given in the early autumn to elderly people and other highly susceptible groups may give them some protection against the winter epidemic, the difficulty being to forecast the antigenic strain of virus likely to be circulating.

In residential institutions for children there may be scope for vaccine trials in outbreaks. Can measles vaccine be given quickly enough to other children to protect them when one or two develop the disease, or is a live dysentery vaccine of use in the face of continued attacks of the disease among the children? New immunization procedures will come with new vaccines, so it is perhaps appropriate to end on a questioning note.

Micro-organism and man

Micro-organisms have a tenacious hold on life. Man with his new techniques, his immunosuppressions, and his ingenious new manipulations of the human body is constantly offering them new territories to explore. They are only too ready to do so and to circumvent obstacles man tries to place in their way. They develop resistance to his drugs or change their antigenic shape. They have more experience in the field than man.

References

Bennett, J. V. and Brachman, P. S. (eds.) (1979). *Hospital infections.* Little Brown, Boston.
Mandell, G. L., Douglas, R. G., and Bennett, J. E. (eds.) (1979). *Principles and practice of infectious diseases.* Wiley, New York.
Christie, A. B. (1980). *Infectious diseases: epidemiology and clinical practice*, 3rd edn. Churchill Livingstone, Edinburgh.
Ramsay, A. M. and Emond, R. T. D. (1978). *Infectious diseases*, 2nd edn. Heinemann, London.

PHYSIOLOGICAL CHANGES IN INFECTED PATIENTS

P. A. Murphy

The physiological responses which are observed in infected patients are generally divided into the local inflammatory response; and systemic features such as fever, neutrophil leucocytosis, and shock. However, it is becoming increasingly clear that this distinction is invalid; bacterial shock simply represents a large scale version of local inflammation, and the same cells and enzymatic cascades participate in both. Detailed knowledge of these processes is still incomplete, but at least one protein synthesized by macrophages stimulates the immune response locally, and causes fever and associated changes when it is liberated into the circulation.

Both the local and the generalized inflammatory response can be triggered by a wide variety of agents. However, it is possible to break them down into three main categories. All bacteria contain polymers in their cell walls which cause inflammation. Bacteria may secrete enzymes and cytolytic toxins, but these are generally of minor importance. Immunological responses, mediated either by antigen–antibody complexes, or by sensitized cells, form a second large category. Drug reactions and auto-immune diseases are the prime examples, but immunological responses contribute in varying degrees to the inflammation caused by bacteria, viruses, fungi, parasites, and tumours. The final category is that of tissue damage. The initial reaction to viral infections is generally attributable to cell death, and the inflammatory response to infarcts and trauma is entirely so caused. Obviously, severe inflammation of any type may be enhanced by cell death. A small minority of cases do not fit into any of these three categories; thus, fever in Hodgkin's disease is attributable to the production of pyrogens by the tumour cells.

Changes caused by particular organisms. There are a few infections where the symptoms and signs are mostly attributable to specific properties of the causative organism. The production of toxin by the diphtheria bacillus or the binding of poliovirus to receptors on spinal motoneurons determine the course of those diseases. Infectious diseases such as these, and others such as measles, tetanus, leptospirosis, and whooping cough have unique and characteristic symptoms and signs, and can be diagnosed simply on the basis of the history, the physical examination, and a thorough knowledge of epidemiology. However, even when there

are distinctive features, some aspects of the illness are shared in common with other infections. Almost always there is fever; generally, inflamed areas hurt.

Infections without specific features. Most of the infections met with in ordinary clinical practice do not have symptoms and signs which enable one to make an organism-specific diagnosis. Rather, the features suggest acute or chronic inflammation in a particular organ or organs. One diagnoses pneumonia, meningitis, urinary tract infection, or endocarditis. The species of organism responsible may be guessed at, but the only safe method of diagnosis is through the laboratory. Competent clinicians cannot diagnose streptococcal sore throat and experienced radiologists shown only an X-ray have great difficulty in deciding whether a pneumonia is due to a bacterium, a virus, or a mycoplasma. The fact is that the lung or the pharynx can react to infection in a rather limited number of ways, and that the symptoms, signs, and pathological appearances are very similar whatever the causative organism.

Importance of bacterial numbers. Both locally and systemically, the crucial variable in determining outcome is the number of microorganisms present. This has been best established for bacterial infections, but the available evidence, as well as common sense, suggests that it must also be true for viral and other infections. Numbers are important because the reactions of bacterial and viral components with host enzymes and cells follow log dose-response laws. A minimum weight of endotoxin or peptidoglycan is required to elicit an inflammatory response; the quantity is of the order of one to ten micrograms. A minimum weight of antigen is required to elicit any immunological response; this varies from a few milligrams for an Arthus reaction to a few nanograms for an IgE mediated mast cell degranulation. In all cases, the required weight greatly exceeds that of one organism (about one picogram for a bacterium). Weights which exceed the minimum produce graded responses: in the case of serum components, more molecules are activated; in the case of cells, the response of each cell is proportional to log concentration, and in addition more cells may become activated.

All bacteria produce very similar inflammatory responses because all bacteria have very similar cell wall constituents, and because we have evolved mechanisms which recognize these constituents as foreign even in the absence of previous experience with the particular species. Bacteria can be divided into Gram-negative organisms, whose major irritant constituent is endotoxin; and Gram-positive organisms, whose major irritants are peptidoglycan and teichoic acids. The inflammatory actions of these polymers can be measured in various ways; endotoxin proves to be more toxic than peptidoglycan by one to three orders of magnitude depending on the test used. Experimental studies in the skin of man showed that dead Gram-negative bacteria caused a standardized inflammatory response when injected in a dose of 10^6 organisms. The species of bacteria was not important, and pathogens produced no more inflammation than non-pathogens. Gram-positive organisms were less effective; they had to be injected in a dose of 10^7 organisms to produce the same histological response. *Lactobacillus casei* was as effective as the pneumococcus. This kind of evidence strongly suggests that the main difference between 'pathogens' and 'nonpathogens' is that pathogens have devices such as capsules and leucocidins which frequently enable them to multiply to a titre which will cause clinically obvious infection. It also accounts for the fact that almost any organism can cause pneumonia, endocarditis, or meningitis on occasion, and that people with grossly compromised defences frequently develop serious or fatal infections with 'non-pathogens'.

A great deal of clinical evidence supports the view that most of the features of bacterial infection are responses to large numbers of organisms, and that species is of little consequence, provided a critical population is attained. The best systemic example is the accidental intravenous infusion of infected fluids. Fluids infected with Gram-negative organisms frequently cause severe shock and sometimes death; fluids infected with Gram-positive organisms cause high fever, but deaths are rare. This observation corresponds to the measured difference in toxicity between endotoxin and peptidoglycan. Many of the bacteria causing these accidents are of unusual, or even unnamed species, which are incapable of causing any kind of spontaneous disease. Furthermore, antibiotics do not ameliorate the symptoms, and if the patient dies there is generally no evidence of bacterial multiplication in the tissues at autopsy. The only important variable is the number of bacteria given to the patient before the situation is recognized and the infusion stopped. If that number is high enough, death will result. A local example of the same phenomenon is respirator-associated pneumonia. If organisms are allowed to multiply in the nebulizer reservoir and large numbers are subsequently blown straight down the trachea, pneumonia will develop even though the organism may be ordinarily non-pathogenic.

Of course, the idea that one bacterium is much the same as another provided an adequate population is attained is something of an exaggeration. There are clinically valid differences between the thick localized pus of *Staphylococcus aureus* and the rapidly spreading thin pus of *Streptococcus pyogenes*. *Bacteroides fragilis* does have a penchant for invading veins. In each case, the organism secretes a specific enzyme which may explain the observed behaviour. But on the whole, the similarities between organisms of the same Gram class are much more impressive than the differences.

Inflammatory reactions of endotoxin. Endotoxin has genuinely complex actions: it damages a number of different cell types *in vitro* in the absence of any serum components; and it activates a number of enzymatic cascades in normal plasma which generate biologically active substances. A bewilderingly large number of actions of endotoxin have been described, ranging from shock to tumour necrosis. There is no agreed view of which, if any, of these actions is responsible for disease or death.

Endotoxin activates complement by the alternate pathway. Small quantities of IgG antibody greatly enhance this process, and IgM, or large quantities of IgG antibody lead to complement fixation by the classical pathway. In either case, the complement factors C3a and C5a cause vasodilation and increased vascular permeability, and C5a is chemotactic. C3b fixed on the organisms surface opsonizes it for phagocytosis. Defects of either C3 or C5 render the local inflammatory process less efficient. Patients with Gram-negative sepsis have been shown to have evidence of systemic complement activation. Whether this contributes to shock is unknown. Systemic complement fixation by the classical pathway does appear to be necessary for thrombocytopenia, at least in the guinea-pig.

Endotoxin also reacts with the Hageman factor (factor XII). This leads to the activation both of blood coagulation and of fibrinolysis. Platelets may be activated either by the action of endotoxin on their 'atmospheres' of clotting factors or by sticking to strands of partially clotted fibrin. Thrombin is a powerful stimulus for platelet degranulation, which provokes further clotting. Fibrinopeptides are strongly chemotactic for neutrophils. Neutrophils confronted with attractive objects too large to phagocytose degranulate on to them. Neutrophil granules contain thromboplastic substances. In addition, proteolytic enzymes from neutrophil granules can split and activate several components of the complement, kinin, clotting, and fibrinolytic cascades.

The upshot of all this is that agglutinated masses of fibrin, platelets and neutrophils form in the bloodstream of people with Gram-negative sepsis, and are filtered off in capillaries, especially pulmonary capillaries. The obstruction of pulmonary capillaries and the liberation of vasoactive substances from platelets and neutrophils cause leaky vessels, with progressive pulmonary oedema and hypoxia. Occasionally, renal arterioles become obstructed, and renal cortical necrosis may result, especially if the patient is pregnant. Bleeding states due to clotting factor depletion or thrombocytopenia do occur, but are comparatively rare.

The Hageman factor also activates the kinin system by converting plasma prekallikrein to kallikrein. This is a protease which liberates bradykinin from a precursor. Bradykinin is a powerful vasodilator, and is thought to be a major cause of vasodilation in local infection and of hypotension in septicaemia. Certainly people with Gram-negative sepsis show evidence both of kinin precursor depletion and of raised plasma kinin levels. Bradykinin also seems to be a major cause of pain in inflamed areas.

Many features of Gram-negative sepsis can thus be explained as resulting from the widespread activation of mechanisms which are clearly protective at the local level. And yet none of the things discussed so far seems to really get to the root of the problem of endotoxin poisoning. Animals can be subjected to systemic fixation of all C3 and later complement components using cobra venom, without shock or death. Generalized intravascular coagulation may go on for months in patients with certain tumours. The thrombocytopenia of endotoxin poisoning does not occur in the C4 deficient guinea pig, yet the LD50 for endotoxin is unchanged. And total depletion of neutrophils is no defence against Gram-negative sepsis in either animals or man. It may be instructive to consider some recent work on the C3H/HeJ mouse.

This mouse arose as a one-step mutant of the C3H/HeN strain. It is highly resistant to endotoxin, apparently because it lacks an endotoxin receptor on its cells. It is not, however, resistant to Gram-negative infections. On the contrary, while the LD50 of HeN mice for *Salmonella typhimurium* is about 10^4 organisms, which is a typical value for most mouse strains, HeJ mice have an LD50 of less than 10 organisms. Apparently, the inability to 'see' endotoxin when the concentration is low and the bacterial population small leads to a fatal delay in mobilizing the inflammatory response.

Rosenstreich irradiated HeN and HeJ mice, and reconstituted them with bone marrow cells from their own or the opposite strain. The chimeras were tested with endotoxin, and it was found that mice reconstituted with HeJ cells were resistant and those reconstituted with HeN cells were sensitive. This experiment at once establishes that complement components, clotting, kinins, and haemorrhage make only minor contributions to lethality, at least in the mouse. Furthermore, since an HeN mouse reconstituted with HeJ bone marrow cells still has HeN cardiac cells, vascular endothelial cells, and so forth, the entire mouse must be irrelevant except for its bone marrow derived cells. This is important because endotoxin in high concentration does directly damage a variety of cells, and it has been thought that the shock of Gram-negative sepsis might be explained either by primary myocardial failure or by endothelial damage.

Of bone marrow derived cells, the one most exquisitely sensitive to endotoxin is the macrophage. A maximal stimulus occurs at 1 ng/ml. Neutrophils become somewhat sticky when treated with endotoxin at 100 µg/ml, but they do not degranulate or show any other morphological changes. T lymphocytes are essentially endotoxin-resistant. B lymphocytes show a polyclonal mitogenic response to endotoxin, and platelets aggregate and degranulate. Both these cells require 10–100 µg/ml endotoxin to demonstrate the responses. It is evident that the macrophage is more sensitive to endotoxin by four or five orders of magnitude than any other bone marrow derived cell.

Macrophages are known to synthesize and release a number of physiologically active proteins when stimulated with endotoxin. These are collectively known as 'monokines' and include colony stimulating factor, interferon, and a protein recently named interleukin I, which will be discussed below. Stimulated macrophages also secrete prostaglandins, and proteolytic enzymes such as collagenase. Whether any, all, or none of these are concerned with the lethal action of endotoxin is at present unknown. However, it seems a promising line of investigation.

Inflammatory reactions provoked by gram-positive bacterial components. The major irritative components of Gram-positive bacteria are peptidoglycan and teichoic acid. Peptidoglycan is quite efficient at causing abscesses: 10 µg in the skin of man is an adequate dose. There is some doubt as to whether it fixes complement by the alternate pathway at all; certainly if it does it is grossly inefficient. However, since all normal sera contain antibodies against peptidoglycan, it does fix complement by the classical pathway. There is no evidence as to whether it activates the Hageman factor. Peptidoglycan is a powerful activating stimulus for macrophages, but concentrations of 10–100 ng/ml are required (compare endotoxin). The active group appears to be N-acetyl muramyl-lala-D isoglutamine (MDP). This compound activates macrophages in solutions of 10–100 µg/ml, and is at least 100 times more active when coupled to an inert carrier. Macrophages activated by MDP secrete the same substances as do macrophages stimulated with endotoxin.

Teichoic acids are efficient activators of complement via the alternate pathway. In addition, antibodies to teichoic acids are present in all normal sera after infancy, sometimes in large quantity. Teichoic acids have many negatively charged groups and therefore ought to activate the Hageman factor. Something about Gram-positive organisms probably promotes clotting, since they are frequently observed adhering to the surface of platelets, and disseminated intravascular coagulation occasionally complicates Gram-positive sepsis.

Inflammation in non-bacterial infections. It is common clinical experience that the local inflammation of viral infections, and the consequences of viraemia, are much less dramatic than those of bacterial infections. The reason appears to be that most of the damage is due to cell death; few viruses contain components which promote inflammation directly. Large particles such as myxoviruses can activate macrophages, but the concentrations required are huge, and the degree of activation achieved is modest. Very large quantities of antigen–antibody complexes are required to produce clinically evident inflammatory changes, and as soon as large quantitiee of antibody are synthesized, viral infections tend to be suppressed, cutting off the supply of antigen. Dengue haemorrhagic fever is thought to be produced by the effects of antigen–antibody–complement complexes on neutrophils. Focal glomerulonephritis appears to be an immune complex disease in which the antigen is often viral. Some cases of periarteritis nodosa are caused by complexes containing hepatitis B antigens. None of these conditions is common compared to the total incidence of infection with those viruses.

The most serious viral infections, like measles and smallpox, are those in which there is widespread activation of cell-mediated immunity. It is probably no accident that sensitized T cells exposed to antigen secrete a lymphokine which is a powerful activating stimulus for macrophages.

Chronic infections with the tubercle bacillus, histoplasma capsulatum and similar fungi, and tissue helminths such as schistosomes are all characterized by little local reaction at first, followed by chronic fibrosing destructive lesions. Especially in tuberculosis, patients may die when the local lesions have not compromised respiration or some other vital function. This 'toxicity' is generally unexplained, but may also be a response to widespread T cell-mediated macrophage activiation.

Shock. As previously discussed, bacteria can cause hypotension in several ways, especially by activating the complement and kinin cascades. Histamine release is important in dogs and rabbits but apparently not in man.

Hypotension in sepsis is also enhanced by the release of endorphins from the anterior pituitary. This occurs apparently because the amino-acid sequences of ACTH and of β endorphin are stored in the pituitary as part of a single, larger, precursor molecule. When ACTH is released as a response to sepsis, β endorphin is also released, molecule for molecule. In several species it is possible to reverse the hypotension of endotoxin poisoning with morphine antagonists such as naloxone.

The release of ACTH in sepsis is clearly useful, because adrenal corticosteroids protect animals against endotoxin poisoning. The fact that this is closely coupled to the release of a powerful vasodila-

tor is food for thought. No one has ever shown that the reversal of hypotension with vasoconstrictors makes any difference to the outcome of Gram-negative sepsis in man. Some of the evidence even suggests that vasoconstrictors are deleterious. And there is evidence in some animals that vasodilators such as phenoxybenzamine may partially protect them from endotoxin poisoning. Perhaps we should concentrate on restoring the intravascular volume of septic patients, and worry less about the tone of the vessels.

Endotoxin also sensitizes the microcirculation to vasoactive amines such as noradrenaline and serotonin. The overall effect early in sepsis appears to be a shuntiung of blood through arteriovenous anastomoses, with stagnation in the true capillaries. If shock is long continued, blood is re-admitted to the capillaries but flow remains stagnant. The capillary walls leak fluid and protein, and there is a progressive loss of intravascular volume. Shocked patients usually, though not always, have evidence of disseminated intravascular coagulation, and small vessels all over the body may be partially obstructed with microscopic thrombi. In the lungs, this process promotes progressive respiratory failure. Vital organs are thus subjected to arterial hypoxia, inadequate cardiac output secondary to hypovolaemia, and partially obstructed blood vessels. Myocardial failure supervenes quite early, probably because the heart normally extracts almost all the oxygen from the blood supplied to it. This compounds the hypoxia of the brain, kidneys, intestine, and liver. Clinically, one sees various degrees of clouding of consciousness, ranging from lethargy to stupor, and from slight disorientation to frank delirium. Urine flow first diminishes and then ceases. Jaundice may occur if the patient survives long enough. Chemically, there is evidence of progressive liver and renal failure. Lactic acid accumulates in the blood because of glycolysis in the anoxic tissues. The serum pH is lowered, and the heart is even further compromised. Lysosomes are destabilized and their enzymes released in many tissues. This vicious circle soon leads to death. It is thought that the final event may be massive endotoxin influx from the ischaemic bowel.

Fever. Endogenous pyrogens were discovered by Beeson in 1948, who made saline extracts from the cells of acute peritoneal exudates in rabbits. These extracts caused fever when injected intravenously, and were clearly distinguishable from endotoxin, which is also pyrogenic, by biological tests. Since over 95 per cent of the cells in these exudates were neutrophils, he naturally thought that neutrophils contained the pyrogen. It was soon found that much more pyrogen could be obtained by incubating exudate cells in short-term tissue cultures. Blood cells did not secrete pyrogen spontaneously, but could be induced to do so if incubated with various stimuli. Effective stimuli included all the bacterial polymers previously discussed, antigen–antibody complexes, T cell lymphokines, myxoviruses, and certain constituents of dead tissue such as DNA. This is the same list of substances as that inducing inflammation. Using similar methods, pyrogens have been obtained from the cells of many mammals, including man, and similar proteins have been found in alleged poikilotherms such as lizards and fish.

In all cases investigated, inhibitors of protein synthesis block pyrogen production by stimulated blood cells. Beeson was successful because the exudate cells became activated in the peritoneal cavity before he removed them for extraction. In rabbits, synthesis of pyrogens was directly proved by stimulating cells in the presence of radiolabelled amino acids, and purifying the endogenous pyrogens to homogeneity. The purified pyrogens were radioactive, and the same pyrogen was obtained whatever stimulus was used to excite the cells.

High fevers occur in diseases such as tuberculosis, where neutrophils are not prominent in the infiltrates, and in patients with agranulocytosis. It was therefore thought likely that macrophages could secrete pyrogens, and this was shown to be the case. A series of workers showed that macrophages secreted pyrogens in response to the same stimuli that activated 'neutrophils', and that pyrogen secretion was blocked by inhibitors of protein synthesis. Other cells were investigated, including lymphocytes, and were found not to secrete pyrogens. It was, therefore, generally agreed that in acute infections neutrophils made pyrogens, and that in chronic infections and immunological responses, macrophages made pyrogens. Fever in patients with malignant disease who were not infected occurred either because of attempts to reject the tumour or because the malignant cells were of the macrophage line and secreted pyrogens spontaneously.

The endogenous pyrogen made by rabbit 'neutrophils' had been purified to homogeneity, and the question of whether macrophage pyrogen was the same or different was addressed. It was found that rabbit macrophages secreted two pyrogens which could be clearly distinguished on biochemical and immunological grounds. One of these was identical with that previously isolated from 'neutrophils'. Since macrophages secreted all the known endogenous pyrogens, neutrophils were reinvestigated. Neutrophils separated from macrophages by density gradient separation responded to chemotactic stimuli, phagocytosed and killed bacteria, and made normal quantities of superoxide. However, they did not make pyrogens. Subject to future discoveries, the present position appears to be that the pyrogens made by exudates containing mostly neutrophils are attributable to the few macrophages which are also present.

In man, pyrogens have been demonstrated in infected pleural and peritoneal fluids. The characteristics of the fevers were quite different from those produced by injections of endotoxin. Transudates due to cirrhosis or nephritis were never pyrogenic. Pyrogen in the circulating blood of infected patients has been difficult to demonstrate, but success was achieved by one heroic experiment in which 200 ml of plasma was removed from each of four patients with Rocky Mountain Spotted Fever, and the entire 800 ml infused into a volunteer.

The mode of action of pyrogens has been worked out in animals, and seems certain to apply also to man. Minute quantities of endogenous pyrogen caused fever when injected into the anterior hypothalamic or pre-optic nuclei of cats or rabbits. These nuclei contain temperature-sensitive neurones, and thermoregulatory responses are obtained if they are warmed, cooled, or stimulated electrically. Other areas of the nervous system were not sensitive to injections of pyrogens. The quantity of endogenous pyrogen required was about 1 per cent of that required to cause fever when injected intravenously. Endotoxin injections caused fever when injected into the same nuclei, but the onset was late, the quantity required was comparable with that required on intravenous injection, and examination of the nuclei when endotoxin fevers were just starting showed that an inflammatory infiltrate was present.

Wit and Wang studied the effect of intravenous injection of pyrogens on the thermal sensitivity of anterior hypothalamic neurones. Neurones were found which increased their firing rate markedly in response to small rises in temperature. Pyrogens abolished the increased firing rate, and aspirin restored it to normal. This suggested that pyrogens might cause fever by stimulating prostaglandin synthesis in the hypothalmic region. This hypothesis is supported by evidence that prostaglandin E_1 levels in cerebrospinal fluid are increased after intravenous injection of pyrogens, and by the fact that small quantities of prostaglandin E_1 are pyrogenic when injected into the anterior hypothalamus. Exactly how increased prostaglandin levels lead to a resetting of the hypothalamic 'thermostat' is not yet clear.

Other systemic changes associated with fever
Changes in plasma proteins. Infected people usually show a stereotyped array of changes in their plasma proteins. The erythrocyte sedimentation rate is raised because of increased synthesis of fibrinogen by the liver. Several other proteins present in normal plasma or serum are also synthesized in increased quantity during infection; they include the haptoglobins and caeruloplasmin. In addition, some proteins which are not present at all in normal serum are synthesized in very large quantity by the liver. Twenty-four hours after the onset of an infection, the concentration of C

reactive protein (CRP) in serum may reach 3 mg per ml. This represents the synthesis of about 15 g of protein in a 70 kg man. Another protein synthesized *de novo* in even larger quantities in the serum amyloid-associated (SAA) protein. Proteins whose concentration increases during infection are known as the 'acute phase reactants'; most have $\alpha2$ globulin mobility, and they are responsible for the increased density of this area in serum electrophoretic strips from infected people.

CRP binds to phosphoryl choline residues; these are commonly present in bacterial cell walls. Both teichoic acids and endotoxins may contain such residues. Bound CRP fixes complement and facilitates phagocytosis of organisms. It is thus a skind of primitive antibody, non-specific and inefficient, but available in large quantity shortly after the onset of infection. SAA is an apolipoprotein, and its relative insolubility may lead to its deposition in tissue as amyloid fibrils in chronic suppurative states such bronchiectasis and osteomyelitis. It presumably has an adaptive function also, but what that might be is unknown. Nor is it clear why increases in fibrinogen and haptoglobins might be useful.

Changes in serum iron. Sick people also show a marked fall in serum iron and serum zinc. The fall in serum iron is clearly adaptive, because all organisms need iron to grow, and the virulence of several pathogenic bacteria can be enhanced by many orders of magnitude if enough ferric iron to saturate serum transferrin is given intravenously. As regards zinc, no evidence is available. Finally, sick people generally show a neutrophil leucocytosis, which again is obviously adaptive.

Mediators of acute phase changes. All these acute phase changes are induced by small proteins obtained from phagocytic cells (macrophages) stimulated by exactly the same substances which induce the synthesis of pyrogens. Indeed, there is very strong evidence, not yet definitive, that these changes *are* induced by pyrogens. All the varied biological activities, from fever to neutrophil leucocytosis, co-chromatograph, co-purify, and are inhibited by antibodies raised against purified pyrogens. Both species of rabbit endogenous pyrogen possess the complete range of activities, although not all are induced with equal efficiency.

Changes during prolonged infections. Several of the acute phase changes reviewed also lead to serious problems if the infection is long continued. Fever raises the metabolic rate approximately 15 per cent for every 1 °C of temperature elevation. Sick people seldom have good appetites, and they tend to eat mostly fluid and carbohydrate. Rarely is the calorie intake sufficient to balance the increased metabolic load, and the protein intake is almost always subnormal. Consequently, amino acids are mobilized from muscle and bone matrix, and are taken up by the liver. Some are used to synthesize acute phase proteins, but most are deaminated and used for gluconeogenesis. The result is a strongly negative nitrogen balance. Muscular wasting is always seen in prolonged infections, and loss of calcium from bone may cause semi-spontaneous fractures or renal calculi.

The iron removed from the plasma during infection is sequestered in the reticulo-endothelial system, and is not available for haemoglobin synthesis. This contributes to the 'anaemia of infection'. Serum albumin synthesis is repressed when the synthesis of acute phase proteins is switched on, and the serum albumin falls progressively if infection is prolonged.

Local actions of pyrogens. Within the last three years, it has been realized that pyrogens have local actions as well as systemic ones. They induce a selective degranulation of neutrophils, with release of lysozyme and lactoferrin extracellularly. Both these proteins are antibacterial and lactoferrin may be a modulator of the immune response.

Pyrogens are also identical with macrophage derived proteins named lymphocyte activating factors (LAF). These have been shown to induce the maturation of immature T cells and to potentiate a large number of T cell dependent immune responses, from antibody synthesis to the generation of cytotoxic cells. All these actions were discovered independently and only gradually did immunologists realize that they were all mediated by the same protein or proteins. (So far, the rabbit is the only species in which two pyrogens have been clearly distinguished; there is preliminary evidence that man has at least two, the mouse appears to have only one.) Because LAF appeared to be the first clearly defined molecule which acted as a messenger between co-operating immune cells, it was recently given the name 'interleukin I'.

Finally, pyrogens are identical with macrophage derived proteins which induce the synthesis and secretion of collagenase from a cell in the synovial membrane of joints. The original authors were interested in the pathogenesis of rheumatoid arthritis; obviously collagenase might account for the destruction of articular cartilage, joint capsules, and ligaments characteristic of that disease. More generally, if cells responding to pyrogens in this way are scattered throughout connective tissue, that could be an important cell-mediated mechanism in the inflammatory response.

Summary. Recent discoveries have made it possible to draw together observations on the local inflammatory response, generalized responses to inflammation, and septicaemia. In bacterial infections, cell wall polymers are recognized as foreign by processes which do not require antibody. In viral infections, the initial insult is usually the death of infected cells, which liberate endogenous inflammatory mediators. Immune responses, mediated either by antigen–antibody complexes or by sensitized lymphocytes become increasingly important in chronic inflammations. Each of these three mechanisms activates the same enzymatic cascades; the complement, kinin, coagulation, and fibrinolytic systems. The crucial cell which is activated appears to be the macrophage.

What happens during an infection is a function of how far the invading organism succeeds in multiplying. Single organisms are disposed of by phagocytosis without any other response, and even a few thousand bacteria cause only microscopic inflammation. A few million organisms incite the generation of substances which cause enough vasodilation, increased capillary permeability, and chemotaxis to be clinically visible as inflammation. Many millions of organisms are required to cause local abscesses; the tissue destruction is actually caused by proteolytic enzymes liberated from dead and dying phagosytic cells.

Macrophages are stimulated by very small quantities of bacterial polymers and other inciting agents. Their secretory products make the local environment less favourable for both bacteria and viruses, and also potentiate the local immune response. It is possible that gross over-stimulation of macrophages contributes to local tissue destruction.

The macrophage protein known variously as endogenous pyrogen, lymphocyte activating factor, interleukin I, and leucocytic endogenous mediator appears to mediate several of the local features of inflammation. When large quantities are formed in the local lesion, it leaks into the circulation and induces fever, the acute phase serum changes, and neutrophil leucocytosis.

Septicaemia occurs when large numbers of organisms enter the bloodstream, and there is systemic activation of the plasma enzyme cascades and of macrophages. Most experimental work to date has concentrated on the plasma protein systems, and certainly these can account for the hypotension, disseminated intravascular coagulation, and progressive pulmonary dysfunction. However, recent evidence makes it seem likely that activation of the large numbers of macrophages lining the circulation is important in causing death.

References

Agnello, V. I. (1978). Complement deficiency states. *Medicine, Baltimore* **57**, 1.

Beeson, P. B. (1948). Temperature elevating effect of a substance obtained from polymorphonuclear leucocytes. *J. clin. Invest.* **27**, 524.

Bodel, P. (1974). Pyrogen release *in vitro* by lymphoid tissue from patients with Hodgkin's disease. *Yale J. Biol. Med.* **47**, 101.

— and Atkins, E. (1967). Release of endogenous pyrogen by human monocytes. *New Engl. J. Med.* **276**, 1002.

Braude, A. I. (1958). Transfusion reactions from contaminated blood. Their recognition and treatment. *New Engl. J. Med.* **258**, 1289.

Breese, B. B. and Disney, F. A. (1954). The accuracy of diagnosis of beta streptoccal infections on clinical grounds. *J. Pediat.* **44**, 670.

Faden, A. I. and Holoday, J. W. (1980). Experimental endotoxin shock: The pathophysiologic function of endorphins and treatment with opiate antagonists. *J. infect. Dis.* **142**, 229.

Fearon, D. T., Ruddy, S., and Schur, P. H., *et al.* (1975). Activation of the properdin pathway of complement in patients with Gram-negative bacteremia. *New Engl. J. Med.* **292**, 937.

Glode, L. M., Mergenhagen, S. E., and Rosenstreich, D. L. (1976). Significant contribution of spleen cells in mediating the lethal effects of endotoxin *in vivo*. *Infect. Immunol.* **14**, 626.

Greisman, S. E. and Hornick, R. B. (1972a). Cellular inflammatory responses of man to bacterial endotoxin. A comparison with PPD and other bacterial antigens. *J. Immunol.* **109**, 1210.

—, — (1972b). On the demonstration of circulating human endogenous pyrogen. *Proc. Soc. exp. biol. Med.* **139**, 690.

Hanson, D. H., Murphy, P. A., and Windle, B. (1980). Failure of rabbit neutrophils to secrete pyrogen when stimulated with staphylococci. *J. exper. Med.* **151**, 1360.

Klempner, M. S., Dinarello, C. A., and Gallin, J. I. (1978). Human leucocyte pyrogen induces release of specific granule contents from human neutrophils. *J. clin. Invest.* **61**, 1330.

Mason, J. W., Kleeberg, V., Dolan, P., *et al.* (1970). Plasma kallikrein and Hageman factor in Gram-negative bacteremia. *Ann. intern. Med.* **73**, 545.

Merriman, C. R., Pulliam, L. R., and Kampschmidt, R. F. (1977). Comparison of leucocytic pyrogen and leucocytic endogenous mediator. *Proc. Soc. exp. Biol. Med.* **154**, 224.

Murphy, P. A., Simon, P. S., and Willoughby, W. F. (1980). Endogenous pyrogens made by rabbit peritoneal exudate cells are identical with lymphocyte-activating factors made by rabbit alveolar macrophages. *J. Immunol.* **124**, 2498.

Rawlins, M. D., Huff, R. H., and Cranston, W. I. (1970). Pyrexia in renal carcinoma. *Lancet* i, 1371.

Snell, E. S. (1962). Pyrogenic properties of human pathological fluids. *Clin. Science* **23**, 141.

Tew, J., Calanoff, C., and Berlin, B. S. (1971). Bacterial or non-bacterial pneumonia: accuracy of radiological diagnosis. *Radiology* **124**, 607.

Wit, A. and Wang, S. C. (1968). Temperature sensitive neurons in the preoptic/anterior hypothalamic region: actions of pyrogen and acetyl salicylate. *Am. J. Physiol.* **215**, 1160.

Principles of antimicrobial therapy

A. Percival

Use and abuse of antimicrobials

During the years of the modern era of antimicrobial therapy, probably the two most dominant features to emerge have been overuse and the appearance and spread of resistant microorganisms. They are, to a large extent, inter-related. The challenges of microbial resistance have, so far, been met by the ability of the pharmaceutical industry to produce new agents, but it can not guarantee to continue to do so. Therefore pleas for more rational prescribing are often made to prolong the life of established and new antibiotics, but all too frequently unheeded.

Only relatively recently has antimicrobial use been subjected to much critical analysis. In 1972, a retrospective study in one American hospital judged only 13 per cent of antimicrobial therapies to have been rational, 21 per cent questionable, and 66 per cent irrational, either because such treatment was unnecessary or an inappropriate agent was given. For approximately half the treatments, the indication was prophylaxis. In one-day prevalence surveys in 43 English hospitals in 1980, 22 per cent of patients were receiving antimicrobials, 29 per cent of them two or more agents. In acute medical wards, 28 per cent of patients were having antimicrobial therapy, and in intensive care 56 per cent. In England and Wales, 20 million courses are given, annually, for respiratory tract infection. There is no evidence that localized soft-tissue infections, such as boils and carbuncles in otherwise healthy individuals, will benefit from antimicrobial therapy. Yet in 1977 95 per cent of patients presenting to their English general practitioners with such infections were given antimicrobials, usually orally. The great majority of these infections are caused by *Staph. aureus*, mostly resistant to penicillins, G and V, and ampicillin or its derivatives. Nevertheless, those antibiotics comprised 50 per cent of the market for these infections, but the more rational β-lactamase stable penicillins, such as flucloxacillin, only 8 per cent. Approximately half the prescriptions for treating chronic ulcerative soft-tissue infections were for either fucidin or gentamicin. These antibiotics can be of great value in the management of life-threatening systemic infections, particularly when caused by bacteria resistant to many other antimicrobials, but are not known to be any more effective, topically, than antibacterials which can not be given systemically. Also, it is in just this kind of lesion that bacterial resistance tends to emerge; the organism may then be introduced into a hospital following admission of a patient so treated. A personally conducted review revealed that 60 of 100 babies had received at least one course of antimicrobial treatment during their first year of life. In 70 per cent of those treated, the indications were trivial and not once was there any attempt made to verify the measure by taking a diagnostic specimen for microbiological investigation.

Even in infections with an established microbiological cause, antimicrobial therapy may not only be of no value but a disadvantage. In 1970, a placebo-controlled trial showed that oral neomycin did not reduce the duration of symptoms in patients suffering from salmonella gastroenteritis but, in fact, prolonged the excretion of salmonella in a higher proportion in those treated. Nevertheless, at least 20 oral preparations containing neomycin or similar related agents continued to be available for treating gastrointestinal infections until regulatory committees tried to restrict this practice.

Thus, there is ample evidence of the widespread use of antimicrobials, often irrationally, even in those countries where such drugs can only be supplied on prescription from a medically qualified practitioner. In many other countries, antimicrobials can be purchased by anybody. It is important to recognize that troublesome resistant micro-organisms often first appear and subsequently become widespread in these countries; this possibility should be considered in treating infections in those who have travelled recently.

Understandably, facilitating the appearance and transfer of resistant organisms is of much less immediate concern to the attendant clinician than relieving a sick patient. However, unnecessary antimicrobial therapy may have other harmful consequences. Some antibiotics, notably penicillins, can produce severe, even fatal, reactions in the sensitized, allergic patient. A number of deaths have followed needless administration of penicillin. Some antimicrobials have other potentially serious side-effects, particularly if the patient's capacity to excrete them is transiently or permanently impaired. Antimicrobials, particularly those with a wide spectrum of activity, alter the normal flora of the body, allowing colonization by and multiplication of resistant micro-organisms. These may then cause secondary infection; for example candidal vaginitis in a healthy woman, or a systemic infection in a highly susceptible patient. Recently, attention has been drawn to a serious complication, pseudomembranous colitis. This is caused by the toxin produced by the anaerobic bacterium, *Clostridium difficile*, which is relatively insusceptible to many commonly used antimicrobials and can multiply when the normal colonic flora is suppressed.

The advantages of antimicrobial therapy have been most clearly seen in those acute bacterial infections which had a high mortality before the introduction of antibiotics. In endocarditis, the mortality was 100 per cent and is still approximately 20 per cent overall, though death usually is due to cardiac failure or embolic complications rather than unsuccessful antimicrobial treatment. In bacterial meningitis, a 90 per cent mortality has been reduced to 8–20 per cent depending on the type of infecting bacterium and in acute osteomyelitis from 50 per cent to less than 1 per cent.

Also, there are many other infections in which morbidity and the serious consequences of spread, both systematically in individual patients and to others within the community, have been considerably diminished. For instance, it is often argued that early treatment of relatively minor upper respiratory tract infection has been the major factor in the declining instance of mastoiditis following acute otitis media and rheumatic and scarlet fevers following streptococcal sore throat.

Conversely, in patients made highly susceptible by underlying diseases, major surgery, instrumentation, cytotoxic, or immuno-suppressive therapy, infection remains a major problem. In such patients, the responsible micro-organisms have often become those which were little encountered in the pre-antibiotic era and the concept of opportunistic pathogens has emerged. Predictably, these organisms prosper because they already are resistant or can readily acquire resistance to commonly used antimicrobials. In addition, some of these organisms survive well in the external environment and episodes of hospital cross-infection caused by them are an increasing difficulty. The commonest cause of hospital-acquired infection now appears to eminate from infected indwelling urinary catheters. Certainly, the patterns of hospital diagnostic microbiology have changed markedly since the introduction of antimicrobial therapy. Infection by Gram-negative organisms such as *Klebsiella*, *Pseudomonas*, *Enterobacter*, *Serratia*, previously rare, have now become common as well as those by the traditional pathogens such as *Staph. aureus*, which also have ability to become antibiotic resistant.

Reasons for inappropriate antimicrobial therapy (Table 1). The most difficult thing for a doctor to do for a patient is nothing, because his prestige and concern and the patient's fear of illness and faith in the doctor demand that some form of treatment be given. It is often said by doctors that the relatively well-informed modern public ask for antimicrobial treatment, but it is probable that doctors themselves, rather than the informative media have induced the public to do so. Nevertheless, withholding antimicrobial therapy for an apparently trivial or presumed viral infection is more difficult than to give antibiotic treatment, particularly for children in domiciliary practice. Here, the doctors' fear of the possibility of relatively rapid deterioration and parents' anxieties

Table 1 Reasons for inappropriate antimicrobial therapy

1. Desire to benefit the patient
2. Fear of missing a treatable condition
3. Misconception that antimicrobials may do good but can do no harm
4. Fear of litigation
5. Insufficient knowledge of antimicrobials
6. Insufficient knowledge or rationalization of the possible aetiological agents
7. Confusion due to multiplicity of similar antimicrobials
8. Expert guidance not readily available or sought

would be likely to increase further consultations if antibiotics were withheld. However, greater reluctance to use antimicrobials unnecessarily is required, both in domicillary and hospital practice, if the selective pressures encouraging the spread of resistant micro-organisms are to be contained. The reality of potential harmful effects of antimicrobial therapy, both short term in individual patients and long term in favouring emergent resistance, needs greater consideration.

Fear of litigation on grounds of failure to give antibiotics is an unhelpful but inevitable development, particularly in the United States. However, concern about being accountable for giving an inappropriate agent ought to stimulate a more rational approach or lead to seeking informed advice.

Despite the circulation to all doctors of much clear guidance on appropriate therapy for most infections and a very full account of the problems of and developments in antimicrobial therapy in all the leading medical journals, adequate knowledge is often lacking. Unfortunately, as with other drugs, there are too many antimicrobials with different proper and trade names but similar antimicrobial properties. Too much emphasis is made in promotional activities of marginal differences both in antimicrobial effects and pharmacological characteristics. The only solution appears to be a greater availability and utilization of informed advice by contact and written guidance policies both within the hospital and for domiciliary practice. In the United Kingdom, this advice usually is provided by medical microbiologists partly because, unlike the United States, infectious-disease physicians are rarely employed in teaching or district general hospitals.

Choice of antimicrobial therapy

In choosing an appropriate antimicrobial for treatment, it is important to recognize that:

1. For every clinical presentation which could be an infection, there is always a variety of different microbial causes, but with varying degrees of probability according to the clinical history and features.

2. No single antimicrobial is likely to be active against all the possible infecting organisms.

3. It is rare for any antimicrobial predictably to be active against every isolate of any particular species.

4. Providing that the causative micro-organism is fully susceptible, most infections respond equally well to a variety of antimicrobials if they reach the infected site in sufficient concentration. Therefore, it is unlikely that there will ever be a predictable, single universal cure all or a single 'best drug' for any particular type of infection.

These generalizations need and should not be a justification for treating every infection with a combination of two or more antimicrobials designed to give total cover against all possible infecting organisms, because such therapy usually is potentially more toxic, has greatest considerable side-effects, is the most exacting to administer and monitor, and is the most costly. The essential features for rational antimicrobial therapy are a knowledge of the likely infecting organisms, their probable susceptibilities to antimicrobials, the confirmation of the identity and sensitivities of the infecting agent in a particular patient *by taking appropriate diagnostic specimens before antimicrobial treatment is started*, and a reasonable understanding of the antimicrobial, pharmacological, and potentially harmful properties of the antimicrobials to be used.

Choice of initial therapy—clinical diagnosis. For life-threatening infections, antimicrobial therapy has to be started as soon as possible and before the nature of the infecting organism and its antimicrobial susceptibilities can be established. Even for less severe infections, generally it is more convenient to do likewise. Therefore, having made the differential diagnosis on clinical grounds, initial treatment is based on probabilities. Obviously, the ranges of possible infecting organisms vary, both in number and type, for different infections.

For some infections, rationalization is straightforward. The bacterial causes of sore throat are few; *Strep. pyogenes*, occasionally *Corynebacterium haemolyticum*, rarely *C. diphtheria*, the remainder being viral. The first three predictably are sensitive to penicillins G or V, or erythromycin, a suitable alternative for the penicillin-allergic. Broad-spectrum penicillins, such as ampicillin, are no more effective but have more side-effects, particularly in patients suffering from glandular fever. Resistance to tetracycline is not uncommon and that type of antibiotic can damage the teeth of infants and children if repeated or prolonged courses are given. Therefore, it is clear what is both suitable and what is not. A urinary tract infection occurring in a patient at home will be caused by *E. coli* (85 per cent), *Proteus mirabilis* (11 per cent), or micrococci (4 per cent), but the sensitivities of these organisms are less predictable. Nitrofurantoin will not be effective against proteus, nor nalidixic acid against micrococci. In many areas 25–30 per cent of *E. coli* now are resistant to sulphonamide or ampicillin, but only 5 per cent to its combination with clavulanic acid; 10 per cent are resistant to trimethroprim or oral cephalosporins. Therefore, none of these agents will be effective against every possible infecting organism but treatment should be started on a best-guess based on local knowledge of prevailing susceptibility patterns. Since the condition rarely is life threatening, failure to respond clinically within 48 hours can be accommodated by modifying treatment at that stage, according to the results of a diagnostic specimen taken before starting therapy. For urinary infections acquired in hospital following instrumentation, operation, or catheterization, the possible infecting organisms are much more numerous and their sensitivities largely unpredictable; hence an even greater need for laboratory investigation to guide the appropriate treatment.

For other infections, rationalization of initial antimicrobial therapy can be much more difficult. A patient presenting with the clinical features of pneumonia and producing no or little sputum may be infected by pneumococci, *Mycoplasma pneumoniae*, chlamydia, legionella, *Cocksiella burneti*, adeno- or influenza virus or even *M. tuberculosis* if the onset of illness was not abrupt. *Staph. aureus*, *H. influenzae*, and *Klebsiella pneumoniae* usually are associated with production of sputum except in the very early stage. In this situation, the clinician must seek and be guided by any leading feature from the history or signs, because there is no other way of early differentiation and the most appropriate therapy varies according to the aetiological agent. The choice will also be influenced by the prognosis, for instance staphylococcal and next pneumococcal infection are most likely to be rapidly fatal, if inadequately treated. Both would be likely to respond to a β-lactamase stable penicillin or cephalosporin, but for most of the other causes erythromycin or tetracycline would be appropriate. Aminoglycosides are ineffective against pneumococcal, chlamydial, and mycoplasma infections, as well as obscuring a possible subsequent search for *M. tuberculosis*.

In lung infection developing in hospital in the seriously ill, after major surgery, and in intensive care, Gram-negative rods, often multiply resistant, and anaerobic bacteria are not uncommonly involved and need to be included in the design of therapeutic cover. Also, in these circumstances pulmonary oedema or infarction are not infrequently mistaken for infection.

For bacterial meningitis, the appearance of β-lactamase producing strains of *H. influenzae* has constrained the use of ampicillin as likely initial treatment and chloramphenicol is preferred for this purpose, except where strains resistant to both antibiotics exist, as in Thailand. Hopefully, new β-lactamase stable cephalosporins, such as cefuroxime and moxalactam, with good activity against *H. influenzae* and relatively improved penetration into the cerebro spinal fluid will resolve this problem as well as that in neonatal meningitis, where Gram-negative rods including gentamicin-resistant strains, or group B streptococci are commonly responsible (see page 5.145).

For suspected bacteraemic infection in a leukaemic patient, particularly without localizing signs of the primary site, the possible infecting organisms are so numerous and sensitivities so unpredictable, that only a combination of antimicrobials has been satisfactory. Usually an aminogylcoside, gentamicin, tobramycin, or more recently amikacin, has been combined with either a penicillin or cephalosporin, the latter often given in high dosage, or clindamycin. The introduction of new β-lactams, with high activity against Gram-negative rods and to a lesser extent against pseudomonas, offers a prospect of single therapy in this clinical situation. However, such agents tend to be less active against *Staph. aureus* than earlier penicillins and cephalosporins and may need to be combined with a β-lactamase stable penicillin.

A similar diversity of infecting organisms exists in severe infections emanating from the lower gastrointestinal and female genital tracts, in chronic middle-ear or sinus infections and in internal abscesses, but often with the additional implication of anaerobic bacteria. Aminoglycosides are inactive against all anaerobes and relatively so against streptococci. Conversely metronidazole is active against all anaerobes but not aerobic bacteria. Therefore a combination of these two agents may need a third component to deal with streptococci. Clindamycin and erythromycin are effective for both streptococci and anaerobes but ineffective against aerobic Gram-negative rods. The combination of clindamycin with aminoglycosides became less attractive when it was suspected that the former component may be associated with greater risk of the complication of pseudomembranous colitis than with other combinations. This possibility may prove to apply also to the recently introduced β-lactams with improved activity against bacteroides (cefoxitin, moxalactam, combinations of penicillins with β-lactamase inhibitors), and others in the developmental stage (penems, thienamycin).

Again, it has to be stressed that a variety of combinations for comprehensive antimicrobial cover appear to be similarly effective, but all have different disadvantages and inadequacies. Large doses of β-lactams cause thrombophlebitis, and some involve administration of considerable sodium loads and may induce hypokalaemia. Rifampicin, which has a wide spectrum of antimicrobial activity including anaerobes, can be used in combination, but may be hepatotoxic when given intravenously to seriously ill patients, and some believe it should be reserved for the treatment of tuberculosis. Chloramphenicol, similarly broad-spectrum and inexpensive, has the well-known, rare but usually fatal complication of marrow aplasia and possibility of antagonistic effect against bactericidal antimicrobials when such activity is desirable.

Confirmation of diagnosis—laboratory investigation

Confirmation of the diagnosis by identifying the causative agent is the only really satisfactory basis for proper management and treatment of infection, as well as for epidemiological and preventive purposes. It is increasingly important the more severe the infection and diverse the possible aetiological agents and appropriate antimicrobial therapies. However, it has also to be acknowledged that for the less severe, well characterized, and understood infections, a doctor without access to diagnostic services may often choose and find it more convenient to do without laboratory aid. Certainly, if every infection in domiciliary practice were to be investigated, the laboratory services in the United Kingdom would be unable to meet the demand.

In a few instances, microscopical examination of stained cerebrospinal fluid, sputum, or exudate is invaluable and will quickly establish the diagnosis and identity of the infecting organism, but not its antimicrobial sensitivities. Virologists have taken to direct electron microscopy for early recognition to identify infections. Otherwise, culture is needed and the answer delayed for two or more days for the less rapidly growing pathogens. Improved selective culture has been invaluable in the recognition of campylobacter and *Clostridium difficile*. Immunological techniques, which identify bacterial antigen in the cerebrospinal fluid, sputum or exudates are relatively rapid and need to be much more developed. Staining with fluorescent antisera has been difficult to interpret due to non-specific staining. Reliance on serological recognition of rising antibody titres suffers the obvious disadvantage of the delay before such antibodies appear and, apart from relatively slowly developing infection, plays little or no part in directing initial therapy. Therefore, limitations in the speed of diagnostic services still exist, currently a good example being the lack of a suitable method for recognizing infection by legionella.

Probably the most troublesome circumstance is when antimicrobial therapy was started without or before taking diagnostic specimens. This almost invariably makes it difficult or impossible to isolate the infecting organism even when response to treatment is incomplete. Then, modification of therapy becomes even more uncertain and speculative. For example, not only do antibiotics often mask the presence of pneumococci or *H. influenzae* in sputum of patients admitted to hospital suffering from lung infection, but promote the appearance of Gram-negative rods, being contaminants from an altered oropharyngeal flora. Therefore, previous antimicrobial treatment not only obscures the true cause of infection but can mislead by producing changes in the endogenous flora contaminating diagnostic specimens.

Failure to respond—changing treatment

Management of unresponsive infection first requires an understanding of the usual rates of response to be expected in the successfully treated. Symptomatic relief from treating a simple urinary infection occurs overnight, but it takes several days for the fever to subside in acute pyelonephritis, pneumonia, or other systemic infections and even longer in a viral infection not influenced by antimicrobial therapy. The temperature record should not be judged without also taking notice of the patient's general condition.

Inadequate response demands a full review of all possible explanations and is precisely why a laboratory-confirmed diagnosis is most helpful. Consideration must include; whether the diagnosis was correct or incomplete; the treatment was appropriate in type, dosage, or mode of administration; a drug reaction occurred; and the presence of a complicating factor such as obstruction, infarction, or abscess formation which requires additional diagnostic procedures or provides a site for secondary infection.

Modification of antimicrobial therapy often is indicated when the infecting organism has been identified, because it may then be possible to change to a more appropriate agent or to discontinue unnecessary ones when combination therapy has been given. In practice, some clinicians are reluctant to do this for the very reason that the initial treatment was so effective. An example would be a pneumococcus isolated from a blood culture from a leukaemic patient progressing well on gentamicin and large doses of a broad-spectrum penicillin. In this instance, benzyl penicillin would be no less effective, potentially less toxic, less likely to contribute to selective pressures in the patient or on the ward for emergence of multiply-resistant potentially infecting organisms, and certainly much less expensive. In highly susceptible patients, it may be helpful to bear in mind that secondary or emerging infection by opportunistic pathogens, such as fungi, are unlikely to prove fatal over a short period but are difficult to diagnose and need repeated cultures.

Dosage, administration, and duration of treatment

The manufacturer's information supplied with an antimicrobial will suggest dosages, for adult or paediatric use, often higher for severe than less severe infection or lower for infection of the urinary tract if the drug is concentrated in the urine, and occasionally according to the nature of the infecting organism. Modification of dosage according to impairment of renal ofunction is usually recommended. Manufacturer's dosage recommendations are not infallible. Examples have been the early directions for gentamicin, which gave inadequate doses presumably from a cautious desire to avoid toxicity, and for excessive dosages of broad-spectrum penicillins designed for pseudomonas infection despite the fact that those due to much commoner organisms required considerably less.

In domiciliary practice in the United Kingdom doses used seem more often to have been insufficient than the reverse, perhaps because of the practice of cost-auditing of prescriptions. Examples are 250 or 125 mg of penicillin V respectively for adult or child with a sore throat when twice these doses is needed, and 250 mg ampicillin for chest infections, inadequate for the commonest infecting baterium, *H. influenzae*. On the other hand, there is an understandable tendency for severe infections, meningitis or endocarditis, to be treated in hospital with excessive doses of penicillins, at least by some doctors (referred to as 'megamaniacs'!).

The desirability of systemic administration for severe infection and when oral adsorption or patient compliance is unsure is obvious. Repeated intramuscular injections may be painful, irritant, and cause febril response, so the intravenous route is often preferred. This is best given by bolus injection rather than slow infusion because the latter initially takes longer to achieve distribution within the body, antimicrobial activity may decline in the infusion solution, and peak blood concentrations achieved after the same doses are lower. For less severe infections, particularly in domiciliary practice, absorption from oral administration is more reliable than by suppository, although metronidazole is well adsorbed by the latter method. Peak blood concentrations, for a particular dose, are always higher when given by intravenous bolus than intramuscularly and are, for most antimicrobials, considerably higher by both routes than when given orally. The manufacturer's instructions on a preparation for dosage and means of administration should always be carefully observed.

Periodicity of administration depends on the rate of excretion or metabolic inactivation of the antimicrobial, indicated by its serum half life. Once or twice daily administration has obvious advantages, and once weekly is useful particularly in prophylaxis, providing there is insignificant risk of allergic response. Because there is such little difference, in practice, between the timing of the second and third doses in a four-times-daily oral regimen, both in hospital and the home, it is increasingly proposed that four-times-daily oral regimens be discontinued.

During the whole period of antimicrobial therapy, the question as to whether a continuous blood concentration might be more effective, at least in some circumstances, than a fluctuating one has remained unresolved. The reality is that very few clinical studies are available on which to decide optimal dosage, periodicity of administration or duration of treatment for almost any infection, except gonorrhoea. Practice has been arbitrary and hallowed by time. However, more recently, duration of treatment has been investigated more thoroughly. For simple urinary infections, treatment for three days has been as effective as for ten days, but single-dose regimens less so. Previously, it had been established that cure rates for pyelonephritis were not improved by prolonging treatment beyond ten days. For tuberculosis, too, trials have justified reduction in the long periods of treatment previously recommended. For subacute bacterial endocarditis, results from 10–14 days treatment with penicillin G combined with streptomycin have been as good as the more traditional 4–6 weeks.

Duration of treatment depends upon the nature of the infecting organism, the site of infection and the aims of treatment. The intracellular *M.leprae* may need treatment for life and *M. tuberculosis* for at least six months, but 10–14 days is effective for other intracellular surviving pathogens, *S. typhi*, brucella, or chlamydia. Chronic infections, for example chronic osteomyelitis and actinomycosis, tend to relapse unless treatment is continued for 4–6 months. Generally, even for severe acute infections, meningitis, acute pyelonephritis, acute osteomyelitis, and pneumonia successful treatment can be achieved by a ten-day period of antimicrobial therapy. Relapse is more likely to be caused by

inadequate dose or a complicating factor, such as insufficient access to the infected site or a mistaken diagnosis than to too short a period of therapy, and is unlikely to respond merely to prolongation of the same form of treatment. For less severe infections, mainly treatment in domiciliary practice, clinical response can be achieved by shorter periods of treatment, as already indicated for simple urinary infection: however, clinical studies have yet to establish that three days therapy would be enough for acute sinusitis, otitis media, exacerbation of chronic bronchitis, or soft-tissue infection with evidence of local extension justifying antimicrobial therapy. Five to seven days treatment depending on the severity and patient response is usually recommended. It is perhaps significant that patient compliance studies in domiciliary practice have usually shown that a large proportion of patients cease to take the antimicrobials after a few days when they feel better. It is well known that gonococcal infection responds to a single injection of penicillin, but this is not so for gonococcal salpingitis. The importance of the infection site is clearly indicated from the finding that infection can be eradicated from the urethra and cervix by single-dosage therapy but is less likely to disappear from the rectum or oropharynx. Other highly sensitive bacteria, *Strep. pyogenes*, meningococci, *C. diphtheriae*, and pneumococci often require 10–14 days therapy for eradication from the oropharynx, although a shorter period may be enough to achieve clinical response. Thus the duration of therapy may vary according to whether the aim is merely symptomatic relief or eradication to prevent spread of infection to others or, for example, rheumatic fever following streptococcal sore throat. There are other occasions when long-term therapy is indicated prophylactically and these are considered below.

Although general guidance in relatively simple terms is required, it is important to remember that the dose, mode of administration and duration of treatment need to be varied according to the individual patient, and how that patient responds to therapy. In this sense, there is no such entity as a standard course of treatment.

Factors affecting antimicrobial therapy—its limitations

The factors influencing microbial therapy are summarized in Table 2. The most important are the type of infecting organism, its susceptibility to antimicrobials, and limiting features in the host.

Susceptibility to antimicrobials—their range of activity and modes of actions. The range of activity of antimicrobials against various micro-organisms traditionally has been referred to as narrow (or limited) or broad (or wide) spectrum. This is an over simplification.

Table 2 Factors influencing antimicrobial efficacy

Nature of infecting micro-organism
    its antimicrobial susceptibilities
    degrees of susceptibility to different antimicrobials
    its rate of division
    numbers present in infected areas
    production of substances with inactivate antimicrobials

Host susceptibilities
    impairment of defence mechanisms, generally or locally
    site of infection
    presence of damaged, avascular tissue or foreign bodies
    presence of obstructive disease

Antimicrobial
    delay in initiation appropriate therapy
    appropriate mode of administration
    levels achieved at infected site
    penetration into different body sites
    margin between effective and potentially toxic concentrations
    failure to give adequate dosage
    duration of treatment
    mode and speed of action
    binding to and inactivation by exudate or tissues

Sometimes the terms have been inappropriately attributed, depending on which groups of micro-organisms have been regarded as the more important or based on degrees of *in vitro* sensitivity unrelated to therapeutically achievable concentrations in the body by high dosage. Gentamicin has been considered as broad-spectrum because of its activity against Gram-negative rods including pseudomonas but is inactive against all anaerobes, streptococci, and chlamydia. Conversely, benzyl penicillin is thought narrow-spectrum despite activity against Gram-positive and negative cocci, many anaerobes and, at the kind of high doses currently employed for so-called broader-spectrum penicillins and cephalosporins, against many Gram-negative rods. Just as the earlier penicillins had greatest effect against cocci but much less against Gram-negative rods, some of latest cephalosporins are the reverse. However, some antimicrobials do have a relatively narrow spectrum of therapeutically useful activity, for example fucidin against only staphylococci, cloxacillin, flucloxacillin, and nafathin against only Gram-positive cocci, polymyxins, nalidixic acid and mecillinan against only Gram-negative rods, and metromidazole against only anaerobes (including protozoa).

The spectrum of activity of an antimicrobial is an indication that all members of certain species innately are insusceptible or 'naturally resistant' and this is predictable. The reasons are either that the species does not have the target site of action for the antimicrobial, can protect the site by having a barrier, the cell wall, impenetrable to the antimicrobial, can produce enzymes which inactivate the antimicrobial before it damages the micro-organism irreparably, or combinations of these. Microbial cell wall permeability barriers and enzymic inactivation can often be overcome,

in vitro, by increasing the antimicrobial concentration but beyond achievable or safe levels *in vivo*. The sites and modes of actions of commonly used antimicrobials are summarized in Table 3. All bacteria have a basic cell wall peptidoglycan structure. The failure of the first penicillin to be more comprehensively active was due to its inability to penetrate through the thicker cell walls of Gram-negative bacilli to reach penicillin-binding proteins in the inner aspect. In addition, some bacterial species, for example *K. aerogenes* and *B. fragilis*, produce penicillin-inactivating enzymes—β-lactamases. Only relatively small amounts of β-lactamase production superimposed upon a cell wall penetration barrier are needed to confer a considerable degree of insusceptibility. All bacteria have protein and nucleic-acid synthesizing mechanisms, hence the broad spectrum of activity of tetracycline, chloramphenicol, trimethoprim, and rifampicin, the last named being also active against RNA viruses. Erythromycin, another protein synthesis inhibitor, cannot penetrate through the cell walls of aerobic Gram-negative bacilli. Entry of aminoglycosides is dependent upon an active transport mechanism energized by oxidative metabolism, hence the resistance of anaerobic bacteria. Gram-positive organisms and proteus lack the cell-wall phospholipids required to bind polymyxins.

Selectivity—therapeutic index. The ideal antimicrobial should harm the parasite but not the host. β-Lactams act upon a cell-wall substance present in bacteria but not mammalian cells. Though possibly allergenic, these agents are not toxic for human cells and can be administered in large doses. Since sensitive pathogens are highly susceptible, there is a large safety factor (or high therapeutic

Table 3 Mode of action of antimicrobials

Site of action	Antimicrobial	Mode of action
Cell wall	β-Lactams (penicillins and cephalosporins)	Interfere with cross-linking of peptidoglycan backbone structure. Cells burst in hypotonic environment; cidal within 4 h. Mammalian cells unaffected
	Vancomycin Bacitracin	Inhibit peptidoglycan formation. Cidal
	Miconazole	Increases permeability, causing leakage of intracellular contents
Cytoplast membrane	Polymyxins	Bind to phospholipid and cause cell lysis. Rapidly cidal
	Polyenes (nystatin amphotericin B)	Bind to sterols causing leakage of intracellular substances. Cidal
Ribosomes	Tetracyclines	Interfere with amino-acid attachment to transfer DNA. Static
	Chloramphenicol	Interferes with messenger RNA translation. Usually static; cidal for a few organisms
	Erythromycin Clindamycin Fusidic acid	All interfere with messenger RNA translation. Usually static but incompletely and slowly cidal against some organisms
	Aminoglycosides (gentamicin, tobramycin, amikacin, streptomycin)	Interfere with attachment of messenger RNA to ribosome. Rapidly cidal (30 min)
Nucleic acid synthesis	Sulphonomides	Competitive inhibition of para-amino benzoic acid. Static
	Trimethoprim	Inhibits dihydrofolate reductase. Cidal
	Rifampicin	Inhibits RNA polymerase. Cidal
	Nalidixic acid Nitrofurantoin	Inhibits DNA linkage. Cidal Damages DNA. Cidal
	Metronidazole	Damages DNA. Cidal
	5-Fluorcytosine	Incorporated into DNA causing synthesis of abnormal protein. Static
	Interferon	Interferes with early stages of replication
	Acycloguanosine	Inhibits DNA polymerase
	Cytosine arabinoside	Inhibits synthesis of nucleic acids

index) between the effective but potentially toxic concentrations within the body. Sulphonamides inhibit an enzyme concerned in the synthesis of folic acid, which mammalian cells can absorb but which bacterial cells have to synthesize from para-aminobenzoic acid; again, toxicity is not a problem though sensitization can be. For most other types of antimicrobials, the metabolism of mammalian cells may be affected, as well as that of antimicrobial cells, but to a lesser extent. For example, the affinity of trimethoprim for the dihydrofolate reductase, which it inhibits, is 20 000 times greater for the bacterial than the mammalian cell enzyme. Unfortunately, the margins for other antimicrobials, chloramphenicol, tetrocyclines, and aminoglycosides, are not nearly so wide. This explains the need for caution in selecting the dosage and duration of exposures to such agents, particularly in the patient with impaired excretory function or metabolic inactivation in the liver.

Bactericidal and bacteriostatic activity—degrees of susceptibility.

Theoretically, it would be desirable always to employ an agent likely to kill invading parasites rather than merely to inhibit their growth. However, for most infections, spontaneous resolution by body defences eventually occurs in the majority of patients. Any contributory inhibitory influence can alter the balance and speed the resolution. In fact, there is little evidence from controlled clinical observations of infections, that a microbicidal effect is essential. In endocarditis, that need is founded on individual experiences of relapse and failed control of infection by bacteriostatic agents and by animal model studies rather than by clinical trial, but the evidence is compelling. In addition, a need for bactericidal activity in patients with severely impaired defences (neutropenia) is rational but unproven. Even in severe life-threatening infections due to Gram-negative bacteria, there is no significant difference in survival of patients receiving bactericidal as compared with bacteriostatic antimicrobials, although more studies on neutropenic patients are required.

Aminoglycosides and β-lactams are bactericidal to all susceptible organisms but some antimicrobials vary in their effect. For example, chloramphenicol is bacteriostatic for staphylococci, Gram-negative bacilli, and pneumococci but kills *H. influenzae* and meningococci but only inhibitory to sensitive staphylococci. In these instances, it could be that bacteriostasis is followed by autolysis of those particular bacteria and the killing effect is not directly caused by the antimicrobial. Antimicrobials usually produce a slowing in rates of increase of viable bacteria *in vitro*, at concentrations below those required completely to arrest measurable multiplication—a so called subinhibitory effect. Again, this could be a significant factor in assisting body defence. However, response to treatment has shown a good correlation with the attainment of inhibitory concentrations of antimicrobials in the appropriate body sites, blood for systemic infection, urine for infection of the urinary tract and cerebrospinal fluid for meningitis. Therefore, it seems prudent to continue to design therapy for that purpose.

Numbers of infecting bacteria and rate of multiplication.

Bactericidal agents generally exert their effects best, or only are active at all, on dividing micro-organisms, an explanation for the prolonged treatment required for the more slowly growing pathogens as in tuberculosis.

In most acute infections, the numbers of bacteria at the infected site, are considerable—10^5 as more per ml of infected urine, 10^7 per ml of homogenized infected sputum or pus. However, in the prophylactic situation, an antimicrobial may need only to deal with relatively few micro-organisms. *In vitro* tests always show an effect at lower antimicrobial concentrations against small bacterial inocula, and this is enhanced if the organism produces enzymes which inactivate antimicrobials. Therefore, an agent with marginal activity against high inocula, *in vitro*, may still be effective prophylactically.

Host and antimicrobial factors (see page 5.3). It is now well established that impaired defence mechanisms predispose to infections which may be caused by micro-organisms which do not cause disease in normal individuals. This may occur in general systemic disorders such as leukaemia or lymphoma, following the use of cytotoxic agents, or may be due to local factors such as the damaged bronchi of the chronic bronchitic, or worse the bronchiectatic. Infecting organisms are very difficult to eradicate from a locally damaged site. Although symptomatic relief can be induced by antimicrobial therapy helping to resolve an episode of associated tissue invasion, relapse often follows cessation of treatment. Experience is similar when infection is associated with or complicated by avascular tissue or foreign bodies, which always have to be removed. Obstruction allows distal infection to become more widespread and severe.

Antimicrobials vary in their ability to penetrate different body sites. Concentrations of β-lactams in the cerebrospinal fluid and sputum are very much below blood levels as are those of aminoglycosides. Conversely ampicillin, cephalixin, rifampicin are concentrated in bile, and numerous agents are concentrated in the urine (β-lactams, aminoglycosides, nalidixic acid, nitrofurantoin, sulphonamides, trimethoprim, tetracycline).

Antimicrobials with a wide distribution throughout the body fluids include chloramphenicol, metronidazole, fucidin, erythromycin, clindamycin, isoniazid, and tetracycline is concentrated within many cells, including white cells. To be active against intracellular organisms, antimicrobials first have to enter affected cells before penetrating the microbial cell wall. The characteristics of mammalian cell membranes and bacterial cell walls differ and, not surprisingly, the abilities of antimicrobials to penetrate both are not the same.

Some antimicrobials bind firmly to certain tissues (polymyxins; aminoglycosides) and are released only slowly. For example, binding to serum albumin usually is associated with proportional loss of antimicrobial activity, *in vitro*, but its role is hindering therapeutic effect, *in vivo* remains uncertain. Highly protein-bound antibiotics such as flucloxacillin and fucidin are therapeutically effective.

However, tissue binding is a factor in toxicity, as with that of aminoglycosides to the renal cortex. Antimicrobial activity can also be reduced by other features at the infected site. The eH and pH of pus are low and aminoglycosides are likely to be affected because their activity is diminished by acidity and is abolished under anaerobic conditions.

Additional treatment and procedures

It follows that generalizations about no cure without draining pus, relieving obstruction, or removing foreign bodies or dead tissue can be rationalized in terms of impaired activities or penetration of antimicrobials. Indeed, inadequate response to an infection of established cause, treated with an appropriate agent at correct dosage, can be a clear indication that further procedures are needed to eradicate the infection.

Some infecting organisms produce exo- or endotoxins and it is their effects which produce the main manifestations of the illness rather than direct tissue invasion by the organism itself. Well-known examples are the exotoxins of *Clostridium tetani* and *welchii* and of *Corynebacterium diphtheriae*. Obviously, antimicrobial therapy alone is insufficient in the management of such infection. The endotoxin of Gram-negative bacilli causes profound pathophysiological effects and further advances in the treatment of severe bacteraemic infection by such bacteria still requires developments in supportive therapy designed to remedy these effects rather than refinements in the antimicrobial component of treatment. The situation is similar for severe infection by some Gram-positive organisms. A better understanding is needed of the factors responsible for the circulatory failure often accompanying staphylococcal bacteraemia, and measures need to be designed to alleviate it. It has been pointed out that the mortality rates encountered in the early period of treatment of pneumococcal bacteraemia remain unchanged despite the introduction of anti-microbial therapy and the very great sensitivity of pneumococci to these agents *in vitro*. For these examples, the efficacy of therapy has not progressed for many years in spite of all the developments in new antimicrobials. A new approach is necessary, in which antimicrobial therapy is combined with measures directed towards the secondary consequences of infection mediated by bacterial products.

References

Ball, A. P. (1982). Clinical use of penicillins. *Lancet* **ii**, 196.

Charlton, C. A. C., Crowther, R. A., Davies, J. G., Dynes, J., Howard, M. W. A., Mann, P. G., and Rye, S. (1976). Three-day and ten-day chemotherapy for urinary tract infections in general practice. *Br. med. J.* **i**, 1378.

Fang, L. S. T., Tolkoff-Rubin, N. E., and Rubin, R. M. (1978). Efficacy of single-dose and conventional anoxycillin treatment in urinary tract infection localized by the antibody-coated bacteria technique. *New Engl. J. Med.* **298**, 415.

Garrod, L. P., Lambert, M. P., and O'Grady, F. (1981). *Antibiotics and chemotherapy*. Churchill Livingstone, London.

Gray, I. R. (1979). The choice of antibiotics, for treating infectious endocarditis. *Q. Jl Med.* **44**, 449.

Sykes, R. B., Bunner, D. P., Bush, K., Georgopapadou, N. H., and Wells, J. S. (1981). Monobactams—monocyclic β-lactam antibiotics produced by bacteria. *J. antimicrob. Chemother.* **8**, Suppl., 1.

— and Matthew, M. (1976). The β-lactamases of Gram-negative bacteria and their role in resistance to β-lactam antibodies. *J. antimicrob. Chemother.* **2**, 115.

Wise, R. (1982). Penicillins and cephalosporins: antimicrobial and pharmacological properties. *Lancet* **ii**, 140.

Practical aspects of antimicrobial chemotherapy

Mary P. E. Slack

The era of antimicrobial chemotherapy now spans more than forty years. During that time many bacterial infections which formerly carried a high mortality, such as puerperal sepsis, tuberculosis, and meningitis have become amenable to treatment with a plethora of potent antimicrobial agents. Antimicrobial therapy has become progressively more complex, largely because of the appearance of acquired resistance among micro-organisms, which has only been partly mitigated by the enormous variety of available compounds. Furthermore, changes in medical practice have made the patient population much more at risk from infection caused by organisms which hitherto were regarded as non-pathogenic. It is hard for clinicians and microbiologists to keep abreast of new developments in this field. No sooner has the role of a new compound been established than a potential alternative is launched. It is extremely difficult to draw conclusions on the rela-tive merits of an array of antimicrobials from many diverse papers. Despite these impediments it is essential that every clinician who prescribes antimicrobials should have a clear understanding of the microbiological and pharmacological properties of these com-pounds and adopt a rational approach to their use. Patterns of antimicrobial use and microbial resistance vary from country to country and even between hospitals, and thus it is almost impos-sible to make dogmatic statements on microbial sensitivities and antimicrobial choice. Empirical therapy should be based on the prevailing patterns of resistance among locally isolated pathogenic organisms, and definitive treatment based on laboratory data of the susceptibility of the particular isolate or isolates. This can only be ensured by close co-operation and consultation between clini-cians and medical microbiologists. The final selection of an agent depends on the underlying state of the patient.

Among the reasons quoted for prescribing antimicrobial agents there are three which may be assumed to have a logical basis: for empirical or 'blind' therapy of presumed infection, to treat bacteriologically proven infection, or as prophylaxis to prevent infection. It should be apparent that different considerations govern the selection of an antibiotic in each of the three situations. An antibiotic may be appropriate in one context but wholly inappropriate in another.

Empirical therapy of presumed infection

Ideally, therapy of infectious disease is based on the results of microbiological cultures and antimicrobial susceptibility testing. In reality antimicrobial therapy is often instituted before the culture results are available. There are a number of reasons for this. 'Blind' therapy is inevitable in areas lacking microbiological facilities. In life-threatening situations, where there is a strong presumption of infection, antimicrobial therapy should be started as soon as all the necessary specimens have been collected. There is *always* time to take some samples for culture before giving antimicrobial agents. For example, blood can be taken for culture as an intravascular line is inserted. The appearance of fever in neutropenic patients should prompt careful clinical evaluation and consideration of empirical therapy. As soon as all the appropriate specimens have been taken the patient should be given a combination of antimicrobials, usually a β-lactam antibiotic and an aminoglycoside. There is much debate on the relative merits of the different aminoglycosides and whether a cephalosporin or anti-pseudomonadal penicillin should be used. There is good evidence that the use of a combination of potentially synergistic antibiotics improves the clinical response of these immunosuppressed patients.

Certain clinical conditions are so clearly associated with particular microorganisms of predictable antimicrobial susceptibil-ity that rational treatment may be based on solely clinical grounds. Examples are scarlet fever and lobar pneumonia. It is still necessary, however, to collect specimens for confirmatory micro-biology before starting antimicrobial therapy.

Empirical therapy is often used for less serious infections, such as cystitis. In general practice 80 per cent of acute urinary tract infections are caused by *E. coli* strains, which are usually sensitive to many broad-spectrum antibiotics. In these instances 'blind' chemotherapy is likely to succeed. Since about half the patients with urinary frequency and dysuria are not suffering from bacterial cystitis, many of the antibiotics prescribed will be unnecessary. Urine samples should always be collected for culture before initiating therapy. Acute otitis media is usually treated empirically in the United Kingdom, since pus from the middle ear is so rarely obtained for culture. Diagnostic tympanocentesis is more com-monly performed in Scandinavia and the United States. This tech-nique has provided valuable data on the bacterial aetiology of this common infection of childhood. Empirical therapy can be selected to cover the pathogens known to cause otitis media in children of the same age.

The patient with an undiagnosed febrile illness is a common clinical problem. When an enormous number of investigations have failed to provide the answer the clinicians may be tempted to try a course of antimicrobials as a quasi-diagnostic test. In practice such a 'trial of therapy' rarely clarifies the situation and indeed may cause even more confusion.

When contemplating 'blind' therapy the clinician should be aware of the value and the limitations of antimicrobial tests. Unlike biochemical tests, very few microbiological results are absolute indices of infection. The isolation of *Neisseria gonorrhoea* is always significant, but the culture of Group A streptococci from a throat swab may indicate acute streptococcal pharyngitis or merely streptococcal carriage. The predictive value of a single test may be low, as for example in screening for bacteriuria. Multiple specimens and semi-quantitative culture techniques increase the predictive value of this particular test. Similarly three blood cultures, taken at different times from different sites, will identify more than 95 per cent of blood-culture-positive cases of infective endocarditis.

Obviously the likelihood of a positive result will tend to increase as the disease progresses.

Clinicians should be also aware of how long laboratory tests take to provide a result. Conventional techniques require periods of incubation to allow micro-organisms to grow to detectable numbers in the cultures. Usually a minimum of 18 hours is necessary. The smaller the number of micro-organisms in the original specimen the longer the delay in achieving a result. Fastidious organisms such as anaerobic bacteria, and slow-growing micro-organisms, for example mycobacteria, will require prolonged culture. More rapid techniques may give a presumptive microbiological diagnosis long before culture results are available. Undoubtedly the most valuable of these is the examination of a Gram-stained smear of the specimen. Other rapid tests which may be useful include the detection of bacterial polysaccharide in body fluids, determination of cerebrospinal fluid lactate levels, electron-microscopy of vesicle fluids, and

Table 1 Laboratory investigations with should be initiated before commencing antimicrobial chemotherapy

		Septicaemia	Febrile episode in neutropenic patient	Meningitis	Neonatal sepsis	Pneumonia	Pyrexia of unknown origin	Notes
(a)	*Microbiology*							
	Blood cultures	+	+	+	+	+	+	Take at least 2 sets at different times from 2 sites
	Cerebrospinal fluid			+[a]	±			Gram-stain, lactate, bacterial antigen detection may give rapid microbiological diagnosis. *N.B.* Measure blood glucose at same time as c.s.f. glucose
	Sputum/trans-tracheal aspirate/bronchial aspirate	+	+		+	+[b]	+	[b]Immunofluorescence for *L. pneumophila* if indicated
	Urine	+	+		+	+[c]	+	[c]Pneumococcal antigen detection
	Culture if applicable { wound swab	+	+		+		+	
	joint aspirate	+	+		+		+	
	abscess aspirate	+	+		+		+	
	intravascular line tip	+	+		+		+	
	Faeces	(+)	+	+[a]			+	
	throat swab		+	+[a]	+		+	
	nose swab		+		+			
	ear swab				+			
	umbilical swab				+			
	gastric/nasopharyngeal aspirate				+			
	rectal swab				+			
(b)	*Serology*							
	Clotted sample of blood	+	+	+	+	+	+	Paired sera to show rising titre or initial high diagnostic titre. Bacterial antigen detection
(c)	*Haematology*							
	Haemoglobin	+	+	+	+	+	+	
	Full blood count	+	+	+	+	+	+	
	Differential white cell count	+	+	+	+	+	+	
	Erythrocyte sedimentation rate	+	+	+	+	+	+	
(d)	*Radiography*							
	Chest X-ray	+	+		+	+	+	

[a] For virology, if indicated

Table 2 Empirical therapy for serious infections: to be used only for emergencies prior to bacteriological culture results

Presumed infection	Associated foci or source of infection	Likely organism	Treatment
Gram-negative septicaemia	urinary tract	*E. coli* *Pr. mirabilis*	aminoglycoside ± broad-spectrum penicillin e.g. gentamicin ± ampicillin
	biliary tract	*E. coli* + other enterobacteria [+*Str. faecalis*]	aminoglycoside + broad-spectrum penicillin e.g. gentamicin + ampicillin
	abdominal or pelvic sepsis	*E. coli* + other enterobacteria *Bact. fragilis*	aminoglycoside + broad-spectrum penicillin + antianaerobic agent e.g. gentamicin + ampicillin + metronidazole
Gram-positive septicaemia	skin sepsis septic arthritis acute osteomyelitis	*Staph. aureus* beta-haemolytic streptococci	penicillin + penicillinase-stable penicillin (+ aminoglycoside) e.g. cloxacillin + benzyl penicillin (+ gentamicin)
	intravascular line pacemaker ventriculo-atrial shunt arterio-venous shunt	*Staph. aureus* *Staph. epidermidis*	penicillinase-stable penicillin + aminoglycoside e.g. cloxacillin + gentamicin
Septicaemia in previously well patient	no obvious source	*Staph. aureus* *E. coli*	penicillin + penicillinase-stable penicillin + aminoglycoside benzyl penicillin + cloxacillin + gentamicin
Febrile episode in neutropenic patient	no obvious source	*E. coli* *Staph. aureus* *Klebsiella* spp. *Ps. aeruginosa*	antipseudomonadal β-lactam + aminoglycoside e.g. ticarcillin + gentamicin
Neonatal septicaemia + or meningitis	<48 h old: maternal birth canal	*E. coli* Group B streptococci *List monocytogenes*	broad-spectrum penicillin + aminoglycoside e.g. ampicillin + gentamicin (+ chloramphenicol if meningitis)
	>48 h old: environment + attendants	*Staph. aureus* Group B streptotocci Resistant enterobacteria *Ps. aeruginosa*	broad-spectrum penicillin + penicillinase-stable penicillin + aminoglycoside e.g. ampicillin + cloxacillin + gentamicin
Meningitis in children less than 6 years old		*H. influenzae* type b *N. meningitidis* *Str. pneumoniae*	chloramphenicol ± ampicillin
Meningitis in older children or adults		*N. meningitidis* *Str. pneumoniae* *List. monocytogenes*	benzyl penicillin
Pneumonia	(a) community-acquired	*Str. pneumoniae* *Mycopl. pneumoniae* *Staph. aureus* *L. pneumophila* } *H. influenzae* } less commonly	broad-spectrum penicillin + erythromycin e.g. ampicillin + erythromycin
	if post-influenzal	consider *Staph. aureus*	add cloxacillin to above
	if history of aspiration	consider anaerobes	add metronidazole to above
	(b) hospital-acquired or immunosuppression	*Str. pneumoniae* *Staph. aureus* *L. pneumophila* *H. influenzae* *K. pneumoniae* other enterobacteria *Ps. aeruginosa*	broad-spectrum penicillin + aminoglycoside + erythromycin e.g. ampicillin + gentamicin + erythromycin
	if history of aspiration	consider anaerobes	add metronidazole to above
Brain abscess	paranasal sinuses middle ear, mastoid, metastatic	*Str. milleri* *Bact. fragilis* + other anaerobes (often mixed infections)	benzyl penicillin + chloramphenicol + metronidazole

Use a cephalosporin in the penicillin-hypersensitive patient

immunofluorescent detection of bacteria and viruses. Once bacteria have been isolated in culture, antimicrobial susceptibility tests can be performed. Conventional tests take a further 18 hours, but more rapid semi-automated tests are becoming available. These newer techniques can give an answer within four to six hours.

Before embarking on a course of empirical therapy the clinician should consider the possible consequences. The therapy may be successful because the correct drug was chosen, the patient overcame the infection without the assistance of the drug, or because the patient was not suffering from an infection at all. The therapy may be harmful because of its innate toxicity or the enhanced susceptibility of an individual patient.

The frequent prescription of blind therapy will inevitably lead to over-use of drugs and needless expense. Empirical therapy necessarily utilizes broad-spectrum antimicrobials. The use of these broad-spectrum agents inevitably carries the risk of selecting out resistant microorganisms, which may superinfect the patient. Finally the use of 'blind' therapy often muddies the diagnostic waters. It may be unclear whether a poor response is due to the use of the wrong drug. In such cases the only chance of making a diagnosis is a positive culture from the specimens taken before initiating therapy. Antimicrobial agents cannot be expected to succeed in the absence of infection.

If after careful consideration empirical therapy is deemed necessary the following course of action is advisable. A carefully taken history and thorough examination will often give some clues to the likely microbial causes of the infection. For example, symptoms of urinary tract infection may suggest a Gram-negative bacteraemia and a purpuric rash may point to meningococcaemia. However, it should be noted that the classical features of Gram-negative septicaemia may be seen in overwhelming staphylococcal or streptococcal infections. A complete microbiological screen should be performed. Obviously this is tailored to suit the clinical problem (Table 1). Blood cultures should always be taken in seriously ill patients and are essential in cases of suspected pneumonia or meningitis. It is worth collecting a specimen of clotted blood at this time. The laboratory can save this 'acute' serum pending any relevant diagnostic serology. An early serum sample is invaluable since most serological tests rely on the demonstration of a rising titre in paired samples of sera. The medical microbiologist should be alerted at this early stage, to discuss optimal specimens for culture. The quality of clinical bacteriology depends on culturing the best possible specimen. For example, trans-tracheal aspirated or bronchoscopy specimens will often yield the causative organism in severe pneumonia, but expectorated sputum may be uninformative.

Empirical therapy should be aimed at the most likely pathogens. The microbiologist can advise on appropriate 'blind' therapy based on the prevailing pathogens and their antimicrobial susceptibility patterns. The empirical therapy must be adapted to suit the individual patient, taking into consideration his age, renal and hepatic function, known drug hypersensitivity, and the probable location of the infection. The antimicrobial should be administered at the full therapeutic dosage, appropriate for the patient. An outline of empirical therapeutic regimens is given in Table 2. It must be emphasized that such information can be no more than a rough guide and modifications in the light of local resistance patterns and prescribing habits are necessary.

There will inevitably be some chinks in the armour of even the most broad-spectrum agent. The second-generation cephalosporins, cefuroxime and cefamanadole, are not active against *Enterobacter* species, *Pseudomonas* species, indole-positive *Proteus* species or faecal-type streptococci. The hospital inpatient who becomes seriously ill is more likely to be infected with resistant Gram-negative bacteria than when the infection is contracted at home. If the patient has recently received a course of antibiotics, the infecting organism may be resistant to this drug and an alternative compound should be used initially.

In all these cases the unnecessary antibiotics should be stopped as soon as the bacteriological results are available. The introduction of rapid semi-automated techniques for the detection of bacteria and antibiotic sensitivity testing will hopefully reduce the need for blind broad-spectrum antibiotic therapy.

Therapy of proven infection

When the microbial aetiology of an infection is known, specific antimicrobial therapy can be instituted. Antimicrobial susceptibility testing is essential since, with a few notable exceptions, the majority of microbial species are no longer uniformly susceptible to antimicrobial agents. Susceptibility to penicillin is mercifully still universal among group A streptococci, but cannot be assumed in *Neisseria gonorrhoeae* or *Strep. pneumoniae*.

Antimicrobial susceptibility testing

Antimicrobial susceptibility tests, correctly performed, and with due regard to their limitations, are the proper basis for chemotherapy. *In vitro* susceptibility tests are designed to predict the clinical efficacy of antimicrobials. To be of maximum value to clinicians they must be as rapid as possible. Semi-automated methods are becoming available which can give results within four hours of isolating the pathogen in pure culture. Most laboratories do not yet possess these new machines and must rely on traditional methods.

Disc diffusion. The technique most often used is to place filter paper discs impregnated with known concentrations of antimicrobials onto an agar culture plate preseeded with the test organism. The degree of sensitivity of the organism to the antimicrobials is assessed by the size of inhibition zones around the discs after overnight incubation. Such tests have been used for many years and in general give a very good guide to relevant antimicrobial chemotherapy. The susceptibility patterns of selected bacteria to some common antimicrobial agents are shown in Table 3. The importance of susceptibility testing the majority of bacterial pathogens should be readily apparent. In contrast there are a number of newly recognized pathogens and 'atypical' microorganisms for which susceptibility testing is neither essential nor practical. These organisms may be confidently treated with the antimicrobial agents recommended in Table 4.

For most microbial species, susceptibility and resistance to antimicrobials are bimodally distributed. The majority of strains are either very susceptible to clinically achievable concentrations of the drug or they are so resistant as to render therapy with that drug ineffective. Strains with an intermediate degree of susceptibility, requiring careful monitoring for successful management, are uncommon. These partially 'susceptible' strains are nevertheless sometimes of great importance.

Clinicians seeking advice on antimicrobial chemotherapy are sometimes confused by the microbiologist's jargon. The terms 'susceptible' ('sensitive') and 'resistant' are rather inexact. To a microbiologist an organism as *'susceptible'* to an antimicrobial if it is killed or inhibited at a concentration which can readily be achieved in the serum of a normal individual given the normal dosage of the drug. The clinical definition of susceptibility relates to the amount of drug necessary to 'cure' the infection. To some extent these two definitions are in conflict. There are instances where the clinical outcome is at variance with the *in vitro* prediction. An infection caused by an apparently sensitive organism may fail to respond for several reasons. Penetration of the antimicrobial to the site of the infection may be inadequate. It may not be possible to predict the effectiveness of antimicrobials in patients with impaired host defence systems or serious underlying disease. The antimicrobial may be inactivated by other organisms in the patients commensal flora, for example, penicillinase producing *Staph. aureus*. Conversely the patient may respond to apparently inappropriate

Table 3   Susceptibility of selected bacteria to antibacterial agents

	Penicillin G/V	Cloxacillin/flucloxacillin/methicillin	Ampicillin/Amoxycillin	Amoxycillin + clavulinic acid	Carbenicillin/ticarcillin	Mezlocillin/piperacillin/azlocillin	Mecillinam	Cephalothin/cephradine/cefazolin	Cefuroxime/cefamandole	Cefoxitin	Cefotaxime/ceftazidime	Cefsulodin	Erythromycin	Lincomycin/clindamycin	Tetracyclines	Fusidic acid*	Rifampicin*	Chloramphenicol	Sulphonamides	Co-trimoxazole	Trimethoprim	Gentamicin/netilmicin/amikacin	Polymyxin/colistin	Vancomycin	Metronidazole
Staph. aureus (pen.-sensitive)	1	0	0	0	0	0		2	0	0	0		2	2	2					2		2		2	
Staph. aureus (pen.-resistant)		1	2					2	0	0	0		2	2	2						2			2	
Group A streptococcus	1	0	0	0	0	0		2	0	0	0		2	2	0	0	0							0	
Pneumococcus	1	0	2	0	0	0		2	2	0	0		2	2	0			2						0	
Str. faecalis			1	0		2							2											2	
N. gonorrhoeae	2	0	1	2	0			0	2	2	0		2	0			0			2					
N. meningitidis	1	0	2	0	0	0		0	0	0	0		0	0				2							
L. monocytogenes	2	0	1	0	0	0		0	2	0	0		0	0	0	0	0	2	0	0	0	2		0	
H. influenzae	0		1	2	0			2	0	0			2		2			1			0	0			
E. coli			1	2			2			2										1	1	2	0		
Klebsiella				2			2			2										1	1	2	0		
Serratia/enterobacter						2	2	2												1	1	2	0		
Proteus			1	2			2													1	1	2			
S. typhi			1		0	0	2	0	0	0	0	0		0		0	0	1		2			0		
Ps. aeruginosa				1	1						2	1			0							1	2		
Acinetobacter											2											1	2		
B. fragilis			2	0							2		2	2				2							1
Other *Bacteroides* spp.	1	0	0	0	0			0	0	2			2	2				2							1
Cl. perfringens	1	0	0	0	0	0		0	0	0	0	2			0		0	2						0	2
L. tuberculosis															0		1			0					

Key

| 1 | susceptible first choice |
| 0 | susceptible not usually recommended |

generally resistant

wide variation in susceptibility. *In vitro* testing important

| 2 | susceptible second choice |

usually susceptible but resistance has been rarely reported.

*resistance readily develops if agent used alone; always use in combination

therapy because very high concentrations are achieved. Despite these examples it remains the case that the use of an antimicrobial when the pathogen has been shown to be resistant *in vitro* is likely to result in treatment failure.

Routine susceptibility testing has other benefits. It will identify rare resistant organisms which pose a threat within the hospital, for example, methicillin and/or gentamicin-resistant *Staph. aureus* and multiply resistant Gram-negative bacilli. Patients harbouring these organisms can be isolated to prevent further dissemination.

The results of susceptibility tests on individual bacteria are often analysed to reveal the local susceptibility patterns. This information can be applied to selecting the most appropriate 'blind' therapy in serious infections. In particular it details any instances where resistance is limiting the potential usefulness of an antimicrobial and can form the basis of a policy for antimicrobial prescribing in that hospital.

Disc sensitivity testing may sometimes fail to identify clinically important resistance. Ampicillin resistance in *Haemophilus in-fluenzae* is usually due to the production of a β-lactamase. Standard disc testing may not detect this and a specific test for β-lactamase should always be performed.

Determination of minimal inhibitory concentrations (MICs). For the majority of infections qualitative disc diffusion tests are an adequate guide to therapy. Sometimes it is advisable to assess quantitatively an organism's sensitivity to antimicrobials. Twofold dilutions of the antimicrobial are prepared in a culture medium, either broth or agar. Each dilution is inoculated with a standard number of organisms and then incubated. The lowest concentration of antimicrobial that inhibits visual growth of the organism is called the minimal inhibitory concentration (MIC). All the tubes lacking visible growth can be subcultured onto antimicrobial-free medium and reincubated to determine the minimum bactericidal concentration (MBC). The MBC is defined as the lowest concentration of antimicrobial that kills 99.9 per cent or more of the initial inoculum. The *in vitro* MIC is subject to many variables. A control organism

Table 4 Antimicrobial chemotherapy of some newly recognized and 'atypical' pathogens

Micro-organism	Disease	Antimicrobial agent
Campylobacter jejuni	gastro-enteritis	erythromycin
Clostridium difficile	antibiotic-associated diarrhoea pseudo-membranous colitis	vancomycin
Gardnerella vaginalis	vaginitis	metronidazole
Legionella pneumophila	legionnaires' disease	erythromycin, rifampicin
Chlamydia psittaci	psittacosis, ornithosis	tetracycline, erythromycin
Chlamydia trachomatis	inclusion conjunctivitis trachoma non-gonococcal urethritis lymphogranuloma venereum	tetracycline, erythromycin
Mycoplasma pneumoniae	pneumonia	erythromycin tetracycline
Coxiella burneti	Q fever	tetracycline

with known MIC and MBC should therefore be included in every test. Generally the MBC of an antimicrobial is two to fourfold greater than the MIC. Some strains of bacteria, such as *Staph. aureus*, may be normally sensitive to the inhibitory effect of the penicillins but are killed only at very much higher concentrations of the antibiotic. This phenomenon is called 'tolerance'. Tolerance may be inferred if the ratio MBC/MIC is 32 or greater.

What are the indications for determining MICs? MICs and more importantly MBCs must always be measured for organisms causing infective endocarditis. They may assist in the management of other septicaemic or serious infections. If a pathogen is re-isolated from a patient during or just after therapy, comparison of the MICs of the two isolates may reveal the emergence of resistance. MICs are generally measured when an organism is of intermediate susceptibility in disc diffusion tests. It is debatable whether determination of MBCs is routinely of great interest except in cases of infective endocarditis or to exclude tolerance. The first requirement of any manufacturer introducing a new antibiotic is to produce tabulations of the MICs for common pathogens, presumably on the assumption that most infections are treated blindly. This is reasonable in general terms but it may be the undoing of a particular critically ill patient. It cannot be emphasized too strongly that therapy should wherever possible be based on sensitivity tests of the patient's own organism.

Recently, the effects of sub-inhibitory concentrations of antibiotics have aroused considerable interest. Sub-inhibitory concentrations of antibiotics may enhance phagocytosis and may interfere with bacterial adherence. A third definition, the minimum antibiotic concentration (MAC), has been proposed. The MAC is the minimum concentration that produces structural or morphological changes in the bacteria or which produces a one-log reduction in the number of viable bacteria. Determination of MACs is at present a cumbersome research technique which is scarcely applicable to the routine laboratory.

Choice of drug

When the microbial aetiology of an infection and the antimicrobial susceptibility of the causative organisms are known, appropriate chemotherapy can be instituted. In selecting an antimicrobial several factors ought to be considered.

1. Bactericidal or bacteriostatic antibiotic? Bactericidal antibiotics, such as the penicillins, cephalosporins, and aminoglyco-sides, kill bacteria at clinically achievable concentrations. Bacteriostatic agents, including the tetracyclines, and macrolides merely inhibit their growth. It should be remembered that the standard antimicrobial disc diffusion tests measure only inhibition of growth, and not microbial killing. There is no doubt that bactericidal drugs should be used in infective endocarditis and probably also in neutropenic patients. In other types of infection there is no convincing evidence that bactericidal drugs are superior to bacteriostatic agents, if the infecting organism is susceptible and adequate blood and tissue levels are achieved.

2. Broad-spectrum or narrow-spectrum therapy? Broad-spectrum antimicrobials, such as ampicillin and the cephalosporins, will have a greater impact on the normal flora than narrow-spectrum agents, such as benzylpenicillin. The use of broad-spectrum agents will effectively destroy much of the patient's normal flora and encourage the proliferation of highly resistant species of Gram-negative bacteria. It is therefore advisable to use a narrow-spectrum drug to treat specific infections. Examples include flucloxacillin for treating *Staphylococcus aureus* wound infections, benzylpenicillin for pneumococcal pneumonia, and oral phenoxy-methyl penicillin for streptococcal pharyngitis. The use of cephalosporins in these three instances is unwarranted, save for the penicillin-hypersensitive patient.

3. Site of infection. The site of an infection may influence the choice of an antimicrobial agent. Penetration into and effectiveness of the drug in the infected tissue or body space is obviously an important consideration. Many antimicrobials penetrate poorly into the brain, prostate, ocular humours, and cerebrospinal fluid. Large aggregations of pus interfere with the activity of some antimicrobials, for example flucloxacillin. The aminoglycosides are virtually inactive in the anaerobic and acid conditions found within abscess cavities. The ability of antimicrobials to penetrate into phagocytic cells and kill intracellular organisms may be important in the therapy of some infections, notably tuberculosis. Rifampicin is effective against viable intracellular bacteria and has been recently recommended for this reason in the treatment of persistent serious staphylococcal sepsis.

4. Relative efficacy and toxicity. The choice is often between a relatively safe but less efficacious drug and a more potent but potentially toxic compound. The clinical severity of the infection will influence the selection. Possible toxic effects should not preclude the use of a highly active antimicrobial for a life-threatening infection.

5. The patient. The underlying state of the patient must always be considered. The patient's age, renal and hepatic function, and previous drug history should be taken into account. Tetracyclines are to be avoided in children since they may discolour teeth. In pregnancy drugs that could damage the fetus must not be used. Fortunately, many penicillins, cephalosporins, and erythromycin can be safely given during pregnancy (Table 5). Renal or hepatic insufficiency will enhance the toxic potential of many antimicrobials. Adjustments in dosage or avoidance of the drug may therefore be indicated (Tables 6 and 7). Alternative therapy must be selected in the patient with known sensitivity to an antimicrobial agent.

6. Drug interactions. When two or more drugs are administered simultaneously there may be undesirable interactions. The concomitant use of frusemide or ethacrynic acid enhances the nephrotoxicity of cephaloridine. Rifampicin, a potent inducer of hepatic enzymes, may enhance the metabolism of oral contraceptives. Contraceptive failure may also occur because of ampicillin-induced diarrhoea. The consequences of combining two antimicrobial agents may be microbiological rather than pharmacological, resulting in potentiation or reduction of the antimicrobial effect.

Table 5 Antimicrobial therapy in pregnancy

Relatively safe	Avoid in first trimester	Avoid at all stages of pregnancy
cephalosporins	chloramphenicol	aminoglycosides
erythromycins	ethionamide	amphotericin B
ethambutol	naladixic acid	chloroquine
metronidazole	rifampicin	5-fluorocytosine
nystatin	sulphonamides (and	griseofulvin
penicillins	avoid after 38 weeks)	isoniazid
(esters may be toxic, e.g.		lincomycin
talampicillin bacampicillin)		nitrofurantoin
sodium fusidate		primaquine
		quinine
		spectinomycin
		tetracyclines
		trimethoprim
		co-trimoxazole
		vancomycin

N.B. Avoid all new drugs in pregnancy

Combination chemotherapy

Single drugs are generally preferable to combinations. Nevertheless, combinations may be justifiable in certain situations. A combination of drugs is often indicated as empirical therapy of serious infections before the culture results are available. It may be necessary to combine antimicrobial agents to prevent or delay the emergence of resistant strains, as in antituberculous therapy. Neither fusidic acid or rifampicin should ever be used alone since resistance too readily occurs in these circumstances. Mixed infections may require combined therapy.

The major indication for using a combination of drugs is to achieve a synergic effect. When two drugs act together *in vitro* they may exhibit 'indifference', that is their combined effect is no greater than that of the more active agent acting alone. Antagonism is observed when the activity of one drug is actually reduced by the other. They may be synergic, in which case their combined action significantly exceeds either acting alone. Minor increases in activity are described as addition. Synergy is certainly demonstrable in the laboratory but rather less clearly *in vivo*. Despite this, certain difficult infections, notably infective endocarditis and septicaemia in immunosuppressed patients are generally treated with combinations of antibiotics displaying *in-vitro* synergy. There is clinical evidence of the need to use a synergic combination, generally a penicillin and an aminoglycoside, in the treatment of enterococcal

endocarditis. In one study, therapy with penicillin alone resulted in a very high bacteriological relapse rate of 72 per cent. When penicillin was combined with streptomycin the relapse rate fell to 15 per cent.

It has been suggested that the effect of a combination of antibacterial agents can be predicted by knowing if the components are bactericidal or bacteriostatic. This is an oversimplification and cannot be applied to all combinations. However, two bactericidal drugs will be synergic or additive in their action. Two bacteriostatic drugs are generally additive. Some combinations of a bacteriostatic and bactericidal compound, such as tetracycline and penicillin, are antagonistic, whereas other mixtures, such as tetracycline and rifampicin, may be synergic. To increase the confusion, erythromycin is said to be bacteriostatic in low concentrations and bactericidal in high concentrations. It is therefore advisable to test the effect of any combination on the patient's own organism *in vitro*. These tests are mainly carried out when managing cases of infective endocarditis, where completely bacteridical therapy is mandatory.

Accessory treatment

Antimicrobial agents may not eradicate infection in the presence of large aggregations of pus or foreign bodies. Abscesses require surgical drainage. Sequestra and calculi should be removed. Medical management including control of diabetes, uraemia, and anaemia will facilitate recovery.

Duration of therapy

The time taken to eradicate infecting organisms varies with the nature and site of the infection. It may take one or two days to eradicate organisms from the bloodstream, and even longer for wounds or respiratory tract infections. In the majority of infections response to therapy is best assessed using clinical rather than microbiological criteria. Repeated cultures are usually unnecessary, but can be valuable in the management of infections that are hard to eradicate, such as infective endocarditis or tuberculosis.

The appropriate duration of therapy depends on several factors, including the choice of drug, the antimicrobial susceptibility of the pathogen, the site and extent of the infection, and the host defence mechanisms. A standard duration of therapy has been established for a reliable cure of some infections, for example streptococcal pharyngitis. In many other infections the duration of therapy has not been properly established. It was customary to treat acute cystitis with a ten- or fourteen-day course of an antibiotic, given in full dosage. Several recent studies indicate that a three-day course or possibly even one dose of antibiotic is adequate for uncomplicated cystitis.

Table 6 Antimicrobial therapy in patients with impaired renal function

Normal dosage	Little modification of dosage required	Major modification of dosage required	Drugs to be avoided
chloramphenicol[1]	ampicillin/amoxycillin	aminoglycosides	carfecillin
cloxacillin	benzyl penicillin	carbenicillin/ticarcillin	cinoxacin
doxycycline	cephalosporins[3]	colistin	cycloserine
erythromycin	clindamycin	ethambutol	hexamine mendelate
flucloxacillin	co-trimoxazole	5-fluorocytosine	naladixic acid
sodium fusidate	isoniazid	P.A.S.	nitrofurantoin
rifampicin	lincomycin		sulphadiazine
amphotericin B[2]	metronidazole		tetracyclines[4]
clotrimazole			vancomycin[5]
miconazole			
griseofulvin			

[1] Inactive metabolites accumulate and may cause bone marrow depression. Only use if no alternative (removed by haemodialysis).
[2] Amphotericin B is nephrotoxic but negligible renal excretion, not dialysable
[3] Except cephaloridine
[4] Except doxycycline
[5] May be given orally to treat pseudomembranous colitis

Table 7 Antimicrobial agents which should be avoided or used with caution in patients with impaired hepatic function

Antimicrobial agent	Dosage modification in liver disease	Comments
Esters of ampicillin e.g. talampicillin	Avoid	Unhydrolysed compound may be hepatotoxic
Chloramphenicol	Avoid	Accumulation of unconjugated drug may cause bone marrow suppression
Clindamycin	Use with caution	
Erythromycin estolate	Avoid estolate	Use other preparations with caution
Fusidic acid	Use with caution	
Isoniazid	Avoid in fast acetylators	Hepatotoxicity enhanced by concurrent rifampicin therapy
Rifampicin	Avoid	
Tetracycline	Avoid	Sulphonamides occasionally hepatotoxic
Co-trimoxazole	Use with caution	

If the patient fails to respond after a reasonable period of treatment the case should be reviewed. Antimicrobials cannot be expected to cure non-infected patients. The wrong antibiotic may have been used or there may have been errors in the dosage, route of administration, or spacing of the doses of the drug. Further cultures are needed to exclude the emergence of a resistant strain or superinfection with another organism. Another possibility is the development of drug hypersensitivity. Finally, a poor response to antimicrobial therapy may indicate the presence of an abscess or persistent focus of infection which requires surgical drainage.

Monitoring antimicrobial therapy

Two types of test may sometimes be of value in ensuring optimum antimicrobial therapy. These are antimicrobial assays in body fluids and the measurement of the bactericidal power of the patient's serum against his own infecting organism.

Antimicrobial assays provide information on the actual amount of a drug present in serum or other body fluids. Serum bactericidal tests give an indication of the adequacy of therapy, reflecting all the antimicrobial factors present in the sample. These tests will give meaningful results only if the correctly timed specimens are taken. The clinician should consult the microbiologist on the local availability of these tests.

Antimicrobial assays. The majority of antimicrobial agents can be safely prescribed for most patients without any need for laboratory monitoring. Antimicrobial assays are indicated for a variety of reasons. Drug assays can verify that treatment is adequate. The critical drug level depends on the site and nature of the infection. For example, a peak serum gentamicin level of 5 mg/l or greater is satisfactory when treating a Gram-negative septicaemia but a level of at least 8 mg/l is required to overcome a similar infection in a neutropenic patient or a pseudomonas pneumonia. Sustained high blood levels may be necessary in the treatment of partially resistant organisms. Antimicrobial assays are also of value when the patient's renal function is unstable, as in the neonatal period, during the diuretic phase of renal failure, or following severe trauma. Dosage adjustments can be based on regular monitoring to avoid inadequate or excessive levels. Patients with acute leukaemia, cystic fibrosis, and those on dialysis are likely to receive repeated courses of potentially toxic aminoglycosides. Regular assays will detect any cumulative toxicity. Antimicrobial assays are obviously an essential part of the evaluation of new compounds.

The results of antimicrobial assays are meaningless unless the time of the sample collection and the time and route of administration of the drug are known. Serum samples should be collected to coincide with expected peak levels to assess adequacy of therapy. Samples collected just before the next dose of drug, so-called 'trough' levels, will reveal accumulation and impending toxicity.

Many laboratories still rely on microbiological assays. It is therefore essential to know if the patient has received any other antimicrobial agents in the preceding 48 hours. An assay organism can then be chosen which is sensitive only to the antimicrobial agent being assayed. A notable example of this problem is the concomitant use of an aminoglycoside and a cephalosporin. The commonly used assay organism *Klebsiella edwardsiae* var altantae is sufficiently sensitive to many of the cephalosporins to give aberrant results unless the cephalosporin is initially destroyed by β-lactamase.

Aminoglycosides The aminoglycosides (gentamicin, tobramycin, amikacin, sisomicin, netilmicin, streptomycin, and kanamycin) are often used to treat serious infections because of their wide spectrum of activity. The initial or 'loading' dose can be calculated from dosage tables or nomograms that take into account age, sex, creatinine clearance, and body weight. The patient is then put onto a 'maintenance' dose. Even when the dose is carefully calculated by the suggested formulae the resulting serum levels show marked variation. Many patients have suboptimal concentrations, while a few have potentially toxic levels. Serum concentrations should be monitored in most patients receiving aminoglycosides, particularly those with impaired renal function, the elderly, the obese, and those receiving other nephrotoxic or ototoxic drugs. The peak level should be taken 15–30 min after an intramuscular dose. Trough levels should be taken immediately before the next dose of the drug. Falsely raised 'peak' levels are obtained if the post-dose specimen is withdrawn from an intravascular line used to administer the drug. Desirable peak and trough levels are shown in Table 8. All the aminoglycosides are potentially ototoxic and nephrotoxic. Ototoxicity is more likely when there is renal impairment, previous or concomitant ototoxic therapy, following prolonged courses of therapy, and when the concentration of aminoglycosides in the serum is raised. High trough concentra-

Table 8 Desirable serum levels of antimicrobial agents to minimize toxicity

Drug	Concentration (mg/l)	
	Trough level	Therapeutic range
Gentamicin	< 2	5–12
Tobramycin	< 2	5–12
Amikacin	< 8	20–30
Sissomicin	< 2	5–10
Netilmicin	< 3	7–15
Streptomycin	< 3	25–30
Chloramphenicol		10–20
Vancomycin	< 5	50
5-Fluorocytosine	> 25	35–70

tions, for example above 2 mg/l for gentamicin, seem to be more important than high peak concentrations. Similarly a relationship exists between elevated trough concentrations and the development of nephrotoxicity.

Chloramphenicol. The use of chloramphenicol has been limited by its toxicity. It has been estimated that an idiosyncratic, potentially fatal aplastic anaemia occurs in 1 in 24 500–40 000 courses of treatment. The grey baby syndrome is dose-related. It generally occurs in premature and full-term neonates who have received more than 100 mg chloramphenicol/kg per day for three to five days. This syndrome may be avoided by reducing the dosage of chloramphenicol for premature infants and neonates and by monitoring the concentration of chloramphenicol in the babies' serum and cerebrospinal fluid. Toxicity may develop when the serum concentration exceeds 25 mg/l. A reversible dose-related bone marrow suppression may occur at any age when the serum trough levels exceed 25 mg/l. This toxic problem is best identified by serial monitoring of the reticulocyte and full blood counts. If marrow suppression develops it may be reversed by stopping the drug.

Serum bactericidal assay. This type of assay is a simple method of ensuring adequate bactericidal therapy and is particularly useful where this is essential for success as in infective endocarditis. If the patient is receiving two or more antibiotics a bactericidal assay can be more informative than separate determinations of individual drug levels in the serum. Samples of the patient's serum are collected just before and shortly after a dose of antibiotic. The serum is double diluted in broth. Each dilution is inoculated with the patient's own organism, which has been stored in the laboratory. The bactericidal titre is the highest dilution that completely kills the organism. It is generally felt that a pre-dose

titre of 1 in 4 or greater and a post-dose titre of 1 in 8 or greater are satisfactory. Dosage or therapy can be modified in the light of the results.

Antifungal chemotherapy

Over the last twenty years there have been far more advances in the prophylaxis and treatment of serious bacterial infection than in preventing and treating fungal infections. Indeed it may be argued that the widespread use of potent broad-spectrum antibacterial agents is one of the factors contributing to the increased problem of opportunistic mycotic infections. Unfortunately it can be exceedingly difficult to make a confident diagnosis of fungal infection and the results of existing serological and cultural techniques are often inconclusive. For these reasons antifungal therapy is often initiated before a firm diagnosis has been made. This is an unfortunate state of affairs, particularly since many of the available agents are potentially toxic. *In vitro* susceptibility testing of fungal isolates is usually performed by reference and specialized laboratories and therefore tends to be retrospective. It is mandatory to check isolates for resistance to 5-fluorocytosine before and during treatment with this compound.

It is important to remember that fungal infections are frequently associated with a defect in host resistance, such as immunosuppression or the presence of a prosthetic heart valve. Antifungal therapy may well fail if the predisposing condition is not removed or ameliorated. Similarly dermatophyte infections may recur unless the animal source is removed or controlled.

The drugs currently used in the treatment of fungal infections fall into four major groups: the polyene antibiotics, 5-fluorocytosine, the imidazoles, and griseofulvin. The recommended therapy for various fungal infections is shown in Table 9.

Amphotericin B and the imidazoles (e.g. miconazole) may

Table 9 Recommended therapy for fungal infections

Infection	Therapy	Route of administration
Superficial mycoses		
Candidiasis	miconazole	topical
	nystatin	topical
	ketoconazole	oral
	povidone–iodine	topical
Chronic mucocutaneous candidiasis	ketoconazole	oral
Dermatophytosis	ketoconazole	oral
	griseofulvin	oral
	Whitfield's ointment	topical
Systemic mycoses		
Candidosis	amphotericin B	i.v.
	5-fluorocytosine	i.v. + oral
	miconazole	i.v.
Urinary candidosis	5-fluorocytosine	oral
	amphotericin B	bladder wash-out
Aspergillosis	amphotericin B	i.v.
	(econazole)	(i.v., oral)
	(?ketoconazole)	(oral)
Cryptococcosis	amphotericin B + 5-fluorocytosine	i.v.
	± i.thecal amphotericin B	
Histoplasmosis	amphotericin B	i.v.
	miconazole	i.v.
	(?ketoconazole)	oral
Blastomycosis	amphotericin B	i.v.
	miconazole	i.v.
Coccidioidomycosis	amphotericin B	i.v.
	miconazole	i.v.
	?ketoconazole	oral
Paracoccidioidomycosis (South American blastomycosis)	amphotericin B	i.v.
	miconazole	i.v.
	ketoconazole	oral
	sulphadiazine	oral

Table 10 Recommended therapy for viral infections

Drug	Viruses inhibited	Route of administration	Clinical applications	Comments
Amantadine	influenza A	oral	chemoprophylaxis for highly susceptible patients during epidemics of influenza ?therapy	
Idoxuridine (IDU)	herpes simplex varicella–zoster	topical	herpetic keratitis topical therapy for shingles (use 35% IDU in DMSO)	
Acyclovir (acycloguanosine)	herpes simplex varicella–zoster	i.v. oral topical	severe primary herpes simplex generalized herpes simplex Herpes simplex encephalitis varicella–zoster in immunosuppressed patients	Is less active against varicella–zoster than Herpes simplex. Little activity against cytomegalovirus
Vidarabine (ara A adenine, arabinoside)	varicella–zoster	i.v.	varicella–zoster in immunosuppressed patients	Bone marrow and neurotoxicity
Human interferons	many	topical parenteral	not yet clinically available	

be antagonistic if used in combination. The combination of amphotericin B and 5-fluorocytosine is frequently synergistic. Use of this regime has the further advantages that resistance to 5-fluorocytosine is less likely to emerge and a smaller dose of amphotericin B can be used.

It is advisable to monitor serum levels of 5-fluorocytosine, especially in patients with impaired renal function. Peak levels should not exceed 100 mg/l and the trough level should be maintained above 25 mg/l.

Antiviral chemotherapy

Antiviral chemotherapy is still in its infancy. Many viral infections have been successfully controlled by specific vaccines. This approach has been far less effective in combating the viruses that cause respiratory tract infections, principally influenza viruses, and the herpes viruses. Influenza viruses are capable of altering their antigenic structure at regular intervals, necessitating new vaccines. Herpes viruses, including cytomegalovirus, herpes simplex types I and II, and chickenpox persist in latent forms in the host, and recurrent infections may occur following reactivation of the virus. These specific problems have stimulated the search for antiviral compounds. A major challenge has been to develop compounds which selectively attack the intracellular virus particles without causing unacceptable damage to the host tissues. A number of substances are now available which have proved therapeutically useful (Table 10). Most of these compounds exhibit specific activity against one or more groups of viruses. Interferons are antiviral proteins produced naturally by cells infected with viruses or other microorganisms. They are relatively species-specific, that is interferon from primate cells is needed to affect human infections. Human interferon is now being prepared from human leucocytes, diploid human fibroblasts, continuous lymphoblastoid cell lines, and from E. coli by genetic engineering. Preliminary results suggest that interferon may prove effective in combating infections caused by a wide variety of viruses including hepatitis B, herpes zoster, and rhinoviruses.

Chemoprophylaxis

From one-quarter to one-half of all antimicrobials used in hospitals are aimed at preventing rather than treating infection, especially on surgical wards. Prophylaxis is one of the most contentious areas of antimicrobial chemotherapy but it is generally agreed that any attempt to 'sterilize' the patient will certainly fail, and would in any event be highly dangerous. If prophylaxis is to be justified there

must be a significant risk of sepsis to the patient: either where sepsis commonly follows a procedure or where it causes considerable morbidity and mortality when it does occur. The potential infection must be caused by one or more known pathogens which have predictable antibacterial sensitivities. However great the risk, prophylaxis should be considered only if normal aseptic techniques cannot prevent access of the organism to those sites at risk. The duration of the risk of infection should be estimated since the prophylaxis must afford effective protection throughout this time. Prophylactic agents should be relatively free from toxicity and must achieve adequate concentrations in those tissues which are at risk. There is unfortunately a paucity of information on the drug concentrations achieved in vulnerable tissues. The statistical risk of infection should also be considered. It is obviously illogical to attempt to protect patients against imagined as opposed to real risks. For example, the use of metronidazole during gastrointestinal surgery to protect against possible Bacteroides fragilis endocarditis is irrelevent, since this organism so rarely causes infective endocarditis.

In devising a prophylactic regimen it is necessary to calculate not only the dosage but also the timing of the doses to achieve the peak tissue concentration at the time of maximum risk. It is particularly important to avoid premature drug administration. This is well illustrated by the use of prophylactic penicillin for dental work in patients with abnormal heart valves. After two days of penicillin, penicillin-resistant strains of viridans-type streptococci appear in the mouth and rapidly predominate over the normally sensitive strains. Overprolonged administration is almost as great an error as premature use of chemoprophylaxis. Lengthy post-operative 'prophylaxis' is really early treatment. There is abundant evidence that a single dose of antibiotic or 24 hours' cover is just as effective as more prolonged therapy. Longer duration merely increases the cost, the risk of adverse reactions, and the emergence of resistant organisms. Whenever possible so-called 'narrow-spectrum' drugs should be used to minimize any alteration of the patient's normal flora and the risk of superinfection with resistant organisms.

Antimicrobial chemoprophylaxis presents obvious complexities and the potential user must be mindful of the indications for its use. Carefully controlled clinical trials have given much valuable information on chemoprophylaxis. Clinicians should be hesitant to institute prophylactic chemotherapy in the absence of evidence from controlled trials that it will be effective.

Conditions in which chemoprophylaxis is of value

In certain situations chemoprophylaxis has been clearly shown to be effective. In other instances chemoprophylaxis is widely believed to be useful but its efficacy has not been clearly established. In the following paragraphs the main indications for chemoprophylaxis are considered.

Following acute rheumatic fever (see page 5.142). Recurrences of rheumatic fever carry a considerable risk of increasing cardiac damage, and chemoprophylaxis should be administered to prevent Group A streptococcal infections in such patients. The most effective method is the administration of 1 200 000 units of benzathine penicillin by intramuscular injection once a month. Oral phenoxymethyl penicillin (penicillin V) 250 mg twice daily is less effective but may be more acceptable to the patient. Patients who are hypersensitive to penicillin may be given sulphadiazine (1 g daily) or erythromycin (250 mg twice daily). The duration of the prophylaxis remains controversial but generally is continued till the age of 17 years or for a period of five years, whichever is the longer.

Infective endocarditis (see page 5.148). It is generally agreed that certain procedures carry a risk of endocardial infection to persons with abnormal heart valves. Such procedures include dental work, urinary catheterization, and instrumental delivery. However, there is a paucity of well-controlled clinical studies demonstrating the efficiency of antimicrobial cover in these situations. Recommendations for antimicrobial prophylaxis are outlined in Table 11.

Bacteraemia may occur with any periodontal procedure associated with gingival bleeding. Viridans-type streptococci predominate in the oro-pharyngeal flora and are the most common species of bacteria isolated from the blood after trauma to the teeth and gums. Oral prophylaxis is suitable for the majority of patients who do not receive a general anaesthetic. High-dose amoxycillin is recommended unless the patient is hypersensitive to penicillin when erythromycin is a reasonable alternative. Parenteral prophylaxis is preferable for patients receiving a general anaesthetic. A single injection of intramuscular fortified procaine penicillin or intravenous vancomycin is sufficient. Another alternative for the penicillin-hypersensitive patient is an intravenous injection of erythromycin followed by two doses of oral erythromycin. Patients who are currently receiving penicillin prophylaxis and those who have recently been treated with this drug should be given oral erythromycin to cover dental procedures. *In vitro* studies suggest that the combination of erythromycin with rifampicin may be more effective in this instance, but to date this finding has not been clinically substantiated. Patients with prosthetic or homograft valves are no more susceptible to endocarditis than patients with damaged natural valves, but it is more difficult to eradicate infection when it does occur. For this reason a bactericidal combination of antibiotics is normally recommended. Parenteral penicillin and gentamicin or vancomycin and gentamicin are recommended cover for dental procedures in patients with artificial heart valves.

Genito-urinary and gastrointestinal surgery is associated with a risk of faecal streptococcal endocarditis. Complicated childbirth, urethral catheterization, cystoscopy, and prostatectomy are four such procedures which may precede endocarditis. Ampicillin and gentamicin given by injection, or vancomycin and gentamicin for the penicillin-allergic patient, would be suitable regimens.

Meningococcal meningitis (see page 5.173). Chemoprophylaxis is effective in limiting meningococcal meningitis in close contacts. It has been shown that the incidence of the disease is 1000 times greater in close household contacts of a case than among the general population. Prophylaxis is therefore advisable for close household contacts, room-mates, pre-school children in day nurseries and others in institutions. A two-day course of oral rifampicin 600 mg b.d. is usually recommended. The dose for children aged 1–12 years is 10 mg/kg b.d. and for children under one year old 5 mg/kg b.d. Where the organism is known to be sulphonamide sensitive, sulphadiazine 1 g b.d. for two days may be given. About half the group A strains and 20–25 per cent of other groups are resistant to sulphonamides and prophylaxis should not be delayed for the results of antibiotic sensitivity testing. Rifampicin resistance has already been observed in meningococci and it is clear

Table 11 Recommended chemoprophylaxis for patients with congenital or valvular heart disease undergoing procedures associated with bacteraemia

Procedure	Likely organism	Routine prophylaxis (natural heart valves)		High-risk prophylaxis (prosthetic heart valves)	
		Standard regimen	For penicillin-allergic patient and patients already taking a penicillin	Standard regimen	For penicillin-allergic patients
Dental procedures associated with gingival bleeding e.g. extraction, scaling	viridans-type streptococci	(a) *Local anaesthetic* oral amoxycillin 3 g 30 min before and 8 hours after procedure	oral erythromycin stearate 1.5 g 1 hour before then 500 mg every 6 hours for 24 hours	fortified procaine penicillin BP (300 mg procaine penicillin + 60 mg benzyl penicillin) i.m. + gentamicin 80 mg i.m. 30 min before procedure	vancomycin 1 g i.v. (slowly over 20 min) + gentamicin 80 mg i.m. 30 min before procedure
Oropharyngeal surgery, tonsillectomy, adenoidectomy, bronchoscopy	viridans-type streptococci	(b) *General anaesthetic* fortified procaine penicillin BP (300 mg procaine penicillin + 60 mg benzylpenicillin) i.m. 30 min before procedure	vancomycin 1 g i.v. (slowly over 20 min) 30 min before procedure *or* erythromycin lactobionate 1 g i.v. 15 min before then oral erythromycin stearate 500 mg every 6 hours for 24 hours	fortified procaine penicillin BP (300 mg procaine penicillin + 60 mg benzyl penicillin) i.m. + gentamicin 80 mg i.m. 30 min before procedure	vancomycin 1 g i.v. (slowly over 20 min) + gentamicin 80 mg i.m. 30 min before procedure
Genito-urinary and gastrointestinal surgery including urethral catheterization	faecal streptococci (enterococci)	ampicillin 1 g i.v. + gentamicin 80 mg i.v. 30 min before procedure and repeated twice at 8-hourly intervals	vancomycin 1 g i.v. (slowly over 20 min) + gentamicin 80 mg i.v. 30 min before procedure	ampicillin 1 g i.v. + gentamicin 80 mg i.v. 30 min before procedure and repeated twice at 8-hourly intervals	vancomycin 1 g i.v. (slowly over 20 min) + gentamicin 80 mg i.v. 30 min before procedure

Normal adult dosage given. Reduce dosage for children as follows (do not exceed adult dose):
  Amoxycillin 1.5 g
  Erythromycin 20 mg/kg orally initially then 10 mg/kg
  Fortified procaine penicillin 10 mg/kg
  Vancomycin 20 mg/kg
  Gentamicin 2 mg/kg

at this may increase with widespread usage of this drug. Minocycline is also effective but many patients experience unpleasant side-effects, notably vertigo. Penicillin is *not* effective prophylaxis. Prophylaxis is unnecessary for medical and nursing personnel unless there have been in very close contact with the patient's respiratory secretions, for example after mouth-to-mouth resuscitation.

Haemophilus influenzae meningitis (see page 5.199). The risk of infection in household contacts of an index case is nearly 600 times greater than in the age-adjusted general population. Several different regimens have been used to attempt to eradicate nose and throat carriage. The most encouraging is oral rifampicin 10–20 mg/kg per day in one or two doses for four days. To date there has not been a controlled study to establish the efficiency of chemoprophylaxis in this disease. There have been reports of haemophilus meningitis occurring in close contacts despite chemoprophylactic rifampicin. It is possible that a combination of rifampicin with trimethoprim might be more effective.

Tuberculosis (see page 5.244). Historically the control of tuberculosis in the United Kingdom has depended on the early identification of active cases and mass immunization. Chemoprophylaxis has been more extensively used in the United States. With the end of mass B.C.G. vaccination in some parts of this country prophylactic chemotherapy may become more widespread. Isoniazid 5 mg/kg daily for 6–12 months has generally been shown to be effective prophylactic therapy. Primary resistance to isoniazid remains surprisingly low. Chemoprophylaxis with isoniazid is indicated for: (a) laboratory staff following self-inoculation with tuberculous material, (b) highly susceptible close contacts who are tuberculin negative and who have not received B.C.G. The most frequent example of this is a baby born to a mother with active tuberculosis. In these instances isoniazid is being used to prevent acquisition of infection. In other cases where the patient is tuberculin positive isoniazid may be used to suppress in apparent infection. This constitutes early treatment rather than chemoprophylaxis.

Prophylactic isoniazid should be avoided in adults aged 35 years or more since drug-induced hepatitis is more frequent in older patients.

Recurrent urinary tract infections (see Section 18). Recurrent urinary tract infections have a high morbidity, causing great distress to the sufferer. Antimicrobials have not been shown to protect the kidney from progressive damage nor do they alter the natural history of the condition but they do reduce the morbidity. The broad indication for chemoprophylaxis is frequent recurrences of infection (more than three attacks per year). The urine should be rendered sterile with an intensive course of antibacterial therapy and maintenance therapy should be instituted *immediately* to prevent any reinfection. In reality this is often suppressive therapy rather than true prophylaxis. Long-term low-dose therapy with co-trimoxazole, trimethoprim, or nitrofurantoin, given at bed-time may be instituted. Many patients have been on long-term therapy for many years with no obvious problems of toxicity or emergence of resistant bacteria. When recurrent infections are associated with sexual intercourse, the patient should be advised to micturate immediately after intercourse. In addition a single small dose of penicillin or nitrofurantoin taken at this time will often be effective in preventing infection.

Prophylaxis is much more difficult when the normal wash-out mechanisms of the bladder are impaired, as for example in the grossly abnormal urinary tract. If the patient is symptomatic, bladder wash-outs with an antiseptic (e.g. noxytiolin or chlorhexidine) or an antibiotic (e.g. neomycin) two or three times a day may succeed in reducing the bacterial count to a low level. Recurrent symptoms may sometimes then be prevented by long-term suppressive chemoprophylaxis.

Influenza A (see page 5.46). Epidemics of influenza A can cause considerable morbidity and mortality, especially in patients with chronic chest or heart disease or in the elderly. Amantidine is a highly specific antiviral agent, being active against influenza A but not influenza B or C. Chemoprophylaxis with amantidine (100 mg b.d.) throughout the period of risk has been shown to reduce the incidence of clinical infection in highly susceptible patients. Too short a course of chemoprophylaxis may merely delay rather than terminate the epidemic. Amantidine and influenza vaccine can be given concurrently. Vaccine-induced immunity can then afford protection after the course of amantidine is completed. This form of chemoprophylaxis is expensive and should be considered only for high-risk groups during established or potential epidemics of influenza A.

Surgery
Cardiac surgery. Mitral valvotomies and prosthetic or homograft valve replacements are at particular risk of endocarditis. The mortality of prosthetic valve endocarditis is an unacceptable 30–40 per cent. The most important causes of early onset endocarditis are *Staphylococcus aureus* and *Staphylococcus epidermidis*, which were implanted at operation or which gained entry to the circulation via intravascular lines. Gram-negative bacteria are far less important. There is no general agreement on the best form of prophylaxis. Parenteral benzyl penicillin, cloxacillin and gentamicin given with the premedication and continued for 48 hours is one acceptable prophylactic regimen. It is important to remove all intravascular lines as soon as possible and it may be justifiable to continue prophylaxis until these hazards are removed. There is much less risk of serious infection following coronary artery bypass grafts.

Surgery on ischaemic legs and in pelvic region. Gas gangrene caused by *Clostridium perfringens* or related organisms constitutes a particular risk in major surgery around the hip or amputations of the leg. *Cl. perfringens* is always present in the normal human intestinal flora and the area of skin over the hips and thigh is often contaminated with clostridial spores. Diabetics are particularly prone to develop gas gangrene. In these patients the gangrene is often of mixed clostridial and non-clostridial origin. One mega unit of benzyl penicillin should be given intramuscularly every six hours for two doses pre-operatively and continued for five days after the operation. Thorough pre-operative cleansing of the skin with iodophor compresses is also recommended.

Prosthetic implant surgery
Total hip replacement. The incidence of deep sepsis following total hip replacement is very low, being 1.5 per cent in a recent multicentre study. As with prosthetic heart valves, the most frequent causes of infection are *Staph. aureus* and *Staph. epidermidis*. For this reason cloxacillin is generally used prophylactically. It should be remembered that cloxacillin resistance may occur in both *Staph. epidermidis* and *Staph. aureus*. The use of an acrylic cement incorporating gentamicin provides a novel approach in orthopaedic surgery. The antibiotic elutes out of the cement over a period of time. To date there have been no reports of adverse effects or of the development of resistance. Whether the antibiotic affects the mechanical strength of the cement remains uncertain. There is, however, no doubt about the value of ultraclean air in operating theatres and whole-body exhaust suits in reducing the incidence of deep sepsis after total joint replacement.
Peripheral vascular surgery. The efficacy of antibiotic cover in peripheral vascular surgery has been questioned. It does seem advisable to give prophylaxis when a prosthetic graft is inserted, since the mortality following graft sepsis is over 25 per cent. The majority of infections are caused by staphylococci and prophylactic cloxacillin would be the logical choice.
Ventriculo-atrial shunts. Colonization of cerebrospinal fluid shunts by *Staph. epidermidis* is a serious problem. The organisms are introduced during the insertion or revision of the shunt.

Peri-operative prophylaxis would seem reasonable, but parenteral antibiotics have not proved effective. Preliminary studies have suggested that peri-operative intraventricular gentamicin may be useful. An alternative approach is the use of silicone rubber shunts impregnated with an antibiotic, for example diethanolamine fusidate or clindamycin hydrochloride. This attractive idea has not yet been evaluated clinically.

General surgery. Nowhere has the question of chemoprophylaxis been more fiercely debated than in patients undergoing general surgical operations. There is some evidence that antimicrobial chemoprophylaxis in general surgery prevents wound infection and in so doing results in more rapid wound healing and discharge from hospital. It is beyond question that good patient-selection and first-class aseptic techniques are of much greater importance. Antimicrobials are never a substitute for hygienic practices. There are many instances where topical antiseptics are at least as effective as chemoprophylaxis and carry much less risk. Prophylaxis may be justified where the risk of sepsis is high, its consequences severe, and a known effective drug can be used. Keighley and Burdon detail the following indications for prophylaxis in general surgery:

(1) operations for gastro-oesophageal carcinoma, reconstructive gastric operations and in achlorhydric patients with gastric ulcers;
(2) cholecystectomy in selected patients who have infected bile;
(3) appendicectomies;
(4) colorectal surgery;
(5) hysterectomies.

Numerous publications attest to the effectiveness of particular drugs in certain surgical procedures, for example, metronidazole in appendicectomy and hysterectomy or metronidazole and gentamicin in colorectal surgery.

There is no doubt that intelligent use of chemoprophylaxis can be life-saving. It may well result in more rapid wound healing and improved patient wellbeing. However, the available evidence does not justify the current scale of prophylaxis in surgery. More rational usage should not only decrease the drug bill but would probably represent in improvement in patient care.

Malaria (see page 5.398). Any discussion of antimicrobial chemoprophylaxis would be incomplete if malaria prevention were omitted.

Every person travelling to a malarious area should be advised to take prophylactic antimalarials in addition to protecting themselves from mosquitos once they arrive. Chloroquine-resistant strains of Plasmodium falciparum have been reported from many parts of the world including south-east Asia, Indonesia, the Philippines, New Guinea, the Indian subcontinent, East Africa, and South America. Clinicians must therefore ascertain the current recommendations for travellers to any particular area. Chloroquine phosphate remains the drug of choice for the suppression of malaria caused by chloroquine-sensitive Plasmodium spp. Primaquine should be taken in addition for two weeks after returning home to eradicate any P. vivax or P. ovale parasites that may be present in the liver. Primaquine is contraindicated in pregnancy or in patients with G6PD deficiency. In these patients subsequent relapses with P. vivax or P. ovale infection may occur and can be treated with chloroquine. In areas with chloroquine-resistant strains of P. falciparum, pyrimethamine–sulphadoxine, pyrimethamine–dapsone, or pyrimethamine–sulphalene may be used. However, the patient should also take chloroquine since some strains of P. vivax are now resistant to pyrimethamine–sulphadoxine. Recently strains of P. falciparum resistant to both chloroquine and pyrimethamine–sulphadoxine have been reported in refugee camps along the Thailand–Kampuchean border. Quinine sulphate is possibly the drug of choice in this single instance. Malaria chemoprophylaxis is not always successful, even if taken diligently, and the diagnosis should be considered in anyone returning from a malarious country.

Conditions in which chemoprophylaxis is of doubtful valu

Neutropenia (see page 5.479). Infection is a major cause of deat in neutropenic patients. The debate on the value of protectiv isolation and prophylactic antimicrobials continues. Several tria have shown that total barrier isolation, food sterilization, and th administration of oral non-absorbable antibiotics reduce the rat of infection in patients with acute leukaemia receiving cytotoxi therapy. However, in general there is no improvement in the rate c remission or in the long-term survival. Laminar flow units ar expensive and not universally available. Oral non-absorbabl antibiotics, for example a mixture of framycetin, colistin an nystatin, do not appear to be beneficial when patients are nursed i conventional wards. Moreover they are often nauseating an distressing.

More recently prophylactic oral co-trimoxazole has bee advocated to prevent colonization of the patient's intestinal tract b exogenous organisms. Some workers have reported good result with this simple regime, but others are less optimistic. Furthe studies are necessary to clarify the value of this regime Prophylactic co-trimoxazole has been used for many years t prevent recurrent urinary tract infections, and the development c antibiotic resistance is not a major problem. Prophylactic co trimoxazole is effective in preventing Pneumocystis carin. pneumonitis in children with acute lymphoblastic leukaemia an should be used in units where this infection is common.

Prophylactic oral nystatin does not seem to be a reliable way c preventing fungal infections in neutropenic patients. Prophylacti chemotherapy with oral ketoconazole or intravenous miconazol are currently being evaluated in neutropenic patients. To date th results of these clinical trials are not conclusive. Early result suggest that either regimen may lead to an increase in coloniza tion by resistant fungi.

Post-splenectomy. Pneumococcal infections are more commo following splenectomy or in patients with a non-functioning splee Children are most at risk and the incidence of pneumococcal seps is greater for the first two years after splenectomy. Prophylacti penicillin or erythromycin for penicillin-allergic patients is advo cated by some clinicians, but there is no convincing proof of it efficacy. The value of polyvalent pneumococcal vaccine i splenectomized patients is currently being assessed.

Cerebrospinal fluid rhinorrhoea. Cerebrospinal fluid rhinorrhoe predisposes the patient to bacterial meningitis, which is usuall caused by pneumococci. Prophylactic penicillin or ampicillin ar often given but the evidence for their efficacy is conflicting. In th absence of meningeal inflammation the cerebrospinal fluid concen trations of these antibiotics well be very low indeed.

Prolonged rupture of membranes. The risk of chorio-amnioniti sharply increases when the membranes are ruptured for more tha 24 hours. Chemoprophylaxis has not been shown to be effective i preventing infection and will inevitably lead to an overgrowth o resistant organisms. A more selective policy should be adopted an antibiotic treatment started at the first sign of maternal or feta infection

Group B streptococcal disease in neonates (see page 5.145) Group B streptococci are an important cause of septicaemia an meningitis in neonates. Early-onset and late-onset disease hav been described. Colonization of the maternal genital tract b Group B streptococci during pregnancy is the most importan factor in early-onset disease. Attempts to reduce the colonizatio rates during pregnancy using prophylactic oral penicillin hav proved unsuccessful. An alternative approach is to give prophylac tic penicillin routinely to the newborn baby shortly after birth. In recent controlled study this regimen reduced colonization an infection rates in neonates, but was associated with an increase number of infections caused by penicillin-resistant organisms in the first year of life. Furthermore, prophylaxis at birth will not modify those infections acquired in utero

Chronic bronchitis (see Section 15). Acute exacerbations in chronic bronchitis are almost always due to *Haemophilus influenzae* or *Streptococcus pneumoniae*. Prophylactic antimicrobial therapy with agents such as ampicillin, tetracycline or sulphamethoxazole–trimethoprim has been extensively used, but there is no evidence that it halts the inevitable decline in respiratory function. The increasing prevalence of resistance to these compounds by *H. influenzae* suggests that prolonged prophylaxis be avoided if possible. Equally good results are obtained if the patient is given an antibiotic and instructed to treat himself at the first sign of an impending infection.

Cystic fibrosis. Children with cystic fibrosis are prone to repeated pulmonary infections caused by *Staphylococcus aureus*, *Haemophilus influenzae*, and *Pseudomonas aeruginosa*. Prompt treatment of acute episodes is probably more effective than continuous therapy.

Pertussis (see page 5.205). A week's course of oral erythromycin has been recommended for children who are close contacts of a case of pertussis, if they are less than one year old or unimmunized and less than seven years old. The value of chemoprophylaxis has never been demonstrated. Active immunization of these children should also be considered. Oral erythromycin should be given to the child with whooping cough since it will eliminate naso-pharyngeal carriage of *Bordetella pertussis*.

Diphtheria (see page 5.133). All household contacts of a case of diphtheria should be given an injection of diphtheria toxoid. Unimmunized or inadequately immunized contacts and carriers are usually given a seven-day course of oral erythromycin. Controlled studies of the value of chemoprophylaxis have unfortunately not been carried out.

Tetanus (see page 5.226). Proper immunization and surgical toilet of traumatic wounds are of paramount importance in the prevention of tetanus. The need for active immunization with or without passive immunization depends on the patient's immunization history and the severity of the wound. Antimicrobial therapy may be indicated to combat wound sepsis but its value in preventing tetanus is debatable. Penicillin will kill vegetative *Clostridium tetani* but will have no effect on spores or on any toxin already present in the wound.

Conditions in which chemoprophylaxis is useless

Prophylactic chemotherapy is of no value in the prevention of urinary tract infections in patients with indwelling catheters. If the catheter is left *in situ* for more than three or four days infection is almost invariable. Of far greater importance are good aseptic techniques at the time of introducing the catheter and the use of a closed drainage system. Similarly there is no place for antibiotic prophylaxis for intravascular cannulae.

There has been much interest in the prevention of pneumonia in patients with tracheostomies, by the administration of local antibiotics as an aerosol. This practice inevitably causes an increase in the level of antibiotic resistance and the emergence of resistant bacteria as pathogens. For these reasons, the prophylactic use of antibiotic aerosols should be avoided though they may be a useful adjunct in the treatment of established Gram-negative pneumonia. Prophylactic antibiotics are of no benefit in preventing pneumonia in unconscious patients and merely encourage the overgrowth of resistant organisms.

Peritonitis is a frequent complication of chronic ambulatory peritoneal dialysis and may be due to an enormous variety of organisms. Early treatment of an infection, based on the results of bacteriological culture of the effluent fluid is preferable to continuous prophylaxis.

Sources of information on antimicrobial chemotherapy

Clinicians are often overwhelmed with information on new and currently available drugs. Much of this data is provided by the manufacturers and is inevitably biased towards their own products. This needs to be counter-balanced by critical independent evaluations. Unbiased reviews and summaries are provided in a number of publications (Table 12). In addition postgraduate teaching on antimicrobials should be regularly offered. This is necessary both to reinforce earlier teaching and also to put the manufacturers' claims for new antimicrobial agents into perspective. Close collaboration between microbiologists and clinicians and continuing education of all who prescribe antimicrobials should encourage a more rational approach to antimicrobial chemotherapy.

Table 12 Sources of information of antimicrobial chemotherapy

Manufacturers' data sheets
British National Formulary (BNF)
Prescriber's Journal
Drugs and Therapeutics Bulletin   } freely available in
Monthly Index of Medical Specialities (MIMS) United Kingdom
Data Sheet Compendium
The Medical Letter   } available in the
A.M.A. Drug Evaluations   United States

Medical microbiologists and infectious disease physicians

References

American Heart Association Committee Report (1977a). Prevention of bacterial endocarditis. *Circulation* **56**, 139A
— (1977b). Prevention of rheumatic fever. *Circulation* **55**, 1.
American Thoracic Society (1974). Preventive therapy of tuberculous infection. *Am. Rev. resp. Dis.* **110**, 371.
Appel, G. B. and Neu, H. C. (1977). The nephrotoxicity of antimicrobial agents. *New Engl. J. Med.* **296**, 663, 722, 784.
Barrett, S. P. and Watt, P. J. (1979). Antibiotics and the liver. *J. antimicrob. Chemother.* **5**, 337.
Collier, L. H. and Oxford, J. (1980). *Developments in antiviral therapy*. Academic Press, London.
Garrod, L. P., Lambert, H. P., and O'Grady, F. (1981). *Antibiotic and chemotherapy*, 5th edn. Churchill Livingstone, Edinburgh.
Hirschmann, J. V. and Inui, T. S. (1980). Antimicrobial prophylaxis: a critique of recent trials. *Rev. infect. Dis.* **2**, 1.
Immunization Practices Advisory Committee (1981). Diphtheria, tetanus and pertussis: guidelines for vaccine prophylaxis and other preventive measures. *Morbid. Mortal. Weekly Rep.* **30**, 392, 401.
Kagan, B. M. (1980). *Antimicrobial chemotherapy*, 3rd edn. W. B. Saunders, Philadelphia and London.
Keighley, M. R. B. and Burdon, D. W. (1979). *Antimicrobial prophylaxis in surgery*. Pitman Medical, Tunbridge Wells.
Kusumi, R. and Kunin, C. (1982). Chemoprophylaxis of infection in medicine and surgery. In *Recent advances in infection*, vol. 2 (eds. D. S. Reeves and A. M. Geddes), p. 185. Churchill Livingstone, Edinburgh.
Lidwell, O. M., Lowbury, E. J. L., Whyte, W., Blowers, R., Stanley, S. J., and Lowe, D. (1982). Effect of ultraclean air in operating rooms on deep sepsis in the joint after total hip or knee replacement; a randomised study. *Br. med. J.* **285**, 10.
Morbidity and Mortality Weekly Report (1982). Prevention of malaria in travellers, 1982. *Morbid. Mortal. Weekly Rep.* **31**, (supplement).
Rubin, R. H. and Young, L. S. (1981). *Clinical approach to infection in the compromised host*. Plenum Medical Book Company, New York and London.
Speller, D. C. E. (ed). (1980). *Antifungal chemotherapy*. John Wiley, Chichester.
Yourassowsky, E. (1978). Indications, interpretation and applications of antibiotic assays. *Infection* **6**, 140.

Specific infectious agents

VIRUSES

Respiratory viruses

J. Nagington and D. Rubenstein

Introduction. Virus infections can involve the entire respiratory tract, from the nasopharynx to the alveoli. They are the most common infections of the community.

It is customary to consider the infections according to the anatomical region mainly affected since each region has one or more virus groups with an affinity for it. This is not a rigidly fixed situation and a virus which usually affects one region to produce symptoms commonly infects adjoining regions and may even produce symptomatic infection at a different site to that usually described when there is a heavy exposure or increased susceptibility.

The conventional subdivision is at the larynx, above which are the upper respiratory infections: rhinitis, pharyngitis and tonsillitis, otitis media, and croup or laryngitis (Table 1), and below are the lower respiratory infections: tracheitis, bronchitis, bronchiolitis, pneumonitis or atypical pneumonia, and pneumonia (Table 2). Combinations of these produce the clinical appearances that are described as coryza, influenza, etc.

These clinical syndromes are also caused by organisms which are not true viruses (i.e. mycoplasma, chlamydia) and should be referred to in the appropriate sections.

The common cold (acute coryza, rhinitis). The rhinoviruses are the major group involved in the production of colds. With the enteroviruses they comprise the picornavirus family (*pico*: small, *RNA* viruses) but unlike enteroviruses they are readily inactivated by moderately acid conditions (i.e. less than pH 5.3) which means that they are unlikely to survive gastric acidity and produce faecal spread. Since they lose infectivity when dried in air, it is assumed that the main route of infection is by droplets from the

Table 1   Upper respiratory viruses, listed in order of frequency

Clinical condition	Virus	Pathogenic serotypes
Rhinitis, coryza, febrile colds	rhinovirus	more than 90 serotypes
	coronavirus	several serotypes of which at least 12 strains associated with coryza
	adenovirus	33 serotypes; 4 and 7, most frequently found
	para-influenza	4 types of which 1,2, and 3 important
	echovirus	types 8, 11, 20, 22, and 25 most often of the 34 serotypes
	respiratory syncytial	several variants distinguishable
	coxsackie A	A21 and A24 are the 'common cold' types of the 24 human serotypes
	influenza A	5 main serotypes of which usually 2 are in circulation with strain variation
	influenza B	1 main serotype with strain variation
	rubella	1 main serotype
	reovirus	3 serotypes but pathogenic significance in doubt
Pharyngitis, tonsillitis	Adenovirus	types 1, 2, 3, and 5 common in children types 3, 4, 7, 14, 21 in adult epidemics
	influenza A and B echovirus, coxsackie A and B, rhinoviruses	
Pharyngo-conjunctival fever	Adenovirus	types 3 and 7, commonly; 1, 2, 5, 6, and 14 less often
Ulcerative pharyngitis, herpangina	coxsackie A	A2, 3, 4, 5, 6, 8, and 10 especially
Hand, foot, and mouth disease	coxsackie A	A16, frequently; A5, 9, and 10 much less frequently
Herpetic ulcers	herpes simplex virus	2 types of which type 1 is most common pharyngeal type
Pharyngitis associated with 'glandular fever'	Epstein–Barr virus	1 main serotype
	cytomegalovirus rarely	1 main serotype
Laryngitis, laryngotracheo-bronchitis (croup)	para-influenza	mainly types 1 and 3
	respiratory syncytial	as for rhinitis
	influenza	as for rhinitis
	rhinovirus	as for rhinitis
	adenovirus	as for rhinitis

Table 2 Lower respiratory viruses, listed in order of frequency

Clinical condition	Virus	Pathogenic serotypes (approximate order of frequency)
Acute bronchitis, acute bronchiolitis	respiratory syncytial influenza A influenza B para-influenza adenovirus rhinovirus coronaviruses coxsackie B	serotypes 1, 2 and 3 4, 7 commonly; 3, 14 less often
Pneumonia	influenza A influenza B adenovirus para-influenza respiratory syncytial (infants only) measles (young children only) varicella-zoster (rare) herpes simplex cytomegalovirus	7, 1, 3 in infants, 4, 7 in adults in the immune suppressed

nasopharynx. However, recent experiments have shown the transmission via nasal secretions on the fingers can occur.

Rhinoviruses can be grown in tissue cultures of primate cells that are maintained in physiological conditions with some semblance to the nasopharynx, i.e. 33 °C, well oxygenated, and slightly lower pH than normal. They destroy infected cells and produce a cytopathic effect similar to that produced by enteroviruses.

Immunity after a cold is very transient, perhaps because of the lack of a common immunizing antigen, the absence of viraemia, localized site of infection, or a combination of these. Since horses and cattle each have their own rhinoviruses man is not unique in his affliction.

The clinical features are the same irrespective of the virus concerned and they are produced by inflammation of the nasal mucosa. Mild inflammation produces snuffles, and more severe inflammation produces nasal secretion and oedema of the turbinates, which may block sinus drainage and the airways, and cause pain from inflamed congested sinuses. Extension to the nasolachrymal duct causes lachrymation and extension to the pharynx a dry uncomfortable throat which is seldom painful. Fever is uncommon in children and in adults.

Severity varies widely within an outbreak due to any one virus and is presumably dependent on the degree of immunity of the individual.

Colds are very common in small children and the frequency declines with age, although adults continue to have one to six colds a year.

Spread occurs by the dispersal of droplets of nasopharyngeal secretion during talking, coughing, and especially sneezing.

The incubation period varies between one to four days, and symptoms often start in a localized region such as the pharynx or one area of the nose and rapidly progress during the next 48 hours until the diagnosis is obvious. During resolution the nasal secretion becomes purulent, evidence of polymorphonuclear exudate, and it is not necessarily related to secondary bacterial infection which occurs in only a minority of cases.

Although disabling for the individual and a scourge of considerable economic importance, there are few sequelae and there is no mortality. The sequelae include acute otitis media.

Diagnosis is invariably made by the patient and differential diagnosis is only of value when associated with a haemolytic streptococcal outbreak, when a swab for bacteriology is worthwhile.

No specific therapy or immunization is at present available. The prospects for a vaccine are poor because of the large number of different strains of rhinovirus which are the predominant aetiologic agent, and the short duration of immunity which appears dependent on local mechanisms.

Treatment. There are many proprietary preparations available for the treatment of colds. Aspirin will relieve headache, and aspirin gargles accompanied by throat lozenges (not those containing antibiotics) will ease a sore throat. Nasal congestion can be reduced by inhalations, drops containing ephedrine or phenylephrine, or enteric-coated atropine preparations. Antihistamines can be used particularly in children at night when their sedative action may encourage sleep. Antibiotics are not indicated unless secondary bacterial infection of the sinuses or middle ear ensue.

Pharyngitis and tonsillitis. The most common presentation of viral pharyngitis is a sore throat, and there may be associated coryza and cervical lymphadenopathy. Fever is common. On inspection the pharynx and tonsils are reddened and there is not usually an exudate. Palatal petechiae are often present but are not pathognomonic. The main clinical need is to distinguish it from a haemolytic streptococcal infection. Haemolytic streptococci can cause up to one-third of sore throats. Even in a known epidemic, it is not possible clinically to distinguish between streptococcal and non-streptococcal infection without a bacteriological culture. If the patient's condition will allow, it is well worth waiting for the results of the culture as this will determine with certainty the need for penicillin, which is otherwise best avoided. Table 1 shows the viruses that have been isolated from patients with acute pharyngitis.

Pharyngo-conjunctival fever. Adenoviruses have a special affinity for the pharynx and some infections, particularly epidemics in closed communities, associated with serotypes 4 and 7, may be characterized by acute conjunctivitis and cervical lymphadenopathy, for which the description 'pharyngo-conjunctival fever' provides an apt description.

Herpangina. Infection with some coxsackievirus A serotypes (especially 2, 3, 4, 5, 6, 8, and 10) produces severe pharyngitis with fever and ulceration. In the early stages small discrete papulovesicular lesions appear on an erythematous base and these break down to ulcers which extend irregularly. The shallow ulcers may be difficult to distinguish from herpes simplex ulceration; if the ulceration becomes severe and multiple, agranulocytosis from marrow suppression by leukaemia or drug toxicity must be considered.

Hand, foot, and mouth disease. Sometimes described as 'vesicular stomatitis with exanthema' the pharyngeal ulcers in this coxsackievirus infection are less severe than in herpangina. There is a typical vesicular eruption on the hands and feet, and sometimes in small children the buttocks. Several coxsackievirus strains can cause the syndrome but A16 is the most important.

Infectious mononucleosis. Infectious mononucleosis (glandular fever) (see below) is a common cause of pharyngitis in young adults, easily confused with haemolytic streptococcal infection. Pharyngeal ulceration also occurs in Behçet's syndrome and the Stevens–Johnson syndrome; tuberculous and syphilitic ulcers are usually single.

Treatment. As with other virus infections antibiotics have no place in the treatment of acute pharyngitis once haemolytic steptococcal infection has been excluded. Symptomatic relief of symptoms can be achieved with aspirin for pain and fever, and aspirin gargles with throat lozenges for the soreness in the throat.

If the pain is sufficiently severe to prevent eating and drinking, transient relief can be obtained from anaesthetic lozenges containing amethocaine or by holding ice-cream and ice in the mouth. This will often allow fluids to be taken, if necessary through a straw, if opening the mouth is too painful. In proven glandular fever, if the pain and tonsillar enlargement prevent swallowing, a short course of steroids (prednisolone 40 mg daily for two days reducing rapidly by 10 mg daily to zero) will rapidly shrink the tonsils and relieve symptoms.

Otitis media. Secondary bacterial infection of the middle-ear is an uncommon complication of virus pharyngitis. *Streptococcus pneumoniae* and, in the under five-year-olds, *Haemophilus influenzae* are the likely organisms and respond to penicillin and ampicillin respectively.

Laryngo-tracheitis. The illness begins with fever and a dry cough followed by hoarseness as the larynx becomes infected. Tracheitis produces a burning retrosternal pain on inspiration and expiration. In rare circumstances respiration becomes progressively laboured and inspiratory stridor a marked feature, i.e. croup. The viruses which most often cause laryngitis are the para-influenza group and tracheitis is a feature of these and the influenza group.

In some cases anoxia is sufficiently severe to require tracheostomy and assisted respiration. The degree to which airways obstruction, laryngitis, bronchitis, and parenchymal lung disease contribute in severe cases is often uncertain.

Croup. Croup is a good descriptive term for the inspiratory stridor or crowing that occurs in infants and small children with acute laryngitis. Oedema of the vocal cords obstructs the airway and produces respiratory distress.

Croup is sometimes difficult to distinguish from whooping cough but the characteristic whoop and coughing attack does not accompany the stridor. Acute epiglottitis has a more sudden onset and rapid development which can be fatal if the airway is not maintained.

The viruses most frequently associated with croup are para-influenza (especially type 1), respiratory syncytial virus (RSV), and influenza, especially influenza A in epidemic years. Acute epiglottitis is due to *Haemophilus influenzae* infection.

Differential diagnosis. Viral tracheitis, laryngo-tracheitis, and croup should be distinguished from bacterial epiglottitis, laryngeal obstruction due to a foreign body and laryngeal diphtheria.

Treatment. There is no specific therapy available for the treatment of virus laryngo-tracheitis. Treatment is aimed at relieving the symptoms and maintaining oxygenation. Inhalation of humidified air may prevent rapid drying of secretions along the airways and may also partially relieve symptoms.

In severe cases of laryngeal narrowing oxygenation may be required initially, and if hypoxia develops, tracheostomy with or without assisted respiration may become necessary.

Except in the rare severe case, the outlook for viral laryngo-tracheitis is excellent.

Acute bronchitis. Acute bronchitis is often a clinically distinct entity, although it also forms part of a more general repiratory infection.

Acute viral laryngitis and laryngo-tracheitis are relatively uncommon, and acute bronchitis common, particularly in smoke-filled atmospheres, especially when this includes the bronchial tree of the smoker. The clinical features are usually mild with a fever, cough, and purulent sputum with varying degrees of airways obstruction, expiratory wheeze, and dyspnoea depending upon the severity of parenchymal lung damage from previous attacks of acute bronchitis. All the lower respiratory viruses can cause bronchitis and so can those more often associated with upper respiratory infections. The extent to which respiratory tract bacteria contribute to episodes of acute bronchitis remains uncertain.

Acute bronchitis can also complicate some systemic virus infections, especially measles, and chickenpox.

Acute bronchiolitis. Acute bronchiolitis is the most common severe respiratory infection of infants. The highest incidence in Britain occurs in babies aged one to three months in industrial areas and in families with siblings so that 24.5 per 1000 of this age group require admission to hospital with the infection. Neonates are commonly infected but have negligible symptoms and children over 18 months of age have relatively mild symptoms. The illness is practically pathognomonic of respiratory syncytial virus (RSV) infection and it has a very marked seasonal incidence. Cases begin early in December in the United Kingdom and then increase to a peak in February then decline to a very few by the end of April.

Clinical features. An upper respiratory infection heralds the acute bronchiolitis which follows abruptly with fever, and rapidly progressive dyspnoea due to obstruction of the bronchioles, producing intercostal and suprasternal retraction with associated anoxia and cyanosis. The anoxia may be first apparent as the infant becomes fretful and irritable. Movement of air is severely limited and the lungs hyperinflated.

Differentiation from severe asthma may be difficult, although this is rare in infants of this age group. The clinical distinction during the acute episode is not critical as the management is aimed at maintaining the airway and relieving anoxia. The mortality rate in hospital admissions is approximately 1 per cent.

Treatment. Inhalation of warmed and humidified oxygen in high concentration may be sufficient to relieve anoxia. Bronchodilators and corticosteroids are of unproven value but in severe cases may be life-saving. Adequate and accurate correction of fluid and electrolyte disturbances is essential.

Influenza. The disease has a brief incubation period of one to three days and the clinical features vary from those of a mild febrile coryzal illness indistinguishable from many other respiratory virus infections to the other extreme of influenza proper.

The main symptoms of uncomplicated influenza are: (*a*) acute onset, often dramatic; (*b*) headache, backache, myalgia, shivering, malaise; (*c*) stuffy nose, dryness of the throat, huskiness of the voice; (*d*) dry unproductive cough; and (*e*) anorexia, nausea, and insomnia.

The main signs are: (*a*) fever, increasing rapidly to 38–40 °C in 24 hours; (*b*) conjunctival infection; (*c*) pharyngeal injection; (*d*) the chest sounds are normal except in bronchitic individuals; and (*e*) the patient is ill, sometimes to the point of prostration.

The acute symptoms persist for about four days and then gradually subside in uncomplicated cases. The longer the illness the longer may be the period of recovery.

The complications of influenza are: (*a*) hyperpyrexia with the production of delirium, convulsions and coma, especially in children and the elderly; (*b*) acute bronchitis with increasing age of patient; (*c*) primary pneumonia especially in patients with prior cardiac or pulmonary disease. Secondary pneumonia from very rapid invasion by bacterial flora, especially *Staphylococcus pyogenes*, which can be disastrous; (*d*) myocarditis in a small number of individuals during some outbreaks; (*e*) exacerbation of pre-existing disease such as diabetes; (*f*) neurological changes including Reyes syndrome in children and post-influenza depression in adults; and (*g*) sudden death in a few previously healthy young adults and in a higher proportion of the elderly—hence the well-known term 'the old man's friend'—although there is no apparent sex discrimination.

Epidemiology of influenza. There are three influenza viruses, A, B, and C, which are distinguished by their internal nucleoproteins. The surface of the virions is coated with spikes of haemagglutinin (H) and an enzyme, neuraminidase (N) which are important for attachment of the virus to the respiratory epithelium of the host and infection of susceptible cells.

The three viruses differ in the extent to which they undergo antigenic change in their surface structure. Influenza A undergoes antigenic 'shift', i.e. major change or mutation in both H and N, together or independently, which is associated with pandemic inections. Between these changes there is minor antigenic 'drift' which appears to help maintain interpandemic incidence of infection.

Influenza B is more stable so that the annual incidence remains more consistent. Influenza C is the most stable with a much lower pathogenicity, and causes mainly subclinical infections. The pandemic strains to date are shown in Table 3.

Table 3 Pandemic influenza strains

Period of prevalence	Colloquial description	Antigenic description
1947–1957	A_1	H_1N_1
1957–1968	Asian	H_2N_2
1968	Hong Kong	H_3N_2
1977	USSR (Russian)	H_1N_1

The reappearance of H_1N_1 in 1977 after an absence of about 20 years exposed a large population to infection who had grown up without encountering this antigenic type.

Emergence of a new strain is followed by an increase in prevalence to a peak in two or three years, so that at any particular time there are two strains of influenza A and one of B which dominate the epidemic scene.

A localized outbreak in the USA in 1976 which was associated with $H_{sw1}N_1$ caused considerable apprehension because this strain, which is endemic in swine, may be related to the strain which caused the lethal 1918–19 pandemic. In fact no further spread was recorded and the strain did not appear to be very pathogenic.

Treatment of influenza. The outlook is usually excellent, although most patients with severe influenza are almost incapable of leaving their beds. An adequate fluid intake should be maintained throughout the illness, and the fever can be reduced and the headache relieved with aspirin.

Antibiotics have no place in the treatment of uncomplicated influenza and should be reserved for secondary bacterial infections of the lung. If suspected, Gram-stain of sputum (which should also be cultured) should be performed, and this may indicate the infecting bacteria. This is usually *Haemophilus influenzae* or the *Streptococcus pneumoniae*, both of which are sensitive to ampicillin or its related drugs, or *Staphylococcus pyogenes*. During epidemics in which secondary staphylococcal pneumonia occurs a penicillin resistant penicillin should be added in large doses (e.g. cloxacillin 8–10 g daily intravenously) as the mortality is very high.

If physiotherapy, hydration, and adequate antibiotic therapy and oxygen are insufficient, as judged by the patients' clinical condition and his blood gas analysis, full intensive care with artificial respiration may become necessary.

Influenza pneumonia. This is fortunately a rare complication of influenza since it carries a very high mortality. Even young fit people can be affected, and soon after onset of the disease they become rapidly and progressively more dyspnoeic, with an associated productive cough and blood-stained sputum. On examination there is cyanosis, and in the chest are heard coarse crepitations and the wheezing of bronchitis.

Radiograph of the chest reveals widespread bilateral patchy consolidation typical of severe virus pneumonia. The white count may be greatly elevated which suggests secondary infection with *Staph. pyogenes*.

The clinical condition of the patient with influenzal pneumonia, with or without secondary staphlococcal infection often deteriorates rapidly with progressive dyspnoea and anoxia leading finally to circulatory collapse and death. An autopsy influenza virus can be recovered from the extensively haemorrhagic lungs.

Treatment. If pneumonia is suspected in anyone with influenza they should be transferred to an intensive care unit. Since there is an increased need for intensive care to be available during influenza

outbreaks it is sensible to ensure that the appropriate staff have been immunized with vaccine.

Oxygen and adequate hydration are the mainstay of therapy, and artificial respiration may be required. If there is any suspicion of secondary bacterial infection with *Staph. pyogenes*, which may be confirmed by Gram stain of the sputum, cloxacillin should be given in high dosage (e.g. 8–10 g daily) intravenously.

There is at present no antiviral drug of proven efficacy for the treatment of influenza. Synthetic primary amines have been explored (amantidine) or are still under evaluation (spiroamantidine, ribavirin). Interferon is not commercially available. The prospects for specific therapy are uncertain since the infection is very rapidly progressive and to be effective such a drug would have to be readily available soon after the onset of the symptoms.

Influenza vaccine. Protection against influenza is provided by current vaccine preparations which are prepared from the two most prevalent epidemic strains of influenza A plus the current strain of influenza B.

The categories of patient for whom vaccine is considered of value are those with: (a) chronic heart, lung or renal disease; (b) diabetes; (c) patients on immunosuppressive therapy or for whom immunosuppression is to be given; (d) nurses and staff of other essential services; (e) patients aged 65 years or more; and (f) some closed communities. There are two forms of vaccine, 'whole' vaccine, which consists of whole virus particles, and 'split' vaccine in which the virus has been fragmented into mainly subunits of haemagglutinin and neuraminidase. A variation of this is 'surface' antigen in which aluminium hydroxide is used as a stabilizer.

'Split' vaccine gives fewer reactions and is recommended for children; 'whole' vaccine is valuable for systemic protection especially in bronchitics, and it is usually only given over the age of 13 years.

Virus pneumonia. Pneumonia and pneumonitis are most frequently caused by myxoviruses, a group which contains the influenza (orthomyxoviruses), para-influenza, and measles viruses (paramyxoviruses), and although most respiratory viruses may occasionally be involved the adenoviruses are probably the next most important (Table 4).

Table 4 Viral pneumonias. The clinical features of cough, sputum, dyspnoea, with or without cyanosis, and patchy consolidation on CXR occur in all

	Additional clinical features of diagnostic help	Differential diagnosis
Diagnosis clinically	*obvious*	
Measles	measles rash	
Chickenpox	chickenpox rash	
Diagnosis clinically not obvious		
Influenza	current epidemic	bacterial bronchopneumonia mycoplasmal pneumonia
Adenovirus	none	tuberculosis Q fever pneumonia
RSV	infants	legionnaires' disease aspiration
CMV	immune-suppressive therapy for renal transplant	as above plus fungi and *Pneumocystis carinii*
Herpes zoster Herpes simplex	leukaemia, etc. e.g. steroids, azathoprine, cyclosporin A	

Chickenpox pneumonia. The respiratory tract is always infected in chickenpox (varicella) and is the major means of spread of infection. Although the lungs must be frequently affected, pneumonia of any clinical severity is extremely rare, and then usually in adults. Two to four days after the onset of the rash, a dry cough develops which may progress to a productive cough with haemoptysis, dyspnoea, and cyanosis. The degree of severity varies from a dry cough with or without dyspnoea, to a rapidly progressive pneumonia, respiratory failure, and death within 36–48 hours. Radiological findings also vary from a small area of consolidation to the widespread bilateral diffuse opacities of bronchopneumonia. The lesions calcify over the next 10–20 years in survivors and radiographs show a typical 'military' appearance.

Treatment. Patients on immune suppressive therapy, i.e. patients with leukaemia and lymphomas, are prone to disseminated chickenpox, and if they develop widespread disease with or without pneumonia the drugs should if possible be stopped.

When possible human zoster immune globulin (ZIG) should be given prophylactically to immunosuppressed patients who have been exposed to infection. When symptoms occur it may still improve the outlook if given early.

Acycloguanosine, although still under trial, appears to be clinically effective against varicella-zoster virus and will probably have a place in the treatment of severe chickenpox pneumonia. Adequate hydration is essential and artificial respiration may be required in serious cases.

Measles pneumonia (giant cell pneumonia). Nearly every child with measles has a dry cough, a few crepitations and wheezes on auscultation of the chest, and many have the diffuse radiological changes of intersitial pneumonitis. The majority recover fully and serious pulmonary complications are rare and invariably caused by secondary invaders, usually *Streptococcus pneumoniae* and *Haemophilus influenzae*. In tropical countries measles accounts for 10 per cent or more of the deaths under two years.

Some children with impaired immune competence, including leukaemia, lymphoma, or on immune suppressive therapy, fail to mount an immune response to the virus, shown by the absence of a rash and the persistence of the virus in the lung tissues and secretions. In these children a rapidly progressive pneumonia may result with subsequent death. For this reason live measles vaccines should not be given to children with serious disease or who are taking steroids, azathioprine, or other immune suppressive agents.

In children with chronic heart and lung disease where measles vaccine may be given, but only with caution, it should be attenuated by the simultaneous administration of a measured low dose of antibody in normal immunoglobulin.

Respiratory syncytial virus (RSV) pneumonia. RSV is a very important cause of bronchiolitis in infants (see above) in the winter and it not infrequently extends to pneumonia, said in some areas to produce 10 per cent of infant pneumonias.

RSV pneumonia may cause severe illness in an infant with bronchiolitis who is febrile, irritable, and listless with tachycardia, rapid respiration with intercostal muscle indrawing, and severe anoxia.

The chest radiograph reveals widespread bilateral patchy consolidation indistinguishable from other severe virus pneumonias. Although the illness is very severe and there is a mortality rate of at least 0.5 per cent in the United Kingdom the majority of children recover fully. Second infections are not uncommon but are less severe.

Treatment is supportive and in the more severe cases depends upon expert nursing care, adequate hydration, and the inhalation of humidified air or oxygen depending upon the degree of anoxia. Artificial respiration is rarely required. Antibiotics should be reserved for proven or strongly suspected secondary bacterial infection.

Virus pneumonia in the immune suppressed. Patients given steroids, azathioprine, or cytotoxic agents are made immunologically less competent both by the drugs and their underlying illness, usually an acute leukaemia or a lymphoma. Such patients are more susceptible to pneumonia caused by the herpes viruses—herpes simplex, varicella-zoster, and cytomegalovirus. Pneumonia is only part of a severe systemic illness which carries a high mortality.

Clinically such patients with virus pneumonia rapidly become ill with increasing dyspnoea, cyanosis from anoxia, progressive and terminal respiratory failure over two to seven days.

The problem is to distinguish between the causes of rapidly progressive respiratory failure in patients on immune suppressive agents, usually impossible on clinical grounds alone. They are all very ill and anoxic with rapid respiration and reduced P_{AO2} and the chest radiograph invariably reveals diffuse bilateral patchy consolidation. Amongst the other organisms which produce this picture are *Pneumocystis carinii*, the fungal infections, aspergillosis and cryptococcosis, and tuberculosis. The presence of herpes simplex or chickenpox skin lesions is a helpful guide but obviously not conclusive evidence that the pneumonia is related.

Accurate and rapid diagnosis is essential if treatment is to be given any chance of success, and examination of sputum, preferably obtained from laryngeal washings, either directly or by pertracheal aspiration, or lung tissue must be performed without delay.

Virus pneumonia in the immune suppressed patient carries a very poor prognosis, although acycloguanosine may offer some hope for patients with herpes virus infections.

In practice, virus pneumonias with the exception of RSV in infants, are uncommon in normal individuals and even less frequently cause serious respiratory damage. They may be impossible to distinguish from the more common bacterial bronchopneumonias: *Mycoplasma pneumonia*, Q fever (*Coxiella burneti*), psittacosis (*Chylamydia psittaci*), or Legionnaires' disease (*Legionella pneumophilia*), although they tend to progress less rapidly. Tuberculous pneumonia may cause confusion, as may an aspiration pneumonia if there has been no obvious precipitatory cause.

Laboratory diagnosis. The need for laboratory diagnosis in respiratory virus infections is restricted to those conditions which are severe, e.g. pneumonia, or of epidemiological importance, such as influenza and RSV, or where the condition is of unusual interest. It is obviously unnecessary to contemplate any other than a selective approach.

Since most viral infections of the respiratory tract produce infection of the nasopharynx, this provides a useful source of material for culture in the first few days of infection. After two or three days successful isolation is less likely to be achieved although diagnosis may be possible for another day or two by demonstration of infected cells, using fluorescence antibody technique. Specimens for isolation should be inoculated into tissue cultures within the shortest possible time after they are taken, not longer than a few hours and virus viability should be preserved by the use of a transport medium and cooling. The time for a result depends on available techniques. Serology is invaluable for diagnosis but cannot provide a rapid answer since antibody production requires about seven days. A high titre after this time is strong presumptive evidence of infection but a rise between paired sera is conclusive. Although the time required is longer it is of great value in the confirmation of a provisional diagnosis, in epidemic situations, and in unusual clinical presentations.

The most appropriate specimens can be summarized as follows:

1. Rhinitis, tonsillitis, pharyngitis, and pharyngeal ulceration: swab in virus transport medium (VTM).

2. Infections of neonates and children under one year old: nasopharyngeal aspirate sent to the laboratory in the aspirate tube or a bottle receiver (when long distances are involved slides may be prepared from an aspirate and then sent for fluorescence microscopy).

3. Bronchiolitis in infants: nasopharyngeal aspirate examination for RSV by immunofluorescence the same day is of value for segregation of infected admissions to hospital. A throat swab is a less effective alternative.

4. Influenza: throat swab in VTM during first three days or 10 ml clotted blood during first three days and second specimen 10–14 days later for serology.

5. Pneumonia: clotted blood initially and repeat in 10–14 days. If the patient not seen until after seven days of illness an initial specimen then may contain a diagnostically high antibody titre but further blood should be taken to see if the titre has risen further and so provide confirmation.

6. Post mortem: trachea or tracheal scrapings and affected lung are the usual approach in suspected influenzal pneumonia.
In all cases specimens should also be taken for bacteriology.

References

Lennette, E. M. and Schmidt, N. J. (1979). *Diagnostic procedures for viral, rickettsial, and chlamydial infections*, 5th edn. American Public Health Association, Washington.

Madeley, C. R. (1977). *Guide to the collection and transport of virological specimens*. World Health Organization, Geneva.

Report to the Medical Research Council (1965). A collaborative study of the aetiology of acute respiratory infections in Britain 1961–1964. *Br. med. J.* **ii**, 319.

— (1978). Respiratory syncytial virus infection: admissions in hospitals in industrial, urban and rural areas. *Br. med. J.* **ii**, 796.

Stuart-Harris, C. H., Pereira, M. S., and Tyrell, D. A. J. (1979). In 'Influenza' (ed. G. C. Schild). *Br. med. Bull.* **35**, 3, 9, 77.

— and Schild, G. C. (1976). *Influenza; the virus and the disease*. Arnold, London

Tyrell, D. A. J. (1965). *Common colds and related diseases*. Arnold, London.

— and Pereira, H. G. (1980). *Influenza—a Royal Society Discussion*. The Royal Society, London.

The herpesviruses

B. E. Juel-Jensen

Herpesviruses are widespread throughout the animal kingdom. They contain double-stranded DNA and measure 100–150 nm in diameter. They have an icosohedral capsid with 162 hollow capsomeres. Characteristically a particular herpesvirus is host-dependent. The cat fish, the iguana, and some snakes (*Bungaris fasciatus* and *Naja naja*) have their own herpesvirus as do many higher vertebrates like the dog, cat, pig, horse, monkey and man. Some, like the cytomegaloviruses which can be isolated only in homologous fibroblast cell cultures, appear to be host-specific, and normally do not cross the host-barrier. Following the primary infection of the host, the virus goes latent and may be reactivated sometimes only many years later. The herpesviruses have probably evolved with their hosts over millions of years. They have come to terms with their host and rarely cause more than relatively trivial disease. When they cross the host-barrier the result can be a devastatingly fulminant disease.

Man is host to four herpesviruses: herpes simplex, varicella–zoster virus, Epstein–Barr virus, and cytomegalovirus. Very occasionally the monkey viruses *Herpesvirus simiae*, and possibly *Herpesvirus tamarinus* cause serious disease in man, but they must be considered as examples of herpesviruses that have crossed to another host by accident.

Some herpesviruses, like that which causes Marek's disease in the chicken, have been proved to be the cause of cancer: among human herpesviruses herpes simplex virus and Epstein–Barr virus have been suspected as being involved in cancer production.

Reference

Kaplan, A. S. (ed.) (1973). *The Herpesviruses*. Academic Press, New York.

Herpes simplex virus infections

Since antiquity medical writers have used the term herpes to describe cutaneous manifestations of infection with herpes simplex virus (HSV) and with varicella–zoster virus. The skin lesions of HSV and of zoster are sometimes similar, and the pathological changes at cellular level are similar, for both viruses produce the same type of intranuclear inclusions; both show an affinity for nervous tissue. Both are DNA viruses with an identical morphological structure. The behaviour of the two viruses is quite distinct in the laboratory, but muddled terminology has not helped the clinician. It was proposed to rename HSV *Herpesvirus hominis* to distinguish it from similar viruses in other species. That only added to the confusion for there are four herpesviruses peculiar to man: herpes simplex, varicella–zoster, cytomegalovirus, and Epstein–Barr virus. So did the proposal to rename varicella–zoster virus *Herpesvirus varicellae*. Much misunderstanding can be avoided if the term herpes is reserved for the manifestations of HSV infection, and not used also to describe zoster, the clinical picture produced by reactivation of latent varicella–zoster virus.

Infection with HSV in man is characterized by the primary infection, that is the invasion of the non-immune host by the virus. Antibodies and cell-mediated immunity develop and normally persist for the remainder of the life of the individual, although complement fixing antibodies may wane with time if recurrences cease. The virus goes latent in ganglion cells, usually of the nerves supplying to the site of the primary infection. In some individuals the virus is subsequently reactivated, in some frequently, giving rise to recurrent clinical disease despite the presence of antibody, presu-

Table 1 Schematic course of untreated HSV disease

mably because of changes in cell-mediated immunity and the local environment. The virus has achieved a remarkable degree of symbiosis with its host; remaining unnoticed in most, but being a minor nuisance in many. In a few it causes serious disease, but death is exceptional. The course of the infection has been set out schematically in Table 1.

Most HSV infections are caused by the so-called type 1 virus which usually is recovered from skin, mucous membrane, or the brain of adults with encephalitis. Type 2 virus is the usual infecting agent in genital lesions and disease of the newborn. The two types can be distinguished in the laboratory by different growth characteristics in tissue cultures under varying conditions, and by differences in neutralizing antibodies. The pocks produced on the chorioallantoic membrane of a fertile hen's egg by the two types are different: type 1 produces small lesions, type 2 much larger lesions. There is no good evidence that a previous infection with type 1 virus protects against type 2, indeed both types of virus have been grown from the same patient at the same time.

Epidemiology. The primary infection often occurs with no or only trivial clinical manifestations which may pass unnoticed. Many people with antibody to HSV deny knowledge of any past illness which could have been the primary infection. A comparable pattern has been found in many surveys. In one such, done in Edinburgh in 1965, there was a high incidence of antibodies in children under the age of six months, falling to 19 per cent in children aged six to eleven months. There was then a rise, reaching 65–69 per cent at 15–25 years with a further slow increase to 97 per cent in those over sixty. The high incidence in the very young results from passive transfer of maternal antibody across the placenta. IgM does not pass the placenta, and the presence of IgM in an infant suggests active disease. The subject is further bedevilled by the fact that it is very difficult technically to distinguish antibodies to type 1 from those to type 2 virus in large surveys.

As in the case of Epstein–Barr virus, there is a difference in the prevalence of antibodies to HSV in different social groups. With increasing standards of living, one would expect the level of passively transferred antibodies in the early months of life to fall as fewer mothers will be herpetic. In the period 1964–8, 33 per cent of 131 British-born Oxford clinical students had antibodies, contrasting with 62 per cent of 42 students born in third world countries and in Germany at the end of the Second World War, and contrasting with those of a comparable age group in the Edinburgh Survey mentioned above. Only a third gave a history of recurrent cold sores or other herpetic manifestations. Table 2 shows that the trend has continued. It will be noted that the incidence of antibodies to cytomegalovirus has dropped over the last five years, possibly because an increasing proportion of students have been to day schools where the incidence of cytomegalovirus is lower than in boarding schools.

Table 2 Incidence of antibodies to herpes simplex virus (complement-fixing), and, for later years, for comparison to cytomegalovirus (complement-fixing) and Epstein–Barr virus (fluorescent antibody) in Oxford clinical students. Figures in brackets show numbers tested.

	1964–8	1976	1977	1978	1979	1980
HSV	32.8%(131)	26.7%(60)	16.9%(65)	16.4%(67)	20.3%(69)	23.5%(85)
CMV		57.4%(61)	38.3%(65)	29.2%(65)	26.9%(67)	16.4%(85)
EBV				60.0%(65)	62.3%(69)	68.2%(85)

Other evidence suggests that people born after the Second World War generally have a much lower prevalence of antibody than those in the older age groups. All figures on prevalence must be treated with caution, for the populations tested are often not comparable. Poor black and white slum populations in America are not comparable with a group of suburban English people. Commonly held views on the relative infectivity of the four herpesvirus diseases should be revised. Varicella–zoster is certainly the most infectious;

Epstein–Barr virus is probably the second most easily transmitted, usually by aerosol; and the term 'the kissing disease' would be more appropriate for herpes simplex than for infectious mononucleosis. The spread of cytomegalovirus disease requires close contact.

In most underdeveloped countries nearly all children will have antibodies to HSV by the age of five. The age at which the HSV infection is acquired is of more than academic interest; the later in life the greater the chance that the patient will have obvious clinical disease.

Primary and recurrent infections due to type 1 HSV. The primary infection may pass completely unnoticed, there may be relatively trivial manifestations, the commonest event, or there may be severe disease, occasionally with a fatal outcome. Any part of the 'envelope' of man may be the site of cutaneous manifestations. Although apparently localized, there are often systemic upsets. The recurrent infection is usually relatively trivial, except in immunosuppressed patients.

Gingivo-stomatitis. *The primary infection.* The mouth and lips are the most frequent sites of the primary infection. In many small children the lesions are trivial (Fig. 1). But with falling incidence of HSV infection in childhood, there has been an increase in the number of young adults with quite severe primary gingivo-stomatitis. Over a four-year period (1964–8) there were 18 cases among 600 medical students and nurses at risk in Oxford. The illness usually starts with a sore throat and associated generalized 'influenza' symptoms: general malaise, muscle and joint aches,

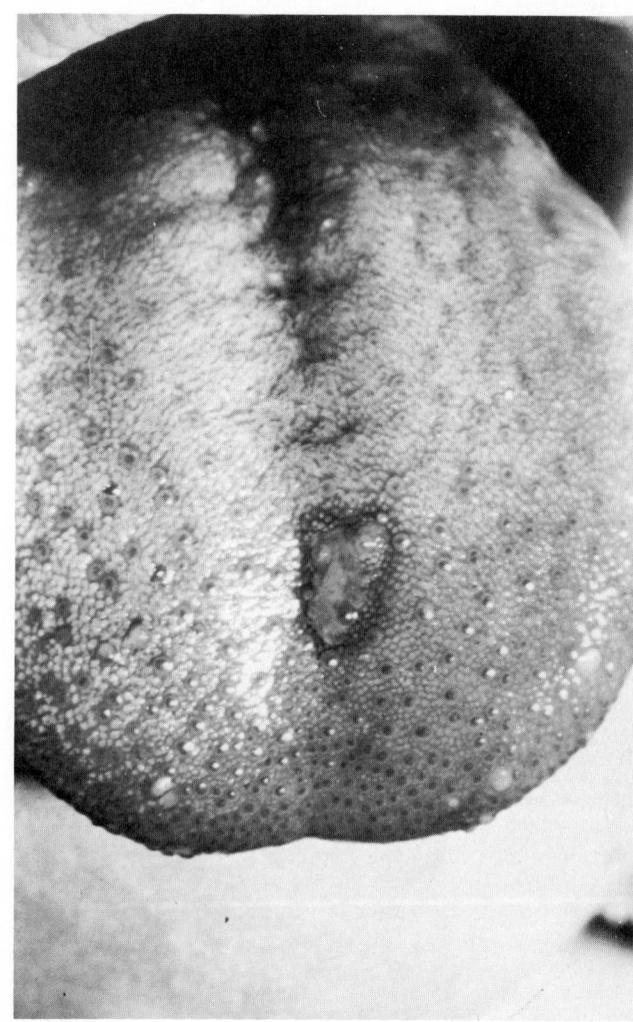

Fig. 1 Primary herpetic stomatitis. A single lesion on the tongue of a six-year-old boy.

sometimes rigors and a fever which for a few days may reach 40.0 °C. There is considerable adenopathy, often generalized, but particularly marked in the neck. The spleen is occasionally enlarged. After a few days lesions, transiently vesicular, but soon bared as shallow ulcers appear on the soft and hard palate, the gums, and usually on the lips (Figs 2 and 3). The ulcers are often painful, there is oedema, and eating becomes difficult or impossible. Left untreated they heal slowly over the following 10 to 14 days. The virus is usually present for two to three weeks and is easily grown from swabs taken from the lesions and sent to the virus laboratory in Hanks's transport medium. Sera should be taken when the patient is first seen and ten days later. Antibodies appear during the second week and the appearance of antibody will confirm that this was a primary infection.

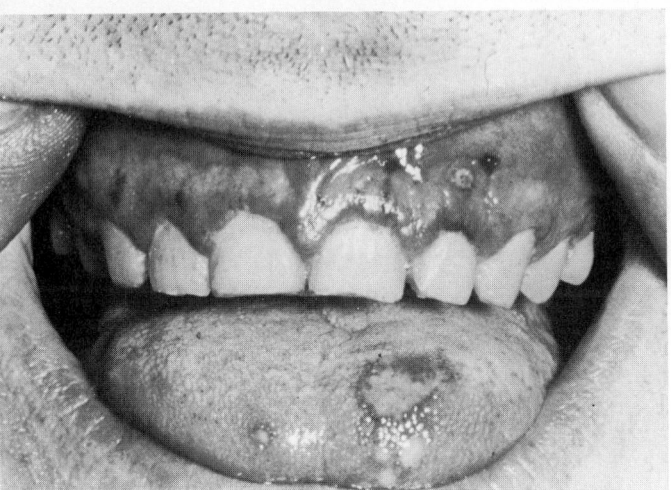

Fig. 2 Primary herpetic gingivo-stomantis in a man of 25. Lesions on the tongue and gums.

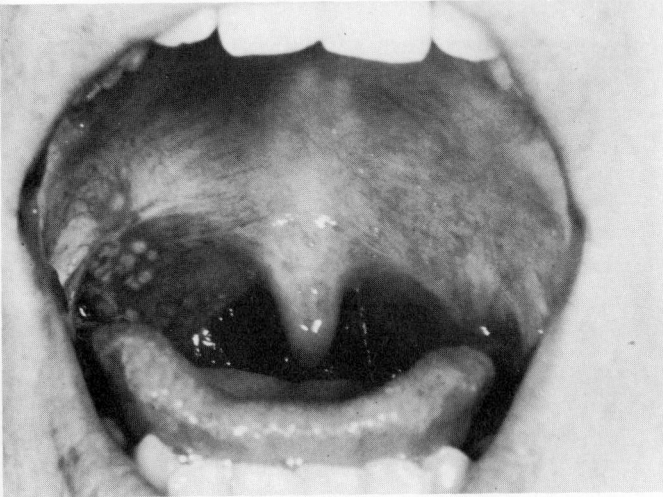

Fig. 3 Primary herpetic gingivo-stomatitis in a woman of 21. The lesions on the soft palate are indistinguishable from the 'Herpangina' in certain coxsackievirus infections.

Differential diagnosis. The oral cavity has only a very limited range of responses to a wide variety of insults, not merely infections, and it can be impossible to tell clinically what the causative agent is without the aid of the laboratory. The correct diagnosis is not made unless HSV is considered. A good many cases of so-called 'Vincent's angina' are probably examples of HSV gingivo-stomatitis. The other three herpesvirus infections must be excluded. Chickenpox (see page 5.57) without a cutaneous eruption is very rare, but zoster of the second branch of the trigeminal nerve

confined to the mouth has caught the unwary (Fig. 4c). It is of course unilateral. Infectious mononucleosis (Fig. 4a) (see page 5.63) may give an identical picture as may cytomegalovirus infection (see page 5.67). Coxsackievirus (Fig. 4b) (see page 5.84) and echovirus infection (see page 5.84) must be excluded, and bacterial disease, particularly diphtheria (see page 5.133) and β-haemolytic streptococcal infection (see page 5.138) should be considered. Severe 'aphthous ulcers' or Stevens–Johnson's syndrome may look like HSV gingivo-stomatitis.

The recurrent infection

The cold sore; herpes labialis, fever blisters. Available evidence suggests that following the primary infection the virus remains latent in the sensory ganglia of the trigeminal nerve. In some, probably only in about a third of all herpetics, one or several of a number of stimuli may provoke recurrences, probably by causing a change in cell-mediated immunity which allows the latent virus to replicate.

Recurrent gingivo-stomatitis is rare, although the primary infection most commonly occurs in the oral cavity. Recurrent lesions usually occur in the cutaneous distribution of the maxillary and mandibular branches of the trigeminal nerve, most commonly on the lips or the skin, round the mouth and in the nostrils: 'cold sores', 'herpes febrilis', and 'fever blisters' are commonly used names.

Recurrences are usually in the same site. They are heralded by itching and tingling, followed, after an interval of a few hours to a day, by the eruption of a cluster of small blisters filled with clear fluid. The lesions may vary in extent, and are often painful. The tops of the vesicles soon come off. The lesions heal by crusting; they may leave scars, particularly if they have become secondarily infected. The average duration to complete healing of the untreated lesion is nine to ten days. The intervals between recurrences are usually unpredictable, but may vary from a few days to years.

A variety of stimuli may provoke a recurrence. Mechanical trauma, such as shaving, and intubation and other manoeuvres during anaesthesia and surgery, including tracheotomy. Ultraviolet light commonly provokes a recurrence: examples are strong sunlight, high altitude, or a visit to the seaside. A rise in temperature from whatever cause is perhaps the commonest form of provocation. 'Herpes febrilis' is not diagnostic of lobar pneumonia or malaria, merely an indication of a good fever from whatever cause in a herpetic. Emotional stress may produce recurrences, probably through the relase of adrenaline. Hyperaemia may be a common mechanism. In some herpetic individuals HSV can be isolated quite frequently from the tears and throat without obvious clinical disease. There is a significant association between trigeminal neuralgia and HSV. If the posterior sensory root of the Gasserian ganglion is cut, 95 per cent of patients develop a herpetic eruption in the mandibular and maxillary divisions of the fifth nerve after two to five days. In one survey, all 61 female patients with trigeminal neuralgia were found to have neutralizing antibody to HSV.

In a few patients, even a trivial recurrence is followed after up to ten days by an attack of erythema multiforme. Perhaps a critical level of antigen triggers the lesion, for in a few cases antiviral treatment at the first sign of a recurrence of the herpetic lesion will prevent erythema multiforme developing.

Differential diagnosis. Usually the diagnosis is easy, but impetigo (see page 5.138) may be mistaken for HSV lesions. Not infrequently, particularly in children, cold sores are secondarily infected with *Staphylococcus aureus*. Small eruptions of zoster may be mistaken for HSV, but zoster hardly ever recurs at the same site. In hand, foot, and mouth disease (see page 5.84) caused by a coxsackievirus there are usually vesicular lesions on the hands and feet also.

The herpetic whitlow.

The herpetic whitlow is an occupational disease of medical students, doctors, dentists, nurses, and physiotherapists. They are mostly recruited from a social group in which a minority are herpetic. In the course of their work, they come into close contact with patients who are particularly likely to be excreting virus: those with high fevers, patients with a tracheotomy, patients who have had surgery and have been anaes-thetized. The skin of the hands is rarely completely intact, and the virus may take. Usually only one finger is involved (Fig. 5a), although adjoining fingers may be affected. Children with primary gingivo-stomatotis may in addition get a whitlow if they are in the habit of biting their fingers. Very occasionally a toe may be affected (Fig. 5b).

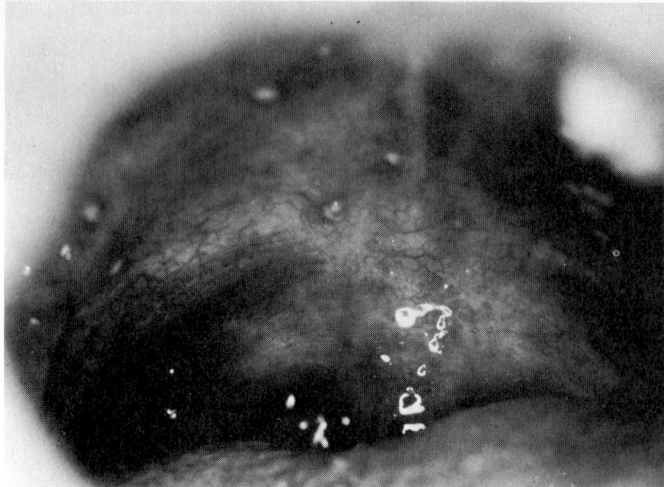

4(a)

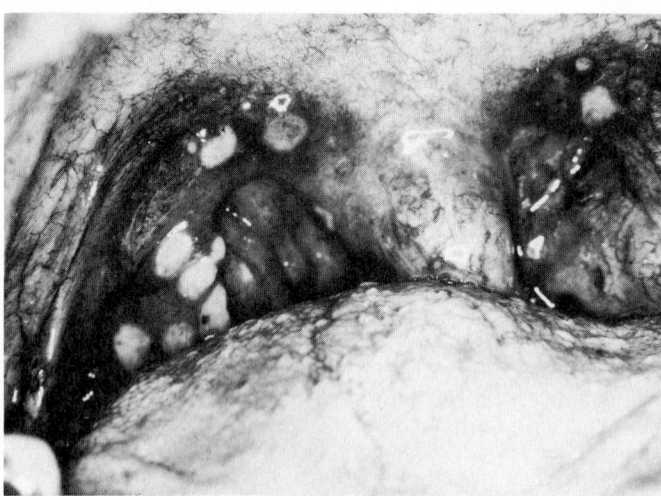

4(b)

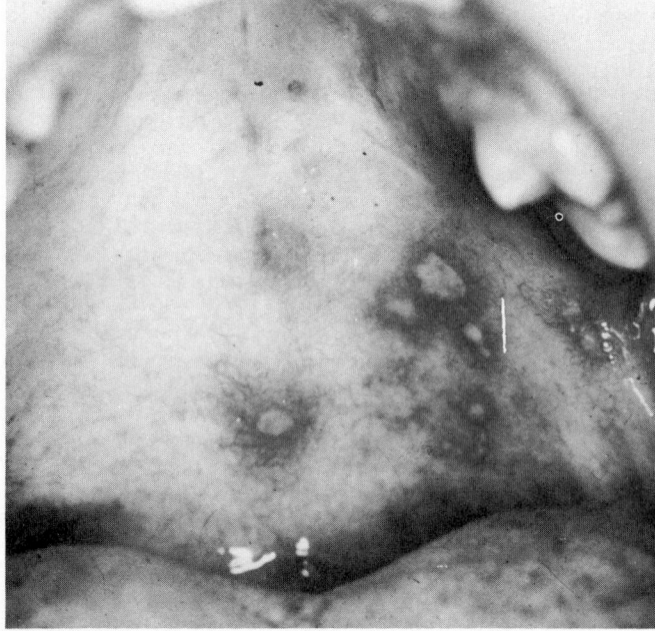

4(c)

Fig. 4   Lesions in mouth of patients with (a) infectious mononucleosis; (b) coxsackie A10 infection; (c) zoster.

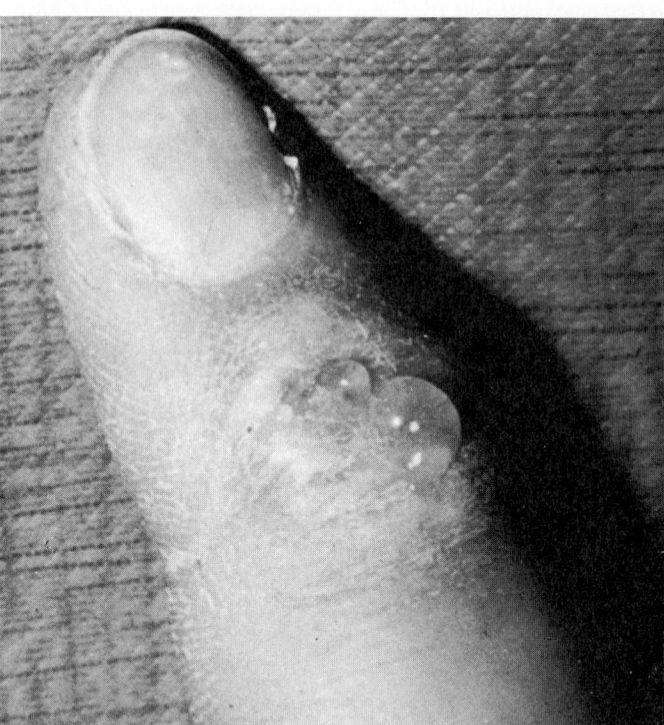

5(a)

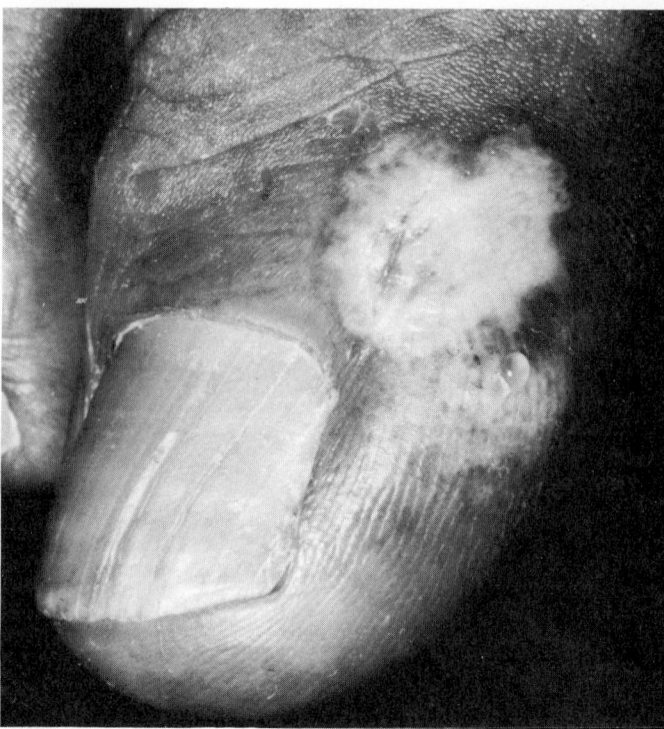

5(b)

Fig. 5   (a) Herpetic whitlow in a woman of 21; (b) Herpetic whitlow of the big toe of a man aged 24.

The herpetic whitlow is extremely painful. The digit swells, and characteristically blisters with clear fluid develop during the first week. The fluid later becomes cloudy with debris. The untreated lesion takes about four weeks to heal, unless it has been incised in which case the virus is spread through the tissues, the agony prolonged and healing delayed. Virus can usually be isolated for three weeks. The infection may recur unless treated actively in the early stages of the infection.

Differential diagnosis. The bacterial whitlow is usually due to *Staphylococcus aureus*; a β-haemolytic streptococcal infection (see page 5.138) might conceivably be mistaken for a herpatic whitlow. The diagnosis should be confirmed by the laboratory. Another not uncommon occupational disease of doctors, vaccinia whitlow, will now probably become a great rarity as vaccination against smallpox ceases. In sheep-rearing country orf (see page 5.72) may cause confusion. Electron microscopy will readily reveal the true nature of the infection.

Herpes gladiatorum; traumatic herpes. From time to time several members of a rugby team, or of some other team game where the participants come into close contact, may get their primary infection on any exposed part of the skin when one member of the team grinds the virus of his active cold sores into his fellow players (Fig. 6). Apart from the different site of the lesion the clinical course is as in gingivo-stomatitis. The lesion may recur if left untreated. Occasionally similar lesions follow trauma: 'traumatic herpes'. The abraded skin has almost certainly become infected with virus from a companion.

Differential diagnosis. The lesions may be mistaken for those of zoster. It is, however, extremely unlikely that several members of a group all develop shingles at the same time.

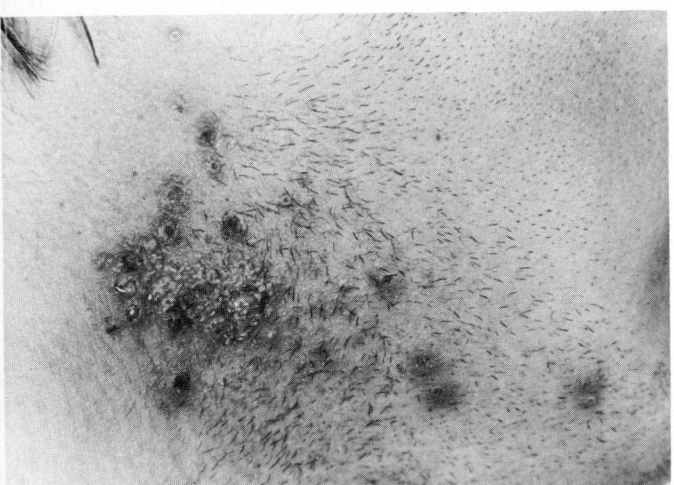

Fig. 6 Herpes gladiatorum in a sixth-form public school rugby football player.

Eczema herpeticum; Juliusberg's pustolosis acuta varioliformis; Kaposi's varicelliform eruption. In patients with eczema and other diseases of the skin (see Section 20) that make it easy for the virus to spread, such as Darier's disease, the primary HSV infection may be alarming with an extensive vesicular rash, most dense where there is particularly active eczema (Fig. 7). As these patients are often on steroid treatment, the spread of the lytic herpes simplex virus is further facilitated. There are usually systemic symptoms: fever, rigor, general adenopathy, and enlargement of the liver and spleen. Untreated, the condition is likely to recur, although the systemic symptoms may be less severe. The term 'Kaposi's varicelliform eruption' as a popular eponym, but should be dropped, not least because Moriz Kaposi was not the first to notice the condition, which he thought was a complication of infantile eczema, possibly caused by fungi. It has been described earlier by Fritz Juliusberg,

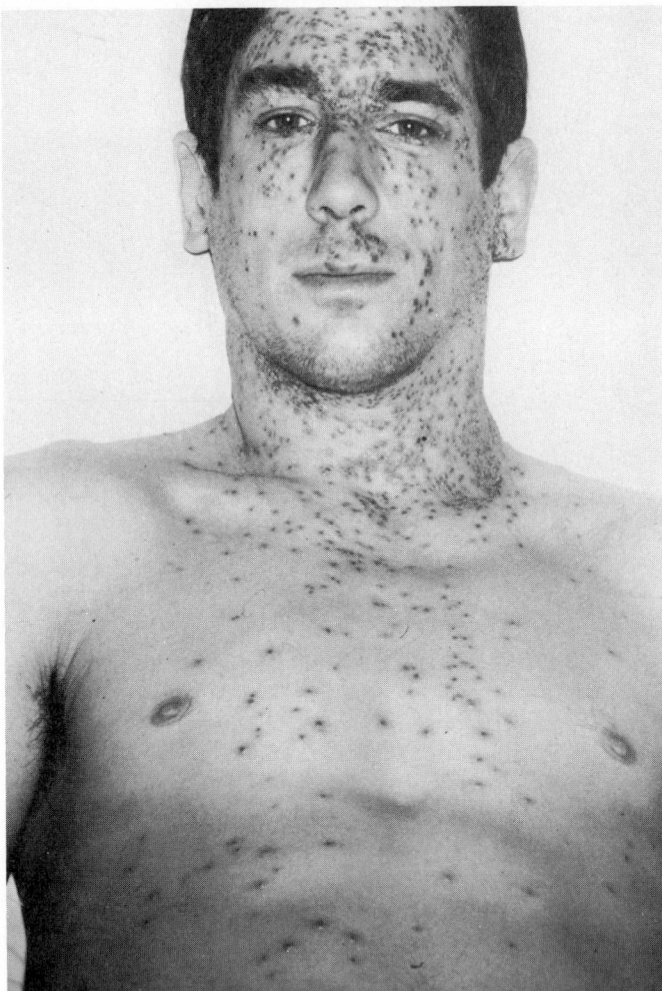

Fig. 7 (a) Eczema herpeticum in a man of 28.

who thought it was caused by staphylococci. The use of an eponym has led to further confusion, for the term 'Kaposi's varicelliform eruption' has without justification been used about eczema vaccinatum. It is as well for the doctor to warn parents of eczematous children to guard them against fond kisses from aunts and other doting admirers with active cold sores.

Differential diagnosis. Eczema herpeticum when severe can be mistaken for smallpox (see page 5.69). The lesions are usually unlike those of the cropping rash of chickenpox (see page 5.57). It is possible to mistake eczema herpeticum for eczema vaccinatum, though, with the decline in smallpox vaccination, this must become rare and other rarities like monkeypox, whitepox, and tanapox (see page 5.72) have to be considered. Electron microscopy will reveal the brick-shaped virus particles of the poxviruses.

Generalized infection; pneumonitis; hepatitis. Severe generalized disease due to Type 1 HSV is uncommon except in immunosuppressed patients. A good many of the cases described in infants and the newborn in the past were probably due to Type 2 HSV. There are reports of fatal disseminated disease in non-white South African children aged 2–25 months. There is a high degree of association with kwashiorkor and measles.

There are several case-reports of severe generalized disease in adults, many of whom were very ill and some died. There was a variable degree of generalized adenopathy, hepatic, and pulmonary involvement. A high fever (38–40 °C) is the rule. Leukopenia and transient thrombocytopenia is usual and occasional atypical mononuclear cells are present. Tests for heterophil antibodies (Paul–Bunnell–Davidsohn and 'monospot' tests) are negative.

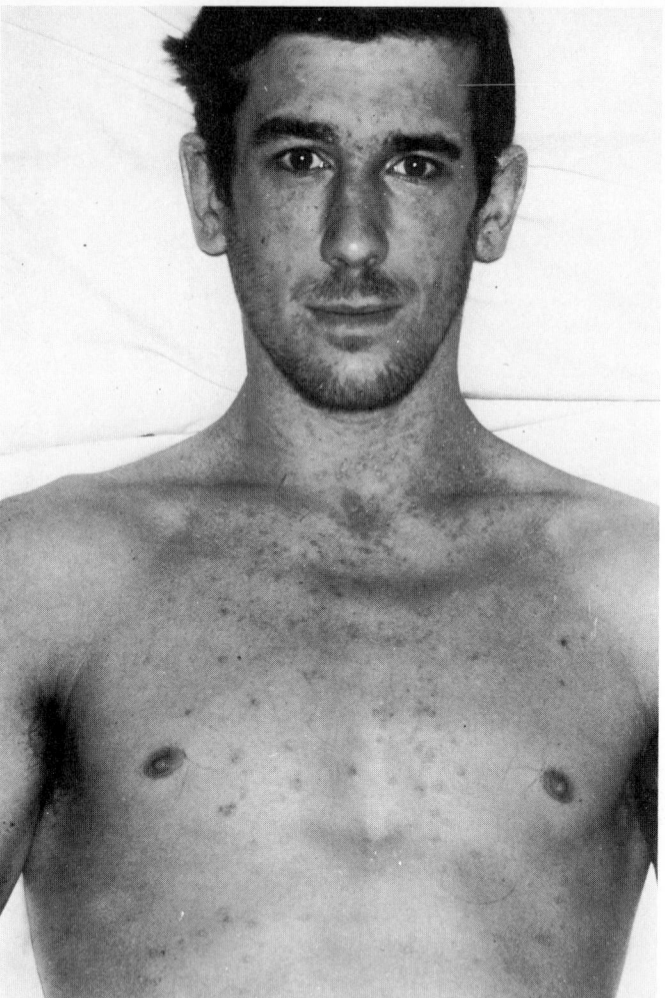

Fig. 7 (b) Appearance of the same patient on the fourth day of treatment with cytarabine.

There is usually a transient rise in the level of liver enzymes (alkaline phosphatase and aspartate transaminase). Severe hepatic involvement with frank jaundice is seen in children with kwashiorkor but very rarely in adults. Occasionally there is clinical and radiological evidence of pneumonitis. The radiological picture is indistinguishable from any of a number of 'atypical viral pneumoniae'—from chickenpox and infectious mononucleosis to Q fever and mycoplasma pneumonitis. It must be appreciated that primary HSV infection is probably always generalized: a strict separation of generalized infection, hepatitis, and pneumonitis as separate entities is artificial.

Differential diagnosis. Septicaemia due to bacterial disease, pneumonia, or hepatitis due to other agents must be considered. There are usually herpetic lesions either on the skin or in the oval cavity which will give one a lead.

Infections of the eye. The primary infection of the eye is usually unilateral, giving rise to a follicular conjunctivitis, often painless though there is chemosis and oedema of the eyelid and regional adenopathy. Unless there is associated disease elsewhere (usually a gingivo-stomatitis), the illness lasts a few days only. The condition is commonest in children in which over half get corneal involvement in the form of coarse epithelial opacities, though dendritic ulceration is rare. Once specific antibodies have formed, recurrences are modified and follicular lesions are rarely seen again.

Recurrent HSV keratitis is a major problem in ophthalmology.

The two main forms of lesion are dendritic ulceration and stromal keratitis. Inappropriate topical treatment of dendretic ulcers with steroids often leads to severe complications such as amoeboid ulcers. Stromal keratitis may be due to a hypersensitivity phenomenon.

Herpes simplex infections of the eye must be seen and treated by experts. Inappropriate use of steroids may lead to permanent blindness or severely impaired vision.

Differential diagnosis. Bacterial conjunctivitis and infection due to other viruses such as adenoviruses (see page 5.45) must be considered; most important: do not label the unilateral painless red eye: 'allergic conjunctivitis' and prescribe steroid. It may be, but if it is due to HSV the doctor may inadvertently endanger the vision in that eye.

Infections of the central nervous system
Meningitis. Herpes simplex meningitis appears to be a benign and self-limiting condition. It presents as a lymphocytic meningitis with a pleocytosis of about 50–100 cells per ml of CSF. The virus is only exceptionally isolated. The diagnosis is made on a fourfold or greater rise in titre complement-fixing or neutralizing antibody in the serum or CSF. No specific treatment is indicated.

Herpes simplex encephalitis. This condition is a serious illness at any age, but particularly after the immediate neonatal period when it is more likely to be due to type 2 virus. The majority of cases are primary infections, and patients with a history of recurrent herpetic lesions at other sites are unlikely to have HSV encephlitis. In most the onset of the disease is moderately dramatic. Fever is nearly always present (40–41 °C) and relatively resistant to antipyretics. Headache is often the earliest symptom and is often severe. Personality changes should arouse the physician's suspicion. Fits are common during the first week. The fully developed picture with neck rigidity, vomiting, and motor and sensory deficits seldom develops during the first week.

The outlook is grave. Although figures differ, the overall mortality is about 55 per cent and perhaps half the survivors have considerable disability. The diagnosis must be considered in any patient who presents with clinical signs suggestive of encephalitis. The commonest differential diagnosis in the adult is that of brain abscess or a neoplasm, but encephalopathy following recent immunizations or recent viral illness such as influenza must be borne in mind. Chickenpox or zoster encephalitis is usually associated with visible lesions on the skin. Lumbar puncture should only be attempted if the clinician is certain there is not significant cerebral oedema, and even so as little CSF as possible should be withdrawn. This nearly always shows an increased number of leukocytes, a normal sugar and a raised protein. It is most unlikely that the virus will be cultured from the CSF, although the finding of HSV antibodies in a titre of 1:4 or greater probably is diagnostic in patients with clinical encephalitis. If possible, a CAT scan should be done as a matter of urgency. It will establish if there is cerebral oedema and may exclude a neoplasm or a cerebral abscess. Carotid angiography is very valuable in skilled hands. The place of electroencephalography is very small. Although a diagnosis of HSV encephalitis may be made on serological investigations, from a four-fold or greater rise in antibody level in the CSF, or a very high titre in the blood, speed is essential if the virus is to be arrested. A brain biopsy, performed by a competent neurosurgeon, carries a low morbidity and is certainly less dangerous than a lumbar puncture which may cause the swollen brain to cone. It is probable that 'post-traumatic epilepsy' following brain biopsy is due to the lesion for which the biopsy was done, rather than to the biopsy. An early biopsy will enable a diagnosis to be made by fluorescent antibody technique within two hours in any competent virus laboratory. The clinician must ensure intensive care of the patients' respiratory, hepatic, and renal functions, with particular attention directed towards reducing cerebral swelling. There is no evidence that steroids influence cerebral oedema in this condition, so administration of mannitol may have to be employed. It is logical to attempt to kill the virus at the earliest possible stage before too many neurones have been destroyed, but antiviral chemotherapy can only be one facet of the care of these patients.

Primary and recurrent infection due to type 2 virus; genital herpes. Although genital herpes has been recognized for a long time, only during the last decade has it been appreciated that the majority of these infections (85–95 per cent) are due to type 2 virus. Genital herpes is usually, but by no means invariably, transmitted through sexual intercourse. In the male, the primary lesion resembles those elsewhere on the skin. It is usually on the glans, in the coronal sulcus, or on the shaft of the penis (Fig. 8). It is generally accom-

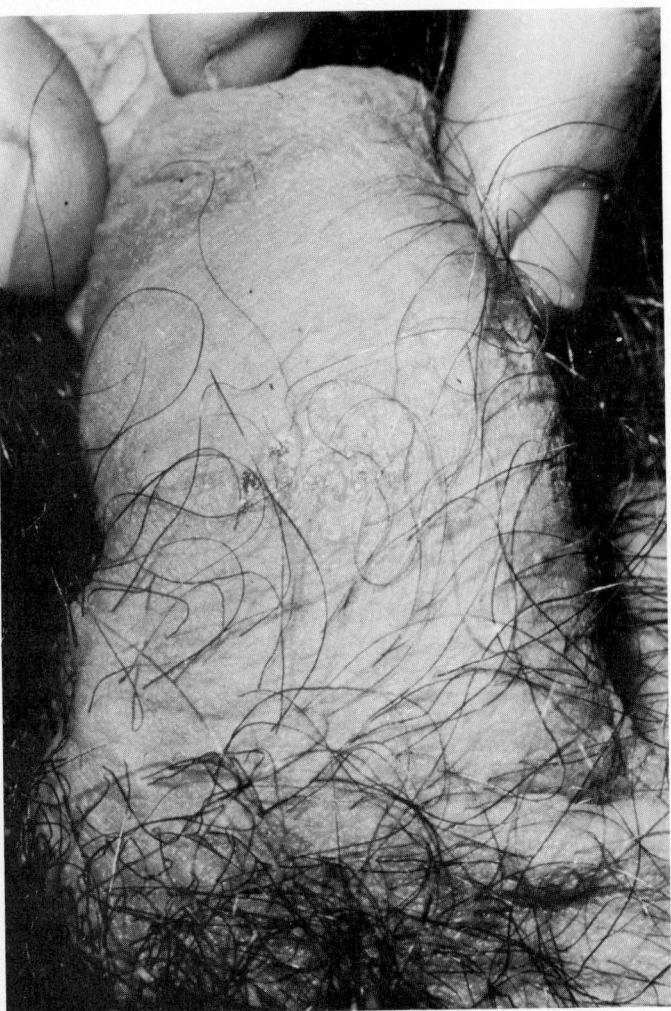

Fig. 8   Primary genital herpes due to type 2 virus.

panied by some systemic symptoms, occasionally severe with lesions elsewhere, in the palms of the hands, on the feet, or in the throat. There is local adenopathy. In the female, the primary attack may be very severe. The labia and vagina are so painful with ulcers that examination can only take place under anaesthesia. The lesions recur in both sexes, probably more often than type 1 infections recur. Intercourse in many seems to provoke a new attack, and the sufferer is often driven to distraction and finds it difficult to appreciate that most doctors do not understand how much he or she is distressed by this relatively trivial complaint.

Occasionally the primary infection involves the central nervous system, and there may be a myelo-encephalitis. This is rare in the adult, but in many, a recurrence is heralded by shooting pains in the distribution of the sacral segments.

Herpes infection of the newborn is rare in the UK (about one per 30 000 births), in some parts of the USA the incidence in poor populations is high. In an analysis of 148 cases of herpes in children of less than a month old, of which 80 per cent were said to be due to type 2 virus, a third had localized lesions and most survived, two-thirds had generalized disease and most died. The overall mortality was 71 per cent. Half of the survivors had no sequelae, the rest had CNS defects, or eye or skin defects. In suspected cases of neonatal herpes, a history of maternal genital herpes during any time of the pregnancy but in particular immediately before or during delivery is suggestive of HSV in the child. Isolation of the virus confirms the diagnosis. If the mother has a past history of type 1 infection, serology in the baby may be confused because of passively transferred antibody to type 1, but the presence of IgM is suggestive evidence of *in utero* or early postnatal infection as IgM normally does not cross the placenta.

Genital herpes near term is an indication for caesarian section.
Differential diagnosis. Genital herpes may coexist with gonorrhoea (see page 5.309), syphilis (see page 5.277) and lymphogranuloma venereum (see page 5.307), and may be mistaken for any of them. Appropriate tests to exclude these venerally transmitted diseases must be carried out. Genital herpes of the buttocks may, when extensive, be mistaken for zoster (Fig. 9). Zosteriform herpes simplex is often bilateral and there is usually a history of recurrences in the same site, a very rare event in zoster.

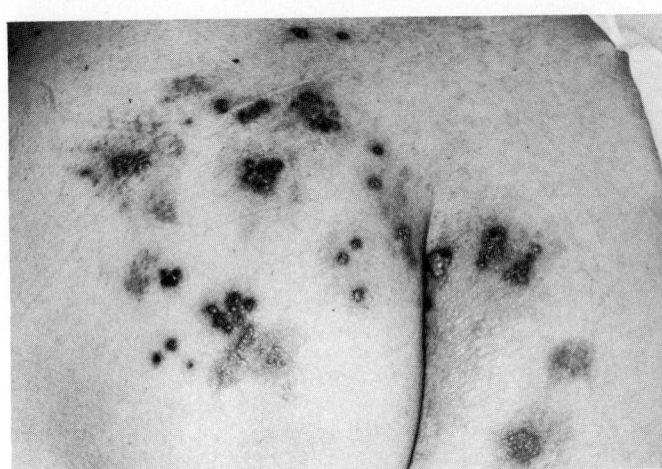

Fig. 9   Recurrent zosteriform herpes due to type 2 virus.

Herpes simplex virus and carcinoma. Herpes simplex virus, and in recent years more particularly type 2 virus, has been implicated as a cause of carcinoma of the cervix. There is an association between HSV and carcinoma of the cervix, but it could be due to at least three sets of circumstances. The virus, or fragments of DNA, might be occasional, innocent passengers. Secondly, cancer of the cervix is induced by a number of factors of which HSV is a major one. Finally the virus might be the only cause of cancer. To date none of these postulates has either been refuted or proven.

Infection in immunosuppressed patients. Herpetic patients in whom the normal immune mechanisms are impaired (see page 5.479) may get severe disease due to luxuriant replication of the herpes viruses—not only HSV but also varicella–zoster and cytomegalovirus.

All patients with lymphoproliferative disease (acute lymphoblastic leukaemia. Hodgkin's disease, multiple myeloma, and other reticuloses), and those on immunosuppressive chemotherapy, such as patients with organ transplants are at risk. In at least one heart transplant patient, the immediate cause of death was overwhelming infection with HSV.

Patients who previously had trivial recurrent cold sores may get

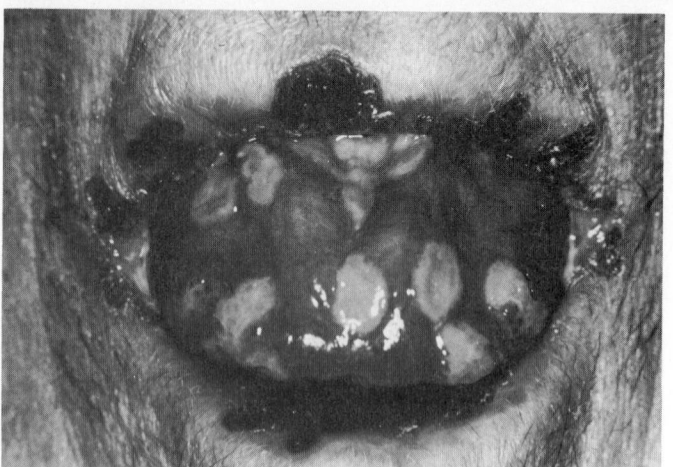

Fig. 10 Severe herpetic stomatitis in woman of 64 on immunosuppressive doses of steroid.

extensive stomatitis (Fig. 10), oesophagitis, pneumonitis, and generalized disease. An *omen malum* in these patients is the disappearance of antibodies when they had been present before.

Vigorous systemic antiviral chemotherapy is often essential in these patients.

Treatment of herpes simplex infections. All sorts of treatments have been advocated and tried for the various manifestations of HSV disease. Most were black magic, which at best prevented secondary infection but probably did little else. Herpes simplex virus is one of the few human virus diseases which has proved responsive to antiviral chemotherapy without significant harm being done to the host.

Herpetic infections of the eye are very accessible, and respond to the very insoluble idoxuridine, whether applied as 0.1 per cent drops or a 0.5 per cent ointment. Unfortunately, prolonged application which is often necessary may sensitize the patient to idoxuridine. Fortunately vidarabine cream is a useful alternative in that site, and more recently acyclovir has proved very effective. Interferon may have a place in the future.

A large number of agents have been tried against HSV. At present only idoxuridine, cytarabine, vidarabine, and acyclovir are of practical importance. Very roughly, the activity of cytarabine is five times, of acyclovir ten times that of idoxuridine whereas vidarabine has only a twentieth of the activity of idoxuridine against several strains of herpes simplex *in vitro*. Phosphonoacetic acid, favoured by some, is even less active, and in some animals has produced bone tumours. There must be and has been increasing understanding between the clinician and the laboratory worker that however excellent a drug may be in the laboratory, it is of little use if it cannot reach the site of infection in the patient.

Although many HSV lesions produce cutaneous lesions, it is unlikely that radical cure with chemotherapy will be achieved unless a systemic drug is given that will reach the virus in the nerve cells, where we know the virus resides in both type 1 and type 2 infections. However good the drug, it will never work satisfactorily delivered only to the skin, except perhaps in the eye.

In relatively trivial recurrent cutaneous lesions, topical idoxuridine will shorten the duration of the lesions and lengthen the intervals between attacks—but only provided it is in a solvent that penetrates the skin, for it is near insoluble in water and has been shown in three double-blind trials to be inactive when applied in cream when compared with a placebo. Dissolved in dimethylsulphoxide (DMSO), a 35 per cent solution applied five times a day to a recurrent or primary skin lesion will shorten the duration of the lesion. Treatment must not be continued beyond three days, for the solvent (which penetrates to the deep fascia within a quarter of an hour) will macerate the skin. At present, topical 35 per cent idoxuridine is perhaps the (imperfect) treatment of choice in recurrent herpes, whether of the face or of the genitals. Primary herpes

gladiatorum responds well to continuous application of 35 per cent idoxuridine in DMSO on lint, renewed daily for four days. Herpetic whitlows treated in the same way with compresses of lint wetted daily with 35 per cent idoxuridine in DMSO for a week will, with a good chance of success, cure the primary lesion. Virus cannot be isolated beyond the first week.

In severe primary and recurrent infections idoxuridine is useless. It cannot be given systemically in adequate doses without causing grave damage to the bone-marrow, liver, and kidneys. It was tried in HSV encephalitis and found to be very toxic without convincing beneficial effect.

On the other hand, cytarabine has been found to reduce significantly the virus shedding in severe HSV infections, except in the very occasional patient who produces high levels of pyrimidine kinase which destroys the drug. Given slowly, intravenously, the drug has maximum adverse effect on the bone-marrow, and it is unlikely a therapeutic level against HSV will ever be achieved. Given as a bolus, the adverse effect on the bone-marrow is minimal in doses of 3–4 mg/kg per day for three to five days. Even doses of 10 mg/kg per day cause only transient suppression of platelets and reticulocytes in the second week after institution of treatment. Therefore, in the treatment of severe, usually systemic primary disease whether gingivo-stomatitis or primary genital herpes, eczema herpeticum or HSV encephalitis, cytarabine which is easily soluble, remains a very useful drug. Acyclovir (acycloguanosine) is less soluble, but also less toxic. In doses of 10 mg/kg given eight-hourly as a bolus there may be problems with temporarily impaired renal function, almost certainly caused by crystalluria. This can be overcome by slow infusion over an hour. Normally only 5 mg/kg eight-hourly will be required in herpes simplex infections. Acyclovir has proved very effective in double-blind controlled trials, used topically in herpetic keratitis, systemically in prophylaxis of HSV infection in bone-marrow transplant recipients, and in patients with genital herpes. The drug depends on its action mainly on the presence in HSV of a thymidine kinase which is avid for acyclovir as a substrate. Thymidine kinase resistant strains have emerged *in vivo*, and the drug should not be used indiscriminately to avoid the emergence of resistant strains. E-5-(2-Bromovinyl)-2'-deoxyuridine (BVDU) is on anecdotal evidence active against HSV keratitis. 2'-Fluoro-5-iodo-arabinosylcytosine (FIAC) is another potentially promising agent against HSV type 1, of low toxicity and easily absorbed by mouth. Vidarabine (Ara-A, adenine arabinoside) which, from *in vitro* evidence, should be a poor agent against HSV, has in practice turned out to be a great disappointment (even though it appears to be very useful against varicella–zoster virus). Very insoluble, it has been used in the treatment of HSV encephalitis. Double-blind controlled trials have on close examination shown that the drug is ineffective.

The greatest challenge is perhaps the case of HSV encephalitis. Too often clinicians are mesmerized by the virus and forget to treat the whole patient. Meticulous intensive care, in an all-out attempt to counteract cerebral oedema, probably with mannitol, even at the risk of causing transient renal failure, and general care is more important than any amount of antiviral chemotherapy.

Extensively used, particularly in the USA, inactivation of HSV by photosensitization has been shown to be ineffective. Neutral red was the usually applied dye. Steroids should be avoided at all costs unless accompanied by simultaneous antiviral chemotherapy.

The role of interferon is still to be determined. By the time a clinical diagnosis of severe HSV infection has been made, circulating interferon levels are probably already so high that added extrinsic interferon will make little difference.

References

Baringer, J. R. (1975). Herpes simplex virus infection of nervous tissue in animals and man. In *Progress in medical virology*, **20** (ed. J. L. Melnick), 1. Karger, Basel.
Juel-Jensen, B. E. and MacCallum, F. O. (1972) *Herpes simplex, varicella and zoster*. Heinemann, London.

Catterall, R. D. and Nicol, S. (eds.) (1976). *Sexually transmitted diseases*, 135 (on genital herpes). Academic Press, New York.

Illis, L. S. and Gostling, J. V. T. (1972). *Herpes simplex encephalitis*. Bristol Scientechnica, Bristol.

Oxford, J. S., Drasar, F. A., and Williams, J. D. (eds.) (1977). *Chemotherapy of herpes simplex virus infections*. Academic Press, New York.

Varicella–zoster virus infections: chickenpox and zoster

B. E. Juel-Jensen

Varicella–zoster virus (V/Z) is of a size and structure similar to that of herpes simplex virus (HSV). The virus may be grown in a variety of primary human tissue cultures, such as fibroblasts and primary human amnion. As no animal other than man has been found readily susceptible to the virus, animal studies of its behaviour, so profuse in the case of HSV, are lacking.

The virus behaves in many ways like its close cousin, the herpes simplex virus. It produces a primary infection in the non-immune host: chickenpox (said to be so called because of its resemblance to chick-pea) or varicella. After the acute, often trivial primary infection, the virus becomes latent in nerve cells, both sensory and motor. Sooner or later when cell-mediated immunity and neutralizing antibody fail to keep the virus in check, it is reactivated in the 'immune' host and reappears as zoster or shingles. All discussion about whether chickenpox and zoster are due to the same virus must now cease. There is overwhelming virological and epidemiological evidence to prove that the two clinical pictures are caused by one virus, in the non-immune and the 'immune' host. There are epidemics of chickenpox, but never of zoster. The skin lesions in both are similar to those caused by HSV. The virus damages the stratum germinativum and stratum spinosum in both, producing fairly superficial vesicles with intranuclear inclusions. In zoster there may be severe inflammatory involvement of the corium, and scarring is common in untreated zoster. Severe systemic involvement in chickenpox is the exception, in zoster the skin manifestations are of secondary importance to the changes in the nerves. There is degeneration of axons and myelin, and virus particles occur in the cytoplasm and nuclei of epidermal cells, in the cytoplasm of perineural cells, and in both cytoplasm and nuclei of Schwann cells. Both cytoplasm and nuclei of ganglion cells are full of virus particles (Fig. 1). The virus presumably spreads peripherally to the skin, and centrally to the posterior columns of the cord and the brain. When there has been extensive inflammation and necrosis, fibrosis follows as has been shown by biopsy at different intervals after the onset of zoster. Inflammatory changes may also involve the anterior horn alone.

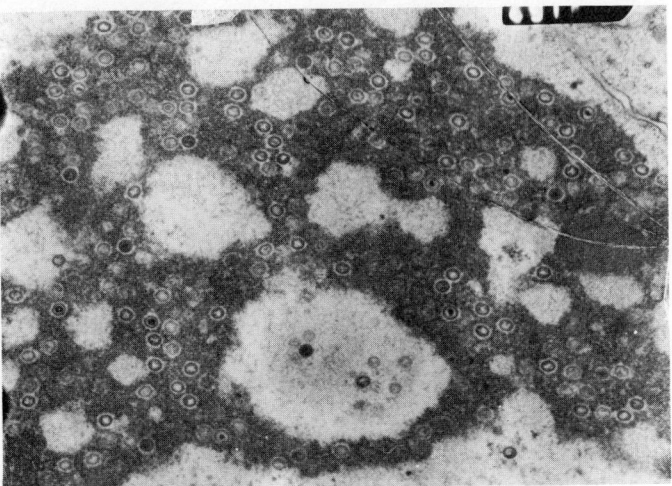

Fig. 1 Varicella–zoster virus in the nucleus of the nerve cell in the Gasserian ganglion four days after the patient developed frontal zoster.

Epidemiology. Varicella–zoster virus is the most infectious of the human herpesviruses. Transmission almost certainly happens by droplets, particularly during the first few days of the illness when the virus is present in the mouth and nose. Vesicle fluid, but not the scabs, is infective, and a non-immune person may contact chickenpox from a patient with shingles. The usual incubation period for chickenpox is about two weeks, with variations from seven to 23 days.

Chickenpox is most commonly a disease of the young; zoster is found with increasing frequency in the elderly, more than 14 times more often in octogenarians than in those under ten. There is no evidence to show that zoster is ever a reinfection. Exceptionally V/Z virus may be implanted and cause the parallel of *herpes gladiatorum* of the skin, e.g. in players in rough football games – one might call it '*zoster gladiatorum*', but elderly ladies rarely play rugger. The increasing frequency of zoster with age may be due to the disappearance of V/Z neutralizing antibody which usually persists for 40 years after the original attack of chickenpox. Presumably children who get zoster lose their neutralizing antibody early.

Chickenpox

Congenital chickenpox. Most women of child-bearing age have had chickenpox, and congenital chickenpox is rare. Intrauterine chickenpox which occurs before the twentieth week of the pregnancy may, apart from skin lesions, lead to cerebral atrophy, optic-atrophy, and choroidoretinitis. Chickenpox caught at the end of pregnancy may be followed by severe chickenpox in the newborn, for the infant is not protected by antibody passed across the placenta. When possible the obstetrician should delay delivery till a fortnight has elapsed from the onset of the rash. Hyperimmune V/Z immunoglobulin should be given.

Chickenpox. Characteristically there are no or minimal prodromal symptoms in children, and the rash is the first manifestation of the illness. It may be so slight—like a few drops of water on the skin—that it is missed. In older children the rash itches, the doctor confirms the diagnosis, calamine lotion is prescribed, and the child gets better without complications.

In adults prodromal signs are much commoner and occasionally they can be so severe that the clinician must worry that he is dealing with smallpox. Severe headache, general aches and pains, severe backache, and extreme malaise are typical. There may, as in smallpox, be a transient pink rash before the vesicles erupt. Because they are more superficial than in smallpox, the vesicles tend to be irregular. Characteristically there are crops of vesicles at different stages of development, macules, papules, vesicles, and scabs. Normally the scabs fall at the end of 10 days.

The rash is characteristically centripital, and dense between the shoulder blades, not like smallpox, which is most in evidence over bony prominences. The limbs are usually relatively spared. Very occasionally there may be a zosterform rash; presumably the virus has travelled by the neurones in a segmental distribution.

Usually the rash is quite characteristic, but if there is uncertainty the diagnosis can be confirmed by paired sera, spaced by about 10 days. The first specimen will have no antibody in the primary infection, and antibody will only appear in the second week. Although, particularly in the elderly, there may be no complement fixing antibody present in zoster, antibody appears after three to four days, demonstrating nicely that the immune mechanism has met the antigen before. Vesicle fluid is best collected in a capillary tube, and the virus grown, e.g. on primary human amnion or fibroblasts. Cytopathic changes take longer to appear, usually three to four days, than in the case of HSV which usually produces changes within 24 hours.

Different diagnosis. Eczema herpeticum could be mistaken for chickenpox. The lesions are usually at the same stage of development, and tend to be densest over flexure surfaces, where the eczema is densest. Coxsackie infection occasionally has a wide-spread vesicular rash, but only very rarely as diffuse as chickenpox.

Although smallpox has been eradicated (but not everyone shares the WHO's optimism that this long-lived virus will never be seen again), the differentiation of atypical chickenpox from smallpox, monkeypox, tanapox, and whitepox will remain important (see page 5.71). Atypical chickenpox can be very similar to smallpox. There may be a centrifugal rash with many lesions on the forearms and legs, in the palms of hands and the soles of the feet, and lesions over pressure points. Cropping may occur in variola, and may not be evident in chickenpox. If there is any doubt the patient must be moved *at once* to an infectious disease unit with staff still actively immunized against smallpox. Vesicle fluid and scrapings must be taken for electron microscopy. The poxvirus will be brick-shaped, V/Z virus has the typical shape of a herpesvirus. That and cross-over immunoelectrophoresis in agar gel and immunofluorescence should provide an answer in one to two hours. Chickenpox may coexist with smallpox of vaccinia.

Complications. Though usually a disease of childhood, chickenpox in some parts of the world is common in older age groups. In a survey in Ceylon one in three of 6000 patients was over 30 and 19 were over 80. In adults it can be an extremely severe illness, the rash is often more intense, and systemic complications are common.

Secondary infection usually with staphylococci of scratched skin lesions is common and may lead to scarring.

Pneumonitis may go unrecognized clinically, but at the other end of the scale may take a rapidly fatal course over a few days with increasing shortness of breath, pulmonary oedema, cyanosis, and chest pain. The latter is the exception, but it is alarming when an otherwise previously healthy person is lost. The picture may be mistaken for carcinomatosis, miliary tuberculosis and/or sarcoidosis. Very occasionally calcified foci may be seen on radiographs subsequently, but this is by no means constant.

Hepatitis is rare, but can be very marked with abnormal liver function tests typical of hepatocellular involvement, and a raised bilirubin corresponding to the jaundice. Atypical lymphocytes are seen on the blood film which may lead to confusion with infectious mononucleosis or infective hepatitis, but neither, of course, has a vesicular rash.

Encephalitis has been described in children preceding the rash by as much as 10 days. In a Canadian series of 57 children half had mainly cerebellar signs and all the children recovered. The CSF usually has a raised leukocyte count and protein.

Purpura fulminans; haemorrhagic chickenpox. At least 20 cases have been described. Following typical chickenpox, ecchymoses appear symmetrically in the lower extremities, and occasionally on the arms (Fig. 2) from five to 18 days after the rash began. Large areas of skin slough, and there is extensive tissue necrosis. Four out of a group of 18 patients died in renal failure, shock, or sepsis, and 11 lost some part of their limbs. There is a low prothrombin and reduced factors V, VII, VIII, and X. Intravascular coagulation takes place in the peripheral vessels, and the picture is one of thrombotic purpura. As in the Shwartzman phenomenon, steroids will aggravate the situation, and they are contra-indicated. Fresh blood and heparin seem to be the most promising supportive measures.

Venous thrombosis with bilateral gangrene of the digits with generalized consumption coagulopathy has been described.

Haemorrhagic chickenpox very occasionally occurs in the absence of obvious blood dyscrasia. The differential diagnostic possibility of smallpox should be borne in mind.

Recurrent chickenpox in otherwise healthy individuals is extremely rare. The writer has seen one family where four brothers had many attacks. The index case, a boy of fifteen, had a second, very severe attack of chickenpox (Fig. 3). A brother of 19 had had two, one of 18 eight and one of 16½ three attacks, all of increasing severity. The parents and two sisters had had only one attack of mild chickenpox. In other respects the boys were normal. Exten-

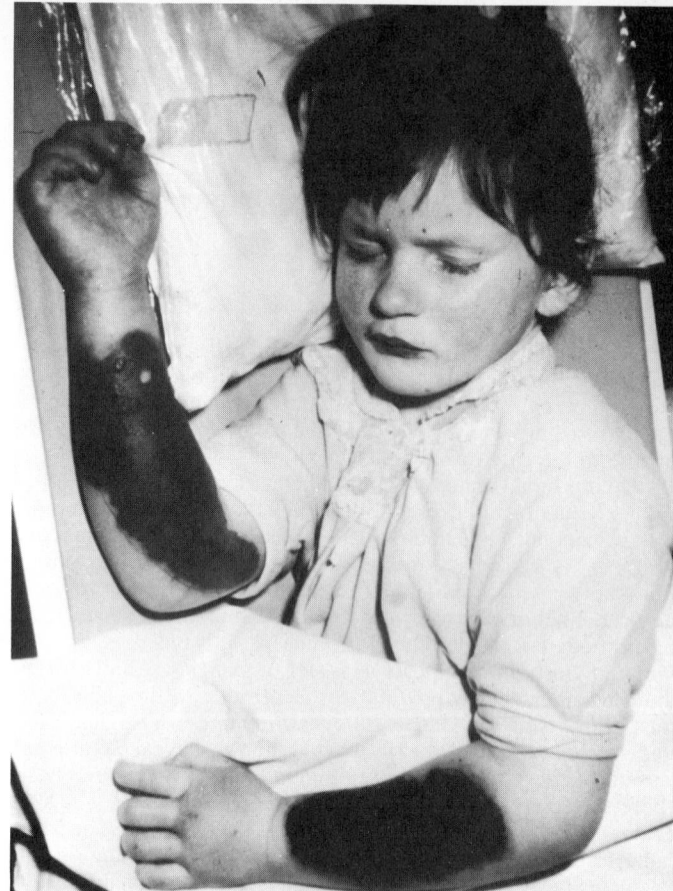

Fig. 2 Purpura fulminans in a nine-year-old girl. (Reproduced by courtesy of Dr A. A. Sharp.)

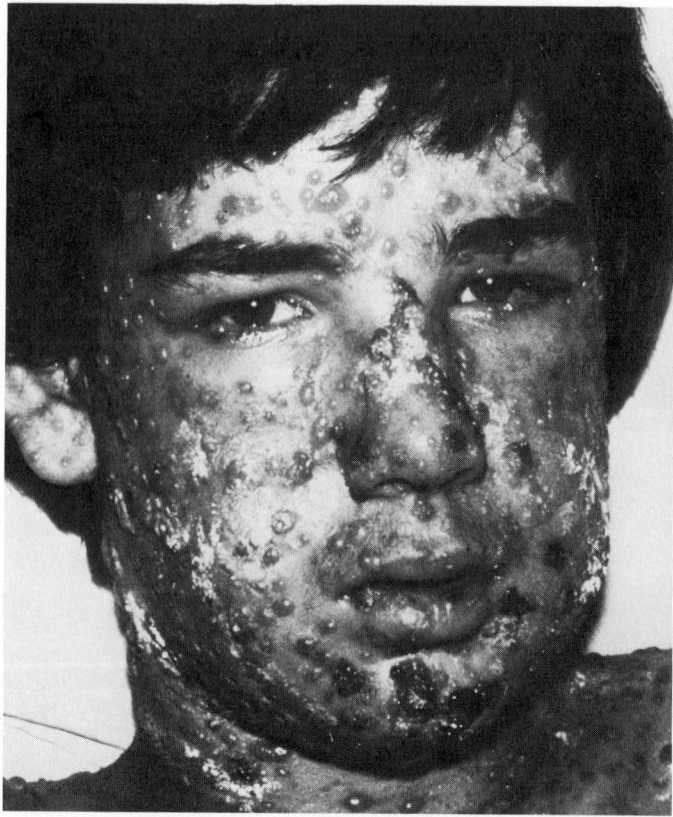

Fig. 3 Severe recurrent chickenpox.

sive investigations failed to reveal genetic or lymphocyte function abnormalities.

Immune deficient states: Patients on long-term steroids and lymphoproliferative disorders have a poor prognosis. In one series 30 of 106 leukaemic children who caught chickenpox died. Vigorous antiviral chemotherapy is mandatory.

Treatment. None is indicated in the average case of chickenpox, except local calamine lotion to relieve the itch and prevent secondary infection.

In adults, and in particular if there is any evidence of pneumonitis or hepatitis, systemic treatment with intravenous vidarabine 15 mg/kg per day for at least four days or acyclovir, 10 mg eight-hourly given intravenously over an hour for at least four days is essential. Similar treatment must be used in the immunosuppressed or in encephalitis and purpura fulminans.

Live vaccine has been developed experimentally. Whether it will find widespread use in leukaemic patients who have not had chickenpox without causing disease, remains to be seen. Preliminary results have been promising.

Zoster

Records from two general practices in the UK suggest that at least 20 per cent of all adults suffer from zoster at some time, but seldom more than once. Reactivation of the latent virus can be caused by a number of insults, physical trauma to the dermatome being perhaps the commonest (38 out of 100 successive cases in one series) though ultraviolet light played a role in a few. Underlying malignancy is found no more often in zoster than in the population at large, but in lymphoproliferative disease (lymphatic leukaemia, Hodgkin's disease, multiple myeloma, and other reticuloses), zoster may recur repeatedly and may be severe.

Zoster and shingles both mean 'a belt'; the Norwegians call it a 'Belt of Roses from Hell', the Danes call it 'Hellfire', a very apt description, for pain is such an important facet of shingles. The eruption is usually preceded by paraesthesiae over the affected dermatome, in most, perhaps two-thirds of all patients by shooting pains which may precede the eruption by as much as three weeks. A proportion of patients get pain at no stage of the illness. Conversely, a few get severe pain but no vesicular eruption: *zoster sine herpete*. The diagnosis can only be made on rising titres to V/Z virus. At least two well documented cases have occurred in doctors.

Pain, the so-called post-herpetic neuralgia may persist for years and make the patient's life unbearable, and is commonest the older the patient. The eruption varies greatly. In the young it is often trivial with a single or a few groups of vesicles and, in particular on the face, it may be mistaken for herpes simplex. In severe cases a whole or several dermatomes may be involved, with an oedematous base and a dense rash covering the entire segment (Fig. 4). The rash is characteristically unilateral and bilateral zoster is very rare, although none of the few seen by the writer died, as popular superstition will have us believe they must.

Much has been written about the occurrence of zoster in different dermatomes. In fact practically all surveys come to the predictable conclusion that shingles is commonest on the trunk—there are, after all, more dermatomes there than over the head and limbs.

In the distribution of the trigeminal nerve, the first division is most commonly affected, probably because the forehead is the part of the head most exposed to trauma.

In about a fifth of elderly patients there will be a variable number of outlying lesions—varying from a few lesions to a dense eruption. These eruptions occur in the early days of the disease before antibodies have reappeared. When the term *generalized zoster* is used is a matter of taste. Except in the immune deficient, dissemination is not necessarily of dire significance. The vesicles normally scab after three to seven days, and all dry scabs have separated at the end of a fortnight. Untreated, the lesions often become infected

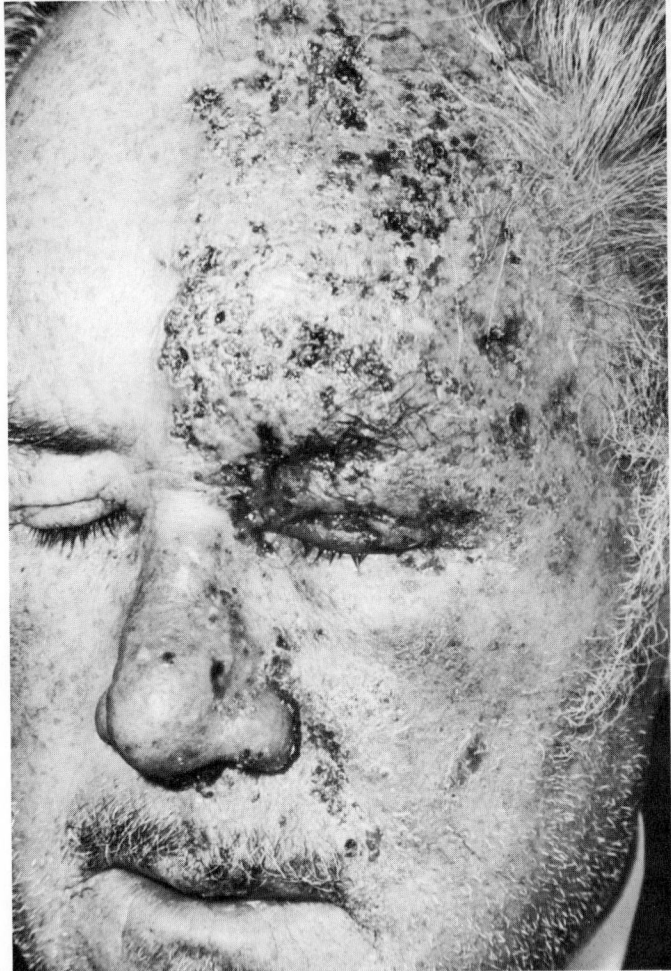

Fig. 4 Frontal and maxillary zoster.

with *Staphylococcus aureus*. If the scabs are levered off, ugly scars may persist.

Differential diagnosis. Zosterform herpes simplex may be mistaken for zoster. A history of recurrence in the same site makes HSV likely. *Zoster sine herpete* may be mistaken for Bornholm disease ('the devil's grip', polymyalgia epidemica), and pain in the prodromal stage before the eruption may, like Bornholm disease, mimic myocardial infarction, gallstones, renal calculi, and appendicitis. Many an appendix has been removed and a distressed surgeon found shingles in his wound the next day. His distress is unjustified. A neglected inflamed appendix is worse than an abdomen opened for a patient with zoster. Simian herpesvirus infection very rarely produces a zosteriform eruption.

Complications.   *Ophthalmic zoster.* The frontal nerve sends the nasoconciliary branch to the eye and the bridge of the nose. When the eye is affected by zoster, conjunctivitis is common. Keratitis occurs from time to time. Optic neuritis with blindness is fortunately rare. Ophthalmic zoster gives rise in many to gross periorbital oedema. The eye on the affected side and sometimes also on the other side are closed, much to the patient's alarm (see Fig. 4).

Sacral zoster. Zoster of S2 and below can be most distressing with acute retention of urine due to parasympathetic paralysis of the bladder and often accompanied by constipation. A haemorrhagic cystitis occurs. Lumbar zoster may be associated with big bowel atony.

Motor zoster. Zoster is not confined to the sensory nerves. The commonest form of motor zoster is facial zoster (Fig. 5). It is usually associated with zoster of the auriculotemporal branch of the

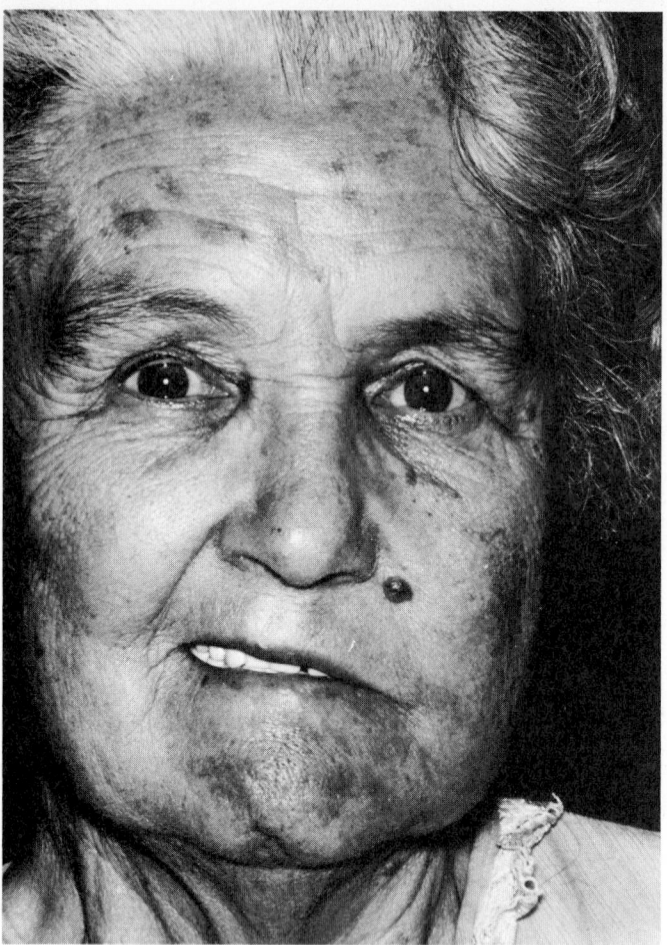

Fig. 5   Motor zoster of the left facial nerve.

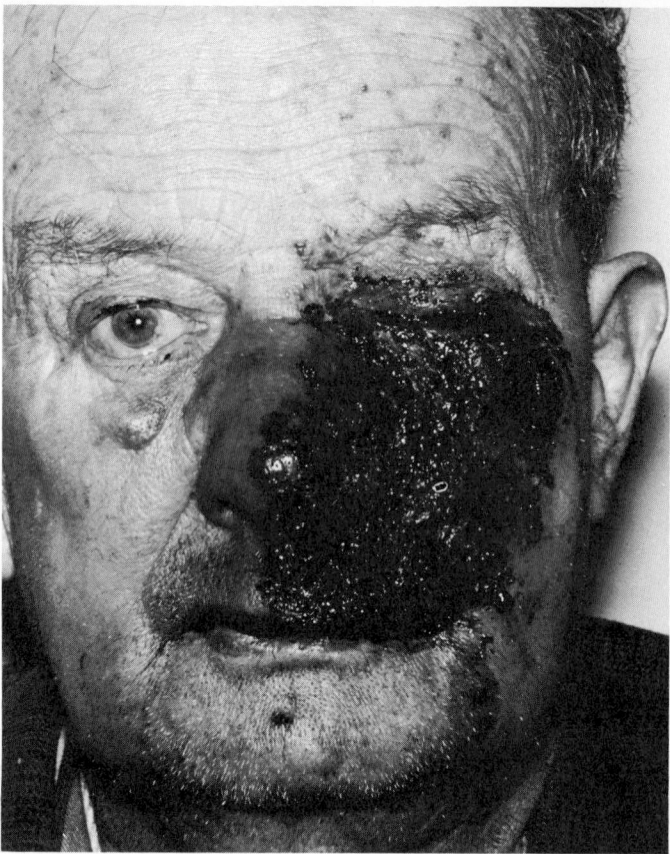

Fig. 6   Purpura fulminans in zoster of the maxillary nerve.

trigeminal nerve or the tympanic branch of the glossopharyngeal, or the auricular branch of the vagus, and of the great auricular and lesser occipital branches of the cervical plexus. The so-called 'Ramsay Hunt syndrome': zoster of the geniculate ganglion, which it was postulated affected vestigial fibres of the seventh cranial nerve, probably does not exist. The recovery, though often slow, is good in most. The facial nerve is swollen in the rigid facial nerve canal and will inevitably be damaged.

Zoster of the cranial nerves III, IV, and VI is not uncommon. We found it in three of 56 patients with ophthalmic zoster. Zoster of C5 and 6 may leady to diaphragmatic palsy, and motor zoster of the upper limb (usually of the deltoid) and lower limbs are occasional complications of sensory zoster at that level.

Zoster encephalomyelitis. This condition is by some thought to have a poor prognosis. In one series of 38, 64 per cent died. We have lost two out of 11 cases under our care. Cerebell involvement is not uncommon.

It is probable that minimal involvement of the CNS is common. Manifestations have varied from the odd cranial nerve palsy to fits, sensory and motor abnormalities in the limbs, and coma. Few data exist on CSF in uncomplicated zoster. It is possible that many cases have an abnormal CSF. It is also likely that motor zoster is a mild local manifestation of encephalomyelitis.

Purpura fulminans in zoster. This very rare condition can lead to alarming tissue loss. It follows a similar course to the condition in chickenpox. In the patient in Fig. 6 the purpura appeared at the end of a week.

Zoster in the immunosuppressed. Patients with lymphoproliferative disease, patients immunosuppressed with cytotoxic chemotherapy and/or with steroids, whether for malignant disease or for organ transplantation will, as they get severe HSV infection, get

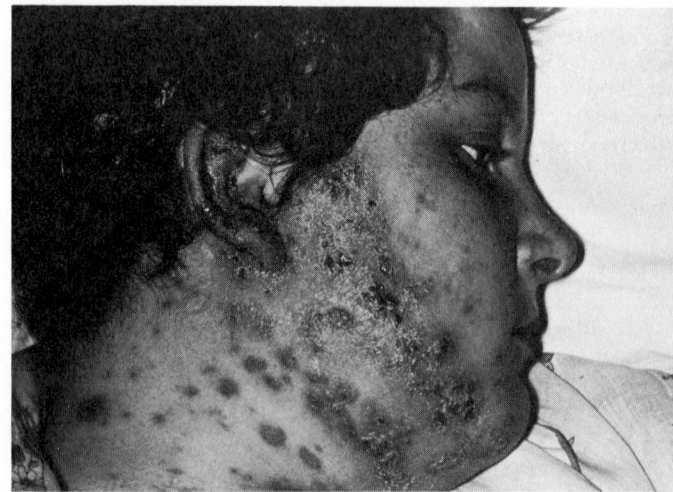

Fig. 7   Zoster of the mandibular nerve with generalized spread in girl following marrow transplantation after whole body irradiation for acute myeloid leukaemia.

severe zoster, which often becomes generalized and may kill. Figure 7 shows a patient who had had a marrow transplant after whole body irradiation for myeloid leukaemia. She developed zoster of the manibular nerve which, despite topical treatment with idoxuridine, became generalized but in the end responded to systemic acyclovir.

Treatment. Doctors often fail to appreciate that the main lesion in zoster is in the nerves, not the blisters of the skin which will heal anyway. Early treatment with antiviral chemotherapy is well worthwhile. It should be emphasized that chemotherapy must be given *early*, within the first three or four days of appearance of the rash, for there to be any hope of arresting the disease. There is *no place* for chemotherapy beyond the acute phase.

Topical idoxuridine in dimethyl sulphoxide applied continuously on lint for four days has in our hands been very useful. Of 300 patients treated with a 40 per cent solution 4.1 per cent had pain for more than seven days, 95.9 per cent for less, and 79.6 per cent for less than four days. The median duration of pain was 2.4 days. All those who had pain for more than seven days were over 65. In a small double controlled trial of 40, 35, and 30 per cent solutions we found that there was little to choose between 40 per cent and 35 per cent solutions. Pain lasted for a median of three days in both, although one patient had pain for 29 days among the seven on 35 per cent; none of the seven on 40 per cent had pain for more than five days. The median for pain in the five on 30 per cent idoxuridine was four days, but one had pain for 60 days. We have therefore settled for 35 per cent.

Systemic chemotherapy is a must in zoster involving the mandibular or maxillary branches (Fig. 8) of the trigeminal nerve, for sacral zoster, for motor zoster, purpura fulminans, encephalomyelitis, and zoster in the immunosuppressed. Two drugs are useful and relatively non-toxic. Vidarabine (Ara-A), which in double-blind controlled trials in immunocompromised patients has been proved effective, should be given in a dose of 10 mg/kg per day for at least four days. It is fairly insoluble and must be given in 4 per cent glucose or normal saline. A few patients develop a transient tremor following the administration of the drug, but this disappears after a few days. Acyclovir has been shown in double-blind controlled trials to be marginally, though not statistically significantly effective on the time to healing of the lesions and on the severity of pain, in the case of low dose (5 mg/kg eight-hourly) treatment on the short-term pain, in the case of high-dose (10 mg/kg eight-hourly) treatment on postherpetic neuralgia. The explanation of this is probably that although VZ virus contains thymidine kinases, these are less avid for acyclovir as a substrate than in the case of HSV thymidine kinase. Acyclovir should therefore be used in a dose of 10 mg/kg eight-hourly. In many trials it has been found to be of low toxicity, provided it is given over at least an hour. This is obviously important, not least in grossly immunosuppressed patients, for instance bone-marrow recipients.

Cytarabine in a dose of 4 mg/kg per day for four days when compared in a double blind controlled trial with 35 per cent idoxuridine in DMSO in early zoster was as effective, but side-effects

(nausea and vomiting), made it less acceptable. Used with antiemetics, there is a place for it if vidarabine or acyclovir are not available.

Post-herpetic neuralgia. This, the aftermath of virus replication in the nerves can be extremely taxing for patient and physician alike. There is no doubt that high dose steroids such as prednisolone 15 mg three times daily will shorten the duration of pain in acute zoster, though some clinicians hesitate to use the drug which occasionally leads to generalized spread. It can be used with success in some cases of postherpetic neuralgia after the acute illness has worn off, the dosage should be decreased over the next few weeks (10 mg three times daily, 5 mg three times daily).

In trigeminal zoster carbamazepine in doses up to 800–1200 mg a day occasionally works.

When hyperaesthesia is a problem, topical 5 per cent lignocaine ointment may give temporary relief.

Surgical division of the peripheral nerve does not normally give relief, no doubt because the spinal cord is also affected.

In leprosy, painful neuropathy has been successfully treated with thalidomide. We have had some promising response in intractible pain to thalidomide 100 mg three times daily for three weeks. The mechanism, one would surmise, is a destruction of sick nerve fibres by the drug, for apart from its notorious effects on the fetus, peripheral neuropathy has been recorded. Naturally thalidomide must not be used in females of childbearing age.

Interferon appears in vesicle fluid in zoster when healing begins. It would be logical to use interferon in the treatment of zoster. In one case it has been used successfully, but until interferon becomes easily and cheaply available through genetic engineering, this treatment is speculative.

Hyperimmune globulin with a complement fixing titre of 1:256 will prevent chickenpox in susceptible children if given in a 2 ml dose within 72 hours of exposure. Ordinary pooled immunoglobulin will not. Obviously this is of value in immunosuppressed children, and children with leukaemia. in adults correspondingly higher doses may be of value when a pregnant woman develops chickenpox. There is no risk from zoster in pregnancy, as low levels of antibody will be present.

References

Taylor-Robinson, D. and Caunt, A. E. (1972). *Varicella virus*. Springer-Verlag, Vienna and New York.
Juel-Jensen, B. E. and MacCallum, F. O. (1972). *Herpes simplex, varicella and zoster*. Heinemann, London.
Christie, A. B. (1980). Chickenpox (varicella). In *Infectious diseases*, 3rd edn., 262. Churchill Livingstone, Edinburgh.

Infectious mononucleosis: Epstein–Barr virus disease

B. E. Juel-Jensen

Until the causative organism was discovered in the late 1960s, infectious mononucleosis was a mystery disease which caused much speculation. The *Drüsenfieber* which Pfeiffer described in 1881 may have included other things, but the name 'glandular fever' stuck. This term should, if used at all, be reserved for a clinical picture of sore throat, adenopathy, and fever, often with splenomegaly, usually with mild hepatic involvement, and a blood picture characterized by a monocytosis with at least 10 per cent of atypical lymphocytes. Although the biggest contributor to that group, infectious mononucleosis shares it with other diseases, such as cytomegalovirus disease and toxoplasmosis. In 1968 the joint work of the Henles, Niederman, McCollum, and Evans made it clear that a herpesvirus, Epstein–Barr virus which Epstein had found in material from children with Burkitt's lymphoma (see page 5.124) probably was the direct cause of infectious mononucleosis, for they found that antibody, absent before the illness, appeared early in

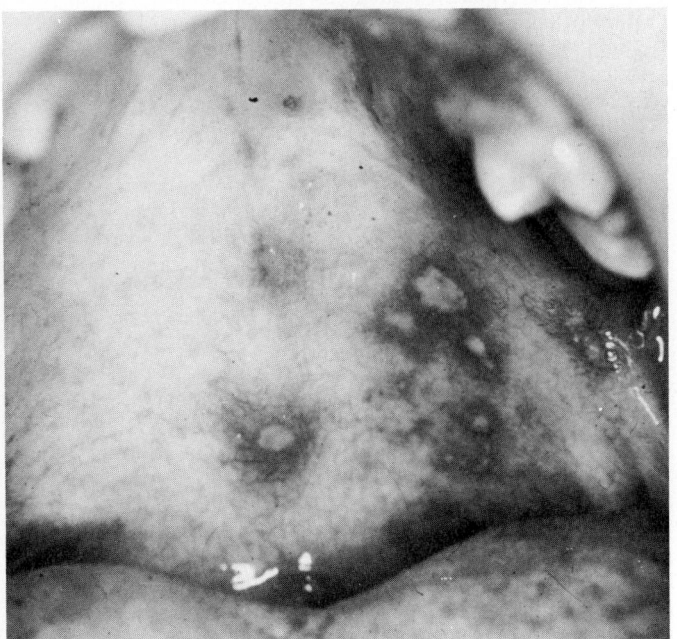

Fig. 8 Maxillary zoster, showing lesions of the palate.

the illness and rose to peak levels within a few weeks and remained raised during convalescence.

Infectious mononucleosis is a disease of young adults, and *par excellence* an illness of students in universities and colleges. In a sample of 1457 students entering British universities and colleges in 1971, 57 per cent had antibody to EB virus. When retested seven months later 12 per cent of the seronegative had acquired antibody. Half developed clinical mononucleosis. At Yale of 362 freshmen bled on entry to college 94 (or 23 per cent) had EB virus antibody. None of them developed infectious mononucleosis during their four years at college, whereas 14 per cent of the seronegative developed the disease. In a small sample at Oxford in 1970, 37 students aged 19–27 had an incidence of EBV antibody of 65 per cent, but in those of 21 or less 52 per cent (or 23) had antibody, whereas 93 per cent of the older students had antibody (13 of 14). In a United States survey of 1400 recruits, two-thirds were seropositive, and over the next four years half the 450 seronegative converted, but only a quarter had typical clinical mononucleosis. As with the other herpesviruses, the incidence of antibody is lower in those from a favoured socio-economic background. They come to university or college with a much higher chance of catching infectious mononucleosis than those from a less favoured background. Surveys of young children have shown that infection is common, but illness rare in children under three. Though heterophile antibodies often are absent, rising antibody to viral capsid antigen (VCA) and to EB virus early antigen as well as the appearance of EB specific IgM antibody are suggestive of recent infection.

There is still uncertainty about transmission; the virus which is present in the mouth may well be spread by aerosol, and not necessarily by close contact (the 'kissing disease' of Hoagland, a term perhaps better reserved for herpes simplex and cytomegalovirus, see page 5.65). The incidence among the very poor in developing countries has been found to be 70–90 per cent in the under threes. But there was no correlation with incidence of Burkitt's lymphoma or malaria. Attempts to transmit the disease by injecting plasma or blood from patients into volunteers have with perhaps one exception been fruitless, and the disease has been transmitted by blood transfusions once only from a donor who was incubating infectious mononucleosis.

The virus. Cultures of leucocytes from peripheral blood of patients with infectious mononucleosis have been shown to be heavily infected with EB virus, which has a growth stimulating effect on the cells. Throat washings from patients with acute infectious mononucleosis will, when added to EB virus-free leucocyte cultures, after incubation, transform the leucocytes into lymphoblasts which contain EB virus. The transforming agent, almost certainly the virus, is found long after the acute phase is over, a parallel with herpes simplex virus. It tends to persist much longer in immunosuppressed patients. The virus can be seen on electron microscopy and is a typical herpesvirus.

Serological tests for the virus. Several antibodies have been identified. Some are of little importance in clinical practice, although one or two can be most useful if the clinician is lucky enough to have access to a good virus laboratory.

Viral capsid antibody (VCA) is an antibody to the EB viral capsid antigen. It rises rapidly at the beginning of the clinical illness and remains elevated for many years. Presence of the VCA merely tells one that the patient has had infectious mononucleosis some time in the past.

Antibody to EB virus/early antigen (EA) appears in the second or third week of the illness only to disappear in the course of the next few months. It may only be present in three out of four patients, perhaps in those with severe illness. If present the antibody is a useful indication of current infection. At least this is true of the D (diffuse) component: the R (restricted) component antibody may persist for years and often in patients with relapsing symptoms.

The EB specific IgM antibody appears early and disappears early.

It is particularly useful in diagnosing current infection. It rises in parallel with heterophile positive tests, but in children, in particular where the latter is negative, the demonstration of EB specific IgM is very helpful.

EB virus associated nuclear antigen (EBNA) is a marker of cells containing EB viral genome, which can be detected by immunofluorescence. Antibody to EBNA appears late and persist for life.

None of these antibodies, which are distinct, appears to be identical to heterophile antibodies. Probably 90 per cent of patients with infectious mononucleosis produce heterophile antibodies.

The heterophile agglutinins for sheeps' red cells are diagnostic for infectious mononucleosis and are used in the *Paul–Bunnell* test. Similar agglutinins occur in people exposed to horse serum and in a variety of conditions from infective hepatitis to Hodgkin's disease and acute leukaemia. They are all of the Forssman type and are absorbed out by tissue rich in Forssman antigen such as guinea pig kidney. The heterophile antibodies of infectious mononucleosis are not absorbed by guinea pig kidney, but react with ox red cells. A positive Paul–Bunnell test should show a titre of sheep cell agglutination after absorption with ox red cells at least fourfold lower than the Paul–Bunnell test for heterophile antibodies, but not more than three times lower after absorption with guinea pig kidney.

A rapid screening test using sheep cells only, or a similar test using formolized horse red cells, which is cheap and which lasts long but may give false positive tests, and may have to be confirmed with EB virus antibody tests, is now widely used. EB virus antibody tests are essential in Paul–Bunnell negative cases.

Pathological findings. *The peripheral blood.* Characteristic is the presence of proliferating mononuclear cells of varying size derived from lymphocytes. They are probably T lymphocytes and contain T lymphocyte specific antigens but lack B cell markers. EB virus infects B cells and causes them to proliferate, but this is controlled *in vivo* by the T lymphocytes. These mononuclear cells usually form at least 10–15 per cent of the white cells. They are not peculiar to infectious mononucleosis but are also seen in other virus diseases such as hepatitis A and influenza. The numbers are usually higher in infectious mononucleosis than in other conditions. These cells infiltrate many organs, notably the spleen and the lymph nodes. The cervical lymph nodes are heavily invaded, and the spleen shows scattered foci of infiltrating mononuclear cells in the pulp and sinuses, which may destroy the architecture and lead to infarcts giving rise to repeated attacks of abdominal pain and at worst rupture of the spleen with bleeding into the abdominal cavity.

The liver is affected in most, but liver biopsy (which is rarely justified) usually shows only infiltration of the sinusoids with T cells, with little evidence of parenchymatous damage. After about five weeks most livers, when re-biopsied, are normal. Acute hepatic necrosis is exceptionally rare.

The heart has been found to have some mononuclear cells in the muscle at post-mortem in patients who have died from a ruptured spleen. There is scant information on the kidney. Severe involvement of the kidney is rare, but it may well be that transient glomerulonephritis is fairly common.

The lungs sometimes show radiological evidence of pneumonitis.

The bone marrow may show a modest infiltration with atypical cells. As in so many viral illnesses, thrombocytopenia is common. Severe *thrombocytopenic* purpura is very uncommon, and may be mediated by an auto-immune process.

Clinical features. It may well be that the clinical picture we see is removed a couple of weeks from the initial replication of the virus. In two or three cases which were followed carefully for other purposes a trivial upper respiratory episode was followed a fortnight later by a fierce attack of infectious mononucleosis. The clinical picture seems to be a violent, almost inappropriate, immune response in some.

Typically, infectious mononucleosis is acquired and passes unnoticed in most young children and in many before the age of 10. In young adults only a proportion, perhaps as few as a quarter to half of those infected, get obvious clinical disease.

By convention, physicians have created categories: the *anginose*, the *glandular*, and the *febrile type*. Gratifying though it may be for the doctor to pigeon-hole disease pictures, the division is artificial. The hospital doctor may get a skewed picture, for he will get only the severe cases. Probably the commonest presentation is that of malaise, a sore throat, a fever, and cervical adenopathy, perhaps influenzal symptoms—that is a glandular picture. The doctor will wonder whether the patient has a β-haemolytic streptococcal throat infection. The throat may be very red, but that can happen in infectious mononucleosis as well as in streptococcal disease. The cervical lymph nodes are enlarged in both. Perhaps a single huge node is commoner in infectious mononucleosis. It is very important to remember that perhaps one in four of all patients with infectious mononucleosis also have an infection with a β-haemolytic strepto-coccus. Most of these patients never reach hospital: at most they will make a university sick bay. This picture merges gradually into one where the oedema of the fauces is more marked, there may be gross oedema, and even membranes that may look like those in diphtheria. This is the *anginose* picture. Most now have seen so little diphtheria that it would be unwise to attempt to distinguish the membranes in infectious mononucleosis from those in diphtheria (which are said to go dark quickly) (Fig. 1). In both forms of infectious mononucleosis a quite characteristic foetor of decaying mold, sickly sweet, is very common. One sometimes sees palatal petechiae (Fig. 2), but they are no more common in infectious mononucleosis than in many other viral illnesses. There may be vesicular lesions on the palate. Oedema of the mucosa of the structures in the nose, mouth, and pharynx is common, making swallowing difficult or impossible. Periorbital oedema, present in perhaps 20 per cent of patients, is quite characteristic.

There is sometimes generalized adenopathy. The spleen is palpable in about every second patient.

The *rash* in infectious mononucleosis is uncommon, it is a transient morbilliform, non-itchy rash—it must not be confused with the drug rash induced by ampicillin and related compounds. The true rash occurs in only a few per cent of all patients.

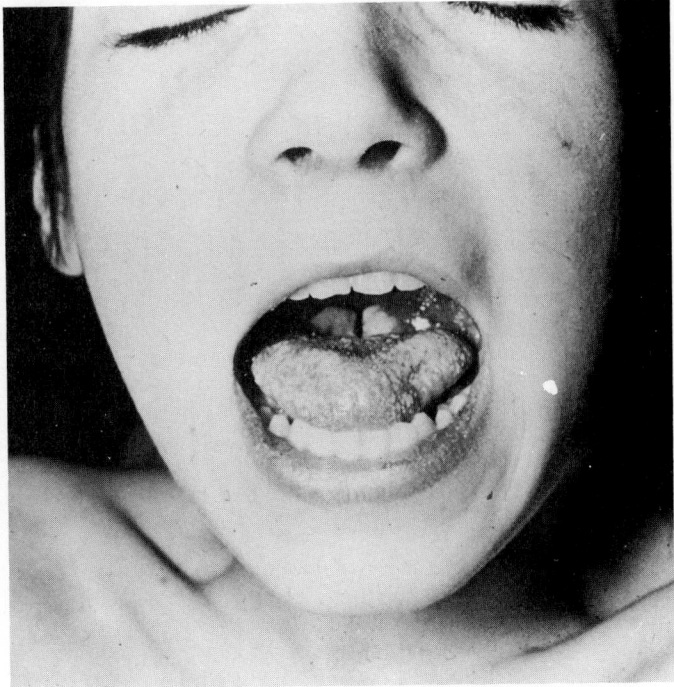

Fig. 1 Infectious mononucleosis. Note membranes on tonsils (Reproduced from Christie, A. B. (1980). *Infectious diseases*, 3rd edn. Churchill Livingstone, Edinburgh, by permission.)

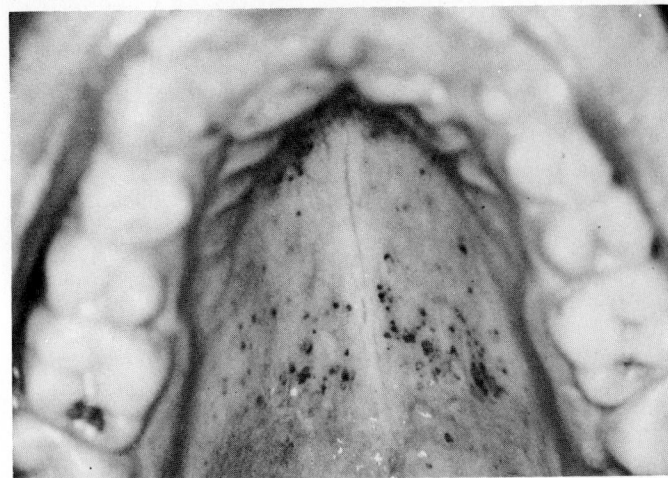

Fig. 2 Petechial haemorrhages on the palate in infectious mononucleosis.

Complications. *Rupture of the spleen.* This uncommon complication is dangerous and accounts for most of the few deaths reported in infectious mononucleosis. It may be heralded by repeated bouts of abdominal pain, due to splenic infarcts. A scintigram of the spleen may show the infarcts. If the spleen ruptures, immediate surgery and replacement of the lost blood is obviously necessary. In the management of patients with infectious mononucleosis, many of whom participate in violent contact games like rugby and football, the doctor must advise abstinence from games for six to eight weeks.

Thrombocytopenia. A minor degree of thrombocytopenia is the rule, but occasionally severe, auto-immune thrombocytopenia may lead to purpura and profuse bleeding. Agranulocytosis is a very rare complication.

Cardiac involvement. Minor T wave changes are relatively common; these changes are found in perhaps ten per cent of patients. Temporary A-V conduction problems have been reported but are very rare. Permanent cardiac damage has not been reported.

Jaundice. Frank jaundice has been reported in up to 25 per cent of cases in some series. The writer would agree with A. B. Christie that it is uncommon, perhaps nearer the 5 per cent mark than the 25 per cent claimed by some authors. However, biochemical hepatitis of the hepatocellular type, reflected in modestly raised alkaline phosphatase, raised aspartate transaminase (AST), or serum gluta-mic oxalacetic transaminase (SGOT) and a near normal bilirubin are common. Liver necrosis is exceptionally rare.

Neurological complications. Perhaps the commonest form of neurological involvement is meningitis. For no very obvious reason there are occasional clusters of cases. The condition is entirely benign.

More alarming is a true encephalitis which in 11 cases carried a 33 per cent mortality.

Single nerve palsies, particularly of the seventh nerve (oedema of the nerve with a long course in a rigid bony canal) are seen occasionally. Acute polyneuritis can be worrying. The patient may be unable to close his eyes and his facial expression has gone. He can hardly lift his arms or legs, and his peak flow drops alarmingly. The physician should in good time plan to have the patient ventilated, for several cases of respiratory paralysis leading to death have been recorded. All respond dramatically to steroids, and there is no excuse for not making every effort to salvage the patient.

Malaise and depression in most disappears after three to four weeks. The long-drawn-out illness is the exception, and in such patients one might find the R component of the antibody to EB virus early antigen. Iatrogenic prolongation of the period of illness is common. Doctors can with success convince the patient that he will feel awful for months.

Pneumonitis. The lungs are occasionally involved, with patchy unilateral and bilateral infiltrations on X-ray. Fibrosing alveolitis has been described but must be very rare.

Ampicillin and amoxycillin reactions. In nearly all patients with acute infectious mononucleosis administration of ampicillin or amoxycillin and related semi-synthetic penicillins leads after eight to 10 days to a distressing maculopapular itchy drug rash. IgG and IgM to the antimicrobial molecule can be demonstrated. It does *not* indicate hypersensitivity to penicillins in general, indeed occurrence of rashes to benzylpenicillin in patients with infectious mononucleosis is less than 1 per cent, identical with that in the population at large. Any acute herpesvirus infection may produce a similar rash.

Nephritis. The present writer has watched the renal function in a large number of young patients with infectious mononucleosis. A transient rise in urea and creatinine is common as is transient showers of red blood cells in freshly passed urine. None of these patients had β-haemolytic streptococcal infection or a rise in antistreptolysin titre. Frank renal failure is extremely rare, and the prognosis is excellent.

Diagnosis. Although infectious mononucleosis is a disease of the young, age does not disqualify. Many physicians have had patients in their seventies with proven infectious mononucleosis, but it is uncommon. The clinical picture should make one suspect the diagnosis. A typical blood picture would make one more certain, but it by no means proves the diagnosis. Hepatic involvement is the rule, so abnormal liver function tests help. A positive screening test for heterophile antibodies gives further support. But it might be a false positive reaction due to, e.g. Hodgkin's disease or syphilis. Many have had antitetanus serum in the past and may have antibodies to horse erythrocytes. A proper Paul–Bunnell test, if still positive, makes the diagnosis nearly certain. The Paul–Bunnell test often does not become positive until the second week of the illness.

In the persistently Paul–Bunnell negative case demonstration of EB specific IgM antibody proves the diagnosis. If that is negative, the patient may have 'glandular fever' due to some other cause of which cytomegalovirus and toxoplasmosis are the two commonest in the United Kingdom. Rise in cytomegalovirus complement fixing titres or in toxoplasma titres will prove the diagnosis. Infectious mononucleosis rarely lasts more than three weeks. If glandular fever lasts longer, the diagnosis should be re-examined. Could the patient have cytomegalovirus or toxoplasma infection? The latter may go on for six to nine months. The rare, but important, differential diagnosis of diphtheria has been mentioned. True lymphoproliferative disorders must be remembered, and practically any respiratory virus disease may present as 'glandular fever'. The physician will of course never forget to ask: 'where have you been?' Trypanosomiasis, collected in East Africa at the end of his long vacation by an Oxford schoolboy, presented as 'glandular fever' and only the finding of the organisms in aspirate from the lymphnodes revealed the true diagnosis.

Many doctors are convinced (in the face of objective evidence to the contrary) that infectious mononucleosis will incapacitate the sufferer for six to nine months. Such is the power of suggestion that the doctor manages to convince the patient. Many a university career has been seriously interfered with because ignorant clinicians have told a student to take six months off quite unnecessarily. Infectious mononucleosis remains one of the great iatrogenic diseases!

EB virus and malignancy. High titres of antibodies to EB virus have been found in most, but not all patients suffering from Burkitt's lymphoma (see page 5.124) and in those with retropharyngeal carcinoma. It is not yet certain what is the role of EB virus in the pathogenesis of these two disparate neoplasms. It could be that EB virus is an opportunist which thrives in the abnormal cells. It could be one of the many contributing factors that cause the neoplasm, or it could be the sole cause. None of these postulates have yet either been proved or disproved.

Treatment. The majority of patients get better with no treatment. High dose, short-term treatment with steroids (e.g. prednisolone, 80 mg the first day, 15 mg three times daily for the next two, 10 mg three times daily for the next two, 5 mg three times daily for the last two) will relieve symptoms dramatically in anginose infectious mononucleosis. It is indicated in neurological complications, where there is pulmonary or hepatic involvement, or when there rarely is purpuric thrombocytopenia. Controlled trials at Harvard and Princeton showed the efficiency and safety of steroids.

A concurrent β-haemolytic streptococcal infection must be treated with erythromycin (500 mg three times daily) which anyway will be appropriate for the rare unrecognized case of diphtheria. Ampicillin or amoxycillin must *never* be used.

The special requirements of patients with neurological problems have been described above.

References

Carter, R. I. and Penman, H. G. (1969). *Infectious mononucleosis*. Blackwell Scientific Publications, Oxford.

Christie, A. B. (1980). Infectious mononucleosis. In *Infectious diseases*, 3rd edn., 890. Churchill Livingstone, Edinburgh.

Hoagland, R. J. (1967). *Infectious mononucleosis*. Grune and Stratton, New York.

L. D. Stauffer (ed.) (1967). *International infectious mononucleosis symposium*. American College Health Association.

Infections caused by simian herpesviruses

B. E. Juel-Jensen

Several true herpesviruses have been isolated from various monkeys. Of these *Herpesvirus simiae* (originally called 'B virus' after Dr 'B'—the first patient from whom the virus was isolated) causes trivial disease, a transient gingivo-stomatitis, in its host under natural conditions. *H. simiae* infects the rhesus monkey (*Macaca mulatta*) and several other Asiatic macaques (including the cynomolgus and Japanese macaque). The African green monkey has been experimentally infected. The virus is extremely virulent in the rabbit. Of the other herpesviruses in monkeys only *H. tamarinus* has once—on serological evidence—been implicated as causing encephalitis in a laboratory worker. Otherwise all human cases described have been due to infection with *H. simiae*. Potentially, other simian herpesviruses such as SA$_8$, isolated from the African vervet monkey, *might* cause disease in man.

Epidemiology. Several surveys of colonies of rhesus monkeys kept for laboratory purposes have shown that a proportion have antibody to *H. simiae*. The older the animals the higher the percentage with antibody. If young animals are kept separate, the incidence is much lower than if they are allowed to mix. In the rhesus monkey colonies (numbering about 300 animals) in Oxford about a third of the animals have antibody, although *H. simiae* was isolated from none of the animals when their mouths were swabbed under anaesthesia. The risk that animals may excrete virus under stress is present. In one series of 400 recently imported monkeys, 2.3 per cent were found to have active infection, in another of 300 newly imported cynomolgus that had not been exposed to rhesus monkeys a 10 per cent incidence of active infection was found. It is likely that recurrent lesions, similar to those in herpes simplex virus (HSV) in man, are rare.

In humans, several surveys have demonstrated that there is naturally occurring antibody to *H. simiae*. An antigenic relationship exists between *H. simiae* and *herpes simplex virus* type 1, which is largely one way. Antiserum to *H. simiae* neutralizes HSV as well or better than homologous antibody. About 50 per cent of HSV positive sera contain antibody to *H. simiae* in low titres. As for HSV antibody, the incidence of *H. simiae* antibody increases with age. There is no evidence that people with antibody have had subclinical infection, although it is possible they have been infected following their primary infection with HSV. Although rabbits infected with HSV or hyperimmunized with inactivated HSV antigen are solidly immune to challenge with *H. simiae*, fatal infection has occurred in at least two persons known to have previously suffered from recurrent HSV skin lesions.

At least 25 possible human cases of infection with *H. simiae* in humans have been described. In 10 of 22 of them the virus was isolated and identified. The possible source of infection was unknown in 10 cases (six of which were confirmed), due to laboratory accidents in two cases (both confirmed), due to certain bites in four (one confirmed), and possibly due to a bite in five. Bites were at one time thought to be the commonest source of infection, but they account for less than half of all reported cases, and only one has been confirmed by isolation of *H. simiae*; four rhesus, three cynomolgus, and one African green monkey were involved. However, all but two had at some time been exposed to monkey colonies although no bites or other accidents had occurred. The virus has been isolated from the trigeminal ganglia in seropositive rhesus monkeys two years after recovery from a typical gingivo-stomatitis. Symptoms appeared three days after a bite in a well documented case while in two others, less well documented, the interval before symptoms was 13 days. In laboratory accidents with broken culture bottles symptoms occurred two and 56 days after exposure.

Clinical manifestations. In patients who have been bitten by monkeys, vesicles have appeared within three to four days at the site, with regional adenopathy. Subsequently blisters may appear in other sites. Muscle pains, abdominal colic, diarrhoea, dysphagia, and neck stiffness may precede or coincide with neurological symptoms, such as paraesthesiae of the limbs, followed by weakness, loss of reflexes, and facial paralysis. Transverse myelitis or a picture like that of herpes simplex encephalitis may be present. With increasing involvement of the central nervous system, the patients rapidly lapse into coma, they have fits, and their respiratory centre fails. Usually the cause of death is due to multisystem failure.

In two patients the illness began with respiratory symptoms, sore throat, cough, aches in the chest, and signs of pneumonitis. Neurological involvement followed, but only after three to four weeks from the onset of symptoms. Both died, one after five days, one three years later. In one patient skin lesions mimicking zoster of the face subsequently spread to the chest and was followed by ascending spinal paralysis.

At post mortem the central nervous system, medulla, and spinal cord show extensive perivascular infiltration of mononuclear cells, necrosis of vessel walls, and necrosis of neurones and supporting glial cells. Demyelinization may occur. The spinal cord may show transverse myelitis. In other organs such as spleen, liver, heart, and adrenals, there is cell necrosis, inflammatory cell infiltration, and intranuclear inclusions may be seen.

Isolation of the virus from any obvious lesion, throat swab, faeces, CSF, and brain biopsy should be attempted. Neutralization tests should be carried out on serum in laboratories with the necessary facilities for handling *H. simiae*. The diagnosis must be considered in anyone who is in contact with Asiatic *macaca* monkeys or other species that have been in transit or housed with macaca monkeys. In all of the 25 reported cases in humans only four lived, three with serious neurological sequelae, only one patient returning to some sort of useful life. A fifth patient lived for 40 months, when he died in coma.

Prevention. A distinguished virologist has said: 'The possibility that inter-species spread of [simian herpes] virus may occur and that this may involve man has to be accepted. It is one of the facts of life. If attention is not paid to guarding against it, it could be a fact of death.'

Clearly it is desirable from several points of view to use for experimental purposes colonies of monkeys free of simian herpesvirus. Whenever possible animals should be bred in captivity from

virus free stock. Serological evidence suggests that about 12 per cent of rhesus monkeys recently imported into Britain had been infected with *H. simiae*. If monkeys are imported, they should be kept separate from one another. Handlers should wear protective clothing. It may be an advantage to employ staff with a known *very high* HSV titre as they have a higher chance of having perhaps protective levels of *H. simiae* antibody.

The Medical Research Council and similar *Guidelines for keeping primates* should be followed.

Treatment. Monkey handlers who are bitten should report at once. A swab should be taken from the wound for herpesvirus culture. The risk of infection is obviously remote if the colony is seronegative, but often this will not be so. The wound is washed and a dressing of lint with 5 per cent acyclovir in dimethyl sulphoxide should be applied daily for three days. Should a herpesvirus be isolated, intravenous therapy should be started. The patient should report at once if untoward symptoms occur within four weeks.

In the established disease, treatment is as for herpes simplex encephalitis, except that cytarabine and vidarabine should not be used, as they, with ribavirin, *in vitro*, have been shown to be ineffective. Acyclovir, however, is active *in vitro* and in experimental animals 15 mg/kg eight-hourly administered over an hour should be given with full supportive therapy.

References

Hull, R. N. (1973). The simian herpesviruses. In *The herpesviruses* (ed. A. S. Kaplan), 389. Academic Press, New York.
Medical Research Council's Simian Virus Committee (1978). *On the management of simians (pro simian monkeys and great apes*. Medical Research Council, London.
Perkins, F. T. and O'Donoghue, P. N. (1969). *Hazards of handling simians*. London Laboratory Animals Ltd., London.

Cytomegalovirus infection

J. O'H. Tobin

The cytomegaloviruses (CMV) are members of the herpesvirus group and are widely distributed in many animal species including monkeys, pigs, rodents, horses, dogs, and sheep. Each virus is specific for its own host and can be isolated only in homologous fibroblast cell cultures. Large characteristic intranucleic inclusions, 'owls eyes', are produced in parotid, kidney, liver, lung, and other organs, as well as in cell cultures. Antigenic heterogenicity exists among human CMV but there is no real evidence yet suggesting separate serological types.

Epidemiology. After infection with human CMV, the virus is excreted for weeks, months, or, in infants, for years even, and is carried in the white blood cells for the life of the individual. Its presence in white cells means that it can be transmitted by blood transfusion and, as it is present in other organs, it can also be transmitted by transplantation. As with other herpesviruses, CMV infection can be reactivated from time to time. This is most often detected in the cervix.

The frequency of infection in relation to age differs from country to country. In western temperate climates, most infection is acquired by direct contact with infected people and probably requires very close contact of mucous membranes. It is thus one of the 'kissing' diseases and, because of its presence in the genital tract, may be transmitted sexually. Infection occurs at a rate of 1 or 2 per cent per year with a slight increase during adolescence and young adulthood up to middle age. The incidence of antibody in women of child-bearing age varies from 40 to 70 per cent in most temperate climates, giving rise to a large number of seronegative pregnant women who are susceptible to infection.

In tropical countries, such as Africa, India, and the Far East, most infection takes place in infancy or early childhood. The newborn infant can be infected by reactivated virus in its mother's genital tract during delivery, or from her milk. In these countries up to 60–70 per cent of children are infected within six months of birth and most of the remainder by the time they are five years of age. This leaves very few women of child-bearing age who have not had CMV infection. In some countries, such as Singapore, half the population appears to have become infected in infancy, with the other half following the western pattern of adolescent and young adult infection. The frequency of antibody is often higher in institutionalized children than in others but the relation of sanitation and socio-economic factors to the prevalence of antibody is not clear.

Table 1 Percentage of individual abnormalities in 88 symptomatic congenital CMV childre

Hepatomegaly	63	Conductive deafness	9
Splenomegaly	60	Sensorineural deafness	7
Jaundice	50	Visual defects:	
Purpura	28	Choroid retinitis	7
Microcephaly	22	Optic atrophy	3
Cerebral palsy	20	Myopia and squint	1
Intracranial calcification	9	Hydrocephalus	5
Epilepsy	9	Speech defect	5
Clumsiness	9	Non-specific retardation	3

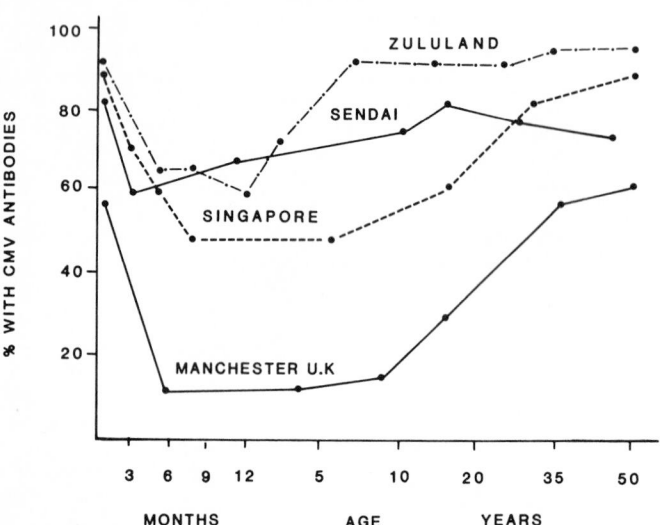

CMV ANTIBODY BY AGE AND AREA

Fig. 1 CMV antibody by age and area. (Reproduced by permission of the Editor, *Annals of the Singapore Academy of Medicine*.)

As congenital infection is considered to be initiated by a maternal primary infection, it is more likely that women in western temperate climates will produce congenitally infected infants than those in tropical climes, where most are immune. In Negroes, it is possible for intrauterine infection to occur following reactivation, but so far this type of disease has not been associated with severe symptoms.

Disease caused by CMV was first brought to general notice by its congenital syndromes, but soon afterwards its importance was recognized in other situations, especially in patients with immunodeficiency diseases or on immunosuppressive drugs. It is now regularly listed in the differential diagnosis of many specific and non-specific syndromes.

Clinical features
Congenital infection. The incidence of congenital infection varies from 1 in 100 to 1 in 500 with the lower level being more common in temperate climates and in 'developed' populations. Congenital CMV infection, unlike rubella, appears to produce defects if it occurs during the first two trimesters and occasionally in the third trimester. It can also cause premature labour in the mother, and the baby may become ill a few weeks after delivery. The most common symptoms encountered by the author are given in Table 1. Signs may be present at birth or develop gradually over months or even years. The prognosis for the child's development depends on the extent of the infection at birth. If the central nervous system is involved, 90 per cent of the infants will be mentally retarded and need special schooling; while, if signs are extra-neural or absent at birth, the chances of permanent central nervous system damage are reduced.

From 25 to 50 per cent of primary maternal infections lead to infection of the fetus, and 45 per cent of such infants will show signs of infection at birth or later. Of these, a third will be severely

affected and the remainder have some disability demonstrable on careful clinical examination.

Short-term symptoms of hepatomegaly, splenomegaly, jaundice, and purpura may occur singly or together, be present at birth, or appear after about six weeks and persist occasionally for as long as one year. Microcephaly, the most common of the long-term sequelae, may rarely be complicated by an encephalocele. Cerebral palsy, which again may not be apparent early in the first year of life, is usually quadraplegic but lesser degrees of involvement can occur. Intracranial calcification is not as frequent as was once thought. Hyperactivity and clumsiness tend to develop after the first year of life and may not be detected until the children go to school. Epilepsy can occur, either as fits or hypsarrhythmia. Visual defects include choroidoretinitis, optic atrophy, and occasionally myopia and squints. Deafness may be conductive due to malformation of the middle ear or sensorineural, usually bilateral. Hydrocephaly is

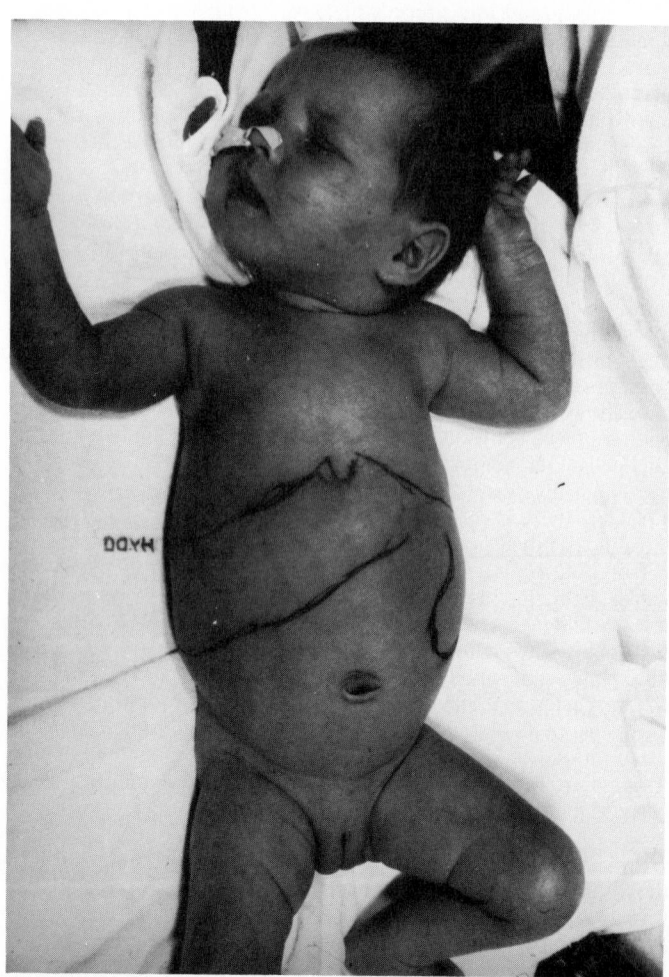

Fig. 2. Cogenital CMV infection. Baby with large liver and spleen, jaundice, and petechiae: later quadriplegia and severe mental retardation developed.

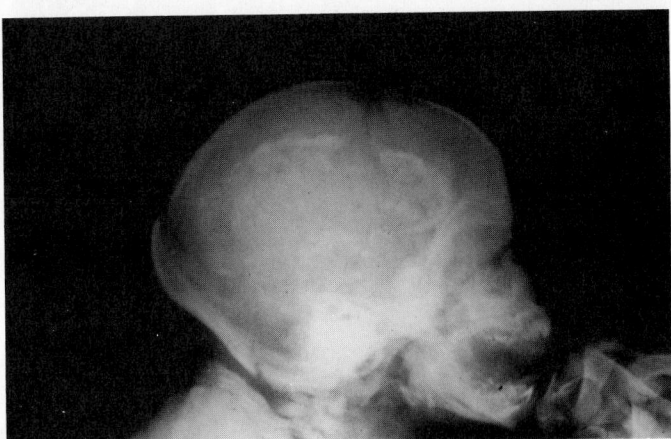

Fig. 3 Congenital CMV infection. Baby with microcephaly and intracranial calcification in roof of lateral ventricules.

more common in CMV infection than in rubella, where it is very rare. Non-specific retardation and speech defects unrelated to deafness may become apparent. Other defects reported include anomalies of the cardiovascular, alimentary, skeletal, and muscular systems (Table 2). Whether all these are actually due to CMV is open to doubt.

Table 2 Other anomalies reported in congenital CMV infection

Alimentary tract	Cardiovascular	Skeletal and muscular
Cleft palate	Septal defects	Club foot
Oesophageal atresia	Patent ductus	Hip dislocation
Biliary atresia	Mitral stenosis	Inguinal hernia
Stenosis of ileum and colon	Tetralogy of Fallot	Hypotonia
Gut perforation		Omphalocele
Megacolon		Abdominal muscle defects
Ascites		Prune belly

CMV disease must be differentiated from congenital toxoplasmosis (see page 5.402), rubella (see page 5.80), herpes simplex infection (see page 5.489), syphilis (see page 5.288), and bacterial disease due to coliforms, group B streptococci (see page 5.146), *Listeria monocytogenes* (see page 5.331), and other pathogenic organisms.

In the United Kingdom it is estimated that 1200 infants with congenital CMV infection are born each year, of whom 200 will be severely affected and another 400 have minor defects.

Acquired infections. Most acquired infections do not give rise to clinical symptoms. Occasionally the case may present as a Paul–Bunnell negative infectious mononucleosis, characterized by fever lasting one to four weeks, a lymphocytosis, often with atypical forms and sometimes lymphadenopathy; the latter two signs are less frequent than in Epstein–Barr virus (EBV) glandular fever. CMV infection can be complicated by hepatitis or polyneuritis, the latter being more common with CMV than with EBV; polyneuritis may be transient with recovery in a few weeks or may persist for months. Other symptoms reported to be associated with acquired CMV infection include hepatosplenomegaly, cranial nerve palsies, encephalitis, and ulcers of the gastrointestinal tract. Infection with CMV is found more often in people suffering from malignant diseases such as leukaemia, lymphoma, and Hodgkins disease, but the exact relation of the virus to the frequency of recurrent respiratory tract infections, fever, rashes, or hepatitis is not known. Changes in CMV antibody levels have been associated with blood transfusions in these patients, rather than to onset of symptoms. Acquired infection can start from the day of birth and no age is exempt, so that signs or symptoms can occur at any age.

Following the transfusion of infected blood to a susceptible recipient of any age the 'post-transfusion mononucleosis syndrome' may occur two to six weeks later. Most infections are symptomless, but approximately 5 per cent are clinically evident and may even prove fatal in premature infants.

Natural neonatal or early infant infection has not yet been shown to be deleterious except in a few instances, but until cohort studies with long follow-ups are carried out, it is not known whether minor damage is inflicted on the developing CNS.

The virus is a common cause of infection in renal transplant recipients both as a primary and a reactivated infection (see page 5.480). In the former, symptoms always occur, and although usually mild, can produce a fever which persists for weeks, and occasionally a severe pneumonia (see page 5.483): this can be fatal, especially if it is accompanied by a second infection with, for example, staphylococci, *Pseudomonas pyocyanea*, fungi, or *Pneumocystis carinii*. CMV pneumonia is more common after bone marrow than renal transplantation and is often fatal. Its incidence may be dependent on the schedule of radiation and the cytotoxic and immunosuppressive drugs used. Although in the normal host acquired CMV infection may cause leucocytosis, the immunologically compromised infection is usually accompanied by leucopenia and thrombocytopenia. The frequency of symptoms in the acquired and reactivated disease is given in Table 3. Severe diffuse ulceration of the alimentary tract following renal transplantation is associated with reactivation of CMV, but the exact role played by the virus in this fatal syndrome is not known. It is, however, a cause of localized ulcers in which the characteristic inclusions can be found and virus isolated.

Table 3 Percentage of symptoms and signs associated with CMV infection in renal transplant patients

Symptoms, etc.	Primary infection (n = 20)	Secondary infection (n = 55)
Fever > 37.5° C	95	16.5
Leucopenia (< 500 WBC × 10⁶ 1⁻¹	65	29
Thrombocytopenia (< 100 × 10⁹ 1⁻¹	60	14.5
Atypical mononuclear cells	50	5.5
Abnormal liver function tests	45	3.5
Lower respiratory tract disease	35	9
Hepatomegaly	20	0
Splenomegaly	30	2
Retinitis	0	2
No abnormality detected	0	51

Primary infection can be avoided in renal transplant patients by using kidneys from donors without CMV antibody for non-immune recipients. Although CMV infection can be associated with graft rejection episodes, no clear relationship between the two events has been demonstrated. CMV infection in renal transplant patients usually appears between the second and third month after transplantation. The onset of the acquired, primary infections occurs after a mean of 42 days, about 10 days earlier than the appearance of symptoms resulting from reactivations. Other herpesviruses may be reactivated in these patients, but these events are independent of CMV reactivity.

CMV infection should be considered as a cause of unexplained fever, lymphocytosis, peripheral nerve disease, retinitis, and in atypical pneumonia, intestinal ulceration or CNS disease, especially if the patient is immunosuppressed.

Laboratory diagnosis. Diagnosis can be made by virus isolation in human embryo fibroblast cell cultures from samples taken from the throat, cervix, urine, blood, or occasionally cerebrospinal fluid. The diagnosis of acute disease cannot be made by virus isolation alone because of the prolonged excretion of the virus after primary infection, especially in infants. For congenital disease to be diagnosed, virus must be found within the first two weeks of life as, after that, neonatal infection may lead to virus excretion and it is then impossible to distinguish between the two by laboratory tests. The virus can take from 24 hours to 6 weeks to produce its cytopathic effect, so virus isolation is by no means a rapid method of diagnosis.

A serological diagnosis can be made more surely and rapidly, for example by the complement fixation test (CFT), which detects IgG antibody. A rise in titre indicates either primary infection or reactivation, but they can be differentiated, as specific CMV IgM antibody is present in primary infections. The tests employed for detecting IgM antibody are immunofluorescence, enzyme linked immunosorbent assay (ELISA), or radio-immunoassay. Specific CMV IgM antibodies persist for a few weeks or a few months, specific IgA antibodies from a few months to about a year and IgG antibodies probably for the whole of an individual's life.

The determination of different classes of antibody may give an indication of the likely time of CMV infection in a particular case. For example, the specific IgM and IgA estimations can often be helpful when the antibody level detected by CFT has risen to its maximum before a laboratory diagnosis is sought.

The presence of specific IgM or IgA in the neonatal period (first two to three weeks of life) is also diagnostic of intrauterine infection; but the production of these antibodies, which may occur independently of each other, can be delayed for up to three months, by which time they could not be distinguished from antibodies produced by post-natal infection. The IgM is more transient in infants than in older people with acquired infection.

In primary infections in transplant patients, the presence of specific IgM antibodies is usually the first laboratory evidence of infection and can frequently be demonstrated three to four days after the appearance of symptoms. CMV reactivation in immunosuppressed patients can also produce a transient IgM response and, in the presence of a steady IgG level, may be the only sign that CMV has become reactivated.

Treatment and prevention

Treatment. Anti-viral drugs, such as idoxuridine, cytosine, and adenine arabinoside have been tried in both congenital and acquired infections, but have not been really successful. There may be a reduction in the amount of virus excreted following treatment; this may reduce the hazard of infection in staff and other case contacts. From laboratory studies, it seems unlikely that acyclovir will be any better. In transplant patients, the use of adenine arabinoside has not been advocated because of toxic side-effects, although these may be due as much to the patient's renal failure as to the drug. Steroids are useful in treating CMV polyneuritis but must be used with caution if more generalized disease is present.

Prevention. Vaccines to CMV are being developed and have been used in non-immune patients awaiting renal transplantation. The outlook is moderately promising as the vaccine sometimes seems to prevent symptoms of primary CMV, even if it fails to stop infection. The use of vaccines for the prevention of congenital CMV is less likely, both because of expense and the difficulty in persuading people of the importance of such an insidious disease. The possibility of producing unit vaccines by genetic manipulation or other means is an aim for the future.

Infection of young non-immune patients undergoing transplantation, exchange transfusions or heart operations and of patients suffering from leukaemia and other immunodeficiency diseases can be eliminated by using CMV-free donors. Immunofluorescence, radioimmunoassay, or ELISA techniques can be used satisfactorily for screening for immunity. Infection during pregnancy can be identified by the detection of specific IgM in antenatal sera. Detection in early pregnancy would be an indication for termination but infections at any stage may be dangerous to the fetus. The iden-

tification of babies at risk would be worthwhile so that the effects of abnormalities could be minimized as far as possible.

As very close contact is needed for spread, danger to nurses and others tending infected individuals is slight, even in maternity units and nurseries. It has been recommended that women of child-bearing age working in special care baby units should be tested for antibody, and, if pregnant and non-immune, they should not nurse known or suspected cases of CMV disease in infancy. It is debatable whether special nursing or isolation procedures should be used for such infants.

References

Benson, J. W. T., Bodden, S. J., and Tobin, J. O'H. (1979). Cytomegalovirus and blood transfusion in neonates. *Arch. Dis. Child* **54**, 538.

Hanshaw, J. B. and Dudgeon, J. A. (1978). *Viral diseases of the fetus and newborn.* Saunders, Philadelphia.

MacDonald, H. and Tobin, J. O'H. (1978). Congenital cytomegalovirus infection: a collaborative study on epidemiological, clinical and laboratory findings. *Dev. med. Child Neurol.* **20**, 471.

Stagno, S., Reynolds, D. W., Pass, R. F., and Alford, C. A. (1980). Breast milk and the risk of cytomegalovirus infection. *New Engl. J. Med.* **302**, 1073.

Warrell, M. J., Chinn, I. J., Morris, P. J., and Tobin, J. O'H. (1980). The effects of viral infections on renal transplants and their recipients. *Q. Jl Med.* **49**, 219.

Poxviruses

K. R. Dumbell

Poxviruses form a family of large and complex DNA viruses; with a characteristic morphology of the virion (Fig. 1). Poxviruses replicate in the cytoplasm of infected cells and therefore need to establish a DNA 'factory' outside the cell nucleus. The virion itself contains enzymes for the transcription of DNA and for the polyadenylation, methylation, and capping of the resultant messengers. This is presumably necessary for the initiation of poxvirus replication, as the viral DNA does not appear to be 'read' by mammalian transcriptases. Poxviruses have also been shown to inhibit the synthesis of host-cell DNA and proteins, so it is not surprising that enzyme activities associated with DNA synthesis are found encoded in poxvirus DNA. Large numbers of mature pox virions are to be found in infected cells. Some of them bud from the cell surface into the surrounding fluids or into adjoining cells. Others often in clumps (Fig. 1) are liberated as the killed cells degenerate.

The poxvirus family is divided into two sub-families and seven genera. The poxviruses of greatest importance in medicine are in the orthopoxvirus genus, but human infections also occur with the parapoxvirus causing *orf* or *contagious pustular dermatitis of sheep* and also with three unclassified poxviruses: *Molluscum contagiosum*, *tanapox*, and *cotia virus*. Each genus is antigenically distinct but within each genus there is extensive sharing of antigens and cross-protection between member species. Among the orthopoxviruses, the degree of antigenic overlap is such that viruses within this genus are difficult to separate by the conventional methods of complement fixation and type specific neutralization tests. Until recently, the identification of a particular orthopoxvirus depended on its behaviour in a number of biological tests, prominent among which was the appearance of the focal lesions (pocks) induced in the chorio-allantois of 12-day-old chick embryos. Cowpox, variola, and vaccinia viruses could quickly be differentiated by this test alone. However, the recent discovery of several more orthopoxviruses has made identification less straightforward and the necessary, additional tests will be described in the section on *monkeypox* (see below).

Smallpox and its eradication

A man in Somalia, who was found to have smallpox in October

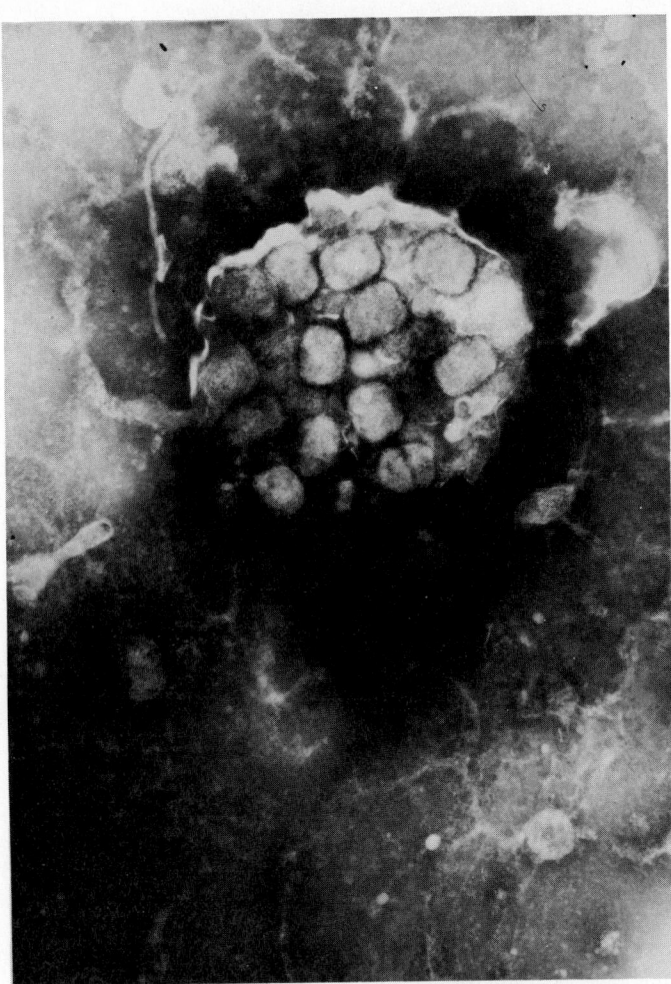

Fig. 1   Electron micrograph of material from smallpox lesion, viewed by negative contrast, showing a clump of poxvirus particles. (By courtesy of the late H. S. Bedson.)

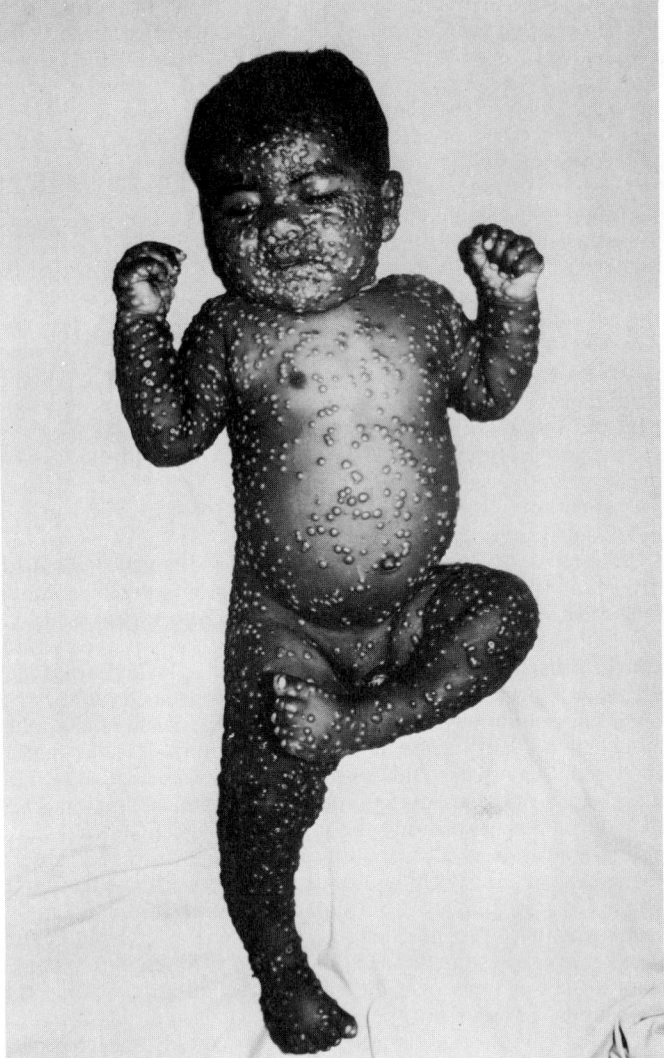

Fig. 2   Smallpox in a nine-month-old boy in Pakistan, photographed on the eighth day of the rash. (By courtesy of the World Health Organization.)

1977, became the last endemic case of this disease which was detected in the Smallpox Eradication Campaign. After two further years of search, a special international commission, set up by the World Health Organization, was able to conclude: (*a*) that smallpox eradication had been achieved throughout the World and (*b*) that there was no evidence that smallpox will return as an endemic disease. This historic announcement has made smallpox a disease of the past, of which it is necessary to give only a brief clinical description. Diagnostic problems concerning smallpox may still arise, because patients may still present, in whom the disease is suspect and the World community must be satisfied that all proper steps have been taken to exclude smallpox and to establish the true diagnosis in any such patient. This will be discussed more fully below.

Clinical smallpox. The incubation period was 10–12 days from exposure to the onset of illness, and during this period the patient appeared to be well. The illness then started abruptly with fever, prostration, and generalized aching; often there would be nausea and even vomiting. On the third day of the illness a maculopapular rash would appear which progressed to a vesicular and then a pustular eruption. The patient usually began to feel better as the eruption developed, and the temperature dropped, only to rise again if there was extensive pustulation. The lesions were tense and firm to the touch, well raised above the surface, but at the same time based deeply into the skin. The developed pustular rash, with its characteristic centrifugal distribution was the classical picture of smallpox (Fig. 2). Scabs formed as the pustular lesions dried, and

over the next two to three weeks the scabs gradually separated leaving depigmented areas. The scarring which subsequently developed was characteristic and could label a person for life as a victim of smallpox. Blindness was another deformity that frequently affected the survivors of severe smallpox.

The above description would cover the majority of patients, but the rash could evolve in other ways, associated with lesser or greater severity of the disease. In smallpox, modified by previous vaccination, the pre-eruptive illness would be less severe and the skin lesions, which might be only few in number, would be more superficial, evolve more quickly, and show less uniformity than those of classical type. The secondary fever might not develop. Such modified disease was never fatal; it could, however, raise many problems in clinical diagnosis.

A grave prognosis could be given when the rash was slower than usual in its evolution and the lesions remained flat and soft. Haemorrhage might develop into the base of the lesions. If, however, the rash was haemorrhagic from the beginning, fatality was almost universal. A particularly severe and prolonged pre-eruptive illness would be followed by slowly developing, dusky macules; or in the most fulminant cases, no distinct rash would develop but generalized haemorrhagic manifestations would appear on the second or third day and the patient would die probably on the fifth to seventh day of illness.

Quite different was the type of smallpox endemic in South America and in parts of eastern and southern Africa during recent years. This disease had a low mortality, even in the unvaccinated and gave rise to much less constitutional disturbance. The rash could be very profuse, but the lesions were more superficial and the resulting pock marks were less characteristic than those following variola major and frequently became inapparent within one to two years after the illness.

Laboratory diagnosis. Laboratory tests were important whenever there was some doubt about the clinical diagnosis. It was seldom necessary to make a formal identification of the variola virus. The demonstration that a suspect case had poxvirus particles or specific orthopoxvirus antigen in the lesions would be sufficient to resolve the difficulty and establish the diagnosis. The most satisfactory test was electron microscopy; this was quick, sensitive, and applicable to lesions at all stages of development. Electron microscopy had the further advantage that it could produce positive evidence to support the most likely, alternative diagnosis of varicella. Diagnosis by culture and identification of a particular poxvirus will be discussed in the section on monkeypox (see below).

Epidemiology

Smallpox, major, minor, and intermediate. Although individual patients in a single outbreak may suffer mild or severe smallpox, there was a tendency for outbreaks themselves to vary in severity. This was particularly pronounced with milder forms of the disease and the occurrence of large outbreaks without a single death led to the general acceptance that there were two distinct varieties of smallpox, one called 'variola major' or 'asiatic smallpox' and the other known as 'variola minor' or 'alastrim'. Variola minor appeared to have a fixed, low virulence and showed no reversion to the severe form, even during an extensive spread to major. This clear distinction has proved to be an over-simplification. Epidemics of intermediate severity were difficult to define when a large percentage of the cases were known to go unreported. The figures in Table 1 were compiled from outbreaks during the eradication campaign where the case-finding was reasonably complete. The case-fatality rates from these raw data cover an hundred-fold range from 20 per cent to 0.2 per cent. Small corrections for differences in vaccination coverage or in age-specific incidence in the different populations would not distort the general pattern that emerges: that there were several variola viruses in circulation, covering a wide spectrum of pathogenicity.

Table 1   Case fatality rates in smallpox

Country	Year(s)	Cases	Deaths	Fatality rate (%)
India	1974–75	2826	575	20.3
Bangladesh	1975	1127	207	18.4
Pakistan	1971	1674	249	14.9
West Africa	1967–69	5628	540	9.6
Indonesia	1969	11 966	950	7.9
Tanzania	1967–70	2232	167	7.5
Uganda	1966–70	1045	54	5.2
Sudan	1970–72	2979	35	1.2
Ethiopia	1972–74	21 250	243	1.1
Brazil	1969	6795	37	0.5
Somalia	1977	3229	12	0.4
Botswana	1972	1059	2	0.2

These figures were collected during the eradication campaign after active surveillance had been organized and from outbreaks where the case finding was reasonably complete; they include all cases, irrespective of vaccination status

Data from World Health Organization (1980). *Report of the Global Commission for the Certification of Smallpox Eradication*. WHO, Geneva

Spread of disease. The most usual incubation period was 12 days during which time the infected person was not infectious to others.

From the onset of disease virus was shed from the throat and mucus membranes and was present in large amounts in the cutaneous lesions. The patient would be presumed infectious until the last scab had separated, but there has never been any evidence

that variola virus could become latent and give rise to a spontaneous recurrence of disease. The virus is stable and survives for some time in dried pustular fluid or in scabs, but there is little evidence that fomites have played any significant role in maintaining the spread of the disease. Subclinical infections did occur, as shown by antibody rises among known contacts but the epidemiological evidence does not suggest that they could transmit the infection. Smallpox has also been a disease confined to the human population and no animal, vertebrate or invertebrate, had played any role in maintaining the existence of the virus.

These features—the obligate human parasite, spreading only from active cases and inducing disease in contacts only after nearly two weeks of non-infectivity—are the ones which permitted an eradication programme to be planned. Furthermore the infectivity was not all that great. During epidemics one infected person would infect from one to five secondary cases but unvaccinated, household contacts would often escape infection. An uncontrolled local outbreak would be relatively long in duration and with only a few chains of transmission operating simultaneously, and this, too aided detection and interruption of transmission.

The eradication of smallpox. Smallpox, almost alone among major infectious diseases, was susceptible to eradication, by the systematic and progressive interruption of the chains of transmission. A potent aid was provided by smallpox vaccine. Jenner had foreseen that the introduction of such an active, immunizing agent would one day result in the elimination of the disease. Liquid vaccine had, however, often lost its potency by the time it came to be used in tropical climates and the provision of stable, freeze-dried vaccine was undoubtedly an important factor in the eradication plan. As surveillance activities were developed, it was found that smallpox transmission often persisted in countries that had achieved 80 per cent or even 90 per cent coverage in mass-vaccination campaigns. The eradication strategy evolved to place more emphasis on a detection and reporting system so that containment activities could be concentrated on the active foci of the disease. It was found that smallpox was not widely and randomly distributed through an endemic area, but that the disease would spread slowly, affecting, at any one time, only a small percentage of towns or villages in the area. Nor would there be explosive outbreaks in these active foci, but rather a slow spread, with a small number of new cases each week. Such outbreaks, once detected could be contained with a relatively modest effort. An efficient detecting and reporting system was thus a vital factor in any national eradication programme.

Confirmation of smallpox eradication. Each previously endemic country was expected to maintain active surveillance for at least two years after the detection of their last case of smallpox and to conduct special studies during this time to establish the validity and sensitivity of their surveillance. These studies varied with the circumstances but included: (*a*) pock mark surveys; (*b*) reports of chickenpox cases; (*c*) submission of specimens for laboratory examination, from suspect cases and particularly from those cases of chicken pox that were severe or that had no vaccination scar; (*d*) surveys of vaccination coverage; (*e*) surveys of public awareness of the disease and of any reward offered for reporting an undisclosed outbreak; and (*f*) assessment of the surveillance coverage and reports.

After two or more years the country would be visited by an independent international commission charged with assessing the evidence produced by the national programme, of making their own assessments, and finally of deciding whether they were satisfied that the national surveillance was sufficiently sensitive and thorough that it would have detected smallpox if any transmission of this disease had occurred since the last recorded outbreak.

The collection of these assessments and of evidence produced by countries that not recently been endemic was evaluated by a global commission set up by World Health Organization and the final conclusion of that commission, that smallpox eradication had been achieved throughout the world, was accepted by the World Health Assembly in May 1980.

Consequences of the eradication of smallpox. *Vaccination policy.* Infection with vaccinia virus undoubtedly induced adequate protection against smallpox. But vaccination itself resulted in occasional complications, some of which were fatal. Now that smallpox has been eradicated there is no longer any justification at all for routine vaccination against smallpox or for international travellers to have a valid certificate of vaccination. The cases of monkeypox (see below) have been so few and in such remote areas that routine vaccination is not justified to protect against this disease. The chance that any patient might have smallpox must now be less than the complication rate following vaccination so that vaccination is contra-indicated even for medical and paramedical personnel. The only remaining justification for vaccination is for those whom the World Health Organization calls 'investigators at special risk'. These would be those studying orthopoxviruses and the members of any mobile team, specifically charged with the task of investigating suspect cases. Some stocks of freeze-dried vaccine will, however, be maintained by the World Health Organization and by many national authorities as a safeguard against unforeseeable events, and it should also be borne in mind that a good degree of post-contact protection against smallpox could be given with anti-vaccinial gamma globulin or with chemotherapy. It is not generally realized what an enormous financial cost underlay the routine protection against smallpox; the abandonment of vaccination should free substantial sums, to the benefit of other health programmes.

Investigation of suspect cases. It is to be expected that suspect cases of smallpox will continue to be reported. This has been the experience even in countries which have been free of the disease for some years. It is therefore important to each country and to the world that any such report be thoroughly investigated.

This investigation is likely to follow the broad lines suggested below, but detailed guidance will be provided by each national health authority and the appropriate local memorandum should be available and its procedures should be strictly adhered to. An expert clinical opinion will be needed, though it is no longer so important that the clinician should have had extensive experience of smallpox for the suspect is all but certain to have some other illness. Should it prove to be a poxvirus infection there must be unusual circumstances and an epidemiological investigation will also be required. The greatest efficiency might be obtained from a mobile team which could be despatched at short notice to the trouble spot to assist not only with the clinical and epidemiologic investigations but also to advise on the necessary control measures. Such a team would be up to date on all relevant information, would maintain and develop their expertise, and would also be regularly revaccinated as 'investigators at special risk'.

Where a suspect case is most unlikely to have the disease in question, management and possible containment decisions can be speeded up by a rapid and sensitive laboratory test. The best one available is undoubtedly electron microscopy (EM) of material from the lesions, which may be done in an hour or so and which has an excellent success rate in all poxvirus infections. This initial examination should be done, using simple containment procedures, but in a way which would permit rapid and effective decontamination should this prove to be necessary. Only in the event that poxvirus particles were seen need the subsequent laboratory investigations be undertaken under more strict containment. This, of course, is on the assumption that smallpox is the only dangerous disease which is suspected in the particular patient.

A suspect case in GP, Surgery, or Casualty department should be held there with the department closed until the EM results are available. If EM is negative for poxvirus (and with good fortune, positive for another agent), the department may be opened and the potential contacts released after record is taken of their names and addresses.

If EM is positive for poxvirus, a final diagnosis of smallpox is still highly improbable. While laboratory investigations are in progress it would be sufficient to maintain the suspect in relatively simple isolation, such as domiciliary confinement, or barrier nursing in a cubicle, might provide.

If poxvirus particles were seen by EM, the specimens should be transmitted, securely packed, to a poxvirus reference laboratory, after appropriate notifications. This reference laboratory will have a containment suite but need not be a laboratory maintaining variola virus. In the future, the identification of poxviruses will largely depend on DNA analysis, and for this, recorded standards can be provided for variola; there will be no need to run comparative biological tests. If further laboratory investigations should reveal either variola, or poxvirus not immediately identifiable, then consideration should be given to transferring the patient to maximum isolation—following the procedures used for suspect viral haemorrhagic fevers; the premises on which he has been should be appropriately decontaminated and the contacts given post-contact protection with gamma globulin. Vaccination at that stage might be extended to certain secondary contacts. The above suggestions have been based on the assumptions that there may be many suspect cases of smallpox, all of which will prove not to be, and that their investigation does not involve a significant degree of hazard. Cover against the totally unforeseen should be based on the availability of effective procedures for decontamination and post-contact protection. Those unfortunate enough to come under suspicion should be investigated with the minimum delay and inconvenience, and it should be borne in mind that vaccination is now a medically unjustified procedure.

Monkeypox

The eradication of smallpox was undertaken on the well-founded belief that there was no non-human reservoir of the virus, and that interruption of transmission in the human population would completely and finally eradicate the disease. During the course of the last few years, the possibility that a potential reservoir of smallpox may after all exist in the animal world has been raised. An orthopoxvirus which is called monkeypox has caused sporadic cases, clinically resembling smallpox. Forty-five such cases have been identified in the ten years 1970–9; all occurred in the tropical rain-forest of West and Central Africa, and most of them in small villages of a few hundred people. Children have been affected more frequently and more severely than adults. Thirty-seven of the 45 cases occurred in children under ten and the seven who died of monkeypox were aged seven years or less. A moderately severe illness in a girl of seven is shown in Fig. 3, from which the resemblance to smallpox is obvious. Unlike smallpox this disease shows little or no tendency to spread in the human population. Sixty-six unvaccinated, household contacts have been identified and only four of these developed the disease. This secondary attack rate of 6 per cent is markedly different from the corresponding 35 to 40 per cent which was characteristic of smallpox; and there has been no evidence of any third generation cases. The virus isolated from these patients is readily differentiated from variola virus after culture in the laboratory. The pocks on the chick chorio-allantois are about the same size as those of smallpox but are slightly haemorrhagic; monkeypox virus is pathogenic for the rabbit and has a higher ceiling temperature for growth than does variola. These additional characters have been used to identify field isolates. Monkeypox virus had originally been isolated from a spontaneous outbreak of exanthematous disease in a captive monkey colony in Copenhagen. The source of this, and other subsequent outbreaks in captive animals has never been identified. There is serological evidence that some monkeys caught in the wild had antibody specific to monkeypox, but the maintenance host of the virus remains unknown.

Culture of tissues of wild monkeys and other animals has not yielded any isolate of monkeypox virus, but a few poxviruses have

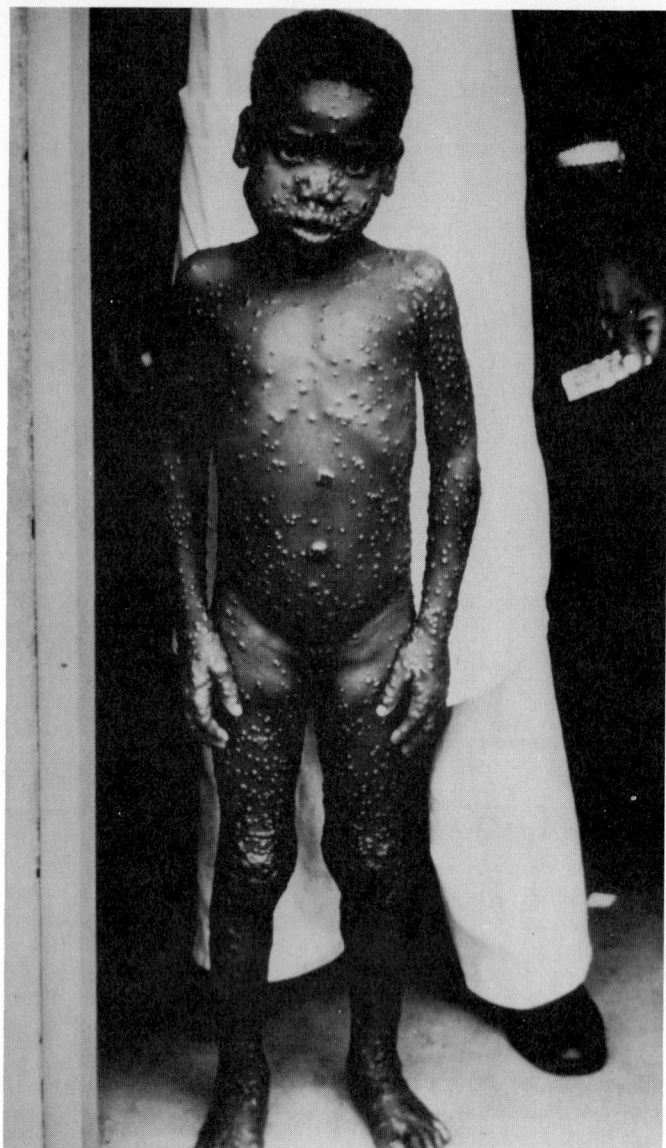

Fig. 3 Moderately severe monkeypox in a girl of seven years from Equateur Province, Zaire. (By courtesy of the World Health Organization.)

been recovered which cannot be distinguished from variola by current laboratory tests. These isolates have, collectively, been called the 'whitepox' viruses and it is clearly important to discover what relationship they have to variola and monkeypox viruses. Recent studies have concentrated on the use of restriction endonucleases to analyse the viral DNAs; this technique examines the structure of the whole genome and is not restricted to those genes being expressed in a particular biological system. Early results have shown clear-cut differences between the DNAs of variola, monkeypox, and vaccinia viruses. It is probable that this technique will rapidly become the main basis for the specific identification of poxviruses.

Cowpox

Cowpox virus, despite its name, does not seem to be endemically maintained in cattle. Occasional outbreaks have been reported in which there were both human and cattle involved and in which virus may have been spread from cow to cow by human. Some of the outbreaks, especially in Holland, were due to vaccinia virus and were almost certainly introduced from a human source.

Cowpox virus can cause moderately severe disease in man. It produces an acutely inflamed local lesion, which may even be suspected as anthrax, with painful enlarged regional lymph nodes and constitutional upset. Sufferers are likely to seek medical aid and some are ill enough to be admitted to hospital. Diagnosis is easily confirmed virologically, once cowpox is suspected, but many patients will give no history of contact with cows. Antibody to cowpox is rare in cattle and the disease is rare in abattoir workers. It is likely that man and cow are only sporadically infected and that the reservoir host for cowpox virus is still to be discovered. Minor variants of cowpox virus have been isolated from fairly severe infections in chance-contact hosts. Thus a cowpox-like virus has been isolated from large felines (lions, pumas, cheetahs) and from elephants in different zoos and also from travelling circus elephants in Europe. The only 'natural' endemic focus of a cowpox-like virus so far described was in the large gerbils in Turkmenistan, USSR. It would seem most likely that the reservour in Britain must be in a small, wild animal, probably a rodent, but no evidence, either serological or by virus isolation, is available to incriminate any particular species. Cowpox virus has not been isolated from outside Europe.

Parapoxvirus infections

A localized lesion, usually on the fingers, may be acquired by those who come in contact with sheep infected with orf (also known as contagious pustular dermatitis) or with cattle infected with pseudo-cowpox (also known as paravaccinia or as bovine papular stomatitis). The two viruses are very closely related and are widely distributed throughout the world. The human infection starts by direct contact through a minor abrasion or cut in the skin. The local lesion runs a protracted course of four to six weeks, starting as a papular lesion which becomes an erythematous nodule which may reach 1 or 2 cm in size, and which slowly regresses. The milker's nodule from cattle usually remains nodular, but the orf lesion produces a weeping ulcer in the second or third week.

Molluscum contagiosum

This infection has a worldwide distribution. It causes papular lesions of the skin with epidermal proliferation, and the papules contain a semisolid, caseous material in which masses of virus particles are imbedded. This material has provided the source of virus for diagnostic and experimental studies for the virus cannot as yet be cultivated in the laboratory. Recent studies of the DNA extracted from virus particles purified from human material indicates the existence of several independent strains of the virus. Transmission is by direct contact and the lesions may persist for months or even years.

Tanapox

This disease was first reported, following an epidemic which occurred in the Tana river valley in Kenya, following unusual flooding. It was considered to be a zoonosis of monkeys, transmitted to man by excessive mosquito activity during the ecological disturbances caused by the floods. Human infections with tanapox have subsequently been discovered in the rain forest areas of central Africa, during searches for any missed foci of smallpox. A closely-related virus has been isolated from epidemics which have occurred in primate colonies in the USA. It must be made clear that the virus is serologically unrelated to monkeypox virus; it is related to the Yaba poxvirus of monkeys and with this seems to form a distinct subgroup of poxviruses.

The disease in man is characterized by a febrile onset lasting a few days with the appearance of one or two skin lesions, which have the characteristics of a poxvirus infection.

References

Baxby, D. (1977). Poxvirus hosts and reservoirs. *Archs Virol.* **55**, 169.

— (1981). *Jenner smallpox vaccine. The riddle of the origin of vaccinia virus.* Heinemann, London.

Dales, S. and Pogo, B. (1981). *The poxvirus.* Springer-Verlag, Berlin.

Dixon, C. W. (1962). *Smallpox.* Churchill Livingstone, London.

Marennikova, S. S. *et al.* (1972). Isolation and properties of the causal agent of a new variola-like disease (monkeypox) in man. *Bull. Wld Hlth Org.* **46**, 599.

World Health Organization (1980). *Report of the Global Commission for the Certification of Smallpox Eradication.* WHO, Geneva.

Paramyxoviruses

Mumps: epidemic parotitis

A. B. Christie

Mumps is a generalized infection. Both the words 'mumps' and 'parotitis' refer only to the swelling of the face: 'to mump' is an old word meaning 'to look glum and weary', which patients with parotitis certainly do. But the swelling of the face is only one of the symptoms of the disease, albeit the commonest one. The virus can infect almost any organ, the salivary glands, the pancreas, the testes or ovary, the brain, the breast, the liver, the joints, and the heart. Parotitis is the outward and visible sign.

Virology

Culture. Mumps virus is a myxovirus. It can be grown in the yolk sac or amniotic cavity of chick embryo, but it produces no lesions there; its presence can be detected only by testing for the haemagglutinin which develops against fowl red blood cells: this haemagglutinin provokes corresponding antibody in a patient's serum. On tissue culture of chick embryo, monkey kidney, human amnion or Hela cells, the virus causes cytopathic changes which may be seen as early as the third day, sometimes later: but immunofluorescence techniques may detect virus in these cultures in hours rather than days. These tissue cultures can be stored ready for use, at 37 °C for seven days. It is not so easy to maintain a supply of embryonated hen eggs.

Resistence of virus. Stored below 10 °C, mumps virus can remain infective for weeks or months; at lower temperatures probably for years. At room temperature the virus may persist for up to three months but seems to lose its infectivity in three or four days. Heating the virus at 55 °C for 20 minutes abolishes infectivity, as does 0.2 per cent formalin at 4 °C for two hours or dilute ether for 30 minutes: intense ultraviolet radiation destroys it at once. None of these processes destroys the antigens responsible for complement-fixation, haemagglutination, or the skin test. But none of all this seems to have any bearing on the epidemiology of the disease: contaminated crockery could perhaps convey infection from a patient to a contact, but all epidemiological evidence shows that transmission depends on close personal contact with a patient who is excreting virus in the saliva.

Source of virus. Mumps virus can be grown in the acute case from saliva, throat washings, or a swab of the Stensen's duct orifice, from urine in every case, and from cerebrospinal fluid when there is meningitis. In the very early stages it can be grown from the blood. It has been grown from breast milk and, in at least one case, from inner ear perilymph at operation. At autopsy it has been grown from brain tissue and it is likely that virus could be isolated from any infected organ. There appears to be only one antigenic type of mumps virus.

A patient excretes virus in the saliva for between two and six days before the parotitis and for up to four days after it. IgA appears in the saliva at about the fourth day and virus thereafter disappears. Virus can be detected in the urine for up to 14 days around the onset of the illness: it can be cultured almost as easily as from saliva, but there is no evidence of spread of the disease by urine. In the blood it can be detected only for a day or two at the onset of the disease. Virus can be isolated from the cerebrospinal fluid for the first three

or four days of the meningeal illness. Spread of the disease seems to depend on the presence of virus in the saliva.

Antibody response to virus. Mumps virus contains several different antigenic components and these provoke distinct antibodies in infected patients. The V and S antigens can each fix complement in the presence of corresponding specific antibody. The V antigen is found mainly in amniotic or allantoic fluid of infected chick embryo; the S, or soluble, antigen is found in embryo tissue, especially in the allantoic and amniotic membranes. They can be separated by centrifugation or adsorption. S antibody is present very early in a patient's serum, rises in the first two weeks, but then declines rapidly. V antibody appears at the end of the first week, usually in high titre: it may persist for years and is an index of past infection. Titration of acute and convalescent sera for V and S antibody is a reliable method of diagnosis, very useful in patients who do not have parotitis. Anomalies do occur: sometimes only the V antibody rises, sometimes the S persists longer than the V; and if the serum is taken late in the disease both V and S antibody may be high, and diagnosis can then be confirmed only if a specimen taken weeks or months later shows a fall in titre.

The V and S antibody tests are both complement-fixing tests (CFT). Haemagglutination-inhibiting (HAI) antibodies also develop in response to the haemagglutinin mentioned above and this HAI response can be readily titrated: there is usually a fourfold rise in HAI antibody during the illness. Neutralizing antibodies also develop, but their titration is too complicated for routine work. But the three tests, CFT, HAI, and neutralization measure different things, and these differences may be important in any work on immunity.

Mumps-specific IgG, IgM, and IgA may also be measured mainly by indirect immunofluorescence tests. IgM fluorescence can be seen in the cytoplasm of cells, IgG only in cell membranes, an important difference, for only IgG can pass through the placenta (see below). IgA can be detected by immunofluorescence in saliva or mouthwashings, and also in the serum early in the disease: the method is as sensitive as culture, and is useful for early diagnosis.

Skin test. Antigen prepared from hen egg or tissue culture produces a tuberculin-like reaction when injected into the skin of persons who have previously suffered from mumps. The test is of no use in diagnosing a clinical attack. The antigen may in fact provoke CF antibody and so confuse rather than aid diagnosis, but is of value in testing for immunity or susceptibility to infection. Inapparent mumps is a common condition, so that the absence of a history of having had mumps is of no value in assessing susceptibility or the need for vaccine: the skin test, if properly prepared, can usually determine susceptibility very accurately. In one investigation 153 of 170 adults exposed to infection but with no history of mumps were shown to be immune: only two did contract mumps, and in both the skin reaction was uncertain.

Virus in the body. *Mode of entry.* It is almost natural to look upon mumps as a disease of the parotid gland which sometimes spreads to other parts of the body, to the testis for example, or to the meninges. But this may be seeing things the wrong way round. Mumps virus may be more like measles virus or smallpox virus in its action, first circulating in the bloodstream and later settling in one organ; in mumps most often in the salivary glands. If mumps virus is injected experimentally into the orifice of the parotid duct, the patient often gets parotitis within eight days, whereas after natural exposure this takes nearer eighteen days, the difference perhaps being in the time the virus takes to get round the body. That may be, and it may be that mumps is excreted by the salivary glands rather than introduced through them. Another possibility is that the parotitis is caused by a reaction between virus and antibody, not by simple inflammation. Antibody is often already present when parotitis develops. In non-parotitic cases, where the virus first declares its presence in the testis or the meninges, there may be a delay in antibody formation, for virus is often present in the saliva some days before the orchitis or meningitis, yet there is no parotitis. The same delay in antibody formation may explain the many cases of inapparent mumps. None of this is certain: further research may make things clearer.

Pathology

Changes in salivary glands. Not many people die during mumps infection, so there is little information about the changes caused in organs by the virus. In the salivary glands there is apparently some lymphocytic infiltration of periductal tissue, and oedematous changes or vacuolar degeneration in the cells lining the ducts. These cells become detached and, with leucocytes and other debris, they block the duct and cause dilatation above the block. Sometimes the whole gland is affected but more often the changes are in some lobules only. The lymphatics in the tissues surrounding and lying over the glands become obstructed, and this produces a gel-like oedema which may spread down over the chest wall especially when the swelling of the salivary glands is severe.

Changes in the genitalia. In mild orchitis there is only oedema and serofibrinous exudate in the interstitial tissues, but when the infection is severe there is intense lymphocytic infiltration and destruction of the cells lining the semeniferous tubules which leads to blocking. Partial atrophy of the testes may follow and the epididymus, spermatic cord, and prostate may all be affected by the inflammatory reaction. All this is bound to affect function, but complete sterility is not a common sequel of mumps (see below). Women sometimes complain of ovarian pain during an attack of mumps, but it is usually mere niggling pain and rarely as severe as in men with orchitis. There is no evidence that it affects fertility. Mastitis is commoner, both in females and males, but it is usually mild and fleeting.

Changes in the nervous system. Mumps virus frequently invades the nervous system: changes can be detected by electroencephalography or by examination of the cerebrospinal fluid (CSF) in at least half the patients with mumps. Some authors have indeed regarded the virus as primarily a neurotropic virus which causes incidental changes in other organs, including the salivary glands. But in most cases with EEG or CSF changes, there are no nervous symptoms or signs. All the same, mumps virus is one of the commonest known causes of lymphocytic meningitis: the virus can be readily isolated from the CSF in the first few days of the meningitis. It is, however, a self-limiting disease so that there are no autopsy reports, but neuronal damage probably does occur and explains the occurrence of quadriplegia or single nerve paralysis in some patients. Apart from transient weakness of the facial nerve, which may be due as much to pressure of a swollen gland as to damage by mumps virus, these complications are all very rare.

Mumps encephalitis is a different entity. CSF is normal and contains no virus. At autopsy there is perivascular demyelination exactly the same as in other forms of post-infection encephalitis: but it is rare after mumps.

Changes in the pancreas and other organs. Mild upper abdominal pain is common in mumps and may be related to viral changes in the pancreas. One author writes of subclinical pancreopathy, but there is little firm evidence of pathological changes in the pancreas in mumps. The amount of amylase in duodenal fluid may be less than normal in patients with mumps who have abdominal pain, and this might be caused by blocking of the ducts in the pancreas, just as in the salivary glands or the testes. But the idea that this leads to backflow of amylase into the bloodstream is not supported by studies of serum amylase in mumps: the level is sometimes high in mild cases, and low in severe cases.

If mumps does affect the pancreas, is there any connection between mumps and diabetes? There are some reports of diabetes occurring after an attack of mumps, but in such cases the virus may simply have stirred into clinical activity a pancreatic defect which, with time alone, would have led to diabetes. This was almost certainly the case, some familial disposition to the disease, when diabetes occurred in a brother and sister within a month or two of

mumps. In other reported cases mumps virus may have damaged pancreatic tissue enough to cause the diabetes. Yet when antibody studies have been done there have been fewer positives for mumps in diabetics than in normal subjects. There may be a connection but it is not a common one.

Mumps virus has been isolated on biopsy from a patient with subacute thyroiditis, and there is a report of several cases in Israel. Myocarditis has been seen in one fatal case, but otherwise the evidence for any heart damage comes from electrocardiographic changes and these are usually fleeting. Mild hepatitic changes have been seen on biopsy of patients with jaundice, a very rare manifestation of mumps. Arthritis is also rare: the CF test may be positive in aspirated joint fluid but nothing is known of any changes in the joint. Mumps virus can probably invade any organ, but, except in the parotid gland, the testes, the meninges, and perhaps the pancreas, it rarely causes other than fleeting damage.

Mumps in the fetus and infant. Mumps vaccine virus has been isolated from placental tissue but, so far, no mumps virus has been found in fetal tissue. Abortion may occur in women with mumps in the first three months of pregnancy, but this is not common; and there is no evidence that it is caused by virus damage in the fetus. The connection between primary endocardial fibroelastosis and mumps is rather vague. Mumps virus has not been isolated from heart tissue at autopsy and these infants have no mumps antibody in their blood. They may show a delayed hypersensitivity response to the skin test. It has been suggested that in these cases, the mother's attack of mumps is a secondary one to which she already has some antibody, and that antibody and virus both pass to the fetus, where their collision in infant tissue causes a hypersensitivity type of reaction. Or there may be some immune defect in the fetus, an absence of B-lymphocyte humoral response perhaps, and that this causes myocarditis and the laying down of the thick layer of collagen and elastic tissue under the endocardium.

In the normal infant maternal IgG does pass to the fetus. This IgG, although it is not detected after the first few months, nevertheless seems to protect the infant against mumps during the first year of life. Such protection has been seen in infant nursery outbreaks, but even in virgin populations, with no previous experience of the disease and so presumably no maternal antibody, mumps in the first year of life is very uncommon: the immaturity of the infant cell may have something to do with this. Orchitis has been reported in infants, and mumps virus may be isolated in vague respiratory infections in infants, but the typical disease of mumps in infants is a rare clinical finding.

Spread of the virus. *Inapparent mumps.* A patient with mumps excretes the virus in his saliva and is infectious for up to ten days. This is true of patients with parotitis, for up to six days before and four days after the gland swells: but it is also true of persons infected with the virus but with no sign of illness at all, those with inapparent mumps. In an outbreak, or in experimental mumps, as many as 30 to 40 per cent of those exposed excrete virus and show a rise of antibody but have no clinical illness. In any assessment of the infectivity of mumps these inapparent excretors must be included, and mumps can then be seen to be a highly infectious condition, comparable perhaps with measles or chickenpox. Spread may seem much slower than in measles; but then the incubation period is longer, and there may be apparent gaps in the spread due to inapparent infections, whereas with measles everyone infected shows signs of the disease. Environment is important: in a classroom the virus spreads readily, as it does in the confinement of a troopship. The host factor too is important, and, like many other infectious diseases, mumps spreads rapidly and causes severe attacks when introduced into an island population with no recent exposure to the virus.

Clinical manifestations

Incubation period. The incubation period seems to lie between 14 and 18 days. Much shorter or longer periods are quoted, but a patient with mumps may have caught the infection not from the last obvious case but from a patient with inapparent or non-parotitic and undiagnosed mumps which could lead to a wrong estimate of the incubation period.

Parotitis. A patient with mumps parotitis is an ill, uncomfortable patient. His temperature may be as high as 40–40.5 °C, though 37.2–38.3 °C is commoner. He feels chilled but does not have rigors, and he has pain near the angle of the jaw. Next day the gland begins to swell, and within another day his face and neck are distorted with swelling. The skin over the gland is hot and flushed but there is no rash as in the swelling of erysipelas. Usually both glands swell, sometimes with a day or two between the sides, but sometimes only one parotid gland is affected. The swelling begins at the zygomatic bone on the face and goes down and back beneath the auricle and into the neck, covering the bony angle of the jaw on the way. One cannot get one's fingers around the swelling in the neck, nor feel the angle of the jaw above or through it, as one can when it is cervical lymph nodes that are swollen from some other cause. If the swelling is severe the patient cannot open his mouth for pain and tightness, and his mouth is dry because the flow of saliva is blocked. The discomfort lasts for three or four days but has usually subsided by the end of a week. Sometimes as one side clears, the parotid on the other side swells and this prolongs the illness.

Submaxillary mumps. The symptoms are similar to those in parotitic mumps, but it is difficult or impossible to distinguish the swelling from other forms of submaxillary swellings. Some of the lymph nodes in the neck lie in contact with the salivary gland, some within its substance. In submaxillary mumps there is sometimes a great deal of oedema of the overlying tissues which may spread down over the sternum, but this is not a constant finding. If the parotid gland is also swollen, diagnosis is easy. Otherwise one must try to examine the fauces for signs of tonsillitis that might cause cervical adentitis. But laboratory tests are needed for definite diagnosis.

Sublingual mumps. The sublingual salivary glands lie below the floor of the mouth on either side of the frenulum of the tongue near the symphysis of the mandible. When they swell, they push up into the mouth below the tongue, forcing it up against the hard palate, and also down under the chin as a very tender swelling. It is an acutely uncomfortable condition, often with severe general symptoms. It usually subsides after a few days, and is fortunately uncommon.

Orchitis. Orchitis may occur four or five days after the onset of parotitis, just when that swelling is beginning to subside and the patient thinks his trouble is over. But quite often it occurs without preceding parotitis. It is an acute condition, and the patient has chills, sweats, headache, and backache, and a swinging temperature as well as severe local testicular pain and tenderness. The scrotum is swollen and oedematous, and one cannot feel the separate testicles. Most often only one testicle is affected but sometimes both: the second testicle may become affected just as the swelling of the first is subsiding. The illness lasts three or four days before the swelling begins to subside.

Orchitis is unusual before the age of puberty, though it has occurred in young boys and even in infants. In adolescent and young adult males it is a common and unpleasant complication. The main problem is whether it leads to atrophy and sterility. Some degree of atrophy of the testicle occurs in at least one-third of patients with orchitis, but this is not the same thing as sterility. Atrophy may be detected by a shrinking and softening of the affected testicle, but it is wrong to make too much of this examination, for the patient is probably already worried. Partial atrophy is not the same thing as azoospermia which alone causes sterility. In one series of 39 patients with atrophy, only one had azoospermia: the others had sperm counts very little different from normal. Moreover azoospermia after mumps may be a temporary condition

only. The fear of sterility after mumps orchitis has been exaggerated. From a study of its incidence one can conclude that mumps is not an important cause of sterility, and the doctor can with a good conscience reassure his patient.

The spermatic cord, the epididymis, and the prostate may be affected though much less often than the testes. Disease in the prostate may have more to do with sterility than infection of the testes.

Meningitis and encephalitis. Mumps is one of the commoner causes of lymphocytic or viral meningitis. It may develop a few days after the onset of parotitis, but almost as often it occurs in a patient with no preceding parotitis. In the cerebrospinal fluid, protein and lymphocytes are both increased and mumps virus can be isolated in the first few days: this last is the only way in which it can be distinguished from other forms of viral meningitis. The meningitis is usually mild and self-limiting. Occasionally the patient develops paralysis of limbs but, unlike poliomyelitis, this usually disappears in time.

Polyneuritis, neuritis of the trigeminal or facial nerve, and retrobulbar optic neuritis have been described in mumps but all are rare.

In encephalitis the outlook is different. The patient is mentally disturbed and may lapse into coma and remain comatose for days, weeks, or months. This is a form of post-infection encephalitis like that which occurs in measles: but it is much rarer after mumps than after measles.

Other complications. Deafness is sometimes reported after mumps: in one outbreak 13 of 298 Finnish soldiers with mumps became deaf but only one of them permanently. Virus has, in one case, been cultured at operation from inner ear perilymph, so that mumps virus can invade the finer structure of the ear. Labyrinthitis has also been reported with tinnitus, vertigo, and nystagmus during outbreaks of mumps, and labyrinthitis has been caused in new-born hamsters by mumps virus. But the complication, if it is caused in a man by mumps virus, is a very rare one. Perhaps in the army outbreak, there were special features connected with dosage or virulence of virus which caused a higher than normal rate of ear complications in the soldiers.

Diagnosis

Diphtheria and other swellings. When there is bilateral parotitis clinical diagnosis is usually obvious. One condition that must be excluded is bull-neck diphtheria (see page 5.133) which can, at a careless glance, look very like mumps. Inflammation of various groups of lymph nodes may cause some difficulty. Those that drain the pinna of the ear and side of the scalp, the pre-auricular group, lie superficial to the parotid, but those draining the front of the scalp and the eyelids lie within its substance: the swelling is less uniform and does not go into the neck. Other groups which drain parts of the pharynx lie deep to the parotid and may swell bilaterally: one must examine the pharynx carefully. Enlargement of the cervical lymph nodes is confined to the neck: one can feel round the swelling and the angle of the jaw is above it. In infectious mononucleosis the glands stand out distinctly and the parotid is not affected. The lymph nodes in contact with the submaxillary and sublingual salivary glands drain the corner of the eye, the side of the nose, the cheeks, the lips, and the floor of the mouth. One must look for lesions there, for otherwise diagnosis from submaxillary or sublingual mumps is difficult.

In septic parotitis there is more tenderness in the parotid, there may be fluctuation, and pus exudes from the orifice of Stensen's duct. Calculus causes spasmodic pain and swelling and may be detected on X-ray. Recurrent parotitis and Miculicz's syndrome are unlikely to be confused with mumps except in the earliest stages, nor are uveoparotid fever and tumours of the gland, for they are chronic conditions. In erysipelas the condition clearly affects the skin and subcutaneous tissue, not the deeper parotid gland.

Orchitis when it occurs without parotitis is difficult to diagnose from gonococcal epididymo-orchitis unless one learns of the contact with mumps, often the patient's child who had parotitis a fortnight earlier. The rare case of orchitis in infancy may resemble torsion of the testis and perhaps it is safer to operate than risk a serious misdiagnosis.

Laboratory diagnosis. Virus isolation and serological tests have already been discussed. In cases without parotitis, especially meningitis, and in the absence of contact history, they are the only means of reaching a firm diagnosis. The skin test and serum amylase levels do not help in diagnosing the acute case.

Treatment. There is no specific treatment. Analgesics may give some relief from pain, but in the severe pain of orchitis, morphia 15 to 30 mg is the only one likely to help: it will not be required for more than a day or two. Corticosteroids are worth trying in severe cases of parotitis, more especially in orchitis. A dose of 300 mg cortisone or its equivalent daily for two or three days sometimes gives dramatic relief from pain though it may not reduce the swelling. There is no need to taper off the dose after such a short course. The action of the drug is uncertain and need not be used in mild cases. The inflamed scrotum should be supported on wads of cotton wool, not wrapped in bandages, for the patient sweats a lot and the bandage becomes sodden.

Prevention
Isolation and immune globulin. Isolation, except in closed communities, is not effective. The patient has been infectious for days before his parotitis, and inapparent cases are not detected at all. Immune globulin has been used in outbreaks but not very successfully. Given in 20 ml doses on the first day of parotitis it may reduce the incidence of orchitis in young male adults.

Vaccine. Killed vaccine is no longer used, mainly because of the need for two injections and the danger of hypersensitivity to live virus in patients only partially immune after killed vaccine.

Attenuated live vaccine gives 95 per cent seroconversion and protection lasts at least for several years. The duration of protection is important because there is no point in protecting a young boy if ten years later his immunity wanes and he gets mumps and orchitis. Mumps virus is however a virus only of man, so that widespread vaccination might lead to the eradication of the disease. Combined with attenuated rubella and measles vaccines, it may well have a place in immunization programmes. Mumps vaccine virus has been isolated from placental but not from fetal tissue so that there may be a risk in pregnant women. Moreover serological tests on unvaccinated adults in London have shown that up to 95 per cent are immune, with or without a history of mumps. There is no point in immunizing the immune: but if mumps can be prevented by vaccine why should any child have parotitis or any adult suffer from orchitis?

References

Annotation (1966). Mumps embryopathy. *Lancet*, **ii**, 692.
Christie, A. B. (1980). *Infectious diseases: epidemiology and clinical practice*, 3rd edn. Churchill Livingstone, Edinburgh.
Gordon, J. E. and Kilham, L. (1949). Ten years in the epidemiology of mumps. *Am. J. Med.*, **218**, 338.
Hanshaw, J. B. and Dudgeon, J. A. (1978). In *Viral diseases of the fetus and the newborn*. W. B. Saunders, Philadelphia.
Henle, W. and Enders, J. F. (1964). Mumps. In *Viral and rickettsial infections of man* (eds. F. L. Horsfall and I. Tamm). Pitman, London.
Robbins, F. C. (1971). Mumps: the problem. In *Proceedings of the international conference on the application of vaccines against viral, rickettsial and bacterial diseases of man*, 216. Scientific publications No. 226, Pan American Health Organization, Washington D.C.

Measles

W. C. Marshall

Measles is an acute, highly transmissible viral infection and is one of the commonest infections of man. There is only one strain of the virus and no evidence of antigenic variation or alteration in virulence. Differences in the severity of measles in different parts of the world are due to host and environmental factors. There is no reservoir of the infection other than man and the evidence of a carrier state. The virus causes a generalized infection: the major clinical features of the disease are due to involvement of the skin, mucous membranes, and respiratory tract. Attack rates in home contacts is of the order of 90 per cent or greater, and subclinical infection is very infrequent. Infection is almost universal in children and only in special circumstances are adolescents or adults affected.

Epidemiology. Measles has a worldwide distribution, and, in the Western world, most susceptible children acquire infection by the end of the first decade of life. In these temperate and developed environments the majority of cases of measles occur in the winter and spring with a bi-annual epidemic pattern (Fig. 1). However, in recent years the epidemicity of measles in some countries has changed, presumably under the influence of immunization programmes. In the USA where the most striking impact of immunization can be seen (Fig. 2) the variation in the annual numbers of notified measles cases is less obvious.

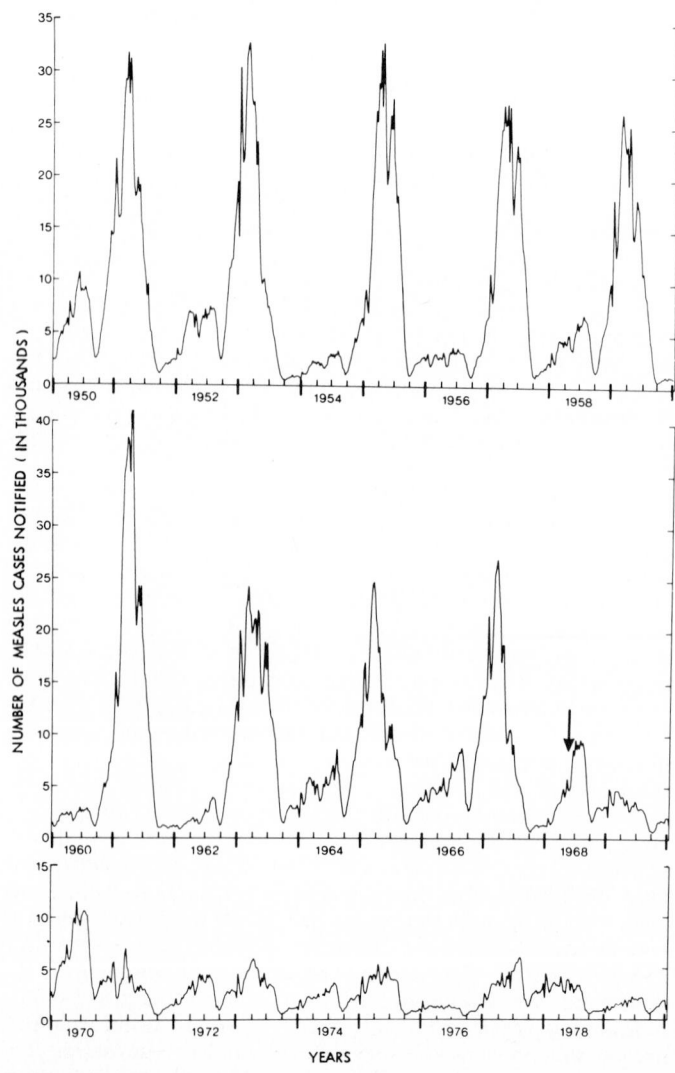

Fig. 1 Measles notification in England and Wales by week (1950–79). Measles vaccination commenced in 1968. (By courtesy of P. E. M. Fine and J. A. Clarkson.)

In tropical countries epidemics are usually annual events, and in some, such as West Africa and India, most cases are seen in the dry months of the year. The infection is considered to be endemic in other areas but this probably reflects a lack of accurate information which may stem in part from cultural attitudes to the disease. Measles behaves differently in isolated communities. The virus spreads rapidly and the attack rate is high. Susceptible persons of all ages are infected as has occurred in the epidemics in the Faroes, in Greenland, and more recently in Tristan da Cunha. The disease in 'virgin soil' epidemics is often of greater severity.

Before the introduction of measles vaccination in the United Kingdom and the USA, measles was most common in the preschool age child, but now age specific attack rates have shifted to older children. Infection is not infrequent under the age of 12 months in tropical countries and is very common during the second year of life. All children are likely to have experienced the infection by the age of two or four years. However, under the age of six months measles is rare in all countries due to the protection afforded by antibody passively derived from the mother.

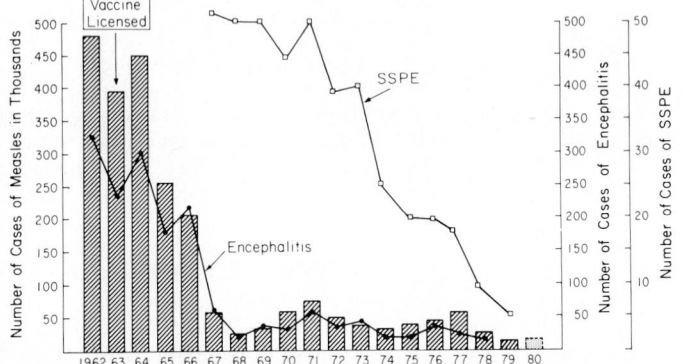

Fig. 2 Incidence of measles, measles encephalitis, and subacute sclerosing panencephalitis in the introduction of live attenuated measles vaccine. (By courtesy of S. Krugman.)

Measles virus, antibody, and cell-mediated immunity. The virus, which is closely related to rinderpest and canine distemper virus, is a single stranded RNA virus which has a pleomorphic appearance on electron microscopy. The size is variable (120–250 nm) and two components can be seen. There is an outer envelope with short projections, and an inner nucleocapsid of a coiled helix of 17 nm diameter composed of the RNA and a glycoprotein. The nucleocapsid possesses an antigen which has complement fixing activity. The envelope is associated with a haemagglutinin but, unlike two other paramyxoviruses, mumps and parainfluenza viruses, does not contain neuraminidase.

Measles is not a very stable virus and cultivation is not easy. It grows slowly in primary cell cultures of human and simian origin. However, laboratory adapted and vaccine strains will grow more rapidly and in a wider range of cell cultures. One of the striking features of the cytopathic effects of the virus is the development of multinucleated giant cells with inclusions in the nucleus and the cytoplasm. These cells can also be seen in tissues in infected individuals. The virus is identified by neutralization of the cytopathic effects or by immunofluorescent techniques using labelled antiserum. Virus can be detected in blood from four to five days before the onset of the rash then disappears within 24–48 hours. During the prerash coryzal stage and for two or three days after the onset of the rash the virus can be isolated from the throat. However, antigen may be detected in pharyngeal cells by immunofluorescent techniques for five to nine days after the onset of the rash.

Antibody can be detected by means of neutralization, complement fixation (CF), haemagglutination inhibition (HI), and haemolysis inhibition and radial haemolysis. The most frequently used tests are CF and HI and antibodies can be detected by all of the above methods within two to four days of the onset of the rash and

reach peak levels in two to three weeks. With the exception of CF antibody in some persons, antibodies are usually detected for life and their presence is associated with solid immunity. It is not known whether the maintenance of antibody is due to persisting antigenic stimulus from latent infection or is periodically boosted by re-exposure to the virus. Although it is considered that some of the manifestations of the disease, especially the rash, are due to delayed hypersensitivity skin test antigens to detect delayed hypersensitivity are not available. That cell-mediated immunity (CMI) is important for recovery from the infection is illustrated by the severity of measles in malnourished children and fatal measles in combined immunodeficiency syndromes in contrast to the occurrence of 'normal' measles in patients with hypogammaglobulinaemia.

Pathogenesis and clinical manifestation. The secretions of the respiratory tract are the principal source of the infection and spread to susceptible contacts is via aerosols; communicability is related to the period when virus can be isolated from the throat. Infection takes place in the nose and respiratory tract. Following a limited local multiplication the virus spreads via leucocytes to the cells of the reticulo-endothelial system where further replication occurs which proceeds the second viraemic phase. Target organs are then infected and the symptoms and signs of measles appear after an incubation period of 10–14 days. The first stage of the illness is fever of gradually increasing severity over three or four days and coryzal symptoms appear within 24 hours of its onset; the conjunctivae become injected and mild cough develops. The rash will appear about four days after the first indication of illness. However, in the 24–48 hours before the rash, Koplik spots may be seen. These are 'small irregular spots of bright red colour in the centre of each spot is seen a minute bluish-white speck'. They are not always easy to see on the buccal mucus membrane and have usually disappeared by the second day of the exanthem.

In the pre-rash period of the illness the total white cell count falls due to depression of the circulating lymphocytes and eosinophils. Suppression of delayed hypersensitivity reactions, including tuberculin, also occurs at this stage and the anergy will persist for six to eight weeks.

The rash of measles first appears on the forehead and the neck as the fever reaches its height. There is spread to involve the trunk and finally the limbs over a period of three to four days. The lesions are initially reddish maculopapules. As the redness diminishes a brownish stain may become apparent and a fine desquamation of the trunk can follow. Extensive desquamation occurs under certain circumstances.

The most important effect of measles is disease of the respiratory tract; however, the central nervous system and the gastrointestinal tract may be affected with varying degrees of severity. The cough is a striking feature; it could be said that the clinical diagnosis of measles must be suspect in the absence of cough. More severe disease of the respiratory tract may occur in the form of tracheo-bronchitis or bronchopneumonia. Otitis media may complicate measles at or soon after this stage. Soreness of the mouth and diarrhoea are frequent features in malnourished children and are discussed below. The cause of the striking irritability and misery of a child with measles is not known. Abnormality in the electro-encephalogram is almost universal in this period suggesting some cerebral dysfunction, but there is no evidence that this is due to acute viral encephalitis as seen in mumps. It is also during the period of high fever, either just before or just after the onset of the rash, that febrile convulsions may occur. In the uncomplicated case, the convalescent period is short, usually lasting less than a week; if fever persists while the rash is fading complications should be suspected.

Complications and measles-associated disorders. Although measles is a universal disease, there is a very wide range of disorders which are due either to the measles virus itself or due to some host or environmental factor. Some are the consequence of measures which have been developed over the past two decades to prevent the infection.

Respiratory tract. Tracheitis and tracheobronchitis should not be considered complications of measles but involvement of other parts of the respiratory tract should be. This may be due to extension of virus causing disease or due to bacterial superinfection or both. Upper respiratory tract obstruction due to severe laryngeal disease occurs early in the infection and is common in tropical countries. It may rapidly cause death unless the obstruction is relieved. Acute bronchiolitis may also be seen in the early stages of the infection in the youngest children. Bronchopneumonia or lobar pneumonia are usually associated with bacterial infections, frequently due to *Streptococcus pneumoniae, Staphylococcus aureus*, or *Haemophilus influenzae*. This complication occurs most frequently during the early convalescent stage. There are no characteristic radiographic findings in these complications but both pneumomediastinum and subcutaneous emphysema may occur. The role of other viruses causing lung complications in measles is not clear, but a severe and often fatal pneumonia occurs when some adenovirus infections follow measles.

Pneumonitis may be due to giant cell pneumonia (Hecht) and is seen in patients with defects in cell-mediated immunity; the child with leukaemia, especially if lymphopenia is present, is particularly vulnerable (Figs. 3 and 4). The lung disease frequently occurs when the patient is in remission from leukaemia and may develop several months following infection. It is not known whether this is a consequence of persistence of the virus or due to reinfection. In most patients the rash of measles is absent and thus the diagnosis may not be suspected if a history of contact is not obtained. As the antibody responses in these patients are variable, the diagnosis must be made by virological and/or histological examination of lung tissue. The mortality rate in these children is very high.

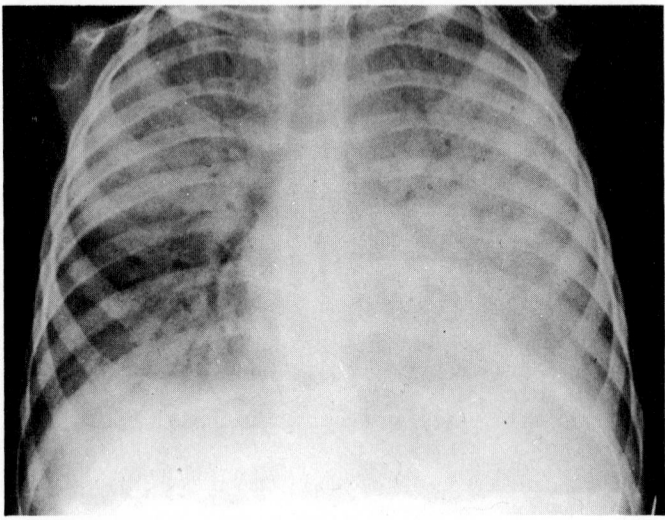

Fig. 3 Fatal measles pneumonia in a child with leukaemia in remission with the disease.

Nervous system. The most common neurological complication is the short generalized seizure which occurs early in the febrile stage of the infection. The rate is of the order of 5–6 per 1000 cases of measles ranging from 7–8 per 1000 during the second year of life to 2 per 1000 in 5–6 year old children. Recovery is usually complete and unless the seizures are prolonged they have no greater significance than simple febrile seizures.

Measles encephalitis on the other hand is often associated with generalized seizures and may be a devastating disorder but one which shows great variability in its clinical course. It occurs in approximately 1–2 per 1000 cases of measles and the risk increases

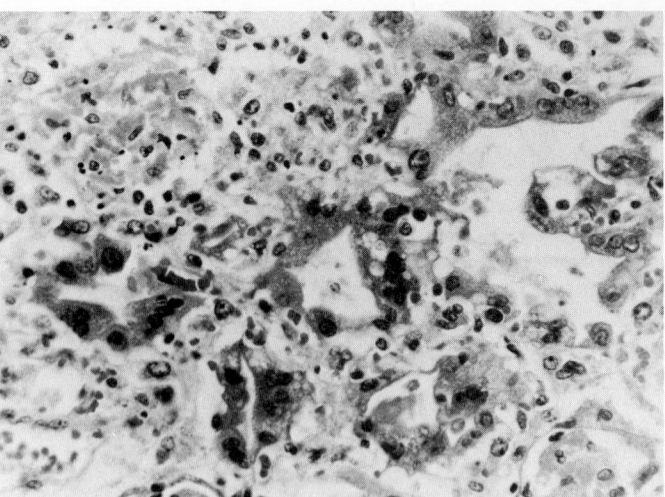

Fig. 4 Histological changes in the lung of a child with measles giant cell (Hecht's) pneumonia. Abundant multinucleated giant cells line the alveoli; these contain intranuclear and intracytoplasmic inclusions. (By courtesy of J. R. Pincott.)

with age. The onset is usually between four and seven days after the rash commences but rarely may occur within 48 hours or up to two weeks of the onset. In addition to the seizures there is often fever, irritability, headache, and a disturbance in consciousness which may progress to profound coma; signs of meningeal irritation are not common. A mild lymphocytic pleocytosis with some elevation of protein is often present in the CSF but the levels of glucose are not abnormal.

It is generally held that the disorder is a 'neuroallergic' process and not the effect of active infection as isolation of the virus from the brain or CSF is rare. This is supported by the histological features which consist of perivascular cuffing, demyelination and gliosis.

Measles encephalitis is a very unpredictable yet serious complication. Mortality is as high as 10–15 per cent and 25 per cent of children will be left with permanent brain damage. However, during the first few weeks of the illness complete recovery is possible even after periods of deep coma and prolonged convulsions over many days. Treatment is supportive and, although dexamethazone is frequently recommended, adequate studies of a beneficial effect are lacking. Neurological disorders may occur following live measles vaccine but many of these will not be causally related to the vaccine. The incidence is only of the order of 1 per million doses of vaccine.

Persistent virus infection is responsible for the development of the slowly progressive disease of the brain known as subacute sclerosing panencephalitis (SSPE). The virus is detected in the brain by electronmicroscopy and by fluorescence methods, and has been isolated only by co-cultivation techniques. It is not yet known whether the cause of this disorder is due to a host abnormality or a defect in the virus itself or even possibly a combination of both. Approximately 0.1–1.4 per million children are affected. The child with SSPE has usually experienced normal measles infection 5–10 years beforehand and often before the second birthday. The first manifestation is a disturbance in intellect and personality; behaviour disorders and deterioration in school work is frequently mentioned. There then follows, over a period of weeks or months, seizures which somewhat resemble myoclonus, signs of extrapyramidal and pyramidal disease, and finally a state of decerebrate rigidity. Death usually follows pneumonia. Arrest or recovery is exceptionally rare. The electroencephalogram shows a characteristic regular series of spikes with also some abnormality between these (Fig. 5). There are very high titres of measles CF and HI antibody in both the serum and the cerebrospinal fluid; the latter is probably produced within the nervous system. Although SSPE has been observed in children who have received measles vaccine, it is 10 times less frequent than SSPE following a history of measles. A decline in the number of cases of SSPE reported in the USA since the introduction of measles vaccine has been observed (see Fig. 2). This figure also shows the benefits of immunization in terms of the decline in the numbers of cases of encephalitis.

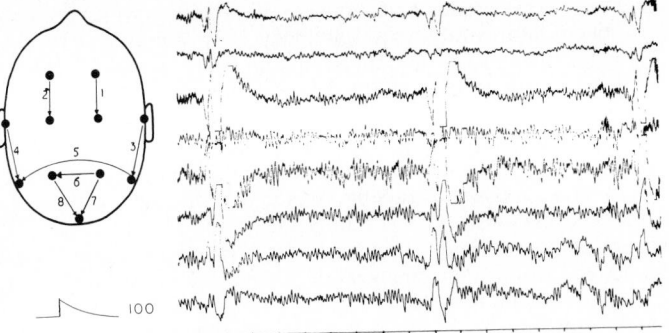

Fig. 5 Electroencephalograph of a 13-year-old boy with SSPE. Periodic phenomena recurring at intervals of about 8 seconds, of large amplitude (over 0.5 mV) with a preponderance in the right hemisphere (calibration: 100 µV; time constant 0.4 s; high frequency cnt 70 Hz; paper speed 1.5 cm/s). (By courtesy of G. Pampiglione.)

Treatments for SSPE have included the use of transfer factor, plasmaphoresis, and the antiviral drug, isoprinosine, but there is no evidence to indicate that the disease can be arrested by any of these measures.

A rare and unusual form of measles encephalitis has been observed in children with acute leukaemia in remission. Very high levels of measles CF antibody are present in serum and CSF similar to those found in SSPE but the clinical features, which includes catatonia in some children, and the EEG do not share the same similarities. Antibody levels of the same type are present in serum and CSF in a proportion of individuals with multiple sclerosis (MS), but there is no known causative or other link between measles and MS.

Other complications of measles include haemorrhagic measles which is now rare. This disorder may have been the consequence of disseminated intravascular coagulation. Thrombocytopenia is an infrequent complication and paroxysmal cold haemoglobinuria has been observed. The clinical importance of the temporary suppression of tuberculin reaction must be stressed but well controlled data to support the often stated adverse effect of measles in patients with pre-existing tuberculosis is scanty.

Measles in the tropics is a disease of the very young. The mortality is high with most deaths occurring in the second year. Severe disease is very closely related to malnutrition, particularly protein energy malnutrition. The skin rash in these children is frequently very florid and extensive desquamation is frequent. Diarrhoea is exceedingly common and anorexia caused by stomatitis is marked; both will exacerbate pre-existing malnutrition. The mouth lesions may be caused by herpes simplex virus as may keratoconjunctivitis which is frequent in children with measles in some tropical communities. However, Vitamin A deficiency probably plays an important role in the eye disease. Prolongation of the excretion of giant cells in the nasopharynx has been shown in malnourished children with measles suggesting that the duration of the infection may be longer.

Measles in the adult was rare but in the USA increased numbers of cases are seen in young adults in whom the disease has been more severe than in childhood. A number of these cases are probably individuals who, have not received vaccine in childhood because of the decline in prevalence of measles. Under usual circumstances measles would not be a risk to the pregnant woman. Information on the role of measles in causation of fetal infection and damage is confined to 'virgin soil' epidemics and is limited. It is possible that fetal damage may result following measles in pregnancy, thus the appearance of measles in the young adult population in the USA may present the problem of measles in a pregnant woman.

Prevention. Passive immunization with human immunoglobulin is highly effective if given within two or three days of exposure in a dose of 0.2 ml/kg. Smaller doses (0.04 ml/kg) may produce modification of the disease without preventing the benefit of the immunity induced by natural infection.

The first measles vaccines which were introduced were inactivated and, although they produced serum antibody, they were of doubtful efficacy. Moreover, a major problem occurred when following live measles vaccine or exposure to natural measles, recipients of the inactivated vaccine developed either a severe local reaction at the site of injection, or a bizarre form of measles. The latter syndrome consisted of an unusual rash which had a tendency to involve the extremities. It was maculopapular but frequently had urticarial, purpuric, and/or vesicular features. Fever was high, oedema of the limbs was not infrequent, and severe pneumonitis occurred. Pleural effusion was also observed. Koplik spots were not present and the disease was not communicable. The cause of this syndrome is not known but an exaggerated reactivity of sensitized lymphocytes probably plays a role in the pathogenesis.

The currently used measles vaccines are live attenuated strains of the virus with low reactogenicity. The optimal age of vaccination is 14–16 months. Fever of moderate severity is infrequent and a mild rash with some signs of upper respiratory tract infection occurs rarely. These manifestations will be observed 7–10 days after inoculation. Approximately 98 per cent of the recipients of the vaccine will develop an antibody response. Hence the very small numbers who fail to respond may subsequently develop measles. The vaccines may also afford protection if administered after exposure. If given within three days of contact almost all individuals will be protected. Thus they may be useful in home, nursery, or hospital exposures. The vaccine should not be given to persons with an intercurrent febrile illness, untreated tuberculosis, or if immunosuppressed by a malignancy especially leukaemia or lymphoma or by drugs such as steroids and antimetabolites. Pregnancy is also a contra-indication. Allergy to eggs is stated by the manufacturers to be a contra-indication but as the fibroblast cultures in which the virus is grown is essentially free of yolk or egg albumen components, children with egg allergy do not react adversely to measles vaccine.

Simultaneous adminstration of immune serum globulin of known measles antibody content (measles vaccine immune-globulin) may be used if it is considered desirable to minimize the risk of a febrile reaction, for example in children with pre-existing brain damage or a previous history of convulsions. This product contains sufficient antibody to reduce the symptoms caused by the vaccine virus but insufficient to neutralize the amount of virus contained in the vaccine.

The use of vaccines in tropical environments presents two special problems; the storage of the vaccine to maintain potency and the early onset of measles before the age of 12 months. The former may be alleviated by the recent introduction of improved stabilizers for the vaccine and the latter may require measles immunization programmes to commence at six to nine months of age. If this policy is adopted a second dose of vaccine at 14–16 months should be introduced if possible.

References

Dossetor, J., Whittle, H. C., and Greenwood, B. M. (1977). Persistent measles infection in malnourished children. *Br. med. J.* i, 1633.

Dudgeon, J. A. (1978). Immunity after rubella and measles viral vaccines. *Am. J. Dis. Child.* **132**, 748.

Fulginiti, V. A., Eller, J. J., Downie, A. W., and Kempe, C. H. (1967). Altered reactivity to measles virus, atypical measles in children previously immunized with inactivated measles virus vaccines. *J. Am. med. Ass.* **202**, 1075.

Guillozet, N. (1979). Measles in Africa: a deadly disease. *Clin. Pediat.* **18**, 95.

Lancet (1979). Measles in adults: annotation. *Lancet* **ii**, 834.

Landrigan, P. J. and Whitt, J. J. (1973). Neurological disorders following live measles-virus vaccination. *J. Am. med. Ass.* **223**, 1445.

Miller, D. L. (1964). Frequency of complications of Measles 1963. *Br. med. J.* **ii**, 76.

Modlin, J. F., Jabbour, J. T., Whitte, J. J., and Halsey, N. A. (1977). Epidemiologic studies of measles, measles vaccine and subacute sclerosing panencephalitis. *Pediatrics, Springfield* **95**, 505.

Pullam, C. R. Noble, C. T., Scott, D. J., Wisniewski, K., and Gardner, P. S. (1976) Atypical measles infection in leukaemic children on immunosuppressive treatment. *Br. med. J.* **i**, 1562.

Rubella

J. O'H. Tobin

The medical importance of rubella infection is not in the usual manifestation of the acquired disease, but in its ability to produce congenital abnormalities in the fetus of women infected in pregnancy. The virus has many of the characteristics of a togavirus, although it is not arthropod borne. There is only one serological type distinct from other viruses.

Epidemiology. Rubella has a world-wide distribution and the frequency of antibodies by age in most countries is very similar, with from 70 to 90 per cent of young adults having antibody. There are a few exceptions, such as in parts of Asia, where the prevalence of immunes is appreciably lower, around 50 per cent. Acquired and congenital rubella have been detected wherever they have been looked for. In temperate climates the acquired disease is most prevalent in the spring and early summer, with increased incidence locally every three to five years, the increase being spread over two years. In large conurbations and nationally, the incidence may appear fairly constant unless peaks in many areas coincide, in which case a major epidemic may be encountered.

Acquired rubella. The incubation period is 14 to 21 days with a mean of 17 days: the disease affects mainly children and adolescents. It is characterized by mild fever, sore throat, enlarged cervical and occipital glands, and a rash; this is usually discrete at first, but the spots may coalesce, giving a general pink flush, especially on the trunk. The face, trunk, and limbs are usually affected in that order, that rash often coming and going every few hours. In adults, arthralgia affecting the ankles, knees, hips, fingers, or the intervertebral joints is common. Other complications are infrequent and include purpura, thrombocytopenia, post-infectious encephalitis, transverse myelitis, and the Guillain–Barré syndrome. Symptoms persist for three to seven days, usually with only mild constitutional disturbance, but the arthralgia may continue for longer. Infection, especially in children, may pass undetected or the symptomatology may be restricted to a fleeting rash or a sore throat, both with a little glandular enlargement. Any symptoms suggestive of rubella, especially during pregnancy, should be treated as such, and laboratory confirmation sought. True rubella cannot be differentiated clinically from the non-teratogenic infections due to picornaviruses, myxoviruses, adenoviruses, streptococci, and glandular fever, all of which may produce a rubella-like illness, especially in children.

Laboratory diagnosis. This can be useful at all ages, but is essential in a pregnant woman with any symptoms suggestive of rubella.

Virus isolation can be attempted but serological methods are now so accurate and quick that they are the methods of choice (Pattison 1981). A blood sample should be taken when the patient is first seen and another five to seven days later. If blood is taken within a day or two of the rash, a rise in haemagglutination inhibiting (HI) antibody titre can usually be demonstrated without difficulty. Occasionally the titre is already high on the day of the rash and no rise can be demonstrated by this method, as the antibody level has reached a plateau. This is a common occurrence if the patient is first

seen five to seven days or more after the onset of symptoms. When no rise in HI antibody is found, specific rubella antibody in the IgM or IgA immunoglobulin classes must be sought. Specific IgM and IgA are usually short-lived following rubella infection, lasting for the three to five weeks, with occasional persistence at low levels for a much longer period. IgM can be demonstrated by a variety of methods including HI or immunofluorescent (IF) estimation of levels in sucrose gradient fractions, or in samples in which the IgG has been removed by staphylococcal protein A. Radio-immunoassay and enzyme linked immunosorbent assay (ELISA) techniques are also satisfactory. The complement fixation test is of little value but when the same principle is employed in the radial–haemolysis technique, it is a most useful method for screening for immunity. More than four weeks following symptoms, or seven weeks after exposure to rubella, the laboratory cannot confirm or refute the diagnosis with certainty unless the HI titre is low or absent. If the contact of a pregnant woman is under five years old, a blood test may refute a diagnosis of rubella in the child and help in deciding if a 'late reporter' is at risk or not. Only 7–10 per cent of children in this age group in the United Kingdom have rubella antibody but they commonly have all sorts of rashes.

Congenital infection. The classical triad, of cataracts and other eye anomalies, heart defects, and deafness, was first described by the late Sir Norman Gregg in Australia in 1941 (see Table 1). Since then, and especially after the epidemic in the United States in 1964, when laboratory methods of diagnosis became available, the full clinical congenital rubella syndrome (CRS) has been defined. Besides the Gregg triad, hepatitis, thrombocytopenic purpura, bone involvement, behavioural changes, microcephaly, and retardation and 'late onset disease' syndromes have been reported. Up to three quarters of symptomless babies are of low birth weight (<2.5 kg). Defects due to congenital rubella may not become evident for months or years, so follow-up of children exposed to intrauterine infection must be continued well into school age. The approximate period of onset of defects is given in Table 2. Gregg's triad is not always present. Abortion and stillbirths can also occur.

Table 1   Gregg's triad in congenital rubella

Cardiovascular defects	persistent ductus arteriosus
	pulmonary stenosis
	aortic and renal artery stenosis
	tetralogy of Fallot
	myocarditis
Eye defects	cataracts
	retinopathy
	microphthalmos
	glaucoma
Deafness	sensorineural
	central imperception

The behavioural and allied syndromes are probably the direct result of rubella virus infecting the central nervous system; the virus can be found in the cerebral spinal fluid, sometimes persisting throughout the first year of life. Very rarely a chronic progressive panencephalitis, stimulating SSPE, with ataxia, spasticity, myoclonic seizures, and intellectual deterioration may occur in adolescents with congenital rubella (see Section 21). The rubella antibody level may be raised in the CSF and virus isolated from the brain by co-cultivation.

The risk of fetal defects depends on the gestational age at which maternal infection occurs. If infection occurs in the first two months of the pregnancy, multiple defects, including the well-known triad are common, together with other signs. After two months, the triad becomes less frequent, and by 12 weeks the commonest defect is sensorineural deafness. The incidence of congenital defects probably exceeds 50 per cent following infection in the first month, is

Table 2 Defects associated with congenital rubella by approximate period of onset

In newborns	hepatosplenomegaly
	jaundice
	thromocytopenia
	purpura
	lymphadenopathy
	osteopathy
	cardiac defects
	eye defects
	hepatitis
In infancy	hypogammaglobulinaemia
	chronic rash
	intestinal pneumonitis
	chronic diarrhoea
	thymic hypoplasia
	growth retardation
In childhood	deafness
	speech defects
	diabetes mellitis
	growth deficiency
	hypothyroidism
	abnormal dermatoglyphics
	autism
In adolescence	panencephalitis

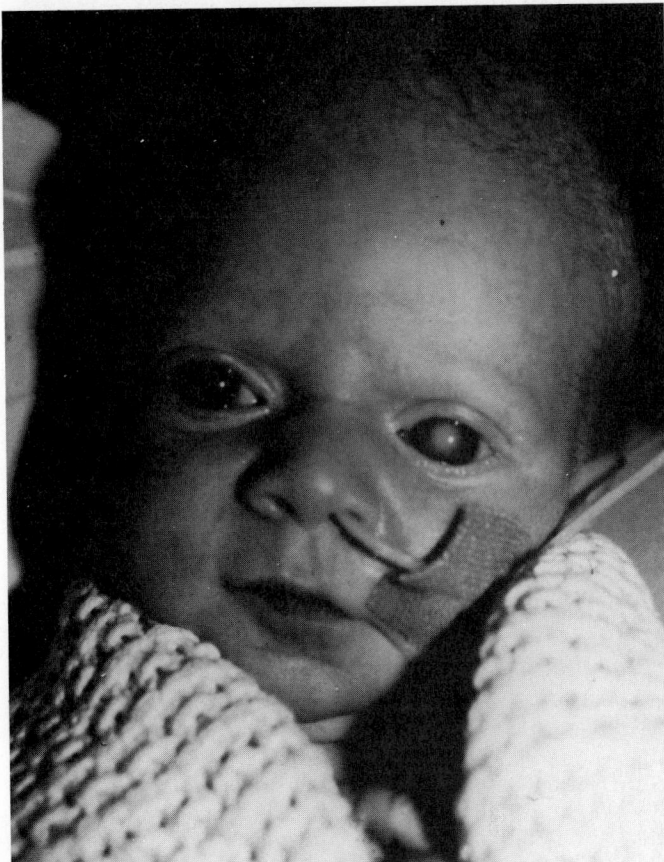

Fig. 1 Congenital rubella. Corneal haze of left eye. (Reproduced by permission of Marcel Dekker Inc.)

about 40 per cent in the second month, 20 per cent in the third and 10 per cent if the disease occurs in the fourth month. After that, it is more difficult to assess the risk of damage to the fetus, although there are occasional reports of deafness and other abnormalities following infection later in pregnancy. The chance of a fetus acquiring intrauterine infection is high: virus can be isolated from over 90 per cent of embryos of infected pregnancies; the infant apparently can cure itself as only 50 per cent of proved maternal rubella infections result in an infant with persistent IgG antibodies or IgM antibodies in the few months following birth. The proportion of infants with serological evidence of intrauterine infection at birth, whose mothers were infected between the 16th and 36th week is appreciably lower, indicating increased resistence to persisting infection.

All children with evidence of congenital rubella or a history of maternal infection during pregnancy should be followed up for defects so that alleviating treatment can be instituted as soon as possible. This is especially important with deafness, which may not be recognized until the child has entered school.

The prognosis for children with severe deformities seems to be better in the Australian experience than in that from the United States or United Kingdom. Modern treatment of cataracts and heart defects have reduced the incapacity due to them, but only those with minor degrees of deafness seem to be able to attend normal schools satisfactorily.

The fetal damage in rubella is due to infection of the placenta, which reduces the blood supply and impairs intrauterine growth; it disturbs normal metabolic activity giving rise to malfunction and diminished organ growth; and causes cellular damage to organs. The persistence of virus produces continuous chronic infection in the ear, eye, and brain and immunological reactions involved in late onset disease syndromes.

Laboratory diagnosis of congenital rubella. After birth, an infant with congenital rubella will excrete the virus from the throat, in urine, and faeces, and it can be found in the CSF, blood, eyes and ears. Excretion usually diminishes slowly and ceases in 70 per cent of cases in six months. The infant is capable of producing an antibody response of its own, so persistence of IgG antibody after the disappearance of maternally transmitted IgG indicates congenital infection. IgG antibody can be detected for up to five years of age and even longer. Maternal antibody has a half-life of three to

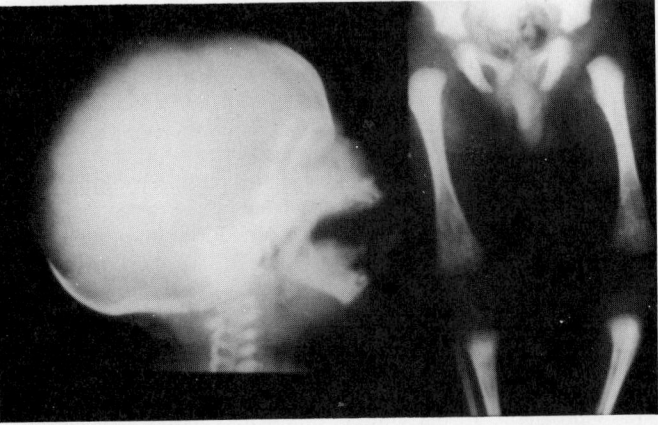

Fig. 2 Congenital rubella. Skeletal changes in skull and large bones of legs. (From Marshall, W. C. In *Practice of pediatric opthalmology*, Marcel Dekker Inc., by permission.)

four weeks and its persistence depends on the level at birth, but it usually takes at least five months to disappear. Rubella-specific IgM, but no IgA, antibody is found in the infected baby for three to nine months, and its estimation is a useful early diagnostic tool, as it is not affected by the presence of maternal antibody.

Other adverse effects of rubella. The toll of rubella results not only from congenital defects in infants due to maternal infection, but also from the loss of normal fetal material by therapeutic abortions because of fear of a damaged child. Most women in the United Kingdom who get rubella in the first three months of pregnancy have a termination, as do a considerable proportion who get infected in the fourth month of gestation. In Britain between 200 and 900 abortions are performed each year because the mother contracts rubella or is in contact with it during pregnancy. Of these 70 per cent are in multipara.

Prevention

Vaccination. Soon after the virus of rubella had been isolated in 1964, progress towards the production of a vaccine was rapid and various strains have been used for this purpose. In the United Kingdom, RA27/3 and the Cendehill strains have been most popular. In the United States, RA27/3 is now used almost exclusively, having superceded the previous monkey/duck embryo (HPV77De5) vaccine which had been used most widely until 1979. These vaccines are not identical, and the choice has to be made depending on the situation in which they are to be used.

As the vaccines contain live virus, derived from wild rubella strains, they can produce the disease in vaccinated hosts. The incidence of sore throats, glandular swelling, arthralgia, and rashes are more common after RA27/3 than after Cendehill, but in compensation, the antibody response tends to be higher and there are very few non-responders. The persistence of antibody depends on the initial response and if this is good, easily detectable antibody will remain for at least 10 years. If the initial response is poor, especially following Cendehill vaccine, a small proportion of those vaccinated will lose detectable antibody within a few months.

The vaccine does not produce enough virus in the upper respiratory tract to be transmitted to other susceptible women, and so it can be used with safety in antenatal and maternity unit personnel. Reinfection with wild virus, followed by a substantial rise in antibody is common after vaccination with Cendehill but rare after RA27/3 or natural infection. It is claimed that immunity after RA27/3 vaccine is similar to that following natural infection, but so far no CRS has been reported in the offspring of any vaccinated woman. How dangerous the vaccines are to the fetus has not yet been determined, but it has been isolated from the products of conception. Two of 65 children born of non-immune women vaccinated early in pregnancy have shown serological evidence of infection, although no defects have been detected so far. The potential danger of the vaccine has meant that women who were pregnant at the time of vaccination or two or three months later, have sometimes been advised to be terminated. Since 1972, in the United Kingdom, over 450 such terminations were said to have been performed for this reason.

The policy for vaccination varies in different parts of the world. In the United Kingdom at present, schoolgirls between the ages of 11 and 14 and postpartum women screened for immunity in pregnancy, are offered vaccination, together with other groups thought to be at increased risk, e.g. staff of special care baby units, day nurseries, and school teachers. Any woman desiring vaccination can have it, but it is recommended that a blood test to discriminate those immune should be done first to reduce the number vaccinated unnecessarily. This minimizes the chance of vaccinating somebody who is pregnant. In the United States, all children from the second year upwards have been offered vaccination to reduce the amount of virus in the community. It is also given to adults on request. The notified cases of acquired and congenital rubella have apparently fallen, although many cases of congenital rubella are still occurring.

In the United Kingdom, the policy of schoolgirl vaccination is unlikely to have any effect until 1985. For this reason, inoculation of primary schoolchildren has been advocated to reduce the amount of circulating virus in schools and so indirectly protect non-immune pregnant women.

Approximately 70 per cent of women who have a termination for rubella, or who have a congenitally infected infant, are in multipara. Postpartum vaccination of women screened during pregnancy and found non-immune, is the most economical method of immunizing the adult population. Vaccination of all women before their first pregnancy is more difficult to accomplish unless they can be 'caught' when they are in some institution such as a college or university, or through their places of employment.

Immunoglobulin after contact. Both hyperimmune and normal immunoglobulin have been used as passive immunotherapy after contact with rubella. Normal immunoglobulin, made from the blood of ordinary donors, does not stop infection but may sometimes render it subclinical. This may reduce the frequency of subsequent congenital defects. Hyperimmune immunoglobulin is prepared from the blood of people who have recently had rubella, or who have high antibody levels. It is claimed to be more effective than normal immunoglobulin, but is not yet available for routine use. One of these preparations should be given to any non-immune woman, less than 16 weeks gestation, who is likely to continue her pregnancy even if infected. The dose is between one and three grams, depending on the product. It should be given within ten days of contact with a case of rubella after laboratory screening for immunity.

References

Cradock-Watson, J. E., Ridehalph, M. K. S., Anderson, M. J., Pattison, J. R., and Kanguo, H. O. (1980). Fetal infection resulting from maternal rubella after the third trimester of pregnancy. *J. Hyg., Camb.* **85**, 381.

Dudgeon, J. A. and Hanshaw, J. B. (1978). *Viral diseases of the fetus and newborn.* Saunders, Philadelphia.

MacDonald, H., Tobin, J. O'H., Cradock-Watson, J. E., Lomax, J., and Bourne, M. S. (1978). Antibody titres in women six to eight years after the administration of RA27/3 and Cendehill rubella vaccines. *J. Hyg., Camb.* **80**, 337.

Pattison, J. R. (ed.) (1982). *Techniques used in the laboratory investigation of rubella virus infection.* PHLS Monograph Series, HMSO, London.

Preblud, S. R. (1980). Rubella vaccination in the United States: a ten-year review. *Epidemiol. Rev.* **2**, 171.

Enteroviruses

N. R. Grist

Enteroviruses are common infectious agents which spread characteristically by the faecal–oral route. They are typical picornaviruses, having a naked virion with cubic symmetry, 32 capsomeres, a diameter of 20–30 nm and single-stranded RNA of molecular weight 2.5×10^6. As befits their gastrointestinal habitat, enteroviruses are relatively stable, resisting treatment with deoxycholate, either and other fat solvents, and acid (pH 3 for one hour). They survive for long periods in water at low temperatures, but are inactivated by drying or by exposure to heat (50 °C for one hour unless stabilized by magnesium chloride) or free residual chlorine (0.3–0.5 p.p.m.). There are numerous types, some infecting mammalian species other than man. The enteroviruses of man were classified as polioviruses (causing paralytic disease in man and monkeys), coxsackieviruses (causing paralytic disease when inoculated into newborn mice: group A types cause generalized severe myositis and group B types cause patchy myositis but severe brain damage in infected mouselets), and echoviruses (isolatable in cell cultures but not usually pathogenic for newborn mice), the antigenic types being distinguished by neutralization tests with specific antisera. Several anomalous enteroviruses were then found to share the properties of more than one of these classical groups. Those enteroviruses more recently discovered are not classified as poliovirus, coxsackievirus, or echovirus but are designated 'higher enterovirus types'. The current known enteroviruses are summarized in Table 1. Other viruses with enteroviral properties are known, but not yet classified, and the list will undoubtedly grow for several more years.

Pattern of infection. Enteroviruses usually infect by the oral route, being resistant to stomach acid, infecting superficial cells in the throat and lower alimentary tract, and being excreted in the faeces

Table 1   The enteroviruses

Poliovirus types	1–3
Coxsackievirus types	A1–A24*
Coxsackievirus types	B1–B6
Echovirus types	1–34*
Enterovirus types	68–71

* Coxsackievirus A23 is the same as echovirus 9; former echovirus 10 is reclassified as reovirus 1; former echovirus 28 is reclassified as rhinovirus 1A

(Table 2). Sometimes they penetrate systemically, with brief viraemia and fever, and may then reach and infect cells in other organs such as the nervous system, heart, and muscles. Some enteroviruses may infect mainly the respiratory tract and can then be transmitted by respiratory droplet infection; others infect the eye and spread mainly by contagion. Recovery is accompanied by development of humoral immunity protective against symptomatic reinfection by the same virus type, both serum antibodies and also secretory IgA 'coproantibodies' inhibitory to reinfection of the gut. The role of cellular immunity is less understood. At the cellular level, the infective process is cytolytic—virus multiplies in the cytoplasm of the cells which burst liberating progeny virus, as seen in infected cell cultures. No clinically effective antiviral agents are available for enteroviral infection, though interferon suppresses enteroviruses *in vitro*.

Table 2   Main pattern of infection by a typical enterovirus

Portals of entry
1. oral
2. respiratory

Primary site of multiplication
1. alimentary tract
2. pharynx

Viraemia
   in some cases

Secondary sites of virus multiplication and damage
1. CNS (meningitis, poliomyelitis, encephalitis)
2. heart (myocarditis, pericarditis)
3. muscles (Bornholm disease)
4. skin and mucosae (exanthem, enanthem)
5. respiratory tract (URI, LRI)
6. liver, pancreas and other viscera, mainly as part of generalized infection in infants

Portals of exit
1. faeces
2. pharyngeal and respiratory secretions

Epidemiology. Enterovirus infections are most prevalent in young children, and under conditions of overcrowding and poor hygiene, especially in warm seasons and hot climates. In these circumstances, spread occurs mainly by faecal pollution of persons and the environment, water, and food, since the virus is stable for long periods in moist organic matter, sewage and contaminated water. In many such communities in warm climates, paralytic poliomyelitis is prevalent at all seasons and every year. In smaller populations and with improved hygiene, transmission of infection is slowed down, and poliovirus and some other enteroviruses then show epidemic activity at intervals of three or, commonly, four years, which allow recruitment into the population by new births of sufficient non-immune young children to support the outbreaks. In large conurbations in temperate climates twenty or more different enteroviruses may be active in a single year with one or two dominating the summer–autumn epidemic season. In sparse and isolated populations, and with high standards of hygiene, infection tends to die out, allowing accumulation of a susceptible population which may then support an epidemic with broad age-incidence. These older and adult non-immune persons often suffer more severe disease than children other than infants, who may develop life-

threatening illness if unprotected by maternal passive immunity to the infecting virus, but most infections are silent or trivial in their effects. Where hygienic standards are high enough to prevent significant faeco-oral transmission, limited spread may still occur by the respiratory route since acute infections involve brief infectivity of nasopharyngeal secretions, but this route is less effective because enteroviruses do not withstand desiccation.

For poliomyelitis, these patterns are altered by the influence of immunization. Since it is improbable that polioviruses can be eradicated from the crowded populations of the tropics and subtropics, unvaccinated groups and individuals will always be at risk of exposure to infection, and in several well-vaccinated countries the few remaining cases of poliomyelitis mainly involve unvaccinated persons and groups. Improved living standards, with postponement of the average age of first infection, probably explain the emergence of epidemic paralytic poliomyelitis first in the advanced countries of northern Europe and Northern America. It is also possible that increased hygiene exerts selection pressure in favour of the more vigorously multiplying strains of poliovirus which are also more virulent. Urbanization of populations from the relatively isolated rural areas of many developing countries provides new opportunities for epidemic spread among persons without previous exposure to a particular enterovirus. The epidemiological situation throughout the world is complex and changing, requiring constant surveillance and efficient use of available poliomyelitis vaccines. Post-infectious immunity to the same type of enterovirus is good. Transient reinfection of the gut by poliovirus of a type for which the individual already has antibody is not uncommon, showing that 'gut immunity' is neither complete nor permanent, but the reinfecting virus does not cause disease. Antibody responses to the first infections in life are type-specific, but cross-reactions are common in older children and adults because of some sharing of antigens by different enteroviruses.

Virological diagnosis. Diagnosis of acute enteroviral infections is best achieved by virus isolation from faeces after inoculation into cell cultures. Inoculation of newborn mice may be required to detect some coxsackieviruses, especially those of group A. Since enteroviruses are stable in faeces, no special refrigeration of the specimen is normally required. From respiratory illnesses, virus may be isolated from a juicy throat swab taken in the early acute stage and sent in buffered virus transport medium. Cerebrospinal fluid (CSF) from the acute stage of neurological illnesses should also be submitted to the laboratory; although polioviruses are very rarely detectable in the CSF of even paralytic cases, many other common and important neuropathogenic enteroviruses are readily detectable, and the significance of the isolation is obviously high as compared with the chance that an enterovirus found in faeces represents coincidental, silent infection irrelevant to the disease.

Virus isolation provides the best opportunity to identify the infecting type of virus by neutralization tests with specific antisera. Primary serological diagnosis is usually impracticable because of the numerous types of virus and the need to perform tests for some of them in newborn mice. Paired sera from the acute and convalescent stages of illness should nevertheless be collected, particularly from suspected poliomyelitis cases, since neutralization tests can be carried out with those viruses particularly suspected, or known from virus isolation, to be involved. In cardiac cases suspected of coxsackieviral aetiology, sera may show unusually high or rising antibody titres to one or more group B coxsackieviruses. Antibody surveys also provide objective monitoring of the immune status of a population to evaluate the need for or effectiveness of vaccination.

DISEASES CAUSED BY ENTEROVIRUSES

Non-specific, febrile, and respiratory illnesses

Most enterovirus infections are silent or cause only minor and transient symptoms, mainly upper respiratory, e.g. sore throat with or without rhinitis, often with fever. In the UK enteroviruses (mainly coxsackieviruses) have been found to make only a small contribution to the total of respiratory infections: in hospital they most often affect preschool children, in the community children of school age; they also cause pharyngitis, tonsillitis, and 'influenzal' fevers in adults. It is notable that rhinoviruses, the classical 'common cold' viruses, are likewise picornaviruses differing from enteroviruses mainly in their inability to grow at temperatures higher than those of the upper respiratory tract mucosa, and in their sensitivity to acid which makes them unable to survive transit through the stomach like enteroviruses. Early studies in the USA showed that enteroviruses, particularly Coxsackieviruses, were often incriminated in 'summer grippe' and similar febrile catarrhs in their summer–autumn season of peak incidence. Even polioviruses can sometimes cause purely respiratory symptoms.

The most clear-cut relationship of enteroviruses to acute respiratory illness is found in young children, among whom the youngest are most vulnerable to more serious lower respiratory tract diseases which can sometimes be fatal. In closed communities and where nutrition and housing conditions are poor, outbreaks of serious disease may occur. Coxsackie B viruses have been particularly associated with outbreaks of upper respiratory disease, rhinorrhoea, pharyngitis, and fever in young children in nurseries, camps, and residential homes. Echoviruses have also been involved in outbreaks, particularly among neonates and infants, in hospitals and institutions causing rhinitis, pharyngitis, bronchitis, and pneumonia. Echovirus type 11 was isolated from children affected predominantly with croup during outbreaks in Sweden, and has been relatively often identified in upper and lower respiratory tract infections in many parts of the world.

During outbreaks of infection with particular enteroviruses clinically notable because of the many cases with characteristic features such as paralysis (poliovirus) or aseptic meningitis (echovirus types 9, 30; coxsackievirus types A9, B5, etc.), many cases of nonspecific minor febrile and respiratory illness due to the same virus will also be found in the community, especially in family contacts of patients with more serious and characteristic disease.

Enanthems and exanthems

Enterovirus infections, particularly with certain types, are sometimes accompanied by skin rashes and/or vesicular oropharyngeal lesions from which the virus can sometimes be isolated as well as from faeces. Each syndrome can be due to any of several enteroviruses each of which can cause a variety of mucocutaneous manifestations as well as other types of disease (Table 3). During an outbreak, most cases are due to one particular enterovirus.

Table 3 The main enteroviruses associated with exanthems and enanthems

Syndrome	Coxsackievirus types		Echovirus types	Others
	A	B		
Herpangina	1–10	1–5	6,9,16,17	
Lymphonodular pharyngitis	10			
Hand, foot, and mouth disease	5,9,10,16	2,5		enterovirus 71
Erythematous rashes	2,4,5,9,16	1,3,4,5	1–7,9,11,14 16, etc.	

Enanthems. These may be considered as more florid and localized forms of the nonspecific respiratory diseases considered in the previous section, but the high titres of mainly IgG antibodies found in the acute-phase sera of some patients suggest the possibility of an underlying Arthus-type reaction due to previous infection with a different but antigenically related type of enterovirus.

Herpangina. This term was introduced by Zahorsky for a form of 'herpetic sore throat' recognized clinically thirty years before coxsackievirus was isolated by inoculating mice with throat secretions from similar cases. It is mainly seen in young children, presenting with rapid onset of fever, headache and painful sore throat. The faucial pillars particularly show inflammation with small, initially vesicular lesions which macerate into punched out aphthous ulcertaions surrounded by reddened areas. These persist for about two days before healing. Lesions may also involve the uvula and palate. The febrile illness lasts usually for two or three days only. Abdominal pain, nausea, and transient neck stiffness are sometimes present. Coxsackieviruses, mainly of group A but sometimes of group B, are the usual causes of herpangina. Echoviruses have been isolated from sporadic cases.

Lymphonodular pharyngitis. This is a similar but uncommon condition from which coxsackievirus A10 was isolated. The yellowish or white oral lesions are nodular instead of vesicular and do not ulcerate.

Hand, foot, and mouth disease. Coxsackievirus A16 is the usual cause of this condition which has been reported in outbreaks or epidemics from many parts of the world. Children are mainly affected, characteristically by rapid onset of fever and sore throat. Small, superficial ulcers develop rapidly from vesicles on the gums, tongue, buccal mucosa, and palate. One or two days after onset, punctate and usually fleeting skin lesions appear—maculopapules and greyish, oval vesicles on the palms of hands and soles of feet, often on nail folds, sometimes on the dorsa of fingers and toes, and occasionally on buttocks, axillae, or other areas. The skin lesions may be few. The fever and rash subside quickly but mouth lesions may take more than a week to disappear. Adults often feel unwell for these one or two weeks.

Exanthems. Various transient and erythematous (rubelliform, maculo-papular, rarely morbilliform or vesicular) skin rashes may accompany infections by echoviruses of many types and occasionally coxsackieviruses, particularly in young children among whom outbreaks of fever and maculopapular rash can occur. Rashes are commonest in infancy and may be petechial or purpuric in severe infections of the newborn.

Echovirus 9. This is the commonest cause of those epidemics of rubella-like disease (see page 5.80) in children during community outbreaks in which others (particularly adults) have 'influenzal' febrile illnesses, and many cases of aseptic meningitis occur. After an incubation period of about five days, the onset is sudden with headache, fever, and often vomiting, illness being most severe in older and adult patients but often trivial in young children in whom the rash may be the first or only notable feature. The rash may present as pink or red maculo-papules, sometimes confined to the face, and also as minute pink or pale papules usually on the trunk and limbs. Cervical, axillary, and inguinal lymph nodes may be enlarged. The illness usually subsides in four or five days. Differentiation from rubella may be difficult or impossible without laboratory investigation, though occurrence during a known epidemic is suggestive. Virological tests comprise attempted virus isolation from throat swab or faeces, plus serological tests to exclude rubella. Unlike rubella, echovirus 9 does not cause fetal damage.

Boston exanthem. This name was given to the first enteroviral eruptive fever to be recognized in children. The maculopapular rash on face, trunk, and extremities tends to appear after defervescence of the fever. Echovirus type 16 is the virus concerned.

Other rashes. Petechial, purpuric, urticarial, and telangiectatic rashes have also been described in children infected usually with echoviruses but sometimes with coxsackieviruses.

Neurological diseases

Paralytic poliomyelitis was the first enteroviral disease to be recognized. Originally isolated in monkeys, poliomyelitis viruses were the first members of the group to be identified. Further studies of paralytic and nonparalytic meningeal illnesses led to isolation of the coxsackieviruses in newborn mice. Later the development and application of cell culture techniques revealed '*enteric cytopathic human orphan*' (echo) viruses and unmasked the characteristic enteric ecology of the group.

The typical course of evolution of a developing country with rising standards of living and hygiene is from an originally hyperendemic or endemic situation, with infection essentially confined to susceptible children under five years of age and a relatively inconspicuous penalty of disease ('infantile paralysis'), past a threshold after which recurrent epidemic paralytic poliomyelitis becomes established as a serious public health problem affecting a wide age range and inflicting a heavy burden of lifelong disability until controlled by vaccination (Fig. 1). Different socioeconomic groups of the same population may simultaneously be at different stages of this evolution (Fig. 2).

The main patterns of neurological diseases caused by enteroviruses comprise acute paralytic poliomyelitis, nonbacterial 'aseptic' meningitis (the commonest syndrome), and encephalitis (Table 4). Intermediate syndromes (meningoencephalitis, polioencephalitis) also occur.

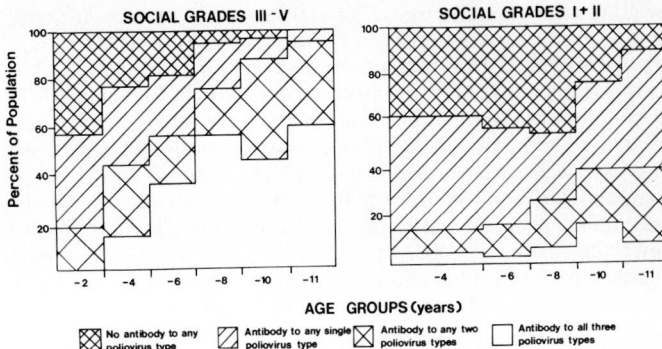

Fig. 2 Poliovirus antibody surveys in western Scotland in 1955–6 before the introduction of vaccination showed marked differences between the lower and higher social grades of the same population. Children in grades III–V show progressive acquisition of immunity during pre-school and school years, most of them acquiring antibodies to at least two or all three types by natural exposure to infection. Those in grades I and II acquired antibodies slowly and incompletely, most of them remaining susceptible to two or three of the poliovirus types. (Data from MacLeod *et al., Scott. Med. J.* (1958) **3**, 76.)

Table 4 Main associations of enteroviruses with acute neurological diseases

Syndrome	Poliovirus	Coxsackievirus	Echovirus	Enterovirus
Paralytic disease	+++ esp. types 1, 3	+ esp. type A7	±	+ types 70, 71
Meningitis	+ types 1, 2, 3	++ esp. types A9 B5, etc.	+++ esp. types 9, 30, etc.	+ type 71
Encephalitis, ataxia	+	++	±	+ type 71

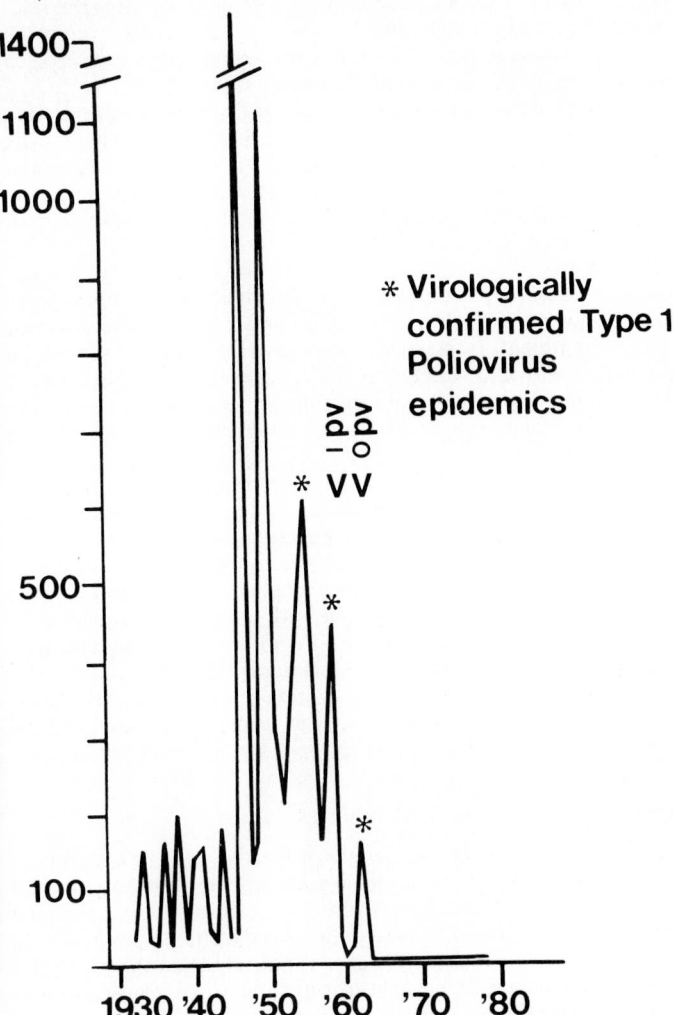

Fig. 1 Poliomyelitis notifications in Scotland from 1932 to 1978 illustrate transition from the stage of endemic 'infantile paralysis' to epidemic paralytic poliomyelitis in 1947, brought under control by vaccination with inactivated vaccine (ipv) from 1958 and oral vaccine (opv) from 1962 up to the present. Virological tests became available in time to identify type 1 poliovirus as the cause of the last three epidemics. (Statistical data from the Information Services Division of the Common Services Agency, Scottish Home and Health Department; virological data from publications of the Virus Laboratory, Ruchill Hospital, Glasgow.)

Paralytic poliomyelitis. Typically, this is a minor prodromal illness lasting several days with fever, sore throat, anorexia, and occasionally nausea, vomiting, and diarrhoea. If the later stages of the disease do not develop, this minor illness is known as 'abortive poliomyelitis': this cannot be diagnosed by clinical criteria alone. With or without a few days of well-being, there is abrupt onset of the major neurological illness. The patient is anxious, irritable, and often sweating, with fever (38–39 °C), headache, stiffness, and pains in the neck, trunk, and limbs. Nuchal rigidity and positive Kernig's sign are present. In about a third of cases which reach this stage, the condition resolves in about a week and is then known as 'nonparalytic poliomyelitis'—aseptic meningitis due to poliovirus. The remaining cases progress rapidly to paralysis which may be preceded by pain and fasciculations in the muscles to be affected. Paralysis usually appears during the fever, rarely afterwards, and may be the first sign of poliomyelitis in infants or very young children. It may evolve rapidly or progress gradually over a week or so. The pattern of paralysis is variable, typically asymmetrical, and usually affects the lower limbs more seriously than other muscles. Bulbar and encephalitic signs may appear. The paralysis is of lower motor neurone type, flaccid with absent tendon reflexes. Paralysis tends to be more severe, extensive, and possibly progressive if there has been strenuous physical exercise during the incubation period. It may also be more severe or localized in a traumatized area, e.g., following an irritating injection of vaccine ('provocation poliomyelitis'), or after tonsillectomy, which may provoke severe bulbar paralysis. Paralysis classically presents as follows.

Spinal form. Muscles innervated by spinal nerves are affected by paralysis which is often preceded by diminution or loss of deep reflexes a few hours before weakness is detectable. The paralysis is more widespread in the early stages than later, due to recovery of function of many temporarily injured anterior horn cells. Some muscle groups usually escape serious damage even in a severely paralysed limb, and slow recovery of function can progress over many weeks or months. In a recent epidemic in Malawi, where three-quarters of the cases were in the first three years of life, severe residual disability involving mainly the lower limbs affected 16 per cent of these but 25 per cent of children over three years old. Most commonly affected, in order of frequency, are: in the lower limb, the quadriceps, tibialis anterior, and peroneal muscles; in the upper limb, the deltoid, biceps, and triceps; in the trunk, abdominal muscles, back, intercostals, and diaphragm. Respiratory paralysis can cause life-threatening impairment of ventilation and is commonly associated with involvement of shoulder muscles.

Bulbar form. This is the most severe and dangerous form of poliomyelitis, resulting from damage in the brain stem, particularly the medulla. Any case of poliomyelitis with unusually rapid and stormy onset and development, drowsiness or marked apprehension, should be carefully watched for signs of medullary involvement which may progress rapidly to death despite therapy. The main patterns are as follows:

1. Cranial nerve nuclei involved: (a) upper group (third to seventh nerve nuclei), with good prognosis and recovery usual; (b) lower group (ninth to twelfth nerve nuclei) with difficulties in such functions as swallowing and clearing secretions from the pharynx, where pooled saliva and mucus can obstruct the airway or be inhaled. Clearance of the airway and maintenance of ventilation are essential to preserve life.

2. Respiratory centre impaired: irregularities of rhythm and rate of breathing lead to respiratory failure which can cause sudden collapse.

3. Circulatory centre impaired: hypertension, peripheral circulatory failure, and hypotension can occur, sometimes with hyperpyrexia.

Multiple neurological signs may coincide with hypoxia and hypercapnia from ventilatory dysfunction, and death may be associated with acute myocarditis. Encephalitic forms of poliomyelitis are often combined with bulbar or bulbospinal features.

In the preparalytic and paralytic stages of poliomyelitis the cerebrospinal fluid is clear, rarely slightly hazy, with increased cells (10–500 per mm³) and lymphocytic predominance; the cell count is maximal in the preparalytic phase when polymorphs may predominate. The protein level is raised, persisting for some time after the cell count has reverted to normal—an example of 'albumino-cytological dissocation' to be distinguished from the Guillain–Barré syndrome.

Aetiology. The commonest cause of the paralytic poliomyelitis syndrome is a poliovirus: type 1 causes the major epidemics and outbreaks before vaccination has been instituted; type 3 tends to predominate among the few cases occurring after general immunization. Type 2, the least neurovirulent poliovirus, both as attenuated vaccine and as 'wild' virus, tends to establish itself in the gut more efficiently than types 1 or 3. A few sporadic cases of similar paralytic disease are caused by other enteroviruses, mainly those of the Coxsackie group: paralysis tends to be milder with more rapid recovery, and encephalitic features may be relatively more prominent. Coxsackie virus A7 caused outbreaks of meningitis, paralysis, and some deaths mainly in children in the USSR and Scotland but has not established itself as a serious threat. Enterovirus 71 likewise has caused large outbreaks in children in eastern Europe with many paralytic, bulbar, and fatal cases. In order to monitor such occurrences, and to distinguish possible failures of vaccination control programmes, it is important for every case of acute paralytic poliomyelitic disease to be investigated as fully as possible, combining attempts to isolate virus from faeces and other specimens with serological tests of paired sera. Epidemiological details should also be recorded including the history of poliomyel-itis immunization and/or contact with recently vaccinated persons, and every case should be notified.

Aseptic meningitis (benign lymphocytic meningitis; viral meningitis). Enteroviruses are the commonest cause of this benign infective form of meningitis, which outnumbers bacterial meningitis except during epidemics of meningococcal disease. Outside the epidemic season for enteroviruses, mumps is the commonest cause, while arboviruses are important in the areas where they are endemic. The general pattern of cases seen during different enteroviral epidemics varies according to the characteristic effects of the particular enterovirus which, either in the meningitis cases or in the associated non-meningeal illnesses of contacts, can produce many infections with, for instance, rash (especially echovirus 9), myalgia (especially coxsackievirus B), etc. Most cases involve children, but the age distribution differs from one outbreak to another with a higher proportion in older and adult age groups for those enteroviruses (e.g. echovirus types 4, 30) which recur in larger epidemics at longer intervals.

The onset is usually sudden or may be preceded by brief prodromal illness. Fever, headache, stiff neck, and often nausea, vomiting, sore throat, myalgia, or photophobia develop, subsiding usually within a few days to a week with complete recovery the rule. Transient, mild encephalitic features or paresis may rarely be noted, and there may be associated extraneural manifestations such as maculo-papular eruptions, especially in infants.

The main clinical feature is nuchal rigidity with fever and often faucial redness. The CSF is clear or cloudy with lymphocytic pleocytosis up to 500 per mm³, though higher counts with polymorph preponderance may be found in the earliest stages especially in echovirus 9 infections. Protein levels are moderately increased, but sugar levels are normal.

Differential diagnosis is important to distinguish the many other possible causes of meningeal irritation, particularly tuberculosis and other types of bacterial meningitis and intracerebral lesions for which treatment is essential. Enterovirus isolation should be attempted with CSF and faeces. Paired sera should be checked for an antibody response to identify mumps, leptospirosis, and other infections. Bacteriological tests including culture should be also performed.

Encephalitis. Encephalitis or ataxia, with or without sequelae, is a rare complication of enteroviral infections and is seen mainly in generalized neonatal coxsackieviral disease. It is usually combined with other features (e.g., meningoencephalitis, polioencephalitis). Coxsackieviruses are commonly involved, and encephalitis was a marked feature of the enterovirus 71 epidemics; cases are also seen during epidemics or paralytic poliomyelitis. The clinical pattern is not specific, and laboratory investigation is required to identify the enteroviral aetiology by isolating virus from faeces, CSF (or postmortem brain), and testing paired sera for antibody responses.

Diseases of the heart and muscles

Coxsackieviruses show myotropic properties both in experimentally infected newborn mice and in man, affecting both skeletal and cardiac muscle. A few echoviruses can rarely do the same and myocarditis is reported in fatal poliovirus infections. In addition to sporadic cases, increased incidence is noticeable during epidemics of, for example, coxsackievirus B5 infection, when many cases may manifest Bornholm disease (epidemic myalgia) and/or acute myocarditis and pericarditis.

Acute myocarditis and pericarditis. The term 'myo-pericarditis' is sometimes used because probably neither myocarditis nor pericarditis of enteroviral origin occurs in a pure form. Nevertheless, in most cases the illness is predominantly myocarditic (especially in young children) or pericarditic (especially in older children and adults). Severe pancarditis can complicate generalized infections of the newborn (see below) with tachycardia, heart enlargement and progressive congestive failure with liver swelling, and sometimes arrhythmias or heart block; mortality in these infants is high but recovery appears to be complete in those who survive the first weeks of stormy illness. The cardiac effects of enteroviruses are shown in Table 5.

Table 5 Effects of enteroviruses on the heart*

1. Nil
2. Transient ECG changes only
3. Myo-pericarditis
   (*a*) acute, with recovery:
       (i) complete recovery
       (ii) residual ECG changes
   (*b*) relapsing (i) with recovery?
       (ii) chronic disease:
              cardiomyopathy
              constrictive pericarditis
              endocarditis?
   (*c*) persisting (iii) fatal ($< 1\%$)
   (*d*) fatal during the acute illness ($< 1\%$)

* Similar effects are also produced by arboviruses in areas where they are endemic

Carditis in early childhood. Prodromal fever and throat congestion may precede the major illness. Weakness, dyspnoea, precordial pain, tachycardia with or without irregularities, feeble pulse, and sometimes heart block are typical features. X-ray examination may show cardiomegaly. ECG examination shows signs of myocarditis, usually without pericarditis unless in later childhood. Death from heart failure may occur in the acute stage or after months of persisting failure, but most children recover fully after a few weeks of serious illness.

Pericarditis can dominate the picture in later childhood, typically with fever and precordial pain like Bornholm disease, with which it may be associated. Dyspnoea and heart failure may become severe as a result of cardiac tamponade by pericardial effusion. Constrictive pericarditis is a rare, late complication.

Carditis in older children and adults. Acute pericarditis is the commonest presentation. There may be prodromal fever and upper respiratory symptoms, though often the onset is rapid with precordial pain, palpitations, dyspnoea, and feelings of weakness and oppression. Bornholm disease may be present at the same time. The pericarditis is detectable by ECG examination and sometimes by clinical signs of friction, and pericardial effusion is often demonstrable by X-ray. There is usually good recovery after an illness of several weeks, but a few patients suffer recurrent episodes of pericarditis with renewed effusions at intervals of a few months for several years. Constrictive pericarditis is a rare late sequel.

Acute myocarditis may also be heralded by fever and perhaps myalgia. Illness can be severe with dyspnoea, congestive failure, tachycardia, arrhythmias, and sometimes heart block, often with associated pericarditis. ECG changes and sometimes enzyme abnormalities reflect the myocarditis which is sometimes difficult to distinguish from myocardial infarction. The stormy, febrile illness may last for several weeks or months. Recovery may be complicated by relapsing or persisting illness. Mortality is low (< 1 per cent), but death can occur either in the acute stage or later.

Virological diagnosis. Virological tests can be helpful, especially for differential diagnosis of acute cases in young adults without previous cardiac illness or signs of previous vascular disease. Faeces should be collected for attempted isolation of virus as early as possible in the illness; a throat swab in viral transport medium may also yield virus but only if collected during the first few days of febrile illness. Pericardial fluid, if available, can also be a source of virus. Since virus has often ceased to be excreted by the time the patient comes under examination, paired acute and convalescent sera should be taken for tests for antibodies to group B coxsackieviruses (it is impracticable to test serologically for the numerous other enteroviruses unless the type has been identified by virus isolation). Virus isolation can also be attempted with fragments of cardiac biopsy tissue, if available, and with post-mortem myocardium or pericardial fluid. Group B coxsackieviruses predominate as the identifiable cause at all age groups, though the importance of group A Coxsackieviruses is probably underestimated because of the special difficulties of testing for most of them in newborn mice; echoviruses are identified in a few cases, especially in young children.

Chronic cardiac disease. Recurrent and constrictive pericarditis have been referred to above. Congestive cardiomyopathy of adults is reported to be often associated with unusually high titres of antibodies to group B coxsackieviruses, inflammatory cells in the myocardium, and defective cellular immunity, suggesting that a minority of patients characterized by this immune defect may be predisposed to develop congestive cardiomyopathy as a result of the infection which in most persons does not lead to heart damage. There are conflicting reports of the possible relationship of these infections to non-streptococcal 'rheumatic' heart disease. Immunofluorescence tests have been reported to show coxsackieviral antigen in diseased endocardium and heart valves, and there are suggestions that the virus may also damage the aorta and coronary vessels. A relationship to myocardial infarction has not been satisfactorily confirmed.

Myositis; Bornholm disease. Bornholm disease is the common term for epidemic myalgia, epidemic pleurodynia, and 'devil's grip' because of the classical description of an early epidemic on the Danish island of Bornholm. Sporadic cases can occur, as well as those during epidemics, usually of coxsackievirus B infection, but sometimes caused by a group A coxsackievirus or rarely echovirus, especially type 6. They affect mostly children but often young adults and may involve any age. The illness usually begins suddenly with severe abdominal or thoracic pain, generally with fever and headache, and sometimes sore throat. In children the pain is commonly abdominal, often periumbilical, or right-sided, suggesting appendicitis, with superficial muscle tenderness but not usually with nausea or vomiting. In adults and older children, the pain is more often thoracic, substernal, or localized on either side, often with local intercostal tenderness and sometimes transient pleuritic friction, and often suggests pneumonia, acute pneumothorax, or cardiac infarction. Definite pericarditis or myo-pericarditis may complicate the disease, and orchitis or aseptic meningitis are less frequent complications. The association between myalgia and myocarditis is close, and a high proportion of patients with myalgia in acute viral infections have been reported to show ECG changes. The illness generally improves in a few days to full recovery in a week or so, but relapses sometimes occur.

If virological diagnosis is required, faeces should be collected for virus isolation and also paired sera for tests for the corresponding antibody.

Diseases of the gastrointestinal tract and associated organs

Diarrhoea. Although it seems reasonable to expect that viruses which infect the gut would cause diarrhoea, there is no clear evidence that enteroviruses as a group, or any particular type of enterovirus, actually do so. From time to time there are reports that an enterovirus has been isolated from the stools of infants or children involved in an outbreak of diarrhoea, and sometimes that the same virus has not been isolated from unaffected controls or not with the same frequency; and there have been reports that a relative excess of or even multiple infections with enteroviruses have been found in diarrhoeal children. But there are also reports to the contrary, and it is possible that these enteroviruses merely reflect a high prevalence of enteric viral infections in these children whose diarrhoea is due to some other cause or undetected agent circulating at the same time in the group, the diarrhoea then helping to disseminate whatever infectious agents happen to be present in the faeces of the victims. Some enterovirus infections may occasionally be accompanied by mild gastrointestinal upset, but perhaps the extent of damage by enteroviruses to the rapidly replaced cells of the gastrointestinal tract is not sufficient to disturb normal function in most persons.

Hepatitis. Echovirus 6 and coxsackievirus A10 have been isolated from patients in outbreaks of hepatitis, but as with diarrhoea (above), these enteroviruses may merely represent 'epidemiological passengers' in hepatitis due to another agent. Hepatitis A virus (see page 5.116) has the properties of an enterovirus and shares the epidemiology of enteroviruses, except for its inability to be cultivated in the laboratory by the methods successful with enteroviruses. Severe and often necrotic hepatitis is a typical feature of the generalized infections, usually with coxsackieviruses, which may affect newborn infants (see below).

Pancreatitis. Acute pancreatitis is a rare manifestation of infection with coxsackieviruses, mainly of type B4 but occasionally of other types. Coxsackie B3 and B4 antibodies have been reported as more prevalent in cases of recent acute pancreatis than in controls, and raised serum and/or urine amylase levels suggesting pancreatic damage were reported in about a quarter of cases in outbreaks of coxsackievirus B5 and A9 infection. Although rarely recognized as a complication of enteroviral infection of man, pancreatitis is a characteristic effect of group B coxsackieviruses in experimentally infected mice.

Diabetes mellitus. Although reports are conflicting, there is growing support for the view, based on finding an excess of coxsackieviral antibodies, that insulin-dependent diabetes mellitus (see Section 10) can be a late consequence of infection particularly with type B4 coxsackievirus. Persons with HLA-A8 or W15 antigens appear to be at higher risk of developing diabetes after coxsackievirus B4 infection. One case has been reported of an infant with acute coxsackievirus B5 infection complicated by glycosuria and hyperglycaemia, with partial remission for a few months and then development of insulin-dependent diabetes; this child had a high-risk HLA haplotype (B18 DRw3). Further work may throw more light on the role of these and possibly other viruses in causing acute onset diabetes, especially in early life.

Acute conjunctivitis

The ability of some enteroviruses to cause infections of the eye was hardly recognized until the sudden pandemic appearance of acute haemorrhagic conjunctivitis in several countries of Africa and Southeast Asia in 1969. Infection spread to many other countries during the next few years but failed to establish itself in northern Europe, Australia, New Zealand or the Americas. From 1970, epidemics of similar disease but due to a different enterovirus were reported from Singapore and Hong Kong, 'Picornavirus epidemic conjunctivitis' has been proposed as a term to cover both these diseases, distinguishing them from epidemic keratoconjunctivitis due to adenoviruses.

Acute haemorrhagic conjunctivitis. This term was applied to a pandemic disease from which a hitherto unknown enterovirus, type 70, was isolated and shown to be the cause. It was characterized by explosive outbreaks in densely populated areas. Spread of the highly contagious infection within the family was common, transmitted mainly via contaminated fingers and fomites, and spread within eye clinics was reported. Onset is sudden after a short incubation period of about 24 hours. A gritty, painful eye with lachrymation becomes red and inflamed with acute subconjunctival haemorrhage complicating the severe, blinding conjunctivitis. Corneal involvement is slight and transient. Both eyes are usually involved. Despite the severe, incapacitating acute illness, complete recovery is usual within a week or two. Neurological complications, mainly acute lumbar radiculomyelopathy, were reported from Bombay. Enterovirus 70 can be isolated from conjunctival swabs or scrapings or sometimes from the throat or faeces by inoculating appropriate cell cultures.

Epidemic conjunctivitis due to coxsackievirus A24. This has been mainly reported from the Far East, sometimes concurrently with enterovirus 70 epidemics. The acute conjunctivitis varies from mild to severe but subconjunctival haemorrhage is unusual. The disease tends to be rather less severe than that due to enterovirus 70 infection and the prognosis is good. Neurological complications have not been reported. The virus spreads like enterovirus 70 by eye–hand–formite routes, and can be isolated from the eye or throat.

Infections of the unborn and newborn child

Viraemic enterovirus infections in pregnancy may reach the fetus, but significant developmental defects rarely ensue. Serological studies in the USA showed somewhat more evidence of coxsackievirus B infections in infants with congenital heart disease than in controls, and also in the mothers of infants with cardiovascular abnormalities than in the mothers of normal controls.

Perinatal and neonatal disease. The effects of intrauterine infection range from a silent process without obvious disease to severe, generalized infection usually due to a group B coxsackievirus and affecting particularly the liver, nervous system, and heart, which is often fatal. Maternity and neonatal units are vulnerable to outbreaks after introduction of infection by a patient or member of staff whose symptoms have often been minor or inapparent. Several such outbreaks with deaths were caused by echovirus 11 in Britain in 1978. Features of severe enterovirus infections can be difficult to differentiate from bacterial sepsis, but a viral aetiology is suggested when birth was not associated with trauma or other factors known to predispose to bacterial infection, when bacteriological tests are negative, when birth took place during a community or hospital outbreak of enterovirus infection, or when the mother has a history of febrile illness within a week of the birth.

Usual presenting features are fever and gastrointestinal disturbances (feeding difficulty, abdominal distension, vomiting, diarrhoea), often with lethargy or irritability and occasionally convulsive seizures. Hepatomegaly may be accompanied by jaundice. A maculo-papular skin rash often appears after a few days; the rash may be petechial with thrombocytopoenia, and this carries a poor prognosis. Disseminated intravascular coagulation and haemorrhages may occur. The throat is often red, and tachycardia and tachypnoea may be observed, suggesting cardiac involvement. Other effects include meningitis or meningoencephalitis, mild or severe respiratory infection including interstitial pneumonitis, carditis, hepatitis, pancreatitis, focal adrenal cortical necrosis, and renal medullary haemorrhage which has been reported particularly in type 11 echovirus infections.

Leucocytosis with polymorph preponderance is common, resembling bacterial infection. The cerebrospinal fluid often shows pleocytosis and virus may be isolable from it, even though clinical signs of meningitis are often absent. Thrombocytopoenia and liver enzyme elevations may be found.

Prematurity, low birth weight, and onset of the illness within the first week of life are factors which increase the risk of the most severe forms of disease. Later in infancy meningitis and acute carditis are the major presentations of enterovirus infections which more often produce only minor febrile or respiratory illness or may be symptomless.

Other diseases due to enteroviruses

Orchitis. Acute orchitis occasionally complicates Bornholm disease due to group B coxsackieviruses but rarely occurs as an isolated syndrome. Coxsackievirus B5 has been isolated from testicular biopsy of a young adult with acute orchitis.

Renal disease. Echovirus 9 and coxsackievirus B4 infections have been found in children with acute glomerulonephritis. Serological evidence of coxsackievirus B5 infection has been reported in patients with acute oliguric renal failure. Evidence of coxsackievirus A4 and group B infections has been found in children with the haemolytic-uraemic syndrome. Renal medullary haemorrhage has been reported in infections with echoviruses of types 6, 19, and particularly type 11. These renal syndromes appear to be rare effects of enteroviruses.

Parotitis. Parotitis has been reported in coxsackievirus B3 infection but it is a rare manifestation of enterovirus infection.

Infectious lymphocytosis. An untyped enterovirus was isolated from children in an institutional outbreak of acute infectious lymphocytosis.

CONTROL OF ENTEROVIRUS INFECTIONS

Personal prophylaxis

Specific vaccines are available for the prophylaxis of poliovirus infections but are impracticable for the numerous other enteroviruses. The only general measures to minimize the risk of infection are adoption of high standards of personal hygiene and avoidance, as far as possible, of the consumption of faecally polluted food or drink unless adequately cooked or boiled or chlorinated, and of contagion from likely excretors such as young and sick children.

Poliomyelitis vaccination. For individual protection, or in any country where paralytic poliomyelitis has become a serious or epidemic public health problem, the essential preventive measure is immunization by vaccine before exposure to virulent virus is likely. Because there are three antigenic types of poliovirus, the vaccine must contain all three antigens. Two effective vaccines exist (Table 6), inactivated (developed by Salk and others) and live attenuated (developed by Sabin and others).

Table 6   Characteristics of poliomyelitis vaccines

Characteristics	Live attenuated vaccine	Inactivated vaccine
Usual seed viruses	attenuated (Sabin strains)	virulent
Usual substrate	human diploid cells	monkey kidney cells
Combined formulation with bacterial antigens	no	possible
Route of administration	oral × 3	injection × 3
Immunity produced:		
systemic	IgA, IgM, IgG	IgM, IgG (IgA)
local (gut)	IgA	no
Later doses required	yes, 'plug gaps'	yes, boosters
Reliability of effect	uncertain in infants in tropics; no effect if already immune	reliable if antigenicity is satisfactory
Spread to contacts	yes	no
Reversion towards virulence	rare and slight	not applicable
Vaccine-associated paralysis*	$0-2 \times 10^{-6}$ in recipients $(0.1-0.6) \times 10^{-6}$ in contacts	not applicable
Use in immuno-deficient persons	contra-indicated	acceptable

* maximal estimates

Inactivated poliovirus vaccine contains all three polioviruses, grown in bulk and inactivated by formaldehyde. It is given as a primary course of three intramuscular injections each of 1 ml with an interval of six to eight weeks between the first two and preferably a longer interval of about six months before the third. Further boosting injections are required at school entry and between 15 and 19 years. The vaccine elicits IgM, IgG, and IgA serum antibodies but no detectable oro-intestinal secretory IgA antibody. It therefore effectively prevents systemic invasion by poliovirus and thus prevents paralytic disease. It decreases shedding of virus from the throat during infection, possibly by inhibiting the access of virus via the antibody-containing bloodstream from the gut to the throat, but does not prevent silent alimentary infection by polioviruses. It may therefore minimize oropharyngeal spread of virus in conditions of good hygiene where the faecal–oral route is less important, but is unlikely to suppress circulation of poliovirus in less favoured populations. Inactivated vaccine poses no threat of potential mutation and reversion towards virulence. It can thus be used to attempt to protect immunodeficient and immunodepressed persons. Because the antigen is injected preformed, it can boost the immunity of persons who already have antibody, even as a legacy of previous alimentary infection with natural or attenuated vaccine virus, who would probably be refractory to infection by, and immune response to, oral live vaccine. Disadvantages of inactivated vaccine are its cost, the need for injection, uncertainty of response and of persistence of protective antibody levels in many recipients which necessitates later booster injections, and the theoretical danger of paralytic consequences if the inactivation procedure were inadequate. In practice, inactivated vaccine is mainly used in a few developed countries which achieve high immunization rates and which have successfully controlled poliomyelitis except for occasional cases or outbreaks involving mainly members of cultural groups which reject immunization or are inaccessible to preventive health care. The primary course of immunization can also be conveniently given by a combined 'quadruple' vaccine available in some countries which includes the diphtheria, tetanus, and pertussis antigens appropriate for infant immunization.

Oral life attenuated vaccine attempts to colonize the gut successively with strains of the three poliovirus types. These are generally given as a convenient mixture of the three on each of three occasions at intervals of not less than a month in order to minimize interference between strains. In some countries the first dose is of monovalent type 1 vaccine in order to ensure early protection against the most virulent of the polioviruses. The vaccine virus elicits formation of IgM, IgA, and IgG serum antibodies but also secretory IgA in the alimentary tract and thus renders the gut refractory to reinfection by virus of the same type. It can thus directly suppress circulation of natural polioviruses in the community, though not necessarily completely since, even after natural infections, transient silent reinfections of the gut can occur.

Infection by vaccine virus leads to a period of excretion of progeny virus which has an opportunity to spread and add to the immunity of unvaccinated contacts. This progeny virus often shows slight reversion towards higher virulence and can rarely cause paralytic disease in non-immune contacts, usually parents of vaccinated children. It is therefore advisable to give oral vaccine at the same time to the parents of a child under immunization, if they have not themselves been previously immunized and their immune status is uncertain, in order that the fully attenuated vaccine virus has the first opportunity to infect and immunize them. Very rare cases of paralysis occur in recipients of vaccine, but these associated illnesses are not necessarily or always due to the vaccine. Every such case should be reported and investigated fully, but international studies to date confirm that 'poliomyelitis vaccines (oral) made from the Sabin attenuated strains are among the safest vaccines in use today' (World Health Organization 1976).

Additional doses of vaccine are recommended at school entry and later, but these do not act as true 'boosts' but merely provide an opportunity for infection by vaccine of any type which has not previously managed to infect and thereby immunize. Oral vaccine confers additional and immediate protection against infection with natural virus through viral interference, and this can be valuable in control of outbreaks. Because of its ease of administration (e.g. as drops on a sugar lump), relative cheapness and stability, oral live vaccine is used in most countries of the world. Unfortunately, in some countries with warm climates it fails to immunize a proportion of recipients, possibly because of interference by pre-existing infection with the prevalent enteric viruses of these areas, but more probably because of immunoglobulin-like inhibitors in infant's saliva. Repetition with additional doses of vaccine combats this problem, which is under study because of its importance in many tropical developing countries where efficient protection of infants is very important. Oral live vaccine is contra-indicated in persons who are immunodeficient or immunosuppressed since paralytic poliomyelitis, chronic progressive poliomyelitis, and prolonged excretion of poliovirus may result. Protection by inactivated vaccine is advisable for these children and their household contacts.

Community preventive measures

General measures. These comprise the usual hygiene and sanitation appropriate to reduce faecal pollution and the spread of enteric infections and to ensure that water supplies are uncontaminated or adequately disinfected, e.g., by chlorination. Enteroviruses survive through many of the sewage treatment procedures devised to reduce or eliminate pathogenic bacteria, and the growth of human populations with limited water supplies which necessitate recycling and reuse of water, often from a supply contaminated by effluent from a community upstream, is a cause of current concern and research in case enteroviruses can thus be transmitted and cause infections or outbreaks in recipient populations.

Immunization policy. Routine vaccination of all infants against poliomyelitis is recommended in countries where epidemic poliomyelitis has emerged. Special efforts may be required to identify and offer vaccine to groups with high susceptibility, e.g. those which have not accepted vaccine through ignorance or prejudice. Antibody surveys help to identify susceptible groups and to direct the vaccination programme generally. Consideration should be given to the advisability of poliomyelitis vaccination for any traveller to an area where 'traveller's diarrhoea' is likely, or where typhoid or cholera vaccination, or passive protection against hepatitis A is considered necessary, if the traveller's immune status is in doubt (e.g. if not previously immunized against poliomyelitis).

Outbreak control. Because silent infections outnumber those with paralysis or meningitis, poliovirus must be considered to have spread more widely than the distribution of clinical cases suggests. One specific measure which can be invoked is administration of attenuated oral vaccine (trivalent or monovalent of the same type as the epidemic strain) to known contacts, to secondary contacts, and to entire communities, with priority to young children (excluding older persons if there are good grounds for considering these older age groups to be immune). Faecal samples for virus isolation should be taken from representative cases and from others in the community before they receive vaccine. If possible, representative blood samples should also be collected for studies of the pre-vaccination antibody status of the population.
Poliomyelitis is one of the diseases under surveillance by the World Health Organization: national administrations should report outbreaks. Within countries, cases of paralytic poliomyelitis should be notified on clinical criteria. Where possible they should be subject to virological investigation (at least by stool culture) and the results of these tests should also be reported. In countries with good facilities, cases of aseptic meningitis should likewise be investigated both by stool culture and serologically. In developing countries, where epidemic poliomyelitis has not yet become a

problem but the use of the vaccine is under consideration, surveys of the crippling sequelae may provide a measure of the impact of poliomyelitis, e.g. 7 per 100 000 schoolchildren equivalent to an annual attack rate of 28 per 100 000 in a recent survey of paralysis in Ghana.

It is important to investigate virologically as far as possible any case of paralysis which involves a recent recipient or contact of poliomyelitis vaccine in order to distinguish those whose illness has some cause other than the vaccine, and to give early warning of defective vaccine (in most countries rigorous testing before release makes this highly improbable).

As mentioned above, antibody surveys can guide the most effective and economic use of vaccine to protect groups shown to require it. Continuing serological surveillance provides a useful check on the success of the vaccination programme after control of the disease has made surveillance by notifying actual cases of poliomyelitis ineffective: in a developed country it should be unnecessary to wait for the appearance of cases to signal an inadequate state of immunity.

References

Grist, N. R., Bell, E. J., and Assaad, F. (1978). Enteroviruses in Human Disease. In *Progress in medical virology* (ed. J. L. Melnick) **24**, 114, Karger, Basel.
La Force, F. M., Lichnevski, M. S., Keja, J., and Henderson, R. H. (1980). Clinical survey techniques to estimate prevalence and annual incidence of poliomyelitis in developing countries. *Bull. Wld Hlth Org.* **58**, 609.
Melnick, J. L. (1978). Advantages and disadvantages of killed and live poliomyelitis vaccines. *Bull. Wld Hlth Org.* **56**, 21.
World Health Organization (1976). The relation between acute persisting spinal paralysis and poliomyelitis vaccine (oral); results of a WHO enquiry. *Bull. Wld Hlth Org.* **53**, 319.

Stool viruses

C. R. Madeley

Introduction. Acute non-bacterial diarrhoea in infants is common throughout the world. A proportion will be due to parasites and non-infective causes, but the majority appear to be infective and, in the absence of demonstrable pathogenic bacteria, a virus (or viruses) is presumed to be the cause. Despite several careful studies, however, no one virus has been found with sufficient frequency to be labelled as the culprit. Nevertheless a variety of viruses has been recovered from stools by isolating them in cell culture, and these include various serotypes of enteroviruses, reoviruses, and adenoviruses. Occasionally echoviruses and adenoviruses have been recovered from common-source outbreaks but the serotypes involved (echovirus types 18 and 19, adenovirus 7) are themselves not uncommon and may have taken the opportunity to spread in a closed community.
The absence of any candidate causative viruses was remedied in the early 1970s by the use of the electron microscope and, initially, complex preparative techniques. Two new viruses were detected: Norwalk agent in 1971 by immune electron microscopy in the USA and rotavirus in sections of duodenal biopsy in Australia. It was soon found that rotavirus could be observed directly in extracts of faeces using the simple negative contrast technique, and a search for these and other viruses began wherever virologists could find an adequate electron microscope.
The list of different new viruses has gradually lengthened, and the search has been helped by similar viruses usually being found sooner or later in the faeces of domestic animals with diarrhoea, sooner in the case of rotaviruses and later with some of the other viruses.
The list of new 'stool' viruses discovered by electron microscopy since 1977 now includes, as well as Norwalk and rotavirus, astrovirus, calicivirus, coronavirus, and a variety of 'small round viruses' (SRVs). All fail to grow in the routine cell cultures in which

enteroviruses, reoviruses, and adenoviruses can be grown readily from stools. The list of new viruses may still be incomplete but some older viruses can also be detected. Occasionally reoviruses, which closely resemble rotaviruses and belong to the same family, are seen but these grow in cell cultures. More frequently, seemingly typical adenoviruses may be found in large numbers but fail to grow in cell cultures. This paradox is discussed further below.

Finally, typical lollipop-shaped bacteriophages are frequently observed in human faeces, sometimes in very large numbers and some of the SRVs may also be bacteriophages. Neither the host bacteria nor the significance of finding them are known.

Disease associated with stool viruses. Viruses have been found in the stools of babies and young children of any consistency between 'normal' stools and severe watery diarrhoea with vomiting. Since there is a considerable spectrum in the severity and extent of any disease present, it is not easy to describe a typical syndrome, although, in the case of rotavirus, this has been attempted by several authors.

With considerable variations in the severity of the disease associated with each of the viruses, it is probably too soon to define exactly the syndrome caused by each. In particular it is important to remember that the severity of disease may vary according to the serotype involved.

Nevertheless, available evidence to date suggests that the viruses are associated with a watery diarrhoea of abrupt onset, often preceded or accompanied by vomiting, and which is normally self-limiting with a peak incidence between 12 and 18 months. Occasionally in temperate climates, and more frequently in tropical ones, babies may become more severely ill with increasing dehydration leading to circulatory collapse and death. There may be a rise in body temperature but this is not invariable and may reflect the amount of tissue damage in the gut although there is no direct evidence for this.

A mild upper respiratory tract infection which may include otitis media has been described by several authors as preceding the presence of rotavirus in the stools. This has not been described with infections due to other viruses and rotavirus has not been observed in nasopharyngeal secretions. It should be remembered however, that the methods available for its detection are not very sensitive.

Viruses involved

Rotavirus. This virus has been known by several names: duovirus, human reo-like virus (BHRLV), orbi-like virus, and infantile gastroenteritis virus (IGV). It is a comparatively large virus (see Table 1) with a characteristic surface structure that can be recognized readily. It has been found to be endemic in every country in which it has been sought and is one of the commonest viruses in man. In faeces, the number of virus particles present is often very large and the ease with which it can be recognized has focused considerable attention on it with possibly some neglect of viruses which are smaller and more difficult to recognize.

Rotavirus has been found much more frequently in the stools of children with diarrhoea than in non-diarrhoeal stools and was originally observed in the epithelial cells of duodenal biopsies taken from children with diarrhoea. The human virus, as well as animal strains, have been demonstrated to cause diarrhoea in experimental gnotobiotic newborn animals, a very artificial system. Adult volunteers may be infected only with difficulty and show little or no disease.

This is as good evidence for pathogenicity as has been obtained with the viruses infecting other body systems. However three additional observations suggest that the story is not quite so simple. Firstly, several papers have reported excretion of rotavirus by normal neonates, particularly at an age when gnotobiotic newborn animals are very susceptible. Such excretion has been reported in both breast and bottle-fed babies, although the bottle-fed infants were more likely to have diarrhoea. Secondly, a small-scale community follow-up study showed that excretion by normal neonates may also be found at home. This finding has also been indirectly confirmed by the third observation. Several serological surveys have found that between 80 per cent and 100 per cent of the population over the age of three years have antibody to rotavirus. The techniques used in these surveys included complement fixation which normally detects only short term antibodies detectable for up to a year after the stimulus. This suggests that infection with the virus is widespread and restimulus (perhaps by subclinical infection) may be common.

The picture of rotavirus ecology that is emerging is of a very common virus repeatedly assailing the body's defences (and thereby restimulating the body to produce antibody) but which comparatively rarely causes overt disease. Certainly a spectrum of disease can be observed; how much of this can be accounted for by different serotypes having greater or lesser pathogenic capacity remains to be seen. The evidence so far is not conclusive, and more work will have to be done.

Astrovirus. This virus is smaller and less easily recognized in the EM. It is less frequently observed and hitherto has not been recorded so widely in the world. The evidence linking it with childhood diarrhoea is both as strong and as weak as that for rotavirus: it is found more commonly in the stools of diarrhoeal patients than normals; it can be present in very large numbers; adult volunteers can be infected but do not develop marked symptoms; a serological survey has shown similar high proportions of antibody positives in different age groups throughout life; and morphologically similar viruses have been found in the stools of neonatal animals (lamb, pig, calf) with diarrhoea.

Table 1 Summary of stool viruses

Virus	Number of human serotypes	Found in stool of normal babies	Animal species with similar viruses	Approx. size (nm)	Infection of adult volunteers	Antibody prevalence in general population (%)
Norwalk	3	NR*	NR	27	diarrhoea	0–60
Rotavirus	4?	yes	many species	60–70	minimal infection; no diarrhoea	80–100
Adenovirus	36	yes	many species†	75	NR	NR
Astrovirus	?	yes	few species; diarrhoea caused	28	minimal infection; no diarrhoea	60–80
Calicivirus	?	yes	few species; no diarrhoea caused	31	NR	NR
SRVs	?	yes	?	25–35	NR	NR
Coronavirus	?	NR	few species; diarrhoea caused	pleomorphic 100	NR	NR
Reovirus	3	yes	many species	70–75	NR	NR

* NR = not reported   † reported widely but association with diarrhoea uncommon

Over a period of four years, astroviruses were observed with about a quarter the frequency of rotaviruses. It is not uncommon to find both viruses in the same stool but there is no evidence that a baby with a dual infection is made more ill as a result, nor that the two viruses are related.

Calicivirus. Unlike the two preceding viruses, the calicivirus was not a 'new' virus discovered by EM. Its morphology was familiar because animal strains had been recognized in cats, pigs, and sea-lions for some years previously, although no strains had been found infecting man. A human virus was first described in 1976 in preparations of faeces from a group of babies, most of whom had diarrhoea. Subsequently, caliciviruses have been found in association with common-source outbreaks of diarrhoea and vomiting as well as in the stools of normal babies. With the exception of outbreaks, the calicivirus appears to be less virulent than rotavirus or astrovirus but this variation, too, may be explained by the existence of more than one serotype.

Norwalk and related agents. Originally described in material from a school outbreak in Norwalk, Ohio, the Norwalk agent differs in at least four ways from the preceding viruses. It includes adults as well as children among those who develop symptoms; it has been found only in outbreaks; no equivalent animal strains have been described; and the amount of virus present in diarrhoeal stools is apparently very much less. This last has meant that it is very much more difficult to recognize in the EM. With a few exceptions, it has been found only in the USA. Nevertheless serological surveys in the USA have shown the gradual acquisition of antibody with age although the percentage positive at each age is appreciably lower (up to the age of 50 at least) than with rotaviruses or astroviruses. This probably means that the virus is more common than its occasional emergence as the cause of an outbreak would indicate but is less widespread than the other two viruses. Its appearance in the EM is not incompatible with its being a calicivirus but no unequivocal calicivirus particles have been observed among the Norwalk virus particles.

Viruses similar in appearance were also found in the stools of diarrhoeal patients in Hawaii and Montgomery County, Maryland. The Norwalk and Montgomery County agents have been shown to be related antigenically but Hawaii is probably unrelated. It is possible that other small round viruses (SRVs) (see below), may be part of the same group, and further investigations will reveal other characteristics in common other than looking similar in the EM.

Small round viruses (SRVs). A variety of virus-like particles may be observed by EM in a proportion of diarrhoeal and, less frequently, normal stools. They are usually convincingly virus-like in appearance and may often resemble enteroviruses in size and shape. However no virus can be grown in culture and their identity is unknown.

They can be divided into two groups by morphology, depending on whether their observed outer margin is smooth or rough. Within each of these two groups there is also some variation in size, although the particles in any one stool are usually consistent. So far, the absence of detectable unifying characteristics and the generally small amounts present in a stool specimen have made it difficult to assess their role in disease. Nevertheless it should not be forgotten that most of the common-source outbreaks in the UK, at least, have involved SRVs and earned them sobriquets like W agent, cockle virus, Ditchling agent, etc. depending on the location or presumed vehicle of infection. Some, such as the cockle virus, may have been concentrated from sewage by molluscs, as has been demonstrated to occur with enteroviruses, and others may be bacteriophages whose host bacteria are among the great variety found in the gut.

Coronavirus. Until recently, coronaviruses in man have been known only as causes of a proportion of the common cold syn-

drome, although similar viruses caused diarrhoeal disease in animals, particularly in pigs and cows. Coronavirus-like particles, similar in general structure to respiratory strains but differing in detailed morphology, have been observed in the stools of adults rather than children in the UK, India, and Australia. Prolonged excretion, lasting up to several months, can be found and this has raised doubts whether they are genuine causes of diarrhoea.

Reovirus. First discovered over 20 years ago, reoviruses remain viruses in search of a disease. They belong to the same family as rotaviruses whom they resemble closely in appearance. They can be distinguished by careful inspection and there is no doubt that the two viruses are different. There are three human serotypes and similar viruses have been isolated from animals and plants. Uncommonly, they may be directly detected in stool extracts by EM but the virus is usually grown without difficulty. In this reoviruses are unusual among the EM-detectable viruses although the numbers seen with the EM in any one stool are generally small. There is no good evidence that they cause diarrhoea.

Adenovirus. These have been left to last since they illustrate well the paradoxes in this topic. Adenoviruses have been regularly isolated from stool specimens since the advent of cell cultures made it possible, but cultured strains are rarely implicated in diarrhoea. Exceptionally adenoviruses have been isolated from common source outbreaks, but in these cases it is not clear whether the virus initiated the outbreak or was spread as a consequence of the diarrhoea. Isolates from faeces have been common serotypes (numbers 1, 2, 5, 6 and 7), and it came as a surprise, with the use of the EM on stool extracts, to find that there were a substantial number of apparently typical adenoviruses which did not grow in cell culture, were often present in very large numbers (up to 10^{11} particles per gram of faeces) and which were sometimes found as the only potentially pathogenic micro-organism common to a number of cases of diarrhoea. Further investigation confirmed that they did not grow in routine cell cultures and, although some grew, albeit not well, in other less frequently used cell types, there remained, and remains, a hard core of non-growing adenoviruses.

A major paradox in this situation is that the more virus there is in the stool, the less likely it is to grow in cell cultures. The reason for this has remained undiscovered but does not appear to be due to antibody on the virus surface, to inhibitors in the stool, or to the virus being incomplete. The most likely explanation seems to be that these non-growing strains form at least one new serotype (or a new subgroup) and there is now evidence that this is so.

About 5–8 per cent of all infant stools contain EM detectable adenoviruses and this makes them arguably the most common human virus. There are 36 different serotypes among the cultivable adenoviruses and it seems unlikely, therefore, that the non-growers will all be the same antigenic type. Their role as pathogens is still under investigation.

Diagnosis. The only method capable of detecting any type of virus in a stool is electron microscopy. This suffers from the disadvantages of being insensitive and unsuitable for screening large numbers. Other methods have therefore been developed, particularly for rotavirus, but they all depend on antibody to that particular virus being available and repeating the test for each kind of virus. These other methods include detection of partial growth in cell culture by immunofluorescence, enzyme linked immunosorbent assay (ELISA), immune adherence haemagglutination (IAHA), radioimmune assay (RIA), solid phase aggregation of coated erythrocytes (SPACE), etc. For the detection of virus, a stool specimen is always necessary and attempts have been made to find virus in other body fluids and secretions. With the exception of Norwalk agent in vomitus, these attempts have not been successful.

Tests for antibody, including those for the different classes of antibody (IgG, IgM, and IgA) are available in some laboratories and seroconversion has been demonstrated, although whether this gives any significant additional information over the recognition of virus in the stool is debatable.

In any case, due to the difficulties of interpreting the results from one stool or one patient, it is important to contact the laboratory before deciding to send the specimens.

Epidemiology. Viruses found in large numbers in the faeces are likely to be spread by the faecal–oral route, if by no other. However the acquisition of virus by neonates, including those only a few days old, makes it likely that other routes may also be involved. It is probable that adults, in particular, may spread rotavirus in respiratory droplets, and it is likely that a large outbreak affecting all ages in a town in Sweden may have been water-borne although this was not demonstrated. The methods available for detecting these viruses are still too insensitive, and we know too little of the viruses themselves for us to draw many conclusions about mechanisms of spread.

Treatment. There is no specific treatment for viruses in the gut. Treatment of any diarrhoea associated with them will be nonspecific with restoration of hydration and electrolyte balance, resting the gut by the use of oral clear fluids (solutions of glucose or sucrose plus electrolytes) and intravenous fluids if necessary, as outlined elsewhere (see Section 12).

Prevention. No vaccine is currently available to protect against any of these viruses. This is due partly to the failure to grow the viruses in cell culture and partly to an uncertainty to whom and when any vaccine should be given. Some progress has been made in obtaining a possible seed virus from the human rotavirus by passage through gnotobiotic piglets. After 13 passages the virus still carried markers for the human virus and would then grow in cultures of African green monkey kidney cells. Similar progress has not been made with the other viruses.

There is evidence from experiments in lambs that pooled human gammaglobulin administered orally gives enough protection against rotavirus to prevent illness without preventing growth of the virus in the gut or induction of seroconversion. This has yet to be tried in man and the circumstances under which it could be used have also to be defined.

References

Clarke, S. K. R., Caul, E. O., and Egglestone, S. I. (1979). The human enteric coronaviruses. *Post-grad. med. J.* **55**, 135.

Gary, G. W., Hierholzer, J. C., and Black, R. E. (1979). Characteristics of noncultivable adenoviruses associated with diarrhoea in infants: a new subgroup of human adenoviruses. *J. clin. Microbiol.* **10**, 96.

Greenberg, H. B., Valdesuso, J., Yolken, R. H., Gangarosa, E., Gary, W., Wyatt, R. G., Konno, T., Suzuki, H., Chanock, R. M., and Kapikian, A. Z. (1979). Role of Norwalk virus in outbreaks of non-bacterial gastroenteritis. *J. infect. Dis.* **139**, 564.

Holmes, I. H. (1979). Viral gastroenteritis. In *Progress in medical virology* (ed. J. L. Melnick) **25**, 1. Karger, Basel.

Madeley, C. R. (1979). Viruses in the stools. *J. clin. Path.* **32**, 1.

Scott, T. M., Madeley, C. R., Cosgrose, B. P., and Stanfield, J. P. (1979). Stool viruses in babies in Glasgow. 3. Community studies. *J. Hyg. Camb.* **83**, 469.

Taylor, P. R., Merson, M. H., Black, R. E., Mizanur Rahman, A. S. M., Yunus, M. D., Alim, A. R. M. A., and Yolken, R. H. (1980). Oral rehydration therapy for treatment of rotavirus diarrhoea in a rural treatment centre in Bangladesh. *Archs Dis. Child.* **55**, 376.

Walker-Smith, J. A. (1978). Rotavirus gastroenteritis. *Archs Dis. Child.* **53**, 355.

Rhabdoviruses: rabies and rabies-related viruses

D. A. Warrell

Virology. The *Rhabdoviridae* are a group of more than 60 rod or bullet shaped RNA viruses found in vertebrates, insects, and plants

(Fig. 1). The prototype is vesiculostomatitis virus of cattle and horses which occasionally causes an influenza-like illness in farmers or laboratory workers. A subgroup or genus of antigenically related and morphologically similar viruses are the rabies or lyssaviruses. Rabies virus itself is 180 × 75 nm. A helical single stranded protein nucleocapsid is surrounded by a protein matrix and envelope bearing surface spikes of glycoprotein about 10 nm long. The virus is readily inactivated by sunlight, ultraviolet radiation, drying, and heating especially at pHs outside the range 5–10; and by lipid solvents, 0.1 per cent trypsin, and a variety of antiseptics, but is relatively resistant to phenol. Virus isolated from naturally infected animals is known as 'street virus' or 'field virus'. Repeated intracerebral passage in rabbits produces 'fixed virus' with an incubation period uniformly shortened from 9–15 to 5–6 days, but reduced pathogenicity for other species. Strains of rabies virus were, originally, separated according to the mammal species from which they were isolated, and by their pathogenicity in different

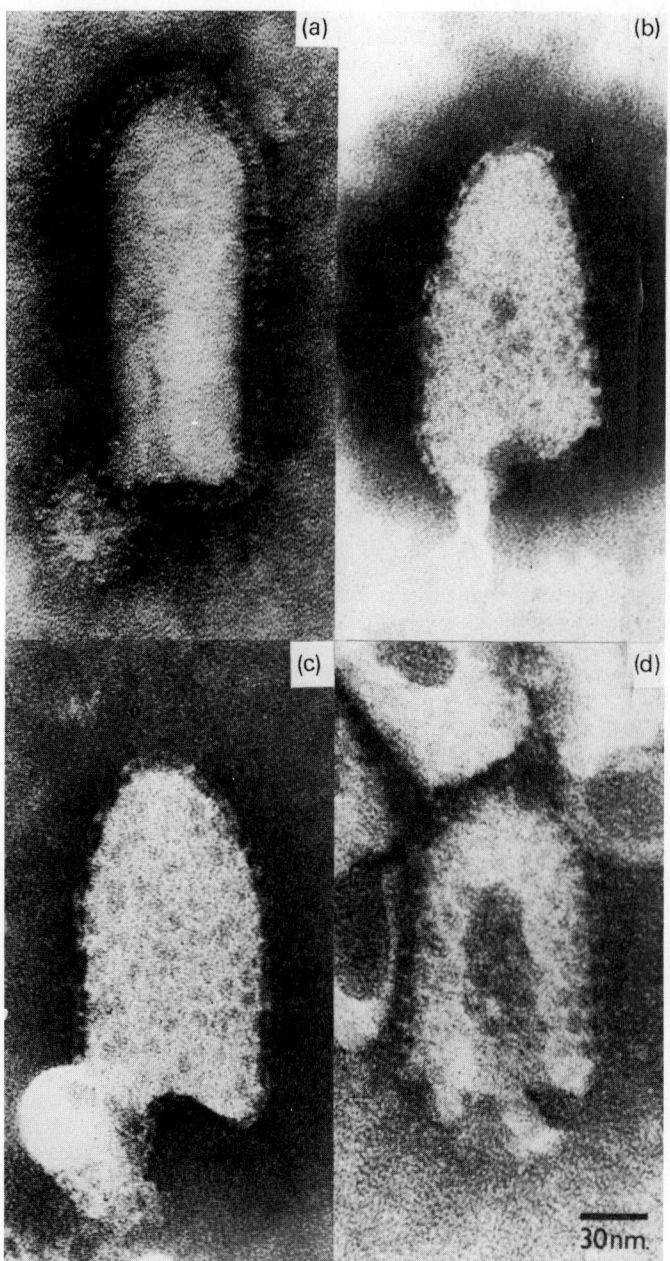

Fig. 1 Rhabdoviruses. Virions of (a) Lagos bat virus; (b) vesicular stomatitis virus; (c) rabies virus; and (d) Nigerian horse virus. (Electron micrographs by courtesy of Dr C. J. Smale and Dr Joan Crick.)

species or when inoculated by different routes; and in the case of laboratory strains by their supposed origin. Recently, the use of monoclonal antibodies against nucleocapsid and glycoprotein antigens, and other techniques have allowed the antigenic characterization of many strains of rabies virus including standard challenge virus CVS, and vaccine strains such as ERA and Flury HEP. Rabies virus is usually isolated in mice but can also be cultivated in embryonated eggs and tissue culture (e.g. BHK 21, Wi38).

Rabies-related viruses. Five rabies-related viruses have now been isolated in Africa. They are serologically related, but distinguishable by neutralization, complement fixation, fluorescent antibody, and vaccine challenge tests. *Lagos bat virus* has been isolated from fruit-eating bats in Nigeria, Central African Republic and South Africa. *Mokola virus* was isolated from shrews in Nigeria and Cameroon and from two children in Nigeria: one died with encephalomyelitis, the other had aseptic meningitis. *Obodhiang virus* was found in *Mansonia uniformis* mosquitoes in the Sudan, and *Kotonkan virus* in *Culicoides* midges in Nigeria. *Duvenhage virus* was isolated from a man who died of a rabies-like illness after being bitten by an insectivorous bat in South Africa.

Epidemiology. Rabies is endemic in most parts of the world. Rabies-free areas include the United Kingdom, Scandinavia (except Denmark), West Malaysia, Taiwan, Japan, Australia, New Zealand, Hawaii, and Antarctica. Primarily a zoonosis, rabies is spread among wild mammals by bites, and to a lesser extent by aerosol in bat caves and by eating infected prey. Each geographical area has its principal wild animal reservoir species: in the USA, skunks in the West, foxes in the East, raccoons in Florida and Georgia, and insectivorous bats in California, Texas, Florida, and elsewhere; in the Arctic, the fox *Alopex lagopus*; in Grenada and Puerto Rico, mongooses; in Trinidad, Mexico, and Central and South America, vampire bats; in most of Africa and Asia, wolves jackals, and small carnivores of the families Viverridae and Mustelidae; and In Europe, foxes, wolves, and raccoon dogs. Rabies in wild rodents has been described in USSR, Germany, Egypt, Nigeria, Thailand, and elsewhere, but its significance is controversial.

In a particular area, transmission may occur predominantly within a single species. For example, in the USA rabies in foxes, skunks, and bats exists in separate ecological compartments. Each vector may have a distinctive virus strain and method of transmission. In many parts of Africa and Asia, and in urban areas elsewhere, domestic dogs are the principal reservoir of rabies. This was the case in the United Kingdom and Japan before rabies was eradicated.

Humans are occasionally infected by wild mammals, but domestic dogs and cats are responsible in more than 90 per cent of cases worldwide. In Western Europe 86 per cent of all isolates of rabies are from foxes, yet about 75 per cent of cases of human exposure result from dog bites, a reflection of the more intimate relationship between dogs and men. Rabies control programmes can reduce the risk of rabies in domestic animals to such an extent that wild animals, such as skunks in the USA, become the major vectors. In Mexico and Central and South America bovine rabies resulting from vampire bites causes a financial loss of more than £100 million each year. In Mexico 100 000 and in Brazil 200 000 head of cattle are lost each year.

Cyclical epizootics of rabies, such as the current fox epizootic in Europe, result from an uncontrolled increase in the population of the key reservoir species. This epizootic started in Poland at the end of the Second World War, since when it has advanced at a rate of about 40 km per year. The fox is the most susceptible species to rabies, but about 3 per cent of animals survive the infection and develop immunity. In Grenada almost half the mongooses have serum neutralizing antibody. Neutralizing antibodies to Kotonkan virus are prevalent in domestic herbivores in Nigeria: it is possible that they afford some cross protection against rabies.

Incidence of human rabies. Only about 700 human deaths attributed

to rabies are reported to the World Health Organization each year, but in India alone an annual mortality of 15 000 seems likely. In Sri Lanka, the Philippines, and Thailand peak annual mortalities of 377 in 1973 (2.9/100 000 population), 383 in 1964 (1.2/100 000 population), and 322 in 1977 (0.8/100 000) respectively were reported. The actual mortalities were probably at least twice these figures. In Cali, Colombia, almost 2 per cent of a large series of autopsies showed evidence of rabies. In the UK, rabies was quite common in dogs and men until 1902 when it was finally eradicated. Since 1946, 15 people infected abroad (mainly in India and Pakistan) have died of rabies in England. Only 4 cases were reported for continental Europe (excluding USSR) in 1978 and 1979, but there were 230 cases in Turkey and 29 in Yugoslavia between 1972 and 1975. In the USA there were more than 25 human deaths each year in the 1940s but since 1960 this has decreased to less than six per year.

Transmission. Virus can penetrate broken skin and intact mucosae. Humans are usually infected when virus-laden saliva is inoculated through the skin by the bite of a rabid animal. Dog bites are common in most parts of the world (see page 6.35). For example, in New York City there are about 40 000 each year. Saliva from a rabid animal can infect if the skin is scratched or already broken. Animals can be infected by eating infected meat, but there is no documented case of this happening in man despite a 4 per cent prevalence of rabies in apparently healthy cattle slaughtered in Mexico City.

Inhalation of rabies virus may be an important mode of transmission among cave dwelling bats. In Texas, two men died of rabies after visiting caves inhabited by millions of insectivorous bats some of which were rabid, and there have been two laboratory accidents in the USA in which infection resulted from inhalation of aerosols of fixed virus. Accidental fixed virus rabies (*rage de laboratoire*) has followed vaccination with live virus, notably in Brazil in 1960 when 18 people died.

Theoretically, rabies should be communicable from person to person, for the saliva, respiratory secretions, tears, and urine of rabies patients contain virus. There have been several unsubstantiated reports in the old literature, but the only virologically documented examples were the five recently reported cases of transmission by corneal grafts in France, USA, Thailand, and Morocco. The donors had died of undiagnosed neurological diseases, Guillain–Barré syndrome, and flaccid quadriplegia. Four of the recipients developed retro-orbital headache on the side of the graft, about one month after surgery, and died of paralytic rabies. Another risk of corneal grafting is transmission of Creutzfeldt–Jacob disease. Patients who die of undiagnosed neurological illnesses are not suitable donors. Transplacental infection has been seen in animals but not in man. There are reports of successful Caesarean section and delivery of healthy babies in mothers with rabies.

Pathogenesis. Virus inoculated by a bite multiplies locally in muscle fibres, accumulates in neuromuscular and neurotendinal spindles, and, after an uncertain interval of days or weeks, gains access to peripheral nerves and is carried centripetally by the flow of axoplasm, to the dorsal root ganglia where further multiplication occurs, and on to the central nervous system where spread also occurs through the cerebrospinal fluid (CSF). This progress can be blocked experimentally by local anaesthetic, metabolic inhibitors, and nerve section. After entering the peripheral nerve, rabies virus is probably inaccessible to humoral defences, except perhaps at the dorsal root ganglion. Within the central nervous system there is viral replication on membranes of neurons and glial cells and direct transmission of virus from cell to cell. Virus also exists free within extracellular spaces. Passive centrifugal spread of virus from the CNS in the axoplasm of many peripheral nerves, including those of the autonomic nervous system, deposits virus in many tissues. These include skeletal and cardiac muscle and adrenal medulla where infection may be clinically significant, kidney, retina, cornea, pancreas, brown fat, and nerve twiglets in the hair follicles. Most important for the further transmission of rabies is the delivery of virus to the salivary and lacrimal glands, taste buds, and respiratory tract. Virus may also be shed in milk and urine. Viraemia has rarely been detected and is not thought to be significant in the pathogenesis or spread.

Immunology

Rabies infection. There is no detectable immune response until after symptoms develop, suggesting avoidance or suppression of the immune system by rabies virus. Neutralizing and fluorescent antibodies became detectable in serum after seven days and in CSF a little later, rising to high levels terminally or in survivors. Most CSF antibody is thought to be produced in the CNS but a late influx of serum antibody due to break down of the blood–brain barrier is possible. Both B lymphocytes or the antibodies they produce, and T lymphocytes acting either as helper cells in the antibody response or by interacting with virus-infected cells have been shown to be important in clearing infection from the CNS. Interferon is induced. In animals, latent infections can be reactivated by corticosteroids and stress.

Rabies vaccination. Serum antibodies appear after about seven days and interferon is induced by some vaccines. Glycoprotein composing the spikes on the surface of the virus is the only antigen capable of inducing neutralizing antibody: other viral components induce complement fixing and precipitating antibodies which are not neutralizing. The conventional view is that neutralizing antibodies are responsible for protection against subsequent challenge with rabies virus. Some experimental work in mice suggests, however, that protection is not related to serum neutralizing antibody titre, but resides in a cell-mediated cytotoxic response which is proportional to the mass of vaccine antigen used. Partially vaccinated humans and animals may die of rabies more quickly than unvaccinated controls. This 'early death' phenomenon may be explained by antibody-mediated enhancement of rabies virus replication in the CNS. Enhancement may be achieved with non-homologous cross reacting antibodies to rabies related viruses (Mokola, Lagos bat) as in the case of flaviviruses.

Rabies in animals. Any warm blooded animal can be infected with rabies, but susceptibility varies in the following decreasing order: foxes and other wild Canidae, skunks, Felidae, Veverridae, rodents, lagomorphs, man, domestic dogs, herbivores, and opossums.

Dogs show an early change in behaviour, but only about 25 per cent develop furious rabies. Clinical features include dysphagia, ptosis, altered bark, paralysis of the jaw, neck, and hind limbs, hypersalivation, congested conjunctivae, pruritus, shivering, trembling, snapping at imaginary objects, pica, and extreme restlessness causing the animal to wander miles from home. Incubation ranges from five days to 14 months, but is usually less than four months, hence the compulsory quarantine of six months imposed on dogs imported to the United Kingdom. Virus may be excreted in the saliva for three days before symptoms appear, and the animal usually dies within the next seven days. There are rare reports of chronic excretion of virus by apparently healthy dogs. Oulou Fato is a clinical variant of canine rabies seen in West Africa. It is probably caused by a strain with reduced virulence for man. The incubation is short. Progressive paralysis and diarrhoea are the dominant features. Survival of dogs may be prolonged. Rabid *foxes* lose their fear of humans and usually develop paralytic rabies. An extreme degree of furious rabies is seen in 75 per cent of affected *cats*. *Cattle* usually have paralytic symptoms with dysphagia, groaning, trembling, colic, and tenesmus. *Horses* often show furious features with sexual excitement. Hydrophobia is never seen in animals.

Clinical features in man

Incubation period ranges from four days to many years, but is between 20 and 90 days in more than 90 per cent of cases. It tends to be shorter after bites on the face (average 35 days) than after those on the limbs (average 52 days).

Prodromal symptoms. The illness usually starts with a few days of non-specific symptoms suggesting an upper respiratory tract or gastrointestinal infection or psychiatric disorder. Fever, chills, malaise, weakness, tiredness, headache, photophobia, and myalgia are common, and there is a change of mood towards anxiety, depression and irritability. A symptom which suggests impending rabies is paraesthesia or pain at the site of the healed bite wound. Subsequently, symptoms of either furious or paralytic rabies will develop, depending on whether the spinal cord or brain are predominantly infected.

Furious rabies is the commoner presentation. Most patients have the diagnostic symptom of hydrophobia: a combination of inspiratory muscle spasm, with or without painful laryngopharyngeal spasm, associated with terror (Fig. 2). Initially provoked by attempts to drink water, this reflex can be excited by a variety of stimuli including a draught of air ('aerophobia'), water splashed on the skin, irritation of the respiratory tract or, ultimately, the sight, sound, or even mention of water. The inspiratory spasm is violent and jerky. The neck and back are extended, the arms thrown up and the episode may end in generalized convulsions with cardiac or respiratory arrest.

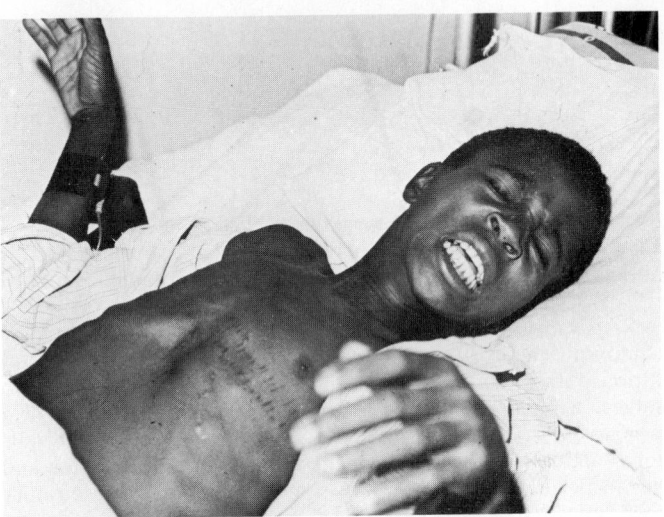

Fig. 2 Hydrophobic spasm in a 14-year-old Nigerian boy with furious rabies. Note the violent contraction of inspiratory muscles: sternomastoids and diaphragm (depressing xiphisternum).

At times there are episodes of generalized arousal, during which patients become wild, hallucinated, fugitive and, sometimes aggressive, alternating with lucid intervals. Despite these dramatic symptoms, attributable to brainstem encephalitis, neurological examination may prove surprisingly normal. Reported abnormalities include meningism, cranial nerve lesions (especially III, VI, VII, IX, X, XI, and XII), upper motor neurone lesions, fasciculation, and involuntary movements. Disturbances of the hypothalamus or autonomic nervous system are reflected by hypersalivation (Fig. 3), lacrimation, sweating, hyper- or hypotension, hyper- or hypothermia, inappropriate secretion of ADH and diabetes insipidus, and, rarely, priapism.

Without supportive treatment, about one-third of the patients will die during a hydrophobic spasm in the first few days. The rest lapse into coma and generalized flaccid paralysis and rarely survive for more than a week without intensive care.

Paralytic or dumb rabies is the form taken by less than a fifth of human cases except in the case of vampire bat transmitted rabies which is invariably paralytic. The largest reported outbreak was in Trinidad between 1925 and 1935, when there were 89 human cases: others have been described from Mexico, Guyana, Brazil, Bolivia, and Argentina. After the usual prodromal symptoms, especially fever, headache, and local paraesthesiae, flaccid paralysis develops, usually in the bitten limb, and ascends symmetrically or asymmetrically with pain and fasciculation in the affected muscles and mild sensory disturbances. Paraplegia and sphincter involvement then develop and finally fatal paralysis of deglutitive and respiratory muscles. Hydrophobia is unusual, but may be represented by a few pharyngeal spasms in the terminal phase of the illness. Even without intensive care, patients with paralytic rabies have survived for up to 30 days.

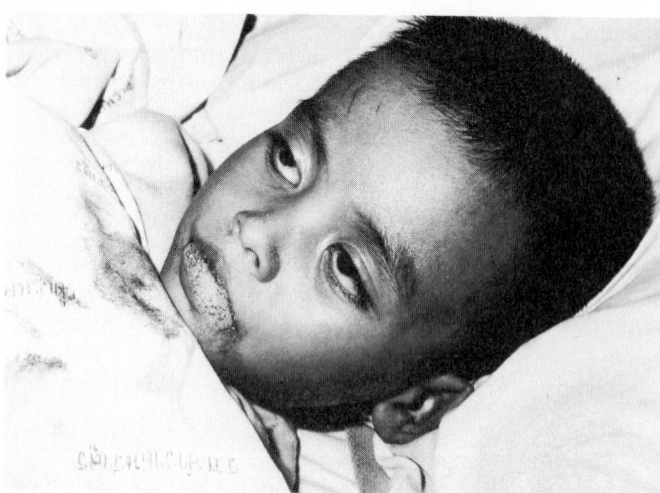

Fig. 3 Hypersalivation, sweating, and haematemesis in a 5-year-old Thai boy with furious rabies.

Other manifestations and complications. The renewed interest recently shown in the treatment of rabies encephalitis has led to better understanding of the systemic manifestations and complications of the disease.

Respiratory system. Asphyxiation and respiratory arrest may complicate the hydrophobic spasms or generalized convulsions of furious rabies, and the bulbar and respiratory paralysis of dumb rabies. Bronchopneumonia is an expected complication, and a primary rabies pneumonitis may occur. Various abnormal patterns of respiration have been described, including cluster and apneustic breathing. There are some similarities to respiratory myoclonus.

Cardiovascular system. A variety of dangerous cardiac arrhythmias has been reported including supraventricular tachycardias, sinus bradycardia, atrioventricular block, and sinus arrest. Hypotension, pulmonary oedema, and congestive cardiac failure are attributable to myocarditis.

Nervous system. Raised intracranial pressure resulting from cerebral oedema or internal hydrocephalus has been reported in a few cases, but spinal fluid opening pressure is usually normal and papilloedema rarely found. Evidence of diffuse axonal neuropathy is consistent with histological appearances of degeneration of peripheral nerve ganglia and axons.

Gastrointestinal system. 'Stress' ulcers and Mallory–Weiss syndrome are possible explanations for the haematemesis often reported in rabies.

Differential diagnosis. Rabies should be suspected whenever a patient develops severe neurological symptoms after being bitten by a mammal in a rabies endemic area. Hydrophobia is pathognomonic of rabies and is unlikely to be mimicked accurately by the hysteric. Inspiratory spasms with associated emotional response are produced by asking the patient to swallow accumulated saliva or by directing a draught of air onto the face. Patients are sometimes misreferred to otolaryngologists or psychiatrists.

Tetanus, which can also follow an animal bite, is similar to rabies in some respects, especially the pharyngeal form of cephalic tetanus

('hydrophobic tetanus'). It is distinguished by its shorter incubation period (usually less than 15 days), the presence of trismus, the persistence of muscle rigidity between spasms, the absence of meningo-encephalitis (CSF is universally normal), and a better prognosis. Hydrophobia does not occur in other encephalitides: the combination of intense brainstem encephalitis and furious behaviour in a conscious patient would be most unlikely except in rabies.

Paralytic rabies can be confused with other causes of ascending (Landry-type) paralysis. Post-vaccinal encephalomyelitis (see below) usually develops within two weeks of the first dose of the older types of rabies vaccines. In poliomyelitis sensory disturbances are absent and fever rarely persists after paralysis has developed. Examination of CSF may help to distinguish acute 'infectious' polyneuritis (Guillain–Barré syndrome). *Herpes simiae* (B virus) encephalomyelitis is transmitted by monkey bites, but the incubation period (3–4 days) is usually shorter than in rabies. Vesicles may be found in the monkey's mouth and at the site of the bite. The diagnosis can be confirmed virologically and the patient treated with acyclovir (see page 5.64).

Pathology. Brain, spinal cord, and peripheral nerves show ganglion cell degeneration, perineural and perivascular mononuclear cell infiltration, neuronophagia, and glial nodules. Inflammatory changes are most marked in the midbrain and medulla in furious rabies, and in the spinal cord in paralytic rabies. Negri bodies which are diagnostic intracytoplasmic inclusions containing virus, are found in up to 80 per cent of cases especially in hippocampal pyramidal cells and in cerebellar Purkinje cells. Neuronolysis is less severe than in some other viral encephalitides, suggesting that the appalling prognosis of rabies is not determined solely by central nervous system damage. There is also focal degeneration in salivary and lacrimal glands, pancreas, adrenal medulla, and lymph nodes. An interstitial myocarditis with round cell infiltration is found in about 25 per cent of cases (Fig. 4).

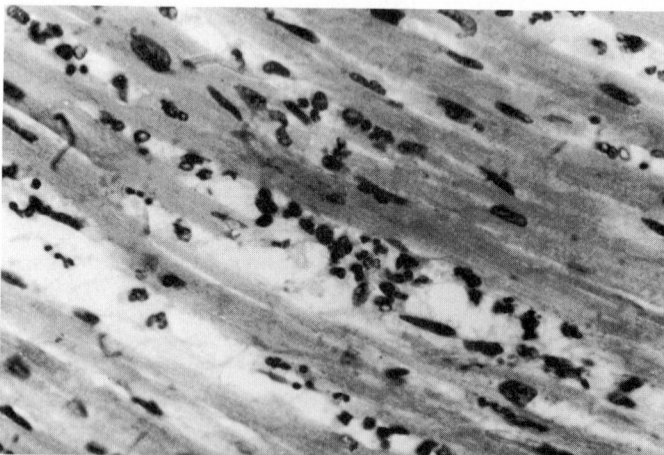

Fig. 4 Interstitial myocarditis in a patient with rabies who presented with supraventricular tachycardia. Myocytes show nuclear swelling and focal degeneration of nuclei and fibres with interstitial mixed inflammatory cell infiltration. Haematoxylin and eosin stain. (× 400)

Laboratory diagnosis. In the animal responsible for the bite, rabies can be confirmed within a few hours by immunofluorescence of brain impression smears or by histological examination for Negri bodies, and in about one week by intracerebral inoculation of mice. Inclusions resembling Negri bodies may sometimes be found in animals suffering from other diseases. In Africa, neutralization tests should be used whenever possible to confirm the diagnosis of rabies, because the rabies fluorescent antibody test is positive with Mokola and Lagos bat viruses.

In humans rabies can be confirmed early in the illness by immunofluorescence of nerve twiglets in skin biopsies, corneal impression smears (Fig. 5), or brain biopsies; but these tests are often falsely negative. During the first week of illness virus may be isolated from saliva, brain, CSF, and urine. Fluorescent and other antibodies are not usually detectable in serum or CSF before the eighth day. The discovery of CSF antibody suggests a diagnosis of rabies rather than post-vaccinal encephalomyelitis.

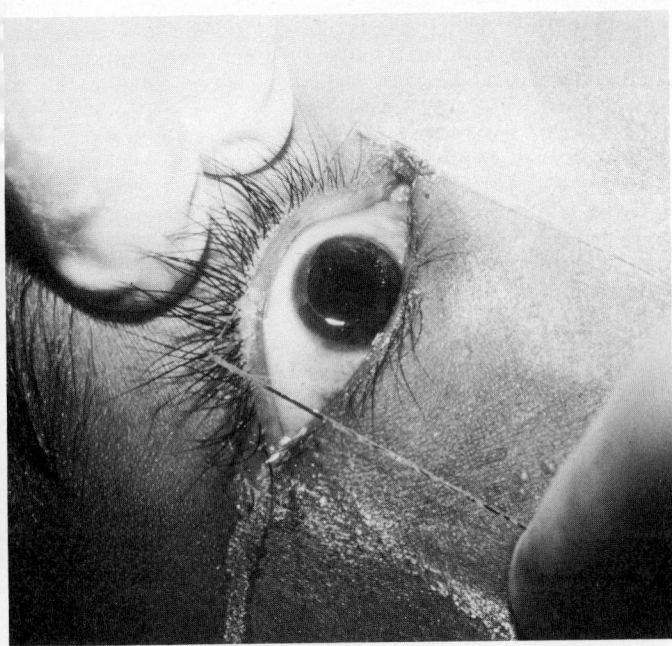

Fig. 5 Technique for obtaining corneal impression smears in which rabies antigen may occasionally be demonstrable by immunofluorescence during life. A glass slide is applied lightly and repeatedly.

Treatment. Patients with rabies must be heavily sedated and given adequate analgesia to relieve their pain and terror. Rabies was formerly regarded as a universally fatal disease, but there have now been three well-documented cases of recovery. The most recent was a New York laboratory technician who inhaled an aerosol of fixed virus. These successes were achieved by intensive care, which is the only known method for prolonging or saving life once rabies encephalomyelitis has developed.

The aim is to prevent complications such as cardiac arrhythmias, cardiac and respiratory failure, raised intracranial pressure, convulsions, fluid and electrolyte disturbances including diabetes insipidus and inappropriate secretion of anti-diuretic hormone, and hyperpyrexia. Antiserum, antiviral agents, corticosteroid, and other immunosuppressants have proved useless.

Prognosis. Despite the limited success of intensive care, the prognosis of rabies encephalomyelitis is still virtually hopeless. At the time of the bite, however, before virus has invaded the nervous system, correct cleaning of the wound (see below) and the use of post-exposure immunization reduce the risk of rabies developing from about 30–50 per cent in untreated cases to less than 5 per cent. The risk varies with the biting species and the site and severity of the bites. It is highest following head bites by proved rabid wolves, when the mortality in unvaccinated people may exceed 60 per cent.

Prevention and control

In countries where rabies is endemic. Control strategy is based on gathering information about the prevalence and host range of rabies in wild and domestic animals. This requires laboratory facilities for confirming the diagnosis. Domestic animals can be protected by yearly vaccination. Dogs are muzzled and kept off the streets, strays are eliminated. People should be discouraged from keeping wild carnivores, such as skunks, raccoons, coatimundis, and mongooses, as pets. Unnecessary contact with mammals

should be avoided (e.g. stroking stray dogs, exploring bat infested caves). Reduction of wild animal reservoir populations may be attempted, but this is difficult to achieve and likely to cause ecological chaos. An alternative approach is to attempt the vaccination of key reservoir species by using live oral vaccines distributed in bait. Rabies is most likely to be controlled or eradicated where the principal reservoir is the domestic dog, as in nineteenth century Britain, Malaysia, and Japan.

Pre- and post-exposure vaccination. Humans who are particularly at risk, such as vets and dog catchers, can be given pre-exposure vaccination, and those bitten by animals must be given post-exposure prophylaxis (see below). Clinics and dispensaries must be adequately supplied with vaccine and antiserum to deal with this problem, but in the developing countries where rabies is most prevalent this may be difficult because of expense, supply, and preservation.

Education and publicity about rabies is always needed. For example, in Bangkok 88 per cent of a series of 328 patients admitted with rabies had not received vaccine, so were presumably ignorant of the risk of dog bite.

In countries where rabies is not endemic. *Pre-exposure vaccination* is needed only by those who handle imported animals before and during quarantine in kennels, stables, farms, zoos, and laboratories; those who work with rabies virus in laboratories; and those who intend to travel to rabies-endemic areas and will be particularly at risk (e.g. veterinarians, cave explorers, naturalists, and animal collectors).

Post-exposure prophylaxis may be required for people who were exposed to the risk of rabies while abroad. Travellers should be educated to seek local medical help if they are bitten, scratched, or licked by animals. Action may then be taken to confirm rabies in the animal, and post-bite prophylaxis can be started promptly, depending on what is known about the local prevalence of rabies.

Many travellers wait until they return to their homeland, sometimes weeks or months after the bite, before asking for medical advice. It is important to determine the precise geographical location of the exposure; when it occurred; its severity—whether it was a bite or lick on broken skin; the nature, appearance, behaviour, and fate of the biting animal and, if possible, whether it had been vaccinated against rabies within the last year. This information may allow proper assessment of risk; but if there is any doubt the patient should be given full post-exposure prophylaxis even if the bite is several months old.

Pre-exposure prophylaxis. Only vaccines without risk of dangerous side effects can be used. Human diploid cell strain vaccine (Merieux) (HDCSV) is the vaccine of choice, given in two doses of 1 ml intramuscularly (or 0.1 ml intradermally), four weeks apart, followed by yearly boosters. The neutralizing antibody response is so predictable that normally it need not be checked in individual cases.

Post-exposure prophylaxis. The aim is to neutralize inoculated virus before it can enter the nervous system. The following measures must be taken as soon as possible.

Wound cleaning is effective in killing virus in superficial wounds and is therefore of great importance, but is often neglected. As first aid, the wound should be scrubbed with soap or detergents and water under a running tap for at least five minutes. Foreign material should be removed and the wound rinsed with plain water. A virucidal agent such as 40–70 per cent alcohol, tincture of iodine, or 0.01 per cent aqueous iodine should be applied liberally. Quaternary ammonium compounds, such as 1 per cent benzalkonium chloride or cetrimonium bromide may become contaminated with pathogens such as *Pseudomonas cepacia* and are no longer recommended. Hospital treatment of wounds involves thorough exploration, debridement, and irrigation of deep wounds, if necessary under local or general anaesthetic. Suturing should be avoided or delayed and the wound should be left without occlusive dressings. Attention should be given to the range of pathogens particularly associated with mammal bites. These include *Clostridium tetani*, *Pasteurella multocida*, *Leptospira* spp., *Spirillium minor*, *Streptobacillus moniliformis*, *Francisella tularensis*, *Yersinia enterocolitica*, *Eikenella corrodens*, *Haemophilus aphrophilus*, *Mycobacterium marinum*, *M. leprae*, *Erysipelothrix indiosa*, *E. rhusiopathiae*, *Actionobacillus lignieresii*, CDCs 'alpha numeric' Gram-negative bacteria, cat scratch fever agent, orf, and *Herpesvirus simiae* (B virus) (see relevant articles for details).

The commoner mammal bite pathogens are sensitive to benzyl penicillin, amoxycillin, or cefoxitin.

Specific prophylaxis consists of active and passive immunization. The indications are given in Table 1.

Table 1 Specific post-exposure prophylaxis for use in a rabies-endemic area

Nature of exposure	Circumstances of bite and species involved	Treatment
Minor exposure Licks of the skin Scratches or abrasions Minor bites (covered areas of arms, trunk, and legs)	(a) unprovoked attack by cat or dog	*start vaccine*: stop treatment if animal remains healthy for five days or if brain fluorescent antibody test proves negative: administer serum upon positive diagnosis and complete the course of vaccine
	(b) attack by wild animal, or domestic cat or dog unavailable for observation	*serum and vaccine*
Major exposure Licks of mucosa Major bites (multiple or on face, head, finger or neck)	(a) or (b) above	*serum and vaccine*: stop if domestic cat or dog remains healthy for five days, or if any animal's brain fluorescent antibody test proves negative

Active immunization. Nervous tissue vaccines introduced by Pasteur in the 1880s and developed by Semple and Hempt are still the most widely used worldwide; 2–5 ml doses of a 5 per cent suspension are given on 14–30 consecutive days: the abdomen is often used as a suitable target for the many subcutaneous injections. These vaccines produce neuroparalytic reactions including post-vaccinal encephalomyelitis in about 1 in 2000 courses (see below). *Duck embryo* vaccine (DEV), which is still recommended in the USA, produced reactions in only 1 in 32 000 courses, with 15 per cent mortality, but the neutralizing antibody response was inadequate in up to 20 per cent of those vaccinated. DEV is given in 21 daily (or 7 twice daily then 7 daily) subcutaneous injections of 1 ml followed by boosters on days 31 and 41. The antibody response should be checked by day 41, especially if passive immunisation has been used. HDCSV is the vaccine of choice, and is now licensed for use in most countries, including the United Kingdom and USA. There is no risk of neuroparalytic complications as the virus is raised in human embryonic lung fibroblasts and is then killed. It induces excellent antibody levels in everyone vaccinated. The post-exposure course is 1.0 ml on days 0, 3, 7, 14, 30, and 90, given intramuscularly. Other vaccines used in some countries are suckling mouse brain vaccine (South America, France, and Thailand) and hamster kidney tissue culture vaccine (USSR and Canada).

In someone who has received a complete course of pre-exposure vaccination with HDCSV, the post-exposure course can be reduced to three doses (0, 7, and 21 days) without immunoglobulin.

Passive immunization. Antirabies serum (ARS) from horses and other animals has proved valuable in neutralizing rabies virus during the first week after initial vaccination, before neutralizing antibody has appeared. The dose is 40 i.u. per kg body weight; 0.1 ml should be given intradermally as a test dose. Hypersensitivity reactions occur in up to 40 per cent of those treated. Human rabies immune globulin (HRIG) has now replaced ARS in all countries which can afford it. The dose is 20 i.u. per kg body weight. Half is given intramuscularly (at a site distant from the vaccine) and half is infiltrated round the bite wound. Passive immunization may cause partial suppression of the response to less potent vaccines (such as DEV), but this can be overcome by giving booster doses.

Post-vaccinal encephalomyelitis and other vaccine-induced neuroparalytic accidents. Approximately 1 in 2000 courses of Semple type (nervous tissue) vaccine and 1 in 32 000 courses of DEV are complicated by a neuroparalytic reaction thought to be an allergic response to myelin-related protein in the vaccine. There seems to be some variation in racial susceptibility: the Japanese are the most vulnerable. Reactions can occur in all age groups, but the incidence is generally higher in adults.

The incubation period ranges from 3 to 35 days after the first injection of vaccine, but in most cases it is between 7 and 14 days. In the late cerebral form peculiar to the Japanese, the incubation is 15 to 125 days. Several forms of the disease have been described. The mildest and probably the rarest or least recognized is *mononeuritis multiplex* involving particularly the facial nerve but also the oculomotor, vagus, radial, brachial, and sciatic nerves. Recovery is rapid and complete. *Dorsolumbar transverse myelitis* develops gradually with a mild initial fever. There is paralysis and sensory loss in the lower limbs with sphincter involvement, loss of tendon reflexes, extensor plantar responses, and severe girdle and thoracic pain. Deaths occur only as a result of complicating infections of bed sores or urinary tract. *Ascending paralysis* (Landry type): after a sudden onset of fever, headache, vomiting, and severe backache there is, progressively, weakness then paralysis of the lower limbs, sphincters, and upper limbs, facial pain, and palsy, and finally in a third of cases, fatal bulbar paralysis. In South America, neuroparalytic complications of suckling mouse brain rabies vaccine have almost always been of this type with Guillain–Barré syndrome. In *meningo-encephalitic* and *meningo-encephalomyelitic reactions* there is impaired consciousness and meningism in addition to paralysis, sphincter involvement, sensory deficit, and cranial nerve lesions. The overall mortality of all reactions is 15–20 per cent. Most survivors make a complete recovery in two to three weeks, but a few are left with permanent neurological sequelae. A moderate lymphocyte pleocytosis and elevated CSF protein is usual. *Pathological changes* consist of swelling and chromatolysis of neurons with extensive perivascular demyelination and lymphocytic infiltration in the spinal cord. These features resemble experimental allergic encephalitis, post-vaccinal encephalomyelitis of smallpox, post-infectious encephalomyelitis, and acute multiple sclerosis. Corticosteroids, for example prednisolone 40–60 mg per day, are thought to be helpful. Vaccination should be stopped as soon as symptoms appear.

References

Baer, G. M. (ed.) (1975). *The natural history of rabies*. Academic Press, New York.

Bell, J. F. and Moore, G. J. (1979). Allergic encephalitis, rabies antibodies, and the blood–brain barrier. *J. lab. clin. Med.* **94**, 5.

Center for Disease Control (1980). Recommendations of the Advisory Committee on Immunization Practices (ACIP) rabies prevention. *Morb. Mort. Wkly Rep.* **29**, 265.

Dibb, W. L. and Digranes, A. (1981). Characteristics of 20 human Pasteurella isolates from animal bite wounds. *Acta path. microbiol. scand.* Sect. B **89**, 137.

Kaplan, C. (ed.) (1977). *Rabies—the facts*. Oxford University Press, Oxford.

Murphy, F. A. (1977). Rabies pathogenesis—brief review. *Arch. Virol.* **54**, 279.

Plotkin, S. A. (1980). Rabies vaccine prepared in human cell cultures: progress and perspectives. *Rev. infect. Dis.* **2**, 433.

Prabhakar, B. S. and Nathanson, N. (1981). Acute rabies death mediated by antibody. *Nature, Lond.* **290**, 590.

Shiraki, H. (1971). Rabies postvaccinal encephalomyelitis. In *Rabies* (eds. Y. Nagano and F. M. Davenport), 155. University Park Press, Baltimore.

Smith, J. S. (1981). Mouse model for abortive rabies infection of the central nervous system. *Infect. Immun.* **31**, 297.

Steck, F. and Wandeler, A. (1980). The epidemiology of fox rabies in Europe. *Epidemiol. Rev.* **2**, 71.

Warrell, D. A., Davidson, N. M., Pope, H. M., Bailie, W. E., Lawrie, J. H., Ormerod, L. D., Kertesz, A., and Lewis, P. (1976). Pathophysiologic studies in human rabies. *Am. J. Med.* **60**, 180.

Wiktor, T. J. and Koprowski, H. (1980). Antigenic variants of rabies virus. *J. exp. Med.* **152**, 99.

World Health Organization (1973). Expert Committee on Rabies, 6th Report. *Wld Hlth Org. Tech. Rep. Ser.* **533**, World Health Organization, Geneva.

Togaviridae

Alphaviruses

D. I. H. Simpson

There are 24 members of the alphavirus group all of which are transmitted by mosquitoes. Eight members produce disease in man (Table 1), and the type of illness produced varies from a mild, febrile illness which may or may not be accompanied by a rash, myalgia and arthralgia, to frank encephalitis. The mild fever, which is often unrecognized, occurs during the initial viraemic stage. This may be followed by a much more serious form of illness at which stage viraemia may have ceased and immunological responses, including the formation of antibodies, have taken place. Generally, only a small proportion of people infected with potentially encephalitogenic arboviruses during epidemics develop encephalitis in the second phase. The great majority develop only the first phase or the infection may be asymptomatic.

Chikungunya. Chikungunya virus was first isolated from patients and mosquitoes during an epidemic in the Newala district of Tanzania in 1952–3. The native name is derived from the main symptom, being 'doubled-up' as a result of excruciating joint pains. Since then chikungunya virus has been frequently isolated from man and mosquitoes during epidemics in India and Southeast Asia as well as in eastern, western, central, and southern Africa. The largest epidemics in recent years have been in cities of the Indian subcontinent, and it has been estimated that there were 300 000 cases of illness in a population of nearly two million in Madras.

Clinical features. Following an infective mosquito bite, there is an incubation period of 3–12 days followed by the sudden onset of fever and crippling joint pains which may incapacitate the patient within a few minutes to a few hours of onset. The pain in the limbs and spine is so severe as to cause patients to be doubled-up and immobile. Headache is usually mild, there is no retro-orbital or eye pain, and patients have anorexia and constipation. The disease has a biphasic course; following one to six days of fever, the temperature returns to normal for one to three days and then there is a second period of fever for a few days. In the second phase of illness, 80 per cent of patients develop a maculopapular, pruritic rash on the trunk and extensor surfaces of the limbs. After six to ten days patients recover completely although, rarely, joint pains can persist. A leucopenia is the only unusual laboratory finding.

In India and Southeast Asia, chikungunya virus has been implicated in outbreaks of haemorrhagic fever, often in association with dengue viruses. 242 cases of Chikungunya fever were reviewed during the Madras epidemic of 1965, and although the infections were mostly mild, 11 per cent of patients had haemorrhagic manifestations, none of which were severe. Chikungunya virus was isolated from 11 patients with haemorrhagic fever during an outbreak in Calcutta in 1963–4; nine had haematemesis and melaena, four had petechiae, and two died of shock. Paired sera from seven of these patients had rising antibody titres against chikungunya and two patients also had dengue virus type 2 antibodies. Chikungunya has been repeatedly isolated, as well as all four dengue serotypes, from patients during haemorrhagic fever outbreaks in Thailand and Singapore, but it has been suggested that if cases displaying 'shock' were the only ones accepted as true haemorrhagic fever, then chikungunya would be excluded. No haemorrhagic complications in chikungunya infections have ever been reported in Africa.

Chikungunya virus is transmitted in Africa by *Aedes africanus* and *Aedes aegypti* while *Ae. aegypti* transmits the disease in the urban centres of India and Southeast Asia. No vertebrate host other than man has been discovered although evidence has been found that monkeys might be a maintenance host in Africa.

Eastern encephalitis. Eastern encephalitis occurs widely along the eastern seaboard states of the USA and South America. Small outbreaks have occurred in the United States, the Dominican Republic, Cuba, and Jamaica. In the USA equine cases occur each summer in coastal regions bordering the Atlantic and the Gulf of Mexico and in other eastern states. Cases in eastern Canada were first recorded in 1972. Outbreaks in man are generally sporadic with only a small number of cases, but in horses and pheasants there is considerable morbidity and mortality. The virus is probably maintained by wild birds and mosquitoes, but the maintenance species in tropical areas have not been elucidated. *Culiseta melanura* seem to be the main mosquito infecting birds in North America; outbreaks are often associated with *Aedes sollicitans* and *Aedes vexans*. In the tropics, *Aedes taeniorynchus*, *Culex taeniopus*, and *Culex nigripalpus* appear to be involved.

Clinical features. In the United States encephalitis occurs mainly in

Table 1 Alphaviruses known to cause human disease

Virus	Probable transmission to man	Geographical distribution of viruses	Other features
Chikungunya	mosquito	tropical Africa, S. and S.E. Asia, Philippines	epidemics E. Africa, India
Eastern encephalitis	mosquito	N. and Central America, Trinidad, Guyana, Brazil, Argentina	? present in S.E. Asia and Philippines; epidemics only in N. America
Mayaro	mosquito	Trinidad, Brazil E. and	
O'nyong nyong	mosquito	W. Africa, Zimbabwe	epidemics E. Africa and Zimbabwe only
Ross River	mosquito	Australasia, Fiji	epidemics of polyarthritis
Sindbis	mosquito	Africa, E. Mediterranean, S. and S.E. Asia, Borneo, Philippines, Australia, Sicily	disease recognized only in Africa
Venezuelan encephalitis	mosquito	Venezuela, Colombia, S. and Central America	
Western encephalitis	mosquito	N. America, Mexico, Guyana, Brazil, Argentina	epidemics only in N. America

young children. Inapparent cases are rare. Onset is abrupt with high fever (39–41 °C), headache, and vomiting followed by drowsiness, coma, and severe convulsions. On examination there is neck stiffness, spasticity and, in infants, bulging fontanelles. Oedema of the legs and face and cyanosis have been described. The CSF is under pressure and contains increased protein and up to 1000 cells/mm. Death can occur within three to five days of onset. Sequelae are common in non-fatal cases and include convulsions, paralyses, and mental retardation. Older patients usually recover more completely.

No vaccine is yet available for human use although a formalin-inactivated vaccine prepared in chick embryos has been found effective in horses.

Mayaro virus. This virus has been isolated from man and various mosquito species in Trinidad and Brazil. The virus causes a two to six day illness in man with fever, headache, conjunctivitis, prostration, joint and muscle pains, and a rash.

O'nyong nyong virus. This virus caused a major epidemic which began in Uganda during 1959 and quickly spread to Kenya, Tanzania, and Malawi involving an estimated 2 million people. This virus is closely related to chikungunya and the disease it produces also resembles this infection. This virus is transmitted to man by *Anopheles gambiae* and *Anopheles funestus* which are predominantly malaria transmitting species.

Clinical features. After an incubation period of up to eight days, illness begins abruptly with fever, rigors and sometimes epistaxis, followed by backache, severe joint pains, headache, pain in the eyes, generalized lymphadenopathy, and an irritating rash beginning on the face and spreading to the trunk and limbs. High fever is uncommon. The rash generally lasts for four to seven days but the joint pains and malaise are protracted. There are no sequelae and no deaths have been directly attributable to the infection.

O'nyong nyong virus is still active in western Kenya, young children having evidence of recent infection, and the virus was again isolated there in 1979.

Ross River virus. This infection has caused epidemics of febrile illnesses with a rash and polyarthritis in Australia, southwestern Pacific Islands and more recently in Fiji. Ross River virus has been isolated from *Aedes vigilax* in Australia and New Guinea and from *Aedes aegypti* in Fiji. Epidemics in the Murray Valley, Australia have involved several thousand people. The patients present with fever, arthralgia of the small joints of the hands and feet, sore throat, skin rash, and paraesthesiae of the palms and soles of the feet. The rash, which sometimes covers the whole body, has sometimes begun as discrete macules, progressed to papules and occasionally to small vesicles. Petechiae and an enanthem have also been seen. Arthritis can last for 2–28 days and in one case lasted for eight months.

Sindbis virus. Although this virus is widely distributed in Africa, India, tropical Asia, and Australia, it has only occasionally been associated with overt human disease. It has been isolated from several *Culex* mosquito species—*C. tritaeniorhynchus, C. pseudovishnui,* and *C. univittatus*—and from wild birds. Five cases in Uganda had fever, headache, and myalgia with slight jaundice in two patients. In South Africa 12 cases of febrile illness with an associated rash have been described, and a more severe illness has been reported in one patient who developed vesicles on the feet. Virus was isolated from fluid taken from the vesicles.

Venezuelan encephalitis virus. This virus causes large epizootics of encephalitis in horses, mules, and donkeys. In man encephalitis occurs in a small proportion of cases but the majority have only a non-fatal 'influenza-like' febrile illness. At least four subtypes of Venezuelan encephalitis are separable on the basis of serological and physiochemical studies. Four antigenic variants can be distinguished with subtype I and are designated IAB, IC, ID, and IE.

Venezuelan IAB and IC viruses have been found in equine epizootics and are more pathogenic for men and horses than the enzootic strains ID and IE and subtypes II, III, and IV. Only about 4 per cent of human cases caused by epizootic viruses develop encephalitis which occur particularly in children below the age of 15 years but the case fatality rate is of the order of 20 per cent. A similar spectrum of disease from inapparent infection with fever to fatal encephalitis is seen in equines. The enzootic strains, ID, IE, II, and III, may occasionally produce sporadic disease but the virulence for equines and man is much reduced.

Epizootic strains of Venezuelan encephalitis appeared in Guatemala and spread in huge epizootic waves reaching north to southern Texas in 1971 and south to Costa Rica. Over 200 000 horses died in this outbreak and there were several thousand human infections.

A wide variety of mosquitoes including *Aedes, Mansonia,* and *Psorophora* species can transmit the virus. Enzootic strains are continually active in subtropical and tropical areas of the Americas having small rodent and marsupial hosts and are transmitted by *Culex* (*melanoconion*) mosquitoes. Birds may also act as hosts.

Clinical features. There is a brief febrile, occasionally 'influenza-like' illness with a sudden onset characterized by malaise, nausea or vomiting, headache which may be severe, and myalgia. Fever lasts up to four days and convalescence may take three weeks with generalized asthenia. A small proportion of patients develop encephalitis which can be severe or fatal.

Vaccines. An effective and safe live attenuated vaccine has been used in laboratory workers. An attenuated vaccine was used extensively to protect horses and mules in the 1969–71 epizootic and was found to be very effective.

A variety of new strains of Venezuelan encephalitis have been reported from time to time some of which cause disease in man. They include Everglades and Mucambo viruses.

Western encephalitis virus. The virus has been isolated in the United States, Canada, Guyana, Brazil, and Argentina, but human disease has been recognized only in North America and Brazil. Epidemics have occurred in the United States where encephalitis in horses is common. Since 1955, 947 human cases have been reported in the USA, the largest recent outbreak occurring in 1975 in North and South Dakota, Minnesota, and adjacent Manitoba. This outbreak was precipitated by extensive flooding in early summer which encouraged the breeding of *Culex tarsalis*. This mosquito is the principal vector in western USA while *Culistea melanura* is more common in the east. The virus has been isolated from a variety of wild birds which appear to be the maintenance hosts at least in North America. Equine epizootics generally precede the appearance of human cases but horses play no part in the transmission cycle. Very little is known about the maintenance cycle of the virus in tropical regions.

Clinical features. The disease varies with age but fever and drowsiness are common at all ages. Convulsions occur in 90 per cent of affected infants and in 40 per cent of those aged between one and four years. Convulsions are rare in adults. Typically there is fever, headache, vomiting, stiff neck, and backache. Restlessness and irritability are commonly seen in children. Drowsiness, severe occipital headache, mental confusion, and coma are seen in up to 40 per cent of adults. In milder cases recovery takes place in three to five days and in severe cases within five to ten days. Convalescence may be protracted. In adults sequelae are rare but become more common with reducing age. In infants almost half are left with convulsions. Mortality varies from outbreak to outbreak from 2 to 15 per cent.

No vaccine is yet available for use in man. A formalin inactivated chick embryo vaccine has been used effectively in horses. In man this vaccine has produced only minor reactions in volunteers.

References

Bartelloni, P. J., McKinney, R. W., Duffy, T. P., and Cole, F. E. (1970). An inactivated eastern equine encephalomyelitis vaccine propagated in chick embryo cell culture. II. Clinical and serologic responses in man. *Am. J. trop. Med. Hyg.* **19**, 123.

Carey, D. E., Myers, R. M., De Ranitz, C. M., Jadhav, M., and Reuben, R. (1969). The 1964 Chikungunya epidemic at Vellore, South India, including observations on concurrent dengue. *Trans. R. Soc. trop. Med. Hyg.* **63**, 434.

Doherty, R. L., Barrett, E. J., Gorman, B. M., and Whitehead, R. H. (1971). Epidemic polyarthritis in eastern Australia, 1959–70. *Med. J. Aust.* **1**, 5.

Pan American Health Organization (1972). *Venezuelan encephalitis.* Scientific Publication no. 243. Pan American Health Organization, Washington, D.C.

Sarkar, J. K., Chatterjee, S. N., Chakravarti, S. K., and Mijram, A. C. (1965). Chikungunya virus infection with haemorrhagic manifestations. *Indian J. Med. Res.* **53**, 921.

Flaviviruses

D. I. H. Simpson

There are just over 60 members of the flavivirus group; 29 are mosquito-borne, 15 are tick-borne while the remainder have no known arthropod vector. Twenty-six flaviviruses can cause human disease (Table 1) but several of them have produced only laboratory-acquired infections or isolated cases of disease in man. The range of clinical manifestations produced by flaviviruses is similar to those of the alphaviruses—febrile illnesses with or without a rash, or encephalitis. In addition, yellow fever, Kyasanur Forest disease, Omsk haemorrhagic fever, and the dengue viruses can cause haemorrhagic signs. Only those viruses which have produced substantial numbers of human infections are discussed in detail.

Murray Valley (formerly) Australia encephalitis. This disease was originally called Australian X disease. The virus causes epidemics in southeastern Australia and southern Queensland and sporadic cases in New Guinea. Outbreaks occur in late summer (February to April) and *Culex annulirostris* is the principal anthropod vector. *Aedes normanensis* and *C. bitaeniorhynchus* may be involved in transmission in enzootic tropical and subtropical areas with birds acting as the vertebrate hosts.

This disease clinically closely resembles Japanese encephalitis. Inapparent infections are common. Several deaths have occurred mostly in children.

Dengue. There are four dengue virus serotypes all of which are endemic throughout the tropics particularly in Asia, the Caribbean, the Pacific, and in some areas of West Africa. The various types (dengue-1, dengue-2, dengue-3, and dengue-4) are closely related and no significant biological differences are known between them. Many of the largest epidemics have been caused by dengue-1 as is the case in the recent outbreaks in the Caribbean. However, in many situations several types co-exist and successive epidemics may be due to different types. Many of the same people may be affected in each outbreak as it has been demonstrated that cross-protection between dengue types in man lasts only a short time.

Epidemics of dengue have been known since the late eighteenth century and waves of urban epidemics occurred in tropical and subtropical regions during the nineteenth and early twentieth centuries. These epidemics seem to have followed the migration of *Aedes aegypti* along trade routes from Africa to India and around the coast of Asia to reach Hong Kong and across the Pacific to Hawaii. Originally, dengue was probably a mainly rural infection in tropical Asia transmitted by indigenous *Stegomyia*. As no virological diagnosis was possible, 'dengue' has been a symptom complex which includes a large number of tropical febrile illnesses.

Dengue is endemic in tropical areas where *Stegomyia* species are constantly active. The boundaries are the winter isotherms for 17.8 °C. Large epidemics occur outside these areas from time to time, e.g. Brisbane (1906), Durban (1927), and Athens (1928).

Table 1 Flaviviruses known to cause human disease

Virus	Probable transmission to man	Geographical distribution of viruses	Other features
Australia encephalitis	mosquito	Australia, New Guinea	
Banzi	mosquito	S. and E. Africa	one case only
Bussuquara	mosquito	Brazil, Colombia, Panama	one case only
Dengue types 1–4	mosquito	S., S.E. Asia, Pacific Is., New Guinea, Caribbean area, Venezuela, Colombia, W. Africa	tropics and subtropics wherever the virus and a *Stegomyia* vector exist
Ilheus	mosquito	Central America, Trinidad, Colombia, Brazil, Argentina	
Japanese encephalitis	mosquito	E., S.E., and S. Asia, W. Pacific	
Kunjin	mosquito	Australia, Sarawak	
Kyasanur Forest	ixodid tick	Mysore, India	laboratory case only
Langat	ixodid tick	Malaysia	only experimental cases proven
Louping ill	ixodid tick	N. and W. British Isles	
Omsk haemorrhagic fever	ixodid tick	Central USSR	
Powassan	ixodid tick	Canada, USA	
Rio Bravo	? bat saliva	USA, Mexico	laboratory cases more severe
Rocio	poss. mosquito	Brazil	epidemics of encephalitis
St Louis encephalitis	mosquito	N. America, Panama, Jamaica, Trinidad, Brazil, Argentina	
Sepik	mosquito	New Guinea	one case only
Spondweni	mosquito	E., W., and S. Africa	
Tick-borne encephalitis (Central European) (Far Eastern)	ixodid tick	Central Europe from Scandinavia to Balkans and from Germany to W. USSR E. USSR and sometimes in W. USSR and Czechoslovakia	
Wesselsbron	mosquito	E., W., and S. Africa, Thailand	
West Nile	mosquito	E. and W. Africa, S. and S.E. Asia, Mediterranean area	disease recognized mainly in Israel and S. France
Yellow fever	mosquito	W. and Central Africa, S. and Central America	periodical epidemics in neighbouring areas, e.g. Ethiopia
Zika	mosquito	E. and W. Africa, Malaysia, Philippines	one case in Uganda

Aedes aegypti is the most important vector particularly in urban areas, but other *Stegomyia* species play a role in rural areas of Asia and the Pacific Islands. These include *Ae. albopictus*, *Ae. polynesiensis*, and *Ae. scutellaris*. There is some evidence that monkeys may play a part in virus maintenance but there is no convincing evidence of a vertebrate maintenance host other than man.

The 'classical' form of dengue fever usually affects adults and older children. Following an infective mosquito bite there is an incubation period of five to eight days followed by the sudden onset of fever, which often becomes biphasic, severe headache, pain behind the eyes, backache, chilliness, and generalized pains in the muscles and joints. A maculopapular rash generally appears on the trunk between the third and fifth day of illness and spreads later to the face and extremities. Lymphadenopathy, anorexia, constipation, and altered taste sensation are common. Occasionally, petechiae are seen on the dorsum of the feet, legs, hands, axillae, and palate late in the illness. In young children, upper respiratory tract symptoms predominate and dengue is rarely suspected. The illness generally lasts for about ten days after which recovery is usually complete although convalescence may be protracted. Laboratory findings show leucopenia, a mild throbocytopenia, and a relative lymphocytosis.

In the past two decades there have been an increasing number of epidemics of a severe disease syndrome caused by dengue viruses throughout Southeast Asia, India, and the western Pacific. It occurs most frequently in young children aged between two and 13 years and is associated with numerous haemorrhagic manifestations and quite often terminates fatally. Since its recognition in the Philippines in 1953, dengue haemorrhagic fever has occurred in Thailand, Burma, Cambodia, Indonesia, Malaysia, Vietnam, Singapore, eastern India, and several western Pacific islands. Outbreaks tend to occur most frequently in primarily affected areas. Over 500 cases a year are admitted to hospital in the Philippines. In the Bangkok–Thonburi area in Thailand, 10 000 cases were hospitalized in the period 1958–63 and all but 25 of these were younger than 14; 694 of these children died—an indication of the severity of the disease. Epidemics continue to occur annually in Thailand, the highest number of cases in a single year being 8288 in 1973 with 310 deaths. Only indigenous populations are involved in these epidemics with neither ethnic origin nor socio-economic conditions apparently having any effect on the incidence of the disease. Outbreaks of classical dengue are uncommon during haemorrhagic disease epidemics but immigrants from non-endemic areas often suffer from classical dengue while haemorrhagic disease occurs in the indigenous population.

Dengue haemorrhagic fever. This syndrome is almost entirely confined to indigenous children, usually orientals, often as young as six months. In the initial phase the child may present with fever, upper respiratory symptoms, headache, vomiting, and abdominal pain. Myalgia and arthralgia are uncommon. This minor illness, during which the child is often not confined to bed, lasts two to four days and many children recover without any further symptoms. In a proportion of children the initial phase is followed by an abrupt collapse with hypotension, peripheral vascular congestion, petechiae, and sometimes a rash. There are varying degrees of shock. The child is often restless, sweating, and has cold, clammy extremities and a hot, feverish trunk. The fourth and fifth days are critical and purpura, ecchymoses, epistaxis, haematemesis, melaena, coma, convulsions, and severe shock indicate a poor prognosis. Should the patient survive this period, recovery is generally complete. Laboratory studies show thrombocytopenia, a prolonged bleeding time, an elevated prothrombin time, a raised haematocrit, hypoproteinaemia, and a positive tourniquet test. The liver is often enlarged, soft, and tender. It has been suggested that the acute onset of shock and the rapid and often dramatic clinical recovery when the shock is treated properly, together with the absence of inflammatory vascular lesions, suggest short-term

vascular lesions. The central role of complement activation with the formation of immune complexes has been demonstrated. C3a and C5a anaphylatoxins, which are products of complement activation, are thought to be the cause of plasma leakage. Their rapid inactivation and elimination from the circulation are consistent with the short duration of shock. There is increased fibrinogen consumption which indicates disseminated intravascular coagulation. Both leucopenia and leucocytosis have been reported. There may be maturation arrest of megakaryocytes in the bone marrow and phagocytic activity of reticulum cells. Immunoelectrophoretic studies of serum proteins has shown the disappearance of the βIC line at the onset of shock suggesting an immunological phenomenon—a massive antigen–antibody reaction. There is a very rapid rise in flavivirus antibody in the early stages of the disease, which suggests that patients may have been previously sensitized to the infecting virus by earlier infection with a closely related virus, probably another type of dengue virus.

Post-mortem studies show that vascular changes predominate with vasodilatation, congestion, oedema, and haemorrhages. Pleural and peritoneal effusions are seen with haemorrhages in the stomach and intestines; there are widespread petechial haemorrhages.

Treatment. It has been maintained that the management of dengue haemorrhagic fever is entirely symptomatic with the basic principle being directed towards correction of plasma leakage. In Bangkok, satisfactory results have been obtained with the following regimen: immediate replacement of plasma loss with isotonic salt solution and plasma or plasma expanders in cases of profound shock; further plasma leakage is continually replaced to maintain the circulation volume for another 12–24 hours to allow extravasated plasma to be reabsorbed; correct the electrolytic and acid–base disturbance; give transfusions of fresh blood in cases of massive bleeding.

Following this regimen the case fatality rate in Bangkok has fallen from 9 per cent in 1964 to 2 per cent in 1974. The use of the microhaematocrit has been claimed to be invaluable as a guideline. Corticosteroids have not been found to be of great benefit, and heparin is not generally indicated in the management of dengue shock syndrome even when there is evidence of disseminated intravascular coagulation.

Control. The control of dengue depends principally on control of the vector, particularly *Ae. aegypti*. A great deal could be done by eliminating the periodomestic breeding places such as flower pots, old jars, and tin cans around houses and by using insecticides carefully. Rural breeding sites are much more difficult to control. No vaccine is yet available although several live attenuated strains are under development.

Ilheus. Ilheus virus is active over a wide area of Central and South America and in Trinidad. It is probably maintained in a forest complex involving birds and mosquitoes. Our knowledge of human disease is limited to five naturally-occurring cases in Brazil and Trinidad and nine cancer patients infected experimentally in 1951. Half of the infections were asymptomatic, three had mild febrile illnesses and four had a more marked illness, with CNS involvement. These patients displayed fever, headache, myalgia, photophobia and signs of encephalitis. No deaths or sequelae have been reported.

Japanese encephalitis virus. This virus occurs over the whole of the eastern seaboard of Asia and the offshore islands from the maritime province of Russia to South India and Sri Lanka. Epidemics have been recognized for years, generally occurring in late summer in more temperate regions but in tropical areas the virus remains enzootic throughout the year. Some of the largest outbreaks in recent years have taken place in India.

Rice-field breeding mosquitoes are the main vectors. They include the *Culex vishnui* complex, especially *C. tritaeniorhynchus*, *C. annulus*, and *C. annulirostris*. In tropical areas, *C. gelidus*, which breeds in close association with pigs and cattle, is also involved. During extensive studies in Japan, it has been shown that there is intense virus activity in the spring among young herons and *C. tritaeniorhynchus*. These mosquitoes then infect pigs which act as amplifying hosts infecting more *C. tritaeniorhynchus* which, in turn, bite man causing outbreaks in late summer. Japanese workers can predict human cases in time and place in any year simply by monitoring abattoir pigs for evidence of infection (antibody conversion, especially IgM) which precedes outbreaks of human disease by two or three weeks. In the tropics, the vertebrate maintenance hosts are not clearly understood but in Sarawak it appears that the principal maintenance hosts are pigs and *C. gelidus*. Following the flooding of padi fields prior to planting, there is intense breeding of *C. tritaeniorhynchus* which produces human infections.

Clinical features. Generally onset is sudden with fever, headache, and vomiting. Fever is usually continuous and subsides after two to four days. Lethargy is a common feature, the face is expressionless, and there are sensory and motor disturbances affecting speech, the eyes, and limbs. There may be confusion and delirium progressing to coma. Convulsions may be the first sign in children. Weakness and paralysis can affect any part of the body, the lesions generally being upper motor neurone in character. Neck rigidity, and a positive Kernig's sign are found, and reflexes are abnormal. An initial leucocytosis is followed by a leucopenia; the CSF is non-turbid and under pressure with increased cells and protein. The duration of illness is very variable. Fatal cases usually die within 10 days. Convalescence is often protracted and sequelae are common especially in young children. They include inco-ordination, tremors, mental impairment, and personality changes. Residual paralysis, aphasia, and cerebellar ataxia can occur. It was estimated in 1956 that only one case of encephalitis occurred in every 500–1000 infections in Japan but the risk may be higher in immigrants.

At post mortem, oedema and congestion of the central nervous system are apparent. Histologically there is neuronal degeneration and necrosis and perivascular cuffing. The Purkinje cells are severely affected.

There is no specific treatment. No really satisfactory vaccine is yet available although formalized vaccines prepared in mouse brain and hamster kidney cultures show some promise. Vaccination of the amplifier hosts, pigs, is worth considering as a means of breaking the infection link to man. An attenuated vaccine for use in pigs is being evaluated in Japan.

Kyasanur Forest disease. This virus, like Omsk haemorrhagic fever virus, is a member of the tick-borne encephalitis complex but only rarely causes disease involving the central nervous system. The virus was first isolated in Mysore State, India in 1957, and human infections, which still occur, are limited to villages surrounding Kyasanur Forest. The virus is now known to be widely distributed in India but human infections do not occur outside Mysore.

Clinical features. After an infectious tick bite there is an incubation period of three to seven days before the sudden onset of fever, frontal headache, severe myalgia, and prostration. This is quickly followed by nausea, vomiting, confusion, and restlessness. The conjunctivae are injected and the palate is suffused and often covered with maculopapular haemorrhagic spots. A generalized lymphadenopathy has been noted. Many patients have bronchiolar involvement. The fever generally lasts for five to 12 days and sometimes follows a biphasic course with a mild meningo-encephalitis seen occasionally during the second phase. Epistaxis, haematemesis, haemoptysis, melaena, and bleeding gums are common and sometimes there may be uterine bleeding. Albuminuria, leucopenia and thrombocytopenia are usual findings. A small proportion of cases may die usually eight to 12 days after the onset of illness developing coma or bronchopneumonia prior to death. The greater majority of cases make an uneventful and complete recovery.

In 1957 there were probably about 500 cases in a 70 square mile area. The death rate was about 10 per cent. Numerous laboratory infections have occurred but there were no deaths.

The virus is transmitted by *Haemaphysalis* ticks, especially *H. spinigera*, and is maintained in small mammals. In Mysore State the silent enzootic situation was dramatically altered by man's need for more grazing land. Cattle were put to graze around the forest and provided the *Haemaphysalis* tick with a new and plentiful source of blood meals which produced a population explosion among the ticks. The abundant ticks fed on other mammalian species such as monkeys and these became infected with Kyasanur Forest disease virus and developed marked viraemia and an illness from which they died. It was noted in 1957 that human infection was preceded by illness and death in forest dwelling *Langur* and *Macacus* monkeys which acted as amplifiers of the virus.

Louping ill. Louping ill is a member of the tick-borne encephalitis complex. It has been known in the United Kingdom for many years as a disease of sheep producing CNS manifestations including paralysis and death. It has never been a serious disease hazard to man with most reported cases being the result of laboratory infections. A few natural infections have occurred in people closely associated with sheep. The illness is generally biphasic with encephalitic involvement in the second phase. The vector is *Ixodes ricinus* and the virus is maintained in rodents and ground-living birds.

Omsk haemorrhagic fever. This virus is also antigenically related to the tick-borne encephalitis complex. An epidemic of severe haemorrhagic fever occurred in Omsk in Novosibirsk Oblast in Siberia between 1945 and 1948. The virus was transmitted by ticks, *Dermacentor pictus*, and by contact with infected muskrats (*Ondrata zibethica*). Most of the more recent cases of human disease appear to have been acquired through direct contact with muskrats. Most infections originate in the northern forest–steppe–lake belt of western Siberia which contains much wet grassland and swamp.

Clinical features. Following an incubation period of three to seven days the illness begins abruptly with fever, which often follows a biphasic course, headache, vomiting, and diarrhoea. An enanthem of the palate, sometimes haemorrhagic, generalized lymphadenopathy, and meningism are common findings. Epistaxis, haematemesis, melaena, and uterine bleeding may occur accompanied by a marked leucopenia and thrombocytopenia and albuminuria. The central nervous system is rarely involved, the case fatality is low (0.5–3 per cent). Convalescence may be prolonged but there are no sequelae.

The precise epidemiology of Omsk haemorrhagic fever virus is still unknown. A biological cycle of unknown complexity, which may involve rodents and ticks, exists. Muskrats which were introduced into the region some 60 years ago for hunting purposes are somehow infected and are capable of transmitting the virus by direct contact.

Powassan virus. This virus is a rare cause of acute viral CNS disease in Canada and the USA. It was first isolated from the brain of a five-year-old child who died in Ontario in 1958. Between 1970 and 1978 eight cases have been seen in the USA, mostly in upper New York State. The clinical manifestation is usually encephalitis and some residual neurological problems have been described in recovered patients. The virus is maintained between ixodid ticks and wild animals (woodchucks and squirrels). Man is very rarely infected; less than 1 per cent of residents of enzootic areas have demonstrable antibodies.

Rocio virus. In February 1975 an acute infective illness affecting the central nervous system appeared in coastal areas in Sao Paulo State, Brazil. This illness was characterized by fever, headache, vomiting, encephalitis, and meningitis. During 1975 and 1976, 825 cases were recorded with 95 deaths. The overall attack rate was 15 per 1000 population and the mortality rate was 2 per 1000; the case fatality ratio was 13 per cent and there was a high incidence in adults.

A newly recognized flavivirus, named Rocio, was isolated from nine patients. It seems most likely that the virus is mosquito-borne and wild birds may be important vertebrate hosts. Only one isolate from mosquitoes has been made—from *Psorophora ferox*—and isolates have also been obtained from sentinel mice and from a wild-caught sparrow.

St Louis encephalitis virus. St Louis encephalitis is the most important mosquito-borne disease in the United States and has caused major epidemics in recent years. It is widely distributed from Canada to Argentina. The virus occurs in endemic form west of the Mississippi whereas in the eastern USA it re-appears in epidemic form especially in the Mississippi–Ohio basin, Texas, and Florida. Outbreaks have also occurred in Canada and northern Mexico. In Central and South America human infections are frequent but epidemics are unknown.

In western USA the important mosquito host is *Culex tarsalis* which breeds in irrigated or flooded dryland areas. It is widely distributed and causes many infections in rural areas. In eastern USA the principal vectors are *Culex pipiens pipiens* and *C.p. quinquefasciatus* which breed in polluted water and produce large populations in urban and suburban areas. In Florida *C. nigripalpus* is the epidemic vector. Wild birds are the major vertebrate host.

There were large outbreaks in the early 1960s in Florida, Houston, Illinois, and the Delaware Valley. After a quiet eight-year period the virus reappeared in epidemic form in 1974 and outbreaks have occurred in each year since particularly in the Ohio–Mississippi basin.

Clinical features. Most patients have a febrile illness with severe headache which lasts a few days and is followed by complete recovery. A variable number of cases develop aseptic meningitis or encephalitis. There is sudden onset of fever, weakness, and nausea, the headache becomes severe and is followed by confusion, drowsiness, and vomiting. There may be convulsions which have a poor prognosis. Fever may last for 3–10 days. A stiff neck is common and the CSF is under increased pressure and has increased cells and protein. There may be muscular weakness, pains, tremors, spasticity, dysphasia, photophobia, and visual disturbances. Occasionally dramatic recovery can occur in even severely ill patients. In the elderly there is a higher incidence of disease, greater severity, and higher mortality; severe sequelae are more frequent.

At post mortem a few haemorrhages are seen in the CNS with neuronal damage occurring particularly in the mid-brain and brain stem together with perivascular cuffing.

No vaccine is yet available.

Tick-borne encephalitis. This disease occurs throughout Russia, eastern and central Europe, and as far west as Alsace. The complex of viruses which make up the group causes illnesses which range from severe paralytic encephalitis, as occurs in Siberia and which is transmitted by *Ixodes persulcatus*, to a less paralytic encephalitis generally following a biphasic course, which occurs in central Europe. This form is transmitted by *Ixodes ricinus*. Agricultural and forestry workers are most frequently affected, as the foci of infection are in and around forest areas, the vertebrate maintenance hosts being rodents and ground-living birds.

The Far East Russian encephalitis. Also known as Russian spring–summer encephalitis, this disease is mainly confined to eastern USSR but a few viruses occur around Leningrad and western USSR. In Czechoslovakia, related strains Absettarov and Hypr have been isolated.

Clinical features. The incubation period ranges from seven to ten days and the illness often follows a biphasic course. The first phase of fever and headache lasts around five to ten days and is followed by an afebrile period of four to ten days. In a proportion of cases the second phase follows with intensive headache and high fever followed by severe CNS manifestations of varying degrees of severity ranging from meningitis to severe encephalitis and death. Flaccid paralysis followed by atrophy is common and there are frequently symptoms due to bulbar involvement. Mortality can be as high as 30 per cent. Nystagmus, vertigo, somnolence, and visual disturbance indicate the development of encephalitis which may cause delirium and coma. In patients who recover, convalescence is prolonged. Headache and debility are common and residual paralysis may persist in 3–5 per cent of cases.

Central European encephalitis. Often called bi-undulant meningo-encephalitis or biphasic milk fever, this infection occurs in central Europe from Scandinavia to the Balkans and from Alsace and West Germany to western Russia. The virus can be transmitted through drinking infected goats' milk. Goats are infected by tick-bite and it has been reported that cases occurring early in the season were due to the drinking of infected milk while later cases were caused by tick bite. Several cases have occurred in campers and picnickers in forested areas of central Europe.

Clinical features. This infection always follows a biphasic course. An afebrile period of four to ten days intervenes between the first 'influenza-like' symptoms and the second phase of meningitis or meningo-encephalitis. Mild or inapparent forms are common. In the more severe cases there may be transient or permanent paralysis and the bulbo-spinal form is often fatal. Generally the disease is not as severe as the Far Eastern form.

Langat virus. This is a member of the group which was isolated from ticks in Malaysia. Its comparatively low pathogenicity for mice and monkeys suggested its possible use as an immunizing agent against the tick-borne viruses. A strain of the virus has been given to over 1000 people with satisfactory results, and an avirulent strain grown in chick embryos gave promising results. Recently low passage strains of Austrian isolates of tick-borne encephalitis have been successfully grown in chick embryo cells and when inactivated with formalin have produced excellent antibody responses in volunteers.

Wesselsbron virus. This virus is widely distributed in Africa and causes epizootics in sheep, producing abortion and death in new-born lambs and ewes. The mosquito vectors are *Aedes caballus* and *Ae. circumluteolus*. Man may also be infected developing fever, headache, muscular pains, and retro-orbital pain. Convalescence may be prolonged. Splenomegaly and hepatomegaly were found in one patient while another had visual disturbances. Several laboratory-acquired infections have occurred.

West Nile virus. This virus has been isolated in many parts of Africa and in Israel, Cyprus, France, India, and Borneo. Recognizable disease due to West Nile virus infection has been observed in Israel where epidemics have occurred between May and October. In France it has caused febrile illness in man and encephalitis in horses. The disease in Egypt is generally a mild febrile illness mainly of young children. The virus is probably maintained by mosquitoes, especially *Culex* species, and wild birds although *Argas* ticks may also play a role in the maintenance cycle.

Clinical features. After an incubation period of three to six days, there is a sudden onset of fever, headache, myalgia, a maculopapular rash mainly on the trunk, and lymphadenopathy. Although most cases recover without untoward effects, the disease is more severe in elderly patients who may develop neurological signs or myocarditis. Death may occasionally result. No vaccine is yet available.

Yellow fever. The first reported outbreak of yellow fever was in Barbados in 1647 and since then innumerable appalling epidemics have occurred in the West Indies, Central and South America, and the southern United States throughout the seventeenth, eighteenth and nineteenth centuries as well as in seaports in more temperate regions of the western hemisphere. This virus is believed to have originated in Africa and to have been carried to the Americas by trading and slaving ships which may have also introduced one of its important vectors, *Aedes aegypti*. Epidemics generally took place in urban conurbations being transmitted from man to man by *Ae. aegypti*. The elimination of this vector almost completely eradicated yellow fever from towns but sporadic cases of the disease continued to occur in rural areas particularly those bordering on forest zones. It was later discovered that yellow fever virus was maintained in a sylvan cycle involving monkeys and forest-dwelling mosquitoes such as *Haemagogus* and *Sabethes* species in South America and *Ae. africanus* in East Africa where *Ae. simpsoni* provides the link between monkey and man; in West Africa a variety of *Aedes* species appear to be involved. In recent outbreaks *Ae. furcifer/taylori* has been strongly implicated.

Yellow fever is still the most important cause of viral haemorrhagic disease being active in several South American and African countries. Two devastating epidemics took place in Africa in the last two decades. The largest of these was in Ethiopia between 1960 and 1962 when there were enormous numbers of cases and between 15 000 and 30 000 deaths. *Ae. simpsoni* was the mosquito host involved in the man–mosquito–man cycle. The other large epidemic occurred in Senegal in 1965 with several thousand cases and several hundred deaths. *Ae. aegypti* was the main mosquito vector. Sporadic cases continue to occur in rural areas in West Africa and South America.

Clinical features. The disease in man varies from an inapparent infection in native Africans to a fulminating disease terminating in death. After an incubation period of three to six days, the illness begins suddenly with fever, rigors, headache, and backache. The patient is intensely ill and restless with flushed face, swollen lips, bright red tongue, and congested conjunctivae, and nausea and vomiting develops. A tendency to bleeding may be seen early in the course of the disease. This stage of active congestion is followed quickly by one of stasis. The facial oedema and flushing is replaced by a dusky pallor, the gums become swollen and bleed easily and there is a marked bleeding tendency with black vomit ('vomito negro'), melaena, and ecchymoses. The pulse rate is slow despite high fever, the blood pressure falls leading to albuminuria, oliguria, and anuria. Death, when it occurs, is usually within six to seven days of onset and is rarely seen after 10 days of illness. The jaundice, which gives the disease its name, is generally only apparent in convalescing patients. Mortality may be quite low, often of the order of 5 per cent. At post mortem the organs most particularly affected are the liver, spleen, kidneys, and heart. Typically a mid-zone necrosis is apparent in the liver involving cells around the periphery of the lobule and sparing the area around the central vein. Hyaline necrosis is evident and typical Councilman bodies have been described.

Treatment. Treatment is largely symptomatic with maintenance of fluid and electrolytic balances. Blood transfusion is sometimes required to correct blood loss through haemorrhage.

Vaccines. Two live attenuated virus vaccines are available; the 17D strain which was attenuated in tissue culture and is prepared in chick embryos; and the French neurotropic strain which was attenuated and is produced in mouse brain. The 17D strain is given by subcutaneous injection and the French neurotropic strain by scarification. During the Senegal epidemic of 1965 about 1.9 million people received the French neurotropic vaccine and almost 120 000 were given 17D vaccine. Of the former group at least 246 subsequently developed encephalitis with 23 deaths. About 90 per cent were children. Only two children developed encephalitis following 17D vaccination and both recovered. Largely as a result of these complications the French neurotropic vaccine is not now used to such a large extent. Immunity following yellow fever vaccination is long-lasting.

Apart from vaccination, control of yellow fever depends on controlling the vectors. In urban areas where *Aedes aegypti* is the vector, peridomestic breeding sites can be controlled, but in rural areas where forest dwelling mosquitoes are the vectors, little can be done to control them.

References

Casals, J., Henderson, B. E., Hoogstraal, H., Johnson, K. M., and Shelokov, A. (1970). A review of Soviet viral haemorrhagic fevers, 1969. *J. infect. Dis.* **122**, 437.
Halstead, S. B. (1970). Observations related to pathogenesis of dengue haemorrhagic fever. VI. Hypotheses and discussion. *Yale J. Biol. Med.* **42**, 350.
Hotta, S. (1978). *Dengue and related tropical viruses.* Susumu Hotta, Kobe, Japan.
Monath, T. P. (1979). Arthropod-borne encephalitides in the Americas. *Bull. Wld Hlth Org.* **57**, 513.
Sabin, A. B. (1952). Research on dengue during World War II. *Am. J. trop. Med. Hyg.* **1**, 30.
World Health Organization (1966). Mosquito-borne haemorrhagic fevers of southeast Asia and the Western Pacific. *Bull. Wld Hlth Org.* **35**, no. 1, 1–103.

Bunyaviridae

J. S. Porterfield

Bunyaviridae are large (90–100 nm in diameter) enveloped, spherical viruses having a genome of single-stranded, negative-sense RNA which is divided into three segments and which together give a total molecular weight of $4–6 \times 10^6$ dalton. About 200 different Bunyaviridae are known, making this family the largest amongst the arboviruses, and indeed probably amongst all animal viruses. All presently recognized Bunyaviridae are arthropod-transmitted, by mosquitoes, ticks, phlebotomines or culicoides.

The family name is taken from that of the type species, Bunyamwera virus; this was isolated in Uganda from *Aedes* mosquitoes collected in Bwamba county (Smithburn *et al.* 1946). As originally defined, the family had only a single genus, *Bunyavirus*, with other possible members (Porterfield *et al.* 1975/6), but recently three additional genera have been proposed. These are *Nairovirus*, named after Nairobi sheep disease virus, *Phlebovirus*, named after the *Phlebotomus*, or sandfly fever viruses, and *Uukuvirus*, named after Uukuniemi virus, an agent isolated in Finland from ticks. This taxonomic approach brings together about 200 different viruses previously classified into some 20 different serological groups, and reveals hitherto unrecognized relationships between viruses, sometimes occurring in quite different habitats and associated with quite different diseases in man or animals. A few Bunyaviridae remain outside the four presently recognized genera. (Bishop and Shope 1979; Bishop *et al.* 1981.) Table 1 summarizes the present taxonomic state of the family, and names those Bunyaviridae that have been associated with disease in man (Figs. 1 and 2).

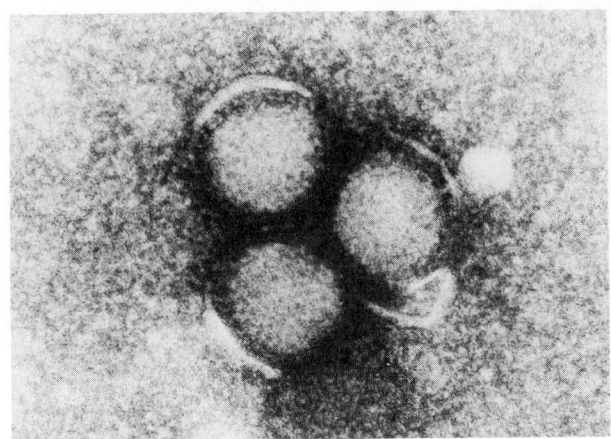

Fig. 1 Electron micrograph of Rift Valley fever virus ($\times$ 200 000). (Electron micrograph by courtesy of Dr D. Ellis.)

Table 1   The family Bunyaviridae, its genera, serological groups, and viruses associated with disease in man

Genus	Serological group	Viruses producing disease in man
Bunyavirus (over 100)*	Anopheles A (10)†	
	Bunyamwera (20)†	Bunyamwera, Calovo, Germiston, Guaroa, Ilesha, Maguari, Tensaw, Wyeomyia
	Bwamba (2)	Bwamba
	C group (13)	Apeu, Caraparu, Itaqui, Madrid, Marituba, Murutucu, Oriboca, Ossa, Restan
	California (11)	California encephalitis, Inkoo, La Crosse, Tahyna, Trivittatus
	Capim (10)	–
	Gamboa (4)	–
	Guama (12)	Catu, Guama
	Koongol (2)	–
	Mirim (2)	–
	Olifantsvlei (3)	–
	Patois (4)	–
	Simbu (22)	Oropouche, Shuni
	Tete (5)	–
Nairovirus (19)	Crimean–Congo (2)	Crimean–Congo H. F., Hazara.
	Dera Ghazi Khan (5)	–
	Hughes (3)	–
	Nairobi sheep disease (3)	Dugbe, Ganjam, Nairobi sheep disease
	Qalyub (2)	–
Phlebovirus (30)	Phlebotomus fever (30)	Candiru, Chagres, Phlebotomus fever, Naples and Sicily, Punta Toro, Rift Valley fever
Uukuvirus (7)	Uukuniemi (7)	Uukuniemi
Other Bunyaviridae (30)		Bhanja, Thogoto

* Approximate number of viruses in genus
† Approximate number of viruses in serological group

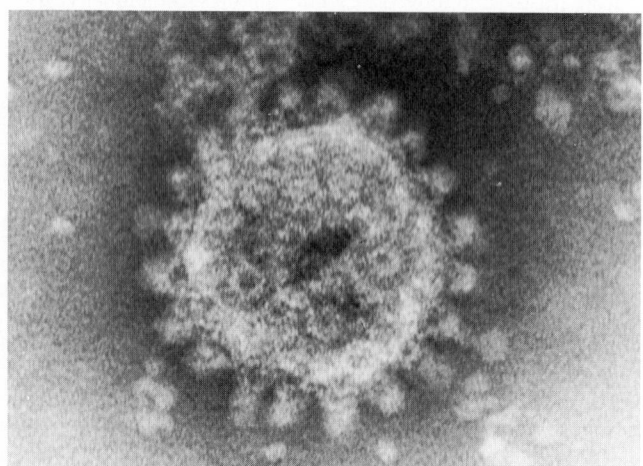

Fig. 2   Electron micrograph of Crimean–Congo virus (× 400 000). (Electron micrograph by courtesy of Dr D. Ellis.)

References
Bishop, D. H. L., Calisher, C. H., Casals, J., Chumakov, M. P., Gaidamovich, S. Ya., Hannoun, C., Lvov, D. K., Marshall, I. D., Oker-Blom, N., Pettersson, R. F., Porterfield, J. S., Russell, P. K., Shope, R. E., and Westaway, E. G. (1981). Bunyaviridae. *Interviriol.* **14**, 125.
—and Shope, R. E. (1979). Bunyaviridae. In *Comprehensive Virology*, vol. 14, 1 (eds. H. Fraenkel-Conrat and R. R. Wagner). Plenum Press, New York.
Porterfield, J. S., Casals, J., Chumakov, M. P., Gaidamovich, S. Ya., Hannoun, C., Holmes, I. H., Horzinek, M. C., Mussgay, M., Oker-Blom, N., and Russell, P. K. (1975/6). Bunyaviruses and Bunyaviridae. *Intervirol.* **6**, 13.
Smithburn, K. C., Haddow, A. J., and Mahaffy, A. F. (1946). Neurotropic virus isolated from Aedes mosquitoes caught in Semliki Forest. *Am. J. trop. Med.* **26**, 189.

Genus *Bunyavirus*

The genus *Bunyavirus* contains at least 12 distinct serological groups of viruses, and includes at least 28 viruses known to infect man of which Bunyamwera virus and seven others are placed within the Bunyamwera serogroup. Bunyamwera, Germiston, and Ilesha viruses occur in Africa; Guaroa, Maguari, Tensaw, and Wyeomyia viruses occur in the Americas, and one virus, described as Calovo virus in Europe, is found also in Asia, where it was originally described as Batai virus.

Serogroup Bunyamwera
Bunyamwera virus. *Definition.* Genus *Bunyavirus*, serogroup Bunyamwera, species Bunyamwera virus.

Epidemiology. Serological surveys indicate that the virus is widespread throughout Africa south of the Sahara, but most infections of man are unrecognized. Virus has been isolated from *Aedes, Culex, Anopheles*, and *Mansonia* species of mosquitoes. The main animal reservoir of infection is not established.

Clinical disease. A mild, febrile illness, sometimes associated with a rash, but more usually with headache, joint and back pains, and occasionally with mild involvement of the central nervous system. Laboratory infections have been recorded.

Calovo virus. *Definition.* Genus *Bunyavirus*, serogroup Bunyamwera, species Calovo virus.

Epidemiology. The type species was isolated in Czechoslovakia from *Anopheles maculipennis* mosquitoes, and serological surveys indicate that the virus is widely distributed throughout Central Europe, including Yugoslavia, and extending to the Ukraine and to Scandinavia. A serologically indistinguishable virus was isolated in Malaysia and was described as Batai virus. Other isolations have been made in India and Thailand. In Europe, transmission is principally by *Anopheline* mosquitoes, whereas in Asia *Culex* mosquitoes are involved.

Clinical disease. A benign febrile illness only.

Germiston virus. *Definition.* Genus *Bunyavirus*, serogroup Bunyamwera, species Germiston virus.

Epidemiology. The type species was isolated from *Culex theileri* and *C. rubinotus* mosquitoes collected at Germiston, South Africa; other isolations have been made in Rhodesia, Mozambique, Uganda, and Ethiopia, and antibody studies indicate the presence of the virus in Botswana and Caprivi.

Clinical disease. A mild three-day fever without a rash. Laboratory infections have occurred, in which a sudden onset of fever has been followed by headache, backache, and mental confusion, symptoms resolving completely after three days.

Guaroa virus. *Definition.* Genus *Bunyavirus*, serogroup Bunyamwera, species Guaroa virus.

Epidemiology. Six isolations of Guaroa virus were made in Colombia from human sera collected from apparently healthy people whilst investigations were being made into an outbreak of fever of unknown origin. About 60 per cent of adults in Colombia have antibodies against Guaroa virus. Isolations have also been made from man in Brazil, several times from individuals with mild fevers, and once from a liver biopsy taken from a man with partial paralysis of the arms and legs. *Anopheles (K) neivai* mosquitoes have yielded virus in Colombia.

Clinical disease. An undifferentiated mild fever with body and joint pains, but no rash.

Ilesha virus. *Definition.* Genus *Bunyavirus*, serogroup Bunyamwera, species Ilesha virus.

Epidemiology. The first three isolations were made from children attending an out-patients clinic at Ilesha Hospital, Nigeria, on account of undiagnosed febrile illnesses. These children had no localizing signs, but occasionally a rash may be present. The vector appears to be *Anopheles gambiae*. Other isolations of Ilesha virus have been reported from Senegal, Central African Republic, Cameroun, Uganda, and Ethiopia.

Clinical disease. An undifferentiated, mild febrile illness, occasionally associated with a rash.

Maguari virus. *Definition.* Genus *Bunyavirus*, serogroup Bunyamwera, species Maguari virus.

Epidemiology. A virus originally isolated in Belem, Brazil, was initially identified as a strain of Cache Valley virus, in the California serogroup, but was later found to be distinguishable from this by neutralization and other tests. Other isolations have been made in Trinidad, French Guiana, Guyana, Guatemala, Argentina, Colombia, and Peru. A variety of different mosquitoes, including *Aedes* and *Culex* species appear to act as vectors. The natural reservoir of the virus is unknown.

Clinical disease. Although serological surveys show that infections of man are common in the Neotropical region, overt disease is rarely recognized.

Tensaw virus. *Definition.* Genus *Bunyavirus*, serogroup Bunyamwera, species Tensaw virus.

Epidemiology. Originally isolated from a pool of *Anopheles crucians* mosquitoes collected from Florida, Tensaw virus has been isolated many times from mosquitoes in Southern Alabama and Georgia. Isolations have also been made from at least one dog, a cotton rat, and from marsh rabbits.

Clinical disease. Serological surveys in south eastern states of USA have shown that up to 25 per cent of normal adults have antibodies against Tensaw virus. For many years overt infections were not recognized, but there is at least one report of a human case associated with neurological disease (McGowan *et al.* 1973).

Wyeomyia virus. *Definition.* Genus Bunyavirus, serogroup Bunyamwera, species Wyeomyia virus.

Epidemiology. The prototype virus was isolated in 1940 from *Wyeomyia melanocephala* mosquitoes collected in Colombia; other strains have been isolated from a variety of different mosquito species in Brazil, French Guiana, Trinidad, and Panama.

Clinical disease. One isolation of virus was made in Panama from the blood of a patient with a low grade fever. Antibody rates in Panama are from 8–17 per cent.

Serogroup Bwamba

Bwamba virus. *Definition.* Genus *Bunyavirus*, serogroup Bwamba, species Bwamba virus.

Epidemiology. From blood samples collected from young adult males working in Bwamba forest, Uganda, Smithburn *et al.* (1941) isolated nine strains of a virus which became known as Bwamba virus. More than 75 per cent of adult human sera collected in Nigeria, and more than 95 per cent of human sera collected in Tanzania and Uganda have antibodies against Bwamba virus. Other isolations of Bwamba virus have been made in Nigeria and in the Central African Republic. A very closely related virus, Pongola, has been isolated many times from a variety of mosquito species in South Africa, Rhodesia, Central African Republic, Kenya, and Uganda, but it is questionable whether or not Pongola virus infects man.

Clinical disease. The original cases showed fever, headache, generalized pains and conjunctivitis. No deaths have been reported, and although no rash was noted in the original description, cases with a rash have been seen in the Central African Republic.

Serogroup C. Eleven group C viruses are known, most of them having been isolated in South America, and more specifically in Brazil, but the distribution of some viruses includes Trinidad and Central America, and at least one virus, Gumbo Limbo, has been isolated as far north as Florida, as well as from Brazil. They are probably all viruses of small rodents in nature, but at least nine viruses are known to infect man, the two exceptions being Gumbo Limbo and Nepuyo viruses.

Apeu virus. *Definition.* Genus *Bunyavirus*, serogroup C, species Apeu virus.

Epidemiology. Virus isolations have been made from man, from sentinel *Cebus* monkeys and from sentinel mice exposed in the Belem forest, from the blood of small rodents, and from *Aedes* and *Culex* mosquitoes. No isolations have been reported from outside Brazil.

Clinical disease. Natural infections appear to be mild, but a moderately severe laboratory infection has been reported (Gibbs *et al.* 1964), with fever, severe headache, joint and muscle pains, and a leucopenia.

Caraparu virus. *Definition.* Genus *Bunyavirus*, serogroup C, species Caraparu virus.

Epidemiology. The prototype virus was isolated in Brazil from the blood of a sentinel *Cebus apella* monkey; other isolations have been made from man and from small rodents as well as a variety of mosquito species, mainly *Culex* species.

Clinical disease. A mild, febrile illness with headache, muscle and joint pains, leucopenia, and sometimes conjunctival inflammation.

Caraparu virus has been isolated in Brazil, Panama, Guyana, and Surinam; serological surveys indicate a wider distribution, including Colombia and Peru.

Itaqui virus. *Definition.* Genus *Bunyavirus*, serogroup C, species Itaqui virus.

Epidemiology. Many isolations have been made in the Belem forest, Para, Brazil, from wild rodents, sentinel monkeys, and *Culex* mosquitoes. A single isolation has been reported from man.

Clinical disease. An undifferentiated febrile illness.

Madrid virus. *Definition.* Genus *Bunyavirus*, serogroup C, species Madrid virus.

Epidemiology. The prototype virus was isolated from the blood of a mosquito catcher who had been exposed in the forest in Bocas del Toro province, Panama. Other isolations were made from sentinel mice and hamsters, *Culex vomerifer* mosquitoes, and *Proechimys semispinosus*.

Clinical disease. The single human case had fever, chills, headache, prostration, and pains in the upper right quadrant.

Marituba virus. *Definition*. Genus *Bunyavirus*, serogroup C, species Marituba virus.

Epidemiology. This was the first group C virus to be isolated, coming from the blood of a sentinel *Cebus apella* monkey exposed in Belem Forest, Brazil. Other isolations have been made from *Culex* mosquitoes, from forest marsupials, and from man.

Clinical disease. A febrile illness with headache, generalized body pains, and pains in the joints.

Murutucu virus. *Definition*. Genus *Bunyavirus*, serogroup C, species Murutucu virus.

Epidemiology. The virus has been isolated many times in the Belem forest, Brazil, from sentinel mice and *Cebus* monkeys, *Culex* mosquitoes, a variety of forest rodents and marsupials, and from man; it has also been reported from French Guiana.

Clinical disease. An undifferentiated febrile illness with headache, fever, myalgia, and arthralgia.

Oriboca virus. *Definition*. Genus Bunyavirus, serogroup C, species Oriboca virus.

Epidemiology. Virus isolations have been made from man in Brazil and Surinam, and from wild and sentinel animals, mosquitoes, mainly *Culex* species; also from Trinidad and French Guiana.

Clinical disease. A febrile illness with headache, myalgia, arthralgia and conjunctival inflammation.

Ossa virus. *Definition*. Genus *Bunyavirus*, serogroup C, species Ossa virus.

Epidemiology. Like Madrid virus, Ossa virus was isolated from the blood of a mosquito catcher working in the rain forest of Panama. Other isolations have been made from *Culex* mosquitoes and from forest rodents.

Clinical disease. An undifferentiated febrile illness with myalgia and prostration.

Restan virus. *Definition*. Genus *Bunyavirus*, serogroup C, species Restan virus.

Epidemiology. Originally isolated in Trinidad from *Culex* (Melanoconion) species, the virus has been isolated from man in both Trinidad and Surinam.

Clinical disease. An undifferentiated febrile illness with generalized body pains, and prostration.

Serogroup California. Four viruses, California encephalitis virus, Inkoo, La Crosse, and Tahyna viruses, have been positively associated with disease in man; a fifth virus, Trivattatus virus, may possibly also infect man.

California encephalitis virus. *Definition*. Genus *Bunyavirus*, serogroup California, species California encephalitis virus.

Epidemiology. The prototype California encephalitis virus was isolated in 1943 from *Culex tarsalis* mosquitoes collected in San Joaquin valley, California. Other isolations were made from *Aedes melanimon (dorsalis)*, *Aedes vexans*, and other mosquito species in California, New Mexico, Texas, and Utah states, USA, and serological evidence pointed to the virus as a possible cause of encephalitis in children, in Kern County, California, in 1945. The virus is relatively rarely isolated, and recent isolates have been from New Mexico, Texas, and Utah, where no overt human disease has been seen.

Inkoo virus. *Definition*. Genus *Bunyavirus*, serogroup California, species Inkoo virus.

Epidemiology. Inkoo virus was originally isolated from a pool of *Aedes* mosquitoes collected in southern Finland but the virus extends throughout the whole of Finland, north of the arctic circle, where the great majority of adult Lapps have antibodies against this virus. Mammals, including cows, reindeer, and moose are frequently infected, as determined by antibody studies, but birds are rarely immune.

Clinical disease. The great majority of infections are probably silent, but children with febrile illnesses associated with some evidence of CNS involvement, such as meningismus, have been found to convert from antibody negative to positive in laboratory studies with Inkoo virus. The virus has not yet been isolated from a human case.

La Crosse virus. *Definition*. Genus *Bunyavirus*, serogroup California, species La Crosse virus.

Epidemiology. In 1964 Thompson *et al.* (1965) isolated a virus from brain tissue which had been removed from a four-year-old girl who had died in 1960 from meningoencephalitis in La Crosse, Wisconsin. The virus was shown to be closely related, but distinguishable from, the previously recognized California encephalitis virus. La Crosse virus is widely distributed throughout the USA, from the east coast westward as far as Utah. There have been many isolations of virus from a variety of mosquito species, *Aedes*, *Culex*, *Anopheles* and *Psorophora*, as well as from horseflies. Transovarial transmission of La Crosse virus in *Aedes triseriatus* mosquitoes has been established, which probably explains how the virus overwinters in the mid-west of the USA. Chipmunks, tree squirrels, cotton tail rabbits, and flying squirrels in the Wisconsin area have very high antibody rates, and are the probable vertebrate hosts for amplification of the virus. Since 1967 about 900 cases of 'California encephalitis' have been recognized in the USA, the great majority of which are attributable to La Crosse virus infections. Most human cases are reported from Wisconsin, Iowa, Indiana, Minnesota, or Ohio, but 20 states have had one or more cases.

Clinical disease. The great majority of diagnosed cases of California encephalitis occur in children, more often males than females, and there is nearly always a history of outdoor exposure in areas where woodland mosquitoes are prevalent. The incubation period is probably five to ten days, and is followed by a gradual onset of symptoms, with fever and headache, mild at first and becoming more severe and usually frontal, leading on to mental confusion and convulsions. Neck rigidity is common, as is nausea and vomiting. General lethargy may progress to coma, and although there may be meningeal signs, paralysis or permanent damage to the CNS are rare. The mortality is probably less than 1 per cent, but four virus isolations from fatal cases were made in 1978, suggesting a possible increase in virulence.

'California encephalitis' is something of a mis-nomer, since only a small minority of those infected with virus develop encephalitis. In parts of Wisconsin, up to 40 per cent of the population may have antibodies against La Crosse virus, so clearly only a small minority of those infected become ill. There is evidence from a prospective study carried out in Minnesota that some children had mild febrile illnesses associated with pharyngitis.

Tahyna virus. *Definition*. Genus *Bunyavirus*, serogroup California, species Tahyna virus.

Epidemiology. Originally isolated in Czechoslovakia from *Aedes caspius* mosquitoes collected in the village of Tahyna, the virus is now known to be widely distributed through a number of European countries including Austria, France, Germany, Italy, Romania, Norway, Yugoslavia, and USSR; a very similar virus, named Lumbo virus, was isolated at a place bearing the name in Mozambique. The principal vectors in central Europe are *Aedes vexans* and *Aedes cantans*, although many other species in at least five genera may play a part in the spread of the virus. The vertebrate hosts include rabbits, hedgehogs, horses, especially in the Camargue region of France, and probably a variety of small, woodland mammals, but birds do not appear to be involved in the natural history of this virus.

Clinical disease. The great majority of human infections are probably silent, in that overt disease is seldom recognized, but immunity rates can exceed 95 per cent in adults in certain areas of Czechoslovakia, and are about 50 per cent in the Rhône valley of France, and near the Danube in the vicinity of Vienna, Austria. There is increasing evidence that Tahyna virus infection may occasionally give rise to a febrile illness, with nausea, anorexia, headache, and, rarely, a non-fatal encephalitis. No deaths attributable to Tahyna virus have been reported.

Trivittatus virus. *Definition.* Genus *Bunyavirus*, serogroup California, species Trivittatus virus.
Epidemiology. Named after *Aedes trivittatus* mosquitoes, from which the first isolations were made, the virus circulates in cotton rats and other small mammals, and several mosquito species in Alabama, Florida, Illinois, Iowa, North Dakota, Ohio, Minnesota, and Wisconsin.
Clinical disease. None has been established with certainty.

Guama serogroup. Two of the eight Guama group viruses are known to infect man, Catu and Guama viruses.

Catu virus. *Definition.* Genus *Bunyavirus*, serogroup Guama, species Catu virus.
Epidemiology. The prototype virus was isolated from serum taken from a man with a febrile illness, in a forest area near Belem, Para, Brazil. Other isolations have been made in French Guiana and Trinidad. The virus circulates in wild forest rodents and marsupials, and is transmitted by *Culex* and *Anopheline* mosquitoes.
Clinical disease. Few cases have been recognized, but infection appears to cause a mild fever, with headache and muscle pains; there is no rash.

Guama virus. *Definition.* Genus *Bunyavirus*, serogroup Guama, species Guama virus.
Epidemiology. This is one of the most frequently isolated arboviruses in the Belem area of Brazil, and circulates in forest mammals, being transmitted by *Culex portesi* mosquitoes, as well as a variety of other Culex species, also *Aedes, Mansonia, Limatus, Psorophora,* and *Lutzomyia* species.
Clinical disease. Few cases have been recognized, but infection appears to cause a mild fever, with headache, muscle pains, and leucopenia.

Simbu serogroup. Two Simbu group viruses, Oropouche and Shuni viruses, are known to infect man; two others, Aino and Akabane viruses, produce congenital deformities (arthrogryposis, hydranencephaly, and anencephaly) in sheep, goats and cattle, but there is no evidence that these two infect man.

Oropouche virus. *Definition.* Genus *Bunyavirus*, serogroup Simbu, species Oropouche virus.
Epidemiology. Oropouche virus was first isolated in Trinidad from the blood of a forest worker who had a mild, febrile illness. In Brazil, isolations were made from the blood of a sloth, *Bradypus tridactylus*, and from *Aedes serratus* mosquitoes, but in 1961 the virus was shown to be responsible for an epidemic of a febrile disease in man in the Belem area involving some 7000 cases. Since then there have been other epidemics in Brazil involving tens of thousands of cases. The natural history of the infection is still imperfectly understood.
Clinical disease. A moderately severe febrile illness, with headache, generalized body pains, backache, moderately high fever (40 °C), prostration, joint pains, no rash, and occasionally neurological involvement progressing to definite encephalitis, but with no reported fatalities.

Shuni virus. *Definition.* Genus *Bunyavirus*, serogroup Simbu, species Shuni virus.

Epidemiology. Shuni virus was originally isolated in northern Nigeria from cattle blood collected at a slaughter house, and from *Culicoides* species collected in cattle sheds. It was subsequently isolated in Ibadan Nigeria, from the blood of an 18-month-old child; clinical details of the illness, if any, are not available. The virus has also been recovered in South Africa from *Culex theileri* mosquitoes.
Clinical disease. Not established.

References

Gibbs, C. J. Jr., Bruckner, E. A., and Schenker, S. (1964). A case of Apeu virus infection. *Am. J. trop. Med. Hyg.* **13**, 108.
McGowan, J. E., Bryan, J. A., and Gregg, M. B. (1973). Surveillance of arboviral encephalitis in the United States, 1955–1971. *Am. J. Epidemiol.* **97**, 199.
Smithburn, K. C., Mahaffy, A. F., and Paul, J. H. (1941). Bwamba fever and its causative virus. *Am. J. trop. Med.* **21**, 75.
Thompson, W. H., Kalfayan, B., and Anslow, R. O. (1965). Isolation of California encephalitis group virus from a fatal human illness. *Am. J. Epidemiol.* **81**, 245.

Genus *Nairovirus*

The genus *Nairovirus* is named after the virus of Nairobi sheep disease, an acute, haemorrhagic, gastro-enteritis affecting sheep and goats in East Africa, which was first described by Montgomery (1917), who correctly attributed the condition to a virus, and pointed out that transmission was due to the tick, *Rhipicephalus appendiculatus*. In addition to Nairobi sheep disease virus, the genus also includes four other viruses known to infect man, namely Crimean–Congo virus and the closely related Hazara virus, Dugbe virus and Ganjam virus. Crimean haemorrhagic fever was described by Chumakov (1946) as an acute, febrile, haemorrhagic disease affecting man in the Crimean region of the USSR, transmitted by ticks and carrying a mortality of 15–30 per cent. In Africa, Congo virus was first isolated in the then Belgian Congo from the blood of a 13-year-old African boy, and it caused a moderately severe laboratory infection in an adult European; related viruses were isolated in Uganda, where more laboratory infections occurred, one of which ended fatally after a severe haematemesis (Simpson *et al.* 1967). In Asia, a virus indistinguishable from Congo virus was isolated from tick pools collected in West Pakistan from a variety of wild and domestic animals, and a related, but serologically distinct virus, Hazara virus, was recovered from *Ixodes redikorzevi* ticks collected from the vole, *Altiocola roylei*, in a subarctic habitat at an altitude of 12 000 feet in the Kaghan valley of Hazara district (Begum *et al.* 1970*a, b*). Casals (1969) demonstrated that Crimean haemorrhagic fever virus was serologically indistinguishable from Congo virus, hence the use of the term Crimean–Congo virus. Shortly after the isolation of Hazara virus, another virus which was named Ganjam virus was isolated from *Haemophysalis intermedia* ticks collected from healthy goats in Ganjam district, Orissa, India, and in Africa, Dugbe virus was isolated from *Amblyomma variegatum* ticks collected from healthy white Fulani cattle at Dugbe market, Ibadan, Nigeria (Boshell *et al.* 1970; Causey *et al.* 1971; Kemp *et al.* 1971). Davies *et al.* (1978) reported that Nairobi sheep disease and Ganjam viruses were almost indistinguishable, and Casals and Tignor (1980) proposed the name Nairovirus for the set of viruses, since recognized as a genus, which included Nairobi sheep disease, Crimean–Congo, Dugbe, Ganjam, Hazara, as well as ten other viruses in three further serogroups known respectively as Dera Ghazi Khan, Hughes, and Qalyub serogroups. There are thus 15 different Nairoviruses, all transmitted by ticks, and all related by neutralization tests but separable by haemagglutination-inhibition and immunofluorescence tests.

Crimean–Congo virus. *Definition.* Genus *Nairovirus*, serogroup Crimean–Congo, species Crimean–Congo virus.
Epidemiology. In USSR, *Hyalomma anatolicum* ticks are principally responsible for virus transmission amongst domestic animals,

whereas *Hyalomma plumbeum plumbeum* ticks are more frequently infected and are concerned in the infection of wild mammals and birds, as well as domestic animals. In Africa, a variety of *Halomma* species, as well as *Amblyomma* and *Boophilus* ticks are known vectors, and in West Pakistan, Iran, and Iraq, *Ornithodorus* and *Hyalomma* species are involved. Vertebrate hosts include cattle, goats, hedgehogs, hares, and a number of bird species including rooks. Human infection mostly occurs in males who work closely with cattle, starting to appear in April, and reaching a peak in mid-summer. Transovarial transmission through ticks has been reported. In addition to transmission by tick bites, airborne infections have occurred in both hospital and laboratory environments.

Clinical disease. The incubation period is about one week. The onset of fever is usually sudden, and fever is usually continuous, although occasionally remittent or biphasic. Signs and symptoms include fever, headache, nausea, vomiting, joint pains, backache, photophobia, together with severe circulatory disorders, thrombocytopenia and leucopenia. Haemorrhagic manifestations are common, with bleeding from nasal, gastric, intestinal, uterine, and renal membranes and into the skin (Fig. 3). Cases may present with acute abdominal pain, mimicking an acute surgical emergency, and operating theatre staff have become infected and have died through contact with infected secretions exposed at operation. The mortality is about 15–30 per cent, but may be as high as 40–80 per cent in hospital or nosocomial outbreaks (Burney *et al.* 1980). There may be neurological involvement, which usually indicates a poor prognosis. Those patients who recover may be left with a polyneuritis which persists for months, but eventual recovery is to be expected. Transient hair loss has been reported.

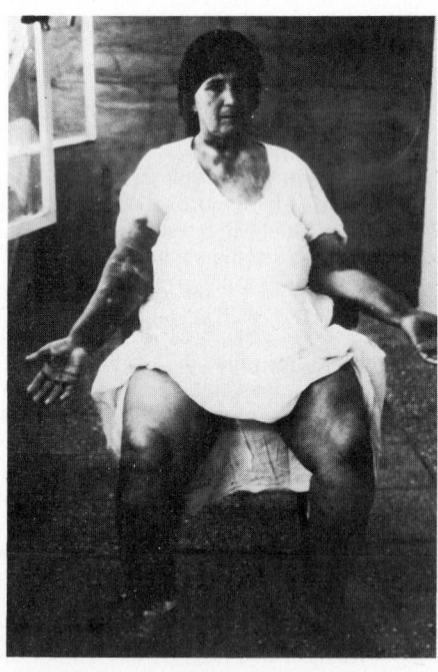

Fig. 3   Patient with Crimean–Congo haemorrhagic fever, showing extensive echymoses on the arms and thorax. (Photograph by courtesy of D. I. H. Simpson.)

Hazara virus. *Definition.* Genus *Nairovirus*, serogroup Crimean–Congo, species Hazara virus.

Epidemiology. The only evidence that this virus infects man is the finding that about 3 per cent of human sera collected in the Hazara district, Karachi, Lahore, and Dacca, had antibodies against this virus.

Dugbe virus. *Definition.* Genus *Nairovirus*, serogroup Nairobi sheep disease, species Dugbe virus.

Epidemiology. Several hundreds of isolations of Dugbe virus have been made in Nigeria from ticks, both *Ixodidae* and *Amblyomma*, but isolations have also been made in Nigeria from man and from *Culicoides*. Dugbe virus has also been detected in Kenya, Uganda, Central African Republic, Cameroun, Mozambique, and South Africa.

Clinical disease. The first known human case of Dugbe virus infection occurred in a laboratory worker in Nigeria who developed a fever, with nausea and prostration. The fever subsided on the fifth day, but the patient remained lethargic for several days; there were no sequelae. Three further cases were seen in children in Ibadan, Nigeria, one of which was accompanied by a fever of 41.3 °C, and with vomiting, but all showed a speedy recovery.

Ganjam virus. *Definition.* Genus *Nairovirus*, serogroup Nairobi sheep disease, species Ganjam virus.

Epidemiology. The original isolation was made in Orissa state, India, from *Haemaphysalis* ticks, but laboratory infections demonstrated the potential pathogenicity of the virus for man. Neither infection was serious.

Nairobi sheep disease virus. *Definition.* Genus *Nairovirus*, serogroup Nairobi sheep disease, species Nairobi sheep disease virus.

Epidemiology. In some outbreaks in East Africa, the mortality in sheep may be 70–90 per cent, both local and imported sheep being susceptible. Goats are less severely affected, but antibody surveys indicate a fairly wide distribution of the virus south of the Sahara as far south as Botswana and parts of South Africa. Herdsmen associated with sheep occasionally show mild, febrile illnesses which may be attributable to the virus, and there have been laboratory infections.

Clinical disease. A mild, febrile illness with conjunctivitis, headache, joint and body pains, but with no sequelae.

References

Begum, F., Wisseman, C. L., Jr., and Casals, J. (1970a). Tick-borne viruses of West Pakistan. II. Hazara virus, a new agent isolated from *Ixodes redikorzevi* ticks from Kaghan valley, West Pakistan. *Am. J. Epidemiol.* **92**, 192.

—, —, and — (1970b). Tick-borne viruses of West Pakistan. IV. Viruses similar to, or identical with, Crimean haemorrhagic fever (Congo-Semunya), Wad Medani, and Pak Argas 461 isolated from ticks of the Changa Manga forest, Lahore district, and of Hunza, Gligit Agency, West Pakistan. *Am. J. Epidemiol.* **92**, 197.

Boshell, J., Desai, P. K., Dandawate, C. N., and Goverdhan, M. K. (1970). Isolation of Ganjam virus from ticks *Haemaphysalis intermedia*. *Indian J. med. Res.* **58**, 561.

Burney, M. I., Ghafoor, A., Saleen, M., Webb, P. A., and Casals, J. (1980). Nosocomial outbreak of viral haemorrhagic fever caused by Crimean haemorrhagic fever–Congo virus in Pakistan, January 1976. *Am. J. trop. Med. Hyg.* **29**, 941.

Casals, J. (1969). Antigenic similarity between the virus causing Crimean haemorrhagic fever and Congo virus. *Proc. Soc. exp. Biol. Med.* **131**, 233.

—, and Tignor, C. H. (1980). The Nairovirus genus: serological relationships. *Interviriol.* **14**, 144.

Causey, O. R., Kemp, G. E., Casals, J., Williams, R. W., and Madbouly, M. H. (1976). Dugbe virus, a new arbovirus from Nigeria. *Niger. J. Sci.* **5**, 41.

Chumakov, M. P. (1946). Crimean haemorrhagic fever. *Vestn. Akad. Nauk. SSSR.* **2**, 19 (In Russian).

Davies, F. G., Casals, J., Jesset, D. M., and Ochieng, P. (1978). The serological relationships of Nairobi sheep disease virus. *J. comp. Path.* **88**, 519.

Kemp, G. E., Causey, O. R., and Causey, C. E. (1971). Virus isolations from trade cattle, sheep, goats and swine at Ibadan, Nigeria. *Bull. epizoot. Dis. Afr.* **19**, 131.

Montgomery, R. E. (1917). On a tick-borne gastro-enteritis of sheep and goats occurring in British East Africa. *J. comp. Path. Ther.* **30**, 28.

Simpson, D. I. H., Knight, E. M., Courtois, Ch., Williams, M. C. Weinbren, M. P., and Kibukamusoka, J. W. (1967). Congo virus: a hitherto undescribed virus occurring in Africa. *E. Afr. med. J.* **44**, 87.

Genus *Phlebovirus*

Six *Phleboviruses* are known to cause disease in man: the Naples and Sicilian strains of Phlebotomus, or Sandfly, fever viruses, Candiru, Chagres, Punta Toro and Rift Valley fever viruses. Some twenty other Phleboviruses have been isolated from rodents, other mammals, or from Phlebotomines, but are not known to infect man.

Candiru virus. *Definition*. Genus *Phlebovirus*, serogroup Phlebotomus fever, species Candiru verus.

Epidemiology. A single isolation of Candiru virus was made in Belem, Brazil, in 1960, from the blood of an adult male who complained of a fever. The virus was shown to be serologically related to, but distinct from other Phleboviruses. Its natural history remains unknown.

Chagres virus. *Definition*. Genus *Phlebovirus*, serogroup Phlebotomus fever, species Chagres virus.

Epidemiology. At least three virus isolations have been made from human blood in Panama, and others have also been made there from *Phlebotomines*.

Clinical disease. A mild, febrile illness, with headache, retro-orbital pains, dizziness, anorexia and nausea.

Phlebotomus fever, Naples and Sicilian viruses. *Definition*. Genus *Phlebovirus*, serogroup Phlebotomus fever, species Naples and Sicilian viruses.

Epidemiology. Pappataci fever, Sandfly fever, or Phlebotomus fever, was recognized as a clinical entity in the Mediterranean area during the nineteenth century, and the association with *Phlebotomus papatasi* midges was clearly demonstrated by Doerr, Franz, and Taussig (1909) who showed that filtrates of human blood would reproduce the disease in human volunteers. For many years it was thought that man was the only vertebrate host, although possible transovarial transmission through phlebotomus flies was demonstrated by Whittingham (1924), but more recently gerbils have been shown to be infected, and antibodies have shown that cattle and sheep may also be infected with these viruses. The Naples virus was isolated by American investigators from human serum collected during an outbreak in Naples (Sabin, Philip, and Paul 1944), and the Sicilian virus was isolated by the same workers from American troops with clinical Sandfly fever in Palermo, Sicily. The two viruses have many common properties, but they are serologically quite distinct. In addition to Italy, infections are widespread throughout Egypt, Iran, Turkey, India, Pakistan, Bangaladesh, Yugoslavia, Greece, and the southern states of USSR.

Clinical disease. The incubation period is from two to six days, and the illness usually starts with general lassitude, malaise, and ill-defined body pains. The temperature rises to its peak of 39–40 °C, usually within 24 hours of the onset. There may be quite severe headache, pains in the eyes, and conjunctivitis, and gastro-intestinal disturbances are also common. There is usually an erythema of the exposed parts of the face, neck and chest, but there is no true rash such as occurs in dengue fever. A bradycar.'ia is usual, as is a moderate leucopenia and a relative lymphocytosis. Fever seldom lasts longer than three days, and symptoms resolve rapidly once the fever abates, but there may be transitory mental depression during convalescence. The condition is never fatal, and there are almost no complications (Bartelloni and Tesh 1976).

Punta Toro virus. *Definition*. Genus *Phlebovirus*, serogroup Phlebotomus fever, species Punta Toro virus.

Epidemiology. Confined to the Canal Zone, Panama, and Colombia, although originally isolated in USA from the blood of a man recently returned from Panama. Transmission is by *Lutzomyia* species, *L. prapidoi* and *L. ylephilator*.

Clinical disease. The single established human case had a febrile illness, with headache, myalgia, retro-orbital pain, liver and splenic

enlargement, with some increased protein in the cerebrospinal fluid, without a pleocytosis.

Rift Valley fever virus. *Definition*. Genus *Phlebovirus*, serogroup Phlebotomus fever, species Rift Valley fever virus.

Epidemiology. Prior to 1977, Rift Valley fever was principally a disease of domestic animals, mainly sheep, which very occasionally spread to farm workers and others handling infected animals. The infection is enzootic in wild game animals in Africa, although seldom recognized in these. In 1977 the virus spread for the first time into Egypt, producing a major epizootic in domestic animals, principally sheep and goats, but also involving cattle and causing some 600 human deaths within a period of about three months. In central Africa, virus has been isolated from a variety of mosquitoes, *Aedes*, *Culex*, *Eratmopodites*, and *Culicoides*, but in Egypt the principal vector appears to have been *Culex pipiens*. The virus was probably introduced into Egypt through the Sudan, by the movement of infected camels. Transovarial transmission through mosquitoes has been demonstrated, and this mechanism may explain the recurrence of the disease in Egypt in 1978 and 1979. There is a high risk of infection in the laboratory, and infection of man may take place by aerosol created when infected animals are killed.

Clinical disease. There is an incubation period of three to six days, followed by an abrupt onset of fever, shivering, nausea and vomiting, epigastric pain, and often severe, generalized headache. The fever may be biphasic, with temperatures between 38 and 40° C, and may remain elevated for at least a week. There is no rash, but small haemorrhages into the skin and mucous membranes may be seen. Photophobia and eye pains are not uncommon: there may be conjunctival inflammation, a central serous retinitis, leading to central scotoma and sometimes to retinal detachment. The fundus may show macular exudates which are slow to disappear. There is often a lymphadenopathy, and although the liver is frequently involved and may be tender, jaundice is rare. Convalescence may be protracted, but is usually uncomplicated. There is no rash, but small haemorrhages into the skin and mucous membrane may be seen. Death from Rift Valley fever was virtually unknown in man prior to the 1977 outbreak in Egypt, and whether the severity of that outbreak resulted from a change in the virus towards increased virulence, or from a sensitization phenomenon similar to that of haemorrhagic dengue, or to a synergism between the virus and endemic schistosomiasis remains unknown.

Control measures are difficult. Vaccines for use in animals have been available for a number of years, and experimental vaccines have been used to protect laboratory workers at high risk, but a safe and potent vaccine for use in man is urgently needed.

References

Bartonelli, P. J., and Tesh, R. B. (1976). Clinical and serologic responses of volunteers infected with Phlebotomus fever virus (Sicilian type). *Am. J. trop. Med. Hyg.* **25**, 456.

Doerr, R., Franz, K., and Taussig, S. (1909). *Das Pappatacifieber*. Deuticke, Leipzig.

Sabin, A. B., Philip, C. B., and Paul, J. R. (1944). Phlebotomus (pappataci or sandfly) fever: a disease of military importance; summary of existing knowledge and preliminary report of original observations. *J. Am. med. Ass.* **125**, 603, 693.

Whittingham, H. E. (1924). The aetiology of Phlebotomus fever. *J. State Med.* **32**, 461.

Genus *Uukuvirus*

No *Uukuvirus* has yet been isolated from man, although antibodies against the prototype virus, *Uukuniemi* virus, or a strain of this virus known as Potepli virus, have been demonstrated in human sera collected in Czechoslovakia and in Estonia. *Uukuniemi* virus was originally isolated in Finland from *Ixodes ricinus* ticks, and other isolations have been made from birds or bird ticks in Norway, Poland, Czechoslovakia, USSR, other European countries, USA, Africa, and the Far East.

Unclassified Bunyaviridae

A number of viruses which are believed to be Bunyaviridae remain outside the four named genera, *Bunyavirus*, *Nairovirus*, *Phlebovirus*, and *Uukuvirus*. At least two such agents, Bhanja virus and Thogoto virus, are known to cause disease in man. Both are transmitted by ticks.

Bhanja virus. *Definition*. Genus unknown, serogroup unknown, species Bhanja virus.

Epidemiology. Bhanja virus was first isolated in India from *Haemophysalis intermedia* ticks collected in Ganjam district, Orissa, India, from goats being investigated for a condition known locally as 'lumbar paralysis of goats' (Shah and Work 1969). Other isolations have been made from cattle and goat ticks in West Africa, and from blood samples collected there from cattle, sheep, ground squirrel, and hedgehog, but no clear relation to disease in man was found in Africa or India. In Italy and Yugoslavia, Bhanja infection of goats is widespread. A laboratory worker handling the virus developed a moderately severe illness with neurological involvement (Calisher and Goodpasture 1975). More recently, there have been reports of at least two naturally acquired infections in Yugoslavia with severe neurological disease and death (Vesenjak-Hirjan *et al.* 1980).

Clinical disease. Laboratory infections have been associated with muscle and joint pains, frontal headache, and photophobia. The headache was accompanied by retro-bulbar pain, nausea, and vertigo. Recovery followed after an illness lasting about 10 days. The serologically confirmed natural infection began with pain in the back, fever, photophobia, and vomiting. The patient was admitted to hospital on the third day, and became semi-conscious, reacting violently to touch, with spinal rigidity, and a positive Kernig sign. The fever persisted for 11 days, and consciousness was disturbed for 16 days, the reflexes being hyperactive during all this time. There were relatively few cells in the CSF, but those present were predominantly mononuclear cells. The clinical picture was that of an acute meningoencephalitis with quadriparesis. The patient was discharged on the 45th day showing only slight muscular hypertonus and increased reflexes.

Thogoto virus. *Definition*. Genus unknown, serogroup Thogoto, species Thogoto virus.

Epidemiology. The original Kenyan isolation was made from *Boophilus* and *Rhipicephalus* ticks; other isolations have been made in Uganda, Nigeria, Egypt, and Sicily from ticks and from camel blood. There have been at least two virus isolations from man in Nigeria, one from an adult African male who had bilateral optic neuritis, and the other from a 14-year-old boy who died of a sickle-cell crisis following a meningitis.

Clinical disease. The adult was admitted to hospital with a history of joint cramps and malaise, followed by blurring of vision. The pupils reacted poorly to light, and there was bilateral papilloedema, but no conjunctival injection, exudate, or haemorrhage; the CSF was clear and colourless with a pressure of 130 mm of water, sugar 64 mg/dl ml, protein 60 mg/dl, some red blood cells, but no white blood cells. Thogoto virus was isolated from the CSF. Five days later he developed pyramidal signs in the limbs, and was diagnosed as a case of Devic's disease. After three months' steroid treatment he made a complete recovery, with full restoration of vision in both eyes.

Virus was isolated from the blood, but not the CSF, of the 14-year-old Nigerian boy, who was admitted to hospital with a history of headache and fever for four days. Two days later he had anorexia, dysphagia, and hepatosplenomegaly. He died on the sixth day. At post-mortem there was a leptomeningitis, but the liver showed extensive focal and mid-zonal eosinophilic necrosis, with marked sickling in the sinusoids (Moore *et al.* 1975).

References

Calisher, C. H. and Goodpasture, H. C. (1975). Human infection with Bhanja virus. *Am. J. trop. Med. Hyg.* **24**, 1040.

Moore, D. L., Causey, O. R., Carey, D. E., Reddy, S., Cook, A. R. Atkinbugbe, F. M., David-West, T. S., and Kemp, G. E. (1975). Arthropod-borne viral infections of man in Nigeria, 1964–1970. *Ann. trop. med. Parasit.* **69**, 49.

Shah, K. V. and Work, T. H. (1969). Bhanja virus: a new arbovirus from ticks *Haemaphysalis intermedia* Warburton and Nuttall, 1909, in Orissa, India. *Indian J. med. Res.* **57**, 793.

Vesenjak-Hirjan, J., Calisher, C. H., Beus, I., and Marton, E. (1980). First natural clinical Bhanja virus infection. In *Arboviruses in the Mediterranean Countries* (eds. J. Vesenjak-Hirjan, E. Artslanagic, and J. S. Porterfield). *Zbl. Bakt.* suppl. **9**, 297.

Arenaviruses

D. I. H. Simpson and E. T. W. Bowen

The arenavirus taxon takes its name from its sand-sprinkled (arenous) appearance when viewed in the electron microscope. Eleven members of the group have been described and almost all of them have rodents as their reservoir hosts.

Arenaviruses are enveloped, single-stranded RNA viruses with the virions seen as round, oval, or pleomorphic structures with diameters between 60 and 350 nm. The prototype member of the group, lymphocytic choriomeningitis virus (LCM), has been known since 1934 and occurs all over the world as a common contaminant of laboratory mice, rats, and hamsters. Eight viruses occur only in the New World and two are confined to Africa. All the New World members, often referred to as the Tacaribe complex, are more or less related by complement fixation tests; LCM and Lassa show only a distant relationship to the Tacaribe group viruses and are not closely related to each other.

Only two major rodent families are associated with arenaviruses. They are Muridae (mice, rats) and Cricetidae (voles, lemmings, gerbils). Lassa, LCM, and a more recent isolate from Mozambique are all found in members of the Muridae family while all the New World viruses are confined to cricetines. Arenaviruses, particularly those which cause human disease, have a capacity to produce a persistent, tolerant infection in their natural reservoir rodent hosts. The infection produces no ill-effects in the host and there is no immune response; virus can be excreted in body fluids during the animal's lifetime. Using laboratory animals, LCM infection of adult mice causes severe disease and death and is the classic example of virus-induced immunopathological disease. In contrast, if mice are infected before or shortly after birth they develop a non-pathogenic, life-long carrier state. In the newborn mouse, being immunologically immature, the virus does not stimulate an immune response and the virus causes no illness. The immunologically mature adult mouse develops an immune response following LCM virus infection and a fatal choriomeningitis results without evidence of neuronal damage. Immunosuppressants, neonatal thymectomy, and anti-lymphocytic serum protect adult mice against fatal LCM infection which suggests that the immune disease is cell-mediated.

Four arenaviruses—Junin, Lassa, LCM, and Machupo—cause significant and often severe disease in man. Pichinde virus may also infect man but no significant human disease has been reported. The mechanisms by which arenaviruses cause disease in man are not fully understood. There is no evidence that either immunopathological or allergenic processes play any part in causing disease, and it appears much more likely that direct viral damage to cells is the cause. It has been suggested that, in man, the virus enters the body either by the upper respiratory tract or by the alimentary route, is taken up in local lymph nodes or lymphoid tissue and replicates there initially; it then invades the reticulo-endothelial system including cells involved in immune and cellular immune responses and damages them, thus inhibiting their responses. The virus damages capillaries either directly or indirectly causing capillary fragility, haemorrhages, and hypovolaemic shock. Various organs may malfunction due to capillary damage and oedema of the parenchyma rather than due to direct cytolytic action. As the disease regresses, since little cell damage occurred, no permanent damage follows. In more severe cases there may be direct cell damage.

Lymphocytic choriomeningitis

Clinical features. The infection in man may present in one of four ways: as an inapparent infection, as an influenza-like, febrile illness, as aseptic meningitis, or as severe meningo-encephalomyelitis. The great majority of LCM infections follow a benign course.

The incubation period has been estimated to be from six to thirteen days. In the influenza-like illness there is fever, malaise, coryza, muscular pains, and bronchitis. In the meningeal form, which is more common, the same symptoms occur together with stiff neck, headache and nausea. These signs and symptoms may remain mild and of short duration and patients recover within a few days, but there can be a more pronounced illness with severe prostration lasting for two weeks or more. Fatalities are fortunately rare but chronic sequelae have been reported on occasions. They include paralyses, headache, and personality changes. The few deaths that have occurred followed severe meningo-encephalomyelitis and occasionally after severe bleeding. One case had a mild pharyngitis and a diffuse erythematous rash followed by haemorrhages and death.

A leucopenia has been a constant finding early in the course of disease with a lymphocytosis later. The cerebrospinal fluid is under increased pressure with slight increase in protein, normal or slightly reduced sugar, and a moderate number of cells (150–400 per mm^3). Virus can be isolated from the blood, CSF and, in fatal cases, from brain tissue.

Man is usually infected through contact with mice. Many infections occur in laboratories where LCM may be a contaminant in laboratory colonies of mice and hamsters. The mechanism of transmission of the virus to man is not fully understood, but it may be airborne through dust contaminated by urine, or through the alimentary tract through the contamination of food and drink. Transmission through skin abrasions may also be a possible route.

Argentinian haemorrhagic fever

This disease has been known since 1943, causing annual outbreaks with between 100 and 3500 cases of severe illness in Buenos Aires, Cordoba, Sante Fe, and La Pampa provinces of Argentina in an area of intensive agriculture known as the 'wet pampa'. The causative virus, Junin, was first isolated in 1958. The mortality rate in individual outbreaks has ranged from 10 to 20 per cent, although the overall mortality is generally 3–15 per cent. The disease is sharply seasonal coinciding with the maize harvest between April and July when rodent populations reach their peak. Agricultural workers, paticularly those involved in harvesting maize, are most commonly affected.

Clinical features. After an incubation period of 7–16 days, the onset of illness is insidious with chills, headache, malaise, myalgia, retro-orbital pain, and nausea followed by fever, conjunctival injection and suffusion, and enanthem, exanthema, and oedema of the face, neck and upper thorax. A few petechiae are most pronounced in the axilla. There is hypervascularity and occasional ulceration of the soft palate and generalized lymphadenopathy is common. After a few days in the more severe cases, the patient's condition becomes appreciably worse with the development of hypotension, oliguria, haemorrhages from the nose and gums, haematemesis, haematuria, and melaena. Oliguria may turn to anuria and pronounced neurological manifestations may develop. Death may result from anaemic coma or hypovolaemic shock caused by plasma leakage rather than blood loss. Most patients recover when the fever falls by lysis and is followed by a pronounced diuresis and rapid improvement. Subclinical infections are extremely rare and man-to-man transmission of the infection has not been recorded.

Treatment. Therapeutic trials with immune plasma have been carried out in Argentina for some time with encouraging results. Provided immune plasma is administered within eight days of the onset of symptoms viraemia levels have been considerably reduced and clinical improvement recorded. One complication of immunotherapy has been the development of late neurological symptoms of an encephalopathic type, but this phenomenon is fortunately rare.

Laboratory findings have included leucopenia, thrombocytopenia, and urinary casts. At post mortem lymphadenopathy with endothelial swelling in capillaries and arterioles in almost every organ have been found together with lymphocyte depletion in the spleen. Focal non-zonal necrosis in the liver with Kupffer cell hyperplasia, erythrophagocytosis, and acidophilic necrosis of hepatocytes have been noted. Other lesions which have been described include tubular necrosis in the kidneys, interstitial pneumonitis, lymphocytic infiltration of the spleen, minimal inflammation of the central nervous system and mycardium, and occasional evidence of intravascular coagulation.

The main reservoir hosts of Junin virus are *Calomys laucha* and *C. musculinus* which live and breed in burrows in the maize fields and in the banks which surround them. Other rodent species may also be involved and include *Akodon, Azarae,* and *Mus musculus.* *Calomys* species have a persistent viraemia and viruria, and virus is also present in considerable quantities in saliva. The mode of transmission of Junin virus to man has not been conclusively established. The virus may be carried in the air from dust contaminated by rodent excreta or may enter via the alimentary tract in foodstuffs similarly contaminated. Infection may also be acquired through skin abrasions.

Vaccine. A live attenuated vaccine against Junin has been under study. A plaque purified mouse brain passaged strain has shown considerable promise producing a good antibody response in voluteers with only minor febrile reactions. Until a suitable vaccine becomes available the best means of control seem to be rodent control and the use of more mechanical systems of farming.

Bolivian haemorrhagic fever

This disease was first recognized in 1959 in the rural areas of the Beni region in northeastern Bolivia. The most notable outbreak affected 700 people in San Joaquin township between late 1962 and the middle of 1964. The mortality rate was 18 per cent. The disease has continued to occur in the Beni region more or less annually in sharply localized epidemics. Transmission from man to man is unusual but a small episode took place in 1971 well outside the endemic zone. The index case, infected in Beni, carried the infection to Cochabamba and caused five secondary cases and four deaths by direct transmission.

Clinical features. The disease is extremely similar to Argentinian haemorrhagic fever. The incubation period ranges from seven to 14 days and the onset is insidious. About one-third of patients have bleeding tendencies with petechiae on the trunk and on the palate and bleeding from the gastrointestinal tract, nose, gums, and uterus. Almost half the patients develop a fine intention tremor of the tongue and hands, and several patients may have more pronounced neurological symptoms. The acute disease can last two to three weeks and convalescence may be protracted with generalized weakness being the commonest complaint. The mortality rate in individual outbreaks has varied from 5 to 30 per cent. Clinically inapparent infection is rare.

Isolation of the responsible virus, Machupo, from acutely ill patients has been difficult. Most isolations have been made from specimens taken seven to 12 days after the onset of illness. Virus has, however, been readily isolated from post mortem lymph nodes and spleen in fatal cases.

The rodent reservoir of Machupo virus is *Calomys callosus*; over 50 per cent of this species caught during the San Joaquin epidemic were found to be infected. The distribution of cases in San Joaquin was associated with certain houses and *C. callosus* was trapped in all households where cases occurred. Transmission to man is probably by contamination of food and water or by inoculation through skin abrasions.

Control is best achieved by rodent control and by improved housing. No vaccine is yet available.

Lassa fever

Lassa fever made a dramatic appearance in Nigeria in January 1969 as a lethal, highly transmissible, hitherto unknown disease. The first victim was an American missionary nurse who was infected at a small mission station in Lassa township in northeastern Nigeria from whence the virus and the disease which it causes derive their names.

The first recognized case became ill on 12 January 1969. The mode of her infection was never determined although it is thought that the disease was acquired through direct contact with a febrile patient in Lassa. In the early stages of her illness the nurse was not acutely ill and she continued to work until 20 January when severe pharyngitis and weakness developed. Her condition thereafter steadily deteriorated and she was flown to the Evangel Hospital in Jos on 25 January and died the following day.

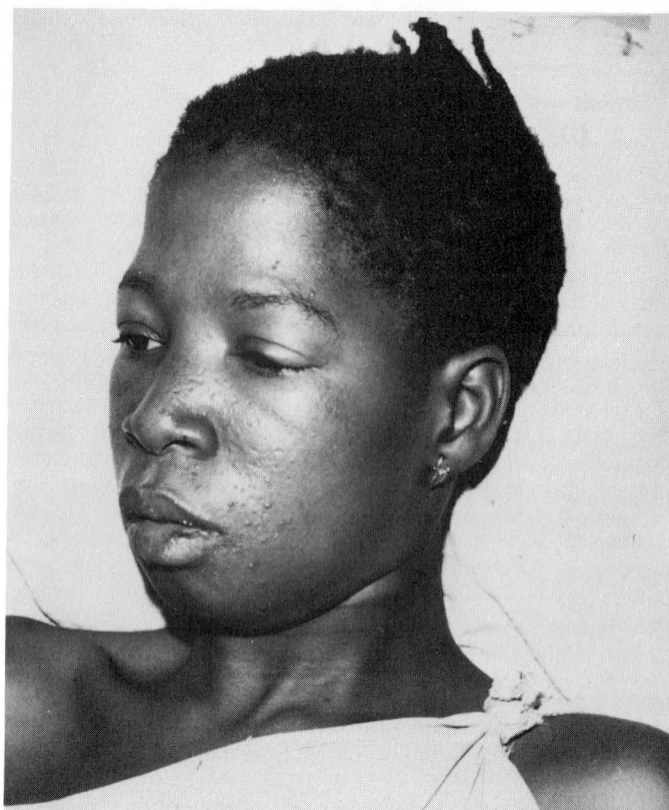

Fig. 2 Lassa fever in a young Sierra Leonean woman. Note characteristic oedema of eyelids and face indicative of increased capillary permeability. (Copyright: Dr D. A. Warrell.)

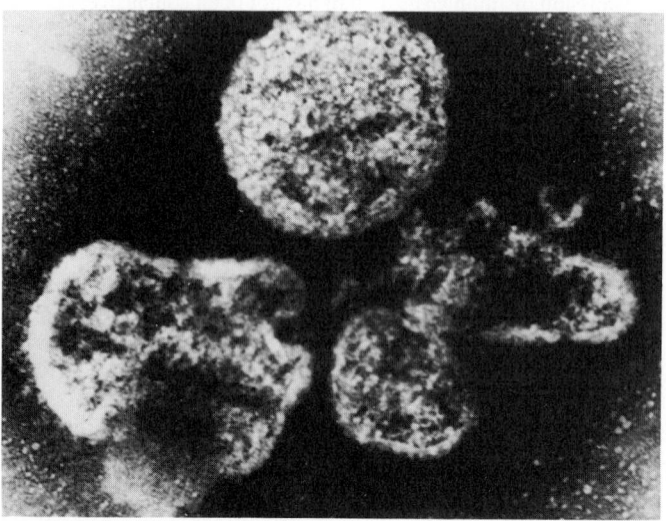

Fig. 1 Lassa virus, one of the arenaviruses (courtesy of Mr G. Lloyd and Dr D. S. Ellis).

While she was in hospital in Jos she was cared for by two other American nurses, one of whom was sequentially infected by direct contact, probably through a skin abrasion. This nurse became unwell after an eight-day incubation period and died after an illness lasting 11 days. The head nurse of the hospital who had assisted at the autopsy of the first patient and had cared for the second patient fell ill on 20 February, seven days after the second patient died. It seems most likely that she was infected while nursing the patient rather than at the autopsy. The third patient was evacuated to the USA by air in the first class cabin of a commercial Boeing 707 airliner with two attendants and screened from economy class passengers by only a curtain. She was admitted to the Presbyterian Hospital, Columbia University, New York, where after a severe illness under intensive care she slowly recovered. A virus, subsequently named Lassa, was isolated from her blood by workers at the Yale Arbovirus Research Unit. One of these virologists became ill on 9 June and survived only as a result of an immune plasma transfusion donated by the surviving third case.

Five months after this infection a laboratory technician in the Yale laboratories who had not been working with Lassa virus fell ill and died. The mode of infection was never elucidated.

This tragic trail of events not unnaturally received considerable

publicity in the world press and earned for Lassa virus a formidable notoriety. This malevolent reputation was sharply enhanced by a second devastating outbreak of Lassa fever in the Evangel Hospital in Jos in January and February 1970, almost exactly a year after the original one. A smaller epidemic took place a few miles away in Vom almost simultaneously. The source of this outbreak is thought to have been a patient admitted with a diagnosis of pneumonia. It seems that during her stay in hospital this patient infected 16 other patients and staff in the ward who in turn transmitted the disease to a further five, as well as infecting one out-patient. The twenty-third case was the American doctor of the hospital who was infected through direct inoculation through a knife wound while carrying out an autopsy. Five further cases occurred outside the hospital through intimate home contacts of patients in the ward. This outbreak involved 28 cases, 27 of them native Nigerians, and 12 deaths including the American doctor who had first recognized the disease.

The third outbreak was in Zorzor, Liberia in March and April 1972 when 11 cases occurred in the obstetric ward of Curran Lutheran Hospital. This was again a nosocomial outbreak, with 11 cases, seven of whom were hospital staff. The remaining three cases were other patients in the obstetric ward. The index case was a pregnant woman admitted with fever and vaginal bleeding. She aborted and underwent dilatation and curettage carried out by an American nurse who subsequently died from her infection. There were no tertiary cases and no spread of the infection beyond immediate ward contacts.

The fourth epidemic was seen in Panguma and Tongo townships, Sierra Leone, between October 1970 and October 1972 involving 64 suspected cases and 24 deaths. This outbreak was not confined to hospitals, although hospital staff were at considerable risk and several were infected. Most of the patients acquired their illnesses in the community and there were several intrafamilial episodes within households.

Lassa fever has continued to occur in West Africa usually as sporadic cases. Since the first report in 1969 and July 1978 there have been 17 reported outbreaks involving 386 cases and 105 deaths, which is an overall mortality rate of 27 per cent. Eleven of the episodes were in hospitals comprising 57 cases and 25 deaths, a case fatality rate of 44 per cent; two were laboratory infections, two were individual community-aquired outbreaks and two were prolonged community outbreaks. Eight patients were flown to Europe or North America. One of them was evacuated with full isolation precautions and the remainder, of whom five were infectious, travelled on scheduled commercial flights as fare-paying passengers. Fortunately no contact cases resulted.

Clinical features. Lassa fever has a wide spectrum of disease from subclinical to fulminating fatal infection. The incubation period ranges from three to 16 days and the illness usually begins insidiously with feverishness, chilliness, malaise, and muscular pains followed by fever, headache, and sore throat. These non-specific early symptoms make clinical diagnosis difficult, and the disease may not be recognized until the later stages when the intensity of the illness increases markedly.

Between the third and sixth days of illness the symptoms dramatically worsen and there is high fever, severe prostration, conjunctival injection, diarrhoea, chest and abdominal pains, dysphagia, and vomiting. One important physical finding is a distinct pharyngitis with or without a sore throat, and yellow-white exudative spots may occur on the tonsillar pillars together with small vesicles and ulcers. The patient appears toxic, lethargic, dehydrated, the blood pressure is low with a narrow pulse pressure and there may be cervical lymphadenopathy and a coated tongue. Chest pain, located substernally and along the costal margins is often associated with tenderness on pressure and is exacerbated by coughing and deep inspiration. There may be puffiness of the face and neck (Fig. 2), blurred vision, deafness, and pleural effusions and occasionally a faint maculopapular rash may be seen during the second week of illness on the face, neck, trunk, and arms. In severe cases, haemorrhages also occur. Relative bradycardia, leucopenia, albuminuria, and granular casts in the urine may be seen. Cough is a common symptom and light-headedness, vertigo, and tinnitus appear in a few patients in the second week of illness. Deafness has been noted in about 20 per cent of patients in the second or third week and may be reversible but is more frequently permanent.

The fever generally lasts for seven to 17 days and is frequently variable; patients in whom the disease is fatal not uncommonly have a high sustained fever. Acutely ill patients suddenly deteriorate between days seven and 14 with a sudden drop in blood pressure, peripheral vasoconstriction, hypovolaemia, and anuria. The patient is restless and apprehensive and there may be pleural effusions and ascites. In addition coma, stupor, tremors and myoclonic twitching can occur. Death is due to shock, anoxia, respiratory insufficiency, and cardiac arrest.

Convalescence begins in the second to fourth weeks when the temperature returns to normal and the symptomatology improves. Most patients complain of extreme fatigue for several weeks. Loss of hair and deafness are often observed and brief bouts of fever can occur.

Laboratory findings. Because of the hazards which might result from contact with blood or other body fluids, few studies have been carried out. In the early stages a leucopenia has been noted but a leucocytosis can occur later in the illness. The differential count has not been particularly helpful but there is usually a neutropenia and a low platelet count. The prothrombin level may be normal or low whilst other blood clotting studies are usually normal. Albuminuria and granular casts in the urine have been noted in several instances. The blood urea is usually raised while lactic dehydrogenase, serum glutamine-oxaloacetic transaminase, and creatinine phosphokinase may be elevated. Serum bilirubin and protein levels are not altered.

Pathology. Only a limited number of autopsies have been carried out. Lassa virus is pantropic and causes lesions or malfunction in liver, kidney, myocardium, lung, brain, skeletal muscle, and pleura. Increased capillary permeability leads to interstitial oedema and haemorrhage while necrotic foci are found in many organs, particularly in the liver where diffuse hepatocellular damage is evident with focal necroses. Changes in the kidneys are minimal, contrasting strangely with the functional impairment. In the spleen atrophy of the Malpighian corpuscles and eosinophilic necrosis of surrounding cells have been described. It is still uncertain whether the cellular damage is caused directly by the virus or by the immunological response to infection.

Diagnosis. The absence of characteristic signs or symptoms in the early stages of infection makes clinical diagnosis difficult unless there is a history of contact with a known case or else there is a local outbreak. The possibility of Lassa fever should be considered whenever a patient from an endemic area presents with an unexplained febrile illness of relatively slow onset. A detailed travel history is very relevant because Lassa fever is only endemic in West Africa. The differential diagnosis in the early acute stage would include malaria, typhoid fever, typhus, influenza, yellow fever, other virus infections, infectious mononucleosis, meningococcaemia, and septicaemia.

The laboratory diagnosis of Lassa fever is confirmed by: (a) isolating the virus from the patient's blood, pharyngeal secretions or urine; or (b) demonstrating a serological response to Lassa fever in serum.

Lassa virus grows readily in Vero cell culture and isolation of the virus can usually be achieved within four days. Virus has been isolated from serum, throat washings, pleural fluid, and urine; virus excretion has been shown in the pharynx for up to 14 days after the onset of illness and in urine for up to 32 days after onset.

Virus isolation should only be attempted in laboratories specially equipped to provide maximum containment to protect the investigator. The most sensitive serological test for the detection of Lassa antibodies is the indirect immunofluorescence reaction. Antibodies can be detected by this method in the second week of illness. Complement-fixing antibodies develop more slowly and are rarely detectable before the third week after onset. On occasions complement-fixing antibodies have failed to develop in patients from whom Lassa virus has been isolated. It may be possible to make an early diagnosis of Lassa infection by detecting Lassa-specific antigens in conjunctival cells by using indirect immunofluorescence but this test system is still under review.

Management and control. Any patient with suspected or confirmed Lassa fever should be immediately placed in isolation. Some hospitals have special facilities which are designed to prevent contamination of the area outside the patient's immediate environment. Lassa fever is generally diagnosed and suspected in medical facilities which have no specialized containment areas. In these cases strict isolation and barrier nursing should be carried out without delay. To minimize the risk of transmitting Lassa virus to medical and nursing staff caring for the patient, several precautions should be undertaken. The patient should be placed in a private room which should only be entered through an anteroom. Ideally the isolation facility should be in a separate building. Hospital staff should wear gowns, full-face respirators with HEPA filters or surgical masks and goggles, gloves, boots and caps. The anteroom should have washing facilities and should have supplies of protective clothing and facilities for disposal of soiled and contaminated articles. Access to the patient's room and anteroom should be limited only to those responsible for the care of the patient. A chemical toilet should be provided for the patient and all excreta treated with Lysol or 0.5 per cent sodium hypochlorite. All objects for removal from the isolation facility should be double-bagged in sealed plastic bags and the outside should be washed down in 0.5 per cent hypochlorite solution before removal.

Therapy. Although the passive administration of Lassa immune plasma may suppress viraemia and favourably alter the clinical outcome of the disease this has not always been found to be true. The simultaneous presence of Lassa virus and naturally-acquired antibodies have been found in patients' blood during the second week of illness. This suggests that some of the pathology may be due to the deposition of antigen–antibody complexes. Administration of Lassa immune plasma may, under certain circumstances, only aggravate the patient's condition.

Treatment is largely symptomatic and supportive. Antimalarials and broad-spectrum antibiotics have been given routinely and the clinical response may be very helpful diagnostically especially if typhoid fever is suspected. If a clinical response is not observed after four to five days, antibiotics may be discontinued. Care should be taken to maintain water and electrolyte balance. If renal failure develops, peritoneal dialysis may be required.

It has recently been reported that ribavirin, an antiviral drug, has been successfully used in the treatment of Lassa-infected rhesus monkeys. Clinical trials with ribavirin are currently being carried out in Sierra Leone.

Epidemiology. In common with other arenaviruses, Lassa virus appears to have a natural cycle of transmission in rodents. Lassa virus has been repeatedly isolated from the multimammate rat, *Mastomys natalensis*, in Sierra Leone and Nigeria. This rodent is a common domestic and peridomestic species and is widely distributed in Africa south of the Sahara. It is a prolific breeder and large populations may be present in the countryside. During the rainy season it may desert the open fields and seek shelter indoors especially where the more aggressive black rat has been eliminated from human dwellings. Some genetic variation has been shown in *Mastomys* populations which may account for the focal distribution of Lassa fever in West Africa. Like other arenaviruses, Lassa produces a persistent tolerated infection in its rodent reservoir host with no ill effects in *Mastomys natalensis* and without any immune response. The animals are infected at birth or during the perinatal period and remain infective during their lifetime freely excreting Lassa virus in urine and other body fluids.

Primary infection in man is thought to be acquired directly from infected rodent urine or indirectly from foodstuffs or dust contaminated by urine. It has been suggested that a low level of sanitation, storage of food within houses, and the ease with which rodents can infest mud-and-thatch houses increase contact between rodents and man. However, the way the virus is spread from person to person is still not clear. Secondary spread from person to person may occur in overcrowded houses but spread of this kind is particularly important in rural hospitals. Medical attendants or relatives providing direct personal care are most likely to contract the infection, and accidental inoculation with a sharp instrument and contact with blood have accounted for a few cases. Airborne spread as well as mechanical transmission can occur. Although in Sierra Leone there has been no evidence of airborne spread in hospital outbreaks, the 1970 outbreak in Jos, Nigeria is believed to have been caused by airborne transmission from a woman with severe pulmonary involvement.

Subclinical infection or mild attacks of Lassa fever seem to be quite common, at least in the endemic areas of Sierra Leone. There, surveys have shown that 6–13 per cent of the population has Lassa antibodies. With rapid air travel, it is all too easy for patients incubating Lassa infection to develop their illnesses in distant countries where the disease and its natural reservoir hosts do not normally exist.

Prevention. There is still no vaccine available for prophylactic immunization. The best means of control might well be in controlling the rodent populations by the use of rodenticides.

References

Carey, D. E., Kemp, G. E., White, H. A., Pinneo, L., Addy, R. F., Fom,

A. L. M. D., Stroh, G., Casals, J., and Henderson, B. E. (1972). Lassa fever. Epidemiological aspects of the 1970 epidemic, Jos, Nigeria. *Trans. R. Soc. Trop. Med. Hyg.* **66**, 402.

Casals, J. (1975). Arenaviruses. *Yale J. Biol. Med.* **48**, 115.

Commission Nacional Coordinadora para Estuido y Lucha Contra la Fievre Hemorragica (1966). Buenos Aires, Argentina.

Elsner, B., Schwartz, E., Mando, O., Maiztegui, J., and Vilches, A. (1970). Patologia de la fievre hemorragica Argentina. *Medicina* **30**, Suppl. 1, 85.

Frame, J. D., Baldwin, J. M., Gocke, D. J., and Troup, J. M. (1970). Lassa fever, a new virus disease of man from West Africa. I. Clinical description and pathological findings. *Am. J. trop. Med. Hyg.* **19**, 670.

Jahrling, P. B., Hesse, R. A., Eddy, G. A., Johnson, K. M., Callis, R. T., and Stephen, E. L. (1980). Lassa virus infection of rhesus monkeys: pathogenesis and treatment with ribavirin. *J. infect. Dis.* **141**(5), 580.

Lehmann- Grube, F. (1971). *Lymphocytic choriomeningitis virus.* Virology monographs, 10. Springer-Verlag, New York.

Mackenzie, R. B. (1965). Epidemiology of Machupo virus infection. I. Pattern of human infection, San Joaquin, Bolivia, 1962. *Am. J. trop. Med. Hyg.* **14**, 808.

Maiztegui, J., Fernandez, N. J., and de Damilano, A. J. (1970). Efficacy of immune plasma in treatment of Argentine haemorrhagic fever and association between treatment and a late neurological syndrome. *Lancet* **ii**, 1216.

Monath, T. P. (1973). Lassa fever. *Trop. Doctor* **4**, 155.

Weissenbacher, M. C., de Guerrero, L. B., and Boxaca, M. L. (1975). Experimental biology and pathogenesis of Junin virus infection in animals and man. *Bull. Wld Hlth Org.* **52**, 507.

Winn, W. C. and Walker, D. H. (1975). The pathology of human Lassa fever. *Bull. Wld Hlth Org.* **52**, 535.

Hepatitis viruses

A. J. Zuckerman

Many viruses may infect the liver of animals and man, and may produce severe hepatitis. In man, the general term viral hepatitis refers to infections caused by at least three different viruses, hepatitis A (infectious or epidemic hepatitis), hepatitis B (serum hepatitis), and the more recently identified form of hepatitis, non-A, non-B hepatitis, which appears to be caused by more than one virus. Indeed, viral hepatitis has emerged as a major public health problem occurring endemically in all parts of the world.

Acute viral hepatitis is a generalized infection with particular emphasis on inflammation of the liver. The clinical picture of the infection varies in its presentation from asymptomatic or subclinical infection, mild gastrointestinal symptoms, and the anicteric form of the disease, acute illness with jaundice, severe prolonged jaundice, to acute fulminant hepatitis. Hepatitis B and non-A, non-B hepatitis may be associated with a persistent carrier state and both forms of infection may progress to chronic liver disease, which may be severe. There is now substantial evidence of a close association between hepatitis B virus and primary hepatocellular carcinoma.

Hepatitis A and hepatitis B viruses have been identified and characterized, and these infections can now be differentiated by sensitive and specific laboratory tests for the antigens and antibodies associated with these infectious agents. The third form of hepatitis is at present the most common type of post-transfusion hepatitis occurring in some areas and an important cause of sporadic hepatitis in adults, although precise virological criteria and specific laboratory tests are not yet available.

Hepatitis A

Hepatitis A occurs endemically in all parts of the world, but the exact incidence is difficult to estimate because of the high proportion of asymptomatic and anicteric infections, differences in surveillance and differing patterns of disease. The degree of under-reporting is believed to be very high. Recent serological surveys have shown that while the prevalence of hepatitis A in industrialized countries, particularly in northern Europe, North America, and Australia is decreasing, the infection is almost universal in most countries.

Incubation period. The incubation period of hepatitis A is usually between three and five weeks with a mean of 28 days. Subclinical and anicteric infections are common, and although the disease has, in general, a low mortality, patients may be incapacitated for many weeks. There is no evidence of persistence of infection and progression to chronic liver damage does not occur.

Mode of spread. Hepatitis A virus is spread by the faecal–oral route, most commonly by person to person contact, and infection is particularly common in conditions of poor sanitation and over-crowding. Common source outbreaks most frequently result from faecal contamination of drinking water and food, but waterborne transmission is not a major factor in industrialized communities. On the other hand, many food-borne outbreaks have been reported. This can be attributed to the shedding of large amounts of virus in the faeces during the incubation period of the illness in infected foodhandlers, and the source of the outbreak can often be traced to uncooked food or food that has been handled after cooking. The consumption of raw or inadequately cooked shellfish cultivated in polluted water is associated with a high risk of hepatitis A infection. However, although hepatitis A is common in the developed countries, the infection occurs mainly in small clusters and often with only few identified cases. Hepatitis A is highly endemic in many tropical and subtropical areas, with the occasional occurrence of large epidemics. This infection is frequently acquired by travellers from areas of low to areas of high endemicity.

Outbreaks of hepatitis A have also been described among handlers of newly captured nonhuman primates, particularly chimpanzees and other apes. Hepatitis A is not transmitted by blood and blood products and rarely if ever by the parenteral route, although this has been achieved experimentally in volunteers and in susceptible nonhuman primates.

Age incidence. All age groups are susceptible to hepatitis A. The highest incidence in the civilian population is observed in children of school age, but in many countries in northern Europe and in north America most cases occur in adults. This shift in age incidence is similar to the change in age incidence which occurred with poliomyelitis during and after the Second World War, reflecting improvement in socio-economic and hygienic conditions.

Seasonal pattern. In temperate zones the characteristic seasonal trend is for an increase in incidence in the autumn and early winter months falling progressively to a minimum during the midsummer. However, more recently the seasonal peak has been lost in some countries. In many tropical countries the peak of the infection tends to occur during the rainy season with a lower incidence during the dry periods.

Pathological changes in the liver. Two features are constant in acute viral hepatitis: parenchymal cell necrosis and histiocytic periportal inflammation. Usually the reticulin framework of the liver is well-preserved except in some cases of massive and submassive necrosis. The pattern of histological changes in the liver is essentially similar in hepatitis types A and B and consists of marked focal activation of sinusoidal lining cells; accumulations of lymphocytes in histiocytes within the parenchyma, often replacing hepatocytes lost by necrosis; mild diffuse hepatocytic changes with occasional coagulative necrosis in the form of acidophilic bodies; and focal regeneration and portal inflammatory reaction with alteration of bile ductules. The lesions in hepatitis A develop earlier, and the duration of morphological changes is shorter, while the lesions in hepatitis B linger on, fluctuate, and regress slowly. There is some difference in the distribution of the lesions: in hepatitis A, the localization of parenchymal changes is predominantly periportal, whereas in hepatitis B the lesions are diffuse and tend to be accentuated around the hepatic vein tributaries, and streaks of focal necrosis may extend from portal tracts to hepatitic vein tributaries.

The nature of hepatitis A virus and laboratory tests. In 1973, small cubic virus particles (Figs. 1 and 2), measuring 27 nm in diameter, were identified by immune electron microscopy in faecal extracts obtained during the early acute phase of illness of adult volunteers infected orally or by the parenteral route with the MS-1 strain of hepatitis A virus. The availability of viral antigen permitted in turn the identification of specific antibody and the development of serological tests for hepatitis A. Human hepatitis A has been transmitted experimentally to certain species of marmosets and to chimpanzees free of hepatitis A antibody, thereby providing an important model of infection and a source of reagents. The infection in nonhuman primates is mild, often subclinical and always anicteric.

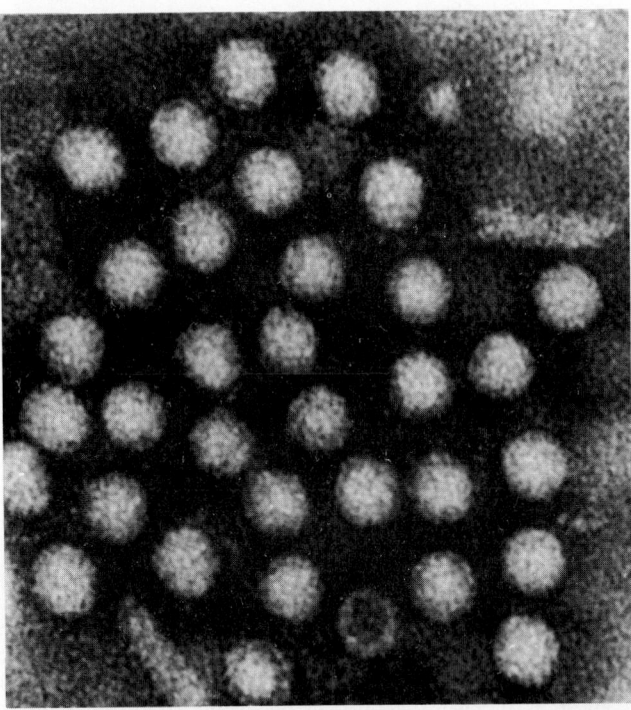

Fig. 1 Electron micrograph showing hepatitis A virus in faecal extracts obtained during the early acute phase of illness. The particles measure about 27 nm in diameter ($\times$ 400 000). (From a series by A. Thornton and A. J. Zuckerman.)

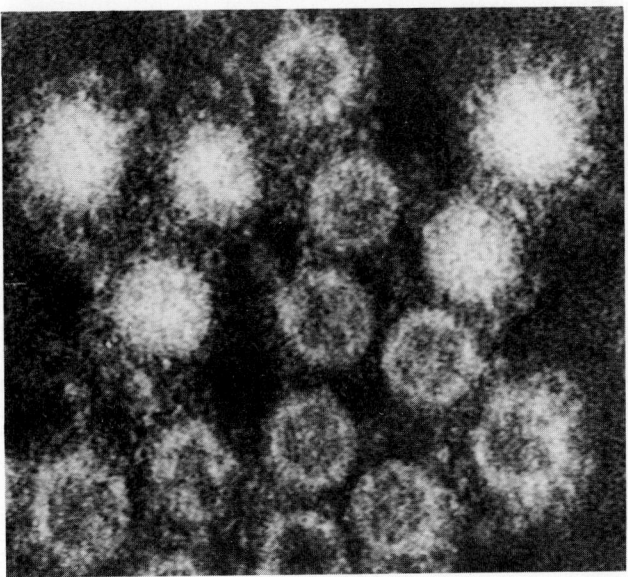

Fig. 2 Electron micrograph showing a large aggregate of hepatitis A virus particles heavily coated with antibody giving the appearance of a 'halo'. Both 'full' and 'empty' particles are shown $\times$ 400 000. (From a series by A. Thornton and A. J. Zuckerman.)

Large numbers of virus particles are found during the incubation period in experimental infection in chimpanzees, beginning as early as nine days after exposure, and shedding of the virus continues usually until peak elevation of serum aminotransferases. Similar observations have been made in the course of experimental and natural infection in man. The virus is also detected during the acute phase of illness, but the number of particles decreases rapidly after the onset of clinical jaundice. Prolonged virus excretion and a persistent carrier state have not been demonstrated. It is interesting to note that in chimpanzees and in man, antibody to hepatitis A virus is found in the serum during the late incubation period of the infection, coinciding approximately with the onset of rising serum aminotransferase levels.

Recent studies on the nature of hepatitis A virus have shown that this virus is unenveloped containing a linear genome of single-stranded RNA with a molecular weight of 1.9×10^6 dalton, and polypeptides with similar molecular weights to the four major polypeptides of the *Enterovirus* genus within the picornaviridae. The virus is ether-resistant, stable at pH 3.0 and relatively resistant to inactivation by heat. It is partially inactivated by heat at 60 °C for one hour, mostly inactivated at 60 °C for ten hours and inactivated at 100 °C for five minutes. Hepatitis A virus is inactivated by ultraviolet irradiation and by treatment with 1:4000 concentration of formaldehyde solution at 37 °C for 72 hours. There is also preliminary evidence that hepatitis A virus is inactivated by chlorine at a concentration of 1 mg/l for 30 minutes.

The successful propagation of hepatitis A virus in 1979 in primary monolayer and explant cell cultures and in continuous cell strains of primate origin opens the way to the detection and assay of the virus *in vitro* and also to the preparation of hepatitis A vaccines.

Specific serological tests for hepatitis A antigen and antibodies have been developed, including immune electron microscopy, immune adherence haemagglutination, radioimmunoassay, and enzyme-linked immunosorbent assay. Hepatitis A antibody is always demonstrable by radioimmunoassay or enzyme immunoassay during the early phase of the illness, and titres increase rapidly. The antibody usually persists for many years and its presence indicates immunity. Since antibody develops very early in the course of the infection, serological diagnosis of recent infection can be established only by titrations of serial samples of serum, or by the demonstration of hepatitis A antibody of the IgM class, which is the simplest and most economical method of establishing the diagnosis. Hepatitis A IgM is detectable in serum for 45–60 days after the onset of symptoms.

Because of the development of serological tests for hepatitis A antibody, it became possible to study the incidence and distribution of hepatitis A infection in different populations and various geographical areas. An early survey of hepatitis A antibody, using immune adherence haemagglutination for testing serum samples from healthy adults, mostly volunteer blood donors, from seven countries, showed that the age-standardized prevalence of hepatitis A antibody was 24 per cent in Switzerland, 41 per cent in the USA, 75 per cent in Senegal, 88 per cent in Belgium, 90 per cent in Taiwan, 93 per cent in Israel, and 97 per cent in Yugoslavia.

Although only one serotype of hepatitis A has been identified in volunteers infected experimentally, in patients from different outbreaks of hepatitis A in different geographical regions, in sporadic cases of hepatitis A, and in naturally and experimentally infected chimpanzees, there is evidence that some antigenic strain differences may occur.

Control. Control of the infection is difficult. Since faecal shedding of the virus is at its highest during the late incubation period and prodromal phase of the illness, strict isolation of cases is not a useful control measure. Spread of hepatitis A is reduced by simple hygienic measures and the sanitary disposal of excreta.

Normal human immunoglobulin, a 16 per cent solution in a dose of 0.02–0.12 ml/kg body weight, given intramuscularly before exposure to the virus or early during the incubation period, will prevent

or attenuate a clinical illness, while not always preventing infection and excretion of hepatitis A virus, and inapparent or subclinical hepatitis may develop. The efficacy of passive immunization is based on the presence of hepatitis A antibody in the immunoglobulin, but the minimum titre of antibody required for protection has not yet been established. Immunoglobulin is used most commonly for close personal contacts of patients with hepatitis A, and for those exposed to contaminated food. Immunoglobulin has also been used effectively for controlling outbreaks in institutions, such as homes for the mentally-handicapped, and in nursery schools. Prophylaxis with immunoglobulin is recommended for persons without hepatitis A antibody visiting highly endemic areas.

Vaccines against hepatitis A are under development.

Hepatitis B

The discovery of Australia antigen in the circulation in 1965, and subsequently its association with hepatitis type B, led to rapid advances in the understanding of this complex infection.

Serological markers of hepatitis B. Infection with hepatitis B virus (Fig. 3) leads to the appearance in the plasma during the incubation period of a specific antigen, hepatitis B surface antigen (originally referred to as Australia antigen), about two to eight weeks before biochemical evidence of liver damage or the onset of jaundice. The antigen persists during the acute illness, and it is usually cleared from the circulation during convalescence. Next to appear in the circulation is specific DNA polymerase associated with the core or nucleocapsid of the virus, and at about the same time another antigen, the e antigen, becomes detectable, again preceding serum aminotransferase elevations. The e antigen is a distinct soluble antigen which is specifically associated with hepatitis B and is located within the core of the virus particle. This marker of infection with hepatitis B virus correlates closely with the number of virus particles and the relative infectivity of the plasma or serum. Antibody to the core is found two to four weeks after the appearance of the surface antigen, and it is usually detectable during the early acute phase of the illness, persisting after recovery.

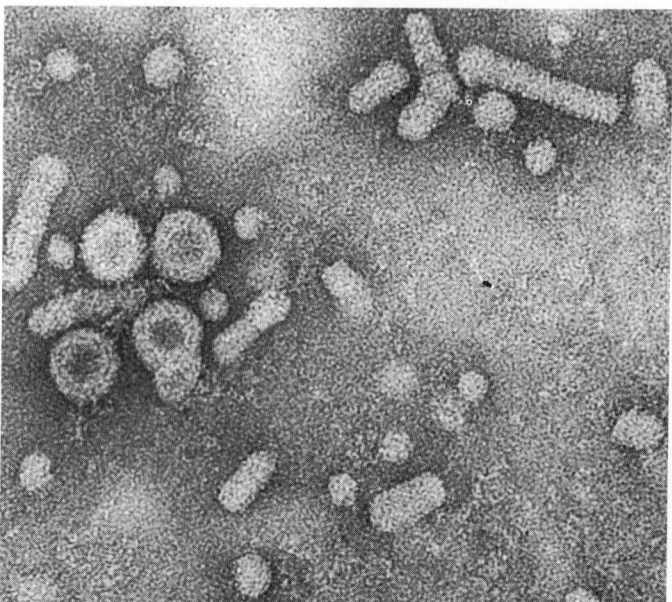

Fig. 3 Electron micrograph of serum containing hepatitis B virus after negative staining. The three morphological forms of the antigen are shown: (*a*) small pleomorphic spherical particles 20–22 nm in diameter (hepatitis B surface antigen); (*b*) tubular structures (a form of the surface antigen); (*c*) the 42 nm double-shelled virus, with a core surrounded by the surface antigen. (× 214 000). (Reproduced with permission from A. J. Zuckerman (1975). *Human Viral Hepatitis*. North Holland, Amsterdam.)

The next antibody to appear in the circulation is directed against the *e* antigen, and there is evidence that, in general terms, anti-*e* indicates relatively low infectivity of serum. Antibody to the surface antigen component, hepatitis B surface antibody, is the last to appear late during convalescence. More recently, precipitating antibodies reacting with specificities on the complete virus particle have been described. These antibodies may be relevant to the clearance of circulating hepatitis B virions and the termination of acute infection. Cell-mediated immunity also appears to be important in terminating hepatitis B infection and, under certain circumstances, in promoting liver damage and in the genesis of autoimmunity.

The availability of hepatitis B serological markers (Table 1) which can now be detected by sensitive laboratory techniques, such as enzyme-linked immunosorbent assay and radioimmunoassay, has proved extremely useful for unravelling the epidemiology of hepatitis B. The use of serological markers has established the global dissemination and public health importance of this infection, led to the routine screening of blood donors for the surface antigen, and resulted in remarkable advances in the knowledge of the virology and pathogenesis of hepatitis B and its associated chronic liver disorders.

Table 1   Interpretation of results of serological tests for hepatitis B

HBsAg	HBeAg	Anti-HBe	Anti-HBc IgM	Anti-HBc IgG	Anti-HBs	Interpretation
+	+	−	−	−	−	incubation period
+	+	−	+	+	−	acute hepatitis B or persistent carrier state
+	+	−	−	+	−	persistent carrier state
+	−	+	+/−	+	−	persistent carrier state
−	−	+	+/−	+	+	convalescence
−	−	+	−	+	+	recovery
−	−	−	+	−	−	infection with hepatitis B virus without detectable HBsAg
−	−	−	−	+	−	recovery with loss of detectable anti-HBs
−	−	−	−	−	+	immunization without infection; repeated exposure to antigen without infection, or recovery from infection with loss of detectable anti-HBc

Hepatitis B virus. Examination of serum specimens containing hepatitis B surface antigen by electron microscopy and immune electron microscopy reveals a remarkable pleomorphism of virus-like particles (Fig. 3) consisting of small roughly spherical particles measuring about 22 nm in diameter, tubular forms of varying length but with a diameter close to 22 nm and large double-shelled particles about 42 nm in diameter. The 42 nm particle consists of a core about 28 nm in diameter with a 2 nm shell and an outer coat approximately 7 nm in thickness. There is substantial evidence that the 42 nm particle is the hepatitis B virus whereas the small particles and the tubular forms are non-infectious surplus virus coat protein.

The core of the virus has a sub-unit structure organized according to the principles of icosahedral symmetry, and an endogenous core antigen-associated DNA-dependent DNA polymerase in close association with a DNA template. Double-stranded DNA has been isolated from circulating virus and also from cores extracted from the nuclei of infected hepatocytes. The DNA consists of circular

nucleic acid molecules with a mean contour length of 0.79 ± 0.09 μm, with a molecular weight of about 2.3×10^6 dalton. The DNA has been characterized by gel electrophoresis and restriction enzyme cleavage, and shown to be a structure approximately 3600 nucleotides in length containing a single-stranded gap of 600–2100 nucleotides. The endogenous DNA polymerase reaction appears to repair the gap, but the relevance of the gapped circular DNA to the mode of replication of the virus is not clear.

The entire DNA of hepatitis B virus has been cloned in *Escherichia coli* with expression of viral antigenic proteins.

Properties of hepatitis B surface antigen. The presence of distinct surface antigenic determinants on particles of hepatitis B virus permits the isolation of the surface antigen from normal serum proteins for immunochemical analysis. The lipoprotein nature of the surface antigen permits its partial separation from the normal serum proteins by virtue of its characteristic buoyant density within the range of one of the two major subclasses of serum high-density lipoproteins (HDL_3: 1.08–1.21 g/ml). The exact buoyant density of hepatitis B surface antigen varies with the serum tested and with the chemical employed in forming the density gradient. Centrifugation of serum in caesium chloride results in separation of the surface antigen at an average density of 1.20 g/ml. The tubular forms are found in the same fraction and some empty or partially full virus particles. Complete or partially full virus particles separate at a density of 1.25 g/ml after equilibrium centrifugation in caesium chloride.

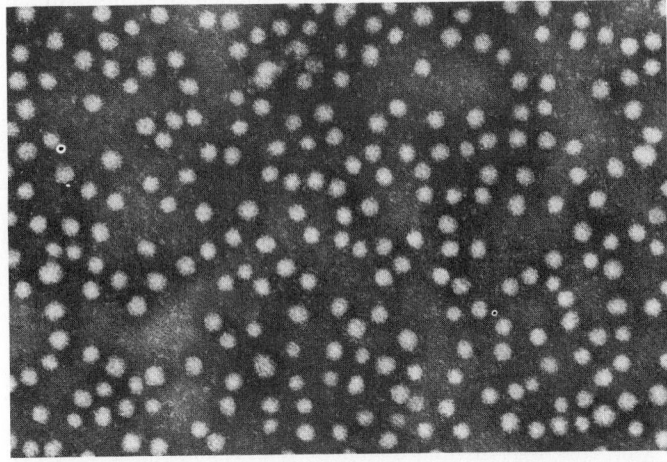

Fig. 4   Low power electron micrograph of purified 22 nm hepatitis B surface antigen particle vaccine (× 126 000).

The small spherical 22 nm particles comprise the bulk of the surface antigen in most sera. The lipid content of the small particles may account for 30 per cent of the total weight, with a predominance of polar lipids and cholesterol, and smaller quantities of nonpolar lipids. Phosphatidyl choline, sphingomyelin, and lyso-phosphatidyl choline are the major phospholipids present. The protein moiety has a substantial content of tryptophan and it is rich in hydrophobic aminoacids, particularly leucine. Several gly-copeptides and nonglycosylated polypeptides have been separated and studied extensively. A significant amount of carbohydrate is also found, estimated at 3.6–6.5 per cent, and at least some of the carbohydrate moiety is present as glycolipid. It has not yet been established whether the carbohydrate helps to preserve the structural integrity of adjacent antigenic sites, or whether it carries a novel haptenic specificity. There is evidence that the surface antigen particles may contain small amounts of normal host serum components, particularly albumin and possibly other host proteins.

The morphological complexity of hepatitis B virus is surpassed by the antigenic heterogenicity of the surface antigen reactivities. Careful serological analysis has shown that the hepatitis B surface antigen particles share a common group-specific antigen *a* and generally carry at least two mutually exclusive subdeterminants, *d* or *y*, and *w* or *r*. The subtypes are the phenotypic expressions of distinct genotype variants of hepatitis B virus. Four principal phenotypes are recognized, *adw*, *adr*, *ayw*, and *ayr*, but other complex permutations of these subdeterminants and new variants have been described, all apparently on the surface of the same physical particles. The major subtypes have differing geographical distribution. For example, in northern Europe, the Americas and Australia subtype *adw* predominates. Subtype *ayw* occurs in a broad zone which includes northern and western Africa, the eastern Mediterranean, eastern Europe, northern and central Asia and the Indian subcontinent. Both *adw* and *adr* are found in Malaysia, Thailand, Indonesia, and Papua New Guinea, while subtype *adr* predominates in other parts of south-east Asia including China, Japan, and the Pacific Islands.

Epidemiology of hepatitis B. In the past, hepatitis B was defined on the basis of infection occurring about 60–180 days after the injection of human blood or plasma fractions, or the use of inadequately sterilized syringes and needles. The availability of specific laboratory tests for hepatitis B confirmed the importance of the parenteral routes of transmission, and infectivity appears to be especially related to blood. However, a number of factors have altered the epidemiological concepts that hepatitis B is spread exclusively by blood and blood products. These include the findings that, under certain circumstances, the virus is infective by mouth, that it is endemic in closed institutions and institutions for the mentally-handicapped, that it is more prevalent in adults in urban communities and in poor socio-economic conditions, that there is a huge reservoir of carriers of markers of hepatitis B virus in the human population exceeding 200 million worldwide, and that the carrier rate and age distribution of the surface antigen varies in different regions.

There is considerable circumstantial evidence for transmission of hepatitis B by intimate personal contact and by the sexual route. At very high risk are the sexually promiscuous, particularly male homosexuals. Hepatitis B surface antigen, a marker of the virus, has been found repeatedly in blood and in various body fluids such as saliva, menstrual and vaginal discharges, seminal fluid, colostrum and breast milk, and serous exudates, and these have been implicated in the spread of infection. The presence of the antigen in urine, bile, faeces, sweat, and even tears has also been reported but not confirmed. It is therefore not surprising that contact-associated hepatitis B is apparently of major importance. Transmission may result from accidental inoculation of minute amounts of blood or fluids contaminated with blood such as may occur during medical, surgical, and dental procedures, immunization with inadequately sterilized syringes and needles, intravenous and percutaneous drug abuse, tattooing, ear piercing and nose piercing, acupuncture, laboratory accidents, and accidental inoculation with razors and similar objects which have been contaminated with blood.

The modes of transmission of hepatitis B in the tropics are similar to those in other parts of the world but additional factors may be of importance. These include traditional tattooing and scarification, blood letting, ritual circumcision, and repeated biting by blood-sucking arthropod vectors. Results of investigations into the role which biting insects may play in the spread of hepatitis B are conflicting. Hepatitis B surface antigen has been detected in several species of mosquitoes and in bed bugs which have either been trapped in the wild or fed experimentally on infected blood, but no convincing evidence of replication of the virus in insects has been obtained. Mechanical transmission of the infection is a possibility, particularly as a result of interrupted feeding in high prevalence areas.

It is clear from the above account that there are different possible ways of transmission of hepatitis B from person to person including spread by parenteral, inapparent parenteral, and non-percutaneous routes. There is also evidence of clustering of this infection within family groups. On the whole, the frequency of serological markers of hepatitis B in family contacts is not in accord with the hypothesis of autosomal recessive inheritance and does not reflect maternal and venereal transmission. The mechanisms of intrafamilial spread of the infection have not been elucidated.

Transmission of hepatitis B virus from carrier mothers to their babies can occur during the perinatal period and appears to be an important factor in determining the prevalence of infection in some regions. The risk of infection may reach 50–60 per cent, although it varies from country to country and appears to be related to ethnic groups. The risk is greatest if the mother has a history of transmission to previous children, has a high titre of hepatitis B surface antigen and/or e antigen. There is also a substantial risk of perinatal infection if the mother has acute hepatitis B in the second or third trimester of pregnancy or within two months after delivery. Although hepatitis B virus can infect the fetus *in utero*, this appears to be rare. The mechanism of perinatal infection is uncertain, but it probably occurs during or shortly after birth as a result of a leak of maternal blood into the baby's circulation, its ingestion or inadvertent inoculation. Most children infected during the perinatal period become persistent carriers.

The carrier state. On the basis of longitudinal studies of patients with hepatitis B, the carrier state has been defined as persistence of hepatitis B surface antigen in the circulation for more than six months. The established carrier state, which may be life-long, may be associated with liver damage ranging from minor changes in the nuclei of hepatocytes to chronic active hepatitis and cirrhosis. A number of risk factors have been identified in relation to development of the carrier state. It is commoner in males, more likely to follow infections acquired in childhood than those acquired in adult life, and more likely to occur in patients with natural and acquired immune deficiencies. A carrier state becomes established in approximately 5–10 per cent of infected adults. In countries in which hepatitis B virus infection is common, the highest prevalence of the surface antigen is found in children aged 4–8 years with steadily declining rates amongst older age groups. Hepatitis B e antigen has been reported to be commoner in young than in adult carriers, while the prevalence of e antibody appears to increase with age.

Survival of hepatitis B virus is ensured by the reservoir of carriers, estimated to number some 200 million. The prevalence of carriers, particularly among blood donors, in northern Europe, North America and Australia is 0.1 per cent or less; in central and eastern Europe up to 5 per cent, a higher frequency in southern Europe, the countries bordering the Mediterranean and parts of Central and South America, and in some parts of Africa, Asia, and the Pacific region as many as 20 per cent or more of the apparently healthy population may be carriers. There is an urgent need to define the mechanisms which lead to the high carrier rate in endemic areas and to introduce methods of interruption of transmission. The management of the carrier state is a complex and vexed issue with considerable personal, social, and economic implications. Guidance in management and general recommendations are to be found in several official reports.

The immune response. The suggestion that hepatitis B virus exerts its damaging effect on liver cells by direct cytopathic changes is inconsistent with the persistence of large quantities of the surface and core antigens in the hepatocytes of many asymptomatic and apparently healthy carriers of the surface antigen in their blood. There is, however, evidence to suggest that the pathogenesis of liver damage in the course of hepatitis B infection is related to the immune response by the host to the various structural components of the virus, as described above.

Immune complexes of surface antigen and antibody may be found in the sera of some patients during the incubation period and acute phase of hepatitis B. Immune complexes have been found in the sera of patients with fulminant hepatitis B, but only infrequently in non-fulminant infection. Immune complexes are also important in the pathogenesis of syndromes characterized by damage of blood vessels in polyarteritis nodosa, in the renal glomeruli in some forms of chronic glomerulonephritis in children, and in infantile papular acrodermatitis. Surface antigen, surface antibody, core antibody, and surface antigen–antibody immune complexes have been found in variable proportions of patients with virtually all the recognized chronic sequelae of acute hepatitis B. Deposits of such immune complexes have also been demonstrated in the cytoplasm and plasma membrane of hepatocytes, and on, or in, the nuclei. It is not clear, however, why only a small proportion of patients with circulating immune complexes develop vasculitis or polyarteritis. It may be that complexes are critical pathogenic factors only when they are of a particular size and of a certain antigen–antibody ratio.

Cellular immune responses are important in determining the clinical features and course of viral infection. Cell-mediated immunity to hepatitis B antigens has been demonstrated in most patients during the acute phase of hepatitis B and in a significant proportion of patients with surface antigen-positive chronic active hepatitis, but not in symptomless hepatitis B carriers. These observations suggest that cell-mediated immune responses may be important in terminating the infection and, under certain circumstances, in promoting liver damage and in genesis of auto-immunity.

Immunopathogenic mechanisms implicated in the progression of acute hepatitis B to chronic liver disease involve the appearance of viral associated antigens on the surface of infected hepatocytes after release of the virus from the cell. T lymphocytes, recognizing these new antigenic determinants, destroy the infected hepatocytes. The T cells also stimulate B cells to produce antibody to liver specific protein, a normal constituent of the hepatocyte cell membrane. The resulting antibody-dependent cell-mediated K cell reaction against normal liver membrane antigens contributes to necrosis of the hepatocytes. Virus released from the cells stimulates antibody directed against the viral components and the antibody complexes with the virus. The immune complex is then removed by the reticulo-endothelial system. With removal of the virus, T cell reaction ceases, as well as the 'helper effect' for the production of autoantibody to liver-specific lipoprotein, which, together with a normally functioning suppressor T cell system, leads to cessation of liver cell necrosis and recovery from acute hepatitis. In surface antigen-positive chronic active hepatitis, as a result of a quantitative or qualitative defect in the production of antibody to the virus, the virus is not cleared and in turn infects other hepatocytes, and both mechanisms of immunological liver cell damage continue. In patients who progress to surface antigen-negative chronic active hepatitis, the production of antibodies directed against the virus is adequate, and the virus is cleared. In these patients the defect probably lies in suppressor T cell function, which is unable to switch off the auto-immune reaction against liver specific protein. A further membrane antigen, liver membrane antigen, seems to be involved. The disease-specific auto-antibody, liver membrane antibody, can be demonstrated in hepatocyte membranes. Genetic factors may also be involved, as indicated by an association with histocompatibility antigens HLA-A1 and B8, the associated high titres of auto-antibodies and viral antibodies, and the increased frequency of serological abnormalities in first-degree relatives.

Hepatocellular carcinoma. Although primary liver cancer is rare in Europe and North America, it is very common in many areas of the world including Africa and Southeast Asia, and it may therefore be among the most common human cancers. Review of many studies shows a highly significant occurrence of markers of hepatitis B infection in patients with hepatocellular carcinoma. Hepatitis B is ubiquitous in areas of the world where macronodular cirrhosis and primary liver cancer are common. It is possible, therefore, that patients with hepatocellular carcinoma are unduly susceptible to hepatitis B infection and to the development of the persistent carrier state. The question has been asked whether the infectious

agent is the driver or the passenger? It has been suggested that an important factor in the possible aetiological association between hepatitis B infection and liver cell carcinoma may well lie in an early age of exposure to infection and high prevalence of persistent hepatitis B carriers. Indeed, in geographical regions where the prevalence of macronodular cirrhosis and primary liver cancer is high, infection with hepatitis B virus and the carrier state occur most frequently in early life, before the defence immune mechanisms have fully developed, and as many as 20 per cent or more of the apparently healthy population may be carriers. It seems likely, therefore, that persistent hepatitis B infection occurs before the onset of chronic liver damage. Another possibility is that persistent infection with hepatitis B virus leads to cirrhosis, and that carcinoma then arises from regenerative nodules by mechanisms in which the virus itself is not involved. However, this sequence does not explain liver cancer associated with persistent hepatitis B infection in about 20–30 per cent of patients in the absence of cirrhosis. More recent laboratory studies have shown the presence of viral DNA sequences in host cells derived from patients with persistent hepatitis B infection and chronic active hepatitis, and also in patients with hepatocellular carcinoma. These findings are consistent with integration of hepatitis B viral DNA into host chromosomal DNA molecules. In addition, several cell lines which produce hepatitis B surface antigen in culture have been derived from primary liver cell tumours. The actual mechanisms involved in the pathogenesis of hepatocellular carcinoma are under study. It is possible that liver cancer is the cumulative result of several cofactors including genetic, nutritional and hormonal factors, mycotoxins, chemical carcinogens, and other environmental factors, and that hepatitis B virus acts either as a carcinogen or a cocarcinogen in persistently infected hepatocytes.

Passive immunization. The availability of laboratory tests for hepatitis B surface antibody permitted the selection of plasma for the preparation of high titre hepatitis B immunoglobulin. This type of immunoglobulin may confer temporary passive immunity under certain defined conditions. Although many studies have been conducted in different countries, the results were frequently inconclusive or conflicting, and the design of many of the trials were faulty in some respects. The major indication for the administration of hepatitis B immunoglobulin is a single acute exposure to hepatitis B virus, such as occurs when blood containing surface antigen is inoculated, ingested, or splashed on to mucous membranes and the conjunctiva. The optimal dose has not been established, but doses in the range of 0.04–0.07 ml/kg have been used effectively. It should be administered as early as possible after exposure and preferably within 48 hours. It should not be administered seven days following exposure. It is recommended that two doses of hepatitis B immunoglobulin should be given 30 days apart.

Hepatitis B immunoglobulin has also been used on a continuing basis for susceptible staff in endemic settings, such as haemodialysis and oncology units, where transmission of hepatitis B virus is known to occur and where preventive hygienic measures cannot be effectively introduced. It should be stressed that passive immunization in such situations does not provide complete protection, and it is not a substitute for strict hygienic and cross-infection control measures.

Preliminary data on the use of hepatitis B immunoglobulin for prophylaxis in babies at risk of infection with hepatitis B virus are encouraging if the immunoglobulin is given within 48 hours of birth, and the chance of the baby developing the persistent carrier state was reduced. In another study the administration of 0.51 ml/kg of hepatitis B immunoglobulin within 48 hours of birth to babies born to carrier mothers, followed by monthly doses of 0.16 ml/kg for six months, appeared promising for interrupting maternal to infant transmission.

Active immunization. A vaccine against hepatitis B is urgently needed for groups which are at an increased risk of acquiring this infection. These groups include individuals requiring repeated transfusions of blood or blood products, prolonged inpatient treatment, patients who require frequent tissue penetration or need repeated access to the circulation, patients with natural or acquired immune deficiency, and patients with malignant diseases. Viral hepatitis is an occupational hazard among health care personnel and the staff of institutions for the mentally-retarded. High rates of infection with hepatatis B occur in narcotic drug addicts and drug abusers, homosexuals, and prostitutes. Individuals working in high endemic areas are also at an increased risk of infection. Women in areas of the world where the carrier state in that group is high are another segment of the population requiring immunization in view of the increased risk of transmission of the infection to their offspring. Consideration will also have to be given to young infants, children, and susceptible persons living in certain tropical and sub-tropical areas where present socio-economic conditions are poor and the prevalence of hepatitis B infection is high. Some authors also include military personnel.

The repeated failure to grow and passage hepatitis B virus serially in tissue culture has prevented the development of a conventional vaccine. Attention has therefore been directed to the use of other preparations for active immunization. The foundation for such hepatitis B immunogens was laid by the demonstration of the relative efficacy of diluted serum containing hepatitis B virus and its antigens heated to 98 °C for one minute in preventing or modifying the infection in susceptible persons. Since hepatitis B surface antigen leads to the production of protective surface antibody, purified 22 nm spherical surface antigen particles have been developed as vaccines (Fig. 4). These experimental vaccines have been prepared from the plasma of symptomless carriers. Although it is generally accepted that the preparations of 22 nm particles, when pure, are free of nucleic acid and therefore non-infectious, the fact that the starting material is human plasma obtained from persons infected with hepatitis B virus means that extreme caution must be exercised to ensure their freedom from all harmful contaminating material. Some concern has also been expressed on the possible induction of harmful immunological reactions to host components, including pre-existing structures of liver cells, which may be present in such vaccine preparations. However, much of the host material is being removed during additional steps of purification.

Human hepatitis B infection has been transmitted to chimpanzees, the only available susceptible non-human primate to this infection. The infection in chimpanzees is mild, but the biochemical, histological, and serological responses in the chimpanzees are very similar to those in man. Susceptible chimpanzees have been shown to be protected by the 22 nm particle vaccines which had been treated with formalin. Small-scale safety tests in volunteers have been completed, and trials on protective efficacy in high-risk groups are in progress.

Considerable advances are also being made in the development of hepatitis B vaccines from the constituent polypeptides of the surface antigen. Such vaccines are more chemically defined and would have an added margin of safety since they would be even less likely to contain infectious virus or contaminating host proteins. These subunit polypeptide vaccines are being tested for safety and efficacy.

The rapidly progressing field of recombinant DNA technology offers the possibility of providing immunizing antigen using a prokaryotic system and indeed hepatitis B antigen proteins have been expressed in clones of *E. coli*. Perhaps one of the most interesting prospects for the future is the development of synthetic vaccines. Detailed immunochemical studies of purified hepatitis B antigens, and determination of the primary amino-acid sequence and three-dimensional structure of the antigens, are essential steps towards developing a synthetic peptide. Once these data are available it should be possible to define by animal immunization the moiety responsible for antigenic activity. There are reports in the literature to support the feasibility of such an approach. For example, studies with tobacco mosaic virus led to the identification of the antigenic determinant and amino-acid sequences responsible for the immunogenic activity of the virus. Such amino-acid moieties can be synthesized and, when coupled to a carrier protein, will induce the production of neutralizing antibody in experimental animals. It has also been shown that it is possible to use a synthetic macromolecule for eliciting antibodies reacting exclusively with a specific region of a native egg-white lysozyme. This was achieved by synthesizing a particular segment of the enzyme from its amino-acid components, attaching the peptide to a carrier, and using the conjugate for immunization. The resulting antibodies to a completely synthetic immunogen reacted with native lysozyme via a unique region which is conformation-dependent. More recently the neutralization of a baterial virus with a synthetic antigen was accomplished.

Thus the conceptual way to synthetic vaccines is now open since, if it can be done for one protein, it should be possible to achieve this with other proteins. With the rapid advances in knowledge of protein chemistry and X-ray crystallography, a similar approach could be employed for at least some viral coat proteins and particularly with viruses such as the hepatitis viruses which cannot be cultivated in tissue culture. It will be necessary, of course, to establish whether antibodies to such synthetic immunogens will be protective, and whether immunity will persist. There will, however, be many obvious advantages in attaining synthetic vaccines to replace current vaccines which often contain many irrelevant microbial antigenic determinants, proteins, and other material that contaminate the essential immunogen and which may lead to untoward side-effects.

Antiviral therapy in chronic hepatitis B infection

Interferon. Interferon is still being evaluated for the treatment of chronic hepatitis B in several centres. A number of reports indicate that the administration of human leucocyte interferon both in man and in persistently infected chimpanzees has an inhibitory effect on replication of hepatitis B virus.

Ribavirin (Virazole). Ribavirin is a synthetic nucleoside analogue of guanosine, and it has a broad spectrum, though modest, antiviral activity. Several clinical studies with ribavirin appeared to yield encouraging results in acute hepatitis B as well as in persistent carriers. However, no significant changes were noted in more recent studies in patients nor in several chimpanzee carriers of hepatitis B virus.

Vidarabine (ara-A, adenine arabinoside): Vidarabine acts as an analogue of the deoxyribonucleoside of adenine, and it has been shown to have significant antiviral activity against several DNA viruses. Several small studies have so far been carried out in patients with chronic liver disease. In most patients there was an immediate loss of DNA polymerase followed by a rebound in many of the patients when treatment was stopped. A similar temporary effect was found in infected chimpanzees treated with vidarabine. Further trials with this potent drug are underway to determine whether prolonged treatment with this drug alone and in combination with interferon will have a more sustained effect on replication. of hepatitis B virus.

The flavonoid, (+)–cyanidanol–3. The use of this drug for the treatment of acute viral hepatitis has shown what appear to be marginal and mainly subjective beneficial effects.

Non-A, non-B hepatitis

The specific laboratory diagnosis of hepatitis A and hepatitis B has revealed a previously unrecognized form of viral hepatitis which is clearly unrelated to either type and which is referred to as non-A, non-B hepatitis. It is now the most common form of hepatitis occurring after blood transfusion and the infusion of certain plasma derivatives, particularly clotting factors, in some areas of the world. The infection has also been transmitted experimentally to chimpanzees. Although specific laboratory tests for identifying this new type of hepatitis are not yet available, and the diagnosis can only be made by exclusion, there is considerable information on the epidemiology and some clinical features of this infection.

Non-A, non-B hepatitis has been found in every country in which it has been sought and it shares a number of features with hepatitis B. This form of hepatitis has been most commonly recognized as a complication of blood transfusion, and in countries where all blood donations are screened for hepatitis B surface antigen by very sensitive techniques, non-A, non-B hepatitis may account for as many as 90 per cent of all cases of post-transfusion hepatitis. Outbreaks of non-A, non-B hepatitis have also been reported after the administration of blood-clotting factors VIII and IX. Non-A, non-B hepatitis has occurred in haemodialysis and other specialized units, among drug addicts, and after accidental inoculation with contaminated needles and other sharp objects. In several countries a significant number of cases are not associated with transfusion, and such sporadic cases of non-A, non-B hepatitis account for 10–25 per cent of all adult patients with recognized viral hepatitis. The route of infection or the source of infection cannot be identified in many of these patients. Males predominate as is the case with hepatitis B. Differences from the epidemiology of hepatitis B include lack of evidence of transmission of non-A, non-B hepatitis in the family setting, and no evidence of transmission by sexual contact either heterosexual or homosexual.

Although in general the illness is mild and often subclinical or anicteric, severe hepatitis with jaundice does occur, and the infection is a significant cause of fulminant hepatitis. There is considerable evidence that the infection may be followed in many patients, and in experimentally infected chimpanzees, by prolonged viraemia and the development of a persistent carrier state. Studies of the histopathological sequelae of acute non-A, non-B infection revealed that chronic liver damage, which may be severe, may occur in as many as 40–50 per cent of the patients.

Clinical, epidemiological, and experimental studies in several laboratories indicate that non-A, non-B hepatitis may be caused by two, or possibly more than two, infectious agents. Clinical evidence is based on the observation of multiple attacks of hepatitis in individual patients. Epidemiologically, short-incubation and long-incubation forms of non-A, non-B hepatitis have been described. The incubation period, however, does not appear to be a reliable index for differentiating between the two non-A, non-B types of hepatitis, and it is likely that differences in the incubation period represent differences in the infective doses. Experimental evidence for the existence of at least two distinct non-A, non-B hepatitis viruses has been obtained from recent cross-challenge experimental transmission studies in chimpanzees, but final confirmation must await the development of specific laboratory tests for non-A, non-B hepatitis and the identification and characterization of the virus(es).

References

Bianchi, L., Gerok, W., Sickinger, K., and Stadler, G. A. (eds.) (1980). *Virus and the liver*. MTP Press, Lancaster.

Krugman, S. and Gocke, D. J. (1978). Viral hepatitis. In *Major problems in internal medicine* (ed. L. H. Smith, Jr.). Saunders, Philadelphia.

Sherlock, S. (ed.) (1980). Viral hepatitis: *Clins. Gastroent.* **9**.

Szmuness, W. (1978). Hepatocellular carcinoma and the hepatitis B virus. Evidence for a causal association. *Progress in Medical Virology* (ed. J. L. Melnick) **24**, pp. 40. Karger, Basel.

World Health Organization (1977). *Advances in viral hepatitis*. Report of the WHO Expert Committee on viral hepatitis. *Tech. Rep. Ser., Wld Hlth Org.* no. 502.

Zuckerman, A. J. (1978). The three types of human viral hepatitis. *Bull. Wld Hlth Org.* **56**, 1–20.

— (1979). Specific serological diagnosis of viral hepatitis. *Br. med. J.* ii, 84.

— (1980). *A decade of viral hepatitis*. Elsevier, Amsterdam and New York.

— and Howard, C. R. (1979). *Hepatitis viruses of man*. Academic Press, London, and New York.

Tumour viruses

R. A. Weiss

Introduction. Several different kinds of virus can cause cancer. The various viruses with oncogenic potential probably act through different mechanisms, and interact with different host factors and environmental cofactors. Malignant disease is usually a rare result of virus infection and may occur many months or years after initial infection, although the viral genome, or part of it, appears to be present in the tumour cells.

Viral oncogenesis has been intensively studied in animals, and there is increasing evidence for the involvement of viruses in certain human cancers. Among the DNA-containing viruses, many herpesviruses, adenoviruses, papovaviruses, and hepatitis viruses elicit tumours in natural or experimental infection, whereas among the RNA-containing viruses, only the retroviruses are known to have oncogenic properties. There is a vast literature on tumour viruses and no attempt will be made to review it here. Several recently published books cover the subject in detail and the reader is referred to these texts: two textbooks, on DNA viruses (Tooze 1980) and on RNA viruses (Weiss *et al.* 1982), provide a comprehensive treatise on tumour viruses; Klein (1980) has edited a volume on selected topics in viral oncology, and the proceedings of a conference on viruses in naturally occurring cancers (Essex *et al.* 1980) broadly covers the natural history, epidemiology, and pathogenesis of the better known tumour viruses.

Human oncogenic viruses. Table 1 lists human viruses associated or implicated as inducing agents or cofactors in oncogenesis. Some of them, e.g. adenovirus strains, or the SV40-like virus BK (see page 5.131), are natural, ubiquitous human infections which, while they have not been associated with specific human malignancies, are known to cause cancer with high efficiency in experimental animals. These viruses are not regarded as carcinogenic for man,

Table 1 Human viruses with oncogenic properties

Virus		Association with human tumors	Experimental induction of tumors or cell transformation
Family	Type		
Herpes	simplex	Ca. cervix?	rodents, human
	EBV	Burkitt's lymphoma Nasopharyngeal ca. Immunoblastic lymphoma in renal transplant patients	marmosets, human
	CMV	Kaposi's sarcoma?	rodents
Hepatitis	B	Ca. liver	
Adeno	2,5,12	none	rodents
Papova	papilloma	warts squamous cell ca.?	
	BK, JC	meningioma? glioblastoma multiforme?	rodents
	SV40	melanoma?	rodents
Retro	HTLV	T-cell lymphoma-leukemia	human

Data assembled from Essex *et al.* (1980) except TCLV (Reitz *et al.* 1981)

but if they were to be considered as chemicals, their molar oncogenicity for rodents would register them as the most potent 'environmental' carcinogens discovered. Some of the viruses listed may be involved in human cancer, but definitive evidence is still lacking. For example, epidemiological studies suggest that carcinoma of the uterine cervix in women may have an infectious aetiology, and both herpes simplex virus type II and a papilloma virus variant are currently under suspicion as transmissable, causative agents of this disease. Hepatitis B virus (see page 5.118) has recently been associated with hepatocellular carcinoma, one of the major cancers in the world, though relatively uncommon in Western countries; a related hepatitis virus of American woodchucks and ground squirrels is providing a useful animal model for liver cancer (Essex *et al.* 1980).

Epstein–Barr virus (EBV) is the agent that causes infectious mononucleosis (see page 5.61), but it is also associated with two quite distinct tumours, Burkitt's lymphoma and nasopharyngeal carcinoma (Essex *et al.* 1980; Klein 1980). EBV belongs to a family of lymphoproliferative and lymphomagenic herpesviruses of primates that share certain viral antigens. It is a very common human infection worldwide. Infection in infancy is usually apathogenic, whereas primary infection in adolescence or adulthood frequently induces infectious mononucleosis. Burkitt's lymphoma is prevalent in regions of Africa and New Guinea where malaria is holoendemic, that is, where children are subject to repeated malarial infection. EBV is implicated in Burkitt's lymphoma because the virus was originally isolated from lymphoma cells in culture, and indeed is present in latent form in the tumour cells, and because an elevation in antibodies to certain EBV antigens presages the development of lymphoma. The role of malarial infection as a cofactor in Burkitt's lymphoma is not yet understood, although its immuno-suppressive effect has been widely discussed. Given the prevalence of EBV infection, but the rarity of Burkitt's lymphoma outside malarial areas, malarial control would appear to be the crucial factor for reducing the incidence of this lymphoma.

EBV can transform B lymphoblasts in culture to an 'immortal' state of indefinite growth which can be regarded as a pre-neoplastic stage of lymphomagenesis. Some patients on immunosuppressive regimens, such as renal transplant patients, develop immunoblastic lymphomatous growths which are probably polyclonal and may be due to the uncontrolled proliferation of EBV-transformed cells. Burkitt's lymphoma, in contrast, is a clonal disease and the lymphoma cells show a specific chromosomal translocation not seen in EBV-transformed cells.

Nasopharyngeal carcinoma cells also contain the EBV genome. This disease is prevalent in people of southern Chinese origin and is associated with a particular histocompatibility type. The role of EBV in this carcinoma is not understood.

Another Herpes virus implicated in human cancer is cytomegalovirus (CMV). Antigens, DNA and RNA related to CMV have been detected in Kaposi's sarcoma cells (Boldogh *et al.* 1981). Kaposi's sarcoma is a rare disease in the Western world occurring mainly in patients of Jewish or Mediterranean ancestry especially in renal transplant recipients (Harwood *et al.* 1979). The tumour is relatively common in parts of Africa. An aggressive form of Kaposi's sarcoma has recently become endemic among homosexual men in the USA and Europe (Durak 1981). These patients are severely immunodeficient and have a variety of fungal, bacterial, and viral infections, including CMV. There also appears to be strong correlation between the disease and inheritance of the HLA-DR5 histocompatibility antigen. Thus the incidence of Kaposi's sarcoma is geographically, ethnically, and behaviourally clustered; it appears to be associated with a ubiquitous virus (CMV), a particular histocompatibility type and immunosuppressed conditions.

The human polyoma-like viruses BK and JC are also ubiquitous viruses which are usually apathogenic and remain latent except in immunosuppressed patients (Tooze 1980; Essex *et al.* 1980). JC is found in the brain and is associated, probably causally, with progressive multifocal leucoencephalopathy. It has also been detected in some meningiomas and in glioblastoma multiforme, but whether it is an aetiological factor or merely a passenger virus is not known. SV40 is a related virus which is common in rhesus monkeys. Several early batches of polio vaccine grown in monkey kidney cells were unwittingly contaminated with live SV40 virus, and a cohort of humans now in their early twenties has thus been inoculated with SV40. Studies of this cohort to date suggest no increased incidence in cancer with the exception of malignant melanoma, but more data are needed.

Because retroviruses are a common cause of leukaemia and lymphoma in animals ranging from fish to apes, they have been sought intensively in relation to human malignancies (Weiss *et al.* 1982). Many prematurely published leads have not held up to more detailed analysis. Recently, however, strong evidence has accrued that a newly discovered retrovirus, HTLV (human T-cell lymphoma virus), is associated with a newly classified type of adult T-cell lymphoma-leukemia previously diagnosed as mycoses fungoides, or Sézary syndrome (Gallo 1981; Catovsky *et al.* 1982). This virus appears to be a rare human infection, although there is a relatively high incidence of T-cell lymphoma in Southwest Japan (The T- and B-cell Malignancy Study Group 1981), and preliminary serological studies indicate that antibodies to the retrovirus are common in that population (Hinuma *et al.* 1981). It would appear that HTLV is endemic in that region of Japan and in the West Indies (reviewed in Weiss *et al.* 1982).

Natural history of tumour virus infections. All tumour viruses can establish persistent infections in their hosts. As malignancy is usually a clonal proliferation from a single infected cell, perhaps years after initial exposure to virus, it can be regarded as a rare though lethal sequela of infection. The persistent infection may remain entirely latent or it may be suppressed to a low level of viral activity by host immune responses. Several latent viral infections tend to become reactivated in immunosuppressed individuals. These include herpesviruses of all kinds, including EBV, and papovaviruses such as BK and JC. Likewise, herpes infections of monkeys are only lymphomagenic in the natural hosts under immunosuppressed conditions, and wild mice in which polyoma virus infection is frequently endemic, do not develop viral tumours except in old age or when immunosuppressed.

The production of neutralizing antibodies to virus particles or cellular immunity to virus-infected cells will markedly cut down the spread of virus within the infected host. There is also some evidence for immunity to neoplasia. For example, one of the greatest success stories in cancer prevention is the control of Marek's disease in chickens by immunization. Marek's disease is a T-cell lymphoma caused by a herpesvirus. Inoculation of newly hatched chicks with a live vaccine prepared from a related, non-pathogenic virus of turkeys protects the chicks from Marek's disease. Curiously, the vaccine does not immunize the chicks to infection by the Marek's agent, but it prevents the development of lymphoma.

The widespread evidence for immunological control of several tumours of known viral aetiology in animals and man has led to the notion that immunological surveillance as a means of natural tumour control is only pertinent to viral tumours. Immunological surveillance is clearly not a general mechanism of cancer prevention because few kinds of tumour show an increased incidence in immunodeficient hosts. In man, an elevated risk of malignancy in immunosuppressed patients has been found for few kinds of tumours, such as immunoblastic lymphoma (reticulum cell sarcoma) probably associated with EBV, and basal cell carcinoma of the skin. Perhaps one should investigate the possibility of a viral aetiology for basal cell carcinoma.

The lack of evidence for immunological surveillance for the majority of human neoplasms does not mean that medical science could not devise immunological methods of cancer treatment. But non-specific means of stimulating the immune response, e.g. inoculation of BCG or *C. parvum*, neither have a rational scientific basis nor empirical evidence for efficacy in preventing, let alone treating, malignant disease.

Papovaviruses and retroviruses may be regarded as the ultimate parasites in that they form persistent infections by inserting viral genetic information into host chromosomal DNA. In the case of retroviruses, the genome in the virus particle is carried as an RNA molecule, but in the infected cell this is copied into DNA by the viral enzyme, reverse transcriptase. The insertion of 'proviral' DNA into host DNA is called integration and leads to the adoption of viral genes as host genetic elements. During vertebrate evolution some strains of retrovirus have become integrated into host DNA of germ cells and have henceforth been carried as host Mendelian traits. Several species, such as cats, mice, chickens, and baboons, carry such 'endogenous' viral genomes, which are typically apathogenic; otherwise they would be rapidly eliminated by natural selection operating on the host.

Retroviruses may also be transmitted vertically by congenital infection. This should be distinguished from genetic transmission in that it requires infectious transmission of virus particles from maternal parent to offspring. Well-known examples of vertical infection are the milk transmission of mammary carcinoma virus in mice and the egg transmission of lymphoid leukosis virus in chickens. Figure 1 shows the natural transmission of leukosis viruses in chickens, which cause B-cell lymphoma and leukaemia arising in the bursa of Fabricius. Malignant disease is common in congenitally infected birds as the chick does not mount an immune response to the virus. However, the bird frequently survives to adulthood and breeds, thus enabling the virus to pass vertically to the next generation as well as horizontally among the flock. In contrast to chickens, horizontal infection of leukosis virus among cats, cattle, and gibbons frequently results in leukaemia. The T-cell lymphoma virus recently discovered in humans is also probably transmitted horizontally, possibly by an insect or helminth vector.

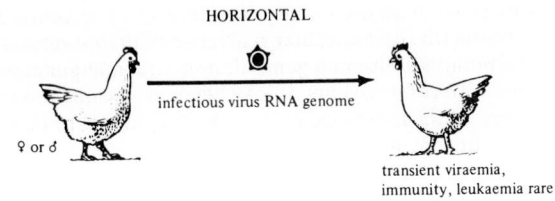

HORIZONTAL

infectious virus RNA genome

♀ or ♂

transient viraemia, immunity, leukaemia rare

VERTICAL

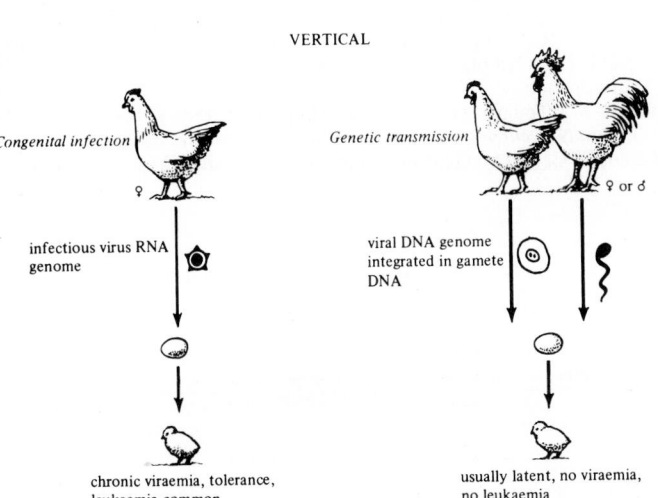

Congenital infection ♀

infectious virus RNA genome

Genetic transmission

♀ or ♂

viral DNA genome integrated in gamete DNA

chronic viraemia, tolerance, leukaemia common

usually latent, no viraemia, no leukaemia

Fig. 1 Horizontal and vertical transmission of leukosis viruses in chickens.

Vertebrate hosts which carry retrovirus genomes as Mendelian traits generally have evolved mechanisms suppressing the horizontal spread from cell to cell and re-infection should the virus become activated. The host cells are not permissive to re-infection either because they do not express surface receptors for the virus or because the replication of the virus is restricted early in the replication cycle. A few inbred strains of mice and chicken are permissive to replication of their own endogenous viruses, and these tend to have a relatively high incidence of malignant disease. It thus appears that viraemia is prerequisite to oncogenesis.

Cells of host species other than the one carrying the endogenous virus may be highly susceptible to infection. This is a phenomenon known as xenotropism, whereby an endogenous virus transmitted vertically as a chromosomal element in one species is only able to infect other species (Fig. 2). There is evidence, too, that an endogenous virus from one host species has been transmitted via an

infectious phase in its natural history to the germ line of another unrelated host, e.g. from primate to cat. One may ask, then, whether commensal animals, such as mice and cats, may act as natural reservoirs of oncogenic viruses infectious for man. However, there is no epidemiological or serological evidence that such zoonoses have occurred.

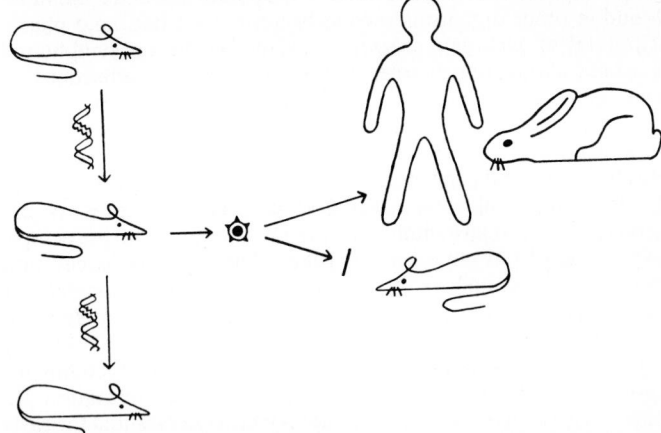

Fig. 2 Transmission of a xenotropic retrovirus. The viral genome is transmitted as DNA integrated into the chromosomes of mouse gametes. If activated to synthesize virus particles, these are not able to re-infect cells of mice, but can infect cells of 'foreign' species such as humans or rabbits.

Mechanisms of viral oncogenesis. How viruses transform cells into a neoplastic state is not yet understood clearly, although remarkable advances have recently been made in probing the molecular genetics of the smaller tumour viruses. With the DNA tumours, such as herpes, hepatitis, or papovaviruses, full replication of the virus is cytopathic so that the infected cell is destined to die rather than transform to malignancy. However, replication is frequently incomplete, either because the infected cell is of a type that does not support the complete viral life cycle (non-permissive cell) or because the virus has lost genetic information essential for later stages of replication (defective virus). With the RNA retroviruses, full replication is not usually cytocidal, so the infected cell may support virus production as well as becoming neoplastic. Nevertheless, many retrovirus infections are non-productive, and the most highly oncogenic retroviruses are defective for viral replication as described below.

Tumour viruses could induce neoplasia by a variety of mechanisms:

1. Non-specific tissue damage inducing regeneration. The chronic cytopathic effects of virus infection may stimulate regeneration or hyperplasia in neighbouring uninfected cells that eventually become neoplastic. One can envisage such events, for example, in liver infected with hepatitis B virus. There is evidence, however, that viral transformation is more specific, as only a small number of cytopathic viruses are oncogenic. Furthermore, in all cases adequately studied, a portion of the viral genome can be found in each of the tumour cells. The persistence of viral genetic information appears to be essential for viral oncogenesis.

2. Tumour viruses as insertional mutagens. As mentioned above, tumour virus DNA is able to integrate into host chromosomal DNA. Integration itself is a recombinational event that causes changes (mutations) in the organization of host genetic information. The sites of viral integration into host DNA has been studied extensively for papovaviruses and retroviruses, and it appears to be almost random, that is, the viral genome integrates at a different site, and often in a different chromosome for each infected cell. Some of these integration events are bound to be functionally mutagenic, and in rare cases could induce neoplasia, analogous to mutagenesis by chemical carcinogens. SV40 is known to be mutagenic and also to induce chromosome breaks and rearrangements.

With retroviruses, there is growing evidence that integration of the viral genome can alter the expression of neighbouring host genes, in particular by switching on their expression ectopically. This is thought to be an important step in viral leukemogenesis. Retroviruses carry signals for gene expression in 'LTR' sequences (Fig. 3a). The LTRs are duplicated at both ends of the proviral DNA and structurally resemble transposable genetic elements found in other organisms such as bacteria, fruit-flies, and maize. The LTR of avian leukosis virus genomes in chicken lymphomas has been shown to promote the transcription of an adjacent host gene important in neoplasia. Of the many millions of bursal cells infected with the virus, a clonal lymphoma is derived from one cell in which the virus has integrated in a suitable position to switch on this particular cell gene. Each strain of retrovirus causing different kinds of tumour appears to switch on different host genes. Where different viruses cause similar neoplasms, they promote the ectopic expression of the same cellular genes. These cellular genes with oncogenic potential are collectively notated *c-onc*, for cellular oncogenes. They have been identified by their close resemblance to viral oncogenes (*v-onc*) discussed below.

3. Viral oncogenes. Many tumour viruses carry genes coding for proteins which are necessary for neoplastic transformation. In papovaviruses like SV40, viral proteins which are essential for early phases of viral replication also play a role in cellular transformation. For instance, the large T antigen of SV40 is required for initiating replication of viral DNA, but it also stimulated cellular DNA synthesis (Tooze 1980). Viral T antigen forms complexes with a cellular protein, called 53K, and it is probably the complex that activates cell replication. The 53K protein is synthesized in normal cells too, just before initiation of DNA synthesis, but it is then rapidly degraded. When complexed to T antigen it persists and triggers uncontrolled cell proliferation. Several tumours not transformed by SV40 also express high levels of unusually stable 53K protein. Thus a transiently expressed cellular protein normally involved in activation of DNA synthesis may induce neoplasia when it is persistently expressed in an uncontrolled way. Its interaction with viral T antigen proved to be a window on a more general phenomenon of cellular control mechanisms.

Some highly oncogenic retroviruses carry transforming genes in place of the virus' normal replication genes (Fig. 3b). These genes have nothing to do with viral replication, indeed they render the virus defective, but they induce cell transformation. They are collectively known as *v-onc* genes and the best studied is the *src* gene of Rous Sarcoma virus. Molecular hybridization studies (see Section 4) show that *v-onc* genes are derived from cellular genes. By recombination into the viral genome they come under viral control signals and may also be packaged and transmitted infectiously when viral replication is complemented by a related non-defective 'helper' virus. The *v-onc* genes of defective, transforming retroviruses represent the converse situation to the *c-onc* genes activated by non-defective retroviruses. Instead of virus causing ectopic gene expression by inserting itself next to the cellular gene, it picks up that gene and carries it as part of the virus. The result is that all the cells that virus infects are likely to become neoplastic. Such transducing oncogenic viruses only occur very rarely outside the laboratory, perhaps because they are defective and so pathogenic that they will not be maintained in natural host populations. However, they are proving to be immensely powerful tools for investigating the molecular biology of cancer. The transduced *v-onc* genes are derived from cell genes that are well conserved in evolution. It is therefore possible to use *v-onc* genes of chicken or mouse retroviruses to probe for the molecular rearrangement and ectopic expression of homologous human genes in non-viral malignancies (Weiss *et al.* 1982). In coming years, it may become possible to exploit our knowledge of these oncogenes for the diagnosis and treatment of human malignant diseases.

References

Catovsky, D., Greaves, M. F., Rose, M., Galton, D. A. G., Goolden, A. W. G., McCluskey, D. R., White, J. M., Lampert, I., Bourikas, G., Ireland, R., Bridges, J. M., Blattner, W. A., and Gallo, R. C. (1982). Adult T-cell lymphoma-leukemia in blacks from the West Indies. Lancet **i**, in press.

Essex, M., Todaro, G. J., and zur Hausen, H. (eds.) (1980). *Viruses in naturally occurring cancers.* Cold Spring Harbor Laboratory.

Gallo, R. C. (1981). Growth of human normal and leukemic T cells: T-cell

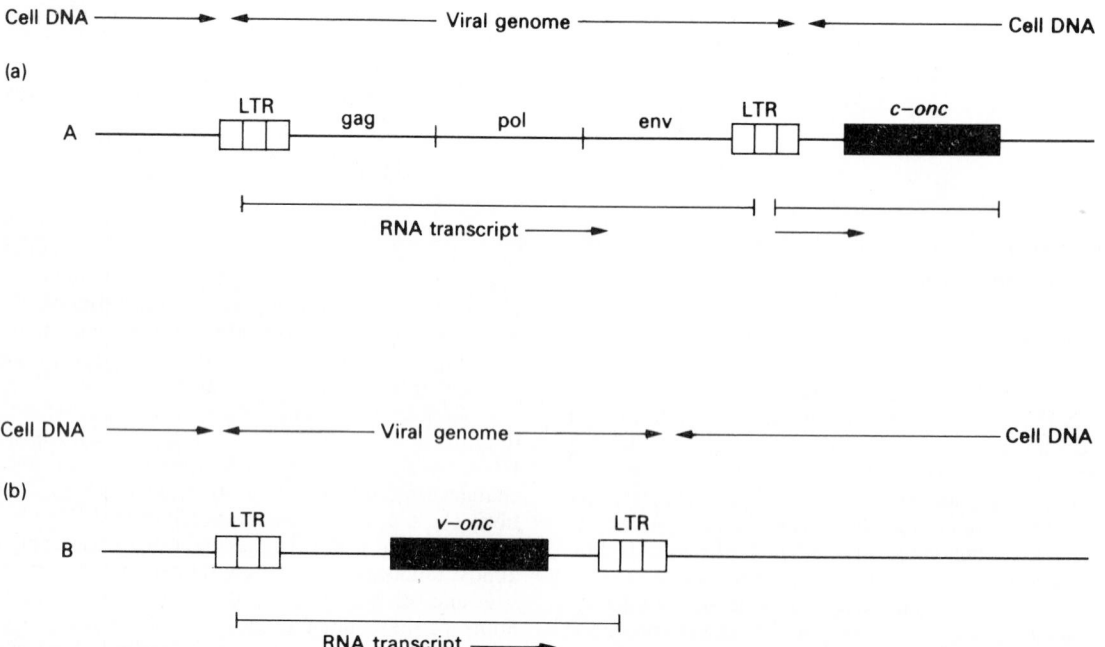

Fig. 3   Oncogenes controlled by retroviruses: (a) a non-defective leukosis virus integrated next to a cellular *c-onc* gene switches on its transcription 'downstream' from the right-hand LTR sequence of the virus in addition to its own genes from the left-hand LTR; (b) a transducing, defective retrovirus carries a *v-onc* gene as part of the viral genome and the transcription in this case starts from the left-hand LTR sequence.

growth factor (TCGF) and the isolation of a new class of RNA tumour viruses (HTLV). *Blood Cells* **7**, 313.

Hinuma, Y., Nagata, K., Hanaoka, M., Nakai, M., Matsumoto, T., Kinoshita, K. I., Shirakawa, S., and Miyoshi, I. (1981). Adult T-cell leukemia: antigen in an ATL cell line and detection of antibodies to the antigen in human sera. *Proc. natl Acad. Sci. USA* **78**, 6476.

Klein, G. (ed.) (1980). *Viral oncology.* Raven Press, New York.

The T- and B-cell Malignancy Study Group (1981). Statistical analysis of immunologic, clinical and histiopathologic data on lymphoid malignancies in Japan. *Jpn J. clin. Oncol.* **11**, 15.

Tooze, J. (ed.) (1980). *Molecular biology of tumor viruses*, 2nd edn., Part 2: *DNA tumor viruses*. Cold Spring Harbor Laboratory.

Weiss, R. A., Teich, N. M., Varmus, H. E., and Coffin, J. M. (eds.) (1982). *Molecular biology of tumor viruses*, 2nd edn., Part 3: *RNA tumor viruses*. Cold Spring Harbor Laboratory.

Marburg and Ebola fevers

E. T. W. Bowen and D. I. H. Simpson

History. Marburg virus disease, sometimes referred to as 'vervet monkey' or 'green monkey' disease, is a severe distinctive haemorrhagic febrile illness of man. It was first recognized in August 1967 when it caused three simultaneous outbreaks in Europe, at Marburg, Frankfurt, and Belgrade. There were 31 cases of which 25 were primary infections; seven of the primary cases died, but there were no deaths among the six secondary cases. All the primary cases were laboratory personnel who had come into direct contact with blood, organs or tissue cultures from one particular consignment of vervet monkeys (*Cercopithecus aethiops*) imported from Uganda. Four of the secondary infections were hospital personnel who had come into close contact with patients' blood. The wife of a Yugoslav veterinary surgeon was infected through blood contact with her husband while the sixth case was the wife of a patient who transmitted the disease during sexual intercourse 83 days after the onset of illness. Marburg virus was detected in his seminal fluid. There were no tertiary cases and no spread of the disease to the community at large.

The disease next appeared in South Africa in 1975 in a young Australian man who had been hitch-hiking through Central and Southern Africa. He died shortly after his admission to a Johannesburg hospital. His female travelling companion and a nurse who looked after him also contracted the disease. Both girls survived. Virological investigations confirmed that the virus isolated from these three cases was morphologically and antigenically identical to Marburg virus.

On 15 January 1980 Marburg re-appeared, this time in Kenya. A 58-year-old male was admitted to the Nairobi Hospital with an eight-day history of progressive fever, myalgia, and backache. On admission he was in a state of peripheral vascular failure and bleeding profusely from the gastrointestinal tract. He died within six hours of admission. Marburg virus particles were seen by electron microscopy in liver and kidney tissues removed at autopsy. On 24 January, a male doctor who had attended this patient and had attempted resuscitation became ill with a similar disease syndrome. He survived after a stormy illness and Marburg infection was confirmed serologically.

Between June and November 1976 outbreaks of severe and frequently fatal viral haemorrhagic fever occurred in the equatorial provinces of the Sudan and Zaire. In the Sudan there were 284 known cases with 151 deaths, a case fatality rate of 53 per cent, whilst in the Zaire outbreak there were 318 known cases with 280 deaths, a case fatality rate of 88 per cent. The virus strains isolated from patients in both these outbreaks were found to be morphologically identical to Marburg virus but antigenically distinct. The name Ebola was given to the new strain.

A second outbreak of Ebola haemorrhagic fever occurred in the southern Sudan during August and September 1979, in the same area as the original 1976 outbreak. There were 34 reported cases of which 22 were fatal. The clinical diagnosis was confirmed by both virus isolation and serology.

Aetiological agent. Electron microscope studies have shown that both Marburg and Ebola viruses are structurally indistinguishable from one another. The virus particles in both instances are pleomorphic, appearing in contrast preparations as either long filamentous forms, 'U' shaped, or circular forms resembling a doughnut or torus. The length of these filamentous forms can vary from 130 nm to more than 2600 nm, and in some preparations virions of almost 14 000 nm in length have been observed. The diameter appears to be fairly uniform at 80–100 nm.

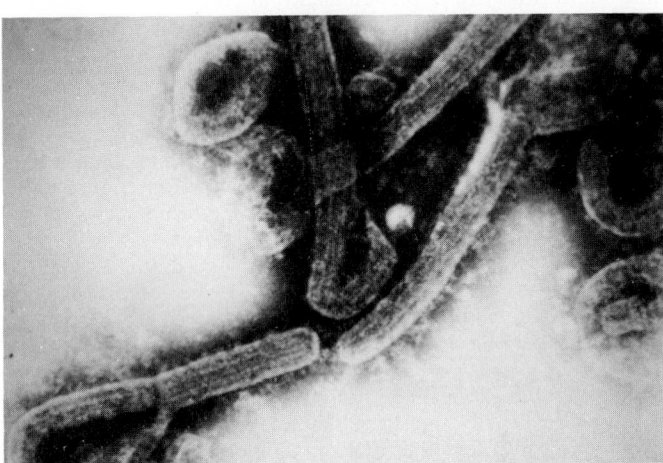

Fig. 1   Marburg virus (courtesy of Dr F. A. Murphy).

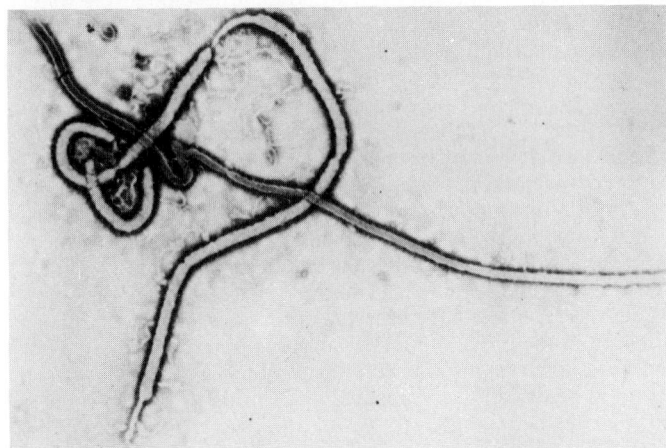

Fig. 2   Ebola virus (courtesy of Dr F. A. Murphy).

Recent studies on chemical composition have indicated that both Marburg and Ebola virions contain four to six proteins including one glycoprotein. The viral genome appears to be a single strand RNA with a molecular weight of approximately 5.6×10^6 dalton.

Information on the stability of these viruses is based on the more extensive knowledge of Marburg virus. The virus is stable when stored at temperatures of $-70\,°C$, and there appears to be very little reduction in infectivity when stored at room temperature for periods of up to five weeks. The virus is completely inactivated by heating at $60\,°C$ for one hour but not at $56\,°C$ over the same period. Rapid inactivation occurs under ultraviolet irradiation. Formalin, acetone, Chloros, diethyl ether, and Tego MGH completely inactivate the virus after one hour's exposure.

Marburg and Ebola viruses grow in a variety of primary and established cell culture systems. In early passage neither produce specific cytopathic effects, but a more obvious cytopathic effect may appear after several passages. Most workers, however, have preferred to base their evidence of cell infection on the appearance of characteristic intracytoplasmic inclusion bodies demonstrated by immunofluorescent staining techniques.

Monkeys and guinea pigs are susceptible to experimental infection with both viruses and Marburg was successfully adapted to baby hamsters after a course of several intracerebral or intraperitoneal passages.

Marburg and Ebola produce an illness in monkeys which in many ways closely resembles that found in man, with high fever, anorexia, haemorrhages, severe weight loss, and a distinctive skin rash, most pronounced on the forehead and face (where it is often confluent), on the chest, and on the medial aspect of the fore and hind limbs. Both viruses predominantly affect the liver, spleen, and lymph nodes and, in addition, Ebola virus has some affinity for the lungs, intestines, and testes. Of particular interest is that the only monkey pancreas examined had high concentrations of virus. This accords well with the clinical observation of pancreatitis in man following Marburg infection during the South African outbreak.

Guinea pigs inoculated with acute-phase blood become febrile (40.5–41 °C) after an incubation period ranging from four to seven days. The febrile illness lasts for about three to four days during which time the guinea pigs fail to thrive and generally look ill. High concentrations of virus are found in the blood during the febrile period. The liver, spleen, and lymph nodes are the organs most consistently affected. Passage of the virus in guinea pigs produces a uniformly fatal illness.

Clinical features. The illness caused in man by Marburg and Ebola viruses are virtually indistinguishable. Both infections have an abrupt onset with severe frontal and temporal headache, followed by high fever and generalized pains, particularly in the back. A relative bradycardia was often one of the early symptoms. The patient rapidly becomes prostrated and some develop severe watery diarrhoea leading to rapid weight loss and dehydration. Diarrhoea, abdominal pain with cramping, nausea, and vomiting often persist for a week. In the Sudanese Ebola outbreak, knife-like chest and pleuritic pain was an early symptom, and many patients complained of a very dry (rather than sore) throat accompanied by cough. On white skin, a characteristic non-itching maculopapular rash appears between five and seven days, lasts three of four days and is followed by a fine desquamation. On black skin the rash, often described as being 'like measles', is not so obvious and can often only be recognized later with the appearance of skin desquamation. Conjunctivitis was a regular feature in all the outbreaks. An exanthema of the palate was reported in the Marburg outbreak in Germany, but was not seen in the three South African cases. In the Sudanese Ebola outbreak, pharyngitis was commonly noted and the throat was found to be dry and accompanied by fissuring with open sores on

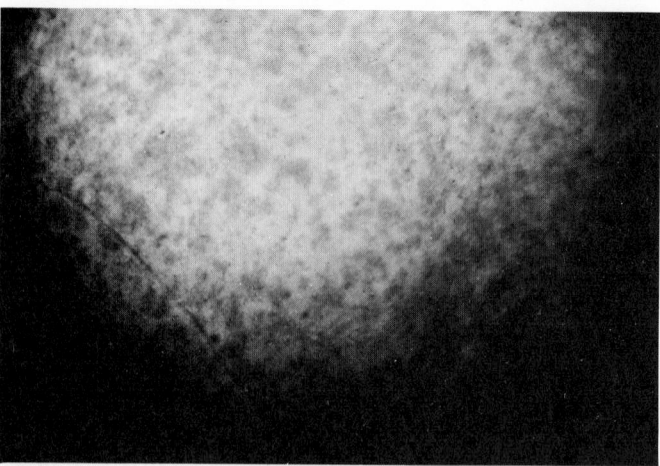

Fig. 3 Ebola fever—maculopapular rash (courtesy of Dr R. T. D. Emond).

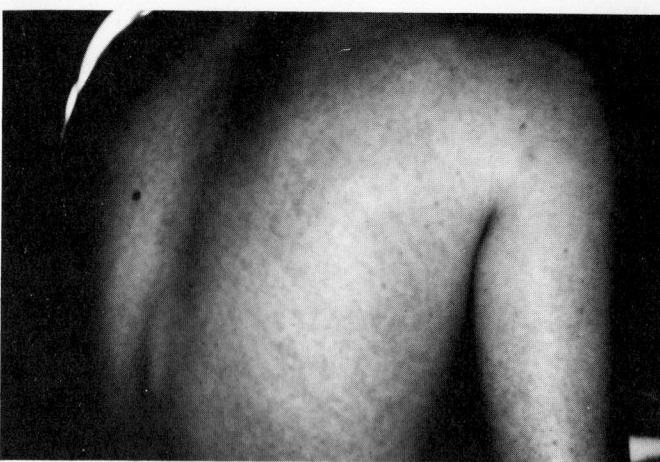

Fig. 4 Marburg fever—maculopapular rash seen on patient in South Africa (courtesy of Professor J. H. S. Gear).

the tongue and lips. Genital involvement with irritation and inflammation of the scrotum or labia majora was frequent and orchitis occurred in a few patients. Pancreatitis occurred in several instances.

In both Ebola outbreaks, patients were generally admitted to hospital on the fifth day of illness and their general appearance was described as 'ghost-like', with drawn, anxious features, expressionless faces, deep-set eyes, a greyish pallor, and extreme lethargy. Central nervous system involvement may be apparent in a number of cases with paraesthesia, lethargy, confusion, irritability, aggression, and signs of meningeal irritation.

A large number of patients in both the Marburg and Ebola outbreaks developed severe bleeding between days five and seven. The gastrointestinal tract and lungs were most frequently involved with haematemesis, melaena, and sometimes the passage of fresh blood in the stools. There was also bleeding from the nose, gums, and vagina, and subconjunctival haemorrhages were common. Petechiae and bleeding from needle puncture sites is also very common. In some cases laboratory investigation suggested a disseminated intravascular coagulation with subsequent kidney failure. In surviving patients recovery is slow with considerable debility persisting for many weeks. Death generally occurred between days seven and sixteen usually preceded by severe blood loss and shock.

Laboratory features. Clinical laboratory studies have necessarily been limited to investigations carried out on patients from the first two Marburg outbreaks. A leucopenia early in the course of illness has been a constant feature; this was followed by a leucocytosis and a low erythrocyte sedimentation rate. The acquired Pelger–Huet anomaly of the neutrophils together with atypical mononuclear cells was a feature in a number of patients. A considerable thrombocytopenia was recorded in most patients from about day three onwards.

Biochemical investigations showed that all patients had severe liver damage with both SGOT and SGPT levels considerably raised. In most of the fatal cases studied the SGOT levels exceeded 2500 u/l. Bilirubin values were only slightly elevated, if at all. Serum alkaline phosphatase and creatinine phospholinase remained normal. Creatine and urea increased only in cases of anuria. ECG changes were compatible with a myocarditis or other damage to the myocardium.

Pathology. Marburg and Ebola viruses are pantropic and produce lesions in almost every organ, with the liver and spleen the most conspicuously affected. Severe degeneration of lymphoid tissue, spleen, and liver result in large accumulations of cellular and nuclear debris.

The pattern of disease is that of stimulation of the reticulo-endothelial system, inhibition of the lymphatic system, and vascular changes leading to vascular occlusions and the formation of thrombi and haemorrhages. Macroscopic findings are similar in all cases. The stomach and parts of the intestines are usually filled with blood. Petechiae are seen in the mucosa of the stomach and the small intestines. In a number of cases the liver and spleen are enlarged and dark in colour. On section the spleen has no follicles and the pulp is soft and mushy. The liver is extremely friable and blood pours out freely on section leaving the organ a light yellow colour. Histologically severe congestion and stasis are obvious in the spleen. There is proliferation of reticulo-endothelial elements in the red pulp with the formation of large numbers of macrophages. Necrosis of the red pulp is accompanied by destruction of lymphoid elements. In the Malpighian bodies lymphocytes are markedly depleted. There is widespread degeneration and necrosis of the liver cells, and hyaline changes are frequently seen. Hyaline-necrotic-eosinophil bodies similar to the Councilman bodies of yellow fever are often seen. The Kupffer cells are swollen and bulging and full of cellular debris and red blood cells. Sinusoids are also full of debris while mononuclear accumulation is seen in the periportal spaces. Even at the height of the necrotic process in the liver there is evidence of liver cell regeneration.

Mononuclear transformation of lymphoid tissue as well as necrotic lesions are found not only in the liver and spleen but also in the pancreas, gonads, adrenals, hypophysis, thyroid, kidneys, and skin.

The lungs show few lesions except for circumscribed haemorrhages and evidence of endoarteritis especially in the small arterioles. Neuropathological changes are confined mainly to glial elements scattered throughout the brain. No lymphocyte reactions have been observed but multiple haemorrhages into the brain have been seen. Glial lesions are either proliferative in the form of glial knots, nodules, and rosettes or degenerative in the form of nuclear pyknosis or karyorrhexis. All glial elements are affected including astrocytes, microglia, and oligodendroglia. Cerebral oedema was found in all the human brain material examined.

Laboratory diagnosis. Specific diagnosis requires isolation and identification of the virus or evidence of antibody development between paired serum samples. The isolation of the virus is best achieved by the inoculation of acute-phase blood intraperitoneally into young guinea pigs and into various tissue culture cell lines. Identification is made by indirect immunofluorescent staining techniques. Attempts to isolate the virus must be carried out in high containment laboratories.

Epidemiology. There is a strong suspicion that the disease is a zoonosis. Monkeys were originally implicated in the three Marburg outbreaks in 1967, but there was no real evidence to suggest that primates were involved in the natural reservoir cycle of the virus. Following the South African outbreak in 1975, an extensive search for a reservoir was carried out without success. In 1977 large numbers of small mammals were caught in the epidemic areas of the Sudan and Zaire and blood and tissues removed for virological investigation in an attempt to throw some light on the natural reservoir for these viruses, again without success.

The disease occurs in all age groups with a predominance in adults. The incubation period was from three to nine days in both the German and South African outbreaks of Marburg disease, but in the two Ebola epidemics a wider range of four to 16 days was recorded.

Virological studies in both these virus infections have shown no evidence of significant virus shedding by any other route other than that of haemorrhage. There appears to be very little virus in the throat or urine but the persistence of virus in some body fluids for periods up to 83 days does pose a risk of late transmission. One of the South African Marburg patients developed a painful right eye.

Uveitis was diagnosed and Marburg virus was cultured from fluid aspirated from the anterior chamber two months later.

The mechanism of transmission of infection in these outbreaks was mainly by direct contact with infected blood, by very close and prolonged contact with an infected patient, or by inoculation by accident or through the use of a contaminated syringe and needle. There was no evidence to suggest that there was any respiratory spread of infection in the community. Both in the Sudan and in Zaire there was serological evidence of small numbers of minor or even sub-clinical infections.

It may be assumed that sporadic cases of Marburg/Ebola virus-like disease occur from time to time and die off spontaneously without secondary spread. Exceptionally as in the outbreaks in the Sudan and Zaire, unusual nosocomial transmission creates an amplifying cycle and causes epidemics. This happened in the Federal Republic of Germany in 1967, whereas the South African cases in 1975 were more illustrative of the sporadic type of infection.

In the two Ebola epidemics the attack rate in infected communities varied from 3.5 per 1000 to 15.3 per 1000 in the Sudan and from 8 per 1000 in the infected community of Yandongi in Zaire to less than 1 per 1000 in neighbouring communities. This has indicated that the virus was not as highly transmissible as previously thought.

The secondary attack rate was about 15 per cent in Zaire. In the Sudan active cases documented showed a secondary spread of 13 per cent, a tertiary spread of 14 per cent, and a quaternary spread of 9 per cent. Transmission stopped spontaneously after four generations, but in exceptional circumstances at least eight generations could be documented. The epidemics were readily brought under control by isolating the patients and instituting strict barrier nursing with gowns, gloves, masks, and the effective treatment of patients' excreta with disinfectants such as formaldehyde and hypochlorite.

Therapy. Therapy for these diseases has mainly been limited to nursing care and supportive measures. No vaccine is yet available. Only in a small percentage of cases has the use of specific therapy in the form of convalescent plasma been successful. The opportunity was taken to study the viraemic response in man following accidental laboratory infection with Ebola virus. Virus was detected early in the disease, $10^{4.5}$ Guinea pig infectious units (GPIU)/ml being detected on the first day of illness. No detectable change in the levels of circulating virus was evident on the day following initiation of interferon therapy. However within twelve hours of administering 450 ml of Ebola immune plasma the viraemia level had fallen to $10^{0.5}$ GPIU/ml. This much reduced level of circulating virus persisted throughout the acute stage of illness and virus became undetectable on the ninth day of illness. As both interferon and immunotherapy were administered together their respective merits cannot be assessed. There is no doubt that viraemia levels were dramatically reduced after the administration of immune plasma, but the patient's clinical condition did deteriorate despite the low virus levels in the blood.

During the South African outbreak attempts were made to prevent the severe haemorrhage experienced in the first patient by giving the other two patients heparin early in the course of the disease and prevent disseminated intravascular coagulation. The results reported suggest that the prophylactic use of heparin in severe viral illnesses associated with haemorrhage may be warranted but only provided that continuous laboratory monitoring can be provided.

References

Emond, R. T. D., Evans, B., Bowen, E. T. W., and Lloyd, G. (1977). A case of Ebola virus infection. *Br. med. J.* **ii**, 541.

Gear, J. S. S., Cassel, G. A., Gear, A. J., Trappler, B., Clausen, L., Meyers, A. M., Kew, M. C., Bothwell, T. H., Sher, R., Miller, G. B., Schneider, J., Koornhof, H. J., Gomperts, E. D., Isaacson, M., and Gear, J. H. S. (1975). Outbreak of Marburg virus disease in Johannesburg. *Br. med. J.* **iv**, 489.

Kiley, M. P., Regnery, R. L., and Johnson, K. M. (1980). Ebola virus: identification of virion structural proteins. *J. gen. Virol.* **49(2)**, 333.

Pattyn, S. R. (ed.) (1978). Ebola virus haemorrhagic fever. In *Proceedings of an International Colloquium on Ebola infection and other haemorrhagic fevers.* North-Holland, Amsterdam.

Siegert, R. (1972). Marburg virus. *Virology monographs 2.* Springer-Verlag, Berlin and New York.

Simpson, D. I. H. (1977). Marburg and Ebola virus infection: a guide to their diagnosis, management and control. *Offset Publication No. 36,* World Health Organization, Geneva.

Slow virus encephalopathies

W. B. Matthews

Within recent years a hitherto unsuspected form of transmissible agent has been detected as a probable cause of human disease. These agents cannot be seen on electronmicrographs and induce no antibody response, so they can be detected only by the production of disease. Their infectivity is resistant to many physical agents used to destroy conventional viruses and bacteria. For example, formalin fixed material may remain infective for many months or perhaps indefinitely and prolonged autoclaving at high pressure is needed to ensure sterilization. It is characteristic that in laboratory transmission, and in instances of natural or accidental transmission in man that can be identified, the incubation period is prolonged, sometimes for as much as several years. In the laboratory transmission is most readily effected by the intracerebral injection of brain material but peripheral tissues are also infective.

Only two human diseases have so far been identified as being transmissible to laboratory animals in the manner described above and presumably caused by these unconventional agents. Transmission was first achieved from the truly exotic disease *kuru*. This appeared to be confined to the Fore people of the almost inaccessible highlands of New Guinea. At first thought to resemble Parkinson's disease, the clinical features were eventually shown to be those of progressive cerebellar ataxia. The disease occurred in both children and adults, more frequently in women, and led to helpless incapacity and death within a year. Dementia was not obvious but the patients became extremely withdrawn. When the disease was discovered, kuru was by far the commonest cause of death among the Fore people.

The second human slow virus encephalopathy to be identified is now generally, but perhaps incorrectly, known as *Creutzfeldt–Jakob disease* (CJD). The original descriptions were indeed difficult to recognize as a distinct entity and for a long time numerous sub-divisions were described or invented, based on minor variations in clinical or pathological features. The form described as *subacute spongiform encephalopathy* presented a more uniform picture that differed in some respects from the original case reports. The transmission of spongiform encephalopathy to a chimpanzee, reported in 1968, drew this hitherto obscure disease into the limelight.

The main reason for heightened interest was that CJD had been considered a purely 'degenerative' disease. The characteristic pathology is that of neuronal degeneration, astrocytic proliferation, and the presence of minute vesicles in both neurones and glial cells—the spongy change. There is no trace of inflammation and no hint from the histological appearances of an infectious disease. The distribution of the neuronal loss varies from case to case but involves the cerebral cortex, basal ganglia, cerebellum, and anterior horn cells to different degrees.

Creutzfeldt–Jakob disease occurs in both sexes most commonly between the ages of 50 and 65 with a range of from 32 to old age with occasional cases being recognized in the second and third decades. In about 90 per cent of cases the disease runs its course to a fatal outcome in less than a year, sometimes within a month. The onset is often abrupt but sometimes vague prodromal symptoms of depression, lack of interest, and dizziness may be described by relatives. The initial symptoms are varied but are usually identifiable as being due to organic brain disease; cerebellar ataxia, localized weakness, hemianopia, cortical blindness, or aphasia. Onset with intellectual deterioration may briefly be misinterpreted as primary psychiatric disease. Advance is usually rapid and whatever the presentation the features in the later stages are often stereotyped. Speech is rapidly lost and swallowing becomes difficult. The limbs adopt the rigid decorticate flexed posture. Plantar reflexes when obtainable are extensor. A characteristic feature is myoclonus consisting of rapid, repetitive contraction of muscles or parts of muscles in the face, trunk, or limbs, increased by startle. Focal or generalized fits occur less commonly. Even when the patient is completely mute and helpless the eyes may remain open and it is not possible to determine the level of consciousness. Death results from the complications of the immobile state.

In the remaining 10 per cent of cases the onset is more gradual and there are other clinical differences. In these more chronic cases cortical blindness and myoclonus are less common and the dominant features are dementia, increased tone in the limbs and muscular wasting and fasciculation. All these signs are also seen in the subacute cases and the pathological findings are the same but the patients may survive for several years. It is possible that in some patients the disease may become arrested but recovery has not been adequately documented.

The cerebrospinal fluid is usually normal but the total protein is occasionally slightly increased. A mild degree of cerebral atrophy can be detected by CT scan or air encephalogram. In subacute cases the EEG nearly always develops a pattern of repetitive slow and sharp wave complexes but in the early stages and in chronic cases this pattern is not seen.

Differential diagnosis in the early stages is from focal brain disease and such patients are often referred to neurosurgeons. The established disease may be confused with *Alzheimer's disease* (see Section 21), where myoclonus is also not uncommon. Progression is, however, slower and speech is retained for much longer. When amyotrophy is present, the distinction from motor neurone disease can be difficult.

Epidemiology. The incidence of Creutzfeldt–Jakob disease is not fully known but in most countries is probably not more than one per million. It probably occurs worldwide. Laboratory transmission has naturally raised the possibility of natural transmission of the agent as the means of perpetuating the disease. Although possible clusters of cases have been found and in particular an unusually high incidence in Israelis of Libyan origin, there is no evidence that Creutzfeldt–Jakob disease is contagious. An animal reservoir, particularly dietary, is an alternative. Scrapie, a disease of sheep, is caused by a similar agent but there is no convincing evidence to incriminate eating mutton as the means of transmission of Creutzfeldt–Jakob disease. However, there seems little doubt that kuru was transmitted by ritual cannibalism and incidence is now rapidly declining. Considerable alarm has been caused by the accidental transmission of Creutzfeldt–Jakob disease by means of a corneal graft and by intracerebral electrodes that formalin had failed to sterilize. As far as is known transmission can only take place if tissue from the donor is implanted in the host. Blood and cerebrospinal fluid are only doubtfully infective and excreta have not been shown to contain the agent. Special care must be taken when handling tissues from known or suspected cases of Creutzfeldt-Jakob disease but the patient can be nursed normally.

Reference

Matthews, W. B. (1978). Creutzfeldt–Jakob disease. *Postgrad. med. J.* **54**, 591.

PAPOVAVIRUSES

S. D. Gardner

General description. Papovaviruses are small, spherical, DNA viruses which are usually host-specific and infect many different animal species including man. These viruses are separated, partly on the basis of their size, into two genera, papillomaviruses and polyomaviruses. Viruses infecting man occur in both.

The *papillomaviruses* have a particle size of about 55 nm. They occur both in domesticated and wild animals causing benign tumours and papillomas. In some animals these papillomas may develop into carcinomas. In man the viruses cause skin and genital warts, and laryngeal and oral papillomas. Papillomaviruses have not yet been grown satisfactorily in cell culture in the laboratory.

The *polyomaviruses* are smaller (45 nm). Human and animal types have been grown in cell culture. Tumours have been induced following inoculation of these viruses into experimental animals, but evidently do not occur in the natural host unless the animal is immunosuppressed. Two polyomaviruses have been isolated from man, *BK* and *JC* viruses (from the initials of the patients from whom they were first isolated) but there may be others. JC virus is the principal aetiological agent of *progressive multifocal leuco-encephalopathy (PML)*, a rare demyelinating disease. An animal virus, simian virus 40 (SV40), also in this subgroup has no association with Creutzfeldt–Jakob disease but was present in early batches of polio vaccine which were inadvertently given to millions of people without any noticeable effect so far. Rarely SV40 has been implicated in human disease: the source of the virus in these cases was not established.

Properties which suggest that the papovaviruses may be important in man are: (*a*) their persistence in the body after the primary infection; and (*b*) their capacity to produce tumours in the natural host or experimental animal. The long-term effect of these persistent infections, both in normal and immunologically compromised patients, needs to be evaluated. Reactivation of the papovaviruses occurs frequently, especially in immunosuppressed patients, and these viruses may have a role in human tumours.

Human papillomaviruses. Warts are common tumours of the skin and mucous membranes which occur at different ages, and are of various clinical and histological types. The infectious nature of the lesions has been established by transmission experiments. The types of lesion recognized are (*a*) common and plantar warts (verrucae vulgares and verrucae plantares), (*b*) juvenile or plane warts (verrucae planae), (*c*) genital warts (condyloma acuminata), (*d*) laryngeal papillomas, and (*e*) oral papillomas. Common, plantar, and juvenile warts occur most frequently in childhood, whereas genital warts, which are sexually transmitted, are seen in young adults. A second high incidence of genital warts has been described in older African males. Laryngeal papillomas are uncommon tumours occurring predominantly in pre-school children aged one to five years but occasionally found in adults. These papillomas are extremely difficult to treat because of their recurrent nature, and may cause acute respiratory obstruction. The antiviral drug vidarabine (adenine arabinoside) has ben used in some patients when papillomas recurred following conventional surgical removal. A possible association between maternal condyloma acuminata and juvenile laryngeal papillomas has been suggested and Caesarian section may be indicated for patients with genital warts at term. A rare, often familial disease *epidermodysplasia verruciformis* (EV) is characterized by an extensive cutaneous eruption of lesions resembling plane warts which persist for years. The disease is associated with a defect in cell mediated immunity; Bowen's disease, or squamous or basal cell carcinomas may develop in the lesions. One patient with a 30-year history of EV who developed multiple tumours was successfully treated in France with the oral aromatic retinoid RO-10-9359 (Roche). The patient received 1 mg per kg body weight per day and after two months most of the flat

warts had disappeared and two tumours not removed surgically had become smaller.

Warts and papillomas generally regress spontaneously but can be present for long periods and may recur. It is likely that the virus persists in the body indefinitely after the lesions have regressed. Evidence for this is suggested by the recurrence of warts in immunosuppressed renal transplant patients and of condylomas during pregnancy.

For many years it was thought that a single virus type was responsible for the various lesions. However, recent work on the viral DNA extracted from different kinds of warts has established that there are at least five types of human papillomavirus (HPV); serological studies have confirmed the biochemical results. The types identified so far have been described and designated HPV 1–5 but there are possibly at least nine types. HPV 1, 2, and 4 have been found in common and plantar warts, whilst HPV 3 and HPV 5 have occurred in the plane warts present in patients with the disease EV, type 5 being associated with lesions which were undergoing malignant change. Insufficient DNA has been obtained so far from condylomas and laryngeal papillomas for detailed study, but DNA hybridization experiments have shown no homology between the viral DNA present in condylomas and HPV 1–3, although there was a low level homology with HPV 5. The aetiological agent of condylomas is therefore different from the viruses causing common and plane warts, and is a probable sixth type, HPV 6. Subtypes of HPV 1 have been described.

A possible relationship has been suggested between HPV infections and malignant disease. The malignant changes occurring in the skin of patients with EV has been mentioned already. Rarely, tumours develop in laryngeal papillomas particularly those which occur in adults. There is also some epidemiological evidence to link HPV infections and carcinomas of cervix, vulva, penis, and perianal area.

Human polyomaviruses. Man was recognized as the natural host of a virus morphologically resembling a polyomavirus in 1965 when virus particles were seen in ultrathin sections of the brains of patients who had died from the rare disease PML (Fig. 1). Six years later in 1971 two polyomaviruses were grown in cell culture in the laboratory. BK virus was isolated in England from the urine of a renal transplant patient and excretion of the virus was largely associated with a heavily infected stenosed ureter which required resection. JC virus was isolated in America from the brain of a

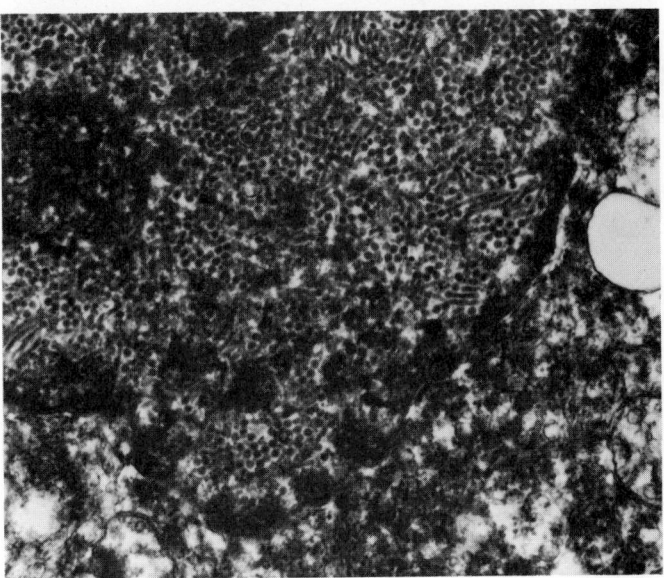

Fig. 1   Electron micrograph showing spherical and filamentous papovavirus particles in the nucleus of a cell from post-mortem brain material of a patient with PML. Thin section 25000. (Micrograph by Dr A. M. Field.)

patient with PML complicating Hodgkin's disease. These two viruses are different serotypes but are distantly related. The human polyomaviruses are known to multiply in the renal tract in the urothelium lining the ureter and renal calyces. Exfoliated inclusion-bearing cells, sometimes in very large numbers may be present in the urine. In the brain the oligodendrocytes and occasionally astrocytes are affected. One report also suggested possible multiplication of a polyomavirus in lymphocytes.

Since the original isolations were made, BK virus has been identified in the urine of patients immunologically compromised either by disease or therapy (Fig. 2). These include patients with renal and bone marrow transplants; with congenital immune deficiency diseases and those undergoing immunosuppressive treatment for malignant and non-malignant conditions. BK virus infections have also been confirmed in pregnant women, in one immunologically normal adult with non-bacterial cystitis, and in two infants, one aged four weeks with multiple dysplasias and hepatosplenomegaly and the other aged 11 months with cerebral atrophy. Apart from being excreted in the urine, BK virus was once reported in a brain tumour (reticulum cell sarcoma) occurring in a child with Wiskott–Aldrich syndrome. BK virus has been implicated in further cases of ureteric stenosis in renal transplant patients. Recognition of these cases is important because the clinical features may be similar to those of rejection and any increase in immunosuppression enhances the polyomavirus infection and may result in unnecessary transplant nephrectomies.

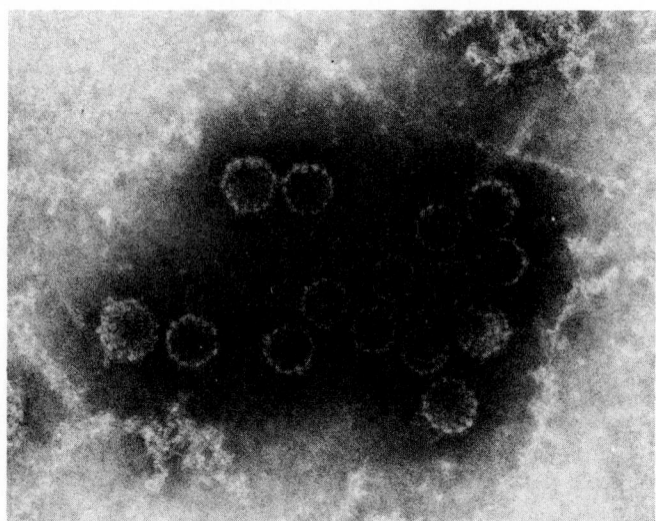

Fig. 2 Papovavirus particles from urine. Negative stain × 150 000. (Micrograph by Dr A. M. Field.)

JC virus has been identified in the brain of at least 46 patients with PML and is now recognized as the principal aetiological agent of this serious disease. In addition JC virus infects the renal tract and has been found in the urine of renal transplant patients, occasional pregnant women, and one patient with PML.

Transplacental transmission of both viruses may occur. Electron microscopic observations of polyomaviruses in urine have also been reported, and of particular importance was one case where virus was present in the urine of an otherwise normal child with acute haemorrhagic cystitis.

The natural history of the two viruses, how they are spread and maintained in the community, and whether there is any illness related to the primary infections is not yet known. Antibody to both viruses is frequently found in healthy people. More than 70 per cent of children in many countries have acquired BK virus antibody by the age of 10 years. Primary infections with JC virus occur later in life; only 17 per cent of English children have acquired antibody by the age of 10 and only 35 per cent by 17 years. Infection may be more common in America where more than 70 per cent of adults

have antibody to JC virus compared with 50 per cent of those in England.

Little is known about the primary infections with these viruses and it is likely that most of them are subclinical. There is some evidence to suggest that infection with BK virus may be associated with a pyrexial illness possibly with respiratory symptoms or neurological involvement. Convulsions and meningitis have been observed in children and the Guillain–Barré syndrome in adults. Infections due to reactivation of virus which persists in the body after the primary infection are mostly subclinical but have been associated with prolonged pyrexia and an influenzal-like illness. There is no evidence yet to linking BK and JC viruses with any human tumours.

Progressive multifocal leucoencephalopathy. This is a rare demyelinating disease (see Section 21) of the central nervous system with a distinct neuropathology which was recognized as a disease entity in 1958. The principal pathological changes consist of small patches of demyelination which fuse together and ultimately involve large areas of brain tissue. Oligodendrocytes are absent from the centre of the lesions but at the periphery these cells are abnormal and have enlarged basophilic nuclei often with eosinophilic inclusions. Astrocytic hyperplasia may be present and the astrocytes are often grossly enlarged and appear neoplastic but do not form tumours. Inflammatory changes, if present, may influence the prognosis. The nuclei of the abnormal oligodendrocytes contain very large numbers of polyomavirus particles; both spherical and filamentous forms may be present (Fig. 1).

PML usually is seen as a late complication in patients with an underlying disease of the reticulo-endothelial system, commonly leukaemia, lymphoma, or sarcoidosis, but also occurs in patients whose immunity is impaired for other reasons. It is normally a disease of adults but on rare occasions has been reported in children, the youngest aged five years, with combined immune deficiency disease. The clinical features reflect the location and extent of the area of demyelination. Predominantly the cerebral hemispheres are involved. Early signs include disorders of speech (dysarthria and dysphasia), visual disturbances (diplopia), impairment of motor function, and hemiparesis. Intellectual deterioration and personality changes are marked. As the disease advances the patient becomes blind, demented, and paralysed. Death occurs within four to six months. The cerebrospinal fluid is usually normal. Radiological investigations and radioisotope scanning are unhelpful in confirming the clinical diagnosis, but the electroencephalogram may be abnormal. A few cases are known where spontaneous remission has occurred. Various antiviral drugs have been used to treat a small number of patients, but a successful outcome has been reported in only two, both treated with cytosine arabinoside (Ara-C). In one of these biopsy-confirmed cases, treatment with Ara-C was continued at three-weekly intervals for several years and the patient was alive without serious sequelae after seven years. Inflammatory changes were present in the brain of this patient who also maintained very high serum levels of JC virus antibody: an immune response which may have contributed to her recovery.

At present, the clinical diagnosis of PML can be confirmed during life only by histological or virological examination of brain biopsy material.

References

Gardner, S. D. (1977). The new human papovaviruses: their nature and significance. In *Recent advances in clinical virology* (ed. A. P. Waterson), 93. Churchill Livingstone, Edinburgh.
— (1977). Implication of papovaviruses in human diseases. In *Comparative diagnosis of viral diseases*, vol. 1 *Human and related viruses*, Part A (ed. E. Kurstak), 41. Academic Press, New York.
Howley, P. M., Law, M.-F., Hellman, C., Engle, L., Alonso, M. C., Israel, M. A., Lowry, D. R., and Lancaster, W. D. (1980). Molecular characterization of papilloma virus genomes. In *Viruses in naturally occurring*

cancers (eds. M. Essex, G. Todaro, and H. zur Hausen), 233. Cold Spring Harbor Laboratory.

Padgett, B. L. and Walker, D. L. (1976). New human papoviruses. *Prog. med. Virol.* **22**, 1.

Takemoto, K. K. (1980). Human polyomaviruses: evaluation of their possible involvement in human cancer. In *Viruses in naturally occurring cancers* (eds. M. Essex, G. Todaro, and H. zur Hausen), 311. Cold Spring Harbor Laboratory.

Walker, D. L. (1978). Progressive multifocal leukoencephalopathy: an opportunistic viral infection of the central nervous system. In *Handbook of clinical neurology*, vol. 34, part II (eds. P. J. Vinken and G. W. Bruyn), 307. North Holland, Amsterdam.

zur Hausen, H. (1977). Human papillomaviruses and their possible role in squamous cell carcinoma. In *Current topics in microbiology and immunology*, vol. 78, 1. Springer-Verlag, Berlin.

BACTERIA

Diphtheria

A. B. Christie

The name of the organism, *Corynebacterium diphtheriae*, is from the Greek and refers to the club-shaped rod which produces a membrane in the throat of its victim. The disease, diphtheria, may also be of some antiquity and not unknown to the Greeks and the Romans. The 'Egyptian disease' of the former may have been diphtheria and the Romans probably knew the disease as one brought back from North Africa by Scipio's legionnaires in the Hannibalian wars. If so, one aspect of the epidemiology of the disease has not changed in 2000 years, for in the Second World War, the soldiers of Rommel's North Africa corps certainly carried the disease back into Germany, while on the other side of the world soldiers carried it from the Solomon Islands to civilians in New Zealand.

The disease is not, however, characteristically one of military campaigns or of movement. Soldiers in the Second World War had not previously been exposed to the diphtheria bacillus and were highly susceptible to infection when they moved into an area where the bacillus was common. They were Schick positive, whereas most of the natives of the countries they moved into were Schick negative, from early childhood exposure to the bacillus. This difference is at the root of the epidemiology of diphtheria, for it is an infection which illustrates very sharply how the virulence of an organism clashes with the immune status of the host; an infection which causes no symptoms in the highly immune, the carrier state, but an overwhelming, often fatal disease in the patient who has no immunity at all.

Bacteriology

Morphology. Corynebacterium diphtheriae is a Gram-positive, non-motile, and somewhat pleomorphic organism. The club-shaped forms are long and slender with swollen ends. Some have swellings along their length: these take stains heavily and look like round dots on the body of the bacillus. Sometimes these dots look like a chain of cocci, especially when stained with methylene blue or Neisser's stain. On a slide from a culture on Loeffler's serum several of these forms will be seen, often arranged in pairs, with the pairs grouped to form clusters. Such a slide can be of diagnostic value to a physician who is familiar with diphtheria and has seen the patient from whom the culture was taken. But one cannot on a slide distinguish between virulent and avirulent *C. diphtheriae*, nor between true diphtheria bacilli and other corynebacteria.

Growth. C. diphtheriae grows readily on ordinary nutrient agar, but much more readily on Loeffler's serum, on a slope culture of which there is a creamy growth within 24 hours. A stained slide from these colonies shows many typical bacilli, and during an outbreak, this is enough to confirm a clinical diagnosis. On blood tellurite agar, the three types of *C. diphtheriae, gravis, mitis*, and *intermedius*, form slightly different colonies and the bacteriologist, if he has the experience, can often tell one from the other. The three types also differ biochemically. All three ferment glucose and maltose, but rarely sucrose; *gravis* in addition ferments starch and glycogen. The diphtheroid, *C. xerosis*, always ferments sucrose, and *C. hofmanni*, a non-pathogenic diphtheroid, ferments no carbohydrate at all. But strains of *C. diphtheriae* may be atypical, and in countries where diphtheria has become a rare disease microbiologists have difficulty in recognizing *C. diphtheriae* with certainty solely on cultural and biochemical tests.

Toxin production. The serious effects of diphtheria in man are caused by diphtheria toxin, and only by testing organisms for toxigenicity can one finally determine that a corynebacterium is a true *C. diphtheriae* and whether it is pathogenic or not. Gel diffusion tests are available but are liable to false negative, false positive, and non-specific reactions. *C. diphtheriae* can be classified into types according to their ability to produce bacteriocine or diphthericin, and this corresponds closely with toxigenicity and can be useful in tracing spread during epidemics. But guinea pig tests are still the most reliable tests for toxin production, either the lethal subcutaneous or the more economical intracutaneous test.

Gravis, mitis, and *intermedius* strains all produce the same toxin. *In vitro*, *mitis* strains may produce as much toxin as *gravis* or *intermedius* strains. Small changes in the medium affect the rate of growth and the amount of toxin produced, especially the amount of iron in the medium. It may be that the conditions in the throat of a patient favour the growth and persistence of *gravis* and *intermedius* more than *mitis* strains and so lead to more production of toxin by the two former strains. Another element may be more important. There appear to be two factors in diphtheria toxin, factor A and factor B. A is the lethal factor, B the spreading factor. A can exert its full lethal effect only when enough B is present, and it seems that *gravis* strains at least are always rich in factor B. Whatever the exact mechanism, very small doses of toxin can cause death: it needs only eight times the lethal guinea pig dose to kill a five-year-old child. It is of interest that factor B, not factor A, is the antigen which calls forth protective antibody.

The action of toxin

Membrane formation. The membrane on the throat or on other parts of the body, the skin for example, is the result of an inflammatory reaction to the presence of multiplying *C. diphtheriae*. Fluid and leucocytes pass from dilated blood vessels on the inflamed surface where the epithelial cells become necrotic. The fluid clots and grips these dead cells, enmeshing at the same time leucocytes, diphtheria bacilli, cellular debris, and sometimes small blood vessels. So is formed the membrane so typical of diphtheria.

Effect on nerves. C. diphtheriae does not normally pass beyond the membrane site, but it has occasionally been seen in organs at autopsy, and it has been isolated, though very rarely, from blood taken from contacts before they have developed membrane in the throat. But there is no doubt that it is toxin that causes the severe damage in diphtheria. It can pass in the bloodstream to the heart and other internal organs and become fixed to cells, but how and where it reaches the nervous system is not so clear. There is evidence to support blood, lymph, and neural spread, and demyelination of peripheral nerves is certainly common. This, and degeneration of sensory and motor fibres, may be seen in the nerves to the eye, the palate, pharynx, larynx, and heart and in the nerves to the muscles of the limbs. Whether the toxin can pass the blood–brain barrier and cause central lesions is not so certain: older and later writers differ on this point.

Effect on heart. The lesions in most organs, the liver, spleen, and kidney for example, are non-specific. In the adrenals the changes are usually slight and barely detectable, very different from the congestion and haemorrhage seen in the guinea pig adrenals. In the heart changes are common: fatty degeneration of cardiac muscle and infiltration of the interstitium with leucocytes, sometimes affecting the conduction fibres, is seen, but necrosis of the parenchyma is rare. Fibrosis and scarring, if severe, may lead to death in late convalescence, but usually, if the patient survives the acute toxaemic state, the heart recovers completely. Mural endocarditis may occur and embolism may then cause hemiplegia, but valvular endocarditis is a very rare finding. In the late paralytic stage of the disease, neuritic changes may be seen in the nerves to the heart.

Antigenic types. C. diphtheriae can be classified serologically into many sub-types, although it is not clear which antigens are responsible for the differences. There are at least 13 *gravis*, 4 *intermedius*, and 40 *mitis* serological types. The organism may also be classified into types by bacteriophage lysing, and all toxigenic strains are lysogenic. Phage types I to III are *mitis*, IV to VI intermedius, VII an avirulent *gravis*, and the rest all *gravis* strains. These phage types are stable. Typing based on bacteriocin or diphthericin production by *C. diphtheriae* has already been mentioned. One serotype may contain variants which differ both in bacteriocin and bacteriophage characters. Typing is useful, and sometimes essential, in tracing the spread of apparently unconnected outbreaks of the disease.

Host immunity and spread of infection

The Schick test. The injection of fluid containing a measured amount of toxin into the skin of the left forearm will cause a red reaction (positive Schick test) unless there is enough antitoxin in the patient's blood to prevent it. In the right forearm the same amount of fluid is injected, heated to destroy toxin. Any reaction on this arm must be due to something in the fluid other than toxin and must, of course, appear on both arms. Fortunately the reaction due to toxin persists for days and increases, while the non-specific reactions fade quickly. This is the basis of the Schick test and it measures susceptibility to diphtheria. How much serum antitoxin is necessary to produce a negative Schick test is not so clear, and figures may differ widely according to the method of assay, whether by passive haemagglutination, cytotoxic inhibition on tissue culture, or radioimmunoassay. But in spite of these figures, the Schick test remains a reliable one: a Schick-negative person is unlikely to get diphtheria, or, if he does, it is likely to be a mild attack and due to a *gravis* or *intermedius* strain, for *mitis* strains do not often cause clinical signs in Schick negative persons. A Schick-positive person on the other hand is susceptible to diphtheria, and his attack may be of any severity, mild or subclinical to fatal.

Schick conversion. Schick negativity is not, however, an inborn state. The new-born child is indeed Schick negative, protected by maternal antibody, but he loses this immunity round about the sixth month and becomes Schick positive. He is then exposed to infection from without and the degree of exposure will, of course, depend on how common *C. diphtheriae* is in the environment. In a highly immunized community *C. diphtheriae* tends to die out, and the child may grow to adult life without encountering the bacillus. This we have already seen was the case among German soldiers in North Africa, and among American soldiers during the Second World War the Schick positive rate before going overseas was between 35 and 45 per cent. In other parts of the world *C. diphtheriae* is a common pathogen and the young child meets it early, maybe becoming a faucial, nasal, or aural carrier. Many children suffer severe or fatal attacks before the age of five years. This is a pattern which may be seen in large subtropical cities lacking an efficient immunization programme.

Spread by skin lesions. In the rural tropical world there is another pattern. Faucial diphtheria is rarely seen, yet older children and adults are Schick negative. Skin diphtheria in the form of sores and ulcers is, however, common, and in crowded, humid, and bacteriologically unhygienic conditions *C. diphtheriae* readily spreads from the skin of one child to the skin of another. Toxin is absorbed only slowly from the skin sores and converts the child without much harm from the Schick positive to the Schick negative state. This is perhaps an over-simplification. When the Schick positive troops went to North Africa or the Solomon Islands, skin diphtheria was certainly a common complaint among them, but so too was severe faucial diphtheria. Their mode of life was scarcely the same as that of the native population, and minor differences in life style can have a major effect on the spread and pattern of a disease. In a London fever hospital in the late 1930s, nurses who joined the staff from London and other big cities were usually Schick negative, while nurses from rural Ireland were usually Schick positive and had to be immunized before going on the diphtheria wards which were then full of diphtheria patients. The city nurses had presumably had subclinical attacks in childhood, but the country nurses had not encountered *C. diphtheriae*.

Fomites, dust, and milk. Diphtheria spreads from person to person, from the acute case or the carrier. Fomites and dust are not important, although the organism resists drying and can be isolated from floor dust in a ward or an infected classroom. Diphtheria has been spread by milk contaminated by a human carrier: animals do not suffer from diphtheritic mastitis nor excrete *C. diphtheriae* in their milk, *C. diphtheriae* is a parasite exclusively of man. Pasteurization kills *C. diphtheriae* as does heating at 58°C for 10 minutes or exposure to most common disinfectants.

Clinical features Infection with diphtheria bacilli may be subclinical, mild (anterior nasal), moderate (tonsillar), or severe and life-threatening (laryngeal or nasopharyngeal). *C. diphtheriae* may attack other sites on the body, the skin, for example, or the eye.

Anterior nasal diphtheria. The main symptom is nasal discharge, thin at first, then thick, purulent and bloody, with soreness of the nostril and the skin above the lip, and crusting or thin membrane inside the nostril. There is little or no absorption of toxin from this site so that the child is not ill, but anterior nasal may coexist with faucial or nasopharyngeal diphtheria, and it is a fatal mistake to miss this. The child is highly infectious: but he is more than a carrier, for a carrier has no signs of infection at all, although he may be pouring *C. diphtheriae* from his nose.

Tonsillar diphtheria. The incubation period is from two to five days and the onset is slow. The child is off-colour, tired but not acutely ill. He may have no sore throat, very unlike a child with acute streptococcal tonsillitis or early scarlet fever. In a day or two he becomes drowsy, pale, and toxic, and takes to bed. He remains ill for a week or two, he may get palatal paralysis about the third week, but he is unlikely to suffer any of the more serious complications of diphtheria.

On the first day of his illness, there may be only a small spot of membrane on his tonsils, a few millimetres wide, yellowish white and with a crinkled edge. No-one is likely to look at the throat at this stage, unless it is a doctor examining contacts. Soon the membrane spreads over most of both tonsils, greyish-yellow, a millimetre thick and all of one piece, not soft and mushy, edged with a rim of redness but confined to the tonsils. The rest of the throat and fauces looks normal. The lymph nodes in the neck are a little enlarged and a little tender. After another day or two the membrane is greenish-black, and later it sloughs off. A typical case of diphtheria and easy to diagnose so long as it is typical. But anyone with experience of diphtheria knows it is dangerous to rely on clinical appearance alone. Tonsillar diphtheria can look very like any other form of tonsillitis.

Nasopharyngeal diphtheria. The onset is more acute, the child soon becoming very ill. The membrane first spreads from the tonsils to the uvula. It may then creep forward across the hard palate almost to the teeth, or up behind the uvula into the nasopharynx and sometimes then down the nose. From the nasopharynx toxin passes readily into the bloodstream and diphtheria has now become a life-threatening disease.

The membrane has a thick edge, and as this advances the earlier parts become necrotic. It is now foul, greenish-black, and smelly: the smell, the *foetor oris*, is not diagnostic, for any foul exudate smells, as, for example, in Vincent's angina or infectious mononucleosis.

The lymph nodes in the neck are now very swollen, but it is not easy to feel them separately because the surrounding tissues of the neck are swollen too. The whole space between the mandibles and the clavicles is bulging with lymph nodes and oedema; this is the bull-neck of severe diphtheria (Fig. 1). A patient with bull-neck diphtheria is gravely ill. He may bleed from his mouth and nose and into his skin. Such a child has little hope of recovery. If he does recover it will only be after a long illness and many dangerous complications.

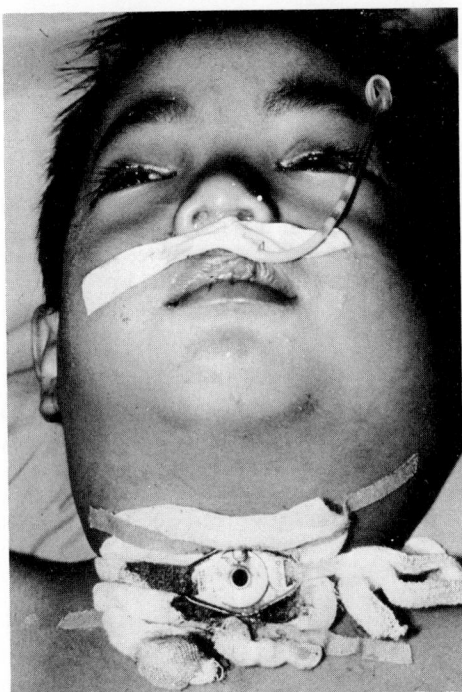

Fig. 1 Diphtheria: bull-neck swelling of pharyngeal diphtheria: tracheotomy for associated laryngeal diphtheria.

Laryngeal diphtheria. Diphtheria of the larynx occurs most often separately from faucial diphtheria. There is often no membrane on the throat at all. Less commonly membrane spreads from the throat to the larynx. The earliest symptom is a feeble, unproductive cough or croup. Obstruction to breathing comes on gradually in the course of 24 hours or so: a child who wakes in the night with sudden croup has probably not got diphtheria. The lower intercostal spaces are sucked in as the child breathes in, showing that enough air is not getting in to fill the lungs. Later the fossae above and below the clavicles, the epigastrium, and the sternum itself are sucked in as the child tries to drag air through the narrowed larynx. The child pulls himself up the side of the cot in his struggle for breath, his face congested, and his lips blue. This may bring on a feeble spasm of coughing and he falls back, grey and exhausted from asphyxia. Without tracheostomy the child will soon be dead.

Tracheostomy brings rapid relief if the membrane is confined to the larynx and upper part of the trachea. In a few cases the membrane has spread down into the bronchi and bronchioles and then tracheostomy helps very little, unless the child coughs up a cast of the bronchial tree. In the pure laryngeal case the relief is dramatic and the child falls into a sound sleep. There is little absorption of toxin from the hard rings of the trachea and the cartilage of the larynx so that serious complications are not common after the relief of the obstruction. Provided, of course, there is no membrane on the fauces.

Complications

Cardiovascular changes. If membrane extends beyond the tonsils cardiovascular complications may occur, usually in the first two weeks. The patient complains of pain in the upper abdomen and may vomit, often the first ominous signs. The pulse is rapid and thready, the blood pressure collapsed. The child is in shock. He may die at this stage or go on to show signs of cardiac failure. The apex beat goes down and out, there are murmurs at all areas, and triple or gallop rhythm. The liver enlarges, urine is scanty. The child has pain over the heart and lies limp and exhausted.

Electrocardiographic changes are common: a flattening or inversion of the T wave, a lengthening of the PR or QT interval, or, in severe cases, bundle branch or complete block. Auricular or ventricular fibrillation may occur. Death is not inevitable, but most deaths from diphtheria occur at this stage. But if the child recovers, the recovery is complete.

Paralyses. Paralyses come on late, usually many weeks after the onset of the illness. Palatal paralysis is common, even after tonsillar diphtheria. It comes on about the third week, causes a nasal voice, allows fluids to come down the nose on swallowing, but usually disappears after a week or so: a minor complication with careful management. A little later the child may have blurred vision from paralysis of accommodation or an internal squint from external rectus paralysis: again a passing inconvenience.

About the sixth or seventh week the dangerous paralyses come on: paralysis of the pharynx making swallowing difficult or impossible; paralysis of the larynx adding greatly to the danger; then paralysis of the breathing muscles. The nerves to the heart may be affected, with tachycardia and great irregularity of rhythm.

These paralyses are all dangerous to life and many children die now, often after several weeks when everything seemed to be going well. Sometimes a child is discharged from hospital when all the throat signs clear up and he seems well, but dies weeks later in his home from what seems a new and unconnected illness. The outlook for a child with late paralysis is not hopeless if skilfully treated; he resembles a child with poliomyelitis, but with this difference, that if he can be kept alive with expert care, the paralyses eventually disappear completely and the child regains normal health, whereas a child with severe poliomyelitis is usually left with some permanent paralysis.

Other clinical types

Skin. In contrast to the severe course of some faucial infections, *C. diphtheriae* often causes chronic but mild infections of the skin. This is especially common in the tropics and has already been mentioned (see page 5.134). Perhaps the temperature and the moisture of the skin and the scanty clothing may have something to do with it. Sores and ulcers are commonest on the legs but may occur anywhere. The sores are indolent and slow to heal. Paralysis may occur, usually of the affected limb, or myocarditis, but both are rare. Absorption of toxin is slow from the skin and leads to seroconversion of the patient rather than to any toxic complication.

The eye. Conjunctivitis is not uncommon. Usually this is no more than a slight, catarrhal condition in a patient with faucial diphtheria. Occasionally membrane forms in the lower conjunctiva and spreads over the cornea causing great destruction of tissue.

The gastrointestinal tract. *C. diphtheriae* may spread to the oesophagus from the fauces causing dysphagia and there are reports of membrane in the stomach and the intestine: but these are pathological curiosities.

Urogenital tract. Diphtheria may be spread on a child's fingers from the throat to the vulva causing local sores: this is not altogether rare. Occasionally *C. diphtheriae* invades the vagina and even the cervix, when there may be serious absorption of toxin, but this is certainly rare. Diphtheria of the glans or coronal sulcus of the penis has occurred in infants after circumcision. In one case the father was a soldier with unrecognized skin diphtheria. Sores on the penis may also occur on men in conditions where diphtheria of the skin is spreading. A report of diphtheria membrane found on the wall of the bladder at operation is probably unique: the patient developed peripheral neuritis and died of heart failure.

Endocarditis. This must be rare, but cases are on record where *C. diphtheriae* has been isolated from heart blood and valves after death, and there is at least one record of a proved case successfully treated with prolonged antibiotics.

Other corynebacteria. C. ulcerans produces two toxins, one of which seems to be the same as diphtheria toxin. It can cause membranous tonsillitis but seems not to cause toxic complications nor to spread from case to case. C. xerosis has been isolated from the blood of patients with bacterial endocarditis and from prosthetic valves at operation. C. haemolyticum has caused outbreaks of tonsillitis with or without a maculo-papular rash, and C. sepsis has caused death in a few patients on immunosuppressive treatment for some other condition. All these, except perhaps C. haemolyticum, are examples of uncommon or rare infecting agents. C. vaginale seems to be a common vaginal commensal, and, when present in large numbers, a frequent cause of vaginitis. It has also been isolated on one or two occasions from the urine of men with cystitis or urethritis and in one case from the blood of a patient after prostatectomy.

Diagnosis

Clinical. In many parts of the world diphtheria is still a common disease, and there one should always think of diphtheria in a child with exudate on the throat. If the exudate is thick and discoloured, the child should be given antitoxin. Elsewhere the idea of diphtheria is unlikely to enter the mind of a doctor who has never seen or heard of a case of diphtheria since he qualified. He knows infectious mononucleosis: there is membrane on the patient's throat and the neck glands are enlarged, but the membrane is white, even after a week, and the neck glands are discrete. It is no great harm to diagnose as diphtheria a case of infectious mononucleosis; but the other way round is a tragic error. Streptococcal or virus tonsillitis cannot be distinguished from mild diphtheria with only a few flecks on the tonsils, but it should not be confused with severe, membranous diphtheria. Peritonsillar abscess, quinsy, can cause great distortion of the tissues of the throat so that one cannot see the surfaces of the tonsils and this can happen too in severe diphtheria, so one must take care. Monilial infection causes soft white exudate and there are usually patches on the cheeks and gums as well. Secondary syphilis in the adult sometimes causes glairy exudate on the tonsils: the patient usually has a rash and laryngitis. Leukaemia and other blood dyscrasias cause foul ulcerations of the fauces, bleeding into the skin and great toxicity in the patient, a picture very like severe diphtheria. In all these conditions only blood counts and bacteriology can lead to a sure diagnosis, if they are done. They would be, if the doctor could only say to himself 'Can this be diphtheria?'.

Laboratory. Direct stained smears from throat swabs, if positive, can help the experienced doctor who has also seen the patient: but only the experienced doctor, and only if he looks at the smears himself. Smears from cultures the next day are more useful, and during an outbreak they meet most needs. In isolated cases or where there is any bacteriological doubt, full cultural, biochemical, immunological, and guinea pig tests must be carried out. Occasionally, with an atypical strain, only a reference laboratory can classify the corynebacterium.

Treatment. Only antitoxin can neutralize toxin, and it can do so only before the toxin reaches and damages tissue cells. So it must be given as soon as possible after C. diphtheriae begins to multiply on a patient's throat; on clinical suspicion, and before bacteriological confirmation. Hypertoxic diphtheria is hypertoxic from the start: it is wrong to believe that only in late cases is there danger to life.

The dosage is simple. If the membrane is confined to the tonsils 20 000 units of antitoxin is enough. If the membrane is beyond the tonsils 50 000 to 100 000 units should be given, half of it intravenously. With highly purified antitoxin the danger from a dangerous serum reaction is much less than the danger of death from hypertoxic diphtheria, but one can, over a period of an hour or two, give small but increasing doses of antitoxin up to the full intramuscular dose, when the intravenous dose can be given. For laryngeal diphtheria 20 000 units is enough, if there is no faucial exudate: the main treatment is in the relief of the respiratory obstruction by tracheostomy.

C. diphtheriae is nearly always sensitive to penicillin and it seems logical to give patients a course of the drug, or of erythromycin if the patient is truly sensitive to penicillin. This will get rid of the organisms in the throat but only antitoxin can deal with any toxin that has passed from them into the bloodstream. Most carriers can be cleared with antibiotics.

For cardiac complications intensive care is needed. Sedation is essential and often the child needs extra oxygen. Digitalis is useful only when there is congestive failure. A cardiac pacemaker has been used to help a child over temporary conduction failure. Expert assessment is valuable, but perhaps the main requirement, and often the only one available, is skilled nursing.

For paralysis expert nursing is again required; for careful suction of pharyngeal secretions which the patient cannot swallow or cough out, and for intragastric or intravenous feeding. When breathing fails, artificial ventilation is essential. The work is demanding but rewarding, for even the child with the most severe paralyses can with care make a complete recovery.

Prevention

Active immunity. Diphtheria is one of the great preventable diseases. With a good immunization programme, there need never be another case. Diphtheria toxoid is usually given, along with tetanus and pertussis vaccine, as DTP to infants between three and six months old. The usual course is of three doses, the first and second separated by at least four weeks, the third after six months. In some countries, because of geographical and many other difficulties, it may be difficult to arrange three visits to or by the vaccinator, but there is evidence that two doses separated by at least two months gives protection. This is not to say that two doses are better than three: simply that in difficult conditions two may be enough. A booster dose of diphtheria tetanus (DT) vaccine at school entry, if there is a school, will ensure prolonged immunity. When such a programme is well organized C. diphtheriae finds it hard to spread in the community and diphtheria is no longer a common disease.

Passive immunity. Contacts of a patient may be protected for two to three weeks by 1000 to 2000 units of antitoxin. This may be useful when there is danger of cross-infection in a ward from a missed case, or in home contacts of a patient. But penicillin given to close contacts may be equally effective. It is certainly the best treatment for carriers.

Control of outbreaks. We have all the tools to control an outbreak in a closed community: the Schick test to detect susceptibles, bacteriology to confirm cases and find the carriers, vaccine to immunize Schick positive children, and antitoxin or penicillin to protect the children while they are acquiring active immunity. The main need is intelligent application. Out in the field or in the villages or in wider epidemics, control is not so easy, but the principles are the same. Eradication lies with active immunization.

References

Ch'in, K. Y. and Huang, C. H. (1941). Myocardial necrosis in diphtheria with a general review of the lesions of the myocardium in diphtheria. *Am. Heart J.* **22**, 690.

Christie, A. B. (1980). *Infectious diseases: epidemiology and clinical practice*, 3rd edn. Churchill Livingstone, Edinburgh.

Gibson, L. F. and Colman, G. (1973). Diphthericin types, bacteriophage types and serotypes of *Corynebacterium diphtheriae* strains isolated in Australia. *J. Hyg., Camb.* **71**, 679.

Helting, T. B. and Zwisler, O. (1976). Breakdown of diphtheria toxin: isolation of a stable immunogenic fragment B derivative. *Behring Inst. Mitt.* **59**, 92.

Liebow, A. A. (1958). Diphtheria and the Schick test in the tropics. *Int. Arcs. Allergy Appl. Immun.* **12**, 42.

— and Bumstead, J. H. (1963). Cutaneous and other aspects of diphtheria. In *History of internal medicine in World War II*, Vol. II, 275. Office of the Surgeon General U.S. Army, Washington.

Robinson, D. T. and Marshall, F. W. (1934). Investigations on the gravis, mitis and intermedius types of *C. diphtheriae* and their clinical significance. *J. Path. Bact.* **38**, 73.

Wilson, S. A. K. (1954). Diphtheria. In *Neurology*, Vol. 11. Butterworth, London.

Pathogenic streptococci

M. T. Parker

Streptococci are Gram-positive cocci that form chains and grow in air, though some of them may require the addition of CO_2 to do this. They are resistant to drying but not to disinfectants or to temperatures exceeding 65° C. Many of them cause disease in man, but the nomenclature of the pathogenic species is somewhat confusing (Table 1). In the past, this was based mainly on two descriptive features of streptococci: their action on blood and the presence of certain cell-wall polysaccharide or teichoic-acid antigens (the Lancefield antigens). Thus, streptococci were described as β-haemolytic when they lysed erythrocytes, α-haemolytic when they caused green discoloration of these cells, and non-haemolytic when they caused no change in them. Also, they were classified into Lancefield groups when the possessed a common cell-wall antigen; but only some of these groups merit recognition as species.

sometimes be β-haemolytic and form the group antigen A, C, F, or G.

The enterococci are somewhat more resistant to heat and other adverse conditions than most other streptococci. Of the two common species found in the gut, *Str. faecalis* and *Str. faecium*, only the former is an important pathogen. All the enterococci belong to Lancefield group D.

A number of other streptococci are members of the normal body flora but seldom give rise to purulent lesions. Their chief medical importance is as causes of endocarditis. Members of two species, *Str. sanguis* and *Str. mitior*, and a number of related strains that are difficult to classify, are usually α-haemolytic and may be referred to as the 'viridans' streptococci. They, and the non-haemolytic *Str. mutans*, are mouth streptococci that often give rise to endocarditis. *Str. sanguis* and *Str. mutans* are particularly associated with the teeth and are concerned in the formation of dental plaque; *Str. mutans* is the most likely cause of dental caries. *Str. salivarius*, a mouth streptococcus not associated with the teeth, very rarely causes disease. *Str. bovis*, another important cause of endocarditis, is found exclusively in the gut. It is the only one of the 'other' streptococci that regularly forms a Lancefield antigen; like the enterococci and *Str. suis* it forms the antigen D.

Table 2 summarizes the distribution of streptococci in the body flora and Table 3 lists the main streptococcal diseases.

Table 1 Streptococci found in man

Division	Common name	Specific name	Haemolysis*	Lancefield antigens
Pyogenic streptococci	group A	*pyogenes*	β	A
	group C	*equisimilis*	β	C
	group G	. . .	β	G
	group B	*agalactiae*	β	B
	group R	*suis*, serotype 1	β	D + R
	pneumococci	*pneumoniae*	α	–
	. . .	*milleri*	$-(\beta, \alpha)$	$-(F,C,G,A)$
Enterococci	faecal streptococci	*faecalis*	$-(\beta)$	D
		faecium	V	D
Other streptococci		*sanguis*	α	$-(H)$
		mitior	α	$-(O,K,M)$
		mutans	–	$-(E)$
		salivarius	–	$-(K)$
		bovis	–	D

In parentheses: less common reactions
* – = non-haemolytic; V = variable

Table 2 The main sites of carriage of streptococci

Streptococci	Throat	Teeth	Other oral	Gut	Vagina
groups A, C and G	(+)	–	–	–	(±)
pneumococci	(+)	–	–	–	(±)
group B	(+)	–	–	(+)	(+)
sanguis, mitior and *mutans*	+	+	+	–	–
salivarius	+	–	+	–	–
milleri	+	+	+	+	(+)
enterococci	–	–	–	+	(+)
bovis	–	–	–	+	–

+ = Normal flora; (+) = frequently carried; (±) = infrequently carried; – = not normally present

Table 3 Diseases associated with streptococcal infection

Streptococci	Diseases
Group A	*local sepsis*: tonsillitis, wound infection, impetigo and others (see text) *systemic infection*: acute septicaemia *other acute manifestations*: scarlet fever, erysipelas *late (non-suppurative) sequelae*: rheumatic fever, acute post-streptococcal glomerulonephritis
Groups C and G	local sepsis and septicaemia
Group B	*neonatal*: early-onset septicaemia, with or without meningitis; late-onset meningitis *adult*: septicaemia (and endocarditis)
Group R	meningitis (occupational zoonosis)
Pneumococcus	pneumonia, otitis media, meningitis, septicaemia, peritonitis
Str. milleri	abscesses in internal organs, notably brain, liver and lung; meningitis, pleural empyema, peritonitis; septicaemia, endocarditis
Faecal streptococci	urinary-tract infection, mild wound sepsis; septicaemia and endocarditis
Str. sanguis, Str. mitior, Str. mutans, and *Str. bovis*	Common causes of endocarditis (*Str. mutans* probably the main bacterial cause of dental caries)

Note: almost any streptococcus can cause endocarditis; only the more common causes are listed

It is customary to describe as 'pyogenic' streptococci several important species that are almost invariably β-haemolytic and are each characterized by the presence of a single Lancefield antigen. Among these, by far the most common human pathogen is *Streptococcus pyogenes*; we shall follow current practice and refer to it as the group A streptococcus, though the group A polysaccharide is also formed by a few strains of a quite distinct species (*Str. milleri*). The group C and G streptococci of man are infrequent causes of disease, but the group B streptococci are responsible for many serious infections. It should be noted that other β-haemolytic streptococci cause diseases in animals, and that some of these possess Lancefield antigens (B, C, or G) similar to those of the human pathogens. However, the animal pathogens are rarely transmitted to man. The one exception is *Str. suis*, serotype 1 (Lancefield group R), a common cause of sepsis in piglets, which occasionally gives rise to meningitis in meat-handlers and pig-farmers.

Several other human streptococci are also responsible for purulent inflammation and thus have claims to be considered 'pyogenic'. These include the pneumococci and *Str. milleri* (see page 5.147). The latter organism occupies an anomalous position in that, though usually non-haemolytic and ungroupable, it may

DISEASES CAUSED BY GROUP A STREPTOCOCCI

Pathogenesis

The group A streptococci are invasive; they enter the body through the mucosa of the upper respiratory tract, through wounds, and possibly under certain circumstances through the unbroken skin. They may then give rise only to a local inflammatory lesion, but in many cases they spread rapidly along lymphatics or tissue planes, soon reaching the bloodstream and causing a severe generalized disease that may be rapidly fatal if appropriate treatment is not given. The means by which the organism penetrates the mucosa is unknown, but adhesion to epithelial cells is said to be mediated by a lipoteichoic-acid component of the streptococcal surface. Once in the tissues, the streptococcus is protected from phagocytosis by the M protein, which is present, along with the lipoteichoic acid, in an outer coat of fine hair-like filaments. Although it is non-toxic, the M protein is undoubtedly the main virulence factor, as is shown by the almost complete protection afforded, in man and in experimental animals, by antibody against M antigen of the infecting type. Once formed, this antibody may persist for a number of years. Some strains also form a non-antigenic capsule of hyaluronic acid, but the role of this as a virulence factor is uncertain.

Some 70 antigenically distinct M proteins have been recognized. The M types differ qualitatively in their pathogenic abilities. Some types frequently cause tonsillitis but almost never impetigo; others are particularly associated with impetigo but seldom give rise to clinical tonsillitis though they may colonize the throat. In general, the M proteins of the former types are more strongly antigenic than those of the latter, but a number are intermediate in character. M types also differ in their ability to cause glomerulonephritis, and probably also rheumatic fever.

In vitro, group A streptococci form an embarrassingly large number of extracellular substances that can be induced to harm laboratory animals. These include two haemolysins (O and S), streptokinase (which initiates fibrinolysis), a proteinase, several DNAases, and a NADase. Culture supernates are leucocidal, an effect probably attributable to streptolysin S. It would be unreasonable to conclude that all of them play a significant part in natural pathogenicity, but several are of importance because the formation of antibody to them provides evidence of recent infection. One extracellular product—the erythrogenic toxin—is responsible for the rash and other symptoms of scarlet fever though, as we shall see, its action may not be as simple as was once thought. In experimental animals it causes profound physiological disturbances: pyrogenesis, suppression of reticulo-endothelial function, and triggering of the Shwartzman reaction.

Cell-wall components may also be toxic; this is not true of the surface proteins and the group polysaccharide, but the mucopeptide skeleton of the cell wall causes a variety of disturbances when given by injection. Delayed hypersensitivity to cell-wall constituents may play a part in the pathogenesis of certain streptococcal diseases.

In addition to the immediate consequences of streptococcal invasion, there are two important late effects—often referred to as 'non-suppurative sequelae'—that develop after a latent period, affect only a proportion of those infected, and are not attributable to the presence of living streptococci in the affected tissues: rheumatic fever and acute post-streptococcal glomerulonephritis. These are unique manifestations of infection with group A streptococci for which there are no parallels in streptococcal infections of other animals.

Acute disease

Infections of the upper respiratory tract.
In Britain we refer to streptococcal sore throat as 'tonsillitis', but there is some justification for the American term 'pharyngitis', because the disease begins as a diffuse inflammation of the pharynx and nasopharynx, and the streptococci are found in large numbers in both nose and throat at this stage. The fully developed picture of acute follicular tonsillitis, as seen in older children and young adults, is as follows: sore throat, pain on swallowing, swollen bright-red tonsils with discrete white spots on the surface, enlargement of the anterior cervical lymph nodes, fever, and leucocytosis; but all of these features are present in only a proportion of cases. All gradations from the typical severe disease through mild sore throat to symptomless infection with antibody response may be seen in the same outbreak. In infants and pre-school children, the signs are less definite, with fever and nasal discharge, often overshadowed by cervical adenitis or otitis media. Severe tonsillitis tends to be more common in outbreaks in residential groups of older children and adolescents, and to affect new entrants.

After the initial mucosal infection, the disease tends to become localized in the pharyngeal lymphatic tissue, from which it may spread directly to adjacent structures, giving rise to a peritonsillar or retropharyngeal abscess, along lymphatics to cervical lymph nodes, or less often through the fascial planes of the neck. A thin purulent nasal discharge usually indicates the presence of sinusitis. Invasion of the bloodstream may occur, but considerably less often than from wound infection.

After the acute signs have abated, the untreated patient may continue to feel unwell, fever may persist, the erythrocyte-sedimentation rate may be raised, and abnormal electrocardiographic signs may be detectable for several weeks. This 'post-streptococcal state' may not be easy to distinguish from mild rheumatic fever.

Infections through the skin
Wound infection. The consequences of introducing group A streptococci into a wound vary from a minimal local inflammation to a rapidly fatal septicaemia. Small puncture wounds, particularly if contaminated at the time of infliction, often lead to acute cellulitis or a rapidly spreading lymphangitis; death from septicaemia may occur within as little as 36 hours of wounding. Infection introduced into deep tissues, e.g. the peritoneum, at the time of surgical operation may be followed in a few hours by a shock-like condition in which the temperature remains subnormal until death. Later contamination of wounds, after healing has begun, tends to give rise to a more localized infection or even to be symptomless. Infection of burns leads to local inflammation of variable severity; septicaemia develops only occasionally, but skin grafts are almost invariably destroyed. The streptococci responsible for invasive infections of wounds usually belong to M types similar to those that cause tonsillitis.

Streptococcal gangrene is a rare but highly fatal disease, usually but not always following trauma, in which dusky discolouration and haemorrhagic bullae appear over an area of cellulitis; ulceration follows, revealing an extensive area of necrosis beneath.

Streptococcal impetigo. This is a common, localized infection of the superficial layers of the skin that shows almost no tendency for invasion of deeper tissues. The lesions are crusted spots seldom exceeding 2 cm in diameter which last for one to two weeks and heal without scarring. They usually affect exposed areas and may appear in succession. In the initial stage there may be a small vesicle, but this soon ruptures and a relatively thick crust develops. The lesions are thus distinguishable from staphylococcal impetigo, in which there is a considerably larger initial vesicle (1 cm or more in diameter); if this breaks, the succeeding crust is paper-thin.

Streptococcal impetigo is a common disease of children in poor socio-economic conditions. It is now much less common in Britain than formerly, but is widespread in many other countries, particularly in association with rural poverty. Many of the areas of high incidence have a warm climate, and epidemics are associated with high atmospheric temperature and humidity, but streptococcal impetigo is in no sense a tropical disease, and occurs at high latitudes in the summer months. The lesions may appear on apparently unbroken skin, but are frequently associated with scabies, insect bites, and minor trauma.

Although predominantly a disease of children, streptococcal impetigo may in certain circumstances be prevalent among adults. It was common among military recruits in Britain during the Second World War and among American troops in Vietnam. Outbreaks may affect members of athletic teams and the workers in slaughterhouses and meat-processing factories.

Amongst the streptococci, it appears that only group A cause impetigo, though the lesions often become secondarily infected with streptococci of groups C and G. Large numbers of *Staphylococcus aureus* are usually present in the older lesions. Colonization with *Corynebacterium diphtheriae* is common in some tropical areas, and some of the strains are toxigenic. In subjects with antitoxic immunity this colonization does not affect the appearance of the lesion, but the patient may be a source for clinical diphtheria in non-immune siblings. Streptococcal strains from impetigo belong to many different M types, but these are in general distinct from those responsible for tonsillitis. Several of these 'skin' types are nephritogenic, and impetigo is the main determinant for post-streptococcal glomerulonephritis in the tropics and subtropics.

Systemic infections. Acute septicaemia is the commonest systemic infection. As we have seen, it usually occurs in association with wound infection (including puerperal sepsis). The local inflammation may not necessarily be prominent and may occasionally be absent. For example, epidemics of septicaemia in geriatric hospitals may result from silent infections in bedsores. It is almost unknown as a complication of streptococcal impetigo. Meningitis and endocarditis, and infections of bones and joints, are rare.

Other septic infections. Puerperal fever due to group A streptococci was once the most feared of the infections associated with childbirth. It may be looked upon as a special case of wound infection. Onset early in the puerperium is usually abrupt, and massive invasion of the bloodstream is the rule. Although probably now less common than in the pre-antibiotic era, its true incidence tends to be concealed by the common practice of beginning specific treatment as soon as fever develops in the puerperium and without previous vaginal swabbing.

Acute purulent vaginitis is not uncommon in children and is almost always a localized infection. This is also true of acute peri-anal cellulitis in children of either sex. Both tend to be associated with family outbreaks of streptococcal tonsillitis.

Serious neonatal group A streptococcal infections are uncommon, but sporadic cases of neonatal meningitis and septicaemia may occur. Investigation often reveals that a number of other babies in the nursery have trivial group A streptococcal infections or are carriers at the umbilical site. There is some evidence that the neonates who suffer invasive infection are those who have not passively acquired antibody against the infecting M type.

Scarlet fever. The symptoms of scarlet fever—pyrexia, headache, vomiting, and a punctate erythematous rash—may be added to those of almost any acute group A streptococcal infection: of the throat, a wound or burn, or puerperal infection. However, scarlet fever is not often associated with streptococcal impetigo.

Pathogenesis. There is no doubt that scarlet fever is caused by the erythrogenic toxin, because its symptoms are reproduced by the injection of filtrates of cultures of group A streptococci isolated from cases of scarlet fever into susceptible human subjects. The intradermal injection of smaller amounts of filtrate leads to a local erythematous reaction; this is the *Dick test*, used in the past to determine susceptibility to the toxin. The injection of serum from a convalescent case of scarlet fever into the skin of a patient in the acute stage of the disease causes local blanching of the rash, the so-called Schultz–Charlton reaction. These observations, and the age-related distribution of a positive Dick reaction (indicating sus-

ceptibility to the toxin), led to the simple hypothesis that scarlet fever was caused by the direct action of erythrogenic toxin in persons who did not have circulating antitoxin—a situation directly analogous to that of the Schick reaction in relation to diphtheria immunity (see page 5.134). Several observations cast doubt on this, notably that the child of a Dick-positive mother may be Dick negative at birth but become positive some months later, and that the blood of 'early' Dick-negative babies may not neutralize toxin.

The alternative view, that scarlet fever is a hypersensitivity reaction, was first advanced over 50 years ago but was not widely accepted. It has recently been revived, with considerable experimental support, in the following form. Erythrogenic toxin is combined in the streptococcal cell with a heat-stable component. Repeated streptococcal infection may result in delayed hypersensitivity to this, and one of the consequences is a hyper-reactivity to erythrogenic toxin. Scarlet fever, then, is a combination of the direct toxicity of the erythrogenic toxin with secondary toxicity caused by hypersensitivity to the heat-stable component. Thus, a person may be Dick negative, and hence insusceptible to scarlet fever, either, as in some neonates, because he is neither hypersensitive nor immune, or, as in some adults after repeated infection, because though hypersensitive he possesses circulating antitoxin. Some such explanation is needed to account for the persistence of insusceptibility to scarlet fever in infants for months or years after the disappearance of maternally acquired passive immunity, and for the steady reduction in the severity of scarlet fever over the last 80 years.

Clinical features. In the latter half of the nineteenth century, scarlet fever was the most common cause of death in children aged over one year, and was often referred to simply as 'the fever'. In Britain, mortality began to decrease before 1900 and had virtually ceased by 1965. Thus, descriptions of 'toxic' or 'malignant' scarlet fever are now of historical interest only. Mild infections are still quite common, but often escape attention and, even more often, official notification. Scarlet fever is characteristically a disease of children of school age.

Cases of moderate severity are usually easy to recognize. They begin abruptly with fever (37.8–39.5 °C) accompanied by a somewhat disproportionate tachycardia, several bouts of vomiting and sometimes by abdominal pain. Coughing is notably absent. In addition to the acute tonsillitis that often is the primary infection, an enathem may develop on the palate some hours before the skin rash appears. This comprises bright red spots superimposed on a general redness of the whole pharynx. Early in the disease the tongue is covered by a white fur through which red-tipped papillae project ('strawberry tongue'). Later, usually after the appearance of the rash, the fur peels off, leaving a raw, red papillate surface ('raspberry tongue'). The spleen may be just palpable, and there may be a mild generalized lymphadenopathy.

The rash usually appears within 24 hours of onset, characteristically first on the chest, neck, and arms, and spreads peripherally; the hands and feet generally escape. It is symmetrical and does not itch. In typical form it consists of a diffuse erythema with superimposed punctate spots approximately 2 mm in diameter, but either of these elements maybe absent and the spots are sometimes larger. In its developed form, the rash is intense on the lower abdomen, the back, the axillae, and groin and the inner aspects of the thighs. Linear petechiae in the elbow flexures (Pastia's sign) and other skin folds may accompany a heavy rash. The face is flushed, but circumoral pallor, though sometimes striking, is not specific to the disease.

In very mild cases fever may be less, vomiting limited to a single episode, and the rash transient and limited in extent. In more severe cases the rash persists for several days. It is followed by the characteristic peeling, either of fine flakes or of larger areas of skin. It may sometimes have to be sought diligently, and may be detectable only on the ears or the tips of the digits. Peeling may occur from 2–3 days to 3 weeks after the appearance of the rash.

Erysipelas. This is an acute disease caused by group A streptococci in which the main clinical manifestations are cutaneous but the primary infection is not always of the skin. Unlike other group A streptococcal diseases, it occurs more often in the later than the earlier years of life, and it tends to recur at the same site, often after months or years.

It begins abruptly with fever (temperature around 39 °C), headache, shivering, and vomiting, often with considerable mental confusion. Within a few hours there may be slight discomfort at the site of the subsequent skin lesion. By the second day there is usually clear evidence of local inflammation in the form of a bright red, somewhat painful area, always with a palpable raised margin. The lesion extends irregularly, often with apparently detached inflamed areas at the periphery. Vesicles and bullae containing clear fluid may appear on the surface, and when these rupture they become crusted. The lesion becomes more and more oedematous as it spreads, but the redness tends to fade at the centre.

The common sites for the appearance of erysipelas are the face, usually around the eye or nose, and the leg. Oedema is particularly severe in facial erysipelas, so that one or both of the eyes are closed. In most cases the lesion regresses after one to two weeks, but elderly patients may die of intercurrent complications such as pneumonia.

Erysipelas lesions may sometimes be seen to have arisen from an adjacent infected wound, and epidemics of erysipelas occurred in surgical wards in the nineteenth century. Even today, a single case of erysipelas may develop in the course of a ward outbreak of surgical wound infection. Sometimes a trivial skin abrasion can be identified as the site of the primary infection. Facial erysipelas often appears to begin from an infection of the upper respiratory tract. In a number of instances, however, the primary lesion is not identifiable.

Bacteriological information about erysipelas is scanty and unsatisfactory. Group A streptococci have been isolated from the skin lesion in a number of instances, but this is not always easy, the numbers isolated are sometimes few, and there are failures. The possibility cannot be excluded that some of the isolations were of 'contaminants' from a primary lesion elsewhere in the body. The evidence that erysipelas is a local inflammatory response to living streptococci is thus not strong. It may be a tissue reaction to fragments of streptococci translocated from the primary lesion.

Epidemiology. Group A streptococci are readily communicable and give rise to epidemics under a variety of circumstances. With rare exceptions the source of infection is human, and may be either a case or a carrier. Broadly there are three main patterns of spread.

Spread by the respiratory route. This occurs through the air. Infectivity by this route falls off progressively at distances exceeding 2 m; this suggests that the infectious particles are the larger of the salivary droplets generated by talking, coughing, and sneezing. Patients in the early stages of tonsillitis have large numbers of group A streptococci in the throat, nose, and saliva and are very infectious, probably by virtue of disseminating large numbers of streptococci in salivary particles. During convalescence, and even if antibiotic treatment is not given, the organisms disappear rapidly from the saliva, and usually also from the nose, and the patient has little infectivity even though throat carriage may persist.

Spread to wounds and the skin. The direct impaction of salivary particles into a wound by a person suffering from an acute infection is an efficient but unusual method of transmission. The throat carrier, who disperses little, is probably also of secondary importance. However, nasal carriers and persons with septic lesions play a leading role, but the routes of dissemination are different from that responsible for respiratory infection, and resemble those of *Staph. aureus*. Particles of dried secretion may be transferred by (*a*) indirect contact, on hands, handkerchiefs, soiled dressings, and so on, or (*b*) aerially, by the liberation of infected particles of dried

secretion or skin scales. Many of these infectious particles are of much smaller size (10–20 μm) and are therefore able to be disseminated for much greater distances through the air (e.g., the length of a hospital ward) than are the particles responsible for respiratory spread.

Carriage on the healthy skin is uncommon in adults, with one significant exception: the perianal skin. Surgeons who were perianal carriers, but had negative nasal and throat swabs, have on several occasions been responsible for epidemics of streptococcal wound infection.

Streptococci dispersed into the air or transferred to inanimate objects persist in gradually diminishing numbers for up to several weeks. There is reason to believe, however, that their infectivity diminishes considerably. Thus, recently contaminated environmental sites are probably of much greater importance than those more remotely contaminated.

There is little doubt that the predominant route of spread in streptococcal impetigo is from skin to skin either directly or indirectly via contaminated objects. In some tropical countries there is in addition evidence of passive transfer on the bodies of nonbiting insects. Colonization of the skin by group A streptococci has been observed in children several days before the appearance of an impetigo lesion at the site of isolation of the streptococci.

In puerperal infection, undue significance has probably been accorded to the throat-carrier midwife who has not suffered a clinical infection. Infection of the mother from her own baby, itself infected in the nursery, has been repeatedly demonstrated.

Food-borne spread. The ingestion of group A streptococci in food may lead to acute tonsillitis. The disease is usually severe, and vomiting tends to be unusually prominent. Numerous outbreaks were described in the first half of the twentieth century in which the vehicle was fresh milk, usually from a single herd. The milk contained the infecting streptococcus in enormous numbers, yet group A streptococci are known to multiply little in milk at ambient temperature. In a number of the outbreaks one of the cows was found to be suffering from mastitis due to the epidemic strain. Group A streptococci very rarely cause septic lesions in animals other than man, but in these instances the cow appears to have been infected from a milker. Milk-borne outbreaks have become exceptionally uncommon in Britain since the introduction of pasteurization.

Food-borne group A streptococcal tonsillitis is nowadays associated with other foodstuffs, and is not very common. The organism grows well in a number of foods, such as custard and sauces, which appear to become contaminated from human cases or carriers.

Diagnosis

Streptococcal tonsillitis. This diagnosis cannot be made with certainty on clinical grounds, and the physician has to decide under what conditions he will seek bacteriological assistance. It is reasonable to expect some 40 per cent of cases of acute sore throat in young persons to be due to group A streptococci, but this figure will vary somewhat with season and locality. In the past, the most compelling reason for taking a throat swab in cases of tonsillitis was to exclude the possibility of diphtheria. This is now a fairly remote possibility in Britain, but the young physician, who has probably never seen a case, will be reassured by a formal exclusion of it. At the same time, some other uncommon bacterial causes of sore throat, for example, *C. ovis* and *C. haemolyticum*, will be excluded, but the bacteriologist will probably not examine the swab for gonococci unless alerted to this possibility in appropriate adult cases. In at least one-half of all cases no bacteriological cause will be found.

In streptococcal tonsillitis, group A organisms will be present in the throat, usually in large numbers, of about 90 per cent of cases; but a carrier of group-A streptococci may suffer from non-bacterial sore throat, so the isolation of the organism is not absolute proof of the presence of streptococcal infection. Throat-carrier rates in children are usually around 10 per cent in the winter months, but are subject to considerable local variation; in adults the rates are rather lower. However, the number of streptococci in the throat is usually considerably less is carriers that in cases. Thus, a moderate or heavy growth can be taken with fair certainty to confirm a diagnosis of streptococcal tonsillitis.

There is little agreement about diagnostic strategy in sore throat because views differ about the importance of detecting and treating all cases of streptococcal tonsillitis. Some authorities argue that this is essential as a means of preventing rheumatic fever (see page 5.144), which may follow streptococcal attacks of all degrees of severity. Others consider that the frequency of rheumatic fever in the area in which they work does not justify the very considerable organization necessary to do this effectively, and give antibiotic treatment, with or without preliminary swabbing, only when they judge this to be necessary for the relief of immediate symptoms.

If the initial symptoms are sufficiently severe, it seems reasonable to begin specific treatment immediately after taking a swab, and to discontinue treatment if streptococci are not isolated. If the infection is mild and the case is seen in the acute stage, it may be justifiable to withhold treatment until a positive swab has been obtained; the laboratory should be able to give a definite report in 24–36 hours, giving sufficient time to begin treatment early enough to prevent a rheumatic attack. This course of action has the disadvantage that it may be difficult to persuade the patient to complete a full course of treatment begun when the symptoms are subsiding.

Serological tests play no part in the diagnosis of acute group A streptococcal infection; if this is to be made in time to influence the outcome of the disease, no significant antibody can be expected; if a bacteriological diagnosis is made and treatment is begun promptly, little antibody will be formed subsequently.

Septic lesions. If the clinical appearances suggest a rapidly spreading cellulitis or lymphangitis, 'best-choice' antibiotic treatment should be begun immediately and revised when the results of wound swabbing and blood culture are obtained. It must be remembered that wounds may be 'silently' infected with group A streptococci. The crusted lesions of impetigo may occasionally give falsely negative cultural results unless a moistened swab is used or the crust is first removed or raised.

Scarlet fever. Recognition is not likely to present difficulties unless the primary streptococcal infection has been missed and the rash is atypical. In measles, the rash is coarser and more blotchy and appears after three to four days of febrile coryza (see page 5.77); the rash of rubella may become scarlatiniform on the trunk but usually remains discrete on the limbs and face (see page 5.80). Scarlatiniform rashes may appear transiently in the prodromal period of several other fevers or after the administration of a variety of drugs. Some epidermolytic staphylococcal infections, notably Ritter's disease in neonates and staphylococcal 'scarlet fever' (see page 5.161), give rise to a rash initially very difficult to distinguish from that of scarlet fever but soon recognizable by the separation *en masse* of the outer layers of the epidermis, leaving a red, raw surface or, if this is less complete, causing the appearance of Nikolsky's sign. Acute exfoliative dermatitis gives a similar appearance but runs a more prolonged course. Scarlatiniform rashes also characterize staphylococcal toxic-shock syndrome (see page 5.162) and Kawasaki's disease (see page 13.124), but in both of these conditions they tend to be associated with high fever, conjunctival reddening, and severe hypotensive shock.

Erysipelas. The appearance of the lesion is usually characteristic. Ophthalmic herpes zoster can usually be distinguished from erysipelas because the lesion stops abruptly at the midline and is confined to the distribution of a single nerve. Cellulitis tends to be more painful and tender and to have an ill-defined edge.

Treatment. Acute group A streptococcal infections respond promptly to treatment with an appropriate antimicrobial agent (Table 4). This is given not only to ameliorate the acute illness but to lessen infectivity and to prevent the subsequent development of non-suppurative sequelae.

Table 4 Use of antimicrobial agents for the treatment or prevention of group A streptococcal infections

Purpose	Agent	Route	Dosage
Short term: (a) treatment of acute infection of normal severity* and prevention of sequelae, and (b) mass chemo-prophylaxis	1. benzathine benzylpenicillin	IM	1.2×10^6 IU (6×10^5– 9×10^5 IU in children); single injection
	2. phenoxymethyl or phenoxyethyl penicillin	O	100–125 mg; 4 times a day; 7–10 days
	3. benzyl-penicillin	O	2×10^5 IU; 4 times a day; 7–10 days
	4. erythromycin	O	250 mg 4 times a day (40 mg/kg a day in children); 7–10 days
Long term: prevention of second and subsequent attacks of rheumatic fever	1. benzathine penicillin	IM	1.2×10^6 IU; 3-weekly in adults (monthly in children)
	2. phenoxymethyl or phenoxyethyl penicillin	O	100–125 mg; twice a day
	3. benzyl-penicillin	O	2×10^5 IU; twice a day
	4. sulphadiazine	O	1 g per day (0.5 g for children)

IM = intramuscular; O = oral; IU = International Units
* For rapidly spreading infections and septicaemia, see text

All group A streptococci are still highly susceptible to benzylpenicillin and the closely related orally absorbable derivatives of this. These are the antibiotics of first choice; their narrow spectrum of activity, and the absence of adverse reaction in cases of glandular fever makes them preferable to ampicillin. For the individual patient, erythromycin is an acceptable alternative if penicillin allergy is suspected, but the occasional strain is resistant to erythromycin (and to the lincomycins) and a few local prevalences of resistant strains have been reported. Tetracycline resistance is sufficiently common to exclude this antibiotic entirely for the treatment of streptococcal infection. Streptomycin and other aminoglycosides, if given alone, are inactive against streptococci.

Severe attacks of tonsillitis are cut short and the development of local septic complications is prevented by as little as four to five days' treatment with an orally absorbable derivative of benzylpenicillin. When so treated, the patient becomes virtually noninfectious within 24–48 hours. However, to prevent the subsequent appearance of rheumatic fever, penicillin treatment must have been begun within six days of onset and must be continued for seven to ten days. A convenient alternative, widely used in the USA, is a single intramuscular injection of 1 g of benzathine benzylpenicillin.

Similar treatments are equally effective for other local septic infections. The presence of penicillinase-forming bacteria in the lesion does not seriously impair the action of penicillin on group A streptococci in most situations, but it may prevent the elimination of streptococci from extensive burns. Lincomycin and clindamycin have therefore been used fairly often for the control of streptococcal outbreaks in burns wards, but on several occasions resistant streptococcal strains have appeared very rapidly. It is then usually necessary to use an appropriate penicillinase-resistant penicillin or cephalosporin even though this may be somewhat less active against the streptococcus.

In rapidly spreading septic infections, or when septicaemia has appeared, very prompt treatment is essential. This should be initially with benzylpenicillin by intramuscular injection or intravenous infusion until there is clear evidence of therapeutic response, when the oral route may be used.

Prevention

Respiratory-tract infection. General hygienic measures are rather ineffective in preventing spread in families and communities. Short-range aerial dissemination—the most important means of spread (see page 5.140)—is favoured by overcrowding. Increased bed-spacing will reduce this if patients are confined to their beds but is unlikely to have much effect if the population is ambulant or semi-ambulant. Moderate increases in natural ventilation and dust-suppressive measures have proved disappointing in effect. It is, of course, desirable to prevent physical contact, and contact mediated by objects used in common, between infected and unifected persons, but these measures are unlikely to be decisive.

The effect of the early penicillin treatment of cases in eliminating sources is undoubted, but patients are usually very infectious for some hours before symptoms appear. Intensive bacteriological search for carriers, and their prompt segregation or treatment *in situ* often fails to halt the spread of infection for a similar reason; by the time that the bacteriological results are available, a fresh crop of infected persons has been generated. Nevertheless, it is worth trying early in an outbreak. Some workers claim success from a limited programme of collecting only nasal swabs and examining all the contacts for nasal and aural discharge; certainly the nasal swab is a good means for the rapid detection of early acute infections.

Dissatisfaction with these methods has led to the advocacy of *mass antibiotic prophylaxis*. An outbreak can certainly be halted by giving oral penicillin for seven to ten days, or one intramuscular injection of benzathine penicillin, to everyone, but the case-incidence has often returned to its original level within a few weeks. Intermittent courses of mass prophylaxis have been widely employed in army camps, but it is uncertain whether they reduced significantly the total number of streptococcal attacks. On the other hand, it has been claimed that giving a single dose of benzathine penicillin to all entrants to such camps, except those with a history of penicillin allergy, produced a greater than ten-fold reduction in morbidity from streptococcal infection.

Wound sepsis and other hospital infections. Here we have to consider the possibility not only short-range droplet infection, but also aerial spread at longer range by smaller particles liberated from nasal and wound discharges and minor skin lesions, as well as infection by direct and indirect contact in the course of medical and nursing procedures. Preventive measures will be similar to those employed for the control of staphylococcal wound infection.

Impetigo. As we have seen (page 5.138), this appears to result from direct or indirect skin-to-skin contact especially when minor skin trauma is frequent. In affluent countries this leads to pockets of infection, notably in institutions, where gross personal neglect has been allowed to occur; the remedies are obvious if not easy to implement. It also occurs in occupational groups in which skin-to-skin contact, or the constant handling of common objects, coexists with a risk of minor skin trauma. Similar troubles were once rife in light-engineering factories and have in large measure been eliminated by an efficient industrial medical service. Only major improvements in living standards, notably in the provision of housing and washing facilities, and the control of biting insects, is likely to be effective in the control of streptococcal skin sepsis in developing countries.

Vaccination. Immunization against group A streptococci is theoretically possible. Vaccines of alum-precipitated, highly purified M protein of single serotypes give good homologous protection against experimental infection in human volunteers. Even more solid type-specific immunity against infection by the respiratory route develops after spraying purified M protein into the throat. However, the difficulties of producing a polyvalent vaccine that gives a sufficiently adequate type coverage are formidable, and it is not likely that such vaccines will be available in the near future.

The non-suppurative sequelae of group A streptococcal infection.

Rheumatic fever and acute post-streptococcal glomerulonephritis develop after a latent period in persons who have had a group A streptococcal infection that was not treated or was treated inadequately in the acute stage. The latent period is on average somewhat longer in rheumatic fever (2½ weeks) than in glomerulonephritis (1½ weeks). The two diseases have the following in common: (*a*) they affect only a proportion of those who have had a streptococcal infection; (*b*) living streptococci are not present in the specific lesions of the disease; and (*c*) irreversible damage to organs (to the heart in rheumatic fever and the kidneys in glomerulonephritis) follows in some of the patients. The diseases differ in one important respect; rheumatic fever enormously increases the chance that a subsequent group A streptococcal infection will be followed by another rheumatic attack, but glomerulonephritis shows no such effect. Rheumatic fever and glomerulonephritis rarely if ever follow the same streptococcal infection.

There is no evidence that group A streptococci play any part in the aetiology of rheumatoid arthritis, and the evidence for a specific association with erythema nodosum or anaphylactoid (Henoch–Schoenlein) purpura is questionable.

Rheumatic fever. This is a loosely associated group of clinical manifestations that may appear in almost any combination: fever; pain with or without swelling in one or more joints; evidence of myocarditis, endocarditis, pericarditis, or pleurisy; subcutaneous nodules; a characteristic skin lesion (erythema marginatum); and an even more characteristic disturbance of central-nervous-system function (chorea). These are all attributable to a single histological lesion, the Aschoff node, comprising a central area of necrosis surrounded by a fan-like arrangement of epithelioid cells and outside this a narrow zone of lymphocytes. In the acute stage these nodes are scattered through the connective tissue of the affected organs; later they undergo fibrosis.

Pathogenesis. Rheumatic fever is uncommon in very young children; high incidences of the disease occur in populations subject to frequent attacks of group A streptococcal infection. This suggests that it is a hypersensitivity reaction to a streptococcal product, but typical Aschoff nodules have not been produced in animals by repeated injections of streptococci. Another possibility is that the lesion is a direct but delayed response to a streptococcal product that persists in the tissues and has been translocated to other organs by phagocytic cells. If cell fragments composed of peptidoglycan and group polysaccharide are injected into animals, remittent granulomatous lesions rather like Aschoff bodies develop at a considerable distance from the site of injection and are attributable to the slow release of the peptidoglycan. Finally, evidence has been produced suggesting that antibodies are produced in response to a cell-membrane component of the streptococcus that cross-reacts with the sarcolemmal membrane of the myofibrils of heart muscle. These three possibilities are mutually exclusive, and the pathogenesis of rheumatic fever is still uncertain.

Clinical feature. In about two-thirds of cases, there is a history of sore throat, of variable severity, 1–5 weeks (average 2½ weeks) before onset; the rest of the cases give no such history. The disease may start insidiously or abruptly. Clinical features of rheumatic fever are described in Section 13.

The course of rheumatic fever is variable, a typical attack lasting six weeks or so, but some attacks may pursue a remittent course for months. It is often difficult to decide when the disease has ceased to be active, because treatment with salicylates or corticosteroids suppresses many of its effects. In the past it was also difficult to distinguish a recrudescence from a further attack triggered by a fresh streptococcal infection, but this is now an unlikely event if effective chemoprophylaxis is given.

Nowadays the average first attack of rheumatic fever in Britain is considerably milder than in former times; death in the acute stage is uncommon, considerably less than one-half of the patients exhibit signs of carditis and many of these do not suffer permanent damage to the heart valves, and chorea is rare. In many developing countries, however, the disease is still of a severity comparable with that experienced in Britain in the nineteenth century, though it is said that chorea, erythema marginatum, and subcutaneous nodules are less frequent.

One attack of rheumatic fever increases many-fold the risk of subsequent attacks. High recurrence rates are favoured by: (*a*) youth; (*b*) a short interval since the last rheumatic attack; (*c*) numerous previous attacks; (*d*) pre-existing rheumatic heart damage; and (*e*) clinical severity of the current streptococcal infection. Thus, the greater the number of rheumatic incidents the greater the certainty of ultimate damage to the heart valves.

Laboratory findings. Early in the disease there is usually a leucocytosis of 10 000–15 000 per mm^3 with a polymorphonuclear predominance. The erythrocyte sedimentation rate (ESR) is considerably raised and the C-reactive protein test is positive in nearly all rheumatic-fever attacks, except those in which chorea is a feature, and except in patients under treatment with salicylates or corticosteroids. None of these findings is diagnostic.

Evidence of a recent streptococcal infection, when obtainable, provides valuable support for a clinical diagnosis of rheumatic fever. However, group A streptococci can be isolated from no more than 15–20 per cent of the patients by the time the disease has appeared. Serological tests may be considerably more helpful. Antibody to several of the extracellular products of group A streptococci appears in the blood towards the end of the first week in untreated streptococcal infections. It disappears progressively during the succeeding months, so that its presence is a reliable indication of a fairly recent infection. It is very rare for an 'acute' serum to have been collected before the appearance of antibody, and a specimen collected at the onset of rheumatic fever must be looked upon as a 'convalescent' serum. Thus, convincing evidence of a rising titre is not often obtained, and the only means of interpretation is to compare the titre in the patient's serum with an arbitrarily determined upper limit for the normal population; but such a population will include some persons who have had a recent streptococcal infection, so some overlap of titres is to be expected. The usual practice is to consider a titre abnormal if it exceeds that found in 80 per cent of the 'normals'. The 'upper limits of normal' for three commonly used tests, the antistreptolysin O (ASO), anti-hyaluronidase, and anti-DNAase tests, as determined in the USA some 20 years ago, are given in Table 5. These are probably still

Table 5 Titres of antibody (units) against group A streptococcal extracellular products in normal persons and in cases of rheumatic fever (modified from Wannamaker and Ayoub 1960)

Antibody	Upper limits* for normal population		Lower limits† for rheumatic fever
	5–12 years	young adults	
Anti-streptolysin O	333	200	250
Anti-DNAase	. . .	80	320
Anti-hyaluronidase	110	80	300

* 80 per cent have titres of this level or lower
† 80 per cent have titres of this level or higher

applicable in most developed countries. If these figures are applied to rheumatic fever, some 80 per cent of cases will give a titre exceeding the upper limit of normal in any one of the tests, but if two of the tests are used, the percentage giving a raised titre in one or both tests rises to around 90 per cent. The tests most commonly used in combination are the ASO and anti-DNAase tests. In some developing countries, the much higher normal levels for streptococ-

cal antibodies in the 'normal' population somewhat reduce the value of these tests in the diagnosis of rheumatic fever.

Another test with a somewhat more specific relation to rheumatic fever is for antibody to the so-called M-associated protein of group A streptococci. Titres exceeding 80 are almost invariable in rheumatic fever; in most normal persons the titre is less than 20. Some uncomplicated streptococcal infections give rise to high titres of this antibody, and these high titres may persist for years, but a negative result in this test is a valuable means of excluding rheumatic fever.

Diagnosis. The most widely accepted means of making a diagnosis of rheumatic fever is the application of the so-called 'modified Jones criteria' (Table 6) in which the evidence is divided into three categories: (*a*) major criteria; (*b*) minor criteria; and (*c*) evidence of preceeding group A streptococcal infection. The presence of two major criteria, or one major and two minor criteria, indicates a high probability of rheumatic fever if there is also supporting evidence of recent streptococcal infection. Thus, the role of the laboratory is seen to be essentially one of exclusion. It must be remembered, however, that some of the Jones criteria may be suppressed by giving salicylates or corticosteroids, and that in chorea, in which the latent period may be very prolonged, the ASO and anti-DNAase titres and the ESR may have returned to normal levels.

Table 6 Revised Jones criteria for the diagnosis of rheumatic fever

(*a*) Major criteria	(*b*) Minor criteria
carditis	previous rheumatic fever or
polyarthritis	rheumatic heart disease
chorea	arthralgia
erythema marginatum	fever
subcutaneous nodules	raised erythrocyte-sedimentation rate or positive test for C-reactive protein
	electrocardiogram: prolonged P-R interval

(*c*) Evidence of recent group-A streptococcal infection
    raised antibody levels
    positive throat swab
    recent scarlet fever

Interpretation: 'high probability' of rheumatic fever if two of (*a*), or one of (*a*) and two of (*b*), are present with any one of (*c*)

Treatment. The patient should be confined to bed for the duration of the acute attack. It is customary to enforce complete rest, but the necessity for this in the absence of carditis is unproven. If cardiac failure develops, specific treatment for this will be needed. Giving penicillin once a rheumatic attack has begun does nothing to limit its severity, but penicillin prophylaxis (see below) should be begun without delay to prevent the possibility of an early second attack.

The acute inflammation can usually be effectively suppressed by the administration of salicylates or corticosteroids, but neither reduces the frequency or severity of the residual heart damage. Both may have unpleasant side-effects. In very mild cases, neither may be necessary if the pain can be controlled by mild analgesics.

In more severe cases, and in all with carditis, one of these drugs should be given. It is best to begin with a salicylate: ordinary aspirin four times a day is usually adequate. It should be given in escalating dosage until the symptoms are suppressed; for example, 60, 90, 120, and 180 mg/kg per day may be given in divided doses respectively on the first, second, third, and fourth days. Treatment with the minimal suppressing dose should be continued for some weeks and then the dose should be reduced cautiously. If desired, the higher dosages may be administered in five or six instalments, and antacids or milk used to control gastric intolerance. If signs of salicylate toxicity develop, the dosage may be reduced cautiously, or the salicylate partially or completely replaced with corticosteroid.

If salicylate fails to suppress the symptoms completely or has to be abandoned, corticosteroid treatment should be begun without delay. Prednisone may be given in an initial daily dose of 40–80 mg according to the size of the patient. If not effective in two days, dosage may be increased up to 120–160 mg daily. A fully suppressive regimen should be continued for at least one week after the ESR has become normal and then progressively reduced.

It is often difficult to decide when to stop treatment with either drug. The general principle is to reduce dosage progressively, watching for the reappearance of symptoms and a rise in the ESR. Short-lived recrudescences of symptoms during withdrawal should not necessarily halt the process. Such 'rebound' effects are particularly common after corticosteroid treatment and may be suppressed by covering the withdrawal by moderate dosage with salicylate.

Prevention. *Primary prevention.* Rheumatic fever can be prevented by early and adequate treatment of the primary streptococcal infection (see Table 3). If treatment is begun within six days of onset, prevention is almost total, but it is worth giving at any time up to the onset of the rheumatic attack.

Secondary prevention. The high probability of second and subsequent attacks in patients who have previously had rheumatic fever makes continuous chemoprophylaxis mandatory. How long to attempt to continue this is a matter of opinion, because patients tend to become less compliant as the years pass. In the absence of damage to the heart, and if no 'breakthrough' has occurred, a period of five years, or until the age of 18 years, whichever is the longer, is a reasonable objective. If either of the two criteria is not met, the period should be extended by several years.

There is no doubt that the most effective means of secondary prevention is a three-weekly intramuscular dose of benzathine penicillin, which gives almost total protection. Alternatively, oral penicillin twice a day (Table 4) may be used, but irregularity in taking the tablets may lead to streptococcal 'breakthrough'. Oral sulphadiazine is almost as effective as oral penicillin and is cheaper. If a streptococcal attack develops while a patient is on prophylaxis, prompt treatment with therapeutic doses of penicillin should prevent another rheumatic attack. Treatment with sulphadiazine will not do this.

Acute glomerulonephritis. This may follow acute group A streptococcal infection of the respiratory tract or the skin, but only strains belonging to a minority of the M serotypes cause it. It develops after an interval of 5 days–6 weeks (average 1½ weeks), and is characterized by the appearance of haematuria and oedema, and, in the more serious cases, signs of renal insufficiency. However, in most cases the symptoms are mild and persist for only a few days; in many the disease is symptomless and detectable only by microscopic examination of the urine.

Pathogenesis. The lesions are mainly in the glomeruli, which show infiltration with inflammatory cells, first polymorphonuclear cells and eosinophils and later lymphocytes and monocytes. The mesangium of the glomerular capillaries is oedematous and infiltrated with inflammatory cells. The epithelium of Bowman's capsule undergoes swelling and some hyperplasia, and cellular 'crescents' are present in a few glomeruli.

In the early stages, areas of electron-dense material ('humps') can be seen on the glomerular basement-membrane. These are generally held to be composed of immune complexes, and gamma-globulin and complement components are readily demonstrable in them; however, a specific streptococcal component has not yet been convincingly identified. Immune complexes are also present in the blood; one hypothesis is that these circulating complexes are deposited in the glomeruli. Alternatively, they may be formed *in situ*, whether by interaction of a streptococcal product previously deposited there with subsequently formed antibody or of a cross-reacting streptococcal antibody with a glomerular antigen; various other possibilities have been mooted, but the question is unsettled. It is conceded, however, that despite the association of nephritogenicity with certain serotypes, the M antigen plays no direct part

in pathogenesis. The inflammatory response to the deposition of the immune complexes eventually heals by fibrosis, with the loss of function of a variable number of glomeruli.

Clinical features. The disease occurs most often in children and young adults; in areas of high incidence, pre-school children are most often affected and the frequency falls off progressively with increasing age.

The most widespread feature, present in nearly all cases, is urinary abnormality. In the mildest cases, the only manifestation is haematuria, which may be detectable only by microscopic examination. This is usually accompanied by RBC casts; granular and leucocytic casts may also be present. In mild but clinically recognizable cases, there is usually frank haematuria, with urine of a dark or 'smoky' appearance, albuminuria of trace or moderate amount, and some oliguria. Oedema may be present, most easily seen on the face.

In cases of moderate severity, oliguria and oedema are more marked, with a raised blood-urea content and hypertension; in the small minority of severe cases, anuria, uraemia, and metabolic acidosis develop. Some 3 per cent of patients admitted to hospital die.

Laboratory tests. In addition to the urinary changes, a blood-urea value of 500–1000 mg/l is usual in cases of moderate severity. Group A streptococci are detectable in the primary lesion in a minority of cases: some 20 per cent in post-tonsillitis and 40 per cent in post-impetigo cases. There is usually serological evidence of recent streptococcal infection (see page 5.140). It should be noted that the ASO titre often does not rise significantly for an attack of streptococcal impetigo, though high titres of anti-DNAase and anti-hyaluronidase are usual. Therefore, in investigations of suspected nephritis associated with skin sepsis, tests for one or other of these antibodies should be added to the ASO test. The most important and specific test for post-streptococcal nephritis is the blood level of the C3 component of complement, which is almost invariably depressed. This is readily determined by means of an immunodiffusion test with a commercially available kit. A level of less than 800 mg l^{-1} is almost diagnostic for the disease.

Renal biopsy. This may be useful in establishing a diagnosis in doubtful cases, and to monitor the course of the disease. The physician may feel, however, that the advantages of this are outweighed by the risks, which are inversely proportional to the experience of the operator; the results obtained are, in any event, unlikely to influence the management of the patient.

Prognosis. In cases of mild or moderate severity, symptoms disappear spontaneously in a few days. Urinary abnormalities decrease progressively during the following weeks or months, and seldom persist for more than 12 months.

The long-term prognosis is still a matter of acute controversy. Nearly all extensive studies in areas of high incidence have shown that 95 per cent or more of children suffer no permanent loss of renal function. Some investigators claim a much higher frequency of permanent and progressive renal disease in adult patients, but their studies have been criticized on the grounds that the initial diagnosis of post-streptococcal nephritis had not always been firmly established.

Second attacks may occasionally occur in high-incidence areas, but with no greater frequency than first attacks, from which they are clinically indistinguishable.

Epidemiology. In general, there are two main patterns of disease: in industrial countries in the temperate zone, nephritis follows tonsillitis and is nearly always associated with M type 12 infections; in poor countries, usually but not exclusively in the tropics or subtropics, it follows impetigo and is associated with certain of the M types that cause this, notably types 49, 55, 57, and a few others. In 'transitional' areas, such as the southern states of the USA, 'winter' nephritis follows tonsillitis and is associated with type 12, but 'summer' nephritis follows impetigo and is associated with other types. Post-impetigo nephritis is now exceptionally rare in Britain, but it appears to have been quite common early in this century; indeed, there is reason to believe that the disease described as 'trench nephritis' in the First World War was of this nature.

Post-streptococcal nephritis is now quite uncommon in Britain, though over 10 per cent of all streptococcal tonsillitis is caused by M type 12 strains. In some tropical countries, as many as 1 in 500 of the child population may suffer from nephritis in an epidemic year. In general, high nephritis rates appear to occur in populations in which there is a high total attack rate for streptococcal infection, whether of the throat or the skin. Nephritis in affluent populations is infrequent and nearly always sporadic; in poor populations it is common and often occurs in epidemics of considerable magnitude. These appear to be determined in part by seasonal and other fluctuations in the incidence of impetigo, and in part to the periodic spread of individual nephritogenic serotypes when the proportion of young children with type-specific immunity has fallen below a critical level.

Prophylaxis and treatment. Early antibiotic treatment of the primary streptococcal infection would be expected, on theoretical grounds, to prevent the development of nephritis. The fact that this has not been convincingly demonstrated in controlled studies suggests that primary prophylaxis would be effective only if begun very early. Once symptoms of nephritis have appeared, giving penicillin will not affect the severity of renal damage. There is no specific treatment for post-streptococcal nephritis, but treatment for uraemia and hypertension may be required in the more severe cases (see Section 21). Patients may be discharged home as soon as the symptoms subside; they are usually kept under supervision, with periodic examination of the urine and blood pressure, for 6–12 months. Antibiotic prophylaxis is not required.

DISEASES CAUSED BY GROUP C AND GROUP G STREPTOCOCCI

These streptococci are found in the throat in healthy persons, but usually considerably less often than group A streptococci; in some parts of Africa group C and G streptococci are very common in the throat. There is reason to believe that both group C and group G streptococci may occasionally cause tonsillitis, though this is very difficult to establish with certainty in the individual sporadic case. Certainly, one extensive food-borne outbreak of tonsillitis due to group G streptococci is on record. Neither streptococcus appears to cause rheumatic fever, and the evidence for an association with nephritis is tenuous.

Group C and G streptococci frequently colonize wounds, and appear on occasion to cause cellulitis. Both streptococci are very common in impetigo lesions in the tropics, but whether they are primary pathogens is uncertain. Streptococci of groups C and G form streptolysin O, and acute infections with them may cause a rise in the titre of antibody to this. Septicaemia, and very occasionally endocarditis, may occur, usually in patients with serious underlying disease or in intravenous users of narcotic drugs. Septic arthritis and osteomyelitis are rare complications.

DISEASES CAUSED BY GROUP B STREPTOCOCCI

The group B streptococcus (*Str. agalactiae*) has been known for over a century as a cause of mastitis in cattle. It attracted little attention as a pathogen of man until the early 1970s, though it had been described as a member of the flora of the human vagina and an occasional cause of severe puerperal fever over 40 years earlier. The recent recognition of group B streptococci as the second most common bacterial cause of death in newborn babies—exceeded in frequency only by *Escherichia coli*—encouraged the belief that severe neonatal infections with this streptococcus had increased

greatly in frequency in the last 20 years. If this is true, no credible explanation of the change has been advanced. Undoubtedly, growing interest in the causes of perinatal death and improved competence in clinical microbiology laboratories have contributed materially to the apparent increase.

Pathogenesis. The usual clinical manifestations of group B streptococcal disease are acute septicaemia and meningitis; purulent lesions in other organs are much less frequent. The organism is very invasive, but seldom gives rise to recognizable acute inflammation at its point of entry into the body; thus, the appearance of a generalized infection is usually unheralded. Profound systemic disturbances appear early in the disease, but these cannot be attributed to the action of any extracellular toxic product.

The chief determinant for virulence appears to be the type antigen. Nearly all human strains form a type-specific cell-wall polysaccharide. In experimental animals, antibody against this confers type-specific protection, and indirect evidence suggests that this may also be true in man. The type polysaccharide, like the M protein of the group A streptococcus, inhibits phagocytosis of the organism and thus is probably a determinant for invasivity. There are four type polysaccharides, Ia, Ib, II, and III; in addition, a cell-wall protein antigen Ic, which also appears to be a virulence factor, is present in some strains, usually in association with the polysaccharide Ia or Ib. Thus there are five common serotypes, with the following (simplified) antigenic structures:

Type Ia: Ia
Type Ib: Ib, Ic
Type Ic: Ia, Ic
Type II: II
Type III: III

However, the Ic protein may sometimes be found in association with antigens II and III, or in the absence of a type polysaccharide.

Members of any serotype may cause severe disease, but there is some association between serotype and the ability to cause meningitis, though this is far from absolute. The percentage of type III organisms among isolates from meningitis is about twice as great as that among isolates from septicaemic infections. In some places, as many as 70–80 per cent of meningitis cases are caused by type III, though in Britain the figure is about 50. Type II strains, on the other hand, form 15–40 per cent of those isolated from cases of septicaemia but rarely cause meningitis.

Clinical appearances

In neonates. The frequency of serious neonatal disease (septicaemia, meningitis, or both) has been variously estimated as between 0.3 and 7.0 cases per 1000 live births. It has therefore been concluded that the incidence shows wide geographical differences, but most of the figures quoted have wide confidence limits. A recent British study of 200 000 neonates gave a figure of only 0.3–0.4 per 1000 live births.

Two fairly distinct clinical patterns of serious neonatal infection can be recognized.

Early-onset disease. This takes the form of neonatal septicaemia (often described as 'neonatal respiratory distress' or 'neonatal shock syndrome') with or without meningitis. Its onset is nearly always in the first seven days of life, and usually in the first five days; in some cases illness develops within a few hours of birth, and exceptionally the baby is seriously ill or dead at birth. Septicaemia is always present, usually accompanied by signs of respiratory distress. Meningitis develops in about one-third of cases. Affected babies usually have a low birth-weight, and many have been born after prolonged labour with ruptured membranes. The mother is almost invariably a vaginal carrier of group B streptococci.

When respiratory distress is a prominent feature, the disease is difficult to distinguish from hyaline-membrane disease. Indeed, at necropsy, the lungs are seen to be filled with such a membrane, which is densely packed with streptococci; there is little inflammatory reaction and pus is seldom seen by the naked-eye. The leading symptoms are rapid respiration, often with episodes of apnoea, pallor, and cyanosis. In other cases, signs of shock predominate. Only about half of the patients are febrile.

The baby is usually very ill within a few hours of onset, and death usually occurs within one to two days. Mortality rates, even with early and intensive treatment, of at least 40 per cent are usual.

Late-onset disease. This is nearly always a purulent meningitis, almost invariably accompanied by septicaemia, but the predominant symptoms refer to the central nervous system. The disease is not clinically distinguishable from other forms of neonatal meningitis. Onset is most commonly in the second to fourth weeks of life, but the disease occurs, though with decreasing frequency, throughout infancy and occasionally in young children.

Late-onset meningitis usually affects babies who were previously healthy, of normal birth-weight, and born after normal labour. In most cases the mother is not a vaginal carrier of group B streptococci. If treatment is prompt and adequate, the mortality rate is about 15 per cent, but many of the survivors suffer serious sequelae, including hydrocephalus and mental retardation. Late-onset meningitis forms no more than one-quarter of all serious neonatal group B streptococcal infections.

In adults. Nearly 80 per cent of all systemic group B streptococcal infections in adults are septicaemic illnesses, in about one-quarter of which endocarditis develops. Some 7 per cent are cases of meningitis and the rest are purulent infections in other internal organs, including peritonitis and purulent arthritis.

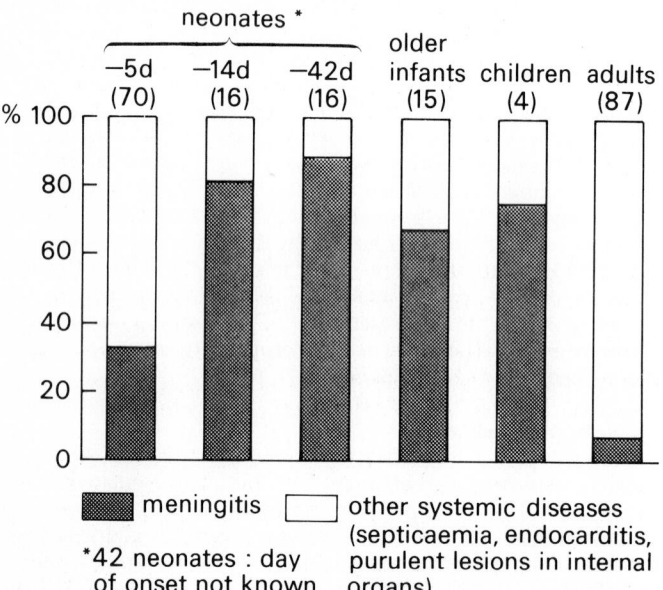

Fig. 1   Percentage of cases of meningitis among systemic group B streptococcal infections at various ages. (Reproduced from the *J. antimicrob. Chemother.* (1979), **5** (suppl. A), 29.)

In over one-half of adults with systemic infections, one or more predisposing factor can be identified: (*a*) a severe underlying disease, notably diabetes mellitus or a reticuloendothelial disease; (*b*) previous damage to a heart valve, in some patients who develop endocarditis; (*c*) trauma or infection at a putative site of invasion by the organism. Infections associated with childbirth, abortion, or gynaecological operations form about one-seventh of all systemic infections. Others follow surgical operations elsewhere in the body or occur in patients with an extensive non-bacterial skin disease or a skin ulcer. Although infections associated with the female reproductive system form a considerable proportion of the cases in young adults, in total more males than females, and more patients over the age of 45 years than under it are affected.

Group B streptococci may be found in septic wounds, and occasionally in pure culture, but it is often impossible to say whether they are responsible for the inflammation. They appear occasionally to cause mild urinary-tract infections in females.

Diagnosis. In cases of suspected septicaemia or meningitis, it is seldom possible to predict the nature of the infecting organism on clinical evidence alone. Culture of the blood and, in appropriate cases, of the cerebrospinal fluid must be made, and a result cannot be expected in less than 24–36 hours. More rapid methods of detecting group B streptococci or their products in the blood and cerebrospinal fluid, or in the amniotic fluid or gastric aspirate in neonates, are urgently needed; several are currently under investigation. Heavy initial contamination of the surface of the newborn baby can best be detected by cultural examination of swabs from the external auditory canal, but the results may be obtained too late to be of use, and if positive do not necessarily indicate an invasive infection.

Epidemiology. The group B streptococci of man resemble closely those of cattle and other mammals, but the balance of evidence suggests that the human and animal strains form distinct populations and that inter-specific transfer of infection is very rare.

Carriage. The organism is often found at a variety of carriage sites in healthy adults. Most attention has been focused on vaginal carriage. Widely differing vaginal carriage-rates, from 3 to over 40 per cent, have been reported. This may be attributed in part to differences in the techniques employed for collecting and examining samples, but true geographical variations probably exist; there are some suggestions of racial differences. High carriage-rates have been recorded for women attending venereal-disease clinics, but an association between sexual promiscuity and carriage has not been established. In general, healthy non-hospitalized women give higher carriage-rates than women admitted to hospital in labour, in whom the rate is generally lower than in members of the staff of the maternity hospital. In Britain, women examined in labour usually give carriage-rates of 3–6 per cent.

Swabs collected from the lower part of the vagina are more often positive than high vaginal or cervical swabs. Serial swabbing shows a notable intermittency of carriage; this suggests that the vagina is often not the primary site of carriage. Urethral swabs, in both males and females, often yield group B streptococci, and several workers have reported higher carriage-rates from the examination of peri-anal swabs than from the vagina. The dynamics of carriage and cross-contamination in the vulva and the ano-perineal region is not yet fully understood. Some 7–10 per cent of normal adults of either sex carry group B streptococci in the upper respiratory tract, but this appears to be independent of urogenital and ano-perineal carriage. Contamination and carriage in the neonate are considered in the next section.

Early-onset neonatal disease. There is no doubt that this infection is acquired from the genital tract of the mother. Occasionally the organism penetrates the intact fetal membranes and multiplies in the liquor amnii, but usually it is acquired by the baby during its passage through the birth canal. Immediately after birth, surface contamination with group B streptococci can be detected in one-half of babies born to mothers with positive vaginal swabs. The organisms can be detected on the skin, in the upper respiratory tract and, most often, in the external auditory canals. They are believed to enter the lungs with contaminated liquor amnii, but there is no direct proof of this. The more profuse the vaginal carriage, the heavier the initial contamination of the baby, but lightly contaminated babies may have become heavy surface-carriers by the second or third day of life.

No more than 1 in 50 contaminated babies develop early-onset disease. There is little doubt that fetal immaturity is the main predisposing factor for this, but some evidence suggests that heavy initial contamination also increases the risk. This may explain the association of the disease with prolonged labour after rupture of the membranes, because multiplication of the streptococci in the liquor amnii during the later stages of labour may increase the dose to which the baby is exposed.

Whether absence of type-specific antibody to the infecting strain (see below) is an important predisposing factor for early-onset disease is uncertain.

Late-onset neonatal disease. This is seldom if ever acquired from the mother before or during labour, and immaturity of the neonate is not a significant predisposing factor. The source of the infecting streptococcus has not been demonstrated directly, but post-natal colonization is known to occur, at rates that appear to vary considerably between hospitals. In a number of instances, spread of a particular strain from one baby to others in the nursery has been demonstrated; in others, several babies have been shown to acquire the same strain from an unknown source. Spread from attendants to babies in hospital, and the acquisition of infection from extra-hospital sources after early discharge, have not yet been studied adequately.

Antibody deficiency as a determinant for neonatal disease. Evidence has been accumulating, particularly in respect of late-onset neonatal meningitis due to type III organisms, that deficiency of antibody against the type polysaccharide is a major factor determining invasion by the streptococcus. Briefly, mothers of babies who developed meningitis were shown not to possess this antibody, but mothers who carried type III organis vagina and subsequently delivered healthy babies often did; and babies who suffered non-fatal meningitis due to type III organisms formed the corresponding type-specific antibody. Information about the relation between carriage and the formation of type-specific antibody is scanty.

Treatment. Group B streptococci are sensitive to the penicillins and usually also to chloramphenicol and the macrolides; they are usually tetracycline resistant. They are resistant to the aminoglycosides, but mixtures of a penicillin and an aminoglycoside have a more potent bactericidal effect than the penicillin alone.

Although penicillins, especially benzylpenicillin, are the drugs of first choice for the treatment of systemic group B streptococcal infections, their minimal inhibitory concentration for these organisms are considerably higher, and their killing-times are longer, than those, for example, for group A streptococci. High parenteral dosage, given two-hourly, is therefore necessary, and treatment should be continued for at least a week. There is a tendency to relapse after penicillin treatment, especially if meningitis is present. For this reason, penicillin plus gentamicin has been advocated, with the addition of intrathecal gentamicin in cases of meningitis.

Early and intensive treatment is essential. Because the treatment must usually be begun before the nature of the infecting organism is known, a 'best-choice' antibiotic regimen is usually employed. For neonates this would probably be ampicillin plus gentamicin; there would be no need to change this if a diagnosis of group B streptococcal infection was made later.

There is some evidence that the prognosis in severe neonatal group B streptococcal infection is improved by the transfusion of fresh whole blood.

Prevention. The following approaches to the prevention of serious neonatal infection with group B streptococci have been advocated, but convincing proof of their efficacy is generally lacking.

Elimination of potential sources of infection. An attempt may be made to detect vaginal carriage and eliminate it before the onset of labour. The intermittency of carriage, and the difficulty of eradicating the organism by the local or systemic use of antibiotics, make this unlikely to be an effective measure. It may be that a temporary reduction in the number of group B streptococci in the vagina during the later stages of labour might be sufficient to exert a significant prophylactic effect. If this could be done by the continuous application of a mild antiseptic, in a cream or on a tampon, the measure could be applied to all women in labour. Quantitative studies of the effects of various antiseptics on the vaginal flora might lead to the development of a suitable regimen.

We cannot hope to eliminate the sources of late-onset neonatal disease until they have been identified.

Prevention of invasion by the prophylactic use of antibiotic. It has been asserted that early-onset disease can be prevented by the administration of a single intramuscular dose of 50 000 units of benzylpenicillin to all babies immediately after birth, but this has not yet been confirmed by controlled trial. Those who consider this form of prophylaxis justifiable, but wish to limit the use of antibiotics, advocate giving penicillin only to babies considered to be at increased risk of early-onset disease, for example, to all babies with a birth-weight of less than 2500 g.

Immunoprophylaxis. If deficiency of maternally acquired antibody against the type polysaccharide is an important determinant for neonatal disease, vaccination of antibody-deficient mothers during pregnancy might reduce its frequency. The protective antibody appears to be that directed against the complete or 'native' form of the polysaccharide. This can be extracted from the streptococci by means of mild chemical agents. Vaccination with purified 'native' type III polysaccharide leads to the production of apparently adequate amounts of antibody in previously antibody-deficient adults. Present evidence suggests that such a vaccine might protect against late-onset meningitis due to type III organisms. Vaccination might have wider applicability if an effective polyvalent product can be prepared, and if antibody deficiency is shown to be of significance also in early-onset disease. Vaccine trials will present formidable difficulties, and it may be doubted whether widespread use of the vaccine could be justified in communities in which the total incidence of serious neonatal infection is less than 1 in 2000 live births.

DISEASES CAUSED BY *STREPTOCOCCUS MILLERI*

This streptococcus, which has become generally recognized only recently, is very widely distributed in the normal body flora; it is found in considerable numbers in the oral cavity, the upper respiratory tract, the gut, and sometimes the vagina. It is an occasional cause of severe and characteristic purulent lesions: abscesses, usually single, in a variety of internal organs, and purulent exudates in serous cavities, but usually does not cause marked acute inflammation at the point of entry into the body. Infections are sporadic and appear to arise by self-infection. The appearance of a purulent internal lesion is often the first indication of disease, but in a considerable proportion of cases this follows a surgical operation or other trauma, a destructive non-bacterial disease, or a local inflammation at or near a carriage-site of the organism in the same region of the body. *Str. milleri* also causes septicaemic illnesses without apparent abscess formation; these also may have been preceded by a similar disturbance at or near a carriage site. Endocarditis forms about 20 per cent of all systemic infections with *Str. milleri*. It is usually of the subacute type and very rarely occurs in patients with purulent lesions. Infections occur at all ages, but are rare in infancy; most affect the middle-aged or elderly; there is a strong predominance of males.

Str. milleri causes brain abscess, localized meningitis, and subdural abscess. It is the predominant cause of these in the frontal but not in the temporal region. Cases have been associated with frontal sinusitis and dental sepsis. The organism is often isolated from abscesses around the jaw and in the upper part of the neck, sometimes in association with *Actinomyces*. It is commonly found in pure culture in pleural empyema and sometimes in lung abscess. However, the most common sites of localization are in the abdomen. Nearly one-half of the intra-abdominal lesions are liver abscesses, from which the organism is often isolated in pure culture. The rest include pelvic peritonitis, and subphrenic and other intraperitoneal collections of pus. A number of these lesions are associated with acute appendicitis or gastro-duodenal ulceration, and *Str. milleri* is often present in them in mixed culture.

Str. milleri is usually quite sensitive to penicillin but is consistently sulphonamide resistant. Cases of pure septicaemia or endocarditis may be treated effectively with antibiotics, but purulent lesions require surgical drainage. The finding of *Str. milleri* in the blood culture of a febrile patient should always lead to an intensive search for an unsuspected collection of pus in an internal organ.

Diseases caused by enterococci

Str. faecalis is the only common pathogen among the enterococci. It may cause mild inflammation in wounds and the urinary tract, but in both situations it is usually present in mixed culture. Urinary-tract infections rarely appear spontaneously, but usually in association with obstruction, catheterization, or surgical operation. Infections appear to be sporadic and from sources in the patient.

The main clinical significance of *Str. faecalis* is as a cause of septicaemia and endocarditis, which tend to occur in relation to urinary-tract infections, operations on other abdominal organs, and childbirth. Although generalized enterococcal infections are less acute than infections with the haemolytic pyogenic streptococci, they are highly fatal and present considerable therapeutic difficulties. Minimum inhibitory concentrations of antibiotics for *Str. faecalis* are a poor guide to treatment. Many strains are inhibited by attainable concentrations of penicillin, ampicillin, chloramphenicol, erythromycin, and tetracycline, but none of these agents can be relied upon to eliminate infection. Although *Str. faecalis* appears to be resistant to the aminoglycoside antibiotics in *in vitro* tests, appropriate mixtures of a penicillin and an aminoglycoside are highly bactericidal. The best combination is probably of ampicillin and gentamicin, but *in vitro* tests of the bactericidal action of this and similar combinations may be needed to determine the optimum regimen.

STREPTOCOCCAL ENDOCARDITIS

Bacterial endocarditis will be discussed in detail elsewhere in this book (see Section 13). Here we will indicate only briefly the role of streptococci. They are still by far the most common cause of this disease, and are responsible for some 70 per cent of cases.

Practically any streptococcus present in the body flora may on occasion cause endocarditis, but some do this much more frequently than others (Table 7). The 'pyrogenic' streptococci are responsible for only a minority of cases of streptococcal endocarditis. The endocarditis they cause is often of the acute form, with rapid destruction of the affected heart valve and a poor prognosis; it may appear in the course of an acute septic infection. Haemolytic members of groups A, C, and G, and pneumococci, are rare causes of

Table 7 Causes of streptococcal endocarditis
Unpublished data on 539 British cases, 1972–6*

Streptococci	Percentage frequency
Group A	0.7
Groups C and G	1.8
Group B	2.2
pneumoniae	0.6
milleri	6.7
Enterococci	5.3
sanguis	17.4
mitior	24.6
Other 'viridans'	7.4
mutans	13.0
bovis	15.8
Other	4.6

* For methods and definitions, see Parker, M. T. and Ball, L. C. (1976). *J. med. Microbiol.* **9**, 275

such an acute endocarditis. Group B streptococcal endocarditis may be of a similar nature, but may be of the subacute form and appear without warning. *Str. milleri* and enterococci are somewhat more common causes of endocarditis.

Over three-quarters of streptococcal endocarditis is caused by organisms that are rarely if ever responsible for septic infections elsewhere, and the disease is almost invariably of the subacute type. Nearly one-half is caused by the 'viridans' streptococci of the mouth, notably *Str. mitior* and *Str. sanguis*. Of the remainder, over 10 per cent are caused by *Str. mutans*, a non-haemolytic streptococcus also found in the mouth, and some 16 per cent by *Str. bovis*, almost exclusively a bowel organism.

The clinical pattern of streptococcal endocarditis has undergone considerable change in the last 30 years. Formerly it was a disease of adolescents and young adults, with a slight predominance of females, affected mainly persons who had suffered from rheumatic carditis or had a congenital heart lesion, and was usually caused by one of the 'viridans' streptococci. Nowadays, infections of middle-aged and elderly males predominate (Fig. 2). These are commonly insidious in onset, and a history of previous chronic heart disease is less often elicited. 'Viridans' streptococci no longer predominate, though they are still important causes of endocarditis.

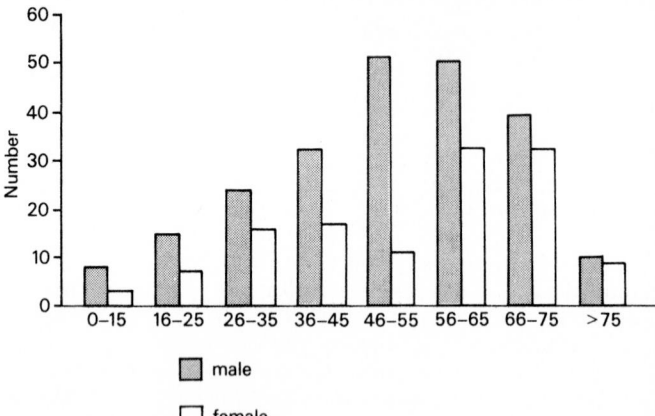

Fig. 2 Age and sex distribution of cases of streptococcal endocarditis. Unpublished data, Britain, 1972–6 (see footnote to Table 7).

There are marked differences in the relative importance of individual streptococcal species as causes of endocarditis in young and elderly patients (Fig. 3). 'Viridans' streptococci are responsible for

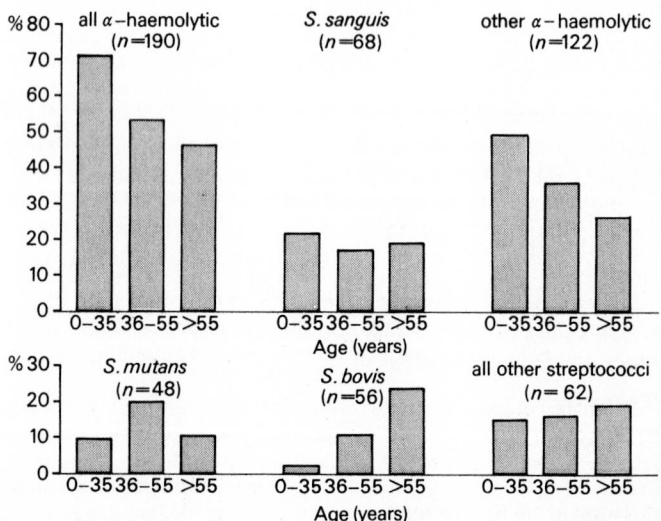

Fig. 3 Age distribution of cases of endocarditis due to various streptococci. Percentage shown is of all cases of streptococcal endocarditis in the stated age group. Unpublished data, Britain, 1972–6 (see footnote to Table 7).

over 70 per cent of the rather small number of infections in young persons, but they cause less than one-half of infections in the elderly; this difference is attributable to a reduced frequency in the elderly of infections with 'viridans' streptococci other than *Str. sanguis*. *Str. mutans* infections appear mainly in the 35–55-year age group, and infections with *Str. bovis* (and *Str. milleri*) mainly in patients over the age of 55 years.

Streptococci reach the heart valves via the bloodstream. In the absence of a septicaemic infection, they are believed to do this as a result of transient episodes of symptomless bacteriaemia, usually the result of minor trauma at or near a site of carriage of the organism. The onset of endocarditis after dental manipulations in persons with damaged heart valves is well known. Transient bacteriaemia has also been demonstrated after tonsillectomy, and manipulations of the urinary and female-genital tracts and the bowel. The mouth is still the most likely source of streptococci in endocarditis, but in a considerable minority of infections, probably amounting to about one-third in elderly persons, the source is probably intra-abdominal. A remarkably close association between *Str. bovis* endocarditis and undiagnosed bowel cancer has been recorded. The fact that most of the elderly patients who develop endocarditis are unaware of any cardiac illness does not exclude the possibility that this may be a predisposing factor. Undetected atherosclerotic damage to heart valves may well render them susceptible to the establishment of a vegetation.

We have already mentioned (see page 5.148) the difficulties of antibiotic treatment in enterococcal endocarditis. Most other streptococci are considerably more sensitive than *Str. faecalis* to benzylpenicillin, and some are very sensitive. This antibiotic has been used alone for the treatment of non-enterococcal endocarditis. However, to reduce the frequency of relapse, it is now customary to add an aminoglycoside. A suitable combination is of benzylpenicillin and gentamicin. Treatment must be controlled by *in vitro* bactericidal tests with antibiotic combinations and the estimation of blood levels of antibiotics. For further information about the treatment of endocarditis see Section 13.

To prevent bacterial endocarditis, patients with known or suspected chronic disease of heart valves should receive antibiotic prophylaxis whenever they are subjected to procedures that may result in transient bacteriaemia. These include not only dental treatment but operations on or manipulations of the throat, urogenital tract, and gut. The prophylactic agent should be chosen after consideration of the organisms (not only streptococci) likely to be disseminated. This matter is discussed further elsewhere (Section 13). In respect of streptococci, the following considerations are relevant. Most mouth streptococci are susceptible to penicillin, but the administration of this agent results in the appearance in the mouth, within as little as one day, of large numbers of penicillin-resistant streptococci. These resistant strains of 'viridans' streptococci normally form a minority population in the mouth but rapidly overgrow the sensitive strains when the antibiotic is given. The administration of other antibiotics may result in the appearance of strains with corresponding resistances. Rapid inter-strain and even inter-species transfer of resistance between mouth streptococci has also been demonstrated. Another effect of administering antibiotics is to encourage the appearance of *Str. faecalis* in the mouth flora, from which in other circumstances it is usually absent. Antibiotic prophylaxis should therefore not be given until just before the procedure is begun; a single parenteral dose is all that is necessary.

References

Baker, C. J. (1977). Summary of the workshop on perinatal infection due to group B streptococci. *J. infect. Dis.* **135**, 137.

Breese, R. B. and Hall, C. B. (1977). *Beta hemolytic streptococcal diseases*. Houghton Mifflin, Boston.

Ginsburg, I. (1972). Mechanisms of cell and tissue injury induced by group A streptococci. *J. infect. Dis.* **126**, 294, 419.

Parker, M. T. (1977). Neonatal streptococcal infections. *Post-grad. med. J.* **53**, 498.

— (ed.) (1979). *Pathogenic streptococci*. Reedbooks, Chertsey, Surrey.

Read, S. E. and Zabriskie, J. B. (eds.) (1980). *Streptococcal diseases and the immune response*. Academic Press, New York.

Shaper, A. G. (1972). Cardiovascular disease in the tropics. I. Rheumatic fever. *Br. med. J.* **ii**, 683.

Skinner, F. A. (ed.) (1978). *Streptococci*. (*Symp. Soc. appl. Bact.* no. 7). Academic Press, London and New York.

Strasser, T. (1978). Rheumatic fever and rheumatic heart disease in the 1970s. *Wld Hlth Org. Chron.* **32**, 18.

Wannamaker, L. W. (1970). Differences between streptococcal infections of the throat and the skin. *New Engl. J. Med.* **282**, 23–31, 78–85.

Wannamaker, L. W. and Matsen, J. M. (eds.) (1972). *Streptococci and streptococcal diseases: recognition, understanding and management*. Academic Press, New York and London.

Wilson, G. S. and Miles, A. A. (1975). *Topley and Wilson's Principles of bacteriology, virology and immunity*, 6th edn., vol. 2, chapter 65. Arnold, London.

World Health Organization (1968). *Streptococcal and staphylococcal infections*. Tech. Rep. Ser. Wld Hlth Org. no. 394. Geneva.

Pneumococcal infection

B. M. Greenwood

Streptococcus pneumoniae (the pneumococcus) is a frequent commensal of the upper respiratory tract and an important cause of pneumonia and meningitis. The organism was first identified in saliva by Pasteur and by Sternberg in 1881. In 1886 Weichselbaum showed that the pneumococcus was an important cause of pneumonia. Despite the discovery of antibiotics which are highly effective against the pneumococcus *in vitro*, pneumococci still cause many deaths and much morbidity in both industrialized and in developing countries.

The organism. The pneumococcus is a Gram-positive bacterium which, in clinical specimens, appears as a lanceolate diplococcus. In culture it may form short chains. It grows rapidly on most bacteriological media, and on blood agar virulent, encapsulated strains form small, shiny colonies which are surrounded by a greenish area of α-haemolysis. Pneumococci grow rapidly in broth but, after some hours of growth, production of autolytic enzymes may lead to death of the culture. In addition to an α-haemolysin, pneumococci produce hyaluronidase and a leucocidin. Pneumococci can be differentiated from other α-haemolytic streptococci by their solubility in bile, and their sensitivity to ethyl hydrocuprein chloride (Optochin), a compound that was once used in the treatment of pneumococcal infection. Mice are very susceptible to many strains of pneumococcal infection, and mouse inoculation can be used to isolate pneumococci from clinical samples.

Virulent strains of pneumococci possess a polysaccharide capsule. At least 83 different serotypes of pneumococci have been identified on the basis of antigenic differences in the composition of their capsular polysaccharides. Two different numbering systems, the Danish and the American, have been employed in serotyping pneumococci; the Danish system is now applied more widely. Pneumococci can be serotyped by the Quellung reaction; exposure to a specific antiserum causes the capsule of the bacterium to swell. Typing can also be achieved by other immunological methods such as counter-current immunoelectrophoresis.

Epidemiology. Pneumonia is associated in the minds of most physicians with winter and cold, but pneumococcal infection is not restricted to countries with a temperate climate: it is one of the commonest causes of admission to hospital in many tropical, developing countries. There are few accurate statistics as to the incidence of pneumococcal disease. It has been estimated that in the United States between 200 000 and 1 million cases of pneumococcal pneumonia occur every year and that pneumococcal infection accounts for between 10 000–50 000 deaths annually. In the United States about 20 per cent of children experience an attack of otitis media by the age of two years; many of these attacks are caused by the pneumococcus. In the United States the disease is recorded more frequently in Blacks than in Whites. In New Guinea an attack rate of over 10 cases per 1000 population per year has been recorded. It is probable that many other developing countries have a similarly high incidence of the infection.

Pneumococcal disease is, in general, an endemic infection but occasionally localized outbreaks occur. Outbreaks have been recorded most frequently in communities where people have been living under crowded conditions such as those prevailing in refugee camps. The incidence of pneumococcal disease is very high among recruits to mining companies in South Africa. Attack rates as high as 100 per 1000 population per year have been reported in these miners.

The presence of capsulated pneumococci in the nasopharynx of up to 50 per cent of healthy subjects has been noted on many occasions but few detailed studies on the carriage of pneumococci have been undertaken. A comprehensive survey of infants in a day-care centre in the United States, carried out over a four-year period, showed that 44 per cent of all nasopharyngeal swabs yielded a pneumococcus. A limited number of serotypes accounted for most infections. Many infants carried a pneumococcus of the same serotype for many months. Studies in families have shown that acquisition of pneumococci is often associated with upper respiratory tract infections. Pre-existing specific antibody does not prevent acquisition but shortens the duration of carriage.

In countries with a temperate climate pneumococcal pneumonia occurs more frequently in winter than in summer. Winter epidemics of viral respiratory tract infections may be one explanation for this seasonal association. However, it is possible that climatic factors have a more direct effect on the incidence of pneumococcal disease. In some tropical countries pneumococcal infection occurs most frequently during the hot, dry time of the year when, as during winter in countries with a temperate climate, absolute humidity is lowest. Perhaps a low absolute humidity impairs local, surface defences against pneumococci.

Individual pneumococcal serotypes show variation in their virulence and in their geographical distribution. In general, pneumococci with a low serotype number are more likely to cause clinical disease, as opposed to a harmless carrier state, than pneumococci with a high number serotype. Type 3 pneumococci have an especially bad reputation. Geographical variations in the distribution of pneumococcal serotypes causing clinical disease are now of considerable practical importance in relation to pneumococcal vaccination, for vaccines can only be effective if they contain the polysaccharide antigens corresponding to those of the pneumococci responsible for most cases of pneumococcal disease in a particular area. Type 5 pneumococci are an important cause of pneumococcal disease in West Africa but type 5 pneumococcal capsular polysaccharide is not present in any of the currently available commercial pneumococcal polysaccharide vaccines. For many parts of the world information on the distribution of pneumococcal serotypes is lacking. Some of this missing data will be provided by a collaborative scheme, organized by the World Health Organization, which is now in progress.

Pathogenesis and immunity. Pneumococci spread from person to person by droplet infection. If local conditions are favourable, inhaled pneumococci become established in the nasopharynx. Local spread of pneumococci from the nasopharynx may cause otitis media (Fig. 1). Clinical observations and studies in experimental animals suggest that most causes of pneumococcal pneumonia result from aspiration of nasopharyngeal secretions containing pneumococci into alveoli. Once established in the lung, pneumococci may spread to adjacent pleura or pericardium. About one-third of patients with pneumococcal pneumonia have a positive blood culture, and bacteria may spread through the systemic circulation to reach the meninges, joints, eyes, or other distant sites. Many patients with extra-pulmonary pneumococcal disease do not

have any signs of pneumonia. Whether bacteraemia arises in such patients from a sub-clinical pulmonary focus or directly from the nasopharynx is uncertain.

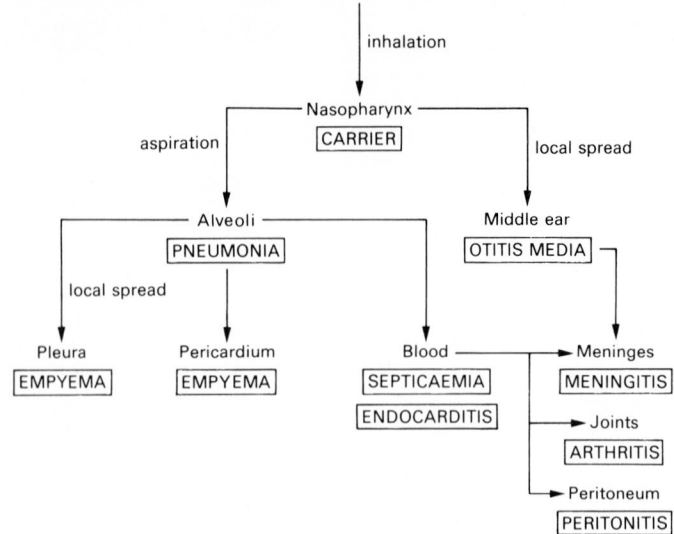

Fig. 1   The pathway of pneumococcal infection.

Pneumococci produce an acute inflammatory reaction characterized by an increase in vascular permeability, oedema, and an accumulation of polymorphonuclear neutrophil leucocytes at the affected site. The endothelium of vessels in affected tissues may be damaged. Several factors contribute to the pathogenesis of this acute inflammatory response. Pneumococci produce a number of enzymes which have a direct toxic effect on polymorphonuclear neutrophil leucocytes, platelets, and vascular endothelium. Some, but not all, pneumococcal capsular polysaccharides activate the alternative complement pathway producing the complement components C3a and C5a which are chemotactic for polymorphonuclear neutrophil leucocytes. Activation of the complement pathway may play a part in initiating the disseminated intravascular coagulation which sometimes occurs in patients with fulminating pneumococcal septicaemia. Immunopathological responses are relatively unimportant in the pathogenesis of pneumococcal infections. Although capsular polysaccharide antigens may persist in the serum for many days after an episode of pneumococcal infection, immune complex disease is a rare complication of pneumococcal infection. A few patients have been described who developed immune complex-mediated glomerulonephritis after a pneumococcal infection but the allergic arthritis and cutaneous vasculitis which often complicate meningococcal infection are not seen.

The pathogenesis of the jaundice detected in some patients with pneumococcal pneumonia is controversial. Some workers believe that it is primarily due to haemolysis and that it is especially likely to occur in those who are glucose 6-phosphate dehydrogenase deficient. Others believe that it is due mainly to liver cell damage; liver biopsy may show liver cell damage and cholestasis. Probably both factors are involved in most jaundiced patients.

Both local and systemic defence mechanisms are involved in protection against pneumococcal disease. In a healthy subject nasopharyngeal secretions are prevented from reaching the alveoli by the epiglottis, the sticky mucus that lines the bronchial tree and the respiratory cilia which ensure that bacteria trapped in this mucus are carried upwards, away from the alveoli, and expectorated or swallowed. Even if pneumococci manage to overcome these mechanical barriers and reach alveoli, they may be destroyed rapidly by alveolar macrophages. Small amounts of antibody and complement are present in alveolar secretions and coating of bacteria with IgG antibody or with C3b may promote their phagocytosis by these alveolar macrophages. Surfactant in alveolar secretions may have some protective effect also.

If these initial defence mechanisms are overcome and an acute inflammatory reaction is set in progress, further protective mechanisms come into play at once. Polymorphonuclear neutrophil leucocytes are brought to the site of infection in large numbers and attempt to ingest pneumococci. This they may be unable to achieve unaided. However, complement components are present in acute inflammatory exudates. Coating of pneumococci with C3b and C5b, as a result of activation of the alternative complement pathway, may help polymorphonuclear neutrophil leucocytes to phagocytose them. Although they may be unable to phagocytose some strains of virulent pneumococci *in vitro*, polymorphonuclear neutrophils may be more successful when they can trap the bacteria against some immobile object such as an alveolar wall. Polymorphonuclear neutrophil leucocytes and non-specific opsonins cannot contain infection with some virulent strains of pneumococci; recovery from infection with these organisms can only be achieved if the untreated patient survives long enough to form specific anticapsular antibodies which agglutinate pneumococci and which are very powerful opsonins. Formation of specific polysaccharide antibodies takes five to seven days. The persistence of capsular polysaccharide antigen in the serum interferes with the appearance of these antibodies in serum, and patients with persistent antigenaemia often have a prolonged and stormy clinical course.

An increase in susceptibility to pneumococcal infection may result from defects in either local or systemic defence mechanisms. Factors that impair the cleansing action of the respiratory cilia favour aspiration of infected nasopharyngeal secretions into alveoli. These include cold, anaesthesia, alcohol intoxication, drug overdose, and viral infection of the respiratory tract. Viral infections, such as influenza or measles, increase respiratory tract secretions, damage the ciliated epithelium of the respiratory tract, and interfere with polymorphonuclear neutrophil leucocyte function. It is, therefore, not surprising that epidemics of influenza are often followed by an increase in the incidence of pneumonia, especially among the elderly. *Mycoplasma pneumoniae* may likewise predispose to pneumococcal pneumonia for, both organisms are isolated from some patients with lobar pneumonia. The presence of pulmonary oedema as a result of heart failure or as a result of chemical, mechanical, or infective irritation of the lung favours the growth of any pneumococci reaching the alveoli and thus predisposes to pneumococcal pneumonia. Mechanical obstruction of a bronchus, for example by a carcinoma, has a similar effect. Damage to the base of the skull predisposes to recurrent invasion of the meninges by pneumococci present in the nasopharynx.

Three groups of patients with generalized immune defects show an increased susceptibility to pneumococcal infections—patients with hypogammaglobulinaemia, patients with complement deficiencies, and patients without a spleen or with a non-functioning spleen. The high incidence of pneumococcal infection in patients without a spleen suggests that this organ plays a very important part in clearing pneumococci from the blood, perhaps by bringing bacteria into close contact with phagocytic cells. Pneumococcal infection in patients without a spleen is often fulminant and has a high mortality. There is some evidence that patients who have had their spleen removed following a traumatic injury are less susceptible to systemic bacterial infections than patients who have had an elective splenectomy for a haematological or neoplastic disease, perhaps because seeding of splenic tissues at the time of rupture results in the formation of small, but functioning, splenunculi—the 'born-again spleen'. Patients with sickle cell disease have an increased incidence of pneumococcal infection. Splenic dysfunction and an abnormality in the alternative complement pathway have been identified as factors predisposing to pneumococcal infection in patients with this condition.

Pathology. Pneumococcal lobar pneumonia has been used to demonstrate the characteristic features of an acute inflammatory reaction to many generations of medical students, for the sequential features of this response can often be observed in the same pathological specimen. The first response to virulent pneumococci lodged in alveoli is an exudation of oedema fluid which helps to carry bacteria into adjacent alveoli. Polymorphonuclear neutrophil leucocytes and red blood cells than accumulate in infected alveoli (red hepatization). Finally the affected part of the lung becomes consolidated with a dense accumulation of polymorphonuclear neutrophil leucocytes (grey hepatization). Centrifugal spread may be observed in an affected lobe with a peripheral oedema zone, a middle area of early consolidation, and a central area of dense consolidation where some resolution of the infection has already begun to take place. This inflammatory reaction may be confined to a lobe or segment of the lung but may spread to a second lobe following aspiration of infected material. The pleura overlying an infected lobe shows an acute inflammatory reaction and a small pleural effusion may form. A remarkable characteristic of pneumococcal lobar pneumonia is the way in which a consolidated lobe can completely recover both anatomically and functionally. Macrophages play an important part in removing dead bacteria and damaged polymorphonuclear neutrophil leucocytes. Occasionally recovery occurs more slowly than usual, a condition termed 'delayed resolution', and some fibrosis of the lung parenchyma may then occur. Necrosis of lung tissue, resulting in a lung abscess, is rare in patients with pneumococcal lobar pneumonia.

For reasons that are not fully understood, the outcome of the acute inflammatory reaction produced by pneumococci at other sites is rarely as favourable as that observed in the lung. Invasion of the pleura or the pericardium by direct or lymphatic spread results in the formation of an effusion which is initially serous or slightly blood stained. However, if treatment is not started rapidly, deposition of fibrin and the accumulation of large numbers of leucocytes in the serous cavity results in the formation of thick pus. The lining walls of the pleural or pericardial cavity become thickened and fibrotic and, if the accumulated pus is removed, dense fibrous scarring may remain. In the case of the pericardium, this may cause constrictive pericarditis. A similar purulent response is observed when pneumococci lodge in the meninges, the synovium, or other peripheral sites. Arteries and veins may be damaged by this acute inflammatory response and cerebral arteritis, sometimes with fibrinoid necrosis, and intracranial thrombophlebitis have been recorded in patients with pneumococcal meningitis.

Clinical features

The clinical features of pneumococcal infection are described most conveniently in realtion to the main clinical syndromes that can be caused by pneumococci. However, these syndromes are not mutually exclusive and many patients with pneumococcal disease have more than one clinical manifestation of the infection, for example pneumonia and meningitis. Some accounts of pneumococcal disease describe conditions such as pneumococcal meningitis and pneumococcal pericarditis under the complications of pneumococcal pneumonia. Whilst this approach may be correct in pathological terms, it can give rise to the misleading impression that these conditions are seen only in those who have, or have recently had, a clinical lung infection. This is often not the case and many patients with pneumococcal meningitis, arthritis, or empyema give no history of a recent chest infection.

Pneumonia. Pneumonia is one of the commonest manifestations of pneumococcal disease. It may occur in subjects of any age, but it is encountered most frequently in the very young and in the old.

Symptoms. The onset of illness is usually sudden, although there may be a history of a recent, preceding upper respiratory tract infection. Fever is usually the first clinical feature of pneumococcal pneumonia and it is frequently accompanied by rigors. The patient feels ill, anorexic, and weak. Headache and myalgia may be severe.

Chest pain usually appears in the course of illness. This pain, which results from involvement of the parietal pleura, is sharp and stabbing and is aggravated by deep inspiration or coughing. The patient may try to obtain relief by splinting the affected side of his chest with his hands or by lying on the affected side. If the diaphragmatic pleura is involved, pain may be referred to the shoulder or the abdomen.

Cough may be absent at the onset of the illness but, in most patients, it becomes a prominent symptom. Cough is initially non-productive and painful. Subsequently it becomes productive of a blood-tinged 'rusty' sputum. Finally the sputum becomes frankly purulent.

Physical signs. Patients with lobar pneumonia are febrile and toxaemic. The rectal temperature is often as high as 40 °C. Oral temperature may be lower because of hyperventilation. When the patient is first examined no abnormal physical signs may be detected in the respiratory system. Later the classical signs of lobar consolidation appear. The patient's breathing is distressed and the nostrils may dilate on inspiration. Cyanosis may be present as a result of diminished alveolar ventilation or shunting of desaturated blood through the consolidated lung. Chest movement is diminished on the affected side. A dull note is obtained on percussion over the affected lobe. On auscultation bronchial breathing is detected and fine crepitations or a pleural rub may be heard.

General examination shows tachycardia and an apical systolic murmur may be detected, as in any patient with a high fever. Examination of the abdomen may show some distension or, when the diaphragmatic pleura has been involved, upper abdominal tenderness and guarding. Jaundice may be present and, if so, should suggest the possibility of an underlying red cell abnormality. Elderly patients with pneumonia frequently become confused and disorientated.

Laboratory findings. A polymorphonuclear neutrophil leucocytosis is usually present; white cell counts as high as $40 \times 10^9/l$ may be recorded. There may be a reticulocytosis. Both conjugated and unconjugated bilirubin levels are raised in jaundiced patients and serum transaminases may be elevated. Serum C3 and properdin levels may be reduced, especially in bacteraemic patients. Blood culture is positive in about one-third of patients. The P_{O_2} is often diminished but the P_{CO_2} is normal unless terminal respiratory failure occurs.

The sputum may show large numbers of Gram-positive diplococci together with polymorphonuclear neutrophil leucocytes and alveolar macrophages.

X-ray of the chest shows diffuse opacification of the affected part of the lung (Fig. 2). Postero–anterior and lateral views are required to make an accurate anatomical diagnosis of the site of the infection. A small pleural effusion can be seen in the costophrenic angle in some patients. Pneumococci can cause either a lobar pneumonia or a bronchopneumonia. The lower lobes are affected more frequently than the upper. In about one-third of patients more than one lobe is involved.

Differential diagnosis. The initial febrile phase of acute pneumococcal pneumonia cannot be differentiated from that of any other acute febrile illness. Once the characteristic respiratory symptoms and signs have appeared, a diagnosis of acute pneumonia can usually be made on clinical grounds but these signs may be absent when the patient is first seen. Many physicians will remember ruefully the febrile patient that, as a house officer, they admitted in the middle of the night, who had no abnormal chest signs but who had classical signs of pulmonary consolidation when examined by their consultant on a ward round the following morning. There are only two major pulmonary conditions that are likely to be confused with acute bacterial pneumonia—pulmonary infarction and pulmonary atelectasis (Table 1). Pulmonary infarction may be very difficult to differentiate from pneumonia. A sudden onset of fever, chest pain, breathlessness, and cough are common to both conditions. Clinical and radiological examination may show indistinguishable patterns

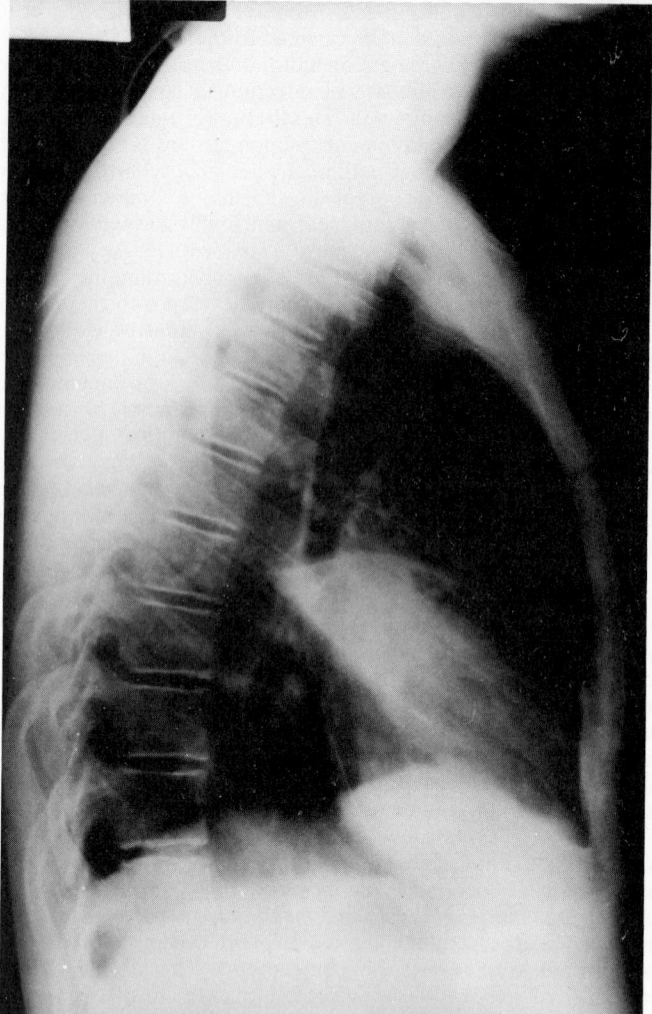

Fig. 2 The characteristic radiological features of pneumococcal pneumonia of the right middle lobe. (Courtesy of Dr J. T. Macfarlane.)

of consolidation and leucocytosis occurs in patients with pneumonia or infarction. Furthermore, infarcts may become infected. Rigors and a very high fever favour a diagnosis of pneumonia as opposed to one of infarction; a very sudden onset of symptoms and frank haemoptysis favour a diagnosis of infarction. Pulmonary atelectasis, resulting from the aspiration of mucus, may give rise to symptoms and signs which are very similar to those of pneumonia. Fever and signs of toxaemia are usually less marked in patients with atelectasis than in patients with pneumonia unless the collapsed area of lung becomes infected.

Table 1 The differential diagnosis of pneumococcal pneumonia, pulmonary infarction, and atelectasis

	Pneumococcal pneumonia	Pulmonary infarction	Atelectasis
Sudden onset	+ +	+ + +	+ +
Haemoptysis	+	+ +	−
Fever	+ + +	+ +	+
Toxaemia	+ + +	+	−
Thrombophlebitis	+ *	+ +	−

* Found most frequently during the recovery phase of the infection

Occasionally sub-diaphragmatic lesions, such as a sub-phrenic abscess or an amoebic liver abscess, cause a clinical picture that mimics that of the lower lobe pneumonia. Conversely lower lobe pneumonia, by producing abdominal pain and guarding, may suggest the diagnosis of an acute abdominal condition such as a perforated peptic ulcer or acute cholecystitis or appendicitis.

Pneumococcal pneumonia can usually be differentiated from viral pneumonias or pneumonia caused by *Mycoplasma pneumoniae* because of its sudden onset, associated severe toxaemia, and accompanying polymorphonuclear neutrophil leucocytosis, but differentiation from other forms of acute bacterial pneumonia cannot usually be made without the aid of microbiological investigations. *Klebsiella* pneumonia, staphylococcal pneumonia, and legionnaires' disease may all produce a similar clinical picture.

Course and prognosis. Without treatment the mortality of acute pneumococcal pneumonia is high, especially when bacteraemia is present. Some patients who survive long enough to make specific anticapsular polysaccharide antibody recover spontaneously by crisis, or by a more gradual lysis, seven to ten days after the onset of their illness. Overall mortality among patients treated promptly with antibiotics is about 5 per cent. Mortality is lowest in healthy fit adults. It is highest among the old and the very young, and among those with an associated underlying illness such as cirrhosis, alcoholism, or heart disease. Lung lesions may be slow to resolve in such patients. Infection with certain pneumococcal serotypes (especially type 3), involvement of more than one lobe of the lung, bacteraemia, leucopenia, jaundice, and persistent pneumococcal polysaccharide antigenaemia are bad prognostic signs. Most deaths from treated pneumococcal pneumonia occur within the first few days of admission to hospital. It is often difficult to establish an exact cause of death in such patients—peripheral circulatory collapse, cardiac arrhythmias, and respiratory failure are some of the contributory factors.

Complications of pneumococcal lobar pneumonia result from local of lymphatic spread of bacteria to adjacent pleura or pericardium, producing pleural or pericardial effusions, or from bacteraemic spread to meninges and other distant foci. The likelihood of one of these infective complications developing is reduced, but not completely abolished, by prompt treatment of the infection with antibiotics.

Pneumococcal pneumonia may precipitate congestive cardiac failure, especially in elderly patients, and can precipitate acute dilatation of the stomach or paralytic ileus. Herpes labialis is a common accompaniment of this condition.

Pleural effusion and empyema. A large pleural effusion or an empyema may occasionally develop during treatment of a patient with established pneumococcal pneumonia. Other patients present with the clinical features of this condition.

Symptoms. Some, but not all, patients give a history suggestive of a previous parenchymatous lung infection. A history of days or weeks of fever, malaise, anorexia, and weight loss is often obtained. Fever may be hectic and accompanied by rigors and episodes of profuse sweating. Patients with a large pleural effusion are breathless and they may complain of dull chest pain on the affected side.

Physical signs. General examination shows persistent fever and tachycardia. The patient may look toxaemic and there may be signs of recent weight loss. Examination of the chest usually shows the characteristic signs of a pleural effusion—diminished chest movement, dullness on percussion and diminished breath sounds over the accumulated fluid. The chest wall overlying an empyema may be tender.

Laboratory findings. A persistent polymorphonuclear neutrophil leucocytosis is nearly always present. Radiographs may be very helpful in localizing a loculated effusion. On aspiration, turbid fluid or thick pus is obtained which contains pneumococci and degenerate white cells.

Differential diagnosis. Association of persistent pyrexia and leucocytosis with abnormal chest signs indicates a chronic pulmonary infection. Absence of copious purulent sputum differentiates the condition from a lung abscess. Differentiation from tuberculosis may be difficult on clinical grounds alone. Diagnosis of an empyema is confirmed by the aspiration of pus from the pleural cavity. Repeated needling with a wide-bored needle, preferably under fluoroscopic control, may be needed to find a loculated empyema.

Course and prognosis. Untreated, an empyema may rupture through the chest wall (empyema necessitatis) or rupture into a bronchus causing a bronchopleural fistula. Even when pus is aspirated and healing achieved, subsequent fibrosis and calcification may seriously restrict expansion of the underlying lung.

Pericardial effusion and empyema. Pneumococci may spread from an infected lower lobe to produce pericarditis. Pericarditis is clinically silent in some patients; in other patients it is manifest only as a transient pericardial rub or as an abnormal electrocardiogram. However, in occasional patients pericardial involvement is the dominant feature of a pneumococcal infection. Only a proportion of such patients give a history suggestive of an initial acute respiratory tract infection.

Symptoms. Patients with a pneumococcal pericardial empyema usually give a history of several days, or even weeks, of persistent fever, malaise, anorexia, and weight loss. They may complain of dull central chest pain and they may have noted swelling of the ankles or of the abdomen.

Physical signs. Many patients with a pneumococcal pericardial empyema are critically ill by the time that they reach hospital. They are febrile and toxaemic. There may be signs of severe pericardial tamponade—a rapid, small volume pulse, pulsus alternans, a low blood pressure, elevation of the jugular venous pressure, and peripheral oedema and ascites. Percussion of the chest may show some enlargement of the area of cardiac dullness but this is an unreliable clinical sign. The heart sounds are usually faint and in some, but not all, patients a pericardial rub is heard.

Laboratory findings. A peripheral blood polymorphonuclear neutrophil leucocytosis is present and blood culture may be positive for pneumococci. A chest X-ray may show globular englargement of the heart and there may be radiological evidence of an associated lung infection. The electrocardiogram shows low voltage potentials and S–T elevation or depression may be present. On aspiration of the pericardium turbid fluid or thick pus is obtained from which pneumococci can be isolated.

Differential diagnosis. Detection of the signs of pericardial tamponade in a patient who is febrile and toxaemic should suggest a diagnosis of pericardial empyema. The condition may be confused with tuberculous constrictive pericarditis, but patients with this latter condition usually have a longer history than patients with a pneumococcal pericardial empyema and are generally less toxic. A pericardial empyema may be confused with a pleural empyema in patients without signs of tamponade. Diagnosis of a pericardial empyema is confirmed by pericardial aspiration. A pneumococcal pericardial empyema is a medical emergency, and pericardial aspiration should be undertaken immediately, if necessary at more than one site, if this diagnosis is suspected.

Course and prognosis. Pneumococcal pericardial empyema is a serious condition with a high mortality, even in treated patients. Patients who survive the initial episode may develop constrictive pericarditis within weeks or months of their acute illness.

Otitis media. Otitis media is probably the commonest form of pneumococcal infection. The condition is seen most frequently in young children but it may also affect adults.

Symptoms. The onset of an attack of acute otitis media is sudden, although there may be a history of a recent, upper respiratory tract infection. Fever and severe pain in the ear are the usual presenting complaints in adults and older children, and patients may complain of deafness and tinnitus. Fever, crying, and extreme irritability are the usual features of the condition in young children in whom febrile convulsions may occur.

Physical signs. On examination of the affected ear, the tympanic membrane is seen to be red and swollen, and it may bulge outwards into the external ear. If perforation has occurred, the external ear may be full of pus and a ragged hole may be seen in the tympanic membrane. The affected ear is usually partially deaf. In children meningism may be present.

Laboratory findings. A polymorphonuclear neutrophil leucocytosis is usually found. If the drum has ruptured pneumococci may be found in the purulent discharge present in the external ear but contaminants are likely to be present also.

Differential diagnosis. A clinical diagnosis of otitis media is rarely difficult provided that the ears of all febrile and irritable children are carefully examined. The aetiology of the condition can often be established by examination of fluid obtained from the middle ear with a fine needle.

Course and prognosis. Prompt treatment is usually followed by a rapid and complete resolution of the infection. However, some patients, especially those in whom rupture of the drum has occurred, are left with partial conductive deafness. When untreated, pneumococcal otitis media can give rise to a chronic discharging ear. Spread of the infection posteriorly may result in acute mastoiditis, and spread of the infection upwards can cause pneumococcal meningitis.

Pneumococcal meningitis. Pneumococcal meningitis may result from damage to the base of the skull, and it can occur as a complication of pneumococcal otitis media or pneumococcal pneumonia. However, many patients with this condition, the proportion varying from series to series, present with the clinical features of acute pyogenic meningitis.

Symptoms. Fever and headache are the usual presenting symptoms of pneumococcal meningitis. Headache usually comes on gradually over a few hours; it is generalized and may be very severe. Nausea, backache, and photobia may develop and convulsions may occur.

Physical signs. Patients with pneumococcal meningitis are febrile and toxaemic. Neck stiffness and a positive Kernig's sign, indicators of meningeal irritation, are usually found in adults and in older children. Some impairment of consciousness is often present which varies in severity from drowsiness and confusion to deep coma. Bradycardia and hypertension may indicate the presence of raised intracranial pressure but papilloedema is rarely seen. Bulging of the anterior fontanelle may be present in infants. Cranial nerve palsies, most frequently of the sixth or of the third cranial nerve, may be present on presentation and, occasionally, other peripheral localizing neurological signs are found.

An associated pneumococcal lesion, such as otitis media or pneumonia, may be detected. Petechiae are rarely seen. Herpes labialis may be present.

Laboratory findings. A peripheral blood polymorphonuclear neutrophil leucocytosis is usually found and a positive blood culture may be obtained. Examination of the cerebrospinal fluid shows a turbid fluid which usually contains an increased number of cells and many bacteria. Most of the leucocytes are polymorphonuclear neutrophils. Cerebrospinal fluid (CSF) bacterial counts are often very high in patients with pneumococcal meningitis; on average bacterial counts are 10 times higher in patients with pneumococcal meningitis than in patients with meningococcal meningitis. Leucocytes are present in only small numbers in the CSF of some patients; in such instances the CSF may still be turbid because of the presence of numerous bacteria. The CSF protein level is increased and its sugar level decreased below that of the corresponding blood value. Gram stain and culture are usually positive for pneumococci. Many other abnormalities have been detected in the CSF of patients with pneumococcal meningitis, as in the CSF of patients with other forms of pyogenic meningitis. These include a fall in pH, an increase in lactic acid concentration, an increase in lactic dehydrogenase level, elevation of IgG and IgM levels, and an increase in levels of fibrin degradation products (FDP). Cerebrospinal fluid FDP levels are considerably higher in patients with pneumococcal meningitis that in patients with meningococcal meningitis.

Differential diagnosis. It is not usually difficult to establish a clinical diagnosis of pyogenic meningitis in adults and older children with pneumococcal meningitis. However, difficulties may arise in the very young and in the very old, for signs of meningeal irritation may be absent in both these groups of patients. Fever and irritability may be the only clinical signs of pneumococcal meningitis in an infant. The appearance of confusion may be the only sign indicating involvement of the meninges in an elderly patient with pneumococcal pneumonia. Any adverse change in the psychological state or in the neurological state of an elderly patient with pneumonia is an indication for lumbar puncture.

On clinical grounds alone pneumococcal meningitis cannot be differentiated with certainty from other forms of pyogenic meningitis. An associated ear infection or pneumonia favours the diagnosis of a pneumococcal infection. If petechiae are found, meningococcal meningitis is more likely.

Bacteriological diagnosis of pneumococcal meningitis is confirmed by examination of the cerebrospinal fluid.

Course and prognosis. The prognosis of patients with pneumococcal meningitis is poor. Many patients make no response to treatment, their conscious level deteriorates progressively, and they die within the first 24–48 hours after their admission to hospital. Other patients make some initial response to treatment but then relapse; their conscious level deteriorates and new neurological signs appear. This deterioration may be due to the collection of pus in the extradural space or brain but, more usually, follows a vascular occlusion. Patients who deteriorate after an initial clinical improvement must be fully investigated by scanning or by arteriography, to exclude the presence of a space-occupying lesion. The clinical course of survivors of the early phase of pneumococcal meningitis is often stormy, being complicated by conditions such as bed-sores, pneumonia, and venous thrombosis. It has been estimated that over one-half of all survivors from pneumococcal meningitis are left with some intellectual impairment or residual neurological disability such as deafness or partial hemiplegia.

Relapses may occur when treatment is stopped. The value of repeated lumbar puncture in monitoring the course of pyogenic meningitis is uncertain, but a lumbar puncture should be performed two or three days after antibiotic treatment has been stopped to ensure that there has been no reactivation of the infection. Pneumococcal antigen may persist in the CSF for one to two weeks after the start of treatment but dead bacteria are seen for only three or four days.

Mortality figures for pneumococcal meningitis varying from 10 per cent to over 50 per cent have been recorded in different series. It is likely that some selection of cases has been employed in many series in which low mortality figures have been recorded, for example cases diagnosed only at post-mortem may have been excluded. It is probable that in industrialized countries the true mortality from pneumococcal meningitis is around 30 per cent. In developing countries mortality figures of approximately 50 per cent have been found consistently. Impairment of consciousness on admission to hospital, associated pneumonia, a low CSF white cell count, and a high CSF bacterial count are poor prognostic features. Death is almost inevitable in patients who are in coma at the time that they are admitted to hospital (Table 2).

Table 2 The influence of conscious level at the time of admission to hospital on the outcome of pneumococcal meningitis

Conscious level	Number of patients	Deaths	Mortality (%)
Fully conscious	19	6	32
Confused	70	28	40
Semi-conscious	69	37	54
Coma	18	17	94

From Baird et al. (1976). Lancet, ii, 1344

Why the prognosis of pneumococcal meningitis is so poor is uncertain. Although there is little difference in the clinical features of patients with pneumococcal or meningococcal meningitis on presentation at hospital and despite the fact that the causative organisms of the two infections have similar in vitro sensitivities to penicillin, death is at least five times more likely in a patient with pneumococcal meningitis than in a patient with meningococcal meningitis. Vascular damage, rapid multiplication of bacteria, and defective leucocyte function have all been suggested as possible causes of the poor outcome of patients with pneumococcal meningitis, but the possible role of these factors has not been clearly documented. The reason for the very poor prognosis of patients with pneumococcal meningitis remains a mystery.

Other clinical syndromes. Acute, fulminating septicaemia is a rare form of pneumococcal infection which is encountered most frequently in patients without a spleen. A sudden onset of fever, peripheral circulatory collapse, and bleeding are the usual presenting features of this condition which is clinically indistinguishable from other forms of overwhelming bacterial septicaemia. In contrast to the findings in other forms of pneumococcal infection, leucopenia is usually found. Bleeding is due to disseminated intravascular coagulation. The mortality of this condition is very high, even when treatment is started promptly.

Acute endocarditis may complicate pneumococcal septicaemia but this condition is now encountered only rarely. Healthy heart valves, especially the aortic valve, may be attacked and rupture of the aortic valve may occur, producing severe aortic incompetence. Emboli derived from cardiac vegetations may reach the brain and other organs. Progression of the cardiac lesion may be very rapid and the prognosis of this condition is poor. Valve replacement may be necessary for those who survive the initial episode.

During the course of pneumococcal septicaemia, with or without endocarditis, bacteria may reach many sites where they can multiply to produce a purulent lesion. Pneumococcal arthritis, opthalmitis, and orchitis may be produced in this way.

Pneumococcal peritonitis is an uncommon condition which is encountered most frequently in patients with the nephrotic syndrome or cirrhosis of the liver, conditions frequently resulting in ascites and generalized impairment in immunity. The condition has been described also in healthy young girls, perhaps as a complication of pelvic infection, and occasionally in neonates. The condition is characterized by a sudden onset of fever and abdominal pain and tenderness. The ascitic fluid is turbid and contains polymorphonuclear neutrophil leucocytes and pneumococci. The general features of an acute infection may not be so obvious in patients with cirrhosis, and peritonitis must be considered as a possible diagnosis in any patient with this condition whose clinical state shows a sudden deterioration. The prognosis of pneumococcal peritonitis is poor in patients with a serious underlying illness.

The bacteriological diagnosis of pneumococcal infections. Detection of pneumococci by Gram stain and culture in pus or in pleural, pericardial, peritoneal, or cerebrospinal fluid establishes a bacteriological diagnosis of pneumococcal infection. However, difficulties arise in the bacteriological diagnosis of pneumococcal pneumonia because of the frequent presence of pneumococci in the upper respiratory tract of healthy individuals. Thus, the isolation of pneumococci from the sputum of a patient with pneumonia cannot be taken as proof that the pneumonia has a pneumococcal aetiology for the bacteria detected may be contaminants from the upper respiratory tract. Demonstration of pneumococci in a blood culture firmly establishes a bacteriological diagnosis in a patient with pneumococcal pneumonia, but positive blood cultures are obtained in only about one-third of patients with this condition. Two techniques are used to obtain respiratory tract secretions which are not contaminated by upper respiratory tract flora—transtracheal aspiration and lung aspiration. Transtracheal aspiration is unpleasant for the patient, may cause localized emphysema and can produce secretions which contain a mixed flora. Lung aspiration is more likely to identify a single pulmonary pathogen, but it frequently results in haemoptysis and may cause a pneumothorax. Thus, the use of these techniques is probably not justified in an uncomplicated case of lobar pneumonia which, on clinical grounds, is thought to be due to a pneumococcal infection. Transtracheal aspiration and lung aspiration are of most value in the investigation of patients with clinically atypical pneumonia, and in the investigations of patients with an underyling immune deficiency which makes them susceptible to infection wtih unusual organisms.

Treatment with inadequate amounts of an antibiotic may make it impossible to culture pneumococci from clinical samples without aborting the progression of the infection. Thus, interest has recently re-awakened in the use of immunological methods for diagnosing pneumococcal infections which depend upon the detection of bacterial products rather than upon the detection of live bacteria. It has been known since the work of Dochez and Avery in 1917 that pneumococcal polysaccharide antigens are frequently present in the urine and in the serum of patients with pneumococcal lobar pneumonia. The recent development of rapid and sensitive methods for the detection of small amounts of bacterial antigens in clinical samples has allowed the successful application of immunodiagnosis to a variety of forms of pneumococcal infection. The two techniques which have been used most widely to detect pneumococcal polysaccharide antigens in clinical specimens are countercurrent immunoelectrophoresis (CIE) and the latex agglutination technique. Countercurrent Immunoelectrophoresis is easy to perform and rarely causes false positive results, but it will not detect type 7 and type 14 antigens, which are positively charged, unless special buffers are used. Latex agglutination tests require a minimum of equipment but care must be taken to exclude false positive reactions caused by rheumatoid-like factors. Pneumococcal polysaccharides can be detected by more sensitive radioimmunoassay and enzyme linked immunosorbent assay (ELISA) procedures but these techniques have so far been little used to analyse clinical samples.

Pneumococcal polysaccharide antigens have been detected by CIE in serum, urine, cerebrospinal fluid, pleural fluid, peritoneal fluid, synovial fluid, and middle ear fluid obtained from patients with pneumococcal infections with a positivity rate comparable to that of culture. Pneumococcal antigen is present in the sputum of nearly all patients with pneumococcal lobar pneumonia. Although positive tests may be obtained in sputum obtained from patients with other forms of respiratory tract infection, the specificity of sputum antigen detection is higher than that of culture in differentiating pneumococcal pneumonia from upper respiratory tract infections (Table 3).

The advantages of antigen detection over culture are that a rapid

Table 3 The specificity of pneumococcal antigen detection in the sputum in the diagnosis of pneumococcal lobar pneumonia

	Sputum culture positive	Sputum antigen positive
Acute bronchitis or sinusitis ($n = 18$)	18	5
Pneumonia ($n = 18$)	18	15

From Perlino and Shulman (1976). *J. Lab. Clin. Med.*, **87**, 496

result is obtained and that a positive test may be obtained in partially treated patients in whom culture is negative. However, antigen detection cannot provide any information on the antibiotic sensitivity of the causative pneumococcus and, if antigen detection is employed in the diagnosis of pneumococcal infections, it should be carried out in parallel with standard microbiological techniques and not as a substitute for them.

Tests for antibody have been little used in the investigation of patients with pneumococcal infection.

Treatment

Antibiotics. Penicillin remains the antibiotic of first choice for the treatment of pneumococcal infections. For patients who are known to be allergic to penicillin, chloramphenicol is an effective alternative, especially for patients with pneumococcal meningitis, as this drug penetrates well into the CSF. Cephalosporins, erythromycin, and lincomycin are effective in the treatment of pneumococcal pneumonia. Aminoglycosides such as gentamicin and kanamycin should not be used to treat pneumococcal infections nor should combinations of antibiotics, such as penicillin and tetracycline, be employed.

Standard doses of penicillin produce serum levels well above the minimal inhibitory concentration (MIC) of most pneumococci. Penicillin diffuses moderately well into inflammatory exudates, and intrathecal therapy or local injection into serous cavities is not usually required. Penicillin levels in the CSF of patients receiving parenteral therapy vary considerably from patient to patient and show marked fluctuations in relation to the timing of intramuscular injections. The temptation to lower the dose of penicillin given to patients with pneumococci meningitis as their clinical condition improves should be resisted for the blood–brain barrier becomes progressively less permeable to penicillin as inflammation of the meninges regresses. Although penicillin is bactericidal to pneumococci, it cannot act on pneumococci in a stationery phase of growth. Pneumococci can thus persist for some time in tissues where the antibiotic concentration is above their MIC. It is probable that in most patients such organisms are destroyed by the host defences, but relapses of pneumococcal infection may occur after a standard course of antibiotic treatment.

The dose and duration of penicillin therapy required for the successful treatment of pneumococcal infections is strongly influenced by the site of the infection (Table 4). Patients with otitis media and pneumococcal pneumonia respond well to low doses of penicillin given for a short period. An effective regimen for adults with pneumonia is crystalline penicillin, 2 million units six-hourly for 24 hours, followed by procaine pencillin, 600 000 units twice a

Table 4 The duration of antibiotic treatment required in different forms of pneumococcal disease

5–7 days	2 weeks	4–6 weeks
Otitis media Pneumonia	Meningitis Septicaemia	Endocarditis Empyema Septic arthritis

day for a further six days. It is probable that shorter courses of treatment would be equally effective. In a study in which patients were given treatment for 24 hours after their temperature had returned to normal, treatment was required for an average of 60 hours. It has been shown in developing countries, where pressure on hospital beds makes the admission to hospital of all patients with pneumonia impracticable, that pneumococcal pneumonia can be successfully managed by outpatient treatment with a single dose of a long-acting penicillin combination.

Patients with pneumococcal meningitis require larger doses of penicillin than patients with pneumonia to ensure that adequate CSF concentrations of antibiotic are maintained. For adults, crystalline penicillin should be given in an initial dose of 16 million units per day, administered intravenously. This form of therapy should be given for at least five days. Patients who respond well to treatment may then be changed to intramuscular therapy but large doses of penicillin are still required, for example 3 million units of crystalline penicillin six-hourly in an adult, to maintain effective CSF levels. Patients with pneumococcal meningitis should receive antibiotics for at least two weeks. An even longer course of treatment is necessary for patients with pneumococcal empyema or with a large collection of pneumococcal pus at another site. For such patients penicillin should be given, for adults, in a dose of 4–8 million units per day for at least four weeks.

The response of patients with pneumococcal lobar pneumonia to penicillin is usually dramatic. The patient's temperature falls to normal within 24–48 hours of the start of treatment and his clinical signs rapidly improve. Within a week or ten days all abnormal clinical signs disappear. However, radiological resolution takes several weeks. Patients with pneumococcal meninigitis respond more slowly but, if improvement is going to occur, it is usually apparent within the first five days after the start of therapy. Failure of a patient with a pneumococcal infection to respond to penicillin suggests that (*a*) the initial bacteriological diagnosis was incorrect; (*b*) the infection was caused by a penicillin resistant pneumococcus; (*c*) a local collection of pus has formed; or (*d*) that the patient has developed a treatment reaction. Each of these possibilities should be investigated.

Until recently it could be assumed that all patients with pneumococcal infections would respond satisfactorily to treatment with penicillin. This is no longer the case. In 1967 it was reported that partially penicillin resistant pneumococci were present in Australia and New Guinea, and such partially resistant organisms have now been identified in many parts of the world. Fortunately infection with such partially resistant strains (which have an MIC to penicillin of between 0.1 and 1.0 µg/ml) usually responds to treatment with a full therapeutic course of penicillin. However, during the past few years an increasing number of cases of pneumococcal disease have been reported in which penicillin failed to control the infection. Some of these cases responded to treatment with amoxycillin or ampicillin. The most worrying reports of antibiotic resistance in pneumococci have come from South Africa. At Durban, three infants died from meningitis caused by pneumococci which were resistant to penicillin and chloramphenicol. At Johannesburg, multiply resistant strains were identified in patients and in the nasopharynx of hospital staff. In this outbreak type 19A strains were identified, which were highly resistant to penicillin (MIC > 4 µg/ml), ampicillin, methicillin, erythromycin, chloramphenicol, cotrimoxazole, and tetracycline. The bacteria were sensitive to rifampicin and fusidic acid. Other type 19 and type 6 pneumococci were identified which were resistant to penicillin or to tetracyline and chloramphenicol. Penicillin resistance was not due to the production of a β-latamase. When rifampicin was used in an attempt to cure carriers, pneumococci rapidly became resistant to this antibiotic. Vancomycin may be an effective alternative.

It seems likely that further outbreaks of infection with multiply resistant organisms will occur, and that penicillin resistance will be detected in pneumococci increasingly frequently. Thus, antibiotic sensitivities must be determined on all pneumococci isolated from patients with clinically important pneumococcal infections, and the possibility of penicillin resistance should be considered in all patients with pneumococcal infection who fail to respond rapidly to treatment with penicillin.

Serum therapy. Serum therapy saved many lives from pneumococcal infection (Fig. 3) although it was not as effective as antibiotics. No comprehensive trials of serum therapy given together with antibiotics have ever been undertaken. As the mortality of certain forms of pneumococcal infection remains very high despite antibiotics, perhaps the use of serum therapy should be reconsidered.

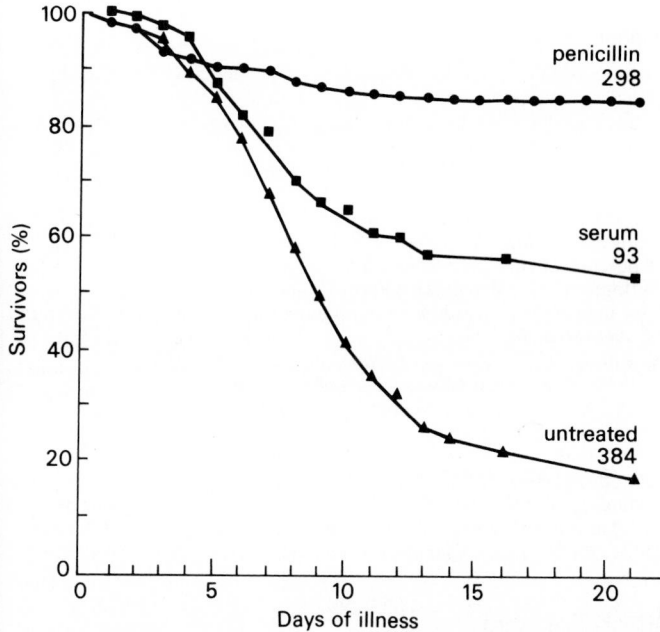

Fig. 3 The effect of antibiotic therapy and immune serum on survival in pneumococcal bacteraemia; figures are based on data from different series. (From Austrian and Gold (1964). *Ann. intern. Med.* **60**, 759.)

Supportive measures

General nursing care. Patients with acute pneumococcal infections are often extremely ill and require careful general nursing care, special attention being paid to fluid balance. Patients with fulminating pneumococcal infections require intensive care facilities. In general, isolation of patients with pneumococcal infection is not necessary but patients with an infection caused by a multiply antibiotic resistant strain should be isolated.

Fluid therapy. Patients with pneumococcal infections are often dehydrated by the time that they reach hospital. Patients with pneumonia may loose large amounts of fluid through the respiratory tract as a result of hyperventilation; patients with pneumococcal meningitis are frequently too confused to drink. For such patients intravenous fluid therapy may be required.

Oxygen and physiotherapy. Patients with pneumococcal pneumonia, especially those with more than one lobe of the lung involved, may be unable to oxygenate their blood adequately and require oxygen therapy. Oxygen can be given conveniently by Venturi mask. If possible the arterial P_{O_2} should be raised to between 60 and 80 mmHg. Physiotherapy, by keeping the larger respiratory pathways clear of secretions, may help in ventilation. Physiotherapy is important in helping the patient to clear tenacious sputum during the recovery phase of the infection.

Careful attention must be paid to the respiratory tract in unconscious patients with pneumococcal meningitis. Intubation and assisted respiration are sometimes employed in patients who have passed into deep coma. The outlook for such patients is so poor that it is doubtful whether these measures are justified.

Analgesics. Local pain may be severe in patients with pneumococcal infections and sufficient analgesics should be given to control this symptom. Analgesics with a central depressant action should be avoided whenever possible.

Other drugs. High doses of dexamethasone may be given to try to reduce cerebral oedema in patients with pneumococcal meningitis but overall corticosteroids are of no benefit in the treatment of pneumococcal meningitis. Heparin is likewise ineffective and may precipitate intracerebral bleeding.

Drainage of pus. Local collections of pus should be removed. Sometimes, for example in patients with an empyema, it may be possible to remove pus by needle aspiration. Repeated aspiration will usually be required. If pus is too thick to be removed from the pleural or pericardial space by aspiration, surgical drainage is necessary. Even when successful drainage is achieved, scarring may be extensive and decortication of a lung or removal of an adherent pericardium may subsequently be required. Burr holes may be needed to drain extradural or cerebral abscesses complicating pneumococcal meningitis.

Prophylaxis

General improvements in living standards in industrialized countries have had much less impact on the incidence of pneumococcal infection than on the incidence of many other infectious diseases. Nevertheless, avoidance, whenever possible, of severe overcrowding in barracks, refugee camps, and similar communities may play a small part in reducing the incidence of the infection.

Chemotherapy. Chemoprophylaxis has been little used in the control of pneumococcal disease because of difficulties in identifying those who are at risk from the infection. Secondary cases are seen only rarely among those who have been in close contact with a patient. Because patients with sickle cell disease have an increased incidence of pneumococcal infection, some paediatricians recommend that children with this condition should be given regular chemoprophylaxis with oral penicillin from the age of six months until they have reached the age of two years, when they should be vaccinated.

Vaccination. Vaccination offers the best hope of controlling pneumococcal infection. Early trials with pneumococcal vaccines, carried out mostly in South Africa, gave equivocal results, but in 1945 McLeod showed quite clearly that vaccination of American Air Force recruits with pneumococcal polysaccharides protected against infection with pneumococci of the corresponding serotype. Two years later Kaufman reported that similar results could be obtained in elderly civilians. Surprisingly, these promising findings evoked little general interest. However, recent appreciation of the fact that antibiotics have had only a limited impact on the morbidity and mortality of pneumococcal disease and the emergence of antibiotic resistance have led to a renewed interest in the development of pneumococcal vaccines and several vaccines are now available commercially. These contain up to 14 purified pneumococcal polysaccharides selected to give protection against approximately 80 per cent of pneumococcal infections in North America and in Europe. However, as mentioned above, there are considerable geographical variations in the distribution of pneumococcal serotypes responsible for pneumococcal disease. Therefore, vaccines devised for use in the USA and in Europe may not necessarily be appropriate for use in other parts of the world.

Pneumococcal vaccines have certain unusual features, in common with other polysaccharide vaccines. Whilst they induce a good antibody response, as measured by radioimmunoassay, in most adults following a single injection, they are poorly immunogenic in young children. Revaccination does not usually have a booster effect in adults and has a variable effect in children. Revaccination in those with persisting high antibody levels may cause a brisk inflammatory reaction at the site of the second injection which is probably the result of an Arthus reaction. The immune response to pneumococcal vaccine is only slightly reduced if influenza vaccine is given at the same time.

The effectiveness of the recently developed pneumococcal polysaccharide vaccines in preventing pneumococcal lobar pneumonia has been demonstrated in controlled trials undertaken in South Africa and New Guinea. A trial of a 13 valent vaccine in South African miners showed a 53 per cent reduction in the incidence of radiologically confirmed cases of pneumonia among vaccinated subjects and a 78 per cent reduction in the incidence of radiologically confirmed cases of pneumonia caused by one of the pneumococcal serotypes represented in the vaccine (Fig. 4). A similar reduction in the incidence of bacteriologically proven cases of pneumococcal pneumonia was obtained in a trial undertaken in New Guinea and overall mortality from pneumonia was reduced by 44 per cent in vaccinated subjects. It has yet to be shown that pneumococcal vaccination prevents pneumococcal meningitis but this would almost certainly be the case. Some protection against otitis media has been demonstrated. However, if vaccination is to be effective in preventing this condition, which occurs most frequently in young children, immunization must be given at an early age when it is least effective.

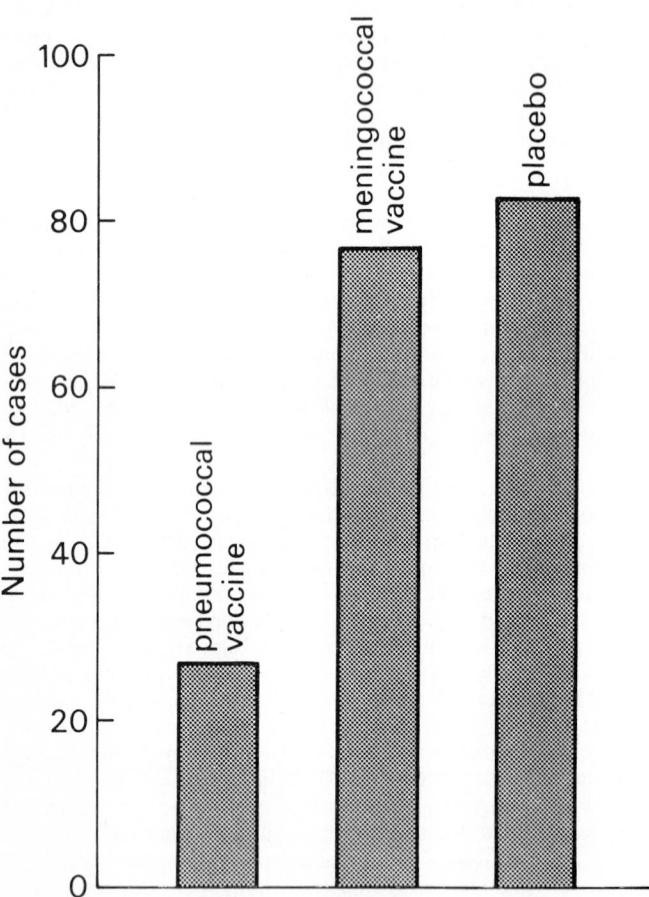

Fig. 4 The effect of pneumoccal polysaccharide vaccine on the incidence in South African miners of pneumococcal pneumonia or bacteraemia caused by pneumococci of the types present in the vaccine. There were approximately equal numbers of subjects in each group. (From Austrian *et al.* (1976), *Trans. Ass. Am. Phycns* 89, 184.)

There is so far little information available as to the duration of the immunity provided by pneumococcal polysaccharide vaccination. In New Guinea clinical protection was observed for at least two years after vaccination and raised antibody levels have been detected in adults five years after immunization. However, in children antibody levels fall faster after immunization than in adults. Until it is known more definitely how long clinical protection persists following vaccination, it is difficult to justify the routine use of

pneumococcal vaccines as part of infant immunization schedules. Thus, pneumococcal vaccines are currently being used primarily to protect those who are known to be most at risk from the infection. These include patients with sickle cell disease, patients who have undergone splenectomy, patients wtih cirrhosis or the nephrotic syndrome, and the elderly. Patients with sickle cell disease or the nephrotic syndrome respond satisfactorily to pneumococcal vaccines but patients who have undergone splenectomy for the staging of a lymphoma may not. A controlled trial has demonstrated the efficacy of pneumococcal vaccination in children with sickle cell disease but, because of the limited number of components to the vaccine, protection is not complete and pneumococcal disease may still occur in vaccinated children.

References

Austrian, R. (1977). Pneumoccal infection and pneumococcal vaccine. *New Engl. J. Med.*, **297**, 938.
— and Gold, J. (1964). Pneumococcal bacteremia with especial reference to bacteremic pneumococcal pneumonia. *Ann. intern. Med.* **60**, 759.
Baird, D. R., Whittle, H. C., and Greenwood, B. M. (1976). Mortality from pneumococcal meningitis. *Lancet* **ii**, 1344.
Jones, D. M. (1979). The rapid detection of bacterial antigens. In *Recent Advances in Infection* (eds. D. S. Reeves and A. M. Geddes), pp. 91. Churchill Livingstone, Edinburgh.
Kauffman, C. A., Watanakunakorn, C., and Phair, J. P. (1973). Purulent pneumococcal pericarditis. A continuing problem in the antibiotic era. *J. Am. Med.* **54**, 743.
The Lancet (1977). Resistant pneumococci. *Lancet* **ii**, 803.
— (1978). Pneumococcal vaccines. *Lancet* **i**, 131.
Likhite, V. V. (1976). Immunological impairment and susceptibility to infection after splenectomy. *J. Am. med. Ass.* **236**, 1376.
Merck, Sharp, and Dohme. (1978). *Pneumococcal pneumonia and polysaccharide vaccines.* Merck, Sharp, and Dohme.
Newhouse, M., Sanchis, J., and Bienenstock, J. (1976). Lung defence mechanisms. *New Engl. J. Med.* **295**, 990, 1045.
Waddy, B. B. (1952). Climate and respiratory infections. *Lancet* **ii**, 674.

Staphylococci

I. Phillips and S. J. Eykyn

The staphylococci and the related micrococci are widely distributed in nature, and some species are among the commonest human and animal parasites. Through all the taxonomic changes that the group has suffered, one organism, *Staphylococcus aureus*, stands out as an important human parasite; its relationship with its host ranging from harmless, or even helpful, commensalism to extreme pathogenicity. The fact that an individual strain may change its relationship with the host from one to the other remains one of the most puzzling problems in infectious diseases.

Taxonomy and nomenclature. Although others had made observations on coccal organisms, Alexander Ogston, a Scottish surgeon, was the first to associate the cluster-forming cocci with pus and over a century ago he presented his classic work, initially in Aberdeen, where it was received with incredulity and then rejected by the *British Medical Journal*, and later in Berlin where its importance was recognized. At the suggestion of the Professor of Greek in Aberdeen, he coined the highly appropriate name 'staphylococcus' for the organism (σταφυλη, a bunch of grapes). Since that time, as the diversity of the organisms in this group has been recognized, they have been given the generic name either of *Staphylococcus* or *Micrococcus* and now both names are in use for two different genera of the family Micrococcaceae. The specific name of Ogston's staphylococcus is now clearly established as *S. aureus* though some still believe that *S. pyogenes* has priority as well as the advantage of greater descriptive accuracy.

Table 1 classifies the Micrococcaceae associated with man. The staphylococci and micrococci are distinguished from each other by the former's ability to utilize glucose anaerobically (although this is difficult to demonstrate with certain species), whereas the latter do so only in the presence of oxygen. In addition, staphylococci have cell walls containing a distinct peptidoglycan with glycine cross-bridges, and ribitol teichoic acids. Finally the nucleic acid contents of the DNA of each genus differ markedly. One may assume that these criteria are sufficient to settle the matter for the foreseeable future. The species are less well characterized and their classification has undergone many changes and still remains controversial. Three major species of medically important staphylococci are identified, *S. aureus*, *S. epidermidis*, and *S. saprophyticus* but there are other species. It has also been proposed that some of the biotypes of *S. epidermidis* and *S. saprophyticus* be given species names. Furthermore certain 'animal' staphylococci are sometimes isolated from man. *S. aureus*, which may produce colonies varying from white to the classical 'gold', is distinguished from other human staphylococci by the production of coagulase, and *S. saprophyticus* is usually resistant to novobiocin. In clinical laboratories, isolates of species other than *S. aureus* are seldom identified and are referred to as coagulase-negative staphylococci or *S. albus*. Among the micrococci only three species are officially recognized, *M. varians*, *M. luteus*, and *M. roseus* though others probably exist.

Table 1　Classification of *Micrococcaceae* associated with man

Family	Genus	Species
	Staphylococcus	
	coagulase-positive	*S. aureus*
	coagulase-negative	*S. epidermidis*
		S. saprophyticus
Micrococcacae		
catalase-positive		other species
spherical Gram-		probably exist but
positive cocci in		await definition
clusters		
	Micrococcus	*M. varians*
		M. luteus
		M. roseus

The ability of *S. aureus* to coagulate plasma is based on two different mechanisms. Coagulase proper is an enzyme that, with a plasma cofactor, possibly prothrombin, has thrombin-like activity. It is detected by the tube coagulase test in which staphylococci are mixed with human plasma in a test-tube. Bound coagulase, or clumping factor, differs in acting directly on fibrinogen, and is detected by the simpler slide coagulase test in which a suspension of staphylococci is mixed with plasma on a slide. The two enzymes usually occur together; the slide test is generally used to screen organisms while the tube test is confirmatory, and of more taxonomic significance.

In common with many other organisms, staphylococci are susceptible to bacteriophages, and schemes for the typing of *S. aureus* are well established and have contributed greatly to epidemiological studies. Table 2 gives details of the International Phage Typing Scheme. There are three major phage groups, I–III, and any individual strain is usually susceptible to one or more phages, from one, or sometimes two groups; for example *S. aureus* phage type 80/81 is susceptible to phages 80 and 81. Some 10–20 per cent of isolates are untypable with the basic set but may be sensitive to supplementary phages. A similar system of phage typing exists for *S. epidermidis*.

Table 2　International phage typing scheme for *S. aureus*

Phage group	Individual phages
I	29; 52; 52A; 79; 80
II	3A; 3C; 55; 71
III	6; 42E; 47; 53; 54; 75; 77; 83A; 84; 85
Unclassified	81; 94; 95; 96

The antigenic structure of staphylococci is complex: *S. aureus* presents a mosaic of antigens, and isolates can be characterized by the identification of the components. Perhaps because of its complexity, the method has seldom been used in epidemological studies. In the past the antibiotic sensitivity pattern of *S. aureus* was useful in the initial detection of cross infection but with the decline of the multiply-resistant 'hospital staphylococcus' it has ceased to be so.

Pathogenicity. *S. aureus* produces toxic extracellular enzymes in variety surpassed possibly only by *Clostridium perfringens* (*welchii*). Coagulase has already been mentioned, but other enzymes include hyaluronidase, phosphatase, deoxyribonuclease, proteases, lipases, catalase, lysozyme, four different haemolysins, α, β, and γ, the Panton–Valentine leucocidin, epidermolytic toxins, and enterotoxins. Alpha-haemolysin disrupts membranes and apart from haemolysis has many potentially harmful properties. It is generally cytotoxic and thus necrotizing, toxic to macrophages and platelets, releases histamine and 5-hydroxytryptamine and it is lethal to certain animals. Delta-haemolysin has similar though less dramatic properties. The Panton–Valentine leucocidin is unique in attacking only polymorphonuclear leucocytes and macrophages.

Perhaps because of the variety of toxic products it has been difficult to establish a role for any of them in the pathogenicity of *S. aureus* For example, α-toxin can be demonstrated in infection, but anti-α-toxin does not prevent disease. Experiments to demonstrate a major pathogenic role for α-toxin have given contradictory results. Epidermolytic toxins and enterotoxins are exceptions to this general rule and have been shown to be involved in well-defined disease entities. There are two epidermolytic toxins, A which is under chromosomal control and B which is plasmid-mediated, that are most commonly produced by certain strains of phage group II staphylococci. These are proteins that produce intra-epidermal cleavage and are responsible for the scaled skin syndrome, usually in infants. A further toxin producing cleavage at or below the basal layer of the epidermis has been described more recently. This toxin is produced by some phage group I strains of *S. aureus* which cause the 'toxic shock syndrome' described initially in children and may be involved later in the syndrome described later in young women, particularly though not exclusively in the USA (see below), and also though rarely in men.

There are at least six enterotoxins, A, B, C_1, C_2, D, and E and their presence in specimens of food, from incidents of suspected staphylococcal food poisoning or in strains of *S. aureus* grown from specimens of vomit or faeces from patients, is usually detected by gel diffusion immuno-assay. Table 3 summarizes the type of enterotoxin produced by strains of staphylococci causing outbreaks of food poisoning in Britain. Enterotoxin A with or without D is

Table 3　Enterotoxin production by strains of *S. aureus* from 255 outbreaks of food poisoning in Britain*

Enterotoxin produced	Positive	
	Number	%
A	127	50
B	0	0
C	4	1.5
D	16	6
E	3	1
A and B	7	3
A and C	5	2
A and D	54	21
C and D	25	10
C and E	1	0.5
None detected†	13	5

* A single representative strain from each outbreak was selected
† Strains did not produce enterotoxins A to E
Data from Dr R. J. Gilbert, Food Hygiene Laboratory, Central Public Health Laboratory, London

responsible for 75 per cent. Staphylococci of phage groups III or I and III are most often implicated. Food poisoning is produced by the ingestion of food contaminated with staphylococci, from the nose or hands, or from a septic lesion on a food handler. The organisms multiply in suitable conditions and elaborate enterotoxin in the food. The enterotoxins are heat-stable proteins and cause vomiting and diarrhoea within one to six hours of ingestion, but it is not clear whether their main site of action is local, in the gut, or central on the vomiting centre. Enterotoxins are produced by many strains of *S. aureus* including those associated with enterocolitis and by those causing the toxic shock syndrome.

Coagulase-negative staphylococci produce a variety of toxic substances including haemolysins, but these organisms are not usually associated with the pathogenic potential characteristic of *S. aureus*.

Normal flora. Staphylococci and micrococci consitute a major part of the normal flora of human skin. The density of these organisms on normal skin varies from about 10^2 to 10^6 organisms per cm^2 depending on the site, and reaches higher levels on diseased skin. The organisms are characteristically present as microcolonies. *S. aureus* is part of this normal flora in some individuals and in them usually colonizes the nose and perineum although it may be found transiently elsewhere, for example, on the hands: it may colonize widely on diseased skin. About 25 per cent of individuals 'carry' *S. aureus* permanently, 25 per cent never do, and the rest do so occasionally. Some individuals, known as 'shedders', lose large numbers of staphylococci into their environment on skin squames and the organisms may survive in a desiccated state for long periods. Other 'carriers' contaminate their environment less readily, but activity such as hand scrubbing or showering increases shedding.

Host factors in staphylococcal disease. Staphylococci are in the broadest sense opportunistic pathogens. Even in the normal individual they often gain access to the tissues, usually from the commensal flora, by way of damaged skin or mucosa. Thus *S. aureus* is the major pathogen in infected traumatic and surgical wounds, and retains this status despite recent renewed attention to Gram-negative bacilli and anaerobes as wound pathogens. These latter organisms are of greater importance only in infections associated with a breach of the mucosa of sites such as the oropharynx, colon, or vagina. In staphylococcal lung infections, predisposing damage to the tissue may be inflicted by a virus such as influenza or a congenital disease such as cystic fibrosis. The presence of foreign material particularly predisposes the patient to infection with staphylococci; examples of this include intravascular catheters, ventriculo-atrial shunts for hydrocephalus, arterio-venous shunts for haemodialysis, heart valves, and hip prostheses amongst others. Finally immunosuppression, whether congenital or acquired, or the result of a disease or its treatment, may increase susceptibility to staphylococcal infection. Thus children with defective granulocyte function as in chronic granulomatous disease may suffer repeated episodes of infection with *S. aureus*, often with the same strain.

The spread of staphylococci. Staphylococci are commonly transferred from one individual to another, either by direct contact or by contaminated fomites. Airborne transfer of organisms on skin squames is also possible. Contamination of food by one of these routes is the initiating factor in staphylococcal food poisoning. The spread of staphylococci in hospitals gave rise to particular problems in the 1950s and 1960s during which time 'hospital staphylococci' evolved. These were strains that spread widely among hospitalized patients and their attendants, in some cases merely colonizing but in others causing overt, sometimes severe, infection. Furthermore, because of the selective pressure from the increasing use of antibiotics these staphylococci became resistant to many antibiotics. There were major outbreaks of staphylococcal sepsis especially in maternity units and surgical wards, and 'hospital staphylococci' were introduced into the community when patients were discharged still carrying the organisms. Such outbreaks still occur but are distinctly less common in most British hospitals, and are as likely to be caused by sensitive as resistant organisms. The resistance patterns for *S. aureus* isolated from patients in one London teaching hospital over a 20-year period (1958–77) are shown in Table 4.

Antibiotic and antiseptic susceptibility of staphylococci. Forty years ago staphylococci were sensitive to a wide variety of antibiotics, including benzylpenicillin. However, even in 1940, a few isolates of *S. aureus* produced a β-lactamase (penicillinase) and were thus resistant to benzylpenicillin. With the increasing use of penicillin, β-lactamase-producing *S. aureus* (and probably also coagulase-negative staphylococci) became more common, reaching their present incidence of about 85 per cent of isolates some 10 years ago. Staphylococcal β-lactamase attacks a number of penicillins including benzylpenicillin, phenoxymethylpenicillin, ampicillin, amoxycillin, carbenicillin, ticarcillin, azlocillin, and mezlocillin. It also attacks cephaloridine, though less readily, but has negligable effect on methicillin, nafcillin, and the isoxazolyl penicillins, such as cloxacillin, which were introduced specifically for the treatment of staphylococcal infection. However, a resistance mechanism for these semi-synthetic penicillins was soon detected. It is a general resistance mechanism involving all penicillins and most, possibly all, cephalosporins, though it is usually referred to as *methicillin* resistance; it is presumed to result from a change in or inaccessibility of the site of penicillin action. Methicillin resistance is, in general, uncommon in Britain, though this is not the case in some countries and troublesome sporadic outbreaks of infection with such strains have been described and continue to be a problem in some surgical and obstetric units. Another mechanism of resistance to β-lactam antibiotics is tolerance, though its distribution and clinical significance have yet to be determined. Tolerant organisms are those which although inhibited by low concentrations of antibiotic, require much more to achieve a bactericidal effect.

As antibiotics other than the penicillins were introduced and extensively used, staphylococci also became resistant to these

Table 4 Antibiotic resistance of *S. aureus* isolated from hospitalized patients: St Thomas' Hospital, London, 1958–77

% isolates resistant to	1958	1959	1960	1961	1962	1963	1964	1965	1966	1967	1968	1969	1970	1971	1972	1973	1974	1975	1976	1977
Penicillin	80	62	75	63	72	63	72	75	62	73	75	72	78	74	79	82	81	79	85	83
Penicillin, streptomycin, tetracyclin*	20	32	35	25	31	32	18	24	14	9	5	7	7	8	5	4	3	0.4	not tested	
Methicillin	not tested							0.1	0.2	0.5	1	2	1	1	1	2	1	0.4	0.4	<0.05
Erythromycin	18	4	4	2	20	24	15	17	4	3	4	9	3	3	2.5	5	4.5	5	6	7
Lincomycin	not tested												0	0.3	0.3	1	0.5	0.4	0.5	
Fusidic acid	not tested												0	2	2.5	2	2	2.6	3.4	4
Number of isolates	202	771	629	762	1089	1133	1240	1397	957	973	935	1109	1128	1414	1759	1476	1441	1348	1748	2305

* the 'hospital staphylococci'

agents. The 'hospital staphylococcus' was characterized by resistance to penicillin, streptomycin, and tetracycline, and resistance to erythromycin, novobiocin, and chloramphenicol was also not uncommon. All these resistance patterns are now less common and hospital isolates are often indistinguishable from community-aquired strains. Some believe that this is a spontaneous event while others attribute it to better control of cross-infection and wiser use of antibiotics in hospitals.

Among the aminoglycosides, streptomycin was the first drug to which *S. aureus* developed resistance, followed by neomycin, especially when this antibiotic was used topically, and then kanamycin. More recently gentamicin resistance has been an increasing problem, again often associated with the topical use of the agent. Resistance is attributable either to reduced uptake and binding of the antibiotic or to the production of aminoglycoside-modifying enzymes, or in some strains to both mechanisms.

Erythromycin resistance is less common today than in the heyday of the 'hospital staphylococcus'. Staphylococci passaged in the presence of this drug or of related macrolides may develop a more or less stable resistance not only to the agent tested but to all macrolides. A type of resistance that has been called 'dissociated resistance' emerges in staphylococci during threatment of patients with erythromycin. Most of the staphylococci in a population developing this type of resistance are initially sensitive to erythromycin, but, if grown on a medium containing the drug, emerge as highly resistant, not only to erythromycin itself but to other macrolides and to the unrelated drugs clindamycin and lincomycin. In the absence of erythromycin the resistance is lost and the organisms appear sensitive.

Resistance of staphylococci to fusidic acid is uncommon but most cultures of *S. aureus* contain a small number of resistant mutants and a fully resistant population can readily emerge both *in vitro* and *in vivo*, the latter being particularly likely after topical use. Vancomycin resistance among staphylococci is rare: we have never encountered such a strain and this may well be related to the limited clinical use of this agent. Rifampicin is extremely active against *S. aureus* but as with fusidic acid, minority populations of resistant cells are found and resistance to this agent readily emerges.

In some contrast to this changing problem of resistance to antibiotics, the staphylococcus has changed little in its susceptibility to other agents. Most disinfectants and antiseptics continue to inhibit or kill the organism. Perhaps most important are the antiseptics: chlorhexidine and hexachlorophane and iodine or iodine-containing compounds such as povidone iodine are probably most used for skin disinfection and when used correctly are highly effective in removing staphylococci from the skin.

Clinical spectrum

The three major staphylococcal species are associated with quite distinct disease spectra and are thus considered seperately. It has become increasingly clear that coagulase-negative staphylococci are not always harmless saprophytes, nor do they merely mimic the more important *S. aureus*.

Staphylococcus aureus

The major inter-relationships between *S. aureus* and man are shown in Fig. 1. Organisms from the patient's own carrier sites or from another individual may give rise to infection which is usually localized but may spread contiguously, or via the lymphatics or blood resulting in bacteraemia and metastatic infection. Staphylococcal food poisoning is an exception to the general rule in that the patient is at no stage infected with the organism.

Staphylococcal food poisoning. This syndrome is caused by the ingestion of enterotoxin preformed in the food. About 5 per cent only of outbreaks of bacterial food poisoning reported to the British Communicable Disease Surveillance Centre for which an aetiological agent is identified are caused by *S. aureus*. The food is usually

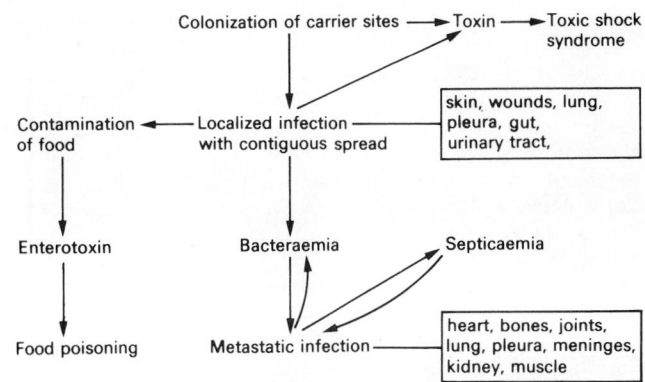

Fig. 1   Inter-relationship between *S. aureus* and man.

contaminated during its preparation by an individual infected with or shedding the organism. Unrefrigerated, protein-rich foods containing meat or milk, are particularly likely to support the growth of staphylococci and the subsequent production of enterotoxin which can then survive cooking. Within a few hours of ingesting the food, the victim feels unwell and soon starts to vomit. Severely affected individuals may have abdominal pain and fever, and may even develop fatal shock, but the symptoms usually subside rapidly and recovery is complete with 24–48 hours. Many patients will have recovered before medical aid can be sought but fluid and electrolyte replacement may be necessary in those severely affected. Antibacterial chemotherapy is not necessary.

Localized infection. *Infection of the skin and appendages. S. aureus* causes skin infections in patients of all ages. Newborn babies may develop skin pustules, or more rarely, pemphigus neonatorum, a severe generalized infection characterized by bullae. They may also develop a purulent discharge from the umbilicus, conjunctivitis or 'sticky eye' (in the newborn very often staphylococcal), or more rarely breast abscess.

The staphylococcal scalded skin syndrome, known as Lyell's disease or, in the neonate, Ritter's disease, also primarily affects young children: a minor staphylococcal infection caused by a strain producing epidermolytic toxin is followed by extensive skin erythema and blistering and the upper layers of the epidermis are shed in sheets. The affected areas show minimal inflammatory response and few staphylococci are found in them. Most affected children eventually recover.

Impetigo is a skin lesion, characterized by blisters that break and become covered with crusting exudate. Most cases are caused by *S. aureus*, usually of phage group II, though others are caused by *Streptococcus pyogenes* and in some both organisms are involved. Children are most commonly affected, especially on the face.

Folliculitis, a superficial infection of the hair follicles, is also usually staphylococcal. Persistent folliculitis of the beard area 'sycosis barbae', is primarily a foreign-body reaction to hair, with secondary infection that is sometimes caused by *S. aureus* but more often by *S. epidermis*. If the subcutaneous tissue becomes involved, a boil or furuncle results. These tend to occur on the neck, axillae (Fig. 2), buttocks, and thighs, are frequently recurrent, and may involve more than one member of a family. Although boils in the perineal region are caused by *S. aureus*, perirectal abscesses, particularly those with an associated fistula-in-ano, are usually caused by colonic bacteria. Occasionally staphylococcal skin sepsis, particularly on the neck, results in the development of a carbuncle, a large indurated painful lesion with several discharging sinuses (Fig. 3). Styes, or hordeola, are staphylococcal infections involving the rim of the eyelid. A rare but serious complication of staphylococcal infection of the face is cavernous sinus thrombosis. Most paronychias are also staphylococcal though streptococci, anaerobes, *Candida albicans* and *Herpes simplex* may cause clinically indistinguishable infection. Staphylococcal breast abscesses usually develop

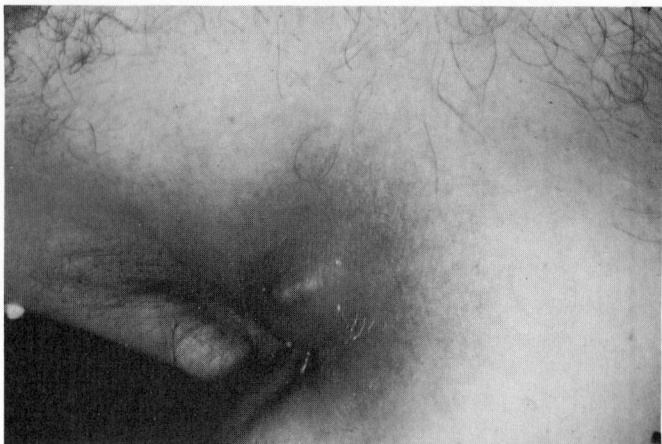

Fig. 2 Axillary abscess.

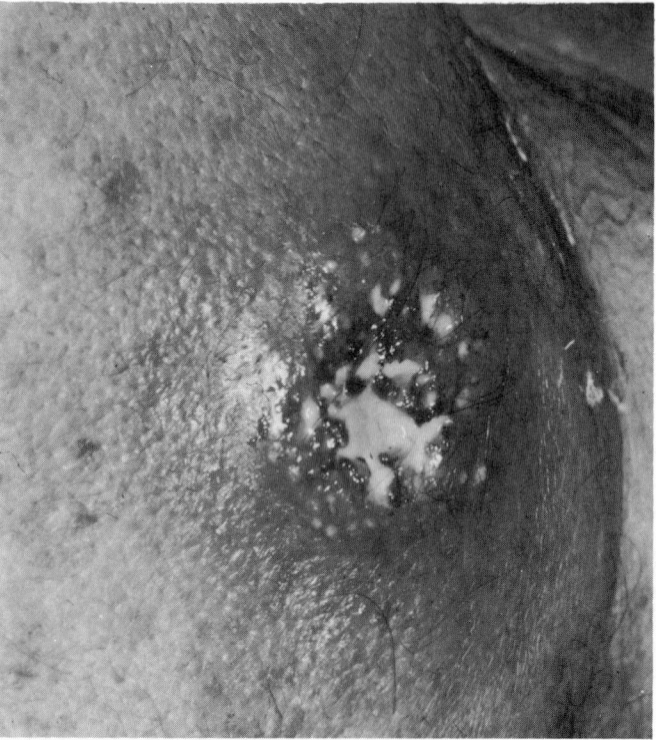

Fig. 3 Carbuncle of neck.

in the puerperium and may be associated with staphylococcal infection of the baby. Staphylococci have been associated with Meleney's synergistic gangrene but the evidence is difficult to assess.

Infections of the ear. S. aureus is commonly involved in otitis externa and sometimes, but much less frequently in otitis media. This latter condition is usually caused by *Str. pyogenes*, *H. influenzae*, or *Str. pneumoniae*.

Wound infection. S. aureus remains the commonest cause of wound infection following surgery or trauma which does not involve mucous membranes with their rich anaerobic commensal flora. The clinical presentation of staphylococcal wound infection ranges from minimal erythema and serous discharge, through small abscesses, often in relation to sutures, to cellulitis with deep pus and wound dehiscence accompanied by systemic illness. Serious staphylococcal sepsis may complicate surgery or trauma involving the central nervous system, bones and joints, and the eye giving rise to problems beyond those of simple wound infections, though the staphylococcus still gains access directly rather than via the bloodstream.

Infection at the site of insertion of intravenous catheters or cannulas, especially those left in place for more than about 48 hours, may present as obvious local sepsis, or more insidiously, as a pyrexia, often severe, with no overt localizing signs. Sudden pyrexia in a patient receiving chronic haemodialysis frequently results from unremarkable staphylococcal sepsis at the site of an arteriovenous fistula.

Pleuro-pulmonary infection. Staphylococcal pneumonia may arise in the previously normal lung that has been seeded by organisms from the blood stream (see below) but far more often arises as a complication of pre-existing lung disease, except in the young infant who can develop a primary staphylococcal pneumonia without predisposing lung disease. Staphylococci from the patient's own sites of carriage are presumed to reach the damaged lung tissue via the trachea and bronchi. Influenza is the most usual predisposing disease in Britain, and S. aureus and Streptococcus pneumoniae are almost equally common secondary invaders, with *Haemophilus influenzae* and *Str. pyogenes* in a few cases. In children, other viral infections of the lower respiratory tract, including severe measles in developing countries, may become secondarily infected by the same group of bacteria. S. aureus is also one of the most important secondary invaders of already damaged lungs and bronchi in patients with cystic fibrosis and it is often the first of many organisms, eventually including *Haemophilus influenzae*, coliforms and *Pseudomonas aeruginosa*.

Staphylococcal pneumonia is characteristically patchy in distribution and is often complicated by abscess formation, empyema, and sometimes by bacteraemia. The patient is usually severely prostrated with high fever and cyanosis and may become disorientated, shocked, and finally comatose. When staphylococcal pneumonia is secondary to influenza, its onset may occur within only a day or two of the initial symptoms with alarming suddenness. The mortality is high, especially in elderly and debilitated patients.

Staphylococcal enterocolitis. This rare disease, acquired in hospitals, is caused by enterotoxin-producing strains of S. aureus that are usually resistant to several antibiotics. In the past when 'hospital staphylococci' were prevalent, it usually arose as a complication of intestinal surgery in a patient given tetracycline. With the disappearance of the 'hospital staphylococcus' the disease too has virtually disappeared. Staphylococcal enterocolitis causes loss of fluid and electrolytes into the gut; the patient may collapse and even succumb before the onset of diarrhoea raises a suspicion of the diagnosis. Fever and abdominal distension are usually present.

Urinary tract infection. S. aureus urinary tract infection is rare. Interestingly, the urinary tract is one of the few sites in which coagulase-negative staphylococci are more important pathogens than coagulase-positive organisms. S. aureus infection probably does not occur in a normal urinary tract other than in the presence of overwhelming septicaemia, but it is found, though infrequently, in patients with abnormal bladder function, usually in association with instrumentation of catheterization. It may also occur occasionally after open prostatectomy in conjunction with an infected wound.

Toxic shock syndrome. This apparently new syndrome, characterized by high fever, diarrhoea, shock, and an erythematous rash, was first described in 1978 in seven children, three boys and four girls, aged between 8 and 17 years. In five of the seven cases, S. aureus of phage group I was isolated from the nasopharynx, vagina, or a localized abscess though not from the blood. Soon after this original description, a similar toxic shock syndrome was described in menstruating women, initially in the USA, but later, though rarely in several other countries. It was shown to be associated with the use of tampons and in the USA with one brand in particular. It has also been described in women who were not menstruating and in men. A mortality rate of around 10 per cent has been reported. The strains of S. aureus isolated from patients with the toxic shock syndrome have been resistant to penicillin, and a penicillinase-resistant antibiotic should be used in an attempt to eradicate the organism. However, since this is a toxin-mediated infection, the

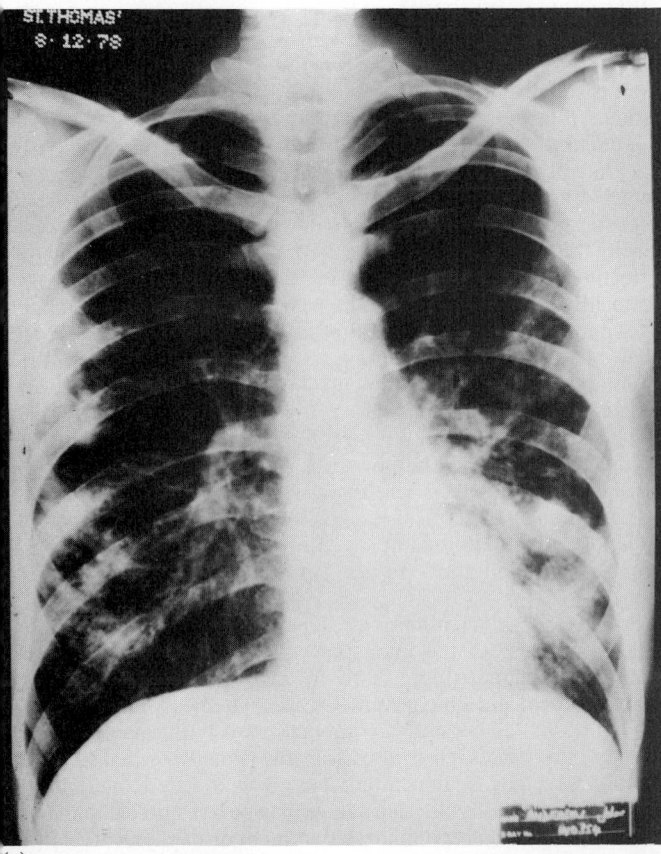

(a)

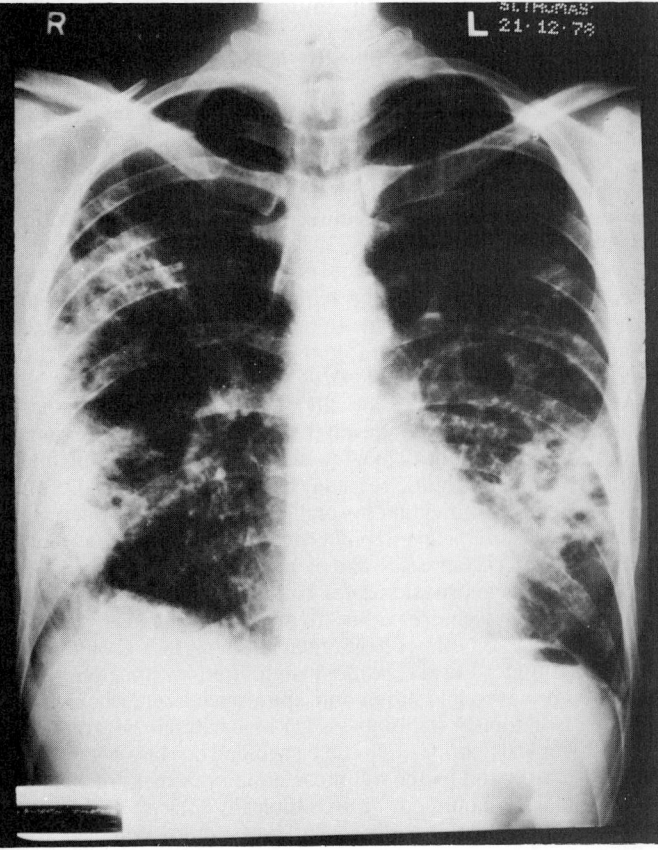

(b)

Fig. 4 Chest radiograph of a 24-year-old man with severe staphylococcal toxaemia (a) on admission; (b) 13 days later. The patient was also suffering from influenza B.

treatment consists primarily of general supportive measures to combat shock.

Bacteraemia and septicaemia. It is possible, though difficult to prove, that staphylococci occasionally gain access to the blood stream from carrier sites. This might explain the occurrence of deep staphylococcal infection without antecedent superficial infection. However, bacteraemia probably does occur not uncommonly as a complication of superficial and often quite minor staphylococcal sepsis, thus providing the usual source of deep infections. Bacteraemia, strictly, merely implies the presence of bacteria in the blood and this may or may not be symptomatic. A symptomatic bacteraemia is usually referred to as a septicaemia. Severe staphylococcal sepsis often gives rise to bacteraemia and *S. aureus* accounts for some 20 per cent of all cases of bacteraemia seen in hospitals.

Metastatic infection. *Endocarditis.* Staphylococcal infection of the heart valves is one of the conditions that may arise without obvious preceding infection or may complicate staphylococcal infection elsewhere. There are four major types. Firstly, *S. aureus* is a rare cause of classical subacute bacterial endocarditis, clinically indistinguishable from the more usual streptococcal infection. Secondly, it is an important cause of endocarditis (usually fatal) associated with intra-cardiac prosthetic surgery. Such infection generally occurs within a few weeks of surgery, often as a complication of sternal wound sepsis. Thirdly, staphylococcal endocarditis is seen in intravenous drug abusers who develop a characteristic right-sided endocarditis with concomitant metastatic lung infection. Finally, *S. aureus* may cause acute endocarditis, usually as a complication of overwhelming septicaemia. Patients with staphylococcal endocarditis have the signs and symptoms characteristic of the disease in general. They usually present with malaise and fever, and are found to have a heart murmur, but occasionally present with the signs of infected emboli, such as brain and kidney abscess, or lung abscesses in those with right-sided infection.

Osteomyelitis. This is mainly a disease of children, particularly boys, who present with a history of minor infection or more commonly trauma, followed by the prompt onset of local pain and tenderness, usually in the leg, with malaise and fever. Chronic infection, with draining sinuses, often supervened in the pre-antibiotic era. Staphylococcal osteomyelitis may occur at other ages including the neonate, and when it involves the vertebrae in the adult it may present with pain and little else, thus often leading to diagnostic difficulty. Overall, *S. aureus* is the commonest cause of osteomyelitis at all ages: it is not however, the only cause.

Septic arthritis. This infection can occur at all ages and involves both previously normal and abnormal joints. Patients with long-standing rheumatoid arthritis treated with steroids are particularly liable to suffer from infection (usually staphylococcal) of an already diseased joint. Such infection may cause diagnostic confusion since it may be mistaken clinically for an acute flare-up of rheumatoid arthritis. Microscopy and culture of the fluid aspirated from such a joint is essential in establishing the diagnosis.

Pneumonia and lung abscess. Staphylococcal bacteraemia may result in metastatic infection in the lungs. In contrast to those with staphylococcal pneumonia complicating viral infections (see above), the patient often presents with lung abscess rather than pneumonia.

Meningitis. Staphylococcal meningitis may result, though rarely, from septic emboli in endocarditis which may first produce brain abscesses, or from bacteraemia.

Renal carbuncle, perinephric abscess. These forms of metastatic staphylococcal infection are rare. A renal carbuncle is an abscess in the cortex, and, although in this infection and in perinephric abscess *S. aureus* may sometimes be isolated from the blood, it is seldom found in the urine. Both infections usually produce fever and localizing signs.

Tropical pyomyositis. In this condition a usually solitary large abscess occurs in one of the major muscles of the trunk or limbs, otherwise an unusual site for staphylococcal infection. The predisposing factors have yet to be identified. This disease is common in certain areas of tropical Africa but is not associated with malnutrition or with preceding skin sepsis.

Diagnosis. *S. aureus* is readily isolated in the laboratory and swabs, pus, or other infected material should be submitted. A Gram-stained film will usually enable a rapid diagnosis of the staphylococcal aetiology to be made: the characteristic clumps of Gram-stained cocci which may be intra- as well as extra-cellular are readily identifiable. This diagnosis can be confirmed by routine culture methods within 24 hours. Staphylococcal bacteraemia is detected by routine blood culture methods, but though the isolation of *S. aureus* is usually indicative of a genuine bacteraemia, this organism may occasionally contaminate blood cultures when it is present on normal or diseased skin. However, such contamination is much less likely with *S. aureus* than with coagulase-negative staphylococci. The diagnosis of staphylococcal food poisoning usually rests on the detection of enterotoxin-producing *S. aureus* in large numbers in the patient's faeces or in food.

Treatment. Drainage of pus where this is present is an essential prerequisite in the management of staphylococcal infection. This may occur spontaneously or with only minor surgical intervention in most superficial infections such as boils, paronychias, and styes. Deep abscesses including osteomyelitis that has progressed to the point of pus formation, require surgical drainage, though in lung abscesses postural drainage accompanied by appropriate chemotherapy will usually suffice. Infection in association with a prosthesis may well necessitate its removal and infection of an intravenous infusion site will rarely resolve until the cannula or catheter is removed.

Antibiotic therapy is indicated if the patient is systemically ill or if the infection shows signs of persisting or spreading. Sometimes antibiotics given early in the course of a potentially localizing pyogenic infection may prevent its progression. Table 5 is a general

guide to the antibiotics useful in staphylococcal infection. The initial choice of agent depends on the patterns of susceptibility of *S. aureus* in the community from which the patient comes. Penicillin itself is the drug of choice only if the isolate can be shown not to produce β-lactamase, and should never be used for the initial 'blind' treatment of staphylococcal infection. Ampicillin and amoxycillin have no place in the treatment of staphylococcal infections. A penicillinase-resistant penicillin such as flucloxacillin is usually appropriate but definitive treatment should be based on *in vitro* sensitivity tests on the patient's own organism whenever possible. Effective drugs include the semi-synthetic penicillins—methicillin, cloxacillin, flucloxacillin, oxacillin, or nafcillin—and the macrolides and related drugs, such as erythromycin, lincomycin, or clindamycin, and one of these latter groups is suitable for the treatment of patients hypersensitive to penicillin. Some would use a cephalosporin under these circumstances but a few patients show hypersensitivity to all β-lactam antibiotics. Fusidic acid is an excellent antistaphylococcal agent, but because of the readiness with which resistance develops, its use is perhaps best reserved for severe infections such as septicaemia, endocarditis, and bone and joint infections. It should then be given in combination with one of the agents mentioned above to prevent the emergence of such resistance.

Staphylococcal meningitis presents considerable difficulties in therapy because of the inadequate penetration into the CSF of many agents that are highly active *in vitro* against *S. aureus* including fusidic acid and clindamycin. Chloramphenicol or flucloxacillin, in high doses, or possibly a combination of both, may be useful.

Aminoglycosides, co-trimoxazole and trimethoprim may also be useful, especially in the initial treatment of severe, initially undiagnosed infections but such agents may be less suitable than those already mentioned for definitive treatment of staphylococcal infections. Gentamicin is better than kanamycin, because resistance to it is less common. Finally useful antibiotics in the face of multiple antibiotic resistance are rifampicin, generally given in combination with other agents because of the likelihood of resistance emerging, and vancomycin. Vancomycin is also particularly valuable for the treatment of staphylococcal infections in patients receiving haemodialysis, as it is excreted almost exclusively by the kidney and is only very slowly removed by dialysis. It is also used as an oral preparation in the treatment of staphylococcal enterocolitis. There is, however, no indication for antimicrobial therapy of any kind in staphylococcal food poisoning.

In all cases the antibiotic should be administered for about two to three days after the patient's temperature subsides or there is obvious clinical improvement. In bone and joint infections, treatment is usually continued for four to six weeks in most cases and in endocarditis for about six weeks.

Antibiotic policies were initially devised in the face of the increasing resistance of the 'hospital staphylococcus'. They seek to limit the use of antibiotics to a few chosen agents, reserving others for difficult and antibiotic-resistant cases. Such policies are often highly specific to individual hospitals or even to individuals.

Recurrent superficial staphylococcal infections may require disinfection of carrier sites and it may be helpful to use hexachloraphane or chlorhexidine for bathing and to apply antiseptic ointment such as chlorhexidine to the anterior nares. Systemic antibiotics may sometimes help eradication but they should not be used as a routine. Local treatment is required for impetigo: crusts should be removed and either antiseptics such as chlorhexidine or clioquinol or topical antibiotics such as bacitracin or gramicidin applied. Topical neomycin should be avoided because of the risk of skin sensitivity, and in general those antibiotics that are available for systemic use should not be used topically because of the risk of resistance.

The role of immunization in the prevention of recurrent infection is difficult to assess. The most widely used preparation in the past was staphylococcal toxoid, but no controlled trials have been undertaken. It is now rarely used.

Table 5 Antibiotics for the treatment of infections caused by *S. aureus*

	Penicillinase-negative strains (< 20% isolates)	Penicillinase-positive strains (> 80% isolates)
Moderate sepsis	penicillin cephalosporin erythromycin clindamycin	flucloxacillin cephalosporin erythromycin clindamycin
Severe sepsis e.g. endocarditis	penicillin and fusidic acid erythromycin and fusidic acid vancomycin	flucloxacillin and fusidic acid erythromycin and fusidic acid vancomycin
Bone/joint infections	penicillin and fusidic acid erythromycin and fusidic acid clindamycin	flucloxacillin and fusidic acid erythromycin and fusidic acid clindamycin
Meningitis	penicillin and/or chloramphenicol intrathecal penicillin gentamicin	flucloxacillin and/or chloramphenicol intrathecal flucloxacillin gentamicin
Sepsis in patients on haemodialysis	vancomycin	vancomycin

Notes

1. In patients hypersensitive to penicillin avoid penicillin, flucloxacillin, and probably the cephalosporins
2. For 'methicillin'-resistant *S. aureus*, choice will be guided by *in vitro* tests but one or more of the non-β-lactam antibiotics listed above will usually be appropriate, with rifampicin or trimethoprim as additional possibilities

Cross-infection control. Many of the aseptic procedures used in hospitals have been found particularly applicable to the control of staphylococcal cross-infection. It is now believed that the main cause of cross-infection is via hands and that there is relatively little transfer via contaminated articles and equipment or via the air. Hand washing is important together with standard 'no touch' techniques in the use of instruments and the wearing of gloves when contact is inevitable. Operating theatre procedures extend these precautions by covering much of the operator with fabric relatively impermeable to bacteria, by restricting activity in the operating room, and by the disinfection of the surgeon's and patient's skin with iodine, or alcohol with or without antiseptics such as chlorhexidine. Similar disinfection of the patient's skin is indicated before the insertion of intravenous cannulae, lumbar puncture, and before numerous other invasive procedures. The strict application of 'no-touch' techniques is difficult in neonatal units and it is usual to apply antiseptics such as alcohol or chlorhexidine to the umbilicus, an important source of cross infection with *S. aureus*. Antiseptics can also be used for bathing babies and in addition mothers can be encouraged to care for their own babies thus minimizing contact with staff.

In the face of persistent cross-infection in obstetric units control has been attained by the inoculation of the new born child's nose and umbilicus with 'avirulent' *S. aureus* 502A, This is not done routinely because the avirulent staphylococcus in fact retains limited pathogenicity and may cause pustules and conjunctivitis and rarely more serious infection.

Staphylococcus epidermidis

This staphylococcus, although often dismissed as a harmless commensal, can be an important pathogen in man. It has a curious predeliction for plastic materials and causes infection in association with intravenous lines, prosthetic heart valves, arteriovenous shunts used for haemodialysis, and ventriculo-atrial shunts used for hydrocephalus. Such infections are unlikely to resolve unless the prosthetic material is removed; an appropriate antibiotic based on *in vitro* sensitivity tests on the organism should also be given. It also commonly produces bacteriuria in the catheterized patient particularly following prostatectomy whether transurethral or open: such infections, whilst frequently asymptomatic and very likely to clear spontaneously on removal of the urethral catheter, are sometimes of clinical significance and may require antibiotic therapy. Very occasionally *S. epidermidis* causes endocarditis, involving rheumatic, degenerative, congenital, prosthetic, or even previously normal valves. Since this organism, together with other coagulase-negative staphylococci found on the skin not infrequently contaminate blood cultures, several will be required to establish the existence of a true *S. epidermidis* bacteraemia, and this is of vital importance in the bacteriological diagnosis of endocarditis.

The antibiotic sensitivity patterns of *S. epidermidis* are varied and unpredictable and resistance to many of the agents so useful against *S. aureus* is fairly common. Many strains produce β-lactamase and a significant number also exhibit resistance to methicillin (and thus to most penicillins and cephalosporins). Resistance to aminoglycosides, in particular to gentamicin, is also common. The antibiotic treatment of any genuine infection caused by *S. epidermidis* should be guided by the laboratory since many agents may need to be tested to determine optimum therapy

Staphylococcus saprophyticus

This curiously named coagulase-negative staphylococcus, although a skin commensal, is also an important urinary pathogen and ranks second only to *Escherichia coli* as a cause of urinary infection in young women. It commonly produces cystitis but may cause infection of the upper urinary tract and has also been isolated from patients with infected calculi. In this latter context the ability of many strains of *S. saprophyticus* to split urea rapidly is of undoubted significance. Most strains are readily identifiable in the

laboratory by their resistance to novobiocin. They are, in contrast to many strains of *S. epidermidis* often sensitive to a wide range of antibiotics and thus their treatment seldom poses problems.

Acknowledgement

We are grateful to Dr R. Marples and Mrs M. de Saxe, Cross-infection Laboratory, and Dr R. Gilbert, Food Hygiene Laboratory, Central Public Health Laboratory, London, for helpful advice.

References

Cohen, J. O. (ed.) (1972). *The staphylococci*. Wiley, New York.
Skinner, F. A. and Carr, J. G. (eds.) (1974). *The normal microbial flora of man*. 1. Academic Press, London.
Williams, R. E. O., Blowers, R. Garrod, L. P., and Shooter, R. A. (1966). *Hospital infection: causes and prevention*, 2nd edn. Lloyd Luke, London.
— and Shooter, R. A. (eds.) (1963). *Infection in hospitals: epidemiology and control*. Blackwell Scientific Publications, Oxford.
Wilson, G. S. and Miles, A. (eds.) (1975). *Topley and Wilson's principles of bacteriology, virology and immunity*, chapter 66, Staphylococcal disease, 1948–1977. Arnold, London.

Meningococcal infection

B. M. Greenwood

Meningococcal disease is caused by infection with a Gram-negative diplococcus, *Neisseria meningitidis*. It is likely that epidemic meningococcal disease is a relatively new condition. Outbreaks were recorded first in Geneva in 1805 and then in New England the following year. Because of the characteristic features of meningococcal disease, it seems unlikely that outbreaks of the infection would have remained unreported, had they occurred at an earlier time. Meningococcal disease was reported in north Africa in 1840, and epidemics were recorded for the first time in sub-Saharan Africa during the first years of the present century. The meningococcus was identified as a cause of meningitis by Weichselbaum in 1887.

The organism. Meningococci usually appear in clinical samples as bean-shaped, Gram negative diplococci. Meningococci are delicate organisms which are very sensitive to chilling or drying; samples must therefore be inoculated and cultured as soon as possible after collection. Transport media, such as Stuart's medium, can be used when this is not possible. Meningococci grow best on enriched media such as Mueller–Hinton medium, incubated at 37° C in an atmosphere containing 5–10 per cent CO_2. Selective media containing antibiotics, such as vancomycin and polymyxin, are useful in identifying meningococci at sites with a mixed flora, such as the nasopharynx.

Structural analysis has shown that meningococci possess an outer polysaccharide capsule, an outer membrane, a cytoplasmic membrane, and an underlying peptidoglycan layer. Some avirulent strains do not possess an outer capsule. Fine pili extend from the outer membrane through the capsule to the outside. On electron microscopy blebs have been observed in the cell wall which contain endotoxin. Three structural components of the meningococcus have been used for serotyping. Structural differences in capsular polysaccharide define eight different serogroups—A, B, C, X, Y, Z, W135, and 29e. The biochemical structure of these different capsular polysaccharides has been defined; that of the group A meningococcus is a polymer of N-acetyl-3-0-acetyl mannosamine phosphate and that of the group C meningococcus a polymer of N-acetyl and o-acetyl neuraminic acid. The capsular polysaccharide of the group B meningococcus, a polymer of N-acetyl neuraminic acid, is very similar antigenically to the capsular polysaccharide of *Escherichia coli* KI, a common cause a neonatal meningitis. Meningococci of the eight different capsular polysaccharide antigen serogroups differ in their virulence and in their geographical distribution. Most cases of meningococcal meningitis are caused by organisms belonging to serogroups A, B, or C. Meningococcal pneumonia is usually caused by organisms belonging to serogroup Y. The outer membrane contains a major outer membrane protein and lipopolysaccharide; both these components have been used to type meningococci. It has been shown by bactericidal assay that a high proportion of group B and group C meningococcal strains isolated from patients with meningococcal disease possess outer membrane protein antigen 2. This serotype antigen is found less frequently among strains isolated from asymptomatic carriers and it is thus a marker of virulence. Polyacrylamide gel electrophoresis has demonstrated heterogeneity among meningococcal lipopolysaccharides but the epidemiological significance of individual antigens has not yet been defined.

Until 1963 nearly all strains of meningococci were very sensitive to sulphonamides but sulphonamide resistance is now widespread among organisms belonging to all the major serogroups.

Epidemiology. The meningococcus has no respect for race or climate and meningococcal disease occurs throughout the world. In areas with a temperate climate the infection is usually endemic. In such areas there is some annual variation in the incidence of the infection but a moderate number of cases are seen every year. At present 500–1000 cases are reported annually in the United Kingdom. Collection of national statistics disguises the fact that even in countries where the infection is endemic, there may be localized areas with a relatively high attack rate. Since the end of the Second World War there have been few major epidemics of meningococcal disease in Europe or north America, perhaps because of general improvements in social conditions. However, the threat of major epidemics of meningococcal disease has not been completely abolished from countries with high living standards, for an extensive epidemic of group A meningococcal meningitis recently occurred in Finland.

At present the major health hazard posed by the meningococcus lies in a belt of sub-Saharan Africa extending from the Sudan in the East to Gambia in the West—the African 'meningitis belt'. Within this area of savanna Africa major epidemics of meningococcal disease occur every 5–10 years. Up to 100 000 people have been affected during individual epidemics and the meningococcus is still responsible for many deaths in this region. Why this geographical area should be so prone to epidemics of meningococcal disease is not known. Within the African 'meningitis belt' epidemics nearly always start in the middle of the dry season, when it is hot and very dry, and end a few months later with the coming of the rains. Epidemics do not extend into the forest regions of West and Central Africa where conditions of very low absolute humidity are never met. In countries with a temperate climate meningococcal disease is seen most frequently during the winter, a time of low absolute humidity. Perhaps low absolute humidity impairs the local surface defences of the upper respiratory tract.

There are considerable geographical variations in the distribution of meningococcal serotypes responsible for cases of clinical disease. In the United States most clinical infections are caused by group C or group B meningococci, whilst in Europe group B meningococci predominate. Recent epidemics in Brazil, Finland, and Mongolia were caused by group A meningococci. Most African epidemics are caused by group A meningococci but outbreaks of group C meningococcal disease have recently been reported in West Africa.

The spread of meningococci is favoured by overcrowding and poor living conditions. Studies in towns affected by an epidemic have shown that the attack rate is highest in the poorest, most crowded areas of the town and lowest in prosperous suburbs. Outbreaks have occurred on many occasions in barracks, hostels, and boarding schools. However, children attending a day school at which there has been a case of meningococcal disease do not have an increased risk of contracting the infection. It is uncertain whether hospital personnel dealing with patients with meningococcal disease, or with their laboratory samples, are at increased risk from infection. Cases of meningococcal disease have been described among hospital staff and in research scientists working with meningococci but, during a recent epidemic in Nigeria, the attack rate among hospital staff was similar to that recorded in the general population living around the hospital.

Only a small proportion of subjects infected with meningococci develop clinical disease; the majority become asymptomatic carriers. Thus, if the epidemiology of meningococcal infection is to be determined in a specific population, carrier studies, as well as case finding studies, must be performed. Many carrier surveys have been undertaken during the course of military and civilian epidemics. On the basis of early surveys, it was suggested that outbreaks were likely to occur only when the carrier rate exceeded a certain level. It is now recognized that this relationship does not necessarily apply and that epidemics may occur when the carrier rate in the general population is low. Conversely clinical cases of disease are often rare in populations with a high carriage rate of a potentially pathogenic strain. As an epidemic progresses, the carriage rate of the epidemic strain increased in the general population.

Only a few carriage studies have been undertaken in non-epidemic circumstances. These have shown that carriage is often prolonged; an average duration of carriage of 9.6 months was observed in a study of American civilians. Detailed studies of carriage in households allow some deductions to be made as to how the infection is usually spread. It appears that in the United States and in Brazil infection is often spread from an asymptomatic carrier father to a young susceptible child in his household who develops clinical disease. In savanna Africa spread from child to child is probably a more usual pathway of infection.

Families of patients with meningococcal disease have an increased risk of contracting the infection. This risk is relatively low (< 1 per cent) when the infection is endemic but may reach a figure as high as 5 per cent during epidemics. Siblings of a patient are the group most at risk. Because many secondary household infections occur within a few days of the onset of illness in the index case, it is probable that some are co-primary infections derived from a common source rather than true secondary cases.

Where meningococcal infection is endemic, most cases of clinical disease are seen among the very young (Fig. 1). In England over three-quarters of all reported cases of meningococcal disease are in children less than five years old. When epidemics occur in industrialized countries, older children and adults are affected more frequently. In the African 'meningitis belt' the disease is seen most often in children age 5–15 years. Children under the age of one year are infected infrequently in this region, perhaps because they are protected by prolonged breast feeding.

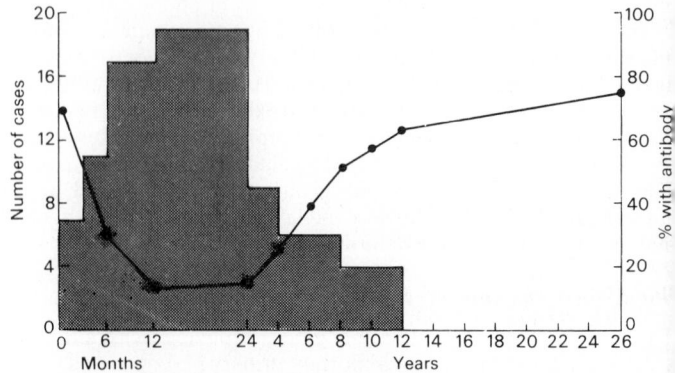

Fig. 1   The relationship between the age at onset of meningococcal disease in American children and the prevalence of bactericidal antibodies in subjects of different ages. Group C meningococcal antibody levels are shown. A similar pattern was obtained for group A and group B meningococcal bactericidal antibodies. (From Goldschneider *et al.* (1969). *J. exp. Med.* **129**, 1307.)

Immunity. There are two main lines of defence against meningococcal infection. Local surface defence mechanisms can prevent colonization of the nasopharynx by meningococci, whilst antibody can ensure that any bacteria reaching the circulation are destroyed.

Little is known about surface immunity to meningococci. It would be anticipated that locally produced secretory IgA antibodies would have a protective role, perhaps by preventing bacterial adherence to epithelial cells, but it has been shown that serum IgA meningococcal antibodies enhance, rather than inhibit, the growth of meningococci, perhaps by blocking bactericidal IgG and IgM antibodies. Meningococci produce a protease enzyme which splits IgA sub-class I molecules, destroying much of their antibody properties. Strains isolated from both patients and from carriers produce this enzyme, but it is not produced by harmless *neisseria*. It has been suggested that damage to the surface defence mechanisms by an upper respiratory tract virus infection or by low absolute humidity predisposes to systemic meningococcal infection but this suggestion is difficult to prove.

The importance of antibody in preventing meningococcal disease has been clearly demonstrated. Patients who have experienced a clinical infection develop bactericidal antibodies against meningococcal polysaccharide and protein components. Formation of such antibodies was probably the means by which some patients recovered from the infection in the days before antibiotics were discovered. Patients who have recovered from a clinical infection are immune to reinfection with meningococci of the same serogroup as the organism that caused their illness and, perhaps, to infection with meningococci of other serotypes. The presence or absence of such serum bactericidal antibodies determines susceptibility to infection. In 1922 Heist and his colleagues reported that blood from more than 95 per cent of adult men was bactericidal to meningococci. Heist, who was one of the few individuals without antibody, died from meningococcal infection. Further evidence for the protective role of antibody has been provided by a classical series of studies carried out in the United States. These investigations have shown that among American children of different ages, an inverse relationship exists between susceptibility to meningococcal infection and the number of children with bactericidal antibodies (Fig. 1). Furthermore, a study of army recruits showed that only 3 of 54 recruits who developed group C meningococcal meningitis in an army camp had a significant titre of anti group C bactericidal antibody when they entered camp whilst over 80 per cent of recruits who did not develop meningitis had bactericidal antibodies at this time. Recruits with group C meningitis had lower antibody titres to meningococci of other serogroups than controls, but it is unlikely that they were generally immunodeficient as they developed a good antibody response to the meningococcus responsible for their acute infection. Why some soldiers had lower initial antibody levels than others was not established. It has been suggested that genetic factors influence susceptibility to meningococcal disease. Study of a small group of Americans showed a relationship between the immune response to vaccination with meningococcal polysaccharide and the possession of certain immunoglobulin allotypes. However, no relation between susceptibility to infection and HLA haplotype or immunoglobulin allotype was found among Nigerian families in whom there had been more than one case of meningococcal disease.

Nasopharyngeal carriage of meningococci induces serum antibody formation and it is therefore likely that the bactericidal antibody found in most healthy adults is produced in this way. Some subjects are immunized by carriage of a potentially pathogenic strain whilst others are immunized by infection with nonpathogenic meningococci or by infection with *N. lactamica*, a bacterium which is very similar to the meningococcus, but which, unlike the meningococcus, ferments lactose. Nasopharyngeal infection with *N. lactamica* is common in young children, reaching a peak at about the age of 18 months. Some children infected with this bacterium develop bactericidal antibodies effective against group A, group B, and group C meningococci.

Complement plays an important part in antibody-mediated killing of meningococci, and patients with complement deficiencies show an increased susceptibility to meningococcal disease. As patients with deficiencies of either early or late complement components are susceptible it is likely that complement enhances both phagocytosis and lysis of meningococci. However, antibody can kill meningococci in the absence of complement by means of an antibody dependent cytotoxicity system which involves K cells.

Patients with meningococcal disease develop cell-mediated immune responses to meningococcal components, but whether these cell-mediated immune reactions have any protective function is not known.

Pathogenesis. To cause disease, meningococci must be able to establish themselves in the nasopharynx. How this is achieved is not fully understood. Encapsulated meningococci with pili adhere strongly to epithelial cells, whilst non-piliated encapsulated strains do not. However, it is unlikely that attachment through pili is the only means by which meningococci can adhere to epithelial cells because non-encapsulated organisms usually attach strongly whether they possess pili or not. Surprisingly, strains isolated from carriers adhere to epithelial cells more readily than strains isolated from patients with meningococcal disease. Perhaps carrier strains are too 'sticky' to pass through the surface barrier and thus cause systemic infection. Meningococci pass through the epithelium of the nasopharynx to give rise to bacteraemia in only a small proportion of infected subjects, perhaps as few as 1 in 500. If systemic invasion is going to take place, it usually does so within a few days of colonization of the nasopharynx. It is likely that in many instances in which bacteria reach the circulation, they are destroyed rapidly by antibody and phagocytic cells before they can cause any tissue damage. However, in a few unfortunate individuals, bacteraemia results in the clinical syndrome of acute meningococcaemia. In other subjects meningococci are cleared from the circulation but lodge in tissues such as the meninges, where they produce local damage. Why some patients develop acute meningococcaemia whilst others develop meningitis is not understood. It is possible that very rapid multiplication of bacteria takes place in the circulation of patients with acute meningococcaemia. Alternatively, such individuals may be especially sensitive to the harmful effects of endotoxin.

The clinical features of acute meningococcaemia are largely those of acute endotoxaemia. Endotoxin diminishes the venous return to the heart and causes a fall in peripheral vascular resistance, thus leading to a diminished cardiac output and to a fall in arterial blood pressure. The plasma volume is initially normal, suggesting that trapping of venous blood is more important than plasma loss through damaged capillaries. Deposition of platelet thrombi in the pulmonary circulation may contribute to the diminished venous return to the left-hand-side of the heart, and myocardial damage may further impair cardiac output. The possible role of acute adrenal insufficiency in the pathogenesis of the peripheral circulatory collapse of fulminating acute meningococcaemia is controversial. Adrenocortical haemorrhage is found frequently at post-mortem in patients with acute meningococcaemia who have died because of circulatory collapse. However, it is found also in patients who have died from acute meningococcaemia without developing hypotension. Furthermore, most patients with acute meningococcaemia have elevated plasma cortisol levels and respond normally to stimulation with adrenocorticotrophin (ACTH). Thus, although acute adrenocortical insufficiency has been documented in a very few patients with acute meningococcaemia, it is probable that, in the majority of patients, peripheral circulatory collapse is brought about by other mechanisms.

Once lodged in the tissues, meningococci produce endotoxin locally and this may contribute to the acute inflammatory response characteristic of acute meningococcal lesions by means of a local Shwartzman reaction or by other mechanisms. It has been shown that meningococcal endotoxin is more potent at producing damage to cutaneous blood vessels than endotoxins isolated from other Gram-negative bacteria.

A proportion of patients with acute meningococcal infections develop arthritis, cutaneous vasculitis, episcleritis, or pericarditis several days after the onset of their illness, at a time when other features of their infection are improving. Such lesions are sterile and are probably produced by immune complexes. Late complications are seen most frequently in patients who are serum meningococcal antigen positive. They appear at the time when antigen disappears from the circulation and at the time when free antibody can first be detected (Fig. 2). Their appearance is associated with a transient fall in serum C3 and with the appearance of complement breakdown products in the plasma. Deposits of meningococcal polysaccharide antigen, immunoglobulin, and complement have been shown by immunofluorescence around damaged cutaneous vessels and within synovial fluid leucocytes obtained from inflamed joints. Serum immune complex levels of patients with allergic complications, although elevated, are no higher than the levels found in patients with uncomplicated acute meningococcal disease. This finding suggests that immune complexes are formed locally at sites such as the skin and synovium, where antigen is trapped during the bacteraemic phase of the infection and suggests that they are not derived from the circulation. This view is supported by the fact that glomerulonephritis is not a usual complication of meningococcal infection.

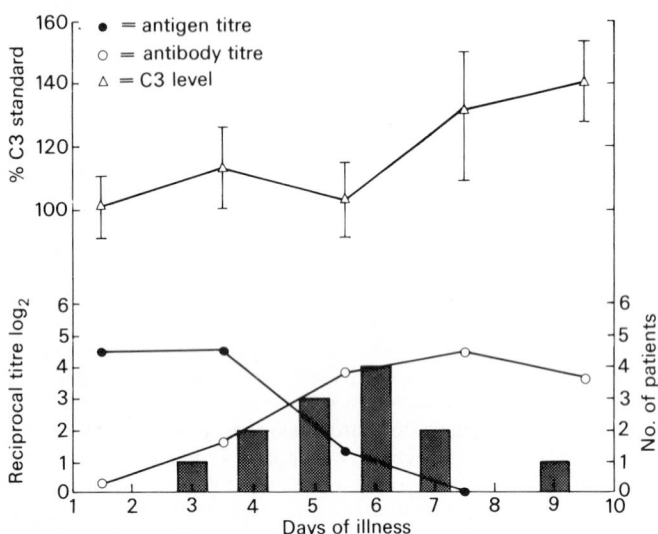

Fig. 2 Serological changes in 13 patients with meningococcal arthritis. (From Greenwood et al. (1976) Br. med. J., i, 797.)

Herpes simplex frequently complicates acute meningococcal disease. Patients with acute meningococcal meningitis show depressed cellular immunity to herpes antigens and to the non-specific mitogen, phytohaemagglutinin (PHA). This transient loss of cell-mediated immunity probably accounts for the high incidence of herpes infection in patients with meningococcal disease.

Pathology. Examination of subjects who have died from acute meningococcal septicaemia shows purpura and more extensive areas of haemorrhage in the skin and in internal organs such as the adrenals. There may be pulmonary and cerebral oedema. Histological examination shows changes in small vessels at sites of haemorrhage. The vascular endothelium is damaged and there may be overlying thrombus. Inflammatory cells are often present within the vessel wall. Meningococci can frequently be cultured from such purpuric lesions.

A fibrinous exudate is present over the surface of the brain of patients who have died from meningococcal meningitis. This response is often most marked around the base of the brain, thus giving rise to an old name for meningococcal meningitis—posterior

basal meningitis. Occlusion of meningeal foramina may result in internal hydrocephalus. Occlusion of damaged cerebral vessels is seen less frequently than in patients with pneumococcal meningitis. Histological examination of inflamed meninges shows fibrin deposition, oedema, vascular dilatation and a heavy infiltration with polymorphonuclear neutrophil leucocytes. Encephalitis is seen in some cases. Acute inflammatory lesions may be present at other sites, such as the joints, myocardium, and pericardium where meningococci have localized.

Some patients with meningococcal disease develop arthritis and skin lesions during the recovery phase of their acute infection. Examination of skin or synovial biopsies obtained from such patients shows a vasculitis with inflammatory cells clustered around a damaged, and sometimes occluded, small vessel. The majority of these inflammatory cells are polymorphonuclear neutrophil leucocytes but large mononuclear cells are more prominent in these lesions than in the vascular lesions seen during the acute phase of acute meningococcal disease.

Clinical features

Meningococci can cause a variety of clinical syndromes, varying in severity from a mild sore-throat to rapidly fatal acute meningococcaemia. It is convenient to consider these syndromes separately but some overlap may occur; for example a patient may have features of both acute meningococcaemia and meningitis.

Nasopharyngeal infection. Most nasopharyngeal infections with meningococci are asymptomatic but it is possible that some subjects develop a mild sore throat at the initial stage of the infection.

Acute meningococcaemia. The proportion of patients with meningococcal disease who develop acute meningococcaemia varies from place to place and from outbreak to outbreak, but it is usually less than 10 per cent.

Symptoms. Acute meningococcaemia is one of the most feared of all infections for it can strike with frightening rapidity; a victim may be well at breakfast time but dead by the same afternoon. Thus delay in making an early diagnosis and in starting appropriate treatment may be disastrous. Unfortunately, the early clinical features of acute meningococcaemia are quite non-specific—fever, general malaise, and headache—and they are indistinguishable from those of many other milder forms of infection. Diarrhoea which may be severe enough to suggest acute gastroenteritis, is sometimes an early feature of the disease.

Physical signs. Initial clinical examination may show no abnormalities apart from fever and tachycardia. However, careful examination may show small petechiae in the skin or in the conjunctivae. The appearance of petechiae is often the first sign which gives a clue as to the underlying diagnosis. Petechiae are seen most readily in dark-skinned subjects in the conjunctivae (Fig. 3) and in the palatal mucosa. Within hours of the onset of illness more extensive haemorrhagic lesions may appear in the skin and there may be bleeding from mucosae. The blood pressure is often normal initially, but then begins on a remorseless fall that is little influenced by treatment. The central venous pressure is low and small vessels are constricted. There may be a gallop rhythm and some patients develop cardiac arrhythmias. The respiratory rate is usually increased. Patients with acute meningococcaemia are often drowsy and confused and they may rapidly become comatose. Impairment of consciousness can occur in the absence of peripheral circulatory collapse and is probably due to encephalitis.

Laboratory findings. Laboratory investigations usually show a peripheral blood polymorphonuclear neutrophil leucocytosis but occasionally, leucopenia is found in fulminating cases. Rarely meningococci can be seen in peripheral blood leucocytes. There is caemia may follow a much more benign course characterized by mild fever and petechiae only. In the African 'meningitis belt' such mild, and sometimes asymptomatic cases, are seen most frequently at the end of an epidemic.

The overall mortality of acute meningococcaemia varies from outbreak to outbreak dependent upon the relative proportion of fulminating and mild cases. However, mortality is always high when patients have peripheral circulatory collapse or impairment of consciousness at the time at which they are first seen. The overall mortality among 47 patients recently studied in Nigeria was 43 per cent, but 93 per cent of patients with shock and impairment of consciousness at the time of presentation died (Fig. 4).

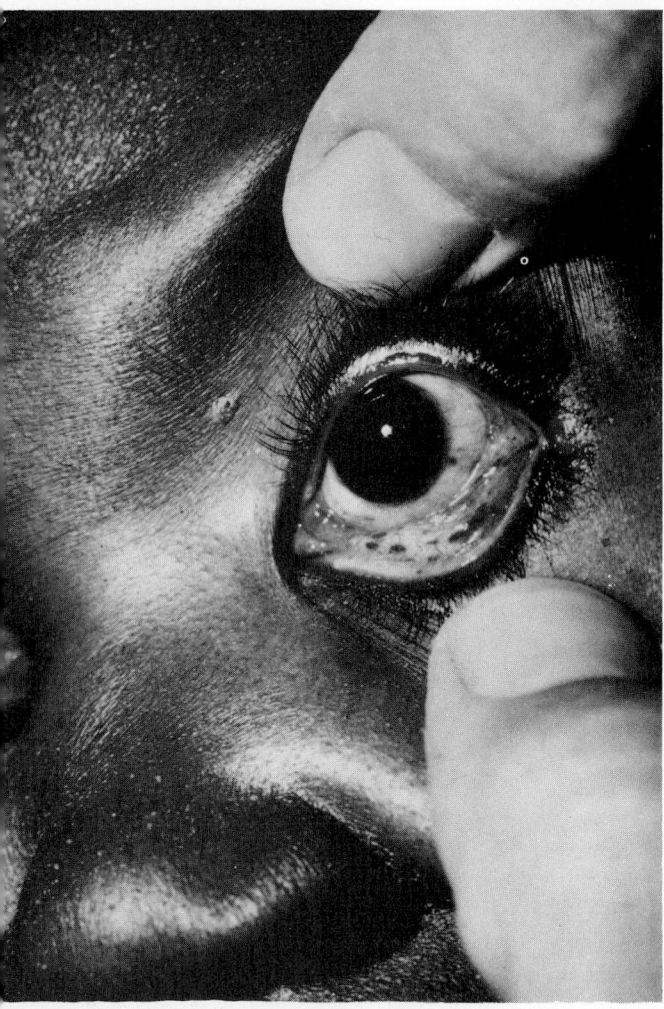

Fig. 3 Petechiae in the conjunctiva of a patient with meningococcal disease. (Photograph copyright Dr D. A. Warrell.)

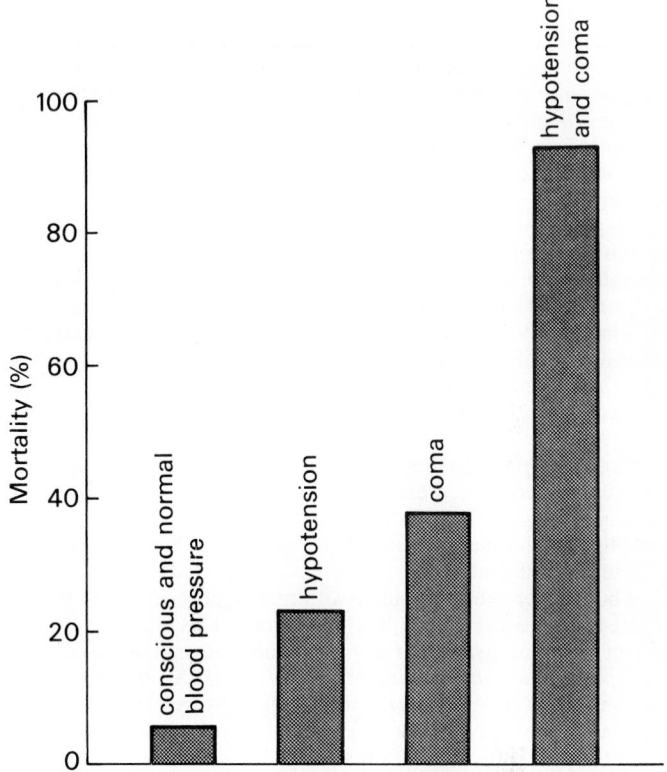

Fig. 4 Prognosis in relation to the clinical features on presentation in 47 patients with acute meningococcaemia. (From Lewis (1979). *Arch. Dis. Child.* **54**, 44.)

usually thrombocytopenia and there may be other signs of disseminated intravascular coagulation such as elevated serum fibrin degradation products (FDP) and a low plasma fibrinogen. Blood culture is frequently positive and meningococcal polysaccharide antigen can usually be detected in the serum. The cerebrospinal fluid (CSF) is clear and contains a normal, or only slightly elevated, number of white cells. However, CSF culture may be positive and meningococcal polysaccharide antigen may be present in CSF even in the absence of an active inflammatory response.

Course and prognosis. Patients with acute meningococcaemia may die within a few hours of the onset of their illness from irreversible peripheral circulatory collapse, haemorrhage, cardiac arrhythmia, or a combination of all three. Patients with acute meningococcaemia who survive the first few hours of their illness sometimes remain unconscious. They may have convulsions and they may develop a variety of localizing neurological signs such as a hemiplegia. These persistent neurological signs are probably the result of an encephalitis. Surviving patients sometimes develop severe pulmonary oedema which may be complicated by a secondary chest infection. Ulceration may occur at the site of haemorrhage into the skin and gangrene of extremities has been recorded. Death may follow from one of these late complications days or weeks after the acute episode of infection has been controlled. Survivors of acute meningococcaemia may develop one or more of the allergic complications of meningococcal infection described in the next section.

The clinical description given above is one of a classical case of severe acute meningococcaemia. However, acute meningococ-

Meningitis

Symptoms. The onset of meningococcal meningitis is generally more gradual than that of acute meningococcaemia. Headache, fever, and general malaise are the usual presenting symptoms. Headache is severe and is usually generalized. Patients may complain also of backache, photophobia, nausea, and vomiting. Convulsions may occur, especially in young children.

Physical signs. On examination the patient is found to be febrile and, in older children and in adults, there are usually obvious signs of meningeal irritation such as a stiff neck and a positive Kernig's sign. Focal neurological signs may be present on presentation; sixth or third cranial nerve palsies are the signs found most frequently but occasionally long tract signs are detected. The presence of raised intracranial pressure may be indicated by bradycardia and hypertension, but papilloedema is rarely seen in patients with acute meningococcal meningitis. Petechiae are present in the skin, conjunctivae, or in the palatal mucosa of up to one half of patients with meningococcal meningitis, a valuable diagnostic sign. Cardiac enlargement, a gallop rhythm, and mild abnormalities on the electrocardiogram are sometimes present, indicating associated myocarditis, but heart failure is rare.

These characteristic clinical abnormalities may be absent in infants with meningococcal meningitis in whom fever, convulsions, and feeding difficulties may be the only abnormal clinical features. Neck stiffness is often absent in such infants but there may be bulging of the anterior fontanelle.

Laboratory findings. Laboratory investigation of patients with acute meningococcal meningitis usually shows a peripheral blood poly-morphonuclear neutrophil leucocytosis. In a few patients blood culture is positive and, in about 10 per cent of patients, menin-gococcal polysaccharide antigen can be detected in the serum. On lumbar puncture a turbid CSF is usually obtained. The CSF white cell count is increased; nearly all the cells are polymorphonuclear neutrophil leucocytes. The CSF protein is increased and the CSF sugar is reduced below the blood sugar level. Meningococci can often be seen both within CSF leucocytes and free within the CSF, and a positive culture can usually be obtained. Meningococcal polysaccharide antigen can be detected in the CSF. Other CSF changes that have been described in patients with meningococcal meningitis include an increase in levels of immunoglobulins G and M, lactic acid, lactic acid dehydrogenase, and fibrin degradation products.

Course and prognosis. Patients with meningococcal meningitis sometimes die suddenly during their first few hours in hospital. It is often difficult to pin-point an exact cause of death in these patients; inhalation of vomit by an unconscious patient and cardiac arrhyth-mias are possible causes. Death is rare in patients who survive their first 24 hours in hospital. Most surveys have shown an overall mortality for meningococcal meningitis of between 5 and 10 per cent.

Most patients with meningococcal meningitis make a rapid and uneventful recovery. Persistence of fever and the appearance of new neurological signs after the commencement of treatment indi-cate the development of sub-dural empyema or the occurrence of a vascular occlusion.

About 5 per cent of patients with meningococcal meningitis, or acute meningococcaemia, develop arthritis. This may be caused by direct bacterial invasion of a synovial joint during the initial phase of septicaemia; synovial fluid obtained from such patients contains meningococci. However, arthritis is seen most frequently about six days after the onset of illness (Fig. 2) at a time when other clinical features of the infection are improving. Its appearance is associated with a secondary rise in fever and its onset is sometimes accom-panied by the appearance of cutaneous vasculitis, episcleritis, or pericarditis. The knee is the joint most frequently affected but any synovial joint or bursa may be involved. Joint signs resolve grad-ually over a period of days or weeks on symptomatic treatment, and progression to a chronic arthritis has not been recorded. The HLA status of patients with meningococcal arthritis has not been deter-mined. Synovial fluid from affected joints is sterile and this form of meningococcal arthritis is probably the result of immune complex formation (see above). The skin lesions of patients with cutaneous vasculitis usually start as blisters; these may rupture to leave exten-sive superficial ulcers (Fig. 5). Pericarditis is usually asymptomatic, being detected on an electrocardiogram or chest X-ray, but accu-mulation of fluid within the pericardium occasionally causes cardiac tamponade.

The prognosis of patients who survive the initial phase of men-ingococcal meningitis is excellent and most patients make a comp-lete recovery. Many of those who leave hospital with a neurological deficit continue to improve during the following weeks and months. However, some patients are left with persistent deafness.

Chronic meningococcaemia. This is a rare condition characterized by persistent meningococcaemia. Episodes of fever, urticarial rashes, arthritis, and splenomegaly are the usual clinical features. The pathological basis of these lesions is a vasculitis and it is probable that immune complexes play a part in the pathogenesis of this syndrome.

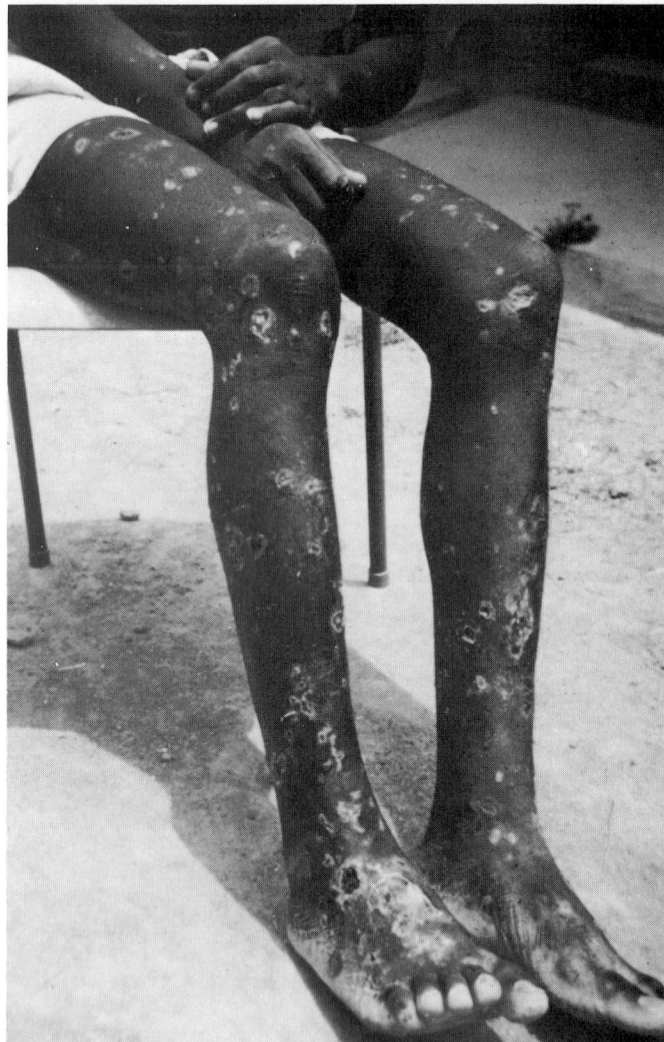

Fig. 5 Cutaneous vasculitis as a complication of meningococcal disease.

Other clinical syndromes. During an episode of meningococ-caemia, bacteria may lodge in many tissues producing acute in-flammatory reaction. Pyogenic arthritis, pericarditis, and pan-ophthalmitis (without associated meningitis) may be produced in this way. Meningococci have been isolated from patients with ur-ethritis, proctitis, or conjunctivitis. It is likely that in such patients the infection has been transmitted sexually. It has recently been appreciated that meningococci can cause pneumonia. Cases were first detected in American military personnel but the condition has now been described in civilians. Most cases of meningococcal pneumonia are caused by meningococci belonging to serogroup Y. Meningococcal pneumonia shows no characteristic clinical fea-tures.

Diagnosis

Acute meningococcaemia. Clinical diagnosis of acute meningococ-caemia is usually impossible during the earliest stage of the infec-tion, unless suspicion is heightened by the knowledge that the patient has been in close contact with a case of meningococcal disease. Meningococcaemia should enter into the differential di-agnosis of all patients with fever and petechiae. Once florid haemorrhagic lesions have appeared and shock has intervened, acute meningococcaemia becomes a likely diagnosis. However, other Gram-negative bacteria, rickettsiae, and some viruses such as dengue, can produce a similar clinical picture.

Diagnosis of acute meningococcaemia is confirmed by a positive blood culture or by the detection of meningococcal polysaccharide antigen in serum by countercurrent immunoelectrophoresis (CIE) or other immunological techniques. Countercurrent immunoelectrophoresis, which allows a rapid diagnosis to be made, is positive in nearly all patients with severe acute meningococcaemia but may be negative in patients with the mild form of the syndrome. Detection of group B meningococcal polysaccharide antigen by immunological techniques can be difficult (see below).

Meningitis. A clinical diagnosis of acute meningitis is usually made readily in adults and older children on the basis of the characteristic history and abnormal physical signs. Differentiation of acute meningitis from meningism, a stiff neck associated with an acute febrile illness such as a streptococcal sore throat, may sometimes be impossible on clinical grounds alone. Signs of meningeal irritation are often absent in infants with acute meningitis. Thus, a possible diagnosis of acute meningitis must be considered in all irritable, febrile infants, especially in those with convulsions. Clinical examination may provide some clue as the causative organism. Detection of petechiae favours a diagnosis of meningococcal meningitis, whilst detection of an associated middle ear infection or pneumonia favours a diagnosis of pneumococcal meningitis.

Confirmation of a clinical diagnosis of acute meningitis requires lumbar puncture. Opinion is divided as to whether all infants with febrile convulsions should be lumbar punctured or not; it is wiser to err on the side of performing too many lumbar punctures rather than too few. Lumbar puncture of a patient with meningococcal meningitis usually reveals a turbid CSF under increased pressure. Occasionally the CSF is clear, for approximately 0.2×10^9 cells per litre must be present before CSF appears turbid to the naked eye. Therefore, a CSF cell count must be made before a diagnosis of meningitis can be excluded. Nearly all the white cells present in an initial CSF sample obtained from a patient with meningococcal meningitis are polymorphonuclear neutrophil leucocytes, thus differentiating the infection from viral meningitides in which lymphocytes predominate. Lymphocytes may be found in the CSF of patients with meningococcal meningitis at follow-up lumbar punctures performed after the start of treatment. Cerebrospinal fluid from patients with meningococcal meningitis has a high protein and a low sugar content, findings characteristic of all forms of bacterial meningitis.

Meningococci can be demonstrated in the CSF by Gram stain or culture in up to 80 per cent of patients. However, because Gram stains can be misinterpreted by inexperienced staff and because culture is often negative in patients who have received antibiotics before coming to hospital, interest has recently reawakened in methods of diagnosis which depend upon detection of bacterial products, rather than viable bacteria, in the CSF. Endotoxin can be detected in the CSF of nearly all patients with meningococcal meningitis by the sensitive Limulus assay, but this test cannot differentiate between meningitis caused by the meningococcus and meningitis caused by other types of Gram negative bacteria such as *Haemophilus influenzae* and *E. coli* which require different treatment. Detection of meningococcal capsular polysaccharide antigen in the CSF by immunological methods is highly specific. Using simple immunological assays such as CIE, latex, or staphylococcal coagglutination tests, the sensitivity of antigen detection is comparable to that of culture (Table 1). Slightly higher positivity rates are obtained when more sensitive techniques such as radioimmunoassay and enzyme linked immunosorbent assays are used and when serum and urine are examined as well as CSF. Group A and group C meningococcal polysaccharide antigens are readily detected by immunological tests; group B meningococcal polysaccharide is more difficult to detect as it is poorly antigenic. Many commercial group B meningococcal antisera are unsuitable for use in antigen detection tests but potent antisera can be prepared. A positive test with a group B meningococcal antiserum cannot differentiate between infection caused by a group B meningococcus and infection caused by *E. coli* type KI as the capsular polysaccharides of these two organisms are antigenically very similar. Bacterial components can be detected in the CSF of patients with meningococcal meningitis by gas liquid chromatography, as well as by immunological methods, but the diagnostic value of this technique has not yet been explored. Antigen detection tests are of value in giving a rapid diagnosis, thus allowing an appropriate antibiotic to be started immediately after lumbar puncture, and in providing a positive diagnosis in patients who have received prior treatment with antibiotics. They also provide some prognostic as well as diagnostic information. Patients with meningococcal meningitis who are serum antigen positive have a higher morbidity and a higher incidence of complications that patients who are serum antigen negative. Prognosis is excellent in patients who are CSF antigen negative. Antigen detection tests should be considered as an adjunct to routine microbiological techniques, and not a replacement for them, as the latter techniques provide valuable information, for example on antibiotic sensitivity patterns, not given by immunological assays.

Table 1   Antigen detection in the diagnosis of meningococcal meningitis. The combined results obtained of ten published series are shown

Samples tested	Number positive		
	Countercurrent immunoelectrophoresis	Latex test	Culture
877	658 (75%)	693 (79%)	710 (81%)

Other syndromes. The presence of meningococci in the nasopharynx is established by culture of a nasopharyngeal swab. Isolation of meningococci is facilitated by use of a selective medium containing antibiotics, such as Thayer–Martin medium, which inhibits normal nasopharyngeal commensals. A diagnosis of chronic meningococcaemia is established by blood culture. Meningococci may be isolated from pus obtained from various metastatic sites. Meningococcal pneumonia is diagnosed by blood culture or by isolation of meningococci from a lung or transtracheal aspirate.

Treatment

Acute meningococcaemia
Antibiotics. The antibiotic of choice for the treatment of acute meningococcaemia is crystalline penicillin which, for adults, should be given in a dose of 4 mega units six-hourly by intravenous injection. Chloramphenicol should be used to treat patients who are known to be sensitive to penicillin. Antibiotics should be given for seven days. There is a theoretical risk that administration of penicillin in a high dosage could initially worsen the patient's clinical state as a result of massive destruction of bacteria and the consequent release of endotoxin, but such a Herxheimer reaction has never been clearly demonstrated in patients with this infection.

Supportive. A wide variety of supportive measures have been tried in patients with fulminating acute meningococcaemia but none have been particularly successful. Whenever possible patients with acute meningococcaemia should be nursed in an intensive care unit. Fluid balance, acid–base status, central venous pressure, and the electrocardiogram should be monitored carefully.

Two main approaches to the control of hypotension in patients with acute meningococcaemia have been adopted—expansion of plasma volume and administration of sympathomimetic amines. Venous return to the heart can be increased by intravenous infusion with plasma or dextran. The central venous pressure should be maintained at between 10 and 15 mmHg if possible. A careful watch must be kept for the development of pulmonary oedema; if pulmonary crepitations appear an intravenous diuretic, such as frusemide, should be given. Administration of a sympathomimetic amine, such as noradrenaline, increases peripheral vascular resistance by causing constriction of the small vessels of the skin, muscles, and spleen, diverts blood to essential organs such as the heart and brain, and helps to maintain arterial blood pressure. Furthermore, it increases myocardial contactility. The drug should be given by slow intravenous injection at a rate which maintains systolic blood pressure at a level of about 100 mmHg. An average dose is 10 μg per minute. Blood pressure can be maintained in most patients with acute meningococcaemia by a combination of plasma expansion and administration of a sympathomimetic amine. However, in some patients, tissue perfusion does not improve on this regimen, perhaps because of intense vascoconstriction of small vessels. In such patients it may be worth trying phentolamine, given intravenously in a dose of between 20 μg and 80 μg per minute, as phentolamine antagonizes the constricting effects of noradrenaline on the microcirculation but does not impair its direct action on the heart. Phentolamine causes dilatation of veins and thus reduces the effective plasma volume. If this drug is used added fluid replacement therapy may be required.

The value of corticosteroids in the management of shocked patients with acute meningococcaemia has never been established by a controlled trial. A few patients have adrenocortical insufficiency which requires replacement therapy. In experimental animals massive doses of corticosteroids protect against endotoxin-mediated shock by stabilizing platelets, polymorphonuclear neutrophil leucocytes, lysosymes, and endothelial cell membranes. Corticosteroids are most effective when given before endotoxin; their value when given to animals with established shock is doubtful. Thus, if corticosteroids are to be used in patients with acute meningococcaemia to prevent shock, they should be given in large doses, for example 1 g of methylprednisone, and they should be given as early as possible.

Digitalis has been used in an attempt to improve myocardial function in patients with acute meningococcaemia but its value has not been clearly established. If cardiac arrhythmias are detected, they should be treated by conventional means.

Bleeding, associated with disseminated intravascular coagulation, may be an important feature of acute meningococcaemia. A beneficial response to therapy with heparin has been reported in individual cases but a controlled trial showed no overall benefit from administration of this drug. If bleeding is severe, blood transfusion may be required.

Treatment of patients with acute meningococcaemia remains unsatisfactory. Although meningococci can be killed rapidly with antibiotics, it has proved difficult to counteract the effects of the endotoxin that they have produced. Before the discovery of antibiotics, immune serum was used to treat patients with meningococcaemia with some success. It is possible that neutralization of endotoxin was an important component of this form of therapy. Perhaps this approach to the treatment of acute meningococcaemia should be re-explored using antisera known to have activity against endotoxin. Plasmapheresis offers another possible way of removing endotoxin and there have been recent reports of individual patients with acute meningococcaemia who have been treated successfully in this way.

Meningitis

Antibiotics. The conventional antibiotic treatment for acute meningococcal meningitis in adults is 3–5 mega units of crystalline penicillin given intravenously or intramuscularly every 6 hours for 5–7 days. Parenteral penicillin given in such a dose produces CSF penicillin levels well above the minimal inhibitory concentration for meningococci and intrathecal antibiotic therapy is unnecessary. Chloramphenicol, given to adults in a dosage of 750 mg 6-hourly, is an effective alternative to penicillin. Chloramphenicol has the advantage that it can be given by mouth as soon as a patient is conscious but, very rarely, it may cause marrow depression. Sulphonamides should not be used for the treatment of meningococcal meningitis unless it is known for certain that the causative organism is sulphonamide sensitive. There is no evidence that combinations of penicillin, chloramphenicol and sulphonamides are any more effective than penicillin or chloramphenicol given alone.

During epidemics large numbers of patients with meningococcal disease become ill at the same time, swamping the available medical resources. At the height of a recent epidemic in northern Nigeria approximately 1000 cases of suspected meningococcal disease presented at one hospital during the course of a single day. Under such circumstances six-hourly penicillin injections are impracticable. Long-acting sulphonamides, given by paramedical staff, were used very successfully to manage such major outbreaks in the past. However, this form of treatment is now no longer reliable because of the widespread prevalence of sulphonamide resistance. A long-acting chloramphenicol preparation (Tifomycine), given in a single injection of 3 g to adults, is a satisfactory alternative to long acting sulphonamides and is as effective as a five-day course of crystalline penicillin, despite the fact that chloramphenicol can be detected in the CSF for only 48 hours after the injection.

The results obtained with Tifomycine suggest that conventional antibiotic regimens for the treatment of meningococcal meningitis involve an unnecessarily long course of treatment and that satisfactory results could be obtained with shorter courses of crystalline penicillin or chloramphenicol. Careful monitoring of patients is essential if new regimens are tried.

Supportive. Unconscious patients with meningitis require careful nursing, particular attention being paid to their airway. Patients with meningitis are often dehydrated, especially in hot countries, because they have a high fever and because they are too confused to drink. Thus, intravenous rehydration may be required. Headache may be very severe and may be an important cause of restlessness. If it cannot be controlled with simple analgesics, pethidine may be needed. Diazepam is of value in quietening restless and violent patients, and in controlling convulsions. If signs of severe raised intracranial pressure are present, dexamethasone or mannitol should be given. Overall, corticosteroids have no beneficial effect on the outcome of the infection.

The development of arthritis or cutaneous vasculitis during the recovery phase of the infection is not an indication for the continuation of antibiotic therapy. Arthritis responds well to treatment with aspirin. Skin ulcers may require dressings for several weeks.

A deterioration in conscious level or the appearance of new focal neurological signs after the start of treatment suggests the development of a sub-dural effusion or empyema, or the occurrence of a vascular occlusion. Patients showing these features should be investigated for the presence of a space-occupying lesion by scanning and/or, arteriography. If a filling defect is found burr holes should be made at the appropriate site. If neurosurgical diagnostic facilities are not available, exploratory burr holes should be made.

Patients with meningococcal meningitis sometimes develop a secondary spike of fever, after making an initial recovery. This may be due to the formation of a local collection of pus, to the development of an allergic complication, to the presence of an organism resistant to the antibiotic being used, to a mistake in the initial bacteriological diagnosis, or to a drug reaction. In such patients, a second lumbar puncture should be performed and the CSF obtained should be recultured. It is doubtful whether it is worthwhile performing repeated lumbar punctures to monitor the course of the treatment in patients who are making an uncomplicated recovery.

Prophylaxis

There are two main approaches to the prevention of meningococcal disease, chemoprophylaxis and vaccination, each of which has its own advantages and disadvantages. Improvement of general standards of living and prevention of overcrowding in barracks and schools also helps to prevent the spread of meningococcal infection.

Chemoprophylaxis. Chemoprophylaxis with sulphonamides has, in the past, proved very effective in preventing meningococcal infection. Sulphonamides protect against clinical disease and eliminate meningococci from nasopharyngeal carriers. A single administration of the drug gives protection for several weeks and, if necessary, this can be repeated. During this period the environmental factors responsible for an outbreak may have disappeared so that stopping chemoprophylaxis does not necessarily result in reactivation of the outbreak of infection.

Unfortunately, many meningococci have become sulphonamide resistant so that sulphonamides can now be used for chemoprophylaxis in only a limited number of outbreaks in which it has been established beyond any doubt that the causative organism is sulphonamide sensitive. Many antibiotics have been tried as prophylactics against meningococcal disease. Although penicillin and chloramphenicol are very effective therapeutic agents, for reasons that are not completely understood, they are ineffective prophylactics unless given in a full therapeutic course. Only two antibiotics have been shown to be consistently effective in preventing spread of meningococci—rifampicin and minocycline. Minocycline has caused an unacceptably high incidence of side effects in some, but not all, studies. Rifampicin has proved less toxic but the drug is too expensive to be used for mass chemoprophylaxis in developing countries. Furthermore, its widespread use is associated with the rapid appearance of rifampicin resistant strains of meningococci, and there is a danger that use of the drug for prevention of meningococcal infection in developing countries might favour the appearance of rifampicin resistant strains of tubercle and leprosy bacilli. The doses of sulphonamides and rifampicin recommended for the prevention of meningococcal infection are shown in Table 2.

Table 2 The recommended dosage of sulphonamides and rifampicin for the chemoprophylaxis of meningococcal disease. Treatment is given for two days

	Sulphadiazine	Rifampicin
Adults	1 g twice a day	600 mg twice a day
Children (1–12 years)	500 mg twice a day	10 mg/kg twice a day
Infants < 1	500 mg a day	5 mg/kg twice a day

Vaccination. Attempts to protect against meningococcal infection by vaccination have been made for at least 50 years. Some success was obtained with early vaccines prepared from whole organisms, but other whole bacteria vaccines were completely ineffective. The discovery in 1969 that purified group A and group C meningococcal capsular polysaccharides were immunogenic and that these preparations consistently gave protection against meningococcal disease opened up an exciting new approach to the control of meningococcal infection. The protective value of both group A and group C polysaccharide vaccines has been demonstrated beyond all doubt by controlled trials (Table 3), and epidemiological evidence

Table 3 Controlled trials of meningococcal vaccine in Africa. These trials were elective studies and were not undertaken as emergency measures to control epidemics

Country	Age group vaccinated (years)	Follow-up (years)	Vaccinated Number	Cases	Controls Number	Cases
Egypt	6–15	3	62 295	0	62 054	15
Egypt	6–15	2	88 263	4	88 383	12
Sudan	All ages	1	10 891	0	10 749	7
Upper Volta	All ages	2	17 300	0	25 700	43
Total			178 749	4	186 886	77

strongly suggests that mass immunization with group A meningococcal vaccine brought under control serious epidemics of meningococcal disease in Finland and in Brazil. Meningococcal polysaccharide vaccines protect against meningococcal disease but it is less certain whether they stop the spread of meningococcal infection. Some studies have shown a significant reduction in nasopharyngeal carriage of meningococci of the relevant serogroup after vaccination but this has not been observed in other investigations. There is no evidence that vaccination against group A and group C meningococci predisposes to infection with meningococci of other serogroups.

Meningococcal polysaccharide vaccines have a number of unusual characteristics. They are poorly immunogenic in young children, an effect which is independent of the presence of maternal antibody. It has been suggested that older children respond better than younger children because they have been primed by natural infection with meningococci of other serogroups. Meningococcal polysaccharides are T lymphocyte independent antigens and, therefore, do not activate T memory cells. Booster responses can be induced by re-immunization but the time interval between doses is important and, under certain circumstances, re-immunization fails to give any enhancement of the antibody response. The duration of the antibody response or the duration of the protective immunity that follows immunization with meningococcal polysaccharide vaccines has not yet been accurately determined. Epidemiological studies suggest that clinical protection lasts for at least three years after vaccination. In adults raised antibody levels are found five years after vaccination, but antibody levels fall faster in children. Detailed studies carried out in the United States have shown that three immunizations are required to maintain group A and group C meningococcal antibody levels at a protective level throughout the first five years of life.

The capsular polysaccharide antigen of the group B meningococcus is poorly immunogenic and cannot be used alone as a vaccine. Attempts have therefore been made to develop a group B vaccine based on outer membrane protein antigens. Some success has been obtained with serogroup 2 protein antigen and with conjugated polysaccharide-serogroup 2 protein vaccines. These vaccines induce an antibody response in volunteers but they have not yet been subjected to clinical trials. Combination of a protein with meningococcal polysaccharide vaccines might increase the duration or protective immunity that these vaccines provide.

Who should be protected and how? No absolute guidelines can be given as to who should be protected against meningococcal disease and how this should be achieved. Some suggestions, based on the risk factor in specific groups, are made in this section and are summarized in Table 4.

Table 4 A scheme for the protection of contacts of patients with meningococcal disease

Organism responsible		Subjects exposed	
Serogroup*	Sulphonamide† sensitivity	Household contacts	Schools, barracks, etc.
A or C	+	vaccination sulphonamides	vaccination sulphonamides
	–	vaccination rifampicin or penicillin‡	vaccination
B	+	sulphonamides	sulphonamides
	–	rifampicin or penicillin‡	? rifampicin

* When the serogroup is not known, the situation should be managed as if the infection was due to a group A or group C meningococcus
† If the sulphonamide sensitivity of the causative organism is not known it should be regarded as sulphonamide resistant
‡ A full therapeutic course of penicillin is required

Household contacts. Those most at risk of contracting meningococcal disease are close household contacts of a patient with the infection. During an epidemic, the risk for siblings sleeping in the same room as a patient may be as high as 1 in 20. Such close contacts should receive the full range of prophylactic measures available. If the organism is know to be a group A or a group C meningococcus, vaccination should be carried out immediately. However, as many secondary, or perhaps coprimary, cases occur within a few days of the onset of illness in the index case, some other form of protection is required to cover the period before vaccination induces protective immunity. If the organism responsible for the outbreak is known to be sulphonamide sensitive, sulphonamides should be given. If the sulphonamide sensitivity of the organism is not known or if it is known to be sulphonamide resistant, two alternatives are available. Either rifampicin can be given or, alternatively, a full therapeutic course of penicillin can be administered.

Residential schools and barracks. When a case of meningococcal disease occurs in a residential school, doss house, or barracks, further cases of the infection are likely. Subjects in close contact with the patient, for example those sleeping in the same small dormitory, should be managed in the same way as household contacts. Subjects with less contact with the patient should be vaccinated, if the causative meningococcus belongs to serogroup A or serogroup C, and they should be given sulphonamides if the organism is known to be sulphonamide sensitive. What, if anything, should be done if the outbreak is due to a sulphonamide resistant group B meningococcus? Mass prophylaxis with rifampicin would probably be effective but would be very expensive.

Hospital personnel. Although the risk of meningococcal disease in hospital personnel is no greater, or only a little greater, that that of the general population, vaccination of all hospital staff coming into regular contact with patients with meningococcal disease or with their laboratory samples is probably a sensible precaution. Research scientists working with meningococci should also be vaccinated.

General population. Mass vaccination can bring an epidemic of group A or group C meningococcal disease under control in a short time. The effectiveness of this approach has been demonstrated at the village, city, and national level. When mass immunization is used to control an outbreak, vaccination must be started as soon as possible. To control an outbreak, it may only be necessary to vaccinate those in the age group most at risk. Thus, in Finland, vaccination was restricted to those under the age of five years, and a recent outbreak in Rwanda was controlled by vaccination of those aged 2–20 years. Restriction of vaccination to the control of outbreaks is a cost effective way of using meningococcal vaccines but this approach fails to protect those individuals whose illness heralds the onset of an epidemic.

An alternative approach to meningococcal vaccination is mass immunization of the whole population by incorporation of meningococcal vaccines into routine immunization schedules. Because of the relatively transient nature of the immune response produced by meningococcal polysaccharides, several injections of vaccine will be required to maintain protective levels of immunity throughout childhood. The cost-effectiveness of such a scheme in industrialized countries has yet to be established. Such a programme is likely to be too expensive for most developing countries to implement. Perhaps, in such areas, routine immunization against meningococcal disease will have to await the development of protein or conjugated polysaccharide vaccines which induce long-lasting protective immunity.

References

Fallon, R. J. (1979). Meningococcal diseases; pathogenesis and prevention. In *Recent advances in infection* (eds. D. S. Reeves and A. M. Geddes), 77. Churchill Livingstone, Edinburgh.

Greenwood, B. M. and Whittle, H. C. (1976). The pathogenesis of meningococcal arthritis. In *Infection and immunology in the rheumatic diseases* (ed. D. C. Dumonde), 119. Blackwell Scientific Publications, Oxford.

Jones, D. M. (1979). The rapid detection of bacterial antigens. In *Recent advances in infection* (eds. D. S. Reeves and A. M. Geddes), 91. Churchill Livingstone, Edinburgh.

The Lancet (1978). Who should be given meningococcal vaccine? *Lancet* ii 1185.

Lapeyssonnie, L. (1963). La méningite cérébro-spinale en Afrique. *Bull. Wld Hlth Org.* **28**, suppl. 3.

Enterobacteria and miscellaneous enteropathogenic and food-poisoning bacteria

M. B. Skirrow

This section describes the large group of intestinal organisms known as the Enterobacteria and other groups of bacteria which cause specific diarrhoeal disease that are not considered elsewhere in this book (see below).

Diarrhoeal disease causes much suffering, particularly among children of tropical and developing countries. In 1975 there were an estimated 500 million episodes of diarrhoea in children under five years old in Asia, Africa, and Latin America resulting in 5–18 million deaths. In recognition of this fact, in 1980, the World Health Organization launched a major attack on diarrhoeal diseases and there are renewed interest in the causes and methods of control of the various agents involved. This section describes *Salmonella* enteritis, *Shigella* dysentery, *Escherichia coli* enteritis, *Campylobacter* enteritis, and food poisoning caused by *Vibrio parahaemolyticus* and *Bacillus cereus*. A sub-section is devoted to the role of Enterobacteria and similar organisms in extra-intestinal infections, and finally the causes and main features of the common types of food poisoning are summarized for easy reference. The following are described elsewhere: Cholera (page 5.195), *Yersinia enterocolitica* infections (page 5.213), staphylococcal (page 5.161) and clostridial (page 5.236), food poisoning, stool viruses (page 5.90). Typhoid and paratyphoid fever, which are among the more serious of the enterobacterial diseases, are described on page 5.183. The reader's attention is also drawn to Section 12 where infections and infestations of the gastrointestinal tract are considered from a clinical standpoint.

THE ENTEROBACTERIA

Definition and general description. The term Enterobacteria strictly denotes bacteria belonging to the family *Enterobacteriaceae*. This is a large family of Gram-negative non-sporing fermentative bacilli that inhabit the intestinal tracts of man and animals; some exist on plants or in the soil. They are capable of growth in both aerobic and anaerobic conditions, and they are easy to cultivate in the laboratory—indeed they often outgrow and mask more fastidious bacteria. Since they are non-sporing organisms, they are killed by moderate heat (60 °C for 20 minutes) but they are in general more resistant than Gram-positive bacteria to chemical disinfectants. They live and multiply in wet conditions but do not readily survive desiccation.

The *Enterobacteriaceae* includes the following genera: *Escherichia, Shigella, Edwardsiella, Salmonella, Citrobacter, Klebsiella, Enterobacter, Hafnia, Serratia, Proteus*, and *Providencia*. The shigellae and salmonellae are the principal pathogens among these and they are described later. The others, except for certain strains of *Escherichia coli*, are not intestinal pathogens, but any of them may cause infections elsewhere in the body given the right opportunity and conditions (see below).

In the laboratory the ability to ferment lactose is traditionally used to distinguish enteropathogenic species. Virtually all salmonellae and shigellae are non-lactose fermenters, whereas most of the other Enterobacteria—with the exception of *Proteus* and *Providencia*—ferment lactose freely. By including lactose and a pH indicator in a culture medium, the colonies of non-lactose-fermenting bacteria stand out pale against the coloured (acid) colonies of lactose-fermenters, hence they can be seen readily and picked out for further study. 'Coliform bacteria' is a clinically convenient term used to denote lactose-fermenting Enterobacteria. The term 'Paracolon' was formerly applied to non-lactose-fermenting Enterobacteria that were not salmonellae, shigellae, or members of the proteus group, but it fell into disuse following the introduction of more precise methods of identification. Such bacteria are usually found to be late-lactose-fermenting strains of *E. coli*, or to belong to the genera *Hafnia* or *Serratia* in which non-lactose-fermenting strains are common.

Antigenic structure. There are three groups of antigens that are important for the identification of Enterobacteria in the laboratory and also for the serological diagnosis of infection, e.g. by the Widal test (see page 5.185). Firstly there are the somatic or O antigens present in the main structure of the bacterial cell wall. These are complexes of lipo-polysaccharide with protein and lipid, and they constitute the endotoxin that triggers the process leading to tissue damage and circulatory collapse in patients suffering from Gram-negative septicaemia, i.e., endotoxic shock (see page 5.21). O antigens tend to be non-specific and shared between otherwise unrelated organisms. Secondly there are surface antigens—sometimes in the form of a capsule (e.g. Klebsiellae)—which, because of their superficial position, may mask the deeper O antigens unless they are first removed or destroyed by heat. One of the best examples of a surface antigen is the Vi factor of the typhoid bacillus, so-called because it is associated with virulence. But the designation K (Kauffmann) is used for the surface antigens of other Enterobacteria. The K antigens of *E. coli* are of three types designated A, B, and L. Thirdly, motile Enterobacteria possess flagellar or H antigens of which there are many types within each group or genus. Salmonellae are unique in showing diphasic variation of the H antigen.

Owing to this complex antigenic structure, it is possible by serological methods to recognize many strains of Enterobacteria, even within a single genus or species (e.g. *Salmonella, E. coli*), and this is of great epidemiological value.

Extra-intestinal infections caused by Enterobacteria and related organisms. Before proceeding to specific diarrhoeal diseases caused by Enterobacteria, a brief account of their infective role elsewhere in the body will be given. It is convenient to include here other non-fastidious Gram-negative bacilli which behave clinically in a similar manner to Enterobacteria and are often found in mixed infections with them. Chief among these is *Pseudomonas aeruginosa (pyocyanea)*, which is notorious as a 'hospital' organism and as a cause of opportunistic and sometimes fatal systemic infection in debilitated or immunosuppressed patients. *Ps. aeruginosa* is naturally resistant to most of the commonly used antimicrobials and also to many antiseptics. Indeed pseudomonads, notably *Ps. cepacia*, are capable of growth in some antiseptic solutions stored at dilute working strengths. Other common opportunistic Gram-negative bacilli are found in the genera *Alcaligenes, Acinetobacter, Aeromonas, Flavobacterium,* and *Chromobacterium*. The term Gram-negative sepsis or septicaemia is used to denote invasive infections with Enterobacteria or these other non-fastidious Gram-negative bacilli.

Since the advent of antibiotics, there has been a progressive increase in serious Gram-negative sepsis, particularly among hospital patients. There are a variety of reasons for this: widespread use (and abuse) of antibiotics, which are generally more effective against Gram-positive bacteria; more adventurous surgery, increasingly performed on old people; more patients fitted with catheters, pacemakers, and prostheses, all of which provide ideal sites for the establishment of infection; and more general use of immunosuppressive and cytotoxic therapy. Enterobacteria, pseudomonads, and similar Gram-negative bacilli easily develop resistance to antimicrobials, which helps them to colonize the hospital environment. Such organisms often replace the normal sensitive bowel flora of patients admitted to hospital, particularly if antibiotics are being given, so the patient's anus then becomes the gateway to colonization and infection elsewhere in the body.

It is against this background that one must consider Gram-negative sepsis, and it is not surprising that these organisms turn up in a wide variety of clinical material. They are frequently found colonizing wounds, sinuses, ulcers, burns, and chronically discharging ears—in fact wherever the body integument is broken. In most cases they are probably of little consequence, but their presence deep in a wound sometimes causes harm by enhancing the growth of anaerobes.

Specific types of infection. *Urinary tract.* This is the most common site for genuine infection as opposed to simple colonization. Such infections range from a simple cystitis to pyelitis, pyelonephritis, and pyonephrosis. Most infections are caused by *E. coli*, but in patients with indwelling catheters or who have undergone genito-urinary surgery, resistant strains of *Klebsiella aerogenes, Proteus* spp., and *Ps. aeruginosa* are more likely to be the infecting agents. In this connection it should be remembered that the removal of a catheter from an infected male patient is likely to cause transient bacteraemia. Proteus infections in male children are commonly associated with a congenital abnormality such as a urethral valve.

Sepsis associated with the intestinal tract. In these infections coliform bacteria are usually found with other bowel flora such as *Bacteroides* spp. and micro-aerophilic streptococci. Peritonitis secondary to a perforated bowel, intraperitoneal abscess (e.g. pelvic, subphrenic, retrocaecal), cholecystitis, cholangitis, and liver abscess are examples of such infections. Remote focal infections such as endocarditis or cerebral abscess may also be caused by coliforms and other bowel flora.

Respiratory tract. Coliform bacteria seldom cause significant respiratory tract infections, but they are often isolated from sputum samples owing to a tendency to colonize the mouths and upper respiratory tract of ill patients, particularly babies. Such colonization is encouraged by antimicrobial chemotherapy. The presence of coliforms in sputum is therefore seldom of any consequence, but a true pneumonia does occasionally occur. The classical type is caused by *Klebsiella pneumoniae* (Friedlaender's bacillus) but this organism accounts for only a tiny proportion of all bacterial pneumonias; most of the Klebsiellae isolated from sputum are of the common aerogenes type and are of no significance. Patients with bronchiectasis or cystic fibrosis are especially prone to Gram-negative bronchial infections, notably with capsulated 'mucoid' variants of *Ps. aeruginosa*.

Klebsiella ozaenae and *K. rhinoscleromatis* are associated with the uncommon nasal diseases ozaena and rhinoscleroma.

Neonatal infections. Newborn babies are especially liable to suffer from serious Gram-negative infections. Gram-negative septicaemia, which usually arises from an infected umbilicus, invariably involves the meninges as an incipient if not overt meningitis. Fortunately such events are rare, but coliforms are the commonest cause of neonatal meningitis, a fact that contrasts sharply with the scarcity of coliform meningitis after the age of one month. *E. coli* is usually responsible, but any of the Enterobacteria may be involved. *Proteus mirabilis* infections, which take the form of a meningo-encephalitis, are particularly severe, and occasionally this common organism, for reasons that are not understood, has caused disastrous hospital nursery outbreaks.

Salmonella infections

Salmonellae are widely distributed in nature as intestinal parasites of vertebrates. They are non-lactose-fermenting members of the *Enterobacteriaceae* and are motile by means of numerous peritrichate flagella. Some bacteriologists include the so-called 'Arizona' group in the genus *Salmonella*; these organisms, which have been found mainly in reptiles and turkeys in the United States but also occasionally in man, differ from the true salmonellae in that many strains ferment lactose, which makes their recognition difficult in the laboratory (see page 5.177). In clinical practice the salmonellae are conveniently divided into those types that cause enteric fever (mainly *Salmonella typhi*, *S. paratyphi* A, B, C, and *S. cholerae-suis*), and those that cause acute enteritis—usually through food poisoning—such as *S. enteritidis* and *S. typhimurium*. Exceptionally food-poisoning strains cause typhoidal illness. The food-poisoning group contains over 1700 serotypes. After White and Kauffmann pioneered their antigenic classification in the late 1920s and early 1930s, it became customary to accord a specific Linnean name to each serotype, a policy that may be taxonomically unsound but convenient in practice. It also became customary to name each new serotype after the place at which it was first isolated. Thus salmonella 1,4,12 : z : 1,7 is *S. indiana* and salmonella 6,8 : e,h : 1,2 is *S. newport* (antigens are listed in the order O : H phase 1 : H phase 2). Strains are divided firstly into some 36 groups according to their main somatic (O) antigens, and then further divided according to their flagellar (H) antigens. Fortunately for the bacteriologist whose task it is to identify salmonellae, most infections are caused by only a small porportion of the 1700 or so known serotypes. In Britain and most other parts of the world *S. typhimurium* (1,4,[5],12 : i : 1,2) is the most prevalent serotype.

Epidemiology

Animal sources. The typhoid bacillus, under natural conditions, is confined to man but the food-poisoning salmonellae are enzootic in a wide range of vertebrates. Salmonella enteritis is therefore a zoonosis. Some salmonella serotypes have preference for a particular host species. For example *S. dublin* is primarily a parasite of cattle, *S. pullorum* of poultry, and *S. cholerae-suis* of pigs, but all may cause illness in man given the opportunity. This epidemiological promiscuity of salmonellae provides many potential sources of infection. Direct contact with infected animals gives rise to sporadic infections. On the farm the source is often cattle (e.g. scouring calves), and in the home, family pets—even reptiles such as turtles and terrapins. But in general, animals are more important as a primary source of infection in the food chain. In technically advanced countries, intensive animal husbandry and mass-production methods have enouraged the spread of salmonellosis: animals are crowded together, and with poultry, bacteria are further spread by mechanized plucking and dressing processes.

Typically the cycle starts with the introduction of a relatively unknown serotype in animal feeds imported from abroad. For example the appearance and subsequent spread of *S. agona* in Britain and the United States in the early 1970s was traced to its introduction in Peruvian fish meal used in poultry and pig feed. Similarly, in the late 1970s, *S. hadar*, formerly unknown in Britain, became well-established in turkey stocks following its introduction in feedstuffs from abroad. Once a strain has become enzootic, it is almost impossible to eradicate, and its prevalence is only likely to diminish when it is displaced by another serotype.

Food sources. The net result of the enzootic state is that poultry and other raw meats at the retail end of the food chain are commonly contaminated with salmonellae of one sort or another. Unsatisfactory though this is, the consequences are not as serious as they at first appear, for the dose of salmonellae required to cause clinical illness is large and only likely to be reached if multiplication is allowed to occur in the food before consumption. Thus correct handling, preparation, and storage of food can prevent infection. Unfortunately this ideal is not always attained: failure to handle cooked foods separately from raw meat or meat products leads to cross-contamination; large frozen joints of meat of carcasses (e.g. turkeys) are given insufficient time to thaw so that cooking becomes inadequate; subsequent storage at ambient temperatures permits multiplication of salmonellae in what is a first-class culture medium. The increase of communal catering involving bulk cooking, and the popularity of warmed take-away foods provide additional opportunities for salmonella food poisoning through failure to observe good hygienic practice. Faulty factory methods can lead to particu-

larly widespread outbreaks corresponding to the distribution of the product. Major incidents have been caused by unpasteurized or improperly pasteurized milk, liquid egg, dried egg, desiccated coconut, chocolate (contaminated cocoa beans from Africa), and meat pies topped up after cooking with jelly from contaminated dispensing machines. The bulk preparation of animal pancreatic extract for the treatment of children with pancreatic insufficiency, a process that precluded the use of sterilizing temperatures, led to a product containing *S. schwarzengrund*.

Human sources. Infection is not readily transmitted from person to person, except among groups of people in closed communities involving the very young, the old, and the debilitated. Salmonellae can be particularly troublesome and dangerous in hospital maternity units.

Pathology. The number of organisms required to produce symptomatic infection is large but it is governed by many factors. Predisposition to infection is seen at the extremes of age and in the debilitated. Also the type and volume of food consumed may influence the outcome by providing a greater or lesser degree of protection from gastric acidity. A pH below 4.5 is lethal to salmonellae. Achlorhydria, the use of antacids, or previous gastric surgery increases the risk of infection. Stress also predisposes to infection, a factor that has special relevance to animal husbandry. The taking of antibiotics may enhance susceptibility by suppression of normal microflora. The newborn are especially prone to salmonella infection but the colonization of the gut by normal flora provides much protection.

The small intestine is the main site of infection, but there may be colonic involvement in some cases which gives rise to dysenteric symptoms. Salmonellae are invasive, usually within the bowel mucosa, but they may penetrate deep to the lamina propria. Occasionally there is generalized invasion which may lead to typhoidal illness, septicaemia, or remote focal infections in almost any organ of the body. Invasion of the bowel causes an acute inflammatory response with polymorphonuclear cell infiltration in the submucosa. Flattening or loss of secretory epithelium occurs adjacent to these inflamed areas. Enterotoxins of both heat-labile and heat-stable types (see page 5.180) are probably formed.

Clinical features. Not everyone who is infected with salmonellae becomes ill. In every food-poisoning outbreak there are unaffected persons who excrete the organism in their faeces. Others suffer a typical attack of acute enteritis lasting two or three days, and there are usually a few who suffer a more severe prolonged attack. The proportion of people who become ill is determined by the extent of contamination of the food and the characteristics of the infecting strain. The incubation period is usually 12–24 hours, but it may range from 6–48 hours depending on the size of the infecting dose. The onset is abrupt with malaise, nausea, headache, abdominal pain, and diarrhoea. Some patients vomit, but seldom more than once or twice. Shivering and fever is common in those that are more than mildly affected. Occasionally there is severe diarrhoea, with fluid green offensive stools that may contain mucus and blood. Dehydration, with cramps, oliguria, and uraemia may occur in the more severe type of illness. This is more likely to be seen at the extremes of age, and a fatal outcome is by no means unknown. Some patients suffer colonic involvement and experience frequent small bloody motions with tenesmus, and tenderness over the sigmoid colon. Salmonella enterocolitis may trigger off an attack of non-specific colitis, acute appendicitis in the young, or mesenteric thrombosis in the elderly. Reactive arthritis is an occasional late sequel of infection, as it is with other forms of acute enterocolitis.

Convalescent excretion. Most patients continue to excrete salmonellae in their faeces for a few weeks after infection—about 4–8 weeks for adults, and 8–24 weeks for infants. The number of organisms in these cases is usually low, but excretors have been found with 10^5–10^7 organisms per gram of faeces. Carriage of salmonellae, other than typhoid or paratyphoid bacilli, for more than six months is rare.

Invasive and focal infections. The clinical picture in one of the invasive types of infection follows the pattern described under pathology: typhoidal, septicaemic, or focal. Focal lesions may be extremely difficult to diagnose because they may only manifest themselves long after an episode of enteritis—or the original bowel infection may have been silent. These focal lesions have a tendency to chronicity and may mimic tuberculosis, particularly in cases of osteomyelitis of a vertebra or paravertebral abscess. Salmonella osteomyelitis or osteo-arthritis is strongly associated with sickle-cell anaemia (see Section 19). Salmonella abscess may develop in the liver, spleen, psoas muscle, uterus (after septic abortion), and in the peritoneal cavity (e.g. subphrenic, pelvic). Cholecystitis, pyelitis, endocarditis, pneumonia, and meningitis are other forms of focal infection. Patients with untreated deep-seated salmonella infections suffer a high mortality.

Laboratory diagnosis. A definitive diagnosis must depend on the isolation of the infecting organism, for salmonella enteritis cannot be distinguished from other forms of enteritis on clinical grounds alone. The culture of salmonellae in the laboratory is a sensitive procedure that allows the detection of small numbers of organisms even when greatly outnumbered by other bacteria. Identification of serotypes can only be done in specialist reference laboratories possessing a full set of antisera, but most clinical laboratories are able to narrow identification down to a short-list by the use of a restricted set of antisera available commercially. Some reference laboratories offer strain identification of *S. typhimurium*, *S. enteritidis*, and *S. hadar* by phage-typing techniques. Patients produce antibody to their infecting strain during convalescence, but this is seldom of diagnostic value. Strains antigenically related to the typhoid and paratyphoid bacilli will cause the Widal test to become partly positive.

Treatment. Nothing more than simple supportive and symptomatic treatment is required for uncomplicated attacks of salmonella enteritis. Specific chemotherapy is contra-indicated: it does not shorten the period of illness, it is liable to prolong excretion of salmonellae, and with ampicillin there is an increased risk of relapse. Patients should be encouraged to take oral fluids, e.g., physiological saline with glucose, to replace what has been lost through diarrhoea and vomiting. Intravenous fluid replacement is likely to be required only for the most severely affected patients and babies.

Invasive salmonellosis is quite a different matter. Here antimicrobials are valuable, even essential. Chloramphenicol, cotrimoxazole, tetracycline, and ampicillin are likely to be the most useful agents and they must be used in full dosage for several weeks, since invasive disease caused by salmonellae other than the typhoid and paratyphoid bacilli tend to be refractory to treatment. It is mandatory to obtain sensitivity results from the laboratory in order to guide chemotherapy, for it is a regrettable fact that many strains of salmonellae possess multiple antibiotic resistance. For a more detailed account of the treatment and management of patients suffering from acute diarrhoea see Section 12.

Prevention and control. Most preventive measures such as the hygienic preparation, handling, and storage of food will be self-evident from the account of the epidemiology of salmonellosis already given. However, since animals form the main reservoir of infection, methods of animal husbandry, marketing, slaughtering, and policies for the disposal of animal and human waste all have an effect on the incidence of the disease in man. Milk and other animal products such as liquid egg should be pasteurized. Compulsory heat treatment of imported or recycled animal feeds would do much to reduce the incidence of salmonellosis in animals. The use of antibiotics in animal breeding, whether as growth supplements or in the treatment of disease, should be restricted, and antibiotics that are of special value for the treatment of human disease, such as chloramphenicol, should be prohibited for animal use. Direct contact with an antimicrobial agent is unnecessary for the salmonellae to become resistant; multiple resistance can be acquired from other non-pathogenic Enterobacteria by means of plasmid transfer.

The importance of a salmonella-excreting food handler as a source of infection has probably been exaggerated. Such a person is more likely to be the victim of handling contaminated animal products during the course of his work than a source of infection. However, it has long been customary to suspend a professional food handler from duty until three consecutive negative stool specimens have been produced, and it would be a strong-minded physician who would be prepared to relax such a rule. But it is probably more important to suspend a food handler who has diarrhoea whatever the cause, for a person with diarrhoea spreads organisms far more readily than a person with formed stools. The occasional long-term excreter constitutes a problem. There is no known way in which the disappearance of the organism can be hastened. The temptation to use antimicrobials should be resisted, as they are likely to prolong the ultimate period of excretion, even though the stools my become culture negative during the course of treatment.

Shigella infections: bacillary dysentery

This genus takes its name from a Japanese, Kiyoshi Shiga, who in 1897 was the first to recognize an association between a certain type of Gram-negative bacillus and epidemic dysentery. The organism became known as *Shigella shigae* or Shiga's bacillus (now *Shigella dysenteriae* type 1). This organism remains the most virulent of the shigellae, and it was probably the cause of much of the severe dysentery that ravaged the soldiers of the Crimean and American Civil Wars. A contemporary writer estimated that in the latter war 1¾ million American soldiers suffered an attack of dysentery or enteritis and 44 000 died—a mortality rate of 2.5 per cent. After a gradual decline during the early part of this century, this organism re-emerged in the late 1960s as a cause of epidemic dysentery in Central America, Mexico, and the Indian sub-continent. In Nicaragua there were an estimated 13 000 deaths in one year, and in Guatemala the monthly death rate reached a peak of 11 000. The situation was aggravated by the appearance in these epidemics of strains with multiple antibiotic resistance, including resistance to chloramphenicol.

Soon after the publication of Shiga's work, Flexner described a similar dysentery bacillus (*Sh. flexneri*), and in 1915 a Dane, C. Sonne, described a third type (*Sh. sonnei*). The most recently described member of the genus (*Sh. boydi*) is named after Boyd who published his work during the 1930s. Thus there are four groups of dysentery bacilli which are differentiated according to biochemical reactions and antigenic structure:

Group A   *Sh. dysenteriae*. Does not ferment mannitol. 10 serotypes: only type 1 ('*Sh. shigae*') and type 2 ('*Sh. schmitzi*') are important human pathogens.

Group B   *Sh. flexneri*. 13 serotypes and subtypes.

Group C   *Sh. boydi*. 15 serotypes.

Group D   *Sh. sonnei*. Serologically homogenous, but strains may be differentiated by phage and colicine typing methods.

Most shigellae, like the salmonellae, are non-lactose fermenters (*Sh. sonnei* ferments lactose late), but they are unusual among the Enterobacteria in being non-motile and, with one minor exception, they are anaerogenic, i.e., they do not produce gas from sugars. *Sh. sonnei* is the least pathogenic and usually causes only minor illness. *Sh. flexneri* and *Sh. boydi* are of intermediate pathogenicity.

Epidemiology. The epidemic potential of *Sh. dysenteriae* and its recent re-emergence in certain parts of the world has already been mentioned. It is an organism that thrives under conditions of overcrowding and squalor, particularly where there are no proper means for sewage disposal; hence its prevalence during times of war and deprivation. It is not endemic in technically advanced countries. *Sh. flexneri* occurs worldwide but is more common in tropical than temperate regions. In Britain and Europe during the 1920s flexner and sonne dysentery were of about equal prevalence, but latterly *Sh. sonnei* has become predominant, and since the Second World War it has accounted for almost all endemic dysentery in these areas.

The epidemiology differs from that of the salmonellae in several fundamental respects. Firstly, man and certain primates are the only natural hosts of the shigellae. Pet monkeys are occasionally a source of infection, but transmission is essentially from man to man by the faecal–oral route. Secondly, the infective dose is very much smaller than it is for salmonellae. In the case of *Sh. dysenteriae* 10–100 bacteria were found to be sufficient to cause disease in 10–40 per cent of volunteers.

Transmission may occur through direct personal contact, mainly by contamination of the fingers, as well as by the consumption of contaminated food or drink. In the latter case, infection does not depend on the organisms multiplying in the food as with salmonella infections; simple contamination is sufficient. So the types of food that are most handled, such as salads, are the likely vehicles of infection, and these tend to give rise to sporadic infections rather than outbreaks. However, large outbreaks have resulted from the faecal pollution of untreated water supplies, and countries that experience regular flooding often suffer a simultaneous increase in dysentery. Flies are also major factors in the spread of organisms from excreta to food, and in many areas the incidence of dysentery parallels fly activity.

Sonne dysentery in temperate zones. Here the pattern of disease is somewhat different, possibly because of improved hygienic conditions and fly control. The highest incidence is in the late winter or early spring, and most infections are in children attending infant or primary schools, or in people in closed institutions such as military barracks. In these circumstances, transmission is mainly by personal contact and by contamination of hands from lavatory seats, flushing handles, taps, door knobs, roller towels, and other fomites. Shigellae may survive on the fingers for several hours. Patients are most infectious when their stools are fluid, for not only are organisms present in abundance, but there is greater opportunity for them to be spread by splashing. Non-syphonic water closets containing liquid faeces have been shown to generate bacteria-carrying aerosols that cause widespread contamination of the environment. Cold, dark, damp conditions favour prolonged survival of shigellae deposited on hard surfaces in this way, and under such conditions organisms have been shown to survive for at least 17 days on wooden lavatory seats.

Pathology. The essential lesion produced by shigellae is an acute locally invasive colitis. This may range from mild catarrhal inflammation of the mucous membrane of the rectum and sigmoid colon, such as is common in *Sh. sonnei* infections, to severe necrotizing lesions involving the entire colon and sometimes the terminal ileum, such as are seen in the worst forms of *Sh. dysenteriae* infections. The bacteria are found in the mucosa, and they may penetrate deep to the lamina propria and even the muscularis mucosae. Generalized invasion and septicaemia, however, is rare and virtually limited to compromised patients. Local mucosal changes consist of oedema, capillary engorgement, and leucocyte infiltration. Small haemorrhages are common and the submucous veins may be engorged or thrombosed. The mucous membrane becomes intensely red and there may be blood-stained mucus. In the severest forms of the disease, areas of mucosa undergo coagulation necrosis which appear as thickened semi-rigid greyish patches. These eventually separate to leave raw ulcerated areas which may ultimately fibrose and cause stenosis. Haemorrhage and perforation may also result from such lesions. Extensive lesions lead to much protein loss, which adds to the severe debility that accompanies these infections. The active agent in this process is thought to

be the somatic antigen of the organism, i.e., endotoxin. Only Shiga's bacillus (*Sh. dysenteriae* type 1) produces an exotoxin, but it does not seem to be an important factor in the disease process. Recent evidence suggests that some shigellae are capable of producing heat-labile cholera-like enterotoxin (see page 5.196) that acts on the upper small intestine, and which accounts for the large-volume watery diarrhoea that some patients suffer in contrast to the more usual frequent sparse stools.

Clinical features. The illness ranges from a triviality, in which the passage of a few loose stools without any constitutional symptoms may be the only manifestation of infection, to fulminating disease as caused by *Sh. dysenteriae*. The incubation period is short, usually about two or three days, but exceptionally it may be as long as a week. Infections of moderate severity are characterized by fever, malaise, headache, and diarrhoea. Faecal material is passed at first, but this is followed by the frequent passage of small quantities of blood-stained mucus ('red-current jelly') and pus. Lower abdominal cramps and tenesmus are common, but usually abdominal pain is not as prominent as it is in salmonellosis or campylobacter enteritis. Exacerbation of haemorrhoids and rectal prolapse may result from rectal oedema and straining at stool. A moderate leucocytosis is usual, but in severe infections there may be leucopenia. The acute disease lasts for a few days and then there is gradual resolution. However, the course of severe Shiga dysentery may be protracted and complicated by failure of other body systems, and sometimes the acute attack is followed by chronic or recurrent bouts of diarrhoea.

Children may develop quite striking meningism which can be misleading to the clinician if it occurs before the onset of diarrhoea. Shigellosis in children may also be associated with acute appendicitis, and in the elderly, mesenteric thrombosis is a recognized complication. Babies are especially prone to the effects of intestinal infections, so that even *Sh. sonnei* can cause serious illness. Dehydration is the particular danger at this age. Occasionally intussusception is a complication in young children. Shigellae can also cause acute vaginitis in children and, since the infection may arise without any history of diarrhoea, it is a condition that can easily pass unrecognized.

Reactive arthritis, Reiter's syndrome, purulent keratoconjunctivitis, and neuritis are uncommon late complications of infection with any of the shigellae. In the case of arthritis the knees and ankles are the joints most commonly affected and this complication is particularly associated with people who possess the human leucocyte antigen (HLA) B27.

Shigellae are usually excreted in the faeces for a few weeks after recovery from illness, and about one in ten patients continue to excrete for more than 10 weeks. Prolonged excretion tends to be more common in young children.

Laboratory diagnosis. It is important to note that shigellae are rather delicate organisms that perish in acid conditions. Since overgrowth of other faecal bacteria may rapidly lower pH, specimens must either be refrigerated or placed in alkaline transport medium if there is to be a delay of more than an hour or two before delivery to the laboratory. Culture techniques are not as sensitive as they are for salmonellae.

Treatment. Mild infections require no treatment, and all but the more severe or complicated infections require only symptomatic and supportive treatment to correct dehydration and electrolyte loss. Antimicrobial drugs should not be used routinely, and certainly not without laboratory control, for strains showing multiple antibiotic resistance are widespread and common. Sulphonamides have traditionally been used for shigellosis, and they are usually adequate provided the infecting strain is sensitive. They must be used cautiously in patients that are dehydrated because of the risk of crystalluria, and this applies even when the so-called non-absorbable types are used. Ampicillin is held by some to be the drug of choice; tetracycline, or co-trimoxazole are alternatives. Purgatives, once advocated for clearing the bowel of 'toxins', should never be used.

Prevention and control. Public health measures, such as the safe disposal of excreta, provision of purified water, and the control of flies, are paramount in the control of shigellosis. Unpurified water can be made bacteriologically safe (though tainted to the taste) by the addition of hypochlorite tablets; salads or fruit can be disinfected by soaking in water containing 80 parts per million of free chlorine.

Outbreaks of sonne dysentery in schools are difficult to control, but measures should be aimed at preventing spread by the hands. Supervised washing and disinfection of hands after defaecation, and frequent disinfection of lavatory seats, taps, and door knobs are effective if rigorously applied. Only disposable hand towels should be provided. It is impracticable to detect and exclude all children excreting shigellae, so exclusion should be limited to those suffering from diarrhoea regardless of whether they are known to be infected.

Food handlers who are suffering from dysentery should be excluded from work until they have produced at least three consecutive negative stool samples taken not less than 24 hours apart and at least two days after cessation of any antimicrobial chemotherapy.

Results of experiments with oral vaccines are encouraging and vaccination may one day be a valuable method of prevention in developing countries.

Enteropathogenic *Escherichia coli* (EPEC): infantile gastroenteritis

The concept that *E. coli*, the common coliform bacillus, might be capable of causing enteritis is not a recent one. In 1895 the German paediatrician, Escherich, suspected that certain strains of '*Bacterium coli*' caused infantile diarrhoea, but attempts to differentiate pathogenic from non-pathogenic strains were unsuccessful, mainly because adequate serological classification was not available at the time. It was not until the development of Kauffmann's serotyping system some 50 years later that progress could be made. It was then noticed that strains of *E. coli* that had been associated with several outbreaks of infantile gastroenteritis studied in Britain between 1945 and 1949 belonged to two serotypes (O 111 : B 4 and O 55 : B 5), and it was not long before other gastroenteritis-associated serotypes were discovered. At least 14 O serogroups are now known to contain such strains (Table 1). These 'EPEC' strains are distinct from strains of *E. coli* found in parenteral infections.

Table 1   O Serogroups in which EPEC strains occur

18	26*	44	55*	86
111*	114	119*	125*	126*
127*	128*	142	158	

* Commonest

From Rowe, B. (1979). The role of *Escherichia coli* in gastroenteritis. *Clins. Gastroent.* **8**, by permission

Epidemiology. Epidemic infantile enteritis was a major problem in hospitals and day nurseries in Britain in the early 1940s. These outbreaks, which were predominant in the winter and early spring, sometimes carried a mortality as high as 50 per cent. Newborn and bottle-fed babies were most at risk. Once the nature of the infecting organism became known, measures were taken to prevent cross-infection and the number of outbreaks fell. Yet there seems to have been an additional unrelated and unexplained decline in the incidence of epidemic EPEC infantile diarrhoea in Britain and North America during the last ten years, but it would certainly be unwise to assume that this trend will continue or not be reversed. The source of such outbreaks can usually be traced to the admission of an infant who is excreting the organism. EPEC gastroenteritis is essentially a disease of children under two years old, but occasional outbreaks involving adults have been reported.

In the tropics, the epidemiology is somewhat different. Infections are more prevalent in the community and the highest incidence is between the ages of 6 and 18 months—the time when children are being weaned. The outbreaks of 'summer diarrhoea' that were common in Britain in the nineteenth and early twentieth centuries were probably caused by EPEC.

Pathology. The pathogenesis is unknown. EPEC do not appear to be invasive (they are rarely isolated from blood cultures) nor do they produce enterotoxins detectable in orthodox test systems for heat-labile and heat-stable toxins. It is probable that they produce toxins of an unknown type. In babies who have died of EPEC infection, the gut is usually dilated, but it otherwise appears essentially normal; there is no gross inflammation or ulceration. The causative organism is found throughout the gut including the jejunum and ileum.

Clinical features. The incubation period is usually one or two days, but with a large inoculating dose it may be as short as eight hours. As with salmonellae the infective dose is high, in the order of 10^5–10^{10} organisms. The onset of diarrhoea may be abrupt or gradual, with a tendency for cases with an abrupt onset to be more ill than the others. Stools become loose and green, then orange-coloured, and eventually watery. Vomiting is common in more severely affected children and it may be projectile. The combination of watery diarrhoea and vomiting quickly leads to dehydration. The child is at first irritable, may have convulsions, and the temperature rises to 39–40 °C. In the absence of prompt fluid replacement, dehydration and metabolic disturbances may be irreversible and the child becomes apathetic and dies. But the disease may be mild and marked only by the passage of a few loose stools without vomiting or general illness; this is the usual pattern in Britain at present. Occasionally the loose stools persist for days or even weeks, but beyond this time it becomes increasingly likely that other factors are involved.

Laboratory diagnosis. Definitive diagnosis of *E. coli* gastroenteritis depends upon isolation of the infecting organism in the laboratory. Faeces should be sent for culture as soon as possible and before any antimicrobial therapy is begun. Since *E. coli* is present in virtually all samples of faeces and colonies of enteropathogenic strains appear similar to non-pathogenic strains, reliance is placed on serological methods of identification. This is done by suspending bacteria from selected colonies in saline and testing for agglutination against a panel of antisera containing antibodies to the common EPEC O serogroups. It should be understood that just because a strain belongs to one of these serogroups it does not necessarily mean that it is enteropathogenic. But the opposite holds true: a strain which is not agglutinated by such antisera is unlikely to be enteropathogenic. A point that helps in the interpretation of cultures is that in EPEC gastroenteritis the infecting strain becomes predominant over others, so all of the *E. coli* colonies are of the one type. The serological screening of cultures is time consuming, so it is usual to restrict the search for such organisms to cultures from children under two or three years old.

Different strains within the same O serogroups can be distinguished by their H or K antigens but typing to this extent, though epidemiologically informative, is a facility available only in reference laboratories.

Treatment. Since the main danger to the infant with gastroenteritis is from the effects of dehydration, immediate efforts should be made to correct fluid and electrolyte loss. If started early, oral therapy—for example with 4.5 per cent glucose in half-strength physiological saline—will usually be adequate, but intravenous or intraperitoneal therapy will be required for those more severely affected. Antibiotics are of doubtful value; they should not be used routinely and certainly not without laboratory control.

Prevention. Firstly, breast feeding should be encouraged, since breast-fed babies are far less likely to suffer from EPEC gastroenteritis than bottle-fed babies. For infants that have to be bottle-fed, the feeds should be prepared aseptically. Infected infants should be nursed in isolation with scrupulous attention to barrier technique. But where infants are concentrated in large units, control of infection is difficult and outbreaks can occur even when all the children are accommodated in cubicles; the environment of a baby suffering from the disease becomes so heavily contaminated that even the best nursing techniques may fail to prevent spread. Outbreaks commonly arise from the admission of a symptomless excreter, often a baby transferred from another hospital or residential institution, so it is a wise policy to isolate all such transferred children until they have been shown to be free from infection.

Enterotoxigenic *E. coli* (ETEC): travellers' diarrhoea

In 1968 a detailed study of an epidemic of diarrhoea in a group of British troops travelling to South Arabia showed that a single serotype of *E. coli* (O 148 : H 28) was present in about half of those affected; it was later shown to produce enterotoxin. This study sparked off a search for other enterotoxigenic strains, and it soon became clear that such strains are a common cause of travellers' diarrhoea. ETEC are prevalent in tropical and developing countries and are uncommon in temperate zones. Thus the infection affects residents of temperate zones moving to countries with warm climates, a pattern that is reflected in the popular names given to the affliction, e.g., Delhi belly, Cairo crud, Montezuma's revenge, Aztec two-step, etc. ETEC have also been responsible for outbreaks of infection from contaminated water supplies. Outbreaks on cruise ships, probably food-borne, have also been reported. ETEC may occasionally cause outbreaks of infantile enteritis, and they probably cause much sporadic diarrhoea among children in endemic areas. Precise information on prevalence is lacking owing to the difficulty of laboratory diagnosis (see below).

Pathogenesis. ETEC may produce one or both of two enterotoxins: heat-labile (LT) and heat-stable (ST) toxins. LT is a protein that is related to the toxin of *Vibrio cholerae*. It stimulates the production of adenyl cyclase in the small intestinal epithelium, which indirectly causes an increased transport of fluid into the bowel lumen. ST is a polypeptide with a lower molecular weight (about 5000) than LT. It too indirectly promotes the transfer of fluid into the bowel but by activation of guanylate cyclase. The dose of bacteria needed to cause disease is large, about 10^8–10^{10}.

Clinical features. The incubation period ranges from one to three days depending on the size of infecting dose; the period is shorter for strains producing ST only. The illness consists of watery diarrhoea and abdominal pain lasting from one to three days. In severe attacks the stools resemble the rice-water stools of cholera.

Laboratory diagnosis. Diagnosis depends on finding an LT or ST-producing strain of *E. coli* in the stools. Unfortunately this involves specialized methods that are unsuitable for ordinary clinical laboratories, and this is the main restriction to progress in our understanding of these infections. The best that can be done at present is to screen cultures serologically in the way that has been described for EPEC strains, except that the antisera used must relate to different serogroups. Such antisera are not yet generally available, mainly because we do not know enough about the range of O serogroups involved or what their geographical distribution might be. So far ETEC have been found in some 26 O serogroups.

Treatment. Supportive and symptomatic treatment is all that is required for what is a short self-limiting disease. Prophylactic chemotherapy for travellers' diarrhoea has its advocates, but there is conflicting evidence concerning its effectiveness; many ETEC show multiple antibiotic resistance. Enterovioform, a once popular 'prophylactic' cocktail, should not be used; there is no evidence that it is efficacious and it contains the potentially toxic compound iodochlorhydroxyquinoline.

Enteroinvasive *E. coli* (EIEC)

Certain strains of *E. coli* that are neither EPEC nor ETEC are associated with diarrhoea which resembles shigella dysentery. These have not been studied in detail and again there is no simple test for pathogenicity. Like shigellae, they invade the colonic mucosa and may cause ulceration. Some of these strains share certain features with shigellae including some antigens. The most important of the group belong to just two serogroups: O 124 and O 164. Six other less important ones have been described but not well evaluated. These organisms are of worldwide distribution, and they tend to affect older children and adults rather than infants. In 1971 there was a widespread and unusual outbreak in the United States caused by *E. coli* O 124 present in a consignment of French cheese.

MISCELLANEOUS ENTEROPATHOGENIC AND FOOD POISONING BACTERIA

Campylobacter

The name *Campylobacter* (Greek, curved rod) was coined by French workers in 1963 for a group of small strictly micro-aerophilic curved or spiral Gram-negative bacteria that were formerly classified as vibrios, but which are now known to be more closely related to the *Spirilla*. They have a single flagellum at one or both poles of the bacterial cell which gives them a characteristic rapid darting motility (Fig. 1). The type species (*Vibrio fetus*—now *Campylobacter fetus*) was first recognized some 70 years ago as a cause of infectious infertility and abortion in cattle and sheep. But it was not until the 1970s that *C. jejuni* and *C. coli* (collectively *C. fetus* subsp. *jejuni* in obsolete American nomenclature) were recognized as a common cause of acute enterocolitis in man. Special selective techniques are required for their isolation from faeces and it is for this reason that they went undetected for so long. *C. fetus* subsp. *fetus* (formerly subsp. *intestinalis*) occasionally infects man, but only as an uncommon opportunist of compromised patients, in whom it causes various forms of systemic infection including an ill-defined febrile illness resembling brucellosis. Here we are concerned only with campylobacter enterocolitis, and in the following text the term 'campylobacter' refers collectively to the two species *C. jejuni* and *C. coli* which are closely related and cause similar illness.

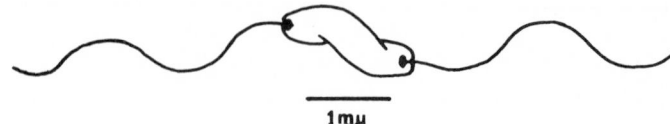

Fig. 1 *Campylobacter jejuni* (from an electron micrograph).

Epidemiology. Like salmonellosis, campylobacter enterocolitis is a zoonosis. Campylobacters are to be found in a wide variety of animal hosts, especially birds in which they appear to form part of the normal intestinal flora. It is a common disease: in 1980 over 9500 campylobacter isolations were reported to the Communicable Disease Surveillance Centre, Colindale, London, and in many laboratories campylobacters are the commonest bacterial pathogens to be isolated from patients with acute enterocolitis. The disease is of worldwide distribution but it has a higher prevalence in tropical and developing countries than in Europe or North America. In the latter regions the disease affects people of all ages with high morbidity in young adults. But in the tropics most infections occur in early childhood, and that adults are relatively unaffected, presumably as a result of acquired immunity or tolerance.

Infection is acquired orally, and the infective dose is small. The infection can be passed from person to person, as with other enteric bacteria, but infectivity is low and most infections probably originate from an animal source. Unfortunately, at the time of writing, we have no satisfactory typing system for campylobacters which makes source tracing difficult, but it is likely that many infections are acquired through the handling or consumption of contaminated food. Chicken carcasses are commonly contaminated with campylobacters, and cross-contamination readily occurs in the kitchen if good hygienic practice is not observed. However, unlike salmonellae, campylobacters do not seem able to multiply in food and thereby cause explosive outbreaks following the consumption of a single meal. On the other hand outbreaks of campylobacter enterocolitis, involving as many as 3000 people have been caused by the consumption of untreated milk or water. Infected dogs and cats have caused family outbreaks, and in such cases the source has almost always been a newly acquired puppy or kitten that itself was suffering from diarrhoea.

Pathology. Campylobacters cause an invasive type of infection, primarily involving the jejunum or ileum but commonly extending to the colon. In the latter site, biopsy material has shown acute inflammation of the mucosa with crypt abscess formation. Campylobacters have not been demonstrated in these lesions, but this is probably a reflection of inadequate technique. Occasionally organisms are cultured from patients' blood; early symptoms certainly suggest bacteraemia, and probably many more such isolations would be made if blood cultures were taken at the onset of symptoms. The ability of campylobacters to produce watery diarrhoea suggests that enterotoxins are implicated, but the test systems currently used for the detection of LT and ST enterotoxins have not shown significant activity. The blood leucocyte count and erythrocyte sedimentation rate are usually raised in patients who are more than mildly affected. Specific agglutinins appear in the blood from about the fifth day of illness and then slowly disappear over several months; complement fixing antibody fades more quickly.

Clinical features. Campylobacter enterocolitis is an acute self-limiting disease that ranges from the inconvenience of a few loose bowel actions to an extremely unpleasant and debilitating attack of acute diarrhoea. A fatal outcome is exceptional and—in developed countries at least—it is limited to the elderly or compromised patient. Symptomless infections are not uncommon.

The incubation period is usually three to five days, but it ranges from one to seven days, and there is some evidence to suggest an even longer period in some cases. Diarrhoea and abdominal pain may be the first signs of illness, but often fever and symptoms of a general nature precede the onset of diarrhoea by a few hours or even days. These prodromal symptoms are influenza-like with malaise, headache, backache, aching limbs, sweating, and sometimes rigors. Fever of 40 °C or more is by no means rare and this may be associated with convulsions in children or delirium in adults. Griping abdominal pains, which may be severe, accompany the diarrhoea, and the stools become fluid, bile-stained, offensive, and sometimes watery. Frank blood is commonly present in the stools of more severely affected patients, and cellular exudate can be detected microscopically in the stools of most patients. Vomiting is not a conspicuous feature of the disease, but almost all patients experience nausea. Severe diarrhoea seldom lasts more than two or three days, but loose stools and abdominal pain often persist for several more days and patients feel washed out and wretched. A brief relapse is not uncommon at this stage and some weight loss is usual. Chronic disease has not been reported, but a few patients may excrete the organism in their stools for up to 12 weeks after recovery; most patients are culture negative by about the fifth week.

Misleading presentations and complications. The abdominal pain can be of a type and severity that suggests acute appendicitis, particularly in older children and young adults, and this is probably the commonest cause of patients with campylobacter enterocolitis being admitted to hospital. If laparotomy is performed, the ileum or jejunum is usually found to be inflamed, oedematous, and associated with mesenteric adenitis, but occasionally there is genuine acute appendicitis. In uncomplicated enteritis, there may be abdominal tenderness but not the classic signs of acute peritonitis.

Some patients may present with symptoms and sigmoidoscopic appearances indistinguishable from non-specific colitis; the danger here is that they might be given steroids. Babies may pass blood-stained motions without obvious diarrhoea, a finding which can lead to a wrong diagnosis of intussusception. An uncommon manifestation of campylobacter infection is acute or acute-on-chronic cholecystitis. Reactive arthritis sometimes follows an attack of campylobacter enteritis, as it may do after other forms of infective diarrhoea.

Laboratory diagnosis. The isolation of campylobacters is not difficult, but it requires special media and conditions for micro-aerobic culture. The precautions recommended for the handling of samples for the culture of shigellae apply to campylobacters, for they are at least as delicate. Rapid presumptive diagnosis can be made microscopically on freshly voided faeces by a skilled observer with the aid of dark-field or phase-contrast illumination: campylobacters are recognizable by their characteristic motility and morphology. This method may be valuable in cases of difficult presentation where an early diagnosis is required.

Treatment. Patients with campylobacter enterocolitis recover without specific treatment, but appropriate chemotherapy seems to be effective in reducing the length of illness and eliminating the organism from the stools. Erythromycin is a logical choice, since most campylobacters are sensitive and it has a narrow spectrum of activity. It is probably the most widely used antimicrobial for this purpose, but furazolidone has also been used successfully; in neither case have controlled trials been done. The choice as to whether to use specific antimicrobial chemotherapy arises less often than might be supposed, for by the time a bacteriological diagnosis has been made the patient is usually recovering. Antimicrobial therapy should be reserved for the more severe infections: erythromycin stearate 500 mg twice daily for five days (40 mg/kg a day of the ethyl succinate for children) is a suitable and safe regimen.

For rare septicaemic or life-threatening infections, gentamicin should be given, since resistance to this antibiotic has not been described. It should be emphasized that campylobacters are naturally resistant to the cephalosporins and most are resistant to ampicillin.

Non-cholera vibrios

Vibrios are curved non-sporing Gram-negative bacilli possessing a single polar flagellum which gives them a characteristic rapid darting or oscillating motility—hence the derivation of their name from the Latin, *vibrare*, to shake. Most vibrios live harmlessly in water, but a few are pathogenic, notably *Vibrio cholerae* (see page 5.195). The only other vibrios of medical importance are the marine or 'halophilic' (salt-loving) vibrios, which are now described.

Vibrio parahaemolyticus. This marine organism was first associated with human disease in Japan in 1963, since when it has come to be recognized as the commonest cause of food poisoning in that country. Seafood is the main source of the organism, and the high incidence of infection in the Far East is doubtless due to the popularity of raw fish food. *V. parahaemolyticus* is most plentiful in warm waters of the world, but it has been isolated from North

Atlantic and Pacific coastlines. Food poisoning has been reported from Europe, America, Africa, south-east Asia, and Australia, and in these regions most of the reported infections have followed the consumption of crabs and prawns. The vibrios can survive inside crabs which have been boiled. With shellfish, poisoning is most likely to arise through contamination after cooking, for a few organisms picked up from a working surface contaminated by the raw product can multiply at atmospheric temperatures. This is one reason why the incidence of infection in temperate regions is higher in summer than winter.

After ingestion, *V. parahaemolyticus* multiplies in the gut and produces an enterotoxin. It is not invasive, nor is toxin pre-formed in the food before consumption. The incubation period is usually 10–20 hours but it spans 2–48 hours. The number of organisms required to cause illness is large and infections are almost always food-borne. Symptoms consist of abdominal colic with watery diarrhoea, sometimes vomiting, and often a mild fever. The illness seldom lasts for more than one or two days and excretion of the organisms generally ceases within 10 days. Tetracycline shortens the period of excretion, but it is hardly justifiable to use antibiotics for a short self-limiting disease. Infected patients are not an important source of infection despite the fact that organisms are excreted in enormous numbers while the patient has diarrhoea.

Laboratory diagnosis. The marine vibrios grow poorly or not at all on media that are not supplemented with extra salt. Therefore if the clinician suspects marine food poisoning, the laboratory must be informed so that appropriate methods can be used. The Kanagawa test (β-haemolysis on medium containing human blood) is sometimes performed as an indication of pathogenicity: most of the strains associated with diarrhoea are Kanagawa-positive whereas many strains isolated from sea water give a negative test.

Vibrio alginolyticus. This marine vibrio is not enteropathogenic, but it can cause opportunistic infection of the external ears of swimmers and in wounds exposed to sea water.

Aeromonas and *Plesiomonas.* These organisms are not true vibrios, but they have several vibrio-like characteristics. Aeromonads are found in water and cold-blooded animals, and some are important pathogens of fish. Only one species, *Aeromonas hydrophila* (syn. *A. liquefaciens*), infects man. It has been associated with acute diarrhoea and it may cause wound sepsis and septicaemia (see page 5.472). Some strains have been shown to produce enterotoxin.

Plesiomonas shigelloides is a vibrio-like organism that has occasionally been associated with diarrhoea, usually of a mild nature, but its causative role is uncertain. Recent work suggests that it produces a heat-stable enterotoxin. Most reports are from the Far East. Many strains share antigens with *Shigella sonnei*, hence the name shigelloides.

Bacillus cereus

This organism is a member of a large group of Gram-positive aerobic spore-forming bacilli of universal distribution. Most of them are of no medical importance, other than as a common cause of food spoilage, but exceptions are the anthrax bacillus (see page 5.217) and *B. cereus* which is a closely related species. Under certain circumstances *B. cereus* can cause food poisoning, and it has also recently become recognized as a cause of wound sepsis. The fact that it is a sporulating organism means that it can survive harsh physical conditions, which include the temperatures reached in many cooking procedures.

Two patterns of food poisoning are caused by *B. cereus*: one, first described in Norway in 1950, is like clostridial food poisoning (see page 5.236) with an incubation period of 8–16 hours and symptoms of abdominal pain and diarrhoea; the other is like staphylococcal food poisoning with a sudden onset of nausea and vomiting within one to five hours of eating the infected food. The former

diarrhoeal type is associated with a wide range of foods ranging from meat and vegetables to dessert dishes and ice-cream. By contrast, the vomiting type, first recognized in Britain in 1971, is almost exclusively associated with boiled or fried rice from Chinese restaurants or 'take-away' shops. In these cases the rice usually yields counts of *B. cereus* in the range 10^6–10^9 per gram. Such astronomically high counts can arise only if the rice is left for long periods at high ambient temperatures after soaking or boiling. Unfortunately it is convenient for such establishments to prepare rice in bulk in advance of demand, so that a batch may be kept for 24 hours or more before it is used up. Refrigeration is unpopular because chilling tends to cause the rice grains to stick together.

The two patterns of food poisoning are usually caused by different serotypes and the toxins involved are distinct. The 'diarrheal' enterotoxin is a relatively unstable protein (molecular weight about 50 000) and it is probably the pyogenic and pyrogenic factor in extra-intestinal wound infections. The 'emetic' toxin is a heat-stable compound of much lower molecular weight (less than 10 000), and it is pre-formed in the food before consumption.

Since *B. cereus* food poisoning is a form of intoxication, symptoms are short-lived, even though they may be dramatic. Diagnosis depends principally on finding counts in excess of 10^6 per gram of *B. cereus* in the suspect food; but if possible the vomitus and faeces of affected persons should also be cultured. Since *B. cereus* is ubiquitous, prevention depends on the observance of correct procedures in food preparation and storage.

FOOD POISONING: A GENERAL SUMMARY

This summary does not purport to be a guide to the investigation of food poisoning outbreaks; for that, the reader is referred to the works listed in the bibliography. Anyone investigating a suspected outbreak of food poisoning should have a thorough knowledge of the behaviour of food poisoning agent, which should include plant and chemical toxins as well as micro-organisms. Strictly, microbial food poisoning refers to outbreaks of infection resulting from the multiplication of organisms in food, but almost any agent capable of causing infection by ingestion may be transmitted by a process of simple contamination. The distinction is not always clear, but from a practical standpoint our chief concern is with agents that cause large outbreaks of infection as opposed to the odd sporadic case. For example there is increasing evidence that certain viruses—which are presumably unable to multiply in food—are implicated in outbreaks of food-borne disease, including viral hepatitis; raw or improperly cooked shellfish have particularly been implicated in such cases. Streptococcal tonsillitis has occasionally been transmitted on a large scale by food, and food-borne out-

Table 2   Characteristics of the principal food poisoning bacteria

Agent	Type of food poisoning	Incubation period	Duration
Salmonella	infection; enterotoxin possibly involved also	6–48 hours (usually 12–24 hours)	1–7 days if uncomplicated
Staphylococcus aureus	intoxication; toxin pre-formed in food	2–6 hours	6–24 hours
Clostridium perfringens	intermediate—see text	8–22 hours	24–48 hours
Clostridium botulinum	intoxication; toxin pre-formed in food	12–96 hours (usually 18–36 hours)	death 1–8 days or slow recovery over 6–8 months
Vibrio parahaemolyticus	infection; enterotoxin also involved	2–48 hours (usually 12–18 hours)	2–5 days
Bacillus cereus vomiting-type diarrhoeal-type	intoxication; toxin pre-formed in food unknown	1–5 hours 8–20 hours	12–24 hours about 12 hours

From Turnbull, P. C. B. (1979). Food poisoning with special reference to salmonella. In *Clins. Gastroent.* **8**, 663 (ed. H. P. Lambert). Saunders, Philadelphia, by permission.)

breaks of disease may even be caused by animal parasites, notably the nematode worm *Trichinella spiralis*.

In microbial food poisoning as originally defined two mechanisms are involved: either a toxin is pre-formed in the food before it is eaten (*Staph. aureus, Bacillus cereus* (vomiting type), *Clostridium botulinum*) or there is actual intestinal infection (*Salmonella, Vibrio parahaemolyticus*, occasionally *Shigella, E. coli*, and possibly *Campylobacter*). *Clostridium perfringens* is of intermediate standing, for toxin is produced when the organisms sporulate in the intestine after ingestion. The main features of food poisoning by these agents is summarized in Table 2. For more detailed accounts of those agents not already described, see page 5.158 (*Staph. aureus*) and page 5.230 (*Clostridium botulinum, Cl. perfringens*).

References

Christie, A. B. (1980). *Infectious diseases: epidemiology and clinical practice*, 3rd edn. Churchill Livingstone, Edinburgh.

Hobbs, B. C. and Gilbert, R. J. (1978). *Food poisoning and food hygiene*, 4th edn. Arnold, London.

Lambert, H. P. (ed.) (1979). Infections of the gastrointestinal tract. *Clins. Gastroent.* **8**, 549.

Reimann, H. and Bryan, F. L. (eds.) (1979). *Food-borne infections and intoxications*, 2nd edn. Academic Press, New York.

Wilson, G. S. and Miles, A. A. (1975). *Topley and Wilson's principles of bacteriology, virology and immunity*. 6th edn. Arnold, London.

Typhoid and paratyphoid fevers

E. B. Adams

These infections are sometimes grouped together as enteric fever. Although time-honoured, the term is somewhat inappropriate since the main manifestations of typhoid and paratyphoid are the result of dissemination of the causative organisms by the blood rather than their effects on the intestines. The most serious complications, however, relate to the bowel—either haemorrhage from erosion of a blood vessel in the wall of an intestinal ulcer or its perforation into the peritoneal cavity.

The name typhoid appears to have come from the Greek 'tuphos' meaning smoke or stupor—the same origin as that of typhus, with which typhoid was once confused. Headache, mounting pyrexia, and mental torpor, which may go on to stupor or a muttering delirium, occur in both conditions, and it was not until the middle of the nineteenth century that their separate identities were established.

Typhoid

A widespread and potentially lethal infection, typhoid follows ingestion of *Salmonella typhi*, with initial lesions in the bowel, bacteraemia, and subsequent affection of many tissues.

Epidemiology. Typhoid fever invariably comes from a human source—another patient with active disease, a patient during convalescence or a chronic carrier. The organisms gain access to the body via contaminated food and water. Usually contamination is from faecal material, but occasionally respiratory secretions, vomitus or other body fluids may be responsible. *S. typhi* may be spread by human hands, by flies, and by other insects, can survive freezing and drying, and may thus be carried to food and drink from the water supply, from sewage, or from less common sources such as dust, ice, and shellfish obtained from polluted water. Of these, the water supply plays the central role. Not only is drinking water essential for man's survival, but many foods are washed in water or mixed with it before being eaten. A safe source providing the consumer with water distributed through a reticulated system of pipes is costly (as is a proper disposal system for sewage). Along with several other water-borne diseases, typhoid is therefore rife in many of the economically underdeveloped countries but somewhat uncommon in the affluent parts of the world. Table 1, compiled from World Health Organization statistics of national notifications, illustrates this contrasting picture. The disparity in prevalence, however, is likely to be much greater than shown since notifications of disease are invariably low when health services are inadequate for the load imposed upon them. Endemic typhoid is a common disease in most of Africa, in Asia, and in Central and South America. It is quite common around the Mediterranean but comparatively rare in northern Europe and North America. In the developing countries, the modern parts of cities and towns are usually almost free of typhoid, general hospitals deriving a large majority of their typhoid patients from slums, peripheral shanty towns, and rural districts where sanitation and the water supply are rudimentary. Working as a clinician in Africa, I have found that one in a hundred patients coming under my care in an adult medical ward has typhoid, while in the same hospital the disease comprises 1.5 per cent of all paediatric admissions.

Table 1 Some national notifications for typhoid

Continent	Country	Year	No. of cases
Africa	Algeria	1976	4746
	Egypt	1976	10040*
	Morocco	1976	3628*
	Togo	1977	1134
America	Chile	1977	11533*
	Colombia	1977	8207*
	United States	1977	372
Asia	Bangladesh	1977	10461
	Sri Lanka	1976	2395
	Thailand	1977	11839
Europe	Belgium	1977	15
	France	1976	1008*
	Spain	1976	2092
	Sweden	1977	14
Oceania	Australia	1977	59
	New Zealand	1977	15
	Papua New Guinea	1977	120

* includes paratyphoid
Compiled from *World health statistics annual* (1979). World Health Organization, Geneva.

In theory, typhoid can be eradicated in any community by a combination of measures: provision of a properly controlled sewage disposal system and a pure water supply; care in the isolation and treatment of typhoid patients; identification and treatment of all carriers; vigilance in the manufacture and distribution of food supplies; ensuring that the disease is not introduced by visitors or immigrants. In practice this ideal has not yet been achieved, although there is now little typhoid in most developed countries with fully-staffed medical services and appropriate public health legislation. Britain is a good example of the potential danger to the community which typhoid presents. Each year some 200 cases are notified, most of them travellers returning from abroad and immigrants coming from countries where typhoid is rife. Apart from such sporadic cases, there is always the risk of an epidemic if one of the public health measures instituted to eradicate the disease proves inadequate, either by its design or in its execution. This was the case in the Aberdeen epidemic of 1964; the source of infection was traced to an imported tin of meat, the fault lying in the process of manufacture in its country of origin.

Pathogenesis. Typhoid is a generalized infection, most of its clinical manifestations reflecting this fact; but the gut is the portal of entry of *S. typhi* and the site of the two main complications. Before the introduction of chloramphenicol for treating typhoid, its duration as a febrile illness was usually between four and five weeks, and it caused profound inanition so that convalescence was likely to be long.

Following ingestion, typhoid bacilli multiply in the second part of the duodenum and infect the mucosa of the bowel, invading its lymphoid tissue and soon entering the blood stream, probably via the thoracic duct. Generalized dissemination thus occurs, many organs being affected, especially the liver, spleen, and reticulo-endothelial system. *S. typhi* may be cultured from the blood during this early stage—the first week or so of the clinically recognizable illness. Organisms pass from the liver to the bile, multiply rapidly, and re-enter the intestinal tract. Although they may be detected in stool specimens early on, this is uncommon until the third week when their growth in the bile is maximal. Heavy reinfection of the gut takes place, the Peyer's patches at the lower end of the ileum being most frequently affected although there may also be lesions in the jejunum and the proximal part of the colon, and the appendix is sometimes involved.

The gut bears the brunt of tissue destruction. The Peyer's patches and solitary lymphoid follicles become swollen from congestion, oedema, and the accumulation of lymphocytes and phagocytes. Similar inflammatory cells may be seen in the lymphatics and in the surrounding tissues of the bowel wall. Polymorphonuclear cells are virtually absent. In the more heavily affected portions of the gut (generally the terminal ileum), this acute inflammatory response is followed by necrosis and separation of dead tissue to produce ulceration and sloughing, but the lesions heal with minimal fibrosis so that strictures do not occur. In some cases, tissue necrosis leads to haemorrhage from erosion of blood vessels, or to perforation of the bowel with resultant peritonitis. These two complications may take place simultaneously. Mesenteric lymph nodes also become swollen from the same inflammatory process, but, although there is tissue destruction, rupture is infrequent. The organisms are now mainly intracellular, explaining why bacteraemia (and therefore a positive blood culture) is uncommon in the later stages of the disease.

Widespread lesions may occur elsewhere. In the liver, apart from cloudy swelling and small globules of fat, typhoid nodules are a characteristic finding. Situated in the hepatic lobule, they consist of collections of macrophages and lymphocytes, sometimes with central necrosis. In them *S. typhi* may be detected. Similar nodules may be seen in the bone marrow and kidney. The spleen is enlarged with marked proliferation of cells in the sinusoids and pulp, and typhoid nodules may also be observed. Rose spots, the characteristic rash of typhoid fever, are papular lesions which on microscopic examination show hyperaemia, monocytic infiltration, and typhoid bacilli. Although *S. typhi* grows readily in bile, acute cholecystitis is most uncommon. However, chronic cholecystitis and the formation of gallstones may occur and are sometimes associated with the carrier state. On rare occasions, typhoid meningitis, endocarditis, orchitis, and osteomyelitis complicate the disease, and there are other pathological manifestations of typhoid which are discussed later.

It was long believed that the continued fever and the various symptoms of typhoid were due to endotoxaemia but this has recently been challenged. In volunteer subjects tolerance to intravenous injections of endotoxin develops early and continued infusions of endotoxin are not accompanied by persistence of fever. Bacteraemia frequently disappears in the second week of typhoid, yet this is when symptoms are most severe. Organisms, however, remain within the cells in various tissues despite their disappearance from the blood; and tissue endotoxin, which enhances inflammatory responses at local sites of multiplication of the organism, is probably the cause of most of the symptoms and of sustained pyrexia.

Recovery from typhoid depends on a number of factors. These include the production of antibodies to the various antigenic components of the organism; the development of cell-mediated immunity (which may be compromised by malnutrition and other diseases); and the sensitivity of the strain of *S. typhi* responsible for the illness to the antibiotic chosen by the clinician. Cell-mediated immunity appears to be a most important factor determining the outcome. Based on the lymphocyte migration inhibition test, a close correlation has been demonstrated between the development of this form of immunity and the patient's recovery. Liability to suffer from complications in typhoid may be largely due to the patient's failure to mount an adequate cell-mediated immune response.

Clinical features. Although no age is exempt, typhoid is a disease of older children and young adults. The sexes are equally affected. The onset is insidious, few patients being able to say with accuracy when their illness started. Most appear to have been indisposed for about a week when first seen but longer and shorter periods are not rare. While some patients are confused and unable to give an account of their complaints, most do so without difficulty, although they often seem to be obtunded.

Headache is the commonest symptom. In adults it is followed in order of frequency by abdominal discomfort or pain, constipation or diarrhoea, generalized aches and pains, cough, malaise, and anorexia. Constipation is said to be commoner than diarrhoea in the initial stages, diarrhoea commoner later on. Both bloody diarrhoea and low backache may occur, but they are uncommon as initial symptoms. Occasionally patients complain of sweating, rigors, abdominal distension, shortness of breath, nose bleeds, and loss of weight. Two of these less common symptoms, dysentery and rigors, are worth further comment. Bloody diarrhoea, which is by no means rare, may be mistaken for bacillary or amoebic dysentery. Rigors usually occur when there are wide variations in body temperature (as in malaria). Their occurrence in typhoid should remind us that, although a stepwise rise in the pattern of pyrexia, with little diurnal fluctuation, has been taken as characteristic of the disease, the temperature may be sustained or intermittent and even hectic at times (hence the rigors). The clinician should therefore not be tempted to rule out the diagnosis on the appearance of the temperature chart.

Headache is also the commonest symptom of typhoid in children—of particular importance when it is remembered that headache is generally uncommon in paediatric practice. Cough, diarrhoea, and abdominal pain are other frequent symptoms in children, who often complain of vomiting, unlike the situation in older patients.

It is worth noting that in both adults and children with typhoid, from the long list of possible symptoms, headache alone occurs in a substantial majority of cases. There is nothing typical about the headache, a symptom in any event common to so many diseases. Nevertheless, in an endemic area an ill-defined pyrexial illness which has lasted a week or more and which is characterized by headache should put typhoid high on the list of possible diagnoses.

Apart from the rash, there are few physical signs which immediately suggest the correct diagnosis. Even so, those clinicians who have seen large numbers of cases of typhoid are familiar with the dull, torpid appearance of the patient, the furred tongue, some degree of abdominal distension (usually slight), and the presence of coarse crepitations or rhonchi on auscultation of the chest. Few physicians can have had more extensive experience of typhoid at the bedside than Osler, nor, at the same time, a greater knowledge of its morbid anatomy based on personal observation. He is therefore worth quoting. At the end of the nineteenth century Osler wrote that 'early in the disease the cheeks are flushed and the eyes bright. Toward the end of the first week the expression becomes more listless, and when the disease is well established the patient has a dull and heavy look.'

The spleen has been said to be palpable in a majority of cases but in my experience this is a generous estimate (27 per cent of 246 consecutive cases of proven typhoid). To have significance it should be soft and not greatly enlarged; large, firm splenomegaly is likely to have an explanation other than typhoid. The spleen is so often not palpable in typhoid that its absence should not detract from making this as a tentative diagnosis. Some degree of liver enlargement is likewise quite common, occurring in about 25 per cent of adults and rather more frequently in children; hepatomegaly therefore has roughly the same clinical significance as splenic enlargement. Relative bradycardia occurs, but in less than half of the patients.

The rash, Osler wrote, 'is very characteristic. It consists of a variable number of rose-colored spots, which appear from the seventh to the tenth day, usually first upon the abdomen. The spots are flattened papules, slightly raised, of a rose-red color, disappearing on pressure, and ranging in diameter from 2–4 mm. They can be felt as distinct elevations of the skin. Sometimes each spot is capped by a small vesicle. The spots may be dark in color and occasionally become petechial. After persisting for two or three days they gradually disappear, leaving a brownish stain. They come out in successive crops, but rarely appear after the middle of the third week. They are present in the typical relapse. The rash is most abundant upon the abdomen and lower thoracic zone, often abounds upon the back, and may spread to the extremities or even to the face.' Most observers now would hasten to modify Osler's otherwise excellent description by pointing out that rose-spots are usually few in number, sparsely distributed on the upper abdomen and lower chest, and rarely abundant. A third of the patients in one large series from the southern United States had this typical rash, the proportion being much higher in light-skinned patients than in those with dark skins; and there were rose-spots in more than half of a series of Mexican cases. In contrast, all over Africa south of the Sahara, where typhoid is endemic and a major cause of morbidity, observers have commented on how rarely rose spots are seen although assiduously sought. Like splenomegaly, relative bradycardia, and a step-wise rise in pyrexia, the rash can be a helpful clinical pointer when present to the diagnosis but is too inconstant to be relied upon.

Headache being a common symptom of many febrile illnesses, there is thus little that may be regarded as characteristic in the history or the physical findings. Nevertheless, where typhoid is endemic the diagnosis is strongly suggested by the combination of an obtunded patient with a history of a rather indefinite malady for the past week or so, headache, abdominal discomfort, pain or tenderness, a slightly distended abdomen, a furred tongue, cough, and scattered rhonchi or crepitations in the chest. Suspicion is increased by information that there are, or have recently been, other members of the family similarly afflicted, especially if the patient comes from an area with a reputation for the disease where the water supply is known to be of dubious quality and the sanitation rudimentary. Untreated, typhoid runs a course lasting about four weeks. For the first half of this period toxicity steadily increases from an insidious start. Wherever it may be encountered, this train of events alone should alert the clinician to the possibility that his patient has typhoid. When the symptoms are also taken into account, as they must be, typhoid becomes a likely diagnosis.

Diagnosis. Those familiar with the disease can probably diagnose typhoid on clinical grounds with about a four in five chance of being correct. This opinion is based on my experience with two series of cases. In one of these, out of 150 patients considered to have typhoid on history and physical signs and admitted on these criteria alone to a randomized clinical trial of two drug regimens, the diagnosis was confirmed by blood culture in 84 per cent. The other series comprised almost 400 routine ward admissions of patients considered to have typhoid as the most likely diagnosis. S. typhi was cultured from the blood in 69 per cent of cases and from the stools and urine in an additional 4 per cent with negative blood cultures. There was a fourfold rise in the Widal titre in a further 11 per cent of patients in whom the organism could not be isolated from blood, stools, or urine, again giving a probability of over 80 per cent of the clinical diagnosis being correct.

These points also serve to underline the dominant role played by blood culture in making a definitive diagnosis of typhoid fever. S. typhi can be cultured from venous blood in some 80 per cent of cases during the first week or ten days of illness. By the third week the chances of obtaining a positive blood culture have roughly

halved. Bone marrow cultures will give even higher yields than blood culture. This method appears to be especially valuable in patients who have already ingested antibiotics, either administered indiscriminately before a diagnosis of typhoid had been entertained, or, being freely available over the counter as they are in some countries, taken by the patient before he sought medical advice.

S. typhi may also be cultured from stools and urine; for diagnostic purposes stool cultures are the more rewarding. They are likely to be positive in only a small minority of patients at the beginning of their illness, but in the third and fourth weeks most patients who have not been treated with an appropriate antibiotic will have positive stool cultures. Stool and urine cultures are less valuable than blood cultures for diagnosing typhoid since they are seldom positive when blood cultures are negative in the early stages of the disease. Nevertheless, specimens of stool and urine as well as blood should be obtained for culture in all cases on suspicion of typhoid. (Stool and urine cultures are mandatory in every case after the completion of what appears to have been a successful course of therapy to exclude convalescent carriers, who, if not treated to eradicate the organisms they continue to excrete, will infect others after discharge from hospital.)

Some help may come from the use of serological tests. The Widal test, which is based on the fact that usually there is an increase in the titre of antibodies against the flagellar (H) and the somatic (O) antigens of S. typhi during the course of the disease, is commonly used. In non-endemic areas elevated titres of H and O of 1 : 80 suggest a diagnosis of typhoid, provided the patient has not previously suffered from the disease or been immunized against it. A rising titre over a week or so, particularly if conspicuous, such as fourfold, adds considerable weight to the suspicion and should be sought in every case if any value is to be placed on the test. It is, however, far from specific, especially in endemic areas. False-positive results may be found in patients previously exposed to other salmonella infections, in those with chronic liver disease giving high serum globulin levels, and in several major immunological disorders. It may remain negative despite bacteriological proof of the diagnosis. The Widal test contributes nothing of diagnostic value in typhoid when the organism has been cultured. Its lack of reliability may be illustrated by the fact that titres of 1 : 320 or more were found only in 74 per cent of a large series of African children with typhoid proved by blood culture. Others have reported rather higher figures than this, but seldom much above 80 per cent. The main value of the test is in suspected cases in which all cultures are negative but the clinical course of the disease and its response to treatment by an antibiotic known to be effective in typhoid are typical. In such cases a conspicuous rise in antibody titre may be taken as diagnostic.

In the past far too much importance has been attached to leucopenia as a diagnostic aid. Leucopenia in fact occurs only in a small minority of patients with typhoid despite a common belief that it is a characteristic feature. This erroneous view has been perpetrated in textbooks of medicine which contain statements such as 'leucopenia is remarkably constant in the acute stage, a total count of over 6000 cells being rare and over 10 000 exceptional', and 'leucopenia of 3000 to 4000 cells per mm³ is characteristic of the febrile phase of typhoid fever'. Leucopenia certainly occurs, but when it does it can at best be regarded as a helpful laboratory finding in a pyrexial illness of unknown cause. Where the belief about leucopenia as a typical feature of typhoid originated is not clear, but it is worth recording that in 1898 Osler, whose experience was extensive, did not hold this view, writing that 'the number of colorless corpuscles varies little from the normal standard (6000 per mm³)'. Most patients with typhoid have white cell counts between 4000 and 11 000 per mm³. Recently the median leucocyte count in children with typhoid was given as 7000 per mm³, which tallies with my finding of a median count of 6400 in a large series of adults. In these patients there was true leucopenia (below 4000 per mm³) on admission to hospital in only 8 per cent. Mild leucocytosis may also occur on occasion but it is never marked. The main value of the white cell count in typhoid lies in the fact that a marked rise makes such a diagnosis most unlikely. As Osler so aptly expressed the point, 'the absence of leucocytosis may be at times of real diagnostic value in distinguishing typhoid fever from various septic fevers and acute inflammatory processes'.

Complications

Haemorrhage and perforation. Each of these occurs in approximately 5 per cent of adults, slightly less in children. They do not always present as dramatic events and sometimes occur together. A clearly-defined episode of haemorrhage may be identified by sudden deterioration in the patient's condition during the second or third week when definite improvement should be taking place on antibiotic therapy. The blood pressure and the temperature drop and the pulse rate rises. Acute perforation is accompanied by sudden abdominal pain, vomiting, and the symptoms of collapse, with tachycardia, hypotension, and rigidity of the abdominal wall. In my experience such major events are uncommon in treated patients, but less well-defined instances of both complications are often seen, making up the majority of the 5 per cent quoted above. It would be surprising if some degree of bleeding did not accompany the sloughing of intestinal ulcers, and indeed such bleeding quite often causes significant anaemia. In other patients abdominal discomfort and distension increase somewhat without clear evidence that perforation has occurred, a situation regarded by some as toxic ileus.

Dramatic events in hospital wards are usually reported promptly, but because these complications, particularly haemorrhage, are more often insidious than dramatic they may easily be missed. Close clinical observation is therefore imperative. A rising pulse rate, increasing pallor, and abdominal distension should be sought for daily. The haemoglobin level should also be determined at regular intervals as a routine investigation because clinical estimation of changes in haemoglobin is notoriously fallible. Increasing anaemia may of course be due to infection and not haemorrhage. The distinction is readily made by looking for polychromasia in the stained blood film or determining the reticulocyte count. The bone marrow is inactive in the anaemia which accompanies long-continued infection so polychromasia is absent and the reticulocyte count is low. In acute post-haemorrhagic anaemia the reverse is found—polychromasia and reticulocytosis are both present.

Pulmonary complications. Scattered rhonchi are commonly audible on auscultation of the chest in patients with typhoid. They represent a mild degree of bronchitis and have no particular significance. Pneumonia on the other hand is a serious complication, especially in children in whom it is usually bronchopneumonic in distribution. Less often children have lobar pneumonia. Lobar pneumonia may occur in adults, although it is rare.

Neuropsychiatric manifestations. When first seen, many patients with typhoid have expressionless faces and are torpid. A minority are confused and disorientated. Some are delirious. In the third week of the disease in untreated cases, profound toxicity may lead to an immobile, semiconscious state in which the patient lies muttering to himself with his eyes open (the coma vigil). In a busy outpatient department there is a risk that such patients might be admitted as psychotic; the presence of pyrexia should suggest the possibility of typhoid.

Occasionally there are other abnormalities in the nervous system. When neck stiffness is present, examination of the cerebrospinal fluid is imperative to exclude typhoid meningitis or infection due to another organism. Usually, however, there are no changes in the spinal fluid in typhoid patients with neck stiffness and the patient is regarded as having meningism. Some reports have given a high incidence of meningism but in my experience it is not common (3 per cent). Rare manifestations include convulsions, encephalitis or diffuse encephalomyelitis, peripheral neuritis, mutism, dysarthria, brisk reflexes, ankle clonus, extensor plantar responses, hemiplegia, extrapyramidal signs, cerebellar ataxia, and myop-

athy. The possible complications of typhoid in the nervous system, in fact, appear to be legion. They generally improve or disappear after treatment with a drug such as chloramphenicol. Their causes are not known but some of them might be vascular in origin, possibly thrombosis of small blood vessels.

Renal complications. Osler remarked on the occurrence of renal lesions in typhoid, particularly acute nephritis coming on in its early stages. In one large series of cases of the disease in children, the incidence of acute nephritis was given as 3 per cent while in another comprehensive report a small number of patients with typhoid needed dialysis for renal failure. Such involvement of the kidney might be an immunological phenomenon in which complexes comprising Salmonella antigen, antibody, and complement form in renal capillary walls. Clearly renal function should be kept under close scrutiny in all cases.

Blood disorders. Apart from leucopenia, leucocytosis, acute post-haemorrhagic anaemia, and the anaemia of chronic infection, to which reference has already been made, several haematological abnormalities may occur during the course of typhoid. One of these is thrombocytopenia, which in adults is seldom of sufficient degree to cause clinical effects but in children may lead to purpura. Others are haemolytic anaemia and disseminated intravascular coagulation, both rare.

Cardiovascular complications. It is most uncommon to find clinical involvement of the heart in adults with typhoid although electrocardiographic changes may be observed. The heart is more often affected in children, particularly those from a poor socioeconomic background. In them congestive cardiac failure sometimes occurs, presumably the result of toxic myocarditis. Deep vein thrombosis, usually of the femoral vein, complicates typhoid in a small number of cases. Infective endocarditis due to *S. typhi* may occur but is a rarity.

Typhoid hepatitis. Jaundice may be observed during the course of the disease, usually the result of intrahepatic cholestasis. In adults, in whom it may be noted in about 1 per cent of cases, it has no clinical significance. In children, however, jaundice, with tender hepatomegaly, occurs rather more frequently (some 5 per cent). It may obscure the true diagnosis since it suggests viral hepatitis. Transaminase levels are raised. This 'toxic' hepatitis appears to be ominous since some children dying in the early stages of typhoid are found at necropsy to have necrosis of the liver. Studies of unselected cases of typhoid have shown that approximately half have biochemical evidence of active liver disease, the liver function tests returning to normal after recovery. Histological examination of biopsy specimens of liver tissue have shown the presence of necrotic liver cells or definite typhoid granulomata.

Other complications. Typhoid increases the risks of abortion in pregnancy, especially in the first trimester. Before the introduction of chloramphenicol, alopecia was a well-known sequel of the disease and occasionally typhoid was complicated by cholecystitis, arthritis, osteitis, and abscess formation in muscle. These and other late manifestations are now rarely seen.

Relapse. A small minority of patients will relapse several weeks or more after apparent cure of their disease. Symptoms and signs return and blood cultures again become positive. The relapse is usually milder and of shorter duration than the initial infection. Before the introduction of specific drug therapy, the relapse rate was of the order of 5 per cent and multiple relapses sometimes occurred. Relapse may still occur after treatment with chloramphenicol, less often with amoxycillin. Multiple relapses are now rare.

Treatment. For many years after its introduction in 1948, chloramphenicol gave excellent results in the treatment of typhoid and came to be regarded as the treatment of choice. It is now apparent, however, that some strains of *S. typhi* are resistant to this drug. Examples of this were first reported in sporadic cases in Britain, Vietnam, and Thailand, and there were many resistant cases in a major epidemic in Mexico. Although small in relation to its expected benefit, there is a risk that chloramphenicol might induce marrow aplasia, either dose-related or on the basis of individual susceptibility. Alternative drugs were therefore sought. Three have been shown to be of value. Ampicillin and co-trimoxazole may be used when chloramphenicol fails, but they are not its equal for the great majority of cases; they are also useful for treating carriers. Only amoxycillin, closely related chemically to ampicillin but producing higher serum concentrations, has emerged from properly-conducted clinical trials as a true alternative to chloramphenicol. There is virtually nothing to distinguish these two drugs as regards time of defervescence, failure to respond, relapse rate, the occurrence of major complications, the chance of becoming a convalescent carrier, and the case-fatality rate. Amoxycillin is less toxic. The great majority of patients with typhoid will do very well on either of these drugs. Nevertheless, its present higher cost makes amoxycillin a second choice to chloramphenicol in most developing countries where hospital drug costs have to be closely scrutinized.

Clinical improvement follows soon after the commencement of therapy and fever should begin to diminish within a few days. Indeed, in a suspected case lacking proof of the diagnosis, the improved well-being and gradual defervescence after starting specific treatment for typhoid is valuable circumstantial evidence in its favour. Despite a common belief that the temperature becomes normal in three to five days in patients treated with chloramphenicol, what has emerged from recent clinical trials is that the median time for the disappearance of pyrexia after commencing treatment with either chloramphenicol or amoxycillin is seven days for adults and eight days for children. Defervescence may occasionally be more rapid, but a precipitate fall in temperature after starting one of these drugs should raise doubts about the accuracy of the diagnosis.

The following are the recommended dosages for routine treatment.

Chloramphenicol. Adults: 1.0 g eight-hourly by the oral route until pyrexia has clearly diminished although the temperature is not necessarily normal (usually four to five days), followed by 500 mg eight-hourly for a week and thereafter 250 mg six-hourly, to give a total duration of not less than 14 days.

Children: 50 mg per kg body weight per day for 21 days.

Amoxycillin. Adults: 1.0 g orally six-hourly for 14 days.

Children: 100 mg per kg per day for 21 days.

If *ampicillin* is used it should be given in doses of 80 mg per kg per day or 6.0 g per day in 4 equal doses, the duration of treatment being 14 days. *Co-trimoxazole* (80 mg trimethoprim and 400 mg sulphamethoxazole per tablet) should be given in a dosage of 2 tablets twice daily for 14 days, or, for children, 6 mg trimethoprim plus 30 mg sulphamethoxazole per kg per day for 14 days.

Acute intestinal haemorrhage calls for immediate blood transfusion. Patients who are restless and show much anxiety should be sedated, preferably with morphine. Any depressant effect on cardiac output which might result from morphine is likely to be more than offset by the reduction in the degree of restlessness and fear which follows its use. Blood transfusions should also be given to those patients whose haemoglobin level steadily drops over a number of days without the dramatic features of acute haemorrhage. A wise precaution in every case after proof of the diagnosis has been obtained is to watch closely for evidence of bleeding, repeat the blood every few days, and in those in whom haemoglobin is dropping, type and cross-match blood for possible transfusion. When perforation occurs in patients already diagnosed as typhoid and on treatment with chloramphenicol or amoxycillin, this complication can be successfully treated conservatively by intermittent aspiration of the gastric contents through a naso-gastric tube combined with intravenous fluid and electrolyte replacement, and is preferred by most physicians. The patient's initial clinical state after perforation and his progress on medical treatment should nevertheless be reviewed in consultation with a surgeon. However, some patients with typhoid first seek medical help because of the symptoms of acute intestinal perforation and are admitted to surgical wards where they are correctly regarded as surgical emergencies. The

diagnosis is generally made at operation or in retrospect on the results of histological examination or blood culture. Wedge resection is preferred to simple closure of the perforation; if there are multiple perforations or if adjacent bowel is thought to show signs of impending perforation, limited resection of bowel is recommended. Surgical treatment is successful in the great majority of such cases.

A small minority of patients will fail to respond to treatment with either chloramphenicol or amoxycillin, or relapse after apparent cure. Since it is rare to find strains of *S. typhi* which are resistant to both drugs, the drug not previously used should be given in such cases. If response is still inadequate it is worth giving ampicillin or cotrimoxazole.

No patient should be allowed to return home until examination of three specimens of stool and urine, taken on consecutive days after drug treatment has ceased, are negative on culture for *S. typhi*. A full course of therapy as outlined above reduces the risk of the patient becoming a convalescent carrier, the state in which the patient continues to excrete *S. typhi* for some weeks while remaining asymptomatic. A course of treatment with a drug not previously used is indicated in such cases.

Typhoid carriers. Convalescent carriers are patients who have recovered from the clinically detectable disease but continue to excrete *S. typhi* in stools or urine for a limited period up to several weeks. Excretion ceases after that, but during the excretory phase in convalescence the situation is potentially dangerous to others since the water supply or food and drink may readily be contaminated and thus spread the infection. Proper medical management of every case of typhoid therefore includes keeping the patient in hospital or in isolation until at least three consecutive specimens of stools and urine are negative for *S. typhi* after the full regimen of drug therapy has been completed. If the organism is cultured from any of these specimens, the patient is a convalescent carrier and a further course of an effective drug should be given, as outlined above.

The chronic carrier is quite distinct from the convalescent carrier. A chronic carrier may be defined as a person who excretes *S. typhi*, usually in the stools, sometimes in the urine, over a period of many years without exhibiting the systemic effects of the disease. The excretion is usually intermittent. Many of these subjects have not to their knowledge had the acute illness, the original infection being subclinical. In such patients *S. typhi* comes from a nidus of chronic inflammatory change in the gall bladder or biliary tract, occasionally the urinary tract.

Chronic carriers clearly pose a health hazard to the community. Identification may be by chance during culture of stools or urine for other purposes, or by design when epidemiological evidence in an outbreak of typhoid points to the existence of a chronic carrier in the community. In the latter case a large number of specimens of stool and urine must be examined from each suspect because of the intermittent nature of *S. typhi* excretion. Eradication of the nidus of infection in a proven chronic carrier is usually difficult. A prolonged course of one of the three drugs, amoxycillin, ampicillin, and co-trimoxazole, is necessary (chloramphenicol being avoided because of its potential dose-related toxicity). If the subject can be demonstrated to have gall-stones or chronic colecystitis, cholecystectomy offers a fair chance of curing the chronic carrier state, but of this there is no guarantee because an intrahepatic nidus of infection may co-exist.

A variant of the chronic carrier is the intravascular shedder, a patient who has similar chronic foci of infection but in whom *S. typhi* is shed intravascularly rather than excreted in stools or urine. Some may do both and are therefore chronic carriers in the usual sense. Generally such intravascular shedders of *S. typhi* are detected by chance in blood cultures during the course of another disease, and this may obscure the correct diagnosis.

Prognosis. Before the introduction of chloramphenicol, the case-fatality rate was high, e.g. 12 per cent in two large series of cases of endemic typhoid admitted to hospitals in Bergen, Norway, and New Orleans, Louisiana. The prognosis is now very much better in countries with well-developed health services, where, in any event, there is little endemic typhoid. Deaths amounted to 0.6 per cent in the extensive epidemic of 1964 in Aberdeen, where epidemiologists and clinicians efficiently tracked down the source of infection and took appropriate measures for the early identification and treatment of new cases. The risk of death from typhoid remains high, however, in most developing countries despite the general availability of drugs effective against *S. typhi*. Death rates of about 7 per cent are often reported, poor nutrition, delay in seeking medical advice, and concomitant disease being common adverse factors.

It is certain that chemotherapy alone is not responsible for the improvement that has taken place in the prognosis of typhoid. Substantial advances have also occurred in the availability and techniques of blood transfusion, and in the monitoring and correction of fluid and electrolyte imbalance. In this regard it is worth noting that 40 per cent of deaths in the Norwegian series referred to above were attributed to intestinal haemorrhage or perforation. Such deaths are now largely preventable.

The prolonged course of typhoid before specific drug therapy became available, so vividly recorded in the writings of Osler, is in striking contrast to the situation now. Unquestionably, a major advance coming from the use of drugs such as chloramphenicol and amoxycillin is that the duration of fever and toxicity in typhoid have been substantially shortened and convalescence greatly curtailed. If diagnosed early and properly treated, typhoid need no longer be a protracted and debilitating disease. But it must be remembered that it remains a dangerous infection. Despite modern hospital facilities, case-fatality rates are still in the range 1–7 per cent; the socio-economic background of the patient, his previous state of health and the stage of illness at which the diagnosis is made playing important parts in determining the outcome.

Prevention. Endemic typhoid can be eliminated only by the provision of proper sanitation, a safe water supply, and public health legislation designed to ensure uncontaminated food and drink, plus a health service which is staffed to carry out these ideals. This is a counsel of perfection quite beyond the capacity of most developing countries. The elimination of typhoid and other diseases carried in a similar way is nevertheless a most important aim to which all health authorities should give the highest priority.

In developing countries the provision of good sanitation and safe water is relatively easy to achieve in cities and towns but difficult or almost impossible in rural districts from which a high proportion of cases of endemic typhoid originates. Where there is much endemic typhoid, its incidence can be reduced by investigating the source of notified cases and doing whatever is feasible to obviate contamination of the water used. Accepting the limitations of the living conditions, much can be achieved by educating the family and neighbours of an affected patient and giving advice about procuring safe water.

There is now relatively little typhoid in industrialized communities with advanced health services, but there is always the danger that typhoid may be contracted from imported cases, travel abroad, foreign visitors, and immigrants providing the sources of infection. Continued vigilance regarding sanitation, the supply of water, and the purity of food, particularly when imported, is therefore mandatory. An outbreak of epidemic typhoid can be contained by prompt action by the health authorities, a good example of which was the Aberdeen epidemic of 1964 when the source of infection of the first case (a can of meat imported from a country where typhoid is common) was identified within three days.

The correct management of proven cases also plays an important part in prevention. Once diagnosed, a case of typhoid must be promptly notified and isolated by barrier nursing from other patients. After apparent cure, no patient must be discharged from hospital until three urine and stool specimens, collected *after* the cessation of treatment, are negative for *S. typhi*. Another measure which will reduce the incidence of typhoid is the reduction of the relapse-rate by prolonging the duration of drug therapy. In children it has been shown that the relapse-rate may be high when chloramphenicol is given for 10–15 days but substantially lower if the drug is continued for 21 days. Amoxycillin seems to be a better drug in this respect.

Much work has been done on the preparation and evaluation of the efficacy of vaccines against typhoid, but it must be acknowledged that no vaccine so far produced will give complete protection. The various measures outlined above must remain the first line of endeavour as regards prevention. This is not the same as saying that vaccination has no place in the control of typhoid. In areas where endemic typhoid is prevalent, a modest degree of protection may be attained for several years by using either acetone-killed or heat-killed-phenolized vaccine. Some have recommended immunizing children in their first year in school, giving them one subcutaneous dose of 0.5 ml and following this by routine booster administration at ages 10 or 11 years. Others advise 0.5 ml of one of the two vaccines given subcutaneously and repeated four weeks later, with boosters every three years where the endemicity of typhoid is high. But the overall evidence suggests that efforts are much better directed towards safeguarding food and water from contamination than embarking on immunization programmes when so much controversy surrounds the degree of possible benefit. Local discomfort and pyrexia may result from vaccination.

Paratyphoid

Three other members of the *Salmonella* group of organisms, *S. paratyphi* A, B, and C, may cause disease closely resembling typhoid. Of these, paratyphoid B is the commonest. Epidemiology and pathology are similar to those of typhoid. The prevalence of paratyphoid was roughly the same as that of typhoid 50 or more years ago, according to data from Norway and statistics about the two diseases in France in the First World War, quoted by Hurst. Both infections were then undoubtedly common. In most countries the prevalence of paratyphoid is now much less than that of typhoid except in parts of Western Europe (see Table 2). Paratyphoid, like typhoid, invariably comes from a human source—a patient with active disease or a carrier. The organisms gain access to the body from contaminated food or drink. There is similar involvement of lymphoid tissue in the small intestine and dissemination to many organs via the blood stream. Ulceration and necrosis in the gut is generally less marked than in typhoid, but there may be catarrhal inflammatory changes over a wide area of the alimentary tract including the stomach, and this may occur without ulceration.

Table 2 Some comparative national notifications for typhoid and paratyphoid

Country	Year	Typhoid notifications	Paratyphoid notifications
Portugal	1977	743	19
Sweden	1977	14	23
Switzerland	1977	27	20
Japan	1977	346	77
Kuwait	1977	397	27
Bolivia	1976	1091	247
Canada	1977	89	30

Compiled from *World health statistics annual* (1979). World Health Organization, Geneva

Paratyphoid usually runs a shorter and milder course than typhoid, with relatively little toxicity. Complications are less frequent and the case-fatality rate lower. Another point of clinical distinction from typhoid is the rash. Although occurring less often than in typhoid, the eruption of paratyphoid may be more extensive and involve the face and limbs as well as the trunk. Hurst wrote that the spots in paratyphoid are 'often larger, more irregular in shape, more raised, and of a deeper red colour than in typhoid fever, and they are sometimes remarkably profuse'. Response is excellent to treatment with the same drugs used for typhoid.

Although paratyphoid is generally regarded as milder than typhoid and covered quite briefly in textbooks of medicine, this should not be taken to imply that it carries no dangers. Paratyphoid may indeed be fatal if the diagnosis is missed or much delayed. Its potential severity and duration in comparison with typhoid may be judged from extensive experience of the two diseases gained in Bergen, Norway, over a period of 50 years before the introduction of chemotherapy. The mean duration of fever in typhoid was 30 days, 20 days in paratyphoid. Relapses occurred in 18.5 per cent of typhoid patients but in only 3.5 per cent of those with paratyphoid. There was gross intestinal haemorrhage in some 12 per cent and intestinal perforation in 14 per cent of typhoid patients, compared with 4 per cent and 9 per cent of paratyphoid cases. The comparative case-fatality rates were 12 per cent and just over 2 per cent respectively. Since the introduction of specific drug therapy and better supportive treatment, the prognosis in paratyphoid has improved considerably, as in typhoid; but there is always a risk, admittedly small, of haemorrhage or perforation, and vigilance during the course of the illness is therefore necessary.

References

Eisman, L. R. and Saunders, S. J. (1978). Liver disease in typhoid fever. *Cent. Afr. J. Med.* **24** (supp. 9), 28.

Gadeholt, H. and Madsen, S. T. (1963). Clinical course, complications and mortality in typhoid fever as compared with paratyphoid B. A survey of 2647 cases. *Acta. med. Scand.* **174**, 753.

Gilman, R. H., Terminel, M., Levine, M. M., Hernandez-Mendoza, P., and Hornick, R. B. (1975). Relative efficacy of blood, urine, rectal swab, bone-marrow, and rose-spot cultures for recovery of Salmonella typhi in typhoid fever. *Lancet* i, 1211.

Gonzalez-Cortes, A., Bessudo, D. Sanchez-Leyva, R., Fragoso, R., Hinojosa, M., and Becceril, P. (1973). Water-borne transmission of chloramphenicol-resistant Salmonella typhi in Mexico. *Lancet* ii, 605.

Hornick, R. B. and Greisman, S. (1978). On the pathogenesis of typhoid fever. *Archs intern. Med.* **138**, 357.

Hurst, A. (1944). *Medical diseases of war.* Arnold, London.

Osler, W. (1898). *The principles and practice of medicine*, 3rd edn. Pentland, Edinburgh.

Osuntokun, B. O., Bademosi, O., Ogunremi, K., and Wright, S. G. (1972). Neuro-psychiatric manifestations of typhoid fever in 959 patients. *Archs Neurol.* **27**, 7.

Pillay, N., Adams, E. B., and North-Coombes, D. (1975). Comparative trial of amoxycillin and chloramphenicol in treatment of typhoid fever in adults. *Lancet* ii, 333.

Sarma, V. N. B., Malaviya, A. N., Kumar, R., Ghai, O. P., and Bakhtary, M. M. (1977). Development of immune response during typhoid fever in man. *Clin. exp. Immunol.* **28**, 35.

Scragg, J. N. and Rubidge, C. J. (1975). Amoxycillin in the treatment of typhoid fever in children. *Am. J. trop. Med. Hyg.* **24**, 860.

—, —, and Wallace, H. L. (1969). Typhoid fever in African and Indian children in Durban. *Archs Dis. Childn.* **44**, 18.

Stuart, B. M. and Pullen, R. L. (1946). Typhoid. Clinical analysis of 360 cases. *Archs intern. Med.* **78**, 629.

Walker, W. (1965). The Aberdeen typhoid outbreak of 1964. *Scott. med. J.* **10**, 466.

Wicks, A. C. B., Holmes, G. S., and Davidson, L. (1971). Endemic typhoid fever. *Q. Jl Med.* **40**, 341.

Anaerobic bacteria

S. J. Eykyn and I. Phillips

Although the description anaerobic infection encompasses all infections associated with anaerobic bacteria, we will not be considering those mediated by the toxins of anaerobic Gram-positive spore-bearing bacilli, which constitute a clinically distinct group and are considered elsewhere (see pages 5.226 and 5.230). Actinomycosis too is considered elsewhere (see page 5.274). It has become fashionable to refer to anaerobes that produce infections unassociated with toxins as the 'non-sporing anaerobes' or the 'non-clostridial anaerobes' but such terms are somewhat misleading for they exclude the genus *Clostridium*. In fact clostridia, including *Cl. perfringens* occur with non-sporing anaerobes, in a variety of infections in which they do not declare their toxic potential. In such a situation their presence or absence makes no difference to the course of the disease.

Anaerobic infections are very common and may affect any tissue or organ in the body and thus will present to all clinicians regardless of speciality. Remarkably, such infections have gone largely unrecognized in the antibiotic era until the last decade, although over 80 years ago French workers, in a classic series of clinical and laboratory investigations, established the significance of anaerobes in a wide variety of human infections. It seems inexplicable that the classic work of Veillon, Zuber, and others should apparently have been forgotten for so many years and that until relatively recently minimal laboratory skill existed for the isolation of anaerobes other than *Clostridium* spp. and the occasional *Bacteroides fragilis*. The credit for 'rediscovering' the anaerobes as important human pathogens must go to American workers, but this 'anaerobic renaissance' rapidly spread to other countries and led to increasing interest in all aspects of the laboratory and clinical diagnosis, management, and prevention of anaerobic infection.

Taxonomic considerations. The classification and characterization of anaerobic bacteria present considerable difficulties, and the many synonyms for these organisms bear witness to this: Finegold quotes over 50 for the organism now classified as *Fusobacterium necrophorum*! Such taxonomic confusion is compounded by the many reports that refer to any Gram-negative obligately anaerobic bacillus as a 'bacteroides' and to those resistant to ampicillin and penicillin as *B. fragilis*. More difficulties arise in differentiating fastidious micro-aerophilic or capnophilic (CO_2-requiring) bacteria from true anaerobes, and this is particularly true of certain streptococci including *Streptococcus milleri*. Such differentiation has therapeutic as well as taxonomic implications as metronidazole, which is so effective against anaerobes, is inactive against most micro-aerophilic and capnophilic bacteria. Table 1 lists some of the major genera and species of anaerobic bacteria associated with man.

Table 1 Major anaerobic genera and species found in man

Gram-positive bacilli	
Spore-forming	*Clostridium perfringens* (*welchii*) *C. botulinum*, *C. butyricum*, *C. difficile*, *C. septicum*, *C. tetani*
Non-spore-forming	*Actinomyces* spp. *Bifidobacterium* spp. *Eubacterium* spp. *Propionibacterium* spp.
Gram-negative bacilli bacteroides: 'fragilis' group	*B. fragilis*, *B. thetaiotaomicron* *B. vulgatus*, *B. ovatus*
Black-pigmented bacteroides	*B. asaccharolyticus* *B. melaninogenicus melaninogenicus* *B. melaninogenicus intermedius*
Other bacteroides	*B. bivius*, *B. ureolyticus* (*corrodeus*) *B. oralis*
Anaerobic cocci	
Gram-positive	*Peptococcus* spp. *Peptostreptococcus* spp.
Gram-negative	*Veillonella* spp.
Spirochaetes	*Borrelia vincenti*

Anaerobic commensal flora of man. The normal commensal flora of man consists largely of anaerobes which are found on all mucosal surfaces: certain species are also found on the skin. The main sites and nature of this commensal flora are shown in Table 2. *B. fragilis* is predominantly found in the large intestine and very seldom at other sites. Although this organism is by far the commonest anaerobe cultured from infections arising from the colonic commensal anaerobes, *B. vulgatus* and *B. thetaiotaomicron* are much more numerous in the colon. Anaerobes are virtually never found in the normal healthy stomach and only in the distal part of the normal small intestine, but when the pH of the stomach contents is increased, as, for instance, in gastric ulceration or carcinoma, anaerobic bacteria, usually of respiratory origin, are found in the stomach. Any condition leading to intestinal stasis will also be associated with overgrowth of colonic bacteria in the small intestine. It is of interest that the extremely oxygen-sensitive anaerobes found in large numbers in the normal colon are not found in clinical infections.

Table 2   Main sites of normal anaerobic flora of man, and anaerobes most frequently found at these sites

	Skin	Mouth naso-pharynx	Intes-tine	Vagina	Urethra
Gram-positive bacilli					
Clostridium spp.			++		
Actinomyces spp.		+			
Bifidobacterium spp.		+	++	+	
Eubacterium spp.		+	++		
Propionibacterium spp.	++				
Gram-negative bacilli					
Bacteroides: 'fragilis' group			++		
Black-pigmented bacteroides		++	+	++	+
Fusobacterium spp.		++	+		+
Others					
Gram-positive cocci		++	++	++	+
Gram-negative cocci		++	+	++	
Spirochaetes		+			

++ = anaerobes present in large numbers   + = anaerobes generally present

Pathogenesis. Anaerobic infections arise endogenously from the normal anaerobic commensal flora, and in many cases occur close to a mucosal surface that supports this commensal flora as with wound sepsis after colorectal surgery or vaginal hysterectomy. Anaerobic pleuropulmonary infection generally occurs after aspiration of oropharyngeal bacteria into the lung, although occasionally it occurs as metastatic foci following an anaerobic septicaemia. Other anaerobic infections, whilst almost certainly of endogenous origin, arise at sites remote from the commensal flora, and the route whereby the commensal bacteria have reached the site of infection is less readily explained unless blood-borne spread has occurred. In view of the fact that anaerobic infections in man are caused by only a small percentage of the several hundred species of commensal anaerobic bacteria, virulence factors are likely to be involved, though few are recognized.

Most anaerobic infections are polymicrobial with either several anaerobic species involved or, more commonly, mixed aerobic–anaerobic infections with multiple species of each again responsible. Thus such infections cannot satisfy Koch's postulates. The curious aerobic–anaerobic interdependence in these infections has not yet been fully elucidated: animal studies show that in intra-abdominal sepsis, where these mixed infections are the rule, the initial stage of acute peritonitis involves aerobes, predominantly *Escherichia coli* and enterococci, and carries a high mortality; the second stage is characterized by the formation of intra-abdominal abscesses in which anaerobes, particularly *B. fragilis*, are found. However, this work was done with a non-capsulated strain of *B. fragilis*, and it was later shown that capsulated strains of this organism cause abscesses when given without an aerobe, and that purified capsular polysaccharide alone is also capable of producing abscesses. Strains of *B. fragilis* isolated from human infections have all been found to possess a polysaccharide capsule which is found in the outer complex of the cell wall. *B. asaccharolyticus* has also been found to have a polysaccharide capsule, but most other bacteroides, including the majority of the colonic commensals, do not. This capsule, which is highly antigenic, appears from the animal studies to be a virulence factor for *B. fragilis* and *B. asaccharolyticus* which, as well as promoting abscess formation, may also render these organisms and others resistant to phagocytosis. It has been shown *in vitro* that a variety of species of obligate anaerobes interfere with phagocytosis and the killing of *Pr. mirabilis* and other aerobic bacteria. The anaerobes most effective in inhibiting phagocytosis are *B. fragilis* and *B. melaninogenicus* (probably actually *B. asaccharolyticus*), presumably encapsulated strains since they were isolated from clinical material. It is probable, however, that capsular polysaccharide may not be the sole virulence factor involved in anaerobic infections since animals protected by an antibody to capsular polysaccharide can apparently still develop abscesses.

Both *B. fragilis* and *B. asaccharolyticus* have a lipo-polysaccharide cell wall that is biologically distinct from that of aerobic Gram-negative bacteria, and it does not function as an endotoxin whereas other Gram-negative anaerobic bacteria, including fusobacteria, possess classical lipo-polysaccharide endotoxins. This is a curious finding in view of the clinical evidence for what appears to be bacteraemic shock in patients with *B. fragilis* bacteraemia. Septic thrombophlebitis is not an uncommon feature of serious anaerobic infection, and it is said to occur particularly, though not exclusively, with *B. fragilis* bacteraemia. The heparinase produced by this organism may be involved; it has also been shown experimentally that both bacteroides and fusobacteria produce accelerated clotting.

Clinical diagnosis. A working knowledge of the nature and whereabouts of the normal commensal anaerobic flora of man is invaluable to the clinician, whatever his specialty, and it also should be remembered that virtually no organ or tissue is immune from infection by anaerobes. Undoubtedly the most helpful clinical indication of the common anaerobic infections is putrid pus or discharge. Where present this is diagnostic: no other group of organisms give rise (by virtue of the products of their metabolism) to such a foul nauseating smell. It must be said, however, that not all anaerobic infections produce putrid pus. For many years foul pus was attributed by surgeons to *Escherichia coli* since that was the organism isolated, laboratory skill being totally inadequate for the isolation of anaerobes. Anaerobic wound sepsis is often associated with cellulitis, which may be readily mistaken for streptococcal cellulitis by the inexperienced, but is seldom accompanied by the profound toxaemia and high fever that *Strep. pyogenes* usually produces. Gas in infected tissues is highly suggestive of anaerobes (not only *Cl. perfringens*) but is not diagnostic since pure aerobic infections may also produce gas. Another useful clinical indication of anaerobes is a laboratory report of 'sterile pus' despite the presence of organisms on a Gram-stained film. Any patient receiving antibiotics inactive against anaerobes (e.g., aminoglycosides or, in the case of the *B. fragilis* group, ampicillin), and still appearing septic, should be suspected of having an anaerobic infection.

Collection and transport of specimens for anaerobic bacteriology
Although all anaerobic bacteria are sensitive to oxygen, they cannot be considered as a homogenous group of organisms in terms of aerotolerance. Some anaerobes, such as *Cl. perfringens* and *B. fragilis*, will tolerate 2–4 per cent oxygen whereas other clinically important organisms, such as *Fusobacterium* spp. and some anaerobic cocci, are much more sensitive to air or oxygen and thus more difficult to grow in the laboratory and much less likely to survive the journey from patient to culture medium. There have been many

recommendations for the collection and transport of specimens for anaerobic bacteriology including some of remarkable complexity unlikely to appeal to any clinician. In practice we have found that pus in a universal container has proved very satisfactory, and even the fastidious anaerobes will survive. If insufficient material is available for collection in this way, a swab should be taken and sent to the laboratory in Stuart's or similar transport medium. Whenever possible, contamination of the specimen by commensal anaerobes should be avoided: this is particularly relevant to anaerobic pleuro-pulmonary infection in which expectorated sputum is unlikely to be a satisfactory specimen and more direct sampling methods are preferred. Vaginal bacteriology too can be difficult to interpret.

Laboratory diagnosis. The putrid smell of the pus in many anaerobic infections has already been mentioned: even swabs will sometimes be noticeably foul when plated out at the bench. Other useful immediate tests for the presence of anaerobes include a Gram-stained smear of the pus, red fluorescence of the pus under ultra-violet light, diagnostic of the presence of black-pigmented bacteroides, and gas–liquid chromatography performed directly on the specimen. Recently specific fluorescent antibody tests have become available for the direct demonstration of *B. fragilis* and the black-pigmented bacteroides. The Gram-stained film is often diagnostic to the experienced microscopist, for example, when a variety of different organisms are seen including pleomorphic Gram-negative bacilli. Filamentous or spindle shaped Gram-negative bacilli are characteristic of the fusobacteria but may be scanty and difficult to see. Gas–liquid chromatography detects volatile fatty acids produced in the pus by anaerobic bacteria. This is an expensive, sophisticated technique capable on occasions of detecting the presence of anaerobes unsuspected by the human nose as well as confirming what is already to the initiated a certain diagnosis. It is by no means an essential requirement for a routine diagnostic laboratory.

Successful culture of anaerobes requires fresh media and a reliable system for maintaining an anaerobic atmosphere which should include 10 per cent carbon dioxide. Whilst the relatively aerotolerant anaerobes such as *Cl. perfringens* and *B. fragilis* will usually grow in 24 hours, many anaerobes take considerably longer for isolation. Fastidious anaerobes require undisturbed anaerobiosis and leaving culture plates on the bench or frequent inspection of cultures are likely to result in failure. The definitive identification of many anaerobes is a lengthy process and their taxonomy has minimal appeal to the clinician. Management of the individual patient will inevitably depend initially on clinical suspicion and perhaps the immediate laboratory investigations. Nevertheless details of the species and sensitivities of various anaerobes isolated in each type of infection provides a useful bank of information on which to draw when devising treatment for the individual. The detection of a specific antibody response to common anaerobes provides an alternative means of diagnosis, especially for closed lesions. Methods are being developed.

Clinical spectrum of anaerobic infection

Infections of the head and neck

Acute necrotizing gingivitis. This condition, variously called Vincent's angina, Plaut–Vincent's infection, trench mouth, and fuso-spirochaetosis is one of the earliest described anaerobic infections. The characteristic symptoms of painful, bleeding gums with the obvious accompanying foul breath and often the presence of a pseudomembrane readily suggest the diagnosis, which can be confirmed in the laboratory on a smear stained with carbol fuchsin in which large numbers of spirochaetes (*Borrelia vincenti*) (see page 5.294) and fusobacteria are seen.

Dental sepsis. The commensal flora of the oropharynx, saliva, and gingival crevice are found, together with the various 'viridans' streptococci, in dental abscesses and in sepsis associated with maxillo-facial surgery. Dental plaque has been shown to be largely composed of anaerobic bacteria, and these organisms, *B. melaninogenicus* in particular, are important in periodontal disease.

Abscesses and cellulitis of the neck or jaw. These are frequently anaerobic and may be accompanied by marked oedema and occasionally cause respiratory embarrassment (Fig. 1). Such infection involving the submandibular space is referred to as Ludwig's angina. Most of these abscesses are associated with dental disease or manipulation, but they may also occur with local tumours. Infection of branchial cysts is also usually anaerobic. *Actinomyces* spp. are often isolated together with other oropharyngeal anaerobes, indeed pus from many cases of clinical actinomycosis involving the jaw or neck will often grow mixed anaerobes as well as *Actinomyces* spp.

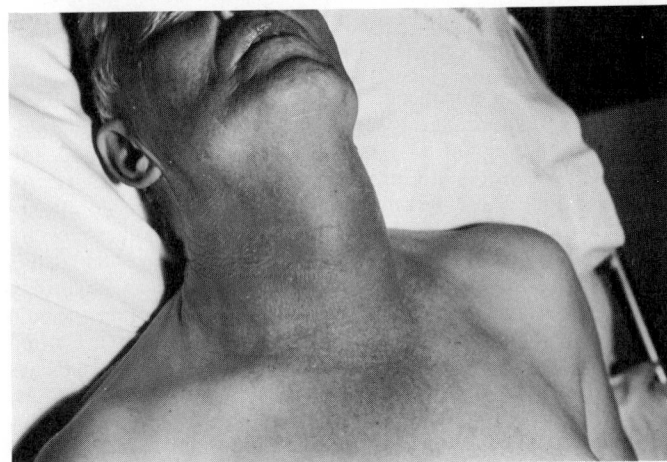

Fig. 1 Spreading cellulitis of the neck resulting from tonsillar sepsis (fatal)—'anaerobic neck'.

ENT infections. Anaerobes, particularly fusobacteria but also other oropharyngeal commensals, are commonly found in infections involving sinuses, middle ear, and mastoid particularly if they are chronic and sometimes if they are acute. This predilection of anaerobes for chronic sinus and middle ear infection is important when considering the bacterial aetiology of brain abscesses arising from such underlying sepsis (see below). Chronic sinus infection occasionally results in acute orbital cellulitis, and this condition is predominantly anaerobic though aerobic oropharyngeal commensals such as *Haemophilus influenzae*, *Str. milleri*, and *Eikenella corrodens* are also commonly isolated. Tonsillar and peritonsillar abscesses are frequently anaerobic, and *F. necrophorum* (see page 5.365) and *B. melaninogenicus* are common, but, unless cultured from pus or blood, they may be presumptive rather than proven pathogens for their presence in a throat swab may indicate little more than normal commensal carriage.

Infections of the central nervous system. Anaerobic bacteria are the major pathogens in cerebral abscess other than those that follow surgery or trauma. Otogenic cerebral abscesses are more common than abscesses arising from chronic sinusitis or other underlying conditions and frequently involve *B. fragilis*. In about half of otogenic abscesses, aerobic bacteria will also be present, particularly *Proteus* spp. but also streptococci, including *Str. milleri*. In contrast, frontal lobe abscesses of sinus or dental origin are most likely to be caused by *Str. milleri*, sometimes alone but more usually with other oropharyngeal aerobes and anaerobes but not *B. fragilis*. Anaerobes can also cause pyogenic meningitis, but such cases are exceptionally uncommon unless associated with a cerebral abscess.

Pleuropulmonary infection. Aspiration of oropharyngeal secretions is the usual mechanism involved in the pathogenesis of anaerobic pleuropulmonary infections, although metastatic infections associated especially with *F. necrophorum* septicaemia also occur. Anaerobic pleuropulmonary infections include aspiration pneumonia, necrotizing pneumonitis, lung abscess, and empyema, as well as secondary infection in underlying conditions such as bronchiectasis. The anaerobes involved are the oropharyngeal commensals as also are the aerobes which are frequently present. *B. fragilis* is found in lung infections, but is distinctly uncommon in most series. Definitive bacteriological diagnosis of anaerobic pleuropulmonary infections can seldom be made by culture of expectorated sputum: invasive procedures are usually required. Transtracheal aspiration, popular in the USA, is seldom performed elsewhere and satisfactory specimens can sometimes be obtained by fibreoptic bronchoscopy. In lung abscess, percutaneous transthoracic aspiration can be particularly useful, firstly to obtain a specimen for bacteriological diagnosis, and secondly to assist in drainage of the pus.

Intra-abdominal infections. These are by far the commonest anaerobic infections, hardly surprising in view of the rich anaerobic microflora of the colon. They may arise *de novo* as in acute appendicitis or acute diverticulitis, or they may follow surgery to the gastrointestinal tract. Most intra-abdominal abscesses and peritonitis are mixed infections with anaerobes predominating. Anaerobes are also found in hepatic abscesses but rather less frequently than is often described: *Str. milleri*, often mistaken for an anaerobe, appears to have a predilection for the liver and is often the sole pathogen. Although a variety of different anaerobes are often isolated from intra-abdominal infections, *B. fragilis* is nearly always present, in contrast to anaerobic infection at most other sites, where it is an infrequent pathogen. Post-operative wound sepsis following colonic surgery and appendicectomy is invariably anaerobic, and wound infection following gastric surgery, particularly for bleeding gastric ulcers or gastric carcinoma, is often caused by anaerobes, although seldom by *B. fragilis* (Figs. 2 and 3).

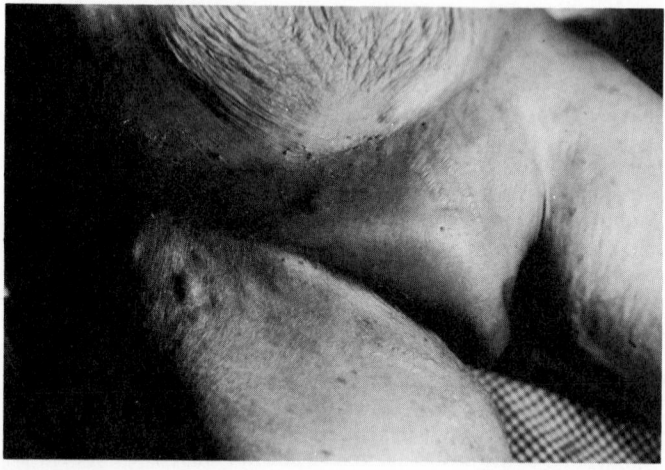

Fig. 2 Necrotizing fasciitis involving perineum, buttock, and thigh three weeks after gastrectomy for carcinoma.

Infections of the biliary tract. In comparison with the frequency of aerobic infections of the gall bladder and biliary tract, anaerobic infections are uncommon, a surprising finding in view of the ability of many anaerobes to grow in bile. In our series of infected gallstones, only 1 of 46 yielded an anaerobe, *B. fragilis*, on culture. Anaerobes are especially likely to be found in wound sepsis following cholecystectomy when a coincidental appendicectomy has been performed, and also in cholangitis following previous biliary surgery which has involved intestinal anastomoses. *Cl. perfringens* seems to have a curious predilection for the bile and is commonly cultured from T-tube specimens of bile following surgery in the absence of symptoms. On rare occasions, however, this anaerobe can cause devastating and usually fatal biliary sepsis.

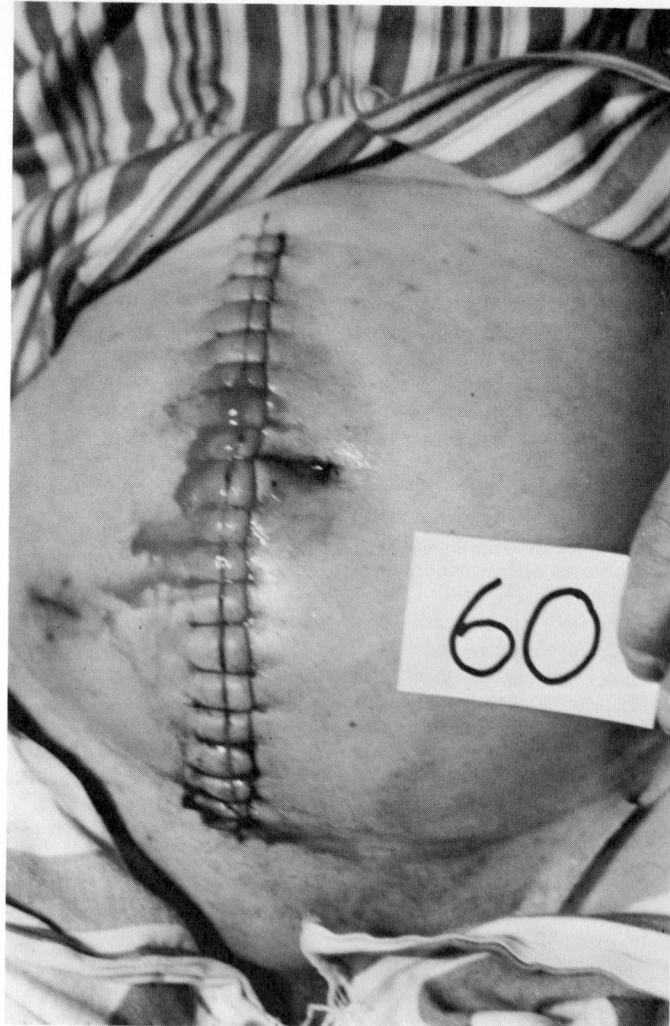

Fig. 3 Wound sepsis following elective colorectal surgery.

Infections of the female genital tract. Anaerobic bacteria are frequently involved in infections of the female genital tract and these infections are often pure anaerobic infections rather than the mixed aerobic–anaerobic infections so common in the abdomen (see Section 12). They include endometritis, tubo-ovarian sepsis, Bartholin's abscess, septic abortion, and infections associated with intra-uterine contraceptive devices. In pregnancy, prolonged rupture of the membranes is associated with anaerobic infection and foul-smelling liquor is often noted, although in the past it was seldom attributed to the presence of anaerobes. In such cases, anaerobes, of vaginal origin, can be cultured not only from the liquor but also from the placenta, which is also invariably foul smelling, and sometimes from the nasogastric aspirate of the baby which may well develop anaerobic pneumonitis. Anaerobic bacteria are an important, though often forgotten, cause of neonatal sepsis. Vaginal hysterectomy carries a high risk of post-operative anaerobic infection, but wound sepsis following abdominal hysterectomy is as likely to be caused by *Staph. aureus* as by anaerobes and should be uncommon with good operative technique. Anaerobic infections of the female genital tract are usually caused by *Bacteroides* species, often other than *B. fragilis*, and particularly black-pigmented bacteroides and *B. bivius* (easily mistaken for *B. fragilis* in the laboratory). *Fusobacterium* spp. and the anaerobic cocci are also commonly found.

Infections of the male genitalia and prostate. The male urethra has a rich commensal anaerobic flora, and these organisms are found in genital infections, including balanoposthitis: the foul odour of anaerobic balanoposthitis is well known to venereologists. Anaerobes also commonly cause secondary infections of penile lesions of varying aetiology, including syphilitic ulcers and condylomata acuminata. Scrotal abscesses are usually anaerobic whether arising *de novo* when they are characteristically recurrent and are almost certainly infections secondary to apocrine blockage, or following surgery to genitalia or urethra.

The rare, potentially lethal condition of Fournier's gangrene, so vividly described over 100 years ago, is a mixed aerobic–anaerobic infection involving the scrotum but also often extending to the perineum, thighs, and abdominal wall. This necrotizing infection is characterized by intense pain and swelling with foul discharge and gas in the tissues. It may arise spontaneously, sometimes in association with a perirectal abscess, or follow trauma or surgery.

Prostatic abscesses may be anaerobic, and it is possible that anaerobes may be important in prostatitis, but the technical difficulties of sampling prostatic fluid uncontaminated by the normal anaerobic flora of the urethra make it difficult to evaluate the role of anaerobic bacteria in this condition.

Infections of the urinary tract.
True anaerobic infection of the urinary tract is very uncommon. When anaerobes are recovered from the urine in heavy growth, the possible explanations are that there is a vesico-colic or vesico-vaginal fistula, or that the urine has been contaminated during collection by vaginal discharge. Conduit urine may become infected with anaerobes.

Bone and joint infections.
Anaerobes are important, if relatively uncommon, pathogens in osteomyelitis and septic arthritis. Many orthopaedic surgeons and rheumatologists are unaware of this and these infections are likely to be misdiagnosed: they require close co-operation between laboratory and clinician. A variety of species may be involved in chronic bone infections, but acute anaerobic infection of bone is likely to be caused by *F. necrophorum* (see page 5.365). A special mention should be made of 'human bite infections' of the hand, for those of the clenched-fist type often penetrate the synovium. Such infections have a well-deserved evil reputation and are invariably anaerobic.

Skin and soft tissue infections
Diabetic foot ulcers. These are frequently anaerobic and may be associated with underlying osteomyelitis and with anaerobic cellulitis, sometimes with gas formation. This condition is readily confused by the inexperienced with clostridial gas gangrene but is not accompanied by the toxaemia and prostration so characteristic of classical gas gangrene.

Decubitus ulcers. These are frequently infected with anaerobes, particularly *B. fragilis* but aerobes, usually several species, are also invariably present.

Sebaceous cysts. Anaerobes, notably the peptococci, are often isolated from infected sebaceous cysts, but many clinically infected sebaceous cysts prove sterile on culture even with adequate techniques for isolation of anaerobes.

Hidradenitis suppurativa. This indolent condition is primarily one of apocrine gland blockage, and thus occurs at any site where these glands occur: commonly the axilla, but also the perineum, thighs, buttocks, and back (Fig. 4). Secondary infection of these blocked glands is always anaerobic, despite being usually attributed to staphylococci. A wide variety of anaerobes is involved including *B. fragilis*, and the method by which they reach the blocked glands is a matter for speculation. The anaerobes are responsible for the foul odour often specifically complained of by these unfortunate patients. Uncomplicated axillary abscesses may also be anaerobic, but they are likely to be recurrent and may ultimately result in overt hidradenitis suppurativa. It is possible that secondary infection of blocked apocrine glands may also be the mechanism involved in anaerobic perirectal sepsis.

Perirectal abscess. These are usually anaerobic, and if faecal

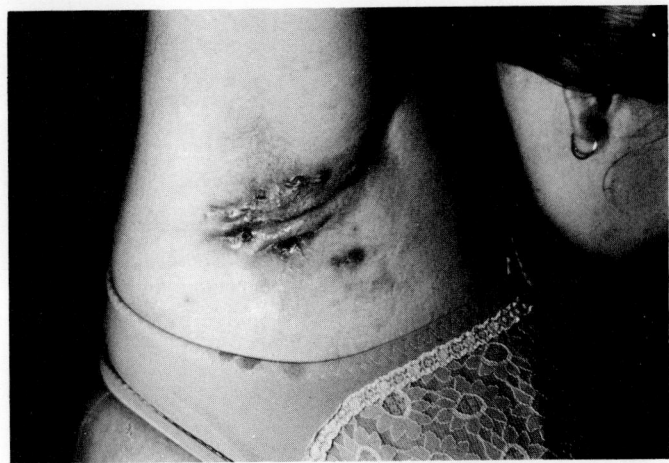

Fig. 4 Hidradenitis suppurativa of axilla.

organisms such as *B. fragalis* are present, there is usually an accompanying fistula. Otherwise the bacteria isolated are similar to those that obstruct the apocrine glands.

Breast abscess. Recurrent breast abscess in the non-peurperal woman, associated with inverted nipples, is a secondary anaerobic infection of an underlying blocked duct, a condition histologically similar to hidradenitis suppurativa. Various anaerobes are involved but not, in our experience, *B. fragilis*. Again one can only speculate on the mode of acquisition of these anaerobes as to whether they arrive via the blood or by local inoculation.

Human bites. These have already been mentioned with reference to infections of the joints of the hand, but they may, of course, involve other parts of the body. A situation similar to a human bite infection also occurs when the victim accidently bites himself. Although animal bites may give rise to anaerobic infections, those involving dog and cat are perhaps more likely to become infected with *Pasteurella* spp. than with anaerobes.

Paronychia. About a third of all paronychias are caused by anaerobes, usually though not invariably occurring with aerobes. The anaerobes are oropharyngeal commensals probably transferred to the fingers by licking or biting. Anaerobic paronychias are usually less acute than those caused by *Staph. aureus* and *Str. pyogenes* but are otherwise clinically indistinguishable.

Bacteraemia and endocarditis.
Anaerobic sepsis at any site may be accompanied by bacteraemia, sometimes producing shock. Anaerobes are recovered from 5–10 per cent of positive blood cultures and laboratory skill is probably the main factor determining this incidence, for anaerobes, in particular those other than *B. fragilis*, are more culturally exacting that most aerobes. In many patients, by the time the laboratory reports the isolation of an anaerobe from a blood culture, the type and site of infection is already established clinically, although gas–liquid chromatography performed directly on blood cultures may detect the presence of an anaerobe much earlier than conventional culture methods. Sometimes the detection of anaerobic bacteraemia is critical in establishing a clinical diagnosis, and this is especially true for fusobacterial bacteraemia.

Anaerobes can cause endocarditis, but such infections seem to be exceedingly rare. It is theoretically possible that it is underdiagnosed in view of the technical difficulties in recovering many anaerobes. It seems curious in view of the abundant commensal anaerobes in the mouth that these organisms have not been more frequently implicated as pathogens in endocarditis associated with dental sepsis and manipulation.

Synergistic infections.
Anaerobic bacteria, usually with aerobes, cause a range of so called 'synergistic' infections: these can involve skin, fascia, or sometimes muscle. The bacteriology in many of the

earlier reports is incomplete but it is clear that many anaerobic species may be involved. Fournier's gangrene, a necrotizing fasciitis, has already been mentioned and Meleney's synergistic infection is almost certainly of similar pathogenesis, although limited to skin and subcutaneous tissues. It is known that these dangerous infections may arise either spontaneoulsy or following surgery or trauma but why they occur remains a mystery.

'Necrobacillosis'. This is a septicaemic infection caused by *F. necrophorum*. Unlike the infections described above, where polymicrobial aetiology is the rule, *F. necrophorum* is usually found alone. Perhaps by virtue of its lipopolysaccharide endotoxin, this bacterium is a virulent organism capable of producing severe toxaemic illness which, in the pre-antibiotic era, was usually fatal. Furthermore, unlike much of the anaerobic infection described in the preceding pages, *F. necrophorum* septicaemia occurs in the previously healthy individual, usually, though not exclusively in the young, and is not associated with trauma, surgery, or underlying disorders as is so frequently the case with other anaerobic infections. The classical syndrome of necrobacillosis is one of the sudden onset of rigors usually associated with a sore throat, sometimes with obvious tonsillar or peritonsillar sepsis. It is further characterized by metastatic abscess formation most often in the lung, sometimes with purulent pleural fluid, but abscesses may occur in other organs including the liver, and septic arthritis and osteomyelitis may also occur. Fusobacterial septicaemia can present diagnostic difficulties for *F. necrophorum* is unlikely to be isolated from the blood or pleural fluid for several days if at all, but the sudden onset of rigors with a sore throat (and often painful neck glands) in a previously healthy young adult with tonsils *in situ* should suggest the diagnosis. Such infections are undoubtedly more common than has previously been realized as *F. necrophorum* is not readily isolated in the laboratory and is exquisitely sensitive to most antibiotics, often given before such patients are referred to hospital. Necrobacillosis was a devastating lethal infection in the pre-antibiotic era, not only in man but also in animals. *F. necrophorum* is also the most important pathogen in calf diphtheria, from which it was first isolated, in bovine hepatic abscess, and is associated with bovine foot rot.

Treatment and prevention

Sensitivity of anaerobic bacteria to antimicrobial agents. The susceptibility of anaerobic bacteria to antimicrobial agents can be tested in the laboratory either by the disc method, which is the easiest and most readily available, or by the more sophisticated techniques that measure the minimum inhibitory or bactericidal concentrations of the drugs. Such investigations are time consuming and seldom of use in the management of an individual patient. It is nevertheless important for laboratories to monitor sensitivity patterns of anaerobes isolated from clinical infections as it is this accumulated information that provides the basis for therapeutic management. Antimicrobial sensitivities of the common anaerobes are shown in Table 3. The 'fragilis' group of *Bacteroides* are resistant to most β-lactam antibiotics including penicillin, ampicillin, and the early cephalosporins, though not to cefotaxime, the cefamycin cefoxitin, and some others under investigation. Most strains have membrane-bound β-lactamases. The substrate profiles indicate that the β-lactamases are predominantly cephalosporinases but with moderate penicillinase activity. An increasing number of isolates of black-pigmented bacteroides have also been shown to produce a β-lactamase that is particularly active against penicillins, but, with the exception of these organisms, other anaerobic bacteria are usually sensitive to penicillins and cephalosporins. Anaerobic bacteria are resistant to aminoglycosides: the mechanism involved is one of failure of active transport of the drug. Tetracycline resistance amongst anaerobes has gradually increased, and this drug is only of limited use. Erythromycin is difficult to assess as sensitivity testing presents technical problems. Chloramphenicol has a wide anaerobic spectrum, and resistance to it is rare and probably mediated by an acetyltransferase and nitroreductase. Clindamycin and lincomycin are active against most anaerobes, but resistance amongst *B. fragilis* is transferable by plasmids. Metronidazole has the widest anaerobic spectrum and only it and the other nitroimidazoles, ornidazole and tinidazole, are selectively active against anaerobes. Resistance has been reliably reported in only one strain of *B. fragilis*, and in this organism there was a block in the uptake of metronidazole by the bacterial cell and a decreased capacity to transform metronidazole to its active intermediates. Lastly, it is probable that co-trimoxazole has useful activity against anaerobes including *B. fragilis*, but sensitivity testing presents problems. It is becoming clear that there are geographical differences in sensitivity, sometimes associated with the common use of individual antibiotics.

Treatment. Much anaerobic infection will require surgical intervention to achieve satisfactory drainage of pus or excision of necrotic tissue, and any antibiotic will be of secondary importance to such procedures. Some infections will respond to antibiotics alone and fusobacterial septicaemia is a good example of this. In the majority of anaerobic infections aerobic bacteria are also present, and in devising appropriate chemotherapy one has to decide firstly which drug is most effective for the anaerobe, and secondly whether it is necessary to treat the aerobes as well. Unquestionably for infections involving the 'fragilis' group, metronidazole is the most logical choice, and it is also appropriate for most other anaerobes. Despite warnings of its potential genotoxicity predicted from animal and bacterial test systems, it has proved safe in clinical practice and highly effective. Penicillins and cephalosporins can be used in the infections not likely to be caused by *B. fragilis* but, with increasing resistance to penicillin amongst *B. melaninogenicus*, they may fail. Clindamycin and lincomycin were used extensively and very successfully until the association between these agents and pseudomembranous colitis was recognized. Chloramphenicol would seldom seem to be justified for anaerobic infection in view of its association with aplastic anaemia, and, although it is particularly valuable in anerobic infection of the CNS, metronidazole provides equal efficacy. Although tetracycline, erythromycin, and perhaps co-trimoxazole are sometimes other possible drugs, in practice they are seldom used.

Table 3 Antimicrobial susceptibility of some common anaerobes

	Penicillin	Ampicillin	Tetracycline	Clindamycin	Metronidazole	Chloramphenicol	Cefoxitin
Bacteroides: 'fragilis' group	R	R	V	VS	S	S	VS
Other bacteroides	VS	VS	VS	S	S	S	S
Fusobacterium spp.	S	S	S	S	S	S	S
Clostridium spp.	S	S	VS	V	S	S	VS
Anaerobic cocci	VS	VS	VS	S	S	S	VS
Actinomyces spp.	S	S	VS	S	R	S	S

S = almost always sensitive   VS = variable but usually sensitive
V = variable   R = almost always resistant

Whether it is always necessary to treat both anaerobic and aerobic components in mixed infections is open to debate. Our clinical studies with metronidazole alone in such infections have convinced us that in abdominal and pelvic sepsis treatment of the anaerobe only (with metronidazole) is all that is necessary. The *in vitro* evidence that anaerobes inhibit phagocytosis in mixed infections would lend support to this hypothesis. However, in pleuropulmonary infection, and in lung abscess in particular, it is necessary to treat both aerobes and anaerobes, and clinical failures with metronidazole used alone in these infections are well documented. For anaerobic infections at other sites insufficient data exists for us to be dogmatic; suffice it to say that the availability of metronidazole has made possible selective treatment of the anaerobic component in mixed infections and provided much information on the relative importance of aerobes and anaerobes in some mixed infections.

Prevention. With the rediscovery of the importance of anaerobes as pathogens, prophylaxis against these organisms became an attractive proposition.

Colorectal surgery. For many years surgeons attempted to 'sterilize the bowel' before colorectal surgery, usually with non-absorbable sulphonamides given alone or with neomycin. These drugs were given to suppress coliforms thought to be the relevant organisms in post-operative sepsis. Despite this almost universal practice many surgeons were unconvinced of the efficacy of such antimicrobial prophylaxis. When prophylaxis was specifically directed against anaerobes, it soon became clear that the appallingly high post-operative wound sepsis rate following elective colorectal surgery could be dramatically reduced. Many different regimens have been used but the concept of bowel sterilization has been replaced by that of an effective tissue level maintained during the operative period. Peri-operative systemic metronidazole either alone or with an antibiotic for the colonic aerobes, is useful and effective.

Appendicectomy. Wound sepsis following appendicectomy is usually anaerobic but is uncommon when the appendix is either normal or only minimally inflamed. It is doubtful whether prophylaxis is indicated in such cases. Where the appendix is found to be gangrenous or where frank pus is present, infection is already present and any antibiotic given is therapeutic as well as prophylactic. In such cases metronidazole alone is almost certainly as effective as regimens including a drug against aerobes. Inadequate drainage is likely to result in further infection whatever antibiotic is given.

Hysterectomy. Whilst anaerobic wound infection can occur after abdominal hysterectomy, it is uncommon and this type of operation probably does not warrant antimicrobial prophylaxis. When such wounds do get infected they are as likely to yield *Staph. aureus* as anaerobes. Prophylaxis against anaerobes is however more certainly indicated for vaginal hysterectomy which carries a much higher risk of infection, invariably with vaginal anaerobes. Such prophylaxis is probably best given during the immediate peri-operative period.

References

Finegold, S. M. (1977). *Anaerobic bacteria in human disease*. Academic Press, New York.

Infection (1980). Diagnosis and therapy of anaerobic infections. *Infection* **8**, suppl. 2.

Phillips, I. and Collier, J. (eds.) (1979). Metronidazole. In *Proceedings of 2nd International symposium on anaerobic infection*. Royal Society of Medicine, London.

— and Sussmann, M. (1974). *Infection with non-sporing anaerobic bacteria*. Churchill Livingstone, Edinburgh.

Reviews of Infectious Diseases (1979). Virulence factors of anaerobic bacteria. *Rev. infect. Dis.* **1**.

Willis, A. T. (1977). *Anaerobic bacteriology: clinical and laboratory practice*, 3rd edn. Butterworth, London.

Cholera

C. C. J. Carpenter

Cholera is an acute illness caused by an enterotoxin elaborated by *Vibrio cholerae* which have colonized the small bowel. In the more severely ill patients, fluid and electrolytes are rapidly lost from the gastrointestinal tract, resulting in hypovolaemic shock, metabolic acidosis and, if untreated, death.

Aetiology and epidemiology. *V. cholerae* are short (0.2–0.4 μm by 1.5–4.0 μm) slightly curved, Gram-negative rods that are readily seen in the excreta of patients with cholera. Rapid presumptive diagnosis can be made by a vibrio immunization test employing dark-field or phase microscopy and type-specific sera.

Cholera has been endemic for two centuries in the Ganges Delta of West Bengal and Bangladesh, has caused multiple epidemics throughout the Indian Subcontinent, and has been responsible for seven global pandemics in the past 160 years. The seventh pandemic, the only pandemic of the twentieth century, began in 1961, extended from Indonesia (Sulawesi) northward to Korea and westward throughout Asia to involve the whole of Africa, Mediterranean Europe and, most recently, the Gulf Coast of the United States. The eltor biotype of *V. cholerae*, which has been responsible for the current pandemic, has almost completely replaced the classical biotype in its endemic home in the Ganges Delta, suggesting that the eltor biotype may have an ecological advantage over its sister biotype.

Man is the only known mammalian host and natural victim of *V. cholerae*. Most major epidemics of this disease have been water-borne, and water plays the major role in the transmission of *V. cholerae* in the endemic rural areas in the Ganges Delta. During major pandemics, however, the direct contamination of food with infectious excreta may be important. Contaminated fresh vegetables appeared to have been a major factor in the transmission of cholera in Israel in the outbreak in 1970, and shellfish were a major factor in the spread of cholera in Naples in 1973, and on the Gulf Coast of the United States in 1978. Shellfish clearly have the capacity to harbour *V. cholerae* in high concentration for long periods of time without obvious damage to the host.

People with mild or asymptomatic infections (contact carriers) may also play a role in the dissemination of epidemic disease. The clinical case : infection ratio with the classical *V. cholerae* biotype is about 1 : 6; with infection by the eltor biotype, this ratio may be as low as 1 : 50. A prolonged gall-bladder carrier state occasionally develops in adult patients convalescing from cholera caused by the eltor biotype, but has never been demonstrated with the classical biotype. The role of such convalescent carriers in the transmission of the disease, if any, has not been clarified. *V. cholerae* does not survive well in fresh water, but may survive for long periods in seawater; this has recently been re-affirmed in association with the 1973 outbreak of cholera in Portugal.

In the cholera endemic areas of Bangladesh and West Bengal, cholera is predominantly a disease of children. Attack rates are ten times greater in the 1–5 age group than in those over 20 years of age. When the disease spreads to previously uninvolved areas, the attack rates are initially at least as high in adults as in children. As the disease becomes endemic in new locations, as has occurred in the Philippines over the past 20 years and in Africa over the past 10 years, the endemic epidemiologic pattern develops, with the disease becoming far more common in young children than in adults.

Pathogenesis. *V. cholerae* causes disease when a large number of viable organisms are ingested, survive passage through the stomach, colonize the small bowel, and produce enterotoxin. The incubation period may vary from 12 hours to as long as six days, but is usually between 24 and 72 hours. Because of the remarkable susceptibility of *V. cholerae* to gastric acid, an enormous number of micro-organisms must be ingested to cause illness in previously healthy individuals. Volunteer studies have indicated that the ingestion of even a thousand million organisms will not consistently produce disease in fasting healthy adults. If, however, gastric acid is neutralized by sodium bicarbonate, or by a high-protein meal, ingestion of one million viable organisms may produce clinical disease in roughly 50 per cent of normal individuals. The individual with relative or absolute achlorhydria is, therefore, abnormally susceptible to cholera; this susceptibility has been re-emphasized by the very sharp increase in incidence of cholera in individuals with total or subtotal gastrectomy in the outbreaks of cholera in Israel and Italy during the last decade.

Once vibrios have colonized the small bowel, a well-defined enterotoxin is produced. This enterotoxin is a protein, with a molecular weight of 84 000 dalton, consisting of two well-defined moieties. The B, or binding, moiety consists of five identical subunits, each of which has a molecular weight of roughly 11 500 dalton, and each of which is capable of combining to a GM-1 monosialoganglioside molecule in the gut mucosal cell wall. The A, or activating, moiety is divided into two unequal subunits; the larger, or A-1, subunit has a molecular weight of roughly 23 000 dalton, and the smaller, or A-2, subunit has a molecular weight of roughly 6000 dalton. The binding subunits of the enterotoxin combine extraordinarily rapidly to the monosialogangliosides in the small bowel epithelial cell wall, and, at body temperature, this binding becomes irreversible within minutes after the initial contact of the binding subunits with the GM-1 monosialogangliosides. The irreversibility of the binding suggests that the binding subunits of the toxin become incorporated in the bacterial cell wall. Following the rapid binding of the toxin to the cell wall, the A-1 subunit migrates through to the inner surface of the epithelial cell, where it stimulates ADP ribosylation of a 42 000 dalton adenylate cyclase component bearing the guanyl nucleotide site. This results in a modification of the GTP binding protein, inhibits the GTP 'turnoff' reaction and thus increases the activity of adenylate cyclase. The resultant increase in intracellular levels of cyclic adenosine 3′,5′-monophosphate (cyclic AMP) leads to rapid excretion of electrolytes into the small bowel lumen.

The net secretion of fluid and electrolytes by gut mucosal cells in cholera reflects dual effect on two different intestinal ion transport sites. In the villus cells the absorption of sodium chloride via the neutral sodium chloride co-transport system is inhibited. In the crypt cells the increased intracellular cyclic AMP results in active stimulation of chloride secretion. The net effect of inhibition of sodium absorption and stimulation of chloride secretion is the rapid outpouring of isotonic fluid in the intestinal lumen at a rate which exceeds the absorptive capacity of the colon, thus resulting in the loss of an isotonic fluid with the electrolyte pattern described in Table 1. In adults with voluminous diarrhoea the electrolyte in cholera stool is remarkably consistent, being nearly isotonic with plasma, with sodium and chloride concentrations slightly less than those of plasma, bicarbonate concentration twice that of plasma, and potassium concentration three to five times that of plasma. In very young children with cholera the mean sodium and chloride concentrations are 15–20 mmol/l less than those observed in older patients.

Table 1 Electrolyte concentrations in cholera stool of adults (mmol/l) (mean values, 38 patients)

	Admission	48 hours after admission
Sodium	116	126
Chloride	100	90
Potassium	30	16
Bicarbonate	40	50

All signs, symptoms, and metabolic derangements in cholera result directly from the rapid loss of these fluids from the gut. All segments of the small bowel participate in the increased secretion of

isotonic fluid, and the resultant fluid lost represents the sum of the contributions of each of the small bowel segments, slightly modified during passage through the colon.

Clinical features. The clinical onset of cholera is generally that of abrupt, painless, watery diarrhoea. Stool volumes vary greatly, and in all epidemics there are large numbers of mild cases in which the fluid loss is not severe enough to require hospitalization. In the more severe cases, however, the initial stool volume may exceed 1500 ml. At variable intervals after the onset of diarrhoea, vomiting ensues; this is also characteristically effortless and productive of rice-watery material. In fulminant cases, severe muscle cramps, most commonly involving the calf muscles, almost invariable develop. Prostration occurs at varying intervals following the onset of symptoms, in direct relationship to the magnitude of the fluid loss.

When first seen by the physician, the severely ill cholera patient presents a characteristic appearance (Fig. 1). He is collapsed, cyanotic, with no palpable peripheral pulses, pinched facies, and scaphoid abdomen. The skin turgor is remarkably diminished. The voice is very weak, high-pitched, and often nearly inaudible. Vital signs include tachycardia, varying degrees of tachypnoea, hypopyrexia, and hypotension, often with no obtainable blood pressure. Heart sounds are faint or inaudible, and bowel sounds are hypoactive or entirely absent. Major alterations in mental status are not common in adults; the adult usually remains well-oriented, although apathetic, even in the face of severe hypovolaemic shock. As many as 10 per cent of small children, however, may have central nervous system abnormalities that range from stupor to convulsions.

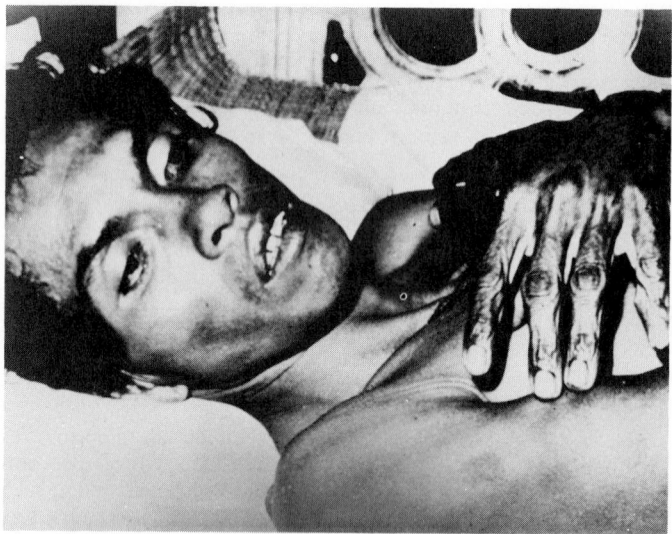

Fig. 1 An acutely ill cholera patient demonstrating the characteristic 'washerwoman's hands', indicative of severe extracellular fluid depletion. (From Carpenter (1972), with permission.)

Laboratory abnormalities are those which would be expected to result from massive gastrointestinal loss of an isotonic, alkaline, virtually protein-free fluid (Table 2). These include increased plasma and whole blood specific gravity, elevated plasma protein, decreased plasma bicarbonate, low arterial pH, normal plasma sodium, slightly increased plasma chloride, and moderately elevated plasma potassium. Since the bicarbonate loss is proportional to stool volume, the decrease in whole blood pH is roughly proportional to the increase in plasma protein concentration at all stages of the untreated disease. The abnormal blood chemical findings are rapidly corrected with appropriate fluid therapy (Table 2).

The illness may last from 12 hours to seven days, and later clinical manifestations depend on the adequacy of therapy. With adequate fluid and electrolyte repletion, recovery is remarkably rapid. If therapy is inadequate, the case mortality rate may exceed 50 per cent. The important causes of death are hypovolaemic shock, un-compensated metabolic acidosis, and renal failure. When renal failure occurs, the characteristic pathologic findings are those of acute tubular necrosis secondary to prolonged hypotension.

Table 2   Blood chemical determinations in 38 adult cholera patients before and four hours after intravenous fluid therapy

	Mean values ± standard deviation	
	Admission	Four hours after admission
Arterial blood pH	7.17 ± 0.06	7.40 ± 0.05
Plasma bicarbonate (mmol/l)	7 ± 4	20 ± 3
Plasma potassium (mmol/l)	5.6 ± 0.4	3.2 ± 0.3
Total plasma protein (g/dl)	14.2 ± 0.8	7.5 ± 0.6

Diagnosis. The working diagnosis of cholera should be made on the basis of the clinical picture; appropriate fluid and electrolyte replacement therapy, as indicated by the physical findings, should be initiated immediately. Although a cholera-like illness may be caused by micro-organisms other than *V. cholerae*, most frequently by enterotoxigenic *Escherichia coli*, the resulting physiologic and metabolic abnormalities are the same, so that identical intravenous and oral electrolyte therapy may be used in all such cases.

After appropriate therapy has been initiated, a geographic history should be obtained. The diagnosis of cholera is unlikely if the patient has not recently been in a known endemic or epidemic area. Stool examination should then be performed. Since the cholera enterotoxin causes neither inflammation nor destruction of intestinal mucosa, neither leucocytes nor erythrocytes are usually seen on a microscopic examination of a fresh cholera stool stained with methylene blue. This, however, is not absolute, as cholera may occasionally be superimposed on other acute or chronic inflammatory bowel disease. With dark-field microscopy, rapid tentative diagnosis can be made by direct observation of the characteristic rapid motility of the comma-shaped bacilli in fresh stool. Group- and type-specific antisera immobilize homologous strains and clearly distinguish them from other vibrios. *V. cholerae*, which are slow lactose fermenters, grow rapidly on a number of selective media, including bile salt agar, glycerine–taurocholate–tellurite agar and thiosulfate–citrate–bile salt–sucrose (TCBS) agar. Of these, TCBS agar has the distinct advantage of not requiring sterilization before use. On TCBS agar, *V. cholerae* can be distinguished from other enteric micro-organisms by a distinct opaque yellow colonial appearance. Distinction between the two major serotypes—Inaba and Ogawa—is made by slide agglutination with type-specific antisera.

Distinction between the two major *V. cholerae* biotypes, classical and eltor, is important for epidemiologic purposes. The eltor is distinguished from the classical biotype by its resistance to polymyin B, resistance to Mukerjee's choleraphage type IV and, with some exceptions, by its ability to haemolyse sheep erythrocytes.

Management. Successful therapy demands only prompt replacement of gastrointestinal losses of fluid and electrolytes.

Intravenous fluids. A 'diarrhoea treatment solution', recommended for intravenous therapy by the World Health Organization, may simply be prepared by adding 4 g sodium chloride, 6.5 g sodium acetate, and 1 g potassium chloride to a litre of sterile, pyrogen-free distilled water. Alternatively, lactated Ringer's solution may be administered. Either of these intravenous fluid preparations should be infused intravenously and rapidly, 50–100 ml, per minute in adults, until a strong radial pulse has been restored. Subsequently the same fluid should be infused in quantities equal to gastrointestinal losses. If these losses cannot be measured accu-

rately, intravenous fluid should be given at a rate sufficient to maintain a normal pulse volume and normal skin turgor. Over-hydration can be avoided by careful observation of the neck veins and by auscultation of the lungs. Close observation of the patient is mandatory during the acute phase of the illness, as an adult patient can lose as much as one litre of isotonic fluid per hour during the first 24 hours of the disease. Inadequate or delayed restoration of electrolyte losses results in a very high incidence of acute renal insufficiency.

In children, complications are both more frequent and more severe. The most serious include stupor, coma, and convulsions (unique to paediatric patients), pulmonary oedema, and cardiac arrhythmias. The central nervous system complications may be due to hypoglycaemia (observed only in paediatric patients), hypernatraemia resulting from the administration of isotonic fluid to the paediatric patient (who, unlike the adult patient, produces stool with a sodium concentration significantly less than that of plasma), or cerebral oedema, presumably secondary to rapid fluid shifts during the administration of intravenous fluids. Pulmonary oedema may result if fluids are given intravenously at too rapid a rate prior to the correction of the metabolic acidosis. Cardiac arrhythmias may result from potassium depletion in children, but rarely occur in adults with cholera. Each of these complications can be avoided by the careful administration of intravenous fluids that are designed to replace the faecal electrolyte losses. The 'diarrhoea treatment solution', recommended by the World Health Organization for cholera as well as for other acute diarrhoeal diseases, has been used successfully to correct the acidosis, hypokalaemia, and hypoglycaemia without provoking hypernatraemia. If lactated Ringer's solution is used in the paediatric patient, perioral supplementation of potassium and glucose is needed. The outcome in paediatric cholera should be essentially as favorable as that in the adult disease, with an overall mortality rate of less than 1 per cent.

Oral replacement fluids. Perioral replacement of water and electrolytes is also remarkably effective in adults, and in children who are alert. An oral glucose-electrolyte solution (prepared by the addition of 20 g glucose, 3.5 g sodium chloride, 2.5 g sodium bicarbonate, and 1.5 g potassium chloride to one litre of drinking water) can be given in mild cholera cases throughout the course of illness, and is also satisfactory in more severe cases once the hypovolemic shock has been corrected by the initial rapid intravenous fluid therapy. When oral therapy is employed, about 1.5 volumes of oral solution are to be given to replace each volume of stool loss. Glucose is an essential component of this solution, in that the success of oral therapy in cholera depends upon enhanced intestinal absorption of sodium in the presence of intraluminal glucose. Although the cholera enterotoxin inhibits neutral sodium chloride absorption by the intestinal mucosal brush border, it does not impair the glucose-facilitated sodium transport across the same membrane. Since, in certain rural areas, glucose is not as readily available as sucrose, sucrose-electrolyte solutions have been evaluated and have been shown to be nearly as effective as glucose-electrolyte solutions in the treatment of cholera. When sucrose is used, 40 g sucrose must be added to each litre of administered fluid, as sucrose is rapidly broken down into equal amounts of glucose and fructose, and only the glucose metabolite is effective in enhancing sodium absorption.

Antimicrobials. Although adequate fluid therapy results in rapid recovery in virtually all cholera patients, the required volume of replacement fluid may be enormous, and in extreme cases, may exceed twice the weight of the patient (Fig. 2). Adjunctive therapy with antimicrobials dramatically reduces the duration and volume of diarrhoea and results in rapid eradication of vibrios from the faeces. Tetracycline in a dose of 40–50 mg per kg body weight daily, given in four equal portions perorally every six hours for two days, was uniformly successful in this regard until 1980, when tetracycline-resistant vibrio strains were isolated in Bangladesh. Furazolidine and chloramphenicol are also effective, and may be used in the case of tetracycline resistance, but are less desirable than tetracycline because of rare, but serious, side effects to both of these antimicrobial agents. Tetracycline, administered in the recommended dosage for 48 hours, should have no adverse effects on dentition in young children.

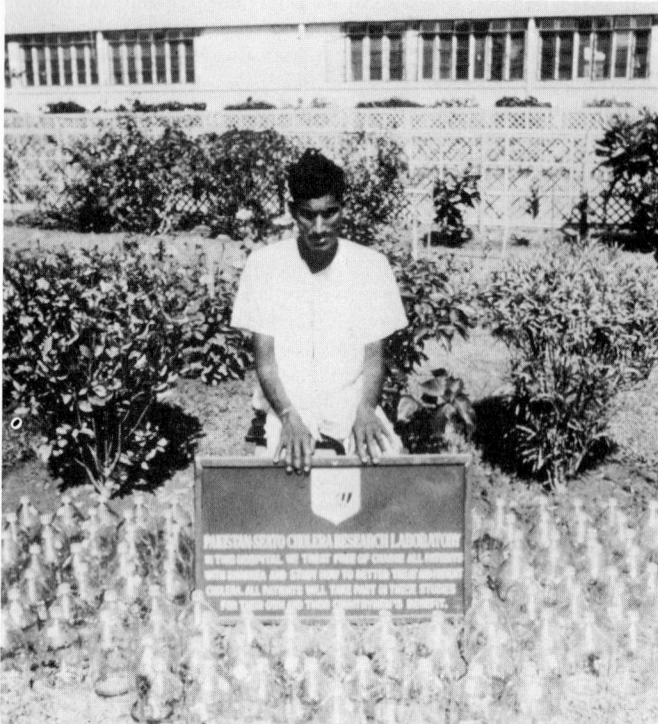

Fig. 2   A convalescent cholera patient, surrounded by the bottles of intravenous fluids which were required to ensure his survival, demonstrates the major logistics problem in treating large numbers of patients, in the absence of adjuvant antimicrobial therapy. (From Carpenter, C. C. J. in Field *et al.* (1980), with permission.)

Immunization and prevention. Immunization using two injections of standard commercial vaccine (containing 1000 million killed vibrios per ml) provides 60–80 per cent protection for 3–6 months to adults in cholera endemic areas. The short duration and relative lack of efficacy of the standard vaccines has led to intense study of immunological mechanisms in cholera over the past few years. Since both the vibrios and the enterotoxin are confined to the intestinal lumen, effective antibodies must be present within the lumen. Patients convalescent from cholera develop high levels of both agglutinating and vibriocidal antibodies against cell-wall constituents of the vibrio, and presumably the short-term protection which follows infection with *V. cholerae* results from the leakage of such immunoglobulin G antibodies into the intestinal lumen. Effective immunity can be produced in experimental animals by repeated intraluminal administration of either holotoxin, the B subunit of the enterotoxin or a glutaraldehyde-inactivated toxoid. Such peroral immunization results in production of antitoxic immunoglobulin A antibodies within the intestinal lumen. However, the large number of doses of oral immunogen which are required makes it unlikely that this approach will prove to be a practical means of conferring immunity against cholera in the near future. Significant immunity can also be developed in experimental animals by parenteral injection of glutaldehyde-inactivated toxoid. However, a recent field trial of immunization by such a toxoid provided significant protection for only a two-month period and was even less effective than the standard whole-cell vaccine. Intensive studies directed toward the development of an effective vaccine continue, but at the present time careful hygiene provides the only certain protection against cholera.

Immunization with current standard commercial vaccines has not proved to be effective in altering the transmission of this disease or in altering the convalescent carriage of *V. cholerae*. Administration of cholera vaccine is therefore no longer recommended by the World Health Organization as a requirement for travellers who have visited cholera endemic areas.

References

Barua, D. and Burrows, W. (eds.) (1974). *Cholera*. W. B. Saunders, Philadelphia.

Carpenter, C. C. J. (1972). Cholera and other enterotoxin – related diarrheal illnesses. *J. infect. dis.* **126**, 551.

Field, M. (1971). Intestinal secretion: effect of cyclic AMP and its role in cholera. *New Engl. J. Med.* **284**, 1137.

—, Fordtran, J. S., and Schultz, S. G. (eds.) (1980). *Secretory diarrhea*. American Physiological Society, Bethesda, Maryland.

Holmgren, L. and Lonroth, I. (1975). Oligomeric structure of cholera toxin: characteristic of H and L subunits. *J. gen. Microbiol.* **86**, 49.

Lindenbaum, J., Greenough, W. B., and Islam, M. R. (1967). Antibiotic therapy of cholera. *Bull Wld Hlth Org.* **36**, 871.

Pierce, N. F., Greenough, W. B., and Carpenter, C. C. J. (1971). *Vibrio cholerae* enterotoxin and its mode of action. *Bacteriol. Rev.* **35**, 1.

Haemophilus

D. C. Turk

Gram-negative bacilli of the genus *Haemophilus* are identified and divided into species mainly on the basis of their special growth factor requirements. Such organisms can be isolated from animals of many kinds, but those which are commensal (mainly in the nasopharynx or mouth) or pathogenic to man are probably always acquired from other humans.

Of the species to be considered here, *H. influenzae* has by far the greatest importance in medicine. It is not the cause of influenza as its discoverer claimed in 1892 and as widely believed for the next 40 years, but it has a wide range of other pathogenic activities. The Koch–Weeks bacillus, identified in 1883 as the cause of outbreaks of conjunctivitis in Egypt and more recently renamed *H. aegyptius*, is now best classified within the species *H. influenzae*. *H. parainfluenzae* (a name under which it is best to include the haemolytic strains that have been classified separately as *H. parahaemolyticus*) is a species commonly found in the human upper respiratory tract but is usually harmless. Carbon dioxide-dependent organisms of the *H. aphrophilus* group, commonly found in the mouth, are being recognized with increasing (but still low) frequency as pathogens in various situations. *H. ducreyi*, the causative organism of the sexually transmitted disease chancroid, is discussed elsewhere (see page 5.305).

Carriage and pathogenicity of *H. influenzae*. Nasopharyngeal carriage of *H. influenzae* is common enough among healthy people to be regarded as normal. It is also common to find that some 3–5 per cent of children and usually a smaller proportion of adults are carrying strains which differ from the rest in being capsulated. Such strains can be divided serologically into six types, a to f. The carriage frequency for type b usually exceeds the total for the other five capsular types. It seems probable that most children carry type b strains for a while at some time during the early years of life. Such carriage is usually asymptomatic, or at least gives rise to no significant illness; but a minority of children are less fortunate in their initial encounter with *H. influenzae* type b and develop meningitis or one of the other bacteraemic diseases described below. Only on rare occasions are strains of any of the other five capsular types incriminated as pathogens. It is also rare for non-capsulated strains to cause any of the severe illnesses; but they can cause some less serious conditions (as do type b strains occasionally), and they have their own quite different form of pathogenic importance, mainly in adults, in relation to acute purulent exacerbations of chronic bronchial diseases.

Haemophilus meningitis

Epidemiology. *H. influenzae* type b is, in many parts of the world and probably in the world as a whole, the commonest cause of bacterial meningitis in children under five years old; indeed, in some countries the number of cases of haemophilus meningitis among such children exceeds the number of cases of meningitis due to all other bacteria among patients of all ages. There is evidence that, in North America at least, haemophilus meningitis has become much more frequent (not just more frequently recognized) during the past 30–40 years. Its recent annual incidence in the United States has been estimated as about 10 000 cases, or 35–50 cases per 100 000 children under five years old. Although it can occur in older children or in adults of any age, the great majority of patients are between three months and four years old—an age-distribution attributable to protection by maternal antibodies in the first months of life and to almost universal acquisition of active natural immunity during the first four or five years. About half of the patients are under one year old, and three-quarters under two years. Some, but not all, surveys have shown higher frequencies among males, among children of black rather than white race, among poorer families, and in winter. Children with haemophilus meningitis have on average more older siblings than do control groups of children of similar age—even than those with other forms of bacterial meningitis; and it seems clear that these siblings, many of whom are nasopharyngeal carriers of *H. influenzae* type b at the relevant times, are the sources of the babies' infections. Despite high carriage rates within the families, second cases of meningitis or other clinically apparent haemophilus infection occur in only 1–3 per cent of families; but even these figures mean that the risk for family contacts, and in particular for those under 2 years old, are several hundred times higher than for the population in general. Small outbreaks of haemophilus meningitis or related infections have been described among children attending day-care centres, and it is common for a group of cases to occur in one area during a short period of time but without any other apparent connection. True epidemics, however, do not happen.

Clinical features. Meningitis due to *H. influenzae* cannot be distinguished with certainty on clinical grounds from that due to meningococci, pneumococci, or other bacteria—although its more restricted age-range may be a help in differential diagnosis. It is usually of acute onset, and sometimes fatal within a few hours; but insidious onset over a few weeks, suggestive of tuberculous meningitis, is seen from time to time, and in some cases is the result of partial antibiotic treatment in the early stages of the illness. Antecedent symptoms of upper respiratory tract infection, in the patient and in family members, and associated otitis media and pneumonia in the patient are common, but so they are in other forms of bacterial meningitis. The association of painful swelling of one or more major joints, due to purulent arthritis, is more suggestive of haemophilus aetiology but is not common. Petechial rashes similar to those of meningococcal infection may occur, and the Waterhouse–Friderichsen syndrome is not unknown. As all of these features imply, haemophilus meningitis is a bacteraemic illness. Perhaps its most distinctive feature, but one that happily is now seldom seen, is the thick yellow-green pus found over the surface of the brain at autopsy.

Laboratory diagnosis. The cytology and chemistry of the cerebrospinal fluid once again fail to distinguish haemophilus meningitis from that due to other bacteria. The leucocytes are increased in number—as a rule markedly so, unless the specimen is collected early in the illness—and are predominantly polymorphs; the protein level is raised; and the glucose level is reduced. In most untreated cases the haemophili are to be seen in suitably stained smears of centrifuged cerebrospinal fluid, sometimes in very large numbers but sometimes requiring a careful search. They may be cocco-bacillary, definitely bacillary, or even filamentous. They are predominantly seen outside cells. Their visibility in Gram-stained films depends on details of staining technique, and therefore they are more commonly missed in such films than are meningococci and pneumococci, for example. Methylene blue staining shows their presence clearly but is less informative about their nature. An experienced observer can usually recognize them with confidence in a good Gram-stained film; but the fact that they almost always belong to capsular type b makes rapid certain identification possible if a good antiserum for that type is available. This can be used either to demonstrate a 'capsule-swelling' reaction of the organisms themselves, as seen microscopically in the cerebrospinal fluid, or to detect the presence of type b polysaccharide in the fluid, by countercurrent immunoelectrophoresis or other means. In the absence of such a typing serum, or on the rare occasions when the *H. influenzae* does not belong to type b, definite identification of the organism has to await its growth from cerebrospinal fluid or blood. Serological demonstration of type b polysaccharide in the patient's cerebrospinal fluid, blood, or urine may be possible even when, after antibiotic treatment, haemophili cannot be seen or grown. Another way of making the bacteriological diagnosis in such circumstances is to demonstrate nasopharyngeal carriage of *H. influenzae* type b among the patient's household contacts.

Antibacterial treatment and prognosis. Before the introduction of type-specific serum therapy in the 1930s, haemophilus meningitis was almost invariably fatal. In contrast, since the first reported use of chloramphenicol for treatment of this disease in 1950, it has been possible to achieve survival rates of 95 per cent or more. However, a few of the survivors are severely damaged, as many as half of them have some degree of detectable permanent defect, and careful testing has shown that even the rest are on average somewhat behind their peers in intellectual performance. Chloramphenicol, in a dosage of 50–100 mg/kg a day intravenously or orally (but not intramuscularly) for 7–10 days, is highly effective for treatment of the infection; but because of fears about its potential toxicity, it was largely replaced for this purpose in the United States and some other countries from 1964 onwards, by ampicillin. However, there were occasional reports of failure of ampicillin to control the infection, or of bacteriological relapse during the treatment period; and from 1974 onwards β-lactamase-producing (and therefore ampicillin-resistant) strains of *H. influenzae*, including type b strains, have appeared and become increasingly common in many parts of the world, whereas chloramphenicol-resistant *H. influenzae* strains fortunately remain very rare. Furthermore, although chloramphenicol is in general merely a bacteristatic drug, it is bactericidal for *H. influenzae* at concentrations readily attainable in the patient, and is more rapidly and reliably so than ampicillin. It therefore remains the drug of choice at present for treatment of this and other life-threatening haemophilus infections. Cefotaxime seems likely to be a suitable alternative when resistance to both ampicillin and chloramphenicol is encountered.

Prophylaxis. The purified polysaccharide of *H. influenzae* type b (polyribosylribitolphosphate), like those of pneumococci and some meningococci, is an effective antigenic stimulus for humans. A single injection results in good levels of type-specific and other antibodies, including those which can be expected to protect against infection. Unfortunately, such antibody responses are much less vigorous in children under two years old, the group who need protection most, than in older children and adults. Attempts to overcome this problem continue.

The high carriage-rate for *H. influenzae* among the household or other close contacts of children with haemophilus meningitis, and the substantially increased risk of serious illness for the young children among them, call for a safe and reliable oral antibiotic regimen for elimination of carriage and for protection of contacts. Trials of ampicillin, rifampicin (rifampin), or trimethoprim plus sulphamethoxazole for these purposes have been only partially successful.

Epiglottitis

Epidemiology. The combination of haemophilus septicaemia and acute obstructive dyspnoea was first reported from France in 1936, having occurred in a middle-aged woman. By the late 1940s this combination, which had been given various names but came to be generally known as *H. influenzae* type b epiglottitis, had become widely recognized in North America, although almost exclusively as a disease of young children. It was known too in Australia, where a paper in 1946 gave a clear account of its occurrence in 15 children and one adult at a single hospital in an 18-month period. In many other countries it was not recognized at all, or only rarely, at that time. Such was the position in Britain up until the early 1970s, except for a few doctors who were particularly interested in and on the look-out for this disease. Its far more frequent and widespread recognition in Britain in recent years is at least in part a reflection of increased awareness and diagnostic accuracy rather than of a true increase in its incidence; and the same may be true in other countries. In some parts of the world it is probably not much less common than haemophilus meningitis.

Whereas haemophilus meningitis is primarily a disease of children under two years old, the maximum incidence of epiglottitis is between the ages of two and four years. In keeping with this age-incidence, the child with epiglottitis is more likely to have one or more younger siblings; and it is therefore not surprising that available evidence suggests a higher risk of secondary cases of serious haemophilus infection in household contacts than is found when the primary infection is meningitis. Meningitis and epiglottitis may occur simultaneously in the same patient, as indeed may any combination of the manifestations of *H. influenzae* type b bacter-aemia. The reported incidence of epiglottitis in adults is much lower than that in children, and bacterial species other than *H. influenzae* have more often been held responsible—though the bacteriological evidence has in general been unconvincing.

Clinical features. In contrast to the position in meningitis, the clinical picture of epiglottitis gives a strong indication of the causative organism, which in the great majority of cases is *H. influenzae* type b. The common story is that a previously healthy child of appropriate age develops symptoms of an upper respiratory tract infection, with nothing distinctive or alarming about them for the

first six hours or so. Then, in many cases quite suddenly, the child becomes much more ill, and around the same time develops dyspnoea with inspiratory stridor, although sometimes the stridor is not obvious if the child is already too ill to fight against the respiratory obstruction. The general illness is due to haemophilus septicaemia; and the dyspnoea and stridor to marked hyperaemia and oedema of the epiglottis and the aryepiglottic and interarytenoid folds. Unless both the septicaemia and the respiratory obstruction are dealt with promptly and effectively, the child may die within the next six hours or so. Clinical features helpful in making the diagnosis of epiglottitis, and particularly in distinguishing it from virus croup, are the severity of the illness, profuse drooling (because swallowing is painful), muffling of the voice rather than hoarseness (because there is supraglottic narrowing of the airway but the vocal cords are not affected), and sometimes a cellulitic swelling of the neck. By depressing the tongue or pulling it forward the large red epiglottis can be made visible; but to do either of these things may provoke a sudden inspiration that sucks the swollen epiglottis into the oedematous ring and causes complete respiratory obstruction. Direct inspection of the epiglottis must therefore be deferred until measures to ensure the airway are in hand. If circumstances permit, the epiglottic enlargement can be demonstrated safely by radiology of the soft tissues of the neck.

Laboratory diagnosis. Polymorphonuclear leucocytosis in the peripheral blood helps to distinguish epiglottitis from virus infections. Swabbing of the throat or epiglottis is dangerous, does not provide bacteriological information soon enough to guide treatment, may fail to give a growth of the relevant organism, and can in any case be useful only if any *H. influenzae* isolates are shown to be capsulated and are typed so as to distinguish them from normal pharyngeal organisms. Blood culture also fails to give any immediate information, though by means of the 'capsule-swelling' procedure it may be possible to demonstrate the presence of *H. influenzae* type b in the broth cultures only six hours or so after they are set up. Blood culture is, however, of value as a means of establishing the diagnosis retrospectively, which allows clinicians to know with certainty the disease with which they have been dealing and so to recognize it more readily on subsequent occasions. As in haemophilus meningitis, demonstration of *H. influenzae* type b polysaccharide in the patient's blood or urine can provide a rapid and definite diagnosis. At autopsy, by which time the supraglottic oedema may be much less obvious than it was in life, the diagnosis can be established by injecting sterile fluid submucosally into the epiglottis and withdrawing it for culture—a difficult procedure if the patient has not had epiglottitis, since the mucosa is then tightly bound down to cartilage, but a reliable way of growing the causative organism if the patient has died of epiglottitis without receiving antibiotics.

Treatment. It is essential that, without delay, an adequate airway is ensured and the bacterial infection is controlled; nearly all patients then make rapid and complete recoveries from this otherwise lethal disease. While it may be possible in some cases to deal with the respiratory problem by humidifying the air and applying local decongestants to the epiglottic area, the consistent advice of all authorities on this disease is that in all but the mildest cases it is wise to insert an endotracheal tube or establish a tracheostomy as soon as possible, without waiting for the situation to become critical. Since the artificial airway is required for only a few days, endotracheal intubation is increasingly preferred to tracheostomy, although it requires more careful supervision. As in the case of haemophilus meningitis, intravenous chloramphenicol is the most appropriate antibacterial treatment, but the doctor who is called to a patient away from hospital is unlikely to have it with him and will have to make do with ampicillin or whatever he has to hand for initial treatment.

Prophylaxis is discussed in the section on haemophilus meningitis.

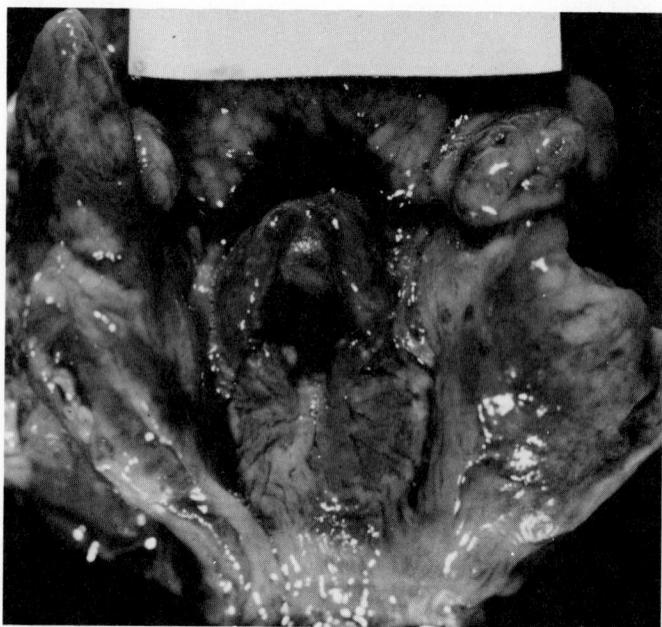

Fig. 1 Haemophilus epiglottis: post-mortem appearances showing intense oedema of epiglottis and aryepiglottic folds. (Photograph courtesy of Dr Derek de Sa.)

Other diseases related to haemophilus meningitis

There are a number of other manifestations of haemophilus infection which resemble haemophilus meningitis and epiglottitis in occurring mainly in young children, in being usually due to type b strains, and in being commonly associated with bacteraemia. Combinations of any of these manifestations, including meningitis or epiglottis, may be seen in the same patient or in the same household. The occurrence of any of them in adults is rather frequently connected with alcoholism, diabetes, or other debilitating conditions. Their laboratory investigation, antibacterial treatment, and problems of prevention are all much as described for haemophilus meningitis.

Pneumonia. This is probably the third commonest manifestion of bacteraemic *H. influenzae* type b infection of children, and often occurs together with others, notably meningitis. It is usually lobar or segmental, but has no clinical or radiological features indicative of the organism responsible. It is commonly accompanied by pleurisy and, if treatment is delayed, by empyema.

Other capsulated types of *H. influenzae* have occasionally been incriminated as causing pneumonia, in children or in adults. The capacity of non-capsulated *H. influenzae* to cause pneumonia is debatable. Many papers contain the assumption that non-capsulated or untyped *H. influenzae* found in the sputa of patients with pneumonia are the cause of the disease. Such an assumption makes no allowance for the frequent presence of this species in the upper respiratory tract and in damaged bronchi (see below).

Cellulitis. A hot tender purplish-red swelling, rather like streptococcal erysipelas but lacking its defined edge, and occurring on the face (sometimes spreading to the neck) or on a limb, is characteristic of haemophilus cellulitis. When it occurs on the face, the patient often also has otitis media on the same side. *H. influenzae* type b can also cause orbital cellulitis, and there is evidence that this is commonly associated with ethmoidal sinusitis.

Suppurative arthritis and osteomyelitis. Haemophilus arthritis is almost exclusively a disease of large joints, usually a single joint, sometimes more. Osteomyelitis is probably a less common manifestation of *H. influenzae* type b infection, though differentiation between the two can be very difficult in a young child, especially if the infection is aborted by antibacterial treatment.

Pericarditis. Purulent pericarditis due to *H. influenzae* is much less common than the conditions mentioned so far. In most reported cases it has been associated with one or more of the commoner conditions, such as pneumonia and pleural effusion. It does not respond satisfactorily to antibacterial treatment alone, and requires surgical drainage.

Some infections commonly due to non-capsulated *H. influenzae* strains

Otitis media. The middle ear is a common site of suppuration in bacteraemic *H. influenzae* type b infections. In some large series of cases of haemophilus meningitis nearly half the children were found also to have otitis media.

However, suppurative otitis media occurs far more often as a separate entity than as part of a serious generalized infection; and *H. influenzae* can be isolated from middle ear fluid in about one-third of all cases that occur in the first few years of life. The strains involved sometimes belong to type b and less often to other capsular types, but most are non-capsulated, i.e. their type-distribution roughly reflects that of normal nasopharyngeal carriage. It is arguable that, in many cases at least, the haemophili did not initiate the trouble in the middle ear but were secondary invaders on the heels of viruses or other primary pathogens; but even if that is so, they need to be eliminated by antibacterial treatment. Chloramphenicol is unsuitable for systematic treatment of relatively minor conditions because of its potential toxicity. The great value of ampicillin and amoxycillin in treatment of otitis media has been reduced by the increasing frequency of β-lactamase-producing strains of *H. influenzae*. Erythromycin and the sulphonamides are alternative oral drugs.

Paranasal sinusitis. Even more than is the case in otitis media, the bacteriological diagnosis of suppurative sinus infections is beset by two problems—difficulty of access to suitable material for culture and overgrowth by normal nasopharyngeal flora. However, there is evidence that *H. influenzae* can be important in sinusitis, and some that suggests involvement of capsular type a strains here, almost the only indication of specific pathogenicity of any type other than b.

Conjunctivitis. Like otitis media, conjunctivitis due to *H. influenzae* can be part of a generalized infection with a type b strain but is far more often a separate entity, usually caused by a non-capsulated strain. It is the only form of haemophilus infection that has been described as occurring in epidemics—in North Africa, the southern United States, and other warm areas. The organism known first as

Table 1 Haemophilus infections

Diseases (not in order of frequency)	Patients		Bacteraemic illness†	Haemophilus influenzae		Other Haemophilus species
	Children	Adults		Capsulated‡	Non-capsulated	
Meningitis Epiglottitis Pneumonia* Cellulitis Suppurative arthritis Osteomyelitis Pericarditis	+++	+	+++	+++	−	−
Otitis media	+++	+	+	+	+++	−
Paranasal sinusitis*	+++	+	+	++	++	−
Conjunctivitis	+++	++	+	+	+++	−
Endocarditis	+	+++	+++	−	+	++ *H. parainfluenzae* ++ *H. aphrophilus*
Exacerbations of chronic bronchitis, etc.	+	+++	−	+	+++	−
Rare infections in various other sites	++	++	+	+	+++	+ *H. aphrophilus*

+++ = most cases
++ = some cases   For *horizontal* comparison only–i.e. within but not between individual diseases
+ = a few cases
− = rare or no cases

* See text for qualification of this entry
† Except in endocarditis, usually due to *H. influenzae* type b
‡ Nearly always of capsular type b

the Koch–Weeks bacillus and later as *H. aegyptius* has been found responsible for some of these outbreaks; but it differs little from the *H. influenzae* strains responsible for other outbreaks and for the great majority of sporadic cases, and can be regarded as belonging within that species. Among the many sporadic cases of haemophilus conjunctivitis are some in infants (and a few in middle-aged women) which are unusually persistent and recur after antibiotic treatment, and which behave in this way because they are basically infections of blocked nasolachrymal ducts. Such cases usually respond satisfactorily to unblocking of the ducts. Chloramphenicol can be used for treatment of haemophilus conjunctivitis, in the form of eye-drops; but now it appears that such use may be encouraging the emergence of chloramphenicol resistance in this species.

Endocarditis

Like many other bacterial parasites of man, *H. influenzae* is responsible for occasional cases of bacterial endocarditis. However, two other members of the genus—*H. parainfluenzae* and *H. aphrophilus*—have been more often incriminated in this disease, and it is probably significant that these two species are found in the mouth more often than *H. influenzae*, which is predominantly a nasopharyngeal organism. The patients have been mostly adolescents or young adults when the organism was *H. parainfluenzae*, and older adults when it was *H. aphrophilus*. Nobody has sufficient experience of any of these forms of haemophilus endocarditis to make firm recommendations about antibacterial drugs, but fortunately it appears that some such combination as ampicillin and an aminoglycoside is as appropriate for them as for other forms of bacterial endocarditis.

Chronic bronchial diseases

The role of *H. influenzae*. By far the largest group of patients who suffer from haemophilus infections are those with chronic bronchitis, bronchiectasis, or fibrocystic disease. The first of these is the commonest, and the simplest as regards bacteriology, in that one species is of predominant importance—*H. influenzae*. There is no evidence that bacteria are responsible for the basic pathological processes of chronic bronchitis; but an important consequence of these processes is that the bronchi lose their power of self-sterilization. *H. influenzae* strains, virtually always non-capsulated and presumably derived from the nasopharynx, establish themselves in such bronchi more readily than other bacteria. In some patients the sputum remains mucoid despite such bronchial colonization; and in those circumstances the haemophili are apparently doing no harm and attempts to eradicate them do the patients no good. *H. influenzae* (still nearly always non-capsulated) is however far more frequently present if the sputum is purulent, and especially when the patient has an acute exacerbation of his bronchitis with increased sputum purulence. Although some exacerbations are probably initiated in most cases by virus infections or other non-bacterial stimuli, it is the haemophili, often assisted by pneumococci, that are responsible for the suppuration. Since this in turn is responsible for the increased respiratory distress and the deterioration in the patient's general condition, he can now be helped by appropriate antibacterial treatment, as outlined below. There is conflicting evidence as to whether such suppurative bacterial infection, in addition to causing immediate distress and illness, adds to the long-term damage to the lower respiratory tract and should therefore be controlled for that reason also.

H. influenzae is often present in large numbers, as the only potential lower respiratory tract pathogen or accompanied by pneumococci, in the sputum of patients with post-operative chest infections. If the patient has a history of chronic bronchitis, such an episode can be seen to be an acute exacerbation induced by anaesthesia or other peri-operative circumstances. Quite commonly, however, there is no such history but the patient is a heavy tobacco smoker. The episode is then presumably a preliminary indication of

bronchial damage. In this connection it is of interest that heavy smokers who have not yet developed chronic bronchitis have been shown to be much more likely than non-smokers to have in their blood *H. influenzae* antibodies of a kind most commonly found in the blood of patients with purulent chronic bronchitis.

H. influenzae plays much the same role in bronchiectasis and fibrocystic lung disease as in chronic bronchitis, but the situations are complicated by the frequent involvement of *Ps. aeruginosa* and coliform bacilli in either of these two conditions and of *Staph. aureus* in fibrocystic disease.

Antibacterial treatment. In this section on haemophilus infections, only the initial (usually oral) treatment of straightforward purulent chronic bronchitis can be legitimately discussed. We are not concerned here with pneumonia (rarely due to *H. influenzae*) superimposed on bronchitis or with the complex microbiological situations that can result from prolonged antimicrobial treatment.

Antibacterial drugs can be used in purulent chronic bronchitis either to inhibit the haemophili and any accompanying pneumococci in the bronchi (bacteristatic treatment) or to kill them (bactericidal treatment). Chloramphenicol is not appropriate for treatment of recurrent infections that carry no immediate threat to life. For bacteristatic treatment, drugs of the tetracycline group are widely and effective used, though they are contraindicated by pregnancy and by impaired renal function. Co-trimoxazole (trimethoprim plus sulphamethoxazole) has also proved useful, though it is probable that only the trimethoprim component achieves effective concentrations in bronchial pus. Ampicillin, potentially bactericidal for *H. influenzae*, passes from blood to the bronchial lumen readily at times of active suppuration, but it ceases to do so as the infection and inflammatory process subside; and therefore at this stage it may achieve only bacteristatic levels for *H. influenzae*, or less, and fail to complete its eradication. High doses of ampicillin (up to 6 g a day by mouth) or corresponding lower doses of one of its better-absorbed esters may achieve bactericidal levels in the bronchi for long enough to be effective, but there is no point in persisting with such dosage for more than about four days. Amoxycillin is comparable to the ampicillin esters in its absorption from the alimentary tract and appears to have the additional advantages of more persistent penetration into the bronchial lumen as the inflammation subsides and possibly a more rapid bactericidal action.

Patients with occasional acute purulent exacerbations of their bronchitis need only temporary help in restoring control in their bronchi, and for this a few days of bacteristatic treatment suffice. Indeed, exacerbations can be prevented or aborted by starting such treatment at the onset of an upper respiratory tract infection or at any other time when it would otherwise be likely to happen in that patient. Those patients whose sputum is persistently purulent, for large parts of the winter or all through the year, may be helped by long-term bacteristatic treatment; but they may then have trouble because of colonization of their bronchi by *Ps. aeruginosa* or coliform bacilli resistant to the drug used. An alternative is to attempt eradication of the haemophili and pneumococci by a short course of bactericidal treatment. If successful, this may give them some months of remission, with improved health and performance.

Infections of the female genital tract and of neonates

H. influenzae strains, usually non-capsulated, have occasionally been incriminated in tubo-ovarian abscesses or other infections of non-pregnant female genital tracts, which in most cases have suffered previous infective or other damage.

Perinatal *H. influenzae* infections of mother, baby, or both are rather more common, though still rare. Some of the strains belong to type b, but most are not capsulated. There may be endometritis, and the amniotic fluid may be turbid and foul-smelling—sometimes only some hours after rupture of the membranes. Some of the mothers are septicaemic, others show no evidence of systemic infection. An affected baby, which in many cases is born prematurely, may be septicaemic at birth or may become so soon afterwards, and frequently has pneumonia, probably from inhalation of infected liquor. Chloramphenicol, the most appropriate antibiotic until the strain has been shown to be ampicillin-sensitive, must be used in carefully calculated dosage for premature infants, because of their inability to conjugate and excrete it.

Other Haemophilus infections

H. influenzae strains, sometimes of type b or other capsular types but usually non-capsulated, are from time to time incriminated as pathogens in various sites other than those already mentioned. This undoubtedly happens more often where their versatility is remembered and therefore culture media suitable for their growth are used for 'improbable' specimens. They have been found to cause urinary tract infections (in the presence or calculi or of anatomical abnormalities), epididymo-orchitis, cholecystitis, and peritonitis, and have been isolated from cases of appendix or other abscesses, and of paronychia. *H. aphrophilus* too is increasingly often (though still rarely) recognized as a pathogen in conditions other than endocarditis, including bacteraemia, abscesses in the brain or around the mouth or elsewhere, and accidental or surgical wounds.

References

Bieger, R. C., Brewer, N. S., and Washington, J. A. (1978). Haemophilus aphrophilus: a microbiological and clinical review and report of 42 cases. *Medicine, Baltimore* **57**, 345.
Dajani, A. S., Asmar, B. I., and Thirumoorthi, M. C. (1979). Systemic *Haemophilus influenzae* disease: an overview. *J. Pediat.* **94**, 355.
Lynn, D. J., Kane, J. G., and Parker, R. H. (1977). Haemophilus parainfluenzae and influenzae endocarditis: a review of forty cases. *Medicine, Baltimore* **56**, 115.
May, J. R. (1972). *The chemotherapy of chronic bronchitis and allied disorders* 2nd edn. English Universities Press, London.
Solotorovsky, M. and Lynn, M. (1978). *Haemophilus influenzae*: immunology and immunoprotection. *CRC crit. Rev. Microbiol.* **6**, 1.
Turk, D. C. (1980). *Haemophili in medical literature, 1883–1978.* Hodder and Stoughton, London.
— (1982). *Haemophilus influenzae.* PHLS monograph, HMSO, London.

Bordetella

C. C. Linnemann, Jr.

The bacteria in the genus *Bordetella* are primarily pathogens of the respiratory tract of man and animals because of their propensity for adhering to ciliated epithelial cells. The only distinctive presentation of *Bordetella* infections is the whooping cough syndrome or pertussis, which is characterized by paroxysmal coughing, an inspiratory whoop, and lymphocytosis. This syndrome is usually caused by *B. pertussis*, although the other two species in the genus, *B. parapertussis* and *B. bronchiseptica*, have occasionally been reported to produce the same syndrome. In the past, pertussis also has been attributed to viral infections. This misconception resulted from two factors—the difficulty of isolating *B. pertussis* from infected patients, and the frequent excretion of adenoviruses (see page 5.44) by patients infected with *B. pertussis*.

Bordetella infections should be suspected when the clinician is confronted either by a patient with a persistent lower respiratory tract infection manifested by paroxysmal coughing, with or without an inspiratory whoop; or by a patient with any respiratory symptoms who has been in close contact with a documented case of *Bordetella* infection. *B. bronchiseptica* is a common pathogen in animals and should be considered in animal handlers with respiratory tract infections. Despite a high index of suspicion, most *Bordetella* infections will go unrecognized because the symptoms are indistinguishable from other respiratory tract infections, and because appropriate diagnostic tests usually are performed only in patients with typical pertussis.

The causative agent. *Bordetella* are small, aerobic, Gram-negative coccobacillary organisms. *B. pertussis* is a fastidious bacterium which is inhibited by a variety of media constituents such as fatty acids. For this reason, cultures must be done on special media containing additives that will inactivate these inhibitors. This organism grows slowly in culture, requiring two to five days to produce recognizable colonies. *B. parapertussis* and *B. bronchiseptica* are less fastidious and faster growing. These organisms will grow on a simple infusion agar or blood agar within one or two days.

Bordetella have been reported to have pili-like surface filaments associated with a haemagglutinin, which may be important in the attachment of the bacteria to cells. *B. pertussis* adheres to ciliated epithelial cells in the respiratory tract, and attachment is followed by ciliostasis and subsequent loss of the ciliated cells. A similar sequence has been observed in dogs infected with *B. bronchiseptica*. Numerous biologically active components and properties have been identified in the *Bordetella*, including toxins, agglutinogens, and a lymphocytosis promoting factor; but there is no direct evidence for the role of these in the pathogenesis of disease in man. Although these organisms are not invasive and usually remain on the surface of the respiratory tract, there are isolated reports of bacteraemia with *B. parapertussis* and *B. bronchiseptica*.

Epidemiology. Man is the only known reservoir of *B. pertussis* and *B. parapertussis*, in contrast to *B. bronchiseptica* which is found in rabbits, dogs, cats, guinea pigs, and other animals. *B. pertussis* is transmitted by droplets from symptomatic patients. Occasionally, asymptomatic infections have been identified, but there is no evidence that these are important in the spread of disease, and there are no chronic carriers. It is assumed that the transmission of *B. parapertussis* is similar to *B. pertussis*. Most *B. bronchiseptica* infections have been reported to be acquired from contact with infected animals, but recently these organisms have been identified in hospital patients with no obvious exposure to animals, which suggests that man may also be a reservoir for *B. bronchiseptica*.

In the pre-vaccine era, epidemics of *B. pertussis* spread through schools, and the schoolchildren carried the infection into their homes. The secondary attack rates in susceptible children were 25 to 50 per cent in schools, and 70 to 100 per cent in homes. The high secondary attack rates at home reflected the intense and prolonged exposure to the organism. Most children developed clinically recognizable disease. Mild infections or re-infections occurred in adults caring for sick children; these illnesses were known as 'grandmother's cough' or 'nurses' cough'.

In the post-vaccine and antibiotic era, major epidemics have disappeared in most developed countries. Mortality from *B. pertussis* was decreasing prior to the introduction of vaccine, but the number of cases was not. The case rate did not decrease significantly until after the vaccines were introduced. This was demonstrated clearly in the United States and Canada, where effective vaccines were used widely (Fig.1). The effect of vaccine was not as dramatic in the United Kingdom, which may have been related to early problems with vaccine efficacy. Pertussis did decrease in the United Kingdom, and the recent resurgence of *B. pertussis* following a decrease in vaccine usage provided a natural experiment demonstrating the effect of vaccine on the epidemiology of the disease.

In a highly vaccinated population, adults may play a more important role in the transmission of disease. In the pre-vaccine era, the source of infection could be identified in most cases as another child. In recent times, it has become increasingly more difficult to trace the source, and, in very young infants, an adult family member frequently appears to be the source. Hospital epidemics have also demonstrated the role adults play in transmission. Physicians or nurses may acquire infection from a patient and then transmit it to other hospital personnel and to patients.

The epidemiology of *B. parapertussis* is similar to that of *B. pertussis* except that it has not been modified by vaccine usage. *B. parapertussis* is widespread in many countries, but it is seldom recognized because of the mildness of the disease. Studies in Denmark have reported that epidemics occur in that country every four years and alternate with epidemics of *B. pertussis*. There is only limited information on the epidemiology of *B. bronchiseptica*. There are no surveys of infections in animal handlers, but in one hospital survey, there were two infections among 1605 patients over a one month period.

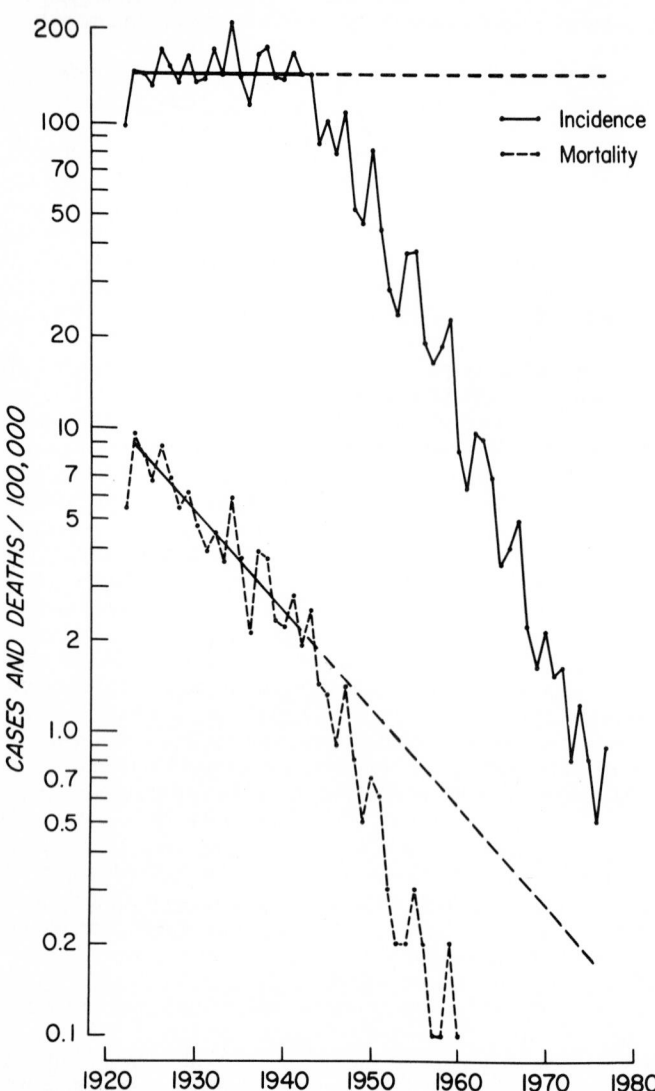

Fig. 1 The effect of pertussis vaccine on the incidence and mortality of pertussis in the United States. The lines superimposed on the graph indicate the trends prior to the vaccine and as projected if vaccine had not been introduced.

Clinical manifestations. After infection with *B. pertussis*, clinical illness begins in 7–10 days with non-specific upper respiratory symptoms, malaise, anorexia, and sometimes a low-grade fever. Traditionally, this is called the catarrhal stage and is indistinguishable from any other mild respiratory infection. Towards the end of this stage a dry, hacking cough appears and becomes progressively worse. Older and presumably partially immune patients may not progress beyond the catarrhal stage. After one to two weeks, the paroxysmal stage begins and continues for several weeks. The cough is now paroxysmal, and prolonged coughing episodes may be followed by the characteristic 'whoop', which is produced by a forced inspiration through a partially closed glottis. In severe cases, the paroxysms of coughing may be followed by vomiting, and may be associated with epistaxis, petechiae, conjunctival or scleral haemorrhages, haemorrhagic myringitis, or perior-

bital oedema. Young infants may not have the whoop, and their paroxysms of coughing may be followed by cyanosis and apnoea. Fever is uncommon at this stage in uncomplicated infections. The convalescent stage begins after two to four weeks, with gradually resolving paroxysms of coughing. The coughing may persist for weeks to months, and exacerbations with whooping may occur with subsequent respiratory viral infections.

The most characteristic laboratory finding is a leucocytosis with lymphocytosis which appears toward the end of the catarrhal stage and continues in the paroxysmal stage. The lymphocytosis is most marked at the time of the most severe coughing. This represents a proportional increase in both T and B lymphocytes, and it has been postulated that it results from a failure of recirculating lymphocytes to re-enter the lymph nodes. The lymphocytosis may not occur in either very young infants or older children and adults.

The appearance of fever suggests a secondary bacterial infection complicating the *B. pertussis* infection. Otitis media and pneumonia are the most common infectious complications, but these seem to have been less frequent in recent years. Atelectasis still occurs as a result of bronchial obstruction by the thick mucous, but bronchiectasis is uncommon. The pressures developed during the paroxysmal coughing probably contribute to the pulmonary, haemorrhagic, and gastrointestinal complications that may include mediastinal and subcutaneous emphysema, pneumothorax, inguinal hernias, and rectal prolapse. The most serious non-infectious complications are neurologic, usually convulsions, but also paralysis, coma, blindness, deafness, and movement disorders. There are no good data on the exact incidence of these complications, but they are extremely rare.

B. parapertussis produces the same respiratory illness as *B. pertussis*, except that most infections are associated with milder clinical manifestations. Twenty per cent or less of children will develop the whooping cough syndrome. This syndrome is even rarer with *B. bronchiseptica* infections. A nondescript bronchitis is probably the most common clinical presentation, although one series of hospital-acquired *B. bronchiseptica* infections suggested that this organism was usually a non-pathogen in the respiratory tract. However, endocarditis has been reported with *B. bronchiseptica*, suggesting that it can be a more invasive organism than the other *Bordetella*.

Diagnosis. *Bordetella* infections are diagnosed by isolation of the organism. Fluorescent antibody staining of material obtained by nasopharyngeal swabs from patients with *B. pertussis* infections will provide a presumptive, but not a definitive diagnosis. There may be considerable observer variation in interpretation of such stains, and good reagents are difficult to obtain. Infections can be diagnosed by antibody responses as measured by assays such as agglutination or immunodiffusion, but few laboratories provide these as routine diagnostic tests. Therefore, the diagnosis depends on recovering the organism from appropriate specimens.

B. pertussis cultures used to be obtained by the cough plate technique, where an open agar plate was held in front of a patient, coughing induced, and the plate sprayed with respiratory secretions. Fortunately, this has been replaced by the nasopharyngeal culture technique. A wire calcium alginate swab is passed through the nose until it touches the posterior nasopharynx, allowed to remain for a few seconds, and removed. Cotton swabs may be used if the cotton has proved to be non-bacteriostatic for *B. pertussis*. The swabs are streaked on to Bordet–Gengou agar plates, both with and without antibiotics such as penicillin or methicillin. Multiple cultures may be useful in increasing the number of patients from whom *B. pertussis* can be recovered. The organism has not been recovered from blood or sites other than the respiratory tract. Since *B. pertussis* is a slow growing bacterium, cultures must be held for six days before being discarded.

B. parapertussis and *B. bronchiseptica* can be recovered on Bordet–Gengou media from patients in whom these organisms were the cause of pertussis, and they also grow on routine media used for recovery of Gram-negative bacteria. There are case reports of both of these organisms being recovered in blood cultures, and *B. bron-chiseptica* has been cultured from urine.

Treatment. Most patients can be managed at home, but very young children may need to be in hospital to ensure good nursing care. Cough medicines are of no value, nor is passive immunization. Some physicians sedate young children, but this should be done carefully, if at all. Steroids have been reported in two studies to shorten the clinical course. In one study, children received betamethasone orally in a dose of 0.075 mg per kg per day, and in another, hydrocortisone sodium succinate intramuscularly in a dose of 30 mg per kg per day for two days, followed by tapering doses for seven to eight days. This may be useful in severe cases in young infants, but more experience with steroid treatment is needed before a general recommendation can be made.

Bordetella are sensitive to a variety of antibiotics, including erythromycin, tetracycline, chloramphenicol, and probably trimethoprim-sulphamethoxazole. Early treatment during the catarrhal stage will shorten the course of the clinical illness, but, if treatment is not started until the paroxysmal stage, antibiotics will have no significant effect. Thus, the only chance that the physician usually has to alter the clinical disease with antibiotic therapy is when he treats symptomatic contacts of patients with diagnosed infections. Even though there is no clinical benefit, patients in the paroxysmal stage should receive antibiotics to render them non-infectious to others. Erythromycin is the antibiotic of choice. Children should receive 40 to 50 mg/kg a day, and adults, 1–1.5 g a day, for 10 to 14 days. Nasopharyngeal cultures will become negative in the first few days of treatment, but the erythromycin should be continued to prevent bacteriologic relapses.

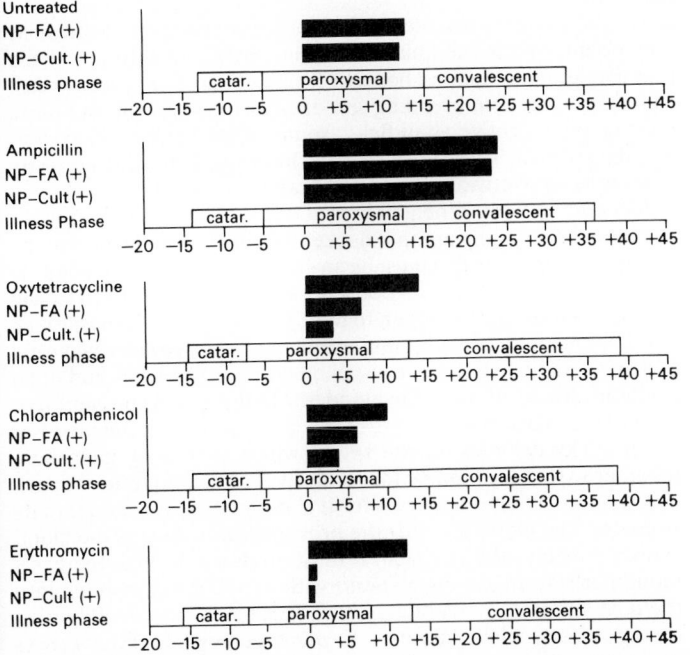

Fig. 2 Duration of excretion of *B. pertussis* as detected by fluorescent antibody staining and culture, and the effect of antimicrobial treatment. The graphs show comparison (group means) of patients treated with anti-microbial agents with untreated control patients. (From Bass, J. W. *et al.* (1969). *J. Pediat.* **75**, 768.)

Prevention. The patient with *B. pertussis* infection should avoid close contact with susceptible individuals to prevent droplet transmission. The untreated patient will remain contagious for weeks, but communicability will decrease rapidly after the initiation of erythromycin therapy. Nasopharyngeal cultures will become negative within 48 to 72 hours after treatment is started, and the patient may be assumed to be non-infectious.

Contacts of patients with *B. pertussis* infections should be managed according to age and vaccination status. Although there are no controlled studies, clinical experience suggests that chemoprophylaxis with erythromycin may be effective. Young children who are not immunized should be treated with erythromycin just like children with disease. If they have been immunized, some recommend that a booster dose of vaccine should be given to children under four years of age in addition to erythromycin. For older children and adults in whom the disease is less severe, the approach is different. The older contacts of patients with pertussis should be treated with erythromycin only if they develop respiratory symptoms.

Prevention of *B. pertussis* infections relies on the use of vaccine. Despite a continuing controversy in the United Kingdom, pertussis vaccine has been shown to prevent disease. The vaccine is associated with frequent local reactions with or without fever, and rare neurological complications. There are only limited data on serious reactions, but these occur less frequently after vaccination than with clinical disease. The vaccine is a killed whole bacterial preparation which can be administered with diphtheria and tetanus toxoids. An effective immunizing schedule includes 12 NIH protective units administered in three injections at one to two month intervals beginning at 6 to 12 weeks of age. A booster dose is given before entry to school. Pertussis vaccines usually are not given after six years of age because of the local reactions, although vaccine has been given to adults to control an institutional outbreak. Immunity after pertussis vaccine is neither complete nor lifelong. In one study, protection against infection was lost by 12 years after vaccination. There are no vaccines generally available for *B. parapertussis* or *B. bronchiseptica*.

References

Bass, J. W., Klenk, E. L., Kotheimer, J. B., Linnemann, C. C., and Smith, M. H. D. (1969). Antimicrobial treatment of pertussis. *J. Pediat.* **73**, 768.

Gardner, P., Griffin, W. B., Swartz, M. N., and Kunz, L. J. (1970). Non-fermentative Gram-negative bacilli of nosocomial interest. *Am. J. Med.* **48**, 735.

Keller, M. A., Aftandelians, R., and Connor, J. D. (1980). Etiology of pertussis syndrome. *Pediatrics, Springfield* **66**, 50.

Linnemann, C. C., Jr. (1977). Pertussis in the adult. *Ann. Rev. Med.* **28**, 179.

— (1979). Host–parasite interactions in pertussis. In *International Symposium on Pertussis* (eds. C. Manclark and J. Hill), 3. U.S. Government Printing Office, Washington, D.C.

Parker, C. D. and Linnemann, C. C., Jr. (1980). Bordetella. In *Manual of Clinical Microbiology* (ed. E. Lennette), 337. American Society for Microbiology, Washington, D.C.

Stuart-Harris, C. H. (1979). Experiences of pertussis in the United Kingdom. In *International Symposium on Pertussis* (eds. C. Manclark and J. Hill), 256. U.S. Government Printing Office, Washington, D.C.

Plague

A. B. Christie

Plague comes from *plaga*, a blow. To the Romans it came as a bolt or blast hurled by one of their angered gods, and later it was accepted by Christians too as an agony sent down on them for their shortcomings. To the Mohammedans it was a martyrdom or mercy related to the *jihad* or holy war. When it gained strength to spread to the West, it was the Black Death or *La Morte Nera*. In modern times it has come under some control, but when it breaks out, it kills again.

Bacteriology

Culture *Yersinia pestis* is a small ovoid bacillus, 1.5 nm by 0.7 nm in size, Gram-negative, non-motile and non-sporing. It stains heavily at both ends but lightly in the centre with Giemsa or

Wayson's stain, and this bipolar staining can be of almost diagnostic value to a doctor in the field if he can prepare and fix smears on the spot from suspect material. But there the simplicity ends. On culture *Y. pestis* becomes pleomorphic, and when grown on serum agar at 37 °C, it forms a capsule. This contains an antigen distinct from the somatic antigen and seems to be concerned with resistance to phagocytosis and so with virulence. The organism forms different colonies on different media, and these may be used to detect different virulence factors. Very slight changes in the *in vitro* environment can lead to variants in the colonies: some are smooth, capsulated, and virulent, others rough, bare, and without virulence. This tendency to vary is not confined to the laboratory. It is a characteristic of plague ecology in the field: a non-virulent *Y. pestis* can persist for long periods in rats with latent plague, and this may have much to do with the persistence of plague in an area.

Virulence factors. Y. pestis contains at least 18 antigenic components: these are found in all strains but may differ in the amounts of each present. Fraction 1 is contained in the capsular antigen: it is specific for *Y. pestis* and has to do with resistance to phagocytosis and so with virulence. Some strains from fatal human cases have nevertheless had very little or no fraction 1: these strains may have survived inside host phagocytes because of two somatic antigens, V and W. These two antigens always exist together, though in different amounts in different strains, and are related to resistance to phagocytosis but also to the ability of *Y. pestis* to survive, if it is phagocytosed, and even to multiply inside host phagocytes.

Temperature may affect the presence or absence of these antigens. A flea is cold-blooded: the temperature in its gut may be around 25 °C, and *Y. pestis* may be detected there apparently without fraction 1 and VW antigens. In that deprived state it can be ingested and destroyed by flea phagocytes; but if instead it is transferred in a bite to a warm-blooded rodent host, where the temperature may be nearer 37 °C, it may undergo what seems like a phenotypic change and regain fraction 1 and VW antigens along with full virulence, a change which may well occur in nature.

There are other factors concerned with virulence. Pesticin 1, a bacteriocin-like substance, is produced by all virulent strains. It is linked, perhaps genetically, with coagulase (C) and fibrinolytic (F) activity, the linkage being denoted by P1–C–F. Virulent colonies appear dark brown on haemin medium, for they absorb pigment (P) from it: on Congo-red agar they appear red. A virulent strain synthesizes purines. If it loses this faculty, it becomes avirulent, but if purines are then supplied to this feeble mutant, it is restored to full virulence. Different laboratory methods are used to detect these virulence factors, and it can be shown that strains lose and regain virulence with changes in environment. This waxing and waning of antigens and virulence is probably a reflection in the laboratory of what occurs in the wild. Certainly strains grown from chronic lesions in rats and apparently avirulent become fully virulent again when injected into normal laboratory animals. A strain of *Y. pestis* may be virulent for one host but not for another: a strain poor in fraction 1 is not virulent for guinea pigs, but it is for mice. Susceptible and resistant animals live side by side in nature, and movement and change like this must be going on all the time, affecting no doubt the rise and fall of the disease in a wild plague focus.

Epidemic varieties. Y. pestis exists in three main varieties, *Y pestis* var *orientalis*, var *antiqua*, and var *mediaevalis*. They differ in their ability to ferment glycerol and to reduce nitrates: *antiqua* does both, *orientalis* reduces nitrates but cannot ferment glycerol, while *mediaevalis* ferments glycerol but cannot reduce nitrates. This is of epidemiological and historical interest, for different rodents harbour different yersiniae, and different varieties are found in different places. *Rattus rattus* and *R. norvegicus* usually carry *orientalis*: so do hares in the Argentine, bandicoots in India, and jack rabbits in California. Marmots in Mongolia and hamsters in S.E. Russia carry *antiqua*, while *mediaevalis* is the common parasite of gerbils in Turkey and Iraq. It was probably *mediaevalis* that caused the Black Death in the fourteenth century. *Antiqua* probably

caused the plague that rocked the Roman empire under Justinian, while *orientalis* escaped from China at the end of the nineteenth century and spread plague across the world in the early twentieth century. There was an outbreak of plague in Western Nepal in 1967. In Uttar Pradesh, a neighbouring Indian province, plague had been present for some time, but the variety there was *orientalis* while the Nepal variety was *antiqua* and probably came down south from the Central Asian *antiqua* focus. To know the variety may help in control.

Epidemiology

Plague foci. *Y. pestis* is the agent that causes the disease, rodents and other animals suffer from the disease, and fleas carry the agent from one animal host to another, thus perpetuating the disease. A very simple cycle. But there are between 2000 and 3000 different fleas, at least 30 of which are proved vectors of plague, and at least 220 different rodents can be infected with *Y. pestis*. Man, another host, is by comparison very homogeneous, and so indeed is *Y. pestis*, but clearly the permutations of host, vector, and parasite can be complicated. Yet number is not the only factor. All the needs and habits of fleas and rodents affect the pattern, and some of these are highly sophisticated. A tuft of grass, a thicket, or a hole in the ground may seem a very humble dwelling, but the rodent selecting it will have had regard to many local amenities—the type of soil and flora, the temperature, rainfall and humidity, the height above sea level perhaps, but especially the foraging potential.

The flea is equally fastidious: it has a large surface area relative to its size, but, being cold-blooded, it cannot regulate its body temperature and can therefore rapidly lose fluid by evaporation and become dehydrated in an atmosphere where temperature and humidity do not suit it. So it has to be careful in selecting its field of operation.

The habits of the two, flea and rodent, must coincide. Some fleas bite rodents only in their burrows while others feed only on rodents that live above ground. The right fleas and the right rodent must come together. The breeding seasons must be related, and there must be plenty active adult fleas around at the peak of the rodent breeding season. There are also many hazards, such as the necessity to be able to overwinter or to withstand starvation.

Blocking of fleas. When all these factors of habit, environment, climate, and foraging are in balance, a stable plague focus may be set up in nature. The flea must be an efficient vector. It must be able to receive *Y. pestis* into its body, to maintain it, and to live long enough to allow the pathogen to multiply in its body. It must block readily. The proventriculus, or oesophagus, of a flea has seven rows of spines, and when the flea sucks blood these interlock and open rhythmically, so allowing the blood first to distend the proventriculus and then to pass into the stomach. If *Y. pestis* is in the blood, it forms sticky colonies on the spines which eventually glue them together so that they can no longer open. The flea continues to suck blood, more avidly than ever, for it is not getting any fluid into its stomach. The blood distends the proventriculus, but, as the blood cannot pass into the stomach, it must go down through the flea's mouthparts again, taking *Y. pestis* with it, and this is injected into the next animal the flea bites. Some fleas block more readily than others, with a smaller dose of *Y. pestis* perhaps, and this makes them more efficient at passing on the infection, provided, of course, that the flea is present in sufficient numbers in the focus, for the life of such a flea is short—it dies of dehydration.

The animal host. The animal host must also be present in sufficient numbers. It must be susceptible to infection with *Y. pestis* but must not be overcome by it, as otherwise the colony will simply be wiped out and plague will come to an end in the area. This happened in Central Colorado where a whole colony of prairie dogs died of plague. (Infected fleas were found in the prairie dog burrows as much as a year later.) Often the balance is held between two animal hosts: one colony, of ground-squirrels perhaps, is highly susceptible and at varying intervals there is an epizootic of plague which kills many ground-squirrels: the other colony, perhaps of voles or field mice, lives alongside in the same plague focus but is more resistant: the voles or mice carry the infection with no sign of illness, they survive the epizootic, and so maintain enzootic plague in the area.

Transfer to man. This is wild plague, a disease of the plains, of rocks, of steppes, and semi-deserts. Fleas, rodents, and plague bacilli mingle there with no great inconvenience to any of them. There is a flare-up every now and then, an epizootic, but it dies down again and the plague grumbles on among the more resistant survivors. There is no danger to man in all this unless he intrudes as a hunter, a shepherd, or a herdsman. In a rural area one of his domestic animals, a goat, a sheep, a camel, or a dog, may become infected. This is rare. The animal is merely a 'sentinel' animal, an index that there is plague somewhere in the area, but occasionally infection may pass from such an animal to a man and his family. But only when man really disturbs the area, as a wandering nomad, or when he sets up a village in the bush, or when man in his complete loss of wisdom invades the area in warfare, only then is there any serious direct threat to men from enzootic plague in the wild. The United States of America contains today one of the greatest and widest plague foci in the world, but it remains a wild rural plague in man, and rarely in any year is there more than a handful of cases of plague in man, and then usually in hunters and others who have handled wild animals, dead or alive.

Rat and flea. Most cases of plague in man, even in the great epidemics, come indirectly to him from the wild. There is an intermediate host. *R. rattus*, the black rat, is a commensal animal: it lives close to man, in his house, his out-buildings or in his work-place, but is rarely out in the field. *R. norvegicus* is the brown rat, though in some parts of the world it is more black than brown; it is a peri-domestic animal, not living quite so close to man, in his sewers perhaps, and liable at times to be in contact both with *R. rattus* and with wild rodents. These are the best-known animal hosts of plague, but only because they are most often seen by man. They are not really efficient hosts, especially *R. rattus*. It could never maintain an enzootic plague focus, for it dies too quickly from the infection. When the rat dies, the flea that gave it plague, *Xenopsylla cheopis*, must find a new living host, and that host may be man, because he is close by—within jumping distance, as a flea cannot fly. Then because *X. cheopis* is full of *Y. pestis*, it gives plague to man. How widespread or how long-lasting the outbreak will be in man depends on the number of rats and fleas that are around.

Epidemic thrust. Just what starts the spread of plague to man, what initiates the periodic surges of activity in a plague focus that lead to contact between the wild and the peri-domestic and commensal animals, and then on to man himself is not clearly understood. It is largely a mystery, just as man's own history of vast uprootings and migrations are not accounted for in full. There is mystery in both, in man's world and its ethnic or economic upheavals, and in colonies of rodents with plague in their midst. Sometimes the cause is clear. Man ploughs up a barren stretch of country and its rodents are driven elsewhere. Or there are floods in the area and the animals are washed out of their burrows. Or a huge warehouse is emptied, and rodents, fleas, and yersiniae are cast out together. But often there is no obvious reason, though there must be a bio-ecological one.

Once the movement starts, and plague spreads to man's rats, it may gather immense epidemic thrust. Man may then be able to follow its spread and pick up its epidemic pattern. He may even nowadays be able to interrupt its progress with his use of insecticides and antibiotics, and his control of ships, docks, railroads, and airports. By counting the number of fleas on rodents in the focus or on his commensal rats—the flea index—or by charting the rise or fall of seropositivity in rodents, he may be able to forecast the likelihood or otherwise of an outbreak. But just what unseen change in the life or microclimate of a focus begins it all still eludes him.

Man to man. Man gets plague, whether in a small household

outbreak or in a world pandemic, by the transfer of fleas from wild rodents to the commensal rat and from that rat to man. *R. rattus* and *X. cheopis* are the commonest or best-known rat and flea, but many other combinations occur. *Mastomys natalis*, a field mouse, is semi-domestic in South Africa and has carried plague to commensal rats via its flea, *X. brasiliensis*. In Java *R. exulans* is a field rat that invades man's dwellings with its flea *Stivalius cognatus*: it shares the dwelling with *R. rattus diardii*, the commensal rat, and, if that rat is now infected with plague, it can quickly pass it on via its own flea, the familiar *X. cheopis*. In the United States many different rodents are infected, ground-squirrels, wood rats, chipmunks, voles, hamsters, and marmosets, and there are several different fleas around, *Malareus telchinum* for example, a poor plague transmitter, and *Histrichopsylla linsdalei*, a highly effective one, but often present only in small numbers. But however plague reaches man, what matters is whether it can then spread from man to man.

A patient with bubonic plague is not himself infectious to anyone else, unless his bubo breaks down when the pus is highly infectious, or unless a flea first feeds on him and then on someone else. A patient with septicaemic plague is not infectious unless, before he dies, *Y. pestis* invades his lungs and is coughed out in his sputum. If someone now inhales these organisms, he is infected with primary pneumonic plague, coughing out *Y. pestis* from the onset of his illness and hence a danger to all around him. But in a plague outbreak in man it is mainly a flea that carries the infection from one patient to another.

Clinical manifestations

Bubonic plague. The word bubo comes from a Greek word meaning the groin, and most patients with a bubo do have it in the groin (Fig. 1). A bubo is a lump caused by a swollen lymph node and oedema of the surrounding tissues. In some patients it is small and difficult to feel, but in most patients it is painful and easily detected, varying from the size of the knuckle of one's thumb up to the size of a small clenched fist. The axilla is the next commonest site, but buboes may appear in the neck or in various lymph nodes, depending on where the flea bites. This may depend on how a man is dressed; in shorts and a hat in some rice field, when he may be bitten anywhere, or swathed in robes in a Middle East desert, when a flea may have difficulty getting in at all. Perhaps when the infection comes from a rat, the bubo is in the groin, but when from a squirrel, it is in the axilla, although it is difficult to see why. A hunter skinning an infected animal may get bitten on the hand and the infection may then travel up to cause a bubo in the axilla, or if he eats infected meat, *Y. pestis* may settle on his tonsil, giving him a bubo in his neck. Some patients have more than one bubo.

The bubo appears in the first few days of the illness. The skin over it becomes hot, turning red or purple. The lump is at first hard and

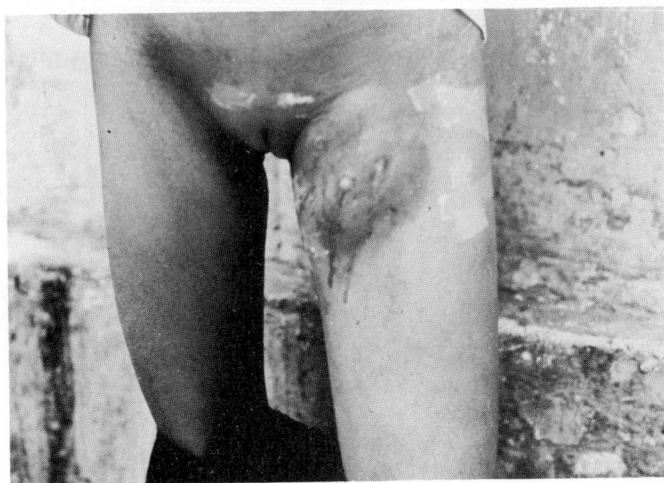

Fig. 1 Plague: a bubo of the groin. (By courtesy of the World Health Organization.)

tense, but it becomes softer and fluctuant. In a severe case it may burst, if the patient lives long enough, and discharge pus full of *Y. pestis* (Fig. 2), but in milder cases, or in patients treated early, it resolves without bursting. There is usually swelling of the tissues beyond the bubo—a bubo in the axilla may cause a swelling below the clavicle, while from a bubo in the neck oedema may spread down over the chest.

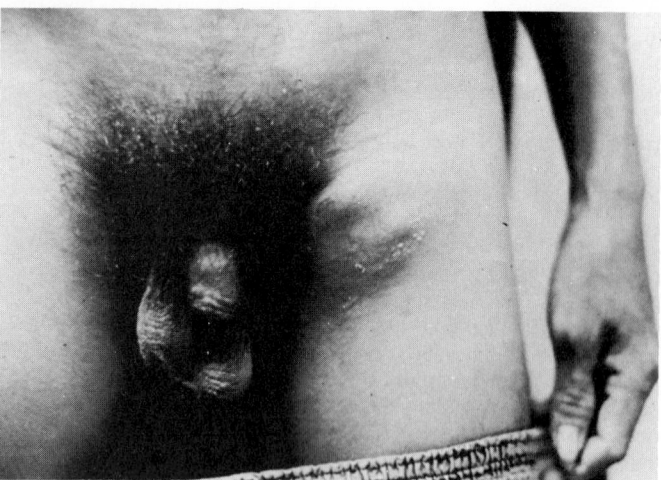

Fig. 2 Plague: a discharging bubo. (By courtesy of the World Health Organization.)

Course of the illness. The onset is usually abrupt, with chills and rise of temperature to 38.8–39.4 °C. Headache is splitting and the patient has pains in the limbs, in his back, and his abdomen. He rapidly becomes restless and confused, often irritable or apathetic, speechless, and unable to sleep, and sometimes almost maniacal. His conjunctivae may be blood-shot and he may bleed into his skin, or internally into his stomach, intestine, or kidney. He becomes prostrate and shocked. His temperature may drop on the third or fourth day and he may for a moment look better, but he is worse the next day and dead very soon after. Most patients die on the third to the sixth day: if a patient is still alive at the end of a week, he may pull through to recovery. So it is an acute febrile illness with nothing to distinguish it from other severe fevers such as typhus, typhoid, or malaria, unless there is a bubo, when it can only be plague. In an outbreak every case of febrile illness is plague until proved otherwise.

Some patients with very severe plague have no buboes or none are discovered. They die before the bubo has time to develop. Their disease is called septicaemic plague, but it differs only in severity from bubonic plague. Some of these patients who live a little longer have signs of chest infection before they die, and these are the patients who cough out *Y. pestis* and infect contacts with pneumonic plague. At the other extreme of bubonic plague are patients who have only a mild illness and a small bubo which they might pay no attention to if others around them were not severely ill with the plague.

Pneumonic plague. A patient catches pneumonic plague not from a flea bite but from the breath of a patient dying of septicaemic plague. The onset is abrupt, with respiratory distress and shock. The temperature is high, the face dusky, and the breathing shallow. Sputum is watery, teeming with *Y. pestis* and soon tinged with blood. It is highly infectious. There may or may not be signs of pneumonia in his chest; more likely there is pulmonary oedema and perhaps a pleural effusion. But the case is not one for physical signs or fine diagnosis. Unless treated immediately, this patient will be dead about the third day, never later than the fifth or sixth.

Pharyngeal or tonsillar plague. In tonsillar or pharyngeal plague the organism may be caught from the breath of a pneumonic case and trapped in the tonsillar tissue, or it may come from eating infected meat, or even from crushing infected fleas with the teeth as may have happened in one outbreak in Ecuador. The patient has a peritonsillar abscess and a bubo in the neck. Some patients are severely ill, some die from spill-over of *Y. pestis* into the lungs, but in others the illness is no more than moderately severe bubonic plague.

Plague meningitis. Meningitis may be the first sign of plague, before the bubo develops and gives the clue to the diagnosis. The patient has all the classical signs of meningitis, and, unless treated early, his chances of recovery are slight. Meningitis during an outbreak is plague until proved otherwise, but penicillin is useless for plague. There are some cases of secondary meningitis on record when the symptoms of meningitis come on later in a patient with bubonic plague, and at least one case where meningeal symptoms persisted for several months before sudden deterioration and death, possibly from a burst abscess. But in most cases, plague meningitis is an early manifestation of a severe attack of bubonic plague.

Plague carbuncle. There is usually no mark at the site of the flea bite in plague, but sometimes a sore develops. This may be an eschar, rather like anthrax, and may occur anywhere on the body: on the face, the neck, the abdomen, the buttocks, the thigh, or the foot. A bubo occurs in the related lymph node area, but often several days after the appearance of the sore, and in this case the outlook may then be fairly good. Sometimes the skin breaks down and there may be necrosis of the tissues down to bone, this being called cellulo-cutaneous plague. Sometimes a small papule develops at the site of the bite, changing to a vesicle and then to an umbilicated pustule. These pustules may be scattered over the body, and they may be the lesions of what was once called plague smallpox or plague blains. None of these skin lesions is now common, except the anthrax type: a misdiagnosis could be dangerous, for penicillin is correct for anthrax, but useless for plague.

Pestis minor. Pestis minor may be fairly common. There are probably cases in every outbreak, but they may be overlooked. The patient is probably still going around or at work in spite of a mild fever. He has one or two swollen glands, in the groin perhaps or in the axilla, but they do not bother him much and they go away without treatment. If samples of his blood are tested early and late in the illness, they show a diagnostic rise in antibody titre, but no one is likely to do this except a doctor investigating an endemic area. Most patients with pestis minor do not know they have had the plague.

Asymptomatic plague. Man can become infected with plague bacilli without becoming ill: this has been shown in several investigations. *Y. pestis* has been grown from throat swabs of household contacts of plague patients, and serological testing in infected villages has shown rises of antibody in healthy people. Such rises occur in endemic areas when cases of plague are occurring, but not in quiescent periods.

Plague in pregnancy. Untreated plague can cause abortion, miscarriage, or death of the fetus in the womb. With early modern treatment a woman can make a good recovery and continue to term with little risk to the baby. But the emphasis is on *early*; early diagnosis and early treatment.

Diagnosis

Clinical diagnosis. In a large outbreak diagnosis is easy: any patient with a swollen lymph node and fever, or any patient with an acute febrile illness probably has plague and should be treated for plague until tests show he has another disease. In a small household outbreak it is more difficult unless one is thinking of plague. Staphylococcal or any pyogenic infection can cause adenitis and fever, as can lymphogranuloma and filariasis, but they do not cause outbreaks, and the patient is not so suddenly and so acutely ill. Tularaemia does cause fever and adenitis, it *is* caused by a bite and it can occur in outbreaks. The illness is not usually so severe, though there have been serious outbreaks. Geographically it tends to occur in the northern rather than in the southern part of the world, but this is not absolute. It is safer to make the more serious clinical diagnosis, plague. The organisms of both diseases, *Y. pestis* and *Francisella tularensis*, are resistant to penicillin but respond to streptomycin. The rare cases of plague with a sore like anthrax are more treacherous, for *B. anthracis* responds to penicillin and might therefore be given when the sore is caused by *Y. pestis* which does not respond. A smear of the lesion directly stained may show bipolar staining of plague instead of the typical anthrax rods.

When a patient is extremely ill with plague, there may be nothing about him to point to the diagnosis other than the severity of his illness. Overwhelming meningococcal infection, Gram-negative septicaemia, typhus, malaria, and the haemorrhagic fevers may all come to mind. If the patient has a painful bubo, then the diagnosis is easier, but a septicaemic, shocked patient may not complain of a local swelling. If there is plague in the area then every ill, febrile patient should be treated as plague until tests prove otherwise.

Laboratory diagnosis. Bipolar staining with Giemsa or Wayson's stain is enough as a first step in the diagnosis of a local outbreak and should be attempted wherever there is a microscope: pus from a bubo, sputum or smears from spleen, liver, or lungs of dead rodents may be examined. If material has to be sent to a distant laboratory, it should go in Carey–Blair or other suitable transport medium: it can then be grown on media and injected into mice or guinea pigs. When a patient dies undiagnosed, smears of liver, spleen, or lungs can be used for culture and inoculation. When autopsy is not permitted, organ puncture, the use of a viscerotome, amputation of a finger digit, or aspiration of heart or venous blood, or of blood-stained nasal froth which is sometimes present at death can yield suitable specimens for the laboratory.

Serological tests are useful for final diagnosis but are far too late for helping with treatment. Agglutinins appear in the blood towards the end of the first week: serum must be absorbed with *Y. pseudotuberculosis* as the test is not otherwise specific for *Y. pestis*. Fraction 1 is tested for in complement-fixing and haemagglutinating tests and these are therefore specific, but antibodies appear later, between the eighth and fourteenth days. The passive haemagglutination test is the best for general use, but it is not a test for the unskilled. A rise in antibody by any of these tests during the illness is diagnostic of plague, but, unless treatment is started early, many patients will be dead before the second sample can be taken.

Prognosis. Without treatment between 30 and 50 per cent of patients with simple bubonic plague will die, and nearly all those labelled septicaemic or pneumonic. Early treatment can save most of the patients with simple bubonic plague, many of those with septicaemic plague, and some of those with pneumonic plague. The critical factor is early treatment: one day can make a difference.

Treatment. Plague infection responds to treatment with streptomycin, tetracycline, chloramphenicol, and sulphonamides. It does not respond to penicillin, and this drug should not be used in any undiagnosed, febrile illness if there is any chance it might be plague. Streptomycin is very effective: 1 g as a loading dose, then 0.5 g every four hours intramuscularly till the fever lessens, then 0.5 g every six hours for a few more days. A loading dose of 3 g tetracycline orally followed by 3 g daily in divided doses is a suitable course: in severe cases a first dose of 0.75 g to 1.0 g may be given intravenously. Chloramphenicol may be used in similar doses. If one is worried by possible Herxheimer type of reaction to streptomycin, a combined course of that drug and tetracycline may be used instead, cutting the doses of each drug by half, or giving each drug alternately. Sulphonamides may be used if antibiotics are not available, but they will not save pneumonic cases. Very high doses have been recommended, but it is safer not to exceed 6 g per day, and 2 to 4 g of sodium bicarbonate should be taken with each dose to keep the urine alkaline.

Safety of staff. Pus from buboes is teeming with *Y. pestis*, even after days of specific treatment. Buboes should therefore not be opened unless this is surgically essential and great care is necessary in handling pus and dressings. Sputum from pneumonic cases and some terminal septicaemic patients is also full of *Y. pestis*, and a pneumonic patient is a danger to staff until he has had at least two days of specific treatment and is obviously responding. A patient with bubonic plague is not a danger provided all fleas have been killed on his person or on his clothing and bedding. Staff looking after a single patient with pneumonic plague should take 500 mg tetracycline every 6 hours during the patient's illness and for some days after his recovery or death. If there is a succession of patients, as is likely, this regime can hardly be followed because, apart from drug reactions, resistant *Y. pestis* might emerge. It may then be wiser for staff not to take the drug but to take their temperature instead three or four times daily and to report any rise at once when treatment, if indicated, can be started.

Prevention and control

Plague vaccine. Two doses of 0.5 ml and 1 ml of killed plague vaccine at four weeks' interval subcutaneously or intramuscularly give useful but not complete protection against plague. A reinforcing dose of 1 ml should be given annually to workers likely to be exposed or to troops in endemic areas. Where life is disrupted by war or other calamity, mass vaccination may be justified in plague areas, but in localized outbreaks vaccines are useless, for plague moves too quickly, whereas antibodies take time to develop.

Control of outbreaks. In small village outbreaks, close contacts may be given tetracycline 500 mg four times daily (less for children) for a week, or sulphonamides 2 to 4 g daily if tetracyclines are not available. Sometimes it may be wise to give all villagers this prophylaxis, but mass indiscriminate prophylaxis is useless.

It is the flea that carries plague to man, and if the flea can be destroyed plague cannot spread. So houses, huts, outbuildings, and tents may be sprayed with an insecticide known to be effective against the local flea. It is not so easy to kill rodents, and this should not even be attempted until the fleas have been dealt with, as otherwise the fleas will just leave the dead rodents for man. But rodent control is a major undertaking. It is easier and more effective to look after human contacts and to kill fleas.

For long-term control expert supervision is required. The whole area must be surveyed: what is the vegetation, climate, and configuration of the area; what kind of animal is common there; how do they live and breed; are they infested with fleas, and, if so, with which species; is there any serological indication of infection and are the titres rising or falling; if *Y. pestis* is around, which variety is it, *orientalis, antiqua,* or *mediaevalis*? A team containing a mammalogist, an entomologist, a microbiologist, and an epidemiologist is required. Such a team can assess the pressure of plague in an area and can forecast the risk of plague breaking out: if it does break out the team can advise on how to act. Away from the field, more general methods of prevention must be applied, but they all relate to the mechanism of spread from rodent through the flea to man. They include the rat-proofing of buildings, of ships, planes, trucks, and trains, and of airports, docks, warehouses, and terminals. Protection depends on informed vigilance.

References

Bahmanyar, M. and Cavanaugh, D. C. (1976). *Plague manual.* World Health Organization, Geneva.
Christie, A. B. (1980). *Infectious diseases: epidemiology and clinical practice,* 3rd edn. Churchill Livingstone, Edinburgh.

—, Chen, T. H., and Elsberg, S. S. (1980). Plague in camels and goats: Their role in human epidemics. *J. infect. Dis.* **141**, 724.

Chosky, K. B. N. H. (1909). The various types of plague and their clinical manifestations. *Am. J. med. Sci.* **138**, 351.

Pollitzer, R. (1960). A review of recent literature on plague. *Bull. Wld Hlth Org.* **23**, 313.

Pollitzer, R. (1954). *Plague.* Monograph series no. 22, World Health Organization, Geneva.

World Health Organization (1973). Technical guide for a system of plague surveillance. *Wkly epidem. Rec.* **14**, 149.

World Health Organization Expert Committee on Plague (1970). Fourth report. *Tech. Rep. Ser. Wld Hlth Org.* **447**.

Tularaemia, glanders, and melioidosis

R. G. Mitchell

Tularaemia

Definition: Tularaemia is an infectious disease caused by *Francisella tularensis*, a Gram-negative bacillus first isolated in 1911 from squirrels, and named after Tulare district in California. It is primarily a zoonosis affecting many animal hosts, mostly rodents, and man is only occasionally and accidentally infected.

Distribution. The disease has been reported in many countries in the northern hemisphere, including North America, Norway, Sweden, mainland Europe, Russia, and Japan, and cases may arrive in non-endemic areas such as Britain. The commonest animal hosts are rabbits and squirrels (USA), hares and voles (Scandinavia), and field mice (eastern Europe). Certain arthropods are vectors of the organism, including various species of ticks (*Dermacentor andersoni, D. variabilis*), the deerfly (*Chrysops discalis*), and mosquitoes (*Aedes cinereus*). Two different strains are recognized: Jellison type A which is highly virulent and found only in North America, and Jellison type B, which is less virulent for man and occurs elsewhere.

Aetiology. The disease is usually acquired by handling infected animals or their carcasses, or from animal or vector bites. The organism enters the body through lesions in the skin, and may perhaps penetrate intact or minimally traumatized skin, mucous membranes, and conjunctivae. Dogs and cats, although themselves immune from the disease, may harbour the organism and transmit the disease to man by bites or scratches. Although the alimentary tract itself is not usually regarded as a portal of entry, the disease is sometimes acquired by the oral route by eating undercooked wild animals, or drinking contaminated water. The organism is infective if inhaled in dust from soil, grain, or silage contaminated with rodent excreta, or in aerosols generated from infected animals. Finally, infections are common among laboratory staff working with the organism. Case-to-case spread among human subjects is surprisingly rare.

Incidence. A bimodal peak incidence of the disease is reported in the USA, attributed to tick bites in the summer months, and the hunting of rabbits in winter. The disease is sporadic, with occasional reports of small common source outbreaks involving parties of hunters or holidaymakers in endemic areas. The incidence of the disease has steadily declined in the USA, where the annual total of cases is now of the order of 100. The disease in adults is much commoner in males, reflecting their greater involvement in outdoor pursuits; it is an occupational disease among hunters, butchers, and allied workers.

Clinical features. The incubation period is about three days (range one to 10 days). The disease usually presents with sudden onset of chills and fever, accompanied by headache, malaise, and muscle pain. The fever may be continuous or remittent, and the liver and spleen may be enlarged and tender. Several different clinical en-

tities are recognized, determined by the mode of infection and presumably by the virulence of the infecting strain.

In the *ulceroglandular* form, a rash appears at the site of inoculation and changes to a papule at about 48 hours. This subsequently breaks down to form an ulcer with ragged edges. The associated lymph nodes become enlarged and painful (bubo), and may suppurate and discharge. The condition is usually self-limiting, the fever continuing for several weeks. Occasionally the ulceroglandular form is accompanied by pharyngitis or develops into the septicaemic or pneumonic forms of the disease.

In the *typhoidal* form there is no history of trauma and no sign of local injury. The non-specific symptoms and signs are those of a septicaemic illness with fever, headache, myalgia, vomiting, diarrhoea, abdominal pains, and sometimes signs of endotoxic shock.

The *pneumonic* form, which usually follows inhalation of the organism but may arise during the course of a septicaemia, presents as a pneumonitis, with fever, dry cough, and chest pain, sometimes accompanied by delirium. It may take the form of bronchopneumonia, or less commonly lobar pneumonia, with or without pleural effusion. Abscess formation is said to be rare. The basic underlying pathological lesion is alveolar necrosis with multifocal areas of bronchopneumonia tending to coalesce. In the more chronic forms of pneumonitis, apical lesions may closely resemble tuberculosis.

The *oculoglandular* form is uncommon, accounting for fewer than 1 per cent of cases: it may be regarded as a specific form of ulceroglandular tularaemia. Introduction of infected material into the eye is followed by purulent conjunctivitis and the formation of yellowish papules on the conjunctiva or cornea which later ulcerate. There is periorbital oedema and painful enlargement of the preauricular and anterior cervical lymph nodes.

Pharyngeal tularaemia may be overlooked if it presents as an exudative tonsillitis or pharyngitis with cervical lymphadenopathy: these features sometimes accompany other forms of the disease. The patient develops sore throat, dysphagia, chills, fever, nausea, and malaise. Examination may reveal an exudative tonsillitis or pharyngitis with membrane formation not unlike that of diphtheria. The disease may extend to involve the trachea, main bronchi, and hilar lymph nodes, giving rise to retrosternal pain and dry cough. The patient, often a young child, is acutely ill and liable to develop tracheal obstruction of septicaemia.

Osteomyelitis and endocarditis have been described, but are rare in this disease.

Prognosis. Overall, the fatality rate in untreated cases of tularaemia is said to be of the order of 5 per cent, falling to 1 per cent or less with treatment. It is much higher in the pneumonic and septicaemic forms, perhaps around 30 per cent. The disease usually confers life long immunity, and relapses are unusual. However, a subsequent infection may give rise to a limited papule or a sensitization rash at the site of the original inoculation.

Differential diagnosis. The differential diagnosis of tularaemia is extensive. The ulceroglandular form must be distinguished from plague, cat scratch fever, lymphogranuloma venereum, granuloma inguinale, chancroid, *Pasteurella multocida* infection, toxoplasmosis, and sporotrichosis. As already stated, the typhoidal form may resemble any septicaemic illness, and has been mistakenly diagnosed as typhoid fever, brucellosis, leptospirosis, glanders, melioidosis, yersiniosis, Rocky Mountain spotted fever, lymphoreticulosis, or various virus infections. Pulmonary tularaemia must be distinguished from other unresolving pneumonias: tuberculosis, mycoplasma pneumonia, Legionnaires' disease, glanders, melioidosis, and pneumonic plague; also psittacosis, Q fever, fungal infections including histoplasmosis and blastomycosis, and malignancy.

Pharyngeal tularaemia is readily confused with streptococcal pharyngitis, glandular fever, and diphtheria.

Diagnosis. Smears from lesions and pus are stained by Gram's method and examined for the presence of small Gram-negative bacilli. The organism may be provisionally identified by immunofluorescence using specific antiserum. Isolation of the organism should be attempted from swabs of lesions, discharges, pus aspirated from buboes, and from sputum, bronchial aspirate, gastric washings, and cerebrospinal fluid where appropriate. Occasionally blood cultures are positive during the first week of the illness. Specimens are inoculated on a selective enrichment medium (glucose-cysteine blood agar and chocolate agar, incorporating penicillin and actidione). Specimens may be inoculated into guinea pigs and attempts made to recover the organism from liver and spleen, but the risk of an epizootic probably rules out this procedure. Histology of diseased lymph nodes shows caseating granulation, and a liver biopsy may show miliary granulomata with scattered areas of necrosis.

Attempts to isolate the organism are frequently unsuccessful and the diagnosis must then rest on serological evidence, using a bacterial agglutination test to demonstrate a rise in titre. The test is usually positive by the second week and may rise from a titre of 80 or so up to a maximum of 5000 by about 8 weeks, remaining positive for many years. High titre sera may show cross-agglutination at a lower titre with *Brucella abortus*, heterophile antigen, and OX-19 antigen. Conversely, a false-positive tularaemia agglutination may occur in brucellosis.

A skin test has been reported upon favourably although the reagent is not generally available. Patients with tularaemia show a delayed hypersensitivity reaction of the tuberculoid type at 48 hours. The skin test is more sensitive in the early and late stages of the disease than is the agglutination test, and it remains positive for many years.

Treatment. The antibiotic most commonly used in the past has been streptomycin given in a dose of 30 mg/kg daily as two intramuscular injections for two weeks. The newer aminoglycosides such as gentamicin are likely to be at least as effective. Tetracycline (2 g daily for two weeks) has been used, and chloramphenicol would be indicated in rare cases of meningitis, but both antibiotics are bacteriostatic and may fail to eliminate the organism.

It is prudent to isolate patients for the first two days, and care should be taken in handling blood, discharges, and excreta, using gloves and disinfectants.

Prevention. Wild animals in endemic areas should be handled with gloves, and the risk of arthropod bites reduced by the use of wrist bands and trouser clips. Animals must be thoroughly cooked before consumption and raw water boiled before use. Swimming should be avoided in endemic areas. Vaccines developed in the USA and Russia afford up to five years protection from the disease, and are essential for laboratory staff working with the organism. The live vaccine strain (LVS) gives complete protection against the typhoidal and pulmonary forms, and results in attenuation of the ulceroglandular form.

Glanders

Definition. Glanders is an infectious disease caused by a non-motile Gram-negative bacillus *Pseudomonas mallei*, first isolated in 1882. It attacks mainly horses, less commonly other animals including sheep, goats, dogs, and cats, and is occasionally transmissible to man.

Equine glanders. Glanders in horses was worldwide in its distribution at the beginning of this century, but has now been eliminated from the Western world as the result of compulsory slaughtering of infected animals, and the general disappearance of the horse from the town and battlefield. The disease is still reported occasionally from eastern Europe, the Middle East, Africa, and Asia. The precise route of infection is often uncertain. Infected material from other animals may be inhaled or inoculated through wounds or abrasions of the skin. Acute or chronic glanders may result, although the distinction is not always clear-cut.

The acute form is characterized by ulceration of the nasal and oral mucosa, trachea, and bronchi, with pneumonia and widespread dissemination of abscesses or granulomatous nodules throughout the viscera. In the chronic form, nodules are present in the lungs, subcutaneous tissues, and muscle, accompanied by ulcerating lesions in the upper respiratory mucosa. A localized form of the disease is called farcy, in which subcutaneous nodules and ulcers develop on the limbs and flanks, accompanied by 'pipestem' thickening of the draining lymphatics and enlargement of the regional lymph nodes. Further nodules may be seeded along the lymphatic pathway. The outcome is very variable, and apparent recovery may be followed by relapse.

Human glanders

Transmission. In man, glanders is an occupational hazard of grooms and others intimately involved with horses. However, the infectivity of infected discharges and excreta is surprisingly low. The disease may be acquired by inhalation, inoculation, or rarely by ingestion of contaminated water or horsemeat. Case-to-case spread has occasionally been reported. By contrast, laboratory staff working with *Ps. mallei* are at considerable risk, and are probably the only group likely to contract the disease in the West.

Clinical features. It is not always possible to distinguish glanders from farcy or the acute illness from the subacute, since intermediate or combined forms of the disease exist, and one form may be followed by another. As with melioidosis, which it closely resembles, glanders may involve any system or organ. The incubation period ranges from a few days to several weeks.

Acute glanders. In the acute disease, the patient is severely ill, with high fever, toxaemia, muscle and joint pains, and occasionally delirium. At the site of inoculation on the limbs or face, an inflamed lesion is often present, which may show ulceration, pustule formation, or localized gangrene, accompanied by lymphangitis and suppurative lymphadenitis. Sloughing of the upper respiratory mucosa occurs, with a purulent haemorrhagic discharge from the nose and mouth, and sometimes deep tissue destruction. Ulceration may extend to involve the pharynx, larynx, trachea, and bronchi. Pulmonary involvement results in cough, purulent sputum, haemoptysis, chest pain, and dyspnoea; it may take the form of bronchopneumonia, empyema, or lung abscess, usually with enlargement of the hilar lymph nodes. Septicaemia results in widespread suppurative lesions, typically subcutaneous or intramuscular abscesses (pyomyositis) which may discharge to form slow-healing sinuses. Pyoarthrosis, osteomyelitis, meningitis, and brain abscess may occur, and endotoxic shock may be a feature of this disease. A generalized skin eruption of ulcerating papules or pustules is characteristic of the terminal stages and may resemble smallpox.

Chronic glanders. In the chronic form of glanders, multiple abscess formation is the rule, with sinus formation and scarring and emaciation. Long-standing suppuration may result in amyloid disease.

A latent or subclinical form of the disease may occur very rarely.

Prognosis. The mortality for glanders in man formerly exceeded 90 per cent.

Diagnosis. In what may present as a non-specific illness, a history of exposure to the disease is crucial to the diagnosis. Attempts should be made to isolate the organism from wound swabs, pus and other discharges, sputum, and urine as appropriate, using selective culture medium. Blood cultures may be positive. Attempts at recovery of the organism by animal inoculation are probably ruled out by the hazards of cross infection. Intraperitoneal injection of infected material into the male guinea pig results in swelling of the tunica vaginalis (Straus reaction).

An intradermal test using mallein, an extract derived from a broth culture filtrate of the organism, analogous to tuberculin, may be used to detect delayed hypersensitivity in horses and man. Since the mallein test itself stimulates antibody production, it should be preceded by a serological test. An indirect haemagglutination test using sensitized horse red cells will detect antibodies to glanders, but it is not entirely specific; it may be positive at low titre in unexposed normal subjects, and is positive in melioidosis. A complement fixation test is also available, antibodies appearing during the second week of the illness and persisting longer than agglutinating antibodies.

Treatment. Sulphonamide therapy was occasionally successful in the treatment of human disease. The disease largely disappeared before the antibiotic era, so there has been little opportunity to evaluate co-trimoxazole and the newer antibiotics. Supportive therapy should be accompanied by surgical drainage where indicated, and any secondary infection treated with appropriate antibiotics.

Melioidosis

Definition. Melioidosis is an infectious disease of man caused by a motile Gram-negative bacillus *Pseudomonas pseudomallei* (formerly *Loefflerella whitmori*). It was first recognized in 1911 in Rangoon by Whitmore who noticed lesions at autopsy which resembled glanders but were caused by a different organism. The first clinical cases were described in 1921 by Stanton.

Distribution. Melioidosis is a sporadic disease of warm climates mostly confined to latitudes within 20° of the equator, principally in Southeast Asia. It is recognized in India, Burma, Malaysia, Thailand, Indo-China, the Philippines, and Papua New Guinea, and affected both Allied and Japanese troops during the Second World War. Servicemen returning from Vietnam probably imported the disease into North Australia; the first cases were reported from Townsville, Queensland, in 1962, followed by cases in Brisbane and the Darwin area. Patients may develop the disease several years after leaving an endemic area. Sporadic cases have occurred in the USA, Panama, Ecuador, and Turkey.

Aetiology. The causative organism occurs as a soil saprophyte and may contaminate muddy surface water such as the rice fields of endemic areas. Certain animals, principally rodents, may acquire the disease and could contaminate water and food with their excreta, but transmission of the disease from animals to man has not been convincingly demonstrated, although melioidosis and leptospirosis may co-exist. Human infections are probably acquired by penetration of the organism through wounds or other skin lesions, by inhalation of dust, or by aspiration or ingestion of contaminated water. Cross-infection in hospital is a possibility, but case-to-case spread appears to be very rare. Laboratory-acquired infections have been described.

Predisposing factors. Overt disease is uncommon even in endemic areas. Predisposing factors include trauma, major surgery, burns, pregnancy, debilitating diseases, such as diabetes mellitus and alcoholism, and acute infections such as pneumococcal pneumonia. The disease is much commoner in males, reflecting their greater exposure risk.

Clinical features. The incubation period may be as short as two days, but sometimes extends to months or years. The disease is characterized by widespread suppuration with the formation of multiple abscesses or 'pseudogranulomata'. Any organ or system may be involved, and the clinical manifestations of the disease and its severity are extremely variable. Melioidosis is conveniently classified as: (*a*) acute or fulminating: septicaemic or pneumonic; (*b*) subacute or chronic; and (*c*) mild, latent, or subclinical.

The *septicaemic* form of the disease presents typically with malaise, high fever, vomiting, myalgia, and sometimes confusion or delirium. Severe diarrhoea is common, although lesions are unusual in the alimentary tract. Examination may reveal anaemia, jaundice, and hepatosplenomegaly. Endotoxic shock and myocarditis are serious complications. Pustular lesions in the upper respiratory tract result in a copious discharge from the nose and mouth and a pustular rash may occur over the trunk or limbs. Subcutaneous abscesses are particularly common; if present on the abdominal wall they may be found to communicate with an intra-abdominal or subphrenic abscess. Suppuration may be associated with lymphangitis and lymphadenopathy. Osteomyelitis and pyoarthrosis are common. Abscess formation may occur throughout the genito-urinary system and involve the kidneys, seminal vesicles, or prostate. Involvement of the central nervous system may result in meningitis, meningoencephalitis, or brain abscess.

In pneumonic melioidosis, the disease may present as a severe pneumonia, possibly as the result of inhalation of the organism, or pneumonia may develop during the course of a septicaemic illness. Typically, fever, cough, dyspnoea, and chest pain accompany expectoration of pink frothy sputum. Examination may show pulmonary consolidation, abscess formation, cavitation or empyema, with corresponding radiological appearances.

Differential diagnosis. Melioidosis should be suspected in any patient with a septicaemic illness or pneumonia who has ever visited an endemic area, and a history of immersion in surface water or of associated trauma should be sought. The differential diagnosis includes glanders, typhoid fever, tuberculosis, cholera, plague, scrub typhus, tularaemia, and formerly smallpox.

Subacute or chronic melioidosis is commoner than the acute forms and usually presents as an unresolving pneumonia, which may closely resemble pulmonary tuberculosis. It may be asymptomatic, or present with fever, cough, dyspnoea, and chest pain. Possible radiological appearances include localized pulmonary infiltration, nodular lesions, consolidation, abscess formation, upper lobe cavitation, generalized mottling throughout the lung fields, and empyema. Hilar lymphadenopathy has been described in association with cervical adenitis and fever. Localized suppuration may involve the skin, bones, joints, and virtually any viscus. There is a great tendency for the disease to relapse, sometimes after an interval of several years.

In childbirth, melioidosis may present as a breast abscess or post-partum septicaemia.

Subclinical or latent infections appear to be common in endemic areas, since up to 20 per cent of healthy agricultural workers show a positive serological test, as did a significant number of healthy American troops stationed in Vietnam for more than six months.

Prognosis. The septicaemic and pulmonary forms of the disease have a mortality rate of up to 90 per cent, despite treatment. Prognosis in the chronic suppurative form of the disease is good, with adequate management and chemotherapy, but the possibility of relapse, even after several years, should always be borne in mind.

Laboratory investigations. Every effort should be made to culture *Pseudomonas pseudomallei* from swabs of wounds, ulcers, skin pustules, pus, blood, sputum, joint fluid, and urine as appropriate. If sputum culture is negative, bronchial or transtracheal aspirate should be submitted for culture. The bacteriologist should be alerted beforehand since the organism is a category BI pathogen in United Kingdom laboratories and its isolation requires special recognition, with prolonged incubation of cultures and the use of selective medium. In pus, the organism is frequently mixed with *Staphylococcus aureus*, which may be mistakenly regarded as the significant pathogen.

The peripheral blood count may show a neutrophil leucocytosis. The ESR is usually raised, in the range 30–120 mm/hr Westergren. Serological tests are of considerable value. The indirect haemagglutination test (IHA), which employs a purified polysaccharide antigen, usually becomes positive towards the end of the first week of the acute illness, with a titre of 40 or more, and reaches a maximum after several weeks. A high IHA titre may persist for years after resolution of the acute illness and complicate later investigations. Seroconversion may not always occur, and titres may sometimes fall during the course of the illness. Complement fixation and bacterial agglutination tests (both positive at a titre of 8) are less specific than the IHA. An indirect fluorescent antibody test is available and may help to distinguish present from past infection: high titres of specific IgM antibody probably indicate active clinical disease.

Treatment. Supportive measures, and treatment of any underlying disease such as diabetes, are combined with surgical drainage of abscesses where appropriate, and a prolonged course of chemotherapy. Barrier nursing is indicated and great care should be taken in the disposal of the patient's dressings, discharges, blood, urine, and faeces. The rational choice of an antibiotic depends on the antibiotic sensitivity of the organism in vitro. Successful treatment of acute cases has been reported with chloramphenicol up to 3 g intravenously every six hours for four weeks; or with tetracycline or doxycycline given intravenously at first, later by mouth. Chloramphenicol and tetracycline may be given together, or either may be combined with kanamycin or novobiocin. Co-trimoxazole is an alternative which seems very suitable for prolonged oral therapy and is specifically indicated for prostatitis. The organism is usually resistant to gentamicin in vitro. Chemotherapy should be prolonged if relapse is to be avoided, possibly continued for 6 or 12 months after resolution of the illness. In an attempt to bolster cellular immunity, levamisole 150 mg twice-weekly for four weeks has been used with apparent success.

References

Tularaemia

Burke, D. S. (1977). Immunization against tularaemia. *J. infect. Dis.* **135**, 55.

Butler, T. (1979). Plague and tularemia. *Pedia. Clins. N. Am.* **26**, 355.

Guerrant, R. L., Humphries, R. K., and Butler, J. E. (1976). Tickborne oculoglandular tularaemia. *Archs. intern. Med.* **136**, 811

Halstead, C. C. and Kulasinghe, H. P. (1978). Tularemia pneumonia in urban children. *Pediatrics, Springfield* **61**, 660.

Hornick, R. B. (1977). Tularaemia. In *Infectious disease* 2nd edn. (ed. P. D. Hoeprich), ch. 133. Harper and Row, New York.

Teutsch, S. M., Martone, W. J., Brink, E. W., Potter, M. E., Eliot, G., Hoxsie, R., Craven, R. B., and Kaufmann, A. F. (1979). Pneumonia tularaemia on Martha's Vineyard. *New Engl. J. Med.* **301**, 826.

Tyson, H. K., (1976). Tularemia—an unappreciated cause of exudative pharyngitis. *Pediatrics, Springfield* **58**, 864.

Wood, J. B., Valteris, K., Hardy, R. H., and Pearson, A. D. (1976). Imported tularaemia. *Br. med. J.* **i**, 811.

Glanders

Howe, C. (1950). Glanders. In *Oxford system of medicine*, vol. 5, 185. Oxford University Press, Oxford.

Howe, C. and Miller, W. R. (1947). Human glanders: report of six cases. *Ann. intern. Med.* **26**, 93.

Melioidosis

Ashdown, L. R. (1981). Relationship and significance of specific immunoglobulin M antibody response in clinical and subclinical melioidosis. *J. clin. Microbiol.* **14**, 361.

—, Duffy, V. A., and Douglas, R. A. (1980). Melioidosis. *Med. J. Aust.* **1**, 314.

Howe, C., Sampath, A., and Spotnitz, M. (1971). The pseudomallei group: a review. *J. infect. Dis.* **124**, 598.

Rode, J. W. (1981). Melioidosis in the Northern Territory of Australia. *Med. J. Aust.* **1**, 181.

Schlech III, W. F., Turchick, J. B., Westlake, R. E., Klein, G. C., Band, J. D., and Weaver, R. E. (1981). Laboratory-acquired infection with *Pseudomonas pseudomallei* (melioidosis). *New Engl. J. Med.* **305**, 1133.

Thin, R. N. T., Brown, M., Stewart, J. B., and Garrett, C. J. (1970). Melioidosis: a report of 10 cases. *Q. Jl Med.* **39**, 115.

Yersiniosis

N. S. Mair

Although the genus *Yersinia* comprises three species, *Y. pseudotuberculosis*, *Y. enterocolitica*, and *Y. pestis*, the term yersiniosis refers to infection with the first two micro-organisms, the age-old name 'plague' being reserved for the disease caused by *Y. pestis* (see page 5.205).

History and aetiology. *Y. pseudotuberculosis* (formerly *Pasteurella pseudotuberculosis*) has long been recognized as a cause of epizootic disease in animals, particularly rodents, since it was first isolated by Malassez and Vignal in 1883 from lesions in a guinea-pig inoculated with pus from a child with tuberculous meningitis. Prior to 1954 it was regarded as a rare cause of septicaemia in man. In that year its role as a human pathogen of some importance was established when it was shown to cause an abscess-forming mesenteric lymphadenitis in children who had been operated on for acute appendicitis. Since then numerous cases of pseudotuberculous mesenteric lymphadenitis have been reported from many parts of the world.

Y. pseudotuberculosis is homogeneous in its biochemical reactions and is divided into six distinct serological types each of which is characterized by thermostable, strictly type-specific O antigens and thermolabile H antigens. Serotypes I, III, and V are specific, but serotypes II and IV share antigens with the salmonella B and D groups respectively, and a common antigen has been identified between serotype VI and *Escherichia coli* O55. In Europe serotype I has been most prevalent in man and animals, although serotypes II and III are not unusual. Strains of serotypes IV and V have been rare while serotype VI has been found only in rabbits in Japan.

The earliest strains of *Y. enterocolitica* were isolated in the USA between 1934 and 1948 from patients suffering from gastroenteritis and skin sepsis. These strains, which resembled *P. pseudotuberculosis*, were described at the time as *Bacterium enterocoliticum* or labelled as unidentified organisms. In 1949 similar strains were isolated in Switzerland from cases of septicaemia. Then in the early 1960s bacteriologists in various European countries obtained a whole series of strains from hares, pigs, sheep, and chinchillas which they named *P. pseudotuberculosis* type b or Pasteurella X. An examination of these strains showed that they resembled the earlier strains isolated from man. In 1964 the name *Yersinia enterocolitica* was proposed for this group of organisms. The first human cases of infection with the new species were diagnosed first in France, Belgium, and Scandinavia in 1964, but since then the infection has been reported with increasing frequency throughout the world. The increase in reported isolations is probably the result of greater awareness about this organism and about its potential role in human and animal disease.

Biochemically, *Y. enterocolitica* is a complex, heterogeneous species divided into five biotypes and an ill-defined group of *Y. enterocolitica*-like organisms. Thirty-four serotypes have been identified but at present only three serotypes, 3, 8, and 9 are of medical importance. Serotypes 3 and 8 are specific while serotype 9 crossreacts strongly with organisms of the *Brucella* group. Serotype 3 is found extensively in Europe, Africa, Asia, and Canada. Serotype 8 is the predominant isolate in the United States where serotypes 3 and 9 are virtually non-existent. Serotype 9 has been observed in several European countries, especially Finland.

Epidemiology. *Y. pseudotuberculosis* is found in a wide variety of mammals and birds, particularly in western and central Europe. The principal reservoirs of infection are rodents and birds, but in fact all species, even the most susceptible experimentally, are capable of harbouring the organism in the digestive tract for a considerable time and of disseminating it around them. It is probable that human infection is by the oral route and is acquired by direct or indirect contact with infected animals. The role of animals as a source of human infection is suggested by the following observations. Human and animal strains of *Y. pseudotuberculosis* have the same cultural, biochemical, and pathogenic characteristics. The majority of animal strains belong to serotype I which is most prevalent in Europe and found most frequently in man. Both the animal and human disease reach their peak about the same time of the year. In western Europe the maximum incidence is between November and February when animals are most exposed to cold and starvation. Under these conditions of stress, *Y. pseudotuberculosis* infection which is latent in many animals may become manifest. In some rural areas where there is a high incidence of animal infection, there is a correspondingly high incidence in humans. Many patients, both in urban and rural areas provide a history of contact with animals. Further evidence has been provided by numerous observations in which antibodies have been found in animals in close proximity to the patient. There is no record of transmission of the disease from one person to another.

The incubation period is uncertain but it would appear to be about ten days.

The epidemiology of *Y. enterocolitica* infection remains obscure. There are numerous reports of isolation of the organism from the environment, water, milk, poultry, meat, vegetables, and from a variety of small rodents like field-mice and shrews, but these strains are biochemically and serologically distinct from those associated with human disease. The pig appears to be the only animal species to harbour the pathogenic human serotype 3 regularly, although there is no evidence to suggest that the organism is pathogenic for the pig itself, nor is there firm evidence to indicate that it is an important source of human infection. Whatever the original source may be, the frequently familial character of the disease in which symptoms of enteritis appear in other members of the family, often at intervals of several days, suggests that contact with clinical cases or symptomless carriers may play a considerable part in the spread of human infection with *Y. enterocolitica*.

The incubation period varies from five to ten days.

Clinical features The diseases caused by both micro-organisms can be regarded as manifestations of a number of primary acute infections and secondary immunological complications (Table 1).

Table 1   Clinical manifestations of yersiniosis

Primary acute infections
  Pseudo-appendicular syndrome
    acute mesenteric lymphadenitis
    acute terminal ileitis
  Enteritis
  Septicaemia
  Far-eastern scarlatiniform fever or
    epidemic pseudotuberculosis
  Localized infections

Secondary immunological complications
  Erythema nodosum
  Arthritis
  Thyroid disease
  Glomerulonephritis

Primary acute infections. *Pseudo-appendicular syndrome.* This syndrome is the most frequent manifestation of infection with *Y. pseudotuberculosis*. About 90 per cent of patients diagnosed as being infected with the organism present as acute mesenteric lymphadenitis with or without an associated terminal ileitis. The disease shows a predilection for males between 10 and 19 years. In *Y. enterocolitica* infection the pseudo-appendicular syndrome is much less frequent, the incidence varying between 15 and 20 per cent.

The clinical picture is that of acute or subacute appendicitis with pain in the middle or right lower quadrant of the abdomen. Vomiting occurs regularly. The temperature rises rapidly to 38–40 °C. Diarrhoea is not infrequent when the causal agent is *Y. enterocolitica* but it is rarely observed with *Y. pseudotuberculosis*. Signs of

peritoneal irritation are often present though no generalized peritonitis has ever been observed. A moderate leucocytosis and a high erythrocyte sedimentation rate are usually present. At laparotomy the peritoneal cavity usually contains some clear fluid. In most cases the appendix appears normal or mildly congested. The mesenteric lymph nodes, especially those in the ileocaecal angle are enlarged and inflamed, and the mesentery shows redness, either diffuse or limited to the region of the affected nodes. The terminal ileum and caecum may be swollen and indurated, and show serosal hyperaemia. In this instance the condition may be mistaken for Crohn's disease (see Section 12). When there is gross involvement of the lymph nodes, the mass of glands extending sometimes to the root of the mesentery, the disease may be mistaken for tuberculosis or neoplasm.

The pathogenesis of the pseudo-appendicular syndrome varies according to the infecting organism. In *Y. pseudotuberculosis* infection the ingested bacteria are arrested in the last part of the ileum where passage is slow, resorption pronounced, and lymphatic drainage at its height. The bacteria pass by way of the lymph vessels to the regional lymph nodes where they give rise to a characteristic necrotizing reticulocytic lymphadenitis. It has been shown that the swelling and redness of the terminal ileum is the result of obstruction of the lymph drainage to the infected lymph nodes. The primary lesion in the intestinal mucosa is rarely found because it is small or because it has already healed at the time of clinical illness. This may explain why *Y. pseudotuberculosis* is seldom isolated from the stools.

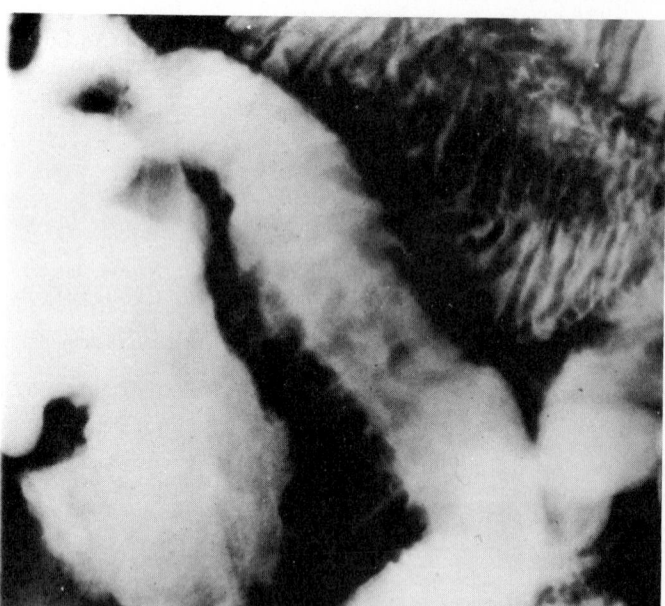

Fig. 1   Appendix, showing characteristic pseudotuberculous reticulocytic granuloma with necrotic centre infiltrated by polymorphonuclear cells.

In *Y. enterocolitica* infection, on the other hand, the ileitis appears to be due to the primary toxic effect of the bacteria on the mucosa and underlying tissue as is the case with other pathogenic enteric bacteria. Indeed, it has been suggested that acute terminal ileitis is the basic lesion and specific manifestation of *Y. enterocolitica* infection, and that mesenteric lymphadenitis can be relegated to the rank of an epiphenomenon. It is true that in *Y. enterocolitica* infection the lesions in the ileum are more severe than those caused by *Y. pseudotuberculosis*, but, nevertheless, the occurrence of mesenteric lymphadenitis and terminal ileitis as separate entities is exceptional. As a rule they are associated with one another, but in each patient one or the other may predominate. Without doubt the stage at which the laparotomy is done influences the findings.

X-ray examinations of patients with *Y. enterocolitica* infection indicate that radiologically demonstrable lesions of the terminal ileum are both common and fairly characteristic without being pathognomonic. The changes are characterized by a thickening of the wall of the terminal ileum as shown by a separation of the adjacent caecum on one side and small intestine on the other, by thickening of the mucosal folds which are increased in number and show a very tortuous course, and by the presence of multiple mural-filling defects (cobblestone effect) probably due to hyperplasia of lymphoid tissue (Fig. 2). These radiological findings differ slightly from those obtained in Crohn's disease where there is no increase in the number of mucosal folds, and the cobblestone effect is more pronounced and of more oval shape. There is no evidence that yersinia ileitis ever results in Crohn's disease. The ulcerations of ileum and colon heal within a few weeks and the radiological abnormalities of the terminal ileum disappear although more slowly.

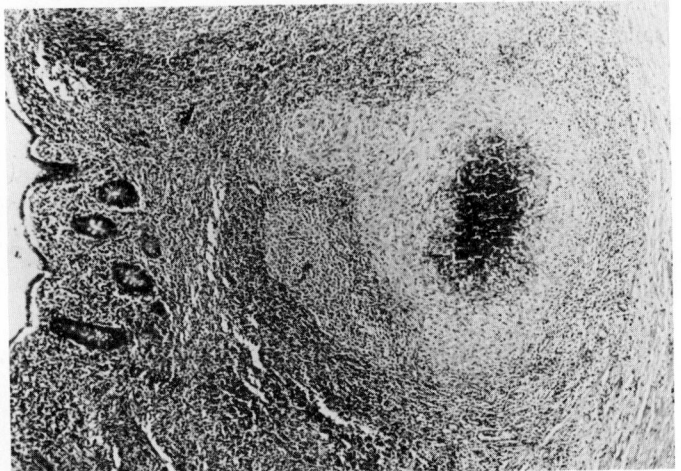

Fig. 2 X-ray film of patient with *Yersinia* ileitis, showing (a) swollen terminal ileum separated from caecum on one side and small intestine on the other, (b) tortuous folds, and (c) filling defects.

Enteritis In recent years enteritis due to *Y. enterocolitica* has become the most commonly recognized form of yersiniosis. More than three-quarters of patients with culturally confirmed *Y. enterocolitica* infection exhibit enteric symptoms. Next in numerical importance are patients with the pseudo-appendicular syndrome. Nearly 80 per cent of all patients with enteritis are under five years, while patients with the pseudo-appendicular syndrome reach their highest frequency among older children and young adults. There is little significant difference in the sex distribution of patients with enteritis. The clinical picture of abdominal pain, fever, diarrhoea, nausea, and vomiting cannot be distinguished from infection by organisms of the *Salmonella* or *Shigella* groups or by pathogenic *E.coli*. Only by stool culture or serological tests can the causative agent be identified.

Septicaemia. Yersinia septicaemia is a rare disease which shows a predilection for elderly subjects. Alcoholism, cirrhosis of the liver, haemachromatosis, and diabetes seem to be predisposing factors. It has been suggested that the liver plays a critical role in the resistance of the host to *Yersinia* infection. In the cirrhotic patient the organisms may bypass the reticulo-endothelial system of the damaged liver, resulting in a bacteraemia and the formation of metastatic abscesses. *Yersinia* septicaemia has also been reported in young children and adolescents suffering from thalassaemia, aplastic anaemia, leukaemia, and sickle-cell anaemia. The occurrence of septicaemia in patients with blood diseases may be related to iron overload which is known to enhance the pathogenicity of certain bacterial species including the *Yersinia*. Instances of opportunistic infection with *Y. enterocolitica* have been reported in patients undergoing haemodialysis, peritoneal dialysis, and immunosuppressive treatment.

The disease takes the form of either a severe typhoid-like illness

of sudden onset with high fever, general malaise, vomiting, diarrhoea, and enlargement of the liver and spleen, or it may present as a localized form characterized by hepatosplenic abscesses which may be mistaken for amoebic hepatitis. In either case the prognosis is poor; despite antibiotic treatment *Yersinia* septicaemia is accompanied by a 50 per cent mortality.

Far-eastern scarlatiniform fever or epidemic pseudotuberculosis. This syndrome is an unusual form of *Y. pseudotuberculosis* infection which appears to be confined to the far-eastern territories of the Soviet Union. The disease was first observed in Vladivostok in 1959 when an outbreak involving some 300 cases was reported. It is characterized by fever, a scarlatiniform eruption, arthralgia and acute polyarthritis, and the development of symptoms indicative of lesions involving the liver and gastrointestinal tract. Sporadic cases and large outbreaks of the disease have been reported in areas where the organism is endemic among rodents. Symptoms of the disease have been reproduced in volunteers after ingestion of cultures of *Y. pseudotuberculosis*.

Miscellaneous localized infections. *Y. enterocolitica* has been implicated in sporadic cases of meningitis, pleurisy, Parinaud's oculo-glandular syndrome, suppurative conjunctivitis, facial abscesses resembling staphylococcal infection, and erysipelas-like eruptions.

Immunological complications. *Erythema nodosum.* As a rule, erythema nodosum occurs after a prodromal period lasting 4 – 14 days. Most cases of erythema nodosum associated with *Y. pseudotuberculosis* infection have been children or young adults, particularly males, in whom acute mesenteric lymphadenitis has preceded the eruption, although high agglutinin titres to *Y. pseudotuberculosis* have also been observed in patients without gastrointestinal symptoms. Erythema nodosum as a complication of *Y. enterocolitica* infection is usually preceded by a bout of diarrhoea and fever, and occurs predominantly in females over the age of 20.

The eruption reaches its maximum in a few days accompanied by moderate fever and fatigue. The nodes, usually confined to the shins, appear in one to three successive crops and disappear with the constitutional symptoms within three weeks. Relapses have not been recorded.

Arthritis. The connective tissue complications which follow infection with *Y. enterocolitica* include the large group of acute reactive arthritis and arthralgia cases covered by the clinical diagnoses: arthralgia, monoarthritis, polyarthritis, acute rheumatoid arthritis, and Reiter's disease (see Section 16). In its various forms, arthritis is the most frequent complication of yersiniosis. According to Scandinavian studies as many as 10 to 30 per cent of adults with confirmed *Y. enterocolitica* infection develop arthritis.

As in the case of erythema nodosum, there is usually a history of gastrointestinal symptoms 4–10 days before. Several joints are affected in quick succession, the pain and swelling fluctuating in intensity from one area to another. The joints most often attacked are the knees and ankles, less frequently the fingers, toes, wrists, elbows, and shoulders, and occasionally the lumbar spine, hips, and sacroiliac joints. Synovial effusions show a polymorphonuclear pleocytosis and are usually sterile. Articular changes are rarely seen in X-ray films.

After one to four months the inflammatory reaction subsides more or less simultaneously in all the inflamed joints, but arthralgia and stiffness of joints may persist for many months and occasionally may progress to chronic joint disease resembling rheumatoid arthritis.

The development of arthritis in patients with *Yersinia* infection is determined by genetic susceptibility. About 90 per cent of patients with *Yersinia* arthritis are tissue-type HLA-B27. Such patients are liable to develop a severe high-titre arthritis of long duration. In addition to the development of arthritis, the presence of HLA-B27 seems to influence the clinical picture of *Yersinia* infections in other respects. Focal inflammatory signs such as iritis, carditis without grave cardiac sequelae, and some urological manifestations are more common in HLA-B27 positive patients, whereas erythema nodosum has a negative correlation with this antigen.

The existence of 'arthritogenic' strains of *Y. enterocolitica* has been postulated to explain the prevalence of *Yersinia* arthritis in Europe and its absence in Canada and the United States. Strains of *Y. enterocolitica* serotype 3 met with in Europe and Canada differ in phage type. European strains belong to phage type 8 and Canadian strains to phage type 9b. In the United States, where serotype 3 is rarely encountered, the dominant strain is serotype 8, phage type 10 which is seldom observed in Europe.

Apart from the arthralgia sometimes seen in erythema nodosum and the polyarthritis said to occur in far-eastern scarlatiniform fever, joint involvement is rarely reported as a complication of *Y. pseudotuberculosis* infection.

Thyroid disease. *Y. enterocolitica* has also come under suspicion as a cause of thyroid disorders (see section 10). In Scandinavia and the United States a high incidence of agglutinating antibodies to *Y. enterocolitica* has been noted in the sera of patients with thyroid disease, especially Graves' disease and Hashimoto's thyroiditis. The meaning of anti-*Yersinia* agglutinins in the sera of patients with thyroid disorders remains obscure. The most probable explanation is that of cross-reactivity between *Y. enterocolitica* antigen and a thyroid antigen against which antibody has been produced. Supporting this possibility is the observation that during the active phase of *Y. enterocolitica* infection, antibodies are formed that react with surface antigens of thyrotoxic epithelial cells. In this regard it has been noted that patients with thyroid disease show cell-mediated immunity to *Y. enterocolitica* serotype 3 measured by leucocyte migration inhibition.

Glomerulonephritis. Cases of glomerulonephritis (see Section 18) of non-streptococcal origin may be due to *Y. enterocolitica* infection. Immunofluorescent techniques have demonstrated the presence of *Yersinia* antigen as well as large granular deposits of IgA in the glomeruli of patients with serological evidence of recent yersiniosis.

Laboratory investigations. The laboratory diagnosis of infection with *Y. pseudotuberculosis* is established by isolation of the organism from the lymphatic glands, by the demonstration of specific antibodies in the serum, by histological examination of the lymph nodes, and by response to a specific skin-test antigen. The diagnosis of infection with *Y. enterocolitica* is made in the majority of cases on the basis of stool culture and serological examination of paired sera taken at an interval of 10 days. In a few cases of *Yersinia* septicaemia the organism has been cultivated from the blood during life, but most often diagnosis has been made at autopsy when the organism has been isolated from abscesses present in liver and spleen.

The laboratory findings differ according to the infecting species and are summarized in Table 2.

Course and treatment. Yersiniosis is a self-limiting disease. Gastrointestinal symptoms usually subside within one or two weeks without antibiotic therapy. Those treated surgically make an uneventful recovery. Occasionally intermittent pain in the right iliac fossa lasting several months may be encountered with *Y. pseudotuberculosis*, and chronic enteritis characterized by periods of diarrhoea and remission with *Y. enterocolitica*.

Table 2　A comparison of laboratory findings in *J. pseudotuberculosis* and *Y. enterocolitica* infection

	Y. pseudotuberculosis	*Y. enterocolitica*
Culture		
Stools	seldom positive	usually positive within 2 weeks of onset; may remain positive for 4–8 weeks; (> 90% of *Y. ent.* isolations)
Lymph nodes	swollen and congested lymph nodes in ileocaecal angle rarely positive	usually positive; lymph nodes at sites other than mesentery
Appendix	seldom positive	occasionally positive (4% *Y. ent.* isolations)
Serology		
Antibody titres		
Acute	high on onset (160–10 240): types I, III, and V specific; types II and IV confirmed by demonstration of residual agglutins after absorption with corresponding groups B and D salmonellae	low or absent
Convalescent	decline rapidly; disappear in 3–6 months if no complications	high (160–10 240); highest in patients with arthritis or erythema nodosum; may persist for years
Histopathology		
Macroscopic		
Appendix	usually normal	usually normal
Mesenteric lymph nodes	multiple, frequently matted, enlarged 1–4 cm diameter; cut surface—fleshy reddish-grey containing yellowish micro-abscesses	enlarged, soft, inflamed may form retroperitoneal mass
Ileum	ileitis not frequent finding (as for *Y. ent*)	ileitis frequent finding: oedematous, congested serosa, hypertrophied Peyer's patches, mucosal ulceration
Microscopic		
Appendix	mild inflammation: occasional micro-abscess	focal ulceration
Mesenteric lymph nodes	characteristic 4-stage micro-abscess formation: 1. lymphoid tissue hyperplasia 2. diffuse reticulocyte (histiocytic) cell hyperplasia 3. multiple epitheloid granulomatous formation with occasional giant cell 4. central coagulative necrosis of granulomas with polymorphonuclear cell infiltration (see Fig. 2)	proliferation of large pyroninophilic cells (basophilic stem cell hyperplasia) correlating with antibody response; no characteristic micro-abscesses or giant cells
Intradermal test	positive: raised, indurated, erythematous zone 1–2 cm diameter	no intradermal test available

Although many cases of *Yersinia* infection do well, the fact that occasionally septicaemia, intra-abdominal sepsis, or severe terminal ileitis may occur points to the need for antibiotic therapy in some cases. Both *Y. pseudotuberculosis* and *Y. enterocolitica* are sensitive to a wide range of antibiotics including tetracycline, streptomycin, chloramphenicol, colisitin, and sulphonamide. Most strains of *Y. pseudotuberculosis* are sensitive to benzylpenicillin, ampicillin, and cephaloridine, while the β-lactamases of *Y. enterocolitica* render it resistant to these antibiotics.

Pasteurella infections

Of the seven species which constitute the genus *Pasteurella* only *P. multocida* is of medical importance. Although both *P. pneumotropica* and *P. ureae* have been cultured from the human respiratory tract, and *P. pneumotropica* from dog bites, their role as human pathogens has not been established.

P. multocida infections in humans have been reported with increasing frequency during the last 15 years, and the majority have been associated with wound infections caused by a dog or cat bite, or following scratches by a cat. The organism forms part of the normal flora of the upper respiratory tract in many animals and is presumably inoculated directly into the bite. In cases unrelated to animal bites, infection of the respiratory tract predominates. Less frequently encountered infections caused by *P. multocida* include septicaemia and bacteraemia, meningitis, otitis, pyogenic arthritis, brain abscess, pyelonephritis, endocarditis, and peritonitis.

Wound infections. Although most cases are not serious, a small proportion of patients have fairly severe infections characterized by considerable cellulitis, a prolonged course, slow healing, and a tendency to underlying bone necrosis despite intensive antibiotic therapy. The local tissue necrosis which is a feature of many of these wounds may leave the patient with an ugly scar. For this reason dog and cat bites should not be treated lightly, especially in the case of children who are liable to be bitten about the face.

Respiratory infections. It is difficult to assess the pathogenic significance of *P. multocida* in respiratory infections. With the exception of a few patients with empyema and lung abscesses, almost all the patients in this category suffer from chronic bronchitis or bronchiectasis. The isolation of the organism from the purulent sputum of such cases is not necessarily an indication of its pathogenicity. It has been suggested that *P. multocida*, like *P. pneumotropica* and *P. ureae*, may be a secondary invader colonizing an already damaged bronchial tree. It is probable, however, that its presence has some effect on the course, severity, and duration of the established disease.

Treatment. Antibiotic susceptibility studies indicate that penicillin G, ampicillin, carbenicillin, cephalothin, tetracycline, and chloramphenicol are the most active drugs against *P. multocida*. Erythromycin, oxacillin, and methicillin are less active than the above agents. However, abscesses, if present, usually do not heal without surgical incision and drainage even if antibiotics are given.

References

Bottone, E. J. (1977). Yersinia enterocolitica: a panoramic view of a charismatic microorganism. *Crit. Rev. Microbiol.* **5**, 211.

Carter, P. B., Lafleur, L., and Toma, S. (eds.) (1979). Yersinia enterocolitica. *Contributions to microbiology and immunology* **5**. Karger, Basel.

Winblad, S. (ed.) (1973). Yersinia, pasteurella and francisella. *Contributions to microbiology and immunology* **2**. Karger, Basel.

Anthrax

A. B. Christie

Anthrax in the Greek means coal, as does charbon in the French, and both words have been used for the disease in man that is characterized by a sore with a coal-black centre. Man may get his anthrax sore directly from his animals, if he lives closely enough to them, goat-herds, or shepherds wandering over arid plains and hills. Or he may get it indirectly, in the more developed world, from hides, wool, hair, or bones sent thousands of miles across the world from animals which died of the disease. We must look at the bacillus of anthrax, how it persists in nature how it then finds its way through commercial and industrial processes from the dead animal to man, and finally, how the bacillus, surviving these hazards, overcomes the resistance of the human host and causes one or other of the clinical forms of anthrax in man.

Bacteriology

Anthrax bacillus. *Bacillus anthracis* is a Gram-positive, non-motile, rod-shaped organism 3–8 μm long and 1–2 μm broad. The ends are sharply cut off and there is a central non-bulging spore. Spores form only in the presence of oxygen. In the animal body the bacilli occur in pairs or short chains, but on agar plates they form long chains like filaments. On serum agar, or in excess CO_2, the bacilli are surrounded by a capsule, and this has to do with virulence. An anthrax sore on man or the blood of an animal is full of bacilli, and they can usually be seen on stained direct smears; this often being enough to confirm a clinical diagnosis. The organisms grow freely on agar forming large rough colonies. In gelatin stab cultures, they grow downwards like an inverted fir tree. Spores do not form on plain agar, but on oxalated agar they form in abundance.

Bacillus and spore. The vegetative bacillus is not a hardy organism, and finds it difficult to survive in nature in competition with true saprophytes, especially the organisms of putrefaction. If an animal dies of anthrax and its body is left lying in summer heat at a temperature of 28–30 °C, no anthrax bacilli will be found in it after three or four days, for the organisms of putrefaction will have overwhelmed *B. anthracis*. But if the temperature is between 5–10 °C, then putrefaction will not have set in, and anthrax bacilli will still be present after three or four weeks. If anthrax bacilli escape from a carcass and the outside temperature is over 20 °C and the humidity high, the bacilli form spores quickly in the free oxygen and will survive in pasture; if the temperature is low they form spores only slowly and are unable to compete with more robust soil organisms. These differences may have much to do with the ability of anthrax bacilli to persist in pasture in hot or cold climates.

The spore is highly resistant and can survive for years. In one investigation spores were still alive in dry soil in a laboratory after 60 years. Out in open pastures there are seasonal changes of temperature and moisture and competition with other organisms, all of which affect survival, but there is no doubt that spores can survive in warm moist pastures and kill animals that graze there the following year. These carcasses can then re-infect the pastures and lead to permanent anthrax districts. A great deal depends also on the standard of animal husbandry. If the carcass is burned or buried deep at once, there is little risk of contamination of pasture: but if the carcass is left where the animal falls, as is common in some parts of the world, anthrax spores are very likely to contaminate the land. Pasteur held that spores could survive on the surface of dry soil for 12 years.

If *B. anthracis* spores can survive for these long periods on dry soil, it is not surprising that they can also survive on animal hair, wool, hides, bones, or any other contaminated material, and the *B. anthracis* can in this way be transported from one side of the world to another, causing disease in man far away in time and place.

Effect of heat and disinfectants. Dry heat at 150 °C for one hour, or boiling for 10 minutes may destroy spores, but the only reliable treatment is autoclaving at 121 °C for 15 minutes, and even then penetration of bulky wool, hair, and bedding must be complete. Spores survive any amount of freezing and thawing. One must be very careful with disinfectants; because some may be bacteriostatic only. Oxidizing agents seem best: potassium permanganate 4 per cent for 15 minutes, or hydrogen peroxide 4 per cent for an hour. Formaldehyde has been used successfully in commercial disinfection. In a stable or cowshed straw, manure, and other organic material can interfere with disinfection, and in a contaminated area these are best burned before chemicals are applied. In hospitals, old bedding and bed clothes should be used for patients and burned after use.

Pathogenesis and disease in animals. Herbivores suffer most often, for they graze the ground where anthrax spores linger. The spores germinate quickly after being swallowed, and the vegetative bacilli emerge and become capsulated. If the animal is fairly resistant, such as the dog, pig, or rat, the bacilli lose this capsule quickly and die, but in susceptible animals, cattle, sheep, and goats, for example, the capsule persists and probably prevents phagocytosis. The capsulated bacilli then produce a lethal factor, which can be demonstrated experimentally in guinea pigs; this lethal factor seems to overcome the defences of the body and allows the bacilli to multiply exceedingly fast and invade many organs, especially the spleen. (In guinea pigs anthrax bacilli may outnumber the animals' red blood cells.) Septicaemia is not the sole cause of death. The toxin or lethal factor seems able directly to affect cerebral electrical activity, including the action of the respiratory centre, and this leads to anoxaemia, hypertension, cardiac collapse, and sudden death. An apparently healthy animal suddenly 'falls' from anthrax. A rare apoplectic form of the disease occurs also in man.

The disease in animals can be of this sudden, dramatic nature for cattle, sheep, and goats. More often it takes a less fulminating form. The animals are excitable at the start, then depressed. They tremble, stagger, or convulse and show signs of cardiac or respiratory distress. They may have swellings on various parts of the body and bleed from any orifice. They are usually dead after a few days, mortality in cattle, sheep, and goats ranging between 70 and 100 per cent. Horses are equally susceptible, but pigs and dogs are more resistant and tend to suffer from a pharyngeal, choking type of illness from which they may recover after a few days. The pig may suffer from a chronic intestinal infection. Cats also suffer and die from choking if they eat contaminated meat.

Animals vary in their susceptibility: elephants have died in zoos and their carcass meat has given the disease to other animals. Bears, tigers, lions, raccoons, and badgers have all been infected and died from anthrax in zoos, usually from being fed contaminated meat. How much of this occurs in the wild is not known. Birds seem to be highly resistant, though they may act as carriers: *B. anthracis* has been grown from the faeces of eagles and from the crops of sparrows. Frogs, toads, and fish can be infected experimentally, but only with difficulty. Mice, guinea pigs, and rabbits are the laboratory animals. They die rapidly from infection, but rats are highly resistant.

Spread from animals. An animal dying of anthrax excretes anthrax bacilli in its faeces, urine, saliva, and any bloody discharges. If its carcass is opened, it can cause heavy contamination of the surroundings, and *B. anthracis* can find its way into pools, ditches, and ponds where it may survive for years as spores. An animal dying in a cowshed or other building can grossly contaminate straw and manure, and *B. anthracis* in this way can get into hay and other feedstuffs and so infect other animals. This can be prevented by good husbandry. In the United Kingdom there may be several hundreds of outbreaks in animals in a year, from imported feed-stuffs, but usually these cause the death of only one animal. Infection does not spread directly from animal to animal.

Man may be infected by close contact with animals. Where anthrax in animals is common, shepherds, goat-herds, and peasants handle sick, dying, or dead animals and may easily rub anthrax bacilli into their skin. Thousands of cases occur annually in some countries in this way. Apart from such close and heavy contamination, man seems highly resistant to infection. As mentioned below workers may carry *B. anthracis* in their nose and have serological evidence of subclinical infection; and in one disinfection station in the United Kingdom, in which *B. anthracis* was regularly isolated from a third of the imported wool and hair handled, men worked

for years without real precautions yet few ever went down with anthrax.

Spread by animal products
Industrial spread. The value of an animal carcass only begins when it dies. Its hide goes to make leather, its wool is turned into clothes, its hair into carpets, mattresses, and paint brushes, its hooves, horns, or bones are crushed to make fertilizer or rendered down to make gelatine and glue. All these parts of the carcass can be contaminated with *B. anthracis* unless the carcass is carefully disposed of. In an advanced agricultural country the carcass will be burned or buried with every precaution, but elsewhere the nomad may skin it where it dies and leave all the parts to dry in the sun. 'Sun-dried' is a commercial term: 'sun-dried' bones are preferred for gelatin and glue production but they may carry anthrax to a distant factory. 'Wet' and 'dry' are also commercial terms for hides: wet hides come from healthy animals killed in abattoirs, dry hides from animals that died in the open, perhaps from anthrax.

There is an enormous trade in hides, wool, hair, and bones: *B. anthracis* spores survive on them and may be transported across the world from arid plains in Iran or China, or from lush pastures in the Argentine to a mill in North America or a tannery in the United Kingdom. Most factory processes kill the spores. Leather, for example, is rarely contaminated, but the raw hides often are. The same is true of the rough wool and hair, terms which cover a wide variety of materials from vastly differing sources, but the finished factory product, the carpet or the cloth, is nearly always free of anthrax bacilli or spores. Bones, hooves, and horns, especially if sun-dried, may be heavily contaminated. There is no good way of sterilizing them before processing, so that workers are exposed to danger from crushed bones or bone dust. The gelatine, glue, and bone charcoal that are produced by processing are sterile, but unprocessed bone meal or hoof and horn meal often are not.

Non-industrial spread. Bone meal and hoof and horn meal are too expensive for widespread agricultural use, but they are commonly used as fertilizers by gardeners and horticulturists, and cases of anthrax do occur in this way. Workers who handle sacks or trucks used for these fertilizers occasionally suffer too. One sculptor probably got the disease from carving statuettes from horse bones. A piano-tuner was said to have been infected from piano keys made of elephant ivory. A plumber was infected by the wadding he used for packing pipe joints. A veterinary student probably infected a cut on his face while examining anthrax slides in the laboratory: live spores were found on some slides stained several years earlier. One man borrowed the scarf of his son who worked in a tannery and was infected on his neck, and there are a few reports of wives contracting anthrax from dust on their husbands' clothes. But most infections in man are from raw, contaminated animal products, and in spite of much exposure, industrial anthrax is an uncommon disease.

Clinical manifestations
Cutaneous anthrax. The anthrax sore begins like an ordinary pimple. This may be all that is seen in a patient who has had anthrax vaccine previously, or in the odd patient with a second attack of the disease. Usually the pimple grows rapidly in two to three days. Its centre ulcerates, but quickly becomes a dry, black, firmly adherent scab, and around it there forms a circle of purplish vesicles (Fig. 1). This is the typical anthrax sore, often called a malignant pustule, although it is neither malignant nor pustular. Indeed if there is any pus the case is almost certainly not anthrax.

There are no other sores quite like the anthrax sore, unless it be the lesion of vaccinia after smallpox vaccination, which comes quite close to it, or the eschar near the flea-bite, which is seen, but very rarely, in plague (see page 5.207).

Oedema. Most anthrax sores are about 2–3 cm across, but some may be up to 6–7 cm. Sometimes, however, the sore may be no more than pin-head in size, as may be the case when there is massive oedema and a tiny sore in its midst. Oedema is typical of anthrax and often extensive. From a primary sore in the neck, oedema may

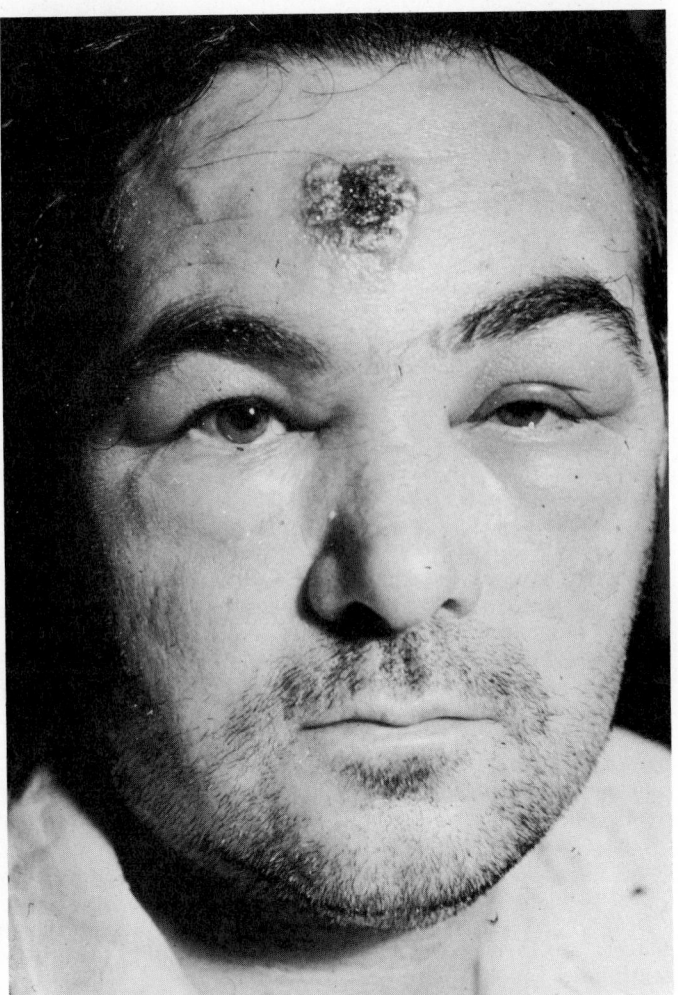

Fig. 1   Anthrax sore showing central eschar and ring of vesicles.

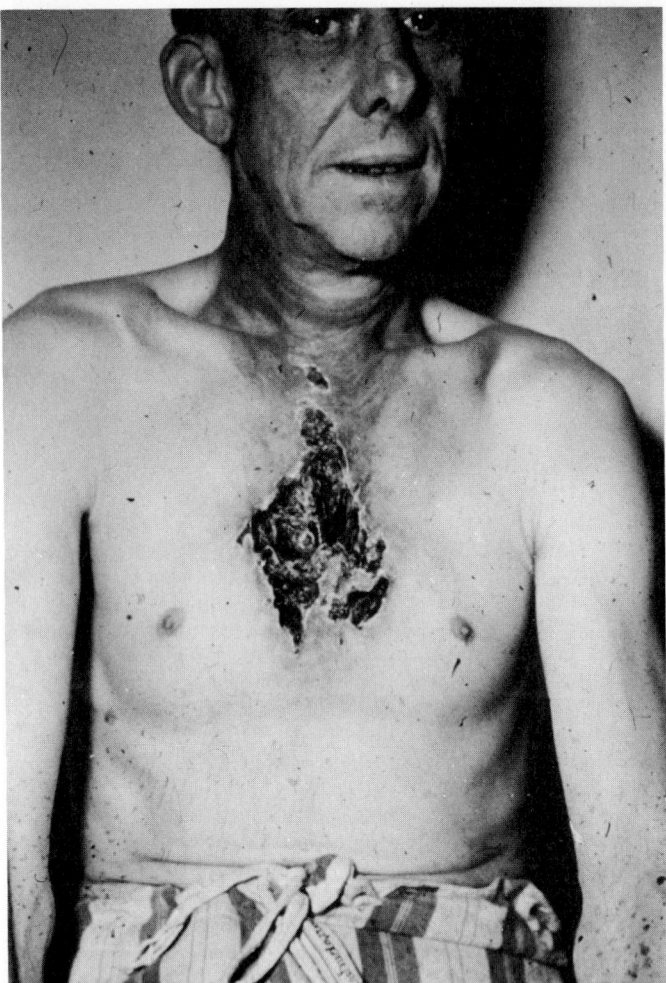

Fig. 2   Anthrax: healing eschar of chest wall. The primary sore was on the back of the patient's neck. Oedema spread from the neck over the chest and abdomen into the scrotum.

spread down over the chest and abdomen, even into the scrotum (Fig. 2). This is the extreme, but there is always swelling around the sore. The oedema is non-pitting, and the skin is usually neither hot nor red. There is no pus beneath the swelling, no abscess to open: the urge to incise it must be resisted. Lymph nodes usually enlarge and may be tender, but here again there is no abcess formation.

Site and type of sores. Sores occur on the part of the body exposed to infection. Porters carrying hides off ships on their shoulders get sores on the head and neck, those who open bales of wool or hair may get them on their forearms. A stiff, sharp hair may pierce a shirt or blouse and cause anthrax on the breast or chest. But the sore may be anywhere. Oddly enough, anthrax on the fingers is uncommon.

Sometimes the vesicles round the sore are large and bullous and filled with blood-stained fluid: the eschar may be quite small. Sometimes there are vesicles but no eschar, and sometimes the vesicles spread widely away from the sore. Sometimes there is an eschar and no vesicles, sometimes only oedema. In the partially immune patient the lesion may look like an innocent pimple. The typical sore, the malignant pustule, looks angry and tender; but usually there is very little local pain.

General symptoms. The amount of illness varies. Chilliness, headache, lack of appetite, and nausea are common. The temperature may be normal, but more often is around 38.3–38.8 °C. In severe cases the patient may have rigors and the temperature reaches 40 °C. A fall to subnormal level in these patients is an ominous sign, as is vomiting, weakness, and a thready pulse. In most cases the illness is not more than moderately severe and responds rapidly to treatment.

Complications. When the sore is on the lower part of the face or on the neck, the oedema may encircle the neck and press on the trachea. Sometimes there is also oedema of the larynx, and these two may make breathing difficult, and tracheotomy must be done to save life. The earlier it is done in such a case the better, for when the oedema is extensive it can be difficult to find the trachea at operation.

Most sores heal and leave little trace, but over the jaw or the eye gangrene may develop, and scarring may be serious and require plastic repair, especially when the eyelid is damaged. Oedema in any part is often very slow to resolve, even when the sore has healed: again the impulse to incise must be resisted. The same is true of the lymphadenitis which may also last a long time.

In cases coming late under treatment and in the rare case that is overwhelming from the onset, collapse of the circulation occurs and the patient bleeds. There may be petechiae on the mesentery and elsewhere, haemorrhagic mediastinitis or massive intestinal haemorrhage. But if a patient comes early under treatment, before he is collapsed and moribund, the illness responds readily to specific treatment. The eschar, on the other hand, may take weeks to separate, though there are no longer anthrax bacilli in it after a day or two of penicillin treatment.

Pulmonary anthrax. In pulmonary anthrax there is no local lesion on respiratory mucous membranes. Anthrax spores are carried in particles of less than 5 μm deep into the lung and from there along lymphatics to mediastinal lymph nodes. There they germinate and

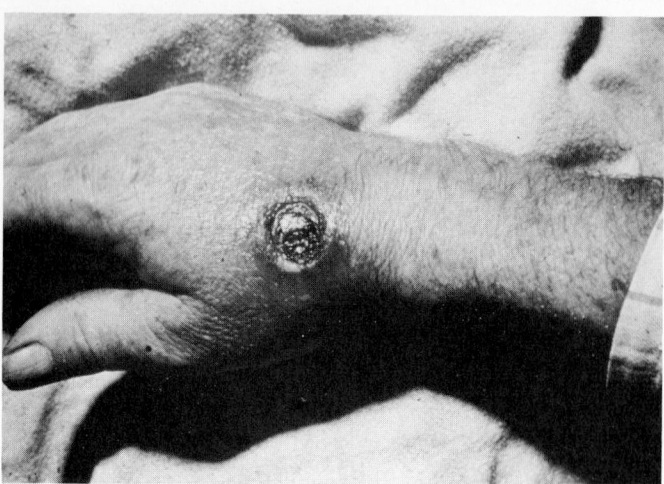

Fig. 3 Anthrax: healing eschar.

release toxin and possibly vegetative bacilli into the bloodstream. Clinically the onset is abrupt with chills and often blood-stained vomit. In an hour or two the patient is dyspnoeic, cyanosed, and acutely ill. His temperature soars, his chest is full of moist sounds, his heart is rapid, and his pulse feeble. His spleen may be enlarged and tender, there may be some tender lymph nodes in the axilla, but there is nothing else to point to the diagnosis, except perhaps his occupation. Untreated he dies in two to three days.

Subclinical cases. It is of course possible that milder cases occur, cases of bronchitis in which the diagnosis of anthrax is not even thought of. Workers in some industries are heavily exposed to anthrax dust: nasal swabs from workers going off duty are often positive for anthrax bacilli and serological tests show that sub-clinical infection must occur.

Intestinal anthrax. Intestinal anthrax may be a cause of acute gastroenteritis, abdominal pain, and prostration, probably from eating the meat of animals which died from anthrax. How common it is in such circumstances is not known, nor how many patients survive, but intestinal anthrax can be a severe and fatal disease. At autopsy glassy oedema of the intestinal wall with an eschar in the centre of it and haemorrhagic swelling of the mesenteric lymph nodes have been seen. At laparotomy on one patient the mesentery was covered with petechiae and there was a typical anthrax sore in the duodenum. This patient recovered; but most patients with severe intestinal anthrax probably die. The literature is scanty.

Other forms of anthrax. Anthrax meningitis is rare. It may occur as the only manifestation of the infection or as a complication of cutaneous anthrax. The meninges are inflamed and in some parts haemorrhagic. Cerebrospinal fluid may be blood-stained and contain anthrax bacilli. The outlook is poor, though with immediate treatment recovery is possible.

In second attacks and in vaccinated patients, the lesion may be less than 3 mm in diameter, there are no vesicles, no eschar, and no oedema. Anthrax bacilli can be isolated from scrapings of the lesion, but unless one knows the patient's occupation and one's awareness of anthrax risk is high, it is unlikely that such examination of a small pimple will be carried out, and the sore will probably heal undiagnosed.

Diagnosis

Clinical diagnosis. An anthrax sore with black eschar and its ring of vesicles should at once suggest anthrax, especially if there is an occupational risk. In its early pimple stage there is nothing to suggest anthrax except occupation. A boil may look like anthrax, especially if the patient knows of the risk of anthrax at his work and has treated the boil with strong antiseptics, but there is always pus in a boil, never in anthrax. Vaccinia can look very like anthrax; one

doctor's receptionist had what looked like a typical anthrax sore on her hand, but she had been cleaning up after a smallpox vaccination session. A young man had a sore like anthrax on his forehead, but it was vaccinia: his doctor had put stitches in a cut there and a few days later removed them, using the same scissors as he had been opening vaccine vials with. When the eschar is tiny and the vesicles profuse the diagnosis can be easily missed unless the occupational risk is known. Orf is a skin condition sometimes seen in abattoir workers: it is a ragged, raw spreading sore with no eschar and no ring of vesicles, but the occupational factor is, of course, the same. The great clinical difficulty is to think of anthrax: the vast majority of doctors never see a case during a life in medicine.

The clinical diagnosis of the pulmonary form depends entirely on the knowledge of the occupational factor. The factory medical officer should think of it at once in a patient with respiratory distress, but another doctor will not, unless the patient tells him of the risk. (In dangerous trades, there should be posters on factory walls about anthrax in workers.) Intestinal anthrax is unlikely to be diagnosed clinically except in outbreaks associated with eating contaminated meat.

Laboratory diagnosis. Stained direct smears of lesions usually show the Gram-positive rods and this is enough for the clinician: he can do the examination himself in a ward sideroom. Smears of sputum in pulmonary cases are often positive too. Immunofluorescence techniques are more sensitive: they will give positive results even on smears from suspected meat. Culture is easy on serum agar or other more selective media. Blood should be added to broth culture at the bedside and the syringe and needle carefully disposed of. Inoculation of mice or guinea pigs will confirm the diagnosis, but this is not usually required in a typical case. Autopsy should not be performed on an animal dead from anthrax: an ear may be cut off and sent with care to the laboratory. Industrial material such as wool, hair, or bone should be soaked in water for several hours. The supernatant is heated to destroy other organisms but not anthrax spores, and cultures are then made, and guinea pig inoculation done with centrifuged sample.

Treatment. Penicillin is the best antibiotic and resistance is rare. A suitable course is benzylpenicillin 250 000 units six-hourly for four or five days: the sore is probably sterile within 48 hours. In severely toxic or late cases the first doses may be given intravenously. *B. anthracis* is usually sensitive to tetracyclines and chloramphenicol, but there is no need to use these drugs, unless the organism is reported as resistant to penicillin or the patient is truly sensitive to it. In the average cutaneous case there is no need for dramatic or heroic measures as the patient responds quickly.

Local treatment for the sore is not required. The eschar takes a long time, sometimes several weeks, to separate and there is no way of hurrying this. There are no live anthrax bacilli in the sore after systemic treatment with penicillin and no need to keep the patient in hospital until the scab separates. There is usually a pale scar left on the skin. Very occasionally there is damage to the underlying tissue, especially the eyelid and this may require plastic surgery.

In pulmonary, intestinal, or hypertoxic cases penicillin is still the best drug, but the patient needs intensive care as well. In experimental animals death may still occur even when antibiotics overcome the septicaemia, and this may be true of the hypertoxic human case as well. Whether anti-anthrax serum, if available, would help in these cases is unknown: it is certainly not required in the average cutaneous case. When there is much oedema of neck tissues and breathing is threatened, it is wise to do tracheotomy early.

Prevention. In highly developed countries anthrax is not an epizootic disease. An animal may die, infected by imported feed-stuff. Its carcass is burned or buried with every precaution, straw and other materials are burned, and the surroundings are disinfected. Everything is supervised by veterinary experts. But where shepherds and herdsmen roam over miles of arid country with their animals, all this is impossible. Animals may die in their thousands in some areas. The only hope here lies in mass vaccination of animals against anthrax, an immense problem in age-old areas of nomadic culture. Millions of animals have been vaccinated and the disease controlled in South Africa, but where husbandry is primitive the disease remains.

In industry. Industrial anthrax can be prevented by pre-treatment of wool, hair, and other materials: no satisfactory treatment of hides is available. But this pre-treatment is an immense economic problem, and industrial anthrax in man is a rare disease. The commercial processing of materials removes the risk of anthrax from finished products. The risk before processing can best be removed by good factory hygiene, by informed occupational medical cover, by awareness on the part of the workers themselves, and corresponding personal precautions. One exception is bone-meal fertilizer. This is often not processed at all: it should be sterilized before it is put on sale.

Specific prevention. When a case occurs in a place of work, other workers may become anxious. They report with all sorts of pimples and sores. Scrapings of these can be examined directly under the miscroscope, and, if positive, treatment begins at once. To allay fears one must sometimes treat patients with no firm evidence of infection. One injection of combined short- and long-acting penicillin can be given, 300 000 units of benzylpenicillin and 900 000 units of benzathine (long-acting) penicillin. Anti-anthrax serum should not be used. It may cause severe reactions, yet give no protection.

Vaccine. A vaccine prepared from a sterile filtrate of *B. anthracis* culture precipitated with alum is available and should be recommended for exposed workers. Two doses of 0.5 ml are given at a six-weeks' interval, a third at six months, and then 0.5 ml once every year. This vaccine protects monkeys against challenge with *B. anthracis*, but it is difficult to assess efficacy in man in such a rare industrial disease. Some figures indicate that it is over 90 per cent effective. The vaccine seems not to cause severe reactions and is certainly worth using in exposed workers. But its use should not interfere with improvements in factory hygiene and animal husbandry.

References

Brachman, P. S., Plotkin, S. A., Bumford, F. H., and Atchison, M. M. (1960). An epidemic of inhalation anthrax: the first in the twentieth century. 2. Epidemiology. *Am. J. Hyg.* **72**, 6.
—, Gold, H., Plotkin, S. A., Felety, F. R., Werrin, M., and Ingraham, N. R. (1962). Field evaluation of human anthrax vaccine. *Am. J. Pub. Hlth.* **52**, 632.
Christie, A. B. (1980). In *Infectious diseases: epidemiology and clinical practice*. 3rd edn. Churchill Livingstone, Edinburgh.
Kohout, E., Sehat, A., and Ashraf, M. (1964). Anthrax: a continuous problem in Southwest Iran. *Am. J. Med. Sci.* **247**, 565.
Report of the committee of enquiry on anthrax. Cmnd. 846, HMSO, London.
Sterne, M. (1959). Anthrax. In *Infectious diseases in animals due to bacteria* (eds. A. W. Stapleforth and I. A. Galloway). Butterworth, London.

Brucellosis

E. Williams

The bacterial cause of Malta fever was identified in 1886 by Sir David Bruce. The genus *Brucella*, named after him, can be defined as small, non-sporing, non-motile, Gram-negative coccobacilli or short rods. They are strict aerobes. Growth is poor on ordinary media and is often improved by carbon dioxide. Six species are recognized on the basis of oxidative metabolism and phage susceptibility (Table 1), and within species a number of biotypes can be distinguished using biochemical and serological tests.

Animal reservoirs of infection. Brucella are primarily mammalian parasites. Their natural hosts and some of the regions throughout the world where brucellosis is encountered are listed in Table 1, although its precise global distribution is not known. Host specificity, furthermore, is not exclusive. *Br. abortus* can cause abortion in sheep, orchitis in dogs, and poll evil or fistulous withers in horses. It has been isolated from ticks, bugs, and fleas, and evidence of infection had also been found in animals in the wild far removed from a bovine source.

In the natural host brucellosis is highly contagious. Only in spreading *Br. suis*, *Br. ovis*, and *Br. canis* infection is the male of the host species significantly involved and transmission by secondary hosts is rare. Bovine brucellosis resulting in abortion, failure to thrive, and a low milk yield is economically the most important and is especially a burden on the resources of developing countries where large dairy production units are being assembled in the process of urbanization. So-called 'flying herds', whose cattle are continually replaced to maintain milk production, are often heavily infected.

Disease in humans. All brucella, with the exception of *Br. suis* type 2, *Br. ovis*, and *Br. neotomae*, are recognized human pathogens. Invasion occurs through the abraded skin, the conjunctiva, or the respiratory or gastrointestinal mucosa.

Occupational brucellosis. This is a disease mostly of farmers, slaughtermen, butchers, meat packers, agricultural engineers, and laboratory technicians. When work involves close contact with animals or carcasses, guarding against exposure is difficult, but

Table 1 Brucellosis in animals

Brucella species	Natural hosts	Distribution
abortus types 1–9	cow	worldwide, excluding the following countries where eradication has been achieved: Northern Ireland, Belgium, Netherlands, Denmark, Norway, Sweden, Finland, Luxembourg, Switzerland, Federal German Republic, Austria, Czechoslovakia, Yugoslavia, Romania, Israel, Tasmania, Japan; campaigns well advanced in Britain, USA, Canada, Australia, New Zealand
melitensis types 1–3	goat, sheep	most Mediterranean countries, Iran, Turkey, India, parts of the USSR, Central and South America, Asia, Africa
suis types 1, 3	pig	mid-western States of USA, Central and South America, SE. Asia
type 2*	pig, hare	Denmark and parts of Central Europe
type 4	reindeer, caribou	Arctic Russia and North America
canis	dog	USA, Central and South America, Japan, Germany, Czechoslovakia
*ovis**	sheep	Australia, South Africa, parts of South America, USA, parts of Central Europe
*neotomae**	desert woodrat	Utah, USA

* Not pathogenic for humans
The list of countries where *Br. melitensis* and *Br. suis* are found is not comprehensive. *Br. abortus* type 8 is no longer recognized

inseminators, who are fastidious about asepsis, are usually spared. For veterinary surgeons involved in eradication schemes, accidental self-inoculation or conjunctival contamination with live brucella vaccine is an added risk, a local reaction, mild or severe, being followed in some cases by symptoms of generalized infection (Figs. 1 and 2). Dead vaccines can also cause severe local tissue necrosis.

The risk to public health. A clean herd, when infected, may show a high initial rate of abortion—the dreaded 'abortion storm'. Cows with long-standing brucellosis, on the other hand, can give birth to healthy calves and the producer–retailer of raw infected milk may be unaware of his transgressions although, regrettably, the reverse is often true. Whereas in the United Kingdom it is widely assumed that all milk supplied in bottles or elegant cartons is above suspicion, bottled or cartoned raw milk is labelled 'untreated' and pasteurized milk is labelled 'pasteurized' or, if ultra heat treated, 'UHT'. Though the sale of raw milk from brucella-ridden herds has, belatedly, been made illegal, sale from brucella-free herds remains a vehicle for other serious pathogens.

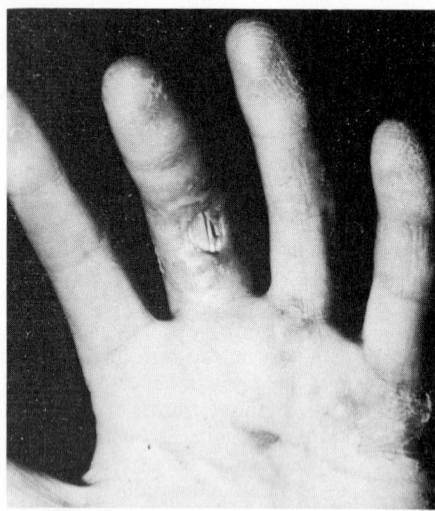

Fig. 1 The hand of a veterinary surgeon after accidental self-inoculation with live brucella vaccine (S19). The tendons of flexor digitorum sublimus and flexor digitorum profundus are exposed. Skin grafting was unsuccessful and the finger was amputated. (From the *Journal of the Royal College of Physicians*, by permission.)

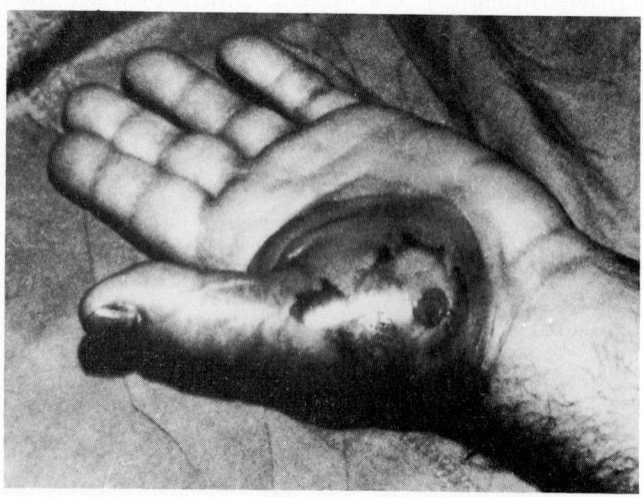

Fig. 2 The hand of a veterinary surgeon 10 days after accidental self-inoculation with brucella S19. A discharging sinus was present for several weeks, and examination five years later showed atrophy of thenar muscles. (From the *Journal of the Royal College of Physicians*, by permission.)

Cream in cartons is now also properly labelled, but when bovine brucellosis was rife in the United Kingdom, clotted cream in buns and doughnuts was a notorious source of human disease. Brucellosis occurs not only in rural areas but in distant towns and cities where infected milk or meat, or their products, are consumed. *Br. abortus* infection acquired in a hotel in central London, for example, was traced to unpasteurized milk supplied from a Hertfordshire farm, and an outbreak of *Br. melitensis* infection, also in London, to imported Italian pecorino cheese. There is no risk of cross-infection and the disease is not sexually transmitted, but it has followed transfusion of blood from infected donors.

The risk from antacids. When brucella are ingested gastric hydrochloric acid is some defence against infection. This is lost by taking antacids. Travellers, known to have achlorhydria or requiring treatment for dyspepsia, therefore, should take extra care in avoiding raw milk, cream, and cheese, especially in regions where caprine brucellosis is enzootic. In such areas antacids should be prescribed only if clearly indicated.

Brucellosis in children. The disease is not rare in children. There is usually a history of contact with animals or farm implements and thus, in the nomadic tribes of Mongolia childhood infection with *Br. melitensis* is common because newborn lambs with adherent placental fragments are brought into tents to be nursed and fondled. Infection, however, can also be acquired from milk, and *Br. melitensis* infection is readily acquired from cheese freshly made from sheep or goat's milk.

Brucellosis and pregnancy. Brucella grow preferentially in the fetal tissues of cow, goat, sheep, and pig because they contain the carbohydrate erythritol. This is not found in the human and abortion or miscarriage in pregnant women, described more often in *Br. melitensis* than *Br. abortus* infection, is arguably no more common than during other severe acute infections.

Brucella, however, are sometimes recovered in products of conception when there is little clinical evidence of maternal disease.

Clinical features. Brucellosis can be acute or chronic in presentation.

Acute brucellosis. The incubation period ranges from under two weeks to several months. In a few patients the illness is short and trivial without immediate or late sequelae, but in the majority it is more severe. Headache, occipital or frontal, intense back pain, and pain in the arms and legs are common, and sweats, typically drenching and dramatic, may be preceded or accompanied by shaking chills and followed by extreme prostration. Even in the absence of sweats, lassitude is a prominent symptom. Other symptoms likely to be misleading, are chest pain worse on breathing, palpitation due to an arrhythmia, abdominal pain with constipation, and confusion with nightmares and somnambulism.

High fever is usual and the spleen is often enlarged and the liver palpable. In *Br. abortus* infection significant lymphadenopathy is an exceptional sign but it may be more common in infection due to other species. Rarely there is a transient erythematous or morbilliform rash, and erythema nodosum has also been described. Symptoms, especially lassitude, may persist for many weeks or months, and convalescence may be slow. Full recovery, however, is likely even from a severe protracted illness and becomes more certain if antibiotics are prescribed.

Relapse can occur after seemingly successful antibiotic treatment. It is sometimes precipitated by another infection or by trauma, accidental or surgical, and, when long delayed, may be indistinguishable from re-infection. In comparing the three main brucella species as human pathogens *Br. suis* and *Br. melitensis* are often more virulent than *Br. abortus*. *Br. abortus* infection, however, can also be fulminating and life-threatening especially when resistance is low. Few examples of *Br. canis* infection have been described. Most of the patients have been laboratory workers, dog owners, or dog handlers, and the illness has been brief and uncomplicated.

Chronic brucellosis. Estimates of the incidence of chronic brucellosis in high risk areas after cursory enquiry can be inaccurate. It is missed when the weary smallholder with demanding cows to milk but without help denies ill-health or seems inarticulate, unable to describe his symptoms properly. But mistakes are less likely if the diagnosis is kept in mind and the patient's family is questioned. The onset may be insidious or it may follow an acute attack, untreated or inadequately treated. Commonly there is a story of recurring 'flu' with lassitude, headache, pain, and sweats. Lassitude is mild, allowing work, or disablingly severe. Mild lassitude, sometimes described as breathlessness, may not seem undue, but on closer questioning the patient owns that he must rest from time to time, especially after heavy tasks, and that in the evening when work is done he sleeps in his chair. In some, a compelling need for sleep after lunch is a significant new symptom. Headache is frontal or retro-orbital, and may be wrongly attributed to sinusitis. Low back pain is common, unassociated with radiological evidence of spondylitis, and limb pain or stiffness is more often muscular than articular, and more often proximal than distal. Sweats occur especially on effort and also at night, and when the diagnosis seems certain but the patient denies nocturnal sweats, his wife should be asked, for it may happen that she alone is disturbed.

Dizziness after a severe sweat is accompanied by faintness and fatigue, but occurring alone its significance as a symptom of chronic brucellosis may not at first be recognized. The victim of long-standing undiagnosed infection has cause to be anxious and dispirited, especially the farmer without help who must also bear the cost of an infected herd. Suicidal depression, however, is rare.

Despite the epithet 'undulant fever' temperature recordings in patients admitted for observation are usually normal. Weight loss is not invariable and the patient may look deceptively well, though usually his appearance suggests serious underlying disease. As in acute brucellosis, moderate splenomegaly is the only noteworthy sign. It is present in a minority, not always the most severely ill, and it may persist long after effective cure. When the spleen is very large—more than four fingerbreadths below the costal margin—another cause must be sought.

Complications. These can occur during either phase of the infection in patients already under surveillance. Many, on the other hand, present with complications. The commonest are skeletal, cardiovascular, neurological, and genito-urinary but no system is immune.

Skeletal. Lesions in bones or joints were found in 10 per cent of patients in one large series. Infection in brucella spondylitis begins anteriorly in an intervertebral disc and spreads to contiguous vertebral bodies. The lumbar spine is usually involved, radiographs showing disc space narrowing with simultaneous bone destruction and repair. Paravertebral abscesses may form and evidence of new bone formation is then helpful in excluding tuberculosis. Spurs on the anterior surfaces of adjacent vertebrae—the parrot's beak sign—are not diagnostic, for this appearance is common also is osteoarthrosis. Other sites of osteitis are the long bones and the bones of the hand. Suppurative arthritis is usually monarticular, involving a hip or some other weight-bearing joint, although in chronic brucellosis a painful swollen knee is more often due to bursitis or synovitis.

Cardiovascular. Cardiovascular complications include thrombophlebitis, which is common, and endocarditis and endaortitis which are rare. Thrombophlebitis in the brain or the eye can be permanently disabling and pulmonary embolism from a femoral vein has resulted in death. Endocarditis and end-aortitis, if untreated, are invariably fatal.

Neurological. Diagnosis is elusive especially when the nervous system is involved. Encephalitis with headache, convulsions, and raised intracranial pressure can masquerade as a brain tumour, and when the patient at first shows no abnormal signs the significance of changes in mood and behaviour due to an organic psychosis may be missed. Rupture of a mycotic aneurysm is a rare cause of sub-arachnoid haemorrhage. Usually the cerebrospinal fluid shows a lymphocytic pleocytosis, an increase in protein and a fall in glucose concentration and it may appear xanthochromic. Tuberculous meningitis can be simulated if symptoms are progressive. On the other hand a long disabling illness, punctuated by unexplained remissions, may be wrongly assumed to be non-infective.

In acute brucella meningitis recovery in response to treatment is rapid. In chronic meningitis with damage to nerve roots by adhesions and inflammatory infiltration also of brain and spinal cord, the outcome is usually less favourable. Paraplegia due to brucella meningomyelitis is sudden or gradual in onset. It can also be due to an extradural abscess, and then the likely source of the infection is the spine. Infective polyneuritis is a rare complication. When symptoms suggest single nerve involvement, other causes must be carefully excluded. Sciatica in patients with chronic brucellosis, for example, will follow protrusion of an uninfected intervertebral disc.

Isolation of *Br. abortus* from a ventriculo-atrial shunt in a child with hydrocephalus has recently been reported. He had presented with fever, the shunt was removed, and his recovery was uninterrupted.

Genito-urinary. Acute unilateral epididymo-orchitis is relatively common. It occurred in six of 102 veterinary surgeons in one reported series, and in two it recurred. Testicular atrophy was not a sequel. Tubo-ovarian infections are rare. When renal failure complicates brucella endocarditis, it is relentlessly progressive. It can also be due to interstitial nephritis or pyelonephritis.

Pulmonary. Pleural effusion or pneumonia is an uncommon manifestation of severe acute infection. A lung abscess may form after pulmonary infarction and consolidation has also been recognized as an incidental finding in the later stages of brucella endocarditis. When chronic lung infection with *Br. suis* becomes localized, it may show on radiographs as a discrete peripheral shadow and differentiation from carcinoma will be required.

Certain other described examples of so-called pulmonary brucellosis are likely to have been coincidental. Thus bilateral hilar adenopathy followed by progressive pulmonary fibrosis, typical of sarcoid, was at one time attributed to brucellosis and a claimed causal relationship between this disease and pulmonary eosinophilia is also unconfirmed.

Ocular. Diplopia or amaurosis is the result of oculomotor or optic nerve damage but disturbance of vision in brucellosis can also be due to direct involvement of the eye. Nummular keratitis, retinal thrombophlebitis, and uveitis are rare complications during the acute or the chronic stage of the illness. When they occur long after recovery in patients showing little or no residual serological evidence of infection, a diagnosis of ocular brucellosis is at best presumptive.

Intra-abdominal suppuration. Suppuration is associated with *Br. suis* infection and occurs usually in the liver or spleen. Another organ or a group of lymph glands can also be the site of abscess formation with spread to surrounding tissues, and cholecystitis, acute or chronic, has been described. Discrete or confluent foci of calcification may appear in chronic abscesses, showing in the spleen on radiographs as typical 'snowflake' or 'target' shadows. Calcification, however, does not signify healing for such lesions of very long-standing have been found to contain viable brucella organisms. In *Br. melitensis* infection demonstrable calcification in areas of necrosis is unusual.

The liver in brucellosis. Although the liver is often palpable in acute brucellosis, clinical or laboratory evidence of functional impairment is rare, and when jaundice occurs it can be a misleading sign. The typical lesion on liver biopsy is a histiocytic granuloma (Figs. 3 and 4). It has no special diagnostic feature although large granulomas undergoing caseation are more in favour of tuberculosis, and extensive hyaline fibrosis of a mature granuloma is characteristic of sarcoid. In acute brucellosis other inflammatory changes include portal tract infiltration and Kupffer cell hyperplasia and, especially in *Br. suis* and *Br. melitensis* infection, there

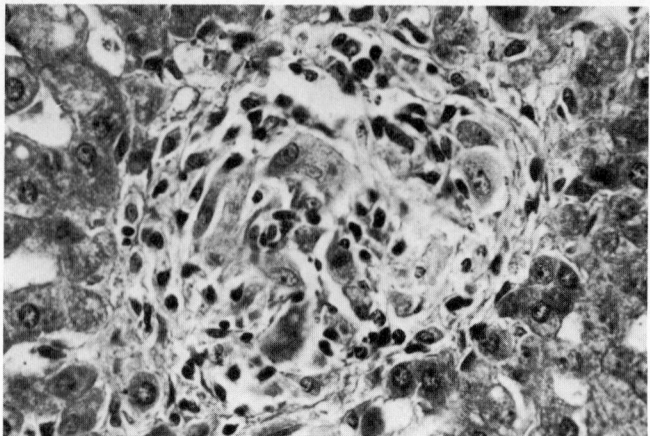

Fig. 3   A liver biopsy showing a small parenchymal granuloma consisting of histiocytes and multinucleate cells with a rim of lymphocytes. The patient was a young veterinary surgeon with mild acute brucellosis (⅗ of ×520.)

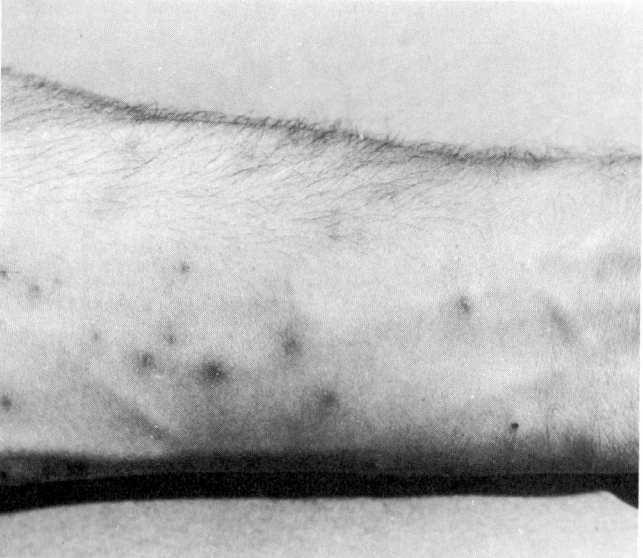

Fig. 5   A veterinary surgeon's forearm three days after he had delivered a stillborn calf. He had not worn protective gloves. Such papular and pustular calving rashes have been attributed to brucella allergy. In this case the cause was *Salmonella dublin* dermatitis.

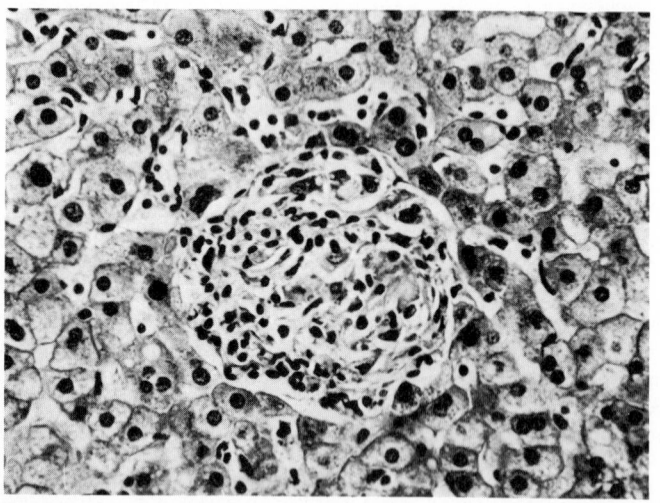

Fig. 4   A liver biopsy showing a small parenchymal granuloma and intrasinusoidal inflammatory cell infiltration. The patient was a farmer ill for eight months with brucellosis (⅗ × 520.)

may be widespread focal necrosis. *Br. suis* is also a cause of liver abscess.

Hepatic granulomas are often found in chronic brucellosis and also sometimes in patients who have become symptom free. When the cause of symptoms is uncertain, therefore, demonstrating scanty granulomas in a liver biopsy is of limited diagnostic value. Mild portal tract fibrosis is common in brucellosis but cirrhosis is rare. Patients who present with cirrhosis addiction to alcohol, itself a risk in long-standing infection, must be excluded.

The skin in brucellosis. The rare exanthems of acute brucellosis have already been mentioned. Papular and pustular rashes on the arms of veterinary surgeons after obstetric procedures have traditionally been attributed to brucella allergy, based on scanty observations made when enrichment and selective media were not available. Some rashes, however, typical of so-called brucella allergy, are infective, due to serious bovine pathogens other than *Br. abortus*—including *Salmonella dublin*, *S. typhimurium*, and *Listeria monocytogenes* (Fig. 5). They are mostly trivial and smaller lesions may not even be recognized unless carefully sought. Their significance is in confirming that man is a potential vector of certain zoonotic diseases.

An infective follicular brucella dermatitis has not been described although *Br. suis* can cause widespread indolent skin ulceration.

Laboratory tests in diagnosis. Mild granulopenia can occur in

acute brucellosis and lymphocytosis in chronic brucellosis. Examination of peripheral blood, however, is usually unhelpful. It is even misleading when, in the acute illness, atypical lymphocytes are wrongly attributed to glandular fever. Rare but important haematological findings are anaemia due to hypersplenism and thrombopenia causing haemorrhage even in otherwise asymptomatic patients. Erythrophagocytosis during severe acute infection has also been observed, with marrow changes mimicking malignant histiocytosis. The erythrocyte sedimentation rate is often moderately raised in acute brucellosis. It is usually normal in uncomplicated chronic brucellosis.

Bacteriological tests. Despite the use of media enriched with essential vitamins and other nutrients, efforts to grow *Br. abortus* from blood, even during severe acute infection, usually fail. Several attempts should be made, however, allowing an incubation period of at least six weeks. The organism can sometimes be isolated from bone marrow when blood culture is unsuccessful, and also from liver obtained by biopsy but this should not be attempted routinely. In *Br. suis* and *Br. melitensis* infection confirmation by blood culture is the rule. Examination of material from lesions in bone and elsewhere has often led to an unsuspected diagnosis, but in all forms of brucellosis when the clinical diagnosis seems certain, treatment should not be delayed to await bacteriological confirmation.

Serological tests. These tests (Table 2) reflect changes in immunoglobulins IgG, IgA, and IgM. IgM and IgG antibodies appear during acute infection, and IgG and IgA but not IgM are present during chronic infection and also when immunity is repeatedly stimulated by exposure to brucella antigen. The four tests commonly used are: (*a*) standard agglutination test; (*b*) standard agglutination test with added 2-mercapto-ethanol; (*c*) antihuman globulin test; and (*d*) complement fixation test. Most agglutinating antibodies are IgM but some are IgG or IgA, 2-mercapto-ethanol destroys the agglutinating ability of IgM, the antihuman globulin test correlates closely with IgG concentration, and both IgM and IgG can achieve complement fixation.

The great majority of patients with acute brucellosis soon show strongly positive results in all four tests. In a few they are negative for several weeks and then (*c*) and (*d*) may become positive before (*a*) and (*b*). Very rarely tests for antibodies are consistently nega-

Table 2 Some examples of serological tests in brucellosis

Standard agglutination	2-mercapto-ethanol	Antihuman globulin	Complement fixation	Remarks
0	0	0	0	farm boy, age 13; acute brucellosis; splenomegaly with fever and abdominal pain of five weeks' duration; two weeks later all tests became strongly positive and liver biopsy showed brucella granulomas
0	0	5120	80	girl, age 9; acute brucellosis; splenomegaly with symptoms of six weeks' duration; later all tests became positive; the daughter of an agricultural engineer, she had played with farm implements
5120	2560	5120	80	head cowman with acute brucellosis, a week after being crushed against an iron gate by a stampeding herd; symptoms recurring for seven years; ? relapse due to trauma
0	0	320	160	veterinary surgeon with fever, headache, and cough productive of purulent sputum; he had psittacosis
1280	1280	> 5120	> 320	farmer's son, age 21; symptom free; his father had presented with acute brucellosis
160	160	> 5120	> 320	practising veterinary surgeon, age 75; he claimed that he had never been ill

The reciprocals of the dilutions are shown

tive even in bacteriologically confirmed infection, although in one such case a response was shown by radio-immunoassay. After treatment tests, especially (c) and (d), may remain positive long after recovery. On the other hand, symptoms may persist when serological evidence of infection has disappeared. Progress, therefore, must be assessed clinically and not according to the laboratory findings.

In individuals still exposed to brucella antigen, serological tests are often strongly positive regardless of symptoms. For example, in veterinary surgeons treating infected animals or administering brucella vaccine, such findings are of no value in diagnosis. Tests are most helpful in acute non-occupational disease especially when antibodies are found in rising titre. There is no advantage in performing all four tests routinely. A combination of the standard agglutination test and the complement fixation test will suffice, and in field surveys a sensitive card test is useful in screening for agglutinating antibodies.

Antigens A and M are common to the three main brucella species. In the typical *Br. abortus* strain (type 5, once confusingly called 'British melitensis' is an exception) there is more A than M, in the typical *Br. melitensis* strain there is more M than A, and *Br. suis* closely resembles *Br. abortus* in its antigenic composition. The prepared antigen for serological testing is a suspension of brucella organisms. Though ideally in all countries it should consist of the predominant species, when another is used an antibody response to infection is unlikely to be missed. When, for example, the cause of the infection is *Br. abortus* type 1, tests with *Br. melitensis* antigen will be positive. Similarly in *Br. melitensis* infection and in *Br. abortus* type 5 infection, an antibody response will be shown to *Br. abortus* type 1 (Table 3). In order to confirm infection with *Br.*

Table 3 The results of serological tests using Br. abortus antigen (a) and Br. melitensis antigen (b)

Tests	Case 1		Case 2		Case 3	
	(a)	(b)	(a)	(b)	(a)	(b)
Standard agglutination	640	320	640	1280	160	320
Antihuman globulin	1280	640	5120	10240	640	1280
Complement fixation	160	0	128	256	16	16

The reciprocals of the dilutions are shown
Case 1 Acute brucellosis due to *Br. abortus*, type 1
Case 2 Fatal brucella endocarditis due to *Br. abortus*, type 5
Case 3 Acute brucellosis due to *Br. melitensis*, type 1
A slight variation in response is shown but the tests are positive using both antigens. (Details of cases 2 and 3 supplied by Dr R. W. D. Turner, Edinburgh and Dr J. H. Ross, Hereford)

canis, on the other hand, an antigen consisting of a suspension of this organism must be used.

Non-specific agglutination has been attributed to the use of suspensions of brucella organisms which are not absolutely smooth and it may then occur even in normal serum. A strong serological cross reaction however exists between smooth brucella strains and *Yersinia enterocolitica* serotype 9 (see page 5.213). It has been noted especially in Finland where yersiniosis is a familiar disease and brucellosis is no longer enzootic. Cholera vaccine is another unusual cause of false positive results in serological tests.

Skin tests. The antigen used to demonstrate delayed cellular hypersensitivity in brucellosis consists either of a sterile filtrate of a culture of brucella organisms (Brucellin) or a purified extract. It is injected intradermally and the test is positive if local redness with induration is present after 24 to 48 hours. This procedure gives no useful information which cannot be obtained from serological tests. Furthermore, later interpretation of these tests is compromised for the antigen can itself provoke an antibody response or a significant rise in a pre-existing response.

Treatment. Brucella are intracellular pathogens relatively inaccessible to agents of proven efficacy *in vitro*. Prolonged treatment may, therefore, be necessary to achieve permanent cure. Most patients will respond to oral tetracycline 0.5 g six hourly for six weeks together with intramuscular streptomycin 1 g daily for the first three weeks, although in severe infection tetracycline should be continued for at least another six weeks. At first a brisk febrile reaction may occur but it is not a reason to alter treatment. An intravenous infusion of cortisol can be given if toxaemia is severe and is essential if the rare complication of thrombopenia is a cause of bleeding.

Treatment with tetracycline is usually well tolerated. Infrequently the dose must be halved to prevent diarrhoea and other gastro-intestinal symptoms, but the advantage of prescribing costly tetracycline derivatives which are more easily absorbed and more able to penetrate cells is unconfirmed. Some are more likely to cause photosensitization. Streptomycin should be withheld in the elderly and in patients with labyrinthine disease and when resistance to this antibiotic is confirmed or suspected another aminoglycoside, for example netilmicin or kanamycin, may be a suitable alternative.

Co-trimoxazole is preferred in many countries where *Br. melitensis* is enzootic. The relapse rate is high when it is given for less than a month and low after a prolonged course of treatment. Co-trimoxazole three tablets twice daily can be given for two weeks followed by two tablets twice daily for a minimum period of six weeks, (each tablet contains trimethoprim 80 mg and sulpha-methoxazole 400 mg). This preparation is effective in some patients who have relapsed after treatment with tetracycline but in others the reverse is true. Side-effects of co-trimoxazole necessitating its withdrawal have been an irritating skin rash and dyspepsia.

Rifampicin has been evaluated in laboratory animals but experience in the treatment of human infection is limited. It is best prescribed in combination with tetracycline or co-trimoxazole.

Experience in Mediterranean and Latin American countries suggests that rifampicin is a valuable addition to treatment. In a dose of 600–900 mg daily it is best combined with tetracycline or co-trimoxazole. As with other drugs, there is a significant chance of relapse when it is given for only three weeks.

When patients whose symptoms have been attributed to chronic brucellosis fail to improve the use of vaccines, levamisole and other agents claimed to enhance immune responses is not recommended. In some it might be advisable to reconsider the diagnosis.

Treatment during pregnancy. Acknowledging that brucellosis may cause abortion or miscarriage, control of infection must be immediate and effective even if symptoms are mild. The toxicity of tetracycline is established but there is no evidence that co-trimoxazole is harmful to the developing human fetus.

Surgical treatment. Complications calling for surgical intervention are osteomyelitis, paravertebral abscess, and various suppurative lesions due to *Br. suis.* Radiographic evidence of splenic calcification is a certain indication for splenectomy and hypersplenism is another. Brucella endocarditis is rarely cured by antibiotics alone. The need to replace the diseased natural or prosthetic valve may become urgent and surgical treatment of aneurysmal brucella aortitis has also been successful.

References

Blobel, H. and Schliesser, Th. (eds.) (1982). *Handbook of bacterial infection in animals.* V. E. B. Gustar Fisher, Jena.

Spink, W. W. (1956). *The nature of brucellosis.* University of Minnesota Press, Minneapolis.

Tetanus

E. B. Adams

Tetanus is a hazard of wounds wherever they may occur because of the wide distribution of the causative organism, *Clostridium tetani.* Like other members of the genus, this Gram-positive bacillus will only grow under anaerobic conditions. Its spores are commonly found in soil and in the faeces of domestic animals; they may also be detected in human faeces. Soil is its main natural habitat, particularly when cultivated and rich in animal manure. *Cl. tetani* may contaminate the human environment from soil or from faeces. Spores can be recovered from clothing, house dust, and even the air of occupied buildings such as hospitals.

The hazard is greatest where ignorance, poverty, poorly developed health services, and a humid climate prevail. These factors may be concerted but often act singly. For instance, there are striking differences attributable to climate alone in the prevalence of tetanus in adjacent parts of southern Africa. The disease is rare in Lesotho, a mountainous region which is dry and cold, but common in coastal Natal, which is hot and humid. In a review of the global situation it was estimated that at least a million people had tetanus during the ten-year period 1951–60 and half of them died. The prevalence is greatest in the developing countries. Large numbers of cases are reported from India, and there are considerable national statistics from elsewhere in Asia, such as 1565 deaths over a two-year period in Indonesia and 445 deaths in one year in Turkey. These figures, and large series of cases emanating from Africa and South America, give some idea of the importance of tetanus as a major killing disease. As might be anticipated from the more advanced immunization programmes practised in many parts

of Europe and in North America, the incidence of the disease is much lower in the developed countries; but other factors such as industrialization, urbanization, the mechanization of agriculture, the replacement of animal dung by chemical fertilizers, and improvements in education, public health services, and standard of living have also played substantial roles in reducing the incidence of the disease. Nevertheless, tetanus remains a danger to life everywhere since the spores of *Cl. tetani* are almost ubiquitous.

After gaining entry to the body, generally following trauma of some sort, and when anaerobic conditions develop in the wound, the organism produces two toxins, tetanospasmin and tetanolysin. Only the former has clinical effects, reaching the spinal cord or brain by several routes, of which blood spread and retrograde axon transport along peripheral nerves have long been recognized. The toxin is selective in its effects and appears to increase reflex excitability in motor neurones by blocking the function of inhibitory neurones. The toxin may also affect medullary centres. Recent work suggests another route of spread. Toxin may pass along sympathetic fibres and lead to overactivity of the sympathetic nervous system, possibly acting by blocking inhibitory neurones to produce its effects, in much the same way as it leads to motor overactivity.

Clinical features. The great majority of patients with tetanus become infected through minor rather than major wounds. This is presumably because those with the latter almost invariably seek medical care and their lesions are properly cleaned and appropriately treated while minor wounds are often neglected. Some 20 per cent of patients with tetanus, however, have no evidence of a recent wound. The finding of only minor lesions or none at all is therefore no bar to the diagnosis.

Two dominant manifestations characterize this disease: rigidity and reflex spasms. Rigidity occurs in every case but spasms may be absent. The cumulative effect of both phenomena continued over many days leads to an overriding danger of respiratory failure. Because of the central role they play in tetanus, these cardinal features are discussed in advance of an account of its natural history. The diagnosis is made on the observation of rigidity and spasms. The role of each must be appreciated if the disease is to be successfully treated.

Rigidity of muscles shows itself in several ways. When the jaw muscles are stiff, the mouth cannot be fully opened (trismus or 'lockjaw'). Stiffness of the facial muscles alters the patient's expression. A peculiar sneering appearance results from pursing of the lips and retraction of the angles of the mouth (risus sardonicus). Involvement of the pharyngeal muscles causes dysphagia, often an early symptom. Simultaneous neck stiffness, abdominal rigidity, and splinting of the muscles of the back, arms, and legs gives rise to a characteristic ram-rod appearance; and when the sardonic smile is added there can be little doubt about the diagnosis. Shortening of the long muscles of the back may be excessive so that the body is curved backwards and the head fully retracted (opisthotonus).

In newborn infants the arms and legs may be held slightly flexed, with the arms partly crossed over the abdomen and the hands clenched. The tip of the thumb may be seen protruding between the index and middle fingers. The cry is stifled, the face wrinkling up at the same time. Pharyngeal stiffness impairs sucking. The cry and this difficulty at the breast are often the first abnormalities noticed by the mother.

A reflex spasm is a sudden exacerbation of underlying rigidity. It may be mild and last only a second or two, but more commonly a spasm in tetanus is an alarming and dramatic event. Suddenly there is simultaneous contraction of whole groups of muscles, agonists as well as antagonists. The posture of the patient is exaggerated for several seconds before relaxation occurs to the previous tonic state of the muscles. The thorax is splinted during a spasm and until it passes off respiration is impeded or becomes impossible. If, as sometimes happens, spasms follow each other in rapid succession, pulmonary ventilation is seriously impaired and cyanosis results.

There are often excessive secretions in the mouth and nasopharynx so that breathing is not only difficult but also noisy and bubbling, to the patient's obvious distress. Such secretions may be inhaled into the lungs when the spasm is over and the patient gasps for air to make up his oxygen debt. Little areas of atelectasis follow; if the plug is bigger a segment of lung collapses. Since the inhaled secretions are often infected, pneumonia supervenes—a major danger of the disease.

Laryngeal spasm is the most dramatic and perhaps the most dangerous event in tetanus. Airway obstruction compromises gaseous exchange or renders it impossible, cyanosis occurs, and death follows if the spasm does not pass off shortly, or if it is not quickly relieved by medical intervention.

Apnoea may follow repeated spasms or succeed a laryngeal spasm. Sometimes, however, the patient stops breathing for no obvious reason. All these events—repeated spasms impeding adequate respiration, laryngeal spasms, the inhalation of secretions, atelectasis, pneumonia, and apnoeic attacks—contribute to the onset of respiratory failure. This, in reality, becomes the central problem in the management of tetanus.

The natural history of tetanus. Trismus, pain in the neck, and muscle stiffness are usually the first symptoms except in the newborn in whom crying or refusal to suck are reported by the mother as the first signs that something is amiss with her baby.

The incubation period, the time in days between the injury and the first symptom, varies considerably. In neonates, cutting of the cord should be regarded as the injury. In all but the mildest cases the incubation period is generally less than 14 days. Short intervals between injury and first symptom of between four and six days are by no means uncommon, especially in neonates. Occasionally the interval may be only one or two days or, in contrast, as long as three months. The shorter the incubation period the worse is the prognosis. Numerous reports bear this out. In my own experience with non-neonatal patients treated conservatively the case-fatality rate was over 60 per cent when the incubation period was less than nine days, but only 25 per cent when it was nine days or more—and the difference was even more striking in the newborn. In many cases, however, one cannot be sure when the contaminated wound occurred. While it may be obvious, the wound causing tetanus is often trivial and soon heals, leaving behind it little or no evidence of a lesion. The incubation period therefore cannot be relied upon as a guide to prognosis.

If spasms occur, the first may follow shortly after the first symptom or take place many days later. The interval in hours between the first symptom and the first spasm is known as the *period of onset*. It is one of the most important observations in tetanus. As in the case of the incubation period, short periods of onset carry the worst prognoses. In a large series of non-neonatal cases in Bombay the case-fatality rate was 63 per cent for periods of onset under 48 hours but only 22 per cent for periods longer than this. Since the period of onset is more readily determined than the incubation period, it is a better index of prognosis. Patients more frequently remember the time of the first spasm (an alarming event) than the date of the wound and, as has been stated, no wound can be found in an appreciable proportion of patients (20 per cent).

Most cases of severe tetanus run a similar course. Within 48 hours of the first symptom a reflex spasm occurs, followed by another within an hour or so. The interval between spasms shortens progressively and less disturbance seems to give rise to a spasm. The march of events usually quickens over the first three or four days. Spasms become more frequent and are feared by the patient, who in addition is often troubled by secretions in the mouth and upper respiratory passages. The disease generally reaches its peak within three days of the first sign and for the next four or five days the patient remains gravely ill. The first eight days are all-important in tetanus. The great majority of deaths occur during this time. The frequency and severity of spasms are much reduced after the tenth day and rigidity slowly diminishes. Most patients who survive

beyond this time have recovered completely within a month to six weeks.

Spasms play a major part in determining the outcome. Patients with rigidity but no spasms ('mild' tetanus) usually recover, whereas those with frequent and severe spasms often die ('severe' tetanus). In an Indian series of over 4000 cases the case-fatality rate was 50 per cent among those with spasms but only 2 per cent when spasms were absent. There are many patients who have an occasional spasm which is not marked in degree ('moderate' tetanus), a situation which is compatible with a good prognosis in patients treated conservatively. Indeed the case-fatality rates in mild and moderate tetanus (spasms absent or infrequent) are similar and always less than 10 per cent. In contrast, when severe cases (those with frequently repeated spasms) are managed conservatively, death occurs in well over 50 per cent of children and adults, and in more than 90 per cent of neonates.

These points about prognosis are made because of their importance when it comes to choosing the method of treatment, but they need some clarification. It must be admitted that the term 'moderate' tetanus is arbitrary and defies precise definition; it is nevertheless useful in practice. Most cases have declared themselves as regards severity by the end of the second day, but an occasional case behaves otherwise. Although judged first to have mild tetanus, a patient may unexpectedly develop laryngeal spasm many days later; or at a late stage frequent and severe spasms may take the place of the occasional spasm observed in the first few days. In both cases the prognosis must be regarded as having changed from good to bad. While the presence of absence of spasms and their frequency and severity are the most important factors determining the outcome, the incubation period and the period of onset must also be taken into consideration.

Complications. *Respiratory complications.* These play a dominant role in tetanus. They are the commonest and most dangerous features of the disease and pose a major problem in its management. They comprise excessive secretions in the mouth and upper respiratory passages; inhalation of these secretions or indeed anything that happens to be in the mouth (such as food) during a bout of severe spasms; atelectasis; pneumonia; and laryngeal and oropharyngeal spasms.

Cardiovascular complications. They may be observed in about half of the patients with severe tetanus. Tachycardia and sweating have long been recognized as features of the disease and were once believed to be due solely to excessive muscular activity. They persist after total curarization, however, a fact which appears to demonstrate that they are the result of direct autonomic involvement by the tetanus toxin. In some patients there are wide variations in the blood pressure, and terminally they may develop hypotension and a cold periphery. This apparent state of shock is not always due to intoxication of the autonomic nervous system. Gram-negative septicaemia may produce the same clinical picture, infection with these organisms being a constant danger in centres where the total paralysis regimen is practised on a large scale.

Fractures. They are virtually confined to the mid-dorsal region of the spine. Their occurrence depends on the presence and severity of spasms. Simultaneous and powerful contraction of the flexors and extensors gives rise to longitudinal compression of the spine as a whole, forcibly increasing the spinal curvatures. The cervical and lumbar vertebrae escape injury, apparently because they are supported on the inside by the neural arches. The thoracic spine, curved as it is in the opposite direction, is forcibly flexed about a fulcrum in the region of the posterior part of the fifth vertebral body or its neural arch. This compresses and fractures the anterior portion of this and adjacent vertebral bodies, which become wedge-shaped. Despite their frequency in patients whose spasms are poorly controlled, they do not appear to be important. They cause no pain, lead to no neurological sequelae, and heal with little or no deformity. They obviously occur early on in the illness when spasms are most severe, and in those patients who survive what is clearly very severe tetanus, healing of vertebral fractures is helped by the prolonged convalescence in bed enforced by the slow diminution of muscular rigidity.

Causes of death. Morbid anatomical lesions do not explain all deaths in tetanus, but the respiratory system is incriminated in most cases treated conservatively. In a large series of cases in New Orleans managed before the introduction of the total paralysis regimen, death was attributed to pneumonia in just under 50 per cent, atelectasis, aspiration, pulmonary oedema, and asphyxia bringing the respiratory causes of death to almost 80 per cent. Others have confirmed these observations about the overriding importance of pulmonary complications, especially in those patients who survive for many days before succumbing to the combined effects of uncontrolled spasms and lung lesions. In a study of newborn infants with tetanus there was surprisingly little at necropsy to account for death in the first two days, whereas the respiratory complications listed above were common among those dying later. Overwhelming tetanus intoxication of the brainstem is another important factor. It produces swelling of the nerve cells, chromatolysis, perivascular glial nodules, and demyelination. Failure of the respiratory centre with apnoea follows and this is probably a major contributor to early death. Other causes in those treated conservatively are uncontrolled spasms and spasm of the larynx, both of which embarrass respiration, leading to cerebral hypoxia.

Since the introduction of the total paralysis regimen which has saved most of the severest cases of tetanus from early death and minimized the risks of pulmonary lesions, cardiovascular instability has emerged as a significant danger to survival. The syndrome appears to be due to tetanus intoxication of the sympathetic nervous system, with attendant tachycardia and wide fluctuations in blood pressure. These compromise tissue perfusion, brain, heart, and kidneys all being affected and, in failing, contributing to death.

The main causes of death, in summary, are respiratory failure in one form or another, pneumonia and septicaemia, damage to medullary centres by toxin, and cardiovascular instability.

Treatment. Current practice is to give human tetanus immunoglobulin in preference to heterologous antitetanus serum (obtained from the horse). All patients with established tetanus should receive 500 units of human tetanus immunoglobulin on diagnosis, given either intramuscularly or intravenously in accordance with the manufacturer's recommendations. If heterologous antitetanus serum is used, preliminary testing for sensitivity is essential. The dosage is 10 000 units. Intravenous administration is better than intramuscular because the peak blood level may be delayed two or three days after the latter. Previously there was much controversy about the value of heterologous serum in the treatment of tetanus, the arguments for and against its use being almost evenly balanced. The suggestion made by Sherrington in 1917 that intrathecal antitetanus serum was beneficial has been revived and tested in recent years following work reported from Turkey in 1972. It has been claimed that after intrathecal antitetanus serum spasms can be reduced or abolished by the use of diazepam with or without steroids and that the death rate is substantially reduced; but again there is much controversy and the claims at present must be regarded as unproven. If the intrathecal route is decided upon, human tetanus immunoglobulin should be given in preference. It should be noted, however, that either form of antitoxin if stabilized, as it is normally, with a phenolic substance may result in convulsions and permanent nerve damage if given intrathecally.

There are two main forms of therapy. These are drug treatment alone (conservative management) and the total paralysis and mechanical ventilation regimen, the spasms being abolished by curarization. The choice depends on the severity of the disease and the hospital facilities available. The most severe cases of tetanus should undoubtedly be treated in intensive care units equipped to manage patients with respiratory failure. Unfortunately this is a counsel of perfection since such facilities seldom exist in places where the disease is common.

Conservative management. Its aim is to control the rigidity and spasms of tetanus by means of drugs which do not seriously affect respiration. Rigidity can usually be reduced and in many cases spasms may be diminished in frequency and severity. Drugs used include paraldehyde, phenobarbitone, mephenesin, meprobamate, chlorpromazine, and diazepam. While there is admittedly little to choose between them, the combination of chlorpromazine with either diazepam or phenobarbitone is easy to manage and is recommended. Chlorpromazine should be administered intramuscularly in dosages not exceeding 50 mg every four hours in the case of children and adults, and 12.5 mg for neonates. If adequate control is not achieved, diazepam or phenobarbitone may be added up to three times a day. Dosages recommended are 5–20 mg diazepam for children and adults, 2 mg for neonates; and 200 mg phenobarbitone for adults, 100 mg for children, 66 mg for neonates. Drug administration should be by the intramuscular route except in the case of mild tetanus and during recovery from severe tetanus when the oral route is used. If either diazepam or phenobarbitone, given three times a day in addition to chlorpromazine, still fail to control spasms, tracheostomy should be done provided facilities for its management are adequate.

In some centres very much higher doses of diazepam and phenobarbitone than those stated above have been used (without chlorpromazine) in an attempt to control spasms in the severest cases and claims of better results have been made. However, these drugs, being central depressants, may so depress ventilation that mechanical ventilation is required. This must be borne in mind if high dosage conservative management is embarked upon.

Muscular rigidity can certainly be reduced and suffering alleviated by these drugs. What is in considerable doubt is their ability to make any difference to the death rate. Many years ago, after much experience with a variety of conservative regimens, New Orleans workers wrote that 'any type of sedative or hypnotic agent when properly administered so as to avoid respiratory depression has the same effect or lack of effect upon the outcome of tetanus': rather strongly expressed views but probably not far from the truth. There is as yet no convincing evidence from properly conducted clinical trials that one form of drug therapy is superior to any other. What is certain, however, is that good nursing and diligent medical vigilance can do much to lessen the risks of the disease. The patient should not be unduly disturbed since repeated physical examination and other tactile stimuli undoubtedly increase the frequency of spasms; a darkened room and avoidance of noise, on the other hand, do not appear to play a significant part in preventing spasms. Excessive oral secretions should be removed and laryngeal spasms should be watched for and treated with 100 mg chlorpromazine intravenously immediately a laryngeal spasm occurs. Nutrition and hydration must be maintained. Despite doubts about the efficacy of drug therapy as means of increasing the patient's chances of survival, it is the clinician's task to relieve symptoms as well as to cure. Conservative management as outlined above should therefore be used for severe tetanus where tracheostomy and the total paralysis regimen cannot be carried out because of lack of facilities and experience. For all mild and many of the moderate cases (an occasional spasm which is short-lived and mild in degree), conservative treatment is the method of choice because the case-fatality rate is generally well under 10 per cent and the procedures involved in treatment by the total paralysis regimen carry inherent risks of the same order, except in highly sophisticated units.

Tracheostomy. This has a number of advantages in patients with tetanus but it also carries risks which are minimal only in experienced hands. Tracheostomy reduces the dead space by about 100 ml and improves pulmonary ventilation. A major advantage is that it obviates the dangers of laryngeal spasm, which occurs particularly in those who have repeated spasms and in those who have dysphagia. Tracheostomy facilitates the removal of secretions which collect in the trachea and bronchi and it isolates the respiratory tract from the digestive system, thus eliminating the dangers in tetanus of aspirating food or gastric juice into the lungs during or after spasms. Atelectasis and aspiration pneumonia should therefore occur less frequently and pulmonary ventilation should be better. Tracheostomy is an essential part of the total paralysis regimen. It should also be performed in all patients in whom there is initial doubt about the severity of their disease since, apart from the advantages discussed above, it enables the total paralysis regimen to be started without delay should the patient's condition suddenly deteriorate, as sometimes happens after an admission assessment of mild or moderate tetanus. In the absence of facilities for the full total paralysis regimen, however, tracheostomy should only be performed if skilled nursing is available and the medical team is experienced in its management.

Feeding. Patients with mild tetanus (who have no spasms) can usually swallow easily and may be fed by mouth. Patients with spasms should be fed intravenously and this should continue until spasms have diminished to one or two a day—a state seldom reached before the sixth or seventh day after the first spasm. Then, under heavy sedation, a nasogastric tube can be passed, usually without causing spasm of pharynx or larynx. A nasogastric tube can also be passed with safety after tracheostomy.

Total paralysis regimen. Intermittent positive-pressure ventilation was introduced by Danish workers for treating respiratory failure in poliomyelitis and later applied successfully to patients with tetanus by paralysing the respiratory muscles with curare. Where facilities are available, this is now the method of choice for treating patients with severe tetanus. In some centres the death-rate has been reduced to under 10 per cent, but in others, despite much experience with the regimen, death still occurs in some 30 per cent of patients. The best results are obtained where tetanus is relatively rare and intensive care facilities can be employed to maximum effect; poorer results are found where the numbers of patients with severe tetanus are high in relation to the intensive care facilities available. Cardiovascular instability and difficulties experienced in its management also contribute to the less favourable results. Nevertheless, in the 20 years since its introduction, the total paralysis regimen has established itself as a major therapeutic advance.

After preliminary intubation, tracheostomy is performed under local or general anaesthesia. Ventilation is maintained by mechanical means and the patient kept paralysed by repeated doses of d-tubocurarine (curare) or nor-allyl toxiferin (Alloferin). Preference is for intravenous or intramuscular nor-allyl toxiferin, 5–20 mg for children and adults, or 1.25 mg for neonates. The paralysing drug is repeated when spontaneous movements appear. The inspired air, enriched by oxygen, must be humidified. The patient's position must be changed from time to time and the air passages cleared by suction. For these tasks the services of a trained physiotherapist are invaluable. Scrupulous attention must be paid to aseptic techniques throughout the total paralysis regimen. Blood gas analyses are a valuable guide to proper ventilation. Microbiological examination of aspirated secretions, and blood culture help in the choice of antibiotics for pulmonary infections.

It should be remembered that the patient's consciousness is not impaired by the disease, nor by the paralysing drug; and that without hypnotic doses of a sedative (recommended as an adjuvant to the regimen), the patient can follow all that is being done to (and for) him. Realizing his dependence on the respirator, he fears the periods when it is disconnected to enable suction to be carried out through the tracheostomy tube. Injudicious remarks about his progress—or lack of progress—must therefore be rigorously avoided. Feeds consist of a high protein, liquid diet given via a nasogastric tube, and intravenous feeding, as outlined below.

The minimum duration of paralysis is 10 days. It is hazardous to attempt to withdraw the paralysing drug earlier because patients can seldom re-establish adequate spontaneous respiration in a shorter time. It is unnecessary to continue paralysis much beyond 10 days in view of the natural history of the disease. When the patient is swallowing well (generally three to seven days after the last dose of curare), an attempt can be made to remove the tracheostomy tube. This is often successful at the first attempt in children and adults. The procedure takes longer in neonates. In some cases repeated attempts at weekly intervals may be required before the patient can breathe normally.

There are other hazards. Vigilance and proper maintenance of machines should eliminate technical faults but respiratory infections cannot always be prevented. Particular importance must be attached to aseptic measures by the attendant staff, and respirators must be carefully disinfected. Penicillin and cloxacillin are usually effective in Gram-positive infections. Gram-negative and anaerobic infections are less readily controlled and carry a high mortality rate. Gram-negative septicaemia probably accounts for some of the instances of shock to which reference has already been made. Useful antibiotics for such infections are the cephalosporins, gentamicin, and metronidazole.

Sympathetic nervous system overactivity is common in patients with severe tetanus. Its clinical manifestations, already alluded to, are episodes of hypertension alternating with hypotension, tachycardia, and intermittent cold extremities. Fluid balance, moreover, is delicately poised in patients with severe tetanus. Electrolytes need constant monitoring and correction when abnormal. Dehydration may be a problem since insensible fluid loss is high even in patients treated on the total paralysis regimen. Hypotension may thus reflect dehydration, sympathetic nervous system instability, or septicaemic shock. It is not always easy to sort these out and indeed two or more may coexist.

Full laboratory facilities are mandatory if this complicated regimen is embarked upon. Cultures of aspirated secretions and blood culture will help to identify an infective cause of apparent shock or unexplained pyrexia. Close scrutiny of fluid and electrolyte balance will enable imbalance to be recognized and corrected in most cases. The average adult on the total paralysis regimen requires more than 3 litres of fluid a day; daily estimations of blood urea, serum and urine osmolarity, and urinary specific gravity will enable fluid requirements to be met. Measurement of central venous pressure is advisable when large amounts of fluid are needed to prevent dehydration. Blood should be transfused when the haematocrit falls below 35 per cent. In patients with tetanus of such severity, intravenous fluids are also essential to supplement nasogastric feeding. At least one third of the daily intravenous fluid under such circumstances should be given as colloid in the form of blood, plasma, or albumin. If colloid is not included in the fluid given, oedema commonly occurs, especially pulmonary oedema.

In some centres cardiovascular instability poses the major threat to the success of the total paralysis regimen; it has been observed to occur in more than half of the patients with severe tetanus. The complexities of its management have recently been reviewed by Kerr. Unexplained tachycardia may be taken as an early indicator of its development. While beta-blockade with a drug such as propranolol can control fast pulse rates, unopposed alpha-stimulation in the form of hypertension of severe degree may be troublesome. A drug combining alpha- and beta-blocking actions appears to be more rational therapy. Labetolol is the adrenergic blocking agent recommended for this purpose. It should be given intravenously, either intermittently (50–100 mg two- to four-hourly) or by continuous infusion (1–2 mg per minute). The smaller dosages should be used initially. Alternatives to this peripheral therapeutic approach are the use of central depressants such as morphine (in either low or high doses) and general anaesthesia.

Prevention. In no other disease is prevention more rewarding nor its lack more calamitous. Simple measures for minor wounds and prompt and thorough care of major trauma go far towards the prevention of tetanus. Ignorance of these facts is the cause of most cases. Nevertheless, some organisms may remain in wounds despite apparently adequate attention. Added safeguards are therefore necessary in those who have not been properly immunized against tetanus or whose immune status is not known. At present there is no finality to the question of whether cloxacillin (500 mg six-hourly for five days) is preferable to passive immunization. Antitetanus serum (1500 units by intramuscular injection) is still in common use, but since it is prepared from the horse it carries an appreciable risk of hypersensitivity reactions, some of which may be fatal. Preliminary testing for hypersensitivity was once in vogue but in itself may be dangerous. Such heterologous antitoxin should therefore be avoided. Although in short supply in many places and more costly, human tetanus immunoglobulin is a much safer form of passive immunization. The dosage is 250 units, given by the intramuscular route.

Active immunization with toxoid is the surest way of preventing tetanus. If proof is required, the high death rate from tetanus in the First World War, when active immunization was not practised, should be compared with the virtual absence of the disease in the British and American Armies in the Second World War, when immunization with toxoid was routine. Three intramuscular injections, each of 0.5 ml toxoid, should be given, preferably with six weeks between the first two injections and six months between the second and the third. Good immunity is also established by the triple vaccination method commonly used in infancy in which the intervals are usually a month each. After such immunization, protection can be regarded as absolute for the first year and there is limited but highly important partial protection for many years, even without booster doses. Despite this statement, a booster dose (also 0.5 ml) is recommended after a tetanus-prone wound (and most wounds, however minor, are at risk) occurring more than a year after the completion of a full immunizing course. A booster need not and should not be repeated earlier than one year after the last dose.

In areas where tetanus neonatorum is common it is worthwhile commencing a course of active immunization during pregnancy. Although there is generally insufficient time for all three injections of toxoid, two have been shown to reduce the chances of tetanus occurring in the infant after birth. The course can be completed later with profit, ensuring lasting protection for the mother.

Two other points are worth stressing. The first is that non-immune patients given passive immunization after wounds should in addition be persuaded to have the first dose of toxoid immediately and to return at the appropriate times for completion of the full course. The other point is that an attack of tetanus does not confer immunity (since the lethal dose of tetanus toxin is less than the immunizing dose) so active immunization should be practised in all who recover from the disease. The first injection of toxoid should be given during convalescence and the other two at the recommended intervals.

References

Adams, E. B., Holloway, R., Thambiran, A. K., and Desai, S. D. (1966). Usefulness of intermittent positive-pressure respiration in the treatment of tetanus. *Lancet* ii, 1176.
—, Laurence, D. R., and Smith, J. W. G. (1969). *Tetanus*. Blackwell Scientific Publications, Oxford.
Bytchenko, B. (1966). Geographical distribution of tetanus in the world, 1951–60. A review of the problem. *Bull. Wld Hlth Org.* **34**, 71.
Creech, O., Glover, A., and Ochsner, A. (1957). Tetanus: evaluation of treatment at Charity Hospital, New Orleans, Louisiana. *Ann. Surg.* **146**, 369.
Hörtnagl, H., Brücke, T., and Hackl, J. M. (1979). Involvement of the sympathetic nervous system in tetanus. *Klin. Wochenschr.* **57**, 383.
Kerr, J. (1979). Current topics in tetanus. *Intensive Care Med.* **5**, 105.
—, Corbett, J. L., Prys-Roberts, C., Crampton-Smith, A., and Spalding, J. M. K. (1968). Involvement of the sympathetic nervous system in tetanus: studies on 82 cases. *Lancet* ii, 236.

Botulism, gas gangrene, and Clostridium gastrointestinal infections

H. E. Larson

Botulism

Definition. Botulism is an acute, symmetrical, descending paralysis of cranial and autonomic nerves produced by the exotoxin of *Clostridium botulinum*. Intoxication usually results from the ingestion of canned, smoked, or fermented foods which *C. botulinum* spores have contaminated. Rarely *C. botulinum* infects wounds or colonizes the intestinal tract of infants and symptoms are produced by toxin absorbed from these sites.

Occurrence. *Clostridium botulinum* is an anaerobic, spore-forming micro-organism which is widely distributed in soil and mud. Food is, therefore, easily contaminated with spores that survive brief periods of heating at 100 °C. Subsequently the same anaerobic conditions required for food preservation suit proliferation of the organism and release of toxin during storage. The occurrence of botulism reflects human customs of food preparation in various countries and among ethnic groups. Cases have been associated with sausage preparation in Europe (Latin *botulus* = a sausage), fermented milk in Africa, home-canned vegetables in North America, fermented stew in Japan, and imported fish in the United Kingdom. Typically outbreaks involve small groups of individuals reflecting the domestic origin and use of the incriminated food product. However, when home-canned peppers were served in restaurants in the United States, two large outbreaks resulted. The prevalence of botulism from home canning may be increased when processing is performed at high altitudes.

Between 1899 and 1973, 9 per cent of reported outbreaks were caused by commercially processed foods, nearly all fish or meat products. Commercially canned mushrooms have been found contaminated with *C. botulinum* but ballooning of the cans gave obvious notice of spoilage and no cases of botulism resulted. Two outbreaks in the UK caused by commercial products include the Loch Maree episode in 1922 where eight persons died after eating duck paste and the 1978 outbreak in Birmingham involving four persons and tinned Alaskan salmon. In the latter case spoilage may not have been noted because gas resulting from bacterial fermentation leaked out of a small defect in the can.

Botulism is rare in the UK, probably because home canning is discouraged and the British are disinclined to eat exotic fermented dishes. Since 1922 there have been only seven outbreaks of botulism in the UK; these occurred in 1932, 1934, 1935, 1949, 1955, and 1978 and involved a total of 18 persons.

In an extensive summary of botulism outbreaks in the USA, 60 per cent involved vegetables, 13 per cent fruit, 12 per cent fish, 7 per cent condiments such as peppers, 3 per cent beef, 2 per cent milk or milk products, and 1.5 per cent each pork and poultry.

Aetiology. Seven types of *C. botulinum* are distinguished (A–G) depending on the serological specificity of the toxin produced. Types A, B, and E account for nearly all human cases; types F and G are rare. Types C and D are chiefly responsible for botulism in domestic and wild fowl and may cause economically significant losses. All serotypes carry bacteriophages, and toxin production by types C and D is contingent on the presence of specific prophages. Strains cured of their prophages cease to produce toxin.

Serotypes A and B have been isolated from 4–8 per cent of soil samples in Britain and types B, C, and E from 70–98 per cent of mud samples from both fresh and salt water environments. Type E is widely disseminated in the area around the Baltic Sea and this and other serotypes have been isolated in the USSR, Japan, Indonesia, Java, and Iran around the Caspian Sea. In the USA type A is found in the West, type B in the East, and type E around the Great Lakes and Alaska. The types implicated in outbreaks of botulism generally parallel the distribution of spores in soil. Type E is nearly always associated with fish. Since outbreaks caused by fish products involve types A and B as well as type E, a serotype cannot be specified from the clinical history.

Spores of *C. botulinum* are more resistant to heating than those of other pathogenic clostridia. They can survive up to two hours of boiling (100 °C), but are killed rapidly at usual autoclave temperatures (120 °C).

The toxin. Clostridium botulinum produces a heat labile, protein neurotoxin that is one of the most potent substances known to man. The lethal dose for mice is in the range of 10 pg. The molecule is composed of two polypeptide chains connected by disulphide bonds with a molecular weight of about 150 000 dalton. The biological activity appears to be dependent upon the dichain structure. Botulinum toxin can be detoxified by treatment with formalin with retention of its ability to elicit antibody formation.

In cultures the toxin first appears as a protoxin which is subsequently activated by a trypsin-like enzyme also produced by the organism. Activation of type E toxin is associated with a change from a single chain molecule to the dichain form. Botulinum toxin is rapidly inactivated by heating at ordinary cooking temperatures. For example it loses activity at 80 °C in five minutes and at temperatures above 85 °C in one minute or less.

Pathogenesis. Botulinum toxin is absorbed directly across mucous membranes, tissue invasion with replicating organisms not being a regular feature of the disease. Locally acting toxin may produce some of the symptoms but cranial nerve paralysis results from distribution of toxin by way of the blood. Cranial nerves are preferentially affected because botulinum toxin binds more rapidly to sites where the cycles of depolarization and repolarization are frequent. Binding is irreversible and once bound the toxin cannot be neutralized by antitoxin. Recovery occurs when nerve terminals sprout from the axon to form new motor end plates.

Botulinum toxin blocks impulse transmission mediated by acetylcholine, such as at myoneural junctions, at autonomic ganglia, and at parasympathetic nerve terminals. Impulse conduction within peripheral nerves and muscle contraction are not affected. Transmission is blocked because the toxin prevents acetylcholine release from the presynaptic membrane. Acetylcholine synthesis and impulse transmission within terminal nerve fibrils remain intact. On the other hand the miniature end plate potentiale spontaneously generated by release of acetylcholine in a resting nerve decrease and eventually disappear in the presence of toxin. If a poisoned nerve is stimulated repetitively, temporary summation of acetylcholine release occurs producing an augmented response (Fig. 1). Labelled toxin localizes at the neuromuscular junction and its specificity for acetylcholine transmitter sites has been used to iden-

tify cholinergic nerves in the small intestine, salivery gland, sino-atrial node, and nerve ganglia.

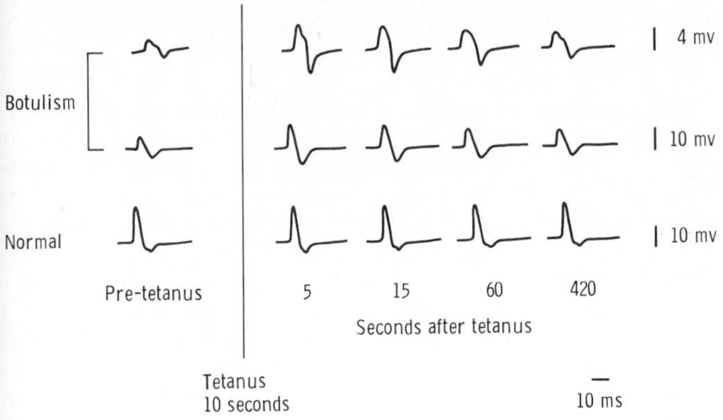

Clinical findings. Botulism varies from mild symptoms unaccompanied by physical signs to fulminating weakness and collapse leading to death within 24 hours. It has been a cause of sudden, unexpected death in previously healthy undividuals. Most patients first note symptoms between 12 and 72 hours after eating. The earliest and commonest symptom is a dry mouth which may be severe enough to cause pain in the tongue and throat. This is closely attended by blurred vision, diplopia, and dizziness or unsteadiness on standing. Other early symptoms are nausea and vomiting; not all patients complain of these but occasionally retching and vomiting are severe. Subsequently patients complain of difficulty with speech or swallowing, then experience progressive difficulty in breathing, generalized weakness and lassitude, weakness or paralysis in the limbs, difficulty holding up the head, abdominal distension, and constipation and urinary hesitancy.

Patients with botulism are invariably conscious although sometimes drowsy. There is no fever. Clinical signs are limited to the motor and autonomic nervous systems. The mouth is dry and the tongue is furrowed. In the eyes lateral rectus weakness produces internal strabismus. Failure of accommodation is common and the pupils may be fixed in midposition or dilated and unresponsive to light. Ptosis, weakness of other extra-ocular muscle movements, inability to protrude the tongue or to raise the shoulders are other early findings. Weakness in the limbs is a flaccid, lower motor neurone type. Facial muscles may be spared. Gag and corneal reflexes and sensory modalities are not lost. Even if not present initially, weakness of the respiratory muscles can develop later and deterioration can be very rapid. Hypotension without compensatory tachycardia, intestinal ileus and urinary retention are evidence of a widespread autonomic paralysis. Patients are described whose symptoms and signs are nearly entirely confined to the autonomic nervous system.

Patients with short incubation periods are likely to have ingested large amounts of toxin. However, clinical attack rates in botulism vary and individuals are known to have ingested large amounts of contaminated food without developing symptoms. The mortality from botulism in the early part of the century was 60–70 per cent, but this has improved to 23 per cent for cases reported between 1960 and 1970 since the use of respiratory support. In a single large outbreak in 1977 there were no deaths among 59 cases.

Diagnosis. The diagnosis in the first case of an outbreak is often missed because cranial nerve symptoms and signs may be ignored in what is apparently a gastrointestinal disturbance. When looked for, the clinical findings are characteristic enough. Competing diagnoses include myasthenia gravis, Guillain–Barré syndrome, diphtheria, tick paralysis, intoxication with atropine or organophosphorous compounds, or basilar artery thrombosis. Patients with variants of acute idiopathic polyneuritis may have symmetrical cranial nerve paralysis and a descending pattern of peripheral nerve involvement. Botulism has been incorrectly diagnosed as pharyngitis and at least once a patient was subjected to exploratory laparotomy because of severe intestinal ileus.

Sometimes patients with other types of poisoning are thought to have botulism. This concern most often arises following an outbreak of staphylococcal food poisoning. Individuals with carbon monoxide poisoning have mistakenly been thought to be poisoned by food, but they invariably have headache and altered consciousness. Poisoning from chemicals or fish produces rapid onset of symptoms. Mushroom poisoning is characterized by severe abdominal pain.

The clinical diagnosis of botulism can be confirmed by testing for botulinum toxin in the patient's serum; 0.5 ml of serum is inoculated intraperitoneally into mice with and without mixing with polyvalent botulinum antitoxin. The mice are then observed for signs of botulism. The specific toxin serotype can be identified by

Fig. 1 Electromyography in botulism. The muscle action potential is markedly reduced, but following tetanic stimulation it is augmented. (From Gutmann, L. and Pratt, L., (1976). Pathophysiologic aspects of human botulism. *Archs Neurol.* **33**, 177, by permission. Copyright 1976, American Medical Association).

repeating the tests using monospecific antitoxins. Free toxin in patient's serum may be detected for as long as 28 days after the onset of symptoms if antitoxin has not been given.

Occasionally electromyography has suggested the diagnosis of botulism. Single or slowly repeated stimuli elicit muscle action potentials that are reduced in amplitude. If tetanic or rapid stimuli are given, a single stimulus following will then elicit an augmented response. This result is also seen in the Eaton–Lambert syndrome, but readily differentiates botulism from the Guillain–Barré syndrome. Patients with botulism may show slight improvement when given edrophonium chloride but this response is very much less than in patients with myasthenia gravis.

Treatment. Patients with botulism may survive if respiration can be successfully supported; in modern times most deaths occur from complications of attempts to do this. Respiratory effort should be monitored carefully using vital capacity or peak flow and the development of arterial hypoxaemia or respiratory acidosis is an indication to assist ventilation. Providing three to four weeks of respiratory support may be a severe test of the resources of even a specialized unit and tracheostomy, repeated bronchoscopy with bronchial lavage, parenteral nutrition, and early treatment of infections (as opposed to colonization) with appropriate antibiotics will be required. Note that some aminoglycoside antibiotics can potentiate neuromuscular blockade. A breathing circuit incorporating intermittent mandatory ventilation can be used to assist breathing in partially paralyzed patients.

Some patients with botulism become profoundly hypotensive; this can be secondary to hypoxaemia, acidosis, and accumulated fluid deficits or be a feature of the autonomic paralysis. The best approach for treatment of the latter is by expansion of the intravascular volume using whole blood, protein and/or saline. The venous pressure should be monitored centrally and kept at 10–15 cmH$_2$O. If this approach fails dopamine infusion can be tried. Initially it should be given cautiously at a rate of 2.5–3.0 µg/kg/minute and titrated to the patient's blood pressure, pulse and urine output.

Trivalent (types A, B, and E) botulinum antitoxin should be administered; half the dose is given intramuscularly and half intravenously. Antitoxin is available from designated regional hospitals in the United Kingdom. Multivalent antitoxin is used since the toxin type cannot be specified from the clinical history and treatment must be initiated before the diagnosis is confirmed by animal tests. The antitoxin available is horse serum and it is customary to give 0.1 ml intradermally as a test dose in case of hypersensitivity. For patients known to be sensitive to horse serum, human botulism immune plasma can be obtained from the Center for Disease Control, Atlanta, Georgia, USA. Except for type E there is no proof that antitoxin alters the course of the illness. However, free circulating toxin may persist in patients' serum for extended periods and use of antitoxin has always seemed a prudent measure.

Some physicians treat with penicillin to eliminate the possibility that toxin might be formed endogenously. Many years ago it was shown that patients dying of botulism carried bacilli in their intestines. The discovery that clinical disease results from toxin formed within the gastrointestinal tract of infants makes antibiotic treatment seem like a more reasonable idea than perhaps was formerly thought.

Drugs capable of reversing neuromuscular blockade have been used to treat patients with botulism. Both guanidine and 4-aminopyridine enhance transmitter release in experimental studies and have been shown to increase the amplitude of evoked muscle action potentials in patients. Clinical effects in patients with botulism include rise in systolic pressure and heart rate, reappearance of bowel sounds, improvement in extraocular muscle movements and strengthened limb power. Not every patient treated with guanidine has shown improvement, however, and neither drug has had any noticeable effect on respiratory muscle weakness or tidal volume. Guanidine given at a dose of 20–35 mg/kg/day for short periods has

not been accompanied by serious side-effects. Experience with 4-aminopyridine is very limited. *In vitro* it is 20–30 times more potent than guanidine but seizures occurred in two patients when 1.5 mg/kg was infused over four hours.

Gastric lavage, repeated high enemas, and cathartics have been given to attempt to remove unabsorbed toxin from the gastrointestinal tract. Nasogastric suction may be indicated in cases with severe ileus and catheter drainage for urinary retention.

Wound botulism. Rarely symptoms and signs of botulism develop in individuals who sustain traumatic injuries. Recognition may be complicated by the presence of fever from septic wound complications or from actual gas gangrene or by the absence of gastrointestinal symptoms. Respiratory failure in a patient receiving kanamycin or gentamicin may be the first event which attracts the physician's attention. The diagnosis has been confirmed by electromyography or by detecting botulinum toxin in serum in about half of the reported cases. *C. botulinum* can be recovered from wounds in the absence of clinical botulism. The incubation period averages seven days with a range of four to 17 days. Clinical findings and management are the same as for patients with food borne botulism.

Infant botulism. Since 1976 botulism has been recognized to occur in infants under six months of age. The cases have been sporadic not connected with ingestion of spoiled food. Previously healthy babies develop constipation which may then progress over three to 10 days to poor feeding, irritability, a hoarse cry, and weakness in head control. Examination shows a generally weak, hypotonic afebrile infant, with cranial nerve paralysis. Abnormalities in eye movements and pupillary reactions are sometimes present and deep tendon reflexes are reduced or absent. The range in severity is considerable, but respiratory failure can develop and there have been several deaths. Most recover completely. The diagnosis can be confirmed by finding *C. botulinum* and toxin in the faeces and by electromyography. Botulinum toxin is not present in the serum.

The disease is thought to follow ingestion of *C. botulinum* spores which then become established in the infant gastrointestinal tract, multiplying and producing toxin. Excretion of *C. botulinum* and toxin may continue following clinical recovery for as long as three months. Honey has been implicated as a source of spores for some cases. Other than supportive measures, no consistent pattern in treatment using antitoxin, antibiotics, cathartics, or enemas has been established.

Gas gangrene

Definition. Gas gangrene is a rapidly developing, spreading infection of muscle by toxin producing *Clostridial* species, especially *Clostridium perfringens* (formerly known as *Clostridium welchii*). It is accompanied by profound constitutional toxicity and is invariably fatal if untreated (see also page 5.472).

Occurrence. Gas gangrene is a rare complication of war wounds, civilian trauma, elective surgery, or intramuscular injections. It also occurs as a primary infection of the perineum and scrotum. The actual incidence of the disease depends upon the conjunction of a number of factors: viable forms of the causative clostridial species must be present and the local environment of the wound must be conducive to their growth. The incidence of gas gangrene after trauma largely reflects the speed with which wounded or injured persons can be evacuated and receive expert surgical debridement. During the Vietnam war there were eight cases among the 139 000 American casualties. In comparison, when a jet airliner crashed in the swamps of the Florida everglades, eight of 77 injured survivors developed the disease. Wounds involving large muscle masses such as the shoulder, hip, thigh, and calf, wounds from high velocity projectiles, damage to major arteries, contamination with dirt, shrapnel, bits of broken bone or clothing, or wounds near faecally ontaminated clothing or skin are all attended by an increased risk f gas gangrene. In civilian life open fractures, crush injuries, urns, amputation for ischaemic vascular disease, hip surgery, and jections of epinephrine are similarly predisposed.

Aetiology. Gas gangrene is caused by certain anaerobic, Gram- ositive, spore forming bacilli capable of producing exotoxins hich damage living tissues. Most cases are caused by *Clostridium erfringens* type A, but in some series 30–60 per cent have been due o *C. novyi* and 5–20 per cent to *C. septicum*. In small numbers of ases *C. histolyticum*, *C. sordellii*, and *C. fallax* have been found. ot uncommonly more than one species is isolated from a case. lostridia occur naturally in the soil and in the gastrointestinal racts of humans and animals. Even toxin producing species are ainly saprophytes and strict conditions for their growth must be net. Oxygen directly inhibits the growth of gas gangrene bacteria nd prevents toxin production as well. However, possession of the nzyme superoxide dismutase can permit the organisms to survive n the presence of small amounts of oxygen. Necrotic tissue, foreign odies, and ischaemia in a wound all operate to reduce the locally vailable oxygen.

The clostridia responsible for gas gangrene elaborate a wide ange of toxic activities with from four to more than twelve separate oxins each described for *C. septicum*, *C. novyi*, and *C. perfringens*. ubtypes of these organisms can be defined according to which oxins are found in culture supernatants. Many of the toxins have een characterized in terms of a specific enzyme, although the toxic nd enzyme activities are not always perfectly correlated. For xample, *C. perfringens* produces lecithinase, collagenase, rotease, hyaluronidase, and deoxyribonuclease. Animal protec- ion experiments using specific antitoxins suggest, however, that he lethality of *C. perfringens* culture filtrates is almost wholly due o the alpha-toxin. This is a phospholipase C for which phosphatidyl holine, sphingomyelin, and phosphatidyl ethanoamine are subs- rates.

Experimental inoculation of culture filtrates reproduces the his- ologic findings of gas gangrene except for oedema and gas. Ex- amination by electron microscopy shows 7.5–18 nm gaps appearing n the plasma membrane as early as one hour after injection. These lasma membrane defects increase with time and are adjacent to oxin molecules labelled with ferritin. This mode of action is consis- ent with the phospholipase activity of alpha-toxin. However, toxin annot be detected in the tissues or serum of patients with gas angrene, possibly because the toxin binds rapidly and irreversibly o tissues.

Clinical findings. The incubation period of gas gangrene is usually ess than four days, often less than 24 hours, and very occasionally s short as one to six hours. Sudden onset of pain at the site of the wound is the first symptom and subsequent evolution of the disease s very rapid. Oedema around the wound soon becomes apparent and a thin serous ooze emerges. Pain steadily increases in severity; the overlying skin becomes stretched and develops a brown or 'bronzed' discoloration. Haemorrhagic vesicles may appear subse- quently and finally areas of frank necrosis. A sweet odour from the wound has been described. In spite of the name gas is not invariably present, especially early in the disease. Later crepitations can be felt and the wound itself becomes exquisitely tender.

Concomitantly with these local events, profound constitutional symptoms develop. The patient becomes sweaty and febrile, and though alert and orientated, very disquieted about his condition. The pulse is elevated out of proportion to the fever which is not necessarily high. Death may occur within 48 hours of onset.

At operation, infected muscle appears dark red with purple discoloration; frank gangrene and liquefaction may even be seen. Involved muscle is devitalized and does not contract after direct stimulation.

According to MacLennan, infections with the various clostridial species show clinical differences. *C. novyi* infection has a longer

incubation period, may begin with a sense of weight in the affected part, and develop without producing gas. Mixed *C. perfringens* and *C. septicum* infections are the most acute. He has also documented the importance of differentiating true clostridial myonecrosis from anaerobic cellulitis and from anaerobic streptococcal myositis. Anaerobic cellulitis is a purulent wound infection where putrifying anaerobic clostridia have colonized muscle and other tissues made necrotic by trauma. Streptococcal myositis is a spreading muscle infection with anaerobic streptococci and either *Streptococcus pyogenes* or *Staphylococcus aureus*. Neither is associated with the pronounced constitutional toxicity characteristic of gas gangrene and neither requires as radical excision. Diabetic patients develop gas gangrene but this is due to their predisposition for ischaemic vascular disease. It is also worthwhile emphasizing that numerous other micro-organisms, both aerobic and anaerobic, can produce gas in tissues.

Diagnosis. The diagnosis of gas gangrene has to be made on clinical grounds as treatment must be initiated urgently. Sudden deterioration in a post-operative patient or following trauma re- quires examination of the wound and surrounding tissue or removal or windowing of a cast. Prompt recognition and treatment improves the prognosis. Cases of primary gas gangrene and cases following elective surgery may have a higher mortality rate because the disease is unexpected and recognition is delayed.

Gram stain of the wound discharge may be a help to the diag- nosis. In gas gangrene this shows many large, plump Gram-positive bacilli, usually without spores (*C. perfringens* in clinical lesions often does not sporulate). Few if any polymorphonuclear leuco- cytes are present. On the other hand both anaerobic streptococcal myositis and anaerobic cellulitis show many leucocytes and the former long chains of Gram-positive cocci.

X-ray has been used to detect small amounts of intramuscular gas in early lesions, but for the reasons given above the absence of gas does not exclude the diagnosis.

Culture of clostridia does not confirm a diagnosis of gas gangrene since simple colonization without clinical disease occurs in up to 30 per cent of wounds.

Treatment. Surgical removal of all affected muscle is essential to recovery from gas gangrene. The decision as to whether to remove only muscle tissue or to amputate is a finely balanced surgical judgement, best when informed by previous experience.

Although not substitutes for surgery, antibiotics, hyperbaric oxygen, and administration of antitoxin have been found to be helpful adjunctive therapies. Penicillin is the drug of choice in doses that offer hope of obtaining diffusion into relatively avascular areas, i.e. 20–30 million units daily. If the patient has a history of angioneurotic oedema or anaphylaxis following administration of penicillin, erythromycin can be substituted at a dose of 1 g every six hours.

Hyperbaric oxygen is widely used to treat gas gangrene. Although an effect on mortality has never been shown by con- trolled trials, its application is well supported by experimental evidence. Proponents claim dramatic relief from the constitutional toxicity and clearer demarcation between involved and uninvolved muscle at operation and this may permit more a conservative resection. One hundred per cent oxygen is given at three atmos- pheres pressure for 60–120 minutes two to three times daily. With this schedule problems with toxicity are minimal. Some workers have achieved comparable mortality rates without using hyperbaric oxygen.

Therapeutic administration of gas gangrene antitoxin is also controversial. Some authorities report abandoning its use many years ago or are cautious of possible reactions to horse serum. On the other hand its use in very toxic cases may be justified and during the Second World War it was said to afford a reduction in mortality.

Patients with gas gangrene need supportive measures to combat shock, blood loss, and dehydration. *C. perfringens* septicaemia in association with gas gangrene is not common. It is heralded by massive haemolytic anaemia and jaundice. Septicaemia with other micro-organisms such as *Escherichia coli* can occur and these should be treated with intravenous gentamicin or as suggested by the results of antibiotic susceptibility testing. Acute renal failure may complicate gas gangrene, resulting from the renal tubular toxicity of free haemoglobin or myoglobin.

Prevention. Gas gangrene is more easily prevented than treated especially since the mortality, even in specialized centres, still ranges between 11 and 31 per cent. Prevention may be achieved either by an attack on the micro-organism itself or by eliminating the conditions which allow it to replicate. Patients undergoing elective operations with an increased risk of gas gangrene, such as amputation for ischaemic vascular disease, should receive penicillin intravenously just before surgery and by mouth post-operatively for five days. Metronidazole may be useful in patients who are hypersensitive to penicillin. Following trauma wounds should be debrided as thoroughly and as early as possible and then dressed open until delayed closure can be performed. In Vietnam soldiers were also given penicillin in large doses.

Experiments with gas gangrene in sheep have shown that both passive and active immunization can confer protection. Antitoxin gave best results when given up to nine hours after wounding but some protection could be seen as late as 18 hours. Active immunization protects but employment of this in humans requires clearly defined risk categories. It is important to know that, if needed, potent toxoids can be prepared for each of the causative species.

Clostridial infections of the gastrointestinal tract

Pseudomembranous colitis

Definition. Pseudomembranous colitis is an acute purulent infection of the colon caused by *Clostridium difficile*. The name derives from plaques of necrotic membrane which adhere to the mucosal surface in the clinically most severe form of the disease (Fig. 2).

Occurrence. Pseudomembranous colitis has been identified as a pathologic entity since before the present century but its clostridial

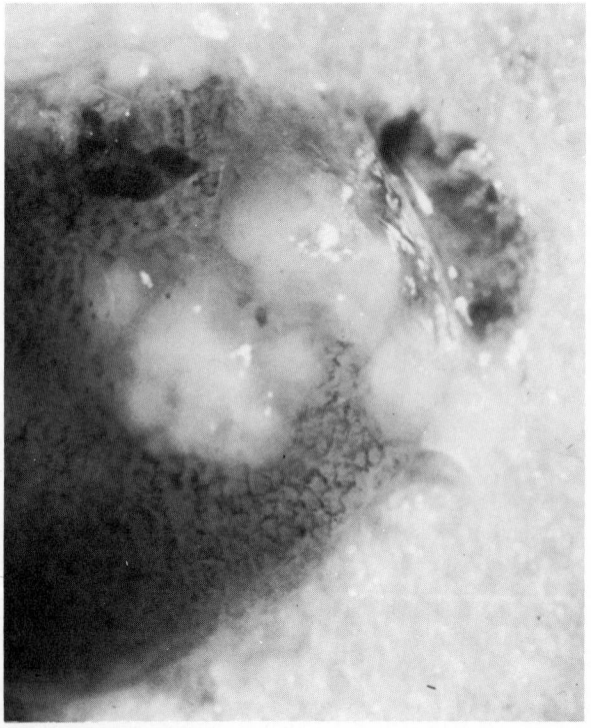

Fig. 2   Pseudomembranes on the rectal mucosa in a patient with *C. difficile* colitis.

aetiology only became known in 1977. Rarely the disease develop spontaneously in otherwise healthy individuals. More often it i secondary to other conditions like chronic colonic obstruction colon carcinoma, leukaemia, or uraemia. Most commonly, how ever, it occurs as a complication of antibiotic treatment. It has been reported to follow every antibiotic in common medical practice, bu association with lincomycin, clindamycin, ampicillin, amoxacillin and cephalosporins is strongest. Most cases are sporadic but clus ters of cases have been reported in hospitalized patients. The disease is more common in older patients but the typical syndrome has been described in persons of all ages including infants.

Aetiology. *C. difficile* is an anaerobic, spore forming, Gram positive bacillus. Strains from patients with colitis produce a potent exotoxin capable of eliciting an inflammatory response in anima tissues. The organism and free toxin can regularly be detected in the faeces of patients with pseudomembranous colitis but not in pa tients with other established causes for diarrhoea. Healthy adult rarely carry *C. difficile*. Infants and young children do so more often, although these strains can be non-toxigenic. The toxin itself i lethal when inoculated into small laboratory animals and a gram o liquid stool from a patient with pseudomembranous colitis may contain thousands of animal lethal doses.

Antibiotic treatment plays an accessory role in the developmen of the colitis. It is probable that antibiotics alter the native resis tance to colonization by *C. difficile*. Since colonization and anti biotic treatment may be separate events, antibiotic susceptible strains of this organism are fully capable of producing disease. In this sense pseudomembranous colitis is an opportunistic infection Culture of *C. defficile* from stools and from environmental site requires differential methods. Toxin is usually assayed by means of its ability to produce characteristic cytopathic changes in cultured cells. The identity of the toxin in unknown specimens can be established by the cytopathic effect and by neutralization with either specific antitoxin or cross-reacting *C. sordellii* antoxin.

Clinical features. The spectrum of colitis caused by *C. difficile* includes mild, self-limited diarrhoea, severe debilitating, pro longed diarrhoea, and an acute fulminating toxic megacolon re sembling acute peritonitis (Fig. 3). The onset of illness may be surreptitious and a persistent diarrhoea may resist all attempts to give symptomatic relief. Sudden onset occurs with a chill, fever and signs of an abdominal catastrophe. It is not unusual for patients with acute findings to be subjected to exploratory laporatomy Severe abdominal pain is not common, and patients only occa sionally report frank blood in the stools. Low fever, a dry furred tongue, and abdominal tenderness sometimes with peritonism are the most common clinical signs. Stools may be watery or of a porridge-like consistency. Many patients show marked polymor phonuclear leucocytosis and leucocytes are present in the faeces. Chemical findings in patients with prolonged diarrhoea include azotaemia and hypoalbuminaemia.

Diagnosis. If clinical findings suggest an acute colitis, every attempt should be made to establish a specific and aetiologic di agnosis. Suspicion of *C. difficile* colitis can be heightened by a history of previous antibiotic therapy. Often this requires direct questioning of the patient since antibiotics may have been self administered, taken for trivial complaints, or used as long as three to four weeks prior to the onset of the diarrhoea. If the tests are available, faeces should be examined for the presence of *C. difficile* and its toxin. If toxin is present, a mechanism for the diarrhoea can be considered to be established. Sigmoidoscopy with rectal biopsy is also helpful as the 0.2–2 mm raised, mucoid to opaque yellow plaques are diagnostic (Fig. 4). Even if the mucosa has a normal appearance, multiple sectioning of a biopsy may reveal microscopic lesions which are also diagnostic. Some patients with *C. difficile* colitis do not have visible pseudomembranes either because lesions are distributed unevenly in the colon or because the illness is mild

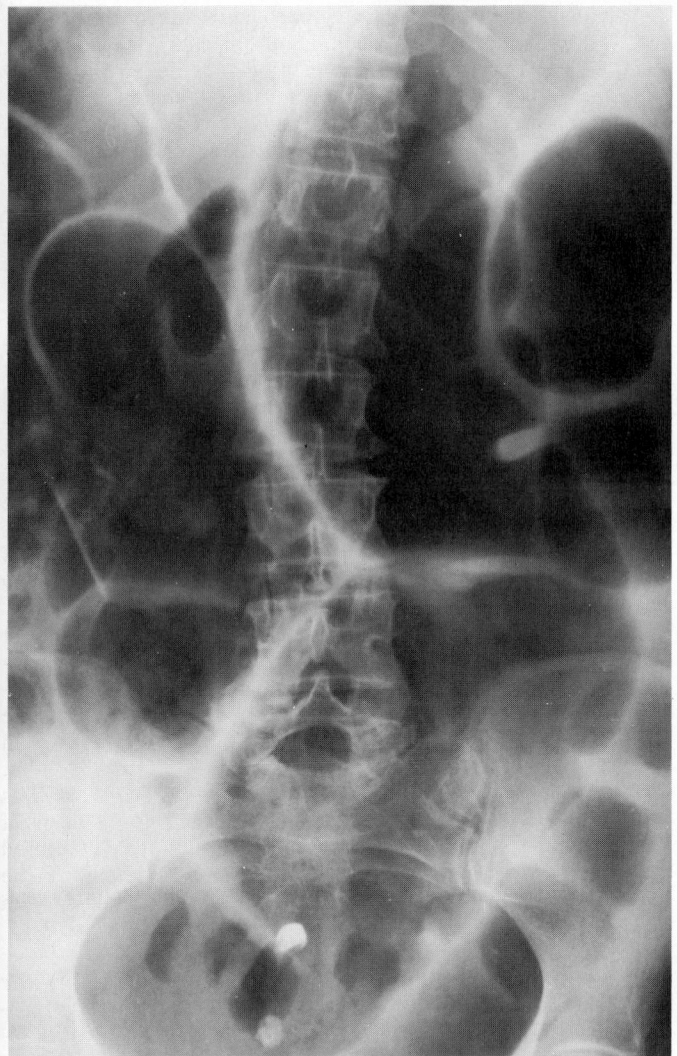

Fig. 3 Acute toxic dilatation of the colon in an elderly lady. She had pseudomembranous colitis.

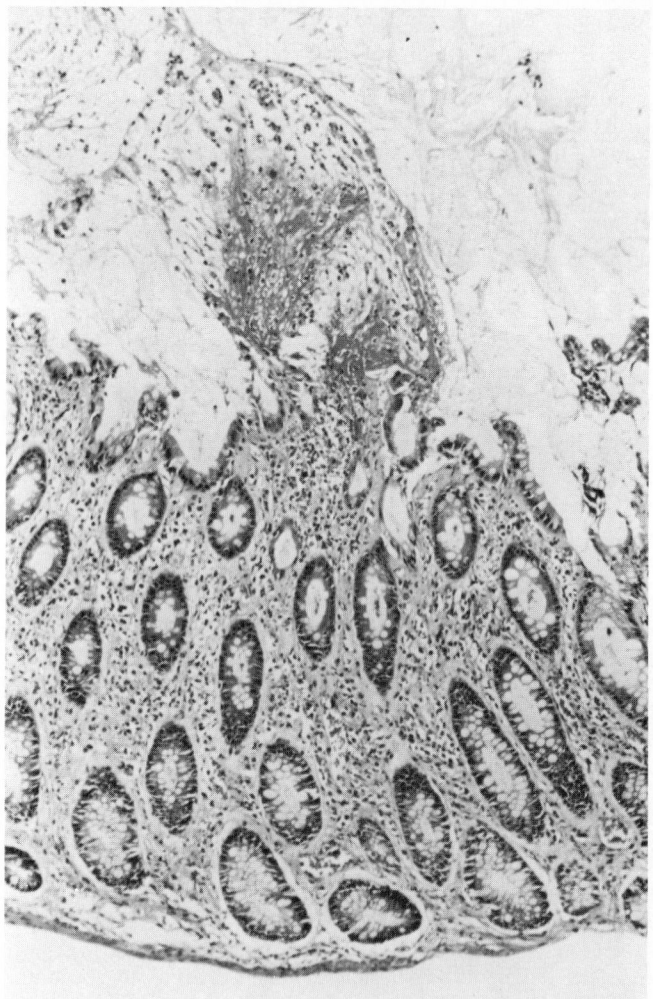

Fig. 4 A rectal biopsy diagnostic of pseudomembranous colitis. There is a flame-like eruption of fibrin and polymorphonuclear leucocytes from a focal area of mucosal necrosis.

and short. In these cases the diagnosis can only be confirmed by testing for toxin and C. difficile.

The differential diagnosis of pseudomembranous colitis includes other forms of antibiotic-associated colitis, diarrhoea due to *Salmonella, Shigella*, and *Campylobacter* species, intestinal amoebiasis, and non-specific ulcerative colitis. All of these can be differentiated by sigmoidoscopy and rectal biopsy or by microscopy and culture of the faeces. Two-thirds or more of patients with simple antibiotic-associated diarrhoea do not have infection with C. difficile. Often they complain of sudden onset of abdominal pain and bloody diarrhoea which subsides within a day or two of stopping antibiotic treatment. Occasionally patients may be infected with C. difficile in addition to another micro-organism capable of causing diarrhoea. Infection with C. difficile has been found to cause exacerbation of symptoms in some patients with non-specific ulcerative colitis.

Treatment and prevention. Treatment specifically directed against C. difficile and resulting in eradication of it and the toxin from the stools has been shown to be accompanied by clinical improvement in a randomly allocated, placebo-controlled trial. The antibiotic of choice is one which is not absorbed following oral administration and one to which C. difficile is susceptible. Vancomycin fulfills both criteria and may be given in doses of 125–500 mg every six hours. Improvement in severe cases is usually apparent after 48 hours of treatment and following this signs and symptoms rapidly return to

normal. Nearly all strains of C. difficile are susceptible to metronidazole but only anecdotal results of treatment with this drug are known. Bacitracin and tetracycline may also prove useful. Treatment failures have attended parenteral administration of both vancomycin and metronidazole. The decision to treat must be made on clinical grounds; in some cases the disease is self-limiting. Patients who are dehydrated need fluid resuscitation, but if the principal findings are constitutional toxicity and peritonism, direct treatment against the cause and the elimination of the toxin should be the chief objectives. Cholestyramine resins bind C. difficile toxin in vitro, but have no effect on the clinical course of the colitis.

Pseudomembranous colitis has been successfully treated by colectomy and patients are often subjected to exploratory laparotomy because the abdominal signs may suggest peritonitis. However, the disease is completely reversible by appropriate antibiotic treatment. If a diagnosis of pseudomembranous colitis has been established, it is appropriate to wait for medical treatment to have an effect in the absence of absolute surgical indications like free abdominal air or complete intestinal obstruction.

Vancomycin-treated patients may suffer relapse of their illness. In some cases the relapse may be clinically more severe than the original. C. difficile remains susceptible and vancomycin can be used to treat relapses if treatment is indicated. It is not certain whether patients relapse because vancomycin treatment does not completely clear them of C. difficile or whether a new exposure to environmental strains has occurred. There is evidence from animal experiments that oral vancomycin itself can induce susceptibility to the disease and it is likely that both reasons for relapses are correct.

Prior to the understanding that pseudomembranous colitis had an infectious aetiology, outbreaks were occasionally reported in particular medical or surgical units. Now it is known that *C. difficile* can be isolated from the environment of patients with diarrhoea and that the spores can persist there for weeks to months. Since clinically mild infections may remain undetected, the chain of infection can be difficult to trace. It is reasonable to assume that infection can be communicated to other patients by means of fomites or air. In any situation where other persons are at risk of becoming infected, for example, a hospital ward with numbers of patients receiving antibiotics, it seems justified to institute barrier isolation for patients with pseudomembranous colitis.

Under certain circumstances it may be necessary to continue the inducing antibiotic when a patient has developed pseudomembranous colitis. There is no evidence to suggest that concurrent therapy with vancomycin will not be successful. Repeat treatment with an inducing antibiotic at some later time is likewise not contraindicated in a patient who has recovered from pseudomembranous colitis.

Necrotizing enterocolitis

Occurrence. Necrotizing enterocolitis refers to a fulminating clinical illness characterized by extensive necrosis of the intestinal mucosa and sometimes the entire wall. Numerous terms have been used to describe geographic variants of the condition such as 'darmbrand', enteritis necroticans, pig bel, or gas gangrene of the bowel. Sporadic cases are regularly reported from Scandinavia, Europe, the United States, and Australia. These tend to occur in patients over 50 and in those recovering from gastric surgery. Outbreaks have been described in post-war Germany and among the highlanders of Papua New Guinea. These follow ingestion of contaminated food or a dramatic change in eating habits, such as occurs when the highlanders engage in pig feasting.

Necrotizing enterocolitis occurs in infants, especially ones with an associated medical condition such as birth asphyxia, respiratory distress syndrome, or umbilical artery catheterization. Cases of neonatal necrotizing enterocolitis have sometimes occurred in clusters.

Aetiology. In the preponderance of adult cases where appropriate pathological and bacteriological investigations have been done, *C. perfringens* (*C. welchii*) has been implicated as the cause of the disease. In sporadic cases this is usually *C. perfringens* type A. Gram stain of the necrotic mucosa and the bowel wall shows many Gram-positive bacilli whose morphology and immunofluorescent staining suggest *C. perfringens*.

However, in the German and especially in the Papua New Guinea outbreaks there is substantial evidence implicating *C. perfringens* type C. This type produces large amounts of beta-toxin which has lethal and necrotizing effects on tissues. New Guinea highlanders have a high prevalence of beta-antitoxin, but antibodies are rare in persons who have lived where the disease is uncommon. Patients with pig bel show rising beta-antitoxin titres and specific passive or active immunization has been shown to prevent the disease. *C. perfringens* type C causes a similar disease in piglets, but it is not clear whether exogenous human infection with these organisms occurs or whether the lesions are produced by the overgrowth of endogenous clostridia. Sweet potato, a local dietary staple, contains an inhibitor of trypsin. Combined with a low protein diet this may impair the ability of the intestine to inactivate endogenously produced beta-toxin. However, the methods used for roasting the pigs offer many opportunities for clostridial contamination.

It has not been proved that clostridia are the cause of neonatal necrotizing enterocolitis.

Clinical findings and course. Symptoms develop suddenly in a person who was previously well. Abdominal pain is severe; colicky at first, it afterwards becomes continuous. Bloody diarrhoea and vomiting may occur. The patient may be extremely toxic and go into shock. On examination there is fever with abdominal distension, localized or diffuse tenderness, and reduced bowel sounds. A tender mass may be palpated. Later intestinal malabsorption or chronic partial obstruction may develop because of scarring. Mild cases recover without surgical intervention, but if surgical indications are present, the mortality ranges from 35 to 100 per cent. Recent studies in Papua New Guinea showed that active immunization with a *C. perfringens* type C toxoid could prevent pig bel.

Clostridium perfringens food poisoning

Occurrence and clinical findings. In the United Kingdom and the United States, food poisoning caused by *C. perfringens* is the third most common type of food-borne illness. Meat and poultry are responsible for at least 90 per cent of the outbreaks which occur where food is prepared in large quantities. Two-thirds of the reported outbreaks are in schools, hospitals, factories, restaurants, or catering establishments, and in a typical outbreak 35 to 40 persons are affected. An estimated 12 000 cases were associated with a single outbreak in 1969.

The circumstances surrounding an outbreak repeat themselves with monotonous regularity. A meat dish is prepared by stewing, braising, boiling, or steaming and then is allowed to stand at ambient temperatures for a period of four to 24 hours. The food is served cold or after desultory rewarming. Six to 12 hours after eating the meal sufferers complain of crampy abdominal pain and then diarrhoea. Vomiting is unusual and fever inconsequential. Twelve to 24 hours later the diarrhoea and pain have subsided. Fatal cases occur rarely; at post-mortem examination they show severe enterocolitis.

Undoubtedly many cases of *C. perfringens* food poisoning occur at home but are not reported because symptoms are self-limited and because documentation requires special bacteriological methods. However, antibodies to the toxin mediating the symptoms are very common and it is likely that nearly everyone has experienced this disease once or more in his lifetime.

Aetiology. *C. perfringens* is a ubiquitous sporulating anaerobe with an unparalleled virtuosity for production of biologically significant toxins. The clinical effects of infection with any particular strain may largely depend on its toxin producing capacity. Strains associated with food poisoning have a number of special characteristics. They are type A although their production of alpha-toxin is variable; they are often heat resistant. Eighty-six per cent of food-poisoning strains produce a specific heat labile factor which fulfills criteria for being an enterotoxin. Toxin production *in vitro* is closely associated with sporulation rather than with the multiplication of vegetative cells. *In vivo* toxin probably acts by causing structural damage to enterocyte membranes. Free enterotoxin has been detected in diarrhoeal stool after *C. perfringens* food poisoning, antibody rises to enterotoxin develop after such a episode, and ingestion of 8 to 12 mg of enterotoxin by volunteers produces abdominal pain and diarrhoea.

C. perfringens is part of the normal human faecal flora, is regularly found in the intestinal tract of domestic animals, often contaminates raw meat, and can be carried by flies. The distribution of enterotoxin producing strains may be more restricted. However, surface contamination of meat with *C. perfringens* is likely to occur commonly and subsequent rolling or grinding will distribute these organisms throughout. Heat-resistant strains survive cooking methods using a maximum temperature of 100 °C. Spores then germinate and multiply to 10^6 to 10^7 cells per gram in the highly advantageous, anaerobic environment afforded when meat cools slowly or stands at ambient temperature. Reheating may be inadequate to kill these cells; when ingested they multiply still further, sporulate, and release their toxin.

References

Botulism

Ball, A. P., Hopkinson, R. B., Farrell, I. D., Hutchison, J. G. P., Paul, R., Watson, R. D. S., Page, A. J. F., Parker, R. G. F., Edwards, C. W., Snow, M., Scott, D. K., Leone-Ganado, A., Hastings, A., Ghosh, A. C., and Gilbert, R. J. (1979). Human botulism caused by *Clostridium botulinum* type E: the Birmingham outbreak. *Q. Jl Med.* **48**, 473.

Das Gupta, B. R. and Sugiyama, H. (1977). Biochemistry and pharmacology of botulinum and tetanus neurotoxins. In *Perspectives in toxicology* (ed. A. W. Bernheimer). Wiley, New York.

Gilbert, R. J. (1974). Staphylococcal food poisoning and botulism. *Post-grad. med. J.* **50**, 603.

Merson, M. H. and Dowell, V. R., Jr. (1973). Epidemiologic, clinical, and laboratory aspects of wound botulism. *New Engl. J. Med.* **289**, 1005.

Palin, R. A. and Brown, L. W. (1979). Infant botulism. *Pediat. Clins. N. Am.* **26**, 345.

Gas gangrene

Altemeier, W. A. and Fuller, W. D. (1971). Prevention and treatment of gas gangrene. *J. Am. med. Ass.* **217**, 806.

Darke, S. G., King, A. M., and Slack, W. K. (1977). Gas gangrene and related infection classification, clinical features and aetiology, management and mortality. A report of 88 cases. *Br. J. Surg.* **64**, 104.

Freer, J. H. and Arbuthnott, J. P. (1976). Biochemical and morphologic alterations of membranes by bacterial toxins. In *Mechanisms in bacterial toxins* (ed. A. W. Bernheimer), 169. Wiley, New York.

MacLennan, J. D. (1962). The histotoxic clostridial infections of man. *Bacteriol. Rev.* **26**, 177.

Gastrointestinal infections

Bartlett, J. G. (1979). Antibiotic-associated colitis. *Clins Gastroent.* **8**, 783.

Hobbs, B. C. (1974). *Clostridium welchii* and *Bacillus cereus* infection and intoxication. *Post-grad. med. J.* **50**, 597.

Lancet (1977). Clostridia as intestinal pathogens. *Lancet* **ii**, 1113.

Larson, H. E. (1979). Pseudomembranous colitis is an infection. *J. Infection* **1**, 221.

Tuberculosis

K. M. Citron and D. J. Girling

Mycobacterium tuberculosis

Mycobacterium tuberculosis was first described by Robert Koch in 1882. The species is, like *M.leprae*, an obligate parasite with no free-living saprophytic forms. But, unlike *M.leprae*, it is a facultative intracellular parasite, capable of either intracellular or extracellular existence. It can infect many wild, farm, and domestic animals, but spread of infection from animals to man is probably exceedingly rare, except by drinking heavily infected milk.

Two main species are recognized, *M.tuberculosis* and *M.bovis*, Bacille Calmette-Guérin (BCG) being a form of the latter. The vole bacillus, which has sometimes been used for vaccinating humans, causes no natural infection in man.

M.africanum, occurring in West and Central Africa, has properties intermediate between *M.tuberculosis* and *M.bovis* and is probably not a distinct species. A heterogeneous group of strains of *M.tuberculosis* is frequently found in India, and less frequently in nearby countries such as Pakistan, Burma, Thailand, and East Africa. This group is characterized by low virulence for the guinea-pig, susceptibility to the bactericidal action of hydrogen peroxide, sensitivity to T2H (thiophen-2-carboxylic acid hydrazide), and absence of certain toxic sulpholipids found in more virulent strains.

The different strains vary in their cultural and biochemical properties, in their geographical distribution, in their virulence, and in the distribution of bacteriophage types within them.

M.tuberculosis is particularly well adapted for parasitism having characteristics which enable it to survive host defences for many years in a balanced relationship. For example, it is a slow-growing organism and is strongly acid-fast, a property which is closely related to the high lipid content of its cell wall, countering host defences. The temperature range in which it can grow is narrow, its nutritional requirements are exacting, particularly with regard to carbohydrates, and it is a strict aerobe. A particularly important feature is its ability to lie dormant for many years. These adaptations result in the inhibition of bacillary growth but not necessarily in bacillary death in the presence of tissue damage. They also provide a basis for bacteriological identification tests.

M.tuberculosis is by far the most important of the mycobacterial pathogens, accounting for almost all cases of human tuberculosis.

Morphology. Tubercle bacilli are long, curved, often beaded or banded rods 4 μm or more in length and about 0.5 μm in diameter. They tend to form long cords. They do not stain easily with Gram stain because of the high cell lipid content, but once stained, for example by Ziehl–Neelsen or fluorochrome procedures, they strongly resist decolorization with acid and alcohol, a characteristic which depends upon the intergrity of the cell wall.

Biological effects of mycobacterial cell components. Mycobacterial cells are rich in lipids, and their biological effects, such as the induction of host defence mechanisms and resistance to them, and adjuvant activity, are related to these lipids. The principle ones are mycolic acids, glycolipids, phospholipids, and mycosides, all of which are found predominantly in the highly complex cell wall (Fig. 1).

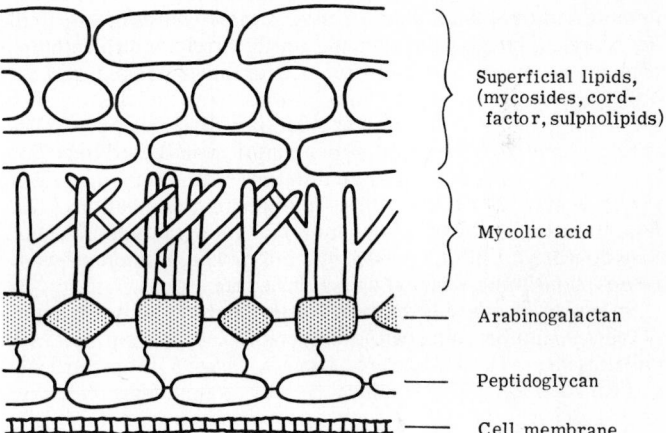

Fig. 1 A diagrammatic representation of the mycobacterial cell wall. Next to the cell membrane is a peptidoglycan (murein) layer, as in other bacteria, giving the cell its shape and rigidity. Attached to this are fairly distinct layers, linked together, of arabinogalactan (a polysaccharide polymer of arabinose and galactan), mycolic acid and superficial lipids. (From Grange, J. M. (1980), by permission.)

Superficial to and within the wall structure are free lipids which can form part of the cell wall because of the lipophilic characteristics of mycoloyl esters. They include mycosides (which are glycolipids or peptidoglycolipids), trehalose 6,6′–dimycolate (cord factor), and sulpho-lipids.

Many of these highly complex cell wall components have important functions in mycobacterial physiology and also affect the host. They determine colonial morphology and agglutination serotype, act as storage compounds, immunogens, antigens, and phage receptor sites, inhibit macrophage migration, immobilize polymorphs, provide protection against digestive lysosomal enzymes of the macrophage, and play a part in inducing granuloma formation. Glycolipids, such as cord factor and the sulpholipids, are toxic and also have adjuvant activity.

Virulence. Unlike other pathogenic bacteria, tubercle bacilli do not produce exotoxins, endotoxins, or extracellular enzymes noxious to the host, and they are rapidly phagocytosed, even in the absence of antibody. Moreover, large numbers of organisms can be injected into animals without causing immediate distress. Indeed the precise mechanism of their virulence is not at all clear.

The virulence for the guinea-pig of different strains of *M.tuberculosis* is closely related to their phage type and to their ability to resist the bactericidal action of hydrogen peroxide, but virulence for the guinea-pig and for man are not necessarily closely correlated. A high sulpholipid content is found in the virulent phage type A strains and may contribute to their virulence, but the equally virulent phage type B strains contain no sulpholipid.

Attenuated strains of tubecle bacilli can be produced by subcultivation on artificial medium, which is how the BCG strain of *M.bovis* is obtained. But attenuated strains of *M. tuberculosis* also occur in human disease. For example, many strains from India and all strains highly resistant to isoniazid are attenuated. These attenuated strains usually have a reduced catalase and peroxidase activity. This renders them highly susceptible to the bactericidal action of hydrogen peroxide, and suggests that the host defence mechanism responsible for killing them involves hydrogen peroxide production by the phagocytic cells.

The ability of tubercle bacilli to adjust their rate of metabolism to compensate for a slow reduction in oxygen tension and become dormant is most marked in the more virulent strains.

Phage type. Some of the bacterial cell wall lipids act as phage receptor sites, and phage typing can be used to subdivide *M.tuberculosis* into four main phage types, namely A, I (intermediate), B, and C, of which type C is very rarely encountered. Approximately a third of the Indian strains of *M.tuberculosis* belong to the intermediate phage type, a finding which correlates well with their comparatively low degree of virulence for the guinea-pig, and only about 5 per cent belong to type B. In contrast, of the strains of bacilli found in the indigenous population of Britain, approximately 55 per cent are of type A, 38 per cent of type B, and only 7 per cent of type I. These phage type differences are useful in studying the epidemiology of tuberculosis in immigrant populations. They have, for example, been used to show that immigrants to the United Kingdom from the Indian subcontinent in whom tuberculosis develops, tend to be infected with Indian-type strains.

Strains of *M.tuberculosis* from Europe and the USA are mainly of types A and B. Almost all strains from West and Central Africa, and those from Hong Kong are of type A. Phage 33D has particular value in identifying BCG in that it lyses all strains of *M.tuberculosis* and *M.bovis* except BCG.

Pathology and immunology

The response of the host to tubercle bacilli is primarily cellular, involving particularly the reticuloendothelial and lymphocytic systems, the characteristic lesion being the tubercle.

Tubercle formation. The basic cellular response to tubercle bacilli is the phagocytosis of the organisms by macrophages. They begin to ingest bacilli within minutes of encountering them. Those which do so are transformed into epithelioid cells. Both macrophages and epithelioid cells can probably form the characteristic giant cells (Langhans cells) by fusion, which probably results most commonly from simultaneous endocytosis of the same material by two or more phagocytes.

Thus within a few days, and before the onset of the acquired immune response, a typical concentric tubercle has formed, with epithelioid and giant cells surrounded by macrophages. The tubercle enlarges; blood monocytes are incorporated; the phagocytes in the lesion multiply locally; adjacent cells are compressed and atrophy, and a network of reticulum fibres, which then undergo transition to collagen, develops. A few lymphocytes may be seen among the epithelioid cells, and the centre of the lesion eventually caseates, as delayed hypersensitivity develops.

Functionally, the circulating monocytes and the tissue macrophages are predominantly phagocytes. Phagocytosis stimulates the secretion of lysosomal and other enzymes. These can kill other tissue cells; they may also have a chemotactic action on other

macrophages, and stimulate macrophage cell division and fibroblast activity. Macrophage proliferation is self-limited by the appearance of chromosomal abnormalities after a few generations and these cells soon die, to be removed by the lymphatic system. The macrophages are stimulated by phagocytosis, by various mycobacterial components, and by sensitized T lymphocytes.

Some of the epithelioid cells retain a certain degree of phagocytic activity, but their role is predominantly secretory, and they contain numerous vesicles. The giant cells function as a disposal system.

The presence of large numbers of lymphocytes at the periphery of a granuloma suggests that its development had been arrested. Little or no caseation suggests minimal bacillary multiplication while the presence of large numbers of dividing bacilli is usually associated with extensive caseation. When bacilli are numerous and caseation extensive, a few polymorphonuclear leucocytes are not infrequently seen.

The primary granulomatous response is an important nonspecific host defensive response. It develops in only a few days, it limits the local spread of infection, and may achieve complete resolution. However, it is a local response, depending upon the accumulation of large numbers of macrophages within a short period.

Bacilli inside macrophages. Phagosomes are the phagocytic vacuoles of macrophages. But for bacilli inside phagosomes to be killed, the phagosomes must fuse with lysosomes which are sacs of enzymes which may kill bacilli and which break up phagocytosed refuse. However, phagosome–lysosome fusion does not invariably lead to bacillary death, although it probably inhibits those virulent bacilli which survive. It results in the production of hydrogen peroxide which, as we have already seen, is probably responsible for killing some bacilli.

Macrophage activation. Before activation, macrophages can probably only kill a minority of virulent bacilli. They become activated largely by being stimulated by sensitized T lymphocytes, that is by specific acquired immunity, but also in response to various mycobacterial components. The first phase of activation if one of excitation, the macrophage showing increased motility and phagocytosis. This is followed by longer lasting changes, notably an increase in the number of lysosomes and increased production of lysosome enzymes and hydrogen peroxide. Some of the lysosomes of activated macrophages move to the cell surface and eject their enzymes thus attacking extracellular bacilli. Macrophages when activated have a greater capacity to destroy bacteria, but they behave non-specifically, and indeed increase the resistance of the host to a large number of micro-organisms.

Specific acquired immune response. Specific acquired immune responses against intracellular parasites such as *M.tuberculosis* are largely cell mediated. That is to say, the macrophages become activated against the parasites primarily under the influence of T lymphocytes which have become sensitized by contact with parasite antigen (Fig. 2). Sensitized T lymphocytes on encountering antigens from tubercle bacilli accumulate at the site, and release a large number of soluble mediators called lymphokines, different lymphocyte populations producing different lymphokines. Some of these lymphokines are important in host defence mechanisms; they activate macrophages, exert a chemotactic influence over them, and inhibit their migration, thereby encouraging these cells to accumulate within the lesion and to be retained there. Some activate non-sensitized lymphocytes. In contrast, other lymphokines have a deleterious effect, suppressing macrophage activity and having a cytotoxic action on other host cells. Thus the balance of many factors determines the degree of host resistance, but it is T lymphocytes from the immunized host which are the cells primarily responsible for mounting the specific acquired immune response to tuberculous infection, the end result of which is an increased capacity of macrophages to kill tubercle bacilli and inhibit their intracellular multiplication.

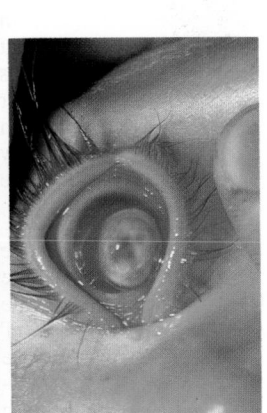

1 Vitamin deficiency: keratomalacia.

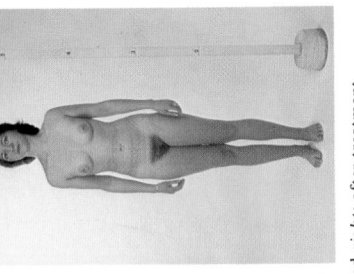
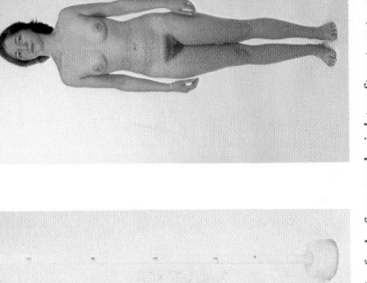
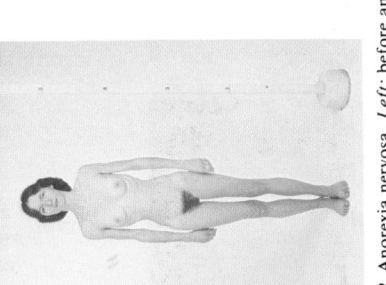
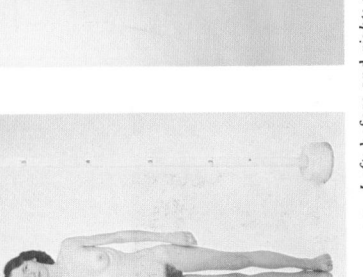
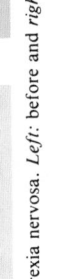

2 Anorexia nervosa. *Left*: before and *right*: after treatment.

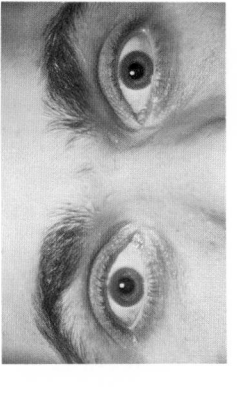

4 The Kayser – Fleischer ring. The brownish gold, occasionally green, discoloration of the cornea due to the deposition of copper in Descemet's membrane.

3 Diabetes

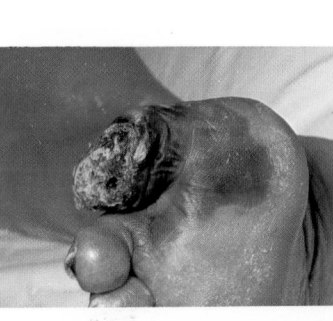
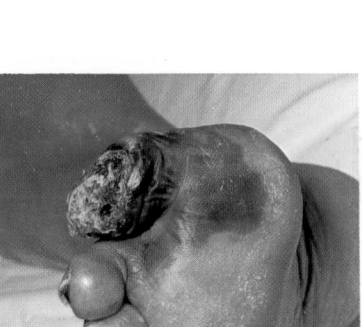

3(a) Diabetic background retinopathy with small numbers of microaneurysms and dot and blot haemorrhages.

3(b) Diabetic retinopathy showing marked peripheral neovascularization as well as soft exudate.

3(c) Diabetic septic foot ulcer. Severe neuropathy, normal blood supply. Complete recovery of skin integrity with debridement, antibiotics and skin grafts.

3(d) Diabetic non-infected gangrene. Macroangiopathy + neuropathy. Amputation at lowest level where blood supply reckoned adequate for healing.

5 Rickettsial diseases

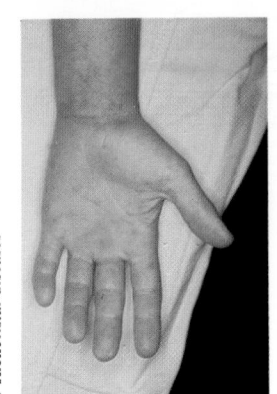

5(a) –(c) Early rash of Rocky Mountain Spotted Fever on the palms and legs.

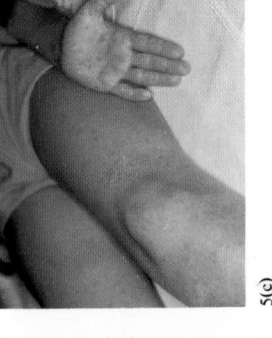

5(b)

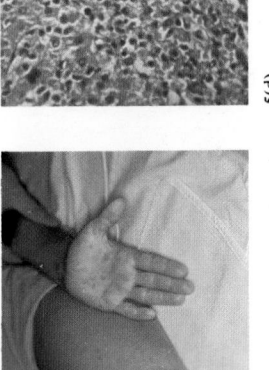

5(c)

5(d) Q fever: acute granulomatous hepatitis in a man with fever, myalgia, and right upper abdominal quadrant pain with no headache, pulmonary signs, or jaundice. Full recovery with chloramphenicol. Note inflammatory reaction and multi-nucleated giant cell. *C. burnetii* were demonstrated by IF technique and CF reaction was positive.

5(d)

6 Bleeding disorders

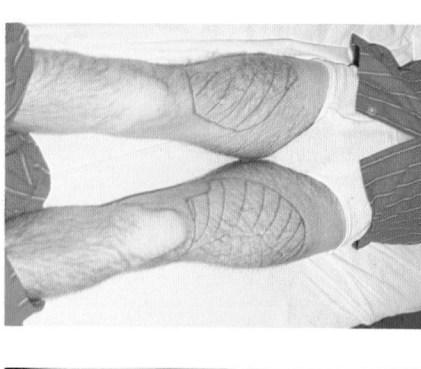

6(a) Haemophilia. The sensory changes secondary to bilateral femoral nerve involvement due to bleeding into the psoas sheath.

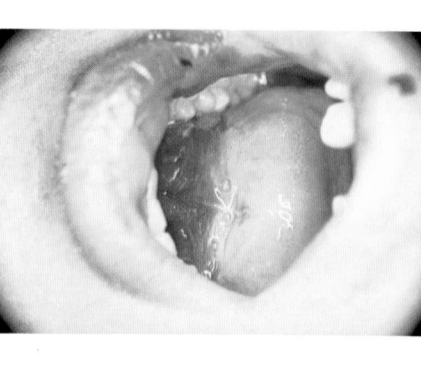

6(b) Haemophilia. A haematoma under the tongue resulting from mild trauma to the jaw.

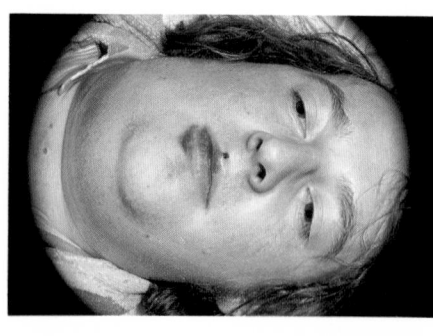

6(c) Haemophilia. The same patient as illustrated in (b) 12 hours later; there has been massive bleeding into the neck leading to asphyxia.

6(d) Idiopathic thrombocytopenic purpura.

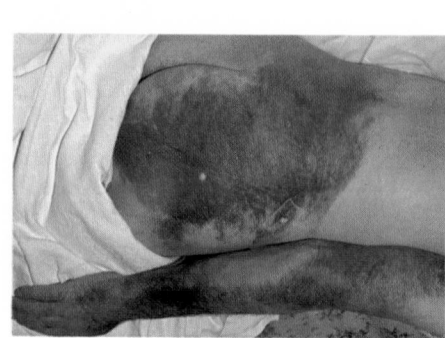

6(e) Disseminated intravascular coagulation secondary to carcinoma of the prostate. The massive haematoma is the result of a posterior iliac crest bone marrow puncture.

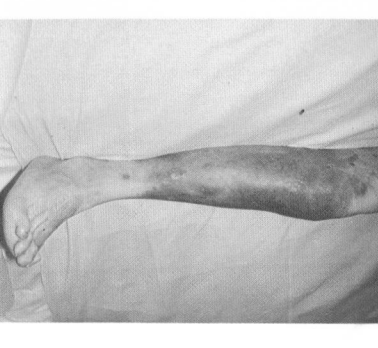

6(f) Scurvy. Extensive subcutaneous bleeding into the lower limb in a 70-year-old patient with severe dietary insufficiency.

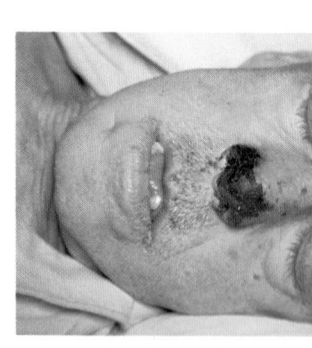

6(g) Purpura gangrenosa. Haemorrhagic necrosis of the tip of the nose in a patient with gram-negative septicaemia.

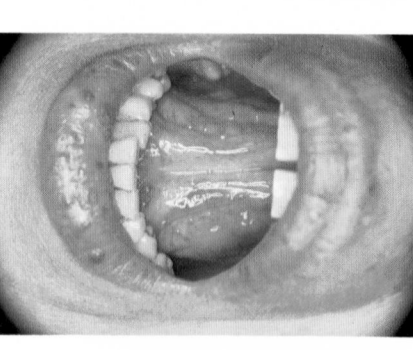

6(h) Hereditary telangiectasia. This patient has chronic iron deficiency anaemia and these typical lesions were disclosed after removal of lipstick.

6(i) Amyloidosis. Typical vascular purpura involving the periorbital region.

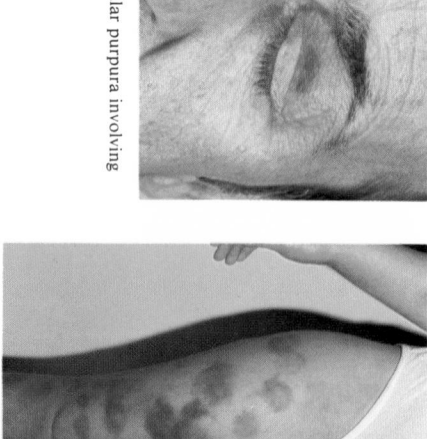

6(j) The painful bruising syndrome. Typical lesions over the limbs in a 21-year-old female.

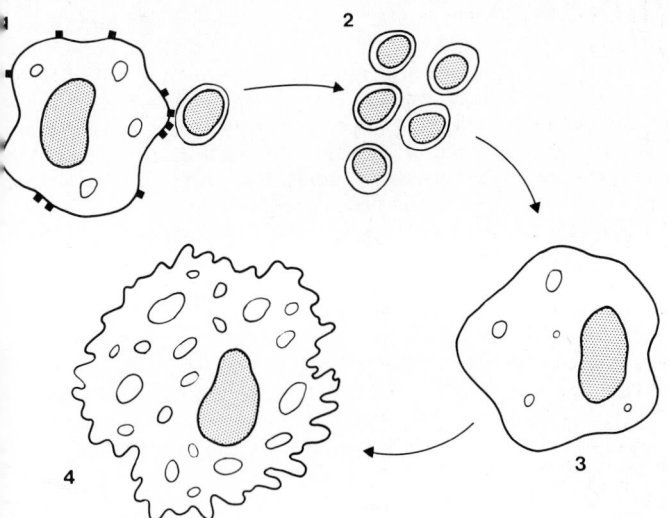

Fig. 2 Macrophage activation: (1) antigen processed by the macrophage is presented to a T lymphocyte bearing specific antigen receptors; (2) the T lymphocyte undergoes blast transformation and divides to form a clone of cells which produce lymphokines; (3) and (4) lymphokines cause the macrophage to transform into an activated macrophage. (From Grange, J. M. (1980), by permission.)

Delayed hypersensitivity. Infection with tubercle bacilli induces in the host delayed hypersensitivity to some of the mycobacterial protein antigens, a state which can be demonstrated by intradermal injection of tuberculoprotein which elicits a local delayed acute inflammatory response. Like the specific acquired immune response described above, delayed hypersensitivity is a cell-mediated host response, involving circulating sensitized T lymphocytes and macrophages. It may cause a considerable amount of local tissue damage. Indeed delayed hypersensitivity probably accounts for much of the tissue destruction which is such a characteristic feature of post-primary tuberculous disease.

In spite of the similarity in the mechanism of delayed hypersensitivity and acquired cellular immunity and their frequent coexistence, these two host responses are not identical. For example, there is no correlation in man or animals between the degree of hypersensitivity and the degree of immunity as indicated by the severity and course of the disease. Indeed, when disease develops, it is more likely to be active and progressive in patients with a high degree of hypersensitivity. It has been argued that hypersensitivity and acquired immunity are separate immune responses directed against different components of the mycobacterial cell. Certainly hypersensitivity is not responsible for acquired immunity. Quite probably the two responses involve different lymphokines, and so different populations of T cells.

Clinical bacteriology

The culture of *M.tuberculosis* from pathological specimens is necessary to confirm a diagnosis of tuberculosis. A clinical bacteriological service of a high standard is required, both for accurate diagnosis and for monitoring chemotherapy.

Collection of specimens. The collection of adequate specimens is essential for reliable bacteriology. Specimens should be collected in sterile wide-mouthed screw-capped 'Universal' containers.

Whenever possible, sputum specimens should be collected overnight and on waking in the morning. The patient should be instructed to cough vigorously after deep inspirations, repeatedly, if necessary, until at least 3 ml of sputum has been produced. Two or more specimens should be collected for initial diagnostic purposes. If sputum cannot be produced, pharyngeal secretions mixed with saliva should be obtained, after clearing the back of the throat. Laryngeal swabs are also sometimes used, but are less reliable.

In children, or patients who are unable to co-operate in providing sputum or pharyngeal secretions, gastric contents may be aspirated through a nasogastric tube in the early morning before food or drink. The patient should be encouraged to cough and swallow immediately before the procedure.

When urine is required, at least three early morning specimens should be collected. Specimens of pleural, peritoneal, or pericardial fluid should be collected into bottles containing sodium citrate to prevent clotting. CSF, pus, and other fluid specimens should be of as large a volume as possible for the laboratory to stand a good chance of isolating the organism.

Biopsy specimens should be divided into two. Half should be sent for bacteriological examination, and half, in formalin, for histological examination. *M.tuberculosis* can rarely be isolated from necrotic tissue or pus; tissue adjacent to necrotic areas should therefore be obtained.

Direct microscopy. Sputum smears are prepared by selecting purulent particles of the specimen and smearing them direct on to a microscope slide using a wire loop. They are then dried, fixed, and stained. Two methods of examining sputum smears or other specimens by direct microscopy are currently in use, bright field microscopy after Ziehl–Neelsen staining and fluorescence microscopy after staining with auramine O or auramine-rhodamine, both of which methods make use of the acid-fastness of mycobacteria. Fluorescence microscopy is the method of choice in technically advanced countries and in all laboratories with a large workload (including those in developing countries examining 100 specimens or more a day) because it is more rapid, more sensitive, and less likely to yield false positive results. However, in peripheral laboratories in developing countries the Ziehl–Neelsen method should be used so that the microscope can be used for other types of microscopy as well.

An adequate direct smear service is an essential part of the antituberculosis programme in all countries; it is much cheaper and provides more valuable information than repeated chest radiography.

Culture. For growth on culture, *M.tuberculosis* requires a nitrogen source such as glutamate or asparagine, either glucose or glycerol as a source of carbon, and essential metals such as iron and magnesium. On liquid media, cultures grow exponentially at first (as is to be expected from division by binary fission) in a veil or pellicle on the surface, or as cords deeper in the medium. In the presence of a dispersing agent, such as Tween 80, exponential growth is followed by linear growth, a consequence of oxygen deprivation. Solid media are usually prepared with egg-yolk or whole eggs. Löwenstein–Jensen medium is a whole-egg medium and, without potato starch, is probably the most widely used medium for culturing tubercle bacilli in standard bacteriological tests.

Sputum specimens should be prepared for culture by concentration and decontamination with sodium hydroxide (the Petroff method); they are usually cultured on Löwenstein–Jensen medium without potato starch, as slopes in screw-capped bottles sterilized by inspissation. Two slopes may be inoculated, one containing pyruvate to increase the size of colonies of *M.bovis*.

Specimens other than sputum, especially those likely to be contaminated with other organisms, should be initially decontaminated with sulphuric acid and cultured not only on Löwenstein–Jensen medium but also on media made selective for *M.tuberculosis* by the addition of antibiotics, for example, selective 7H-11 oleic acid–albumin agar and selective Kirchner's medium.

A good culture service should be available in all countries because it can increase the proportion of bacteriologically confirmed tuberculosis by 35–50 per cent. At least one pretreatment specimen should be sent for culture. For a high standard of testing to be maintained some degree of centralization of the culture service is necessary.

Identification tests. The cultural and metabolic properties of *M.tuberculosis* distinguish it from other mycobacteria. Thus, *M.tuberculosis* is characterized by colonial morphology, slow growth, failure to produce pigment, oxygen preference, absence of growth on Löwenstein–Jensen medium containing 500 mg of p-nitrobenzoate (PNB) per litre, and by absence of growth at 25 °C. On Löwenstein–Jensen medium colonies of *M.tuberculosis* are large and heaped up (eugonic) while those of *M.bovis* are small and flat (dysgonic), although their growth is stimulated by pyruvate, making the colonies larger. Colonies of *M.tuberculosis* lie on the surface while those of *M.bovis*, because they can tolerate lower oxygen tension, extend into the surface layers. *M.tuberculosis*, unlike *M.bovis*, produces nicotinamide (niacin), reduces nitrate to nitrite, is resistant to T2H, and is sensitive to pyrazinamide, unless resistance has been acquired.

Positive cultures should be screened to find out whether they are *M.tuberculosis* or *M.bovis*, or another mycobacterial species. The recommended screening tests, apart from demonstrating acid-fastness and noting the morphology and pigmentation of colonies, are incubation at 25 °C and on slopes containing PNB, and testing for niacin production (Table 1). The full identification of non-tuberculous mycobacteria involves specialized procedures.

Table 1   Screening tests for identifying cultures of Mycobacteria

Organism	Growth at 25 °C	Growth on PNB	Niacin production
M. tuberculosis	–	–	+
M. bovis	–	–	–
Other mycobacteria	+	+	–

Sensitivity tests. Sensitivity tests are most commonly done by the indirect method in which cultures from specimens are tested. Indirect tests are of three main types, the MIC (minimal inhibitory concentration) method, the RR (resistance ratio) method, and the proportion method.

Tests for isoniazid, rifampicin, and ethambutol are very stable, being unaffected by minor variations in laboratory conditions or methods, but tests for streptomycin and ethionamide are less stable. A method involving different pH values is necessary for pyrazinamide. All sensitivity tests should be calibrated regularly, and good quality control in the laboratory is important if results are to be consistent and reliable.

In the MIC method, measured quantities of the primary culture are sub-cultured on to media containing an appropriate range of drug concentrations. The minimal concentration of the drug which inhibits growth is assessed, growth being defined as 20 or more colonies on a slope, because all strains contain a few resistant mutants. In the RR method, the MIC of the test strain is divided by the MIC of a standard strain, usually H37Rv. In the proportion method the actual proportion of resistant bacilli in the strain is measured, by comparing the number of colonies on medium containing a concentration of the drug just sufficient to begin inhibiting sensitive organisms with the number on drug-free medium. The MIC and proportion methods are slightly better than the RR method in distinguishing between sensitive and resistant strains.

The results of indirect tests do not become available until seven to eight weeks after receipt of the specimen in the laboratory. For this reason, direct tests (so called because they are done directly on the specimen and not on a culture) are sometimes used, particularly if a patient has had previous unsuccessful treatment and urgently requires further treatment. Results are available four weeks after receipt of the specimen. Such tests, and the even more rapid slide-culture test, can only be done if the sputum is heavily infected.

Drug resistance. Resistance has been defined as a decrease in sensitivity of sufficient degree for it to be reasonably certain that the strain concerned is different from a sample of wild strains which have never come into contact with the drug. In the laboratory, strains which are predominantly sensitive and strains which are predominantly resistant are compared, and a definition of resistance is chosen which best distinguishes between these two populations. However, it is very important to realise that a laboratory definition of resistance in a culture grown from a pretreatment specimen does not necessarily imply that there will be a poor therapeutic response to the drug concerned.

Clinically, resistance can be 'primary', 'initial', or 'acquired'. *Primary resistance* is resistance which has not resulted from treatment of the patient with the drug concerned. It includes natural resistance, that is resistance in strains which have never come into contact with the drug (wild strains), and acquired resistance occurring as a result of exposure of the strain to the drug, but in another patient. *Initial resistance* is resistance in patients who give a history of never having received chemotherapy in the past; it includes resistance due to previous treatment concealed by the patient or of which he was unaware. *Acquired resistance* results from exposure of the strain to the drug and the consequent selecting out of resistant mutant bacilli. 'Transitional resistance' is a term used to describe a resistant culture (usually of only a few colonies) obtained during successful chemotherapy, due to the isolation of a persistent resistant mutant which is not actively multiplying in the lesions. Such cultures are usually obtained early in treatment, just before the sputum cultures became negative.

Definitions of resistance. Commonly accepted definitions of resistance with the MIC method and proportion method of sensitivity testing are shown in Table 2. However, there is variation from one laboratory to another, and, with the less stable tests, within the laboratory. With the RR method, a strain with an RR of between two and four is usually regarded as borderline resistant, one with an RR of more than four as resistant, and one with an RR of eight or more as highly resistant.

Table 2   Definitions of resistance to the main antituberculosis drugs with the MIC and proportion methods

Drug	MIC (mg/l)	Proportion method	
		Drug concentration (mg/l)	Minimal proportion of resistant bacilli (%)
Isoniazid	1	0.2	1
Streptomycin	32	4	10
Rifampicin	64	40	1
Pyrazinamide	100*	100	10
Thiacetazone	2	2	10
PAS	8	0.5	1
Ethambutol	5.6	2	10
Ethionamide	80	20	10

* The test is set up at pHs of 4.75, 4.85, and 4.95. The MIC on the most acid medium on which heavy growth occurs on drug-free medium is used. On reading the MIC, the 10-colony end-point is used.

Clinical significance of initial resistance. The incidence of initial resistance varies greatly in different countries. For example, initial resistance to isoniazid, streptomycin, or both these drugs, is found in about 4 per cent of patients in the United Kingdom, 8 per cent in the USA, 10 per cent in France, and 20 per cent in Hong Kong. Initial resistance to rifampicin, pyrazinamide, and ethambutol is, in contrast, rare.

It used to be assumed that if a patient was found to have sputum cultures initially resistant to one or more of the drugs of his prescribed regimen, the drugs to which his organisms were resistant should be replaced by others to which they were sensitive. However, a study in Hong Kong carried out in the 1960s showed that such a policy is inadvisable, because standard chemotherapy with streptomycin, isoniazid, and PAS (the regimen then in use) was successful in the treatment of the great majority of patients with strains initially resistant to one, two, or even all three of these drugs. By far the most important reason for failure of chemotherapy is poor patient compliance, not drug-resistance.

Patients' treatment should not be changed solely on the basis of the results of sensitivity tests on pretreatment sputum cultures. Indeed, routine sensitivity testing of pretreatment cultures is unnecessary. Only if the patient is responding unsatisfactorily to treatment should a change of regimen be considered. In this way, a considerable amount of unnecessary altering of treatment (often to less potent, more toxic, and more expensive regimens) can be avoided.

Clinical significance of acquired resistance. If the sputum cultures remain positive and drug-sensitive during treatment with an ad-

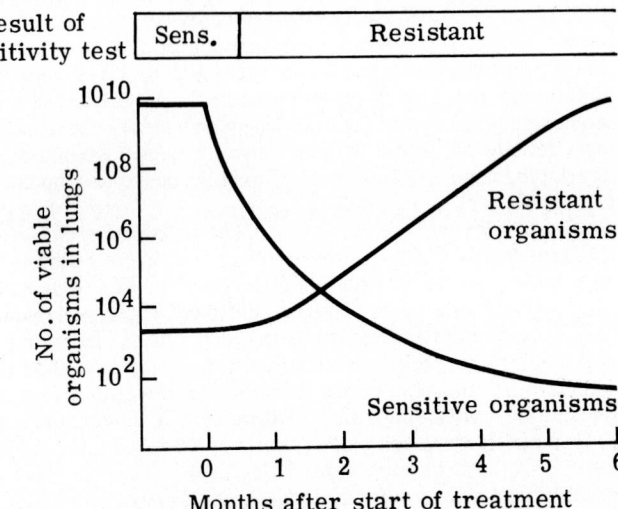

Fig. 3 Diagrammatic representation of the emergence of resistance in the lungs of a patient treated with isoniazid. As treatment proceeds, the sensitive organisms are killed and replaced by the growth of resistant mutants. As soon as the proportion of resistant to sensitive organisms changes from its usual value of about 1 in 10^6 to about 1 in 10^4, the strain can be shown to be resistant in a sensitivity test. (From Mitchison, D. A. (1968). *Recent advances in respiratory tuberculosis.* Churchill Livingstone, Edinburgh, by permission.)

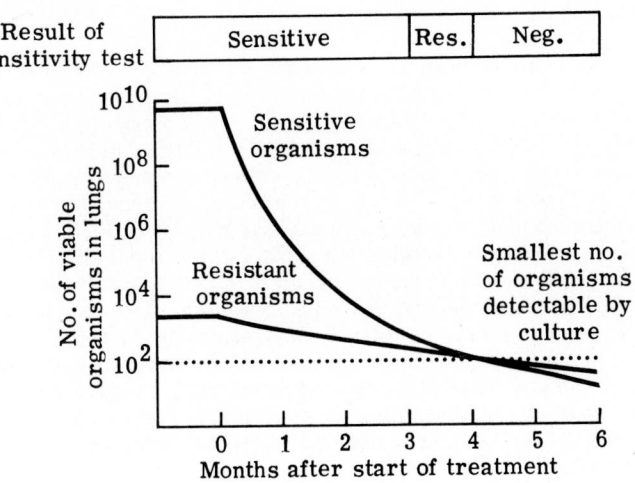

Fig. 4 Diagrammatic presentation of transitional resistance during successful chemotherapy. The resistant mutants are killed more slowly than sensitive organisms. Just before sputum conversion to culture negativity occurs, the few viable organisms may appear resistant. (From Mitchison, D. A. (1968). *Recent advances in respiratory tuberculosis.* Churchill Livingstone, Edinburgh, by permission.)

equate regimen it is almost certain that the patient is not ingesting his drugs. The persistence or recurrence of positive cultures when chemotherapy is being received is almost invariably associated with the emergence of acquired resistance. This can occur if a patient is prescribed an inadequate regimen (such as isoniazid alone) or fails to take all his drugs regularly, thus allowing the number of viable resistant mutants to increase while that of sensitive organisms falls (Fig. 3). This is very different from the situation in which transitional resistance may emerge because resistant mutants are being killed less rapidly than sensitive organisms (Fig. 4). When chemotherapy fails, with the emergence of acquired resistance, the regimen must be changed; if transitional resistance occurs, the regimen should not be changed.

When bacteriological relapse occurs after the end of chemotherapy, the relapse cultures usually have the same pattern of sensitivity and resistance as the pretreatment cultures.

At present, the main roles of sensitivity testing are: (*a*) in research, to help elucidate the mechanisms of chemotherapy; (*b*) to study the epidemiology of drug resistance in a community, and so provide information useful in the planning of antituberculosis programmes; and (*c*) to determine the best retreatment regimen for a patient whose primary chemotherapy has failed.

Epidemiology

Tuberculosis has been a major affliction of man since ancient times. In the United Kingdom during the industrial revolution of the eighteenth century, a tuberculosis epidemic claimed so many victims that it became known as 'the white plague'. Subsequently the disease declined steadily, even in the absence of control measures. The reasons for this may have been related to diminution in the risks of infection associated with reduced overcrowding and also improved nutrition and social conditions, leading to better host resistance. The use of effective case-finding and chemotherapy contributed to the rapid decline occurring in the last few decades in the United Kingdom and other technically advanced countries. By contrast, in many developing countries, control measures have as yet had little impact on tuberculosis, which remains a major cause of illness and death.

Epidemiological studies of tuberculosis are concerned both with tuberculous infection and with tuberculous disease. Tuberculous infection may be defined as a state in which the tubercle bacillus is established in the body without symptoms or detectable evidence of disease. Tuberculous disease is a state in which one or more organs of the body become diseased as shown by bacteriological, radiographic, or other clinical means. Most people in Europe and North America were, until recently, infected by tubercle bacilli at some time in their lives. In contrast, among the younger generation, infection is now uncommon. In developing countries, however, infection is the rule.

The great majority of infected people remain well, the only detectable evidence of infection being a positive tuberculin test. It has been estimated that only about 5–15 per cent of infected persons will develop tuberculous disease. Clinical tuberculosis commonly involves the respiratory system but non-respiratory tuberculosis occurs in 10–30 per cent of patients. The risk of developing tuberculous disease after infection depends on the size of the infecting dose and host factors. The most important host factors include:

1. Age. Infants and children under five have a high risk of progression to disease.

2. Ethnic group. Infection occurring in populations who, because of geographical remoteness, have been exposed to tuberculosis more recently, for example North American Indians and Eskimos, are likely to have a high risk of developing fulminating, acute, rapidly fatal disease. Other races who have experienced tuberculosis for a long time appear to have better host resistance and it has been suggested that this may result from natural selection. Some ethnic groups have a comparatively high risk of tuberculosis. Immigrants from a high-prevalence to a low-prevalence coun-

try may experience an incidence of tuberculosis comparable to that of their country of origin. This appears to occur in spite of adequate screening on entry to the country and persists for some time after entering the country of lower prevalence.

3. Debilitating illness, alcoholism, poor nutrition, immunosuppressants, gastrectomy, and diabetes mellitus are well recognized risk factors.

Source of infection. It has been estimated that one undiagnosed, smear-positive case of pulmonary tuberculosis infects about ten persons during one year. In some developing countries, most of these cases remain undetected and die of tuberculosis, having infected on average more than twenty other people. Raw milk was previously an important source of bovine infection for man. The use of pasteurized milk and the establishment of tuberculosis-free herds of cattle has virtually eradicated bovine tuberculosis from most technically advanced countries. In developing countries the consumption of cow's milk is low and bovine tuberculosis is therefore of minor importance.

Epidemiological indices. Various measures have been used to estimate the impact of tuberculosis on communities. These include statistics of mortality, notification, surveys of the prevalence of patients excreting tubercle bacilli demonstrable by direct smear sputum examinations, mobile chest radiographic surveys, and estimation of the annual tuberculosis infection rate. The latter is the best single indicator for evaluation because, unlike all the other methods mentioned, it is independent of the procedures of the tuberculosis programme in the community, such as the accuracy of notification and mortality rates and the efficiency of case-finding.

Mortality. It is estimated that tuberculosis causes three million deaths annually throughout the world, more than three-quarters occurring in the developing countries. However, mortality is an unreliable measurement of the disease. In the prechemotherapy era, the ratio of mortality to incidence was about one to two. Now, in technically advanced countries, the use of chemotherapy has reduced this ratio to about one to ten. In spite of this, statistics from some technically advanced countries reveal the surprising fact that between 20 and 50 per cent of the total cases dying of tuberculosis were undiagnosed during life.

Morbidity. *Notification rates.* Tuberculosis is a notifiable disease in many technically advanced countries, and notification rates provide useful indices of the tuberculosis problem within each country. Strict comparisons of rates between different countries may, however, be invalid because of differences in local diagnostic and reporting systems. An indication of the difference between technically advanced and developing countries is obtained by noting that for Western Europe and North America rates per 100 000 are of the order of 20 or less, whereas for some developing countries in Southeast Asia and Africa, they are five to ten times greater, even though many cases in developing countries are never detected or notified.

In the United Kingdom, notification rates have declined rapidly since the introduction of effective chemotherapy. Currently the rate is declining at approximately 10 per cent per annum. The rate of decline varies according to age and sex, being steepest in the younger age groups. In men over 55 years of age there has been little fall. These older men represent a cohort most of whom were infected much earlier in their lives and the high morbidity now is likely to be due to endogenous breakdown. The low morbidity in young persons is a reflection of the reduced risk of infection. A survey of notifications for 1978–9 in England showed an estimated annual notification rate of 16 per 100 000, the rate for respiratory tuberculosis being 13, and for non-respiratory five. Among patients of Indian sub-continent origin respiratory disease was 30 times more common than in white patients; non-respiratory disease was 80 times more common. Notifications in Indian sub-continent chil-

dren born in the United Kingdom were 22 times and for those born abroad 51 times those of white children. Non-respiratory disease in Indian sub-continent patients involved most often the cervical or mediastinal lymph nodes, and in white patients the genito-urinary system.

Differences in the incidence and type of tuberculosis among various ethnic groups in the same community may result from differences in the strain of *M.tuberculosis* as shown by phage typing, the stresses of recent emigration, immunological factors and the balance between exogenous and endogenous infection. The major source of infection in the United Kingdom remains the white male aged 55 or more. For every infectious sputum smear-positive patient from the Indian sub-continent there were four patients of white ethnic origin in the 1978–9 survey.

Prevalence of sputum smear-positive cases. The prevalence of sputum smear-positive cases is a measure of the size of the source of infection in a community. It is an indirect measure of the prevalence of the disease. It can easily be assessed by surveys carried out by paramedical staff trained in sputum smear examination. Surveys in developing countries reveal that from 0.2 to 1 per cent of the population are expectorating tubercle bacilli demonstrable by direct smear examinations. Surveys of pulmonary tuberculosis by mass mobile miniature radiography in selected communities in developing countries show disease in between 0.5 and 5 per cent of the population.

Annual tuberculosis infection rate. The annual tuberculosis infection rate is obtained from the results of tuberculin testing surveys. Tuberculin surveys are carried out at intervals in a representative sample of subjects of the same age, tested by the same techniques, excluding those who have received BCG. From the information obtained, the annual tuberculosis infection rates are calculated. This rate is a measure of the risk of tuberculosis in a community and, unlike other epidemiological indices, is independent of the procedures of the tuberculosis programme. In the United Kingdom in 1971–3 the estimated annual risk of infection for children of parents born in the United Kingdom was 0.07 per cent. For children born in the United Kingdom of Asian parentage it was 0.5 per cent and for children born abroad of Asian parentage 1.56 per cent. The risk of infection in the United Kingdom is declining at the rate of about 10 per cent per year. It is likely that in the future tuberculosis will be virtually eradicated in most technically advanced countries during the first half of the next century. In contrast, in most developing countries the present risk of tuberculous infection is 20 to 50 times higher. The trend in the risk of infection varies but in many developing countries has remained constant or has decreased only very slowly over the years (Fig. 5).

The tuberculin test. The tuberculin test is used to detect people infected by the tubercle bacillus. Unfortunately a reaction to tuberculin does not always indicate infection by *M.tuberculosis*. Studies of populations in different parts of the world using PPD tuberculin have shown important variations between communities. By plotting the percentage of reactors against the size of the Mantoux test tuberculin reaction, different patterns emerge (Fig. 6). Sometimes the distribution is bimodal, there being clearcut separation between the distribution of reactions smaller than 10 mm and that of larger reactions due to infection by *M.tuberculosis*. However, in other communities there is no such clear distinction, the distribution being continuous (Fig. 6). The small reactions are evidently non-specific and are probably associated with infection by non-tuberculous mycobacteria. The proportion of a population showing non-specific reactions varies greatly, from 80 per cent or more in some parts of East Asia and India to less than 10 per cent in Denmark and North America. In England it is below 30 per cent and is probably due to infection with *M.avium*. The use of doses higher than 5 TU (tuberculin units) in the Mantoux test or the use of the multiple puncture (Heaf) test increases the frequency with which non-specific reactions are observed. In the UK, using the Mantoux test 5 TU PPD, reactions above 10 mm are likely to

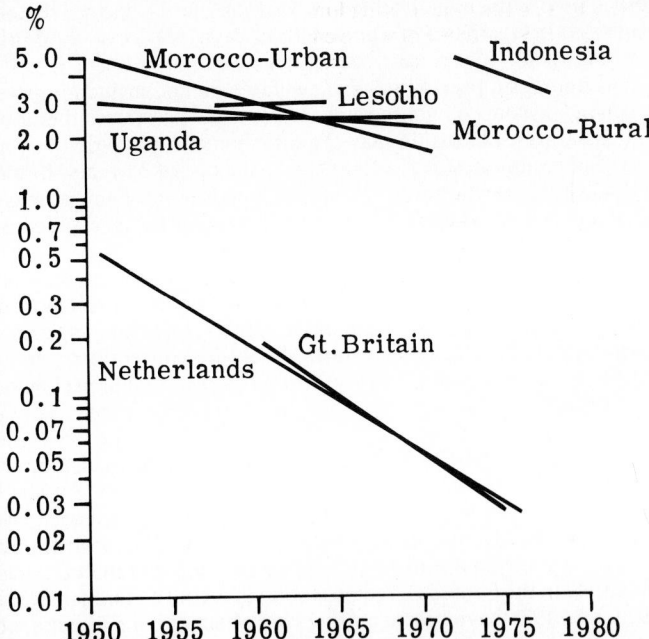

Fig. 5 Estimated annual risks of tuberculous infection in some high-prevalence and low-prevalence countries. (Reproduced by permission of Dr K. Styblo and the International Union Against Tuberculosis.)

indicate tuberculous infection. Most patients with pulmonary tuberculosis have reactions of this size. However, severely ill or malnourished patients may fail to react to 5 TU; these usually become tuberculin positive after their condition has been improved by treatment.

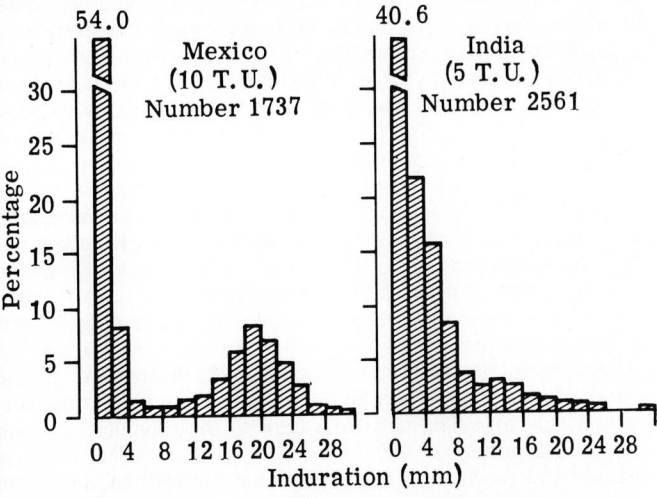

Fig. 6 Size of tuberculin reactions to intradermal testing with 10 TU in Mexico and with 5 TU in India. (Reproduced by permission of the Editor of the *Lancet*.)

Techniques of tuberculin testing. OT (old tuberculin) has been replaced by PPD (purified protein derivative). PPD varies according to its source. Developing countries use a single batch of tuberculin RT23 distributed by the World Health Organization. For tuberculin surveys 5TU of PPD stabilized in Tween 80 is commonly used.

The Mantoux test. In the Mantoux test, 0.1 ml of a solution containing 1, 5, 10, or 100 TU of PPD are injected strictly intradermally. If the technique is correct, a wheal of at least 5 mm should be raised. The reaction is read 48 to 72 hours later and the diameter of induration is measured. The criteria for positivity are mentioned above.

Multiple puncture (Heaf) test. The multiple puncture test is a very convenient technique which is rapid and simple. An instrument which has six needles arranged in a circle is used to puncture the skin through a special, highly concentrated solution containing PPD 2 mg per ml. The reaction may be read between three and ten days later. Reactions are read as follows. Grade 1, four or more discrete papules. Grade 2, confluent papules to form a ring. Grade 3, a disk of induration. Grade 4, induration greater than 10 mm. In Britain grades 1 and 2 are likely to indicate non-tuberculous infection, grades 3 or 4 tuberculous infection.

Other forms of tuberculin testing, including the tine test and scratch test, are not recommended as they are less reliable than the above tests.

Tuberculosis control. The control of tuberculosis depends upon:
1. Case-finding, that is the detection of individuals with tuberculosis in order to render them non-infectious by chemotherapy. This is by far the most important and effective method of control.
2. The detection of individuals who are infected but have not yet developed tuberculous disease in order to prevent them from developing tuberculosis by the use of chemoprophylaxis.
3. The detection of uninfected persons in order to prevent them from acquiring infection by immunizing them with BCG.

Case-finding. Case-finding may be passive, in which patients themselves seek medical help. In developing countries this is usually the only case-finding method used. It can be supplemented by propoganda to encourage symptomatic patients to report for investigation. Case-finding may be active, in which high risk groups are screened.

In the United Kingdom the following high risk groups are actively sought and investigated:
Tuberculosis contacts. About 10 per cent of family contacts of patients with smear-positive pulmonary tuberculosis develop the disease. In most contacts with disease, this is detected on the initial chest radiograph and clinical examination. However, among Asian contacts who eventually develop the disease, in about one-third it takes one or two years after detection of the index case to become clinically evident. Contacts should be tuberculin-tested. Young persons who have a positive tuberculin reaction are probably recent tuberculin convertors and should receive chemoprophylaxis. Tuberculin-negative contacts should receive BCG. However, tuberculin-negative contacts of patients whose sputum is positive on direct smear should not be given BCG immediately but should have their tuberculin test repeated in two months, since they may be in the process of converting. If they remain tuberculin-negative on retesting, they should receive BCG vaccination. Patients whose sputum is negative on smear are very unlikely to have infected their family contacts.
African and Asian immigrants. These immigrants have a high risk of tuberculosis for 10 or more years after arrival in the United Kingdom. They should be screened for tuberculosis soon after arrival in the country, and their medical attendants should take the opportunity of referring those who have escaped this screening on arrival for examination at a later date to exclude tuberculosis and to protect the uninfected by BCG vaccination.

Mass mobile radiography of large numbers of apparently healthy persons, previously used as a method of active case-finding in developed countries, has now been abandoned because, with the decline of tuberculosis, it is no longer cost-effective. However, selective miniature radiography is widely used in the United Kingdom and is based on static miniature camera units situated in chest clinics and district general hospitals. These units screen rapidly and relatively cheaply large numbers of persons referred from general practitioners and other sources.

In the United Kingdom, the following groups are especially worth screening for tuberculosis by chest radiography:
1. Middle-aged and elderly males who develop respiratory symptoms. Unfortunately many of these have chronic respiratory symp-

toms due to cigarette smoking and as a result, the onset of pulmonary tuberculosis produces no obvious change in their symptoms so that the diagnosis may be made late or missed.

2. Individuals with persistent respiratory symptoms, for example a cough of more than three months' duration.

3. Inmates of common lodging houses and psychiatric hospitals and chronic alcoholics.

4. Tuberculin-positive school children.

Tuberculin tests are performed on school children aged 11 to 13 years prior to BCG vaccination. Weak positive reactions are not usually due to tuberculosis infection but strong positive reactors (Mantoux reaction greater than 10 mm, or Heaf test grade 3 or 4) are referred for investigation.

Chest radiography is recommended for people who, though not at high risk from tuberculosis, are working in occupations which bring them in contact with susceptible persons, particularly children. These people include workers in schools, nurseries, and hospitals.

Chemoprophylaxis. *Primary chemoprophylaxis* refers to the use of antituberculosis drugs in uninfected tuberculin-negative individuals in order to prevent infection. It has been used, for example, to prevent infection in infants breast fed by tuberculous mothers. *Secondary chemoprophylaxis* refers to the use of anti-tuberculosis drugs in infected but healthy people who have no clinical evidence of tuberculous disease, in order to prevent the development of disease.

The efficacy of isoniazid in chemoprophylaxis has been validated in several large trials in various countries. These have shown that the incidence of clinical tuberculosis in the treated groups was about two-thirds less than in the placebo groups and that the protective effect lasted for many years. The dose of isoniazid is 300 mg daily in adults (5–10 mg per kg daily in children) continued for 12 months. Six months of treatment is probably as effective as 12 months. The risk of isoniazid-induced liver disease is small and age-related. In the USA, a large study showed that progressive liver damage was rare in subjects under 20 years of age, occurred in 0.3 per cent or less of subjects aged 20 to 34 years, in 1.2 per cent aged 35 to 49 years, and in about 1.7 per cent of persons aged 50 years or more. Liver dysfunction is usually reversible on stopping isoniazid. Up to 20 per cent of persons receiving isoniazid will have some asymptomatic elevation of serum hepatic enzyme concentrations which usually normalize without discontinuing the drug. However, chemoprophylaxis is contra-indicated in subjects with liver disease and in people who take alcohol regularly. Patients receiving isoniazid chemoprophylaxis should be seen at monthly intervals, but routine liver function tests are not recommended, only being undertaken when patients have symptoms suggestive of hepatotoxicity.

There is considerable disagreement about the indications for chemoprophylaxis. The decision to give chemoprophylaxis depends upon the consideration of: (*a*) the risk of developing tuberculosis; (*b*) the risk of isoniazid-induced hepatitis; and (*c*) the likelihood of patient compliance.

Chemoprophylaxis is usually recommended for the following groups in technically advanced countries:

1. Recently infected persons, about 10 per cent of whom can be expected to develop tuberculosis within one year. These include recent tuberculin convertors and tuberculin-positive persons in close contact with infectious tuberculosis.

2. Tuberculin-positive children under the age of five years, whose risk of developing tuberculosis, including miliary tuberculosis and meningitis, is known to be high.

3. Strongly positive tuberculin reactors among other groups known to be at high risk, for example recent immigrants and refugees from countries with a high prevalence of tuberculosis.

The use of chemoprophylaxis in the following groups remains contentious:

1. Children aged 11–13 years with a strongly positive tuberculin

test. The occurrence of tuberculosis in this group in the United Kingdom is less than 1 per cent in five years. This very small risk does not justify the routine use of chemoprophylaxis.

2. Immunosuppressed patients. Some patients, including those receiving prolonged immunosuppressive or corticosteroid therapy and renal transplantation may require chemoprophylaxis.

3. Tuberculin-positive patients up to the age of 35 years. In the USA, where the control programme depends upon chemoprophylaxis rather than on BCG vaccination, chemoprophylaxis is recommended for this group.

Care should be taken not to give chemoprophylaxis to subjects who may have active tuberculous disease, for whom treatment with at least two antituberculosis drugs is necessary. In developing countries with limited facilities, efforts should be concentrated upon efficient treatment services for tuberculosis rather than on chemoprophylaxis.

BCG vaccination. BCG vaccine consists of an attenuated strain of the bovine bacillus developed by Calmette and Guérin which, when injected into man, confers considerable immunity against tuberculosis. The effectiveness of the BCG has been clearly demonstrated in several controlled studies, but appears to vary in different communities. In the United Kingdom studies in school children in 1952, 1973, and 1978 have shown a protective effect of over 70 per cent persisting for 15 years, and studies elsewhere have shown similar protective effects. Some other studies, however, have shown less protection and some none at all. Apparently unsatisfactory results from BCG have been reported most often from communities where infections with non-tuberculous mycobacteria are common. These non-tuberculous infections convey some protection against tuberculosis. Administration of BCG to these already partly immune subjects blunts the effect of BCG. When such partly immune subjects have been excluded by tuberculin tests using 100 TU, BCG vaccination has been shown to be highly effective. Other factors that may be responsible for low efficacy include low potency and incorrect administration of the vaccine, and poor nutritional status and unfavourable genetic factors in the vaccinated subjects.

Indications. BCG is recommended for the following groups:

1. Persons repeatedly exposed to tuberculosis such as medical students, doctors, nurses, laboratory technicians and other hospital workers.

2. Travellers to high prevalence areas.

3. Contacts.

4. People living in communities where there is a high incidence of infection, such as Asian communities in the United Kingdom.

5. School children aged 11–13 years. In the United Kingdom mass vaccination of these children is undertaken and remains cost-effective. However, the risks of infection are declining by 10 per cent per year.

The policy for the last group is being periodically reviewed with a view to discontinuing vaccination when infection risks become appropriately low. The need to vaccinate the other groups will continue indefinitely.

Mass BCG vaccination in developing countries must be given before infection has taken place, preferably at birth or in infancy. In communities where this policy has been efficiently implemented the mortality and morbidity from tuberculosis in childhood have fallen greatly.

BCG vaccination technique. In technically advanced countries, subjects for BCG are first tuberculin tested using the Mantoux or the Heaf test. In the United Kingdom, those who react with less than 6 mm of induration to 5 TU or whose reaction to the Heaf test is grade 0 or 1 are given BCG. In developing countries, BCG vaccination may be given without preliminary tuberculin testing since reactions to BCG in tuberculin-positive subjects are rarely severe. Freeze-dried BCG vaccine is stable and convenient. It is best administered by syringe and needle intradermally. Percutaneous vaccination with a multiple puncture apparatus delivering 40 punctures using a specially concentrated vaccine is also effective nd rapid, and its use requires minimal skill. Administration by jet ajector is less effective and may cause severe local reactions.

Adverse reactions to BCG are rare. A small ulcer may occur at ne site of injection. Large ulcers or abscesses usually result when BCG is injected too deeply. Local lymphadenitis may occur, particularly in infants. Bad local reactions may be controlled with oniazid. BCG osteomyelitis has recently been reported in Scandinavia. The very few deaths reported from BCG appear to have een confined to immunologically deficient subjects.

Pathogenesis

Tuberculosis is almost always spread by the airborne dissemination of droplet nuclei, each measuring about 2–10 μm in diameter and ontaining one or two viable bacilli, which are inhaled and deosited in alveoli. However, tuberculous disease develops in only a roportion of individuals infected. Whether disease develops, and ts extent when it does, are influenced by the patient's immune tatus, particularly the balance between hypersensitivity and imnunity, the virulence of the infecting strain, the size of the infecting lose of organisms, the route of infection, and the host's age, native esistance, and general level of health and nutrition.

Primary infection. Primary infection usually occurs through the ower respiratory tract so that the lung is almost invariably the first organ involved. Primary infection of the gastrointestinal tract causng disease of the tonsils or of the intestine and the associated nodes s now uncommon since the virtual eradication of bovine tuberculosis. Inoculation may result from accidents in laboratories or utopsy rooms.

Because there is at this stage no acquired immunity, the bacilli nultiply rapidly, eliciting an exudative inflammatory response in which polymorphonuclear leucocytes and monocytes predominate, and, within a few hours to a few days, there is widespread haemaogenous and lymphatic dissemination to other parts of the lungs and to most other tissues, particularly lymph nodes, bones, and kidneys, bacilli multiplying most rapidly in the lungs. Also, because hypersensitivity has not yet developed, there is no tissue destrucion and no cavitation. Primary infection is essentially a widespread nfection of the reticulo-endothelial system, the bacilli multiplying rapidly within mononuclear phagocytes. It may be associated with fever and mild illness, but these are usually so trivial that patients do not usually present at this stage.

In spite of the widespread nature of the primary infection it rarely causes widespread disease. Indeed, in the majority of subjects it resolves spontaneously within a few weeks; the rate of multiplication of bacilli rapidly decreases in all sites as acquired immunity develops, and dissemination ceases. The inflammatory reaction resolves, the initial site of infection and its related lymph nodes may calcify, and any surviving bacilli become dormant and remain so indefinitely, particularly in the apical and subapical regions of the lungs (Simon's foci). At the same time tuberculin sensitivity develops, demonstrating the presence of specifically sensitized T lymphocytes. Thus, in the majority of subjects, primary infection is rapidly and effectively controlled by the host's immune response, which also greatly modifies the response to subsequent reinfection or to the reactivation of a primary focus (post-primary tuberculosis).

In children, the initial lesion of primary infection usually remains small, but the associated lymph nodes become greatly enlarged, forming the well-known primary (Ghon) complex. In contrast, node enlargement is usually much less evident in adult patients, especially in the white races. Indeed, primary infection in the tuberculin-negative white adult may closely resemble post-primary tuberculosis. These differences probably reflect differences in immunological competence and in degrees of exposure to other mycobacteria.

Although the commonest course of primary infection is healing and calcification, in a few patients it progresses. This may occur by continued haematogenous and lymphatic dissemination causing seeding of disease in other organs or generalized miliary disease. Alternatively, as hypersensitivity develops, the initial lesion may become destructive and extend locally.

A heavy infection during the first few months of life is particularly liable to lead to widespread and rapidly progressive disease. Pulmonary disease can also progress rapidly during adolescence, particularly in girls.

Post-primary tuberculosis. The alteration to the host's immune status which occurs during primary infection greatly modifies the response to the reactivation of a primary lesion or to reinfection. Post-primary tuberculosis occurs in spite of acquired cellular immunity and is therefore characteristically localized without regional lymph node enlargement or lymphatic or haematogenous dissemination. It usually results from the reactivation of one or more primary lesions. Histologically the lesions are characterized by granuloma formation with giant cells and central caseation. There may be extensive tissue destruction and necrosis, reflecting hypersensitivity to tuberculoproteins, and healing occurs by fibrosis rather than by calcification. Once necrosis has occurred, cellular immunity is locally abolished, because macrophages and lymphocytes cannot function in unoxygenated necrotic tissue.

The most commonly affected sites of post-primary tuberculosis are the apical and subapical regions of the lungs, probably because of the high intra-alveolar oxygen tension, but any of the sites of the original primary haematogenous dissemination may be involved.

Tubercle bacilli can remain viable but dormant for many years. The immune response greatly inhibits multiplication of bacilli in post-primary tuberculosis, but it does not necessarily kill them. Any condition which compromises cellular immunity makes the reactivation of a previous lesion more likely. Such conditions include severe malnutrition, old age, diabetes mellitus, any debilitating disease, and immunosuppressive therapy. It is also important to realize that active tuberculosis itself depresses cellular immune responses, which recover within about eight weeks with effective antituberculosis chemotherapy.

CLINICAL COURSE

Clinical features of the primary infection

The natural history of primary tuberculosis is summarized in Fig. 7.

Four to eight weeks after the initial infection, tuberculin hypersensitivity appears and may be detected by tuberculin testing. This immunological event is not usually associated with symptoms but some individuals may have malaise and fever, symptoms which soon subside without treatment. Occasionally, erythema nodosum and phlyctenular conjunctivitis occur as an allergic manifestation.

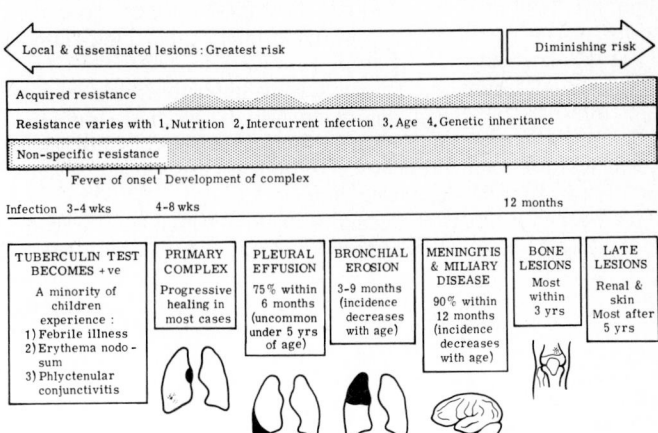

Fig. 7 The natural history of untreated primary tuberculosis. (Adapted from Miller, F. J. W. (1963) and (1981). *Tuberculosis in children*. Churchill Livingstone, Edinburgh, by permission.)

The most serious sequel to the primary infection is disseminated tuberculosis, which is almost always rapidly fatal if untreated. The risk is greatest when infection occurs in infancy and early childhood.

Primary pulmonary tuberculosis. The pulmonary component of the primary intrathoracic complex consists of a lesion which is usually close to the pleura, most commonly in the lower two-thirds of the lungs, where ventilation is greatest and hence the deposition of airborne infection most likely, but some observers report a bias to upper zones in adolescents and young adults. The draining peribronchial and hilar lymph nodes soon become involved. In young children, lymph node involvement tends to be prominent and easily seen on the chest radiograph, on which the lung component may be small or invisible. Bronchial complications due to lymph node enlargement, such as compression, erosion, and the bronchial aspiration of caseous material are a greater risk in young children than in older patients.

In older children and adults, the lung component is the most obvious part of the primary complex and the lymph node component may be small or invisible. Under these circumstances, primary tuberculosis is indistinguishable from post-primary tuberculosis, except when tuberculin conversion is known to have occurred recently.

Symptoms and signs. Primary pulmonary tuberculosis is usually symptomless, and discovered as a result of the routine screening of contacts of an infectious patient. The symptoms comprise cough, which is usually dry, fever, reduced appetite, and, in children, failure to thrive. More severe symptoms may arise as a result of involvement of the trachea and bronchi by caseating parabronchial or paratracheal lymph nodes, the rupture of which into the air passages causes severe respiratory distress. Pressure on the bronchi produces a paroxysmal cough, which may be mistaken for pertussis. Wheeze, due to bronchial narrowing, may be confused with asthma. Valvular obstruction resulting in obstructive emphysema is best seen on chest radiographs taken in expiration. Bronchial compression by lymph nodes may result in lobar or segmental collapse. Resolution is usual but bronchiectasis may develop distal to the obstruction.

When the primary lesion is sited in the upper lobes, severe sequelae are unlikely to occur because the drainage is good. However, involvement of the middle lobe, or lingular or apical segments of the lower lobe is more likely to result in subsequent sputum retention and troublesome symptoms of infected bronchiectasis. Involvement of the wall of the bronchus by caseating lymph nodes may result in permanent damage and fibrous stricture. This is particularly likely to occur at the orifice of the middle lobe. Patients so affected may present years later in adult life with middle lobe pneumonia, lung abscess, or appearances mimicking bronchial carcinoma. However, the presence of calcified lesions close to the middle lobe orifice, suggests previous primary tuberculous infection at that site (Brock's syndrome).

Lymph nodes may heal yet contain living bacilli which remain latent for years but eventually reactivate and discharge into the bronchus. Patients so affected present with haemoptysis and other clinical features, and bronchoscopic appearances closely resembling those of bronchogenic carcinoma.

Homogeneous lobar or segmental shadows which resolve without treatment are a well-recognized feature of childhood primary pulmonary tuberculosis and have been referred to as epituberculosis. This is thought to result from the inhalation of tuberculous material from lymph nodes, which in the presence of hypersensitivity to tuberculoprotein results in an intra-alveolar hypersensitivity reaction which clears as hypersensitivity diminishes.

In spite of the long list of possible complications, it must be stressed that primary pulmonary tuberculosis is usually a mild illness which resolves spontaneously without sequelae. In general it is only in infants and in children under five years of age that the disease is likely to have serious immediate consequences.

Diagnosis. Primary pulmonary tuberculosis is usually diagnosed during routine radiographic examination of the contacts of tuberculous patients and rarely as a result of symptoms. The tuberculin test is almost always strongly positive (positive Mantoux to 1 or 10 TU or multiple puncture test grade 3 or 4). Previous BCG vaccination does not usually result in a strongly positive tuberculin test. Radiographic appearances may be suggestive if there is evidence of the lung and/or the lymph node component of the primary complex. The radiographic appearances of epituberculosis have been noted above.

Bacteriological confirmation should be sought by culture of available material (sputum, pharyngeal secretions, laryngeal swab, or gastric lavage). It is reasonable to assume that children who have not received BCG and who have a strongly positive tuberculin test and compatible lung shadows, have primary pulmonary tuberculosis unless an alternative cause for lung shadows is evident.

Treatment. Chemotherapy should be given to all cases of primary pulmonary tuberculosis in order to prevent complications and progression of the pulmonary lesion and dissemination of tuberculosis to other organs. A combination of two drugs should be used, since the number of organisms may be great and there is risk of acquired resistance if monotherapy is given. This contrasts with the policy for individuals in whom the only evidence of infection is a positive tuberculin test and who have no clinical evidence of tuberculous disease, for whom chemoprophylaxis with isoniazid alone is recommended.

Chemotherapy with daily isoniazid, 5–10 mg/kg, and rifampicin 10 mg/kg is well accepted by children. Isoniazid may be given as crushed tablets and the rifampicin as a palatable syrup, both drugs being given in a single daily dose. This treatment is given for nine months. Sodium PAS is a cheaper alternative to rifampicin as a companion drug to isoniazid and is given in a dose of 300 mg/kg per day. However, when PAS is used, chemotherapy should be continued for a minimum of one year, extending to 18 months for extensive or slowly resolving lesions. Ethambutol is not recommended in children because of difficulty in detecting eye toxicity should it occur.

It is important to enquire into the probable source of infection. If this is likely to be a patient harbouring bacilli resistant to one of the drugs being used, then chemotherapy may need to be modified appropriately. If a third drug is required because of the possibility of drug resistance, streptomycin 20 mg/kg per day should be given by intramuscular injection.

Children with primary pulmonary tuberculosis are often asymptomatic or rapidly lose their symptoms. The need to continue with prolonged medication needs careful explanation to parents.

Tracheal and bronchial complications may need additional treatment. The rupture of lymph nodes into the trachea or bronchi may require emergency bronchoscopy to clear the airway. Massive lymph node enlargement which jeopardizes the airway may justify surgical draining of the nodes to prevent rupture or obstructive emphysema. The place of corticosteroids in treating the bronchial complications is unestablished, but their use is probably justified before resorting to surgery unless the condition is critical. Damage to the bronchi from caseating lymphadenitis often heals satisfactorily during chemotherapy, but occasionally severe bronchial stenosis may jeopardize the function of otherwise normal lobes and require correction by appropriate reconstructive surgery.

Bronchiectasis, which may follow primary tuberculosis, rarely requires special treatment since it is usually asymptomatic.

Erythema nodosum. Erythema nodosum is a skin rash associated with allergic hypersensitivity and occurs in a wide variety of disorders, including tuberculosis.

The dermal lesions consist of a perivascular inflammation involving veins and arteries, and also fat and connective tissues. The lesions are thought to be associated with high levels of circulating immune complexes. Erythema nodosum due to primary tubercuosis infection has been reported in between 1 per cent and 15 per cent of these infections in Caucasians; it is said to be rare in dark-skinned races. It is more common in girls than boys and in older than in younger children. The eruption appears within a few weeks of the primary infection, although occasionally occurring much later, or in association with post-primary tuberculosis.

The principle clinical feature of erythema nodosum is a rash on the front of the legs below the knee. The lesions are red, nodular, usually multiple, discrete, but sometimes confluent. They may also occur on the front of the thighs and on the extensor aspects of the forearms. Lesions usually resolve within three weeks but sometimes crops of nodules recur over several weeks. Systemic symptoms include prolonged fever in association with arthralgia involving the larger joints, particularly the ankles and knees, with swelling, heat, and tenderness of the joints. These severe systemic symptoms occur most often in adult females.

The diagnosis of the cause of erythema nodosum may be difficult because it is associated with a wide variety of disorders, including tuberculosis, leprosy, haemolytic streptococcal infection, coccidio-idomycosis, histoplasmosis, cat-scratch disease, rheumatic fever, drug allergy, and sarcoidosis. In Britain, sarcoidosis is by far the commonest cause. Tuberculous erythema nodosum is invariably associated with a strongly positive tuberculin test and there may be characteristic radiographic appearances of primary tuberculosis. A negative or weakly positive tuberculin test suggests other causes, and if bilateral hilar node enlargement is present, sarcoidosis is almost certainly the cause. Evidence of streptococcal infection or drug allergy should be sought.

Tuberculous erythema nodosum should be treated with anti-tuberculosis drugs. When the chest radiograph shows evidence of primary pulmonary tuberculosis or when there is evidence of a primary focus elsewhere, two antituberculosis drugs should be used. When there is no clinical evidence of tuberculosis but the tuberculin test is strongly positive, and when there is no evidence of another cause for the erythema nodosum, isoniazid chemoprophy-laxis is given in order to prevent tuberculosis from occurring later.

Phlyctenular conjunctivitis. This form of conjunctivitis is associated with tuberculous allergic hypersensitivity. It is now very rare in Britain. It occurs most often in children within a year of primary infection. The characteristic appearance is of small, multiple, yellow or grey conjunctival nodules near the limbus with a sheaf of dilated vessels radiating outwards. Lesions subside in a few days but may recur at intervals. Treatment is with chemotherapy for the associated tuberculous lesion, and local treatment with atropine ointment, to dilate the pupil, and hydrocortisone drops, to relieve symptoms.

Miliary (disseminated) tuberculosis. Miliary tuberculosis is characterized by the occurrence of tuberculous granulomata in many organs of the body following the widespread haematogenous dissemination of tubercle bacilli. A grave illness results which, if untreated, is almost invariably fatal.

The epidemiology and clinical features of miliary tuberculosis vary greatly in different communities. In developing countries, where tuberculosis is frequent, it is mainly a disease of young children in whom it occurs within a year of the primary infection. The illness is of rapid onset and is acute and rapidly fatal (acute miliary tuberculosis). By contrast, in the United Kingdom and other technically advanced countries, the pattern has changed greatly and it now tends to afflict the elderly, in whom it is an insidious and chronic disease (cryptic disseminated tuberculosis). The diagnosis is all too often missed and revealed only at autopsy. In Asian immigrants to the United Kingdom, prolonged pyrexia may be the only clinical feature preceding the appearance of clinically evident disseminated lesions.

Disseminated tuberculosis is a hazard in patients with lymphomas and leukaemias and in other situations associated with immunosuppression. Under these circumstances the lesions are often of the non-reactive variety in which many tubercle bacilli are seen in areas of necrosis which do not show any typical tuberculous granulation tissue. Surgical procedures on tuberculous organs may result in miliary dissemination and hence antituberculosis chemotherapy should precede surgery or follow surgery as soon as possible if the diagnosis is made at surgery.

Clinical features. The onset in the young is usually acute, in the elderly insidious. General symptoms are fever, weakness, malaise, loss of weight, dry cough, and breathlessness. Associated tuberculous meningitis may cause the presenting symptoms.

A pathognomonic sign is the presence of choroidal tubercles which, if carefully sought, are often found to be present. Hepatosplenomegaly usually occurs. The chest radiograph classically shows uniformly distributed nodules, occasionally with a reticular pattern in the more chronic cases. However, the radiograph may be normal. Pleural effusions, if present, offer the opportunity of diagnosis by finding tuberculous granulation tissue in the pleura obtained by needle biopsy.

Diagnosis. Diagnosis depends upon the finding of tubercle bacilli or characteristic tuberculous granulation tissue. However, in the non-reactive type of disease the histology is not specific but acid-fast bacilli are usually plentiful. Sputum and urine may yield *M. tuberculosis* on smear or culture. Biopsy of liver, lymph node, or bone marrow, or of any suspicious bone or skin lesion, may yield tuberculous granulation tissue or acid-fast bacilli. Transbronchial lung biopsy using the fibre-optic bronchoscope is valuable in cases in which miliary pulmonary shadows occur. The tuberculin test is usually positive, but in elderly or the immunosuppressed may be negative. The white blood count is usually normal. However, in the elderly, blood dyscrasias of a wide variety may occur; they include anaemia, leucopenia, thrombocytopenia, pancytopenia, leucoerythroblastic anaemia and polycythaemia, and disseminated intravascular clotting. These reactions may occur as a result of bone marrow involvement, hypersplenism, or hypersensitivity effects on the marrow. Biochemical abnormalities include hypokalaemia and also hyponatraemia due to inappropriate secretion of antidiuretic hormone.

In the elderly with cryptic disseminated disease, and in Asian immigrants to Britain who present with prolonged pyrexia, the diagnosis is often missed because the possibility of tuberculosis is not thought of. All too often chronic fever and ill health in the aged are erroneously attributed to some coexistent chronic disease or presumed occult tumour. Diagnosis is particularly difficult because choroidal tubercles are often absent, miliary pulmonary mottling may not be seen on chest radiography, and the tuberculin test may be negative. Patients must be adequately investigated, bacteriologically and by biopsy of liver, lymph node or bone marrow. Should all these tests in addition to other investigations for possible causes of pyrexia prove negative, a therapeutic trial of isoniazid with ethambutol or PAS should be given. Other antituberculosis drugs which may affect other causes of pyrexia should be withheld initially. When fever is due to tuberculosis, pyrexia will usually begin to respond within a week.

Treatment. Chemotherapy should be started without delay, once bacteriological and biopsy specimens have been obtained, even if the diagnosis has not yet been confirmed. Initial treatment is with three or four drugs as recommended for pulmonary tuberculosis (see page 5.246). Continuation therapy should be maintained up to 18 months since there is no evidence from controlled clinical trials about the efficacy of short-course chemotherapy in disseminated tuberculosis.

In severely ill patients corticosteroid drugs should be added. Prednisolone 40–60 mg daily suppresses fever and improves the condition of the patient. Thereafter, the dose is reduced to the minimum required to prevent the return of pyrexia or other symptoms, continuing for six to eight weeks.

In countries with a higher prevalence of tuberculosis, BCG vaccination at birth or in infancy is important in preventing miliary tuberculosis and meningitis in childhood.

Post-primary pulmonary tuberculosis

The lungs are the commonest site of post-primary tuberculosis and provide the main source of spread of infection. A person in whose sputum bacilli are present on direct smear may cough up over 1000 million bacilli daily.

Post-primary pulmonary tuberculosis in Britain usually results from reactivation of a pulmonary primary infection acquired by the patient many years before. This is the usual reason for the occurrence of the disease in middle aged and elderly men, who provide the majority of cases seen in this country. Exogenous reinfection and haematogenous spread to the lung are uncommon mechanisms. Post-primary pulmonary tuberculosis may also result from a direct progression of the pulmonary primary infection. This is seen particularly in young Asian immigrants in Britain but rarely occurs in the white native-born population. The course of pulmonary tuberculosis varies greatly. At one extreme is an acute caseating lesion with gross cavitation (galloping consumption). This type is seen particularly in Africans and in people from the Indian subcontinent. At the other extreme the disease may be very chronic, grumbling on for many years, healing spontaneously by fibrosis in some some areas, while spreading in others and forming chronic cavities as the long fight between bacilli and host continues over many years.

Clinical features. Pulmonary tuberculosis may give rise to no symptoms for a considerable time during which it is detectable only by routine chest radiography. The early symptoms usually have an insidious onset and are general in nature; they include malaise, weight loss, fever, night sweats, anxiety, depression, anorexia, and dyspepsia.

Among the respiratory symptoms cough is the commonest and when it is productive, sputum tends to be produced in the morning, and is purulent and sometimes blood-stained. Chest pain may be aching or pleuritic in character. Rarely patients present with an acute pneumonia.

Common presenting features of patients in Britain are as follows:
1. Persistent cough. In middle-aged smokers with tuberculosis this symptom may have been attributed to smokers' cough thus delaying diagnosis.
2. Pneumonia which fails to respond to antibiotics. Under these circumstances sputum should always be examined for tubercle bacilli.
3. Haemoptysis. This is usually recurrent and minor.
4. Unexplained chronic ill health.
5. The radiographic detection of pulmonary lesions during examination of high incidence groups including people with respiratory symptoms and recent immigrants from Asia and Africa.

Physical signs are often absent, even though shadows are obvious on chest radiography. Crackles occur, especially after cough. Chronic fibrotic disease may produce a variety of chest signs including diminished movement, dullness, bronchial breathing at the apex, and tracheal deviation.

Radiology. There are no absolutely diagnostic radiographic appearances. The following findings support the diagnosis:
1. Nodular or patchy shadows in the upper lobes, particularly in the posterior and apical segments.
2. Bilateral upper zone shadows.
3. Cavitation in the upper lobes.
4. Calcification.
5. Linear shadows indicating fibrosis in the upper lobes associated with soft shadows suggesting an active process.

Pulmonary shadows may be associated with pleural effusion. Mediastinal lymph node enlargement may be very prominent in post-primary tuberculosis in Asian immigrants to Britain. Single or multiple pulmonary nodules and diffuse reticular or miliary shadows present special diagnostic problems.

Bacteriology. Growth of M. tuberculosis from sputum specimen provides proof of diagnosis. Microscopy of sputum smears gives a rapid diagnosis but bacilli can be seen in only about half the total number of patients treated for pulmonary tuberculosis. Examination of direct smears by fluorescence microscopy is a rapid and cheap technique. Culture examination by standard techniques requires between three and eight weeks to grow bacilli. Spontaneously produced sputum is the best material for examination (see page 5.239). If the patient has no sputum, secretions may be stimulated by the inhalation of ultrasonically nebulized water. Alternatively, specimens may be obtained by aspirating resting early morning gastric juice or by taking laryngeal swabs. Bronchial lavage using a fibre-optic bronchoscope taken from appropriate sites close to the radiographic lesion is especially likely to yield positive results and can be combined with bronchial or transbronchial biopsies for histological and bacteriological examination.

The blood count usually shows a normal total white cell count, a raised ESR, and sometimes anaemia due to deficiency of iron and folic acid. Liver function tests are quite commonly impaired due to toxic effects on the liver or the presence of tuberculous granulomata. Liver function generally improves during chemotherapy.

The tuberculin test is usually strongly positive but may occasionally be negative. The diagnostic value of the test is limited by the fact that a positive reaction may occur in the absence of active tuberculous disease and may result from previous infection with M. tuberculosis or BCG vaccination, and small reactions may be due to non-tuberculous mycobacterial infections.

Differential diagnosis. Pulmonary tuberculosis may mimic many other diseases and difficulty in diagnosis may arise under the following circumstances:
1. Bronchogenic carcinoma may be suggested in middle-aged smokers by evidence of collapse in the upper lobes or the presence of a solitary round focus. Tomograms showing central cavitation, calcification, or the presence of satellite lesions, though favouring tuberculosis, may also occur in carcinoma. In the absence of a positive sputum, confirmation of diagnosis may require histological evidence from bronchial biopsy, transbronchial or needle biopsy of the lung, or occasionally thorocotomy. Even the finding of tubercle bacilli does not exclude carcinoma since both diseases may coexist and falsely positive sputum cytology may occur in the presence of active pulmonary tuberculosis.
2. In acute pneumonia and lung abscess, examination of sputum for acid-fast bacilli should not be forgotten, especially if these conditions do not respond to antibiotics. Chronic pneumonia due to staphylococci, Klebsiella pneumoniae, or anaerobic organisms can result in an illness resembling tuberculosis. The presence of much foul sputum suggests a pyogenic abscess.
3. Sarcoidosis. Patients typically have few symptoms and negative tuberculin tests. Confirmation by biopsy of lymph node, Kveim test site, or lung establish the diagnosis. It should be remembered that tissue taken from the periphery of caseating tuberculous lesions may show non-caseating granulomata histologically indistinguishable from sarcoidosis.
4. Allergic bronchopulmonary aspergillosis of long standing gives rise to fixed upper zone shadows resulting from bronchiectasis and fibrosis, the appearances closely resembling tuberculosis. Patients are usually asthmatic and have characteristic immunological evidence of allergic aspergillosis.
5. Extrinsic alveolitis, especially avian lung, gives upper lobe shadowing but should be distinguished by a history of exposure to organic antigens and by immunological tests.
6. Pneumoconiosis, especially that due to silica or coal, may be complicated by tuberculosis and requires investigation by careful sputum examination.

7. The chronic constitutional symptoms associated with pulmonary tuberculosis may be mistaken for those produced by many other disorders, including psychoneurosis, diabetes mellitus, hyperthyroidism, and in the elderly may simply be attributed to old age. Tuberculosis should never be forgotten as an important cause of fever of obscure origin.

8. Gross mediastinal lymphadenopathy associated with post-primary pulmonary tuberculosis is a feature of tuberculosis in immigrants to the United Kingdom from Asia and Africa. In distinguishing this from lymphadenopathy due to lymphoma or sarcoidosis a strongly positive tuberculin test is helpful but lymph node biopsy by mediastinoscopy may occasionally be necessary.

Complications of pulmonary tuberculosis. *Pleural effusion.* The release into the pleural space of tuberculoprotein from a lung lesion in a host who is hypersensitive to tuberculoprotein gives rise to a vigorous inflammatory reaction in the pleura and the formation of a pleural effusion. Pleural effusions may occur in primary or post-primary disease. Pleural effusion occurring within six months of primary tuberculous infection used to be common in the United Kingdom, particularly in adolescents and young adults, but is now rare since the introduction of mass BCG vaccination of schoolchildren. It is still seen in Asian immigrants. The primary complex may not be evident on chest radiography. Recognition of the tuberculous aetiology of the pleural effusion is important because, although the effusion tends to resolve spontaneously, patients commonly develop pulmonary tuberculosis within the subsequent five years, an event prevented by giving antituberculosis chemotherapy at the stage of the effusion. Pleural effusions may result from post-primary pulmonary tuberculosis, which is usually evident on chest radiography. Diagnosis of the tuberculous nature of the pleural effusion is best made by obtaining pleura by needle biopsy. Tuberculous granulation tissue is seen in about 80 per cent of cases investigated by this method. The pleural exudate is usually lymphocytic but rarely contains tubercle bacilli on smear or culture. The tuberculin test is positive except in acutely ill, febrile patients.

Tuberculous pleural effusions usually resolve on treatment with antituberculosis drugs. Prednisolone is a useful aid to the absorption of fluid and for the prevention of pleural thickening, and is indicated when effusions are massive and slow to absorb, or when there is evidence of the onset of pleural thickening. Multiple aspirations of pleural fluid are seldom needed, because antituberculosis drugs with prednisolone are usually very effective at dealing with large or slowly absorbing effusions.

Tuberculous empyema. Rupture of a cavity or large caseous lesion into the pleura produces an empyema and pneumothorax (pyopneumothorax) with bronchopleural fistula. Tubercle bacilli are usually found on direct smear of the pleural pus. Treatment requires adequate drainage and antituberculosis drug therapy.

Haemoptysis. Bleeding arising from ulceration of the bronchial mucosa is usually slight or moderate in amount. Occasionally a pulmonary artery within a tuberculous cavity is eroded and this may cause massive and sometimes fatal haemoptysis.

Aspergilloma. Study of British patients with open healed tuberculous cavities showed that about one-third of them had serological evidence of aspergillus infestation but were without clinical evidence of pulmonary disease due to the fungus. Another 15 per cent had radiological evidence of an aspergilloma (aspergillus fungus ball) within a pulmonary cavity. Whilst most of these aspergillomas are innocuous, about 10 per cent of them result in recurrent, severe, or life-threatening haemorrhage. When haemorrhage is a feature, pulmonary resection should be undertaken for removal of the aspergilloma if respiratory function permits this operation to be performed safely. Aspergillomas rarely occur in the presence of active tuberculosis.

Tuberculosis of bronchi and larynx. Bronchi are frequently damaged by tuberculosis or its fibrotic healing process. Upper lobe bronchiectasis rarely gives rise to symptoms because it is well drained, but in the lower portions of the lungs, symptoms of infected bronchiectasis may result and require treatment. Haemoptysis in the absence of active tuberculosis may arise from post-tuberculous bronchiectasis. Tuberculous endobronchitis may cause tubercle bacilli to appear in the sputum in the presence of a normal chest radiograph. Tuberculous laryngitis occurs in advanced smear-positive pulmonary tuberculosis and gives rise to hoarseness of the voice, pain, and dysphagia.

Lymph node tuberculosis

Lymph node tuberculosis in the United Kingdom is predominantly a disease of African and Asian immigrants who contribute about 75 per cent of all cases. Lymphadenitis, occurring predominantly in the cervical region, contributes more than half the non-respiratory tuberculosis occurring in this ethnic group. At the beginning of the century the disease in Europe was frequently due to the bovine organism. Now *M. tuberculosis* is most commonly isolated. *M. scrofulaceum* and *M. avium-intracellulare* are found occasionally, and bovine organisms rarely. In Asians, *M. tuberculosis* is predominant and this is often of the intermediate phage type (see page 5.238).

Cervical lymphadenitis (scrofula). Cervical adenitis in African and Asian immigrants in the United Kingdom is often associated with tuberculosis in the lungs or elsewhere. Usually of insidious onset, lymph node swelling may progress to the formation of abscesses and chronic discharging sinuses, which leave unsightly scars. Bacteriological confirmation is hindered by the fact that there is a low isolation rate (60 per cent) on culture from biopsy or pus aspirated from specimens which, on biopsy, show histological evidence of tuberculosis. Reasons for this include a very small population of organisms within the lymph nodes, or the absence of any living organisms within the node, which becomes enlarged as a result of a hypersensitivity response to tuberculoprotein. The behaviour of lymph nodes during chemotherapy is notoriously unpredictable, as was shown by observation of 108 patients (mainly Asian) given 18 months of isoniazid with either rifampicin or ethambutol plus an initial supplement of streptomycin. During chemotherapy, palpable lymph nodes enlarged or new nodes appeared for the first time in 25 per cent of the patients. Formation of abscesses, discharging sinus, or scar breakdown occurred in 22 per cent, and 19 per cent required surgery or aspiration procedures. However, the final outcome was excellent, since by the end of chemotherapy only 13 per cent still had node enlargement and all these were asymptomatic. Eighteen months after the end of chemotherapy, over half of these nodes had resolved, but in 7 per cent of patients lymph nodes had enlarged transiently after the end of chemotherapy.

The reasons for deterioration during chemotherapy are not understood but may include hypersensitivity to tuberculoprotein released at intervals from disrupted macrophages. Corticosteroids have been used with the aim of suppressing these reactions but the place of the drug in treatment remains contentious. Chemotherapy is recommended for 18 months; nine-month regimens are currently under evaluation in controlled studies. Routine excision of enlarged cervical lymph nodes is unnecessary since chemotherapy alone ultimately achieves satisfactory results, surgery being reserved for diagnostic biopsy or, when necessary, abscess drainage.

Mediastinal lymphadenitis. Transient unilateral enlargement of hilar lymph nodes is commonly seen in primary tuberculosis. Very different clinical features occur in the massive mediastinal lymph node enlargement seen particularly in Asian immigrants in the United Kingdom. A survey of these people showed that among those notified as suffering from respiratory tuberculosis almost 20 per cent had mediastinal lymph node enlargement in the absence of pulmonary shadows, though the sputum of some of them contained tubercle bacilli. In the differential diagnosis, sarcoidosis, lymphoma, and carcinomatous metastases must be considered. Confirmation by lymph node biopsy obtained by mediastinoscopy may be required. However, in an Asian immigrant with a strongly positive tuberculin test, the diagnosis is so likely that biopsy confirmation is rarely needed. As with cervical nodes, response during chemotherapy is unpredictable and mediastinal abscesses with involvement of the trachea, bronchi, and superior vena cava may need urgent surgical drainage.

Genito-urinary tuberculosis

Genito-urinary tuberculosis has declined much more slowly than pulmonary tuberculosis in white British subjects, in whom it comprises about one-third of all non-respiratory notifications. It is rare in Asian immigrants. The lesions, which originally result from the haematogenous dissemination of the primary infection, do not usually become clinically manifest for many years, usually between five and 20 years later. It is, therefore, mainly a disease of adults. Early lesions occur in the cortex of the kidney where the high oxygen tension may favour the persistence and growth of tubercle bacilli. Progression of disease results in ulcerocavernous lesions with eventual ulceration into the renal pelvis and spread of infection down the ureter to the bladder. Ureteric obstruction may result in hydronephrosis, which is more often the main cause of renal function impairment and destruction of the kidney than is the effect of tuberculosis within the kidney itself. Tuberculosis of the bladder results in ulceration, fibrosis, and shrinkage. Tuberculosis of the male genitalia may be the result of spread from the urinary tract.

Tuberculosis of the urinary tract
Clinical features. The commonest presenting symptoms are frequency and dysuria, which are the result of cystitis. Frank haematuria may occur but microscopic haematuria is more usual. Other symptoms include ureteric colic, loin pain, and backache. Advanced cases may present with a cold abscess in the loin or, when renal destruction is advanced, with the symptoms of chronic renal insufficiency. The classical constitutional symptoms of tuberculosis are usually absent.

Diagnosis. The occurrence of haematuria or, especially, pyuria in the presence of apparently sterile urine, should always suggest tuberculosis. Bacteriological confirmation is the cornerstone of diagnosis. Culture of early morning specimens is best. Microscopic examination of urine for acid-fast bacilli may be helpful but confirmation by culture should be carried out, since non-tuberculous mycobacteria from the genital tract may contaminate urine specimens. Routine examination of urine in all tuberculous patients is recommended, since this may enable renal tuberculosis to be diagnosed in an early pre-symptomatic stage before irreversible damage has occurred.
Intravenous pyelography is essential in initial investigation and in monitoring progress. It enables the site and extent of lesions in the kidney and bladder to be assessed and also reveals ureteric obstruction and hydronephrosis which need special management. These investigations should always be carried out before the start of treatment. Isotope renography is helpful for the same purpose. Cystoscopy may sometimes be indicated to reveal the state of the bladder, and retrograde pyeloureterography is required when excretion urography is unsatisfactory. Renal function may be impaired as a result of hydronephrosis or tuberculosis of the kidney. Information about renal function is important in the selection and dosage of antituberculosis drugs used in treatment.

Treatment. Chemotherapy starting with a daily three-drug regimen followed by a two-drug continuation phase is used, as for pulmonary tuberculosis. However, in the presence of renal impairment, streptomycin and ethambutol should be avoided or given intermittently. Rifampicin, isoniazid, and pyrazinamide are safe given in conventional dosage (see page 5.252). Drugs should be continued for a minimum of 12 months, preferably for 18 months. The use of short-course regimens can not be recommended until they have been further evaluated in renal tuberculosis.

Ureteric obstruction due to inflammatory oedema or fibrous stricture may be present initially or may occur during treatment, as healing takes place, resulting in the loss of kidney function. Excretion urography should be repeated routinely six weeks after the beginning of chemotherapy. When obstruction is present it should be treated with prednisolone initially in a dose of 20 mg daily and continued for three months, progress being monitored by repeated urography. The ureteric obstruction will be relieved in the majority of cases, but if it is not significantly relieved after about six weeks, other methods for its relief should be used including cystoscopic ureteric dilatation or other surgical techniques. Nephrectomy is rarely required; it is used only for the removal of a functionless kidney giving rise to symptoms, for recurrent urinary tract infections, or in an attempt to relieve hypertension in the presence of a unilateral functionless kidney.

Genital tuberculosis
In the male. Involvement of the genital tract is secondary to renal tuberculosis from which bacilli may reach seminal vesicles, prostate, and epididymis. Hence the genital tract should always be routinely examined in renal tuberculosis. Symptoms are usually of insidious onset, with scrotal pain and swelling. Nodularity of the epididymis, vas deferens, seminal vesicles, and prostate are the usual clinical findings. Sinus formation with resulting involvement of skin is common.

In the female. The Fallopian tubes and endometrium are the usual sites of disease. Association with renal tuberculosis is less common than in the male. Infertility is usually the only symptom. Other symptoms include pelvic pain, menstrual disorders, dyspareunia, and vaginal discharge. Spread to peritoneum causing pelvic abscess and peritonitis is rare. Diagnosis is usually made by histological and bacteriological examination of endometrial curettings.

Bone and joint tuberculosis

In developing countries, orthopaedic tuberculosis remains one of the most common crippling diseases. In the United Kingdom it has become uncommon among the native-born white population but is being seen especially among African and Asian immigrants, who may present with bizarre features unfamiliar to many doctors, a circumstance leading to late diagnosis. The spine is involved in about half the cases, other less common sites being knee, ankle, and hip, but any bone can be involved, and multiple sites are frequent. Infection usually begins at the ends of long bones, forming an abscess in the bone which bursts into the subperiosteal space from which infection may spread into the surrounding tissue to form a cold abscess. These abscesses originating from bones, may present in unusual ways, such as vulval abscesses from the bones of the pelvic girdle. Tuberculosis of the bones of the hands and feet may be misdiagnosed as ingrowing toenails, whitlows, or ganglions. Subacute or chronic non-traumatic synovitis or tenosynovitis, especially at the wrist, should lead to a suspicion of tuberculosis.

A remarkably low bacterial population is a feature of bone tuberculosis. Abscesses arising from bone contain few bacilli and positive cultures are found in only 40 per cent of aspirates. It follows that bone biopsies should be generous in size in order to allow for the chance of obtaining positive culture from the specimens.

Spinal tuberculosis (Pott's disease). Patients present in childhood or adult life with a wide variety of symptoms. Back pain is an early symptom. Paravertebral abscesses in the thoracic region may present as lumps on the chest wall or as pleural effusion or empyema. Tracking downwards, they may present in the groin as a psoas abscess. Late cases present with kyphosis with or without paraparesis or paraplegia.
The usual radiographic appearance of the early lesion is that of an infective spondylitis starting in the anterior part of the vertebral bodies. However, atypical appearances with lesions in the posterior

art of vertebrae are sometimes found in Africans and Asians in the United Kingdom.

Progression occurs with narrowing of the intravertebral disc space, bony destruction of one side of the space, and eventual destruction of two or more adjacent vertebrae with wedge-shaped collapse and the development of paravertebral abscess. This appearance can also result from other infections or from malignant disease. Diagnosis is made by surgical exploration of the lesion with bone biopsy or aspiration of abscesses.

Treatment by chemotherapy alone has been shown to be effective in most cases. Controlled clinical trials with a five-year follow-up have shown that outpatient ambulant chemotherapy with isoniazid and PAS for 18 months with or without the initial addition of streptomycin is highly effective. No extra benefit is to be gained by bed rest, by a spinal plaster of Paris jacket, or by surgical debridement, or radical resection of all affected bone followed by anterior spinal fusion with a bone graft (the Hong Kong operation), as assessed by physical activity, radiographic quiescence of the disease, and residual damage to the central nervous system. However, the Hong Kong operation, in skilled hands, has the advantage of producing more frequent and earlier bone fusion, less vertebral destruction, and slightly less residual deformity. Clearly, the early diagnosis of the disease and adequate chemotherapy are of the highest priority. Controlled studies using rifampicin and isoniazid in short-course chemotherapy are currently being made and are giving encouraging results. Severe paraparesis, though often responding to chemotherapy, is generally treated by surgical decompression of the spinal cord because of the rapid relief produced.

Abdominal tuberculosis

Tuberculosis of the intestinal tract, including enteritis, ileocolitis, and fistula-in-ano, is often associated with cavitatory pulmonary tuberculosis. Diarrhoea, abdominal pain, and rapid weight loss result. Peritoneal tuberculosis is not usually associated with pulmonary tuberculosis. It originates from mesenteric lymph nodes, infected fallopian tubes, or from haematogenous dissemination. Symptoms are usually insidious with chronic or recurrent abdominal pain, bowel irregularity, abdominal swelling, or subacute intestinal obstruction, fever, night sweats, weakness, and weight loss. In the United Kingdom, chronic and atypical abdominal symptoms in tuberculin-positive Asian immigrants should be particularly suspect. Ascitic fluid is an exudate containing lymphocytes. Diagnosis is made by bacteriological and histopathological examination of biopsy specimens obtained by laparotomy, laparoscopy, or percutaneous needle biopsy.

Tuberculous pericarditis

Tuberculous pericarditis arises usually as a result of spread from adjacent mediastinal lymph nodes, which may not be radiographically evident, but it is sometimes a feature of a widespread disseminated cryptic tuberculosis which is sometimes seen in Asian immigrants in the United Kingdom. Clinical features may be those of dry pericarditis or, alternatively, pericarditis with effusion which may produce cardiac tamponade. Presentation may be delayed until constrictive pericarditis has occurred.

Dry pericarditis is manifest by substernal pain, pericardial friction, and ECG abnormalities. Pericarditis with effusion usually presents insidiously with clinical, radiological, ECG, and echocardiographic signs of pericardial effusion with or without tamponade. The aetiology may be clear because of tuberculosis elsewhere, or suspected because of fever, constitutional symptoms and a strongly positive tuberculin reaction. Confirmation is obtained by surgical pericardial biopsy, which in case of tamponade may be combined with a drainage procedure.

Treatment is with antituberculosis drugs. In addition it is possible that corticosteroids may speed resolution of the effusion, reduce the incidence of arrhythmias, and reduce the risk of subsequent constrictive pericarditis.

Constrictive pericarditis may follow tuberculous pericarditis with effusion within a few weeks or months in spite of treatment. Alternatively it may arise years later after tuberculous pericarditis has healed. The clinical features include dyspnoea, high venous pressure, hepatosplenomegaly, and oedema. Paradoxical pulse, inspiratory rise in venous pressure, a small quiet heart, a lack of pulmonary engorgement, the ability of the patient to lie flat without dyspnoea, and the disproportionate enlargement of the liver with ascites, are striking physical signs which should prevent confusion with other causes of congestive heart failure, cardiomyopathy or cirrhosis of the liver. Treatment is by surgical resection of the pericardium. The pericardium removed may show histological evidence of tuberculosis, but there may be non-specific fibrobis and calcification only.

TREATMENT

The very great advances in the treatment of tuberculosis which have been achieved since the early 1950s have come through the discovery and development of highly effective antituberculosis drugs and drug combinations, and through the application of controlled clinical trials to the study of treatment in all its aspects, supported by appropriate *in vitro* and *in vivo* laboratory work. Many important questions still remain to be answered, however, particularly concerning the management of extrapulmonary tuberculosis, and the applicability of new treatment regimens to routine tuberculosis service conditions, especially in developing countries, where the incidence of the disease is usually high, and where the diagnostic and treatment services are often limited.

The aims of chemotherapy are not only to cure patients and prevent death from tuberculosis, but also to avoid relapse, to prevent chronic disease and its complications, to prevent the emergence of acquired drug resistance and the spread of drug-resistant infection to contacts, and to reduce the level of infectivity in the community.

The antituberculosis drugs

The drugs used for previously untreated patients, the first-line drugs, are isoniazid, rifampicin, streptomycin, pyrazinamide, ethambutol, thiacetazone, and *p*-aminosalicylic acid (PAS). Additional reserve drugs, which may be used in treating patients whose first-line treatment has failed, are ethionamide or prothionamide, cycloserine, kanamycin, capreomycin, and viomycin. Tetracycline in high dosage may occasionally be used to treat patients with multiple acquired drug-resistant infection.

The clinically important characteristics of the drugs are described separately below, including the important adverse reactions to each. Serious adverse reactions to antituberculosis regimens are uncommon, but trivial or mild cutaneous and gastrointestinal reactions are not infrequent. All the drugs can cause or contribute to cutaneous reactions, generalized hypersensitivity reactions, and hepatitis, and so these reactions are discussed separately below. The dosages of the drugs are summarized in Table 3.

All strains of *M. tuberculosis* contain some drug-resistant mutants, and active tuberculosis, however limited its extent, should never be treated with a single drug because of the risk that acquired resistance will emerge.

Isoniazid. Isoniazid (isonicotinic acid hydrazide) is the main drug in the treatment of all forms of tuberculosis. It is bactericidal for *M. tuberlosis* and has no activity against non-mycobacterial pathogens. There is no cross-resistance with other antituberculosis drugs. It is very well absorbed from the gastrointestinal tract, a peak serum concentration being obtained about one to two hours after a single oral dose. Similar peak concentrations are achieved by all patients, but four to six hours after administration, the serum concentrations differ according to the rate at which individuals metabolize the drug, there being a genetically determined bimodal distribution of

Table 3　Dosages of the antituberculosis drugs

Drug	Dosages for adults			Daily doses for children
	Weight	Daily	Intermittent	
Isoniazid		300 mg	15 mg/kg	10 mg/kg
Rifampicin	less than 50 kg 50 kg or more	450 mg 600 mg	600–900 mg 600–900 mg	10–20 mg/kg
Streptomycin	less than 50 kg 50 kg or more	750 mg 1 g (750 mg if over 40 years of age)	750 mg 1 g	20 mg/kg
Pyrazinamide	less than 50 kg 50 kg or more	1.5 g 2.0 g	3 times a week, 2.0 g twice a week, 3.0 g 3 times a week, 2.5 g twice a week, 3.5 g	40 mg/kg
Ethambutol		25 mg/kg for 2 months, then 15 mg/kg	3 times a week, 30 mg/kg twice a week, 45 mg/kg	as for adults if aged 12 years or more
Thiacetazone		150 mg	–	4 mg/kg
PAS (sodium salt)		10–15 g	–	300 mg/kg
Ethionamide	less than 50 kg 50 kg or more	750 mg 1 g	–	15 mg/kg
Prothionamide	less than 50 kg 50 kg or more	750 mg 1 g	–	15 mg/kg
Cycloserine		500 mg	–	–
Kanamycin		500 mg–1 g	–	–
Capreomycin		1 g (15 mg/kg)	–	–
Viomycin		1 g	twice a week, 2.0 g	–

slow and rapid acetylators of the drug, giving mean serum half lives of about 1.4 hours for rapid acetylators and three hours for slow acetylators.

Isoniazid diffuses into all body cells and fluids, including the CSF, with significant quantities detectable in pleural and ascitic fluids. It is eliminated mainly by acetylation in the liver, and its half-life may be prolonged in patients with gross hepatic impairment.

It is very acceptable to patients and rarely causes serious toxicity. However, it forms a hydrazone with pyridoxine and can inhibit enzymes in the synthesis of nicotinamide from tryptophan; it can thereby cause or exacerbate pyridoxine and, more rarely, niacin deficiency. Alcoholic patients may be prone to develop hepatotoxicity and peripheral neuritis, and it is advisable to administer pyridoxine 10 mg per day to these patients during isoniazid therapy.

Adverse reactions. Peripheral neuropathy, optic neuritis, or mental symptoms are uncommon forms of chronic toxicity, and probably result from pyridoxine deficiency. They are less common among rapid than among slow acetylators, and among well nourished than among poorly nourished patients.

Giddiness and, very rarely, convulsions can occur as acute toxicity within a few hours after the peak serum concentration is attained.

Convulsions respond to anticonvulsants together with pyridoxine 100 mg intravenously. They hardly ever recur. Other neurological reactions respond well to pyridoxine 20 mg daily by mouth and can be prevented by giving 10 mg of pyridoxine with each dose of isoniazid. Hepatitis occurs in less than 1 per cent of adult patients, the risk increasing with age. Cutaneous reactions are uncommon. Rare adverse reactions include haemolytic and aplastic anaemia, agranulocytosis, pellagra (related to niacin deficiency), lupoid reactions, arthralgia, and gynaecomastia.

Dosage. The daily dosages are 300 mg for adults and 10 mg/kg for children. There is no advantage in giving larger doses except, perhaps, in the initial treatment of meningitis or miliary disease, for which double these dosages may be given. The dosage in intermittent regimens is 15 mg/kg with pyridoxine 10 mg per dose to prevent neurotoxicity.

Rifampicin. Rifampicin is bactericidal for M. tuberculosis and for many other pathogens. It is an excellent companion drug for isoniazid in first-line regimens, and is also useful in reserve regimens when it has not already been used. There is no cross-resistance with other antituberculosis drugs (except other rifamycins). It is readily absorbed from the gastrointestinal tract, peak serum concentrations being reached one to three hours after an oral dose. However, absorption is delayed after a fatty meal, and it is usual to give the drug half an hour before a meal, although this is not essential if inconvenient. A high proportion is bound to plasma proteins but the unbound moiety diffuses readily into all body tissues and fluids, including the CSF.

Rifampicin is mainly metabolized to desacetyl-rifampicin which is biologically active and which is excreted predominantly in the bile. About 10 per cent is excreted in the urine, which is stained red. The drug may accumulate in patients with severe liver disease or biliary obstruction.

Rifampicin induces hepatic microsomal enzymes, and hence reduces the serum half-lives and the clinical efficacy of corticosteroids, digoxin, coumarin anticoagulants, oral contraceptives, oral antidiabetic agents (sulphanylureas and biguanides), narcotics and analgesics (methadone, morphine, and phenobarbitone), and dapsone, if given concurrently. It is teratogenic in very high doses for rats and mice, but there is no convincing evidence that it is harmful to the human fetus. Patients should be warned that it may turn their urine, and occasionally other body secretions, red.

Adverse reactions. Rifampicin rarely causes serious toxicity, but should be used with care in treating patients with chronic liver disease. Cutaneous, gastrointestinal, and hepatic reactions and thrombocytopenic purpura may occur during daily or intermittent administration of the drug. Intermittently administered rifampicin may also induce the 'flu' syndrome, shortness of breath, shock, haemolytic anaemia, and acute renal failure.

Cutaneous and gastrointestinal reactions are usually mild and self-limiting. If gastrointestinal symptoms are troublesome, they can often be stopped by giving the drug during or after a meal. Hepatitis occurs in less than 1 per cent of patients.

The 'flu' syndrome of fever, chills and malaise, sometimes with dizziness, headache, and bone pain coming on two to three hours after an intermittent dose and lasting for up to eight hours is common only if high dosages (more than 20 mg/kg) are given once a week. It is less common when the drug is given twice a week and very uncommon when it is given three times a week or daily. It is uncommon and usually mild when the intermittent dosages stated in Table 3 are used. The mechanism of the 'flu' syndrome is almost certainly immunological, and circulating rifampicin-dependent antibodies can often be detected in patients with the syndrome.

Thrombocytopenic purpura, shock (sometimes with shortness of breath), acute haemolytic anaemia, and acute renal failure are all rare, but many occur when rifampicin administration is resumed after an interval, or if a patient is irregular in taking a regimen prescribed to be taken daily. If one of these reactions occurs, the drug should be withdrawn immediately and never given again. All these potentially serious reactions are usually reversible. Of the reported cases of acute haemolytic anaemia, all those tested were found to have rifampicin-dependent antibodies in high titre.

Dosage. The daily dosages are 450 mg for adults weighing less than 50 kg and 600 mg for heavier patients, and 10–20 mg/kg for children. The dosage in intermittent regimens is 600–900 mg.

Streptomycin. Streptomycin, one of the aminoglycoside antibiotics, is bactericidal for M. tuberculosis, particularly at neutral or alkaline pH, and for many other pathogens. It is used as a companion drug for isoniazid and other bactericidal drugs. Partial cross-resistance occurs with kanamycin and viomycin. After oral administration it is not absorbed from the gastrointestinal tract. After parenteral administeration the serum half-life is about three hours, unless renal function is impaired, when it may be greatly prolonged. It is distributed throughout the extracellular fluid and penetrates fairly well into the peritoneal and pleural fluid, but less well into pericardial fluid and synovial fluid, and hardly at all through normal meninges. It crosses the placenta.

It is excreted unchanged by the kidney, by glomerular filtration; small amounts are excreted into the bile. The biological half-life is considerably longer in newborn babies and in adults over about 40 years of age than in older children and young adults.

It should be avoided in the treatment of patients with ear disease because of its ototoxicity, patients with myasthenia gravis because it is a weak neuromuscular blocker, and pregnant women because it may occasionally damage the eighth nerve of the fetus. It is rarely given intrathecally to patients with tuberculous meningitis. The intrathecal dosage is 1 mg/kg to a maximum of 50 mg per daily dose by slow infection until the CSF is normal.

Adverse reactions. Cutaneous reactions to streptomycin are quite common and can be severe. Transient giddiness and numbness (especially around the mouth) are not uncommon at the time of peak serum concentrations. If they are troublesome the dose size should be reduced. Severe and persistent giddiness, vertigo, tinnitus, ataxia, and deafness can occur due to eighth nerve toxicity, and can become permanent. If such symptoms occur, streptomycin should be withdrawn. The risk of ototoxicity depends upon the age of the patient. It is especially high in patients aged more than 40 years, in whom, also, recovery from ototoxicity is slower and less often complete than in younger patients. Ototoxicity can occur in the fetus whose mother is given the drug.

Rare reactions include renal damage, lupoid reactions, aplastic anaemia, and agranulocytosis.

Dosage. The dosage is 750 mg for patients weighing less than 50 kg or more than 40 years of age, 1 g for heavier patients less than 40 years of age, and 20 mg/kg for children. Because of the risk of acute toxicity, the dosage cannot be increased in intermittent regimens.

Pyrazinamide. Pyrazinamide (pyrazinoic acid amide) is bactericidal for M. tuberculosis, particularly when growth of the organism is inhibited by an acid environment (for example, within microphages), and has no activity against non-mycobacterial pathogens. There is no cross-resistance with other antituberculosis drugs. It is readily absorbed from the gastrointestinal tract, peak serum concentrations occurring about two hours after an oral dose, and the serum half-life is about 10 hours. It diffuses readily into body tissue and fluids, including the CSF.

Pyrazinamide is mainly eliminated by metabolism, about 30 per cent being excreted in the urine as pyrazinoic acid and only about 4 per cent as unchanged pyrazinamide.

Pyrazinoic acid (the main metabolite) inhibits the renal tubular secretion of uric acid causing the serum uric acid concentration to rise; this is much more marked during daily than during intermittent administration of the drug. Exceptionally, high serum uric acid concentrations may precipitate acute gout in patients with the disease.

Adverse reactions. Pyrazinamide may cause flushing, mild degrees of anorexia, nausea, and, less commonly, vomiting. It may also cause arthralgia, possibly associated with the high serum uric acid concentration. Arthralgia is less common during intermittent than during daily administration of the drug, and usually responds well to symptomatic treatment, for example with aspirin.

With present dosage schedules (Table 3) it does not often cause clinically evident hepatitis, a toxic effect which is dose-dependent, but care should be taken in treating patients with chronic liver disease or alcoholism.

Rare reactions include sideroblastic anaemia and photosensitization of the skin.

Dosage. The daily dosages are 40 mg/kg for adults and children. The intermittent dosages are 50 mg/kg three times a week, and 75 mg/kg twice a week. In practice, adults weighing less than 50 kg should be given 1.5 g daily, 2.0 g three times a week, and 3.0 g twice a week, and heavier patients 2.0 g daily, 2.5 g three times a week, and 3.5 g twice a week.

Ethambutol. Ethambutol is bacteriostatic for M. tuberculosis, and is used in antituberculosis regimens to prevent the emergence of strains resistant to other drugs. It is inactive against non-mycobacterial pathogens. There is no cross-resistance with other antituberculosis drugs. It is well absorbed from the gastrointestinal tract and is mostly excreted unchanged in the urine. It should be avoided in the treatment of patients with impaired renal function, because it can accumulate and cause serious eye toxicity. It should not be given to children, because appropriate dosage schedules are not yet known and because of the difficulty in detecting eye toxicity, nor to patients with ocular disease, because it can cause optic neuritis.

Adverse reactions. Ethambutol can cause a dose-related retrobulbar neuritis with a reduction in visual acuity, central scotoma, impaired red-green colour vision and peripheral field defects. These effects are reversible if administration of the drug is stopped as soon as they are detected, but they can progress to optic atrophy and permanent blindness if administration of the drug is continued. All patients given ethambutol should be warned of the danger of visual complications asked to report to the doctor immediately they notice any deterioration. This warning should be recorded in the case notes.

The drug causes mild hyperuricaemia in the majority of patients. Hepatitis is uncommon. It may rarely cause peripheral neuropathy.

Dosage. The dosages are 25 mg/kg for two months and then 15 mg/kg (or 15 mg/kg from the start) daily, 30 mg/kg three times a week, and 45 mg/kg twice a week. The difference between a therapeutically inadequate and a toxic dose size is small, and it is therefore essential that these dosages be correctly calculated; they very rarely cause retrobular neuritis, provided that renal function is normal.

Thiacetazone. Thiacetazone is a thiosemicarbazone which is bacteriostatic for *M. tuberculosis*. It is widely used, particularly in Africa, the Indian subcontinent, and South America, because of its cheapness, as a companion drug to isoniazid. It is inactive against non-mycobacterial pathogens. Cross-resistance can occur with ethionamide and prothionamide. It is well absorbed from the gastrointestinal tract, and is partly metabolized, about 15 per cent of an oral dose being excreted unchanged in the urine. It should not be given to patients with liver disease because of its hepatotoxicity.

Adverse reactions. Thiacetazone is well tolerated in some communities but not in others, for reasons which are not understood. It is particularly poorly tolerated by patients of Mongolian ethnic origin, but there are large geographical as well as racial variations in the frequency and severity of its adverse effects. Its toxicity in a community should therefore be determined before it is widely used. It may commonly cause gastrointestinal disturbances, vertigo, blurred vision, and conjunctivitis. The main potentially serious reactions are erythema multiforme, hepatitis, agranulocytosis, and haemolytic anaemia.

Dosage. The dosage is 150 mg daily for adults and 4 mg/kg daily for children. It is usually given in a combined preparation with isoniazid (Thiazina) each tablet containing 50 mg of thiacetazone and 100 mg of isoniazid. Children weighing less than 10 kg should be given half a Thiazina tablet daily, 10–24 kg one tablet, 25–39 kg two tablets, and heavier children and adults three tablets daily. However, children given only half a tablet of Thiazina should also be given an additional 100 mg tablet of isoniazid.

PAS. PAS (para-aminosalicylic acid and its salts) is bacteriostatic for *M. tuberculosis* and is used as a companion drug to isoniazid. It is inactive against non-mycobacterial pathogens. Because it frequently causes gastrointestinal reactions and is bulky and unpleasant to take, it has now largely been replaced by other drugs in technically advanced countries, but is still widely used in developing countries because it is cheap. There is no cross-resistance with other antituberculosis drugs.

It is readily absorbed from the gastrointestinal tract, peak serum concentrations occurring about two hours after an oral dose. It diffuses well into body tissues and fluids, but does not reach the CSF in therapeutic concentrations unless the meninges are inflamed.

It is partly metabolized and partly excreted unchanged in the urine. If possible, it should not be given to patients with impaired renal function and the sodium salt should not be given when a restricted sodium intake is necessary.

Adverse reactions. PAS commonly causes gastrointestinal disturbances, which may occasionally be severe enough to cause steatorrhoea. Febrile cutaneous reactions, hepatitis, and hypokalaemia can occur. Rare reactions include acute renal failure, mild hypoprothrombinaemia, haemolytic anaemia, and thrombocytopenia. Prolonged administration can lead to hypothyroidism and goitre.

Dosage. The dosage is 10–15 g for adults and 300 mg/kg for children, divided into two doses because of gastrointestinal intolerance. Aqueous solutions are unstable, polymerizing to form toxic compounds. They must not be used if they are darker in colour than the freshly prepared solution.

Ethionamide (and prothionamide). The use of ethionamide and prothionamide (propyl ethionamide) is limited by their adverse effects, notably gastrointestinal irritation. However, this tends to be less severe in children. Both drugs are well absorbed from the gastrointestinal tract and diffuse readily into the CSF. They are almost entirely metabolized. Cross-resistance can occur with thiacetazone.

Adverse reactions. Ethionamide and prothionamide cause the same adverse reactions, but prothionamide may be the better tolerated of the two. Gastrointestinal reactions, including excessive salivation and a metallic taste, are common. Cutaneous reactions and hepatitis can occur. Rare reactions include alopecia, convulsions, deafness, diplopia, gynaecomastia, hypotension, impotence, mental disturbances, menstrual irregularity, hypoglycaemia, and peripheral neuropathy.

Dosage. The dosage of ethionamide and prothionamide is 750 mg for adults weighing less that 50 kg, 1 g for heavier patients, and 15 mg/kg for children. The drugs may be given as a single dose last thing at night to avoid nausea during the day.

Cycloserine. Cycloserine is considerably less potent than the first-line drugs and its use is further limited by the quite frequent mental disturbances which it can cause. It should not be given to patients with a history of epilepsy or psychiatric disturbance. It is well absorbed from the gastrointestinal tract.

Adverse reaction. Adverse reactions to cycloserine are common and are mainly dose-related neurological reactions, including dizziness, headache, slurred speech, confusion, tremor, convulsions, depression, and psychosis. The possibility of suicide must be born in mind. Cutaneous hypersensitivity and hepatitis are uncommon reactions.

Dosage. The dosage is 500 mg daily; up to 1 g may be given divided, toxicity depending on peak serum concentrations.

Other aminoglycosides. Kanamycin, capreomycin, and viomycin are aminoglycosides which can be used as alternatives to the more potent streptomycin in patients hypersensitive to streptomycin or who are infected with strains resistant to first-line drugs. Complete cross-resistance occurs between capreomycin and viomycin, and partial cross-resistance between these two drugs and kanamycin; partial cross-resistance can also occur between kanamycin, viomycin, and streptomycin. All three drugs are poorly absorbed from the gastrointestinal tract and are therefore given parenterally. They are excreted predominantly unchanged in the urine.

Adverse reactions. These drugs can cause cutaneous hypersensitivity reactions which are usually less severe than with streptomycin. Severe and irreversible damage to the eighth cranial nerve can occur, kanamycin affecting predominantly the auditory division, capreomycin the vestibular division, and viomycin affecting both divisions equally. They can also cause renal damage. It is advisable to monitor serum electrolyte concentrations during treatment (especially with capreomycin and viomycin) because hypokalaemia and hypocalcaemia may occur.

Dosage. These drugs are given in a dosage of 1 g (15 mg/kg). Capreomycin is given daily; kanamycin and viomycin may be given three or four times a week; viomycin may be given as two injections of 1 g on two days per week.

Cutaneous and generalized hypersensitivity reactions. Mild cutaneous reactions to an antituberculosis regimen may be self-limiting and require only symptomatic treatment without interrupting or altering the regimen.

Generalized hypersensitivity reactions usually occur during the first one or two months of chemotherapy. They consist of a rash, sometimes accompanied by periorbital swelling and conjunctivitis, and by systemic symptoms and signs such as fever, malaise, vomiting, aching limbs, headache, generalized lymphadenopathy, hepatosplenomegaly, and occasionally transient jaundice.

The principles of management are:

1. Stop all chemotherapy until the reaction has subsided.

2. Identify the drug or drugs responsible.

3. Resume adequate chemotherapy as soon as possible, using not less than two drugs to which the patient is not hypersensitive.

The patient should be desensitized to the drug or drugs responsible for the reaction only if this is necessary for the resumption of adequate chemotherapy.

Once the reaction has subsided, daily challenge doses to the drugs of the prescribed regimen should be started, the aim being to challenge the patient first to drugs which are *unlikely* to have caused the reaction, so that administration of these can be resumed with the minimum of delay, while (if necessary) challenge doses and desensitizing doses of other drugs are administered. Challenge doses of each drug of the regimen should be given in the sequence in which they occur in Table 4, until a reaction occurs. If no reaction occurs to either of the challenge doses shown in Table 4, administration of that drug should be continued in full dosage. If the reaction was a particularly severe one, smaller initial challenge doses should be used before the dosages shown under day 1. These should be approximately one tenth of the dose shown under day 1.

Table 4 Challenge doses for detecting cutaneous or generalized hypersensitivity

Drug	Challenge doses	
	Day 1	Day 2
Isoniazid	50 mg	300 mg
Rifampicin	75 mg	300 mg
Pyrazinamide	250 mg	1.0 g
Ethionamide, prothionamide	125 mg	375 mg
Cycloserine	125 mg	250 mg
Ethambutol	100 mg	500 mg
PAS	1.0 g	5.0 g
Thiacetazone	25 mg	50 mg
Streptomycin or other Aminoglycoside	125 mg	500 mg

Challenge doses of the drugs of the regimens should be given in the sequence in which they are shown. The drugs near the bottom of the list are the ones that are most likely to cause a reaction. If the reaction was a severe one, smaller initial challenge doses should be given (approximately one-tenth the doses shown for Day 1).

Once a patient has been shown to be hypersensitive to a drug and if it is considered necessary to desensitize the patient to this drug, it is important to achieve this under cover of at least two antituberculosis drugs to which the patient is not hypersensitive, to prevent the emergence of drug resistance. If the reaction was a severe one, if the patient is hypersensitive to more than one drug, or if administration of the drug concerned needs to be resumed rapidly because of severe disease, desensitization should be carried out under steroid cover, the steroids being tailed off on completion of the desensitizing course. No attempt should be made to desensitize (even under steroid cover) patients with severe exfoliative dermatitis or renal reactions.

Patients can usually be rapidly desensitized. If the patient had a reaction to the second challenge dose but not to the first, start the desensitization course with a dose equal to that of the first challenge dose. If a reaction occurred after the first challenge dose, start the course with a dose approximately one-tenth that of the first challenge dose. Desensitizing doses should be given, on an inpatient basis if possible, at least twice a day in steadily increasing dose sizes until the full dose is reached. This can often be done by making each dose double the previous dose. If a reaction occurs during desensitization, reduce the dose again, and increase the doses thereafter more gradually.

Hepatitis. It is not necessary to do liver function tests as a routine during antituberculosis chemotherapy, unless the patient has liver disease. Mild, transient, and symptomless increases in serum hepatic enzyme concentrations are usual during the early weeks of treatment, whatever the drugs of the regimen, and on no account should treatment be interrupted or altered because of them. However, if clinically evident hepatitis, with anorexia, nausea, vomiting, hepatic enlargement and tenderness, and jaundice, occurs all drugs should be stopped and supportive treatment given while impaired liver function is confirmed by appropriate tests. If the hepatitis has been caused by the drug regimen, liver function usually returns to normal once administration of the regimen has been halted. Treatment with the same drugs can often be resumed uneventfully, but liver function should be carefully monitored. The aim should be to resume treatment, either with the originally prescribed regimen, or with an alternative regimen, as soon as possible.

Modern regimens including all three of the drugs isoniazid, rifampicin, and pyrazinamide, in the dosages shown in Table 3, carry no greater risk of hepatotoxicity than the old standard regimens given for 12 months or longer; this risk has been found to be of the order of 1 per cent, even in studies which included, severely malnourished and ill patients, some of them with liver disease. Rapid acetylators of isoniazid are not exposed to an increased risk, although this has sometimes been claimed, and even patients with chronic liver disease and alcoholics are not exposed to an unacceptable risk. On the rare occasions when patients have died from presumed drug-induced hepatitis, other predisposing factors such as severe malnutrition or other known liver disease, have almost always been associated.

Scientific basis of chemotherapy

The drugs of an antituberculosis regimen are selected such that they will kill tubercle bacilli efficiently and prevent the emergence of drug-resistant strains without causing unacceptable levels of toxicity to the patients. In the older regimens, given for 12 months or longer, this was achieved by giving two effective drugs for an adequate period of time, a third drug being added initially in case of initial resistance to one of the drugs. The inclusion of rifampicin and pyrazinamide in modern regimens increases the rate at which tubercle bacilli are killed in the early weeks of treatment, and leads to the killing of special portions of the bacillary population relatively unaffected by other antituberculosis drugs. This means that such regimens can be highly effective when given for only six months, even in the presence of initial resistance to isoniazid and streptomycin.

The antituberculosis drugs vary in their ability to prevent the emergence of resistant strains and in their bactericidal activity.

Preventing the emergence of resistant strains. Drug-resistant tubercle bacilli emerge by mutation (and hence occur in wild strains), the number of resistant mutants depending upon the size of the bacillary population, the frequency of cell division, and the drug. If monotherapy is given to patients with a large and actively dividing bacillary population, the relatively small number of resistant mutants already present overgrow the drug-sensitive bacilli, which are inhibited by the drug during treatment. One or more additional drugs must therefore be given to inhibit mutant bacilli. The effectiveness of drugs in doing this can be assessed from their ability to prevent bacteriological failure due to the emergence of drug resistance during chemotherapy in patients with severe disease. Of the first-line drugs, isoniazid and rifampicin are highly effective in this role, streptomycin and ethambutol less so, and PAS, thiacetazone, and pyrazinamide least effective of all.

Bactericidal activity. The bactericidal activity of drugs can be assessed from their ability to sterilize lesions in experimental animals, from their effect on *in vitro* cultures of tubercle bacilli, and from their contribution to the bactericidal activity of antituberculosis regimens in man. Rifampicin and pyrazinamide are the two most potently bactericidal drugs in sterilizing lesions in the mouse and in preventing bacteriological relapse after short-course chemotherapy in man. Isoniazid is less effective than rifampicin and pyrazinamide in sterilizing experimental lesions, although it is at least as effective as these two drugs against *in vitro* cultures in the logarithmic phase of growth. It has a particularly potent bactericidal action in man as measured from the viable counts in sputum when given alone for 14 days before the start of conventional treatment. When assessed in this way, rifampicin is less effective that isoniazid, and streptomycin and pyrazinamide even less so. This suggests that isoniazid is a particularly potent bactericidal drug against that part of the bacillary population which is actively multiplying.

The apparent discrepancies in the results of assessing the bactericidal activity of drugs according to the method used can probably best be explained in terms of the action of the individual drugs against different components of the total bacillary population in lesions.

Components of the bacillary population. Not all the bacilli in the lesions of untreated patients are likely to be metabolizing and multiplying at the same rate. Some will be rapidly multiplying; at the other extreme others will be almost completely dormant. Bacilli in open cavities with a plentiful supply of oxygen and isolated from the host's acquired immunological defences are likely to be growing rapidly, while those in closed lesions, deprived of oxygen, or within activated macrophages are likely to be growing slowly or may be completely dormant. It has been suggested that bacilli which are growing rapidly and continuously are killed most quickly by isoniazid and somewhat less quickly by rifampicin and streptomycin, the bactericidal activity of isoniazid falling as the rate of bacillary growth declines. Pyrazinamide, unlike the other antituberculosis drugs, is bactericidal only against bacilli whose growth is inhibited by an acid environment, and is therefore active against a portion of the bacillary population which is not susceptible to other drugs—possibly bacilli within the phagosomes or phagolysomes of macrophages. Rifampicin is unique among the antituberculosis drugs in beginning to kill bacilli within only about 15 minutes of their exposure to the drug; it is therefore probably active against bacilli which are dormant but which have occasional short periods of active metabolism and growth, and which are not susceptible to other drugs because they take longer to begin to kill bacilli. Completely dormant bacilli are unlikely to be killed by any drug.

If the above hypothesis is correct, it explains why isoniazid, rifampicin, and pyrazinamide have been found to be such important drugs in short-course chemotherapy.

It was at first assumed that the serum concentrations of orally administered drugs should be maintained above their minimal inhibitory concentration for tubercle bacilli throughout the 24 hours, and as a consequence these drugs used to be given in two to four doses each day. However, a controlled clinical study showed that 400 mg of isoniazid alone was more effective when given as a single dose each day than when given as two doses of 200 mg, even though the latter schedule maintained a serum concentration above the minimal inhibitory concentration whereas the former did not. The drugs of a regimen should therefore be given together as a single dose each day.

Chemotherapeutic regimens for pulmonary tuberculosis

Daily long-term regimens. Daily long-term regimens consist of isoniazid given with a companion drug which is included to prevent the emergence of acquired isoniazid resistance. The companion drug may be ethambutol, rifampicin, PAS, or thiacetazone. During the initial phase of treatment, a third drug is given because of the possibility of there being initial resistance to one of the drugs. This initial phase of three-drug chemotherapy is given for one to three months. The third drug is commonly streptomycin. However, in the

treatment of older patients, likely to suffer streptomycin toxicity, or in situations in which daily injections are inconvenient, rifampicin is a useful alternative third drug when ethambutol, PAS, or thiacetazone are being used as the main companion drug to isoniazid.

The continuation phase of chemotherapy, consisting of isoniazid and a single companion drug, is continued until a total of at least 12 months of chemotherapy has been given, and it should be continued up to 18 months if the risk of relapse after the end of treatment is to be minimized. Ethambutol or rifampicin is commonly used as the companion drug to isoniazid in technically advanced countries (although if rifampicin is used, nine months of treatment is adequate—see below) because they are both very well tolerated. PAS or thiacetazone is generally used in developing countries because they are both cheap.

All the drugs of the regimen are given together as a single dose each day except for PAS, which is often given as two divided doses because of gastrointestinal toxicity. The regimens are given mainly on an outpatient basis, and patients must be carefully instructed to medicate themselves regularly and to continue doing so long after they feel well. The drug dosages are shown in Table 3.

Results of long-term chemotherapy. With the many drugs now available which are effective against *M.tuberculosis* it is possible to treat all patients with tuberculosis successfully, except those few whose disease is already too advanced at the time they present for treatment. In spite of this, the results obtained by routine chest services with standard long-term daily regimens of chemotherapy (Table 5), often fall a long way below the very high success rate which is possible, particularly in developing countries. Treatment surveys have established the main reasons for this. They are as follows:

1. Patients terminate their treatment prematurely or take it irregularly.
2. The infection is drug-resistant initially.
3. The regimen prescribed is inadequate.
4. Drug toxicity leads to interruptions or changes in treatment.

Table 5   Results obtained by routine chest services in treating pulmonary tuberculosis with standard regimens of chemotherapy for 12 months or longer

Area and year of survey	Status of patients at 1 year	
	Had stopped attending	Disease quiescent
South India (1969)	50%	52%
Kenya (1970)	72%	63%
Paris (1970)	22%	unknown
Scotland (1976)	6%	93%

Of these, the first is by far the most important; it has been found to account for a treatment failure rate in previously untreated patients of between about 5 per cent, in highly organized and efficiently run services in technically advanced countries, to about 50 per cent or even more in some developing countries. All too often patients stop taking their treatment once their symptoms improve; or they may become irregular in taking it or stop taking it if they experience adverse reactions to their regimen, even if these are not serious. Two ways have been developed of improving patient compliance. The first of these is the use of intermittent chemotherapy. The doses are given three times or twice a week, every dose under full supervision, so that irregularity in drug-taking is immediately evident to the service staff who can take appropriate action. However, this approach can only be applied when the patients live near a centre for supervision; in practice this usually limits it to urban communities. The second method of improving patient compliance is to shorten the total duration of chemotherapy to periods of six to nine months. It is also important that the patients themselves should be well-motivated and properly supervised by well-trained staff.

Intermittent supervised chemotherapy

Scientific basis. The finding that 400 mg of isoniazid was more effective when given as a single daily dose than when divided into two 200 mg doses 12 hours apart raised the important possibility that large doses of antituberculosis drugs, with their correspondingly high peak serum concentrations, given even less frequently than once a day might be just as effective and perhaps even more effective than smaller doses given daily. It led to a large number of clinical studies of twice-weekly and once-weekly regimens, and to the experimental demonstration that single exposures of cultures of tubercle bacilli to bactericidal drugs could inhibit cell division for several days, and that in the treatment of experimental tuberculosis in guinea-pigs, isoniazid, streptomycin, rifampicin, ethambutol, and ethionamide, but not thiacetazone, were just as effective when given at intervals of two or four days as one day, provided the drug dosages were increased such that the total amount of drug given remained the same. Indeed, isoniazid, rifampicin, and ethambutol were more effective when given intermittently up to once every four days; at intervals of eight days, rifampicin and ethambutol, but not isoniazid, remained more effective than when given daily. However, ethambutol was much less effective than either isoniazid or rifampicin in curing guinea-pig disease. More recently, pyrazinamide also has been shown to be highly effective when given intermittently to guinea-pigs at intervals of up to eight days.

The reasons for the efficacy of intermittent drug administration and for the differences between the drugs studied are not known, but this sort of work provides an experimental basis for intermittent chemotherapy in man. From the findings, one would expect drugs such as isoniazid, rifampicin, pyrazinamide and ethambutol, the dose size of which can be increased as the interval between doses is increased, to be effective in intermittent regimens, and this has in general proved to be the case in clinical studies. The dose size of intermittent streptomycin cannot be increased above the daily dose size, because of acute toxicity.

Practical advantages and organization of intermittent supervised regimens. The main advantage of intermittent regimens is that they can far more easily be given under full supervision on an outpatient basis than daily regimens. Every dose, even of orally administered drugs, is given under the supervision of the health service staff, patients being seen to swallow their drugs. If a patient fails to attend for a dose of his regimen, immediate action can be taken. For example, he can be visited at home and the dose that is due can be administered there, the reasons for his failure to attend can be discovered and he can be encouraged to attend regularly in the future. These regimens are particularly suitable for the treatment of patients, such as alcoholics and vagrants, who are unlikely to be reliable in taking self-administered medication daily, and also in communities, such as many developing countries, in which self-medication has been shown to be unsuccessful.

Intermittent regimens in general cause considerably less chronic drug toxicity than daily regimens, and have the additional advantage of being cheaper than daily regimens based on the same drugs because the total quantity of drug is smaller. Because treatment is fully supervised, it is known when a patient has received adequate treatment, and follow-up after chemotherapy is unnecessary.

The organization of fully-supervised intermittent chemotherapy must be flexible so that it is convenient for the patients, who should be able to receive their doses of chemotherapy at centres near their home, near their place of work, or on their way to work, and to choose the facility most convenient for them. The centres used include chest clinics, general practitioners' surgeries, dispensaries, welfare clinics, hospitals, factory clinics, rural health units, and special treatment stations (for example on market days in rural areas). The overall management of the patient, of course, remains in the hands of the physician.

Twice-weekly regimens. The intermittent regimens shown in Table 6, the drug dosages for which are shown in Table 3, are all twice-weekly regimens with an initial daily phase of chemotherapy. All of them have been shown to be very highly effective in controlled clinical trials, and the twice-weekly streptomycin and high-dosage (15 mg/kg) isoniazid regimens in particular are widely used in service programmes. All of them should be given for a total duration of 18 months except for the regimen containing rifampicin in the intermittent phase, which should be given for 12 months.

Table 6 Twice-weekly regimens of at least 12 months' duration

Initial daily phase		Twice-weekly phase	Total duration of regimen	Cost for 50 kg patient (UK prices, 1981)
Drugs*	Duration			
SHE (SHP)	2–3 months	HS	18 months	£82–£98 (or £59–£70)
SHT	3 months	HS	18 months	£54
SHR	3 months	HS	18 months	£129
SHE (SHP)	2–3 months	HE	18 months	£190–£199 (or £166–171)
SHR	2 weeks	HR	12 months	£100

* H = isoniazid, S = streptomycin, E = ethambutol, T = thiacetazone, P = PAS, and R = rifampicin.

For drug dosages see Table 3. Note that the twice-weekly dosages of isoniazid, rifampicin, and ethambutol are higher than the daily dosages.

Short-course chemotherapy

Scientific basis. The mechanisms of chemotherapy and the roles of the different antituberculosis drugs in preventing the emergence of resistant strains and in killing various components of the bacillary population in lesions have been discussed above. The most effective short-course regimens very rapidly reduce the bacillary load and so halt mutation to resistant strains, and also eliminate those portions of the bacillary population which, because of their environment or slow rate of metabolism, are relatively unsusceptible to isoniazid and which are therefore potentially capable of giving rise to relapse after the end of chemotherapy.

For the reasons discussed above, evidence for which has been obtained in many controlled clinical trials, the combination of isoniazid, rifampicin, and pyrazinamide has proved to be particularly effective in short-course chemotherapy, isoniazid because of its ability to kill rapidly multiplying bacilli, rifampicin and pyrazinamide because of their ability to prevent relapse by killing portions of the bacillary population relatively unaffected by other drugs. Other bactericidal drugs, such as streptomycin, contribute to the killing of actively dividing bacilli, and the bacteriostatic drugs, such as thiacetazone and ethambutol, probably help to prevent the emergence of drug resistance.

In the treatment of patients with smear-positive pulmonary tuberculosis, six-month regimens based on isoniazid, rifampicin, and pyrazinamide are the shortest regimens capable of curing virtually all patients. In the treatment of patients with smear-negative disease, three months of treatment has proved to be inadequate, and such patients should be treated for the same duration as those with smear-positive disease.

Practical advantages of short-course chemotherapy. The main advantages of short-course regimens are that although given for only six to nine months, they are very highly effective even for patients with very extensive disease, and for those with strains initially resistant to isoniazid, streptomycin, or both these drugs. Their short duration and their acceptability to patients mean that the patient's daily life is disrupted as little as possible. Follow-up, particularly after fully supervised short-course chemotherapy, is unnecessary, and relapse, if it occurs, almost invariably does so soon after the end of treatment and without the emergence of drug-resistant strains (or of additional resistance if the initial strains were resistant). This means that patients who relapse can be identified rapidly and retreated successfully with the drugs of the primary regimen. They also have the important advantage that they cure patients rapidly, so that even early defaulters are more likely to have been cured than would have been the case if they had been prescribed a longer and less intensive regimen. These advantages should make it easier to persuade patients with symptoms to seek medical advice, and to persuade those who require treatment to comply with it.

Short-course regimens. Short-course regimens are now recommended for use in many countries including the United Kingdom, the United States, France, Hong Kong, and Singapore. Those regimens shown in Table 7 have been shown to be very highly effective in the treatment of patients with initially drug-sensitive strains of tubercle bacilli, and the four-drug regimens, particularly those containing rifampicin throughout, are also equally effective in the treatment of patients with bacilli initially resistant to isoniazid, streptomycin, or both these drugs.

Choice of regimen

Technically advanced countries. In technically advanced countries, the incidence of tuberculosis is, in general, much lower than in developing countries, the level of initial resistance is low, medical services are plentiful, and drug costs are not a limiting factor. In many countries a daily regimen of isoniazid and rifampicin for nine months, with ethambutol or streptomycin as well for the first two months (Table 7) is currently recommended. This regimen has the advantage of causing very few adverse reactions. Its disadvantages are that it is not given under full supervision and it may not be adequate for patients with isoniazid-resistant bacilli.

When self-medication is unlikely to be successful, for example in the treatment of alcoholics, a fully supervised twice-weekly regimen (Table 6) may be used, or a fully supervised short-course intermittent regimen (Table 7). The short-course regimens containing all three of the drugs isoniazid, rifampicin, and pyrazinamide have the advantage that they are highly effective for patients with initially resistant infection.

Developing countries. In developing countries, the incidence of tuberculosis is high, medical services are limited, and the availability of some drugs is limited by their cost. Indeed, the choice of regimen is often determined primarily by the cost of the component drugs. In many countries, daily isoniazid and thiacetazone for 12 months or longer, with up to three months of daily streptomycin initially, is still used because it is so cheap, although it is somewhat less than 100 per cent effective. When given for 12 months and with three months of streptomycin, it costs less than £20 per patient. But in most countries patients have to be admitted to hospital during the period of streptomycin administration. This is expensive for the service and often disruptive for the patient. Also, as already discussed, this regimen achieves poor results in practice. Choosing the cheapest regimen may be a false economy.

In urban areas, which are usually better provided with medical services than rural ones, and where most patients live or work near appropriate medical facilities, a fully-supervised regimen based on twice-weekly isoniazid and streptomycin (Table 6) is likely to prove more successful and less toxic. Moreover, such a twice-weekly regimen, with a three-month initial daily phase is not unduly costly, although the additional cost of providing an injection service must be considered.

Alternatively, a fully-supervised partially or completely intermittent short-course regimen (Table 7) might be preferred. If the aim is to admit patients to hospital for the first one to two months, a partially intermittent regimen should be chosen. An eight-month regimen of daily streptomycin, isoniazid, rifampicin, and pyrazinamide for one month followed by twice-weekly streptomycin, isoniazid, and pyrazinamide, costs only £76.

If full supervision on an entirely outpatient basis from the start of chemotherapy is the aim, so saving the cost of admission to hospital, then one of the completely intermittent regimens should be used. All of them contain isoniazid, rifampicin and pyrazinamide. If an injectable is considered desirable, for example to encourage patient compliance, one of the streptomycin-containing regimens should be selected. The completely oral regimen of ethambutol, isoniazid, rifampicin, and pyrazinamide three times a week for six months is equally effective, but costs more.

In large, sparsely populated, rural areas it is rarely possible to organize fully supervised chemotherapy. In this case a daily short-course regimen (Table 7) may be selected, the patient being admitted to hospital for the initial intensive phase, and then discharged to continue with self-administered chemotherapy coming to a clinic once a month to renew supplies. An eight-month regimen of streptomycin, isoniazid, rifampicin, and pyrazinamide for two months, followed by isoniazid and thiacetazone is not costly. The six-month regimen, containing rifampicin throughout is more expensive.

In populations with a high level of initial drug resistance, four-drug regimens should be used because of their effectiveness in the treatment of patients with bacilli resistant to both isoniazid and streptomycin. The emphasis must be on curing as high a proportion of patients as possible with their primary regimen. High failure rates, the need for alternative second-line regimens, and high levels of chronic active disease greatly add to the costs and complications of treatment.

The treatment of patients in renal failure

With the success of modern methods of treating renal failure, many patients with impaired or even absent renal function are being kept alive. Their treatment may include the administration of corticosteroids or immunosuppressant drugs, rendering them vulnerable

Table 7   Short-course regimens

Initial intensive phase		Continuation phase	Total duration of regimen	Cost for 50 kg patient (UK prices, 1981)
Drugs* and rhythm	Duration	Drugs* and rhythm		
Daily regimens				
EHR daily	2 months	HR daily	9 months	£261
SHR daily	2 months	HR daily	9 months	£242
SHRZ daily	2 months	HR daily	6 months	£178
SHRZ daily	2 months	HT daily	8 months	£ 80
Partially intermittent regimen				
SHRZ daily	1–2 months	SHZ twice a week	8 months	£76–£109
Completely intermittent regimens				
EHRZ 3 times a week	6 months	–	6 months	£140
SHRZ 3 times a week	6 months	–	6 months	£104
SHRZ 3 times a week	2 months	HR 3 times a week	6 months	£ 79
SHRZ 3 times a week	4 months	SHZ twice a week	8 months	£ 90

* S = streptomycin, H = isoniazid, R = rifampicin, Z = pyrazinamide, E = ethambutol, and T = thiacetazone
For drug dosages see Table 3

to tuberculosis. For these reasons they not uncommonly require antituberculosis treatment.

The adjustment of dosage of an antituberculosis drug required for such patients depends upon the extent to which the drug is normally excreted unchanged in the urine and on the degree of renal impairment. Drugs such as isoniazid, rifampicin, pyrazinamide, ethionamide, and prothionamide which are eliminated primarily by routes other than renal, namely by metabolism or by biliary excretion, should be given in normal dosage, whatever the degree of the renal failure. Fortunately the most potent drugs are also the safest for patients with impaired renal function, namely isoniazid and rifampicin.

The aminoglycosides are excreted exclusively, and ethambutol predominantly by the kidneys as the parent compound. If they are to be given to patients with impaired renal function their dosages must be adjusted according to the degree of impairment. Thus, 0.75 g of streptomycin should be given at intervals such that the trough serum concentrations do not exceed 4 µg per ml. For patients on regular dialysis, 0.75 g should be given four to six hours before dialysis. Ethambutol should be given in a dosage of 25 mg/kg three times a week to patients with a creatinine clearance of between 50 and 100 ml per minute, and twice a week to patients with a creatinine clearance of between 30 and 50 ml per minute. For patients being dialysed three or more times per week, 25 mg/kg should be given four to six hours before dialysis. This should be increased to 45 mg/kg for twice-weekly dialysis and to 90 mg/kg for once-weekly dialysis.

Thiacetazone and PAS are partly excreted unchanged in the urine and are partly metabolized. Both are weak antituberculosis drugs. The difference between a toxic and a therapeutically inadequate dose of thiacetazone is small, and the gastrointestinal effects of PAS can potentiate or exacerbate acidosis in patients with impaired renal function. Both drugs should therefore be avoided if possible.

The treatment of pregnant women

If a woman becomes pregnant while she is receiving antituberculosis chemotherapy, the pregnancy is not likely to be diagnosed before fetal organogenesis has started; the fetus is therefore at risk from any teratogenic effects of drugs being given to the mother. However, none of the antituberculosis drugs has been proved to have teratogenic effects in the human fetus, although rifampicin has such effects when given in very high dosages to rats and mice. If a woman is already known to be pregnant when tuberculosis is diagnosed, the pregnancy is likely to have advanced beyond 12 weeks by which time there is little risk of any teratogenic damage to the fetus. Some physicians may, nevertheless, wish to avoid giving rifampicin to women who are likely to become pregnant, or who are less than 12 weeks pregnant. If a woman becomes pregnant during rifampicin administration there is no need to alter the treatment; the patient should be reassured that there is no good reason to suppose that the fetus has been damaged. Patients who are more than 12 weeks pregnant can be treated normally with the single exception that streptomycin, which can cause toxic damage to the eighth nerve of the fetus, should not be given at any stage of a pregnancy, and should be withdrawn immediately if a woman becomes pregnant during its administration.

General management of patients during chemotherapy

Even the best chemotherapy regimen is likely to fail if it is incorrectly administered or if the patient does not take it as prescribed. The successful treatment of tuberculosis is largely an administrative problem, requiring well-trained and highly motivated staff. Facilities for treatment vary greatly between the technically advanced and developing countries. The recommendations made in this section relate to technically advanced countries and may not always be applicable to developing countries with a shortage of staff and finance.

Hospital treatment. Rest, good food, and nursing care given in hospital were previously thought to be essential in treatment when recovery depended on the host's defence against the tubercle bacillus. With the use of effective chemotherapy these are not required. Treatment of tuberculosis is predominantly undertaken as an outpatient procedure. This enables developing countries to concentrate their economic resources on providing chemotherapy and good supervision. Initial treatment in hospital is reserved for a few selected patients which include (a) seriously ill patients; and (b) patients with special treatment problems such as alcoholics, psychiatrically disturbed patients, or those with drug-resistant disease. Such patients usually benefit from initial chemotherapy under hospital supervision. The first few weeks of treatment is a time when the bacterial population is greatest and hence the risk of acquired drug resistance emerging due to irregular unsupervised self-administration of drugs is greatest. Nevertheless, even in these difficult patients intermittent fully supervised regimens administered in the patients' homes or near their place of work, can be a very satisfactory alternative to hospital treatment. There is no evidence suggesting that the patients who have been treated initially in hospital subsequently self-administer their drugs better than those who have never been treated in hospital; indeed, the reverse may be the case.

In addition, infectious patients may be admitted to hospital to segregate them from their contacts. Only patients in whose sputum acid-fast bacilli can be demonstrated on direct smear need be regarded as infectious. Chemotherapy renders such patients rapidly non-infectious, usually within one month of the start of chemotherapy, especially when rifampicin is used with isoniazid. Controlled studies suggest that segregation during this short stage of infectiousness conveys little extra protection to home contacts, and, domiciliary chemotherapy is acceptable under almost all circumstances. However, in most technically advanced countries, smear-positive patients whose home contacts include young children or other persons likely to be at risk of infection are often segregated in hospital for the first few weeks of treatment.

Outpatient management. Outpatient management is mainly concerned with the supervision of chemotherapy. This requires specially trained nursing or paramedical staff under specialist medical supervision.

Management of chemotherapy. The first essential step is to instruct patients in the drugs required, when and how to take them, and the need for regular medication throughout the total duration of chemotherapy, long after they feel better. Both verbal instructions and written and illustrated leaflets are useful in educating the patient. Also relatives or home contacts may help in the supervision of home chemotherapy. Drugs should be provided by the clinic rather than through the patient's general practitioner who may prescribe alternative pharmaceutical preparations which may give rise to confusion. If possible, the drugs should be provided in combined pills so that one drug cannot be taken without the other. Rifampicin–isoniazed pills are conveniently provided on cards labelled with the day of the week as an aid to memory. Drugs are taken in a single daily dose before or with meals. This should become a ritual in which the patient may be reminded of his medication by a relative eating with him, thus reducing chances of forgetfulness. Rifampicin colours urine red and this is a useful reminder to the patient that medication has been taken that day.

The patient attends the clinic at intervals when enquiry is made about symptoms, the regularity of self-administration of drugs, and any difficulties or toxicity arising. The patient's statement about self-medication may be checked by urine tests which are easily made if the patient is receiving rifampicin, the urine being red in colour four hours after taking this drug. Paper-strip test can be used to detect isoniazid, the test being positive between half an hour and twelve hours after taking the drug.

Detecting irregular self-medication. Irregular self-medication is usually the result of forgetfulness or a failure to appreciate that chemotherapy needs to be continued long after the patient feels well. It is most likely to occur in alcoholics, drug addicts, mentally disturbed people, or those with emotional pressures. Irregularity of self-medication of patients on daily regimens may be suspected if there is admitted forgetfulness or unexplained negative urine tests for drugs, if sputum smears do not show the expected diminution in the number of organisms, or when pill counts in the clinic or at home suggest that drugs are not being taken as prescribed. Such patients may respond to reinforcement of advice about regular self-medication or involvement of the family in supervision, but often it is best to change to intermittent fully supervised treatment.

Bacteriological surveillance. The success or failure of chemotherapy is evaluated on bacteriological evidence. However, frequent bacteriological tests during treatment are unnecessary. Two sputum cultures at the third month and at the end of chemotherapy are valuable. The third month cultures, the results of which will be available before the end of chemotherapy, will usually be negative, as will the cultures at the end of chemotherapy. However, if one of the cultures is positive, another culture should be taken, and only if this is also positive, or if the patient shows radiographic or clinical evidence of relapse should retreatment be started, preferably not before the results of sensitivity tests are known.

Sputum smears may remain positive for a considerable time during treatment, after the cultures have become negative, the patient expectorating dead bacilli. However, serial sputum smears usually show progressive diminution in the number of organisms. A fall in the number of organisms seen in successive sputum smears followed by a rise usually means that the patient has stopped taking the drugs, or less commonly that drug resistance has emerged. Pretreatment drug sensitivity tests are not required routinely in previously untreated patients and repeated sensitivity tests during chemotherapy are usually unhelpful. Drug resistance is frequently observed at the point in treatment at which sputum cultures are beginning to go negative (transitional resistance). This does not indicate failure of treatment and should not lead to change of chemotherapy (see page 5.240).

Radiographic surveillance. An initial chest radiograph and one at the end of chemotherapy is all that is required. Chest radiography is of limited value as a guide to progress. Persistence of a large residual cavity at the end of treatment does not indicate increased risk of relapse and there is no need to prolong or change chemotherapy, providing good chemotherapy has been prescribed and taken by the patient.

Management of relapse and acquired drug resistance

Relapse occurs very rarely when good chemotherapy is well administered by efficient treatment services. In some developing countries with poor treatment services, it is a common problem. Relapse occurs for one of two main reasons, first, because the patient having taken drugs regularly defaults before the end of treatment and so relapse occurs with organisms fully sensitive to the drugs of the primary regimen; secondly, because the patient takes drugs irregularly for much of the time. Relapse then usually occurs with organisms resistant to one or more of the drugs used in the primary regimen. About half the patients relapsing after long-term chemotherapy are of this sort.

Patients must be carefully appraised before retreatment. A single new drug should never be added to a previously failing or suspect regimen because this may lead to the emergence of further drug resistance. Appraisal is made in the following ways:

1. A detailed history is taken of chemotherapy, including drugs used, their dosage, duration, and the compliance of the patient with the regimen. Often a reliable estimate of the likelihood of resistance to drugs can be obtained from this history. When patients are unaware of the drugs received, every effort should be made to obtain details from the physicians who treated them.

2. Drug-sensitivity tests are done on relapse cultures. These tests require specialized laboratories for reliable results and the tests require seven to eight weeks before results are available. The physician may be faced with a very difficult problem in regard to sick patients who are known to have received many drugs previously; for these patients few effective drugs may remain. It is better to wait for the results of sensitivity tests so that a wise decision can be made, rather than to start inappropriate therapy which may lead to further resistance, and the loss of the patient's remaining hope of cure. However, some patients are so ill that delaying the resumption of chemotherapy may be unacceptable. It may be evident from the history that only a limited number of drugs had been given so that alternatives are available. Unfortunately in developing countries where drug resistance is most common, these expensive drugs may not be available.

When it is confirmed, or is highly likely, that acquired resistance has emerged, the following principles should guide the retreatment of the patient:

1. At least three antituberculosis drugs which have not previously been received and to which organisms are likely to be sensitive should be used. This is particularly important when the only suitable drugs are the less potent or bacteriostatic drugs, ethionamide, cycloserine, ethambutol, thiacetazone, PAS, and the aminoglycosides other than streptomycin. The choice may be influenced by considerations of cross-resistance with other drugs previously received by the patient and by the adverse reactions to drugs. Drugs previously used but about which there is doubt in regard to the sensitivity of the organism may be used in addition. It is not unusual to use five or six drugs initially.

2. All drugs are given in a single dose daily except for cycloserine and PAS, which are given in two divided doses.

3. Patients suspected or known to have been unco-operative in the past, should be given fully supervised therapy, and should not be relied upon to medicate themselves. Treatment in hosptial initially is usually required since treatment with multiple reserve drugs is often toxic or unpleasant and careful monitoring and great encouragement are required to maintain the patient on effective treatment. Change of drugs is often required, because of adverse reactions. In technically advanced countries patients with drug-resistant infection are often alcoholic or psychiatrically disturbed patients or drug addicts and a close and good doctor–patient relationship is essential in order to guide the patient through difficult treatment. Close bacteriological monitoring is required.

The problem of poor complicance among alcoholics has been tackled on a pilot basis with considerable success in the United Kingdom by providing, under the supervision of the local chest clinic, a special centre for tuberculous homeless alcoholics where medication is fully supervised by lay staff and where the arrangements are such as to tolerate continued drinking, providing the antituberculosis drugs are taken regularly.

When organisms prove to be resistant to all the main drugs (isoniazid, rifampicin, and streptomycin), the chance of permanent cure is reduced. Surgical excision should be considered for pulmonary lesions if these are suitably localized.

DISEASES CAUSED BY NON-TUBERCULOUS MYCOBACTERIA

Introduction. The main species of the genus mycobacterium which can be pathogenic in man, or which can colonize human lesions, are shown in Table 8. The mycobacterial environmental saprophytes which are capable of facultative parasitism include some important human pathogens, notably, *M.kansasii*, *M.avium*, including the intracellulare variant, and *M.scrofulaceum*. Most of the species and their variants have been taxonomically defined, but it is sometimes convenient to refer to them in broad groupings based on their culture characteristics. Thus, among the slow growers, *M.kansasii* and *M.marinum* are photochromogens, producing orange or yellow carotenoid pigments when exposed to light, *M.scrofulaceum*, *M.szulgai*, and *M.gordonae* are scotochromogens, producing pigment in the dark, and *M.avium-intracellulare*, *M.xenopi*, and *M.ulcerans* are usually monchromogens. *M.chelonei* and *M.fortuitum* are rapid growers.

Table 8 Main species of *Mycobacteria* and their pathogenicity in man

Pathogenicity in man	Species	Usual type of disease in man
Obligate parasites	*M. leprae*	leprosy
	M. tuberculosis	tuberculosis
	M. bovis	tuberculosis
Environmental saprophytes, occasional facultative parasites	*M. kansasii*	pulmonary, rarely extrapulmonary
	M. avium	pulmonary, rarely extrapulmonary
	M. intracellulare	pulmonary, rarely extrapulmonary
	M. scrofulaceum	lymphadenitis, rarely pulmonary
	M. xenopi	pulmonary, rarely extrapulmonary
	M. szulgai	pulmonary, rarely extrapulmonary
	M. simiae	pulmonary
	M. fortuitum	pulmonary
	M. chelonei	pulmonary
	M. marinum	cutaneous
	M. ulcerans	cutaneous
	M. gordonae	rarely pulmonary
Non-pathogenic environmental saphrophytes	*M. gastri*	
	M. terrae complex	
	M. triviale	
	M. flavescens	
	M. vaccae	
	M. phlei	
	M. smegmatis	

The parasitism of these mycobacteria is often opportunistic, involving the colonization of tissues already damaged or rendered susceptible by necrosis or by some other disease, but it is important to realize that many of them can also cause disease in previously healthy subjects.

The types of disease they produce closely resemble tuberculosis clinically, and for this reason the diagnosis can usually only be confirmed bacteriologically by culturing and identifying the causative organism, although differential skin tests may be helpful in some circumstances. Even so, these mycobacteria are primarily saprophytes and culturing them from clinical material does not necessarily imply that they are causing any harm. They may be laboratory contaminants, particularly in some tropical laboratories. A definite diagnosis must therefore include appropriate clinical or radiographic evidence of disease. The commonest forms of disease attributable to non-tuberculous mycobacteria are chronic pulmonary disease and lymphadenitis. Cutaneous infections are not uncommon, but bone and joint disease, genito-urinary disease, meningitis, and disseminated disease are rare.

Disease is virtually never the result of direct transmission from man to man, although close family contacts of patients excreting these mycobacteria in the sputum may become sensitized to their specific proteins, indicating that they have been infected subclinically.

Geographical distribution. The non-tuberculous mycobacteria are widely distributed in the environment, for example in the soil, in house dust, and in tap water, and may infect many wild, farm, and domestic animals. However, comparative incidences of disease vary in different parts of the world, although apparent geographical differences may sometimes be due to more thorough studies in some areas than in others. *M.kansasii*, the natural reservoir of which is unknown, is particularly prevalent in the USA and western Europe, where it is found in tap water. *M.avium*, which infects

birds (including poultry), pigs and some other animals, is prevalent in the south eastern USA, the United Kingdom, western Australia, Czechoslovakia, and Japan. *M.scofulaceum* is prevalent in the USA, Canada, Australia, and Europe. *M.xenopi*, originally isolated from the toad, is found mainly in coastal areas and near tidal estuaries, possibly because it can infect sea birds. The rapid growers such as *M.chelonei* and *M.fortuitum* are very widely distributed throughout the environment. *M.ulcerans* occurs in tropical regions, particularly central Africa, but has never been isolated from the environment.

The incidence of disease caused by these organisms does not appear to be changing, and so in countries where the incidence of tuberculosis is falling, the relative frequency of non-tuberculous mycobacterial disease is rising.

Chronic pulmonary disease. Chronic pulmonary disease can range from mild self-limiting trivial disease to severe, progressive, and fatal disease accompanied by extensive cavitation. The commonest pathogens are *M. kansasii* and *M. avium-intracellulare*, but *M. xenopi* and, rarely, *M. gordonae*, *M. szulgai*, *M. scrofulaceum*, *M. chelonei*, and *M. fortuitum* may be involved. *M. avium-intracellulare* and *M. chelonei* are particularly liable to cause severe, progressive disease.

There may be a history of other long-standing pulmonary disease such as chronic obstructive airways disease, tuberculosis, silicosis or other pneumoconiosis, bronchiectasis, cystic fibrosis, arc welders' disease, or chronic aspiration pneumonia, but in many cases there is no such history nor any evidence of immunological deficiency.

The pathogenesis is obscure, but infection almost certainly occurs from the environment, and direct transmission from man to man is probably very rare.

Because these organisms are only facultative parasites, it is important to confirm the diagnosis bacteriologically. A single isolation by culture from the sputum is unlikely to be clinically significant, since this is not uncommon even in normal healthy subjects, and these organisms can occur in the upper respiratory tract without causing disease. At least two cultures of pure growth from specimens obtained at least one week apart, accompanied by radiographic deterioration are usually considered to be necessary to be certain of the diagnosis. Highly specific differential skin tests may prove to be useful diagnostic aids in the future. There are no reliable radiographic or histological differences between chronic lung disease caused by *M. tuberculosis* or by other mycobacteria.

The treatment depends upon the organism involved. *M. kansasii* is sensitive to rifampicin and ethambutol, and is partly sensitive to isoniazid. Infection will usually respond well to these three drugs given daily for two years. It is also usually sensitive to streptomycin, kanamycin, capreomycin, pyrazinamide, and ethionamide. *M. avium-intracellulare* and *M. scrofulaceum* are, in contrast, highly resistant to the antituberculosis drugs. It is usually recommended that patients should be given daily treatment with an aminoglycoside and four or five of the drugs rifampicin, pyrazinamide, isoniazid, ethambutol, ethionamide, and cycloserine, treatment with at least four drugs being continued for two years from the time the sputum becomes smear-negative. However, it has also been claimed that daily treatment with isoniazid, rifampicin, and ethambutol is just as effective. Even with intensive chemotherapy the disease will continue to progress to an eventual fatal outcome in about 20 per cent of patients. *M. xenopi* usually responds well to isoniazid, rifampicin, and streptomycin, and *M. szulgai* to rifampicin, ethambutol, ethionamide, and streptomycin. *M. chelonei* and *M. fortuitum* may be relatively sensitive in laboratory tests, some strains, particularly of *M. fortuitum*, being sensitive to one or more of the drugs ethionamide, viomycin, kanamycin, capreomycin, and erythromycin, but in spite of this, they tend not to respond well to treatment. Indeed, laboratory sensitivity tests are of little value in planning chemotherapy regimens for disease due to non-tuberculous mycobacteria.

When pulmonary disease does not respond well to chemotherapy, surgical removal should be considered, particularly when the lesion is well localized.

Lymphadenitis. Non-tuberculous mycobacterial lymphadenitis occurs mainly in young children. It most commonly involves the cervical nodes, but may also affect other groups, such as inguinal, femoral, and axillary nodes. Characteristically, a group of nodes becomes swollen and matted together without pain, tenderness, or systemic disease. Rupture and sinus formation commonly occur with periods of regression and deterioration, but the most usual eventual outcome is gradual healing accompanied by fibrosis and calcification. The organisms most commonly involved are *M. avium-intracellulare* and *M. scrofulaceum*; *M. kansasii* may be involved, particularly in some parts of the USA; *M. szulgai*, *M. chelonei*, and *M. fortuitum* are rarely responsible.

The pathogenesis is unclear. Inguinal or axillary adenitis may follow local trauma, and cervical adenitis may follow infection of the mouth, throat, teeth, tonsils, or adenoids. In many countries where the incidence of tuberculosis is low, mycobacterial lymphadenitis is much more frequently non-tuberculous than tuberculous.

The differential diagnosis includes other causes of lymphadenitis, such as tuberculosis, sarcoidosis, pyogenic infection, cat scratch disease, and infectious mononucleosis, and also malignant disease. The precise diagnosis can only be confirmed by culturing and identifying the organism responsible, but differential skin tests—comparing reactions to tuberculin PPD, PPD-Y, prepared from *M. kansasii*; PPD-A, from *M. avium*; PPD-B, from *M. intracellulare*; and PPD-G, from scotochromogens—may be helpful but are not conclusive. Infections with *M. avium-intracellulare* and *M. scrofulaceum* will usually produce weak reactions to tuberculin PPD and stronger but similar reactions to all three of the non-tuberculous PPDs, A, B, and G. *M. kansasii* infection will usually produce equally positive reactions to both tuberculin PPD and PPD-Y.

Since most cases are caused by *M. avium-intracellulare* or *M. scrofulaceum*, they respond poorly to chemotherapy. Therefore, if the disease does not regress and heal spontaneously, the involved nodes should be totally excised. Discharging sinuses should be treated initially by curettage and debridement, followed later by total excision. Surgical treatment is almost invariably successful, although there is a very remote risk of progressive, disseminated, and eventually fatal disease.

Soft tissue infections. Apart from sinuses draining underlying nodes, or very rarely underlying osteomyelitis, and causing local cutaneous infection (scrofuloderma), primary cutaneous, subcutaneous, and soft tissue infections can occur. The organisms most commonly involved are *M. ulcerans*, *M. marinum*, *M. fortuitum*, and *M. chelonei*.

M. ulcerans causes cutaneous and subcutaneous ulceration, and is described on page 5.273. *M. marinum*, which infects much marine life, can infect man from the sea, rivers, lakes, swimming pools, fish tanks, and aquariums. Mild abrasions of the skin can lead to a warty, granulomatous cutaneous lesion which is usually limited to the skin because *M. marinum* requires a temperature lower than 37 °C to grow, and which may closely resemble sporotrichosis or cutaneous leishmaniasis. Papules may break down to form shallow ulcers, but the lesions almost invariably heal spontaneously in a few months and no specific treatment is necessary. However, *M. marinum* may occasionally infect deeper structures of the hand such as synovial sheaths, tendons, and bone. In such circumstances, treatment with rifampicin and ethambutol has been claimed to be of benefit, or with trimethoprimsulphamethoxazole, tetracycline, or minocycline. *M. chelonei* and *M. fortuitum* may infect any site of trauma in which the skin is broken, including garden accidents and war wounds, but also including surgical incisions and injection sites. These organisms characteristically cause local abscesses, but may

give rise to serious disseminated disease in renal transplant recipients and patients on dialysis. They have also infected porcine replacement heart valves and can cause extensive damage after open heart surgery through a sternum-splitting incision, with mediastinal abscesses and osteomyelitis of the sternum. When they are responsible for chronic pulmonary disease, there is almost always a history of a previous pulmonary lesion. Because they are highly drug-resistant, serious infection usually has to be treated by surgical excision.

Rare infections. Rare, serious infections can occur, but usually only after appropriate predisposing events. For example, osteomyelitis, and infection of associated tendons, tendon sheaths, joints, and bursae can follow trauma, including open heart surgery referred to above. Carious teeth can become secondarily infected. Genito-urinary disease, resembling genito-urinary tuberculosis, can rarely occur. However, disseminated disease, including endocarditis and meningitis, is only likely to occur in the patient who is immunosuppressed by disease or by drugs, or who has an underlying haematological disease such as leukaemia. In such circumstances, disseminated disease is usually fatal. Serious infections following open heart surgery or renal transplantation have mainly affected adults and have involved predominantly *M. chelonei* and *M. fortuitum*. Otherwise, disseminated disease has usually occurred in young children already seriously ill with some other underlying disorder, and has most frequently involved *M. kansasii*, and *M. avium-intracellulare*.

References

Crofton, J. and Douglas, A. (1981). Tuberculosis. In *Respiratory diseases*, 3rd edn., Blackwell Scientific Publications, Oxford.

Fox, W. (1979). The chemotheraphy of pulmonary tuberculosis: a review. *Chest* **76**, suppl., 785.

— (1980). Short course chemotheraphy for tuberculosis. In *Recent advances in respiratory medicine* (ed. D. C. Flenley), 183. Churchill Livingstone, Edinburgh.

Girling, D. J. (1978). The hepatic toxicity of antituberculosis regimens containing isoniazid, rifampicin and pyrazinamide. *Tubercle, Lond.* **59**, 13.

Grange, J. M. (1980). In *Current topics in infection: mycobacterial diseases* (ed. I. Phillips). Arnold, London.

Griffiths, D. Ll. (1980). Tuberculosis of the spine: a review. *Adv. Tuberc. Res.* **20**, 92.

Mitchison, D. A. (1979). Basic mechanisms of chemotherapy. *Chest* **76**, suppl. 771.

— (1981). The mycobacteria. In *Scientific foundations of respiratory medicine* (eds. J. G. Scadding and G. Cumming), 371. Heinemann, London.

Rouillon, A., Perdrizet, S., and Parrot, R. (1976). Transmission of tubercle bacilli: the effects of chemotherapy. *Tubercle, Lond.* **57**, 275.

Styblo, K. (1980). Recent advances in epidemiological research in tuberculosis. *Adv. Tuberc. Res.* **20**, 1.

Wolinsky, E. (1979). Nontuberculous mycobacteria and associated diseases. *Am. Rev. resp. Dis.* **119**, 107.

Particular problems of tuberculosis in developing countries

M. Aquinas and D. Todd

'The predicament in public health today is the vast areas of unfulfilled expectations of people, too vast to be tolerable, in the greater part of the developing world. We live in a world in which in one part 50 per cent of all deaths occur over the age of 70, and in another 50 per cent of all deaths occur under the age of five. There is a large gap between what medicine can do and what it is actually doing; between the possession of knowledge and the ability to translate that knowledge into the reality of the local setting. The former does not mean that the latter will follow automatically and as a result many advances in knowledge are not being applied' (Ramalingaswami in an address to the WHO in 1976).

From an economic or technical point of view we tend to label countries under one of two general headings, 'developed' or 'developing' and we attempt to explain different standards of health, education, etc., accordingly (see Section 3). And so it is in the case of tuberculosis. From the information available it is accepted that the highest prevalence, morbidity, and mortality rates are to be found in parts of Asian, African, and South American countries.

Control programmes. The basic essentials of a tuberculosis control programme are time-honoured and theoretically very simple and do not require the assistance of highly specialized skills and equipment. On the one hand we have case-finding and chemotherapy and on the other, preventive measures—largely BCG vaccination and health education. Of course treatment also has a major contribution to make in the field of prevention, for every case that is made non-infectious by treatment a source of spread is removed. The actual implementation of these formulae is, however, frequently beset with obstacles that are often outside the power of health authorities to remove. The impediments may range from political and cultural to social, economic, or even medical. In some countries the presence of many other pressing problems makes it understandable that a chronic disease like tuberculosis should occupy a very low rung on the ladder of national priorities. Even in the health field a high prevalence rate of tuberculosis could not compete with outbreaks of such diseases as cholera, plague, or smallpox for immediate attention.

According to official estimates about 20 million people suffer from tuberculosis today. It has also been established that the annual infection rate decreases by about 10 per cent a year in low prevalence countries, while the decrease, if at all, has been very much slower in high prevalence areas. And we know that more than two-thirds of the world's population live in Asia, Africa, and South America where the disease may, in certain areas, be even on the increase. It is important to bear in mind that methods of recording the disease lack uniformity on an international level, and indeed on a national level and even from doctor to doctor. This makes it difficult to obtain accurate or reliable figures concerning any aspect of tuberculosis.

The diagnosis and treatment of tuberculosis is based on two avenues of approach: on individual patient presentation, or on a community-wide basis. In the case of the individual patient who presents at an office or clinic because of symptoms, the diagnosis and treatment is a relatively simple medical matter. In the case of whole communities, however, one has deliberately to organize programmes to find and to treat the patients. It is with this aspect that developing countries are now concerned as the developed countries passed through this stage decades ago. The success of case-finding in developing countries will depend on the presence or absence of enthusiasm on the part of authorities; the finances available and the amount allocated to tuberculosis; and health education programmes and the participation of the community in the overall control activities. In order to be effective it is obvious that a control programme for a communicable disease like tuberculosis should be nationwide. Probably one of the errors of the past, however, was to separate this disease from the mainstream of medicine. Now the idea is to steer its management back into that of the general medical care system and so to integrate it into the overall health services of a country. In order to maintain a balanced national health service the World Health Organization for more than two decades has been emphasizing the importance of such integration of health programmes as opposed to the purely specialized attempts to handle tuberculosis on its own. This latter approach, which isolated tuberculous patients and their physicians from the rest of medicine, suffered in the same way as psychiatry did and for the same reason. Both specialities now have an uphill struggle to claim a place within the orbit of medicine in general.

Before an effective, integrated tuberculosis programme can function, there should be an infrastructure of basic health services which covers the whole country and are so located that such facilities are readily accessible to everybody. Many countries in the developing world do not have such a basic requirement or at least do not have a satisfactory one. More than three-quarters of whatever facilities and resources exist are often found concentrated in the urban areas even though three-quarters of the population live in rural areas.

Control agencies. There are usually two agencies involved in the programme for the control of tuberculosis. One is the national government operating through its ministry of health and which represents the official agency. It is ultimately responsible for the control of infectious diseases and for providing the financial resources. Governments can get assistance with their control programmes from the World Health Organization in Geneva, which has been responsible for many national and international health campaigns during the past 40 years. The other agency involved in the tuberculosis control programme represents the voluntary sector. Almost every country has a voluntary agency—a national Tuberculosis Association which is a member of the main voluntary association, the International Union Against Tuberculosis (IUAT) with its headquarters in Paris. These voluntary associations have a common emblem, the double-barred Cross of Lorraine which was arbitrarily chosen as a battle-standard in the fight against tuberculosis at the very beginning of this century. There are regional branches of IUAT in the Middle East, Europe, the Far East, South America, etc. Regional and/or international meetings take place every year, and in this way an attempt is made to co-ordinate the international effort.

Case finding. The object of case-finding is to identify the sources of infection in a community. There has been considerable controversy over what actually constitutes a 'case of tuberculosis'. From the point of view of preventing the spread or further spread of infection and disease, it is a person who is discharging tubercle bacilli in his sputum. It is paramount therefore to find these patients first. Side by side with the discovery of infectious cases treatment must be provided, otherwise there is little point in just informing patients that they are suffering from an infectious disease. And as treatment is by chemotherapy which is specific for the tubercle bacilli, arrangements must be made to have an adequate supply of antituberculosis drugs available. In its ninth report the World Health Organization expert committee summarized the situation when it said 'the first priority would be to provide facilities for direct smear examination of sputum from persons, who, of their own volition, present with symptoms and to provide treatment for those who are found to excrete tubercle bacilli'. The most infectious patients are usually the most symptomatic and so they are the most likely to seek medical attention whenever facilities are available. To provide facilities for examination of sputum in large rural areas can be a major undertaking in many countries but more especially in areas where no health facilities exist. One of the difficulties in the delivery of any medical care is the absence of an adequate health infrastructure throughout a country. Simple as it may seem, it can be a vast undertaking for some areas to provide these basic facilities. However, all countries do not present a homogeneous picture either in the absence of such facilities or in the presence of an adequate medical care structure. Most are in the process of building up as good a system as is possible within the limits of their own economic resources.

Sputum examination. The diagnosis and treatment of tuberculosis is a simple matter once the principles are grasped. Many countries are now trying to set up a network of simple laboratories for direct smear examination of the sputum. Where possible these are located in the same building as the general health clinic in the peripheral areas. To operate these centres, bright young people from the villages are selected and trained, usually at a central bacteriological department or at provincial centres for a period of about one year, after which they are posted back to a peripheral centre near where they live. Periodically, supervisors from the provincial or central departments visit the peripheral stations and check on the technique of collecting sputa, preparing the slide specimens, identifying the acid-fast bacilli, and recording the results. Through health education programmes, symptomatic patients present themselves at the health centre and are asked to bring sputum specimens for examination. Those who are found to be positive are advised on the diagnosis and start immediately on treatment. At its simplest the health campaigns aim at picking out the symptomatics and use such slogans as 'if you have a cough for a month or so, attend the clinic for a check-up, you may have tuberculosis'. Patients who are coughing are much more likely to be spreading tubercle bacilli into the atmosphere than those who are not coughing, and therefore it is vital that these patients are discovered without delay and treated early. And so the first step in the diagnosis of tuberculosis is the direct smear examination under the microscope at the peripheral health centre. Non-specialized staff given training are capable of providing satisfactory service especially when periodically reviewed by the staff from the provincial or central department. Naturally, the skill and enthusiasm of the technician as well as the ability to get the symptomatic patients to have their sputum checked will vary from place to place. The handling of sputum, however, especially in the case of an infectious disease like tuberculosis, is not always carried out without objections and technicians are sometimes loath to restrict themselves to this unpleasant task.

Despite the limitations of direct smear examination, however, it remains the first step and sometimes the only one in the diagnosis of patients in many developing countries. To identify *M. tuberculosis* and to differentiate it from other mycobacteria, it is essential to perform cultures. And where resources and personnel are available culture facilities should be and undoubtedly are encouraged. However, it must be remembered that in spite of the many advantages of cultures, especially the much higher possibility of finding positive results when sputum specimens contain only small numbers of bacilli, operational disadvantages are much greater. Apart from the skilled personnel and special equipment, the necessity for permanent supplies of more basic requirements such as electricity, water, and air-conditioning in hot climates makes the possibilities for cultures of good standard out of reach of many peripheral health centres. Probably the great disadvantage of the culture method is the length of time it takes, usually six weeks, to obtain a result. The greatest advantage of the direct smear examination is the fact that the results can be available on the same day. This is of paramount importance in many rural areas where treatment can be started before the patient leaves the centre, for he may not return. It is also very useful in identifying those patients who are coughing large numbers of bacilli into the atmosphere, and are the most serious sources of infection in the community. Direct smear microscopy can be performed practically anywhere as long as there is a technician, a microscope, sputum, and the appropriate staining materials.

It is well known that the vast majority of the patients with progressive tuberculosis usually have symptoms of cough, fever, and haemoptysis, and so present themselves at any health facility within reach. While finding and treating the most infectious cases is a vital first step, it remains just the first step, and is a long way from detecting and treating the patient at a much earlier stage of the disease, at a time when he may not have any symptoms but when the bacilli are multiplying or beginning to do so.

Radiography in the diagnosis of tuberculosis. In the technically advanced parts of the world and in big cities generally, it is now unthinkable to diagnose and treat tuberculosis without the assistance of radiography. Indeed more emphasis may be put on radiographic findings than is warranted. We believe that a considerable number of patients treated for tuberculosis are done so on the basis of radiographic findings and never have the disease confirmed bacteriologically. There is no doubt that many of these patients do

in fact need treatment as bacteriological proof may be found several months later if they are maintained on an 'observation' programme instead of a treatment one. While there can be no denying the contribution of radiography in chest diseases, it is a facility that is not universally available. The microscope is one of the first pieces of equipment to be provided where resources are limited and where the need is to check the presence of active and infectious disease by finding those patients who are smear-positive and treating them as soon as possible.

Mass mobile radiography. There has been more controversy over the use of mass mobile radiography (MMR) than of any other measure associated with case-finding in tuberculosis. Even now there is far from universal agreement on its place in the programme. Having been introduced to Europe after the Second World War, it had a boom period when there was a high prevalence of the disease and large numbers of cases were easily discovered. However, with the passage of time and as tuberculosis came under control in Western countries, it was becoming obvious that this method of case-finding was costing too much to make it worthwhile. The current recommendation is that mass radiography as a means of discovering tuberculosis is not worth the expense involved. This advice is particularly relevant to developing countries which can ill afford to purchase such X-ray units and where the cost of operating, maintaining, supplying spare parts, or finding engineers to repair them, not to mention the lack of roads or electricity, make their presence of little practical value. Furthermore the interpretation of the radiographs themselves requires considerable skills which are not always readily available in many of the areas concerned.

There are times and areas where mass radiography does have a place. Travel is increasing at such a rate that no country is immune to tuberculosis. In particular, there is the risk associated with mass migration of peoples, either immigrants or refugees moving from one country to another, bringing with them tuberculosis and other indigenous diseases. Immigrants or refugees frequently congregate in groups and are readily accessible to health teams. Screening for tuberculosis is one of the main concerns of the health authorities and for two reasons. Firstly because of the importance of discovering and treating an infectious disease in people living in such close proximity to one another, secondly because many of the countries which eventually accept refugees stipulate that they should be free from tuberculosis.

Treatment. A major development in treatment policies is that hospitals or sanatoriums for tuberculosis patients are now a thing of the past. Except in very occasional instances lung surgery for the disease has also disappeared. This relieves high prevalence areas of a very large financial and medical burden.

With the advent of chemotherapy and its current state of near perfection, the aim is that the lifestyle of the average patient should be barely disturbed during treatment or indeed by the fact that he is suffering from tuberculosis. The cure of the disease revolves around two factors: (*a*) providing an adequate drug regimen, and (*b*) making sure that the patient does in fact take the adequate drug regimen. This formula presents no real difficulty within the existing medical setting found in most Western countries. But if there is an inadequate framework through which treatment can be delivered to the patient, then it is clear that much more is necessary than just a simple drug prescription in order to implement a cure on a country-wide basis. The questions at issue are how to apply the knowledge that is now available to countries that are economically deprived, and how the various obstacles can be removed so that tuberculosis patients throughout the world can have access to treatment. It is 100 years since the tubercle bacillus was discovered and about 40 years since a chemical cure became available. Knowing both the cause of the disease and how to cure it and yet being unable to achieve substantial success in eliminating it because of socio-economic obstacles make the whole project an unenviable challenge. The treatment of tuberculosis is thus more a problem of administration and organization than an entirely medical problem. However desirable an ideal chemotherapeutic regimen may be, the fact is that each country or area has to decide on a regimen which is within its own resources and facilities to provide. When the per capita expenditure on the overall health services may be about 1 per cent of that in a technically advanced country, there is little point in trying to prescribe an expensive drug regimen. Indeed the cost of such a regimen may be more than 30 times that of a less effective but more feasible and applicable one.

While most drugs are available to individual doctors and individual patients (who can pay) in practically any country, it is the national programme that matters for the control of an infectious disease. Therefore it is what the particular country can afford in money, manpower, and management for the control and treatment of tuberculosis in its own territory that is important.

It can be said that if isoniazid and rifampicin were available to all countries, it would be much easier to organize the delivery of treatment to patients and to guarantee a cure. This oral regimen has proved to be virtually 100 per cent successful when given for nine months. Treating patients for a short period of six to nine months is much more acceptable to patients as well as to the staff. Probably most countries could afford isoniazid, which is one of the least expensive drugs on the market, but unfortunately the cost of rifampicin remains so prohibitive that it cannot be considered in the parts of the world that are most in need of it. Therefore these countries must attempt to provide their own drug regimens which are usually given for treatment of about one year's duration. The longer the duration of treatment, the greater the dropout rate. In order to be effective it must not only be a good regimen but it should be provided free to the patients. There is much too much experience of patients who cannot afford the whole treatment programme, paying for a few weeks and then being obliged to abandon the treatment because they cannot afford to continue paying for it. Indeed, patients often do this without reference to medical advice at all as in some countries drugs, even the most expensive ones, are readily available across the counter. In this case, it is easy to understand why a patient could jeopardize his treatment not only by the haphazard use of the medication but also by an unauthorized dosage system that must inevitably occur. This practice makes it more difficult to control the disease later, even with other treatment regimens, as it is likely that drug resistance will have emerged to the most effective drugs.

It is common practice in remote areas in some countries to appoint a village elder or an accepted leader in the community to supervise the treatment of the patients in the district and to collaborate with the medical personnel in gaining patient co-operation in drug-taking as well as in all other aspects of health education. The medical team may not even be resident in the village and may in fact have to cover many such districts away from base in the course of a month. It is here that the community participation is so important. The scarcity of qualified professionals, doctors, nurses, social workers, and dispensers, would make it impossible to achieve any success without the assistance of a considerable number of reliable lay people who are thoroughly familiar with the district and who have the respect and confidence of the community they serve.

The difficulties encountered in the control and treatment of tuberculosis are by no means uniform in the economically developing parts of the world. They vary from country to country, from urban to rural areas, and from the highly educated to the most illiterate.

Clinical presentation of tuberculosis. While tuberculosis remains an outpatient disease for the vast majority of those needing treatment, some patients find their way into hospitals, though not always with a ready-made diagnosis. In general hospital practice, the entire spectrum of tuberculous disease is still seen, although the more acute forms in the young are becoming rare. Pulmonary tuberculosis remains the most common variety. Prolonged cough, with or without dyspnoea and blood-streaked sputum, may be the result of tuberculosis rather than chronic bronchitis, especially in the elderly. As the majority of the population will have been exposed to tuberculosis in early childhood, reactivation can be expected in patients suffering from diabetes mellitus, chronic alcoholism, drug addiction, severe malnutrition, haematological malignancies, or immunological defects. Tuberculosis is one of the most common complications of therapy with corticosteroids or with immunosuppressive agents, and pulmonary lesions may become radiologically evident over as short a period as two weeks.

Tuberculosis is still one of the most common diseases which present as pyrexia of unknown origin (PUO). In early miliary tuberculosis, radiological examination of the lungs may reveal no lesions and tuberculosis of intra-abdominal or pelvic organs, the pericardium, vertebrae, or meninges can be difficult to diagnose. The tuberculin skin test is often negative in widely disseminated disease, in chronically ill and undernourished patients, and in those who are immunologically suppressed. In miliary tuberculosis, aspiration of liver or bone marrow trephine biopsy may be diagnostic and repeated examination of the optic fundi may reveal choroidal lesions. Often invasive diagnositic procedures cannot be carried out, as in the case of patients with severe thrombocytopenia, and under these circumstances a therapeutic trial with antituberculous drugs may be warranted. However, pyrexia which responds to agents such as rifampicin or streptomycin need not have been due to *M. tuberculosis* infection.

While rare, the adult respiratory distress syndrome is occasionally encountered in disseminated tuberculosis. Nodular lesions are seen on radiological examination of the lungs and there may be clinical and laboratory evidence of disseminated intravascular coagulation. The mortality rate is high.

BCG vaccination. An antituberculosis programme, like any health programme, includes various measures. These measures should be considered simultaneously in order to present a balanced effort and to make it possible to provide the greatest impact on the disease. In the early 1950s the WHO/UNICEF launched BCG campaigns in many countries that had high levels of transmission of tuberculosis. It was believed that this specific preventive method would give the highest epidemiological profit per dollar spent. When available resources are limited, as they invariably are in countries with a high prevalence rate, it becomes vital to produce the most practicable cost-effective programme possible. BCG vaccination does not prevent an infection with tubercle bacilli from actually taking place but its effect is rather to prevent the bacilli from multiplying at such a rate that they result in disease. It should therefore be most effective in persons who are infected with virulent tubercle bacilli soon after getting vaccinated. The general recommendation was that in areas with a high exogenous infection rate, vaccination with BCG should have the widest possible coverage as early in life as feasible. Hong Kong might serve as an example of an ideal country in which to test or to use BCG. A prevaccination tuberculosis survey in 1952 revealed that over 90 per cent of the population at the age of 15 years was tuberculin positive, and in its report the WHO showed that the level of tuberculin reactions in Hong Kong was 116 per cent above the general level in Asian countries. Moreover at this time in Hong Kong 34 per cent of all deaths from tuberculosis occurred under the age of 5 years. A BCG campaign was initiated in 1952 and it was aimed largely at newborns and young children. In the early 1960s the coverage of newborns had increased to virtually 100 per cent and has continued at that level since. It was not compulsory but with health education campaigns BCG was readily accepted.

After nearly 30 years use in Hong Kong can anything be attributed to BCG? All that can be said is that it does appear that BCG in newborns has made a considerable contribution to the decline in serious forms of tuberculosis in young children (Fig. 1). In 1952 the death rate from tuberculosis was 3.5 per 1000 live births and in the 1970s practically nil. This decline in deaths from tuberculosis was much more marked than the death rate from other causes in the same age group. Simultaneously with the use of BCG, however, there were other contributory factors operating in the control programme—specific chemotherapy and marked improvements in the general standard of living. Currently there are two questions to be asked about BCG vaccination. The first is how good is it and the second who should be vaccinated? It is accepted from vast experience that it is generally one of the safest vaccinations. Much more work has yet to be done is assessing the value of BCG in newborns especially with reference to the immunological response present in the first few days of life. While it may be more effective to perform the vaccination some months later, it may be adminstratively much more difficult. If deliveries generally take place in institutions or maternity homes, it is obviously much easier to organize a vaccination programme while the newborn is in the institution.

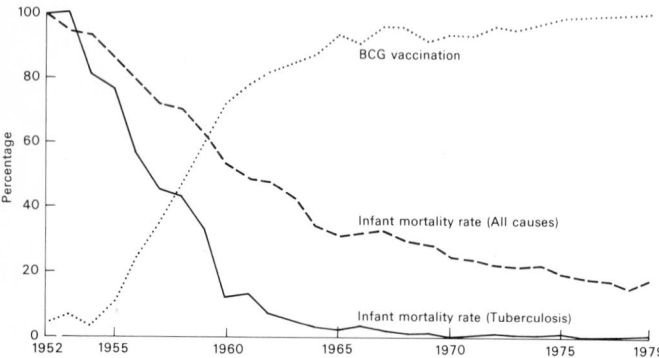

Fig. 1 Infant mortality rates in Hong Kong from all causes and tuberculosis (expressed as a percentage of 1952 rates) and BCG vaccination of newborns, 1952–79.

Concerning the efficacy of BCG vaccination we know that the controlled trial in British schoolchildren conducted by the Medical Research Council produced a 77 per cent reduction in the incidence of the disease when followed up to 20 years. This was in 1950, but with the continued decline in the risk of infection since then, it may now be more costly to continue the programme than to treat the small numbers that might develop the disease if the vaccination were to stop.

Several other clinical trials including the most recently controlled study in South India give a wide variation in the percentage protection offered by BCG vaccination. It is difficult to apply the results obtained in one country to those of another where many fluctuating factors may operate and so, for the time being, it is advisable that each country adopt its own policy. In so far as BCG continues to be recommended in the preventive field then it is obvious that those eligible are newborns, children, and others at risk in areas of high prevalence. As with any other measure involved in the antituberculosis programme BCG vaccination, though seemingly very simple, is liable to a multitude of pitfalls. These include the vaccine itself. (whether liquid or freeze-dried), the potency, the dosage, the methods used (oral, intradermal, or percutaneous), the skill of inoculators, as well as many others. It is necessary that every step in the whole procedure be constantly monitored and assessed. In order to make an impact in preventing the disease it has been agreed that about 80 per cent of the susceptible population should be vaccinated and this involves a nationwide effort. It also means that it is largely a matter of organization and training inoculators. In a city like Hong Kong, which for practical purposes has no rural area, there is no problem, but for countries with largely rural areas, as in most developing countries, the situation is much more difficult. However, tremendous efforts have been made to make a BCG programme nationwide. This has been successful especially in countries where governments and voluntary agencies have made concerted and sustained efforts to organize an effective programme and to provide trained vaccination teams.

References

Chest Service of the Medical and Health Department (1979). *Annual report* Hong Kong Government Printer, Hong Kong.
Farga, V. (1978). Proceedings of the XXIVth World Conference of the IUAT *Bull. Int. Union Tuber.* **53**, 228.
Fox, W. (1979). The current status of short-course chemotherapy. *Tubercle, Lond.* **60**, 177–98.
Nsanzumuhire, H., Lukwago, E. W., Edwards, E. A., Stott, H., Fox, W., and Sutherland, I. (1977). A study of the use of community leaders in case-finding for pulmonary tuberculosis in Kenya. *Tubercle, Lond.* **58**, 117.
Rouillon A. (1979). Editorial. *Am. Rev. resp. Dis.* **120**, 1203.
WHO Expert Committee on Tuberculosis (1974). Ninth report. *Technical Report Series* no. 552. World Health Organization, Geneva.

Leprosy

M. F. R. Waters

Synonym. Hansen's disease, Hanseniasis.
Definition. Leprosy is a chronic inflammatory disease of man caused by *Mycobacterium leprae*, which displays a wide clinical 'spectrum' related to host ability to develop and to maintain specific cell-mediated immunity (CMI). In high resistant 'tuberculoid' leprosy, localized signs are restricted to skin and peripheral nerve, whereas low resistant 'lepromatous' leprosy is a generalized bacteraemic disease involving many systems, with widespread lesions of skin, peripheral nerves, upper respiratory tract, the reticuloendothelial system, eyes, bone, and testes. Common complications include immunologically mediated inflammatory episodes ('reactions'), secondary inflammation in the anaesthetic areas which result from nerve damage, and deformity of face, hands and feet.

Aetiology. *M. leprae*, discovered by Hansen in Norway in 1873, is an intra-cellular, rod-shaped organism, 1–7 µm long and 0.25 µm in width, more acid- and less alcohol-fast than *M. tuberculosis*, which it resembles. Despite repeated claims to have grown *M. leprae in vitro*, none has been confirmed to date, although incorporation of tritiated thymidine by bacilli in short-term culture, without multiplication, has been obtained. Successful experimental transmission was not achieved until 1960, when Shepard reported limited infection in mouse footpads, and subsequently similar infections have been claimed in hamster and rat footpads and the ears of hamsters and mice. A footpad inoculum of 5000 or 10 000 bacilli yields 10^6 after six to eight months, but in normal mice no subsequent increase occurs. During the log phase of multiplication, the generation time is 12–13 days, the longest of any known bacterium. In thymectomized-irradiated mice multiplication continues, yields of 10^9 per footpad being not uncommon with lepromatous histology, and systemic spread occurs; this enhancement may, however, be largely prevented by transfusions of syngeneic lymphocytes. Lepromatous leprosy may also be obtained in nude mice and in a proportion (around half) of immunologically normal nine-banded armadillos inoculated with leprosy bacilli. Such armadillos are now the main source of *M. leprae* for immunological and biochemical studies and for the preparation of a possible vaccine.

M. leprae is most easily detected in the skin lesions of patients by Wade's 'scraped incision' method. After cleansing, the skin is pinched to exclude blood, and a small cut made in the skin fold some 5 mm long and 2–3 mm deep. One side of the cut is then scraped with the back of the scalpel point. The tissue pulp collected on the blade is spread on a glass slide, dried, fixed, and stained by the Ziehl–Neelsen method, care being taken never to overheat the carbolfuchsin. Leprosy bacilli are very scanty in tuberculoid lesions, and are often not detected by routine methods. They become more numerous as the spectrum is crossed and are present in huge numbers in lepromatous lesions. A lepromatous patient may have as many as 10^{12} bacilli in the body. Many untreated lepromatous patients excrete leprosy bacilli in their nasal secretions. Therefore 'nose-blows', collected in polythene handkerchiefs, can be smeared and examined for acid-fast bacilli. It should, however, be remembered that saprophytic mycobacteria may occasionally be present in the upper respiratory tracts of healthy people. The density of bacilli in smears or tissues is termed the bacterial index (BI), which is best scored on Ridley's logarithmic scale, at one end of which the finding of one to nine leprosy bacilli in 100 oil immersion fields is graded 1+ and at the other end the finding of over 1000 bacilli in a single oil immersion field is graded as 6+.

In lepromatous tissues, the bacilli are characteristically in 'cigar-bundle' groups, and in large aggregates or 'globi', the latter situated in multinucleate Virchow giant cells derived from histiocytes. The cytoplasm of many bacilli is fragmented; such bacilli are dead. Dead bacilli are only slowly broken down, and may remain in tissues for many months or years, probably only very slowly releasing their antigens. The percentage of solid-staining, presumed viable, bacilli in smears or tissues is termed the morphological index (MI).

A standardized, autoclaved suspension of *M. leprae*, extracted either from human or from armadillo lepromatous tissue, is used as an intradermal skin test, the 'lepromin' test, which gives an assessment of specific sensitization in leprosy patients. The early (Fernandez) reaction is similar to a tuberculin reaction and is read at 48 hours. The late (Mitsuda) reaction is read at three to five weeks and gives an accurate assessment of specific CMI; it is negative in lepromatous and strongly positive in tuberculoid patients. The test is not, however, diagnostic as it is often positive in non-leprosy patients including those who have never visited leprosy-endemic areas, and shows some cross-reactivity with tuberculin. A specific delayed-type hypersensitivity (DTH) skin test read at 48 hours is being developed by the IMMLEP (Immunology of Leprosy) Committee of WHO, using cell-wall free extract standardized for protein content of sonicated armadillo-derived *M. leprae*.

There is no known animal reservoir of leprosy, although infection of wild armadillos in a limited area of the United States of America, has recently been discovered, and one naturally-occurring infection in a captive chimpanzee has been reported.

Epidemiology From Governmental returns submitted to the World Health Organization in 1975, a conservative estimate was made of a world total of 10.6 million leprosy patients, although many consider 12 million to be a more accurate figure. The importance of leprosy lies not only in numbers but also in the chronicity of the disease, which frequently disables but now seldom kills. Therefore it makes disproportionate demands on the health services and economies of developing countries. Leprosy occurs in almost all tropical and warm temperate climate regions, including Japan and Korea, parts of southern Europe, and several States of the United States. It has only recently died out in certain Northern European countries and Canada and, perhaps surprisingly, does not appear to have become re-established as an endemic disease despite the widespread immigration from the tropics which has occurred over the last 30 years. Leprosy is associated particularly with overcrowding, and as living standards rise, the disease becomes less common.

The main source of infection in the community consists of untreated or relapsed lepromatous patients, who may shed 10^8 leprosy bacilli in 24 hours in their nasal secretions. *M. leprae* is also secreted in the breast milk of untreated lepromatous mothers, although few bacilli are excreted through intact skin. Bacilli from dried nasal secretions remain viable after being kept in the dark or in shade for at least 24 hours and sometimes for more than seven days, and thus could be largely responsible for the spread of leprosy which appears to have many similarities to the spread of tuberculosis. Nevertheless, the exact mode of infection remains unknown. Entry via the upper respiratory tract, the most likely route, is supported by the finding of microlesions in nasal biopsy specimens obtained from healthy contacts. Entry through the contaminated skin remains a possibility, as does via the gastrointestinal tract in babies. Insects are known to carry bacilli but in such small numbers that significant spread by bites appears unlikely. Transplacental infection is unproven.

Unfortunately, hitherto there has been no simple, specific skin test, comparable to the Mantoux test in tuberculosis, which could be used for studying the spread of subclinical infection in the community. Small-scale studies employing specific lymphocyte transformation tests (LTT) have confirmed sensitization due to subclinical infection. The IMMLEP specific skin test is undergoing extensive evaluation.

Opportunity for contact with the disease, especially in childhood, appears important in the spread of leprosy. The incidence of disease among household contacts of lepromatous leprosy is five to 10 times, and among those of tuberculoid leprosy about twice as high as in the general population; this does not necessarily indicate that tuberculoid leprosy is infectious; it may merely reflect the tuberculoid family's contact with an unidentified lepromatous case. Only perhaps 5 per cent of spouses of lepromatous patients acquire the disease. Susceptibility to tuberculoid leprosy may be weakly but significantly linked to the HLA region of the chromosomes. Although there is some evidence from early work that lepromatous disease is a host-determined characteristic possessed by a small fixed proportion of all people, studies in like twins have failed to show complete concordance. Further twin studies are required, using modern genetic markers and accurate classification of the type of leprosy developed.

The incubation period is measured in years, being longer in lepromatous than tuberculoid leprosy. In leprosy-endemic areas, the overall peak incidence occurs in the 20–35 years age group, although that for tuberculoid leprosy usually occurs in the 10–19 years age group. In a group of American servicemen sent to the tropics, the tuberculoid incubation period averaged four and the lepromatous 10 years, although the range was wide in both types of leprosy. The incidence of tuberculoid leprosy is higher than for lepromatous leprosy. In most races, at least from puberty onwards, the incidence of leprosy is higher in males than in females.

Pathology and clinical features Whatever the portal of entry of *M. leprae*, the target organ for the invading bacilli is probably the endoneurium, an immunologically protected site. Once leprosy bacilli have been engulfed by Schwann cells, their subsequent fate and the type of disease which ensues, is decided by the speed and degree of resistance developed, and maintained, by the infected individual. This in turn may be related to the route of antigen presentation and load of antigen presented to the immune system, as well as to variations in non-specific CMI.

Indeterminate leprosy. Child contacts may develop a single (rarely two or three) hypopigmented macule, 2–5 cm in diameter, which when fully developed shows hypoaesthesia and decreased sweating. The majority of such lesions are self-limiting, fading after some months, but about a quarter may evolve to one of the determinate 'spectrum' types of leprosy to be described. Histological changes are slight and nonspecific, consisting of lymphocytic cuffing around the dermal appendages and neurovascular bundles. After careful searching, an acid-fast bacillus may eventually be found within a cutaneous nerve.

The spectrum of leprosy Apart from its extreme chronicity, leprosy has two special features. One is the invasion by *M. leprae* of certain superficial nerves, which may become thickened and firm. The other is the wide range of clinical and histological manifestations, reflecting the intricacies of the host–parasite relationship. The spectrum of leprosy was first defined by Ridley and Jopling (1966) who proposed a five-group system of classification according to certain immunological features. These included the cytology of the host cells of the macrophage-histocyte series (whether histiocytic or epithelioid), the degree of infiltration by lymphocytes, and the bacterial density. The five groups are, in order across the spectrum, tuberculoid (TT), borderline-tuberculoid (BT), borderline (BB), borderline-lepromatous (BL), and lepromatous (LL). This classification enables most patients to be diagnosed accurately from their clinical features, although the intermediate 'borderline' (dimorphous), BT, BB, and BL groups are relatively unstable; they tend to move towards lepromatous in the absence of treatment and toward tuberculoid after the institution of effective chemotherapy.

Skin lesions, which are best seen in good oblique light, may occur anywhere, although they only very rarely involve the hairy scalp, axillae, and perineum. The nerves of predilection, which should always be palpated, include the ulnars at and above the medial epicondyle of the humerus, the superficial radials and medians at the wrist, the great auriculars at the posterior edge of the sternocleidomastoid muscle usually running about 1 cm above the external jugular vein, the lateral popliteals at the neck of the fibula, and the posterior tibials posterior to the medial malleolus. The surals, the superficial peroneals, and the supra-orbitals are sometimes palpably enlarged. When nerves of predilection are affected, both appropriate regional anaesthesia may develop and appropriate muscle weakness and wasting may occur resulting in claw hand (ulnar and/or median), foot drop, and claw toes. Branches of the facial and trigeminal nerves, although not palpable, may also be involved, leading to lagophthalmos and to corneal anaesthesia respectively. Wrist drop from radial nerve involvement is comparatively rare. Tendon reflexes are preserved.

Tuberculoid leprosy (TT). When a high degree of CMI is developed, the infection remains very localized and asymmetrical. Only a small number of skin lesions develop, usually one to three, although the cutaneous sensory nerve supplying the skin of the lesion is frequently thickened. Typically, a tuberculoid skin lesion is large and annular, with a sharply-raised outer edge and a thin erythematous rim which slopes gradually to a hypopigmented, flattened centre. In profile, it resembles a saucer the right way up. The surface is dry with loss of sweating, sometimes scaley, and usually with a diminished number of hairs; established lesions are always markedly anaesthetic, save for some situated in the mid-line of the face or forehead. Sometimes the lesion is a plaque or a hypopigmented macule. The nerves of predilection are little involved, either none or only one being enlarged; rarely, however, symptoms and signs may be purely neural, related to a single thickened nerve. Histology of the active edge of the skin lesion reveals a tuberculoid granuloma, consisting of whorls of epithelioid cells enclosed by lymphocytes, surrounding neurovascular elements and extending up to the epidermis without leaving the papillary zone clear. The epidermis may be eroded, acid-fast bacilli are so scanty as to be seldom found, and cutaneous nerves within the granuloma are unrecognizable. Caseation is absent in the skin, but may occur in nerves. The lepromin test and the specific LTT are strongly positive. The lymph node draining the skin lesion area is free from paracortical infiltrate but immunoblasts may be present.

Borderline-tuberculoid leprosy (BT). The skin lesions, which may be very few to moderate in number, resemble those of TT leprosy, although they are usually smaller in size, or else small 'satellite' lesions may be present near the periphery of the larger lesions. Sharp-edged papules may also appear. Cutaneous sensory nerves are not usually enlarged, whereas asymmetrical enlargement of the peripheral nerves of predilection is common although caseation only rarely occurs. Therefore BT leprosy is often associated with deformity of one or both hands and/or feet. A patient may present with burns or infection of anaesthetic fingers or with a plantar ulcer in an anaesthetic foot. Lagophthalmos may result in exposure keratitis. Although the skin histology resembles that of TT leprosy, the tuberculoid granuloma tends to be more diffuse and there is usually a free, although narrow, subepidermal zone and no epidermal erosion; although many cutaneous nerves are destroyed, some may still be seen, swollen and infiltrated, and small numbers of leprosy bacilli may be detected, usually in Schwann cells or in the erectores pilae muscle. Draining lymph nodes often have an epithe-

lioid cell, sarcoid-like paracortical infiltrate. The LTT and lepromin tests are moderately positive.

Borderline leprosy (BB). The skin lesions are rather numerous, though asymmetrical, vary markedly in size, and are erythematous or hypo- or hyperpigmented. Papules and plaques may occur but the most characteristic lesion is annular with a broad rim. The outer edge is often flattish and irregular; it rises to a thick inner edge overlooking a sharply 'punched-out' hypopigmented anaesthetic centre. In profile, the lesion resembles a saucer the wrong way up, save that where the cup should sit is a deep central depression. Satellite lesions are common. Widespread, usually moderate enlargement of the nerves of predilection may occur with or without associated muscle weakness and wasting. Histologically, the skin lesion consists of a diffuse epithelioid infiltrate with small numbers of scattered lymphocytes; some dermal nerves are visible; bacilli are present in moderate numbers, especially in Schwann cells and epithelioid cells; there is a sub-epidermal clear zone. Lymph nodes show diffuse epithelioid-cell paracortical infiltrate. The specific LTT and lepromin tests are usually negative.

Borderline-lepromatous leprosy (BL). The skin lesions are moderate to many in number, although still usually somewhat asymmetrical in distribution, and the intervening skin appears normal. They consist of erythematous or hyperpigmented papules, often dimpled in outline, nodules, or plaques which are moist and succulent, and which possess normal or near normal sensation. Indefinite-edged hypopigmented macules may also be present, somewhat asymmetrical and, in particular, variable in size. Often the first one or two lesions to develop have the characteristic appearance of punched-out BB annular lesions, indicating progression (downgrading) from BB leprosy. Nerves of predilection close to the latter may be markedly enlarged; elsewhere they may be only slightly enlarged. Ear lobes may appear normal, or may be asymmetrically or, more rarely, symmetrically enlarged. The eyebrows and nasal cartilage and bones are unaffected. Although bacilli are very numerous in the lesions, they are often undetected in the normal-looking skin. Histological examination of a skin lesion reveals a diffuse histiocytic granuloma, dermal nerves are visible often with an 'onion-skin' perineurium, and there are many bacilli present both in the histiocytes and in Schwann and perineurial cells. Lymphocytes are either rather scanty or else present in considerable numbers in some segments of the granuloma; in the latter case, they are B lymphocytes. Lymph nodes show diffuse histiocytic infiltrate in the paracortical region, with some hypertrophy of the germinal centres. The specific LTT and lepromin tests are negative.

Lepromatous leprosy (LL). The early manifestations are dermal, never neural. At this stage, the skin lesions consist of very numerous, small, symmetrical, vague-edged, hypopigmented macules with erythematous, smooth, shiny surfaces, which are neither anaesthetic nor anhydrotic, and small papules with indefinite edges. The nerves of predilection may show little thickening though in more advanced cases they are symmetrically enlarged. Thickening of the nasal mucosa often occurs early, eventually giving rise to nasal blockage and blood-streaked discharge. With time, plaques and nodules develop, and the skin progressively thickens as lepromatous infiltrate increases; the lines on the face coarsen and deepen giving a 'leonine facies' and the ear lobes enlarge. Nodules may occur in the mucosa of the palate, on the nasal septum, and even on the sclera. The lips often swell, and the eyebrows and eyelashes become scanty and are lost.

Iritis and keratitis are common. The nasal cartilage and bones may be gradually destroyed, resulting in saddle-nose deformity. Lepromatous laryngitis may cause hoarseness or stridor. Oedema of the extremities sometimes occurs and the skin of the lower part of the legs often becomes firm and waxy in appearance and ulcerates easily. The lymph nodes are often enlarged, especially the supratrochlear and axillary, and testicular involvement may lead to atrophy and occasionally to gynaecomastia. In the absence of treatment, the dermal nerves are gradually destroyed, leading to a progressive pseudo 'glove-and-stocking' anaesthesia; light touch, pain, and temperature sensation are eventually lost over most of the body except the hairy scalp, axillae, perineum and groins, but position sense is well preserved. Therefore patients can continue to use their hands almost normally (unless there is motor weakness), but because of the peripheral anaesthesia, some patients repeatedly traumatize their fingers and toes; as a result, the digitis progressively shorten, and in addition, secondary infection may occur leading to local osteitis and tissue damage. X-rays of the hands of untreated LL patients may rarely reveal asymmetrical phalangeal 'cysts', presumed to be due to lepromatous infiltrate. In some long-standing cases, whether treated or untreated, there is absorption of the terminal phalanges, and typical 'pencilling' of the heads and shafts of the metatarsals. X-ray of the face may reveal atrophy of the nasal spine and of the maxillary alveolar process, the latter often being associated with loss of the upper central incisors (Fig. 1).

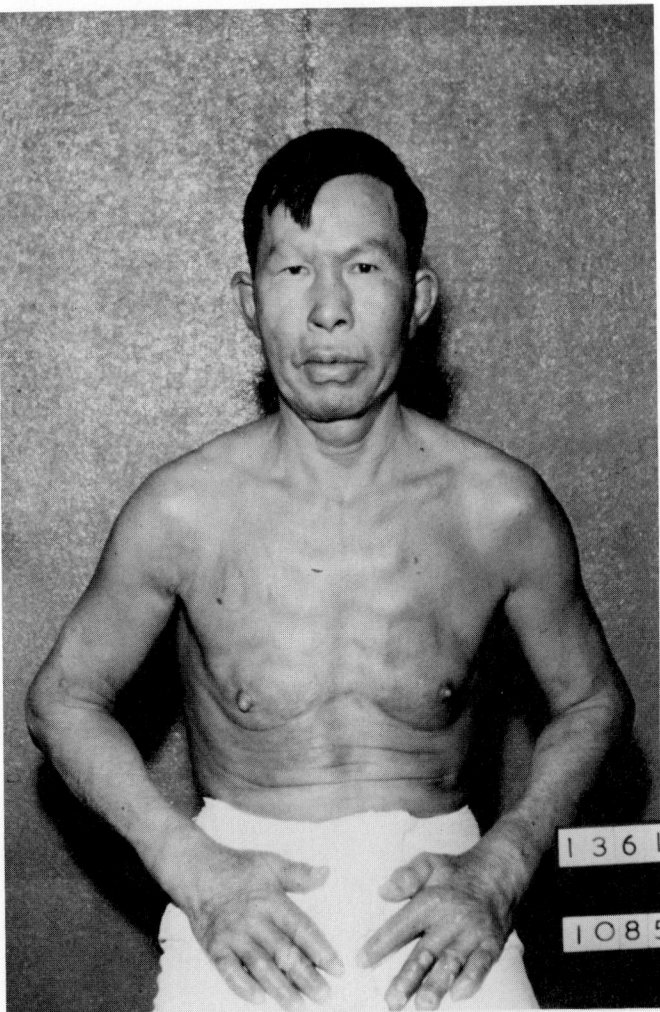

Fig. 1 Active, untreated lepromatous leprosy, showing generalized infiltration of the skin, swelling of fingers and lips, and thinning of eyebrows and eyelashes. The residual annular lesion visible in the left pectoral region indicates that this patient has 'downgraded' from borderline.

Many lepromatous cases originate as borderline, and in these 'sub-polar lepromatous' (LLs) patients, a small number of residual BB-type or more rarely BT-type lesions with central anaesthesia may be found, with associated increased enlargement of the neighbouring nerve or predilection. In Central America, some lepromatous patients develop diffuse infiltrate with no nodules, plaques, or papules (primary diffuse lepromatous leprosy). Should an LL patient relapse, whether from failure to take treatment or from developing drug resistance, his new lesions are initially usually asymmetrical; in addition, they are often more rounded and more discrete from the surrounding skin than typical lepromatous papules and nodules and such relapse lesions are described as 'histoid'.

Histologically, the dermis is massively and diffusely infiltrated with foamy histiocytes full of leprosy bacilli and globi-containing Virchow giant cells. In contrast, bacilli are only rarely found either in the epidermis, which is thinned with flattening of the rete ridges, or in the 'clear zone' immediately below the epidermis. In polar lepromatous (LLp) leprosy, which has not been down-graded from borderline, lymphocytes are very scanty, and nerves appear near-normal in the infiltrate apart from the bacilli within them. In LLs patients, small numbers of lymphocytes and plasma cells are scattered in the lepromatous infiltrate and cutaneous nerves may show lamination of the perineurium. Untreated lepromatous patients suffer from bacteraemia and bacilli are present often in large numbers in the reticulo-endothelial system especially in the spleen, the Kupffer cells of the liver, and the lymph nodes, especially those draining the skin. These are frequently enlarged with hypertrophy of the germinal centres, numerous plasma cells at the cortico-medullary junction, and almost complete replacement of the paracortical area with histiocytes laden with acid-fast bacilli. Bacilli are also present in the testes in large numbers, although they are scanty in the kidneys, and the central nervous system, heart, and lungs appear to be unaffected.

Reactions. The active multiplication and spread of *M. leprae* clinically causes no more than a mild erythema of skin lesions. Nevertheless, episodes of acute or chronic inflammation, known as 'reactions', may occur in any type of leprosy except indeterminate. The majority of reactions occur in patients receiving effective chemotherapy, and there is evidence that they are immunologically-mediated. Unless they are adequately treated, they may result in crippling deformity. Although terminology has not yet been standardized, nearly all reactions can be classified into two main groups.

Non-lepromatous lepra reactions (reversal reactions). These occur very frequently in treated BT, BB, and BL, and more rarely in LLs leprosy, the reactions commencing within a few weeks of the start of treatment in BT but usually only after several months of treatment in BL and LLs patients. They may also occur in untreated BT patients. Over the course of a few days or weeks, the leprous lesions themselves become markedly swollen, erythematous and often scaly, new skin lesions may appear, and the hands and feet and sometimes the face may become oedematous. The viable skin lesions may ulcerate, leading to unsightly scarring. Painful neuritis may develop in one or more nerves of predilection, especially in those already enlarged, and may rapidly result in (further) functional nerve damage. The reaction usually lasts for several months before gradually fading. By then, many but by no means all patients are found to have changed in classification towards tuberculoid. The histological picture is variable, but usually shows oedema, proliferation of fibroblasts, and the presence of giant cells of the foreign body type. In those patients who become more tuberculoid, an increase in the numbers of lymphocytes eventually occurs.

Clinically similar reactions may very rarely occur in untreated or ineffectually treated (for example, as the result of the development of drug resistance) BT, BB, or BL patients which, when they subside, lead to a change of classification towards lepromatous. Such reactions are known as 'downgrading reactions'.

Erythema nodosum leprosum (ENL); lepromatous lepra reaction. ENL occurs only at the lepromatous end of the leprosy spectrum, more than 50 per cent of treated LL patients and the occasional untreated LL or treated BL suffering from one or more episodes of this type of reaction. Over the course of a few hours, a crop of painful erythematous papules develops, typically on the extensor surfaces of the limbs, but in severe attacks over much of the body except the scalp. In BL patients, most papules erupt in juicy plaques or nodules in which the concentration of leprosy bacilli is highest. The papules become more purple over two or three days and then gradually subside, leaving dark staining of the skin. The episodes are usually associated with general malaise and with high afternoon fever, the temperature on waking being sub-normal, and sometimes with bone pain. They may be of all degrees of severity, in some patients being isolated and almost unnoticed and in others occurring continuously over months or years, leading, if untreated, to gross prostration, weakness, and occasionally death. In severe ENL, the papules may form sterile pustules and ulcers. Other systems may also be involved; the most frequent complication is painful neuritis, usually of the ulnar, median, or lateral popliteal nerves, which may result in increasing muscle weakness and anaesthesia of appropriate distribution, but acute lymphadenitis, iridocyclitis, and epididymoorhitis may also occur, and more rarely, nephritis and large joint arthritis. Episodes of ENL usually commence a few months after the start of effective treatment and are sometimes precipitated by intercurrent infection or by physical or mental stress. Histologically, ENL resembles the Arthus phenomenon, with vasculitis and polymorphonuclear infiltrate on a background of resolving lepromatous granuloma with fragmented leprosy bacilli.

The Lucio reaction. Untreated Central American patients suffering from diffuse lepromatous leprosy may develop irregularly-edged erythematous lesions of their skin, especially on the lower limbs, which scab and ulcerate, eventually healing with typical ragged scars. Histologically, there is vasculitis leading to small infarcts of the skin. Unlike ENL, the condition usually subsides once effective antileprosy treatment has been commenced.

Haematology and immunology. In LL and BL leprosy, mild normocytic normochromic anaemia may occur. This may become more marked in chronic ENL. During episodes of ENL, a polymorphonuclear leucocytosis is usually present.

Reversal of the albumen–globulin ratio occurs in many LL and some BL patients and IgG is almost always raised, although IgM and IgA are more variable. Such patients often give false positive tests for syphilis, and long-standing LL patients may also give positive tests for thyroglobulin antibodies, LE cells, antinuclear factor, and cryoglobulin.

In untreated LL and BL patients, there is gross specific depression of CMI for *M. leprae*, as evidenced by the negative specific LTT and lepromin tests, although the former may be a better measure of DTH rather than CMI. In addition, there is variable non-specific depression of CMI, which gradually improves with treatment. The depression of specific CMI very rarely alters in LL patients, almost all of whom remain lepromin negative after more than 20 years of therapy, and should they relapse at this stage, almost invariably relapse with lepromatous or histoid lesions; very few have been reported to relapse with BT or BB-type lesions and with weak positive lepromin tests. There is a relative and absolute depression in the number of circulating T lymphocytes in the blood of untreated LL patients, and suppressor cells have also been detected. What factor or factors initiate the gross depression of CMI in lepromatous leprosy remains uncertain, although Shepard has recently shown that the pre-priming of experimental mice with intravenous *M. leprae*, one week before the intradermal inoculation of *M. leprae*, prevented the subsequent development of specific sensitization. Early lepromatous leprosy was also obtained in a single experimental gibbon, whose infecting dose of *M. leprae*, given 15 years earlier, was administered largely, although not entirely, intravenously.

From LTT studies, reversal reactions are thought to be due to increase in DTH usually associated with increase in CMI. They may be produced experimentally in thymectomized-irradiated mice which have already developed lepromatous leprosy, by the administration of syngeneic lymphocytes. There is no experimental model for ENL. This type of reaction is believed to be due to immune complex formation; IgG and complement have been detected in acute ENL papules but methods for demonstrating mycobacterial antigen have not yet been satisfactory. It is thought that the antigen is derived from the cytoplasm of dead leprosy bacilli and the antibody from the markedly elevated serum immunoglobulin levels which occur in LL leprosy. Most of the manifestations of the ENL syndrome could be explained by the local formation of immune complexes, although the systemic manifestations (e.g. fever) and the glomerulonephritis are presumed to be due to circulating immune complexes. Intradermal immune complexes have been detected in the lesions of the Lucio reaction.

Diagnosis and differential diagnosis. The diagnosis of leprosy should always be considered in any patient with skin or peripheral nerve lesions who has resided in an endemic area. It should especially be suspected when skin or nasal symptoms persist despite routine treatment; in idiopathic foot drop; in unusual presentations of arthritis and erythema nodosum; in chronic plantar ulceration; and in painless burns or injuries to the hands and feet. The discovery of one or more of the following three findings is almost pathognomonic for spectrum leprosy: (*a*) anaesthetic skin lesions, which are present in almost all TT, BT, and BB patients, and in many BL and LLs patients; (*b*) the finding of thickening of one or more nerves, either of predilection or cutaneous sensory – nerve enlargement is found in some TT, many BT, and the great majority of BB, BL, and LL patients; and (*c*) the presence of acid-fast bacilli in skin smears which are positive in many BT and in all untreated BB, BL, and LL patients. Therefore skin lesions should be tested for anaesthesia, peripheral nerves systematically palpated for thickening, and skin smears taken from both ear lobes and up to four typical skin lesions. The diagnosis should be confirmed by biopsy of the skin, the whole depth of the dermis being included in the specimen. In pure neural leprosy, a thickened sensory nerve can be safely biopsied, e.g. the superficial radial at the wrist, the superficial perineal in front of the ankle or the great auricular in the neck. The diagnosis of indeterminate leprosy is especially difficult; biopsy examination may not be possible, especially if the single lesion is on the face, and sensory testing may be difficult to interpret in children. The finding of lack of sweating in the lesion is particularly helpful; alternatively, a histamine test may be performed as the flare is often impaired or absent in a leprosy macule, due to damage to the cutaneous sympathetic nerves.

Leprosy is the only common cause of peripheral nerve thickening and its finding will exclude almost all other neurological conditions; it may, however, occur in direct peripheral nerve injury, in which there will be an appropriate history and residual signs of trauma; primary systemic and, rarely, secondary amyloidosis, in which amyloid may be detected in an appropriate organ biopsy; and in familial progressive hypertrophic interstitial neuritis of Dejerine and Sottas, which can be differentiated from leprosy by the familial history and by the absence of skin lesions and of acid-fast bacilli. The anaesthesia of TT and BT leprosy differentiates tuberculoid lesions from vitiligo, mycotic skin infections, lupus erythematosis, and psoriasis as well as from lupus vulgaris and sarcoidosis, and histological examination of the two last conditions will reveal the presence of normal cutaneous nerves in the otherwise very similar granuloma. Certain conditions bear a superficial resemblance to lepromatous leprosy, including diffuse cutaneous leishmaniasis, secondary syphilis, neurofibromatosis, mycosis fungoides, and dermal deposits in Hodgkin's disease, but may be easily differentiated by the absence of nerve thickening and the failure to find acid-fast bacilli in skin smears.

Treatment. In leprosy, as much as in any other disease, it is necessary to treat the 'whole patient'. This is because of the strong sense of stigma still persisting needlessly in many cultures, the extreme chronicity of the infection and the liability to relapse after many years, the high incidence of reactions occurring in patients receiving correct chemotherapy, and the continuing possibility of damage to anaesthetic hands and feet even after the infection with *M. leprae* has been cured.

Treatment of the infection — chemotherapy. Effective chemotherapy with the sulphone drugs was introduced in 1943, and dapsone, slowly effective but cheap and usually non-toxic, has been the drug of choice since 1947. Since then for 30 years, monotherapy was recommended for, unlike tuberculosis, drug resistance was very slow to make its appearance. But relapse off treatment was quickly recognized and therefore the recommended duration of treatment became increasingly prolonged. Expert Committees of WHO ruled that paucillary (indeterminate, TT, and BT) leprosy should be treated until it became inactive and then for at least another 18 months, but although inactivity usually only took 3–18 months to achieve, few patients were released from therapy in under five years. In multibacillary (BB, BL, and LL) leprosy, it was recommended that treatment should be continued for at least 10 years after smear negativity had been achieved; therefore BB leprosy was usually treated for 12–13 years, BL around 15 years, and LL for 20 years or longer. But secondary dapsone resistance, first proven in 1964, has been found to be increasing steadily and probably exponentially in incidence in LL and BL patients. Therefore drugs known to be of value in the treatment of leprosy were carefully studied under experimental conditions and those found to be bactericidal for *M. leprae* on mouse footpad testing are listed in Table 1. Since 1976 it has been recommended that all newly diagnosed multibacillary patients should receive treatment with two or more drugs. Moreover, the increasing incidence of primary dapsone resistance, which can occur in any type of leprosy, detected over the last five years has also caused serious concern and the WHO Study Group on Chemotherapy of Leprosy for Control Programmes (1982) has now recommended that all leprosy patients should receive multi-drug therapy. In addition, poor compliance among patients receiving monotherapy together with the high rate of failure to complete the recommended course of treatment has directed attention to the possibility of multi-drug therapy of limited duration which should improve cost effectiveness as well as lessen the burden on patients and leprosy control schemes.

Table 1 Minimum inhibitory concentrations against *M. leprae* (MIC), peak serum concentrations, durations of coverage, and bactericidal activities of antileprosy drugs (adapted from: Ellard, G. A., 1980, *Leprosy Review* **51**, 200).

Drug	Human dosage (mg)	MIC in mice (ng/ml)	Ratio PSC/MIC*	Duration which serum concentrations exceed MIC (days)†	Bactericidal activity‡
Rifampicin	600	300	30	1	+++
Dapsone	100	3	500	10	+
Ethionamide	375	50	60	1	++§
Prothionamide	375	50	40	1	++§
Clofazimine‖	100	?	?	?	+

* Ratio of PSC (peak serum concentration) in man after a single dose to MIC determined in the mouse
† Serum concentrations in man after a single dose
‡ Relative degrees of bactericidal activity (+, ++, +++)
§ Not yet assessed clinically in this dosage
‖ Because clofazimine is deposited in cells, the significance of serum concentrations is uncertain

Dapsone (4–4′ diaminodiphenyl sulphone). This drug is as cheap as aspirin and may be administered by mouth or parenterally. Clinical improvement is detected from about three months after starting dapsone in LL and BL patients (often earlier in TT, BT, and BB leprosy), and from around this time bacilli from nose and skin will no longer infect normal mice; the MI reaches zero by six

months, although the BI takes many years to become smear negative. Small numbers of viable, presumed physiologically dormant, bacilli have been detected persisting in a number of tissue sites in LL patients treated continuously for at least 10 years, and it is thought that these 'persisters' could cause a patient to relapse if treatment is stopped. The relapse rate, however, among 362 LL and BL patients treated for around 20 years with supervised dapsone therapy only totalled 8.8 per cent (1 per cent per annum) for the succeeding nine years off treatment.

The recommended standard adult dose is 100 mg a day (6–10 mg/kg body weight per week) by mouth. This dosage gives a peak blood level about 500 times the serum minimal inhibitory concentration (MIC) which explains why drug resistance was seldom seen in the early days of dapsone chemotherapy. Dapsone resistance, which develops in a step-wise manner, has been detected 2–33 years after the start of treatment, sometimes long after the patient has become smear negative. New active usually asymmetrical lesions, typically histoid or else papules and small plaques with high BI and MI, are found on a background of resolving or resolved lepromatous leprosy. Bacilli from the relapse lesions will grow in the footpads of mice treated with dapsone mixed in their diet. Low dosage dapsone and irregular treatment predispose to the development of secondary dapsone resistance. Estimates of its prevalence in various countries and areas range between 2 and 24 per cent; in West Malaysia it has risen from 0.2 per cent in 1966 to 10 per cent of all registered LL and BL patients in 1981. Proven primary dapsone resistance has already been reported from six countries.

The important toxic side-effect of dapsone is drug allergy, which may occur in one of several hundred patients. Three to seven weeks after commencing dapsone, the patient develops fever, pruritis, and dermatitis, and sometimes also jaundice and psychosis; the dapsone must be stopped immediately and prednisolone given for several weeks. Other rare side-effects include dose-related sulphaemoglobinaemia and haemolytic anaemia.

Rifampicin is so rapidly bactericidal that a single dose of 600–1200 mg renders an LL patient a minimal public health risk within a few days, bacilli obtained from the skin or from nasal secretions four days after the dose failing to multiply in the footpads of normal mice.

Clinical improvement commences within 7–14 days after starting rifampicin and the MI falls to zero within six weeks. Nevertheless, the BI falls no faster than with dapsone and persisting viable bacilli have been detected after five years of treatment in the dosage of 600 mg daily. The recommended dosage is 10–15 mg/kg body weight, that is 600 mg to those weighing 40 kg or over, preferably given on an empty stomach. Rifampicin may be given daily or, because of the prolonged generation time of *M. leprae*, monthly; indeed monthly rifampicin (600 mg given on two consecutive days every four weeks) has been used safely since 1973 and has proved as effective as daily dosage. Under field conditions, monthly rifampicin is not only much cheaper but also easier to supervise than daily rifampicin; weekly rifampicin is not recommended because of the high incidence of toxic side-effects which have been reported in tuberculosis patients. A single dose of 600 mg gives a peak blood level about 30 times the MIC. As rifampicin resistance has already been reported in lepromatous leprosy, rifampicin should always be used in combination with at least one other effective antileprosy drug. Rifampicin is a potent microsomal enzyme inducer when given daily, and its possible effect on the metabolism of other drugs given concurrently should always be remembered.

Clofazimine is a rimino-phenazine dye which is fat soluble and deposited in fat and other cells; therefore its MIC cannot be measured, although the minimum effective dose preventing multiplication of *M. leprae* in mice is very low, of the order of 0.0001 per cent in the diet. In the dosage of 100–200 mg daily it kills leprosy bacilli at about the same speed as dapsone. Various intermittent dosages, from 100 mg three times a week to 600 mg on two consecutive days every four weeks are also effective but give a slightly slower rate of kill. In high dosage, the drug is also anti-inflammatory, and it has been widely used in dark-skinned races in a dose of 100 mg three times a day to control ENL reactions, though several weeks elapse before its full anti-inflammatory effect is produced; as prolonged high dosage may cause serious diarrhoea, the dose should be reduced after three to six months. In the dose of 100 mg daily, the drug is relatively non-toxic, its chief disadvantage being that it causes a reddish-brown pigmentation of the skin which is objectionable to most light-skinned patients. Clofazimine resistance has not yet been reported. Capsules containing 50 mg clofazimine have recently been marketed.

Ethionamide and prothionamide are interchangeable and give cross resistance with each other and also with the bacteriostatic drug thiacetazone. Ethionamide probably kills *M. leprae* at least as fast as dapsone although certainly more slowly than rifampicin, but has been studied in only a very few lepromatous patients. The standard dosage of 500 mg daily gives about a 10 per cent incidence of dose-related gastric intolerance and nausea and a few cases of jaundice have also been observed. A dose of 375 mg ethionamide gives a peak blood concentration about 60 times, and of prothionamide about 40 times, the MIC. Resistance to ethionamide has been reported after five to eight years of monotherapy. Prothionamide has been more widely used in the dosage of 350 mg daily but only in combined chemotherapy. Ethionamide, or prothionamide, remains the only alternative to clofazimine in those patients requiring triple drug therapy who will not accept clofazimine pigmentation.

Recommended regimens. *Multibacillary leprosy.* Three groups of patients have to be considered, namely, those newly diagnosed with active untreated leprosy who may or may not be suffering from primary dapsone resistance, those who have undergone active relapse either from failure to take treatment with the resulting multiplication of persisters or because of the emergence of secondary dapsone resistance, and those who appear to be responding normally to treatment but who could well relapse in the future from the development of dapsone resistance. Therefore the chemotherapeutic aims are to prevent the emergence of secondary dapsone resistance, both in the newly diagnosed patients and in those now under apparently successful treatment with dapsone monotherapy; to prevent the emergence of secondary resistance to any other antileprosy drug used in each regimen, especially rifampicin; to treat effectively and immediately any patients who have relapsed suffering from secondary dapsone resistance; and to treat effectively all newly diagnosed patients whether or not they are suffering from primary dapsone resistance. Therefore it is essential to give a minimum of three drugs, assuming one of the three is dapsone, so as to prevent the emergence of resistance to a second drug should dapsone resistance, whether primary or secondary, be present.

As mouse footpad diagnosis of dapsone resistance is only available in a limited number of centres, and takes 6–12 months to complete, the WHO Study Group (1982) designed a single regimen to cover all types of multibacillary patients. It is equally effective in both treated and untreated and in dapsone sensitive and dapsone resistant patients. This regimen is designed for maximum supervision of the more expensive drugs, particularly rifampicin. The regimen consists of:

1. Rifampicin 600 mg once monthly (or every four weeks) supervised.
2. Clofazimine 50 mg daily, unsupervised, plus 300 mg (supervised) every month or four weeks.
3. Dapsone 100 mg daily, unsupervised.

The WHO regimen was designed for field conditions. Where more complete supervision is possible or when compliance is known to be good, it may be preferred to double the dose of rifampicin, the patient being given 600 mg on two consecutive days each month or every four weeks. Under these conditions, the supervised 300 mg dose of clofazimine may be omitted.

Although this regimen has been recommended for all three main groups of patients already enumerated, its duration depends upon the individual patient's group and leprosy classification. It is recom-

mended that the regimen should always be given for a minimum period of two years, and that it should be continued until a patient reaches smear negativity. Therefore untreated LL patients may receive 8–10 years' triple-drug treatment before all therapy is stopped when smear negativity is achieved, whereas, for example, smear negative patients treated hitherto with dapsone monotherapy would receive two years' treatment. Relapse rates after stopping triple-drug therapy are as yet unknown, but are unlikely to be unacceptable and those patients who do relapse are likely to relapse with drug-sensitive bacilli.

Patients who find clofazimine completely unacceptable, should be given 250–375 mg self-administered daily doses of ethionamide or prothionamide.

Paucibacillary leprosy. It is important to treat effectively, in the shortest possible time, all tuberculoid and indeterminate patients, whether suffering from dapsone-sensitive or from primary dapsone-resistant leprosy, even though the latter could only normally be diagnosed by failure to improve after a period of treatment with dapsone monotherapy. Short-course chemotherapy with rifampicin (either eight weekly doses of 900 mg or 14–21 daily doses of 600 mg) appears to provide fully effective treatment in tuberculoid leprosy on a two to three year follow-up. Therefore short-course rifampicin therapy in paucibacillary leprosy is both practical and acceptable. The recommended regimen (WHO 1982) consists of rifampicin, 600 mg monthly for six doses, each dose being carefully supervised, plus dapsone 100 mg daily unsupervised for six months. Subsequent relapse rates off treatment, which are likely to be very low, should be carefully noted and reported. In those tuberculoid patients receiving steriod therapy for reversal reactions beyond six months after commencing treatment, it is recommended that dapsone therapy should be continued until steroid therapy is stopped. Because the bacterial load is usually so tiny in paucibacillary leprosy, resistance to rifampicin is unlikely to develop should the patient be suffering from primary dapsone resistance. When a brief interruption in treatment occurs, the patient should continue his course where he left off; when the interruption is prolonged (say, more than six months), then the patient should recommence a full six months' course. Should a patient be unable to come every month for his supervised dose of rifampicin, then either the rifampicin may be given unsupervised or it should be given whenever the patient is able to attend, at intervals of not less than one month, until six doses have been given, sufficient unsupervised dapsone being provided to cover the whole period of treatment.

Treatment of reactions. It is essential to continue the course of antileprosy chemotherapy unchanged in patients suffering from reactions.

ENL. The symptoms of mild ENL may usually be controlled with paracetamol or soluble aspirin, supported when necessary by a course of stibophen, 2 ml daily parenterally for five days. The treatment of severe ENL is best commenced in hospital. ENL is graded severe if there is high fever and severe general malaise, or if moderate fever lasts more than four weeks; if the papules become pustular and/or ulcerate, or if they coalesce; if there is lymphadenitis; if the nerves become painful or if there is any loss of nerve function; or if there is iridocyclitis, orchitis, or arthritis; or if urine examinations reveal persistent albuminuria with red cells present on microscopy. There are three alternative regimens. Prednisolone usually rapidly suppresses ENL in an initial dose of 30–40 mg daily which can often subsequently be lowered. But not infrequently steroid therapy proves to be prolonged, and severe steroid toxicity may occur. Therefore steroids are best reserved for short courses to control episodic ENL, or for short-term cover for operations, childbirth, and similar situations. The drug thalidomide is equally effective in controlling ENL and in general is safer than steroids, but its use is contraindicated in women of child-bearing age because of its teratogenic properties. Nevertheless, it is the drug of choice in males and post-menopausal females. The initial dosage is 200 mg twice daily; subsequently it is progressively lowered to a maintenance dose, usually of 50–100 mg nightly, which may be continued for years. Thalidomide peripheral neuropathy has not yet been reported in ENL patients although regular neurological checks are indicated in those receiving long-term therapy. The third alternative is clofazimine 300 mg daily for an initial period of three to six months and subsequently the dosage is progressively lowered. Clofazimine is the safest drug for pre-menopausal women, but it does not appear to be so powerful as thalidomide or prednisolone and it takes four to six weeks to achieve its full ENL-suppressive action; therefore if a very rapid action is required, it may need to be combined initially with prednisolone. In iridocyclitis, local treatment with steroid and homatropine eye drops is also recommended.

Reversal reactions. Mild reactions can usually be controlled with paracetamol or soluble aspirin, with or without stibophen. In severe reactions, the signs of inflammation should be suppressed with prednisolone. Reactions are graded severe if there is marked fever and malaise; if there is oedema of the hands and feet; if the skin lesions ulcerate; or if there is nerve pain and tenderness or loss of nerve function. The initial dose of prednisolone required is usually 30–40 mg daily; this may be reduced during the subsequent three to four weeks but maintenance therapy with dosage of the order of 15–20 mg daily may be required for several months before the prednisolone can be finally tailed off and stopped. An acutely painful nerve should be rested by splinting of the appropriate limb. Serial voluntary muscle and sensory nerve tests are often of help in assessing whether successful control of neuritis has been achieved.

Ancillary treatment. It is essential to educate patients to protect their anaesthetic limbs which they should inspect daily for injuries and secondary infection. Callosities over pressure points should be regularly softened by soaking in water, and trimmed. Well fitting shoes with microcellular rubber insoles help to prevent plantar ulceration. A plantar ulcer requires rest or the application of a below-knee walking-plaster splint. Injured or infected anaesthetic hands may also require splinting to prevent the patient from using his injured, but pain-free limb. Patients suffering from lagophthalmos or paralysis of hands or feet require physiotherapy and may be helped by reconstructive surgery. Facial deformity may be improved by plastic surgery.

Prognosis. Before the advent of specific chemotherapy, LL patients used to die from intercurrent infection, laryngeal obstruction, or amyloid nephritis, and blindness was common. Some BT and most BB and BL patients, tended to lose CMI so that their disease became more lepromatous. Patients with TT leprosy, however, and about three-quarters of those with indeterminate leprosy, eventually cured themselves. With early diagnosis and correct treatment, the prognosis is now excellent. Death from LL leprosy is rare, although secondary amyloidosis still occasionally occurs, especially in inadequately-treated ENL. Widespread nerve damage may still develop in BT and BB patients, either if diagnosis is delayed, or if reversal reactions are inadequately treated. Patients who fail to care for anaesthetic limbs may develop increasing deformity and amputation may become necessary for chronic osteomyelitis. Iridocyclitis may cause impairment of vision or blindness and cataract is common in LL patients.

Prophylaxis. The strategy of leprosy control still rests on early case finding and treatment of infectious LL and BL patients. Prophylactic dapsone is seldom justified. Vaccination of young children with BCG may be of some slight value in protecting against early leprosy. A vaccine consisting of irradiated-killed *M. leprae* derived from armadillos combined with live BCG has been developed by the IMMLEP (Immunology of Leprosy) Committee of WHO. This vaccine is able to protect animals against infection with leprosy, but its evaluation in human populations will take at least a decade.

References

Ellard, G. A. (1981). Editorial: Drug compliance in the treatment of leprosy. *Leprosy Rev.* **52**, 201.
Kirchheimer, W. F. and Storrs, E. H. (1971). Attempts to establish the armadillo (*Dasypus novemcinctus* Linn.) as a model for the study of leprosy. *Int. J. Leprosy* **39**, 693.
Rees, R. J. W., Waters, M. F. R., Weddell, A. G. M., and Palmer, E. (1967). Experimental lepromatous leprosy. *Nature, Lond.* **215**, 599.
Ridley, D. S. and Jopling, W. H. (1966). Classification of leprosy according to immunity: A five-group system. *Int. J. Leprosy* **34**, 255.
Shepard, C. C. (1960). The experimental disease that follows the injection of human leprosy bacilli into foot pads of mice. *J. exp. Med.* **122**, 445.
— (1981). A brief review of experiences with short-term clinical trials monitored by mouse-foot-pad inoculation. *Leprosy Rev.* **52**, 299.
Waters, M. F. R., Rees, R. J. W., Pearson, J. M. H., Laing, A. B. G., Helmy, H. S., and Gelber, R. H. (1978). Rifampicin for lepromatous leprosy: nine years' experience. *Br. med. J.* **i**, 133.
WHO Expert Committee on Leprosy (1977). Fifth Report. *Wld Hlth Org. Tech. Rep. Ser.* no. 607.
WHO Study Group on chemotherapy of leprosy for control programmes (1982). *Wld Hlth Org. Tech. Rep. Ser.* (in press).

Mycobacterium ulcerans infection

M. F. R. Waters

Synonyms. Bairnsdale ulcer, Buruli ulcer.
Definition. A skin disease, caused by *Mycobacterium ulcerans*, which usually commences as an indurated nodule which breaks down to form a chronic expanding ulcer with a necrotic base and a deeply undermined edge; the lesion may heal spontaneously, often with extensive scarring.

Aetiology. *M. ulcerans*, first described by MacCallum and his colleagues in 1948, is a rod-shaped acid-fast bacillus, 2–6 μm long and 0.2–0.35 μm in width, with rounded ends and parallel sides, which occurs singly and in groups in the necrotic base and undermined edge of the ulcer (not in the growing outer edge of the lesion). Many bacilli are extracellular, some are intracellular in macrophages. *M. ulcerans* grows best at 33 °C. On primary isolation, usually rather poor growth occurs at 30 °C or 33 °C, and none at 37 °C, on solid media such as Löwenstein-Jensen's and Petragnani's. Growth usually improves on passage when the cream or pale yellow colonies take three to four weeks to appear, the generation time being about 24 hours. Primary isolation is sometimes more easily achieved by the inoculation of infected material into the hind feet of mice. After four to six weeks the footpads swell and may ulcerate; at 8 to 10 weeks some mice develop a spreading, generalized oedema, which suggests that an exotoxin may be secreted. On intravenous inoculation of *M. ulcerans* in mice, lesions develop on the cold extremities, namely, the nose, tail, ears, feet, and scrotum.

In vitro, *M. ulcerans* is able to degrade hydroxyproline. It is usually sensitive to streptomycin, and often to rifampicin and clofazimine, but resistant to isoniazid, thiacetazone, and PAS.

Immunodiffusion studies reveal at least 12 antigenic compounds, of which five are species specific.

An extract of sonicated *M. ulcerans*, standardized for protein content, known as 'Burulin' is used for a specific skin test; it is positive in patients during the reactive phase of the infection.

Epidemiology. Although first identified in Bairnsdale, Victoria, Australia, most known centres of *M. ulcerans* infection are in tropical rural areas near rivers, including the Congo in Zaire, the Buruli district (upper Nile and Lake Kyoga) in Uganda, the river Nyong in the Cameroons, the Kumusi river in Papua New Guinea, and near lowland swamp jungle in Malaysia. One case has been reported from Mexico.

The incidence is usually higher in children than in adults, and in some areas women are more affected than men; tuberculin negative individuals may be more liable to the disease than tuberculin positive reactors.

The method of transmission is unknown, although it is assumed that the infection is introduced through a skin abrasion or by an insect bite. No reservoir or vector has been detected, nor has *M. ulcerans* as yet been isolated from the environment. Subclinical infections are thought to occur.

Pathology. In early, non-ulcerated lesions, there is a vague-edged, indurated, opaque area of necrotic fat with no functional capillaries, situated in the lower dermis and subcutaneous adipose tissue. Microscopically, the faint outline of the dead fat cells may be made out in some places, swollen, lacking in nuclei, and separated from each other by amorphous eosinophilic material. Inflammatory cells are not conspicuous and, at the junction of the viable and necrotic tissue, there is also a lack of any significant vascular or inflammatory cell response, although a few macrophages, lymphocytes, and plasma cells may be present. Colonies, clumps, and individual *M. ulcerans* are found concentrated in the centre of the necrotic zone, in which scattered calcification may occur. As the area of non-inflammatory necrosis expands, the corium is undermined and ulcerates, and secondary infection may develop. In self-healing ulcers, the induration eventually softens, the necrotic tissue separates, non-caseating epithelioid granulomata are laid down, and acid-fast organisms become very scanty, and are usually intracellular.

Clinical features. After an incubation period probably of 3–12 weeks, a painless, small, well-demarcated, indurated subcutaneous swelling develops, attached to the skin but not to the deep tissues. The lesion is almost always single, and most occur on the limbs, often near joints, although the site is more variable in young children. There is little or no systemic upset or fever, and the regional lymph node is not enlarged. In most cases, the lesion increases steadily in size, the overlying skin desquamating and becoming hyperpigmented before eventually ulcerating at the centre (Fig. 1). The ulcer edge is characteristically overhanging, and may be undermined to a distance of 5–15 cm. Satellite ulcers or lesions may also appear, but metastatic spread is rare. Once ulceration has occurred, secondary pyogenic infection may take place, and a foul-smelling slough forms. Some lesions remain unchanged for months; others grow rapidly in size, within a few weeks covering much of a limb or the trunk. Even so, there is little pain or tenderness or, save for slight fever, evidence of systemic upset. In the absence of treatment, healing slowly occurs, resulting in widespread scarring and often contractures and deformities.

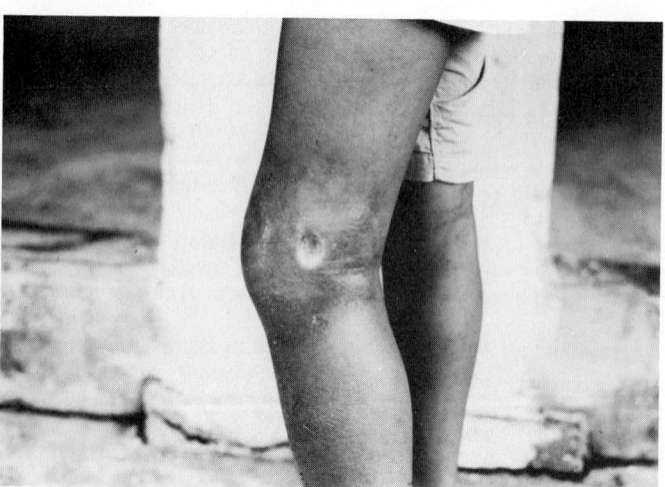

Fig. 1 *Mycobacterium ulcerans* ulceration of the knee, showing the necrotic sloughing ulcer base and the indurated, desquamating, undermined surrounding skin. (Patient of Dr A. B. G. Laing and Dr A. H. Smelt.)

The diagnosis is suggested by the characteristic appearance of the swelling and ulcer, the absence of pain or of lymph-node enlargement, and the failure to respond to standard tropical ulcer therapy. It is confirmed by the finding of acid-fast bacilli in the necrotic ulcer base, the isolation of *M. ulcerans* in culture at 33 °C or in mice, and by the histological appearance of the lesion.

The differential diagnosis at the pre-ulceration stage includes boils, foreign-body granuloma, infected sebaceous cyst, low-grade fibrosarcoma, and tumours of the skin appendages; at the ulcerating stage, tropical, mycotic, parasitic, and malignant ulcers and yaws.

Treatment. Treatment with antibiotics such as streptomycin, clofazimine, or rifampicin, to which sensitivity of the strain of *M. ulcerans* has been confirmed, has little healing effect by itself although it is usually given to cover surgery. Early nodular lesions should be totally excised, followed, if possible, by primary closure of the incision. In ulcerated lesions, all diseased tissue is best excised, followed by skin grafting; all dead tissue must be removed, otherwise grafting will fail with delayed healing and increased scarring. Before surgery, secondary pyogenic infection should be controlled with antibiotics, and the ulcer irrigated with saline. The value of the application of local heat is being investigated.

Prognosis. The severity of resulting scarring is greatly improved by early diagnosis and adequate surgical treatment.

Prevention. In areas of high risk, health education should lead to early presentation and diagnosis; BCG vaccination of children may afford some protection.

References

Connor, D. H. and Lunn, H. F. (1965). *Mycobacterium ulcerans* infection (with comments on pathogenesis). *Int. J. Leprosy*, **33**, 698.

MacCallum, P., Tolhurst, J. C., Buckle, G., and Sissons, H. A. (1948). A new mycobacterial infection in man. *J. Path. Bact.* **60**, 93.

Ravisse, P. (1977). Skin ulcer due to *Mycobacterium ulcerans* in Cameroun. I. A clinical, epidemiological and histological study. *Bull. Soc. Path. exot.* **70**, 109.

Actinomycosis

R. G. Mitchell

The actinomycetes are members of the order Actinomycetales. They are filamentous, branching, Gram-positive bacteria which grow in the form of a mycelial network resembling that of filamentous fungi; indeed both groups of organisms may cause very similar infections such as mycetomas (see page 5.374). However, actinomycetes differ from fungi in their cell wall composition, notably in the lack of chitin, and their filaments or hyphae exceed 1μm in diameter, tending to fragment into bacillary forms of subculture. They are susceptible to several antibacterial agents but not to the usual antifungal drugs. The two genera of actinomycetes which cause infections in man are *Nocardia* and *Actinomyces*. Another genus, *Streptomyces*, includes several species which produce antibiotics of medical importance.

Actinomycosis is an infection caused by anaerobic or microaerophilic actinomycetes, principally *Actinomyces israelii*, occasionally *A. naeslundii* and other species. *A. bovis*, the cause of actinomycosis in cattle, does not appear to cause human disease. *A. israelii* typically occurs as a filamentous, branching, Gram-positive, non-acid-fast organism which readily fragments in tissues and in culture into short bacillary or diphtheroid forms. In tissues, compact mycelial growth results in the formation of characteristic colonies of 'ray fungus' in which a filamentous network is arranged around an amorphous centre and acquires a fringe of radially arranged 'clubs'.

Habitat. *A. israelii* is worldwide in its distribution. It is a commensal of the human oropharynx, and is found in the periodontal flora, usually in association with dental caries, and in the tonsillar crypts. 'Silent' colonies are sometimes found in routine sections of tonsils.

General description. Actinomycosis is an endogenous infection and case-to-case transmission is only likely to occur through human bites or bare knuckle injuries by opponents' teeth. It is a subacute or chronic granulomatous disease which progresses to fibrosis and suppuration with the formation of external sinuses. Compact bodies containing mycelium may be extruded from the sinuses as pale buff 'sulphur granules'. *A. israelii* is frequently associated with other organisms, such as *Actinobacillus actinomycetemcomitans*, bacteroides, and *Streptococcus milleri*, which may behave as synergistic pathogens. The disease is commoner in males, and in the young, and the somewhat higher incidence in country dwellers is usually attributed to traumatization of gums by straw-chewing.

Clinical entities. Cervicofacial, thoracic, and abdominal forms of the disease formerly made up 95 per cent of cases of actinomycosis; currently pelvic actinomycosis is probably the commonest form of the disease.

Cervicofacial actinomycosis (lumpy jaw) is associated with dental caries and usually follows dental extraction or some other form of local trauma. Presumably the resulting necrosis forms a nidus for anaerobic multiplication of the organism as a prelude to invasion. Within a few days a painful intra-oral swelling forms at the site of trauma; this slowly expands to present as a firm external lump over the angle of the jaw, cheek, or submandibular region, often with surrounding inflammation and oedema. Suppuration and sinus formation follow, and the mandible, salivary glands and other adjacent structures may be eroded or destroyed.

Abdominal actinomycosis is usually acquired by ingestion of the organism which penetrates the gut wall at a site where it is diseased or traumatized. Thus, actinomycosis may follow appendicitis, drainage of an appendix abscess, elective appendicectomy, gastroectomy, and other bowel operations, or external trauma to the abdominal wall. Inflammatory masses are formed inside the abdomen which may involve mesentery, gut wall, or other viscera. Most commonly the disease develops in the ileocaecal region, causing discomfort or pain in the right iliac fossa. The resulting mass may simulate an appendix abscess, ileocaecal tuberculosis, Crohn's disease, neoplasm, or mesenteric lymphadenitis. Complications include the formation of external sinuses and faecal fistulae, intestinal obstruction, and extension to other viscera. Occasionally *A. israelii* is isolated from anorectal abscesses.

Hepatic actinomycosis may account for up to 15 per cent of cases of actinomycosis. It can be primary, or secondary to pre-existing abdominal disease, the organism reaching the liver via the portal venous circulation. Alternatively the liver may be involved by direct extension of adjacent disease, or very rarely bacteraemic spread may occur via the hepatic artery. Usually a solitary abscess is formed, resulting in a tender enlarged liver with fever and rigors, jaundice, elevated peripheral white count and ESR, and abnormal liver function tests. Sinus formation may occur in the upper abdomen. Less commonly, the liver may be extensively involved by infiltration, diffuse granulomata, or micro-abscesses.

The kidney may be involved either by local extension or by bacteraemic spread, resulting in pyonephrosis or perinephric abscess.

Pulmonary actinomycosis arises by aspiration of the organism into a previously damaged lung, or by infiltration through the oesophageal wall. Chest radiographs typically show a slowly expanding discoid lesion readily mistaken for neoplasm or tuberculosis, but the condition may present as an abscess cavity or diffuse pneumonitis. Symptoms include productive cough, haemoptysis, fever, and weight loss. Complications arise by extension: empyema, pericarditis, mediastinitis, chest wall sinuses, and rib erosion, and haematogenous spread of infection may follow.

Pelvic actinomycosis may arise by extension from an abdominal lesion but occurs most commonly in women fitted with plastic intra-uterine devices, notably the Dalkon shield, worn for several years. The pathology ranges from cervicitis and endometritis to salpingitis and tubovarian abscess. It is uncertain whether actinomyces is a normal resident of the genital tract or is sexually transmitted. Symptoms include vaginal discharge, 'spotting', or irregular menstrual bleeding, followed by low abdominal or pelvic discomfort or pain. Severe sepsis may be accompanied by anorexia, weight loss, vomiting, and fever. The signs are those of pelvic inflammatory disease, including uterine or adnexal tenderness.

Disseminated bacteraemic actinomycosis is rare and may involve any organ or system. It may be accompanied by generalized painful red nodules in the skin which become fluctuant.

Cerebral actinomycosis arises either from bacteraemia or by extension of lesions in the paranasal sinuses and middle ear. Solitary, multiloculated or multiple thick-walled abscesses develop, sometimes with basilar meningitis. Meningitis without abscess formation occurs very rarely.

Diagnosis. Purulent exudates should be carefully examined for sulphur granules which are identified by Gram stain. All pathological material submitted is examined for the presence of isolated Gram-positive filaments. These cannot be differentiated from other organisms such as nocardia on morphology alone, although it may be possible to identify *A. israelii* at this stage by specific immunofluorescence. Cultures are set up and incubated aerobically and anaerobically with additional CO_2 for a prolonged period.

In histological sections stained with haematoxylin and eosin, the bacterial filaments are stained by haematoxylin, and any peripheral 'clubs' are eosinophilic.

Gram stain of sputum smears may show aggregates of branching Gram-positive rods. Since these may be confused with oropharyngeal commensals, it is advisable to use more invasive techniques to secure an uncontaminated specimen such as transtracheal, broncheal, or even percutaneous lung aspiration.

Pelvic actinomycosis is most commonly diagnosed by the cytologist when examining cervical smears by Papamicolaou stain. Fluffy aggregates are seen which represent mycelium with other mixed organisms. They can be identified by PAS and Gram stain, and confirmed as actinomyces by fluorescent microscopy using specific antiserum. Attempts may be made to isolate the organism by anaerobic culture from such specimens as cervical biopsy tissue, endometrial curettings, pus from pelvic abscesses, adnexal tissue obtained at operation, and intra-uterine devices.

Hepatic actinomycosis is diagnosed by percutaneous liver biopsy or from swabs or biopsies taken at operation.

Blood culture may be indicated in disseminated disease.

Serology. Agglutination, haemagglutination, precipitin, and complement fixation tests are available, but are of little value in diagnosis.

Prognosis. This is favourable if the disease is treated early before serious extension or dissemination, although cicatrization may still lead to complications such as intestinal obstruction.

Treatment. The antibiotic of choice remains benzyl penicillin given in high dosage and continued for several weeks after clinical resolution. Alternatives in case of penicillin hypersensitivity include the cephalosporins, erythromycin, clindamycin, tetracycline, and isonicotinic hydrazide. Appropriate therapy for any associated organism should be given for a shorter period. Surgical drainage or excision should be carried out if indicated. Replacement of an intra-uterine device should not be attempted until the infection has been eradicated.

Actinomyces odontolyticus. This is a mouth commensal associated with dental caries. It forms small reddish colonies after prolonged anaerobic incubation. It has been isolated from subcutaneous and pulmonary abscesses, and in mixed culture from a brain abscess.

Actinomyces viscosus. This is present in the normal periodontal flora of older children and adults. Reported infections by this organism include cervicofacial abscesses, ulceration of the chest wall with osteomyelitis of the ribs, lobar pneumonia and empyema, and endocarditis associated with a dental apical abscess.

Investigation and treatment are as for *A. israelii*.

References

Baron, E. J., Angevine, J. M., and Sundstrom, W. (1979). Actinomycotic pulmonary abscess in an immunosuppressed patient. *Am. J. clin. Pathol.* **72**, 637.

Hutton, R. M. and Behrens, R. H. (1979). *Actinomyces adontolyticus* as a cause of brain abcess. *J. Infect.* **1**, 195.

Meade, III, R. H. (1980). Primary hepatic actinomycosis. *Gastroenterology.* **78**, 355.

Spence, M. R., Gupta, P. K., Frost, J. K., and King, T. M. (1978). Cytologic detection and clinical significance of *Actinomyces israelii* in women using intra-uterine contraceptive devices. *Am. J. Obstet. Gynaec.* **131**, 295.

Thadepalli, H. and Rao, B. (1979). *Actinomyces viscosus* infections of the chest in humans. *Am. Rev. resp. Dis.* **120**, 203.

Nocardiasis

R. G. Mitchell

Definition. Nocardiasis is a systemic infection caused by species of *Nocardia*, usually *N. asteroides* but rarely *N. brasiliensis* and *N. caviae*.

Nocardia is a Gram-positive, filamentous, branching bacterium which ramifies in tissues to form loose aggregates of narrow, irregularly staining interlacing hyphae, with a tendency to break up into shorter bacillary or diphtheroid forms. It is aerobic, moderately acid fast, and grows readily on ordinary culture media.

Habitat. *Nocardia* is a soil saprophyte present in decomposing vegetation and in the air. It is not a commensal of the oropharynx, but is acquired by inhalation, so that the lungs are usually the site of primary infection. Rarely the disease may be acquired by direct inoculation of the organism into the skin, as with mycetomas, or by ingestion. Infections are characterized by necrosis and abscess formation, with minimal surrounding granulation or fibrosis. Consequently there is a tendency for haematogenous spread, resulting in metastatic lesions in the brain as well as in other organs and in the skin. Sinus formation is uncommon in this disease. Although sulphur granules are not formed, pus is occasionally noted to be flecked with minute reddish or orange granules.

Predisposing factors. Strains of nocardia are heterogeneous and appear to differ in virulence. Nocardiasis affects males at least twice as commonly as females and usually occurs in the age range 20–50, the mean age being around 45. It may affect subjects who were in previous good health, but more commonly occurs as an opportunistic infection in patients with impaired immune defence mechanisms, including defects of cell-mediated immunity, leucocyte function, and immunoglobulin production. The following disorders may be associated with nocardiasis:

1. Malignancies, including cancer, leukaemia, and the reticuloses
2. Auto-immune disease; collagen diseases, notably SLE
3. Hypogammaglobulinaemia, dysproteinaemia, intestinal lipodystrophy, and chronic granulomatous disease
4. Pre-existing pulmonary disease
5. Treatment with steroids and cytotoxic drugs; organ transplantation.

Clearly in many patients, multiple predisposing factors may operate.

Clinical features. Mycetoma caused by *Nocardia* spp. is described elsewhere (see page 5.374). Pulmonary infections are recognized in at least 75 per cent of cases of nocardiasis. Symptoms are variable, as is fever and leucocytosis, but cough with tenacious purulent sputum is usually present, and the clinical features are usually those of a lung abscess. The course of the disease may be acute and fulminating or chronic. Chest radiograph appearances are non-specific and include segmental or lobar infiltrations, widespread bronchopneumonia, nodular lesions, abscess cavities, or miliary lesions, usually without hilar lymphadenopathy or calcification. The infection may spread locally to involve the pleura, with resulting empyema, or the pericardium, or may invade the chest wall, ribs, and dorsal vertebrae and diaphragm. Occasionally *N. asteroides* is isolated from the sputum of patients who are not considered to have nocardiasis. Further, it is claimed that a mild form of nocardia pneumonitis may occur with fever, minimal respiratory symptoms without signs, and positive sputum cultures, the illness resolving spontaneously without chemotherapy. Conversely, sputum cultures are sometimes negative in patients with pulmonary lesions and established nocardiasis.

Disseminated nocardiasis. Haematogenous spread is common, particularly following overt pulmonary disease. The brain is the site of metastasis in about 25 per cent of cases. In this respect nocardiasis resembles bronchial carcinoma with which it may indeed be associated, and nocardia brain abscesses may co-exist with primary or secondary neoplastic brain lesions. Curiously the organism is rarely recovered from the cerebrospinal fluid. Primary nocardia meningitis has been reported but is extremely rare. The organism may spread to the skin and soft tissues, forming dark coloured subcutaneous abscesses. In widespread dissemination almost any organ or tissue may be involved, including liver, kidneys, eyes, lymph nodes, and bone.

Prognosis. This depends on several factors, not the least being delay in diagnosis if the disease is unsuspected. Disseminated nocardiasis involving at least two different organs or systems carries a bad prognosis irrespective of the nature of any underlying debilitating disease. Involvement of the central nervous system is usually fatal. Localized pulmonary nocardiasis has an overall mortality of perhaps 20 per cent but the outlook is more favourable if the patient was previously healthy or is not receiving immunosuppresive therapy. The prognosis is worse in acute disease of very short duration. In contrast nocardiasis limited to the skin or subcutaneous tissues is said to be benign and self-limiting. Adequate therapy appears to prolong survival in ultimately fatal cases. Rapid diagnosis and immediate chemotherapy greatly improve the prospects for survival.

Diagnosis. Pus and swabs are submitted for microscopy and culture. In Gram-stained smears, individual filaments of nocardia cannot be reliably distinguished from *Actinomyces* spp. Nocardia is moderately acid-fast when stained by a modified Ziehl–Neelsen method. Tissue secretions should also be Gram-stained: nocardia is not stained by haematoxylin and eosin.

Cultures are set up on ordinary media for prolonged incubation. *N. asteroides* grows aerobically as orange-pigmented, star-shaped colonies. The organism is sometimes isolated from routine Löwenstein–Jensen slopes after about seven days' incubation.

If pulmonary nocardiasis is suspected, sputum should be obtained and purulent portions examined. Since other Gram-positive filaments may be present as commensals in the oropharynx, and patients may fail to produce sputum, it would seem justifiable to obtain specimens by more invasive techniques which bypass the upper respiratory tract such as transtracheal aspiration, bronchial aspiration, transbronchial or pulmonary brush biopsy, or even percutaneous lung aspiration or open lung biopsy. Nocardiasis may co-exist with other lung pathogens such as *Pneumocystis carinii* and legionella and these should be considered at the time.

Since dissemination of nocardia is haematogenous, blood cultures should be obtained, for which a diphasic medium of the

Casteneda type using brain heart infusion agar and broth may be suitable. Urine, pleural fluid, and cerebrospinal fluid are cultured as appropriate. Skin tests and serological tests for nocardia are not helpful in diagnosis, but serological tests may be of value in following the course of an established case on treatment.

Treatment. Sulphonamides such as sulphadiazine or sulphafurazole are still the mainstay of treatment, given in a dose of 4–8 g daily to achieve a peak blood concentration of about 150 mg/l. Treatment should be continued for several weeks after clinical resolution, and prolonged in disseminated disease. Co-trimoxazole may be superior, but the component ratio may not be optimal for nocardia and prolonged therapy could carry a risk of folic acid depletion. Minocycline, amikacin, ampicillin, cycloserine, or fusidic acid may be considered as additives or as alternatives if sulphonamide is not tolerated, the choice depending on carefully standardized *in vitro* tests.

Surgical drainage may be required, especially of cerebral lesions. *N. caviae*, a widely distributed soil saprophyte is usually isolated as a cause of mycetoma (see page 5.374) but has occasionally been implicated in pulmonary and disseminated nocardiasis, with a terminal pustular rash involving forehead and trunk.

Prevention. The clustering of cases in renal transplant and cancer units and the isolation of nocardia from ward air and dust suggests the possibility of common source outbreaks or cross infection. In such circumstances, cases should be isolated to protect other immunosuppressed patients.

Although the differences between actinomyces and nocardiasis have been stressed, similarities are sometimes encountered, and the two diseases may have been confused in the past:

1. Nocardiasis has been reported after dental extraction, resulting in cervicofacial lesions with dissemination.

2. The alimentary tract may be a portal of entry for nocardia. Thus, removal of a gangrenous appendix may be followed by intra-abdominal abscess formation due to nocardia, sometimes associated with an extensive sinus network in the abdominal wall.

3. Nocardia has been isolated from ischiorectal abscesses.

4. As with actinomyces, external trauma may determine the localization of nocardia lesions.

References

Arroyo, J. C., Nichols, S., and Carroll, G. F. (1977). Disseminated *Nocardia caviae* infection. *Am. J. Med.* **62**, 409.

Beaman, B. L., Burnside, J., Edwards, B., and Causey, W. (1976). Nocardial infections in the United States, 1972–1974. *J. infect. Dis.* **134**, 286.

Curry, W. A. (1980). Human nocardiosis. *Archs intern. Med.* **140**, 818.

Frazier, A. R., Rosinow, III, E. C., and Roberts, G. D. (1975). Nocardiosis – A review of 25 cases occurring during 24 months. *Mayo Clinic. Proc.* **50**, 657.

Gorevic, P. D., Katler, E. I., and Angus, B. (1980). Pulmonary nocardiosis. Occurrence in men with Systemic lupus erythematosius. *Archs intern Med.* **140**, 361.

Houang, E. T., Lovett, I. S., Thompson, F. D., Harrison, A. R., Joekes, A. M., and Goodfellow, M. (1980). Nocardia asteroides infection – a transmissible disease. *J. hosp. Infect.* **1**, 31.

Palmer, D. L., Harvey, R. L., and Wheeler, J. K. (1974). Diagnostic and therapeutic considerations in *Nocardia asteroides* infection. *Medicine* **53**, 391.

Spirochaetes

Syphilis

G. W. Csonka

Synonyms. Lues, the great pox, morbus gallicus.

Definition. Venereal syphilis is a systemic contagious disease of great chronicity caused by *Treponema pallidum* and capable of being congenitally transmitted. The natural host is man. It has an incubation period of around three weeks at the end of which a primary sore develops usually on the genitalia, associated with regional lymphadenitis. In most patients this is followed by the secondary bacteraemic stage characterized by a symmetrical rash, generalized lymphadenopathy, and other lesions. After a latent period of many years this is terminated in 40 per cent by a destructive and potentially dangerous late stage which may involve the skin, mucous membranes, skeleton, CNS, eyes, hearing, and above all the aorta. Occasionally other organs are also affected. Any of these stages may be absent or so inapparent as to be overlooked.

The introduction of penicillin has profoundly changed the course and prognosis of syphilis and has made it the most curable of all sexually transmitted diseases.

Distribution. Venereal syphilis, unlike non-venereal syphilis has a worldwide distribution and knows no climatic, racial, or geographical barriers.

History. At the end of the fifteenth century a pandemic of syphilis known as the great pox, as distinct from smallpox, spread through Europe and Asia soon after the return of Columbus and his crew from the New World in 1493. The infection was very virulent and many people died during the then malignant secondary stage. It was only much later that it was realized that the infection was sexually transmitted, and later still that it was a chronic disease which could involve the skin, the CNS, aorta, and other organs.

Surprisingly, syphilis, chancroid, and gonorrhoea were for long believed to be the same disease and this received support in the eighteenth century when John Hunter inoculated himself with gonococcal pus and developed gonorrhoea and syphilis. It is now thought that whilst he conducted this experiment, he did not in fact inoculate himself!

It is in this century that spectacular advances were made and some of the milestones are:

1903 Metchnikoff and Rowe inoculated primates with syphilis.

1905 Schaudinn and Hoffmann discovered *T. pallidum*.

1906 Landsteiner used dark-field microscopy for its demonstration.

1910 Wassermann elaborated the first serological test for syphilis which he erroneously believed to be specific.

1910 Paul Ehrlich and Hata discovered Salvarsan, the 606th preparation tried, which proved to be the first effective drug against syphilis and also initiated the era of chemotherapy.

1917 Wagner–Jauregg used malaria in the treatment of neurosyphilis.

1928 Sir Alexander Fleming discovered penicillin which after its introduction in the treatment of syphilis in 1943 changed the prognosis of this disease and his discovery is arguably the most significant made in this century.

1949 Nelson and Mayer reported their work on the *Treponema pallidum* immobilization (TPI) test, the first truly specific serum reaction in the diagnosis of syphilis and is still used as the highest standard test against which other and newer procedures are compared. Because of its complexity and expense it is now only performed in a very few centres.

Aetiology. *T. pallidum* is a bacterium which belongs to the *Treponemataceae* which include three groups pathogenic for humans. They are: *Leptospira* which causes leptospirosis (rat-bite fever). *Borrelia* which includes *B. recurrentis* (recurrent fever) and *B. vincenti* (Vincent's angina). *Treponema* which includes *T. pallidum* (venereal syphilis, non-venereal endemic childhood syphilis, bejel, njovera), *T. pertenue* (yaws), and *T. carateum* (pinta). *T. cuniculi* produces rabbit syphilis.

There are a number of non-pathogenic treponemes such as *T. microdentium* and *T. macrodentium* in the mouth. They are difficult to distinguish from *T. pallidum* and for that reason dark-field examination of mouth lesions should be avoided because of the danger of misdiagnosis.

Other treponemes of low pathogenicity reside in the genital tract such as *T. balanitidus* and others which can together with fusiform bacilli under anaerobic conditions superinfect genital lesions producing 'fusospirochaetosis'. These treponemes are unlike *T. pallidum* and unlikely to be confused.

T. pallidum is a delicate, pale, motile spiral organism, 6–15 μm long and 0.2 μm wide. It has a three-layered cell membrane which is enveloped by the periplast which gives it the characteristic rigidity. The spiral structure is maintained by six fibrils which wind around the axis of the organism and are believed to be responsible for the motility of *T. pallidum*. The organism has also the unique ability to bend in the middle to form a V-shape. *T. pallidum* including all the other pathogenic treponemes has not yet been cultured in the laboratory and has to be propagated by the inoculation of laboratory animals for use in serological tests such as the TPI and FTA-ABS and for research.

The organism is seen in the wet-preparation by dark-field microscopy and shows a steady 'deliberate' linear progression. It can be detected from fluid taken from open lesions in early syphilis and failing that in the needle aspirate from affected regional lymph nodes. In late lesions the organism is no longer demonstrable by microscopy but occasionally can be grown by inoculating material into the testicle of rabbits. It divides by binary fission every 30–32 hours and contains the lipid cardiolipin which cross-reacts with the host tissue antigen and is the basis of the invaluable, though non-specific, serological 'reagin' tests.

The pathogenic treponemes which cause syphilis, non-venereal syphilis, yaws, and pinta cannot be morphologically differentiated from each other, give rise to the same serological reactions, produce similar lesions in laboratory animals, and are susceptible to penicillin. Clinically, however, the conditions show important differences with pinta being purely a skin condition and least like the other treponematoses. There are two major theories trying to account for these difficulties:

The Columbian theory. As briefly mentioned, at the end of the fifteenth century, a dramatic pandemic of venereal syphilis swept through Europe and Asia believed to be a new infection introduced by Columbus and his crew from the New World. In support of this idea it is often quoted that no convincing clinical description of syphilis existed in Europe before this time, but there are some objections to this theory. Evidence is accumulating that the infection did exist in these regions for many centuries before by finding skeletons with signs suggesting late syphilitic lesions and that earlier writing going back to Hippocrates makes reference to a disease which may have been syphilis. In the Columbian theory venereal syphilis is considered a disease apart from other treponematoses. If the Columbian theory is rejected, the difficulty still remains to explain the sudden emergence of the virulent spread of syphilis.

Unitarian theory. The rival theory has been put forward by Hudson when working in Syria where he described bejel, a non-venereal childhood treponematosis and evolved the unitarian theory. He suggests that all treponemes have a single ancestor and therefore refers to venereal syphilis, yaws, bejel, and the rest as *treponematosis*. The original disease was probably pinta which was then prevalent in Africa and Asia. Clinical differences developed in time due to adaptation of the organism to changing climatic factors, especially humidity and temperature and improvement in hygiene with wearing of clothes and less frequent intimate contacts between children. Yaws evolved and spread throughout the tropical belt, pinta was forced to retreat into remote and primitive communities in South and Central America, and non-venereal childhood syphilis such as bejel and similar conditions was found widely in the Middle East, Africa, Yugoslavia, Scotland, Ireland, and Scandinavia. These were all benign and involved the skin, mucous membranes, and bones but not the CNS, aorta, or other internal organs. Congenital transmission did not occur as it was essentially a childhood infection and by the time these children were old enough to have their own offsprings, the disease had become non-infectious. The treponeme which caused *venereal syphilis* was obliged to seek shelter in the protected, warm, and moist regions of the genitalia and so became a sexually transmitted infection. It spread throughout the world as an adult disease and acquired the ability to invade the CNS, aorta, and other organs and could be transmitted to the next generation. There are also objections to this ingenious theory, thus non-venereal treponematosis and venereal syphilis can exist side by side in tropical and sub-tropical regions and it does not explain satisfactorily the reason why this organism has changed so profoundly as to produce the potentially fatal late stage of venereally acquired syphilis.

The issue will probably be finally settled when the organism(s) can be cultured and fully investigated.

Epidemiology

Transmission. Sexual transmission is the rule in adult patients. Asexual transmission by close contact with an open lesion of early acquired or congenital syphilis is a rare event. Other unusual modes of transmission are by direct blood transfusion with blood from an infectious individual and contact with infected fomites. Congenital syphilis which was not uncommon last century has become very rare.

Incidence. There has been a steady decline in the incidence of syphilis in the Western world since the 1860s, interrupted only by major wars. Since 1940 there has been a 99 per cent drop in admissions of general paresis of the insane (GPI) and congenital syphilis in the USA, and the trend is similar in the UK and Europe. There has also been a sharp reduction in other forms of late syphilis and the gumma has almost disappeared. Early syphilis does not share this decline to the same degree since the Second World War. In the USA it reached a low in 1956, with 6576 reported cases, but has since risen to around 24 000. This pattern is also found in most European countries. Thus in England the number of early infectious syphilis cases was 1187 in 1971 against 1447 in 1978. This increase is largely due to an increased rate of infection in homosexual men; in 1971, homosexual males accounted for 50 per cent of early syphilis, and in 1980 the figure was 58 per cent. It is therefore important to keep these increases in perspective. They occur to an important degree in a circumscribed group and are not diffused throughout the population. For unknown reasons this trend has not been so evident in the USA; but this may be due to differences in reporting and contact tracing and not due to true epidemiological reasons. In other parts of the world, notably in the Far East, infected prostitutes may play an important part in the spread of early syphilis.

The changing clinical presentation of syphilis. There is clinical evidence that syphilis is becoming milder and less typical. This has been especially noted in neurosyphilis and the virtual disappearance of the gumma. The widespread use of antibiotics for unrelated conditions may be responsible. This is supported by finding that meningovascular syphilis has not shown the dramatic decrease of GPI and tabes dorsalis, possibly because the latter two conditions take many more years to develop giving cumulative chances of antibiotics being given. It is also possible that the disease is tending to become milder and less typical as a result of 'natural' changes which appear to have started long before the antibiotic era. For whatever reasons syphilis is apparently becoming clinically less clearcut. Its exclusion by serology and other tests becomes more important in patients attending the dermatologist, neurologist, ophthalmologist, the ENT specialist, or cardiologist with conditions of uncertain pedigree.

Sex. There is good evidence that early syphilis is less florid in women than men and is almost asymptomatic during pregnancy. Cardiovascular syphilis is at least twice as common in men than women where it is more severe and appears earlier. Neurosyphilis is also more common in men than women. The reasons for these differences are not known.

Race. Caucasians suffer more commonly from neurosyphilis than Negroes and they in turn are much more prone to develop cardiovascular syphilis than Caucasians.

Infectivity. The estimated figures for infectivity vary but is commonly assumed to be around 50 per cent. After a single exposure the figure is nearer 25 per cent.

Some control measures. The main source of case finding is the more intensive use of serological tests for syphilis as already mentioned. Another valuable control measure is contact tracing, which is very variable in different countries, but should be standard practice everywhere. Its use across international borders should be developed with proper safeguards to preserve confidentiality. Other measures which should prove valuable are the education of the young without inducing anxiety, the education of doctors, and encouraging regular check-ups of high-risk individuals such as homosexual men and prostitutes. The obligatory antenatal blood test for syphilis should continue. A more controversial suggestion is to treat contacts of infectious syphilis epidemiologically in certain situations, e.g. promiscuous individuals, known defaulters, and those who may infect their regular consort if not treated.

These measures can be expected to uncover up to 75 per cent of all cases of syphilis.

Persistence of treponemal forms. Persistence of *T. pallidum*-like forms in the CSF, aqueous humour, lymph nodes, and other tissues in penicillin-treated patients with late or late latent syphilis has been reported from several centres. The same phenomenon is the basis for relapses after penicillin treatment in borreliosis (see page 5.295). In some cases, the forms may have been non-pathogenic treponemes or artifacts, but in others rabbit inoculation confirmed them to be pathogenic *T. pallidum*. These treponemes appeared to be fully sensitive to penicillin in animal experiments.

Their presence in the aqueous humour or CSF might be explained by the low concentration of antibiotics in these locations. This is not the case in lymph nodes and other tissues and as yet there is no explanation for their persistence. As these cases are very rare there appears to be no need to change our ideas about treatment or prognosis.

The natural course of untreated syphilis. *T. pallidum* penetrates the abraded skin and intact mucous membrane. Within hours it becomes disseminated via the blood stream and lymphatics and is beyond any effective local treatment. The incubation period is traditionally given as 9–90 days but in practice it is around three weeks (range: two to six weeks). The time depends on the size of the inoculum, sexual practice, and hygienic measures. A single treponeme leads to the longest incubation period. The primary lesion develops at the site of contact and heals in two to six weeks. In a proportion of patients a secondary stage appears six weeks after the primary lesion has healed but there may be an overlap of the healing primary and the onset of the secondary stage. In some cases the period between these stages can be prolonged to several months. The main characteristic of the secondary stage is a generalized, symmetrical, painless, and non-irritating rash. In about 20 per cent infectious relapses occur during the following year (range: one to four years). In the rest, the latent asymptomatic period follows and may persist for life in at least 60 per cent. In 30–40 per cent a third late destructive stage develops. Its more benign form involves only the skin, mucous membranes, and bones. In the serious form the CNS, aorta, and other internal organs are affected. The major events are shown in Figs. 1 and 2.

The course of untreated syphilis has been investigated in the now famous Oslo study (1891–1951) when almost 2000 patients with early syphilis were left untreated and studied. Approximately 1000 patients were finally analysed with the following results: relapsing secondary syphilis was observed in 25 per cent; cardiovascular syphilis was diagnosed in 10.4 per cent; CNS lesions in 6.5 per cent; and gumma of the skin, mucous membranes, or bone in 16 per cent. A total of 23 per cent died as a direct result of syphilis. Serious late syphilitic complications were twice as common in men than women.

This study is open to several criticisms. The study was completed before all the patients had died and thus some late complications

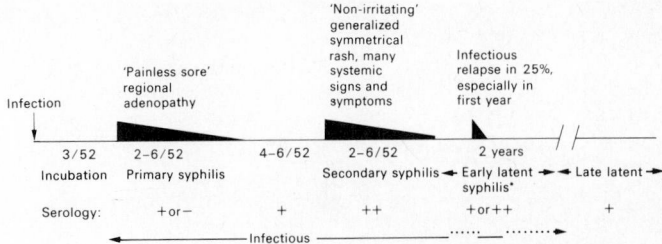

Fig. 1 The course of untreated early acquired syphilis.

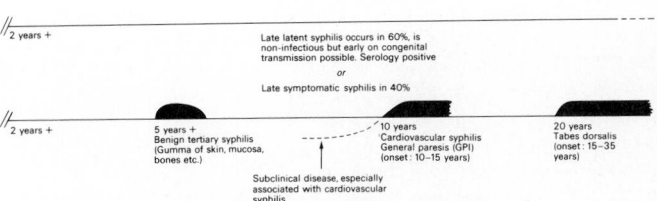

Fig. 2 The course of untreated late acquired syphilis.
Asymptomatic neurosyphilis is present in 20 per cent and 20 per cent of these develop clinical neurosyphilis.
Cardiovascular syphilis starts subclinically many years earlier and when clinically apparent, it is in fact in an advanced state.
Prognosis: Gumma heals spontaneously in a few years. Cardiovascular syphilis is usually fatal without treatment. Neurosyphilis: general paresis has a poor prognosis without treatment, meningvascular syphilis commonly responds well to penicillin, tabes progresses slowly but penicillin has no obvious influence.
Overall mortality of untreated syphilis: 20–30 per cent.

may have escaped inclusion. The study took place at a time when many patients died young mainly due to tuberculosis and once again late complications may have been underestimated. Finally, the disease was already changing as noted elsewhere and the change was particularly marked in the incidence and severity of the late stage. If a similar study could be undertaken at present, the results might be quite different, and the Oslo study is by now of greater historical interest than of practical value in predicting the fate of patients with untreated syphilis.

In the more recent Tuskegee study of Negro males with latent syphilis, it was found that one third died of late syphilis, mostly due to cardiovascular lesions. In post-mortem investigations aortitis was present in 40–60 per cent, far in excess of the clinical diagnosis, supporting the view that the cardiovascular lesion is the most important and lethal late syphilitic complication. Though the death rate directly attributed to late syphilis is around 30 per cent in several studies, the incidence may be higher as there is some evidence that the patients are more prone to other diseases including hypertension. In all the more recent reports the incidence of CNS syphilis and gumma is lower than in the Oslo study, confirming that a change is taking place in the evolution of the disease.

Clinical features

Primary syphilis. The first sign is a small, painless papule which rapidly ulcerates. The ulcer (chancre) is usually solitary, round or oval, painless, and often indurated (Fig. 3). It is surrounded by a bright red margin. It is not usually secondarily infected, a feature of all open syphilitic lesions of any stage. The reason for this might repay investigations. *T. pallidum* can be demonstrated in the serum from the sore which is easily obtained after slightly abrading the base. In heterosexual men the common sites are the coronal sulcus, the glans, and inner surface of the prepuce but may be found on the shaft of the penis and beyond. In homosexual men the ulcer is usually present in the anal canal, less commonly in the mouth (Fig. 4) and genitalia. In women most chancres occur on the vulva, the labia, and more rarely the cervix when it is liable to be overlooked.

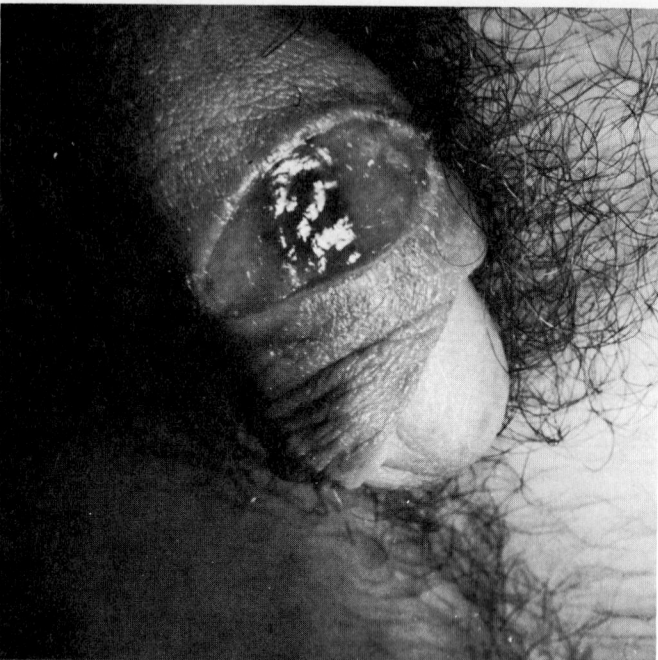

Fig. 3 Large primary sore. Note the even shape and the absence of secondary infection.

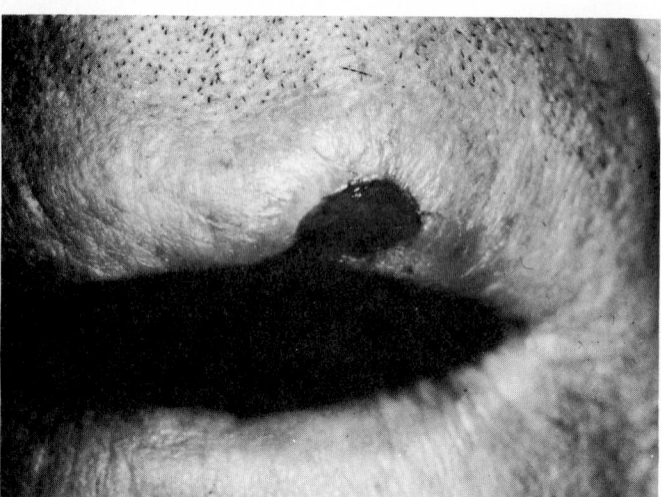

Fig. 4 Healing primary sore of the lip with some induration around it.

Extragenital chancres usually involve the lips when they become large and associated with some oedema, other sites are the mouth, buttocks, and fingers. The regional lymph nodes are invariably enlarged a few days after the appearance of the chancre and with genital sores they are *bilaterally* involved. The lymph nodes are painless, discrete, firm, and not fixed to surrounding tissues.

Atypical primary sores are not uncommon and depend on the size of the inoculum and the immunological status of the patient; thus a small inoculum usually produces a small atypical ulcer or papule and looks trivial. This may also be the case in patients who had previously treated syphilis and may be dark-field negative.

Histologically the chancre shows perivascular infiltration with plasma cells and histiocytes, capillary proliferation, and olbiterative endarteritis and periarteritis. The affected lymph nodes contain numerous treponemes, a depletion of lymphocytes, follicular hyperplasia, and histiocytic infiltration. If *T. pallidum* cannot be recovered from the primary sore, it may be possible to demonstrate it from the needle aspirate of the regional lymph node.

Differential diagnosis. All genital sores must be regarded as syphilitic until proven otherwise, especially when they are solitary and painless.

Genital lesions which must be differentiated from primary syphilis are:

1. Genital herpes (see page 5.327), which is much more common than syphilis in either sex. It is characterized by a crop of painful or irritating vesicles which develop into shallow erosions. In the first attack there is also painful inguinal adenitis.

2. Traumatic sores. These are painful, irregular and may become secondarily infected.

3. Erosive balanitis. These are inflammatory, irregular erosions which may become purulent in the uncircumcised.

4. Fixed drug eruptions. These are macules or occasionally ulcers following various drugs, especially tetracyclines.

5. Chancroid (see page 5.305). This is mostly seen in the tropics, presents as painful, superficial, 'soft chancre', which is often multiple with painful suppurative regional adenitis.

Other conditions which may have to be considered are scabies, Behçet's syndrome, granuloma inguinale, and lymphogranuloma venereum.

Secondary syphilis. The lesions are numerous, variable, and affect many systems. Inevitably there is a symmetrical, non-irritating *rash* and generalized painless *lymphadenopathy*. *Constitutional symptoms* are mild or absent; they include headaches, which are often nocturnal, malaise, slight fever, and aches in joints and muscles. The rash is commonly macular, pale red, and sometimes so faint as to be appreciable only in tangential light. It may be papular and sometimes squamous (Fig. 5). Pustular and necrotic rashes are rarely seen in temperate climates but still occur in tropical regions. The later the secondary rash develops, the more exuberant it becomes. The distribution of the rash can be of great diagnostic help. It usually covers the trunk and proximal limbs, but when it is seen on the palms, soles, and the face, syphilis should always be high on the list of probable causes (Figs. 6 and 7). In warm and moist areas such as the perineum, external female genitalia, perianal region, axillae, and under pendulous breasts, the papules enlarge into pink or grey discs, the *condylomata lata,* which are highly infectious (Fig. 8). *Mucous patches* in the mouth and genitalia are painless greyish-white erosions forming circles and arcs ('snail-track ulcers'). They too are very infectious.

Meningism and headache are due to low-grade meningitis which can be confirmed by a raised cell count and raised protein in the CSF.

Less common lesions include *alopecia* and *laryngitis. Syphilitic hepatitis* is usually associated with a marked rise in serum phosphatase. There are non-specfic inflammatory changes in liver biopsy material which are quite unlike those found in viral hepatitis. A *nephrotic syndrome* may develop and glomerular immune-complex deposits have been observed.

Pain in the bones, often worse at night, is usually due to *periostitis. Uveitis* may be seen both in secondary and tertiary syphilis.

In about one fifth of patients *recurrent infectious episodes* occur especially during the first year after the secondary stage.

All these lesions disappear spontaneously and leave no evidence behind. It was repeatedly suggested in the older literature that extensive skin lesions had a protective effect and that late lesions of the CNS or aorta were less likely in such cases. It was believed that this was due to elaboration of significant amounts of protective antibodies by the skin lesions but no formal proof of this interesting idea has been presented. If true, one might further speculate that the extensive and prolonged skin lesions so prominent in all types of non-venereal syphilis may be a factor protecting these patients from the severe complications of the late stage.

Latent syphilis. By definition the patient is asymptomatic with normal CSF findings but positive serology for syphilis. It is arbitrarily divided into *early* and *late latent* syphilis. Infectiousness does not stop with the advent of latency as women may continue to give

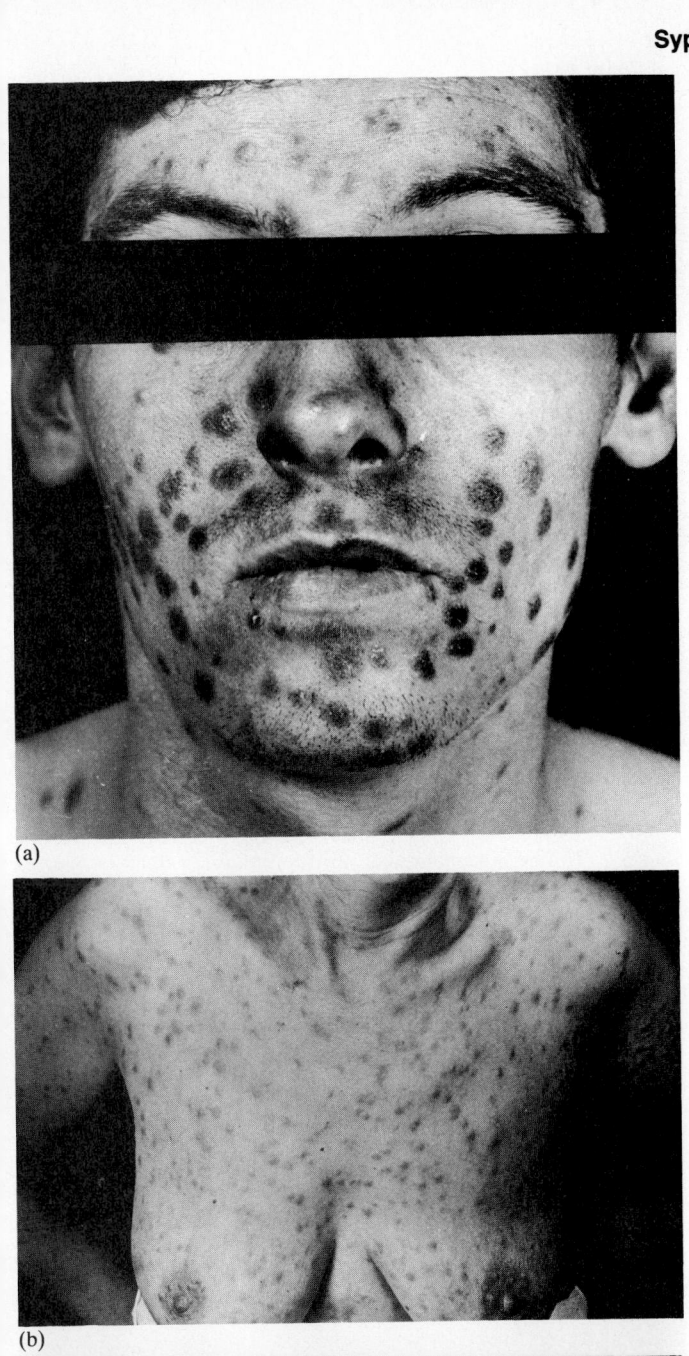

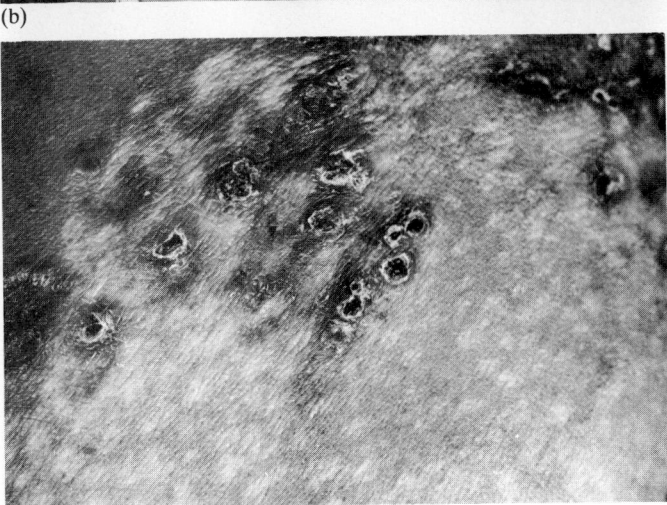

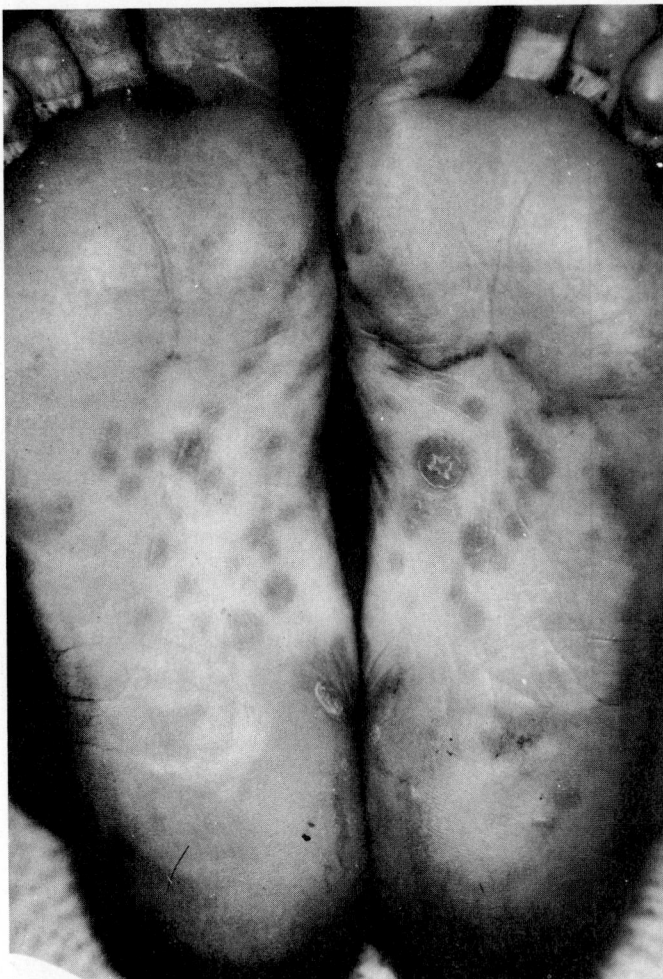

Fig. 6 Secondary papulosquamous rash of the soles.

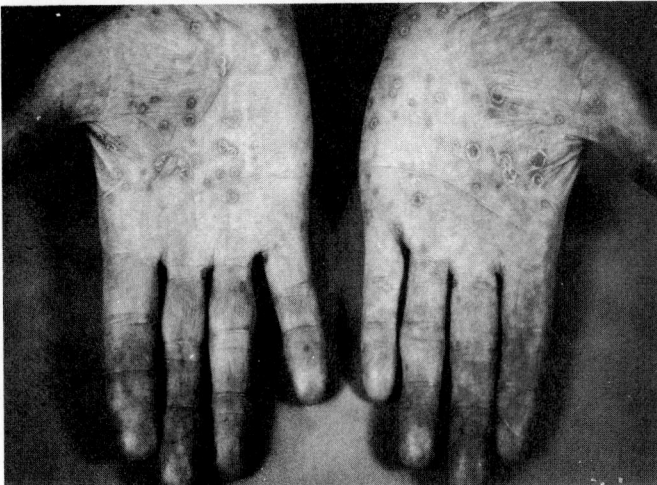

Fig. 7 Secondary rash of the palms.

Fig. 5 (a) and (b) Secondary papular syphilitic rashes; (c) Late secondary/early tertiary papulosquamous lesions.

birth to congenitally infected infants during the early latent stage and for at least two years into the late latent stage. Approximately 60 per cent of patients remain latent for the rest of their lives, the only evidence of syphilis being positive serology with a usually low titre. The rest develop clinical late syphilis but autopsy studies indicate that a higher proportion has subclinical infection especially of the cardiovascular system.

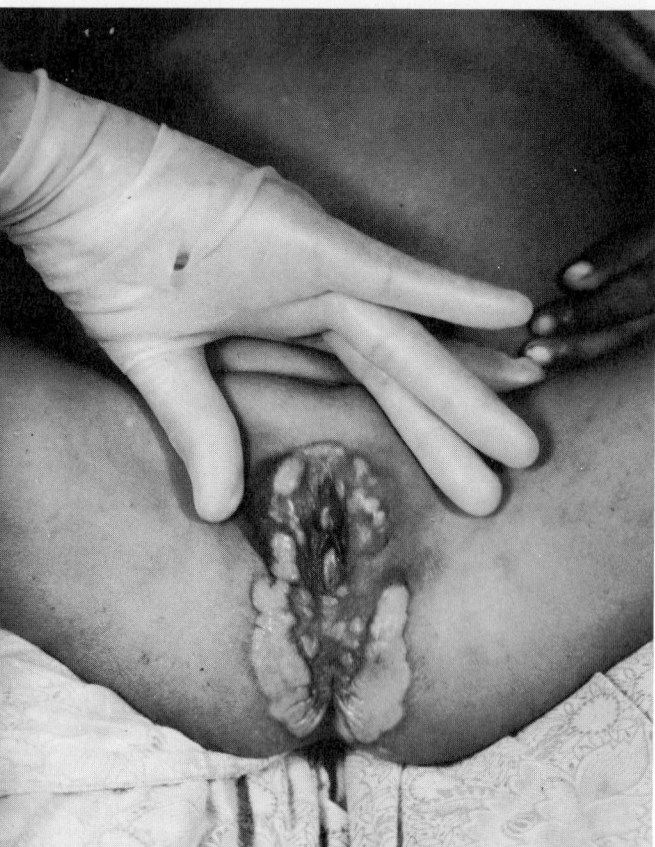

Fig. 8   Condylomata lata.

Late syphilis (tertiary syphilis). This includes late latent syphilis already referred to, benign tertiary syphilis, involvement of viscera, the CNS, and the aorta.

Benign late syphilis. *1. Cutaneous gumma.* The gumma is a chronic granulomatous lesion which is usually single but may be multiple or diffuse (Fig. 9). Histologically there is central necrosis with peripheral cellular infiltration of lymphocytes, plasma cells, and occasional giant cells with perivasculitis and obliterating endarteritis. *T. pallidum* is present and can be demonstrated by rabbit inoculation. Clinically it starts as a slowly progressive painless nodule which becomes dull red and breaks down into one or several indolent punched-out ulcers. The base has a 'wash-leather' appearance and is remarkably free from secondary infection (Fig. 10). It often resembles other granulomatous conditions. It heals slowly from the centre, which may become depigmented, whilst the periphery shows hyperpigmentation. Eventually a paper-thin scar forms. This combination of pigmentation, depigmentation, and atrophic scars can be of considerable retrospective diagnostic help. The sites preferentially involved are the face, legs, buttocks, upper trunk, and scalp. The process may be more superficial producing papulosquamous lesions which include the palms and soles. It too heals with the typical scars already described.

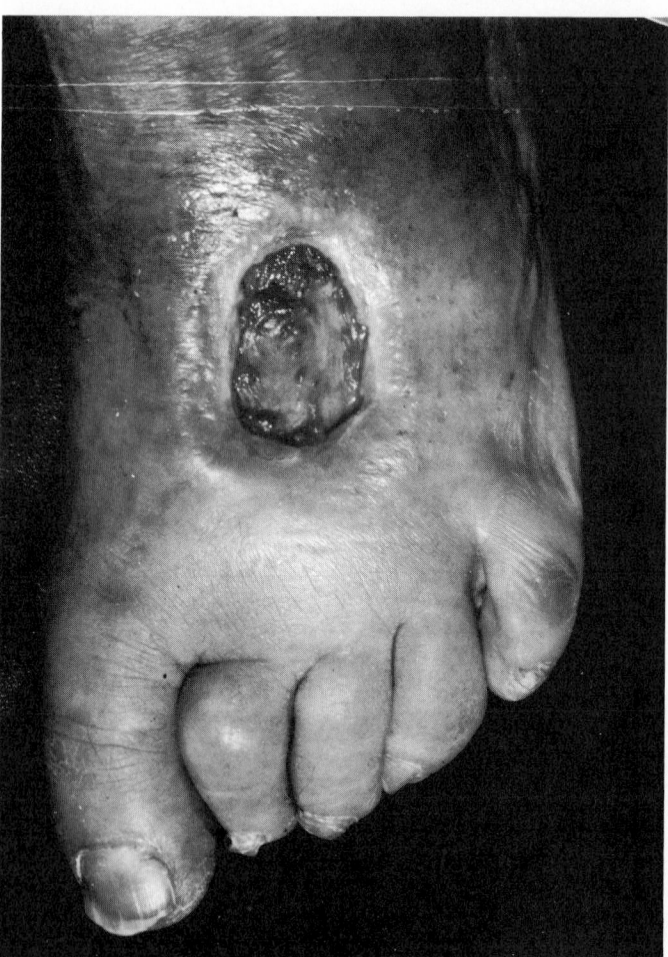

Fig. 10   Single gumma. Note the punched-out ulcer and absence of secondary infection.

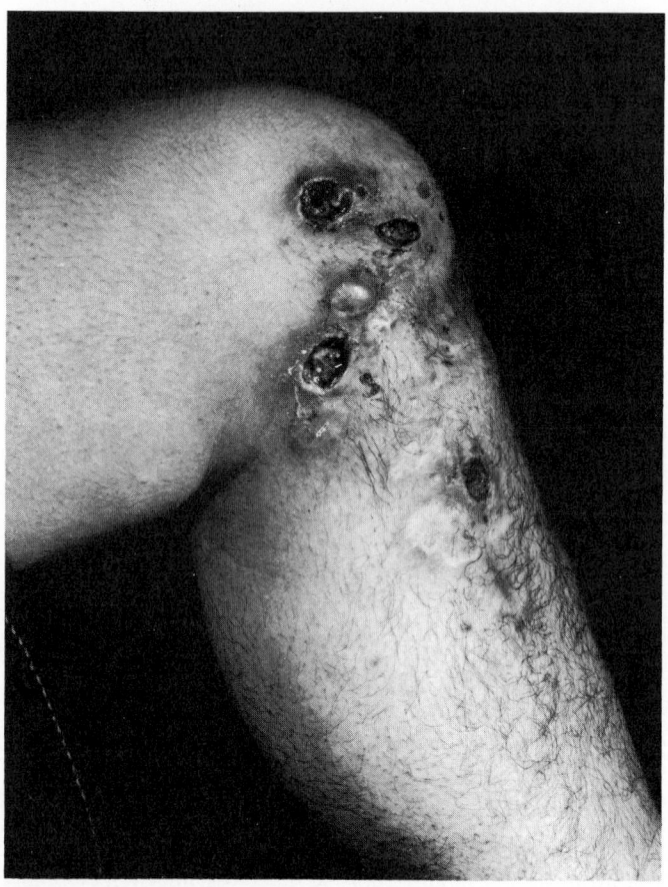

Fig. 9   Multiple gummatous ulcers. This is a typical site.

2. Mucosal gumma. These are most commonly seen in the oropharynx and involve the palate, pharynx, and the nasal septum. They tend to be destructive causing perforation of the hard palate and the nasal septum. In the pharynx and larynx they tend to lead to severe scarring. The most serious lesion is the diffuse gummatous infiltration of the *tongue* leading first to a general swelling of the organ, then due to loss of papillae to a smooth red surface (Fig. 11). After a while the poor blood supply produces necrotic white patches on the dorsum of the tongue and this leucoplakia has a strong tendency to become malignant: thus regular check-ups with biopsy are necessary (Fig. 12). Penicillin has no effect on the progress of syphilitic glossitis at this late stage.

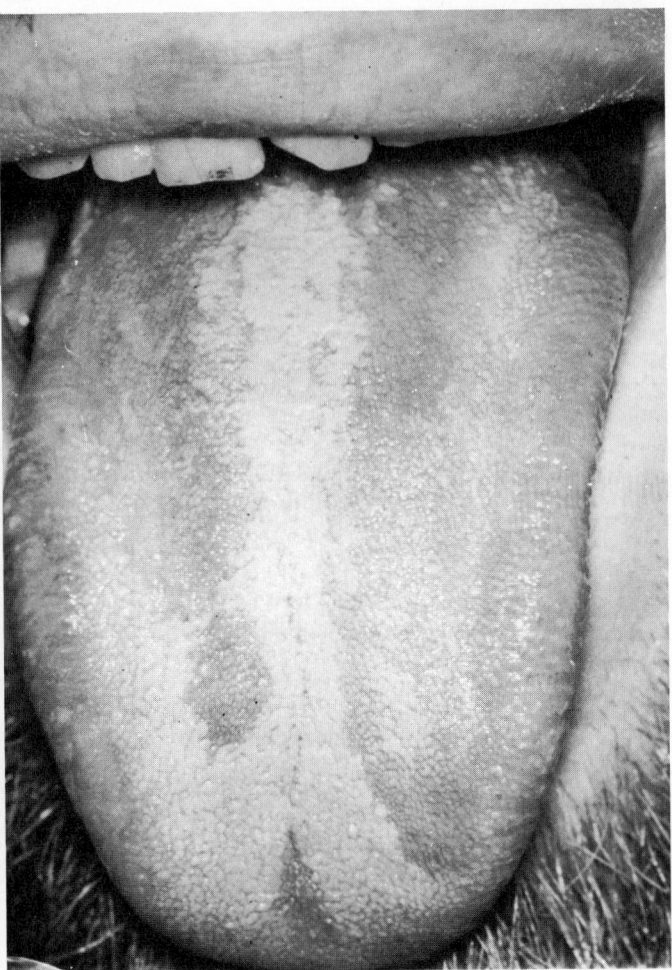

Fig. 11 Late syphilitic glossitis, early stage.

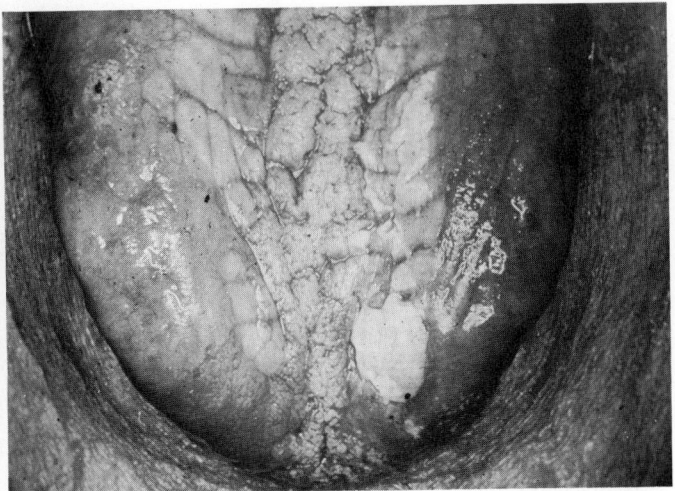

Fig. 12 Syphilitic leucoplakia of the tongue; premalignant.

3. *Late syphilis of bones.* Osteoperiostitis of long bones such as the tibia and fibula causes thickening and irregularities which may be diffuse as in the 'sabre tibia' or localized and evident as a circumscribed bony swelling. Unlike most other syphilitic lesions, those of the bone are often painful, the pain being worse at night. Very rarely the process breaks through the skin producing a chronic 'syphilitic osteomyelitis'. Lesions of the palate, nasal septum, and the skull are destructive leading to bone defects of the hard palate and nasal septum, and multiple osteolytic lesions of the skull.

Differential diagnosis. 1. Mucocutaneous gumma. The superficial skin lesions may have to be differentiated from fungal skin lesions, psoriasis, and bromide and iodide rashes. The deep gummata may resemble deep mycoses, sarcoidosis, tuberculosis, leprosy, granuloma inguinale, lymphogranuloma venereum, reticulosis, and epithelioma of the skin.

Serological tests for syphilis, which must include specific reactions such as the FTA-ABS, prompt response to penicillin, and possibly evidence of syphilis elsewhere should clarify the diagnosis.

A case history might serve to illustrate an important principle: A woman of 55 had a large painless ulcer overlying the tibia. The lesion was secondarily infected. All the blood tests for syphilis were positive and a diagnosis of gumma was made (in spite of the bacterial infection which is unusual). Penicillin cleared the bacterial infection but there was no further progress. Biopsy showed it to be an epithelioma.

It is not uncommon to see patients with ulcers or nodes of the skin or various organs and a positive serology for syphilis. A diagnosis of syphilis is made, treatment is given, and only after obvious therapeutic failure is the diagnosis reconsidered and malignancy found. Positive blood tests for syphilis may be coincidental and as late *symptomatic* syphilis is rare whereas malignancy is not this differential diagnosis should always be taken into account.

2. Late syphilis of bones. Conditions to be considered include primary and secondary carcinoma, Paget's disease, chronic osteomyelitis, tuberculosis, and leprosy. All forms of non-venereal syphilis except Pinta give rise to similar lesions.

Visceral syphilis. This is not common and response to treatment is variable. Late syphilis may involve the liver, eyes, stomach, lungs, and testes.

1. Liver. Multiple gummata of the liver give rise to irregular hepatomegaly ('hepar lobatum'), which may be asymptomatic. Symptoms may result from pressure on bile ducts or blood vessels or destruction of liver parenchyma. Antisyphilitic treatment is reported to lead to accelerated fibrosis with distortion of the liver architecture and an increase in symptoms ('therapeutic paradox'), but the available data are too scanty to confirm this.

2. Eyes. Uveitis, choroidoretinitis or optic atrophy may sometimes be the sole feature of late syphilis. Uveitis can also develop during early syphilis. Response of the late form to penicillin is poor. Optic atrophy is further discussed under neurosyphilis.

3. Stomach. Single or diffuse gummatous infiltrations of the stomach have been described and are said to respond to antisyphilitic treatment.

4. Lungs. Single or multiple gummata are rare and respond to treatment.

5. Testis. Gummatous infiltration and dense fibrosis may produce smooth painless enlargement of a testis. Testicular sensation is lost. In the only case seen by us penicillin had no effect.

6. Paroxysmal cold haemoglobinuria. Syphilis is a rare cause of this haemolytic anaemia (see Section 19).

It is often claimed by patients who had recent treatment for late latent syphilis that it improved their well-being. This may be a psychological reaction but it is also possible that it is due to an effect on subclinical visceral lesions. The warning given earlier against undue delay in the diagnosis of malignant disease because of misleading positive serology for syphilis which is coincidental, applies even more strongly in this section.

Neurosyphilis

1. Asymptomatic neurosyphilis. There are no neurological manifestations but the CSF shows abnormalities such as a raised cell count (5 or more cells/ml), raised protein (over 40 mg/ml), and commonly a positive FTA-ABS test. The VDRL is less reliable and if it is the sole abnormality, it is probably due to passive transfer and not due to intrinsic production of antibodies in the CNS. However, if there are atypical neurological signs as well it is safest to treat as neurosyphilis.

Asymptomatic neurosyphilis occurs in about 20 per cent of untreated patients and 20 per cent of these will progress to symptomatic neurosyphilis in the absence of treatment.

Neurosyphilis of any kind is more common in Caucasians than Negroes and at least twice as common in men than women.

Experience shows that if the CSF is normal two years after untreated infection, neurosyphilis will not develop. If the serology for syphilis becomes negative, that too effectively rules out neurosyphilis.

2. Symptomatic neurosyphilis

Meningovascular syphilis. *Pathology.* The essential lesion is vascular and perivascular inflammation leading to endarteritis obliterans. The perivascular space is infiltrated with lymphocytes, plasma cells, and fibroblasts and the impaired blood supply produces necrosis of neighbouring tissue with gumma formation surrounded by a zone of fibrotic reaction. Treponemes may be seen at the periphery. Gummatous leptomeningitis involves mainly the basal meninges but can spread to cover the hemispheres. The pia and arachnoid form an adherent and thickened membrane. If cerebral endarteritis involves main cerebral arteries, it will cause focal symptoms corresponding to the area of the brain supplied by the vessel. The process may extend to the spinal cord.

Clinical features. Meningovascular syphilis is the earliest neurosyphilis to cause symptoms. These may start five years after infection. *Cerebral pachymeningitis* is rare and causes cortical irritation with headaches, focal convulsions, and paresis of the limbs. *Cerebral leptomeningitis* may give rise to diffuse or focal symptoms such as an isolated cranial nerve palsy. In the commoner diffuse type with basal meningitis, there are headaches which are worse at night. Papilloedema may develop. Mental changes are usual with impaired memory and loss of concentration. If the patient is anxious and nervous, he is usually diagnosed as being neurotic. In the more severe case there is apathy and eventually severe mental deterioration leading to a state of semi-stupor. The cranial nerves are often damaged including the optic chiasma leading to defects of the visual field or even optic atrophy. The third nerve is most commonly involved followed by the sixth, seventh, and fifth nerves. Occasionally the patient presents with only an isolated cranial nerve palsy. If the eighth nerve is damaged there may be vertigo and deafness. Pupillary changes showing some elements of the Argyll Robertson pupil may be present. Before complete occlusion of a cerebral artery, there are episodes of transient sensory and motor symptoms (cerebral arteritis). Finally, thrombosis leads to infarction. The middle and posterior cerebral arteries are most involved. The resulting unilateral hemiplegia has a rapid onset with headache but no loss of consciousness.

Differential diagnosis. The symptomatology is so extensive and covers so many alternative neurological disorders that the diagnosis must in the end depend on the serological evidence of syphilis and associated changes in the CSF which include increased cells and protein and positive FTA-ABS test. With purely syphilitic vascular lesions, the CSF may be normal or show only minor abnormalities. Routine serology for syphilis should be performed in all neurological disorders especially as there is some evidence that neurosyphilis is becoming less typical and less florid. Suspicion of syphilis should be aroused when hemiplegia develops in a comparatively young person. Mental changes may imitate a variety of psychoses, and in the mild case, neuroses. When papilloedema is present, space-occupying lesions especially brain tumours must be considered,

however, the protean manifestations of cerebral syphilis are of help. If there is only a focal lesion, brain tumour should not be ruled out in the presence of positive serology. In epileptiform attacks occurring for the first time in adults, syphilis should always be excluded. Due to the multitude of symptoms, disseminated sclerosis may cause a diagnostic problem. In disseminated sclerosis pupillary reflexes are normal, on the other hand, nystagmus and incoordination of the limbs without sensory loss are not found in cerebral syphilis. The knee jerks are exaggerated in disseminated sclerosis and often diminished or lost in cerebral and spinal syphilis.

Prognosis. With early treatment of meningitic neurosyphilis the prognosis is very good. If there are severe mental disturbances, some residual impairment is the rule. With cerebrovascular syphilis improvement can only be expected before complete thrombosis has occurred. Hemianopia due to posterior cerebral thrombosis is permanent.

Spinal syphilis. This is an extension of meningovascular syphilis and shows the same histological changes.

Spinal pachymeningitis. This occurs in the cervical region (cervical hypertrophic pachymeningitis) and may also a non-syphilitic aetiology. At first there is pain due to compression of the posterior roots by the thickened dura. The pain occurs in the neck, shoulders, and upper limbs. This is followed by atrophy of muscles innervated by the anterior roots. Finally, compression and endarteritis of the cord result in progressive spastic paraplegia and sensory loss below the level of the lesion.

Meningomyelitis. The severity of this condition varies and may involve the small muscles of the hands or the shoulder girdle, causing atrophy. In the more severe form the dorsal cord is involved giving rise to pain in the back and trunk followed by weakness of the lower limbs. In the most severe cases flaccid paralysis develops with urinary retention and complete loss of sensation below the level of the lesion. Eventually severe flexor spasms appear. The CSF changes are the same as found in cerebral syphilis.

Prognosis. The response to treatment is good provided it can be given before irreversible damage has occurred. Even in patients with complete paraplegia, some degree of recovery can be expected, once the spinal shock and oedema have disappeared and the inflammatory tissue responded to treatment.

General paresis (GPI, dementia paralytica). The name is strictly not correct as these patients are not paralysed but only appear to be so in advanced cases due to their mental inability to carry out certain motor functions.

Pathology. The brain is shrunken ('walnut brain') with compensatory hydrocephalus. Atrophy is most marked in the anterior two-thirds of the cortex where most of the histological changes are found. There is infiltration with lymphocytes and plasma cells. The ganglion cells of the cortex show varying degrees of degeneration. The changes are found in the layers of the small and medium-sized pyramidal cells. Demyelinization of cortical fibres is focally distributed. Gliosis is always present. With appropriate staining treponemes may be found in the cortex. Similar but less marked changes may involve other parts of the cortex. If tabes dorsalis is also present, the condition is known as taboparesis. Aortitis and occasionally gummata may be associated.

Clinical features. General paresis was once a common disease and mental hospitals always had a number of such patients. Nowadays it has become very rare. It usually develops 10–20 years after the initial infection, its onset being gradual over a period of many months. Occasionally the onset is abrupt with mental confusion, hallucinations, delusions, and severe intellectual defects.

1. Mental symptoms. In the slow-onset form there is impaired intellectual efficiency and lapses of memory which lead to deterioration at work. This becomes apparent to members of the family and friends but not to the patient. The old aphorism that 'everyone suffers in general paresis but not the patient' is still true. Speech and writing show the same deterioration and eventually

communication becomes impossible. The patient has no insight into his condition and often has a vacant expression or a fatuous smile. A degree of inappropriate boastful euphoria is present in a minority of patients but more common is progressive dementia until a state is reached where the patient is unable to feed himself, is incontinent and bedridden, and leads a vegetative existence. In some patients anxiety, irritability, and episodes of violence predominate which may lead to alcoholism and causes diagnostic and social difficulties.

2. Physical symptoms. There is an irregular coarse tremor, made worse on voluntary movement, which involves the lips, tongue, and outstretched fingers. Epileptiform fits without loss of consciousness occur in at least one-third of patients. Apoplectiform episodes with transient hemiplegia, aphasia, and hemianopia occur with brief loss of consciousness. The tendon reflexes are exaggerated, the abdominal reflexes lost, and plantar reflexes are extensor. The pupils may show the classical Argyll Robertson abnormalities or are contracted with sluggish reaction to light. If inco-ordination develops it will impede normal gait.

The cerebrospinal fluid is of the greatest diagnostic help in general paresis. It is never normal. The cells are increased up to 100 mm³, protein is raised over 50 mg/ml, Lange's gold curve is of the first zone (paretic) type e.g. 5554321000, and the FTA-ABS is positive. Serology for syphilis is always positive.

Differential diagnosis. Were it not for the characteristic CSF changes and positive serology for syphilis, diagnosis of general paresis on clinical grounds, especially early on would be impossible.

Early paresis may give identical symptoms to neurosis. Later on psychoses may cause difficulties and include manic-depressive psychosis, presenile and senile psychoses, alcoholic dementia, toxic effects of drug addiction, and liver disease. Other conditions needing consideration are epilepsy, frontal lobe tumour, carcinomatosis, and encephalitis.

Prognosis. Before Wagner–Jauregg introduced malarial treatment, general paresis was always fatal. His treatment greatly improved at least 50 per cent of patients.

Since the advent of penicillin the outlook is very good in early cases and more variable later on when irreversible mental changes may have taken place. However, there is now no mortality in this disease.

Tabes dorsalis (locomotor ataxia). Tabes dorsalis affects males four times more often than females and accounts for about 30 per cent of neurosyphilis. It develops later than the other types of neurosyphilis, between 15–35 years after the initial infection. Thus the patient is usually aged between 35–55 years.

Pathology. Macroscopically there is atrophy of the posterior columns in the dorso-lumbar-sacral regions (tabes dorsalis=dorsal wasting). The posterior columns look grey and translucent. Microscopically there is degeneration of the posterior nerve roots with ascending degeneration in the posterior column and secondary gliosis. The cause is uncertain and it has been suggested that the lesions are due to the thickened pia compressing the posterior root fibres at the point of entry into the dorsal column. The autonomic nervous system is also impaired. Degenerative changes can occur in any sensory nerve including the trigeminal and glossopharyngeal nerves. Optic atrophy is often associated with tabes but the cause is uncertain and may be due to primary degeneration in the retinal ganglion cells or be secondary to syphilitic inflammation of the interstitial tissues. The mechanism which produces the Argyll Robertson pupil is also uncertain. Association of tabes with general paresis, meningovascular syphilis, and aortitis may occur.

Clinical features. Tabes is a disease of many signs and many symptoms (Fig. 13). The *onset* is generally insidious and the disease may take years to develop. Due to the slightness of the initial sensory changes the patient may wait until he develops lightning pain, ataxia, impotence, gastric crisis, or optic atrophy before consulting a doctor.

The most startling symptom is *'lightning pain'* which is well

named. It is sharp, intense, stabbing, and repetitive, and often involves a small area of a leg or foot. The attack ceases as abruptly as it started, after a few hours or days, with symptom-free intervals of weeks or many months. The severity of the pain varies from mild (when it is commonly thought to be due to 'rheumatism') to one of the most agonizing pains known in medicine. There are similarities to *gastric and other crises* during which the patient has severe epigastric pain often with vomiting which brings him to the point of collapse. It too stops suddenly and may repeat itself after variable periods. Few patients with this symptom have escaped the surgeon's knife, but nothing is found. Laryngeal, rectal, and vesicle crises are similar in nature. *Girdle pains* are an unpleasant sensation of a tight band around the upper abdomen. Many patients complain of a numb feeling in their feet when walking, as if walking on cotton wool.

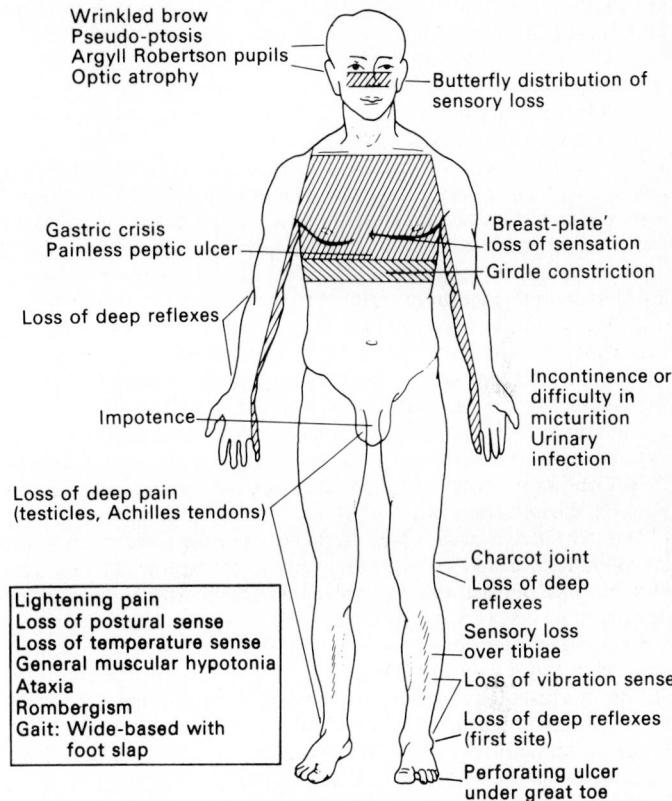

Fig. 13 Symptoms and signs of tabes dorsalis.

1. Objective sensory changes. One of the first sensations to be impaired is appreciation of vibration sense, followed by recognition of posture and passive movement. The lower limbs are affected before the upper ones. Sensation of deep and superficial pain is reduced or lost. Thus compression of the Achilles tendon or testis is painless. Pain sensation of the skin is lost preferentially in certain sites as shown in Fig. 13.

2. Ataxia. This is partly due to loss of postural sensibility and partly due to loss of afferent impulses regulating posture and movement. Initially there is some unsteadiness on walking and this can be compensated for by vision. Such patients become unsteady in the dark and may fall when they close their eyes ('Romberg's test'). As ataxia increases the patient walks with a wide base and brings his foot down too forcibly ('footslap'). Finally he can walk only when supported on both sides. In the most severe cases the trunk muscles become ataxic and the patient is unable to sit up unaided. Ataxia of the upper limbs can be recognized by clumsiness and by the finger–nose test.

3. Reflexes. Degeneration of afferent nerve fibres leads to the loss of tendon reflexes. The ankle-jerk is lost before the knee-jerk,

the abdominal reflexes may become brisk. The upper limb reflexes are diminished and later lost. The plantar reflexes remain flexor.

4. Muscular hypotonia. The muscles, deprived of afferent impulses, become hypotonic allowing joints to hyperextend and hyperflex.

5. Impotence. This may be one of the first symptoms and cause of presentation.

6. The bladder. If the sacral roots are involved, the bladder may become atonic and the patient experiences incontinence or difficulty in urination. Residual urine is inevitable as is urinary infection which needs priority treatment and attention to prevent progression to pyelonephritis.

7. The rectum. Sensation may be lost and in combination with atony, constipation or faecal incontinence develops.

8. Eyes. Pupillary abnormalities are the rule. The complete Argyll Robertson pupil may not be present early. When fully developed the pupils are irregular, contracted, off centre, and do not react to light but react to accommodation. In blue-eyed tabetics the iris takes on a faded blue because of loss of pigment.

Optic atrophy may be mild and not progressive. If the patient complains of progressive visual loss, optic atrophy will become complete with blindness.

9. Trophic changes. A Charcot's joint is a completely disorganized joint with osteoarthritis, subluxation, and extensive osteophytes. The exact mechanism is not known but some consider it due to repeated trauma affecting an insensitive joint. The knee is most commonly involved, followed by the hip. Other joints including the shoulder and intervertebral joints may be affected.

Trophic ulcer beneath the great toe, also called perforating ulcer, may develop. It may extend down to the bone and is painless.

The cerebrospinal fluid. There is an increase in cells which is usually below 50/mm^3. Protein is normal or slightly raised. The FTA-ABS may be positive or more rarely negative. The reagin blood tests for syphilis are negative in about 20 per cent especially in 'burnt out' cases when the CSF may also be normal. The serum FTA-ABS is almost always positive.

Differential diagnosis. Once ataxia has developed the diagnosis is usually simple as many of the other signs and symptoms of tabes are also present. Difficulties may be experienced with a number of neurological diseases including:

1. Diabetic neuropathy. There are many features in common with tabes but the calf muscles are tender when squeezed and the laboratory tests for diabetes will clarify the diagnosis.

2. Alcoholic neuropathy. This may closely resemble tabes but the peripheral muscles are weak, giving rise to wrist and foot-drop and the calf muscles are tender on pressure.

3. Disseminated sclerosis. The patient is younger. The ataxia is associated with spasticity, increased ankle-jerks, and extensor plantar response. Nystagmus is usually present.

4. Friedreich's ataxia. There is ataxia as in tabes with loss of ankle-jerks, but the patient is younger, has nystagmus, extensor plantar responses, dysarthria, and scoliosis.

5. Infectious polyneuritis.

6. Lead and arsenic poisoning.

7. Subacute combined degeneration of the cord.

8. Gastric crisis. One must always exclude gastric ulcer which may co-exist. It is noteworthy that *painless perforation* of a peptic ulcer may occur in tabes as it did in one of our patients who had no gastric symptoms and suddenly died. Autopsy revealed perforation of an unsuspected gastric ulcer which was the cause of death. Cholecystitis and other painful intra-abdominal conditions may also have to be excluded. *The atonic bladder syndrome* must be differentiated from prostatic hypertrophy or carcinoma.

9. Charcot's joint may also develop in syringomyelia when it affects the upper limb.

10. Lightning pain. Lesser degrees of lightning pain are often diagnosed and treated for a considerable time as rheumatic in origin.

11. Trigeminal neuralgia. Other causes may have to be excluded.

12. Optic atrophy. Other causes may have to be excluded.

Prognosis. The prognosis in tabes varies; the longer the pre-ataxic period, the milder the subsequent course. The pre-ataxic stage may last from months to five years. In some patients ataxia never develops and in others the disease 'burns out' with no further progression. Response to penicillin is not easy to assess but when given early there is some evidence that it may arrest the disease and lead to some improvement.

Conscientious bladder drill, avoidance of constipation, and re-education of ataxic limbs are helpful. It is essential to treat infections vigorously, especially those of the urinary and respiratory tracts.

If there is associated symptomatic cardiovascular syphilis, this will dominate the prognosis.

Syphilitic deafness and vertigo. The eighth nerve may be involved in basal meningovascular syphilis resulting in vertigo and deafness. The prognosis for hearing loss is uncertain but it appears that when it is advanced it becomes permanent. Syphilitic nerve deafness may also develop in late syphilis as a single lesion and in our experience the prognosis is poor.

Follow-up examination in neurosyphilis. As in other forms of late syphilis with symptoms, the follow-up should be for life to monitor clinical progress. The traditional repetition of serological tests for syphilis is unlikely to contribute much to the management of the patient.

Cardiovascular syphilis (see also Section 13). The main lesions in cardiovascular syphilis are: (*a*) uncomplicated aortitis; (*b*) aortic regurgitation; (*c*) coronary ostial stenosis; and (*d*) aneurysm of the aorta.

Symptomatic lesions develop in 10 per cent of untreated syphilis some 10–40 years after initial infection. Autopsy data suggest that the incidence of subclinical lesions is considerably higher. In Negroes up to 50 per cent of lesions were found; it is much more common in Negroes than other racial groups and in men than in women.

Pathology. Macroscopical appearance of syphilitic aortitis is characterized by intimal plaques, longitudinal grooves, and a sharp demarcation of lesions at the origin of vessels in the neck, the diaphragm, or the renal vessels. They do not occur below the level of the renal arteries. The ascending aorta is most extensively involved, followed by the arch and descending aorta. Lesions are found in only 10 per cent in the upper abdominal aorta. The ascending aorta is widened, the wall is irregular with thickened and thinned portions and there are intimal scars.

Microscopically the primary changes are seen in the vasa vasorum which show endarteritis obliterans and perivascular cellular infiltration with lymphocytes and plasma cells. The consequence is destruction of the muscular and elastic layers of the aortic wall and replacement with functionally inert scar tissue. The fact that the vasa vasorum are the primary target of the syphilitic lesion explains the anatomical distribution of cardiovascular syphilis as the ascending aorta is most richly endowed with vasa vasorum. The ostial stenosis of the coronary arteries appears to be due to their involvement whilst traversing the aortic wall.

Clinical features. *Uncomplicated aortitis.* This may be undiagnosable during life. There are no symptoms. The most characteristic siear calcification confined to the ascending aorta. This is especially significant under 40. The loud bell-like second sound which was thought to be characteristic of syphilitic aortitis, occurs also in hypertension.

Aortic regurgitation. This is three times as common as aneurysm. It follows extension of aortitis with widening of the commissures between the cusps and eversion of the free edges of the cusps which become rolled, retracted, stiff, and shortened. Eventually the left ventricle enlarges and hypertrophies. The coronary ostia are encroached upon by the raised intimal plaques and are also involved within the wall of the aorta which results in ostial stenosis and angina pectoris. Sudden death may occur in these patients.

The early features are chest pain and dyspnoea. Angina due to ostial stenosis is similar to that produced by coronary arteriosclerosis. For a long period the condition is well compensated though there may be palpitations, pounding in the ears, and pulsation felt in the neck. Eventually heart failure develops partly because of the strain on the left ventricle and partly because of coronal ostial stenosis. Paroxysmal dyspnoea at night ('syphilitic asthma') is an early symptom. Later there is dyspnoea on exertion and eventually orthopnoea with cough, weakness and right-sided heart failure.

The apical impulse is heaving and displaced downwards and markedly to the left. Radiographs will confirm the enlarged left ventricle. On auscultation the characteristic sign is a soft diastolic murmur with its intensity diminishing (diminuendo). It has been likened to the musical cooing of the seagull ('seagull murmur'). It often lasts throughout diastole. Generally the longer the diastolic murmur, the more severe the regurgitation. It is best heard over the mid- or lower sternum and to the right of the sternum and over the aortic area. If there is a haemic systolic murmur as well, one hears the 'to-and-fro' sound. A rough presystolic apical murmur (Austin–Flint) may be accompanied by a diastolic thrill. In practice it is rarely present. Peripheral signs include a low diastolic blood pressure and high pulse pressure. The diastolic pressure is 50 mmHg or even nil and the pulse pressure which is normally 30–50 mmHg is 80 mmHg or more. The pulse at the wrist strikes the finger sharply and briefly (Corrigan's pulse, collapsing pulse, waterhammer pulse). Visible arterial pulsation may be found in the neck, the temporal arteries, and also in the capillaries in the nail bed, the fundus, and the lips when it can be demonstrated by pressing a glass slide lightly against the lips. The 'pistol shot' femoral sound is a booming noise heard with each pulse over the femoral artery and is probably due to vibrations.

Coronary ostial stenosis. This may have to be considered in patients with uncomplicated syphilitic aortitis or aortic incompetence who also suffer from angina pectoris. In older patients, angina may be due to concomitant arteriosclerotic coronary disease. If surgery is contemplated, coronary angiography will differentiate between the strictly localized ostial stenosis of syphilis and arteriosclerotic coronary artery disease.

Aneurysm of the aorta. This may remain asymptomatic for years until pressure symptoms arise or it ruptures.

1. Aneurysm of the ascending aorta. This is also called 'aneurysm of signs'. It extends forward, upward and to the right and exerts pressure on the right bronchus, right lung, superior vena cava, and the second and third rib. It may attain large proportions and occasionally is seen and felt as a pulsatile mass in the chest wall. The diagnosis usually depends on radiographic findings. It may compress the lung and cause dullness on percussion. If it erodes the sternum or upper ribs, there will be pain. Pressure on the pulmonary artery may produce right heart failure. As the ascending aorta is mostly inside the pericardial sac, it may rupture into the pericardium.

2. *Aneurysm of the arch.* Also called 'aneurysm of symptoms'. The symptoms are due to compression of the various structures around the convex part of the arch and include the trachea, oesophagus, left recurrent laryngeal nerve, the sympathetic chain, and various blood vessels. Symptoms occur early and the patient may consult a laryngologist, gastroenterologist, or a chest physician. Chest pain is often constant due to pressure on nerves and erosion of bones. A brassy dry cough is due to pressure on the trachea or main bronchus and can lead to bronchiectasis and lung abscess. Dyspnoea is either due to pressure on the trachea or main bronchus and often causes an inspiratory stridor. Hoarseness is a consequence of pressure on the left recurrent laryngeal nerve. Haemoptysis follows erosion of the trachea or pulmonary infection. Dysphagia is associated with pressure on the oesophagus. Horner's

syndrome (myosis, enophthalmos, slight ptosis) is due to pressure on the sympathetic chain and is one of the many signs. They include also visible and palpable pulsation in the suprasternal notch, a pulsatile expanding mediastinal tumor seen on fluoroscopy, and a characteristic suffusion of the upper chest, neck, and face because of pressure on large vessels. Over the aneurysm there is a systolic thrill and diastolic shock. A tracheal tug is felt with every heart beat. The pulse at the wrists is often unequal, the right pulse being diminished and often delayed. The blood pressure is correspondingly lower on the right side because of pressure on the innominate artery. Death may occur from rupture into the trachea, pleura or mediastinum.

3. *Aneurysm of the descending aorta* is often silent and may attain huge proportions but it does not often rupture. Eventually symptoms develop due to pressure, giving rise to chest pain, dyspnoea, and cough. A sign often overlooked is visible pulsation posteriorly around the scapula.

4. *Abdominal aortic aneurysm.* This too may remain asymptomatic for years. Eventually a pulsating abdominal mass is felt. Symptoms are a very ominous feature as they are soon followed by rupture. The leading symptom is pain due to pressure on vertebrae and retroperitoneal nerves.

As radiology gives commonly the first evidence of an aortic aneurysm, a plain radiograph of the chest must be routinely performed in all patients with late syphilis.

Prognosis. The prognosis of aortic regurgitation and aneurysm was once considered to be universally bad with a life expectancy of three years after the diagnosis was made. It now appears that the prognosis is less gloomy. Lesions of cardiovascular syphilis are not infrequently found at autopsy in selected populations as a chance finding. It is estimated that in those with cardiovascular lesions, 30 per cent died as a direct result of it.

Syphilitic aortitis. The prognosis is good and only a few progress to aortic regurgitation. It has also been found that simple syphilitic aortitis was correctly diagnosed in only 5–10 per cent during life.

Syphilitic aortic regurgitation. The latent compensated period lasts between two and 10 years (average six years); 60 per cent die within 10 years.

Syphilitic aortic aneurysm. The latent period varies with the site and factors such as heavy manual labour. It is shortest with aneurysm of the arch, followed by aneurysm of the ascending aorta, and then descending aorta. The symptomatic stage lasts on average five years.

Bad prognostic points are:

1. Angina pectoris.

2. Congestive heart failure. Patients usually die in their third attack within two to three years from the first attack.

3. Aneurysmal pressure signs. Once it develops, the patient usually dies within a year.

4. Sudden unexpected death is associated with aortic regurgitation and syphilitic angina.

5. The prognosis is worse in Negroes.

6. It is also worse in patients continuing in a physically demanding job.

A rare *favourable* factor is the development of an organized clot in an aneurysm which will protect the vulnerable aortic wall from the blood pressure. Such patients may continue to live a fairly normal life.

The effect of treatment on the prognosis. The value of penicillin in cardiovascular syphilis has not been properly assessed. It has been suggested that it prevents progression and prolongs life though clearly cannot influence past mechanical damage which may be the deciding factor.

Congestive heart failure responds to the customary treatment and should be given before penicillin is administered, but the outlook remains poor.

According to some physicians syphilitic angina responds to the usual treatment as well as angina due to arteriosclerotis, others maintain that the response in syphilitic angina is inferior.

Cardiac surgery has already saved a number of patients's lives and is the most positive advance in the prognosis of established cardiovascular syphilis.

Congenital syphilis (see also page 5.487). Syphilis is transmitted to the fetus throughout pregnancy by the infected mother but lesions will only develop after the fourth month *in utero* when immunological competence of the fetus becomes established. The more recently the mother became infected, the more severe the infection of the fetus because treponemal bacteraemia of the mother will be at its height. The risk of fetal infection in this situation is about 90 per cent, it then decreases, but is still present for at least four years after the secondary stage in the mother. Treatment of the mother before the fourth month of pregnancy will ensure an undamaged and uninfected infant as the infection was cured before any permanent lesions may have developed in the fetus. If the mother remains untreated, early congenital syphilis may occur in a proportion of pregnancies. In later years, the infant may be born apparently healthy but develop late congenital syphilis or escape infection altogether. In these later years, a healthy baby may be born between two infected ones, probably because the maternal bacteraemia becomes sporadic and an uninfected infant may be the result of a pregnancy occurring between episodes of bacteraemia. Third generation syphilis has been reported but appears to be an unlikely event as the natural course of the untreated disease is such that by the time the patient with congenital syphilis is old enough to have her own child, she is non-infectious. Once a woman has been treated she is cured and cannot infect any subsequent fetuses.

Prevention depends largely on blood tests taken during pregnancy, especially as the clinical manifestations of syphilis are suppressed during pregnancy. The ideal would be to test the blood early in pregnancy and again in the last trimester in high-risk patients to diagnose syphilis acquired since the first test. As a compromise it is usual (and obligatory in the UK and in many other countries) to have one blood test, usually taken at the first antenatal attendance.

The incidence of congenital syphilis has dropped throughout the Western world and is now at a very low rate. A fair proportion of such cases occur when the mother comes to hospital in labour without having had any previous antenatal care.

The outlook for a baby when treatment is given late in pregnancy of an actively infected mother is variable. If the infection has already damaged the fetus, it may be irreversible and show itself as late symptomatic congenital syphilis. If infection occurs just before birth and no treatment is given to the mother, the baby may have fulminant congenital syphilis with a poor prognosis or much more likely to have early infection of moderate severity which responds very well to treatment. If the mother does receive treatment, the results are very good.

Most commonly the baby was infected sometime during early pregnancy and appears healthy at birth and develops signs of late congenital syphilis two years or more after birth. A considerable number escape all active signs of syphilis, but remain seropositive for many years or life—latent congenital syphilis.

Early congenital syphilis
1. Fulminant congenital syphilis at birth. Prognosis is poor. Rare.
2. The baby appears healthy at birth and develops signs of secondary syphilis 2–10 weeks after birth. Occasionally the onset may be delayed for months.
Clinical features. There is no primary sore. Commonly there is a symmetrical rash which may be bullous or papulosquamous. The bullous lesions contain a highly infectious fluid. The rash is especially prominent on the palms, soles, distal parts of the limbs, and face around the mouth and nose. The lesions become eroded on the face and condylomata lata may develop at the angle of the mouth.

Eventually the lesions heal leaving linear scars radiating from the angles of the mouth and each side of the nose('rhagades'). In the most severe cases there is also marasmus and failure to thrive giving the infant an 'old-man look'. The scalp hair may show alopecia or be overabundant. The nails are often shed and eye brows and eyelashes are absent. In the fulminant case the baby dies of intercurrent infection, hepatitis, or pulmonary haemorrhage.

Mucus patches occur in the nasopharynx and are highly infectious as are all open lesions at this stage. Nasal lesions give rise to rhinitis ('snuffles') and occurs early. The septum may be destroyed and give rise later on to the saddle nose.

Visceral lesions include hepatosplenomegaly producing an enlarged abdomen and more rarely a nephrosis with deposits of immune complexes on the glomeruli. Choroiditis may develop and produce the 'pepper and salt' appearance found later. It is sometimes associated with optic atrophy diagnosed in later years.

Meningitis is a rare complication and is usually mild.

Osteochondritis appears early and involves the metaphysis. It may lead to separation of the metaphysis and is usually seen after six months. Periostitis is more common and unlike osteochondritis which clears spontaneously within a few months, may remain active for much longer. Dactylitis is a very characteristic lesion involving the proximal phalanges of fingers and toes.

As mentioned, the open lesions are very infectious and *T. pallidum* can be easily demonstrated from them. Of the serological the FTA-IgM is the most valuable test as it may be positive at a very early time before any clinical manifestations of infection (but see later for its limitations). The VDRL may show a higher titre in the infant than in the mother in the presence of active disease.

Differential diagnosis. This is mainly from other infections such as rubella, cytomegalovirus infection, or toxoplasma infection.

Late congenital syphilis.   *Definition.* Lesions appearing for the first time two years or more after birth make up symptomatic late congenital syphilis. These lesions are not infectious. In over 60 per cent the conditions remains *latent* with a fixed positive serology which declines but may remain positive for life.

Clinical features. The cardiovascular system is rarely if ever involved. The reason for this is unknown. It extends to syphilis acquired in children below the age of 10. On the other hand CNS lesions are at least twice as common as in adult syphilis and have a much worse prognosis. Lesions not seen in acquired syphilis are interstitial keratitis (IK) and Clutton's joints. Eighth nerve deafness and optic atrophy occur in both acquired and congenital syphilis but appear to be more common in the latter. The age range is 2–30 and females appear to be more commonly seen with symptomatic or late latent syphilis. This may be misleading due to the fact that women are far more liable to have blood tests for syphilis as it is obligatory during pregnancy and may uncover unsuspected cases. Gumma of the skin is very unusual in congenital syphilis except in the oropharyngeal region where mucocutaneous gummata do occur and if they involve the palate or nasal septum, may produce perforations. The long bones may show osteoperiostitis with dense irregular new bone being deposited and producing, e.g. the sabre tibia. This is not due to bowing so much as rather due to accretion of bone over the middle third of the tibia which becomes wide with palpable irregularities along the shin. Local osteoperiostitis of the frontal and parietal bones of the skull produces bumps known as Parrot's nodes.

Interstitial keratitis (IK) is bilateral and may have its onset between 5–30. It starts with photophobia, lachrymation, discomfort, and soon one sees a circumcorneal injection with vessels growing into the deeper layers of the cornea. As it heals it may leave behind a ground-glass appearance and sometimes a dense white scar. If the scars are situated over the pupils, vision is grossly impaired or lost (Fig. 14).

Clutton's joints is a symmetrical painless synovitis of the knees which clears spontaneously. Eighth nerve deafness and optic atrophy: the mechanism of these lesions is unknown. Treponema-

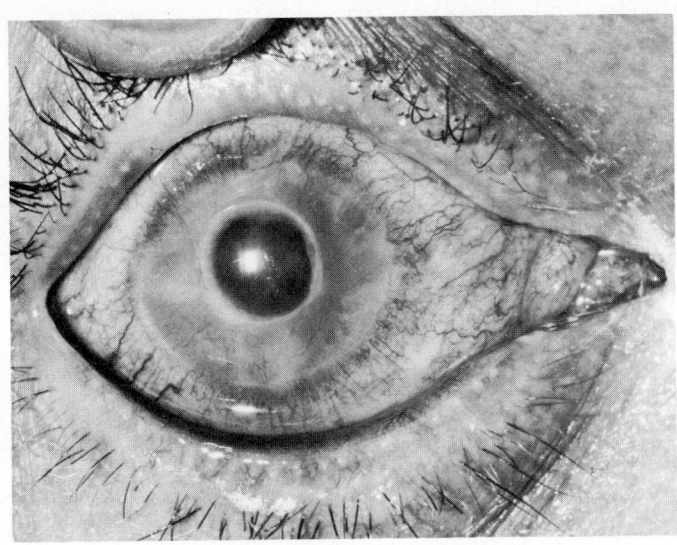

Fig. 14 Congenital syphilis: interstitial keratitis after corneal grafting.

like organisms have been found in the aqueous humour but their significance is uncertain. It has often been suggested that immune defects may play a part in their development. This receives some support by the fact that whilst penicillin has no effect on these lesions, corticosteroids are most effective in suppressing the symptoms of IK and thus saving sight.

Neurosyphilis. At least 15 per cent of children with late congenital syphilis develop neurosyphilis. This may take the form of asymptomatic neurosyphilis as in adults, vascular neurosyphilis (very rare) which may lead to cranial nerve palsies, monoplegia, or hemiplegia with minimal changes in the CSF, and the parenchymatous forms: GPI usually arises between 8–15 years and is much more intractable than the acquired type. It has been suggested that a special neurogenic treponeme is involved, as a significantly higher proportion of neurosyphilis is seen in a parent of such a child. The clinical features are similar to the adult GPI except that simple mental deterioration is particularly common and progressive. Epileptiform fits are also seen. *Locomotor ataxia* (tabes dorsalis) is very rare and occurs between 12–20. The pupils show a variety of abnormalities but the classical Argyll Robertson pupil is less frequent. It may be associated with eighth nerve deafness often with labyrinthitis. At first, appreciation of high frequency notes is lost and it may progress to total deafness. When congenital syphilis was common, the combination of nerve deafness, optic atrophy, and mental deficiency was recognized as a triad; this appears to be now only of historical interest.

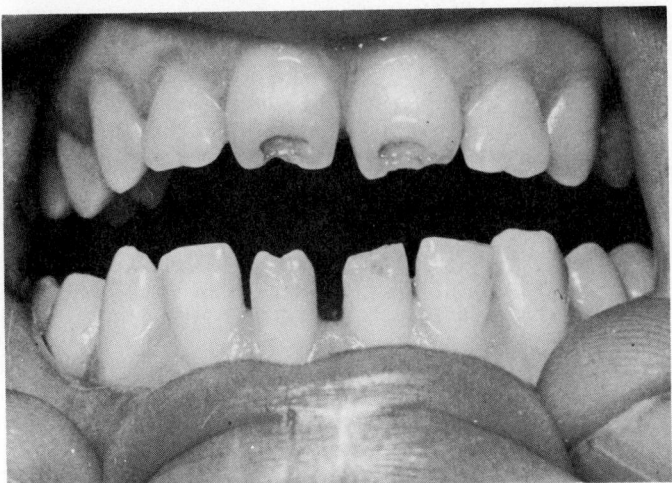

Fig. 15 Hutchinson's teeth in congenital syphilis. Note the gaps between the incisors.

The stigmata. Some stigmata are due to intrauterine infection, others are the result of lesions occurring after birth.

1. The entire skeleton is underdeveloped with poor moulding and with defects. The stature is small.

2. Hutchinson's teeth: there is central notching of the central upper incisors due to defective development of the middle column of cells of the permanent incisors *in utero*. The result is not only the notch, but also a narrowing of the biting surface (peg-shaped teets) and a widening of the gaps between the teeth (Fig. 15).

3. Moon's molar. The first molar show poorly shaped cusps. The teeth are generally defective and rarely last for more than 20 years.

4. The face. This is characteristically flat due to underdeveloped maxillae. In addition there may be the frontal bosses (Parrot's nodes), a saddle nose, Hutchinson teeth, and rhagades (linear scars radiating from the angle of the mouth and side of the nose). This gives such congenital children a family resemblance.

5. As the pelvis is often underdeveloped, this may cause obstetric difficulties in later life: and as the vertebrae and intervertebral discs are poorly developed in some of these individuals, lumbar puncture can be quite difficult.

It is generally found that children with congenital syphilis, even if asymptomatic, do less well in school and work than their unaffected siblings, a fact which may lead to considerable difficulties in the family.

Serology. The FTA-ABS is the most constantly positive test followed by TPI and VDRL.

Laboratory diagnosis of syphilis

Dark-field microscopy. Dark-field microscopy of wet-mounted material from the chancre or open lesions of early acquired or congenital syphilis should show the *T. pallidum* without difficulty. Sometimes it is negative in the presence of lesions. This may be due to recent use of antiseptics on the lesion, to a small number of treponemes being present, or in cases of reinfection. In any case, the examination should be repeated two to three times before accepting a negative result. Needle aspirates from regional lymph nodes may be successful when direct examination of the sore is difficult or when the sore has healed. In view of the excellent serological tests available, this procedure is now rarely used.

Animal inoculation. Animal inoculation with material from late lesions or in cases of 'persistent *T. pallidum*-like forms' is usually reserved for research purposes.

Serology. Two classes of antibodies are found: (*a*) non-specific reagin antibodies (IgG and IgM); and (*b*) specific antitreponemal antibodies.

The reagin antibodies act on lipoidal antigen which results from action on *T. pallidum* on host tissue. The antigen used contains cardiolipin, cholesterol, and lecithin.

The specific antigen is derived from *T. pallidum*. The specific tests do not differentiate between past or present infection and are therefore of no value to assess activity.

The interpretation of the tests is given in Table 1.

Currently used serological tests for syphilis. *Reagin antibody tests*
1. Rapid plasma reagin (RPR) test. This can be automated and is useful for screening purposes.

2. VDRL test. This is a quantitative test and as the titres reflect activity, it is of great value for this purpose. It may, for example, be the only evidence of re-infection in a patient with previous syphilis whose VDRL was either negative or weakly positive after treatment. A sharp sustained rise of the titre four-fold or higher even in the absence of clinical signs is good evidence of active infection. False positive VDRL is usually of a low titre (1:8 or less). It becomes positive during the primary stage and rises to its maximum during the secondary stage (1:32 or more). After successful treatment, the titre declines (1:4 or less), and if treatment was given

Table 1 Interpretation of serological tests in syphilis

Diagnosis	VDRL	Titre	TPHA	FTA–ABS IgG	FTA–ABS IgM	Comment
Early untreated primary syphilis	+or−	rising	+or−	+	+	FTA–ABS is the first test to become +. VDRL − in 30%
Untreated late primary or secondary syphilis or reinfection or untreated or recently treated late syphilis	+	high or rising	+	+	+	
Untreated latent syphilis	+or−	moderate	+	+	+	
Treated early syphilis	−		+or−	−	−	
Treated latent syphilis	+or−	low	+or−	−	−	
Neurosyphilis any type, treated or untreated or cardiovascular syphilis	+or−	varies	+or−	+	+	CSF: FTA–ABS often +. VDRL − in 30%
Active gumma (skin, mucosa, bone)	+	varies	+	+	+	
Early congenital syphilis	+	rising	+	+	+	in some infants, tests may be negative for weeks until immunologically more mature
Passive transfer of maternal antibodies	+	same or lower than mother	−	+	−	FTA–ABS IgM: see also text under congenital syphilis
Late congenital syphilis	+	low or moderate	+	+	+	
Biological false positive reaction	+	low	−	−	−	FTA–ABS may be weakly positive

False positive reaction: VDRL will be of low titre. TPHA may give false positive results in 2 per cent. FTA–ABS may give borderline positive in pregnancy and systemic lupus. TPI negative in such problem sera.

early in the disease it often becomes negative. An occasional small and transient rise in titre is of no significance.

Specific antitreponemal tests

1. *T. pallidum* immobilization (TPI) test. This was the first truly specific test in which live treponemes are used. When the organism is mixed with serum from a patient with syphilis, at least 50 per cent of the *T. pallidum* are immobilized (i.e. killed as seen under the microscope). It is still the most specific of all serological procedures and sets the standard against which other specific tests are compared. It is the last to become positive in early syphilis but remains positive for long periods of time after successful treatment. It is therefore of no use to evaluate activity. The test is complex, cumbersome and expensive and is now only performed in a few specialized centres.

2. The *T. pallidum* haemagglutination (TPHA) test is a very valuable and simple test using an indirect haemagglutination method with red cells sensitized by sonicated *T. pallidum* extract. It is almost as specific as the TPI but is less sensitive than the FTA-ABS. False positive reactions occur in up to 2 per cent. The micromethod is particularly suitable for screening purposes. Together with the VDRL it is probably the best combination for routine use. In cases of doubt the FTA-ABS is added. TPHA can be adapted for automation.

3. The FTA-ABS test. This uses the indirect fluorescent technique with killed *T. pallidum* as antigen. The organisms are fixed on a slide to which the serum is added. The antibody in the serum will unite with the treponemes and this can be made visible by adding anti-human globulin conjugated with a fluorescent stain which attaches itself and produces fluorescence of the treponemes seen by fluorescent microscope. The test has been made more specific by absorbing the group antibodies with Reiter's treponemes. The test is then called FTA-ABS. The FTA-ABS is the most sensitive test available and is also specific. It becomes positive earlier during the primary stage of syphilis than other procedures. It is not suitable to assess activity as it persists long after successful treatment. The FTA-ABS-IgM may prove to be better in this respect but not all the difficulties have been removed. It may be positive in biologically false reactions.

When the routine serology includes the VDRL and TPHA, the FTA-ABS may be added in cases of problem sera.

4. The FTA-ABS-IgM test in the diagnosis of congenital syphilis. IgG is a small molecule and passes through the placenta, thus the baby may inherit maternal IgG but not necessarily the infection. Tests such as the VDRL may therefore be positive in the newborn

by passive transfer and may take three months to disappear. IgM is a large molecule and does not pass through the placenta, thus if it is found in the neonate, it must be assumed that it is produced by the infected infant. When this test was introduced there were great expectations that neonatal syphilis could be diagnosed rapidly and at a very early period. This promise has not been entirely fulfilled as the immune mechanism of the infant may be immature leading to a delay of IgM production, furthermore IgM-anti-IgG may be elaborated by the infant with rubella, toxoplasmosis, and cytomegalovirus infections giving a false positive reaction. This somewhat limits the value of this test, and in cases of doubt it is best to treat the infant rather than await events.

Biological false-positive tests for syphilis. They concern mainly the reagin tests and are classified as acute if they become negative within six months. They are associated with a number of bacterial and viral infections including mycoplasma pneumonia, infectious mononeucleosis, and following smallpox vaccination. They are chronic if they persist for longer than six months and occur in about 20 per cent of drug addicts, auto-immune disease when they may precede the symptoms by years, leprosy, and in a small proportion of people over 70. The TPI is always negative and the other specific tests are either negative or weakly positive.

The management of syphilis

Suggestions for drug treatment of syphilis are given in Table 2. As soon as a diagnosis of infectious syphilis has been made, the patient should be interviewed by the social worker regarding all sexual contacts. In the case of primary syphilis this should cover the previous three months, in patients with secondary syphilis this should be extended to one year, and in patients with *early* latent syphilis to two years because of the possibility of infectious relapses during that period. The patient is warned against intercourse during treatment and for a further two weeks. Experience suggests that advice for longer abstinence will be disregarded in many cases and is almost certainly unnecessary.

If the patient gives no history of penicillin allergy, it is the first choice for the treatment of all stages of the disease. Sir Alexander Fleming predicted that penicillin would continue to be effective against syphilis even if not necessarily for other infections and he has proved to be right. Penicillin is as effective now as it was almost 40 years ago when first introduced. If there is penicillin allergy, the alternative drugs are tetracycline and erythromycin. Cephalosporins are also effective but there is cross-allergy with penicillin in

5–7 per cent of patients and it is therefore not advised. These alternative drugs have not been fully evaluated or compared with penicillin to assess their value and some of their drawbacks, notably the poor concentration in the brain and in the fetus are briefly mentioned in the table on treatment.

Table 2 Recommended treatment for syphilis

Diagnosis	Treatment
Primary, secondary, latent syphilis and early re-infections	aqueous procaine penicillin G 900 000 units/day × 8 days; some advise 1 million units/day × 8 days i.m. *If allergic to penicillin*: erythromycin stearate 1 g twice daily × 14 days *or* tetracycline hydrochloride 2 g daily × 14 days *If pregnant and allergic to penicillin*: erythromycin as above
Asymptomatic or symptomatic neurosyphilis*	aqueous procaine penicillin G 900 000 units/day × 14 days i.m. *or* aqueous penicillin G 12–24 million units/day × 10 days i.v. *If allergic to penicillin*: erythromycin stearate 1 g twice daily × 30 days *or* tetracycline 2 g daily × 30 days
Cardiovascular syphilis or benign tertiary syphilis*†	aqueous procain penicillin G 900 000 units/day × 10 days i.m. *If allergic to penicillin*: erythromycin or tetracycline as above
Early congenital syphilis (including *suspected* early congenital syphilis)	aqueous penicillin G 50 000 units/kg × 10 days i.m. (use only penicillin in congenital syphilis). If mother received erythromycin during pregnancy, treat the infant with a course of penicillin
Late congenital syphilis	aqueous penicillin G—dose according to age and equivalent to acquired syphilis of the same stage
Interstitial keratitis	0.5% prednisolone eye drops, 1 drop 1–2 hourly until condition controlled
Optic atrophy (congenital or acquired)	penicillin as for late stage
Eighth nerve deafness	penicillin as for late stage + corticosteroid
Iridocyclitis (early or late)	penicillin as for the appropriate stage + 1% atropine eye drops; consult ophthalmologist
Syphilis of the tongue	penicillin as for late syphilis and consult ENT specialist for regular follow-up

* In patients with gumma of the larynx, late neurosyphilis, especially general paresis, and cardiovascular syphilis, especially with angina try to minimize any Herxheimer reaction by covering the first injection of penicillin with corticosteroid started the day before injection

† In patient diagnosed as symptomatic cardiovascular syphilis consult cardiac surgeon from the start with a view to possible cardiac surgery (removal of coronary ostial stenosis, aortic valve replacement, repair or replacement of aneurysmal aortic segment). If there is congestive heart failure treat it before giving penicillin

The optimal dose or duration of treatment with penicillin or the other drugs has not been established and therefore a great variety of treatment schemes have been put forward but the results appear to be similar. This suggests that a fair degree of variation is permissible. The general tendency is to treat with larger doses and over a longer period of time in the later stages of syphilis and some prefer to repeat the course. There is no convincing evidence that large, much extended or repeated courses give any added benefit.

There is good experimental evidence that serum concentrations of penicillin should be at least 0.03 µg/ml and should be maintained for 7–10 days and that troughs in the concentration should not exceed 15 hours.

Some physicians prefer a single injection of the long-acting benzathin penicillin (2.4 million units) for the sake of simplicity, but the concentration reached is low and does not give a useful level in the CSF, also the injection is quite painful. Others repeat this dose a week later. We prefer not to use this preparation; in exceptional circumstances where a patient is unable to attend more than once and is unable to continue treatment elsewhere, it may be justified but as an alternative one could give the full course of erythromycin or tetracycline.

Procaine penicillin has several advantages over other penicillin preparations and is preferred by many. In some centres the course is 1 million units/day for 10 days in others it is given for 20 days though evidence that such a prolonged course gives better results is lacking.

Procaine penicillin in 2 per cent aluminium monostearate (PAM) has a prolonged action and was used extensively by the WHO in their mass campaign against non-venereal syphilis with good results. It is still being used for venereal syphilis in a few centres.

Penicillin reactions. All patients receiving penicillin injections should be kept in the clinic for 15–20 minutes as severe reactions needing immediate treatment will develop well within this period. An emergency tray to deal with anaphylactic penicillin reaction must be readily available wherever penicillin is given. It should contain ampoules of 1:1000 adrenaline solution, syringes and needles, intravenous hydrocortisone, injectable antihistamine, aminophylline, an airway, respirator (Ambubag or Brooke's respirator), and oxygen with face mask or nasal catheter.

Prevention of penicillin reactions. Some 3–5 per cent of the population in the UK are allergic to penicillin and it is essential to enquire about this and if there is a history, penicillin must not be given. This fact should be displayed prominently on the cover of the medical notes and the patient told to inform any doctor who may wish to give this antibiotic. Careful history taking may, however, show that the 'allergy' to penicillin is doubtful, e.g. the rash antedated the giving of penicillin and may have been due to one of the childhood infections. It is quite common to be told that patients who apparently did have a penicillin reaction, had no problems when the antibiotic was inadvertently given subsequently. In such cases we still prefer to avoid giving penicillin.

Clinical features. The most serious reaction is *anaphylactic shock* appearing immediately or within a minute or two after the injection. The more immediate the onset, the more severe the attack. The patient becomes unconscious, stops breathing, and becomes pulseless. Very rarely the patient dies immediately. A fatal outcome is estimated to occur one or two times per 100 000 injections. In the more moderate reaction the patient feels faint with acute anxiety and a feeling of impending death; there may be oedema of the face, possibly with an asthmatic attack, soon followed by urticaria. Arthralgia and some pyrexia may develop. The urticaria is liable to last one to two weeks.

The commonest form is the delayed reaction when urticaria appears days after injection or oral penicillin. Arthralgia and fever may develop.

Sometimes a local reaction around the injection site is seen. It can be urticarial but is more commonly a painful red swelling and usually responds to rest. It is best to discontinue the course as recurrences are otherwise common.

In some patients a hysterical episode follows an injection and may be due to procaine or possibly inadvertant intravenous injection. It passes off spontaneously.

Treatment of the anaphylactic reaction. The patient is laid flat with feet up and head down. Blood pressure and pulse are monitored throughout. Adrenaline 1:1000 (0.5–1.0 ml) is given intramuscularly without delay. If bronchospasm develops, 250 mg aminophylline in 10 ml water is administered by slow intravenous injection. Intravenous hydrocortisone may also be tried (Efcortesol, Solu-cortef) and may be repeated. Some prefer intravenous antihistamine (Piriton injection 10–20 mg). Adrenaline, nevertheless, is the mainstay of treatment. If there is no response, the cardiac arrest team is summoned. If recovery is slow, the patient should be admitted as recurrences may occur occasionally. In any case the patient must be kept under observation for several hours. Later, urticaria develops in most patients and antihistamines by mouth are indicated.

Treatment of the delayed reaction. The leading feature is urticaria, possibly with oedema of the face, arthralgia, and some fever. Such patients respond to oral antihistamines such as chlorpheniramine (Piriton) 4 mg four times daily or promethazine (Phenergan) 25 mg twice daily until the condition is controlled. If it is very severe, prednisolone 10 mg four times daily may be added for a few days, reducing it as soon as possible. Penicillinase is not recommended as it may produce reactions of its own.

Vasovagal attacks. This occurs most commonly in young men following intramuscular injection or after having blood taken. The patient looks very pale and may faint. He may slump to the floor and occasionally go stiff and have jerky movements. The most important diagnostic sign is a slow pulse. Recovery is rapid once he is laid flat on a couch. There is a tendency for recurrence in the same individual under similar circumstances and this can easily be prevented by giving injections or taking blood whilst the patient is lying down.

The Jarisch–Herxheimer reaction. This systemic reaction is believed to be due to the release of endotoxin when large numbers of *T. pallidum* are killed by antibiotics. It is mainly associated with early syphilis. The incidence of the reaction appears to be related to the total number of the organism in the body. The mechanism may not be straightforward as it is not a feature of neonatal syphilis or non-venereal syphilis in childhood.

It can be expected in 50 per cent of primary syphilis, 90 per cent of secondary syphilis, and in 25 per cent of early latent infection. It is very rare in late syphilis.

The reaction begins 4–12 hours after the first injection, lasts for a few hours or up to a day, and is not seen with subsequent treatment. There is malaise, slight to moderate pyrexia, a flush due to vasodilation, tachycardia, leucocytosis, and existing lesions become more prominent. In some patients with early syphilis, a secondary rash may become visible which was absent before treatment.

In early syphilis the reaction is only a minor nuisance. In late syphilis it can on very rare occasions be more serious. Thus in neurosyphilis it may lead to a rapid irreversible progression, and in general paresis it can cause exacerbation amounting to temporary psychosis. Sudden death has been reported in cardiovascular syphilis. In laryngeal gumma, local oedema may necessitate tracheotomy.

It is customary to give corticosteroids in late symptomatic syphilis starting a day before the first penicillin injection and tailing it off the day after injection. This does not prevent the Herxheimer reaction but is said to ameliorate it.

We never withold penicillin in late syphilis because of the remote chance of a reaction, nor do we give small initial doses as it is not dose-related. The patient with early syphilis should be warned about the possibility of mild indisposition on the day of the first injection and be advised to go to bed and take some aspirins.

Follow-up. It is generally sufficient to perform blood tests 1, 3, 6, and 12 months after treatment of *early syphilis.*

In *late symptomatic syphilis,* surveillance is for life. The frequency of attendance must be adapted to the condition; thus in patients with leucoplakia of the tongue, a regular check-up every three months is recommended or at any time between, should the lesions increase. In symptomatic cardiovascular syphilis regular radiological and clinical examination is essential to determine any change which might suggest the need for cardiac surgery. In neurosyphilis the follow-up varies with individual needs and an annual review might be adequate. There is no consensus of opinion about the follow-up in *latent syphilis.* However, if there is a satisfactory serological response, a period of two to three years seems reasonable. In *early congenital* syphilis the observation time should be similar to that of early acquired syphilis. In *late symptomatic congenital syphilis* follow-up varies individually. In *late latent congenital syphilis* no further attendance is necessary unless symptoms of interstitial keratitis or other lesions not prevented by penicillin develop.

In high risk patients such as male homosexuals and prostitutes a regular check-up every three months for syphilis and other sexually transmitted diseases is advised. In special circumstances the interval may have to be much shorter. If such patients have had syphilis, the VDRL should have become negative or of a low titre after treatment, if the titre suddenly rises fourfold or more, re-infection must be assumed and treated accordingly.

Prophylaxis and abortive treatment. In the USA it is recommended to treat asymptomatic contacts of early syphilis as there is a 50 per cent chance of infection. Such pre-emptive treatment is likely to reduce the spread of infection in the promiscuous or those likely to infect their spouses or regular sexual partners and is also indicated in persons known to be unreliable attenders. Such patients, however, should be impressed to keep to the simple follow-up schedule of early syphilis. We follow this practice and believe that this is an important measure in certain communities in reducing the spread of infection. It is only fair to state that opinion in the UK is divided and some feel strongly that treatment before diagnosis is 'second-rate medicine'.

The proper use of condoms will do much to prevent infection of all forms of sexually transmitted diseases and should be recommended to all those most likely to get infected. It is unfortunately these very people who often find this advice unacceptable.

Various vaginal chemical spermicidal creams give a small degree of protection but are quite unreliable in this respect.

References

Abel, E., Marks, R., and Wilson-Jones, E. (1973). Secondary syphilis: A clinico-pathological reappraisal. *Br. J. Derm.* **89,** suppl. 9, 19.

Csonka, G. W. (1975). Sudomotor reaction in neurosyphilis. *Br. J. vener. Dis.* **33,** 168.

Felton, W. F. (1973). Estimate of annual incidence of undiagnosed syphilis. *Br. J. vener. Dis.* **49,** 249.

Hager, W. D. (1978). Transplacental transmission of spirochaetes in congenital syphilis: A new perspective. *Sex. transmitted Dis.* **5,** 122.

Harris, J. R. W. (ed.) (1981). Clinical syphilis. In *Recent advances in sexually transmitted diseases.* Churchill Livingstone, Edinburgh.

Harter, C. A. and Benitschke, K. (1979). Fetal syphilis in the first trimester. *Am. J. Obstet. Gynaec.* **124,** 705.

Kiraly, K. and Prerau, H. (1974). Evaluation of the *T. pallidum* haemagglutination (TPHA) test for syphilis on 'problem sera'. *Acta derm.* **54,** 303.

Luger, A., Schmidt, B. and Spendlingswimmer, I. (1977). Quantitative evaluation of the FTA-ABS IgM and VDRL test in treated and untreated syphilis. *Br. J. vener. Dis.* **53,** 287.

Luxon, L., Lees, A. J. and Greenwood, R. J. (1979). Neurosyphilis today. *Lancet* **i,** 90.

McCracken, G. H. and Kaplan, J. M. (1974). Penicillin treatment for congenital syphilis. A critical reappraisal. *J. Am. med. Ass.* **228,** 855.

Traviout, E. C. (1976). Persistence of *Treponema pallidum* following penicillin G therapy. Report of two cases. *J. Am. med. Ass.* **236,** 204.

Turner, T. B., Hardy, P. H., Newman, B. and Nell, E. E. (1973). Effect of passive immunization of experimental syphilis in the rabbit. *Johns Hopkins Med. J.* **133,** 241.

Wilkinson, A. E. (1981). Routine diagnostic procedures in treponemal diseases. In *Recent advances in sexually transmitted diseases* (ed. J. R. W. Harris). Churchill Livingstone, Edinburgh.

Willcox, R. R. (1974). Changing pattern of treponemal disease. *Br. J. vener. Dis.* **50,** 169.

Yoder, F. W. (1973). Penicillin treatment of neurosyphilis. Are recommended dosages sufficient? *J. Am. med. Ass.* **232,** 270.

Rat bite fevers

D. A. Warrell

Rat bites occur in most parts of the world. In some places they are quite common. For example, in Baltimore, USA, between 1948 and 1952, 322 bites were reported in a population of 900 000 people. Sixty per cent of the victims were less than six years old and 25 per cent less than one year old; 80 per cent were bitten while asleep. During that period the following rat-related diseases occurred in Baltimore: endemic typhus, sodoku, Haverhill fever, leptospirosis, and *Pasteurella multocida* infection. Two different pathogens, commonly transmitted by rodent bites, give rise to acute severe and relapsing febrile illnesses, both known as rat bite fever.

Streptobacillus moniliformis **infection, rat bite fever, Haverhill fever.** *Streptobacillus moniliformis* (synonyms include *Actinomyces muris*, *Actinobacillus muris*, and *Streptothrix muris ratti*) can be recovered from the nasopharynx, middle ear, and saliva of up to 50 per cent of wild and laboratory rats. Many of these animals seem to be healthy carriers but the organism can produce severe illnesses in rodents with septicaemia, pneumonia, polyarthritis, and abortion. The organism has also been isolated from mice, squirrels, and turkeys, and animals which feed on rodents such as cats, dogs and weasles.

S. moniliformis derives its name from the filaments and chains with yeast-like swellings seen in mature cultures on solid media. It is a Gram-negative, non-motile, pleomorphic rod, 1–5 μm long which requires blood, serum, or ascitic fluid for growth. L_1 variants occur which lack a cell wall and are therefore resistant to penicillin. The organism has been cultured from patients' bite wound, blood, synovial fluid, pericardial fluid, and from abscesses. In blood cultures, fluffy-ball-like growths appear at the surface of the sedimented red cells after three to eight days incubation.

Epidemiology. The disease occurs worldwide as a result of bites by rodents or their predators, or contact with live or dead mammals. Laboratory staff who work with rats are at special risk. The risk of infection following bites by wild rats is thought to be about 10 per cent. Haverhill fever, named after a town in Massachusetts, results from drinking milk contaminated by rats.

Clinical features. After an incubation period of less than 10 days there is sudden high fever with rigors, headache, and myalgia. A few days later a diffuse macular or purpuric rash develops which may involve the palms and soles. There is migratory arthralgia or arthritis, usually involving the knees and often resulting in effusions. The bite heals permanently and is not associated with much local lymphadenitis or lymphadenopathy. There is no recurrent inflammation or breakdown of the bite wound during the febrile illness. Fever and symptoms subside in a few days in treated cases and in one to two weeks in untreated ones. Bacteraemia can result in abscess formation (including cerebral abscess), pneumonia, endocarditis, pericarditis, and anaemia. Haverhill fever (erythema arthriticum epidemicum) follows the same clinical course after the patient has drunk unpasteurized milk. The untreated mortality is 10–13 per cent. Relapses are less common than in sodoku but may occur at intervals of a few weeks for several months.

Diagnosis. The diagnosis can be confirmed by cutting the organism and by detecting a high or rising titre of agglutinins, complement fixing, or fluorescent antibodies.

Spirillum minor, **sodoku, sokosha.** *Spirillum minor* (formerly known as *S. minus*) is a thick, tightly coiled, spirochaete 5 μm long which darts about under the power of its polar flagella. The organism has been found in blood and conjunctival discharge of up to 25 per cent of rats. Continuous culture on artificial media has not yet been achieved, but the organism can be demonstrated by inoculating material from the bite wound, regional lymph nodes or blood, intraperitoneally in mice or guinea pigs.

Epidemiology. Sodoku is a worldwide infection which results from bites or other wounds inflicted by rodents or their predators, including pigs.

Clinical features. After an incubation period of 5–30 (average 7) days there is sudden fever, reaching its height in three days, and resolving by crisis after a further three days. Acute symptoms include rigors, myalgia, and prostration. At the start of the illness the healed bite wound becomes inflamed and breaks down with lymphadenitis and tender local lymphadenopathy. A macular or papular exanthem is generalized or most marked near the bite wound. Arthralgia may be severe but there are no joint effusions. Meningitic or encephalitic symptoms develop in 10 per cent of cases. Relapses of fever and symptoms lasting three to six days may occur between remissions of a week or so, or even up to a year, and recur on six to eight occasions. The untreated mortality is about 6 per cent. Severe manifestations outside the central nervous system include endocarditis, myocarditis, and involvement of liver, kidney, and other organs.

Diagnosis. This can be confirmed by examining aspirate from the bite wound, lymph node, exanthem, or blood by dark field, or by staining with Giesma. Spirochaetes can be detected in the blood, peritoneal fluid or heart muscle of inoculated rodents. No serological test is available: false positive serological tests for syphilis and reactions with proteus OXK are common.

Differential diagnosis of rat bite fevers. An acute, severe febrile illness following rat bite, or other contact with rodents, should raise the possibility of other rodent-related infections such as *Pasteurella multocida,* plague, tularaemia leptospirosis, murine, typhus, and arenaviruses such as lymphocytic choriomeningitis and Lassa viruses. In the cases where rodent contact was not apparent the differential diagnosis is broadened to include other rickettsial diseases such as Rocky Mountain spotted fever, meningococcaemia, chlamydial, and viral infections.

Treatment. Penicillin is the drug of choice for *Spirillum minor* and *Streptobacillus moniliformis* infections. For adults, procaine benzyl penicillin 600 000 units should be given 12-hourly for 7–14 days. Streptomycin or tetracycline can be used for penicillin-resistant L variants of *Streptobacillus moniliformis*. Erythromycin, chloramphenicol, and cephalosporins are also effective. Patients with endocarditis should be treated with a daily dose of 8–24 million units of benzylpenicillin intravenously for four to six weeks. A Jarisch–Herxheimer reaction may follow the antimicrobial treatment of *Spirillum minor* infection.

Prevention. These infections can be prevented by eradicating rats, by preventing rat bites to laboratory workers by ensuring correct handling techniques and the use of gloves, and by cleaning all rodent bite wounds and giving penicillin.

References

Brown, R. McP. and Nunemaker, J. C. (1942). Rat-bite fever: a review of the American cases with re-evaluation of etiology: report of cases: *Bull. Johns Hopkins Hosp.* **70**, 201.

Roughgarden, J. W. (1965). Antimicrobial therapy of rat bite fever; a review. *Archs intern. Med.* **116**, 39.

McCormack, R. C., Kaye, D., and Hook, E. W. (1967). Endocarditis due to Streptobacillus moniliformis. *J. Am. Med. Ass.* **200**, 77.

Borrelia infections

D. A. Warrell

The borreliae are large, loosely coiled, motile spirochaetes. *B. vincenti* has, with *Fusobacterium (Bacteroides) fusiforme,* been implicated in acute necrotizing ulcerative gingivitis and Vincent's angina. *B. recurrentis* is the cause of louse-borne relapsing fever, while tick-borne relapsing fever is caused by a number of species or groups of *Borrelia*, for example *B. duttoni* and *B. crocidurae* in Africa, and *B. hermsi*, *B. turicatae*, *B. parkeri*, and *B. mazzotti* in the USA.

Vincent's angina and acute necrotizing ulcerative gingivitis

B. vincenti is 4–20 μm long with three to eight coils and 10 axial filaments. The spirochaetes can be demonstrated, often accompanied by large banded fusiform bacilli, in pus from ulcerative and necrotic lesions on the gums, oropharynx, tonsils, glans penis, skin (cancrum oris), and lung abscess, and sputum from patients with bronchiectasis. Smears can be stained with dilute carbol fuchsin or Romanovsky stains or examined under dark ground. The organisms can be cultured under anaerobic conditions in digest broth enhanced with ascitic fluid. *B. vincenti*, *B. buccalis*, and a small oral treponeme were found to have weak endotoxin activity. Penicillin is the treatment of choice for these borreliae. A Jarisch–Herxheimer reaction is described. Clinical details are given in the sections on oral and dental infections.

References

Mergenhagen, S. E., Hampp, E. G., and Scherp, H. W. (1961). Preparation and biological activities of endotoxins from oral bacteria. *J. infect. Dis.* **108**, 304.

Williams, R. H. (1941). Fuso spirochaetes. Recovery of the causative organisms from the blood, with report of two cases. *Archs intern. Med.* **68**, 80.

Relapsing fever

The borreliae which cause relapsing fever are spirochaetes 8–40 μm long and 0.2–0.5 μm thick with 3–10 coils and a number of axial filaments. Flagella have been described in some strains. These motile organisms divide by transverse binary fission. They can be stained in blood films (Fig. 1) by a wide variety of routine methods including Giemsa, Leishman, and Romanovsky stains. Wright's stain is rapid and convenient. Dark ground examination can also be used. Five species of *Borrelia* including *B. recurrentis* have now been cultured in an artificial medium. *Borrelia* can also be cultured on chick chorioallantoic membrane and perpetuated in rodents and ticks.

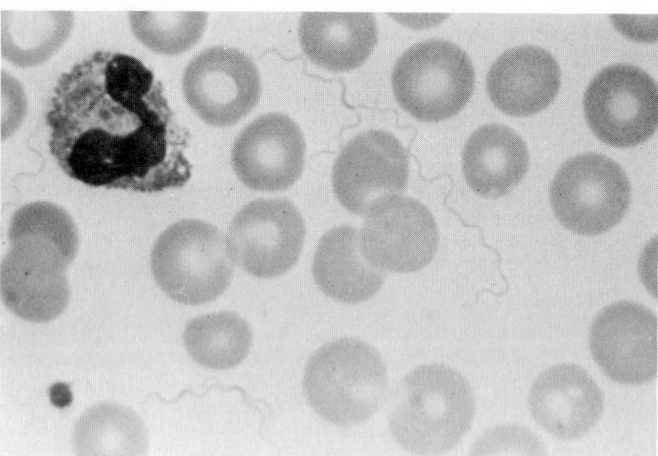

Fig. 1 *Borrelia recurrentis* spirochaetes in a Giemsa-stained thin blood film from a patient with louse-borne relapsing fever. (Photograph copyright Dr D. A. Warrell)

Epidemiology

Louse-borne (epidemic) relapsing fever. The human body louse, *Pedunculus humanus*, the sole vector, becomes infected while feeding on blood from a human patient. The louse's infected haemolymph may be inoculated through the skin by scratching, but spirochaetes can also penetrate intact skin: in this way a new infection can arise. Lice move from person to person when there is crowding and poor hygiene. When the host's surface body temperature deviates far from 37 °C, as a result of death, fever or exposure, or if infested clothing is discarded, the louse is forced to find a new host. The chaos of war, famine, and other disasters favours the spread of lice and epidemic louse-borne infections such as relapsing fever and typhus. The yellow plague in Europe in AD 550 and the famine fevers of the seventeenth and eighteenth centuries were probably relapsing fever. During the first half of the present century it is estimated that there were at least 50 million cases with a 10 per cent mortality. Epidemics occurred in Europe, the Middle East and the northern third of Africa, starting in 1903, 1923, and 1943. The major endemic focus of the disease persists in the highlands of Ethiopia where there is an annual epidemic coinciding with the cool, rainy season, when people are forced to wear lice infested clothes and crowd together into shelters. An annual incidence of 10 000 cases in Ethiopia seems likely. Recent outbreaks have occurred in the Sudan, West Africa and Vietnam. Other endemic foci may exist in the Balkans, Peruvian Andes, and China.

Tick-borne (endemic) relapsing fever. There is a close, but not exclusive, relationship between the species of *Borrelia*, their soft (argasid) tick vectors and reservoirs (genus *Ornithodoros*), and mammal reservoir species. For example, in Africa, the domestic tick *O. moubata* transmits *B. duttoni* between humans, and in the western USA *O. hermsi*, a parasite of chipmunks and other tree squirrels, transmits *B. hermsi* to humans. Tick-borne relapsing fever has occurred in most continents except Australasia and the Pacific region. Cases are usually isolated and sporadic but in 1968, 11 out of a group of 42 boy scouts were infected on Browne Mountain, Washington, USA while camping in rodent-infested cabins, and in 1973 there were 62 cases amongst people staying in the log cabins along the north rim of the Grand Canyon in Arizona, USA. 280 cases of tick-borne relapsing fever have been identified in the USA during the past 25 years.

In Jordan from 1959 to 1969 there were 723 cases of tick-borne relapsing fever with four deaths. Spirochaetes enter the tick in its blood meal from infected humans or animals. Unlike *B. recurrentis*, they invade the tick's salivary and coccal glands and genital apparatus, and so can be transmitted when the tick feeds on a new host and transovarially to the tick's progeny. Thus ticks are reservoirs of *Borrelia* while lice are not. Ticks infest the burrows, caves, tree stumps, and roughly built shacks which harbour their mammal hosts—rodents, insectivores, lagomorphs, bats, and small carnivores.

Clinical features. The illness starts suddenly with rigors, and a fever which mounts to nearly 40 °C in a few days. Early symptoms are headache, dizziness, nightmares, generalized aches and pains often focused in the lower back, knees, and elbows, anorexia, nausea, and vomiting. Later there is upper abdominal pain, cough, and epistaxis. Patients appear severely ill. Most are confused. Hepatic tenderness is the commonest sign (about 60 per cent). The liver is palpably enlarged in about 50 per cent of cases. Splenic tenderness and enlargement are slightly less common. Jaundice has been reported in between 10 and 80 per cent of cases. A petechial or ecchymotic rash is seen in between 10 and 60 per cent of cases: the lesions occur particularly on the trunk (Fig. 2). Elsewhere spontaneous bleeding occurs as epistaxis in 25 per cent, and less commonly as haemoptysis, gastrointestinal bleeding, and as subconjunctival and retinal haemorrhages (Fig. 3). Many patients have tender muscles. Meningism occurs in about 40 per cent of patients: other neurological features include cranial nerve lesions, monoplegias, flaccid paraplegia, and focal convulsions attributable, perhaps, to focal haemorrhages in the central nervous system.

Time course. The incubation period is between 4–18 (average 7) days. In untreated cases of the louse-borne disease, the first attack of fever resolves by crisis in 4–10 (average 5) days. There follows an afebrile remission of 5–9 days and then a series of up to five relapses. No petechial rash occurs during the relapses which are

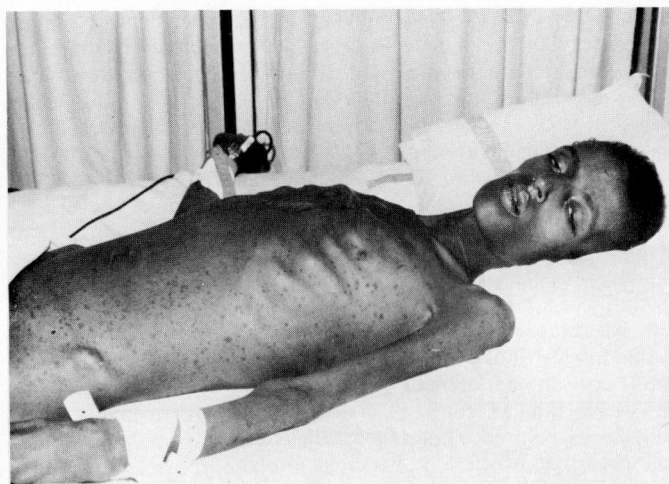

Fig. 2 Ethiopian patient with severe louse-borne relapsing fever. Note emaciation and petechial rash. (Photograpoh copyright Dr D. A. Warrell)

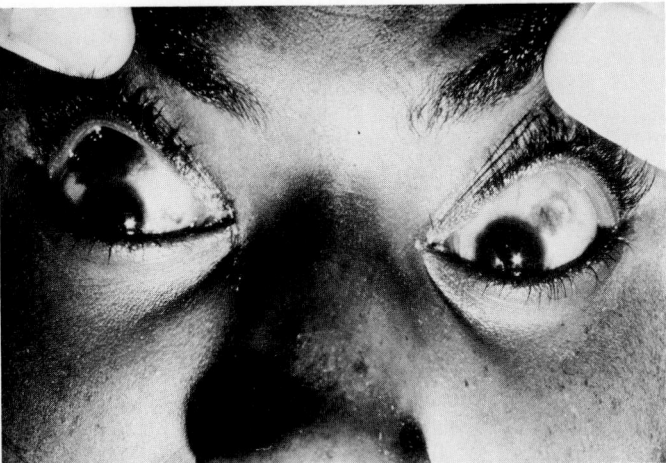

Fig. 3 Subconjunctival haemorrhages in louse-borne relapsing fever. (Photograph copyright Dr D. A. Warrell)

generally less severe than the initial attack. Iritis or iridocyclitis and severe epistaxis may, however, occur during the relapses.

Differences between louse-borne and tick-borne relapsing fever. The tick-borne disease is generally milder and less drawn out. The initial fever lasts only about three days but there may be up to 13 relapses. The incidence of some symptoms and signs in the two diseases appears strikingly different. For example, in some series of cases, only 7 per cent of patients with tick-borne relapsing fever were jaundiced and neurological signs were more common than in the louse-borne disease.

Severe manifestations are myocarditis presenting as acute pulmonary oedema, liver failure, and severe bleeding attributable to thrombocytopenia, liver damage, and disseminated intravascular coagulation. Typhoid, typhus, malaria, and tuberculosis have been described in association with relapsing fever.

The spontaneous crisis and Jarisch–Herxheimer reaction. Whether or not treatment is given, an attack of relapsing fever usually ends dramatically. About one hour after intravenous tetracycline, or on about the fifth day of the untreated illness the patient becomes restless and apprehensive and suddenly begins to have distressingly intense rigors which last 10–30 minutes. The ensuing phenomena have features of a classical endotoxin reaction. During the chill phase temperature, respiratory and pulse rates, and blood pressure rise strikingly. Delirium, gastrointestinal symptoms, cough and limb pains are associated. Some patients die of hyperpyrexia at the peak of fever. The flush phase which last several hours is characterized by profuse sweating, a fall in blood pressure, and slow decline in temperature. Deaths during this phase follow intractable hypotension or the development of acute pulmonary oedema, and are attributable to myocarditis.

Pathophysiology. Spirochaetes are present in the blood, sometimes in enormous numbers (up to one million per mm³). The role of borrelial endotoxin is controversial. Although spirochaetes contain little or no endotoxin, endotoxin-like activity has been detected in patients with relapsing fever, syphilis, and other spirochaetal infections. In the case of louse-borne relapsing fever, patients' plasma proved pyrogenic to normal but not to endotoxin-refractory rabbits, and the Limulus assay was occasionally positive, but in other studies there was evidence of a non-endotoxin particulate pyrogen. In mice infected with *B. duttoni*, the Limulus assay for endotoxin became positive during a Jarisch–Herxheimer reaction precipitated by ampicillin. Sonicates of the borreliae could produce a generalized Shwartzman reaction. In human patients, spirochaetes disappear from the blood just before the spontaneous crisis or Jarisch–Herxheimer reaction. Silver staining by Dieterle's method has revealed intense phagocytosis by circulating neutrophils. There is marked leucopenia at the height of the reaction. Spirochaetes may be found in the organs which bear the brunt of the infection (liver, spleen, myocardium, and brain), but it is not known how their pathological effects are produced. The petechial rash is not a vasculitis, but results simply from thrombocytopenia.

The cardiorespiratory and metabolic disturbances in relapsing fever are principally the result of persistent high fever, dramatically accentuated by the Jarisch–Herxheimer reaction or spontaneous crisis.

Immunology. Patients and animals infected with borreliae develop a variety of antibodies of which the immobilizins and lysins seem to be the most important in ending an attack and preventing or ameliorating a new infection. Residents of an endemic area are said to suffer less severe attacks than newcomers. During the afebrile remissions between relapses, spirochaetes disappear from the blood but persist in tissues such as the central nervous system. The relapse is the result of antigenic variation by the spirochaete in answer to the host's immune response. Plasma levels of Hageman factor and prekallikrein are decreased. Immune complexes have been detected in about half the patients: their significance is not clear.

Diagnosis. In the febrile patient spirochaetes can usually be demonstrated in thin or thick blood films stained with Giemsa or Wright's stain counterstained for 10–30 minutes with 1 per cent crystal violet, or by dark-field examination (see Fig. 1). Towards the end of the attack, during remissions, and particularly in children with tick-borne disease, spirochaetaemia may not be detectable. In these cases blood or CSF can be injected intraperitoneally into young mice which will develop spirochaetaemia within 14 days. Serological methods are not generally used. The serum of patients with relapsing fever may give positive reactions with *Proteus* OXK, OX19, and OX2 and false positive serological responses for syphilis in 5–10 per cent of cases.

Differential diagnosis. In a febrile patient with jaundice, petechial rash, bleeding, and hepatosplenomegaly, the differential diagnosis will include falciparum malaria, yellow fever, rickettsial infections especially louse-borne typhus, and leptospirosis. The diagnosis can be quickly confirmed by examining a blood smear, but the possibility of a complicating infection, particularly typhoid, should not be forgotten.

Prognosis. The mortality in treated cases is less than 5 per cent.

During major epidemics of louse-borne relapsing fever mortalities of 40 per cent or higher have been reported. Deaths during relapses are most unusual: they occur only in the tick-borne disease.

Pathology. Spirochaetes are usually confined to the lumen of blood vessels but tangled masses are also found in the characteristic splenic miliary abscesses and infarcts and within the central nervous system adjacent to haemorrhages. A perivascular histiocytic interstitial myocarditis is found in the majority of cases and may be responsible for conduction defects, arrhythmias, and myocardial failure resulting in sudden death. Splenic rupture with massive haemorrhage, cerebral haemorrhage, and hepatic failure are other causes of death. The liver shows hepatitis with patchy mid-zonal haemorrhages and necrosis. There is meningitis and perisplenitis: most serosal cavities and surfaces of viscera are studded with petechial haemorrhages (Fig. 4). Thrombi are occasionally found occluding small vessels, but the peripheral gangrene sometimes found in patients recovering from louse-borne typhus, is not seen.

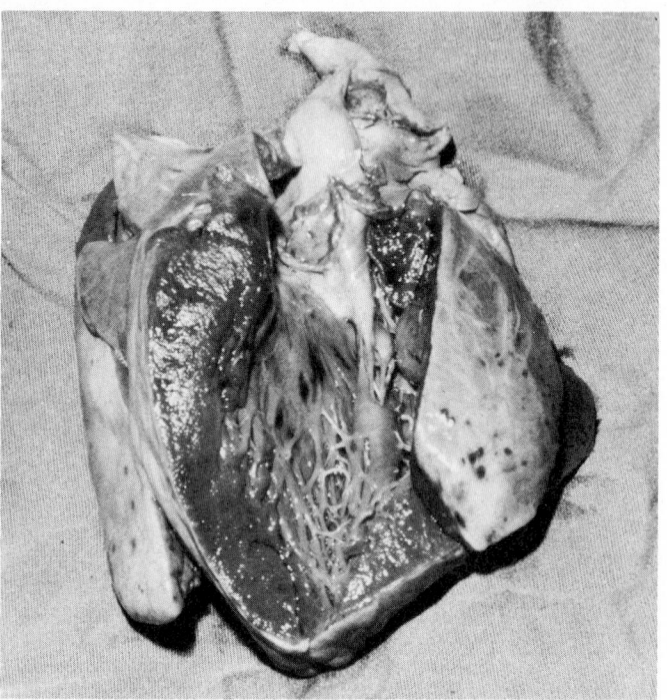

Fig. 4　Epicardial and endocardial haemorrhages in a victim of louse-borne relapsing fever. (Photograph copyright Dr D. A. Warrell)

Treatment

Antimicrobials. Although tick-borne relapsing fever is usually milder than the louse-borne variety, it is more difficult to treat because spirochaetes persist in tissues, such as the central nervous system and eye, and produce relapses. Oral tetracycline, 500 mg six-hourly for 10 days is, however, effective. Oral erythromycin can be given to pregnant women (500 mg six-hourly for 10 days) and children (125–250 mg six-hourly for ten days). In patients unable to swallow tablets, treatment can be initiated with intravenous tetracycline hydrochloride 250 mg, or erythromycin lactobionate 300 mg.

Louse-borne relapsing fever is readily cured with a single oral dose of 500 mg of tetracycline or 500 mg of erythromycin stearate. Few patients with severe louse-borne relapsing fever are able to swallow the tablets without vomiting them up: a more reliable treatment is a single intravenous dose of tetracycline hydrochloride 250 mg or, for pregnant women and children, a single intravenous dose of erythromycin lactobionate 300 mg (children 10 mg/kg body weight). In mixed epidemics of louse-borne relapsing fever and louse-borne typhus a single oral dose of 100 mg of doxycycline has been effective.

Benzylpenicillin (300 000 units), procaine penicillin with benzylpenicillin (600 000 units), and procaine penicillin with aluminium monostearate (600 000 units), all by intramuscular injection, have been used but they may fail to prevent relapses, and the long-acting preparations produce only slow clearance of spirochaetaemia. Chloramphenicol is effective in tick-borne relapsing fever in a dose of 500 mg six-hourly for 10 days in adults and 250 mg six-hourly for 10 days in older children; and in louse-borne relapsing fever in a dose of 500 mg by mouth or intravenous injection in adults.

Jarisch–Herxheimer reaction. Antimicrobials have reduced the mortality of relapsing fevers from 30–70 per cent to less than 5 per cent, but drugs such as tetracycline which rapidly eliminate spirochaetes from the blood and prevent relapses, usually induce a severe Jarisch–Herxheimer type of reaction which may occasionally prove fatal. Clearly, in a disease with such a high natural mortality, treatment cannot be withheld, especially as severe spontaneous crises, which may also prove fatal, occur in a large proportion of louse-borne cases after the fifth day of fever. There is no evidence, however, that the shorter and more intense reaction following tetracycline is more dangerous than the more prolonged but apparently milder reaction following slow-release penicillin. Hydrocortisone, in doses up to 20 mg/kg, and paracetamol, fail to prevent the reaction but reduce peak temperature, hasten the fall in temperature, and lessen the fall in blood pressure during the flush phase. It is extremely interesting that the ampicillin-induced Jarisch–Herxheimer reaction in murine *B. duttoni* infection is prevented by naloxone and very high doses of hydrocortisone (2 mg per 15 g mouse).

Supportive treatment. Patients must be nursed in bed for at least 24 hours after treatment to prevent postural hypotensive collapse and the precipitation of fatal cardiac arrhythmias. Hyperpyrexia should be prevented with antipyretics and vigorous fanning with tepid sponging. Although patients with acute louse-borne relapsing fever have an expanded plasma volume, most are dehydrated and relatively hypovolaemic. Adults may need four or more litres of isotonic saline intravenously during the first 24 hours. Infusion should be controlled by monitoring of jugular venous, central venous, or pulmonary artery wedge pressures. Particularly during the flush phase of the Jarisch–Herxheimer reaction or spontaneous crisis, acute myocardial failure may develop. This is signalled by a rise in central venous pressure above 15 cmH$_2$O; 1 mg digoxin should be given intravenously over 5–10 minutes. Because of the intense vasodilatation, diuretics may accentuate the circulatory failure by causing relative hypovolaemia. Oxygen should be given during the reaction, particularly in severe cases. Vitamin K should be given in all cases with prolonged prothrombin times. Heparin is not effective in controlling coagulopathy and should not be used. Complicating infections—typhoid, bacillary dysentery, tuberculosis, typhus and malaria—must be treated appropriately.

Delousing. Patients with louse-borne relapsing fever are infectious until they have been thoroughly deloused by washing with soap or 1 per cent lysol solution, and dusting with 10 per cent DDT or 1 per cent lindane. Their clothes, instinct with infected lice, are disinfected by heat. Ticks should be searched for and removed but they are rarely found by the time the patient presents with tick-borne relapsing fever.

Prevention. Tick control can be attempted by spraying buildings with insecticides such as 2 per cent benzene hexachloride or 0.5 per cent malathion, and by reducing the number of rodent vectors. Lousiness is prevented by improved hygiene and use of DDT powder.

References

Anderson, T. R. and Zimmerman, L. E. (1955). Relapsing fever in Korea. A clinicopathologic study of eleven fatal cases with special attention to association with salmonella infections. *Am. J. Path.* **31**, 1083.

Bryceson, A. D. M. (1976). Clinical pathology of the Jarisch–Herxheimer reaction. *J. infect. Dis.* **113**, 696.

—, Parry, E. H. O., Perine, P. L., Warrell, D. A., Vucotich, D., and Leithead, C. S. (1970). Louse-borne relapsing fever. A clinical and laboratory study of 62 cases in Ethiopia and a reconsideration of the literature. *Q. Jl Med.* **39**, 129.

Butler, T., Aikawa, M., Habte-Michael, A., and Wallace, C. (1980). Phagocytosis of *Borrelia recurrentis* by blood polymorphonuclear leukocytes is enhanced by antibiotic treatment. *Infect. Immun.* **28**, 1009.

Felsenfeld, O. (1965). Borrelia, human relapsing fever and parasite–vector–host relationships. *Bacteriol. Rev.* **29**, 46.

— (1971). *Borrelia*. W. H. Green, St Louis.

Johnson, R. C. (ed.) (1976). *The biology of parasitic spirochetes*. Academic Press, New York.

Warrell, D. A., Pope, H. M., Parry, E. H. O., Perine, P. L., and Bryceson, A. D. M. (1970). Caridorespiratory disturbance associated with infective fever in man: studies of Ethiopian louse-borne relapsing fever. *Clin. Sci.* **39**, 123.

Wright, D. J. M. (1980). Reaction following treatment of murine borreliosis and Shwartzman type reaction with borrelial sonicates. *Parasite Immunology* **2**, 201.

— (1981) The fall in circulating leucocyte and platelet counts after endotoxin: an adrenergic opioid interaction. *Neuropeptides* **1**, 181.

Leptospirosis

V. Sitprija

Leptospirosis is an infectious disease caused by the *Leptospira interrogans* complex. The disease is characterized by a broad spectrum of clinical manifestations including fever, chills, headache, conjunctivitis, and muscular pains. In mild cases the disease may be subclinical. Jaundice and renal failure are seen in severe infection known as Weil's syndrome.

Aetiology. Leptospires are spirochaetes belonging to the order Spirochaetales and family Treponemataceae. The organism is tightly coiled, thin and flexible, 5–20 μm long and 0.1–0.2 μm wide with bending at one end. It is highly motile with a corkscrew motion. Leptospires are demonstrable by dark field examination and silver impregnation stain. The organisms are easily cultivated aerobically at 28–30 °C in buffered alkaline 2 per cent nutrient agar containing peptone or serum enrichment. Noguchi's ascitic fluid medium, membranes of developing chick embryo, and synthetic media containing inorganic salts are other media used for culture.

Leptospira interrogans is the only species of leptospires. It is divided into two complexes: the interrogans complex which is pathogenic, and the biflexa complex which is saprophytic. Definite antigenic difference is noted between the two complexes. The interrogans complex has 18 serogroups and 130 serotypes. The 18 serogroups consist of *andomana*, *australis*, *autumnalis*, *ballum*, *bataviae*, *canicola*, *celledoni*, *cynopteri*, *grippotyphosa*, *hebdomanis*, *icterohaemorrhagiae*, *javanica*, *panama*, *pomona*, *pyrogenes*, *semaranga*, *shermani*, and *tarassovi*. All serotypes are serologically related with cross reactivity in serologic tests, indicating overlapping in the antigenic structure. Two kinds of antigens have been identified. The surface antigen contains protein polysaccharide and is serotype-specific, while the somatic antigen contains lipopolysaccharide and is genus-specific. The organisms possess haemolysin which is soluble, non-dialyzable, thermolabile, and oxygen stable. Various enzymes including catalase, transamidase, lipase, hyaluronidase, and oxidase are present. The presence of endotoxin has been shown in certain serotypes.

Epidemiology. Rodents, especially rats, are the most important reservoir. *Rattus norvegicus* and *Mus musculus* carry a broad spectrum of serotypes. The other hosts include cattle, pigs, goats, hamsters, mice, dogs, jackals, voles, gerbils, coypus, hedgehogs, foxes, mongooses, shrews, civets, skunks, raccoons, and marsupials. Isolation of leptospires from birds and reptiles has been documented. The organisms may exist in the animal host without causing pathological damage. Leptospires may be isolated from urine, blood, and brain of seronegative rats. Rodents usually do not succumb to leptospiral infection. Their alkaline urine pH and renal tissue pH are favourable for the organism's survival, permitting permanent colonization and urinary shedding. On the other hand, animals susceptible to infection are only temporary urine shedders.

The major vectors to man are rodents. Transmission occurs by direct contact with blood, tissue, or urine of infected animals or exposure to an environment contaminated by leptospires. The moisture, warmth, and optimum pH of soil or surface water in tropical and temperate climates are suitable for the organisms, and they may survive for weeks. Dry climate, excessive sunlight, and chemical pollution tend to kill the organisms.

Leptospires enter a host through abrasions in the skin or through the intact mucous membranes including conjunctiva, vagina, and nasopharynx. Entrance through the intact skin is unlikely, although prolonged exposure of the skin to contaminated water may provide an opportunity for invasion. Infection via the intestinal mucosa can occur when leptospiral-contaminated food is ingested in quantity.

People working in an environment infested by rats or other animals, or where there is infected material or water are prone to infection. Some serotypes may be traced to certain animal hosts. *Icterohaemorrhagiae* can be traced to rat exposure, *gryppotyphosa* to vole contact, *seroje* to pig, *canicola* to dog, and *pomona* to cattle exposure.

Pathogenesis. Once entry has been gained, leptospires are transported by the blood stream to all organs. Multiplication occurs in both blood and tissues. Within 24 hours the organisms can be isolated in most tissues except brain, skeletal muscles, and aqueous fluid. After 48 hours they are recovered in all tissues. Multisystem involvement is due to bacterial invasion and toxic reactions. Clearance of the organisms is accomplished by phagocytosis and humoral mechanism. Leptospires rapidly disappear from the blood after the appearance of agglutinins. After the septicaemic period, which lasts from four to seven days, the organisms can only be recovered in the renal and ocular tissues. Leptospiruria continues for one week to four weeks.

Three mechanisms are involved in the pathogenesis of leptospirosis. These include direct bacterial invasion, non-specific inflammatory factors, and immunologic reactions.

Direct bacterial invasion. Tissue damage in the acute phase of infection is related to bacterial multiplication. The presence of leptospires is necessary for the development of the lesions in the early stage of the disease. It is not clear whether the lesions are caused by bacterial migration *per se* or by factors inherent in bacterial virulence such as bacterial enzymes, metabolites, or toxins. In general, it is felt that both are involved. Hyaluronidase, which may assist in bacterial penetration, cytotoxic factor, and haemolysin have been identified. Vascular endothelial damage with haemorrhage is attributed to the cytotoxic factor derived either from bacteria or interaction between leptospires and the host cells. The role of haemolysin in human disease is not clear. Haemolysis is not an important feature in human leptospirosis although it may occur in certain cases. Leptospiral infection is interesting in that in the early stages multiplication of the organisms is very rapid, resulting in acute and intense organ dysfunction. The fact that there is marked peripheral leucocytosis in the absence of neutrophilic infiltration in the tissue is worth pointing out, and suggests the role of toxins in the pathogenesis of the disease. Several clinical features in leptospiral infection resemble endotoxaemia. Yet, endotoxin is present only in certain serotypes. Serum C3 may be decreased in the early stage of the disease, presumably due to complement activation through the alternative pathway by either leptospires or endotoxin.

The kidney and the liver are most affected by leptospires. In the kidney, leptospires initially cause glomerular injury, and by haematogenous spread, the organisms reach peritubular capillaries (Fig. 1) and migrate to the interstitium (Fig. 2), renal tubules and tubular lumen causing interstitial nephritis and tubular necrosis. Cellular infiltration is predominantly mononuclear. Polymorphonuclear cells may appear in the early stage of glomerular injury. In the liver, there is centrolobular necrosis with the proliferation of Kupffer cells being responsible for jaundice. Since severe pathologic changes occur at a time when leptospires are hardly found in the lesion, it seems plausible that the toxin released by the organisms is responsible for liver injury. It remains puzzling, however, that leptospires are present in the cerebrospinal fluid and the aqueous fluid early in the course of the disease without causing damage.

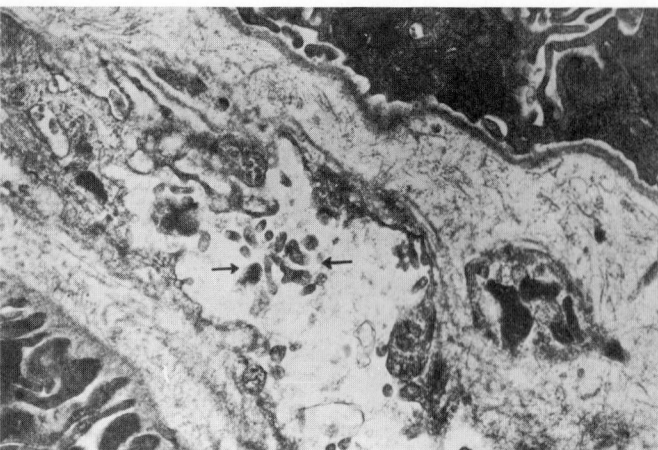

Fig. 1   Demonstration of leptospires (arrowed) in the peritubular capillary in a hamster three hours after inoculation. (Courtesy of Dr V. Boon-pucknavig.)

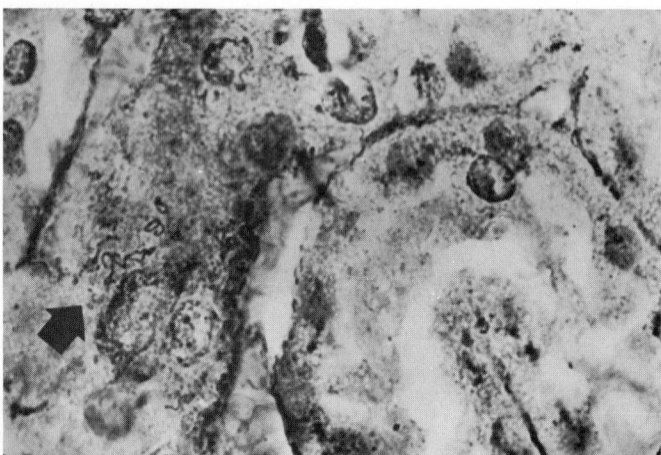

Fig. 2   Demonstration of leptospires (arrowed) in the renal interstitium of a hamster six hours after inoculation. (Levaditi's stain) (Courtesy of Dr V. Boonpucknavig.)

Non-specific inflammatory factors. Certain pathophysiological changes that occur in infection also play a contributing role in causing organ dysfunction. These changes include hypovolaemia, blood hyperviscosity, and intravascular coagulation. Hypovolaemia in leptospirosis is attributed to decreased fluid intake, increased insensible fluid loss, and increased vascular permeability due to the effects of chemical mediators released during inflammation. Increased blood viscosity is accounted for by increased plasma fibrinogen and hypovolaemia. A low-grade intravascular coagulation is also observed, evidenced by the presence of fibrin degradation products in the serum. These factors can compromise the microcirculation, leading to capillary stasis and tissue anoxia. Capillary permeability is therefore further increased, resulting in fluid leakage, haemoconcentration, and further rise in blood viscosity, creating a vicious cycle. Hypoperfusion in severe infection may also be the result of cardiac dysfunction. Although these non-

specific factors do not play the primary role in the development of the lesions, they contribute to organ dysfunction. In fact, they are important in the pathogenesis of renal failure in leptospirosis. Impaired renal function is both toxic and ischaemic in origin.

Immunologic mechanism. In leptospiral infection, IgM antibodies are produced earlier, followed by the appearance of IgG which persists for a longer period of time. However, the IgM response is usually higher than the IgG response, and may last for several months. The immune response is effective in clearing the organisms, but may also produce inflammatory reactions. The evidence is convincing in certain animal species. In canine leptospirosis, renal lesions with immunoglobulin deposition have been shown. The disease runs a chronic course and may lead to chronic renal failure. This has not been observed in man. The role of cell-mediated immune response has not been established. Interstitial and glomerular changes are rather non-specific inflammatory reactions to leptospires, and in hamsters these changes occur a few hours after inoculation of organisms. It is interesting that the rise in antibody titre coincides with certain inflammatory lesions such as meningitis and uveitis. Many authors agree that meningeal inflammation is not due to leptospire invasion. The fact that leptospires are consistently isolated from the cerebrospinal fluid but disappear during the onset of meningeal signs following antibody formation suggests an immunological mechanism as being responsible for the development of meningitis. The suggestion of the immunologic role in uveitis is based on the prolonged presence of leptospires in the ocular fluid and the demonstration of agglutinins in the aqueous fluid.

Pathology. Leptospires cause primarily vascular changes. The cytotoxic factor produces damage to the vascular endothelium causing haemorrhage in the mucous membranes, skin, lungs, kidneys, and other organs. Haemorrhage occurs early in the acute stage during the febrile period.

Liver. Liver lesions consist of focal centrolobular necrosis with focal lymphocytic infiltration and disorganization of liver cell plates, but seldom with fatal results. Proliferation of Kupffer cells with cholestasis associated with scanty round cell infiltration in the periportal areas are often noted. Microscopic changes in the liver are in general not diagnostic and correlate poorly with the degree of functional impairment. With electron microscopy there is mitochondrial destruction. Histochemically, the activity of succinic, isocitric, glutamic, and lactic dehydrogenases is reduced along with functional changes. Jaundice is cholestatic in type with elevation of alkaline phosphatase out of proportion to the mild rise in transaminases. In animals liver lesions are noted within 24 hours of inoculation of leptospires since the liver is the primary site of leptospire multiplication. However, in man it is of interest that severe pathological changes occur at the time when it is hard to show leptospires in the tissue.

Kidney. Renal changes occur early in the course of the disease although functional changes may not be noticeable. The kidneys are grossly swollen with pale cortex and congested medulla. Mesangial proliferation with polymorphonuclear cell infiltration is noted early during bacterial invasion. Focal thickening of the basement membrane and fusion of foot processes are noted by electron microscopy. There is deposition of C3 in the arteriolar wall and in the glomeruli. Interstitial nephritis may be observed without any alteration of renal function and forms the basic renal lesion in human leptospirosis (Fig. 3). Cellular infiltration consists of mononuclear cells and a few eosinophils. Tubular necrosis is seen in cases with acute renal failure. Proximal tubular degeneration is common, and distal tubules are affected when the disease progresses. Basement membrane disruption may be noted. Although tubular necrosis and interstitial nephritis are observed in renal failure, interstitial nephritis chronologically precedes tubular necrosis since leptospires migrate through the peritubular capillaries to the interstitium and then to renal tubules. Renal tubular enzymuria may antedate the histological lesions.

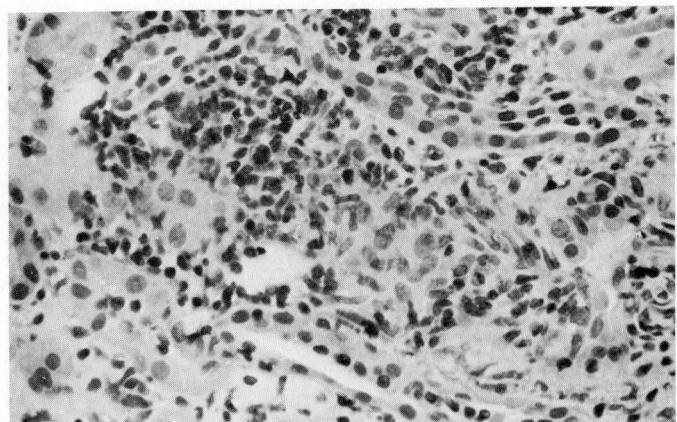
Fig. 3 Demonstration of interstitial nephritis with mononuclear cell infiltration in a patient with leptospirosis.

Heart. Epicardium, endocardium, and myocardium may be involved. Myocardial changes may be focal or diffuse, characterized by interstitial oedema with infiltration of mononuclear cells and plasma cells. Necrosis may be associated with neutrophil infiltration. Focal haemorrhage in the myocardium may also be noted. Endocarditis has been described.

Striated muscle. Vacuolation of the myofibril cytoplasm is noted early in the course of the disease. The other changes consist of loss of cellular detail and fragmentation resulting in homogenous or irregular acidophilic masses. Polymorphonuclear cell infiltration is minimal. Leptospiral antigen is demonstrable in the muscle. In most cases myopathy resolves completely within less than two weeks as leptospiral antibodies develop.

Central nervous system. The meninges show some thickening with a slight increase in the number of arachnoid cells and mononuclear cells. Although leptospires can be isolated from cerebrospinal fluid and meninges, they disappear rapidly following the onset of meningeal irritation which occurs during the second week. It is believed that meningitis is due to immunological mechanism and not to the invasion of the meninges by leptospires. Encephalitis, myelitis, radiculitis, and peripheral neuritis are uncommon. Perivascular infiltration of blood vessels in the spinal cord, basal ganglia, hippocampus, and white matter of the cerebellum has been described.

Other organs. Haemorrhage in the gastrointestinal tract attributable to endothelial damage may occur. Haemorrhage is also noted in the lungs, pleura, and tracheobronchial tree. Adrenal haemorrhage is rare, and may be responsible for shock state. Interstitial oedema and mononuclear cell infiltration have also been noted in the testes. Acute ocular inflammation may occur. Persistence of leptospires in the aqueous fluid may be responsible for chronic, recurrent and latent uveitis. Haemorrhage in the pancreas has also been shown.

Clinical manifestations. The incubation period varies from 7–12 days, but may range from 2–20 days. The duration of the incubation period bears no prognostic significance. The variability of symptoms reflects the dose of the organisms and the host factors. In mild form the disease may be subclinical and can be diagnosed only by serological tests. Leptospirosis may present as Weil's syndrome with jaundice and multi-organ involvement or as an acute but anicteric form with milder clinical symptoms. Ninety per cent of cases are anicteric. In general, both anicteric and icteric cases follow a biphasic course.

Septicaemic phase. The initial septicaemic phase is characterized by fever with chills, myalgia, headache, abdominal pain, skin rash, vomiting, and conjunctival injection lasting from four to seven days. Since leptospires are present in all tissues, the symptoms are systemic. Renal involvement is invariably present ranging from urinary sediment changes and mild proteinuria to renal failure. Leucocyturia, more than 5 cells/high power field, haematuria, and granular casts are often noted. Total urinary protein excretion is often less than 1 g per 24 hours. Renal failure occurs in 67 per cent of cases. Jaundice with impairment of liver function may be present in severe cases. Among the symptoms, headache, myalgia, fever, and chills are most common occurring in over 85 per cent of cases. The other symptoms include diarrhoea, arthralgia, cough, sore throat, bone pain, splenomegaly, lymphadenopathy, and hepatomegaly.

Headache is usually intense, sometimes throbbing, and often not controlled by analgesics. It is commonly frontal, and may be associated with retrobulbar pain. Persistent headache may indicate meningitis. On occasions, mental disturbances including delirium, hallucination, and psychotic behaviour may be observed. Tachycardia is common, but relative bradycardia may occur.

Myalgia, either localized or generalized, is one of the hallmarks in leptospiral infection. Calf, abdominal and lumbosacral muscles are often affected. After the septicaemic period myalgia disappears.

Conjunctival suffusion, photophobia, ocular pain and conjunctival haemorrhage are frequently observed.

Abdominal pain, especially when associated with nausea and vomiting, present a difficult problem in differential diagnosis, and may even lead to abdominal exploration. Splenomegaly is noted in 15–25 per cent of cases.

Pulmonary involvement frequently occurs, and is manifested by a dry cough, occasionally with blood-stained sputum. There may be rales on physical examination. Pleural rub and pericardial rub are rare. A variety of patterns shown by a chest X-ray include small patchy lesions, confluent infiltration or even consolidation. The lesions are prevalent in the periphery of the lung.

Skin rashes may be macular, maculopapular, erythematous, urticarial, or haemorrhagic, and are confined largely to the trunk; but any area may be involved. Pretibial erythematous eruption have been noted in patients with *autumnalis* infection.

Pharyngitis occurs in 23 per cent of anicteric cases. Lymphadenopathy is seen in 15–45 per cent. Parotitis, orchitis, epididymitis, prostatitis, otitis media and arthritis rarely occur.

Mild bleeding may be seen in leptospirosis especially in icteric cases, and epistaxis may occur. Hypotension and congestive heart failure may be observed in severe cases.

Immune phase. The second or immune phase varies from 4–30 days. Fever has already subsided with disappearance of leptospires from most tissues except for the kidney and aqueous fluid. This period coincides with the rise in circulating antibody titres. There may be no symptoms in 35 per cent of cases. Meningitis, uveitis, rash, and secondary fever may occur. Hepatic and renal manifestations which continue from the first phase are still present, and may even be more severe in some patients. Meningeal reactions are found in 80–92 per cent of cases, but less than 50 per cent are symptomatic. Meningeal symptoms disappear within a few days, but rarely may persist for two weeks. Cerebrospinal fluid pleocytosis may last as long as 80 days, but usually disappears within two weeks. Cerebrospinal fluid pressure is not always elevated, and is usually less than 200 mmH$_2$O. In the early stage polymorphonuclear cells predominate, but later mononuclear cells account for most of the cells. Encephalitis, focal weakness, spasticity, paralysis, nystagmus, seizures, visual disturbances, peripheral neuritis, cranial nerve paralysis, radiculitis, myelitis, and Guillain–Barré syndrome are rare findings.

The anterior uveal tract may be affected by the third week of illness. It is characterized by iritis, iridocyclitis, and chorioretinitis. Uveitis may be unilateral or bilateral.

Jaundice, impaired renal function, changes in consciousness, and sometimes vascular collapse occur in Weil's syndrome. Any leptospiral infection, not specific in serotype, in its severe form can produce the syndrome. Jaundice, cholestatic in type, occurs without significant hepatocellular destruction. The serum bilirubin is often less than 20 mg/dl, but may be as high as 80 mg/dl. Jaundice may last from a few days to several weeks. Renal dysfunction, haemorrhagic complications, and cardiovascular collapse occur more frequently in patients with severe jaundice.

Renal manifestations are common in Weil's syndrome although it also occurs in anicteric leptospirosis. Renal failure is hypercatabolic in type. Hyperuricaemia and hyperphosphataemia are occasionally observed. Severe oliguria or even anuria may be seen in the patient with hyperbilirubinaemia.

Diagnosis. Leptospirosis should be differentiated from other febrile illnesses such as malaria, enteric fever, rickettsial diseases, glandular fever, brucellosis, viral hepatitis, influenza, dengue fever, relapsing fever, atypical pneumonia, and aseptic meningitis.

There is usually leucocytosis with neutrophilia although leucopenia may also occur. The erythrocyte sedimentation rate is elevated along with a rise in plasma fibrinogen which is often noted early in the course of the disease. Plasma fibrinogen of over 1000 mg/dl has been reported. Blood viscosity is increased. Thrombocytopenia is observed in occasional cases. Increased serum fibrin degradation products are often observed. Mild intravascular haemolysis may occur but is uncommon. There may be mild anaemia. Serum C3 may be decreased during the early stage of the disease, presumably due to complement activation through the alternative pathway. Rarely haemolytic-uraemic syndrome evidenced by the presence of fragmented or distorted erythrocytes, reticulocytosis, thrombocytopenia, haemolysis, and intravascular coagulation may be noted.

Urinalysis shows abnormalities. Mild proteinuria and cellular elements in the urinary sediment are often observed. Elevation of blood urea nitrogen and serum creatinine is noted in 67 per cent of cases. In severe renal failure there may be hyperuricaemia and hyperphosphataemia.

Jaundice is cholestatic in type with increased serum alkaline phosphatase and serum bilirubin accompanied by modest elevation of serum transaminases. Serum creatine phosphokinase is often increased due to muscular involvement.

Pleocytosis is observed in cerebrospinal fluid with early rise in polymorphonuclear cells which is later followed by mononuclear cells. Cerebrospinal fluid sugar is normal, and protein is very slight.

Culture. Isolation of leptospires from blood or cerebrospinal fluid can be made only during the first 10 days of clinical illness. Urine culture becomes positive after the second week until one month. For routine use Fletcher's semisolid medium and Stuart's medium are recommended. Multiple cultures should be obtained. Blood specimens should be collected during the leptospiraemic stage prior to antimicrobial treatment. Growth of leptospires in Fletcher's semisolid medium usually does not occur until several weeks after inoculation. Animal inoculation may be used especially when the specimen is contaminated. Dark field microscopy of body fluids for leptospires can be made by experienced clinicians. Fluorescent antibody techniques may be applied to detect leptospires in the urine and tissue preparation.

Serology. Serological diagnosis is very helpful during the second week of the disease. In macroscopic slide agglutination test killed or formalinized antigens are used, but in microagglutination test live antigens are used. Macroscopic slide agglutination is often performed as a screening test. The test can be performed rapidly and easily, and is designed to provide serogroup specificity. When positive results are obtained, the titre and specific serotype are determined by microscopic agglutination. Other serological tests include complement fixation, an erythrocyte sensitizing substance test, a haemolytic test, and an indirect immunofluorescent test. These tests may become positive earlier than the agglutination tests. They also revert to negative earlier, and therefore are of limited value in the diagnosis. The haemagglutination test offers an

advantage of detecting antibodies as early as four days after the onset of illness. It is genus-specific and is less time consuming than the microscopic agglutination test.

The serologic criteria for diagnosis includes a fourfold or greater rise in titre during the course of the disease. Elevated microscopic agglutination titres are commonly noted by the tenth day of illness. A slow rise in antibody titre has been observed in the patient with severe infection and in severe uraemia. In leptospirosis a single microscopic agglutination titre of 1:100 is sufficient to warrant a diagnosis of previous infection.

Treatment. Penicillin, streptomycin, tetracycline, and erythromycin are among the antibiotics capable of killing leptospires. Although the beneficial role of the antimicrobial agents in human leptospirosis is controversial, most investigators agree that, to be effective, penicillin or tetracycline should be given within four to seven days of the onset of the disease. Parenteral aqueous penicillin G at a dosage of 1 mega unit at six-hour intervals for a period of one week is recommended in adults. The dose may be modified when there is renal failure. For the patients with penicillin hypersensitivity, tetracycline at a dosage of 2 g daily is recommended provided that renal function is normal.

Fluid and electrolyte balance must be maintained especially when the patient is febrile. In renal failure this problem is even more critical. Haemodialysis or peritoneal dialysis may be needed when renal failure is severe. Since renal failure is catabolic in type, dialysis may have to be performed frequently. In hyperbilirubinaemic renal failure exchange blood transfusion is fruitful in reducing the serum bilirubin and improving the renal function.

Prognosis. Favourable prognosis is usual in most cases. Mortality is greater in the elderly patients and in those with severe jaundice and renal failure. However, dialysis has much reduced mortality in such cases. The long-term follow-up of those with renal failure shows good recovery of renal function. Interstitial fibrosis with permanent renal tubular dysfunction is rare, and this is in contrast to canine leptospirosis in which chronic renal failure may occur. Iridocyclitis may persist for several years. Fetal mortality is high when leptospirosis is associated with pregnancy.

Prevention. Vaccines are effective in preventing the disease in animals. Its use in man is impractical due to the presence of many serotypes. However, vaccination against a specific serotype prevalent in the area has been shown to be effective. The other methods include surface decontamination, the wearing of protective clothing, and the eradication of the animal reservoir.

References

Adler, B. and Faine, S. (1978). The antibodies involved in the human immune response to leptospiral infection. *J. med. Microbiol.* **11**, 387.

Berman, S. J., Tsai, C., Holmes, K., Fresh, J. W., and Walten, R. H. (1973). Sporadic anicteric leptospirosis in South Vietnam. A study in 150 patients. *Ann. intern. Med.* **79**, 167.

Bhamarapravati, N., Boonyapaknavig, V., Viranuvatti, V., Tuchinda, U., Bunnag, D., and Nye, S. (1966). Liver changes in leptospirosis; a study of needle biopsies in 22 cases. *Am. J. Proctol.* **17**, 480.

Feigin, R. D. and Anderson, D. C. (1975). Human leptospirosis. CRC Crit. Rev. Clin. Lab. Sci. **5**, 413.

Finco, D. R. and Low, D. G. (1967). Endotoxin properties of *Leptospira canicola*. *Am. J. vet. Res.* **128**, 1863.

Knight, L. L., Miller, N. G., and White, R. J. (1973). Cytotoxic factor in the blood and plasma of animals during leptospirosis. *Infect. Immun.* **8**, 401.

Morrison, M. I. and Wright, N. G. (1976). Canine leptospirosis: an immunological study of interstitial nephritis due to *Leptospira canicola*. *J. Pathol.* **120**, 83.

Sitprija, V. and Evans, H. (1970). The kidney in human leptospirosis. *Am. J. Med.* **49**, 780.

—, Pipatanagul, V., Mertowidjojo, K., Boonpucknavig, V., and Boonpucknavig, S. (1980). Pathogenesis of renal disease in leptospirosis: clinical and experimental studies. *Kidney Int.* **17**, 827.

Turner, L. H. (1973). Leptospirosis. *Br. med. J.* **i**, 537.

Non-venereal treponemes: yaws, endemic syphilis, and pinta

P. L. Perine

Yaws is one of the endemic treponematoses, a group of chronic, granulomatous diseases caused by spirochaetes belonging to the genus *Treponema*. Yaws occurs in children living in rural areas in warm, humid climates between the Tropics of Cancer and Capricorn. About 10 per cent of untreated cases develop late destructive or crippling lesions of skin, bone, and cartilage.

Aetiology. Yaws is caused by *T. pertenue*, a spirochaete which is morphologically identical to *T. pallidum*, the cause of venereal and non-venereal syphilis, and to *T. careteum*, the cause of pinta. These treponemes share common antigens so that infection by one species produces varying degrees of cross-immunity to the others. No serological test exists that differentiates the antibodies produced, and none of these organisms grows *in vitro*. The only means of differentiating yaws, syphilis and pinta is their epidemiological characteristics and the pattern of infection produced by the respective treponemes in man and experimentally infected laboratory animals (Table 1).

The treponemes of yaws, syphilis, and pinta are fragile and readily killed by exposure to atmospheric oxygen, drying, mild detergents, or antiseptics. They prefer temperatures below 37 °C, which may explain their predilection for the skin and bones of the extremities. These organisms cannot penetrate intact skin and gain entry to the body through small abrasions and lacerations.

The pathogenic treponemes are small, corkscrew-shaped organisms measuring 0.5 μm in width and 7–20 μm in length. Because of their small mass, they cannot be seen by the ordinary microscope unless a darkground condenser is used.

Epidemiology. Yaws is transmitted by direct contact with an infectious lesion. Yaws transmission is enhanced by a crowded environment with poor sanitation and personal hygiene. The disease is usually acquired in childhood between the ages of 5–15. Statistically, there are no racial or sex differences which distinguish those who become infected, and in endemic areas more than 80 per cent of the population are infected.

Climatic conditions influence the type of yaws lesion and its transmission. In humid, warm environments the early lesion tends to proliferate and teems with spirochaetes, thus increasing the infectious reservoir; whereas in dry, arid climates or seasons the reverse is true.

Yaws and the other endemic treponematoses have undergone dramatic changes in prevalence over the past three decades. The first change was a precipitous decrease in cases brought about by mass penicillin treatment campaigns in the 1950s and 1960s sponsored by the World Health Organization. An estimated 152 million people were examined and 46.1 million clinical cases, latent infections, and contacts were treated. The yaws reservoir was reduced to a few areas in West and Central Africa, Central and South America, and Oceania. Recently, however, yaws has been resurgent in several West African countries because of limited surveillance and premature dismantling of the control programme. To cope with this resurgence, new campaigns of mass treatment were initiated in 1980.

Some African nations, previously rendered yaws-free by mass treatment campaigns, have experienced a sharp rise in the incidence of venereal syphilis. This increase in venereal syphilis may represent a decline of herd-immunity to yaws, and thereby, to syphilis.

Endemic syphilis is also transmitted by non-venereal contact among children. In contrast to yaws, transmission of infection by contaminated drinking vessels may be more common than by direct contact with infectious lesions, and the disease tends to be familial with spread of infection from children to adults rather than communal as in yaws. Endemic syphilis lesions are virtually indistinguishable from early yaws, and the two diseases may occur at different times in the same population but not in the same person. Moreover, venereal syphilis can be acquired by children through social contact with adults suffering from venereal syphilis and then be spread by non-venereal person-to-person contact if the level of sanitation and personal hygiene are low.

Several variants of endemic syphilis are recognized by their geographic distribution. Although each is caused by the same organism, different strains of endemic *T. pallidum* and different factors modify disease expression. Examples are *bejel* of the Eastern Mediterranean and North Africa; *njovera* or *dichuchwa* of Africa; and the now extinct *sibbens* of Scotland, *radesyge* of Nor-

Table 1 Major features of the treponematoses

Feature	Venereal syphilis	Endemic syphilis	Yaws	Pinta
Organism	*T. pallidum*	*T. pallidum*	*T. pertenue*	*T. carteum*
Age of infection	15–40	2–10	5–15	10–30
Occurrence	worldwide	Africa; Middle East	Africa, South America, Oceania, Asia	Central and South America
Climate	all	dry, arid	warm, humid	warm, rural
Transmission				
Direct:				
Venereal	common	rare	no	no
Non-venereal	rare	rare	common	common
Congenital	yes	unproven	no	no
Indirect:				
Contaminated utensils	rare	common	rare	no
Insects	no	no	rare	no
Reservoir of infection	adults	infectious and latent cases	infectious and latent cases; ? subhuman primates	infectious cases
Ratio infectious: latent cases	1:3	1:2	1:3–5	?
Late complications				
Skin	+	+	+	+
Bone, cartilage	+	+	+	no
Neurologic	+	unproven	no	no
Cardiovascular	+	unproven	no	no

way, and *skerjevo* of Yugoslavia. Bejel is the only type of endemic syphilis still prevalent, and it is found in mainly semi-nomadic people living in the Saharan regions of Africa. Improved standards of living and mass penicillin treatment campaigns have greatly reduced disease prevalence.

Pinta is restricted to the Western Hemisphere and is found today only in a few parts of Central and South America, principally in the semi-arid region of the Tepalcatepec Basin in Southern Mexico and focal areas of Columbia and Venezuela. Active surveillance and treatment programmes have greatly decreased the prevalence of pinta.

Pathogenesis. The lesions of yaws and the other treponematoses are largely due to the immune response of the host to the treponeme. As far as can be determined, none of these treponemes carries or produces toxic substances. They have the ability to invade living cells without causing apparent injury. Cell destruction and tissue damage are probably due to the action of immune cells that injure normal tissue in the process of killing treponemes.

Host immunity reaches its highest level after several months of infection, just before disseminated lesions heal and latency begins. Thereafter the host is immune to reinfection and is not contagious, but since not all treponemes are killed, infectious lesions may reappear as immunity wanes over time. Most yaws patients experience two or three infectious relapses during the first 5 years of infection.

In venereal and possibly endemic syphilis, infection is systemic and late lesions may develop in any organ or tissue of the body. In yaws, *T. pertenue* produce lesions only in skin and osseous tissue, although it is certain that periodically the organism spreads systemically; *T. careteum* resides only in the skin. This peculiar tissue tropism is unexplained. It is probably an inherent property of the treponeme, acting in concert with climatic factors.

Clinical features. The clinical course of yaws and endemic syphilis resembles that of venereal syphilis with division of infection into primary, secondary, and tertiary or late stages, each stage separated by a quiescent or latent period. None of the endemic treponematoses, however, progresses by these clearly defined stages of infection as does venereal syphilis. In yaws, lesions are described as *early*, comprising those of the primary (initial) and secondary (disseminated) stage, and *late*, which correspond to the tertiary stage.

The initial lesion in yaws usually appears on the extremities after an incubation period of three to five weeks. Characteristically it is a papule; a painless lesion which appears at the site of infection, enlarges, forming a raspberry-like, vegetative lesion called a papilloma. The papilloma is round to oval-shaped, elevated and not indurated, ranging in size from 1–3 cm in diameter. The surface teems with spirochaetes and is often covered by a thin yellow crust which is easily removed. The papilloma may ulcerate as it enlarges and becomes secondarily infected with other micro-organisms. Lymph nodes draining the initial lesion may enlarge and become tender, but systemic symptoms are rare.

Secondary or disseminated papillomata appear after two to six months, often without an intervening latent period, on the skin of moist areas such as the axillae, joint flexures, genitalia, and the gluteal cleft (Fig. 1). They also occur on the soles and palms and, because they are tender, may interfere with gait and use of the hands. Papillomata in different stages of development persist for six to eight months and heal without scar formation, unless they become secondarily infected. Despite the size and number of lesions, children with generalized papillomata experience little discomfort or other constitutional symptoms.

Slightly raised, scaly, pigmented, macular yaws lesions measuring from 1–4 cm in diameter commonly occur when the climate is dry and arid. These lesions have the same distribution as papillomata and may appear together with lesions of different morphology in the same patient (maculo-papular yaws).

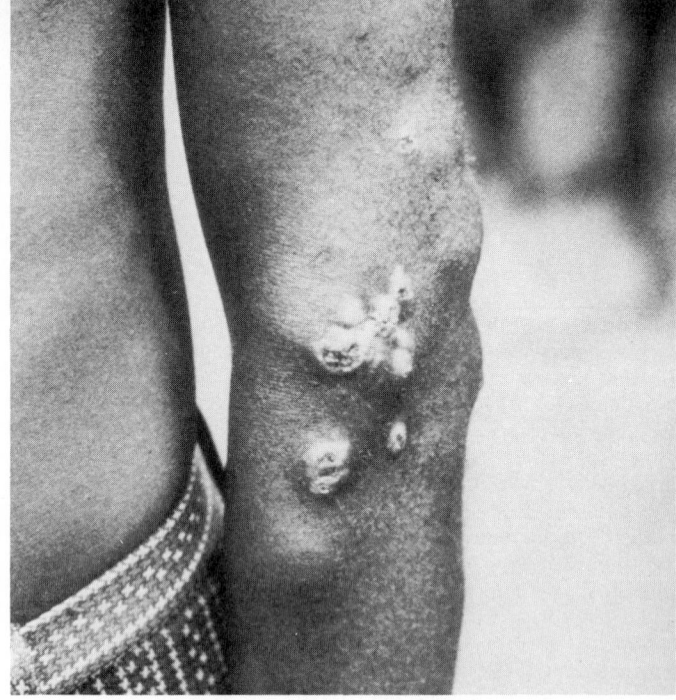

Fig. 1　Early yaws: juxta-articular nodular and cutaneous papillomata in a young man.

The periosteum and osseous tissue of the bones of the extremities are frequently inflamed during early yaws, causing swelling, pain, and tenderness. Scaly, tender, hyperkeratotic lesions of the palms and soles also occur and may be incapacitating. Hyperkeratotic and bone lesions are not contagious, and macular lesions are only minimally so.

One or more relapses of secondary-type lesions usually occur during the first five years of infection, each separated by period of latency. Late yaws lesions occur thereafter in about 10 per cent of untreated cases.

Late yaws lesions are not infectious because they contain few treponemes. Cutaneous plaques produce atrophic scars; subcutaneous granulomatous nodules erode skin and produce deep ulcers that destroy underlying tissue and disfigure. Hyperkeratotic palmar and plantar yaws are incapacitating and often prevent the use of hands, or the ability to walk normally. The weight is placed on the sides of the feet, which produces a gait much like that of a crab ('crab' yaws).

The granuloma of late yaws have a histological appearance like the gummata of syphilis. These proliferative lesions may involve the palate and destroy the soft tissues of the nose, causing a terrible disfiguration called gangosa. Gummatous periostitis of the skull, fingers, and long bones is erosive and often retards or stops growth. Active periostitis is occasionally found in young and middle-aged adults who had yaws in childhood.

The clinical differentiation of yaws from endemic syphilis may not be possible. The initial lesions of endemic syphilis usually appear at the mucocutaneous borders of the mouth or on the oral mucous membranes (mucous patches) as the result of transmission by contaminated drinking vessels (Fig. 2). Although mucous patches are very rare in yaws, ulcero-papillomata around the mouth are common, and the axillary and anogenital papillomata of yaws are indistinguishable from the condylomata lata of venereal and endemic syphilis. Late ulcero-nodules and osteoperiostitis are seen in late endemic syphilis, but cardiovascular and neurologic complications either do not occur or are extremely rare.

The lesions of pinta are easily differentiated from yaws and syphilis. The initial papule appears on the skin of the extremities and enlarges slowly over a period of several weeks or months to form an erythematous plaque. Satellite papules form at the edge of the lesion and undergo a similar type of evolution. The plaques coalesce to form violaceous pigmented plaques which in several years, slowly dispigment from lighter shades of blue to white, leaving atrophic depigmented scars.

Ulcero-nodular skin lesions of yaws and endemic syphilis resemble tropical ulcers. Yaws lesions are not as painful, necrotic, nor as deep as tropical ulcers, which are usually singular and restricted to the lower one-third of the leg.

Plantar warts are frequently confused with plantar papillomata of yaws and both conditions may occur in the same patient.

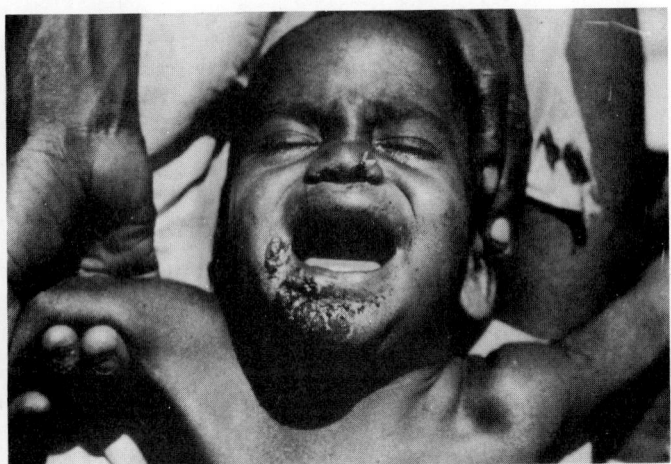

Fig. 2 Endemic syphilis: mucocutaneous lesions in a young child.

Diagnosis. The diagnosis of yaws is made by a combination of clinical assessment, of positive dark-ground examination of lesions, and of reactive serologic tests for syphilis. Early and late yaws should be diagnosed with caution unless there is evidence that the patient resides or has lived in a yaws-endemic area.

The diagnosis of early yaws, or endemic syphilis, is not difficult in endemic areas where the disease has existed for centuries. The local population in such areas is usually well-informed about the different types and characteristics of yaws lesions. The most difficult diagnostic problem arises when a person who had yaws as a child emigrates to an area of the world where the disease never existed. Such a person usually has reactive serological tests for syphilis and may have a few atrophic scars suggestive of earlier infection. What are the chances that this patient has or has had venereal syphilis? Should he be treated for latent yaws or syphilis?

The patient's social and medical history should be carefully reviewed. Clinical findings suggestive of old yaws (scars, inactive tibial periostitis), and the absence of stigmata of congenital and venereal syphilis support the diagnosis of inactive or treated yaws.

If the patient has a reagin titre of less than 1:8 dilutions, he probably does not have active latent yaws or syphilis. If he received at least one therapeutic dose of long-acting penicillin in his native country during a yaws campaign, he requires no furthe. treatment for evaluating yaws. On the other hand, if the patient is a contact of a case of infectious venereal syphilis, he should be treated as potentially infected with syphilis, because *T. pallidum* occasionally superinfects people who have had yaws as children. If treatment is given, the patient should receive a certificate stating the drug and dosage used and the results of his serological tests for future reference. Otherwise, some of these patients will be re-treated unnecessarily by each new physician they consult.

Treatment and prevention. Long-acting penicillin G given by intramuscular injection is the recommended treatment for all the endemic treponematoses. The preparation used in previous mass treatment campaigns was penicillin aluminium monostearate (PAM), but benzathine penicillin is currently recommended because it is no longer acting and more readily available than is PAM. Active infections and non-infectious cases should be given 2.4 mega units in a single intramuscular injection; children under 10 years of age receive 1.2 mega units. Patients allergic to penicillin may be given tetracycline or erythromycin, 500 mg by mouth four times daily for two weeks; children under 10 years of age should be given erythromycin in dosages adjusted for their age.

Prevention of yaws in a community requires elimination of the reservoir of infection by penicillin treatment. This reservoir comprises both incubating and early latent cases, the latter being the more important because of their tendency to relapse with infectious lesions. The experience of the yaws mass treatment campaigns indicated that the entire population should receive penicillin when the prevalance of clinically active yaws was over 10 per cent in the community (total mass treatment); that active cases, all children under 15, and obvious adult contacts of infectious cases should be treated when the prevalance of clinically active yaws was between 5–10 per cent (juvenile mass treatment); and that only active cases, household, and other obvious contacts need be treated when less than 4 per cent of the population has clinically active yaws. Contacts receive the same dose of penicillin as active cases.

The yaws control programmes sponsored by the World Health Organization attempted to create an ever-enlarging yaws-free area by carefully planned and conducted mass treatment campaigns. The consolidation phase of these campaigns required long-term, expensive, active surveillance for yaws to prevent its reintroduction or resurgence in a community. The costs of maintaining these programmes have increased enormously, with the growth in population, the expensiveness of vehicles, drugs, and of personnel. The tragic result has been a curtailment of yaws control activities and a resurgence of the disease in many parts of the world.

References

Edmundson, W. F., Rico, A. L., and Olansky, Sidney (1952). A study of pinta in the Tepalcatepec Basin, Michoacan, Mexico. *Am. J. Syph. Gonor. vener. Dis.* **37**, 201.

Grin, E. I. (1956). Endemic syphilis and yaws. *Bull. Wld Hlth Org.* **15**, 959.

Guthe, T. (1969). Clinical, serological and epidemiological features of framboesia tropica (yaws) and its control in rural communities. *Acta. derm.-Vener.*, Stockh. **49**, 343.

Hackett, C. J. and Loewenthal, L. J. A. (1960). *Differential diagnosis of yaws.* World Health Organization, Geneva.

Granuloma inguinale

P. L. Perine

One of the less prevalent venereal diseases, granuloma inguinale is a slowly progressive, granulomatous disease of the skin and subcutaneous tissues of the inguinal and ano-genital region. Also known as *granuloma venereum* and *Donovanosis*, it shows little tendency towards healing. It mutilates the genitalia, and may predispose to cancer.

Aetiology. The putative cause is the Donovan body, once thought to be a protozoan but now classified as a member of the *Brucellaceae* with the name *Calymatobacterium granulomatis*. In infected tissue it is found within the cytoplasm of large mononuclear cells. There is no satisfactory method for isolating *C. granulomatis* in culture and its biologic characteristics are poorly understood. The organism is not pathogenic for laboratory animals.

Epidemiology. Granuloma inguinale occurs sporadically throughout the world and is endemic in southern India, parts of the South Pacific and the Caribbean. It is seen in relatively high prevalence in New Guinea. The disease occurs predominantly in males, in dark-skinned races, and in individuals of low socio-economic status who practise poor personal hygiene. Women tend to have more extensive infections than men, and pregnancy accelerates the pathological process.

Granuloma inguinale is classified as a venereal disease because of the genital location of most lesions and because the age of peak incidence corresponds to the age period of maximum sexual activity. Transmission of infection to steady sexual partners, however, is very rare and calls into question the idea of a sexual mode of transmission. On rare occasions *C. granulomatis* has been cultured from stools which suggests that ano-genital contact may facilitate transmission. An increased incidence of genital carcinoma has been attributed to granuloma inguinale, but this association needs further clarification.

Pathogenesis. Granuloma inguinale is auto-inoculable provided the skin is first traumatized. This suggests that *C. granulomatis* invades the host through small skin abrasions, including those caused by sexual activity. Infection incites a granulomatous inflammatory response in the skin and subcutaneous tissue. On histologic examination, the majority of the organisms are found within the cytoplasm of histocytes. The lesion spreads locally by direct extension, destroying skin and underlying tissues. Secondary infection by other micro-organisms is common and contributes to tissue destruction. The vegetative granulomatous response may compromise the vasculature and cause gangrene. The regional lymphatics are seldom invaded but may become obstructed and produce elephantiasis of the genitalia. Systemic infection and death have also been reported.

Lesions of granuloma inguinale show little tendency towards healing. Although the number of organisms in lesions tend to decrease with time, they can usually be found within macrophages in the depths of relatively old lesions. Persistence of *C. granulomatis* suggests some problem in phagocytic killing.

Clinical features. The incubation period is not known; estimates range from several days to months. In men, the initial lesion occurs most frequently on the prepuce or coronal sulcus of the penis; in women, the initial lesion is usually on the labia or in the posterior fourchette. The lesion begins as a painless papule which slowly enlarges and erodes the skin forming a spongy, ulcerative lesion. The borders are sharply demarcated, the edges are rolled and the surface covered with smooth, glistening granulating tissue. The surface bleeds easily and becomes more uneven with time. The lesion extends locally along the inguinal creases for over a period of several months and becomes painful when secondarily infected. Secondarily infected lesions discharge seropurulent, foul-smelling material; this deepens the ulceration, and may produce a fistula. On occasion, the granulomatous hypertrophic process forms spectacular, beefy-red, vegetative growths extending several centimetres from the surface of the lesion.

Extragenital lesions occur in about 10 per cent of cases and are invariably secondary to long-standing genital granuloma. Primary infection of the inguinal region occurs in about 5 per cent of patients. Inguinal lesions involve subcutaneous tissue only, but resemble the lymphadenopathy seen with lymphogranuloma venereum until the ulcero-vegetative stage develops. This early inguinal lesion is termed a 'pseudobubo' (Fig. 1).

Diagnosis. The diagnosis of granuloma inguinale is based on finding typical intracellular organisms on Wright's or Geimsa stained scrapings taken from infected tissue, or aspirated by needle and syringe from pseudobuboes. A small wedge biopsy taken from the edges of a lesion, or scrapings from a clean granulomatous surface, are placed between two glass slides, crushed and spread. Typical *C. granulomatis* are found in varying numbers within the cytoplasm of large macrophages. They are encapsulated and have a 'safety-pin' shape because of densely staining polar bodies at each end.

No culture or serological method is available for diagnostic use. Repeated examination of infected tissue, including use of silver

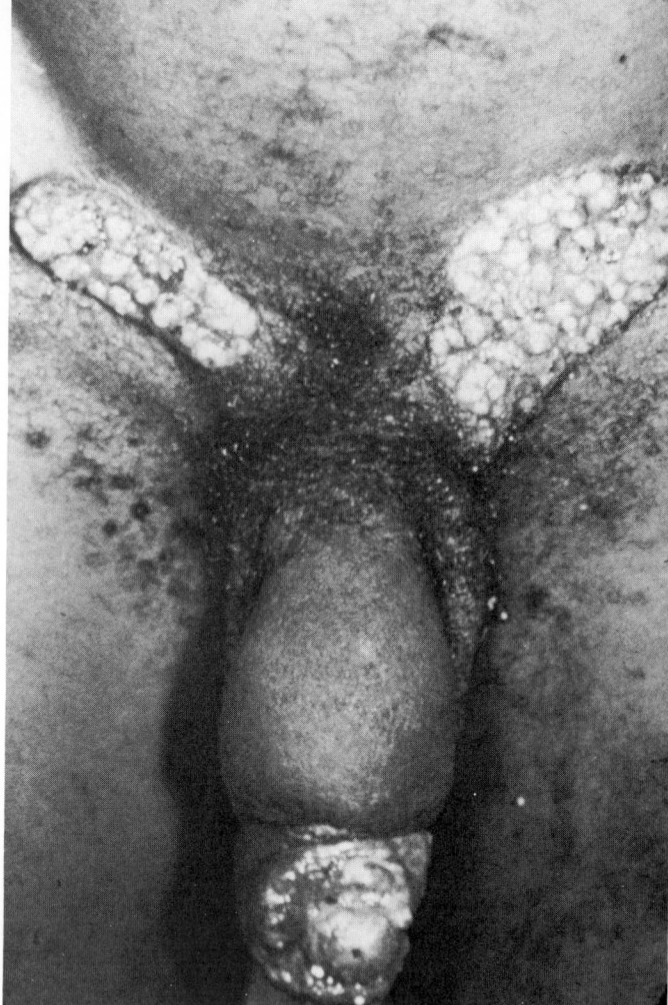

Fig. 1 Granuloma inguinale: pseudobubo with penile ulceration.

impregnation stains, may be necessary, particularly in chronic granuloma lesions and in those patients partially treated with antibiotics.

Granuloma inguinale can be differentiated from syphilis by a negative dark-ground microscopic examination and by syphilis serology tests; from lymphogranuloma venereum by biopsy and serologic tests; from chancroid by culture of lesion material for *H. ducreyi*; and from ano-genital cutaneous amoebiasis by serological tests and biopsy (see Tables 1 and 2, page 5.306). These diseases, however, may coexist with granuloma inguinale.

Treatment and prevention. Tetracycline, chloramphenicol, streptomycin, gentamicin, and co-trimoxazole are effective treatments for granuloma inguinale. Penicillin is ineffective. Recent reports from New Guinea indicate that an unacceptable number of patients fail to be cured with streptomycin in a dose of 2 g twice daily by intramuscular injection for five days. Better results are obtained by treatment with chloramphenicol, 500 mg by mouth four times a day for a minimum of 10 days. Applying compresses soaked with a dilute solution of potassium permanganate (1:4000) to contaminated lesions facilitates healing.

Duration of therapy depends on the clinical response. Complete healing usually takes several weeks and leaves a scar. Reconstructive surgery for elephantoid masses and deforming scars may be required but should not be attempted until antibiotic treatment is completed to prevent auto-inoculation and extension of disease. Relapses are common and usually reflect inadequate duration of therapy.

Granuloma inguinale is transmitted with such a low frequency that it should be easy to control if the reservoir of infection can be identified and treated. In endemic areas, the prevalence of disease appears to be inversely related to the level of sanitation, education, and economic development. Prevalence should decrease with improved standards of living.

References

Kuberski, T. (1980) Granuloma inguinale (Donovanosis). *Sex. trans. Dis.* **7**, 26.

Rajam, R. V. and Rangiah, P. N. (1954). *Donovanosis*. WHO monograph series, no. 24, World Health Organization, Geneva.

Chancroid

P. L. Perine

Chancroid is a sexually transmitted disease caused by the bacillus *Haemophilus ducreyi*. This organism invades small abrasions of the skin and produces painful ulcerations at the site of infection. Auto-inoculation and the formation of painful, suppurative inguinal buboes is characteristic. Chancroid tends to be self-limiting with no systemic complications, but superinfection of genital ulcers by other bacteria can produce large, locally destructive lesions that may persist for several weeks or months. Untreated ulcers heal by scarring and despite evidence of delayed hypersensitivity to *H. ducreyi*, the patient is susceptible to re-infection.

Aetiology. *H. ducreyi* is a short, pleomorphic, Gram-negative rod discovered by Ducrey in 1889. As it grows, the organism forms chain-like patterns in infected tissue and cultures which may resemble a shoal of fish. The Ducrey bacillus is fastidious and difficult to culture from ulcers or buboes unless a culture medium containing special growth supplements and vancomycin is used. With this method, about two-thirds of chancroid ulcers and a much lesser percentage of bubo aspirates are culture positive for *H. ducreyi*.

Pathogenesis. The Ducrey bacillus cannot penetrate intact skin or mucous membranes, but any small abrasion, laceration, or excoriation may serve as the portal of entry. Once the epithelium has been breached, the organism multiplies and incites an inflammatory reaction in the dermis leading to formation of a pustule which soon ruptures and forms a shallow ulcer. The edges of the ulcer are undermined by an acute inflammatory process, giving the lesion a 'soft' consistency, as compared to the indurated chancre of primary syphilis. Most chancroid ulcers become superinfected with aerobic and anaerobic bacteria which may accelerate tissue necrosis and bubo formation.

No toxic or virulent factors have been identified in *H. ducreyi*. The organism may cause genital ulceration without bubo formation, and chancroid buboes are often sterile and Gram stain negative despite the isolation of *H. ducreyi* in a genital ulcer. Intradermal inoculation of the bubo aspirate or culture-purified *H. ducreyi* causes typical chancroid lesions in the skin of rabbits, apes, and human volunteers. Infection is normally limited to skin, subcutaneous tissue, and local lymphatic tissue.

Local and systemic immunity limits the extent of the chancroid lesion and it heals by granulation with scar formation. This immunity does not prevent re-infection. Patients become sensitized to *H. ducreyi* early in the course of infection and may demonstrate a tuberculin-like skin reaction to the intradermal injection of heat or phenol-inactivated *H. ducreyi* for several years thereafter.

Epidemiology. Chancroid occurs sporadically throughout the Western Hemisphere, Europe, and Australia, but it is highly prevalent and endemic throughout most of sub-Saharan Africa and south-east Asia. Before sulphonamides, chancroid was the most common cause of genital ulceration in the world, and it remains so in endemic areas.

Clinical disease is recognized much more frequently in men than in women, because lesions are not as apparent in women. The Ducrey bacillus has been isolated from the smegma of uncircumcized men, who also have a higher risk of becoming infected. It is suspected, but not proven, that uncircumcized men are the reservoir for the Ducrey bacillus. Sporadic epidemics usually occur among the economically deprived elements of society whose standards of personal hygiene are low. Whether or not these people are more common carriers of *H. ducreyi* is unknown.

The risk of infection following exposure to *H. ducreyi* is not known. In older medical literature it was said that a man exposed to a woman suffering from both gonorrhoea and chancroid became infected much more readily with chancroid than with gonorrhoea. About 25 per cent of chancroid patients have another venereal infection, the most common being gonorrhoea.

Clinical features. The typical chancroid ulcer begins as a papule, after an incubation period averaging seven days (range, 1–21 days). The papule enlarges over one to three days to become a pustule which ruptures to form a shallow ulcer. In men, the most common locations of lesions in decreasing order of frequency are the prepuce, the coronal sulcus, the glans, and the penile shaft. In women, the most common sites of lesions are the labia minora, fourchette, perianal area, and the thighs. Cervical lesions are rare. The majority of both men and women will have more than one ulcerative lesion (Fig. 1).

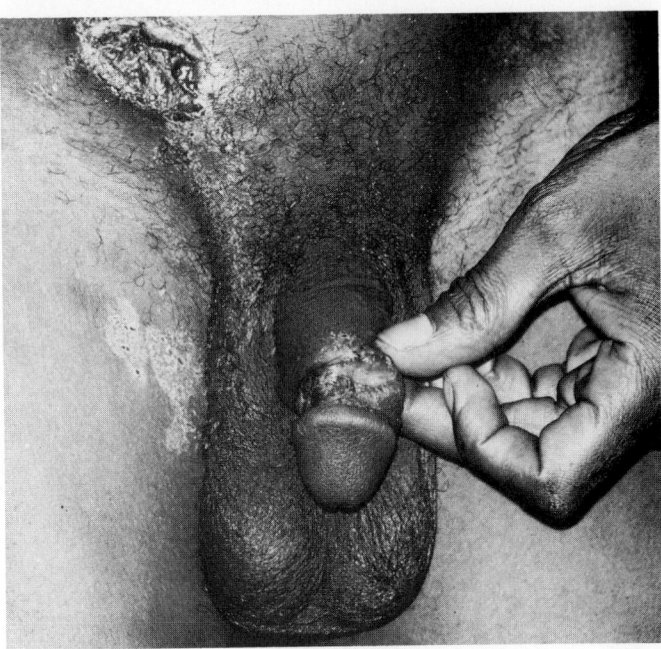

Fig. 1 Chancroid: multiple penile ulcerations and a broken-down inguinal bubo.

The initial chancroid ulceration is sharply circumscribed, painful, and tender. It rapidly enlarges to reach a diameter of 1–2 cm. The edges are ragged and undermined, and the base of the ulceration consists of uneven, purulent, granulation tissue. The lesions are vascular and bleed easily when manipulated. Because of the frequent involvement of the prepuce, phimosis and paraphimosis are common complications.

Women may have asymptomatic chancroid lesions or complain only of external dysuria, or tenesmus if the lesions involve the anus. Perianal lesions due to direct inoculation or to contamination by infectious vaginal secretions are common. These lesions are exquisitely painful and may be confused with ulcerated, thrombotic haemorrhoids.

In 50–70 per cent of chancroids, the regional lymph nodes enlarge unilaterally and become tender shortly after the lesion appears. In 30–50 per cent of cases, the lymph nodes fuse together and form a painful bubo. Buboes greater than 5 cm in diameter usually suppurate, become fluctuant, and will rupture spontaneously unless aspirated. Bubo formation and size, however, do not correlate with the size, number, or duration of chancroid lesions.

Healing usually takes place after the bubo ruptures or resolves, but in a few unfortunate cases, a large, rapidly destructive 'phagedenic' ulcer forms which spreads peripherally by contiguous auto-inoculation. These lesions may mutilate the genitalia. They heal by granulation and months may elapse before healing is complete.

Diagnosis. Chancroid ulcers and buboes must be differentiated from other causes of genital ulceration and bubo formation. Three diagnostic methods are used to diagnose chancroid: Gram stain, auto-inoculation, and culture but only culture of *H. ducreyi* is specific.

The characteristic pleomorphic Gram-negative bacilli can be identified in about 50 per cent of smears taken from the edges of a suspect ulcer. The morphological characteristics of the Ducrey bacillus are common to other Gram-negative organisms that frequently superinfect chancroid lesions, which limits the specificity of this procedure. Identification of *H. ducreyi* by Gram stain of bubo

aspirate makes the diagnosis of chancroid more secure, but this happens only rarely

The classical method of differentiating chancroid from other causes of genital ulceration and bubo formation was by auto-inoculation of bubo aspirate or, less commonly, by producing typical chancroid lesions in the forearm of a volunteer by intradermal inoculation of bubo aspirate. This technique was not without hazard and has no use today.

The definitive diagnosis rests on isolation of *H. ducreyi* in culture from genital ulcerations or bubo aspirates. Only a slight majority of clinically diagnosed chancroid patients, however, are culture positive.

Hammond and his colleagues proposed levels of diagnostic certainty for clinical chancroid; the first is confirmed by culture isolation of *H. ducreyi*; a second includes probable cases who have no laboratory evidence for syphilis or herpes virus but who are sexual contacts of a proved chancroid case; and a third, suspect category includes those who are dark-ground and serologically negative for syphilis but in whom herpes infection and other causes of genital ulceration are not exluded by laboratory tests.

None of the venereal ulcers or buboes is so clinically distinct as to preclude the need for careful laboratory evaluation (Tables 1 and 2). A recent example in Atlanta is illustrative: several patients

Table 1   Differential diagnosis of venereal genital ulcers

Type	Pain	Size	Edges	Induration	Evolution	Scar tissue	Bubo formation	Diagnostic tests
Primary syphilis	rare	0.5–2 cm	smooth, elevated	present	2–6 weeks	no*	very rare	dark-ground serology
Chancroid	frequent	0.5–5 cm	ragged, undermined	no	6 days–6 months	yes	yes	culture, smear for the Ducrey bacillus
Granuloma inguinale	rare	variable	smooth, rolled elevated	present	2–6 months	yes	pseudo-bubo	tissue biopsy, smears for Donovan bodies
Lymphogranuloma venereum	no	0.2–2.5 cm	smooth	no	1–5 days	no	yes	culture, serology for chlamydia
Genital herpes	frequent	0.2–2 cm	irregular	no	2–6 weeks	no*	yes	culture, serology for herpes simplex
Gonorrhoea	yes	variable	irregular, undermined	no	1–2 weeks	no*	very rare	culture, smear for gonococci
Trauma	frequent	variable	smooth or irregular	no	rapid	variable	no	negative other tests

* Unless superinfected by other bacteria

Table 2   Differential diagnosis of venereal buboes

	Occurrence	Site	Pain	Genital lesion	Usual size	Consistency	Suppuration	Diagnosis
Primary syphilis	rare	usually bilateral	painless	present	<5 cm	rubbery, firm	absent	dark-ground examination of genital lesion and bubo aspirate for *T. pallidum*; serology
Chancroid	70% cases	usually unilateral	moderate to severe	present	<5 cm	unilocular, soft	common, with spontaneous rupture	culture of genital lesions and bubo aspirate for Ducrey bacillus
Granuloma inguinale	pseudobubo in 50% cases	variable	mild	often very extensive	variable	not involved, unless secondarily infected	ulcerates overlying skin	smears and biopsy for Donovan bodies
Lymphogranuloma venereum	very common	⅓ bilateral	moderate to severe	absent	>5 cm	multilocular, soft; later fluctuant	common with multiple sinus tracts	culture of bubo aspirate and serologic tests for chlamydia
Genital herpes	rare	bilateral	mild to moderate	present	<5 cm	firm, discrete	absent	smear and culture for herpesvirus
Gonorrhoea	very rare	unilateral	moderate to severe	rare	>5 cm	unilocular, soft	common	cultures and smears for gonococci

diagnosed clinically as granuloma inguinale had negative tissue biopsies for *C. granulomatis*, but the biopsies grew almost pure cultures of *H. ducreyi*.

Treatment. Tetracycline and sulphonamides have been recommended for treatment of chancroid for several decades. The recommended doses are tetracycline hydrochloride, 500 mg by mouth four times a day for seven days, or sulphisoxazole, 1 g four times a day for seven days. Treatment should be extended if buboes enlarge during treatment or if the genital sores have not healed within one week.

Other drugs such as doxycycline, 300 mg by mouth in a single dose, or ampicillin have been used to treat chancroid. The therapeutic response to doxycycline is good if the chancroidal lesion is small and the bubo is less than 5 cm in diameter. The efficacy of this regimen as well as the tetracycline regimen is uncertain. Recent reports indicate that *H. ducreyi* isolated in Southeast Asia and East Africa are relatively resistant to tetracycline.

Kanamycin, 500 mg by intramuscular injection twice daily for 7–14 days was used successfully to treat sulphonamide- and tetracycline-resistant chancroid in South Vietnam. Co-trimoxazole (80 mg trimethoprim and 400 mg sulphamethoxazole) tablets given four times a day for 7–10 days has shown some promise in treatment of 'resistant' chancroid.

Dual infections of gonorrhoea and chancroid, or of syphilis and chancroid should be treated as separate infections. Penicillin has only limited activity against *H. ducreyi* and several recently isolated strains have elaborated a β-lactamase which inactivates benzylpenicillin and ampicillin.

Prevention. Cleaning the genitalia with soap and water or douching with a mild antiseptic solution immediately after sexual exposure will prevent chancroid in most instances. Identification of sexual contacts of a suspect or proven cases of chancroid and providing prophylactic antibiotic treatment to such contacts will contain epidemics.

Control of chancroid where the disease is endemic will be difficult given the low levels of sanitation and personal hygiene that usually exist. A reservoir of infection among prostitutes might be eliminated if contact tracing were possible. Chancroid will, in all likelihood, decrease in prevalence as living standards improve in endemic areas.

References

Hammond, G. W., Slutchuk, M., Scatliff, J., *et al* (1980). Epidemiologic, clinical laboratory and therapeutic features of an urban outbreak of chancroid in North America. *Rev. infect. Dis.* **2**, 867.

Nsanze, H., Fast, M., D'Costa, L. J., *et al.* (1981) Genital ulcer in Kenya: a clinical and laboratory study of 97 patients. *J. vener. Dis.* (in press).

Marmar, J. L. (1972). The management of resistant chancroid in Vietnam. *J. Virol.* **107**, 807.

Tau, T., Rajan, V. S., Koe, S. L., *et al.* (1977). Chancroid: a study of 500 cases. *Asian J. infect. Dis.* **1**, 27.

Stamps, T. J. (1974). Experience with doxycycline (Vibramycin) in the treatment of chancroid. *J. trop. Med. Hyg.* **77**, 55.

Lymphogranuloma venereum

P. L. Perine

Lymphogranuloma venereum (LGV) is a systemic venereal disease caused by certain bacterial strains of *Chlamydia trachomatis*. It is primarily a disease affecting lymphatic tissue, with acute manifestations which include an inguinal syndrome with painful swelling of inguinal, femoral, and deep iliac lymph nodes, and an anorectal syndrome characterized by an ulcerative proctitis. Late complications include genital elephantiasis, rectal stricture, penile and rectovaginal fistula formation.

Aetiology. The *Chlamydiae* (see also page 5.346) and a group of obligatory intracellular parasites with a unique, complex, reproductive cycle. Small in size (0.2–0.4 μm), they are non-motile, Gram-negative, coccoid bacteria that differ from viruses by having a cell wall, by an ability to synthesize both DNA and RNA, and by being susceptible to antibiotics. The two species, *C. psittaci* and *C. trachomatis*, share a common complement-fixing antigen but differ in their susceptibility to sulphonamides, synthesis of glycogen, and host range. *C. trachomatis* are supha-sensitive and infect only man. They multiply within the cytoplasm of infected cells and form compact, glycogen-rich inclusions which stain brown with iodine.

Fifteen strains of *C. trachomatis* are differentiated through a fluorescent antibody technique into serotypes designated by the letters A to K. Serotypes A, B, Ba, and C cause trachoma; types D to K infect the genito-urinary tract and cause urethritis, cervicitis, salpingitis, and neonatal pneumonia; and types with designations L1, L2, and L3 cause LGV. Serological cross-reaction is observed between other types of *C. Trachomatis*. The LGV chlamydae are more invasive than the other serotypes and cause disease primarily in lymphatic tissue.

Epidemiology. LGV is found worldwide, but its major incidence is limited to endemic foci in tropical and sub-tropical Africa, Southeast Asia, South America and the Caribbean. All races are equally susceptible to infection, but the reported sex ration is usually greater than 5:1 in favour of men. This is because early clinical LGV recognized much more frequently in men than in women, who may not be diagnosed until late complications have developed.

In North America and Europe LGV is usually diagnosed in travellers, seamen, and military personnel returning from endemic areas, and male homosexuals. The reservoir of infection is presumed to be asymptomatically infected women and male homosexuals. The frequency of infection following exposure is not known, but the coincidence of LGV in sexual partners indicates that transmission occurs much less often than is the case in gonorrhoea and syphilis.

Pathogenesis. The process by which LGV chlamydiae invade the host is not known, but it probably involves attachment to epithelial cells and their phagocytosis in the urogenital tract and rectosigmoid colon. Chlamydiae multiply, destroy cells, and are carried to regional lymph nodes whence they may spread systemically. Host immunity presumably limits chlamydial multiplication, cell destruction, and the progression of disease in the majority of cases, but it may not eliminate organisms from the body. Latent infection occurs, but its mechanism is poorly understood.

Although a small, evanescent, genital lesion may be the first sign of infection, the pathology is largely restricted to the regional lymph nodes. These rapidly enlarge. Inflammation of the capsule causes the nodes to mat together. Multiple minute abscesses form in the parenchyma, and in the absence of treatment they may coalesce and form sinus tracts which rupture through the overlying skin.

Scar tissue may obstruct lymphatic flow causing lymphoedema and elephantiasis of the genitalia. Patients become sensitized to chlamydial antigens, and the chronic inflammatory response to their presence in tissue causes hyperplasia and necrosis. The end result may be strictures, ulceration, and fistula formation.

Clinical features. Three stages of infection designated primary, secondary, and tertiary, are usually recognized. Following an incubation period of 3–21 days, the primary lesion appears on the external genitalia. It occurs in fewer than 25 per cent of cases and may escape notice. It is a small, painless vesicular or ulcerative lesion that disappears spontaneously within a few days and leaves no scar.

Extragenital primary lesions are rare. A small ulcerative lesion usually appears at the site of infection and invariably causes regional lymphadenitis.

The manifestations of the secondary stage are conventionally separated into *inguinal* and the *genito-anorectal* syndromes. The more common inguinal syndrome is usually seen in men and is manifested by acute, painful bubo formation of the inguinal lymph nodes. The skin overlying the bubo is stretched taut and has a bluish discoloration. The lymphadenopathy is unilateral in two-thirds of cases, and in a rare instances it may be so extensive that the inguinal mass is cleaved by the inelastic Poupart's ligament—the almost pathognomic 'groove sign' of LGV. Buboes are accompanied by fever, malaise, chills, arthralgia, and headache. About 75 per cent of buboes suppurate and form cutaneous sinus tracts. Sinus drainage may persist for several weeks or months and, occasionally, an indurated inguinal mass forms which may persist for a lifetime.

In women, the external and internal iliac lymph nodes and the sacral lymphatics are involved more frequently than are the inguinal lymph nodes. Fever, chills, and malaise occur and may not be associated with LGV unless the pelvis is examined. Signs include a hypertrophic cervicitis with discharge of pus from the cervical os, backache, and adnexal tenderness due to enlarged retroperitoneal lymph nodes. None of these findings, however, is specific for LGV.

In both sexes, a genito-anorectal syndrome characterized by a haemorrhagic proctitis or protocolitis may occur, a result of chlamydial invasion of epithelial cells lining the intestinal tract. But it is found more frequently in women, probably as the result of contamination of the anal area with infectious vaginal secretions or by spread of infection by the pelvic lymphatics. The rectal mucosa may be directly infected by chlamydiae in homosexual men practising rectal intercourse. The mucosa is friable and hyperaemic. Scattered, 1–2 cm diameter ulcerations with granular bases are seen by proctosigmoidoscopic examination. The inflammatory process is limited to the rectosigmoid colon and is accompanied by fever, a mucopurulent or bloody anal discharge, tenesmus, and diarrhoea. The process usually resolves spontaneously after a period of several weeks.

Early proctocolitis is rarely complicated by rectal abscesses, fistulain-ano, rectovaginal, rectovesical, and ischiorectal fistulas. Late in the course of disease, a rectal stricture located 2–6 cm from the anal orifice and extending proximally for several centimetres may develop.

Rare manifestations of the secondary stage of LGV are acute meningoencephalitis and follicular conjunctivitis. The latter is usually the result of auto-inoculation of infected material from buboes, the vagina, or rectum to one or both eyes. Although it may cause enlargement of the maxillary and post-auricular lymph nodes (Parinaud's oculoglandular syndrome), the follicular conjunctivitis is self-limiting.

The lesions of the tertiary stage appears after a period of latency of several years, during which the only evidence of infection is scars from secondary lesions and positive serologic tests for LGV. Late complications are rarely seen today because they can be prevented by treatment with a variety of broad-spectrum antibiotics, which may coincidentally cure LGV when given to the patient for other infections.

Genital elephantiasis caused from a combination of lymphoedema, hyperplasia, and necrosis is the most common tertiary complication. It occurs predominantly in women as a sequel to the genito-anorectal syndrome and is very rare in men. The elephantiasis may be accompanied by polypoid growths which, when they occur in the perianal area, resemble haemorroids ('lymphorrhoids'). Fistulae occur frequently in association with elephantiasis. These lesions are often very painful and interfere with normal functions of the affected parts. Secondary bacterial infection is usual and accelerates tissue necrosis.

Rectal stricture is the most serious tertiary lesion and is found almost exclusively in women. Symptoms include constipation, tenderness, and pain. Complete obstruction may lead to bowel perforation. Recto-vaginal fistula formation is common.

Diagnosis. Three different categories of diagnostic tests are used to diagnose LGV. They are the Frei skin test, the identification of LGV chlamydiae from infected tissue, and serological tests. The now outdated classical Frei skin test for LGV used a suspension of elementary bodies grown in yolk sac, inactivated by treatment with formalin and phenol. A standard concentration of this material in 0.1 ml was inoculated intradermally on one forearm, and a control inoculation of normal, formalin-phenol treated yolk sac was placed on the other forearm. The diameter of induration was read at 48 hours; a positive response had a diameter of not less than 5 mm, with a negative control. The Frei test has fallen into disfavour because it is neither highly sensitive nor specific for LGV. As a result, Frei antigen is no longer commercially produced.

LGV chlamydiae can be identified in infected tissue when special stains and microscopic techniques are used, or by isolation in the yolk sac of embryonated hen eggs or in tissue culture. Chlamydiae tissue culture is more sensitive and practical than is microscopic examination of infected tissue, but only 25–40 per cent of LGV patients have positive cultures of bubo aspirate, endo-urethral or endocervical scrapings, or other infected material. Yield can be improved by culturing specimens from a variety of sites.

Several serological tests detect chlamydial antibody in serum. The oldest and most widely used test is the complement fixtation (CF) test which uses an antigen common to all chlamydiae, and is, therefore, not specific for LGV. However, the titre of CF antibody in acute LGV infections is usually greater than 1:64. Although a fourfold or greater incrase in CF titre between acute and convalescent sera renders the diagnosis of LGV more certain, this is rarely observed. The CF titre usually declines rapidly after adequate treatment.

The different serotypes of *C. trachomatis* can be distinguished by the micro-immunofluorescent (micro-IF) test. In the micro-IF test, the different strains of *C. trachomatis* are placed separately or in groups on microscope slides and reacted with varying dilutions of the patient's serum in an indirect fluorescent antibody assay. Micro-IF antibody titres are frequently greater than 1:256 in acute sera from patients with LGV. Because of the broad cross-reactivity seen in the micro-IF test between different strains, it may not be possible to determine which of the LGV types is responsible for a given infection.

When possible, a serum specimen should first be tested by CF and then, if strongly positive, in by micro-IF. The combination of a positive CF and micro-IF in high-titre in a patient with typical signs and symptoms is diagnostic of LGV.

Other diseases that must be considered in the differential diagnosis of the inguinal LGV syndrome are genital herpes infection, syphilis, chancroid, extrapulmonary tuberculosis, cat-scratch fever, plague and malignant lymphoma. Lymphadenitis of the deep iliac nodes may mimic appendicitis or pelvic inflammatory disease (see page 5.319). Many surgeons, ignorant of LGV, have mistaken an LGV bubo for an incarcerated inguinal hernia and realize their error only at the time of surgery.

Primary genital herpes infection (see page 5.327) provides the greatest diagnostic confusion. Constitutional symptoms are similar in both infections, and herpetic lesions may be occult. Herpetic patients often have tender, discreetly enlarged inguinal lymph nodes, but those seldom reach the size seen in LGV. The inguinal lymphadenitis common in primary syphilis and the suppurative inguinal buboes characteristic of chancroid occur at the same time as genital chancres or ulcers, but the combination is seldom found in LGV. Nevertheless, dark-ground examination and serological tests for syphilis, as well as cultures of genital ulcers and bubo aspirates for *Haemophilus ducreyi* and *Neisseria gonorrhoeae* should be part of the diagnostic evaluation of any patient with genital lesions and lymphadenitis. One or more of these diseases may occur simultaneously in the same patient. The proctitis of the genito-anorectal syndrome of LGV may be indistinguishable from that seen at the onset of chronic ulcerative, acute amoebic, or antibiotic-associated colitis. Every patient with haemorrhagic proctitis should, therefore, be carefully evaluated by proctosigmoidoscopic and radiologic examination, rectal biopsy, culture, and other tests of stool for both bacterial and parasitic pathogens.

Patients with ulcerative colitis and regional ileitis may have positive CF chlamydial serological tests in high titre and a positive micro-IF test. Only in rare instances, however, have LGV chlamydiae been isolated from an inflamed bowel, and, despite circumstantial evidence, no causal relationship has been proved to exist between LGV and these diseases. Positive chlamydial CF tests are also seen occasionally in patients with cat-scratch fever.

Tuberculosis and certain parasitic and fungal infections of the genital tract cause lymphoedema and elephantiasis of the genitalia. Tissue biopsy and special culture techniques may differentiate elephantiasis due to LGV from other causes.

Treatment. Of the several antimicrobial drugs active against LGV chlamydiae in tissue culture, only a few are used to treat LGV patients. Oral tetracycline, 1–2 g daily or a sulphonamide such as sulphadiazine 4 g daily, are usually recommended. There is little evidence to support the choice of one drug rather than another, and only marginal evidence that antimicrobial treatment is better than symptomatic treatment alone in acute inguinal LGV. Fever and bubo pain rapidly subside after antimicrobials are started, but buboes may take several weeks to resolve. Suppuration and rupture of buboes with sinus tract formation is usually prevented by antimicrobials. It is not known how long treatment need be continued to prevent relapse and progression of disease. A minimum of two weeks is recommended. The patient's sexual partner should be treated at the same time, to prevent reinfection. Unruptured, fluctuant buboes should be aspirated with a syringe through a large bore needle. This prevents sinus tract formation. Surgical incision and drainage is neither necessary nor recommended. Buboes that are draining should be covered with dressings soaked in antiseptic solution until drainage ceases, in order to prevent auto-innoculation and nosocomial infection.

The fistulae, strictures, and elephantiasis of chronic LGV may require plastic repair. Surgery should not be attempted until the patient has received several weeks or months of antibiotic treatment which often reduces the degree of inflammation and necrosis so that healing proceeds normally and only limited surgical repair is necessary.

Prognosis. The early manifestations of LGV are self-limiting. Late sequelae are rarely seen today, even in areas of the world where the disease is still common. At one time, rectal fibrosis was thought to predispose to carcinoma, but there is little supportive evidence that such is the case today. In the pre-antibiotic era, rectal stricture causing complete bowel obstruction, perforation, and death were reported.

Genital elephantiasis, recto-vaginal, and other types of fistulae are significant social and medical problems in several lesser developed nations in Africa and Asia. Whether or not LGV plays a significantly aetiologic role in these problems is unknown.

References
Alergant, C. D. (1957). Lymphogranuloma inguinale in the male in Liverpool, England, 1947 to 1954. *Br. J. vener. Dis.* **33**, 47.
Dunlop, E. M. C., Vaughan-Jackson, J. D., and Darougar, S. (1972). Chlamydial infection: improved methods of collection of material for culture from the urogenital tract and rectum. *Br. J. vener. Dis.* **48**, 421.
Greaves, A. B., Hilleman, M. R., Taggart, S. R., Bankhead, A. B., and Feld, M. (1957). Chemotherapy in bubonic lymphogranuloma venereum. *Bull. Wld Hlth Org.* **16**, 227.
Perine, P. L., Andersen, A. J., Krause, D. W., Awoke, S., Wang, S. P., Kud, C. C., and Holmes, K. K. (1980). Diagnosis and treatment of lymphogranuloma venereum in Ethiopia. In *Current chemotherapy and infectious disease*, 1280. American Society of Microbiology, Washington, DC.
Schachter, J. (1977). Lymphogranuloma venereum and other nonocular *Chlamydia trachomatis* infections. In *Nongonococcal urethritis and related infections* (eds. D. Hobson and K. K. Holmes), 91. American Society of Microbiology, Washington, DC.

Gonorrhoea

G. W. Csonka

Definition. Gonorrhoea is an infection of the mucosa of the genito-urinary tract due to *Neisseria gonorrhoeae* usually transmitted by sexual intercourse, but can be asexually acquired by young children and by infants of infected mothers during birth. Man is the natural host. Sites which may be involved apart from the genital tract are the rectum, oropharynx, the eyes, the epididymis, the Fallopian tubes, and perihepatic tissue. Dissemination of the infection may produce lesions in joints, skin, and rarely the meninges and endocardium.

Aetiology. The causative organism, *N. gonorrhoeae* is fastidious in its environmental and nutritional requirements and dies quickly outside the body. It is a Gram-negative diplococcus found typically in a group inside the cytoplasm of polymorphonuclear leucocyctes (Fig. 1). In appearance it is identical with *N. meningitidis* and non-pathogenic *neisseria*. Five colony types have been recognized, of which type 1 and 2 are virulent and characterized by having appendages called pili which play a part in the mechanism of attachment to epithelial cells and probably in increasing resistance to phagocytosis.

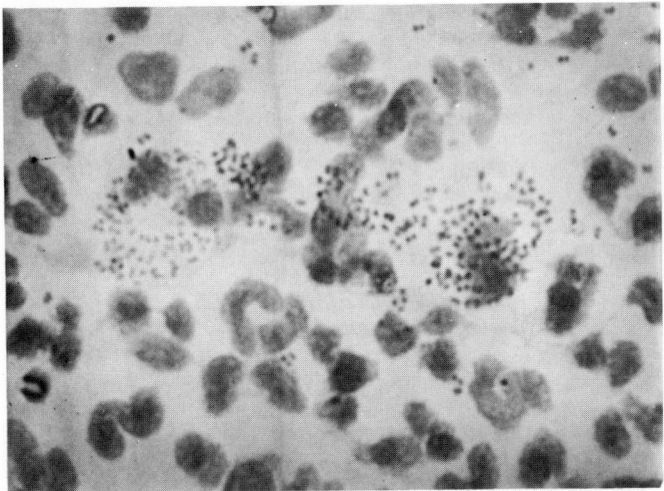

Fig. 1 Gram-stained urethral smear showing intracellular and extracellular diplococci.

There are a number of different strains but no simple method of typing is available. Classification according to nutritional requirements (auxotyping), immunological characteristics, and antibiotic sensitivity pattern have all been used. The strains isolated in disseminated gonorrhoea are highly sensitive to penicillin and have other features which separate them from the rest.

Pathogenicity. The gonococcus involves the columnar epithelium of the genitalia, rectum, and conjunctivae, while stratified squamous epithelium is much more resistant to the organism. It invades the mucosal cells and, after penetration, colonizes the subepithelial tissues. Inside polymorphonuclear cells they multiply but are eventually phagocytosed, and the infection terminates spontaneously, though significant protective immunity does not develop.

Misuse of antibiotics, especially penicillin, in Asia and elsewhere has been responsible for the emergence of penicillin-resistant strains. Such strains show often cross-resistance to other antibiotics and make control more difficult. Some strains produce penicillinase (β-lactamase) which destroys penicillin and renders the organism completely resistant to this antibiotic.

Strains producing β-lactamase. In 1976 β-lactamase producing gonococci were reported in USA servicemen who had returned from the Philippines. At the same time a localized outbreak of 76 such cases occurred in Liverpool. The infection almost certainly originated in West Africa. Cases have now been reported from many parts of the world. The majority were initially contracted from the Far East and West Africa but recently an increasing proportion of cases found in Europe, notably in the Netherlands, were infected locally, indicating that the infection has become established outside the endemic areas. One should keep the problem in perspective; whilst of major significance in the endemic areas, in Europe and the USA the strains have so far not spread as fast as was feared. Thus, in the UK there were 15 cases in 1977, 31 in 1978, and 104 in 1979 out of a total of over 61 000 cases in that year. Continued epidemiological assessment is essential.

Epidemiology. In the UK the incidence was low before the Second World War and as expected, increased sharply during the War followed by a steep fall after 1945. The figures started to rise in the mid-fifties up to 1977. This was the first time that a sustained rise in the incidence had occurred in peace time. The most significant factor was probably a change in sexual behaviour. Other causes which encouraged the spread of the infection were the increasing use of oral contraception which may have encouraged casual sexual relationships and at the same time reduced the need for condom protected intercourse, the increased mobility of large number of people into foreign countries and away from stable home conditions, movements of many from rural areas to towns where opportunities for infection are greater, and the increase of homosexuality which accounts for a large number of infections in the cities. There is a suggestion that this prolonged upward trend may have reached its peak as in 1978 and 1979 the number of new cases of gonorrhoea in the UK has decreased from 65 963 in 1977 to 61 616 in 1979. The experience in the USA and elsewhere is similar but it remains to be seen whether this downward trend will continue.

The incidence of some of the more serious complications has significantly decreased. Severe systemic gonorrhoea and gonococcal ophthalmia neonatorum have decreased in incidence, but PID appears to be on the increase and is now the most important major complication of gonorrhoea.

Men with gonorrhoea have greatly outnumbered women attending clinics but this too is changing. Thus the male/female ratio in the USA dropped from 2.4:1 in 1960 to 1.5:1 in 1977. In Sweden the difference has almost disappeared with a ratio of 1.1:1 in 1976 and in the UK from 4:1 in 1961 to 1.5:1 in 1978. This change in the relative incidence of the sexes does not necessarily reflect solely an increase of infection amongst women but is probably due to several factors, one of which is the increasingly successful contact tracing, the effect of control programmes directed mainly at women, and the greater willingness of young women to attend clinics.

Homosexual men contribute a considerable number of gonococcal infections in some areas, but there are no national figures available. It would be of considerable help to have reliable statistics on gonorrhoea, syphilis, hepatitis B, and other sexually transmitted diseases commonly found in this group to provide a sound basis to evaluate epidemiological, prophylactic, and therapeutic measures.

Clinical features

Uncomplicated gonorrhoea in heterosexual males. The incubation period is short—on average three to five days (range: 1–12 days). It starts with mild dysuria and a purulent urethral discharge. The first voided urine will show a haze due to pus. In the UK 90–95 per cent have marked urethritis but 5–10 per cent may be asymptomatic and therefore especially prone to spread the infection unwittingly. The asymptomatic form is more common in men whose female partner

develops pelvic inflammatory disease and in men who suffer from gonococcal epididymitis or systemic gonococcal infection.

Local complications are rare now that prompt and effective treatment is the rule. They include abscess formation of urethral glands such as the para-urethral ducts near the meatus, tysonitis which is infection of small parafrenal glands, abscess formation of glands along the medial ventral raphae of the shaft of the penis, and peri-urethral abscesses which can become large and painful and usually burst into the urethra, or more rarely externally to produce a sinus. Infected Cowper's glands cause pain in the perineum, giving rise to a very tender swelling which can be felt between a finger in the anus and one on the perineum. This complication must be differentiated from perianal and ischiorectal abscess.

The most important though still rare local complication is *gonococcal epididymitis*. It is an ascending infection, usually unilateral and though a number of provoking factors have been suggested, such as trauma and sexual intercourse, generally no initiating factor is found. It starts fairly acutely with painful swelling and redness of one side of the scrotum sometimes with some overlying oedema. On gentle palpation the lower pole of the epididymis feels enlarged and is very tender. The spermatic cord is often palpable and thickened. A secondary hydrocele may be mistaken for testicular involvement. Malaise and low-grade fever may be present. Urethritis is often minimal or has cleared by the time epididymitis develops. After recovery which may take a few weeks, residual fibrosis of the globus major may prompt quite unnecessary investigations and treatment. In the very unusual patient with bilateral epididymitis, sterility may follow.

Differential diagnoses includes:

1. Non-gonococcal epididymitis. The absence of gonococci in the urethral discharge and good response to tetracycline but not penicillin are characteristic. In general, the epididymitis tends to be milder than the gonococcal form.

2. Testicular torsion. The patient is commonly a teenager, the onset is hyperacute with intense pain and rapid swelling of the scrotal content. This is a surgical emergency and the patient should be operated on without delay.

3. Tuberculous epididymitis. The onset is more insidious, the epididymis feels hard and craggy, and the two-glass urine test often shows pus in both glasses due to renal involvement. Full bacteriological and urological examination is called for if this complication is suspected.

4. Malignant tumour of the testis. Any undiagnosed enlargement or nodule in the scrotum in a young person, especially if the swelling involves the testis and there is no evidence of urinary infection must be investigated by surgical exposure.

5. Trauma. The history usually makes the diagnosis clear.

Urethral stricture used to be a dreaded and not uncommon late complication of gonorrhoea in the pre-antibiotic era. Nowadays it may be found in remote areas of the world where treatment for gonorrhoea is not readily available. It develops years after the original infection with symptoms of progressive urinary obstruction, such as poor urinary stream, delay in starting urination, straining at micturition, and dribbling. Ultimately urinary retention may develop sometimes precipitated by large intake of alcohol. Urinary infection is almost invariably present.

Post-gonococcal urethritis (PGU). This is non-gonococcal urethritis which develops after successful cure of gonorrhoea and is discussed on page 5.317.

Uncomplicated gonorrhoea in homosexual males. The infection is often asymptomatic. Sometimes there is an abrupt onset of proctitis with anorectal discharge and discomfort. On proctoscopy the appearance may be normal or the mucosa is inflamed with streaks of mucopus or frank discharge. If there are ulcers, tests for genital herpes and syphilis must be undertaken. As syphilis is relatively common in these patients one may consider using a drug such as co-trimoxazole which will not mask this infection. In any case serological tests for syphilis should be taken at the outset and again two or three months later.

Oropharyngeal gonorrhoea is more common in homosexual men than other groups of patients and throat cultures are the only means to make this diagnosis.

Uncomplicated gonorrhoea in females. The commonest sites involved are the endocervix, followed by the urethra and rectum; the latter can be the only site yielding gonococci. Before puberty the vaginal epithelium can support the growth of gonococci but after puberty the fornices may be the only area of the vagina capable of being infected; however, there is no consensus of opinion on this. Trichomonas vaginitis is commonly associated with gonorrhoea when the profuse discharge may overshadow gonococcal infection, therefore patients with trichomoniasis should be carefully screened for gonorrhoea.

Clinically, at least half the women have no symptoms and little or nothing abnormal is seen on examination. The rest have a variable discharge which is not characteristic. Some patients complain of dysuria and some have proctitis. The majority of women seek medical attention because their sexual partner has gonorrhoea.

Screening women at risk for gonorrhoea is of proven value in detecting and treating asymptomatic carriers and thus reducing the infectious pool.

Local complications. Occasionally the paraurethral glands (Skene's glands) are infected. More important is involvement of Bartholin's glands producing unilateral *Bartholinitis*. The gland and its short duct is situated in the posterior third of each labium majus. The duct becomes infected and often obstructed when an abscess forms. It is seen as a forward projection of the vulva and the inflamed mass eventually becomes fluctuent and will burst through the inner surface of the labium minus unless the patient can be treated.

Vulvitis is more characteristic in children with gonorrhoea. Signs of mild *trigonitis* may be present.

Pelvic inflammatory disease (PID).This is the commonest and most important complication of gonorrhoea in women. Gonococcal PID appears to be much more frequent in the USA than in the UK, possibly reflecting the differences in the incidence of gonorrhoea in the two countries. Gonococcal PID is more readily recognized than the non-gonococcal form and is estimated to occur in 10–15 per cent of untreated women with gonorrhoea. Whether this estimate is correct is uncertain when one recalls that more than half of women with gonorrhoea are asymptomatic and may not seek medical advice and an unknown number have minimal PID which is unsuspected and discovered by chance during investigation for infertility. In a proportion of women with chronic vague lower abdominal pain due to PID, clinical examination is unhelpful and the diagnosis can only be made on laparoscopy.

The infection ascends from the cervix through the uterus to the mucosa of the Fallopian tubes which it colonizes, producing a purulent exudate which accumulates and may spill into the peritoneum. The Fallopian tubes enlarge and become oedematous. If the infection is not checked early on, the mucosa of the tube is irreversibly damaged. This acute salpingitis is the basis of PID.

Clinical features are more clear-cut than in non-gonococcal PID (see page 5.319) and the disease is usually more acute. The onset is sudden with:

1. Lower abdominal pain and tenderness which is often bilateral.
2. Reflex spasm of the lower abdominal muscles.
3. Fever which is usually over 38 °C.
4. Leucocytosis of over 20 000/ml.
5. An onset which commonly occurs during or immediately after a period which may be more severe and prolonged than usual and can be regarded as already part of the illness.
6. Examination reveals marked tenderness in one or both iliac fossae.

7. At pelvic examination, movement of the cervix from side to side induces pain in *both* tubes (unilateral infection is unusual).
8. Bimanual palpation of the lateral fornices elicits severe pain and at a later stage when a tubal abscess has formed, the tubes can be felt as smooth sausage-shaped structures, and later still if pus collects in the pouch of Douglas, this too can be felt as a boggy mass.

There are, however, a number of patients in whom symptoms and signs are indefinite and the diagnosis can only be made by laparoscopy. The gonococcus may be isolated from the cervix and other genital sites but this is not always the case. If there are grounds for suspecting a gonococcal aetiology e.g. if the sexual partner had gonorrhoea recently, one should treat without delay. Luckily if the patient is diagnosed as non-gonococcal PID when in fact the gonococcus is the cause, the treatment is likely to include antibiotics which are effective in both types.

Treatment. This is essentially medical: (*a*) bed rest until fever and pain have disappeared, which means admission of most patients to hospital; (*b*) penicillin in large doses. Details of drug treatment are given in Table 2; and (*c*) watch for bowel obstruction in the early days.

Generally the patient improves in 48 hours of antibiotic therapy and should be clear within two weeks. If there is no rapid response to medical treatment, the patient should be re-assessed in consultation with the gynaecologist.

Surgery is rarely needed. Indications are: (*a*) doubt about the diagnosis. Especially when appendicitis cannot be excluded, laparotomy should be performed. If salpingitis is confirmed, the abdomen is closed; (*b*) when rupture of a pyosalpinx is suspected; (*c*) intestinal obstruction; and (*d*) development of a pelvic abscess which should be drained early to reduce the incidence of severe chronic PID.

Late complications. These are more common when treatment has been delayed or was inadequate and in severe bilateral infection. They include reduced fertility, infertility, greater tendency to tubal-pregnancy, recurrence of salpingitis because the damaged mucosa is non-functional and cannot keep the tubes clear; the infections are no longer due to the gonococcus which has been eliminated during the original course of antibiotics. Chronic PID, sometimes with acute exacerbations, is essentially characterized by chronic lower abdominal pain and deep dyspareunia. If such a patient fails to respond to repeated courses of antibiotics, radical surgical clearances may have to be considered.

Differential diagnoses include tubal pregnancy, acute appendicitis, acute pyelonephritis, infected ovarian cyst, septic abortion, endometriosis, intestinal obstruction, and non-gonococcal salpingitis.

Oropharyngeal gonorrhoea in both sexes. Infection at this site is getting more common due to an increase in orogenital sexual contact especially in homosexual males where incidence figures of 10–20 per cent have been reported. It is usually asymptomatic though some patients have signs of pharyngitis or tonsillitis. The diagnosis rests on a positive culture.

Disseminated gonococcal infection in both sexes. The incidence varies greatly in different regions of the world. It is uncommon in the UK and frequent in the USA. Women, especially pregnant women, are slightly more often affected than men. The *gonococcal strains* responsible differ in important respects from other strains by being exceptionally sensitive to penicillin and to the complement mediated bactericidal action of normal serum and by belonging to a limited number of autotypes. These strains are frequently associated with asymptomatic gonorrhoea in men. Host factors are also involved as strains causing disseminated gonorrhoea do not usually give rise to disseminated disease in sexual contacts and in some patients a deficiency of the sixth, seventh, and eighth components of complement is present.

Clinically there is a wide spectrum of symptoms ranging from the mildest transient arthralgia with some malaise and fever of short duration, to a severe destructive arthritis with marked constitutional upset. The arthritis is asymmetrical and may involve a knee or an ankle, the wrist, fingers, shoulder, sternoclavicular, and temporomandibular joints. In some patients arthritis is limited to a single joint. Tenosynovitis is a common feature. In about 30 per cent a characteristic painful rash develops. It may be papular, petechial, pustular, or necrotic. The lesions contain gonococci and it has been suggested that their endotoxin produce the skin lesions. Favourite sites are the distal parts of the limbs, including hands and soles. The rash is scanty with rarely more than 10–15 lesions present, often in various stages of their development at the same time. The severe form with septic arthritis is a medical emergency as delay or inadequate treatment can lead to the destruction of the joint with eventual ankylosis.

Nowadays, gonococcal meningitis, endocarditis or myopericarditis are very rarely seen in patients with disseminated infection. Endocarditis should be suspected if heart murmurs, embolic phenomena, ECG abnormalities, and unusually profuse skin lesions are present and blood cultures are repeatedly positive.

Diagnosis. Many patients do not have obvious urogenital or anorectal gonococcal infection and cultures from these sites may be negative. Culturing from all involved sites may also be unproductive. Blood cultures for gonococci should be performed within three days of onset, preferably whilst the temperature is still raised. Synovial fluid cultures are more often positive at a later stage. In pus from the skin lesions, Gram staining or immunofluorescence are superior to cultures. All patients with suspected septic arthritis must have their synovial fluid cultured.

Differential diagnoses include Reiter's disease, septic arthritis, meningococcal septicaemia, and rheumatic fever.

The presence of conjunctivitis, stomatitis, or keratoderma blennorrhagica points to a diagnosis of Reiter's disease even in the presence of the gonococcus.

Perihepatitis. This is usually seen associated with PID but can occur in men and may be mistaken for cholecystitis. There is pain in the right hypochondrium and sometimes a rub is heard over the liver. Apart from the gonococcus, other genital pathogens such as chlamidiae may be the causative micro-organism.

Vulvovaginitis in girls before puberty. The vulva is usually red and sometimes swollen and there is a variable amount of vaginal discharge due to true gonococcal vaginitis. The condition is often first noticed by the mother. It is rarely due to sexual assault but rather due to close contact with an infected parent, commonly the mother who shares a bed or a flannel with the child. Pharyngeal, rectal, and urethral infections have been reported amongst children from lower socio-economic groups. Sexual assault was not considered to be a significant factor.

Laboratory diagnosis
Microscopy of Gram-stained smears (see Fig. 1). In men with urethral gonorrhoea this simple method is almost 100 per cent diagnostic though confirmation by culture is desirable. If only extracellular diplococci are seen, culture is essential. In asymptomatic men the urethral smear will show fewer gonococci and once again culture is advisable. In women, direct microscopy is far less reliable and at best only 70 per cent accurate. The cervix gives the highest yield of positive results and culture is mandatory in women. In homosexual males the rectal smear is also less reliable than culture. In oropharyngeal gonorrhoea the smear has no diagnostic value whatever.

Culture. Cultures are therefore essential in women, homosexual men, in oropharyngeal infections, and are recommended in men with urethritis. They are of less value in skin lesions found in disseminated gonorrhoea. The Thayer–Martin selective medium which contains antibiotics to suppress contaminants allows the growth of gonococci and meningococci only and is satisfactory as is the more recent 'improved New York City medium'.

Oxidase test. Tetramethyl-p-phenelenediamine dihydrochloride stains gonococcal colonies and those of other neisseria purple and is used to pick out such colonies for further tests.

Gram-stained smears from suspected colonies. All *Neisseria* spp.

Table 1   Treatment of uncomplicated gonorrhoea

Diagnosis	Treatment	Comment
1. Uncomplicated gonorrhoea in men and women	oral ampicillin 3.5 g plus probenecid 1.0 g *or* procaine penicillin 2.4 million units i.m. plus probenecid 1.0 g	single dose treatment; cure rate is over 95% in the UK; not suitable in areas where β-lactamase producing strains are endemic or where penicillin resistance is high
2. Gonorrhoea due to β-lactamase producing strains	spectinomycin 2.0 g i.m. *or* cefuroxime 1.5 g i.m. plus probenecid 1.0 g	cure rate 99% cross allergy to penicillin in about 5%
3. Patients allergic to penicillin	co-trimoxazole 4 tabs b.d. × 2 days *or* doxycycline 300 mg single dose *or* minocycline 300 mg single dose *or* erythromycin stearate 1.5 g at once followed by 0.5 g q.i.d. × 4 days	cure rate 95%; evidence of some cross resistance with penicillin; advantage: does not mask syphilis nausea may occur vertigo in 5% In some areas erythromycin and tetracycline give poor results; advantage: longer course reduces incidence of PGU
4. Pregnant women allergic to penicillin	spectinomycin 2.0 g i.m. *or* erythromycin as above	
5. Anorectal or pharyngeal gonorrhoea, both sexes	ampicillin or co-trimoxazole as above	cure rate 95%
6. Post-gonococcal urethritis (PGU)	tetracycline 250 mg q.i.d. *or* equivalent × 7 days	

Table 2 Treatment of complicated gonorrhoea

Diagnosis	Treatment	Comment
1. Acute gonococcal PID *mild*	procaine penicillin 2.4 million units i.m. plus probenecid 1.0 g followed by oral ampicillin 0.5 g q.i.d. × 8 days	
2. Acute gonococcal PID *severe*	aqueous crystalline penicillin G 10 million units/day i.v. until improving (usually 48 hours) then: ampicillin by mouth 0.5 g q.i.d. × 8 days *or* procaine penicillin 2.4 million units b.d. until improving (approx. 48 hours) then ampicillin as above	*none of the treatments used in gonococcal PID are ideal* a case can be made for giving tetracycline as well as penicillin in the treatment to deal with mixed infections of gonococcal plus non-gonococcal PID
3. PID in patient allergic to penicillin	spectinomycin 2 g *or* cefuroxime 2 g i.m. t.i.d. until marked improvement followed by doxycycline 100 mg t.i.d. × 8 days *or* co-trimoxazole tabs. 2 t.i.d. × 8 days *or* erythromycin lactobionate 600 mg i.v. t.i.d. until marked improvement followed by erythromycin stearate orally 500 mg t.i.d. × 8 days	cephalosporins: cross allergy with penicillin in about 5%
4. Chronic severe PID	if repeated courses of antibiotics are ineffective radical surgical clearance should be considered but with every effort to save at at least part of an ovary	
5. Perihepatitis	as for PID which is commonly present	
6. Bartholinitis	ampicillin 0.5 g q.i.d until resolved; aspirate if abscess has formed; if that fails, marsupialize	treat as early as possible to prevent abscess formation
7. Disseminated gonorrhoea, *mild*	ampicillin 3.5 g orally plus probenecid 1.0 g orally followed by ampicillin 0.5 g q.i.d. × 8 days	highly sensitive to penicillin: if clinical picture suggests disseminated gonorrhoea but the organism is not isolated, treat just the same; prompt response supports the diagnosis
8. Disseminated gonorrhoea, *severe*	aqueous crystalline penicillin G 5–10 million units/day i.v. until improved (usually 48 hours) followed by ampicillin 0.5 g orally q.i.d. × 8 days *or* benzyl penicillin 1.2 million units i.m. q.i.d. × 2 days followed by oral ampicillin as above	
9. Disseminated gonorrhoea but patient allergic to penicillin	doxycycline 100 mg t.i.d. × 8 days *or* co-trimoxazole tabs. 2 t.i.d. × 8 days	
10. Gonococcal meningitis or endocarditis (may be part of 9)	crystalline penicillin G i.v. 10–20 million units daily until clear	highly sensitive to penicillin
11. Acute gonococcal epididymitis	ampicillin 0.5 g orally q.i.d *or* doxycycline 100 mg t.i.d. *or* co-trimoxazole tabs. 2 t.i.d. } until resolved (average 7–10 days)	if ambulant, to wear scrotal support during the day
12. Urethral stricture	should be under the care of the urologist who may decide to treat conservatively by regular urethral dilatation or by plastic restorative surgery	

Table 3 Treatment of gonorrhoea in infants and children

Diagnosis	Treatment	Comment
1. Gonococcal ophthalmia neonatorum	locally with penicillin eye drops (10 000 units/ml) at once and then after every feed plus procaine penicillin 300 000 units/day i.m. × 5 days	isolate infant with mother to prevent cross infection of other infants; start treatment without delay; treat mother and trace and treat her sexual contact
2. Gonococcal arthritis neonatorum	procaine penicillin 300 000 units/day i.m. × 5 days	treat mother and trace and treat her sexual contact
3. Vulvovaginitis of girls under the age of puberty	ampicillin syrup or paediatric suspension 250 mg t.i.d. × 5 days in children under 10 years; over 10 years: 500 mg t.i.d. × 5 days	test and treat the parent or person responsible for the infection

are Gram-negative and for final identification the *carbohydrate fermentation test*, preferably the new rapid method, is necessary. We also suggest that screening for β-lactamase production should be routinely employed to allow speedy contact tracing and appropriate treatment of all patients and their contacts infected with β-lactamase-producing strains.

Delayed fluorescent antibody staining (DFA). Staining smears from suspected colonies provides another method of identifying gonococci but is complex and requires many safeguards to be entirely reliable. For these reasons it is not entirely satisfactory for routine work.

Results incorporating all these procedures can be expected within three days.

Antibody sensitivity tests should be performed periodically to recognize sensitivity changes in a community. If any hitherto successful treatment fails to cure 95 per cent of uncomplicated gonorrhoea a change of treatment is indicated.

Serum tests for gonorrhoea. The GCFT and many newer serological methods have not much to offer in routine laboratory work.

Treatment. There are differences in the type of antibiotics used, the favoured mode of administration, and dosage schemes between individual clinics in a country and even more markedly between countries though the antibiotic sensitivity patterns are comparable. The results, however, appear to be similar. This suggests that a fair degree of latitude is permissible in the treatment of gonorrhoea.

Another factor which forces one to vary treatment is the ability of the versatile gonococcus to increase its resistance to a variety of unrelated compounds. The treatment suggested in Tables 1, 2, and 3 is based on experiences at many centres but may need frequent up-dating.

Follow-up examination. *In the male with uncomplicated gonorrhoea*. The patient is asked to return if the signs do not clear promptly after treatment and at any time should they reappear. Otherwise he is examined one week after treatment for gonococcal and non-gonococcal urethritis. If at that time there is no evidence of gonorrhoea it is unlikely to return unless the patient is reinfected. If there is PGU, this is treated. A final test which includes a second blood test for syphilis is performed two months later.

In practice many patients default once the symptoms and signs have disappeared.

In the female with uncomplicated gonorrhoea. Cure is indicated by two sets of negative cultures taken at weekly intervals after treatment and a final test including the second blood test for syphilis two months later. If rectal gonorrhoea was also found initially, rectal cultures should be repeated at every attendance as persistence of gonococci at this site may occur.

In patients of either sex with rectal or pharyngeal infection two negative cultures taken at weekly intervals after treatment and a second blood test for syphilis two months later are satisfactory. Thus on average patients with uncomplicated gonorrhoea need attend the hospital only three or four times.

With high risk patients such as promiscuous homosexual males and female prostitutes the same routine is followed. Three-monthly check-ups are recommended.

Prognosis. At present all patients with uncomplicated gonorrhoea can be cured. If they fail on one antibiotic an effective alternative can be found. Routine screening for β-lactamase-producing organisms will ensure that patients infected with such strains will receive the appropriate treatment at the earliest opportunity. Non-gonococcal infections associated with gonorrhoea may cause problems. Post-gonococcal urethritis responds to tetracycline as readily as NGU alone but there have been no large-scale studies comparing recurrence rates or those of complications between PGU and NGU. Reiter's disease can follow PGU.

The prognosis in complicated gonorrhoea is good except in the case of pelvic inflammatory disease and the rare gonococcal

meningitis and endocarditis which are potentially fatal diseases. In gonococcal endocarditis the valves may be rapidly destroyed and valve replacement may become necessary.

Some control measures. Measures which are of proven value in containing the infection include:
1. Contact tracing by fully trained personnel.
2. Readily available, accessible and well-publicized clinics in strategic positions dealing specifically with sexually transmitted diseases.
3. Large-scale screening programmes of women. These have been remarkably successful in the USA in finding new cases and reducing the infectious pool. They may be valuable in regions with endemic gonorrhoea but may have less scope elsewhere.
4. Health education: studies have shown a wide-spread ignorance amongst young people but also of young doctors due to lack of teaching the subject.
5. Epidemiological treatment, especially of women and homosexual men. This proved valuable in our experience and is also the policy in the USA.
6. Regular check-ups of high risk individuals.

References

Csonka, G. W. and Knight, G. J. (1967). Therapeutic trial of trimethoprim as a potentiator of sulphonamides in gonorrhoea. *Br. J. vener. Dis.* **43**, 161.
Hager, W. D. and Wiesner, P. J. (1977). Selected epidemiologic aspects of acute salpingitis: A review. *J. reproduct. Med.* **19**, 47.
Holmes, K. K., Counts, G. W. and Beaty, H. N. (1971). Disseminated gonococcal infection. *Ann. intern. Med.* **74**, 979.
Jacobson, L. and Westrom, L. (1969). Objectivized diagnosis of acute pelvic inflammatory disease. *Am. J. Obstet. Gynec.* **105**, 1088.
Owen, R. L. and Hill, J. L. (1972). Rectal and pharyngeal gonorrhoea in homosexual men. *J. Am. Med. Ass.* **220**, 1315.
Pariser, H., Farmer, A. D., and Marino, A. F. (1964). Asymptomatic gonorrhoea in the male. *Southern med. J.* **57**, 688.
Thompson, S. E. (1981). The clinical manifestations of gonococcal infections. In *Recent advances in sexually transmitted diseases* (ed. J. R. W. Harris). Churchill Livingstone, Edinburgh.
Wiesner, P. J. and Thompson, S. E. (1979). Gonococcal diseases. In *Disease-a-month* (ed. H. P. Dowling). Year Book Medical Publishers, Chicago.

Genital candidiasis

G. W. Csonka

Definition. Genital candidiasis (candidosis, moniliasis, thrush) is an infection usually due to *Candida albicans* causing vulvovaginitis in women, balanitis or balanoposthitis in heterosexual men, and anorectal infection in homosexual males.

Aetiology. In 98 per cent *C. albicans* is responsible, in the rest one of the other *Candida* species are isolated. The yeast grows as a non-capsulated oval blastophore which reproduces by budding. *In vivo* and in culture, elongated thin hyphae may develop.

Epidemiology. The fungus can be found anywhere on the human body but most commonly in the mouth, nails, vagina, and anorectal canal. *C. albicans* is an opportunist and exists often as a saprophyte becoming pathogenic under certain host conditions which include pregnancy, diabetes, administration of antibiotics, corticosteroids, and possibly oral contraceptives. The wearing of nylon pantihose creates a moist, warm environment which encourages fungal growth. In a proportion of women none of these factors is found.

It is apparent that in many female patients, genital candidiasis is not sexually initiated though it may subsequently be transmitted sexually to the male partner. In men, sexual transmission is the rule.

Prevalence. The infection is worldwide and appears to be increasing. The number of infections reported from sexually transmitted disease (STD) clinics in the UK in 1979 is 42 667. It is the third most common specific infection seen in women. Willmott (1981) found *Candida* in the rectum of 44 per cent of homosexuals. Vaginal smears from up to 30 per cent of asymptomatic or oligosymptomatic women attending STD clinics show *Candida* species.

Relationship to sexually transmitted diseases. Any STD may coexist with *Candida* infection, but with *Trichomonas* vaginitis it is rare, possibly because the vaginal pH of 4, usual in candidiasis, is inimical to trichomonads which prefer a pH of 5–8. Gonorrhoea is also uncommon though the reason for this is not clear.

Histology. There is invasion of the epithelium by hyphae. Polymorphonuclear leucocytes kill *Candida* species *in vitro* and are likely to be of major importance in the host's defence against the infection.

Clinical features

In the female. The characteristic picture is vulvovaginitis with marked pruritus, often worse at night and sometimes accompanied by a vaginal discharge. Characteristically it consists of a curdy material best seen during late pregnancy. The vulva is usually erythematous and the inflammation may spread to the perineum, inguinal folds (especially in obese women), and adjacent skin. In severe cases, oedema of the vulva is present, often with scratch marks due to the intense irritation. The patient may also complain of burning, dysuria, frequency, and dyspareunia. The vagina can appear normal or show white patches ('thrush plaques') with underlying shallow erosions which tend to bleed. In severe cases the inflammation of the vulva spreads by satellite lesions of the adjacent skin.

Recurrences of vulvovaginal candidiasis may be infrequent or become a most troublesome feature. In some women with frequent recurrences and none of the known provoking factors, immune defects have been reported but no clear pattern has emerged.

In the male. Symptomatic candidiasis is much less common than in women. Balanitis or balanoposthitis are the principal signs with eroded maculopapular lesions on the glans penis. Occasionally there are white thrush plaques which tend to coalesce. Intertrigo of the groins may develop. If the condition becomes chronic it may spread to the skin of the scrotum which shows some flaking and later a shiny appearance.

A small number of patients develop balanitis within hours after intercourse with a consort carrying *C. albicans*. The organism is rarely found in the male and it is probable that this is a true allergy to the fungus. It generally resolves in a day or two without specific treatment. The female partner should be investigated and treated. *Candida* urethritis is exceedingly rare: the discharge is said to be profuse. In homosexual men, *Candida* is frequently present in the anorectal canal and some complain of anal irritation. In all patients with *Candida* balanitis it is essential to exclude diabetes.

Differential diagnosis. Gonorrhoea in women does not produce pruritus and if there is any discharge it is more copious and yellow than that of candidiasis. *Trichomonas* vaginitis gives a characteristic yellow, foamy, offensive discharge and skin lesions are not prominent.

Vulvovaginitis in little girls may be due to threadworms, intravaginal foreign bodies, primary herpes, masturbation, or be associated with measles or scarlet fever.

'Recurrent infections' with no yeast detectable have been associated with psychosexual difficulties (Willmott 1981).

Laboratory diagnosis. In symptomatic patients, vaginal, subpreputial or anal smears (in homosexual men) stained by Gram's method will usually show the Gram-positive fungal elements. In addition, culture markedly increases the yield of positive results. *C. albicans* can also be identified by the outgrowth of germ tubes in serum within a few hours and this simple and rapid procedure can be used as an alternative to formal cultures.

Treatment

In the female. A number of local antifungal preparations are available including polyenes (nystatin) and the numerous imidazole derivatives. The immediate cure rate with nystatin is 80 per cent or less. Imidazoles are successful in about 90 per cent but whichever drug is used, recurrences are common. Nystatin pessaries and cream are given as 1 vaginal pessary at night for 14 nights and the cream is used for vulvitis and lesions of the adjacent skin. Clotrimazole is now available as 200 mg vaginal pessaries (1 pessary nightly for three nights), miconazole pessaries (one or two pessaries nightly for seven nights), and miconazole tampons are used morning and night for five days. Econazole pessaries are given one a night for three nights. Tampons give very good results and due to their absorbency, they are less messy, and therefore more acceptable to the patient. They have the added advantage of being readily used during periods. Ketoconazole (Nizoral) is a new synthetic imidazoledioxolane derivative and is the first systemic oral fungicide which is at present undergoing clinical trials.

Most physicians do not treat women who are asymptomatic carriers but Hurley (1977) feels that the presence of candida in the vagina is abnormal and should be eliminated.

Women with frequent recurrences pose an unsolved problem and if no underlying factor such as diabetes or frequent courses of antibiotics are found, miconazole tampons for use during each period have been found to help.

Opinions vary on whether clearing the anorectal reservoir of *Candida*, by giving oral antifungal therapy, such as nystatin tablets which are active in the intestine but are not absorbed, reduces the chances of relapse by auto-infection.

Fungicidal pessary-cover may be given to women with a history of recurrent candidosis and who need antibiotics for any reason.

Women in the last trimester of pregnancy with symptomatic *Candida* vaginitis should be treated partly for their own comfort and partly to prevent neonatal infection.

In the male. *Candida* balanitis, balanoposthitis, intertrigo, and scrotal fungal infection will respond to a course of antifungal cream which should be used until the lesions have completely cleared.

In homosexuals with anal irritation due to candida infection, antifungal creams are effective.

Contacts of *Candida* vaginitis are traditionally given antifungal cream to be smeared lightly on the glans penis for a few days.

References

Hurley, R. (1977). Trends in candidal vaginitis. *Proc. R. Soc. Med.* **70**, suppl. 4, 1.

— (1978). Diagnosis of candida vulvovaginitis. *J. clin. Path.* **31**, 98.

Morton, R. S. and Rashid, S. (1977). Candida vaginitis. *Proc. R. Soc. Med.* **70**, suppl. 4, 3.

Willmott, F. E. (1975). Genital yeasts in female patients attending a VD Clinic. *Br. J. vener. Dis.* **51**, 119.

— (1981). Candidiasis. In *Recent advances in sexually transmitted diseases* (ed. J. R. W. Harris). Churchill Livingstone, Edinburgh.

Clinical approach to non-gonococcal urethritis (NGU)

G. W. Csonka

Synonym. Non-specific urethritis (NSU).

Non-gonococcal urethritis (NGU) in men is the most frequent condition seen in clinics dealing with sexually transmitted diseases (STD) in the UK.

Definition. NGU in heterosexual men is an infection of multiple aetiology and is clinically much better defined than NG infections in women or homosexual men. The presumptive infectious agents include *Chlamydia trachomatis, Ureaplasma urealyticum,* and a number of other organisms some of which are only rarely isolated. In a proportion of cases no micro-organism has been identified. As the clinical appearance, course, complications, and response to antibiotics is similar whether these organisms are isolated or not, it is possible that the apparently 'sterile' cases of NGU will also be found to have bacterial causes. Complications include Reiter's disease, acute epididymitis, and chronic prostatitis. In homosexual men NG proctitis may be the equivalent of NGU seen in heterosexual men, and in women the complications of NG infection pelvic inflammatory disease. A proportion of cases of non-gonococcal ophthalmia neonatorum is due to agents transmitted from the genital tract of the mother during birth. For details of Reiter's disease see page 5.321, and pelvic inflammatory disease, page 5.319.

Epidemiology

Incidence. The conditions occur worldwide and in some countries may be amongst the commonest infections of young adults. NGU in men is about twice as commonly seen as gonorrhoea in STD clinics in the UK. The figures suggesting that in women gonorrhoea and non-gonococcal genital infections occur with similar frequency, are unreliable because of diagnostic difficulties leading to substantial under-reporting of both conditions. The latest figures (1978) from the STD clinics in England and Wales give an incidence of 76 826 cases of NGU in men and 19 738 non-gonococcal genital infections in women. However, these figures should not be taken as more than indicating a trend which is of value mainly in comparing them with previous years. They are probably less accurate than those for gonorrhoea as more patients with NG genital infections belong to a higher socio-economic class than those with gonorrhoea and often seek private treatment and thus are not included in the statistics. Furthermore, a sizeable number have such minor symptoms that they do not see a doctor. The annual statistics for NG infections may also be distorted in the opposite direction because, unlike gonorrhoea, these infections are prone to relapse within a year.

Transmission. There is good evidence that transmission is by sexual intercourse. One is sometimes handicapped in individuals with NGU when neither they nor their regular female partner can be shown to carry pathogens and especially when the female consort is asymptomatic. There are other situations which are difficult to explain, e.g. a married man may acquire NGU from an extra-marital source and has repeated sexual contact with his wife before treatment and yet his wife, who may remain untreated throughout, does not re-infect her husband. It is also common experience that one female sexual source of NGU may not cause infection in any of her other sexual contacts, nor is the well-known chain of infection seen in gonorrhoea at all common in NGU. There may be several explanations for this which includes the possibility that host factors may play a part, that infectiousness of these conditions is low, and that NG infections may give rise to so few signs as to be easily overlooked.

Race. No race is exempt though it appears that NGU and its complications are more frequent in Caucasians than in Negroes.

Marital status and age. Compared with gonorrhoea, male patients with NGU are more often married and the patients tend to be older.

Seasonal variation. We noticed a significant peak of NGU in late summer and a trough in winter, identical with that of gonorrhoea. This seasonal pattern is common to all sexually transmitted diseases in the Western hemisphere. We concluded that this regular swing in NGU points to sexual transmission.

Aetiology. The micro-organisms thought to be aetiological agents of NGU include *Chlamydia trachomatis, Ureaplasma urealyticum, Trichomonas vaginalis, Corynebacterium genitalium,* herpes simplex virus, and very rarely *Mycobacterium tuberculosis.*

C. trachomatis has been isolated from about 40 per cent of cases, and there is convincing evidence that it is pathogenic (see page

5.353). The role of ureaplasmas is less clearly defined and the proportion of infections caused by them is uncertain. For evidence of the pathogenicity of unreaplasma see page 5.358.

An organism which was first isolated from patients with NGU, *Corynebacterium genitalium* (Furness and Csonka 1966) has also been recovered from patients with epidymitis, cervicitis, and conjunctivitis (Furness and Kaminski, 1975), but its significance remains uncertain.

Trichomonas vaginalis may produce urethritis in men in about 3 per cent of cases but there is need to be cautious before accepting this diagnosis. In patients with NGU who do not respond to tetracycline, *T. vaginalis* should be looked for in a wet preparation and if found, it is possible that the patient will respond to metronidazole. In other patients *T. vaginalis* may be seen initially and there is no response to metronidazole; such patients are probably suffering from NGU which is cleared with tetracycline and the trichomonad is only a transient non-pathogenic passenger which disappears spontaneously.

Primary genital herpes simplex can produce urethritis in up to 20 per cent of such cases. It is unlikely to do so in recurrent attacks.

Tuberculosis of the urinary tract can produce a chronic urethritis which does not respond to tetracyclines, although this is rarely seen nowadays.

Mycoplasma hominis is not considered to be a cause of NGU, but does appear to cause pelvic inflammatory disease and related conditions (see page 5.360).

Bacteroides fragilis may be a cause of pelvic infection in women and *Gardnerella vaginalis* (formerly known as *Haemophilus vaginalis*) is a coccobacillus of low virulence, believed to cause vaginitis, and a few cases of male urethritis have been reported.

Clinical features

NGU in men. The incubation period varies from a few days to two months. The onset is less acute than in gonorrhoea and the patient presents with mucupurulent discharge and dysuria. There may be discomfort in the shaft of the penis or meatus. At times the discharge is seen only first thing in the morning after accumulation overnight and before being washed away by the first urination and may be ignored by the patient and not seen by the doctor. Cystitis is not a feature except for the very rare 'abacterial haemorrhagic cystitis' which has a hyperacute onset with the patient complaining of frequency of urination every 15 minutes or so, dysuria, and malaise. The urine contains a great deal of pus and macroscopically visible blood. The condition is sometimes followed by Reiter's disease. The diagnosis of NGU depends on clinical findings but above all on microscopy of the Gram-stained smear and culture to exclude gonorrhoea. The all-important smear shows polymorphonuclear leucocytes, epithelial cells and usually no organisms (Fig. 1). There is no agreement about the minimal number of polymorphs for the diagnosis of NGU; some feel that they should be entirely absent in a normal preparation, others make a diagnosis if there are five or more such cells in several high-power microscopical fields. In the average case 20–40 pus cells are present, but it is most unusual to see the sheets of pus found in gonorrhoea where epithelial cells are usually absent. If one sees such a specimen without finding gonococci, culture is obligatory otherwise gonorrhoea may well be missed.

Course. If untreated, the discharge will eventually cease but this may take weeks, rarely even months. If treated with tetracycline there is a rapid response within a week in 80–90 per cent of cases; if given a placebo there is a similar response in about 20 per cent. However, this difference becomes less as time goes on and at three months may be only 10 per cent in favour of tetracycline because of recurrences during this period. NGU has a marked tendency to recur and it is often impossible to decide whether one is dealing with a new infection or a recurrence of the old one. Even when the regular sexual partner has been treated with the same drug, at the same time as the patient, recurrences do occur. Some claim that if such treatment is given to couples carrying *C. trachomatis* the recurrence rate is greatly reduced. Our own experience suggests that a more cautious attitude is appropriate as we have seen many failures.

In homosexual men, the rectal Gram-stained smear shows large numbers of polymorphonuclear leucocytes and chlamydia are isolated from only a minority. Cultures must always be taken as otherwise gonorrhoea may be easily missed.

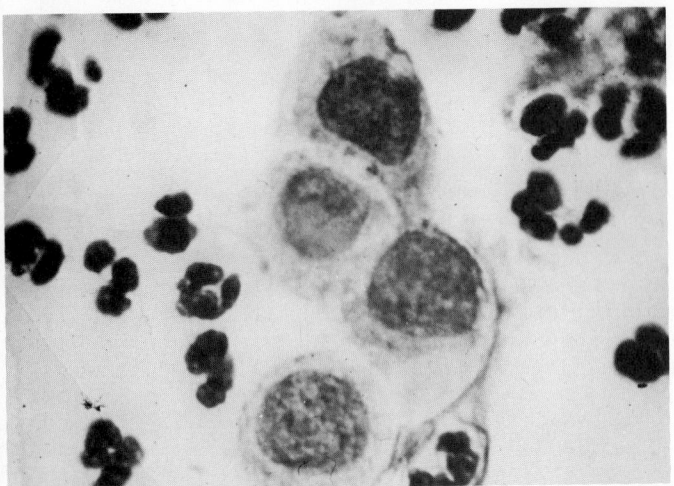

Fig. 1 Typical urethral smear showing polymophonuclear leucocytes and epithelial cells.

Post-gonococcal urethritis (PGU). After successful treatment of gonorrhoea with penicillin 35–50 per cent of patients develop PGU. Their urethritis recurs and an excess of polymorphonuclear leucocytes are seen but *N. gonorrhoeae* is no longer isolated. It is assumed that these patients have a double infection of gonorrhoea and NGU. PGU can be greatly reduced by using tetracycline in the treatment for gonorrhoea given for several days. Thus in one such study the incidence of PGU was only 6 per cent. If co-trimoxazole is given (4 tablets twice daily for two days) which is as effective as penicillin in the treatment of gonorrhoea, PGU was reduced from 36 per cent after penicillin-treated gonorrhoea to 18 per cent after co-trimoxazole. It may be of interest to note that whilst tetracycline is effective against both chlamydia and ureaplasma, co-trimoxazole has an effect on chlamydia only. This may in part explain the less effective prevention of PGU by co-trimoxazole than by tetracycline. Chlamydia is isolated in up to 50 per cent of cases of PGU. The role of ureaplasma in PGU is less well documented.

Local complications of NGU and PGU. Cowperitis, littritis, and tysonitis can occur but even more rarely than in gonorrhoea and a much milder disease occurs. On the other hand *chronic prostatitis* is much more commonly associated with NGU or PGU than with gonorrhoea. The diagnosis of chronic prostatitis is a difficult one and fraught with uncertainties. Probably the most significant feature is 'prostatic pain' which is compounded of perineal pain or discomfort, discomfort in the groins, thighs, and suprapubic region. There may be painful ejaculation. Other features are sheets of pus, often with clumping, in the expressed prostatic fluid and flakes and heavy threads in the first glass of the two-glass urine test in patients with recurrent urethritis. Treatment is unsatisfactory. Antibiotics which are most likely to be beneficial, at least in the short-term, are those which are known to penetrate into the prostate such as doxycycline and erythromycin. The response is better if there is also some urethritis present. Prostatic massage has no place in the treatment of prostatitis (sexual intercourse will achieve more effective emptying of the prostate!). Some patients are very sensitive to alcohol, so alcohol consumption may have to be curtailed. Patients are usually very worried and it is worth making time for a simple explanation and reassurance coupled with a full examination to allay their anxiety. Many will not voice their worries about the possibility of their disease leading to impotence, infection of their sexual partner, sterility, infecting their children-to-be, and the possibility of developing cancer of the prostate. The laboratory has little to offer, as in the majority of patients with chronic prostatitis no organisms are isolated. This is also the experience in the majority of chronic or frequently recurring NGU and may explain the indifferent results of antibiotic treatment. It is important to distinguish chronic prostatitis from *prostatorrhoea* where the patient gives a typical history of seeing clear or white urethral discharge which is acellular and occurs only on straining at defaecation. A simple explanation is usually sufficient to put the patient's mind at rest. *Urethrophobia* is an anxiety state similar to that found with chronic prostatitis but it must be admitted that even repeated reassurance after full negative examination may give disappointing results. Sometimes feelings of guilt due to infidelity, fear of VD, and sexual difficulties are uncovered. Such patients with reactive anxiety should only rarely be referred to a psychiatrist as they loose all confidence in the referring doctor and in any case often fail to turn up to see the psychiatrist but rather go to another clinic. The outlook is best in reactive anxiety where a response to simple supportive explanation and reassurance is successful in up to 75 per cent. It is far less good in anxiety neurosis and endogenous depression.

Haemospermia brings a number of worried young people to the clinics. It is of no consequence and often disappears in a few weeks. It is however, essential to take blood pressure readings as in a small proportion severe, sometimes malignant hypertension is the provoking condition. In patients over 40 it is advisable to seek the advice of a urologist.

Epididymitis occurs in about 1 per cent of patients with NGU and is almost invariably unilateral. NG epididymitis is an ascending infection, less acute than gonococcal epididymitis and due to a variety of micro-organisms. Furness *et al.* (1973) aspirated the epididymis through the scrotum in 20 young people with unselected epididymitis and found that the aspirate was sterile in 11, four contained *Corynebacterium genitalium* in pure culture, three grew gonococci, one had genital mycoplasma, and one *Mima polymorpha*. Chlamydia were not looked for. In another series, chlamydia were isolated from the aspirate in a proportion of patients. In patients over 35, *Escherichia coli*, *Pseudomonas aeruginosa*, *Proteus* ssp., and other urinary pathogens may be responsible and should be treated with the appropriate antibiotic.

The onset of NG epididymitis is acute, and any associated urethritis has usually disappeared by the time the patient is seen. There is acute pain, swelling, and redness of the scrotum on one side. There may be an overlying hydrocele. The process starts at the lower pole and may eventually involve the whole body and the spermatic cord becomes tender and thickened. The urine will show some pus and threads in the first glass only. In epididymitis due to *E. coli* or other urinary pathogens there is no urethritis but both glasses of urine in the two-glass urine test show turbidity due to pus. NG epididymitis tends to clear within a week or two after treatment but a palpable, painless and indurated epididymis may persist for a long time and needs no treatment.

The differential diagnoses are the same as for gonococcal epididymitis.

Treatment. The drug treatment of NGU and its complications are given in Table 1.

Systemic complications of NGU and PGU. *Reiter's disease* (see page 5.321) develops in about 1 per cent of these patients in the UK.

Non-gonococcal genital infections in women. These conditions are far less well defined than in men. Many sexual partners of men with NGU have no signs or symptoms. They may carry *C. trachomatis*, mycoplasmas, and other organisms including anaerobes but even when these are eliminated by treatment, the male partner may

Table 1 Treatment of non-gonococcal urethritis

Diagnosis	Treatment	Comment
1. NGU	oxytetracycline 250 mg 4 times daily × 7 days *or* minocycline 100 mg twice daily × 7 days *or* doxycycline 100 mg/day after food × 7 days *or* triple tetracycline ('Deteclo') tablets, 1 twice daily × 7 days *or* erythromycin stearate 500 mg twice daily × 7 days	if patient fails on tetracycline, look for *T. vaginalis*, if found give metronidazole 400 mg twice daily × 7 days; if not found, change to erythromycin or repeat tetracyline; minocycline may give rise to transient vertigo in 5%; doxycycline may cause photo-sensitization—avoid in the tropics; dairy products should be avoided with all tetracyclines except doxycycline
2. Female contacts of NGU	As for NGU (erythromycin if pregnant); add antifungal pessary (clotrimazole or equivalent) one pessary/night	antifungal preparation is given to avoid producing candidosis and is especially important in patients with a history of candidosis
3. NG proctitis in homosexual men	As for NGU	condition is not clearly defined
4. Post-gonococcal urethritis (PGU)	As for NGU	
5. Chronic prostatitis	course of doxycycline or erythromycin as above	treatment difficult; patience and reassurance essential; do not overtreat
6. Acute NG epididymitis	as for NGU + scrotal support during daytime	
7. Reiter's disease	see page 5.321	
8. NG cervicitis, urethritis, proctitis	as for NGU + antifungal pessary; metronidazole 400 mg twice daily × 7 days may be added	Results variable and often disappointing
9. PID	see page 5.319	
10 NG bartholinitis	as for NGU but give antibiotics for at least two weeks	treat early; if abscess forms, repeat needle aspiration as necessary; if that fails, marsupialize
11. *Gardnerella* vaginitis	metronidazole 400 mg twice daily × 7 days	causal relationship probable but needs confirmation
12. Urethrophobia	full examination, if negative enquire about possible psychological causes, explain, and reassure	generally do not refer to a psychiatrist but continue to give supportive help when necessary; outlook best in reactive anxiety

continue to suffer from recurrent attacks of NGU. In our present state of incomplete knowledge, it is probably advisable to treat *all* female contacts irrespective of bacteriological findings in the hope of preventing complications in themselves and to reduce recurrences in their male partners. There is good evidence that anaerobes such as *Bacteroides fragilis* may be involved in pelvic inflammation, as the evidence was obtained by isolation during laparoscopy. Though the cervix and vagina may be the site of many of the opportunist micro-organisms, their isolation from these sites is not a sound basis on which to determine the cause of pelvic infection; isolation from material obtained at laparoscopy is the only certain way for bacteriological diagnosis. This is not true for the gonococcus, whose presence on the cervix correlates well with inflammation beyond. Some women develop a vaginal discharge when their partner has NGU and chlamydia may be isolated from both the cervicitis and the urethritis in the male. More far-reaching are the possible complications which may lead to chronic and severe 'pelvic invalidism'.

Gardnerella vaginitis. There is as yet no agreement about the role of *G. vaginalis* but evidence is accumulating that it causes a distinct and common clinical entity and presents as a malodorous vaginitis with a pH of 5.5 (normal: 4.2–4.9). There are few polymorphonuclear leucocytes but the epithelial cells which are studded with *G. vaginalis* are called 'clue cells' and are of diagnostic value. Diagnosis is further helped by the simple 'amine test': a drop of 10 per cent potassium hydroxide is added to a drop of vaginal secretion and when positive, an immediate 'fishy' odour develops which is fleeting. Whilst metronidazole is effective according to most authorities in clearing both the organism and the vaginitis, its mechanism may be more subtle than previously believed. Metronidazole is only moderately effective against *G. vaginalis* but is very effective against all known anaerobes. However, its acetic acid metabolite is

highly effective against *G. vaginalis* and less against anaerobes. It is therefore possible that the therapeutic effect is due to a metabolite or alternatively that the effect is due to a combination of metronidazole and its metabolite against anaerobes and *G. vaginalis* which may be both involved in producing symptoms.

Complications of NG infections in women. *Bartholinitis.* This is a rare local complication, similar to gonococcal bartholinitis though generally milder. *M. hominis* has been isolated from a few cases. The duct and small gland is situated in the posterior third of the labium majus. When infected, an abscess may develop and if untreated is likely to burst through the labium minus. This must be avoided by early and energetic antibiotic therapy. Once an abscess has formed, needle aspiration may help. If it does not, marsupialization should be considered in preference to excision. Recurrences do occur but the content of the swelling is sterile and more in the nature of a cyst.

Pelvic inflammatory disease (see page 5.319) is the most important complication and it is estimated that there are between 10 000 and 20 000 chronic cases in the UK.

Reiter's disease (see page 5.321) associated with NG genital infection is occasionally seen in women.

References

Balston, M. J., Taylor, G. E., Pead, L., and Maskall, R. (1980). Corynebacterium vaginale and vaginitis: A controlled trial of treatment. *Lancet* i, 501.

Csonka, G. W. (1965). Non-gonococcal urethritis. *Br. J. vener. Dis.* **41**, 1.

— and Atkin, W. (1981). Comparison of the incidence of post-gonococcal urethritis following treatment with co-trimoxazole or penicillin.

—, Williams, R. E. O., and Corse, J. (1966). T-strain mycoplasma in non-gonococcal urethritis. *Lancet* i, 1292.

Dunlop, E. M. C. (1981). Chlamydial infection: terminology, disease and treatment. In *Recent advances in sexually transmitted diseases*. (ed. J. R. W. Harris). Churchill Livingstone, Edinburgh.

— (1981). Chlamydial infection: local complication and systemic diseases. In *Recent advances in sexually transmitted diseases* (ed. J. R. W. Harris). Churchill Livingstone, Edinburgh.

Furness, G. and Csonka, G. W. (1966). Isolation of diphtheroids from non-gonococcal urethritis. *Br. J. vener. Dis.* **42**, 185.

— and Kaminski, Z. (1975). Asymptomatic bacteriuria, bacteremia and other infections due to NSU corynebacteria. *Invest. Urol.* **13**, 227.

—, Kamat, M. H., Kaminski, Z., and Seebode, J. J. (1971). The etiology of idiopathic epididymitis. *J. Urol.* **106**, 387.

Holmes, K. K., Handsfield, H. H., Wang, S. P., Wentworth, B. B., Turck, M., and Andersen, J. B. (1975). Etiology of nongonococcal urethritis. *New Engl. J. Med.* **292**, 1199.

Prentice, M. J., Taylor-Robinson, D., and Csonka, G. W. (1976). Non-gonococcal urethritis. A placebo-controlled trial of minocycline in conjunction with laboratory investigations. *Br. J. vener. Dis.* **52**, 269.

Richard, S. J. and Clarke, S. K. R. (1977). Problems of assigning a causal role to chlamydia isolated in nongonococcal urethritis. In *Nongonococcal urethritis and related infections* (eds. D. Hobson and K. K. Holmes). American Society of Microbiology, Washington DC.

Schachter, J. and Dawson, C. R. (1978). *Human chlamydial infections*. PSG Publishing Company, Littleton, Massachusettes.

Stimson, J. D., Hale, J., Bowie, W. R., and Holmes, K. K. (1981). *Ann. intern. Med.* **94**, 192.

Taylor-Robinson, D., Csonka, G. W., and Prentice, M. J. (1977). Human intra-urethral inoculation of ureaplasmas. *Q. Jl. Med.* **46**, 309.

— and MacCormack, W. M. (1980). The genital mycoplasmas. *New Engl. J. Med.* **302**, 1063.

Clinical approach to pelvic inflammatory disease (PID)

G. W. Csonka

Definition. Pelvic inflammatory disease (PID) is a common and complex group of diseases of sexually active young women in which pathogenic micro-organisms ascend from the endocervix via the normally sterile uterus into the Fallopian tubes which they colonize to cause salpingitis. The infection often spreads beyond the tubes to involve neighbouring pelvic tissues.

It is convenient to divide these infections into gonococcal and non-gonococcal (NG) PID either of which may be acute or become chronic. Sometimes mixed gonococcal and non-gonococcal infections develop. Gonococcal PID is more acute and better defined than NG PID which may be due to a variety of micro-organisms. In at least a third of cases, PID may be followed by far-reaching complications.

Aetiology. *Gonococcal PID* has its onset soon after the woman becomes infected. In most cases the gonococcus can be isolated from the endocervix and the tubes. The gonococcal strain differs from that isolated from uncomplicated gonorrhoea, in that it produces a high proportion of genitally silent infections in *both* women and gonococcal PID and their male sexual partners. On occasion the organism disappears entirely from the urogenital tract and the diagnosis rests on clinical history, epidemiological data, and a prompt response to penicillin.

Table 1   Organisms associated or causing non-gonococcal pelvic inflammatory disease (NG PID)

Conditions	Organisms	Comment
Acute NG PID	*Chlamydia trachomatis*	is isolated from a varying proportion of Fallopian tubes and pelvic abscesses on laparoscopy; a specific serum antibody response is commonly associated; evidence for a causal relationship is strong; the disease tends to be mild
	Mycoplasma hominis	the same comments apply as for *C. trachomatis*
	Ureaplasma urealyticum	although this organism is closely associated with some cases of NGU, its significance in PID is less assured; it has been isolated from some patients during laparoscopy; much more work is needed to determine its role in PID
	Corynebacterium genitalium	sporadic laparoscopic isolations have been reported but causality has not been proved
Acute NG PID	Anaerobes: *Bacteroides fragilis*, peptostreptococci, and others	anaerobes have a profound destructive effect on the ciliated endothelium of the tubes and have been repeatedly isolated alone, or more frequently with other potential pathogens in PID; they may be primary or secondary invaders; they appear to be important and it may be worth adding metronidazole to the conventional therapy to eliminate them; this might be considered even when facilities to obtain bacteriological proof of their presence is lacking
	Actinomycosis israelii	this organism has either a low pathogenicity or none; it is commonly associated with IUCD and if it appears to cause inflammation, the device is best removed
	Mycoplasma pneumoniae, *Escherichia coli*, and a number of enteric and urinary pathogens have occasionally been isolated on laparoscopy	these organisms have been recovered from single or very few cases and their significance has not yet been evaluated
	no organism isolated	in a number of patients no organisms have been found; this may be due to the original agent(s) having spontaneously disappeared or our inability to grow them
Chronic NG PID	no organisms isolated	abscesses and inflamed tissue tested on laparoscopy or laparotomy are usually sterile
	Mycobacterium tuberculosis	the incidence of genital tuberculosis varies with the social status and environment of the patient and is now rare in the UK; in endemic areas it occurs in up to 10% of patients with post-pubertal pulmonary tuberculosis; the tubes are involved, the endometrium frequently; often there are no symptoms but chronic pelvic pain may occur; it should be suspected in virgins with chronic pelvic pain and in others with primary infertility in endemic areas

The many and sometimes contradictory reports suggest that apart from the gonococcus, the tubercle bacillus, and probably anaerobes, only *C. trachomatis* and *M. hominis* are consistently associated with a fair proportion of acute PID. The role of the other organisms listed has yet to be evaluated. Owing to significant differences and shifting pattern of isolation according to time and place of the agents thought to be potential causes of PID one cannot generalize and single out any one as heading the field and it is concluded that PID is a multi-aetiological condition

Cervical isolation of potential pathogens in *NG PID* is far less reliable. The main contenders as causal agents in NG PID are *Chlamydia trachomatis* and *Mycoplasma hominis*, but there are many others (Table 1). Isolation of these organisms from the cervix does not necessarily indicate a causative role in PID and laparoscopy may be necessary to confirm the diagnosis of PID and aid in establishing the responsible microbial agent. Culdocentesis is of doubtful value as the isolates may be vaginal contaminants. NG PID is often milder than the gonococcal form, and tends to become chronic. Serum antibodies are detectable in *C. trachomatis* and *M. hominis* infections. Anaerobes, such as *Bacteroides fragilis*, may be primary or secondary pathogens. *Mycobacterium tuberculosis* is no longer common in the Western world, but is still an important cause in some developing countries. In some patients *no* pathogen is recovered: the more chronic the condition, the less likely will isolation attempts be successful. It is worth noting that the isolation rates of the various organisms associated with PID vary greatly between countries and even between communities in the same country.

Incidence. Published figures are merely rough estimates applicable to the country and time when the study was undertaken. In gonococcal PID it has been repeatedly estimated that 10–15 per cent of untreated patients develop PID. Chronic PID, probably mostly of the NG type, is thought to involve between 10 000 and 11 000 patients a year in England. Gonococcal PID appears to be more common in the USA than in the UK. *C. trachomatis* is most frequently reported from Sweden. Mixed PID is commonly found in the USA. PID of unknown aetiology is very common in parts of Africa. PID appears to be universal and common.

Pathogenesis. Factors which may aid ascending infections include minor gynaecological procedures such as dilatation and curettage, termination of pregnancy, the insertion of an intra-uterine contraceptive device, and a history of previous PID, but in most cases no factors are found.

The ciliated tubal endothelium is capable of supporting the colonization of the gonococcus with the production of a purulent exudate which may spill into the peritoneum and produce an abscess in the pouch of Douglas. The tubal lining is partially destroyed and this, together with internal tubal adhesions, will slow the passage of the fertilized egg in the future and may lead to tubal pregnancy. If the fimbriated ends become obstructed, sterility will result. These complications are less likely with gonococcal PID than with NG PID, as the former is usually treated early and more effectively.

M. hominis and *C. trachomatis* can also survive in the Fallopian tubes but do not destroy the endothelial lining. Anaerobes, on the other hand, have a profoundly destructive effect on the endothelium and this should be borne in mind when treating NG PID.

Other complications in neglected cases are pyosalpinx, hydrosalpinx, and pelvic abscess. Eventually, multiple sterile abscesses, adhesions, a fixed uterus, and acute-on-chronic salpingitis may lead to chronic pelvic invalidism.

Clinical features

Gonococcal PID. Details will be found in the section on gonorrhoea (see page 5.311).

Acute NG PID. The illness is less acute than gonococcal PID and when associated with *C. trachomatis* is often mild. Symptoms usually start during or soon after menstruation, in the puerperium, or less commonly after some gynaecological procedure. Previous PID predisposes to subsequent attacks.

The patient complains of constant lower abdominal pain which is characteristically felt below the iliac crests in a sausage-shaped area. There may also be low backache. A variable degree of tenderness is present in one or both iliac fossae with some muscular guarding. In at least 10 per cent pain may be minimal. Systemic symptoms are less than in gonococcal PID with temperature only slightly raised, normal, or with minor elevation of ESR and a leucocytosis of under 20 000/ml. On pelvic examination, moving the cervix usually elicits pain in *both* tubes. The extent of misdiagnosis can be gauged by the fact that clinically diagnosed NG PID is confirmed in only 60 per cent on laparoscopy. In gonococcal PID the diagnosis is much more commonly correct and laparoscopy is not normally required. On the other hand unexpected NG PID is found in 20 per cent of laparoscopies. Pelvic abscess is more likely to develop in NG PID than in that due to gonococci and needs draining. It can be felt as a tender mass on palpating the rectovaginal pouch. Pain suggesting salpingitis can occur without any anatomical evidence of tubal inflammation. Its mechanism is unknown.

Differential diagnoses include tubal pregnancy, appendicitis, miscarriage, mittleschmerz, endometriosis, ruptured ovarian cyst, acute pyelonephritis, and intestinal obstruction.

Indication for laparoscopy. Although laparoscopy is being increasingly used and is safe in skilled hands, there is a morbidity of around 5 per cent and a mortality of 0.1 per cent due to gas embolism, anaesthetic mishaps, and burns. It is indicated in this

Table 2 Complications of pelvic inflammatory disease

Early (E) or late (L)	Complication	Comment
E	Tubal abscess (pyosalpinx)	
E	Pelvic abscess	
E	Perihepatitis	often associated with PID but may occur on its own
E or L	*Recurrent salpingitis*	less likely in gonorrhoea; once tubes damaged and non-functional almost any vaginal microorganism may infect the tube(s)
E or L	*Sterility/subfertility*	may occur even in asymptomatic PID; if fimbriated ends obstructed, sterility will result
E or L	Hydrosalpinx	
E or L	*General illhealth with marked psychological overtones*	anxiety, depression, and tension may become dominant especially when the illness becomes chronic and there is little progress
E or L	*Multiple miscarriages*	
L	Adhesions	may be of little importance but if intraluminal and the tube is obstructed or kinked, may facilitate ectopic pregnancy
E or L	*Ectopic pregnancy*	less likely in gonococcal form; chances of ectopic pregnancy increase from about 1:150 to 1:25
L	*Chronic pelvic pain*	there may or may not be organic changes; even with gonococcal PID with its better prognosis, 20% develop chronic pelvic pain
L	Deep dyspareunia	
L	*Severe distortion of pelvic organs with sterile abscess formation and fixed retroverted uterus*	such patients who also suffer from deep dyspareunia may have to be considered for radical surgery as a last resort
L	*Premalignant changes of the cervix*	as with other sexually transmitted diseases associated with promiscuity, such cervical changes are more common than in the general population

The complications in italics are considered to be more troublesome and potentially serious. The division between 'early' and 'late' complications is often arbitrary as some may develop at varying times after an attack. The patient with mild, gonococcal PID which is treated early stands the best chance to escape complications

Table 3 Treatment of non-gonococcal pelvic inflammatory disease (NG PID)

Diagnosis	Treatment	Comment
Acute NG PID	doxycycline 100 mg twice daily × 10 days or equivalent with food; avoid antacids; add metronidazole 400 mg four times daily × 7 days plus antifungal pessary to prevent candida infection whilst on tetracycline	
Perihepatitis associated with NG PID	treatment for NG PID will suffice	often due to *Chalmydia trachomatis*
Chronic gonococcal or NG PID	there is no satisfactory treatment; try repeated and prolonged courses of doxycycline (2–3 weeks) or equivalent plus metronidazole plus antifungal pessary cover; erythromycin and co-trimoxazole are alternatives as under non-specific urethritis	results are often disappointing; psychological problems arise frequently in these long-standing cases and need careful attention; surgery for infertility often not successful; in patients with severe chronic pelvic pain with or without acute exacerbations and with deep dyspareunia, surgical clearance with preservation of part of an ovary may be the last resort; it should not be lightly undertaken in younger women

context *whenever the diagnosis of PID is in doubt*, if there is no response to medical treatment, in older women less likely to suffer from sexually transmitted diseases, and in recurrent cases. It has little relevance in gonococcal PID but is important when chronic or acute-on-chronic PID is suspected. Bacteriological specimens taken at laparoscopy should include tests for gonococci, *C. trachomatis*, and mycoplasmas if possible, and both for aerobic and anaerobic organisms. The gonococcus is sometimes unexpectedly isolated when it had not been recovered from other sites.

Chronic NG PID. This condition is arbitrarily diagnosed when the pain has lasted for at least three months. Most patients are aged 20–40. It is rare below or above this age group.

Clinical features. Commonly there is a dull intermittent lower abdominal pain, sometimes associated with sacral backache. Menstrual periods are heavy and frequent. The uterus is retroverted, fixed, and the adnexae are thickened and irregular on both sides. Some patients give a history of multiple miscarriages, others suffer from infertility. Sooner or later psychological features become dominant especially when little or no progress is made after repeated attempts of medical treatment.

In a proportion of cases there are no symptoms and clinical examination shows no abnormality; the diagnosis is then established by laparoscopy undertaken, e.g. for the investigation of infertility.

Chronic PID poses major diagnostic, therapeutic, and prognostic problems. None of the treatments conventionally used are really satisfactory and it is not surprising that the disappointed patient often becomes anxious and depressed. Laparoscopy may confirm chronic PID, endometriosis, a combination of both, or of some other relevant pathology in 30–50 per cent of cases.

Complications associated with chronic PID are shown in Table 2.

Differential diagnoses include endometriosis, mobile retroversion of the uterus, irritable colon syndrome, and abdominal malignancy.

Treatment. Some principles are already mentioned in several sections but details of drug treatment are summarized in Table 3. The patient with acute PID should generally be admitted to hospital and always if there is any doubt about the diagnosis, the patient is pregnant, or has social and psychological difficulties which may make it impossible for her to rest or comply with therapy.

Prognosis. Patients with gonococcal PID have a more abrupt onset which brings them earlier to the doctor than those with NG PID and the combination of early treatment which is also more effective in gonorrhoea than with other infections improves the prognosis. Many of these patients remain fertile and a smaller proportion develop pelvic pain or other complications at a later date.

References

Lemcke, R. and Csonka, G. W. (1962). Antibodies against pleuro-pneumonia-like organisms in patients with salpingitis. *Br. J. vener. Dis.* **38**, 212.

Mårdh, P. H., Lind, I., Svensson, L., Weström, L., and Møller, B. R. (1981). Antibodies to *Chlamydia trachomatis, Mycoplasma hominis*, and *Neisseria gonorrhoeae* in sera from patients with acute salpingitis. *Br. J. vener. Dis.* **57**, 125.

Møller, B. R., Weström, L., Ahrons, S., Ripa, K. T., Svensson, L., von Mecklenburg, C., Henrikson, H., and Mårdh, P. H. (1979). *Chlamydia trachomatis* infection of the Fallopian tubes. *Br. J. vener. Dis.* **55**, 422.

Paavonen, J., Saikku, P., Vesterinen, E., and Aho, K. (1979). *Chlamydia trachomatis* in acute salpingitis. *Br. J. vener. Dis.* **55**, 203.

Renaer, M. (ed.) (1981). *Chronic pelvic pain in women.* Springer-Verlag, Berlin.

Taylor-Robinson, D. and Csonka, G. W. (1981). Laboratory and clinical aspects of mycoplasma infections of the human genitourinary tract. In *Recent advances in sexually transmitted diseases* (ed. J. R. W. Harris). Churchill Livingstone, Edinburgh.

Thomas, M., Jones, M., Ray, S., and Andrews, B. (1975). *Mycoplasma pneumoniae* in a tubo-ovarian abscess. *Lancet* **ii**, 774.

Treharne, J. D., Ripa, K. T., Mårdh, P. H., Weström, L., and Darougar, S. (1979). Antibodies to *Chlamydia trachomatis* in acute salpingitis. *Br. J. vener. Dis.* **55**, 26.

Venereologist's approach to Reiter's disease

G. W. Csonka

See also Section 16 for further discussion of Reiter's disease.

Definition. Reiter's disease (RD) is a condition of uncertain aetiology characterized by an association of non-gonococcal urethritis (NGU) or post-gonococcal urethritis (PGU), sero-negative arthritis, conjunctivitis, and a number of less frequent symptoms in various combinations. It may also follow enteric infections such as bacillary dysentry, salmonellosis, and yersiniosis. In a proportion of post-dysenteric Reiter's disease no organisms have been isolated.

History. Post-dysenteric RD was first described by Stoll in 1776 and that associated with sexually transmitted urethritis by Brodie in 1818 who gave a superb description of six male patients. In 1916 Hans Reiter published a case history of a soldier serving at the Western Front on the German side with post-dysenteric arthritis, urethritis, and conjunctivitis. Almost simultaneously Fiessinger and Leroy reported their patient on the French side of the same front. More recently, Paronen (1948) published the largest series of 344 patients with post-dysenteric RD during a dysentery epidemic following the Russo-Finnish War. In 1958 Csonka reported on 185 patients with 'Venereal' RD attending a London Hospital. Brewerton (1973) and Aho (1974) independently demonstrated the existence of the long suspected genetic factor when they found a remarkably close association of the genetic marker HLA-B27 with RD.

Epidemiology

Incidence. In one London clinic for sexually transmitted diseases, the incidence of RD was 0.8 per cent. This figure has proven valid for the whole country. The incidence figure is almost certainly an underestimate as mild cases are either not recognized or not referred to the hospital clinics. Moreover they may be seen in departments dealing with one of the features of RD and be lost to statistical analysis.

With the worldwide increase of urethritis there is every likelihood that the number of RD cases will also increase.

Geographical and racial distribution. RD has been reported from many parts of the world. However, the sexually acquired form predominates in the UK and USA and the post-dysenteric type in North Africa, India and parts of Europe.

In a clinic in London with approximately 40 per cent coloured patients, RD was six times more common in Caucasian patients than in coloured immigrants or their offspring. It might be relevant to study the distribution of the genetic marker HLA-B27 as well as NGU and PGU in these racial groups to see whether there are differences to account for differences in the incidence in RD.

Age and sex. RD associated with NGU is most commonly found in young men aged between 20–30 years of age. In the UK statistics the sex ratio is 13 men to 1 woman; this may underestimate the incidence in women where the disease is unexpected and therefore more reluctantly diagnosed. In the post-dysenteric series there seems to be also a preponderance of young male adults but far less marked than in the urethritis form; moreover, children and even infants have been repeatedly reported to suffer from post-dysenteric RD.

Heredity and the histocompatibility antigen HLA-B27. As with many other rheumatic diseases, hereditary factors might be expected to play a part in RD. A familial aggregation has been noticed on a few occasions and an increased family history of ankylosing spondylitis has been found which has certain similarities with RD. The hereditary factor was strikingly demonstrated by Brewerton (1973) and Aho (1974) independently when they found a close association of the histo-compatibility antigen HLA-B27 which is a genetic marker with RD in 80–90 per cent against 7 per cent in the general population in the UK and 14 per cent in Finland respectively. It is therefore fascinating to note that whilst in the UK the incidence of RD amongst the urethritis patient is a constant 1 per cent it is exactly double that in Finland which may be a reflection of the difference in the prevalence of the hereditary factor B27. This association was present whether the disease followed NGU, bacillary dysentery, yersinia or salmonella infections. Ankylosing spondylitis has the closest relationship to B27 (90–100 per cent) followed by RD (65–100 per cent). A number of other conditions which have certain characteristics in common such as psoriatic arthritis are also related to the possession of the B27 antigen.

There is a practical side to this; a patient who carries B27 and acquires NGU runs a 20–25 per cent risk of developing RD against less than 1 per cent in the unselected population with urethritis. It has also been shown that if both parents are B27-positive, familial aggregation of RD may result. Against this it should be noted that positive reactors in the presence of one of the triggering infections do not always develop RD and that B27-negative individuals can develop RD, thus B27 is not essential for the disease to occur and clearly other factors may also operate. B27 has, however, some prognostic value, the more severe and complete the disease, especially if there is also sacroiliitis and anterior uveitis, the higher the incidence of B27; in other words, a negative B27 is a favourable prognostic sign in RD.

Aetiology. In the UK, USA, and several other countries urethritis is the commonest precursor of RD. In North Africa and Asia shigella dysentery precedes many cases of RD, but in all areas both forms co-exist.

Of the various organisms believed to be of aetiological importance, chlamydia has been most extensively studied, but the isolation rate in RD urethritis is the same as in uncomplicated urethritis, the only important difference being a rise in serological titre to chlamydia antigen during active RD. This by itself does not confirm a causal relationship and Koch's postulates have not been fulfilled.

Yersinia has been firmly associated with arthritis in patients with a significantly high carrier rate of B27. A number of other micro-organisms have been implicated at one time or another but in a fair proportion of patients no micro-organisms have been isolated from the urethra or other sites involved in RD yet clinically the disease is indistinguishable from cases when one or other of these organisms have been found (Table 1). Even the route of entry of these organisms is uncertain except that recent studies have exonerated the commonly held importance of chronic prostatitis as the port of entry (which is not surprising once it was shown that females also develop RD).

Table 1　Micro-organisms suspected to be associated with the development of Reiter's disease

Chlamydia trachomatis
Shigella
Salmonella
Yersinia
Ureaplasma urealyticum
Corynebacterium genitalium
Infection with unidentified organisms

At present we must conclude that the cause(s) of RD as indeed all other members of the group of seronegative spondarthritides remains unknown.

Clinical features. Table 2 gives the spectrum and incidence of the main clinical findings in RD in 410 consecutive cases seen in three London clinics.

Sequence of symptoms. It is to be noted that many of the symptoms and signs may give rise to minimal, transient discomfort and are therefore easily overlooked. They include NGU, PGU, balanitis, stomatitis, and even minor degrees of keratoderma and conjunctivitis.

The majority have NGU (cervicitis in women) followed within a few days by arthritis and in one third by conjunctivitis. Balanitis and stomatitis tend to occur early while keratoderma and anterior uveitis develop weeks or months after the onset of arthritis.

The onset of arthritis is typically abrupt and precedes other symptoms. If only two symptoms are present such as urethritis and conjunctivitis or urethritis and balanitis, a definite diagnosis cannot be made unless years later, arthritis develops making a retrospective diagnosis possible. Involvement of the attachment of fascia and tendons to bone such as plantar fasciitis and Achilles tendonitis occur fairly early and tend to persist. Spinal ligamentous lesions develop gradually and become radiologically evident only after years. Radiological changes due to sacroiliitis, spondylitis, and destructive lesions of joints and bones of the feet may take months or years to become demonstrable.

Individual symptoms. *Non-gonococcal urethritis or post-gonococcal urethritis.* They appear to be no different clinically, microbiologically, or as regards therapeutic response from the uncomplicated variety. Sometimes urethritis is minimal and has to be carefully sought. It may only be evident in the early morning. In recurrent attacks, NGU or PGU may be absent, in others a fresh attack of urethritis is followed again by features of RD and in some patients not every appearance of urethritis is followed by other symptoms.

Table 2   Major clinical features of Reiter's disease in 410 consecutive cases

Lesions	Patients (%)
Genitourinary infections	
NGU	314 (76.5)
PGU	66 (16.0)
Gonorrhoea	30 (7.3)
Peripheral joint lesions	
Polyarthritis	360 (87.8)
Monoarthritis	23 (5.6)
Arthralgia	12 (2.9)
Sacroiliitis	45 (10.9)
Spondylitis	4 (1.0)
Eye lesions	
Conjunctivitis	141 (34.4)
Anterior uveitis	30 (7.3)
Keratitis	5 (1.2)
Keratoderma blennorrhagica	55 (13.4)
Circinate balanitis	105 (25.6)
Stomatitis	45 (10.9)
Plantar fasciitis	80 (19.5)
Achilles tendonitis	50 (12.2)
Cardiovascular lesions	
Incomplete heart block	15 (3.6)
Transient pericarditis	2
Complete heart block	1
Aortic incompetence	8 (1.9)
Thrombophlebitis of calf	19 (4.6)
Nervous system	
Meningo-encephalitis	2
Seventh nerve palsy	1
Amyloidosis	1
Hepatitis	1

NGU = non-gonococcal urethritis; PGU = post-gonococcal urethritis

Cystitis and 'haemorrhagic cystitis'. Symptoms suggesting cystitis with pus in the urine but no organisms on routine bacteriological tests is not uncommon but 'haemorrhagic cystitis', which was occasionally seen years ago, appears to be very rare now. Clinically it is a hyperacute cystitis with the patient complaining of severe dysuria, severe frequency, malaise, and often NGU. The urine shows macroscopically a large amount of pus and blood and on routine testing is sterile. Nevertheless, it responds to antibiotics. Most, but not all develop RD. This has been seen in both sexes.

In the female, urethritis, cystitis, the urethral syndrome, and cervicitis are less clearly associated with RD, but in some patients a definite urogenital phase precedes arthritis by a few days.

Arthritis. Asymmetrical polyarthritis is the most prominent, constant, and disabling feature. The onset is usually acute and develops rapidly to its greatest intensity within a week. Generally one joint at a time becomes painful and swollen. The smaller joints are often red and hot. Resolution varies greatly from days to months. The joints of the lower limbs are involved about three times as often as those of the upper limbs. The shoulder and hips are rarely affected unlike in ankylosing spondylitis. The commonest joints involved are the knees and ankles followed by toes and tarsal joints. In the upper limbs the wrists are most frequently affected. The arthritis is markedly asymmetrical. In large joints, synovial fluid accumulation is the rule.

Plantar fasciitis, Achilles tendonitis. These cause chronic painful feet which can disable long after all other symptoms of RD have disappeared. Calcaneal spurs and calcified attachment of the Achilles tendon are eventually seen radiologically. Other tendons, including those of the forearm and around the elbow are more rarely involved. In severe cases permanent foot deformities such as pes cavus with hammer toes or pes planus develop. Lateral deviation of

the foot often associated with destruction of toe joints are a possible additional handicap.

Sacroiliitis and spondylitis. A few patients develop a condition resembling ankylosing spondylitis, however, over the years, the progressive spinal rigidity of classical spondylitis was not seen in any of our patients. The radiological appearances of the spine in RD are characteristic and are described below. Sacroiliitis is much more common and similar to that seen in ankylosing spondylitis. If associated with recurrent anterior uveitis, the combination is almost invariably B27 positive and the condition tends to become chronic.

Eye lesions. Bilateral conjunctivitis is the commonest eye lesion (Fig. 1). It is usually mild and of short duration. Anterior uveitis occurs later, and is frequently unilateral though in subsequent attacks alternate eyes may be involved. It tends to recur and become the dominant symptom.

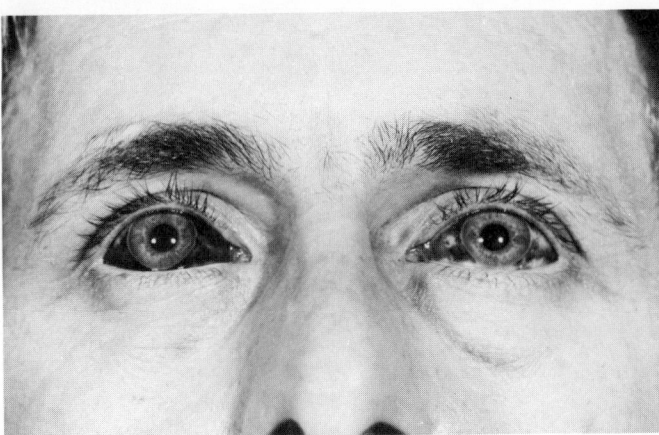

Fig. 1 Marked bilateral conjunctivitis with some subconjunctival haemorrhage; painless.

Balanitis. If the patient is circumcised, the lesions are dry and the scaly macules are sharply demarcated from their surroundings. In uncircumcised men the lesions are glistening, moist, red elevated macules which become confluent and are given the descriptive name of 'circinate balanitis' (Fig. 2). The condition is remarkably painless and sometimes unnoticed by the patient. Similar lesions on the vulva in a woman with RD has been recently reported.

Stomatitis. This may involve the palate, buccal mucosa, and tongue and is probably more frequent than reported as it is usually painless and may go unnoticed.

Keratoderma blennorrhagica. This is the most characteristic single lesion of RD. The soles are most commonly affected but the lesions may spread over the dorsum of the feet, involve the shaft of the penis, palms, trunk, and the scalp when differentiation from pustular psoriasis may become impossible. Keratoderma appears first as brown macules on both soles and within a day or two develops into hard papulovesicles with an opaque yellow content (Fig. 3a and 3b). Eventually layer upon layer of scale is heaped up giving sometimes rise to limpet-like scaly masses (Fig. 3c). Minor degrees can be very difficult to distinguish from keratinized skin due to chronic pressure but the latter is usually much harder. Keratoderma clears in about a month but may persist longer.

Nails. The nails of toes and fingers may be affected showing a gross dystrophy of the whole nail plate which lifts as subungual debris accumulates under its distal half (Fig. 4). Eventually the nail is shed and grows again within three months.

Histologically the lesions of the skin and mucous membranes are non-specific and bear a resemblance to each other. They have also in common the remarkable absence of pain or irritation.

Cardiovascular system. Transient *pericarditis* with or without chest pain appears to be benign and in our experience has not led to constrictive pericarditis. *Myocarditis* is associated with a first

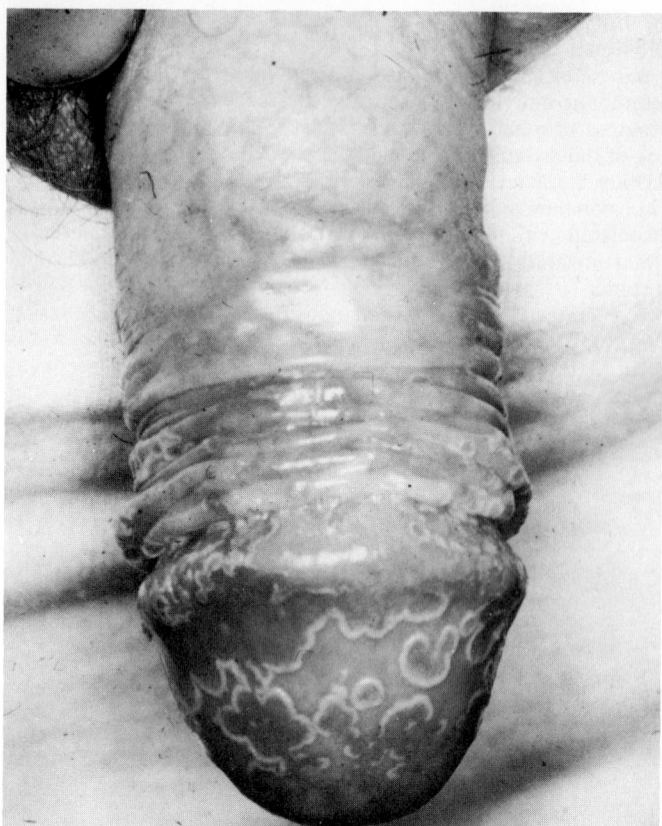

Fig. 2   Circinate balanitis; painless.

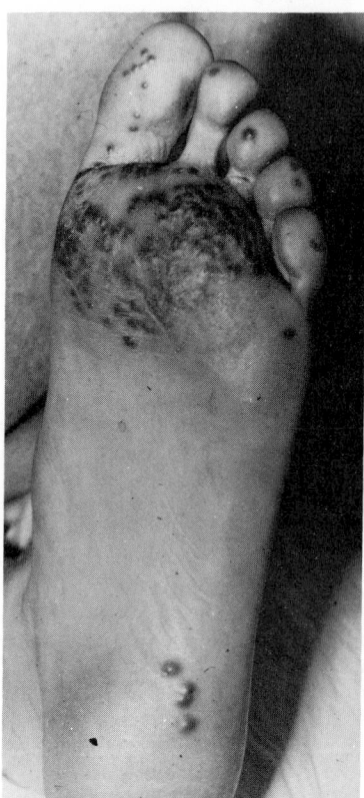

3(a)

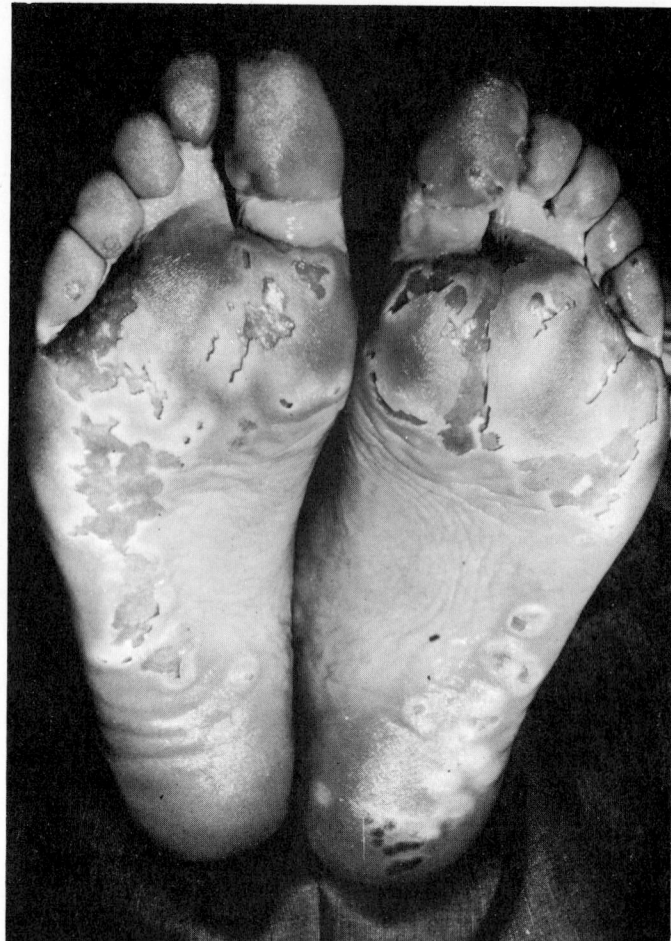

3(b)

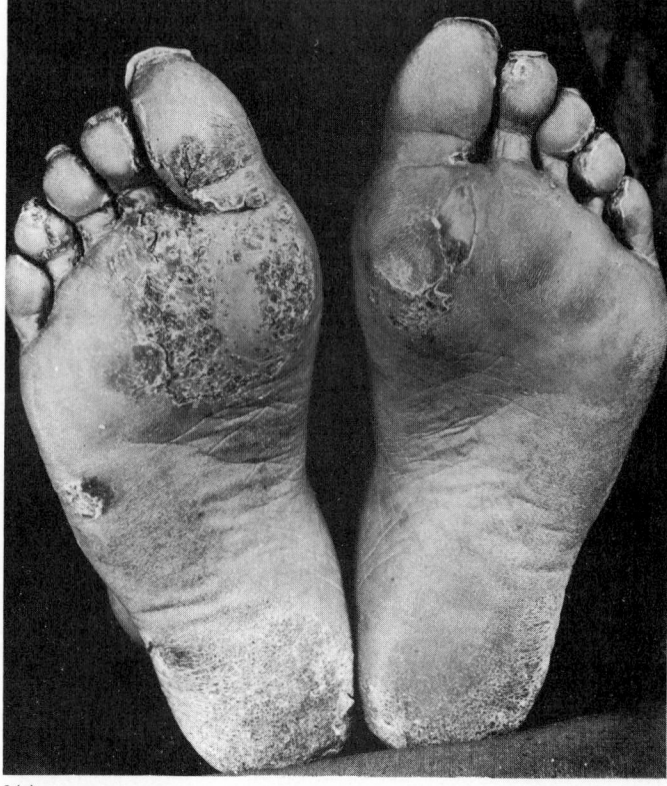

3(c)

Fig. 3   Keratoderma blennorrhagica showing (a) the typical indolent deep-seated brown papules; painless; (b) later stage with peeling of plantar skin; and (c) marked hyperkeratosis; painless.

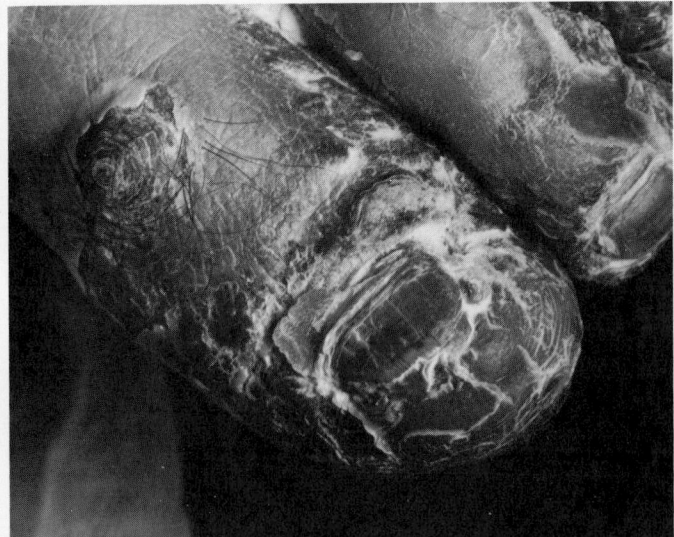

Fig. 4 Keratoderma blennorrhagica and involvement of the nails; nodular and hyperkeratotic lesions.

degree heart block, and this too is usually benign, however, in one of our patients complete heart block developed.

Aortic incompetence is a rare complication.

Nervous system. A variety of abnormalities have been reported but are very rare. They include meningo-encephalitis, amyotrophic lateral sclerosis, and peripheral neuropathy. In one of our patients Bell's palsy developed early in an attack and recurred during the next episode. It cleared each time within a few weeks.

Thrombosis of the deep veins of the legs. This was present in 4.6 per cent of our patients early in the attack. Recovery was rapid and uneventful.

Respiratory system. Paronen reported pleurisy in a number of patients with post-dysenteric RD.

Amyloidosis. A few cases of amyloidosis have been recorded in severe RD with fatal outcome.

Course and prognosis. Some patients apparently experience only one attack which clears completely in between a few weeks and several months; in others the acute phase clears up to a point but continues as a low-grade illness with chronic painful feet resulting in invalidism. Such patients often experience partial remissions and exacerbations. The possibility of *recurrences* is a constant threat for many years (Fig. 5). The risk of a first recurrence in a group of 144 patients followed for up to 10 years was 15 per cent annually. During this period 63 per cent had more than one attack. Patients with early involvement of feet and ankles are more liable to suffer from continuous or recurrent symptoms. The combination of sacroiliitis and anterior uveitis was also associated with a poor prognosis.

The later complications can be divided into those with recurrences without residual damage, those who suffer from painful feet with or without deformity, those with recurrent uveitis and some visual loss, a small group with spondylitis few of which are akin to classical severe ankylosing spondylitis, and a very small group with lesions of the aorta or the nervous system.

The type and incidence of late morbidity in patients followed for up to 20 years is similar whether the RD was venereal or post-dysenteric. Thus about half of the patients had some disability which interfered with work or leisure and 18 per cent were severely affected and unable to work.

Mortality. The mortality of patients with serious cardiovascular disease was 22 per cent in our series and might be reduced by judicious aortic valve replacement. The overall mortality was under 1 per cent and this too might be lessened by avoiding potentially dangerous drugs such as phenylbutazone.

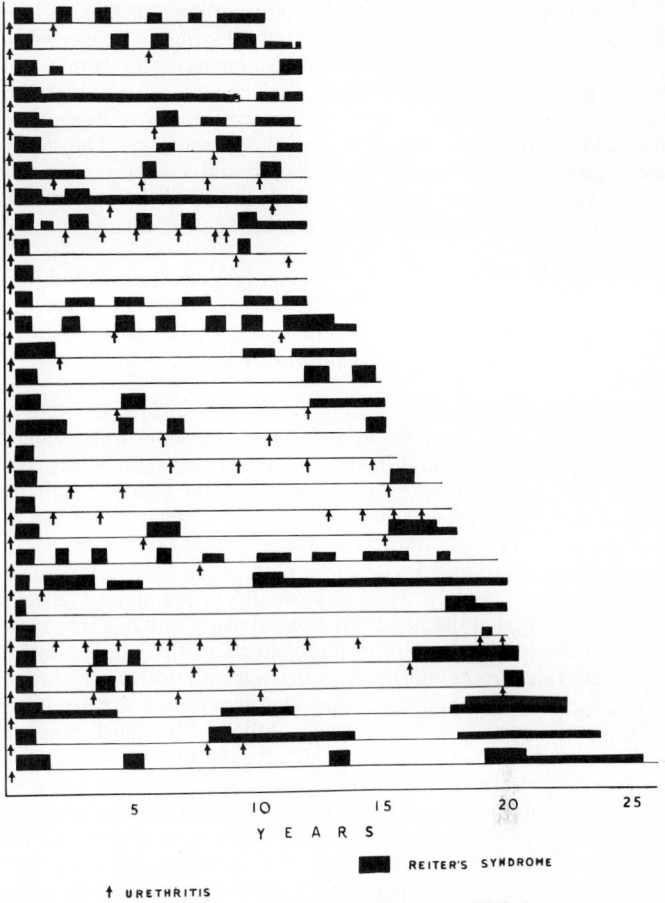

Fig. 5 30 patients were observed for 10–26 years and show the unpredictability of the relationship between urethritis and recurrent Reiter's disease. Many episodes of urethritis occurred and were not followed by Reiter's disease, in others recurrent Reiter's disease was not associated with urethritis. These variations were seen in the same individuals. There was also a wide range in the symptom-free intervals between attacks. In a few, the disease continued from the beginning on a chronic course.

Multiple cases. Multiple cases are common in post-dysenteric RD but rare in sexually acquired RD and in the latter group infectivity is very low.

Laboratory tests. There are no specific laboratory tests for RD but the results of some investigations have characteristic features, which by accumulation are of real help in diagnosis. They are useful in excluding other similar diseases and by monitoring activity.

The *erythrocyte sedimentation rate* (ESR) is the most valuable single test to assess activity and is also of diagnostic help. The ESR is usually markedly raised in the presence of active arthritis and values over 100 mm/hour (Westergren) are not uncommon even in the patient who is generally well except for arthritis which may be mild. During convalescence values fall slowly and may be normal in three months. In 10–20 per cent a slightly elevated ESR may persist for many months.

In severe cases a mild normocytic, normochromic *anaemia* is found which improves spontaneously as the attack draws to an end. A mild *neutrophil leucocytosis* may be present in a third of acute attacks.

As in other infections, the alpha globulin fraction of the *plasma proteins* is elevated. More recently we found raised levels of a beta globulin in patients with NGU and RD but not in those with gonorrhoea or in healthy controls; their significance is not known. The rheumatoid factor is present in the same proportion as in the general population and therefore RD is classified as one of the 'seronegative' arthropathies.

Aspiration of *synovial fluid* from a large effusion such as is often found in the affected knee joint is not only of differential diagnostic value to exclude septic arthritis, but also increases the comfort of the patient. In RD the synovial white cell count is raised and varies between 1000 and 5000 × 10⁶/l and consists mainly of neutrophil leucocytes which are later replaced by lymphocytes. The aspirated fluid is yellow, may clot spontaneously and is sterile on conventional media. The protein content is high (40–50 g/l against the normal 10–20 g/l) and the sugar concentration is usually normal (4.0 mmol/l).

Cell-mediated immunity to analogous IgG has been found in a minority of patients with RD. The haemolytic complement activity is normal or raised. So far immunological studies have failed to provide an answer to the mechanism of RD.

Radiology. Initially there is only evidence of soft tissue swelling seen well in the plantar fascia and Achilles tendon. Later radiological changes are found in the metatarsophalangeal joints, the interphalangeal joints of the toes, particularly the great toe, and the posterior aspects of the calcaneal bone, where reactive sclerosis at the insertion of the plantar fascia causes 'plantar spurs' (Fig. 6). In severe cases there may be localized destruction of metatarsophalangeal joints (Fig. 7). Hips and shoulders are almost always spared. Changes in the hands are less extensive and less frequent. Though the terminal interphalangeal joints of the hands may be involved, this is more markedly associated with psoriatic arthritis. Radiological abnormalities in the sacroiliac joints are frequent (Fig. 8). They start as fluffy changes followed by 'hard' reactive sclerosis and eventually ankylosis. Unlike the rest of the skeleton where changes are asymmetrical, those of the sacroiliac joints may be bilateral. In the majority of patients with sacroiliitis, spondylitis is absent or minimal. When spondylitis develops, it can mimic *ankylosing spondylitis* in a few, but the majority show asymmetrical lateral bony bridges between vertebral bodies. The intervertebral discs are usually normal. Typically, some of the spinal segments are 'skipped'. Most of the patients with these spinal lesions are asymptomatic.

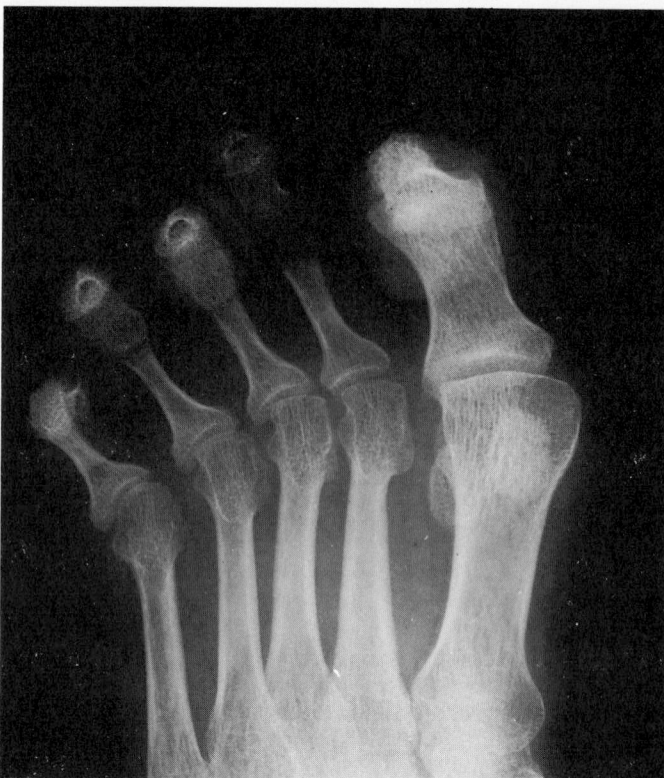

Fig. 7 Distruction of distal phalanges, lesions of interphalangeal joints, and marked lateral deviation.

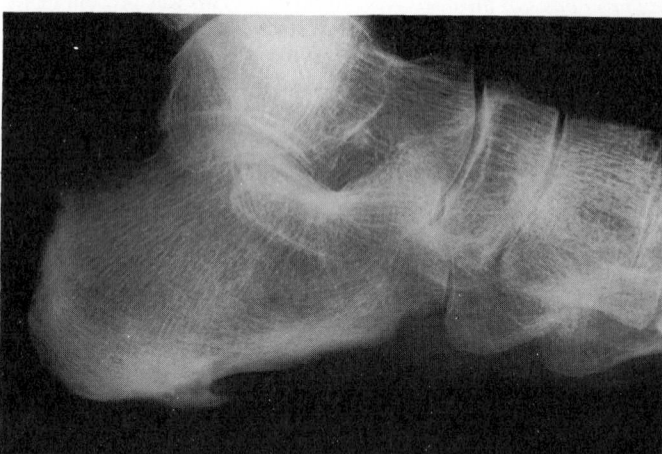

Fig. 8 Bilateral sacroiliitis; obliteration of sacroiliac joints and some bony sclerosis.

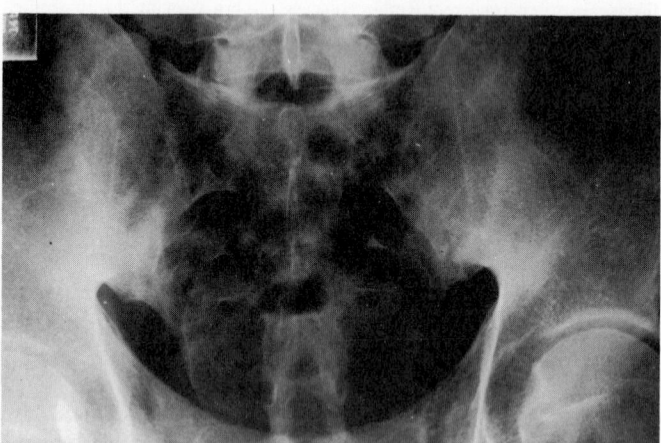

Fig. 6 Calcaneal spur formation.

Whilst it cannot be claimed that a positive diagnosis can be made by radiological changes, the combination of some or many of the changes mentioned can point towards the correct diagnosis. A summary of the main characteristics are given in Table 3.

Diagnosis. The most important factor in reaching the proper diagnosis is to consider the possibility in any young adult with unexplained arthritis. In cases with the three principal features present the diagnosis is not in doubt; if there are fewer signs the most immediate differential diagnosis is *gonococcal arthritis* because gonorrhoea may occur coincidently with RD. The presence of non-gonococcal conjunctivitis and mucocutaneous le-

Table 3 Radiological features characteristic of RD

Severe involvement of the feet with relative sparing of the hands
Predilection for the calcaneus, interphalangeal joint of the great toe, and metatarsophalangeal joints
Periosteal bone apposition near affected joints
Sacroiliac arthritis, especially when asymmetric
Asymmetric, often large, bridging syndesmophytes involving mainly the lateral aspects of the vertebral bodies with relative sparing of the anterior surfaces

After Martel (1979)

sions of RD are not associated with gonococcal arthritis. If the diagnosis is still in doubt, a therapeutic trial with penicillin should rapidly settle the issue as gonococcal arthritis always responds dramatically to penicillin whilst RD does not.

Other differential diagnoses which should be excluded are rheumatoid arthritis, ankylosing spondylitis, psoriatic arthritis, brucellosis, other seronegative arthritides (see Section 16), and trauma.

It is always helpful to remember that only in RD is one likely to see circinate balanitis and keratoderma blennorrhagica. Conjunctivitis, however, is of less value as it may appear in several conditions mentioned particularly psoriatic arthritis.

Diagnostic difficulties are certain to arise when there is an overlap of RD with ankylosing spondylitis, psoriatic arthritis, or seronegative rheumatoid arthritis. Sometimes features of both conditions are seen together or else sequentially.

Treatment. Bed rest is necessary in all but the mildest case but strict immobilization is to be avoided as it will speed muscle wasting especially of the quadriceps and seriously delay convalescence. As soon as the patient can bear it, active movement of the affected limbs should be started. Aspiration of grossly swollen joints, usually the knee, relieves the painful pressure and is often followed by rapid recovery of the joint. Tetracycline is given for the urethritis as detailed in the section on NGU (see page 5.315), but it will not influence the rest of the syndrome. For arthritis and other locomotor symptoms we usually give indomethacin 25 mg three or four times daily after food. Side-effects are gastrointestinal upsets (not dose-related), persistent headaches, hallucinations, and dizziness (dose-related). If there is marked early nocturnal pain or morning stiffness, a 100 mg indomethacin suppository administered at night or 75 mg in retard form with food on retiring are valuable. Naproxen 250–500 mg morning or flurbiprofen 50 mg three or four times daily are some of the alternatives. Although there is little to choose between many of these non-steroidal anti-inflammatory drugs, individuals vary greatly regarding tolerance and efficacy. If any of these drugs has no appreciable effect after one week, an alternative preparation should be tried. They are essentially symptom-relieving drugs. None should be given to patients with an active or recent peptic ulcer and only very cautiously to those with a history of peptic ulcers. We do not recommend phenylbutazone because of the high incidence of side-effects some of which, although rare, can be fatal.

For acute tenosynovitis around the wrist or elbows, local injection of corticosteroids has been found very effective. Systemic corticosteroids are disappointing but may have to be tried in the most severe cases.

Conjunctivitis is self-limited and usually needs no treatment.

Anterior uveitis is best managed by the ophthalmologist. In principle mydriasis is obtained by 1 per cent atropine eye drops and steroids are given by frequent use of prednisolone eye drops (0.5 per cent Predsol). Exceptionally, iridectomy may be required.

Keratoderma and circinate balanitis may need only hygienic measures though 1 per cent hydrocortisone cream appears to shorten the course of balanitis.

In patients who develop aortic incompetence which may appear late or surprisingly early, the cardiologist and cardiac surgeon should be consulted with a view to valvular replacement.

In thrombophlebitis a supporting elastic stocking and early mobilization are suggested.

Prophylaxis. We are unaware of any serious effort to investigate the possibility of prophylaxis. Ideally, individuals known to carry B27 antigen should avoid getting NGU, PGU, or dysentery. There are clearly enormous practical difficulties to consider but suggestions can be made to patients with past RD who wish to prevent recurrences. Protected intercourse may be helpful, but since some recurrences develop apparently unprovoked by sexual intercourse, this might at best be only partially successful. The earliest possible treatment of any subsequent NGU infection seems reasonable, but as yet there is no knowledge whether it would protect, and the treatment of all sexual partners with tetracycline, in the hope of reducing recurrences of NGU, should be encouraged.

A simple step, though probably of modest impact, would be to treat all patients with past sexually acquired RD who develop fresh gonorrhoea, with tetracycline (500 mg four times daily for five days) which would significantly reduce the incidence of PGU.

References

Aho, K., Ahvonen, P., Lassus, A., Sievers, K., and Tii; ikainen, A. (1974). HL-A27 in reactive arthritis. *Arthritis Rheum.* **17**, 521.

Brewerton, D. A. (ed. (1975). Symposium on histocompatibility and rheumatic disease. *Ann. rheum. Dis.* suppl. 1, 34.

— (1979). Many genes, many clinical features. *Ann. rheum. Dis.* suppl., 145.

—, Coffrey, M., Hart, F. D., Walter, D., Oates, J. K., and Jones, D. C. O. (1973). Reiter's disease and HIA-A27. *Lancet* **ii**, 996.

Brodie, B. C. (1818). *Pathological and surgical observation on disease of the joints.* Longman, Hurst, Rees and Brown, London.

Csonka, G. W. (1958). The course of Reiter's disease. *Br. med. J.* **i**, 1088.

— (1965). Reiter's syndrome. *Ergeb. Med. Kinderkht.* **23**, 139.

— (1969). Multiple cases in Reiter's syndrome. *Br. J. vener. Dis.* **45**, 157.

— (1979). Clinical aspects of Reiter's syndrome. *Ann. rheum. Dis.* suppl., 4.

— (1979). Long-term follow-up and prognosis of Reiter's syndrome. *Ann. rheum. Dis.* suppl., 24.

—, Bassett, E. W., and Furness, G. (1974). Raised levels of an unknown beta globulin in the serum of patients with non-specific urethritis and Reiter's disease. *Br. J. vener. Dis.* **50**, 17.

Durel, P. and Siboulet, A. (1954). *Non-gonococcal urethritis in males.* WHO monograph, WHO/VDT/126, 2. World Health Organization, Geneva.

Lassus, A. and Kousa, M. (1981). Reiter's disease. In *Recent advances in sexually transmitted diseases.* (ed. J. R. W. Harris). Churchill Livingstone, Edinburgh.

Martel, W. C. (1979). Radiological manifestations of Reiter's syndrome. *Ann. rheum. Dis.* **38**, 12.

Paronen, I. (1948). Reiter's disease. A study of 344 cases observed in Finland. *Acta med. scand.* suppl. 212, 131.

Sairanen, E., Paronen, I., and Mahonen, H. (1969). A follow-up study of Reiter's syndrome. *Acta med. scand.* **185**, 57.

Venereologist's approach to herpes simplex infection

G. W. Csonka

Definition. Two types of herpes simplex virus are recognized—type 1 (HSV–1) and type 2 (HSV–2). Genital herpes is usually caused by HSV–2 and far less frequently by HSV–1. Following the primary episode, the virus persists in the presacral ganglia in a latent form and may be reactivated to cause recurrent infections. Genital herpes is potentially a far more serious condition in women than men because of the risk of their transmitting the infection to their infants, the suggestion that the virus is directly or indirectly a cause of cervical carcinoma and, least important, the greater severity of the primary attack.

Incidence. In the United Kingdom the incidence of genital herpes is increasing. In 1979 over 9000 new cases were reported from the VD clinics. This is four to five times the number of cases of early infectious syphilis. Genital herpes is the most common cause of genital ulceration seen in our clinics.

The incidence in women is about 30–35 per cent of that in men, but this proportion may not reflect the true position. The lesions in women are often more difficult to see, may be atypical, and, when confined to the cervix in primary attacks, are commonly misdiagnosed. There is evidence that genital herpes with minimal symptoms may accompany gonorrhoea and other sexually transmitted diseases (STD). Because genital herpes is often unsuspected, a number of well conducted studies will be needed to clarify the incidence of symptomatic and asymptomatic genital herpes and the ratio between the sexes.

Transmission. Genital herpes is transmitted by sexual intercourse. The danger period for infection is still considerable after the painful lesions become painless and the patient is assumed to be non-infectious, yet virus shedding may continue for up to two weeks. Asymptomatic shedding of virus from the cervix has been found especially in prostitutes, who may form an infectious reservoir of HSV-2 infection. This may also be true for anorectal infection of homosexuals. Autoinoculation and spread of herpes by fingers occurs, and patients should be warned about this. An infected mother can transmit herpes to the neonate during delivery. Whether the fetus can be infected *in utero* is uncertain. The frequency of neonatal infections is much higher with primary maternal infection than with recurrences.

Recurrences. A high proportion of patients will have further attacks. The incidence of recurrences is uncertain. In one study the median time to the first recurrence in women was 118 days compared with 59 days in men. The period between attacks can vary from days to years. Recurrences are milder than the initial attack.

After an attack the virus retreats via the sensory nerve axons to the presacral ganglia. Factors believed to precipitate recurrences include sexual intercourse, immunosuppression, corticosteroids, intercurrent infection, menstruation, and stress or fatigue.

In some patients recurrences are so frequent that they almost match the periods of freedom from symptoms. These patients are understandably distressed because of the adverse effect on their sexual activity, anxiety about infecting their sexual partners, and the doctor's obvious inability to influence the course of the infection.

Clinical features. The incubation period is two to four days but can be longer. Prodromata occur in about half the cases and may be of the same type in individual patients with every recurrence. They include pain, burning or numbness corresponding to the distribution of S1 to S5, and subsequently the site of herpetic lesions.

Genital herpes in heterosexual men. The lesion starts as a patch of erythema followed rapidly by one or several groups of papules or vesicles which break down to form shallow ulcers (Fig. 1). These crust over and after separation of the crust heal usually without scarring. The lesions are painful and irritating—an important diagnostic feature. Regional tender inguinal adenopathy is associated with the primary attack but rare in recurrences. The commonest sites for the lesions are the glans penis, coronal sulcus, penile shaft, and occasionally the scrotum and adjacent skin. Less typically there are only one or two lesions present. In severe cases involving the glans penis, phimosis and necrotizing balanitis occur. In the circumcised patient, genital herpes is distinctly uncommon.

Genital herpes in homosexual men. In the passive partner, the site of the lesion is the anal canal. In primary attacks, severe proctitis with extension to the anus and surrounding skin may develop. However, symptoms are sometimes slight and as the lesions can be difficult to demonstrate, the true cause is liable to be overlooked.

Genital herpes in women. There are important differences between primary and recurrent attacks (Table 1). Prodromata are similar to those recognized in men except that dysuria is more prominent. The usual site for the lesions is the vulva and surrounding area of skin. Vaginal discharge may be present with severe cervicitis. In some patients the cervix is covered by necrotic ulcers and the patient feels unwell. In many patients with primary infection, the dominant early feature is dysuria leading to acute retention of urine, which may be due to fear of urination because of severe pain, but may also be the result of involvement of the sacral nerve roots causing temporary paresis of the bladder.

Disseminated infections in both sexes. Disseminated infections with HSV-2 virus in adults are luckily very rare but are potentially fatal.

Neonatal herpes. This usually develops 2–12 days after birth. It is rare in the UK but more common in the USA as indeed is adult

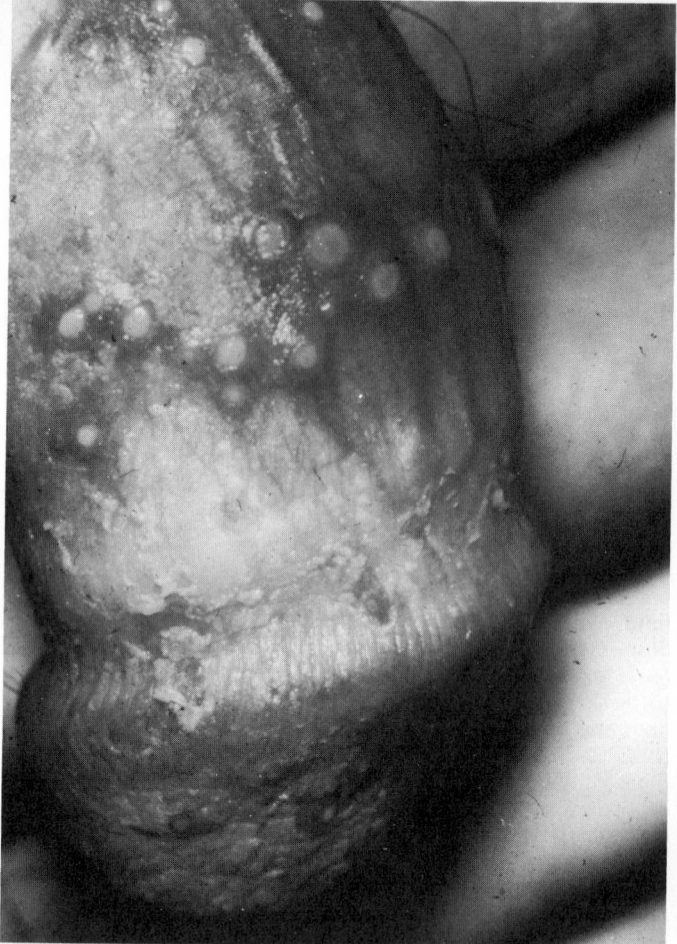

Fig. 1 Herpes genitalis.

genital herpes. Neonatal herpes occurs more readily with primary maternal infection than with recurrent attacks, but even with the latter the risk is still present. It is thought by some that herpes can be transmitted during pregnancy but most observers believe that most cases of neonatal herpes are acquired *during* labour when the infant passes through the infected birth canal. The emphasis in the literature is mainly on the serious and fatal clinical aspects of the

Table 1   Characterization of primary versus recurrent attacks of genital herpes in women

	Primary attack	Recurrent attack
Severity and duration of attack	3 weeks; severe	5–10 days; milder
Dysuria, dyspareunia, urinary retention	+++	–
Painful inguinal adenitis	+	– or ±
Pain of herpetic lesions	severe and prolonged	less severe but rarely absent
Involvement of cervix	+	–
Systemic symptoms (malaise, fever, occasionally meningism)	+	–
New lesions developing	for approx. 10 days	for approx. 3–4 days
Average duration of virus shedding = infectivity	10–12 days	4–5 days
Antibody response in serum	+	–
Danger of infecting neonate intrapartum	+++	+

infection. Yet, infants with minimal lesions are probably not uncommon. To give an example, a nappy rash may in fact be a herpetic rash which will not be appreciated unless the appropriate tests are undertaken. The largest published series showing the clinical spectrum and outcome is shown in Table 2.

Table 2   Outcome in 302 cases of neonatal herpes

Clinical groups	No.	Died	Mortality (%)
Disseminated			
Without CNS lesions	98	92	84
With CNS lesions	97	71	
Localized			
CNS	52	38	
Eye	16	—	39
Skin	34	3	
Mouth	3	—	
A symptomatic	2	—	
Total	302	204	68

After Nahmias *et al.* (1976)

Laboratory diagnosis. Infection is best diagnosed by viral isolation. Herpes virus is comparatively easy to grow in tissue culture and results can be expected within three days.

Blood should be taken at the same time as culture and repeated in two weeks to differentiate between primary and recurrent attack. In primary infection the first sample may contain little or no antibody by the complement fixation test, the second sample should show a marked rise in titre. In recurrent attacks both samples usually have a similar low titre.

When culture is not possible, cervical cytology smears stained with Papanicolaou stain provide a simple, rapid, but less sensitive alternative. Characteristically, multinucleated giant cells with eosinophilic inclusions are present.

Differential diagnosis. Syphilis must be excluded in every patient by dark-field microscopy of the erosions and by serology. In endemic areas chancroid and other ulcerative venereal diseases may have to be considered. Genital ulcers may be self-inflicted, traumatic, allergic, due to a fixed eruption often associated with tetracycline, Vincent's infection, Behçet's syndrome, or part of erythema multiforme. Herpetic urethritis and cervicitis must be differentiated from other causes of these conditions.

Treatment and prophylaxis. So far no effective and acceptable treatment is generally available. Idoxuridine (IDU) in DMSO is at best of marginal value in HSV–2 infections. It appears that the new drug acyclovir, which is at present undergoing clinical trials, will prove of value in shortening individual attacks though it appears not to prevent recurrences. If pain is present, simple analgesics are adequate. Topical corticosteroids are completely contra-indicated as they aggravate the infection. In women with a severe primary attack associated with dysuria and retention of urine, admission to hospital for a few days is usually necessary.

Annual checks of cervical cytology are advisable until there is proof that genital herpes is not associated with the development of malignant changes of the cervix.

Pregnant women who have had sexual contact with a partner with active genital herpes should be repeatedly examined for herpes clinically and virologically especially towards the end of pregnancy.

Management of pregnancy in women with genital herpes. Suspicion of maternal genital herpes should be confirmed by repeated viral cultures of the lesions and the cervix. If a primary attack develops *after the 36th week* of pregnancy, Caesarean section should be considered as it may reduce the incidence of neonatal infection from over 50 per cent to around 5 per cent. If the lesions have healed and virus is no longer isolated, vaginal delivery is indicated. If, however, lesions are detected just before or during labour while the membrane is still intact, Caesarean section is the safest course. If primary HSV–2 infection occurs *early* in pregnancy, the fetus may be infected and permanently damaged. The indications for a later Caesarean section are therefore uncertain.

Men with genital herpes must be warned not to have sexual contact during the active phase of the infection and for some days after.

Neonatal herpes. In the *localized form* (skin, eye, mouth) topical acyclovir is probably best. In the *disseminated form* systemic antiviral therapy is necessary. The drugs used include IDU (very toxic) and adenosine arabinoside (Ara-A) which is less toxic. Acyclovir is least toxic and may supersede the older preparations.

One has to face the dilemma that should the baby survive with treatment, crippling brain damage is a fearsome possibility.

References

Corey, L. (1980). Natural history and therapy of genital herpes simplex virus (HSV) infection. *Third International meeting on sexually transmitted diseases.* Antwerp.

Hurley, R. (1978). In *Towards the prevention of foetal malformations* (ed. J. B. Scrimgeour). Edinburgh University Press, Edinburgh.

Longson, M. and Bailey, A. S. (1977). In *Recent advances in clinical virology* (ed. A. P. Waterson). Churchill Livingstone, Edinburgh.

Nahmias, A. J., Josey, W. E., Naib, Z. M., and Visinitine, A. M. (1976). In *Sexually transmitted diseases* (eds. R. D. Catterall and C. S. Nicol). Academic Press, London.

Roizman, B. and Frenkel, N. (1976). Does genital herpes cause cancer?—a midway assessment. In *Sexually transmitted diseases.* (eds. R. D. Catterall and C. S. Nicol.) Academic Press, London.

Listeria

R. Hurley

Listeria monocytogenes

Current evidence from numerical taxonomy, serological, and DNA base pairing studies points to *Listeria* as a separate genus grouped with the lactobacilli and the streptococci in the family *Lactobacillaceae*. It is distinct from *Erysipelothrix*, but shares antigens with staphylococci, enterococci, *Escherichia coli* and *Corynebacterium pyogenes*. Although taxonomists have sought to introduce other species, notably *L. grayi*, the genus contains only one undoubted species, *L. monocytogenes*, which is probably a ground saprophyte, multiplying in soil and infecting man and animals through the ingestion of contaminated food. The short, motile, aerobic, and micro-aerophilic Gram-positive bacilli grow sparsely on nutrient, McConkey, and blood agar, usually surrounded on the latter by a narrow zone of β-haemolysis although non-haemolytic strains occur. Growth is improved in the presence of carbon dioxide, and the microbe is of few pathogens that can form colonies at 4 °C. Selective media are available, and, with prolonged cold incubation, are recommended for cultivation. Morphologically, *L. monocytogenes* resembles a diphtheroid, from which it is distinguishable by its characteristic tumbling motility from cultures grown at 18–20 °C. It is catalase positive.

At low temperatures it can survive in culture media for up to 12 years, also surviving in nature in hay, straw, milk, and earth for many months. It is resistant to salt, tolerating concentrations of up to 20 per cent, and remaining viable in 16 per cent salt for up to a year. It can withstand 40 per cent bile and, possibly, pasteurization. Thus, it is a relatively hardy microbe. Growth is inhibited by penicillin, ampicillin, erythromycin, tetracycline, and sulphadiazine, but high concentrations of penicillin and ampicillin are required for killing. Chlorination of effluents destroys it and such treatment may interrupt the cycle of transmission from infected faeces to soil and thence, again, to the gastrointestinal tracts of man and animals.

At least four main serotypes are distinguishable by flagellar and somatic antigens, the primary distinction being based on flagellar antigens A, B, C, and D and, secondarily, on somatic antigens i to ix. In this way, some 10 serotypes can be recognized. There is no genuine tendency towards zoological or geographical distribution of serotypes, although types 1a and 4b have been reported most frequently from man. The grouping obtainable by phage typing agrees closely with that of serological typing.

The definition of the genus includes the property, demonstrated by *L. monocytogenes*, of producing a monocytosis in rodents, keratoconjunctivitis in rabbits, and septic lesions in various organs of warm-blooded animals. The disease, as described in rabbits in 1926, was characterized by large celled mononucleosis.

Listeriosis

Carriage, habitat, and transmission to man. *L. monocytogenes* has been isolated from some 50 species of domestic and wild animals and from some 20 species of birds, fish, insects, and crustaceans. It can be isolated regularly from sewage, water, mud, fodder, silage, and the earth. Survival is poor in acid soil or silage, but good in grass, soil, or silage of near neutral pH. The infective cycle is probably based on its survival in soil or vegetation, multiplication in silage, establishment of carrier or diseased state in animals or fowls and, for man, growth in food derived from these sources which is consumed after inadequate heating. Cold prepared foods may also, presumably, become contaminated and multiplication of the bacteria may proceed under refrigerated conditions. Certainly, it has been recovered from lamb meat held at 0 °C for 24 days and will grow in lamb, beef, pork, and egg at 4 °C. The portal of entry is thus, predominantly, the gastrointestinal tract. Overt disease of the gastrointestinal tract is unlikely to ensue, although there is suggestive evidence that ingestion of heavily contaminated food may cause acute diarrhoea both in man and animals.

Carriage in man, as in animals, is widespread, *L. monocytogenes* having been isolated from the faeces of 0.6–29 per cent of healthy persons. In the majority of cases, carriage is unrelated to the person's work or profession, although some believe it to be higher in slaughterhouse workers and shepherds. The event of carriage may be of no clinical significance whatever, merely indicating the recent consumption of contaminated food. Carriage is likely to be transient, the microbes being excreted for no longer than a month. Over half the chickens consumed in United Kingdom homes contain *L. monocytogenes* inside or on the surface, although adequate cooking will destroy the bacteria. In man, the seasonal incidence of carriage is highest in the early summer, whereas in cattle the incidence both of carriage and disease is greatest in late winter and early spring.

Strains isolated from the faeces differ markedly in virulence, and high carrier rates may be associated with low virulence. However, in the majority of infections, the distal alimentary tract must be regarded as the proximate reservoir from which the organism is able to invade the tissues when defence mechanisms become impaired. The microbe, which is an intracellular parasite capable of multiplying not only in the cytoplasm but in the nucleus of the host cell, localizes in the intestinal wall, especially in Peyer's patches whence it invades the bloodstream or passes to the liver and other organs producing micro-abscesses. The incubation period is not known, but it is at least as long as seven days, and up to 30 days, in experimental infections of large animals. The nasopharynx may be the portal of entry in the anginose glandular form and, perhaps, in the meningoencephalitic form. The microbe does not survive long in the throats of healthy persons, but it has been suggested that it reaches the meninges via branches of the trigeminal nerve after penetration of the buccal mucosa in the vicinity of minor lesions. The nasopharynx may become contaminated through the ingestion of contaminated liquids, such as milk, the infected droplets reaching the meninges by way of the olfactory nerve. Experimentally, fatal meningitis and septicaemia have been induced

in calves in this way, using a nebulizer to deliver a fully virulent strain. Listeria can be harboured in the genital tract for long periods, suggesting the possibility of venereal transmission. The route of infection in listeric neonatal sepsis is deemed to be twofold: by way of haematogenous transplacental transmission or by intrapartum infection as the newborn traverses the birth canal. In either event, the infection is maternally derived. *L. monocytogenes* has been isolated from human as well as cow's milk, and breast feeding cannot be discounted as a potential source of infection. Cross infection, with person to person spread is also possible.

Types of disease in man. Although described as lately as 1933, over 2000 cases of listeric infection had been described in Germany alone by the 1960s. Most reported cases emanate from temperate zones but the disease is worldwide in distribution. Attack rates are highest at the extremes of life, during pregnancy, and in those with serious underlying disease. *L. monocytogenes* may cause disease of the throat, the eyes, the skin, the lymph nodes, the central nervous system, or the pregnant uterus, or it may give rise to a syndrome resembling typhoid fever. In the newborn, it is often a multisystem disease, with pulmonary and central nervous system symptoms predominating. Reports vary on the relative frequency of the types of listeric infection, but conviction is growing that cases of maternal and perinatal disease outnumber those of listeric meningoencephalitis. The great majority of cases are believed to be mild and inapparent or subclinical.

Anginose-septic, oculoglandular, and other focal forms of listeric infections. The anginose form of listeriosis may be confused with glandular fever, although *L. monocytogenes* may be isolated from the bloodstream. It is sometimes accompanied by conjunctivitis, which may arise in consequence of accidental inoculation following exposure to infected animals or as part of the primary infection. The oculoglandular form is characterized by purulent discharge from the conjunctiva and by enlargement of the parotid and submandibular glands, which may occasionally suppurate, with secondary infection and the formation of fistulae. *L. monocytogenes* can be isolated from pus or from a biopsy specimen. Conjunctivitis may also be associated with meningoencephalitis. Acute anterior uveitis may be caused by listeria.

Focal manifestations of listeric infection, such as those above and others, are rare. Infective endocarditis, involving principally the left heart and occurring more often in the male than the female, and usually in those with defective heart valves, has been recorded. Arthritis, osteomyelitis, cholecystitis, peritonitis, and brain and spinal cord abscesses attributable to listeria are all known. A chronic form of listeric infection of the genital tract, characterized by urethritis with purulent discharge, also occurs.

Cutaneous form. This is an occupational hazard of veterinary surgeons or others in close contact with diseased animals, especially at parturition. Within 48–72 hours of exposure, maculopapular lesions, progressing to pustules, appear on the hands and forearms. Constitutional disturbance is slight, but there may be headaches, dizziness, fever and slight axillary lymphadenopathy. The condition responds rapidly to antibiotic treatment.

Listeric infection in pregnancy. Characteristically, infection in pregnant women is associated with two or more febrile episodes (see page 5.485). The first, recognized in retrospect as the primary infection, is associated with malaise, headache, fever, backache, pharyngitis, conjunctivitis, diarrhoea, and abdominal or loin pain. The condition may be diagnosed as pyelonephritis, for the kidneys may be involved in the listeric process, but the true nature of the infection will be recognized if the often slow growing *L. monocytogenes* is actively sought in cultures of blood and of other sites, such as the genital tract and urine. Resolution of fever may occur if antibacterial therapy has been given, but relapse is likely. Within 1–20 days of delivery, often of an infected, premature baby, there is a further febrile episode, regarded as a manifestation of re-infection from the placenta. In about 40 per cent of cases, fever is not marked at any time, the disease presenting as an influenza-like illness or being completely unremarked by the patient. There is evidence that recurrent or persistent genital listeric infection may be a cause of habitual abortion in man, as in domestic or wild animals. Due to difficulties in isolation of the microbe, and, until recently, in the performance and interpretation of serological tests, the aetiological diagnosis may be difficult to substantiate in abortion.

Perinatal listeric infection. The incidence of listeric infection in the perinatal period in the United Kingdom is about 1 in 37 000 births and in the United States about 1 in 1 000 000 population. Neonatal septicaemia may occur in epidemic form in cattle, and epidemics in man have been reported from East Germany and New Zealand. Cross-infection in neonatal units has also occurred.

Listeric infection of the newborn occurs in two forms: the early onset type results from infection *in utero*, whether by the haematogenous transplacental route or following the inhalation of contaminated amniotic fluid, and is manifest as septicaemia within two days of birth. There is meconium staining of the amniotic fluid, and the usually prematurely born infant has signs of respiratory distress and, sometimes, a rash; the late form of the disease presents predominantly as a meningo-encephalitis, sometimes with slow hydrocephalus, after the fifth day. This type of the disease may be transmitted from the environment. About a third to a quarter of babies with early onset disease are born dead, necropsy demonstrating the typical appearances of granulomatosis infantiseptica, with miliary micro-abscesses and granulomata in the liver, spleen, adrenal glands, lungs, pharynx, gastrointestinal tract, central nervous system and skin. The disease is more frequent in continental Europe than in the British Isles, and *L. monocytogenes* ranks third, after *Escherichia coli* and the group B streptococcus as the cause of neonatal sepsis in France.

Meningo-encephalitis. As well as infecting the pregnant, *L. monocytogenes* has a predilection for infecting the central nervous system, and the majority of cases of listeric meningo-encephalitis occur in the newborn, as late onset sepsis, and in immunosuppressed adults. The onset of the disease is undramatic in both, fever being low grade. In adults, some of whom may have been previously healthy, focal neurological signs may develop, with cranial nerve palsies or hemiparesis, as well as insidious disturbance of consciousness leading to coma. *L. monocytogenes* is probably the most common cause of meningitis in compromised hosts, particularly in those undergoing therapy that affects the thymus-derived lymphocyte–mononuclear phagocyte system, and, since it also affects the previously healthy, it should always be considered in the differential diagnosis of meningitis. Save in cases of cerebritis, brain stem infection, or brain abscess, examination of cerebrospinal fluid usually shows an increase in lymphocytes and polymorphonuclear leucocytes, either of which may predominate. The protein concentration is usually raised. Glucose levels may be normal. *L. monocytogenes* can usually be isolated.

Sepsis of unknown origin: typhoid-pneumonic type. The patients are adults or neonates with chills or spiking fever of acute onset repeated over several weeks. On rare occasions, the peripheral blood shows a monocytosis, and the patients may be hypotensive showing signs of septic shock. During the typhoidal course, focal pneumonic infiltrates, pulmonary cavitation, and empyema may occur. There is suppuration in distant organs and septicaemia. Blood cultures are positive.

Diagnosis. A high index of suspicion is necessary for early diagnosis. Specimens from affected sites, including the throat, conjunctiva, skin, cerebrospinal fluid, vagina, placenta, meconium, urine, faeces, bloodstream, purulent discharges, and collections of pus should be sent for examination. Isolation of the causative microbe may be facilitated by 'cold enrichment', a process in which specimens are stored at 4 °C for at least four weeks and subcultured weekly to selective media. The isolation of 'diphtheroids' from such specimens should be regarded with suspicion, and the microbes carefully examined. As there is a high frequency of natural antibodies cross-reacting non-specifically with *L. monocytogenes*, serological diagnosis has, hitherto, been unsatisfactory, having as yet no unequivocal place in routine diagnostic practice although demonstration of rising titres and of listeria-specific IgM may help. The serum fibrinogen may exceed 340 mg/100 ml in neonatal listeriosis.

Management and treatment. *L. monocytogenes* is susceptible to ampicillin, penicillin, erythromycin, and tetracycline. The treatment of choice is ampicillin, penicillin G being less consistently effective. Synergistic activity is demonstrable between ampicillin or penicillin and streptomycin or gentamicin, and combination therapy with both drugs may be considered for serious listeric disease. A suitable dosage schedule is ampicillin 200–400 mg/kg body weight per day divided in four doses, and gentamicin 5–6 mg/kg per day divided in three doses. Treatment should be continued for one week after the fever subsides. Oral erythromycin or tetracycline may be used to treat the oculoglandular or cutaneous forms.

Prognosis. Formerly, mortality rates of 90 per cent were recorded for infantile listeriosis, but given early diagnosis and prompt treatment with bactericidal agents in high dosage, an overall mortality of 50 per cent is more likely. If the surviving infant was more than 36 weeks of gestation at birth, there are unlikely to be adverse sequelae. The prognosis for other forms of listeriosis, other than listeric meningo-encephalitis, is good, complete cure being achieved. The overall mortality of all forms of the disease reported in the United Kingdom in recent years has been of the order of 20 per cent.

References

Bojsen-Moller, J. (1972). Human listeriosis: diagnostic, epidemiological and clinical studies *Acta path. microbiol. scand.* Section B, supplement no. 229.

The Lancet (1980). Perinatal listeriosis. *Lancet* **i**, 911.

Relier, J. P., (1979). Listeriosis. In *Perinatal and neonatal infections*, (ed. R. Hurley, J. de Louvois, and F. Drasar) *J. antimicrob. Chemother.* **5**, 51.

Wilson, G. S. and Miles, A. (eds.) (1975). *Topley and Wilson's Principles of Bacteriology, Virology and Immunity* 6th edn. Arnold, London.

Woodbine, M. (ed.) (1975). *Problems of listeriosis.* Leicester University Press, Leicester.

Legionnaires' disease

J. O'H. Tobin

In 1976 an outbreak of pneumonia occurred among American Legionnaires who had attended a convention in a Philadelphia hotel. There were 182 cases of 'Legionnaires' disease' with 29 deaths. Initially there was some difficulty in determining the cause, but subsequently it was shown by workers at the Center for Disease Control, Atlanta, that a newly identified organism, *Legionella pneumophila* was responsible. Following this discovery retrospective and prospective outbreaks, as well as sporadic cases were identified in the United States, the United Kingdom, and elsewhere, so that the infection is now recognized as one form of bacterial pneumonia. There are at least six serological groups of *L. pneumophilia* of which serogroup 1 is the most frequently encountered in human infections.

The organism has also been associated with a syndrome called 'Pontiac fever', which is possibly related to 'humidifier fever'.

More recently other legionella species besides *L. pneumophila* have been associated with sporadic respiratory infections in man. The legionella species and where they were found are listed in

Table 1. It has been suggested recently that the legionellae should be divided into three genera, Legionella, Tatlockia, and Fluoribacter within the family Legionellaceae. An association of legionellae with Bushy Creek and Fort Bragg Fevers has not been susbtantiated, the latter being caused by a leptospira. The guinea pigs inoculated were probably the source of the organism as in the isolation from a case of pityriasis rosea.

Table 1   *L. pneumophilia* and other legionella-like organisms (LLO)

Species	Strains	Sources
L. pneumophilia Serogroup 1	Philadelphia Pontiac, ODLA, Kingston, etc.	Human respiratory tract, post mortem lung Pontiac Fever
2	Togus 1, etc.	air conditioning systems, i.e. cooling towers etc.
3	Bloomington 2, etc.	
4	Los Angeles 1, etc.	water systems, i.e. showers, taps, tanks, etc.
5	Dallas, Cambridge 2, etc.	lakes, streams, and mud
6	Chicago 2, Oxford 1 and 2, etc. Oxford P183, etc.	
Others		
L. micdadei	Tatlock, HEBA, Pittsburgh	Fort Bragg (pretibial) fever, lung, pneumonias
L. pittsburgensis	pneumonia agent (PAA), etc.	pityriasis rosea
L. bozemanii	WIGA, MI15	lung, pneumonias
L. dumoffii	NY23, Tex KL	cooling tower, lung
L. gormanii	L13	wet soil
L. longbeachae	Long Beach 4, Los Angeles 24, etc.	lung pneumonias
L. jordanii	–	river water

Epidemiology. The natural habitat of *L. pneumophila* is possibly moist soil and it has been found in mud and water from streams and lakes. It has been found in waters with temperatures varying from 5 °C to 62 °C and with pH of 5.4 to 8.2. It has not been found in salt water as it is inhibited by sodium chloride.. In the initial Philadelphia outbreak, the air-conditioning system came under suspicion as the source of infection, as most of the cases were associated with congregating in the hotel lobby; this suspicion was not confirmed microbiologically, and other cases also occurred among pedestrians in the street outside who had not been associated with the hotel itself, the so-called 'Broad street disease'.

The outbreak of 'Pontiac fever' in 1967, in which 95 per cent of the staff of a US Health Department office suffered from an acute non-pneumonic respiratory disease, was shown to be due to a leak between the ducts of the evaporative condenser cooling system, in which *L. pneumophila* was growing, and ventilation systems.

Infected water from evaporative condensers and cooling towers of air-conditioning systems have been shown repeatedly to be infected with legionellae whether associated with clinical cases of Legionnaires' disease or not. These condensers and towers emanate in their cooling air streams, fine drops of water (known as 'drift') containing bacteria, which can be carried short distances in the vicinity of these structures. The temperature of the water in cooling systems is usually 30–38 °C which is optimal for legionella growth. The organism multiplies only very slowly at temperatures below 25 °C. The presence of other micro-organisms in cooling water may augment the growth of legionellae; algae and amoebae have been

implicated in this synergism. The legionellae may grow intracellularly in amoebae and this habitat may be part of a regular life cycle.

Two cases of Legionnaires' disease in an Oxford transplant unit were associated with infected shower water. Subsequently, the organism has been found in many water systems of hospitals and hotels in the United Kingdom and the United States, often associated with outbreaks of Legionnaires' disease. Hot water systems are usually more often infected than cold water ones with bacteria being found in such systems from taps through to the calorifier.

It seems, therefore, that wherever water is held at temperatures over 25 °C the organism may multiply, and if in large enough quantities, may be inhaled in droplets into the respiratory tract causing pneumonia. The relative importance of infected cooling towers and tap and shower water has yet to be determined but currently it appears that droplets produced by showering, washing, and bathing are the more important. Although infected cooling towers of air conditioning systems have almost certainly been the source of infection in at least three outbreaks, Legionnaires' disease has occurred in establishments without this amenity, but with infected water systems. One large hospital outbreak *was not controlled by* cleaning the cooling towers *but was by* chlorinating the water supply.

There is a higher incidence of Legionnaires' disease in August and September in temperate climates. About a third of cases diagnosed in the United Kingdom are infected while on holiday in southern Europe. In tropical countries, the disease should have no obvious season incidence. Infection by the gastrointestinal route is a possibility, but of much less consequence than by the respiratory route. Infection seems to be environmental with little evidence for case to case spread.

Clinical features. The main clinical caused by *L. pneumophila* are Legionnaires' disease pneumonia and 'Pontiac fever', but it is likely that it can cause other mild respiratory illnesses not yet clearly defined. It has been suggested that Legionella pneumonia be the term used to describe pnemonia due to *Legionella* species and reserve Legionnaires' disease for outbreaks similar to that in Philadelphia.

Legionnaires' disease pneumonia. The incubation period is 2–10 days with a mean of 7 days with males being three times more likely to be infected than females. Cases have been reported from infancy upwards, but three-quarters of the cases are in the 40–70 year old age group, with a mean of 57 years of age. The mortality, 8–30 per cent in different series, is higher in those over 55 years of age, and is highest in those with chronic cardiac, pulmonary, or renal disease, in the immunosuppressed, and in diabetics. Forty per cent of cases reported are patients undergoing renal transplantation, or on immunosuppression for cancer, and the infection is often nosocomial.

Characteristically, the patient with Legionnaires' disease presents with malaise, myalgia in the muscles of the back, limbs, or neck, headache, and a fever of 38.5–40.5 °C. Chills and mild diarrhoea with abdominal pain are common, and the patient may show signs of prostration.

Within a few days, a dry cough develops with or without haemoptysis, and chest pain and dyspnoea are present. The patient appears acutely ill, tachopneic, often disorientated and confused. Haematuria may occur and the illness may be complicated by renal failure, pleural effusions, and, occasionally, apparent CNS involvement. Ataxia, aphasia, tremors, peripheral neuropathy, slurred speech, memory defects, lethargy, emotional outburst, hallucinations, delirium, and retrograde amnesia have all been reported.

Gastrointestinal symptoms, such as nausea, vomiting, abdominal pain, distension, and bleeding can occur and may sometimes dominate the early stages of the illness in which respiratory symptoms may be minimal.

On physical examination, the patient is usually ill and febrile with some dehydration, tachycardia, and tachopnea. Rhonchi and crepitations can be heard, and signs of consolidation are present in

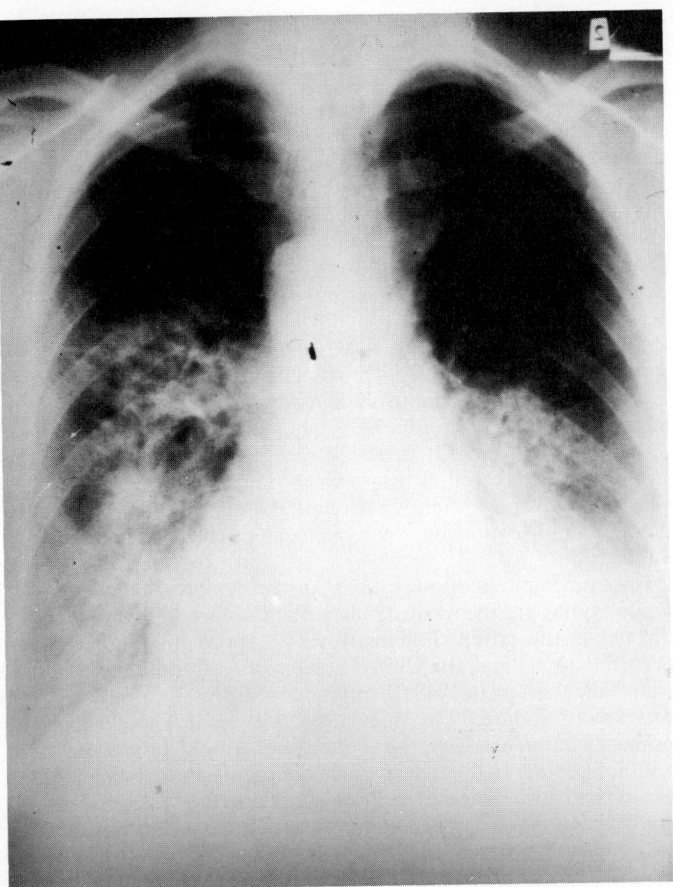

Fig. 1 Radiograph of bilateral lung involvement in a woman aged 60 taken one week after the start of clinical recovery.

about one third of patients when first seen. A pleural rub may be detected. Diffuse abdominal tenderness may be present and rarely, an enlarged but not tender, liver may be felt.

Sputum is sparse and mucoid initially but later may become purulent and more plentiful. Radiological signs of consolidation are present in over 90 per cent of cases when first seen, and may be limited to one lobe, may already have involved both lobes, or be patchy in distribution. During the illness, consolidation usually spreads.

Eighty per cent of patients probably recover spontaneously. The more severe symptoms last for five to seven days unless the pneumonia continues to spread or renal failure occurs. Radiological signs may only resolve slowly.

Laboratory findings. There is a moderate polymorphonuclear leucocytosis usually from 10 000–15 000/mm³, often associated with a lymphopenia of less than 1000/mm³. Total cells are rarely above 15 000 and there may be a shift to the left. Thrombocytopenia is rare unless associated with some underlying illness. A plasma sodium of less than 130 mmol/l or a calcium equal to or less than 1.9 mmol/l is found in half the patients, and liver function tests may be abnormal. Routine bacterial cultures of blood, sputum, urine, or CSF are usually negative.

Microbiological diagnosis. A serological diagnosis can be made by immunofluorescence, complement fixation, haemagglutination, radioimmunoassay or ELISA techniques. Immunofluorescence, using formalized or heat-killed preparations of all or some of the legionella serogroups, grown in the yolk sac of chick embryo, is the usual test employed.

Antibodies start to appear 5–10 days after onset of illness and reach maximum titres in 2–4 weeks. The initial response is usually in the IgM class of antibody followed by an IgG rise, although variations in the pattern of immunoglobin response occur. For definite serological diagnosis, an early and convalescent sample are

required, but a titre of more than 1:250 in a convalescent sample is suggestive of recent infection in a patient with an unidentified pneumonia. Antibody can disappear within a year, or persist at low levels for a longer period. In immunosuppressed patients, antibody may have reached its maximum level within 36 hours of onset of the disease as the prodromal symptoms may be masked by their therapy.

L. pneumophila can sometimes be seen in sputum, in fibre-optic bronchoscopy specimens and transtracheal washouts , in lung puncture, or biopsy specimens, either by using modified Gram stains, silver stains, or by immunofluorescence. Fibre-optic and lung puncture specimens are the samples of choice, especially in cases not progressing satisfactorily.

Isolation on special media or by guinea pig inoculation has been successful from respiratory tract samples and from blood, although it may take from 4 to 20 days to become positive.

Differential diagnosis. In the absence of a specific laboratory diagnosis, Legionnaires' disease should be suspected in a patient whose pneumonia does not respond to antibiotic therapy, is on immunosuppression, has been abroad to warmer climates immediately prior to the onset of the illness, or has been in hospital during the incubation period of the disease.

Patients with fever of more than three days before being seen, who are confused, have haematuria, a low lymphocyte count, or low plasma sodium and calcium levels, have a spreading consolidation and abnormal liver function tests should be treated as having Legionnaires' disease.

Treatment. Erythromycin, 4 g per day, preferably intravenously for the first week and continued for three weeks, is the antibiotic therapy of choice. If the patient does not respond, and the diagnosis is still likely, rifampicin should be added, 150–300 mg twice daily. Patients may seem to be recovering and therapy stopped only for relapses to occur often with fatal results.

Supportive therapy, including the use of a respirator may be necessary. If there is any doubt about the seriousness of the patient's condition, he should be artificially ventilated as soon as possible: there is evidence that early ventilation may be life saving.

Prognosis. The prognosis depends on the patient's age, perhaps on smoking and drinking habits, and on the presence of underlying disease. Hodgkin's disease patients have a poor prognosis compared with other cancer patients.

Pathology. In fatal cases, the lungs are the only organs showing any definite changes. The pneumonia is often lobar in distribution with fibrinous exudate and polymorph and macrophage infiltration into alveoli. Involvement of the bronchioles is common, and often the normal alveolar architecture is lost. In some cases red and grey hepatization may be seen. Fibrosis occurs later in the illness, and, in immunosuppressed patients, abscesses and cavity formation may occur. Organisms can be seen using silver stains or immunofluorescence.

'Pontiac fever'. This syndrome is a short febrile illness lasting two to five days with an incubation period of about 36 hours. Chills, fever up to 40 °C, headache, myalgia, dizziness, cough, photophobia, nausea, and vomiting are the main symptoms. Sore throat, mid-sternal pain, and a constrictive sensation in the chest can occur. Less often, confusion, poor co-ordination, insomnia, and nightmares develop. Usually the illness is self-limiting, but insomnia, poor memory, general irritability and weakness may occasionally persist for weeks or months. Physical signs are scarce and radiological evidence of chest involvement very rare. No deaths have been reported.

Antibodies to *L. pneumophila* are present but may not show a significant rise in level in convalescence, or be as high as in Legionnaires' disease itself.

Pontiac fever is thought by some to be related to humidifier fever and associated with the release of legionellae antigen from inhaled amoebae containing these organisms.

Prevention. In nosocomial infection in hospitals or other defined outbreaks elsewhere, the environmental source of infection should be sought, but until this is identified, no specific antimicrobial measures should be undertaken except to enforce adequate routine maintenance of cooling towers or other water systems. No steps should be taken until all requisite samples for microbiological tests have been obtained. These include water from cooling towers (5 l), from showers and taps (15–25 l), and from humidifiers (1–5 l), as well as other epidemiologically likely sources.

The organism is isolated and identified in these samples by (*a*) filtering them through bacteria-retaining cellulose filters; (*b*) washing off the deposit from the filter into distilled water, (*c*) inoculating four- to six-week-old guinea pigs intraperitoneally, (*d*) culturing the blood, spleen, liver and peritoneal fluid from animals ill, or killed on the fourth or fifth day after inoculation, either on special media, or in five- to seven-day-old chick embryo yolk sacs.

The optimal treatment of infected cooling towers has yet to be determined, but chlorination may give a short-term respite to harassed administrators. Infected water supplies may need continuous chlorination to produce 1 to 4 parts per million free chlorine at all outlets to control infection or keeping hot water at higher temperatures than usual. This requires knowledge of the exact location of the organism in the water systems if money and monitoring services are to be carried out most economically. The long-term effects of control measures on the organisms' survival and on the materials used in water systems has yet to be determined but already eradication of Legionellae has proved very difficult.

References

International symposium on Legionnaires' disease (1979). *Ann. intern. Med.* **90**, 489–713.

Lattimer, G. L. and Ormsbee, R. A. (1981). Legionnaires' disease. Marcel Dekker, New York.

McKinney, R. M., Poischen, R. K., Edelstein, P. H., Bissett, M. L., *et al.* (1981). *Legionella longbeachae* species nova, another aetiological agent of human pneumonia. *Ann. intern. Med.* **94**, 739.

Meyer, R. D. and Finegold, S. M. (1980). Legionnaires' disease. *Ann. rev. Med.* **31**, 219–32.

Tobin, J. O'H., Swann, R. A., and Bartlett, C. R. (1981). Isolation of *Legionella pneumophila* from water systems. *Br. med. J.* i, 515.

Wing, E. J., Schefer, F. J., and Pasculle, A. W. (1981). Successful treatment of Legionella micdadei (Pittsburg pneumonia agent) pneumonia with erythromycin. *Am. J. Med.* **71**, 836.

Rickettsial diseases

T. E. Woodward

Introduction. The human rickettsioses are of relative minor clinical importance throughout the world, but it is clear that at least one rickettsial disease is present in most countries whenever attempts are made to identify them. They occur sporadically and occasionally in epidemic numbers when epidemiologic conditions are favourable. Since causative rickettsiae are well established in their natural habitat, it is essential for physicians to recognize the diseases clinically so that appropriate treatment and control measures be applied.

The most important rickettsial infections are Rocky Mountain spotted fever (RMSF), epidemic, murine, scrub typhus, and Q fever. Rickettsial-pox and Brill–Zinsser disease occur sporadically in certain areas. Practitioners of medicine must be familiar with these infections in their own countries, such as in England or the United States, as well as those which might be encountered elsewhere under appropriate environmental conditions. A compendium of information on the rickettsial diseases is presented in Table 1.

Rocky Mountain spotted fever in the United States and São Paulo typhus are the most significant and clinically severe types of the tick-borne group. For many years, approximately 500 cases occurred annually in the United States, and, after the introduction of specific therapy in 1948, the number of infected cases decreased to a low of about 200 in 1959, 1960, and 1961. This decline was primarily influenced by the widespread use of broad spectrum antibiotics early in the illness which led to under-reporting and the use of pesticides. Since 1969, there has been a gradual increase with approximately 900 cases reported in 1975 and 1976, and cumulative totals of 1115, 1011, and 1070 in 1977, 1978, and 1979, respectively. Transformation of farms into housing developments and recreation of children and adults in wooded areas probably accounts for the added exposure to infected ticks, particularly in the South Atlantic states where the largest number of cases occur.

In the Eastern Hemisphere and elsewhere, the tick-borne rickettsioses are milder and known variously as *fièvre boutonneuse*, South African, North Asian, Kenya, Indian, or Siberian fever, or Queensland tick typhus and other names. Mite-borne rickettsial-pox with its rodent reservoir is troublesome rather than important.

Table 1   Rickettsial diseases

Disease	Agent	Geographic distribution	Arthropod	Mammal	Principal means of transmission to man
Spotted fever group					
Rocky Mountain spotted fever	*R. ricketsii*	western Hemisphere	ticks	wild rodents, dogs	tick bite
Fièvre Boutonneuse	*R. conorii*	Africa, Europe, Middle East, India	ticks		
Queensland tick typhus	*R. australis*	Australia	ticks	marsupials, wild rodents	tick bite
North Asian tick-borne rickettsioses	*R. siberica*	Siberia, Mongolia	ticks	wild rodents	tick bite
Rickettsialpox	*R. akari*	United States, Russia, Africa	mite	house mouse, other rodents	mite bite
Typhus fever group					
Endemic (murine)	*R. mooseri*	worldwide	flea	small rodents	infected flea faeces into broken skin
Epidemic	*R. prowazekii*	worldwide	body louse,	humans, flying	infected louse
	R. canada	North America	ticks	squirrels	faeces into broken skin
Brill–Zinsser disease	*R. prowazekii*	worldwide	recrudescence years after original attack		of epidemic typhus
Scrub	*R. tsutsugamushi*	Asia, Australia, Pacific Islands	trombiculid mites	wild rodents	mite bite
Other rickettsial diseases					
Q Fever	*C. burnetti*	worldwide	ticks	small mammals, cattle, sheep, goats	inhalation of dried infected material

Rats, fleas, and crowded populations, particularly in port cities, favour the presence of murine typhus fever. Its close relative, epidemic louse-borne typhus fever, has ravaged humans during wars, famine, poverty, or during periods of privation and now exists in the cold environments of Europe, Africa, the Asian subcontinent, Latin and South America. Louse-borne typhus fever remains an important cause of morbidity where environmental and socioeconomic conditions allow proper interplay between the microbe, susceptible populations, and the vector. During 1976, a total of 8065 cases with 106 deaths were reported to the World Health Organization with principal foci in the highlands of central Africa, including Burundi, Rwanda, and southern Uganda. A few cases were reported from Nigeria and Algeria. Bolivia, Ecuador, and Peru reported a total of 223 cases with eight deaths. Ethiopia has reported no cases since 1971. Patients with Brill–Zinsser disease are the reappearing ghosts of typhus fever and serve as human reservoirs of *Rickettsia prowazekii*. It now appears that flying squirrels and possibly other mammals serve as reservoirs.

Scrub typhus fever (Tsutsugamushi disease) occurs in Japan, China, Australia, the Southwest Pacific Islands, Malaysia, Indonesia, Burma, Thailand, and the Asian subcontinent. It is mite-borne with a rodent reservoir and can be mild or fatal.

Q fever is the lone rickettsial infection unassociated with an exanthem which is usually mild and associated with a characteristic pneumonitis unless manifested in the chronic forms of hepatitis or endocarditis which are increasingly becoming clinically significant.

The rickettsioses consist of a variety of clinical disorders with certain basic similarities such as a febrile course ranging from one to three weeks, headache, a body rash (except in Q fever), signs of central nervous system involvement in some, and appearance of specific antibodies or agglutinins to the proteus organisms during convalescence. The causal agents, the rickettsiae, are obligate, intracellular parasites about the size of bacteria which are pathogenic for man and capable of existing in nature within arthropods as well as in animals and man. Most of the rickettsiae are maintained in nature by a cycle which involves an insect vector and an animal reservoir. Unlike smallpox, said to be virtually eliminated, human rickettsial diseases will persist because rickettsiae and their animal vector hosts have adapted to a firmly established existence with man as an accidental sporadic victim.

Pathogenesis, pathology and laboratory diagnosis

Pathogenesis. Rickettsia gain access to man via the skin, mucous membranes, and the respiratory tract. Rickettsial-laden faeces of the tick, louse, flea, or mite which cause RMSF, epidemic, murine and scrub typhus, respectively, are deposited in the skin through the bite of the arthropod at the time of feeding. After tick attachment for several hours or feeding by other arthropods, infection is acquired through abrasion in the skin contaminated by infected faeces or juices. Local lesions (eschars) develop at sites of arthropod attachment and initial multiplication of rickettsiae, with considerable rapidity in scrub typhus, the tick-borne rickettsioses of the eastern Hemisphere, rickettsialpox and occasionally in RMSF. In tick-borne tularaemia (see page 5.210), an eschar occurs as an initial lesion and may confuse the diagnosis. Q fever results following inhalation of rickettsiae as an aerosol derived from dried infected tick or animal excretions or the drinking of contaminated milk. *Coxiella burnetii*, like other rickettsiae, is particularly hardy and maintains viability in infected hides and when dried for prolonged periods. Inhalation or deposition of infected dried arthropod faeces on mucous membranes may occasionally account for RMSF, murine typhus, and epidemic typhus.

After infection, illness occurs in periods varying from three to twenty days. The mean varies for each rickettsial infection. A short incubation period usually indicates a more serious infection, particularly for RMSF and epidemic typhus. Studies in volunteers have shown that patients with Q fever, murine typhus, or scrub typhus have rickettsaemia late in the incubation period prior to onset of fever. Similar events probably occur in all rickettsial diseases; circulating rickettsiae can be detected during the early febrile period in RMSF, rickettsialpox, murine and epidemic typhus, and Q fever. Little is known about the pathogenesis of infection during the mid-incubation period. Volunteers infected with murine typhus showed febrile rises late in the incubation period prior to actual onset. Presumably during this time in most rickettsioses, a transient, low-grade rickettsaemia results from release of organisms which multiply at the initial site of infection wich then seeds further rickettsia throughout the vascular system.

Following entry of rickettsiae into the blood from the initial site, i.e. skin, or lungs, organisms undoubtedly circulate and enter endothelial cells everywhere, although the mechanism of entry into the endothelial cell is unknown. Vascular lesions which develop at these parasitized sites presumably account for the pathologic abnormalities including the rash. There are reports of transmission of RMSF and Q fever by blood transfusion from donors whose blood was inadvertently taken during the incubation period of their illnesses.

Pathological abnormalities. Small blood vessels are the usual sites of involvement with characteristic swelling of endothelial cells, cellular proliferation, and degeneration with thrombus formation and partial or complete occlusion of the vascular lumen in patients with RMSF and epidemic typhus. Muscle cells of arterioles undergo degenerative changes of swelling, fibrinoid infiltration with invasion of the adventitia by mononuclear leucocytes, lymphocytes, and plasma cells. The vasculitis may be widespread involving localized areas of arterioles, veins, and capillaries with normal architecture preserved throughout most of the vascular system. In murine and epidemic typhus, the endothelial and adventitial changes are similar to RMSF although thromboses are rare and degenerative changes in the musculature unusual. There are parenchymatous abnormalities throughout the body adjacent to the vascular lesions, most conspicuous in the brain, cardiac and skeletal musculature, lung, and kidneys. Cerebral glial nodules which represent a cellular response in an area adjacent to a capillary or arteriole occur in patients with murine, or epidemic typhus, RMSF, and scrub typhus (see Fig. 1).

Small micro-infarcts, which represent areas of anaemic necroses caused by intimal reaction and thrombotic occlusion, develop in most tissues including the myocardium.

Rickettsial pneumonitis may occur in patients with RMSF and typhus and is a characteristic pathologic change in many patients with Q fever. The reaction is primarily interstitial resembling the type found in pneumonia caused by mycoplasma, influenza virus, or legionella. There are patchy areas of congestion and oedema with greyish consolidation; the alveoli in these consolidated areas are filled with fibrinocellular exudate containing lymphocytes, plasma cells, large mononuclear cells, and erythrocytes, but few polymorphonuclear leucocytes. In Q fever, the alveolar epithelium is hyperplastic and the interalveolar septa and the peribronchial and perivascular tissues are thickened by accumulation of leucocytes such as are found within the alveolar lamina. Utilization of specific fixation and staining techniques, including immunofluorescence, reveals rickettsia (or legionella, with which they may be confused) in endothelial cells of various tissues, including lung, skin, and muscle obtained by biopsy or at post mortem.

Nature of the vasculitis. An abnormal antigen–antibody reaction (immune complex) may explain certain aspects of the vasculitis late in illness since extensive haemorrhagic skin necroses tend to occur when humoral antibody titres are present; in RMSF, the administration of hyperimmune convalescent serum was observed to cause capillary leakage and tissue oedema. However, in early stages of RMSF no abnormalities of complement levels have been noted which would tend to refute this concept. Cell-mediated immunity may be an important mechanism useful for inhibition and eradication of rickettsiae in tissues; patients convalescent from various

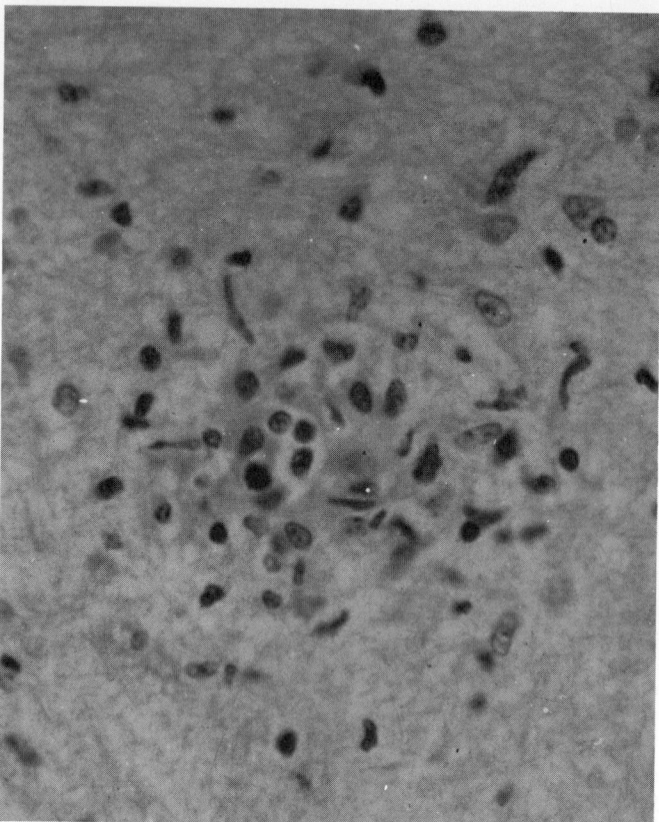

Fig. 1 Epidemic typhus fever. Typhus nodule in brain of patient (death about twelfth day) showing proliferative cellular reaction surrounding a small cerebral vessel. (From *Med. Clins N. Am.* **43**, 1512 (1959) by permission.)

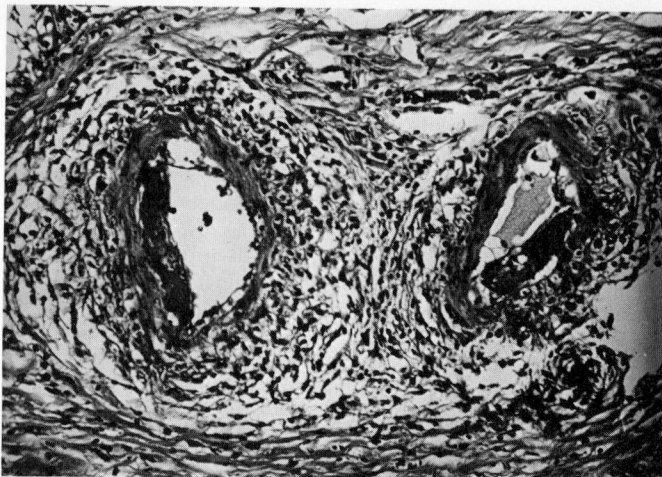

Fig. 2 RMSF. Classic lesion of endoangiitis in patient, showing diffuse changes of endothelial swelling, perivascular proliferation of mononuclear cells, fibrinoid changes of vessel wall, and thrombus formation.

rickettsioses exhibit delayed hypersensitivity reactions to injected rickettsial antigens. Such reactions of hypersensitivity could also contribute to the vasculitis.

Various investigations have shown a specific toxic action in the capillaries of animals resulting in vasoconstriction, plasma leakage, haemoconcentration, and the unusual finding of an unaltered reactivity to epinephrine. Wolbach, in his classic treatise on RMSF, described the histologic lesions and attributed the vasculitis to the presence of the parasite: 'an acute specific endoangiitis chiefly of the peripheral blood vessels'. He attributed the character and evolution of the rash, the skin necroses, and gangrene to the angiitis. Sixty years later, there is little to add to Wolbach's explanation except that a toxin is known to promote capillary leakage and that vascular abnormalities may result from either immune complex or cellular immune (hypersensitivity) reactions or both. A typical lesion of vasculitis is shown in Fig. 2.

General laboratory results. In all rickettsioses, including RMSF and typhus, routine laboratory tests are not diagnostic and merely reflect the severity of organ involvement. Normocytic anaemia occurs in patients severely ill with rickettsial diseases; the blood leucocyte count is usually within the normal range, i.e., 6000 to 10 000/mm. Leucopenia is occasionally observed and, in the presence of complications such as superimposed infections and extensive vascular lesions, moderate leucocytosis occurs. The differential count is usually normal. In severely ill patients in whom there are extensive areas of haemorrhagic necroses and renal involvement, there may be azotaemia, hyponatraemia, hypochloraemia, and hypoalbuminaemia. Appropriate laboratory tests may be used to demonstrate these abnormalities. As a sequel to the vasculitis and capillary leakage, plasma, water, sodium, chloride, and albumin diffuse from the vascular system into the extravascular space. The development of disseminated intravascular

coagulopathy with significant depression of platelets, fibrinogen, and prolongation of prothrombin and partial thromboplastin coagulation times is very troublesome.

Specific laboratory diagnosis. Rickettsia may be isolated from the patient's blood during the early stages of illness or from postmortem tissues by inoculation of animals and subsequent growth in fertile hens' eggs or tissue culture systems. The techniques are time consuming, expensive, and often hazardous to laboratory personnel. In ordinary practice, the currently available serological tests are adequate for the laboratory confirmation of the clinical diagnosis in each of the rickettsioses.

Serological tests, to be useful, require two and preferably three serum samples during the first, second, and fourth to sixth weeks of illness in order to demonstrate a rise in titre of specific antibody during convalescence.

Weil–Felix test (WF). The Weil–Felix test using *Proteus* strains of OX19 gives positive results in patients with RMSF, murine, epidemic typhus and negative or non-specific results in those with rickettsialpox, Q fever and scrub typhus. In Brill–Zinsser disease (recrudescent typhus), *Proteus* OX 19 titres are usually negative or low. *Proteus* OXK agglutinins are present in over 50 per cent of patients with scrub typhus. The *Proteus* reaction does not distinguish between the spotted fever and the typhus groups but is a dependable screening test for the presence of certain rickettsioses. A single convalescent serum titre of 160 to 320 is usually diagnostic, but the demonstration of a rise in titre is of greater value. *Proteus* OX 19 agglutinins fail to appear in approximately 10 per cent of patients with spotted fever or typhus, and, when antibiotics are given early during the first week of illness, the titre may be delayed but usually reaches diagnostic levels.

There may be false positive reactions in such conditions as urinary tract infections or bacteraemia caused by *Proteus* organisms, enteric, relapsing, and rat-bite fevers, leptospirosis, brucellosis, and tularaemia.

Complement fixation reaction. These tests which use group-specific soluble rickettsial antigens provide data which clearly differentiate the rickettsial disease groups (the typhus fevers, spotted fevers, and Q fever). With type-specific, washed rickettsial antigens, it is possible to distinguish between the various member diseases of the spotted fever group (RMSF, rickettsialpox, *fièvre boutonneuse*, North Asian tick-borne rickettsiosis, and Queensland tick typhus). Both types of antigens are prepared from yolk sacs heavily infected with *R. rickettsii*. CF antibodies appear during the second or third week in patients who receive no specific therapy but may be delayed in those whose illness is shortened by vigorous antibiotic treatment initiated within several days after onset of fever. Under these circumstances, a blood specimen should be taken four to six weeks after convalescence.

Antibodies after response to a primary infection of RMSF and typhus are usually 19S globulins. In Brill–Zinsser disease, antibodies appear rapidly several days after onset of illness and are primarily of the 7S type. Q fever antigens are specifically diagnostic. In acute Q fever infections, antibodies to phase II antigens appear; phase I antibodies indicate chronic infection, such as hepatitis or endocarditis.

Other serological tests. Specific diagnoses of RMSF, other tick-borne rickettsioses, and the typhus fevers may be achieved by the rickettsial micro-agglutination (MA), the indirect fluorescent antibody (IFA) and haemoagglutination (HA) reactions. These are

Table 2 Serological reactions in the rickettsioses

| Type | Proteus | | CF* | MA† | IFA‡ |
	OX19	OXK			
RMSF	+	0	+	+	+
Rickettsialpox	–	0	+	+	+
Tick-borne (eastern hemisphere)	+	0	+	+	+
Epidemic typhus	+	0	+	+	+
Recurrent typhus (Brill–Zinsser disease)	low or neg.	0	+(7S)	+	+
Murine typhus	+	0	+	+	+
Scrub typhus	0	+	+	+	+
Q fever	0	0	+ (strain specific)	+	+

* CF = complement fixation
† MA = microscopic agglutination
‡ IFA = immunofluorescent antibody

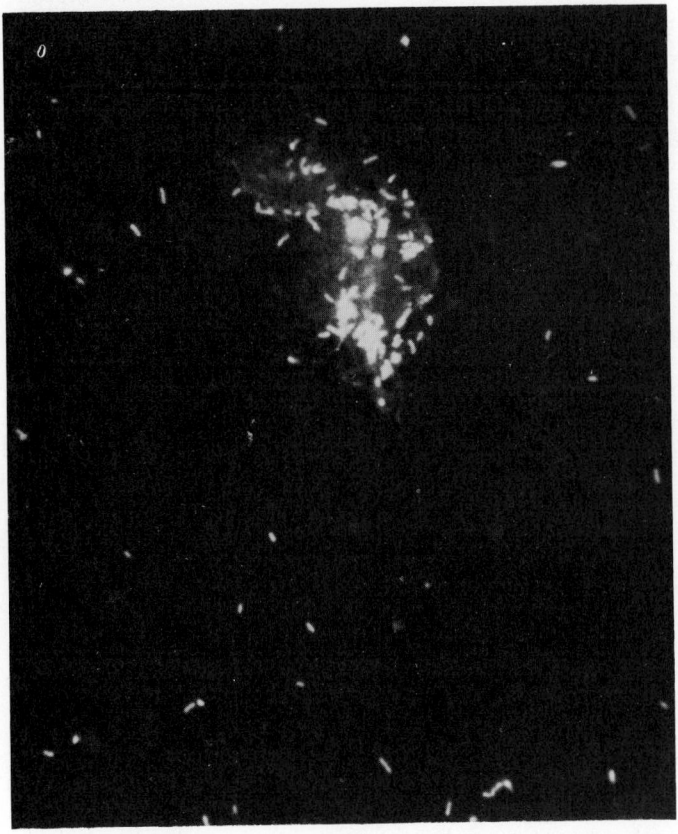

Fig. 3 RMSF. IF technique showing *R. rickettsii* in skin lesion obtained by biopsy on about seventh day of illness. Note presence of small coccal and bacillary-like forms in cytoplasm and nucleus of cell.

developing as standard procedures and are more reliable than the WF or CF tests.

Early diagnosis (identification of rickettsiae in tissues). IF techniques will show identifiable *R. rickettsii* and *R. prowazekii* in tissues of chick embryos, guinea pigs, and vector ticks. Rickettsiae have been seen in pink macular skin lesions of patients with RMSF obtained by biopsy as early as the third day or from ecchymotic lesions as late as the ninth day. They have an identifiable morphology and staining properties. Rickettsiae may be stained by IF technique of formalized tissue (Fig. 3). Heart valves of patients with endocarditis caused by *C. burnetii* show the organism.

Major coverage will be devoted to RMSF; similarities and distinguishing features will be described in appropriate sections for all of the rickettsioses.

References

Fuller, H. S. (1959). Biologic properties of pathogenic rickettsiae. *Archs Inst. Pasteur (Tunis)* **36**, 311.
Greisman, S. E. and Wisseman, C. L., Jr. (1958). Studies of rickettsial toxins. Cardiovascular functional abnormalities induced by Rickettsia mooseri in white rats. *J. Immunol.* **81**, 345.
McDade, J. E., Shepard, C. C., Redus, M. A., Newhouse, V. F., and Smith, J. D. (1980). Evidence of *Rickettsia prowazeki* infections in the United States. *Am. J. trop. Med. Hyg.* **29** (2), 277.
Parker, R. T., Menon, P. G., Merideth, A. M., Snyder, M. J., and Woodward, T. E. (1954). Persistence of *Rickettsia rickettsii* in a patient recovered from Rocky Mountain spotted fever. *J. Immunol.* **73**, 383.
Smadel, J. E. (1959). Status of the rickettsioses in the United States. *Ann. intern. Med.* **51**, 421.
Sonenshine, D. E., Bozeman, F. M., Williams, M. S., Masiello, S. A., Chadwick, D. P., Stocks, N. I., Lauer, D. M., and Elisberg, B. L. (1978). Epizootiology of epidemic typhus (*Rickettsia prowazekii*) in flying squirrels. *Am. J. trop. Med. Hyg.* **27**, 339.
Walker, D. H. and Cain, B. G. (1978). A method for specific diagnosis of Rocky Mountain spotted fever on fixed, paraffin-embedded tissue by immunofluorescence. *J. infect. Dis.* **137**, 206.
Wisseman, C. L., Jr., Batawi, Y., Wood, W. H., and Noriega, A. A. (1967). Gross and microscopic skin reactions to killed typhus rickettsia in human beings. *J. Immunol.* **98**, 194.
Wolbach, S. B. (1919). Studies on Rocky Mountain spotted fever. *J. med. Res.* **41**, 1.
Woodward, T. E. (1959). Rickettsial diseases in the United States. *Med. clin. N. Am.* **43**, 1507.
—, Pedersen, C. E., Jr., Oster, C. M., Bagley, L. R., Romberger, J., and Snyder, M. J. (1976). Prompt confirmation of Rocky Mountain spotted fever. Identification of rickettsiae in skin tissues. *J. infect. Dis.* **134**, 293.

Rocky Mountain spotted fever (RMSF)

RMSF, known also by the following names: spotted fever, *fiebre maculosa.* São Paulo typhus (Brazil), *fiebre manchada* (Mexico), *fiebre petequial* (Colombia), or tick typhus (England), is an acute febrile illness caused by *Rickettsia rickettsii*, transmitted to man by ticks. It is characterized by sudden onset with headache, chills, and fever which persists for two to three weeks. The rash, which is generally present, appears first on the extremities and trunk about the fourth day of illness. Like other anatomical manifestations, it stems from scattered focal areas of endoangiitis throughout the body. Delirium, shock, and renal failure mark the severely ill. *Proteus* OX19 agglutinins and specific antibodies of the CF, MA, and IFA-type appear in the patient's serum during the second to third week of illness. Chloramphenicol and the tetracyclines are highly specific in therapy.

Historical sketch. To Ricketts belongs credit for clearly incriminating the tick as the vector and demonstration of rickettsemia by transfer of infection to animals with the patient's blood. Soon to follow was evidence of transovarial transmission or rickettsia to the offspring of infected female ticks and a vaccine made from inactivated infected tick tissues. Wolbach defined the endoangiitis in his monograph in 1917. With the advent of better cultural methods and chemical methods to purify antigens, specific serological tests made it possible to distinguish between the various rickettsioses and within the spotted fever and typhus groups. With the advent of specific broad spectrum antibiotic therapy in 1948, first chloramphenicol and then the tetracyclines, mortality from these illnesses was drastically reduced.

Aetiology and epidemiology. *R. rickettsii*, the cause, is the prototype for the rickettsial group. They are minute micro-organisms, resembling bacteria about 1 µm in length and 0.2–0.3 µm wide which stain purple with Giemsa, pink with Macchiavello, and red with Geminez stains. They grow in pairs and possess a cell wall which is the locus of antigens and an endotoxin-like substance. *R. rickettsii* in a tissue culture cell are shown in Fig. 4.

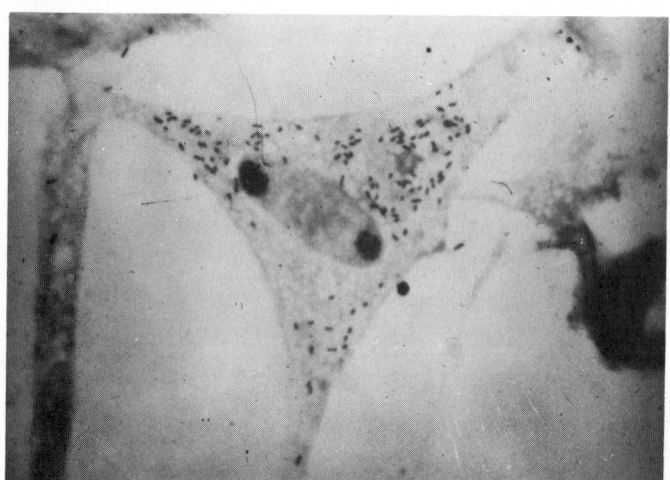

Fig. 4   RMSF. Shown are the coccal and bacillary forms of *R. rickettsii* in tissue culture cell. Note localization of rickettsia in nucleus and cytoplasm. (Courtesy Dr C. L. Wisseman, Jr.)

Rickettsiae grow in the nucleus and cytoplasm of infected cells of ticks, mammals, embryonated eggs, and cell cultures. The intranuclear habitat is shared by other members of the spotted fever group but not by rickettsia of the typhus group. Cross-immunity tests in guinea pigs and specific serological tests such as CF, IFA, and MA, using antigens prepared from infected yolk sac tissues or cell culture readily distinguishes agents causing typhus fever as well as between members of the spotted fever group.

Distribution and incidence. The first reports of RMSF were in Idaho and Montana late in the nineteenth century. Practically all states in the United States report cases as well as Canada, Mexico, Panama, Costa Rica, Colombia, and Brazil. Related members of the spotted fever group occur in other continents; RMSF is particularly limited to the western Hemisphere. From 1977 to 1980, there were about 1000 cases in the United States with more than one-half occurring in the south Atlantic and south central States with the greatest number in North Carolina, Virginia, Georgia, Maryland, Tennessee, and Oklahoma. Most cases occur during the period of maximal tick activity, i.e., late spring and early summer, and 60 per cent occur in persons under the age of 20. Mortality rates increase with age. In about one-quarter of cases, there is no history of a tick bite.

Vector. Two species of ticks, the wood tick, *Dermacentor andersoni*, and the dog tick, *Dermacentor variabilis*, are the principal vectors in the western and eastern United States respectively. The tick serves as a natural vector and also as a reservoir since it survives the infection and transmits the agent readily to its offspring; ticks remain infected for life. Small wild animals may spread rickettsia in nature by infecting other ticks which feed on them. Most natural hosts show only inapparent infection and no diagnostic gross le-

sions. Other ticks of importance are *Amblyomma americanum* in Texas and Oklahoma, the brown dog tick, *Rhipicephalus sanguineus*, In Mexico and the United States (this is the tick which serves as vector and reservoir of *fièvre boutonneuse* and others), and *Amblyomma cajennense* in Brazil and Colombia.

Man usually acquires infection from the bite of an infected tick which must remain attached for several hours early in the season; later, in the warm months, the time of feeding and transmission is shorter. Spencer and Parker described this phenomenon of 'reactivation' as a change from a non-virulent resting phase to a virulent phase brought about by ingestion of fresh blood which changed the microbes' metabolism after a winter's hibernation in the cold earth. Infection may be acquired through abrasions in the skin which become contaminated by infected tick faeces or tissue juices. Hence, ticks should not be crushed between the fingers on removal. The agent has been transmitted accidentally to humans by infusion of blood taken from a donor just before onset of illness.

Incubation and prodromata

Clinical manifestations. Either a history of a tick bite or exposure in a wooded area is elicited in most cases and illness ensues after an incubation of about seven days, range 3–12. A more serious infection usually follows short incubation periods. General malaise and headache with feverish and chilly reactions may precede the actual onset.

Onset and symptoms. In susceptible persons, sudden onset of severe headache, shaking chills, prostration, and myalgic pain involving the back and leg muscles occur. Nausea with vomiting and fever of 39.4–40 °C are common within the first few days. Pain in the abdominal and leg muscles is noted on forceful palpation; arthralgia occurs. Occasionally, the onset in children and adults is mild and vague associated with irritability, lethargy, insomnia, anorexia, headache, and low-grade fever similar to other infectious diseases.

Pyrexia. In severely ill patients, fever may last for 15–20 days at a high sustained level with lower morning remissions, not reaching normal. Fever of 40.7 °C or more signifies a more severely ill patient, although death can occur with normal temperatures associated with vascular collapse. The fever generally abates by slow lysis over several days; crises are uncommon. Recurrence of fever is uncommon except when secondary pyogenic complications occur or when specific antibiotic treatment is initiated very early (in the first few days). The recurrent rickettsial infection responds to treatment and rickettsiae do not become resistant to the specific antibiotics.

The headache is usually severe, intense, and localized over the forehead. It may persist during the first and most of the second week. Malaise, irritability, and indifference to questioning and examination characterize the first week (Fig. 5).

Rash (Plate 5(a)–(c)). Most patients develop a characteristic exanthem by the fourth febrile day (range, two to six days) which should alert the physician. Initially, the lesions are 2–6 mm in diameter, flat, delicate, pink, on the palms, soles, wrists, forearms, and legs, and fade on light pressure. A warm compress to an extremity will make them more visible and they are observed better when the temperature is high. In a day or less, the rash spreads to the buttocks, axilla, trunk, neck, and face and may become faintly maculopapular. In a few days, they are deeper red, petechial, fail to fade on pressure, and in untreated patients, they coalesce to form haemorrhagic legions and large ecchymotic blemishes simulating acute meningococcaemia (Fig. 6).

With recovery, these latter lesions slough, form indolent, slow healing ulcerations and scars. The smaller haemorrhagic lesions form brown pigmented discolourations which disappear. In mild cases, the rash does not become haemorrhagic or purpuric, and the macules may disappear in a few days, particularly after antibiotic treatment. In a few patients, particularly in those with dark skin, a rash may not be noted.

Application of a tourniquet for several minutes (Rumpel–Leede reaction) will provoke additional petechiae which is evidence of

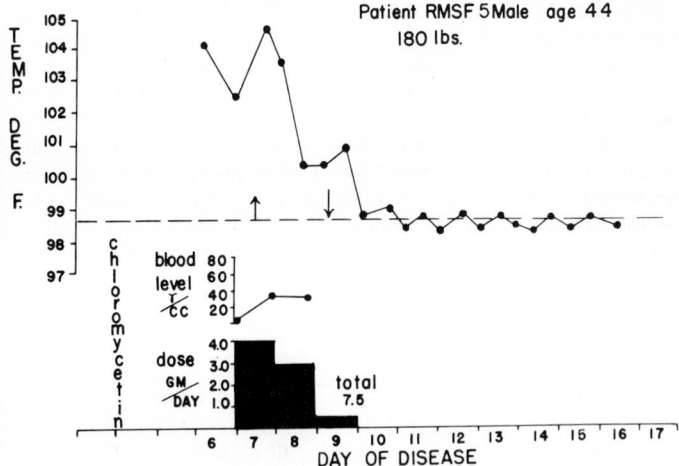

Patient RMSF 5 Male age 44
180 lbs.

Rickettsiemia	+		
complement fixation			1/32
Proteus ox 19	C 1:80 P 1:160	1/1280	
W.B.C. thousands	7.05		

Fig. 5 RMSF. Course of illness in a moderately ill patient first treated on seventh day of illness. Note defervescence in three days and confirmation by demonstration of rickettsemia and positive WF and CF reaction. (From *Med. Clins N. Am.* **43**, 1528 (1959) by permission.)

enhanced capillary fragility secondary to angiitis and, if present, thrombocytopenia.

Cardiovascular and respiratory manifestations. Early in illness, the pulse is full and regular, and accelerates with elevation of temperature; the blood pressure is sustained. In seriously ill children and adults, the pulse becomes rapid, weak, and hypotension develops at the peak of illness (7–10 days). Long sustained circulatory failure with associated anorexia and cyanosis leads to agitation and confusion, and contributes to formation of ecchymoses and gangrene of fingers, buttocks, scrotum, ear lobes, and nose. Measurements of venous pressure at this stage do not show elevations indicative of congestive heart failure *per se*, nor is the venous pressure unduly elevated following the judicious administration of intravenous fluids. At this stage, there is a mild reduction of circulating blood volume and evidence of non-specific myocardial changes, i.e., low voltage of ventricular complexes, minor ST segment deflections and delayed AV conduction time. These changes are usually transient and simulate those encountered in pneumonia, typhoid fever, uraemia, etc. In these severely ill patients, there may be a puffy appearance to the face, and oedema of the feet, hands, arms, and legs indicative of an expanded extravascular space (see Fig. 6). Occasionally, a severe and fatal myocarditis occurs with various arrhythmias and cardiac arrest.

The respiratory rate is normal in the early stages, and later accelerates with an harassing, non-productive cough in some patients indicative of bronchitis or broncholitis. Pulmonary consolidation is unusual as is pulmonary oedema except when intravenous fluids are given injudiciously.

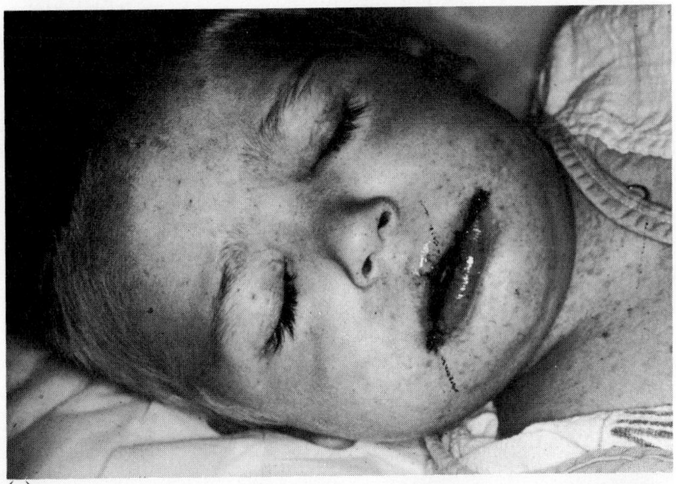

(a)

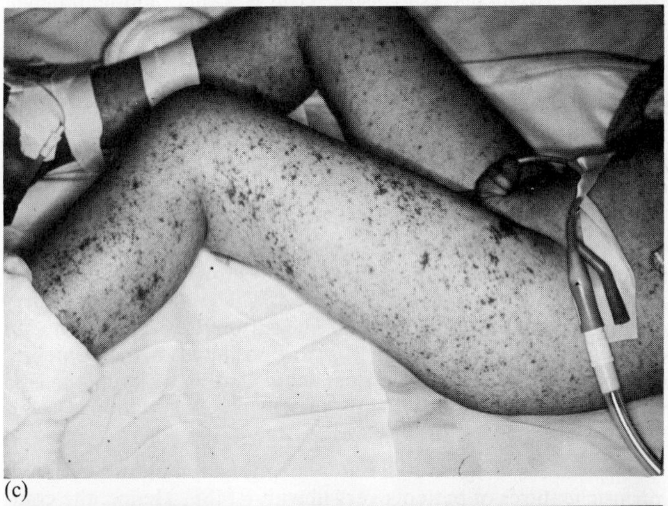

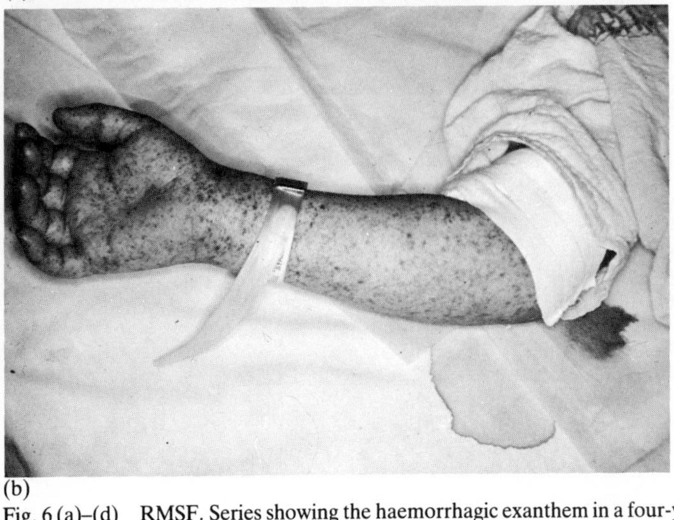

(b)

(c)

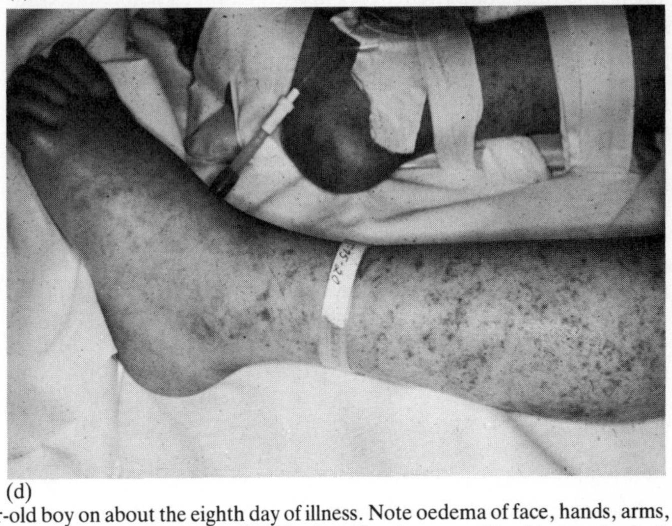

(d)

Fig. 6 (a)–(d)   RMSF. Series showing the haemorrhagic exanthem in a four-year-old boy on about the eighth day of illness. Note oedema of face, hands, arms, and feet, and bleeding from mouth. There was evidence of disseminated intravascular coagulation (DIC). Specific therapy with chloramphenicol, glucocorticoids for several days, and *no* heparin. Recovery complete.

Table 3 Haematological data for patient shown in Fig. 6 suffering from RMSF

Day of disease	Platelets	Prothrombin time (%)	PTT	Fibrinogen (mg %)
8	16 300	<5	120	80
Cloramphenicol, no heparin				
10	11 500	<5	190	15
12	10 000	14	60	12
Afebrile				
15	33 000	45	42	90
17	78 000	100	36	20
19	162 000			

Hepatic and renal manifestations. Usually there is little clinical evidence of dysfunction of the liver or kidney in the mild or moderately severely ill patient. Hepatomegaly occurs; jaundice is uncommon. When present, there is elevation of the alkaline phosphatase and liver enzymes. Oliguria and anuria associated with hypotension and extensive cutaneous haemorrhagic necrosis in very ill patients is associated with azotaemia, often very high. In these patients, who often have tissue oedema, there is hypoalbuminaemia. Splenomegaly occurs in about one-half of patients; the spleen is firm and non-tender.

Neurologic manifestations. Headache, restlessness, irritability, and varying degrees of insomnia typify most severely ill patients as does myalgia, muscle rigidity, and stiffness of the back and neck. Athetoid movements, convulsive seizures, coma, and hemiplegia are grave signs indicative of rickettsial encephalitis. The cerebral spinal fluid is usually clear, with normal dynamics, a mild pleocytosis, and normal chemical levels. During the acute stages and for several months, deafness is noted and, as a rule, all neurologic abnormalities abate without serious residuals. Peripheral neuropathy is a rare result. The electroencephalogram may show signs of diffuse involvement which may not abate for a year or more.

Other physical manifestations. Dryness of the lips, gums, and tongue with hot dry skin are indicative of dehydration before the stage of skin ecchymoses and vascular collapse. The conjunctivae are frequently injected and the eyes pink and suffused. Patients complain of photophobia, and petechiae are often noted in the palpebral conjunctivae and retinae. Abdominal distention without localized tenderness is associated with intestinal ileus. Constipation is usual.

Complications; prognosis. The aforementioned manifestations are intrinsic features of patients very ill with RMSF. Hence, the complications are those associated with secondary bacterial infections, such as otitis media, parotitis, bronchopneumonia, and indolent skin ulcers. Gangrene of a digit or a portion of an extremity results from thromboses of blood vessels and attendant vascular decompensation. All of the abnormal elements of disseminated intravascular coagulation (DIC) contribute to anoxia and gangrene in the limbs and organs. There is no evidence that heparin therapy is useful (Table 3).

Prior to the advent of specific antibiotic treatment, the overall mortality was 20 per cent; when corrected for age, more than half of those adults over age 50 died. Few deaths occur with chloramphenicol or tetracycline used in conjunction with the application of careful support of the circulation and renal output, based on precise measurement of the physiologic abnormalities. Fatalities occur when there is too much delay and subsequent organ failure, and occasionally a severe arrhythmia associated with myocarditis results in sudden death.

Therapy for the rickettsial diseases. The measures advisable for all rickettsioses are here described; variations will be described in specific subsections.

Patients seriously ill with the typhus-spotted fever group of rickettsial diseases manifest physiochemical changes which merit understanding in planning a therapeutic regimen. Often there is circulatory collapse, oliguria, anuria, azotaemia, anaemia, hyponatraemia, hypochloraemia, hypoalbuminaemia, oedema, and coma. In mildly and moderately ill patients, these alterations are absent, making management less complicated. Those principles necessary for treatment of all rickettsioses are (*a*) specific chemotherapy and (*b*) supportive care. Attention to each is mandatory for the late, seriously ill patient. During the first week in patients who are moderately ill, specific therapy combined with general supportive care suffices.

Specific treatment. Chloramphenicol and the tetracyclines are specifically effective; they are rickettsiostatic and not rickettsicidal. Prompt alleviation of clinical signs occurs when therapy is initiated during the early stages coincident with appearance of the rash. Response is less dramatic when therapy is delayed until the rash becomes haemorrhagic and diffuse.

Optimal antibiotic regimens are: chloramphenicol, an initial oral dose of 50 mg/kg body weight or tetracycline, 25 mg/kg body weight. Subsequent daily doses are calculated as the initial oral dose, divided equally and given at six to eight hour intervals. Antibiotic treatment is given until improvement and the patient has been afebrile for about 24 hours. Intravenous preparations are employed for the loading and subsequent doses in patients too ill to take oral medication. All patients with rickettsioses respond promptly to antibiotic treatment when it is initiated early in illness before serious tissue changes have occurred. Obvious clinical improvement is noted in 36–48 hours with defervescence in two to three days. In scrub typhus, the response is even more dramatic. In those patients first treated during the latter stages, clinical improvement is slower and fever extends over longer periods. Large, single oral doses of chloramphenicol (50 mg/kg) have been effective in patients with RMSF and scrub typhus, although this regimen is not recommended. A single oral dose of 200 mg doxycycline (a lipotropic tetracycline derivative which produces sustained high blood and tissue levels) has been shown to be practically effective for treatment of louse-borne typhus fever under field conditions.

Steroid treatment. In critically ill patients first observed late in the course of severe illness, large doses of adrenal cortical steroids given for about three days, in combination with specific antibiotics, are recommended. The temperature abates more rapidly than usual, as do the toxic manifestations. For mild or moderately ill patients, glucocorticoids are not recommended.

Supportive treatment. Proper mouth care with swabbing of the oral cavity and use of mouth washes may help prevent gingivitis and

Table 4 Effect of specific antibiotics on the course of rickettsial diseases

Disease	Mean duration of fever (days)	Average mortality (%)	Mean duration of fever after RX (days)	Mortality (%)
RMSF	16 (8–20)	20*	3	6‡
Rickettsialpox	7 (3–12)	0	2	0†
Other tick-borne rickettsioses	16 (7–16)	2	3	0†
Epidemic typhus	14 (8–20)	20	2	2
Brill–Zinsser disease	9 (7–12)	0†	2	0†
Murine typhus	12 (8–18)	2	2	0‡
Q fever	10 (3–20)	1†	3	1§

* Fatality varies with age, virulence of causative rickettsia, etc.
† Fatal cases unusual
‡ Occasional fatality with delays of treatment
§ Rare fatality with chronic types such as endocarditis

parotitis. Frequent turning of the patient will help avert pressure sores over bony prominences and prevent aspiration pneumonia. In order to avoid negative nitrogen balance, a generous intake of protein supplements with frequent feedings is useful. Protein intake of 3–5 g protein per kg normal body weight with adequate carbohydrate and fat sufficient to make the diet palatable, is usually well-tolerated. In unco-operative patients, when there is *no* abdominal distention, hourly liquid protein feedings by gastric tube are helpful, but such measures are usually obviated by proper intravenous alimentation. Care must be taken to avoid a fluid overload.

In critically ill patients with enhanced capillary permeability, oedema, and vascular decompensation, attention is given to parenteral alimentation with glucose and amino acid supplements. Small whole blood transfusions are indicated when anaemia is present. The judicious use of serum albumin may favourably improve the circulation. With oliguria, anuria and azotaemia, the circulation should not be overloaded; results of laboratory tests and clinical judgement guide therapy. Dialysis is indicated if there is clear-cut evidence of acute tubular necrosis.

References

Aikawa, J. K. (1966). *Rocky Mountain spotted fever*. C. C. Thomas, Springfield, Illinois.
Burgdorfer, W. and Brinton, L. P. (1975). Mechanisms of transovarial infection of spotted fever in ticks. *Ann. N.Y. Acad. Sci.* **266**, 261.
—, Sexton, D. J., Gerloff, R. K., Anacker, R. L., Philip, R. N., and Thomas, L. A. (1975). *Rhipicephalus sanguineus*: Vector of a new spotted fever group of rickettsia in the US. *Infect. Immun.* **12**, 205.
Harrell, G. T. (1949). Rocky Mountain spotted fever. *Medicine* **28**, 333.
Hattwick, M. A. W., O'Brian, R. J., and Hanson, B. F. (1976). Rocky Mountain spotted fever: epidemiology of an increasing problem. *Ann. intern. Med.* **84**, 732.
Wells, G. M., Woodward, T. E., Fiset, P., and Hornick, R. B. (1978). Rocky Mountain spotted fever caused by blood transfusion. *J. Am. med. Ass.* **239**, 2763.
Woodward, T. E., and Jackson, E. B. (1965). Spotted fever rickettsiae *In Viral and rickettsial infections of man*, 4th edn. (ed. Horsfall and Tamm), 1095. Lippincott, Philadelphia.

Differential diagnosis of rickettsial diseases

The physician should have a high index of suspicion of Rocky Mountain spotted fever in any patient with fever, prostration, headache, and a history of tick bite while engaged in work or recreation in a rural or wooded area of endemicity. During the early stages of infection before the rash has appeared, differentiation from other acute infections is difficult. Meningococcaemia and measles are the most common mistaken diagnoses.

The rash of meningococcaemia resembles Rocky Mountain spotted fever, and louse-borne typhus fever in certain aspects, since it is macular, maculopapular, or petechial in the acute or subacute forms, and petechial (confluent or ecchymotic) in fulminant type. The meningococcaemia skin lesion is tender to palpation, haemorrhagic, and often necrotic. It develops with extreme rapidity in the fulminant form, whereas the rickettsial rash occurs on about the fourth day of disease and gradually becomes petechial. High blood leucocyte counts are common in meningococcal infections.

Measles, which occurs often during the autumn and winter, is associated with coryza, cough, conjunctival injection, and photophobia with a characteristic cephalocaudal progression of the rash. It appears in about three days after onset, first on the face and neck as pink macules which soon become maculopapular, and spreads within a day or two to the trunk and extremities. Petechiae or ecchymoses may occur; Koplik spots are characteristic. In rubella (German measles), the rash is frequently a flush, like scarlet fever, which soon spreads from the face and neck to the trunk and extremities. It is less extensive and more evanescent than measles with mild constitutional manifestations. Post-auricular adenopathy and absence of Koplik spots suggest rubella.

The exanthem of varicella or variola is first erythematous and later becomes vesicular. The rose spots of typhoid fever are usually on the lower chest or upper abdomen and remain delicate, without haemorrhagic character. Rocky Mountain spotted fever skin lesions, in contrast to typhoid, begin on the periphery of the body and later become petechial. The rash of infectious mononucleosis (uncommon except when associated with drugs) is usually morbilliform on the trunk and rarely becomes petechial. Angina, lymphadenopathy, and atypical lymphocytes in the blood are differentiating features.

Murine typhus is a milder disease than Rocky Mountain spotted fever and epidemic typhus; the rash is less extensive, non-purpuric and non-confluent; renal and vascular complications are uncommon. Not infrequently, differentiation of these three rickettsial infections must await the results of specific serologic tests. Epidemic typhus fever is capable of causing all of the pronounced clinical, physiologic, and anatomic alterations noted in cases with Rocky Mountain spotted fever (hypotension, peripheral vascular failure, cyanosis, skin necrosis, and gangrene of digits, renal failure with azotaemia, and neurologic manifestations). However, the rash of classic typhus occurs initially in the axillary folds and on the trunk and later extends peripherally, rarely involving the palms, the soles, or the face.

The serologic patterns in these three diseases are distinctive when specific rickettsial antigens are employed in tests, such as the IFA and MA reactions. Moreover, louse-borne typhus is not recognized in the United States except in the form of Brill–Zinsser disease (recurrent typhus fever). Epidemic typhus associated with contact with flying squirrels is a new finding. It is usually milder than classical typhus. An illness simulating RMSF is caused by *Rickettsia canada*, a member of the typhus group. Rickettsialpox, although caused by a member of the spotted fever group of organisms, usually is readily differentiated from Rocky Mountain spotted fever by the initial lesion, the relative mildness of the illness, and the early vesiculation of the maculopapular rash. The Weil–Felix reaction is positive in Rocky Mountain spotted fever and in murine and epidemic typhus but is negative in rickettsialpox.

Control of rickettsial diseases

Vector control. Great strides were made during the Second World War in the conquest of rickettsial diseases with the highly successful attack on the insect vectors, i.e., lice, mites, fleas, and ticks. All were made possible through development of chemical compounds which either destroyed or repelled arthropods. The application of DDT to clothing successfully controlled louse infestation and culminated in the total arrest of epidemics of typhus fever, such as in Naples, Italy, and in concentration camps for the first time in medical history. Application of insecticides to the person and clothes helped control scrub typhus fever which was a major military problem in the Pacific area. Prevention of murine typhus was attained by reducing the natural reservoir and vector through application of measures for eliminating rodents and employing DDT or other insecticides in rat-infested areas to control fleas.

Adherence to the general measures of avoiding or reducing the chance of contact in tick-infested areas of known endemicity is the principal preventive measure for spotted fever. When this is impractical, area control of spotted fever ticks may include the following prophylactic measures: spraying the ground with dieldrin or chlordane for tick control. Although there are environmental objections to the use of residual insecticides, under special conditions, such procedures may be warranted.

Useful measures include application of repellents, such as diethyltoluamide or dimethylphthalate to clothing and exposed parts of the body, or in very heavily infested areas, the wearing of clothing which interferes with the attachment of ticks, i.e., boots and a one-piece outer garment preferably impregnated with repellent.

There should be daily inspection of the entire body, particularly in children, including the hairy parts, to detect and remove attached ticks. Care should be taken in removing attached ticks to avoid crushing the arthropod with resultant contamination of the bite wound. Touching the tick with petrol or whisky encourages detachment, but gentle traction with small forceps applied close to the mouth parts allows ready extraction. The skin area should be disinfected with soap and water or other antiseptics such as alcohol. These precautions should be employed in removing engorged ticks from dogs and other animals because infection through minor abrasions in the hands is possible.

Immunization. An inactivated vaccine consisting of whole *R. prowazekii* effectively prevented or reduced the severity of typhus fever in Allied forces during the Second World War. This type of vaccine is commercially available for prevention of typhus but not for RMSF. Improved vaccines are now under development for RMSF which have been prepared using tissue culture techniques. A new vaccine, consisting of rich suspensions of purified whole rickettsiae, should soon be available for use in those exposed to great risk, such as persons frequenting highly endemic areas and laboratory workers exposed to the agent. A vaccine containing a viable strain of *R. prowazekii* which gives protection to man against epidemic typhus is not available for general use but has been effectively field tested.

Q fever is preventable by using inactivated vaccines made from phase I rickettsiae which are potent and afford considerable protection to slaughterhouse and dairy workers, herders, rendering plant workers, wool sorters, tanners, laboratory workers, and others at risk. Measures should be taken to avoid exposure to infected aerosols; milk from infected domestic livestock must be pasteurized or boiled.

The question is often raised whether antibiotics should be given prophylactically after human exposure to virulent rickettsiae, such as *R. rickettsii*. In guinea pigs, a single dose of oxytetracycline prevents the disease when the antibiotic is given shortly before expected onset of illness. Furthermore, relapses occur when treatment precedes expected onset by 48 hours or more. This regimen is not recommended for prevention of RMSF or other rickettsial diseases, such as epidemic typhus. After a tick or louse bite in a known endemic area, an exposed person should be observed for signs of fever, headache, prostration, and rash; therapy is very effective at the early stages of illness.

There is no vaccine available for the prevention of scrub typhus. Chemoprophylactic regimens may be used when there is known exposure and probable infection. Chemoprophylactic studies conducted in volunteers exposed in mite-infested areas showed that single 1.0 oral doses of chloramphenicol given every five days for a total of 35 days (seven doses with five-day intervals) prevented scrub typhus and resulted in active immunity. This procedure is recommended only under special circumstances. A long acting tetracycline (doxycycline) has been shown to serve the same purpose.

References

Ascher, M. S., Oster, C. N., Harber, P. I., Kenyon, R. H., and Pedersen, C., Jr. (1978). Initial clinical evaluation of a new Rocky Mountain spotted fever vaccine of tissue culture origin. *J. infect. Dis.* **138**, 217.
DuPont, H. L., Hornick, R. B., Dawkins, A. T., Heiner, G. G., Fabricant, J. B., Wisseman, C. L., Jr., and Woodward, T. E. (1973). Rocky Mountain spotted fever: A comparative study of the active immunity induced by inactivated and viable pathogenic *Rickettsia rickettsii*. *J. infect. Dis.* **128**, 340.
Huxsoll, D. L. (1981). Scrub typhus chemoprophylaxis. Personal communication.
Smadel, J. E., Ley, H. L., Jr., Diercks, F. H., Paterson, P. Y., Wisseman, C. L., Jr., and Traub, R. (1952). Immunization against scrub typhus: duration of immunity in volunteers following combined living vaccine and chemoprophylaxis. *Am. J. trop. Med. Hyg.* **1**, 87.

Other rickettsial diseases

Other tick-borne rickettsioses. The tick-borne rickettsioses are caused by rickettsiae which are related closely to each other and to RMSF and are termed variously according to their geographic presence (*fièvre boutonneuse*, South African tick typhus, Mediterranean Marsielles fever, Indian tick typhus, Kenya tick typhus, North Asian tick-borne rickettsioses, Queensland tick typhus, and others). Much additional work on their specific antigenic structure, immune relationships, ecological, and epidemiological characteristics is required. Otherwise, they are regarded as related diseases and *fièvre boutonneuse*, North Asian tick-borne rickettsioses, and Queensland tick typhus are the currently accepted prototypes.

Illness is transmitted to man by the bite of an ixodid tick; the illnesses are mild to moderately severe characterized by an initial lesion (eschar or *tache noir* in *fièvre boutonneuse*), fever of several days to two weeks, a generalized maculopapular, erythematous eruption appearing first on about the fifth febrile day involving the palms, soles, and adenopathy satellite to the eschar. Agglutinins to *Proteus* OX 19 and specific CF antibodies to spotted fever antigens confirm the diagnosis.

Aetiology and epidemiology. The aetiological rickettsiae of *fièvre boutonneuse* (*R. conorii*), North Asian tick-borne rickettsioses (*R. siberica*), and Queensland tick typhus (*R. australis*) possess group antigens common to *R. rickettsii* and *R. akari* which are demonstrable by agglutination, complement fixation, microscopic agglutination, and immune fluorescent antibody reactions.

R. conorii, which causes *fièvre boutonneuse*, can be regarded as the prototype for this group of infections although further laboratory work will clarify whether the agents and the diseases they cause merit unification or separation.

The epidemiology of the tick-borne rickettsioses resembles that of RMSF in the western Hemisphere; ixodid ticks, small wild mammals and dogs maintain the rickettsiae in nature. When humans intrude accidentally into the cycle, they simply represent a dead end in the transmission chain. In some areas, particularly in Mediterranean countries, the cycle of *fièvre boutonneuse* involves domestic environments with the brown dog tick, *Rhipicephalus sanguineus*, as the dominant vector. Several species of ixodid ticks are known vectors of *R. sibericus* and *R. australis*. There is serological evidence of spotted fever group rickettsiae in Thailand, Malaysia, Europe, Israel, India, and Pakistan.

Clinical manifestations. After an incubation of about one week, clinical manifestations of the tick-borne rickettsioses are usually milder than RMSF; there is a shorter febrile course and fewer severe complications. Fatalities are minimal except in the aged or disabled. An initial lesion is present in most cases at the febrile onset; it is an erythematous lesion which vesiculates, ulcerates, and forms a scab with surrounding enlarged lymph glands. The rash, which begins on the fourth febrile day (range three to five), is red, maculopapular, noted on the arms and rapidly involves the trunk, face, palms, and soles. It is distinctly papular and may become haemorrhagic. Conjunctival injection is common. The febrile course is usually remittent or constant for a week to ten days. Headache is moderate to severe. Recovery is the rule and there are few residuals.

Diagnosis, treatment, and control. See sections on pages 5.340–5.342.

Rickettsialpox. Rickettsialpox, also called vesicular rickettsiosis and vesicular and varioliform rickettsiosis (gamaso-rickettsiosis vesiculosa), is caused by *Rickettsia akari*. It is transmitted to humans by mites, and is characterized by an initial lesion or eschar, a febrile course of about a week, and a sparse papulovesicular rash resembling varicella. The Weil–Felix reaction is negative; specific CF, MA, and IFA antibodies appear during convalescence.

Aetiology and epidemiology. The first cases were reported in New York City in 1946, and later from several sites in New England, Philadelphia, Pittsburgh, and Cleveland. In 1949–50, cases were reported in the Soviet Union and were designated 'vesicular rickettsioses'. For a few years, 180 cases were reported annually in New York City alone. The disease is uncommon perhaps because of under-reporting, better control of mouse infestation, or failure to confirm the diagnosis.

The agent simulates other rickettsiae morphologically and biologically; it is distinct from, but antigenically related to *R. rickettsii*, stains well with Giemsa and Macchiavello techniques, and grows well in the cytoplasm and nucleus of cells. Mice, fertile hens' eggs, and guinea pigs support growth of *R. akari*. Diagnostic antigens for serologic reactions are prepared from infected yolk sacs.

The vector is a colourless, blood sucking mite, *Allodermanyssus sanguineus*. *R. akari* has been isolated from mites, the house mouse (*Mus musculus*), rats, and voles. In the United States, the mouse–mite–mouse cycle involves man as an accidental participant, particularly in congested housing developments where there is dense mouse infestation, improper incineration, and crowding. *R. akari* is probably transmitted by mite bite.

Clinical manifestations. The primary eschar appears about a week after the mite bite; it is a firm reddish papule, 1–1.5 mm in diameter, which vesiculates in a few days and is surrounded by a red halo. Soon a black scab forms and the local nodes are enlarged. The eschar is non-painful, heals slowly, and leaves a small scar.

Fever develops several days after the initial lesion, reaches 39.4–40.0 °C, and lasts for about a week with morning remissions. Chills, headache, malaise and myalgia, anorexia, and photophobia occur but are milder than RMSF. The characteristic rash is maculopapular, with a central unilocular vesicle; it may be sparse over the trunk or abundant. Oral lesions occur, but the palms and soles are usually spared. The vesicles dry and disappear without scar formation. Constitutional symptoms are usually mild and the illness is uncomplicated. No fatalities have been reported.

Diagnosis, treatment and control. See sections on pages 5.340–5.342.

Epidemic typhus fever. Epidemic or the classical form of typhus fever also called European typhus, ship fever, jail fever, *Dermatypho* (Italy), *tifus exanthematico*, *tabardillo* (Spain), and *Fleckfieber* (Germany), is caused by the transmission of *R. prowazekii* to man by the body louse. Characteristically, there is intense headache, prostration, continuous high, slightly remittent fever for two weeks, a macular skin eruption noted first on about the fifth febrile day, malaise, myalgia, and vascular and neurologic abnormalities. Diagnosis is confirmed by demonstration of agglutinins to *Proteus* OX 19 and specific CF, IFA, and MA antibodies late in illness or during convalescence. Chloramphenicol and the tetracycline antibiotics are highly effective.

Aetiology and epidemiology. *R. prowazekii*, which is antigenically closely related to *R. mooseri*, which causes murine typhus, enters the body via rickettsia-laden faeces usually contaminating the skin at the site of attachment of louse, *Pediculus humanis corporis*. The louse, which is the only important human vector, dies of its infection and fortunately fails to transmit infection to its offspring. Flying squirrels are infected with *R. prowazekii* and undoubtedly their ectoparasites are also infected. The natural cycle of the agent probably involves man–louse–man, and new epidemics can originate from patients with Brill–Zinsser disease when lice may become contaminated during active infection. Pathogenic rickettsiae reside for months or years in patients convalescent from epidemic typhus, RMSF, and scrub typhus. Hence, a recurrent form of illness in these other rickettsioses is possible. The dried faeces of lice, fleas, and ticks infected with *R. prowazekii*, *R. mooseri*, and *R. rickettsii* remain viable for long periods, and inhalation of such dust containing aerosols can cause infection. The finding of *R. prowazekii*

infection in squirrels does pose a serious question regarding the man–louse–man concept as the sole cycle for maintenance of this infection naturally.

Louse-borne typhus has occurred in all countries, and, when uncontrolled due to privation and poor health standards, epidemics usually occurred in susceptible populations over a three year period. The first year of an outbreak usually seeded the infection broadly, in the second year, the epidemic reached its peak and in the third year, the infection tapered off because the majority of persons had developed a natural immunity. Summer months witnessed a decline because of bathing and cleanliness which favoured better louse control. The illness is now restricted to a few countries but its potential for spread persists; it appears occasionally in eastern Europe and sporadically in central Africa, Ethiopia, southern Africa, Afghanistan, northern India, Mexico, Central America, and the South American Andes.

Clinical manifestations. The clinical manifestations are very similar to those of RMSF (see page 5.338). The incubation period is about seven days. A dusky or smoky appearance is occasionally noted in typhus patients. A significant distinguishing feature is the rash. It becomes apparent on about the fourth to fifth day (a little later than RMSF), and it is first apparent in the axillary folds and on the trunk. It is initially macular and pink and in a day or so becomes red, petechial and does not fade on pressure. In later stages, it becomes confluent, haemorrhagic, and occasionally necrotic. Its spread is centrifugal from the trunk to the extremities, just the reverse of RMSF (see Fig. 7). Rarely does it involve the palms, soles, or face. The neurologic, cardiovascular, and other manifestations, including superimposed infections, that present in severe cases of RMSF also occur in typhus.

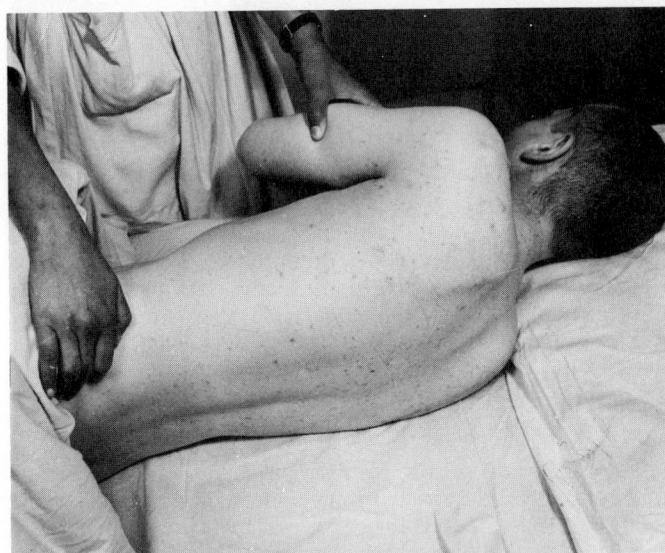

Fig. 7 Epidemic typhus fever. Typical body rash in louse-borne typhus on about eighth day of illness showing diffuse, discrete haemorrhagic lesions.

Epidemic typhus has reached mortality rates of 60 per cent in uncontrolled epidemics. With specific chemotherapy and supportive care initially, it can be virtually eliminated and the course of illness sharply reduced.

Differential diagnosis, treatment, and control. See sections on pages 5.340–5.342.

Recrudescent typhus (Brill–Zinsser disease). Persons who have recovered from epidemic louse-borne typhus fever may develop recurrent fever and other characteristic clinical manifestations of typhus months or years after their initial infection in known endemic areas. The causative *R. prowazekii* have been isolated during recurrence from the blood or from lice fed on patients during the active stage of their recurrent illness. Unlike epidemic typhus, the Weil–Felix test using *Proteus* OX 19 is usually negative or these agglutinins are present in low titre. CF, IFA, and MA antibodies to *R. prowazekii* are present and appear in several days after onset of the recurrence. These antibodies are primarily of the 7S type in contrast to 19S antibody which characterizes the initial infection.

Clinical manifestations. The clinical manifestations, including the rash, resemble those of murine typhus, mild RMSF or epidemic typhus fever (Fig. 8). Occasionally the course may be more severe and the circulatory, neurologic, hepatic and renal changes simulate those observed in severe RMSF or epidemic typhus. Full recovery is the rule and the clinical course is usually mild.

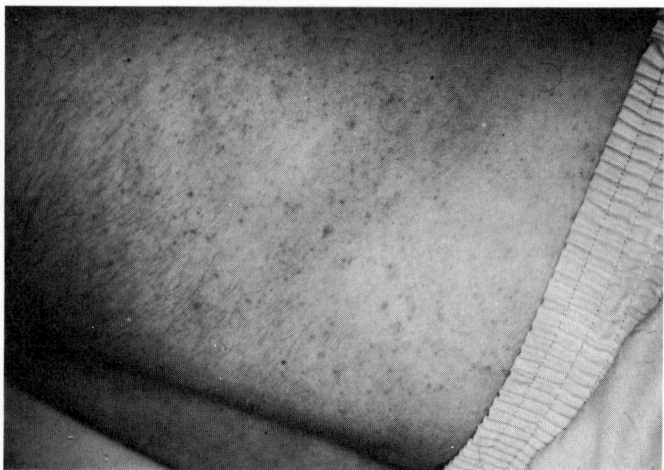

Fig. 8 Brill–Zinsser disease (recrudescent typhus). Note (pink) macular rash on body. Illness in an adult whose initial illness with typhus occurred 30 years earlier in Poland. Second attack occurred a week after appendectomy. Full recovery.

Diagnosis, treatment, and control. See sections on pages 5.340–5.342.

Murine typhus fever. Murine typhus, also called endemic typhus, urban or shop typhus, and flea-borne or rat–flea typhus, is a junior counterpart of epidemic louse-borne typhus. It is an acute febrile illness caused by *Rickettsia mooseri* (typhi) transmitted to man by fleas and characterized by fever for 9–14 days, headache, a pink maculopapular rash, myalgia, and prostration. The Weil–Felix (*Proteus* OX 19) reaction is positive and special serologic tests are diagnostic.

History. In spite of its existence since ancient times, murine typhus was not clearly differentiated from epidemic louse-borne typhus until the 1930s. Maxcy, in 1926, on purely epidemiological evidence, surmised that typhus in the United States had its reservoir in rodents and was transmitted to humans by ticks or fleas. Confirmation of this hypothesis was obtained in 1930, when Dyer and his associates isolated rickettsiae from brains of rats obtained in the vicinity of several patients in Baltimore, and soon incriminated the flea as a vector. Mooser, Castaneda, and Zinsser confirmed these findings from brains of rats trapped in Mexico City the same year. Previously, the illness had been erroneously called Brill's disease or endemic typhus in the southeastern United States. It then became apparent that murine typhus was global in its distribution and was generally prevalent in those countries where louse-borne typhus occurs.

Aetiology and epidemiology. *R. mooseri* (typhi) resembles other rickettsiae in morphological, staining properties and intracellular parasitism. It differs from *R. rickettsii* in that it always multiplies within the cytoplasm of cells.

Rats (*Rattus rattus* and *Rattus norvegicus*) and mice are normally infected with *R. mooseri*, and, although the rodent disease is non-fatal, viable rickettsiae persist in the brain for variable periods. The rat flea (*Xenophyllus cheopis*) becomes infected by feeding on a rat during the acute stage of infection. The flea, once infected, discharges rickettsiae in its faeces throughout its life; the flea is the natural human source of infection. Dried flea faeces may infect the conjunctiva or respiratory tract.

Fleas other than *X. cheopis*, such as *Pulex irritans*, are susceptible to infection and human body lice, experimentally infected with *R. mooseri* cause a resulting illness similar to epidemic typhus. Whether this occurs in nature is unknown.

Guinea pigs are readily susceptible to murine typhus after intra-abdominal inoculation and from them infection may be transferred to other animals, fertile hens' eggs, or tissue culture cells.

Murine typhus is one of the mild rickettsioses and is widespread in its prevalence, although sporadic in incidence. The disease commonly occurs among persons working in proximity to granaries or food depots and in those whose activities bring them in contact with rats and their fleas.

Clinical manifestations. The incubation period is 8–16 days (average 10) with prodromata of headache, backache, arthralgia, chilly sensations, and transient temperature elevations. Actual onset is usually clear-cut with a spiking chill, repeated rigors, severe frontal headache, and fever. All other manifestations except the exanthem simulate those of epidemic typhus or RMSF (although milder). Fever lasts usually for 10–12 days reaching 38.9–40.0 °C with slow lysis. Some patients experience low-grade fever.

The early rash is sparse, discrete, and hidden in the axillae or inner surface of the arms or trunk. Most patients then develop a generalized, dull red, macular rash on the upper abdomen, shoulders, chest, arms, and thighs. It may become maculopapular. It usually appears by the fifth febrile day, ordinarily does not become haemorrhagic like RMSF or epidemic typhus, persists for about four to eight days, and fades at defervescence or before. Fatality is low except in the debilitated or elderly.

Differential diagnosis, treatment, and control. See sections on pages 5.340–5.342.

Scrub typhus fever. Scrub typhus fever, also called Tsutsugamushi disease, rural typhus, Japanese fever, flood fever, mite-borne typhus, is an acute febrile illness. It is characterized by fever of almost two weeks, a primary lesion with local adenitis at the site of an infected mite attachment, and a cutaneous rash appearing first on about the fifth day. Its cause is *Rickettsia tsutsugamushi* (*Rickettsia orientalis*). Rickettsaemia is present during the acute stage, agglutinins to *Proteus* OXK appear in most cases, but sero diagnosis is best confirmed by the IFA test.

Aetiology and epidemiology. *R. tsutsugamushi* simulates other rickettsiae in morphology but differs from them in antigenic structure, vector, and reservoir. It possesses no known antigens in common with other rickettsiae, but shares an antigen with *Proteus* OXK. Unfortunately, there are multiple serotypes which produce effective homologous immunity but transient cross-protection in man which has precluded development of an effective vaccine.

Larvae of several species of mites, especially *Leptotrobidium* (trombicula) *akamushi* and *L. deliense* become infected by attaching themselves to the skin of wild rodents and ultimately to man as an accidental host. Typhus infection is well-established in nature, often as 'typhus islands' in a cycle involving mites and small rodents and probably by transovarial transmission in mites. Man invades these habitats which vary from river banks, semi-deserts, disturbed rain forests, sea shores, and terrain undergoing secondary vegetation. Rats, field mice, voles, and shrews serve as secondary hosts.

Clinical manifestations. Ten to 12 days after infection, chills, fever, and headache abruptly usher in the illness. Injected conjunctivae and a small lesion present at the febrile onset first appears as an erythematous indurated spot 1–2 mm in diameter with surrounding adenopathy. The eschar is surrounded by multi-loculated vesicles which ulcerate in a few days to be covered by a black crust. These are the principal clinical features: the remainder of the findings, including headache and myalgia, simulate those described for RMSF and epidemic typhus.

The pink-red, macular rash begins on the trunk on about the fifth day, spreads to the extremities, occasionally becomes maculopapular and fades in a few days. Therapy with chloramphenicol and tetracycline is remarkably effective.

Interstitial myocarditis is said to be a common feature of scrub typhus but careful follow-up studies have failed to reveal serious sequelae.

Differential diagnosis, treatment, and control. See sections on pages 5.340–5.342.

Q Fever (Balkan grippe). Q fever is characterized by an abrupt onset of fever, headache in most cases, general malaise, and weakness, and usually interstitial pneumonitis simulating 'atypical pneumonia'. Rickettsaemia to *C. burneti* is present during the febrile course, specific antibodies to phase II antigens appear during the acute illness and phase I type antibodies in chronic forms of illness such as hepatitis or endocarditis. There is no exanthem.

Aetiology and epidemiology. Derrick and Burnett of Australia, and Cox of the United States, independently described the clinical illness, and identified and characterized the agent (*Coxiella burneti*) isolated from patients and ticks. It is a diplobacillary, spherical micro-organism, 1.5 μm in length and 0.2 μm wide which has a wide host range in nature; guinea pigs and embryonated eggs are the laboratory hosts employed for its propagation.

Clinical manifestations. After a long incubation of 14–26 days (average 19), fever, headache, chilly sensations, malaise, myalgia, and anorexia begin abruptly. The fever ranges from 38.3–40.3 °C for several days, and the entire remittent febrile course averages about a week, often extending to two weeks and occasionally longer. Headache is usually severe and the fever may fluctuate widely. In a few days, there is a hacking dry cough with chest pain when rales are usually audible. The chest X-ray shows findings indistinguishable from 'atypical pneumonia', 'mycoplasma pneumonia', or 'legionella infection' on the third of fourth days of illness. They appear first as patchy areas of consolidation involving a portion of the lobe showing a ground-glass appearance. Such respiratory manifestations persist beyond the febrile period and occasionally patients may be unaware of their presence.

Q fever, like other rickettsial infections, is a systemic disorder and not solely a pneumonic infection. Under artificially induced infection by aerosol in humans, X-ray evidence of pneumonitis occurred in less than one-half of those infected. In this study, the development of pneumonitis was unrelated to the size of the infecting dose.

Coincident with deffervescence, the appetite returns and convalescence progresses slowly for several weeks associated with weakness. Some patients may lose 7 kg or more during illness; in about 20 per cent of cases, the course may be protracted with fever persisting for four weeks or more, particularly in elderly patients. Complications are uncommon although relapse occurs, especially in patients treated with antibiotics during the first several days of illness.

Hepatitis. Approximately one-third of patients develop either acute or chronic protracted hepatitis. A low level of jaundice, fever, malaise, hepatomegaly, and right upper abdominal quadrant pain with absence of headache and respiratory signs are indicative of an acute granulomatous hepatitis. Liver biopsy specimens show diffuse granulomatous changes with multinucleated giant cells, scattered infiltrations of polymorphonuclear leucocytes, lymphocytes, and macrophages (Plate 5(d)). *C. burneti* are demonstrable with IF staining in such specimens. A chronic type of hepatitis is said to occur in a significant number of patients. Q fever must be included in the differential diagnoses of conditions associated with hepatic granulomas, such as sarcoid, syphilis, tuberculosis, mycoses (particularly histoplasmosis), brucellosis, and other causes.

Endocarditis. Whenever there are clinical manifestations of subacute bacterial endocarditis and negative blood cultures, infection caused by *C. burneti* should be suspected. A previously damaged aortic valve is most commonly involved. Classical signs of endocarditis are usually present, the epidemiological history may suggest exposure to the agent, and antibodies to phase I *C. burneti* antigens are present. Once the diagnosis is suspected or confirmed, prolonged chemotherapy with either tetracycline or chloramphenicol is indicated; operative intervention with replacement of damaged valves is usually necessary because the vegetations are usually large and bulky, and the effective antibiotics are not rickettsicidal.

Pneumonia caused by *Legionella pneumophila* may simulate the rickettsial pneumonia caused by *C. burneti* including morphologic similarities of the two micro-organisms, particularly when Giemsa stain is used. IFA techniques are definitive for each.

Prognosis. There are few fatalities except in those patients with endocarditis. Hepatitic involvement may lead to protracted illness. The course is generally benign and uncomplicated.

Diagnosis, treatment and control. See sections on pages 5.340–5.342.

References

Brill, N. E. (1910). An acute febrile illness of unknown origin. *Am. J. med. Sci.* **139**, 484.

Dyer, Rumreich, A. and Badger, L. F. (1931). A virus of the typhus type derived from fleas collected from wild rats. *Pub. Hlth Rep.* **46**, 334.

Elsom, K. A., Beebe, G. W., Sayen, J. J., Scheie, H. G., Gammon, G. D., and Woodward, F. C. (1961). Scrub typhus: A follow-up study. *Ann. intern. Med.* **55**, 784.

Maxcy, K. F. (1929). Typhus fever in the United States. *Pub. Hlth Rep.* **44**, 1735.

Tigertt, W. D. Studies in Q fever in man. In *Symposium of Q fever. Med. Sci. Pub.* no. 6, WRAIR, 39. U.S. Govt Printing Office, Washington, D.C.

Urso, F. P. (1980). Deceived but described Legionellosis masquerading as Rickettsia pneumonia. *Am. J. clin. Path.* **74**, 364.

Trench fever

Trench fever, also called His–Werner disease, Quintan fever, shin bone fever, and Volhynian fever, is characterized by sudden onset with fever, headache, and pain in muscles, bone, and joints. It is a non-fatal, louse-transmitted illness.

Aetiology and epidemiology. The agent, *Rochalimeae* (rickettsia) *quintana*, grows extracellularly in the louse gut; it is excreted in louse faeces. Humans become infected by inoculation of contaminated faeces into abraded skin or the conjunctiva. The organisms multiply extracellularly and are not transmitted transovarially to other lice, which acquire infection by ingestion of blood from an infected person. At least one strain may be cultivated on blood agar and typical trench fever has been induced in volunteers. *R. quintana* may be recovered periodically from human blood for several years after convalescence from an acute attack.

Trench fever exists in Mexico, Tunisia, Eritrea, Poland, the USSR, and possibly in China. There is serological evidence of its presence in Bolivia, Bermuda, and Ethiopia.

During the First World War, the illness was very prevalent in western Europe, and in the Second World War, it recurred in large numbers in eastern Europe.

Clinical manifestations, prognosis. The incubation period varies from 10–30 days, the onset may be insidious or abrupt, and the manifestations of trench fever may range from a mild febrile illness to a protracted clinical course with numerous relapses. Characteristically, in the acute type, there is malaise, headache, fever, and bone and body pain especially severe in the shins. Occasionally, one febrile peak occurs; in others, there may be fever from five to seven days with a saddleback-like pattern; in others, there is an initial febrile episode lasting one to three days followed by relapses which characteristically occur at four to five day intervals. In some patients, fever and manifestations are continuous for two to three weeks. Splenomegaly and a red macular rash occur in approximately 70 per cent of cases. With each febrile relapse, myalgia usually occurs.

R. quintana persists in the blood throughout the initial attack, during relapses, and often during asymptomatic periods between relapses. Recurrences have been reported 10 years after the initial illness.

Trench fever is non-fatal; the clinical course is variable with 80 per cent of patients fully recovered in two months. About 5 per cent of patients become chronic and there may be delayed recovery in the aged or debilatated.

Differential diagnosis. Under epidemic conditions, the illness is readily diagnosed based on the clinical manifestations. Those other illnesses which are suggested are influenza, typhoid, typhus, malaria, dengue, leptospirosis, and relapsing fever which are confirmed by specific laboratory tests. The causative *R. quintana* may be cultivated on blood agar; a serological test is not in general use.

Treatment and control. Although there is no reliable data, it is *likely* that the broad spectrum antibiotics, tetracycline and chloramphenicol, would be therapeutically helpful particularly in preventing chronic or lingering forms of illness. Palliative care with bed rest and salicylates or codeine for relief of pain usually suffice.

Those methods to control lice for prevention of epidemic typhus apply to control of trench fever.

References

Vinson, J. W. (1964). Etiology of trench fever in Mexico, In *Industry and tropical health*. vol. 5. Harvard School of Public Health, Boston.
—, Varela, G., and Molina-Pasquel, C. (1969). Trench fever III: induction of clinical disease in volunteers inoculated with *Rickettsia quintana* propagated on blood agar. *Am. J. trop. Med. Hyg.* **18**, 713.

Chlamydial infections

S. Darougar
M. A. Monnickendam
J. D. Treharne

Chlamydiae, known previously as the Bedsonia or psittacosis–lymphogranuloma–trachoma group of agents, are common pathogens of man and many other species of mammals and birds. They were first recognized in 1907 by Halberstaedter and von Prowazek in conjunctival scrapings from patients with trachoma and experimentally infected orang-utans. In the past 20 years there have been considerable advances in our knowledge of chlamydiae and the diseases they cause. In this chapter, we discuss ocular, genital, and systemic infections in man.

Microbiology

Classification. Organisms of the family *Chlamydiaceae* are obligate intracellular parasites. They are classified as bacteria because they possess both RNA and DNA, a discrete cell wall similar to that of Gram-negative bacteria, primitive enzyme systems, and are susceptible to some antibiotics (e.g., rifampicin, tetracycline, erythromycin).

The genus *Chlamydia* is divided into two species; *Chlamydia trachomatis* which has iodine-staining polysaccharide in its inclusion bodies, and is sensitive to sulphadiazine; and *Chlamydia psittaci* which has inclusion bodies that do not stain with iodine, and is resistant to sulphadiazine. *C. trachomatis* is commonly divided into trachoma inclusion conjunctivitis (TRIC) strains and lymphogranuloma venereum (LGV) strains.

Life cycle. The chlamydial life cycle is complex and not yet fully understood. The infectious elementary body is DNA-rich, relatively stable, approximately 250 nm in diameter and initiates the developmental cycle when it enters a susceptible cell by phagocytosis. Some hours later, it undergoes reorganization to form the non-infectious, large (400–1000 nm), labile, metabolically active, reticulate or initial body. This has an increased RNA content, and divides a number of times by binary fission, ultimately producing new elementary bodies. The whole cycle is completed in 36 to 48 hours.

Chemical and biological properties. The molecular weight of chlamydial DNA is $470–660 \times 10^6$ dalton, which is about four times larger than that of vaccinia virus DNA and one quarter of *Escherichia coli* DNA. It contains sufficient genetic information for the coding of several hundred different proteins. DNA homology studies show considerable differences in the nucleotide sequences of *C. trachomatis* and *C. psittaci*, and remarkable similarities between different strains of the same species.

Biological differences between strains of *C. trachomatis* isolated from chlamydial ocular and genital infections (TRIC strains), lymphogranuloma venereum (LGV strains), and strains of *C. psittaci* can be demonstrated in animal pathogenicity studies. *C. psittaci* and LGV organisms are generally lethal when inoculated into the mouse brain, whereas TRIC organisms are rarely lethal. TRIC agents cause a follicular conjunctivitis when inoculated into the eyes of non-human primates, but *C. psittaci* and LGV strains do not. Such studies are, however, of limited value because responses are dose-dependent, and influenced by host factors. Other biological differences between TRIC and LGV strains are shown in HeLa cell cultures. The growth of TRIC strains is enhanced by pretreatment of cells with the poly-cation DEAE-dextran, whilst the growth of LGV organisms is not affected. Conversely, the growth of TRIC strains in HeLa cells is inhibited by the addition of neuraminidase, whereas LGV is not inhibited, suggesting that different receptor sites are involved in the phagocytosis of TRIC and LGV particles.

The complement fixation (CF) test shows that the two species have a common group specific antigen which is heat stable. The indirect micro-immunofluorescence (micro-IF) test divides *C. trachomatis* into several serotypes, and there is an interesting link between different serotypes and various diseases. Serotypes A, B, and C are associated with hyperendemic trachoma of eye-to-eye transmission whereas serotypes D, E, F, G, H, I, J, and K are associated with paratrachoma (ocular infections of sexually transmitted origin) and genital infections. There are also three LGV serotypes, L1, L2, and L3. There is no equivalent classification of *C. psittaci* strains, although the mouse toxicity prevention test shows that isolates from the same host species tend to be more similar to one another than to those isolated from other hosts.

Studies in cell culture demonstrate that the most effective drugs against *C. trachomatis* are rifampicin, tetracyclines, and macrolides. No such tests have been made on *C. psittaci* agents, although clinical studies indicate that they are sensitive to the same chemotherapeutic compounds (with the exception of sulphonamides).

CLINICAL FORMS

Ocular infection

Chlamydial ocular infections can be divided into three groups:

1. Hyperendemic trachoma of eye-to-eye transmission, caused mainly by *C. trachomatis* serotypes A to C.
2. Paratrachoma of sexually transmitted origin, caused mainly by *C. trachomatis* serotypes D to K.
3. Infections of animal origin caused by *C. psittaci*.

Hyperendemic trachoma. Hyperendemic trachoma is a chronic follicular conjunctivitis associated with scarring of the palpebral conjunctiva, pannus, and scars in the cornea. The disease is hyperendemic in rural communities of the Middle East, Asia, Africa, and South and Central America. Over 500 million people have trachoma, and approximately 5–10 million have resulting blindness.

Epidemiology. From the public health viewpoint, trachoma is divided into blinding and non-blinding disease. Blinding trachoma is distinguished by a high prevalence of severe disease, causing blinding complications. Non-blinding trachoma may also be endemic, but it is a mild disease which does not generally produce potentially blinding lesions. The distinction between blinding and non-blinding trachoma is important in determining the priorities of programmes for the prevention of blindness.

Blinding trachoma is generally associated with over-crowding, lack of sanitation, substandard levels of hygiene and medical care, and poor standards of living. Under these conditions, babies may become infected at two to three months, and at three to five years of age, most children have moderate to severe disease. After this, the prevalence and severity of active trachoma declines and at 15–20 years old, only a small proportion, mainly those who live in large families with young children, show signs of active disease. Children with moderate to severe trachoma are the main reservoir of infection. They harbour most infectious particles in their conjunctivae, and shed the greatest numbers of viable organisms in their eye secretions. It has been suggested that the excessive amounts of mucoid or muco-purulent ocular discharges caused by trachoma, or associated bacterial conjunctivitis, can protect the infectivity of chlamydia particles. These particles are transmitted by flies, fingers, towels, or bedclothes. House flies, particularly *Musca sorbens*, may play an important role in transmitting infection from one child to another. *C. trachomatis* has been isolated from flies which have fed on the eye secretions of patients with active trachoma. We have shown that flies can carry viable *C. trachomatis* (serotypes A and B) on their proboscises and legs and in their intestines for up to six hours. They can also transmit guinea pig inclusion conjunctivitis (GPIC) agent from the eyes of one guinea pig to another.

Clinical features. Trachoma is a chronic follicular conjunctivitis associated with papillae, follicles, and scars in the palpebral conjunctiva, and pannus, keratitis, and scars in the cornea (Fig. 1). The incubation period of trachoma is unknown, but in experimentally infected human volunteers it was one to three weeks.

Trachoma is a bilateral disease which is occasionally associated with rhinitis, otitis media, upper respiratory tract infection, and pre-auricular lymphadenopathy. Symptoms are generally mild and include watering, discharge, redness, swelling of lids, and ptosis in one or both eyes. Clinical signs occur in the bulbar and palpebral conjunctiva and in the cornea.

The bulbar conjunctiva may show a mild or moderate hyperaemia, a mild diffuse infiltration and occasionally follicles, mainly in areas adjacent to the upper and lower fornices.

In the palpebral conjunctiva, a papillary reaction occurs in the whole conjunctiva—upper tarsus, upper fornix and the lower lid—but it is most severe in the upper tarsal conjunctiva. Follicles may also be present over the whole conjunctiva; in the upper tarsal area

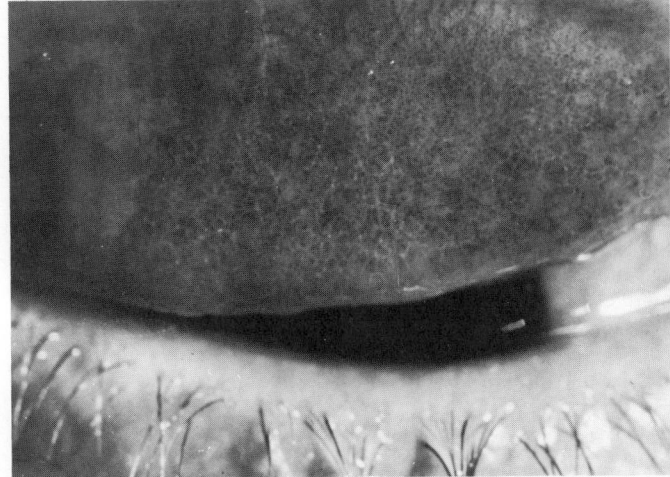

Fig. 1(a) Hyperendemic trachoma: upper tarsal conjunctiva showing papillae and small follicles.

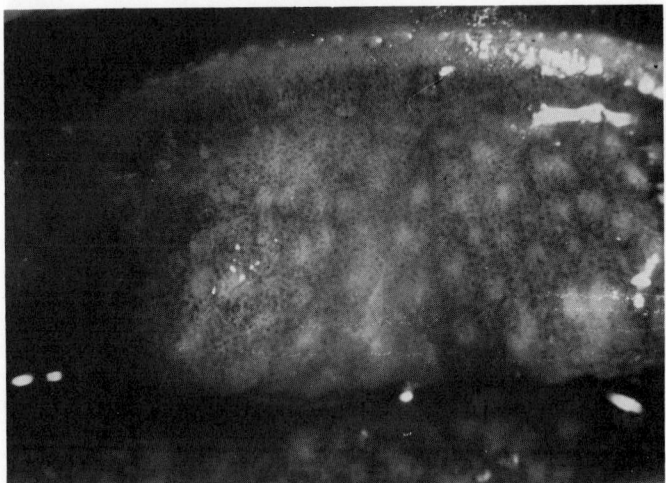

Fig. 1(b) The same as Fig. 1(a) but with large follicles.

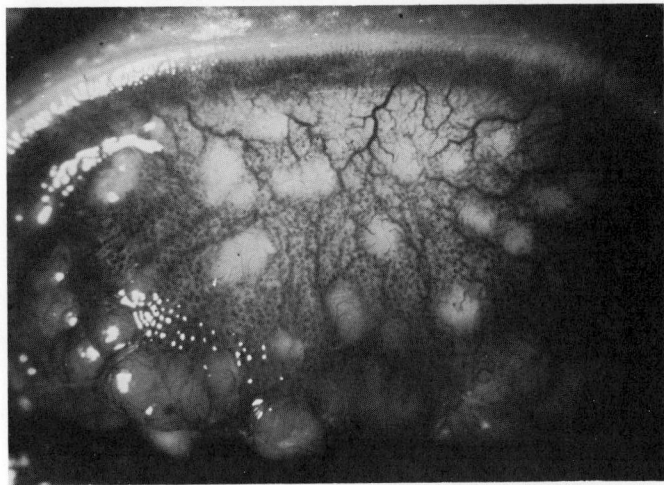

Fig. 1(c) The same as Fig. 1(a) but with mature follicles.

they are elevated yellowish or grey-white lesions against a background of red papillae, and vary from 0.2 mm to 3 mm in diameter. Large follicles may occasionally become necrotic or soft (mature follicles) and rupture under light pressure. In the upper fornix and the lower lid, the follicular response is more severe, and follicles are larger. Conjunctival scarring in mild disease appears as fine, focal (stellate) or linear scars (Fig. 2). In more severe cases, larger linear or diffuse scars develop, and it is these patients who are likely to develop the potentially blinding complications of trachoma.

Corneal signs in trachoma include limbal follicles with resultant scars (Herbert's pits), epithelial and sub-epithelial punctate keratitis, and pannus (Fig. 3). Fine epithelial punctate keratitis may develop in the periphery in severe trachoma. Coarse epithelial infiltrates are associated with pannus. Sub-epithelial punctate keratitis, similar to that seen in paratrachoma of sexually transmitted origin or in adenovirus ocular infection, may occasionally develop. The opacities are coarse, may be visible with the naked eye, and are more common in the upper half of the cornea. The pannus consists of superficial vascularization of the cornea and associated diffuse and punctate epithelial infiltrates. It is more marked in the upper part of the cornea, but circumcorneal pannus is also found.

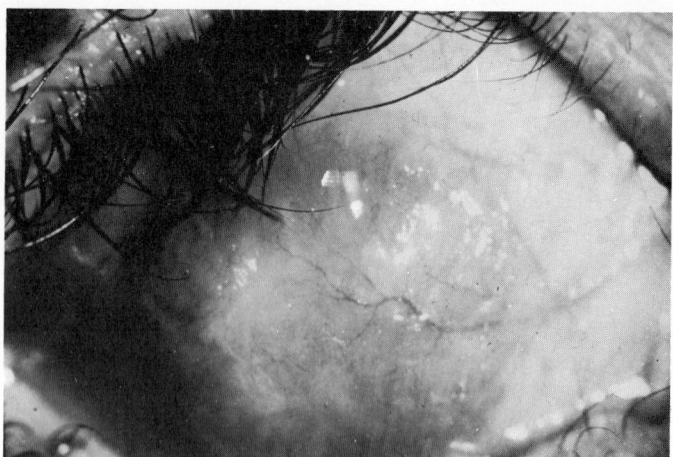

Fig. 4 Hyperendemic trachoma: trichiasis and corneal scarring.

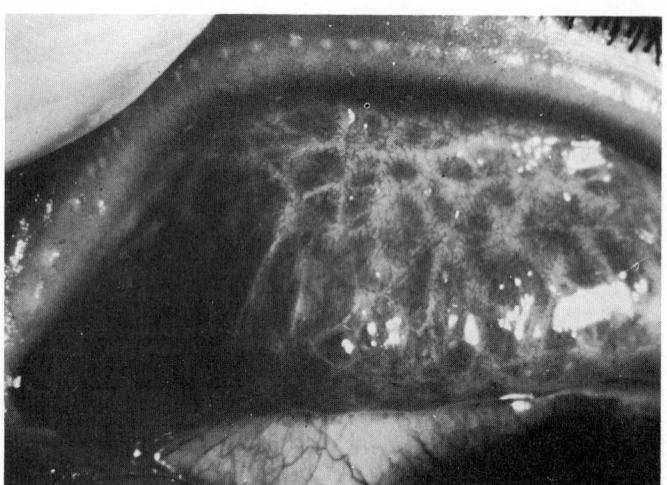

Fig. 2 Hyperendemic trachoma: scarring of upper tarsal conjunctiva.

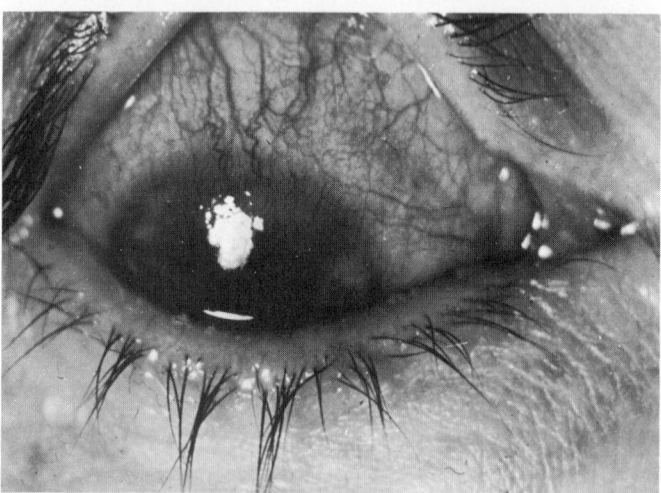

Fig. 3 Hyperendemic trachoma: showing vascularization and infiltration of the cornea (pannus).

The potentially blinding complications of trachoma are severe scarring of the tarsal conjunctiva leading to trichiasis and entropion. The resultant misdirected lashes cause constant abrasion of the cornea leading to corneal ulcers, scarring, and loss of vision (Fig. 4). These complications generally occur in older people (over 35–40 years), although they are occasionally found in young adults, particularly mothers of children with severe trachoma.

Trachoma may present in various clinical forms. In babies, it appears as a moderate or severe papillary conjunctivitis with some follicles in the upper fornix and the lower lid but no pannus. In young children, the disease presents in its classical form with

varying degrees of papillary and follicular responses in the upper tarsal conjunctiva, and active pannus. In older children and young adults, conjunctival scarring and inflammatory responses may be seen together.

The clinical course of trachoma was divided into four stages by McCallan, representing a single cycle of infection. This classification is of limited value because it does not measure degrees of severity of inflammation or blinding complications. A proposed new method of grading conjunctival inflammatory responses and potentially blinding complications (Dawson *et al.* 1975) is much more satisfactory.

Diagnosis. The clinical diagnosis of active trachoma can be made when follicles are present in the palpebral conjunctiva together with one of the following signs; conjunctival scarring, pannus, limbal follicles, or Herbert's pits. In the early stages, a differential diagnosis should be made from bacterial, viral, and allergic conjunctivitis. Laboratory tests, particularly the demonstration of chlamydial inclusions in conjunctival scrapings and isolation of chlamydiae, are helpful (Table 1).

Table 1   Comparison of laboratory tests for the diagnosis of chlamydial infections

Clinical	Cytology/ histology (direct demon-stration)	isolation (cell culture)	Serology		CF Serum
			Micro-IE		
			Serum	local secretions	
Hyperendemic trachoma	++	+++	+	+++	–
Adult ocular paratrachoma	++	+++	++	+++	–
Neonatal conjunctivitis	+++	+++	+	++	–
Neonatal pneumonitis	?	++	+	+	?
Cervicitis	–	+++	+	++	+
Salpingitis	?	+	++	++	+
Urethritis	–	++	+	–	–
Lympho-granuloma venerum	–	+++	++	?	++
Psittacosis/ ornithosis	–	+++	++	?	++

– = no value, + = poor, ++ = fair, +++ = good, ? = unknown

Treatment and prevention. Topical therapy with tetracycline, rifampicin, or erythromycin eye ointment three times daily for at least five weeks is highly effective. Systemic treatment, with tetracycline or erythromycin (15 mg/kg body weight), doxycycline (1.5 mg/kg) or sulphamethoxazole (30 mg/kg) daily for three weeks, is equally effective.

In blinding trachoma, intermittent topical therapy with tetracycline eye ointment twice daily for seven days each month for a period of four to six months; or systemic treatment with doxycycline (5 mg/kg) given as a single dose once a month for at least six months, reduces the severity of trachoma and the shedding of the agent. These methods of therapy reduce the reinfection rate and hence the possibility of developing potentially blinding complications.

In recent years, attempts have been made to produce a vaccine for the prevention of trachoma. The results of several clinical trials in the field have shown that vaccines only produce short-lived partial immunity, and may also induce hypersensitivity. The prospects of producing a useful vaccine in the near future are poor.

Paratrachoma. Paratrachoma, or chlamydial ocular infection of sexually transmitted origin, comprises neonatal chlamydial ophthalmia and adult chlamydial ophthalmia which may present as inclusion conjunctivitis, TRIC punctate keratoconjunctivitis, or trachoma.

Neonatal chlamydial ophthalmia (NCO). Chlamydial ocular infection in new-born babies (TRIC ophthalmia neonatorum) is an acute conjunctivitis which is acquired during passage through the infected cervix of the mother.

Epidemiology. The incidence of NCO depends on the prevalence of chlamydial genital infection in sexually active women. In the United States where the prevalence of chlamydial cervical infection is estimated to be 5–13 per cent, NCO may occur in 2–6 per cent of newborn babies. In London, approximately 3 per cent of women are infected, and the rate of NCO is less than 1 per cent. Prospective studies have shown that 50 per cent of babies born to mothers with microbiologically proven cervical chlamydial infection develop NCO.

Clinical features. The incubation period of NCO is usually 5–14 days, but it can vary between 1–40 days. Infection is acute, and usually involves both eyes. It is associated with watering, profuse muco-purulent discharge, and swelling and erythema of the eyelids. The bulbar conjunctiva is generally hyperaemic and oedematous. The palpebral conjunctiva is also hyperaemic and may show severe diffuse infiltration and papillae (Fig. 5). Follicles can occur after several weeks and a pseudomembrane may develop in more serious cases. The cornea usually remains normal. After this, the disease may become chronic and last for months or years and follicles, pannus, and scarring may develop. Mild and sub-clinical forms of NCO have been reported.

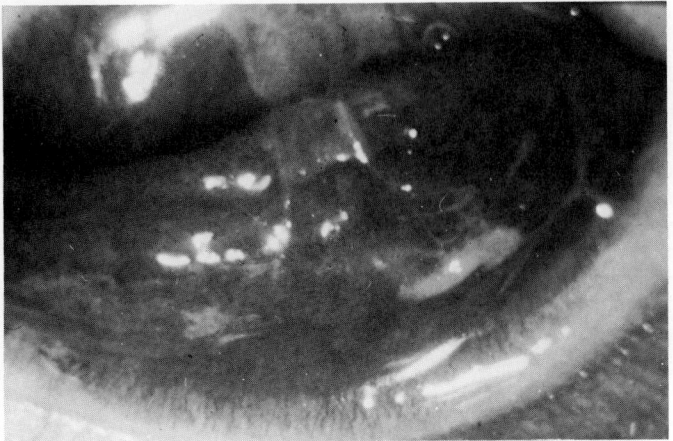

Fig. 5 Neonatal chlamydial ophthalmia: lower conjunctiva showing discharge, oedema, infiltration, and papillae.

Babies with NCO may develop chlamydial infection of the upper respiratory tract (rhinitis and pharyngitis), lung (pneumonitis) and the genital tract (vulvovaginitis).

Diagnosis. The clinical features of NCO—copious discharge, lid swelling, and acute papillary conjunctivitis— are similar to those of neonatal bacterial and viral ophthalmia. The direct demonstration of chlamydial inclusions in conjunctival scrapings and isolation of chlamydiae are the most useful laboratory tests (Table 1).

Treatment and prevention. Topical therapy with tetracycline, rifampicin, or erythromycin eye ointment three times daily for a minimum period of five to six weeks is effective. Unfortunately, because of the difficulty which parents have in applying ointment to the eyes of babies, the failure rate of topical therapy is very high. Systemic therapy with erythromycin syrup for a period of three weeks is highly effective. The application of silver nitrate solution to the eyes of newborn babies advocated by Credé does not appear to prevent NCO. The increasing prevalence of cervical chlamydial infection in women may make it advisable to check for such infection in pregnant women using isolation and serological tests, and to carry out isolation tests on all babies who develop sticky eyes.

Adult chlamydial ophthalmia (ACO). ACO of sexually transmitted origin is a chronic follicular conjunctivitis of acute or sub-acute onset. It may present as inclusion conjunctivitis, TRIC punctate keratoconjunctivitis, or trachoma.

Epidemiology. ACO is commonly found amongst young adults aged 15–40. It can also occur in young children and in older people.

The infection is usually transmitted from the genital tract to the eye, although eye-to-eye transmission may occur. The role of swimming pools in transmission is uncertain. The main reservoir of infection is women with chlamydial genital infection. Chlamydiae have been isolated from the cervices of almost all women with ACO, and in nearly half of female consorts of men with ACO. Patients are sexually active, often have multiple sexual partners, and a history of other sexually transmitted diseases.

ACO is common in the urban communities of developed countries and its incidence is likely to increase in parallel with the growing incidence of chlamydial genital infections.

Clinical features. Inclusion conjunctivitis is the commonest form of ACO. It presents as an acute follicular conjunctivitis. The incubation period is generally between one and two weeks. The infection is unilateral in about 70 per cent of patients, and common symptoms include: mild to moderate lacrimation, mucopurulent discharge, lid swelling, redness, photophobia, and foreign body sensation in the eye. Conjunctival signs consist of a mild to moderate hyperaemia and oedema in the bulbar conjunctiva, moderate or severe hyperaemia, diffuse infiltration, and papillary and follicular reactions in the palpebral conjunctiva. The papillary reaction is more severe in the upper tarsal conjunctiva, but the follicles are generally more numerous and larger in the upper fornix and the lower lid (Fig. 6). The cornea may remain unaffected, but occasionally fine punctate epithelial keratitis develops. Inclusion conjunctivitis may also be associated with pre-auricular lymphadenopathy, upper respiratory tract infection, or otitis media.

TRIC punctate keratoconjunctivitis resembles inclusion conjunctivitis, with the addition of sub-epithelial punctate keratitis. The keratitis may develop two or three weeks after the onset of conjunctivitis and appears as large discrete infiltrations in the superficial stromal area of the cornea. The infiltrations are occasionally visible to the naked eye, and may resemble the sub-epithelial opacities associated with keratoconjunctivitis caused by adenovirus types 8, 10, and 19. These corneal opacities usually appear in the upper and lower zones of the cornea and may remain for several months.

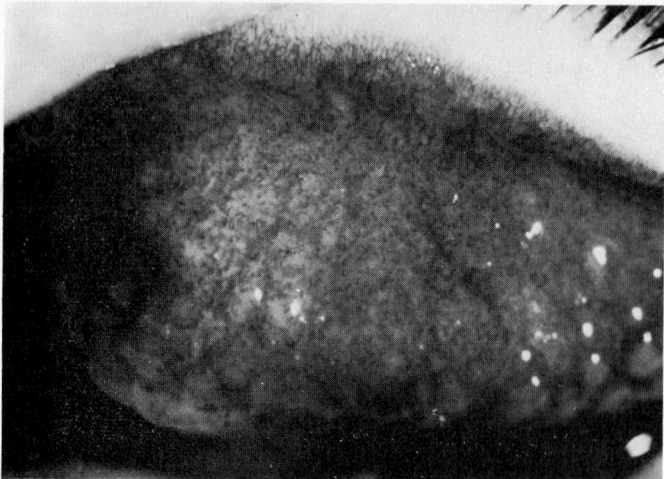

Fig. 6(a) Adult chlamydial ophthalmia: papillae and follicles in the upper tarsal conjunctiva.

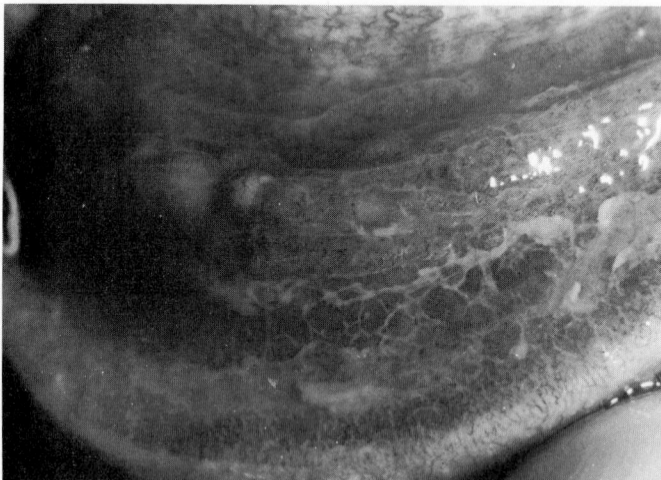

Fig. 6(b) Adult chlamydial ophthalmia: follicles and papillae in the lower conjunctiva.

The classical forms of trachoma—follicular conjunctivitis associated with pannus and/or scarring—have been reported in association with concurrent chlamydial genital infections caused by serotypes D to K. Studies in London suggest that inclusion conjunctivitis, TRIC punctate keratoconjunctivitis, and trachoma of sexually transmitted origin are different manifestations of one disease. Some cases of inclusion conjunctivitis develop punctate subepithelial keratitis, and progress to typical trachoma, whereas in other cases, inclusion conjunctivitis may be present in one eye and trachoma in the other.

Patients with ACO occasionally complain of symptoms of genital infection.

Diagnosis. The clinical features of ACO, particularly the presence of a follicular reaction with large numbers of follicles in the upper and lower fornices, help in the diagnosis. But the differential diagnoses of viral, allergic, and bacterial conjunctivitis should be considered. Laboratory tests are helpful, particularly isolation and micro-IF tests on eye secretions and blood (Table 1).

Treatment and prevention. Topical therapy with tetracycline, rifampicin, or erythromycin eye ointment three times daily for a minimum of five weeks is highly effective. Because of the concurrent genital infection, systemic treatment with tetracycline (15 mg/kg body weight), erythromycin (15 mg/kg), doxycycline (1.5 mg/kg) or sulphamethoxazole (30 mg/kg) daily for three weeks is preferable.

To prevent ocular re-infection, it is imperative to seek for chlamydial genital infections, both in patients and their sexual consorts, and to treat them accordingly.

Ocular infections of animal origin. Some strains of *C. psittaci* can cause ocular infection in man. The psittacosis agent produces an acute but transient papillary conjunctivitis. Feline keratoconjunctivitis (FKC) agent causes a chronic follicular conjunctivitis similar to paratrachoma caused by *C. trachomatis* serotypes D to K. The source of this infection is domestic cats with conjunctivitis and rhinitis, whose ocular and nasal discharges are heavily infected with FKC agent. In London, this micro-organism has been isolated both from the affected eyes of patients and of their domestic cats. Studies of cats in a large cattery in London have shown a high prevalence of feline keratoconjunctivitis. The clinical features of the disease in cats vary from an acute papillary conjunctivitis in young kittens, to a chronic follicular conjunctivitis in young adults and a trachoma-like syndrome in older cats with scarring of the palpebral conjunctiva, pannus, and scarring of the cornea. The FKC agent can also be isolated from the genital tract of female cats, suggesting that genital infection may be the reservoir.

In recent years, a few strains of *C. psittaci* have been isolated from the eyes of patients with follicular conjunctivitis or keratoconjunctivitis. These isolates differ serotypically from other strains of *C. psittaci* known to be pathogenic for man.

Genital infections

Chlamydial genital infections are divided into three groups:
1. Urethritis and associated diseases in men caused mainly by *C. trachomatis* serotypes D to K.
2. Cervicitis and associated diseases in women mainly caused by *C. trachomatis* serotypes D to K.
3. Lymphogranuloma venereum caused by *C. trachomatis* LGV serotypes L1, L2, and L3 (see page 5.307).

Urethritis in men. Chlamydial urethritis is an inflammatory disease transmitted sexually. *Citrachomatis* is the commonest cause of non-gonococcal urethritis (NGU), non-specific urethritis (NSU), and post-gonococcal urethritis (PGU).

Epidemiology. NGU is the commonest sexually transmitted disease in urban populations of developed and developing countries. Recent studies suggest that its incidence is two to three times higher than that of gonococcal urethritis (GU). *C. trachomatis* (serotypes D to K) has been isolated in up to 70 per cent of patients with overt NGU and in up to 80 per cent of those with PGU. Other findings, such as the presence of antichlamydial antibodies in the blood of patients with NGU or the isolation of *C. trachomatis* from the genital tract of their female sexual consorts, suggest that chlamydiae may be responsible for an even higher proportion of NGU. The prevalence of chlamydial urethritis is not known. In London, about 1 per cent of male blood donors have antichlamydial antibodies.

Chlamydial urethritis is common amongst promiscuous adults with a history of other sexually transmitted diseases. Women with chlamydial cervicitis are probably the major reservoir of infection.

C. trachomatis has also been isolated from up to 50 per cent of patients with GU, and 80 per cent of those with PGU, indicating that the two infections are closely associated.

The combination of promiscuity, low standards of personal hygiene, and inadequate treatment of sexually transmitted diseases promotes repeated infection, the development of chronic chlamydial urethritis, and occasionally urethral scarring.

Clinical features. The clinical features of chlamydial urethritis have not been fully described. The results of limited studies in man and in experimentally infected non-human primates have shown that the incubation period is from one to three weeks.

Some patients complain of mild dysuria, frequency of urination and discharge, but many are asymptomatic. In these, the infection may be detected because they develop ocular symptoms or because their sexual partners have a symptomatic infection. The clinical signs may consist of slight swelling and erythema of the glans associated with hyperaemia, diffuse infiltration, and papillary reaction in the urethra. Untreated, the urethritis commonly lasts for a few weeks and may resolve spontaneously. Occasionally, it becomes chronic, lasting for several months, and can be associated with follicles. In patients with repeated recurrences of re-infections, a chronic but mild urethritis develops, lasting for many years. *C. trachomatis* can rarely be isolated at this stage.

Patient's with chlamydial urethritis occasionally develop chlamydial conjunctivitis, pharyngitis, epididymitis, orchitis, prostatitis, or Reiter's syndrome.

Diagnosis. The diagnosis of chlamydial urethritis depends on the isolation of chlamydiae from the urethra (Table 1). A patient's first infection may be diagnosed by a rising titre of serum antibody, detected by the micro-IF test.

Treatment and prevention. Systemic treatment with tetracycline (15 mg/kg body weight), minocycline (3 mg/kg), doxycycline (1.5 mg/kg), erythromycin (15 mg/kg), or sulphonamides (35 mg/kg) daily for a period of three weeks is effective. Simultaneous treatment of the sexual partners of these patients prevents re-infection.

Cervicitis. Chlamydial cervicitis is a mild or asymptomatic sexually transmitted disease. It is one cause of the syndrome of non-specific genital infection (NSGI).

Epidemiology. Chlamydial cervicitis is common amongst women attending clinics for sexually transmitted diseases. *C. trachomatis* has been isolated from the cervix in up to 31 per cent of these women. Significantly higher isolation rates are found in women with gonorrhoea (62 per cent), in sexual consorts of men with NGU (68 per cent), in mothers of babies with NCO (90 per cent), and in women with ACO (90 per cent). The prevalence of chlamydial genital infection in different countries is not known. In the United States, it is estimated that 5–13 per cent of adult sexually active women are infected. In London, approximately 3 per cent of adult women have antibodies against *C. trachomatis* serotypes D to K. Clinical chlamydial cervicitis is commonly found amongst promiscuous women, who are major sources of infection in the community.

Clinical features. The incubation period is unknown. The onset of disease is insidious, and the majority of patients are asymptomatic. Occasionally, patients complain of a mild vaginal discharge, irritation, and discomfort. The clinical signs in the cervix in the majority of patients, with or without symptoms, are mucopurulent discharge in the endocervical canal, hyperaemia, hypertrophic erosions, follicles, and occasionally scarring. The disease generally persists for several months, and *C. trachomatis* has been re-isolated from the cervix for as long as one year. Occasionally, chlamydiae have been isolated from apparently normal cervices.

Patients with chlamydial cervicitis may develop urethritis, proctitis, and pelvic inflammatory disease. *C. trachomatis* has been isolated in the urethra in up to 50 per cent of women who were shown to harbour the organism in their cervix. They may complain of mild dysuria, frequency of urination, and discharge from the urethra. The clinical signs in the urethra may consist of hyperaemia, diffuse infiltration, and papillary reactions. Occasionally cystitis may develop.

Chlamydial infection of the rectum may occur in one-third of patients with cervicitis. Proctitis is generally asymptomatic, although in the majority, clinical signs such as mucopurulent discharge, hyperaemia, diffuse infiltration, and occasionally follicles may be seen in the rectum.

Pelvic inflammatory disease (PID) develops in association with chlamydial cervicitis. *C. trachomatis* has been isolated from the Fallopian tubes of up to 30 per cent and from the cervix in up to 36 per cent of patients with acute PID. High titres of antichlamydial antibodies are found in the blood of up to 73 per cent of patients with PID, and in fluid aspirated from the pouch of Douglas in up to 67 per cent.

Diagnosis. Because of the lack of distinctive signs, clinical diagnosis of chlamydial cervicitis is not possible. Laboratory diagnosis is made by the isolation of chlamydiae or, rarely by the detection of a rising titre of antichlamydial antibodies in the blood or the presence of antibodies in endocervical discharge (Table 1).

Treatment and prevention. Chlamydial cervicitis responds satisfactorily to a three-week course of the following: tetracyclines, (15 mg/kg body weight), minocycline (3 mg/kg), doxycycline (1.5 mg/kg), erythromycin (15 mg/kg), or sulphonamides (35 mg/kg). It is important to avoid treating pregnant women with tetracyclines and their derivatives.

In order to prevent re-infection, it is imperative to treat sexual consorts of patients in parallel. The transmission of chlamydial genital infection may be reduced by detecting and treating infected women, particularly those attending sexually transmitted diseases or family planning clinics.

Systemic infections

Systemic chlamydial infections are divided into:
1. Psittacosis (ornithosis) caused by *C. psittaci*.
2. Pneumonitis, Reiter's disease, perihepatitis, and endocarditis caused by *C. trachomatis*.

Psittacosis. Psittacosis is an infection of psittacines (parrots and related birds) which can be transmitted to humans. Ornithosis is a similar disease of other avian species.

Epidemiology. Psittacosis is a serious hazard to people who keep pet birds or who work in the poultry industry. Approximately 130 species of birds harbour chlamydiae, but psittacine species, poultry, and pigeons are the major sources of human infection. Domestic animals and lower mammals which harbour their own strains of *C. psittaci* may occasionally transmit infection to man. Transmission from man to man is rare. Humans acquire infection by exposure to infected animals, possibly through inhaling dried excreta.

Psittacosis is more common amongst adults. The disease is generally sporadic, but occasionally, outbreaks of infection occur. Psittacosis may constitute 20–25 per cent of cases of atypical pneumonia. The high prevalence of antichlamydial antibodies amongst people working in the poultry industry, veterinaries, and those who handle exotic birds, and who have no history of psittacosis, suggests that mild and sub-clinical forms of disease are common.

Clinical features. The incubation period is generally one to two weeks. The onset may be acute or insidious. Symptoms include high fever, headache, muscular pain, chills, and coughing. Clinically, acute psittacosis presents in two major forms. The first form is pneumonitis (atypical pneumonia) associated with high fever (37.8–39.5 °C) and extensive focal or lobal pneumonia. The second form has features suggestive of a toxic or septic condition: high fever, chills, enlargement of liver and spleen, but only a mild pneumonitis. The severity of clinical signs may decline in the second week, but the course of psittacosis is often prolonged and relapses are not uncommon. The fatality rate in some outbreaks of psittacosis is rather high particularly in older patients. Myocarditis and rarely endocarditis may occur in association with severe or mild psittacosis.

Diagnosis. The clinical features of psittacosis are similar to those of viral pneumonia, typhoid, and protracted influenza. Serological tests necessary to confirm the diagnosis of psittacosis include: the CF test, to detect high levels of antichlamydial antibodies (1:128 or more) or a fourfold rise in titre; and the micro-IF test, to detect type-specific IgM or high levels of type-specific IgG (1:64 or more) in blood.

Treatment and prevention. Systemic therapy with tetracycline (15 mg/kg body weight) daily for a minimum of three weeks is recommended. Shorter courses of treatment may result in relapse of infection. Erythromycin is an effective alternative.
To control psittacosis, it is imperative to:
1. Identify diseased birds, which may have ruffled feathers, conjunctivitis, or diarrhoea, and then to treat or destroy them.
2. Eradicate psittacosis in breeding stocks by feeding them medicated seed for at least 30 days, and supplementing their food with vitamins and tetracycline.
3. Provide clean and secure premises for parakeets.
4. Quarantine imported psittacines and treat them with medicated seed for 30 days.

Pneumonia in infants. C. trachomatis is a major cause of pneumonia in infants in the United States, where the incidence is estimated to be three to four cases per 1000 newborn babies. In the United Kingdom, the incidence is very low. The disease occurs in infants under the age of three months and is normally associated with NCO, and a high level of antichlamydial antibodies in blood. Chlamydia can be isolated from the upper respiratory tract and occasionally from the lung.

The affected infant is commonly afebrile, has slight breathing difficulty, a characteristic cough (closely spaced staccato coughs separated by a brief inspiration), and a diffuse pneumonia. The disease generally resolves without intervention, but severe disease and death occasionally occur.

The clinical diagnosis is suggested when pneumonia is associated with conjunctivitis. The isolation of chlamydiae from the eye or respiratory tract, and detection of high levels of antichlamydial antibodies in blood confirm the diagnosis.

Systemic therapy with erythromycin or sulphonamides for a minimum of three weeks is recommended.

Reiter's disease. The main features of Reiter's disease are arthritis, urethritis, and keratoconjunctivitis. The arthritis is generally asymmetric and involves the large joints. Occasionally, phalangeal arthritis and ankylosing spondylitis may develop. The urethritis presents as (NGU) with discharge, frequent urination, and dysuria. In the eye, papillary conjunctivitis, punctate epithelial keratitis, stromal keratitis, and occasionally anterior uveitis may develop. The signs do not always occur together. Generally arthritis and urethritis appear together, preceded by conjunctivitis.

Reiter's disease occurs in an epidemic form and a sporadic form. The latter is common amongst young men who have a history of venereal disease or who are contacts of patients with these diseases. The sporadic form develops in about 1 per cent of patients with NGU. C. trachomatis may be a cause of the disease because it has been isolated from the urethra in up to 30 per cent of patients, and because the majority of patients have high levels of antichlamydial antibodies in their blood. C. trachomatis has not yet been isolated from synovial fluid.

Perihepatitis. Perihepatitis, associated with peritonitis and pelvic inflammatory disease (Curtis Fitz-Hugh syndrome), may occur as a complication of sexually transmitted diseases. The isolation of C. trachomatis from the genital tract of some of these patients, and the presence of high levels of antichlamydial antibodies in their blood suggest that C. trachomatis is a cause of this syndrome.

Endocarditis. Recently, a case of endocarditis caused by C. trachomatis has been reported. A young, pregnant woman, with a history of genital infection, developed fever, nausea, pericarditis, aortic murmur, and transient hemiparesis. Necropsy showed a haemorrhagic cortical infarct, acute bronchopneumonia, exudate in the pericardial sac, left ventricular hypertrophy, and fingerlike projections on the ventricular surface of the left coronary cusp. The fingerlike projections resembled those seen in endocarditis caused by C. psittaci. Electron microscopy of the tissue showed the presence of chlamydial elementary and reticulate bodies. Micro-IF tests on blood collected at 15 and 10 days before death showed a 16-fold increase in the level of IgM against C. trachomatis serotype G.

Host–parasite relationships

The clinical manifestations of chlamydial disease depend on the pathogen, the site of infection, and host responses. In human ocular infection, there are considerable differences between the clinical features of trachoma, associated with C. trachomatis serotypes A to C and paratrachoma, associated with serotypes D to K. These differences are evidently not due to the differences between serotypes because experimental ocular infection of human volunteers with strains isolated from trachoma or paratrachoma produce similar, acute, self-limiting diseases, and do not cause scarring or pannus. It is, therefore, considered likely that immune responses are important in the pathogenesis of trachoma.

Immune responses

Humoral immune responses. Infection leads to the appearance of antibodies in blood and local discharges. In the majority of humans with chlamydial infection, serum antibody titres are low. High titres are only found in the comparatively uncommon systemic infections. Repeated infection does not produce further increases in antibody titres.

Cell-mediated responses. Infection induces cell-mediated responses which can be demonstrated by skin tests or *in vitro* techniques. Surveys of cell-mediated responses in various groups of people have produced conflicting results. Some studies have found positive skin tests or *in vitro* tests in both infected and also uninfected people with no history of chlamydial infection, whilst others have observed a disappointing lack of response in patients with microbiologically proven infection. This variability in results suggests that in some instances, the tests lack specificity, and in others, they lack sensitivity.

Experiments in a guinea pig model (see below) have shown that the number of chlamydial particles required to elicit skin responses is rather high, and it is possible that the lack of response in some studies may be due to the use of an insufficient dose of antigen.

The role of immune responses. Evidence from animal models, experimental human infections, and field studies suggest that immune responses to Chlamydia may have some protective effect, but also contribute to the pathogenesis of trachoma.

Studies of human experimental ocular infection with various serotypes of C. trachomatis have shown that whilst primary infection is a moderate, self-limiting disease which does not cause blinding damage, re-infection causes more severe, long-lasting disease, and the development of pannus and scarring.

Studies of experimental infection of primates with C. trachomatis have shown that pannus develops only in animals which have had previous exposure to Chlamydia. The mode of exposure (eye infection or immunization) and strain (homologous or heterologous) is unimportant.

Studies in the guinea pig, infected with its own ocular pathogen, GPIC agent, have produced a range of ocular diseases. Primary ocular infection is an acute, self-limiting disease which does not cause permanent damage to the eye. Many chlamydial inclusions are found in conjunctival epithelial cells, and many polymorphonuclear cells are present. Re-infection produces more severe disease which is also self-limiting. There are fewer inclusions and many more mononuclear cells compared with primary infection. Repeated re-infection produces severe, chronic inflammatory diseases, and the development of follicles, scarring of the conjunctiva, lid deformities, and pannus. There are many mononuclear cells, but no chlamydial inclusions. Re-infection requires only slightly more chlamydial particles than primary infection, showing that there is no good protective immunity.

Field studies in Iran have shown that trachoma is a multicyclic disease. Young children have active inflammatory disease, but they rarely have blinding complications. These complications are commonly found in adults who rarely have acute disease. However, mothers in large families with several young children have a higher incidence of active disease and blinding lesions. The results of these clinical, experimental, and epidemiological studies suggest that inclusion conjunctivitis and trachoma represent the two ends of a spectrum of disease, and that the development of trachoma results from a high rate of re-infection associated with hypersensitivity.

Latency. Chlamydial infection of psittacine birds is not normally apparent and often goes undetected until humans are infected. It is when these birds are kept in crowded and insanitary conditions that they commonly develop overt disease. It has therefore been suggested that they have a latent infection. In the absence of thorough clinical and microbiological studies of healthy birds captured in the wild, it is not possible to decide whether they have mild, persistent infection, are carriers, or have latent infection.

It has also been suggested that latency occurs in trachoma and chlamydial genital infection. The evidence is by no means convincing since clinical examinations are often inadequate, and the microbiological methods used are not the most sensitive. For example, in studies of trachoma, clinical examination is often limited to the upper tarsal conjunctiva, which may be free of active disease whilst the fornices exhibit signs of active infection. Cytological diagnostic methods are commonly used, which demonstrate only the presence of growing, replicating *C. trachomatis*, and cannot detect free elementary bodies. In studies of chlamydial genital infection, clinical examination is often not carried out, and negative isolation results are not a sufficient basis on which to propose latent disease.

We therefore consider it unlikely that true latent chlamydial infection occurs in humans. Thorough clinical examination coupled with the most sensitive laboratory techniques may establish that mild persistent infections are common, and that some individuals may be carriers.

Laboratory diagnosis

Cytology. The direct demonstration of chlamydial inclusions in exfoliated cells is still a useful test, particularly in ocular infections (Fig. 7). The collection of conjunctival cells is generally preceded by topical anaesthesia. Cells are collected on a sterilized metal spatula, which is applied to the everted conjunctiva with firm, even strokes. Plastic impression spatulae, to which cells adhere, can be used without local anaesthesia.

Methods of collection of specimens from the genital tract vary, but generally, after cleaning the meatus, urethral cells can be collected with a specially designed curette. Cervical scrapings are collected from the marginal area of the os after exposing the cervix with a speculum.

Scrapings are spread thinly and evenly on to clean microscope slides and allowed to dry. They are stained with iodine, Giemsa, immunofluorescent antibody, immunoperoxidase or immunoferritin.

In NCO, cytology, with Giemsa staining provides a sensitive, simple and rapid diagnostic test. In trachoma, immunofluorescent staining gives a much more sensitive test than Giemsa staining. In genital infection, cytology is of little value.

Isolation. Specimens are usually collected by swabbing. In the eye, specimens are taken by firmly swabbing the whole palpebral

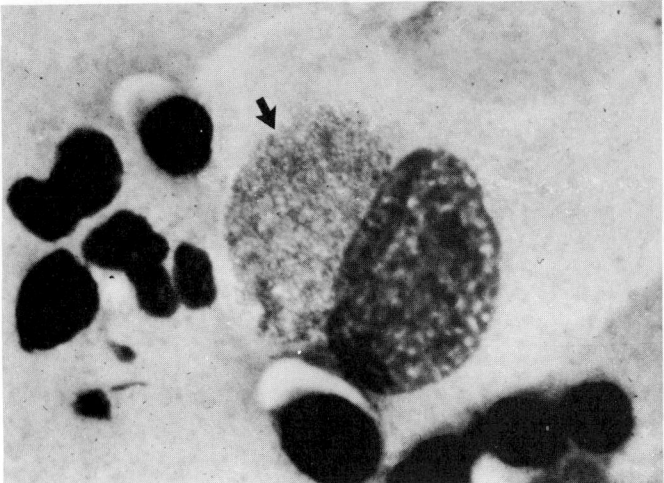

Fig. 7 *Chlamydia trachomatis* inclusions in exfoliated conjunctival epithelium, stained with Giemsa.

conjunctiva with a dry, sterile cotton swab. Urethral specimens are collected by inserting a swab into the endourethra and gently rotating it before withdrawal. Cervical specimens are collected in a similar fashion from the endocervical canal. Specimens from the Fallopian tubes may be collected with a swab attached to a catheter during laparoscopy. Specimens from patients with psittacosis may include sputum, pleural fluid, blood, and lung biopsies, all of which should be handled with caution to avoid spreading infection to laboratory personnel.

Specimens should be placed in a suitable transport medium such as sucrose phosphate containing antibiotics (e.g. streptomycin and vancomycin) to suppress the growth of other bacteria. The best isolation results are achieved when specimens are inoculated within a few hours of collection. However, if this is not possible, specimens should be frozen as soon as possible after collection and stored at −70 °C or in liquid nitrogen until inoculation.

Several cell culture systems are used, all of which require centrifugation of the inoculum on to treated cells. The most commonly used systems are McCoy cells, pretreated with ionizing radiation or 5-iodo-2-deoxyuridine, or treated after inoculation with cycloheximide (Fig. 8a, b, and c). These methods are probably equally sensitive.

Inoculated cell cultures are incubated for 48–72 hours, and then stained with iodine, Giemsa, or immunofluorescent techniques. Giemsa staining followed by dark-field microscopy is more sensi-

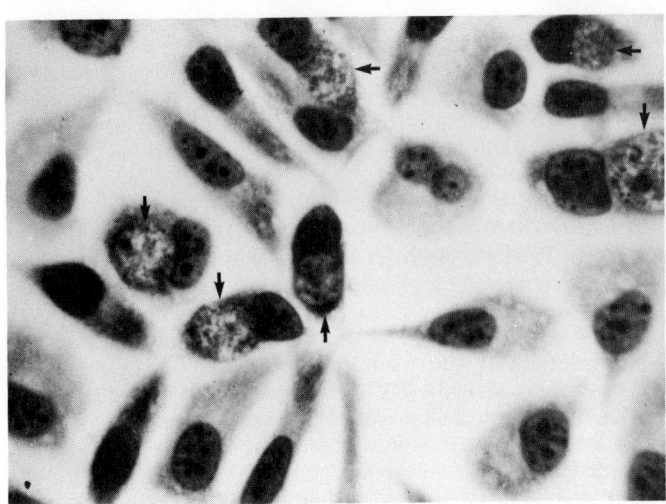

Fig. 8(a) Chlamydia trachomatis inclusions in cycloheximide-treated McCoy cells, stained with Giemsa and viewed by bright-field illumination.

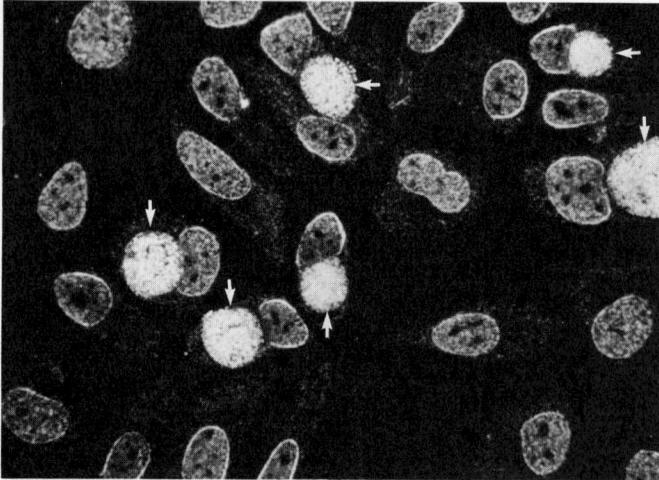

Fig. 8(b)   The same as Fig. 8(a) but viewed by dark-field illumination.

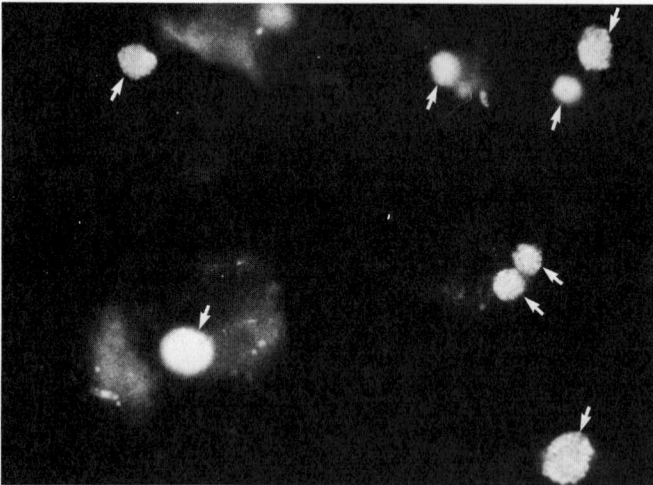

Fig. 8(c)   The same as Fig. 8(a) 24 hours after inoculation, stained using an indirect fluorescent antibody technique.

tive than iodine staining for the detection of *C. trachomatis*. *C psittaci* is not stained by iodine, but is visible when stained with Giemsa and examined under bright-field illumination.

Using immunofluorescence or immunoperoxidase staining methods, inclusions can be detected in cell cultures within 24 hours of inoculation, providing a very rapid and sensitive diagnostic test.

In London, using irradiated McCoy cells, chlamydiae have been isolated from 90 per cent of patients with neonatal and adult chlamydial ophthalmia; from 73 per cent of those with severe hyperendemic trachoma; from 68 per cent of men with severe NGU; and from 90 per cent of cervical specimens collected with women from ACO.

Serology. The CF test is used in the diagnosis of LGV and psittacosis. The test, which detects a group-specific antibody, is not sufficiently sensitive for the serodiagnosis of ocular and genital infections.

The micro-IF test is used extensively in studies of ocular and genital infection. It is very sensitive and detects type-specific antibodies. Fifteen serotypes of *C. trachomatis* have been characterized, but the use of all these serotypes makes the test laborious. A modification has been introduced, in which these serotypes are combined into three pools, and a pool of representative strains of *C. psittaci* added. This simplifies the test without sacrificing speci-

ficity or sensitivity. The collection of whole blood from finger pricks, or local discharges, using dry cellulose sponges further simplifies the technique.

It is usually impossible to demonstrate the classical four-fold increase in antibodies in acute and convalescent specimens because the onset of genital infection and trachoma is generally insidious, and because in ACO, genital infection precedes ocular infection.

In ACO, the presence of antichlamydial IgG or IgA in eye secretions, or specific IgG at a titre of 1:64 or more, or Specific IgM in serum correlates well with clinically active disease from which *C. trachomatis* can be isolated.

In men with NGU or PGU, the presence of antichlamydial IgG in serum at a titre of 1:20 or greater may be suggestive of active infection although some men with isolation-positive urethritis have no antibody. It is sometimes possible to find seroconversion, or specific IgM after PGU.

In women with non-specific genital infection, the presence of antichlamydial antibodies in local discharges or specific IgM or IgG in serum at a level of 1:64 or more, are indicative of active chlamydial cervicitis. Women with acute salpingitis often have levels of IgG in blood in excess of 1:128 and antibodies detectable in aspirates from the Fallopian tubes or the pouch of Douglas.

Patients with LGV infections have very high levels of antibodies which cross-react with most serotypes of *C. trachomatis*. High levels of antibodies against *C. psittaci* are found in patients with psittacosis, using the modified micro-IF test.

References

Becker, Y. (1974). *The agent of trachoma.* Monographs in virology vol. 7. Karger, Basel.
Darougar, S., Kinnison, J., and Jones, B. R. (1971). Simplified irradiated McCoy cell culture for isolation of chlamydiae. In *Trachoma and related disorders* (ed. R. L. Nichols), 63. Excerpta Medica International Congress Series 223.
Darougar, S., Monnickendam, M. A., El-Sheikh, H., Treharne, J. D., Woodland, R. M., and Jones, B. R. (1977). Animal models for the study of chlamydial infections of the eye and genital tract. In *Non-gonococcal urethritis and related infections.* (eds. D. Hobson and K. K. Holmes), 186. American Society for Microbiology, Washington, D.C.
—, and Treharne, J. D. (1981). Chlamydial infections: laboratory aspects. In *Recent advances in sexually transmitted diseases*, vol. 2 (ed. J. W. R. Harris), 141. Churchill Livingstone, Edinburgh.
Dawson, C. R., Jones, B. R., and Darougar, S. (1975). Blinding and non-blinding trachoma. The assessment of intensity of upper tarsal inflammatory disease and disabling lesions. *Bull. Wld Hlth* **52**, 279.
Dunlop, E. M. C. (1980). Chlamydial infection: clinical aspects. In *Recent advances in sexually transmitted diseases*, vol. 2 (ed. J. W. R. Harris), 101, Churchill Livingstone, Edinburgh.
Jones, B. R. (1974). Ocular syndromes of TRIC virus infection and their possible genital significance. *Br. J. vener. Dis.* **40**, 3.
— (1975). The prevention of blindness from trachoma. *Trans. ophthal. Soc. U.K.* **95**, 16.
Monnickendam, M. A., Darougar, S., Treharne, J. D., and Tilbury, A. M. (1980). Development of chronic conjunctivitis with scarring and pannus, resembling trachoma, in guinea pigs. *Br. J. Ophthal.* **64**, 284.
Muller-Schoop, J. W., Wang, S. P., Munzinger, J., Schlapfer, H. U., Knoblanch, M. and Ammann, R. W. (1978). *Chlamydia trachomatis* as a possible cause of peritonitis and perihepatitis in young women. *Br. med. J.* **i**, 1022.
Schachter, J., and Dawson, C. R. (1978). *Human chlamydial infections.* PSG Publishing, Littleton, Massachusetts.
Storz, J. (1971). *Chlamydia and chlamydia-induced disease.* C. C. Thomas, Springfield, Illinois.
Taylor-Robinson, D. and Thomas, B. J. (1980). The role of *Chlamydia trachomatis* in genital tract and associated diseases. *J. clin. Path.* **33**, 205.
Treharne, J. D., Darougar, S., and Jones, B. R. (1977). Modification of the micro-immunofluorescence test to provide a routine serodiagnostic test for chlamydial infection. *J. Clin. Path.* **30**, 510.
Van der Bel-Kah, J. M., Watanakunakorn, C., Menefee, M. G., Long, H. D., and Picter, R. (1978). *Chlamydia trachomatis* endocarditis. *Am. Heart J.* **95**, 627.

Mycoplasmas

D. Taylor-Robinson

Characteristics of mycoplasmas. Mycoplasmas, originally called pleuropneumonia-like organisms (PPLO), are the smallest free-living micro-organisms. They lack a cell wall so that they are resistant to penicillins and other antimicrobials which act on this structure. Instead, they are bounded by a pliable unit membrane which encloses the cytoplasm, DNA, RNA, and other metabolic components necessary for propagation in cell-free media. Mycoplasmas have a number of other characteristics which also distinguish them from bacteria, chlamydiae, and viruses (Table 1). Furthermore, they are not related to the L-phase variants of bacteria.

Table 1   Characteristics of mycoplasmas compared to those of bacteria, chlamydiae and viruses

Characteristic	Mycoplasmas	Bacteria	Chlamydiae	Viruses
Size (diameter)	$0.3\ \mu m$*	$1–2\ \mu m$	$0.3\ \mu m$	$< 0.5\ \mu m$
Lack a cell wall	yes	no	no	yes
Contain both DNA and RNA	yes	yes	yes	no
Multiplication on cell-free medium	yes	yes	no	no
Multiplication dependent on host cell nucleic acid	no	no	no	yes
Usually require sterol and native protein for propagation	yes	no	no	no
Intrinsic energy metabolism	yes	yes	yes	no
Usually narrow range of host specificity	yes	no	no	yes
Growth inhibited by specific antibody alone	yes	no	yes	yes
Resistant to cell-wall active antibiotics (e.g. penicillins)	yes	no	no	yes
Resistant to antibiotics which inhibit metabolism (e.g. tetracycline)	no	no	no	yes

* Smallest organisms capable of propagation

Despite the general similarity among mycoplasmas, they comprise a heterogeneous group of micro-organisms which differ from one another in DNA composition, nutritional requirements, metabolic reactions, antigenic composition, and host specificity. Taxonomically the mycoplasmas are divided into three families (Table 2), the Mycoplasmataceae, which require sterol for growth, the Acholeplasmataceae, which do not, and the Spiroplasmataceae which also require sterol but, in addition, have a characteristic helical structure. The mycoplasmas isolated commonly from humans belong to the Mycoplasmataceae. This family comprises the genus *Mycoplasma*, which contains organisms that do not hydrolyse urea, and the genus *Ureaplasma*, the organisms of which do hydrolyze urea. The latter originally were termed T-strains or T-mycoplasmas because of the tiny colonies they form on agar medium.

The small size of the mycoplasma genome restricts their metabolic capabilities. Nevertheless, apart from their importance in man, certain mycoplasma species are of economic importance because of the pneumonia, arthritis, keratoconjunctivitis, and mastitis they cause among livestock and poultry in Africa, Australia, and other parts of the world. Furthermore, a number of mycoplasma species are a laboratory nuisance as occult contaminants of cell cultures.

Occurrence of mycoplasmas in man. Twelve mycoplasma species constitute the normal flora or are pathogens of humans (Table 3). Most of them are found in the oropharynx. There is no information, as yet, about the distribution or significance of *M. genitalium*, which has been discovered recently in the genito-urinary tract.

Respiratory infections

The relationship of mycoplasmas to respiratory disease. Evidence that any mycoplasma, apart from *M. pneumoniae*, is implicated in acute respiratory disease is lacking. Although adult male volunteers given large numbers of *M. hominis* organisms orally, developed a mild exudative pharyngitis accompanied by an antibody response, attempts to demonstrate that this mycoplasma is a cause of naturally occurring sore throats in children and adults have been unsuccessful.

In the late 1930s non-bacterial pneumonias were first recognized and brought under the heading of primary atypical pneumonia (PAP) to distinguish them from typical lobar pneumonia. Gradually PAP was recognized to be aetiologically heterogeneous and, in one variety, cold agglutinins often developed. It was from this form of disease that an infectious agent was isolated in embryonated eggs. This micro-organism, the 'Eaton agent', produced pneumonia in cotton rats and hamsters, and for a number of years was thought to be a virus. However, serious doubts about this arose when it was found to be affected by chlortetracycline and gold salts, and its mycoplasmal nature was finally established by cultivation on a cell-free agar medium. The agent was subsequently called *M. pneumoniae* and its ability to cause respiratory disease was estab-

Table 2   Classification of and some distinguishing features among members of the Mycoplasmatales

Classification		Distinguishing features				
		Sterol required	Genome size (dalton)	NADH oxidase	Urea metabolized	Helical organisms
Class:	Mollicutes					
Order:	Mycoplasmatales					
Family I:	Mycoplasmataceae	yes	5×10^8	in cytoplasm		no
Genus I:	*Mycoplasma*				no	
	About 50 species					
Genus II:	*Ureaplasma*				yes	
	Single species, *U. urealyticum* with at least 14 serotypes					
Family II:	Acholeplasmataceae	no	1×10^9	in membrane		no
Genus I:	*Acholeplasma*				no	
	6 species					
Family III:	Spiroplasmataceae (proposed)	yes	1×10^9	in cytoplasm		yes
Genus I:	*Spiroplasma*				no	
	Single species, *S. citri*					

Table 3　The biological features, occurrence, and disease association of mycoplasmas isolated from human subjects

| Mycoplasma | Metabolism of | Preferred atmosphere | Haemadsorption | Frequency of isolation from the | | | | | Cause of disease |
				Respiratory tract	Genito-urinary tract	Rectum	Eye	Blood	
M. buccale	arginine	anaerobic*	no	rare	–†	–	–	–	no
M. faucium	arginine	anaerobic	yes‡	rare	–	–	–	–	no
M. fermentans	glucose, arginine	anaerobic	no	–	rare	–	–	–	no
M. hominis	arginine	aerobic	no	rare	common	common	rare	very rare	yes
M. genitalium	glucose	anaerobic	yes	?	?	?	?	?	?
A. laidlawii	glucose	anaerobic	no	rare	–	–	–	–	no
M. lipophilum	arginine	anaerobic	no	rare	–	–	–	–	no
M. orale	arginine	anaerobic	yes‡	common	–	–	–	–	no
M. pneumoniae	glucose	aerobic	yes	rare§	very rare	–	–	–	yes
M. primatum	arginine	anaerobic	no	–	rare	–	–	–	no
M. salivarium	arginine	anaerobic	no	common	rare	–	–	–	no
U. urealyticum	urea	anaerobic	serotype 3 only	rare	common	common	rare	very rare	yes

* 5% CO_2, 95% nitrogen.
† No reports of isolation.
‡ With chick erythrocytes only.
§ Except in disease outbreaks.

lished fully by studies based on isolation, serology, volunteer inoculation, and vaccine protection.

M. pneumoniae disease manifestations. M. pneumoniae produces a spectrum of effects from inapparent infection, mild afebrile upper respiratory tract disease to severe pneumonia. Clinical manifestations often are not sufficiently distinctive to permit an early definitive diagnosis of mycoplasmal pneumonia. Indeed, the latter shares the features of other non-bacterial pneumonias in that general symptoms, such as malaise and headache, often precede chest symptoms by one to five days, and radiographic examination frequently reveals evidence of pneumonia before physical signs, such as rales, become apparent. Usually, only one of the lower lobes is involved and the radiograph most often shows patchy opacities. About 20 per cent of patients suffer bilateral pneumonia, but pleurisy and pleural effusions are unusual. The course of the disease is variable, but often it is protracted. Thus, cough, abnormal chest signs, and changes in the radiograph may persist for several weeks and relapse is a feature. The organisms also may persist in respiratory secretions despite antibiotic therapy, and this is particularly so in hypogammaglobulinaemic patients where excretion may continue for months or years rather than weeks. Although a few very severe infections have been reported, occurring usually in patients with immunodeficiency or sickle cell anaemia, death has occurred rarely. In children, infection has been characterized occasionally by a prolonged illness with paroxysmal cough followed by vomiting, thus simulating the features of whooping cough (see page 5.203).

Extrapulmonary manifestations. Illness caused by M. pneumoniae is limited usually to the respiratory tract, but a wide variety of extrapulmonary clinical conditions may occur during the course of the respiratory illness or as a sequel to it. These complications and an estimation of the frequency of their occurrence are shown in Table 4. Haemolytic anaemia with crisis is brought about by the development and action of cold agglutinins (anti-I antibodies). There is dispute about the mechanism of their production but the organisms may alter the I antigen on erythrocytes sufficiently to stimulate an auto-immune response. It is possible that some of the other clinical conditions, such as the neurological complications, may arise in a similar way. However, invasion of the central nervous system cannot be discounted as there is one report of the isolation of M. pneumoniae from cerebrospinal fluid. Furthermore, M. hominis has been isolated from the cerebrospinal fluid of neonatal infants suffering from meningitis.

Diagnosis. Mycoplasmas are Gram negative but are not recognizable in Gram-stained smears. The diagnosis depends, therefore, on culturing specimens and/or performing a specific (complement fixation) or non-specific (cold agglutinin) serological test. The usual medium employed for isolation of M. pneumoniae consists of PPLO broth, 20 per cent horse serum and 10 per cent (v/v) fresh yeast extract (25 per cent w/v). However, it seems that a more sensitive medium is that used for the isolation of spiroplasmas, comprising essentially a conventional mycoplasma broth medium with fetal calf serum and a tissue-culture supplement. Either medium is supplemented with thallium acetate, penicillin, and glucose with phenol red as a pH indicator. Such fluid medium inoculated with sputum, throat washing, pharyngeal swab, or other specimen is incubated at 37 °C and a colour change (red to yellow), which occurs usually within 4 to 21 days, signals the fermentation of glucose (Table 3) with production of acid due to multiplication of the organisms. This preliminary identification may be confirmed after subculturing to agar medium. Since erythrocytes of any animal species adsorb almost uniquely to M. pneumoniae colonies (Table 3), haemadsorption provides a presumptive identification which may be confirmed by demonstrating inhibition of colony development around discs impregnated with specific antiserum.

Table 4　Extra-pulmonary manifestations of M. pneumoniae infections

System	Manifestation	Estimated frequency
Cardiovascular	myocarditis, pericarditis	< 5%
Dermatological	erythema multiforme; Stevens–Johnson syndrome; other rashes	some skin involvement in about 25%
Gastrointestinal	anorexia, nausea, vomiting and transient diarrhoea	14–44%
	hepatitis	?
	pancreatitis	?
Genitourinary	tubo-ovarian abscess	insignificant
	acute glomerulonephritis	?
Haematological	cold agglutinin production	about 50%
	haemolytic anaemia	?
	thrombocytopenia	?
	intravascular coagulation	50 reported cases
Musculoskeletal	myalgia, arthralgia	14–45%
	arthritis	?
Neurological	meningitis, meningoencephalitis, ascending paralysis, transient myelitis, cranial nerve palsy, poliomyelitis-like illness	6–7%

Since culture and identification is slow, it is used usually only as a research tool or in special circumstances. Antibody is detectable by a variety of procedures but many are not practical for most laboratories. However, a complement-fixation test is undertaken easily and a four-fold or greater rise in antibody titre with a peak at about three to four weeks indicates a recent infection. The test is positive in this way in about 80 per cent of cases. An antibody titre of 1:128 or greater in a single serum is suggestive of a recent infection; a four-fold or greater fall in antibody titre perhaps over six months may be helpful but sometimes it may be difficult to relate it to a particular prior illness. Cold agglutinins, detected by agglutination of O Rh-negative erythrocytes at 4 °C, develop in about half the patients. Although they are occasionally induced by a number of other conditions, a titre of 1:128 or greater is suggestive of a recent M. pneumoniae infection. When the test is negative, it should be repeated perhaps after a week because a rise in the titre of cold agglutinins is meaningful.

Epidemiology

Relationship to age. M. pneumoniae affects children and adults, the consequence of infection depending upon age. Thus, about a quarter of infections in persons 9–14 years old result in pneumonia while about 7 per cent of infections in young adults do so. Thereafter, pneumonia is even less frequent, but generally is more severe the older the patient.

Relative importance of M. pneumoniae. Although M. pneumoniae causes inapparent and mild upper respiratory-tract infections more commonly than severe disease, it is responsible for only a small proportion of all upper respiratory-tract disease, most of it being of viral aetiology. Acute pharyngitis, occurring mostly in adolescents and younger persons, is due mainly to group A streptococci and rarely to M. pneumoniae. However, the mycoplasma plays a relatively greater part in producing pneumonia. Although bacteria still cause most cases of pneumonia, in certain groups of people pneumonia caused by M. pneumoniae ranks high and outweighs in frequency that caused by respiratory viruses. Thus, it has been calculated that in a large general population, the proportion of all pneumonias due to M. pneumoniae is about 15 per cent and in certain populations, for example military recruits, it may be responsible for as much as 40 per cent of acute pneumonic illness. There is very little evidence that other infections predispose to infection by M. pneumoniae or vice versa. The occurrence of *Haemophilus influenzae* pneumonia soon after infection by M. pneumoniae seems to be a rare event.

Distribution and spread of infection. M. pneumoniae infections have been reported from every country where appropriate diagnostic tests have been undertaken. Infection is endemic in most areas and occurs during all months of the year with a predilection for late summer and early autumn. However, epidemic peaks have been observed about every four years in some countries. The incubation period ranges from two to three weeks and spread from person to person occurs slowly, usually where there is continual or repeated close contact, for example in a family, rather than where there is only casual contact.

Immunopathological factors in the development of *M. pneumoniae* pneumonia.

Several observations indicate that immune mechanisms play a role in the development of M. pneumoniae pneumonia in man. Death due to it has been reported rarely so that the histopathological picture is derived mainly from experimental infection of hamsters and natural mycoplasmal disease in other animals. The pneumonic infiltrate is predominantly a peribronchiolar and perivascular cuffing by lymphocytes, most of which are thymus-dependent. The importance of cell-mediated immune mechanisms in the pathogenesis of M. pneumoniae pneumonia is indicated by the fact that immunosuppression of hamsters, in a variety of ways, results in ablation of the pneumonia or a decrease in its severity. The development of a cell-mediated immune response to M. pneumoniae has been shown further by positive lymphocyte trans-

formation, macrophage migration-inhibition and delayed hypersensitivity skin tests. A polysaccharide-protein fraction of the organisms is involved in this response rather than the glycolipid which is the main antigenic determinant in complement fixation and other serological reactions. The initial lymphocyte response is followed by a change in the character of the bronchiolar exudate with polymorphonuclear leucocytes and macrophages predominating. The rather slow development of these events on primary infection contrasts with accelerated and often more intense host response seen on reinfection. To at least some extent, therefore, the pneumonia caused by M. pneumoniae is an immunopathological process. Children two to five years of age often possess mycoplasmacidal antibody suggesting infection at an early age, although it remains to be determined whether this antibody is induced primarily by M. pneumoniae infection or by related glycolipids in bacteria and plants. Nevertheless, it is tempting to suggest that the pneumonia which occurs in older persons is an immunological over-response to reinfection, the lung being infiltrated by previously sensitized lymphocytes.

Treatment. Mycoplasmas are indifferent to the penicillins, cephalosporins, and other antibiotics that affect cell wall synthesis, but they are generally sensitive to those antibiotics which inhibit protein synthesis. Thus, M. pneumoniae, like other mycoplasmas, is most sensitive to the tetracyclines but more sensitive to erythromycin than the other mycoplasmas of human origin. The value of tetracyclines was shown first in a controlled trial of dimethylchlortetracycline in US marine recruits, a dose of 300 mg three times daily for six days significantly reducing the duration of fever, pulmonary infiltration, and other signs and symptoms. Since then other trials also have provided evidence for the effectiveness of various tetracyclines, as well as erythromycin and josamycin. Planned trials provide the most favourable conditions for determining the value of antibiotics but in civilian practice they have proved less effective, probably because disease is often well-established before treatment is instituted. Despite this, it is worthwhile treating with an antibiotic. For pregnant women and children it is advisable to use erythromycin rather than a tetracycline, and the former antibiotic has sometimes proved more effective than a tetracycline in adults. Successful treatment of clinical disease, however, is not always accompanied by early eradication of the organisms from the respiratory tract, probably because the drugs only inhibit their multiplication and do not kill them. This is a possible reason for relapse in some patients and a plausible reason for recommending a two-to-three week course of antibiotic treatment. It is a moot point whether early treatment would prevent some of the complications but nevertheless it should commence as soon as possible. Since laboratory confirmation of M. pneumoniae infection may take several weeks, it would seem wise to start antibiotic treatment on the basis of the clinical evidence and a cold agglutinin and/or complement-fixing antibody titre of 1:128 or greater in a single serum sample.

The true value of corticosteroids is in doubt although, in conjunction with antibiotics, they appear to have been helpful in patients with severe pneumonia and erythema multiforme.

Prevention

Resistance to disease. One of the best ways of assessing the relative importance of cell-mediated and humoral immune mechanisms in resistance is to determine the ability of lymphocytes and of serum from immune animals to confer immunity when they are transferred to recipient non-immune animals. Most of the information on the protective capacity of 'immune' cells and serum has been obtained not from the M. pneumoniae hamster model but from another mycoplasmal pneumonia model, namely M. pulmonis infection of mice. Serum from mice infected up to five weeks previously protects recipient syngeneic mice against respiratory disease, whereas spleen cells do not. This suggests that humoral immune mechanisms are relatively more important than cell-mediated ones in resistance. However, serum antibody to *M. pneumoniae* does not confer complete protection against infection or disease since they may occur despite high titres of, for example, serum mycoplasmacidal antibody. Furthermore, mycoplasmal infection of the respiratory tract of laboratory animals may stimulate only a weak antibody response and yet induce greater resistance to reinfection and disease than parenteral inoculation of organisms which stimulates much higher titres of serum antibodies. Such observations have led to the belief that local immune factors are crucial in resistance. The correlation between the resistance of adult volunteers to *M. pneumoniae* disease and the presence of IgA antibody in respiratory secretions is consistent with this contention. This antibody could provide the first line of defence by preventing attachment of the organisms to respiratory epithelial cells.

Vaccination. The efficacy of inactivated *M. pneumoniae* vaccines in preventing pneumonia caused by this mycoplasma has ranged from 45 per cent to 67 per cent in field trials. Some protection is consistent with the known ability of transferred serum antibody to suppress the development of *M. pulmonis*-induced pneumonia in the mouse model. The failure of killed *M. pneumoniae* vaccines to protect fully may have been due to poor antigenicity of some of them. Others, however, induced serum antibody levels similar to those that develop after natural infection, which suggests that the relatively poor protection afforded by the vaccines may have been due to their inability to stimulate local antibody production. With this in mind, live attenuated temperature-sensitive mutants of *M. pneumoniae* have been produced which multiply at the temperature of the upper, but not the lower, respiratory tract. Some of these mutants have produced pulmonary infection of hamsters without causing pathological changes, and infection of human volunteers without causing disease. In so doing the mutants have induced significant resistance to subsequent challenge with virulent wild strains of *M. pneumoniae* but whether they can be made sufficiently stable and attenuated for human vaccination on a large scale remains to be seen. Even if this is feasible, their ability to induce permanent protection would seem unlikely since the occurrence of re-infections and second bouts of *M. pneumoniae* pneumonia suggests that naturally-acquired *M. pneumoniae* infection does not provide life-long immunity. Furthermore, it is possible that live mutants could trigger the immunopathological events that seem to be important in the development of disease.

Chronic respiratory disease. Since mycoplasmas of animals are frequently involved in chronic illnesses, the possible role of mycoplasmas in human chronic respiratory disease, particularly chronic bronchitis, is worthy of consideration.

M. pneumoniae infections. The isolation of *M. pneumoniae* from some patients experiencing an acute exacerbation of chronic bronchitis, in addition to a serological response, suggests that this mycoplasma apart from viruses, is sometimes responsible for the exacerbation. The occurrence of complement-fixing antibody to *M. pneumoniae* more frequently in the sera of patients suffering from chronic bronchitis than in those of normal subjects is in keeping with this suggestion. However, the real contribution of *M. pneumoniae* in this situation is difficult to assess because it is also evident that patients with chronic bronchitis sometimes acquire mycoplasmal infections without an apparent worsening of their disease.

M. pneumoniae frequently persists in the respiratory tract long after clinical recovery and occasionally the respiratory disease it causes has a protracted course. Furthermore, tracheobronchial clearance is very much reduced soon after infection and there is a tendency for slower clearance, in comparison with that in healthy subjects, even one year later. Despite this, however, there is no evidence that *M. pneumoniae* is a primary cause of chronic bronchitis, or that it is responsible for maintaining chronic disease other than by possibly causing some acute exacerbations.

Other mycoplasmal infections. There is no doubt that *M. salivarium*, *M. orale*, and perhaps other mycoplasmas present in the oropharynx of healthy persons spread to the lower respiratory tract of some patients suffering from chronic bronchitis. There is no evidence that these mycoplasmas are a cause of acute exacerbations. However, antibody responses to them occur more frequently in association with acute exacerbations than at other times which suggests that the organisms, normally associated with silent infections, are more antigenic during exacerbations. This is probably due to increased mycoplasmal multiplication and participation in tissue damage brought about primarily by viruses and bacteria, and it is tempting to believe that in this way the mycoplasmas play some part in perpetuating a chronic condition.

Genitourinary infections

Clinical conditions which the evidence strongly suggests are caused, at least in part, by mycoplasmas will be considered in some detail. These and other diseases in which the evidence for a mycoplasmal cause is weak and/or contentious are mentioned briefly in Table 5.

Diagnosis. Swabs from the urethra or vagina provide a more sensitive means of collecting specimens for mycoplasmal isolation than urine specimens. The basic medium is similar to that described for the isolation of *M. pneumoniae*. Advantage is taken of the metabolic activity of the mycoplasmas (Table 3) in order to detect their growth. Clinical material is added to separate vials of liquid medium containing phenol red and 0.1 per cent glucose, arginine, or urea. *M. hominis* and *M. primatum* convert arginine to ammonia, and ureaplasmas possess a urease which breaks down urea to ammonia. In each case, the pH of the medium increases and there is a colour change from yellow to red. Subculture to agar medium results in the formation of colonies of about 200–300 μm diameter by all genital mycoplasmas except ureaplasmas. Their colonies are small (15–30 μm) and, on medium containing manganous sulphate, are brown in colour and therefore more easily detected. On ordinary blood agar, *M. hominis*, but not ureaplasmas, produces non-haemolytic pinpoint colonies, the nature of which can be established by the methods outlined above. The metabolism-inhibition technique is used most frequently to detect antibodies to *M. hominis* and the ureaplasmas. Specific metabolites (arginine for *M. hominis* and urea for ureaplasmas) are incorporated in liquid medium containing phenol red, organisms, and antibody. The antibody inhibits multiplication and metabolism of homologous organisms thus preventing a change in colour of the pH indicator. The indirect-haemagglutination technique is useful for detecting antibody to *M. hominis* but other tests such as the ELISA are, at the moment, research tools only.

Non-gonococcal urethritis (NGU). There have been many studies concerned with the role of large-colony-forming mycoplasmas. It is clear that *M. fermentans* and *M. primatum* (Table 3) cannot be considered as significant causes of NGU because they are isolated so rarely from the genito-urinary tract either in health or disease. Furthermore, although *M. hominis* may be isolated from about 20 per cent of patients, the results of numerous studies have failed to implicate this mycoplasma as a cause. On the other hand, several lines of investigation, discussed below, have provided results which indicate *Ureaplasma urealyticum* organisms (ureaplasmas) as one of the causes of NGU.

Isolation studies. One of the difficulties in assessing the significance of ureaplasmas in NGU is that they are only one of the potential causes and they need to be evaluated in relation to other micro-organisms, such as chlamydiae. Earlier workers were unaware of this complex situation but contemporary investigators should not fail to take into account other micro-organisms. Another difficulty is the selection of controls, and the study of inappropriate subjects as controls has probably contributed most to the difference between the result of one investigation and another.

Table 5 The association of genital mycoplasmas with human genitourinary and perinatal disease

Disease	Evidence suggesting a causal relation of		Comments on the relationship and proportion of disease attributable to mycoplasms
	M. hominis	*U. urealyticum*	
Non-gonococcal urethritis	none	strong	the proportion of NGU caused by ureaplasmas is unknown
Urethro-prostatitis	weak	some	ureaplasmas may cause some acute disease; *M. hominis* is associated with a few cases of chronic disease, but a causal relation is unproved
Epididymitis	none	none	mycoplasmas not important
Urinary calculi	none	very weak	experimentally, ureaplasmas cause bladder calculi in male rats but so far no convincing evidence for a cause of natural human disease
Pyelonephritis	strong	none	*M. hominis* causes some cases of acute pyelonephritis and exacerbations
Reiter's disease	none	none	the significance of ureaplasmas should be assessed further
Abscess of Bartholin's gland	very weak	none	doubtful whether *M. hominis* involved
Vaginitis and cervicitis	none	none	*M. hominis* often associated with disease, but a causal relation is unproved
Pelvic inflammatory disease	strong	weak	*M. hominis* causes some cases, but the proportion is unknown
Postabortal fever	strong	none	*M. hominis* is responsible for some cases, but the proportion is unknown
Postpartum fever	strong	none	*M. hominis* may be a major cause
Involuntary infertility	none	none	ureaplasmas are associated with reduced sperm motility, but a causal relation is unproved
Repeated spontaneous abortion and stillbirth	none	none	maternal and fetal infections associated with spontaneous abortion, but a causal relation is unproved
Chorio-amnionitis	none	some	an association exists, but a causal relation is unproved
Low birthweight	none	some	an association exists in some studies, but a causal relation is unproved

Ureaplasmas have been isolated significantly more frequently from patients suffering from NGU than from subjects apparently free of disease in about half the investigations, whereas the rate of isolation in these two groups has been about the same in the other studies. Certainly their failure to provide a clear-cut answer to the problem of ureaplasmal pathogenicity should deter future investigators from pursuing this approach, unless the studies are designed to be quantitative in nature. Most studies have not been so, isolation rates, but not the number of organisms isolated from individual patients, having been documented. If ureaplasmas are involved in the pathogenic process, it would be reasonable to expect them to be present in larger numbers than if they were behaving only as commensals and, indeed, a few workers have provided quantitative data to support this idea.

Antibiotic therapy. Antibiotics have been used in the following ways to assess the role of ureaplasmas in NGU: (*a*) sub-optimal doses of doxycycline have caused a temporary disappearance of both symptoms and ureaplasmas from the urine, the return of symptoms being accompanied by re-appearance of the organisms in numbers similar to those found before treatment. (*b*) Placebo controlled trials of tetracycline in conjunction with comprehensive microbiological investigations have been few, but in one such trial there was a significant association between minocycline therapy and the resolution of symptoms and signs in patients from whom only ureaplasmas had been isolated. The association was only a little less convincing than that seen between therapy and resolution of disease in patients from whom only chlamydiae had been isolated and it provided some evidence for the pathogenicity of ureaplasmas. (*c*) Antibiotics which differentiate between ureaplasmas and other potentially pathogenic micro-organisms have been used as an approach to understanding the role of ureaplasmas in NGU. Urethritis in men who harbour chlamydiae and ureaplasmas is unaffected by treatment with aminocyclitols (streptomycin and spectinomycin) which eradicate ureaplasmas only, and, similarly, treatment with sulphafurazole, which eliminates chlamydiae only, is ineffective. Patients have been treated also with minocycline or rifampicin, the former being active against both micro-organisms but the latter against chlamydiae only. A greater proportion of patients respond to minocycline than to rifampicin, and those infected with ureaplasmas fail to respond to rifampicin significantly more often than those who are not infected. These findings suggest, therefore, that ureaplasmas as well as chlamydiae cause NGU, and, indeed, they would be difficult to explain if ureaplasmas were not involved at all. (*d*) Currently, about 10 per cent of ureaplasmas are resistant to tetracyclines and the urethritis of some patients infected by them is cured only by treatment with antibiotics, such as erythromycin, to which the organisms are susceptible.

Animal models and human experimentation. Some ureaplasma strains, unpassaged in the laboratory, have produced urethritis and an antibody response in chimpanzees when inoculated intraurethrally. Human experimentation is more difficult. It does not seem reasonable or ethical to seek volunteers for this purpose. However, three investigators have inoculated themselves intraurethrally and each developed urethritis. In one detailed study, two of them received 5×10^4 ureaplasma organisms, identified subsequently as serotype 5, which had been isolated from patients with NGU in whom no other potentially pathogenic micro-organisms could be detected. The first subject developed urethritis characterized by dysuria, frequency, urethral discomfort, and pyuria. Ureaplasmas were isolated consistently from urine, but they and the associated symptoms and signs disappeared during treatment with minocycline. The second subject also had evidence of mild urethritis and, like the first, a transient antibody response, but the predominant feature was the appearance of urinary threads in which polymorphonuclear leucocytes were observed regularly. The threads persisted for at least six months after treatment with minocycline which eliminated the organisms from meatal, urine, and semen samples. Analysis of fractionated semen samples indicated that the ureaplasmas had infected the prostate. These results indicate that some ureaplasmas are likely to be pathogenic under natural conditions and that they may be capable of initiating chronic disease. In this regard, it is interesting to note that some hypogammaglobulinaemic patients develop a chronic urethro-cystitis and that they have persistent ureaplasmal and/or *M. hominis* infections.

Interpretation of the findings in NGU. *C. trachomatis* infection (see page 5.353) accounts for probably no more than 50 per cent of cases of NGU and the question arises of whether ureaplasma infection fills part of the remaining gap. It would not seem reasonable to take the view that all the results of the studies outlined above are entirely spurious. It seems more rational to believe that these cumulative data are indicative of a pathogenic role for ureaplasmas in the male genital tract. On the other hand, this suggestion has to be reconciled with at least two counter arguments which may be expressed as follows. Since ureaplasmas exist frequently in the female genital tract so that sexually active men must be exposed to them often, why, if they are pathogenic, is NGU not even more common? Further, if ureaplasmas are a cause of NGU, why is it possible to recover them so often from men who do not have urethritis? There are a number of possible explanations. It may be that: (*a*) only certain serotypes are pathogenic. Serotype 4 was recovered in one study twice as frequently from men with NGU as from those who were symptom-free. There may be some substance, therefore, in the idea that serotypes are important but the situation is complex because mixtures of serotypes may exist within one isolate and pathogenic and non-pathogenic strains could belong to a single serotype. (*b*) Ureaplasmas involve only the prepuce and meatus in a non-disease producing capacity but under some circumstances invade the urethra to cause NGU. Procedures have not, so far, distinguished between the different sites of colonization or infection in men with and without disease. (*c*) Ureaplasmas produce NGU which resolves spontaneously but the organisms then persist. (*d*) Ureaplasmas produce NGU but those within the prostate and para-urethral glands are not always eliminated by treatment. These do not cause subsequent disease but are sometimes detected in the urethra. (*e*) Ureaplasmas cause only the first or early episodes of NGU, later encounters resulting in colonization without urethritis. It is not possible to predict which of these suggestions, if any, is most likely to be correct, and, of course, they may not be mutually exclusive. It is clear, however, that studies designed to resolve the situation should take into account all potential pathogenic micro-organisms and be quantitative rather than qualitative in nature. In the meantime, it is important to emphasize that there is no virtue in testing for ureaplasmas on a routine basis since positive results, so easy to obtain, are difficult for the clinician to interpret and use in patient management.

Pyelonephritis. *M. hominis* has been isolated, sometimes in pure culture, from the upper urinary tract of about 9 per cent of patients with acute pyelonephritis. In addition, antibody to *M. hominis*, measured by the indirect-haemagglutination technique, has been demonstrated in the serum and urine of some of these patients. In contrast, the mycoplasma has not been found in the upper urinary tract of patients with non-infectious urinary diseases nor has antibody been detected in their urine. The data suggest that *M. hominis* causes a few cases of acute pyelonephritis or acute exacerbations of chronic pyelonephritis and that ureaplasmas are involved less often if at all.

Pelvic inflammatory disease (PID). Micro-organisms present in the vagina and lower cervix may ascend to the normally sterile upper genital tract and cause inflammation of the Fallopian tubes and adjacent pelvic structures. Like NGU, non-gonococcal PID does not have a single cause and the possibility that infection by genital mycoplasmas might be one cause has engaged the attention of numerous investigators. Three sorts of evidence indicate that this is so.

Isolation studies. M. hominis has figured prominently among more than a dozen reports of the isolation of large-colony-forming mycoplasmas from inflamed Fallopian tubes, tubo-ovarian abscesses, and pelvic abscesses or fluid. The most revealing studies have been those of Swedish workers because they confirmed the diagnosis and collected specimens by laparoscopy. *M. hominis* was isolated directly from the Fallopian tubes of about 10 per cent of women with salpingitis but not from the tubes of women without signs of salpingitis. In addition, *M. hominis* has been isolated significantly more often from the cervix and urethra of patients with salpingitis than from those without disease.

Ureaplasmas have been studied less intensively, but they have been isolated directly from the Fallopian tubes of a very small proportion of patients with acute salpingitis, from pelvic fluid, and from a tubo-ovarian abscess. *M. pneumoniae* has been isolated also from such an abscess. The significance of these findings is unclear but it seems that ureaplasmas are likely to be of less importance than *M. hominis.*

Serological studies. Several workers have found *M. hominis* complement-fixing antibody titres to be greater in the sera of some patients with salpingitis than in those of other women serving as controls. The more sensitive indirect-haemagglutination technique was used by the Swedish workers to examine the sera of patients in whom they had sought *M. hominis.* Antibody to this mycoplasma was found in about half the patients with salpingitis but in only 10 per cent of healthy women. Furthermore, a significant rise or fall in antibody titre occurred during the course of disease in more than half the women who had *M. hominis* in the lower genital tract.

Antibody responses to *U. urealyticum* have been detected less often than responses to *M. hominis* in patients with PID. This is consistent with the impression that ureaplasmas are less important than *M. hominis* in this disease, but the greater difficulty of detecting antibody responses to ureaplasmas has to be recognized.

Organ culture and animal models. Organ cultures, in which tissues can be maintained in a condition similar to that *in vivo*, provide a valuable means for examining the relationship between micro-organisms and the epithelial cell surface. Fallopian tube organ cultures are particularly useful in this respect because ciliary activity may be assessed and used as an index of cell viability. In such cultures, *Neisseria gonorrhoeae* destroys the epithelium, whereas *M. hominis* organisms, although multiplying, produce no more than swelling of some of the cilia. No damage has been caused by ureaplasmas of human origin. This gradation of effect may be a true reflection of the pathogenic potential of these micro-organisms *in vivo*. However, failure to demonstrate damage does not mean necessarily that the organisms are avirulent because tissues in organ culture are separated from host immune systems which may play an important part in pathogenesis. Studies in intact animals may be helpful in elucidating this aspect. It is of interest, therefore, that the introduction of *M. hominis* into the oviducts of grivet monkeys has resulted in a self-limiting acute salpingitis and parametritis with an antibody response, whereas ureaplasmas have had no effect.

These various data, in particular those concerning *M. hominis*, indicate that mycoplasmas have a primary pathogenic role in some cases of acute PID.

Postabortal fever. The results of early studies and more recent observations suggest an important role for *M. hominis* in fever after abortion (see page 5.486). Thus, this mycoplasma has been isolated from the blood of about 10 per cent of women who had fever after abortion but not from afebrile women who had abortions, nor from normal pregnant women. In addition, a rise in the titre of antibody to *M. hominis* has been detected in half the women who become febrile but in only a small proportion of those who have abortions and remain afebrile. Thus, the evidence indicates that *M. hominis* causes some cases of postabortal fever but there is none to suggest that ureaplasmas do likewise. Patients recover whether or not they receive appropriate antimicrobial treatment.

Postpartum fever. Like other micro-organisms in the vagina, genital mycoplasmas have been found transiently in the blood after normal vaginal delivery. In one study, the blood of about 8 per cent of women contained mycoplasmas, mostly ureaplasmas, a few minutes after delivery, but the organisms did not persist and were not associated with postpartum fever. However, there have been many reports of individual postpartum fever patients from the blood of whom *M. hominis* has been isolated a day or more after delivery, and in whom an antibody response has been detected. In fact, the organisms, which are serologically diverse, may be isolated from the blood of 5–10 per cent of such women. Since genital mycoplasmas are seldom recovered from the blood of afebrile postpartum women, it appears that *M. hominis* induces postpartum fever, presumably by causing endometritis. The patients have a low-grade fever for a day or two after delivery, are not severely ill, and recover uneventfully without antibiotic therapy. Further studies are needed to define more fully the contribution of *M. hominis* relative to other micro-organisms as a cause of contemporary postpartum fever.

Joint infections

Rheumatoid arthritis. The knowledge that mycoplasmas cause several animal arthritides, and that gold salts inactivate mycoplasmas and have a beneficial effect on rheumatoid arthritis, provided the impetus to search for mycoplasmas in the joints of persons suffering from this disease. However, attempts over almost 40 years by more than 20 investigators to detect mycoplasmas in rheumatoid synovial fluids or tissues have failed or produced inconsistent and unrepeatable results. There seems no doubt that the rheumatoid joint is not the source of those mycoplasmas (*M. hyorhinis, M. hominis*) which have been recovered by means of tissue-culture techniques, and there are logical reasons for believing that the claims for isolation of mycoplasmas from synovial samples by direct or indirect inoculation of mycoplasmal medium are not valid. The case made in the late 1960s and early 1970s for the probable importance of *M. fermentans* in the pathogenesis of rheumatoid arthritis has not been substantiated.

M. pneumoniae and other mycoplasmal infections. A feature of the mycoplasmal arthritides of animals is that the mycoplasmas isolated from the joints are found also in the respiratory tract. The question must arise, therefore, of whether the known respiratory pathogenic mycoplasma of man, namely *M. pneumoniae*, causes arthritis. In this regard, there is no doubt that infection is often accompanied by non-specific arthralgia or myalgia (Table 4) during the acute phase, and occasionally it leads to migratory polyarthritis in adults affecting middle-sized joints. There is also recent evidence to implicate *M. pneumoniae* in some cases of Still's disease, either as an initiating factor or in exacerbations of existing disease. The association is based on the demonstration of a fourfold or greater rise in antibody titre or a single high titre and not on isolation of *M. pneumoniae* organisms from joints, although in immunologically deficient patients isolation has been achieved (see below).

M. hominis has been isolated from septic hip joints which have developed in patients after childbirth. The arthritis responds to tetracycline therapy and the diagnosis should be considered in a postpartum arthritis which is unaffected by penicillin.

Reiter's disease. (See also page 5.321 and Section 16.) Several investigators have considered the possibility that arthritis or arthritis and conjunctivitis, following or concomitant with sexually transmissible NGU, might be due to mycoplasmal infection. It is clear, however, that the problems encountered in defining the role of mycoplasmas in NGU are no less apparent when considering these complications. A major difficulty in investigating Reiter's patients is that often they have been treated with antibiotics before microbiological investigations can be attempted. Despite this, several workers have isolated *M. hominis* and/or ureaplasmas from the genital tract of such patients as frequently as from those suffering from uncomplicated NGU, although this does not indicate that the organisms are a cause of the complications. A further problem is the involvement of *C. trachomatis* which is apparently capable of initiating the pathological events in about 50 per cent of genetically predisposed men who develop sexually-acquired Reiter's disease, that is in those who are HLA-B27 antigen-positive. The initiating factor in the others is unknown but the possible role of ureaplasmas should not be ignored in view of their implication in uncomplicated NGU. In this respect, arthritis has been seen to develop in untreated NGU patients from whom ureaplasmas, but not chlamydiae, were isolated from the urethra. The organisms have not been isolated from

synovial fluids or tissues although cells, probably lymphocytes, sensitized to ureaplasmas have been found in the fluids of some patients. This, however, in the absence of other isolation or serological data, is insufficient to establish convincingly a link between ureaplasmas and Reiter's disease.

Arthritis in hypogammaglobulinaemic patients. Arthritis of mycoplasmal aetiology should be considered in hypogammaglobulinaemic patients (see Section 4) who develop an abacterial septic arthritis. Thus, *M. pneumoniae, M. hominis* and ureaplasmas have been isolated from synovial fluids of a small proportion of these patients. The organisms were recovered in such a way as to indicate that they derived from the inflamed joints and were not spurious laboratory contaminants. The arthritis responds to tetracyclines or other antibiotics to which the organisms are sensitive, an indication that they are a cause of the disease, although intravenous therapy may be required.

References

Cassell, G. H., and Cole, B.C. (1981). Mycoplasmas as agents of human disease. *New Engl. J. Med.* **304**, 80.

Murray, H. W., Masur, H., Senterfit, L. B., and Roberts, R. B. (1975). The protean manifestations of *Mycoplasma pneumoniae* infections in adults. *Am. J. Med.* **58**, 229.

Taylor-Robinson, D. and McCormack, W. M. (1980). The genital mycoplasmas. *New Engl. J. Med.* **302**, 1003, 1063.

— and Taylor, G. (1976). Do mycoplasmas cause rheumatic disease? In *Infection and immunology in the rheumatic diseases* (ed. D. C. Dumonde), 177. Blackwell Scientific Publications, Oxford.

Tully, J. G., Rose, D. L., Whitcomb, R. F., and Wenzel, R. P. (1979). Enhanced isolation of *Mycoplasma pneumoniae* from throat washings with a newly modified culture medium. *J. infect. Dis.* **139**, 478.

— and Whitcomb, R. F. (eds.) (1979). *The mycoplasmas*, vol. 2, *Human and animal mycoplasmas*. Academic Press, London.

Bartonellosis

D. A. Warrell

Bartonellosis (Oroya fever, Carrion's disease, verruga peruana, or Guaitara fever) is caused by *Bartonella bacilliformis* a 2–3 × 0.2–0.5 μm intracellular flagellate bacterium which is weakly Gram negative but stains deep red or purple with Giemsa. Organisms may be seen within the red cells of patient's blood, up to 10 per cell, in vascular and lymphatic endothelial cells, reticulo-endothelial tissue, skin lesions, and in lymphocytes in the cerebrospinal fluid. Electron microscopy confirms that the organisms are intra-erythrocytic but they have also been demonstrated in shallow depressions on the surface of the red cell. Branching rods and chains are seen early in the illness, but when recovery begins the organisms become coccoid. *Bartonella* is easily cultured in semi-solid medium, containing rabbit serum and haemoglobin or proteose peptone, at 28 °C under aerobic conditions. Chick chorioallantoic membrane and tissue culture may also be used.

Epidemiology. Bartonellosis is endemic in narrow river valleys and canyons on both sides of the Andes, at altitudes between 800 and 3000 metres and between latitudes 2° North and 13° South in Peru, Ecuador, Colombia, Bolivia, and Chile. The disease has also been reported from Guatemala and the Amazonian basin. Clinically similar infections associated with intra-erythrocytic bacteria have been described from the USA, Sudan, Niger, and Thailand. Large epidemics have occurred: during the building of the Lima–Oroya Railway in the 1870s there were 7000 deaths, and, most recently, in 1959, there was an epidemic with 200 deaths in Anco, Peru.

Infection results from the bite of female sandflies. *Phlebotomus (Lutzomya) verrucana* and other species. The reservoir may be human asymptomatic or convalescent cases. In the endemic area a proportion of healthy people have positive blood cultures. No animal reservoir is known. Transmission is greatest towards the end of the rainy season (January to April).

Pathogenesis. There are two forms of the disease. *Oroya fever* is an acute severe infection which occurs during the first two years of life in residents of the endemic area, and in non-immunes who enter the area. There is invasion and multiplication in red cells, endothelium, and cells of the reticulo-endothelial system which have phagocytosed infected cells. The results are severe haemolytic anaemia and blockade of the reticulo-endothelial system leading to complicating infections by enterobacteria and other pathogens. A few months after the acute illness has subsided, the mild persistent cutaneous form, *verruga peruana*, develops. The vascular skin lesions show endothelial proliferation, histiocytosis (the cells containing organisms), and later fibrosis and necrosis.

Clinical features. After an incubation of 8–100 (average 21) days following the sandfly bite, non-specific prodromal symptoms appear: these last for up to a week. High fever may develop rapidly or build up over a few days. It is accompanied by sweats and rigors. Common symptoms include severe headache, pain in joints and long bones, and confusion. The clinical picture is dominated by severe haemolytic anaemia: the patients rapidly become pale and jaundiced. Other signs include hepatosplenomegaly, generalized lymphadenopathy, a fine vesicular or petechial rash, mononeuritis multiplex and meningo-encephalomyelitis. Fever persists remittently for 7–20 (average 14) days. After a week or so there may be some signs of improvement but, in up to 45 per cent of cases, the illness may then be complicated by secondary infection with *Salmonella typhi*, other enteric bacteria, amoebiasis, malaria, or tuberculosis. The mortality is between 10 and 50 per cent: deaths occur during the first three weeks of illness.

Verruga peruana develops *de novo* or 30–60 days after acute Oroya fever. Nodular yaws-like lesions appear on the face and extensor surfaces of the limbs during a period of one to two months and persist for three months or more. There is accompanying mild fever, arthralgia, and myalgia. The red or purplish skin lesions vary from papules a few millimetres in diameter to pedunculated or plaque-like lesions a few centimetres across. They are painless and prone to bleeding, secondary infection, and ulceration. The appearance resembles yaws, haemangioma, granuloma pyogenicum, Kaposi's sarcoma, or fibrosarcoma. The lesions eventually dry up and slough off, the large ones leaving permanent scars. Apart from the skin, mucous membranes of the mouth and nose, serous cavities and the gastrointestinal and genito-urinary tracts may be involved, leading to obstructive symptoms, such as dysphagia or bleeding.

Investigations. *Bartonella* can be cultured from the blood during the prodrome. As fever develops, intra-erythrocytic bacteria are visible in thick and thin film stained with Giemsa. At the height of the infection up to 90 per cent of the red cells may contain bacteria. Organisms can also be seen and cultured in the skin lesions of verruga peruana.

Haematology. The haemolytic anaemia is Coomb's test negative: no agglutinins or haemolysins have been demonstrated. The blood picture is macrocytic and hypochromic with polychromasia and poikilocytosis. Reticulocytosis may reach 50 per cent. Howell–Jolly bodies and basophil granules are seen in the red cells. The marrow is hyperactive and megaloblastic with erythrophagocytosis. The white cell count is not elevated unless there is secondary infection. Thrombocytopenia is quite common. After the crisis the intracellular organisms become coccoid and then disappear, the white cell count rises, and there is lymphocytosis followed by eosinophilia.

Immunology. Complement fixing antibodies and agglutinins develop during the acute infection. There is cross-reaction with *Proteus* OX19, OXK, and OX2. Verruga peruana results from persistent infection modulated by partial immune response. Experimentally, a reversion to the non-immune state, with recrudescence of the acute septicaemic illness, is precipitated by splenectomy.

Treatment. Chloramphenicol, penicillin, streptomycin, and tetracycline are dramatically effective, usually eliminating the fever in less than 48 hours. Because of the common association with typhoid, chloramphenicol is the treatment of choice in an adult dose of 2 g/day for seven days. Supportive treatment includes blood transfusion. Large necrotic and infected skin lesions should be excised. Corticosteroids are contra-indicated: they seem to promote the skin lesions.

Prevention. Sandflies can be eliminated from homes by spraying inside and out every few weeks with 5 per cent DDT in kerosene. Bites always occur after dusk. They can be prevented by insect repellants, sleeping inside fine mesh nets, or by avoiding sleeping in the endemic area. There have been some promising early attempts at vaccination.

References

Cuadra, M. (1981). Bartonella bacilliformis. In *Medical microbiology and infectious diseases* (ed. A. I. Braude), 510. W. B. Saunders, Philadelphia.
— and Takano, J. (1969). The relationship of *Bartonella bacilliformis* to the red blood cells as revealed by electron microscopy. *Blood* **33**, 708.
Dooley, J. R. (1980). Haemotropic bacteria in man. *Lancet* ii, 1237.
Hennemann, H. H. (1963). Oroya-fieber (carrionsche Krankheit): eine akute erworbene hamolytische Anamie. *Deutsche Med. Wschr.* **88**, 1759.
Trelles, J. O. and Trelles, L. (1978). Neurological manifestations of verruga peruana (Carrion's disease, Oroya fever, neurobartonellosis). In *Handbook of clinical neurology*, vol. 34 (eds. P. J. Vinken and G. W. Bruyn), 659. North Holland, Amsterdam.

'Newer' and lesser known organisms causing infection in man

R. G. Mitchell

This is an arbitrary list based on recent publications, and omits fungi. Some of the infections, listed are extremely rare, others are acquired extensively in hospital, and the intention is to emphasize the importance of precise bacterial identification and classification in the study of infection. The distinction between Isolations and Infections is often arbitrary, since the significance of a bacterial isolate from a clinical specimen is not always clear. For a systematic account of the 'newer' Gram-negative bacteria, the reader should consult the *Manual of clinical microbiology*, third edition (ed. E. H. Lennette, A. Balows, W. J. Hausler, and J. P. Truant), chapters 20, 21 *et seq.*, which include an authoritative account of the so-called alphanumeric designated series of bacteria which have not so far been assigned to particular genera.

Abbreviations. CSF, cerebrospinal fluid; CSOM, chronic suppurative otitis media; CSU, catheter specimen of urine; IP, incubation period; i.v., intravenous; LRTI, lower respiratory tract infection; SBE, subacute bacterial endocarditis; URT, upper respiratory tract; UTI, urinary tract infection; (1) single case report only.

Organism	Habitat	Isolations	Infections	Predisposing factors	Treatment	References
Achromobacter xylosoxidans	Aquatic	Ear, throat, sputum, urine, blood, CSF Disinfectants and parenteral fluids	Peritonitis associated with dialysis; bacteraemia, pneumonia, ventriculitis after neurosurgery	Immunodeficiency Broad spectrum chemotherapy Contaminated parenteral fluids	Carbenicillin Co-trimoxazole	1, 2
Acinetobacter calcoaceticus (*A. anitratus*; *Bacterium anitratum*)	Soil and water Hospital environment	Hospital equipment: disinfectants, bowls, respiratory equipment, urine utensils Skin, hands of patients and attendants CSU, URT, faeces	UTI, septicaemia, meningitis, pneumonia, acute and subacute endocarditis	Cross infection Broad spectrum chemotherapy Urethral catheterization, intubation, and other invasive procedures Immunodeficiency Debility	Aminoglycosides Carbenicillin Co-trimoxazole	3, 4, 5
Actinobacillus actinomycetemcomitans (HB–3, HB–4)	URT		Actinomycosis (± *Actinomyces israelii*), soft tissue infections, endocarditis (major emboli, heart failure, high mortality), brain abscess, pneumonia, UTI	Dental manipulation	Penicillin *or* Ampicillin *and* Gentamicin	6, 7
Actinobacillus lignieresii	Rumen of sheep and cattle		Meningitis, abdominal wound sepsis following trauma, suppurative pneumonia with metastatic abscess formation, endocarditis, mesenteric lymphadenitis, conjunctivitis, lumbar abscess with osteomyelitis	Animal contact or bites	Ampicillin *and* Gentamicin	8, 9
Aerococcus viridans	Air, vegetation, occasionally URT and skin	Mouth, surface wounds	SBE, UTI, empyema	Previous tissue damage	Penicillin	10, 11
Aeromonas hydrophila	Fresh water lakes and streams, fish, soil Hospital environment	Refrigerated blood products, contaminant in clinical specimens, faeces	Wound infections (extensive necrosis of muscle, soft tissue, or skin), septicaemia (ecthyma gangrenosum), endocarditis, CSOM, LRTI, corneal ulceration in contact lens wearers, meningitis following neurosurgery, acute diarrhoea	Injuries in contact with soil or water (e.g. fish-fin or hook injuries) War wounds Septicaemia in immuno-compromised patients	Aminoglycosides Chloramphenicol	12, 13, 14, 15
Aeromonas sobria	Aquatic	Blood, sputum, faeces, lung tissue at autopsy	Wound sepsis in a diver (1)			16
Arachnia propionica	Oropharynx	Periodontal scrapings	Actinomycosis, brain abscess, lacrimal canaliculitis	Dental sepsis and trauma Human bites	Penicillin	17, 18
Babesia bovis, microti (piroplasma), a protozoal blood parasite	Tick-borne disease of wild and domestic animals Red water fever in in cattle		Rare human cases reported from USA, mainland Europe, Eire, Scotland Europe: infections with *B. bovis* in splenectomized patients; severe malaria-like illness with haemolysis, jaundice, and renal failure, usually fatal USA: Nantucket Island and Martha's Vineyard: mild or latent infections with *B. microti* in patients with intact spleen; IP 7–28 days; anorexia, fever, sweating, rigors, myalgia, splenomegaly, haemolytic anaemia	Infected tick bites in endemic areas Adults only Asplenism	Chloroquine 4–4 diazo-amino benzamidine (climinazene)	19, 20, 21, 22
Bacillus cereus	Aerial saprophyte	Common ward and laboratory contaminant	Traumatic and surgical wounds, especially war wounds, non-clostridial gangrene, panophthalmitis, otitis media, pneumonia, lung abscess, puerperal sepsis, UTI, septicaemia, endocarditis (may follow i.v. drug abuse), meningitis following LP or spinal anaesthetic, brain abscess, haemodialysis reactions due to contaminated equipment, osteomyelitis	Tissue damage Instrumentation Systemic infections in immuno-compromised subjects	Aminoglycosides Erythromycin Clindamycin	23, 248

Organism	Habitat	Isolations	Infections	Predisposing factors	Treatment	References
Bifidobacterium	Mouth, intestine, vagina	Usually isolated in mixed culture, evaluation difficult	Obstetric and gynaecological sepsis, intra-abdominal sepsis and peritonitis, pleuro-pulmonary infections, UTI, bacteraemia, SBE	Dental manipulation Parturition Disease of bowel	Penicillin	25, 26
Bordetella bronchiseptica (*B. bronchicanis*, *Alcaligenes bronchiseptica*)	Oropharynx of wild and domesticated animals	URT	Coryzal illness in animal attendants, para-pertussis, pneumonia, septicaemia, SBE; meningitis following kick from horse, peritonitis associated with CAPD (1), wound infections	Childhood Animal contact Immunodeficiency, debility in adults	?Co-trimoxazole ?Erythromycin	27, 28, 29
Branhamella catarrhalis (*Neisseria catarrhalis*)	URT, occasionally vagina		Bronchopneumonia, acute otitis media, sinusitis, septicaemia, SBE, meningitis neonatal conjunctivitis	Chronic bronchitis in coal miners Post-operative pneumonia Immunodeficiency	Amoxycillin Cefuroxime (if penicillinase-producing strain)	30, 31, 32
Capnocytophaga ochracea (DF–1)	Periodontal	URT, bronchial aspirate, pleural fluid, CSF, eye, female genital tract	Periodontal infection, septicaemia with ulcerative stomatis	Granulocytopenia in malignant disease	Minocycline Clindamycin Carbenicillin	33
Cardiobacterium hominis (II–D)		URT	SBE (normal and prosthetic valves; major emboli, heart failure common: mortality 25%)	Dental manipulation	Penicillin	34, 35, 36, 37
Chromobacterium violaceum	Soil and water of tropical and sub-tropical regions; Florida, SE Asia		Localized skin lesion ± adenitis followed by severe septic illness with liver abscess, pustular rash, UTI	Minor skin trauma ?Ingestion	Chloramphenicol Carbenicillin *and* gentamicin	38, 39
Citrobacter koseri 40, 41, 42 (*C. intermedius*, *C. diversus*, *Levinea malonatica*)	Intestine	Frequently isolated as a contaminating 'coliform'	Wound sepsis, UTI, cholecystitis, septicaemia, neonatal meningitis and brain abscess	Cross infection in neonatal units	Appropriate β-lactam antibiotic *and* gentamicin	40, 41, 42
Corynebacterium bovis (*C. pseudotuberculosis*)	Soil, sheep (also horses, cattle, goats, deer) Australia (also Africa and South America) Caseous lymphadenitis broncho-pneumonia of sheep		Suppurative granulomatous lymphadenitis, mainly involving axillary and inguinal glands (± fever, malaise, myalgia, arthralgia, hepatomegaly, transient blood eosinophilia) Eosinophilic pneumonia (1)	Contact with sheep (mainly rural Australia) ? Ingestion of raw milk	Penicillin Erythromycin Surgical drainage excision of infected nodes	43, 44
Corynebacterium haemolyticum (*C. pyogenes var. hominis*)	URT		Membranous tonsillitis with scarlatiniform rash, leg ulcer infection, brain abscess, septicaemia		Penicillin Erythromycin	45, 46, 47, 48, 49
Corynebacterium ulcerans	Zoonosis in cattle		Mild tonsillitis, ± generalized rash; or severe diphtheria-like illness with toxaemia, nerve palsies, and myocarditis	Consumption of contaminated milk	Penicillin Erythromycin Diphtheria anti-toxin	50
DF–2 (dysgonic-fermenter group)	Oropharynx of dogs		Cellulitis, septicaemia, endocarditis, meningitis, arthritis, pulmonary infiltrations, Friderichsen–Waterhouse syndrome	Dog bites or contact Immunodeficiency Splenectomy	Penicillin	51, 52, 53
Edwardsiella tarda	Aquatic: fish, lizards, sea mammals Cattle, pigs	Association with *Entamoeba histolytica*?	Traumatic wound sepsis with cellulitis or abscess formation; gastrointestinal symptoms, peritonitis and septic shock, perirectal abscess, liver abscess, cholangitis; typhoidal illness, septicaemia, meningitis	Injuries in contact with water or fish	β-lactam antibiotic *and* gentamicin	54

Organism	Habitat	Isolations	Infections	Predisposing factors	Treatment	References
Eikenella corrodens (HB–1)	Oropharynx, intestine, genitourinary tract	Usually isolated in mixed culture	Sinusitis, otitis media, neck abscess, pulmonary infections, empyema, intra-abdominal abscess, SBE, meningitis, subdural abscess, osteomyelitis, septic arthritis	Trauma to oropharynx, oesophagus, dental manipulation Amphetamine abuse Selection by previous chemotherapy Human bites	Penicillin Gentamicin	55, 56
Enterobacter agglomerans (Erwinia agglomerans, Herbicola-lathyri bacterium)	Plant crops	Urine, faeces, URT, mixed cultures from wounds	Traumatic wound sepsis in agricultural workers (USA), septicaemia due to contaminated i.v. fluids, post-operative wound sepsis, post-partum bacteraemia, vaginal discharge, UTI, meningitis, brain abscess	Occupational	Appropriate β-lactam antibiotic and gentamicin	57
Erysipelothrix rhusiopathiae (E. insidiosa)	Meat, game, fish		Cutaneous erysipeloid (mild and local, or severe and generalized), septicaemia, arthritis, acute or subacute endocarditis (often previously normal valves, high mortality)	Occupational, especially butchers	Penicillin	58
Eubacterium	Soil and water Mouth, intestine, vagina	Skin, bacteraemia	Post-operative wounds, furuncles, obstetric and gynaecological sepsis, peritonitis, intra-abdominal abscess, pleuropulmonary infections, SBE	Dental manipulation Parturition Bowel lesions	Penicillin	26, 59
Flavobacterium meningosepticum	Soil and water	Hospital environment: sinks, basins, parenteral fluids, disinfectants (especially chlorhexidine), respiratory equipment, URT	Epidemic neonatal meningitis, adult meningitis, post-operative bacteraemia, SBE (in a drug addict)	Immature infants Immunocompromised adults	Rifampicin, Erythromycin, Chloramphenicol ?Newer β-lactam antibiotics	60, 61
Flavobacterium multivorum (Group 11 K–2)			Spontaneous bacterial peritonitis		β-lactam antibiotics	62, 63
Fusobacterium necrophorum (Sphaerophorus necrophorus)	Oropharynx, periodontal, intestine, vagina		Vincent's angina, dental abscess, exudative pharyngitis, peritonsillar abscess, aspiration pneumonia, lung abscess, intra-abdominal abscess (appendix, liver, tubovarian), Lemierre's post-angina septicaemia (oropharyngeal infection with local septic thrombophlebitis, bacteraemia, and metastatic septic foci), arthritis, meningitis, SBE	Tonsillectomy	Penicillin Chloramphenicol Clindamicin Metronidazole Surgical drainage	64, 65, 66
Gardnerella vaginalis (Haemophilus vaginalis)	Vagina, urethra		Greyish, malodorous vaginal discharge, pH 5.0–5.5 without pus cells or inflammatory changes; neonatal bacteraemia, bacteraemia following Caesarean section, episiotomy, abortion, or hysterectomy	Sexually transmitted	Metronidazole Ampicillin Tetracycline (Treat consort also)	67, 68
Haemophilus aphrophilus (HB–2)	Oropharynx, periodontal, in man and dogs		Actinomycosis (with A. israelii), soft tissue infections, wound sepsis, otitis media sinusitis, bronchopneumonia, empyema, brain abscess, arthritis, osteomyelitis, cholecystitis, SBE (major emboli and heart failure common; 50% mortality)	Dental manipulation Human and dog bites	Penicillin Ampicillin	69
Haemophilus equigenitalis	Equine genital tract	A recently recognized cause of equine metritis, a venereal disease of horses	Male patients with non-specific urethritis show a high incidence of serum agglutinins to the organism, which has not so far been isolated from human subjects			70, 71

Organism	Habitat	Isolations	Infections	Predisposing factors	Treatment	References
Haemophilus parainfluenzae	URT, occasionally genital tract	Commonly isolated from sputum	SBE (major emboli common), puerperal and neonatal septicaemia, peritonitis, meningitis, rarely UTI	Ear or sinus infections Dental manipulation	Ampicillin Cefuroxime Chloramphenicol	72, 73, 74
JK	Skin	Frequently in mixed culture when isolated as a 'diphtheroid'	Skin and wound sepsis, cellulitis, abscesses (especially perineal and inguinal sites) SBE following cardiac surgery, bacteraemia, thrombophlebitis, pneumonia, peritonitis, pyelonephritis	Percutaneous instrumentation. Neutropenia complicating malignant blood dyscrasias Males 70%	Vancomycin Erythromycin	75, 76
Kingella kingae, denitrificans (*Moraxella kingae*)	URT	Nose, throat, blood, joint aspirate, bone	Pharyngitis, laryngitis, eyelid abscess; septicaemia with arthritis and skin lesions in leukaemia (1), SBE, osteomyelitis, invertebral disc infection (1)		Carbenicillin *and* gentamicin	77, 78, 79, 80
Kurthia bessonii	?URT, urethra, vagina	Faeces, sputum, pilonidal cyst, eye	SBE		Penicillin	81, 82
Lactobacillus	Vagina, mouth, intestine	Bacteraemia, intra-abdominal abscesses	Dental caries, obstetric and gynaecological sepsis, SBE	Dental manipulation Parturition Bowel lesions	Penicillin Gentamicin	26, 83, 84
Megasphaera elsdenii	Intestine	In mixed culture from tracheal aspirate, lung abscess, rectal drainage, frontal lobe abscess	SBE (1)		Metronidazole	85
Moraxella osloensis			Conjunctivitis, wound sepsis, vaginal discharge, UTI, meningitis, brain abscess, septicaemia, SBE, arthritis, haemorrhagic stomatis (1)		Penicillin	86, 87
Pasteurella multocida (*P. septica*)	Oropharynx of wild and domestic animals and birds, especially cats and dogs	Oropharynx, sputum (role in chronic bronchitis uncertain)	Cat and dog bites and scratches (± lymphadenopathy, bacteraemia, osteomyelitis), sinusitis, pneumonia, lung abscess, empyema, septicaemia, puerperal sepsis, peritonitis, SBE, neonatal meningitis, adult meningitis following head injury, brain abscess, arthritis, UTI	Elderly Pre-existing lung disease Immuno-incompetence Animal contact	Penicillin, Tetracycline Erythromycin Clindamycin	88, 89, 90
Peptococcus magnus	Skin, oropharynx, intestine, genito-urinary tract	Common in mixed anaerobic cultures from wounds, soft tissue abscesses, sebaceous cyst, endometritis, prostatitis; bacteraemia	Osteomyelitis, arthritis, post-operative wound sepsis	Orthopaedic and vascular surgery; prostheses, fractures	Penicillin Metronidazole	91
Propionibacterium acnes (*Corynebacterium acnes*)	Skin, especially of scalp	Frequent contaminant of blood cultures	Acne vulgaris, wound abscess, post-neurosurgical sepsis, meningitis, CSF shunt infections, SBE, osteomyelitis, granulomata of liver (botyromycosis) (1)		Penicillin Tetracycline	92, 93
Prototheca wickerhamii, zopfii (*achlorophyllous algae*)	Soil, water, and vegetation	Occasionally, faeces Africa, China, Vietnam, USA, Spain	Cutaneous or subcutaneous granulomata of skin ± lymphadenopathy; olecranon bursitis; disseminated disease (1): cutaneous nodule and rash, septicaemia granulomata of liver and peritoneum	Males traumatic implantation	Excision, Oral and systemic amphotericin B	94, 95, 96
Providencia stuartii (closely related to *Proteus rettgeri*)		Skin, throat, and faeces (±) Commonly mixed with *Proteus* spp.	UTI, septicaemia, burn infections, post-operative sepsis, pneumonia	Urinary catheterization Previous chemotherapy Debility Immuno-suppression Nosocomial spread by contact	Appropriate β-lactam antibiotic or aminoglycoside	97, 98, 99

Organism	Habitat	Isolations	Infections	Predisposing factors	Treatment	References
Pseudomonas cepacia (*Ps. multivorans*, EO–1, IV–d)	Soil, water, and vegetation	Aqueous disinfectant solutions especially chlorhexidine	Wound sepsis, foot rot, UTI, pneumonia septicaemia, ecthyma gangrenosa, SBE	Debility Prolonged hospitalization, Contaminated i.v. equipment, i.v. solutions, disinfectants, i.v. drug abuse Urethral catheterization Swamp training	Co-trimoxazole *and* gentamicin	100, 101, 102, 103
Pseudomonas denitrificans			Bacteraemia and meningitis (1)		Co-trimoxazole Ticarcillin	104
Pseudomonas maltophilia	Environmental, water, milk, animal faeces	Nosocomial acquisition, commonly found in mixed culture when isolated; URT, faeces	Wound sepsis, ear and eye infections, pneumonia, UTI, bacteraemia during haemodialysis and open heart surgery, SBE (prosthetic valves)	Debility Previous chemotherapy Contaminated equipment and solutions	Co-trimoxazole Chloramphenicol	4, 105, 106
Pseudomonas paucimobilis (II K-biotype 1)	Environmental (moist sites)	Tap water, dialysis fluid, respirators Wound swabs, abscesses, trachea, vagina, cervix, urine, blood, CSF	Septicaemia (2), leg ulcer (1), meningitis (1), UTI (1)	Nosocomal acquisition	Appropriate β-lactam antibiotics	107, 108, 109, 110
Pseudomonas pickettii (Va – biotype 2)		Hospital environment Sputum, blood	Bacteraemia	Intravenous catheterization	Co-trimoxazole Cephalosporins Minocycline	111
Rothia dentocariosa (*Actinomyces dentocariosus*)	Oropharynx	Throat, nose, sputum, postoperative wounds, blood, urine	Appendix abscess ('abdominal actinomycosis') pilonidal cyst (1), SBE (2)	Dental manipulation	Penicillin *and* gentamicin	86, 87
Serratia marcescens	Water, soil, foodstuffs, animals, man	Skin, sputum, urine, faeces (±) Nosocomial spread: (a) common source outbreaks due to contaminated solutions or equipment (b) hand carriage by by attendants	Wound and burn sepsis; pneumonia, lung abscess, empyema UTI, red diaper syndrome, septicaemia, liver abscess, peritonitis, meningitis, arthritis, osteomyelitis, SBE (i.v. drug abuse, prosthetic valves)	Debility Immunosuppression Prolonged hospitalization Previous chemotherapy Invasive procedures especially involving urinary tract and airways	Appropriate β-lactam antibiotic *and* aminoglycoside	88
Tatumella ptyseos (*enterobacterium*) (EF–9)		Throat, sputum, tracheal aspirate, urine, faeces, blood	Bacteraemia			115

References

1. Igra-Siegman, Y., Chmel, H., and Cobbs, C. (1980). Clinical and laboratory characteristics of *Achromobacter xylosoxidans* infection. *J. clin Microbiol.* **11**, 141.
2. Holmes, G. L., Snell, J. J. S., and Lapage, S. P. (1977). Strains of *Achromobacter xylosoxidans* from clinical material. *J. clin. Path.* **30**, 595.
3. French, G. L., Casewell, M. W., Roncoroni, A. J. Knight, S., and Phillips, I. (1980). A hospital outbreak of antibiotic-resistant *Acinetobacter anitratus*: epidemiology and control. *J. hosp. Infect.* **1**, 125.
4. Cohen, P. S., Maguire, J. H., and Weinstein, L. (1980). Infective endocarditis caused by Gram-negative bacteria: a review of the literature, 1945–1977. *Prog. cardiovasc. dis.* **22**, 205.
5. Rosenthal, S. L. and Freundlich, L. F. (1977). The clinical significance of *Acinetobacter* species. *Health Lab. Sci.* **14**, 194.
6. Geraci, J. E., Wilson, W. R., and Washington II, J. A. (1980). Infective endocarditis caused by *Actinobacillus actinomycetemcomitans*. Report of four cases. *Mayo Clinics Proc.* **55**, 415.
7. Ellner, J. J., Rosenthal, M. S., Lerner, P. I., and McHenry, M. C. (1979). Infective endocarditis caused by slow-growing, fastidious, Gram-negative bacteria. *Medicine, Baltimore* **58**, 145.
8. Orda, R. and Wiznitzer, T. (1980). *Actinobacillus lignieresii* human infection, *J. R. Soc. Med.* **73**, 295.
9. Dibb, W. L., Digranes, A., and Tønjum, S. (1981). *Actinobacillus lignieresii* infection after a horse bite. *Br. Med. J.* **283**, 583.
10. Janosek, J., Eckert, J., and Hudáč, A. (1980). *Aerococcus viridans* as a causative agent of infectious endocarditis. *J. Hyg. Epidemiol. Microbiol. Immunol.* **24**, 92.
11. Colman, G. (1967). Aerococcus-like organisms isolated from human infections. *J. clin. Path.* **20**, 294.
12. Smith, J. A. (1980). Aeromonas hydrophila: analysis of 11 cases. *Can. med. Ass. J.* **122**, 1270.
13. Davis, W. A., Kane, J. G., and Garagusi, V. F. (1978). Human *Aeromonas* infections :a review of the literature and a case report of endocarditis. *Medicine, Baltimore* **57**, 267.

14. Wolff, R. L., Wiseman, S. L., and Kitchens, C. S. (1980). *Aeromonas hydrophila* bacteremia in ambulatory immunocompromised hosts. *Am. J. Med.* **68**, 238.
15. Young, D. F. and Barr, R. J. (1981). *Aeromonas hydrophila* infection of the skin. *Archs Derm.* **117**, 244.
16. Daily, O. P., Joseph, S. W., Coolbaugh, J. C., Walker, R. I., Merrell, B. R., Rollins, D. M., Seidler, R. J., Colwell, R. R., and Lissner, C. R. (1981). Association of *Aeromonas sobria* with human infection. *J. clin. Microbiol.* **13**, 769.
17. Riley, T. V. and Ott, A. K. (1981). Brain abscess due to *Arachnia propionica*. *Br. med. J.* **i**, 1035.
18. Brock, D. W., Georg, L. K., Brown, J. M., and Hicklin, M. D. (1973). Actinomycosis caused by *Arachnia porpionica*. *Am. J. clin. Path.* **59**, 66.
19. Entrican, J. H., Williams, H., Cook, I. A., Lancaster, W. M., Clark, J. C., Joyner, L. P., and Lewis, D. (1979). Babesiosis in man: report of a case from Scotland with observations on the infecting strain. *J. Infect.* **1**, 227.
20. Symposium on human babesiosis (1980). *Trans. R. S. trop. Med. Hyg.* **74**, 143.
21. Ruebush, T. K., Juranek, D. D., Spielman, A., Piesman, J., and Healy, G. R. (1981). Epidemiology of human babesiosis on Nantucket Island. *Am. J. trop. Med. Hyg.* **30**, 937.
22. Spielman, A., Etkind, P., Piesman, J., Ruebush, T. K., Juranek, D. D., and Jacobs, M. S. (1981). Reservoir hosts of human baesiosis on Nantucket Island. *Am. J. trop. Med. Hyg.* **30**, 560.
23. Turnbull, P. C. B., Jorgensen, K., Kramer, J. M., Gilbert, R. J., and Parry, J. M. (1979). Severe clinical conditions associated with *Bacillus cereus* and the apparent involvement on exotoxins. *J. clin. Path.* **32**, 289.
24. Tuazon, C. U., Murray, H. W., Levy, C., Solny, M. N., Curtin, J. A., and Sheagren, J. N. (1979). Serious infections from Bacillus sp. *J. Am. Med. Ass.* **241**, 1137.
25. Wilson, W. R., Martin, W. J., Wilkowske, C. J., and Washington, II, J. A. (1972). Anaerobic bacteremia *Mayo Clinics Proc.* **47**, 639.
26. Bourne, K. A., Beebe, J. L., Lue, Y. A., and Ellner, P. D. (1978). Bacteremia due to bifidobacterium, eubacterium, or lactobacillus: twenty-one cases and review of the literature. *Yale J. Biol. Med.* **51**, 505.
27. Ghosh, H. K. and Tranter, J. (1979). *Bordetella bronchicanis* (bronchiseptica) infection in man: a review and a case report. *J. clin. Path.* **32**, 546.
28. Dale, A. J. D. and Geraci, J. E. (1961). Mixed cardiac valvular infections: report of case and review of literature. *Mayo Clinics Proc.* **36**, 288.
29. Byrd, L. H., Anama, L., Gutkin, M., and Chmel, H. (1981). *Bordetella bronchiseptica* peritonitis associated with continuous ambulatory peritoneal dialysis. *J. clin. Microbiol.* **14**, 232.
30. Ninane, G., Joly, J., and Kraytman, M. (1978). Bronchopulmonary infection due to *Branhamella catarrhalis*: 11 cases assessed by trantracheal puncture. *Br. med J.* **i**, 276.
31. McNeeley, D. J., Kitchens, C. S., and Kluge, R. M. (1976). Fatal *Neisseria (Branhamella) catarrhalis* pneumonia in an immunodeficient host. *Am. Rev. resp. Dis.*, **114**, 399.
32. Garvey, R. J. P. (1981). Ophthalmia neonatorum due to *Branhamella catarrhalis*: case reports. *Br. J. vener. Dis.* **57**, 346.
33. Forlenza, S. W., Newman, M. G., Lipsey, A. L., Siegel, S. E., and Blachman, U. (1980). Capnocytophaga sepsis: a newly recognised clinical entity in granulocytopenic patients. *Lancet* **i**, 567.
34. Savage, D. D., Kagan, R. L., Young, N. A., and Horvath, A. E. (1977). *Cardiobacterium hominis* endocarditis: description of two patients and characterisation of the organism. *J. clin. Microbiol.* **5**, 75.
35. Geraci, J. E., Greipp, P. R., Wilkowske, C. J., Wilson, W. R., and Washington II, J. A. (1978). *Cardiobacterium hominis* endocarditis. Four cases with clinical and laboratory observations. *Mayo Clinics Proc.* **53**, 49.
36. Midgley, J., Lapage, S. P., Jenkins, B. A.G., Barrow, G. I., Roberts, M. E., and Buck, A. G. (1970). *Cardiobacterium hominis* endocarditis. *J. med. Microbiol.* **3**, 91.
37. Rönnevik, P. K. and Neess, H. C. (1981). Septicaemia caused by *Cardiobacterium hominis*. A case report. *Acta path. microbiol. Scand.* **89B**, 243.
38. Tucker, R. E., Winter, W. G., and Wilson, H. D. (1979). Osteomyelitis associated with *Chromobacterium violaceum* sepsis : a case report. *J. Bone Joint Surg.* **61**, 949.
39. Victoria, B., Baer, H., and Ayoub, E. M. (1974). Successful treatment of systemic *Chromobacterium violaceum* infection. *J. Am. med. Ass.* **230**, 578.
40. Altman, G., Sechter, I., Cahan, D., and Gerichter, C. B. (1976). *Citrobacter diversus* isolated from clinical material. *J. clin. Microbiol.* **3**, 390.
41. Gwynn, C. M. and George, R. H. (1973). Neonatal citrobacter meningitis. *Archs Dis. Childn.* **48**, 455.
42. Graham, D. R., Anderson, R. L., Ariel, F. E., Ehrenkranz, N. J., Rowe, B., Boer, H. R., and Dixon, R. E. (1981). Epidemic nosocomial meningitis due to *Citrobacter diversus* in neonates. *J. infect Dis.* **144**, 203.
43. Goldberger, A. C., Lipsky, B. A., and Plorde, J. J. (1981). Suppurative granulomatous lymphadenitis caused by *Corynebacterium ovis* (pseudotuberculosis). *Am. J. clin. Path.* **76**, 486.
44. Keslin, M. H., McCoy, E. L., McCusker, J. J., and Lutch, J. S. (1979). *Corynebacterium pseudotuberculosis*. A new cause of infectious and eosinophilic pneumonia. *Am. J. Med.* **67**, 228.
45. Ryan, W. J. (1972). Throat infection and rash associated with an unusual corynebacterium. *Lancet* **ii**, 1345.
46. Fell, H. W. K., Nagington, J., Nayler, G. R. E., and Olds, R. J. (1977). *Corynebacterium haemolyticum* infections in Cambridgeshire. *J. Hyg., Camb.* **79**, 269.
47. Jobanputra, R. S. and Swain, C. P. (1975). Septicaemia due to *Corynebacterium haemolyticum*. *J. Clin Path.* **28**, 798.
48. Wickremesinghe, R. S. B. (1981). *Corynebacterium haemolyticum* infections in Sri Lanka. *J. Hyg., Camb.* **87**, 271.
49. Green S. L. and LaPeter, K. S. (1981). Pseudodiphtheritic membranous paryngitis caused by *Corynebacterium haemolyticum*. *J. Am. med. Ass.* **245**, 2330.
50. Meers, P. D. (1979). A case of classical diphtheria, and other infections due to *Corynebacterium ulcerans*. *J. Infect.* **1**, 139.
51. Chandhuri, A. K., Hartley, R. B., and Maddocks, A. G. (1981). Waterhouse–Friderichsen syndrome caused by a DF–2 baterium in a splenectomised patient. *J. clin. Path.* **34**, 172.
52. Butler, T., Weaver R. E., Venkata Ramani, T. K., Uyeda, C. T., Bobo, R. A., So Ryh, J. I., and Kohler, R. B. (1977). Unidentified Gram-negative rod infection: a new disease of man. *Ann. intern. Med.* **86**, 1.
53. Martone, W. J., Zuehl, R. W., Minson, G. E., and Scheld, W. M. (1980). Post splenectomy sepsis with DF–2: report of a case with isolation of the organism from the patient's dog. *Ann. intern. Med.* **93**, 457.
54. Clarridge, J. E., Musher, D. M., Fainstein, V., and Wallace, R. J. (1980). Extraintestinal human infection caused by *Edwardsiella tarda*. *J. Clin. Microbiol.* **11**, 511.
55. Maia, A., Goldstein, F. W., Acar, J. F., and Roland, F. (1980). Isolation of *Eikenella corrodens* from human infections: report of six cases. *J. Infect.* **2**, 347.
56. Geraci, J. E., Hermans, P. E., and Washington II, J. A. (1974). *Eikenella corrodens* endocarditis: Report of cure in two cases. *Mayo Clinics Proc.* **49**, 950.
57. Pien, F. D., Martin, W. J., Hermans, P. E., and Washington II, J. A. (1972). Clinical and bacteriologic observations on the proposed species, *Enterobacter agglomerans* (the Herbcola–Lathyri bacteria). *Mayo Clinics Proc.* **47**, 739.
58. Baird, P. J. and Benn, R. (1975). Erysipelothrix endocarditis. *Med. J. Aust.* **2**, 743.
59. Sans, M. D. and Crowder, J. G. (1973). Subacute bacterial endocarditis caused by *Eubacterium aerofaciens*: report of a case. *Am. J. Clin. Path.* **59**, 576.
60. Thong, M. L., Puthucheary, S. D., and Lee, E. L. (1981). *Flavobacterium meningosepticum* infection: an epidemiological study in a newborn nursery. *J. Clin. Path.* **34**, 429.
61. Werthamer, S. and Weiner, M. (1972). Subacute bacterial endocarditis due to *Flavobacterium meningosepticum*. *Am. J. Clin. Path.* **57**, 410.
62. Dhawan, V. K., Rajashekaraiah, K. R., Metzger, W. I., Rice, T. W., and Kallick, C. A. (1980). Spontaneous bacterial peritonitis due to a group 11k–2 strain. *J. Clin. Microbiol.* **11**, 492.
63. Holmes, B., Owen, R. J., and Weaver, R. E. (1981). *Flavobacterium mutivorum*: a new species isolated from human clinical specimens and previously known as group 11K-biotype 2. *Int. J. Syst. Bact.* **31**, 21.
64. Vogel, L. C. and Boyer, K. M. (1981). Metastic complications of *Fusobacterium necrophorum* sepsis. *Am. J. Dis. Childn.* **134**, 356.
65. Nastro, L. J. and Finegold, S. M. (1973). Endocarditis due to anaerobic Gram-negative bacilli. *Am. J. Med.* **54**, 482.

66. Lanby, M. (1981). Septicémie post-angineuse à *Fusobacterium necrophorum* avec métastases. *Méd. Mal. Infect.* **11**, 451.

67. Gardner, H. L. (1980). *Haemophilus vaginalis* Vaginitis after twenty-five years. *Am. J. Obstet. Gynecol.* **137**, 385.

68. Venkataramani, T. K. and Rathbun, H. K. (1976). *Corynebacterium vaginale* (*Haemophilus vaginalis*) bacteremia: clinical study of 29 cases. *Johns Hopkins Med. J.* **139**, 93.

69. Elster, S. K., Mattes, L. M., Meyers, B. R., and Durado, R. A. (1975). *Haemophilus aphrophilus* endocarditis: review of 23 cases. *Am. J. Cardiol.* **35**, 72.

70. Taylor, C. E. D. (1979). A recently recognised venereal disease of horses and its causative organism. *J. Infect.* **1**, 81.

71. Taintturier, D. J., Delmas, C. F., and Dabernat, H. J. (1981). Bacteriological and serological studies of *Haemophilus equigenitalis*, agent of contagious equine metritis. *J. Clin. Microbiol.* **14**, 355.

72. Jemsek, J. G., Greenberg, S. B., Gentry, L. O., Welton, D. E., and Mattocx, K. L. (1979). *Haemophilus parainfluenzae* endocarditis: two cases and review of the literature in the past decade. *Am. J. Med.* **66**, 51.

73. Lynn, D. J., Kane, J. G., and Parker, R. H. (1977). *Haemophilus parainfluenzae* and *influenzae* endocarditis: a review of forty cases. *Medicine, Baltimore* **56**, 115.

74. Greenspan, J., Noble, J. T., and Tenenbaum, M. J. (1981). Cure of *Haemophilus parainfluenzae* endocarditis with chloramphenicol. *Archs intern. Med.* **141**, 1222.

75. Gill, V. J., Manning C., Lamson, M., Woltering, P., and Pizzo, P. A. (1981). Antibiotic-resistant Group JK bacteria in hospitals. *J. Clin. Microbiol.* **13**, 472.

76. Pearson, T. A., Braine, H. G., and Rathburn, H. K. (1977). Corynebacterium sepsis in oncology patients. *J. Am. med. Ass.* **238**, 1737.

77. Redfield, D. C., Overturf, G. D., Ewing, N., and Powars, D. (1980). Bacteria (? bacteraemia), arthritis, and skin lesions due to *Kingella kingae*. *Archs Dis. Childn.* **55**, 411.

78. Goldman, I. S., Ellner, P. D., Francke, E. L., Garvey, G. J., and Squilla, N. (1980). Infective endocarditis due to *Kingella denitrificans*. *Ann. intern. Med.* **93**, 152.

79. Ödum, L. and Frederikson, W. (1981). Identification and characterisation of *Kingella kingae*. *Acta path. microbiol. scand.* **89B**, 311.

80. Vincent, J. (1981). Septic arthritis due to *Kingella* (*Moraxella*) *kingii*: case report and review of the literature. *J. Rheum.* **8**, 501.

81. Elston, H. R. (1961). *Kuthia bessonii* isolated from clinical material. *J. Path Bact.* **81**, 245.

82. Pancoast, S. J., Ellner, P. D., Jahre, J. A., and Neu, H. C. (1979). Endocarditis due to *Kurthia bessonii*. *Ann. intern. Med.* **90**, 936.

83. Isenberg, D. (1977). Lactobacillus infective endocarditis. *Proc. R. S. Med.* **70**, 278.

84. Pinon, G. (1981). Lactobacilli and urinary tract infections. *Lancet* **ii**, 581.

85. Brancaccio, M. and Legendri, G. G. (1979). *Megasphaera elsdenii* endocarditis. *J. Clin. Microbiol.* **10**, 72.

86. Feigin, R. D., San Joaquin, V., and Middelkamp, J. N. (1969). Septic arthritis due to *Moraxella osloensis*. *J. Pediat.* **75**, 116.

87. Butzler, J. D., Hansen, W., Cadranel, S., and Henriksen, S. D. (1974). Stomatitis with septicemia due to *Moraxella osloensis*. *J. Pediat.* **84**, 721.

88. Nelson, S. C. and Hammert, G. S. (1981). *Pasteurella multicoda* empyema: case report and review of the literature. *Am. J. med. Sci.* **281**, 43.

89. Patton, F., Dumas, M., and Cannon, N. J. (1980). *Pasteurella multocida* septicemia and peritonitis in a cirrhotic cock trainer with a pet pig. *New Engl. J. Med.* **303**, 1126.

90. Francis, D. P., Holmes, M. A., and Brandon, G. (1975). *Pasteurella multicoda* infections after domestic animal bites and scratches. *J. Am. med. Ass.* **233**, 42.

91. Bourgault, A-M., Rosenblatt, J. E., and Fitzgerald, R. H. (1980). *Peptococcus magnus*: a significant human pathogen. *Ann. intern. Med.* **93**, 244.

92. Maniatis, A. and Vassilouthis, J. (1980). *Propionibacterium acnes* infection complicating craniotomy. *J. hosp. Infect.* **1**, 261.

93. Schlossberg, D., Keeney, G. E., Lifton, L. J., and Azizhkan, R. G. (1980). Anaerobic botryomycosis. *J. Clin. Microbiol.* **11**, 184.

94. Ahbel, D. E., Alexander, A. H., Kleine, M. L., and Lichtman, D. M. (1980). Protothecal olecranon bursitis. *J. Bone Joint Surg.* **62A**, 835.

95. Sudman, M. S. (1974). Prototheosis: a critical review. *Am. J. Clin. Path.* **61**, 10.

96. Cox, G. E., Wilson, J. D., and Brown, P. (1974). Prototheosis: a case of disseminated algal infection, *Lancet* **ii**, 379.

97. Edwards, L. D., Cross, A., Levin, S., and Landau, W. (1974). Outbreak of a nosocomial infection with a strain of *Porteus rettgeri* resistant to many antimicrobials. *Am. J. Clin. Path.* **61**, 41.

98. McHale, P. J., Walker, F., Scully, B., English, L., and Keane, C. T. (1981). Providencia stuartii infections: a review of 117 cases over an eight year period. *J. hosp. Infect.* **2**, 155.

99. Penner, J. L., Hinton, N. A., Hamilton, L. J., and Hennessy, J. N. (1981). Three episodes of nosocomial urinary tract infections caused by one O-serotype of *Providencia stuartii. J. Urol.* **125**, 668.

100. Noriega, E. R., Rubinstein, E., and Simberkoff, M. S. (1975). Subacute and acute endocarditis due to *Pseudomonas cepacia* in heroin addicts. *Am. J. Med* **59**, 29.

101. Phillips, I., Eykyn, S., Curtis, M. A., and Snell, J. J. S. (1971). *Pseudomonas cepacia* (multivorans) septicemia in an intensive-care unit. *Lancet* **i**, 375.

102. Speller, D. C. E., Stephens, M. E., and Viant, A. C. (1971). Hospital infection by *Pseudomonas cepacia. Lancet* **i**, 798.

103. Taplin, D., Bassett, D. C. J., and Mertz, P. M. (1971). Foot lesions associated with *Pseudomonas cepacia. Lancet* **ii**, 568.

104. Fiscler, R. A., Doern, G. V., and Cheeseman, S. H. (1981). *Pseudomonas denitrificans meningitis. J. Clin. Microbiol.* **13**, 1004.

105. Holmes, B., Lapage, S. P., and Easterling, B. G. (1979). Distribution in clinical material and identification of *Pseudomonas maltophilia. J. Clin. Path.* **32**, 66.

106. Fisher, M. C., Long, S. S., Roberts, E. M., Dunn, J. M., and Balsara, R. K. (1981). *Pseudomonas maltophilia* bacteremia in children undergoing open heart surgery. *J. Am. med. Ass.* **246**, 1571.

107. Slotnick, I. J., Hall, J., and Sacks, H. (1979). Septicemia caused by *Pseudomonas paucimobilis. Am. J. Clin. Path.* **72**, 882.

108. Hajiroussou, V., Holmes, B., Bullas, J., and Pinning, C. A. (1979). Meningitis caused by *Pseudomonas paucimobilis. J. Clin. Path.* **32**. 953.

109. Crane, L. R., Tagle, L. C., and Palutke, W. A. (1981). Outbreak of *Pseudomonas paucimobilis* in an intensive care facility. *J. Am. med. Ass.* **246**, 985.

110. Southern, P. M. and Kutscher, A. E. (1981). *Pseudomonas paucimobilis* bacteremia. *J. Clin. Microbiol.* **13**, 1070.

111. Fujita, S., Yoshida, T., and Matsubara, F. (1981). *Pseudomonas pickettii* bacteremia. *J. Clin. Microbiol.* **13**, 781.

112. Pape, J., Singer, C., Kiehn, T. E., Lee, B. J., and Armstrong, D. (1979). Infective endocarditis caused by *Rothia dentocariosa. Ann. intern. Med.* **91**, 746.

113. Shafer, F. J., Wing, E. J., and Norden, C. W. (1979). Infectious endocarditis caused by *Rothia dentocariosa. Ann. intern. Med.* **91**, 747.

114. Yu, V. L. (1979). *Serratia marcescens*: historical perspective and clinical review. *New Engl. J. Med.* **300**, 887.

115. Hollis, D. G., Hickman, F. W., Fanning, G. R., Farmer III, J. J., Weaver, R. E., and Brenner, D. J. (1981). *Tatumella ptyseos* gen. nov., sp. nov., a member of the family Enterobacteriaceae found in clinical specimens. *J. Clin. Microbiol.* **14**, 79.

FUNGAL INFECTIONS (MYCOSES)

R. J. Hay and D. W. R. Mackenzie

Introduction. The fungi are a specialized group of saprophytic or parasitic organisms which are normally assigned to the phylum Protista. They have the complex subcellular organization seen in both animal and plant cells as well as highly organized genetic material. The fungal cell wall is a distinctive feature and contains complex macromolecules such as cellulose or chitin. The arrangement and reproduction of individual cells is also characteristic. Certain fungi form new cells terminally, but remain connected to form chains of cells, hyphae (the mould fungi). Others reproduce in a similar manner but each new cell separates from the parent by a process of budding (the yeast fungi). It is a feature of certain fungi to be yeast-like during one phase of their life history but to form hyphae at another, a phenomenon known as dimorphism. In culture mould fungi usually form a cottony growth on laboratory media while yeasts normally have a smooth shiny appearance.

Fungi adversely affect man in a number of ways. They cause

disease indirectly by their contribution to the spoilage and destruction of food crops and subsequent malnutrition and starvation. Secondly, many of the common moulds produce and release spores which may act as airborne allergens to produce asthma or hypersensitivity pneumonitis. Thirdly many fungi elaborate complex metabolic by-products, some of which are useful to man, e.g., the penicillins. However others are toxic. Disease caused by the ingestion of fungal toxins includes both poisoning by eating certain mushrooms (mycetism) and damage caused by the ingestion of minute quantities of toxin (mycotoxicosis) for instance in contaminated grain. The contribution of the latter mechanism to human disease remains largely unexplored. Finally fungi may invade human tissue. Medical mycology is largely concerned with this last group.

Invasive fungal diseases are normally divided into three groups—the superficial, subcutaneous, and deep mycoses. In superficial infections invasion of skin and mucous membranes is seen. The dermatophyte or ringworm infections and thrush (superficial candidosis) are examples. Extension deeper than the surface epithelium is rare. Most of the subcutaneous infections are tropical and the main site of involvement is within subcutaneous tissue, although secondary invasion of adjacent structures such as bone or skin may occur. In deep or systemic infections deep viscera such as lung, spleen, or brain are invaded. This classification is based on the main 'sphere of involvement' by the relevant organisms, but there are rare exceptions. For instance in chromomycosis, normally a subcutaneous infection, brain involvement has been recorded in exceptional circumstances.

The fungi causing systemic mycoses are often classified in two groups—the opportunists and the pathogens. The former cause disease in compromised individuals. These contrast with the true pathogens which cause infection in all subjects inhaling airborne spores. However, in the vast majority the infection is usually controlled in an asymptomatic illness.

References

Emmons, C. W., Binford, C. H., Utz, J. P., and Kwon-Chung, K. J. (1977). *Medical Mycology*. Lea and Febiger, Philadelphia.
Rippon, J. W. (1974). *Medical mycology*. W. B. Saunders, Philadelphia.

Superficial fungal infections

The major superficial mycoses are the dermatophyte infections, superficial candidosis, and tinea versicolor which are common and widespread in distribution. Rare superficial infections include tinea nigra, and black or white piedra.

Dermatophyte infections

Aetiology. The dermatophyte or ringworm infections are caused by a group of organisms which are capable of existing in keratinized tissue such as stratum corneum, nail, or hair. Mechanisms of pathogenicity are thought to be linked to production of extracellular enzymes. For instance *Trichophyton mentagrophytes* produces three distinct keratinases, but other proteases may also be involved.

Epidemiology. Some dermatophyte fungi have a worldwide distribution. Others are more restricted. The commonest and most widely distributed is *T. rubrum*, which causes different types of infection in different parts of the world. It is commonly associated with athletes foot (tinea pedis) in temperate areas and tinea corporis (body ringworm) in the tropics. This distinction is not based solely on climatic factors as immigrants from tropical countries, particularly the Far East, may still have tinea corporis caused by *T. rubrum* when living in northern Europe. However, certain dermatophytes are limited to defined areas. For instance tinea imbricata caused by *T. concentricum*, is found in hot humid areas of the Far East, Polynesia, and South America. Scalp ringworm tends to occur in well-defined endemic areas in Africa. In different regions

different species of dermatophytes may predominate. Thus in North Africa, the commonest cause of tinea capitis is *T. violaceum*, in southern parts of the continent the major agents may be *Microsporum audouinii*, *M. ferrugineum*, and *T. soudanense*. Not all dermatophyte infections are endemic and dominant species may disappear to be replaced by others. *Microsporum audouinii* once endemic and common in the United Kingdom has largely disappeared as a cause of scalp ringworm, probably because of improved treatment and detection of carriers. Conversely dermatophytes common to an immigrant group may be introduced into their new society.

Dermatophytes may be passed from man to man (anthropophilic infections), from animal to man (zoophilic), or soil to man (geophilic). Sources of zoophilic organisms in Europe include cats and dogs, cattle, hedgehogs, and small rodents. Rarer sources include horses, monkeys, and chickens. Lesions produced by zoophilic species may be highly inflammatory.

Factors governing the invasion of stratum corneum are largely unknown. However heat, humidity, and occlusion have all been implicated. Recently it has been suggested that the carbon dioxide tension at the skin surface may be a critical factor.

Clinical features. The clinical features of dermatophyte infections are best considered in relation to the site involved. Often the term tinea, preceded by the Latin name of the appropriate part (e.g. *corporis*—body) is used to describe the clinical site of infection.

Tinea pedis. Scaling or maceration between the toes, particularly in the fourth interspace is the commonest form of dermatophytosis seen in temperate countries. Itching is variable but may be severe. Sometimes blisters may form both between the toes and on the soles of the feet. The causative organisms are commonly *T. rubrum* and *T. interdigitale*.

'Dry type' infections of the soles and palms. These are normally caused by *T. rubrum*. The palms or soles have a dry scaly appearance which in the latter may encroach on to the lateral or dorsal surfaces of the foot (Fig. 1). The palmar involvement is often unilateral, an important diagnostic feature. Nail invasion is often seen (see below). Itching is not prominent.

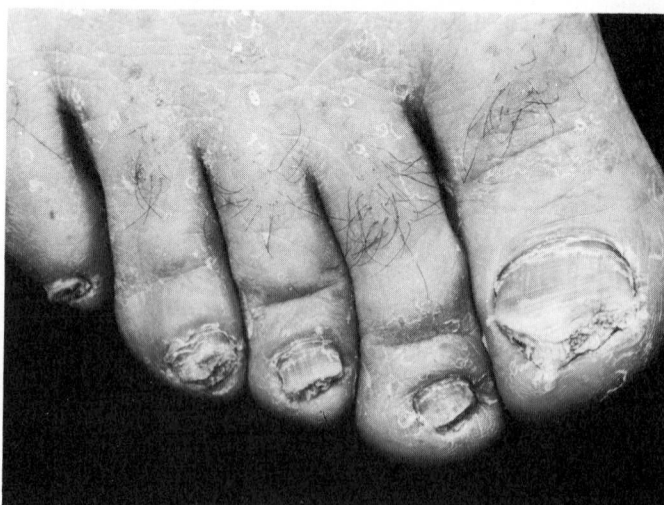

Fig. 1 *T. rubrum* infection involving both nails and dorsum of foot.

Tinea cruris. Infections of the groin most often caused by *T. rubrum* or *Epidermophyton floccosum* are relatively common. They occur in both tropical and temperate climates, although in the former the infection may spread to involve the whole waist area in both males and females. Tinea cruris in females is uncommon in Europe. An erythematous and scaly rash with a distinct margin extends from the groin to the upper thighs or scrotum. Itching may be severe.

Onychomycosis (caused by dermatophytes). Invasion of the nail plate is most often seen with *T. rubrum* infections. The plate is invaded distally and becomes enlarged and friable. Onycholysis may be seen. More rarely, and most often with *T. interdigitale*, the dorsal surface of the plate is invaded—superficial white onychomycosis.

Tinea corporis (body ringworm). Dermatophyte or ringworm infection on the trunk or limbs may produce the characteristic annular plaque with a raised edge and central clearing. Scaling and itching is variable. Lesions caused by zoophilic organisms may be highly inflammatory, and in certain cases, particularly those caused by *T. verrucosum*, intense itching, oedema, and pustule formation, a kerion may develop. This reaction is seldom secondarily infected by bacteria but is a response to the fungus on hairy skin. Infections of the beard, tinea barbae, are often highly refractory to treatment.

On the legs an unusual variant, nodular folliculitis, may superficially resemble erythema nodosum. A hot tender dermal nodule is formed on the shin or lower leg. However close inspection usually reveals its relation to a hair follicle and some scaling. *T. rubrum* is the usual cause.

Facial dermatophyte infections may mimic a variety of non-fungal skin diseases including acne, rosacea, and discoid lupus erythematosus. However the underlying annular configuration can usually be distinguished.

Tinea capitis (scalp ringworm). In the United Kingdom the commonest cause of scalp ringworm is *Microsporum canis* originating from an infected cat or dog. Scalp ringworm is mainly a disease of childhood with rare infections occurring in adult women. Spontaneous clearance at puberty is the rule. *M. canis* causes an 'ectothrix' infection where spores form on the outside of the hair shaft and the scalp hair breaks above the skin surface. Scaling, itching, and loss of hair occur. Other causes of ectothrix infection include *M. audouinii*, which is now rare in Europe, but still seen in the tropics. This infection can be spread from child to child and cause serious social handicap. The infection may occur in epidemic form, particularly in schools. By contrast infections with *M. canis* are acquired from a primary animal source rather than by spread from human lesions.

In endothrix infections, where sporulation is within the hair shaft, scaling is less pronounced and hairs break at scalp level, black dot ringworm, *Trichophyton tonsurans* and *T. violaceum* being examples. The latter is most prevalent in the middle East, parts of Africa and India, although it is recognized with increasing frequency in Europe.

Favus, now most often seen in the tropics, is a particularly chronic form of scalp ringworm where hair shafts become surrounded by a necrotic crust or scutulum. Individual crusts coalesce to form a pale, unpleasant smelling mat over parts of the scalp. Such infections may cause extensive and permanent hair loss.

Tinea imbricata (Tokelau). This infection, endemic in parts of the Far East, South Pacific, and areas in central and South America, is caused by *T. concentricum*. In many cases the trunk is covered with scales laid down in concentric rings producing a 'ripple' effect. The infection is often chronic and may constitute a serious social handicap.

Laboratory diagnosis. The mainstays of diagnosis are direct microscopy of skin scales mounted in potassium hydroxide (20 per cent) to demonstrate hyphae, and culture. Scalp hairs may also be examined in a similar way and the site of arthospore formation, inside or outside the shaft, recognized. Further tests, such as the ability to penetrate hair, may be used to separate similar cultures.

When large numbers of children are involved, screening of scalp infections with a filtered ultra-violet (Wood's light) lamp is useful. Certain species cause infected hair to fluoresce with a vivid greenish light. *M. canis* and *M. audouinii* behave in this manner. Scalps can also be screened for invasion by passing a sterile brush through the hair and plating this directly on to an agar plate.

Treatment. The treatment of dermatophyte infections depends to an extent on the nature and severity of infection. Topical therapy is usually reserved for circumscribed infections such as athletes foot or tinea corporis, not involving hair or nail keratin. Scalp and nail infections, severe or widespread ringworm, and failures on topical therapy are usually treated orally with griseofulvin.

Older treatments, such as Castellani's paint, which contains magenta and resorcinol, are still employed with some success. However the commonest and cheapest preparation is Whitfield's ointment (benzoic acid compound). The half strength preparation is well tolerated and can be applied twice daily to localized lesions. More specific antifungal drugs in topical form are more expensive and there is no clear evidence that they are more effective although they are better tolerated and may be quicker in action than Whitfield's ointment. The important compounds in this group are miconazole, clotrimazole and econazole which are imidazole derivatives, undecenoic acid, tolnaftate, and haloprogin. They are all very similar in their clinical efficacy. Adverse effects from these compounds are rare.

Griseofulvin is the only orally effective agent widely used against dermatophytes. It is normally given in doses of 0.5–1.0 g daily in adults or 10 mg/kg daily in children. The treatment should be continued for at least three weeks. The griseofulvin tablets are prepared in a microcrystalline form and are probably best absorbed when given with a meal. Side effects are not common, but include headache, nausea, and urticaria. The drug can also precipitate acute intermittent porphyria in predisposed subjects.

Griseofulvin is normally highly effective except in certain cases of 'dry type' infection caused by *T. rubrum* and toe-nail infections. Cure is obtained in only 50–70 per cent of the latter. The newer imidazole drug, ketoconazole, is also active orally against dermatophytes, but its precise role has yet to be determined.

References

Jones, H. E., Reinhardt, J. H., and Rinaldi, M. G. (1974). Immunologic susceptibility to chronic dermatophytosis. *Archs Dermatol.* **110**, 213.
Rebell, G. and Taplin, D. (1970). *Dermatophytes: their recognition and identification.* University of Miami Press, Miami.
Roberts, S. O. B. and Mackenzie, D. W. R. (1979). In *Textbook of dermatology* (eds. Rook, Wilkinson, and Ebling), 775. Blackwell Scientific Publications, Oxford.
Zaias, N. (1972). Onychomycosis. *Archs Dermatol.* **105**, 263.

Hendersonula and Scytalidium infections. Two organisms, *Hendersonula toruloidea* and *Scytalidium hyalinum*, can cause a superficial scaly condition which resembles the 'dry' type of dermatophyte infection on the palms or soles (page 5.370). Nail plate destruction may also occur (Fig. 2). The disease has been seen in Europe almost invariably in immigrants from the tropics particularly the Caribbean, West Africa, and India or Pakistan. In skin scrapings the

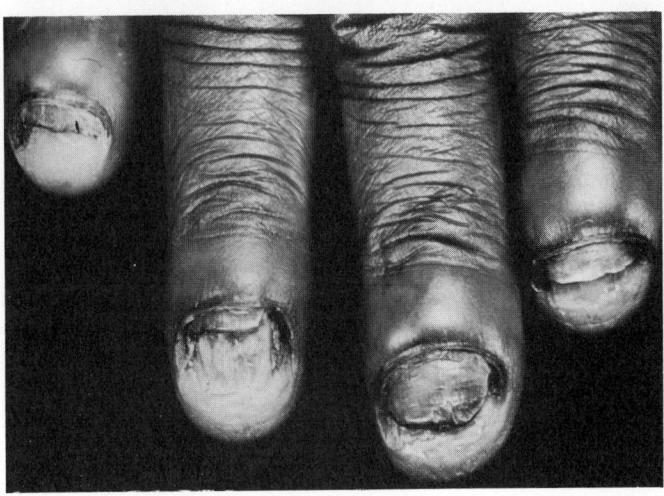

Fig. 2 Onychomycosis caused by *H. toruloidea*.

tortuous hyphae may resemble those of a dermatophyte but the organisms do not grow on media containing cycloheximide, which is often incorporated into agar for dermatophyte isolation.

Treatment is difficult, but some improvement may follow the use of keratolytic compounds such as salicylic acid. The organisms do not respond to griseofulvin.

Reference

Campbell, C. K., Kurwa, A., Abdel-Aziz, A. H. M., and Hodgson, C. (1973). Fungal infection of skin and nails by *Hendersonula toruloidea. Br. J. Derm.* **89**, 45.

Miscellaneous nail infections. Occasionally fungi other than dermatophytes, *Hendersonula*, or *Scytalidium* are isolated from dystrophic nails. These include *Scopulariopsis brevicaulis, Cephalosporium* species and certain types of *Aspergillus*. These infections are usually seen in the elderly and it is often difficult, particularly with *Aspergillus* species to establish that the organism is playing a pathogenic role.

Tinea versicolor (pityriasis versicolor)

Aetiology. Tinea versicolor is a superficial infection caused by *Malassezia furfur*. Commonest in tropical countries, it has a worldwide distribution. Dermal penetration does not occur.

M. furfur is probably the parasitic form of a common saprophytic yeast *Pityrosporum orbiculare* which is found on normal skin. Its conversion from saprophytic to parasitic phase has been observed following renal transplantation. It is likely that the state of host immunity plays some role in pathogenesis, and depression, for instance, by endogenous or exogenous corticosteroids produces the disease in some individuals. However, it is also commonly seen in normal individuals. There is no effective animal model for this disease.

Epidemiology. Tinea versicolor is very common in the tropics where it may be widespread on the body. Its incidence in temperate climates has increased over the last 20–30 years.

Clinical features. The rash of tinea versicolor is asymptomatic or mildly pruritic. It presents with scaling confluent macules on the trunk, upper arms, or neck. These may be hypo or hyperpigmented (Fig. 3). In some individuals and in the tropics other areas including face, forearms, and thighs may be involved.

The diagnosis is rarely confused with other complaints, although eczema or ringworm infections are sometimes considered. Patients are often anxious to exclude leprosy but the two are unlikely to be mistaken.

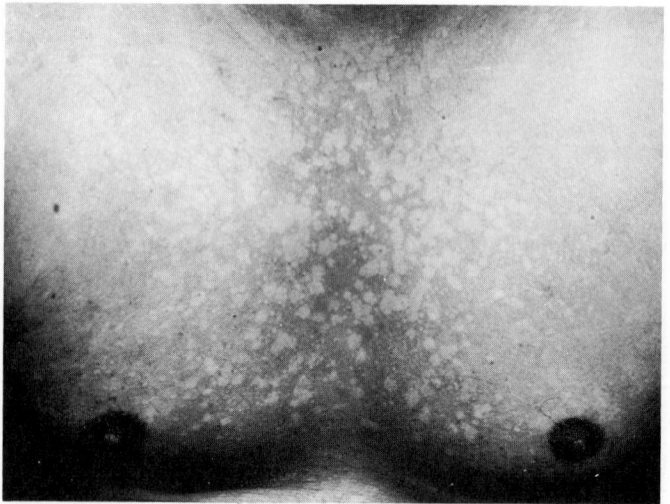

Fig. 3 Tinea versicolor.

Laboratory diagnosis. The diagnosis is made by scraping and demonstration of the yeasts and hyphae of *M. furfur* in skin scales. Culture is difficult and unnecessary.

Treatment. Treatment with keratolytics including sulphur or Whitfield's ointment may be effective. More usually 1 per cent selenium sulphide or 20 per cent sodium thiosulphate lotions are used. Alternatively topical miconazole, clotrimazole, or econazole are also effective.

Reference

Roberts, S. O. B. (1969). Pityriasis versicolor: A clinical and mycological investigation. *Br. J. Derm.* **81**, 315.

Superficial candidosis (candidiasis)

Aetiology. Superficial candidosis is a term used to describe a group of infections of skin or mucus membranes caused by species of the genus *Candida*. They range in severity from oral thrush to chronic mucocutaneous candidosis, a chronic infection refractory to conventional treatment.

Candida albicans is the organism most frequently involved. It is a saprophytic yeast often found as a commensal in the mouth and gastrointestinal tract and commonly present in the vagina. Several factors may influence the incidence of carriage. For instance, oral colonization is commoner in hospital staff than in equivalent non-hospital subjects. Vaginal carriage is commoner in pregnancy. Other factors (Table 1) are known which predispose to conversion from a commensal to a parasitic role with the causation of disease candidosis. The list includes factors which influence host immunological response such as carcinoma or cytotoxic therapy, those which disturb the population of other micro-organisms, e.g., antibiotics, and those which affect the character of the epithelium, e.g., dentures.

Table 1 Predisposing factors in superficial candidosis

1. Local epithelial defects, occlusion etc.,
      e.g. damaged nail folds, beneath dentures
2. Defects of immunity (primarily T cell or phagocytosis)
      (a) Primary immunological disease, e.g. chronic granulomatous disease
      (b) Immunodefects secondary to intercurrent illness, e.g. leukaemia
      (c) Immunodefects secondary to therapy, e.g. cytotoxic therapy in organ transplantation
3. Drug therapy, e.g. antibiotics
4. Carcinoma or leukaemia
5. Endocrine disease
      (a) Diabetes mellitus
      (b) Hypothyroidism, hypoparathyroidism, hypoadrenalism
            (in chronic mucocutaneous candidosis)
6. Physiological changes, e.g. infancy, pregnancy, old age
7. Miscellaneous disorders, e.g.
      (a) Iron deficiency
      (b) Malabsorption

Other species of *Candida* may also cause superficial infections but are less common. They include *C. guilliermondii, C. tropicalis, C. pseudotropicalis,* and *C. parapsilosis*.

Epidemiology. Superficial *Candida* infections are seen in all countries.

Clinical features. There are a number of clinically distinct types of superficial infection caused by *Candida* species.

Oral candidosis (thrush). Oral infection by *Candida* is fairly common particularly in infancy and old age, or in association with antibiotic or cytotoxic therapy, or in diseases where the immune response may be impaired. In the older age group the wearing of dentures is a predisposing factor. The lesions present with discomfort both in the mouth and at the corners of the lips (Fig. 4). The mouth and buccal mucosa show a patchy or confluent white adherent plaque. Angular cheilitis usually accompanies the oral lesions. In long-standing cases the plaque may become hypertrophic with oedema of the mucosal surfaces or the mucosa may appear glazed and raw.

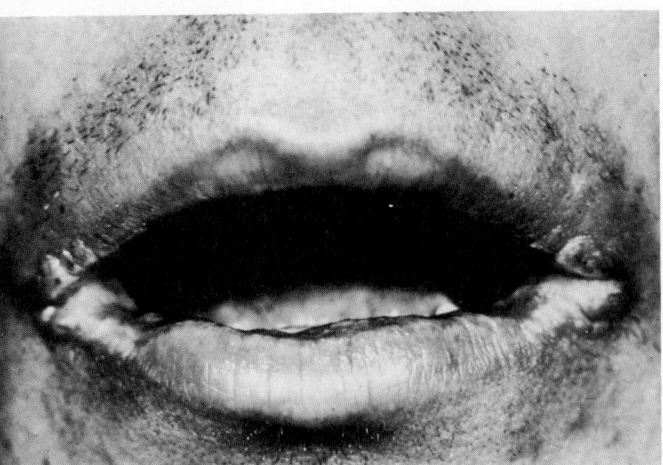

Fig. 4 Angular cheilitis in a patient with oral candidosis.

The diagnosis is made by the demonstration of yeasts and hyphae of *Candida* in smears, and by culture.

Vaginal candidosis (thrush). A similar infection can occur in the vagina with secondary spread to the vulva. This is seen in normal women as well as in pregnancy or in association with diabetes mellitus. Vaginal candidosis has been diagnosed increasingly in recent years and this may reflect upsurge of the disease. It has been suggested that some of this increase may be due to the use of the contraceptive pill.

As with oral candidosis, soreness is the main symptom although irritation may occur. A creamy discharge is also common. The diagnosis is confirmed principally by direct microscopy and secondarily by culture.

Secondary spread to the vulva is common with the development of a red scaling rash. Beyond its edge small satellite scales and pustules are seen and these are typical of superficial *Candida* infections.

Paronychia. Infection around the nail fold is seen in housewives or patients with eczema or psoriasis. In some cases this is caused by bacterial infection but *Candida* may also be a primary cause. The condition presents with painful red swelling of the nail fold. Pus may be discharged. Secondary invasion of the lateral border of the nail plate may occur from this site.

Candida intertrigo. Infection of the moist folds of the skin in the groin or under the breasts causes itching and discomfort. The area becomes macerated and erythematous. *Candida* may contribute to this condition but is certainly not the only factor. It may also superinfect the nappy area in infants where there is pre-existing nappy dermatitis.

Direct invasion of toe web folds by *Candida* closely resembles 'athlete's foot' caused by dermatophytes. A similar erosive infection may occur in the finger webs and is seen most commonly in the tropics.

Laboratory diagnosis. All these infections are diagnosed by microscopy and culture. When associated with the condition *Candida* cells are always evident on microscopy. Culture establishes the specific identity, but, as a rule, is of less value than direct microscopy.

Chronic superficial candidosis. Chronic *Candida* infections of the mouth, vagina, and nail present problems in management. Predis-

posing causes should be searched for. The most serious of this group of infections is chronic mucocutaneous candidosis, a rare condition, in which chronic skin, nail, and mucosal infection co-exist (Fig. 5). A series of underlying genetic, endocrine (hypoparathyroidism or hypothyroidism), and immunological abnormalities have been found. Other superficial viral or fungal infections may

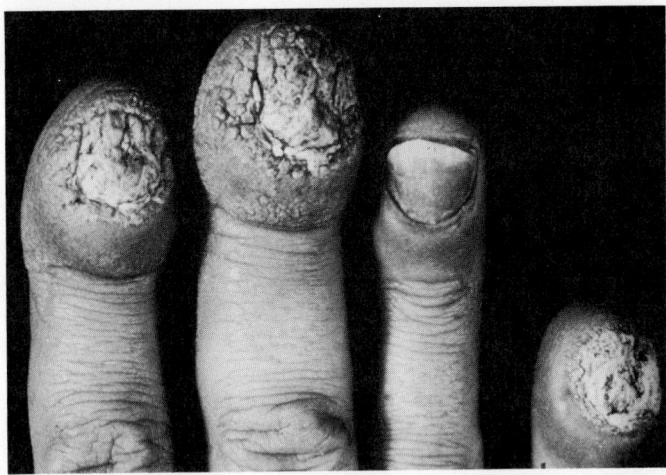

Fig. 5 Chronic mucocutaneous candidosis—nail dystrophy.

also be present in thse patients whose condition is normally diagnosed in childhood.

Treatment. Two groups of drugs are effective in topical creams or ointments against superficial *Candida* infections. The first, the polyene antibiotics, contain drugs such as amphotericin B and nystatin. The second is the imidazole group, particularly miconazole, clotrimazole, and econazole. For resistant infections ketoconazole (200–400 mg daily), can be given orally although its precise role has not yet been determined. Chronic mucocutaneous candidosis may respond to the latter. Alternatives include intravenous miconazole or low dose amphotericin B, intermittent oral clotrimazole, and transfer factor.

For vaginal infections topical cream should be combined with a pessary or medicated tampon containing a polyene or imidazole drug. Where treatment fails, thought should be given to the possibility of faecal carriage or infection of the male partner. In many cases treatment of vaginal candidosis for as little as 3 days may be sufficient. However, if this fails, longer courses are necessary.

References

Higgs, J. M. and Wells, R. S. (1972). Chronic mucocutaneous candidiasis: associated abnormalities of iron metabolism. *Br. J. Derm.* **86**, Suppl. 8, 88.
Winner, J. I. and Hurley, R. (eds.) (1966). *Symposium on candida infections.* Livingstone, Edingburgh.

Miscellaneous superficial mycoses. There are a number of relatively rare superficial fungal infections such as tinea nigra, and black or white piedra. They never cause invasive disease and are mainly confined to the tropics.

Tinea nigra. Tinea nigra is a superficial infection confined to the epidermis of the palms or soles, and more rarely elsewhere. Each lesion is a dark macule without scaling which resembles a brown stain on the skin. The disease is normally asymptomatic.

On scraping brown pigmented hypae can be seen by direct microscopy and the causative organism, *Exophiala werneckii* isolated. The lesion responds to Whitfield's ointment.

Black piedra. Black piedra is a disease of the tropics in which small dark nodules form on hair shafts in the scalp or, less commonly, elsewhere. There are no symptoms. Each nodule consists of a dense mat of hyphae containing the sexual spores (ascospores) of the fungus.

The diagnosis is made by direct microscopy of infected hair and the isolation of *Piedraia hortae*. Treatment using formalin solution or amphotericin B lotion is usually effective.

White piedra. White piedra occurs in both temperate and tropical climates and is rare. It produces pale nodules on the hair of the beard, groin, or scalp. The hair shaft may fracture. The nodule consists of hyphae, arthrospores (spores formed by fragmentation of hyphae), and blastospores (budding yeast cells). The organism *Trichosporon beigelii* can be readily cultured. The treatment is similar to that used for black piedra.

The subcutaneous mycoses

Subcutaneous infections caused by fungi are rare and are mainly seen in the tropics. It is assumed that the organism gains entry via the skin, although there is good evidence for this only in the case of mycetoma. However, the majority of the causative organisms in this group of infections can be isolated from vegetation or soil, and involvement of deep viscera is rare. Attempts to establish experimental infections which resemble the human disease have been largely unsuccessful. A clearer understanding of their pathogenesis therefore awaits such a model system.

Mycetoma (Madura foot):

Aetiology. Mycetoma is a chronic infection involving subcutaneous tissue, bone, and skin, in which colonies of infecting fungi or actinomycetes, 'grains', are found in a network of burrowing abscesses and sinuses.

A list of the commoner organisms which cause mycetoma is shown in Table 2. By tradition the organisms are divided into two groups, the actinomycetomas and the eumycetomas, caused by actinomycetes and fungi respectively. The colour of the grain (red, pale, or dark) serves as a further clue to indentification. The organisms are found in the natural environment and some have even been indentified in Acacia thorns in an endemic area. The infection is initiated when an infected thorn is left implanted in deep tissue. However, many years may elapse before the growth of a mycetoma.

Table 2   Causes of mycetoma

1. *Fungi*
   Madurella mycetomatis
   M. grisea
   Petriellidium boydii
   Exophiala jeanselmei
   Leptosphaeria senegalensis
   Species of *Acremonium, Aspergillus, Fusarium*

2. *Actinomycetes*
   Nocardia brasiliensis
   Actinomadura madurae
   A. pelletieri
   Streptomyces somaliensis

Epidemiology. The disease is again seen primarily in the tropics although rare cases, apart from imported ones, may occur in temperate areas. Countries with the most reported cases included Sudan, India, Senegal, Mexico, and Venezuela. However, the disease is widely distributed in the tropics, particularly to the south and east of the Sahara Desert in Africa.

The pattern of prevalence of infections caused by certain organisms differs strikingly in different parts of the world. For instance *Streptomyces somaliensis* is commonest in the Sudan and Middle East. Altogether about 60 per cent of reported infections are caused by actinomycetes.

Clinical features. Early mycetomas may present as a circumscribed area of subcutaneous thickening. Later sinus tracts open on to the skin surface and grains may be discharged along with serosanguinous fluid (Fig. 6). Bone erosion and destruction leading to deformity may occur. However, severe pain is rarely a problem. Local lymph node invasion may occur but more widespread involvement is rare.

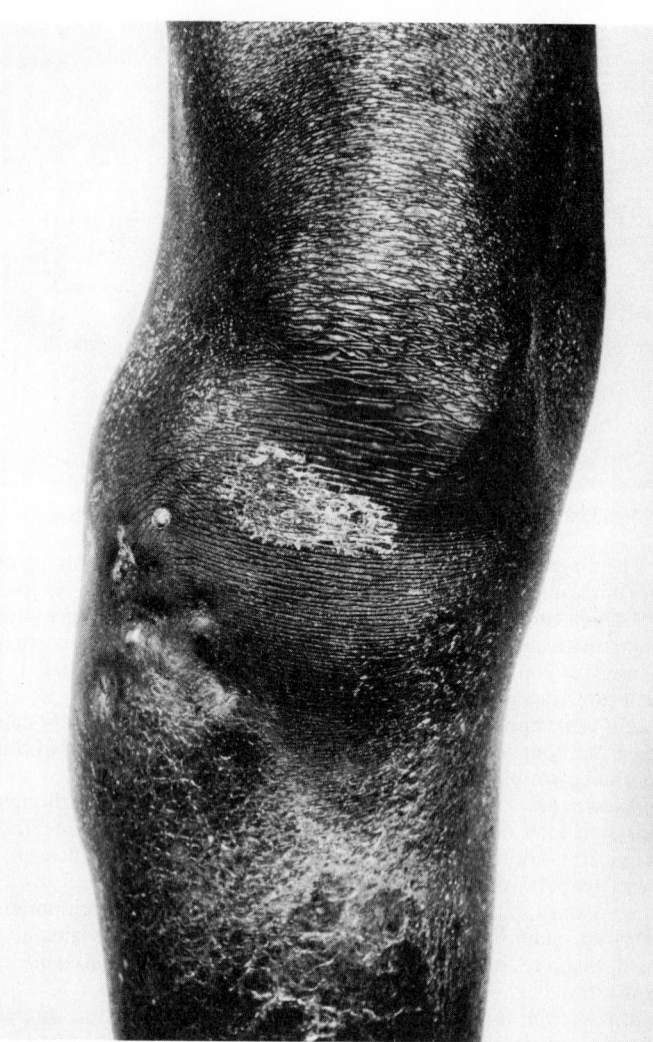

Fig. 6 Mycetoma (eumycetoma): right knee.

The foot and lower legs are the commonest areas involved, but the arm, buttocks, chest, and head may all be sites of infection. Mycetoma caused by *Nocardia brasiliensis* may occur in any site, but one favoured area is the chest wall.

The radiological features of mycetoma are cortical erosion followed by the development of lytic deposits in bone. Periosteal proliferation and destruction leading to deformity may follow.

Laboratory diagnosis. The diagnosis is made by the demonstration and identification of grains obtained from the sinus openings by gentle pressure or curettage. These can be mounted by potassium hydroxide and examined microscopically. Grains containing filaments 3–4 μm in diameter or more are caused by true fungi (eumycetomas), and those with filaments less than 1 μm by actinomycetes (actinomycetomas).

The morphology of grains fixed, sectioned and stained with haematoxylin and eosin is typical. Grains can be used for culture although several attempts at isolation may have to be made. Serology, e.g., immunodiffusion, can also be helpful particularly when cultures are difficult to obtain.

Treatment. Actinomycetomas may respond to sulphones such as dapsone (50–100 mg daily) or sulphonamides such as suphadiazine. The treatment of choice for many is long-term co-trimoxazole (two tablets twice daily) with an initial 2–3 months of streptomycin. Treatment may have to be continued for many months or years. Dapsone is an effective and cheaper alternative to co-trimoxazole. Extensive actinomycetomas may respond poorly, although generally marked improvement is obtained even when lytic bone lesions are well established.

The eumycetomas rarely respond to antifungal therapy. On very rare occasions griseofulvin, amphotericin B, and miconazole have produced remission or cure. Trial of therapy may be attempted where the patient can be monitored closely in outpatients. Otherwise radical surgery or amputation is usually necessary. Local excisions are rarely successful.

Mycetoma is slowly progressive and increasingly disabling. However wider dissemination is very rare, and, therefore, cases are seldom fatal except where the skull is involved.

Reference

Mahgoub, E. S. and Murray, I. G. (1973). *Mycetoma*, Heinemann, London.

Chromomycosis (chromoblastomycosis)

Aetiology. Chromomycosis is a chronic subcutaneous infection characterized by the presence of round pigmented fungal cells demonstrable in histology. Epidermal proliferation occurs and may lead to extensive warty plaque formation on the skin.

The agents of chromomycosis are four fungi of the genus *Phialophora*—(*P. pedrosoi*, *P. compacta*, *P. dermatitidis*, and *P. verrucosa*) and *Cladosporium carrionii*. There is some controversy over the correct designation of the Phialophora species, and some of them have been assigned to other genera such as Fonsecaea. Although the organisms are widely distributed, certain species are most commonly found in certain areas. For instance, Australian cases of chromomycosis normally grow *C. carrionii*. *P. dermatitidis* is mainly seen in Japan. The organisms have been found in nature mainly in association with soil or vegetation, particularly tree bark. It is presumed that they enter the dermis via an abrasion, and people whose work brings them into contact with the appropriate habitat, e.g. forestry or agricultural workers, are the group mainly affected.

Epidemiology. Chromomycosis is mainly a disease of the tropics, particularly areas with forest and high humidity. Southern Africa (particularly Madagascar), Central and South America, and northern Australia are the areas with the highest incidence. However, sporadic cases may also be seen in north America and Europe (e.g. Finland).

Clinical features. The early lesion of chromomycosis is a raised cutaneous nodule. Progressive warty proliferation and outward extension occur over a number of years. The lower legs and lower arms are the commonest areas affected.

Over a number of years extensive areas may be involved and some lesions develop a flat atrophic appearance. Scar formation also occurs. Secondary satellite lesions locally or in distal sites may follow scratching and, possibly, biopsy or attempted surgery. One characteristic feature of many cases of established chromomycosis is the smell associated with secondary bacterial infection.

Early leisons may resemble verrucose tuberculosis, squamous carcinoma, or extensive warts. Very extensive lesions have to be distinguished from 'mossy foot' which follows chronic lymphatic obstruction.

Laboratory diagnosis. The diagnosis is confirmed by the demonstration of pigmented round cells in the dermis or in epidermal abscesses. The former is best shown by biopsy. However, direct microscopical examination of skin mounted in potassium hydroxide may demonstrate the typical fungal cells. Culture of lesions may be helpful, but identification of the organisms requires the services of a specialist laboratory. Serology is helpful but has not yet found an important place in diagnosis.

Treatment. Treatment is often difficult. It has been suggested that surgery may spread lesions and it should probably be reserved for circumscribed nodules as an adjunct to chemotherapy.

5-fluorocytosine given by oral route is probably the treatment of choice. It is given in a dose of 150–200 mg per kg body weight daily divided into four doses. Resistance may occur particularly in extensive lesions or where low doses are used and in these amphotericin B (intravenous) should be added for the first 2–3 months of therapy. Treatment with 5-fluorocytosine may have to be continued for up to two years.

Patients rarely die from chromomycosis although there have been occasional instances of secondary brain involvement. However, treatment may be only palliative in advanced cases. Repeated topical applications of heat may be effective in some patients.

References

Bayles, M. A. H. (1971). Chromomycosis. *Archs Derm.* **104**, 476.
Mauceri, A. A., Cullen, S. I., Vandevelde, A. G., and Johnson, J. E. (1974). Flucytosine and effective oral treatment for chromomycosis. *Archs Derm.* **109**, 873.

Sporotrichosis

Aetiology. The most common clinical form of sporotrichosis is a subcutaneous infection which may spread proximally from its initial site in a series of nodules along the course of a lymphatic. More rarely systemic involvement is seen, e.g., in the lung (see under systemic mycoses).

The causative organism *Sporothrix schenckii* can be found in soil, vegetation, or in association with wood or bark. People who develop the subcutaneous infection may have contact with material which harbours the organism, such as moss or flowers (e.g. florists). It is assumed that the pathogen gains entry via an abrasion, and in some endemic areas there is often a preceding history of a scratch or insect bite.

Epidemiology. Although sporotrichosis was once prevalent in Europe, particularly France, non-imported cases are now rare in this area. However the disease is seen in the USA, Mexico, Central and South America, and Africa. In the late 1930s there was a remarkable epidemic of sporotrichosis in workers in the Witwatersrand gold mines. The source of infection was a large number of pit props contaminated with the organism. Other smaller 'epidemics' have been described in certain groups such as Mexican pottery workers packing ceramics in straw. Normally, however, cases are sporadic in incidence.

Systemic sporotrichosis is much rarer and cases have mainly been described from the USA.

Clinical features. There are two main clinical types of cutaneous sporotrichosis. The first, the fixed type, presents with a solitary cutaneous ulcer or nodule. However, other variants include the psoriasiform or verrucose types, or a superficial granuloma which resembles lupus vulgaris. The fixed type does not spread along lymphatics. It has been suggested that it is commonest in children, and it has been described most frequently in Central and South America.

In the lymphangitic form an initial nodule forms on an extremity such as a finger. This may break down and ulcerate. Subsequently one or more secondary nodules develop along the draining lymphatic channel, and these may also ulcerate through the skin.

Rarer forms include secondary spread via scratching, which may present with multiple widespread ulcers or cutaneous lesions secondary to systemic disease.

Fixed type sporotrichosis may resemble many other forms of

cutaneous ulceration. However, in endemic areas a major source of confusion is cutaneous leishmaniasis. The lymphangitic variety may also resemble other infections notably atypical mycobacterial infections, particularly fish tank granuloma, or 'sporotrichoid' leishmaniasis.

Treatment. Some cases of sporotrichosis may heal spontaneously. However, treatment is usually advised to prevent scar formation. The treatment of choice is potassium iodide adminstered in a saturated aqueous solution. The starting dose is 0.5–1.0 ml given three times daily and this is increased drop by drop per dose to 3–6 ml three times daily. The mixture is more palatable if given with milk. Treatment should be given for a month after clinical resolution.

Recently miconazole and ketoconazole have been shown to be effective, but more work with these drugs is necessary in order to clarify their role.

Reference

Lurie, H. I. (1971). In *The pathologic anatomy of the mycoses*; 662. Springer-Verlag, Berlin.

Subcutaneous phycomycosis. Subcutaneous phycomycosis is an infection primarily seen in children in Africa or the Far East (Indonesia). It is characterized by the development of swelling of the limbs or trunk. The swelling is rarely inflammatory but has a well defined leading edge and is hard. Progression is slow. The causative organism *Basidiobolus haptosporus* can be cultured or demonstrated histologically in biopsy material.

Although resolution has been recorded without treatment, therapy is normally given. Potassium iodide solution is the treatment of choice and is given in as high a dose as possible (cf. sporotrichosis).

Reference

Harman, R. R. M., Jackson, H., and Willis, A. J. P. (1964). Subcutaneous phycomycosis in Nigeria. *Br. J. Derm.* **76**, 408.

Rhinoentomophthoromycosis. Rhinoentomophthoromycosis is a similar infection confined to subcutaneous tissue and presenting with painless swelling. The infection is mainly seen in West Africa but a case has been seen in the Caribbean. However, there are important differences between it and subcutaneous phycomycosis. The disease is commonest in young adults and is confined to facial tissues around the nose, the forehead, and the upper lip. The initial site of infection is in the region of the inferior turbinate in the nose. The diagnosis is established by biopsy or culture.

The treatment of choice is high-dose potassium iodide and co-trimoxazole.

Lobo's disease (lobomycosis). Although Lobo's disease is best regarded as a subcutaneous infection, the organism, in tissue, bears some resemblance to *P. brasiliensis* (see page 5.379). It has a tendency to form chains of four to six yeast cells with prominent nucleoli. However, the organism has never been cultured from human cases and is demonstrated by biopsy and histology. The disease is seen in countries of South America around and north of the Amazon basin and cases are also seen in Central America. Often exposed sites, e.g., ear lobes, are invaded and small nodules develop which may resemble keloids. These contain the organisms. More diffuse plaques may also be seen although deep invasion has not been documented. The treatment is excision.

Systemic mycoses

The systemic or deep visceral mycoses include some of the rare and more serious groups of the fungal infections. There are two main types of infection in this group, those caused by organisms which invade normal hosts, the pathogens, and those which only cause disease in compromised patients, the opportunists. The fungi associated with these two types of infection differ in their innate levels of pathogenicity, but an element of opportunism (i.e. host susceptibility) is usually recognizable in all cases of systemic mycoses. The systemic pathogens cause infections such as histoplasmosis or coccidioidomycosis. These diseases have well-defined endemic zones, and the majority of those exposed are symptomless but develop positive skin tests. However, in certain patients chronic lung or disseminated disease may occur. In the systemic infections caused by the opportunists, there is usually a serious underlying abnormality in the patient such as carcinoma or lymphoma. Such infections are worldwide in occurrence and, where tissue invasion occurs, the mortality is high. Cryptococcosis, a systemic yeast infection, has features of both types of systemic disease and occurs in both normals and the immunosuppressed.

The systemic pathogen infections are histoplasmosis, coccidioidomycosis, blastomycosis, and paracoccidiodomycosis. The significance of various laboratory tests in these infections in shown in Table 3.

Histoplasmosis. There are two forms of histoplasmosis. In the first, small-form or classical histoplasmosis, the organism is present in tissue in its yeast phase. The diameter of the cells is between 3–4 μm. The infection is commonest in the USA, but sporadic cases are reported widely from Central and South America, Africa and the Far East. By contrast, large-form or African histoplasmosis is seen in Central Africa, roughly between the southern Sahara and north of the Zambezi river. Yeast forms in infected tissue are much larger, 10–15 μm in diameter. Both infections are clinically distinct (see below) but cultural isolates are indistinguishable.

Histoplasmosis (classical or small form)

Aetiology. Histoplasmosis is a systemic infection caused by *Histoplasma capsulatum*. The main route of infection is pulmonary. The majority of those exposed are sensitized without overt signs of infection, but more rarely chronic pulmonary or disseminated forms of the disease are seen.

The organism, *H. capsulatum*, can be found in soil in endemic areas. Its growth is facilitated by the presence of bird excreta, for instance in old chicken houses, bird roosts, and barns. In tropical and some temperate areas bat guano plays a similar role although there is evidence that the bat, unlike birds, may carry and be infected by the organism. Exposure to a suitable source is most often recorded in acute epidemic histoplasmosis (see below). It is rarely identified in more slowly evolving cases.

The disease was first diagnosed in Panama in 1904 by Darling, who thought that the organism was a protozoan. It was subsequently shown to be fungus in 1934 by de Monbreun. These early cases were examples of disseminated disease. However, in later years, it was recognized that *H. capsulatum* could also cause chronic lung disease, similar to tuberculosis. The condition of the host is extremely important in determining the clinical manifestations of histoplasmosis. Disseminated disease may occur in normal individuals. However, infants, the elderly, or those with certain neoplastic disorders appear to be more likely to develop the more rapidly progressive forms of disseminated infection.

Epidemiology. The major endemic area as shown by skin testing is in the central region of the USA around the Ohio and Mississippi valley basins. The states of Tennessee, Kentucky, and Ohio are involved in particular. Up to 95 per cent of those skin tested in certain parts of these areas, have positive delayed reactions to intradermal histoplasmin (cf. Mantoux test). Scattered cases of active disease, healed calcified foci in chest X-rays, and post-mortem foci representing inactive histoplasmosis also provide evidence of spread within this area. However, the disease also occurs in other parts of the USA, Mexico, Central and South America, Africa, the Far East, and Australia. There is a small focus in central Italy. In all these areas human cases are extremely rare

Table 3   Laboratory tests in systemic mycoses

	Direct microscopy	Significance of positive culture	Serology*	Histology
Histoplasmosis				
1) classical (small form)	sometimes positive	significant	ID, CIE, CF	yeasts (3–4 μm)
2) African	positive in pus (valuable)	significant	ID, CF	yeasts (10–15 μm)
Coccidioidomycosis	positive in pus, sputum, etc. (valuable)	significant (handle with caution)	ID, CF, TP, CIE	spherules (50–150 μm)
Blastomycosis	positive in pus, sputum, etc. (valuable)	significant	ID, CF, CIE (unreliable)	yeasts (4–10 μm) broad-based buds
Paracoccidioidomycosis	positive in pus, sputum, etc. (valuable)	significant	ID, CF, TP	yeasts (5–15 μm) multiple buds
Cryptococcosis	often positive in CSF (rare in urine, pus) n.b. Indian ink	significant	ID, CF, WCA, IF, latex agglutination (antigen)	yeasts (5–10 μm) mucicarmine positive
Systemic candidosis	positive in oral smears, sputum, etc. (interpret with caution)	significance depends on site and presence of positive microscopy	ID, CF, WCA, CIE, ?role of antigen detection	yeast (5–10 μm) and hyphae
Invasive aspergillosis	rarely positive	depends on site. +ve sputum cultures not always significant	ID, CIE (rarely positive)	hyphae—dichotomous branching
Invasive phycomycosis (mucormycosis)	rarely positive	depends on site	ID, CIE (rarely positive)	hyphae—broad and aseptate

* ID = immunodiffusion, CIE = counterimmunoelectrophoresis, CF = complement fixation test, TP = tube precipitation, WCA = whole cell agglutination, IF = immunofluorescence

and much of the evidence of the endemicity comes from positive skin tests or the presence of the organism in selected sites such as caves.

Although there has been considerable discussion on the nature of soil factors responsible for the growth of *H. capsulatum*, the conditions limiting it to certain areas are largely unknown.

Clinical features. The clinical forms of histoplasmosis can be placed in several clinical groups:
1. Asymptomatic;
2. Acute symptomatic pulmonary: (*a*) acute epidemic; (*b*) acute reinfection;
3. Chronic pulmonary;
4. Disseminated (acute, subacute and chronic);
5. Primary cutaneous (by inoculation).

Asymptomatic infection. Over 99 per cent of patients becoming infected in endemic areas record no overt symptoms but develop a positive skin test.

Acute (symptomatic) pulmonary histoplasmosis. (*a*) Acute epidemic histoplasmosis. Groups of individuals exposed to a source of infection, for instance during cave exploration, or those who may have inhaled a large infecting dose, often develop a symptomatic illness, 12–21 days after exposure. The main features are pyrexia, cough, chest pain, and malaise. Flitting arthralgia and, less commonly, erythema nodosum or multiforme may occur. The radiological appearance may be much more severe than would be supposed from the symptoms, and hilar lymph node enlargement and patchy consolidation suggesting pneumonitis may occur. These patients develop precipitating or complement fixing antibody but this often follows the peak of illness. Likewise skin test conversion is often too late to be of diagnostic value and its use is normally contra-indicated as a single histoplasmin test may cause the development of false positive serological results. Cultures are often negative. The symptoms and history of exposure to a suitable source combined with a rising antibody titre is often the best evidence of infection.

The majority of cases require no specific therapy apart from rest. Those with severe or prolonged symptoms or impaired gas exchange require intravenous amphotericin B. The lung lesions often heal to leave multiple scattered pulmonary calcifications.

(*b*) Acute reinfection histoplasmosis. Acute exposure in sensitized individuals causes a less severe infection associated with bi-

lateral pulmonary infiltrates. The incubation period, 5–10 days, is shorter than with acute epidemic histoplasmosis.

Chronic pulmonary histoplasmosis. Chronic pulmonary disease caused by *H. capsulatum* is mainly seen in the USA. It is commoner in males and smokers, and there is often underlying pulmonary emphysema. Early cases may develop pyrexia and cough, but later malaise and weight loss occur. Initially lesions may heal but relapse is common leading to established consolidation and cavitation. The common radiological appearance of early lesions is of unilateral wedge-shaped segmental shadows in the apical zones. Subsequently the disease may become bilateral with fibrosis and cavitation. In some cases extensive destruction of lung tissue may occur.

Culture and serology are both helpful in this form of histoplasmosis, but repeated attempts may be required before positive results are obtained for either.

In early cases resolution may occur on rest alone. However, relapse occurs in 25 per cent of cases and these may require amphotericin B therapy. Although chemotherapy may virtually sterilize lesions, fibrosis persists and relapse may occur. Surgical excision or lobectomy is sometimes effective.

Solid lung tumours may persist after the primary infection. These may be single (coin lesion) or multiple and have to be distinguished from carcinomas. The diagnosis is normally made at surgery although the presence of calcification may give a clue to the nature of the lesion (histoplasmoma).

Disseminated histoplasmosis. There is considerable variation in the rate of progression of histoplasmosis which persists beyond the initial focus in the lung. In acutely disseminated cases widespread infiltration of reticulo-endothelial cells of bone marrow, spleen, and liver may occur. Gastrointestinal lesions, endocarditis, and meningitis are less common, and the latter is more usually associated with a slower course of disseminated disease. Infants, the elderly, or immunosuppressed patients are more susceptible to acute dissemination. The most prominent symptoms are fever and weight loss with accompanying hepatosplenomegaly. Extensive purpura and bruising secondary to thrombocytopenia may occur. The blood picture may reflect marrow infiltration with organisms.

It is particularly important to consider histoplasmosis in such patients and not to ascribe the clinical features to any underlying disease. Cultures, including sputum or bone marrow, should be taken and serology is often positive with high titres occurring in some patients.

A much more slowly progressive form of disseminated histoplasmosis may present with persistent oral ulcers, chronic laryngitis, or adrenal insufficiency. Such cases may present up to 30 years after the patient has left an endemic area. In the United Kingdom this form is the most widely recognized presentation of histoplasmosis, often occurring in Europeans who have worked in Africa or the Far East. Such imported cases are nevertheless rare.

The diagnosis is made on culture or biopsy of affected areas. Sera may only be positive in low titres and in all cases adrenal involvement should be looked for.

In all forms of disseminated histoplasmosis, treatment is required with intravenous amphotericin B. A mean total dose of 2 g is often used.

Primary cutaneous histoplasmosis. Primary infection may sometimes follow accidental inoculation of viable organisms in a laboratory or post-mortem room. This type of infection is normally associated with a chancre at the site of inoculation and regional lymphadenopathy. The condition is self-limiting.

African histoplasmosis. The normal portal of entry of this form of histoplasmosis is not known particularly as overt pulmonary involvement is rare. The most common presenting features are skin lesions (papules, modules, abscesses, or ulcers) or lytic bone deposits. Solitary or multiple foci may be present, and in the latter instances rapid progression and death may occur.

The diagnosis is normally made by culture, smear, or biopsy. The organism *H. capsulatum* var. *duboisii* is identical to that causing classical histoplasmosis in culture.

In some cases local excision of a nodule may be curative but in most cases a course of amphotericin B is advisable. Sulphonamides are less active. A skeletal survey should be performed to detect occult foci of bone infection as these may be asymptomatic.

References

Cockshott, W. P. and Lucas, A. O. (1964). Histoplasmosis duboisii. *Q. Jl Med.* **33**, 223.

Goodwin, R. A. and des Prez, R. M. (1973). Pathogenesis and clinical spectrum of histoplasmosis. *Sth. med. J., Nashville* **66**, 13.

Goodwin, R. A., Owens, F. T., Snell, J. D., Hubbard, W. W., Buchanan, R. D., Terry, R. T., and des Prez, R. M. (1976). Chronic pulmonary histoplasmosis. *Medicine, Baltimore* **55**, 413.

Larabee, W. F., Ajello, L., and Kaufman, L. (1977). An epidemic of histoplasmosis on the isthmus of Panama. *Am. J. trop. Med.* **27**, 281.

Symmers, W. St.C. (1972). Histoplasmosis in Southern and South-eastern Asia. A syndrome associated with a peculiar tissue form of histoplasma. A study of 48 cases. *Ann. Soc. belge. Méd. trop.* **52**, 435.

Coccidioidomycosis

Aetiology. Coccidioidomycosis is a systemic mycosis caused by a soil organism *Coccidioides immitis*. Acute or chronic lung infections, meningitis, and disseminated disease are seen.

The causal agent is a mould fungus which grows in arid and semi-desert conditions. It infects wild and domestic animals as well as man. People in close contact with soil, such as agricultural labourers or oil rig crews, are often exposed to infection although severe dust storms may extend the disease to other groups. The route of infection is almost always pulmonary.

Epidemiology. The endemic zone is confined to North and South America. The main areas are parts of the south-western USA and arid zones in Guatemala, Honduras, Colombia, Argentina, and Uruguay.

Clinical features. The clinical forms of coccidioidomycosis are similar in their general pattern to those seen in histoplasmosis.

Asymptomatic infection. Up to 80–90 per cent of people living in an endemic area may develop positive skin tests without overt disease.

Acute pulmonary coccidioidomycosis. Acute respiratory infection (Valley fever) may follow infection with *C. immitis* in the endemic area. It is characterized by fever, malaise, and cough. Arthralgia and toxic erythema or erythema nodosum or multiforme are also commonly associated. As with histoplasmosis, culture is sometimes positive or patients develop complement fixing or precipitating antibodies. The latter are raised earlier in the disease.

Most cases are self-limiting requiring rest only and no specific chemotherapy. However, some ethnic groups such as Negroes, Mexican or American Indians, or Filipinos, as well as pregnant women are at risk from dissemination. Signs of this include persistent symptoms or pulmonary shadowing, prolonged high titres of precipitating antibody, and a negative skin test. Progressive pulmonary disease may also develop, particularly in diabetics or the immunosuppressed.

The 'at risk' groups may require amphotericin B therapy.

Chronic pulmonary coccidioidomycosis. Solid coin lesions (cf. histoplasmosis) may follow primary infection. Alternatively cavitating coccidioidomycosis may occur. Cough with sputum production is common and serious complications, such as pneumothorax or bronchopleural fistula, may develop. The cavity is characteristically regular and thin-walled. It may also contain a fluid level. In such cases serology and culture are helpful in diagnosis of the tissue phase of *C. immitis*, the spherule (Fig. 7) may be seen in sputum smears. Amphotericin B therapy may be required in some cases, possibly in conjunction with surgery. However, in asymptomatic cases observation without specific therapy may be the best course of action.

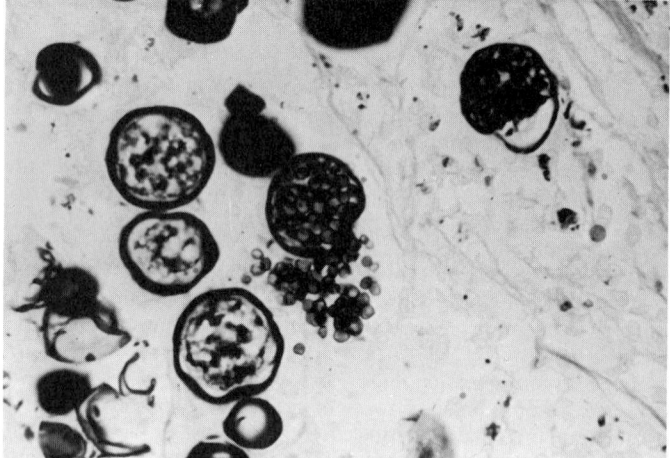

Fig. 7 Coccidioidomycosis: mature and immature spherules in lung (GMS).

Disseminated coccidioidomycosis. Rapid or slow extrapulmonary dissemination may occur with this disease. Favoured sites of involvement include skin, bone, meninges, and joints but other organs including lung may be involved. Meningeal involvement and its main complication, hydrocephalus, is particularly difficult to correct. The symptoms, headache, fever, and confusion, are those commonly seen with chronic meningitis. Smears, cultures, or serology are all helpful in diagnosis or monitoring the course of the infection. Systemic amphotericin B therapy supplemented by intrathecal or intra-articular injections as indicated is required. In recalcitrant disseminated or meningeal cases intravenous miconazole or oral ketoconazole are possible alternative drugs and in some instances transfer factor may be used. Neither of these latter methods have been fully evaluated.

Primary cutaneous coccidioidomycosis. Inoculation by laboratory workers has been described and the clinical lesions are similar to hose seen in histoplasmosis (see page 5.377). Similarly local infec-ion may occur at sites of injury in agricultural workers presumably ollowing inoculation of contaminated soil. In rare instances sys-emic spread may occur from the cutaneous site.

Laboratory hazard. The main laboratory risk from *C. immitis* fol-ows inhalation of the infective particles—the arthrospores. For hese reasons suspected cultures should be handled with a bio-ogical safety cabinet preferably by specialized laboratories.

Prophylaxis. Recently an antigen derived from spherules of *C. immitis* has been shown to protect against dissemination in mice. It s currently being evaluated as a vaccine in human disease.

References

Drutz, D. J. and Cantanzaro, A. (1978). Coccidioidomycosis Parts I and II. *Am. Rev. resp. Dis.* **117**, 559, 727.
Einstein, H. E. (1971). Coccidioidomycosis. In *Management of Fungus Diseases of the lungs*, 86. C. C. Thomas, Springfield, Illinois.

Blastomycosis. Blastomycosis (North American blastomycosis) caused by *Blastomyces dermatitidis* is a systemic fungal infection in which skin and lung involvement are common features.

The infective organism *B. dermatitidis* has only been isolated from the environment on rare occasions. Positive sites have in-cluded soil and rotten timbers. The organism infects man and domestic animals particularly the dog.

Epidemiology. Blastomycosis was originally thought to be confined to the USA where it occurs sporadically throughout the south and east central area and in areas of central Canada. 'Epidemics' of acute disease are rare and where these occur a source of infection is rarely demonstrated.

More recently, cases have been found in Africa. Again these are widely scattered from the north coast to the southern parts of the continent, and are rare in all areas.

Clinical features. The clinical forms of blastomycosis differ from histoplasmosis in a number of important aspects. The presence of asymptomatic variants is larely conjectural, although likely, because there is no reliable skin test. Acute or grouped infections are rare and the features are often similar to histoplasmosis (acute pulmonary). However specific serological tests may be negative in at least 50 per cent of cases. The demonstration of the organisms in sputum and positive cultures are more reliable diagnostic criteria. Although some cases undoubtedly resolve without sequelae, some physicians advise chemotherapy with a short course of ampho-tericin B in acute cases.

Chronic pulmonary blastomycosis. Chronic consolidation or cavitation of the upper or mid zones occur with chronic pulmonary infections. Fever, malaise, and cough with sputum are seen. Weight loss may be prominent. Again culture is the most reliable method of diagnosis.

The mainstay of treatment is amphotericin B, given in a total dose of 2 g or more.

Disseminated blastomycosis. Although generalized infiltration in skin, lungs, and liver may occur over a short period leading to rapid death, more chronic signs of extrapulmonary dissemination are more usual.

The skin is an area which is frequently involved (chronic cutaneous blastomycosis). The face or forearms and hands are common sites for skin lesions. These are slow spreading verrucose plaques with central scarring. The initial lesion is often a dermal nodule. Many of such cases have underlying pulmonary consoli-dation, or cavities. The diagnosis is established by biopsy and culture.

Bone deposits in the form of lytic lesions, and involvement of the genitourinary tract are also seen in chronic disseminated blasto-mycosis. Unlike tuberculosis, the kidneys themselves are often

spared the infection which involves the epididymis in particular.

In slowly progressive forms of blastomycosis, amphotericin B given by intravenous route is the most effective method of treat-ment. However in patients who are elderly or in those who cannot tolerate the drug the aromatic diamidine 5-hydroxystilbamidine may be given instead. The drug is given by intravenous route in two courses of 8 g daily. Relapse is commoner after this regimen than with amphotericin B and the initial results of treatment are not as good. However there are fewer side effects.

References

Abernathy, R. S. (1959). Clinical manifestations of pulmonary blasto-mycosis. *Ann. intern. Med.* **51**, 707.
Lockwood, W. R., Allison, F., Batson, B. E., and Busey, J. F. (1969). The treatment of North American blastomycosis: ten years' experience. *Am. Rev. resp. Dis.* **100**, 314.

Paracoccidioidomycosis (South American blastomycosis)

Aetiology. Paracoccidioidomycosis is an uncommon infection caused by *Paracoccidioides brasiliensis*. The commonest clinical manifestations include lung involvement and ulceration of the mucosal surfaces and adjacent skin.

The causative organism, *P. brasiliensis*, has never been convin-cingly demonstrated in the environment nor does it appear to infect animals commonly although it has rarely been isolated from bats. The usual victim of the infection is the agricultural or forestry worker although sporadic cases are known in city dwellers.

Epidemiology. Paracoccidioidomycosis has been described in most of the countries of South America apart from Chile and Guyana. Cases have also been seen in Central America and southern Mex-ico. As with the other systemic mycoses, skin testing has shown that there is evidence of exposure in a proportion of the normal popu-lation. For instance between 6 and 13 per cent of those tested in two cities in Colombia had positive paracoccidioidin tests. Although males with overt paracoccidioidomycosis outnumber females by ratios sometimes in excess of 25:1, skin test surveys nevertheless show that males and females are infected in equal numbers.

Many workers believe that the main portal of entry is the lung, and there has been some histological confirmation of this view in post-mortem studies, which have shown the organism in lung nodules in asymptomatic patients. However, the prevalence of mucosal lesions has led to the alternative hypothesis that direct introduction into the mucosa is also possible.

Clinical features. Paracoccidioidomycosis has a number of clinical forms similar to histoplasmosis although acute pulmonary infec-tions are rare. There are three main clinical types, chronic pulmon-ary and acute or chronic disseminated disease.

Chronic pulmonary paracoccidioidomycosis starts from an in-filtrating lesion mainly in the upper lobes which may spread to the other parts of the lung. Subsequent progress is variable. Cavitation may occur or progressive fibrosis. Alternatively a coin lesion may be formed. The symptoms are pyrexia and cough. Tuberculosis must be considered in the differential diagnosis and the two infec-tions may even co-exist.

Often pulmonary lesions are found with other clinical variants of paracoccidioidomycosis such as oral ulcers (mixed form).

Acute dissemination is normally accompanied by multiple skin pauples, gastro-intestinal infiltration with accompanying diarrhoea and bleeding, and lymphadenopathy. Weakness may follow muscle invasion and hepatosplenomegaly may occur. This form of disease follows a rapid downhill path to death. More commonly dissemi-nation is slower and the process may pick out one or more sites. Chronic ulceration of the mouth, tongue, palate, or anterior nose and adjacent skin is a well-recognized clinical pattern (mucocu-taneous form). Acneiform papules or vegetations may also de-velop. Alternatively lymph nodes may enlarge and discharge pus mimicking tuberculosis. The cervical chain of nodes is often affected. Both these forms may have accompanying pulmonary infiltration and, in the rapidly progressive variety, miliary spread in the lungs may be seen.

Laboratory diagnosis. The diagnosis is confirmed by demonstrating the organisms and their characteristic pattern of multiple bud formation (Fig. 8) in smears or sputum. The organism is relatively easy to culture, and serology, immunodiffusion, or complement fixation is specific and helpful in monitoring disease activity.

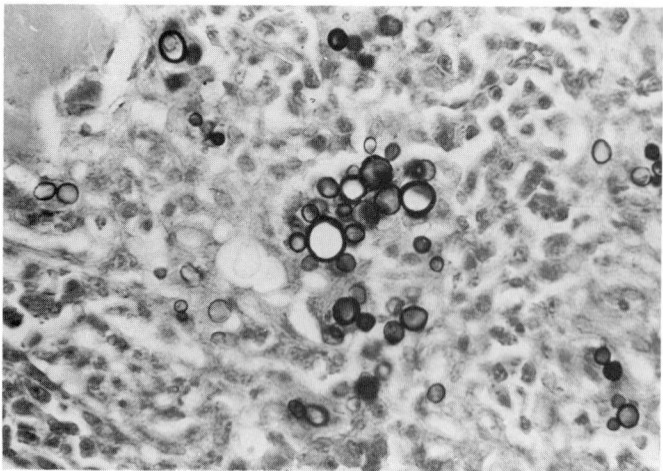

Fig. 8   Paracoccidioidomycosis: a 'multiple budding' yeast in nasal mucosa (GMS).

Treatment. The treatment of choice is probably amphotericin B given in a course of 2 g or more. The sulphonamides are also active and these may be given concurrently and used as maintenance therapy subsequently. For instance, sulphadiazine 3–4 g daily is an average dose. The relapse rate after combined therapy is less than that obtained by using sulphonamides alone. However, most patients should be followed up indefinitely.

Recently intravenous miconazole (1 g three times daily) and oral ketoconazole (200–600 mg daily) have both been found to be effective.

Reference

Restrepo, A., Robedo, M., Guitierrez, F., San Clemente, M., Castaneda, E., and Calle, G. (1970). Paracoccidioidomycosis (South American blastomycosis). A study of 39 cases observed in Medellin, Colombia. *Am. J. trop. Med. Hyg.* **19**, 68.

Cryptococcosis

Aetiology. Cryptococcosis is a systemic infection caused by *Cryptococcus neoformans*. Its commonest clinical feature is meningitis but pulmonary, cutaneous, and widely disseminated forms of the infection are also recognized.

C. neoformans is a yeast which can be isolated from the environment although it is most often found in pigeon extracts. Its growth from soil appears to be enhanced by certain nitrogenous compounds such as creatinine in the pigeon droppings. The birds are not infected although their crops may be heavily colonized. Very large quantities of the organism, e.g. 1×10^7 yeasts per gram of droppings may be found in densely populated urban areas.

The portal of entry is usually the lung from whence the organism spreads to involve other organs or sites such as the meninges. Although many natural isolates are relatively small in appearance, one feature of invasion is the development of a large mucoid capsule *in vivo*, a feature which may confer some protection on the organism. Infections caused by *C. neoformans* are seen in both normal or immunocompromised hosts. The main underlying processes are sarcoidosis, Hodgkin's disease, collagen disease, carcinoma, or the administration of systemic corticosteroid therapy.

Epidemiology. Cryptococcosis has been recorded from most countries although it is most prevalent in the USA, and Australia. In the USA, approximately 50 per cent of cases occur in normal persons. By contrast in the United Kingdom 85 per cent of cases are found in patients with underlying disorders (see above). There is no skin test reagent widely available, but some pilot studies in the USA suggest that workers exposed to the organism, e.g. in laboratories, are more likely than other groups to have a positive skin test without any overt sign of infection. It is probable, therefore, that there is an asymptomatic form of cryptococcosis (c.f. histoplasmosis). Additional evidence for the existence of subclinical infection is provided by the repeated isolation of *C. neoformans* from individuals without evidence of disease.

Clinical features. *Pulmonary cryptococcosis*. Acute or subacute respiratory disease caused by *C. neoformans* is rare in most parts of the world but is well recognized in the USA. The disease consists of a chest infection with fever and cough and scattered, often with circumscribed, areas of pulmonary infiltration seen on X-ray. In some patients no treatment is required and the whole process resolves, although it is probably advisable to give chemotherapy to those with prolonged disease or underlying abnormalities. The laboratory diagnosis is made by biopsy or culture. Serological tests for antibody or capsular polysaccharide antigen (latex test) are often positive. In treated cases, a short course of amphotericin B is advised depending on the clinical response.

Isolated cryptococcal granulomas (cryptococcoma) may present as coin lesions and are removed surgically to exclude carcinoma. Once the correct diagnosis is made, many workers advise a short course of amphotericin B as there is a small risk of dissemination to other organs following surgery.

Disseminated cryptococcosis. The best recognized form of extrapulmonary cryptococcosis is meningitis. This may present with signs of acute meningism. However, more usually the features are less specific. Pyrexia, headache, and mental changes such as confusion or drowsiness occur. The latter probably follows the development of hydrocephalus. Blurring of vision and papilloedema may also occur. Cranial nerve involvement is less common.

The cerebrospinal fluid (CSF) shows pleocytosis which is highly variable. Often there are excessive numbers of lymphocytes, but sometimes polymorphonuclear leucocytes abound. In some cases only small numbers of white cells (4–10) are seen. Characteristically the glucose concentration falls and protein rises, but again there is variation. Cryptococci can be seen in some cases in an Indian ink preparation which is used to highlight the capsule. A spun sediment is best for this purpose. The organism can also be cultured from the CSF. The latex test for antigen is usually positive for CSF in titres over 1:8 but on rare occasions this is negative. The antigen titre has both diagnostic and prognostic value. Initial high (> 100) titres are likely to correlate with relapse following therapy and with a poor prognosis. Extrameningeal disease should be looked for by sputum or urine culture and serology in patients presenting with meningitis.

The prognosis of untreated meningitis is poor with death ultimately occurring. However, the progression may be very slow over several years.

Therapy of meningitis. The current treatment is a combination of oral 5-fluorocytosine (150–200 mg/kg body weight daily) and intravenous amphotericin B (0.3–0.5 mg/kg body weight daily). This should be continued for at least six weeks and longer if necessary. The CSF picture and antigen levels can be used to monitor treatment. Alternatively amphotericin B may be given on its own in full dosage (0.8–1.0 mh/kg) and this is often supplemented by intrathecal or intraventricular instillation. Miconazole has been used with success on a few occasions but, as with amphotericin B, may have to be given into an Ommaya reservoir. In every treatment regime relapse may occur and long-term follow up is advised.

Other sites. Cryptococci may disseminate to other sites including liver and spleen, kidney, skin, or bone. The latter are particularly found in sarcoidosis. In every case underlying deep disseminated lesions, e.g., meningitis, may be found. The methods of diagnosis and treatment are similar to those seen with meningitis. Only a small proportion of cases of cryptococcosis may have detectable antibody (15–30 per cent) and this may occur late in the course of therapy.

It is important in all cases where cryptococcosis presents with lesions in an extrameningeal site to exclude occult meningitis by performing a lumbar puncture.

References

Cambell, G. D. (1966). Pulmonary cryptococcosis. *Am. Rev. resp. Dis.* **94**, 236.

Spickard, A. (1973). Diagnosis and treatment of cryptococcal disease, *Sth, Med. J., Nashville* **66**, 26.

Diamond, R. D. and Bennett, J. E. (1979). Prognostic factors in cryptococcal meningitis. *Ann. intern. Med.* **80**, 176.

Systemic sporotrichosis. In addition to causing cutaneous disease *Sporothrix schenckii* may be responsible for a systemic mycosis. The infection is rare and has been mainly reported from the USA. Involvement may be confined to one organ such as lung or a joint, or it may be multifocal. Cavitation in the lung associated with weight loss and pyrexia is probably the commonest variety of systemic sporotrichosis. Unlike the cutaneous variety systemic sporotrichosis responds poorly to potassium iodide, and amphotericin B is the treatment of choice.

Rare systemic infections. These include pulmonary invasion by *Geotrichum candidum*—geotrichosis and adiaspiromycosis, a respiratory infection caused by *Emmonsia crescens* or *E. parva*. Isolated examples of human disease caused by fungi are consistently reported and almost always occur in the immunosuppressed host. In these patients many fungi which are normally saprophytes in the environment may invade and cause disease.

Systemic mycoses caused by opportunistic fungi. The opportunistic mycoses are a worldwide problem although fortunately rare in most countries. In recent years they have been recognized more frequently with the increase in the use of transplantation of organs such as heart or bone marrow and in the more effective but immunocompromising regimens of cancer chemotherapy. Opportunistic invasion by organisms such as *Candida* or Zygomycetes (*Mucor, Absidia*) may also occur in cases of malnutrition.

The opportunist presents particular problems in diagnosis and management. Because many of the organisms are normally saprophytic, it has to be positively established that they have assumed an invasive role. Mere isolation may not be present even in normal hosts. The significance of various laboratory tests in these infections is shown in Table 3. Treatment is also difficult, and it is important in most cases to attempt to reverse the process which led to the establishment of the infection. This may mean interrupting courses of cytotoxic therapy or risking loss of a transplant by reducing immunosuppressive therapy.

Systemic candidosis

Aetiology. In addition to the role of yeasts of the genus *Candida* in superficial infections, they may also cause invasive systemic disease. The clinical forms described range from a temporary candidaemia, to disseminated invasive disease, and involvement of a single organ or body cavity (deep focal candidosis), as may occur in endocarditis or meningitis. Urinary tract infections may also be caused by *Candida* species.

The factors underlying systemic *Candida* infections are shown in Table 4. All these factors are important in disrupting the balance by which *Candida* is maintained as a saprophyte. Intravenous or central venous pressure lines may serve as a portal of entry or as a nidus for circulating yeasts in candidaemia. Antibiotic therapy may upset the balance by inhibiting potentially competitive bacterial flora.

Table 4 Predisposing factors in deep *Candida* infections

1. Local defects, foreign bodies, e.g. prosthetic heart valves, intravenous lines
2. Defects of immunity (primarily T cell or phagocytosis), e.g. cytotoxic therapy, systemic lupus erythematosus
3. Drug therapy, e.g. antibiotics
4. Carcinoma or leukaemia
5. Endocrine disease, e.g. diabetes mellitus in urinary tract candidosis
6. Physiological changes, e.g. infancy, old age, and pregnancy (urinary tract)
7. Miscellaneous disorders, e.g.
   (a) malnutrition
   (b) surgery such as gastrointestinal resections

C. albicans is the commonest species involved but other species may be isolated, particularly in cases of endocarditis, e.g. *C. parapsilosis, C. pseudotropicalis*, or *C. guilliermondii*. Portals of entry include the gastrointestinal tract (common), skin, and urinary tract (rare). However, superficial candidosis or saprophytic colonization of mouth skin, or airways may also occur in compromised patients and does not necessarily indicate systemic invasion.

Epidemiology. Systemic infections caused by *Candida* species are worldwide in distribution.

Clinical features

Candidaemia. The isolation of *Candida* in blood culture may follow any of the factors listed in Table 4. Common predisposing features are the presence of intravenous lines, previous surgery (mainly gastrointestinal), antibiotic therapy, or neutropenia. Patients develop a swinging fever and feel generally unwell. Clinical shock may occur.

Many such cases resolve following removal of predisposing factors, particularly the intravenous lines. However, a careful watch should be made to exclude the presence of established invasive disease. Other sites should be searched for evidence of infection, e.g. urine by culture or the presence of white cells. Signs of muscle invasion (tenderness) or metastatic skin nodules should be excluded. Other signs of invasion include the development of new cardiac murmurs or of soft white retinal plaques caused by *Candida*. Persistently positive blood cultures or high antibody titres may also indicate possible deep invasion.

Disseminated candidosis. Although multiorgan invasive candidosis may follow candidaemia, at least 50 per cent of disseminated infections develop in patients without initially positive blood cultures. The features of some forms of invasive candidosis are listed above (under Candidaemia), Although *Candida* may be isolated from the sputum in these patients, there is rarely objective evidence of lung invasion. Moreover there is no radiological appearance which is diagnostic of pulmonary candidosis and, indeed, chest X-rays may even appear normal.

Laboratory diagnosis of disseminated candidosis. The diagnosis may be made by culture and repeated attempts to isolate should be made where cultures were initially negative. Numerous techniques have been used to detect antibody in disseminated candidosis. However, ideally more than one procedure should be used, e.g. whole cell agglutination combined with a more sensitive method such as counter-immunoelectrophoresis. Changes of titre are often more significant than single values particularly where antibody levels are low. None the less 20 per cent or more of genuine cases may not have detectable antibody. Attempts to detect antigenaemia by immunological methods or gas–liquid chromatography are currently being examined.

By themselves positive cultures, particularly from sputum, or the presence of antibodies do not necessarily prove the existence of deep-seated candidosis. A positive isolation may simply indicate the presence of colonization and normal individuals may have low titres of antibody to *Candida*. If there is a readily accessible lesion to biopsy such as a skin nodule or even a pulmonary infiltrate, this may provide the best evidence of invasion, although such procedures may carry their own risk.

Treatment of disseminated candidosis. Untreated disseminated candidosis is normally progressive and fatal. The signs must be separated from, for instance, a bacterial septicaemia which may co-exist with the *Candida* infection.

The treatment of invasive candidosis is intravenous amphotericin B given until there is a clinical and mycological response. This may take between 2–20 weeks depending on the site of infection. Although there is no objective evidence as yet to support the addition of 5-fluorocytosine in doses of 150–200 mg/kg body weight daily, it may give an additional advantage in serious infections or where cure may be hampered by poor penetration of amphotericin B such as in the eye. Miconazole may also be effective in this type of candidosis.

Deep focal candidosis. *Candida* infections in the peritoneum or meninges most often follow direct implantation after dialysis or surgery. Alternatively secondary invasion from the middle ear or a perforated bowel are also possible. The signs and symptoms are similar to bacterial meningitis or peritonitis but *Candida* is isolated. Sometimes these infections clear spontaneously but normally treatment is instituted with amphotericin B or miconazole, given locally. Alternatively 5-fluorocytosine may be used provided the organism is sensitive and the length of the course is under two to three weeks.

Candida endocarditis. Invasion of heart valves, mainly the mitral or aortic valves, most commonly follows homograft replacement, but it may occur *de novo* in leukaemics or drug addicts. The symptoms are similar to bacterial endocarditis. However, *Candida* vegetations may reach considerable size. Embolic phenomena may involve obstruction of large vessels including the femoral artery or large cerebral vessels. The presence of large vegetations using an echo-scanning device, particularly in cases with negative blood cultures, should raise the possibility of fungal endocarditis. Blood cultures are usually positive at some stage in the illness but repeated sampling may be necessary. High antibody titres are usually seen in such cases and serological tests are therefore of considerable value.

Untreated *Candida* endocarditis in uniformly fatal. There is also a high mortality associated with cases in which early surgical intervention is precipitated by impending heart failure. Normally treatment consists of amphotericin B given intravenously and valve replacement. There is no evidence as yet to suggest that the addition of 5-fluorocytosine to the regimen increases the effectiveness. However the relapse rate is high and combination treatment may therefore be a reasonable approach on theoretical grounds.

Urinary tract candidosis. *Candida* species may be isolated from the urine particularly in conditions associated with urinary stasis such as neurogenic bladder or where there is an indwelling catheter. Maturity onset diabetes mellitus is another factor. There is no information on the value of using the presence of pyuria or quantitative yeast colony counts to assess the significance of infection. Treatment is normally given where there are symptoms such as dysuria or frequency, or where there is a potential risk of invasion such as in immunosuppressed patients.

Trial of conservative therapy, such as the removal of a urinary catheter, should be attempted before chemotherapy is started. 5-fluorocytosine penetrates urine in adequate amounts and, provided the organism is sensitive, should be given for two weeks. Alternatively local instillations of amphotericin B or miconazole may be administered.

References

Ellis, C. A. and Spivak, M. L. (1967). The significance of candidemia. *Ann. intern. Med.* **67**, 511.

Krick, J. A. and Remington, J. S. (1976). Opportunistic invasive fungal infections in patients with leukaemia and lymphoma. *Clinics Haemat.* **5**, 249.

Taschdjian, C. L., Kozinn, P. J., Cuesta, M. B., and Toni, E. F. (1972). Serodiagnosis of candidal infections. *Am. J. clin. Path.* **57**, 195.

Turnier, E., Kay, J. H., Bernstein, S., Mendez, A. M., and Zubiate, P. (1975). Surgical treatment of candida endocarditis. *Chest* **67**, 262.

Aspergillosis

Aetiology. There are a number of different disease states caused by fungi of the genus *Aspergillus*. These range from allergic disorders to invasive disease. As a rule the organism affects predisposed hosts.

In the majority of diseases caused by *Aspergillus*, *A. fumigatus* is the causative organism. *A. flavus* may cause invasive disease, primarily in the USA, or an erosive paranasal granuloma in tropical countries. Both these species together with *A. niger* may also cause an intracavitary fungus ball or aspergilloma. Rarely other species are involved. Otomycosis, an infection of the external ear, may be caused by species of *Aspergillus*, but *A. niger* is the commonest organism isolated. *Aspergillus* species are common in the environment in dust, soil, or vegetable material. They are common laboratory contaminants. They may also be isolated from sputum in patients with diseased airways e.g. chronic bronchitis, although in the United Kingdom they are not often cultured from this source in other patients including leukaemics. The significance of the isolation of the organism in sputum may therefore vary with the nature of the underlying disease.

Epidemiology. *Aspergillus* infections are sporadic but ubiquitous, and invasive disease or aspergilloma are found in all countries. The former is commoner where transplantation and intensive cytotoxic therapy are undertaken. There are other regional trends in aspergillosis. The destructive paranasal granuloma normally caused by *A. flavus* is most often seen in the tropics or in patients who originate from these areas. *A. nidulans* has been found to be a rare cause of mycetoma in the Sudan. Otomycosis appears to be commoner in the tropics.

Clinical features

Colonization by Aspergillus. *Aspergillus* species are not infrequently isolated from patients with chronic obstructive airways disease. Such positive cultures can rarely be correlated into clinical symptoms except in certain specific conditions, described below.

Allergic bronchopulmonary aspergillosis. Allergic bronchopulmonary aspergillosis is associated with persistent endobronchial growth of *Aspergillus*, usually *A. fumigatus*. In predisposed subjects, such as atopics, an immunological response to the organism probably involving both type I and type III hypersensitivity may contribute to the disease. The condition may start in childhood or early adult life.

Symptoms of reversible airways obstruction, e.g. asthma, are seen in early cases. However, where extensive bronchial damage has occurred patients may present with breathlessness and a chronic productive cough.

In many cases the chest X-ray shows scattered linear shadows in the peripheral lung fields. In order to establish the diagnosis a positive *Aspergillus* prick test, eosinophilia, the presence of *Aspergillus* in sputum, and weakly positive precipitins in serum are all helpful.

Treatment is difficult particularly in late cases. Attempts to remove the organism from the airways using antifungal therapy, if successful, are normally of only temporary benefit. Therapy is therefore aimed at the inflammatory response rather than the organism and bronchodilators, where appropriate, or corticosteroids are given.

Aspergilloma. The development of a fungal ball in an existing pulmonary cavity is most commonly associated with *Aspergilli* although other organisms including *Petriellidium boydii*, *Coccidioides immitis*, and *Candida albicans* may also produce this condition. Frequently there are no symptoms apart from intermittent cough. However, haemoptysis of varying severity may develop. The condition is diagnosed by positive cultures and the presence of high titres of specific antibody in serum. Radiologically an opacity can be demonstrated in a cavity and this can usually be shown to move with changes of posture.

In some cases the fungal mass is expectorated and no action is required. However where a decision to treat is reached the most reliable approach is surgical excision. For instance recurrent or severe haemoptysis would be an indication for intervention. Parenteral antifungal therapy is rarely successful. Local instillation of antifungal drugs is attended by a high frequency of relapse, and to be effective, they have to be delivered by cannula under radiological control into the cavity.

Invasive aspergillosis. In severely compromised individuals, particularly patients with leukaemia, neutropenia, collagen disorders, or those on immunosuppressive regimens, *A. fumigatus* and less commonly, *A. flavus* may invade tissue. The initial site is normally the lung, but extrapulmonary dissemination may occur particularly to the brain, kidney, liver, and skin. Symptoms such as pyrexia and cough are often masked by the patient's poor general state and other fungal or bacterial infections often co-exist. Although a variety of X-ray appearances may be seen, the rapid development of a discrete focus of pulmonary consolidation which may appear to cavitate should arouse suspicions, particularly in the presence of a positive *Aspergillus* culture. Often, however, both culture and serology are negative and biopsy offers the best chance of establishing the diagnosis.

Treatment should not be delayed. Intravenous amphotericin B in full dosage (1 mg/kg body weight daily) is the recommended treatment. The newer imidazole drugs, particularly clotrimazole or econazole, may be active *in vitro* against *Aspergillus* species. Their clinical use has not been fully investigated. However, if possible, predisposing factors such as neutropenia should be corrected, e.g. by granulocyte transfusions or interruption of cytotoxic therapy.

There are two rarer types of invasive disease caused by *Aspergillus*. Endocarditis is uncommon but usually follows homograft valve replacement and may be accompanied by myocardial invasion. Secondly, an erosive granuloma containing *Aspergilli* within the paranasal sinuses, paranasal aspergilloma, may invade the orbit or brain.

The mortality of all invasive forms of aspergillosis, even with treatment is high.

References

Bodey, G. P. (1966). Fungal infections complicating acute leukaemia. *J. chron. Dis.* **19**, 667.

Kilman J. W., Ahn, C., Andrews, N. C., and Klassen, K. (1969). Surgery for pulmonary aspergillosis. *J. thorac. cardiovasc. Surg.* **37**, 642.

Young, R. C., Bennett, J. E., Vogel, C. L., Carbone, P., and de Vita, V. T. (1970). Aspergillosis: The spectrum of disease in 98 patients. *Medicine* **49**, 147.

Invasive phycomycosis (mucor-mycosis, zygomycosis)

Aetiology. Invasive disease caused by mucor-like fungi is rare. In the compromised host it may lead to paranasal destruction, necrotic lung or skin lesions, and disseminated disease.

The causative organisms commonly belong to three genera *Absidia*, *Rhizopus*, and *Mucor*. More rarely other organisms such as *Cunninghamela* or *Saksenaea* have been implicated. Most of these fungi are organisms associated with decaying vegetable matter and are common airborne moulds. The route of infection is highly variable and they may invade via the lungs, paranasal sinuses, gastrointestinal tract, or damaged skin. The predisposing illness may in some way determine the site of clinical invasion. Underlying factors include diabetic ketoacidosis (rhinocerebral involvement), leukaemia and immunosuppressive therapy (lung and disseminated infection), malnutrition (gastrointestinal infection), and burns or wounds (cutaneous invasion). These patterns are not always strictly followed.

Epidemiology. Invasive phycomycosis is rare but has a worldwide distribution. Its invasive nature, particularly the tendency to involve blood vessels, and its selection of compromised hosts distinguish this form of infection from subcutaneous phycomycosis which is also caused by zygomycete species (see page 5.376).

Clinical features. The characteristic of this type of infection is extensive necrosis and infarction which may follow blood vessel invasion leading to thrombosis. A similar type of invasion may occur with invasive aspergillosis but is usually less prominent. Invasive phycomycosis follows a number of patterns.

The infection may initially localize in one of several sites. The commonest is in the paranasal sinuses and this is most often seen in diabetic patients with ketoacidosis. The patient presents with fever and unilateral facial pain. Subsequently there may be facial swelling with nasal obstruction and proptosis. Invasion into the orbit leading to blindness, to the brain, and to the palate may occur. Palatal ulceration should be searched for. Subsequently widespread dissemination with infarction of major organs or limbs may occur. A similar pattern of invasion of surgical wounds or burns may occur and has on occasions been associated with contamination of dressing packs. The infection is initially localized causing extensive necrosis around the original wound. Gastrointestinal invasion may be heralded by perforation of viscera, diarrhoea, or haematemesis or melaena.

Alternatively a patient may present with established pulmonary or widespread dissemination. Such patients are usually leukaemics or are severely immunosuppressed. Neutropenia is often seen.

Once infection has spread beyond the original site, invasive phycomycosis is almost invariably fatal with or without treatment.

Laboratory diagnosis. The diagnosis is suggested by the combination of infection and extensive infarction particularly if it occurs in any of the sites mentioned. The organisms may be difficult to culture even from biopsy, and histology is often the quickest way of establishing the diagnosis. Serology is frequently negative.

Treatment. Treatment should be initiated as soon as possible and extensive surgical debridement combined with intravenous amphotericin B in maximum daily dosage offers the best chance of success. Local instillations of amphotericin B may also be used where appropriate, e.g. nasal sinuses. Some physicians also recommend anticoagulation with heparin to forestall thrombosis. Despite therapy the mortality remains high.

Reference

Meyer, R. D. and Armstrong, D. (1973). Mucormycosis. In *Critical reviews in clinical laboratory sciences* (eds. King and Faulkner), vol. 4, 421, Cleveland.

Rhinosporidiosis. Rhinosporidiosis is an infection found in India, Sri Lanka, and South America. It is characterized by polypoid growth from the nose or conjunctiva. The causative organism can be demonstrated in tissue and consists of aggregates of large sporangia containing spores in various phases of development. However, they have never been successfully cultured and their fungal nature has only been assumed from their morphological appearance in histology.

The treatment is surgical excision.

Otomycosis and oculomycosis. External otitis is often multifactorial, but in some cases dense fungal colonization can contribute to the picture. In severe cases, the external ear may be plugged by a dense mat of mycelium. *Aspergillus* species are the commonest organisms cultured, particularly *A. niger*, but *Candida*, *Penicillium*, and *Mucor* may all contribute. Intensive ear toilet may eradicate the infection without recourse to antifungal agents.

Infections of the eye, particularly the cornea, caused by fungi (oculomycosis) are rare. They often follow penetrating injuries to the globe or contamination of lacerations. An opacity develops within the cornea with associated pain and chemosis. An exudate is usually present in the aqueous humour. Prompt treatment with intensive topical instillation of drugs containing an antifungal drug such as miconazole or econazole is necessary every two to four hours. Perforation of the eye may occur in advanced cases.

Chemotherapy in systemic mycoses. There are very few drugs which are effective in systemic fungal infections and those which are used should always be accompanied by supportive measures and, if possible, an attempt to revise any predisposing conditions. For instance, if their condition permits, a patient who has developed a candidaemia while a central venous line is in place should receive a trial without antifungal chemotherapy involving removal of the line for 24–72 hours.

The polyene group of antifungal antibiotics which includes natamycin and nystatin are normally only used in topical preparations. Amphotericin B is the only drug in this group which is given parenterally. It forms a fine colloidal suspension and must be freshly made up. The drug is given in a 5 per cent dextrose infusion not containing additional drugs, if possible. A test dose of 1–5 mg is given over two hours and this is followed by gradually increasing doses over the next three to nine days to the normal maximum of 0.8–1.0 mg/kg body weight daily. In some cases this slow approach may help the patient to tolerate the drug better or define the dose at which side effects such as pyrexia start. In severely ill cases the full dose may be given initially, usually under hydrocortisone cover. Side effects include thrombophlebitis, nausea, hypotension, and pyrexia. Renal clearance may fall in the initial period but this usually returns to normal after a temporary halt in therapy. More permanent renal tubular damage may follow a total dose of 4 g or more. Amphotericin B does not enter urine, CSF, or peritoneal fluid in significant concentrations. So, for instance, in cases of fungal meningitis, local instillations of 0.5–1.0 mg of amphotericin dissolved in CSF may be given in addition to intravenous therapy, although a total of 15 mg is normally not exceeded. Arachnoiditis and sensory or motor disturbances may follow intrathecal injection of amphotericin B. An indwelling (Ommaya) reservoir is sometimes used for instillation of the drugs into the cerebral ventricles, but its insertion carries serious peri- and post-operative complications, particularly secondary infection.

Amphotericin B is normally given until clinical or mycological cure is induced. This is often difficult to judge accurately and in many of the mycoses caused by the systemic pathogens a course of at least 2 g is often used on an empirical basis. In the opportunistic infections lower total doses are probably effective and the length of treatment should depend on the clinician's judgement.

5-fluorocytosine is an effective antifungal agent which is primarily active against yeasts such as *Candida* and *Cryptococcus*. It is well absorbed after oral administration and is given in four divided doses totalling 150–200 mg/kg body weight daily. It enters urine, CSF, and peritoneal fluid. Its excretion is reduced in renal failure and the daily dose should be reduced accordingly and blood levels monitored. The drug can also be given intravenously.

The main disadvantage of 5-fluorocytosine is the development of either primary or secondary drug resistance in a significant number of isolates, and, when given in toxic doses, it may cause bone marrow depression. The serum level should not be allowed to rise above 100–120 µg/ml. The drug is mainly used in urinary or peritoneal candidosis, or chromomycosis. An important use is its combination with amphotericin B (see below).

Combination treatment with amphotericin B and 5-fluorocytosine may offer a highly effective method of therapy. Theoretically where the drugs synergize, the dose of amphotericin B may be reduced. In cryptococcal meningitis combination therapy using a dose of 0.3 mg/kg body weight of amphotericin B with the normal dose of 5-fluorocytosine is more effective at sterilizing the CSF and preventing relapse. In other forms of systemic infection such as candidosis there is little evidence that it is more effective than amphotericin B, although this may in time prove to be the case.

Of the synthetic imidazole drugs, miconazole is the one most commonly used in systemic fungal infections. Its penetration into CSF and urine is poor but it has proved to be effective in cases of paracoccidioidomycosis, coccidioidomycosis, candidosis, sporotrichosis, and cryptococcosis. The drug is less toxic than amphotericin B, the main side-effects being thrombophlebitis, rash, and pruritus. It is given intravenously in a dose of 600–1000 mg three times daily by infusion. More critical studies of its use are needed, before its value can be accurately assessed. It is probably best reserved as a second line of treatment at present.

Other imidazoles which have been used include thiabendazole in chromomycosis and the newer oral drug ketoconazole in paracoccidioidomycosis, histoplasmosis, and candidosis. More studies of the latter compound are currently in progress.

Other agents which are used in specific systemic infections include 2-hydroxystilbamidine in blastomycosis and sulphonamides in paracoccidioidomycosis.

Immunotherapy has been used in certain systemic infections, for instance transfer factor or leucocyte transfusions in coccidioidomycosis. The use of the former has been sufficiently encouraging in anergic forms of this infection to warrant more detailed studies.

References

Bennett, J. E. (1974). Chemotherapy of systemic mycoses. *New Engl. J. Med.* **290**, 30, 320.
Hildick-Smith, G., Blank, H., and Sarkany, I. (1964). *Fungus diseases and their treatment.* Little, Brown, Boston.
Speller, (ed.) (1980). *Antifungal chemotherapy.* Wiley, Chichester.
Stevens, D. A., Levine, H. B., and Deresinski, S. C. (1976). Miconazole in coccidioidomycosis. II. Therapeutic and pharmacologic studies in man. *Am. J. Med.* **60**, 190.

PROTOZOA

Amoebic infections

R. Knight

The amoebae that infect man. The structure and life cycles of parasitic amoebae are simple compared with the other protozoans infecting man. The motile feeding stages are called trophozoites, they have no fixed shape and the cell is bounded only by a unit membrane. The cytoplasm is differentiated into a clear external ectoplasm, that surrounds the more granular endoplasm which contains the nucleus, food vacuoles, and other organelles. The cytoplasmic proteins can interchange their physical state between a colloidal sol in the endoplasm and a colloidal gel in the ectoplasm; the ectoplasmic gel is contractile and provides the propulsive force needed to form pseudopodia during movement and feeding. A pseudopodium is produced when an area of ectoplasmic gel becomes a sol and endoplasm streams into the defect which becomes lined with newly formed gel. Food vacuoles are formed when pseudopodia completely envelope a portion of the surrounding medium.

The trophozoite nucleus is almost always single and its detailed structure is of great importance in species identification. Its general form is described as vesicular for the nuclear chromatin is partly concentrated in a central endosome while the remainder lines the nuclear membrane as the 'peripheral chromatin'; between lies a clear nuclear sap. Trophozoites multiply by simple binary fission and this can continue indefinitely under favourable conditions. Under specific environmental conditions, however, the trophozoites of most amoebic species can form cysts. The organisms round up and secrete a relatively rigid cyst wall which is resistant to many environmental conditions that would destroy trophozoites. In many species one or more nuclear divisions occur before the cyst becomes fully mature. After escaping through the cyst wall the mass of cytoplasm divides to surround each nucleus and forms uninucleate trophozoites. For each species the nuclear structure is similar in the trophozoite and the cyst.

The amoebic species infecting man fall ecologically into two very different groups.

The amoebae of the alimentary tract. These are all obligate parasites and their trophozoites cannot survive for long in the external environment. There are eight species in this group and, with the exception of *Entamoeba gingivalis*, which occurs in the mouth, they are normally found in the lumen of the large bowel. They are all anaerobes and live commensally adjacent to the mucosal surface as a continuously replicating population of trophozoites feeding upon bacteria, exfoliated epithelial cells, and other tissue debris. Six of the seven intestinal species form cysts and these are the transmissive form of the parasite enabling direct or indirect faeco-oral spread to occur.

Only one of these species, *E. histolytica*, the cause of amoebic dysentery and amoebic liver abscess, has undisputed pathogenicity. However, two others, neither of which form cysts, appear to have some pathogenic potential. *E. gingivalis* is normally found in tooth pockets, carious dental cavities, and in the tonsillar crypts. It probably contributes to periodontal disease by causing immunologically mediated inflammatory responses. Prevalence rates may reach 25 per cent and transmission is mainly by kissing and shared drinking vessels, eating utensils, and tooth brushes. The colonic species *Dientamoeba fragilis* is now believed to cause a relatively mild and usually self-limited diarrhoeal illness, although tissue damage has never been proven histologically. Unlike all other parasitic amoebae, the trophozoites of this species are mostly binucleate, being in a state of arrested telophase. Transmission is probably direct or possibly within the eggs of the threadworm *Enterobius vermicularis* (see page 5.435).

Free-living soil amoebae. Several species of 'soil amoebae' are known to produce cytopathic changes in tissue cell monolayers and to cause progressive tissue destruction after intranasal inoculation into mice and other animals; they may also 'contaminate' and feed upon bacterial cultures grown upon agar plates. The cytopathic effects of one of these amoebae upon monkey kidney monolayers was thought initially to be due to a virus and was named as the Ryan virus—a classic example of failure to use the microscope. Since 1965 it has been realized that some of these amoebae can produce serious human disease and well over 150 cases have now been documented. Since these organisms are cosmopolitan in nature, it is surprising that so far very few cases have been reported from the tropics; it is likely that many are missed.

These amoebae live in the soil and in muddy water, especially when it is contaminated by bacteria. They multiply in warm water and can survive chlorination. They have also been found in tap water, the warm water of health spas, and the humidifier units of air-conditioning systems. Under dry conditions the trophozoites form resistant cysts that permit survival and also air-borne dispersal. Unlike the parasitic gut amoebae, the soil amoebae are aerobic and their endoplasm contains mitochondria, a Golgi complex, and contractile vacuoles. They may easily be grown in culture upon agar plates seeded with a bacterium.

Most human disease is caused by two species *Naegleria fowleri* and *Acanthamoeba culbertsoni*; their biology and clinical effects differ and they will be considered separately. A shared feature of both these genera is that the nucleus contains a very large central endosome, quite unlike that of the invasive gut species *E. histolytica*. The soil amoebae infecting man are a classical example of facultative parasitism—the adoption of a parasitic life style by a free-living organism.

These species also account for the so-called 'coprozoic amoebae' found in faecal specimens, especially when they are not fresh. Their presence results either from contamination of the specimen, or the excystation of cysts that have passed through the gut following accidental ingestion.

N. fowleri and related organisms are now known to be one of the causes of 'humidifier fever', a form of extrinsic allergic alveolitis presenting with fever, cough, and sometimes progressive pulmonary fibrosis and dyspnoea. The amoebae grow readily in the warm water of the cooling units of air-conditioning systems; the patient's sera show high antibody titres to the amoebae.

Although many amoebic species are now known to infect man, the unqualified term amoebiasis is, by convention, normally limited to infections by *E. histolytica*.

Entamoeba histolytica infection

Biology and pathogenicity. In most persons infected with *E. histolytica*, the parasite lives entirely as an intraluminal commensal; most of these amoebae, which divide mitotically every eight hours, are located adjacent to the muscosa of the proximal colon and caecum. When examined microscopically commensal amoebae measure between 10–20 µm in diameter, the endoplasm appears granular and contains many bacteria and particles upon which the organism is feeding; the pseudopodia are relatively blunt and movement rather sluggish. The transmissive cystic form of the parasite is derived entirely from this population of commensal trophozoites. Encystment occurs within the colonic lumen and never outside the body. The cysts are spherical and measure between 10–15 µm in diameter. When immature they contain a single nucleus and a glycogen vacuole that stains brown with iodine. Later, two nuclear divisions produce four nuclei, during the maturation process the glycogen vacuole is lost and large refractile cigar-shaped rods appear in the cytoplasm; these are chromatoid bodies and they constitute a ribosome store. Mosts cysts passed in the faeces contain four nuclei, but some may have only one or two, or more rarely three; maturation can continue outside the body. The chromatoid bodies slowly disappear as the cysts age, and they are best seen in the cysts from fresh faecal specimens. Intestinal hurry from any cause, including the use of laxatives, can lead to the appearance of commensal trophozoites in the faeces.

When *E. histolytica* trophozoites invade the colonic muscosa, their appearance and behaviour becomes very different from that of their commensal progenitors. Invasive trophozoites may reach 30–40 µm in diameter, and they are usually very active with apparently purposeful unidirectional movements during which they become considerably elongated. Diagnostically their most important characteristic is the frequent presence of host erythrocytes within the endoplasm, which otherwise appears relatively clear and contains no bacteria. Invasive trophozoites containing red blood cells are described as haematophagous. The evident size difference between commensal and invasive trophozoites has led to their designation as 'minuta' and 'magna' forms respectively, but these terms are now rarely used. Invasive amoebae appear to damage host cells only by direct contact which induces the release of membrane-bound cytolytic enzymes from dendritic plasmalemmal processes. Progression through the tissues is by active movement, facilitated perhaps by secreted hyaluronidase; leucocytes are drawn chemotactically towards the amoebae but are rapidly destroyed on contact.

Besides intact red blood cells, the food vacuoles of invasive amoebae contain ingested tissue debris and cell fragments. The factors which trigger the transformation of the harmless commensal into a dangerous invasive pathogen remain largely unknown, yet this is the key to our understanding of the disease. Both host and parasite factors affect the likelihood of tissue invasion.

When injected intracaecally into rats, strains of *E. histolytica* isolated from patients with invasive colonic amoebiasis are usually more pathogenic than those isolated from symptomless carriers. Virulence often declines after prolonged *in vitro* culture but can be restored by animal passage. Attempts to characterize strains biochemically and antigenically have so far been largely unsuccessful, although recent studies with isoenzyme patterns appear promising. A very small number of 'atypical' or *E. histolytica*-like strains have now been isolated. These grow at room temperature, can survive in hypotonic media, and differ antigenically from normal strains; they are not pathogenic in animals nor apparently, in man. With this one exception all strains of *E. histolytica* must be regarded as potentially virulent.

Host factors that increase susceptibility include protein energy malnutrition, steroid therapy given systemically or locally into the rectum, and cytotoxic therapy. Severe bowel infections are particularly common in late pregnancy and the puerperium. Before puberty both sexes are equally susceptible to hepatic amoebiasis but after puberty this condition is at least seven times more common in males. Local disease can also favour tissue invasion; thus amoebic ulceration may be superimposed upon colonic and rectal cancers, and colonic invasion is favoured by co-existent infection with *Trichuris trichiura* and intestinal schistosomiasis. Overt or latent non-specific colitis, and probably *Shigella* infections predispose to amoebic colitis. Hepatic lesions appear to be more common in the presence of liver cell damage, including that due to alcoholism.

Epidemiology. About one tenth of the world's population are infected with *E. histolytica*, and in some tropical countries the prevalence exceeds 30 per cent. In most European countries and the more temperate parts of North America the overall prevalence is usually now well below 2 per cent, although foci with higher rates are not uncommon. At any one time the majority, probably at least 95 per cent, of infections are non-invasive.

Apart from the very rare sexually acquired infections, transmission is exclusively by ingestion of cysts. Excystment occurs in the lower ileum and caecum. Under optimal conditions cysts remain viable for two months. Symptomless or convalescent carriers are the main source of infection; patients with dysentery normally pass only trophozoites in their stool, and therefore they are non-infectious. The daily cyst output in the faeces of a carrier can reach 45 million but is usually much lower; the number varying from day to day, and excretion may be intermittent; some persons give persistently higher cyst counts than others. The minimal infective dose is unknown, although in volunteers 2000 or more cysts give 100 per cent infection and a prepatent period of between four and eight days. The duration of an infection varies greatly and can exceed 20 years. However, the rate of spontaneous loss of infection appears to be a random process with a half life of two to three years. Tissue invasion can occur at any time during an infection, but it is most common in the first four months, although the incubation period is rarely less than three weeks. Serological evidence suggests that mild self-limited tissue invasion is commoner than previously supposed, and symptomatic bowel disease may sometimes undergo spontaneous remission; recurrent tissue invasion, with or without symptoms, is probably common in some predisposed persons.

Amoebiasis is normally a stable endemic infection and a typical age prevalence curve shows a steady rise in prevalence with age until a plateau is reached in adolescence or early adult life; such curves suggest that the rates of gain and loss of infection are often relatively constant and independent of age. However, under insanitary conditions, an early peak in prevalence is commonly observed in early childhood. All the modes of faeco-oral transmission occur in amoebiasis; of special importance is the infected food handler. Vegetables may be contaminated when human faeces are used as fertilizer, or when sewage polluted water is used for irrigation or for 'freshening' vegetables before sale in the market place; fly-borne infection is common. More or less direct spread between infants, and within institutions for children and the mentally subnormal, is common and can produce outbreaks of infection. Household clustering is common; hand-fed infants are frequently infected from the fingers of their mother. Water-borne infection frequently occurs by contamination within the home; infection from piped water supplies is rare and previous epidemics attributed to this source were probably due to other pathogens. True epidemics of amoebiasis are likely to go unrecognized because of the low morbidity rate of *E. histolytica* and the variable incubation period. The

incidence of disease does not necessarily correlate with the prevalence of infection; invasive disease is especially common in Southeast Asia, Natal, the west coast of Africa, Mexico, and parts of South America.

Although rats, dogs, and certain monkeys are sometimes found to be infected with *E. histolytica*, it is exceptional for them to be a source of infection to man.

Pathology. The basic lesion in amoebiasis is a lytic tissue necrosis, which, by creating relatively anoxic and acidic conditions, favours the further penetration of amoebae into the tissues. Secondary bacterial infection is uncommon except in amoebic lesions of the bowel wall and skin; its main pathological significance may be an enhancement of amoebic proliferation due to the physio-chemical conditions that are created. In tissue sections amoebae are often surrounded by a clear space due to shrinkage. They stain rather indistinctly with haemotoxylin and eosin but with periodic acid-Schiff stain they appear bright red; iron haematoxylin staining is necessary to show nuclear detail. In the absence of secondary bacterial infection, the inflammatory cell response comprises a mild or moderate local accumulation of lymphocytes and polymorphs. Most amoebae are seen at the advancing edge of the lesion, but some may be seen beyond this in apparently healthy tissue.

Intestinal amoebiasis. The initial lesions are small, discrete, superficial mucosal erosions. These later cross the muscularis mucosae and expand laterally to produce lesions that are typically flask-shaped in cross-section. Further lateral spread leads to a coalescence of lesions and denudation of the overlying mucosa. Deeper penetration can extend through the muscle coats of the bowel and lead to intestinal perforation. Blood vessels involved in the disease process undergo local thrombosis or may bleed freely. Amoebic ulceration is most common in the rectosigmoid and caecum but can occur anywhere in the large bowel, and much less commonly in the appendix or terminal ileum.

Amoebomas are granulomatous tumours of the colonic wall measuring up to several centimetres in length; they are commonest in the caecum and may be multiple. Histologically there is considerable tissue oedema and a prominent round cell infiltration. Rarely amoebomas can initiate an intussusception. Amoebic strictures are narrower annular bands of granulation tissue that are most frequent in the anorectal region.

Hepatic amoebiasis and its sequelae. It is likely that very few of the amoebae, reaching the liver passively via the portal vein from the gut wall, ever succeed in establishing themselves. Possibly a nidus of tissue necrosis is necessary, and this could result from local thrombosis or embolism. Once initiated, however, the amoebic lesion extends progressively in all directions to produce the liver cell necrosis and liquifaction that constitute the so-called amoebic 'liver abscess'. The lesions are commonly solitary, and are most frequently located in the upper part of the right lobe of the liver; multiple lesions are more common in children and in patients with severe coexistant amoebic bowel ulceration. Liver abscesses are sharply demarcated from surrounding liver tissue, which shows hyperaemia, oedema, and a moderate inflammatory cell response; a fibroblastic reaction occurs only in long-standing lesions. There is no pathological basis for a diffuse form of amoebic hepatitis, although this term is sometimes used by clinicians. Non-specific hepatic inflammatory changes are quite common in uncomplicated intestinal amoebiasis, and in many patients with amoebic dysentery, this accounts for the mild hepatomegaly that may be found clinically; its pathogenesis is similar to that seen in other inflammatory bowel diseases.

Nearly all amoebic abscesses eventually extend into adjacent structures and a variety of complications are produced in this way. Less commonly the lesions may compress intrahepatic bile ducts or the portal vein. Rarely amoebae are carried, after the lesion erodes into the hepatic veins, by the blood stream to distant organs, usually the lung but occasionally the brain.

Cutaneous and genital lesions. Skin lesions are commonest in the perianal area and can result from ruptured ischiorectal abscesses or be a direct mucosal extension of rectal ulceration; they also occur at colostomy stomas, laparotomy scars, or by rupture of a liver abscess through the skin. In the female, genital involvement results from faecal contamination, the extension of perineal lesions, or by the formation of internal fistulae from the gut; the latter occasionally involve the bladder. The uterine cervix is sometimes extensively involved. In the male, genital lesions usually follow rectal coitus, the lesion beginning as a balanoposthitis and progresses rapidly.

Immunological responses. Commensal intraluminal amoebae do not evoke an immune response. Invasive amoebiasis evokes both humoral and cellular immune responses. Most detectable amoebic antibody is IgG and it may persist for several years after successful therapy. In active disease IgM antibody may be found. Immediate skin sensitivity to amoebic antigen, presumably mediated by IgE antibody, occurs in some patients with active disease. Lymphoblast transformation to amoebic antigen can be demonstrated in many patients with active disease.

There is no evidence that these immune responses shorten the duration of intraluminal infections. Similarly they do not control severe invasive disease, particularly that of the liver. However it is likely that mild self-limited tissue invasion is controlled by these mechanisms. Clinical relapse is quite common unless the infection is eliminated from the gut lumen, even in the presence of antibody. Using sensitive techniques 25 per cent of symptomless carriers have detectable antibody.

Although histological features of amoebic lesions do not suggest that cellular immunity is important, it should be remembered that self-limiting lesions are rarely biopsied and that many of the host factors that increase susceptibility are those that depress cellular immunity.

Clinical manifestations
Invasive intestinal amoebiasis. The clinical features show a wide spectrum from mild changes in bowel habit to severe dysentery. Lesions may be limited to a small part of the large bowel or extend through its length. A relapsing course is common.

Amoebic dysentery. Dysentery, the passage of loose or diarrhoeal stools containing fresh blood, occurs when there is generalized colonic ulceration, or when more localized lesions are located in the rectum or rectosigmoid. The constitutional upset is initially mild and the patient often remains ambulant; mild or moderate abdominal pain is common and is often colicky and maximal over the affected parts of the gut. Tenesmus is infrequent even when the rectum is involved. Stools vary in consistency from semiformed to watery, they are often malodorous and always contains some visible blood together, usually, with mucus; even when watery, some faecal material is nearly always present. Symptoms frequently wax and wane over a period of weeks or even months. Eventually the patient can become very debilitated and wasted. In a few patients the disease runs a fulminating course.

The most frequent physical sign is abdominal tenderness which may be generalized, but most frequently is localized to one or both iliac fossae; affected areas of gut may be palpably thickened. A low-grade fever is common; there may be some hepatomegaly especially when the colonic lesions are widespread. Dehydration is infrequent. Abdominal distension occurs in the more severely ill patient who sometimes passes relatively small amounts of stool; some patients progress to toxic megacolon.

Stool microscopy usually shows large trophozoites, many of them haematophagous. Numerous bacteria are present together with moderate numbers of leucocytes, most of them macrophages; free red cells are often agglutinated and may show degenerative changes. When no haematophagous amoebae are found on stool

microscopy, then sigmoidoscopy should be performed, unless the patient has severe dysentery. In the latter situation sigmoidoscopy can occasionally cause bowel perforation if the ulcers are deep; nevertheless proctoscopy is essential whenever the diagnosis is in doubt. The endoscopic appearances of amoebic ulcers are non-specific but the presence of normal looking intervening mucosa between them is suggestive; early lesions are often elevated with a pouting opening that may be only 1 or 2 mm in diameter. Scrapings should be taken from all types of ulcerative lesions with a sigmoidoscopic spoon or curette; more solid lesions should be sampled with a curette or biopsy forceps.

Complications of amoebic dysentery. The most important local complication is peritonitis. Sometimes this is localized and leads to signs of acute peritonitis or more rarely to a pericolic abscess or retroperitoneal faecal cellulitis. More commonly perforation occurs in patients with toxic megacolon, the bowel being grossly diseased and perforating at many points. These patients show progressive abdominal distension, vomiting, and dehydration. Bowel sounds are absent and there may be no localized tenderness, guarding, or rigidity; free gas in the peritoneum on an erect X-ray film confirms the diagnosis. Profuse haemorrhage due to erosion of a large blood vessel is a rare complication. After successful chemotherapy a few patients develop fibrous strictures of the gut, or have persistent internal fistulae. A far larger number develop symptoms of an irritable colon syndrome that can persist for many months. A rare complication is post-dysenteric colitis, and in these patients dysentery continues despite parasitological cure. Sigmoidoscopy shows a reddened oedematous mucosa with superficial erosions. The condition is distinct from simple ulcerative colitis and is usually self-limiting over a period of months, amoebic antibody titres remaining very high.

Non-dysenteric colonic disease. When ulceration is limited to the caecum or ascending colon, it rarely produces dysentery; similarly mild or localized ulceration elsewhere in the colon may give no dysenteric symptoms. The patients complain of frequent changes in bowel habit and sometimes notice occasional blood staining of the stool, that may be wrongly attributed to haemorrhoids; flatulence is common and may be associated with colicky pains. Often the only physical sign is tenderness in the right iliac fossa or elsewhere along the course of the colon. Sigmoidoscopy is often normal when the distal bowel is not involved. These patients are difficult to evaluate as even a barium enema can be virtually normal. The most important diagnostic measure is repeated stool examination for haematophagous amoebae; cysts alone will often be found and also sometimes commensal trophozoites if there is intestinal hurry. The administration of a saline purge is occasionally helpful. The most important complication of this form of disease is progression to amoebic dysentery. However, some patients eventually undergo complete remission.

Amoebomas present as an abdominal mass, frequently in the right iliac fossa. The lesion may be painful and is often tender, and fever is quite common. Bowel habit is often altered and some patients have intermittent dysentery; commonly the lesions are multiple. Clinically, simple appendicitis or an appendiceal abscess may be closely simulated. Sometimes a true amoebic appendicitis occurs as an extension of caecal ulceration or when an amoeboma blocks the appendiceal lumen.

Both amoebomas and granulomatous strictures can cause colicky abdominal pains and intermittent obstructive symptoms; complete obstruction occurs when an amoeboma initiates an intussusception.

The stools of patients with amoebomas and granulomatous strictures may contain cysts, commensal trophozoites, or haematophagous trophozoites depending upon the site of the lesion. When lesions are within reach of the sigmoidoscope they should be biopsied and the material examined as a fresh wet preparation, and by histology. The appearances of these lesions on barium enema can closely resemble neoplasms.

Differential diagnosis. Amoebic dysentery must be differentiated from bacillary dysentery and non-specific ulcerative colitis; other conditions causing confusion are intestinal salmonellosis, heavy infections with intestinal schistosomiasis and *Trichiuris trichiura*, and balantidiasis. More chronic amoebic disease of the bowel can resemble carcinoma, diverticulosis, and Crohn's disease. It must always be remembered that *E. histolytica* can invade carcinomas and the finding of this parasite should not delay the search for other possible diagnoses. Caecal amoebomas may resemble ileocaecal tuberculosis and anorectal amoebic strictures can be confused with lymphogranuloma venereum. Therapeutic trials with amoebicides can be difficult to interpret, and sometimes cause unnecessary delay.

Hepatic amoebiasis. In about 70 per cent of patients, the liver abscess is solitary; only about half of all patients give a history of preceding dysentery, the time interval being anywhere between a week and several years.

The condition normally presents with fever, sweating, and liver pain. Fever is often remittent with a prominent evening rise, rigors are brief, but sweating is often very profuse. Liver pain is initially poorly localized but may later become pleuritic or referred to the right shoulder tip. Most patients present within one to four weeks of the onset of symptoms, but in some the progress is much slower; the onset is usually insidious. Constitutional upset is considerable and weight loss is often prominent. An anaemia develops within a few weeks.

The most important clinical finding is liver enlargement with localized tenderness. When liver enlargement is mainly upwards beneath the right hemidiaphragm, it can be difficult to detect hepatomegaly by abdominal palpation; left-sided lesions present as an epigastric mass, and there may be bulging of the right chest wall. Local tenderness should be searched for in the right hypochondrium and along all the intercostal spaces overlying the liver; pain on liver compression or heavy percussion may be considerable but this is not a specific sign. An elevation of the right hemidiaphragm is a frequent early finding and may be associated with crepitations at the right lung base and a dry cough. Jaundice is rare unless the lesions are multiple or very large.

An important radiological finding is a raised or localized upward bulging of the right diaphragm which is immobile on screening. Radiology may also reveal areas of lung collapse or consolidation above the diaphragm and sometimes a pleural effusion. A neutrophil leucocytosis is almost invariably present, the erythrocyte sedimentation rate is raised, and there is often a normochromic normocytic anaemia. Liver function tests are frequently completely normal although there may be some increase in serum transaminase or alkaline phosphatase, and less commonly the serum bilirubin is raised. For reasons that are not understood an intestinal infection can only be demonstrated in about 60 per cent of patients; positive stools commonly only contain cysts but haematophagous trophozoites may be found, or sometimes commensal ones. Liver scanning to demonstrate a filling defect is of great value; the findings with ultrasound and with isotope scanning, made upon the same patient, do not always correspond, and, when there is doubt, both methods should be employed. When available, computerized axial tomography will demonstrate the lesion.

Complications. The three most common complications of liver abscess are rupture into the right chest, the peritoneum, and the pericardium. Lesions that extend upwards usually produce adhesions, between the liver, the diaphragm, and the lung; as a result subphrenic rupture and an amoebic empyema are rare; a small or moderate right serous effusion is, however, not uncommon. Most commonly the disease process progresses upwards through lung tissue until a bronchus is reached. A hepatobronchial fistula results and the patient may cough up large quantities of brownish necrotic liver tissue, the so-called 'anchovy sauce' sputum. Rupture into the peritoneum is sometimes the mode of presentation of an amoebic liver abscess, the cause of the peritonitis being discovered only at laparotomy. Amoebic pericarditis usually results from upward extension from the left lobe of the liver but it may derive from a right lobe lesion or a lung abscess. Intially there is a serous effusion but this is a prelude to suppurative amoebic pericarditis. Patients may present in shock due to cardiac tamponnade, or with a more gradual onset of pericardial signs; retrosternal pain is common and also a friction rub. The diagnosis is most difficult when the underlying liver abscess is not previously apparent.

Less commonly the lesion extends through to the skin producing a sinus and cutaneous lesion. The gut, stomach, vena cava, spleen, and kidney can also occasionally be involved by direct spread. Blood-borne spread to the lung produces a lesion resembling an isolated pyogenic lung abscess, but this is rare. More than 100 amoebic brain abscesses due to *E. histolytica* have now been reported, so far almost all patients with this diagnosis having died and all having had an amoebic liver abscess. Rarely a large abscess causes an obstructive jaundice by compressing the common bile duct. Alternatively multiple abscesses can cause jaundice by compressing several intrahepatic bile ducts. Rupture into a bile duct is rare but can cause haemobilia. Portal vein compression occasionally produces portal hypertension and congestive splenomegaly.

Differential diagnosis. In tropical countries the condition causing most diagnostic difficulty is primary hepatocellular carcinoma; malignant secondary deposits in the liver produce similar problems. Other conditions to be distinguished include pyogenic hepatic and subphrenic abscesses, lesions of the right lung base and right pleura, viral and alcoholic hepatitis, cholecystitis, septic cholangitis including that caused by aberrant *Ascaris* worms, and liver hydatid cysts.

Serology and scanning techniques have now greatly simplified diagnosis. However, the previously widely practised diagnostic needle aspiration of the liver is still sometimes necessary. A medium bore chest aspiration needle (about 1.5 mm in diameter), attached via a three-way tap to a 50 ml syringe should be used, preceded by premedication and local anaesthetic. If the lesion is pointing, the needle should be inserted through adjacent healthy tissue. When an area of localized tenderness has been located in an intercostal space, this should be the site for aspiration. Lesions of the left lobe should only be aspirated percutaneously if they are superficial. When there is no definite clinical evidence as to the site of the lesion, the eighth or ninth intercostal space in the mid-axillary line should be selected, provided of course, that the site is dull to percussion. A depth of 7.5 cm should not be exceeded in an adult and usually not more than three attempts should be made, pointing the needle in a slightly different direction each time. The colour of the aspirate is not necessarily the classical reddish brown, but may be yellow or cream, especially in old lesions; compared with a bacterial abscess the odour is slight. The main complication of this procedure is introduced bacterial infection, an event suggested by the finding, on later aspiration, of a thinner, malodorous, or frothy aspirate. Haemorrhage is very uncommon after aspiration when the diagnosis is amoebic liver abscess, because the right diaphragm is immobile and adhesions form between the liver and the chest wall. In contrast, attempted aspiration of a hepatoma commonly produces a brisk haemorrhage.

Cutaneous and genital amoebiasis. Skin ulceration due to *E. histolytica* produces deep, painful, and foul smelling lesions that spread rapidly. Secondary bacterial infection is common. Lesions are most frequently located on the abdominal wall, perianal area, and perineum; the external genitalia may be rapidly destroyed in both sexes. Spread to the uterine cervix gives rise to ulcerative lesions resembling carcinoma. This diagnosis is often missed or delayed especially when they occur at laparotomy scars or colostomy stomas.

Laboratory diagnosis

Microscopy and culture. The identification of live haematophagous trophozoites of *E. histolytica* in temporary wet mounts is of prime importance because it confirms the diagnosis of invasive amoebic disease. No other human intestinal amoebae ingest red blood cells.

They should be sought in dysenteric stools, bowel wall scrapings, in the last portion of aspirate from a liver abscess, in sputum, and in material obtained from suspected skin lesions; the latter should be incised and the scrapings taken from the sides of the incision. In non-dysenteric stools, flecks of mucus or pus should be looked for and examined. The amoebae remain active for about 30 minutes at room temperature but if delay is unavoidable the specimen may be kept for up to four hours at 4 °C and then rewarmed. In non-intestinal lesions haematophagy by *E. histolytica* is less evident but this is of little importance because other amoebic species are not found at these sites. If necessary, the material should be diluted with saline, preferably buffered to pH 6.8. If stained permanent preparations are needed, the material should be fixed in Schaudinn's solution and stained with Gomori trichrome or Heidenhain's iron haematoxylin; however, these techniques are rather complex and lengthy and are not much used for routine diagnosis. They can, however, be usefully applied to preserved specimens kept in polyvinyl alcohol fixative. Commensal *E. histolytica* trophozoites can only be distinguished from the other intestinal commensal amoebic species in permanent stained preparations, but differentiation, which depends upon details of nuclear structure, is difficult.

In contrast the cysts of *E. histolytica* are fairly easy to recognize in wet mounts made from faecal specimens. Direct mounts are made by emulsifying a small portion of stool in 1 per cent eosin and another portion in Lugol's iodine solution. Provided the eosin preparations are thin enough, cysts stand out as round or oval white objects against a pink background. Nuclear structure cannot be seen but the refractile chromatoid bodies can be made out. The iodine preparation stains the nuclei and the glycogen vacuoles. The probability of detecting *E. histolytica* cysts in one stool specimen from an infected person using direct mounts is only about 30 per cent, therfore concentration methods, which increase diagnostic sensitivity to about 70 per cent are usually used; either formol–ether sedimentation or zinc sulphate flotation can be used. The concentrate is examined as a wet mount stained with Lugol's iodine. Three negative stool concentrate examinations on different days will miss only about 3 per cent of infections.

Four species of *Entamoeba* infect man; they all have a similar nuclear structure with a small central karyosome and a ring of peripheral chromatin. Three other amoebic species inhabit the human colon, one, *Dientamoeba fragilis*, produces no cysts and the remaining two, *Iodamoeba buetschlii* and *Endolimax nana*, have very large karyosomes. The three *Entamoeba* species other than *E. histolytica* may be briefly described as follows. *E. coli* is a common species; mature cysts have eight nuclei, inconspicuous finely pointed chromatoids and measure 14–20 μm. *E. hartmanni* closely resembles *E. histolytica*; it is usually less common, the mature cyst having four nuclei, cigar-shaped chromatoids, and measuring 6–10 μm, *E. polecki* is primarily a pig parasite and is very rare in man except where he lives in close association with pigs; the mature cyst has only one nucleus, the chromatoids are inconspicuous, and the cysts measure 10–14 μm. The only reliable criterion distinguishing the cysts of *E. hartmanni* and *E. histolytica* is size, the dividing line being 10 μm. In the past *E. hartmanni* has sometimes been referred to as the 'small race' of *E. histolytica*, but there is no evidence that it is ever pathogenic.

Human intestinal amoebae can be cultivated relatively easily, with bacterial associates, in suitable media such as that developed by Robinson. However fixed stained preparations of the cultured amoebae must be made to determine their specific identity. Furthermore, when applied to faecal specimens, the method will not distinguish invasive *E. histolytica* infections from symptomless commensal infections with this species. Positive cultures from extra intestinal sites are more useful, since they must be *E. histolytica*; in liver aspirates, particularly, amoebae are often difficult to find microscopically.

Serological tests. Although a variety of serodiagnostic methods have been applied to amoebiasis, it is suspected that these do not necessarily detect the same antibody since their correspondence is not complete; it may therefore be useful to perform more than one test. The most sensitive methods are indirect haemagglutination, enzyme-linked immunosorbent assay (ELISA), indirect immunofluorescence, and counter immunoelectropheresis. Latex agglutination and gel diffusion precipitation tests are also used, the former being available commercially as a slide test, taking only minutes to perform.

Seropositivity does not distinguish current tissue invasion from past disease, and in endemic areas many normal persons give positive tests, although usually at low titres. Positivity may persist for two years or more after successful therapy. However using sensitive tests over 95 per cent of liver abscess patients are seropositive, as are between 60 and 80 per cent of those with invasive bowel disease. A negative test is therefore quite strong evidence against a diagnosis of liver abscess. Patients with amoebomas are usually seropositive.

Treatment

Amoebicidal drugs. Some drugs destroy invasive amoebae in the tissues, others act upon those in the bowel lumen; they are known as tissue (systemic) and luminal amoebicides respectively; some compounds, like metronidazole act at both sites. Parasitological cure implies that the intraluminal commensal infection has been eliminated.

Metronidazole. When given by mouth metronidazole is rapidly absorbed and reaches all tissues. Most of the drug is excreted by the kidney, mainly as inactive metabolites. Some is secreted into the colonic lumen, and there is an enterohepatic circulation. It acts upon *E. histolytica*, as it does upon anaerobic bacteria, because the drug's very low redox potential traps electrons, halting the production of hydrogen from pyruvate and so depleting the organism of NADH and NADPH. The nitro-ring becomes cleaved in the process producing a toxic substance that hastens cell death. In short courses metronidazole is very safe but some patients complain of nausea, a metallic taste in the mouth, and dizziness; a few develop rashes, weakness, and mild transient ataxia. Prolonged courses can cause leucopenia and peripheral neuropathy. Recent evidence of oncogenicity in animals and mutagenicity in bacteria has caused concern, but the risks in man appear to be very small, and it is generally agreed that in invasive amoebiasis its effectiveness outweighs these potential dangers. Metronidazole has been widely used in pregnancy for trichomoniasis and there is so far no evidence of fetal damage.

The usual dose for adults is 800 mg thrice daily for five or eight days (paediatric dose 35–50 mg/kg in three divided doses). Lower doses, such as 400 mg thrice daily in adults, are frequently effective in invasive disease but may fail to eliminate the intraluminal infection and so clinical relapse can occur. The parenteral preparation, 500 mg as an 0.5 per cent aqueous infusion, is given over eight hours and may be useful in severely ill patients, but it has not yet been properly evaluated in amoebiasis.

Several other nitroimidazoles have been tested in amoebiasis, the most promising is tinidazole (Fasigyn), especially in children. It is given as a single daily dose of 50–60 mg/kg for three to five days. Parasitological cure rates may be lower than with metronidazole and the drug has yet to be shown to be more effective.

Emetine. Emetine hydrochloride is the most potent tissue amoebicide, and, despite its potential toxicity, it continues to be a life saving drug when properly used in appropriate situations. Given parenterally it has very little activity within the colonic lumen. The drug is cumulative and slowly excreted into the gut and urine: high concentrations may build up in the liver, heart, and other viscera. Emetine is given by daily intramuscular or deep subcutaneous injections (1 mg/kg daily, maximum 60 mg) for a maximum of 10 days and the course should not be repeated within 28 days. Local pain and tenderness at the sites of injection are common, and a local myositis can cause weakness; skin necrosis can occur if injections are too superficial. General side-effects include nausea, diarrhoea, weakness, and moderate hypotension; some of these effects are due to autonomic blockade, and occasionally a generalized myopathy results from neuromuscular block. Cardiovascular toxicity is potentially the most serious side-effect and may be heralded by tachycardia, dyspnoea, and retrosternal pain. ECG changes are common and not necessarily serious; they include flattening and inversion of T waves, prolongation of the PR interval, widening of QRS complexes, and alterations in rhythm. Bed rest is essential during treatment. Emetine is contra-indicated in heart disease except amoebic pericarditis, and must be used cautiously in the presence of renal disease or gross debility.

The synthetic derivative racemic 2-dehydroemetine was introduced in 1959 and has become established as an alternative to emetine. It is released more rapidly from most body organs, including the heart, than emetine, and is excreted more quickly in the urine, the daily dose is therefore somewhat higher at 1.25 mg/kg (maximum 90 mg). Its efficacy is similar to that of emetine and its toxicity is almost certainly less, hence dehydroemetine is generally to be preferred to emetine when both drugs are available.

Chloroquine. This drug becomes strongly bound to host proteins within the liver, lung, and kidney; its usefulness in hepatic amoebiasis results from this tissue binding which also accounts for the long half-life (6–7 days) of the drug in the body, and the necessity of giving a loading dose when treatment is started. The standard course of treatment in adults is chloroquine base 150 mg four times daily for two days followed by 150 mg twice daily for 19 days (paediatric dose 10 mg base per kg daily). Side-effects are exceptional at this dosage and the minor ECG changes are of no significance; unless the patient has been taking long term chloroquine previously there is no risk of retinopathy. Patients being treated for invasive intestinal disease with drugs other than metronidazole or emetine should receive a two-week course of chloroquine to prevent the development of hepatic lesions. Chloroquine has no effect upon intraluminal amoebae or amoebae invading the intestine.

Antibiotics. Tetracycline is a useful drug in invasive intestinal amoebiasis but has no action within the gut lumen. Its direct amoebical action is weak and its effectiveness is mainly due to antibacterial effects upon secondarily infected gut lesions. Because of its wide antibacterial spectrum, tetracycline is especially valuable in patients with gut perforation and peritonitis, to whom it can be given parenterally. The adult dose is 1–2 g daily in divided doses for 5 to 10 days. Because of potential toxicity, tetracycline should be avoided in late pregnancy and in infants and young children.

Erythromycin can be used in invasive intestinal disease. Its actions are similar to those of tetracycline but somewhat less effective; however, it has a wide margin of safety and is especially useful in infants and young children; it is a poor luminal amoebicide.

Paromomycin (Humatin) is a poorly absorbed aminoglycoside that was first used in amoebiasis in 1959. It has been used mainly for mild or moderately severe invasive intestinal disease but is also a useful luminal amoebicide. The usual dosage for adults and children is 25–35 mg/kg daily in three doses for 5 to 10 days.

Diloxanide furoate. This dichloroacetanilide derivative is marketed as Furamide or entamide furoate; it shows strong amoebicidal activity *in vitro*. Absorption from the gut is poor and side-effects are minimal, flatulence being the most common. It is used only as a luminal amoebicide, the standard dosage in adults being 500 mg thrice daily for 10 days (paediatric dose 20 mg/kg daily in three divided doses).

5-hydroxyquinolines. Several compounds in this group have been widely used as luminal amoebicides, and for the treatment of very mild invasive intestinal disease; they are believed to act upon amoebae, as they do upon many other micro-organisms, by chelating ferrous iron ions that are essential for microbial metabolism. Diiodohydroxyquin (Diodoquin) has been the most consistently used hydroxyquinoline in amoebiasis; only about 5 per cent of an oral dose is absorbed. The usual dosage schedule in adults is 650 mg thrice daily for 20 days (paediatric dose 30–40 mg/kg in three divided doses to a maximum of 2 g daily). Side-effects are usually mild and include headache, nausea, rashes, and pruritus ani; they are partly attributable to iodine sensitivity. Of far greater concern is the association between the related compound iodochlorohydroxyquin (Clioquinol) and subacute myelo-optic neuropathy first reported in Japan, and later in Europe and USA. Although most of these cases resulted from prolonged drug usage without prescription, the reports led to a withdrawal of these compounds by many manufacturers. Diodoquin had previously been the most widely used luminal amoebicide and was regarded as very safe although optic neuritis has very occasionally been reported.

Patient management. *Intestinal amoebiasis: amoebic dysentery.* In patients with uncomplicated disease, metronidazole for five days will be the first choice in most patients. If follow-up stool examination cannot be performed to assess parasitological cure, it is wise to extend treatment to eight days; alternatively a five-day course of metronidazole can be followed by diloxanide.

Supportive management plays a predominant role in patients with complicated amoebic dysentery with emphasis on fluid and electrolyte replacement, gastric suction, and blood transfusion as necessary. Gut perforation carries a very poor prognosis; in the less common presentation of acute perforation, surgical repair should be considered; when the colon is diffusely dilated with multiple leaks, management is medical. Before the advent of metronidazole, patients with peritonitis were treated with emetine and a parenteral broad spectrum antibiotic, usually intravenous tetracycline, to be followed later by a lumicide. In patients unable to take oral medicines parenteral metronidazole offers the dual advantage of potent tissue amoebicidal activity and action against anaerobic bacteria in the peritoneum and blood stream. When this preparation is available it should be tried in such situations. However, until its efficacy has been proven, it is wise to give emetine as well. In addition another antibiotic must be given to cover aerobic bacteria leaking from the gut. Even in patients without proven perforation, many physicians would recommend the use of emetine in addition to oral metronidazole in seriously ill patients with dysentery who threaten to progress to toxic megacolon; in such circumstances it is normally only necessary to give emetine for three to five days and the risks of cardiovascular toxicity are very small.

Intestinal amoebiasis: non-dysenteric colonic disease. This will normally be treated as for uncomplicated amoebic dysentery. Emetine is known to be effective in amoebomas and amoebic strictures and, although reports so far with metronidazole are favourable, it may be wise to use combined treatment to achieve a more rapid response. Whatever treatment is used, a slow response should arouse suspicion that the amoebic lesion is superimposed upon other pathology, particularly a carcinoma.

Intestinal amoebiasis: non-invasive carrier state. The decision to treat carriers will depend upon the context. Patients who have had invasive disease must always be parasitologically cured otherwise they frequently relapse. Food handlers must be treated. In temperate countries and where the chances of reinfection are small, most physicians recommend the treatment of all detected carriers to prevent transmission to others and future invasive disease.

Diloxanide is currently the drug of choice. Metronidazole is also effective when given at full dosage for eight days, and is the drug of choice in combined *Giardia lamblia* and *E. histolytica* infections. Until the possible risks of metronidazole are resolved, many physicians, particularly in the USA, consider that this drug should not be used for the generally benign carrier state. When available diiodohydroxyquin is effective and almost certainly completely safe; when not available the other safe and effective alternative is paromomycin.

Hepatic amoebiasis. In simple uncomplicated liver abscess metronidazole will usually be the drug of choice, given for five or eight days according to response. Even though not detected, a luminal gut infection must always be presumed to be present and eliminated. It is wise to give diloxanide even when an eight-day course of metronidazole is used, it should always be given after a five-day course.

Several failures have now been reported with metronidazole given for liver abscess, and in a very small number of patients, liver abscesses have appeared soon after metronidazole treatment for dysentery. Some of these failures may be due to liver reinvasion from the gut, and in others the outcome might have been more favourable if therapeutic aspiration had been performed. Many physicians feel that metronidazole is somewhat less effective than emetine in some patients, particularly those with large or multiple abscesses; in such circumstances both drugs can be given together and if the response is good, emetine can be stopped after five to seven days.

Therapeutic aspiration does not appear to affect the outcome when abscesses are small or of moderate size, and in such circumstances the resolution time may not be affected. In large abscesses and those threatening rupture, therapeutic aspiration does affect the outcome, and if the percutaneous route is unsuccessful or anatomically contraindicated, then surgical help should be sought; failure to improve after five days medical treatment is another indication for therapeutic aspiration. Many physicians experienced in this disease recommend aspiration in all patients in whom local tenderness can be elicited or whose lesions cause severe pain. Therapeutic aspiration is carried out in the same manner as diagnostic aspiration except that a wider bore needle may be necessary to remove thick 'pus'.

Multiple abscesses are commonest in children and in patients with concurrent amoebic dysentery. Adequate drainage of all the lesions is rarely feasible, even at laparotomy, and reliance must be placed upon intensive chemotherapy with metronidazole plus emetine. Ruptured liver abscesses present a wide variety of surgical problems; extension into the pleural or pericardial cavities necessitates drainage of these structures, together with aspiration of the liver lesion. Amoebic pericarditis or serous pericarditis adjacent to an amoebic lesion may present as cardiac tamponnade requiring immediate drainage. Combined treatment with emetine plus metronidazole must be considered in all seriously ill patients with ruptured abscesses. Parenteral metronidazole is particularly useful in patients who have undergone laparotomy.

When metronidazole is not used in hepatic amoebiasis, for whatever reason, the combination of emetine plus chloroquine is at least equally effective. Even chloroquine alone, in non-critical situations, has a place in management when other drugs are contraindicated; however a course of 10 weeks therapy would be indicated in this circumstance. Diloxanide or another lumicide must, of course, be given when metronidazole is not used.

In a few patients it may be justifiable to do a therapeutic trial for suspected hepatic amoebiasis; in this circumstance it is worth noting that emetine is specific for amoebic lesions, having no antibacterial activity, whereas metronidazole has a wide spectrum of activity against anaerobic bacteria. The differentiation between amoebic and bacterial abscesses is sometimes very difficult.

Invasive amoebiasis at other sites. Cutaneous and genital amoebiasis respond well to metronidazole, perhaps because these lesions often contain anaerobic bacteria; whenever these lesions are very extensive or involve critical structures then emetine should be given as well. Amoebiasis at other sites is nearly always secondary to hepatic amoebiasis and the chemotherapy will be the same. Isolated amoebic lung lesions without hepatic involvement are extremely rare, but chemotherapy is the same as for hepatic lesions. Amoebic brain abscesses are nearly always fatal; since both emetine and metronidazole cross the blood–brain barrier, they should be used together in this desperate situation.

Prognosis. Uncomplicated invasive intestinal disease and uncomplicated hepatic amoebiasis should normally have a mortality rate of less than 1 per cent. In complicated disease the mortality is much greater and may reach 35 per cent for amoebic peritonitis with multiple gut perforation. Prognosis is usually better in centres where the disease is common and more likely to be recognized early. Late diagnosis increases the probability of complicated disease and the mortality rises accordingly.

Unless parasitological cure is achieved, and the gut completely freed of *E. histolytica*, clinical relapse is quite common and certain host factors, such as mild non-specific colitis, may be relevant. There is so far no evidence of naturally occurring strains of *E. histolytica* which are resistant to the normally used drugs. Hepatic scanning suggests that liver abscesses normally disappear within two to four months; little scar tissue remains but if the lesion was secondarily infected bizarre hepatic calcification may be seen years afterwards. Within the bowel healing is nearly always complete after successful chemotherapy; fibrous scars are most unusual.

There is no reason why a person from a temperate country should not return to the tropics after successful treatment for amoebiasis.

Prevention. In tropical and developing countries the incidence of amoebiasis will fall as sanitary measures are introduced to combat other faeco-orally transmitted infections. Repeated mass chemotherapy with metronidazole or diloxanide has been used in Mexico and elsewhere where invasive disease is common, and may sometimes be justified in temeperate countries when prevalence is high, for example among institutionalized persons. Chlorination of water supplies does not destroy amoebic cysts, but adequate filtration will remove them. All food handlers and domestic staffs involved in food handling should regularly have their stools examined.

Visitors to the tropics should not attempt chemoprophylaxis, in particular long-term unsupervised use of hydroxyquinoline compounds must be strongly deprecated. Simple hygienic measures provide considerable protection. Boiling water for five minutes kills cysts. Cooked foods should not be purchased from markets or street vendors, or from places where flies are prevalent. Fruit that can be peeled should be safe. Salad vegetables can be soaked in a dilute solution of sodium hypochlorite and then rinsed in boiled water. A weak solution of iodine is a more potent cysticide than chlorine.

In temperate countries, routine stool examinations are recommended for returning visitors from the tropics and for new residents coming from such countries.

Naegleria fowleri infection

Biology and epidemiology. *N. fowleri* is an amoebo-flagellate, and in its normal free living state there are two forms of trophozoite, one amoeboid and the other a non-dividing flagellate. Transformation into the flagellate form occurs in hypotonic media and these free swimming forms are believed to facilitate dispersal. Nearly all patients give a history of swimming or diving in fresh water between two and 14 days before the illness begins. Several small outbreaks have occurred, especially during warm summer months in temperate countries, affected persons having swum in the same water.

Pathology. The basic lesion is an acute necrotizing meningoencephalitis; at autopsy the brain is oedematous and there is blood-stained purulent exudate in the subarachnoid space, especially within the basal cisterns. Areas of cerebral softening are located in midbrain, pons, medulla, and inferior surfaces of the frontal lobes; the olfactory bulbs are always grossly damaged. Microscopically amoebae are seen at the advancing edge of the necrotic lesion and extending into healthy tissue, particularly along perivascular routes. There is little local inflammatory reaction around the amoebae, but a neutrophilic inflammatory reaction often extends into the grey matter from the subarachnoid space. The necrotic tissue shows petechial haemorrhages, vascular congestion, demyelination, and neuronal degeneration. As a terminal event amoebae may be disseminated throughout the body. Cysts are never formed in the tissues.

Naegleria trophozoites are presumed to cross the human cribriform plate from the nasal mucosa, as they do in experimental animals after intranasal insufflation, to reach the olfactory bulbs and subarachnoid space. During swimming, especially diving, these amoebae initially invade the mucosa and establish themselves on the roof of the nasal cavity.

Clinical features and diagnosis. Nearly all patients have previously been in good health, many are young adults or children. Initially upper respiratory symptoms and headache are common but within a few days patients become severely ill with fever, neck rigidity, coma, and, later, convulsions; localizing neurological signs are uncommmon. Many patients die within five days of the onset of the meningitic illness but some have been kept alive for longer periods with mechanical ventilation. In some patients the nasal and faucial mucosae are oedematous and inflamed. It is possible that some patients experience only a mild self-limited illness.

Lumbar puncture reveals a purulent, turbid, and frequently blood-stained cerebrospinal fluid. Microscopy reveals numerous red cells and neutrophils, the protein level is very high and the glucose level often low. The amoebae are frequently mistaken for macrophages, counts of several hundred amoebae per cubic millimetre are not unusual. They must be specifically looked for in fresh wet preparations of cerebrospinal fluid and the centrifuged deposit, many contain ingested red cells; amoeboid activity will be greatest between 25 and 37 °C, phase contrast microscopy is the preferred method. The clinical and cerebrospinal fluid changes much resemble those of bacterial meningitis, in Gram-stained preparations the amoebae appear as ill-defined smudges. However, if fixed preparations are stained with iron haematoxylin, full details of nuclear structure can be seen. For further confirmation the amoebae can easily be cultured aerobically upon a confluent growth of *Escherichia coli* on an agar plate.

Although so far only about 120 cases have been documented since the first human infection was reported in 1965, it is likely that many cases are missed; some are only discovered at necropsy. At least three cases have been diagnosed retrospectively from preserved pathological material. Specific antisera can be raised in rabbits, and after incubation with tissue sections, the amoebae can be recognized by labelling with flouorescein-tagged antiglobulin. Besides acute bacterial meningitis, this condition has been confused with tuberculous meningitis, and cryptococcal and other mycotic meningitides. The key to early diagnosis, which is essential if there is to be any hope of recovery, is the immediate microscopic examination of warmed, wet cerebrospinal fluid specimens. Serological diagnosis has not yet proved of value.

Treatment. The only drug known to be effective in this condition is amphotericin B which should be given by daily intravenous infusion and by intrathecal injections with the dosage regimens used for crytococcal meningitis. So far very few patients have survived but this may partly be due to delays in diagnosis. Drugs active against *E. histolytica* are of no value in this condition. Recently another antifungal drug, clotrimazole has been shown to be active against *N. fowleri in vitro* and this drug could be tried in man.

Acanthamoeba infections

Biology and epidemiology. These soil amoebae have no flagellate forms. The amoeboid trophozoites are usually covered by small tiny pseudopodia known as acanthopodia. Their cysts are very thick walled and buoyant so that they are readily wind-borne. Man probably becomes infected by swallowing or inhaling the cysts, but sometimes the amoebae apparently contaminate wounds or corneal abrasions; rarely the mode of infection is similar to that of *Naegleria*.

Acanthamoeba species are not uncommonly isolated from throat or nasal swabs in patients with minimal symptoms. They may also be cultured from stool specimens, the cysts having passed through the gut after accidental ingestion.

Clinical features, pathology, and diagnosis. The disease manifestations of this organism are much more protean than those of *Naegleria*. In most patients there is some local or systemic condition that predisposes to tissue invasion by these ubiquitous amoebae. Thus many are suffering from lymphomas or other malignancies, diabetes mellitus, or have experienced trauma, especially to the face and orbit. Pathologically the lesions are granulomatous and relatively slow growing, unless a body space such as the subarachnoid is invaded.

Lesions have been described from the lung, skin, orbit, scalp and underlying skull, middle ear, and the gastric wall. In addition cerebral lesions have been reported resembling chronic bacterial abscesses; some of these appear to have developed at the site of vascular infarcts. Meningeal involvement can result from rupture of these cerebral abscesses, extension of scalp or orbital lesions into the skull, or by the transnasal route by which *Naegleria* reaches the brain. Recently it has been appreciated that some indolent corneal ulcers are caused by *Acanthamoeba*; possibly wind-borne cysts are deposited upon a damaged cornea, and local steroid therapy may favour establishment by the amoebae.

Unless these amoebae are found in wet preparations of corneal ulcer scrapings, or in cerebrospinal fluid, the diagnosis of the diverse pathology caused by these organisms will be based upon histology. Even if histological material is examined, the organisms can easily be missed unless special strains, such as iron haematoxylin are used. As with *Naegleria* the most important diagnostic characteristic of these amoebae is the large central endosome. Indirect immunofluorescence, using specific antisera, can also be used to locate the amoebae in the tissue. Cultural diagnosis can be made from fresh biopsy material in the same manner as for *Naegleria*. Present evidence from cultures and fluorescent staining suggests that most human infections are caused by *A. culbertsoni*, although corneal lesions are usually due to *A. polyphaga*. Unlike both *E. histolytica* and *Naegleria*, *Acanthamoeba* trophozoites do sometimes encyst in human tissues. Serodiagnosis may be of some help in the diagnosis of these conditions but some normal persons show antibody to *Acanthamoeba*, suggesting that mild and self-limiting infections can occur.

Since clinically evident infections occur mainly in predisposed persons, *Acanthamoeba* should be regarded as an opportunistic parasite as well as a facultative one.

Treatment. As for *Naegleria* infections, amphotericin B is the drug of choice. For corneal ulcers this drug need only be used locally. *In vitro* sulphonamides are active against *Acanthamoeba* and there is now clinical evidence to support their use, in conjunction with amphotericin.

References

Entamoeba histolytica infection

Adams, E. B. and MacLeod, I. N. (1977). Invasive amoebiasis. I. Amebic dysentery and its complications. II. Amebic liver abscess and its complications. *Medicine, Baltimore* **56**, 315, 325.

Barbour, G. L. and Juniper, K., Jr. (1972). A clinical comparison of amebic and pyogenic abscesses of the liver. *Am. J. Med.* **53**, 323.

Elsdon-Dew, R. (1968). The epidemiology of amoebiasis. *Adv. Parasit* **6**, 1.

Knight, R. (1980). The chemotherapy of amoebiasis. *J. antimicrob. Chemother.* **6**, 630.

Krogstad, D. J., Spencer, H. C., Healy, G. R., Gleason, N. N., Sexton, D. J., and Herron, C. A. (1978). Amebiasis: Epidemiologic studies in the United States, 1971–1974. *Ann. intern. Med.* **88**, 89.

Robinson, G. L. (1968). Laboratory diagnosis of human parasitic amoebae. *Trans. R. Soc. trop. Med. Hyg.* **62**, 285.

Wilmot, A. J. (1962). *Clinical amoebiasis*. Blackwell Scientific Publications, Oxford.

World Health Organization (1969). Report of a WHO Expert Committee. *Tech. Rep. Ser. Wld Hlth Org.* **421**, 1.

Naegleria and *Acanthamoeba* infections

Carter, R. F. (1972). Primary amoebic meningo-encephalitis. *Trans. R. Soc. trop. Med. Hyg.* **66**, 193.

Culbertson, C. G. (1971). Pathogenic soil amoebae. *Ann. Rev. Microbiol.* **25**, 231.

Griffin, J. L. (1978). Infections with pathogenic soil amoebae. In *Parasitic Protozoa*, vol. 2, (ed. J. P. Kreier), 507.

Symmers, W. St. C. (1969). *Br. med. J.* **iv**. 449.

Malaria

L. H. Miller

Malaria is caused by four species of *Plasmodium*, *P. falciparum*, *P. vivax*, *P. ovale*, and *P. malariae*, each with its own morphology, biology, and clinical characteristics (Table 1). Of the four, *P. falciparum* causes the most morbidity and mortality and presents the therapeutic problem of chloroquine resistance. Accordingly, early diagnosis and treatment are essential, and require immediate and repeated examination of blood films in any febrile patient who has travelled in countries endemic for malaria or who has received a blood transfusion.

The infection can be divided into three phases: (*a*) an asymptomatic period following the inoculation of sporozoites and their development within hepatic parenchymal cells, (*b*) the asexual erythrocytic cycle which causes the disease, and (*c*) the gametocytes, sexual erythrocytic parasites, which are infectious to Anopheline mosquitoes but cause no disease.

Life cycle in man. Infection is initiated when female Anopheline mosquitoes inoculate sporozoites druing a blood meal. Sporozoites disappear from the circulation within one hour, and by unknown mechanisms enter liver parenchymal cells where they proliferate into thousands of individual merozoites. Development in liver cells requires about one week for *P. falciparum* and *P. vivax*, and two weeks for *P. malariae*. In *P. vivax* and *P. ovale* infections, some parasites (hypnozoites) remain dormant in liver cells for months to years before undergoing proliferation (see section on Relapses). Upon rupture of a liver cell containing a mature parasite, merozoites pour into the blood stream to invade red cells. This initiates the asexual erythrocytic phase of infection.

Development of the intra-erythrocytic parasite follows one of two pathways: asexual proliferation or differentiation into sexual parasites, the gametocytes. Asexual parasites divide into 6 to 24 merozoites, the number determined by the species of malaria. Merozoites, on release from infected red cells, attach to other red cells by specific receptors, form a junction between the anterior end of the merozoite and the red cell membrane, and move within a vacuole as the junction moves around the parasite. In the case of *P. vivax*, the receptor is associated with the Duffy blood group system.

Parasites proliferate until they are controlled or terminated by the host's immune response or antimalarial drugs. Throughout the asexual infection, some parasites differentiate into gametocytes that, after full maturation, await ingestion by the mosquito. *P. falciparum* gametocytes mature for nine days within the spleen and bone marrow, and then retun to the peripheral circulation as mature, crescent-shaped parasites where they may survive for two to three weeks. *P. vivax* gametocytes require about 36 hours for maturation. Mature gametocytes of *P. vivax* survive for not more than two to three days.

P. falciparum infects red cells of all ages. The resultant high parasitaemia accounts for the high morbidity and mortality of falciparum malaria. *P. vivax* and *P. ovale* invade primarily reticulocytes; *P. malariae* is limited to older red cells. Because these three

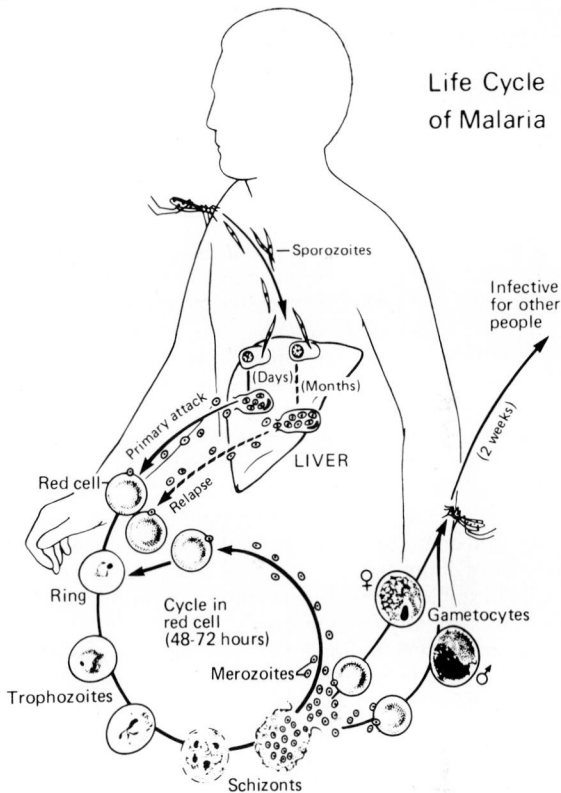

Fig. 1 Life cycle of malaria. (From Miller (1975). In *Transmissible disease and blood transfusion* (eds. Greenwalt and Jamieson), Grune and Stratton, New York, with permission.)

Table 1 Summary of clinical and diagnostic features

	P. falciparum	*P. vivax*	*P. ovale*	*P. malariae*
Clinical features	high parasitaemia, severe anaemia, renal failure, cerebral malaria, pulmonary oedema, death	anaemia, splenic rupture		RBC infection persists for years; nephritis
Chloroquine resistance	yes	no	no	no
Incubation period*	8–25 days (av. 12)	8–27 days (av 14)	9–17 days (av. 15)	15–30 days
Asexual cycle	48 hours	48 hours	48 hours	72 hours
Relapse†	no	yes	yes	no
Characteristic on thin	rings predominate; multiply-infected RBCs; rings with thread-like cytoplasm, double nuclei; banana-shaped gametocytes	enlarged RBC with Schüffner's dots; trophozoite cytoplasm amoeboid; 12 to 24 merozoites in mature schizont	oval RBC with fringed edges; Schüffer's dots; trophozoite cytoplasm compact 6–16 merozoites in mature schizont	trophozoite cytoplasm compact (band forms) 6–12 merozoites in mature schizont

* Incubation period: interval from mosquito bite until clinical symptoms (fever). Chemoprophylaxis may suppress initial attack of *P. falciparum* for months and of *P. vivax* and *P. ovale* for months to years.

† Relapse: recurrent red cell infection derived from latent parasites in liver parenchymal cells after a mosquito-induced infection.

malarias are limited to a subpopulation of red cells, they rarely reach high parasitaemia and usually do not cause serious disease or death.

Each malaria induces characteristic ultrastructural changes on the infected red cell membrane. As *P. falciparum* asexual parasites mature, knobs, 100 nm in diameter, appear on the red cell membrane and are the points of attachment of falciparum-infected red cells to venular endothelium. Thus young falciparum parasites, ring forms, predominate in the peripheral blood; red cells with more mature parasites sequester along venules. Malarial antigens localized over these knobs may be recognized by the immune system. During pregnancy, red cells containing mature parasites concentrate in the villous spaces of the placenta. Multiple vesicles form around membrane invaginations on *P. vivax-* and *P. ovale*-infected red cells and appear as eosinophilic stippling over infected red cells on Giemsa-stained blood films (Schüffner's dots).

Epidemiology. Most malaria patients seen in Europe and the United States are infected in countries in Africa, Asia, and Latin America. Programmes for eradication of malaria in these tropical countries have mostly failed, although the mortality from malaria in countries such as India has been greatly reduced. The presently available methods that include lavriciding, spraying houses with residual insecticides, and antimalarial drug treatment of patients can only reduce transmission and therefore must be applied indefinitely. These methods are expensive, administratively demanding, and become less effective each years as drug and insecticide resistance becomes more widespread. New tools are being sought, such as biological control of mosquitoes and vaccination, but these methods are at present a dream for the future.

Characteristics of the vector mosquito, environmental conditions, and man's habits determine the endemicity of malaria. In sub-Sahara Africa where some members of the *Anopheles gambiae* complex feed primarily on man, the people are infected repeatedly every year and immunity develops until those over five years of age have disease of diminished severity. Malaria under these conditions is considered stable since epidemics do not occur. However, young children suffer greatly from malaria.

In other areas, such as South Asia, epidemics occur when there are unusual climactic conditions which markedly increase the vector populations. The peoples in these regions are relatively non-immune during periods between epidemics.

Since complete development of the parasite in the mosquito cannot occur at low temperatures, transmission of malaria rarely happens above 2200 m.

Vector capacity and host factors determine the distribution of malarial species. *P. falciparum* predominates in Africa, Haiti, and New Guinea. *P. vivax* occurs more frequently than *P. falciparum* in South Asia and Central America. *P. falciparum* and *P. vivax* are both prevalent in Asia, South America, and Oceania. *P. ovale* largely replaces *P. vivax* in Africa, as black Africans lack red cell receptors for *P. vivax* and are thus resistant to this species. *P. malariae* occurs throughout the tropical world.

Mosquito vectors capable of transmitting malaria still exist in countries where malaria has been eradicated (e.g., *Anopheles freeborni* in the western United States). In these areas, episodes of transmission have occurred following infection of local mosquitoes by individuals infected in the tropics. Other causes of infection in non-endemic areas include blood transfusion, communal use of syringes by drug addicts, and congenital infection. The single most important factor in preventing transfusion malaria is the development of rules for blood donor selection that are practical and easily understood by blood bank personnel. Since infections in donors are usually asymptomatic, donors who have lived or travelled in endemic areas must be excluded until their risk of infection is negligible. Most falciparum-infected individuals undergo self-cure in three years. *P. vivax* and *P. ovale* may persist for three to five years. *P. malariae* may persist as an asymptomatic, erythrocytic infection for decades, although infection with this parasite is rarely serious.

Host resistance factors. Host resistance to malaria results from innate (genetically determined) characteristics and immunity. The immune response to malaria may be controlled in part by immune response genes.

Innate resistance to malaria. Sickle-cell trait reduces the level of *P. falciparum* parasitaemia and in this way markedly decreases the morbidity and mortality from falciparum malaria. It has no effect on the prevalence of the infection in the population. *P. falciparum* in sickle cell trait red cells grows poorly *in vitro* under conditions of low O_2 tension because K^+ loss from the red cell leads to parasite death. Consequently, reduced parasitaemia probably results from adherence of *P. falciparum*-infected red cells to venous endothelium, an anoxic environment. Because children with SA haemoglobin have a survival advantage in falciparum endemic areas over either homozygote (SS or AA), the frequency of genes for S and A haemoglobin reaches a fixed level called balanced polymorphism.

Other genetically determined red cell abnormalities, glucose 6-phosphate dehydrogenase (G6PD) deficiency and thalassaemia, occur frequently in regions of the world endemic for falciparum malaria. Proof that these characteristics reduce severity of *P. falciparum* is lacking. Resistance to malaria may require another environmental factor such as the interaction of favism and G6PD deficiency, since oxidant stress reduces the survival of the parasite in culture in G6PD-deficient red cells. Oxidant stress also reduces the growth of *P. falciparum* in thalassaemia red cells in culture. Vitamin E protects the parasite from oxidant stress in B-thalassaemia red cells. Histocompatibility and immune response genes also may affect survival.

Unlike the sickle-cell trait that reduces the severity of falciparum malaria, many black Africans are completely refractory to *P. vivax*, although they are susceptible to the other three species of malaria. The vivax resistance factor is a blood group determinant, the Duffy negative genotype *FyFy*. All other populations in the world are either *Fy*a or *Fy*b and are susceptible to infection by *P. vivax*. A Duffy blood group associated determinant is probably involved in attachment between vivax merozoites and red cells, an early step in the internalization of the parasite within the red cell.

Immunity in malaria. Immunity to sporozoites and asexual erythrocytic parasites is species-specific. For example, immunity to *P. falciparum* does not protect against infection with *P. vivax*. Immunity to asexual erythrocytic parasites of *P. falciparum* is also strain-specific. Immunity develops only after prolonged or repeated infection. The mechanism by which the parasite has evolved to evade immune response is poorly understood and may involve antigenic variation and immune suppression. Immunity is predominantly directed against asexual erythrocytic parasites. The effector mechanisms may kill intra-erythrocytic parasites in immunologically specific and non-specific ways or block merozoite invasion of red cells by antibodies. The spleen is of primary importance in host survival; thus, splenectomy puts the individual at grave risk from subsequent malarial infections. The passive transfer of IgG from immune adults markedly reduces *P. falciparum* parasitaemia in non-immune children, although the site of action for this immune IgG is unknown.

Pathogenesis. The symptoms and pathology are a direct result of the asexual erythrocytic cycle. The disease can be classified into: (*a*) general symptoms including fever, (*b*) anaemia, (*c*) reduced blood flow to tissues, and (*d*) immunopathology.

Fever and the associated symptoms of headache, nausea, and muscular pain occur at the time that schizont-infected red cells (the mature parasites) rupture and release merozoites invasive to other red cells. Although it is presumed that pyrogens and other toxins are released from the ruptured schizont, none have been identified to date. Fever develops at lower parasitaemia in the non-immune than in the partially immune patient.

Intravascular haemolysis of infected red cells causes the anaemia of malaria. However, in studies on experimental animals, the anaemia usually exceeds that explained by parasitaemia alone. The mechanisms of this excessive anaemia are unknown. Coombs-positive haemolytic anaemia rarely occurs and usually results from quinine sensitivity.

Tissue hypoxia and organ damage (renal failure and cerebral malaria) develop in patients who are heavily infected with *P. falciparum*. Malaria is one of many diseases that cause acute renal insufficiency. The mechanisms include severe haemolytic anaemia, haemoglobinuria, hypovolaemia, and possibly splanchnic vasoconstriction. Pathologic findings in the kidney are often minimal.

The pathology of the diffuse cerebral disease is unique to malaria. Parasitized red cells obstruct cerebral capillaries, the brain becomes oedematous, and ring haemorrhages develop around obstructed capillaries. Schizont-infected red cells which sequester along venular endothelium at low parasitaemia are found in the peripheral blood of heavily infected patients and become trapped in capillaries of the brain and other organs. The decreased deformability of infected red cells and their tendency to adhere to vascular endothelium probably causes the plugging of capillaries by these cells.

P. malariae infection in some children produces chronic progressive nephritis. Immune complexes deposit in the glomerular capillary walls. The antibody in the complexes is specific for *P. malariae*. The majority contain the C3 component of complement and 25 per cent have *P. malariae* antigen. The reasons only *P. malariae* initiates this kidney disease and only a small percentage of the infected children develop the disease are unknown.

Clinical features

The acute attack. Symptoms are caused only by asexual infection of red cells. Sporozoites from the mosquito, parasites in liver cells, and gametocytes, sexual stages within red cells, produce no symptoms or disease. The parasitaemia (concentration of asexual parasites in red cells), at which symptoms occur, differs from patient to patient. Semi-immune patients generally develop higher parasitaemia than non-immune patients before symptoms occur.

The incubation period, the time from mosquito infection to the first symptoms, is about 10 to 16 days. The incubation period is longest for *P. malariae*. Drug prophylaxis may suppress the initial attack of *P. falciparum* for weeks to months and of relapsing malarias (*P. vivax* and *P. ovale*) for months to years.

No sign or symptom is pathognomonic of malaria. Since delay in treatment of *P. falciparum* increases mortality, the diagnosis should be considered in any febrile patient who has travelled in an endemic area or who has received a blood transfusion. Fever is not always associated with paroxysms and is usually not periodic, especially in malignant falciparum malaria and during the initial attack of *P. vivax*.

Characteristic malaria paroxysms have three stages: cold stage (rigor, chill), hot stage (high fever), and sweating stage (defervescence). The paroxysm begins with a chilly feeling, bedshaking chills, and a rise in temperature (cold stage). Ths skin appears pale with cyanosis of the lips and nail-beds. The patient experiences headache, nausea, and may vomit. Within one to two hours, the temperature rises towards 39–40.5 °C, the patient feels hot, and his skin is warm and dry (hot stage). As the temperature falls, sweating begins and drenches the clothes. The patient feels fatigued and weak and often sleeps. This description is most typical of benign malarias; fever may persist and symptoms are prolonged in malignant falciparum malaria.

Fever results from schizont rupture and release of unidentified pyrogens. Periodicity of fever or paroxysms occurs only in synchronized infections when the majority of infected red cells contain mature schizonts and rupture at the same time. This occurs at intervals determined by the length of the asexual erythrocytic cycle. The cycle in *P. vivax* and *P. ovale* takes 48 hours and thus the paroxysms occur every other day. *P. malariae* matures in 72 hours and causes paroxysms every third day. Broods of parasitized red

cells may rupture daily in any species of malaria and cause daily fever. Irregular fever, as is often the case in malaria, reflects an asynchronous infection.

The pulse is rapid but not commensurate with the fever. A non-productive cough during fever may occur. Orthostatic hypotension is common in falciparum malaria and weakness may persist for weeks. Splenomegaly occurs frequently and hepatomegaly less frequently. Tenderness on palpation of liver and spleen may be due to sudden stretching of their capsules. The absence of hepatosplenomegaly does not exclude the diagnosis of malaria. Labial herpes are often present. Rashes and lympadenopathy are uncommon and point to diagnoses other than malaria.

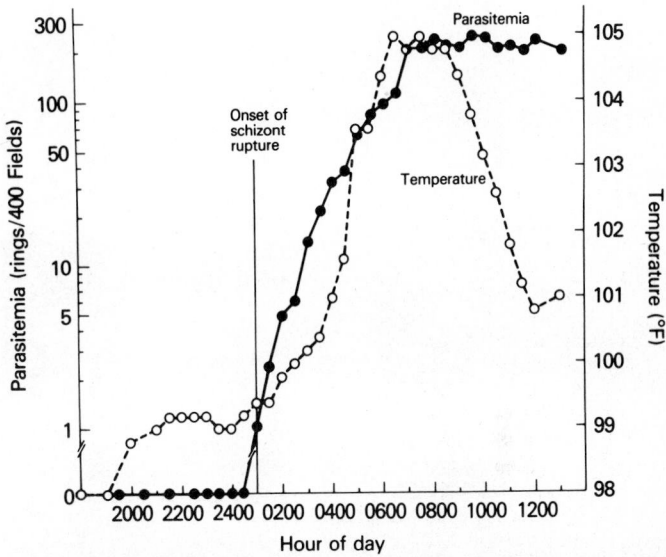

Fig. 2   Relation between schizont rupture (appearance of rings in red cells) and fever. (From Miller (1975). In *Transmissible disease and blood transfusion* (eds. Greenwalt and Jamieson), Grune and Stratton, New York, with permission.)

Abnormalities in routine laboratory tests in uncomplicated malaria include normochromia, normocytic anaemia, leucopenia due to a decrease in granulocytes and lymphocytes, thrombocytopenia, and minimal albuminuria. Biologic false positive VDRL may occur.

Complications of malaria. *P. falciparum*. High parasitaemia in *P. falciparum* accounts for the severe morbidity and mortality. When parasitaemia rises above 100 000 infected red cells per mm³ and the haematocrit falls below 30 per cent, the patient is at grave risk. Hyponatraemia, one of the complications in seriously ill patients, is caused by salt depletion and water retention. Disseminated intravascular coagulation may occur, but its role in pathogenesis has not been established. A rare and serious complication of falciparum malaria, algid malaria, is caused by increased capillary permeability leading to hypovolaemic shock.

Severe haemolytic anaemia is usually associated with high parasitaemia and may result in haemoglobinuria. Erythrophagocytosis by the reticulo-endothelial system is common. Few instances of Coombs-positive haemolytic anaemia have occurred. In the past when quinine was administered repeatedly for malarial suppression, quinine allergic haemolytic anaemia occurred. Drugs in patients with G6PD deficiency may cause severe haemolysis.

Acute renal insufficiency is usually associated with high parasitaemia, severe a haemolysis, and haemoglobinuria (blackwater fever). Haemolysis from quinine sensitivity may also cause blackwater fever. Renal failure may occur in the absence of severe haemolysis and may be associated with hypovolaemia. It may occur with normal urine volume. Azotaemia may not indicate renal failure but may reflect an increased catabolic rate.

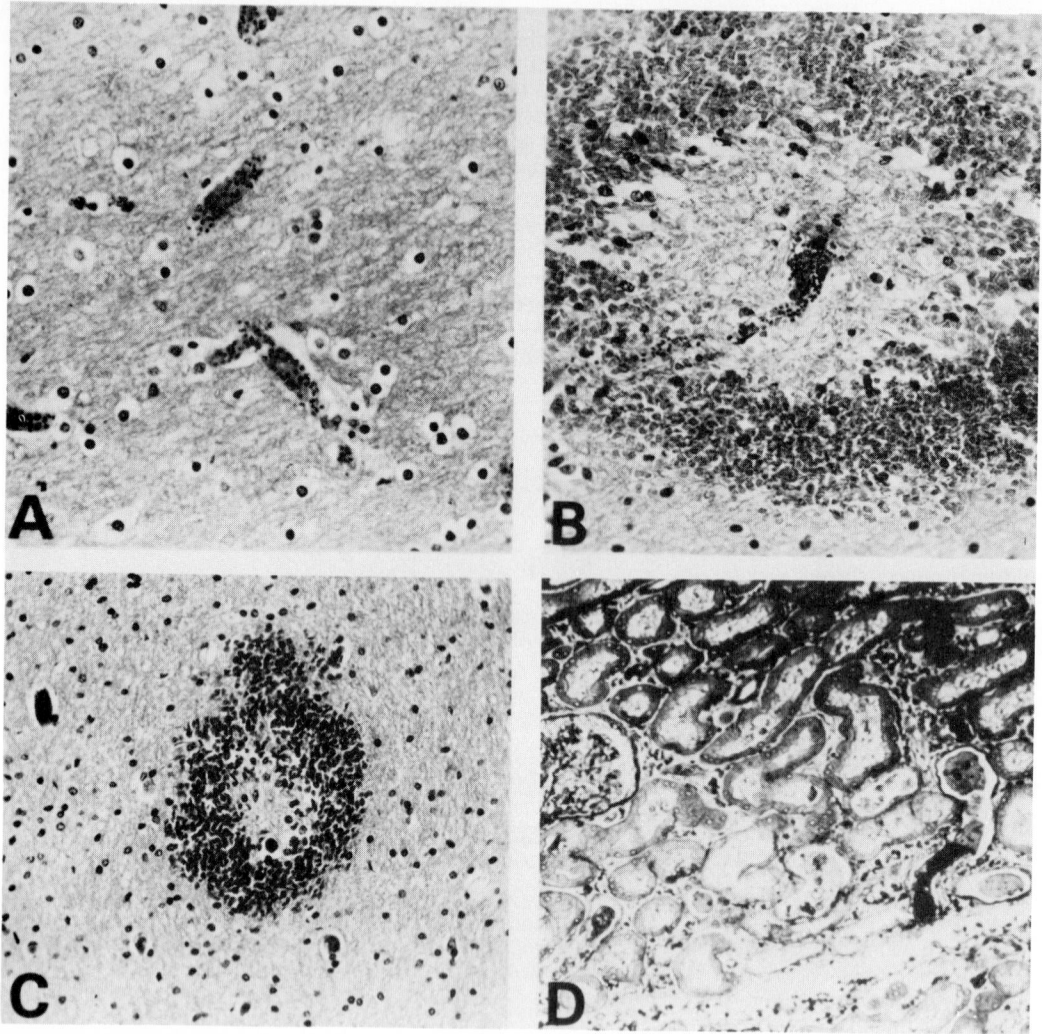

Fig. 3 Complications of falciparum malaria. (A) Cerebral malaria showing cerebral vessels obstructed by parasitized red cells. (From Armed Forces Institute of Pathology (AFIP), Washington, DC, AFIP 66–7680, with permission.) (B) Cerebral malaria showing ring haemorrhage surrounding a vessel obstructed with parasitized red cells. (From AFIP 66–6871, with permission.) (C) Cerebral malaria showing a ring haemorrhage. (From AFIP 66–7191, with permission.) (D) Renal failure. (From C. Canfield, Walter Reed Army Institute of Research, Washington, DC, with permission.)

Cerebral malaria presents as disturbances in consciousness ranging from somnolence to coma, psychosis, and major motor seizures which in young children are impossible to distinguish from febrile seizures. Neurological examination may reveal hyperreflexia and bilateral Babinski signs, but focal findings are uncommon. The findings in the cerebral spinal fluid include an elevated pressure and concentration of protein, rarely accompanied by pleocytosis. The cerebral capillaries are obstructed by *P. falciparum*-infected red cells because of their reduced deformability and tendency to adhere to vascular endothelium. Cerebral oedema, ring haemorrhages, and necrosis occur throughout the brain.

Greatly elevated bilirubin and transaminase occur rarely in association with centrilobular necrosis of the liver. Another unusual complication, pulmonary oedema, may be associated with fluid overload. The lungs have microvascular congestion, interstitual oedema, and hyaline membrane formation.

P. vivax. Moderate anaemia may result from a chronic, undiagnosed infection. Splenic rupture, a rare and serious complication, occurs most commonly from *P. vivax* infections.

P. malariae. Chronic infection with *P. malariae* in children may produce progressive nephritis which responds poorly to treatment.

Diseases associated with falciparum malaria. *Tropical splenomegaly syndrome*. Patients living in endemic regions of Africa and New Guinea develop massive splenic enlargement and hepatic sinusoidal lymphocytic infiltrates. They respond to chronic antimalarial chemoprophylaxis with decrease in spleen size and reversal of liver pathology. Splenectomy is generally contra-indicated as it exposes these patients to the risk of severe malaria.

Burkitt's lymphoma. This tumour occurs in areas of Africa hyperendemic for *P. falciparum* and is believed to be an atypical response to Epstein–Barr virus infection.

Asymptomatic infection, recrudescence, and relapse. Partial therapy or immunity reduces parasitaemia and symptoms may disappear. Despite persistent erythrocytic infection during these asymptomatic periods, parasites are difficult to locate on blood films. Periodic rises in parasitaemia causes recurrent clinical attacks (recrudescence). The total duration of erythrocytic infection varies for each malaria. Most falciparum infections are eliminated in one year; a few persist for up to three years. *P. malariae* may persist as an asymptomatic infection for the life of the patient. How *P. malariae* evades the immune response for years while infecting new red cells every 72 hours remains a mystery. Ths asymptomatic erythrocytic infection poses two potential risks to others. Firstly, donated blood induces malaria in the recipient. Secondly, the asymptomatic patient can infect vector mosquitoes.

Relapse differs from recrudescence in that the parasite that induces the relapse originates from the hepatic parenchymal cells rather than from red cells. Some sporozoites inoculated by mosquitoes fail to develop after entering hepatic parenchymal cells but remain as small, dormant parasites with a single nuclei called hypnozoites. The recurrent attacks (relapses) occur when these latent parasites (hypnozoites) begin to divide within liver cells months to years after the original bite of the infected mosquito. The mature parasites then rupture into the circulation and invade red cells. Subsequent multiplication within red cells causes the clinical attack. Relapses occur only in *P. vivax* and *P. ovale*. Different strains of *P. vivax* have their own characteristic patterns of relapse. Some strains (e. g., from New Guinea) relapse monthly after the primary attack. Others relapse six months or longer after the primary attack or may not have a primary attack. Drugs that cure the latent infection in the liver differ from those that destroy asexual erythrocytic parasites (see Treatment section). Relapses never occur from a blood-induced infection (e.g., transfusion malaria) as the asexual erythrocytic parasite cannot infect liver parenchymal cells.

Diagnosis. The definitive diagnosis is made from examination of blood films in the laboratory. Because malaria parasites may be overlooked in the course of a routine differential count, the clinician must specifically request thick and thin blood films in a febrile patient who has travelled in the tropics or who has recently received a blood transfusion. Blood examinations should be obtained immediately and repeated at 6–12 hour intervals as the number of parasites may fluctuate throughout the day. Symptoms may precede detectable parasitaemia by a few days during the initial attack. Although young parasites (rings) appear in the circulation during the paroxysm as schizonts rupture and release merozoites, the clinician should not wait for a paroxysm to obtain a slide, since delay in diagnosis and treatment of *P. falciparum* increases the risk to the patient. If malaria is strongly suspected on clinical grounds in a patient with repeatedly negative smears, a therapeutic trial may be instituted.

Well-prepared and properly stained thick and thin blood films simplify diagnosis. A cleaned slide should be labelled with the patient's name, the date, and time. For the thick film, one drop of blood at one end of the slide should be evenly spread in a circular motion to a diameter of 1 cm with the edge of another slide. A second drop of blood should be spread on the slide for the thin film as for routine blood cell examination. After the blood films are dry, the thick film should be lysed in water and the thin film should be fixed with absolute methanol. Both should be stained with Giemsa at pH 7.0–7.2.

Once malaria parasites are identified on the blood film, the most important distinction is whether the patient has *P. falciparum*, as this will influence treatment. All other malarial species are initially treated with chloroquine. Criteria suggestive of *P. falciparum* include predominant small ring forms, double nuclei, multiple infection, appliqué form, and the diagnostic crescent-shaped gametocytes. There is no enlargement or pink stippling (Schüffner's dots) of the infected red cells. Except at high parasitaemia, trophozoites and schizonts are rarely seen, as they adhere to venular endothelium. If more than 5 per cent of the red cells are infected, *P. falciparum* should be suspected.

Artefacts such as platelets on red cells, precipitated stain, and dirt may be confused with malarial parasites. *Babesia* spp. in red cells resemble *P. falciparum* rings but can be differentiated by an experienced microscopist.

Serologic tests have no place in the diagnosis of the acutely ill patient. The indirect fluorescent antibody test is useful in identifying infected donors in cases of transfusion malaria.

Treatment

P. falciparum. Prompt diagnosis and early treatment are essential. Delay in chemotherapy increases morbidity and mortality. All patients should be placed in a hospital and treated as medical emergencies. Patients who appear stable on admission may deteriorate rapidly.

The decision on drug regimen will depend on the origin of the infection, for chloroquine resistance occurs in certain regions of the world. Drug resistance is divided into three types: RI, disappearance of parasites on blood films and clinical recovery followed by recrudescence weeks later; RII, reduction in parasitaemia and clinical symptoms followed by a rise in parasitaemia; and RIII, no response to therapy. Since treatment failure may occur with any drug regimen, the course of parasitaemia must be followed at

12-hour intervals. Failure to reduce parasitaemia in the first 24–48 hours of treatment should raise the possibilty of parasite resistance to that treatment. No asexual parasites should be detectable on smears four to five days after completing a course of chloroquine; persistence after the fifth day indicates drug failure. A simple method for estimating parasitaemia from the thin blood film is as follows: at low parasite densities, the number of infected red cells in 25 oil emersion fields is counted; at high parasite densities, the number of infected red cells per 500 red cells is counted. Gametocytes may persist in the blood for weeks after asexual forms have been successfully eliminated. Gametocytes do not cause disease and their presence does not indicate treatment failure.

RI-resistant parasites recrudesce up to two months after treatment in the non-immune. The patient should be warned that any febrile episode weeks to months after treatment may indicate drug failure and he should return for evaluation.

Chloroquine resistance is widespread. It extends from India through Asia to New Guinea and from Panama to South America (Table 2). Although a few cases of RI resistance have been reported from East Africa, *P. falciparum* from Africa should generally be treated with chloroquine and the response followed closely. Because RI resistance to quinine (i.e., response followed by recrudescence) occurs in Southeast Asia and other areas, quinine is never used alone in treatment. Resistance to Fansidar, a fixed-drug combination of pyrimethamine and sulfadoxine, has been reported in Southeast Asia and South America.

Table 2 Worldwide distribution of chloroquine resistance of *P. falciparum*

Latin America	Africa	Asia
Brazil	East Africa	Bangladesh
Colombia		Burma
Ecuador		India
Guyana		Indonesia
Panama		Kampuchea
Surinam		Laos
Venezuela		Malaysia
		New Guinea
		Philippines
		Thailand
		Vietnam

Symptomatic and supportive measures. As in other infectious diseases, symptomatic and supportive measures should be instituted as indicated. Headaches, muscular pain, and other symptoms of malaria associated with high fever can be ameliorated by lowering the temperature below 38.9 °C. Treatment includes acetaminophen, sponging with tepid water, and fanning to increase evaporation. Orthostatic hypotension, usually observed early in infection, is an indication for complete bed rest. The patient may not recover full strength for weeks after completion of therapy.

Patients should be observed closely for complications that include severe haemolytic anaemia, renal failure, fluid imbalance, and pulmonary oedema. Packed red cells or whole blood should be infused slowly in severe anaemia. Platelet transfusion are generally not indicated for thrombocytopenia, as the platelets rapidly return towards normal during specific chemotherapy. Renal failure may progress rapidly because of the high catabolic rate and is an indication for early haemodialysis. Administration of excessive fluids may aggravate cerebral symptoms or precipitate pulmonary oedema. Pulmonary oedema is usually not associated with a rise in central venous pressure during intravenous fluid administration and often results in death despite treatment.

Although splenic tenderness is common in acute malaria, evidence of peritoneal and diaphragmatic irritation may indicate splenic rupture. This life-threatening complication is more common in *P. vivax*.

Treatment of chloroquine-sensitive P. falciparum. Chloroquine-sensitive strains occur in Western Asia, Africa, and Central America (except Panama). These patients should be treated with chloroquine or amodiaquine. The recommended oral dosage regimens for adults are either chloroquine phosphate, 1000 mg initially, 500 mg six hours later, and 500 mg on each of two succeeding days; or amodiaquine hydrochloride, 780 mg initially and 520 mg on each of the two succeeding days.

Because of the possibility of chloroquine resistance, the parasitaemia should be followed closely during treatment (see above) and alternative drugs instituted if indicated. Fever occurring weeks after therapy may indicate a recrudescence.

Treatment of chloroquine-resistant P. falciparum. Patients who have acquired *P. falciparum* malaria in an area of known chloroquine resistance (Asia east of Pakistan, South America, and Panama) or who have transfusion falciparum malaria (source of infection unknown) should not be given a course of chloroquine or amodiaquine. The drug regimen combines three drugs: quinine sulphate, 650 mg every eight hours for ten days; pyrimethamine, 25 mg twice daily for three days; and a sulphonamide (sulphisoxazole or sulphadiazine), 0.5 g every six hours for five days. Occasionally, after treatment with this regimen, the patient may suffer a subsequent recrudescence. Treatment failures should be treated with the following regimen: quinine sulphate, 650 mg every eight hours for three days, plus tetracycline hydrochloride, 250 mg every six hours for ten days.

If quinine is not immediately available, treatment should be instituted with a sulphonamide plus pyrimethamine and quinine added when available.

Cinchonism (nausea, vomiting, tinnitus, and vertigo) commonly results from treatment with quinine and is not an indication to alter or discontinue therapy. A rare complication of quinine therapy, Coombs-positive haemolytic anaemia, is an indication for immediate withdrawal of the drug.

Mefloquine, a new antimalarial drug developed by the Walter Reed Army Institute of Research, is highly effective against chloroquine-resistant *P. falciparum*. As more data becomes available on its relative safety, it may become the treatment of choice for *P. falciparum*.

Treatment of severe and complicated malaria. Patients with *P. falciparum* who have parasitaemia greater than 100 000 per mm³, marked anaemia, cerebral complications, or are vomiting repeatedly should be treated with intravenous quinine dihydrochloride. Quinine dihydrochloride, 600 mg dissolved in 250 ml of 5 per cent dextrose water, should be infused slowly over eight hours. This should be repeated every eight hours until oral medication is tolerated. Since quinine is excreted by the kidneys and metabolized by the liver, the dosage in patients with renal failure and hepatic disease should be decreased by at least half.

Cerebral malaria is considered by some physicians as an indication for glucosteroids. In a double-blind trial, however, dexamethasone was deleterious in cerebral malaria and should no longer be used. Heparin is contra-indicated even in patients with disseminated intravascular coagulation because of the risk of haemorrhage.

P. vivax, P. ovale, and P. malariae. Acute attacks with any of these species should be treated with chloroquine or amodiaquine (see regimen under Treatment of chloroquine-sensitive *P. falciparum*).

P. vivax and *P. ovale* infections acquired by mosquito bites may have persistent hepatic forms and these must be eliminated to prevent relapses. After completion of chloroquine treatment, primaquine phosphate, 26.6 mg daily for 14 days, is administered. Primaquine causes haemolysis in patients with G6PD deficiency. Patients who have a mild G6PD deficiency may be treated under close supervision as the haemolysis is self-limited. Severe G6PD deficiency is a contra-indication to the use of primaquine, each relapse requiring retreatment with cloroquine. Primaquine is not indicated in the treatment of transfusion malaria because erythrocytic parasites of blood-induced infections do not infect the liver.

Site of action of antimalarial drugs. Of all the drugs used against malaria, only the sites of action of pyrimethamine and sulphonamide are known. Pyrimethamine has a greater affinity for parasite than host dihydrofolate reductase and blocks folate metabolism. Sulphonamides block utilization of para-aminobenzoic acid (PABA). It has been suggested that chloroquine interferes with enzymatic digestion in the parasite's food vacuole. Red cells containing chloroquine-resistant *P. falciparum* take up less chloroquine than red cells containing sensitive strains.

Prevention. While physicians will seldom see malaria patients, they will frequently be asked for advice by travellers to endemic areas. Because of chloroquine-resistant *P. falciparum* in many areas of the world (see Table 2), an ideal chemoprophylaxis is no longer available. Therefore the patient should be warned that fever during or following travel in endemic areas may be caused by malaria, even though the patient was on drug suppression. If mefloquine, an experimental drug, proves safe for prolonged administration, it may become the replacement for chloroquine in areas of chloroquine resistance.

Prevention of malaria can usually be accomplished in adults by the ingestion of chloroquine phosphate, 500 mg once weekly, or amodiaquine hydrochloride, 520 mg once weekly. The drug should be continued for six weeks after leaving an endemic area. Travellers who were heavily exposed to malaria and are not G6PD deficient should receive primaquine, 26.6 mg daily for 14 days, on return from an endemic area to eliminate hepatic forms of *P. vivax* and *P. ovale*.

Fansidar, each tablet of which contains pyrimethamine, 25 mg, and the long-acting sulphonamide sulphadoxine, 500 mg, is effective for prevention of chloroquine-resistant *P. falciparum*, although Fansidar resistance occurs in Southeast Asia. The dose is one tablet weekly. Long-acting sulphonamides, but not sulphadoxine, have been rarely associated with Stevens–Johnson syndrome.

In addition to drug prophylaxis, the traveller should be advised to prevent contact with night-biting Anophelines. The traveller should use netting over the bed, insecticides, and mosquito repellents such as *Off* (*N,N*-diethyltolnamide).

Chemoprophylaxis in pregnancy. Drugs in pregnancy always present a potential risk to the fetus, especially for prolonged use as in chemoprophylaxis. Chloroquine is considered generally safe when used at the recommended dosage. Chemoprophlyaxis in areas of chloroquine-resistant *P. falciparum* presents a more difficult problem. Fansidar, the drug of choice, contains pyrimethamine which produced teratogenicity in some animal experiments. Although there are no documented cases of fetal abnormality during human pregnancy, a low frequency of congenital defects could have been missed. Therefore the physician and patient must decide on the best course: delay travel until after pregnancy, use of chloroquine which has the risk of breakthrough of resistant *P. falciparum*, or use of Fansidar which poses a potential, although not documented, risk to the fetus.

Acute malaria because of its risk to mother and child should be treated according to the regimens outlined above (see Therapy). Primaquine should not be used during pregnancy for the treatment or prevention of relapsing malarias (*P. vivax* and *P. ovale*).

References

Boyd, M. F. (ed.) (1949). *Malariology*. W. B. Saunders, Philadelphia.
Center for Disease Control (1978). Chemoprophylaxis of malaria. *Morbidity and Mortality Weekly Report* **27**, 81.
Friedman, M. J. (1979). Oxidant damage mediates variant red cell resistance to malaria. *Nature* **280**, 245.
Garnham, P. C. C., (ed.) (1966). *Malaria parasites and other haemosporidia*. Blackwell Scientific Publications, Oxford.
Miller, L. H. (1977). Current prospects and problems for a malaria vaccine. *J. infect. Dis.* **135**, 855.
Spitz, S. (1946). The pathology of acute falciparum malaria. *Milit. Surg.* **99**, 555.

World Health Organization (1969). Parasitology of malaria. *Wld Hlth Org. Tech. Rep. Ser.* no. 433.
— (1973) Chemotherapy of Malaria and resistance to antimalerials. *Wld Hlth Org. Tech. Rep. Ser.* no. 529.
— (1975) Developments in malaria immunology. *Wld Hlth Org. Tech. Rep. Ser.* no. 579.
Wyler, D. J. and Miller, L. H. (1979). Malaria. In *Principles and practices of infectious diseases* (eds. G. L. Mandell, R. G. Douglas, and J. E. Bennett), chapter 223. Wiley, New York.

Pneumocystis carinii

W. T. Hughes

The disease caused by *Pneumocystis carinii* is currently recognized solely as an extensive pneumonitis occurring almost exclusively in the immunosuppressed, immunodeficient, or otherwise compromised host (see page 5.481). A unique feature of the infection is that, with rare exceptions, both the disease and the organism remain localized to the lungs, even in fatal cases in severely immunosuppressed individuals. Furthermore, 'latent' *P. carinii* organisms have been identified in the lungs of a large variety of healthy lower animal species, as well as man, with no evidence of disease.

Aetiology. While the taxonomy of *P. carinii* has not been clearly defined, its tinctorial and morphological characteristics have been precisely described. Three forms of the organism can be identified in infected lungs. The cyst is a rounded or slightly pleomorphic structure measuring about 4–6 µm in diameter. Smaller cells within the cyst are termed sporozoites, which are 1–1.5 µm in diameter, and as many as eight may occupy a single cyst. The *trophozoite* is a thin-walled extracystic form, believed to represent the excysted sporozoite and varies from 1–5 µm in diameter.

P. carinii can be propagated *in vitro* in chick epithelial lung cells or Vero cells. However, the natural habitat and mode of transmission are unknown.

Host susceptibility. *P. carinii* pneumonitis was first recognized as interstitial plasma cell pneumonitis in European infants following the Second World War. Although studies were limited, the debilitated, premature, and under-nourished infants in maternity institutions were prime victims. Since then the disease has occurred in children and adults with malignancies, congenital immune deficiency disorders, and organ transplantation, and those receiving immunosuppressive therapy. The pneumonitis has occurred in patients with collagen-vascular disorders, aplastic anaemia, haemolytic anaemia, and thrombotic thrombocytopenic purpura. The infection can be provoked by severe protein energy malnutrition. It is reasonable to expect that any individual with impaired humoral or cell-mediated immunity or combined deficiencies is susceptible to *P. carinii* pneumonia. Although one method of immunosuppressive therapy has not been implicated to a greater extent than another, the intensity of the immunotherapy is clearly a determinant. For example, cancer patients receiving four immunosuppressive drugs have been found to have a much higher incidence of *P. carinii* pneumonitis than similar patients receiving only one of the drugs for maintenance chemotherapy.

Since about three-quarters of normal healthy individuals have humoral antibody to *P. carinii* by the age of four years, subclinical infection appears to be highly prevalent.

Pathology. *P. carinii* pneumonitis in immunocompromised adults and children is characterized by an extensive desquamative alveolitis. The organisms are clustered in the alveolar lumen, some in various stages of phagocytosis and digestion by alveolar macrophages and others not associated with host cells, but tending to localize along the septal wall. The 'foamy exudate' described in earlier studies actually represents unstained clusters of cysts and alveolar cells with cytoplasmic vacuoles, since *P. carinii* does not stain well with the standard haematoxylin and eosin stains. With severe infections inflammatory infiltrates may be prominent in the alveolar septae but the organisms are contained almost entirely in the lumen.

In the infantile form of the pneumonitis the alveolar lumens contain large numbers of organisms. However, a prominent feature in infants is an extensive interstitial plasma-cell infiltration which distends the alveolar walls from 5 to 20 times the normal thickness. Little fibrinous exudate is evident.

Only rarely has the organism been found outside the lung.

Clinical features. Tachypnoea is the most constant sign of *P. carinii* pneumonitis and the respiratory rate may exceed twice that of the normal. Cough is usually non-productive. Fever is almost always present in children, rarely present in infants, and present in about one-half of adults with the pneumonitis. Occasionally, coryza or diarrhoea may precede the pneumonitis. The illness progresses to pronounced dyspnoea with flaring of the nasal alae, intercostal retractions, and cyanosis. Although pneumonitis may be evident by X-ray at the onset of symptoms, signs and symptoms often precede radiographic densities by a day or so.

The chest X-ray typically reveals diffuse, bilateral alveolar disease. The infiltrate originates at the hilus and progresses peripherally, appearing granular with halo emphysema surrounding the non-aerated infiltrates. The apical portions of the lungs are usually spared until late in the course of the disease. Rarely, the infection may appear as lobar or solitary coin lesions.

The arterial oxygen tension (P_{AO_2}) is reduced, usually less than 80 mmHg while breathing room air. The arterial pH may be increased and the arterial carbon dioxide tension may be low or normal, indicating an uncompensated respiratory alkalosis.

The white blood cell count is not influenced in any consistent way by *P. carinii* pneumonitis. If the patient is undernourished, the serum albumin level may be below the range of normal.

Diagnosis. The identification of *P. carinii* in lung tissue is essential for a definitive diagnosis. The most dependable approach is to sample the lung with an open biopsy. The specimen obtained permits an appraisal of the histopathology and the extent of disease. Other invasive approaches include percutaneous transthoracic needle aspiration of the lung, cutting needle biopsy, trephine biopsy, transbronchial biopsy, and endobronchial brush biopsy techniques. Tracheal aspirates, sputum specimens, gastric aspirates, and hypopharyngeal secretions have on occasion yielded *P. carinii* organisms. However, these sources are not dependable and their use should not delay a more direct approach with an invasive procedure.

If a biopsy specimen is obtained touch imprints on to microscope slides should be done before the specimen is placed in the fixative. Imprints and sections should be prepared with Gomori's methenamine silver nitrate, toluidine blue O, and a polychrome stain, such as Giemsa, Gram–Weigert, or polychrome methylene blue. With the Gomori and toluidine blue O stains, the cyst wall is impregnated but the intracystic structures and small trophozoites are not stained. The cyst wall stains brownish-black with Gomori and lavender-blue with toluidine blue O stains (Fig. 1). The polychrome stains reveal the intracystic sporozoites and the eztracystic trophozoites but the cyst wall stains poorly, or not at all (Fig. 2). The cytoplasm stains blue and the nuclei reddish-blue. The organism is Gram-positive by the Gram–Weigert strain and cannot be identified with the haematoxylin and eosin stain.

Serological tests for antibody to *P. carinii* are not useful for diagnosis of the pneumonitis in adults and children, since by four years of age about 70 per cent of healthy individuals have antibody titres of 1:16 or greater. On the other hand, the complement fixation test has been helpful in the diagnosis of the infantile type in Europe. Unfortunately, the antigen preparations have not been standardized for either the complement fixation or the immunofluorescent test.

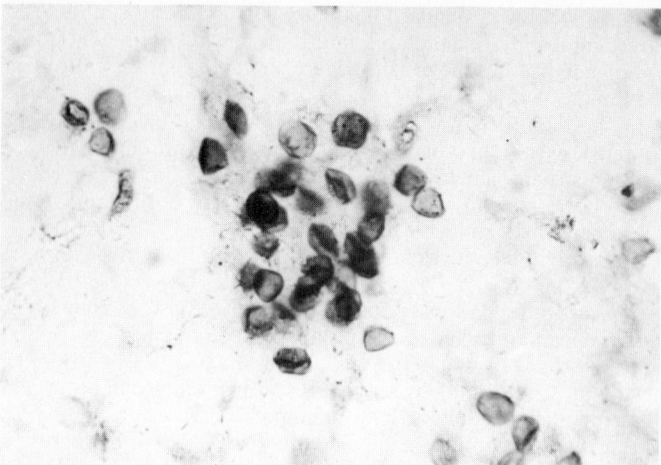

Fig. 1 *P. carinii* cysts stained with Gomori's methenamine silver nitrate stain. The cysts measure about 5 μm in diameter and appear as brownish-black cells against a green background.

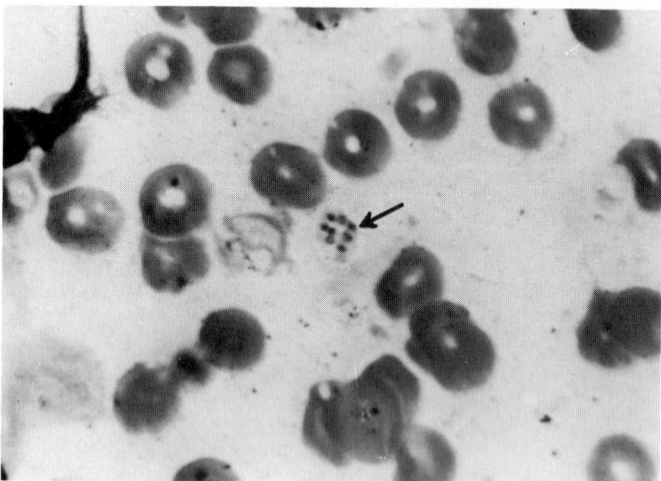

Fig. 2 *P. carinii* in lung aspirate prepared with Giemsa stain (arrow). The cyst wall does not stain. The sporozoites are intracystic and measure 1–2 μm in diameter. As many as eight sporozoites may occupy a single cyst. The red blood cells in the photomicrograph provide a comparison for perspective in size.

Treatment. Two antimicrobial agents are equally effective in the treatment of *P. carinii* pneumonitis. However, the adverse effects of trimethoprim–sulphamethoxazole (co-trimoxazole) are considerably less frequent and less severe than those incurred from pentamidine isethionate.

Trimethoprim–sulphamethoxazole is administered orally or intravenously in the dosage of 20 mg trimethoprim and 100 mg sulphamethoxazole per kg per day divided into four parts and given at six-hour intervals. Usually a course of 14 days is adequate. The dosage is larger than that recommended for bacterial infections. Although adult doses calculated on a body weight basis are considered adequate and safe, it is recommended that serum levels be monitored at intervals. The two-hour post-dosage serum levels should be from 3–5 μg/ml for trimethoprim and 100–150 μg/ml for sulphamethoxazole. The adverse effects are essentially those known to occur with sulphonamides.

Because of the high prevalence of untoward and toxic effects of pentamidine it must be considered a second choice to trimethoprim–sulphamethoxazole. The drug is administered intramuscularly as a single dosage of 4.0 mg/kg per day for 10 to 14 days. The total dosage should not exceed 56 mg/kg. It is advisable to filter the drug through a 0.22 μm pore size filter immediately before injection to ensure sterility in the immunosuppressed host. The adverse

effects include nephrotoxicity in 24 per cent, hepatotoxicity in 10 per cent, haematologic abnormalities in 4 per cent, injection site reactions in 18 per cent, hypoglycaemia in 6 per cent, hypotension in 10 per cent, rashes in 2 per cent, and hypocalcaemia in 1 per cent of the patients.

Most patients will require oxygen therapy to maintain the P_{AO_2} above 70 mmHg. The fraction of inspired oxygen (F_{IO_2}) should be kept below 50 volumes per cent, it at all possible, to avoid oxygen toxicity. In some cases assisted or controlled ventilation is required. This should be considered when an F_{IO_2} of 50 volumes per cent is inadequate to maintain the P_{AO_2} at 60 mmHg or greater. Efforts should be made to discontinue the use of immunosuppressive drugs if possible.

Prognosis. Untreated the fatality rate is near 100 per cent in children and adults with *P. carinii* pneumonitis. Treatment with either trimethoprim–sulphamethoxazole or pentamidine reduces the fatality rate to about 25 per cent. Of the patients who recover approximately 15 per cent are expected to have a second episode.

Prevention. The disease is preventable by the use of chemoprophylaxis with trimethoprim–sulphamethoxazole. Patients at unusually high risk for the pneumonitis should be maintained on 5.0 mg trimethoprim and 25 mg sulphamethoxazole per kg per day in two divided doses. The prophylaxis is dependable only so long as the drug is administered, since the organism is not completely eliminated even with therapeutic doses.

References

Burke, B. A. and Good, R. A. (1973). *Pneumocystis carinii* infection. *Medicine, Baltimore* **52**, 23.

Hughes, W. T. (1980). Pneumocystis pneumonia: a plague of the immunosuppressed. *Johns Hopkins med. J.* **143**, 184.

—, Feldman, S., Chaudhary, S. C., Ossi, M. J., Cox, F., and Sanyal, S. K. (1978). Comparison of pentamidine isethionate and trimethoprim-sulphamethoxazole in the treatment of *Pneumocystis carinii* pneumonia. *J. Pediat.* **92**, 285.

—, Kuhn, S., Chaudhary, S., Feldman, S., Verzosa, M., Aur, R. J. A., Pratt, C., and George, S. L. (1977). Successful chemoprophylaxis for *Pneumocystis carinii* pneumonitis. *New Engl. J. Med.* **297**, 1419.

—, Price, R. A., Kim, H. K., Coburn, T. P., Grigsby, D., and Feldman, S. (1973). *Pneumocystis carinii* pneumonitis in children with malignancies. *J. Pediat.* **82**, 404.

Price, R. A. and Hughes, W. T. (1974). Histopathology of *Pneumocystis carinii* infestation and infection in malignant disease. *Human Pathol.* **5**, 737.

Walzer, P. D., Perl, D. P., Krogstad, D. J., Rawson, P. G., and Schultz, M. G. (1974). *Pneumocystis carinii* pneumonia in the United States. *Ann. intern. Med.* **80**, 83.

Singer, C., Armstrong, D., Rosen, P. P., Walzer, P. D., and Yu, B. (1979). Diffuse pulmonary disease in immunosuppressed patients. *Am. J. Med.* **66**, 110.

Toxoplasmosis

W. Kwantes

Toxoplasmosis is a worldwide infection of man and animals caused by the protozoon *Toxoplasma gondii*. It was first identified in 1908 by Nicolle and Manceaux in a North African rodent, the gondi, and named after it. The organism attracted attention as a cause of disease in warm-blooded animals, and it has since been found in almost all of them. In 1923 the first recognized case in humans was described by Janku, an ophthalmologist from Prague, who found parasitic cysts in the retina of an 11-month-old child with congenital toxoplasmosis. During 1937, toxoplasmosis was established as a human disease when Wolf and Cowen reported a fatal case of infantile granulomatous encephalitis which they believed was caused by a protozoon. This was confirmed as being due to *Toxoplasma* by Sabin who had encountered the disease in guinea pigs. The real impact on medicine came in 1948 when Sabin and Feldman discovered a serological test, the dye test, which enabled investigators to study the epidemiological aspects of the disease.

In 1967 Hutchison discovered that a sexual cycle took place in the gut of cats and that this resulted in the excretion of infectious oocysts. An important role for cats in the transmission of the disease was thus demonstrated.

The organism. *Toxoplasma* can be found in three different forms, the trophozoite or proliferative form, the tissue cyst, and the oocyst.

The trophozoite is crescent shaped, approximately 2–4 μm wide and 4–8 μm long, with one end tapered and the other rounded. This form of the organism is employed in the Sabin–Feldman dye test. Electron microscope studies reveal that the parasite is enclosed in a double membrane. It contains a nucleus, which is approximately central, and a complicated system of organelles. It has no flagella or cilia: locomotion is by body flexion. It proliferates by endodyogeny, multiplying intracellularly in any nucleated cell including red corpuscles of birds.

Following invasion, the organism multiplies within the vacuoles of the cell filling it with a rosette of trophozoites. The cell subsequently disrupts, and the released organisms invade adjacent cells. Colonies of trophozoites may be produced in tissues, forming tissue cysts. Retina, brain, skeletal, and heart muscle are the most commonly affected tissues. Cysts may contain hundreds or even thousands of organisms which can persist in living tissues for many years.

The oocyst is the result of a sexual cycle occurring in the intestine of members of the cat family, following ingestion of tissue cysts from infected mice, birds, or other animals. Schizogeny and gametogeny occur throughout the small intestine and after about a week oocysts appear in the faeces; as many as 10 million may be excreted in a single day. Sporulation takes place in two to three days at 20 °C but may take longer at lower temperatures. After sporulation the oocysts become infectious if ingested. They have been shown to survive in the soil for many months.

There is a variation in the virulence of *Toxoplasma* strains, some killing mice and rabbits in 7–10 days whereas others cause chronic infection.

Epidemiology. Toxoplasmosis is a zoonosis. The cat is the definitive host and all mammals and birds may become infected. Only the cat family excrete oocysts in their faeces and so contaminate the soil. This is a source of infection for both humans and animals. The natural cycle is as follows: the cat eats infected mice or other animals and, after a developmental stage in the intestine, *Toxoplasma* oocysts are excreted in the faeces. After a period of a few days these become infective and the cycle is complete when mice or other animals ingest them.

Infection in man occurs after the ingestion of either the infectious oocysts or of tissue cysts in infected meat, particularly mutton. Following ingestion, the cyst or oocyst is disrupted and the released sporozoites invade the intestinal epithelium and spread via the blood stream to all organs in the body. They multiply to form tissue cysts which are found particularly in the brain, heart, and skeletal muscle.

The disease is of considerable importance in sheep farming because it is a cause of ovine abortion which may affect the whole flock and so result in economic loss.

Serological surveys have shown that the prevalence of *Toxoplasma* infection in humans varies according to age, geographical locations, and dietary habits. In the United Kingdom about 10 per cent of persons have been infected and have *Toxoplasma* antibody by the age of 10, 20 per cent by the age of 20, and approaching 50 per cent by the age of 70. The figures are similar in the United States, but in France there is a much higher incidence, about 80 per cent of French people have been infected by the age of 20 years. This is probably due to the fact that far more raw or under-cooked meat is consumed there.

There is an association between the prevalence of human toxoplasmosis and the presence of cats. *Toxoplasma* antibody in humans and animals is found more frequently on those Pacific atolls on which cats live, than on those where they are absent.

The sex distribution of toxoplasmic lymphadenopathy in Europe is interesting. In childhood, boys are affected three times as commonly as girls. During adolescence the sexes are about equally affected, but during adulthood women are affected three times as commonly as men.

Clinical features. The disease can be divided into four clinical patterns, the acquired disease, the disease in the immunologically compromised patient, congenital infection, and ocular disease.

Acquired toxoplasmosis. It must be stressed that the vast majority of acquired human *Toxoplasma* infections do no harm, are not recognized, and so do not demand medical attention. When there are clinical signs they usually present as a lymphadenopathy, with or without malaise and fever. This is sometimes accompanied by a headache and sore throat. One or more lymph nodes may be enlarged in one or more groups. Those most commonly affected are in the upper deep cervical chain, but axillary and inguinal nodes may also be enlarged as part of a generalized lymphadenopathy. The lymph nodes are not tender, and are rubbery in consistency. Splenomegaly and hepatomegaly may be present and occasionally there is a maculopapular rash. A diagnosis of infectious mononucleosis is usually considered first. When this diagnosis has been excluded, the possibility of malignancy may lead to a lymph node biopsy.

The histology of the lymph node in toxoplasmosis is characteristic and is now recognized by histopathologists. Typically, the architecture of the node is retained and there is follicular hyperplasia. The characteristic feature is the presence of collections of enlarged epithelioid cells with abundant pale cytoplasm, vesicular nuclei, and prominent nucleoli. These collections range in size from two or three cells to a mass 100 μm in diameter and are most often seen at the periphery of the node. Caseation is not seen and the organisms are rarely found (Fig. 1). The diagnosis of toxoplasmosis is confirmed by finding a high or rising *Toxoplasma* antibody titre.

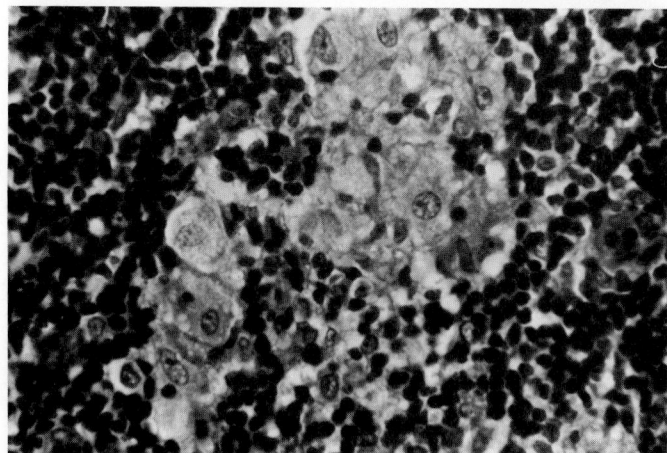

Fig. 1 Photomicrograph of the lymph node on toxoplasmosis. (Reproduced from *The laboratory diagnosis of toxoplasmosis*, PHLS monograph no. 13, with the permission of the Controller of Her Majesty's Stationery Office.)

The illness follows a variable course: malaise, fatigue, and glandular enlargement may last from a few weeks to several months, but there is practically always a complete recovery.

Occasionally, myocarditis may complicate the clinical picture, and so an electrocardiogram should be carried out. The patient should be treated if any abnormality is found as this condition is sometimes fatal.

Encephalitis is a rare complication of toxoplasmosis, but if untreated is often fatal. It may occur with or without glandular enlargement and, in the acute stage, may present with disturbances of consciousness or coma. The chronic stage may mimic multiple sclerosis, or present with neurological signs of a localized lesion in the brain.

Toxoplasmosis in the immunocompromised host. Toxoplasmosis, being a common infection, will every now and then affect a patient who is on immunosuppressive drugs or suffering from Hodgkin's disease, lymphoma, or other malignancy. There is then a dual pathology and it is important that this should be recognized. Antibody studies will suggest toxoplasmosis but there may be an underlying immunological disturbance from some other condition. There is then the possibility of progression to toxoplasmic encephalitis with headache, disorientation, and coma which, if untreated, may end fatally within a few days.

Congenital toxoplasmosis. Congenital toxoplasmosis occurs only in the infants of about one third of women who contract infection during gestation. Those who have Toxoplasma antibody before conception will not bear an infant with congenital toxoplasmosis. Similarly there is no recorded instance of a mother having more than one such infant. About 20 per cent of women in the UK and USA have been infected before their first pregnancy and can therefore be considered immune.

This leaves 80 per cent who are at risk in these countries. Their chances of becoming infected will vary according to their hygiene and cooking habits which directly influence their chances of acquiring infection either from oocysts in the soil or from tissue cysts in meat. Because of the high prevalence of infection in France, an English or American woman moving to France has a much higher risk of contracting infection during pregnancy than the indigenous population.

Infections contracted during pregnancy are usually asymptomatic. A few women notice enlarged posterior cervical glands.

If infection is acquired early in pregnancy, it may result in abortion of the fetus. Severe congenital infection is more likely if infection takes place in the first trimester than in the second, but congenital infection may still be apparent if infection takes place during the third.

An infant born with congenital toxoplasmosis may present in one of two ways.

Firstly, the disease may be easily recognizable at birth. The classic tetrad of signs described by Sabin, namely, internal hydrocephalus or microcephaly, chorioretinitis, convulsions, and cerebral calcifications are present in fully developed cases, but any combination of these may be found. If clinically recognizable at this stage, the disease is always severe, neurological damage is extensive, and the neonates often die.

Secondly, the disease may be discovered later. These cases comprise the majority of infants who, although asymptomatic at birth, develop sequaelae such as chorioretinitis, strabismus, hydrocephaly, or microcephaly, convulsions, spasticity, mental retardation, or deafness. The signs may become apparent during the first few months of life or take years to appear. There is, unfortunately, no way in which the outcome of the disease can be predicted, but there is usually some improvement with treatment. When the eyes are affected a white mass may be seen against the pale orange background of the fundus. An inflammatory exudate may cloud the vitreous; this clears when the inflammation subsides. The vast majority of lesions are near the posterior pole of the retina. A diagnosis cannot be made with absolute certainty, but the clinical signs supported by laboratory evidence, are strongly suggestive. A necrotizing chorioretinitis can occur in both syphilis and tuberculosis, and these diseases should be excluded.

Ocular toxoplasmosis. This almost always follows congenital infection and is a common cause of posterior uveitis in adults. Almost invariably the infection is confined to the posterior segment of the eye involving primarily the retina and then the underlying choroid. One or both eyes may be affected and to a different extent. The diagnosis is often made during the second decade of life, the patient typically presenting with blurred vision and an aching eye. The clinical picture is fairly characteristic. Ophthalmoscopic examination shows one or more areas of acute focal chorioretinitis. Initially, inflammatory exudate may cloud the vitreous making examination difficult. The focus of infection appears as a fluffy cotton-wool-like patch in the fundus. As the acute process subsides the vitreous clears, and a sharply demarcated chorioretinal scar is left.

After the inflammation has resolved, the organisms may remain dormant and a recurrence can occur many years later. This is presumably due to encysted colonies of parasites rupturing and as a result, fresh satelite lesions of active chorioretinitis appear near the margins of the old scar.

Lesions may be seen for the first time when the eyes are examined for other conditions. They appear as old healed foci, often bilateral, usually near the posterior pole, but sometimes peripheral. They do not cause the patient any trouble.

Toxoplasma antibody titres are frequently low and tend to remain at the same level. Their complete absence excludes toxoplasma infection.

Laboratory Investigations. Isolation of the parasite provides absolute proof of infection. This is most frequently achieved from lymph nodes and cerebrospinal fluid, but muscle, brain, and eye tissue or products of conception may be used for attempted isolation. The material should be transported to the laboratory in saline, containing 100 µg of penicillin and 100 µg of streptomycin per ml. Freezing or contact with formalin must be avoided. Several mice are inoculated and if infected, their brains show typical tissue cysts after four to six weeks and toxoplasma antibodies are present in their blood.

Serological tests are most commonly used for diagnosing Toxoplasma infection. The most widely used are the Sabin–Feldman dye test (DT), the indirect fluorescent antibody test (IFA), the indirect haemagglutination test (IHA), and complement fixation tests (CF) with either soluble or cuticular antigens. Other tests available are the direct agglutination test, the precipitin test, the latex agglutination test, and the enzyme linked immunosorbent assay (ELISA). The DT is considered to be the reference test but is only carried out in a few laboratories because of its complexity and the need to use live toxoplasma which present a risk of laboratory infection.

Infection with Toxoplasma results in cell-mediated immunity which can be demonstrated with the toxoplasmin skin test. This becomes positive several months after infection and is therefore of little use in the diagnosis of acute toxoplasmosis. Its main use has been for epidemiological studies.

Laboratory diagnosis in acquired infection. If lymphadenopathy is present and a biopsy of a lymph node has been made, the histology may suggest infection. The parasite can also be isolated from fresh biopsy material by animal inoculation and so confirm the infection.

The diagnosis of toxoplasmosis can also be established by demonstrating rising titres. However, this is often not possible, a single high titre being the usual finding when the patient first sees a physician. A high titre (1:500 or higher) may be present for several years and although such a titre is suggestive it is not diagnostic of current infection.

The dye test, CF test with cuticular antigen, and the IFA test measure the same antibody and the titre reaches a maximum a few weeks after the onset of infection. On the other hand the IHA test and the CF test, using a soluble antigen, measure a different antibody and the titre may take several months to reach a maximum. If the dye test or IFA titres are high and the IHA or CF titres are low, this is suggestive of an early infection.

Recent infection can also be investigated by examining for IgM antibody. This can be determined either by ELISA, the IFA test, or by sucrose density centrifugation of the serum followed by tests on the fractions. It may be present for several months in adult infection and when present, confirms the diagnosis. Figure 2 shows the changes in antibody titre of the different tests at various times after acquired infection.

Patients who are immunodeficient present a problem because the consequences can be serious. IgM antibody should be looked for and efforts should be made to identify the parasite in CSF, brain biopsy, lung biopsy, or bone marrow aspirates as determined by the clinical conditions.

ANTIBODY TITRES AT VARIOUS TIMES AFTER ACQUIRED INFECTION

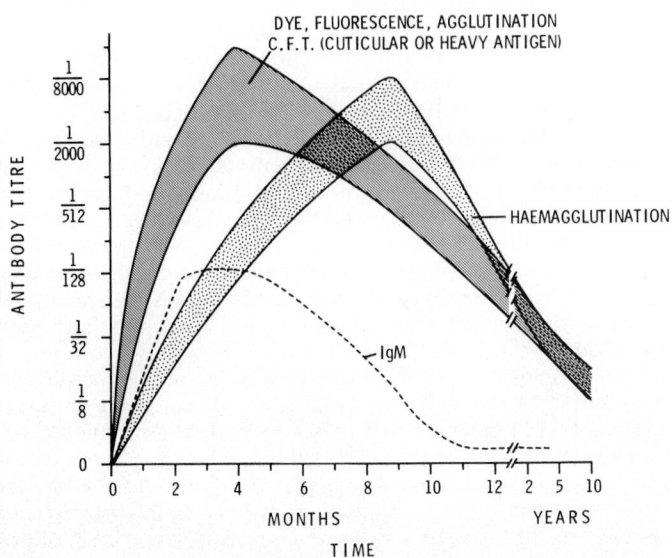

Fig. 2 Antibody titres at various times after acquired infection. (Reproduced from *The laboratory diagnosis of toxoplasmosis*, PHLS monograph no. 13, with the permission of the Controller of Her Majesty's Stationery Office.)

Laboratory diagnosis in congenital infection. A presumptive diagnosis can be made if the characteristic clinical signs, such as cerebral calcifications, chorioretinitis, and CSF abnormality are present and the infant also has an elevated *Toxoplasma* antibody titre. If the antibody titre remains persistently elevated for at least six months then the diagnosis becomes definite.

The presence of a positive IgM, ELISA or IFA test in the cord blood suggests infection but it must be remembered that this could be caused by a placental leak and a repeat sample from the infant must be examined to exclude this possibility. A negative IgM test does not exclude congenital toxoplasmosis.

Sometimes there is a history of *Toxoplasma* infection of the mother during pregnancy and in such cases it is worthwhile attempting to isolate *Toxoplasma* from the placenta by animal inoculation.

Laboratory diagnosis in ocular infection. The diagnosis rests almost entirely on the clinical findings together with the presence of *Toxoplasma* antibody. The level of the antibody titre does not correlate with the degree of chorioretinitis making diagnosis more difficult. The absence of antibody, however, excludes *Toxoplasma* infection.

Treatment. Acquired toxoplasmosis is often so mild clinically that treatment is unnecessary. Treatment is indicated when the disease is active and there is a rise in temperature, severe malaise, widespread glandular involvement, or involvement of the myocardium or central nervous system.

In children treatment consists of a combination of pyrimethamine (Daraprim) 2 mg/kg per day, for three to four days then 1 mg/kg per day for three weeks together with sulphadiazine 100 mg/kg per day in divided doses. Adults should receive pyrimethamine, 25–50 mg three times a day for three to five days, then 25–50 mg daily for three to four weeks. This should be administered in combination with sulphadiazine, 4–6 g per day. The

same dose of other sulphonamides such as sulphadimidine or triple sulphonamide may be substituted.

Pyrimethamine and sulphonomides act synergistically against *Toxoplasma* and the simultaneous use of both drugs is therefore indicated. However, pyrimethamine may cause depression of haemopoiesis because of its antagonism to folic acid; blood and platelet counts should therefore be carried out twice a week during treatment.

In the event of leucopenia or a low platelet count treatment should be stopped and folinic acid, 15 mg daily should be given.

Pyrimethamine should not be administered during the first three months of gestation because of its possible teratogenic effect. After this period treatment may help to reduce the incidence of congenitally infected infants.

Spiramycin, a macrolide antibiotic, is a less toxic alternative which has been used extensively in France and is devoid of teratogenic effects. A three week course of 2–3 g per day, in four divided doses, was given to women who acquired toxoplasmosis during pregnancy. This effectively reduced the incidence of transplacental infection but it was not possible to show a reduction in clinically apparent congenital disease. It may be of value in treating the immunodeficient patient with toxoplasmosis because it does not depress bone marrow activity.

Patients with ocular lesions should not be treated with spiramycin. Treatment with pyrimethamine and sulphonamides is effective in some cases. Small acute lesions of the retina sometimes benefit, but this treatment appears to have little effect on chronic elevated lesions. In active lesions oral corticosteroids given in combination with the antimicrobials are of value in suppressing the inflammation.

Congenital toxoplasmosis, whether clinical or subclinical, should always be treated with pyrimethamine and sulphonamides in the dosage schedule mentioned previously for children. Folinic acid, in doses of 5 mg, should be given twice weekly in addition.

Treatment should be started as soon as the diagnosis is made. It may be considered necessary to give three or four courses during the first year of life and these can be interspersed with six week courses of spiramycin, 100 mg/kg per day.

Prevention. The known sources of *Toxoplasma* are tissue cysts in meat and oocysts from cats faeces. The prevention of infection must therefore be related to the elimination of these two sources.

Tissue cysts in meat can be killed by heating to 60 °C or freezing at −20 °C but, as most domestic freezers do not reach this low temperature, raw meat in the home is a definite risk. Meat for human consumption should therefore be well cooked, and pregnant women should certainly avoid eating rare steaks or hamburgers. The handling of meat in the kitchen constitutes a risk of infection, by contamination of cuts or abrasions. Hand washing with soap and water after handling meat is therefore essential.

Cats become infected when they first start catching mice or birds, and they should be discouraged from hunting and be fed with dry, canned, or cooked meat. Rubber gloves should be worn when litterpans are cleaned. This should be carried out daily so that any oocysts that may be present will not have had time to sporulate. The faeces should be incinerated or flushed down the toilet and the litterpan sterilized with boiling water. Pregnant women should preferably avoid handling cats altogether.

Children may contract infection from soil contaminated with oocysts and sandpits should be covered when not in use to prevent cats defaecating in them.

References

Fleck, D. G., and Kwantes, W. (1980). *The laboratory diagnosis of toxoplasmosis*. PHLS Monograph no. 13. HMSO, London.
Hentsch, D. (1971). *Toxoplasmosis*. Huber, Berne.
Remington, T. J. and Klein, J. O. (1976). *Infectious diseases of fetus and newborn infant*. W. B. Saunders, Philadelphia.
Symposium on Toxoplasmosis (1974). *Bull. N. Y. Acad. Med.* **50**, 107.

Giardiasis, balantidiasis, sarcocystosis, and isosporiasis

S. G. Wright

Giardiasis

Parasitology. *Giardia lamblia* is a flagellate parasite infecting the small intestine of man. The trophozoite usually lies with its ventral sucker disk on the microvillous border of the epithelial cells. It is a pear-shaped organism measuring 9–21 μm long, 5–15 μm wide and 2–4 μm thick. It has two nuclei, one on either side of the mid-line. The dorsal surface is convex and most of the concave ventral surface forms the sucker disc. Two flagella emerge close to the mid-line on the ventral surface and the other six emerge symmetrically around the periphery. Trophozoites encyst in the gut lumen, and cysts, the infective form of the parasite, are passed in the faeces. The cyst is ovoid or ellipsoid in shape and measures 8 μm long, 12 μm wide and 7–10 μm thick. It contains an easily recognized median body and four nuclei are seen in the mature cyst. Cysts can remain viable outside the body for up to two months in cold water but at higher temperatures fewer cysts remain viable.

Epidemiology and transmission. *G. lamblia* has a worldwide distribution. It is most common in the tropics and sub-tropics but the countries of Eastern Europe and Leningrad, USSR, are endemic areas. In tropical regions infection occurs as a result of ingestion of cysts in contaminated food and water. Inadequate or non-existent sanitation, faecal contamination of the environment, and untreated water supplies are important factors in transmission. In North America epidemics of giardiasis have occurred because of defective water-treatment plant and because of leakage of untreated sewage into pipes carrying domestic water supplies. In one outbreak beavers were found to harbour the parasite and were contaminating a surface water source. Person-to-person spread can occur as a result of atypical sexual practices and giardiasis is not infrequent among homosexuals. The importance of low standards of personal hygiene in transmission is borne out by the frequent occurrence of giardiasis in residents of homes for the mentally sub-normal.

In endemic areas young children are most often infected and symptomatic, possibly reflecting close contact with the contaminated environment around the home and first infection with the parasite. The lower prevalence of infection among adults may indicate some degree of resistance to reinfection. Volunteer feeding studies have shown that a comparatively small number of cysts is required to produce the infection, but even those fed large numbers of cysts developed only minor gastrointestinal symptoms. Spontaneous eradication of the infection was the rule.

Pathogenesis. It is likely that a number of factors contribute to mucosal damage in giardiasis. There is electron microscopic evidence of damage to the brush border and microvilli of epithelial cells beneath trophozoites, and this damage to the functional surface of the epithelium may be most important. The severity of damage may be proportional to the number of trophozoites present. In patients with persisting symptoms and impaired intestinal absorption, there may be abnormalities of the mechanisms that normally lead to natural eradication of the infection or at least to a considerable reduction in parasite numbers. These mechanisms probably include mechanical washing out of the parasites as well as the secretion of specific antibody, IfA and IgM, directed against the parasite. Immunologically mediated damage to the mucosa may result from responses to absorbed giardial antigens and to trophozoites which opportunistically invade the mucosa. Mucosal invasion is an uncommon finding. The upper small bowel is normally sterile but enterobacterial colonization has been found in patients with giardiasis and marked malabsorption. Though these organisms secrete enterotoxins and alcohol, which can impair func-

tion, they are not affected by metronidazole which produces rapid resolution of giardiasis and so do not play a primary role in pathogenesis.

Clinical features. The incubation period is usually about two weeks though it can vary between extremes of three days and six weeks. The first symptom is diarrhoea of sudden onset with yellowish, watery stools that have a very offensive smell; bowel actions are accompanied by the passage of foul-smelling flatus. A smaller number of patients notice a more insidious change in bowel habit. Additional symptoms are anorexia, nausea, weight loss, abdominal distension, and abdominal discomfort. Chills and low grade fevers have been attributed to giardiasis but have not been observed by the present author in acute cases. In most patients symptoms resolve over seven days. In a comparatively small number of patients gastrointestinal symptoms persist for weeks or months. Lassitude is common among this group. Some patients fail to regain lost weight and may continue to lose weight. Milk and dairy produce, alcohol, and spicy foods usually exacerbate intestinal symptoms. Children may be brought to medical attention because of failure to thrive. Physical examination does not reveal any specific physical signs but there may be obvious weight loss with muscle wasting around the shoulder and pelvic girdles, abdominal distension, and increased bowel sounds.

The diagnosis is made in most cases by stool microscopy. Trophozoites are sometimes found in diarrhoeal stools on direct examination of faecal smears, while formed stools contain cysts. Concentration techniques, such as the formol–ether method, improve the yield of positive results particularly when there are few cysts in the stool. Cyst excretion varies considerably from day to day. A single stool sample will reveal the diagnosis in up to 75 per cent of cases so that several stool examinations may be necessary. If repeated stool examinations have not revealed cysts and giardiasis is suspected, trophozoites may be found in jejunal fluid, in impression smears made from the epithelial surface of a fragment of a jejunal biopsy specimen, and in stained sections of the jejunal biopsy where trophozoites may be seen on the surface of epithelial cells and in the intervillous spaces. A further technique for sampling the upper gastrointestinal tract uses a fine thread coiled inside a weighted plastic capsule. The free end of the thread is taped to the patient's cheek and the capsule is swallowed and passes through the stomach into the small intestine. After several hours the thread is pulled out and the bile-stained fluid is squeezed out for microscopy.

Intestinal absorption is usually abnormal in symptomatic patients and impaired absorption of fat, D-xylose and, vitamin B_{12} is found

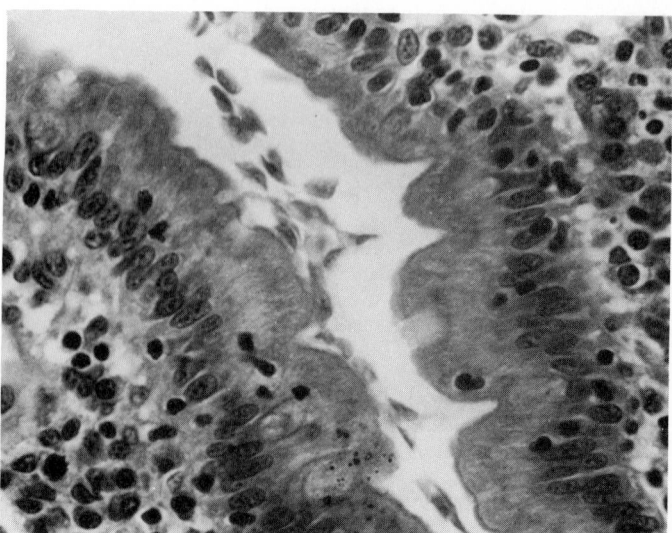

Fig. 1 Giardia trophozoites lying in the intervillous space in a jejunal biopsy section. A number of trophozoites are lying on the brush border of epithelial cells.

in those with severe symptoms. Acquired lactose intolerance is common. There is a considerable range of changes in the jejunal mucosa from almost normal appearances on dissecting microscopy and in histological sections in patients with minimal symptoms, to a ridged or convoluted mucosa with thickened villi and obvious histological abnormalities—shortened villi and deepened crypts containing increased numbers of cells in mitosis and a considerable increase in the lamina propria infiltrate of plasma cells and lymphocytes—in patients with marked symptoms and functional changes. A completely atrophic mucosa is rarely seen in giardiasis and should raise the possibility that the patient has coeliac disease as well as giardiasis. Megaloblastic anaemia due to folate deficiency occurs occasionally when severe symptoms have been present for several months. Radiological changes in the small bowel on barium follow-through examination are non-specific and comprise dilatation of small bowel loops and mucosal oedema. Again these are most often found in patients with marked symptoms.

Treatment and course. Treatment produces rapid relief in symptomatic patients. Asymptomatic cyst excreters represent a source of infection to others and should also be treated. Pregnant women represent an exception to this rule as the safety of the drugs used is not established and the benefits of treatment must be weighed against the possible harmful effects of the drugs on the fetus.

Mepacrine was the first effective drug for the treatment of giardiasis and gives cure rates of 90 per cent after courses of 100 mg thrice daily for five to ten days. Reduced doses are given to children. The disadvantages are thrice daily dosage for a week or more, occasional gastrointestinal side effects comprising nausea and vomiting, and the production of a yellowish discolouration of the skin which fades after stopping treatment. Toxic psychosis occurs rarely. Mepacrine is contra-indicated in patients with psoriasis. The nitroimidazole compounds, metronidazole and tinidazole are both effective in giardiasis. Metronidazole can be given as a single daily dose of 2.0 g with breakfast for three successive days. Children over 10 years old can be given the adult dose. Those between seven and ten years can take 1.0 g as a single dose for three days. Children between three and seven years can take 600 mg daily for three days, and 500 mg daily for three days can be given to children between one and three years old. Tinidazole can be given as a single dose of 2.0 g to adults and in appropriately reduced doses to children. Both of these compounds have disulfiram-like interactions with alcohol and so patients should be told not to drink alcohol while they are taking these drugs. Impaired concentration and drowsiness are side-effects which may occur in patients on high dose treatments and so patients should be advised that they should not ride bicycles, drive cars, or operate dangerous machines such as power tools while on high dose treatments. Those who cannot tolerate high doses of these drugs can be given metronizadole, 200 mg thrice daily for 14 days, or tinidazole, 150 mg twice daily for seven days. Reduced doses are given to children.

The response to treatment is rapid with diarrhoea stopping over a seven to ten day period after treatment and subsequently the other symptoms resolve. Functional and histological changes resolve over one to three months. Lactose intolerance is usually temporary but a low lactose diet is helpful. Avoidance of alcohol and spicy foods may also help in controlling persisting abdominal symptoms after eradication of the parasite. Where possible a stool sample should be examined six to eight weeks after treatment to ensure eradication of the parasite.

Balantidiasis

Balantidium coli is the largest protozoan parasite of man, measuring up to 300 μm by 100 μm, and is usually found as a commensal in the lumen of the colon. It is motile through the beating of cilia arranged in longitudinal rows. Organisms encyst in the lumen, and cysts are passed in the faeces. The parasite has a wide geographical distribution from Scandinavia and northern USSR to the tropics and sub-tropics, where it is most common. Pigs are an important animal reservoir for human infection but rodents are thought to be the animal reservoir in predominantly Muslim countries. An epidemic of human balantidiasis occurred on the Pacific Island of Truk in the wake of a typhoon because pig faeces contaminated water for domestic use. Balantidiasis occurs in residents of homes for the mentally retarded as a result of poor personal hygiene.

Most infected patients are asymptomatic but dysenteric disease of varying degrees of severity can occur. Rarely this may be acute in onset with diarrhoea containing blood and mucus, abdominal pain, nausea, and vomiting. Fulminant cases can pursue a rapidly deteriorating course with death from blood loss and intestinal perforation. In most symptomatic cases there is less severe diarrhoea with blood and mucus in the stools. Pathological changes are usually limited to the caecum and ascending colon though a greater length of the bowel is affected in severe cases. The surface epithelium is ulcerated and there is necrotic slough in the bases of the ulcers. There is a prominent infiltrate of lymphocytes and eosinophils in the mucosa, and trophozoites can usually be seen in sections stained with haematoxylin and eosin. Haematogenous spread to other organs does not occur even though organisms may penetrate through to the serosa. The diagnosis is made by finding trophozoites or cysts in the stools or organisms in biopsies of affected colonic mucosa. The disease is often self-limiting after several weeks. Tetracycline is the best drug available for treatment in doses of 250–500 mg four times daily for seven to ten days in adults. Metronidazole has been used with varying degrees of success. Nitrimidazine is also effective.

Sarcocystosis

Sarcocystis hominis, *S. suihominis*, and *S. lindemani* are coccidian parasites that can infect man, though their pathogenicity is uncertain. These parasites have two hosts, and man is a definitive host of the first two and an intermediate host for the third. After ingestion of undercooked beef (*S. hominis*) or pork (*S. suihominis*) containing parasite sporocysts, sporozoites are released and these invade the epithelial cells of the intestine to replicate asexually by schizogony. Merozoites are released and they carry on the same sequence in other epithelial cells. Some merozoites develop into gametes which fuse and after sprorulation form oocysts which are shed into the gut to be passed in the faeces. Oocysts are infective for the intermediate host but not for the definitive host. Anorexia, nausea, vomiting, and abdominal pain have been ascribed to infection with these two species but volunteer feeding studies have failed to produce any symptoms. The diagnosis is made by finding oocysts in the stools. *S. lindemani* can infect man as its intermediate host. Occasional cases with a local myositis and nodules due to the sporocysts in muscles have been reported.

Isosporiasis

Human infection with the coccidian parasite *Isospora belli* is relatively uncommon. The parasite has a complex life cycle involving only one host infected by ingestion of oocysts from which sporozoites are liberated. These invade intestinal epithelial cells where they undergo asexual schizogony. Merozoites are released and invade other cells to replicate asexually or become gametes which fuse and sporulate to produce oocysts which are shed into the gut lumen. Many of these are passed in the faeces, but it is thought that some may mature and excyst in the lumen to allow further infection of the same host. A range of severity of infection has been described from a mild self-limiting disease to a protracted gastrointestinal illness with diarrhoea, weight loss, and low-grade fever. In such cases malabsorption and a severe degree of villous atrophy have been described. The diagnosis is made by finding oocysts in the stools or duodenal aspirate or by finding forms of the parasite in jejunal biopsy specimens. Treatment with pyrimethamine and sulphadiazine produced rapid and permanent resolution of the infection in one well-documented case.

References

Knight, R. (1978). Giardiasis, isosporiasis, and balantidiasis. *Clins Gastroent.* **7**, 31.

Trier, J. S., Moxey, P. C., Schimmel, E. M., and Robles, E. (1974). Chronic intestinal coccidiosis in man: intestinal morphology and response to treatment. *Gastroenterology* **66**, 923.

Wolfe, M. S. (1978). Giardiasis. *New Engl. J. Med.* **298**, 319.

Wright, S. G., Tomkins, A. M., and Ridley, D. S. (1977). Giardiasis: clinical and therapeutic aspects. *Gut* **18**, 343.

African trypanosomiasis

B. M. Greenwood

African trypanosomiasis, or sleeping sickness, occurs in two forms: Gambian or West African sleeping sickness due to infection with *Trypanosoma brucei gambiense*, and Rhodesian or East African sleeping sickness due to infection with *Trypanosoma brucei rhodesiense*. *Trypanosoma brucei brucei*, the third *T. brucei* sub-species, causes trypanosomiasis in cattle but does not cause disease in man.

Throughout the first half of the twentieth century many parts of tropical Africa were affected by major epidemics of sleeping sickness which caused hundreds of thousands, and possibly millions, of deaths. During the past twenty years the incidence of the disease has declined progressively and now only about 5000 cases are recorded annually. How much of this decline is the result of active control measures and how much results from a natural change in the behaviour of the infection is uncertain. At present Zaire accounts for most reported cases of sleeping sickness but some cases are detected each year in most African countries (Fig. 1). Sleeping sickness thrives under conditions of strife and civil disturbance and there has been a recent resurgence of the infection in Uganda. Although sleeping sickness is not, at present, a major health problem, the potential threat of further large scale epidemics remains as long as transmission continues in small active foci.

The organism. Trypanosomes of the *T. brucei* group are elongated parasites, around 10–30 µm in length, which have a promi-

nent nucleus and kinetoplast. They are actively motile and possess a flagellum which projects from their anterior end. Blood forms show some variation in morphology; some trypanosomes are elongated whilst others occur in a short, stumpy form. The three sub-species of *T. brucei* cannot be differentiated morphologically. However, *T. b. rhodesiense* can usually be distinguished from *T. b. brucei* by the blood incubation test because *T. b. rhodesiense*, but not *T. b. brucei*, survives on incubation in human serum. Isolates of *T. b. rhodesiense* and *T. b. gambiense* can usually be differentiated by electrophoretic analysis of their iso-enzymes. Electron microscopy shows that trypanosomes of the *T. brucei* group are coated with amorphous material. This material contains the surface variant antigens which play an important role in allowing the parasite to escape the host's immune response.

Epidemiology. Sleeping sickness usually follows from a bite by an infected tsetse fly but the infection can be caused by direct inoculation with infected material. African trypanosomiasis has occurred as a result of laboratory accidents with infected samples and it can follow blood transfusions. A few cases of congenital trypanosomiasis have been recorded following infection *in utero*.

When a tsetse fly of a suitable species bites a patient with parasitaemia, trypanosomes are sucked up into the gut of the fly with the blood meal. Within the gut they pass around the peritrophic membrane and penetrate the wall of the proventriculus to reach the salivary glands where they develop into infective metacyclic forms. Metacyclic trypanosomes are morphologically similar to blood forms but they are usually smaller. Development within the fly takes between two and five weeks.

Although both Gambian and Rhodesian trypanosomiasis are spread by tsetse flies, which are found only in Africa, the epidemiology of the two forms of sleeping sickness differs in a number of important respects (Table 1). Gambian sleeping sickness is primarily a human infection whilst Rhodesian sleeping sickness is a zoonosis.

Table 1   The contrasting epidemiological features of Gambian and of Rhodesian sleeping sickness

	Gambian	Rhodesian
Trypanosome	*T. b. gambiense*	*T. b. rhodesiense*
Source of infection	man (? pig)	game (occasionally man)
Vector	riverine tsetse (*G. palpalis, G. tachynoides*)	savannah tsetse (*G. morsitans*)
Distribution	West and Central Africa	East Africa
Clinical course	chronic	acute

Gambian sleeping sickness is spread by riverine tsetse flies, especially *Glossina palpalis* and *G. tachynoides*. These flies live and breed in the vegetation bounding rivers and streams in many parts of the West African savannah. Such areas are frequently visited by man for the collection of water and for washing, thus providing favourable conditions for transmission of the infection. Under such conditions of close man–fly contact, a small number of flies can cause an extensive local outbreak of the disease. Although major epidemics of Gambian sleeping sickness have occurred in the past, the infection is now encountered most frequently in small, localized outbreaks. Gambian sleeping sickness is spread predominantly from human to human but the occasional occurrence of an isolated case in an area where there has been no other case of the infection for many years suggests that some patients derive their infection from an animal reservoir. The recent isolation from Liberian pigs of trypanosomes with iso-enzyme patterns very similar to those of *T. b. gambiense* suggests that the pig could act as such a reservoir.

In contrast to *T. b. gambiense*, *T. b. rhodesiense* is primarily a

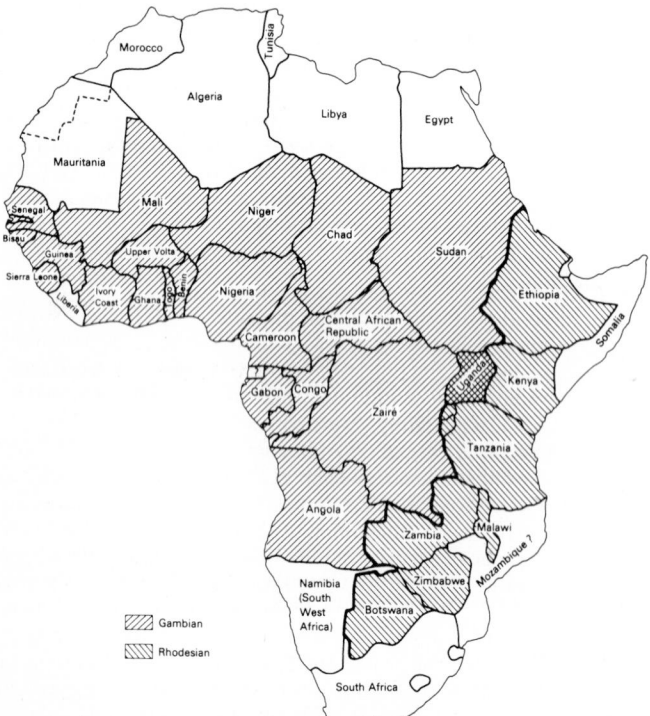

Fig. 1   Countries reporting cases of sleeping sickness in 1975. (From *The African trypanosomiases, Wld Hlth Org. Tech. Rep. Ser. no. 635.*)

parasite of game, especially the bushbuck, and man enters the transmission cycle only occasionally. Rhodesian sleeping sickness is transmitted by species of tsetse fly, such as *G. morsitans*, which inhabit open savannah. Thus, those most at risk from this infection are people such as hunters, fishermen, and tourists whose activities take them into the bush. Although Rhodesian sleeping sickness is usually spread from animal to man it is possible that human to human transmission occurs under epidemic conditions.

Pathology. The pathological features of sleeping sickness were well described in the early years of this century by Mott but there have been few recent histopathological studies. Such studies would be of interest now that a great deal more is known about the immunological importance of pathological changes in various parts of the lymphoid system.

The lymph nodes of patients in the early stage of Gambian sleeping sickness are swollen and infiltrated with large numbers of lymphocytes, plasma cells, and pale staining mononuclear cells. Similar changes occur in the spleen. Later, affected lymph nodes become shrunken and atrophic.

Following invasion of the central nervous system, which probably occurs through the choroid plexus, the meninges become congested and infiltrated with lymphocytes, plasma cells and large vesicular cells—the morular cells of Mott. Morular cells are plasma cells grossly distended with vesicles of immunoglobulin. Inflammatory changes extend from the surface of the brain into the Virchow–Robin spaces, producing a characteristic picture of perivascular cuffing (Fig. 2). Finally inflammatory cells invade the substance of the brain and there is proliferation of glial cells. These changes may be prominent in the basal ganglia. Demyelinization of nerve fibres has also been described.

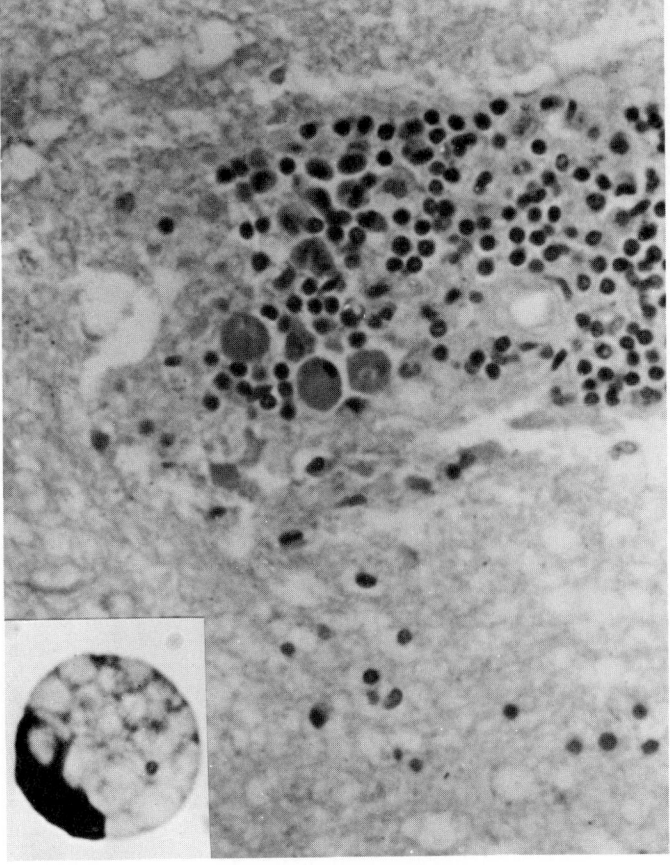

Fig. 2   The brain in advanced Gambian sleeping sickness showing perivascular infiltration with lymphocytes and morular cells (haematoxylin and eosin × 350). The insert shows a morular cell in greater detail (Giemsa × 875).

The pathology of Rhodesian sleeping sickness is similar to that of Gambian sleeping sickness but infiltration of the myocardium with lymphocytes, plasma cells, and morular cells is often a prominent feature of this form of the infection.

Pathogenesis and immunity. The pathogenesis of the characteristic lesions of sleeping sickness is little understood. It is likely that they are produced as a result of some form of immunopathological reaction, for they are poorly developed in immune deprived animals infected with African trypanosomes, but what type of immunopathological reaction is involved is uncertain. High levels of immune complexes are found in sera of most patients with sleeping sickness, but the absence of polymorphonuclear neutrophil leucocytes from the lesions in the brain and heart makes it unlikely that these are a result of immune complex mediated tissue damage. Infection with African trypanosomes causes polyclonal activation of B lymphocytes resulting in the production of large amounts of IgM and in the production of autoantibodies. Proliferation of B lymphocytes may contribute to the lymphadenopathy and to the lymphocytic infiltration of the brain and heart characteristics of sleeping sickness, but how this proliferation is induced is uncertain. Proliferation of B lymphocytes is associated with the impairment of some specialized lymphocyte functions. This impairment of immunity may be one factor contributing to the increased susceptibility to secondary bacterial infections shown by patients with sleeping sickness. Current speculations as to the pathogenesis of sleeping sickness are summarized in Fig. 3.

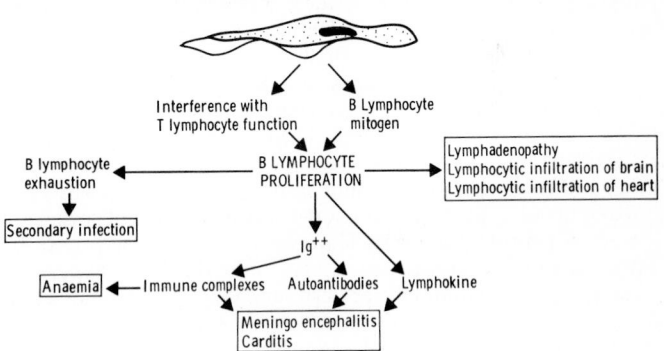

Fig. 3   Possible ways in which trypanosomes may bring about the clinical features of sleeping sickness (from Greenwood, B. M. and Whittle, H. C. (1981). *Trans. R. Soc. trop. Med. Hyg.* **74**, 716.

Despite a vigorous immune response, patients with sleeping sickness fail to control their infection. This failure follows from the ability of trypanosomes of the *T. brucei* group to change their surface antigens, thus enabling them to keep one stage ahead of the immune response of the host. How this process of antigenic variation is achieved is not fully understood, but it is likely that each trypanosome possesses the genetic potential to form a variety of surface antigens, a switch to the synthesis of a new antigen being precipitated by exposure to an altered environment such as that resulting from the formation of antibody. The ability of *T. brucei* trypanosomes to change their surface antigens accounts for the fact that infection does not confer protection against subsequent reinfection and has greatly impeded attempts to produce an effective vaccine.

Clinical features

Gambian sleeping sickness. The clinical features of Gambian sleeping sickness can be divided conveniently into three stages: an initial lesion at the site of a bite by an infected tsetse fly, an early phase associated with generalized dissemination of trypanosomes, and a late or advanced stage which follows invasion of the central nervous system.

Two to six weeks after a bite by an infected tsetse fly a nodular lesion may appear at the site of the bite from which trypanosomes can be isolated. This lesion, one of several designated as a chancre, has been noted most frequently in infected Europeans. Among the population of endemic areas it is rarely distinguished from the many other cutaneous lesions prevalent in these areas.

Weeks or months after having been bitten, the patient develops fever and general malaise, the first clinical features indicating systemic invasion with trypanosomes. Febrile episodes are frequently separated by periods during which the patient feels quite well. Examination of patients in the early phase of Gambian sleeping sickness usually reveals lymphadenopathy and, sometimes, a modest degree of splenomegaly. The posterior cervical group of lymph nodes are preferentially affected but other lymph glands are sometimes involved. Affected nodes are firm and discrete; they are not usually tender. Cervical lymph nodes may be enlarged sufficiently to produce an obvious swelling (Winterbottom's sign) but, more often, the enlarged nodes can be detected only on palpation. This procedure is best carried out with the examiner standing behind the patient. Clinical signs of cardiac damage are encountered infrequently in patients with Gambian sleeping sickness, but an electrocardiogram often shows minor abnormalities. Some patients develop an urticarial rash. After a period of months, fever subsides and lymphadenopathy regresses without treatment. A symptom-free period lasting for months or even years may then ensue.

Following invasion of the central nervous system new symptoms and signs appear. The first features of advanced sleeping sickness are often a personality change and the adoption by the patient of unusual patterns of behaviour such as an abnormal interest in religion. In some endemic areas these features are well-recognized by the local population as early features of sleeping sickness. Disturbance of the normal sleep rhythm is another early feature of invasion of the central nervous system. Excessive sleepiness during the day is the usual pattern, thus giving rise to the common name of the disease, but this is not invariable and mania may occur. At this stage of the infection patients often complain of headache, neckache, and backache. Examination of patients with these early features of invasion of the central nervous system may not reveal any abnormal neurological signs. However, as the disease progresses extrapyramidal signs such as chorea, athetosis, and hypertonia usually appear. Pyramidal tract signs and cranial nerve palsies are found much less frequently. Convulsions may occur. Impotence or amenorrhoea are common features of advanced Gambian sleeping sickness and obesity is sometimes encountered. Obesity probably results from an endocrine disturbance but the nature of this endocrine abnormality has not been defined. In the last stages of their illness patients with Gambian sleeping sickness stop eating and become stuporose and cachectic. Death often follows from an intercurrent infection such as pneumonia.

Rhodesian sleeping sickness. The clinical features of Rhodesian and Gambian sleeping sickness are similar but the clinical course of Rhodesian sleeping sickness is usually more rapid than that of Gambian sleeping sickness, with less demarcation between the early and late stages of the infection. Cardiac involvement is a more prominent feature of Rhodesian sleeping sickness than of Gambian sleeping sickness and death from cardiac failure may occur before neurological signs have appeared. Many patients have a moderate degree of haemolytic anaemia and a few are jaundiced. Bleeding associated with disseminated intravascular coagulation has been recorded.

Laboratory abnormalities. During the early, systemic phase of the infection anaemia and thrombocytopenia are usually present; these abnormalities are more marked in patients with Rhodesian sleeping sickness than in patients with Gambian sleeping sickness. The anaemia is predominantly haemolytic and it is usually associated with a reticulocytosis. In some patients positive Coombs tests have been obtained with anti-gammaglobulin and anti-complement antisera. In patients with Gambian sleeping sickness thrombocytopenia is probably a reflection of increased recticuloendothelial activity.

Thrombocytopenia may be associated with other laboratory features of disseminated intravascular coagulation in patients with Rhodesian sleeping sickness. Serum IgM levels are raised during the early phase of the infection in patients with both types of sleeping sickness.

Following invasion of the central nervous system, the cerebrospinal fluid (CSF) shows abnormalities. A moderate increase in CSF cell count is found; this is usually in the range of $50–500 \times 10^9$ cells/l. About 90 per cent of these cells are lymphocytes, predominantly B lymphocytes. The remainder are plasma cells and morular cells. The CSF total protein is increased, usually within the range of 0.5–2.0 g/l; much of this protein is IgM. Trypanosomes may be present.

Diagnosis. Clinical diagnosis of the early stage of sleeping sickness is difficult, unless it is realized that the patient comes from, or has recently visited, an endemic area or has been exposed to the infection in a laboratory, for the early features of fever and lymphadenopathy are indistinguishable from those of many other infectious and neoplastic disorders. A careful geographical history must be taken from any patient with an unexplained febrile illness. If the patient has recently visited an area known to be endemic for trypanosomiasis (Fig. 1), a diagnosis of sleeping sickness must be considered a possibility. Trypanosomes can usually be detected in blood smears obtained from patients with early Rhodesian sleeping sickness. Patients with early Gambian sleeping sickness infrequently have demonstrable parasitaemia unless special concentrating techniques are used, and diagnosis is established most readily by gland puncture in this form of infection. To carry out this technique a venepuncture needle is inserted into an enlarged gland, the drop of gland juice obtained expelled by a syringe on to a clean slide, and the wet preparation examined immediately for motile trypanosomes. Gland puncture is diagnostically more helpful than gland biopsy which may show only non-specific reactive changes.

Clinical diagnosis of the advanced stage of sleeping sickness is not usually difficult, provided that it is realized that the patient has been exposed to the infection. A diagnosis of a functional psychosis may be made in patients presenting with florid psychological changes, and there is a danger that such patients will be admitted to a mental hospital without a lumbar puncture having been performed. A definitive diagnosis of advanced sleeping sickness can nearly always be established by examination of the CSF. In about one half of patients trypanosomes can be seen, provided that the specimen is examined immediately after the CSF sample is collected and provided that scrupulously clean glassware is used. A high CSF IgM is found in most patients with advanced sleeping sickness. Detection of a high CSF IgM (average 50 IU/ml) in the face of only a modest increase in the CSF total protein is strong presumptive evidence for the presence of sleeping sickness and, in association with a suggestive clinical picture, is an indication for treatment, even if trypanosomes cannot be found.

Treatment
General measures. Patients with advanced sleeping sickness are sometimes in a poor general condition by the time that they reach hospital. Such patients should receive a short period of general rehabilitation, during which any associated infections are diagnosed and treated, before they start on specific chemotherapy, unless they are critically ill with advanced neurological disease, in which case specific chemotherapy should be started straight away.

All patients with sleeping sickness must have a lumbar puncture performed before treatment as the chemotherapy of early and of advanced disease differs in a number of important respects. If any CSF abnormalities are found (an increase in cells or an increase in protein), a patient must be treated as a case of advanced disease, even if there are no clinical signs of central nervous system involvement.

Chemotherapy of early disease. Suramin is the drug most widely recommended for the treatment of early Gambian and early Rhodesian sleeping sickness. Suramin is a white powder which is dissolved in sterile distilled water immediately before intravenous injection. The drug is given in a dose of 20 mg/kg. A course consists of 5–10 injections given at five-day intervals. Because a small number of patients, especially those with associated onchocerciasis, collapse when given suramin, it is customary to start a course with a test dose of 0.2 g (adults). Suramin can cause renal damage and the urine should be tested for protein before each injection is given. A trace of proteinuria can be safely ignored, but if heavy proteinuria or a raised blood urea are found, treatment with suramin must be stopped and an alternative drug should be given.

Melarsoprol (Mel B) is highly effective in the treatment of early sleeping sickness. Only a short course of four injections, given over a one week period, is needed (see Table 2). This is a major advantage over suramin, for which a much longer course of injections is required, especially when patients must be treated in remote areas with limited health resources. Despite the generally high toxicity of melarsoprol (see below), few complications have been encountered when the drug has been used in this way.

Table 2 A schedule for the use of melarsoprol (Mel B) in the treatment of early and advanced Gambian or Rhodesian sleeping sickness. Adult dosages are given. (Early sleeping sickness can be treated effectively with suramin.)

Day	Early sleeping sickness	Advanced sleeping sickness
1	melarsoprol 2.5 ml	suramin 0.2 g
3	melarsoprol 2.5 ml	
5	melarsoprol 5.0 ml	suramin 1.0 g
8	melarsoprol 5.0 ml	melarsoprol 2.5 ml
10		melarsoprol 2.5 ml
12		melarsoprol 5.0 ml
		rest
22		melarsoprol 5.0 ml
24		melarsoprol 5.0 ml
26		melarsoprol 5.0 ml
		rest
36		melarsoprol 5.0 ml
38		melarsoprol 5.0 ml
40		melarsoprol 5.0 ml

Chemotherapy of advanced disease. Once invasion of the central nervous system has occurred, suramin is no longer effective, for it penetrates poorly into the CSF, and melarsoprol must be used. Melarsoprol is dispensed as a 3.6 per cent solution in propylene glycol. This solution is very irritant and frequently causes thrombophlebitis at the site of an intravenous injection and severe cellulitis if it leaks outside a vein. The full dosage of melarsoprol is 3.6 mg per kg which must be given by intravenous injection. Several different schemes for administering melarsoprol have been tried but there have been few controlled trials to compare their relative efficacies. A schedule which the author has found effective in the treatment of Nigerian patients with advanced Gambian sleeping sickness is shown in Table 2. Other schemes build up to full dosage more gradually. It is customary to give one or two injections of suramin before starting treatment with melarsoprol to prevent the severe febrile reaction sometimes produced by a first injection of melarsoprol in patients who have received no previous treatment. Melarsoprol is a very toxic drug. It can cause renal damage, rashes, and bone marrow depression, but its most serious side effect is the production of an encephalopathy which occurs in about 5 per cent of patients receiving a full course of treatment with the drug. This complication occurs most frequently at the time of the third or fourth injection. The onset of encephalopathy may be sudden or gradual. Severe headache, fever, convulsions, and coma may ensue and death occurs in about one half of the patients developing this complication. The pathogenesis of melarsoprol encephalopathy is not understood. It is not known whether it is due to poisoning with the arsenic present in the compound or whether it is due to some form of allergic response to trypanosomes killed in the brain by the drug. On the assumption that the encephalopathy is due to arsenic poisoning, dimercaprol (BAL) has been used in its treatment but the efficacy of this approach has never been clearly substantiated. Melarsoprol encephalopathy is not prevented by prophylactic administration of corticosteroids.

Treatment of relapses. A relapse of advanced Gambian or Rhodesian sleeping sickness treated initially with melarsoprol should be treated with a further three courses of melarsoprol (total 40 ml for an adult given in combination with nitrofurazone. Nitrofurazone is given by mouth; the adult dosage is 0.5 g three or four times a day for seven days. Nitrofurazone is another very toxic drug which can cause peripheral neuropathy and haemolytic anaemia, the latter complication being especially likely in those who are glucose 6-phosphatase dehydrogenase deficient.

Other chemotherapeutic agents. Tryparsamide, once widely used in the treatment of sleeping sickness, should no longer be given because resistance to the drug is widespread and because it can cause optic neuritis. Mel W is soluble in water, and therefore does not need to be given intravenously, but is as toxic as melarsoprol and is of unproven efficacy in Rhodesian sleeping sickness. Berenil has been used successfully to treat Rhodesian sleeping sickness.

A new, effective drug which is safer than melarsoprol is urgently needed. Experimental studies have indicated several ways of interfering with the metabolism of African trypanosomes. Thus haem, and some related porphyrins, are trypanocidal because they split endogenously produced hydrogen peroxide into toxic-free radicals. Unfortunately the commercial prospects of a new drug for the treatment of sleeping sickness are poor. Development of any promising new compound by a pharmaceutical company is unlikely to take place unless non-profit-making agencies offer financial support.

Course and prognosis. The clinical course of sleeping sickness is very variable. Some patients with Rhodesian sleeping sickness die from cardiac failure within weeks of the onset of symptoms whilst many patients with Gambian sleeping sickness remain relatively well for many years. However, once the central nervous system has been invaded death is inevitable unless treatment is given.

Most patients with early sleeping sickness make a rapid and complete recovery following treatment. However, a few patients who have been treated with suramin subsequently develop neurological signs, probably because they had undetected invasion of the central nervous system at the time that they were first seen. Patients with early sleeping sickness should, therefore, be followed up carefully for at least one year after treatment and their cerebrospinal fluid should be re-examined at the end of this period.

Parasitological cure is achieved in at least 90 per cent of patients with advanced sleeping sickness treated with melarsoprol. Clinical cure is often achieved but, unfortunately, some patients are left with permanent neurological sequelae. These residual neurological signs may be confused with those produced by a parasitological relapse requiring further treatment. Persistence of a high CSF IgM for longer than one year after treatment strongly suggests reactivation of the infection, even if trypanosomes cannot be found in the CSF.

An attack of sleeping sickness does not induce any protective immunity, and reinfection may follow successful treatment of an initial episode.

Prevention. Many different approaches have been made to the control of sleeping sickness; these are summarized in Fig. 4. Some control campaigns have resulted in a marked fall in the incidence of the infection. However, it is sometimes forgotten that in other areas where no control programmes have been undertaken the disease has disappeared equally dramatically.

Gambian sleeping sickness   Rhodesian sleeping sickness

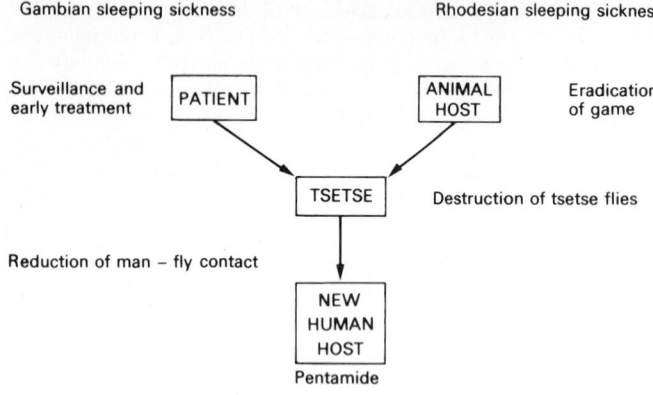

Surveillance and   PATIENT   ANIMAL   Eradication
early treatment   HOST   of game

TSETSE   Destruction of tsetse flies

Reduction of man – fly contact

NEW
HUMAN
HOST

Pentamide

Fig. 4   Methods for controlling sleeping sickness.

In West Africa extensive surveillance schemes have been employed to detect and treat cases of sleeping sickness as soon as possible, thus reducing the reservoir of the infection. Such schemes have been very effective but, when the incidence of the infection falls to a very low level, they are no longer cost effective. In East Africa attempts have been made to reduce the reservoir of infection by destruction of game but the effectiveness of this approach is uncertain. Game destruction is very unpopular with nature conservationists and commercially undesirable in countries with an important safari tourist industry.

Elimination of tsetse flies is now being attempted in several parts of Africa in order to control animal trypanosomiasis. As an added bonus such control schemes also destroy the vectors of human sleeping sickness. Methods of eliminating tsetse flies range in scope from hand catching to extensive aerial spraying with insecticides.

Pentamide, given by intramuscular injection in a dose of 4 mg/kg every three months, can prevent Gambian sleeping sickness; but its prophylactic value in Rhodesian sleeping sickness has not been clearly shown. However, there is a risk that pentamide used in this way will produce cryptic infections. The drug can cause diabetes and peripheral neuritis. Thus, pentamidine prophylaxis can be recommended only for those who are going to be exposed to a high risk of infection for a short period.

The ability of *T. brucei* trypanosomes to undergo antigenic variation makes the development of a vaccine against sleeping sickness very difficult and there has, so far, been little progress in this field.

References

Ford, J. (1971). *The role of African trypanosomiases in African ecology.* Clarendon Press, Oxford.

Greenwood, B. M. and Whittle, H. C. (1981). The pathogenesis of sleeping sickness. *Trans. R. Soc. trop. Med. Hyg.* **74**, 716.

The Lancet (1978). New leads for trypanosomiasis chemotherapy. *Lancet* **ii**, 1190.

Mulligan, H. W. (1970). *The African trypanosomiases.* Allen and Unwin, London.

Vickerman, K. (1978). Antigenic variation in trypanosomes. *Nature, Lond.* **273**, 613.

World Health Organization and Food and Agriculture Organization (1979). *The African trypanosomiases. Wld Hlth Org. Tech. Rep. Ser. no. 365.*

American trypanosomiasis: Chagas' disease

P. D. Marsden

No eponym is more richly deserved, for Carlos Chagas in the decades after his discovery was announced in 1909 described the life cycle and the principle manifestations in man of *Trypanosoma cruzi* infection.

Restricted to North and South America the cycle of transmission of *T. cruzi* between blood sucking triatomine bugs (Fig. 1) and mammals is longstanding in evolutionary time. This is reflected in

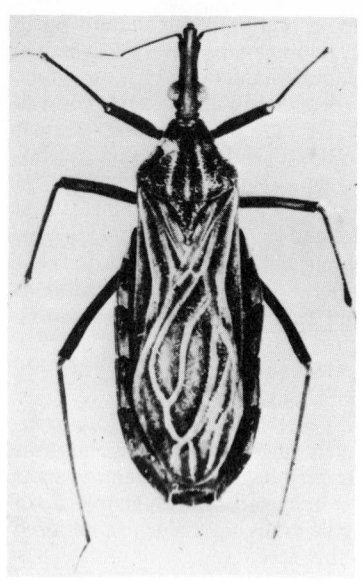

Fig. 1 *Rhodnius prolixus* adult (approximately three times natural size. (By courtesy of the Wellcome Museum of Medical Science.)

documentation of more than 100 mammalian reservoirs. *T. cruzi* does not infect birds or reptiles. The majority of vector bugs are linked with these sylvatic cycles but several species have adapted to live with man, possibly because blood meal sources became scarce and man is a large blood reservoir. Bug-infested houses are of poor quality with cracks in the mud walls providing hiding places for the bugs (Fig. 2). Bugs tend to localize in the house fabric near blood meal sources (e.g. over beds). They are nocturnal feeders and, once having ingested an infected blood meal, can remain infected for their natural lives (two years). Transmission is by contamination with bug faeces containing infected trypanosomes. With a rise in intra-abdominal pressure during feeding, many bugs defaecate while on the skin. Like African trypanosomiasis Chagas' disease transmission usually in remote rural communities. Although many bug species are vectors, the three most important ones are *Triatoma infestans* (Argentina, Chile, and central and southern Brazil), *Rhodnius prolixus* (Venezuela and Columbia), and *Panstrongylus megistus* (northeast Brazil). Transmission of *T. cruzi* to man has occurred in all South and Central American countries, Mexico, and in the state of Texas in the United States. Countries where it constitutes a big public health problem are Brazil, Argentina, Venezuela, Chile, Peru, and Bolivia. In Brazil transmission to man is almost unknown in the Amazon basin since the few bug species present are sylvatic, and an Indian house, having no walls, is unsuitable for bug colonization.

Different geographical regions show differences in the pathogenicity to man of the *T. cruzi* strains present in the area.

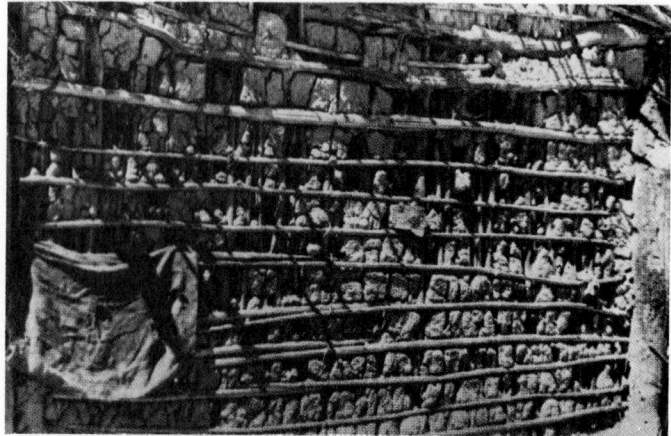

Fig. 2   A wall made of wooden lath and mud—an ideal bug habitat. (By courtesy of the Wellcome Museum of Medical Science.)

Examples are the high prevalence of symptomatic acute cases in northern Argentina. Megasyndromes are common on the Brazilian Central Plateau but absent in Venezuela. Cardiomyopathy is common in both these countries but relatively rare in Chile. Positive seroreactors in central Brazil have more electrocardiographic changes than those in the extreme south of that country. *T. cruzi* strains from Argentina and Chile respond better to antitrypanosomal drug therapy than those of Brazil. Using new biochemical taxonomic methods (isoenzyme, buoyant density of DNA) these strain differences are being currently investigated.

While the great majority of new infections occurring yearly are in children in the first decade of life living in bug infested houses, interest is now being shown in transmission by blood transfusion and congenital infections. The importance of these is still not clear. In general documentation of the size of the problem of American trypanosomiasis in each country is improving. For instance Venezuela estimates one million infected people and Brazil has recently completed a nationwide serological survey giving an estimate of six million human infections. In some states of Brazil up to 20 per cent of the population has positive serology. A distinction must be made, however, between positive serology, indicating evidence of *T. cruzi* infection, and Chagas' disease where there is clinical evidence of organ damage. To establish the prevalence of the latter, a nationwide electrocardiographic survey in positive seroreactors is in progress in Brazil.

Pathogenesis. *Trypanosoma cruzi* can be seen directly in the peripheral blood only in the acute phase of the disease. In fact its presence is the best definition of the acute phase since all other signs are variable. It is a trypanomastigote with a very large kinetoplast (a DNA organelle characteristic of this family). Multiplication only occurs in the amastigote phase which grows a variety of tissue cells especially muscle. Chronic inflammation of the heart muscle and the smooth muscle of the gut is the basis of the pathology, the infiltrate being mainly of lymphocytes and plasma cells. Early in the infection such infiltrates in the heart muscle are associated with amastigote nests but in chronic cases parasites cannot be found. An auto-immune process has been suggested to explain this finding. There is some evidence that *T. cruzi* shares a common antigen with heart muscle stimulating sensitized lymphocytes to destroy non-parasitized muscle fibres. A circulating auto-antibody (endothelial-vascular-interstitial antibody or EVI) has been detected in chagasic patients but the titre of this antibody does not correlate well with the presence of cardiomyopathy.

The Chagasic heart at autopsy shows a thinning of the ventricular muscle and frequently an apical aneurysm. Many muscle fibres are fragmented and the infiltration of lymphocytes and plasma cells is associated with areas of oedema, degeneration, and haemorrhage.

After the initial wave of parasitaemia the number of circulating trypanosomes falls below detectable levels. IgM and IgG antibodies, however, usually appear within a month. The presence of IgM antibodies assists in confirming congenital Chagas' disease in the neonate. However, as in the treponematoses, small numbers of viable organisms persist in the tissues probably for life. Decades after the childhood infection the chronic cardiomyopathy may result in heart muscle failure or conduction disturbances due to inflammation of the Purkinje fibres. A similar inflammation around parasympathetic ganglia in the smooth muscle of the gut wall leads to inco-ordinated peristalsis. Solid residues accumulating in the oesophagus and colon give rise to megasyndromes.

Clinical presentation and diagnosis. Patients usually know the triatomid bugs well. It is very important to ask for a past history of living in a bug-infested house and to have a specimen of the bugs to show the patient available in the outpatient department.

There are three phases of the infection. The acute phase usually passes unnoticed but there may be a inflamed swelling or chagoma at the site of entry of the trypanosomes. Romañas sign is when this swelling involves the eyelids. Such clinical evidence of local para-

sitic multiplication occurs in about half of the detected cases. Reticulo-endothelial activation is evidenced by hepatosplenomegaly and lymphadenopathy. There is less than a 5 per cent mortality in this phase; either from acute heart failure or meningo-encephalitis. Congenital Chagas' disease is acute Chagas' disease in the neonate and clinically can closely resemble other neonatal infections such as toxoplasmosis, cytomegalic inclusion disease, and syphilis. Abortions are more frequent in infected pregnant women. Laboratory investigation detects the circulating trypanosomes in fresh blood smears. Failing this the strout technique, where the supernatant from clotted blood is examined, is usually positive. There is a lymphocytosis and often a false positive unabsorbed Paul Bunnel test. Blood cultures, mouse innoculation, and xenodiagnosis all reveal circulating *T. cruzi*.

The term intermediate phase is useful to emphasize that, after infection in early life, decades may pass before clinical syndromes appear. During this time the patient has evidence of infection but not disease, the definition of this phase. Detection is based on serology which has improved greatly in recent years. Ideally complement fixation, indirect fluorescent antibody, and indirect haemagglutination tests should all be done on the same sera and usually there is close concordance. Fifty per cent of these patients have small numbers of circulating trypanosomes detectable by xenodiagnosis, a technique where uninfected bugs are fed on the patient and subsequently examined 30 days later for infection. Xenodiagnosis tends to be more frequently positive in younger patients in this phase.

From the field study in São Felipe, Bahia, comes information on the outcome of this phase. In 10 years follow-up of 400 patients 96 (24 per cent) developed electrocardiographic abnormalities and 5 clinically detectable megaoesophagus. In many patients with positive serology disease never appears. The most famous case is Berenice who at age two was diagnosed in the acute phase by Carlos Chagas himself. Now an old woman she has no detectable heart or gut pathology.

The chronic phase of Chagas' disease appears decades after infection but a rare subacute form has been described where heart muscle failure supervened months after the acute phase. Chagasic cardiomyopathy has two principle manifestations, heart muscle failure and conduction defects. Bilateral ventricular failure is the rule since a panmyocarditis is the pathology. Therefore patients usually have little pulmonary oedema but marked congestive failure. Intraventricular thrombi are common, and systemic or pulmonary emboli may be the initial sign of this disease. Heart size is variable but it is frequently greatly enlarged with feeble pulsation on screening. There are no organic valvular lesions, only functional mitral or tricuspid incompetence. Complete right bundle branch block with left anterior hemiblock is a very characteristic ECG finding but extrasystoles and any form of AV conduction defect may be present. Left bundle branch block and atrial fibrillation are rare. Complete heart block with Stokes–Adams attacks may cause the patient's admission to hospital. Repeated heart failure, massive embolus, or cardiac arrest are common causes of death. Severe heart disease is commoner in males 30–50 years old (possibly due to increased cardiac work in this sex).

Megaoesophagus has been classified into four degrees of severity depending mainly on oesophageal diameter on barium swallow. In the most severe grades (III and IV) difficulty in swallowing may lead to wasting and parotid gland hypertrophy (the 'cat face'). Food residue overspill may produce lung infections and bronchiectasis. The patient gives a clear history of swallowing difficulty and with each mouthful may need water to accomplish deglution. Likewise megacolon is associated with abnormal constipation (weeks). Faecal impaction, sigmoid volvulus, and toxic megacolon with *E. coli* septicemia are side effects of megacolon.

The role of parasympathetic denervation producing other gastrointestinal, endocrine, and renal abnormalities has to be further defined. Absence of patellar reflexes in seropositive patients suggesting peripheral neuropathy has been recently described.

Laboratory diagnosis relies heavily on positive serology as in the treponematoses. Xenodiagnosis is only indicated as a specialized investigative procedure since serology is now reliable. Serology should be checked by one of the central reference laboratories if the laboratory concerned has little experience with the tests. Patients with leishmaniasis may have positive titres. Apparently no cross reaction occurs with *T. rangeli*.

Treatment and prevention. It is generally agreed that the acute stage should be treated with an antitrypanocidal drug since parasympathetic ganglia damage is thought to occur in the acute stage and theoretically the parasitaemia reduction achieved with such drugs should be advantageous. Two drugs are in common use nifurtimox (Lampit) is given in an oral dose of 8 mg per kg body weight for 60 or 90 days. The longer course of 120 days shows no better results on follow-up and is prone to more side-effects especially convulsions and psychosis. Benzimidazole (Rochagan) is given in an oral dose of 6 mg per kg body weight for 30 or 60 days. A serious side-effect, fortunately rare, is an exfoliative dermatitis. Both drugs produce anorexia, weight loss, headache and dizziness, gastric irritation, and in 12–30 per cent peripheral neuritis.

There is no evidence that patients in the intermediate or chronic phase benefit from such drug therapy. Evolution of the disease with or without these drugs in such studies as are available at the present time appears to be the same. Control of heart failure with digitalis and diuretics is of benefit but the response is frequently not good. Digitalis sensitivity is common especially in the presence of hypokalaemia. Anti-arrhythmia drugs must be used with caution. Procaine amide and lignocaine may help in ventricular tachycardia or multiple extrasystoles. Beta-adrenergic blocking agents may produce bradycardia and shock, and propranalol is contra-indicated.

Pacemaker implantation to relieve severe heart block has a better prognosis if the heart is of normal size. Patients with embolization may benefit from anticoagulation. Early megaoesophagus can be relieved by balloon dilatation but established severe megaoesophagus and megacolon require surgery. Cardiotomy is giving good results in megaoesophagus. Half the patients with megaoesophagus have abnormal electrocardiograms.

Congenital Chagas' disease and transfusion acute disease require Lampit or Rochagan therapy. Transfusion infection can be prevented by either rejecting seropositive potential donors or, failing this mixing the blood with gentian violet for 24 hours (dilution 1:4000). We have so many donors in our hospital in Brasilia with positive serology that we cannot afford to reject them. Using gentian violet we have never had a case of transfusion infection.

The effectiveness of residual insecticides in controlling domestic bug population was first reported in the 1940s. Since then widespread campaigns have been conducted in many South American countries. Obviously fresh infections occurring yearly in children pose a problem for hospital medical services in the future. Although the economic impact of this disease cannot be calculated, it must be considerable both in terms of morbidity and mortality in farming communities and in the strain it poses on hospital services. Chagas' disease is the commonest cause of admission to our medical service in Brasilia.

Since reduviids are often resistant to DDT, hexachlorocyclohexane (BHC or HCH), or hexachlor-dimethanonaphthelene (Dieldrin) are the chlorinated hydrocarbon residual insecticides most frequently used. HCH (Gammexane) is used in a dose of 500 mg per square metre of wall and dieldrin 1 g per square metre. The walls and roof of a house are sprayed as are out-houses with permanent animals such as chicken houses. Domestic animals may show toxicity. Care must be taken to avoid contamination of water sources, food, cooking utensils, and infant bedding. The frequency of retreatment depends in the insecticide and surface treated. Residual activity on mud walls of HCH in tropical climate conditions is only two to three months. The survival of eggs and bugs in the wall necessitates repeated spraying. Often this has been carried on for years although there is evidence in the literature that two sprayings

three months apart may be sufficient. The emergence of resistance to these insecticides in *Rhodnius prolixus* and *Triatoma maculata* in Venezuela underlines the necessity for proceeding with all possible speed in the spraying of still virgin areas of transmission. It might be asked why this has not already been done? Often areas of active transmission are remote and roads only passable in the dry season. Also the cost is a governing factor. Many years ago Pinotti estimated that it cost US$2 to spray a house.

Apart from insecticide spraying, house improvement is also important. In endemic areas in Venezuela many new houses have been built but this is expensive. Walling up the bugs with new plaster is initially effective until this too cracks or the bugs escape into the the roof. A third factor is community participation, and a householder actively killing bugs and reporting their presence after a spraying control programme will have a noticeable effect.

An economic control programme will utilize all three factors together. Certainly in Brazil, the country with the largest infected population, the situation will continue to improve as a result of Ministry of Health control programmes. However, for decades a large number of patients with cardiomyopathy and megasyndromes will continue to be seen in the hospital outpatient service due to the long period of evolution of a *T. cruzi* infection acquired in childhood.

References

Brener, Z. and Andrade, Z. (1979). *Trypanosoma cruzi e doença de Chagas*. Ed. Guanabara Koogan, Rio de Janeiro.
Koberle, F. (1968). Chagas' disease and Chagas' syndromes: the pathology of American trypanosomiasis. In *Advances in Parasitology*. (ed. B. Dawes), vol. 6. 63.
Marsden, P. D. (1971). South American trypanosoamiasis (Chagas' disease). *Int. Rev. trop. Med.* **4**. 97.
PAHO. (1975). *American trypanosomiasis research*, 318. PAHO Scientific Publication, no. 318, Washington, DC.
Prata, A., Andrade, Z., and Guimarães, A. (1974). Chagas' heart disease. In *Cardiovascular disease in the tropics* (ed. A. C. Shaper, M. S. R. Hutt, and A. Fejfar). British Medical Association, London.
Trypanosomiasis and leishmaniasis with special reference to Chagas' disease (1974). *Ciba Foundation Symposium*, no. 2 (new series). Associated Scientific Publishers, Amsterdam.
World Health Organization (1974). Immunology of Chagas' disease. *Bull. Wld Hlth Org.* **50**, 459.

Leishmaniasis

P. E. C. Manson-Bahr

Leishmaniasis is a communicable disease caused by protozoa of the genus *Leishmania* which have an intracellular (*amastigote*) form in man and other mammals, and an extracellular flagellate (*promastigote*) form in various species of sandfly whose bites are responsible for transmitting the infection from host to host. Infections by *L. tropica* and *L. mexicana* are limited to the skin; infection by *L. braziliensis* to the skin and mucous membranes; and *L. donovani* infects the entire reticuloendothelial system causing kala azar.

Aetiology. The leishmanial amastigote or Leishman–Donovan body (Fig. 1) is an ovoidal or rounded body about 2–3 μm in length which lives intracellularly in monocytes, polymorphonuclear leucocytes, and endothelial cells. Its cytoplasm stains pale blue with Giemsa and Wright's stains. The large round nucleus is seen as a mass of red staining granules and the characteristic *kinetoplast*, a round body in the cytoplasm, stains bright red or reddish purple. The cultural or flagellate form is a pear shaped, or slender spindle shaped, body 15–25 μm in length and 1.5–3.5 μm in width, with a single flagellum 15–28 μm long. Material such as skin, spleen pulp, sternal marrow, or blood may be cultured on a biphasic medium of agar and fresh rabbit blood, Novy–Nicolle–McNeal medium (NNN), or Schneider's insect medium. Promastigotes take up to 21 days to appear in NNN, but three to five days on the insect medium. Hamsters are very susceptible to leishmaniasis. They die three to six months after the intraperitoneal injection of infected material, and are useful for detecting very small numbers of leishmania in biological material.

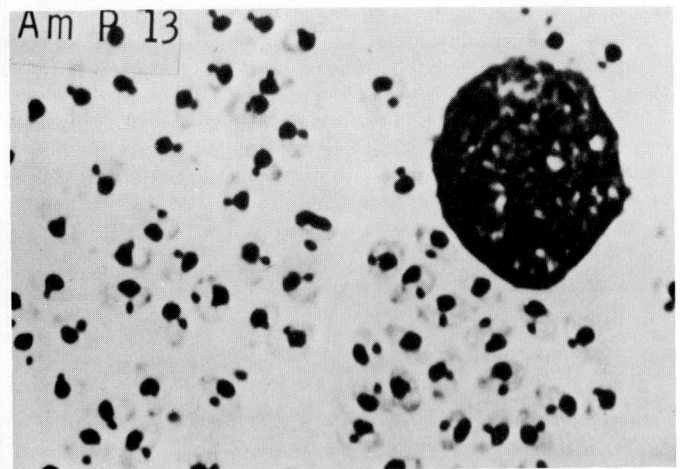

Fig. 1 Leishman-Donovan bodies (× 3200).

Epidemiology. Leishmaniasis is essentially a zoonosis. It can be found in an environment varying from the humid rain forests of South and Central America (*L. mexicana* and *L. braziliensis*) to the dry savannah of Africa south of the Sahara, and deserts of the Middle East (*L. tropica* and *L. donovani*). The reservoirs, rodents and canine, vary; and transmission to man is by sandflies, and in the case of kala azar rarely by blood transfusion, and transplacentally. Female sandflies are infected by feeding on mammals with leishmaniasis. In the anterior portion of the gut ingested amastigotes develop into the infective promastigote forms which move to the salivary glands in about 10 days and are inoculated into a susceptible host at the second feed. Sandflies require a humid microclimate with decomposing organic matter for breeding. Their life cycle lasts from 1½ to 2 months in summer and warm climates, but is extended in colder climates. The adults are normally nocturnal but some bite during the day especially if disturbed. They can fly from a few to hundreds of metres.

Leishmania tropica (Oriental sore). *Leishmania tropica* is the cause of cutaneous leishmaniasis of the Old World and is a parasite of rodents, principally the giant gerbil (*Rhomobomys opimus*) in Central Asia and the Middle East. In some areas other small rodents (*Meriones*) play a part. A high percentage of gerbils may be infected and small lesions on the tail or ear are usual. Transmission of infection to man by sandfly bite occurs when communal gerbil burrows exist near (3–5 km) villages or when people visit desert areas frequented by gerbils. Rural or moist cutaneous lesihmaniasis (*L. major*) results. In other parts of the Middle East dogs are the reservoir and the infection is transmitted mainly in cities causing urban or dry cutaneous leishmaniasis (*L. tropica*). In endemic areas children are mainly infected and almost every adult in the Middle East has a scar of an Oriental sore. Non-immune adults from non-endemic areas can become infected; and epidemics may occur if the number of non-immunes is sufficient.

Leishmania mexicana. *Leishmania mexicana* is the cause of cutaneous leishmaniasis of the New World which is confined to the skin and occurs in Central America and northern South America. It is an infection of small forest rodents (white-tailed mouse, spiny rat, and others) in which the infection may be inapparent or cause small indistinct lesions on the tail. Transmission is by forest sandflies in small enzootic foci in the humid rain forest areas of Guatemala and Mexico: humans are infected when they enter the forest as

woodcutters or to collect gum (chicle) hence the name 'chiclero's ulcer'.

Leishmania braziliensis. *Leishmania braziliensis* is the cause of New World mucocutaneous leishmaniasis (espundia) which is a zoonosis found in the neotropics of South America, chiefly in Amazonian Brazil. The hosts are small forest rodents; transmission takes place in well-defined enzootic areas in the forest. When the forest is disturbed for development or road building, devastating epidemics may occur which have led to the failure of these projects. Espundia is a destructive mucocutaneous lesion of the nose and mouth which is a major cause of ill health and low morale in construction camps and settlements in the Amazon region.

Leishmania donovani. *Leishmania donovani* is the cause of kala azar. It is an infection of the domestic dog, wild canines (foxes and jackals), and also some small rodents. In the Mediterranean, Middle Asia, and Middle East it is an urban and peridomestic infection, with the dog as the reservoir; or it may be rural with jackals as reservoirs in the Middle East, and foxes in southern Europe. Infants under five years of age are the chief victims (infantile kala azar), but non resident (non-immune) adults can also be infected. The disease is sporadically endemic, and not epidemic. The vast majority of infections are inapparent.

In Africa (Sudan and East Africa) rodents may be a source of infection. Inter-human transmission also occurs, and epidemics lasting up to 10 years occur every 15 years, and are a cause of depopulation and social disturbance. Young adults are chiefly affected.

In India, where transmission is exclusively interhuman, cessation of insecticidal spraying for malaria eradication has led to the reappearance of kala azar in epidemic form.

In South America (northeast Brazil) the reservoir is the dog and fox, but interhuman transmission and epidemics occur resembling those in East Africa.

Immunity. The introduction of infective promastigotes from a sandfly bite initiates a cellular immune response, similar to that of tuberculosis and leprosy, and the infection is eradicated in the majority of cases. The essential pathological change is the formation of a granuloma. In the majority of cases, at least with *L. donovani*, the infection is inapparent: the parasite is eradicated and a permanent immunity to reinfection develops. This immunity is to a homologous strain, but strains vary in their cross immunity. *L. major* protects against *L. tropica* but not vice versa. *L. braziliensis* protects against *L. mexicana* but not the reverse. None protects against *L. donovani* except the homologous strain. The development of immunity and delayed hypersensitivity is shown by the *leishmanin* skin test which is similar to the tuberculin test. Leishmanin is a suspension of washed promastigotes in 0.5 per cent phenol saline; 0.1 ml (1 000 000 organisms) is injected intracutaneously. A positive result is shown at 48–72 hours by the development of an indurated area which can be measured in the same way as the tuberculin reaction. The reaction is not intraspecific and can be induced by any species of leishmania; it denotes previous infection and can be used epidemiologically as well as diagnostically. Leishmanin testing on an age-related basis in a community can be useful in demonstrating the endemicity of leishmanial infection.

Immunopathology. In cutaneous leishmaniasis the infection is confined to the skin. The reaction is a granuloma surrounding macrophages containing amastigotes. The spectrum of reaction varies, as in leprosy, from a well-marked granulomatous reaction with few or no parasites, to a widespread infection with numerous macrophages containing amastigotes and little cellular reaction (diffuse cutaneous leishmaniasis and kala azar). Humoral immunity is not important, but specific antibodies are found in kala azar and espundia. In kala azar, large amounts of IgG are produced by the hypertrophied parasitized reticulo-endothelial system. This is neither protective nor specific, but is responsible for the great increase in gamma globulin in this condition.

Clinical features

Cutaneous leishmaniasis of the Old World (Oriental sore). The clinical features vary with the degree of host resistance and strain of parasite.

L. major typically causes single or multiple lesions with a short incubation period, rapid growth, considerable tissue reaction, and scanty parasites. These heal in less than a year.

L. tropica causes a single ulcer with a longer incubation period, less tissue reaction, and more parasites. Ulcers last longer than a year.

The *incubation period* can be days, weeks, or months and has been as long as three years. The local lesion (Fig. 2) begins as a minute itching papule that expands as a shotty, congested infiltration of the dermis. After a few days or weeks the papule becomes covered with fine papery scales that later become moister, brown, and adherent. A crust is formed which, on falling off or being scratched off, uncovers a shallow ulcer with a raised indurated base. Histologically the appearance is that of a non caseating granuloma with varying numbers of amastigote, filled macrophages, and superficial secondary infection. Micro-abscesses do not occur. The sore extends by erosion at its edge and by satellite lesions (Fig. 2). After two to 12 months or more, healing sets in, often beginning in the centre while the ulcer continues to extend at its edge. Ultimately a depressed white or pinkish scar forms; contraction may cause unsightly deformities especially on the face. Oriental sores may be single or multiple: two or three are not uncommon, and in rare instances as many as 150 have been found on one patient. Because of the site of inoculation, ulcers are mostly situated on the face, hands, feet, arms and legs, occasionally on the tip of the nose or lower lip, and rarely on the upper eyelids (ocular leishmaniasis). Sometimes the initial papule subsides without ulceration. Oriental sore does not cause death but is troublesome and unsightly. In many parts of the Middle East, especially Iraq and Iran, most adults bear the typical scar of a healed sore contracted in childhood.

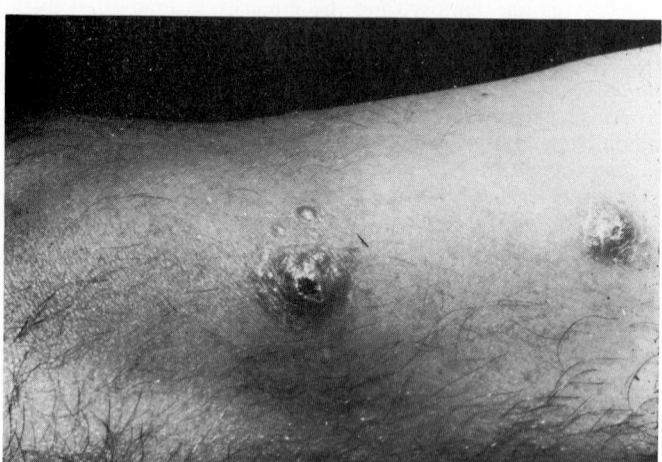

Fig. 2   Cutaneous leishmaniasis. *L. major* lesion on forearm. Well-marked satellite lesions. Mali, West Africa.

American cutaneous leishmaniasis. Two main types of cutaneous leishmaniasis are found in the New World. *L. mexicana* causes a single non-metastasizing skin lesion (chiclero's ulcer), which subsides spontaneously in about six months. *L. braziliensis* causes a single or primary skin lesion which heals but later metastasizes to other areas of the skin and mucous membranes (espundia).

Chiclero's ulcer; bay sore; forest yaws. The lesion is found on exposed areas of the body, usually the face and commonly on the pinna of the ear (chiclero's ear) where it causes a very chronic destructive lesion which may persist for 20 years and cause destruction of the pinna. Elsewhere the lesion is small and self-limiting, healing spontaneously in less than six months.

Espundia. The lesion begins as a nodule or ulcer on an exposed area of the skin or mucous membranes of the nose or mouth. It heals in a few months leaving a characteristic scar. After an interval of months, or in some cases years, intractable fungating ulcers break out on the tongue, buccal or nasal cavities (Fig. 3) destroying and obstructing them, and leading to eventual death from secondary infection after years of suffering. The histological changes are those of a granuloma with varying degrees of necrosis and micro-abscesses. The lymph glands may be involved but the viscera escape.

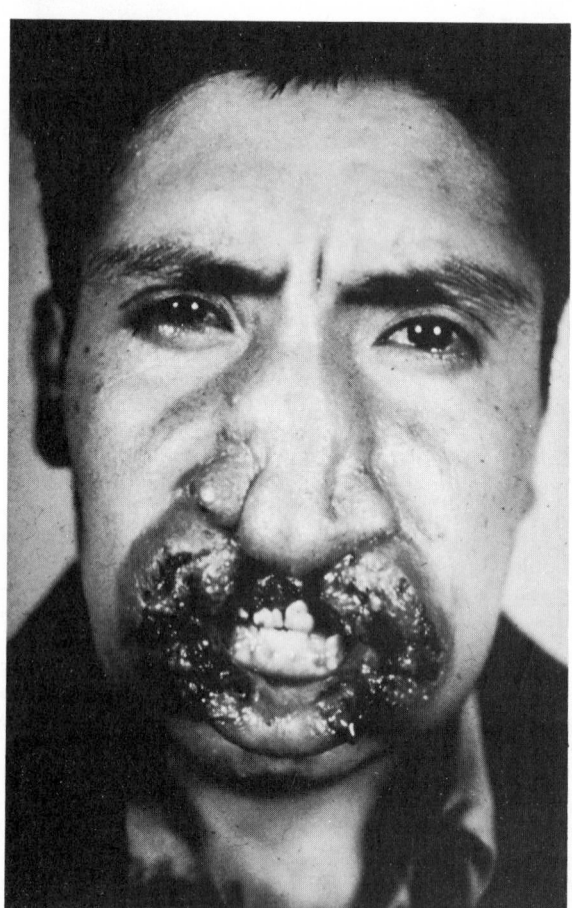

Fig. 3   Espundia (mucocutaneous leishmaniasis) (courtesy of Professor P. D. Marsden, Brazil).

When a primary sore develops, it cannot be predicted whether it will metastasize or not: the incidence of metastasis varies from 2 per cent in Panama to 80 per cent in Paraguay. Destruction of the nasal septum produces a characteristic 'tapir' nose and ulceration may extend to the pharynx.

Unusual forms of cutaneous leishmaniasis

Leishmaniasis recidiva. This form is found chiefly in Iraq, Iran, and Anatolia. The cellular immune response is not sufficient to eradicate the infection completely and a chronic relapsing tuberculoid type of lesion occurs, closely resembling lupus vulgaris. Relapses occur after preliminary healing, and a scar forms in the centre with nodules and papules extending at the periphery. Amastigotes are impossible to demonstrate in the 'apple-jelly' nodules and this form of leishmaniasis is extremely resistant to treatment. The leishmanin test is strongly positive indicating a high degree of delayed hypersensitivity.

Diffuse cutaneous leishmaniasis. In parts of Venezuela and in the Ethiopian Highlands a very chronic form of cutaneous leishmaniasis may be found in areas where typical cutaneous leishmaniasis is by far the commonest form.

The lesion begins as a nodule which never ulcerates but gradually spreads to involve the whole body. It specially affects the nose but, unlike lepromatous leprosy which it otherwise closely resembles, does not destroy the nasal septum. Amastigotes are numerous in macrophages in the lesions, which show little cellular reaction. This variety is a result of failure of the specific host's cell-mediated immunity. The course may extend for 20 years or more and resists any form of treatment, with the occasional exception of repeated courses of pentamidine.

Kala azar (visceral leishmaniasis). All the geographical forms of kala azar are generally similar in their clinical features. A primary skin lesion is found in Africa and in Middle Asia. Amastigotes are common in the skin in the African, American, and Chinese forms. Post kala azar dermal leishmanoid is common in India, less common in Africa, and unknown elsewhere.

Pathology. The pathological changes depend upon the level of resistance in the host. The self healing forms show a cell-mediated esponse in which multiple granulomas are found in the liver, spleen, and lymph glands. Parasites are few or absent. Since the great majority of infections are inapparent, these changes are rarely seen. In the *kala azar syndrome*, where there is little or no immune response, the liver, spleen, lymph glands, and bone marrow are filled with amastigote laden histiocytes especially in the portal tracts of the liver. The spleen is grossly enlarged due to reticuloendothelial hypertrophy and a considerable portion of its substance is composed of amastigotes. There are usually numerous infarcts and in more resistant cases granulomatous nodules with few or no demonstrable parasites. But in fatal cases the portal tracts are packed with amastigote-filled Küpffer cells. The intestinal villi may be hypertrophied with reticuloendothelial proliferation and swollen with parasitized cells.

The *lymphatic glands* may contain numerous amastigote-filled histiocytes or show granulomata without parasites: these appearances closely resemble tuberculosis. The tonsils are commonly involved in a similar manner. The kidneys may show amyloid changes.

Haematological changes in kala azar are described below.

Clinical features. The primary lesion at the site of the infective bite is usually so small as to be undetectable. In the Sudan more extensive lesions have been described resembling epitheliomata.

The incubation or prepatent period is usually four to six months but up to 10 years has been described. With extension of the infection to the reticulo-endothelial cells of the spleen, liver, bone marrow and lymph glands the infection becomes apparent.

Symptoms. The onset may be abrupt or, more commonly in the inhabitants of endemic regions, insidious. Cough is frequent and pneumonia may be the cause for admission to hospital. Diarrhoea and even dysentery may be the presenting symptom, and epistaxis and fever are also common.

An insidious onset is associated with a chronic wasting disease with pain beneath the left costal margin resulting from an enlarging spleen. In cases with an acute onset the fever starts suddenly reaching 40 °C: rarely, there is a characteristic pattern with two maxima in the 24 hours. In spite of the fever the patient is ambulant and seems surprisingly well. In more chronic cases there is little or no fever. Lymph glands may show enlargement, especially in the inguinal region, or in the cervical region in the case of the tonsillar form found in the Mediterranean.

The spleen enlarges gradually so that eventually it may reach right into the right iliac fossa; at first it is soft but soon becomes hard. The liver enlarges but not to the same extent as the spleen: jaundice is found in about 10 per cent of patients.

Parasites may be found in the skin in the absence of any lesions. In India the skin acquires a strange earthy grey colour which gave rise to the Hindi name 'kala azar' or 'black fever'. Cutaneous lesions are not common but polymorphic and wartlike lesions may be associated with active infection in Africa, and in India post kala azar dermal leishmanoid occurs (see below).

The concentration of polyclonal IgG in the serum may reach 4 g/dl (Fig. 4) and is responsible for the positive formol gel test. Proteinuria is found in some patients to a greater degree than can be accounted for by the fever.

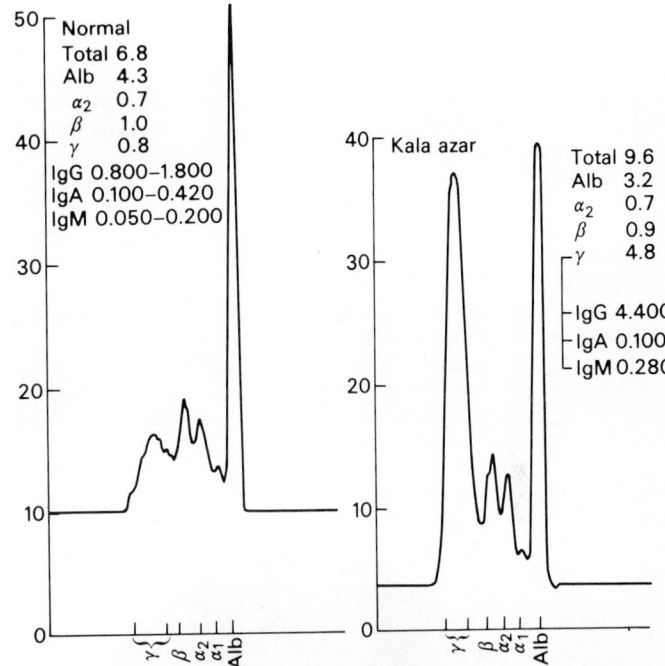

Fig. 4 Immunoglobulins in kala azar: IgG is greatly increased.

Haematological changes. Pancytopenia related to spleen size and duration of infection is a frequent finding in kala azar; and most of the changes can be accounted for by hypersplenism. There is a moderate to severe anaemia which is normocytic and normochromic. Haemoglobin values of 8 g/dl or below are common. There is a reduction of the life span of both autologous and homologous labelled RBCs with increased sequestration of cells in the spleen. The marrow is hypercellular with increased numbers of macrophages, and haemopoietic cells, and erythroid hyperplasia. Reticulocytosis is, however, usually mild and not appropriate to the severity of the anaemia. Leucopenia is usually mild to moderate (white count $2-4 \times 10^9$/l) and is usually due to neutropenia with a normal or reduced absolute lymphocyte count and relative monocytosis. Myelopoiesis shows a reduced number of mature neutrophils with numerous myelocytes.

There is moderate thrombocytopenia, the most common manifestation of which is epistaxis, which is rarely severe enough to be life threatening. The platelet count is usually $90-150 \times 10^9$/l but may rarely be as low as 20×10^9/l. Megakaryocytes are normal in number but show poor platelet formation.

Although the above changes implicate hypersplenism in the pancytopenia of kala azar, some patients present with a positive direct antiglobulin test with anti-complement sera, and others have an increased plasma clearance of radio-iron but with reduced iron incorporation. These observations suggest that additional factors, such as haemolysis and ineffective haemopoiesis, may also play a part in the anaemia or pancytopenia.

The pancytopenia of kala azar always responds to specific antiparasitic therapy.

Inapparent infection. In areas where kala azar is endemic, many of the inhabitants develop a positive leishmanin skin test although they have never had clinical kala azar. In these areas the leishmanin rate increases with age. Some other individuals recover after a short illness. In a population in Italy the attack rate, as measured by the leishmanin skin test, was 44 per cent; but clinical illness developed in only 3 per cent of those infected.

Unusual forms. *Acute toxic kala azar.* This form is rare and occurs mainly during epidemics. The course is short and often fatal with high fever, little or no splenic enlargement, and haemorrhagic manifestations. There may be extensive liver necrosis.

Lymphatic forms. Kala azar, especially in the Mediterranean, may present with general lymphatic glandular enlargement without any fever or other signs of visceral involvement. In one form the tonsils are involved with enlargement of the cervical lymph glands, giving the appearance of a tuberculous infection. Granulomatous changes in the glands add to the difficulty in diagnosis.

Nasopharyngeal and oral forms. Mucocutaneous espundia-like lesions of the mouth and nose, and warty tumours of the nasopharynx and larynx are found in the African form. These granulomatous lesions may or may not be associated with visceral disease and usually contain few amastigotes.

Post kala azar dermal leishmanoid (Fig. 5). This skin eruption appears from a few months to up to two years (in India) after recovery from kala azar. There are two constituents, a macular depigmented eruption found mainly on the face, arms, and upper trunk; and a warty papular eruption mainly on the face, which contains a varying number of amastigotes. At the time of the eruption there is no longer any visceral infection and the condition must be distinguished from lepromatous leprosy.

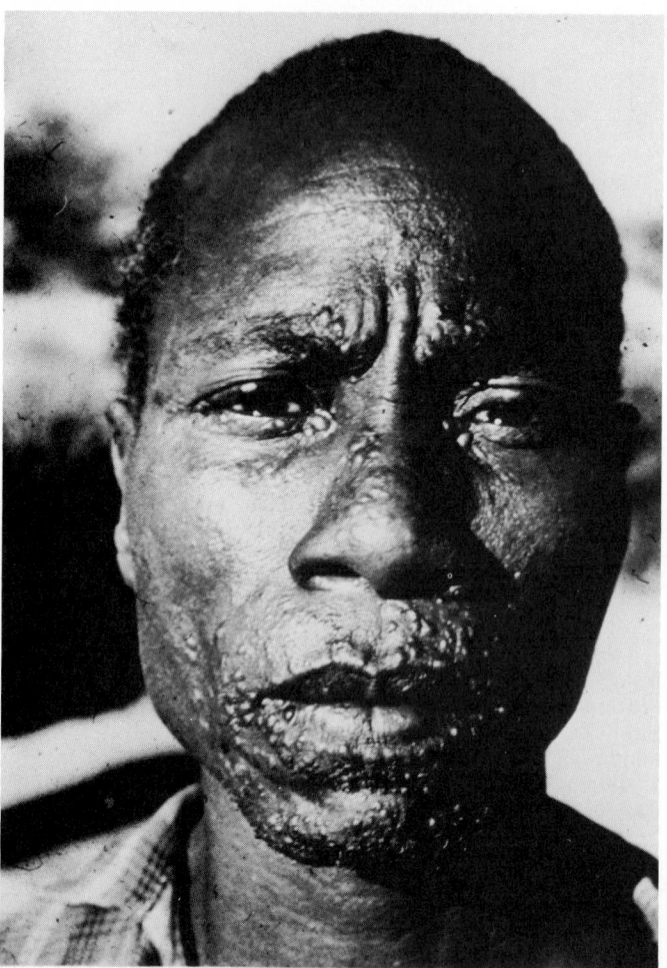

Fig. 5 Post kala azar dermal leishmanoid; papular eruption.

Diagnosis. The diagnosis is best made by demonstration of the parasites in smears of skin, spleen, bone marrow, liver, or lymph glands; culture on special media (NNN, Schneider's insect medium); or by intraperitoneal inoculation of hamsters (positive result takes six months).

In kala azar, spleen puncture is used when the spleen is large and firm and the prothrombin time normal. An 18–20 gauge or smaller needle is thrust through the anterior abdominal wall into the border of the spleen, the edge of which held by the left hand. The thumb of the right hand is then used to occlude the end of the needle, which is withdrawn, and the spleen pulp blown onto a slide and washed out with saline for culture and intraperitoneal inoculation of a hamster. The material on the slide is spread like a blood smear, stained with Giemsa, and examined for LD bodies. Sternal puncture is safer and more usually performed, but is not so productive. Splenic puncture is contra-indicated in children under five, in early cases, and where there is a haemorrhagic tendency. Liver biopsy is useful, but lymph gland puncture is only about 60 per cent effective. In cutaneous lesions a small portion of the whole of the edge of the lesion is biopsied and an impression smear is made before placing it in formol saline for histology.

Serology. *Leishmanin skin test* (see Immunopathology). This is a test of delayed hypersensitivity and cellular immunity to any species of leishmania. It becomes positive *par passu* with the development of delayed hypersensitivity, and denotes some form of immune response. In cutaneous leishmaniasis it becomes positive about two to three months after infection, but before complete healing has occurred. It remains positive for life and denotes exposure to some form of leishmaniasis in the past. It can be used for diagnosis of cutaneous leishmaniasis both of the Old and New World. In *Leishmaniasis recidiva* it is strongly positive but parasites are few so it is very useful. It is negative in kala azar until six to eight weeks after recovery, by which time all parasites have been eradicated.

Formol gel test. This is a measure of the globulin level of the blood. Blood is allowed to clot and the supernatant serum is drawn off. To 2 ml of serum 2 drops of 40 per cent formalin are added. The mixture is shaken and allowed to stand for 20 minutes. In a positive result the serum becomes solid with an opacity like the white of a hard-boiled egg. False positives may be found with a lesser degree of opacity whenever the immunoglobulins are increased to a significant degree, such as in African trypanosomiasis (IgM), chronic malaria, hepatosplenic schistosomiasis, and in multiple myeloma. The reaction is negative in cutaneous and mucocutaneous leishmaniasis.

Complement fixation test (CFT). Complement fixing antibodies are found only in kala azar. An antigen prepared from an acid-fast bacillus (Kedrowsky's bacillus) is used, and titres of 1:20 or over are significant. These appear early in kala azar when the disease is active but disappear within six months of cure. They are a good test of active infection.

Immunofluorescence. Fluorescent antibodies (FAT) appear early in kala azar and persist for two to three years after recovery. Titres of over 1:20 are significant and 1:28 diagnostic of active infection. Both the CFT, but more usefully the FAT, can be used to demonstrate the presence of inapparent infection. Cross reactions occur with African and American trypanosomiasis. In espundia the FAT becomes positive in the mucocutaneous state and can be very useful in diagnosis. The FAT is negative in all other forms of cutaneous leishmaniasis.

Differential diagnosis. Kala azar must be distinguished from other prolonged fevers of the tropics—malaria, typhoid, liver abscess, miliary tuberculosis, disseminated histoplasmosis, brucellosis, and reticuloses. The wasting may suggest starvation, pulmonary tuberculosis (which often accompanies kala azar), or malignant disease. The raised IgG levels may resemble myeloma, other macrogammaglobulinaemias, and collagen diseases. The splenomegaly must be distinguished from that of portal hypertension, especially hepatosplenic schistosomiasis, chronic malaria (tropical splenomegaly), myelogenous leukaemia, lymphatic leukaemia, some haemoglobinopathies, and other severe anaemias associated with splenomegaly.

Cutaneous and mucocutaneous leishmaniasis may resemble fungal, tuberculoid, syphilitic, or leprotic lesions and epitheliomata. The leishmanin test is useful and biopsy may confirm the diagnosis.

Prognosis. The natural course of cutaneous leishmaniasis due to *L. tropica* or *L. mexicana* is self limiting, but scarring is likely to be disfiguring especially where the lesions are on the face or are secondarily infected. The mucocutaneous lesions (espundia) caused by *L. braziliensis* may extend to secondary sites, become secondarily infected, and can cause death where there is extensive involvement of the nasopharynx and larynx. Most infections with *L. donovani* are inapparent, and others are self limiting and rarely diagnosed. Without treatment the kala azar syndrome is usually fatal for there is little resistance on the part of the host. African kala azar may run an acute course terminating in five months with severe anaemia, or fine lobular cirrhosis of the liver may develop. Haemorrhages can occur from any part of the body. Death results from exhaustion or intercurrent infection. *Noma* (gangrene of the face) is common in advanced cases. Other sequelae are pulmonary tuberculosis, and in advanced cases amyloid disease with amyloid nephrosis.

Treatment. Most of the simple cutaneous lesions require no treatment. The more sophisticated methods of applying heat locally with suitable prostheses and maintenance of an intralesional temperature of between 37 and 43 °C for twelve hours at a time have been very successful. All cases of kala azar and metastatic South American leishmaniasis need specific treatment, as do cutaneous lesions which are growing or likely to lead to metastases. For specific treatment, pentavalent antimony preparations, aromatic diamidines, and amphotericin B are the most effective agents.

Sodium stibogluconate and N-methylglucamine antimoniate. These drugs are given daily by intravenous or intramuscular injection as a solution containing the equivalent of 100 mg pentavalent antimony per ml. In adults the dose is 10 mg/kg daily for 30 days with a maximum of 600 mg (6 ml) a day. For children the dose is 15 mg/kg or 400 mg (4 ml) aged 4–12 and never less than 200 mg (2 ml) daily for 30 days. Pentostam (sodium stibogluconate) is active in both kala azar and cutaneous leishmaniasis. Side effects are few (nausea and vomiting).

Urea stibamine. This is a compound of urea with stibamine used in India. It is given intravenously, 3 mg/kg daily, for three courses of 10 days with seven-day intervals. A total of six injections is often sufficient for Indian kala azar. This drug is not active in cutaneous leishmaniasis.

Hydroxystilbamidine isethionate. This is given intravenously 3–5 mg/kg daily for 10 days for three courses for kala azar. 10 mg promethazine hydrochloride three times a day is necessary to control the fall in blood pressure. Diamidines are used when pentavalent antimonials have failed and are of no use in cutaneous leishmaniasis. Pentamidine has been used but is liable to cause hypoglycaemia.

Amphotericin B. This is reserved for cases which do not respond to antimony. It is active in both kala azar and metastasizing leishmaniasis. A total dose of 2.0 g is sufficient. Apparent antimony resistance in kala azar is due to faulty batches of the drug or sometimes an inability of the host to metabolize it correctly. The spleen should subside and the dysproteinaemia resolve within six months. Failure of the spleen to subside is often the result of portal hypertension but associated pulmonary tuberculosis should also be suspected. Relapses are not common, but can take place up to two years after apparent cure. Post kala azar dermal leishmanoid responds to further courses of antimony. Very rarely kala azar is resistant to all forms of treatment in which case splenectomy followed by another course of antimony is often successful.

Prevention. Cutaneous leishmaniasis in Asia has been controlled by the destruction of gerbil colonies, by poisoning the burrows within a radius of 7 km from villages . In India mass treatment of the only known reservoir, man, has produced a fair degree of control. In Brazil, dog destruction has been successful.

When the sandfly vector is anthropophilic and lives in close contact with man, residual DDT spraying, as for malaria, has stopped transmission. But the sandflies return if the spraying is stopped, so six-monthly spraying is probably necessary to maintain permanent interruption of transmission.

Inoculation of living promastigotes of *L. major* to prevent later infection has been practised with success both in the USSR and the Middle East. A small lesion is produced on a covered area of the body and, after three months, immunity is conferred for life. Successful vaccination against American mucocutaneous leishmaniasis and kala azar has not yet been achieved.

References

Bryceson, A. D. M. (1969). Diffuse cutaneous leishmaniasis in Ethiopia. 1. The clinical and histological features of the disease. Trans. R. Soc. trop. Med. Hyg. 63, 708.

Cartwright, G. E., Chung, H., and Chang, A. (1948). Studies on the pancytopenia of kala azar. Blood 3, 249.

Garnham, P. C. C. (1971) American leishmaniasis. Bull. Wld Hlth Org. 44, 521.

Hiçsönnez, G. and Özsoylu, S. (1977). Studies of the anaemia of kala azar in 68 childhood cases. Clin. Paediat. 16, 733.

Hoogstraal, H. and Heyneman, D. (1969). Leishmaniasis in the Sudan Republic, 30. Final epidemiologic report. Am. J. trop. Med. Hyg. 18, 1091.

Knight, R., Woodruff, A. W., and Pettitt, C. E. (1967). The mechanism of anaemia of kala azar: a study of two patients. Trans. R. Soc. trop. Med. Hyg. 61, 701.

Lainson, R. and Shaw, J. J. (1972). Leishmaniasis of the New World: taxonomic problems. Br. med. Bull. 28, 44.

Moskovskij, S. D. and Duhanina, N. N. (1971). Epidemiology of the leishmaniases. General considerations. Bull Wld Hlth Org. 44, 529.

Musumeci, S., Romeo, M., and d'Agata, A. (1974). Red cell survival and iron kinetics in kala azar. J. trop. Med. Hyg. 77, 106.

Pampiglione, S., Manson-Bahr, P. E. C., Giungi, F., Guinti, G., Parenti, A., and Ganestri Trotti, G. (1974). Studies on Mediterranean leishmaniasis. 2. Asymptomatic cases of visceral leishmaniasis. Trans. R. Soc. trop. Med Hyg. 68, 447.

—, —, la Placa, M., Borgatti, M. A., and Musemeci, S. (1975). Studies in Mediterranean leishmaniasis. 3. The leishmanin skin test in kala azar. Trans. R. Soc. trop. Med. Hyg. 69, 60.

Ridley, D. S. (1979). The pathogenesis of cutaneous leishmaniasis. Trans. R. Soc. trop. Med. Hyg. 73, 150.

Woodruff, A. W., Topley, E., Knight, R., and Downie, G. C. B. (1972). The anaemia of kala azar. Br. J. Haemat. 22, 319.

Trichomoniasis

G. W. Csonka

Trichomoniasis is a common cause of vaginitis in women and occasionally of urethritis in men. It is caused by the protozoan *Trichomonas vaginalis*. The condition is localized and considered to be sexually transmitted in the majority of patients. As the parasite can survive outside the body in a moist environment, extracorporeal transmission by fomites is a theoretical possibility. A proportion of women, especially in the older age groups, are asymptomatic carriers, in others the vaginitis ranges from mild to severe. In men, trichomoniasis is not commonly recognized; this may be due to the infection being mild or asymptomatic, or because the parasite is not regularly looked for even in the presence of urethritis. It is also possible that *T. vaginalis* is commonly inhibited from colonizing the male urethra for any length of time.

Aetiology

The organism. *T. vaginalis* is a motile protozoan of round or oval shape. It is on average 10–12 μm in length and 8–10 μm in width. It has four anterior flagella, an undulating membrane, a posterior axostyle which projects as a spine, and a large oval nucleus. Abnormal forms of *T. vaginalis* have been repeatedly reported, especially in men. It is actively motile with jerky movements impelled by the flagella and the undulating membrane. The smaller and rounder the organism the more motile it is. Phagocytosis and pinocytosis (ingestion of small particles and large molecules) is an essential characteristic of the trichomonads. Reproduction is by binary fission. It is anaerobic and needs carbohydrate as a source of energy which is abundantly present in the vagina in the form of glycogen.

Epidemiology. Although transmission is generally assumed to be by sexual contact the demonstration of *T. vaginalis* in male contacts of trichomonas vaginitis is often unsuccessful. Reports of positive isolation range from under 20 per cent to 69 per cent. Male patients harbouring the organism may act as reservoir of further infections. Vaginal trichomonads have also been found in infants, children and virgins.

In support of the idea of sexual transmission is the age incidence of trichomoniasis which is maximal in the sexually most active second and third decades of life, and the common association of gonorrhoea with trichomonas vaginitis.

Incidence. The reported incidence of around 19 000 new cases per year from the VD clinics in the United Kingdom is similar to that of gonorrhoea in women and has shown no significant change for several years. In men, the reported incidence is about a tenth of that in women. *T. vaginalis* has been occasionally demonstrated in infants infected by their mothers but infection appears to be transient.

Racial incidence. Several reports suggest that Negro women are more prone to trichomonas vaginitis than Caucasian women but this difference may be a reflection of differences in promiscuity rather than a true racial one.

Pathology. Trichomonas vaginitis is considered by most observers to be strictly localized to the lower urogenital tract. Histologically there is marked epithelial hyperplasia with polymorphonuclear infiltration. The parasites cluster around degenerating squamous epithelial cells which are later replaced by polymorphonuclear leucocytes. In carriers, histological changes are minimal or absent.

Clinical features

Trichomoniasis in the female. There may be no symptoms and only a scanty vaginal discharge to suggest trichomonal infection. However, many patients have florid vaginitis with profuse, purulent, frothy, offensive yellow discharge with itching and soreness. Sometimes there is vulval swelling and excoriation of the adjacent skin. There may be red spots on the vaginal wall and cervix ('strawberry' appearance). The patient with such severe vaginitis may also complain of dyspareunia, frequency, and dysuria. The vaginal pH tends to become more alkaline (pH 5–8) than normal (pH 4–5).

Trichomoniasis and carcinoma of the cervix. Trichomonas vaginitis is sometimes associated with endocervical hyperplasia and increased patchy vascularity ('strawberry cervix') which reverts to normal after successful treatment. Cervical smears stained with Papanicolaou stain which also shows the trichomonads, has usually to be repeated some three months after elimination of the infection to allow correct interpretation of the smear. It has been suggested that trichomoniasis, especially if chronic and untreated, may lead to carcinoma of the cervix. More recent evaluation seems to suggest that the changes are *not* indicative of cervical malignancy.

Trichomoniasis in the male. The majority of male contacts appear not to be infected. Those infected may (*a*) be asymptomatic carriers of the organism in the urethra; (*b*) suffer from trichomonas urethritis; or (*c*) have non-specific urethritis with additional transient *T. vaginalis* present.

Thus *T. vaginalis* may be found in the urethra or urethral secretions but specific antitrichomonal therapy will not be effective in patients with non-specific urethritis as the basic disorder.

Laboratory diagnosis. Direct microscopy of fresh secretions preferably by dark-field illumination is generally adequate for routine diagnosis. Staining has so far not been found to have any advantages over the simpler and more rapid procedure. Cultures using various media such as that of Fineberg and Whittington, Johnson and Trussel, or the modified Bushby medium give good results, and the combination of direct microscopy and cultures is superior to either of them alone.

Treatment. Oral metronidazole (Flagyl) which was introduced in 1959 is very effective and our treatment of choice. It can be used in a variety of treatment schemes ranging from the single dose of 2 g, which set the fashion for the use of short therapies in a variety of sexually transmitted diseases, to 200 mg three times daily for seven days; all giving satisfactory results. The shorter courses are preferable because of more ready acceptance by the patient and possibly, by reducing the total dose given, may minimize the as yet hypothetical long-term adverse effects of the drug (see below). If the sexual partner is also treated concurrently, the cure rate is marginally improved. Alternative drugs are nitroimidazole (Naxogin) and its numerous derivatives. These are given either in a single dose of 2 g or 500 mg to 1 g at 12 hourly intervals for three to four doses.

Metronidazole is thought to have an antabuse effect and therefore alcohol should be disallowed.

Whichever of these drugs are used, one can expect an immediate cure-rate of over 90 per cent and relapses appear to be very rare.

Carcinogenicity and mutagenicity of metronidazole. It has been reported from animal and bacterial genetic studies that metronidazole can induce tumours in mice using, however, doses far in excess to those given in patients and that mutations can be induced in some bacteria. Such effects have *not* been confirmed in man. However, the American Medical Association counsels caution in using metronidazole in human beings. As an alternative it suggests that in simple cases povidone-iodine (Betadine) douches be used followed by insertion of povidone-iodine gel nightly throughout the menses and repeated during the next two periods. This is a very cumbersome and messy treatment which has not yet been fully evaluated.

Treatment failure. Provided the preparation was taken as prescribed and reinfection can be ruled out, failure to respond to metronidazole or nitroimidazole may be due to: (*a*) poor absorption; (*b*) inactivation of the drug by a variety of vaginal micro-organisms; or (*c*) exceptionally, due to partially drug resistant strains.

Poor absorption can usually be overcome by giving larger doses and longer treatment. Microbiological inactivation of the compound in the vagina can be treated by using antibiotic vaginal pessaries prior to a further course of metronidazole and the few reported cases with partially drug resistant trichomonads usually responded to more intensive treatment with nitroimidazole or metronidazole. High doses are not recommended during pregnancy or lactation.

Treatment of the male contact. The sexual partner(s) should receive a short course of metronidazole whether symptomatic or not as it appears to reduce the small failure rate in females even further, suggesting that some of the recurrences are due to reinfection. However, as the benefit is small we do not insist on this if it might cause social or psychological upset.

References

Csonka, G. W. (1971). Trichomonal vaginitis treated with one dose of metronidazole. *Br. J. vener. Dis.* **47**, 456.

Durel, P., Roiron, V., Siboulet, A., and Borel, L. J. (1959). Essai d'un antitrichomonas derive d'l'imidazole. *Soc. Fr. gynaecol.* **29**, 36.

John, J. and Squires, S. L. (1978). Abnormal forms of *Trichomonas vaginalis*. *Br. J. vener. Dis.* **54**, 84.

Keighley, E. E. (1970). Trichomonas in a closed community: efficacy of metronidazole. *Br. med. J.* **i**, 207.

Babesia

T. K. Ruebush II

Babesia are tick-borne intra-erythrocytic protozoan parasites of wild and domestic animals which occasionally cause infections in man. The disease caused by these organisms is known as babesiosis or piroplasmosis and ranges from asymptomatic to severe, often fatal illnesses characterized by fever, haemolytic anaemia, jaundice, haemoglobinuria, and renal failure. Babesiosis is of historical interest because *Babesia bigemina* was the first organism shown to be transmitted by an arthropod.

Epidemiology. *Babesia* infections are common in both domestic and wild animals in many parts of the world, particulary the tropics and subtropics. In some areas these infections are responsible for serious economic losses in livestock. More than 70 different species of *Babesia* have been described in a variety of vertebrate hosts e.g. *B. divergens* (probably identical to *B. bovis*) and *B. bigemina* (cattle), *B. caballi* (horses), *B. canis* (dogs), and *B. microti* (rodents).

Ixodid, or hard-bodied ticks, are the only known vectors of *Babesia* spp. Parasites are ingested by the trick when it feeds on an infected host; the organisms then divide and spread throughout the body of the tick. In some species of ticks *Babesia* organisms enter the ovaries and are passed transovarially through the egg to the developing larval stage. The parasite is then transmitted to its vertebrate host during the next blood meal. Other tick species ingest the organisms during one stage and then transmit the infection after they have moulted to the subsequent stage (transtadial transfer).

Babesiosis is a zoonotic disease. Man is infected accidentally when he intrudes on the cycle between the tick and its vertebrate host and probably plays no role in the transmission of the infection in nature.

Since the first case of human babesiosis was described in 1957, approximately 40 additional cases have been reported. Two organisms, *B. divergens* and *B. microti*, have been responsible for the majority of cases. Human infections with *B. divergens*, an organism which normally parasitizes cattle, have been reported from Yugoslavia, France, Russia, Ireland, and Scotland. The vector of the parasite to man is unknown; *Ixodes ricinus* transmits the organism among cattle. *Babesia divergens* appears to have a narrower host range than *B. microti* and, thus far, infections have reported only in persons who have had previous splenectomies. The absence of a spleen is thought to have increased these patients' susceptibility to infection.

All of the reported cases of human *B. microti* infections have been acquired along the northeast coast of the United States. *Babesia microti* is a parasite of rodents which is transmitted by *Ixodes dammini*, the tick thought to be responsible for transmission to man. Unlike *B. divergens*, *B. microti* is capable of infecting persons with intact spleens. The reason for the limited geographic distribution of human *B. microti* infections is unknown since infections in rodents are widely distributed in the United States and Europe. *Ixodes dammini*, however, appears to have a more restricted range and this may explain the relatively small number of human cases which have been identified.

Cases of human babesiosis caused by organisms whose species could not be indentified have been reported from Mexico and western and southern parts of the United States.

Babesia organisms can also be transmitted by blood transfusion. This route of transmission is particularly likely with *B. microti* because of the tendency of this organism to produce prolonged asymptomatic parasitaemia.

Pathogenesis. When ticks infected with *Babesia* feed on a vertebrate host, the parasites apparently enter red blood cells directly without a preliminary exoerythrocytic stage such as occurs in malaria. Within the red cell the organisms multiply by budding, forming two or four daughter cells. When the infected cell ruptures, the parasites are liberated and other erythrocytes are invaded repeating the cycle.

Asymptomatic *Babesia* infections in animals can persist for several years and in humans infected with *B. microti* parasitaemia has been recorded for up to four months after the initial illness. These prolonged parasitaemias are probably due to the ability of *Babesia* organisms to change their surface antigens so as to avoid the hosts' immune defences, a phenomenon known as antigenic variation.

The spleen apparently plays an important role in resistance to *Babesia* infections since persons who have had previous splenectomies tend to higher levels of parasitaemia and more severe illnesses than persons with intact spleens. Moreover, in animals infected with *Babesia*, splenectomy months or even years after the intial infection may lead to a recurrence of parasitaemia.

The age of the host can also influence its response to *Babesia* infections. In animals *Babesia* infections which are acquired early in life tend to be mild or asymptomatic with much lower mortality rates than in older animals. A similar association between age and severity of illness has been noted in many of the cases of human *B. microti* infection. Symptomatic infections are most common in persons more than 40 years old; younger individuals usually have mild or subclinical infections. No such relationship has been observed in splenectomized persons infected with *B. microti* or in human *B. divergens* infections.

Clinical features. The severity of a case of human babesiosis seems to depend primarily on the species of *Babesia* causing the infection. However, the presence or absence of a spleen and the patient's age may also influence the course of the disease.

Patients infected with *B. divergens* usually present with a one to three day history of fatigue, malaise and occasional nausea, vomiting and diarrhoea. This is rapidly followed by high fever, rigors, jaundice, and the production of small amounts of dark or blood-stained urine. The incubation period is unknown. All of the patients who have been identified thus far have had previous splenectomies for reasons which included trauma, surgical accidents, portal hypertension, and Hodgkin's disease.

The major findings on physical examination are fever, hypotension, and jaundice. Anaemia is due to haemolysis and is generally severe with elevated reticulocyte counts and nucleated red blood cells on blood smear. Leucocyte counts range from normal to more than 40 000/mm^3 with an increase in juvenile and mature polymorphonuclear neutrophils. Marked elevations of bilirubin, liver enzymes, blood urea nitrogen, and creatinine are found in most patients. The course of illness is characterized by progressive haemolytic anaemia, haemoglobinaemia, haemoglobinuria, jaundice, and renal insufficiency. In spite of aggressive therapy with blood transfusions, renal dialysis, and various antiprotozoal drugs, the majority of patients infected with *B. divergens* have died.

Human *B. microti* infections are characterized by a gradual onset of anorexia, fatigue, fever, chills, and generalized myalgia beginning one to four weeks after a tick bite. The acute illness may last from a few weeks to a month or more; thereafter, malaise and weakness often persist for several months. The majority of patients infected with *B. microti* have no history of splenectomy. Patients who have had previous splenectomies tend to have more severe illnesses with higher levels of parasitaemia.

The only findings on physical examination are fever and occasional mild hepatosplenomegaly. Most patients have a mild to moderately severe haemolytic anaemia, with low to normal white blood cell counts. Slight elevations of liver enzymes and bilirubin are noted in about half of the patients. Asymptomatic *B. microti* parasitaemia may persist for several months after clinical recovery.

Evidence from serologic surveys in the northeastern United States suggest that asymptomatic human *B. microti* infections may be quite common in areas where infection is endemic in the rodent population. It is not known whether *B. divergens* can produce asymptomatic infections in man.

Diagnosis. The diagnosis of babesiosis should be considered in any patient with a fever and a history of tick bite. Although cases of human babesiosis have been reported only from Europe and North America, the diagnosis should not be ruled out in persons from other areas, since *Babesia* infections in animals are worldwide in distribution. In *B. divergens* infections the rapid onset of haemolytic anaemia, jaundice, haemoglobinuria, and renal insufficiency should suggest the diagnosis. In contrast, human *B. microti* infections can easily be mistaken for a variety of viral or bacterial illnesses because of their non-specific clinical presentation.

Babesia parasites are most easily recognized in thin or thick blood smears stained with Giemsa. The organisms are variable in morphology and are frequently mistaken for malaria parasites. *Babesia divergens* ranges from round, oval, or piriform in shape to small ring forms. Dividing forms usually consist of two daughter cells held together by a thin strand of cytoplasm. *Babesia microti* parasites tend to resemble *Plasmodium falciparum* rings. *Babesia* can be distinguished from malaria parasites by the absence of pigment in erythrocytes infected with the older stages of *Babesia*.

Inoculation of a susceptible laboratory animal, such as a hamster, has been a useful technique in the diagnosis of human *B. microti* infections. Patent infections usually appear within two to four weeks in inoculated animals. Although *B. divergens* seems to have a narrower host range than *B. microti*, the organism has been successfully isolated in gerbils, and this technique may be useful in cases in which parasites are difficult to detect by direct microscopic examination of the patient's blood.

Serologic tests may also be helpful in diagnosis although they are not widely available. An indirect immunofluorescent test has been used in several of the patients infected with *B. microti*. Serum antibody titres rise within the first two to four weeks after the onset of illness and then fall gradually over the next 6–12 months. Serologic cross-reactions with malaria occur occasionally; but titres are generally highest to the infecting organism.

Treatment and prevention. There are no generally effective drugs for the treatment of human babesiosis. In infections caused by *B. divergens* a drug such as pentamidine, which has been shown to be effective against various species of *Babesia* in animals, is a logical choice as a chemotherapeutic agent although there is evidence to suggest that it may simply reduce parasitaemia without eliminating it completely. Chloroquine has been used successfully in the treatment of two patients with *B. divergens* infections but it was not clear whether their recovery was related to drug therapy or to the supportive treatment they received. Chloroquine appears to have no effect against infections in animals. In patients with severe *Babesia* infections chemotherapy should be combined with aggressive supportive treatment including blood transfusion and renal dialysis if necessary.

Since most human *B. microti* infections are self-limited, symptomatic therapy is recommended for all but the most severely ill patients. A drug such as pentamidine should be reserved for patients with progressive anaemia who fail to respond to symptomatic treatment.

The only effective means of preventing *Babesia* infections is by avoiding areas infested with ticks. Insect repellents are probably of little value. Since it appears that *Babesia* organisms are transmitted to vertebrate hosts only after the vector has been feeding for several hours, prompt removal of attached ticks may help to prevent or reduce the risk of infection.

References

Garnham, P. C. C. (1980). Human babesiosis: European aspects. *Trans. R. Soc. trop. Med. Hyg.* **74**, 153.

Hoare, C. A. (1980). Comparative aspects of human babesiosis. *Trans. R. Soc. trop. Med. Hyg.* **74**, 143.

Ruebush, T. K., II. (1980). Human babesiosis in North America. *Trans. R. Soc. trop. Med. Hyg.* **74**, 149.

NEMATODES

Filarial infections and diseases

B. O. L. Duke

General principles

The various pathogenic filarial parasites of man affect some 300 million people living in tropical countries. In addition to their clinical importance they thus present an enormous public health problem.

There are nine recognized species of filariid for which man is the normal definitive host. Five commonly cause disease *Wuchereria bancrofti*, *Brugia malayi*, and *B. timori*, the widespread lymphatic-dwelling filarial worms responsible for filarial fever, adenolymphangitis and elephantitis; *Onchocerca volvulus* causing cutaneous onchocerciasis and river blindness; and *Loa loa*, which produces Calabar swellings. The four others, *Tetrapetalonema streptocerca*, *T. perstans*, and *T. semiclarum*, and *Mansonella ozzardi*, are, with rare exceptions, non-pathogenic and may be regarded as common but incidental parasitoses.

Some other filariids (e.g. *Dirofilaria* spp.), which normally parasitize other animals, are occasionally transmitted to man, in whom they may undergo partial or aberrant development and thus give rise to disease.

Certain general features of filarial infections need to be borne in mind by clinicians who are called upon to diagnose and treat the diseases which they may produce.

Geographical distribution. In the tropics the clinician must know which parasites occur in the country where he is practising. In non-tropical practice he must know which filarial parasites are endemic in the area from which the patient comes or to which he has paid a visit.

Life-history of the parasite and its vectors. It is essential, as an aid to diagnosis and prognosis, that the clinician should know the probable duration of life of the various stages of the parasite, and that he should appreciate which stage or stages of each parasite are responsible for the manifestations of disease. Likewise he needs to know which insects are vectors of the various parasites so that he can warn the patient of the dangers of re-exposure and give simple advice as to avoidance of reinfection.

Adult filarial worms inhabit the lymphatic system, the subcutaneous and deep connective tissues, or the serous cavities, according to species. Their lifespan extends for many years. The fertilized females produce a continuous supply of living motile embryos, known as microfilariae, which are found in the blood or in the skin. The lifespan of microfilariae is of the order of 6–24 months and they do not develop further unless they are ingested by a blood-feeding female insect capable of acting as the vector or intermediate host of the parasite concerned. The microfilariae of some species living in the blood exhibit periodicity, i.e. they are only found in the peripheral blood at a certain period of the 24 hours which coincides with the biting activity of their vector. Inside the vector the microfilariae develop, without multiplication, for 6–15 days to become infective (third stage) larvae, lying mainly in the head and proboscis of the insect. When the insect again bites man they enter the human host through the wound made by the proboscis. Development of the parasite to the adult stage in man, with production of detectable microfilariae, requires 3–18 months according to species.

Intensity of infection. Filarial parasites do not multiply in the vector, nor do they do so in the human host except in so far as the production of microfilariae is concerned. One infective larva inoculated into man remains as one worm, male or female and, when adult, it requires to meet another worm of the opposite sex before microfilariae can be produced. Although one fertile female can produce large numbers of microfilariae continually throughout her life, these organisms develop no further in man. It follows that repeated exposure to infective larvae is necessary before infections of high intensity (whether in terms of adult worms or of microfilariae) can build up in the human host.

Infection versus disease. In areas where filarial parasites are endemic it is very likely that almost the whole population will be infected. But only a proportion will have infections that are detectable parasitologically, and a smaller proportion still will show signs and symptoms of filarial disease. Not everyone who harbours a filarial infection is in need of treatment and usually it is only those who have disease, or who are at risk of developing disease, that merit treatment.

In endemic areas it is generally the heavily infected persons who are most likely to show severe signs and symptoms of filarial disease. Unfortunately such patients are often the most difficult to treat for they may suffer severe reactions when large numbers of parasites die in their tissues as a result of treatment. On the other hand it may not be necessary to get rid of all the filarial parasites in a heavily-infected patient in order to reduce the risk of disease developing. A light residual infection may be well tolerated in place of a heavy disease-producing infection.

Immunological factors and exposure in early life. The immunological status of the patient *vis à vis* his filarial parasites may also be of great importance in the production of disease. Patients who are first exposed in adult life frequently suffer severely from relatively light infections. It is also true that certain patients born and bred in endemic areas appear to mount an above-average immunological response to their parasites, and such a high degree of intolerance may give rise to severe disease syndromes.

Nutritional status and concomitant disease. Patients born and bred and living in rural areas in the tropics are often malnourished and may harbour a large number of other helminthic, protozoan or bacterial infections. To this extent treatment of their filarial disease may present a vastly more difficult clinical problem than does treatment of an otherwise healthy and well-nourished expatriate who has acquired a light infection during a short spell in the tropics.

Multiple infections with filarial parasites. In some tropical countries multiple infections with filarial parasites are common. In Africa, for example, *O. volvulus*, *L. loa*, *W. bancrofti*, *T. perstans* and *T. streptocerca* may be found in the same patient. Reactions to a concomitant infection may complicate the treatment of the parasite that is causing clinical disease, especially if both are susceptible to the same drug.

Diagnosis. The diagnosis of filariasis has to be made largely on clinical and/or parasitological grounds. Immunological tests have a limited role to play, owing to the present lack of specific and sensitive antigens. In puzzling cases, if all filarial immunological tests (usually IFAT or a skin test) are negative using currently available heterologous antigens, the diagnosis of filariasis (*sensu lato*) becomes unlikely. By contrast a positive result, while consistent with the diagnosis of filariasis, does not prove it.

Chemotherapy. Specific filaricides are few and far from satisfactory. Diethylcarbamazine citrate (DEC-C), along with suramin as a macrofilaricide for the treatment of onchocerciasis, are the only drugs that can currently be recommended. DEC-C is believed to act largely by 'unmasking' filarial parasites so that they become recognized as foreign bodies to be destroyed by the host's defence system.

Arsenical compounds, such as melarsonyl potassium, should not be used on account of the danger of encephalopathy. Antimonials should be avoided as being toxic and uncertain in their action. Levamisole and metrifonate appear to have no advantages over DEC-C. The use of mebendazole at high doses is still at the stage of research.

Most of the reactions to treatment are due to the death of parasites in the tissues, and much of the skill in treatment consists in damping down these reactions by the use of anti-inflammatory compounds and by using low doses of the filaricide at the outset.

The lymphatic filariases

These include infections with *Wuchereria bancrofti*, *Brugia malayi*, and *B. timori*, all of which inhabit the lymphatic tissues and may be considered together. The main difference between the two genera is that *Wuchereria* is very prone to attack the genital lymphatics (especially in males), whereas *Brugia* never does so.

Geographical distribution and vectors. *Bancroftian filariasis* is the most widespread human filarial infection. Most of the world's infected persons live in Asia, particularly India, Sri Lanka, Bangladesh, Burma, Thailand, Malaysia, Indonesia, China, Philippines, and Papua New Guinea. Infections are also found in: the tropical parts of East, Central, and West Africa; Malagasy and neighbouring islands; Egypt and countries of the East Mediterranean and around the Red Sea; northern South America; parts of central America; and the West Indies. In all these places, and in the Pacific Islands west of Buxton's line (approximately longitude 170° E), the infections show a nocturnal microfilarial periodicity. The only exception is in Thailand where the microfilariae are nocturnally subperiodic. The main vectors are *Culex* mosquitos in urban environments, and anopheline mosquitos in rural environments. East of Buxton's line, in the more easterly Pacific Island countries, the parasite is diurnally subperiodic and is spread by *Aedes* mosquitos.

Brugian filariasis is more restricted in distribution and overlaps in some places with Bancroftian filariasis. *B. malayi* is found in Indonesia, Malaysia, India, southern China, Thailand, Vietnam, Philippines, and South Korea. The parasite occurs in two forms. One is nocturnally periodic, without an animal reservoir, and is spread by *Mansonia* and *Anopheles* mosquitos. The other is nocturnally subperiodic, is spread by *Mansonia*, and has a reservoir in domestic cats, monkeys, and some other wild animals.

B. timori, closely allied to *B. malayi*, is localized to the lesser Sunda Islands in eastern Indonesia, is nocturnally periodic, and is spread by *An. barbirostris*.

Life cycle of the parasites and pathology. The adult worms are thin, whitish, and thread-like, the females reaching up to 10 cm in length and the males up to 4 cm. They live in the lymphatic vessels and nodes. The infective larvae, after inoculation by the vector mosquito, pass fairly rapidly to the adult sites and complete their development to the stage of microfilarial production in a period of three to six months. The sheathed microfilariae have a maximum life span of about 12 months, but the adult parasites can live for many years (up to 40 as a record).

The adult worms and the immature forms are the cause of most of the disease manifestations. They settle down in the lymph vessels and nodes draining the limbs; and sometimes in the para-aortic vessels, or in those draining the breast. *W. bancrofti* also shows a predeliction for the lymphatics of the scrotum, testis, epididimis, and spermatic cord; its role in the corresponding female lymphatics has not been well studied. According to the amount of host reaction a degree of inflammation is set up in the affected lymphatics which may lead to intermittent attacks of adenolymphangitis, sometimes with suppuration, and eventually to chronic granulomatous reactions and fibrosis. Although this may kill some of the worms, it often results in incompetence and leakage of the lymph valves and in obstruction of the lymph flow. Thus lymphoedema and elephantiasis develop. Secondary bacterial infection may hasten the process.

If blockage occurs in the thoracic duct or its afferent branches, stasis of the abdominal lymphatics occasionally results in a lymph fistula developing in the pelvis of the kidney or more rarely in the bladder. This will give rise to chyluria or lymphuria.

The blood-dwelling microfilariae are responsible for very little pathology apart from contributing to tropical pulmonary eosinophilia (see below). Their death and destruction in the liver or other deep organs under the influence of DEC-C may give rise to short-lived reactions of fever and malaise.

Clinical picture

Filariasis of the lymphatic system. The normal clinical picture of the disease as it affects the lymphatic system can be divided into early acute and late chronic manifestations. Prompt treatment of the former will usually prevent development of the latter.

Acute manifestations. In endemic filarial areas these may commence in early childhood, but in previously unexposed adults they may come on as early as three months after first infection, when inflammatory reactions begin to occur around the immature and adult worms in the lymphatics. They are characterized by recurrent episodic attacks of fever and lymphadenitis, usually affecting a single superficial lymph node. This may heal by itself after two to three days; or it may progress to a retrograde lymphangitis; or it may spread to the neighbouring tissues leading to acute cellulitis, abscess formation, and suppuration in the lymph node, followed by ulceration and scar formation or lymphoedema. The whole process may last from two weeks to three months. The distribution of the affected area in the extremities is usually along the saphenous drainage system or along the pathway of the median nerve. Sometimes the affected nodes appear in crops; the proximal ones healing while the distal ones are still developing. If an abscess forms and suppurates, the resulting ulcer is relatively clean with some sero-sanguineous fluid dripping out. This is in contrast to bacterial infections. The lymphatic inflammation is usually accompanied by high fever, but sometimes the clinical picture is dominated by fever with little local inflammation, or vice versa. The episodic attacks are quite frequently precipitated by hard labour, leading to periodic inability to work. The oedema usually regresses completely after an acute episode, but when the attacks recur the affected part remains more and more permanently swollen after each acute attack is over, and eventually the chronic stage develops.

In *Bancroftian filariasis* the affected lymphatics are usually in the region of the spermatic cord and testis, giving rise to severe attacks of funiculitis, epididymitis, and orchitis; and fluid may begin to collect in the tunica vaginalis. Recurrent attacks of adenolymphangitis may also involve the limbs, usually the inguinal region and the legs, and to a lesser extent the arms.

In *Brugian filariasis* the inguinal region is most commonly affected, and the arms to a lesser extent. Paradoxically when elephantiasis develops, it is always below the knee or below the elbow. Genital involvement has never been well documented.

Chronic manifestations. Under conditions of prolonged exposure to infection, repeated acute attacks give rise to signs of chronic inflammation and failure of lymph flow in the affected parts. Occasionally obstructive signs develop without previous acute attacks. In other persons the acute attacks subside and decline in frequency, leaving no serious after-effects.

Both in Bancroftian and Brugian filariasis varices may develop in the fibrosed and incompetent lymphatics of the limbs. The lymph nodes become enlarged, sometimes remaining discrete, sometimes becoming matted as a result of abscess formation and subsequent scarring. Oedema develops, soft and pitting at first, but becoming gradually hard after a year or two. Lymph fluid, with its high protein content, initiates fibroblastic activities, leading to the formation of fibrotic subcutaneous tissue. The skin epithelium may hypertrophy and the underlying muscles atrophy. Full development may take years. The final size of the affected part depends on the amount of fibrotic tissue that has accumulated and how far the elasticity of the skin permits it to stretch. Children below 10 years rarely develop elephantiasis, but previously unexposed adults migrating from non-endemic to endemic filarial areas may develop elephantiasis within a year or two.

In *Bancroftian filariasis* the most common sign is hydrocoele. It is rarely painful, except when the size is so huge that it is a real burden for the patient. However, it is always associated with some mental stress, especially among the younger age group.

Elephantiasis may involve the whole lower limb (usually unilaterally), the scrotum, arm, vulva, or breast in decreasing frequency. Thickening of the spermatic cord and funicocoele are sometimes observed. Lymphatic varices in the abdomen may rupture through to the pelvis of the kidney or to the bladder leading to chyluria or lymphuria.

In *Brugian filariasis* elephantiasis always involves the limb below the knee or the arm below the elbow. Genital lesions have never been recorded with certainty.

Tropical pulmonary eosinophilia (TPE). This clinical syndrome, most common in India and Southeast Asia, is now known to be associated with occult infection by *W. bancrofti* or *Brugia* spp. The syndrome has been produced experimentally in man following infection with *B. pahangi* from animals. TPE occurs mainly in adults who have not previously been exposed to infection in early life, or in those who have been lightly exposed and who have become sensitized.

It is characterized by persistent cough, mainly at night, accompanied by wheezing and shortness of breath resembling an asthmatic attack. There is persistent eosinophilia of at least 3000 and up to 50 000 cells per mm³, the IgE levels are high, the ESR is raised, there are variable pulmonary shadows on X-ray, and the IFAT for filariae found, reference should be made to textbooks of parasitology. peripheral blood but are almost certainly present in the lung. In some patients, particularly in *B. malayi* areas, there is associated lymphadenopathy and splenomegaly.

The diagnosis can only be made with certainty by finding remnants of microfilariae (Meyer–Kouwenaar bodies) in the liver, lymph nodes, or spleen. However, the condition responds well to DEC-C at 10 mg per kg per day in three divided doses for five days, and a favourable clinical response to this treatment, accompanied by a falling eosinophilia, confirms the diagnosis. Relapses should be retreated.

Diagnosis. The diagnosis of lymphatic filariasis can only be made with certainty by finding the parasite. It is dangerous to remove lymph nodes in attempts to find adult worms since such biopsies may further upset lymph drainage. Therefore the diagnosis depends on finding the microfilariae in blood films, which should be taken at the time of peak periodicity. Where the microfilariae are nocturnally periodic and it is impractical to take blood films at night, a provocative dose of 100 mg DEC-C may be given by day and the blood examined 45 minutes later for microfilariae which have been provoked to leave the lung capillaries and enter the peripheral blood. At least 60 mm³ blood should be smeared as a thick film to be dehaemoglobinized, fixed, and stained with Mayer's haemalum or Giemsa. For the specific identification of microfilariae found, reference should be made to textbooks of parasitology. Microfilariae may be very scanty, and positive results will be obtained more often if 1–3 ml venous blood are examined by a filtration technique, such as Nuclepore or Millipore, or by Knott's method (take the blood into 10–20 ml of 2 per cent formalin in distilled water, centrifuge for five minutes and examine the deposit). Denham (1978) gives details of all these methods.

Unfortunately many patients with clinical filariasis, including most with advanced elephantiasis, do not show patent microfilaraemia. This is especially true of infections acquired by temporary residents in filarial areas. The diagnosis has therefore to be made largely on the clinical history and signs. However, since DEC-C is in itself almost devoid of toxicity, there is almost no risk in undertaking trial therapy. An initial and characteristic reaction to treatment, followed by improvement, may indeed serve to make the diagnosis.

Differential diagnosis. Acute attacks of retrograde filarial adenolymphangitis have to be distinguished from the ascending lymphangitis and adenitis resulting from local bacterial infection at the periphery. The diagnosis of filarial lymphangitis is something that has to be thought of in puzzling cases and becomes more probable as the patient's degree of exposure to filariases increases. Acute attacks of funiculitis, epididymitis, and orchitis may have to be distinguished from gonorrhea (which may coexist) by the history, the presence of a discharge, and bacteriological examination.

Filarial elephantiasis has to be differentiated from elephantiasis due to other causes, e.g. familial, post-operative, and the obstructive lymphopathy of the peripheral lymphatics in barefooted people who absorb aluminosilicate particles from red clay soils through the skin of the feet (see page 6.97). Chyluria and lymphuria, with their predominance of lymphocytes, can easily be differentiated from pyuria by microscopic examination.

Treatment

Chemotherapy. Chemotherapy with diethylcarbamazine citrate (DEC-C) is usually effective. The drug kills the microfilariae and many, but not always all of the adult worms. It is probably also effective against the immature worms, but this is not yet proven. By eliminating the parasites, it prevents the recurrence of acute filarial attacks and the subsequent development of chronic lesions, but it cannot be expected to cure the chronic lesions which result from fibrous changes in specialized tissue. Cases must therefore be treated early, either before, or as soon as, the first signs of acute disease develop; and many may have to be retreated subsequently if they continue to be exposed to infection. Even in the early stages of elephantiasis, treatment with DEC-C may be beneficial since the changes may still be reversible.

For *W. bancrofti* DEC-C is usually given at 6 mg/kg per day in two or three divided doses after food; and treatment is continued for 10–12 days (total dosage 60–72 mg/kg). For *Brugia* infections 3 mg/kg per day is usually given over the same period (total dosage 30–36 mg/kg). Two to four such courses at intervals of a month or more may be necessary to eliminate all the adult worms and prevent continued clinical attacks.

In order to decrease reactions to the death of microfilariae, it may be advisable to start treatment with low doses for the first few days, e.g. for an adult: 50 mg on day 1; 2 × 50 mg on day 2; 2 × 100 mg on day 3; and then proceed to full dosage.

Reactions during DEC-C treatment. DEC-C *per se* at the doses used in treatment occasionally causes nausea, dizziness, and sleepiness. These can be avoided by taking the drug after food or before going to sleep at night.

Reactions to the death of microfilariae occur within a few hours of the first dose and are usually over by the fifth day of treatment. Fever, headache, aches and pains in the joints, muscles, and especially in the back, and general malaise, are the commonest manifestations. Reactions are usual in patients with microfilaraemia, and the greater the microfilarial density the more severe the reaction. However, similar reactions may occur in patients whose blood films are microfilariae-free but who presumably harbour microfilariae in the deep organs of the body.

Death of adult worms, and the cellular reaction associated therewith, may cause lymphangitis, lymphadenitis, and lymph abscesses, usually in the limbs or around the scrotum and spermatic cord. Such reactions are commonest from the third day of treatment onwards and may last for as long as 10 days.

Before commencing treatment it is important to warn patients of the likelihood of reactions. Aspirin may help to reduce them. Usually the reactions are more common and more severe in Brugian infection than with *W. bancrofti*.

Treatment of chronic lesions. Elephantiasis of the limbs, etc., may be alleviated by pressure bandaging or treated more radically by surgery. Hydrocoeles require surgical intervention. Chyluria or lymphuria may respond to DEC-C, to douching with silver nitrate solution, or they can be dealt with surgically. For these procedures surgical textbooks should be consulted.

Prophylaxis. Causal and/or clinical chemoprophylaxis with DEC-C may well be possible but has never been proven (see under Loiasis for a possible dosage schedule).

Prevention of infection is by avoiding the bites of infective mosquitoes. Mosquito screening of houses or sleeping rooms, burning of repellent coils, use of bed nets, and wearing long trousers and long-sleeve shirts all go a long way towards this.

Onchocerciasis

Geographical distribution and vectors. Transmission of *Onchocerca volvulus* occurs mainly near the fast-flowing watercourses where the *Simulium* vectors (black-flies) breed. In Africa infection may be acquired from members of the *S. damnosum* complex across the tropical sub-Saharan belt in Senegal, Mali, Upper Volta, Niger, Guinea Bissau, Guinea, Sierra Leone, Liberia, Ivory Coast, Ghana, Togo, Benin, Nigeria, Cameroon, Chad, Central African Republic, Gabon, Congo, Zaire, Equatorial Guinea, Rwanda, Burundi, Angola, Sudan, Ethiopia, Uganda, Kenya, Tanzania, and Malawi. Species of the *S. neavei* complex are important vectors locally in parts of east and central Africa. There is also a focus in Yemen.

In America *S. ochraceum* is the main vector in Guatemala and Mexico, and smaller foci occur in Venezuela (*S. metallicum*), Brazil (*S. amazonicum/sanguineum* group), and Colombia (*S. exiguum*).

Life cycle of the parasite and pathology. The adult worms (males 5 cm long, females 50 cm long) live in fibrous nodules and have a life-span of up to 15 years. Some nodules are subcutaneous and palpable; many others lie deep and impalpable, between the muscles, and against the capsules of joints (especially the hip joint) or the periosteum of the long bones. The nodules may be unsightly or inconvenient. Occasionally they suppurate, and they have been recorded rarely as eroding the skull; but usually they cause no clinical manifestations *per se*.

The microfilariae are large (300–320 µm long). They can live for 12–24 months, and they cause almost all the pathology of onchocerciasis. They invade the skin, where initially their presence, and especially their death, provoke small granulomatous reactions infiltrated with eosinophils, which lead to itching and a rash. Prolonged and heavy infection of the skin leads later to fibrosis, scarring of the papillae, replacement of dermal collagen by hyalinized scar, and atrophic changes. When microfilariae invade the eye, either directly from the skin to the conjunctiva and cornea, or via the sheaths of the posterior ciliary vessels to reach the interior of the globe, they give rise to all the ocular lesions of the disease. The pathology of the anterior segment lesions centres on microfilarial granulomata; that of the posterior segment lesions is not well understood.

The pre-patent interval or 'incubation period' between the inoculation of infective larvae by *Simulium* and the first appearance of symptom-producing microfilariae in the skin is usually 9–18 months.

Clinical picture. The clinical picture in heavily-infected patients varies from one geographical area to another. In the hot Sudan-savanna zones of Africa severe eye lesions are common and the overall blindness rate in the community may reach 15 per cent. In the forest zones of Africa blindness rates are generally lower but skin changes and lymphatic lesions may be marked. In Mexico and Guatemala head nodules are very common and, if untreated, may be associated with blindness; but skin lesions are generally mild. In South America the disease pattern is not severe and there are few serious eye lesions. In Yemen, an exaggerated cutaneous and lymphatic form of the disease is common. It usually affects one limb and is known as 'sowda' (black).

Nodules. Probably the number of deep impalpable nodules exceeds those that are superficial. Those which are subcutaneous and palpable normally lie over bony prominences, especially the knees, trochanters, iliac crests, ribs and scapulae. Those on the head are particularly dangerous as they provide a source of microfilariae which can readily reach the eye. They must therefore be searched for carefully, and removed. The patient should be asked to help in locating them, and it is sometimes necessary to shave the head in order to find them. A common site for small nodules is behind the ear.

Skin lesions. *'Acute' lesions.* Lightly and recently infected persons, among whom may be classed most expatriates and others who become infected for the first time in adult life or later childhood during temporary residence in an area of transmission, are those most commonly presenting for treatment. They do so on account of the pruritic cutaneous lesions of onchocerciasis (*gâle filarienne*).

Typically such cases harbour an adult worm or worms (often impalpable) in the subcutaneous or deep tissues on one side of the limb girdle concerned. Microfilariae then invade the skin, predominantly over the same anatomical quarter, and give rise to a persistent and variously itchy rash of typically lop-sided distribution. It usually involves the buttock, thigh, and leg on one side with extensions to the opposite buttock and up the back; or the shoulder and arm on one side with extensions down the back, across to the other shoulder or up the same side of the neck. The rash comprises numerous small discrete papules, 1–3 mm in diameter, which show red on a white skin. Wheals, vesicles, scratch marks, and secondary skin infection may be superimposed. The skin fold is thickened on the affected side, and the skin may be blacker than normal in negroes or reddened in white subjects. Sometimes a slightly thickened and lichenified skin is seen without accompanying pruritus or rash. Usually there is some enlargement of the inguinal or axillary lymph nodes on the affected side. Deep-seated aches and pains may be felt in the limb concerned.

Chronic lesions of the skin and lymph glands. Chronic, disfiguring and sometimes disabling skin lesions, resulting from long-standing heavy infection with *O. volvulus* microfilariae, are most often seen in adult Africans living in the areas where onchocerciasis is endemic. The lower limbs, where the highest concentrations of microfilariae are found, are usually worst affected. There is gross lichenification and thickening of the skin with hyperpigmentation, giving way later to the atrophy and slackness of 'lizard' skin; and a mottled depigmentation, especially common over the shins. The skin is poorly nourished, and heals badly. Indolent tropical ulcers often develop following minor abrasions. The femoral and inguinal lymph glands enlarge and may hang in pockets of loose skin (hanging groins), conditions which may predispose to herniae. Elephantiasis of the lower limbs or of the scrotum may develop. Microfilariae are usually abundant in the skin, unless the infection has 'burnt out'; and nodules are frequent.

Ocular lesions. The eyes are affected by serious lesions most often in patients with heavy microfilarial infections and/or with nodules on the head. Microfilariae (not the adult worms) can invade all tissues of the eye except the lens. The main ocular lesions can be divided according to the seriousness of their import.

Lesions of less serious import. Punctate keratitis. This is composed of so-called 'snowflake' opacities, which are cellular aggregates around dead microfilariae in the cornea. They vary in number from 1 to 100 or more, have a tendency to be peripheral and/or interpalpebral in distribution, and are of diameter up to 0.5 mm. Usually they are symptomless but sometimes there is associated photophobia and watering. They are characteristic of light and recent infections. They resolve spontaneously, usually without vascularization, but may be succeeded by new lesions, and are not *per se* of serious import. DEC-C treatment, by killing the microfilariae in the cornea, will eventually lead to their resolution.

Lesions of serious import. The ocular lesions of serious import usually develop in cases of heavy and often long-standing infection, particularly in children with head nodules.

Sclerosing keratitis. This lesion is characteristic of heavy infection

with abundant microfilariae in the cornea, and is particularly common in the African savannahs. the limbus is often swollen (limbitis) and a chronic interstitial keratitis develops from the sides and below. It is headed by a slowly advancing zone of milky opacification in the corneal stroma, behind which develops a scantily vascularized and commonly pigmented 'pannus'. The clear segment above may contain many hundreds of visible microfilariae. The affected area of the cornea becomes opaque and finally the pupillary area may be obscured.

Anterior uveitis. Acute episodes of uveitis are superimposed on a chronic inflammatory process. The pigment ruff of the pupil is lost and the pupil becomes distorted, often pear-shaped, with or without posterior synechiae. Secondary glaucoma and cataract may follow, the former being a common cause of blindness.

Fundus lesions. Choroidoretinal lesions may develop, sometimes terminating in the classical Hissette-Ridley fundus. Typically the lesions are bilateral. They start temporal to the macula and involve primarily the retinal pigment epithelium. Large well-defined patches of choroidoretinal degeneration develop, involving much of the posterior fundus. Within these areas the retinal elements (excluding the vessels) and the choriocapillaris disappear, and the choroidal vessels appear bright orange, pink, or white. Irregular pigment masses are seen and the optic disc often shows a consecutive atrophy. The surrounding retina appears healthy.

Optic neuritis. In other cases a post-neuritic optic atrophy is seen. There is often sheathing of the retinal vessels for a varying distance from the optic disc and narrowing of the retinal arteries. The visual field is often grossly reduced, with only tubular vision remaining. Loss of twilight- and night-vision is also common.

Diagnosis. Firm diagnosis depends on seeing microfilariae in a skin snip or in the eye, or on finding a nodule containing adult worms. Skin snips are usually positive in patients with advanced lesions. They are best taken from the iliac crests or the lateral calf in Africa, or from the scapula in Latin America.

In patients with acute pruritic skin lesions a presumptive diagnosis can be made on clinical grounds, especially if the rash is predominantly unilateral. There is often a mild eosinophilia but this cannot be considered as diagnostic.

Skin snips. Confirmatory parasitological diagnosis may be made by finding the microfilariae of *O. volvulus* in skin snips taken from the affected area of skin. To take a skin snip the skin is cleaned with spirit, a suitable needle is inserted horizontally into the epidermis to raise up a small cone-shaped fold of skin, and the top of this fold is sliced off with a safety razor blade or a sharp scalpel to remove a piece of skin 2–3 mm in diameter and 0.5–1.0 mm deep, which should be bloodless on removal. The snip is placed in a drop of normal saline on a slide and is examined at intervals over 30 minutes, using a ×10–×50 magnification, for the presence of motile microfilariae of *O. volvulus*. If negative after 30 minutes, it may be kept in a moist chamber overnight and then re-examined. *O. volvulus* microfilariae are relatively large and sturdy organisms 300–320 μm in length, without a sheath. They have a slightly bulbous head and a pointed tail, and they exhibit vigorous lashing and wriggling movements. In practice, they have only to be distinguished in Africa from those of the much rarer *T. streptocerca* which are thinner, have shepherd's-crook tails, and make shivering and stretching movements; and in South America from the shorter and smaller microfilariae of *M. ozzardi*, which are sometimes found in the skin. If there is doubt as to the identity of fresh specimens, the slide should be dried, fixed, stained (Mayer's haemalum or Giemsa) and compared with the illustrations in standard works on parasitology.

Mazzotti test. In lightly-infected patients microfilariae are often very hard to find. If two to four snips fail to reveal microfilariae, rather than continuing to take more, it is better to perform a Mazzotti test. For this 50 mg of DEC-C is given by mouth. The test is positive if, within 30 minutes to 24 hours, there develops an acute exacerbation of the itching and of the rash centred on the previously ffected parts but extending also further afield. Sometimes the ffected area of skin becomes swollen, hot, and itchy without a papular rash appearing. These changes are due to inflammatory eactions around microfilariae which have been 'unmasked' and illed in the skin.

Microfilariae in the eye and elsewhere. In the eye microfilariae can be seen with a slit-lamp at a magnification of ×20–×25. In the cornea they may be either alive (translucent) or dead (straight and opaque often with cellular reaction around them). In the anterior chamber they can be seen as shining bodies floating and wriggling in the aqueous humour, and the numbers visible can often be increased by making the patient sit for one minute with the head inverted between the knees before the examination is carried out.

Microfilariae are sometimes also found in urine, blood, sputum, CSF, and hydrocoele fluid, especially in heavily infected patients during the first days of DEC-C therapy.

Differential diagnosis. The differential diagnosis of early pruritic cutaneous onchocerciasis is from (*a*) scabies, which often coexists in Africans; (*b*) streptocerciasis (q.v. relatively rare) by identification of the microfilariae of *T. streptocera*; (*c*) prickly heat; (*d*) contact dermatitis; and (*e*) insect bites. Bites of *Culicoides* or *Simulium* may cause great irritation to persons newly arrived in the tropics, although most eventually become desensitized. The itching 'rash' of bites may give rise to fear of having acquired 'the filaria' long before the pre-patent interval of *O. volvulus* can have had time to elapse.

Treatment

Indications for treatment. Not all persons require treatment for infection with *O. volvulus* and each case should be judged individually. Many who have been born and bred in areas where the parasite is lightly or moderately endemic strike an asymptomatic balance with their parasites. If they have no complaint that can be related to the infection, and their eyes are not at risk, it is better to leave them untreated. Over-enthusiastic doctors in endemic areas who take unnecessary skin snips and demonstrate the wriggling microfilariae found therein are likely to be faced with overwhelming numbers of worried patients clamorous for a long and difficult course of treatment, which is not without hazards, which may be totally unnecessary, and which may have to be repeated if reinfection occurs later on in zones where there is no *Simulium* control. There is also little point in treating those who are already blind. Their eye lesions are irreversible and the only indication for treating them would be severe pruritus.

Those who do require treatment fall broadly-speaking into three groups.

'Acute' pruritic skin eruptions. This group includes (*a*) most expatriate cases of the sort commonly presenting to physicians in temperate climates; (*b*) cases of the 'sowda' type, with scanty microfilariae but with maximum skin reaction, among persons resident in endemic areas; and (*c*) a proportion of cases with heavy microfilarial loads.

Threat of severe eye lesions and blindness. Such patients will be mainly natives of the endemic area, and will usually be heavily infected. Dangers signs are:

1. Presence of a head nodule;
2. More than five microfilariae in a skin snip taken at the outer canthus of the eye;
3. More than five microfilariae in the anterior chamber;
4. More than 20 microfilariae in the cornea;
5. Evidence of night blindness or peripheral field loss;
6. Presence of any serious lesion of ocular onchocerciasis at an early stage.

Persons with any of these signs are at increased risk of developing severe eye lesions and blindness, even though their eyes may still be clear at the time of examination.

Disabling skin and lymph node lesions. Persons with extreme and disabling skin and lymph node lesions (hanging groins, herniae,

elephantiasis of the scrotum or lower limbs, etc.) may require surgical treatment for the relief of these conditions, whether or not specific therapy for onchocerciasis is considered necessary.

Aims and methods of treatment. The aim of treatment is to get rid of the microfilariae without doing further damage to specialized tissues in the process, and to kill or permanently sterilize the adult worms from which they come. To be fully effective it must therefore be carried out before specialized tissues have been irreparably damaged to fibrotic scarring and degenerative processes. Treatment is usually by chemotherapy, but in certain circumstances it may be supplemented by nodulectomy.

Nodulectomy. Head nodules should always be removed as early as possible, and in Mexico and Guatemala this measure alone may be of great value. Other nodules may be removed if they are unsightly or a nuisance to the patient, but remembering that almost certainly many deep nodules will remain to produce microfilariae.

Nodulectomy should be done under local analgesia (2 per cent lignocaine), preferably without adrenaline. After incising the skin the nodule can usually be shelled out using curved blunt-pointed scissors. Before suturing the operator should feel the wound for 'seed' nodules. Removal of nodules deep in the chest wall or around the knee joint requires especial care.

Chemotherapy. There are still only two drugs used in treatment and both have disadvantages. Diethylcarbamazine citrate or DEC-C (Banocide, Hetrazan, Notézine) is in itself non-toxic but it brings about such a rapid destruction of microfilariae that it often produces violent and even dangerous reactions in the process. Unfortunately, it usually has no effect on the adult worms. Suramin (Bayer 205 or Germanin, Moranyl, Antrypol) is effective against the adult worms, but is potentially toxic and can also excite reactions by its microfilarial action. The course of chemotherapy requires three months or more for its completion; it demands supervision by a medical practitioner at least on an outpatient basis; and it becomes increasingly difficult the more heavily the patient is infected, especially if there are microfilariae in the eyes.

Suramin medication is better tolerated if there are few microfilariae in the body. DEC-C should therefore be given first to reduce the initial load of microfilariae and should start with low doses which are gradually increased. This is especially important in patients with heavy microfilarial loads or with microfilariae in the eye, to whom it should be given under corticosteroid cover (unless there is some absolute contra-indication, e.g. concurrent untreated tuberculosis). Betamethasome (1 mg three or four times daily) should be started two days before the first dose of DEC-C and should be continued until the patient is through the worst of the reaction. The dosage with betamethasone can then be tailed off by reduction to 0.5 mg three times a day for two days and then to 0.25 mg three times a day for two days. A suggested sheme of DEC-C dosage (which can be modified in the light of the patient's response) for an adult would be: day 1, 25 mg; day 2, 25 mg morning and evening; day 3, 50 mg morning and evening; day 4, 100 mg morning and evening; day 5, *et seq.* (until the microfilarial count has been reduced to near zero) 200 mg daily in a single dose. Usually 7–10 days treatment suffices. Special care must be taken in heavily infected patients to avoid accidents resulting from postural hypotension and vertigo. Antihistamines (e.g. antazoline HCl 100 mg 6-hourly) have previously been recommended for control of the sometimes intense itching, but recent controlled trials have shown them to be ineffective. Aspirin and codeine help to relieve the fever and pain in the skin, glands, head, and joints.

Suramin treatment should begin within a few days of the end of the first course of DEC-C. The powder should be stored in the dark and should be mixed within 30 minutes of injection as a 10 per cent solution in pyrogen-free distilled water. The drug should be given slowly by intravenous injection. The standard course in the past has been to give an initial dose of 0.1 g to test for very rare idiosyncrasy, and to follow this by 1.0 g weekly for adults of 60 kg or more to a total of 4–7 g, depending on the patient's tolerance. Recent trials in Africans indicate that a course of weekly doses at 0.2 g, 0.4 g, 0.6 g, 0.8 g, 1.0 g, 1.0 g for an adult of 60 kg or more, may be better tolerated and have a considerable effect on the adult worms. The doses for children and adults under 60 kg should be reduced in proportion to their weight.

Persons with disease of the liver or kidneys should not be treated with suramin, nor should pregnant women, or the old and weak. The urine should be examined for albumin and casts before each injection. Suramin excretion is almost invariably accompanied by some albuminuria; and in low degrees this may be ignored, but a heavy albuminuria and the presence of many granular casts are indications to interrupt treatment for a week or to stop it altogether.

Minor manifestations of the drug itself may be: (a) tenderness of the soles and palms; (b) polyuria and increased thirst; (c) slight tiredness, anorexia, and malaise. Most severe toxic signs which indicate stopping treatment are: (a) severe prostration; (b) ulceration of the mouth and tongue; (c) exfoliative dermatitis; (d) chronic diarrhoea; (e) high fever and bronchitis; (f) swelling, pain, and immobilization of limb joints.

Reactions from the effect of suramin on the adult worms include: (a) tenderness, swelling, and even abscess formation in subcutaneous nodules; (b) deep abscesses centred round worms lying between the muscles; (c) painful immobilization of the hip in a semi-flexed position, presumably due to reaction around deep nodules near the joint capsule.

Reactions due to the effect of suramin on any remaining microfilariae include: (a) itching and inflammation of the skin with or without papular or vesicular eruptions and desquamation; (b) iridocyclitis and/or the development or exacerbation of an optic neuritis. Betamethasone may be necessary to prevent or to reduce any of the above reactions.

After the course of suramin the adult worms are likely to have been sterilized and most will be moribund; but they may take some weeks to die, and living microfilariae may continue to escape from their uteri for three to four months. If pruritus or other signs of microfilarial pathology continue after the suramin injections are completed, a further short course or courses of DEC-C should be given (200 mg twice a day for three days) at intervals of a month, until such time as DEC-C can be taken without exciting any skin reactions (i.e. the Mazzotti test is negative).

In patients who cannot tolerate suramin, the possibility of using DEC-C as a microfilarial suppressant may be tried, at a weekly dose of 50–200 mg or a daily dose of 25–50 mg, whichever produces least pruritic reaction.

Symptomatic treatment of reactions in the eye during chemotherapy. The development of a red eye during treatment usually indicates an onchocercal iridocyclitis. This requires immediate recognition and careful treatment to avoid the development of synechiae. Atropine sulphate drops (1 per cent) should be instilled, with due regard to the possibility of provoking mydriatic glaucoma; and corticosteroid drops or ointment should be instilled at least three-hourly until the inflammation is controlled. In patients showing temporarily increased intraocular pressure, acetazolamide may be of use.

In cases with large numbers of intraocular microfilariae or with early posterior segment lesions, specialized opthalmic supervision may be needed to detect and prevent, as far as possible, the risk of damaging inflammatory reactions developing in the retina and optic disc.

Prophylaxis. There is no practically effective chemoprophylactic for *O. volvulus* infection. Personal exposure to *Simulium* can be reduced by wearing clothing that protects the body areas most exposed to bites, i.e. long trousers, stockings, and shoes help against *S. damnosum* s.l., *S. neavei* s.l. and *S. metallicum*; long-sleeved shirts, and a hat and veil help against *S. ochraceum*.

Loiasis

Geographical distribution and vectors. Transmission of *Loa loa* is confined to the Central African forest belt east of the Dahomey (Benin) gap. Infections are commonly acquired in southern Nigeria, Cameroon, Gabon, Equatorial Guinea, Congo, and Zaire; they occur less frequently in southern Chad, Central African Republic, Sudan and Uganda, and Angola. *L. loa* is spread by tabanid flies of the genus *Chrysops*, known as 'red-flies'.

Life cycle of the parasite and pathology. Development from infective larvae to fertile adult worms takes about five months. The adult worms (males 3–4 cm long; females 5–7 cm long) are freely motile in the subcutaneous tissue and along the fascial planes, and they may live for up to 15 years. They cause the fugitive Calabar swellings and may be seen migrating across the conjunctiva. Their death under the skin may excite inflammatory reactions.

The sheathed microfilariae (225–300 μm long) are relatively large and show a diurnal periodicity. They probably live for about a year and are non-pathogenic except that, when present in high densities, their death under DEC-C treatment may block the capillaries of the brain or retina.

Clinical picture. Infective *Chrysops* bites may cause very severe swelling and itching. The infective larvae of *L. loa* are large (2 mm long) and often very numerous in a single fly. Discrete papules may develop in the skin in association with the larvae as they move away from the site of entry over the ensuing week or more.

Adult worms moving under the skin cause prickling and itching sensations; those moving deeper in the fascial planes cause shifting aches and pains and parasthesiae. Allergic, oedematous, subcutaneous Calabar or 'fugitive' swellings, 5–10 cm or more in diameter, may develop anywhere but are common on the back of the hand or on the arm. They last from some hours to several days and are often brought on by local muscular activity. The overlying skin may be red, hot, and painful, resembling cellulitis; and it may also itch. The swellings can be very large and temporarily incapacitating. Sometimes the worm can be seen moving under the skin.

The adult worm may also cross the conjunctiva, where it becomes visible for a matter of 5–30 minutes and may be removed by prompt surgical intervention. Its passage is accompanied by reddening, swelling of the eyelids and conjunctiva, watering, and photophobia, and the periorbital tissues may swell so as to close the eye.

It is often lightly- and recently-infected persons who suffer most from Calabar swellings and who seek treatment. The swellings may cause a significant loss of working time in labour forces in endemic areas and this is a good reason for treatment. Persons with heavy infections of long standing may be entirely asymptomatic and, if so, are probably best left untreated.

Diagnosis. The diagnosis is made on the clinical picture, which has only to be distinguished from the effects of insect bites and stings, and septic cellulitis. Marked eosinophilia (up to 10 000/mm) is almost invariable and may help to distinguish a Calabar swelling from cellulitis. Finding the microfilariae in day blood, or sight of an adult worm, will confirm the diagnosis, but in many patients with Calabar swellings no microfilariae can be found.

Treatment. Diethylcarbamazine citrate (DEC-C) is effective against the microfilariae, the immature worms, and a good proportion of the adult worms. The standard course for killing the adult worms is 6 mg/kg daily, in three divided doses after food, continued for three weeks. Courses of seven days duration at the same daily dosage and repeated at intervals of a month may sometimes be more effective, but some infections remain resistant to treatment even after repeated courses. The adult worms often surface and become visible under the skin when they die.

In all cases it is wise to start treatment with a low dose of DEC-C (25–50 mg) in order to see whether there is a severe reaction to death of *Loa* microfilariae in the blood, or a reaction to coincident infection with *O. volvulus*. Depending on the clinical response the dosage may then be increased towards the 6 mg/kg per day level. In cases with heavy microfilaraemia (200–1000 mm/kg³) very severe febrile reactions may be expected, with danger of capillary blockage by microfilariae in the brain and meninges (leading to a meningo-encephalitic syndrome), retina, and elsewhere. Dosage with DEC-C should then be given under coverage with betamethasone (started two days before the first dose of DEC-C). The dose of DEC-C should be not more than 12.5 mg on the first day and should only be increased gradually (such as doubling up each day) with due regard to the clinical response and to the fall in microfilaraemia.

Prophylaxis. DEC-C has a chemoprophylactic action against *L. loa*. For an adult a course of 200 mg twice daily for three consecutive days once each month will probably kill all infective larvae and immature worms inoculated during the previous month, and this at the expense of a minor papular reaction in the skin around dead parasites. Prevention of *Chrysops* bites may be achieved in large measure by wearing long trousers and by fly-screening dwellings.

Other filarial infections

Streptocerciasis. *Tetrapetalonema streptocerca*, causing streptocerciasis, occurs in the more humid parts of Ghana, Togo, Nigeria, Cameroon, Gabon, Congo, Equatorial Guinea, and Zaire. Transmission is by *Culicoides* (especially *C. grahamii*), commonly but erroneously known as 'sandflies'.

The adult worms and microfilariae are found in the skin, mainly on the torso. Infections are normally asymptomatic but occasionally give rise to a chronic itching rash composed of very small urticarial papules, not unlike the acute rash of onchocerciasis. Hypopigmented macules, probably associated with the adult worms, may be seen in dark-skinned patients. Diagnosis is by finding the characteristic crook-tailed microfilariae in skin snips.

DEC-C kills both microfilariae and adult worms, but the reactions are never so violent as in onchocerciasis. A course of 2 mg/kg three times a day for 7–10 days should suffice for an adult.

Perstans filariasis. *Tetrapetalonema perstans* is found in tropical Africa south of the Sahara, in parts of South America, and in Algeria, Tunisia, and New Guinea. Transmission is by *Culicoides* spp. *T. semiclarum*, described from Zaire, is a similar parasite.

The adult worms live in the serous cavities, in the mesentery and retroperitoneal tissue. The microfilariae are non-periodic and are found in the blood.

These parasites are generally considered to be non-pathogenic although a high proportion of persons in endemic areas may be infected. Normally no treatment is necessary. However, cases of infection with a microfilaria identical to, or closely resemblimg *T. perstans* have been found in Zimbabwe in association with meningeal symptoms (microfilariae in the CSF), and general malaise. Such infections may be a virulent form of *T. perstans*, but it has also been suggested that they may be caused by the monkey parasite *Meningonema peruzzi*. DEC-C is ineffective but some success in treatment has been reported following combined dosage with mebendazole (100 mg three times daily p.c.) and levamisole (100 mg twice daily).

Mansonelliasis. *Mansonella ozzardi* is confined to South America, Central America, and the West Indies. Transmission is by *Simulium* spp. in South America and by *Culicoides* in the Caribbean. Little is known of the adult worms, but the microfilariae occur in the blood and are non-periodic. They may also be found in skin snips and should not be confused with *O. volvulus*.

In the West Indies infections are considered to be non-pathogenic. In the Amazon region, joint pains, fever, lymphadenopathy, and headache have been attributed to this parasite. Treatment with DEC-C is variously reported as being ineffective against

the parasite but effective in reducing the allegedly-associated symptoms.

Dirofilariasis. Infections with *Dirofilaria immitis*, the dog heartworm, with *D. repens* (from dogs or cats) or with *D. tenuis* (from the racoon in America) are occasionally transmitted by their mosquito vectors to man. Case reports come from USA, Japan, Australia, Europe, Africa, Asia, and South America.

In man *D. immitis* usually ends up in the lung giving rise to infarction vasculitis and the formation of a granuloma. This may be discovered as a silent 'coin lesion' on chest X-ray or may be associated with chest pain, cough, haemoptysis, and fever. There is no certain way to make a correct prospective diagnosis, for there is never any microfilaraemia. Hence the differential diagnosis from bronchial carcinoma, secondary neoplasms, or systemic fungal infections in the lung can only be made with certainty after removal and histopathological examination.

D. tenuis and *D. repens* can give rise to a subcutaneous granuloma anywhere on the body or under the conjunctiva. Surgical removal is the only treatment, and subsequent histological examination makes the diagnosis.

References

Binford, C. H. and Connor, D. H. (eds.) (1976). Diseases caused by filarial nematodes. In *Pathology of tropical and extraordinary diseases*. Section 8. vol. 2, 340.

Buck, A. D. (ed.) (1974). *Onchocerciasis—symptomatology, pathology, diagnosis*. World Health Organization, Geneva.

Denham, D. A. (1978). *Counting and identifying microfilariae*. London School of Hygiene and Tropical Medicine, London.

Sasa, M. (1976). *Human filariasis—a global survey of epidemiology and control*. University Park Press, Baltimore.

Guinea worm disease (dracunculiasis, dracontiasis)

B. O. L. Duke

Infection with the guinea worm (*Dracunculus medinensis*) is a localized, rural, tropical disease of remote and backward areas, causing much disability. It is characterized by the rapid onset of focal dermatitis and an ulcer, from which the long female worm extrudes.

Geographical distribution. The disease occurs in hot and often dry parts of Africa and Asia, chiefly around open water points. It is found in Mauritania, Mali, Senegal, Upper Volta, Benin, Guinea, Ivory Coast, Nigeria, Niger, Chad, Cameroon, Sudan, and the Nile valley. In Asia it occurs in the Arabian peninsula, western India, Pakistan, Afghanistan, Iran, and Turkey. Rare reports come from the West Indies and South America.

Life cycle of the parasite and pathology. The male worms die after mating and are rarely seen. The females are 70–120 cm long and about 2 mm wide. When mature the anterior end protudes from the skin and releases up to a million rhabditoid larvae (250–700 μm long) over the course of about two weeks before the worm dies. The larvae emerge especially on exposure to water. They penetrate into species of *Cyclops* (small 'water fleas' just visible to the naked eye), wherein they develop over two weeks to infective larvae. When a person drinks water containing infected *Cyclops*, the infective larvae emerge, penetrate the gut, pass to the tissues and complete their development to the gravid adult stage in 9–12 months. Transmission tends to be seasonal during the rains (farming season), and infections acquired one year become patent the next. There is no immunity to reinfection.

Clinical picture. Cases occur almost exclusively in rural tropical populations with inadequate water supplies and a low degree of health education. Few patients report to hospitals unless secondary infection supervenes, for the treatment available there is prolonged and often provides little advance on traditional methods.

The infection is usually silent until the gravid female reaches the subcutaneous tissue. Some worms may die and calcify without emerging. Normally, however, a papule forms over the anterior end of the female, leading on to a blister and finally to an ulcer, from which the anterior end of the worm extrudes, sheds its larvae over two weeks or so, and then dies. Sometimes the coiled body of the worm may be seen under the skin, and there may be some generalized allergic reaction just before the worm emerges. Delayed hypersensitivity responses may develop locally from the presence of the worm of the larvae in the tissues. These cause considerable pain and swelling and may immobilize the patient. Usually an attempt is made to extract the worm by winding it out onto a small stick a few centimetres each day. This process or other trauma may rupture the worm's uterus, releasing larvae into the subcutaneous tissues. Secondary infection often develops along the track of the worm, giving cellulitis or abscess formation; and the ulcer may be the site of entry for *Clostridium tetani*. Multiple infections are common, the worms coming out one after another or several at one time.

Female worms may extrude anywhere on the surface of the body but the commonest sites are on the legs or scrotum. Reactional effusions into one or more joints may occur, particularly when the worms extrude near the joint capsule. More rarely the worm may extrude into a joint cavity. The joint lesions can be very painful and incapacitating. Occasionally a disoriented worm may end up anywhere in the body causing a bizarre local lesion. Extrusion of the worm is associated with two to four weeks disability, but if secondary complications arise, the patient may be out of action for several months.

Diagnosis. The emergence of the worm is usually self evident. Adding some water to the exudate of the ulcer and examination under the microscope will reveal the motile larvae. Diagnosis of pre-patent infections by immunological means has not been evaluated in man.

Treatment. There is no specific chemotherapeutic treatment. The affected part should be rested and wet compresses may be applied for one or two days in order to hasten expulsion of the larvae. Thereafter the ulcer should be kept clean and covered with a mild antiseptic dressing, and the old-fashioned method of winding the worm out onto a stick should be tried. This must be done gently, taking care not to burst the uterus into the tissues and not pulling too hard. A few centimetres a day may be extracted, and the worm comes out more easily when it is dead, or if it can be partially paralysed by immersing the affected part in ice-cold water.

Various chemotherapeutic agents will facilitate the extraction of the worm. They do not kill the worm (which is already near the end of its life when it extrudes) but appear to act by reducing the associated inflammation and tissue reaction, thus speeding up the extraction. Treatment should start as soon as the first signs of worm emergence appear. Metronidazole (400 mg daily for an adult for 10–20 days) is probably the most effective. Niridazole (25 mg/kg daily for 7–10 days) or thiabendazole (50 mg/kg daily for 3 days) are also effective.

Secondary infection and abscess formation will require antibiotics and drainage. The possibility of tetanus should be borne in mind.

Prophylaxis. Prevention is by avoidance of drinking water sources infested with *Cyclops* or, if this is impracticable, then the water should be filtered through a cloth to extract the *Cyclops*, or should be boiled before it is drunk. The disease disappears as soon as safe water supplies are installed. Applications of temephos (Abate) granules will kill *Cyclops* in contaminated ponds, wells, etc. and keep them free for up to two months.

Reports that diethylcarbamizine citrate prevents the development of the young worms in man require confirmation.

Hookworm and strongyloides

P. A. J. Ball

The nematodes of the orders Rhabdiasoidea, Strongyloidea and Trichostrongyloidea are small fine worms, 2 cm or less in length, whose adults live in the lumen or wall of the small bowel of mammals. The two human hookworms *Necator americanus* and *Ancylostoma duodenale* (Strongyloidea), and *Strongyloides stercoralis* (Rhabdiasoidea) are common and important causes of disease in people who live, or have at some time lived, under the conditions of subsistence farming in the tropics, and will be discussed in detail in this section. *Strongyloides fülleborni* is a parasite of primates in Central Africa which can also affect man, as can *Oesophagostomum apiostomum* (Strongyloidea). Various species of the genera Trichostrongylus and Ostertagia (Trichostrongyloidea), which are primarily parasites of bovines, may be transmitted to people who live in close association with camels, goats, or sheep in the Middle and Far East. *Ancylostoma braziliense* and *A. caninum*, hookworms of carnivores, affect cats and dogs in the tropics and subtropics: they do not mature in man, but often cause lesions where their larvae penetrate the skin.

The hookworms

Distribution. *N. americanus* and *A. duodenale* are the common hookworms of man. *N. americanus* is indigenous to the moist tropics, where transmission is possible the year round, while *A. duodenale* is adapted to seasonally dryer or colder areas. Both were formerly restricted to the Old World, but their distribution has been altered by local extinction and human migration, so that *A. duodenale* now occurs with *N. americanus* in the Indian subcontinent, and alone in Egypt and its last stronghold in southern Europe (the Po valley). *N. americanus* occurs alone or nearly so in sub-Saharan Africa and the Americas. *A. duodenale* was formerly important in northern Europe in such artificial environments as the St Gothard tunnel during its construction and in the Cornish tin mines. *N. americanus* has declined where the economic conditions of subsistence farmers have improved, particularly in the southern United States since the 1930s and recently locally in Africa, or following organized campaigns of commercial plantations, as in Sri Lanka and Central Amercia. *A. duodenale* declined earlier in Europe, and more recently in Japan, for similar reasons.

Necator americanus. Most experimental work has been carried out on this species, which is therefore discussed in greatest detail.

Diagnosis. The diagnosis of hookworm depends upon finding eggs in the stools, and of hookworm as the cause of disease upon counting them. There is no specific serological test available for hookworm infection, or indeed for any of the parasites discussed in this section. Hookworm eggs are oval, about 50×35 μm, and in a fresh stool contain a four- or eight-celled morula (Fig. 1). A simple quantitative technique is that of Stoll: NaOH 0.1 mol/l is added to 1 g of faeces to a total volume of 15 ml, preferably stood overnight, and then thoroughly mixed. Then 0.15 ml is taken in a haematological pipette and the total number of eggs is counted under a large coverslip. Multiplication by 100 gives eggs per g of faeces. The number of worms present can be estimated from the egg output, as each female worm lays about 6000 eggs daily, irrespective of the heaviness of the infection or the clinical state of the patient.

Many techniques exist for concentrating eggs in stools to enable diagnosis when they are scanty. They are useful in surveys of prevalence, but do not help in the differential diagnosis or management of a patient.

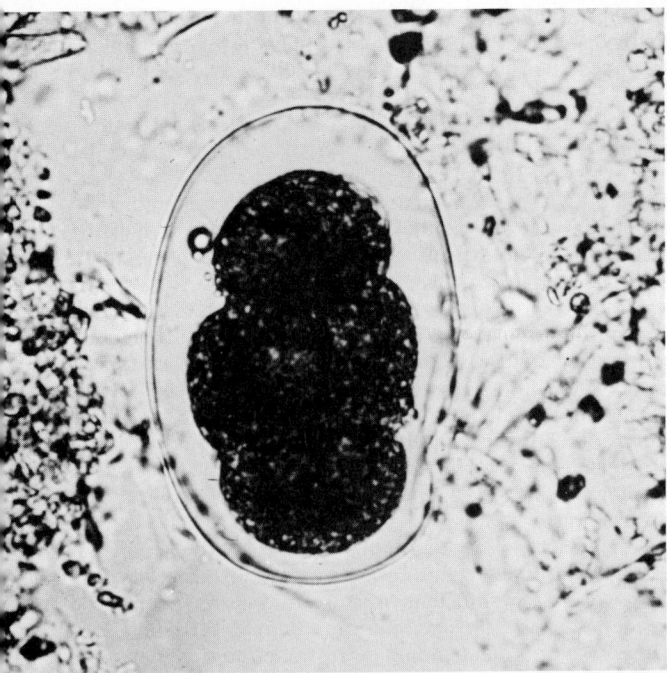

Fig. 1   Ovum of *Necator americanus*.

Pathology. Adult hookworms live in the lumen of the duodenum below the ampulla of Vater, and in the upper jejunum. They attach themselves to the mucosa by enclosing a villus in their pharynx, which has shearing jaws, and suck actively a mixture of blood and interstitial fluid (Fig. 2). Their chief source of nutrition is dissolved protein, not red cells, and the stimulus to continue sucking requires the presence of high molecular weight globulins. Disease results from depletion of iron and albumin. Each worm sucks red cells equivalent to about 0.03 ml of venous blood daily, and perhaps twice the equivalent amount of protein. Given that about 50 per

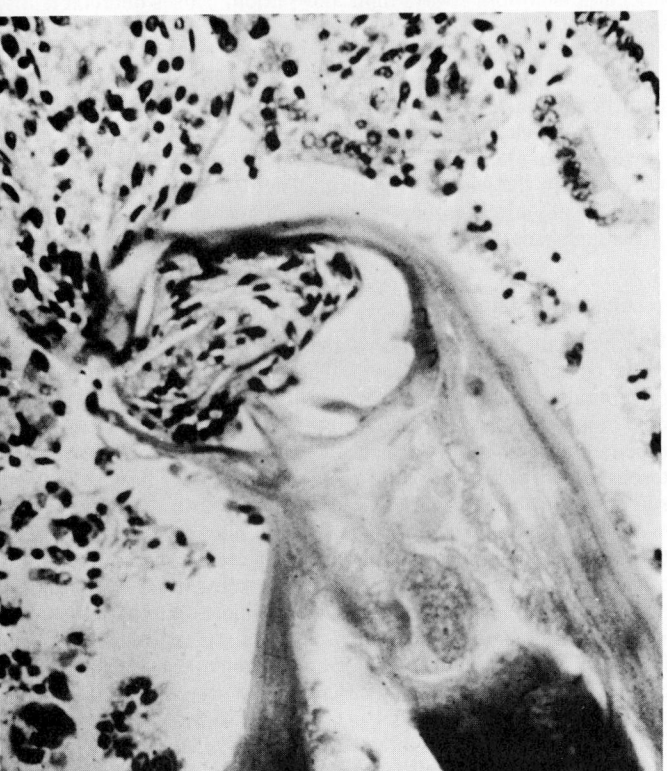

Fig. 2   *Necator americanus*: adult worm showing relationship of its pharynx to a jejunal villus.

cent of the iron removed is absorbed in a patient who is iron depleted and whose small bowel is otherwise normal, it is possible to calculate net iron loss from a knowledge of the number of worms present. It has thus been possible to define a threshold, expressed either crudely as eggs per g or more accurately as total egg output based on 24 hour stool collections, above which progressive iron depletion may be expected to occur, and below which the presence of hookworms is not a sufficient cause for anaemia. This threshold will vary with the patient's sex, and from place to place according to the iron content of the diet and the presence or absence of tropical enteropathy as a limiting factor in iron absorption. It is important to know the local threshold where the patient is seen if other sources of intestinal blood loss are not to be overlooked, and the more so since patients with hookworm are usually not available for later follow-up. The threshold egg count varies from 0 where a low iron content in the diet combines with tropical enteropathy to make spontaneous iron deficiency widespread, for example in rural Bengal or Puerto Rico, through a threshold count of about 4000 eggs per g in men and 2000 in women in South America, to about 20 000 in sub-Saharan Africa, where iron intake exceeds 30 mg daily and tropical enteropathy is rare.

It has been recognized for more than a century that patients with hookworm anaemia, and especially children, are often disproportionately oedematous, and hookworms have come to be recognized as a cause of protein-losing enteropathy as well as blood loss. In children loss of albumin is often sufficient to overtake the synthetic capacity of the liver before they have become anaemic. In adults this seldom happens until the haemoglobin level has fallen below about 5 g/dl unless some other disease is present to cause additional protein loss or to compromise synthesis: perhaps the commonest such associated conditions in practice are tropical enteropathy, damage to the large bowel by *Schistosoma mansoni*, and cirrhosis of the liver. In addition opportunistic infections may act to increase hypoalbuminaemia in the late stages of hookworm anaemia. Frequent examples are strongyloidiasis, mesenteric glandular tuberculosis, and salmonellae infection.

Where they penetrate the skin, filariform larvae cause small blisters which itch intensely: in previously exposed subjects, or, as with *A. brasiliense* or *A. caninum*, when the worms are in an abnormal host, they wander under the skin before moving on or dying, and give rise to tortuous tracks up to 5 cm long. In the lungs the larvae cause an interstitial pneumonitis: as a cause of symptoms it has been recorded much less often than the seasonal pneumonitis of ascariasis, and only in people massively exposed for the first time.

During their fourth instar the larvae enter the submucosa of the duodenum. In a first infection they give rise there to local inflammation sufficient to cause pain, which resembles that of duodenal ulcer, and radiologically visible thickening and rigidity of the mucosal folds. The patient may have diarrhoea, and occasionally fever and albuminuria. The eosinophil count begins to rise while the larvae are still in the lungs, and reaches a peak during their fourth instar. Symptoms subside and the eosinophil count falls shortly before egg laying begins, and coincidentally with the first appearance of circulating antibodies. Any subsequent infection is associated with an increase in circulating antibody titres but no further symptoms referable to the larvae or increase in eosinophilia.

Adult worms live for about 15 years, and excite no further visible immune reaction. In fact, the only obvious evidence of a response to the presence of adult *N. americanus* is a steady rise in the serum IgE level, which takes place over some years, even in the absence of further exposure. Much of this IgE is specific, though there is evidence that the presence of hookworms potentiates the production of IgE in response to other antigens also.

The mechanism by which adult worms isolate themselves from the host's immune response is not known, but evidence from animal models and human filariasis suggest that they fail to elicit an effective antibody response, perhaps in part due to a direct stimulation of specific suppressor T cells.

The evidence that repeated infection induces protective immunity is circumstantial, or based upon experiments upon related worms in animals. Such immunity is likely to be directed entirely against larvae in the tissues. The circumstantial evidence derives from the stability of infections in people repeatedly exposed, as opposed to their reaccumulation of parasites after treatment. Evidence from animal models suggests that there is a delay of at least months after first infection before protective immunity can develop: the epidemiology of hookworm infection supports this concept, in that in areas of intense transmission the heaviest infections are seen in people whose first exposure has been recent, notably children when they first start farm work and immigrant labourers entering endemic areas.

Ancylostoma duodenale. This worm's life history is more complicated than that of *N. americanus*, and varies with the seasons. The filariform larvae may enter the host either through the skin, or, less often, by ingestion. Those that do so during the early rainy season mature directly and lay eggs after about seven weeks: those entering in the later part of the rains undergo a period of suspended development or diapause, probably within the host's muscles. Studies of related worms in animals have shown that the occurrence or otherwise of diapause is decided by the temperature or humidity to which the free living larvae are exposed, though this has not been demonstrated directly for *A. duodenale*. After several months the larvae resume development, migrate, and mature, so that eggs start to be laid just before the first rains allow transmission of infection. As the intensity of infection rises during the wet season, the rising number of larvae in the tissues induce a humoral immune response intense enough to initiate the rejection of most of the worms in the gut, but which spares larvae in the tissues. This process is known in veterinary practice as 'self-cure'. The result is that the host enters the cold or dry season, when transmission is not possible, with only a few adult worms and a store of metabolically undemanding larvae.

The process of self-cure ensures that *A. duodenale* is not a cumulative infection over more than one season. Because of the possible presence of larvae in diapause and the fall in egg output which accompanies the earlier stages of self-cure, the number of eggs in a sample of stool is not necessarily proportionate to the number of adult worms actually or potentially present. Even in the absence of further infection the adults of *A. duodenale* do not live more than three years. On the other hand they suck much more blood than *N. americanus*, about 0.5 ml per worm daily, and have a much higher potential egg output, about 50 000 daily. Superimposed on the annual variation in worm load is a progressive protective immunity which is acquired during adolescence and presumably acts upon the developing larvae; as a result in any area peak egg output during the rains tends to be highest in children.

Treatment. Treatment requires removal of the worms and replacement of iron losses. Serum albumin levels rapidly return to normal except in patients who have associated illnesses and in young children who receive insufficient protein. Anaemia should not be treated by transfusion, which, even under better conditions than usually apply, carries a risk of heart failure. The best immediate treatment is with rest and a diuretic such as frusemide to cover the period until iron begins to take effect. Patients with hookworm disease are almost always illiterate and live far from hospitals, and so are unable or reluctant to receive long courses of treatment. Replacement of total exchangeable iron by a single dose is the ideal, but intravenous iron is often unsafe in severely anaemic patients whose iron binding capacity is reduced due to intestinal loss of transferrin. It should only be given if the serum albumin exceeds 35 g/l or if the iron binding capacity of the serum has been shown to be high. Recently preparations of iron for intramuscular use have been recommended which require only a small number of injections. They are probably safe when used without the precautions necessary for intravenous replacement. Folic acid, 5 mg daily,

should always be given for at least the first month to cover the erythropoietic response: a majority of patients in endemic areas fail to correct their haemoglobin levels fully and develop macrocytosis if this is not done.

The benzimidazole drugs, thiabendazole and mebendazole, are effective against both species of hookworm, thiabendazole in an oral dose of 25 mg/kg and mebendazole 2 mg/kg, both twice daily for two days. Thiabendazole, at least, is not predictably active against larvae, and neither drug affects larvae in diapause. Both drugs may be too expensive for therapeutic use in endemic areas or for mass prophylaxis. There tetrachlorethylene in a single fasting oral dose of 0.1 ml/kg (to a maximum of 5 ml) or bephenium hydroxynaphthoate 5 g orally while fasting on three consecutive mornings, may be used instead. The latter is the safer in very sick patients, in whom liver failure has occasionally been recorded after tetrachlorethylene, but is less certainly effective against *N. americanus*. Treatment with tetrachlorethylene should be preceded by piperazine, since adult *Ascaris* may be caused to migrate, with an attendant risk of cholangiitis, pancreatitis, or, in children, intestinal obstruction.

It is not always easy to decide whether to treat an infected patient who is not iron deficient. Patients who have been shown to have a hookworm load sufficient to cause disease in time, and patients resident outside an endemic area should certainly be treated. Otherwise treatment should be restricted to organized campaigns designed to reduce transmission.

Thiabendazole cream has been reported as being effective in the local treatment of ground itch due to *A. caninum* and *A. braziliense*.

Infections of local importance

Trichostrongyles. The ova of trichostrongyles are larger than those of hookworms (about 80 × 50 μm) and the morulae much more segmented by the time the stools are passed. Their life history is identical to that of *A. duodenale*. The adult worms behave similarly to hookworms. Although a majority of the population is affected in some areas, for example Azerbaijan and parts of Korea, human infection is almost always light and seldom causes detectable disease.

Oesophagostomum apiostomum. This parasite occasionally infects man in Central Africa, but is probably always transmitted from primates. In its natural host the adult worm is found in the small bowel, but in man it is usually single and enclosed in a granulomatous mass in the wall of the colon. The diagnosis is usually made histologically after surgical resection of a suspected carcinoma or paracolic abscess.

Strongyloides stercoralis

Worms of the genus *Strongyloides* differ in one very important respect from the others considered here. They undergo a succession of generations within their host, so that heavy infection may build up when conditions are favourable for them without the need for repeated transmission. As a result patients may die of fulminating disease many years after leaving an endemic area, having had few symptoms in the interval.

Strongyloides stercoralis is patchily endemic throughout the tropics and sub-tropics. People at risk in temperate countries are those who were born into, or have at some time lived under, peasant farming conditions in an endemic area. In the United Kingdom the main sources of potential patients are immigrants from the West Indies, Pakistan, and Bangladesh, an unknown, though certainly large, proportion of whom are infected. In addition it has been estimated that 15 per cent of former prisoners of war in the Far East were still infected 30 years after their return to this country.

Life history. The adult females are about 3 mm long. There are many fewer males than females in the gut, and it is thought that the parasitic females are largely parthenogenetic. When infection is light the worms are confined to the mucosal crypts of the duodenum and jejunum and feed on tissue which has been prepared by partial exodigestion. Eggs either hatch before the stools are passed, or are fully embryonated and contain a motile larva. They are the same size and shape as hookworm eggs. Larvae reaching the soil may moult to produce an infective stage, as do hookworms, or go through one or more free living generations before producing filariform larvae. Exactly how development as free living or parasitic stages is determined is still unknown, though anaerobic conditions seem to favour parasitic development. In all patients occasional larvae become infective before the stools are passed, and penetrate the bowel wall, or more rarely the peritoneum, to reach the lungs and mature. Under certain conditions infective larvae penetrate the sub mucosa in enormous quantities: a large proportion go on to migrate and so to augment the number of adults.

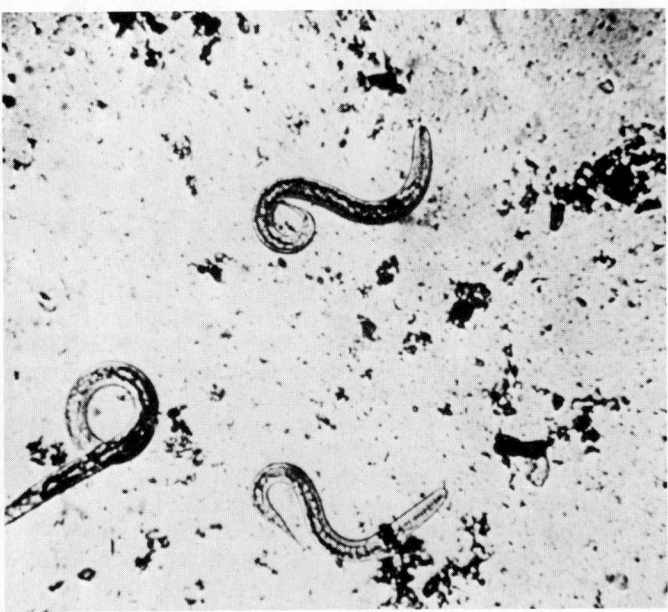

Fig. 3 *Strongyloides stercoralis*: first stage larvae in stool.

The commonest circumstances in which such cumulation occurs in temperate countries are diabetic ketosis, treatment with immunosuppressive drugs—especially doses of steroids equivalent to 45 mg or more of prednisone daily—and Hodgkin's disease, of which symtomatic strongyloidiasis may be the first indication. In the tropics it has been described as selectively complicating measles, lepromatous leprosy, disseminated tuberculosis, amoebiasis, and burns, but has to be suspected as a factor when diarrhoea complicates any severe illness. This list of associated diseases suggests that in a healthy host the penetration of the larvae and their subsequent survival are checked by immune responses, and that the integrity of thymus-derived lymphocytes is critical.

In animals both strongyloidiasis and ancylostomiasis, and in man strongyloidiasis certainly, and ancylostomiasis possibly, may be transmitted from mother to child in colostrum. In strongyloidiasis the number of migrating larvae is increased, and in ancylostomiasis the breaking of diapause is in some way conditioned, by parturition and lactation.

Pathology. The migration of larvae under the skin is accompanied by urticarial wheals overlying their course: this condition, called cutaneous larva migrans, affects most chronically infected patients from time to time. Larvae where they penetrate the skin cause ground itch. In heavy infections larvae in the lungs may cause asthma, and in fulminating disease patients may die of massive alveolar haemorrhage.

Bowel symptoms are commonly absent in light infections, though most patients will recall over the years a series of episodes of bulky motions, vague upper abdominal pain, and distension. During these episodes the clinical and radiological picture closely resembles that of symptomatic giardiasis. The stools usually contain both larvae and embryonated eggs, and jejunal biopsy shows eggs and larvae free on the mucosal surface, larvae in the submucosa, a degree of villous atrophy, dilatation of villous lymphatics, and a mixed interstitial infiltration with inflammatory cells. Very heavy infections cause a profuse and painless watery diarrhoea. It probably results from infiltration of the wall of the ileum and consequent interference with the absorption of water. The patient may also develop ileus which is disproportionate to any potassium depletion that may be present. It is easy to overlook the extent to which diarrhoea is contributing to extracellular fluid depletion and impaired renal perfusion in a sick patient, and particularly in diabetic ketosis, and even if the diagnosis of strongyloidiasis is considered, the stools may be wrongly reported as free of parasites unless they are examined fresh. This is because in such fulminating disease the stools usually contain only larvae, which are relatively scanty due to dilution, and are hard to identify once dead. Eosinophilia is usually absent, and, as already said, there is no specific serological test for strongyloidiasis.

Fulminating disease is often accompanied by Gram-negative septicaemia. It has been suggested that the migration of larvae disseminates bacteria, though it is difficult to prove the point because so many patients are at risk by virtue of their primary illness. Reports of meningitis associated with larvae in the brain suggest that in this case at least they play a direct role. Similarly, disseminated intravascular coagulation quite commonly complicates fatal strongyloidiasis, even when septicaemia is not present (or is overlooked). Disseminated intravascular coagulation may also contribute to the severity of the alveolar haemorrhage already mentioned, which, after fatal fluid depletion and septicaemia, is perhaps the most frequent cause of death.

Prophylaxis and treatment. Thiabendazole and mebendazole are both effective against adult worms, though neither predictably kills migrating larvae. All patients, whether they have symptomatic infection or are being treated prophylactically, should therefore receive further courses of treatment two and four weeks after the first and have their stools examined monthly for at least three months before cure is assumed. Patients with chronic strongyloidiasis may need replacement treatment with folic acid, iron, and vitamins D and K. Fulminating disease demands urgent extracellular fluid replacement, a search for or presumptive treatment of Gram-negative septicaemia, and a watch for evidence of disseminated intravascular coagulation.

Strongyloides fülleborni. *Strongyloides fülleborni* is an enzootic of primates in Central Africa, but is also almost certainly transmitted directly from man to man. Most cases have been reported from Zimbabwe and Zaire, where in some areas a large proportion of the rural population is infected. The same species appears to be present in Papua also. If so it is certainly truly endemic there, as non-human primates are absent, and must either have had some other animal reservoir or have accompanied the original Melanesian migrations to that island.

References

Ball, P. A. J. and Bartlett, A. (1969). Serological reactions to infection with *Necator americanus*. *Trans. Soc. trop. Med. Hyg.* **63**, 362.

Brown, R. C., and Girardeau, M. H. F. (1977). Transmammary passage of *Strongyloides* spp. larvae in the human host. *Am. J. trop. Med. Hyg.* **26**, 215.

Carvalho-Filho, E. (1978). Strongyloidiasis. *Clin. Gastroent.* **7**, 179

Gill, G. V. and Bell, D. R. (1979). *Strongyloides stercoralis* infection in former Far East prisoners of war. *Br. med. J.*, **ii**, 572.

Gilles, H. M., Watson-Williams, E. J., and Ball, P. A. J. (1964). Hookworm infection and anaemia. *Q. J Med.* **33**, 1.

Rivera, E., Maldonado, N., Valez-Garcia, E., Grillo, A. J., and Malaret, G. (1970). Hyperinfection syndrome with *Strongyloides stercoralis*. *Ann. intern. Med.* **72**, 199.

Roche, M. and Layrisse, M. (1966). The nature and causes of 'hookworm anaemia'. *Am. J. trop. Med. Hyg.* **15**, 1032.

Schad, G. A., Chowdhury, A. M., Dean, C. G., Kochar, V. K., Nawalinski, T. A., Thomas, J., and Tonascia, J. A. (1973). Arrested development in human hookworm infections: and adaptation to a seasonally unfavourable external environment. *Science* **180**, 502.

Pathogenic, free-living nematodes

D. A. Warrell

Micronema deletrix and possibly some other species in this genus are minute nematodes (length 400–500 μm), free-living and saprophytic in soil, humus, and manure. In horses and other equines they can cause local infections in the nasal cavity and maxillary bones and sometimes spread to the central nervous system and invade and multiply in viscera such as the kidney and lung. Three fatal cases have been described in humans who developed meningo-encephalitis and, in one case, involvement of liver and heart. Contamination of multiple deep wounds with manure was assumed to be the cause of the infection in one case, while another had extensive deep decubitis ulcers.

Reference

Gardiner, C. H., Koh, D. S., and Cardella, T. A. (1981). Micronema in man: third fatal infection. *Am. J. Trop. Med. Hyg.* **30**, 586.

Other gut nematodes

V. Zaman

Ascariasis

Ascariasis is an infection caused by *Ascaris lumbricoides*. Normally, the adult worms are located in the small intestine. In unusual circumstances such as fever, irritation due to drugs, anaesthesia, and bowel manipulation during surgery, the worms may migrate to ectopic sites where they may give rise to severe disease.

Geographic distribution. The distribution is cosmopolitan but the parasite occurs more frequently in moist and warm climate. In some rural tropical areas, the infection rates may reach 100 per cent of the population. In relative terms, it is more common in children who also carry higher worm loads.

Morphology. A mature worm is cylindrical in shape with tapering ends. It is creamy white to light brown in colour. The female measures 20–35 cm in length and 3–6 mm in breadth. The male measures 12–31 cm in length and 2–4 mm in breadth and has a curved tail. The head has three lips at the anterior end which carry minute teeth or denticles along their margins. The lips can be closed or extended allowing the worm to ingest food. In cross section, the worm reveals a thick cuticle, adjacent to which is the hypodermis which projects into the body cavity in form of lateral chords (Fig. 1). The somatic muscle cells are large and elongated and lie adjacent to the hypodermis. The worm is able to maintain its portion in the small intestine by the activity of these muscles. If the somatic muscles are paralysed by anthelmintics, it is expelled by the normal peristaltic movement.

The fertilized eggs are avoidal and measure 60–70 mm by 30–50 mm. When freshly passed they are not infective and contain a single cell. In the soil, the infective larva develops and only then they become infective. The cell is surrounded by a thin vitelline membrane. Around the membrane is a thick translucent shell which in turn is surrounded by an irregular albuminous coat. The albuminous coat is sometimes lost or can be removed by chemical treatment, when it is called a decorticated egg. In the lumen of the intestine, the eggs acquire brownish colour from the bile pigments. The unfertilized eggs are 88–94 mm by 40–44 mm and have disorganized contents. The larvae of *Ascaris lumbricoides* may be seen in infected lungs and measure up to 2 mm in length, and 75 mm in diameter. They have a central intestine, paired excretory columns and prominent lateral alae.

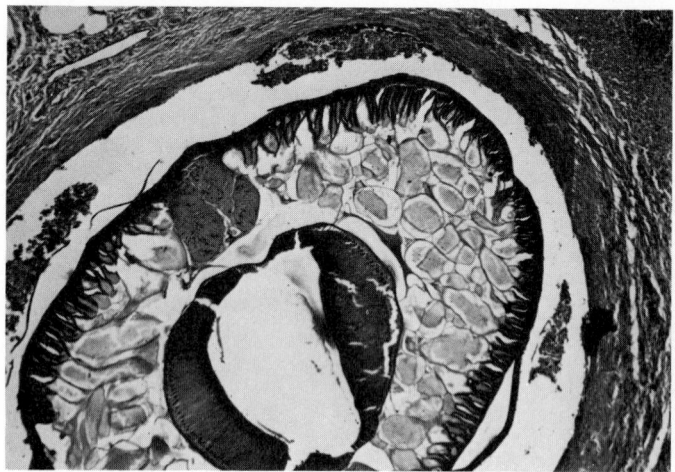

Fig. 1   *Ascaris lumbricoides* in the bile duct (× 250).

Life cycle. (See Fig. 2.) The gravid female produces 200 000–250 000 eggs daily. These take three or four weeks to develop into the infective stage. Recent studies indicate that this may be third stage and not second stage larva as was previously thought. The eggs are resistant to chemicals and low temperature and may remain viable for years in moist soil. On ingestion, the infective larva hatches out in the small intestine and penetrates the intestinal wall to enter the portal circulation. From the liver it is carried to the heart and via the pulmonary artery to the lungs. In the lungs, it breaks out of the capillaries into the alveoli and undergoes another moult to become fourth stage larva. From the lungs the larva moves up the bronchi and then crawls over the epiglottis to enter the digestive tract. In the intestine, it moults again to become a sexually mature worm. The life span of adult worm is approximately one year, after which it is spontaneously expelled. In hyperendemic areas, children are being continuously infected so that as some worms are being expelled, others are maturing to take their place.

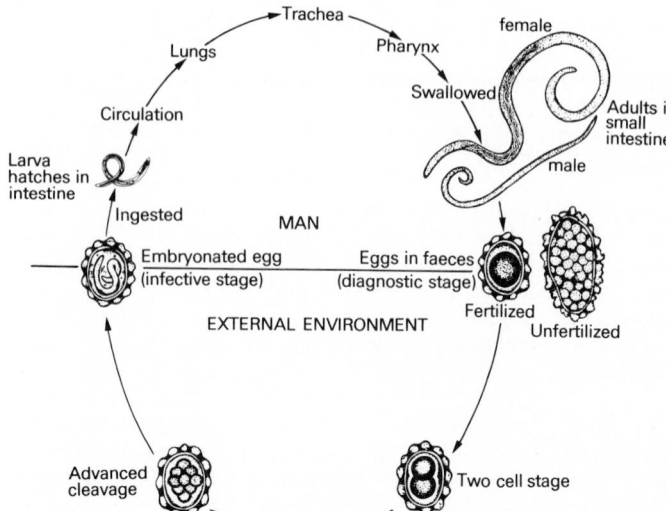

Fig. 2   Life cycle of *Ascaris lumbricoides*. (Adapted from Center for Disease Control, Atlanta, Georgia, USA.)

Clinical aspects. In majority of cases, the infected individual remains asymptomatic. However, there is considerable evidence to indicate that the presence of *Ascaris* causes nutritional problems and hinders the normal development of children. Occasionally, patients may develop fever, malaise, urticaria, intestinal colic, nausea, vomiting, diarrhoea, and central nervous system disorders.

The larval migration of *Ascaris* through the lungs may produce varying degrees of pneumonitis and bronchospasm which is known as Loeffler's syndrome. Chest radiographs may show diffuse mottling and increased prominence of peribronchial markings. There is generally high eosinophilia and the condition subsides in 7–10 days time unless re-infection occurs. The larvae of *A. suum* (pig *Ascaris*) may also produce severe pneumonitis and bronchospasm in areas where pig farming is common.

Occasionally, *Ascariasis* can manifest as severe life threatening disease. This could happen in the following situations:

1. When large number of worms get entangled to form a bolus and block the intestinal lumen producing signs and symptoms of acute intestinal obstruction.

2. In ectopic migration resulting in the entry of the worm into appendix, common bile duct, and pancreatic duct. In the case of the entry of the worm into the biliary tract, there is severe colic often followed by suppurative cholangitis and multiple liver abscesses. Suppuration occurs as a result of the disintegration of the trapped worm and secondary bacterial infection. The disintegration of the female worm releases large number of eggs in the liver which can be recognized on histological examination.

Diagnosis. This is usually made by detecting *Ascaris* eggs in the faeces. Sometimes, the patient brings developing or adult worms which have been passed in the faeces or have emerged from the anus or the nose in a sick child. Occasionally, adult worms are outlined in the intestines during barium meal examination.

Treatment. Whenever possible, all positive cases, irrespective of the worm load, should be treated as even a few worms can undergo ectopic migration with dangerous consequences:

1. Pyrantel pamoate: a single dose of 10 mg per kg body weight is effective in curing over 90 per cent of cases. Side reactions are mild, if any, and the drug is well tolerated. It has the advantage of being active against *Enterobius vermicularis* and hookworms. This wide-spectrum activity is a useful factor in endemic areas where multiple nematode infections are common.

2. Mebendazole: this drug is also a wide-spectrum anthelmintic with good host tolerance. It is given as 100 mg twice daily for three days, irrespective of age. Unfortunately, a few cases of ectopic migration, induced by the drug have been reported.

3. Levamisole hydrochloride: this is probably the most effective anti-*Ascaris* agent and produces rapid paralysis of the worm. It is administered as a single dose of 150 mg for adults and 50 mg for persons under 10 kg. Side reactions are more common than pyrantel and mebendazole. Prolonged therapy with this drug has occasionally resulted in blood dyscrasias when it was used in treatment of auto-immune diseases and rheumatoid arthritis.

4. Piperazine salts: these are widely used because of their low cost and high degree of efficacy which includes *Enterobius vermicularis*, but not hookworm. The dose is 75 mg/kg (maximum of 3.5 g) given as a single dose daily for two consecutive days. Prior fasting is not required. Occasionally, symptoms involving the central nervous system such as unsteadiness and vertigo have been reported.

Prevention and control. As *Ascaris* eggs can survive in the soil for many years, prevention and control in the endemic areas is difficult. Mass chemotherapy given at intervals of six months along with environmental sanitation can break the cycle. Prevalence rates of *Ascariasis* and other soil-transmitted helminths are greatly reduced by improvement in housing. At a personal level, infection is prevented by eating only cooked food and by avoiding green vegetables and salads in countries where human faeces is used as a fertilizer.

Anisakiasis

Anisakiasis is an infection caused by the larvae of nematodes belonging to the family *Anisakidae*.

Geographic distribution. The adult worms are commonly found in sea mammals in many parts of the world. Human infections occur wherever raw or improperly cooked fish is consumed. The incidence is highest in Japan followed by Holland, Scandinavia, and countries along the pacific coast of S. America.

Morphology. This is a large group of parasites and complete speciation of adults and larvae has not been done. The larval stages which are found in man can be recognized as those belonging to the family *Anisakidae* only, by the presence of large bulbous lateral chords in cross sections.

Life cycle. Adults live in the lumen of the intestine of marine mammals, eggs are passed in water, second stage larvae are ingested by crustaceans, which are then ingested by fish or squid where they enter the muscles; marine mammals and humans get infected by eating fish. In humans, larvae do not develop into maturity but attach themselves to the muscosa of stomach or intestine.

Clinical aspects. The majority of patients present with gastric symptoms which develops within 12–24 hours after eating infected fish. The symptoms are due to the ulceration produced by the larvae as they burrow into the mucous membrane. In addition to epigastric pain, nausea and vomiting, there may be haematemesis during the acute stage of the disease.

Diagnosis. Gastroscopy often reveals the lesion and the presence of larvae which are attached to the mucous membrane. X-ray examinations may show the presence of single or multiple ulcers. Serological tests are now available in some specialized centres.

Treatment. In acute infection, an attempt should be made to remove all the larvae through a gastroscope. In chronic cases, surgical removal of the ulcerated area may be required. No effective chemotherapy is available. Infection is prevented by avoiding ingestion of raw fish in the endemic areas.

Capillariasis

Capillariasis is an infection by parasites belonging to the genus *Capillaria*. Two species infect humans, *C. philippinensis*, which produces intestinal capillariasis, and *C. hepatica*, which produces hepatic capillariasis.

Geographic distribution. *C. philippinensis* has been described from the Philippines and Thailand. In the Philippines, the distribution of the disease includes the western and northern coastal areas of Luzon and the northeast of Mindanao. In Thailand, the infection is mostly sporadic and widely scattered. *C. hepatica* is a rare parasite of humans but is commonly found in rodents in many parts of the world.

Morphology. The adult *C. philippinensis* are thin, small worms measuring 2.5–4.3 mm in length. They have a row of stichocytes at the anterior end, as in the case of *Trichuris*. The eggs measure 36–45 μm in length and 19–21 μm in breadth and have bipolar plugs also like *Trichuris* (Fig. 3). However, unlike *Trichuris*, the eggs are not barrel shaped and the plugs do not protrude from the lateral ends. The adults of *C. hepatica* measure 52–104 mm in length and the anterior region contains the stichocytes. The eggs measure

48–66 μm by 28–36 μm and have bipolar plugs. The egg shell is thick and distinctly striated.

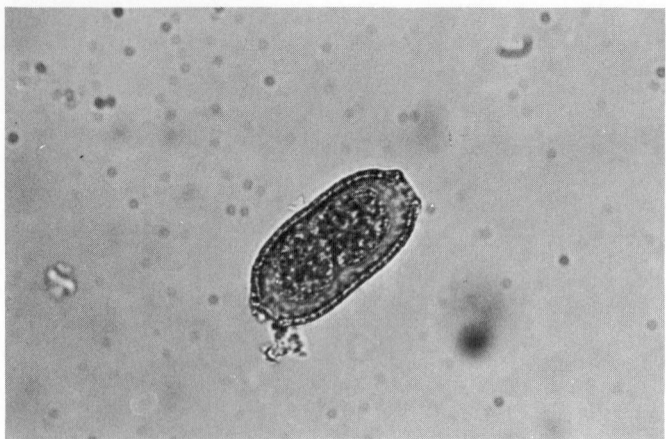

Fig. 3   *Capillaria philippineses* egg (× 1400).

Life cycle. The life cycle of *C. philippinensis* has not been completely worked out, but man is infected by eating fresh-water fish containing the infective larvae, and fish-eating birds act as natural or reservoir host. In nature, therefore, there is a fish–bird–fish cycle with man getting only accidentally involved. The main danger with this infection lies in the possibility of auto-infection which leads to very heavy worm loads.

C. hepatica is found in the liver of rodents and other mammals. The eggs are discharged in the liver tissue and remain there until the animal dies (Fig. 4). They eventually reach the soil by the decay of the carcass. Humans are infected by accidentally swallowing embryonated eggs from the soil.

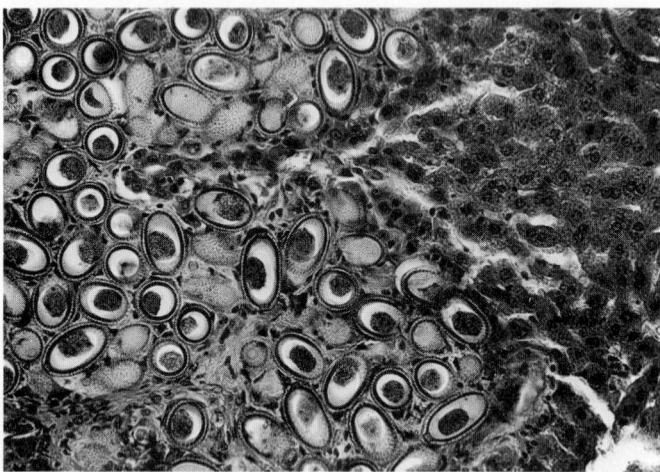

Fig. 4   *Capillaria hepatica* eggs in the liver (× 250).

Clinical aspects. *C. philippinensis* can produce severe disease which may lead to death. In the beginning, patients often present with abdominal pain, diarrhoea, and borborygami. As the worm load increased due to auto-infection, diarrhoea becomes most severe with anorexia, nausea and vomiting. Prolonged diarrhoea leads to cachexia and muscular wasting. There may also be signs of hypotension and cardiac failure. In untreated cases, the mortality rate is close to 20 per cent.

In *C. hepatica* infection, symptoms of visceral larva migrans may be present. The patient may have enlarged tender liver with low-grade fever and eosinophilia.

Diagnosis. In the case of *C. philippinensis*, diagnosis is made by

finding the typical eggs in the faeces. In *C. hepatica*, diagnosis is made by identifying the parasite or eggs in the biopsy of liver.

Treatment. All cases of *C. philippinensis* should be treated with mebendazole, in a dose of 400 mg per day until the symptoms subside and the eggs disappear from the faeces. Supportive measures to overcome malnutrition and diarrhoea will be required in severely ill patients. There is no specific treatment for *C. hepatica* infection. Infection with *C. philippinensis* is prevented by not eating raw fish in the endemic regions of southeast Asia.

Trichinosis

Trichinosis is an infection caused by *Trichinella spiralis*.

Geographic distribution. The infection is endemic in many parts of the world where pork is consumed. These areas include central and eastern Europe, central, south, and north America, and parts of Africa and Asia. Infection is also endemic in the Arctic regions resulting from eating boar meat.

Morphology. The adult males are small nematodes measuring 1.4–1.6 mm. The female is viviparous and about twice as long as the male. The anterior part contains a row of glandular cells (stichocytes) as in *Trichuris trichiura*. The male worm lacks a spicule but has two conical papillae on sides of the cloacal opening.

Life cycle. (See Fig. 5.) Humans become infected by eating improperly cooked pork or pork products such as sausages. In some parts of the world, wild boars are heavily infected. After ingestion,

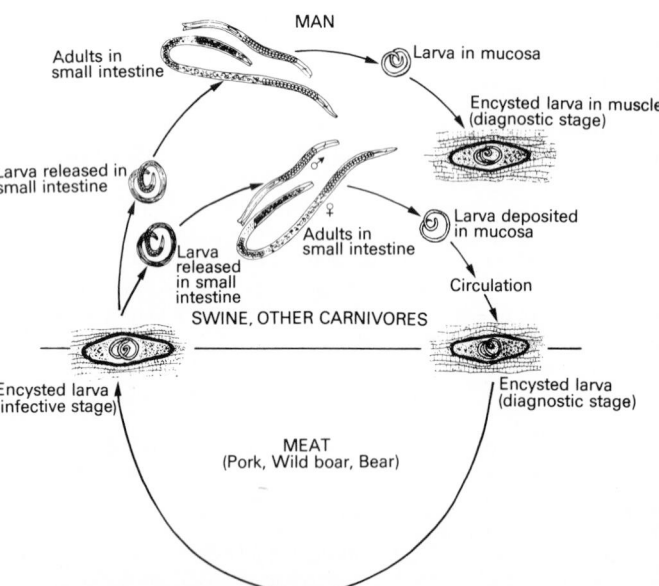

Fig. 5   Life cycle of *Trichinella spiralis*. (Adapted from Center for Disease Control, Atlanta, Georgia, USA.)

the larvae are liberated in the small intestine and mature into adults. The female deposits larvae in the intestinal tissues from where they find their way into the the blood circulation and then into the striated muscles of the body (Fig. 6). The most heavily parasitized muscles are the diaphragm, tongue, larnygeal, and abdominal muscles. After penetration, the larva undergoes three moults and coils into a spiral which eventually becomes enclosed in a thick-walled cyst. In this form, the larva may remain viable for many years.

Pigs become infected by eating infected scrap and garbage from slaughter houses or farms. Occasionally, they become infected by eating carcases of infected rats.

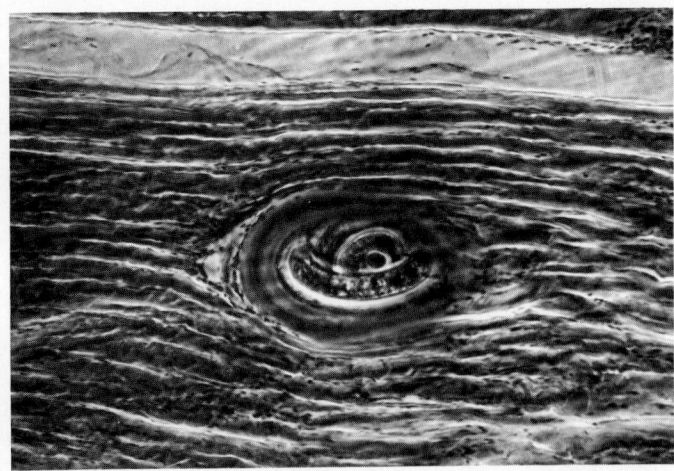

Fig. 6 *Trichinella spiralis* in human muscle (× 1000).

Clinical aspects. The majority of individuals with light infection remain asymptomatic. In cases of heavy infection, disease manifests in three clinical stages:

1. The invasion stage. This is seen during the first week of infection and is due to juveniles and adults burrowing into the intestinal tissues. The patient complains of abdominal pain, nausea and vomiting, and diarrhoea of varying intensity. There may be fever, profuse perspiration, and tachycardia.

2. The migration stage. This usually begins after the first week of infection. During this period, the larvae are liberated into the circulation by the gravid female and find their way to the muscles. Symptoms occur due to the toxic effects of the larvae and a hypersensitivity reaction occurs as a result of the liberation of parasite antigens. There is oedema of the face and periorbital tissues, fever, muscular tenderness, and hypereosinophilia. Complications involving the myocardium, lungs, and the central nervous system may occur due to the migrating larvae. However, the larvae do not encyst in the myocardium.

3. The encystment stage. This usually begins after the third week of infection. There is usually a gradual recovery from the symptoms. In a few cases with heavy infection, the symptoms may get worse and death may occur due to myocardiac failure, and respiratory and central nervous system involvement. All serological tests become positive during this stage.

Diagnosis. This is based on a combination of clinical and epidemiological evidence. In a characteristic case, the patient will give a history of gastrointestinal disturbances (invasion stage) within 48 hours of eating pork products, wild boar, or bear meat. If the patient comes in the later stage (migration stage), there is periorbital oedema, irregular fever, and hypereosinophilia.

Amongst the various serological tests which become positive during the encystment stage, the two most commonly used are the skin test and the slide flocullation test. Recently ELISA has also been used. The skin test antigen is made from larvae and gives an immediate type reaction in positive cases. The test is very good for surveys but unsuitable for the detection of acute disease as it remains positive for many years after infection. The slide flocullation test is also prepared from larval antigen which is attached to cholesterol particles. In a positive reaction, flocullation is seen under the microscope. The test remains positive for about 10 months after infection. Serum enzymes such as oxalacetic, glutamic, and pyruvic transaminases are elevated. Muscle biopsy is positive in approximately 90 per cent of clinically positive cases.

Treatment. The prognosis is good and majority of patients recover after the larvae have encysted. In case of myocarditis and severe myalgia, oral prednisone for three to five days (0.5–1.0 mg/kg per day) is useful and provides symptomatic relief. The drug should not be used for a longer period as it may interfere with the development of immune response and encystment. In experimental animals, thiabendazole is able to kill encysted larvae. In humans, its efficacy against larvae is doubtful but it provides symptomatic relief. The dosage of 25–50 mg/kg per day for two to five days is given and this usually brings down the fever and eosinophilia.

Control and prevention. *Trichinosis* in the pig population can be greatly reduced or eliminated by hygienic rearing methods. Larvae in pork can be killed by freezing at −18 °C for 24 hours. Thorough cooking of pork is the best safeguard against infection in all endemic areas.

Enterobiasis

Enterobiasis is an infection caused by *Enterobius vermicularis*.

Geographic distribution. This is one of the few parasites which is more prevalent in the temperate regions of the world than in the tropics. Children are more often involved than adults. It occurs in groups such as families living together, inmates of hostels, army camps, etc.

Morphology. The male is approximately 5 mm long with a diameter of 0.1–0.2 mm. The female is approximately 13 mm long with a diameter of 0.3–0.5 mm. The gravid female has two distended uteri which practically fill the whole body. The male has a single spicule and a curved tail. The cuticle has cervical alae which enable its easy recognition. The eggs are generally flattened on one side and measure approximately 50–60 mm in length and 20–30 mm in breadth. They have a thick transparent shell. The eggs are unembryonated when passed but become infective within a few hours.

Life cycle. The adults are mainly located in the caecal region (Fig. 7), and the female deposits its eggs on the anus and perianal skin. Direct human-to-human infection occurs by inhalation and swallowing of the eggs. In addition, auto-infection occurs by contamination of fingers. There is no visceral migration and the larva matures into an adult in the lumen of the intestinal tract. The life cycle of the parasite is completed in about six weeks.

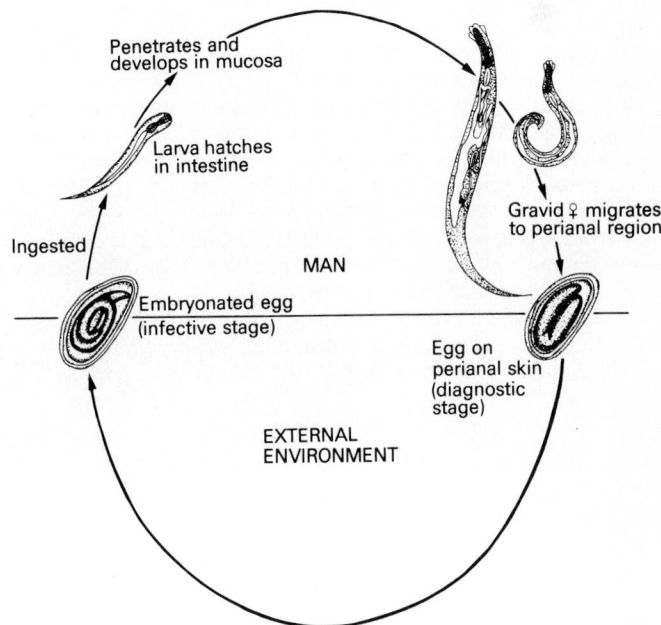

Fig. 7 Life cycle of *Enterobius vermicularis*. (Adapted from Center for Disease Control, Atlanta, Georgia, USA.)

Clinical aspects. The most common presenting symptom is pruritis ani. This can be very troublesome and occurs more often during the night. Persistent itching may lead to inflammation and secondary bacterial infection of the perianal region. Infected children may suffer from insomnia, emotional disturbance, anorexia, weight loss, and enuresis. Occasionally, adult worm undergoes ectopic migration and may enter the female genital tract. Inside the uterus or the Fallopian tube it may get encapsulated and produce symptoms of salpingitis. The parasite may also get lodged in the lumen of the appendix leading to appendicitis (Fig. 8). The life span of the parasite is three to six weeks.

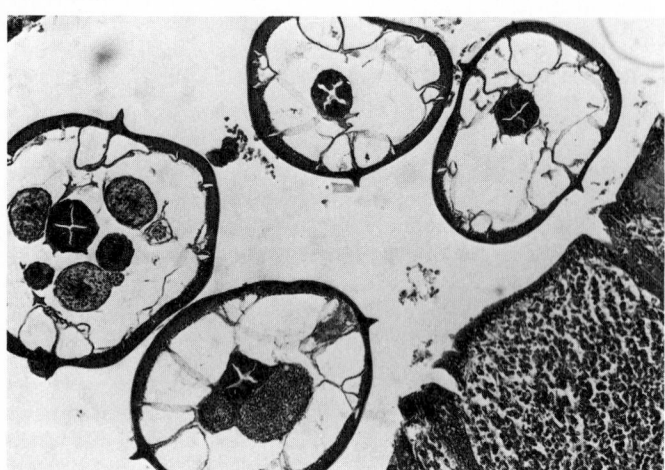

Fig. 8 *Enterobius vermicularis* in the lumen of the appendix (× 250).

Diagnosis. The eggs are not usually found in the faeces. The best method to look for their presence is around the anus. This is done by taking a swab or using cellulose adhesive tape. The anal examination for eggs should be done before defecation or bathing. Sometimes intact worms are passed out in the faeces and can be easily recognized by their size and shape.

Treatment. Attention to personal hygiene is an important part of treatment and prevention. The patient should be instructed to keep nails short and wash hands with soap and water after going to the toilet. The bed cover and sleeping garments should be changed every day and the floor in the bedroom kept clean. With these simple hygienic measures, infection will disappear on its own due to the short lifespan of the parasite.

Many drugs are available to treat the infection and it is advisable to treat all the children in the same household at the same time.

1. Piperazine citrate is given in a dose of 65 mg/kg for seven days. The course is repeated after two weeks. Piperazine is contra-indicated in renal and liver disease and epilepsy.

2. Pyrantel pamoate is equally effective in a single dose of 10 mg/kg (maximum 1 g) and its side-effect profile is better than piperazine. The drug is repeated after two weeks.

3. Mebendazole is effective in a single dose of 100 mg, repeated after two weeks. This drug is contra-indicated in pregnancy.

4. Pyrvinium pamoate is specific for *Enterobrius vermicularis* and is given in a single dose of 5 mg/kg (maximum 350 mg), repeated after two weeks. The main disadvantage of this drug is that it stains garments and skin.

Trichuriasis

Trichuriasis is an infection caused by *Trichuris trichiura*.

Geographic distribution. It has a worldwide distribution and is the most common intestinal nematode in some tropical regions such as southeast Asia.

Morphology. The adult male measures 30–45 mm and the female 35–50 mm in length. The parasite is commonly known as the whipworm because the anterior three-fifths is thin and elongated and the posterior two-fifths is bulbous and fleshy. One important feature of this group of worms is the possession of a thin elongated oesphagus which is surrounded by gland cells known as stichocytes. The adults are mainly located in caecum and produce barrel-shaped eggs which have a length of 22–50 mm. At the lateral ends, eggs have a transparent blister-like plug and are single celled when freshly passed. In the soil, the eggs become infective in about three weeks.

Life cycle. (See Fig. 9). Infection occurs by the ingestion of the embryonated egg. The larva does not undergo visceral migration but penetrates the gut wall for a short period before returning to the lumen to mature into adult stage. The worms attach themselves to the large intestine by threading their anterior end into the epithelium (Fig. 10). The posterior end hangs free in the lumen of the bowel. The whole period of development in the host takes about three months to complete.

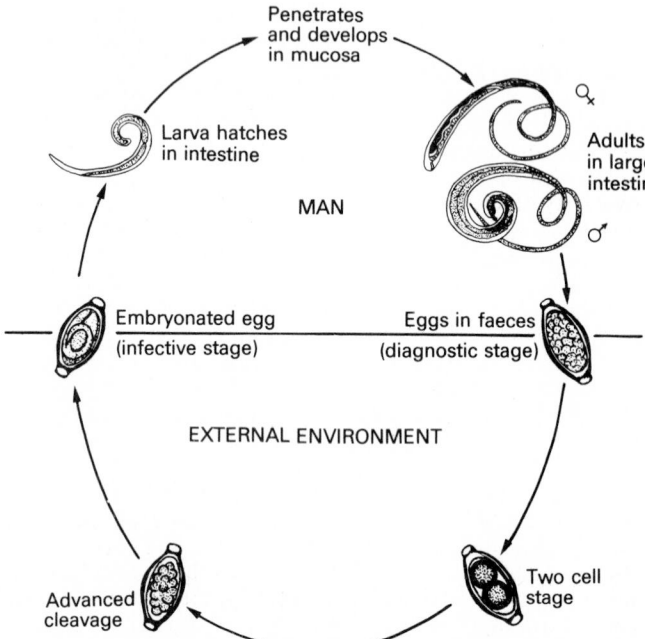

Fig. 9 Life cycle of *Trichuris trichiuria*. (Adapted from Center for Disease Control, Atlanta, Georgia, USA.)

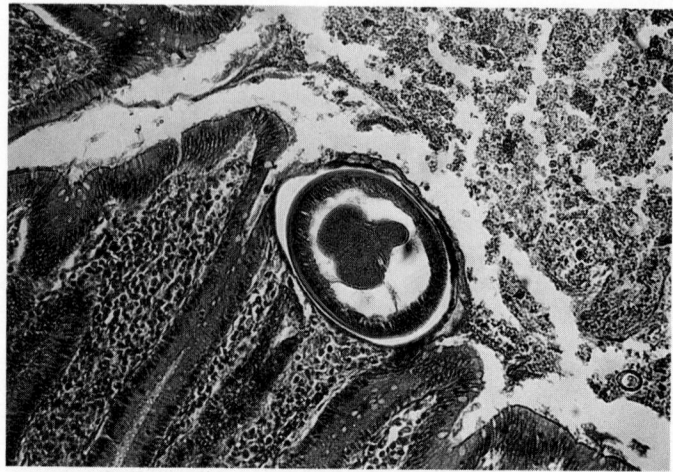

Fig. 10 *Trichuris trichiuria*: anterior end embedded in the superficial layer of intestine epithelium (× 250).

Clinical aspects. Light infections are generally asymptomatic. In heavy infections, there is colitis with the passage of blood and mucus in faeces. Heavy infection in children leads to anaemia resulting in oedema, dyspnoea, and cardiac failure. The anaemia is probably due to bleeding from the damaged and inflamed mucous membrane rather than sucking of blood by the parasite itself. In some cases, prolapse of the rectum occurs, probably due to constant irritation produced by the worm and the weakness of the levator ani muscle. Occasionally, the worm may lodge itself in the lumen of the appendix and cause acute appendicitis.

Diagnosis. This is based on finding characteristic barrel-shaped eggs in the faeces. Eosinophils and Charcot–Leyden crystals are often present. Sigmoidoscopy or proctoscopy may show worms attached to the mucous membrane and sometimes intact worms may be passed out in the faeces.

Treatment. Two very effective chemotherapeutic agents are now available:

1. Mebendazole is a synthetic benzimidazole derivative which is active against other intestinal nematodes in addition to *Trichuris*. During therapy, abnormal *Trichuris* eggs are produced as the drug interferes with embryogenesis. Side effects are few and it is well tolerated. Dosage is 100 mg twice daily for three days irrespective of the age of the patient. Mebendazole is contra-indicated in pregnancy.

2. Oxantel puls pyrantel pamoate. This combination is effective against *Ascaris lumbricoides*, *Enterobius vermicularis*, hookworm and *Trichuris trichiura*. Dosage is 10–20 mg/kg body weight of each component as a single dose. In heavy infections, the drug may be repeated two or three times.

Preventive measures are same as in *Ascariasis*.

Toxocara and visceral larva migrans

D. R. Bell and M. J. Clarkson

Ascarid worms are common in many animals but the overwhelming evidence is that *Toxocara canis* is the main 'animal' ascarid causing disease in man.

Life cycle

Dog. The adult worms live normally in the intestine of dogs and foxes and very rarely in other hosts, including man. Large numbers of sticky eggs are passed out in the stools of pups and it takes about two weeks before the eggs are infective, when they contain a larva. The eggs are swallowed and hatch in the intestine and bore their way through its wall to reach the blood. They migrate through the body, their route varying with the age of the dog. In young pups they break into the alveoli of the lungs, are coughed up and swallowed and become adult in about five weeks. In older dogs, the larvae migrate through many organs and can remain alive for years in the muscles. In the bitch, these larvae are reactivated from the fortieth day of pregnancy and cross the placenta where they infect the pups in the uterus. The larvae travel to the lungs of the pup and only continue their migration to the intestine when the lungs become expanded after birth. Since the life cycle is partly completed in the uterus, adult worms are found in pups as early as three weeks after birth. Pups may also become infected by larvae in the milk of the bitch. Although adult dogs may pass small numbers of eggs in their stools, it is the pup which is the important source of infection. As larvae are reactivated at each pregnancy, it is best to assume that every pup is infected and adopt measures to destroy the worms.

Man. Man becomes infected by swallowing infective eggs from the coat of pups, from soil or sand-pits, or possibly from food contaminated by dog faeces (salads), or by eggs transferred by flies. The larvae migrate through the liver and lungs, and sometimes reach the eye. They typically give rise to an eosinophil-rich granuloma, and the clinical picture is related to the intensity of infection, and the sites where the larvae are most numerous. The larvae die naturally in about one year, so the infection is self-limiting.

Disease. When a clinically recognizable disease occurs, the condition is called visceral larva migrans (VLM); for every recognized case of VLM, there are many clinically inapparent infections. There are two recognizable clinical syndromes.

Ocular toxocariasis. The most important syndrome is produced when a larva in the eye causes a granuloma. If this is near the macula, it will interfere with vision, and retinal granulomas can be seen with the help of an ophthalmoscope. The condition is almost entirely confined to childhood, the average age at diagnosis being about six years. The commonest presenting features are complaints about vision in one eye, and squint.

Diagnosis is difficult, because eye lesions are seldom accompanied by more generalized manifestations of VLM, eosinophilia is usually absent, and even the most sensitive serodiagnostic tests may be negative. It used to be thought that only identification of the larva in histological sections of the enucleated eye could be accepted as definitive diagnosis. It now seems that high antibody titres in the aqueous humour may occur in such cases, and specific antigen might also be identified in future. Despite the dangers of paracentesis of the anterior chamber, they may seem preferable to the irrevocability of enucleation.

The gross VLM syndrome. This is most often identified in very young children with a massive exposure to *T. canis* eggs by virtue of pica, or in others at especially high risk, such as the mentally defective. The clinical manifestations are the result of the invasion of the viscera by numerous migrating larvae. The main features are fever, eosinophilia, asthma or cough, and hepatomegaly. The diagnosis is suggested by the clinical picture, confirmed by the finding of the larvae in granulomas revealed at liver biopsy, by the accompanying eosinophilia, and by a variety of serodiagnostic tests.

The human syndromes: the lack of overlap. The rarity of ocular lesions in those with gross VLM is well-documented, to the extent that the syndromes seem almost mutually exclusive. This could be explained by a different aetiology, such as gross VLM being due to ingestion of numerous eggs, and ocular toxocariasis being due to a late reactivation of an infection acquired *in utero* via the placenta, or even by the ingestion of larvae taken in with mothers' milk. No one has investigated the antibody titres in the mothers of children who develop ocular toxocariasis, or the infant-feeding practices of these mothers. Such studies might throw new light on an old problem.

Serodiagnosis. Toxocara is not the only cause of the gross VLM syndrome, but, probably, the most common cause in northern Europe. Elsewhere, a similar clinical picture can be produced by a variety of invasive helminth infections such as *Ascaris lumbricoides*, *Strongyloides stercoralis*, and various schistosomes. So one would expect an efficient test for *Toxocara* antibodies to be positive in almost all such cases in the United Kingdom. Unfortunately, this is not so. The reasons remain obscure, but it might be that other zoonotic helminth infections—such as *Toxascaris* spp.—infect man with similar results.

Treatment of human toxocariasis. This is unsatisfactory. The gross VLM syndrome often responds temporarily to a course of diethylcarbamazine (DEC) or thiabendazole but usually relapses occur when medication is stopped. The killing of the larvae in granulomas of ocular *Toxocara* might be expected to enhance the inflammatory response, and so make the condition worse. For this reason, steroids—locally, systemically, or both—are usually employed. As ophthalmologists cannot agree on the criteria needed to establish the diagnosis, there is no consensus on the effectiveness of this approach.

The importance of toxocariasis in man. Compared with infection by *Toxoplasma gondii*, *Toxocara* is probably a relatively unimportant cause of blindness; it is certainly a far less important cause of other morbidity. A large number of asymptomatic members of populations throughout the world possess antibodies to *Toxocara* but this has nothing to do with the frequency of *disease* related to the organism. Nor has the finding of environmental contamination with *Toxocara* eggs any inevitable implications for human disease.

Control. There is no need to recommend that families should not have pet dogs or that pups should be destroyed to avoid the slight risk to man associated with *T. canis* as there are many efficient drugs available to remove the worms. Piperazine is a cheap drug which removes adults only and therefore should be given when pups are 3, 5, and 8 weeks old. Since most pets are acquired at 8 weeks old, they should be wormed then, again at 12 weeks when vaccinated against distemper, at six months old and then every year. Other drugs such as dichlorvos, mebendazole, and nitroscanate are effective against migrating stages and might therefore be given less frequently to young pups, but they are much more expensive than piperazine. Recent work suggests that some antihelmintics may destroy larvae in the bitch which might lead to a method of producing pups which were not infected. For example, one suggested regimen is to dose bitches daily from the 45th to the 50th day of the pregnancy with fenbendazole.

Sensible hygiene like hand washing and the separation of dog exercising areas from children's playing areas are logical measures to assist in control.

References

British Medical Journal (1979). Visceral larva migrans again. *Br. med. J.* i, 435.

Glickman, L. T., Schantz, P., Dombroske, R., and Cypess, R. H. (1978). Evaluation of serodiagnostic tests for visceral larva migrans. *Am. J. trop. Med. Hyg.* **27**, 492.

Jacobs, D. E., Pegg, E. J., and Stevenson, P. (1977). Helminths of British dogs: *Toxocara canis*—a veterinary perspective. *J. small Anim. Pract.* **18**, 79.

Zinkman, W. H. (1978). Visceral larva migrans. A review and reassessment indicating two forms of clinical expression: visceral and ocular. *Am. J. Dis. Child.* **132**, 627.

Angiostrongyliasis

S. Punyagupta

Cerebrospinal and abdominal angiostrongyliasis are the two clinical diseases in man caused by accidental infections with two species of rat nematode: *Angiostrongylus cantonensis* and *Angiostrongylus costaricensis* respectively. *A. costaricensis* is also known as *Morerastrongylus costaricensis*.

Cerebrospinal angiostrongyliasis, also known as eosinophilic meningitis (see Section 21), is prevalent in many Asian-Pacific countries including Hawaii, Tahiti, Cook Island, Caroline Island, New Hebrides, American Samoa, New Caledonia, the Philippines, Indonesia, Malaysia, Thailand, Vietnam, Taiwan, Japan, and Australia. Abdominal angiostrongyliasis, characterized as eosinophilic enteritis, is an important disease in Central and South America, from Mexico, Costa Rica, El Salvador, Panama, Honduras, Venezuela, Columbia, and Brazil.

Angiostrongyliasis cantonensis

Eosinophilic meningitis is a clinical entity characterized by central nervous system involvement associated with eosinophilic pleocytosis. It was rarely recognized until the major South Pacific outbreaks during the Second World War. Since the discovery of *A. cantonensis* in a human brain by Rosen and colleagues in 1962, there have been at least 32 parasitologically-proven cases, and thousands of clinically diagnosed cases.

Adult *A. cantonensis* reside in the pulmonary arteries of rats; the first stage larvae hatch from the eggs lodged in terminal vessels, and migrate along the air passages and intestine. Various slugs, snails and crustacea serve as intermediate as well as transporting hosts, by picking up the larvae from the soil. The infective third stage larvae then develop. Man is infected when he eats apple snails (*Pila* spp.), giant African snails (*Achatina fulica*), and possibly shrimps, fish, and vegetables, contaminated with these larvae.

The parasites are neurotropic, both in men and rats, and so migrate to the brain. After moulting to become fourth and fifth stage larvae, they leave the brain and reach the adult state in the pulmonary arteries of rats. The period of brain involvement covers roughly four weeks. The fate of all fifth stage larvae in man is not certain. Some die in the brain and spinal cord, some reach the eyes, and a very few are found in the lungs.

Clinical features. The disease is usually benign and self-limiting with complete recovery. Yet it may be severe, resulting in permanent neurological deficit or even death. The degree of clinical severity probably depends on the number of infecting worms, which varies from a few to hundreds. There is evidence that some human infections are subclinical. The incubation period varies from 3–36 days with an average of two weeks. Nausea, vomiting, abdominal discomfort, and urticarial rashes were noted in a few cases soon after ingestion of the suspected source of infection. Acute intermittent unbearable occipital or bitemporal headache is the main complaint and the only constant symptom throughout the clinical course. Patients may experience neck stiffness: meningeal irritation can be elicited in only about 15 per cent of mild cases, but more in severe cases. Nausea and vomiting are frequent during the first week. Disturbances of consciousness of varying degree are uncommon except in children or in very severe cases. Some patients present with convulsions or psychosis. One useful feature is the absence of marked fever in most cases, except those with severe cerebral symptoms.

Cranial nerves are sometimes involved, particularly the optic, facial, and abducens nerves. Paraesthesia of the trunk or extremities, indicating peripheral nerve injury, may be observed. Generalized motor weakness is sometime noted in severe cases, but paraplegia due to spinal cord damage is very rare. Mild constitutional symptoms, such as malaise, anorexia, and general aching are usual.

Pulmonary symptoms, such as cough, audible rales, and radiographic features of pneumonitis have been recognized in some very severe cases and autopsies revealed *A. cantonensis* in the lung tissue.

A. cantonensis has so far been recovered from the eye chambers in seven cases: lumbar punctures done in three of these cases showed concomittent eosinophilic meningitis. Retinal haemorrhages and detachment are important complications. Bilateral or

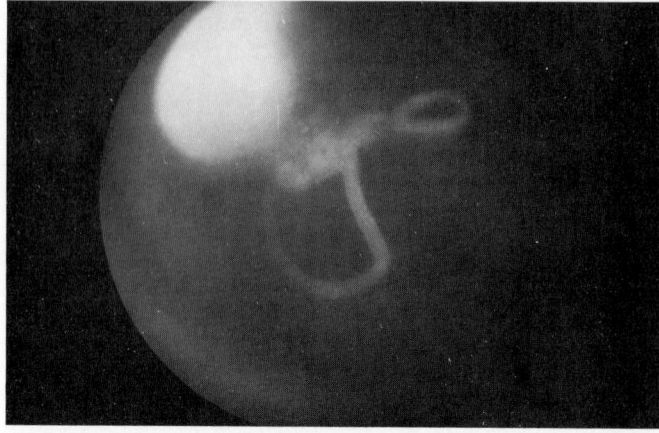

Fig. 1 A living *A. cantonensis* larva in the posterior chamber of a patient's eye.

unilateral amblyopia of varying degree, associated with abnormal fundi, is not uncommon. Diplopia, abnormal visual fields, optic atrophy, and periorbital oedema are seldom seen.

Laboratory findings. The peripheral blood usually shows slight leucocytosis with eosinophilia of 10–50 per cent persisting for about three months.

Lumbar puncture, the single most useful diagnostic test, must be performed in all suspected cases. The pressure is usually high, in some cases over 500 mm of water. The fluid may be clear, colourless, and turbid or slightly xanthochromic but not purulent. The white cell count is usually in the range 500–2000 per mm³. Red blood cells may be seen occasionally. Eosinophilic pleocytosis varies from 10 per cent to over 90 per cent. The predominant cells may, however, be lymphocytes, and some neutrophils may also be found. Eosinophilic pleocytosis reaches a peak around the second week after the first symptom and gradually disappears over three months. In a few cases, the pleocytosis may recur during the second month with return of some symptoms. The protein concentration is high but the sugar concentration is normal. Spinal fluid must be examined closely under a bright light with the help of a hand lens to detect small moving larvae.

Other investigations including biochemical tests, electroencephalogram, brain scan, and cerebral angiography are of no value.

temporarily, after each lumbar puncture. The tap should therefore be repeated at intervals of three to seven days until there is a definite clinical as well as laboratory improvement. Analgesics and sedatives are helpful. Based on the immunopathological concept, corticosteroids, such as prednisolone, in a dose of 30–60 mg daily, have been advocated in critical cases with cerebral depression, or those with cranial nerve involvement, but no benefit has been confirmed in milder cases. Although clinical symptoms persist for only two to four weeks, the neurological deficit may last longer.

Ocular *Angiostrongylus* should be removed surgically, but complications are inevitable if the posterior chamber is involved.

Fatality rate is low: 3 per cent in Taiwan, 0.5 per cent in Thailand, and none in Tahiti. Patients die in coma between two and four weeks after the onset. Energetic neurological and cardiopulmonary intensive care during the acute stage can be life saving.

Angiostrongyliasis costaricensis

Eosinophilic gastroenteritis is a clinical syndrome of unknown aetiology. Parasites, such as *Eustoma rotundatum*, *Anisakis*, *Gnathostoma*, and *A. costaricensis* are, however, capable of producing eosinophilic gastroenteritis or granuloma.

A. costaricensis lives in the mesenteric arteries of cotton rats (*Sigmodon hispidus*), *Rattus rattus*, and some other rodents. First

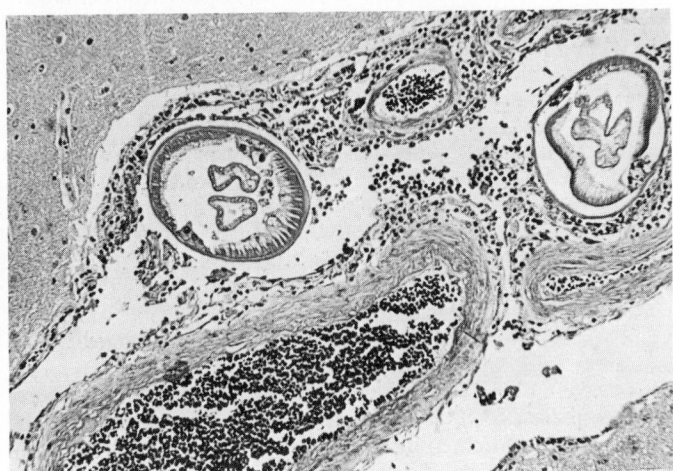

Fig. 2   Cross-sections of an *A. cantonensis* larva in the cerebral vein with eosinophils and mononuclear cells infiltration.

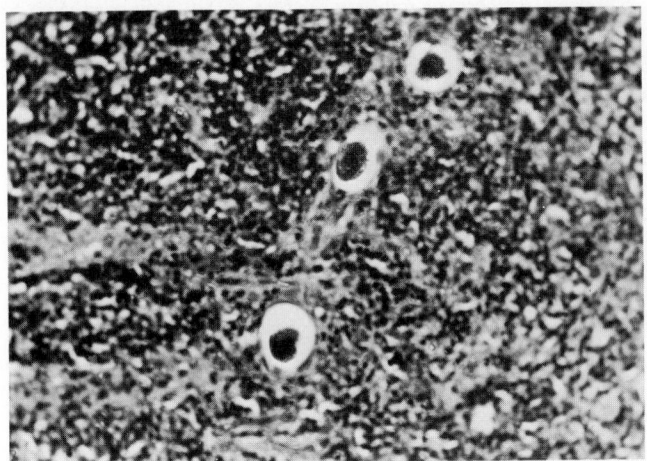

Fig. 3   Section of a human caecum showing three ova of *A. costaricensis* with cellular infiltration mostly of eosinophils. (By courtesy of Dr Pedro Morera, University of Costa Rica.)

Diagnosis. Cerebral angiostrongyliasis should be suspected if a patient from the known endemic area presents with a history of typical symptoms and eosinophilic pleocytosis within one month of eating snails, shrimps, etc. A definite diagnosis can only be made by recovering *A. cantonensis* larvae from the spinal fluid or ocular chambers, or at autopsy. Recently, the use of enzyme linked immunosorbent assay, with antigen prepared from fourth stage larvae, has shown promising results.

Differential diagnosis. In some countries in the Far East, eosinophilic pleocytosis associated with neurological involvement has been found in patients infected with other parasites, including *Gnathostoma spinigerum*, *Paragonimus westermani*, and *Schistosoma*. Of these, gnathostomiasis (see page 5.440) is most frequently encountered, and should be suspected if the patient develops paralysis of the extremities following radiculitis or impairment of sensorium with haemorrhagic or xanthrochromic spinal fluid and eosinophilic pleocytosis.

Treatment and clinical course. The effective anthelminthic, even if available, should not be given because the reaction to the dead worms in the brain can be disastrous, leading to clinical deterioration or even death. Headache usually subsides dramatically, but

stage larvae hatch from eggs in the intestinal capillaries and enter the intestine. Slugs (*Vaginulus plebeius*) which ingest the larvae in rat's faeces, serve as intermediate hosts in which second and third stage larvae develop. Man accidentally ingests vegetable leaves smeared with mucous secretion of slugs containing infective larvae. Man is not a definitive host, yet the female worms are capable of producing fertile but unhatched eggs.

Clinical features. The disease mainly attacks children. The incubation period is unknown. Patients experience high fever for two to four weeks, anorexia, vomiting, and right-sided, particularly right iliac fossa, abdominal pain resembling that of acute appendicitis. Some present features of partial or complete intestinal obstruction. Physical examination reveals tenderness or a tender mass in the right inferior quadrant and tenderness on rectal examination. Leucocytosis of $10–50 \times 10^9/l$ with 11–82 per cent eosinophilia is a constant finding. Radiographs may show spasticity, filling defects, and irritability at the caecum and ascending colon. Serodiagnosis may be helpful in chronic as well as acute cases.

Diagnosis and treatment. The diagnosis should be considered in children with features of appendicitis, inflammatory bowel disease, or ileocaecal mass associated with blood eosinophilia. Definitive diagnosis and treatment are best achieved by surgical exploration and resection of affected bowel. The lesions are confined to the ileocaecal region. Oedema and thickening of the intestinal wall with miliary yellowish granulomatous inflammation of the appendix, terminal ileum, caecum, or ascending colon are observed. Regional lymph nodes, liver, omentum, and testicles are occasionally involved. Arteritis or thrombosis of arteries by the 2–4 cm long filiform adult worms may be noted. Microscopy of the lesions shows eosinophilic infiltration and characteristic thin-walled eggs or larvae of *A. costaricensis*. Medical treatment with thiabendazole has achieved inconclusive results. In the majority of cases appendectomy, ileocolonic resection, right hemicolectomy, or colostomy were performed. Mortality was observed in two out of 114 reported cases who received both surgical and medical treatment.

References

Loria-Cortes, R. and Lobo Sanahuja, J. F. (1980). Clinical abdominal angiostrongylosis. A study of 116 children with intestinal eosinophilic granuloma caused by *Angiostrongylus costaricensis*. *Am. J. trop. Med. Hyg.* **29**, 538.
Morera, P. (1973). Life history and redescription of *Angiostrongylus costaricensis*. Morera and Cespedes, 1971. *Am. J. trop. Med. Hyg.* **22**, 613.
Punyagupta, S., Juttijudata, P., Bunnag, T., and Comer, D. S. (1968). Two fatal cases of eosinophilic myeloencephalitis, a newly recognized disease caused by *Gnathostoma spinigerum*. *Trans. R. Soc. trop. Med. Hyg.* **62**, 801.
—, (1975). Eosinophilic meningitis in Thailand. Clinical studies of 484 typical cases probably caused by *Angiostrongylus cantonensis*. *Am. J. trop. Med. Hyg.* **24**, 921.
Yii, C. Y. (1976). Clinical observations on eosinophilic meningitis and meningoencephalitis caused by *Angiostrongylus cantonensis* in Taiwan. *Am. J. trop. Med. Hyg.* **25**, 233.

Gnathostomiasis

P. Suntharasamai

Gnathostomiasis in man is an extra-intestinal infection with larval or immature *Gnathostoma spingerum*, a nematode parasite of feline and canine stomachs. The disease is characterized by intermittent and migratory space-occupying lesions in the skin and less commonly in the internal organs, due to inflammation or haemorrhage. It is also known by the following local names: *tau-chid* (Thailand), *choko-fushu*, (Japan), and Yangtze oedema (China).

Aetiology. The adults of *G. spinigerum* live in the stomach of definitive hosts including dog, cat, tiger, leopard, golden cat, leopard cat, jungle cat, ocelot, lynx, lion, otter, opossum, mink, and raccoon. *Cyclops*, the first intermediate host, ingests the sheathed first stage larvae which hatch in water from ova shed with the host's faeces. The third-stage larvae are found in visceral walls and muscles of second intermediate hosts—including fish, frog, snake, lizard, chicken, duck, rat, and mongoose—which have ingested the infected cyclops or the infected flesh of another second intermediate host. Only the consumption of the third-stage larvae by a definitive host can lead to the development of mature male and female worms in the stomach.

Man usually acquires the infection by eating the undercooked flesh of second intermediate hosts, and sometimes by applying the flesh as a poultice. Paratenic transmission is extremely rare. The parasites recovered from man are larvae, immature females, or mature males. The stages of development of parasites in man are not correlated with the duration of clinical illness. Infection with more than one larva is rare.

Geographical distribution. Human gnathostomiasis is endemic in Thailand and Japan, and sporadic in Australia, Burma, China, India, Indonesia, Laos, Mexico, the Philippines, and Vietnam.

Animal infections also occur in Bangladesh, Palestine, USA, USSR, and Zimbabwe.

Pathology and pathogenesis. After being ingested, the larva penetrates the gut wall and migrates to the liver before wandering, perhaps randomly, through almost any tissue except bone. The migration appears to be facilitated by production of enzymes and by the organism's cuticular architecture and musculature.

As the worm migrates, the tissue is destroyed producing track-like spaces together with varying degrees of haemorrhage and eosinophil-associated acute inflammation which may be the result of immunological reaction and toxic products of the parasite. Oedema is prominent in some skin lesions, while large and multiple areas of haematoma are typical of brain and spinal cord involvement.

In a more stationary lesion the eosinophil-associated zone will be surrounded by granulomatous changes, occasional multinucleated cells, and histiocytes filled with Charcot–Leyden crystals. Onion-like perivascular fibrous thickening of small arteries, and eosinophilic endarteritis with thrombosis are also observed. The draining lymph nodes show follicular hyperplasia with marked eosinophilic infiltration within medullary cords and sinusoids.

Symptoms and signs result from space-occupying effects and tissue destruction or disruption of blood supply, and vary according to the sites and sizes of the lesions induced intermittently along the migratory route.

Clinical features. After consumption of infected flesh, nausea, vomiting, and abdominal pain may occasionally be noted within one or two days, and a syndrome consisting of fever, pain in the right upper quadrant of the abdomen, chest pain, dry cough, and hypereosinophilia may develop within one to two weeks. The incubation period is, however, unknown in most cases and patients usually present with only one of the following forms of the infection.

Cutaneous forms.   *Gnathostomal creeping eruption.* This is extremely rare. The serpentine track is similar to, but bigger than, that due to dog or cat hookworm larva.
Cutaneous migratory swelling. Swellings can occur anywhere, and may recur close to the original site or at a distance. When the parasite moves into the forearm or leg, swellings are usually at, or distal to, the knee or elbow.

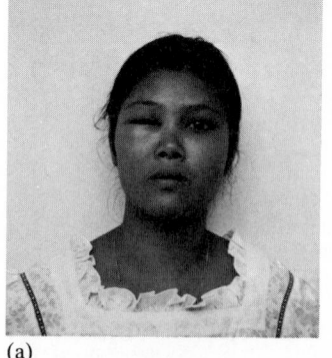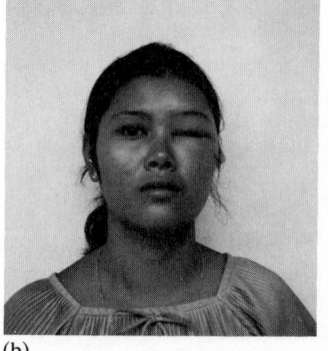

(a)   (b)

Fig. 1 Gnathostomal cutaneous swelling in a 23-year-old Thai woman. The swelling in the right eye (a) lasted five days and was followed after an interval of one week by swelling around the left eye (b).

Swelling develops rapidly and usually lasts for about one week. Frequently it is large and widespread involving the whole wrist or hand. Swelling of the digits or plantar surfaces can be very painful and incapacitating, but pain is unrelated to the size of the swelling. Itching is the major associated symptom. The overlying skin is normal in colour or occasionally erythematous. Regional lymphadenitis and fever are absent. When the swelling occurs in the eyelid, chemosis and conjunctival haemorrhage may be observed. The worms can escape spontaneously through the skin or the conjunctiva. The interval between episodes of swelling varies from a few days to months. The illness may recur for 20 years. In cases where reinfection could be excluded, persistence of infection for $3\frac{1}{2}$ years has been observed. The youngest patient with proved infection was three days old.

Visceral forms. *Spinocerebral gnathostomiasis*. Involvement of the central nervous system commonly starts with intermittent agonizing and shooting pain with paraesthesia of a limb or a segment of trunk followed by paraplegia with urinary retention and, rarely, quadriplegia. Sensation is correspondingly impaired and the Brown–Séquard syndrome is sometimes seen. A few cases present with severe headache and vomiting, followed very quickly by coma, cranial nerve palsies, and hemiplegia, resembling a cerebrovascular accident. Physical findings, other than the usual signs of meningeal irritation, depend on the site and size of the lesion, but the rapidly advancing or changing pattern of neurological deficit is characteristic of the infection. Cutaneous migratory swelling precedes or follows the episode only in a few of these cases. Eosinophilic meningitis without focal neurological deficit can be seen occasionally in association with the cutaneous migratory swelling.

Ocular gnathostomiasis. The gnathostoma can be found in the anterior chamber, in the vitreous humour, and on the retina. Inflammation and destruction markedly impair vision. The parasite usually migrates through the sclera or the cornea, but may die in the vitreous humour.

Intra-abdominal and oral gnathostomiasis. The parasite can induce intestinal obstruction, melaena, or a painful intra-abdominal mass. It is very likely that some of the worms may escape into the lumen of the gastrointestinal tract, for spontaneous escape through the mucosa of oral cavity has been observed.

Pulmonary gnathostomiasis. The parasite has been found in the sputum of patients with eosinophilic pneumonitis, or following symptoms indicating irritation of the upper respiratory tract.

Genitourinary gnathostomiasis. The parasite has been found in blood-stained urethral discharge, accompanying haematuria, in the glans penis, or in the uterine cervical mucosa. Venereal transmission is thus theoretically possible.

Auditory gnathostomiasis. In a case with involvement of the seventh and eighth cranial nerves, a gnathostoma larva was found in the external auditory meatus.

Diagnosis
General. The diagnosis of this infection is suggested by clinical characteristics, and geographical and dietary history. It is supported by finding eosinophilia and excluding other causes, and is proved if the worm is identified.

Immunodiagnosis is of limited use. Immediate skin hypersensitivity using crude extracts of adults and larvae appears to be nonspecific. An immunoenzyme test for IgG antibody against antigen from an aqueous extract of the third-stage larvae has been developed. A titre of 1:1600 is indicative, while a titre of 1:400 is only suggestive of this infection.

Laboratory features. Blood eosinophilia occurs in practically all cases and hypereosinophilia of up to 90 per cent is sometimes seen. However, the degree of eosinophilia does not correlate with the clinical severity. With spinocerebral involvement the CSF can be bloody, xanthochromic, or slightly turbid with a minor increase in protein content. The proportion of eosinophils is higher than expected from haemorrhage *per se*. Neutrophil pleocytosis is sometimes noted, but eosinophil pleocytosis is almost always found in the spinocerebral form of the infection.

Differential diagnosis. The commonly found cutaneous migratory swelling needs to be differentiated from contact dermatitis and urticaria. Calabar swellings (caused by *Loa loa*) occur only in the Central African forest belt and are associated with microfilariae in the blood. With a first episode of swelling, the relatively mild symptoms and absence of signs of acute inflammation, the presence of eosinophilia, and the absence of regional lymphoadenitis and fever suggest gnathostomiasis in patients in or from the endemic area. Stationary swellings must be differentiated from other infections such as fascioliasis, sparganosis, and dirofilariasis, and from non-infectious causes. *Paragonimus heterotremus* infection was found in one case with cutaneous migratory swelling after pneumonitis and empyema, but this infection is confined to a small area about 100 km northeast of Bangkok. Diseases most likely to be confused with gnathostomal creeping eruption are those caused by dog or cat hookworm, in which the track is smaller and the affected area has been exposed to contaminated materials.

Gnathostomal aetiology is highly likely if rapidly advancing myelitis follows shooting or root pain, or if features of cerebral or subarachnoid haemorrhage occur in a person who is otherwise healthy but for a history of cutaneous migratory swelling and blood eosinophilia. Eosinophilic pleocytosis is essential for the diagnosis, and the exclusion of non-helminthic encephalomyelitis and of Guillain–Barré syndrome. Eosinophilic meningo-encephalitis caused by *Angiostrongylus cantonensis* can produce severe headache, meningeal irritation, cranial nerve palsies, and impaired consciousness, but the development of symptoms is less dramatic. Development of meningo-encephalitis after eating poorly cooked freshwater snails favours the diagnosis of *A. cantonensis* infection. Rarely, Angiostrongylus larvae can be identified in the CSF. In the case of intra-ocular infections, the larvae of *A. cantonensis* can be distinguished by being thinner, longer, and folding: they appear in the eyeball two to three weeks after the manifestation of eosinophilic meningo-encephalitis. The much smaller microfilariae of *Onchocerca volvulus*, found only in Africa and America, can be seen in the anterior chamber by slit lamp examination.

The diagnosis of visceral gnathostomiasis depends mainly on the identification of the worm in surgical specimens and secretions such as sputum, urine, or vaginal discharge. The presence of eosinophils in tissue sections and the migratory phenomenon strongly suggests the diagnosis.

Treatment. Surgical removal of the parasite is curative, but rarely possible. Various antiparasitic agents such as chloroquine, diethylcarbamazine, levamisole, mebendazole, quinine, and thiabendazole have been tried without convincing effect. Metronidazole in a dose of 400 mg thrice daily for 21 days significantly reduces the recurrence rate, the duration of swelling, and the eosinophil count in the blood, but is not curative. Efficacy of ultrasonic application for an apparently superficial infection needs proper evaluation. Supportive, symptomatic, and anti-inflammatory treatments are preferable to surgical attempts.

Prognosis. Fatality can occur in cerebral gnathostomiasis and blindness is usual in intra-ocular gnathostomiasis. The probability of central nervous system or intra-ocular involvement is less than 1 per cent in cases with cutaneous migratory swelling. Intestinal obstruction may prove fatal if it is complete and prolonged, but more frequently the patient will lose a segment of his gut because of, perhaps unnecessary, operation.

Prevention. The infective larvae in the flesh of second intermediate hosts can be killed by adequate heat or by chemicals. In the endemic area all dishes that contain raw or poorly cooked flesh of animals, particularly those of freshwater fish or chicken, must be avoided.

References

Boongird, P., Phuapradit, P., Siridej, N., Chirachariyavej, T., Chuahirun, S., and Vejjajiva, A. (1977). Neurological manifestations of gnathostomiasis. *J. neurol. Sci.* **31**, 279.

Daengsvang, S. (1968). Further observations on the experimental transmission of *Gnathostoma spinigerum. Ann. trop. Med. Parasit.* **62**, 88.

— (1980). *Monograph on the genus Gnathostoma and gnathostomiasis in Thailand.* Southeast Asian Medical Information Centre, International Medical Foundation of Japan, Tokyo.

Miyazaki, I. (1960). On the genus *Gnathostoma* and human gnathostomiasis, with special reference to Japan. *Exp. Parasit.* **9**, 338.

Sirikulcharjanonta, V. and Chongchitnant, N. (1979). Gnathostomiasis, a possible etiologic agent of eosinophilic granuloma of the gastrointestinal tract. *Am. J. trop. Med. Hyg.* **28**, 42.

Swanson, V. L. (1971). Gnathostomiasis. In *Pathology of protozoal and helminthic diseases with clinical correlation.* (ed. R. A. Marcial-Rojas, 871. Williams and Wilkins, Baltimore.

CESTODES

Hydatid disease

A. J. Radford

Echinococcosis, hydatidosis, and hydatid disease are synonyms for infection with the dog tapeworm, *Echinococcus granulosus.*

E. granulosus infection is a cyclozoonosis, that is, a parasitic disease that man shares with other vertebrates but which requires at least one other vertebrate (and no invertebrate) host for completion of its life cycle. Less common species infecting man include *E. multilocularis* and *E. vogeli.*

'Hydatidosis is not a tropical disease and it is unwise to dismiss (it) as a curiosity' (*Lancet*). Nor has it been recently recognized. Hippocrates noted that 'when the liver is filled with water and bursts . . . the belly is filled with water and the patient dies'. In 1773 John Hunter made an accurate description of hydatid disease nothing that large and small hydatids were 'uniformly round and filled with clear water . . . in a transparent bag . . . of two coats . . . the inner surface covered with small hydatids . . . not so large as the heads of pins'.

Epidemiology. Although it is decreasing in prevalence in many countries, the worm is alive and well and living in many parts of the world. Its global prevalence is illustrated in Fig. 1. It is widespread throughout the whole Euro-Asian landmass except Scandanavia, in northern and eastern Africa as well as southern and western South America, much of Canada, and in Australasia. Overall there is evidence of an increasing pandemic. *E. multilocularis* is common in North America, the USSR, Japan, parts of central Europe, and Turkey.

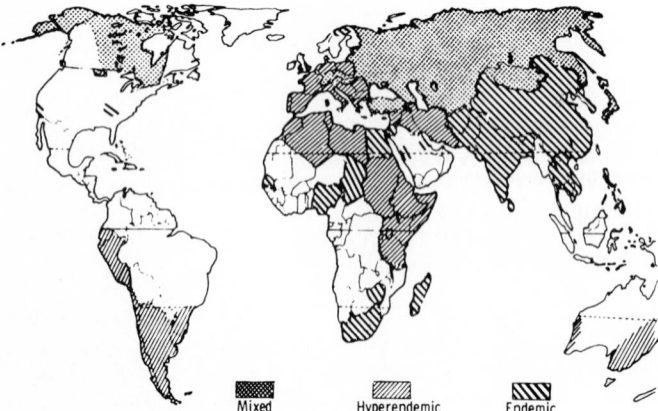

Fig. 1   Distribution of hydatid disease. (From Matossian *et al.* (1977). Bull. Wld Hlth Org. **55**, 449, by permission.)

Man is usually an intruder ('accidental host') in the life cycle of *E. granulosus* and represents a 'dead end' for the parasite whose most usual cycle is between sheep and dogs. Other animals, including

camels, swine, buffaloes, kangaroos, deer, pigs, goats, and rodents, may also be intermediate hosts. Hydatids occur both in domestic and sylvatic (wild) forms but the disease is principally an enzootic of dogs. The life cycle is shown in Fig. 2. Some forms of *E. granulosus* in horses are probably unable to establish themselves in man. Definitive hosts other than dogs also exist and include foxes, wolves, and jackals.

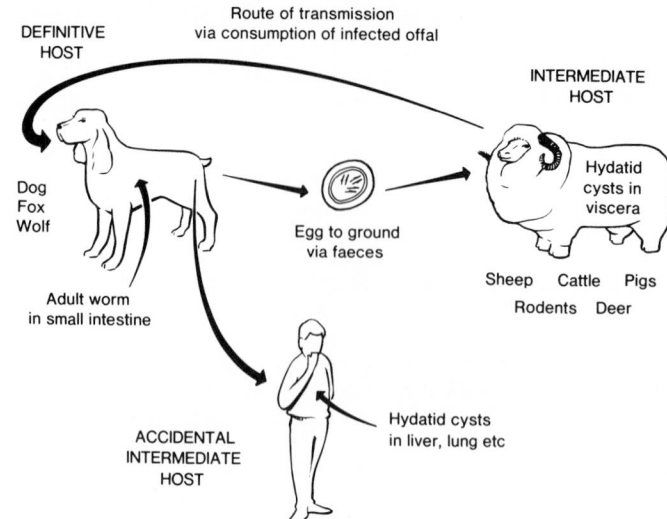

Fig. 2   Life cycle of *E. granulosus.*

Infection rates have been reported in excess of 50 per cent in horses in England, 50–90 per cent of cattle in Italy, and over 20 per cent of some Eskimo dog packs. A major factor in the appearance of hydatidosis in countries previously free from it is the importation of infected livestock in which diagnosis is difficult clinically and in which serological cross-reactions occur with closely related tapeworms such as *Taenia ovis* and *T. saginata.*

Wales has an annual incidence of 1.5 per million of the population, almost ten times that of England. Rural Tasmania, prior to its campaign in 1960, had an annual hospital incidence of 274 per million per year. Rural rates are almost always higher and in certain areas specific cultural patterns result in high prevalence rates, as in the Maoris of New Zealand (up to six times that of Europeans), and in the seasonally mobile sheep ranchers in the western United States. Higher numbers of dogs per person, an easy familiarity with dogs, and ignorance of, or indifference to, the significance and prevalence of the disease are important epidemiological factors in maintaining infection rates in man.

Life cycle. The adult cestode (flat) worm is 3–9 mm long with three or four segments (proglottids). There may be several thousand adults in the jejunum of an infected animal. The terminal segment is the longest and broadest, giving the adult tapeworm a tapered bottle shape. This segment is gravid and shed every two weeks; on rupture it releases 500–800 eggs into the intestine. These are passed in faeces on to the ground where herbivores incidentally ingest them while grazing. Man most commonly ingests them after handling dogs with contaminated hair, or by consuming contaminated vegetables or water.

In the intermediate host eggs hatch in the alkaline duodenum and the emergent hexacanth embryo (with its three pairs of cephalic hooks) passes through the intestinal wall into the portal and lymphatic systems and thence most commonly to the liver or lungs, but may pass on from the lungs to any other organ of the body. When it settles, the embryo develops into a cyst with an outer elastic layer, the laminated membrane, and a more fragile inner germinal membrane of epithelial cells from which bud brood capsules. Growth is slow, taking three months to reach 4–5 mm diameter and five to six months to become 20 mm in size and infective. In the case of *E.*

granulosus the cyst is single and filled with clear fluid, but for *E. multilocularis* the cyst is an 'alveolar' or honeycombed structure.

Carnivores acquire the parasite by consuming the infected viscera of intermediate hosts. For *E. granulosus* this most commonly occurs when dogs devour sheep livers, and for *E. multilocularis* when foxes or cats consume infected rodents.

Clinical features. There are no specific local or general symptoms and signs of hydatid disease. Its distribution and manifestations are both ubiquitous and protean, but liver and lung involvement is most common, and in only about 10 per cent of patients are neither organ involved. Almost every organ has been involved from brain, heart, spleen, biliary tract, thyroid and parotid to tongue, tooth, bone, broad ligament, prostate, bladder, tonsil, pulmonary artery, and inferior vena cava. Of 1802 patients in an Australasian Hydatid Register (now discontinued), 63 per cent of lesions were in the liver, 25 per cent in the lung, 25 per cent in muscle, 3 per cent in bone, 2 per cent in kidney, 1 per cent each in spleen and brain. In 20 per cent of patients multiple organs were involved. In other series pulmonary lesions are more frequent.

Man is remarkably tolerant to the effects of hydatid infection and walls off the laminated cyst of the parasite which calcifies in about 3.5 per cent of patients. Many lesions are picked up at autopsy having been asymptomatic during life. The latent period may vary from one to two years to over half a century. The growth of some cysts is slow and sometimes is arrested. The largest lesion described contained over 50 litres.

The diagnosis is usually made in young adults and in most cultures there is a preponderance of males, which can be attributed to their greater relationship to infected dogs. The majority of infections are diagnosed following incidental findings at X-ray examination for non-related complaints. The commonest symptoms and signs are secondary to the progressive expansion of cysts and are either those of a space-occupying lesion, or obstructive features secondary to direct pressure, or due to embolization.

Pulmonary lesions are most commonly found incidentally. When present, symptoms consist of a cough in 60 per cent of cases, with or without haemoptysis. Coughing up pieces of ruptured membrane and a salty taste from cyst fluid occurs in 20 per cent of patients. Multiple lesions occur in 40 per cent and are bilateral in 20 per cent of cases. Lower lobe is more common than upper lobe involvement, the posterior segments more frequently involved than the anterior and the right lobe more commonly than the left.

Similarly, in the case of liver disease most lesions are silent but, when present, pain and discomfort are the commonest symptoms. Where lesions are near the surface, fluctuation and a 'hydatid thrill' may be elicited. The right lobe is involved in 75 per cent of cases and about one third of cysts are solitary. Up to 2–3 per cent of intracerebral lesions in endemic regions are hydatid cysts. Presentation of such lesions relates to a rise in intracranial pressure with signs and symptoms progressing over two to six months according to the site of localization.

Complications are the commonest form of presentation of hydatid disease. At the time of diagnosis 36–40 per cent of hepatic cysts and 27–67 per cent of pulmonary ones have ruptured or become secondarily infected. *E. multilocularis* infections are more invasive. Anaphylaxis, which may be fatal, can follow rupture but broncho-pulmonary or hepatobiliary obstruction and fistulae are commoner complications of infection. Long bone lesions may result in spontaneous fractures. Bladder involvement with hydatiduria may also occur. Fifty years ago over 30 per cent of these complications were fatal.

Diagnosis. 'Where were you born and where have you been living over the past several decades?' are important components of the clinical history. The absence of an appropriate geographical history and no contact with dogs makes the diagnosis unlikely.

Over 90 per cent of pulmonary diagnoses can be made by radiography which indicates well-defined solitary or multiple lesions.

Lesions are usually round and uniform unless surrounding pneumonitis or atelectasis occurs, but occasionally they calcify if the parasite dies. Polycystic lesions of *E. multilocularis* infections show notching and budding of cyst walls from 1–20 cm in diameter. Various, almost pathognomonic signs may occur. These give rise to 'crescent', 'double arch', or 'water lily' signs as a result of broncho-pulmonary fistula formation and collapse of the cyst wall. A fluid level may be present after rupture. Thin or thick-walled cavitation may occur requiring a differential diagnosis from other pulmonary abscesses. A pleural reaction occurs in about one third of cases. Sputum microscopy may reveal invaginated or evaginated protoscolesces, even when immunodiagnostic tests are negative. A plain X-ray of the abdomen reveals about a third of cases of hepatic disease, and may reveal 'white line' images for almost the full circumference of the walled cyst. Intralesional gas-bubbles may be present if hepatobronchial fistula formation has occurred. The right hemidiaphragm is deformed and elevated in almost half of liver lesions. Skull X-ray may show signs of increased intracranial pressure with asymmetrical growth or thinning of the underlying bone in intracranial lesions.

Next to plain X-ray, computerized tomography (and to a lesser extent ultra sound) is the best aid to diagnosis. The appearances are usually pathognomonic and by accurate localization and identification of the number, size, and most external sites this technique minimizes the chance of accidental tapping or tearing of cysts at surgery. In the case of liver lesions it usually differentiates hydatid cysts from malignant metastases, hepatomata, angiomata and abcesses. In the case of intracranial lesions the appearances are cystic, spherical with a sharp border, a central absorptive value similar to CSF, no perifocal oedema, and usually with significant ventricular distortion and a shift of midline structures. There is a lack of enhancement and of the perifocal oedema seen in cerebral abcesses or of solid portions and perifocal oedema seen in cystic tumours.

Immunodiagnosis. Since the first complement fixation test in 1906 an immense array of immunodiagnostic techniques has been developed to assist in individual diagnosis and epidemiological surveys of hydatid disease. With every method the single intact pulmonary cyst gives the fewest positive results, because apparently the concentration of antibodies is close to zero until the cyst leaks or ruptures.

The intradermal Casoni test (first developed in 1911) is the best known. It has a wide range of positivity reported variously from less than 40 to over 90 per cent. Up to 15 per cent false positives are reported, especially in the presence of taeniasis, leishmaniasis, carcinomatosis, cirrhosis, and collagen disease. Diluted antigen decreases sensitivity but increases specificity, while low nitrogen concentration increases sensitivity. The 'intermediate' reaction is read as positive if induration is over 25 mm in diameter at 20–30 minutes and is more reliable than the 'delayed' reaction.

At present the immuno-electrophoresis test (IEP) is the most specific and the most sophisticated test in general use. Its sensitivity is lower than some other tests but is improved by concentration of serum. False negative reports of up to 20 per cent occur, mainly in cases with intact cysts for the reasons stated above. Although precipitin bands at points 3 and 4 occur, it is the Arc 5 band which is used as the marker. Whole sheep hydatid cyst fluid is the best source of antigen. Reactions also occur with *E. vogeli* and *E. multilocularis*. False positives also are rare but include a few taeniid species such as the dog tape-worm, *Taenia hydatigena*, which does not usually infect man. Positives occur only if active disease is present or within 12 months after surgery; a few remain positive even longer. The complement fixation test (CFT) gives up to 80 per cent positive results and also usually returns to normal within a year of surgery whereas the indirect haemagglutination (IHA) test may continue to remain positive even after two years. The latex agglutination (LA) test is a good screening test with high specificity and few false positives.

Radio-immunoassay (RIA) and ELISA tests will improve in the future and may eventually differentiate IgM and IgG fractions. At present the Casoni skin test and LA test (or IHA test) as a screen and the IEP (or CFT or indirect fluorescent antibody test) as a confirmation test appear the best tools to specific diagnosis. Eosinophilia occurs in only 20 per cent of patients.

Management. Surgery is the main line of treatment and in some cases is technically very demanding. It carries a mortality rate of up to 3 per cent. Rupture on cyst enucleation is reported in up to half of the cases after which anaphylactic shock may occur immediately as may infection in the days or weeks that follow. Several techniques have been used to sterilize the contents of the cysts before enucleation is attempted by a small aspiration followed by the injection of a scolicide. Formalin, alcohol, and 20 per cent hypertonic saline have been used but the least absorbable and least toxic is 1 per cent aqueous iodine or 0.5 per cent silver nitrate solution. Low viscosity of the iodine solution gives rapid diffusion and complete sterilization with a few minutes. A technique to minimize rupture and allow controlled evacuation of all parasitic material by strengthening the friable outer layer has developed by freezing it using CO_2 gas in a steel cone over the incision site. In pulmonary disease simple enucleation, cystectomy, wedge or segmental resection, lobectomy, or pneumonectomy may be required. Cystectomy with or without resection may be done for liver disease and the common bile duct should always be explored in these cases. In intracerebral lesions limited but significant expansion of the brain occurs postoperatively.

There may be a place for medical treatment at some future date. The benzimidazole derivatives mebendazole, fluoromebendazole, and combendazole have undergone clinical trials. None has consistently demonstrated either its efficiency in the human or its safety at prolonged high dosage, though occasional reductions in size of lesions with mebendazole are reported using doses of 10–50 mg/kg for 4–13 months.

Control. Some of the world's most successful public health measures against any communicable disease have been hydatid programmes. It may be significant that all the effective campaigns have been carried out on islands with relatively small populations, namely Iceland, New Zealand, Tasmania, and Cyprus. During the nineteenth century Iceland had the world's highest prevalence of hydatidosis with a quarter to one-third of all autopsies showing evidence of disease. It is now hydatid-free except for incidental calcifications found in the elderly. Tasmania, which based its programmes on that of New Zealand, has reduced the annual incidence from about 15 cases per 100 000 before 1965 to 1.4 per 100 000, the annual prevalence in dogs from 12.7 to 0.4 per cent and that of aged sheep from 52 to 7.9 per cent over the same period. This campaign had one principal objective—'to prevent dogs from getting offal'—thereby interrupting the life cycle of the parasite (see Fig. 2). It started by an intensive education campaign based on geographically defined areas with maximum community involvement. In due course the Department of Agriculture was able to use the power available under the stock diseases legislation in what was correctly seen as a response to public opinion. Used late in the campaign to mop up resistant pockets of 'delinquent human behaviour', these measures were highly effective and popular.

Effective control measures include:

1. The prevention of infestation of dogs by their exclusion from slaughtering areas and the installation of deep offal pits or incineration systems.

2. Raising the level of public and, especially, farmer awareness and participation in the project with literature, media, and school programmes.

3. On-site farm visits with individual contacts and the demonstration of dogs' infection by purgation with arecoline hydrobromide (15–30 mg). Such purgation does not constitute treatment (which

may be effected by praziquantel, mebendazole, nitroscanate, or bunamidine).

4. Control of stray dogs is also important in some areas.

5. Legislation which may be preceded or accompanied by incentives but is probably always necessary to effect control or eradication.

6. Dog immunization as a real possibility for the future.

Other hydatiform cysts. Other important taeniid larval infections of man which may cause the development of bladder-like structures in the tissues include *Cysticercus cellulosae*, the larva of *Taenia solium* (see page 5.446), *C. bovis*, the larva of *T. saginata* (see page 5.445) and *Coenurus cerebralis*, the larva form of *T. (Multiceps) multiceps* in sheep and which appears to be morphologically indistinguishable from the larvae of *M. Serialis* of rabbits and rodents and *T. brauni*, one of the tapeworms of African dogs.

Coenurus—the 'gill' worm—is a common parasite of dogs which causes blind staggers in its intermediate host, sheep. Transmission to dogs occurs by eating infected brain. Most human reports are from Africa, but occasionally it is seen in the United Kingdom, the USA, and France. It is more common in children. There are some variations in clinical presentation. The cerebral forms produce effects due to raised intracranial pressure or focal signs, and may involve the spinal cord. They are usually unilocular but occasionally huge cysts develop which look like a bunch of grapes, most of which are sterile. On rupture cysts are said to produce signs of a toxic psychosis. Many African patients present with solitary and asymptomatic subcutaneous lumps, usually on the chest wall, which are probably caused by a different species. They are slow-growing, may be present for months and require differentiation from sebaceous or epidermal cysts and lipomata. On section cysts show a narrow zone of fibrous tissue with infiltration by lumphocytes and eosinophils. Lesions may also occur in the eye, and especially with *M. serialis* whose cysts bud both externally and internally, in muscle layers.

References

Abbassioun, K., Rahmat, H., Ameli, N. O., and Tafazouli, M. (1978). Computerized tomography in hydatid cyst of the brain. *J. Neurosurg.* **49**, 408.

Beard, T. C. (1969). Hydatid control. A problem in health education. *Med. J. Aust.* **2**, 456.

— (1973). The elimination of echinococcosis from Iceland. *Bull. Wld Hlth Org.* **48**, 653.

Capron, A., Vernes, A., and Biguet, J. (1967). *Journées Lyonnaises d'Hydatidologie.* SIMEP ed., Lyon.

Little, J. M. (1976). Hydatid disease in Royal Prince Alfred Hospital, 1964 to 1974. *Med. J. Aust.* **1**, 903.

Matossian, R. M. (1977). The immunological diagnosis of human hydatid disease. *Trans. R. Soc. trop. Med. Hyg.* **71**, 1, 101.

—, Rickard, M. D., and Smith, J. D. (1977). Hydatidosis: a global problem of increasing importance. *Bull. Wld Hlth Org.* **55**, 499.

McConnell, J. D. and Green, R. J. (1979). The control of hydatid disease in Tasmania. *Aust. Vet. J.* **55**, 140.

Saidi, F. (1977). A new approach to the surgical treatment of hydatid cyst. *Ann. R. Coll. Surg. Eng.* **59**, 115.

Templeton, A. C. (1968). Human *Coenurus* infection: A report of 14 cases from Uganda. *Trans. R. Soc. trop. Med. Hyg.* **62**, 251.

Wainwright, J. (1957). *Coenurus cerebralis* and racemose cysts of the brain. *J. Path. Bacteriol.* **73**, 347.

Gut cestodes

V. Zaman

Taeniasis

Taeniasis is an infection caused by tapeworms known as *Taenia saginata* and *Taenia solium*.

Geographic distribution. Infection with *T. saginata* occurs in many parts of the world where raw or improperly cooked beef is eaten. This includes North, South, and Central America, parts of Asia, and Africa. The most highly endemic part of the world is East Africa where the prevalence rates are close to 10 per cent of the general population.

T. solium is endemic in all parts of the world where pork and pork products are consumed in raw or improperly cooked form. Endemic areas include South Africa, Central and South America particularly Mexico, parts of the Indian subcontinent, some regions in Southeast Asia, most recently West Irian (West New Guinea) where a major outbreak took place.

Morphology. The tapeworms are segmented parasites. Each segment is known as a proglottid. In between the head or the scolex and the first segment is a narrow zone known as the neck. The scolex is the principal means of locomotion and attachment to the host tissue (Figs. 1 and 2).

All medically important tapeworms are hermaphroditic and each segment contains a complete set of male and female reproductive

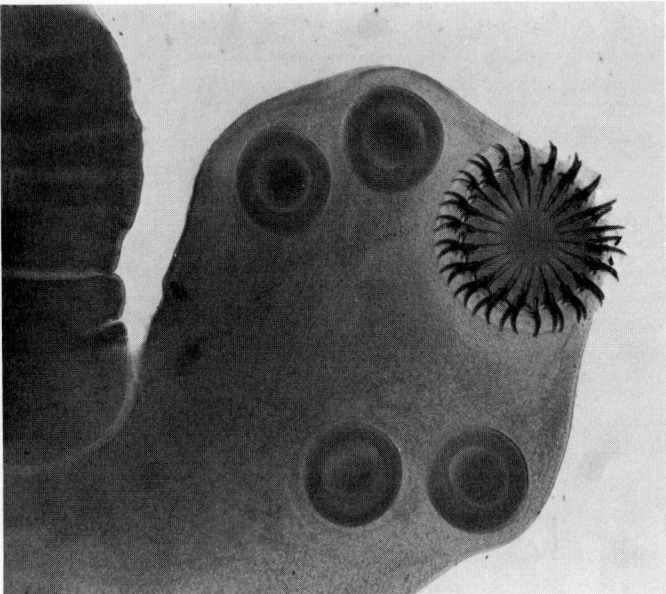

Fig. 1 Taenia solium showing scolex with four suckers and a row of hooks (× 250).

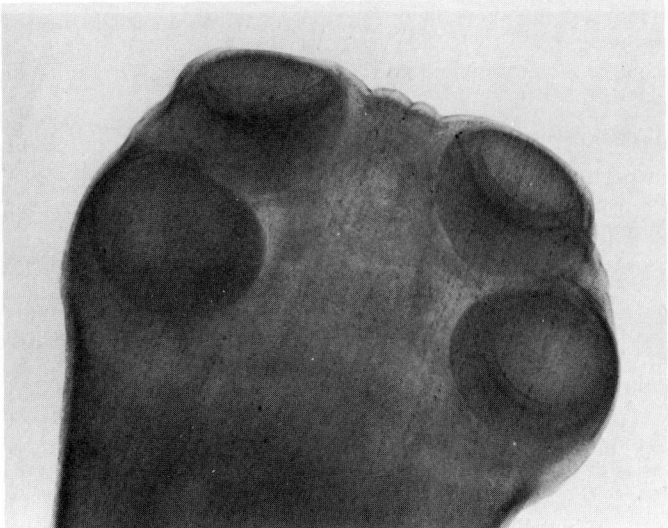

Fig. 2 *Taenia saginata* showing scolex with four suckers and no hooks (× 250).

organs. In *Taenia*, the uterus ends blindly so the eggs can only be dispersed by the disintegration of the segment.

The eggs of *T. saginata* and *T. solium* are indistinguishable. They are spherical and brown in colour measuring 31–43 μm in diameter. The egg shell proper known as the embryophore is thick-walled and radially striated. The embryophore is surrounded by a sac-like membrane which is often lost when the eggs are found in the faeces. The embryophore contains the juvenile parasite known as the oncosphere which has three pairs of hooklets. Differences between the two species are shown in Table 1.

Table 1 Characteristics of *T. saginata* and *T. solium*

	T. saginata	*T. solium*
Scolex	4 suckers no hooks	4 suckers rostellum with hooks
Egg	radially striated embryophore	radially striated embryophore
Mature segment Ovary	2 large lobes	1 small and 2 large lobes
Testes	small follicular testes 300–400	small follicular testes 150–200
Gravid segment Uterine branches	15–30	7–12

Life cycle. Man is the only definite host of *T. saginata* and *T. solium* and the adult worms are located in the small intestine. The gravid segments become separated from the main body of the worm and migrate out of the anus or are discharged in the faeces. The evacuated proglottids disintegrate in the soil freeing the eggs which find their way into the intermediate host. In the intermediate host, which is cattle for *T. saginata* and pigs for *T. solium*, the hexacanth embryos enter various organs of the body where they transfer into the larval (cysticercus) stage. The larval stage in case of *T. saginata* is known as *Cysticercus bovis*, and in case of *T. solium* as *Cysticercus cellulosae*. Sometimes humans become infected with the larval stages of *T. solium* when the condition is known as *cysticercosis* (Figs. 3 and 4).

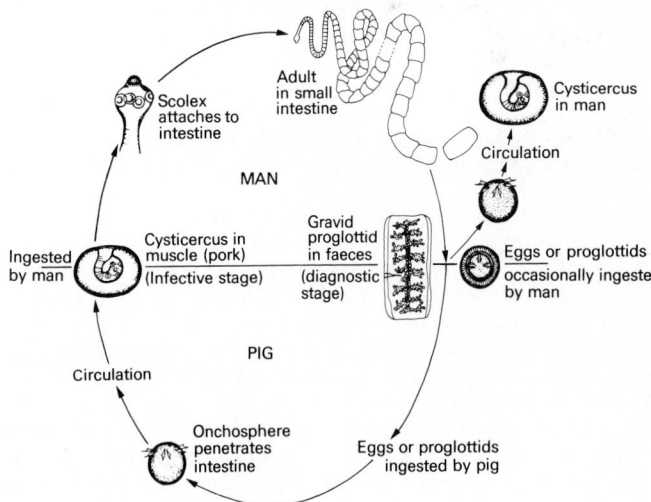

Fig. 3 Life cycle of *Taenia solium*. (Adapted from Center for Disease Control, Atlanta, Georgia, USA.)

Clinical aspects. In majority of cases, these parasites do not produce any major clinical disturbances. There is sometimes gastrointestinal disturbances, nausea, loss of weight, nervousness, and pruritis ani. The most common complaint is the discharge of segments from the anus. The patient is often aware of a crawling sensation in the perianal region while this happens and may bring the segment to the doctor. The adult worms may survive in the intestine for many years.

Diagnosis. This is usually made by finding the segments in the faecal sample. Eggs may not be found in faeces and perianal swabbing is more useful in diagnosis than microscopic examination of the faeces.

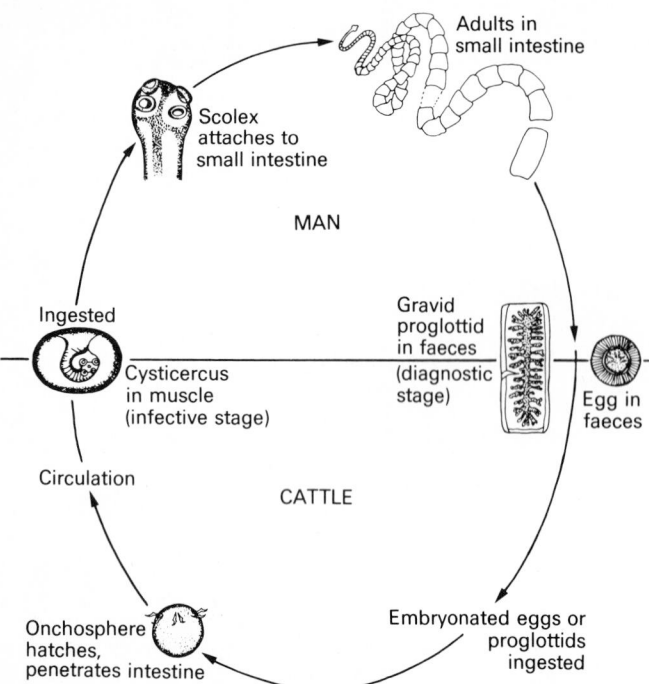

Fig. 4   Life cycle of *Taenia saginata*. (Adapted from Center for Disease Control, Atlanta, Georgia, USA.)

Treatment. Niclosamide is generally regarded as the drug of choice. The cure rate is about 90 per cent after a dose of 2 g (adults) which is given in two equally divided doses with a one hour interval. Each tablet consists of 0.5 g which is chewed and swallowed on empty stomach with minimum of water to attain high concentration in the duodenum. A saline purge is given two to three hours later. The worm is partially digested during therapy and therefore, may not come out intact. The success of treatment cannot be assessed immediately and the patient should be asked to report back for another course if the segments reappear in two to three months time.

Alternatively, mepacrine can be given in a dose of 1 g (adults), also on an empty stomach. It is followed two to three hours later by a saline purge. The whole worm is expelled intact but yellowish in colour due to absorption of mepacrine. Sometimes, the worm is passed out on the next day of therapy.

Finally the advantage of dichlorophen is that no special preparation of the patient is required. It causes disintegration of the worm, and the success of the treatment cannot be assessed immediately. The patient should be asked to report back for another course if the segments reappear in two to three months. The drug is administered in a single dose of 12 tablets (0.5 g each) for adults before breakfast along with a drink. No purgation is required as the drug has a laxative effect.

Infection with *T. saginata* and *T. solium* can be prevented by not eating improperly or uncooked pork and beef in the endemic areas.

Cysticercosis

Cysticercosis is the name given to human infection with the cysticercus stage of *Taenia solium*, which is normally found in pigs. It occurs in all areas where *T. solium* is present.

Morphology. It is typically a semi-transparent fluid-filled ovoid structure with an average size of 10 × 5 mm. In sections, an invaginated scolex is visible which carries four suckers and a row of hooks.

Life cycle. Human infection occurs by the accidental ingestion of eggs from patients harbouring the adult worm, as a result of contamination of food and water. In addition, there is a possibility of retro-infection in which it is assumed that the gravid segments are regurgitated into the stomach, resulting in the liberation of eggs and development of cysticercosis in the same individual.

Clinical aspects. Symptoms occur mainly due to the invasion of the central nervous system by cysticerci. It was previously thought that neuropathology results only from calcification and death of the cyst. Recent studies in West Irian, however, indicate that living cysts can also produce profound neurological symptoms. The symptoms vary from mild nervous manifestations to severe epileptiform attacks, which could be of Jacksonian or grand mal type. If grand mal attacks occur, patients may fall and injure themselves. In West Irian, many cases sustained burns by falling into fire during such attacks. Other symtoms include headache dizziness, eye complaints such as blurred vision, photophobia and diplopia, personality changes, localized anaesthesia, aphasia, amnesia, lethargy, and weakness. Sometimes death occurs from hypocephalus following blockage of the circulatory pathway of cerebrospinal fluid by cysticerci.

Diagnosis. Cysticercosis should be suspected in all adult patients presenting with epilepsy who have not been previously epileptic. These patients may have subcutaneous nodules and a thorough search of the body should be made to locate such swellings. X-ray examinations of the limbs may show calcified cysts but a negative X-ray examination does not exclude cysticercosis. Serological tests commonly used are haemagglutination and complement fixation. However, these tests cross-react with hydatid antigen and also give false positives to patients harbouring the adult worms only. The specificity of complement fixation test is greatly increased if CSF rather than the serum is employed.

Treatment. There is no specific chemotherapy for cysticercosis at present. Patient should be warned about the possibility of injuring himself during an epileptic attack so that appropriate preventive measures are taken. Mebendazole in large doses have given encouraging results in hydatid disease. It may have beneficial effects in cysticercosis but as yet there are no reports of its use in human cases.

Praziquantel has been shown to be effective in a single dose of 50–100 mg/kg body weight against larval *T. saginata* in cattle. It requires to be evaluated against human cysticercosis.

Hymenolepiasis

Hymenolepiasis is an infection caused by tapeworms belonging to the genus *Hymenolepis*. Two species infect man, *H. nana* and *H. diminuta*.

Geographic distribution. *H. nana* has a cosmopolitan distribution and is a common parasite in children in Central Asia, North India and Pakistan, the Middle East, Mediterranean countries, North Africa, and some parts of South and Central America. *H. diminuta* is common parasite of rats but is only occasionally seen in humans.

Morphology. *H. nana* is the smallest tapeworm infecting man. It varies in length from 25 to 40 mm, with approximately 200 segments. The eggs are ovoidal measuring 20–47 μm in diameter. They have two membranous shells. The inner shell has two poles, and from each pole four to eight filaments arise. Inside the egg is the oncosphere or the hexacanth embryo which carries six hooks.

H. diminuta measures 20–60 cm in length and may have up to 1000 segments. The eggs are spherical and measure 76–86 μm in diameter. Unlike *H. nana*, they do not possess polar filaments.

Life cycle. In case of *H. nana*, infection occurs by the swallowing of the egg as a result of faecal contamination of food and water. The oncosphere penetrates the villi of the small intestine where it transforms into a cysticercoid larva. The cysticercoid emerges from the villus and develops into an adult worm (Fig. 5).

In case of *H. diminuta* (Fig. 6), the eggs passed in faeces are ingested by anthropods, usually a flour beetle or a rat flea. In the body cavity of the anthropod it develops into the cysticercoid stage. If the infected anthropod is accidentally swallowed by a rodent or a human, the larva develops into maturity in the small intestine.

Clinical aspects. Light infections with *H. nana* and *H. diminuta* generally do not produce any symptoms. In heavy infections, gastrointestinal disturbances such as diarrhoea, anorexia, and vomiting may be present. Patients sometimes complain of restlessness, dizziness, weakness and insomnia. Presumably these symptoms are caused by the waste products of the parasite and allergic response to its presence.

Diagnosis. This is based on the identification of eggs in the faeces. Unlike *Taenia* spp. The segments disintegrate in the small intestine and are not passed out in faeces. Patients may have high eosinophilia.

Treatment. Niclosomide is generally used, which is given at a dosage of 80 mg/kg daily for five to seven days. If the infection still persists, the course is repeated after two weeks. Recently, praziquantel, an isochinolinpyrazin compound, has been shown to be highly effective. Parasitological cures were obtained in 98.5 per cent of children given a single oral dose of 25 mg/kg body weight. Drug tolerance was good and no clinical side effects were observed.

Dipylidiasis

Dipylidiasis is an infection caused by the common dog tapeworm, *Dipylidium caninum*.

Geographic distribution. It is found in dogs and cats in many parts of the world. Human infection has been reported from Asia, Europe, Africa, and the United States.

Morphology. The adult worms measure 20–40 cm in length. The gravid proglottids contain eggs in clumps known as egg packets or capsules. These are ingested by the larvae of dog and cat fleas and develop in their body into cysticercoids (Fig. 7). Man gets infected by accidentally ingesting fleas.

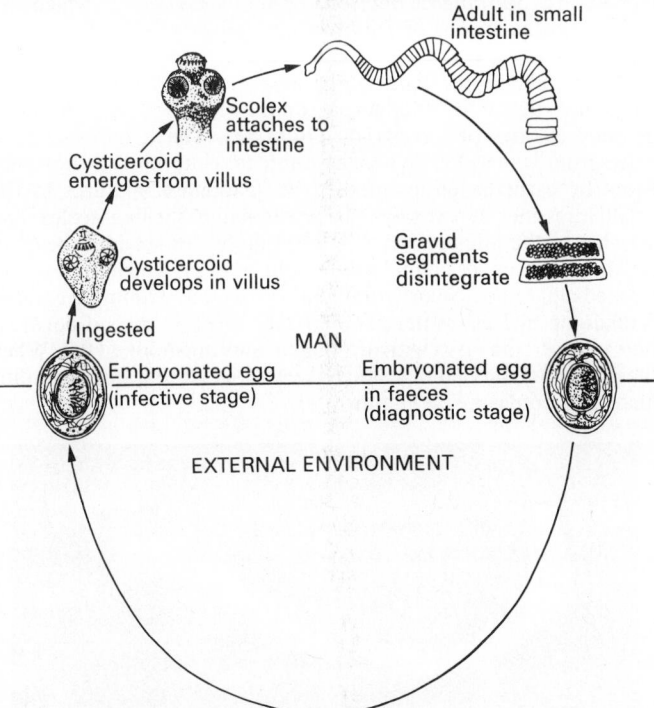

Fig. 5   Life cycle of *Hymenolepis nana*. (Adapted from Center for Disease Control, Atlanta, Georgia, USA.)

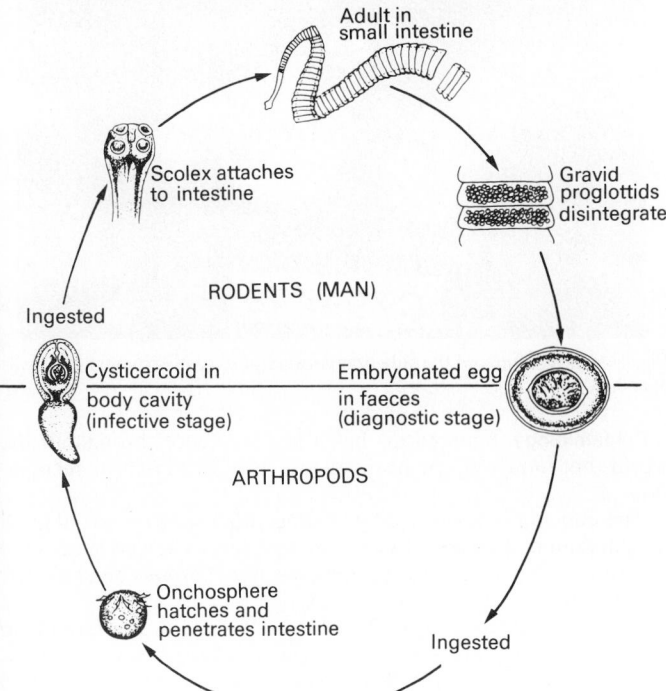

Fig. 6   Life cycle of *Hymenolepis diminuta*. (Adapted from Center for Disease Control. Atlanta, Georgia, USA.)

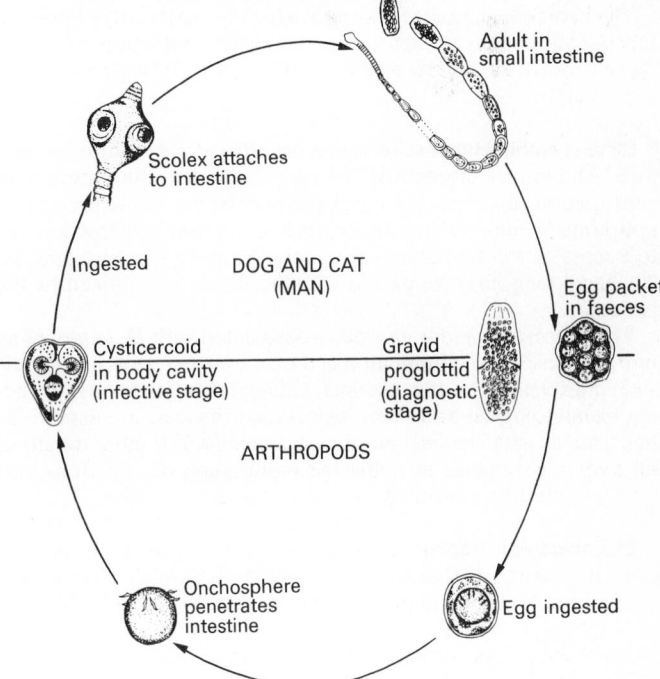

Fig. 7   Life cycle of *Dipylidium caninum*. (Adapted from Center for Disease Control, Atlanta, Georgia, USA.)

Clinical aspects. Infection is more common in children and the infected child may present with gastrointestinal disturbances with or without allergic manifestations such as urticaria and fever.

Diagnosis. This is based on the detection of gravid proglottid or the egg packet in faeces. Eosinophilia may be present.

Treatment. This is same as for Taeniasis.

Diphyllobothriasis and sparganosis

S. Y. Cho

Diphyllobothriasis

Diphyllobothriasis is an intestinal infection with tapeworms belonging to the genus *Diphyllobothrium*. The most important species is *D. latum*, which is commonly called 'fish-tapeworm' or 'broad-tapeworm'.

Biology and epidemiology. Human diphyllobothriasis is contracted by consuming raw fish such as pike, burbot, perch, and other salmonid fish which are sometimes infected with hundreds of plerocercoid larva. In the human intestine these larvae develop into adult worms which may reach 20–25 m in length and 2–3 cm in width, and produce millions of eggs each day. The eggs are operculated, and $65 \times 45 \mu m$ in size: they develop into coracidia which are freely swimming in fresh water. The coracidium is taken up by fresh water zooplankters such as *Cyclops strenuus* and *Eudiaptomus gracilis* and develop into a procercoid. This larva is transferred to small fresh water fish such as sticklebacks which, in turn, are eaten by large salmonid fish in which the plerocercoid develops. It is 1–1.5 cm long and 1 mm wide, and is found as a white, transversely-wrinkled larva in muscle and in the peritoneal cavity.

The highest incidence of human cases is in the Baltic region, especially in Finland, Leningrad, and throughout Siberia. Villages used to exist where 80 per cent of the population were infected. In Switzerland, northern Italy, arctic and lake regions of North America, Chile, Manchuria, Korea, and Japan, cases are not uncommon. Eskimoes may be infected with various species of *Diphyllobothrium*.

The habit of eating sliced raw fish, which is particularly popular in Finland and Japan, creates the opportunity for infection. The Russian custom of eating raw pike roe and Jewish *gefüllte fisch* also lead to infection.

Clinical manifestations. Infection usually results in little discomfort. Abdominal discomfort, fatigue, diarrhoea alternating with constipation, dizziness, and urticaria may be the vague presenting symptoms. Vomiting up a tapeworm and intestinal obstruction due to a mass of worms occurs very rarely. Strips of gravid segments, 20–30 cm long, may be passed with the stools and noticed by the patient.

Tapeworm pernicious anaemia is associated with *D. latum* infection. In these cases, elimination of the tapeworm results in progressive improvement of the anaemia. Clinical manifestations, including haematological and neurological disturbances, are essentially the same as with classical pernicious anaemia. For more details of tapeworm pernicious anaemia the monograph of von Bonsdorff (1977) should be consulted.

Diagnosis and treatment. Clinical symptoms are rarely responsible for raising the suspicion of diphyllobothriasis. Racial and geographical origin and predilection for raw fish provide the clues to a diagnosis which can be easily confirmed by identifying the characteristic eggs, or long chains of worm segments in faeces.

In endemic areas all patients with pernicious anaemia should have their stools examined.

Treatment is relatively simple and effective. In the Baltic region, oleoresin of male fern is still used. Atabrine, niclosamide, bithionol, dichlorophen, paromomycin, and praziquantel are all good vermifuges effective in over 80 per cent by single treatment. Niclosamide, in a single adult dose of 2 g, is the drug of choice. Identification of an expelled scolex confirms a complete cure.

Prevention is achieved by freezing fish at $-18\,^{\circ}C$ for one day.

Sparganosis

Sparganosis is a zoonotic infection caused by the larval stage of tapeworms, *Spirometra mansoni* or *S. mansonoides*, which are taxonomically cousins of *Diphyllobothrium*.

Biology. The white, slender, ribbon-shaped tapeworm larva without round suckers is called a sparganum when it is found in tissue or body cavities of terrestrial vertebrates. The length of larvae varies from 1 cm to 1 m. When larva-infected intermediate hosts are eaten by carnivorous mammals, the sparganum matures in the small intestine. It extrudes the invaginated slit-like scolex and attaches to the intestinal mucosa. Within five or six days the adult worm produces operculated immature eggs which mature to hooked ciliated embryos (coracidia). When the swimming embryo is taken up by fresh water zooplankters, *Cyclops* spp., it develops into a procercoid larva with prolonged body and hooked tail. When the procercoid larva is ingested by terrestrial vertebrates, including man, it becomes a sparganum.

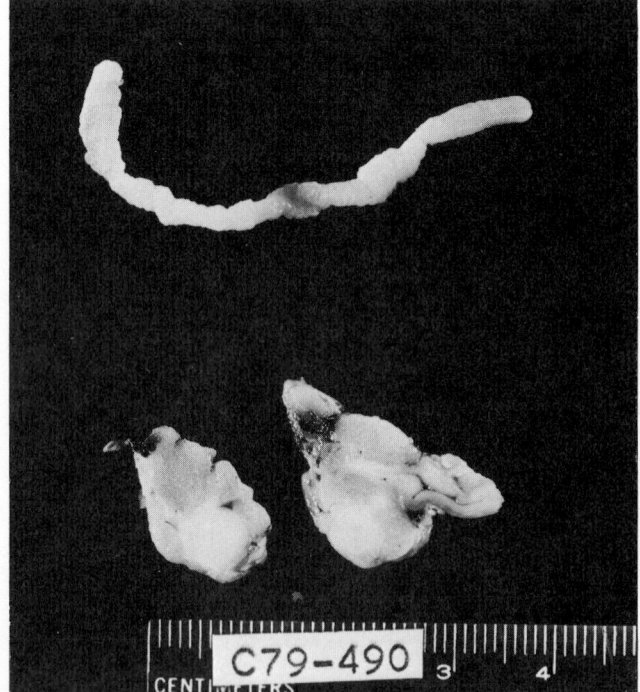

Fig. 1   Sparganum and the subcutaneous adipose tissue from which it was expelled.

Epidemiology. Sparganosis has a low incidence throughout the world, but improved medical services have increased its recognition.

The infection is contracted by eating either the procercoid larva or sparganum. The procercoid larva may be swallowed in infected *Cyclops* when people drink untreated water in brooks or lakes near camp sites.

The most endemic areas for sparganosis are in the Orient, in countries such as Japan, Korea, China, and Vietnam, where traditional habits contribute to the relatively high incidence. Poultry and snakes are important sources of infection. Some people believe that eating these animals raw is beneficial for physically feeble children and victims of tuberculosis and arthritis. Others believe that live vipers are a tonic! Raw pork is a source of sparganosis as well as *Taenia solium* infection. The practice of poulticing an inflamed eye or abscess with frog or snake skin was common in the pre-antibiotic era in southern China and Vietnam. In these instances, the sparganum in the herpetile's skin could invade the eye directly through conjunctiva or friable abscess wall.

Thus sparganosis is mainly a disease of rural people or of those who seek the rural life.

Pathology and clinical manifestations. The procercoid larva or sparganum ingested by a human actively penetrates the intestinal wall to reach the peritoneal cavity, whence it begins to migrate systemically. The worm usually lodges in subcutaneous tissue or muscle in the chest or abdominal walls, limbs, or scrotum. Orbital sparganosis is also common even in those not using poultices. Urinary tract, pleural cavity, pericardial sac, abdominal viscera, brain, and spinal canal are other reported sites where severe symptoms of inflammation or obstruction are produced.

The worm may slowly migrate within the body. A lump appears then spontaneously disappears, only to reappear some weeks or months later at a site remote from the first. There is redness and itching of overlying skin, and local bleeding, and acute suppurative necrosis may complicate the sparganosis.

The characteristic pathological finding is focal necrosis along the tortuous track of migration. These tracks are surrounded by zones of necrotic debris and lymphohistiocytic reaction. Heavy eosinophilic infiltration with occasional Charcot–Leyden crystals are usually found. The inflammatory reaction often extends into surrounding muscle or fat tissue particularly during the acute phase. Part of the dead worm may be found in the tissues, leaving its characteristic calcospherules which are engulfed by histiocytes.

Diagnosis and treatment. Pre-operative diagnosis of sparganosis is rarely made. Past history of eating raw animals together with detection of a migrating mass is almost diagnostic, particularly in endemic areas. In most cases the definitive diagnosis is made by recovering the worm from various lesions at surgery. The sparganum is, characteristically, a white, ribbon-shaped, moving worm with transverse wrinkling and an actively protruding head. If the collected worms are naturally branched, they are called *Sparganum proliferum*.

The excision of a mass or removal of a worm from the lesion is therapeutic in itself. Sometimes repeated surgical intervention is needed when the patient has multiple lesions or the worm is rapidly changing its site. No drugs are known to be effective for sparganosis.

Except for the case of *Sparganum proliferum*, only a few worms infect each patient. Prognosis of sparganosis is excellent in almost all cases unless the vital organs have been irreversibly damaged by the worms.

References

von Bonsdorff, B. (1977). *Diphyllobothriasis in man*. Academic Press, London.

Nelson, G. S., Pester, F. R. N., and Rickman, R. (1965). The significance of wild animals in the transmission of cestodes of medical importance in Kenya. *Trans. R. Soc. trop. Med. Hyg.* **59**, 507.

Swartzwelder, J. C., Beaver, P. C., and Hood, M. W. (1964). Sparganosis in southern United States. *Am. J. trop. Med. Hyg.* **13**, 43.

TREMATODES

Schistosomiasis

K. Warren

Schistosomiasis (bilharziasis) is a chronic trematode infection of at least 200 000 000 people in Asia, Africa, the Caribbean, and South America caused largely by three species, *Schistosoma mansoni*, *S. japonicum*, and *S. haematobium*. Infection occurs on entry into fresh water containing infective larvae (cercariae) emitted by the snail intermediate host. These cercariae penetrate the skin and the immature parasites (schistosomula) migrate via the lungs and liver to their final habitat in the veins of the intestines or urinary bladder. The 1–2 cm long adult male and female worms, which remain *in copulo* for many years, do not themselves multiply within the human definitive host, but produce large numbers of eggs, many of which are trapped within the tissues, primarily in the intestines and liver, or the urinary tract. Immunological reactions to the eggs result in granulomatous inflammation and fibrosis obstructing blood flow within the liver or urine flow from the ureters. Eggs excreted in the urine and faeces which reach fresh water hatch into ciliated miracidia which penetrate into snails, multiply, and develop into cercariae, the infective form for man.

Aetiology. The cercariae of many avian and mammalian schistosome species penetrate human skin, but there are three major species that complete their life cycles in man and are thus capable of causing systemic disease: *Schistosoma mansoni*, *japonicum*, and *haematobium*. These three species have similar life cycles: as digenetic trematodes they alternate between a sexual phase of reproduction in the human definitive host and an asexual reproductive phase in the snail intermediate host. There are differences among each of the species, however, of importance to the epidemiology, pathogenesis, and clinical aspects of the disease syndromes associated with these parasites.

The schistosomes are members of the class Trematoda of the phylum Platyhelminthes or flat worms. The adult male worms are 10–20 mm in length and 0.5–1 mm in width and have cleft bodies within which the longer and thinner females are clasped (see Fig. 1f, page 5.456). The life span of the worms within man may be as long as 30 years, but it is now believed that their mean longevity is three to eight years. The adult *S. mansoni* and *S. japonicum* reside in the venules of the large and small intestines and those of *S. haematobium* in the ureteric and vesical venules.

The worms take up nutrients via their intestine and integument. Their energy metabolism is dependent largely on anaerobic glycolysis, and the schistosomes utilize one fifth of their dry body weight of glucose per hour converting 80 per cent of it to lactic acid. As the worms contain a proteolytic intestinal enzyme that breaks down globin, their ingestion of red blood cells may be of nutritional significance. The schistosome intestine terminates blindly and the remaining insoluble haematin-like pigment is regurgitated. The rapid metabolic rate of the schistosomes may in part be related to their continual output of many eggs, estimated at 1400 to 3000 per day for *S. japonicum* and one tenth that number for *S. mansoni*. The eggs of *S. mansoni* are released singly, while those of *S. japonicum* and *S. haematobium* are deposited in large aggregates. They embryonate over a period of six days and reach a mean size of 66×155 µm for *S. mansoni*, 60×143 µm for *S. haematobium* and 67×89µm for *S. japonicum*. The shape of the eggs is distinctive, *S. mansoni* being ellipsoidal and having a lateral spine; *S. haematobium*, also ellipsoidal but with a terminal spine; and *S. japonicum*, spheroidal with a tiny knob. The eggs live for approximately 21 days after laying, during which time they absorb nutrients from the host and secrete enzymes which facilitate their passage from the blood vessels through the tissues and into the lumen of the excretory organs. A large proportion of the eggs, however, either remain in the intestinal and urinary tract tissues or break free in the bloodstream and are carried into the liver and lungs.

Eggs that leave the body in faeces or urine and reach fresh water hatch rapidly into free-swimming ciliated miracidia. Those of *S. mansoni* are negatively geotropic and positively phototropic; those of *S. haematobium* appear to be the opposite. Their average life span is about six hours. On encountering a snail the miracidium will attempt penetration by means of vigorous movements and enzymatic secretions. The organism can complete its life cycle, however, only if certain genera and species of snails are entered: the genus

Biomphalaria for *S. mansoni*, *Bulinus* for *S. haematobium*, and *Oncomelania* for *S. japonicum*. *Biomphalaria* and *Bulinus* are aquatic, *Oncomelania*, amphibious. The miracidium develops into a mother sporocyst close to the site of penetration. About ten days later, daughter sporocysts begin to migrate into the hepatopancreas of the snail and about five weeks from penetration by the miracidium, free swimming cercariae produced by the daughter sporocysts begin to be shed by the snail. Maximal stimulus for shedding of *S. mansoni* and *haematobium* cercariae is provided by light, but darkness seems to favour the output of *S. japonicum* cercariae. Mean daily cercarial output of *S. mansoni* and *S. haematobium* is about 700, but that of *S. japonicum* is only about two. The cercariae may live for two to three days under ideal conditions, but their infectivity is lost by 20 hours; under field conditions both their life span and their infectivity are greatly reduced. The fork-tailed schistosome cercariae are about 125–200 μm in length by 50–75 μm in width. *S. mansoni* and *S. haematobium* cercariae move vertically, alternating between active movement towards the surface and slowly sinking; they can move laterally towards certain stimuli. In contrast, *S. japonicum* cercariae attach themselves to the surface film where they tend to remain at rest unless disturbed. When cercariae encounter mammalian skin, they attach themselves with suckers, and by vigorous movement aided by enzymatic secretions, the heads penetrate, leaving the tails behind. This process occurs during immersion in water or while the skin remains moist (drying kills the organisms if not fully penetrated), and takes four to ten minutes for *S. mansoni*, but only a few seconds to three minutes for *S. japonicum*.

Immediately on skin penetration the cercarial integument is drastically altered, the cercaria becomes tolerant of a saline environment and its metabolism shifts from an efficient tricarboxylic acid cycle to glycolysis, the organism being transformed into a schistosomulum. It should be emphasized that each cercaria that penetrates the skin can develop into only one worm. Many schistosomula die in the skin, however, and in the best of experimental hosts only about 60 per cent of the *S. mansoni* organisms reach maturity. Within a few hours to days the schistosomula migrate to the lungs, mainly by the bloodstream. After a few days in the pulmonary vessels the schistosumula pass to the liver, largely by the bloodstream. This phase takes ten to twelve days for *S. mansoni*, a somewhat shorter period for *S. japonicum*, and a longer one for *S. haematobium*. Once in the intrahepatic portal venules the worms rapidly reach maturity, mate, and move against the blood flow to their final habitats. Egg output is detectable at five to six weeks for *S. japonicum*, seven to eight weeks for *S. mansoni*, and ten to twelve weeks for *S. haematobium*.

Epidemiology. In endemic areas infection first occurs when children begin to make consistent contact with water, playing or doing chores. Reinfection will continue as long as there is significant water contact and is related both to the time and degree of exposure. As the schistosomes do not multiply within the definitive human host, complete immunity apparently does not occur, and the worms live for many years, the worm burden being essentially determined by the amount of exposure to the infectious organisms in the water. The system is not highly efficient, however, and the incidence of schistosomiasis in most endemic areas is low, and the build-up of worm burdens takes many years. Under these circumstances of gradual acquisition of schistosomes and relative longevity of the worms, the prevalence of the infection may build up to massive proportions in some individuals.

The prevalence of schistosomiasis worldwide is now estimated at over 200 000 000 cases. It is known to be endemic in 71 countries that have a total population of about 2 000 000 000.

Both *S. haematobium* and *S. mansoni* are widespread in Africa. Only the former species occurs in Tunisia, Algeria, Morocco, Mauritania, Guinea-Bissau, Niger, the Congo Republic (Brazzaville), Somalia, and the island of Mauritius. Both species are found in all other countries, including the Malagasy Republic. Sixty per

cent of Africans live in areas where exposure to schistosomes is possible, and 40 per cent of these are infected.

In Southwest Asia, *S. haematobium* is endemic in Aden, Saudi Arabia, Yemen, Israel, Iraq, Iran, Syria, Turkey, and Lebanon. *S. mansoni* occurs in the first four of these countries, and is particularly prevalent in Yemen, where half the population are thought to be infected. The highest prevalence rate for *S. haematobium* occurs in Iraq, where 20 per cent of the exposed population is infected.

Only *S. mansoni* is found in endemic areas of the New World where over 20 000 000 people are estimated to be exposed. Brazil has the largest number of cases, estimated at 8 000 000, but a major control campaign is now being waged. Schistosomiasis also occurs in Venezuela, where it is apparently on the wane, and in Surinam. It is endemic in the following Caribbean islands: Puerto Rico, Vieques, Dominican Republic, Antigua, Guadeloupe, Martinique, and St Lucia. The parasite has not been found in any of the Central American countries.

The one tiny focus of schistosomiasis in Europe, *S. haematobium* in southern Portugal, is no longer existent.

S. japonicum is the species occurring in the Orient and is found in China, Japan, Taiwan, the Philippines, and the Celebes. The prevalence in China was estimated at 32 000 000, but it has been reduced by approximately 70 per cent by massive control campaigns. The prevalence of schistosomiasis in Japan has been markedly decreased by decades of control efforts, but a principal effect has been ascribed to general development. The infection seems to be spreading in the Philippines with irrigation projects. Small foci of schistosomiasis japonica have recently been discovered in Thailand and Laos. A tiny focus of *S. haematobium* in Maharashtra State, India has apparently been eliminated.

The presence of susceptible snails is necessary for the establishment of the life cycle of schistosomiasis. While the infection is prevalent on the West Indian island of St Lucia, St Vincent, only 80 km away, is completely free of the parasite. There are several hundred thousand infected Puerto Ricans living in the continental United States but they cannot transmit the infection as there are no susceptible intermediate hosts. Prevalence rates in endemic areas may vary from close to 100 per cent to almost zero. This is governed by the interaction of many local ecological factors relating to both the snail and human populations. Another important factor in the epidemiology of schistosomiasis is the variation in geographic strains of the species; for example, *S. japonicum* in Taiwan is highly infective to domestic and wild animals but not to man.

Animal reservoirs are of major significance in maintaining the life cycle of *S. japonicum*—in particular, cows, dogs and probably rats. Natural *S. mansoni* infections have been found in rodents, baboons, and insectivores in Africa and South America, but it is generally believed that they do not play a significant role as reservoirs. *S. haematobium* is rarely encountered in animals.

Transmission patterns differ among the three species of schistosomes, but there is little doubt that for each species agricultural development because of irrigation usually leads to marked increases in the prevalence of schistosomiasis. A major epidemic occurred in Egypt after the construction of the low Aswan dam, and in Zimbabwe after the development of large-scale irrigation schemes.

Schistosomiasis is an insidious disease, thus making it difficult to determine morbidity and mortality. It was only recently that field and autopsy studies using quantitative methods (i.e. counting of eggs in measured tissue, faecal, or urine samples) revealed a high degree of correlation between intensity of infection and manifestations of disease, primarily hepatomegaly and splenomegaly in *S. mansoni* and *S. japonicum* infections, and bladder abnormalities and hydronephrosis in *S. haematobium*. Virtually all investigations of morbidity based on educational attainment or work capacity have provided negative results until a very recent study using quantitative methodology demonstrated a reduction in work capacity by bicycle ergometry, but only in those with very heavy *S. mansoni* infections.

As the worms do not multiply in man, the intensity of infection in populations is related to degree of water contact and perhaps the occurrence of partial immunity. Under these conditions, schistosomes have an overdispersed distribution in which most members of the host population bear low worm burdens. As far as has been determined, little or no morbidity occurs in the large majority of the population carrying infections of low intensity. Though the proportion of heavily infected individuals is small, when this figure is multiplied by the vast number of cases of schistosomiasis, it becomes obvious that this helminthic infection constitutes a major global problem. In addition, there is no question that in all of its forms schistosomiasis is potentially lethal—Katayama fever in *S. japonicum* infections, portal hypertension with haematemesis in both schistosomiasis japonica and mansoni, uraemia in *S. haematobium* infection and cor pulmonale in all three. That schistosomiasis may also potentiate the development of other diseases such as hepatitis, hepatoma, cirrhosis, and cancer of the urinary bladder has been suggested by both clinical and experimental studies.

Pathogenesis and clinical manifestations. Certain facts are basic to an understanding of the disease processes in schistosomiasis: the schistosomes do not multiply in man; complete immunity does not follow initial infections; repeated infections usually occur; the worms are relatively long lived; most individuals have low worm burdens, but many worms may accumulate in some; and a large proportion of schistosome eggs are not excreted but remain within the body. Disease is correlated with the intensity of infection and is related not only to the presence of the various stages of the schistosomes in the body tissues and their secretions and excretions, but to the inflammatory responses of the host to them.

Three distinct syndromes occur at different stages of schistosome infection. Within one day of cercarial penetration, swimmer's itch, a pruritic papular rash, may appear. Several weeks later Katayama fever, a self-limited but possibly fatal illness resembling serum sickness, may develop. Finally, after many years, during which the infection is largely asymptomatic, fibrosis of the periportal areas of the liver may result in the signs and symptoms of portal hypertension in schistosomiasis mansoni and japonica. Fibrosis of the ureters and bladder in schistosomiasis haematobia may result in changes associated with bladder malfunction and obstruction to urine flow.

Schistosome dermatitis. Schistosomiasis begins with penetration of the skin by cercariae. These organisms will indiscriminately penetrate the skin of most animals, susceptible or insusceptible, living or dead. Schistosomes of animals or birds all die on entering human skin. Even in highly susceptible experimental hosts many *S. mansoni* cercariae perish in the skin and perhaps in the lungs. In the highest primate thus far studied, the chimpanzee, only 4–8 per cent of *S. mansoni* cercariae, 14–40 per cent of *S. haematobium* cercariae, and 1–48 per cent of *S. japonicum* cercariae were recovered as adult schistosomes.

The death of cercariae in the skin leads to the development of a pruritic papular rash known as swimmer's itch. This syndrome occurs in its most severe form after exposure to animal schistosomes, and has been shown to be a sensitization phenomenon, rarely occurring on primary exposure. Papules appear in sensitized persons at five to fifteen hours, and there is massive round cell invasion of the dermis and epidermis, suggesting a delayed hypersensitivity response. A rash has been demonstrated in infected individuals experimentally re-exposed to *S. mansoni* and *S. haematobium* cercariae. A mild form of swimmer's itch appears to occur in patients exposed to *S. japonicum* cercariae, but the rice paddy dermatitis of the Far East is caused mainly by avian schistosomes.

Acute schistosomiasis. The next clinical phase of schistosomiasis begins 20–60 days after exposure and has been known in Japan as Katayama fever since the mid-nineteenth century. This syndrome occurs most frequently and is most severe in *S. japonicum* infections; in schistosomiasis mansoni it is less commonly found; it is rarely if ever seen in schistosomiasis haematobia. The patient suffers from fever, chills, sweating, anorexia, headache, diarrhoea, and cough. Hepatosplenomegaly is frequent, and generalized lymphadenopathy and urticaria are often seen. Eosinophilia occurs in most cases, averaging about 40 per cent. The fever may last for several weeks; when it subsides the other signs and symptoms of infection also disappear in spite of the fact that egg output in the stools may continue to remain high. Death may occur in the Katayama fever stage of schistosomiasis japonica, and has been recorded in *S. mansoni* infection. At autopsy, massive infection is usually found, with large numbers of eggs in the liver and intestines; 1608 worm pairs were demonstrated in a Brazilian child. Katayama fever, which usually appears on initial infection, begins at about the time of onset of egg-laying by the worms, although some cases have been reported to appear prior to the onset of oviposition. A strong correlation has been shown between the severity of acute schistosomiasis and the number of eggs in the stools. It has been suggested that this serum sickness-like syndrome may be a form of immune-complex disease.

Chronic schistosomiasis. There is a good correlation between the size of the worm burden and the occurrence of chronic disease as demonstrated by the quantity of worms found at surgery and at autopsy. Virtually all of the patients with hepatosplenic disease had moderate to heavy infections. Occasionally, relatively low worm burdens are seen in hepatosplenic schistosomiasis, but this is probably related to the fact that the disease is usually not seen until the later teens or early adulthood after water contact has declined. It is highly unlikely that patients who have never had more than light infections will ever develop significant disease, the exceptions being central nervous system disease or possibly an occasional blockage at the ureteric–vesical junction.

It has been claimed that patients with chronic schistosomiasis mansoni or japonica complain of fatigue, abdominal pain, and intermittent diarrhoea or dysentery. Nevertheless controlled trials in school children or villages in highly endemic areas have revealed few such signs and symptoms, even in heavily infected individuals. On sigmoidoscopy, particularly in Egypt, granulomatous nodules or polyps may be observed. In *S. haematobium* infection, terminal haematuria, and, occasionally, dysuria and frequency are found. Mild chronic blood loss has been measured by radioisotope labelling in both *S. mansoni* and *S. haematobium* infections, but anaemia is not usually seen in areas where there is normal iron intake. All the aforementioned signs and symptoms are related to the passage of eggs through the mucosa of the intestines and the urinary bladder.

A large proportion of the eggs do not leave the body; in laboratory animals less than half of them are excreted. Over a period of ten years, for each *S. mansoni* worm pair producing eggs at a rate of 300 per day, at least 500 000 eggs will remain in the body. The figure for each *S. japonicum* worm pair, which produce 3000 eggs per day, will be 5 000 000.

In infection with the schistosomes of the intestines, *S. mansoni* and *S. japonicum*, some of the eggs remain in the submucosa of the gut, but many of them break free in the circulation and are carried into the liver. In schistosomiasis haematobia many eggs remain in the tissues of the bladder and adjacent organs, but some (usually too few to cause significant disease) enter the lungs via the inferior vena cava as well as the liver via the portal system. Granulomatous inflammation develops around the eggs trapped in the tissues. The *S. mansoni* granuloma has been demonstrated to be an immunological response of the delayed hypersensitivity type. This is based on numerous studies in experimental animals demonstrating the following: (*a*) on secondary exposure to eggs an anamnestic inflammatory reaction occurs in which the granuloma becomes much bigger much more rapidly; (*b*) this reaction is specific; (*c*) it can be transferred with lymphoid cells and not with serum; (*d*) it correlates with delayed skin reactions and *in vitro* correlates of cellular immunological reactions; (*e*) the early granuloma secretes lymphokines but not immunoglobulins; (*f*) it is suppressed by inhibitors of cellular but not humoral immunological reactions. Less extensive studies suggest a similar mechanism for the *S. haematobium* egg granuloma, but it appears that the *S. japonicum* lesion has a different aetiology, perhaps due to immune complexes. These findings strongly suggest that schistosomiasis is essentially an immunological disease.

It must be realized, however, that the development of disease is related to two factors, the number of eggs in the tissues and the size of the inflammatory reaction around them. The quantity of eggs in the tissues is determined not only by the numbers produced by the worms but by the rate of egg destruction by the host. The size of the lesions is determined by the rapid onset of the anamnestic response. This, however, is gradually modulated in chronic infections by the development of suppressor cells and blocking antibodies. Thus, the presence of few eggs will not result in disease no matter how large the reactions, and massive numbers of eggs with virtually no reactions will also not result in disease. There will be disease, however, when there are very large numbers of eggs in the presence of moderate reactions. The optimal conditions for the development of disease, of course, are large numbers of eggs plus large granulomas. The proliferative inflammatory lesions and the eventual fibrosis are the determinants of disease. In schistosomiasis mansoni and japonica this leads to hepatosplenic disease and in schistosomiasis haematobia to urinary tract disease.

Hepatosplenic schistosomiasis. The clinical consequences of this syndrome relate primarily to granulomatous inflammation and portal fibrosis (Fig. 1). Pathophysiologically this results in an intrahepatic block to portal blood flow and the development of portal hypertension and portal-systemic collateral circulation. The lesion is presinusoidal, thus intrasplenic and portal pressures are markedly elevated, while wedged hepatic vein pressure is normal. Total liver blood flow tends to remain within normal limits owing to a compensatory increase in arterial flow. As the liver parenchyma is relatively unharmed by the pathological processes and liver perfusion is maintained, liver function tests remain within normal limits, and the physiological and biochemical abnormalities associated with cirrhosis of the liver are rarely seen.

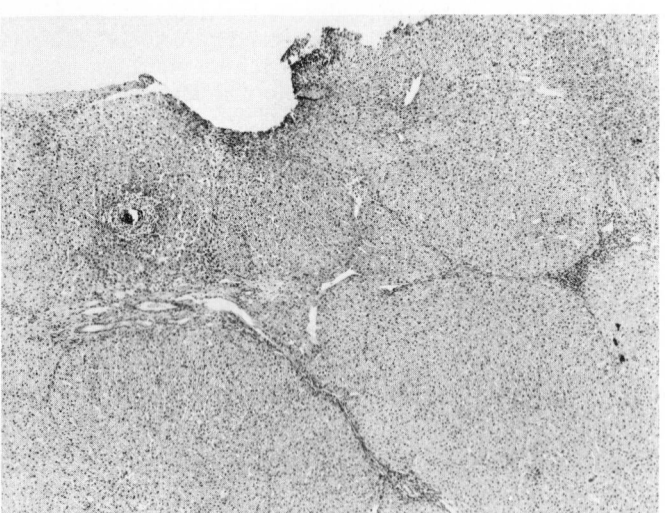

Fig. 1 Wedged liver biopsy from a patient with hepatosplenic schistosomiasis mansoni. Schistosome egg granuloma and mild periportal liver fibrosis.

Clinically, the earliest sign of significant liver involvement is hepatomegaly. With progression, the spleen enlarges and becomes firm in consistency. Eventually it may extend to well below the umbilicus (Fig. 2). At this point the patient tends to be in good

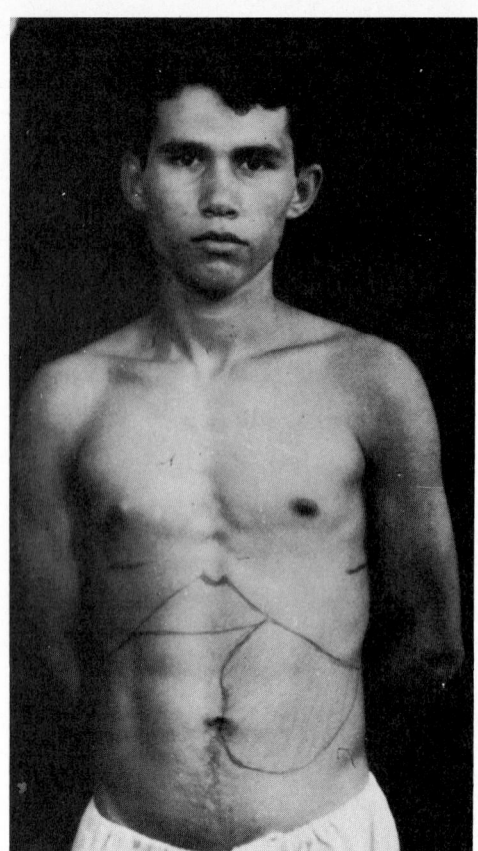

Fig. 2   Twenty-two year old patient from Bahia, Brazil with hepatosplenic schistosomiasis mansoni.

general health, but may consult a physician because of a dragging feeling in the left upper abdominal quadrant. The other major factor bringing the patient to the attention of the physician is a sudden haematemesis due to bleeding oesophageal varices (Fig. 3). Such an episode may not reappear for many years or may recur at fairly frequent intervals. The consequences of haematemesis in schistosomiasis are very different from those in cirrhosis of the liver: the blood ammonia concentration tends to remain normal, hepatic coma rarely occurs, and fatalities are few, being due primarily to exsanguination. This is consistent with relatively normal liver function. Jaundice is almost never seen in uncomplicated schistosomiasis, and the levels of both conjugated and unconjugated bilirubin are usually normal. Serum albumin concentration is normal or only slightly decreased, and globulin is somewhat elevated. As a consequence, ascites and oedema are rarely encountered. Even sulphobromophthalein retention is often normal in these patients. Stigmata of chronic liver disease such as palmar erythaema, spider angiomas, altered hair distribution, and gynaecomastia are rare. Patients may suffer multiple severe haematemeses; but aside from temporary changes, liver function tends to remain relatively normal.

In spite of moderate chronic and occasional severe acute intestinal blood loss, a significant degree of anaemia rarely occurs in uncomplicated schistosomiasis. The white blood count is usually within normal limits, but there may be a moderate eosinophilia. Splenomegaly, however, may result in hypersplenism, the patient developing leucopenia, thrombocytopenia, and anaemia with decreased red blood cell life span.

In hospitals in endemic areas patients may be seen with so-called decompensated hepatosplenic schistosomiasis characterized by liver parenchymal malfunction and all of the physical stigmata of this state, including jaundice and ascites. Pathologists have stated that it has not been possible to prove the transformation of advanced schistosomal fibrosis into true cirrhosis. There is little question, however, that patients with schistosomiasis might concomitantly have other forms of liver disease. Finally, it must be recognized that all those infected with *S. mansoni* and *S. japonicum* perforce have some degree of liver involvement, and that the effects of malnutrition, hepatotoxins, and hepatitis may be potentiated; such interrelationships have been demonstrated in laboratory animals.

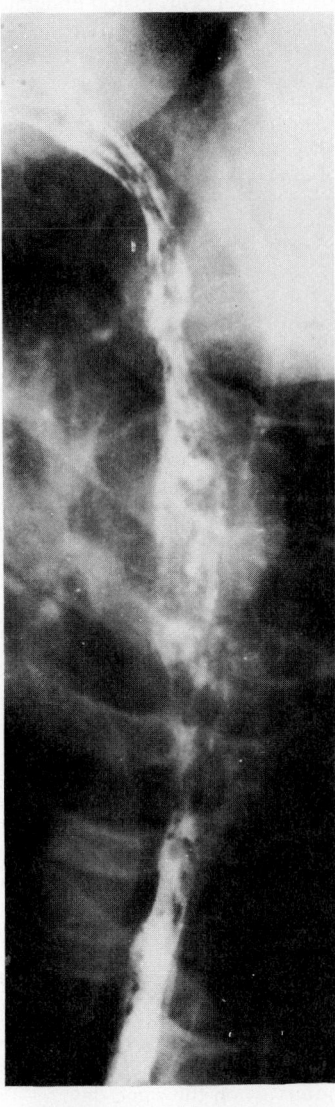

Fig. 3 Barium swallow revealing oesophageal varices in a patient with schistosomiasis mansoni.

Pulmonary schistosomiasis. Although the lungs are frequently involved in schistosomiasis due to embolization of the eggs, its most severe state, characterized by signs and symptoms of cor pulmonale, is a complication of hepatosplenic schistosomiasis. Portal-systemic collateral circulation enables large numbers of eggs to bypass the liver, and they are trapped in the pulmonary capillary bed. Arteritis occurs and there is obstruction to pulmonary blood flow. Pulmonary hypertension is found in every case, but cardiac output usually remains within the normal range. Arterial oxygen saturation is usually normal, and cyanosis is rare. The lungs are often involved in schistosomiasis haematobia because of the passage of the eggs from the vesical plexuses into the inferior vena cava, but egg embolization appears to be relatively light, and significant disease is uncommon.

Urinary tract schistosomiasis. Both in the early and late phases of *S. haematobium* infection, severe urinary tract disease may occur. Initially there may be ureteral obstruction owing to proliferative granulomatous inflammatory reactions to the eggs in both the ureters and the bladder; these lesions appear to be highly reversible after antischistosomal therapy. Later in the course of the disease irreversible fibrosis may occur. Bladder fibrosis and calcification lead to frequency and dysuria. On cystoscopy, so-called sandy patches may be seen on the bladder walls; these are made up of large numbers of schistosome eggs with little reaction around them. The disease may progress through hydronephrosis, secondary infection, and finally uraemia. An association between cancer of the bladder and urinary schistosomiasis has been suggested.

In the past decade there has been a growing impression among Brazilian clinicians and pathologists that there is an increased frequency of renal disease in patients with schistosomiasis mansoni. Initially proteinuria was noted in patients with hepatosplenic schistosomiasis, and then, at autopsy, the renal glomeruli of similar patients were found to have pathologic changes. This was followed by ultrastructural and immunocytochemical studies which revealed electron-dense deposits in the glomerular basement membranes which contained immunoglobulins. Similar deposits have been observed in laboratory animals. The significance of these findings remains to be established.

Central nervous system schistosomiasis. Central nervous system involvement in schistosomiasis, while relatively rare, is a severe complication of the infection. *S. japonicum* usually involves the brain, whereas *S. mansoni* and *S. haematobium* tend to affect the spinal cord. Schistosomiasis japonica is reputed to be one of the important causes of focal epilepsy in the Far East. The disease may also present as a space-occupying lesion or occasionally as a generalized encephalitis. Cerebral schistosomiasis japonica may appear at any time in the course of infection from the first three weeks on. At autopsy the lesions almost always consist of large collections of eggs in the venous circulatory system, suggesting the presence of adult worms, although they have never been found. *S. mansoni* and *S. haematobium* in the spinal cord may be associated with a transverse myelitis-like syndrome; at surgery or autopsy large granulomas made up of eggs are usually found.

Diagnosis. The diagnosis of schistosomiasis in non-endemic areas should always begin with the question 'Where have you been?' If the patient has been in an endemic area it is essential to determine whether any significant contact with fresh water has occurred (clean chlorinated swimming pools and ocean bathing are safe). It is unlikely that the patient will report either a 'swimmer's itch' or a Katayama fever-like syndrome, but a history of these reactions would be suggestive. *S. mansoni* and *S. japonicum* village studies in endemic areas do not suggest any significant generalized or abdominal symptoms. *S. haematobium* infection may be associated with terminal haematuria, dysuria, and perhaps frequency.

Definitive diagnosis can be made only by finding schistosome eggs in the excreta (faeces or urine) or in a biopsy specimen, usually rectal. Eggs may not be present in the early stages of acute schistosomiasis. Schistosome eggs are relatively large, and are easy to identify because of their distinctive shape. Direct faecal smear is too insensitive, but techniques which provide both concentration and quantitation of eggs in the faeces have been developed. This is important, because correlations between egg output and intensity of infection have been made. The Kato thick smear technique is a simple and highly effective method for faecal egg counting. A small portion of stool (schistosome eggs are distributed randomly in faeces) is passed through 105-mesh stainless steel bolting cloth and 50 mg is added to a tared glass slide and covered with a cellophane cover slip impregnated with 50 per cent glycerin. The slides are inverted and pressed on to a bed of filter paper, turned face up, and left for a period of 24 hours during which the faecal matter clears. Although the embryo within the egg also clears, the characteristic shape of the egg shell can be easily seen. After counting all of the eggs in the sample, multiplication by 20 provides the number of eggs per gram of faeces. A more rapid diagnosis may be made by using 20 mg of faeces; the slide can then be read in 15 minutes and the results are multiplied by 50.

If schistosomiasis cannot be detected by faecal examination, the patient perforce has a very light and thus innocuous infection (the rare exception is central nervous system involvement). If diagnosis is deemed imperative, however, rectal biopsy is a highly efficient method both for *S. mansoni* and *S. japonicum* infection, and will often help detect *S. haematobium* eggs. Through a proctoscope, snips are taken from the valves of Houston (8 to 10 cm from the anus), pressed between glass slides, and examined immediately under a microscope. Sometimes only opaque dead eggs are observed, suggesting a burnt-out or successfully treated infection. Liver biopsy has been suggested as a means of diagnosis, but will only rarely detect an infection not revealed by the aforementioned methods.

For the diagnosis of schistosomiasis haematobia, urine is collected at mid-day, because a diurnal variation in egg output has been demonstrated. The urine specimen is centrifuged and the sediment examined. For quantitative data a 10 ml aliquot of urine collected between 1100 and 1300 hours is passed through a Nuclepore Filter (13 mm in diameter with a pore size of 10 μm) held in a PT-013 chamber. The filter is removed, placed face down on a microscope slide, examined immediately at × 40 magnification, and the terminal-spined eggs counted.

Immunodiagnosis via either skin or serological tests has suffered in the past from lack of sensitivity and specificity. This has been due largely to the use of crude antigens. Via immunochemistry, however, antigens are now being purified which give great promise for the future. MSA_1 (major serological antigen$_1$) from *S. mansoni* eggs, a glycoprotein of molecular weight 50 000 is now being used in a highly specific and sensitive radioimmunoassay. Antigens have also been isolated from *S. japonicum* eggs that look promising in an ELISA test.

For determining the severity of intestinal disease, sigmoidoscopy and barium enema are of value. The extent of liver disease may be estimated by liver biopsy, barium swallow, oesophagoscopy, and especially splenoportography with measurement of intrasplenic pressure. In schistosomiasis haematobia, cystoscopy and intravenous pyelography are useful techniques.

Treatment. Individual antischistosomal treatment should never be instituted without proof of infection by the demonstration of living eggs in excreta or biopsy specimens, except in the rare case of suspected schistosomiasis of the central nervous system. A positive serological or skin test does not provide a definitive diagnosis. With the more effective and less toxic drugs available today, cure of schistosomiasis is a reasonable goal for those in non-endemic areas. In endemic areas where reinfection may occur, complete cure is not necessary and indeed is not always desirable in schistosomiasis because disease is related to intensity of infection, surviving worms do not multiply, and immunity may be premunitive, i.e. dependent on the presence of living organisms. The recent use of quantitative egg counts has shown that in cases in which cure is not achieved by the full course of treatment with an established drug, egg output is usually reduced by over 90 per cent. Thus striving for cure by increasing the drug dosage or repeating the course of treatment is rarely necessary and, because of the toxicity of the antischistosomal drugs, may actually be harmful.

No specific treatment is available for swimmer's itch; although it has been claimed that antihistaminic ointment may be of some value. Treatment of Katayama fever is difficult, because none of the drugs now available for human use have any effect on the schistosomes during their early migratory phases in the body (the first three to six weeks). Steroids have been used to suppress the clinical manifestations during this stage of the infection.

For the chronic stages of schistosomiasis the three schistosome species vary considerably in their response to drugs, *S. haematobium* being the most susceptible and *S. japonicum* the most resistant. Furthermore, some of our better drugs will treat only one of these species while having little or no effect on the others. One drug is effective against two species and a few are effective against all

three. In recent years the armamentarium for schistosomiasis has been greatly improved by the addition of new drugs. Because of the different susceptibility of the organisms, however, this means the use of different drugs for the different parasites in different localities as shown in Table 1. Metrifonate is the drug of choice for treating *S. haematobium* infection. In endemic areas a single oral dose of 10 mg/kg has provided a cure rate of 22 per cent and a reduction in egg output of greater than 90 per cent. In non-endemic areas the standard regimen of 7.5 mg/kg given three times, two weeks apart has provided a cure rate of about 50 per cent and a reduction in egg output of greater than 90 per cent.

Table 1   Treatment of schistosomiasis*

	Dose	Route	Regimen
Schistosoma mansoni			
Americas and Caribbean			
oxamniquine	15 mg/kg	oral	single dose
Africa and environs			
hycanthone	1.5 mg/kg	intra-muscular	single dose
Schistosoma japonicum†			
praziquantel	20 mg/kg × 3	oral	administered in one day
Schistosoma haematobium			
Endemic area			
metrifonate	10 mg/kg	oral	single dose
Non-endemic area			
metrifonate	7.5 mg/kg × 3	oral	administered at 2-week intervals

* For the USA, antischistosomal drugs are available at the Parasitic Drug Service of the Center for Disease Control, Atlanta, Georgia, 30333. These include niridazole, astiban and metrifonate

† When available, praziquantel may well be the treatment of choice for all three species in patients in non-endemic areas. In endemic areas cost may be a significant factor

A geographic difference in susceptibility of *S. mansoni* in the Americas and Africa results in the following recommendations. For South America and the Caribbean, oxamniquine is given orally in a single dose of 15 mg/kg for adults, but children should receive 20 mg/kg divided into two equal doses of 10 mg/kg given on the same day. Because the African strains require two to four times higher dosages of oxamniquine than the American strains, hycanthone is recommended for Africa and environs in a single intramuscular dose of 1.5 mg/kg.

Schistosoma japonicum should be treated with a new drug praziquantel in an oral dose of 60 mg/kg divided into three equal doses of 20 mg/kg delivered at four hour intervals on the same day.

The only drugs available in the USA can be obtained from the Parasitic Drug Service of the Center for Disease Control, Atlanta, Georgia 30333. These drugs include metrifonate, niridazole, and astiban; instructions for use are provided.

In general, the surgical treatment of schistosomiasis should be approached with caution. Many of the apparently irreversible lesions of urinary tract schistosomiasis will resolve completely after antischistosomal treatment, particularly in young patients. Cerebral schistosomiasis japonica is frequently cured or markedly ameliorated by drug therapy. Finally, prophylactic portacaval shunts should never be performed in hepatosplenic schistosomiasis, because haematemesis is not invariable and is unpredictable in onset, and, when it occurs, mortality is low. If the creation of a shunt by surgery is necessitated by repeated bleeding episodes, splenorenal shunt, or other similar operations, are preferable to portacaval shunt because of a much lower incidence of chronic portal-systemic encephalopathy. Prior to shunting, however, antischistosomal therapy is necessary to prevent prolonged passage of eggs into the lungs which may lead to the development of cor pulmonale.

Prognosis. Many patients with schistosomiasis never have symptoms or signs of disease, or have only mild ones. Epidemiologically, both the infection and the disease reach their peak in early adult life and decline with age. Disregarding the factor of death among heavily infected patients, this may be due to decreased exposure to infection, gradual death of the worms, slow development of immunity, and diminution in the inflammatory response to the parasite and its products.

The early stages of hepatic or urinary tract disease appear to be reversible after antischistosomal therapy. Although late disease seems relatively irreversible, progression may be halted and gradual improvement may follow drug therapy. In hepatosplenic schistosomiasis the prognosis in patients suffering a haematemesis is far better than in those with cirrhosis, because the former do not tend to go into hepatic coma. Patients with cerebral schistosomiasis japonica may show remarkable improvement after antischistosome therapy.

Prevention and control. Prevention of infection by an individual entering an endemic area is based on the avoidance of contaminated fresh water. Both sea water and chlorinated swimming pools are safe. If fresh water must be entered, boots should be worn; if contaminated water reaches the skin, rapid drying or rubbing with alcohol will prevent infection. Storage of water for more than 24 hours will ensure the death of cercariae, as will the boiling of drinking water. Repellents are of no great value, and vaccines or prophylactic drugs are not available.

The three principal methods for the mass control of schistosomiasis are the provision of water supplies and sanitary facilities to break the man–snail exposure cycle, the use of molluscicides to kill the snails, and the use of chemotherapy to kill the schistosomes within the human host. Water supplies and sanitation are extremely costly and rarely can be justified for the control of schistosomiasis alone. Furthermore, it has been shown that it is necessary to bring the plumbing directly to each home, to have a good maintenance system, and to carry out a major health education campaign. Destruction of the snail is primarily based on the use of molluscicides such as the various copper salts, sodium pentachlorophenate, Bayluscide, and n-trityl-morpholone. Molluscicides, however, are quickly inactivated by sunlight and adsorption to mud and organic matter; they pass rapidly through running water or are diluted in vast bodies of still water, and they often destroy other aquatic fauna and flora. Also, although molluscicides may appear to be highly effective, they rarely kill all the snails; only a few survivors can repopulate an area in a matter of a few months. The snails that transmit *S. japonicum* are amphibious and are frequently found along the banks of water courses; their eradication can necessitate the use of earth-moving equipment and flame throwers. When the snails are 'buried' in this way, as in the campaigns in the People's Republic of China, it appears to reduce the infectivity of the environment.

Mass chemotherapy has been rendered feasible in recent years with the development of rapid quantitative field diagnostic methods, with the understanding that light infections usually do not require treatment and that a reasonable goal of treatment is to reduce heavy to light infections, and with the advent of new, less toxic, single dose, treatment regimens. It must also be appreciated that the rate of reinfection in terms of attaining worm burdens that may result in disease is so slow in most endemic areas that retreatment may be necessary at only three to five year intervals.

With respect to cost, water supplies and sanitation are by far most expensive with maintenance costs alone exceeding those on a per capita basis of the other measures. Chemotherapy is the least costly of the control measures.

Finally, the goal of control campaigns must be considered. Will there be an attempt at eradication, control of infection, or control of disease? Eradication will, of course, require the use of all three of the principal methods of control simultaneously. This will not only be extremely costly, but it is this author's belief that with the tools available today, it is impossible to achieve in most areas of the world. Control of disease by mass chemotherapy alone, directed toward the most susceptible segment of the population, the school children, using low, non-toxic drug doses to drastically lower worm burdens would be relatively inexpensive and has been shown to be efficacious.

References

Awad El Karim, M. A., Collins, K. S., Brotherhoood, J. R., Dore, C., Weiner, J. S., Sukkar, M. Y., Omer, A. H. S., and Amin, M. A. (1980). Quantitative egg excretion and work capacity in a Gezira population infected with *Schistosoma mansoni*. *Am. J. trop. Med. Hyg.* **29**, 54.

Cheever, A. W., Kamel, I. A., Elwi, A. M., Mosimann, J. E., and Donner, R. (1977). *Schistosoma mansoni* and *S. haematobium* infections in Egypt. II. Quantitative parasitological findings at necropsy. *Am. J. trop. Med. Hyg.* **26**, 702.

Hiatt, R. A., Sotomayor, Z. R., Sanchez, G., Zambrana, M., and Knight, W. R. (1979). Factors in the pathogenesis of acute schistosomiasis mansoni. *J. infect. Dis.* **139**, 659.

Jordan, P. (1977). Schistosomiasis—research to control. *Am. J. trop. Med. Hyg.* **26**, 877.

Lehman, J. S., Jr., Farid, Z., Smith, J. H., Bassily, S., and El-Masry, N. A. (1973). Urinary schistosomiasis in Egypt: clinical, radiological, bacteriological and parasitological correlations. *Trans. R. Soc. trop. Med. Hyg.* **67**, 384.

Siongok, T. K. A., Mahmoud, A. A. F., Ouma, J. H., Warren, K. S., Muller, A. S., Handa, A. K., and Houser, H. B. (1976). Morbidity in schistosomiasis mansoni in relation to intensity of infection: Study of a community in Machakos, Kenya. *Am. J. trop. Med. Hyg.* **25**, 273.

Warren, K. S. (1973). Regulation of the prevalence and intensity of schistosomiasis in man: Immunology or ecology? *J. infect. Dis.* **127**, 595.

— (1978). The pathology, pathobiology, and pathogenesis of schistosomiasis. *Nature, Lond.* **273**, 609.

—, Reboucas, G., and Baptista, A. G. (1965). Ammonia metabolism and hepatic coma in hepatosplenic schistosomiasis. Patients studied before and after portacaval shunt. *Ann. intern. Med.* **62**, 1113.

World Health Organization (1980). Epidemiology and control of schistosomiasis. Report of a WHO Expert Committee. *Wld Hlth Org. Tech. Rep. Ser.* no. 643.

Liver fluke diseases of man

N. Bhamarapravati, W. Thamavit, and A. Limsuwan

Taxonomy. Two major groups of liver flukes are found to infect humans and result in significant disease. The first is the *Opisthorchis* group, namely *O. felineus* and *O. viverrini*, which have cats as their definitive hosts and man as an accidental host. The second is the *Clonorchis* group. The genus *Opisthorchis* was established for the elongate distomes with small suckers, unbranched caeca, lateral vitellaria, and posterior lobed testes situated one behind the other. The genus *Clonorchis* was for larger flukes which have branched testes. Some authorities now classify these flukes in the one genus, *Opisthorchis*.

Geographical distribution and prevalence. *O. felineus* infection has been reported from Central and Eastern Europe, eastern USSR, India, Vietnam, Korea, Japan, and the Philippines. *O. viverrini* is the most important liver fluke infection of humans in northeast Thailand and Laos. The prevalence of the infection based on one survey of ova in the stool was as high as 87.7 per cent of the population. *C. sinensis* (*Opoisthorcis sinensis*) is found in humans in China, Korea, Japan, Taiwan, Hong Kong, and Vietnam, and rarely in Malaysia, Singapore, Thailand, and perhaps in other countries to which the Chinese have migrated. The prevalence of this fluke varies, according to the community, up to 34 per cent in some reports from Taiwan. Forty per cent of livers in autopsy material from Hong Kong were reported to show gross and microscopic evidence of liver fluke infection. Some authors consider man to be the definitive host of *C. sinensis*.

Life cycle. Adult liver flukes usually inhabit the intrahepatic bile passages and gall bladder and occasionally the pancreatic ducts. Detailed description of the adult flukes of both genera can be found in any standard textbook of parasitology (Fig. 1). The mature eggs are ovoidal, measuring 26–30 μm by 15–17 μm for *Clonorchis*; while those of *Opisthorchis* are slightly smaller. There is a cap or operculum at one end. The wall of the egg is about 5 μm in thickness and is usually yellowish brown in colour. After the fully embryonated eggs have been passed with the faeces, they remain unhatched until they are ingested by snails (important species are *Bulimus* and *Parafossarulus* for *Clonorchis*; and *Bithynia* for *Opisthorchis*). The miracidia, which are ciliated, emerge from the ova in the snail's digestive tract, and change into sporocysts in the snail's perirectal and the peri-oesophageal spaces. The sporocysts change into sac-like structures which later evolve into cercariae. These cercariae leave the snails and swim freely in the water until they find the second intermediate hosts, of which cyprinid fish are the most common. They penetrate the skin of the fish, leaving their tails outside and finally encyst in the muscles and develop into metacercariae. The metacercarial cysts are about 0.1–0.2 nm in diameter and contain moving larvae. The cycle of the liver fluke is completed when man or another definitive host eats the raw flesh of fish containing metacercariae. The metacercariae excyst in the duodenum and are attracted towards the ampulla of Vater by some obscure mechanism (possibly pH), and then migrate upward into the liver. Within one week after the infection the metacercariae develop into juvenile flukes with rudimentary reproductive systems. These change into adult flukes with mature reproductive systems. The adults begin to lay eggs around four weeks after the infection.

Pathology. Liver flukes can live for a long time in the host: the pathological changes result both from cumulative effects of host parasite interaction and from some secondary effects such as malnutrition and bacterial infection. Very few studies have been made to define factors such as the number of infecting parasites, chronicity, effects of vitamin A, or protein deficiency which may affect the severity of the lesions, and which only become apparent when the individuals come to the autopsy table after a long period of liver fluke infection. At this time, the livers infected with liver flukes show an increase in weight, and cut with varying resistance depending on the degree of peribiliary fibrosis or biliary cirrhosis. The bile ducts are dilated, sometimes to cystic proportions. Studies using transcutaneous cholangiography have shown that the dilatation of the bile duct in opisthorchiasis can be mulberry-like, saccular, cystic, or a combination of these. Thousands of parasites along with muddy bile may be expressed from the lumen of these ducts which have thickened walls due to peribiliary fibrosis. The gall bladder, common bile ducts, and cystic ducts may also show dilatation and thickening of their walls. Microscopic examination shows areas of hyperplasia of biliary mucosa with occasional areas of atrophy. There is an increase in the number of goblet cells suggesting mucinous metaplasia. Glandular formation is prominent in many places. There is acute or chronic inflammatory reaction around the bile ducts with varying degrees of fibrosis. Thickening of the walls of the vessels, especially portal veins, can be seen. Rarely granulomata can also be observed in biopsies but these are even less frequent in autopsy material. Complications of liver fluke infection include cholangitis and abscess formation. Biliary calculi have been reported to be frequent in clonorchiasis but very rare in opisthochiasis.

One important finding, that has been reported in several series of autopsy cases with liver fluke infection, is associated bile duct carcinoma. This has been found in both clonorchiasis and opisthorchiasis. The livers of patients who have bile duct carcinoma usually show a large single mass of tumour in non-cirrhotic livers but with manifestations of liver fluke infection such as dilated bile ducts with thickened walls, cystic gall bladders, and the presence of adult flukes in the bile.

Pathogenesis. In his classical study of the pathology of clonorchiasis, Hou maintained that flukes produced lesions in the bile duct either by mechanical or chemical effects or both. We have added a third factor, based on recent experiments; an immunopathological mechanism. Liver flukes cause loss and atrophy of biliary epithelial cells leading to increase in cellular division hyperplasia and mucinous metaplasia. Provided the bile duct mucosa is intact the fluke and the host's bile duct coexist without harm to one another, but if the bile duct become ulcerated a cellular reaction develops, involving macrophages and lymphocytes, and the flukes are killed. The reaction, which becomes granulomatous, destroys the wall of the bile duct, and extends into the peribiliary tissue, can be considered immunopathological in nature. Granulomata, observed in the hamster model, are of at least three kinds: non-specific, or directed against adult flukes or against ova or their contents. Fluke antigens can apparently pass through the bile duct wall to sensitize the host's humoral immune system, for immunoglobulin deposits around the fluke, the ova, and occasionally the embryos have been demonstrated. While the walls of ova appear to be impermeable, unlike those of schistosomes, we have seen immunoglobulins passing through the operculum into the ovum. In the hamster model, large amounts of immune complex can be found in the glomeruli.

Clinical features. Liver fluke infection is usually symptomless and is recognized only when ova are found in the stools. The symptoms and signs merge with those of other liver diseases common in the same geographical areas where liver fluke exists, and may be related to the number of adult flukes in the liver. The nature of the infection, in which patients eat relatively small numbers of metacercariae periodically, makes the definition of the clinical syndrome difficult. When a large number of flukes is ingested, three clinical stages are recognizable. Early manifestations consist of fever, eosinophilia, leucocytosis, and epigastric discomfort or pain. These features must be distinguished from those of other parasitic infections, visceral larval migrans, and hepatic amoebiasis. A more advanced stage is characterized by diarrhoea, progressive hepatomegaly, anorexia, prolonged low-grade fever, episodes of jaundice, and hepatic tenderness. Jaundice is more likely to be associated with biliary obstruction due to biliary 'sand', which consists of muddy concretions of flukes, mucin, and bile. The most advanced cases are said to develop ascites, cachexia, and acute or chronic pancreatitis, with further enlargement of the liver. Clearly, some of this group may have malignancy of the bile duct. Suppurative cholangitis can be an important complication. A thorough clinical study of liver fluke disease is still needed. The disease is recognized when the clinician elicits a history of eating raw fresh water fish from a patient in or from the endemic areas for this infection. This information together with the protean liver manifestations may provide clues leading to further investigation of the patient.

Diagnosis. Specific diagnosis can be made only by identifying ova in a well prepared, concentrated specimen of stool. Ova can sometimes be recognized in needle biopsies of the liver. Immunological diagnosis based on the detection of precipitating antibody has been described by some authors, but the methods have not been standardized and are not generally available. A pre-beta globulin pattern on serum protein electrophoresis is said to be related to fluke infection, but its diagnostic value is uncertain. In a large group of individuals in the northeast of Thailand, no differences in biochemical profile were found between those with and without liver fluke ova in their stools. Abnormalities were noted in both groups implicating local environmental, toxic or infective factors exerting damaging effects on the liver of the whole population.

At the clinical level, the assessment of bile duct pathology can be made by percutaneous cholangiography, percutaneous needle biopsy, or surgical biopsy of the liver after exploratory laparotomy.

Treatment. Several drugs, such as dithiazanine iodide, chloroquine phosphate, hexachlorparaxylol, Hetol (1,4-bis-trichloro-methylbenzol), and bithionol have been tried and claimed to be effective, at times, against liver flukes; but it is generally agreed that until recently, there was no good drug against the parasite which was safe enough to use. Praziquantel, which was originally intended for the treatment of schistosomiasis, has, however, proved effective with relatively few side-effects. The drug can be used in a dose of 25 mg/kg bodyweight for either one or two days.

References

Bhamarapravati, N. and Thamavit, W. (1978). Animal studies on liver fluke infestation, dimethylnitrosamine, and bile duct carcinoma. *Lancet* i, 206.

—, —, and Vajrasthira, S. (1978). Liver changes in hamster infected with a liver fluke of man *Opisthorchis viverrini. Am. J. trop. Med. Hyg.* **27**, 787.

Bunnag, D. and Harinasuta, T. (1980). Studies on the chemotherapy of human opisthorchiasis in Thailand. I. Clinical trial of praziquantel. *S.E. Asian J. trop. Med. publ. Hlth* **11**, 528.

—, — (1981). Studies on the chemotherapy of human opisthorchiasis. III. Minimum effective dose of praziquantel. *S. E. Asian J. trop. Med. publ. Hlth.* **12**, 413.

Gibson, J. B. and Sun, T. (1971). Clonorchiasis, In *Pathology of protozoal and helminthic diseases with clinical correlation* (ed. R. A. Marcial-Rojas), 546. Williams and Wilkins, Baltimore.

Hou, P. C. (1955). The pathology of *Clonorchis sinensis* infestation of the liver. *J. path. Bact.* **70**, 53.

Komiya, Y. (1966). Clonorchis and clonorchiasis. In *Advances in parasitology*, vol. 4 (ed. B. Dawes), 53. Academic Press, New York.

Markell, E. K. and Voge, M. (1981). *Medical parasitology*, 5th edn., 140. W. B. Saunders, Philadelphia.

Sadun, E. H. (1955). Studies on *Opisthorchis viverrini* in Thailand. *Am. J. Hyg.* **62**, 81.

Strauss, W. G. (1962). Clinical manifestations of clonorchiasis. A controlled study of 105 cases. *Am. J. trop. Med. Hyg.* **11**, 625.

Thamavit, W., Bhamarapravati, N., Sahaphong, S., Vajrasthira, S. and Angsubhakorn, S. (1978). Effects of dimethylnitrosamine on induction of cholangiocarcinoma in *Opisthorchis viverrini* infected Syrian golden hamsters. *Cancer Res.* **38**, 4634.

Viranuvatti, V. and Stitnimakarn, T. (1972). Liver fluke infection and infestation in South East Asia. In *Progress in liver diseases*, vol. 4. (eds. H. Popper and F. Schaffner), 537. Grune and Stratton, New York.

Other liver flukes

See also opisthorchiasis and chlonorchiasis.

Fascioliasis

Life cycle. Adult flukes of *Fasciola hepatica* are up to 3 cm long. They live in the biliary tract of domestic sheep, cattle, lagomorphs, other herbivores, and men. *F. gigantica* flukes are up to 7.5 cm long and are found in cattle, water buffalo, and man. Ova are discharged with the faeces and remain viable for up to nine months in moist conditions. They hatch in water releasing miracidia which invade amphibious snails of the family *Limnaeidae*, in which they pass through phases of mother sporocyst, rediae, and daughter rediae during the next 30 days. Cercariae leave the snail and encyst as metacercariae on water plants such as watercress which are eaten by the definitive host. Metacercariae develop into larvae in the gut and burrow through the gut wall producing necrotic foci and microabscesses. They cross the peritoneal cavity, penetrate Glisson's capsule, and enter the liver where they mature and live for several years. The ova are large (130 × 150 μm) yellowish and operculated.

Epidemiology. *F. hepatica*, the sheep liver fluke and cause of sheep liver rot, is worldwide in distribution being most prevalent where sheep are grazed on water-logged lowland pastures. Human infections are most common where salad is a popular dish; in Europe (the United Kingdom, France, Germany, Russia), the Caribbean (Cuba), and South America (Chile, Uruguay, Argentina). In the United Kingdom, outbreaks seem to follow wet summers. Six cases were reported in Ringwood, Hampshire in 1960, and 44 in Chepstow, Monmouthshire in 1969, following consumption of raw watercress. Human infection with *F. giganica* has been reported from Hawaii, Asia, and Africa.

Pathogenesis. The presence of flukes in the bile ducts excites hyperplasia and necrosis of the epithelium, distension thickening and tortuosity of the ducts with proliferation of minor ducts, pericholangitic exudate (neutrophils and eosinophils) and cholecystitis, and periportal fibrosis with compression of liver parenchyma. These changes rarely occur except in heavy infections and there is no evidence that cirrhosis and portal hypertension can result. Malignant change has not been reported. Migration of larval flukes through the parenchyma leads to some necrosis, fibrosis, and inflammatory reaction. Rarely a fluke may block the common bile duct. Larval flukes may migrate to other parts of the body including brain, orbit, lung, bladder, and subcutaneous tissues.

The acute nasopharyngitis, known as halzoun in Lebanon or marrara in Sudan, may be an allergic response to larval flukes eaten in raw sheep or goat liver. It can also be caused by the pentastome *Linguatula serrata* (see page 5.468), by the catfish fluke *Isoparorchis hypselobagri*, and by leeches such as *Limnatis nilotica* and *Dinobdella ferox* (see page 6.47).

Clinical features. Intermittent fever with night sweats, dyspepsia, vomiting, diarrhoea, malaise, myalgia, weight loss, right subcostal pain, mild jaundice, tender hepatomegaly, cough, and urticaria have been described. Migratory subcutaneous nodules, which are tender and itchy, may occur.

Diagnosis. The characteristic ova (similar to those of *Fasciolopsis buski*) may be scanty in the stool but can usually be found in aspirate from the duodenum or bile duct. Ova may be found in the stools of uninfected patients who have eaten raw infected sheep liver. Blood leucocytosis with eosinophilia, and elevated ESR are usually found. 'Liver function tests' are nearly always abnormal.

Intradermal and complement fixation tests have been used. Liver biopsies show marked eosinophil infiltration.

Differential diagnoses include infection by other biliary flukes, cholangitis, cholecystitis, amoebic liver abscess, and right lower lobe pneumonia or pleurisy. The presence of eosinophilia may suggest hydatid disease or Hodgkin's disease. Differential diagnoses of obstruction of the common bile duct include gallstone, carcinoma of the duct or head of the pancreas, hydatid, or nematodes such as *Ascaris*.

Treatment. Bithionol is effective, given as in paragonimiasis. Praziquantel, emetine hydrochloride (adults 30 mg by intramuscular injection daily for 18 days) and chloroquine (children 5 mg per kg/day by mouth for three weeks) have also been used successfully.

Prevention. Sheep pastures should be drained and treated with molluscicides such as copper sulphate and Frescon (Shell) to eliminate the snail hosts. Watercress that is to be eaten raw should not be grown near sheep or cattle pastures.

References

Biggart, J. H. (1937). Human infestation with *Fasciola hepatica. J. Path. Bact.* **44**, 488.

Facey, R. V. and Marsden, P. D. (1960).Fascioliasis in man: an outbreak in Hampshire. *Br. Med. J.* **ii**, 619.

Hardman, E. W., Jones, R. L. H., and Davies, A. H. (1970). Fascioliasis—a large outbreak. *Br. med. J.* **iii**, 502.

Janssens, P. G., Fain, A., Limbos, P., De Muynck, A., Biemans, R., Van Meirvenne, N. and De Mulder, P. (1968). Trois cas de distomatose hepatique à Fasciola gigantica contractés en Afrique centrale. *Ann. Soc. Belg. Méd. trop.* **48**, 631.

Neghume, A. and Ossandan, M. (1943). Ectopic and hepatic fascioliasis. *Am. J. trop. Med.* **23**, 545.

Pantelouris, E. M. (1964). *The common liver fluke.* Pergamon Press, Oxford.

Dicrocoellasis. Adult flukes of *Dicrocoelium dentriticum* are about 1 cm long. They live in the biliary tract of sheep, goats, and other domesticated and wild herbivores, and have been found rarely in man in Europe, Egypt, Iran, Nigeria, Ivory Coast, and China. Unlike other trematodes their ova passed in the faeces do not need water but are eaten by land snails such as those of the genus *Hellicella*. In wet weather masses of cercariae are discharged from the snail's respiratory apparatus in slime balls which are eaten by the second intermediate host, ants such as *Formica fusca* and *F. rufibarbis*. Mammalian definitive hosts acquire metacercariae by eating ants. Up to 200 metacercariae may be found in one ant.

The effects of *D. dendriticum* on the liver are similar to those of *F. hepatica*: there is fibrous thickening of the portal tracts. *Diagnosis* is confirmed by finding the small thick-shelled, embryonated ova (approximately 40×30 μm) in faeces or duodenal or biliary aspirate. People who eat raw infected sheep or goat liver may pass ova in their stools without being infected. Symptoms are usually mild and the same as in fascioliasis, but progressive obstructive jaundice has been reported. Treatment has not been adequately studied. By analogy with fascioliasis and *D. lanceolatum* infection in animals; bithionol, hexachloroparaxylene (Hetol), and thiabendazole might prove effective.

References

Mandoul, R., Demartial, L., Pestre, M., and Moulinier, C. (1966). La distomatose hepato-biliare à petit douve. (A propos d'un nouveau cas.) *J. Med. Bordeaux* **143**, 685.

Roche, P. J. L. (1948). Human dicrocoeliasis in Nigeria. *Trans. R. Soc. trop. Med. Hyg.* **41**, 819.

Other hermaphrodite flukes parasitic in man

D. A. Warrell

Apart from the genera *Clonorchis* and *Opisthorchis* dealt with above, the following species of flukes are parasitic, in their adult stage, in the biliary tract: *Fasciola hepatica*, *F. gigantica*, and *Dicrocoelium dendriticum*. Intestinal species include *Fasciolopsis buski*, *Heterophyes heterophyes*, *Metagonimus yokagawai*, *Echinostoma ilocanum*, *Echinochasmus perfoliatus*, and *Plagiorchis javanensis*. Adults of the species of the genus *Paragonimus* and *Achillurbainia nouveli* inhabit the lungs and other sites.

The adult flukes are oval or leaf-shaped, range in length from 2 to 75 mm when laid flat, and are hermaphrodites. Sexual reproduction at the adult stage and asexual multiplication in the snail intermediate host is typical of these digenetic flukes.

Lung flukes

Paragonimiasis

Life cycle. The definitive hosts of flukes of the genus *Paragonimus* are wild carnivores (including large felines such as tigers and leopards, viverrids, and mustelids), domestic pigs, dogs, cats, and men. Adult flukes live in the lungs: ova discharged into the airways are coughed out or swallowed and passed in the faeces. If the ova reach water, they develop after about three weeks into miracidia which invade the heads of various species of fresh water snail, the first intermediate hosts. They undergo asexual division (mother sporocyst, rediae, daughter rediae) in the snail and after about three months cercariae emerge which invade the gills or joints of fresh water crabs, crayfish, and shrimps, the second intermediate hosts, and encyst as metacercariae until the host is eaten by a mammal. Larval flukes develop in the small bowel and migrate to the lungs by crossing the peritoneal cavity, diaphragm, and pleural cavity.

Adult flukes are 1–2 cm long. They are oval, brownish, and translucent (Fig. 1a). 43 species have been described, of which 10 are known to infect man. Species are distinguished by the arrangement of cuticular spines, the shape of the ovary, the relative size of the oral and ventral suckers, and the characteristics of the ova. Bisexual and hermaphroditic (parthenogenetic) forms are known.

Epidemiology. There are three main endemic areas for paragoni-

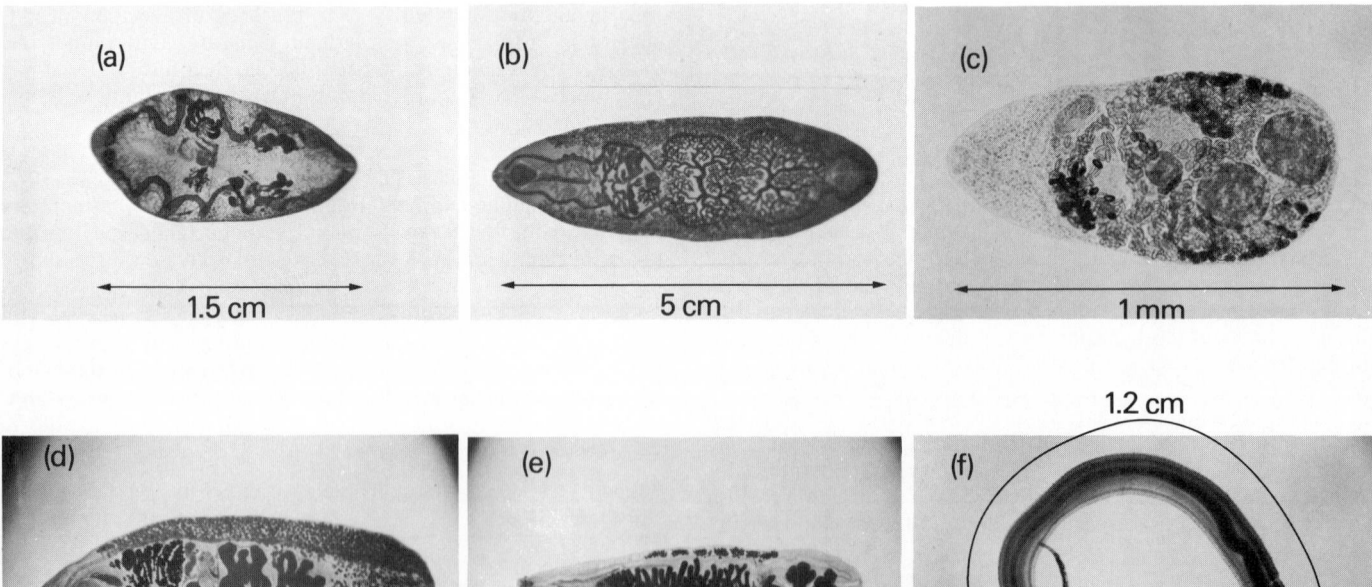

Fig. 1 Adult flukes of (a) *Paragonimus heterotremus*; (b) *Fasciolopsis buski*; (c) *Metagonimus yokogawai*; (d) *Echinostoma malayanum*; (e) *Opisthorchis viverrini*; and (f) *Schistosoma haematobium*. (By courtesy of Mr Prayong Radomyos, Bangkok.)

miasis. In Asia the infection is particularly prevalent in Korea, China, and Taiwan, and also occurs in India, Sri Lanka, Malaysia, Indonesia, Papua New Guinea, Thailand, Laos, Vietnam, Philippines, and Japan. The principal species are *P. westermani* (named after a director of Amsterdam Zoo, in whose Bengal tigers it was first detected by Kerbert in 1878), *P. (szechuanensis) skjabini*, and *P. heterotremus*. In Africa paragonimiasis is endemic in eastern Nigeria, Cameroons, Benin, The Gambia, Zaire, and elsewhere. *P. uterobilateralis* (Nigeria) *P. africanus* (Cameroons), and *Poikilorchis congolensis* (Zaire) have been identified. In Central and South America the affected countries include Mexico, Costa Rica, Guatemala, Peru, Colombia, Paraguay, Ecuador, and Venezuela: species include *P. mexicanus*, *P. peruvianus*, and *P. caliensis*.

Various species of fresh water snails can act as first intermediate hosts, notably *Semisulcospira (Melania) libertina*, and the crustacean second intermediate hosts are fresh water crabs (e.g. *Eriocheis* and *Potamon* species) and crayfish (*Cambarus*, *Cambaroides*, and *Procambarus* species). Infection is acquired by eating raw or inadequately cooked crustaceans, by contamination of other food by utensils used to cut them up, and by the use of their raw juices as medicines for fever, measles, diarrhoea, and other illnesses in Korea, Japan, and elsewhere. Death of infected crustaceans may release metacercariae into sources of drinking water. Ingestion of these cysts may also lead to infection.

In some paratenic mammalian hosts such as rat, mouse, pig, and wild boar, the larval fluke cannot mature but remains in the larval stage in muscles. In southern Kyushu, Japan, humans have been infected by eating these larvae in uncooked meat of the wild boar.

The prevalence of paragonimiasis, as assessed by intradermal testing with fluke extract, ranged from 0.3 to 78.0 per cent in different parts of South Korea. In areas around the Cross and Imo Rivers in eastern Nigeria the prevalence was between 5 and 10 per cent in people under the age of 40 years. There was an epidemic increase in the incidence of paragonimiasis in eastern Nigeria during the Nigerian civil war, when shortage of protein forced people to eat fresh water crustaceans. In parts of Peru the prevalence of skin test reactions to *P. peruvianus* antigen was 15 per cent.

Pathogenesis. Larval flukes, which develop from encysted metacercariae ingested in the muscle or viscera of crustaceans, create a necrotic haemorrhagic and eventually fibrotic track through the tissues, during their migration to the lung and elsewhere. In the lung, the fluke settles a few centimetres deep to the pleural surface and initially causes local necrosis and haemorrhage of the gas-exchanging tissue followed by inflammatory exudate and fibrous encapsulation. Ova excite a granulomatous reaction. Flukes may move about producing transient shifting radiographic opacities. One or two flukes occupy a capsule which eventually ruptures into the bronchial tree allowing discharge of ova, together with blood and brownish necrotic material which is coughed up in the sputum. Granulomatous inflammatory reaction and secondary infection with abscess formation are common. The lung is assumed to be the ideal habitat for the fluke, but they may end up in almost any tissue. Flukes can migrate from the lungs, through jugular and carotid foramina at the base of the skull, to reach the temporal and occipital lobes of the brain where they cause necrosis and an eosinophilic granulomatous reaction. The fluke dies within two years and becomes calcified or perhaps returns to the lung. The spinal cord may be invaded through an intervertebral disc. Flukes produce cysts and abscesses in the gut wall and other abdominal viscera: ova may be discharged into the lumen of the gut. Other reported sites for adult flukes are the psoas and other muscles, testis, scrotum, spermatic cord, and uterine and vaginal wall. Migratory subcutaneous swellings are particularly common with *P. skjabini* infection in China. Fibrous and inflammatory adhesions of peritoneal and pleural cavities and subarachnoid space may be extensive. Ova have been found at the centres of small eosinophilic granulomata in a variety of organs and tissues including liver, pericardium, and meninges.

Cinical features.   *Pulmonary paragonimiasis*. The average incubation period between eating the infected crustacean and the first respiratory symptom is about six months (range one to 27 months). Chronic cough is productive of rusty, mucopurulent sputum or there is frank haemoptysis. Sputum is usually produced on waking or after exertion. Episodic pleuritic pain is common. About half the patients complain of breathlessness on exertion and some notice wheezing. Physical signs are not usually impressive. There may be mild fever. Digital clubbing is reported. Rales may be audible and occasionally there is evidence of pleural effusion, pleural thickening, or consolidation. Empyema and haemothorax are uncommon. Secondary bronchopneumonia and lung abscess may develop and pulmonary tuberculosis may coexist. Milder symptoms have been observed in patients in the Heilongjiang province of China, attributed to a particular species, *P. westermani ichunensis*.

Chest radiographs are normal, at some stage, in up to one fifth of proven cases. The early lesions are ill-defined migratory opacities (Fig. 2). Later changes include multilocular cavities, cysts or ring shadows without fluid levels, abscess cavities, fibrosis, calcified foci, pleural thickening, and effusions.

Cerebral and spinal paragonimiasis. Cerebral lesions occur in less than 1 per cent of patients with paragonimiasis in the community, but in 25 per cent or more of hospitalized cases in parts of Asia. They are particularly common in South Korea where 7500 cases of cerebral paragonimiasis were said to exist in 1966, and where this disease is the commonest cause of cerebral tumour. The disease progresses from an early meningitic phase characterized by inflammatory reaction, through a necrotic granulomatous phase with tumour formation, to the late stage of calcification when the patient has epilepsy, dementia, or hemiplegia.

Symptoms include fits which are sometimes Jacksonian, headache, visual disturbances, vomiting, nausea, and hemihypoaesthesia. Homonymous hemianopia, decreased visual acuity, optic atrophy, facial palsy, hemiplegia, and paraplegia are common findings. Plain skull radiographs show signs of raised intracranial pressure or cerebral calcification. The cysts can be demonstrated by computerized axial tomography, air encephalography, or angiography. Blockage of the subarachnoid space or interventricular foramina may be found. Spinal paragonimiasis is rare. It may cause transverse myelitis.

Abdominal paragonimiasis. Features include abdominal pain and tenderness, bloody diarrhoea, nausea, vomiting, and palpable nodules.

Subcutaneous paragonimiasis. Migratory, subcutaneous nodules occur in 20–60 per cent of patients with *P. skjabini*, and 10 per cent with *P. westermani* infection. They are up to 6 cm in diameter, firm, slightly mobile and tender, and often give rise to mild pain or irritation. The commonest sites are lower abdomen, inguinal region and thigh. Cysts may also occur behind the ear in the orbit and elsewhere in the head. In West and Central Africa and China the flukes *Poikilorchis congolensis* and *Achillurbainia nouveli* have been discovered in retro-auricular subcutaneous cysts.

Diagnosis. The characteristic brown operculated ova ($80 \times 50\,\mu m$) may be found in sputum, stool, pleural fluid, and cerebrospinal fluid. Very rarely adult flukes may be coughed up, or discovered in excised subcutaneous nodules or other surgical specimens.

There may be a blood leucocytosis with eosinophilia. Eosinophils may also be found in cerebrospinal fluid and pleural aspirate. Intradermal tests have been used epidemiologically, but their specificity is insufficient for diagnosis and they remain positive for years after cure. Complement fixation and other serological tests have proved useful. Countercurrent immunoelectrophoresis is probably the most satisfactory. Most treated cases become seronegative after about six months.

Differential diagnoses of pulmonary paragonimiasis include tuberculosis (which may coexist in some cases), lung abscess, chronic pulmonary infection of other causes, and bronchial or secondary carcinoma.

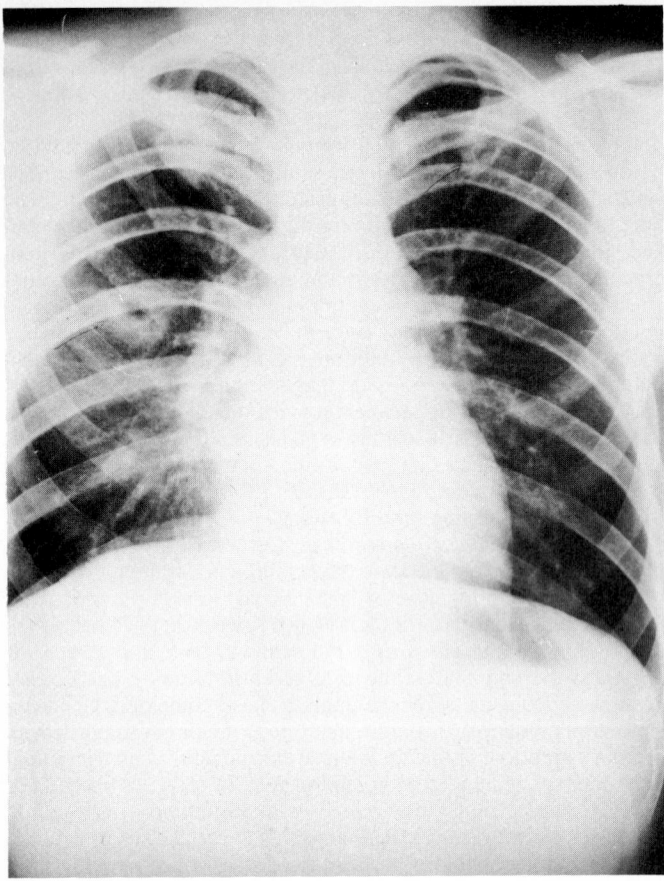

(a)

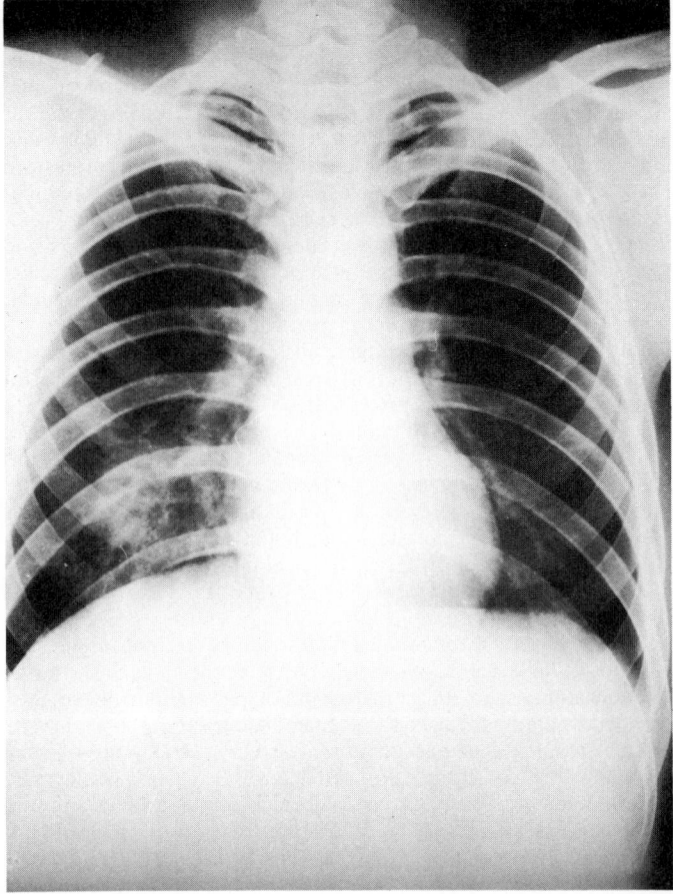

(b)

Fig. 2 Chest radiographs of patients with proven paragonimiasis: (a) nodular and ring shadows; (b) poorly defined opacity with multiple cavities; and (c) Chronic paragoniamiasis. Calcification (C), multilocular cyst (M), fibrosis (F), pneumonic infiltration (I), cavity and connected nodular lesion (N) and abscess cavity (A). (By courtesy of Dr Sirivan Vanijanonta, Bang-kok.)

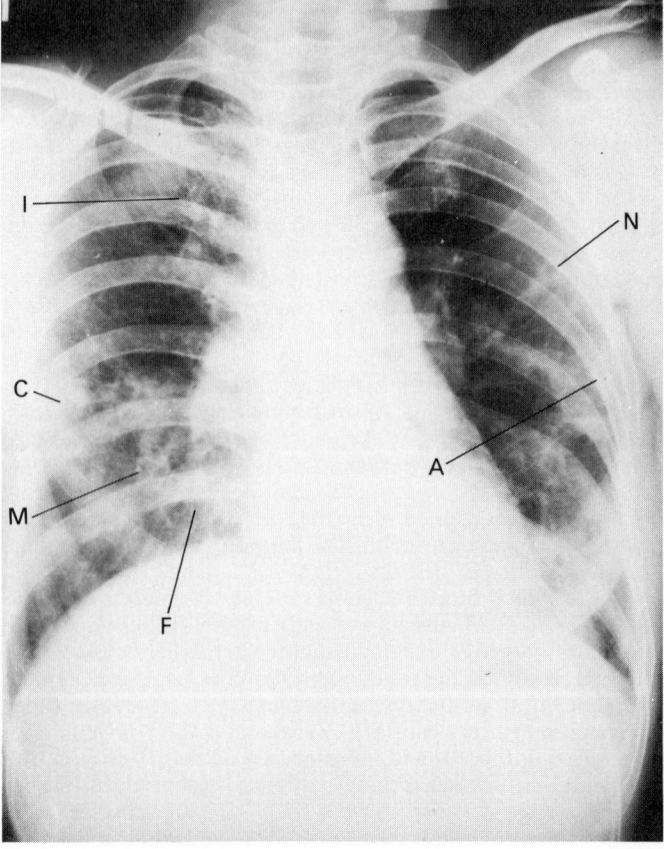

(c)

Cerebral and spinal paragonimiasis must be distinguished from abscess, other granulomata such as tuberculoma, other helminth infections of the CNS including fascioliasis, *Schistosoma japoni-cum*, cysticercosis, and hydatid disease. Eosinophilic meningitis may result from angiostrongyliasis and gnathostomiasis. The differential diagnosis of epilepsy includes cerebral malaria, tumour, encephalitis and cysticercosis.

Abdominal symptoms could be mistaken for diarrhoea of other causes (amoebiasis, shigellosis), and other causes of peritonism and acute abdomen (appendicitis, strangulated hernia, and ectopic pregnancy). Subcutaneous paragonimiasis may be confused with gnathostomiasis, sparganosis, and even ochocerciasis.

Treatment. Three drugs are recommended. *Bithionol* (Bitin, Actamer) is 2,2'-thiobis (4,6-dichlorophenol). It is the drug of choice, but is not available in some countries, e.g. Thailand. A dose of 30–50 mg/kg, given by mouth on alternate days for 10–15 doses, has cured 80–100 per cent of cases of pulmonary paragonimiasis in Asia and Africa. Cure is indicated by disappearance of symptoms, radiographic lesions, and ova, from sputum and faeces. Serological tests become negative over six months. Repeated courses may be required for cerebral and subcutaneous paragonimiasis. Bithionol is dramatically effective in the early meningitic stage of cerebral paragonimiasis and is also useful in the granulomatous tumour stage but not for the chronic calcified stage. Side-effects include nausea, vomiting, abdominal pain, diarrhoea, urticaria, and rare hepatic, renal, and cardiovascular toxicity.

Niclofolan or menichlopholan (Bayer 9015, Bilevon) is 2,2'-

dihydroxy-3,3'-dinitro-5,5'-dichlorodiphenyl. A single dose of 2 mg/kg by mouth proved 73–90 per cent effective in Nigeria and Korea. Side-effects include sweating, joint and body pains, and morbilliform rash. Higher doses can produce severe toxicity.

Praziquantel (Embay 8440) has proved effective in human pulmonary paragonimiasis in South Korea and Thailand. A dose of 25 mg/kg is given three times a day by mouth. Cure rate increases from about 70 to 100 per cent as the course is increased from one to three days. There are few side-effects.

Surgery is indicated for granulomatous tumours in the central nervous system and subcutaneous nodules.

Prognosis. Pulmonary paragonimiasis is rarely fatal: even without treatment flukes die or disappear within 10 years. Cerebral paragonimiasis carries a 5 per cent mortality: most deaths occur during the first two years, but there is chronic morbidity from epilepsy, dementia, and other neurological sequelae.

Prevention. Paragonimiasis could be completely prevented if fresh water crabs and crayfish and their juices were thoroughly cooked before being eaten. Unfortunately lightly-cooked, raw, pickled, and marinated crustaceans are regarded as delicacies in many Asian countries, and their raw juices are believed to have medicinal properties.

References

Chen-kang, L. and Tao-nien, L. (1963). The pathologic anatomy of paragonimiasis. *Chinese Med. J.* **82**, 650.
Chung, H.-L., Hsu, C.-P., and Kao, P.-C. (1978). Preliminary studies on paragonimiasis in Ichun, Hokiang and Mutankiang areas of Heilungkiang Province with observations on a new subspecies of *Paragonimus westermani—Paragonimus westermani ichunensis. Chinese Med. J.* New series **4**, 349.
Hung-Tien, C., Chi-Wu, W., Chich-Fei, Y., Chi-Fa, H., and Jung-Ch'üan, F. (1958). Paragonimiasis. A clinical study of 200 adult cases. *Chinese Med. J.* **77**, 3.
Kim, J. S. (1970). Treatment of *Paragonimus westermani* infections with bithionol. *Am. J. trop. Med. Hyg.* **19**, 940.
Miyazaki, I. (1974). Lung flukes in the world. Morphology and life history. In *A symposium on the epidemiology of parasitic diseases*, 101. International Medical Foundation of Japan, Tokyo.
— and Nishimura, K. (1975). Cerebral paragonimiasis. In *Topics in tropical neurology* (ed. R. W. Hornabrook), 109. F. A. Davis, Philadelphia.
Nozais, J. P., Doucet, J., Dunan, J., and Assale N'Dri, G. (1980). Les paragonimoses en Afrique Noire. A propos d'un foyer recent de Côte-d'Ivoire. *Bull. Soc. Path. exot.* **73**, 155.
Nwokolo, C. (1972). Epidemic paragonimiasis in eastern Nigeria. Clinical features and epidemiology of the recent outbreak following the Nigerian civil war. *Trop. geograph. Med.* **24**, 138.
— and Volkmer, K. J. (1977). Single dose therapy of paragonimiasis with menichlopholan. *Am. J. trop. Med. Hyg.* **26**, 688.
Oh, S. J. (1978). Paragonimiasis in the central nervous system. In *Handbook of clinical neurology*, vol 35 (eds. P. J. Vinken and G. W. Bruyn), 243. North Holland, Amsterdam.
Sadun, E. H. and Buck, A. A. (1960). Paragonimiasis in South Korea—immunodiagnostic, epidemiologic, clinical, roentgenologic and therapeutic studies. *Am. J. trop. Med Hyg.* **9**, 562.
Yokogawa, M. (1969). Paragonimus and paragonimiasis. *Adv. Parasit.* **7**, 375.

Intestinal flukes

Fasciolopsiasis. *Fasciolopsis buski* is a very large fluke (about 2–7.5 cm long) (Fig. 1b) which lives in the duodenum and jejunum, and sometimes the pylorus or colon of pigs, men and, less commonly, domestic dogs or lagomorphs. Large numbers of variable-sized, usually 130×80 μm, ova are passed in the faeces, perhaps 25 000 per fluke per day. Those dropped into water hatch, releasing miracidia after three to seven weeks. Miracidia invade aquatic snails; in which they become sporocysts, rediae, and daughter rediae; and 30–50 days later cercariae emerge and encyst on aquatic plants. The metacercariae can survive for more than a year under moist conditions. When eaten by the mammalian definitive host, they develop into larval flukes which attach to the gut wall and mature in a few months.

Epidemiology. Fasciolopsiasis is a most prevalent infection in eastern Asia. 10 million people are thought to be infected in the Far East. The disease has been reported from central and southern China, eastern India, Bangladesh, Burma, Malaysia, Thailand, Laos, Kampuchea, Vietnam, Indonesia, Taiwan, and Europe. The prevalence is about 5 per cent in China and up to 50 per cent in parts of Assam.

Snail hosts are members of the genera *Segmentina*, *Hippeutis*, *Gyraulus*, and *Planorbis*. The most potent sources of human infection are artificial ponds in which edible water plants such as red water caltrop (*Trapa natans*), water chestnut (*Eliocharis tuberosa*), and watercress are cultivated. The ponds are fertilized with human and pig faeces. Other commonly infected plants are lotus, water hyacinth, and water bamboo. The stems, bulbs, tubers, and fruits of many of these plants are peeled with the teeth and eaten raw. The practice of keeping the plants fresh in water until they are eaten promotes the survival of encysted matacercariae.

Pathology. Where the flukes attach to the gut mucosa, there are areas of ulceration, inflammation, abscess formation, and haemorrhage. Heavy infections with thousands of flukes may produce intestinal stasis or even obstruction.

Clinical features. Many of the lighter infections are probably asymptomatic. Abdominal pain simulating peptic ulcer, and alternating diarrhoea and constipation are common symptoms. Severe infections may lead to nausea, vomiting, anorexia, abdominal pain, cachexia, and the passage of green or pale offensive stools. Malabsorption is suspected but has not been convincingly demonstrated. Oedema of the face and dependent areas and ascites have not been explained: protein-losing gastroenteropathy is a possible mechanism. There is a small mortality.

Diagnosis. Flukes and ova are passed in the stool or may be vomited up. They must be distinguished from those of other large species such as *Fasciola hepatica* and *F. gigantica*. Leucocytosis and eosinophilia are common.

Differential diagnosis. The symptoms associated with heavy infections might be confused with those of giardiasis, massive gut nematode infection, peptic ulcer and other causes of bowel obstruction. Generalized oedema might suggest nephrotic syndrome and other causes of hypoproteinaemia.

Treatment. Hexylresorcinol (Crystoids anthelminthic) is recommended in a single dose of 400 mg for children under seven years old and 1 g for others. The drug must be swallowed and washed down with water or it will cause burns in the mouth or oesophagus.

Tetrachloerythylene, bephenium and piperazine are also effective.

Prevention. Water plants should be cooked or else grown in ponds that are not contaminated with human or pig faeces. Molluscicides could be used to eradicate the snail vectors.

References

Cross, J. H. (1969). Fasciolopsiasis in Southeast Asia and the Far East. In *Schistosomiasis and other snail-transmitted helminthiasis*. (Ed. C. Harinasuta). Proc. 4th S.E. Asian Seminar on Parasitology and Tropical Medicine, 177, Bangkok.
Plaut, A. G., Kampanort-Sanyakorn, C., and Manning, G. S. (1969). A clinical study of *Fasciolopsis buski* in Thailand. *Trans. R. Soc. trop. Med. Hyg.* **63**, 470.

Heterophyiasis. *Heterophyes heterophyes* is a tiny intestinal fluke parasitic in fish-eating mammals including cats, dogs, foxes, and men. Human infections are common in the Philippines, Indonesia, Japan, central and southern China, western India, South Korea, Taiwan, and in North Africa (Tunisia and the Nile delta). Other species have been identified in Japan (*H. katsuradai*) and the Philippines (*H. brevicaeca*).

The first intermediate hosts are snails and the second, fresh water or estuarine fish especially mullets. Definitive mammalian hosts are infected by eating raw fish.

Pathology. Flukes attach to small bowel mucosa producing shallow ulcers and a mild inflammatory response. Ova deposited in the bowel wall may enter blood vessels and embolize to the heart and central nervous system. In the Philippines severe cardiac damage has been described. The heart is dilated, there are subepicardial haemorrhages and myocardial damage due to occlusion of vessels by the ova. Ova stick to the mitral valve which becomes thickened and calcified.

Clinical features. Dyspepsia and gastroentero-colitis with mucous diarrhoea are common. Cardiac involvement may produce chronic congestive cardiac failure or there may be sudden death due to massive coronary embolization. This disease was said to be responsible for more than 14 per cent of cardiac deaths in the Philippines.

Diagnosis. Small ova, similar to those of *Chlonorchis* are found in the stool. There may be blood eosinophilia.

Treatment. Hexylresorcinol, tetrachloroethylene, and bephenium are effective.

References

Africa, C. M., De Leon, W., and Garcia, E. Y. (1935). Heterophyidiasis: II. Ova in sclerosed mitral valves with other chronic lesions in the myocardium. *J. Philipp. Med. Ass.* **15**, 583.

—, —, —. (1936). Heterophyidiasis: III. Ova associated with a fatal haemorrhage in the right basal ganglia of the brain. *J. Philipp. Med. Ass.* **16**, 22.

—, —, — (1936). Heterophyidiasis: IV. Lesions found in the myocardium of eleven infected hearts including three cases with valvular involvement. *Philipp. J. Publ. Hlth.* **3**, 1.

—, —, — (1937). Heterophyidiasis: VI. Two cases of heart failure associated with the presence of eggs in sclerosed valves. *J. Philipp. Med. Ass.* **17**, 605.

Kean, B. H. and Breslau, R. C. (1964). Cardiac heterophyidiasis. In *Parasites of the human heart*, 95–103, Grune and Stratton, New York.

Sheir, Z. M. and Aboul-Enein, M. El-S. (1970). Demographic, clinical and therapeutic appraisal of heterophyiasis. *J. trop. Med. Hyg.* **73**, 148.

Metagonimiasis. *Metagonimus yokogawai*, which resembles *Heterophyes heterophyes*, is the smallest human fluke, being scarcely 1 mm long (Fig. 1c). It is also a parasite of other fish-eating mammals (dogs, cats, pigs) and birds (pelicans). Infection is very common in the Far East (China, Japan, Korea, Taiwan) and is also reported from the USSR, Spain, and the Balkans. The first intermediate hosts are snails such as *Semisulcospira (Melania) libertina*, and the second, freshwater salmanoid and cyprinoid fish such as the oriental trout. Human infection results from eating the raw fish. Larval flukes invade the small bowel wall where they or their ova excite a granulomatous reaction. The ova may embolize to other organs as in heterophyiasis. Mild mucous diarrhoea is the usual symptom. Diagnosis is confirmed by finding the 25×15 μm ova in the faeces.
Treatment is the same as for heterophyiasis.

Echinostomiasis. *Echinostoma ilocanum* (China, Philippines, Java), *E. malayanum* (Singapore, Malaysia) (Fig. 1d), *E. lindoensis* (Lake Lindu, Sulawesi), *Echinochasmus perfoliatus*, and a few other related species of small spiny-collared flukes pass through molluscan first and second intermediate hosts in fresh water.

Metacercariae are ingested in snails and mussels by humans, rats, and pigs. Diarrhoea, abdominal pain, and eosinophilia may occur. Treatment is the same as for heterophyiasis.

Gastrodisciasis. This is a large bowel infection by *Gastrodiscoides hominis*, prevalent in eastern India (Assam), Burma, Southeast Asia, and Guyana. The fluke is up to 1 cm long and has a very large ventral sucker disc or acetabulum. Mouse deer and pigs are the mammalian hosts. Diarrhoea is the only known symptom. Treatment is the same as for heterophyiasis.

Alariasis. In North America, various species of *Alaria* are parasites, in their adult fluke stage, in the gut of wild carnivores such as wolves, foxes, bobcats, martens, and skunks. Ova passed in faeces hatch in water, invade snails (genus *Helisoma*) from which cercariae eventually emerge and infect frog tadpoles. One fatal human infection with *A. americana* was assumed to have resulted from eating raw frogs' legs and another eye infection to direct penetration by the infective mesocercarial stage while frogs were being prepared for the table. Treatment has never been attempted, but bithionol or niridazole might prove effective.

References

Freeman, R. S., Stuart, P. F., Cullen, J. B. *et al.* (1976). Fatal human infection with mesocercariae of the trematode *Alaria americana*. *Am. J. trop. Med. Hyg.* **25**, 803.

Fernandes, B. J., Cooper, J. D., Cullen, J. B. *et al.* (1976). Systemic infection with *Alaria americana* (Trematoda). *Canad. med. Ass. J.* **115**, 1111.

Other minor genera of intestinal flukes, occasionally reported as human infections, include *Hypoderaeum*, *Prosthodendrium*, *Phaneropsolus*, *Haplorchis*, *Stellantchasmus*, *Procercovum*, *Spelotrema*, *Plagiorchis*, *Didymozoids*, and *Isoparorchis*.

General References (fluke infections)

Cross, J. H. (1974). Diagnostic methods in intestinal fluke infections: a review. In SEAMEO-TROPMEO Technical Meeting: *Diagnostic methods for important helminthiasis and amebiasis in Southeast Asia and the Far East*. Tokyo, 5–8 February, 87.

Faust, E. C., Beaver, P. C., and Jung, R. C. (1975). *Animal agents and vectors of human disease*. Lea and Febiger, Philadelphia.

Hunter, G. W. Swarzwelder, J. C., and Clyde, D. F. (1976). Trematodes exclusive of schistosomes. In *Tropical medicine*, 569–92. W. B. Saunders, Philadelphia.

Markell, E. K. and Voge, M. (1981). *Medical parasitology*, 5th edn., 140, W. B. Saunders, Philadelphia.

NON-VENOMOUS ARTHROPODS

A. Radford

The non-venomous arthropods of medical interest include the insects—flies, lice, fleas, and bugs—and the arachnid mites. Most are infestations transmitted by direct contact and with various degrees of symbiosis occurring between man and these ecto-parasites. With the exception of the flies, they are most commonly transmitted between children and their friends and families, or during sexual intercourse.

Myiasis

Myiasis is the infestation of an organ or tissue by dipterous (fly) larvae. Such infestations can be accidental, facultative (i.e. normally free-living) or obligatory (i.e. necessary for part of the life cycle of the species concerned). Although human myiasis is relatively uncommon, it is frequent in many other vertebrates and serious economic consequences can occur in domestic stock.

Several dozen species are involved. The commonest lesions are non-specific and caused by the house, stable, or one of the bot (warble) flies depositing their maggots into orifices or on to open epithelial surfaces of sleeping or debilitated persons. Alternatively, their eggs fall off from their oviposition on the abdomens of carrier flies or mosquitoes and effect transmission. Sites most commonly involved are the eye, mouth, and wounds, and in children nasal and genital orifices or the sites to which the larvae can wriggle or be carried, such as the middle ear, nostril, bladder, trachea, pulmonary system, or intestine. In one large series almost 30 per cent were situated in the ear. In another almost 80 per cent of ENT involvement was nasal; two-thirds of these patients had pre-existing atrophic rhinitis or sinusitis. Each site gives rise to definitive terminology such as intestinal, cutaneous, and external or internal ophthalmomyiasis. Intestinal infestation may lead to genuine or pseudomyiasis—in the latter form ingested larvae do not feed and develop in the digestive tract. Other descriptions are made from the character of the lesion with results such as 'furuncular myiasis' and 'creeping eruption'.

Accidental myiasis is most commonly due to one of the house or screw worm flies (*Muscidae* and *Sarcophagidae* spp.), 'facultative myiasis' to one of the blow flies (*Calliphoridae*), and obligatory myiasis to one of a large number of families including the bot and warble flies. Only one is a blood-sucker—the Congo floor maggot (*Auchmeromyia luteola*) which is nocturnal, hiding in floor crevices or bed matting by day.

Cases are recorded from all continents but infestations are more common in warmer climates and in eastern Europe, as well as in travellers who return from these places.

Clinical features. Signs and symptoms are variable. In some species infestation is benign and may be symptomless with the larvae confined to superficial necrotic tissue—a feature used for surgical debridement by many New and Old World healers for centuries. Invasion of living tissue may be painful and involve specific organs. In the case of conjunctival myiasis (usually with *Oestrus* spp.) this may be acute catarrhal conjunctivitis accompanied by irritation, burning, photophobia, epiphora, and oedema of the lids with or without secondary bacterial infection. Deeper invasion of orbit with iridocyclitis, endophthalmitis, and even retroretinal invasion with characteristic visible 'tracks' may occur. In the case of aural involvement pain and discharge is almost always present, with two-thirds of patients giving a history of otitis media, but up to a third have an intact drum. Invasion of other organs such as the bladder may give temporary haematuria, frequency and/or obstruction. The primary screw worm larvae (such as *Cochliomyia*, *Cordylobia*, *Dermatobia* and *Chrysomya* spp.) feed on living flesh and are directly invasive. Pain and discomfort can be severe with such lesions.

Where superficial creeping eruptions occur, they represent attempts by maturing larvae to gain access to the surface of their abnormal host to form the final 'boil' stage ('the warble') where the larvae point to the surface with a visible grey-white central aperture. Maturation occurs over one to three months before extrusion occurs and the larvae fall to the ground to complete their life cycle. Lesions are erythematous, raised, and indurated and may have a seropurulent discharge. They are usually situated on the thigh, head, or neck. Pruritis may be intense. A transient eosinophilia may occur, as may secondary infection.

Management. The characteristic multiple black hooklets on the head of screw worm larvae make removal difficult. Direct application of turpentine or ether drops may encourage extrusion. Larvae are removed by gentle surgical extraction under local anaesthetic when direct removal or expression cannot be effected. Species diagnosis has little clinical relevance and usually requires the assistance of a zoologist or veterinarian to whom larvae should be sent,

preserved in 10 per cent formalin or 70 per cent ethyl alcohol.

References

Gordon, R. M., and Lavoipierre, M. M. J. (1962). *Entomology for Students of Medicine*, Blackwell Scientific Publications, Oxford.

Harwood, R. F., and James, M. T. (1979). Myiasis. In *Entomology in human and animal health*, MacMillan, New York.

James, M. T. (1948). *The flies that cause myiasis in man*. Miscellaneous Publication No. 631, U.S. Department of Agriculture, Washington DC.

Lee, D. J. (1968). Human myiasis in Australia. *Med. J. Aust.*, **1**, 170.

Scott, H. G. (1964). Human myiasis in North America (1952–1962 inclusive). *Fla. Entomol.* **47**, 255.

Zumpt, F. (1965). *Myiasis in man and animals in the old world*. Butterworth, London.

Lice

Order. Acarina. *Family*. Anoplura : Pediculidae

These ectoparasites have associated with man for a long time and have been found on ancient mummies in Egypt. Once known as 'pearls of poverty', they were regarded as a sign of sainthood—Thomas à Becket's clothes were noted to crawl with them after his death.

The two varieties of human pediculosis (Latin: *louse*) are morphologically quite distinct. Although they may co-exist, there is no correlation between the density of one with the other, that is, they are spatially and ecologically isolated. Where double infection occurs, the areas of overlap are less than 1 per cent, indicating that the habitat of one is unsuitable for the other. The pubic louse, pthirus (Greek: *louse*) from the Family *Pthiridae*, is usually incorrectly spelt 'phthirus'.

Head louse infestation (*Pediculus humanus capitis*). An increasing prevalence, up to 25 times, has been reported throughout Europe during the last two decades. It is lower before preschool age but is by no means uncommon in adults. In some cultures infestation is not only regarded as normal, it has specific social significance (Fig. 1). Widely varying prevalence rates have been reported in Britain from a high 30 per cent in the early 1940s, and 23 per cent in the lower socio-economic groups of Teeside in the 1970s, 4–10 per cent in Glasgow and slightly less in Northern Ireland, to current estimates of 2–3 per cent for the United Kingdom as a whole. Female rates outnumber male ones almost 3:1. In the New World rates of 22.5 per cent in females and 17 per cent for males in Chile and an average for whites of 7 per cent in males and 10 per cent in females in the USA, with a lower rate in blacks, have been noted.

Head lice, like scabies, have no respect for class. The rise in

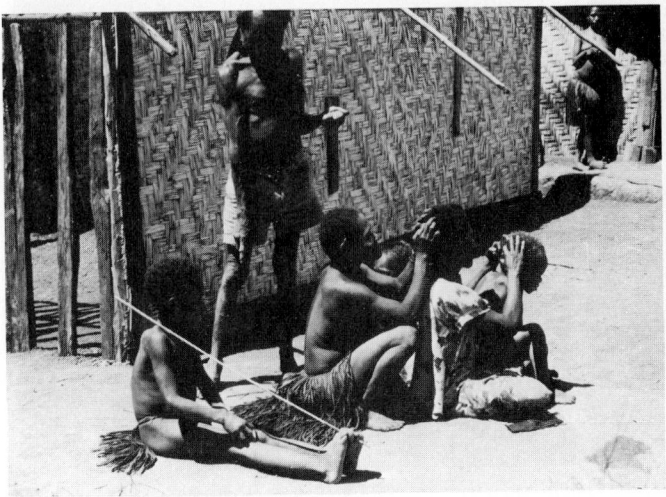

Fig. 1 Delousing—a family affair in Papua New Guinea.

prevalence in Europe may reflect increasing resistance to DDT and/or increased social mixing between groups in society.

Lice are blood, not debris, feeders. Studies show that hygiene, or rather lack of it, is not a principal factor in their epidemiology, nor is the length of hair. A persistence of these beliefs is a barrier to control. Other possible factors, largely unproven, include ignorance, apathy of authorities, increased tourism, migrant labour, and communal living. While most transmission is in younger age groups, and is usually effected by direct contact or by shared combs and brushes, lice can be transmitted during sexual intercourse. There is little evidence that lice are significant reservoirs for infections other than pyogenic skin bacteria, though they can be experimentally infected with the organisms of typhus and relapsing fever. Extensive community education and ready access to treatment is essential as control can be expensive in terms of personnel.

Biology. Adult lice are 3–4 mm long with colour variations from dirty white to grey-black (Fig. 2). They are scalp rather than hair dwellers, living very close to the scalp where food, moisture, warmth, and ovipositing sites are readily available. They attach to the hair base by strong, crab-like claws and suck blood through a stylet. An anticoagulant in saliva provides increased flow and may, together with the sensation caused by the movement of the arthropods, be the cause of irritation. Adults are very difficult to dislodge but once damaged tend to die quickly. They readily resist washing by closing over their breathing apparatus. An average infestation is 10 lice per head. Eggs are produced at a rate of six to eight per day and are well dispersed over the scalp. Immature forms (nymphs) pass through three instars (moults) over 7–16 days. The warmer the

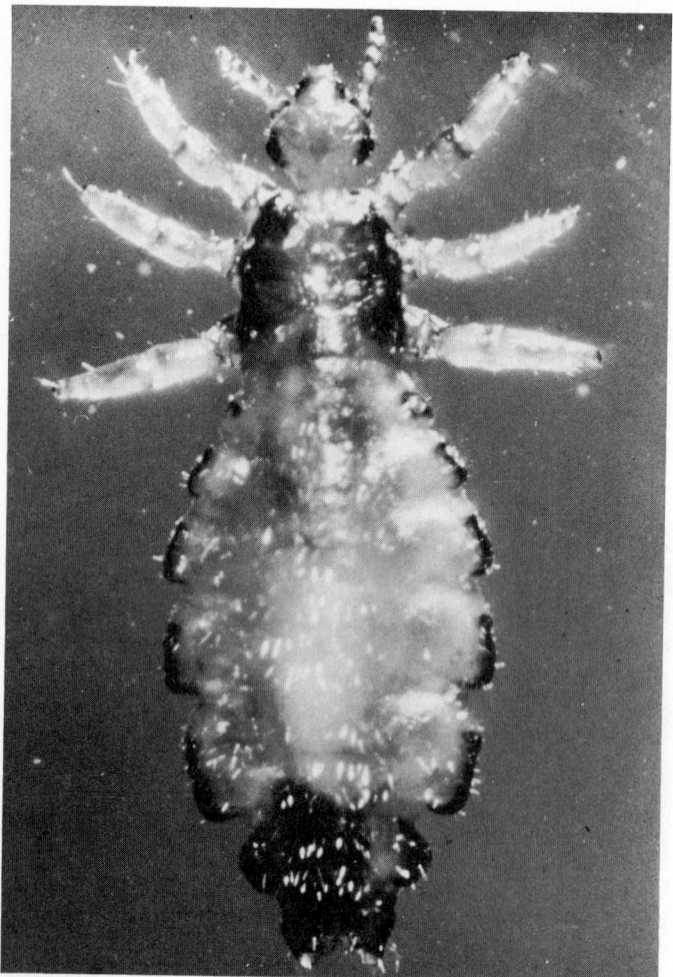

Fig. 2 Adult specimen of *Pediculus humanus*. (Reproduced by courtesy of R. V. Southcott, Adelaide, South Australia.)

environment the shorter the incubation period. During a lifetime of 30–40 days up to 300 eggs are laid. These are laid within 1 cm of the scalp and are strongly cemented to the base of the hair, growing out at a rate of 1 cm a month. The duration of infection can be measured by the distance of the ovoid egg containers, 'nits', from the scalp.

Clinical features. Variable but often intensive itching is the predominant symptom. Therefore inattention or observation of persistent scratching of the scalp by teacher or parent may alert one to the diagnosis. Secondary infection can lead to impetigo or furunculosis and consequent cervical adenitis may lead one to a diagnosis. Occasionally a 'cap' of debris may form over the scalp with the lice attached to the base of hairs underneath.

Differential diagnosis includes seborrhoeic scales ('dandruff'), hairspray, soap flakes, and hair casts, all of which readily brush off. Diagnosis is most commonly confirmed through finding the white empty nits firmly adherent to hairs and a more careful inspection will reveal the lice attached to hairs near the scalp.

Body louse infestation (*Pediculus humanus humanus*). Unlike its loftier, smaller relative, body lice may be associated with the transmission of serious infections. These include the often fatal louse-borne or epidemic typhus (*Rickettsia prowazekii*) (see page 5.343), the less serious trench fever (*Rochalimaea quintana*) (see page 5.345), and epidemic relapsing fever (*Borrelia recurrentis*) (see page 5.294). Body lice may also play a role in the spread of salmonella infections and some of the taenias such as the dog tapeworm *Dipylidium caninum*. Rickettsiae, spirochaetes, and tubercule bacilli have been shown experimentally to be capable of multiplication in lice. Evidence is less convincing for *Bartonella bacilliformis* and *Toxoplasma gondii* transmission. Man is infected through inoculation by contaminated faeces being scratched into the skin, or through mucous membranes or conjunctivae. Less common inoculation occurs through crushing of lice into the skin. With rickettsial infections the epithelial cells of the louse mid-gut are involved, and once infected the louse remains infected for life. On rupture of these cells into the digestive tract, large numbers of pathogens are released.

They are a clothing rather than a body infestation and are found especially on the socially deprived and the mentally defective, giving rise to the synonym 'vagabond's disease'.

Although eggs are most commonly found on the seams of clothing, where there is greatest access to body contact thus facilitating the feeding of young, they may also be found on body hair. The incubation period is from six to 15 days. Adults are 10–20 per cent larger than head lice. Gregarious by nature, they are said to be attracted to each other by smell. Feeding points produce pin-point macules, which may provide portals of entry for pyogenic bacteria by excoriation, and resolve leaving pigmented scars.

Pubic or crab louse (*Pthirus pubis*). Sexual intercourse is the most common form of transmission of pthirus, giving rise to the synonym 'butterfly of love', which also indicates its triangular shape (Fig. 3). Fomite transmission is rare as adults rarely leave the body unless damaged or dying. Transmission from toilet seats, whilst possible, is therefore most unlikely.

Children may be affected by direct contact with infested adults or other children, and about 1 per cent of head lice in their age group are *Pthirus* spp. Adults live about one month. They are broader in the upper abdomen than other lice and their second and third pairs of legs are stouter. They vary in colour from dirty white through yellow to grey. Pthirus is a voracious feeder, taking up to 12 meals a day, largely of tissue fluid.

Clinical features. Itching and irritation are the major presenting symptoms, especially in the inguinal, pubic, lower abdominal, and perineal hair areas. Axillary, arm, and leg hair infestation also occurs but is less common. Skin lesions may appear as blue-grey macules, or, if excoriated, as reddish pustules. Involvement of eyebrows and eyelashes has given rise to the term 'pthirus palpeb-rarum'; it is more common in childhood infestations and gives rise to a typical blepharoconjunctivitis, sometimes with a blood-stained discharge at the eyelid margins. Careful observation with a loop reveals adult lice towards the roots of lashes.

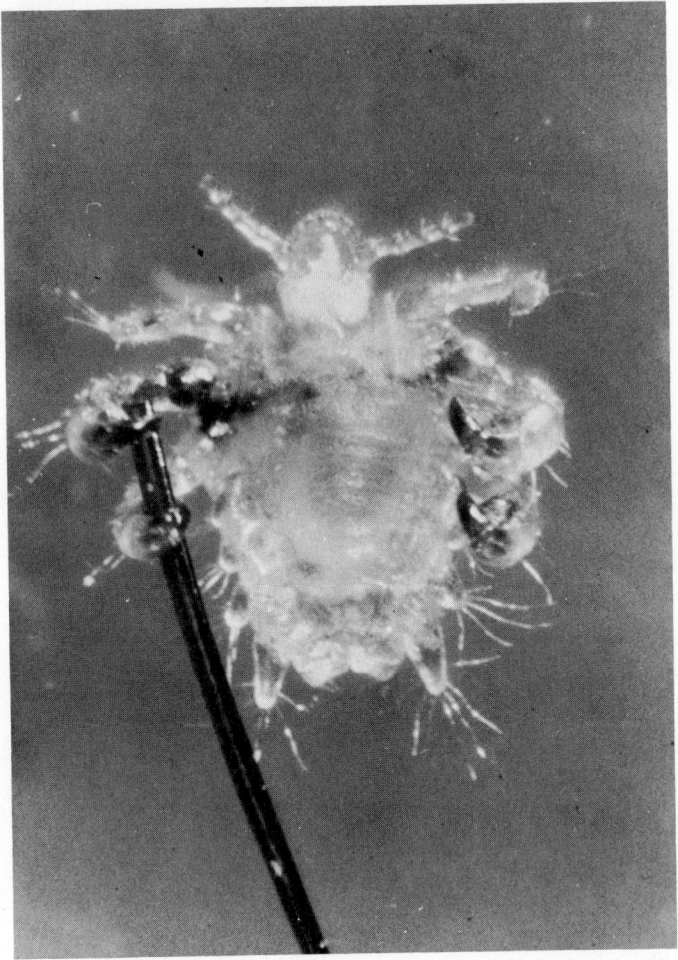

Fig. 3 Adult specimen of *Pthirus pubis*. (Reproduced by courtesy of R. V. Southcott, Adelaide, South Australia.)

Management *For head lice.* In many parts of Europe increasing resistance of head lice to the chlorinated hydrocarbons (DDT) has made organophosphorous insecticides the drug of choice. An additional advantage of malathion as an 0.5 per cent alcohol lotion or shampoo with or without dicophane, and carbaryl 0.5 per cent liquid is that they are ovicidal as well as pediculicidal. Their chemical binding properties with hair ensure that there is a persistence of action for four weeks. Head shaving is not necessary. With lotions, sprinkle into the palm of the hand and, avoiding the eyes, work well into the scalp. Repeat until the whole head is moist and allow to dry naturally. Avoid artificial heat as it will denature malathion which is also inflammable. With shampoos, wet the hair, lather and work well into the scalp, leave five minutes and repeat. Wash the head in 12 hours and use a tight comb while the hair is wet to assist in nit removal. In areas of non-resistance, DDT 2–5 per cent emulsion or 10 per cent powder and 1 per cent gamma benzene hexachloride (BHC) shampoo can be used but require a repeat application one to two weeks later to kill recently hatched immature forms. Malathion should be avoided in pregnancy.

Topical antimicrobials, such as chlorhexidine and, where substantial local infection and adenitis have occurred, systemic antibiotics or co-trimoxazole are required. Treatment failure is often due to re-infection from within the family up to a third of whom may

be infected. Therefore a thorough inspection of family and close contacts is necessary.

For body lice. Malathion, DDT, or gamma benzene hexachloride as for head lice is effective. Clothes are readily disinfected by boiling or hot water machine laundering and ironing.

Pubic lice. As for head and body lice, shaving affected areas is not necessary. Mechanical removal of adults by forceps may be done but is often difficult because of their strong attachment to hair by claws. Yellow oxide of mercury ointment may be used for eyebrow/lash involvement. Its usual method of spread should alert the physician to exclude other concomitant venereal diseases, especially asymptomatic gonorrhoea. All sexual partners and, for children, adult family contacts require inspection and treatment as necessary.

Parasitophobia. Parasitophobia is the erroneous and unshakeable belief in skin infestation with a parasite. Rarely severe forms may present as toxic psychosis, dementia praecox, involutional melancholia, or paranoia and require specific psychiatric management. Much more common is the stigma attached (especially by parents and teachers) to the false belief of the relationship of infestation with poor hygiene. Sympathetic explanation of the ubiquity of lice, their method of spread, and the effectiveness of simple treatment may be required—indeed it should be an integral part of management, as the worry is often unvoiced.

References

Busvine, J. R. (1978). Evidence from double infestations of the specific status of human head lice and body lice. *Syst. Entom.* **3**, 1.
Donaldson, R. J. (1976). The head louse in England. *R. Soc. Hlth J.* **96**, 55.
The Lancet (1979). Head lice in the seventies. *Lancet* **ii**, 130.
Maunder, J. W. (1977). Parasites and man. Human lice—biology and control. *R. Soc. Hlth J.* **97**, 29.
Morley, W. N. (1977). Body infestations. *Scott. med J.* **22**, 211.

Fleas

Order. Siphonoptera. *Family.* Pulicidae. There are 2000 species of these temporary obligate blood-sucking parasites of many animals which include rats, cats, dogs, poutry, horses, and pigs as well as man. Over 20 species attack man. Ovipositing usually occurs among the hairs of the host (or in its nest). The incubation period varies from one to three weeks. *Pulex irritans* is the most common offender. The most common manifestation of flea infestation is their bite. However, they can also be vectors to man of the plague, especially by *Xenopsylla* spp., the milder murine typhus (*R. typhi*), Q fever, listeriosis, salmonellosis, and the dog tape worm, *Diphlidium caninum*. The usual presentation is a small series of linear erythematous papules accompanied by varying degrees of itchiness. Pathogens are most commonly transmitted by scratching organisms from flea faeces into excoriated skin lesions or into mucous membranes.

Family. Tungidae.

The most troublesome flea to man is *Tunga penetrans*, the 'chigoe', 'jigger', 'chigger', or 'sand flea' found in the tropical Americas and Africa. Normally only 1 mm in length, the reddish brown gravid female may swell to almost 1 cm across, after burrowing into the skin. Irritation may be extreme. Under the toe nails (very painful), between the toes, and the soles of the feet are the sites of predilection. Secondary infection and ulceration may occur and tetanus or gangrene are occasional complications. The female may become completely embedded except for a minute aperture. Surgical enucleation is required.

Bed bugs

Order. Hemiptera. *Family.* Cimidae.

The common bed bug, *Cimex lenticularis* (Fig. 4), has been an annoying companion of man for a long time. Both *C. lenticularis* and its virtually identical tropical relation *C. hemipterus* occur in both hemispheres. A second genus *Leptocimex boneti* is found in tropical Africa. They are nocturnal bugs which hide in the crevices of beds by day and sally forth at night, often in great numbers. Transmission can also occur from clothing contact, for example, when sitting next to someone in public transport. The young are white-yellow and the adults red-brown in colour. Through a long stiletto mouthpiece they can complete a meal in less than 10 minutes.

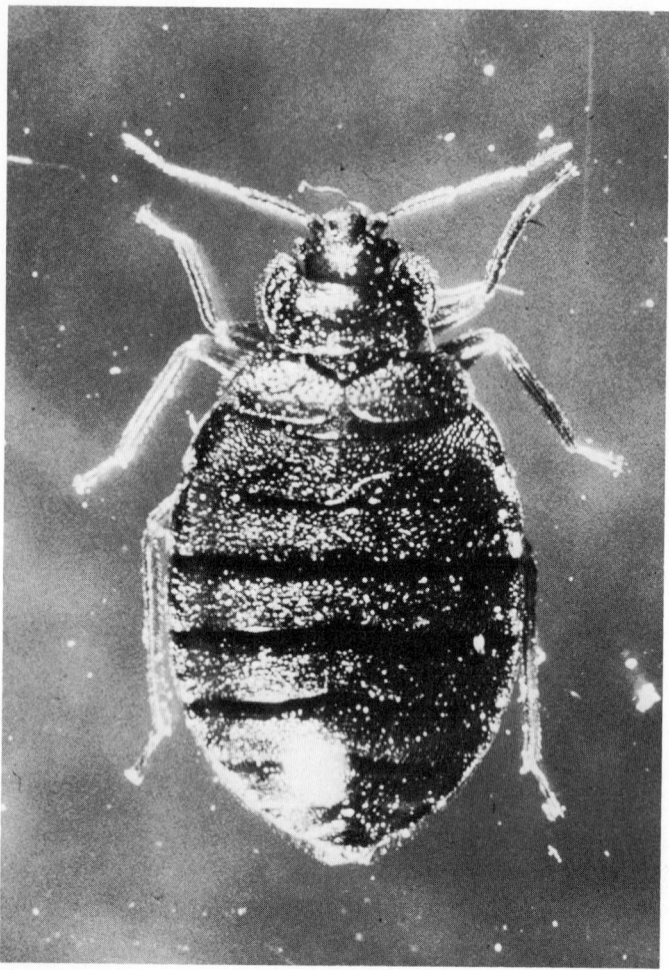

Fig. 4   Adult specimen of *Cimex lenticularis*. (Reproduced by courtesy of R. V. Southcott, Adelaide, South Australia.)

As with fleas there is a great variation in the effect of bites from minimal to marked irritation and swellings secondary to sensitization by saliva. While *Cimex* has been shown to a vector to pathogens experimentally, it has not proven to be so naturally. Other *Cimex* species may also attack man.

No specific therapy is necessary, other than calamine lotion or a short course of antihistamines when local reaction is marked.

Cimex can facilitate the transmission of relapsing fever (*Borrelia recurrentis*) and probably hepatitis viruses with which it has been infected experimentally.

ARACHNIDS

Order. Acarina. *Family.* Sarcoptidae.

Scabies (*Sarcoptes scabei*, the itch mite)

Epidemiology. Bonomo in 1687 first drew attention to the causal relationship between mite and itch, so scabies is probably the first infection for which the known cause was found.

Two pandemics, each lasting about 15 years have occurred this century with peaks in 1918 and 1945. Each had a 30-year cycle. We are currently experiencing a third pandemic.

Explanations for the above pattern are not clear. Scabies is a disease of the clean and the dirty. Herd immunity levels do not provide a satisfactory explanation as epidemics would take about 45 years to build up a non-sensitized population and this would produce 60-year not 30-year cycles. While the greatest peaks occurred at the end of the World Wars, the epidemics both started in Europe beforehand and also occurred in countries not significantly involved. The increase during the last decade is worldwide.

Denmark is one of the few countries in which scabies is a notifiable disease and almost a million cases have been reported there since 1900. The prevalence in Denmark today is identical to that at the turn of the century—about 2 per 1000—despite a marked improvement in the standards of living, so the oft-quoted poor standard of living as a significant aetiological factor has little basis. Similarly, in a recent US naval study, rates increased eight-fold in less than a decade without any concomitant change in the prevalence of gonorrhoea, syphilis, or body lice. Thus, while scabies may be transmitted during intercourse, promiscuity is unlikely to be the major factor in the current epidemic. Armed forces personnel also have very high standards of hygiene and diet. Prevalence in the West is usually under 5 per cent but may reach 30 per cent in selected groups in less developed countries. The prevalence in the United Kingdom today is between 2 and 4 per cent and the incidence rate in US dermatological practice is similar.

Transmission is greater where there is a great density of infestation. Winter levels exceed those of summer in northern Europe but the provinces in Denmark show no greater prevalence than the capital. Higher rates occur in the tropics where the disease is usually endemic and where poorer living conditions, greater illiteracy, and lower resistance exist but also where much greater skin-to-skin contact occurs especially between siblings. Fomites appear to play little role as repeated experiments with volunteers have failed to facilitate transmission. Nosocomial infections occur in nursing homes and mental hospitals, especially when staff are unfamiliar with the less known but more infectious Norwegian form of the disease.

Scabies is most commonly a 'family affair' with a reported secondary attack rate within families of 38 per cent. There is a fairly uniform age distribution until about age 45 after which there is a marked fall in prevalence (Fig. 5). Friends are the commonest point source and the greater tendency of girls to hold hands may be the significant factor in the greater prevalence in females, which outnumbers that in males 3:2 in industrial countries.

Direct transmission from dogs, pigs, horses, and cats is not uncommon and occurs especially from external ear, periorbital, back, and abdominal lesions to points of contact. Zoonotic scabies

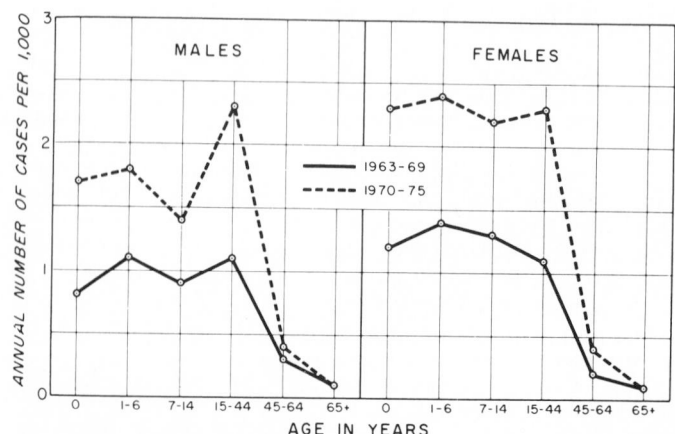

Age pattern of scabies, 1963 to 1969 and 1970 to 1975.

Fig. 5   Age pattern of scabies 1963–9 and 1970–75, Denmark. (From Christophersen, J. 1978. *Archs Derm.* **114**, 749, by permission.)

has a shorter incubation period and is usually self-limiting over a few months because the mite does not propagate on human skin. *Sarcoptes scabei* var. *humanus* is indistinguishable morphologically from var. *canis*, var. *equi* and var. *suis*. *Notoedres cati* is smaller, rounder, and rarely affects man. Animal sources can initiate mini-epidemics within families.

Life cycle. The female mite averages 0.4 × 0.3 cm in size and is about twice the size of the male. It is virtually headless apart from its 'jaws' (Fig. 6). There are four pairs of legs—the front two end in suckers and in the female the third and fourth pair are 'trailers'. In the male, the fourth pair also has suckers. Adults can move at the rate of 2.5 cm per minute.

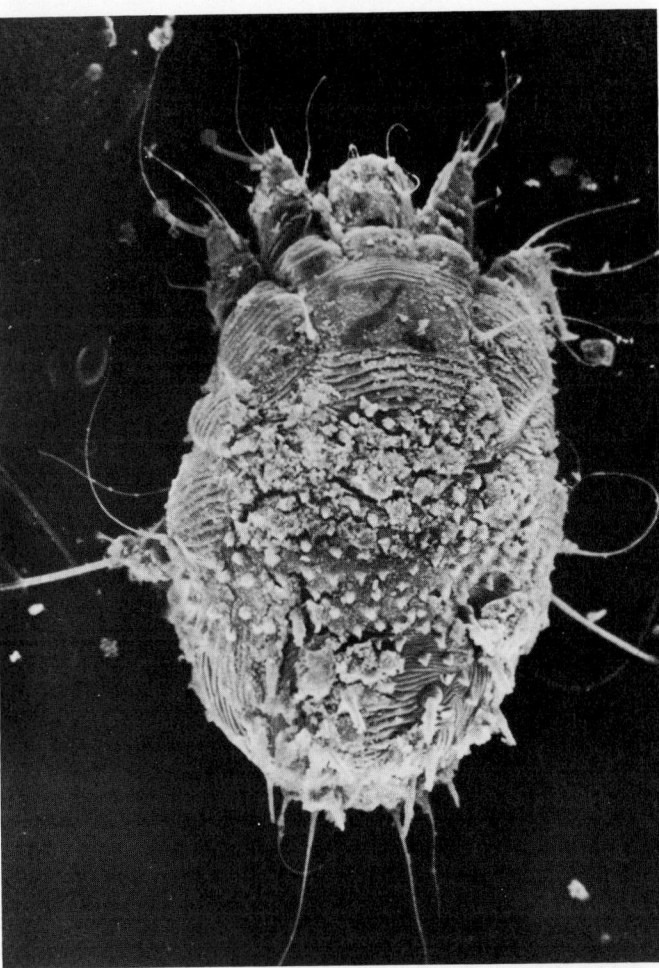

Fig. 6 Adult specimen of *Sarcoptes scabei*. (Reproduced by courtesy of R. V. Southcott, Adelaide, South Australia.)

Only the adult female of the human variety burrows. This she does under the cornified layer to its junction with the stratum granulosum, continually extending her burrow about 2 mm a day, leaving eggs (two or three per day) and faecel pellets in her wake. The eggs hatch in three to four days producing six-legged larvae that evolve into eight-legged nymphs three days later. These moult once or twice before reaching adulthood—the whole process taking 10–14 days. Less than 10 per cent of eggs mature into adults which survive about 30 days.

Almost all initial infections 'take' but there are generally no symptoms and few signs for the first four to six weeks during which period sensitization occurs. Over ensuing weeks and months a measure of immunity builds up as only 60 per cent of re-infestations establish themselves and then with lower density loads. With re-infestation irritation is almost instantaneous. The sensitization is due to mite saliva, faecal material, or both. Infestations in temperate countries are relatively light with 50 per cent having less than six adults and only 4 per cent having greater than 50 in the United Kingdom reports.

Clinical features. Itching is the hallmark symptom of scabies infestation. It is often worse at night or after a hot shower, possibly due to activation of the mite. The itch can be excruciating. Scabies is a very polymorphic disease. Lesions tend to be symmetrical and papulovesicular lesions with or without eczematous dermatitis are the commonest form. The vesicles are 2–3 mm in diameter. Macules, pustules, and scaly plaques also occur. Lesions are confined to the dorsal surface of the interdigital spaces and to the flexor surface of wrists in two-thirds of cases and at least one lesion is found here in 85 per cent of patients. Lesions may also occur around the elbows, anterior axillary folds, the breasts, periumbilicus, belt line, lower buttocks, thighs, penis (including glans), and the scrotum. The face and the palms of the hands and feet are usually involved only in infants in whom lesions may also be bullous.

The characteristic burrows are from 3–15 mm long and irregular in direction. They may be difficult to identify and are said to be less common in the current epidemic in industrial countries. (In scabies transmitted from animals they are absent and areas involved tend to be more localized.) There are usually many more lesions than burrows as larval mites do not burrow, only imbed. Periumbilical lesions tend to be eczematous and spokelike in distribution. Scrotal and penile lesions are reddish and nodular but never discharge unless secondarily infected. In adults, especially where there has been recent contact with an unstable partner and where perineal lesions are present, other venereal diseases should be excluded–up to 15 per cent of infected adult females have been shown to have asymptomatic gonorrhoea.

The nodular variety may persist for months or years and the Norwegian form even longer. The Norwegian variety is more commonly found in the elderly, the incapacitated, and the mentally retarded (especially in Down's syndrome patients), and at any age in the tropics. In all these groups presentation for treatment is often delayed. In this form thick white or yellowish scales or plaques may be widespread and may involve the palms and the soles. Nail dystrophy is common. The diagnosis is occasionally masked in immunosuppressed patients in whom the Norwegian form is now a recognized complication. It is so named because it was first described in Norwegian leprosy patients. A less common syndrome of recurrent vesicles and pustules which persists for many months, despite repeated treatments, has recently been described in some Asian refugees.

Diagnosis. The characteristic appearance is often sufficient, especially in an epidemic. A hand lens may assist in teasing a female adult out of her burrow with a needle. Alternatively, a drop of oil placed on the lesion, half a dozen brisk scrapes with a scalpel blade and application of the material to a slide will reveal faecal pellets and eggs on microscopy. Scrapings are often negative in zoonotic forms because adults do not burrow. Biopsy is rarely necessary but reveals characteristic histopathology.

Histopathology. There is a perivascular cellular infiltrate in both the superficial and deep layers of the epidermis. Histocytes, lymphocytes, and eosinophils are found in varying proportions. Polymorphonuclear leucocytes are also present when excoriation and secondary infection occur.

Spongiotic vesiculation occurs in the papulovesicular type, a dense cellular reaction in the nodular variety and a hyperkeratotic psoriaform dermatitis characterized by ortho- and parakeratosis with intra-epidermal pustules related to mites and eggs is seen in the Norwegian form of the disease. Eggs, larvae, and adults are abundant in this variety, episodic in papulovesicular biopsies, and rare in the nodular form. IgE is sometimes found in the walls of upper dermal blood vessels using direct but not indirect immuno-fluorescence and some humoral immune responses have been described. Histopathological differentiation from lymphoma, erythema multiforme, and drug eruption is essential.

Differential diagnosis. Scabies, like syphilis, has been called 'a great imitator'. Any of the pruritic dermatoses needs to be considered and especially papular urticaria in children. Other diagnoses to be excluded are dermatitis herpetiformis (both shoulder and buttock lesions occur eventually), reticuloses (especially nodular lymphomas), Paget's disease of the breast, drug eruptions, insect bite reaction, atopic eczema, keratosis follicularis, necrotizing vasculitis, and, when considering Norwegian scabies, psoriasis and erythroderma.

Complications. The most common complication is local secondary bacterial infection with or without secondary adenitis. The most serious but uncommon sequela is glomerulonephritis following colonization of lesions by nephritogenic streptococci. While this complication may be more common in the tropics it also occurs in temperate zones. *Staphylococcus aureus* and *Corynebacteria diphtheriae* may also be associated with scabies infections.

Treatment. After soaking in a hot bath to soften vesicles, scrub the lesions with a firm brush to remove the tops. Where secondary infection is present the scrubbing is unnecessary due to epidermal maceration. To decrease percutaneous absorption, dry and cool the skin before applying benzyl benzoate 25 per cent emulsion or gamma benzene hexachloride (BHC) 1 per cent as cream or alcoholic lotion. Apply thinly from the neck down but rub well into burrows. Wash off after 24 hours. Because of some percutaneous absorption BHC is best avoided in pregnant woman and infants. Repeat in one week. About 30 g is required for an adult. Other effective medicaments include crotamiton 10 per cent cream or lotion and monosulfiram 25 per cent diluted with 2 to 3 parts of water. Repeat with a second application two or three days later. The former is occasionally irritating and with the latter alcohol consumption needs to be avoided due to its similarity to disulfiram ('Antabuse').

The itchiness can be troublesome and may require an oily calamine solution or even a systemic anti-histamine preparation. Itching may persist for some time after basic therapy. Very rarely a short course of corticosteroids, such as prednisolone 40 mg daily for three to seven days, may be required. Family and sexual contacts need careful checking and treatment as necessary. Where secondary bacterial infection occurs, local antimicrobials are necessary. Where such lesions are confluent or where adenitis occurs, a course of systemic antibiotics is needed.

For the crusted Norwegian form a strong keratolytic agent such as salicylic acid may be required before using a scabicide. When nodules persist for some time a nightly application of targel may help.

Acarinophobia. Acarinophobia (phobia about mites) will affect some patients who will require reassurance that scabies is a non-respector of persons and that its treatment is easy and effective. Clothing and bedding are not significant factors in transmission, but hot water washing machines, dry cleaning, and ironing will kill any mites.

Follicle mite
Family. Demodicidae
Demodex folliculorum and *D. brevis* are found in man, but the role of these obligatory parasites as the cause of any definitive pathology is still disputed. The former aggregate around hair follicles whose orifices they may plug, whilst *D. brevis* usually appears solitarily in sebaceous glands. They are very small (0.1–0.4 mm long) and are most commonly found on the nose, in the nasolabial folds, and on the eyebrows. Infestation rates vary from 10 to 100 per cent and increase with age.

Blepharitis, with or without the loss of eye lashes, a seborrhoeic dermatitis, perioral rosacea, and granulomatous acne are all said to occur with these mites. In summary, both (species) seem minor pathogens—merely harvesting the cells of their respective habitats.

References

Christopherson, J. (1978). The epidemiology of scabies in Denmark, 1900 to 1975. *Archs Dermatol.* **114**, 747.

Church, R. E. and Knowelden, J. (1978). Scabies in Sheffield: a family infestation. *Br. med. J.* **i**, 761.

Fernandez, N., Torres, A., and Ackerman, A. B. (1977). Pathologic findings in human scabies. *Archs Dermatol.* **113**, 320.

Harwood, R. F. and James, M. T. (1979). *Entomology in human and animal health.* Macmillan, New York.

Mellanby, K. (1972). *Scabies*, 2nd edn. Classey, Hampton Middlesex.

Melton, L. J., Brazin, S. A., and Damm, S. R. (1978). Scabies in the United States Navy. *Am. J. publ. Hlth* **68**, 776.

Nutting, W. B. and Green, A. C. (1976). Pathogenesis associated with hair follicle mites (*Demodex* spp.) in Australian aborigines. *Br. J. Derm.* **94**, 307.

Orkin, M. and Maibach, H. I. (1979). Scabies, a current pandemic. *Postgrad. Med. J.* **66**, 52.

PENTASTOMIASIS (POROCEPHALOSIS)

D. A. Warrell

Degenerate annelid-like arthropods of the class *Pentastomida* are variously known as pentastomes, pentastomids, linguatulids, or tongue worms. Members of two genera, *Linguatula* and *Armillifer*, cause disease in man.

Linguatula serrata has been reported from Europe, the Middle East, and South America. The adults which are multi-segmented, legless creatures 1–2 cm long, are found in the nasopharynx of the definitive hosts; mammals such as wild and domestic canines and herbivores. Eggs are shed in the saliva and faeces and picked up by the intermediate hosts which are reptiles, especially snakes, and mammals. Larvae hatch in the lumen of the gut of these intermediate hosts, burrow into the tissues and encyst. When the intermediate host is eaten by the definitive host, nymphs hatch from the cysts and migrate to the lungs and nasopharynx where they mature.

Clinical features. If humans ingest *Linguatula* eggs, the resulting cysts, which are usually found in the liver, do not cause symptoms unless they obstruct or compress, for example the filtration angle of the anterior chamber of the eye, biliary or respiratory tracts, or brain.

Ingestion of cysts in raw liver or lymph nodes of sheep, goats, cattle, and lagomorphs result in acute nasopharyngitis, known as Halzoun or Marrara syndrome. This has been reported from the Middle East (especially Lebanon), Greece, and the Sudan. A few hours after eating the infected viscera there is intense irritation of the upper respiratory and gastrointestinal tracts associated with coughing, sneezing, retching, vomiting, lacrimation, rhinorrhoea, haemoptysis, epistaxis, cervical lymphadenopathy, transient deafness, and difficulty in speaking, swallowing, and breathing. Patients usually recover in one to two weeks but deaths have followed acute upper airway obstruction. These features suggest a hypersensitivity reaction. Halzoun has also been attributed to flukes (*Fasciola hepatica*) ingested in raw sheep and goat liver, and to the leeches *Limnatis nilotica* and *Dinobdella ferox*.

Armillifer (Porocephalus) armillatus, A. grandis, A. moniliformis, and A. crotali. These are reported to have caused human disease in West, Central, and East Africa, Southeast Asia, China, Japan, and the USA. The worm-like bodies of the adults contain a series of rings and are 3–12 cm long (Fig. 1). They live in the respiratory and digestive tracts of snakes, especially pythons and, in West Africa, giant vipers of the genus *Bitis,* cobras, and mambas. Humans are infected when they eat snake meat, especially the raw meat which is a feature of ju-ju rituals, or drink water contaminated by snakes. Ingested eggs hatch in the gut releasing larvae which burrow into the tissues where they develop into nymphs. Wriggling nymphs

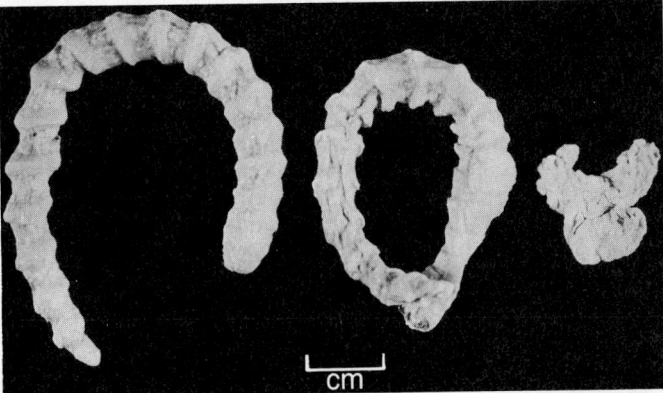

Fig. 1 *Armillifer armillatus*. Left: two adults found in the lungs of a Gaboon viper (*Bitis gabonica*). Right: calcified nymph from the mesentery of a Ghanaian patient. (By courtesy of Dr G. M. Ardran.)

have been discovered beneath the visceral peritoneum during laparatomy.

Clinical features. The commonest evidence of *Armillifer* invasion is the discovery of calcified nymphs on radiographs of the abdomen and chest (Fig. 2). These appear as discrete crescent-shaped soft tissue calcifications, 4 × 4 mm in size. In West Africa they are seen particularly in the right upper quadrant and are situated beneath the peritoneum covering the liver. In Ibadan, Nigeria these shadows were seen in 2 per cent of adult males and 4 per cent of adult females. Encysted nymphs have been found at autopsy in the liver, gut wall and lumen, lungs, serosal cavities, central nervous system and elsewhere in 27 per cent of cases in the Congo, between 6 and 13 per cent in Cameroon, and in 45 per cent in Malaysian Orang Asli. Often there is no tissue reaction round the cysts but sometimes there is granuloma formation, necrosis, and fibrosis. *Armillifer* is said to be the third commonest cause of hepatic fibrosis in Ibadan, Nigeria.

Armillifer infection is usually symptomless but serious inflammatory and obstructive effects have been described in the gut, lungs, central nervous system, biliary tract, pericardium, and anterior chamber of the eye. Severe acute reactions may be related to hypersensitivity or perhaps to massive infection such as might follow ingestion of a gravid female. Fatalities have occurred. There is some evidence from Nigeria and Zaire that *Armillifer* infection may be associated with malignancy.

Diagnosis. Pentastome nymphs can be distinguished from helminths when found in tissue sections. In infected patients antibodies to *Armillifer* have been detected by fluorescent technique.

Other infections transmissible from reptiles to man include salmonellosis, sparganosis, capillariasis, strongyloidiasis, Q fever and *Aeromonas shigelloides* infection, the mite *Ophionyssus natricis*, and possibly some togaviruses and herpesviruses.

Treatment. There is no specific treatment for pentastomiasis. Obstruction and compression should be relieved surgically. Hypersensitivity phenomena could be treated with adrenaline, anti-

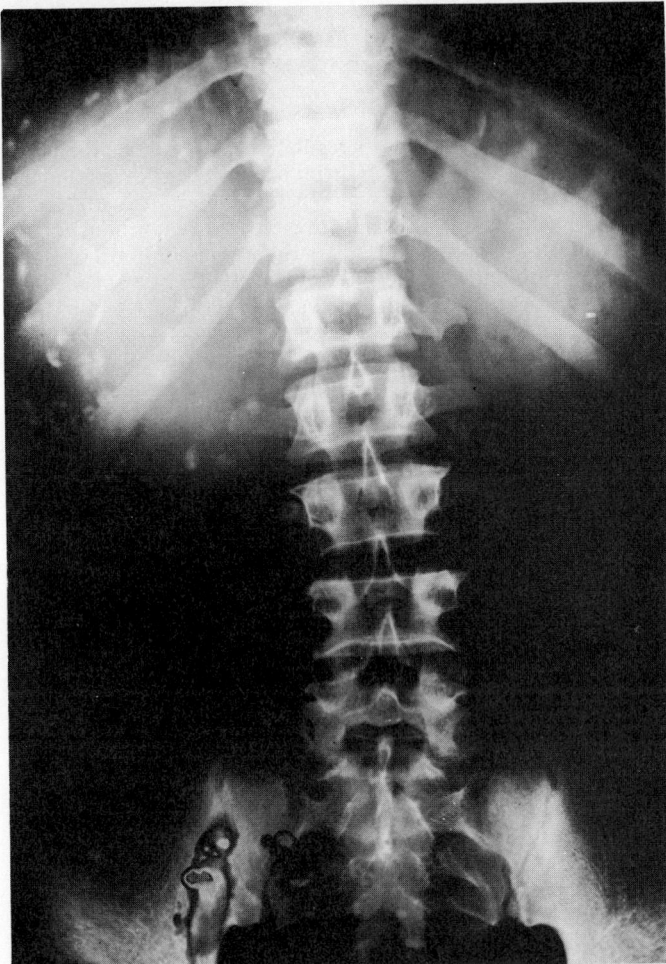

Fig. 2 Typical radiographic appearance of calcified nymphs of *Armillifer armillatus* in the abdominal cavity of a Ghanaian patient. (By courtesy of Dr G. M. Ardran.)

histamines, and corticosteroids. The infection can be prevented if all meat is thoroughly cooked.

References
Ardran. G. M. (1948). *Armillifer armillatus*. A note of three cases of calcification in man. *Br. J. Radiol.* **21**, 342.
Fain, A. (1960). La Pentastomose chez l'homme. *Bull. Acad. R. Med. Belg.* **24**, 516.
— (1975). The Pentastomida parasitic in man. *Ann. Soc. Belg. Med. trop.* **55**, 59.
Self, J. T., Hopps, H. C., and Williams, A. O. (1975). Pentastomiasis in Africa. *Trop. geog. Med.* **27**, 1.
Schacher, J. F., Saab, S., Germanos, R., and Boustany, N. (1969). The aetiology of halzoun in Lebanon: recovery of *Linguatula serrata* nymphs from two patients. *Trans. R. Soc. trop. Med. Hyg.* **63**, 854.
Prathap, K., Lau, K. S., and Bolton, J. M. (1969). Pentastomiasis: a common finding at autopsy in Malaysian aborigines. *Am. J. Trop. Med. Hyg.* **18**, 20.

Infectious disease syndromes

PYREXIA OF UNCERTAIN ORIGIN

P. B. Beeson

In this chapter the words 'pyrexia' and 'fever' will be used inter-changeably, to indicate abnormal elevation of body temperature resulting from disease. By that definition we avoid inclusion of such physiological events as transient rise in core body temperature that may occur after strenuous exertion such as rowing or playing squash, when the huge energy expenditure generates more heat than the body's dissipating mechanisms can balance. Pyrexia is a non-specific clinical manifestation, comparable to elevation of the erythrocyte sedimentation rate.

Pathogenesis of fever. Smooth regulation of the core temperature of the body is a function of hypothalamic centres containing temperature-sensitive neurones. When the body temperature is tending to fall, these centres initiate increased heat production by acceleration of action currents of striated muscle fibres. At the same time blood flow to the surface of the body is lessened, thus reducing dissipation of heat. Conversely, when a positive heat balance is threatened, muscle fibre activity diminishes, more blood is brought to the skin, and sweating occurs, to faciliate loss by evaporation. There is a normal diurnal cycle of body temperature, the lowest level being reached in the late hours of sleep towards morning. Then follows a gradual rise throughout the day and a decline beginning in the late evening. In pyrexial patients central thermoregulation is affected: control of the diurnal variation is less smooth, and the core temperature of the body tends to be set at a higher-than-normal level, especially in the afternoon or evening. This may then be followed by a precipitous decline during sleep, likely to be manifested by sweating—one of the hallmarks of fever. When there are hectic swings of body temperature, the muscular activity causing increased heat production may be manifested by a rigor, with such diminution of cutaneous blood flow that the skin is cold and cyanotic. The commonest cause of a rigor is liberation of bacteria or, say, malarial parasites, into the circulating blood. Rigors also occur in some viral infections such as influenza, and even occasionally in neoplastic disorders, e.g. hypernephroma or Hodgkin's disease.

The mechanism of disturbed thermoregulation in fever is thought to be by the action of products of tissue injury, called endogenous pyrogens. These are present in polymorphonuclear leucocytes, monocytes, and fixed macrophages such as Kupffer cells, but have not been demonstrated in lymphocytes. Endogenous pyrogens appear to be proteins, with molecular weights in the neighbourhood of 13 000–15 000 dalton. For details of present thinking about their nature and mode of action in the brain, the review by Bernheim can be consulted.

Approach to diagnosis. Elucidation of the cause of prolonged pyrexia can be a frustrating and tantalizing clinical challenge, because fever develops as a manifestation of so many kinds of injury, in every organ or tissue. The causes include not only infections, but also neoplasms, immunogenic disorders, vascular insufficiencies, etc.

The present discussion will deal with the diagnostic approach to illness characterized by prolonged fever, i.e. more than three weeks, and will exclude the common short self-limited infectious pyrexias that are most often caused by viral infections. Long lists of disorders capable of causing fever could be compiled, but they would serve no purpose here. Instead, emphasis will be placed on the three major categories into which obscure febrile illnesses tend to fall: infections, neoplastic diseases, and immunogenic diseases. Brief mention will also be made of some miscellaneous causes of prolonged fever, mainly to remind the reader of the great diversity of possibilities that have to be considered in the diagnostic search.

Three points deserve to be stressed at the outset. First, most cases of prolonged obscure fever are instances of well-known diseases manifesting themselves atypically. Secondly, the actual pattern of the graphic record is so variable that it is not helpful in pointing to specific diagnoses. Thirdly, an aggressive diagnostic effort is usually justified, because curative or palliative measures can so often be brought into use once the diagnosis has been achieved.

Infections. Despite the great advances that have been made in the diagnosis and treatment of many kinds of infection, this general

class of diseases is still the largest single cause of prolonged fever of uncertain origin. It is worth emphasis, however, that one general exclusion can be made, i.e. infections by filterable viruses. Although these often cause *acute* febrile illnesses, such as respiratory tract infections, the illnesses usually run their courses, or cause death of the patient, in a shorter time than the arbitrary three-week limit established for the subject of this chapter. There are a few exceptions: the hepatitis viruses may cause chronic febrile illness, and in rare instances the febrile phase of infectious mononucleosis persists more than three weeks. But as a general rule, intensive search for evidence of viral infection is not likely to be productive in a patient with prolonged pyrexia of obscure origin.

Infectious agents that may be difficult to verify are those which cause granulomatous inflammations. Tuberculosis heads this list, even today. The lesions of miliary tuberculosis may not be discernible in the chest X-ray until the disease is well advanced, and even greater diagnostic difficulty can be encountered when there is active tuberculosis in an extra-pulmonary site, such as kidney or the tubo-ovarian structure. Other kinds of chronic pyogenic or granulomatous infections that should be thought of include actinomycosis. candidiasis, histoplasmosis, coccidioidomycosis, and toxoplasmosis.

Persons residing in, or travelling through, tropical areas may acquire infections caused by parasites not indigenous to the developed countries of the world, e.g. schistosomiasis, trypanosomiasis, amebiasis, and malaria.

In addition to the foregoing, there are specific bacterial infections featured by prolonged pyrexia without distinctive localizing manifestations; these include salmonellosis and brucellosis.

Deep-seated bacterial abscesses sometimes cause fever, with few or no localizing symptoms and physical findings. Examples are subphrenic or perinephric abscesses, and purulent infection involving the large bowel or the female pelvic organs. A long-standing area of osteomyelitis, thought to be sterile, can become reactivated.

Bacterial endocarditis is always mentioned as a cause of prolonged obscure fever, but this infection is nearly always disclosed by repeatedly positive blood culture. True enough, endocarditis does occur rarely without demonstrable bacteraemia, notably when caused by organisms that do not grow in conventional blood culture, e.g. that of Q fever or aspergillus. In such cases, when other features point to this possibility, serological tests may be helpful. A non-infectious disease, atrial myxoma, can be confused with 'abacteraemic bacterial endocarditis'.

Patients with pyorrhoea alveolaris do not usually exhibit fever, even in the presence of extensive sepsis in the gums. Now and then, however, a periapical abscess can give rise to fever, even though the patient does not complain of local pain. Its presence may be revealed by X-rays, or a physical sign that may be helpful is elicitation of tenderness on percussion over individual teeth.

Neoplastic disease

Lymphomas. Hodgkin's disease and allied disorders of the lymphatic system are well-known causes of fever. When the lesions are deeply situated, as in the retroperitoneal nodes, spleen, and liver, the aetiology of the pyrexia may be uncertain for weeks or months. Endogenous pyrogenic materials have been extracted from homogenates of lymph nodes affected by Hodgkin's disease.

Leukemias. Fever is commonly encountered in all forms of leukemia, especially during treatment. Although it is undoubtedly true that occasional instances of untreated acute leukemia can be manifested only by fever, this is probably comparatively rare, because infectious complications are so common in this group of diseases. As methods for the demonstration of infectious agents have improved, and as knowledge has been gained about the characteristics of infection in immunocompromised hosts, clinical experience suggests that most pyrexias in leukemic hosts should be regarded as evidence of complicating infections. This is particularly true of the myelogenous forms, and of chronic lymphocytic leukemia; also in any case where therapy has greatly reduced the number of phagocytic cells.

Solid tumours. In rare instances solid tumours, such as hypernephroma, pancreatic carcinoma, and various sarcomas, can cause fever. Tumours of the gastrointestinal tract may be responsible, when there is extensive metastatic invasion of the liver. Such tumours may release pyrogenic products, or they may cause fever by reason of tissue necrosis and phagocytic ingestion of debris. As with the leukemias, proof that fever is due to the neoplasm and not to accompanying infection, is often difficult. For example, some pyrexias that once would have been attributed to lung cancers are now thought usually to be caused by associated pulmonary infection. In the 1960s reports from cancer clinics described fever as a manifestation in 40–50 per cent of cases of bowel or lung cancer, but it now appears that not more than about 5 per cent of such pyrexias should be attributed to the neoplastic process itself.

Collagen-vascular (immunogenic) diseases.

Pyrexia may be the only clinical manifestation of one of this group of conditions for weeks or months, before there is evidence of localized disease in any organ. Examples are acute rheumatic fever, rheumatoid arthritis, disseminated lupus erythematosus, polyarteritis nodosa, cranial arteritis/polymyalgia, and the juvenile form of rheumatoid arthritis (Still's disease). The special diagnostic tests applicable to this group of disorders are considered in more detail elsewhere in this text. Special attention is drawn here to the likelihood of rheumatoid arthritis, and to a kindred disorder in young adults, usually males, that may present with obscure pyrexia over a period of weeks or months, and only later manifest myalgia, stiffness, and arthritis, the clinical syndrome resembling that of Still's disease in children.

Miscellaneous causes

Chronic granulomatous hepatitis. This disease, quite apart from cases due to tuberculosis, brucellosis, or sarcoidosis, can be the cause of prolonged fever, with striking debility and weight loss, but without jaundice. It occurs most often in males in the fourth and fifth decades of life. There may or may not be a history of alcoholism. Liver function tests are usually, though not always, abnormal. The diagnosis can only be made by liver biopsy. In most instances these patients can be greatly benefited by prolonged steroid therapy.

Recurrent pulmonary thrombo-embolism. Fever is a common and usual accompaniment of a large pulmonary embolus, but should subside within a week. Nevertheless, occasional instances of prolonged puzzling fever appear to result from a *series* of pulmonary infarctions, which may not be causing distinctive clinical manifestations.

Drug fever. In today's era of polypharmacy, one of the commonest causes of pyrexia of uncertain origin is idiosyncracy to a drug. Almost any drug can be responsible, even a simple inorganic compound such as potassium iodide. Of the agents in common use today, some of the most frequent offenders are the penicillins, the barbiturates, the sulphonomides, procainamide, and diphenylhydantoin. Drug fever may be accompanied by dermatologic manifestations, changes in numbers of circulating blood elements, especially eosinophilia, and evidence of organ injury, perhaps in the kidneys and lungs. As is described more fully in Section 16, a syndrome closely resembling systemic lupus erthyematosus can be associated with administration of certain drugs, such as procainamide and hydralzine. It should be mentioned that although drug fever usually appears within two weeks of the initiation of therapy, it may not begin until after several months or years of treatment with an agent such as diphenylhydantoin. In nearly all instances, drug fevers subside within a few days of discontinuing therapy.

Sarcoidosis. Fever is commonly present in the form of sarcoidosis that resembles erythema nodosum, i.e. with skin lesions, arthralgias, arthritis, and hilar adenopathy, but it may also accompany less distinctive forms of that disease when the principal involvement is in such organs as the lungs, the liver, the meninges, or the joints.

Cirrhosis of the liver. Pyrexia is present in a substantial proportion, perhaps a third, of patients admitted to hospitals because of advanced active Laennec's cirrhosis. This appears to be independent of infection and there may be difficulty in its interpretation, because these patients are susceptible to many kinds of infection.

Central nervous system lesion affecting thermal regulation. This item is mentioned only to emphasize its extreme rarity. Although hyperpyrexia may accompany heat stroke, or be a terminal event in cerebral vascular accidents, such states do not fall within the scope of the present discussion.

Inflammatory bowel disease. In rare instances, patients with Crohn's disease, ulcerative colitis, or Whipple's disease, can exhibit pyrexia at a time when there are unimpressive complaints of diarrhoea and abdominal pain.

Factitious fever. Sometimes patients employ trickery to simulate illness with 'fever'. They can accomplish this in many ways, but to be successful, some familiarity with hospital routine is needed; consequently the most successful ruses have been enacted by nurses, orderlies, and doctors. Where mercury thermometers are being employed, the commonest manoeuvre is to have an extra thermometer, artificially raise its temperature reading, and substitute that for the one that has been placed in the mouth or rectum. Circumstances pointing to factitious fever are variations in temperature unaccompanied by appropriate changes in pulse rate, sweating, chilling, anaemia, or alterations in leucocyte count or erythrocyte sedimentation rate. Patients who do this are often willing to re-enforce their simulation by submitting to unpleasant and painful diagnostic procedures, even exploratory laparotomy. If this possibility is considered by the attending team, it can usually be exposed relatively easily.

A more serious and threatening variant of the problem is provided by patients who inject irritating substances into themselves. This may give rise to subcutaneous inflammations, or to septicaemia. They may deliberately inoculate themselves with materials containing bacteria—including faecal suspensions. Life-threatening bacteraemic shock can result. This practice can usually be exposed by looking for syringes and needles among the private belongings, while the patient is away from the bed for some lengthy diagnostic procedure.

Patients with factitious fever have serious psychological problems and are in need of skilful and sympathetic treatment. Direct confrontation may take away all possibility of help. The need is for counselling or psychiatric guidance, to assist the patient to cope with situations that have been regarded by him as intolerable. Rumans and Vosti have reviewed this subject in some detail.

Habitual hyperthermia. There are people, most often young adult women, who have imperfect thermoregulation and may, over long periods of time, be found to have core temperature up to 0.5 °C above the normal level; yet they do not have other systemic signs of disease such as weight loss, anaemia, elevated sedimentation rate, etc. The term 'habitual hyperthermia' has been applied in such cases. The important thing is to recognize this entity, reassure the patient, and counsel against endless attempts to determine the cause of 'fever'.

Diagnostic approach to patients with prolonged pyrexia of uncertain origin.

It is assumed that patients will not be considered as belonging in this category until the more-or-less routine tests carried out on all patients admitted to a general hospital have been completed. They include blood count, urinalysis, blood culture, the usual battery of blood chemistry tests, and chest X-ray. Assuming that they have not yielded helpful information, the question is how to proceed to determine the cause of the patient's continued temperature elevation. The number of kinds of disease that have to be considered is sufficient that a routine systematic study is not justified. Special diagnostic procedures must be carried out based on clues provided by careful observation and study of the clinical picture. The achievement of correct diagnosis demands all the faculties of the good physician: factual knowledge, tenacity, and willingness to spend time on the problem.

Stress should be laid on the need to repeat examinations done during the first day or two of the study. Too often a consultant scores, simply because he or she asks questions, or finds something on physical examination, that was not asked about or looked for initially. Sitting down and talking with the patient in an unhurried manner is perhaps the most important of all. In no group of diseases are we more likely to confirm Trotter's famous dictum: 'Disease often tells its secrets in a casual parenthesis . . .'

Foreign travel, contact with pets or domestic animals, occasional bouts of mild diarrhoea, a non-prescription drug for headache or constipation, a previous attack of pleurisy—all these are worth special inquiry. But even more important is to let the patient talk, and to listen carefully.

The physical examination must be done again and again with care, searching for appearance of the skin lesions, lymph node enlargement (special attention to the retroclavicular area), an enlarging spleen or liver, and repetition of the rectal and vaginal examinations. As already mentioned, a consultant may find something on physical examination simply because the primary doctor had not repeated the procedure.

Naturally, thoughts about the likelihood of various possibilities will be influenced substantially by the age and sex of the patient. One does not look for cranial arteritis and polymalgia in people under 50 years of age, and in people over 50 years of age one tends to give greater weight to the possibility of neoplasm. One searches more carefully for evidence of endocarditis in people with cardiac valvular anomalies. In young adults special attention is given to the possibility of venereally acquired infection.

A very high neutrophil count, more than 25 000, should suggest the possibility of occult neoplasm. A high eosinophil count can be accepted as strong evidence against presence of infection by any class of agent except the metazoan parasites.

The diagnosis of fungus infection, neoplastic disease, and immunogenic disorders can often be made only by the use of special tests, or by biopsy of tissues. It is more or less routine to test for rheumatoid factor, anti-nuclear antibody, and antistreptolysin if there is a suspicion of immunogenic disease.

Witholding of drug ingestion can sometimes solve the mystery of unexplained pyrexia. If the patient is receiving several drugs, and if there are good indications for their use, it may be advisable to discontinue one at a time, waiting 48 to 72 hours after each one, to see whether the pyrexia has abated.

Since the cause of many puzzling pyrexias lies within the abdominal cavity, special attention, not only in the history and physical examination, but in other diagnostic procedures, must be given to this part of the body. This may include barium studies of the gastrointestinal tract, intravenous pyelogram, scans of the liver, spleen, and kidneys, and use of ultrasound and CT imaging of this region.

Needle biopsy of the liver may yield handsome dividends in the diagnosis of tuberculosis, granulomatous hepatitis, or neoplastic disease. It is particularly likely to be helpful when liver function tests are deranged, especially when the alkaline phosphatase level is elevated; nevertheless, such diagnoses as metastatic malignancy and granulomatous hepatitis have been achieved by this procedure in patients whose liver function tests fell within the normal ranges.

At times, with the availability of superb diagnostic aids such as CT scanning and ultrasound, there is a tendency to defer exploratory laparotomy. Yet this procedure may be thoroughly justified if the history and physical findings point to presence of intra-abdominal disease, even without foreknowledge of its exact site.

A large proportion of all diseases causing prolonged obscure fever can now be treated or palliated, and a search for the correct diagnosis should continue stubbornly, though not mindlessly, until the process has either subsided spontaneously or the diagnosis is clear. At times, however, it is good practice to discontinue the diagnostic search for a period, allowing the patient to spend some time at home. During the interval, new symptoms or new findings may have developed which will point to the correct diagnosis.

References

Bernheim, H. A., Block, L. H., and Atkins, E. (1979). Fever: pathogenesis, pathophysiology, and purpose. *Ann. intern. Med.* **91**, 261.

Bujak, J. S., Aptekar, R. G., Decker, J. L., and Wolff, S. M. (1973). Juvenile rheumatoid arthritis presenting in the adult as fever of unknown origin. *Medicine* **52**, 431.

Jacoby, G. A. and Swartz, M. N. (1973). Fever of undetermined origin. *New. Engl. J. Med.* **289**, 1407.

Klastersky, J., Weerts, D., Hensgens, C., and Debusscher, L. (1973). Fever of unexplained origin in patients with cancer. *Eur. J. Cancer* **9**, 649.

Petersdorf, R. G. and Beeson, P. B. (1961). Fever of unexplained origin: report on 100 cases. *Medicine, Baltimore* **40**, 1.

Rumans, L. W. and Vosti, K. L. (1978). Factitious and fraudulent fever. *Am. J. Med.* **65**, 745.

Simon, H. B. and Wolff, S. M. (1973). Granulomatous hepatitis and prolonged fever of unknown origin: a study of 13 patients. *Medicine, Baltimore* **52**, 1.

SEPTICAEMIA

P. A. Murphy

Septicaemia is not a term which is easy to define precisely. It is used to denote those clinical states in which bacteria are present in the bloodstream and give rise to serious systemic symptoms such as fever and shock. It shades on one side into bacteraemia, in which organisms are present in the blood without causing symptoms. On the other side, it shades into pyaemia, when the patient is desperately ill, and multiple abscesses develop under the skin and in various internal organs such as the liver or brain. Septicaemia is an acute condition; most cases of infective endocarditis or miliary tuberculosis would not be included, even though many of the symptoms and signs are the same. Lastly, septicaemia has a connotation of urgency; unless the right things are done quickly, the patient is likely to die.

Aetiology. Almost any bacterium known to man may cause septicaemia on occasion. However, some organisms do so regularly in healthy people, while others need considerable assistance even to cause disease in sick people. Anything is possible, but not everything is equally frequent, and useful clinical information can be gained from a consideration of the circumstances under which the septicaemia arose. This matters because the initial therapy must usually be undertaken in the absence of bacteriological information, and it is important to guess right.

All septicaemias start from some kind of infected focus. If that focus is obvious clinically, one regards the septicaemia as 'secondary'. Finding the focus is important for several reasons. If Gram stains of pus, sputum, urine, and so forth are positive, that provides early information about the species probably responsible for sepsis. Even if stained smears are not helpful, the site of primary infection enables one to make a better guess at the aetiology of sepsis. Removal or drainage of the focus will go a long way towards curing the septicaemia. In fact, if an undrained focus of infection is allowed to persist, the patient will probably remain septicaemic even though the organisms in the abscess and the bloodstream are completely susceptible to the antibiotics being used. Such patients generally die. Lastly, if a focus really cannot be found, that influences both the intensity and duration of therapy. With Gram-negative rods, one would be reassured, and treat for five to seven days. With *Staphylococcus aureus*, one would assume that the patient probably had endocarditis, and would treat for at least four weeks. This may sound curious, but is based on the fact that Gram-negative endocarditis is rare, and need not be considered in the absence of compelling clinical evidence. On the other hand, about half of patients with staphylococcal sepsis and no evident focus prove eventually to have endocarditis.

Almost any organism may cause a secondary septicaemia. Some are high grade pathogens such as the pneumococcus, following its usual path of nasopharyngeal colonization to pneumonia to sepsis. At the other end of the spectrum are organisms such as *Pseudomonas thomasii*, which causes disease only if it is allowed to grow in intravenous fluids, and then is infused into the patient. The essence of secondary septicaemia is that some circumstance allows the generation of a large local population of organisms, which may be virulent, but do not have to be. From the local lesion, organisms are fed into the bloodstream.

'Primary' septicaemias are those without a clinically obvious focus of infection. Of course, there always is a portal of entry, but it may be subtle. Meningococcal nasopharyngitis, trivial staphylococcal folliculitis, or the intestinal ulcers which develop in people on chemotherapy are examples. Since there is no large local population, the organisms have to be capable of maintaining themselves in the bloodstream. In one kind of primary septicaemia, high-grade capsulated extracellular pathogens infect reasonably normal people. In the other kind, organisms of low virulence invade persons whose defences have been abrogated by disease or its treatment.

Primary septicaemia acquired in the community. Most patients in this class are not in the best of health. They are old, alcoholic, malnourished, or suffer from various debilitating diseases such as cirrhosis or diabetes. Nonetheless, they have some defenses, and a relatively few organisms cause most of the septicaemias (Table 1). This list refers to adults: a paediatric list would be headed by the pneumococcus and *H. influenzae*, and a neonatal one by Gram-negative rods and group B streptococci. The list is in approximate order of frequency for times when salmonellae and meningococci are not epidemic. The pneumoccocus is third on the list only because the pneumonia is generally apparent in adults with pneumococcal sepsis. Noteworthy is the position of the Gram-negative rods so common in hospitals: if there is no urinary tract infection or other local pathology, these are rare causes of sepsis acquired outside hospital. Primary fungal septicaemia in patients outside hospital is virtually unheard of.

Table 1   The common causes of community-acquired 'primary' septicaemia in adults

Neisseria gonorrohoeae
Staphylococcus aureus
Streptococcus pneumoniae
Streptococcus pyogenes, Groups A–T
Non-typhoidal salmonellae
Streptococcus faecalis
Neisseria meningitidis
Listeria monocytogenes
Escherischia coli, pseudomonas, etc.

Gonococcal septicaemia is common in young people, but is usually mild and subacute. Septicaemia with shock acquired in the community by a healthy young person is a great rarity. One should think of infection with unusual, very virulent organisms such as those of plague, anthrax, and tularaemia. If these can be ruled out, then the most likely culprits are *Staph. aureus* and the meningococcus. Persons who inject themselves with illegal drugs frequently develop acute infective endocarditis, which may be right-sided and difficult to diagnose. The most common cause is *Staph. aureus*, followed by yeasts, pseudomonas, and serratia.

Community-acquired septicaemia with a local focus. Common foci for the origin of sepsis are listed in Table 2, along with the classes of organisms most likely to be responsible. Well over half of urinary tract infections are caused by *Escherischia coli*, and most of the rest by other aerobic Gram-negative rods. A Gram stain of the spun urinary sediment is a reliable guide to those few cases where enterococci or *Staph. aureus* are responsible.

Skin ulcers and areas of cellulitis generally have a mixed Gram-positive flora of staphylococci and streptococci. Lesions around the perineum may be contaminated by aerobic Gram-negative rods. However, if there is frank cellulitis of the perineum, or a decubitus ulcer, anaerobes such as *Bacteroides fragilis* are the only organisms present in the blood stream in half the cases, and are one component of the mixture in the others. One should never forget that *Clostridium perfringens* is normal human faecal flora and may also cause buttock cellulitis. The skin often shows haemorrhagic blebs, and Gram stains of exudate show large Gram-positive rods. The ischaemic or diabetic foot is usually infected with a mixed flora dominated by anaerobes.

Table 2   Common sites from which septicaemia arises in relatively normal patients

Site	Likely bacterial causes of sepsis
Urine	aerobic Gram-negative rods (90%)
	aerobic Gram-positive cocci (10%)
Skin	Gram-positive cocci
Respiratory	*Streptococcus pneumoniae*
Abdominal	
Gall bladder	aerobic Gram-negative rods, *Str. faecalis*
Bowel perforations	aerobic Gram-negative rods
Pelvic inflammatory disease	*Neisseria gonorrhoeae*
	mixed anaerobes

When pneumonia is the obvious focus, and the patient has not been treated with antibiotics, the pneumococcus is the most frequent cause. Klebsiella pneumonia may occur primarily in alcoholics; most other Gram-negative rod pneumonias occur in patients with bronchitis who have received tetracycline or other antibiotics. Staphylococcal pneumonia is commonest as a complication of influenza. Both staphylococcal and Gram-negative rod pneumonias are easily diagnosed on Gram stain, and neither commonly causes a lobar infiltrate. Occasionally *Haemophilus influenzae* causes pneumonia and septicaemia in an adult, and another organism seen from time to time is acinetobacter. In both cases, sputum Gram stains show Gram-negative cocco-bacilli.

If the respiratory focus is a nasal sinus or the middle ear, more organisms need to be considered. Acute otitis media is a rare disease in adults; the most usual causes are the pneumococcus, and other streptococci, and spread to the bloodstream is exceptional. Acute sinusitis is very common in adults; again the pneumococcus is the most usual cause and again septicaemia is rare. Much more likely as causes of sepsis are chronic otitis media and chronic sinusitis. Complications such as cholesteatomas and infective necrosis of bone are usually present, and the sepsis is precipitated by invasion and thrombosis of one of the cerebral venous sinuses. The bacterial flora is usually mixed anaerobes, and the most likely aerobes are staphylococci and Gram-negative rods.

Abdominal catastrophes usually present as such. However, cholecystitis can be completely silent, especially in an old person, and may give rise to septicaemia with Gram-negative rods or enterococci. Similarly, diverticulitis or appendicitis in an old person may cause few local symptoms. Despite the very large numbers of anaerobes in colonic contents, the organisms in the blood stream are usually Gram-negative aerobic rods. However, if the patient has an abscess, bacteroides or other anaerobes may cause septicaemia.

Young women may acquire septicaemia because of pelvic inflammatory disease. Gonorrohea is probably the most frequent single cause. Infected abortions are now uncommon, but infections of intra-uterine devices are quite frequent. Post-partum infections due to retained products of conception are also seen. Most pelvic infections cause septicaemia with *E. coli* or anaerobic cocci. Often several organisms infect the bloodstream simultaneously.

Septicaemia in hospitalized patients. Septicaemia in patients in the hospital is no different in principle from sepsis in the community. However, it is vastly more frequent, for a number of reasons. The most important reasons from the diagnostic point of view are the portals of entry for organisms which are provided by surgical wounds, urinary and vascular catheters, and the other impedimenta of modern medicine. General factors such as old age, steroid treatment, or diabetes make it more likely that patients will get septicaemia but do not greatly influence the route. However, patients with severe neutropenia are so susceptible to infection that bacteria may invade from trivial local lesions, or from no visible lesion at all.

The commonest focus of infection is the urinary tract; it is estimated that 10 per cent of all hospitalized patients have an indwelling urinary catheter, and that even with the best care, 25 per cent of those will be infected by the fourteenth day. The commonest organism is still *E. coli*, but because of the strong selective pressure of antibiotics, it now causes only one third of cases. Other Gram-negative rods such as klebsiella, proteus, serratia, and pseudomonas account for most of the remaining cases, and the enterococcus is the most common Gram-positive species. In forming an opinion of the likely cause in any particular patient, there are two main considerations. First, if the patient's urine is known to be infected with, say, *Enterobacter cloacae*, then that organism is the most likely cause of the sepsis. Secondly, in most hospitals particular organisms are troublesome on particular wards at particular times. If it is known that three patients on a particular urology ward developed septicaemia with *Serratia marcescens* in the last 10 days, then when a fourth patient on that ward develops sepsis, *S. marcescens* is probably the culprit.

The next most common source of sepsis is probably the surgical wound. Included in this category are deep-seated processes such as mediastinitis, leaking intestinal anastomoses, vaginal cuff infections, and infections of the renal transplant bed. In any of these, there may be no evidence of infection in the surface incision. If the patient has recently had an operation, one should be very loathe to consider any other source of sepsis. The bacteria likely to be responsible vary with the site of the incision; one expects *Staph. aureus* after cranial surgery, and *E. coli* or mixed anaerobes after a gynaecological operation.

Intravenous line sepsis is rare if the device has been in place less than 24 hours, and is uncommon before 48 hours. Lines maintained for long periods, such as hyperalimentation lines, inevitably become infected unless cared for by special teams. The most troublesome area for line sepsis in most hospitals is the intensive care unit. It is not uncommon for a patient to have a peripheral line, a central line, a Swan–Ganz catheter, and an arterial line, all inserted in haste under conditions of dubious sterility, and all maintained for several days.

There are several distinct types of intravenous line sepsis. Sometimes the infusion fluid is contaminated, especially if additives have been necessary. In bottles containing glucose as the only nutrient, the organism is almost always klebsiella, enterobacter, or serratia, since these organisms can grow fairly well in such solutions. Hyperalimentation solutions support the growth of yeasts such as *Candida albicans* and *Torulopsis glabrata*.

In other types, the fluid is sterile, but there is cellulitis of the puncture wound, infection of the plastic catheter, or septic thrombophlebitis. The risk of septicaemia from a peripheral line is highest for cutdowns, and least for steel needles (Table 3). *Staph. aureus* accounts for about a third of cases with a demonstrated cause; most of the remaining cases are due to *Staph. epidermidis*, klebsiella, pseudomonas, and *Candida albicans* in roughly equal proportions.

A very common source of sepsis in patients in hospital is the chest. Some cases have straightforward illnesses such as post-influenzal pneumococcal pneumonia, which are entirely analogous to the same diseases developing in the community. Most cases, however, develop in patients who aspirate pharyngeal contents for one reason or another. Many are weak or obtunded, others have had abdominal operations and are recumbent with nasogastric

tubes in place. Nosocomial pneumonia is particularly frequent in patients on respirators. Most such patients have been treated with antibiotics, and pneumonia with septicaemia is almost always caused by aerobic Gram-negative rods.

Table 3   Incidence of intravenous line sepsis with various devices

Device	Incidence of sepsis (%)
Hyperalimentation line	12
Cutdowns	6.5
Subclavian plastic cannula	3.8
Peripheral plastic cannula	0.5
Steel needle	0.2

Modified from Rhame, Maki, and Bennet (1979)

On obstetric and gynaecological wards, sepsis is usually associated with infection of the pregnant or recently pregnant uterine cavity. Attempts to induce abortion by intra-ammiotic injections of urea or saline, prolonged labour with ruptured membranes, or the retention of products of conception are the usual predisposing factors. The most dangerous organism is the group A *Streptococcus pyogenes*, but this has become rare. Most cases now are caused by other streptococci, including Group B, viridans, and enterococcal strains, anaerobic cocci, and aerobic Gram-negative rods such as *E. coli*, klebsiella, and proteus. Serratia and pseudomonas are very uncommon; *Bacteroides fragilis* is a major pathogen occasionally.

Burned patients are very susceptible to septicaemia because the dead skin rapidly becomes colonized with bacteria, often in concentrations of 10^8 organisms per gram. The organism causing septicaemia is almost always that most prominent in the burn at the time, and on good burn units this information is available. There is a predictable progression in the species of organism which colonize the burn. In the first week after injury, sepsis is usually caused by Gram-positive cocci. Later, Gram-negative rods such as pseudomonas or *Providencia stuartii* cause most cases. If the burn remains unhealed for weeks, *Candida albicans* and other yeasts may take over.

A very important patient population is those who do not have normal defences against infection. By far the most important defect is the lack of mature neutrophils; septicaemia becomes progressively more common as the absolute neutrophil count falls below 1000 per mm³. Such patients are susceptible to all the usual hospital acquired infections, but in addition are constantly in danger of being overwhelmed by their own flora. They often have several episodes of septicaemia. The initial ones are generally caused by organisms such as *E. coli* and klebsiella which are normal enteric flora. Antibiotics select out resistant organisms, and subsequent episodes are due to organisms such as enterobacter or pseudomonas which are rarely found in the faeces of normal people. Fungaemias due to candida species or to *Torulopsis glabrata* also become common. At all stages of the illness, 10–20 per cent of septicaemias are caused by Gram-positive species such as *Staph. aureus*.

Prevention of septicaemia. Septicaemia is a dangerous illness, with an appreciable mortality even in fundamentally healthy people. We have no control over cases arising in the community, but most of the cases arising in hospital are preventable. Infection control is humdrum, devoid of excitement, and essential. It is best not left to physicians, since few of them are temperamentally suited to carry it out. However, physicians should be made to follow the rules. They must not take down septic wound dressings with bare hands and move to the next patient without washing. They must not irrigate urinary catheters in 30 seconds between other commitments. They must not be allowed to flout the rules about isolation of infected patients. Every study ever done has shown that physicians ignore protocol far more often than nurses or other personnel. Physicians can make a major contribution to infection control by reducing the number of invasive procedures used, and especially by restricting their duration. Surgeons can contribute by following the fundamental principles of surgery in clean procedures, and by the proper use of drains and antibiotics when infection is probable. If it is known that a patient will be aplastic for some time, the incidence of septicaemia can be reduced somewhat by protective isolation coupled with the use of oral antibiotics to reduce the populations of bowel flora.

Clinical features. Sepicaemia is one of the very few clinical situations in which the patient can give little useful information. He may complain of fever, rigors, or headache, may simply feel awful, or may be too obtunded to complain of anything. Frequently, septicaemia develops in a patient already gravely ill from some other process, and incapable of communicating with his attendants. The responsibility therefore rests squarely on the doctor.

Septicaemia should be suspected whenever there is an acute change in the patient's condition. Almost all patients develop some fever, and those in reasonably good condition usually exceed 39 °C. Failure to develop a temperature greater than 37.6 °C is a bad prognostic sign and patients whose body temperature stays subnormal virtually all die. Chills and rigors simply mean that the temperature is rising rapidly, they have no independent significance, and the number of rigors gives no clue to the organism.

If the patient is closely observed, certain signs may be seen even before fever. Unexplained apprehension, lethargy, and clouding of consciousness are commonly noticed by alert relatives or nurses. Tachypnoea and respiratory alkalosis is another early sign. Occasionally, someone will notice that the patients hands are unusually warm.

Hypotension usually follows fever, but if a large number of organisms has been suddenly introduced into the circulation, it may be the initial sign. As judged by microscopic observation of the circulation in animals, sepsis initially causes a shunting of blood away from the true capillaries through arteriovenous anastomoses. Later, blood is re-admitted to the capillaries, but plasma leaks out through their walls, the lumina are blocked with masses of sludged red cells, and flow is not restored. In man there may be a phase of 'warm shock' early in sepsis in which the cardiac output is raised and the peripheral resistance is low. Presumably this corresponds to the arteriovenous shunting phase described above. Most patients are pale, cold, and clammy by the time they come under observation, with an elevated peripheral resistance.

Haemodynamic measurements in cold, clammy patients make it perfectly clear that the major cause of the hypotension is loss of fluid from the circulation. The cardiac output is initially elevated, and remains elevated or normal till late in the disease. Cardiac failure does occur terminally and the output drops below normal, but that is pretty clearly secondary to anoxia and acidosis. The central venous pressure is normal or low throughout.

The pulmonary vascular resistance is persistently elevated, and very early on the arterial oxygen tension becomes subnormal. At least some of this pulmonary vascular dysfunction is due to obstruction of vessels with microthrombi; much of the rest appears to be due to leaky pulmonary capillaries. Severe forms of pulmonary dysfunction are associated with gross hypoxaemia, visible infiltrates on chest X-rays, and other features of the adult respiratory distress syndrome. There is also disorder of the microcirculation in non-pulmonary tissues; the oxygen consumption is subnormal from the outset, and becomes grossly so terminally. However, the mixed venous P_{O_2} is generally normal, so tissues are failing to take advantage of what oxygen is available.

If the patient is already severely ill, septicaemia may present as unexplained deterioration. Bleeding, thrombocytopenia, or leucocytosis may be noticed. Leucopenia may also occur if the patient's marrow reserves of neutrophils become exhausted. Oliguria or anuria, jaundice, or cardiac failure, may follow inadequate perfusion of those organs. Organic psychoses of many varieties may occur for the same reason. Some cases present with ecthyma gangrenosum or other skin lesions. One case was discovered because a house physician noticed an anion gap which turned out to be secondary to lactic acidosis.

Management. The essentials in the management of septicaemia are to cut off the inflow of organisms to the bloodstream, to kill or inhibit those already there, and to restore the perfusion of vital organs. All other considerations are secondary, and time should not be wasted on them initially. Bleeding, delirium, pulmonary and renal failure will generally take care of themselves if the essentials have been achieved. Operationally, the initial steps are the removal or drainage of the source of sepsis if that is possible, the selection of a suitable antibiotic or antibiotics, and the infusion of large quantities of fluid intravenously.

Clinical assessment. The experienced clinician makes a gestalt assessment of the severity of the patient's state, taking many factors into consideration, often unconsciously. The bedside chart shows the height of the fever and the speed of its rise. The pulse rate and blood pressure are measured if not charted. A look at the patient from the foot of the bed may show apathy, clouding of consciousness, or tachypnoea. Other associated findings may include skin rashes or jaundice. A rapid search for the source of the infection follows. In a patient from outside the hospital, one looks for signs of cutaneous ulcers, pneumonia, local or generalized peritonitis, pyelonephritis, and pelvic inflammatory disease. In a patient already in the hospital, one thinks first of intravascular catheters and monitoring devices, urinary catheters, surgical wounds and deep infections of recent operative sites, pneumonia, and decubitus ulcers. Parenthetically, one should not forget common non-infectious problems such as drug reactions and pulmonary emboli. This rapid assessment should take no more than 30 minutes. A tentative diagnosis is made, together with a guess at the responsible organism. The most useful diagnostic specimens are taken for culture; these will always include two blood cultures, together with urine, sputum, CSF, etc. as appropriate. Treatment must be started immediately. X-rays, sonograms, CT scans, and other time-wasting investigations should be deferred until the patient's condition stabilizes.

Differential diagnosis. There is a very large number of causes of fever, and if there is no evidence of shock it may be reasonable to consider drug reactions, viral infections, and various other non-urgent diagnoses, even to the point of deferring treatment. But the more acute the onset of fever, the higher the value it reaches, and the sicker the appearance of the patient, the more likely is it that bacteria are in the bloodstream. Treatment should not be delayed, unless bacterial sepsis is thought to be an improbable explanation of the patient's state. Even then, the patient should be closely observed for evidence of deterioration until the situation clarifies. If the patient is neutropenic, there is no case for delay. It is true that only about half of the febrile episodes occurring in neutropenic patients can be shown to be due to bacterial infection. But untreated sepsis in such patients is generally fatal within 24 hours.

If the patient suddenly develops both fever and shock, he should be treated for septicaemia unless there is clear evidence of some other cause. One can imagine circumstances where pulmonary embolism or myocardial infarction might present in this way. Intraperitoneal or retroperitoneal bleeding, or even bleeding into the gastrointestinal tract might cause confusion. But the shock must be treated in any event, and two days of antibiotic therapy is unlikely to be harmful. If one attempts to be always correct in urgent situations, the likely result is that patients will deteriorate irreversibly while time is frittered away.

Antibiotic selection. It is important not to waste too much time on this. Most organisms are somewhat sensitive to most antibiotics. Even in leukaemic patients, antibiotic regimes which are theoretically unsuitable for the organism which eventually grows out of the bloodstream, often lead to clinical improvement. It is better to do anything than to do nothing.

The initial choice is made by a judicious appraisal of the information available. If the focus of infection is known, the nature and antibiotic sensitivity of the probable cause may also be known. Patients generally become septicaemic with the organism which is most prominent in the urine, sputum, burn, wound, etc. Neutropenic patients often become septic with the most prominent organism in the faeces. Data on the organisms colonizing the patient is most useful for predicting antibiotic resistance; for example, if the pseudomonas in the burn is resistant to gentamicin, it would be logical to use amikacin in the initial treatment of sepsis. However, one should not neglect to cover other possibilities just because a patient is known to be colonized.

If no such information is available, or if the patient is from outside the hospital, one attempts to cover the most likely bacterial flora. A young woman with non-gonococcal pelvic inflammatory disease will probably respond to penicillin or ampicillin, plus kanamycin. An old man with an ischaemic foot should receive cloxacillin to cover *Staph. aureus* and an aminoglycoside to cover Gram-negative rods. He may well have anaerobes in his blood, but they will probably be peptococci or peptostreptococci, and while cloxacillin is not ideal, it will do for the present. A boy with a ruptured appendix had best receive cefoxitin until more information is available. Ampicillin alone might be adequate for a housewife septic from a urinary source.

If one has absolutely no idea, one uses a combination of a penicillin-like drug and an aminoglycoside. In a neutropenic or burned patient there is a reasonable probability of pseudomonas, and one should use carbenicillin or ticarcillin with gentamicin, tobramycin, or amikacin. The choice would be influenced by knowledge of the antibiotic sensitivities of the local Gram-negative rods. For other patients, cefamandole plus gentamicin would probably be adequate. A previously healthy young person with overwhelming sepsis should be given penicillin G as well as a cephalosporin and gentamicin because neither of the two latter drugs penetrates the meninges well, and the meningococcus is a real possibility.

A few treatable organisms are completely resistant to cephalosporins and aminoglycosides. Rickettsiae can cause septic shock, and both typhus and Rocky Mountain Spotted Fever should be thought of in the right parts of the world. Occasionally, psittacosis presents with very high fever and few or no pulmonary signs. Chlamydial and rickettsial infections respond to tetracycline. Malaria should be specifically excluded by the examination of blood smears if it is conceivable that the patient might have acquired it by any route, including transfusion. *Candida albicans* can cause intravenous line sepsis in normal patients or septicaemia in debilitated ones. Fungal sepsis is seldom immediately lethal, and most oncology units do not treat for it in the first instance, particularly since amphotericin B is so toxic. Viral haemorrhagic fevers are not treatable with antibiotics. However, if the patient has been to Africa, or works with monkeys, they are worth remembering because several of them pose an infection hazard to the attendants.

Whatever antibiotic regime is chosen, it should be given intravenously in large doses. There is no place for half measures in the treatment of septicaemia.

Intravenous fluid therapy. A large bore intravenous line should be inserted as soon as possible. Through it one gives fluid until the patient improves, or until there is evidence of fluid overload. Under most circumstances, when the patient is not desperately ill, this process can be monitored by ordinary clinical methods. The pulse rate, blood pressure, and respiratory rate should be measured and recorded at regular intervals. In most patients it is best to catheterize the urinary bladder to provide accurate information about urine flow. One watches the jugular veins and regularly listens for crepitations at the lung bases.

A good starting dose of fluid would be 1 litre of 0.15M sodium chloride in the first hour. If marked hypotension is present, it could be given faster and rapidly followed by a second litre. One would then reassess the patient. If the blood pressure has risen to normal, the pulse has slowed somewhat, respiration is no faster, the patient is alert and oriented, and urine flow exceeds 75 ml per hour, well and good. One would slow the rate of fluid administration to perhaps 1 litre every six hours and await events.

If the patient remains hypotensive and there is no evidence of fluid overload, more fluid should be given. It would be reasonable to correct any obvious electrolyte abnormalities, especially acidosis. It would also be reasonable to give plasma or albumin in the hope that more fluid would be retained in the vascular system. Whole blood would be appropriate if the patient were severely anaemic. The arterial oxygen should be measured, and if there is substantial desaturation while the patient breathes room air, supplemental oxygen should be given by whatever means is available.

If the patient fails to respond to simple management, or is desperately ill to start with, the full resources of an intensive care unit should be used if available. One can install a central venous catheter, a Swan–Ganz catheter, and a radial artery catheter. The arterial, central venous, and pulmonary capillary wedge pressures should be regularly monitored, and regular samples of arterial blood for pH, oxygen and carbon dioxide, and venous blood for electrolytes should be taken. The cardiac output should be measured from time to time using dye dilution or radioisotopic methods. If the patient's respiratory function is unsatisfactory, intubate the trachea and supply room air enriched with oxygen, varying the Fi_{O_2}, the tidal volume, the end-expiratory pressure and the respiratory rate, as appropriate. A urinary catheter is installed to measure hourly urine flow.

With all this equipment, fluid therapy can be much more aggressive. Fluid is given until the cardiac output plateaus or the pulmonary capillary wedge pressure exceeds 18 mmHg. If pulmonary oedema develops, the end-expiratory airway pressure is increased cautiously until the oedema goes away. There are conflicting opinions about the use of albumin; the oedema often improves temporarily, but since the pulmonary capillaries are leaky, much of the albumin may pass into the alveoli and the pulmonary oedema may recur later.

Steroids. Adrenocorticosteroids clearly protect animals from endotoxin poisoning. Also, steroids plus antibiotics have sometimes been shown to allow animals infected with Gram-negative rods to survive when antibiotics alone were ineffective. In man, there are many uncontrolled studies which suggest that very large doses of steroids may be helpful in bacterial shock, and there is at least one controlled study which says the same thing. This study has been heavily criticized, but no-one has shown that steroids are harmful, and the animal data is well controlled. Pending further information, it seems reasonable to give patients with septicaemia and shock one dose of 30 mg/kg of methylprednisolone at the outset, and to repeat that dose after four hours if hypotension continues. There is no evidence which suggests that continuing adrenal steroids beyond four hours would be useful.

Vasoconstrictor and inotropic drugs. These drugs should only be considered when the patient has been given antibiotics and steroids, and has failed to respond to maximum fluid repletion. Acidosis and anoxia should also have been corrected as far as possible. It is usually wise to give bicarbonate until the plasma pH is 7.2 or 7.3, rather than attempt a total correction. As regards anoxia, any arterial oxygen tension over 60 mmHg is adequate, and frequently one must accept less. If the patient is hypotensive but tissue perfusion is adequate as judged by urine flow and cerebral function, vasoconstrictors are unnecessary. However, if the patient remains in shock, they should be used.

There is general agreement that dopamine is greatly superior to strong general vasoconstrictors such as norepinephrine. Dopamine has substantial inotropic activity at doses between 2 and 10 µg/kg/min, and even at doses of 1–2 µg/kg/min, it causes vasodilatation in the cerebral, coronary, and renal vascular beds. Providing there has been adequate volume replacement, dopamine improves the cardiac output and raises the blood pressure while greatly increasing blood flow to vital areas. It seems probable that this is useful, though no controlled studies are available. It is usual to start at 5 µg/kg/min and increase the rate until a satisfactory response is obtained or the maximum of 50 µg/kg/min is reached. Beyond 20 µg/kg/min dopamine acts as a powerful general vasconstrictor, and while the blood pressure may rise temporarily, the patient generally dies.

Other measures for circulatory support. Patients who have not responded to all the above measures are usually in irreversible shock and rapidly go on to die. Other measures are sometimes used; digoxin and/or calcium to strengthen the heart beat, lidocaine to suppress ventricular arrhythmias, naloxone to antagonize the effects of endorphins. None is of proved benefit.

Removal of septic foci. If a patient in hospital develops septicaemia and no other source is evident, it is advisable to remove all intravascular devices. If they must be replaced, completely new systems should be inserted in vessels far removed from the old sites. If there is evidence of suppurative thrombophlebitis, the affected segment of vein must be removed surgically, or the septicaemia will probably continue.

Localized collections of pus such as empyema or subphrenic abscess should be drained. Foci that are acutely infected but where there is no frank abscess formation are usually left alone in the first instance. Cholecystitis, pneumonia, sinusitis, and pelvic inflammatory disease will all generally respond to antibiotic therapy. If an operation is thought necessary, it can be done later when the patient's condition is stable and the local inflammation has subsided.

Anticoagulation. Disseminated intravascular coagulation is common in Gram-negative sepsis, and also occurs in Gram-positive infections. However, there is no evidence that preventing it by the use of heparin makes any difference to the outcome of sepsis. Antifibrinolytic agents such as E amino caproic acid are contraindicated on theoretical grounds, because if they are used while clotting continues, renal vessels may become seriously obstructed with thrombi. However, heparin therapy is life-saving for septic pelvic thrombophlebitis in women. Antibiotic therapy alone does not cure these patients; they continue to have septic pulmonary emboli, abscesses, and empyemas. The addition of heparin generally leads to cure.

Other supportive measures. Septicaemic patients are usually already gravely ill with some other process. They will need all the usual measures for their underlying condition. They may also develop organ failure because of sepsis. It may be necessary to manage post-operative ileus, epileptic fits, and hepatic, renal, or pulmonary failure.

Prognosis. It is important not to be unreasonably optimistic, particularly when talking to relatives. In all infections, there is a 'point of no return' after which antibiotic therapy ceases to influence the outcome. Even with the best care, many patients die.

The most important single factor is the patient's general condition. The mortality rises with age; most of the excess death are attributable to cardiac and pulmonary problems, and to tumours. The effect of general condition was first shown by McCabe and Jackson (1962) and every study since has confirmed it. The species of organism is of some consequence; *Pseudomonas aeruginosa* consistently causes high mortality, probably because of its exotoxin. Other Gram-negative rods, including bacteroides, cause mortalities in the 25–40 per cent range in most series, and there is little difference between species. Gram-positive sepsis may be overwhelming, but overall the mortality is lower, perhaps 10–20 per cent.

When death is attributable mainly or entirely to infection, it is often due not so much to the septicaemia as to the consequences of infection in the primary site. Extensive pneumonia, meningitis, or widespread intraperitoneal infection may be impossible to deal with, or may lead to such debilitation that the patient expires of the diseases of the bed-ridden—bedsores, pulmonary emboli, and bronchopneumonia.

The presence of shock suggests a large dose of organisms, and not surprisingly, mortality in shocked patients is two or three times that of comparable patients with normal blood pressure. This applies whatever the species of organism. The excess mortality almost always occurs in the first 48 hours, and is directly attributable to septicaemia. A normal or subnormal temperature in the presence of septicaemia is also a very bad prognostic sign.

The effect of antibiotic therapy on prognosis is discernible, but not as great as might be expected. Patients treated with antibiotics to which the organisms are sensitive do survive better than those in whom the initial treatment was not appropriate. However, the general condition and the presence or absence of shock are powerful independent variables.

Septicaemia persisting in the face of therapy. If the patient remains febrile and sick after 48 hours of therapy, a total reassessment should be made. The most important is a complete physical examination looking for infectious foci which might have become apparent since admission. Examination should be detailed, including the fundi, the entire skin surface, and rectal and vaginal examinations. New blood cultures, and cultures of anything else which might be helpful, should be obtained.

If the original blood cultures were positive, and the antibiotic therapy was inappropriate, it should be changed. If the original blood cultures were positive and the organisms were sensitive to the antibiotics employed, then it is probable that the patient has undrained pus somewhere, and search for that should be made by X-rays, sonograms, CT scans, or [111]Indium scans, as seem appropriate. The antibiotic regimen should be reviewed to make certain that the route, frequency, and dosage are adequate; sub-therapeutic doses are particularly common with aminoglycosides and are best excluded by determining blood levels. Neutropenic patients, and those with large infected tissue foci may respond very slowly, even when the antibiotic regime is adequate. In such patients, it may be right to persist with the same therapy provided one is reasonably certain that there are no other adverse factors. If compatible granulocytes are available, they may assist severely neutropenic patients to control their septicaemia.

If the original blood cultures are negative, and the patient remains febrile, the antibiotics should be discontinued, and two new ones substituted. The only exception to this rule is if some acceptable non-infectious cause of the symptoms has declared itself. A search for deep infected foci should be made as outlined above. In neutropenic patients, one should probably add amphotericin B at this stage since candida and other yeasts may take some days to grow out of the original blood cultures.

Failure to respond to two different antibiotic regimes, with no evidence of local sepsis and no response to antifungal drugs suggests that the diagnosis of septicaemia was wrong. Many fevers in hospitalized patients are caused by drug reactions, tumours, or viral infections of diverse types. High spiking fever may persist for months in alcoholic hepatitis. The best way of managing such situations is to withdraw antibiotics while carefully observing the patient, and reculturing as indicated.

References

Altemeier, W. A., Burke, J. F., Pruitt, B. A., and Sandusky, W. R. (eds.) (1976). *Manual on control of infections in surgical patients*. J. B. Lippincott, Philadelphia.

Bodey, G. P., Buckley, M., and Sathe, Y. S. (1966). Quantitative relationships between circulating leukocytes and infection in patients with acute leukemia. *Ann. intern. Med.* **64**, 328.

Corrigan, J. C. and Kiernat, J. F. (1975). Effect of heparin in experimental Gram-negative septicaemia. *J. infect. Dis.* **131**, 138.

Duma, R. J., Weinberg, A. W., Medrek, T. F. and Kung, L. J. (1969). Streptococcal infections: A bacteriologic and clinical study of streptococcal bacteremia. *Medicine, Baltimore* **48**, 87.

Dutcher, J. P., Schiffer, C. A. and Johnston, G. S. (1981). Rapid migration of [111]Indium labelled granulocytes to sites of infection. *New Engl. J. Med.* **304**, 586.

Galpin, J. E., Chow, A. W., Bayer, A. S., and Guze, L. B. (1976). Sepsis associated with decubitus ulcers. *Am. J. Med.* **61**, 346.

Kreger, B. E., Craven, D. E., and McCabe, W. R. (1980). Gram-negative bacteremia. Re-evaluation of clinical features and treatment in 612 patients. *Am. J. Med.* **68**, 344.

Kunin, C. M. (1979). Urinary tract infections. In *Hospital infections* (eds. J. V. Bennett and P. S. Brachman), 239. Little, Brown, Boston.

Ledger, W. J. and Peterson, E. P. (1970). The use of heparin in the management of pelvic thrombophlebitis. *Surg. Gynec. Obstet.* **131**, 1115.

Louie, T. J., Bartlett, J. G., Tally, F. P., and Gorbach, S. L. (1976). Aerobic and anaerobic bacteria in diabetic foot ulcers. *Ann. intern. Med.* **85**, 461.

McKay, D. G. and Müller-Burghaus, G. (1967). Therapeutic implications of disseminated intravascular coagulation. *Am. J. Cardiol.* **20**, 392.

McCabe, W. R. and Jackson, G. G. (1962). Gram-negative bacteremia. Clinical, laboratory and therapeutic observations. *Archs intern. Med.* **110**, 856.

Maki, D. G., Goldman, D. A., and Rhame, F. S. (1973). Infection control in intravenous therapy. *Ann. intern. Med.* **79**, 867.

Monif, G. R. G. and Baer, H. (1976). Polymicrobial bacteremia in obstetric patients. *Obstet. Gynec. N.Y.* **48**, 167.

Nolan, C. M. and Beatty, H. N. (1976). Staphylococcal bacteremia: current clinical patterns. *Am. J. Med.* **60**, 495.

Rhame, F. S., Maki, D. G., and Bennett, J. V. Intravenous cannula-associated infections. In *Hospital infections* (eds. J. V. Bennett and P. S. Brachman), 433. Little, Brown, Boston.

Schumer, W. (1976). Steroids in the treatment of clinical septic shock. *Ann. Surg.* **184**, 333.

Singer, C., Kaplan, M. H., and Armstrong, D. (1977). Bacteremia and fungemia complicating neoplastic disease: A study of 364 cases. *Am. J. Med.* **62**, 731.

Stein, J. M. and Pruitt, B. A. (1970). Suppurative thrombophlebitis. A lethal iatrogenic disease. *New Engl. J. Med.* **282**, 1452.

Weil, M. H. (1977). Current understanding of mechanism and treatment of circulatory shock caused by bacterial infections. *Ann. clin. Res.* **9**, 181.

INFECTION IN THE COMPROMISED HOST

Christopher Bunch

Recent decades have witnessed a significant change in the pattern of infection in hospital patients. The advent of antibiotics has reduced the mortality of many common infections, and in an increasing number of patients, infection is related to underlying impairment of host defences. This has led to the concept of the 'compromised host' in whom a primary disease or its treatment has reduced resistance to infection. Such patients may develop not only those infections to which all are prone, but also 'opportunistic' infections caused by organisms which would normally be considered non-pathogenic.

In general, the risk and severity of infection is proportional to the degree of impairment of host defences. However, environmental factors play an important part in determining the pattern of infection, and it has become increasingly apparent that the hospital environment may be particularly unfriendly in this respect. This is no doubt partly fortuitous in that hospitals attract sick and debilitated patients, but they also encourage dangerous antibiotic-resistant organisms to flourish, and invasive diagnostic and therapeutic procedures afford these pathogens ample access. In this respect, all hospital patients may be compromised to some extent.

The mechanisms of host defence are discussed in detail on page 5.3, and it is not difficult to envisage how their impairment may lead to infection ranging, for example, from a simple catheter-site infection to an overwhelming infection with a normal commensal organism such as *Candida albicans* in a child with severe congenital immune deficiency. The pattern of infection encountered in disorders commonly associated with impaired defences is shown in Table 1, and some of the potential sources of such infection in Table 2. In some instances impaired defences are a direct consequence of a primary underlying disorder, as illustrated by the frequency with which bronchial obstruction by tumour or other lesion is associated with pneumonia. In other instances impairment may be a result of treatment, for example marrow depression produced by cytotoxic drugs given to eradicate malignant cells. In this example, immunosuppression is an unwanted side-effect of treatment, whilst in transplantation, it is quite intentional and is employed, often intensively, to prevent rejection of the transplanted tissue.

Bacterial infections. Bacterial infections occur most commonly in patients whose mechanical barriers are in some way disrupted and in those with phagocytic defects. However, the defences against certain bacteria involve the humoral and/or cell-mediated limbs of the immune response and thus virtually all compromised patients have an increased susceptibility to infection by bacteria. As the vast majority of bacterial infections are potentially curable with antimicrobials, investigation and treatment of possible infective episodes should be undertaken without delay. It is frequently necessary to start antibiotic therapy before the results of bacteriological investigations are known and the choice of antibiotic must be guided by knowledge of the common patterns of infection seen in different clinical situations (Table 1). Patients who become infected in hospital have usually acquired the responsible organisms from the hospital environment, where Gram-negative antibiotic-resistant strains predominate. On the other hand, common Gram-positive organisms such as streptococci, pneumococci, and staphylococci are more commonly responsible for infection acquired in the home environment.

Table 1   Patterns of clinical infection associated with defects in host-defences

Defence mechanism	Clinical examples of deficiency	Pattern of opportunistic infection
Mechanical barriers	various, e.g. penetrating injuries, obstruction of hollow viscus, i.v. cannulation, cytotoxic drugs	various, e.g. abscess formation, pneumonia, empyemia, etc., phlebitis
Phagocytic system	neutropenia	bacterial infections: septicaemia; skin, oral and perineal abscesses, pneumonia. Candidal infections
	impaired neutrophil function	increased incidence of bacterial sepsis; chronic granulomatous disease. Candidal and fungal infections
Humoral immunity*	myeloma, B-cell lymphomas, chronic lymphatic leukaemia	bacterial infections, particularly pneumococcal
Cell-mediated immunity*	Hodgkin's disease, cytotoxic drugs, radiation, tissue transplantation	viral infection, particularly reactivation of herpesviruses; interstitial pneumonia, e.g. CMV, pneumocystis; deep-seated fungal infection; *Mycobacteria*, *Listeria*

* Rarely presented as an isolated defect

Table 2 Sources of infection in immune-compromised patients

Source	Potential pathogens
Air	
Air conditioners, building materials	staphylococci, aspergilli varicella–zoster, Gram-negative bacteria
Water	
Tap water, showers, humidifiers, sinks, toilets, baths and drains, cut flowers	*Pseudomonas* and other Gram-negative bacilli, *Legionella*
Food	
Various, particularly dairy products, salads, cold meats, fruit, etc.	Gram-negative bacilli, staphylococci, streptococci
Invasive procedures	
i.v. therapy and transfusion, urinary catheters, endoscopy	staphylococci, *Candida*, Gram-negative bacilli, CMV, *Toxoplasma*, hepatitis B virus
Personal contact	
Other patients, staff, visitors	staphylococci, streptococci, *Pseudomonas*, *Serratia*, herpesviruses, respiratory viruses
The patient	
Own bacterial flora	*Enterobacteraciae*, staphylococci
Reactivation of latent infection	herpes simplex, varicella–zoster, CMV, tuberculosis, mycotic infection

Note that many infections may be readily contracted from the hospital environment, or hospital organisms may colonize and augment the patients' normal flora
After Pizzo, P. A. (1981). *Am. J. Med.* **70**, 631

Infection associated with phagocytic defects. *Neutropenia.* There is an inverse relationship between the absolute neutrophil count and the risk of bacterial infection (see page 5.3). Infection is usually caused by organisms colonizing the skin or gastrointestinal tract, and this flora is readily modified by antibiotic-resistant organisms from the hospital environment. Organisms particularly associated with infection in neutropenic patients are listed in Table 3. Local infection may occur in the mouth (particularly when there is poor oral hygiene or dentition), the perianal area, skin, or in the lungs. The inflammatory response is deficient as pus cannot form without neutrophils, and thus surgical drainage is not usually appropriate. Fever is often the earliest manifestation of infection in neutropenic patients and may herald a severe and fulminant septicaemia. The management of this important clinical problem is discussed below.

Functional disorders of neutrophils occur in a wide variety of clinical disorders including alcoholism, diabetes mellitus, renal failure, and collagen vascular diseases, but are usually minor and although susceptibility to infection may be increased, it is not usually a significant problem. More serious are the rare inherited neutrophil defects that involve the ability to kill ingested bacteria, and which produce the clinical picture of *chronic granulomatous disease*. These patients are particularly prone to infection with catalase-positive organisms such as staphylococci, serratia, candida, and aspergillus. Catalase-negative organisms such as streptococci and most Gram-negative bacteria are unable to inactivate endogenous peroxides and are killed normally.

Table 3 Bacterial infections in neutropenic patients

Common	Uncommon
Gram-negative	*Salmonella*
Enterobacteriacae	*Haemophilus influenzae*
Pseudomonas	Bacteroides spp.
Klebsiella	*Clostridium perfringens*
Serratia	*Clostridium septicum*
Gram-positive	*Bacteroides cereus*
Stapyhylococci	*Nocardia*
Streptococci, including *Strep. faecalis* and pneumococci	*Listeria monocytogenes*

Tuberculosis. An increased incidence of tuberculosis in patients with Hodgkin's disease has been recognized for many years. This condition is associated with pronounced impairment of cell-mediated immunity and patients are usually unreactive to tuberculin skin testing. Infection is more common in patients with advanced, resistant disease and in the elderly. Less well appreciated is the association between disseminated 'cryptic' miliary tuberculosis or atypical mycobacterial infection with myeloproliferative disorders such as chronic myeloid leukaemia and myelosclerosis. The association is complicated as the haematological changes of miliary tuberculosis may in the presence of fever, malaise, and weight loss, suggest a primary myeloproliferative disorder. The diagnosis of mycobacterial infection may be difficult, and skin tests are usually negative. A trial of antituberculosis therapy may be warranted if a definitive diagnosis cannot be made from sputum examination. In disseminated infection liver biopsy may be of value. Infections due to atypical mycobacteria are often resistant to antituberculosis therapy.

Nocardia infections are more frequent in patients with leukaemia or lymphoma than in the general population. Infection may be confined to the lungs, where it may cause lobar pneumonia, empyema, or multiple abscesses with cavitation. Disseminated infection occurs in about one third of patients producing widespread abscesses, notably in the skin and in the brain. Long-term sulphonamide treatment, 4–8 g daily, is the treatment of choice, although minocycline may be given to patients unable to tolerate sulphonamides. *Listeria monocytogenes* may occasionally be a cause of bacterial meningitis.

Anaerobic organisms. Infections with anaerobic bacteria are uncommon despite great efforts made to isolate these organisms. *Clostridium perfringens* and *C. septicum* septicaemias have occurred in some patients and carry a high mortality. The majority of anaerobic organisms are sensitive to penicillin, with the notable exception of bacteroides which are sensitive to clindamycin and chloramphenicol.

Viral infections. Viral infections occur commonly in patients with impairment of cell-mediated immunity. They are not usually a problem in the presence of a pure phagocytic defect, but in many patients with neutropenia treatment of the underlying condition with cytotoxic drugs affects cell-mediated immune processes and viral infections may result. Common upper respiratory viral infections are no more frequent than in the general population and are not usually serious, although a diagnostic problem may result if associated fever is marked. The most troublesome infections are caused by herpesviruses; these have been described in detail elsewhere (see page 5.49) but relevant details are summarized here.

Herpesvirus infections. Herpesvirus infections in the immunosuppressed may represent reactivation of latent virus or a new infection. Herpes simplex infections are extremely common but fortunately usually localized. The usual manifestation is a typical vesicular eruption or 'cold sore' on the face, or an ulcerating stomatitis. Local lesions may be severe and haemorrhagic, particularly in the presence of thrombocytopenia. Active lesions are contagious, and spread to the staff where the development of painful herpetic whitlows may occur. Dissemination to other sites may occur in the profoundly immunosuppressed but is otherwise uncommon. The diagnosis can be confirmed if necessary by electron microscopy of vesicle fluid followed by culture, and local treatment of isolated lesions with idoxuridine 35 per cent in DMSO is worthwhile if started early. Systemic infections should be treated with vidarabine (adenine arabinoside) or acyclovir.

Varicella–zoster infections have been noted in nearly one half of patients surviving at least six months after marrow transplantation and are fairly common in patients with Hodgkin's disease during therapy. They are seen less commonly in patients with non-Hodgkin's lymphoma unless intensive and prolonged chemotherapy has been employed. In the majority of instances the clinical signs are of typical but severe shingles. Generalized spread (varicella–zoster) occurs in about one third of patients or may occasionally be present at the outset. Localized zoster is caused by reactivation of latent virus which may subsequently disseminate to areas beyond the distribution of the affected nerve. In previously uninfected patients, severe chicken pox (varicella) may occur. Mortality is higher in the immunosuppressed than in the normal population; in marrow transplant recipients the infection is fatal in 8 per cent of affected patients and in 27 per cent of those with varicella. Treatment is discussed on page 5.61 but is only effective if started early. Examination of vesicular fluid under the electron microscope can confirm the presence of a herpesvirus within a few hours; differentiation between zoster and herpes simplex infections, if not possible on clinical grounds, requires culture of the virus. However, when the clinical picture is that of disseminated infection, treatment with vidarabine or acyclovir should not be delayed. Recovery follows the development of specific antibody. Specific immunosuppressive or cytotoxic therapy should be withheld for the duration of the infection.

Cytomegalovirus (CMV) Infections. CMV infection is endemic in the community and specific antibody is demonstrable in a high proportion of the population. Most infections are subclinical, but the virus may produce an illness clinically indistinguishable from infectious mononucleosis. Infection in the immunocompromised host may be due to reactivation of latent virus, or the virus may be newly acquired from blood transfusion or a transplanted organ. Subclinical reactivation occurs in the majority of previously seropositive patients and most moderately immunosuppressed patients shed virus in their urine or saliva at some time. Generalised disease may occur in the severely compromised, and the illness tends to be more severe in previously seronegative patients, when it is a primary infection. It is often difficult to determine whether clinical infection in CMV-seropositive patients is caused by a primary or a secondary infection, unless serum has been stored since before the onset of symptoms. The presence of previous antibody indicates reactivation of latent infection or reinoculation of virus in a previously infected patient. These two possibilities may be distinguished only by typing the virus using restriction enzyme techniques.

The clinical manifestations are varied and range from a mild febrile illness to a rapidly fatal condition with generalized organ involvement affecting particularly the lungs and liver. Interstitial pneumonitis (see below) is a common complication of organ transplantation and has been associated with CMV infection in about one half of cases. The diagnosis of CMV infection can be difficult, especially in seropositive patients who may shed the virus without having a clinically obvious infection. Biopsy, with demonstration of typical inclusions, or culture of the virus remains the mainstay of diagnosis, but the picture is often complicated by the coexistence of other infections. There is no satisfactory treatment for disseminated CMV infection; vidarabine or acyclovir should be tried but the results are often disappointing. In those patients who are CMV seronegative, strenuous efforts should be made to avoid transfusion of fresh blood products from seropositive donors. Indeed this may be a sensible policy for all profoundly immunosuppressed patients irrespective of CMV-antibody status. When feasible, a CMV seronegative organ donor should be chosen for seronegative recipients.

Other viral infections. *Viral hepatitis* is uncommon in immunocompromised patients other than narcotic addicts, except in areas where transmission by blood transfusion is a significant risk. In centres where blood for transfusion is regularly obtained from commercial blood banks employing 'professional' donors, circulating hepatitis B surface antigen (HBsAg) is found in 10–12 per cent of leukaemic patients compared with 0.1 per cent of normals. Antigenaemia may persist for months or years but clinical evidence of liver damage is infrequent, although these patients may be hazardous to others. Outbreaks of hepatitis A, B or non-A, non-B

varieties have occurred in some centres. Compromised patients exposed to hepatitis A should be given pooled immunoglobulin, whilst specific immune globulin is indicated for patients exposed to hepatitis B.

Measles may occur in susceptible patients. The illness may follow a similar course to that in the normal population or it may be severe and fulminating with pneumonitis, nephritis, hepatitis, or encephalitis. Neutropenic patients are particularly at risk from secondary bacterial pneumonia and otitis media, and widespread bleeding may occur in the presence of thrombocytopenia. There is no specific therapy but cytotoxic chemotherapy should be interrupted and hyperimmune gammaglobulin administered to patients at risk who are exposed to infection. Vaccination with live attenuated measles virus is absolutely contra-indicated in immunosuppressed patients.

Rubella, mumps, and influenza are not major hazards but immunosuppressive therapy should be interrupted in patients at risk who are exposed to these infections. Secondary bacterial infections are common following influenza and are more dangerous than the primary infection. For this reason it is advisable to administer killed influenza vaccine to patients at risk each autumn.

Smallpox vaccination should not be performed in immune-compromised patients as there is a serious risk of fatal generalized vaccinia. Furthermore, patients should avoid contact with recently vaccinated persons.

Mycotic infections. Opportunistic fungal and yeast infections are particularly likely to occur when phagocytosis and cell-mediated immunity are severely impaired. They are fortunately uncommon during brief periods of neutropenia but are more troublesome when the defect is severe or prolonged as may occur in aplastic anaemia, following transplantation, or after repeated and intensive courses of chemotherapy for relatively resistant malignant disease. The exact incidence is hard to establish as the diagnosis often has to be made on clinical grounds without microbiological confirmation, but infection has been found in 13–69 per cent of autopsy studies of patients with acute myeloid leukaemia. However, many of these patients died with resistant leukaemia following prolonged periods of drug-induced immunosuppression and such figures probably overestimate the true magnitude of the problem. Nevertheless, as it seems likely that the control of invasive fungal infection depends upon early diagnosis and treatment, a high index of suspicion is essential if treatment is to be effective.

Diagnosis. The definitive diagnosis of deep invasive mycotic infection depends upon the demonstration of the organism in otherwise viable tissue, or its isolation from uncontaminated body fluids other than blood or urine. This almost always implies an invasive diagnostic procedure, the advisability of which may be questioned in ill patients whose underlying disease may itself carry a poor prognosis. Unfortunately the mainstay of treatment—amphotericin B—is at best unpleasant and at worse extremely toxic, so it behoves the physician to consider carefully the implications that a diagnosis, however presumptive, of mycotic infection may have for his patient.

Candidiasis. *Candida* spp., are by far the most common agents responsible for mycotic infection in the immunosuppressed, and they account for at least half such infections in patients with acute leukaemia. *Candida albicans* is an obligate commensal on the skin and gastrointestinal tract, and deep-seated infection may result from direct invasion at sites of injury or follow haematogenous spread to remote tissues. The most common portal of entry is the gastrointestinal tract: oral candidiasis occurs at some time in the majority of patients with acute leukaemia but is usually trivial. Oesophageal invasion is more sinister and presents with retrosternal discomfort and dysphagia; the diagnosis is confirmed by endoscopy and biopsy but may be suggested by typical radiographic appearances after barium swallow. Involvement of other parts of the gastrointestinal tract is difficult to diagnose clinically but is commonly found at autopsy. Disseminated candidiasis must involve haematogenous spread. Candidaemia alone is not necessarily significant, however, in the absence of clinical evidence of deep seated infection, particularly when an indwelling intravenous catheter is *in situ*. Pulmonary involvement may follow aspiration or haematogenous spread. The diagnosis of opportunistic lung infection is discussed below. Endocarditis may be caused by infection of previously damaged, artificial or otherwise normal valves. Embolization is common and peripheral mycotic arterial aneurysms may result.

Aspergillosis. Infection with genus *Aspergillus* accounts for up to one half of invasive fungal infections in the immunosuppressed. Probably any member is capable of producing infection but *A. fumigatus* and *A. flavus* account for the majority. The lungs are most commonly affected although generalized invasion is occasionally seen. Infection most often follows inhalation of spores but activation of endogenous spores may occur, particularly in patients with existing chronic lung disease. Corticosteroids and broad spectrum antibiotic administration may also predispose to infection. Environmental contamination with spores has been a problem in some institutions particularly where pigeons inhabit air conditioning intake ducts or in new buildings where heavily contaminated building materials have been used.

The clinical manifestations are variable but there is commonly evidence of generalized pulmonary infection with fever, cough, tachypnoea, and rales. Radiological changes are often unimpressive unless focal abscess or cavity formation occurs. The diagnosis rests on the demonstration of hyphae in otherwise viable tissue obtained by biopsy, with subsequent confirmation by culture. For practical purposes it may be adequate if the branching organism can be demonstrated in material obtained by percutaneous lung aspiration or less reliably, from the sputum. Disseminated aspergillosis may follow haematogenous spread but blood cultures are useless and serology unhelpful.

Cryptococcosis. Cryptococcosis is caused by invasive infection with *Cryptococcus neoformans*. The disease has a worldwide distribution but the vast majority of cases in the United Kingdom occur in immunosuppressed individuals. There is a particular association with Hodgkin's disease but it is occasionally seen in other heavily immunosuppressed patients. The clinical picture is varied and infection may be confined to the lungs or be disseminated. Meningitis is common and the onset may be insidious with headache, fever, and altered consciousness. Focal neurological signs may be present and small white or yellow retinal lesions are typical. The diagnosis of pulmonary cryptococcal infection requires biopsy but encapsulated yeasts may be demonstrated in India ink-stained preparations of CSF in patients with meningitis. Alternatively, cryptococcal antigen may be detectable in the CSF or serum.

Phycomycosis (mucormycosis). The phycomycoses are caused by invasion of viable tissue with organisms of the genus *Phycomycetes*, particularly *Rhizopus* or *Mucor*. This infection is rare in the United Kingdom but not uncommon in North America. Mucormycosis involving the nasopharynx is particularly associated with diabetes mellitus, and most often involves the lungs in patients with leukaemia or lymphoma. A characteristic feature is invasion of large blood vessels with extensive tissue infarction.

Treatment of mycotic infections. The mainstay of treatment for systemic invasive mycotic infection is amphotericin B. This must be given intravenously but side-effects are common. It is usual to start with a dose of 1 mg in 500 ml of 5 per cent dextrose (not saline) infused over 30 minutes, and to increase the dose gradually by 4–5 mg a day up to 0.6 mg/kg/day. Fever, rigors, nausea, and vomiting are common and generally require symptomatic relief. Nephrotoxicity is a major problem but may be reduced by giving 12.5 g mannitol intravenously before each dose. Renal function should nevertheless be monitored closely. The duration of therapy required to eradicate systemic mycotic infections varies widely and total doses of 1–2 g are not unusual in severe cases.

Flucytosine may be effective in the treatment of some patients with candidiasis or cryptococcosis. Resistance develops commonly, and the drug should thus only be given to those patients whose organism is fully sensitive. Amphotericin should be given concurrently in the presence of severe infection. Toxicity is less and the drug distributes well throughout the tissues including the CSF. An initial dose of 50 mg/kg six-hourly is suitable. It may be given by mouth but in severe infections intravenous administration is preferred.

The imidazoles miconzole, econazole, and ketoconazole are newly available antifungal drugs whose efficacy is severe mycotic infections has yet to be defined. They may be given by mouth or intravenously, and their main indication at present is for patients who are intolerant of amphotericin. Toxicity appears to be minimal and, if effective, these drugs may well replace amphotericin as first-line treatment for severe infections.

Protozoan infections. Protozoan infections have been discussed in detail on pages 5.384–420. The infections most commonly encountered in the immunosuppressed are *toxoplasmosis* and *Pneumocystis carinii pneumonitis*. Toxoplasmosis may present a clinical picture resembling infectious mononucleosis or it may cause more disseminated disease with a predilection for the central nervous system. Diagnosis is made by identification of the organism in lymph node or tissue specimens, CSF, blood or marrow aspirate, or after innoculation of mice with infected material. Serological tests are often useful; the dye test is positive in 20–40 per cent of normal adults in titres between 1:8 and 1:128, but higher titres are suggestive of recent infection and a rising titre is diagnostic.

The diagnosis and management of *Pneumocystis carinii* pneumonia is discussed below and on page 5.399.

Management problems

Fever in the neutropenic patient. Fever is common in patients with neutropenia and should always arouse suspicion of infection, particularly of a bacterial nature. Non-infective causes include underlying disease such as leukaemia or lymphoma, and transfusion or drug reactions. Viral infections may be transmitted by transfusions, reactivated during periods of immunosuppression, or may be contracted in the usual way. Finally, opportunistic yeast or fungal infections may occur when immunosuppression is profound or prolonged and particularly during administration of broad-spectrum antibiotics.

Unfortunately one of the commonest causes of fever in neutropenic patients is a bacterial infection or septicaemia, which may overwhelm the patient within a matter of hours. There is a clear inverse relationship between the absolute neutrophil count and the likelihood of bacterial infection, which becomes increasingly likely with neutrophil counts below 1.0×10^9/l. Urgent investigation and treatment is required and there is little point in trying to be clever diagnostically. There is no doubt that a well-defined protocol for the management of this situation is essential, and most units specializing in the treatment of haematological malignancies employ a similar approach, though details may differ according to the particular pattern of infecting organisms seen by each unit.

Most of bacterial infections are caused by organisms carried by the patient himself on the skin or in the gastrointestinal tract, and the likelihood of infection is obviously increased if these barriers are broken, perhaps as a result of the underlying condition or its treatment. Table 3 shows the commonest organisms producing infections in patients with marrow failure. It is worth remembering that the 'normal' flora is readily supplemented by hospital organisms within a few days of admission; these are usually acquired from hospital food, particularly salads, and may involve multiple antibiotic resistant organisms.

In general, the presence of neutropenia *per se* is not an indication for hospitalization. If the patient is well and has no sign of infection, he or she may be safer at home, but clear instructions should be given to contact the ward *directly* should any symptoms arise, and there should be minimal delay in seeing any patient who becomes ill. If admission for specific or supportive treatment is required, the patient is best nursed in a side ward or at least away from other infected patients. Strict barrier nursing is unnecessary, but a high standard of hygiene should be maintained by the patient and all his attendants. Total isolation in a protected environment with vigorous decontamination of endogenous flora and the provision of a strict diet can reduce the incidence of infection, but does not generally alter the prognosis of the underlying condition and its considerable cost and inconvenience are rarely justified. Similarly, routine bacteriological surveillance (e.g. taking cultures in the absence of clinical signs of infection) is time consuming and unproductive. Efforts should be directed towards obtaining adequate diagnostic samples when the need arises.

Provided that the patient feels well and has no focal or general sign of infection, a temperature of less than 38 °C can be ignored. However, should there by any suspicion of infection, perhaps due to a sudden rise in temperature, a rise above 38 °C or the development of specific symptoms or signs or any other change in clinical condition, a careful physical examination should be performed without delay with particular attention to mouth, throat, venepuncture sites and the perianal area. Rectal examination should be avoided if possible as this may precipitate bacteraemia or perianal sepsis. Bacteriological samples should be taken from suspicious sites, urine and sputum should be examined and cultured, and one or more blood cultures drawn. A chest X-ray should be obtained as pneumonia is common and clinical signs may be absent in the early stages (see below).

At this stage it can be difficult to exclude infection absolutely, but if there are no signs other than fever, and a blood transfusion is in progress, it is probably safe to suspend the transfusion temporarily and to review the situation an hour or two later. In other instances empirical broad-spectrum antibiotic cover should be started without waiting for bacteriological confirmation as rapid clinical deterioration may otherwise occur. The choice of antibiotics should be guided by previous experience and knowledge of the likely organisms (Table 3). In any event a consistent policy should be persued and the use of an aminoglycoside such as gentamicin (2 mg/kg eight-hourly) plus ticarcillin (40–50 mg/kg four-hourly) is recommended. All antibiotics should be given intravenously. A cephalorsporin (e.g. cefuroxime 20 mg/kg eight-hourly) may be included if there is reason to suspect a staphylococcal infection or if past experience on the ward dictates the need for additional cover. It may also be used in place of ticarcillin in patients with a clear history of penicillin allergy. Gentamicin blood levels should be obtained regularly to ensure adequate blood levels but particular care should be exercised in the presence of impaired renal function. A good fluid intake is required, preferably intravenously: large amounts of potassium supplements are often required, occasionally up to 200 mmol/day.

Antibiotic cover may be subsequently modified if indicated by bacteriological cultures. More often than not, however, these are negative, and if this is the case and the fever subsides, there is little point in continuing antibiotics for more than five days as there is an increasing risk of superinfection with resistant organisms. If an organism has been isolated, appropriate antibiotic cover should be continued until recovery from the neutropenia is evident, as the infection may otherwise relapse. If established infection fails to respond to adequate antibiotic therapy within 48 hours, the use of granulocyte transfusions (see Section 19) should be considered. These are most likely to be effective when given daily for at least three days, when obtained from a donor histocompatible with the patient (usually a relative), and when marrow failure is likely to persist for longer than a week but has a good chance of eventual recovery.

The difficult problem not infrequently arises of the patient in whom infection has not been confirmed bacteriologically but whose fever persists despite empirical antibiotic therapy. Other causes of fever should be considered as indicated above, and cultures should be repeated. No firm guidelines can be given and each patient must be managed individually. If bacterial infection is still thought likely, then further antibiotics may be added. However, if this fails to produce a response then all antibiotics should probably be withdrawn for a period to allow further cultures to be taken. It is unusual for any patient to perish from bacterial infection before its nature becomes evident. Fever is occasionally due to a drug reaction and may subside on withdrawal of antibiotics. If it is thought to be due to the underlying disease, then it may respond to specific chemotherapy or to steroids, although it should be remembered that these drugs may produce further immunosuppression. Significant viral infections generally produce specific signs although CMV infections (see above) may produce only fever. Evidence for fungal infection (see above) should be carefully sought, particularly in patients in whom immunosuppression has been prolonged or severe.

Infection following splenectomy. One of the most important roles of the spleen is to remove particulate foreign matter from the bloodstream (see Section 19). Many serious infections such as meningitis, septicaemia, and endocarditis follow the haematogenous spread of a few bacteria, and prompt removal of blood-borne organisms is an important function of the reticulo-endothelial system as a whole, and the spleen in particular. This ability to recognize and remove circulating foreign material is independent of the ability to produce specific antibody, and thus the presence of a normally-functioning spleen is even more critical to the infant or young child in whom antibody-producing mechanisms may not be fully developed, or who may have had limited opportunity to produce antibody from previous exposure.

It is well recognized that asplenic individuals are prone to develop serious and fatal bacterial septicaemia, and that the risk of this occurring is greatest in the first five or so years of life and in patients whose underlying disease or treatment may have suppressed their defences in other ways. The commonest organisms responsible are the pneumococcus and *Haemophilus influenzae* type B, and it should be emphasized that infection may develop without warning in otherwise well patients, and that it may be fulminant. Interestingly, the risk of infection is not increased in adults or older children who have undergone splenectomy for traumatic rupture, as seeding of splenic tissue into the peritoneal cavity may occur at the time of injury or operation and promote the subsequent return of at least some splenic function. In contrast, the risk of infection appears to be particularly high when splenectomy has been performed in children with Hodgkin's disease and similar conditions in which other disorders of the immune system may coexist. Occasionally one encounters non-splenectomized patients presenting with severe infection and whose blood film shows the changes of hyposplenism (see Section 19). This may rarely be due to congenital asplenia but is more commonly acquired and may be associated with coeliac disease, sickle cell disease, essential thrombocythaemia, or systemic lupus erythematosus.

Because of the rapidity with which infection may develop in these patients, it is generally recommended that long-term prophylactic penicillin should be taken, but it is difficult to advise for how long such prophylaxis should continue. Children should certainly persevere well into their teens, but there is no age at which prophylaxis can logically be stopped. Vaccination with polyvalent pneumococcal polysaccharide vaccines is currently under trial and, if safe may prove useful.

Pneumonia. The mucous membrane lining the respiratory tract has a surface area 40 times that of the skin, or about the size of a tennis court, and each day is exposed to some 10 000 litres of inspired air (enough to fill a swimming pool) which may contain various harmful dusts, chemical or micro-organisms. The defences are necessarily elaborate (Table 4) and are fully discussed elsewhere (see Section 15). Infection is likely to occur if any of these mechanisms are impaired whether as a result of local processes or as part of a more generalized suppression of the immune response, and it is not surprising that the lungs are by far the most frequently infected organ in the compromised patient. Local disturbances of pulmonary defences such as neoplasia, cystic fibrosis, and Kartagener's syndrome are discussed in detail in Section 15.

Table 4 Pulmonary defence mechanisms

Mechanical
    Tortuous nasal passages; nasal hairs; sneezing, coughing, nose-blowing; mucociliary action; epithelial barrier
Secretory
    Mucus; immunoglobulin (secretory IgA; serum IgS); lysozyme; surfactant; interferon; complement
Cellular
    Alveolar macrophages; neutrophils, monocytes; cell-mediated (T cell) responses: direct cellular cytotoxicity and lymphokines

Clinical pulmonary infection in the immunosuppressed may present with a lobar or patchy bronchopneumonia, abscesses with or without cavitation, or with non-specific fever, tachypnoea, an unproductive cough, and clinical and radiological signs limited to a few rales and some patchy infiltrate. This picture is usually caused by infection but tumour infiltration may be responsible, and thrombocytopenic pulmonary haemorrhage may produce a similar radiological appearance. Furthermore, a similar picture is occasionally seen during treatment with radiation and certain drugs such a methotrexate and busulphan (Table 5). Unfortunately differentiation between these various aetiological factors and identification of any resposible infectious agent may be difficult or impossible and a pragmatic approach is usually required.

Table 5 Causes of radiological pulmonary 'infiltrate' in the immune-compromised patient

Infection
    Bacterial: various including *Legionella* and Pittsburgh pneumonia agent
    Protozoan: *Pneumocystis carinii*, *Toxoplasma*
    Viral: CMV, herpesvirus, measles
    Mycotic: *Candida*, *Apsergillus*, *Cryptococcus*
Infiltration due to underlying malignancy
    Leukaemia; lymphoma; lymphangitis carcinomatosa
Pulmonary haemorrhage
    Thrombocytopenia
Cytotoxic agents
    Methotrexate; busulphan; bleomycin
    Radiation
Other
    Pulmonary embolism may occur even in the presence of thrombocytopenia

In general, profoundly suppressed patients may be infected with virtually any organism but in neutropenic patients with acute myeloid leukaemia bacteria are usually responsible, unless marrow suppression has been prolonged when the likelihood of candidal or fungal infection increases. *Pneumocystis carinii* infections are usually confined to patients with acute lymphoblastic leukaemia who are receiving intensive maintenance therapy and to transplantation patients. Pneumocystis and viral pneumonias produce the clinical picture of 'interstitial pneumonitis' in which dyspnoea, tachypnoea, and tachycardia are out of proportion to signs in the chest and radiological changes. Blood gases show severe hypoxia and hypocapnia which may not be fully corrected by oxygen administration. *Legionella* infections have been particularly associated with new hospital buildings. However, the organism is ubiquitous and although infection is uncommon, the diagnosis should always be considered as it is often rapidly fatal in the immunosuppressed.

If pulmonary infection is suspected, blood and sputum cultures should be obtained without delay. Transtracheal aspiration should be employed if an adequate sputum sample is not forthcoming. Broad spectrum antibiotics should be started but there is no general agreement of the choice of agents. Gentamicin and ticarcillin should be given to neutropenic patients as discussed above, and the addition of erythromycin (for *Legionella*) and co-trimoxazole (for *Pneumocystis*) should be considered. In any event, adequate cover for pneumococcal infection is essential. If there is no response, mycotic or viral infection becomes increasingly likely and alternative, invasive diagnostic procedures may be contemplated in patients whose underlying condition otherwise carries a good prognosis. Open surgical lung biopsy undoubtedly offers the highest yield but is not well tolerated by the sick patient with pneumonia. Percutaneous needle aspiration and drill biopsy are more acceptable but less effective alternatives. Platelet transfusion cover will be required for any thrombocytopenic patient undergoing these procedures. Unfortunately, even with an aggressive approach, a positive diagnosis will be obtained in less than a half, and may not be apparent even at autopsy. Rather than subject patients to unpleasant diagnostic procedures, it may be reasonable simply to administer high doses of co-trimoxazole on the presumption that infection may be due to *Pneumocystis*. However, it may be difficult to exclude candidal or fungal infection, and in view of the toxicity of amphotericin it is better to obtain a positive diagnosis before commencing treatment with this drug (see above).

Transplantation. The success of organ transplantation may be largely ascribed to the development of immunosuppressive therapy to a point where rejection of the transplanted tissue occurs in only a minority of patients. The immunological processes involved in rejection are complex and incompletely understood but they comprise all branches of the immune response and the effector mechanisms are largely the same as those involved in the defence against infection. When discrete organs, such as the kidney or heart, are transplanted, immunosuppression is required indefinitely to prevent rejection. For marrow transplantation, massive immunosuppression is employed prior to grafting and successful graft subsequently repopulates not only the haemopoietic system but also the entire immune system, including alveolar macrophages. This process takes several months, during which there is extreme susceptibility to all forms of infection but particularly to those caused by herpesviruses and pneumococci. Interstitial pneumonitis has complicated up to half the transplants in some centres; the most commonly associated organism is CMV, but in one half of cases no aetiological agent has been demonstrated. The process of immune reconstitution may be severely retarded by graft versus host disease.

Transplanted patients are thus prone to any of the infections discussed in this section, and much of the success achieved by transplantation programmes is due to the fact that patients have been treated in specialized units sufficiently experienced to recognize, diagnose, and treat such infections without delay.

References

Allen, J. C. (ed.) (1976). *Infection and the compromised host*. Williams and Wilkins, Baltimore.

Betts, R. F. and Hanshaw, J. B. (1977). Cytomegalovirus (CMV) in the compromised host(s). *Ann. Rev. Med.* **28**, 103.

Dick, G. (ed.) (1979). *Immunological aspects of infectious diseases*. MTP Press, Lancaster.

Feldman, S. and Cox, F. (1976). Viral infections and haematological malignancies. *Clinics Haemat.* **5**, 311.

Green, G. M., Jakob, G. J., Low, R. B., and Davis, G. S. (1977). Defense mechanisms of the respiratory membrane. *Am. Rev. resp. Dis.* **115**, 479.

Hughes, W. T. (1976). Protozoan infections in haematological diseases. *Clinics Haemat.* **5**, 329.

Krick, J. A. and Remington, J. S. (1976). Opportunistic invasive fungal infections in patients with leukaemia and lymphoma. *Clinics Haemat.* **5**, 249.

Levine, A. S., Schimpff, S. C. Graw, R. G., Jr., and Young, R. C. (1974). Hematologic malignancies and other marrow failure states: progress in the management of complicating infections. *Semin. Hemat.* **11**, 141.

Neiman, P. E., Reeves, W., Ray, G., Flournoy, N., Lerner, K. G., Sale, G. E., and Thomas, E. D. (1977). A prospective analysis of interstitial pneumonitis and opportunistic viral infection among recipients of allogenic bone marrow grafts. *J. infect. Dis.* **136**, 754.

Winearls, C. G., Lane, D. J., and Warrell, M. J. (1979). Infectious complications after renal transplantation. In *Kidney transplantation* (ed. P. J. Morris), 285. Academic Press, London.

Winston, D. J., Gale, R. P., Meyer, D. W., and Young, L. S. (1979). Infectious complications of human bone marrow transplantation. *Medicine, Baltimore* **58**, 1.

INFECTION IN PREGNANCY

R. Hurley

Any of the acute or chronic specific infectious diseases may be contracted during pregnancy or the puerperium, and conception may occur in women already harbouring infection. (See also Section 11 on Reproductive Medicine.) Pregnancy predisposes to certain specific infections, for example, to candidosis and listeriosis, and its co-existence may aggravate the risk to maternal life of the more serious infections. Diseases such as varicella (see page 5.57) which are, ordinarily, not life-threatening in previously healthy adults may prove lethal during pregnancy, and acquired infectious disease may have further grave consequence, constituting a hazard to the fetus or the newborn. Fetal death may result from contagion, for some viruses, bacteria, and protozoa are able to cross the placental barrier, or it may be caused by placental insufficiency, hyperpyrexia, maternal exhaustion, or toxaemia. The newborn may contract a transmissible disease from close contact with an infected mother shortly after birth, or, as a result of maternal infection, it may be born in a sickly and marasmic condition, soon to succumb to intercurrent infection. During birth and in the early part of the puerperium, parturient women are susceptible to serious infections of the genital tract, and childbed fever has always been one of the leading causes of maternal death. Pyelonephritis, 'pyelitis of pregnancy', was, formerly, one of the most frequent and important medical complications of pregnancy and early detection and treatment of asymptomatic urinary tract infections is a dominant feature of modern obstetric care (see Section 18).

The incidence of infections of all types is greatest in malnourished and unhygienic communities and in areas where serious epidemic and endemic microbial diseases are rife. Many of these diseases are preventable. Rigorous campaigns to improve the general standard of hygiene, and the introduction of measures specifically designed to control communicable disease are accompanied by lessening of the maternal, fetal, and perinatal mortality and morbidity rates. The importance of the public health services to maternal and fetal life and health cannot be exaggerated and a good service provides the soundest basis for the development of high standards of obstetric care and practice.

Acute fortuitous infections. Casual or chance infections during pregnancy range from mild illnesses to the major microbial infections.

In the Far East and in other parts of Asia, in Africa, and in South America, pregnant women may be exposed to diseases such as cholera, plague, dysenteries, the enteric fevers and various forms of viral hepatitis. Control of these epidemic infections can have far reaching effects on populations. Variolation for the smallpox and its efficacy in preventing the deaths of young children and women in childbirth was probably the major cause of the great increase in population in western Europe which began during the first half of the eighteenth century. Smallpox has now been eradicated globally. Though under partial control, pandemic viral infections, with high untreated mortality, such as influenza, still occur and may be worldwide in distribution. A high perinatal mortality rate is

believed to be attendant on pandemic influenza. Abortion or premature birth may occur in the course of such illness and the baby, if born alive, may be sickly and weak. In parts of Africa, and the Americas, severe, systemic fungal infections such as coccidioidomycosis, histoplasmosis, and North and South American blastomycosis occur, and, rarely, may be transmitted to the fetus. Parasitic infestations with hookworm or tapeworm, schistosomiasis, and other diseases are common in many parts of the world, and it should be borne in mind that as a world producer of death and morbidity, malaria is second to none. Exotic infections including a considerable range of tropical and semi-tropical infections may be imported into temperate zones through population movements and air travel.

Although serious microbial disease is well controlled in the West, mothers of young children, particularly of those at school, are exposed to the specific infectious diseases of childhood and, in addition to the common upper respiratory tract infections, may contract mumps, chickenpox, measles, rubella, scarlet fever, acute bacterial tonsillitis, whooping cough, dysentery, or viral diarrhoeas. As young adults, the mothers may contract toxoplasmosis or poliomyelitis. Some of these diseases have important consequences in obstetric practice.

The sexually transmitted diseases may be contracted at any time during pregnancy or the puerperium, and those that could have fatal or crippling effects on the fetus are sought during the antenatal period. Routine serological tests for treponemal disease are performed during pregnancy, usually at the first visit. The other venereal diseases, gonorrhoea, chancroid, granuloma inguinale, lymphogranuloma venereum, and herpesvirus hominis infection are sought at antenatal examination by eliciting the medical and social history, by physical examination, and by appropriately chosen laboratory tests. Vaginal discharge, accompanied by pruritus, signifies infection by *Trichomonas vaginalis* or *Candida species*. The latter infection is extremely common.

Exacerbation of caries and dental sepsis occurs during pregnancy and women with valvular disease of the heart, particularly those with rheumatic mitral regurgitation, either pure or with stenosis, are at risk of infective endocarditis at delivery, or if dental surgery becomes necessary.

The clinical stigmata of fortuitous acute infections, such as viral hepatitis, varicella, or primary herpesvirus hominis infection may occur at term, or in the puerperium and, again, may have deleterious consequence for the newborn.

Chronic fortuitous infections. Pregnancy may occur in the course of a chronic infection, or chronic infection may first be diagnosed during pregnancy. Its detection is one of the purposes of the general medical examination made at the first antenatal visit. Clinical and radiographic examination of the chest to diagnose or exclude pulmonary tuberculosis is standard practice in the United Kingdom, as is the performance of screening tests for treponemal disease. Other chronic infections are less frequently encountered, but other sexually transmitted diseases, actinomycosis, leprosy, brucellosis, and chronic fungal and parasitic disease do occur. If the infection is open and communicable, women with these diseases should be segregated from other patients, and from the newborn under certain circumstances.

Infections associated with pregnancy and the puerperium. These are all acute infections, though recrudescence of chronic infection may occur. None is peculiar to pregnancy, but their incidence is increased in pregnant as compared with non-pregnant women. Infections of the urinary tract afflict some 4–7 per cent of pregnant women, occurring also with increased frequency during the puerperium. Any part of the renal tract may be involved, and with modern bacteriological techniques infection by significant numbers of organisms can be detected before the onset of symptoms. The infections may be acute and primary, or recrudescences of chronic infection; they range from urethritis to acute pyelonephritis, which, in former days, was sometimes accompanied by bloodstream infection ('catheter fever'). The usual causes during pregnancy are members of the *Enterobacteriaceae* (see page 5.175) and other Gram-negative rods, as well as the pathogenic Gram-positive cocci. The relationship of the less flagrant forms of urinary tract sepsis to abortion, prematurity, low birth weight, and stillbirth is not established with certainty.

The incidence of vulvovaginitis increases in pregnancy, being occasioned largely by infection with members of the genus *Candida*, notably *C. albicans*, the fungus of thrush. Trichomonadic vulvovaginitis does not increase. Candida vulvovaginitis is the most frequent of all the specific infections encountered, affecting 10–17 per cent of pregnant women. Thrush of the newborn, and systemic candidosis in sickly and low birth weight infants may arise in consequence. The former is common but the latter rare.

Infection with *Listeria monocytogenes* is more often diagnosed in pregnant women than in other healthy adults. It may be transmitted to the fetus or newborn and is the cause of serious perinatal disease.

The hepatitis viruses (A, B, and non-A, non-B) (see page 5.116) may cause acute disease fortuitously in pregnant women, but there is no evidence of increased incidence. Some pregnant women, in consequence of previous infection with hepatitis B virus, are chronic carriers and may transmit virus to their unborn or newly born children. In most cases, this is of little moment other than in the maintenance of a reservoir of virus in nature by vertical transmission, but chronic liver disease and primary liver tumours may conceivably be the long term outcome in some.

The infections associated with the puerperium are all acute, the most notorious being infection of the genital tract, which formerly accounted for a great number of deaths and is still the most important cause of death from infection in obstetric practice. Inflammation and suppuration of the lactating breast may also occur, and urinary tract infections are fairly frequent. Wound infection and bronchopneumonia are important post-operative complications. All are common causes of elevation of the body temperature in the lying-in period.

Congenital and perinatal infections. Certain bacteria, viruses, protozoa, and fungi can pass the placental barrier, causing congenital infection or malformation, and, sometimes, abortion or death *in utero*. Well known for transmission by this route are *Treponema pallidum*, rubella virus, and cytomegalovirus and *Roxoplasma gondii*. Congenital deformity may follow intrauterine infection with the last four named agents.

The fetus may be infected directly during operative procedures, such as intrauterine blood transfusion, and is prone to infection via the amniotic fluid when the membranes have been ruptured longer than 24 hours, for it is able to gasp and may swallow contaminated liquor amnii. It may also become infected as it traverses the birth canal, which is thought to be the usual mode of acquisition of inimical microbes such as *Neisseria gonorrhoeae*, group B streptococci, or herpesvirus hominis type 2.

The newborn is unduly susceptible to certain infections, and is less well able to localize them than is the adult. Its immunological status is the resultant of two systems: the first is active, depending on its own capacity to develop immunity; the second is passive, the result of the transfer of maternal antibody during gestation. In addition to the physiological dysglobulinaemia of immaturity, the cellular response to infection is probably less brisk and less effective than that of the older child or adult. Infections such as rubella, cytomegalic inclusion disease, toxoplasmosis, herpes, and listeriosis may disseminate widely and fatally in the newborn, and there is a proclivity towards severe infections with organisms that, in the adult, are of little virulence, such as some staphylococci, or *Flavobacterium meningosepticum* which causes menigitis only in the newborn.

The commonest source of infection in the newborn, and the only frequent source in the fetus, is the mother. Most serious disease manifests as neonatal sepsis, that is, as meningitis or septicaemia,

or both, with septicaemia either of early onset or late onset type predominating. The early onset type is more often associated with prejudicial peripartum factors, and the source of infection is the maternal genital tract. In late onset disease, presenting, usually, after the first week of life, infection from a wider environment including human contacts or contaminated fomites is probable. The mortality from the latter is lower at 10–20 per cent than in early onset disease, in which it varies from 20–50 per cent. While *Escherichia coli* and other coliforms still remain the most important causes of neonatal sepsis, having replaced *Staphylococcus aureus*, group B streptococci have become increasingly implicated in neonatal meningitis, and in early and late onset septicaemia.

Microbes associated with late onset disease, such as *Pseudomonas aeruginosa* or *Staph. aureus*, reflect, epidemiologically, the distribution of pathogens at large in a particular nursery or intensive care baby unit. Theoretically, therefore, late onset disease is preventable. Its control is complicated, however, by the intensive care of very low birthweight babies (≤ 1500 g), who are more subject to serious infection of both types, the rates being 5 to 100 times higher in babies weighing less than 2500 g than in others. Paradoxically, as the ever widening frontier of neonatal medicine pushes back the gestational age and the birthweight at which survival is to be expected, so, too, do the number of serious infections in neonatal units rise.

Strict attention to regimens of personal and ward hygiene, use of disposables, and scrupulous care in the preparation of bottle feeds in nurseries lowers the incidence of both superficial and systemic microbial disease. It is plain that the danger of nurses and nursery personnel acting as vectors can be diminished greatly by the imposition of rigorous standards of hygiene. There is general agreement that prematurity and low birthweight, prolonged labour, prolonged rupture of the membranes, vigorous manipulative or operative delivery, and maternal infection all predispose to infection in the newborn. These are regarded by many physicians as indications for prophylaxis with antibacterial antibiotics.

Types of infections and specific infections

Since some broad categories of infection, for example, wound and puerperal infection, urinary tract infection, ophthalmia neonatorum, and neonatal sepsis are caused by diverse microbes, a general account of them precedes that of specific infections. The only specific infections discussed will be those that have important sequelae for the newborn.

Non-specific maternal infections

Urinary tract infections. Urinary tract infections are more common in women than in men and are particularly likely to occur during pregnancy, labour, and the puerperium. Infections of all grades of severity are encountered and any part of the urinary tract may be involved. Thus the infections range from asymptomatic bacteriuria, through mild urethritis and cystitis, to pyelitis and pyelonephritis with possible risk of chronic irreversible kidney damage.

Pyelonephritis, or 'pyelitis of pregnancy' was, once, the most frequent and important of the medical complications of pregnancy, with an incidence of just over 1 per cent and a maternal mortality of 3–4 per cent at the beginning of the antibiotic era. Fetal loss, from premature termination of the pregnancy, was 16–30 per cent. The complete clinical picture of frank pyelonephritis is seen far less frequently nowadays, almost certainly owing to early diagnosis and the prompt administration of antibiotics. Characteristically, the onset of the acute disease is about the fifth or sixth month of pregnancy, or in the first week of the puerperium. The symptoms include fever, rigors, headache, pain in the renal angle, dysuria, and frequency. Examination of the urine usually shows that it is strongly acid, loaded with organisms and pus cells and, sometimes, with frank blood. Proteinuria also occurs, and bacteria are present in significant number. Subacute or low-grade infections are far more common.

Most studies have shown that 4–7 per cent of women examined during pregnancy have significant bacteriuria, figures not unlike those recorded for the adult female population in general, a small but definite proportion of whom have bacteriuria. Pregnancy itself need not cause any increase in prevalence of bacteriuria, though few would dispute the relationship of asymptomatic bacteriuria during early pregnancy to the subsequent development of symptoms referable to urinary tract infection. Acute pyelonephritis is particularly liable to develop in bacteriuric women, early treatment substantially reducing its incidence. For this reason, many antenatal clinics send urine to be screened for bacteriuria by quantitative methods. The term 'significant bacteriuria' implies that bacteria are multiplying in the bladder urine and, therefore, that infection as opposed to microbial contamination is present. Under these circumstances, the bacterial population, usually of known urinary pathogens, will ordinarily exceed 100 000 per ml of urine. The specimen must be taken correctly and either processed promptly, or stored at 4 °C for examination later on the same day.

The principal route of infection is probably an ascending one, and the risk of introducing infection by catheterization has long been recognized. Much hospital acquired infection, following catheterization or operations on the bladder, is associated with organisms that are being disseminated in the wards. Another route of infection is the lymphatic system, for the right kidney has a direct connection, via the lymphatics, with the ascending colon, to which it is directly related. Infection may be blood borne, and blood cultures are often positive in pyelonephritis, as a result of blood borne or of ascending infection. Experimentally, the intravenous injection of some urinary pathogens into laboratory animals causes localized disease of the kidney, but in the case of *Escherichia coli*, the ureter must have been ligated or the kidney previously damaged, suggesting that local anatomical anomaly, or malfunction, is important in its genesis.

In the female, the proximity of the urethral orifice to the rectum and the moist environment of the perineum favours growth of microbes, including pathogens of the urinary tract. The distal 4 cm of the urethra is colonized by bacteria. Local minor trauma such as that occasioned by sexual intercourse may favour bacterial multiplication, and, during pregnancy, increased concentrations of amino acids and lactose are believed to encourage growth of *Escherichia coli* in the urine.

Mechanical factors, expecially those that obstruct urinary flow, are important in promoting bacterial infection, and the immediate predisposing cause of urinary tract infections during pregnancy is stasis. Progesterone causes dilation of the ureters, and oestrogens cause muscular hypertrophy at a time when changing anatomical relationships in the pelvis lead to compression of the right ureter. Complete bladder emptying is important, for present evidence suggests that bacteria coming into contact with the mucosa are killed. Interference with normal micturition, such as may occur during delivery or in operations to repair the pelvic floor, promotes infection. Ureteric valve incompetence leading to reflux has been postulated but not demonstrated during pregnancy.

Most of the infections that occur sporadically in the population are caused by *Esch. coli* which is also most frequently isolated in obstetric and gynaecological practice. Organisms less frequently isolated include *Proteus* spp., *Str. faecalis*, *Klebsiella* supp., staphylococci, and *Ps. aeruginosa. Micrococcus* spp. and *Staph. epidermidis* as well as *Enterobacteriaceae* carried in the introitus are associated with the 'frequency–dysuria' or 'urethral' syndrome, in which patients have symptoms suggestive of cystitis.

The bacteriological diagnosis of urinary tract infection depends on quantitative examination of freshly voided urine. Care must be taken in collection of specimens from women, and catheterization should be avoided. If the results of culture are equivocal, or if there is persistent contamination, the urine may be sampled directly by suprapubic aspiration, which is quite safe in pregnant women. The

presence of 100 000 organisms per ml is generally accepted as the criterion of infection within the urinary tract, and special methods, including serotyping may serve to distinguish relapse from reinfection.

Sulphonamides, ampicillin, cephalexin, and nitrofurantoin are all used in treatment. Co-trimoxazole is also effective, though not generally recommended because of the theoretical risk of fetal damage.

With early diagnosis and prompt and successful treatment, the long-term prognosis in terms of chronic infection and renal damage is good. However, it is prudent to follow the outcome in those who have responded slowly or only partially to treatment, and further urine examinations and intravenous pyelography, the latter carried out not less than three months post partum, may be required.

Puerperal sepsis and wound infections. Peurperal sepsis includes a series of febrile disorders of the lying-in period that share the common aetiology of being wound infections of the genital tract. It may occur after delivery or abortion and is occasioned by several genera of pathogenic bacteria, of which the most notorious and dangerous are *Clostridium* and *Streptococcus*. In the great majority of fatal cases, the microbes are introduced from without, and such infections are preventable. Endogenous microbes, harboured in the vagina, such as *Enterobacteriaceae* and *Staphylococcus* cause less severe forms of sepsis in general.

The contagiousness of childbed or milk fever was postulated before the promulgation of the theory of 'vegetable parasitism' by bacteria and was, in part, demonstrated. The pioneer epidemiological studies of Semmelweis in Vienna and Oliver Wendell Holmes in the United States in the mid-nineteenth century showed that infection could be carried from the dead house, and was conveyed by the unclean hands of the attendant accoucheur. The use of antiseptic solutions and attention to general hygiene, particularly that of the hands, diminished the ravages of puerperal sepsis long before the aetiological agents were discovered in the era of scientific bacteriology. In the time of Semmelweis, epidemics, with high mortality, occurred, and, in the late twenties and early thirties of this century, the overall mortality from all forms of puerperal sepsis was as high as 11 per cent.

Since the establishment of rigid schedules of asepsis and antisepsis in maternity units over the last century and since the introduction of chemotherapeutic agents and antibiotics, the aetiological pattern of puerperal sepsis has altered. Formerly, exogenous microbes accounted for the majority of fatal cases, being mainly Lancefield group A β-haemolytic streptococci originating from the attendants, the patient's own body outside the genital tract, and from visitors; they spread to the parturient patient by droplet infection, infected dust, infected hands, and contaminated fomites, such as instruments and dressings. Nowadays, aerobic non-haemolytic steptococci, anaerobic steptococci, members of the *Enterobacteriaceae*, occasionally staphylococci, *Cl. welchi, Str. faecalis* (Lancefield group D), or haemolytic steptococci of other groups are encountered. As well as having extrinisic origins, all can be isolated from the vagina regularly. *Bacteroides, Mycoplasma*, and other genera may be implicated in puerperal sepsis, as in other infections of the genital tract, but their causal relationship to disease therein has been less thoroughly studied.

Puerperal sepsis is a wound infection, which may involve any part of the parturient genital tract, from infected episiotomies, perineal or cervical lacerations, metritis and endometritis, to involvement of the uterine appendages, with local or generalized peritonitis and invasion of the bloodstream. Disease localized to the genital tract proper does not run a fatal course, but the prognosis is poor if peritonitis or bloodstream infection supervenes as it is very likely to do if the causative agent is an unchecked streptococcus. The factors predisposing to infection include premature rupture of the membranes, repeated examination of the vagina, instrumentation and internal monitoring of labour, lacerations of the birth canal, episiotomy, manual rotation, and forceps delivery. An increased rate of postpartum endometritis follows caesarean section. Factors tending to lower general resistance, such as malnutrition, intercurrent disease, anaemia, haemorrhage, and maternal exhaustion also promote infection. The retention of blood clot, or of fragments of membrane or placenta encourages infection by providing a nidus wherein bacteria may multiply. The basis of prevention is scrupulous hygiene, with a short labour and few internal examinations, followed by an uncomplicated vaginal delivery.

Fever is the cardinal sign of puerperal sepsis, and may arise before, during, or after labour. Puerperal pyrexia occurring in the 48 hours succeeding delivery or abortion may also be caused by urinary tract infection, administration of contaminated intravenous infusions, aspiration pneumonia, or retained products of conception. Septic thrombophlebitis, 'third day fever', infection of an abdominal wound, breast engorgment with or without incipient mastitis or breast abscess, drug fevers, surgical misadventure with swabs or other foreign bodies, and fortuitous infection in sites remote from the genitourinary tract should all be considered, especially when fever arises later in the puerperium. Patients with streptococcal endometritis appear acutely ill, with temperatures up to 40 °C. The induration and purulent uterine discharge associated with less severe and more localized disease are usually absent, being replaced by diffuse slight pelvic tenderness and clear cervical discharge, in which Gram-positive cocci can be seen on staining. Treatment must be instituted without awaiting laboratory reports. Low grade endometritis is characterized by diminution in the lochial flow before the onset of fever, uterine tenderness, and a foul-smelling discharge from the endocervical canal.

The diagnosis of puerperal sepsis is made on clinical grounds, and the identity of the infecting microbes is established by the laboratory. Direct Gram-stained smears of exudate from the cervix, or from within the uterus, are examined and the specimen is cultured. The nature and the sensitivity of the pathogen to antibiotics is usually established in less than 48 hours. The patient is treated with appropriate antibiotics, penicillin with an aminoglycoside being used for incipient severe infection, and safe, broad spectrum antibiotics being used for low-grade infections if the aetiological diagnosis is completely unsuspected. Metronidazole or clindamycin, active against anaerobes, are often added to the regimen of therapy. Surgical measures are used as indicated, and supportive therapy including bedrest, fluids, and oral and nasal hygiene is given. Isolation of the patient may be necessary.

Septic abortion and shock. The availability of contraceptive techniques and the legalization of abortion has led to diminution in the number of women with septic abortion, but the diagnosis should be suspected in every febrile woman who is bleeding in the first trimester of pregnancy. In the majority of cases the cervical os is open, and there is evidence of the passage of the products of conception. High, spiking fevers and the presence of hypertension are bad prognostic signs. Pelvic examination, with assessment of uterine size is important, for most serious infections follow attempts to terminate pregnancy in women beyond the twelfth week of gestation. As in puerperal sepsis following delivery (Table 1) extension of the infection beyond the uterus is attended by correspondingly grave risk for the patient. Plain X-rays of the abdomen with the patient both in the supine and the upright positions may demonstrate the presence of intraperitoneal or myometrial gas. Exploratory laparotomy may be required. Myometrial gas suggests *Cl. welchi* (perfringens) infection, and operative intervention may be required. Foreign bodies such as an intrauterine contraceptive device, may require removal. Many patients respond successfully to curettage and antibiotic therapy. Many antibiotics have been used, but the most favoured regimen is a combination of intravenous penicillin with intramuscular aminoglycoside in high dosage. The blood pressure and urinary output should be measured at regular intervals, and aminoglycosides, if administered, should be assayed.

The microbes causing septic abortion are similar to those causing

post-delivery sepsis, but non-sporing anaerobes, such as *Bacteroides fragilis*, may be implicated and with Gram-negative aerobes, such as *Esch. coli* and *Klebsiella* spp. are related to endotoxic shock.

Table 1   Relationship of mortality in puerperal fever to morbid anatomical extent of the lesions. Based on 251* cases of puerperal fever of whom 23* died (11.2 per cent)

	(%) Mortality
Infection limited to vagina, perineum, or uterus	nil
General peritonitis	68.2
General peritonitis (*Str. pyogenes*)	78.0
Septicaemia	70.0
Septicaemia (*Str. pyogenes*)	98.0
All infections with *Str. pyogenes* irrespective of extent of lesions	21.1

* *Str. pyogenes* was isolated from 36 per cent of all patients and from 68 per cent of those who died
From Colebrook's data, 1932

Shock may be defined as a state of widespread, inadequate perfusion of the tissues which, if prolonged, leads to general impairment of cellular function. It is usually accompanied by hypotension, but this sign is not invariable. Septic shock usually follows bacteraemia with members of the *Enterobacteriaceae* and seems to have been afforded little recognition before the late fifties of this century. It may also occur with Gram-positive cocci, such as streptococci and pneumococci, with *Bacteroides fragilis* and with *Pseudomonas aeruginosa*. The syndrome is due to the release of lipopolysaccharides from the cell walls of the bacteria into the circulation, and bacteraemia is not invariable. Increased peripheral vascular resistance consequent on direct toxic effect on small blood vessels with the effect of local acidosis leads to pooling of blood in the pulmonary, splanchnic, and renal capillary beds, with leaking of plasma and anoxia of the tissues. There is decrease in the circulating blood volume, reduction of the cardiac output, and hypotension. Metabolic acidosis and severe tissue damage lead to an irreversible state, if perfusion of vital organs remains defective. The endotoxin also produces fibrin thrombi in capillaries, on which fibrin-platelet aggregates, typical of advanced shock, form. Deficiency of clotting factors, due to consumption coagulopathy leads to disseminated intravascular coagulation (DIC). Different patterns of septic shock have been described, and the clinical state is variable. Renal and cardiac failure may both ensue in the course of shock and death occurs from respiratory failure (shock lung). The onset of bacteraemia is accompanied by fever, rigors, nausea, vomiting, diarrhoea, and prostration. With the development of septic shock, tachycardia, tachypnoea, hypotension, usually with cool, pale extremities and often with peripheral cyanosis, oliguria, and mental confusion, are added.

For the laboratory diagnosis and management of shock, see page 5.475.

Wound infections. The organism most frequently isolated from septic wounds in obstetric practice is *Staphylococcus aureus*, followed by members of the *Enterobacteriaceae* and streptococci. Infection by *Ps. aeruginosa* may occur. Opinions differ on the relative importance of operating room or ward as the source of most infections, but consideration must be given to the personal and surgical hygiene of the operating team, fomites surrounding the patient, theatre ventilation, and the patient's own skin. Inexpert and clumsy surgery may well be a contributing factor.

Specific infections during pregnancy that lead to congenital defect or illness

Syphilis. Caused by *Treponema pallidum*, syphilis (see page 5.288) alone amongst the treponematoses is transmissible as a prenatal infection any time after the formation of the placenta, that is, after the third month of intrauterine life. The disease may be transmitted long after the mother had ceased to be infectious by the sexual route, but, in general, the more recent the infection in the mother, the more severe will be the infection in the fetus. In untreated maternal syphilis, after the passage of many years healthy non-infected children may be born, but, commonly, miscarriages, still-births, living syphilitic children, or healthy babies are interspersed. The eighteenth week of gestation is the earliest age at which spir-ochaetes have been detected in fetal tissues, and the incidence of fetal death ascribable to syphilis is greatest at the twenty-sixth week.

The clinical manifestations of congenital syphilis are divided into three groups. Those of early, infectious congenital syphilis re-semble, in some ways, those of secondary acquired syphilis, with skin rashes, abnormal distribution of scalp hair, 'snuffles' with mu-cous patches in the nose, throat, mouth, and larynx, abnormalities of the nails, hepatosplenomegaly, lymphadenopathy, syphilitic osteo-chondritis and the syphilitic pseudo-paralysis of Parrot, other bony anomalies, and severe anaemia. Active neurosyphilis occurs in about 10 per cent of cases. The diagnosis is established by the demonstration of *T. pallidum* on dark-ground examination of serum from lesions of the skin, mucous membranes, or in the nasal discharge. Serological tests must be interpreted with caution, but the presence of specific IgM antibody in the infant's blood denotes infection. Infants born to untreated mothers should be kept under observation for at least six months, and those born to treated mothers for at least three months. Even if untreated, the majority of infants survive, the signs of active disease disappear, and the disease becomes latent.

The late, non-infectious manifestations of congenital syphilis including gummata, interstitial keratitis, nerve deafness, Clutton's joints, and juvenile tabes dorsalis or general paresis of the insane occur after the second year of life. The stigmata of congenital syphilis are due to structural damage caused by *T. pallidum* in intrauterine life. Scars and deformities ascribable to the lesions of early congenital syphilis, such as rhagades, may be present, as may the 'hot cross bun' skull, 'saddle nose', and the 'bulldog' facies which, together with interstitial keratitis, the commonest late lesion, lead to a look of sustained perplexity called Stokes facies. The permanent dentition may be deformed, with Hutchinson's teeth and Moon's molars, Hutchinson's triad, consisting of intersti-tial keratitis, Hutchinson's teeth, and eighth nerve deafness, is pathognomonic of congenital syphilis.

Pregnancy masks the early stages of syphilis, and the primary chancre may appear as little more than an abrasion, which if situ-ated on the cervix or located extragenitally may be overlooked. Serological tests are of paramount importance in diagnosis and, because of the danger of untreated syphilis to the fetus, are in-cluded in the routine tests made on pregnant women at the first booking visit. The *Treponema pallidum* haemagglutination test detects specific antibody, is easy to perform and read, and is used increasingly as a screening test in general laboratories. More than one screening test is usually performed.

Toxoplasmosis. Toxoplasmosis (see page 5.400) is probably unique amongst the infectious diseases of man in that its congenital form was recognized before that of post-natally acquired infection. The reported incidence of the congenital disease in the United King-dom, though not so high as in France, exceeds that of congenital syphilis. The coccidian parasite exists in three forms, the tropho-zoite, the tissue cyst, and the cat-associated oocyst, the two latter being the principal forms implicated in transmission.

The parasite is widely distributed in mammals, some birds and, probably, some reptiles. In man antibody acquisition, signifying acquired infection, is related to age, and there is a tendency towards geographical distribution, acquisition rates being lower in colder zones and in hot, dry, or high areas than in warm, moist regions. There is little difference in the prevalence rates between sexes

although, clearly, the disease is more important and more fre-quently diagnosed in women of childbearing age. There are few data from which to derive morbidity, mortality, or case fatality rates.

Clinically, toxoplasmosis presents in three forms, the congenital, the postnatally acquired, and the ocular. The last may be congenital or acquired. In the postnatally acquired form, caused by ingestion of tissue cyst infected meat or oocysts derived from cat faeces, there is a wide spectrum of disease running from symptomless subclinical infection, which is most frequent, to fulminating pneumonitis and fatal encephalomyelitis. In western Europe, the peak incidence lies between 25 and 35 years, and, during pregnancy, rates for acute toxoplasmosis vary from 1 to 140 pregnancies in France to 1 in 400 overall in the United Kingdom. In the United States, for a mean period of five months observation, the frequency was calculated at 6.4 per 1000, approximately 1 in 160.

Although placental transmission has been demonstrated in chronically infected mice, in man congenital infection is believed to follow primary infection and the prognosis for subsequent pregnan-cies is good. The risk to the fetus appears to be related to the gestational age at which primary maternal infection occurs, trans-mission being less likely in the first trimester, but resulting in more severe disease should it occur. Infection leading to stillbirth or neonatal death, or to survival with ocular and cerebral involvement occurs only in the offspring of mothers who acquire infection in the first or second trimester. The data suggest that the placenta bars the transmission of the parasites, with some 80 per cent efficacy during the early months of pregnancy, but less than 40 per cent efficacy at or about term. Once the placenta has become infected, it remains so for the duration of pregnancy, but there may be delay in trans-mission of the parasites to the fetus, the so called 'prenatal incuba-tion period'. Persistence of maternal parasitaemia beyond the stage of delivery of a congenitally infected infant and into the next pregnancy has been reported, and uterine tissue cyst formation can be inferred from serological and cultural studies in some women. It is not clear whether either is related to repeated abortion or still-birth, or to further congenital infection in the course of chronic infection, although the latter seems unlikely. Toxoplasmas have been isolated from vaginal secretions of seropositive women who were otherwise asymptomatic, and infection during passage through the birth canal has been postulated.

Congenital infection thus results from what is usually an acute asymptomatic infection in the mother, and may cause spontaneous abortion, prematurity, stillbirth, or the live birth of a congenitally infected baby. The most severe form of congenital disease is char-acterized by fever, hydrocephalus or microcephaly, hepatospleno-megaly, jaundice, convulsions, chorioretinitis, and cerebral calci-fication. The cerebrospinal fluid may show xanthochromia and increased concentration of mononuclear cells, and there may be grossly elevated protein concentration in the ventricular fluid. The most frequent form of congenital infection has been shown by prospective study to be an inapparent infection, and not a fulminant one. Thus, although transmission rates as high as 33 per cent have been reported following primary maternal infection, 72 per cent of the infected newborn were spared overt clinical infection. Such asymptomatic infants may suffer no serious consequences, or they may, later, develop chorioretinitis, blindness, strabismus, hydro-cephaly or microcephaly, cerebral calcification, psychomotor or mental retardation, epilepsy, or deafness. Children known to have had congenital toxoplasmosis must, therefore, be kept under observation for months or years. The available data are insufficient to support or to refute the hypothesis that *T. gondii* causes mal-formations during the period of organogenesis. The infected infant should be treated with spiramycin, or pyrimethamine/sulphona-mide and folinic acid.

Very little has yet been achieved in the systematic prevention of congenital toxoplasmosis, although various approaches are poss-ible. The infected mother may be treated with spiramycin, or, with caution, with pyrimethamine, sulphonamide, and folinic acid.

Since maternal infection is predominantly asymptomatic, this approach implies mass screening of pregnant women by serological tests, a formidable undertaking in terms of cost and expertise. Vaccines are, as yet, unpromising. Since ingestion of tissue cysts of oocysts is the most probable route of infection in the postnatally acquired disease, pregnant women may be cautioned to eschew the consumption of raw or undercooked meats, and to avoid unhygienic handling of cats and cat litter during pregnancy.

The diagnosis of congenital toxoplasmosis is established by serological tests (see pages 5.400–4).

Listeriosis. Listeriosis is discussed in detail on page 5.330–1.

Viral infections. Nearly a fifth of all perinatal deaths are ascribed to congenital malformations, especially those of the central nervous system. Although the majority of maternal viral infections cause little harm, some may result in severe damage to the fetus. Very careful prospective studies performed on large cohort populations and other studies have failed to establish, unequivocally, teratogenic potential in viruses other than rubella virus and cytomegalovirus, although a strong case can be advanced linking varicellazoster infection with specific defect. There are many case reports, retrospective analyses, and partly controlled epidemiological studies attempting to link congenital malformations with maternal infection with mumps, influenza, varicella–zoster, hepatitis viruses, Epstein–Barr virus, herpesvirus hominis, Coxsackie A4 viruses and measles. There is also considerable evidence linking the cardiotropic coxsackie B3 and B4 viruses with fetal myocarditis, but the relationship to congenital heart disease cannot, as yet, be regarded as proven.

Leaving aside teratogenic effects, that is, malformations consequent on infections blighting the fetus during the period of organogenesis, there is evidence of increased rates of abortion and stillbirth in intrauterine rubella, and in cytomegalovirus infection, and fetal and perinatal death has been reported in the course of maternal herpesvirus hominis infections, varicella–zoster, hepatitis, mumps, poliomyelitis, variola or vaccinia, measles, and influenza. Fetal wastage is not necessarily caused by viral invasion, but may be the result of maternal exhaustion and toxaemia.

Neonatal illness and congenital infection may result following infection with rubella, cytomegalovirus, herpesvirus hominis, varicella–zoster, variola or vaccinia, poliovirus, Coxsackie B viruses, the myxoviruses, and the hepatitis viruses. In general, neonatal infection is more likely to follow maternal infection at or about the time of delivery.

Even if maternal infection with a virus known to be noxious to the fetus is proved, it is important for the obstetrician to be aware of the relative risks and likely magnitude of fetal damage at the different stages of gestation, the better to advise his patient. The probable risks are well established for rubella (see page 5.80) and transmission, with crippling consequence, is more likely to occur during the first trimester of pregnancy. The data of Swan (Table 2) are helpful, based as they were on clinical rubella in the mother and the occurrence of severe, multiple defects in the infant. With more certain gnosis based on laboratory tests, other subtle defects, and defects appearing relatively late in infancy or in early childhood, have been recognized (Table 3). It is important to understand that the fetus may be spared deleterious consequence, and that this outcome is more likely the later in pregnancy that maternal rubella occurs. The corollary, that children born to women who have had rubella at any stage of pregnancy must be kept under observation until the time they attend school, must also be realized.

Table 3 Incidence of congenital abnormalities due to rubella in relation to gestational age

Month of gestation	Incidence (%)
1	15.3
2	24.6
3	17.5
4	6.4
5	1.7

From Hanshaw, J. B. and Dudgeon, J. A. (1978) *Viral diseases of the fetus and newborn* W. B. Saunders, Philadelphia
Based on five prospective studies from 1960–71

Diagnosis of congenital virus infection is based on serological tests that indicate primary infection in the mother, and active infection in the newborn. virus culture is helpful.

Only in the case of rubella has a concerted attempt been made to prevent congenital defect or disease. Rubella virus vaccine is used to immunize children of both sexes in the United States, and female children in the United Kingdom. The vaccine may also be given to adult women, provided that pregnancy is avoided.

Table 2 Incidence of congenital abnormalities due to rubella in relation to gestational age

Month of gestation	Incidence (%)
1	17.9
2	30.6
3	21.3
4	8.3
5	<1
6	<1
7	<1
8	<1
9	<1

From Swan, C. (1949). *J. Obstet. Gynaec. Br. Emp.* **56**, 341

References

Brumfitt, W. and Condie, A. P. (1977). Urinary infection. In *Scientific foundations of obstetrics and gynaecology* (eds. E. E. Phillip, J. Barnes, and M. Newton), 754. Heinemann, London.

David, C. and Finland, M. (1973). *Obstetric and perinatal infections*. Lea and Febiger, Philadelphia.

Davies, P. A. (1977). Infection of the fetus and newborn. In *Contemporary obstetrics and gynaecology* (ed. G. Chamberlain), 68. Northwood Publications, London.

Hanshaw, J. B. and Dudgeon, J. A. (1978). *Viral diseases of the fetus and newborn*. W. B. Saunders, Philadelphia, London, and Toronto.

Hurley, R. (1977). Viral diseases in pregnancy. In *Contemporary obstetrics and gynaecology* (ed. G. Chamberlain), 68. Northwood Publications Ltd., London.

— (1977). Microbiology. In *Scientific foundations of obstetrics and gynaecology* (eds. E. E. Phillipp, J. Barnes, and M. Newton), 727. Heinemann, London.

—, De Louvois, J., and Drasar, F. (1979). Perinatal and neonatal infections. *J. antimicrob. Chemother.* **5**, Supplement A.

Ledger, W. J. (1977). *Infection in the female*. Lea and Febiger, Philadelphia.

Remington, J. S. and Klein, J. O. (1976). *Infectious diseases of the fetus and newborn infant*. W. B. Saunders, Philadelphia, London and Toronto.

Possibly infectious diseases

SARCOIDOSIS

J. G. Scadding

The concept of sarcoidosis as a systemic disease arose from the recognition that certain affections of the skin initially described as separate 'diseases' were often associated with changes in internal organs; that in all involved tissues a similar histological pattern of non-caseating epithelioid-cell granulomatosis could be found; and, later, that various combinations of organ involvement of this sort occurred more frequently without than with skin changes. No infective or other agent uniquely causing this sort of granulomatosis has been conclusively demonstrated, although evidence, discussed below, of an agent transmissible to mice has recently been obtained. There is no convincing evidence of person-to-person transmission, and in the absence of an established infective agent, it is uncertain whether sarcoidosis should be grouped with infectious diseases.

History. The earliest reports of cases that would now be categorized as sarcoidosis related to patients with skin eruptions of various types. In 1889, the French dermatologist Besnier described lupus pernio, an eruption involving the nose and the central area of the face, the lobes of the ears and the fingers. This combined the swelling and erythema associated with chilblains (*pernio*) with the 'apple-jelly nodule' appearance seen under vitropression in lupus vulgaris, then a common form of tuberculosis of the skin. Histologically, it showed non-caseating tuberculoid granulomas. In 1898, the English surgeon, Hutchinson, described 'Mortimer's malady', named after the first patient in whom he had observed it. This had some resemblance to lupus pernio, but also more widespread elements resembling the 'multiple benign sarcoids' described in the following year by the Norwegian dermatologist, Boeck. These consisted of slightly elevated spots and patches of a yellow-brown colour with slight scaling on the limbs and trunk as well as the face, without ulceration, though larger spots became slightly flattened and atrophic centrally. Epitrochlear, axillary, and inguinal lymph-nodes were enlarged. Biopsy of the skin showed foci of epithelioid cells with some giant cells. Boeck at first interpreted this as a benign tumour of connective tissue and therefore proposed the name 'sarcoid'. However, he soon recognized that it was in fact a tuberculoid granuloma resembling that seen in lupus vulgaris, and suggested that the name should be changed to 'lupoid', but this was not widely adopted. It is ironic that the name now generally used, both for the skin changes and for the systemic disease of which they are a manifestation, arose from a soon-corrected histological error. Later, Boeck described involvement of lymph-nodes, nasal mucosa, lungs, spleen, bones of the hands and feet, and conjunctiva in patients with multiple benign sarcoids or lupus pernio. The Swedish dermatologist Schaumann in a series of publications from 1914 onwards showed for the first time that changes in internal organs having a similar histological pattern frequently occurred without skin changes. In 1909, a Danish ophthalmologist, Heerfordt, described a syndrome of irido-cyclitis, parotid gland enlargement, and facial palsy which he called 'sub-chronic uveoparotid fever'; and later parotid glands in patients with this syndrome were shown to be infiltrated with non-caseating tuberculoid granulomas. This complete syndrome is rare, but one or two of its features, especially uveitis, often occur with granulomatous changes in lymph-nodes, skin, lungs, and other internal organs. In 1941, Kveim reported from the Dermatological Department in Oslo the reaction that now bears his name; the gradual development of a granulomatous nodule at the site of intradermal injection of a suspension of sarcoid tissue in patients with active sarcoidosis. From 1946 to 1953, Löfgren, working in the same Stockholm hospital as Schaumann, showed that the syndrome of bilateral hilar lymph-node enlargement (BHL), with or without erythema nodosum, is to be regarded as an early manifestation of sarcoidosis.

Pathology

The characteristic granuloma of sarcoidosis consists of well-formed and sharply demarcated collections of epithelioid cells with little cellular reaction around them (Fig. 1). Multinucleate giant cells are generally found in moderate numbers, but may be very sparse or very numerous. Inclusion-bodies of three sorts, crystalline, conchoidal, and asteroid, may be seen in them. Crystalline and conchoidal bodies occur more frequently in sarcoidosis and in chronic beryllium disease than in other granulomatous conditions. Crystalline inclusions do not take up stains, are birefringent to polarized light, and are composed of crystalline calcium carbonate. Conchoidal bodies, first described by Schaumann, are shaped like an oyster-shell and are basophilic, staining with haematoxylin. They are probably formed by the deposition of protein impregnated with amorphous calcium salts around a small crystalline body, and are not birefringent. Star-shaped asteroid bodies within vacuoles in giant-cells and staining pink with eosin, are no more frequent in sarcoid than in other granulomas.

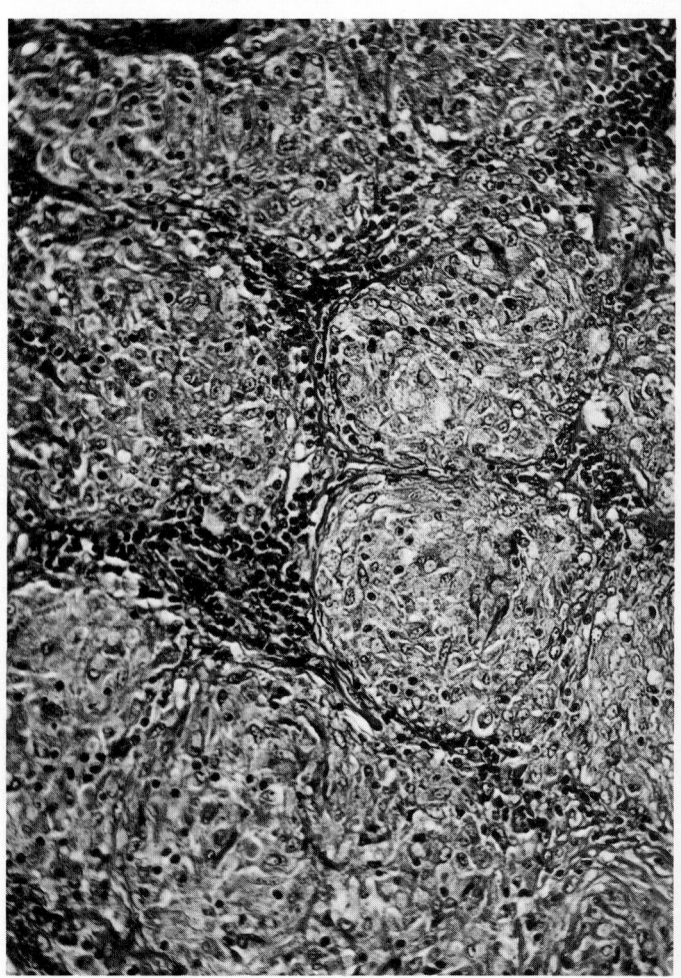

Fig. 1   Typical sarcoid granuloma in a lymph-node.

The granulomas of sarcoidosis do not caseate like those of myco-bacterial tuberculosis, though some fibrinoid necrosis may be seen at the centres of dense aggregations. They persist for a variable, sometimes prolonged, time in a cellular state and are capable of resolution. If they do not resolve, they gradually become replaced, at first peripherally, by hyaline fibrosis (Fig. 2), in which remnants of the granuloma may eventually be hard to find; sometimes con-choidal bodies persist as the only recognizable residue.

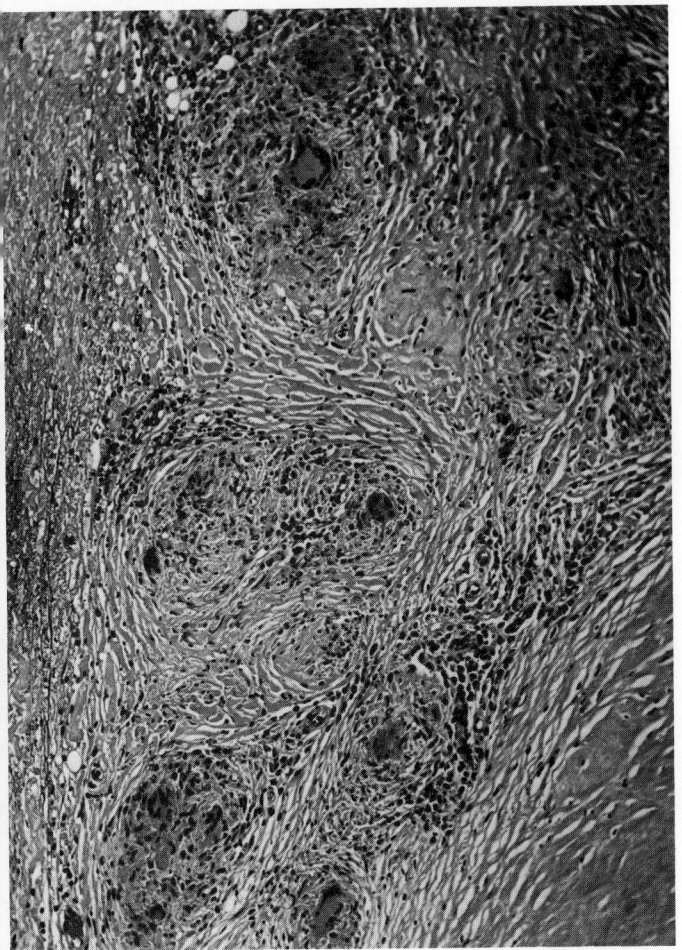

Fig. 2 Hyaline fibrosis developing in a sarcoid lymph-node.

Definition

Since no agent specifically causing sarcoidosis has been identified, sarcoidosis cannot at present be defined aetiologically. In the final analysis, doubt about the correctness of a diagnosis of sarcoidosis can be dispelled only by evidence that characteristic histopatholo-gical changes are widely disseminated. This leads to the definition of sarcoidosis as 'a disease characterized by the presence in all of a number of affected organs of epithelioid-cell tubercles, without caseation though some fibrinoid necrosis may be present, proceed-ing either to resolution or to hyaline fibrosis'. To this may be added a note that the organs most frequently affected are lymph-nodes, lungs, skin, eyes, liver, spleen, small bones of the hands and feet, and salivary glands, though every organ with the possible exception of the adrenal glands has been reported to be involved; and that no unique causal agent has been identified.

Incidence and modes of presentation

Both the initial symptoms and the subsequent course of sarcoidosis are very varied. In many patients, constitutional symptoms are slight or absent. Some have an initial acute stage in which non-granulomatous inflammatory changes, such as erythema nodosum

(EN), arthropathy, and anterior uveitis may occur, sometimes with fever. The liability of granulomatous infiltrations to cause symp-toms depends upon the organs involved, upon the profusion and location of granulomas within these organs, and upon whether they evolve towards resolution or fibrosis. Involvement of the lung and hilar lymph-nodes may cause no symptom, and come to light only because of a chest radiograph. Liver biopsy in the active stages of sarcoidosis shows granulomas in up to 70 per cent of cases, but very few patients have symptoms or signs referable to the liver. On the other hand, infiltrations of the skin are very likely to be noticed; and in some of the organs less often affected—e.g. the heart and the central nervous system—a small collection of granulomas may be so placed as to cause obvious symptoms.

Because of this very varied clinical presentation and of the con-siderable number of asymptomatic cases, of which many proceed to spontaneous resolution, it is difficult to determine the true in-cidence of sarcoidosis in a community. In a study in which special efforts were made to record all possible cases in four selected areas of the United Kingdom, the annual incidence of new diagnoses of sarcoidosis ranged between 3.0 and 4.5 per 100 000. The propor-tions of patients presenting with various features in this and in a series in London are listed in Table 1. Over half present with intrathoracic changes with or without symptoms, discovered by radiography. The 'EN–arthropathy–BHL syndrome' is the earliest clinical feature in a proportion of cases varying between different areas: in several European studies it has been reported in up to one-third of the patients, but in the United States it seems to be much less frequent, especially in blacks. Sarcoids of the skin and eye changes, principally uveitis, are the next most frequent presenting features; and a few patients first notice enlargement of superficial lymph-nodes or of salivary glands. Very rarely the first symptoms are caused by changes in another organ or by the hyper-calcaemia that occurs in a few patients.

Table 1 Percentages of patients with sarcoidosis first seeking medical advice for various reasons in two series

	Scadding (1967)* (%)	BTTA (1969)† (%)
Abnormal chest radiograph	34	31
Respiratory and constitutional symptoms	31	21
Erythema nodosum, febrile arthropathy	14	32
Ocular symptoms	10	4
Skin sarcoids	5	7
Superficial lymphadenopathy	4	3
Other	1	1

* Scadding (1967): 275 patients in London 1946–66
† BTTA (1969): 567 patients in four areas in Great Britain 1961–6

Nearly all studies of incidence in defined populations and of large numbers of clinical records have shown more cases in women than in men. In the study of four areas in the United Kingdom the incidence in women ranged from 1.1 times that in men in the most southerly to 1.7 in the most northerly area. In both sexes, the incidence is highest between the ages of 20 and 35 years, and, in some populations, has shown a small increase later in the 50 to 60 years age-group, especially in women. A few cases occur in child-hood and in old age, but the incidence at the extremes of life is difficult to determine, for two reasons. Reported cases include a high proportion with unusual manifestations, liable to cause di-agnostic difficulty; and in most countries asymptomatic individuals in these age-groups are less frequently submitted to chest radiog-raphy than are young adults, and thus symptomless sarcoidosis proceeding to spontaneous resolution is likely to remain unde-tected. It is relevant that in Hungary and in Japan where radio-graphic surveys of school-children are carried out, symptomless BHL has been reported in children as in adults.

Other estimates of incidence in defined populations include those for Denmark, based on notifications from chest clinics, of 7 per 100 000 per year, and for the United States Army, based on diagnostic records, of 11 per 100 000. The Danish figures excluded some cases not known to chest clinics, and it was thought that the inclusion of these might have raised them by about one-fifth. They are thus higher than those found in the areas studied in the United Kingdom; but the differences between areas in Denmark were greater than those in the UK, the range being from 2 to 18 per 100 000. The figure for the US Army refers to a male population with a high proportion of the most susceptible age-group, young adults, and of blacks, among whom in the United States the incidence of sarcoidosis has been found to be 12 to 14 times that among whites. There are probably differences between other geographic areas and ethnic groups, but these have been less completely studied. In the United Kingdom, the incidence of symptomatic sarcoidosis appears to be especially high among West Indians, and of BHL with or without erythema nodosum among recent young immigrants from Ireland. On the other hand, the Chinese appear to be relatively infrequently affected anywhere, as do Africans in Africa.

Clinical syndromes and organ involvement

Table 2 shows the proportions of patients in a co-operative study from various parts of the world who at any time showed some of the commoner clinical manifestations.

Table 2 Frequency of some clinical manifestations among patients with sarcoidosis reported from London, Paris, New York, Los Angeles and Tokyo. Numbers of patients in brackets

	London* (275) (%)	London† (537) (%)	Paris† (379) (%)	New York† (311) (%)	Los Angeles† (150) (%)	Tokyo† (282) (%)
Lungs, hilar nodes	98	84	92	90	93	87
Peripheral lymph-nodes	31	29	23	37	31	23
Eyes	14	27	11	20	11	14
Skin	17	25	12	19	27	17
Spleen	11	12	6	18	15	1
Parotid	2	6	6	3	6	5
Central nervous system	1	7	6	4	6	5
Bones	4	4	3.5	9	4	2
Erythema nodosum	14	31	6.5	11	9	4

* Scadding (1967)   † Siltzbach et al. (1974)

Erythema nodosum, febrile arthropathy. The clinical features of erythema nodosum (EN) are described in Section 20.

EN associated with sarcoidosis is nearly always the first overt manifestation of the disease.

The proportion of cases of EN attributed to sarcoidosis in a population depends upon the incidences not only of sarcoidosis but also of mycobacterial, haemolytic streptococcal and some other bacterial infections and of such fungal infections as coccidioidomycosis and histoplasmosis; and upon clinical awareness and diagnostic criteria. To quote figures from two countries with similar medical standards, the proportion of a series of patients with EN thought to have sarcoidosis was 13 per cent in Scotland, and 47 per cent in Finland. In reported series of patients with sarcoidosis, the proportions in which EN was observed vary even more. In the British study, mentioned above, it ranged between 24 and 32 per cent, and similar proportions have been reported recently from Sweden, Finland, and Belgium. In earlier studies in London and in Germany, only 10 to 12 per cent of patients with sarcoidosis had had

EN. These studies concerned populations almost entirely Caucasian. In the United States, where blacks constitute the majority of patients with sarcoidosis, EN is found in a higher proportion of white than of black patients. Among blacks, the proportion of sarcoidosis patients with EN is very low, so that the proportion in large series including blacks and whites is as low as 3 per cent.

Fever is usual, but is of very variable degree and duration. Some patients complain only of the eruption on their shins and are afebrile, while others have moderate fever which may last for several weeks.

In most areas, more women than men with sarcoidosis present with EN, though the reported sex-ratio, like the overall incidence, varies widely. In the British study of four areas, the proportions of women with EN ranged between 3.0 and 1.3 times those for men. In Stockholm, EN was recorded in 34 per cent of women and 5 per cent of men with sarcoidosis; in London in 16 per cent of men and 5 per cent of women; and in Philadelphia, where most of the patients were black, in only 4 per cent of women and no men.

Arthropathy. Most patients with EN associated with sarcoidosis have some joint-pains, especially in ankles and knees, though other joints may be affected. The severity of the joint symptoms is very variable. In some cases, swelling of periarticular tissues with redness and tenderness is evident. In a few, mostly men, the painful joint swellings are more prominent than the skin eruption, and in rare cases may occur without EN. In some of these cases, especially if the patient has remained ambulant, a rather characteristic brawny periarticular swelling of the ankle-joints is seen.

Diagnosis of the EN–BHL syndrome. The investigation of a patient with erythema nodosum is discussed in Section 20, and the diagnosis of sarcoidosis in general on page 5.499. Here it is appropriate to consider the clinical, radiographic, and laboratory findings in a patient with EN and/or febrile arthropathy favouring a diagnosis of sarcoidosis.

1. EN in sarcoidosis nearly always occurs as an early, often the first, clinical manifestation, and at a time when BHL is present. Very occasionally, BHL becomes evident soon after EN; and in some cases it is accompanied by mottled opacities in the lung fields. The association of EN with BHL is virtually diagnostic of sarcoidosis.

2. Evidence of sarcoidosis may be found in accessible extrathoracic sites. Uveitis, sarcoid infiltration of the skin, including old scars, and enlargement of superficial lymph-nodes should be sought.

3. Negative tests for infection by agents known to be possible causes of EN, such as haemolytic streptococci, M. tuberculosis, Coccidioides, and Histoplasma increase the probability of sarcoidosis, but positive tests do not exclude it. For instance, although a negative tuberculin test excludes primary tuberculosis as a cause of EN, a positive test does not exclude sarcoidosis. Moderate sensitivity to tuberculin is found in some, and high sensitivity in a few cases associated with sarcoidosis; and among sarcoidosis patients the general level of tuberculin sensitivity is higher at the early EN–BHL stage than in the later more chronic stages. In cases associated with primary tuberculosis, unilateral hilar lymph-node enlargement, sometimes with various sorts of lung shadow, may be seen.

4. The histology of the EN itself is similar, no matter what its cause, and gives no clue to possible association with sarcoidosis.

Management. An onset with EN has generally been found to be of good prognostic in sarcoidosis. EN itself and the arthropathy that may accompany it resolve spontaneously, though after a variable duration. Symptoms can generally be controlled by non-steroidal anti-inflammatory drugs. Joint pain may be controlled by aspirin in the milder cases; if this is not sufficient phenylbutazone is usually effective; and in severe cases indomethacin may be required. These drugs should be continued only as long as they are needed for the control of symptoms. EN and arthropathy are not an indication for the use of corticosteroids.

Respiratory system. Many patients with sarcoidosis, in some series one-quarter or more, come to light because of an abnormal chest radiograph. About the same proportion present with banal respiratory symptoms.

In most, but not all, cases the early stage of pulmonary sarcoidosis is accompanied or preceded by BHL. It is therefore convenient to consider the radiological and clinical features of BHL and of pulmonary sarcoidosis together. There is a convention that three radiologically descriptive groups (*a*) BHL alone, (*b*) BHL and lung changes, and (*c*) lung changes alone should be called stages I, II, and III, with an added stage O for those cases in which the chest radiograph is normal. This carries the unjustified assumption that these appearances represent a necessary temporal sequence. Preferably, descriptions of various combinations of lung and hilar lymph-node changes should be dissociated from estimates of chronicity and extent of fibrosis, which can be separately assessed.

BHL. *Radiology.* The enlarged hilar and mediastinal lymph-nodes of sarcoidosis usually cast roughly symmetrical radiographic shadows, though that on the right tends to appear larger, both because there is a larger number of bronchopulmonary nodes on the right and because the left hilar shadow is partly obscured by the heart. Characteristically the outer border of the enlarged hilar shadow in sarcoidosis is clearly defined with multiple smooth contours, suggesting discrete enlargement of individual nodes; and there is often a clear transradiant band between the inner border of the lower part of the lymph-node shadow and the heart shadow, most evident on the right (Fig. 3). Paratracheal nodes are frequently involved, and are detectable radiographically on the right side in about half the cases; very occasionally they may be more prominent than the hilar group. In rare cases, the hilar node enlargement is predominantly unilateral, usually on the right side: it may become bilateral later. Foci of calcification, presumably due to old primary mycobacterial infection, have been found in the enlarged nodes in a few cases; this must be distinguished from the development of calcification in the late stage of hyaline fibrosis, described below. Tomography may be useful in the few cases in which it is difficult to decide whether enlarged hilar shadows are due to lymph-nodes or to dilatation of pulmonary blood-vessels. With grossly enlarged lymph-nodes there may be tomographically evident narrowing of major bronchi and widening of the carinal angle.

Prognosis. Evidence from lung biopsy suggests that, in patients with BHL, granulomas are present in the lungs, even though these appear normal radiographically. In about half of them, the hilar lymph-nodes subside spontaneously, the lungs remaining clear. In the rest, the granulomas in the lungs become profuse enough to cause radiographically evident changes, usually as the nodes subside. The prognosis for these is similar to that of patients who have both BHL and lung changes when first seen. With or without lung changes, BHL in most cases subsides within three years, sometimes quite rapidly; but rarely it persists for many years. In such cases, it is likely that the nodes have undergone massive hyaline fibrosis.

Lungs. Many patients with sarcoid granulomas in the lung profuse enough to cause changes in the chest radiograph have no or trivial symptoms. Some present with cough, perhaps after an upper respiratory infection, and a few with malaise, fever, usually slight, cough, and some dyspnoea, usually less than might be expected from the radiographic changes. The later development of fibrosis leads to gradually increasing dyspnoea on exertion. The fibrosis of sarcoidosis is rarely associated with clubbing of the fingers, contrasting sharply in this respect with cryptogenic fibrosing alveolitis.

Radiology. The commonest radiographic appearance is widespread mottled or stippled shadowing, distributed more or less uniformly, or tending to be denser in the middle zones (Fig. 4). The individual elements in the mottling usually have ill-defined borders and vary in diameter from 1 to 5 mm. In some cases areas of local confluence give rise to localized uniform shadows, and in a few, very fine stippling, dense in places and sparse elsewhere, causes a cloudy appearance (Fig. 5).

Pulmonary infiltration without BHL is the earliest radiographic finding in some cases, and in a few of these a recent normal radiograph provides evidence that there has been no preceding BHL. Thus radiographically evident BHL though a frequent is not a necessary event in the evolution of pulmonary sarcoidosis; and

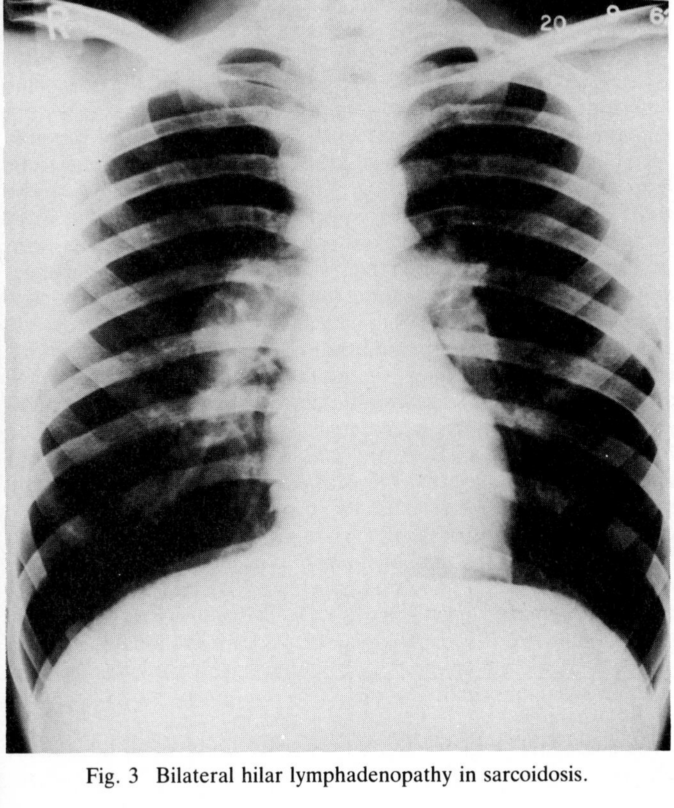

Fig. 3   Bilateral hilar lymphadenopathy in sarcoidosis.

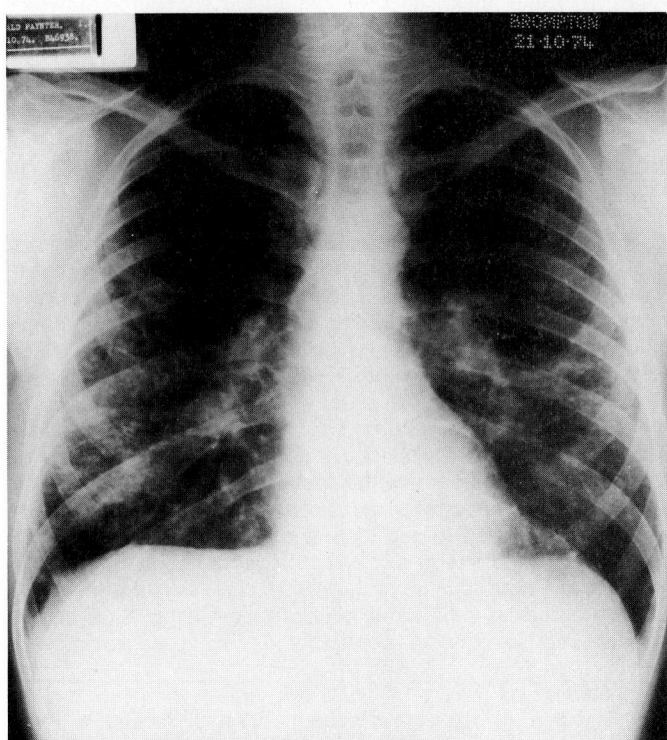

Fig. 4   BHL and sarcoid infiltration of the lung.

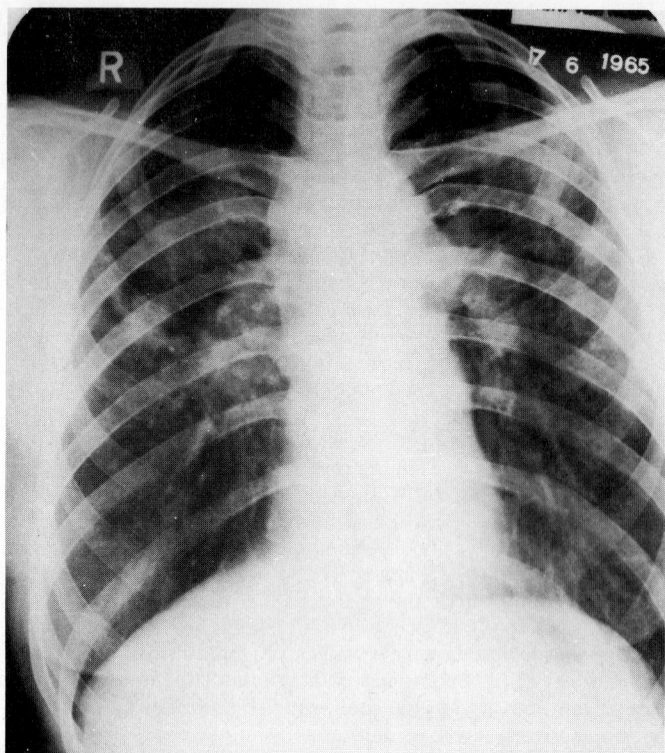

Fig. 5 Cloudy shadowing due to sarcoid infiltration of the lung.

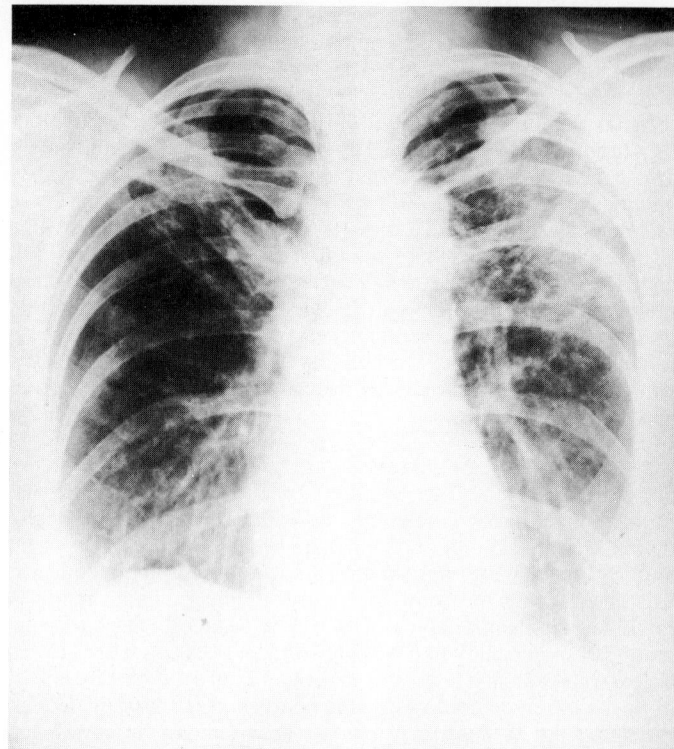

Fig. 6 A characteristic pattern of late sarcoidosis of the lung with fibrosis.

there is some evidence that patients presenting with pulmonary infiltration without preceding BHL differ from those with BHL not only in a lower incidence of EN and of uveitis at the onset, but also in a more chronic course and less favourable prognosis for the lung changes.

Late stages. Many of those developing fibrosis show a rather characteristic pattern of radiographic changes. Mottling becomes denser in the middle or middle and adjacent parts of the upper zones. Irregular linear shadows then appear, extending outwards from the hila (Fig. 6). Later, the hila become raised, mottling tends to clear, the linear shadows become more prominent, and localized dense shadows, presumably due to confluent fibrosis, may appear. At this stage, the lower and sometimes the upper zones show areas of transradiancy suggesting emphysema, sometimes bullous; and air-containing spaces may be evident, especially on tomography, in the densely opaque areas. At necropsy, these have been shown to have dense fibrous tissue walls, without epithelial lining. Occasionally, these spaces become colonized by *Aspergillus*, giving rise to a 'fungus ball', with characteristic radiographic appearance (see Section 15).

Not all patients developing fibrosis show this pattern of predominantly middle and upper zone changes. In a few, the disseminated granulomas undergo focal fibrosis, without confluence or distortion of the macroscopic vascular pattern in the chest radiograph. The mottling may become less dense, individual elements diminishing in size and possibly giving place to a reticular pattern, while disability becomes more severe, with increasing dyspnoea.

Calcification. In about 5 per cent of patients with pulmonary sarcoidosis followed for prolonged periods, foci of calcification develop in a characteristically symmetrical fashion in hilar lymphnodes, and, less frequently, in the lungs. This calcification is dystrophic, occurring in the hyaline fibrosis which is the end-stage of sarcoid granulomas, and is not associated with hypercalcaemia (see below).

Bronchi. In the early stage of pulmonary sarcoidosis accompanying BHL, granulomas are often present even in macroscopically normal bronchial mucosa. In most cases these resolve, but in a few

cases they persist and progress to cause localized bronchial narrowing at first due to granulomatous thickening of the mucosa and later irreversibly fibrotic. These narrowings typically occur in large bronchi, especially at the orifices of segmental bronchi. Patients with these bronchial stenoses have prolonged and noisy inspiratory as well as wheezy expiratory breath-sounds.

Pleura. Pleural changes are rare. A few cases of pleural effusion, at both the early BHL and the later chronic granulomatous stages have been recorded.

Pulmonary function. As would be expected from the foregoing description of the clinical, radiological, and pathological aspects of pulmonary sarcoidosis, the effects on pulmonary function are very variable. With a few exceptions, the functional deficit tends to be less than the severity of radiographic changes might suggest. The commonest pattern consists in a restrictive ventilatory defect (small total lung capacity with proportionate reduction in its subdivisions, possibly diminished compliance, and normal airflow resistance) and a gas transfer defect (arterial oxygen pressure tending to be low at rest and falling on exercise, with a normal or low CO_2 pressure, and reduced carbon monoxide transfer factor). With a prefibrotic infiltration, these tests may give results within normal limits. If they are abnormal at this stage, ventilatory restriction tends to be more prominent than gas transfer defect; changes of this sort may be found in patients with BHL and radiologically normal lungs. With the development of fibrosis, tests especially of gas transfer become more abnormal. Some patients, especially those with fibrotic changes, show expiratory airflow limitation: in such cases the possible role of cigarette-smoking must be considered. In patients with the rather rare multiple proximal bronchial stenoses described above, evidence of inspiratory as well as expiratory airflow limitation is found. In a few patients with widespread focal fibrosis, a severe defect in gas transfer may be found with a relatively minor radiographic abnormality.

Prognosis. In half to two-thirds of patients, pulmonary sarcoidosis resolves to leave radiographically clear lungs. This favourable course is especially likely in those who initially have no respiratory disability. It usually starts within two years, but in patients who remain symptom-free substantial resolution is possible at any time, and only minor non-progressive fibrosis may result. But among those who are breathless with persistent extensive granulomatous changes, some will be left with extensive irreversible fibrosis likely to shorten life. In one prospective study, 6 of 27 patients with established fibrotic sarcoidosis of the lung died of it during five years' observation; and from this and from the proportion of patients first observed at a pre-fibrotic stage who developed fibrosis, it was estimated that the eventual mortality from radiographically evident pulmonary sarcoidosis was likely to be 6–7 per cent.

Upper respiratory tract. Symptomatic involvement of the upper respiratory tract is relatively rare.

Granulomatous changes in the nasal mucosa are often associated with sarcoidosis of the skin of the face, especially of the lupus pernio type, but may occur without it. They cause such symptoms as nasal obstruction and discharge, crusting and dryness, and epistaxis. The bridge of the nose may be swollen even though the skin appears normal. The nasal mucosa is thickened, submucous nodules may be seen, and polypoidal masses may develop in the nasal cavity and sinuses, and the post-nasal space. Rarefactions of the nasal bones may be detected radiographically.

The larynx may be affected, nearly always with other parts of the upper respiratory tract. The extent varies from no more than local infiltration of the epiglottis, an ary-epiglottic fold or a vocal cord, to progressive involvement of the whole larynx, extending even into the trachea. In very rare instances, polypoidal masses and later scarring lead to laryngeal obstruction requiring surgical relief if it does not respond to corticosteroid treatment.

Skin. Sarcoids of the skin are described in Section 20. Their place in the overall picture of sarcoidosis can be indicated by the findings in 500 cases of sarcoidosis followed by a physician for prolonged periods. Skin sarcoids were the reason for first consultation in 5.2 per cent, were found incidentally at the first examination in 4.6 per cent, and appeared later in 6.6 per cent. Small sarcoids and infiltrations of old scars occurred mainly in the early active stage, and tended to be transient, whereas large persistent infiltrations of unscarred skin, such as lupus pernio, were a feature of chronic sarcoidosis, and were generally accompanied by fibrosing changes in the lungs.

Eyes. The most frequent affection of the eyes in sarcoidosis is uveitis. Others include infiltrations of the conjunctiva and of the lachrymal glands, kerato-conjunctivitis sicca due to the consequent deficiency of tears, and the effects of hypercalcaemia on the cornea and bulbar conjunctiva.

Uveitis has been reported in from 15 to 25 per cent of cases in various large series of patients with sarcoidosis. However, the proportion of the very large number of cases of uveitis referred to eye clinics found to be a manifestation of sarcoidosis is small, as low as 2 per cent. Two sorts of uveitis can be recognized. Early in the course, there may be an anterior uveitis which often resolves without permanent damage; it seems to be cognate with EN and febrile arthropathy. Later a granulomatous uveitis may involve the posterior as well as the anterior part of the uveal tract as part of the picture of chronic sarcoidosis. It tends to be persistent, usually fails to respond to local treatment, and may cause irreversible changes, threatening sight. These include posterior synechiae, keratic precipitates, corneal opacification, cataract, fibrotic changes in the anterior chamber leading to glaucoma, and choroidal changes. Ophthalmoscopically it is rarely possible to distinguish with certainty between sarcoid and other sorts of uveitis, and diagnosis depends upon the recognition of other manifestations of the disease.

Although infiltration of the conjunctiva with sarcoid granulomas hardly ever causes symptoms, careful examination in patients with sarcoidosis may reveal appearances suggestive of sub-mucosal follicles, especially in the lower fornix; and biopsy of these may show typical granulomas. These are not necessarily associated with uveitis and are likely to be found only in patients with widespread extrathoracic and intrathoracic sarcoidosis. Thus conjunctival biopsy is unlikely to be helpful in obscure cases.

Some patients with sarcoidosis complain of dryness, soreness, and redness of the eyes. The probable cause of this is sarcoid infiltration of lachrymal glands, though these are rarely palpable; lack of tears leads to degeneration of epithelial cells of the cornea and conjunctiva, especially the exposed parts, with consequent inflammation. Milder cases of this kerato-conjunctivitis sicca can be detected only by slit-lamp microscopy after rose bengal staining. Its reported frequency varies with the assiduity with which it is sought from 66 per cent in an intensively investigated series, to 3 per cent for one in which only symptomatic cases were noted. Its association with other features of sarcoidosis distinguishes such cases from the locally similar kerato-conjunctivitis of Sjögren's syndrome (see Section 16).

The hypercalcaemia that occurs in some patients with sarcoidosis, described below, can lead to deposits of calcium salts in the cornea and the conjunctiva. Bands of corneal calcification are best displayed by slit-lamp examination. Very occasionally small white nodules of calcification develop in the exposed part of the bulbar conjunctiva, usually with inflammatory congestion of blood-vessels.

A few cases of exophthalmos due to sarcoid infiltration of the orbit have been reported; some of these have been associated with granulomatous leptomeningitis at the base of the brain. In such cases, the optic nerve is likely to be involved (see below).

Lymphadenopathy. Superficial lymph-nodes in one or more groups are palpable in many patients with sarcoidosis. The proportion is as high as 80 per cent in some series from the United States including many blacks; in those from Europe it is around 30 per cent. The cervical nodes, especially in the posterior triangle above the clavicle, are most commonly affected, followed by the axillary, the epitrochlear and the inguinal. Isolated nodes anywhere may be enlarged. Occasionally, enlarged nodes noticed by the patient are the presenting feature. Sarcoid lymph-nodes are discrete, firm and elastic, not adherent, and usually painless and not tender. In the neck, they may simulate those of Hodgkin's disease. The removal of a node for biopsy is safe and simple and should not be delayed if diagnosis is not evident from associated features.

Very occasionally, abdominal lymph-node enlargement gives rise to palpable masses, and these may be tender and give rise to pain.

Liver. Liver biopsy shows sarcoid granulomas in up to 70 per cent of patients with active sarcoidosis, but clinical evidence of liver involvement at this stage is hardly ever found. In most cases these granulomas resolve as the disease regresses. In a very few, they persist, increase in number and may eventually undergo hyaline fibrosis; and the liver becomes an important site of persistent sarcoidosis. In such cases, clinical and biochemical evidence of liver dysfunction appears. Both portal hypertension and jaundice may occur, separately or together.

When liver biopsy shows well-defined non-caseating granulomas and there are overt evidences of sarcoidosis elsewhere, diagnosis presents no difficulty. But if no evidence of granulomatous change in other organs can be found, and especially if, as is often the case, the hepatic granulomas are less clearly defined and accompanied by chronic inflammatory changes a large number of possible causes of granulomatous change in the liver must be considered. These include infections such as tuberculosis, histoplasmosis, chronic brucellosis, Q fever, and infectious mononucleosis; chronic beryllium disease; Hodgkin's disease; and biliary cirrhosis. In many cases, associated features and relevant tests resolve the problem; but for some cases, in which investigation is inconclusive, provisional categorization as granulomatous hepatitis must be accepted.

Spleen. The spleen, like the liver, probably contains scattered granulomas in most patients with active sarcoidosis. It has been reported to be palpable in from 10 to 25 per cent of patients with sarcoidosis. Gross splenomegaly is rare; it may be accompanied by depression of marrow function leading to low counts of erythrocytes, polymorphs, or thrombocytes. In a few cases, the spleen becomes large enough to cause abdominal discomfort. Even very large spleens may regress to become impalpable if their increased size is due entirely to dense infiltration with sarcoid granulomas. Splenomegaly may also be due partly or principally to portal hypertension secondary to fibrosing sarcoidosis of the liver.

Blood. During the active stages of sarcoidosis, the lymphocyte count in the peripheral blood is low: this has immunological implications, and is discussed below.

In a few patients with sarcoidosis, thrombocytopenia and purpura have been observed. The spleen may or may not be palpably enlarged, but has usually been found when removed to be infiltrated with sarcoid granulomas. Improvement may follow corticosteroid treatment, but the response is unpredictable; when it does not, splenectomy generally leads to a rise in platelet count and relief of purpura. The association of pancytopenia with splenic enlargement in sarcoidosis has been noted above. A very few cases of haemolytic anaemia in patients with sarcoidosis have been reported, but the relationship of the haemolysis to sarcoidosis is uncertain.

Bones. The most frequently observed changes in the bones in sarcoidosis occur in the hands and feet, usually in phalanges or metacarpals or metatarsals. They are strongly associated with skin sarcoids especially of the lupus pernio type. There may be swelling of the digit around affected phalanges, with or without changes in the overlying skin, and movement of adjacent joints may be painful and limited. Dystrophic changes may be seen in the nails. But in some cases, the changes in the bones cause no symptoms and are discoverable only by radiography. The appearances are of two sorts: a lattice-like pattern of multiple rarefactions in a diffusely expanded phalanx, which may be accompanied by clinically evident swelling and changes in the skin; and localized rounded or oval rarefactions suggesting unilocular or multilocular cysts, usually at the ends of affected bones, and clinically silent. Characteristically there is no periosteal reaction, and joints are affected only when there is very extensive bone destruction. With spontaneous regression of sarcoidosis, or suppression by corticosteroids, a remarkable return towards normal bone structure may occur.

In rare cases, the bones of the carpus, the tarsus and the adjacent bones of the forearm and leg show similar rarefactions, usually in association with changes in the hands or feet.

Involvement of the nasal bones in association with intranasal sarcoidosis has been mentioned above. A few cases of rarefactions, usually well-defined, in the bones of the skull have been reported: some were associated with changes in the overlying skin. Even more rarely, vertebral bodies have been affected in patients with other evidences of sarcoidosis and biopsy has shown sarcoid granulomas.

Joints. The transient arthropathy that occurs, sometimes with erythema nodosum, as an early feature of some cases of sarcoidosis has been described above. In the few cases in which biopsies have been performed, non-granulomatous inflammation has been found. This arthropathy is generally of limited duration, rarely more than two or three months; in a very few it is more persistent or even recurrent.

As noted above, joints in the hands and feet may be involved when the adjacent bones are severely affected.

In a few patients with chronic sarcoidosis, persistent polyarthritis affecting large as well as small joints has been shown to be associated with granulomatous changes in synovial biopsies. This granulomatous arthropathy may simulate rheumatoid arthritis, or in children, Still's disease. Most of the recorded cases have been in North American blacks with widespread sarcoidosis.

Muscles. Random muscle biopsies have been reported to show granulomas in a high proportion of patients with active sarcoidosis, especially those with EN and BHL. Thus it is likely that symptomless infiltration of muscles is frequent at this stage, resolving uneventfully in nearly all cases. Symptomatic involvement of muscles is rare. The muscles most commonly affected in this way are those of the proximal parts of the limbs and the limb-girdles. In most cases, the clinical findings are wasting and weakness of affected muscles, which must be distinguished from other sorts of proximal myopathy, especially that caused by corticosteroids. In some cases, affected muscles show clinically obvious changes, such as palpable nodules, general induration, or even pseudo-hypertrophy. The diagnosis is easily established by biopsy.

Although most of the reported cases have been in patients with widespread sarcoidosis, in a few the granulomatous myopathy has been the principal or even the only clinical finding.

Heart. The heart may be affected in sarcoidosis directly by granulomatous infiltration, or indirectly by the effects of pulmonary hypertension secondary to extensive, usually fibrotic, changes in the lungs. The proportion of known cases in which either of these becomes clinically evident is very small.

Cor pulmonale. Extensive pulmonary sarcoidosis with respiratory insufficiency may lead to pulmonary hypertension, right ventricular hypertrophy, and eventually failure; this cor pulmonale does not differ from that due to other forms of chronic pulmonary disease (see Section 13). It will not be considered further here, except to note that it occurs rather infrequently in pulmonary sarcoidosis and that when it does, airflow limitation is often a complicating factor.

Myocardial sarcoidosis. A very few cases of isolated rhythm disturbances, notably heart block, have been reported in patients with sarcoidosis and an otherwise unremarkable course. The most plausible explanation of these is interruption of conducting tissues by an unluckily sited granuloma in the general dissemination of granulomas in active sarcoidosis, though the frequency of involvement of the heart in this is unknown.

In those cases of symptomatic cardiac sarcoidosis in which information about pathology is available, confluent granulomatous replacement of parts of the myocardium as well as irregularly scattered foci have been found. Pericardium and endocardium are generally less involved. In the myocardium, the most frequent site of massive involvement is the left ventricle, including its papillary muscles, followed by the interventricular septum and the right ventricle, the atria being least affected.

The clinical features, as would be expected from the variable extent and distribution of the morbid changes, are diverse. They include arrhythmias, principally ventricular; various degrees of atrioventricular and bundle branch block; congestive heart failure simulating congestive cardiomyopathy; mitral incompetence of rapid onset from papillary muscle dysfunction; and left ventricular aneurysm. Sudden death, presumably due to ventricular tachycardia, was the first evidence of disease in a high proportion of reported cases.

Nervous system. Sarcoidosis affecting the nervous system can present difficult diagnostic problems, especially if it is the principal clinical manifestation. Its features can be grouped for description into granulomatosis of the central nervous system and neuropathy. These may occur together or separately. Peripheral and cranial neuropathies tend to occur at the early acute stage of sarcoidosis, with such inflammatory phenomena as erythema nodosum, arthropathy, and anterior uveitis. Granulomatous changes in the brain, spinal cord, and meninges tend to follow a prolonged course and may be accompanied by florid manifestations of sarcoidosis elsewhere, though sometimes they constitute the only clinical evidence of the disease. In many cases, neuropathies are transient, and in these it seems unlikely that the nerves are infiltrated with granulomas; but in some cases, it is probable that cranial nerves are involved in granulomatous basal meningitis.

Cranial nerves. Of the cranial nerves, the facial is the most frequently affected. Facial palsy, uveitis, and salivary gland enlargement constitute the syndrome of uveo-parotid fever; this is rare, but facial palsy occurs much more frequently either alone or with only one of the other features of this syndrome. As in other lower motor neurone facial palsies, ageusia may accompany the palsy. The facial palsy of sarcoidosis is usually transient, even though other manifestations of sarcoidosis remain active. It usually starts on one side, but in a third or more of the cases the contralateral side is involved after a variable interval. Transient facial palsy affecting the two sides of the face successively should lead to a search for evidence of sarcoidosis.

The optic nerve may be infiltrated with sarcoid granulomas, usually in association with similar changes in the basal meninges, causing visual field defects or loss of vision and optic atrophy. In other cases, raised intracranial pressure due to involvement of the brain and meninges causes papilloedema.

The eighth nerve, both auditory and vestibular divisions may be affected, causing deafness, tinnitus, and dizziness.

The trigeminal nerve is involved more frequently in its sensory than in its motor functions: diminution of sensation on the face and loss of corneal reflexes are more frequent than weakness of the muscles of mastication.

Anosmia due to involvement of the olfactory nerve and dysphagia due to weakness of the pharyngeal and palatal muscles innervated by the glossopharyngeal and vagus nerves may occur, often in association with uveitis and/or facial palsy. The oculomotor nerves, the third, fourth, and sixth nerves, are relatively infrequently involved.

Peripheral nerves. Peripheral nerves may be affected either with or separately from cranial nerves, with varying combinations of sensory and motor defect usually in the form of a mononeuritis multiplex but sometimes a symmetrical polyneuropathy.

Brain, spinal cord and meninges. Sarcoidosis of the brain, spinal cord, and meninges is usually accompanied by obvious evidences of sarcoidosis elsewhere, but occasionally leads to the first clinical evidence of the disease. Although certain sites—e.g. the basal meninges and the adjacent parts of the brain—are specially liable to be affected, local granulomatous deposits may occur in any part of the brain and, less often, the spinal cord. Thus clinical findings of diverse sorts may result. Changes at the base of the brain may involve cranial nerves, the hypothalamus, and the pituitary gland, and lead to raised intracranial pressure and obstructive hydrocephalus. Diabetes insipidus, somnolence, and central alveolar hypoventilation may occur. Local deposits in the brain may lead to focal epilepsy, or simulate cerebral tumours. In the spinal cord, they may simulate tumours or cause transverse myelitis, though such cases are rare.

Cerebrospinal fluid (CSF). The CSF in general shows changes to be expected from the site and character of the lesions. Local deposits in the brain may cause little change in CSF cells or protein, but usually lead to some increase in both. With meningeal changes, both are raised, sometimes to high levels; the glucose level may be low. When the spinal cord is affected, the changes depend upon whether there is obstruction to the flow of CSF. The reported findings in patients with neuropathies vary widely, particularly for protein content, which may be very high especially with peripheral polyneuropathy.

Gastrointestinal tract. Sarcoidosis of the gastrointestinal tract producing symptoms is rare, though there is evidence that in active sarcoidosis scattered granulomas may be present in the mucosa, especially of the stomach, without causing symptoms.

Recorded cases of sarcoidosis of the stomach fall into two groups. One consists of those in which, after operation for peptic ulcer presenting no unusual macroscopic appearances, histology has shown sarcoid granulomas in the submucosa and mucosa, and often lymph-nodes. These seem to be incidental associations of peptic ulceration and sarcoidosis. The other consists of those cases in which sarcoid infiltration of the stomach has caused symptoms. Most of these have shown clinical and radiological evidence of pyloric stenosis, possibly simulating carcinoma of the linitis plastica type; pathologically there is thickening of the gastric wall with profuse granulomas, and in most cases histological and clinical evidence of involvement of lymph-nodes, liver, and various other organs has been found when sought. In some cases, achlorhydria was found pre-operatively, increasing the suspicion of carcinoma. In a few cases, laparotomy for severe dyspeptic symptoms without diagnostic radiological changes in patients with sarcoidosis has shown diffuse infiltration of the gastric mucosa with granulomas.

Symptomatic involvement of the intestine is extremely rare, though a few cases in which at laparotomy parts of the small intestine were found to be infiltrated with granulomas of sarcoid type without convincing evidence of generalized granulomatosis have been recorded. There is a granulomatous element in the complex histology of Crohn's disease, and some Kveim test suspensions cause granulomatous responses in some patients with this disease (see below); any clinical association between it and sarcoidosis is therefore likely to attract attention. Only two cases in which there was convincing evidence of the co-existence of these two diseases have been recorded. Moreover, it is the stomach that was affected in nearly all recorded cases of involvement of the alimentary tract in generalized sarcoidosis, whereas the stomach is very rarely affected in Crohn's disease. Thus, these two diseases are likely to differ pathogenetically.

Endocrine glands. Although granulomas have been found incidentally in most of the endocrine glands in patients with sarcoidosis, the only endocrine disorders which are at all commonly attributable to sarcoidosis are those caused by involvement of the neurohypophysis and hypothalamus.

Pituitary and hypothalamus. Of these, diabetes insipidus is the commonest. The diagnosis is based upon extreme polydipsia and polyuria in a patient with sarcoidosis and without evidence of renal disease, responding to treatment with antidiuretic hormone. Many of the reported cases have occurred in patients with extensive sarcoidosis, notably the uveo-parotid syndrome. In differential diagnosis, it must be remembered that the nephropathy associated with the hypercalcaemia that occurs in a few patients with sarcoidosis (see below) may give rise to polyuria. Other problems are presented by patients with diabetes insipidus and a widespread lung infiltration. This combination of findings may occur not only in sarcoidosis, but also in histiocytosis X; if the diagnosis is not apparent from changes in other organs, lung biopsy may be required to establish it. And patients with diabetes insipidus may develop extrinsic allergic alveolitis (see Section 15) causing widespread lung shadows, as a result of prolonged treatment with pituitary snuff.

Other evidence of hypothalamic involvement, such as somnolence, alveolar hypoventilation, and impotence, and of infiltration of adjacent structures such as the optic tracts causing visual field defects, and the olfactory nerves causing anosmia may occur in sarcoidosis, with or without diabetes insipidus. Rarely, galactorrhoea from hyperprolactinaemia has been reported in women with sarcoidosis.

Depressed anterior pituitary function, which may or may not be accompanied by diabetes insipidus has been shown in a very few cases to be due to sarcoid infiltration of the gland.

Other endocrine glands. Granulomas have been found in the thyroid gland in a few patients with sarcoidosis who presented with hyperthyroidism, or more rarely, myxoedema, as have localized nodules of confluent granulomas usually without evidence of thyroid dysfunction. The concurrence of sarcoid infiltration with disordered function is probably no more frequent than would be expected by chance.

Although the incidental finding of a few granulomas in the parathyroids has been reported, there is no record of sarcoid infiltration of these glands disturbing function. Inter-relations between the function of these glands and the hypercalcaemia that occurs in a few patients with sarcoidosis are discussed below.

The adrenal glands seem to be relatively refractory to infiltration by sarcoid granulomas. In a few cases in which destruction of the adrenals led to adrenal insufficiency in patients with sarcoidosis, the changes in the adrenal glands were shown to be due to tuberculosis or to histoplasmosis at necropsy.

Genital system. In the male genital system, granulomatous nodules may be found in the testis, the epididymis, the seminal vesicles, or the prostate, usually in patients with extensive sarcoidosis and as incidental findings. In the female, the uterus, both endometrium and myometrium, and the Fallopian tubes may be involved. The number of reported cases is small, especially in relation to the frequency of endometrial curettage and of hysterectomy in women of the age-group most frequently affected by sarcoidosis.

There is no evidence that sarcoidosis in its more usual manifestations affects fertility or the course and outcome of pregnancy. In women with active pulmonary sarcoidosis, the radiographic changes often show improvement or even complete clearing during pregnancy and relapse within a few months of delivery.

Kidneys. It is probable that in the active stage of sarcoidosis, many patients have scattered granulomas in the kidneys, as in the lungs and liver, without symptoms, and eventually resolving. This can cause diagnostic difficulty if a patient during the sometimes prolonged active stage develops unrelated renal disease, and a biopsy shows a few granulomas as well as the histological changes of the renal disease.

A very few cases in which extensive granulomatous changes in the kidneys have caused renal failure in patients with sarcoidosis have been recorded, and even fewer in which transient acute interstitial inflammatory changes have occurred in an early acute stage of sarcoidosis with bilateral hilar lymph-node enlargement.

The commonest cause of impaired renal function in sarcoidosis is the hypercalcaemia which occurs in a few patients.

Calcium metabolism. Hypercalcaemia and hypercalciuria are observed in some patients with sarcoidosis. Reports of the proportion so affected vary greatly, especially those based upon deviations from 'normal' ranges of biochemical values. These variations are probably due partly to differing standards of 'normal', partly to variations in intake of vitamin D and calcium, and partly to real differences between different populations. In most studies of unselected large series of patients with sarcoidosis, not more than 2–3 per cent have shown symptoms attributable to hypercalcaemia.

These symptoms are similar to those of other hypercalcaemic states: anorexia, nausea, vomiting, polydipsia and polyuria, weight loss, and eventually renal failure from hypercalcaemic nephropathy. Calcinosis of soft tissues, including band keratopathy, may occur, as may renal stone formation, with colic and haematuria. The factors determining differences in liability to hypercalcaemia are not known. There is a general association with extensive chronic active sarcoidosis. Since in such cases granulomas are likely to be present in the kidneys, it is not surprising that in studies of

renal function, some patients have been found to have both hypercalcaemic nephropathy and granulomas in renal biopsies; and that occasionally the relative contribution of these to impairment of function is difficult to assess. There is a slightly higher incidence of hypercalcaemia in males. In most cases, the disordered calcium metabolism returns to normal after a variable, sometimes prolonged course.

The biochemical pattern resembles that of hypervitaminosis D. The serum calcium is elevated, sometimes to 4 mmol/l or even more; phosphate is usually normal, and phosphatase normal or slightly elevated. Urinary calcium excretion is moderately elevated, usually within the range 10–20 mmol daily; and faecal calcium excretion is low. Blood urea is generally raised; initially this returns to normal with control of hypercalcaemia, but later there may be irreversible impairment of renal function. At this stage, urinary calcium excretion is likely to diminish.

Patients with this syndrome are extremely sensitive to vitamin D, intake of amounts as small as 10 000 IU daily that have no evident effect on normal persons or insusceptible patients with sarcoidosis causing anorexia, nausea, and vomiting with sharp rises in serum calcium. Levels of vitamin D activity in the blood have been found to be normal, and of parathormone, low in patients with hypercalcaemic sarcoidosis.

In differential diagnosis, hyperparathyroidism, hypervitaminosis D, the milk-alkali syndrome, and the hypercalcaemia associated with malignant disease and with Hodgkin's disease must be considered. The hypercalcaemia of sarcoidosis, like that of hypervitaminosis D, responds rapidly to corticosteroids. A test with 50 mg cortisone or 40 mg hydrocortisone 8-hourly for 10 days has been proposed to distinguish between hypercalcaemic sarcoidosis and hyperparathyroidism, in which calcium levels are not lowered. A few cases of sarcoidosis in which parathyroid adenomas were found to be the cause of hypercalcaemia, perhaps rather more than might be expected by chance, have been described. In these there was no response to the cortisone test; and blood parathormone levels when measured were high.

Immunology

Patients with sarcoidosis, as a group, show a combination of depression of some aspects of T cell function with enhanced or normal ability of B cells to produce humoral antibodies.

T cell function. There is both a low level of delayed skin reactions to 'recall' antigens—i.e. those to which a substantial proportion of the population is hypersensitive as a result of previous infection or contact; and a low capacity to become sensitized by artificial infection, e.g. with BCG, or by contact, e.g. with dinitrochlorobenzone (DNCB). The earliest evidence of this was the finding of a high proportion of negative tuberculin tests in patients with sarcoidosis at a time when the large majority of adults were positive reactors. Not all failed to react, however, and it was found that reactivity was less depressed in patients at the early BHL stage than in those with chronic active sarcoidosis. With reduction in the proportion of positive reactors to tuberculin in a population, antigens such as Candida and mumps virus, to which the great majority of adults are sensitive, may be more useful as tests of depression of previously acquired hypersensitivity.

Skin-test responses to recall antigens are paradoxically restored by local or systemic corticosteroids in some non-responding sarcoidosis patients.

The depression of ability to acquire or express delayed-type hypersensitivity is not associated with deficiency of the protective aspect of T cell function: patients with sarcoidosis show no special liability to fungal or viral infections.

The abnormality of T cell function has been intensively investigated. The number of lymphocytes, both T and B, in the blood is low in active sarcoidosis. A high proportion of T cells appears to be activated, both morphologically and as shown by spontaneous transformation *in vitro*, but response to mitogens is diminished. The proportion of circulating T cells with suppressor effects on responses to mitogens and antigens is increased, and sarcoid sera contain factors inhibiting the response of normal lymphocytes. Studies of cells obtained from the lung by broncho-pulmonary lavage have shown that in pulmonary sarcoidosis the number of lymphocytes washed out from the alveoli is increased and that many of them are activated T cells, suggesting that T cells may be sequestered in active granulomas. It thus seems that the commitment of T lymphocytes to granuloma formation, relative increase in suppressor cell function, and humoral suppressor activity contribute to T cell dysfunction in sarcoidosis, but the relative importance of these factors is unclear, and there may be others to be discovered.

Antibody production. Levels of antibodies to common infective agents in the sera of sarcoidosis patients are higher than or similar to those found in control group. To staphylococcus and mumps virus they have been reported to be similar, and to EB virus, rubella, para-influenza, and mycoplasma to be higher. Response to bacterial vaccines is similar, and iso-agglutinin levels after small injections of mismatched blood rather higher. In active sarcoidosis, there is a general increase in immunoglobulin levels, especially in blacks, and more in females than in males. IgM tends to be elevated in patients with EN, and IgM and IgA to return to normal levels before IgG with the end of the active stage. Levels of rheumatoid factor are higher than in control groups. Thus there is a tendency to enhanced B-cell function associated in a general way with extent and activity but not with any special feature of sarcoidosis.

Immune complexes. Circulating immune complexes have been found in the blood in the early acute stage of sarcoidosis, especially with EN and BHL.

Angiotensin-converting enzyme. Serum levels of angiotensin-converting enzyme (ACE) are elevated in cases of active sarcoidosis and some other granulomatous diseases, and large amounts of ACE have been found in sarcoid lymph-nodes. Serum levels in sarcoidosis correlate generally with the activity of the disease, and there is evidence that cells in the granuloma synthesize ACE.

HLA grouping. Studies of the distribution of HLA groups in sarcoidosis have shown no consistent associations, except that among patients with sarcoidosis HLA-8 has been reported to correlate with EN and with a good prognosis.

The Kveim reaction. The Kveim reaction has been intensively studied, both as a diagnostic test and for its pathogenetic implications.

Kveim test suspension. The only source of effective test suspensions is human sarcoid tissue. Such tissues vary widely in capacity to induce granulomatous reactions selectively in sarcoidosis and in liability to cause banal inflammatory reactions. These properties of a sarcoid tissue are not correlated with its histology, and its value as a source of test material can be assessed only by tests in patients with sarcoidosis and in control subjects, preferably in parallel with a validated suspension. This makes it desirable to start with a large amount of tissue; and of this the usual source is a spleen enlarged by sarcoid granulomas, removed either surgically for valid indications, or at necropsy. The test suspension of very fine particles is derived from a crude 10 per cent aqueous tissue suspension prepared in a mechanical blender.

The active component of Kveim test suspension is insoluble in water and in fat solvents. It is resistant to proteolytic enzymes and nucleases, and to heating to 100 °C for short periods, but is inactivated by alkali. It may be a lipoprotein, but has not been chemically identified.

Performance of the test. The test is performed by intradermal injection of 0.15 ml of the test suspension. In reactive individuals, a small papule appears gradually, reaching its maximum in four to six weeks; it may be visible and of a dull red colour, but may be palpable only. Biopsy is required for two reasons: some macroscopically evident papules show only non-specific inflammatory or banal foreign-body reactions, and some granulomatous reactions are not visible or palpable.

Results of the test. The proportion of patients with sarcoidosis giving granulomatous reactions varies with the stage of the disease. Early, especially with BHL and EN, from 85 to 90 per cent react in this way; as the disease becomes more chronic the proportion diminishes, until at the chronic stage at which patients tend to present with predominant involvement of one organ—e.g. the lung—no more than 30–40 per cent react; and reactivity tends to disappear when the disease becomes inactive. Some well-validated test suspensions, giving the expected responses in sarcoidosis, cause granulomatous reactions in up to 50 per cent of patients with Crohn's disease, and in some with various sorts of lymphadenopathy, including tuberculous, but not in Hodgkin's disease.

Pathogenetic implications. The implications of the Kveim reaction for the pathogenesis of sarcoidosis are unclear. It is unlike any skin-test for infection with a known micro-organism, not only in its time-course and its histology, but in the limitation of reactivity to the active stage. It has analogies with the Mitsuda test in leprosy. This is a slowly-developing granulomatous reaction to a suspension of lepromatous tissue, and is an indicator among those infected with *M. leprae* of the sort of reactivity associated with a tuberculoid pattern of leprosy.

Diagnosis

A diagnosis of sarcoidosis implies that the observed abnormalities are related to a widespread non-caseating epithelioid cell granulomatosis. In the living patient it depends upon the recognition of a compatible pattern of symptoms and signs, the exclusion of other possibilities, and an amount of support from histology varying inversely with the degree of confidence with which the clinical picture is recognized. Some patterns are almost pathognomonic: among these may be listed the EN–arthropathy–BHL syndrome, entirely symptomless BHL, BHL accompanying uveitis, and the rare uveo-parotid syndrome. In such cases, the diagnosis of sarcoidosis is almost certain, and confirmatory histology from one site establishes it beyond doubt, as does a clinical course either to resolution or the appearance of a pulmonary infiltration as the BHL subsides. But with a less characteristic clinical picture, or with evident involvement of only one organ, doubt may remain even after biopsy from the involved organ has shown granulomas, and it is desirable to establish at least the probability of granulomatous changes at another site before accepting the diagnosis of sarcoidosis.

Biopsy. The skin should be searched for possible sarcoid infiltrations, which may be small and inconspicuous, and for changes in old scars, which may become infiltrated and assume a keloid-like appearance in active cases of sarcoidosis, with a view to biopsy which is safe and simple. Similarly, all superficial lymph-node groups should be surveyed for enlarged nodes suitable for biopsy.

A number of sites at which it is known that symptomless infiltration occurs in a substantial proportion of cases of active sarcoidosis have been suggested as useful sources of biopsy material. These include liver, skeletal muscle, and bronchial mucosa. But it is in those cases in which one organ is predominantly involved that diagnostic difficulty is greatest, and in these it is usually best to proceed directly to biopsy of the obviously affected organ if it is accessible.

In patients presenting with hilar and mediastinal masses, the removal of a lymph-node for biopsy by mediastinoscopy should be considered as soon as it becomes evident that the differential diagnosis between sarcoidosis, Hodgkin's disease and other lymphomas, secondary malignant disease, tuberculous lymphadenitis, and mediastinal tumours cannot be decided by less invasive procedures. Similarly, if the lung is the predominantly involved organ, lung biopsy is likely to be the most productive procedure. Fibre-optic bronchosopy provides the means by which both bronchial and lung biopsies may be performed; in many cases, the small fragment of lung obtained provides sufficient histological evidence, but in a few instances the difficulty of histological interpretation makes it desirable to proceed to open lung biopsy.

All biopsies should be examined for micro-organisms after appropriate staining, and whenever possible, a portion of fresh material should be cultured, especially for mycobacteria. In assessing the significance of granulomas in lymph-nodes, the occasional occurrence of granulomas of sarcoid pattern in lymph-nodes as a reaction to a malignant tumour in the area which they drain should be borne in mind.

Significance of the Kveim test. The Kveim test is most usefully assessed in terms of the degree to which a granulomatous response increases, and a 'negative' (non-granulomatous or absent) response diminishes the likelihood of sarcoidosis. This requires knowledge of the proportion of patients with sarcoidosis presenting a clinical picture like that of the patient under investigation who gave a granulomatous response to the test suspension used. A 'negative' response cannot exclude a diagnosis of sarcoidosis, since even at the early reactive stage, 10–15 per cent of known patients fail to react, and this percentage becomes larger in the later stages. A granulomatous response increases the likelihood of sarcoidosis, and may be considered diagnostically equivalent to the finding of granulomas on biopsy of an organ not symptomatically involved.

Tests of immunological reactivity. A number of findings that are frequent in sarcoidosis may help in discrimination from some other diseases while their absence does not conflict with a diagnosis of sarcoidosis. These include cutaneous anergy to recall antigens to which many normal adults react—e.g. Candida, trichophytin, mumps virus, and in some areas tuberculin, histoplasmin, and coccidiodin; increase in immunoglobulin levels; and high ACE levels in the blood.

Some special problems. A few patients present a mixture of features of sarcoidosis and of mycobacterial tuberculosis. They may show various combinations of lymphadenopathy, lung infiltration, sarcoid-type skin infiltrations, and possibly uveitis and changes in other organs; histologically rather more granular necrosis than is usually regarded as acceptable for sarcoidosis, possibly with acid-fast rods or a single positive culture for mycobacteria; usually low or absent tuberculin sensitivity; and granulomatous reactions to Kveim tests. Contention about the diagnostic categorization of such patients will cease only when the aetiology of sarcoidosis is known.

Chronic beryllium disease (see page 6.99) may mimic chronic pulmonary sarcoidosis. As in sarcoidosis, the lung changes may be accompanied by granulomatous infiltrations of the skin, though these are small and never of the florid lupus pernio type; the spleen and liver may be slightly enlarged; and similar serum protein changes and hypercalcaemia may occur. Differences from sarcoidosis include no or only slight hilar lymph-node enlargement and a chronic, usually non-remittent course, and absence of liability to initial EN, to uveitis, or to changes in the bones of the hands and feet.

Aetiology

No more definite statement can be made than that at present it seems likely that sarcoidosis results from interaction between a subject with unusual immunological responses and an infective agent, or possibly one of a number of agents. Whether the immuno-logical abnormality precedes or follows contact with the infecting agent is unknown, as is the role of genetic predisposition and of exposure to infective agents and other environmental factors in its causation.

Sarcoidosis and mycobacterial infection. Some definitions of sarcoidosis require that infection with mycobacteria or fungi known to cause granulomatous disease must be excluded. But in a few patients, whose clinical course otherwise conforms to that of sarcoidosis, mycobacterial tuberculosis precedes or follows sarcoidosis; or mycobacteria have been isolated while the clinical picture has been that of sarcoidosis, with anergy to tuberculin and possible granulomatous response to Kveim tests. These border on others in which undoubted tuberculosis follows a very indolent course, tubercle bacilli are scanty, tuberculin sensitivity is low, and response to antimycobacterial drugs slow. The possibility that in at least some cases of sarcoidosis, mycobacterial infection may be a causal factor should not be rejected, even though most patients show no overt evidence of such infection.

It has been suggested that mycobacterial infection might interact with infection by a virus or one of several viruses, as yet unidentified; this could account for the immunological findings in sarcoidosis, mycobaterial infection stimulating B cell function, and viral depressing T cell function.

Specific transmissible agent. In spite of many attempts, no transmissible agent specifically causing sarcoidosis has yet been identified.

Mitchell and Rees have recently reported the slow development of granulomas in mice injected with fresh sarcoid tissue homogenates, and serially in mice injected with homogenates of the resulting mouse granulomatous tissue. Some of the injected mice gave granulomatous responses to Kveim tests. The fresh homogenate was inactivated by heat or by irradiation. The presumed transmissible agent has not been characterized.

Treatment

Since no pathogenetic factor that can be corrected or eliminated has yet been discovered, it is not surprising that there is at present no specific treatment for sarcoidosis. Symptoms of the early inflammatory changes that occur in some cases can be controlled by anti-inflammatory drugs, as discussed above. Active granulomatous elements can be suppressed by corticosteroids, but often recur when these are withdrawn. It is probable that, except in a few circumstances noted below, the final outcome is little affected by this temporary suppression, patients who do not relapse on withdrawal of treatment being those who, untreated, would have proceeded slowly to resolution. The indications for the use of corticosteroids vary with the clinical presentation.

BHL. BHL in itself requires no treatment.

Pulmonary infiltration. Corticosteroid treatment of pulmonary sarcoidosis is indicated principally for the relief of symptoms, of which the chief is breathlessness on exertion. This correlates well with tests of function, which therefore constitute a helpful guide to progress. Radiographic appearances of pre-fibrotic infiltrations correlate poorly with symptoms and functional deficit, and thus are not a good guide to the need for treatment, but since they generally show a prompt response to corticosteroid treatment, they are often more sensitive than tests of function as an index of response.

Corticosteroid treatment. In most cases, 30 mg daily of prednisolone is sufficient to secure an initial response. This should be continued until maximal symptomatic and radiographic improvement has been attained, and then very gradually reduced to find the dose that maintains this. The 'maintenance' dose is generally in the range 7.5 mg to 20 mg daily. After 6 to 12 months of effective suppression, the dose should be reduced in very small steps at monthly intervals with careful observation for recurrence of symptoms and deterioration in functional and radiographic findings. If these occur, the effective suppressive dose should be re-instituted. This 'trial and error' procedure is the only way of determining how long treatment, once instituted, needs to be continued. Although the short-term effect on symptoms, radiographic appearances, and functional changes in labile pulmonary sarcoidosis is undoubted, it is not known whether long-term treatment can prevent the development of fibrosis in unfavourable cases. A few patients present with rapidly progressive pulmonary sarcoidosis shown by lung biopsy to include acute inflammatory changes in alveolar walls as well as granulomas; the effect of corticosteroid treatment in these is often dramatic and probably improves prognosis for life as well as suppressing the immediate manifestations of the disease.

Hypercalcaemia. Hypercalcaemia and hypercalciuria require prompt control because of the danger of renal damage. The intake of milk and cheese should be checked and, if excessive, reduced; if the patient is taking vitamin D or sun-bathing, these must be stopped. If controlling these factors does not reduce calcium levels, corticosteroid treatment is urgently required. Fortunately the dosage required, which must be found for each case, is usually moderate, of the order of 10 mg of prednisolone daily once control has been established. It must be continued until the hypercalcaemic phase, of variable duration, is over.

Uveitis. Uveitis calls for ophthalmological advice. In general, the early, mainly inflammatory, anterior uveitis may respond to local treatment; if it does not, and for posterior and chronic granulomatous uveitis, systemic corticosteroid treatment is generally needed, since its proper use diminishes the risk of loss of vision.

Other organs. Because of the very varied course and relative rarity of sarcoidosis of other organs it is difficult to generalize about their treatment. It is reasonable to suppose that corticosteroids have their usual suppressive effects on granulomatous changes, but clinical response is unpredictable. In the central nervous system, granulomatous leptomeningitis usually responds; massive granulomatous deposits may be less responsive, and focal epilepsy may be aggravated. Similarly, when it is possible to diagnose sarcoidosis of the heart during life, the effect of corticosteroid treatment can be assessed only by trial: it may be disappointing, especially if arrhythmia is an important feature.

The treatment of skin sarcoids is discussed in Section 20.

Other drugs. The antimalarial drug chloroquine has been found to have some suppressive effect on labile sarcoid infiltrations of the lung and on skin sarcoids, slower and less marked than that of corticosteroids. Side-effects—gastric discomfort, amounting to intolerance in a few patients, and, on prolonged administration, corneal clouding and occasionally irreversible retinal degeneration—greatly limit its usefulness. Hydroxychloroquine tends to be better tolerated than chloroquine: appropriate dosage is 200 mg of the sulphate twice daily, which should not be continued longer than six months, under opthalmological supervision. Its use might be considered in exceptional cases in which corticosteroids are contraindicated, but suppression of the granulomatous process seems essential.

There is some evidence that the cytotoxic or immunosuppressive drugs, chlorambucil, methotrexate, and azathioprine have suppressive effects on the sarcoid granuloma, and it has been suggested that they may be effective in cases apparently resistant to corticosteroids. Indications for a trial of such therapy must be exceptional.

Antituberculosis drugs. Antituberculosis drugs do not affect the course of sarcoidosis. They are required in those cases in which there is a concurrent active mycobacterial infection confirmed by the isolation of *M. tuberculosis*, and should be considered as 'cover' for corticosteroid treatment when dosage of 15 mg or more daily of prednisolone is required in a patient giving a skin reaction of 10 mm or more to 5 TU in an intradermal tuberculin test.

References

British Thoracic and Tuberculosis Association (1969). Geographical variations in the incidence of sarcoidosis in Great Britain: a comparative study of four areas. *Tubercle* **50**, 211.

Crick, R., Hoyle, C., and Smellie, H. (1961). The eyes in sarcoidosis. *Br. J. Ophthal.* **45**, 461.

Daniele, R. P., Dauber, J. H., and Rossman, M. D. (1980). Immunologic abnormalities in sarcoidosis. *Ann. intern. Med.* **92**, 406.

Delaney, P. (1977). Neurologic manifestations of sarcoidosis. *Ann. intern. Med.* **87**, 331.

Fleming, H. A. (1974). Sarcoid heart disease. *Br. Heart J.* **36**, 54.

Gumpel, J. M., Johns, C. J., and Shulman, L. E. (1967). The joint disease of sarcoidosis. *Ann. rheum. Dis.* **26**, 194.

Hedfors, E. (1975). Immunological aspects of sarcoidosis. *Scand. J. resp. Dis.* **56**, 1.

Israel, H. L. and Goldstein, R. A. (1973). Hepatic granulomatosis and sarcoidosis. *Ann. intern. Med.* **79**, 669.

McKelvie, P., Gresson, C., Pokhrel, R. P., and Jackson, P. (1968). Sarcoidosis of the upper air passages. *Br. J. Dis. Chest* **62**, 200.

Mitchell, D. N. and Rees, R. J. W. (1969). A transmissible agent from sarcoid tissue. *Lancet* **ii**, 81.

—, —, and Goswami, K. K. A. (1976). Transmissible agents from human sarcoid and Crohn's disease tissues. *Lancet* **ii**, 761.

—, and Scadding, J. G. (1974). Sarcoidosis. *Am. Rev. resp. Dis.* **110**, 774.

Neville, E., Carstairs, L. S., and James, D. G. (1977). Sarcoidosis of bone. *Q. Jl. Med.* **46**, 215.

Roberts, W. C., McAllister, H. A., and Ferrans, V. J. (1977). Sarcoidosis of the heart. *Am. J. Med.* **63**, 86.

Scadding, J. G. (1967). *Sarcoidosis.* Eyre and Spottiswoode, London.

Siltzbach, L. E., James, D. G., Neville, E., Turiaf, J., Battesti, J. P., Sharma, O. P., Hosoda, Y., Mikami, R., and Odaka, M. (1974). Course and prognosis of sarcoidosis round the world. *Am. J. Med.* **57**, 847.

Silverstein, A., Feuer, M. M., and Siltzbach, L. E. (1965). Neurologic sarcoidosis: study of 58 cases. *Archs Neurol.* **12**, 1.

Winnacker, J. L., Becker, K. L., and Katz, S. (1968). Endocrine aspects of sarcoidosis. *New Engl. J. Med.* **278**, 427, 483.

Whipple's disease

H. J. F. Hodgson

Whipple's disease is a rare condition which may affect virtually every organ. The clinical picture is usually dominated by small intestinal involvement leading to malabsortion, but this may have been preceded by years of systemic complaints such as arthralgia and fever. Affected tissues are infiltrated with foamy macrophages and contain rod-shaped bacteria. There is usually a good response to prolonged antibiotic therapy.

Pathology and aetiology. Whipple's initial description of a fatal case emphasized fatty deposits in the small intestine and mesenteric lymph nodes, leading to the alternative name for the disorder, *intestinal lipodystrophy*. The small intestine is thick and oedematous, with dilated lacteals, and the villi are stubby or absent. The lamina propria is stuffed with macrophages, which stain brilliantly with periodic-acid-Schiff (PAS) reagent (diastase-resistant) and similar PAS-positive material is found extracellularly (Fig. 1). Apart from the macrophages, there is little inflammatory infiltrate, and the enterocyte layer is virtually normal. Mesenteric nodes contain fatty masses, occasional granulomata, and similar abnormal macrophages. In autopsy series most cases also show extraintestinal involvement, with foamy macrophages in spleen, lymph nodes, central nervous system, liver, lung, and heart. Cardiac involvement often leads to endocarditis with vegetations.

Both within and between the abnormal macrophages abundant rod-shaped bacteria are regularly identified in untreated cases. Electron microscopic studies show them to be 1–2 μm in length, occasionally dividing, and probably the source of the PAS-positive material identified histologically. They have been found in gut, lymph nodes, joints, liver, brain, and other tissues. Culture techniques have not yielded a specific bacterium, and various authors have isolated different species of Corynebacteria, Haemophilus, normal or cell-wall deficient Streptococci, brucella-like, nocardia-like, and other organisms from jejunum or lymph nodes. It seems probable that the bacteria enter the body via the small intestine, which appears to be virtually always involved, and then spread both via lymphatics and haematogenously to affect other regions. The failure to identify a specific infectious agent has led to the suggestion that the primary abnormality is an immunological deficiency in the host, so that a variety of bacteria of low virulence persist and cause disease. Deficiencies of both macrophage and T cell function have been documented in patients, but the findings have not been consistent.

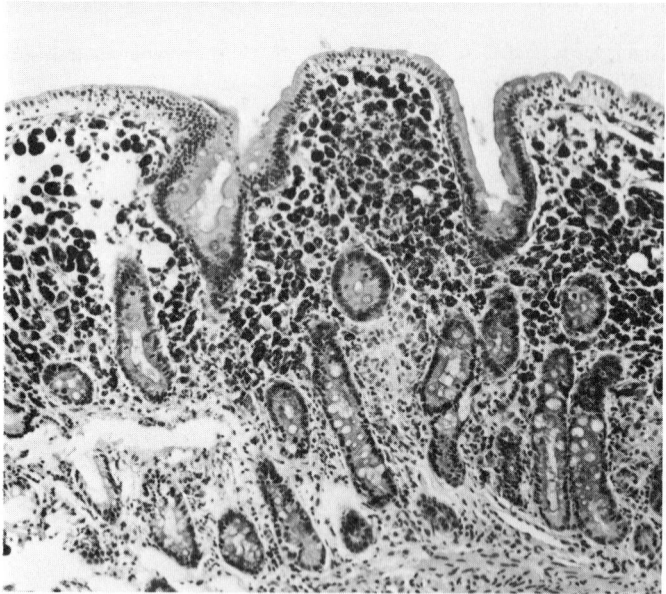

Fig. 1 Jejunal biopsy specimen from 50-year-old male with Whipple's disease showing stunted villi and infiltration of lamina propria with densely staining macrophages (PAS × 150).

Clinical features and diagnosis. The condition is most frequently diagnosed in middle-aged males, but women and infants may be affected. The patient with advanced disease presents with malaise, weight loss, diarrhoea, and arthritis, and examination shows marked pigmentation, lymphadenopathy, anaemia, finger clubbing, hypotension, and oedema. In such cases investigation of an obvious malabsorptive state leads to the diagnosis. Recognition is far more difficult if symptoms are limited to fever, or to the arthritis, which is transient, migratory, non-deforming, and affects peripheral joints. Other early features, which may be present for several years without obvious intestinal disease, include respiratory symptoms with pleurisy and pulmonary infiltrates, pericarditis, and iritis. Chylous or serous ascites, endocarditis, cardiac conduction defects, and myopathy may occur with progression of the condition. A variety of central nervous system manifestations are also reported, including depression, dementia, supranuclear ophthalmoplegia, ataxia, myoclonus, and papilloedema.

Diagnosis depends upon suspicion and the demonstration of the classic histological picture. Whether or not clinical intestinal involvement is present, peroral jejunal biopsy is a convenient and safe means of obtaining affected tissue. Very occasionally jejunal involvement is patchy and multiple biopsies may be required. Rectal biopsy is not an adequate substitute as normal colonic tissue may sometimes contain PAS-positive macrophages.

Other investigations are of use in indicating the presence of intestinal disease or involvement of other organs, but not of diagnostic value. Radiology of the gut characteristically shows oedema-

tous and dilated small bowel. The sedimentation rate is elevated, and anaemia due to iron or folate deficiency may be present. Occasionally eosinophilia and thrombocytosis have been noted. Steatorrhoea, hypocalcaemia, deficiencies of fat-soluble vitamins, and an elevated serum alkaline phosphatase level occur with advanced gut disease, as do hypoproteinaemia and protein losing enteropathy. The total IgA level however may be high.

Treatment and prognosis. Untreated Whipple's disease progresses slowly but is eventually fatal. The condition responds to antibiotic therapy, but in severely ill patients replacement of nutritional deficiencies and short-term treatment with corticosteroids may be required. Many different oral and parenteral antibiotic regimes have been successfully employed, including penicillin alone, penicillin and streptomycin, tetracycline, and co-trimoxazole. In the absence of bacteriological data on the organisms, the approach must be empirical, and for example, failure to respond to tetracycline has been reported. Although clinical improvement occurs in a few days, treatment for many months is required. Parenteral penicillin and streptomycin for two weeks, followed by doxycycline 100 mg daily for a year, is one appropriate regimen. The gut mucosa returns to normal within a few months, although a few PAS-positive macrophages may persist. Even after prolonged treatment relapse may occur when antibiotics are discontinued; in particular central nervous system manifestations may progress in the absence of systemic symptoms, suggesting that the initial therapy should provide adequate antibiotic concentrations on both sides of the blood–brain barrier. Usually return of the bacteria in intestinal tissues precedes clinical relapse, and offers a means of early diagnosis of recurrent disease.

Reference

Maizel, H., Ruffin, J. M., and Dobbins, W. O. (1970). Whipple's disease: a review of 19 patients from one hospital and a review of the literature since 1950. *Medicine, Baltimore* **49**, 175.

Cat scratch fever

C. M. P. Bradstreet

Cat scratch fever (CS fever) is usually a mild illness characterized by regional lymphadenitis occurring two to three weeks after an injury to the skin drained by the affected lymph node. A history of a bite or scratch from a cat is often given, and a skin lesion may be seen as a small macule, vesicle, or pustule. Lymphadenitis does not develop between the skin lesion and the enlarged node. Suppuration of the gland occurs in less than half the cases; after aspiration or surgical removal, healing of the gland is usually rapid but may be protracted. Occasionally complications occur, but a fatal outcome is extremely rare.

Aetiology and epidemiology. Despite extensive microbiological research in laboratories throughout the world since the disease was first described in 1950, no causative agent has yet been found.

Before techniques for virus isolation were widely established, the histopathology of the diseased gland suggested that the causative agent might belong to the chlamydial group of organisms. Subsequently, a number of serological studies in which the complement fixation test was employed supported this theory because of the frequent findings of higher than normal antibody levels to a chlamydial group antigen in sera of patients with CS fever. However, other findings failed to confirm these results or showed similarly raised antibody levels among healthy controls. In more recent antibody surveys on CS fever patients, indirect immunofluorescence methods and additional chlamydial group antigens were used, but again the results were inconclusive. The chlamydial theory fails to be substantiated also by the negative results of the Frei skin test obtained in patients with CS fever.

Most patients are found to have normal levels of serum globulins and immunoglobulins as well as normal antibody levels to brucella, tularaemia, herpes simplex, and Epstein–Barr virus. However, in *in vitro* lymphocyte transformation studies, it appears that during the acute illness CS fever patients have a transient state of lymphocyte unresponsiveness similar to that observed in patients with a variety of illnesses caused by viruses and mycoplasmas.

Attempts to isolate an agent have generally been made from pus and affected lymph nodes of benign cases in which a positive skin test has been obtained. All the common viral, bacteriological, and mycological techniques have been used, including inoculation into chick embryos, tissue culture cells of human and animal origin, laboratory animals, and experimental volunteers.

Pasteurella or other bacteria cultured were presumed to have been contaminants, and patients from whom acid-fast photochromogenic bacilli were isolated were generally thought to be suffering from an atypical mycobacterial infection analogous to the disease in cattle where tuberculin reactors are infected with acid-fast bacteria normally saprophytic.

The frequent history of a cat association has encouraged much research into feline pathogens for the cause of the human infection.

Feline pneumonitis virus. Feline pneumonitis is a chlamydial infection common in cats, with a lymph node lesion resembling that of lymphogranuloma venereum in humans. The fact that the organism survives poorly at 4–20 °C would explain the difficulty experienced in isolating it. Although sensitive to many antibiotics, it is thought that this organism might nevertheless be responsible for some of the cases of CS fever.

Feline herpesvirus. A haemagglutinating virus isolated from a case of CS fever contained a cross-reacting antigen to *F. herpesvirus* but was not pathogenic to chick embryos, and caused no cytopathic effect in tissue culture cells or herpetic-type lesions when inoculated on to corneas of rabbits. These bodies were also found in pus and lesions in patients with other diseases.

Feline infectious peritonitis virus. This organism causes histopathology in cats similar to that found in humans with CS fever. However, it was not possible to infect cats with material from CS fever patients, and these inoculations gave no protection against a subsequent infective dose of feline infectious peritonitis virus. Cats showed no immunological reaction to CS fever skin test antigen.

Other feline viruses not yet implicated or excluded are those that multiply in lymphoid tissue, e.g. feline panleukemias and feline leukemia viruses.

Failure to isolate may result from difficulty in obtaining material sufficiently early in the infection. Most cases are single incidences, and diagnosis is made late or retrospectively; at this stage the agent may no longer be viable in pus or lymph nodes. Isolation may be more successful when the illness has been prolonged with severe complications; such cases may fail to eliminate the organism rapidly and provide a wider range of suitable pathological material. Alternatively, if other members of the family contract the disease, they may be a source of material for isolation if specimens are taken before lymphadenitis and pus formation have fully developed, and before the skin test has become positive. Many new laboratory techniques which enhance the isolation of an agent are now available and should be applied to these possibly more suitable pathological specimens.

CS fever has been reported from most parts of the world. The incidence is not known, but since the skin test antigen is not always or everywhere available, it certainly occurs more frequently than it is diagnosed. It occurs more often during the autumn and winter months and among young persons up to the age of 20–30 years; it occurs equally in both sexes. Although single infections are commonest, family outbreaks of two to five cases are reported, usually within a few weeks of each other, occasionally after a year or more.

Pathology. In the early stages the microscopic appearance of affected lymph nodes is characteristic but not pathognomonic, and must be distinguished from tuberculosis, brucellosis, and tular-

aemia. There is hyperplasia of the reticulum and an increase in the number and size of lymphoid follicles and germinal centres. Later epithelioid cell granulomas are seen surrounded by lymphocytes, plasma cells, eosinophils, and neutrophils. Infiltrating cells and granulomas degenerate into eosinophilic microabscesses, which may enlarge and coalesce to form larger abscesses. The small and large abscesses are surrounded by epithelioid cells in which lymphocytes predominate. Healing occurs with fibroblastic proliferation and scarring.

Clinical features. In typical cases the subacute regional lymphadenitis arises about three weeks after the initial cutaneous lesion, by which time the latter has often disappeared. The axillary, cervical, epitrochlear, and inguinal nodes are most commonly affected. Although 60 per cent of cases show enlargement of only a single node, it is quite rare to have the epitrochlear gland involved without the axillary. Occasionally there is bilateral lymphadenitis or generalized lymphadenopathy; rarely the liver and spleen are also involved. Infection of the mesenteric lymph gland may simulate an acute abdominal problem.

The most common variant of the disease is the oculoglandular syndrome of Parinaud, in which a single granulomatous lesion of the conjunctiva is accompanied by pre-auricular lymphadenitis.

All parts of the respiratory tract may be affected, the most severe cases with bilateral lymphadenopathy.

Variations in skin lesions are numerous but not common. Erythema nodosum is least rare. Others include erythema multiforme, papulovesicular or maculopapular rashes, and thrombocytopenic purpura.

Encephalitis, the most serious of the uncommon complications, develops three to six weeks after the onset of lymphadenopathy, but it usually resolves without sequelae. A fatal outcome is extremely rare.

Diagnosis. Since the causative agent of CS fever is not known its diagnosis is never certain. The following criteria are commonly accepted: (*a*) negative laboratory results for other causes of lymphadenopathy; (*b*) a characteristic histopathology of a biopsied lymph node; (*c*) a positive result with CS fever skin test antigen (Hangar–Rose test). Additional helpful criteria are a history of a (cat) scratch or other identifiable inoculation mark, or contact with a cat. Of these the result of the skin test often plays a decisive part.

The antigen is prepared from purulent lymph gland material which has yielded no bacteria on culture, from patients diagnosed as having CS fever. Material collected from individuals is usually small in quantity, and in making the antigen it is common practice to pool the pus from many patients. It is widely known that patients with CS fever show marked variation in the skin reaction to Hangar–Rose antigens from different sources, and that a single antigen may give positive results in some diagnosed cases and negative in others. These findings are to be expected since neither the number nor the potencies of specific antigens are known. The antigens cannot, therefore, be accurately standardized. In addition, confusion arises because positive skin test results have been found among healthy family contacts (18 per cent), veterinary personnel (23–30 per cent), and healthy controls (4 per cent). Rarely a positive result is not obtained for a week or longer. Skin reactivity persists for many years after an infection.

Thus, where the clinical features make the diagnosis possible and laboratory tests indicate no alternative, CS fever may be confirmed with some certainty by a positive skin test, for only 5 per cent of positive results are false, whereas the diagnosis of CS fever is excluded with slightly less certainty by a single negative skin test, for about 10 per cent of negative results are false.

Treatment. No specific treatment is available. Spontaneous resolution of the infected node is common, but aspiration or surgical removal of the gland may be necessary. Healing is usually rapid.

References

Carithers, H. A. (1970). Cat scratch disease. Notes on its history. *Am. J. Dis. Child.* **119**, 200.

Griesemer, R. A. and Wolfe, L. G. (1971). Cat scratch disease. *J. Amer. vet. med. Assoc.* **158**, 1008.

Margileth, A. M. (1968). Cat scratch disease: nonbacterial regional lymphadenitis. The study of 145 patients and a review of the literature. *Pediatrics, Springfield* **42**, 803.

Warwick, W. J. (1967). The cat-scratch syndrome, many diseases or one disease? *Progr. med Virol.* **9**, 256.

Benign myalgic encephalomyelitis

W. B. Matthews

Benign myalgic encephalomyelitis, also known as *Royal Free disease* or *Icelandic disease* is an epidemic febrile disease with systemic and neurological symptoms of presumed viral origin, but without established pathology.

Epidemiology. Most identified outbreaks have occurred in relatively closed communities, particularly in those in association with hospitals, such as nurses' homes, hence the name 'Royal Free disease' after a much-publicized outbreak, but spread to the general population may also occur. Assuming an infective cause, an incubation period of up to one week has been postulated, the mode of transmission being unknown.

Clinical features. Symptoms have varied in different outbreaks. The onset is usually abrupt, with headache, upper respiratory symptoms, and a low fever. Lymph nodes may be tender but are not enlarged. Sporadic examples of palpable enlargement of the spleen, jaundice, or a rash occur in patients apparently suffering from the same disease, but are never constant features.

The neurological symptoms consist of fluctuating weakness, paraesthesiae, and marked muscular pain and tenderness. Weakness, when present, is often intermittent, imparting a jerking character to the movement, and is not accompanied by unequivocal changes in the tendon reflexes and is very rarely followed by wasting. Cutaneous sensory loss of unusual distribution is often prominent. Mental symptoms, including depression, panic states, hallucinations, amnesia, and inability to concentrate are prominent in some epidemics.

No fatal case has been described, but symptoms may be extremely persistent and relapse is common. Patients who claim to have persistent symptoms derived from presumed Royal Free disease in the past are usually found to have recurrent depression without physical signs. Treatment of the acute episodes and the possible sequelae can only be symptomatic.

Investigation. The cerebrospinal fluid was normal in victims of the Royal Free Hospital outbreak, and no consistent change in the white blood count has been observed. No virus has been incriminated after intensive search.

Pathogenesis. It is by no means certain that all outbreaks categorized as benign myalgic encephalomyelitis have been the same disease. Unequivocal evidence of organic nervous disease is absent in the great majority of patients and epidemic hysteria, at one time linked to a natural fear of poliomyelitis in those exposed to this infection, is still considered by some authorities to be the cause of some epidemics. In the complete absence of pathology or of established infective cause, no definite opinion on this question can be advanced.

References

Dillon, M. J., Marshall, W. C., Dudgeon, J. A., and Steigman, A. J. (1974). Epidemic neuromyasthenia: outbreak among nurses at a children's hospital, *Br. med. J.* **i**, 301.

McEvedy, C. P. and Beard, A. W. (1970). Concept of benign myalgic encephalomyelitis, *Br. med. J.* **i**, 11.

Section 6
Chemical and physical injuries
Climatic and occupational diseases

Poisoning with chemical substances

GENERAL PRINCIPLES IN THE MANAGEMENT OF ACUTE POISONING

G. N. Volans

Whenever poisoning is mentioned there is a general belief that treatment will be based upon the use of a specific antidote. This is not so, for there are, in fact, very few effective agents of this kind. Instead, a common pattern of basic management is applicable to all forms of acute poisoning.

History. Although an adequate history is as important in the effective management of acute poisoning as it is in any other form of clinical medicine, urgency may dictate that this be deferred pending the institution of emergency resuscitative measures. The information moreover may be less readily available than in ordinary medical practice, since the patient may be unconscious and a certain amount of 'detective work' is often required. Valuable details may often be obtained from relatives, workmates, the police, the ambulance crew, or others and it is important to question them before they leave the hospital. Evidence of the suspected poison may have been present where the patient was found and, where necessary, every effort should be made to obtain the remaining material and/or its container. Suicide notes and information on past and recent mental and physical health are obviously important and a detailed description of the scene where the patient was found can provide vital clues, e.g. in accidental carbon monoxide poisoning (see Table 1).

Examination. In the first instance this should be summarily performed so as not unduly to delay treatment. There are very few clinical signs which are diagnostic for particular poisons.

In the conscious patient the history usually suggests the diagnosis and thus the likely signs, or there may be some form of abnormal behaviour, as in the effects of amphetamine or LSD, in which case the differential diagnosis will include a range of psychiatric problems. Occasionally a patient with salicylate intoxication will be too distressed to give a history, but hyperventilation, pyrexia, flushing, and tachycardia suggest the diagnosis, which can then be confirmed by the laboratory with little delay.

The unconscious patient has to be considered by the differential diagnosis of coma from all causes (see Section 21). Pin-point pupils and depressed respiration suggest the effects of a narcotic drug. Habitual drug abusers may have evidence of needle marks on the skin and often shallow skin ulcers from drugs accidentally introduced into the tissue around the vein. There may also be evidence of skin infection from injections under unsterile conditions, but it must be remembered that not all drug abuse is by injection and sniffing is becoming increasingly popular. Dilated pupils and cardiac arrhythmias (most commonly a sinus tachycardia), sometimes with convulsions and extensor plantar responses, in a patient whose respiration *appears* adequate will most commonly indicate the anticholinergic effects of the tricyclic antidepressants, but it must also be remembered that many other drugs have anticholinergic properties too. The breath will smell of alcohol in many patients (up to 70 per cent in some series), but intoxication due to ethanol alone is much less common and most patients have taken significant quantities of other drugs. The breath may also smell of solvents such as toluene, acetone, or xylene as the result of abuse by 'sniffing' glues, cleaning agents, or other preparations which are

Table 1   Summary of the main groups of poisonous agents (see page reference for details)

Corrosives and irritants	page 6.11
Pesticides	6.12
Arsenic, strychnine, nicotine and phosphorus	6.14
Salicylate	6.15
Paracetamol	6.17
Non-steroidal anti-inflammatory (NSAI) drugs	6.18
Opiates and opiate derivatives	6.19
Barbituates	6.19
Non-barbiturate hypnotics	6.20
Sedatives and tranquillizers	6.20
Anticonvulsants	6.21
Tricyclic antidepressants	6.22
Quadricyclic antidepressants	6.23
Monoamine oxidase inhibitors (MAOI)	6.23
Lithium carbonate	6.23
Cardiorespiratory drugs	6.23
Alcohols	6.25
Glycols	6.26
Hydrocarbons	6.27
Solvent abuse	6.29
Ammonia	6.30
Carbon disulphide	6.30
Carbon monoxide	6.31
Chlorine	6.31
Cyanide	6.32
Hydrogen sulphide	6.32
Anticholinergic drugs	6.33
Hypoglycaemic agents	6.33
Iron	6.33
Metoclopramide	6.34
Non-catecholamine sympathomimetic drugs	6.34
Phencyclidene	6.34
Rifampicin	6.35

freely available. 'Barbiturate blisters' on the skin may in fact be caused by other drugs, including glutethimide and the antidepressants. They often occur at sites where two skin areas have been in contact, e.g. inner aspects of the knees, but not at sites of maximum pressure. Burns around the mouth or in the buccal cavity and pharynx indicate ingestion of corrosives amongst which must be included paraquat.

In most patients, therefore, the signs of acute poisoning are non-specific and the initial diagnosis is often based upon probability, since acute poisoning is the most common cause of coma in young adults and is not uncommon in the elderly. This matters little however, since the emergency management follows similar lines in all cases.

Emergency treatment. Emergency treatment of acute poisoning has as its main aim the preservation of the vital functions, since it is well established that supportive measures will be all that are required in the majority of cases.

Respiratory function. Maintenance of adequate respiration is of paramount importance and must be the first objective in any treatment for acute poisoning. The comatose patient is liable to obstruction of the pharynx by the tongue falling back. This can be prevented in the first instance by holding the jaw forward and turning the patient into a semi-prone position. An oropharyngeal airway should then be inserted as soon as practicable and further assessment made of the patient's ventilation. Tidal volume and minute volume should be checked, for many poisons reduce the depth of respiration without necessarily reducing the rate.

No matter how severely respiration is depressed, *respiratory stimulants should never be used*. There is no good evidence that they are ever beneficial in acute poisoning and in the days when they were used extensively they were associated with a higher mortality than that seen with supportive therapy alone. The opiate antagonist, naloxone, is safe and should be used whenever there is the slightest suspicion that an opiate has been ingested (see page 6.19). Even if it is given inappropriately, it will not have any adverse effects.

When there is no response to an adequate dose of naloxone, blood gases should be assessed in all patients where there is grade III or IV coma (Table 2), or where other features suggest inad-

Table 2   Assessment of consciousness

Grades of coma	Description
I	Drowsy but responds to vocal command
II	Unconscious but responds to minimal stimuli
III	Unconscious and responds only to maximal painful stimuli
IV	Unconscious and no response whatsoever

equate gas exchange. Oxygen should be given when indicated clinically and/or an irritant gas has been inhaled and, above all, it is imperative for carbon monoxide poisoning. However, adequate ventilation with air is preferable to attempting to compensate for impaired ventilation by increased inhaled oxygen concentrations. Mechanical ventilation, if indicated, should never be delayed.

Cardiovascular function. Severe acute poisoning is often associated with shock due to expansion of the venous capacitance bed, causing a relative or absolute deficiency of the circulatory fluid volume. In addition, where admission has been delayed many hours after ingestion of poisons, the patient will be dehydrated. Young patients are generally not at risk of cerebral or renal damage unless the systolic blood pressure falls below 80 mmHg, whereas in the elderly a fall below 90 mmHg systolic should be regarded seriously. The immediate action should be to raise the foot of the bed, followed by the commencement of intravenous fluids. Except where dehydration is thought to be the major factor (e.g. in salicylate poisoning, see page 6.16) colloids (human serum albumin or hydroxethyl starches) are more appropriate than crystalloids (0.9 per cent saline or 5 per cent dextrose). Potent vasoconstrictors, such as mataraminol or noradrenaline, are no longer used since they have little effect in increasing the blood pressure and they decrease the blood supply to vital organs. In the relatively few cases where fluid replacement does not correct hypotension, the newer positive inotropes dopamine and dobutamine may be tried. Dopamine is generally preferred since it is less likely to reduce renal blood flow.

When cardiac arrhythmias occur in acute poisoning it is important not to use anti-arrhythmic drugs unnecessarily. These drugs all have narrow therapeutic ratios and all of them may disturb myocardial function in their own right. Thus if an anti-arrhythmic drug is added to a situation where the poison is already affecting the heart, there is a danger of a serious interaction.

Many cardiac arrhythmias in acute poisoning respond to correction of hypoxia and/or acidosis (e.g. with tricyclic antidepressants), and drug therapy should be considered only in persistent life-threatening arrhythmias with consequential impairment of cardiac output. In that situation the drugs used should be selected according to the arrhythmia, their duration of action and their relative toxicity. Thus lignocaine is the class I antiarrhythmic of choice since its short half-life permits rapid adjustment of dosage.

Convulsions. Intravenous diazepam is the drug of choice for the control of repeated convulsions. If adequate doses are used, it is highly effective and alternatives are seldom needed. Where the response is poor, or not sustained, intravenous chlormethiazole may be tried, or intravenous phenytoin may be started with a view to longer control. All of these drugs may depress respiration and thus may further complicate the management of the unconscious patient. In difficult cases measurement of plasma anticonvulsant levels may be of benefit (see page 6.10).

Hypothermia. Many poisons impair temperature regulation and hypothermia is common, especially when admission is delayed. A low reading thermometer must be used or this important observation will be missed and, in the severe cases, peripheral and core temperatures should be monitored. Treatment should include the provision of a warm moist atmosphere (27–29 °C) and a heat-conserving 'space blanket' to minimize heat loss. Cold intravenous fluids should be avoided and the bottles for use should be stored in the room, or the lines should pass through a heating device.

Antidotes. Thus far, in the normal sequence of events for the supportive management of acute poisoning, only two antidotes have been mentioned, naloxone for opiates and oxygen for carbon monoxide. These are, indeed, the only antidotes commonly needed in the unconscious patient. Methionine and *N*-acetycysteine are also used frequently (for paracetamol poisoning) but in these cases the patient is usually conscious and frequently has little in the way of symptoms (see page 6.17). Other antidotes of proven value are used rarely but may be life-saving. Table 3 lists these antidotes and gives brief details of dosage. In some instances the antidotes are toxic in their own right and the reader is recommended to seek further advice in their use as given elsewhere in this book, or via a poisons information service (see page 6.10).

Antivenoms for snake bites are discussed on page 6.40.

Prevention of absorption of the poison. Once a diagnosis of poisoning by ingestion has been made and, where necessary, adequate resuscitation achieved, it is appropriate to consider the use of measures designed to limit further absorption of the poison. Three methods are available, gastric lavage, emesis, and oral adsorbants. Each has its advantages, its contra-indications, and its adverse effects, and it is important to emphasize that none of these treatments should be used unnecessarily.

Gastric lavage. *Indication*. This procedure, more correctly called gastric aspiration and lavage (Table 4) is widely used in accident and emergency departments and indeed is probably overused. One survey has suggested that up to 50 per cent of patients subjected to gastric lavage did not meet the accepted criteria (Table 5) and that in these cases the treatment was given, either as an unthinking routine, or in the belief that it will provide an unpleasant experience which will deter the recipient from any further episodes of self-poisoning. Whilst the study in question probably overstated the case, there is no doubt that many of the drugs now taken in overdose are less toxic than earlier drugs, such as barbiturates, and there is no evidence to support the use of gastric lavage as a deterrent. The decision to use lavage should therefore be taken only after consideration of the individual case and an indication of a real possibility that a toxic dose of poison has been ingested.

Having said this, it is a surprising fact that there is relatively little evidence available to support the efficacy of gastric lavage. In one study carried out during the 1960s on barbiturate and salicylate overdoses the amounts of the drugs removed were determined. It was found that clinically significant amounts of barbiturate were removed only if the procedure was used within four hours after ingestion of the drug, whilst in the case of salicylates the tablets tend to adhere together in the stomach and large amounts of the drug may be removed much later. More recent evidence suggests that drugs with anticholinergic effects (notably the tricyclic antidepres-

Table 3   Antidotes of proven value in acute poisoning due to drugs and chemicals

Toxic substance	Antidote	Dose	Comments
Carbon monoxide	oxygen	100%	continue until blood carboxyhaemoglobin is reduced below danger level
Cyanide First aid Hospital treatment	amylnitrite dicobalt edetate (Kelocyanor) or sodium nitrite plus sodium thiosulphate	1 ampoule inhaled every 5 minutes 600 mg i.v. over 1 minute followed by further 300 mg i.v. if no immediate recovery 10 ml of 3% sodium nitrite i.v. followed by slow i.v. injection of 25 ml of 50% sodium thiosulphate	use in severe life-threatening poisoning only; in patients who have only mild symptoms or who have survived more than 1 minute after exposure supportive therapy is adequate and the antidotes, especially dicobalt edetate may produce serious adverse effects
Arsenic Gold Mercury	dimercaprol (BAL)	2.5–5 mg/kg by deep i.m. injection 4-hourly for 2 days; 2.5 mg/kg twice on the third day, then once daily	see page 6.14
Copper Lead Mercury Zinc	penicillamine	250 mg–2 g orally per day (children 20 mg/kg body weight)	see page 6.13
Iron	desferrioxamine	gastric lavage 2 g in 1 l warm water; leave 5 g in 50 ml water in the stomach; 2 g i.m. followed by slow i.v. infusion 15 mg/kg/hour (maximum 80 mg/kg in 24 hours) or 2 g i.m. twice daily	whilst lavage is in progress send blood for plasma iron level: > 90 μmol/l (5 mg/l) in a child; or > 145 μmol/l (8 mg/l) in an adult indicates the need for further parenteral therapy
Lead	sodium calcium edetate (EDTA)	50–70 mg/kg daily by i.v. in 250 ml 0.9% saline by slow i.v. infusion; continue for 5 days	oral sodium calcium edetate would increase lead absorption dimercaprol 5 mg/kg i.m. 4 times in 24 hours may be given simultaneously
Opiates—morphine and analogues including diphenoxylate (in lomotil) and dextropropoxyphene (in distalgesic)	naloxone	adults 0.4–1.2 mg i.v. children 0.005–0.01 mg/kg i.v.; much larger (up to 10 times these doses) may be needed in severe cases	expect to use the maximum recommended dose; if there is a response, it is safe to give much larger doses and to repeat doses as needed
Organophosphorus insecticides (cholinesterase inhibitors)	atropine pralidoxime mesylate (P$_2$S)	2 mg i.v. repeated as necessary to produce and maintain full atropinization 30 mg/kg body weight i.v. or i.m. 4-hourly for 24 hours	atropine is often the only antidote required; P$_2$S (cholinesterase reactivator) supplies are held in certain centres only; identify these via pharmacy or Poisons Information Services (see page 6.10)
Paracetamol	methionine N-acetylcystine	oral 2.5 g 4-hourly to a total of 10 g 150 mg/kg i.v. over 15 min, 50 mg/kg in 500 ml 5% dextrose over 4 hours, and 100 mg/kg in 1000 ml 5% dextrose over 16 hours; total dose 300 mg/kg over 20 hours	these antidotes are usually fully effective if given within 10 hours after ingestion of paracetamol; they may have a small effect between 10 and 16 hours after ingestion of paracetamol and thereafter are probably dangerous (see page 6.18)
Thallium	prussian blue	10 g orally twice daily via stomach tube	continue until faeces clear of thallium or until urinary excretion of thallium falls below 0.5 mg/24 hours; thallium poisoning is very rare in the United Kingdom

sants) are also retained longer in the stomach and that lavage can be useful up to 8–10 hours after ingestion. In many cases, however, the time of ingestion is not known and the patient is unconscious. In this situation lavage can be justified, since it is obvious that a toxic dose has been ingested and the gastrointestinal stasis which often accompanies deep coma can markedly delay the passage of the poison from the stomach.

Contra-indications, precautions, and adverse effects. In the unconscious patient gastric lavage may easily result in aspiration of fluid into the lungs. The use of a cuffed endotracheal tube is then

Table 4   Gastric aspiration and lavage procedure

1. Place the head of the patient over the end or side of the bed so that the mouth and throat are at a level lower than the larynx and trachea
2. Use a wide-bore, soft rubber tube (Jacques gauge 30) lubricated with vaseline or glycerine. In the adult, 50 cm will reach the stomach. Make sure that the tube is not in the trachea
3. Aspirate first, then use 300 ml water for the first washing. Repeat this process using 300–600 ml at a time for at least 3 or 4 times. Save all washings in case they are needed for analysis

mandatory and it must be acknowledged that aspiration may still occur in some cases, even in the most experienced hands. With petroleum distillates, moreover, the risk of aspiration pneumonia is such that gastric lavage is definitely contra-indicated. When caustic poisons have been ingested, there is the danger that the rubber tube will perforate the oesophagus or the stomach, and in most cases

Table 5   The correct use of gastric aspiration and lavage

Indications	Contra-indications
1. A potentially toxic dose of poison has been ingested	1. Petroleum distillates
2. Treatment can be given within 4 hours of ingestion (longer for salicylates and anticholinergic drugs including tricyclic antidepressants)	
3. Patient unconscious and time of ingestion not known	
4. Cautious use if danger of systemic toxicity from corrosives, e.g. concentrated paraquat solutions or formic acid	

lavage is best avoided. However, there are instances where the danger of systemic toxicity outweighs the risk of perforation (e.g. concentrated solutions of paraquat or formic acid), and in such circumstances cautious use of the procedure is recommended. Caution is also indicated when gastric lavage is considered in alcoholic patients, since if oesophageal varicies are present there is a real danger that perforation will cause life-threatening haemorrhage.

Emesis. *Indications.* As with gastric lavage, emesis should only be considered when it is thought that a potenially toxic dose of poison has been ingested and when it is likely that significant amounts of the poison remain within the stomach.

Contra-indications. Emesis should not be used when there is impairment of consciousness or when petroleum distillates have been ingested, since both situations carry a high risk of aspiration into the lungs. Corrosive substances also contra-indicate emesis since the danger of perforation of the oesophagus would be increased by the retching and the repeated contact of the corrosive with the oesophageal mucosa. When anti-emetics have been ingested, it is normally suggested that emetics should not be used. However, there are many cases recorded where emesis was successful in such cases and few records of failure and/or toxicity due to the emetic. It is obvious therefore that the dose/response relationship in such cases is complex. It seems reasonable, therefore, to give a single dose of an emetic when anti-emetic is thought to have been ingested. However, if this fails, it is not advisable to give further doses of emetic since the risk of systemic toxicity is then much greater.

Five methods of inducing emesis have been recommended: pharyngeal stimulation, sodium chloride, copper sulphate, apomorphine, and ipecacuanha.

Pharyngeal stimulation. Elicitation of the gag reflex by stimulating the pharynx with the fingers is the simplest method of inducing emesis. It is widely practised, particularly in the treatment of children, and does not appear to carry any particular risks, providing the general contra-indications to the induction of emesis are observed. However, its efficacy is probably limited since some patients will not gag sufficiently to vomit. In one study a series of poisoned children were first gagged by the parents before arrival at hospital. Subsequently, the same children were first gagged by the physician and then given syrup of ipecacuanha. Out of 30 cases, only four gagged, (two at home, two in hospital) whilst all 30 vomited after ipecacuanha. In the four children who were successfully gagged the volume of vomitus produced was much greater after ipecacuanha than on gagging. Thus, whilst pharyngeal stimulation can be recommended as a first-aid measure its use should normally be supplemented by further emesis or lavage once the patient reaches hospital.

Sodium chloride. Sodium chloride is widely thought of by the public as an emetic which can be used as first-aid for poisoning. In practice, however, it is a poor emetic and is toxic in its own right. The latter is a very real problem since in the desire to treat the original poison it has often been given in excessive amounts with the result that there are many recorded cases of deaths due to hypernatraemia. Several such cases are listed in Table 6, and it can be seen that in each case there was little danger of death from the original overdose. In view of these findings the Federal Register in the United States has banned the recommendation of salt emesis from product labels and in the United Kingdom several organizations (including the Department of Health and Social Security, the Chemical Industries Association, the Red Cross, and St John Ambulance Association) have made firm recommendations that the use of salt as an emetic can no longer be advised. In spite of this, there were at least two deaths from this cause in England during the first part of 1980. It is important, therefore, that all doctors should be aware of the problem, and that they take steps to prevent further cases if they discover that any manufacturers or parents are still recommending saline emetics.

Copper sulphate. Copper sulphate is a more effective emetic than

sodium chloride. However, its use carries a definite risk of absorption of toxic amounts of copper and at least one death has been recorded. Its use is not recommended.

Apomorphine. Apomorphine is the most rapid acting of emetics under consideration, principally because it is the only one to be given parenterally. However, since it has to be given by intramuscular injection, it is less convenient to use than syrup of ipecacuanha. Furthermore, it causes depression of the central nervous system and, therefore, if given as treatment for a poison with similar CNS effects, it may lead to serious impairment of consciousness in a patient who is vomiting. For this reason its use is not recommended.

Table 6   Deaths due to use of a saline emetic

Age (years)	Overdose	Maximum plasma sodium (mmol/l)	Risk from overdose
74	Perphenazine, imipramine	174	slight
35	Thioridazine	184	slight
2	Dextropropoxyphene	189	dextropropoxyphene not detected
23	Chlordiazepoxide	214	slight
3	Acetylsalicyclic acid	186	plasma salicylate 270 mg/l
26	Anadin	172	plasma salicylate 171 mg/l
35	Acetylsalicyclic acid	200	plasma salicylate 540 mg/l
21	Amitriptyline, chlorpromazine Diazepam, nitrazepam	227	slight

Reproduced by permission of the Editor, *Proceedings of the Royal Society of Medicine*

Ipecacuanha. Ipecacuanha is an extract prepared from the dried root, or rhizome, of *Cephaelis ipecacuanha* or *C. acuminanata*, both of which grow in South America. It contains several alkaloids including cephalline and emetine which are the active ingredients. Both alkaloids act by irritating the gastrointestinal tract and stimulating the medullary vomiting centre. In large doses they cause CNS depression and are cardiotoxic, but for induction of emesis small doses only are needed and emesis further reduces the absorption of the alkaloids.

It was at one time suggested that ipecacuanha was too slow acting to be an effective emetic for the treatment of poisoning. However, several well-documented studies have attested to its efficacy with successful induction of vomiting in 95 per cent or more cases within 30–45 minutes. Only one death has been recorded after the use of syrup of ipecacuanha and this occurred in a child with a congenital defect of the diaphragm in whom the repeated vomiting resulted in the herniation of the stomach. It seems reasonable to conclude that this death could not be directly attributed to the emetic. Deaths have also been recorded when ipecacuanha fluid extract (14 times the strength of syrup of ipecacuanha) was administered by mistake. Since the fluid extract is not dispensed as such, that mistake should not occur again. The overall evidence therefore suggests that syrup of ipecacuanha is the emetic of choice and it is possible to define its correct usage (Table 7).

Emetics versus lavage. When these two techniques have been compared in animal studies using barium or dye markers, emesis has invariably appeared the more effective. Extrapolation of these findings to man is difficult and there have been no controlled studies where recovery of the poison has been recorded. Nevertheless, it is possible to suggest general guidelines on the choice of treatment.

In children The use of gastric lavage is generally so traumatic for all concerned that it is now widely accepted that syrup of ipeca-

Table 7 The correct use of syrup of ipecacuanha for emesis

Indications	Dosage	Contra-indications	Precautions
1. A potentially toxic dose of poison has been ingested 2. Treatment can be given within 4 hours of ingestion (longer for salicylates and anticholinergic drugs including tricyclic-antidepressants)	Ipecacuanha paediatric emetic draught BPC or ipecacuanha syrup, Adelaide Children's Hospital formula: 6–18 months, 10 ml Older children, 15 ml Adults, 30 ml Taken with a glass of water or fruit juice; repeat after 20 minutes if emesis has not occurred	1. Poisoning due to petroleum distillates 2. Poisoning due to corrosives 3. Impairment of consciousness	Poisoning due to anti-emetics (see text)

cuanha is the treatment of choice unless definite contra-indications are present (Table 6).

In adults the contra-indications to emetics (Table 6) are found much more frequently such that lavage is the only appropriate procedure in the majority of cases. For the remainder, however, there is evidence that emesis is effective and in these cases its use is increasing.

The role of lavage and syrup of ipecacuanha in hospital treatment is thus well defined. It remains, however, to consider the use of these treatments in first-aid outside of hospital. We would consider that their use other than by fully trained personnel could be dangerous. Thus we would not normally recommend that ipecacuanha should be available in the home, or in first-aid units. Exceptions might be made for full-time first-aid units in industrial settings where there is considered to be a high risk of ingestion of poisons, and the staff have received appropriate training. In the home, however, we have noted a large series of cases reported from the USA where the use of ipecacuanha was probably unnecessary in most cases, and there was a greater than 9 per cent incidence of vomiting which continued for longer than one hour. In our opinion this represents an excessive effect from the ipecacuanha and we believe that treatment given in this situation need only produce one serious complication in a patient who was not at risk before the whole treatment programme becomes untenable. Exceptions might be made when the patients are at a considerable distance from a doctor, but in an urban setting we would not recommend the free availability of ipecacuanha.

Oral adsorbants. For the poison that has not been removed by emesis or lavage, or when these procedures are contra-indicated, it is worth considering the use of orally administered adsorbants to reduce absorption further. Numerous adsorbants have been recommended including attapulgite, evaporated milk, fuller's earth, bentonite, activated charcoal, and the so-called 'Universal Antidote'. Fuller's earth and bentonite have a particular role in the treatment of paraquat poisoning (see page 6.13) but the value of the others is still disputed.

Activated charcoal. Such evidence as can be found favours the use of activated charcoal. It is a more effective adsorbant than most and it lacks the toxic hazards of the 'Universal Antidote' (a melange of tannic acid 1 part, magnesium oxide 1 part, and activated charcoal 2 parts). The term 'activated' in this context implies no special chemical attribute, but simply that the charcoal concerned consists of fine particles of low mineral content which meet BP or USP specifications for adsorbance.

Efficacy. Many papers on activated charcoal have been published but few contain any evidence to support its efficacy in clinical practice. The vast majority of reports concern the *in vitro* determination of adsorbance and serve only to confirm that activated charcoal is an effective adsorbant for a wide range of drugs and chemicals. *In vivo*, its usefulness is much more difficult to demonstrate. Experiments using toxic doses of drugs in animals *and using therapeutic doses of drugs in man* have shown that activated charcoal used within one hour of ingestion can reduce the adsorbance of most drugs commonly in overdosage, e.g. paracetamol, salicylates,

barbiturates and tricyclic antidepressants. If given later than one hour, its efficacy appears to be much reduced.

Clinical trials of activated charcoal in the treatment of drug overdosage are known to be in progress both in the UK and the USA, but the problems of obtaining matching patient groups are enormous and at present published observations are limited to anecdotes and a demonstration of the acceptability of the charcoal to children.

Adverse effects. Oral activated charcoal appears to be free from serious toxicity. Some preparations are in the form of granules or biscuits which are difficult to swallow dry and not much easier to take in water. More finely ground preparations taken in water are more palatable, but even these may be vomited. Certain oral 'antidotes', e.g. methionine, are strongly adsorbed and the charcoal should not be administered along with these drugs. Syrup of ipecacuanha is also strongly adsorbed and, therefore, any use of oral charcoal should be delayed until emesis is complete. Charcoal colours the stools black and this should not be mistaken for melaena.

Recommended use. In spite of the limited evidence for its value, we believe that oral activated charcoal is the safest of the adsorbants so far studied and that it is possible to offer practical advice on its use. Most importantly, it must be considered as an adjunct to gastric lavage or emesis and it in no way replaces their use. It is easiest to administer as a finely divided powder in water and will be better tolerated if given via a naso-gastric tube. To be effective, the *in vitro* studies suggest that the ratio of charcoal to estimated dose of poison must be of the order of 10:1. Activated charcoal is therefore most likely to prove useful for poisons where small amounts produce large effects, e.g. tricyclic antidepressants (see page 6.22) or theophylline derivatives (see page 6.25), where a 5–10 g dose of charcoal should be adequate. It is unlikely to be of any real value where large amounts of poison are required before there is any risk of serious toxicity: for 50 aspirin tablets (15 g) or 30 paracetamol tablets (15 g) 150 g of charcoal would be required and few if any patients would tolerate this dose. Although its effectiveness probably declines rapidly with time after ingestion of the poison, administration later than one hour after ingestion may still be worthwhile since in practice clinically significant amounts of the drug may remain in the stomach, e.g. due to anticholinergic effects as with tricyclic antidepressants (Fig. 1), or may remain unabsorbed in the intestine due to a slow release formulation (e.g. theophylline derivatives).

Active elimination techniques. Once a poison has been absorbed and providing there is no antidote, it is reasonable to consider treatments designed to speed its elimination (Table 8). It must be stressed, however, that all the techniques under consideration carry considerable hazards in their own right and that for almost all forms of poisoning supportive therapy will be all that is required. Thus before one of these procedures is commenced there should be convincing evidence that: (*a*) the poison can be removed by the technique; (*b*) the clinical condition of the patient suggests that he is at risk of death, or serious morbidity, if treatment is not instituted; and (*c*) there is confirmation from the laboratory that the poison

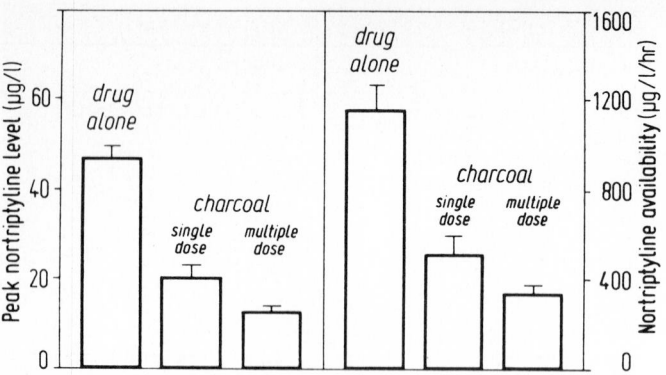

Fig. 1   The effect of single and multiple doses of activated charcoal on peak (mean ± SEM) plasma nortriptyline levels and nortriptyline availability (mean ± SEM) after a single dose of 75 mg of nortriptyline in healthy volunteers.

concerned is present at levels such that clinically significant amounts will be removed by the technique. In practice there will sometimes be a delay in obtaining the laboratory results and the decision to start treatment may have to be made solely on clinical grounds. This is sometimes reasonable if the clinical risks appear to be extreme and the use of the procedure can be reviewed within a few hours, upon receipt of the laboratory results. However, the literature abounds with the descriptions of the use of active elimination methods where the clinical indications of risk were slight, or where the laboratory results showed that no clinically significant amounts of the poisons were removed. Even worse are the instances where claims for the value of the technique are substantiated neither by controlled clinical observations nor laboratory measurements! To emphasize this point the authors (through the London National Poisons Information Service) receive requests for advice on the management of more than 25 000 cases of suspected acute poisoning per year. In spite of this, we have at no time found it necessary to institute charcoal haemoperfusion in more than a dozen or so cases per year. Against this background, each treatment is discussed in turn, and it must be borne in mind that in no case can we turn to data from fully controlled trials to indicate their effectiveness. We believe, however, that theoretical arguments and well reported uncontrolled studies justify the conclusions that we have reached.

Table 8   Active elimination techniques for the removal of absorbed poisons and the poisons for they *may* be considered

Techniques	Poisons removed*
Forced diuresis	
Alkaline	barbitone, phenobarbitone, salicylates
Acid	quinine, amphetamines (?)
Peritoneal dialysis	ethylene glycol, lithium
Haemodialysis	barbitone, ethyl alcohol, lithium, methyl alcohol, phenobarbitone, salicylates
Haemoperfusion	all barbiturates, ethchlorvynol, glutethimide, meprobamate, trichloroethanol, ethyl alcohol, salicylates, theophylline

* This list is not exhaustive but contains only those poisons where we consider the value of the treatment to be well established or where there is a current interest in the problem (see text). In some instances these techniques may be useful for other forms of poisoning but we would suggest that in these cases their use should only be undertaken after discussion of the problem with a Poisons Information Service (see Table 10)

Forced diuresis. Drugs that are normally excreted by the kidney either unchanged, or as active metabolites, may be removed in increased quantity by increasing urine flow. Most drugs are partly reabsorbed from the urine as it flows through the renal tubules. Absorption here, as elsewhere in the body, is confined to the un-ionized, lipid-soluble form of the molecule. If, therefore, the proportion of ionized drug present in the urine can be increased, it is possible to reduce reabsorption and thus increase elimination. Thus for drugs with a weakly acid pKa an increased proportion of ionized drug will present in alkaline urine (pKa is the pH at which the drug is present in equal proportions of ionized and un-ionized molecules). Thus the effectiveness of forced diuresis may be increased in some circumstances by controlling the urine pH. It must be noted, however, that most drugs are either degraded by the liver to non-toxic metabolites, or have a large volume of distribution such that there is insufficient active drug accessible to the kidneys for forced diuresis to be of any clinical value. Most notable amongst these are the short or medium acting barbiturates, which are excreted in the urine mainly as inactive metabolites produced in the liver. A small amount of active drug is eliminated in the urine in these cases and it is possible to show a dramatic increase in amount of active drug (e.g. amylobarbitone) eliminated by a forced alkaline diuresis. However, when the weight of active drug removed is calculated, the amount is insignificant compared to that removed by hepatic metabolism. The practical considerations in the use of forced diuresis are considered in Table 9.

Table 9   Practical considerations in the use of forced diuresis

Indications
1. The poison or its active metabolites must be excreted in the urine
2. There is evidence that supportive therapy alone may not be adequate

Precautions
1. Prove beyond reasonable doubt that the poison is present. (It is not always possible to wait for laboratory measurement of the poison before starting treatment.) In this situation laboratory results must be sought as soon as possible and the treatment reviewed in the light of these results
2. Monitoring plasma electrolytes and fluid balance is essential

Contra-indications
1. Impaired renal function
2. Hypotension which persists after correction of dehydration and use of plasma expanders. (A very cautious diuresis may be possible in patients whose blood pressure is adequate only on treatment with positive inotropic agents, providing that renal function is good.)
3. The poison is known to cause pulmonary oedema

Adverse effects
1. Potassium depletion
2. Pulmonary oedema

Forced alkaline diuresis in practice is commonly used only for poisoning due to salicylates (see page 6.15), phenobarbitone and barbitone (see page 6.19), and lithium (see page 6.23). Several regimens have been suggested and it is difficult to determine whether any one has claim to be more effective.

At least one regimen has claimed to minimize problems with sodium and potassium balance and to reduce the need for monitoring electrolytes. In our experience this advice cannot be accepted and we would suggest that electrolytes be monitored two to four hourly whatever the regimen. A suitable plan is the intravenous infusion of 500 ml bottles of 0.9 per cent saline; 5.0 per cent dextrose; and 1.26 per cent sodium bicarbonate in rotation up to a maximum of 1500–2000 ml per hour.

The urinary pH should be monitored and treatment adjusted to maintain it between 7.5 and 8.5 by substituting bicarbonate for saline or vice versa. A fall in serum potassium concentration is inevitable and supplements should be added to each bottle from the start with subsequent adjustment according to level. At the start of treatment most patients will be dehydrated so that an initial negative fluid balance is to be expected. A central venous pressure line should be inserted in order that rehydration may be monitored. Subsequently fluid intake and output must balance and the use of a diuretic, usually frusemide or mannitol, may be considered. It must be noted, however, that diuretics will tend to reduce the urinary pH and that their use may be hazardous in lithium poisoning.

Forced acid diuresis is most likely to be considered in poisoning due to quinine and related compounds (see page 6.24) since these drugs are widely used and can cause serious toxic effects. In theory it could also be used for a number of other drugs, including amphetamine and related compounds (see page 6.34) but serious cases are unusual. A suitable regimen would be the intravenous infusion of 500 ml bottles of 5 per cent dextrose plus 1.5 g ammonium chloride; 5 per cent dextrose; and 0.9 per cent saline in rotation up to a maximum of 500–1000 ml/hour.

The urinary pH should be maintained below 7.0 and a further 1.5 g ammonium chloride may be added to the second bottle in the cycle if necessary. As with alkaline diuresis, regular monitoring of the electrolyte levels and appropriate correction is essential. In practice this technique is seldom necessary and the evidence for its effectiveness is limited.

Dialysis in the treatment of acute poisoning is most commonly indicated for the treatment of renal failure and is only infrequently used to increase elimination of the poison. That is not to say that these techniques have not been used in acute poisoning, but that experience of their use has shown that for most poisons relatively little is removed in the dialysate. The rate of removal of the poison across the dialysis membrane is dependent upon a number of variables including molecular weight, protein binding, concentration gradient, pH of blood and dialysate, etc. With so many variables, any assessment of dialysis in acute poisoning needs to be fully documented and controlled as carefully as possible. Most published reports do not meet these requirements. We would advise the use of dialysis only for the following:

Peritoneal dialysis is particularly useful in the removal of lithium sodium chlorate, and ethylene glycol (see page 6.26). It may also be used instead of haemodialysis when renal failure complicates poisoning due to phenobarbitone or salicylates and when haemodialysis is not available or impracticable, e.g. in a young child.

Haemodialysis is of value in the removal of salicylates and the long-acting barbiturates, in which cases it is more effective than peritoneal dialysis. However, since these drugs are also removed by forced diuresis, its use is reserved for those cases where renal failure prevents the use of that technique (see Section 18 for a detailed discussion of dialysis techniques).

Haemoperfusion. The failure of dialysis as a technique for removal of most poisons led to further research in which the blood was passed through columns of materials known to be highly adsorbant for drugs and other chemicals, so-called haemoperfusion. *In vitro* tests soon demonstrated the effectiveness of activated charcoal and certain resins in removal of drugs from the blood, but the clinical use of haemoperfusion was delayed by problems with removal of blood platelets, embolization of the adsorbant, and pyrogenic reactions. In time, these problems were overcome and the last seven years has seen the accumulation of a considerable body of evidence on the use of haemoperfusion in the treatment of acute poisoning.

Procedure. The circuit is set up as in Fig. 2 and an arteriovenous shunt is established. A range of columns is available (Fig. 3) mostly using charcoal coated with some form of membrane (e.g. acrylic hydrogel) which permits adsorption of the poison whilst reducing the unwanted removal of blood platelets. Prior to use the circuit is primed with heparinized saline and heparin is given as a bolus at the start of treatment followed by a slow infusion to maintain a plasma heparin concentration of 2.5–5.0 ml/min. The total volume of the circuit is small ($x - y$ ml) and so that any tendency for the blood pressure to fall is easily corrected with intravenous fluids, whilst at the end of the procedure the blood may be returned to the patient by flushing with 5.0 per cent dextrose, without risk of overload.

For effective removal of the poison a blood flow through the column of 100–200 ml/min is advised and the progress should be monitored both by the clinical condition of the patient and by the plasma level of the poison. For adequate evaluation of the technique it is vital that flow rate, together with both arterial and venous concentrations of the poison are recorded, since from these both

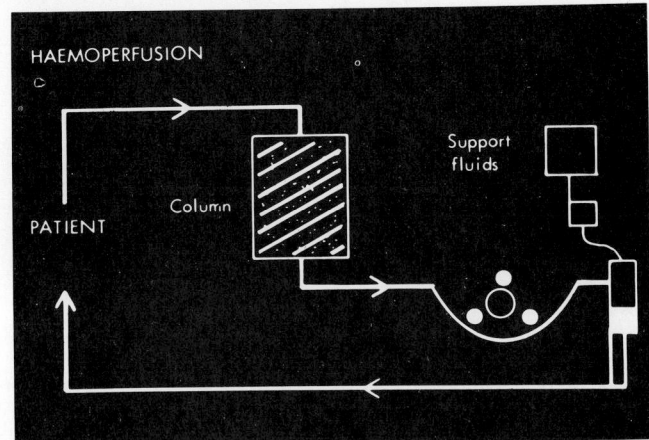

Fig. 2.

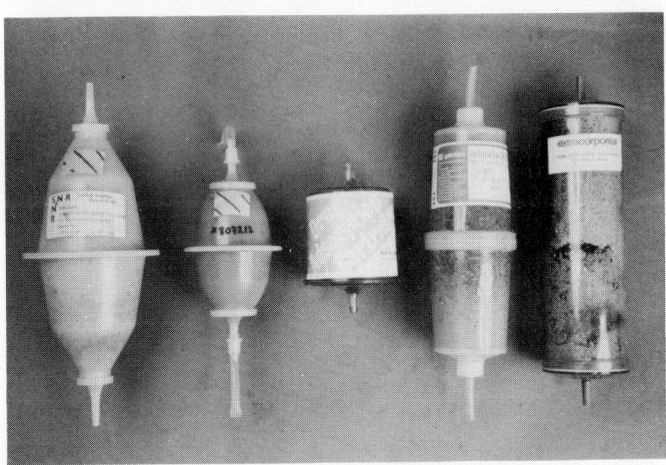

Fig. 3.

the clearance and the actual amount of drug removed can be calculated. The amount of poison removed equals:

$$\tfrac{1}{2}(t_y - t_x) \times [(C_1 - C_2) + (C_3 - C_4)] \times F$$

where $(t_y - t_x)$ is the time interval between samples in minutes, C_1 and C_2 are the inlet and outlet plasma drug concentrations at time t_x, C_3 and C_4 are the corresponding concentrations at time t_y, and F is the blood flow-rate in ml/min. These results are usually not urgent during the procedure since the initial levels provide the indication for treatment and clinical improvement of the patient indicates that treatment may be stopped. When brain death is suspected, however, evidence for the complete, or near-complete removal of the poison may be needed before treatment is discontinued.

Complications. With most columns the blood platelet count will fall by approximately 25–40 per cent but this does not seem to be associated with bleeding problems. Bleeding is more likely to result from excessive heparinization and can be minimized by monitoring heparin levels or, if necessary, by stopping the procedure and giving protamine. Removal of other molecules from the blood, e.g. urea, creatinine, or urate, does not present problems, but it must be remembered that haemoperfusion, unlike dialysis, will not influence electrolyte balance and that this will need separate attention. Pyrogen reactions, leucopenia, and loss of fibrinogen are not problems with the present equipment.

Uses. Like the other active elimination techniques haemoperfusion is being abused. There is, however, good evidence for its use in poisoning due to the causes listed in Table 8, subject to the criteria listed in Table 10. This technique is a major advance in treating some of the most serious cases of poisoning, but its use must be based on adequate criteria and it should be confined to units with experience of its operation, or of the operation of haemodialysis.

Table 10 Criteria for the use of haemoperfusion

Plasma drug levels (mg/l) not less than:	
Phenobarbitone and barbitone	100
Other barbiturates	50
Glutethimide	40
Methaqualone	40
Ethchlorvynol	150
Meprobamate	100
Theophylline	60
Trichloroethanol	50
Salicylates	800*

Plus at least one of the following clinical features:

Severe clinical intoxication, e.g. grade IV coma, hypotension, hypothermia, hypoventilation

Progressive deterioration or failure to improve in spite of good supportive management

Prolonged coma with complications, e.g. pneumonia, chronic respiratory disease

* or at 500 mg/l if arterial pH is < 7.34 more than 4 hours after ingestion

Poisons Information Services. The general principles of management of acute poisoning as outlined in this section and in those which follow should provide adequate guidelines for the treatment of most poisoned patients. It is not difficult to realize, however, that in many cases there may be additional problems which are not immediately answered, e.g. what action is needed in poisoning from more than one agent? Should an antidote or an elimination technique be used in a particular case? What is the toxicity of an unusual poison?

To answer these and other problems associated with poisoning many countries have developed special advisory centres and, in particular, there are National Poisons Information Services available in the UK and Eire (Table 11). Each offers a full 24-hour service, seven days a week. Initially the enquirer is provided with information for his own use but when necessary, expert medical

Table 11 Addresses of Poisons Information Centres

United Kingdom

London	National Poisons Information Service	01-407 7600
	New Cross Hospital	Ext. 4001
	Avonley Road	
	London SE14 5ER	
Edinburgh	Scottish Poisons Information Bureau	031-229 2477
	The Royal Infirmary	Ext. 2233
	Lauriston Place	
	Edinburgh 3	
Cardiff	Poisons Information Service	0222-492233
	Cardiff Royal Infirmary	Ext. 200
	Cardiff CF2 1SZ	
Belfast	Poisons Information Service	0232-40503
	Royal Victoria Hospital	Ext. 2140
	Grosvenor Road	
	Belfast BT12 6BB	

Republic of Ireland

Dublin	Poisons Information Service	0001-72 3355
	Jervis Street Hospital	
	Dublin 1	

The above five centres all use a common information base

Europe

There are many poisons information services in European countries. Most of these are members of the European Association of Poisons Control Centres, from whom further details, including a full list of member centres, may be obtained. The postal address of the Association is: Centre Belge anti-Poisons, rue Joseph Stallaert N⁰ 15, Brussels 1060, Belgium

USA

Information on Poison Control Centres in the United States of America may be obtained from the National Clearinghouse for Poison Control Centers, Food and Drug Administration, Division of Poison Control, 5600 Fishers Lane, Rockville, Maryland 20857, USA

opinion can also be obtained, again on a 24-hour basis. Together these centres handle in excess of 40 000 enquiries per year and the reader is therefore encouraged to make use of their experience. Similar facilities are available in many other countries.

THE ROLE OF THE LABORATORY IN ACUTE POISONING

G. N. Volans and B. Widdop

For most poisoned patients, measurements of physiological status (blood gases, electrolytes, serum enzymes) are far more important than the detection and measurement of the toxin. Most hospital clinical chemistry laboratories offer analyses only for iron, salicylates, barbiturates, and paracetamol. Analyses for other poisons, which can be complex and require considerable expertise, are rarely justified on clinical grounds since the therapy used will not be influenced by the results. Nevertheless, there are situations where more searching analyses for poisons can be of considerable value. These include: (*a*) differential diagnosis of coma; (*b*) diagnosis of brain death; (*c*) diagnostic problems in children including detection of non-accidental poisoning; (*d*) monitoring of drug abuse; and (*e*) influence on active therapy for poisoning. Thus, it is prudent to collect samples (Table 1) for possible analysis in all except the most mild cases of poisoning so that they are available if the subsequent clinical course justifies their use, or in the event of medicolegal enquiries. If these cannot be dealt with by the local laboratory, arrangements should be made to convey the specimen to the nearest laboratory specializing in toxicological analyses.

Table 1 Sample collection for possible toxicological analyses

1. Samples of the suspected poison found on or near the patient
2. Containers (including syringes/needles) thought to have been in contact with the suspected poison
3. For ingested poisons: vomitus, gastric aspirate, or lavage (50 ml). Ideally, the first sample of aspirate should be collected before dilution with the lavage fluid
4. Ingested or injected poisons: urine (50 ml) should be collected in a clean container with no preservatives. Catheterization should only be undertaken if justified on clinical grounds
5. Blood (5–10 ml) collected into plain or lithium heparin tubes. (Analysis of plasma is technically easier for most poisons. Do not use lithium heparin tubes in suspected lithium poisoning. Where ethyl alcohol intoxication is thought to be a major factor use sodium fluoride tubes to guard against changes in alcohol content brought about by extraneous organisms)
6. Metals: for these elements the sample requirements are variable and the advice of the analyst should always be sought prior to despatching specimens

Application of toxicological analyses

Differential diagnosis of coma. There are many causes for coma and the diagnosis is often far from obvious. Acute poisoning is essential to the differential diagnosis and its confirmation may influence therapy, especially when neurosurgical procedures are otherwise being considered. The urgency with which drug analyses are required for patients in coma will vary considerably from case to case according to clinical conditions; in a life-threatening situation an emergency analysis can be justified; in less serious cases or where the diagnosis is not entirely certain even after recovery, a 'routine' analysis is acceptable; and when recovery accords well with the history and clinical findings, analysis is not required. The overall value of such analyses can be seen in one series of 208 patients presenting with coma of unknown aetiology, 108 of whom were shown to be intoxicated by drugs.

Diagnosis of brain death. In cases where brain death is suspected and the decision to withdraw life-support is under consideration, it must always be remembered that drugs taken before admission or given during hospital treatment could be causing CNS depression, even to the extent of suppressing an electroencephalographic record. Whenever there is the slightest chance that this is so, toxicological analyses should be undertaken in addition to the careful neurological assessment (see Section 21). Obviously in these cases there is no requirement for an emergency analytical service, but a comprehensive and sensitive range of tests is required. A positive result almost always indicates that the diagnosis 'brain death' is not yet established.

Diagnostic problems in children. Acute illnesses in children often present diagnostic problems and in recent years it has become increasingly apparent that poisoning, usually from drugs, can account for some cases where the diagnosis was otherwise not established. Children presenting with coma or convulsions are obvious cases where poisoning must be considered, but there are many other cases where altered behaviour or even organ damage could be due to a toxic effect. Where poisoning is suspected, the child often cannot give a history and the diagnosis is based entirely on circumstantial evidence. Without laboratory analyses, such diagnoses are often difficult to sustain and experience has shown that the clinical diagnosis is inaccurate in many cases. Laboratory analyses are of even greater importance in those cases where child abuse by drugs is suspected. Prompt diagnosis can lead to action by the social services, or the courts, whilst delay in recognition of the problem may result in prolonged morbidity, or even death.

Monitoring drug abuse. Drug abusers are unreliable historians and, in particular, they are likely to lie about their drug intake. On the one hand, the abuser who is seeking a prescription may exaggerate his need, either for fear of withdrawal symptoms or because he wishes to sell the drugs which he does not need. On the other hand, an abuser who is undergoing withdrawal therapy may not admit to using drugs which have not been prescribed. In the United Kingdom some addicts attend special treatment centres and thus the laboratory can provide valuable information for their management. In addition, the laboratory can help to identify the drugs used when these were bought in the street, either by analysis of the material involved, or by testing biological fluids.

Influence on active therapy for poisoning. As discussed on page 6.7, all forms of active therapy for removal of absorbed poisons carry inherent risks. Thus they should not be used without evidence that the poison can be removed by the technique concerned and that significant amounts of the poison are present in the individual patient. This situation, therefore, presents the strongest of all the cases for the use of laboratory analyses since these must influence both the decision to start treatment and, when the poison has been shown to be removed, the decision to stop. In practice, it is not always possible to wait for the results of plasma or urine concentrations before starting therapy and the decision to use the treatment may have to be made on clinical grounds alone. However, even in these cases it should be possible to review the need for the treatment as soon as the laboratory results are available.

References

Helliwell, M., Hampel, G., Sinclair, E., Huggett, A., and Flanagan, R. J. (1979). Value of emergency toxicological investigations in the differential diagnosis of coma. *Br. med. J.* ii, 819.

Rogers, D., Tripp, J., Bentovim, A., Robinson, A., Berry, D. J., and Goulding, R. (1976). Non-accidental poisoning: an extended syndrome of child abuse. *Br. med. J.* i, 793.

Widdop, B. (1979). Laboratory diagnosis of intoxication. In *Therapeutic relevance of drug assays* (eds. F. A. de Wolff, H. Mattie, and D. D. Breimer). Boerhaave series, vol. 14. Leiden University Press, Leiden.

POISONING FROM CHEMICALS

R. Goulding

Corrosives and irritants

Of the many chemicals used in the world today, quite a large proportion are found to be endowed with irritant or corrosive properties. Their potential for contributing to poisoning is, there-

fore, immense. Epidemiological study nevertheless suggests that the incidence of poisoning from such agents is, in most countries, fairly low. Occupationally an increasing awareness of the related dangers has led to precautions that mitigate the harm to workers. Yet it is still possible for adults to procure strong corrosives and irritants for suicidal acts, though the tendency nowadays is for those intent upon self-immolation to choose less aversive products, chiefly drugs.

Accidents with excoriating chemicals can still beset adults, nevertheless, and substances of this kind are still left within the reach of small children who may ingest them.

Mode of action. Corrosives and irritants behave as necrotizing and protein-coagulating agents upon living tissue and the resulting hazards can be considered under two headings.

1. External. On the skin, according to the nature of the chemical and its concentration, there may be reddening, inflammation, blistering, ulceration, and penetrating necrosis, with pain at the site. The trauma may, however, remain localized. Similarly, in the eye, there may be conjunctival and/or corneal irritation and ulceration, with or without penetration, and more profound tissue disorganization. In other instances the chemical may give rise not only to circumscribed physicochemical changes, but in addition it may be absorbed from the portal of entry and set up systemic toxicity.

2. Internal. The primary impact of corrosives and irritants by mouth is upon the lips, tongue, mouth, pharynx, oesophagus, and stomach. Depending on the degree to which this advances there may be reactionary oedema, for which the larynx is a prime target, serous exudation, and even perforation. Eventually healing may come about by cicatrization and stenosis. Again, superimposed upon these primary anatomical lesions, the chemical may be absorbed to demonstrate its toxicity upon other organs and tissues.

Mineral acids. Among these are hydrochloric, sulphuric, and nitric acids. On the skin they behave characteristically as corrosives. Treatment of such acid burns consists of liberal irrigation with water, or saline, and the application of dressings as for a thermal burn. Where the affected area is extensive, skin grafting may be necessary later. No systemic consequences are to be expected.

Similarly, an eye into which acid has found its way should be irrigated at once, preferably with saline or else with water, the instillation of a local anaesthetic sometimes being indicated to relieve pain locally and to overcome blepharosphasm. Thereafter, specialist ophthalmic advice should be sought.

By mouth, as little as 10–20 ml of these acids in concentrated form has proved fatal. There is often excruciating pain orally, pharyngeally, substernally, and epigastrically, with dysphagia, and clear evidence of corrosive lesions circumorally and within the mouth and throat. These signs may be accompanied by vomiting and haematemesis, respiratory distress (mainly from laryngeal oedema), collapse, and renal failure. Perforation of the oesophagus and/or the stomach may also ensue. Survival from this acute stage may be succeeded by stenotic changes in the upper alimentary tract.

Treatment is always of extreme urgency. Gastric aspiration and lavage are advisedly withheld and the presentation of weak alkalis on the mistaken principle that they will help neutralize the acid should never be condoned. Instead, water or milk should be given liberally by mouth, mainly as a diluent. Strong analgesics by injection may be warranted to relieve the pain and, with the onset of hypotensive collapse owing to fluid loss, an active supportive regimen should be instituted. Occasionally to preserve the airway, an endotracheal catheter may have to be introduced, or even tracheostomy may need to be undertaken. Observation should be unremitting to detect the performation of any viscus, when surgery is imperative.

Endoscopy should be restrained and cautious, once the immediate emergency is passed. Whether the use of systemic corticosteroids to allay excessive cicatrization is worthwhile remains debatable.

Of notable interest is *formic acid*, strong solutions of which are to be found in many homes in domestic bath cleaners and destaining preparations, for besides bringing about the direct effects seen with mineral acids, only probably more markedly, there is a likelihood of general absorption, evidenced by systemic acidosis, haematuria, and renal damage. So, in addition to the usual treatment, special measures are called for to remedy these complications.

Outstanding, though, among the corrosive poisons in this context is *hydrofluoric acid*. Inhalation of the hydrogen fluoride vapour is intensely irritating to the respiratory tract, with coughing, dyspnoea, and pulmonary oedema. Oxygen therapy and bronchial toilet must be initiated.

On the skin, hydrofluoric acid burns can be excessively painful and they can be insidiously penetrating. Irrigation should be prompt and should be followed by subcutaneous injections of sterile calcium gluconate solution (10 per cent) or, better still, the application of a proprietory calcium gluconate gel.

Hydrofluoric acid burns of the eye demand immediate and liberal irrigation, and often the instillation of local anaesthetic eye drops as well, after which specialist ophthalmic consultation should not be delayed.

Taken by mouth the corrosive injury brought about by this acid can be devastating, with the additional burden of acute, systemic fluorosis, for which intravenous calcium gluconate has been recommended.

Phenol, or as it was once more commonly named 'carbolic acid', is another intense corrosive which does not feature in suicide at the present time as commonly as it did in the past. Its presence is nearly always recognizable by its odour and, distinctively, the pain to which it gives rise is much less than might be expected. This is due to its damage to the afferent nerve endings. On the skin, deep ulceration may be seen covered with conspicuous white eschars. Uptake by the body is common, with systemic phenol poisoning, indicated by coma, convulsions, haemolysis, markedly pigmented urine, and renal failure.

By mouth, there is the usual clinical picture of corrosive poisoning, with the identifying odour and eschars and, again, systemic phenol toxicity. Olive oil, or any other bland vegetable oil, by mouth may inhibit absorption and serve as some protective to the alimentary tract. Affected eyes and skin should, of course, be irrigated. For the general body reactions, diuresis is advised initially, with haemodialysis for renal failure and orthodox supportive care.

Alkalis. The common alkalis are still widely distributed for household as well as for industrial use. The clinical features of exposure, whether locally or orally, mimic those caused by mineral acids, though they tend to be even more severe. Any attempted neutralization by exhibiting weak acids is just as misplaced as the reverse procedure for dealing with mineral acid corrosion, and, in cases of ingestion, gastric aspiration and lavage is probably more hazardous than helpful. What is more, extensive erosion of the oesophagus and stomach can occur without any arresting warning signs in the mouth or pharynx.

The treatment for alkali injury locally or by the oral route, is just the same as for mineral acids.

Sodium hypochlorite is worthy of special mention, for in solution it is widely sold as a bleaching agent. In the stomach it gives rise to hypochlorous acid. Such is its concentration in most domestic brands, however, that symptoms are usually minor, or negligible, unless huge quantities of the undiluted formulation are deliberately swallowed. Then the line of treatment should follow that for other corrosives and irritants.

Lime, or quicklime, can prove very troublesome if particles get into the eye. The local reaction in the conjunctiva and cornea is that to be expected from any alkali. Irrigation alone, however, may not be sufficient, for any particulate lime adherent to the surface of the eye must be physically removed, advisedly under local anaesthetic cover.

Another relatively common chemical that can be incriminated as a corrosive poison is *methylene chloride* (dichloromethane), for it is widely employed as a paint-stripper and so is readily available. To the usual reaction by the body to local contact or ingestion can be added dizziness, bronchopneumonia, toxic myocarditis, liver damage, and haemolysis. Moreover, breathing an atmosphere of methylene chloride can induce carboxyhaemoglobinaemia (see page 6.31).

Pesticides

Medically to refer to 'pesticide poisoning' is somewhat inaccurate and certainly imprecise, for the chemicals deployed to control pests exhibit a wide diversity of purpose, of molecular structure and, above all, of toxic activity. At one end of the scale is the anticoagulant rodenticide, warfarin, utterly different in its biological properties from an organophosphorus insecticide such as parathion. So each case of pesticide poisoning, or suspected poisoning, should be approached as a distinct diagnostic exercise, and accordingly in this section, the clinical toxicology of some of the commoner pesticides will be briefly described, group by group.

Organochlorine compounds. These are included more for historical reasons than for their current clinical significance, for over recent years they have been progressively phased out, mostly to avoid environmental contamination. The group includes DDT (dicophan), aldrin, dieldrin, and a number of related compounds. Effective principally as insecticides they are chemically very stable and biologically persistent. It is this latter character which, from an environmental point of view, has led to their condemnation.

For man they have a fairly low acute toxicity. Very occasionally, by intent or misadventure, a large quantity of one of these substances has been taken by mouth. Symptoms have been confined to the central nervous system, with excitement, tremors, and convulsions, and, so long as these can be suppressed by injections of, for example, diazepam 5 to 10 mg intravenously and provided respiration has been safeguarded during the time that the chemical has become sequestered in the body fat, recovery is invariably complete and without sequelae.

By extrapolation from animal experiments, however, disquiet has been nurtured by the idea that continuing exposure to organochlorine compounds of this kind can underlie reproductive disorders, teratogenicity, and malignancies, but there is as yet no convincing evidence in the human to confirm these suspicions.

Organophosphorus compounds. Increasingly in pest control the organophosphorus compounds have displaced their organochlorine counterparts and today the former are among the most widely used pesticides throughout the world. They owe their origin to the so-called 'nerve gases' conjured up during the Second World War for military use, but it must be emphasized that every one of the derivatives in commercial circulation for pest control should have been subjected to animal tests to demonstrate its freedom from neurotoxicity.

Common to all these substances, nevertheless, is a specific mode of action upon the autonomic nervous system, in so far as they inactivate the body complement of cholinesterase, thereby bringing about a surfeit of acetylcholine at all the autonomic ganglia, at the post-ganglionic parasympathetic nerve endings, and at the neuromuscular junctions. This explains the clinical picture of organophosphorus poisoning, incorporating as it does headache, a sense of exhaustion, weakness, vomiting, colicky abdominal pain, profuse cold sweating, and hypersalivation. Thereafter come muscular twitchings and fasciculations, diarrhoea, tenesmus, convulsions, urinary incontinence, dyspnoea, bronchoconstriction, bronchial hypersecretion, and meiosis. Ultimately there may be respiratory depression, mental confusion, coma, and death.

There is a wide difference in toxicity between the various organophosphorus compounds. Nevertheless, the appearance of a concatenation of the above signs in anyone who has been in contact with one or more of these compounds is virtually diagnostic. Treatment is urgent. The patient should be kept at rest, rendered free from any further contamination by way of the skin and clothing and given an immediate injection of atropine in a dose of 2 mg, this being repeated until full 'atropinization' is achieved and maintained. Further, within the first 12–18 hours of the onset of the disorder, the attempt should be made to reactivate the cholinesterase. Among the drugs designed to deconjugate the union of the enzyme and chemical, pralidoxime is probably the one with which experience has been greatest. This is given in a dose of 1 g intravenously in 5 ml water, repeating this once or twice if the response to the first is disappointing. There is no point in continuing oxime therapy after 24 hours. Even in the absence of convulsions, moreover, diazepam in intravenous injections of 5–10 mg seems to have an ameliorating effect centrally by a mechanism so far unexplained.

The customary supportive care should also be provided as needed.

The diagnosis can be confirmed by estimating the cholinesterase content of the blood and this laboratory test is also valuable for monitoring workers who are repeatedly handling these pesticides.

Carbamate insecticides. Chemically distinct though they are from the organophosphorus insecticides, the carbamates nevertheless display precisely the same mode of action in man, but their affinity for cholinesterase resolves spontaneously. Symptomatic cases require atropine, but oximes are contra-indicated.

Dinitro compounds. These, including DNOC and dinoseb, are not so commonly used now as pesticides, though they still find favour to some extent as winter washes on fruit trees and, in stronger solutions, as defoliants and haulm destroyers, commonly in the warmer weather. It is just this latter circumstance that heightens their hazards.

All of these substances exhibit a facility for staining the skin yellow and this serves as a warning sign to overexposure, so that the protective ritual must be reviewed, even if clinical poisoning is not at that stage evident.

The dinitro compounds are readily taken up percutaneously, as they are from the stomach, and in the body they act biochemically by uncoupling oxidative phosphorylation. In this manner they augment tissue metabolism regardless of the thyroid gland. Poisoning is evinced by undue lethargy, remarkably noticeable sweating, and thirst, along with insomnia, tachycardia, hyperpnoea, dehydration, and collapse.

There is no specific treatment, but the patient should be kept at absolute rest, the respiration should not be allowed to deteriorate, and cold sponging or spraying should be directed on to the patient. Dehydration should be corrected by fluid and electrolyte replacement under laboratory control.

The diagnosis and the severity of the condition can be confirmed by determining analytically the blood levels of the chemical and 5 mg per ml should be regarded as the upper limit of normal.

If recovery comes about, this is usually complete.

Allied to the dinitro compounds are other phenolic agents, notably *pentachlorophenol*, widely used as a timber preservative, which likewise perform as uncouplers of oxidative phosphorylation. The hazards and toxic manifestations of pentachlorophenol emulate those of the dinitro compounds, yet without the yellow staining of the skin. Management of poisoning should follow the same lines.

Chlorophenoxyacetate herbicides. These are probably some of the most widely encountered weed-killers at the present time and the penetrating smell that surrounds their spraying, if not altogether unpleasant, is enough to create concern among people in the vicinity. On dicotyledonous plants they interfere specifically with photosynthetic processes and so they have been termed 'hor-

monal' weed killers. They have no corresponding action in man. Indeed, in human terms their toxicity is low and occupational poisoning is almost unknown, serious overdose occurring only in patients who have intentionally imbibed the concentrated liquid formulation. Then the symptoms and signs comprise hypersalivation, stomach cramps, vomiting, diarrhoea, transient myotonia, muscle weakness with areflexic coma and death.

The stomach should be emptied and treatment then is entirely symptomatic. It is suggested that the elimination of the toxin from the body can be accelerated by forced alkaline diuresis.

Widespread controversy has been generated over one member of this group, namely 2,4,5-T, with allegations of its fetal toxicity, teratogenicity, and carcinogenicity, linked in some degree to the residual dioxin that can be detected in commercial samples of the chemical. These assertions have not so far been validated.

Bipyridilium herbicides. Among these are diquat, morfamquat, and paraquat. They are all 'total' weed killers, destroying all green plant growth indiscriminately, but it is the third member of this trio that has attracted so much notoriety toxicologically. So long as a few simple precautions have been respected there have been no mishaps occupationally with paraquat, and carelessness in handling has led to no more distress to workers than mild epistaxis and some reversible changes in the beds of the finger nails. By mouth, on the other hand, a mere 10–15 ml of the concentrated solution can prove fatal. Larger doses can bring about death in the course of a few hours by multi-organ failure. Lesser quantities may first set up oral and pharyngeal inflammation which, after a few days, may resolve on its own. Then monitoring may detect toxic myocarditis electrocardiographically and transient alterations in renal and hepatic functions, all of which tend to improve. More sinister, after a week or so, is the onset of changes in pulmonary function and in the radiographic appearances in the lung, signalling interstitial pulmonary oedema which proceeds to proliferative alveolar changes, going on to an advancing fibrosis culminating in death.

Since no specific antidote has been contrived, therapeutic efforts are directed at removing the chemical from the body with all expediency. The prognosis can be forecast by measuring the plasma levels of paraquat and relating these to a suitable nomogram—a procedure that unfortunately is as yet within the competence of few clinical laboratories. When there is reason to expect a downward course, the stomach is emptied by gastric aspiration and lavage and a bentonite or kaolin suspension is then introduced as an adsorbent. Vigorous purgation is promoted by mannitol, or similar means, and haemodialysis or haemoperfusion is applied over several days. Unfortunately it is doubtful whether this heroic therapeutic attack is ever really life-saving, except perhaps in a few borderline cases.

Triazine herbicides. This class of chemicals, among which simazine is numbered, have the economic virtue of killing all plant growth so they are convenient for controlling weeds on paths, drives, railway tracks, etc. Their record is of almost total innocuity to man.

Chlorates. Like the triazines, the chlorates of sodium and potassium are total weed killers, but in their handling there are risks of fire and explosion and, if taken internally, they can prove highly toxic, about 15 g being lethal for an adult and proportionately for a child, with prior symptoms of vomiting, diarrhoea, methaemoglobinaemia, haemolysis, and kidney damage.

Poisoning calls for gastric aspiration and lavage, with diuresis being encouraged at the outset, but when renal failure comes about, haemodialysis is obligatory. Survival after the first 24 hours is said to signal a favourable outcome.

Organic mercurials. Some organic mercury compounds are reliable fungicides and consequently form the basis of many seed dressings, as well as being utilized to eradicate moulds and mildews elsewhere. They can be inhaled and are readily absorbed through the skin, so workers must be protected against them occupationally, but the most tragic poisonings have beset man when these substances have been inadvertently ingested by, for instance, the injudicious diversion of treated seed grain as human feed. The alkyl and the alkoxy compounds are more toxic than their aryl counterparts. On the skin they are irritant and, systemically, they cause fatigue, loss of memory and mental concentration, paraesthesia, ataxia, tremors, dysarthria and constriction of the visual fields, going on to blindness. Other more dramatic neurological changes can also emerge.

The action at a cellular level is believed to relate to sulphydril groupings, but dimercaprol and N-acetyl pencillamine have proved disappointing in treatment which, in practice, can be little more than palliative.

Inorganic mercurials. These, such as mercurous and mercuric chlorides, are likewise fungicidal and are almost alone among the remedies that can be confidently recommended to rid lawns of moss. It is by the oral route that they are conspicuously toxic, when they behave as corrosives. Treatment should be for this class of poisons (see page 6.11), though specific chelation by dimercaprol and N-acetyl pencillamine has been advocated in addition.

Rodenticides. The commonest rodenticides currently are the *anticoagulants* and, within this group, warfarin is still the most popular. Low concentrations are incorporated into rat and mouse baits and when the vermin take such a diet over some days their blood coagulability is so depressed that they succumb to fatal haemorrhages. So low is the level of the active principle in the baits as supplied commercially, even in the concentrates, however, that to be any danger to man, or child, extremely large quantities would have to be devoured. There is practically no risk from dermal contact or inhalation.

In the event of a gross overdose of rodenticide bait being swallowed the coagulation status of the patient should be checked and, if it is subnormal, vitamin K$_1$ is the antidote.

A domestic alternative for killing rats and mice is *alphachloralose* which derives its action from the chloral hydrate moiety, depressing the central nervous system. Once more, though, the content of active principle in the baits is fairly low so that a substantial quantity must be eaten by man to prove deleterious. There have been incidents, nevertheless, of children taking sponge cake baits embodying alpha-chloralose and being rendered drowsy and unresponsive. The treatment then is the same as that for any hypnotic overdose.

At some special sites, e.g. main sewers or ships' holds, rats can be abated only deploying highly poisonous substances, of which the fluoroacetic acid derivatives are the best example, phosphorus no longer being used. With these, there is some possibility of percutaneous absorption, but the main risk is of the fluoroacetates getting into the mouth, for as little as 30 mg orally can be fatal. First there is a falsely reassuring latent period of about a half to two hours, after which the patient rapidly displays apprehension, muscle twitching, tremors, cardiac irregularities, convulsions, and death, all due to the fluoroacetate expressly interfering with carbohydrate metabolism via the tri-carboxylic acid cycle.

Lacking any specific antidote, all that can be done is by way of gastric aspiration and lavage and symptomatic care.

In this class, too, the *cyanides* (see page 6.32) may be considered, though they are more often directed against rabbits than rats and mice. Serious accidents have overtaken rabbiters in the field.

Fumigants. Particularly in food storage the ravages of pests can be minimized often by means of toxic fumigants, sometimes singly or otherwise in combination. The principal compounds used in this manner are methyl bromide, carbon tetrachloride, ethylene dichloride, ethylene dibromide, chloropicrin, and phosphine. Some of these are narcotic, many of them are irritating to the eyes and

more so to the lungs, and in some instances they may cause nerve, hepatic and renal damage.

Anyone overcome by these gases should be moved into the fresh air, respiratory function should be accorded prior attention, and thereafter the management should be symptomatic, the facilities of an intensive care unit being preferred.

Summary. The pesticides to which reference has so far been made constitute only a proportion of those actually turned to account commercially. Those named are nevertheless the more common and include those that create the major toxic hazards. Only for a few are specific treatments practicable and, in the main, managment of overexposure is based upon supporting the vital functions.

There are nowadays few countries without some sort of official regulatory scheme for testing, evaluation, and control of pesticides. In this way all of the chemicals so marketed have been toxicologically characterized and it is usually the rule for commercial products to be labelled so as to disclose the identity of the active constituent(s), the precautions to be adopted for the welfare of workers and others, and an indication of the action to be taken if overexposure or poisoning should happen. That is why, in dealing with any such patient, it is essential to find out the name of the chemical likely to have been involved, most explicitly by retrieving the container and its label.

Another advantage of getting these particulars is to be able to quote them whenever guidance is sought from a Poisons Information Service, or Poisons Control Centre.

Arsenic, strychnine, nicotine, and phosphorus

Arsenic. Over past centuries arsenic has been the poison most frequently chosen for homicide, and it has thereby gained a sinister forensic reputation. Medically, industrially, and agriculturally its use has gradually given way to alternatives, so that toxic incidents with it have now become uncommon.

In one of its most dangerous forms, arsenic trioxide, it still appears in chemistry laboratories and a few industries. This is a soluble powder with an acute lethal dose for man of the order of 60–120 mg. In the mouth it imparts a slightly gritty sensation and, after swallowing, there may be no overt response for an interval of time that may extend from about 15 minutes to a few hours. Then poisoning is signalled by vomiting and choleraic diarrhoea, which can quickly result in dehydration and collapse. Meanwhile, the arsenic ion, which has reached the internal organs and tissues, may disorganize vital enzyme systems based on sulphydril groupings.

Whereas the diagnosis can be verified by chemical analysis of gastric contents, faeces, etc., treatment should never be postponed for this preliminary. At once the depleted fluid and electrolyte status of the body should be restored by the parenteral route and, to counteract the systemic biochemical abnormalities, dimercaprol should be administered.

Chronic arsenical poisoning may still be seen industrially, environmentally, and by malicious acts. The patient so afflicted presents with ongoing vomiting and diarrhoea, loss of weight, a skin rash of the so-called 'raindrop' pattern, hyperkeratosis of the palms of the hands and the soles of the feet, and polyneuropathy. Diagnostic validation is afforded to some extent by measuring the arsenic in the urine, the normal values seldom rising above 0.3 mg/l, though in symptomless workers levels of 3 mg/l have been found. More precise is the determination of the arsenic content of the nails and hair by neutron activation, a technique that is available at only a few specialized centres.

Treatment, besides the customary supportive care, should be addressed to disposing of the overload of arsenic in the body by chelation with dimercaprol.

Another form of arsenical poisoning that can still quite frequently and mystifyingly come to light is that from *arsine*, AsH$_3$. This gas is an essential reagent in certain industrial processes, in which context its capacity for harm is well respected. More disconcertingly it can be evolved unsuspectingly when metal, or dross, harbouring arsenical residues, reacts with nascent hydrogen that may be liberated simply by wetting or acidifying. Despite what should be a warning alliacious odour with this gas, a low though dangerous ambient level may prevail without being noticed. Those breathing such an atmosphere absorb the arsine via the lungs, when its major effect is to produce haemolysis. The patient shivers, feels pain especially in the loins, and finds that his urine is deeply coloured. Toxic haemolytic anaemia is the escort to renal damage. The liver and spleen may become palpable, the skin and sclerae take on a yellow metallic hue, mild organic dementia may be noticed, and the blood picture reveals peculiar changes in the erythrocytes.

Apart from terminating any further exposure, treatment converges upon preventing kidney damage and turning to haemodialysis, if this ensues, coupled with exchange blood transfusion, and dimercaprol.

Chronic exposure to arsenic over a period of years may predispose to cancer, principally of the skin but also involving other body organs.

Strychnine. This alkaloid, which is extracted from the *Strychnos nux-vomica* plant, was at one time prescribed liberally as a 'tonic'. It is still the only dependable agent for destroying moles in agriculture. Recently, too, it has been exploited deviantly by the 'drug culture', being 'shot' intravenously.

Its action centres on the central nervous system, where it indiscriminately facilitates transmission through the synapses, in consequence of which it heightens awareness, intensifies the visual impressions, and, more devastatingly, sets up fierce convulsions of the spinal type, mimicking tetanus with the 'risus sardonicus', all without any clouding of consciousness.

The patient should be nursed quietly in a darkened room with all external stimuli reduced to a minimum. The convulsions may be abated by giving diazepam, but often the only satisfactory course is to induce a state of neuromuscular blockade ('curarization') at the same time as the respiration is maintained mechanically.

Since the drug is fairly rapidly metabolized, this regimen seldom has to be prolonged for more than a few hours.

Nicotine. The nicotine response from smoking seldom attains a degree that demands treatment, for abstention is usually sufficient. Moreover, the uptake from chewing tobacco, or from children eating cigarettes, generally falls short of toxic amounts. Yet nicotine itself is still manufactured from tobacco leaves, in which industry the workers are said to develop a tolerance to its effects, as with habitual smokers.

The pure substance finds a limited use in agriculture, chiefly as an insecticide and, as such, it is extremely toxic, for about 50 mg constitutes a lethal dose. First it stimulates and then paralyses the ganglionic synapses throughout the autonomic nervous system. Mild poisoning is illustrated by nausea, giddiness, headache, salivation, vomiting, and weakness, going on to excessive sweating, tachycardia, abdominal pain, irregular respiration, and hypotensive collapse.

Whenever nicotine has been taken by mouth, the stomach should be emptied and activated charcoal given orally as an adsorbent. Otherwise there is no treatment apart from intensive and symptomatic support.

Phosphorus. The red, granular form of phosphorus is relatively safe, but the waxy material known as yellow phosphorus, used in the manufacture of fireworks, etc., and, rarely now, as a rodenticide, is extremely toxic. Small doses can bring about nausea, vomiting, diarrhoea, hypotensive collapse, acidosis, and liver damage, with jaundice and acute hepatic failure.

If taken by mouth, gastric aspiration and lavage is advisable, intensive supportive therapy should be embarked upon, vitamin K

should be given, and liver and renal failure should be treated appropriately.

On the skin, yellow phosphorus can produce burning and the affected area should be washed, it is said, with 1 per cent copper sulphate and then dressed as for a thermal burn.

POISONING FROM ANALGESIC DRUGS

T. J. Meredith, J. A. Vale, and G. N. Volans

Salicylate

Despite the introduction of alternative 'mild' analgesic agents in recent years, aspirin (acetylsalicylic acid) is still used commonly and is found in most household medicine cabinets. It is not surprising, therefore, that aspirin poisoning is a common cause for admission to hospital. Although accidental consumption of aspirin by young children has been reduced in both the United Kingdom and the United States, probably as a result of new legal requirements for child resistant packaging, *iatrogenic* overdose in children is not uncommon. Moreover, aspirin remains the drug of choice for many adults who choose deliberately to poison themselves. Indeed, approximately 200 deaths occur each year in England and Wales from salicylate poisoning. Although ingestion of aspirin tablets represents the most frequent cause of salicylate poisoning, salicylic acid (a keratolytic agent), and methyl salicylate ('oil of wintergreen') are occasional causes of salicylate toxicity.

Mechanism of toxicity. In therapeutic doses, aspirin is absorbed rapidly from the stomach and small intestine but, in overdose, absorption may occur more slowly and blood levels of aspirin may continue to rise for up to 24 hours.

The frequency with which therapeutic overdosage occurs is because the most important biotransformation pathways, the formation of salicyluric acid and salicyl-phenolic glucuronide, are saturable. Furthermore, as metabolic pathways of elimination become saturated, renal excretion of salicylic acid becomes increasingly important and this pathway is extremely sensitive to changes in urinary pH.

From the clinical point of view, the most important pathophysiological consequences are acid–base disturbance and fluid and electrolyte imbalance (Fig. 1). In overdose, salicylates directly stimulate the respiratory centre and so cause a respiratory alkalosis. In an attempt by the body to compensate, bicarbonate is excreted in the urine and this is accompanied by sodium, potassium, and water: dehydration and hypokalaemia result. The loss of bicarbonate diminishes the buffering capacity of the body and allows a metabolic acidosis to develop more easily.

Metabolic acidosis develops not only because of the presence of salicylic acid itself, but because of interference with carbohydrate, lipid, protein and amino-acid metabolism by the salicylate ions. Inhibition of citric acid cycle enzymes causes an increase in circulating lactic and pyruvic acids. Salicylates stimulate fat metabolism and cause increased production of the ketone bodies, β-hydroxy butyric acid, acetoacetic acid, and acetone. Starvation and dehydration also contribute to the development of ketosis. Protein catabolism is accelerated, protein synthesis diminished, and aminotransferases (responsible for the interconversion of amino acids) inhibited. The result is increased circulating blood levels of amino acids together with aminoaciduria; this latter feature is further enhanced by inhibition of active tubular reabsorption of amino acids. The aminoaciduria increases the solute load on the kidneys and thereby increases water loss from the body.

Salicylates also uncouple oxidative phosphorylation, so that ATP-dependent reactions are inhibited and oxygen utilization and carbon dioxide production increased. Energy normally used for the conversion of inorganic phosphate to ATP is dissipated as heat. Hyperpyrexia and sweating result and further dehydration occurs.

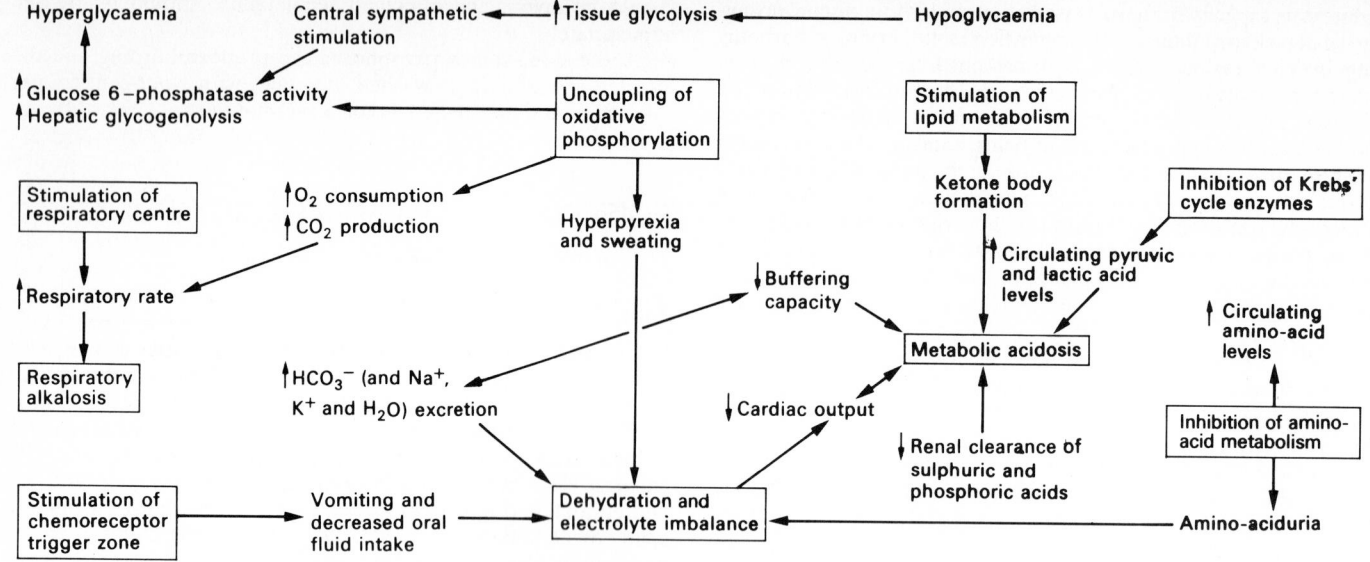

Fig. 1   The pathophysiology of salicylate toxicity.

Fluid loss is enhanced because salicylates stimulate the chemoreceptor trigger zone and induce nausea and vomiting and, thereby, diminished oral fluid intake. If dehydration is sufficiently severe, the low cardiac output and oliguria result in reduced clearance of sulphuric and phosphoric acids from the body; this aggravates the metabolic acidosis already present which, if severe, can itself diminish cardiac output.

Glucose metabolism also suffers as the result of uncoupled oxidative phosphorylation because of increased tissue glycolysis and peripheral demand for glucose. This is seen principally in skeletal muscle and may cause hypoglycaemia. However, CNS glucose depletion (neuroglycopenia) can occur in the presence of a normal blood sugar level. Increased metabolism and peripheral demand for glucose activates hypothalamic centres resulting in increased adrenocortical stimulation and release of adrenaline. Increased glucose 6-phosphatase activity and hepatic glycogenolysis contribute to the hypoglycaemia which is sometimes seen following the ingestion of large amounts of salicylate. Increased circulating adrenocorticosteroids further contribute to the electrolyte and fluid imbalance seen in salicylate overdose.

Clinical features (Table 1). The dose of salicylate ingested and the age of the patient are the principal determinants of the severity of an overdose, but prior therapeutic administration of aspirin will increase the toxicity of an acutely ingested overdose. The plasma

Table 1   Clinical features of salicylate poisoning

Nausea, vomiting, and epigastric discomfort
Hyperpyrexia and sweating
Irritability, tremor, tinnitus, and deafness
Tachypnoea, hyperpnoea, and pulmonary oedema
Dehydration, hypokalaemia, and hyper- or hyponatraemia
Respiratory alkalosis followed by metabolic acidosis
  (except in children)
Hyper- or hypoglycaemia and hypoprothrombinaemia

salicylate level should be determined six hours after ingestion of an overdose, but it is important to repeat it several hours later to make sure that the level is not continuing to rise because of slow absorption. Generally speaking, plasma salicylate levels that lie between 300 and 500 mg/l six hours after ingestion of an overdose are associated with only mild toxicity, levels between 500 and 750 mg/l are associated with moderate toxicity, and levels in excess of 750 mg/l confirm severe toxicity.

In the early stages of moderate to severe salicylate poisoning, hyperpyrexia and sweating, vomiting and epigastric pain, and tinnitus and deafness may all occur. Early loss of consciousness does not occur following the ingestion of a salicylate overdose, unless a hypnotic or sedative drug has been taken as well.

Young children quickly develop a metabolic acidosis following the ingestion of aspirin in overdose but, by the age of 12 years, the usual adult picture of a respiratory alkalosis followed by a metabolic acidosis is seen. Dehydration and electrolyte imbalance occur quickly due to the combination of factors outlined above.

To some extent, the presence of an early respiratory alkalotic phase affords protection against serious salicylate toxicity because, at an alkaline pH, salicylate molecules are ionized and unable to penetrate cell membranes easily. Development of a metabolic acidosis allows salicylate molecules to penetrate tissues more easily and leads, in particular, to CNS toxicity, which is associated with a poor prognosis.

The features of CNS toxicity seen in salicylate poisoning include tremor, hallucinations, delirium and, rarely, drowsiness and stupor. Coma is exceptionally rare in salicylate poisoning.

Pulmonary oedema is seen occasionally in salicylate poisoning, and although this is often due to fluid overload as a result of treatment, it can occur in the presence of hypovolaemia. In these circumstances, the pulmonary oedema fluid has the same protein and electrolyte composition as plasma, suggesting increased pulmonary vascular permeability. It is possible that an effect of aspirin on prostaglandin synthesis and platelet function is responsible for the increased microvascular leak of proteins and fluid.

Although aspirin overdose is associated with inhibition of platelet aggregation and hypoprothrombinaemia, gastric erosions and gastrointestinal bleeding appear to be uncommon following salicylate overdose. Oliguria is sometimes seen in patients following the ingestion of salicylates in overdose. The most common cause is dehydration but, rarely, acute renal failure or inappropriate secretion of antidiuretic hormone may occur.

The urinary pH is usually alkaline in the early stages of salicylate overdose and then subsequently becomes acid. Measurement of arterial blood gases, pH, and standard bicarbonate may show a respiratory alkalosis in the early stage of salicylate intoxication followed by the development of a metabolic acidosis. However, it is more usual to find a mixed acid–base disturbance. Hypokalaemia is usual, but the plasma sodium concentration may be either high or low depending upon the principal source of fluid loss and the type of replacement therapy given. The blood sugar may be high or low and the prothrombin time prolonged.

Treatment (Table 2). Gastric aspiration and lavage may prevent the absorption of significant amounts of salicylate up to 12 and possible 24 hours after ingestion. Insoluble preparations of aspirin may form a large mass in the stomach and can remain there despite vigorous gastric lavage. Young children, who have ingested aspirin tablets accidentally, may be given ipecacuanha paediatric emetic draught BPC, 10–15 ml, rather than being subjected to gastric lavage. Fluid and electrolyte replacement is particularly important and special attention should be paid to potassium supplementation. Sedatives and respiratory depressant drugs should be avoided because they may hasten the development of metabolic acidosis and CNS toxicity.

Table 2   Treatment of salicylate poisoning

Gastric aspiration and lavage or, in a child, ipecacuanha paediatric
    emetic draught BPC, 10–15 ml
Correction of dehydration either orally or parenterally
Correction of hypokalaemia
Correction of severe metabolic acidosis with cautious administration of
    intravenous bicarbonate
Tepid sponging for hyperpyrexia
Intravenous vitamin K for hypoprothrombinaemia
Forced alkaline diuresis if blood salicylate level > 750 mg/l
    and marked clinical features or acidosis present
Consider haemoperfusion of haemodialysis if blood salicylate level
    > 1000 mg/l

Pulmonary oedema occasionally complicates salicylate toxicity. Fluid overload should be excluded so far as possible but, if increased pulmonary vascular permeability is suspected, measurement of the pulmonary artery wedge pressure may be needed both for confirmation of the diagnosis and to monitor subsequent fluid administration. Positive-end-expiratory-pressure ventilation appears to be beneficial in this form of pulmonary oedema.

Mild cases of salicylate poisoning may be managed with either oral or parenteral fluid and electrolyte replacement only. Patients who exhibit marked symptoms or signs of salicylism and whose blood salicylate levels are in excess of 750 mg/l (or lower if acidosis is present) should receive specific elimination therapy. A forced alkaline diuresis is most often used for this purpose (see page 6.8). Although the volume of the diuresis achieved is important, the pH of the urine is of far greater significance. The urinary pH should be in excess of 7.5 and should ideally lie between 8.0 and 8.5. If it proves difficult to achieve this degree of urinary alkalinization without causing the blood pH to rise above 7.6, then any potassium deficit should be fully corrected. Very rarely, severely poisoned patients prove refractory to forced alkaline diuresis despite full potassium supplementation. Haemodialysis or haemoperfusion may then prove necessary to remove salicylate from the body (see page 6.9).

References

Levy, G. (1981). Comparative pharmacokinetics of aspirin and acetaminophen. *Archs intern. Med.* **141**, 279.
Meredith, T. J. and Vale, J. A. (1981). Salicylate poisoning. In *Poisoning: diagnosis and treatment* (eds. J. A. Vale and T. J. Meredith). Update Books, London; MTP Press, Lancaster.
Temple, A. R. (1981). Acute and chronic effects of aspirin toxicity and their treatment. *Archs intern. Med.* **141**, 364.

Paracetamol (acetaminophen)

Paracetamol has a justified reputation as an effective analgesic which, in therapeutic doses, is thought to be safer than aspirin. Although it was first synthesized at the end of the 19th century, it has been actively marketed in the United Kingdom only since 1956, although in the United States it has been available since 1952. The major advantage of paracetamol over aspirin lies in its lack of gastrointestinal side-effects; other known adverse effects,

thrombocytopenia, haemolytic anaemia, and skin rashes are extremely rare. In overdosage, paracetamol causes liver necrosis and may lead to death from fulminant hepatic failure.

Mechanism of toxicity. The toxicity of paracetamol is related to its metabolism (Fig. 2). In therapeutic doses, 60–90 per cent is metabolized by conjugation to form paracetamol glucuronide and sulphate. A much smaller amount (5–10 per cent) is oxidized by the mixed function oxidase enzymes to form a highly reactive compound which is then immediately conjugated with glutathione and subsequently excreted as cysteine or mercapturate conjugates. Only 1–4 per cent of the drug is excreted unchanged in the urine. In overdose, larger amounts of paracetamol are metabolized by oxidation because of saturation of the glucuronide and sulphate conjugation pathways. As a result, liver glutathione stores become overwhelmed so that the liver is unable to 'deactivate' the toxic metabolite. The reactive metabolite has a high affinity for cell protein and binds to liver cell macromolecules to cause hepatic necrosis. The activity of the mixed function oxidase enzyme system and the capacity of the liver glutathione stores may be modified both experimentally and clinically by pharmacological means (Fig. 2).

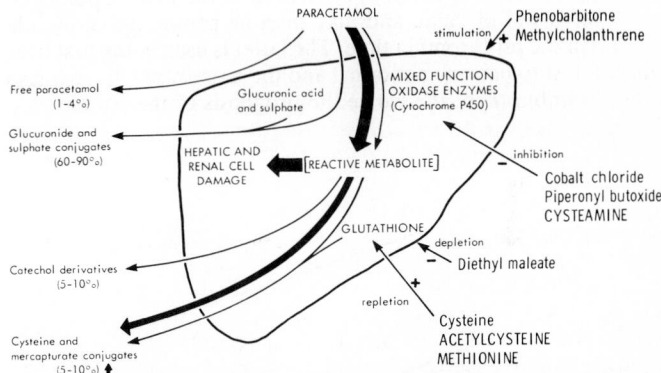

Fig. 2   The metabolism and mechanism of hepatotoxicity of paracetamol.

Clinical features. As would be expected from the mechanism of toxicity, the severity of paracetamol poisoning is dose-related, with a dose of 15 g or more being potentially serious in most patients. There is, however, some variation in individual susceptibility to paracetamol-induced hepatotoxicity and patients with pre-existing liver disease and those with a high alcohol intake in particular should be considered to be at greater risk.

Following the ingestion of a paracetamol overdose, patients usually remain asymptomatic for the first 24 hours or, at the most, develop anorexia, nausea, or vomiting. Liver damage is usually not detectable by routine laboratory liver function tests until at least 18 hours after ingestion of the drug, and hepatic tenderness and abdominal pain are seldom exhibited before the second day. Hepatic failure, manifested by jaundice and encephalopathy, may then develop between the second and seventh day with the rate of clinical deterioration giving an indication of the severity of the overdose. Renal failure due to acute tubular necrosis may be seen in a small percentage of patients and this is thought to be related to the metabolism of paracetamol by mixed function oxidase enzymes in the kidney parenchyma (Fig. 2). Other features of paracetamol toxicity may include hypoglycaemia, metabolic acidosis and cardiac arrhythmias, but all may occur with other causes of liver failure and are probably best regarded as a part of this problem.

Prediction of liver damage. In the early stages following ingestion of a paracetamol overdose, most patients have few symptoms and no physical signs. There is thus a need for some form of assessment which estimates the risk of liver damage at a time when the liver function tests are still normal. Details of the dose ingested may be used but, in many cases, the history is unreliable and even when the dose is known for certain, it does not take account of individual variation in response to the drug. Since the mechanism of toxicity is related to paracetamol metabolism, some measure of the rate of metabolism is likely to be of more value.

The plasma half-life of unchanged paracetamol provides such a measure since prolongation can be demonstrated in those patients who later develop liver damage. This is due to saturation of the glucuronide and sulphate conjugation pathways rather than early liver damage *per se*. Unfortunately, calculation of the half-life requires two measurements of the plasma paracetamol concentration separated by at least four hours and by the time that the second result is available, it may have delayed treatment by an unwarranted period.

It has now been shown that a single measurement of the plasma paracetamol concentration is an accurate predictor of liver damage provided that it is taken not earlier than four hours and not later than 12 hours after ingestion of the overdose. The information gained from several large studies has enabled the production of a graph which may be used for prediction of liver damage and thus serves as a guide to the need for treatment (Fig. 3). A paracetamol assay is now established in most hospital laboratories and, in addition, a kit is available for bedside use. When more than 12 hours have elapsed after ingestion of an overdose, the plasma paracetamol level is still of value and may then be considered alongside changes in the prothrombin time. The latter is usually the first liver function test to become abnormal and the more rapid the increase in prothrombin time, the worse the prognosis of the patient.

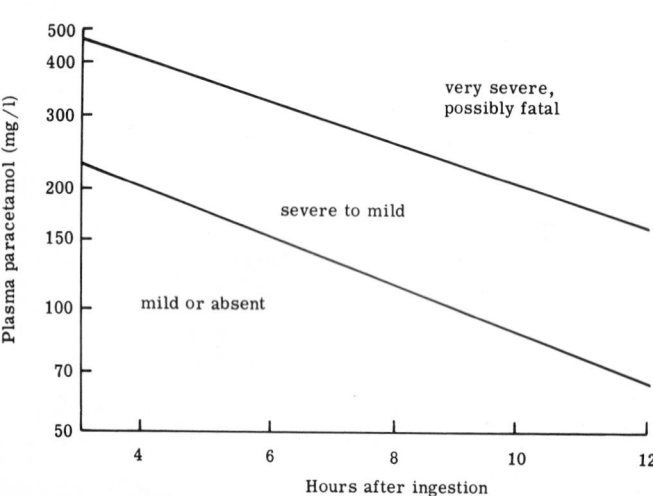

Fig. 3 Graph for use in prediction of liver damage caused by paracetamol.

Treatment (Table 3). Gastric lavage or syrup of ipecacuanha should be used if the patient presents within six hours of ingestion, since good recovery of paracetamol and improved prognosis has been demonstrated up to that time. From knowledge of the mechanism of toxicity, it may be predicted that replenishment of glutathione stores or inhibition of hepatic oxidation would be of value. Both approaches, using several different compounds, have now been tested as antidotes (Fig. 2). Two substances, methionine and N-acetylcysteine, have emerged as safe and effective protective agents, provided that they are administered within 12 hours of ingestion of the overdose. Both act as glutathione precursors and, in addition, N-acetylcysteine may act as a source of inorganic sulphate for simple conjugation. Both agents may be given orally, or parenterally, although methionine appears less effective when given intravenously than when administered orally, whilst *oral* N-acetylcysteine induces vomiting in most patients. Thus, the ideal choice of treatment lies between oral methionine and intravenous N-acetylcysteine and this choice should be dictated by clinical considerations. (In the USA in 1981 only oral N-acetylcysteine is available for use as an antidote in the treatment of paracetamol poisoning.) If the patient vomits intractably, or presents in coma,

Table 3   Treatment of paracetamol poisoning

1 The prevention of gastrointestinal absorption
   Gastric lavage or 'syrup of ipecacuanha' (ipecacuanha paediatric emetic draught BPC). 10–15 ml in children (15–30 ml in adults)
2 'Antidotes'
   Methionine orally 2.5 g stat., then 2.5 g 4-hourly for a further three doses. Total dose 10 g methionine over 12 hours
   N-Acetylcysteine intravenously (i.v.) 150 mg/kg i.v. over 15 minutes, then 50 mg/kg in 500 ml of 5% dextrose i.v. in the next 4 hours and 100 mg/kg in 1000 ml of 5% dextrose i.v. over the ensuing 16 hours. Total dose 300 mg/kg over 20 hours
   N-Acetylcysteine orally 140 mg/kg stat., then 70 mg/kg orally every 4 hours for 17 additional doses
3 Supportive measures
   5% dextrose solution to correct dehydration
   Correction of electrolyte imbalance
   Vitamin K 10 mg intravenously for 3 days if the prothrombin time is prolonged
4 Treatment of hepatic failure

then the intravenous antidote is indicated. Otherwise, oral methionine, which is both cheaper and easier to administer, should be given. In practice, both antidotes are safe and if treatment is started within eight hours of ingestion of the paracetamol it is usually fully effective. Between eight and 16 hours after ingestion of the overdose, the efficiency of the antidotes falls off rapidly, but it appears that there is still advantage to be gained provided that there is no evidence of liver damage. Fortunately, relatively few patients first present more than 16 hours after ingesting a serious overdose of paracetamol but, in these circumstances, the correct treatment is that intended to prevent or support hepatic failure (see Section 12).

References

Gillette, J. R. (1981). An integrated approach to the study of chemically reactive metabolites of acetaminophen. *Archs intern. Med.* **141**, 375.

Meredith, T. J. and Goulding, R. (1980). Paracetamol. *Post-grad. med. J.* **56**, 459.

Prescott, L. F. (1981). Treatment of severe acetaminophen poisoning with intravenous acetylcysteine. *Archs intern. Med.* **141**, 386.

Rumack, B. H., Peterson, R. C., Koch, G. G., and Amara, I. A. (1981). Acetaminophen overdose. *Archs intern. Med.* **141**, 380.

Vale, J. A., Meredith, T. J., and Goulding, R. (1981). Treatment of acetaminophen poisoning. *Archs intern. Med.* **141**, 394.

Non-steroidal anti-inflammatory (NSAI) drugs

NSAI agents other than aspirin and paracetamol are seldom taken in overdose. NSAI agents may be divided into four main groups—anthranilic acid derivatives (fenamates, flufenamic and mefenamic acids), phenylacetic (arylacetic) acid derivatives (diclofenac, fenclofenac), propionic acid derivatives (e.g. fenbrufen, fenoprofen, flurbiprofen, ibuprofen, ketoprofen, and naproxen), and pyrazole derivatives (azapropazone, feprazone, oxyphenbutazone, and phenylbutazone). Diflunisal, indomethacin, and sulindac are further NSAI agents which do not fall into these categories.

Clinical features. Anthranilic acid derivative (fenamate) poisoning is associated with nausea, vomiting and, occasionally, bloody diarrhoea. Drowsiness, dizziness, and headaches are common and hyper-reflexia, muscle twitching, and convulsions have been reported.

Phenylacetic (arylacetic) acid derivative poisoning is less serious and headache, dizziness, nausea, and abdominal discomfort are the most common clinical features. It is possible, though; that gastrointestinal bleeding may also occur.

Propionic acid derivative poisoning causes headache, tinnitus, ataxia, stupor, and, rarely, coma. Hypoventilation, bronchospasm, and hypotension occur, and, more importantly, gastrointestinal haemorrhage is a rare but reported complication.

Pyrazole derivative poisoning is more serious. Nausea, vomiting, abdominal pain, haematemesis, and diarrhoea are typical features. Hyperventilation, dizziness, coma, and convulsions occur, and, more recently, hepatic and renal damage have been reported. Further possible complications are sodium and water retention and bone marrow depression.

The ingestion of *diflunisal*, *indomethacin*, and *sulindac* in overdose is associated with nausea, vomiting, abdominal pain, headaches, drowsiness, and dizziness; indomethacin and sulindac may induce gastrointestinal bleeding, and coma has been reported following the ingestion of large doses of diflunisal and sulindac.

Treatment. In all cases of NSAI drug poisoning treatment should include either emesis or gastric lavage, if appropriate, followed by supportive measures. Activated charcoal is known to adsorb propionic acid derivatives and may reasonably be left in the stomach after gastric lavage in other forms of NSAI drug poisoning. Diazepam, 5–10 mg intravenously, should be given for convulsions and cimetidine, 200 mg four to six hourly intravenously, is often administered prophylactically, though there is no definite evidence that its use prevents the development of gastrointestinal bleeding in cases of NSAI drug poisoning.

References

Balali-Mood, M., Critchley, J. A. J. H., Proudfoot, A.T, and Prescott, L. F. (1981). Mefenamic acid overdosage. *Lancet* i, 1354.
National Poisons Information Service Monitoring Group (1981). Analgesic poisoning: a multi-centre, prospective survey. *Human Toxicol.* **1**, 7–23.

Opiates and opiate derivatives

Acute opiate overdose occurs typically in 'addicts', in whom the presence of infected venepuncture marks and thrombosed veins in the arms and legs is characteristic. The opiate group of drugs is large and includes apomorphine, buprenorphine, codeine, dihydrocodeine, dextromoramide, dextropropoxyphene, diamorphine (heroin), dipipanone, diphenoxylate, methadone, morphine, pentazocine, and pethidine.

Clinical features. The cardinal signs of opiate overdose are pinpoint pupils, respiratory depression (often accompanied by cyanosis), and coma. The depressant effects of opiates are exacerbated by the concomitant ingestion of alcohol and, for example, the ingestion of *dextropropoxyphene* in overdose together with alcohol may be followed by sudden, severe respiratory depression. Hypotension is uncommon in opiate overdose and occurs in less than 10 per cent of cases, and it is then due to peripheral vasodilatation. Paradoxically, hypertension may accompany *pentazocine* overdose.

Heroin (diamorphine) is the opiate most frequently abused. It is self-administered by either intravenous injection (main-lining) or inhalation (snorting). The usual features of opiate overdose may sometimes be accompanied by hypothermia and hypoglycaemia. As many as 50 per cent of heroin overdose victims develop non-cardiogenic pulmonary oedema, the majority of whom, in turn, develop bacterial pneumonia. The prognosis is particularly poor in this group of patients. Other opiates associated with the occurrence of non-cardiogenic pulmonary oedema when taken in overdose are *codeine*, *dextropropoxyphene*, and *methadone*.

Although skeletal muscles are usually flaccid in opiate overdose, *apomorphine*, *codeine*, *dextropropoxyphene*, and *pethidine* cause increased muscle tone, twitching, and convulsions.

Diphenoxylate poisoning may also be associated with convulsions, but tendon reflexes in these circumstances are usually diminished and are sometimes absent. Diphenoxylate is used as an antidiarrhoeal agent in conjunction with atropine and paediatric poisoning due to the ingestion of this antidiarrhoeal preparation is not uncommon. The combination of diphenoxylate and atropine causes marked reduction of gastric emptying and intestinal motility. Symptoms may be delayed for up to 12 hours following ingestion of an overdose and it is wise to continue observation for 48 hours. Relapses occur commonly during the course of recovery. The major complication of diphenoxylate poisoning is respiratory depression and a gradual reduction in respiratory rate is typically followed by total apnoea. Vomiting, abdominal pain, drowsiness, and coma also occur. The small amount of atropine contained in these proprietary antidiarrhoeal agents is often toxic to children, who exhibit variable sensitivity to the drug. Tachycardia, anxiety, restlessness, and flushing may be seen but the pupils are more often constricted (due to diphenoxylate) than dilated.

Treatment. The treatment of choice in opiate overdose is naloxone, a pure narcotic antagonist with no intrinsic agonist activity (unlike nalorphine). Nevertheless, gastric aspiration and lavage are of value if an opiate has been *ingested* in overdose and the patient remains conscious (opiates delay gastric emptying and increase antral tone).

Naloxone is used to reverse severe respiratory depression and coma due to opiate poisoning—the adult dose is 0.4–0.8 mg, given either intravenously or intramuscularly; the dose in children is 5–10 μg/kg body weight. If the diagnosis of opiate poisoning is correct, the patient should improve within minutes with an increase in respiratory rate, an improvement in the level of consciousness and dilatation of the pupils. In severe opiate poisoning, larger initial doses of naloxone may be required to obtain the desired response. The duration of action of naloxone (one to four hours) is often less than that of the drug taken in overdose and, for this reason, careful observation of the patient is necessary. Repeated doses of naloxone may be given as required. *Buprenorphine*, a narcotic antagonist analgesic similar to pentazocine, is unusual in that the analgesic and respiratory depressant effects of the drug are only partially reversed by naloxone. Although doxapram may be used to stimulate respiration, assisted ventilation may be required in cases of severe buprenorphine poisoning.

In opiate dependent subjects, even small doses of naloxone will precipitate a withdrawal syndrome similar to that seen after the abrupt withdrawal of opiates (except that it occurs within minutes of administration of the naloxone). The severity and duration of the syndrome are related to the dose of the antagonist and the degree of dependence but it usually subsides within two hours.

References

Curtis, J. A. and Goel, K. M. (1979). Lomotil poisoning in children. *Archs Dis. Childn.* **54**, 222.
Duberstein, J. L. and Kaufman, D. M. (1971). A clinical study of an epidemic of heroin intoxication and heroin induced pulmonary edema. *Am. J. Med.* **51**, 704.
Schaaf, J. T., Spivak, M. L., Rath, G. S., and Snider, G. L. (1973). Pulmonary edema and adult respiratory distress syndrome following methadone abuse. *Am. Rev. resp. Dis.* **107**, 1047.

POISONING FROM SEDATIVES, HYPNOTICS, AND ANTICONVULSANTS

T. J. Meredith and J. A. Vale

The mortality in England and Wales from barbiturate and non-barbiturate hypnotic drug poisoning has fallen in recent years. At the same time, as the result of changes in prescribing habit, deaths due to other sedative, tranquillizing, and anticonvulsant agents have risen. Even so, barbiturates either alone or in combination with other drugs are associated with approximately 20 per cent of the deaths due to drug poisoning which occur each year in England and Wales (1979).

Barbiturates

A large number of barbiturates remain available on prescription and these include amylobarbitone, barbitone, butobarbitone, cyclobarbitone, heptabarbitone, hexabarbitone, pentobarbitone, phenobarbitone, and quinalbarbitone. They are sometimes combined in proprietary hypnotic preparations, for example amylobarbitone and quinalbarbitone. The conventional classification of barbiturates into those which are short, medium, and long acting has little merit so far as the treatment of overdose is concerned, except that the more lipid-soluble, shorter-acting preparations are commonly associated with more serious poisoning than longer-acting preparations.

Clinical features. Impairment of the level of consciousness, respiratory depression, hypotension, and hypothermia are typical of barbiturate poisoning. In common with all forms of hypnotic overdose, the depressant effects are exacerbated by the presence of alcohol. Hypotension is due not only to peripheral venous pooling but also to direct myocarcial depression. In very severely poisoned patients, there may, in addition, be an element of central medullary depression. Although the overall mortality of barbiturate poisoning is approximately 3–6 per cent, the mortality of patients admitted in grade IV coma may be as high as 32 per cent. The majority of these deaths are due to respiratory complications and, in particular, to the adult respiratory distress syndrome ('shock-lung').

Bowel sounds are often absent in barbiturate poisoning and, when they return during the course of recovery, a relapse in the clinical condition of the patient may occur as further drug is absorbed. Renal failure is now a less common accompaniment to barbiturate overdose than it once was as a result of modern management of hypotension and shock. There are no specific neurological features of barbiturate overdose, and the behaviour of the pupils, tendon reflexes, and plantar responses are variable. Although fixed, dilated pupils may be found in severe barbiturate poisoning, the possibility of cerebral anoxic damage should also be considered.

Hypothermia and poor perfusion of skeletal muscle account for the elevated plasma creatine phosphokinase levels seen during recovery. For the same reason, it is common to observe a peak of temperature during recovery in response to muscle necrosis. Bullous lesions of the skin occur in approximately 6 per cent of cases of barbiturate poisoning, although they may also be found in other forms of drug overdose. Bullae are most often found between the fingers, the knees, and the ankles.

Treatment. Gastric aspiration and lavage and intensive supportive therapy should be administered as appropriate. Forced alkaline diuresis (see page 6.8) is effective only in case of barbitone and phenobarbitone poisoning. It has no place in other forms of barbiturate intoxication and, for this reason, it is important to use specific analytical techniques for the detection and measurement of barbiturates in the blood. Haemoperfusion should be considered in severely poisoned patients.

Non-barbiturate hypnotics

Chlormethiazole. Coma, respiratory depression, reduced muscle tone, hypotension, and hypothermia may all occur as a result of chlormethiazole overdose. Excessive salivation is sometimes a prominent feature and the characteristic odour of chlormethiazole is often detected on the breath and in gastric lavage fluid. Treatment is supportive with pharyngeal suction and assisted ventilation as necessary.

Ethchlorvynol. Ethchlorvynol has a pungent odour often detectable on the breath and in gastric lavage fluid. The clinical features resemble those of overdosage with other hypnotic drugs, but coma is often prolonged and respiratory depression may be severe. Bradycardia, hypotension, and hypothermia are common, and non-cardiogenic pulmonary oedema has been reported. Treatment is supportive but haemoperfusion is of value in very severe poisoning.

Glutethimide. A prominent feature of glutethimide poisoning,

which otherwise closely resembles barbiturate intoxication, is a characteristic fluctuation in the level of consciousness. This may be due to formation of the active metabolite, 4-hydroxy-glutethimide, but alternative explanations include further absorption of drug from the intestine after recovery from an ileus, enterohepatic circulation of glutethimide and its metabolites, and release of the drug from lipid stores during the course of recovery.

The pupils are often dilated and unreactive to light in glutethimide poisoning as a result of the anticholinergic activity of this drug. Papilloedema, cerebral oedema and sudden apnoea may also occur. Treatment is essentially supportive, but intravenous dexamethasone or mannitol should be given for cerebral oedema and haemoperfusion considered in seriously poisoned patients.

Methaqualone. Methaqualone has been used as a hypnotic and sedative drug both alone and in combination with diphenhydramine. Pyramidal signs are a prominent feature of methaqualone overdose. Depression of the level of consciousness is accompanied by hypertonia, increased tendon reflexes, and extensor plantar responses. Papilloedema and convulsions also occur, tachycardia is common, and acute pulmonary oedema has been reported. Treatment is supportive, but haemoperfusion is effective in severely poisoned patients.

Trichloroethanol derivatives. Chloral hydrate, dichloralphenazone and triclofos are converted by the liver enzyme alcohol dehydrogenase, to the active metabolite, trichloroethanol, which, in turn, is further metabolized to the inactive substances, trichloroacetic acid and trichloroethanol glucuronide. The clinical features of acute overdosage with chloral hydrate and its derivatives are similar to those of barbiturate poisoning, although patients may, at an early stage, complain of a retrosternal burning sensation accompanied by vomiting. Cardiac arrhythmias have been described following chloral hydrate overdose, but it is important to exclude respiratory depression and hypoxia as the underlying cause. Treatment should consist of gastric aspiration and lavage, where appropriate, together with intensive supportive therapy. Haemoperfusion should be considered in severely poisoned patients.

Sedatives and tranquillizers

Antihistamines. Antihistamines are employed in the treatment of anaphylaxis, allergy, and motion sickness as well as being used as sedatives. Many antihistamines possess anticholinergic activity and some act as local anaesthetics. An ethylamine moiety is common to all antihistamines but, otherwise, their chemical structure is likely to differ: antihistamines may be derived from an alkylamine, ethanolamine, ethylenediamine, a piperazine, or a phenothiazine moiety. It is not surprising, therefore, that several hundred preparations of antihistamines are available but those encountered most commonly are antazoline, brompheniramine, buclizine, carbinoxamine, chlorpheniramine, cinnazarine, clemastine, cyclizine, cyproheptadine, diphenhydramine, diphenylpyraline, embramine, meclozine, mepyramine, methapyrilene, orphenadrine, pheniramine, pyrrobutamine, tripelennamine, and triprolidine.

The anticholinergic properties of antihistamines are most prominent in cases of mild poisoning with dryness of the mouth, headache, nausea, tachycardia, and urinary retention being evident. The central effects of antihistamines become important in serious overdosage and they may either stimulate or depress the nervous system. In small children the dominant effect is that of excitation: hallucinations, excitement, ataxia, inco-ordination, athetosis, and convulsions may all be seen. Fixed dilated pupils, a flushed face, and hyperthermia are common and produce a syndrome similar to that induced by atropine poisoning. Subsequently, coma and cardiorespiratory depression may develop, and death can occur within two to 18 hours after ingestion of the overdose. Fever and flushing are uncommon in the adult and a phase of excitement leading to convulsions is often preceded by a period of drowsiness and coma.

Treatment should consist of gastric aspiration and lavage and supportive measures as appropriate. Diazepam may be required for the treatment of convulsions.

Benzodiazepines. The benzodiazepines are used widely as mild tranquillizers and sedatives. Compounds encountered in clinical practice include bromazepam, chlordiazepoxide, clonazepam, desmethyldiazepam, diazepam, flunitrazepam, flurazepam, lorazepam, medazepam, nitrazepam, prazepam, and temazepam. Many have active metabolites which account for their sometimes prolonged sedative effect.

The consequences of benzodiazepine overdose are usually mild, but it now cannot be said that overdosage with these drugs is never without harm. Dizziness, ataxia, and slurred speech are common. Coma, respiratory depression, and hypotension are usually mild, but may be more prominent when alcohol has also been taken.

Gastric aspiration and lavage together with supportive therapy are the only necessary measures to be taken.

Butyrophenones. The butyrophenones (benperidol, haloperidol, and triperidol) are used as antipsychotic and neuroleptic agents. Overdosage may result in drowsiness and hypotension, but extrapyramidal effects are common and include akathisia and tardive dyskinesia. Treatment is supportive but benztropine (2 mg intravenously or intramuscularly) may be used to control extrapyramidal features.

Meprobamate. Meprobamate and other carbamates are still used as sedative and tranquillizing agents. Coma, respiratory depression, and hypotension are the usual features of overdosage. Hypotension may be marked and pulmonary oedema has been reported in some patients. Gastric aspiration and lavage should be performed where appropriate. Treatment is otherwise supportive, although haemoperfusion may be necessary in very severely poisoned patients.

Phenothiazines. The phenothiazines are used principally as antiemetic and antipsychotic drugs. Members of this group include chlorpromazine, perphenazine, prochlorperazine, promethazine, promazine, stelazine, thioridazine and trimeprazine. Phenothiazines have complex pharmacological actions—they block peripheral cholinergic and α-adrenergic receptors, re-uptake of amines and the effects of histamine and 5-hydroxytryptamine.

The clinical features of phenothiazine overdosage include impairment of the level of consciousness, extrapyramidal signs (rigidity, tremor, hyperreflexia and dyskinesia), marked restlessness, and convulsions. Hypotension is common, but respiratory depression is seen only in severe poisoning. Tachycardia, ECG changes (prolongation of Q–T interval and T wave abnormalities) and arrhythmias may also occur. Hypothermia may be present and can be profound.

Treatment is supportive and gastric aspiration and lavage should be performed where appropriate. Benztropine (2 mg intravenously or intramuscularly) may be necessary to control the extrapyramidal features and diazepam should be given for convulsions.

Anticonvulsants

Carbamazepine. Carbamazepine possesses anticholinergic activity, being structurally related to the tricyclic antidepressants. For this reason, overdosage may result in drowsiness, a dry mouth, coma, and convulsions. Relapse into coma has been described during the course of recovery. Treatment should include gastric lavage, if appropriate, and supportive therapy. Diazepam may be required to treat convulsions.

Ethosuximide and methsuximide. The ingestion of either agent may cause anorexia, nausea, vomiting, drowsiness, dizziness, ataxia, and coma. Treatment is supportive and gastric lavage should be performed if appropriate.

Paraldehyde. Paraldehyde is now only rarely used as either a hypnotic or an anticonvulsant agent. It causes marked gastrointestinal irritation with nausea and vomiting when ingested by mouth, and it imparts a characteristic odour to the breath. Coma, respiratory and circulatory failure, and metabolic acidosis may occur in overdose. Hepatic and renal damage have also been reported. Treatment is supportive and gastric lavage should be performed if appropriate.

Phenytoin and hydantoin derivatives. Acute overdosage of phenytoin results in nausea, vomiting, headache, tremor, loss of consciousness, cerebellar ataxia, and nystagmus. Respiratory depression may also occur. Treatment should include gastric aspiration and lavage, where appropriate, together with supportive therapy.

Primidone. Primidone is converted to the two active metabolites, phenobarbitone and phenylethyl malonamide. The clinical features and management of primidone poisoning are as for barbiturate poisoning.

Sodium valproate. The ingestion of sodium valproate in overdose causes impairment of the level of consciousness together with respiratory depression. Gastric lavage is of limited value because of the rapid absorption of the drug. Treatment is symptomatic and supportive.

Sulthiame. Sulthiame is a sulphonamide derivative and possesses weak carbonic anhydase inhibitory activity. Overdose results in headache, vomiting, ataxia, vertigo, and hyperventilation. Hyperreflexia, clouding of consciousness, and catatonia may also develop, and renal tubular obstruction due to crystalluria (in acid urine) has been reported. Treatment is supportive but the urine should be kept alkaline to avoid renal impairment.

References

Allen, M. D., Greenblatt, D. J., and Noel, B. .J. (1977). Meprobamate overdosage: a continuing problem. *Clin. Toxicol.* **11**, 501.

Angle, C. R., McIntire, M. S., Zetterman, R. (1968). CNS symptoms in childhood poisoning *Clin. Toxicol.* **1**, 19.

Arieff, A. I. and Friedman, E. A. (1973). Coma following non-narcotic drug overdosage: management of 208 adult patients. *Am. J. med. Sci.* **266**, 405.

Benowitz, N., Abolin, C., Tozer, T., Rosenberg, J., Rogers, W., Pond, S., Schoenfeld, P., and Humphreys, M. (1980). Resin hemoperfusion in ethchlorvynol overdose. *Clin. Pharmac. Ther.* **27**, 236.

Bruce, A. M. and Smith, H. (1977). The investigation of phenobarbitone, phenytoin and primidone in the death of epileptics. *Med. Sci. Law* **17**, 195.

Davis, J. M., Bartlett, E., and Termini, B. A. (1968). Overdosage of psychotropic drugs: a review. *Dis. nerv. Syst.* **29**, 157.

De Zeeuw, R. A., Westenberg, H. G. M., Van der Kleijn, E., and Gimbrere, J. S. F. (1979). An unusual case of carbamazepine poisoning with a near-fatal relapse after two days. *Clin. Toxicol.* **14**, 263.

Gill, D. G. and Sowerby, H. A. (1975). Orphenadrine poisoning in childhood. *Practitioner* **214**, 542.

Greenblatt, D. J., Allen, M. D., Noel, B. J., and Shader, R. I. (1977). Acute overdosage with benzodiazepine derivatives. *Clin. Pharmac. Ther.* **21**, 497.

Hansen, A. R., Kennedy, K. A., Ambre, J. J., and Fischer, L. J. (1975). Glutethimide poisoning. A metabolite contributes to morbidity and mortality. *New Engl. J. Med.* **292**, 250.

Heinonen, J., Heikkila, J., Mattila, M. J., and Takki, S. (1968). Orphenadrine poisoning. *Archs Toxicol.* **23**, 264.

Illingworth, R. N., Stewart, M. J., and Jarvie, D. R. (1979). Severe poisoning with chlormethiazole. *Br. Med. J.* **ii**, 902.

Jay, S. J., Johanson, W. G., Jr, and Pierce, A. K. (1975). Respiratory complications of overdose with sedative drugs. *Am. Rev. resp. Dis.* **112**, 591.

Karch, S. B. (1973) Methsuximide overdose. *J. Am. med. Ass.* **223**, 1463.

Matthew, H. (1975). Barbiturates. *Clin. Toxicol.* **8**, 495.

McKown, C. H., Verhulst, H. L., and Crotty, J. J. (1963). Overdosage effects and danger from tranquilizing drugs. *J. Am. med. Ass.* **185**, 425.

Sangster, B., Van Heijst, A. N. P., Zimmerman, A. N. E., and De Vries, H. W. (1977). Intoxication by orphenadrine HCL; mechanism and therapy. *Acta pharmac. toxicol.*, suppl. 2, 129.

POISONING FROM ANTIDEPRESSANTS

J. A. Vale and T. J. Meredith

Over the last decade there has been a considerable increase in the mortality from antidepressant poisoning. In 1979, the last year for which statistics are available, 282 of the 3952 patients who died from acute poisoning in England and Wales had taken an antidepressant drug, either alone or in combination with other agents. There are two main reasons for this increase. Firstly, the number of prescriptions for antidepressant drugs has risen markedly over the last decade. In 1977, for example, nine-and-a-half million prescriptions for antidepressants were issued in England and Wales by general practitioners. As a result, these drugs became readily available to those attempting either suicide or a parasuicidal gesture. Secondly, antidepressant drugs are given to patients who are depressed and who are, therefore, intrinsically more likely to poison themselves.

Tricyclic antidepressants

Tricyclic antidepressants are believed to act in three main ways. Firstly, they block the re-uptake of noradrenaline and/or 5-hydroxytryptamine into intracerebral neurones thereby increasing the concentration of these monoamines in certain areas of the brain. Secondly, they block the parasympathetic nervous system, and, thirdly, they block the peripheral re-uptake of noradrenaline. In addition, tricyclic antidepressants have a complex action on the heart. These diverse pharmacological properties account for the variety of adverse affects that complicate the therapeutic use of tricyclic antidepressants and cause their toxicity when taken in overdose.

Clinical features. In patients who are only mildly poisoned, drowsiness, sinus tachycardia, dry mouth, dilated pupils, increased reflexes, and extensor plantar responses are the most common clinical features. The morbidity and mortality in those who are severely poisoned are due largely to the cardiorespiratory depressant action of these drugs which produces hypoxia and either respiratory or metabolic acidosis. Grade IV coma and convulsions may also complicate the clinical picture in severe poisoning.

Symptoms typically appear within 30 to 60 minutes after ingestion of an overdose, except when a slow-release preparation has been taken, and they usually reach maximum intensity in four to 12 hours. It is uncommon for coma to last for more than 24 hours and even severely poisoned patients should recover completely within 48 hours. Delirium may be a troublesome complication during the recovery phase.

In the past, cardiac side-effects of tricyclic antidepressants have been attributed to their anticholinergic activity, with potentiation of circulating noradrenaline and consequent cardiac arrhythmias. However, it has been shown recently that tricyclic antidepressants have a dose-related quinidine-like action on the heart, which results in decreased myocardial contractility and increased conduction time. This quinidine-like activity probably accounts for the bizarre ECG changes that may be seen in overdose. In very severely poisoned patients, the blood pressure and cardiac output may fall progressively. At the same time, the QRS complex becomes wider and P waves diminish in amplitude. This may make differentiation between sinus rhythm with prolonged intraventricular conduction and ventricular or supraventricular rhythms difficult, if not imposs-

ible. In common with hypnotic drugs taken in overdose, there may be either a relative or absolute hypovolaemia which contributes to the hypotension seen.

Treatment

Gastric aspiration and lavage. Gastric aspiration and lavage should be performed in all adults when more than 250 mg of the drug has been taken. In children, emesis should be induced with syrup of ipecacuanha (ipecacuanha paediatric emetic draught BPC, 10–15 ml, repeated once if necessary). Tricyclic antidepressants delay gastric emptying and large quantities of tablets may therefore remain in the stomach for a considerable time. For this reason, gastric lavage or emesis may be useful up to 12 hours after ingestion of an overdose.

Activated charcoal. Absorption of drug from the GI tract may be further reduced by the oral administration of activated charcoal. It can be given as a drink, provided the patient is still conscious, or left in the stomach after gastric lavage. The optimum charcoal: drug ratio is 10:1, and a dose of 10–20 g should be sufficient to adsorb most of the drug left in the gut even after a large tricyclic-antidepressant drug overdose. Activated charcoal may be given conveniently as two sachets of 'Medicoal' dispersed in 200–300 ml of water.

Cardiorespiratory support. When taken in overdose, tricyclic antidepressant drugs decrease myocardial contractility and increase conduction times. If there is evidence of poor tissue perfusion (cold extremities, poor urine output, and hypotension) after correction of hypovolaemia, acidosis, and hypoxia, then a positive inotropic drug, e.g. dobutamine 5–20 μg/kg/min intravenously, should be used.

A variety of arrhythmias may occur in those who are severely poisoned. Although there is a natural inclination to use an anti-arrhythmic drug to treat a tachycardia, it should be remembered that disopyramide, lignocaine, and beta-adrenergic blocking drugs have been shown to potentiate tricyclic-antidepressant induced cardiotoxicity in animals and in man. Moreover, tachycardias which occur in this type of poisoning do not appear to have the same prognostic significance as similar arrhythmias occurring after a myocardial infarction. In the majority of cases, therefore, anti-arrhythmic drugs are not only contra-indicated but are not required.

The role of sodium lactate and sodium bicarbonate in the correction of arrhythmias has not been established.

Patients poisoned with tricyclic antidepressants are as likely as those with barbiturate poisoning to become hypoxic. This may be due either to depression of ventilation, aspiration of stomach contents, or to the development of 'shock lung'. Supplemental oxygen and mechanical ventilation may be required.

Convulsions. Fits, especially if repeated, may not only cause cerebral anoxia but may also precipitate cardiac arrest. For this reason, prompt treatment is necessary with either diazepam, 5–10 mg intravenously (which may be repeated), or with an intravenous infusion of chlormethiazole. However, these drugs may further depress respiration. If drug therapy proves ineffective, and particularly if the patient has evidence of impaired cardiac function, mechanical ventilation and muscle paralysis should be instituted without delay. Ventilated patients should continue to receive anticonvulsants (e.g. phenytoin, chlormethiazole) and their progress should, if possible, be observed using a cerebral function monitor.

Physostigmine. The intravenous injection of physostigmine (1–4 mg) may lessen the depth of coma in those poisoned with tricyclic antidepressants. Unfortunately, this effect, if it is seen, is short-lived and the patient usually lapses into coma again after a few minutes. Furthermore, although physostigmine has been shown to have a positive inotropic action in animal experiments, this effect is also short-lived and, moreover, is unpredictable in man. Delirium, choreoathetosis, and tremor may sometimes be reversed by physostigmine, but because of its short duration of action these all recur.

The majority of clinical toxicologists believe that physostigmine has no place in the treatment of tricyclic antidepressant poisoning, not only because its action is transient, but because it may precipitate convulsions, bradycardia, and involuntary defaecation.

Active elimination techniques. As only a relatively small proportion of the body load of tricyclic antidepressants circulates in the vascular compartment, forced diuresis and haemodialysis are able to remove only small amounts of the drug from the body. More recently, haemoperfusion with XAD–4 resin has been claimed to be effective in reversing coma and cardiotoxicity. Although plasma clearance is high, only small amounts of drug are removed by this technique as would be expected from the large volume of distribution.

None of these active procedures mentioned above can be recommended.

Quadricyclic antidepressants

Maprotiline. Although maprotiline is related to the tricyclic antidepressants, the presence of a bridge across the central ring converts it into a three-dimensional tetracyclic structure. It therefore shows many of the pharmacological and toxicological properties of the tricyclic antidepressants and treatment should be according to the principles outlined above for this latter group of drugs.

Mianserin. Mianserin has a four-ringed structure and it is believed to act in depression by increasing noradrenaline turnover. Drowsiness is a common side-effect of overdose but convulsions, cardiotoxicity, and respiratory depression have not been reported, except when other drugs have been taken in addition. Treatment is symptomatic, but gastric lavage should be performed if a substantial overdose has been ingested.

Nomifensine. This drug blocks re-uptake of both noradrenaline and dopamine into intrecerebral neurones. Drowsiness, tremor, and sinus tachycardia are the most common features of overdose, anticholinergic effects, convulsions, and more serious cardiotoxicity have not been reported. Treatment is symptomatic.

Monoamine-oxidase inhibitors (MAOI)

These drugs are now used infrequently in the treatment of depression and overdoses from these agents are, correspondingly, very uncommon. Symptoms may be delayed for some hours after acute overdosage and are due principally to increased sympathetic activity: they include excitement, pyrexia, increased tendon reflexes, convulsions, coma, sinus tachycardia, and either hypo- or hypertension. Treatment of MAOI overdosage is essentially supportive. Hypotension should, in the first instance, be treated by fluid replacement to restore a normal circulating blood volume. If possible, sympathomimetic drugs should be avoided in the treatment of hypotension due to MAOI overdosage lest their pressor effect be potentiated. Hypertension should be treated by the administration of an alpha-blocker, such as phentolamine or phenoxybenzamine. Sedatives such as diazepam or chlormethiazole may be required for patients with marked excitement.

Lithium carbonate

The therapeutic range of lithium is small and toxicity may be either iatrogenic or the result of deliberate overdosage. Symptoms of overdosage include thirst, polyuria, diarrhoea, and vomiting, and, in more serious cases, there may be impairment of consciousness, hypertonicity, and convulsions. Measurement of the plasma lithium concentration will confirm the diagnosis: levels greater than 1.5 mmol/l indicate toxicity. Treatment consists of supportive measures, the use of anticonvulsants, and active elimination techniques. The decision to use the latter is based on the severity of symptoms and a plasma lithium level of greater than 3 mmol/l. Forced alkaline diuresis is effective but peritoneal dialysis or haemodialysis may be needed if renal function is inadequate, if there is severe electrolyte imbalance, or if the patient is very severely poisoned.

References

Biggs, J. T., Spiker, D. G., Petit, J. M., and Ziegler, V. E. (1977). Tricyclic antidepressant overdose. *J. Am. med. Ass.* **238**, 135.

Crome, P. and Newman, B. (1979). Fatal tricyclic antidepressant poisoning. *J.R. Soc. Med.* **72**, 649.

Hansen, H. E. and Amdisen, A. (1978). Lithium intoxication. *Q. Jl Med.* **47**, 123.

Nicotra, M. B., Rivera, M., Pool, J. L., and Noall, M. W. (1981). Tricyclic antidepressant overdose: clinical and pharmocologic observations. *Clin. Toxicol.* **18**, 599.

Park, J. and Proudfoot, A. T. (1977). Acute poisoning with Maprotiline hydrochloride. *Br. med. J.* **i**, 1573.

Starkey, I. B. and Lawson, A. A. H. (1980). Poisoning with tricyclic and related antidepressants—a ten year review. *Q. Jl Med.* **49**, 33.

Thorstrand, C. (1974). Cardiovascular effects of poisoning by tricyclic antidepressants. *Acta med. scand.* **195**, 505.

— (1976). Clinical features in poisoning by tricyclic antidepressants with special reference to the ECG. *Acta med. scand.* **199**, 337.

POISONING FROM CARDIORESPIRATORY DRUGS

J. A. Vale and T. J. Meredith

Beta-adrenergic blocking drugs. Beta-adrenergic blocking drugs antagonize the effects of endogenous catecholamines on the heart and other tissues by competitive inhibition at beta-adrenergic receptors. In overdose these drugs exhibit a marked negative inotropic action.

Clinical features. Cardiovascular and neurological effects include bradycardia, hypotension, low output cardiac failure, drowsiness, delirium, unconsciousness, fits, and cardiorespiratory arrest (asystole or ventricular fibrillation). Bronchospasm and hypoglycaemia occur rarely.

Treatment. Gastric lavage, if appropriate, and supportive measures should be undertaken in all cases. If bradycardia and hypotension are present, give atropine 0.6–3 mg (50 µg/kg in children) intravenously, glucagon 50–150 µg/kg intravenously over one minute followed by an infusion of 1–5 mg/hour and commence a dobutamine infusion (2.5–20 µg/kg/min). It is thought that glucagon activates myocardial adenyl cyclase by a different mechanism from beta-adrenergic catecholamines. This effect is not blocked by beta-adrenergic blocking drugs. If bronchospasm supervenes salbutamol (albuterol) by nebulizer should be employed. Hypoglycaemia should be corrected with intravenous glucose (not glucagon).

Clonidine. Clonidine exerts its hypotensive action by reduction of sympathetic tone mediated by a central effect on postsynaptic alpha-receptors in the medulla. Clonidine decreases heart rate, cardiac output, and total peripheral resistance. In the presence of high plasma clonidine concentrations, peripheral α-agonistic activity predominates and accounts for those instances of vasoconstriction and hypertension reported following clonidine overdose.

Clinical features. A review of 170 cases indicates that poisoning with this drug may be severe and life-threatening, particularly in children, though no deaths occurred in their series. In contrast to other reports, peripherally mediated alpha-sympathomimetic effects (such as hypertension and severe vasoconstriction) were unusual, while bradycardia, hypotension, coma, and respiratory depression (due to the central effects of the drug) were common (Table 1).

Treatment. Gastric lavage or emesis, if appropriate, and supportive measures should be undertaken. Bradycardia should be re-

Table 1   Clinical features of acute clonidine overdosage in 133 children aged under 10 years (mean age 2 years 8 months) and in 37 adults (mean age 29). Mean clonidine dosage: children 0.509 mg (range 0.025 to 3.000 mg), adults 2.096 mg (range 0.250 to 7.000 mg).

Signs and symptoms	No. (%) of children	No. (%) of adults
Impaired consciousness	113 (85)	29 (78)
Pallor	36 (27)	6 (16)
Bradycardia*	32 (24)	18 (49)
Cardiac arrhythmias	6 (5)	
Cardiac arrest		1 (3)
Hypotension†	28 (21)	12 (32)
Depressed respiration	20 (15)	2 (5)
Apnoea	3 (2)	
Miosis	18 (14)	3 (8)
Unreactive pupils	7 (5)	
Hypotonia	14 (11)	2 (5)
Irritability	14 (11)	1 (3)
Hyporeflexia	5 (4)	1 (3)
Extensor plantar reflex	4 (3)	
Hypertension	3 (2)	4 (11)
Dry mouth	3 (2)	4 (11)
Mean duration of effects (h)	16.2 (range 3.5–48.0)	15–96
Mean period of hospitalization (h)	32.5 (range 1.0–72.0)	24–96

* Bradycardia defined as a pulse of <80/min, age 1–4 years; <75/min, age 4–6 years; <70/min, age 6–10 years; <60/min, age >10 years

† Hypotension defined as a systolic blood pressure of <75 mm Hg, age 1–2 years; <80 mm Hg, age 2–40 years; <90 mm Hg age >40 years

From Stein and Volans (1978), reproduced by kind permission of the authors and the Editor of the *British Medical Journal*

versed by atropine 0.6–2 mg intravenously. In addition, alpha-adrenergic blocking drugs (tolazoline or phentolamine) have been advocated and used in severely poisoned patients in order to block both the peripheral and central actions of clonidine. Although forced diuresis has been employed in the treatment of clonidine poisoning, there is no evidence that it is effective.

Digoxin and digitoxin. Digitoxin poisoning is characterized by the same clinical signs that are seen with digoxin.

Clinical features. Nausea and vomiting are common. Cardiac arrhythmias, notably supraventricular arrhythmias with or without heart block, bradycardia, and ventricular premature beats often supervene. Hyperkalaemia occurs due to inhibition of the Na^+–K^+ activated ATPase pump. The diagnosis may be confirmed by measurement of the serum digoxin concentration.

Treatment. Gastric aspiration and lavage should be employed in all patients with a history of a substantial overdose. Supportive measures and specific treatment for arrhythmias should be given as follows: atropine for digoxin-induced heart block and bradycardia (an artificial pacemaker may also be necessary); phenytoin to suppress ventricular ectopic beats and improve conduction through the atrioventricular node; lignocaine and beta-adrenergic blocking drugs to suppress ventricular arrhythmias, but, as they are negatively inotropic, they should be avoided if the cardiac output is low. Hyperkalaemia should be corrected with a glucose and insulin infusion or, if severe, by the use of sodium resonium ion-exchange resins, or dialysis. Haemodialysis and haemoperfusion are unlikely to remove significant quantities of digoxin from the body because of the large apparent volume of distribution of the drug (350 l). The use of digoxin-specific Fab antibody fragments is under evaluation.

Disopyramide. Disopyramide not only possesses membrane-stabilizing activity but it also prolongs the action potential of normal cardiac cells. Anticholinergic effects are common even in therapeutic dosage.

Clinical features. Following a severe overdose of disopyramide, a

steady decline in cardiac output is seen, although the blood pressure is relatively well maintained until sudden circulatory collapse occurs. Typically, respiratory depression and serious arrhythmias do not occur until after circulatory collapse has supervened. The mortality is high in those who are severely poisoned.

Treatment. Gastric lavage, if appropriate, and supportive measures including the correction of any acidosis and hypokalaemia should be employed in all cases. An indwelling arterial cannula is often useful in that it provides immediate warning of cardiovascular collapse. An isoprenaline infusion (5–50 μg/min) should be given if hypotension is present and cardiodepressant drugs such as quinidine, and procainamide should be avoided for the treatment of arrhythmias as they may increase mortality. If asystole occurs, transvenous pacing should be tried but the ventricular response is often poor. Haemoperfusion may be of value in those who are severely poisoned.

Mexiletine. Mexiletine depresses the maximum rate of depolarization of cardiac muscle with little or no modification of resting potentials or the duration of action potentials.

Clinical features. Nausea, vomiting, drowsiness, confusion, dizziness, diplopia, nystagmus, dysarthria, ataxia, tremor, paraesthesiae, convulsions, hypotension, sinus bradycardia, and atrial fibrillation.

Treatment. In addition to the use of gastric lavage, if appropriate, and supportive measures, atropine 1–2 mg intravenously should be given if bradycardia occurs. If severe hypotension develops, an infusion of isoprenaline or dobutamine should be commenced. Transvenous cardiac pacing has been attempted in some severely poisoned patients but the ventricular response is usually poor.

Quinine and quinidine. Quinine and quinidine are optical isomers and share many pharmacological properties, although the latter compound is more toxic. Both alkaloids depress skeletal and cardiac muscle function.

Clinical features. These include ringing in the ears, headache, nausea, vomiting, diarrhoea, abdominal pain, blurred vision, disturbed odour perception, photophobia, diplopia, night blindness, constricted visual fields, scotomata, and, in severe cases, optic atrophy. Collapse with impairment of consciousness, shallow rapid breathing, sinus tachycardia, hypotension, and cardiac arrhythmias may follow.

Treatment. Gastric lavage should be employed if the patient presents within four hours of ingestion. The most important measure in those who have taken a substantial overdose is to perform a bilateral stellate ganglion block to prevent blindness. In severe cases, supportive measures and forced acid diuresis (see page 6.9) may be required. Dialysis does not substantially increase the elimination of either quinine or quinidine.

Verapamil. Verapamil has a specific inhibitory effect on the transmembranal passage of calcium ions in the myocardial cell and reduces the activity of calcium-dependent adenosine triphosphatase. In addition, verapamil diminishes peripheral resistance and so relieves the work load on the heart.

Clinical features. In overdose, verapamil causes dizziness, nausea, vomiting, atrioventricular conduction defects, and hypotension. The ingestion of a large overdose is associated with a poor prognosis in those with ischaemic heart disease and in those who are taking beta-adrenergic blocking agents therapeutically.

Treatment. Gastric lavage should be performed in patients who present early. Supportive measures, including the use of a dobutamine or dopamine infusion are required in severe cases. In addition, it has been suggested that a bolus of calcium gluconate 10–20 ml of a 10 per cent solution should be given.

Beta-2 adrenoceptor stimulant drugs. Beta-2 adrenoceptor stimulant drugs—salbutamol (albuterol) and terbutaline—are used widely in the treatment of obstructive airways disease and, less commonly, in the management of premature labour.

Clinical features. In overdose, these drugs cause tremor, agitation, a 'bursting feeling' in the head, palpitations, sinus tachycardia, peripheral vasodilatation, and, rarely, lactic acidosis, hyperglycaemia, and hypokalaemia.

Treatment. If a substantial overdose has been ingested and presentation is early, gastric lavage should be performed. A cardioselective beta-adrenergic blocking drug should be given if rate-related chest pain or arrhythmias occur.

Theophylline. Iatrogenic poisoning from theophylline and its derivatives, often by the intravenous route, is not uncommon. For this reason, it is important to monitor plasma drug levels during theophylline therapy. Iatrogenic poisoning can generally be managed symptomatically and supportively while the drug is eliminated by metabolic pathways. In cases of severe poisoning, with marked cardiovascular and neurological effects, more rapid removal of the drug may be necessary.

Clinical features. These include nausea, vomiting, abdominal discomfort, diarrhoea, thirst, palpitations, cardiac arrhythmias, hypotension (which may be marked), agitation, tremor, convulsions.

Treatment. In addition to gastric lavage, if appropriate, activated charcoal should be left in the stomach. If the patient is severely poisoned (plasma theophylline level greater than 60 mg/l) charcoal haemoperfusion should be instituted along with intensive supportive measures. Convulsions may be treated with diazepam 5–10 mg intravenously.

References

Conner, C. S. and Watanabe, A. S. (1979). Clonidine overdose: A review. *Am. J. hosp. Pharm.* **36**, 906.

Elkins, B. R. and Watanabe, A. S. (1978). Acute digoxin poisonings: review of therapy. *Am. J. hosp. Pharm.* **35**, 268.

Frishman, W., Jacob, H., Eisenberg, E., and Ribner, H. (1979). Clinical pharmacology of the new beta-adrenergic blocking drugs. Part 8. Self-poisoning with beta-adrenoceptor blocking agents: recognition and management. *Am. Heart. J.* **98**, 798.

Hansteen, V., Jacobsen, D., Knudsen, K., Reikvam, A., and Skuterud, B. (1981). Acute massive poisoning with digitoxin: report of seven cases and discussion of treatment. *Clin. Toxicol.* **18** 679.

Hayler, A. M., Holt, D. W., and Volans, G. N. (1978). Fatal overdose with disopyramide. *Lancet* **i**, 968.

Helliwell, M. and Berry, D. (1979). Theophylline poisoning in adults. *Br. med. J.* **ii**, 1114.

Neuronen, P. J., Elonen, E., Vuorenmaa, T. and Laasko M. (1981). Prolonged Q–T interval and severe tachyarrhythmias, common features of severe sotalol intoxication. *Eur. J. clin. Pharmacol.* **20**, 85.

Smith, T. W. (1980). Treatment of advanced digitalis toxicity with specific antibodies. *Europ. J. clin. Invest.* **10**, 89.

Stein, B. and Volans, G. N. (1978). Dixarit overdose: the problem of attractive tablets. *Br. med. J.* **ii**, 667.

POISONING FROM ALCOHOLS AND GLYCOLS

T. J. Meredith and J. A. Vale

Methyl alcohol (methanol). Methanol is used widely as a solvent and to denature ethanol. It is also found in antifreeze solutions, paints, duplicating fluids, paint removers, and varnishes. The ingestion of as little as 10 ml of pure methanol has caused permanent blindness and 30 ml is potentially fatal, although individual susceptibility varies widely. Toxicity may also occur as a result of inhalation or percutaneous absorption. Methylated spirits consists of 5 per cent methanol and 95 per cent ethanol and, contrary to popular opinion, toxicity is due mainly to the presence of the latter component.

Mechanism of toxicity. In man, methanol is metabolized by alcohol dehydrogenase and catalase enzyme systems to formaldehyde and formic acid. The principal clinical features of methanol poisoning are visual toxicity and a marked metabolic acidosis. It is not certain whether the visual toxicity of methanol is due to the local formation of formaldehyde in the retina by alcohol dehydrogenase (required for the utilization of vitamin A) or to interruption of axoplasmic flow in the optic nerve as a result of inhibition of cytochrome oxidase activity by formate ions. Although the metabolic acidosis of methanol poisoning has not been fully explained, formate ion has been shown to account for half of the increased anion gap and inhibition of cytochrome oxidase activity by formate ions may cause accumulation of other organic acids.

Clinical features. Methanol causes mild and transient inebriation and drowsiness when ingested alone. After a latent period of eight to 36 hours, nausea, vomiting, abdominal pain, headaches, dizziness, and coma supervene. Blurred vision and diminished visual acuity may occur and the presence of dilated pupils, unreactive to light, suggests that permanent blindness is likely to ensue. A severe metabolic acidosis is found in serious cases of methanol poisoning and this may be accompanied by hyperglycaemia and a raised serum amylase. A blood methanol level greater than 500 mg/l confirms serious methanol poisoning.

Treatment. The treatment of methanol poisoning should include gastric aspiration and lavage provided that the alcohol has been ingested within the preceding four hours. Bicarbonate should be given intravenously as a matter of urgency to correct any metabolic acidosis. Competitive inhibition of the metabolism of methanol to formaldehyde and formic acid is achieved by administration of ethanol (a loading dose of 50 g orally followed by an intravenous infusion of 10–12 g/hour) in order to achieve circulating ethanol levels of 1000–2000 mg/l. Haemodialysis is indicated if the blood methanol level exceeds 500 mg/l, the metabolic acidosis cannot be corrected, mental, visual, or fundoscopic complications develop, or if more than 30 ml of methanol have been ingested. The infusion of ethanol will need to be increased by at least 7–10 g/hour during haemodialysis because this substance, too, is readily dialysable. Peritoneal dialysis is less effective than haemodialysis, but ethanol may be added to the dialysate in a concentration of 1–2 g per litre. 4-Methyl-pyrazole (4-MP) has been used successfully to treat methanol poisoning in monkeys and it is possible that 4-MP may eventually be used in the treatment of severe methanol poisoning in man. This substance inhibits alcohol dehydrogenase activity by forming a ternary complex with the enzyme and the cofactor, nicotinamide adenine dinucleotide (NAD). An alternative approach employed recently in the treatment of experimental methanol poisoning in monkeys has been the administration of folinic acid to enhance the metabolism of formate to carbon dioxide by means of a folate-dependent, one-carbon pool pathway.

Ethyl alcohol (ethanol). Ethyl alcohol is commonly ingested in beverage form either prior to, or concomitant with, the deliberate ingestion of other substances in overdose. Ethyl alcohol is also used as a solvent and it is found in cosmetic and antiseptic preparations. Ethanol is rapidly absorbed through the gastric and intestinal mucosae and approximately 90 per cent of an ingested dose is oxidized via acetaldehyde and acetic acid to carbon dioxide and water at a rate of about 10–20 ml/hour.

Mechanism of toxicity. Ethyl alcohol acts as a central nervous depressant which in small doses interferes with cortical function, but which in large doses may depress medullary processes. The effects of alcohol exacerbate those of other central nervous system depressants, in particular, hypnotic agents. The fatal adult dose of ethyl alcohol when taken alone lies between 300 and 500 ml, if this is ingested in less than one hour (strong spirits, such as whisky and gin, contain 40 to 55 per cent ethanol).

Clinical features. The clinical features of ethanol intoxication are well known and are related to blood alcohol levels: *mild intoxication (500–1500 mg/l)*: emotional lability, slight impairment of visual acuity, muscular co-ordination, and reaction time; *moderate intox-*

ication (1500–3000 mg/l): Visual impairment, sensory loss, muscular inco-ordination, slowed reaction time, slurred speech; *severe intoxication (3000–5000 mg/l):* marked muscular inco-ordination, blurred or double vision, sometimes stupor and hypothermia, and occasionally hypoglycaemia and convulsions; *coma (5000 mg/l):* Depressed reflexes, respiratory depression, hypotension, and hypothermia. Death may occur from respiratory or circulatory failure or as the result of aspiration of stomach contents in the absence of a gag reflex.

Severe hypoglycaemia may accompany alcohol intoxication due to inhibition of gluconeogenesis. This occurs more commonly in children than in adults. Typically, alcohol-induced hypoglycaemia occurs within 6 to 36 hours of ingestion of a moderate to large amount of alcohol by either a previously malnourished individual or one who has fasted for the previous 24 hours. The patient is often in coma and hypothermic; the usual features of hypoglycaemia, such as flushing, sweating, and tachycardia, are frequently absent.

Treatment. The treatment of ethanol poisoning should include gastric aspiration and lavage where appropriate together with intensive supportive therapy. Naloxone (0.4–1.2 mg intravenously) has recently been shown to improve the level of consciousness in a proportion of patients with ethanol-induced coma. Hypoglycaemia should be treated with either oral or intravenous glucose (glucagon is ineffective in the treatment of ethanol-induced hypoglycaemia). The administration of fructose may be useful in the treatment of severe alcohol poisoning because fructose metabolism increases the conversion of $NADH_2$ to NAD, the supply of which may be rate-limiting for ethanol metabolism. However, the use of fructose may be accompanied by retrosternal and epigastric discomfort and, more importantly, metabolic acidosis. Haemodialysis and haemoperfusion are efficient means of removing alcohol from the body and the use of one of these techniques may occasionally be necessary in very severe alcohol poisoning.

Isopropyl alcohol (isopropanol). Isopropyl alcohol is used as a sterilizing agent and as rubbing alcohol. It is also found in aftershave lotions, disinfectants, and window-cleaning solutions. The symptoms and signs of isopropanol toxicity are similar to those of ethyl alcohol, although it is at least twice as potent as the latter agent because of a slower rate of metabolism. Ten to 15 per cent of an ingested dose of isopropyl alcohol is metabolized to acetone, and ketonuria is found commonly in isopropyl alcohol poisoning. Isopropyl alcohol is readily dialysable and haemodialysis is indicated in severely poisoned patients. In most instances, however, gastric lavage and supportive therapy suffice.

Ethylene glycol. Ethylene glycol has a variety of commercial applications though it is most commonly used as an antifreeze fluid in car radiators. Its sweet taste and ready availability have contributed to its popularity as a suicide agent and as a poor man's substitute for alcohol.

It is thought that the minimum lethal dose of ethylene glycol is about 100 ml for an adult, although recovery after treatment has been reported following the ingestion of up to 1 litre. Deaths from ethylene glycol are uncommon in England and Wales: only 32 cases have been reported in 26 years (1954 to 1979), though 15 of these occurred in one year (1977).

Mechanism of toxicity. Ethylene glycol itself appears to be non-toxic. Until metabolized it has no effect on respiration, the citric acid cycle, or other biochemical pathways. Metabolism takes place in the liver and kidneys and proceeds as shown in Fig. 1. The toxicity of ethylene glycol may be explained on the basis of accumulation of the following four metabolic products:

1. Aldehydes, which inhibit oxidative phosphorylation, cellular respiration and glucose metabolism, protein synthesis, DNA replication and ribosomal RNA synthesis, central nervous system respiration, and serotonin metabolism. Aldehydes also alter central nervous system amine levels. (Cerebral symptoms occur six to

12 hours after the ingestion of ethylene glycol and coincide with the maximum production of aldehydes.)

2. Glycolate which, in monkeys and in rats, has been shown to be largely responsible for the development of the marked acidosis in overdose.

3. Oxalate, which causes renal damage and acidosis. It is thought, however, that only about 1 per cent of an ingested dose of ethylene glycol is converted to this substance. The production of oxalate is also important in that it chelates calcium ions to form insoluble calcium oxalate crystals: hypocalcaemia may result. As well as renal intratubular obstruction, impairment of cerebral function follows deposition of calcium oxalate in the brain.

4. Lactic acid is produced as the result of large amounts of nicotinamide adenine dinucleotide being formed during breakdown of ethylene glycol. In addition, some of the condensation products of glyoxylate metabolism inhibit the citric acid cycle, increasing lactic acid production (Fig. 1).

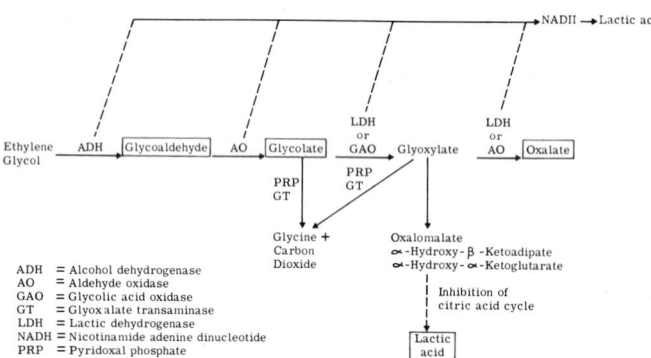

Fig. 1 Pathways for metabolism of ethylene glycol showing mechanism of production of lactic acidosis.

Clinical features. The clinical features of ethylene glycol poisoning may be divided into three stages depending on the time after ingestion (Table 1). The severity of each stage and the progression

Table 1. Clinical features of ethylene glycol poisoning

Stage 1 (30 min–12 hour): gastrointestinal and nervous system involvement
Patient appears intoxicated with alcohol (but no alcohol on breath)
Nausea, vomiting, haematemesis
Coma and convulsions (often focal)
Nystagmus, ophthalmoplegias, papilloedema, optic atrophy, depressed reflexes, myoclonic jerks, tetanic contractions

Stage 2 (12–24 hour): cardiorespiratory system involvement
Tachypnoea
Tachycardia
Mild hypertension
Pulmonary oedema
Congestive cardiac failure

Stage 3 (24–72 hour): renal involvement
Flank pain
Costovertebral angle tenderness
Acute tubular necrosis

from one stage to the next depends on the amount of ethylene glycol ingested. Death may occur during any of the three stages. Ethylene glycol poisoning should be suspected if any of the following occur:

1. An apparently inebriated patient with no alcohol detectable on the breath.

2. Coma associated with a metabolic acidosis, a large anion gap (serum bicarbonate may be less than 10 mmol/l) and, sometimes, hypocalcaemia, leucocytosis, and hyperkalaemia.

3. Urinalysis demonstrating calcium oxalate (monohydrate or dihydrate) crystalluria, microscopic haematuria, low specific gravity, and proteinuria.

4. Gastric lavage fluid with the appearance of antifreeze solution.

Ethylene glycol poisoning may be confirmed by measurement of ethylene glycol levels in the blood.

Treatment. Early diagnosis and appropriate therapy significantly reduces the mortality from ethylene glycol poisoning. In addition to gastric lavage to prevent further absorption and to confirm the diagnosis, supportive measures to combat shock, respiratory distress, hypocalcaemia, and metabolic acidosis should be instituted. Thereafter, treatment has two main aims. Firstly, the use of ethyl alcohol as a competitive inhibitor of ethylene glycol metabolism, and, secondly, the use of dialysis to increase elimination of the substance from the body.

Ethyl alcohol. Ethyl alcohol inhibits the oxidation of ethylene glycol by liver alcohol dehydrogenase enzymes. It has been suggested that it is necessary to maintain a plasma ethanol level of 1000–2000 mg/l to inhibit breakdown of glycol but, as the affinity of the enzyme alcohol dehydrogenase for ethyl alcohol is many times that for ethylene glycol, a much lower plasma ethanol level may be sufficient to inhibit glycol metabolism.

The half-life of ethylene glycol is about three hours in man and, for this reason, an ethanol infusion should be commenced as soon as possible after ingestion of the overdose. It should be continued until ethylene glycol can no longer be detected in the blood. The amount of ethanol required to maintain a plasma alcohol level of 1000–2000 mg/l is dependent upon the patient's previous ethanol intake. A loading dose of 50 g ethyl alcohol orally, followed by an infusion of 10 to 12 g/hour, should be satisfactory, but it is important to measure blood alcohol levels regularly. If haemodialysis is employed, the infusion rate should be increased to 17–22 g/hour because ethanol is readily dialysable. Alternatively, ethanol may be added to peritoneal dialysate fluid, 1–2 g per litre of dialysate.

Dialysis. Ethylene glycol and its aldehyde metabolites may be removed by either peritoneal or haemodialysis. Oxalate, however, is poorly dialysable. In addition, it may be necessary to treat the uraemic complications of ethylene glycol poisoning with dialysis and to use haemodialysis/ultrafiltration to correct the sodium overload that can result from over-judicious correction of the metabolic acidosis with sodium bicarbonate. Dialysis should be continued until ethylene glycol is no longer detected in the blood.

References

Beasley, V. R. and Buck, W. B. (1980). Acute ethylene glycol toxicosis: a review. *Vet. human Toxicol.* **22**, 255.

Bennett, I. L., Jr, Cary, F. H., Mitchell, G. L., Jr, and Cooper, M. N. (1953). Acute methyl alcohol poisoning: a review based on experiences in an outbreak of 323 cases. *Medicine, Baltimore* **32**, 431.

Billings, R. E. and Tephly, T. R. (1979). Studies on methanol toxicity and formate metabolism in isolated hepatocytes. *Biochem. Pharmac.* **28**, 2985.

McCoy, H. G., Cipolle, R. J., Ehlers, S. M., Sawchuk, R. J., and Zaske, D. E. (1979). Severe methanol poisoning. Application of a pharmacokinetic model for ethanol therapy and hemodialysis. *Am. J. Med.* **67**, 804.

Naraqi, S., Dethlefs, R. F., Slobodniuk, R. A., and Sairere, J. S. (1979). An outbreak of acute methyl alcohol intoxication. *Aust. N.Z. J. Med.* **9**, 65.

Parry, M. F. and Wallach, R. (1974). Ethylene glycol poisoning. *Am. J. Med.* **57**, 143.

Schneck, S. A. (1979). Methyl alcohol. In *Handbook of Clinical Neurology*, vol. 36 (eds. P. J. Vinken and G. W. Bruyn). North Holland, Amsterdam.

Vale, J. A. (1979). Ethylene glycol poisoning. *Vet. human Toxicol.* **21**, suppl. 118.

Wacker, W. E. C., Haynes, H., Druyan, R., Fisher, W., and Coleman, J. E. (1965). Treatment of ethylene glycol poisoning with ethyl alcohol. *J. Am. med. Ass.* **194**, 1231.

POISONING FROM HYDROCARBONS, SOLVENTS AND OTHER INHALATIONAL AGENTS

J. A. Vale and T. J. Meredith

Hydrocarbons

The aliphatic hydrocarbons include both saturated (a single bond between the carbon atoms) and unsaturated (multiple bonds between the carbon atoms) compounds which are derived almost exclusively from petroleum or petroleum processing. The aromatic hydrocarbons contain one or more benzene rings. Additional aromatic hydrocarbons are derived by substituting groups on the benzene ring. Benzene rings may be condensed together to form polynuclear hydrocarbons which, on halogenation, yield the corresponding halogenated polynuclear hydrocarbon.

Poisoning from hydrocarbons may be occupational or accidental (such as that which occurs in the home) and it may result from solvent abuse or a suicidal or parasuicidal attempt. It has been estimated that in the United States there are more than 30 000 cases of accidental hydrocarbon poisoning annually. Between 1969 and 1973, 327 deaths followed hydrocarbon inhalation or ingestion in the United States. In contrast, the incidence in Britain is much lower, and only 210 deaths have been reported between 1945 and 1979.

Alkanes (paraffins). Natural gas contains methane and ethane, and LPG (liquefied petroleum gas, 'bottled gas') contains propane and butane. Methane and ethane are pharmacologically inert and can be tolerated in high concentrations without the production of any toxic effects. Both gases, however, may produce asphyxia, as a result of oxygen deprivation, in poorly ventilated areas. Propane and butane produce no more than drowsiness even at high concentrations.

Paraffin oil (kerosene). Paraffin oil has two chemical properties which account for its toxicity. First, its low surface tension means that, following aspiration of paraffin oil into the lungs, there is rapid spread of the hydrocarbon throughout both lung fields. Secondly, the low vapour pressure of paraffin oil means that inhalational poisoning is unlikely under normal conditions of use.

Clinical features. Repeated local application to the skin will result in dryness and dermatitis. Following ingestion, irritation of the mucous membranes, vomiting, diarrhoea, chemical pneumonitis, and depression of the nervous system (lethargy, confusion, coma, and convulsions) occur. Death is usually due to pulmonary rather than neurological complications.

Pulmonary toxicity may occur within one hour of ingestion and is characterized by pyrexia, cough, tachypnoea (often with an associated tachycardia), basal crepitations, and cyanosis. Radiologically, non-segmental consolidation and/or atelectasis is seen involving the middle and lower zones predominantly and often bilaterally. Rarely, a pneumatocoele, pneumothorax, pleural effusion, and pulmonary oedema may occur.

There is now good evidence based on observations in both animals and man to suggest that pulmonary lesions follow aspiration, rather than being due to a direct toxic effect following absorption from the gut, though the latter effect may occur if the ingested dose is high.

Treatment. Gastric lavage and emesis should be avoided because of the increased risk of chemical pneumonitis. In addition, there is no evidence that steroids and antibiotics reduce mortality, respiratory complications, or radiological and pathological changes.

Petrol. Petrol is a complex mixture of hydrocarbons containing a small proportion of non-hydrocarbon additives such as anti-knock agents, antioxidants, rust inhibitors, and dyes.

Acute poisoning. The inhalation of high concentrations of petrol, such as those encountered by workmen cleaning storage tanks or those sniffing petrol, may cause immediate death. It is possible that these hydrocarbons so sensitize the myocardium that circulating adrenaline (epinephrine) precipitates ventricular fibrillation. In addition, high concentrations of petrol vapour may lead to death from acute respiratory failure.

Clinical features. Following the inhalation of petrol, dizziness, irritation of the eyes, nose, and throat may occur within five minutes followed by euphoria, headache, and blurred vision. If inhalation continues, or significant quantities of petrol are ingested, then excitation and depression of the nervous system occurs: incoordination, restlessness, excitement, confusion, disorientation, hallucinations, ataxia, nystagmus, tremor, delirium, coma, and convulsions may be seen. Cardiorespiratory arrest may be the end-result in cases of severe poisoning.

Treatment. Supportive measures, following removal from exposure, provide the basis of treatment as gastric lavage and emesis may increase the risk of chemical pneumonitis.

Chronic poisoning. Chronic exposure to petrol (gasoline) vapour, such as occurs in men engaged in cleaning storage tanks or in children who habitually sniff gasoline, may lead both to chronic hydrocarbon and to organic lead poisoning. Tetraethyl lead (the 'anti-knock' additive) is non-toxic, but this substance is converted in the liver to the toxic metabolite, triethyl lead. In addition, triethyl lead may further be degraded to inorganic lead.

Clinical features. Chronic exposure to the hydrocarbon content of petrol leads to gastrointestinal (anorexia, nausea, vomiting, and diarrhoea), cardiovascular (relative bradycardia and hypotension), neurological (muscle weakness, brisk reflexes, extensor plantar responses, tremor, chorea, and convulsions), and neuropsychological (insomnia, irritability, restlessness, anxiety, loss of short-term memory, mania, and suicidal tendencies) disease. Hepatorenal damage has been described occasionally. In addition, the lead content of petrol may give rise to anaemia, cerebellar dysfunction, myoclonus, and encephalopathy.

Treatment. In the case of occupational exposure to petrol, scrupulous attention to hygiene, the provision of industrial clothing, and facilities for these to be laundered, and adequate washing and showering facilities are all essential. The treatment of lead poisoning is described on page 6.5. Solvent 'sniffers' will require intensive psychosocial support though it must be said that such measures rarely change the behaviour of those so addicted (see solvent abuse page 6.29).

Benzene poisoning. Benzene is a colourless, volatile liquid with a pleasant odour. It is an ingredient in many paints and varnish removers and some petrols. It is also the primary raw material for styrene (used in the production of synthetic rubber), for phenol, for nylon intermediates, and for synthetic detergents of the alkylauryl sulphonate type.

Acute poisoning. Acute poisoning results when benzene is ingested or inhaled with suicidal or parasuicidal intent, and is also encountered when workmen enter storage tanks for the purpose of cleaning.

Clinical features. These include euphoria, dizziness, weakness, headache, blurring of vision, mucous membrane irritation, tremor, ataxia, chest tightness, respiratory depression, cardiac arrhythmias, coma, and convulsions.

Treatment. Following removal from the contaminated atmosphere, treatment should be directed to symptomatic and supportive measures. Even if the patient presents soon after ingestion, gastric lavage is probably too hazardous as aspiration is likely to occur.

Chronic poisoning. The toxic effects of chronic poisoning may not become apparent for months or years after the initial contact and, they may, indeed, develop after all exposure has ceased.

Clinical features. Anorexia, headache, drowsiness, nervousness, and irritability are well described. Anaemia (including aplastic anaemia), leucopenia, thrombocytopenia, pancytopenia, leukaemia (particularly of the myelomonocytic type), lymphomas, chromosome abnormalities, and cerebral atrophy have been reported.

In chronic poisoning a steady decrease in the cellular elements of the blood or bone marrow indicates a poor outcome. However, patients have recovered after as long as a year of almost complete absence of formation of new blood cells.

Treatment. Treatment is symptomatic and supportive.

Toluene poisoning. Toluene has a much lower volatility and toxicity than benzene. Certain industrial solvent mixtures containing predominantly toluene have been reported to cause bone marrow failure. It is now thought though, that these mixtures were contaminated with benzene and that this was the cause of the bone marrow depression. Animal studies have failed to demonstrate a convincing myelotoxic effect of toluene.

Clinical features. Acute poisoning results in euphoria, excitement, dizziness, confusion, lacrimation, headache, nervousness, nausea, tinnitus, ataxia, tremor, and coma. Hepatorenal damage (including renal tubular acidosis), cerebellar degeneration, and cerebral atrophy, have been described after chronic poisoning.

Treatment. If poisoning resulted from inhalation (whether accidentally or intentionally as in solvent abuse), the patient should be removed from the contaminated environment. Thereafter treatment is symptomatic and supportive.

Chlorinated hydrocarbons. Chlorinated hydrocarbons have a widespread and essential role in the chemical industry and in a variety of manufacturing operations, including the production of plastics and pesticides. These compounds are also used as solvents (dry cleaning and surface degreasing agents) and as vehicles for paints, varnishes, and other industrial coatings. The more important chlorinated hydrocarbons include: tetrachloromethane (carbon tetrachloride), 1,1,1-trichloroethane (methyl chloroform), trichloroethylene, tetrachloroethylene (perchloroethylene), and trichloromethane (chloroform). The clinical features are summarized in Table 1. Treatment consists of symptomatic and supportive measures.

Methylene chloride. Methylene chloride is a common ingredient in paint removers. It has now been shown that its toxicity is due to the fact that it is rapidly metabolized in the body to carbon monoxide. For example, a six-hour exposure to paint stripper in an unventilated room produced carboxyhaemoglobin levels of 40 per

Table 1   Clinical features of poisoning due to chlorinated hydrocarbons

Local effects on the skin
Drying and fissuring
Inhalation or ingestion
Dizziness, euphoria, confusion, drowsiness
Nausea and vomiting, abdominal pain
Visual disturbances, coma, convulsions
Respiratory depression

Circulatory failure and sudden death due to ventricular fibrillation (because of sensitization of myocardium to endogenous catecholamines)
Hepatic dysfunction (in order of decreasing hepatotoxicity): carbon tetrachloride, chloroform, tetrachloroethane, 1,1,2-trichloroethane, tetrachloroethylene, trichloroethylene, methylene chloride, 1,1,1-trichloroethane

Renal impairment: Carbon tetrachloride, chloroform, 1,1,2-trichloroethane, tetrachloroethylene, 1,1,1-trichloroethane, trichloroethylene

Cerebellar dysfunction, cerebral haemorrhage (carbon tetrachloride)
Peripheral neuropathy (tetrachloroethylene, trichloroethylene)
Cranial nerve palsies (trichloroethylene)
Pulmonary oedema (tetrachloroethylene, trichloroethylene)
Aplastic anaemia, haemolytic anaemia (carbon tetrachloride)

cent in one subject more than 12 hours after exposure had ceased. The addition of methanol to paint removers extends the biological half-life of carboxyhaemoglobin derived from methylene chloride. Patients with ischaemic heart disease are particularly at risk from carboxyhaemoglobin levels of more than 5 per cent and so the mortality is higher in such subjects exposed to methylene chloride. Treatment is described under carbon monoxide (see page 6.31).

References

Baldachin, B. J. and Melmed, R. N. (1964). Clinical and therapeutic aspects of kerosene poisoning: a series of 200 cases. *Br. Med. J.* ii, 28.

Clayton, G. D. and Clayton, F. E. (eds.) (1981). *Patty's industrial hygiene and toxicology*, 3rd revised edn., vol 2A and B: *Toxicology*. Wiley, New York.

Committee on Toxicology of the National Research Council (1976). *Health effects of benzene—a review*. National Technical Information Service PB 254 388, 1, US Department of Commerce, Washington, DC.

Feldman, R. G. (1979). Trichloroethylene. In *Handbook of clinical neurology: intoxications of the nervous system (part 1)* (eds. P. J. Vinken and G. W. Bruyn). North Holland, Amsterdam.

Gerarde, H. W. (1959). Toxicological studies on hydrocarbons. V. Kerosine. *Toxicol. app. Pharmacol.* **1**, 462.

Hayden, J. W., Peterson, R. G., and Bruckner, J. V. (1977) Toxicology of toluene: review of current literature. *Clin. Toxicol.* **11**, 549.

National Institute of Occupational Safety and Health. (1973). *Criteria document: Toluene*. US Department of Health, Education, and Welfare, Washington, DC.

— (1973). *Criteria for a recommended standard document: trichloroethylene*. US Department of Health, Education, and Welfare, Washington DC.

— (1974). *Criteria for a recommended standard document: benzene*. US Department of Health, Education, and Welfare, Washington, DC.

— (1975). *Criteria for a recommended standard document: Carbon tetrachloride*. US Department of Health, Education, and Welfare, Washington, DC.

— (1976). *Criteria for a recommended standard document: tetrachloroethylene*. US Department of Health, Education, and Welfare, Washington, DC.

— (1976). *Criteria for a recommended standard document: 1,1,1-trichloroethane*. US Department of Health, Education, and Welfare, Washington, DC.

von Oettingen, W. F. (1955). *The halogenated hydrocarbons: toxicity and potential dangers*. Public Health Services publication no. 414, US Government Printing Office, Washington, DC.

Recknagel, R. O. (1967). Carbon tetrachloride hepatotoxicity. *Pharmac. Rev.* **19**, 145.

Smith, G. F. (1966). Trichloroethylene: a review. *Br. J. ind. Med.* **23**, 249.

Stewart, R. D. (1968). The toxicology of 1,1,1-trichloroethane. *Ann. occup. Hyg.* **11**, 71.

Sub-committee on Accidental Poisoning (1962). Co-operative kerosene poisoning study. *Pediatrics, Springfield* **29**, 648.

Di Vincenzo, G. D. and Kaplan, C. J. (1981). Uptake, metabolism, and elimination of methylene chloride by humans. *Toxicol. app. Pharmacol.* **59**, 130.

Solvent abuse

Solvent abuse may be defined as the intentional inhalation of volatile organic chemicals other than conventional anaesthetic gases. This definition includes the inhalation of vapours of organic solvents (whether pure or in combination with other non-volatile ingredients), hydrocarbon mixtures, such as petrol (gasoline), and aerosol propellants.

Solvent sniffing is by no means a recent phenomenon, nor is it without harm. The misuse of nitrous oxide, ether, and chloroform by adults was fashionable in the 19th century. Since 1970, there have been more than 50 deaths in the United Kingdom alone due to solvent abuse.

Solvents are either 'bagged' (sprayed into a plastic bag, and then inhaled until the subject passes out) or 'huffed' (sprayed onto a cloth held to the mouth). The composition of products commonly abused is shown in Table 2. Most solvent abusers are male and adolescent and indulge in the habit as a group activity. Some young

Table 2   Solvent composition of products commonly abused

Product inhaled	Chemical constituents
Glues/adhesives	toluene, benzene, xylene, acetone, *n*-hexane
Cleaning fluids	trichloroethylene, tetrachloroethylene, 1,1,1-trichloroethane, carbon tetrachloride, toluene
Petrol/gasoline	hydrocarbons, tetraethyl lead
Aerosols	fluorocarbons
Lighter refills	butane
Acrylic paint	toluene
Paints, varnishes, lacquers	trichloroethylene, methylene chloride, toluene
Polystyrene cements	acetone, toluene, trichloroethylene
Dyes	acetone, methylene chloride
Nail polish remover	acetone, amyl acetate

sniffers progress to regular and heavy drinking within a short period of time after becoming addicted or habituated to solvents. When a group of abusers were questioned about the subjective experience of solvent abuse, most agreed that marijuana provided somewhat similar effects, although vivid hallucinations were an added effect of solvent abuse. Solvent abuse should be suspected if groups of adolescents or individuals behave as if they are drunk. The hair, breath, or clothing may smell of solvent and the clothing is often stained. Unexplained listlessness, anorexia, and marked moodiness are suggestive of solvent abuse.

'Glue' sniffing. Glues are volatile semi-liquid preparations, which usually contain an aromatic hydrocarbon as the vehicle. Fortunately, benzene itself has now been replaced by toluene and other aromatic hydrocarbons in most commercially available products. For this reason, glue sniffing is now attended by fewer short and long-term complications than previously was the case. The inhalation of glues, however, remains hazardous and it can be fatal. Moreover, neurological damage may occur after 'sniffing' of less than one year's duration and symptoms may progress for up to three months after the habit has been abandoned. For example, glues containing *n*-hexane and toluene have been associated with the development of muscle weakness and atrophy and sensory impairment of either the 'glove and stocking' or sensorimotor type, with or without muscle atrophy. It is not certain whether the polyneuropathy is due to *n*-hexane alone or to the combination of *n*-hexane and toluene.

Petrol (gasolene) sniffing. The toxicity of petrol is related to the composition of the mixture, which in turn, is dependent upon the origin of the petroleum from which the petrol is derived and the molecular modifications incurred during refining. The saturated hydrocarbons from C_4–C_8 have strong narcotic properties and cause nausea, ataxia, and loss of consciousness. The unsaturated hydrocarbons in the mixture (e.g. butylenes and isoprenes) are mild anaesthetic agents. As a result of the high hydrocarbon content of petrol, inhalation produces giddiness, vertigo, headache, and stupor.

Abusers of petrol have reported that 15 to 20 breaths of the vapour is sufficient to produce intoxication for three to six hours. Due to the lipid solubility of the components of petrol, there is rapid absorption from the lungs and onset of symptoms occurs within three to five minutes.

The euphoria of mild intoxication may be accompanied by nausea and vomiting. After prolonged inhalation, or rapid inhalation of highly concentrated vapour, the 'sniffer' may experience a phase of violent excitement followed by loss of consciousness and coma. While unconscious, the subject may exhibit convulsive movements and the pupils may become fixed and dilated, or unequal. Nystagmus and conjugate deviation of the eyes may be observed.

Death from inhalation of petrol vapour is rare, but may occur due either to respiratory depression or to ventricular fibrillation from cardiac sensitization by the aromatic fractions of petrol. Cerebral and pulmonary oedema and renal and hepatic damage have been noted at post mortem following death from petrol inhalation. The greatest danger from petrol 'sniffing' is related to possible long-term effects of chronic exposure. Abusers of petrol often inhale the vapour daily for many years. Chronic inhalation may result in loss of appetite and loss of weight, neurasthenia, muscle weakness, and cramps. Abnormal EEGs have been reported in chronic abusers of petrol and there is some evidence that permanent neuropsychological damage may develop. Encephalopathy due to organic lead poisoning may also occur in petrol sniffers due to tetraethyl lead added to petrol as an 'anti-knock' agent. The deliberate abuse of hydrocarbon mixtures other than petrol is unusual, although a 'huffers' neuropathy, similar to the Guillain–Barré syndrome, has been described following inhalation of a lacquer thinner.

Chlorinated hydrocarbon abuse. Inhalation of chlorinated hydrocarbons causes a sense of euphoria and, sometimes, excitement associated with headache, dizziness, nausea, vomiting, stupor, coma, and convulsions.

Abuse of carbon tetrachloride may lead to acute renal failure and centrilobular hepatic necrosis. Trichloroethylene abuse has, on rare occasions, led to similar effects and it has also been associated with cranial nerve damage, particularly affecting the optic and trigeminal nerves. Both carbon tetrachloride and trichloroethylene sensitize the myocardium to circulating catecholamines and fatal ventricular arrhythmias may result.

Toxicity due to aerosol inhalation. The most commonly used aerosol propellants are the fluorinated hydrocarbons (Freons) of which those most widely employed are trichloromonofluoromethane (Fluorocarbon 11), dichlorodifluoromethane (Florocarbon 12), and dichlorotetrafluoroethane (Fluorocarbon 114).

Sudden death following inhalation of fluorocarbon aerosol propellants was first described in 1968. Since then several hundred further deaths have occurred in teenagers from this causes. Initially, deaths associated with aerosol inhalation were thought to be due to suffocation by the plastic bags used for inhalation. However, a study in 1970 of 110 cases of sudden 'sniffing' death without plastic bag suffocation showed that trichloroethylene and fluorocarbons were involved more frequently than other agents. Death often followed 'sniffing' accompanied by some form of exercise or stress. In eight eye-witnessed deaths, there was a brief interval prior to death in which the 'sniffer' suddenly dashed for a distance of several hundred feet before collapsing. No anatomical abnormalities to account for death could be found in any of the cases at post mortem.

Animal experiments have shown that fluorinated hydrocarbons readily sensitize the heart to asphyxia-induced sinus bradycardia and asystole, an effect which persists after exposure to the fluorocarbon ceases. At the same time, fluorocarbons sensitize the heart to circulating catecholamines, and ventricular tachycardia and fibrillation may occur as a consequence.

Possible long-term effects of solvent abuse. There is concern that minor components of petrol, such as benzene and xylene, may have as yet unrecognized long-term effects. Petrol may contain up to 6–8 per cent benzene and, in one report, 18 of 50 cases of acute non-lymphocytic leukaemia had a history of occupational exposure to petroleum products. Trichloroethylene and a number of commonly used chloroethanes are carcinogenic in rodents, although, as yet, there is no evidence that this is so in man.

Diagnosis and management of solvent abuse. The clinical features described above and the circumstances in which patients are found usually point to the diagnosis, but confirmation may be obtained by detection of solvents in blood and tissues by gas–liquid chromatography.

Prevention is by far the most important aspect of management of solvent abuse and every opportunity should be taken to educate teenagers about the serious short and long-term hazards of 'sniffing'. Emergency treatment consists of removal of the patient from the contaminated atmosphere and administration of oxygen. Respiratory depression and cardiac arrhythmias should be treated conventionally and renal and hepatic failure may necessitate further supportive measures and dialysis.

References

Bass, M. (1970). Sudden sniffing death. *J. Am. Med. Ass.* **212**, 2075.
Hayden, J. W., Comstock, E. G., and Comstock, B. S. (1976). The clinical toxicology of solvent abuse. *Clin. Toxocol.* **9**, 169.
King, M. D., Day, R. E., Oliver, J. S., Lush, M., and Watson, J. M. (1981). Solvent encephalopathy. *Br. med. J.* **283**, 663.
Oliver, J. S. and Watson, J. M. (1977). Abuse of solvents 'for kicks': a review of 50 cases. *Lancet* i, 84.
Poklis, A. and Burkett, C. D. (1977). Gasoline sniffing: A review. *Clin. Toxicol.* **11**, 35.
Watson, J. M. (1978). Clinical and laboratory investigation in 132 cases of solvent abuse. *Med. Sci. Law* 18, 40.

Ammonia

Ammonia is used in organic synthetic reactions and as a fertilizer. It has a direct caustic action on cells and produces painful irritation of all mucous membranes.

Clinical features. Inhalation of ammonia causes irritation of the eyes, upper respiratory tract and pharynx. High concentrations result in dyspnoea and pulmonary oedema as well as intense irritation of the mucous membranes and eyes.

Treatment. The casualty should be removed from the contaminated area. The eyes should be irrigated with water or saline (0.9 per cent) for 15–30 minutes and an ophthalmic opinion sought as permanent blindness may result. The pulmonary complications should be treated with humidified supplemental oxygen and bronchodilators. There is no conclusive evidence that diuretics and corticosteroids alter the prognosis. Patients who survive for 24 hours are likely to recover.

Reference

National Institute of Occupational Safety and Health (1974). *Criteria for a recommended standard document: ammonia.* US Department Health, Education, and Welfare, Washington, DC.

Carbon disulphide

Carbon disulphide is used as a fumigant for grain and as a solvent in industry. Although this liquid has a foul odour, this is insufficient to give adequate warning of hazardous concentrations.

Clinical features. Local contact causes reddening, burning, cracking, and peeling of the skin, and a burn may occur if contact continues for several minutes. Splashes of carbon disulphide in the eye causes immediate and severe irritation. Acute inhalation results in irritation of the mucous membranes, blurred vision, nausea and vomiting, headache, coma, convulsions, and respiratory arrest. Chronic industrial exposure may be atherogenic and diabetogenic. Sleep disturbances, fatigue, anorexia, and weight loss are not uncommon complaints, and intellectual decline, depression, and stereotype behaviour have been described.

Treatment. Treatment involves removal from exposure, washing of affected skin area, irrigation of the eyes with water, and symptomatic and supportive measures.

References

Brieger, H. and Teisinger, J. (eds.) (1967). *Toxicology of carbon disulfide.* Excerpta Medica, Amsterdam.
Coppock, R. W. and Buck, W. B. (1981). Toxicology of carbon disulfide: a review. *Vet. human Toxicol.* **23**, 331.
Davidson, M. and Feinlieb, M. (1972). Carbon disulfide poisoning: a review. *Am. Heart J.* **83**, 100.
Hanninen, H. (1971). Psychological picture of manifest and latent carbon disulphide poisoning. *Br. J. ind. Med.* **28**, 374.

Carbon monoxide

Carbon monoxide is produced by the incomplete combustion of organic materials. It is produced endogenously in man from the α-methane carbon atom of the protoporphyrin ring during the catabolism of haemoglobin. Normal endogenous production of carbon monoxide is sufficient to maintain a resting carboxyhaemoglobin (COHb) level of 1 to 3 per cent.

Although the mortality due to carbon monoxide poisoning has fallen since the introduction of natural gas to domestic households, 1000 deaths still occur annually in England and Wales from this cause. Carbon monoxide is the main cause of death from poisoning in children in the United Kingdom. Common sources of carbon monoxide are the exhaust from automobiles, improperly maintained and ventilated heating systems, smoke from all types of fires, and household gas (if supplies have not been converted to natural gas).

The affinity of haemoglobin for carbon monoxide is approximately 240 times greater than that for oxygen and the symptoms and signs which follow inhalation of carbon monoxide are primarily the result of tissue hypoxia. Carbon monoxide combines with haemoglobin to form carboxyhaemoglobin. If carbon monoxide is inhaled, a certain number of oxygen binding sites on the haemoglobin molecule become occupied and the total oxygen-carrying capacity of the blood is reduced. This in itself results in a shift of the O_2 dissociation curve to the left, i.e. more avid oxygen binding. However, the binding of one or more carbon monoxide molecules to a molecule of haemoglobin also induces an allosteric modification in the remaining oxygen binding sites. The affinity of the remaining haem groups for oxygen is increased and the O_2 dissociation curve is therefore distorted as well as being shifted to the left. The degree of tissue anoxia that results is thus far greater than that which would result from simple loss of oxygen-carrying capacity.

Clinical features. The severity of poisoning following exposure to carbon monoxide depends on the concentration of carbon monoxide in the inspired air, the length of exposure, and the general health of the exposed individual (elderly patients and those with pre-existing cardiorespiratory disease are more 'at risk'). The clinical features are summarized in Table 3.

Treatment. The basis of treatment of carbon monoxide poisoning with oxygen lies in the fact that carboxyhaemoglobin readily dissociates when the partial pressure of carbon monoxide in the alveolar air falls below that in mixed venous blood. This state may be obtained by reducing the partial pressure of inspired carbon monoxide to zero, increasing alveolar ventilation and increasing the inspired oxygen tension. The half-life of elimination of carbon monoxide is 250 minutes when breathing room air but this is reduced to 50 minutes when 100 per cent oxygen is inspired at sea level. Hyperbaric oxygen at 2.5 atmospheres pressure further reduces the half-life to 22 minutes. In addition, hyperbaric oxygen increases the amount of oxygen dissolved in the blood and at 2 atmospheres pressure, for example, the amount of oxygen dissolved increases from 0.25 volumes per cent to 3.8 volumes per cent. However, it usually takes too long to transfer a patient to a hyperbaric oxygen chamber and then to achieve full working pressure to make the use of hyperbaric oxygen practicable in most cases of carbon monoxide poisoning.

Table 3 Immediate and late clinical features of carbon monoxide poisoning

Agitation, mental confusion, headache (usually frontal and band-like, sometimes occipital)
Nausea and vomiting, incontinence (occasionally), haematemesis, melaena
Pink skin and mucosae (i.e. there is no sign of cyanosis) because of the carboxyhaemoglobin in the blood
Hyperventilation, pulmonary oedema, respiratory failures, Cheyne–Stokes respiration
Bullous lesions
Hyperpyrexia
Loss of consciousness, hypertonia, hyper-reflexia
Extensor plantar responses, papilloedema, convulsions
Monoplegia or hemiplegia, peripheral neuropathies
Cerebral, cerebellar and mid-brain damage (Parkinsonism, akinetic mutism)
Arrhythmias (ECG changes: atrial fibrillation, prolonged PR interval AV block, bundle branch block, ventricular extrasystoles, prolonged QT interval, ST depression)
Decrease in light sensitivity and dark adaption
Hearing loss (central type)
Acute renal failure
Muscle necrosis
Thrombotic thrombocytopenic purpura
Late neuropsychiatric sequelae

It has been suggested that 5–7 per cent carbon dioxide (CO_2) be added to the inspired oxygen because this further reduces the half-life of elimination of carbon dioxide at one atmosphere (sea level) to about 12 minutes. This effect of carbon dioxide is thought to be due to stimulation of alveolar ventilation and to the development of an acidaemia which promotes dissociation of carboxyhaemoglobin. However, the latter effect exacerbates the acidosis found in severe carbon monoxide poisoning and the use of added carbon dioxide as a routine measure is not recommended.

References

Finck, P. A. (1966). Exposure to carbon monoxide: review of the literature and 567 autopsies. *Milit. Med.* **131**, 1515.
Garland, H. and Pearce, J. (1967). Neurological complications of carbon monoxide poisoning. *Q. Jl Med.* **36**, 445.
Gilbert, G. J. and Glaser, G. H. (1959). Neurologic manifestations of chronic carbon monoxide poisoning. *New Engl. J. Med.* **261**, 1217.
Norman, J. N. and Ledingham, I. McA. (1967). Carbon monoxide poisoning: investigations and treatment. *Prog. Brain. Res.* **24**, 101.
Smith, J. S. and Branden, S. (1973). Morbidity from acute carbon monoxide poisoning at three year follow-up. *Br. med. J.* **i**, 318.

Chlorine

Chlorine gas is commonly used in industry as a reagent and for bleaching cloth and paper, as well as in water purification. It is also a common by-product in chemical plants. Exposure to the gas usually follows a leak from a storage tank and may, therefore, result in a large number of casualties.

The extent of injury from chlorine gas is proportional to the concentration of the gas, the duration of exposure, and the water content of the tissue exposed. Cellular injury is due to the formation of hypochlorous and hydrochloric acid which, together with elemental chlorine and the potent oxidizing effect of nascent oxygen (produced when chlorine and water combine), react with sulphydryl groups and sulphur bonds in proteins. Chlorine gas has been reported to have a cellular toxicity 10–30 times that of hydrochloric acid.

Clinical features. Skin exposure may result in partial or total thickness burns. Conjunctivitis, keratitis, pharyngitis, burning chest pain, coughing, dyspnoea, and haemoptysis (due to bronchiolar constriction and pulmonary oedema) are common. Cardiac arrest may occur secondary to hypoxia.

Treatment. The casualty should be removed from the contaminated environment. (The rescuer may minimize his exposure by using a make-shift gas mask consisting of a water-soaked cloth held to the face). The eyes should be irrigated with copious amounts of saline after topical anaesthesia. A fluorescein stain will indicate the presence or absence of corneal abrasions. Cutaneous burns should be washed with saline and a topical burn cream applied. Bronchodilators and humidified oxygen will alleviate bronchospasm and hypoxia. The use of corticosteroids, diuretics, and antibiotics seems to confer no advantage.

References

Decker, W. J. and Koch, H. F. (1978). Chlorine poisoning at the swimming pool: an overlooked hazard. *Clin. Toxicol.* **13**, 377.
Hedges, J. R. and Morrissey, W. L. (1979). Acute chlorine gas exposure. *J. Am. Coll. Emerg. Phycns* **8**, 59.
National Institute of Occupational Safety and Health (1976). *Criteria for a recommended standard document: chlorine.* US Department of Health, Education, and Welfare, Washington, DC.

Cyanide

Hydrocyanic acid (prussic acid) and its sodium and potassium salts are present in insecticides, rodenticides, metal polishes, electroplating solutions, and fumigant mixtures. In addition, cyanides are used in certain metallurigical processes.

Most deaths from cyanide have been due to suicide or homicide, but some have arisen from accidental exposure in industry, the ingestion of apricot fruit seeds containing cyanogenic glycosides, or the use of 'Laetrile' as a non-approved anticancer agent. 'Laetrile' is a cyanogenic glycoside prepared from the seeds of apricots, prunes, and peaches. Amygdalin is the major cyanogenic constituent which may be cleaved by the gastrointestinal flora to produce the disaccharide gentiobiose, benzaldehyde, and hydrogen cyanide.

Cyanide reversibly inhibits cellular oxidizing enzymes which contain iron in the ferric state, e.g. cytochrome oxidase. This enzyme is the terminal member of the mitochondrial electron transport chain which traps electrons liberated in the tricarboxylic acid cycle and then transfers them to mediate the formation of water from oxygen and hydrogen. In the presence of cyanide, electron transfer is blocked, the tricarboxylic acid cycle is paralysed, and cellular respiration ceases.

The ingestion by an adult of 50 mg of hydrogen cyanide, or 200–500 mg of one of its salts, is likely to prove fatal. The onset of poisoning is hastened by the presence of an empty stomach and high gastric acidity, but symptoms may be delayed for up to four hours if the poison is taken on a full stomach. Inhalation of hydrogen cyanide may produce symptoms within seconds and death within minutes.

Clinical features. Acute poisoning is characterized by dizziness, headache, palpitations, anxiety, a feeling of constriction in the chest, dyspnoea, pulmonary oedema, confusion, vertigo, ataxia, coma, and paralysis. Cardiovascular collapse, respiratory arrest, and metabolic acidosis are seen in severe cases. Cyanosis does not occur and the skin colour may be 'brick-red'. In addition, there is sometimes an odour of bitter almonds on the breath.

Chronic poisoning results predominantly in neurological damage which can include ataxia, peripheral neuropathies, optic atrophy, and nerve deafness. Dermatitis may also occur. Toxic amblyopia associated with heavy cigarette smoking has been attributed to the cyanide content of tobacco.

Treatment. There are five possible approaches to treatment.
Thiosulphate. The principal route to detoxification of cyanide in the body is by conversion to thiocyanate by the enzyme rhodanase. Thiosulphate is required for the conversion of cyanide to thiocyanate and the presence of this substance appears to be the rate-limiting factor for the reaction. Unfortunately, thiosulphate is not

very effective when used alone because it penetrates cell membranes more slowly than cyanide and it is difficult, therefore, to achieve sufficiently high tissue concentrations of the antidote.

Amyl nitrite and sodium nitrite. An alternative and more rapid way of inactivating cyanide is to convert a portion of the body's haemoglobin to methaemoglobin, which contains iron in the ferric rather than the ferrous state. Almost 40 per cent of the haemoglobin in the body may be converted to methaemoglobin without ill-effect. This represents about 300g haemoglogin or 1 g iron, which theoretically can chelate 500 mg of cyanide ion. Inhalation of amyl nitrite has, in the past, been recommended to produce methaemoglobinaemia, but it is poorly tolerated and only low circulating levels of methaemoglobin may be achieved before profound hypotension occurs. Methaemoglobinaemia is best achieved, therefore, by the intravenous administration of sodium nitrite.

Traditionally, a combination of intravenous sodium nitrite and sodium thiosulphate is used in the treatment of cyanide poisoning. Experiments in dogs have shown that the LD_{50} for cyanide may be increased three-fold by sodium thiosulphate alone, five-fold by sodium nitrite alone, and 18-fold by the use of the two antidotes together. In practice, a 3 per cent solution of sodium nitrite (10 ml) and a 50 per cent solution of sodium thiosulphate (25 ml) are given intravenously if there is no response to dicobalt edetate, the preferred antidote.

Dicobalt edetate. Cobalt compounds form stable inert complexes with cyanide (colbalto-cyanides and cobalti-cyanides). Dicobalt edetate (Kelocyanor) is now the treatment of choice for cyanide poisoning and should be given intravenously in a dose of 300–600 mg over one minute, with a further 300 mg if recovery does not occur within one minute. It should be administered only if the diagnosis is certain because, in the absence of cyanide, this drug may cause serious side-effects including vomiting, tachycardia, hypertension, chest pain, and facial and palpebral oedema. These reactions are usually self-limiting.

Oxygen. It is possible to bypass the effect of cyanide poisoning by the administration of oxygen. Experiments in mice using ^{14}C-labelled CO_2, to determine the switch from aerobic to anaerobic metabolism in experimental cyanide poisoning, have shown that oxygen has a synergistic antidotal action when used in combination with sodium thiosulphate and sodium nitrite. The mechanism for this is not known.

Hydroxocobalamin. Hydroxocobalamin could, theoretically, be used in the treatment of cyanide poisoning for a minor route of cyanide metabolism involves the formation of cyanocobalamin (vitamin B_{12}) from hydroxocobalamin. One mole of hydroxocobalamin inactivates one mole of cyanide but, on a weight-for-weight basis, 50 times more hydroxocobalamin is needed than cyanide because hydroxocobalamin is a far larger molecule. Concentrated solutions of hydroxocobalamin are not yet freely available in the United Kingdom and use of the dilute 1 mg/ml solution used in the treatment of pernicious anaemia is not practical.

References

El Gwawabi, S. H., Gaafar, M. A., El-Saharti, A. A., Ahmed, S. H., Malash, K. K., and Fares, R. (1975). Chronic cyanide poisoning: a clinical, radioisotope and laboratory study. *Br. J. industr. Med.* **32**, 215.
Montgomery, R. D. (1979). Cyanogenetic glucosides. In *Handbook of clinical neurology: intoxications of the nervous system.* (eds. P. J. Vinken and G. W. Bruyn), p. 515.
Vogel, S. N., Sultan, T. R., and Ten Eyck, R. P. (1981). Cyanide poisoning. *Clin. Toxicol.* **18**, 367.

Hydrogen sulphide

Hydrogen sulphide is a potential hazard in petroleum refining, the gas industry, tanning, and the chemical industry. It is also found in sewers and mines and it is liberated from decomposing fish—a hazard in fishing boats if the hold is filled with 'trash' fish used for making fishmeal.

Clinical features. Exposure to low concentrations of this substance leads to blephanospasm, pain and redness in the eyes, blurred vision, and coloured haloes round lights. With exposure to higher concentrations, cyanosis, confusion, pulmonary oedema, coma, and convulsions are common. The mortality is in the region of 6 per cent in this group, largely as a result of respiratory arrest.

Treatment. It is thought that the toxicity of hydrogen sulphide is due to inhibition of cytochrome oxidase and, in this respect, it resembles cyanide poisoning (see page 6.32). It has been shown in mice that the efficacy of nitrite (which converts haemoglobin to methaemoglobin) is superior to that of oxygen alone in the treatment of acute hydrogen sulphide poisoning. Hence, it would seem logical to give the casualty an injection of 10 ml of a 3 per cent sodium nitrite solution intravenously over two to three minutes (see treatment of cyanide, page 6.32). Because of the risk of sudden respiratory arrest, it is essential that the rescuer dons breathing apparatus prior to moving the casualty to the fresh air from a heavily contaminated industrial site. If respiratory arrest supervenes, then full cardiopulmonary support should be commenced.

References

Burnett, W. W., King, E. G., Grace, M., and Hall, W. F. (1977). Hydrogen sulfide poisoning: review of five years' experience. *Can. med. Ass. J.* **117**, 1277.
Smith, R. P. and Gosselin, R. E. (1979). Hydrogen sulfide poisoning. *J. occup. Med.* **21**, 93.

POISONING FROM MISCELLANEOUS DRUGS

J. A. Vale and T. J. Meredith

Anticholinergic drugs

Anticholinergic drugs act principally at post-ganglionic cholinergic (parasympathetic) nerve endings but they also block the direct effect of acetylcholine on blood vessels and in the central nervous system. Some anticholinergic drugs have other actions, e.g. an H_1 blocking action. The naturally occurring anticholinergic drugs are alkaloids of the belladonna plants but many semisynthetic compounds, usually quarternary ammonium derivatives, have been developed. In addition, there are a large number of synthetic compounds with structures unrelated to those of the naturally occurring belladonna alkaloids. Some of these compounds block nerve transmission at autonomic ganglia and skeletal neuromuscular junctions, as well as exerting an anticholinergic action.

Infants and young children are particularly susceptible to the belladonna alkaloids. Indeed, poisoning has occurred after conjunctival instillation, systemic absorption occurring from the nasal mucosa after the drug has traversed the nasolacrimal duct. In addition, serious poisoning may follow the accidental ingestion of berries or seeds containing belladonna alkaloids. In recent years, asthma remedies containing stramonium have been abused for their hallucinatory effects.

Clinical features. These are well recognized and include dry mouth, nausea, vomiting, fixed dilated pupils, blurred vision, photophobia, mental confusion, ataxia, excitement, hallucinations, tachycardia, cardiac arrhythmias, hyperpyrexia, urinary urgency, and retention.

Lomotil (atropine plus diphenoxylate) poisoning is an important potential cause of serious poisoning in children in the United Kingdom. The initial clinical features due to atropine are followed by those of diphenoxylate, i.e. cardiorespiratory depression and an impaired level of consciousness. (Naloxone should be given to reverse the effects of diphenoxylate, see page 6.19.)

Treatment. In addition to gastric lavage or emesis, if appropriate, and the use of supportive measures, physostigmine may rarely be indicated. However, it is itself toxic and it has the further disadvantage of possessing a very short duration of action (see page 6.22 for a fuller discussion).

References

Penfold, D. and Volans, G. N. (1977). Overdose from Lomotil. *Br. med. J.* **ii**, 1401.
Welbourn, R. B. and Buxton, J. D. (1948). Acute atropine poisoning: Review of eight cases. *Lancet* **ii**, 211.

Hypoglycaemic agents

Intentional overdose with hypoglycaemic agents is uncommon and is often difficult to recognize. Despite the massive doses of insulin frequently associated with intentional poisoning, the degree of hypoglycaemia is sometimes surprisingly mild, though it may persist for several days.

Of 16 patients reported in the literature who deliberately ingested a sulphonylurea drug, six died. Chlorpropamide has been the agent most commonly ingested and, because of its long half-life, it may, in overdose, induce hypoglycaemia for a considerable period of time.

In all cases of poisoning with hypoglycaemic agents, prompt diagnosis and treatment is essential if death or cerebral damage from neuroglycopenia is to be prevented.

Clinical features. In overdose, these may include nausea and vomiting, abdominal pain, haematemesis and melaena (rarely), drowsiness, coma, twitching, convulsions, depressed limb reflexes, extensor plantar responses, hyperpnoea, pulmonary oedema, tachycardia and circulatory failure. Hypoglycaemia, hyperkalaemia, and metabolic acidosis may also occur. Cholestatic jaundice has been described as a late complication of chlorpropamide poisoning.

Treatment. If the patient presents early, and is not hypoglycaemic, after the ingestion of an oral preparation, gastric lavage should be performed. In addition to intravenous glucose (50 ml of 50 per cent), glucagon 1–2 mg intravenously may be given to correct the hypoglycaemia. A continuous infusion of glucose will be required in severe cases.

Reference

Selzer, R. S. (1972). Drug-induced hypoglycaemia – a review based on 473 cases. *Diabetes* **21**, 955.

Iron

Acute iron poisoning was once a common cause of severe poisoning and death in young children. An increased awareness of the potential seriousness of the problem, changes in the forms of packaging, and use of the chelating agent, desferrioxamine, have together resulted in a decline in the mortality from acute iron poisoning. Indeed, in the 12-year period, 1968 to 1979, only 10 deaths were officially attributed in the United Kingdom to the ingestion of iron preparations by children under 15 years of age. Even so, iron poisoning is extremely dangerous, especially in young children, and particularly when more than 150 mg/kg body weight is ingested. The absorbed iron rapidly exceeds the binding capacity of transferrin and free serum iron accumulates.

Clinical features. Epigastric pain, nausea, vomiting, and haematemesis may all occur within several hours of ingesting iron, complicated by circulatory collapse if the haematemesis is severe. Subsequently, black tarry stools may be passed and any one, or all, of the following complications may develop: acute encephalopathy (headache, confusion, convulsions, and coma), cyanosis and pulmonary oedema, metabolic acidosis, acute renal failure, circulatory collapse, and death. If the patient survives, then hepatic necrosis may develop sometimes proceeding to hepatic coma and death. Late development of pyloric stenosis has been described in a few patients following recovery from severe iron poisoning. Severe poisoning is indicated by serum levels in excess of 90 μmol/l (5 mg/l) in a child and 145 μmol/l (8 mg/l) in an adult.

Treatment. Desferrioxamine mesylate (Desferal) should be given as follows in the treatment of acute iron poisoning. Firstly, 2 g of desferrioxamine (in 10 ml sterile water) should be injected intramuscularly. Gastric aspiration and lavage should then be performed using a solution of 2 g desferrioxamine in each litre of warm water; when this procedure has been completed 5 g of desferrioxamine (in 50–100 ml water) should be left in the stomach. Following this, either a slow infusion of desferrioxamine should be administered at a rate not exceeding 15 mg/kg body weight/hour (maximum 80 mg/kg body weight in 24 hours), or further intramuscular injections (2 g in 10 ml sterile water) should be given at 12-hourly intervals.

The patient's progress should be checked with the aid of serial serum iron determinations. The effectiveness of treatment is dependent on an adequate urine output in order that the chelate, ferrioxamine, is excreted from the body. Therefore, if oliguria or anuria develop, peritoneal dialysis or haemodialysis may become necessary to remove the ferrioxamine complex.

References

Barr, G. D. B. and Fraser, D. K. B. (1968). Acute iron poisoning in children: role of chelating agents. *Br. med. J.* i, 737.

Greengard, J. (1975). Iron poisoning in children. *Clin. Toxicol.* **8**, 575.

Robertson, W. O. (1970). Treatment of acute iron poisoning. *Med. Treatment* **8**, 552.

Whitten, C. F. and Brough, A. J. (1971). The pathophysiology of acute iron poisoning. *Clin. Toxicol.* **4**, 585.

Metoclopramide

Metoclopramide, a chlorbenzamide derivative, is used as an antiemetic agent. Extrapyramidal side-effects have been reported in children receiving the 'recommended dose' and in those who have taken the drug in excess.

Clinical features. Drowsiness, nausea, and tachycardia may occur prior to the development of more alarming extrapyramidal signs, which include opisthotonos, torticollis, increased muscle tone, oculogyric crises, facial grimacing, conjugate deviation of the eyes, diplopia, trismus, nystagmus, and rhythmic protrusion of the tongue. Rarely, these features may be followed or accompanied by agitation, anxiety, oedema of the tongue and periorbital oedema.

Treatment. In addition to measures to prevent absorption, if these are appropriate, benztropine in an adult, 1–2 mg given intravenously should be given if extrapyramidal features are present.

Reference

Low, L. C. K. and Goel, K. M. (1980). Metoclopramide poisoning in children. *Archs Dis. Child.* **55**, 310.

Non-catecholamine sympathomimetic drugs

Amphetamine. Amphetamines are readily absorbed both from the gastrointestinal tract and from parenteral sites. Excretion is pH-dependent and is increased considerably if the urine is acid; about 50 per cent of an administered dose may be recovered in the urine as unchanged drug.

Clinical features. In overdose, these may include restlessness, tremor, irritability, insomnia, dryness of the mouth, nausea, vomiting, diarrhoea, abdominal pain, flushing, sweating, hyperpyrexia, cardiac arrhythmias, marked hypertension, tachypnoea, circulatory collapse, delirium, hallucinations, coma, and convulsions.

Treatment. In the majority of cases supportive treatment and the use of chlorpromazine 50–100 mg intravenously, or droperidol 5–15 mg intravenously, in an adult is all that is required. Only rarely is it appropriate or necessary to use forced acid diuresis (see page 6.9).

Pemoline. Pemoline is a central nervous system stimulant drug which is structurally different from the amphetamines though pharmacologically similar.

Clinical features. As for amphetamine poisoning. In addition, frequent sucking movements of the tongue and choreiform movements have been described.

Treatment. As for amphetamine except that there is no evidence that forced acid diuresis is effective.

Ephedrine. Ephedrine differs from adrenaline (epinephrine) in several respects. It has a much longer duration and exerts more pronounced central effects, although it is of lower potency. The cardiovascular effects are similar to those of adrenaline but persist for much longer, whereas bronchial muscle relaxation is less prominent than with adrenaline.

Clinical features. These may include nausea, vomiting, irritability, fever, tachycardia, sweating, praecordial pain, palpitations, dilated pupils, blurred vision, paranoid psychosis, delusions and hallucinations (auditory and visual), convulsions and coma, respiratory depression, and hypertension.

Treatment. Supportive measures provide the cornerstone of treatment. Gastric lavage should be performed if the patient presents early after a substantial overdose. A cardioselective beta-adrenergic blocking drug should be given if a supraventricular tachycardia supervenes.

Fenfluramine is rapidly and completely absorbed after the oral administration of therapeutic doses in man. Eighty per cent is excreted within 48 hours and elimination is complete 72 hours after ingestion. Excretion is considerably higher when the urine is acid.

Clinical features. In acute overdosage, the clinical features are similar to those of amphetamine: excitability, restlessness, sweating, hyperpyrexia, redness of the face, mydriasis, sluggish or absent pupillary reaction to light, nystagmus, tachycardia, tachypnoea, hyper-reflexia, tremor, clonus, convulsions, and coma. In a recent review of 53 cases of fenfluramine poisoning there was a 20 per cent mortality (10 patients). In nine out of 10 patients who died, cardiac arrest occurred one to four hours after ingestion. None of the surviving patients developed major symptoms later than four hours after ingestion.

Treatment. Activated charcoal adsorbs fenfluramine and may be left in the stomach after gastric lavage has been performed. Supportive measures are required in those severely poisoned. Although forced acid diuresis may enhance renal elimination, the amount recovered in the urine is often disappointing. Diazepam, 5–10 mg intravenously, should be given for convulsions, excitability, and restlessness. Chlorpromazine may be used if marked hyperthermia occurs, though this drug should be avoided in patients who are convulsing.

References

David, T. and Vale, J. A. (1981). Pemoline poisoning. *Archs Toxicol.* **48**, 205.

Espelin, D. E. and Done, A. K. (1968). Amphetamine poisoning: effectiveness of chlorpromazine. *New Engl. J. Med.* **278**, 1361.

Gary, N. E. and Saidi, P. (1978). Methamphetamine intoxication: a speedy new treatment. *Am. J. Med.* **64**, 537.

Smith, D. E. and Fischer, C. M. (1970). An analysis of 310 cases of acute high-dose methamphetamine toxicity in Haight-Ashbury. *Clin. Toxicol.* **3**, 117.

Von Muhlendahl, K. E. and Kreinke, E. G. (1979). Fenfluramine poisoning. *Clin. Toxicol.* **14**, 97.

Phencyclidine

The illicit use of phencyclidine ('angel dust') was first described in the United States in 1967, a decade after the product had been withdrawn as a general anaesthetic because of post-operative psychotic reactions. Phencyclidine abuse has not been reported in the United Kingdom and it is rare in Western Europe. Phencyclidine may be 'snorted' (nasal inhalation), smoked with either parsley or marijuana, ingested, or injected.

Clinical features. In significant overdose, phencyclidine gives rise to agitation, confusion, blurred vision, nystagmus, tremor, hyper-reflexia, muscle rigidity, ataxia, opisthotonos, acute dystonia, hallucinations, coma and convulsions. Hypertension, cardiac arrhythmias, and increased bronchial and salivary secretion are seen frequently. Rhabdomyolysis and acute renal failure are uncommon complications.

Treatment. Gastric lavage, if appropriate, followed by oral activated charcoal will reduce absorption. Supportive measures and careful nursing care to prevent self-injury are the most important aspects of treatment. Forced acid diuresis increases renal elimination of phencyclidine quite markedly.

References

Burns, R. S. and Lerner, S. E. (1976). Perspectives: acute phencyclidine intoxication. *Clin. Toxicol.* **9**, 477.
Done, A., Aronow, R., Miceli, J., and Cohen, S. (1979). Pharmacokinetic bases for the treatment of phencyclidine (PCP) intoxication. *Vet. hum. Toxicol.* **21**, suppl. 104.
Liden, C. B., Lovejoy, F. H., Jr, and Costello, C. E. (1975). Phencyclidine: nine cases of poisoning. *J. Am. med. Ass.* **234**, 513.

Sioris, L. J. and Krenzelok, E. P. (1978). Phencyclidine intoxication: a literature review. *Am J. hosp. Pharmac.* **35**, 1362.

Rifampicin

Poisoning with the antibiotic rifampicin results in the so-called 'red man syndrome', which can be fatal. The skin, and subsequently the sclera, become yellow/orange in colour. The skin discolouration may be removed by washing with water. Nausea, vomiting, abdominal pain, pruritus, and convulsions have been reported in the few cases of overdose so far described. Sudden death following a cardiorespiratory arrest has also been recorded in two patients.

Treatment is supportive and symptomatic and should be preceded by gastric lavage when appropriate.

References

Broadwell, R. O. and Broadwell, S. D. (1978). Suicide by rifampin overdose. *J. Am med. Ass.* **240**, 2283.
Plomp, T. A., Battista, H. J., Underdorfer, H., van Ditmarsh, W. C., and Maes, R. A. A. (1981). A case of fatal poisoning by rifampicin. *Archs Toxicol.* **48**, 245.

Venoms and toxins of animals and plants

INJURIES, ENVENOMING, POISONING, AND ALLERGIC REACTIONS CAUSED BY ANIMALS

D. A. Warrell

MECHANICAL TRAUMA: ATTACKS BY LARGE ANIMALS

In those rapidly dwindling areas of the world that can still support populations of large wild animals, attacks on man are occasionally reported. Mammals that have killed or severely mauled humans include lion, tiger, leopard, hyena, bear, elephant, hippopotamus, buffalo, wolf, and wild pig. There are about 100 shark attacks reported each year, 50 of them fatal. Most occur between latitudes 30° North and 30° South. Other fish capable of causing severe mechanical trauma are barracuda, Moray and conger eels, garfish, and gropers. Crocodiles are responsible for about 1000 deaths per year in Africa (*Crocodilus nilus*): in Asia the most important species is the salt water crocodile (*C. porosus*). There are well-authenticated reports of attacks and fatalities caused by giant pythons: *P. reticulatus* in Indonesia, and *P. sebae* in Africa.

In the more developed countries, attacks by animals, are, if anything, more common than in the tropics. Domestic species, particularly dogs, bite, maim, and occasionally kill. In Los Angeles, USA, the incidence of animal bites was 664 per 100 000 population in 1956. It is estimated that about 600 000 people are bitten by dogs each year in the United States. In Israel the incidence of bites was 447 per 100 000 population. In Canberra, Australia 184 children per 100 000 attended hospital after dog bites in 1977–8, and in two cities in the north of England the incidence of bites was about 500 per 100 000 population. In Britain there were 701 injuries and 10 deaths attributed to animals in 1975. Reports of 11 deaths from dog bite were collected in a two-year period in the United States. Deaths have also been caused by domestic cattle, sheep, pigs, and even ferrets.

Clinical features. Teeth, tusks, claws, and horns produce lacerating, penetrating, and crushing injuries. Severe facial and eye injuries are common, and pneumothorax, haemothorax, bowel perforation, and compound fractures are also recorded. There is a high risk of secondary infection with the wide range of micro-organisms including anaerobic bacteria (*Clostridium tetani, Clostridium perfringens*, etc.), for teeth and claws may be contaminated with rotting meat. Large bovines may trample and kneel on the victim, producing severe crush injuries.

Treatment. Emergency surgery may be required with replacement of blood loss and attention to local mechanical complications such as tension pneumothorax. Infection should be prevented with a combination of a penicillin, aminoglycoside (such as gentamicin), and metronidazole in the case of major contaminated wounds. Tetanus and rabies prophylaxis must be considered. Other animal bite pathogens are listed in the discussion of rabies (see Section 5).

References

Bass, P. G. (1982). Injuries caused by garfish in Papua New Guinea. *Br. med. J.* **284**, 77.
Caras, R. A. (1975). *Dangerous to man.* Holt, Rinehart and Winston, New York.
Castle, W. M. (1971). A survey of deaths in Rhodesia caused by animals. *Central African J. Med.* **17**, 165.
Coppleson, V. M. (1958). *Shark Attack.* Angus and Robertson, Sydney.
Karcola, K., Möttönen, M., and Raekallio, J. (1973). Deaths caused by animals in Finland. *Med. Sci. Law* **13**, 95.
Shattock, F. M. (1968). Injuries caused by wild animals. *Lancet* i, 412.

VENOMOUS ANIMALS

For predation or defence, some animals elaborate venoms which are injected into the prey or enemy through fangs, stings, spines, hairs, nematocysts, or other specialized venom organs, or squirted on to absorbent mucous membranes by spitting snakes, scorpions, and millipedes. As well as suffering direct effects of envenoming, humans may become sensitized to specific venoms and suffer allergic reactions. Although widely distributed throughout the animal kingdom, venoms of only the following are of real medical importance: fish, snakes, lizards, coelenterates, molluscs, sea urchins, insects, spiders, scorpions, centipedes, millipedes, and ticks.

Snakes

Fewer than half of the species belonging to the three venomous families *Viperidae*, *Elapidae*, and *Hydrophiidae* have been responsible for clinically severe envenoming ending in death or permanent disability. Recently a number or species from a fourth family, the *Colubridae*, usually regarded as non-venomous, have produced severe symptoms or death. The distinction between venomous and non-venomous species is ill defined. Bites by any snake should be avoided, and patients bitten by any species should be carefully assessed.

Distribution of venomous snakes. Venomous snakes are distributed throughout warm continents and oceans except at altitudes above 3000 meters, in the Antarctic, in a number of islands such as Ireland, Iceland, New Zealand, Madagascar, and most islands of the Caribbean and Pacific. The adder, *Vipera berus*, occurs within the Arctic Circle. Sea snakes occur in warmer oceans.

Classification. Medically important snakes always possess one or more pairs of fangs in the upper jaw, which penetrate the skin of their victim and conduct venom into the tissues through a venom channel.

Colubridae. The short fangs are at the back of the mouth. Most of the common and familiar non-venomous species belong to this large family, for example the British grass snake and smooth snake. Two African species, the boomslang (*Dispholidus typus*) and vine, twig, or bird snake (*Thelotornis kirtlandi*), and the Japanese yamakagashi (*Rhabdophis tigrinus*) have been responsible for the deaths of a few people who handled them carelessly. A number of other species have caused envenoming. Two species of African burrowing snake, formerly regarded as vipers, *Atractaspis microlepidota* and *A. irregularis*, have caused human deaths, and a number of other species have been responsible for severe envenoming.

Elapidae. Includes cobras, kraits, mambas, and coral snakes, which have short fixed anterior fangs. Three African and one Asian species (the ringhals and spitting cobras) are able to eject their venom from the tips of the fangs as a fine spray for a distance of several metres into the eyes of an aggressor.

Hydrophiidae. Includes all the medically important sea snakes and the Australian venomous snakes. The anterior fangs are short and fixed.

Viperidae. The anterior fangs are very long, curved, and capable of a wide range of movement. Members of the sub-family *Crotalinae*, the New World rattlesnakes, moccasins, and lance-headed vipers, and Asian pit vipers, possess a heat sensitive pit organ behind the nostril.

Incidence and importance of snake bites. Snake bite is a neglected problem of the rural tropics; its incidence is usually underestimated because of the paucity of epidemiological data. In India and Pakistan, 22 480 people (10.3 per 100 000 population) and 3793 cattle died from snake bite in 1889; during the last few years more than a thousand people have died of snake bite each year in Maharashtra State alone. The most important species in India are cobra (*Naja naja*), saw-scaled viper (*Echis carinatus*), Russell's viper (*Vipera russelli*), and common krait (*Bungarus caeruleus*). In Burma, Russell's viper is the most important species. There were about 2000 human deaths per year during the 1930s: in Sagaing District near Mandalay the annual mortality was 37 per 100 000. In Brazil there are at least 2000 deaths per year, and in Venezuela about 1000 bites occur each year with 100 deaths. The Fer de Lance (*Bothrops atrox*) and rattlesnake (*Crotalus durissus*) are responsible for most of the cases. In the Amami and Okinawa Islands of Japan the habu (*Trimeresurus flavoviridis*) inflicted an average of 610 bites with 5.6 deaths per year during the 1960s. In Africa the saw-scaled or carpet viper (*Echis carinatus*), puff adder (*Bitis arietans*), and spitting cobra (*Naja nigricollis*) are the most important species. In the Benue Valley of Northeastern Nigeria *E. carinatus* causes some 947 bites per 100 000 population per year with a 12.2 per cent mortality, and in Northern Ghana the same species is responsible for 86 bites per 100 000 population with a 28 per cent mortality. *E. carinatus*, whose geographical range extends from West Africa to India,

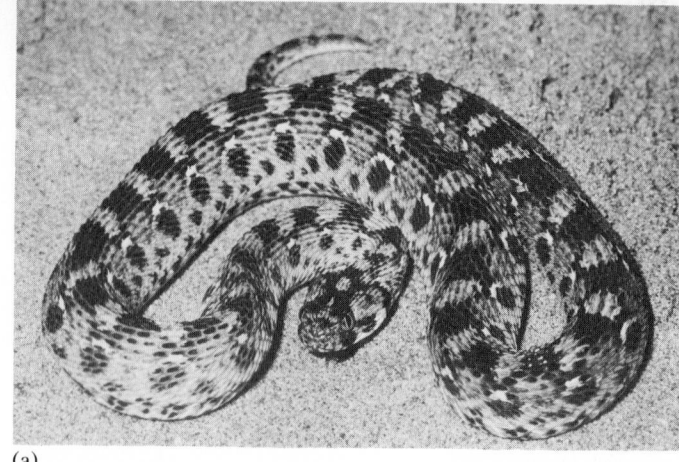

(a)

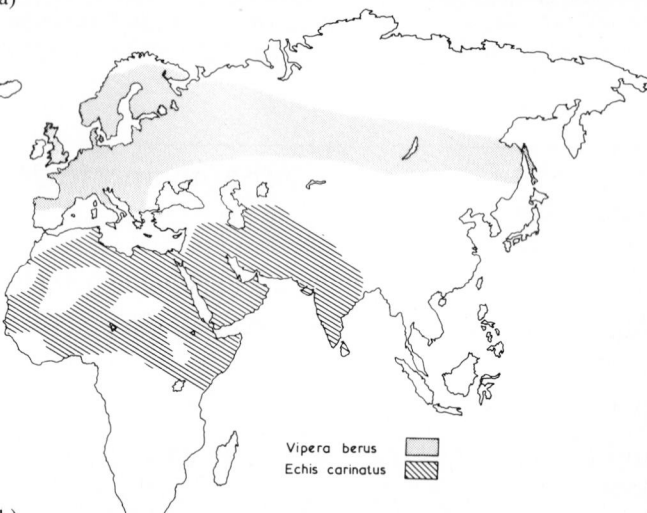

(b)

Fig. 1 The saw-scaled or carpet viper (*Echis carinatus*) which probably accounts for more snake bite morbidity and mortality than any other species. (a) Threatening posture: the coils are rubbed together producing a rasping sound which is often the last thing patients hear before they are bitten. (b) World distribution of *E. carinatus* compared with that of the European adder or viper (*Vipera berus*) which also occurs in Korea.

probably bites and kills more people than any other species of snake (Fig. 1).

The highest snake bite mortalities are suffered by hunter gatherer tribes of Venezuela, Equador, Tanzania, and Papua New Guinea: 2–4 per cent of adult deaths may be attributable to snakes.

In the United States of America there are approximately 45 000 bites per year, 7000 of which are caused by venomous species, with 9–14 deaths per year. The most important species are rattlesnakes (genus *Crotalus*), cottonmouths (*Agkistrodon piscivorus*) and copperheads (*Ag. contortrix*). Most of the fatalities are caused by the Eastern and Western diamond-back rattlesnakes (*Crotalus adamanteus* and *Cr. atrox*). In Britain, the adder or viper (*Vipera berus*) is the only venomous species. More than 100 people are bitten each year but only 14 deaths have been reported during the last 100 years. In Finland this species caused 21 deaths in 25 years with an annual incidence of bites approaching 200.

Epidemiology. Most snake bites occur on the lower limbs of farmers, herdsmen, and hunters in the rural tropics. Often the snake is trodden on at night. Some species such as the Asiatic kraits (*Bungarus*) and African spitting cobra (*Naja nigricollis*) live in and around houses and bite people who are asleep. Snakes do not bite without provocation though this may be an inadvertent tread or touch. In Europe and North America snakes are becoming popular pets: most bites occur on the hands when the snake is picked up. In the USA 25 per cent of bites result from snakes being attacked or handled. Serious bites by back-fanged (colubrid) snakes have occurred only under these conditions. A marked seasonal variation in the incidence of snake bite is usually attributed to changes in farming activity in relationship to seasonal rainfall and to the yearly reproductive cycle of the snake. Severe flooding, by flushing out and concentrating the snake population, has given rise to epidemics of snake bite in Pakistan and India. Development of jungle areas for new highways and irrigation or hydroelectric schemes resulted in epidemics of snake bite in Brazil and Sri Lanka. On rare occasions snake bite or injection of snake venom have been used as a means of suicide.

Venom apparatus. The venom glands lie behind the eye surrounded by compressor muscles (Fig. 2). A venom duct opens within a sheath at the base of the fang, and venom is conducted towards the tip in a fang canal. The quantity of venom injected at a strike is highly variable, and a proportion of bitten patients will suffer negligible envenoming. In species such as the Malayan pit viper (*Calloselasma* (*Ankistrodon*) *rhodostoma*) more than half of those bitten show only trivial effects. The snake uses only a fraction of the content of its venom gland at each strike, and there is no support for the popular belief that snakes are less dangerous after they have eaten.

Venom properties. Snake venoms consist mainly of protein in the form of peptide toxins, non-toxic protein, and enzymes. Metals such as zinc are associated with enzymes such as ecarin, the procoagulant enzyme of *Echis carinatus* venom. Carbohydrate is present in glycoproteins such as Arvin/Ancrod, the procoagulant of *Calloselasma rhodostoma* venom which has been used to treat thrombotic disorders. Snake venoms are a rich source of enzymes: the activity of phospholipase A2 (lecithinase) may contribute to toxic effects such as neurotoxicity, cardiotoxicity, haemolysis, and lethality. The bright yellow colour of some viper venoms is due to L-amino acid oxidase.

Polypeptide toxins (neurotoxins). The unique components of snake venoms are the polypeptide toxins. Their amino acid sequence, and three-dimensional structure and its relationship to toxicity has been established in many cases (Fig. 3).

Pharmacological effects. The toxic polypeptides of *Elapidae* and *Hydrophiidae* are relatively small molecules which are absorbed rapidly into the blood stream, whereas the much larger molecules

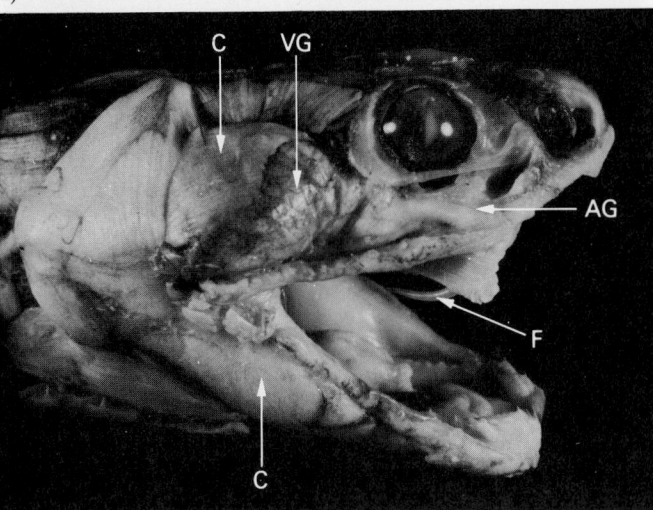

(a)

(b)

Fig. 2   Venom apparatus of viperine and crotaline snakes. (a) Venom gland of Palestine viper (*Vipera xanthina palaestinae*) (b) Venom gland of Western rattlesnake (*Crotalus viridis*). C = compressor glandulae muscle; VG = venom gland; AG = accessory glands; F = fang. (Dissection by Professor E. Kochva, reproduced from Gans, C. and Gans, K. A. (eds.) (1978). *Biology of the reptilia*, vol. 8. Academic Press, London, by permission.)

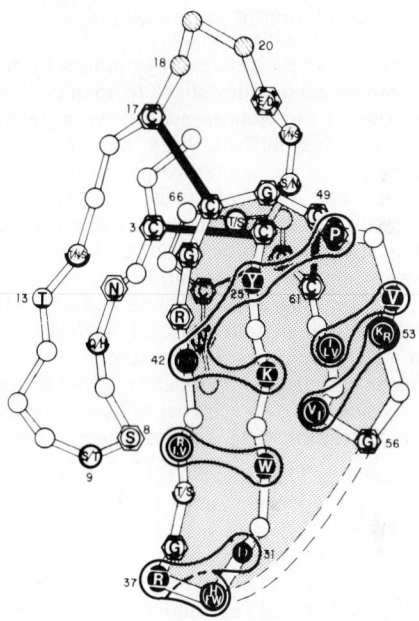

Fig. 3   Three-dimensional structure of the post-synaptic neurotoxin erabutoxin b from the venom of the sea snake *Laticuada semifasciata*.

View of the structure of the erabutoxin b molecule, looking down into the concavity of the reactive site region, which is shown cross-hatched. The reactive site is shaped like a cupped hand. Turn the page upside-down and compare the drawing with your cupped left hand where the thumb forms a loop touching the index finger and this loop is almost at right angles (vertical) to a second loop formed by joining the two middle fingers at their extremities. Thus, the thumb corresponds to the peptide chain region 49–56, and the two middle fingers correspond to the peptide chain region 25–44. The features of this region are presented as prototype for both long and short chain toxins. Within the cross-hatched region are thirteen residues which appear to be involved in toxin–receptor binding interactions. These residues, all of which are pointing upwards from the concavity toward the reader, are identified by one-letter codes. They are either: (a) invariant in both series, for example, R37 (arginine) and D31 (aspartic acid) or (b) conservatively substituted hydrophobic residues, for example, I L V 59 (isoleucine, leucine, and valine). There are close interactions between certain of these residues, e.g. the distance between the quarternary nitrogen of Arg37 and the carbonyl of Asp31 mimics that in acetylcholine.

The reactive site may, therefore, be divided into five functional groupings as indicated in the heavy contoured outlines; alternatively, the whole site may be considered as one continuous region. (By courtesy of Professor Barbara W. Low, Modified from Low, B. W. (1979). In *Advances in cytopharmacology* (ed. B. Ceccarelli and F. Clementi), Vol. 3, p. 141. New York.)

of *Viperidae* venoms are taken up more slowly through lymphatics. Presynaptic neurotoxins such as beta bungarotoxin found in the venom of some kraits (genus *Bungarus*) have an action similar to botulinus toxin, interfering with the release of acetylcholine at the neuro-muscular junction. Post-synaptic neurotoxins such as alpha bungarotoxin bind specifically and irreversibly to acetylcholine receptors on the motor end plate. The lethal effect of these neuro-toxins is respiratory paralysis. Cardiotoxin, originally isolated from Indian cobra (*Naja naja*) venom damages cell membranes including those of cardiac muscle. *In vitro* haemolysis was one of the earliest and most widely studied of venom activities but it is rarely of significance in human envenoming. Haemorrhagin activity is found in a number of *Viperidae* venoms. It causes spontaneous haemor-rhage by opening up endothelial junctions of small blood vessels or creating holes in these cells (Fig. 4). Defibrination and associated platelet abnormalities are rarely responsible for spontaneous haemorrhage in the absence of haemorrhagin. The cause of local swelling, blistering, and necrosis, which is such a prominent feature of envenoming by *Viperidae* and some cobras, is a cytotoxic venom component. Autopharmacological effects of venoms, mainly of *Viperidae*, include the release and potentiation of bradykinin, his-tamine, 5-hydroxytryptamine, and adenosine triphosphate from platelets, and the inhibition of angiotensinase.

Clinical features. Fear is a dominant symptom in many cases of snake bite. Physiological manifestations of anxiety, and even frank hysteria, may confuse the clinical picture. Even patients who are not envenomed may feel flushed, dizzy, and breathless with con-striction of the chest, and may notice palpitations, sweating and acroparaesthesiae. The terror of snake bite may even precipitate angina pectoris, myocardial infarction, or a cardiac arrhythmia. The evolution of signs of envenoming depends on the nature of the venom, the dose, and the site of injection. Pain is usually felt immediately, swelling may start in a few minutes, total defibrin-ation can develop in half an hour and fatal respiratory paralysis has occurred within 20–30 minutes. It is extremely unusual, however, for death to occur earlier than hours after elapid or sea snake bite and days after viper bite. The clinical effects of envenoming are considered here in relationship to the main types of venom activity.

Cytotoxic envenoming. This is characteristic of bites by the *Viper-idae* including the pit vipers subfamily *Crotalinae*, and cobras such as *Naja nigricollis* and *N. mossambica* in Africa and *N. naja* in Asia. Tender swelling spreads from the site of the bite and there is early tender enlargement of lymph nodes draining the bitten area. With-in a few hours bullae may appear under the epidermis filled with serosanguinous fluid. With elapid bites, blistering is usually fol-lowed by superficial tissue necrosis, whereas bullae caused by *Viperidae* bites may dry up and slough without the development of necrosis (Fig. 5). A pale, anaesthetic, demarcated area of skin with a characteristic odour of putrefaction indicates necrosis. Necrotic tissue is susceptible to secondary infection by bacteria including anaerobes. Occlusion of major blood vessels in tensely swollen limbs could result from compression in fascial compartments, such as the anterior tibial compartment; or thrombosis due to high local concentrations of venom procoagulant. It may be difficult to di-agnose vascular occlusion in an oedematous limb which feels cold and in which pulses are impalpable. Measurement of interstitial fluid pressure has been advocated as an aid to the diagnosis of compartmental syndrome. An important result of massive swelling of the bitten limb is loss of circulating volume: a swollen limb can accommodate several litres of blood. The result may be hypotension due to hypovolaemia.

Procoagulant and haemorrhagin. This combination is characteristic of vipers such as *Vipera russelli* and *Echis carinatus*, pit vipers such as *Calloselasma rhodostoma*, *Crotalus viridis*, and *Bothrops* spe-cies, and some Australian snakes such as *Notechis scutatus*, *Oxy-uranus scutellatus* and *Tropidechis carinatus*. Spontaneous bleeding is most frequently detected in the gingival sulci (Fig. 6). The most

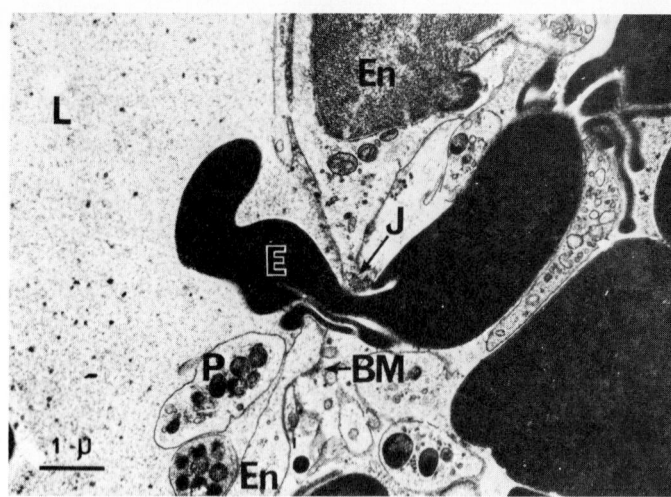

Fig. 4 Haemorrhagin activity. An erythrocyte (E) spurting through an open endothelial junction (J) between endothelial cells (En) from the lumen (L) of a rat mesenteric blood vessel, five minutes after exposure to habu (*Trimeresurus flavoviridis*) venom. Note extensive destruction of the basement membrane (BM), and failure of the platelet (P) to undergo viscous metamorphosis. (Courtesy of Dr. A. Ohsaka and Academic Press, from Ohsaka, A., Suzuki, K., and Ohashi, M., 1975. *Microvasc. Res.* **10**, 208.)

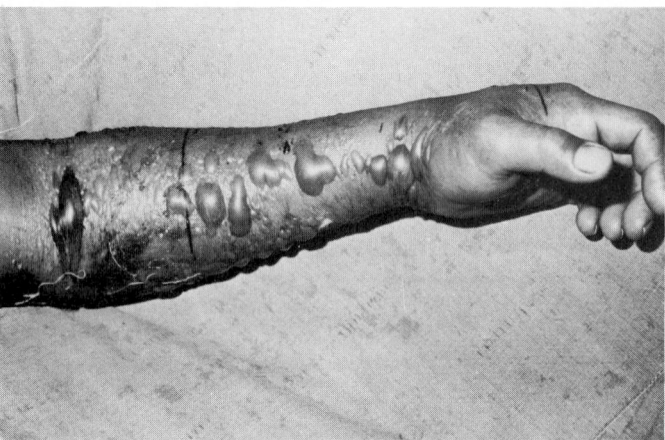

Fig. 5 Extensive cytotoxic effects of a bite on the wrist by the Malayan pit viper *Calloselasma rhodostoma*. The patient was treated with antivenom. The blisters eventually sloughed off without necrosis of underlying tissues.

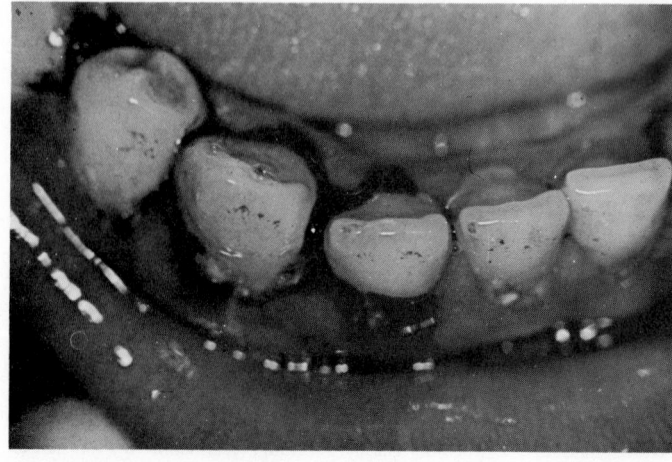

Fig. 6 Haemorrhagin activity. Bleeding from gingival sulci in a patient bitten by *Echis carinatus*.

dangerous forms of haemorrhage are intracerebral, gastrointestinal, and retroperitoneal.

Cardiotoxicity. Cardiac arrhythmias, ECG abnormalities, and hypotension which responds rapidly to intravenous antivenom is the clinical picture of cardiotoxicity. This is seen particularly in *Viperidae* envenoming, for example by the adder *Vipera berus*, puff adder *Bitis arietans*, Malayan pit viper *Calloselasma rhodostoma*, and diamond-back rattlesnakes *Crotalus adamanteus* and *Cr. atrox*. Patients with severe neurotoxic envenoming by elapids sometimes die a cardiac death even though their respiration is adequately supported.

Neurotoxicity. This is a feature of envenoming by elapids, Australian snakes, sea snakes, and a few of the *Viperidae* such as the Mojave rattlesnake (*Cr. scutulatus*), South American rattlesnake (*Cr. durissus terrificus*), and berg adder (*Bitis atropos*). Typically, neurotoxic symptoms develop within one or two hours. The extra-ocular muscles seem to be most sensitive to neuromuscular blockade by the neurotoxin and in some patients the only feature of envenoming is ptosis and ophthalmoplegia (Fig. 7). More serious effects are dysphagia, dysphonia, and paralysis of muscles of deglutition and respiration. Impaired consciousness is sometimes wrongly inferred from closed eyes due to ptosis or exhaustion, but coma and convulsions do occur: cerebral hypoxia resulting from respiratory or circulatory failure may contribute. Neurotoxicity is completely reversible: in some cases acutely in response to specific antivenom or anticholinesterase, in others slowly and spontaneously.

Myotoxicity. The neurotoxins of some *Hydrophiidae* (sea snakes and Australian venomous snakes) cause negligible local reaction at the site of the bite but systemic rhabdomyolysis. The symptoms are muscle pain and stiffness with trismus and respiratory muscle paralysis. Myoglobinuria and hyperkalaemia may result.

Nephrotoxicity. Most snake venoms are concentrated and excreted by the kidney. Some venoms appear to have a direct nephrotoxic effect: vasculitis of the glomerular capillaries, interstitial glomerulonephritis, and tubular damage. More often acute renal failure is a result of acute tubular necrosis secondary to haemorrhagic shock. Complete defibrination, for example by the carpet viper *Echis carinatus*, can occur without any disturbance of renal function, but envenoming by some species has been associated with fibrin deposition in the glomerular capillaries. Myoglobinuria and haemoglobinuria damage the kidney only if the urine is acid, but the associated hyperkalaemia in sea snake bites may cause renal dysfunction. Antivenom may cause immune complex nephritis as part of the late reaction occurring seven days or more after treatment.

Autopharmacological effects and venom hypersensitivity reactions. Patients bitten by a few species—*Vipera berus*, *V. xanthina palaestinae*, *Atractaspis engaddensis*, and some Australian snakes—may develop angioneurotic oedema, diarrhoea, abdominal colic, and anaphylactic shock very soon after the bite. This is thought to be the result of autopharmacological release by the injected venom of vasoactive amines. Laboratory workers who handle venom are prone to become sensitized and may develop conjunctivitis, rhinitis, asthma, and dermatitis on exposure.

Venom ophthalmia caused by spitting cobras. The ringhals (*Hemachatus haemachatus*) and spitting cobras (*N. nigricollis* and *N. mossambica*) of Africa, and some populations of Asian cobra *N. naja*, can eject venom in a fine stream. If the venom enters the eye, there is intense conjunctivitis. Since most patients make an uneventful recovery these injuries used to be thought trivial; but the slit lamp reveals corneal erosions in a large proportion of cases. There is a risk of secondary infection as with any corneal injuries

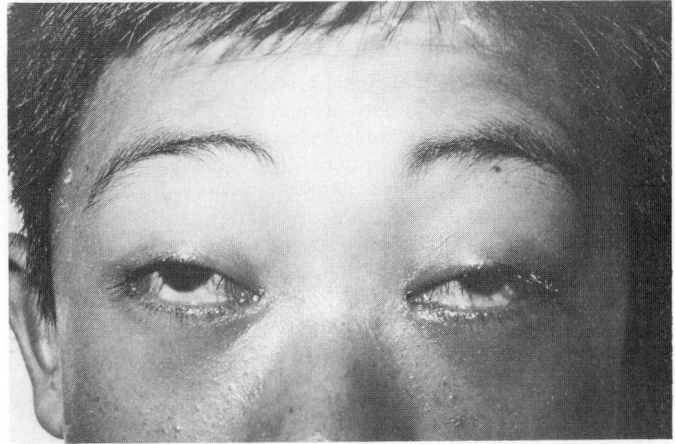

Fig. 7 Severe neurotoxic envenoming by the Malayan krait (*Bungarus candidus*). The patient, who required artificial ventilation for 48 hours, is attempting to look upwards. Note ptosis.

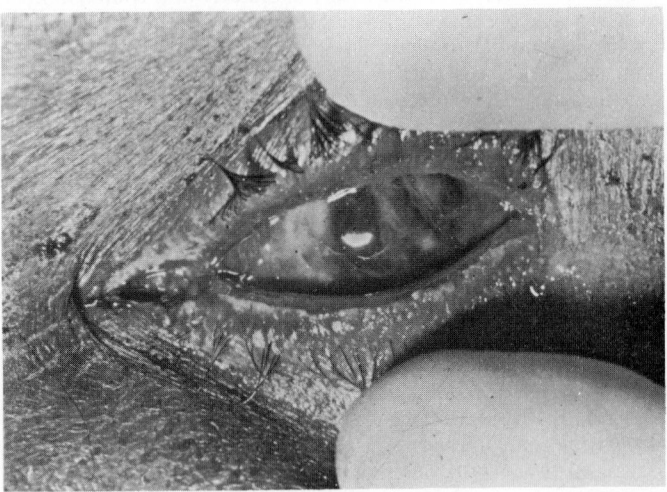

Fig. 8 Venom ophthalmia caused by the black-necked spitting cobra (*Naja nigricollis*). The corneal injury was neglected and so secondary infection developed and led to the loss of the eye.

(Fig. 8). This leads to permanent blindness in some cases. The venom may also be absorbed into the anterior chamber resulting in hypopyon and anterior uveitis.

Laboratory investigations. The peripheral white cell count is raised in severely envenomed patients. Anaemia results from bleeding or, much more rarely, from haemolysis. The South American rattlesnake (*Cr. durissus terrificus*) causes significant haemolysis with methaemoglobinuria. Venoms containing procoagulant may produce thrombocytopenia: this is common following bites by the Malayan pit viper (*Calloselasma rhodostoma*), and Pacific rattlesnake (*Cr. viridis helleri*), but relatively rare after carpet viper (*Echis carinatus*) bite. Useful tests for venom induced defibrination are the simple whole blood clotting and clot quality tests. A few ml of blood are placed in a clean, dry, glass test-tube, left undisturbed for 20 minutes, and then tipped to assess clotting. The tube is again examined after about 12 hours to assess the size of the clot. Non-clotting blood may be diagnostic of a particular species (e.g. *E. carinatus* in Africa), and indicates systemic envenoming. Serum potassium is elevated by the generalized rhabdomyolysis of sea snake envenoming. Serum enzymes such as aspartate and alanine aminotransferases and creatine phosphokinase are mildly elevated in patients with local tissue damage, but grossly raised in sea snake victims. Electrocardiographic changes such as inverted T wave, raised ST segment, prolonged QT_c interval, and arrhythmias are seen in patients bitten by *Viperidae*. The urine commonly contains red blood cells, polymorphs, and granular casts. Dark urine should be tested for haemoglobin/myoglobin.

Immunodiagnosis. Specific snake venom antigens have been detected in wound aspirate, wound biopsies, blood, urine, CSF, and other body fluids by a variety of techniques including immunodiffusion, countercurrent immunoelectrophoresis (CIE), passive haemagglutination, radioimmunoassay, and enzyme-linked immunosorbent assay (ELISA). ELISA appears to be the simplest and most sensitive technique. The Commonwealth Serum Laboratories in Australia (CSL) have recently issued venom detection kits based on this principle. In some cases the ELISA and CIE may produce a result quickly enough to guide clinical management, but the main value of these new techniques is probably in the investigation of the pathophysiology and epidemiology of snake bite, and for forensic purposes in people suspected to have died from snake bite. Venom antibody is also detectable by ELISA and may persist for many years after the bite.

Management of snake bite

First aid treatment. The patient should be reassured and moved to the nearest hospital or dispensary as quickly and comfortably as possible. The bitten limb should be immobilized as far as is practicable with a splint or sling. Paracetamol tablets can be given for pain. Aspirin is not suitable for it may lead to persistent gastric bleeding in defibrinated patients. All traditional 'boy scout' remedies should be avoided. Local incisions and suction are more likely to introduce infection and give rise to persistent bleeding than to remove significant amounts of venom from the wound. Potassium permanganate and ice packs may potentiate local necrosis. The value of tourniquets has not been adequately investigated in human patients. A broad, firm, but not tight, constricting band may temporarily delay the spread of viper venoms along lymphatics, but this is not necessary unless the journey to hospital is likely to take more than about 30 minutes. A tight (arterial) tourniquet is effective in preventing venous return from the occluded limb and delays death in animals given some elapid and viper venoms. Such tourniquets are potentially very dangerous, and have been responsible for gangrenous limbs. Their use is only justified in the case of bites by dangerously neurotoxic elapids, sea snakes, and Australian snakes, when the delay in reaching medical care is likely to be more than 30 minutes but less than two hours. In these particular circumstances the tourniquet may delay the development of respiratory paralysis or cardiovascular collapse until some medical help is available. The arterial tourniquet must be released for 15 seconds every 30 minutes and should, on no account, be applied for more than two hours. Recent studies in restrained monkeys have shown that crepe bandaging and splinting of the injected limb is effective in delaying the spread of snake and spider venoms.

Patients being transported to hospital should be laid on their side to prevent aspiration of vomit. Persistent vomiting can be treated with chlorpromazine by intravenous injection (for an adult 25 mg). Angioneurotic oedema and shock can be treated with chlorpheniramine maleate, 10 mg by intravenous injection, and adrenaline 0.5–1.0 ml of 0.1 per cent solution by subcutaneous injection.

Hospital treatment. In most cases of snake bite there are uncertainties about the type, quantity, and quality of venom injected that can only be resolved by admitting the patient for at least 24 hours observation. Tourniquets should be released. Local swelling is almost always detectable within 15 minutes of significant pit viper envenoming, and within two hours of viper envenoming but does not develop in patients bitten by some neurotoxic species (especially kraits, sea snakes, and coral snakes). Tender enlargement of regional lymph nodes draining the bitten area is an early sign of envenoming by *Viperidae*, some *Elapidae*, and Australian snakes. Buccal and lingual aspects of all tooth sockets should be examined meticulously for bleeding which also occurs at venepuncture sites, from partially healed wounds, nose, conjunctivae, and elsewhere. Hypotension is an important sign of hypovolaemia or cardiotoxicity

in patients bitten by vipers, pit vipers, and cobras. Ptosis is the earliest sign of neurotoxic envenoming. Respiratory muscle power should be assessed objectively, for example by measuring vital capacity. If a procoagulant venom is suspected, haemostasis should be checked at the bedside by the simple whole blood clotting test.

Antivenom treatment. Antivenom, which is made by immunizing horses with whole venom or toxoid, is the only specific treatment for envenoming. The *British National Formulary 1981* states, quite incorrectly, that 'the adder bite itself may be less dangerous than the so-called specific snake bite antiserum which is therefore *not recommended*'. Although the clinical testing of antivenoms has been relatively neglected, there is now sufficient evidence to support the use of specific antivenoms in seriously envenomed patients. For example, *E. carinatus* antivenom has reduced the mortality from 20 per cent to less than 3 per cent, Zagreb *Vipera berus* antivenom is dramatically effective in restoring the blood pressure in shocked patients, and Bangkok *Agkistrodon (Calloselasma) rhodostoma* antivenom has also proved highly effective.

Indications. Antivenom is indicated if there are signs of severe systemic envenoming such as hypotension or other signs of cardiovascular toxicity, neurotoxicity, myotoxicity, impaired consciousness, spontaneous systemic bleeding, or incoagulable blood. Supporting evidence of severe envenoming is a peripheral leucocytosis of more than 20 000/mm^3, abnormal ECG, elevated serum enzymes such as creatine phosphokinase and aspartate and alanine aminotransferases, haemoglobinuria, myoglobinuria, or methaemoglobinuria, severe anaemia or haemoconcentration, uraemia, and oliguria. In the absence of systemic envenoming, local swelling, involving more than half the bitten limb following bites by species known to cause necrosis, is an additional indication for antivenom. Special indications have been described for particular species. In the case of bites by North American rattlesnakes, especially the most dangerous species (*Cr. atrox, Cr. adamanteus, Cr. durissus subspp., Cr. scutulatus, Cr. viridis subspp.*, and *Cr. horridus*), antivenom should be given early, before systemic envenoming has become obvious. Rapid spread of local swelling is considered an indication for antivenom. Similarly, with bites by several species of North American coral snake (genera *Micrurus* and *Micruroides*) antivenom is recommended in all cases of definite bites in which there is immediate pain and any other symptom or sign of envenoming. In Australia the Commonwealth Serum Laboratories (CSL) recommend that antivenom should be given in any patient with a proved or suspected snake bite if there are tender regional lymph nodes or any other evidences of systemic spread of venom, and in any person effectively bitten by an identified highly venomous snake.

It is never too late to give antivenom: sea snake envenoming has been reversed up to two days after the bite, and blood coagulability restored in victims of *Echis carinatus* 10 days or more after the bite.

Selection and administration. All but one of the world's antivenom manufacturers refines the horse serum by ammonium sulphate precipitation, pepsin digestion, dialysis, or ultrafiltration. Expiry dates quoted on ampoules tend to be very conservative, particularly if storage has been at 4 °C, but opaque solutions should always be rejected. Only antivenom whose stated range of specificity includes the species responsible for the bite should be given. Some antivenoms, such as CSL 'Tiger-Sea Snake Antivenom', have a wide range of specificity. Polyspecific (polyvalent) antivenoms are used in many countries because of the difficulty in identifying the species responsible. For example South African Institute for Medical Research (SAIMR) 'Polyvalent Antivenom' is raised against the venoms of 10 species and has paraspecific activity against a further five.

Antivenom should be diluted in isotonic saline to a total volume of 200–500 ml and given by intravenous drip over about one hour, starting at 2 drops per second, then speeding up after 15 minutes; 0.5 ml of 0.1 per cent adrenaline must be drawn up in readiness. At the first sign of a reaction (see below) antivenom should be stopped and adrenaline given by subcutaneous injection. Once the symptoms of the reaction have subsided, antivenom infusion can be continued slowly. Intravenous chlorpheniramine maleate 10 mg is given to prevent recurrent urticaria and to calm the patient. Corticosteroids are not indicated, except for late, serum-sickness-type reactions.

Antivenom reactions are not reliably predicted by conjunctival or intradermal test doses. Although there are no absolute contraindications to antivenom treatment, patients known to be hypersensitive to horse serum and those with a history of atopy should not be given antivenom unless the effects of envenoming are severe and thought to be immediately life-threatening. Pretreatment with adrenaline and antihistamines may be partially effective in preventing reaction. 'Rapid desensitization' is not recommended.

Dose. The initial doses suggested in antivenom manufacturers' literature are usually based on mouse protection tests and are unreliable. Few clinical trials have been performed to establish the appropriate starting dose and in most countries antivenom is used empirically. Many hospitals in the rural tropics give a standard dose of one or two ampoules to every patient who claims to have been bitten, irrespective of clinical severity. This practice squanders the limited supply of antivenom and exposes many non-envenomed patients to the risks of reactions. Some suggested initial doses are given in Table 1. *The dose for children should be the same or greater than that for adults.*

Response. Often there is marked symptomatic improvement soon after starting intravenous antivenom. In shocked patients the blood pressure may rise and consciousness return. Dramatic responses of neurotoxic effects are less common. Spontaneous systemic bleeding usually stops within 15–30 minutes and blood coagulability is restored within six hours of antivenom, provided that an adequate dose has been given. Further antivenom should be given if severe signs of envenoming are not reversed after one to two hours, or if blood coagulability is not restored within about six hours. Some effects of envenoming are unlikely to be reversed by antivenom. For example, post-synaptic neurotoxins such as alpha-bungarotoxin are irreversibly bound to the motor end plate.

Recovery in these cases probably depends on the growth of new receptors.

Antivenom reactions. Early (anaphylactoid) reactions develop, in up to 20 per cent of cases, usually within 10–20 minutes of intravenous injection of antivenom or within half to three hours of starting intravenous infusion of diluted antivenom. Restlessness, cough, itching of the scalp, nausea, vomiting, a feeling of heat, or an increase in pulse rate is followed by the appearance of urticaria, generalized pruritus, fever, tachycardia, and autonomic manifestations. In a few patients dangerous hypotension, airflow obstruction, and angioneurotic oedema may develop. The mortality of antivenom reactions is exceedingly low but individual cases, such as the asthmatic boy who died from anaphylactic shock due to antivenom in England in 1957, have been widely publicized and have led to an unreasonable prejudice against antivenom treatment. The incidence of early reactions is highest when large doses of relatively unrefined antivenom are given by intravenous injection. The assumption that these reactions are always the result of immediate (type I) hypersensitivity to equine serum may not be correct. Complement activation, and other mechanisms may also be involved. Pyrogenic reactions, which may not be immunological in nature, may occur within an hour or two of antivenom treatment and can precipitate febrile convulsions in children. Late reactions of serum sickness type may develop five to 24 days after antivenom. A high incidence of these reactions related to the dose of antivenom given, has been reported in North America. Clinical features include fever, urticaria, subcutaneous and periarticular swellings, polyarthritis, lymphadenopathy, mononeuritis multiplex and other neurological symptoms, and proteinuria.

Adrenaline is the effective treatment for early reactions. 0.5–1.0 ml of 0.1 per cent solution is given by subcutaneous injection. The dose may be repeated if the reaction is not controlled. Patients with profound hypotension, severe bronchospasm, or laryngeal oedema can be given adrenaline by slow intravenous injection. Pyrogenic reactions are treated by cooling the patient and giving antipyretics. Late reactions respond to oral prednisolone 5 mg six-hourly for five to seven days and oral chlorpheniramine 2–4 mg six-hourly.

Table 1   A guide to initial dosage of some important antivenoms

Species			
Latin	English	Manufacturer, antivenom	Approximate initial dose
Acanthophis antarticus	death adder	CSL, monospecific	3000–6000 units
Bitis arietans	puff adder	Behringwerke, SAIMR, polyspecific	80 ml
Bothrops atrox *B. jararaca*	lance headed vipers	South American Institutes Bothrops, polyspecific	40 ml 40 ml
Calloselasma (Agkistrodon) rhodostoma	Malayan pit viper	Thai Red Cross (Saovabha) Bangkok, monospecific	50 ml
Crotalus adamanteus *Cr. atrox* *Cr. viridis* subspp.	diamond back rattlesnake western rattlesnake	Wyeth Crotalidae, polyspecific	30–100 ml 30–100 ml 30–100 ml
Echis carinatus	saw-scaled viper	SAIMR, Echis Behringwerke, Bitis–Echis–Naja	20 ml 100 ml
Naja naja	Asian cobra	Kasauli, polyspecific Haffkine, monospecific Thai Red Cross, monospecific	100 ml 50–100 ml 50–100 ml
Notechis scutatus *Pseudonaja textilis*	tiger snake eastern brownsnake	CSL, monospecific	3000–6000 ml 300–600 ml
Vipera berus	European adder	Imunološki Zavod-Zagreb, vipera polyspecific	10 ml
V. xanthina palaestinae	Palestine viper	Rogoff Medical Research Institute, Tel Aviv Palestine viper monospecific	50–80 ml

Supportive treatment. *Neurotoxic envenoming*. Bulbar and respiratory paralysis may lead to death from aspiration, airways obstruction, or respiratory failure. A clear airway must be maintained, and if respiratory distress develops, tracheostomy should be performed. Most patients with neurotoxic envenoming remain fully conscious with intact sensation. Once it is clear that respiratory muscle power is inadequate, ventilation must be assisted. Patients have recovered from respiratory paralysis after being manually ventilated by relays of relatives and nurses for up to 10 days. All effects of neurotoxic envenoming are fully reversible and so artificial ventilation should always be attempted. Many patients have died of respiratory paralysis because no attempt was made to ventilate them.

Anticholinesterases have a variable but potentially useful effect in patients with neurotoxic envenoming. A test dose of edrophonium chloride, 10 mg by intravenous injection after 0.6 mg of atropine, should be given to all patients with severe neurotoxic envenoming. If there is a convincing response, neostigmine methyl sulphate 50–100 µg per kg body weight with atropine should be given every four hours by continuous infusion.

Circulatory collapse. This may be due to direct effects of the venom on heart and vasculature, hypovolaemia resulting from the leakage of blood and plasma into the envenomed limb or to haemorrhage elsewhere, or to release of endogenous vasodilators by the venom. Antivenom should be given followed by a plasma expander (ideally, fresh whole blood). Monitoring of jugular or central venous pressures or pulmonary wedge pressure (via Swan–Ganz catheter) is very useful in preventing volume overload and pulmonary oedema.

Local necrosis. Once definite signs of necrosis have appeared, surgical debridement, immediate split skin grafting, and broad spectrum antibiotic cover are indicated. Occasionally, thrombosis of a major vessel or neglected local necrosis may necessitate amputation of a limb. This results from inadequate antivenom treatment or inadvisable treatment such as cryotherapy. On rare occasions, increased pressure within a tight fascial compartment, such as the pulp space in the digits and anterior tibial compartment, may contribute to necrosis. In view of the dangers of fasciotomy especially in patients with incoagulable blood, it is important that objective evidence of the compartmental syndrome should be obtained by the use of Doppler untrasound probes, measurement of tissue pressure, or angiography.

Renal failure. Some snake bite victims admitted with oliguria and elevated blood urea and creatinine are simply dehydrated. Acute tubular necrosis resulting from hypotension is the commonest cause of renal failure in snake bite. Urine output should be measured and the patient treated conservatively by strict fluid balance or, if necessary, by peritoneal or haemodialysis. Generalized rhabdomyolysis following sea snake bite causes hyperkalaemia and myoglobinuria. The urine should be kept alkaline to prevent renal damage from myoglobin, and hyperkalaemia corrected by the usual methods.

Other drugs. Heparin, antifibrinolytic agents such as epsilon amino caproic acid, corticosteroids, clotting factors, and a large range of herbal and other remedies have been advocated in snake bite. There is no adequate evidence, based on properly controlled trials, that any of these agents is other than harmful. In particular, heparin has exaggerated bleeding and contributed to the death of snake bite victims.

Management of snake venom ophthalmia. When cobra venom is 'spat', first aid consists of irrigating the eyes with generous volumes of water or other bland liquid. Corneal abrasions should be excluded by slit-lamp examination or fluorescein staining. An antimicrobial should be applied locally and the eye closed with a pad.

Prognosis. Untreated mortality is said to exceed 50 per cent following bites by sea snakes and a few other species such as the South American rattlesnake (*Cr. durissus terrificus*). Untreated bites by *E. carinatus*, *V. russelli*, *B. atrox*, and *N. naja* are probably fatal in 10–25 per cent of cases. The variable proportion of bitten but non-envenomed cases (more than 50 per cent following bites by *Calloselasma rhodostoma*), and the bias towards more severe cases in hospital statistics undoubtedly influences these figures. Antivenoms have reduced mortality by a factor of five or six, and in Australia appear to have virtually eliminated snake bite deaths.

Prevention of snake bite. To reduce the risk of bites, snakes should never be disturbed, attacked, or handled even if they are said to be a harmless species or appear to be dead. In snake infested areas boots, socks, and long trousers should be worn for walks in undergrowth or deep sand. A light should always be carried at night. Collecting firewood, dislodging logs and boulders with the bare hands, pushing sticks into burrows, holes, or crevices, and climbing rocks and trees covered with dense foliage are particularly dangerous activities. Unlit paths and roads are specially dangerous after heavy rains.

It is pointless and ecologically undesirable to attempt the extermination of dangerous species of snake.

References

Bhat, R. N. (1974). Viperine snake bite poisoning in Jammu. *J. Indian med. Ass.* **63**, 383.

Bücherl, W., Buckley, E. E., and Deulofeu, V. (eds.) (1968, 1971). *Venomous animals and their venoms*, vol. 1 and 2. Academic Press, New York.

Campbell, C. H. (1964). Venomous snake bite in Papua and its treatment with tracheotomy, artificial respiration and antivenene. *Trans. R. Soc. trop. Med. Hyg.* **58**, 263.

Efrati, P. and Reif, L. (1953). Clinical and pathological observations on sixty-five cases of viper bite in Israel. *Am. J. trop. Med. Hyg.* **2**, 1085.

Gans, C. and Gans, K. A. (eds.) (1978). *Biology of the reptilia*, vol. 8. Academic Press, London.

Lee, C-Y. (ed.) (1979). *Snake venoms. Handbook of experimental pharmacology*, vol. 52, Springer-Verlag, Berlin.

Reid, H. A., Thean, P. C., Chan, K. E., and Baharom, A. R. (1963). Clinical effects of bites by Malayan viper (*Ancistrodon rhodostoma*). *Lancet* **i**, 617.

Warrell, D. A., Davidson, N. McD., Greenwood, B. M., et al. (1977). Poisoning by bites of the saw-scaled or carpet viper (*Echis carinatus*) in Nigeria. *Q. Jl Med.* **46**, 33.

—, Greenwood, B. M., Davidson, N. McD., et al. (1976). Necrosis, haemorrhage, and complement depletion following bites by the spitting cobra (*Naja nigricollis*). *Q. Jl Med.* **45**, 1.

World Health Organization (1981). *Progress in the characterization of venoms and standardization of antivenoms*. World Health Organization Offset Publication no. 58, Geneva.

Lizards

Two species, the Gila monster (*Heloderma suspectum*) and Mexican beaded lizard or escorpion (*H. horridum*), are venomous. They occur in southwestern USA and western Mexico and reach half a metre in length. Venom is secreted by glands in the lower jaw and is conducted along the grooved lower teeth. It contains a toxin, enzymes, and 5-hydroxytryptamine. Pharmacological effects in animals include respiratory paralysis, myocardial depression, spontaneous haemorrhage, autonomic stimulation, and release of kinins and other mediators.

Humans are occasionally bitten while handling these lizards, which cling on with a bulldog-like grip. Severe local pain develops almost immediately with tender swelling and regional lymphadenopathy. Systemic symptoms include weakness, dizziness, hypotension, syncope, sweating, rigors, tinnitus, nausea and vomiting, leucocytosis, and ECG changes.

Treatment. The animal should be prised off as soon as possible. No more humane method has been devised than to apply a flame to the underside of the jaw. Multiple tooth punctures are produced. Some may contain shed teeth. There is no specific treatment. Powerful analgesia may be required with symptomatic treatment of shock. A number of fatal cases of *H. suspectum* bite has been reported in the literature up to the 1930s, but none is totally convincing.

References

Albritton, D. C., Parrish, H. M., and Allen, E. R. (1970). Venenation by the Mexican beaded lizard (*Heloderma horridum*): report of a case. *S. Dakota J. Med.* **23**, 22.
Bogert, C. M. and Martin del Campo, R. (1956). The Gila monster and its allies. *Bull. Am. Mus. nat. Hist.* **109**, 1.
Roller, J. A. (1977). Gila monster bite: a case report. *Clin. Toxicol.* **10**, 423.
Russell, F. E. and Bogert, C. M. (1981). Gila monster, venom and bite—a review. *Toxicon.* **19**, 341.

Fish and shellfish poisoning

Illness following the ingestion of seafood is usually the result of infection by pathogens, such as *Vibrio parahaemolyticus* (see Section 5), *Salmonella* spp. (see Section 5), and hepatitis A virus (see Section 5), but in some cases symptoms are attributable to toxins. Two main syndromes are described.

Paralytic syndrome. Acute nausea, vomiting, and diarrhoea are associated with paraesthesia of the lips, tongue, mouth, throat, and extremities, distorted temperature sensation so that cold objects impart a burning sensation, ataxia, muscle weakness progressing to respiratory paralysis in some cases, and cardiovascular disturbances. Important causes of this syndrome are:

1. *Ciguatera poisoning.* Symptoms develop about six hours (range: minutes to 30 hours) after eating fish such as red snapper, barracuda, grouper, amberjack, and more than 400 other species occurring between latitudes 35° North and South. The toxin, ultimately derived from planktonic dinoflagellates such as *Gambierdiscus toxicus*, is concentrated in the liver, viscera, and gonads especially of large fish. Symptoms may persist for more than a week. The mortality is less than 10 per cent.

2. *Tetrodotoxin poisoning.* Scaleless toad and puffer fish (order *Tetraodontiformes*) are relished in Japan (fugu) where 50 cases of tetrodotoxin poisoning occur each year with 60 per cent mortality. Symptoms develop five minutes to three hours after ingesting the poison which is especially concentrated in the fish's ovary. There may be cardiovascular, autonomic, and haemorrhagic manifestations.

3. *Paralytic shellfish poisoning.* Bivalve molluscs such as mussels, clams, oysters, and scallops may acquire a neurotoxin, such as saxitoxin, from dinoflagellates of the genus *Gonyaulax* which occur between latitudes 30° North and South. These dinoflagellates may be sufficiently abundant during the months of May to October, when sea temperature is highest, to produce a 'red tide'. The dangerous season is signalled by the deaths of large numbers of fish and seabirds. Symptoms develop within thirty minutes and may progress to fatal respiratory paralysis within twelve hours.

Histamine-like syndrome. The flesh of scombroid fish such as tuna, mackerel, bonito, and skipjack, and of tinned non-scombroid fish like sardines and pilchards may be decomposed by the action of certain bacteria such as *Proteus morgani* to produce histamine and unidentified toxins. About four hours after ingestion (range from minutes to hours) flushing, burning, urticaria, and pruritus of the skin, headache, abdominal colic, nausea, vomiting, diarrhoea, and bronchial asthma may develop. Scombroid poisoning is prevented by refrigerating the fish and eating it fresh.

Treatment. Gastrointestinal contents are eliminated by emetics and purges. No specific treatment is possible but atropine, anticholinesterases, and calcium gluconate have been helpful in some cases of paralytic syndrome. In scombroid poisoning, antihistamines and bronchodilators should be used. In cases of respiratory paralysis endotracheal intubation and mechanical ventilation have proved life-saving in many cases. The toxins responsible are heat stable, so cooking does not prevent poisoning.

References

Bagnis, R. A. *et al.* (1979). Clinical observations on 3009 cases of Ciguatera (fish poisoning) in the Southern Pacific. *Am. J. trop. Med. Hyg.* **28**, 106.
Halstead, B. W. (1978). *Poisonous and venomous marine animals of the world*, revised edn. Darwin Press, Princeton.
Hughes, J. M. and Merson, M. H. (1976). Fish and shellfish poisoning. *New Engl. J. Med.* **295**, 1117.

Venomous fish

More than 100 species of fish have proved dangerous to man by their ability to sting by injecting venom through spines placed in front of the fins or tail, incorporated into dorsal and pectoral fins, or situated on the gill covers. The richest venomous fish fauna is in the Indo-Pacific region and other tropical waters, but venomous species such as sharks, chimaeras, and weevers also occur in the more temperate northern oceans. The most important groups are shown in Table 2.

Table 2   The most important groups of venomous fish

Chondrichthyes, cartilaginous fish
  Squaliformes,* sharks, dogfish, skates, and rays
  Chimaeriformes, chimaeras
Osteichthyes, bony fish
  Siluroidei,* catfish
  Trachinidae,* weever fish
  Scorpaenidae,* scorpion fish
  Batrachoidiformes, toad fish
  Uranoscopidae,* stargazers

*Human fatalities reported

Epidemiology. The incidence of fish sting is unknown. Weever fish stings are a common accident around the coasts of the United Kingdom in the summer months, and 58 cases were seen at a hospital in Pula, Yugoslavia in 13 years. It has been estimated that 1500 stings by rays occur each year and 300 stings by scorpion fish in the United States. In four years 81 cases of stonefish (*Synanceja*) sting were seen in Pulau Bukom Hospital in Singapore. Zebra, lion or turkey fish (genus *Pterois*) are popular aquarium pets and cause large numbers of stings none of which has yet proved fatal.

Clinical features. Pharmacological effects of fish venoms include hypotension, myocardial depression, neuromuscular paralysis, and local necrosis. Human victims suffer immediate intense local pain and swelling which may persist for several days and may be complicated by necrosis and secondary infection particularly if the spine remains in the wound. Systemic effects include vomiting, diarrhoea, sweating, bradycardia, hypotension, cardiac arrhythmias, muscle spasms, flaccid paralysis, respiratory distress, and convulsions.

Treatment. The venomous spine, which may be barbed, should be removed as soon as possible and the stung limb immersed in water as hot as can be borne by the patient. Magnesium sulphate should be added as an anaesthetic. Alternatively, 1 per cent lignocaine may be injected, for example as a ring block in the case of stung digits. Systemic effects must be treated symptomatically. Severe hypotension may respond to adrenaline and bradycardia may be treated with atropine. Specific antivenom for stonefish (*Synanceja*) sting is manufactured in Australia and Yugoslavia.

Prevention. Fish sting can be prevented by employing a shuffling gait when wading, by handling all live and dead fish with caution and by avoiding unnecessary contact with fish especially in the vicinity of tropical reefs.

References

Edmunds, C. (1975). *Dangerous marine animals of the Indo-Pacific region.* Diving Medical Centre, Mosman, New South Wales.

Evans, H. M. (1943). *Sting fish and seafarer*. Faber, London.
Halstead, B. W. (1971). Venomous fishes. In *Venomous animals and their venoms* (eds. W. Bücherl and E. E. Buckley), 587, Academic Press, New York.
Maretić, Z. (1973). Some epidemiological, clinical and therapeutic aspects of envenomation by weever fish sting. In *Toxins of animal and plant origin* (eds. A. De Vries and E. Kochva), 1055. Gordon and Breach, New York.
Russell, F. E. (1965). *Marine toxins in venomous and poisonous marine animals*. Reprinted by TFH Publications, 1971.

Venomous marine invertebrates

Coelenterata (jellyfish, Portuguese man-of-war, hydroids, sea anemones, and corals). The tentacles of the *Cnidaria* are armed with stinging capsules or nematocysts which can produce lines of painful irritant weals on the skin of swimmers unlucky enough to make contact with them. Venoms contain or release substances such as 5-hydroxytryptamine and histamine which cause immediate excruciating pain, inflammation, and urticaria. Rarely there are severe systemic effects including rigors, vomiting and diarrhoea, hypotensive collapse, respiratory muscle paralysis, and convulsions. Local necrosis may develop. Dangerous species include *Chironex fleckeri* (box jellyfish, cubomedusoid, sea wasp, or indringa) which has caused at least 55 deaths in the Indo-Pacific region during the last 100 years; *Chiropsalmus* spp. (sea wasps) and *Carukia barnesi*, the cause of Irukandji sting in Australia. The Portuguese man-of-war, *Physalia* species, can also cause severe systemic symptoms but no deaths have been adequately documented. The imprint of nematocyst stings on the skin may have a diagnostic pattern. Many stings could be prevented if swimmers were particularly cautious during those seasons when jellyfish are swept inshore.

Treatment. The aim is to prevent further discharge of nematocysts on fragments of tentacles stuck to the skin. Methyl alcohol, the traditional remedy, has been shown to have the deleterious effect of causing massive discharge of nematocysts. Commercial vinegar or 4–6 per cent acetic acid are, however, very effective. Application of tourniquets proximal to the stung area may produce a useful delay in the absorption of venom. Specific 'sea wasp' antivenom for *Chironex fleckeri* stings is made in Australia. Cardiorespiratory resuscitation has proved effective.

Echinodermata. Starfish and sea urchins possess venomous spines and grapples (pedicellaria) which can cause local pain and swelling and rarely systemic effects such as cardiac arrhythmias and respiratory paralysis which may prove fatal. Spines and grapples should be removed from the wound after softening the skin with 2 per cent salicylic acid ointment.

Mollusca (snails, slugs, cones, and octopuses) The venomous radula tooth of the cone shell, a kind of sea snail, produces local paraesthesia and numbness, and paralysis which may progress to fatal respiratory paralysis.
The blue-ringed octopuses *Hapalochlaena (Octopus) maculosa* and *H. lunulata* of the Australian region can cause serious systemic envenoming by introducing toxic saliva into wounds inflicted by their beaks. Generalized and fatal paralysis may develop within 15 minutes of the bite.
No specific treatment is available for mollusc envenoming.

References

Hartwick, R. *et al.* (1980). Disarming the box-jellyfish. Nematocyst inhibition in *Chironex fleckeri. Med. J. Aust.* **1**, 15.
Southcott, R. V. (1975). The neurologic effects of noxious marine creatures. In *Topics on tropical neurology* (ed. R. W. Hornabrook), 165. F. A. Davis, Philadelphia.
Williamson, J. A. *et al.* (1980). Serious envenomation by the Northern Australian box-jellyfish (*Chironex fleckeri*). *Med. J.* Aust. **1**, 13.

Venomous arthropods

Hymenoptera (bees, wasps, yellow jackets, hornets, etc.) Venom introduced by the sting of these insects contains amines, kinins, specific toxic peptides, such as apamin and melittin in the case of the honey bee *Apis mellifera*, and enzymes such as phopholipase A2 and hyaluronidase. Bee venom contains interesting inflammatory and anti-inflammatory peptides, such as peptide 410 which may have beneficial effects in arthritis. In addition, wasp (*Vespa vulgaris*) venom contains 5-hydroxytryptamine, bradykinin, catecholamines and cholinesterase.

Stings usually produce only local effects—pain, redness and swelling—due to histamine, 5-hydroxytryptamine, and other substances which are introduced or released. The lethal dose for an unsensitized human usually requires hundreds of stings: but as few as 30 stings have killed and as many as 2243 have been survived. In the rare cases of massive envenoming from many simultaneous stings, the clinical effects are those of histamine overdose (vasodilatation, hypotension, vomiting, diarrhoea, headache and coma). Haemolysis, rhabdomyolysis, myoglobinuria and renal failure have also been described. Rare effects of hymenoptera stings include myasthenia gravis and thrombocytopenic purpura.

In contrast, about 0.5 per cent of the population is hypersensitive to bee or wasp venom and could be killed by a single sting. In England and Wales between 1959 and 1972 there were 61 deaths from insect stings, and in the USA 50–100 people die each year from this cause.

Clinical features of hymenoptera venom allergy. Clinical suspicion of venom hypersensitivity arises when there are progressively severe local reactions to successive stings, or systemic symptoms following a sting. These may consist of tingling scalp, flushing, dizziness, hypotension, and wheezing within a few minutes of the sting, or the development over about 20 minutes of generalized urticaria, angioneurotic oedema, oedema of the glottis, bronchial asthma, hypotensive collapse, and coma. The sooner the symptoms develop, the more severe the reaction is likely to be, and in extreme cases the patient could die within minutes of being stung. In a few cases serum sickness develops a week or more after the sting. Atopy does not predispose to sting allergy, but asthmatics who are allergic to venom are likely to suffer particularly severe reactions.

Diagnosis of venom hypersensitivity. The whole body extracts (WBE) of bees and wasps which were used for many years for skin testing do not discriminate between hypersensitive patients and controls. Intradermal testing with various dilutions of dialysed freeze-dried pure specific venoms have, however, proved reliable.

Treatment. Stings which are left embedded in the skin should be scraped out with a blade or finger nail but not grasped with fingers or tweezers which may inject more venom. It has been claimed that domestic meat tenderizer (Papain) diluted roughly 1 in 5 with tap water can produce dramatic relief of pain. Bee keepers have found that aspirin is a particularly effective analgesic: this may have something to do with its inhibition of prostaglandin synthetase. Local antiseptics are acceptable but topical antihistamines should not be used as they promote sensitization.

The most effective treatment for sting anaphylaxis is adrenaline 0.1 per cent in a dose of 0.5–1 ml given subcutaneously, or, if the patient is unconscious or pulseless, by intravenous or even intracardiac injection. Patients who develop sting anaphylaxis may be discovered unconscious. It is helpful if they can wear an identifying tag, such as provided by Medic Alert. They should always carry with them the equipment for self-injection of adrenaline. Adrenaline delivered by a pressurized inhaler ('Medihaler-epi') will relieve bronchospasm, but insufficient is absorbed to combat other effects of anaphylaxis. Injection of an antihistamine such as chlorpheniramine maleate, 10 mg by intravenous or intramuscular route, may alleviate the mild urticarial symptoms. Severe reaction may require full cardiorespiratory resuscitation. Respiratory tract obstruction is responsible for most deaths. Stings in the mouth may cause serious airways obstruction even in people who are not hypersensitive to venom.

Prevention. Desensitization with WBE has been practised for many years but has not been subjected to controlled trials. Many experienced allergists believe it to be effective, but there is no sound theoretical basis and the immunization programmes may induce early or late (serum sickness) reactions. Desensitization with pure specific venoms has, however, been showed to be significantly more effective than placebo or WBE in preventing anaphylactic reactions to sting challenge.

References

Ackroyd, J. F. (1981). Treatment of severe anaphylactic reactions to insect stings. *J. R. Soc. Med.* **74**, 567.

Frankland, A. W. and Lessof, M. H. (1980). Allergy to bee stings: a review. *J. R. Soc. Med.* **73**, 807.

Golden, D. B. K., Valentine, M. D., Kagey-Sobotka, A., and Lichtenstein, L. M. (1980). Regimens of hymenoptera venom immunotherapy. *Ann. intern. Med.* **92**, 620.

Hunt, J. J., Sobotka, A.K., Valentine, M. D., Yunginger, J. W. and Lichtenstein, L. M. (1978). Sensitization following Hymenoptera whole body extract therapy. *J. Allergy clin. Immunol.* **61**, 48.

—, Valentine, M. D., Sobotka, A. K., Benton, A. W., Amodie, F. J., and Lichtenstein, L. M. (1978). A controlled trial of immunotherapy in insect hypersensitivity. *New Engl. J. Med.* **299**, 157.

—, —, —, and Lichtenstein, L. M. (1976). Diagnosis of allergy to stinging insects by skin testing with hymenoptera venoms. *Ann. intern. Med.* **85**, 56.

Morris Owen, R. M. (1978). Sting allergy: the problem of desensitization. *Br. J. clin. Pract.* **32**, 309, 339; **33**, 7.

Ants, beetles, and caterpillars. Various species of ants, such as the fire ants *Solenopsis richteri* and *S. invicta*, and harvester ant (*Pogonomyrmex badius*), vesicating, cantherides, or blister beetles (*Meloidae*), rove beetles (*Paederus cruenticollis*), and hairy caterpillars (larvae of *Lepidoptera*) can cause local pain, inflammation, urticaria or blistering on contact.

References

Rhoades, R. B. (1977). *Medical aspects of the imported fire ant.* University of Florida, Deansville.

Southcott, R. V. (1978). Lepidopterism in the Australian region. *Records Adelaide Child. Hosp.* **2**, 87.

Allergic responses to non-venomous arthropods. A very large number of species of arthropods and their larval forms have now been implicated in the development of allergic reactions ranging in severity from dermatitis, conjunctivitis, and rhinitis to bronchial asthma. Skin testing, detection of specific IgE, and bronchial challenge tests have suggested that the house dust mites (*Dermatophagoides pteronyssinus* and *D. farinae*) are the major cause of allergic asthma throughout the world. A fascinating example of widespread allergic disease caused by arthropods is the bronchial asthma resulting from chironomid midges (green nimitti) in the Sudan.

Reference

Cranston, P. S., Gad El Rab, M. O., and Kay, A. B. (1981). Chironomid midges as a cause of allergy in the Sudan. *Trans. R. Soc. trop. Med. Hyg.* **75**, 1.

Spiders (Araneae). All but one family in this enormous group are venomous, but very few species are dangerous to man. Spiders bite with a pair of small fangs, the chelicerae, to which the venom glands are connected. There are four important genera.

Latrodectus (widow spiders). *L. mactans tredecemguttatus* lives in fields in the Mediterranean countries and has been responsible for a series of epidemics of bites. 500 bites were reported in Italy between the years 1946 and 1950.

L.m. hasselti, the Australian red back spider, causes up to 340 reported bites each year in Australia. Bites cause a minimum of local signs but intense pain, pain in the local lymph nodes, generalized muscle pain, cramps, sweating, hyperaesthesia, spasms, swollen eyelids, trismus, and autonomic disturbances. A fine erythematous rash may develop on the fourth day. A mortality of up to 6 per cent has been described but this probably reflects selection of severe cases.

Loxosceles. *L. laeta* is widely distributed and causes many bites in Central and Southern America especially in Chile where the mortality ranges from 1–17 per cent.

L. reclusa, the brown recluse spider, was responsible for at least 200 bites and 6 deaths in the United States this century. More than 60 cases were reported in Texas between 1959 and 1962. Bites by *L. rufescens* have been reported from Israel.

Loxosceles bites occur most often in bedrooms while people are asleep or dressing, and in the USA a number of men were bitten on the genitals while they sat on outdoor lavatories in which the spiders had spun their webs. There is burning pain at the site of the bite, oedema, and development of a violacious plaque which, over the course of a few days, becomes a black eschar which sloughs in a few weeks sometimes leaving a necrotic ulcer. Systemic effects occur in about 13 per cent of bites: these include haemoglobinuria and jaundice resulting from haemolytic anaemia, fever, and loss of consciousness. Mortality is about 30 per cent among patients with systemic envenoming.

Phoneutria nigriventer, the banana spider, causes bites and deaths in South American countries such as Brazil. These spiders may be exported in bunches of bananas to temperate countries where they have been responsible for a few bites and deaths. Effects of envenoming are mainly neurotoxic as with *Latrodectus*. There is intense local pain, hypertension, tachycardia, sweating, hyper or hypothermia, and signs of autonomic stimulation including priapism.

Atrax robustus, the Sydney funnel web spider, occurs only in the environs of Sydney, Australia. The aggressive male has a dangerous bite which has caused 11 deaths since 1927. Early symptoms include nausea, vomiting, and diarrhoea, followed by sweating, hypersalivation, lacrimation, dyspnoea, hypertension, muscle fasciculation, trismus, and coma.

First aid treatment. In the case of bites by spiders with rapidly active potent venom, e.g. *Atrax robustus*, a tight tourniquet or crepe bandaging of the bitten limb may delay venom spread until the patient reaches hospital.

Specific treatment. Antivenom for *Latrodectus* bite is made in Australia, USA, Italy, Yugoslavia, and South Africa; for *Loxosceles* in Peru; and for *Loxosceles, Phoneutria*, and *Lycosa* in Brazil. Neurotoxic araneism seems to be more amenable to antivenom than the necrotic type.

Supportive treatment. Calcium gluconate (10 ml of 10 per cent solution given by slow intravenous injection) is said to relieve pain dramatically in *Latrodectus* bite. Muscle relaxants such as diazepam, antihistamines, corticosteroids, beta-blockers, and atropine have also been advocated.

References

Bettini, S. (ed.) (1978). *Arthropod venoms. Handbook of experimental pharmacology*, vol. 48, 121. Springer-Verlag, Berlin.

Maretić, Z. and Lebez, D. (1979). *Areneism with special reference to Europe.* Novit, Pula-Ljubjana, Yugoslavia.

Newlands, G. (1975). Review of the medically important spiders of southern Africa. *S. Afr. med. J.* **49**, 823.

Southcott, R. V. (1976). Arachnidism and allied syndrome in the Australian region. *Records Adelaide Child. Hosp.* **1**, 97.
Zumpt, F. (1968). Lactrodectism in South Africa. *S. Afr. med. J.* **42**, 385.

Scorpions. Scorpions are widely distributed throughout the tropics. Dangerous species occur in South Africa (*Parabuthus*); North Africa and Asia (*Leiurus, Buthacus, Buthotus, Buthus,* and *Androctonus*); USA, Mexico, and Central America (*Centruroides*); and South America and Trinidad (*Tityus*).

Epidemiology. Scorpion stings are relatively common in tropical countries but severe envenoming is rare except in parts of North Africa, Mexico and South America, the Caribbean, and India. In southern Libya there were 900 stings and 7 deaths per 100 000 population in 1979. In Mexico there are between 1000 and 2000 deaths from scorpion stings each year, 10 times as many as snake bite deaths, with a rate of 84 deaths per 100 000 per year in Colima State. Mortality is about 50 per cent in children up to four years old. In Brazil there are many hundreds of stings by *T. serrulatus* and *T. bahiensis*. Mortality increases from around 1 per cent in adults to 15–25 per cent in children less than six years old. *Buthotus tamulus* is the most dangerous scorpion in India.

Symptoms. Scorpion venoms produce autopharmacological effects by releasing transmitters such as acetylcholine and catecholamines, and direct neurotoxic effects on nerve and muscle. Local intense pain is the commonest symptom. There may be slight local oedema and tender enlargement of regional lymph nodes. Systemic symptoms may develop within minutes or hours of the sting. Features of autonomic nervous system excitation include dilated pupils, hypersalivation, sweating, vomiting, diarrhoea, priapism, and loss of sphincter control. Cardiovascular disturbances include hyper- and hypotension, cardiac arrhythmias, ECG changes suggesting myocarditis, pulmonary oedema, and heart failure. Neurotoxic effects are manifest by muscle fasciculation or spasms and respiratory paralysis. Acute pancreatitis and disseminated intravascular coagulation are also described.

Treatment. Specific antivenom should be given by intravenous infusion as with snake bite (see above). A dose of 5–25 ml is usually required to control the symptoms. Antivenoms are manufactured in Arizona, USA, (*Centruroides sculpturatus*), Mexico (*Centruroides* spp.); Brazil (*Tityus* spp.), Iran (six local species), Turkey (*Androctonus crassicauda*), Algeria (*Androctonus australis, Buthus occitanus*), Egypt (*Leiurus quinquestriatus*), and South Africa (*Parabuthus*). Supportive treatments which have been recommended include atropine, local anaesthetic, anticonvulsants, corticosteroids, and calcium gluconate. Local injection of emetine at the site of the sting is said to cure the pain but may cause necrosis.

Prevention can be partially achieved by precluding scorpions from homes by incorporating a row of ceramic tiles around the outside wall, making the door steps at least 20 cm high and killing scorpions with residual insecticides such as 1 per cent lindane or dieldrin powders. Prophylactic vaccination with scorpion venom toxoid is contemplated in Mexico.

References

Bettini, S. (ed.) (1978). *Arthropod venoms. Handbook of experimental pharmacology*, vol. 48, 279, Springer-Verlag, Berlin.
Keegan, H. L. (1980). *Scorpions of medical importance*. University Press of Mississippi, Jackson.
Bücherl, W. and Buckley, E. E. (eds.) (1971). *Venomous animals and their venoms*, vol. 3, 311. Academic Press, New York.
Mazzotti, L. and Bravo-Becherelle, M.A. (1963). Scorpionism in the Mexican Republic. In *Venomous and poisonous animals and noxious plants of the Pacific region*. (eds. H. L. Keegan and W. V. MacFarland), 119. Pergamon Press, Oxford.

Tick paralysis. Ticks, with mites, form a subgroup of the class *Arachnida*. Adult females of about 30 species of hard tick (family *Ixodidae*) and immature specimens of six species of soft ticks (family *Argasidae*) have been implicated in human tick paralysis. The tick's saliva contains neurotoxic activity causing presynaptic neuromuscular block and decreased nerve conduction velocity.

Although tick paralysis has been reported from all continents, most cases occur in western North America (*Dermacentor andersoni*), eastern USA (*D. variabilis*), and Australia (*Ixodes holocyclus* known as the scrub or dog tick). In British Columbia there were 305 cases with 10 per cent mortality between 1900 and 1968. About 120 cases have been reported in the USA, and in New South Wales there have been at least 20 deaths this century.

Ticks are picked up in the countryside or from domestic animals, particularly dogs, in the home. A majority of patients and almost all fatal cases are children. After the tick has been attached for about five or six days a progressive ascending, lower motor neurone paralysis develops with paraesthesiae. Often a child, who may have been irritable for the previous 24 hours, falls on getting out of bed first thing in the morning, and is found to be weak or ataxic. Paralysis increases over the next few days: death results from bulbar and respiratory paralysis and aspiration of stomach contents. Vomiting is a feature of the more acute course of *Ixodes holocyclus* envenoming.

This clinical picture is often misinterpreted as poliomyelitis, although in North America the peak incidence of tick paralysis is earlier in the year than the epidemic season for poliomyelitis. Other neurological conditions including Guillain–Barré syndrome, paralytic rabies, Eaton–Lambert syndrome, myasthenia gravis, or botulism may also be suspected. Diagnosis depends on finding the tick, which is likely to be concealed in a crevice, orifice, or hairy area of the body. The scalp is the commonest place. Fatal tick paralysis has been caused by a tick attached to the tympanic membrane.

Treatment. The tick must be detached without being squeezed. It can be painted with ether, chloroform, paraffin, petrol, or turpentine, or prized out between the partially separated tips of a pair of small iris scissors. Following removal of the tick there is usually rapid and complete recovery; but in Australia, patients have died after the tick has been detached. An antivenom, raised in dogs, is available in Australia. This is recommended for severely affected or very young patients; 20–30 ml are given intravenously.

References

Murnaghan, M. F. and O'Rourke, F. J. (1978). Tick paralysis. In *Arthropod venoms. Handbook of experimental pharmacology*, vol. 48 (ed. S. Bettini), 419, Springer-Verlag, Berlin.
Pearn, J. (1977). The clinical features of tick bite. *Med. J. Aust.* **2**, 313.

Millipedes (Diplopida). Most species possess glands in each of their body segments which secrete, and in some cases squirt out, irritant liquids for defensive purposes. These contain hydrogen cyanide and a variety of aldehydes, esters, phenols, and quinonoids. Members of at least eight genera of millipedes have proved injurious to man. Important genera are *Rhinocricus* (Caribbean), *Spirobolus* (Tanzania), *Spirostreptus* and *Iulus* (Indonesia), and *Polyceroconas* (Papua New Guinea). Children are particularly at risk when they handle or try to eat these large arthropods. When venom is squirted into the eye, intense conjunctivitis results and there may be corneal ulceration and even blindness. Skin lesions are initially stained brown or purple, blister after a few days, and then peel. First aid is generous irrigation with water. Eye injuries should be treated as for snake venom ophthalmia (see above).

References

Eisner, T., Alsop, D., Hicks, K., and Meinwald, J. (1978). Defensive secretions of millipedes; In *Arthropod venoms. Handbook of ex-*

perimental pharmacology, Vol. 48 (ed. S. Bettini), p. 41. Springer-Verlag, Berlin.

Radford, A. J. (1975). Millipede burns in man. *Trop. Geogr. Med.* **27**, 279.

Centipedes (Chilopoda). Many species can inflict painful bites producing local pain, swelling, inflammation, and lymphangitis. Systemic effects such as vomiting, headache, cardiac arrhythmias, and convulsions are extremely rare and the risk of mortality was probably greatly exaggerated in the older literature. The most important genus is *Scolopendra* which is distributed throughout tropical countries. Local treatment is the same as for scorpions stings. No antivenom is available.

Leeches. These annelids (Class *Hirudinea*, family *Hirudinidae*) attach themselves to humans and animals, introduce an anticoagulant, hirudin, and engorge themselves with blood. Two groups are important causes of human morbidity and even mortality particularly in tropical countries.

Land leeches. Species of the genera *Haemadipsa* and *Phyrobdella* are a few centimetres long. They infest, often in enormous numbers, the floor and low vegetation of rain forests, choosing particularly trails and watering places. These leeches usually attach themselves to the lower legs or ankles and seem adept at penetrating such defences as long trousers tucked into socks and laced up boots. The bite is usually painless and the infested person may not realize what has happened until he hears a squelching sound, notices that his feet feel warm and wet, and sees blood welling over the tops of the boots. Land leeches ingest about 1 ml of blood before dropping off, but the wound continues to bleed for some time because of the anticoagulant.

Aquatic leeches (genera *Hirudo*, *Limnatis*, and *Dinobdella*) attack swimmers and attach to the mouth, nostrils, conjunctivae, vulva, vagina, or male urethral meatus. The leeches may penetrate to the bronchi or oesophagus. They ingest 5–10 ml of blood and give rise to bleeding—haematemesis, epistaxis, and vaginal bleeding.

Treatment. Leeches may be pulled off or made to detach by application of a lighted match or cigarette, salt, alcohol, or vinegar. Local bleeding can be stopped by applying a styptic such as silver nitrate. Aquatic leeches which have penetrated the respiratory, upper gastrointestinal or genitourinary tracts must be removed via an endoscope. Spraying with cocaine or dilute (1 in 10 000) adrenaline may cause the leech to detach in the larynx, trachea, and oesophagus, while irrigation with concentrated salt solution may be effective in the genitourinary tract. Leeches do not transmit pathogens but may give rise to severe anaemia, secondary infection, and persistant itching.

Prevention. This can be achieved by applying insect repellants, such as dibutyl phthalate and diethyltoluamide, to skin and clothing. Invasion of footwear during jungle walks can be prevented, rather messily, by rolling a rope of tobacco in the tops of the socks and keeping the feet well soaked with water.

Reference

Keegan, H. L. (1963). Leeches as pests of man in the Pacific region. In *Venomous and poisonous animals and noxious plants of the Pacific region* (ed. H. L. Keegan and W. V. Macfarlane), 99. Pergamon Press, Oxford.

POISONOUS PLANTS AND FUNGI

L. G. Goodwin

Plants

Many plants accumulate biologically active, complex organic chemicals in their tissues; the function of these substances is a mystery. It has been suggested that they may play a part as intermediate or end-products of metabolism because they frequently vary in concentration in step with the growth and maturation of the plant. High concentrations are often found in roots, rhizomes, and bark at the end of the growing season, in leaves when photosynthesis is at its peak, in flowers just before pollination, in unripe fruits, and in mature seeds. However, this hypothesis loses force in the light of the fact that flourishing healthy plants of the same species, grown in different places, and also different genetic variants of a species, often contain widely disparate amounts of these substances. Cultivated variants of cucumbers and beans entirely lose their original intense bitterness or toxicity. The two varieties of *Artemisia maritima*, one with reddish stems and the other grey, are indistinguishable at maturity; only the form with young red stems produces santonin.

Whatever their metabolic functions may be, the elaboration by clever chemistry, of substances that are attractive, unpleasant or toxic to vertebrate and invertebrate animals undoubtedly has an influence on the success and survival of the plant as a species. Perfume and sweetness in flowers attract pollinating insects and in fruits, attract birds and mammals that eat them and 'vernalize' and distribute their seeds after passage through the gut. Stinging hairs, irritant, bitter, and poisonous substances in leaves, and unripe fruits deter animals from eating them.

In temperate areas, plant poisoning occurs mainly in children who eat berries, chew flowers, leaves, or seeds of wild or houseplants, or drink water from vessels that have contained flowers. Some poisonous seeds, such as the jequirity bean (*Abrus*) and castor-oil bean (*Ricinus*) are used to make decorative necklaces and are sometimes chewed by children. In adults, poisoning occurs through the mistaken identity of wild salad plants and the use of herbal remedies.

In tropical countries, where plants containing potent substances are common, where food gathered from the wild provides an important item of diet, and indigenous medicines are widely used, poisoning occurs more frequently.

Poisoning is sometimes caused by plants used as foods; potatoes that have turned green through exposure to light, like the foliage of the potato and of other solanaceous plants, contain the toxic steroid alkaloid, solanine; wilted leaves of species that manufacture cyanogenetic glycosides may contain enough hydrocyanic acid to kill domestic stock. Carelessly washed or inadequately cooked cassava (*Manihot utilissima*) may also contain residual hydrocyanic acid, and some forms of yam (*Dioscorea*) need to be prepared and washed free from toxic dioscorine. In those areas in which flour is made from the root stocks of cycads (*Cycas* or *Zamia*), poisoning may occur as a result of residues of the glycoside cycasin, which causes lesions of the central nervous system and is a liver carcinogen. The aril of the unripe fruit of the akee (*Blighia sapida*), a native of W. Africa, widely naturalized in Jamaica, contains the poisonous alkaloid hypoglycin and has been responsible for many fatalities from 'vomiting sickness'.

There is a considerable variation in individual tolerance to plant poisons.

Plants that contain toxic substances usually produce them in variety—not only families of alkaloids or glycosides with similar pharmacological effects, but compounds of different chemical types with different actions. The results of eating them are therefore seldom the effects of a single, purified active substance. Nevertheless, plants may be broadly classified into eight groups producing:

1. Dermatitis (chemical or allergic)
2. Irritation of the alimentary tract
3. Cardiovascular disturbance
4. Nicotine-like actions
5. Atropine-like actions
6. Central nervous effects
7. Effects caused by hydrocyanic acid
8. Toxicity to the liver.

Dermatitis. Contact with the stinging hairs of *Urtica* (nettles) or

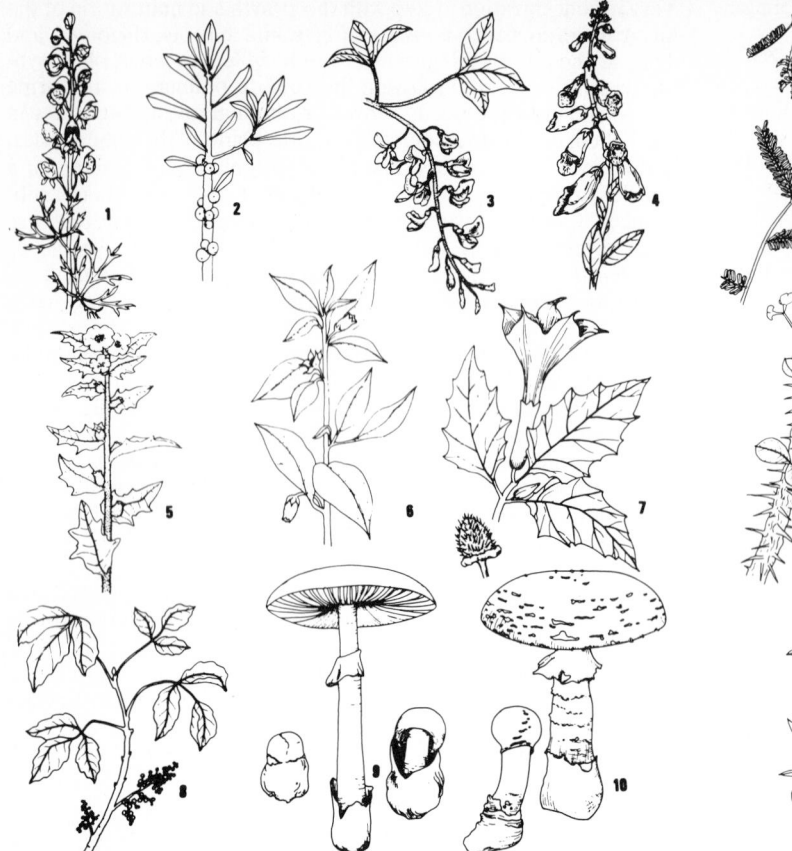

Fig. 1 Poisonous plants and mushrooms.

1. Monkshood (*Aconitum napellus*): perennial, 1 m tall; flowers dark blue.
2. Spurge laurel (*Daphne mezerium*): shrub with clusters of lilac or white flowers; scarlet berries.
3. Laburnum (*Laburnum anagryoides*): small tree with bunches of golden-yellow pea-shaped flowers.
4. Foxglove (*Digitalis purpurea*): biennial, 1 m tall; flowers whitish-lavender to purple, interior often spotted.
5. Henbane (*Hyoscyamus niger*): hairy erect biennial, 0.75 m tall; flowers pale yellow with purple veins and throat.
6. Deadly nightshade (*Atropa belladonna*): perennial, 1 m tall; flowers dark blue-purple; shiny black berries.
7. Thornapple (*Datura stramonium*): annual, 1 m tall; flowers white.
8. Poison ivy (*Rhus toxicodendron*): climbing or trailing shrub; flowers inconspicuous.
9. Death cap (*Amanita phalloides*): cap 8–13 cm broad, slimy and pale olive to amber in colour.
10. Fly agaric (*Amanita muscaria*): cap 8–20 cm broad, orange-red with whitish warts.
11. Jequirity bean (*Abrus precatorius*): slender woody vine with brilliant scarlet and black seeds.
12. Castor-oil plant (*Ricinus communis*): shrub, up to 5 m tall. Seeds black, mottled white or brown.
13. Akee (*Blighia sapida*): tree, growing to 12 m. Fruit bright red at maturity with yellow interior, containing large black seeds and a fleshy white aril.
14. Crown of thorns (*Euphorbia milii*): spiny undershrub about 0.5 m tall.
15. Hemlock (*Conium maculatum*): biennial, 1.5 m tall. Stems usually spotted with purple.
16. Dumb cane (*Dieffenbachia sequine*): decorative house plant. Leaves splotched with ivory marbling.
17. Oleander (*Nerium oleander*): evergreen shrub up to 6 m tall. Flowers white, yellow or red.
18. Yew (*Taxus baccata*): evergreen tree up to 7 m tall. Seed surrounded by a bright red, fleshy aril.

From Lampe and Fagerstrom (1968), by kind permission of authors and publishers.

the irritant latex of *Euphorbia* (spurges) produces an immediate skin reaction. Many other species, notably *Toxicodendron* (poison ivy), *Euphorbia* spp., and *Primula*, cause sensitization followed by allergic dermatitis five or more days after initial contact.

Treatment. The source should be identified and avoided, and relief from itching and inflammation provided.

Irritation of the alimentary tract. The plants found in temperate zones most commonly associated with injury to the alimentary tract are listed in Table 1.

Treatment. The aim should be to remove the ingested material as completely and gently as possible and to keep a sample for identification.

Demulcents are given to assist the healing of the injured mucosa. Systemic effects that may result from the absorption of toxic substances must be anticipated and steps taken to preserve life until the poisons are eliminated.

Cardiovascular disturbance. Plants containing glycosides of the digitalis group or alkaloids related to aconitine or veratrine (Table 2) affect cardiac conduction, rhythm, and vasodepressor reflexes; the effects of poisoning resemble those of overdosage of the digitalis glycosides used in clinical practice (see page 6.24).

Treatment. Ingested material should be removed and cardiovascular function restored. Poisoning with aconite should always be treated as an emergency.

Nicotine-like actions. Nicotine, lobeline, coniine, and cytisine stimulate and then paralyse autonomic ganglia, and the effects of ingesting plants that contain these alkaloids (Table 3) resemble those of classical nicotine poisoning (see page 6.15).

Treatment. Plant residues should be removed by gastric lavage with dilute (1:10 000) potassium permanganate solution and charcoal administered in water or milk. Preparation should be made to assist respiration and to manage convulsions. Poisoning of children

Table 1 Plants that irritate the alimentary tract

	Plant species	Toxic agents	Symptoms and signs	Treatment
Irritation of mouth and throat	*Dieffenbachia* (dumb cane) *Arum* (cuckoo pint) and other aroids	calcium oxalate needles and irritant resins	burning sensation, dysphagia, salivation, oedema	intense pain in the mouth may need relief with pethidine; liquid and soft foods
Irritation of stomach	Amaryllidaceae (*Narcissus* etc.) *Wisteria*	lycorine unknown	vomiting	gastric lavage
Irritation of intestine	*Aesculus* (horse chestnut) *Hedera* (ivy)	Saponins	Salivation, vomiting, colic diarrhoea; effects on CNS, renal and cardiovascular systems if absorbed	remove plant material by gastric lavage; demulcents (egg albumin, milk); correct electrolyte and fluid balance and prevent severe hypotension (especially with yew poisoning); haemodialysis if necessary
	Daphne (spurge laurel) *Arum* (cuckoo pint) *Iris*	Resins		
	Taxus (yew)	Taxine		
	Anemone *Caltha* (marsh marigold) *Clematis* *Ranunculus* (buttercup)	Protoanemonin		
	Allamanda *Chelidonium* (greater celandine)	Chelidonin		
	Ilex (holly) *Ligustrum* (privet) *Lonicera* (honeysuckle)	unknown		
Delayed gastroenteritis	*Abrus* (jequirity bean) *Ricinus* (castor-oil bean) *Robinia* (black acacia)	toxalbumins (lectins)	symptom-free for one hour to two days; severe vomiting and bloody diarrhoea followed by disturbance of CNS, cardiovascular, and renal function	Cautious gastric lavage; demulcents, magnesium trisilicate; allow diarrhoea to remove toxic gut contents but adjust fluid and electrolyte balance; control abdominal pain if necessary with pethidine; assist respiration; haemodyalysis if necessary
	Solanum spp (potato, bittersweet, black nightshade)	solanine		
	Rumex (sorrel, dock) *Psedera* (virginia creeper)	oxalic acid		
	Colchicum (autumn crocus) *Gloriosa* (glory lily)	colchicine		

Table 2 Plants that cause cardiovascular disturbance

Plant species	Toxic agents	Symptoms and signs	Treatment
Digitalis (foxglove) *Convallaria* (lily-of-the-valley) *Nerium* (oleander) *Thevetia* (yellow oleander) *Scilla* (squill)	cardiac glycosides	local irritation of mouth, vomiting, diarrhoea, abdominal pains and headache; cardiac arrhythmias	gastric lavage; give potassium if hypokalaemia occurs; monitor ECG and give anti-arrhythmic agents if necessary; (see overdosage with digoxin (p. 6.24)
Aconitum (monkshood) *Delphinium* (larkspur)	aconitine	tingling, burning, and numbness of mouth and lips; dysphagia, salivation, nausea, and vomiting; tingling and formication in fingers and face; headache, blurred vision, bradycardia, muscular weakness, and dyspnoea; death within 1–6 hours	**Emergency** evacuate stomach immediately; atropine, anti-arrhythmic agents and the intravenous infusion of calcium and magnesium salts have been recommended; assist respiration if necessary
Veratrum (American hellebores)	protoveratrines	epigastric burning, salivation, and prompt emesis; sweating, confusion, bradycardia, and hypotension.	atropine; vasoconstrictor drugs if hypotension is severe
Zygademus (death camas) *Kalmia* (mountain laurel) *Rhododendron*	veratrine andromedotoxin	As for protoveratrines but vomiting may be delayed; drowsiness and coma	gastric lavage; vasoconstrictor drugs; assist respiration if necessary

Table 3 Plants with nicotine-like effects

Plant species	Toxic agents	Symptoms and signs	Treatment
Nicotiana (tobacco) *Lobelia* *Conium* (hemlock) *Laburnum*	nicotine lobeline coniine cystisine	irritation of the mouth, salivation, nausea, and persistent vomiting; vertigo, headache, thirst, and cold sweat; confusion, delirium, hallucinations, fasciculation, and convulsions; massive doses produce paralysis and coma	gastric lavage with 1:10 000 potassium permanganate; charcoal in water or milk; assist respiration, manage convulsions, and give anti-hypotensive drugs

who have eaten laburnum flowers or seeds, or carried twigs in their mouths is not uncommmon in Britain.

Atropine-like actions. The belladonna alkaloids antagonize the muscarinic actions of acetylocholine. The effects of poisoning by plants containing them (Table 4) resemble those of atropine, but vary with the proportion of scopolamine, which does not cause peripheral dilatation, fever, or excitement.

Treatment. The stomach should be emptied and washed promptly because absorption is rapid, and the effects of atropine antagonized with anticholinesterases such as physostigmine 1–4 mg given intravenously (see page 6.22).

Central nervous system. Plants that contain convulsant substances are listed in Table 5. Cicutoxin and strychnine block inhibitory reflexes in the brain and spinal cord; excitatory mechanisms are exaggerated and convulsions ensue. Plants containing thujone have been used for many years in the preparation of herbal teas, employed as anthelmintics or in the belief that they were abortifacients. Poisoning is usually associated with the prolonged use of such preparations.

Plants that contain hallucinogenic compounds are either smoked (*Cannabis* and *Vinca*) or the seeds are chewed (*Ipomoea* and *Myristica*) for self-intoxication. Peyote (*Lophophora williamsii*) is taken by chewing dried slices of the cactus.

Treatment. Convulsions caused by cicutoxin or strychnine must be controlled and respiration supported; it will then be possible to wash out the stomach safely. Patients who have taken hallucinogens should not be left alone; reassurance and support is needed for a 'bad trip'.

Hydrocyanic acid. Many plants contain cyanogenetic glycosides and are dangerous to domestic stock. Human poisoning by plant cyanogens is caused by eating the broken seed kernels of *Prunus spp.* (almond, apricot, cherry, peach) or of *Eriobotrya japonica* (loquat); or as a result of the daily ingestion of *Manihot* (cassava) flour, containing residues of hydrocyanic acid. The symptoms and signs are vomiting, ataxia, dyspnoea, weakness, fibrillary twitchings, stupor, convulsions, and loss of consciousness.

Treatment. This is the same as for cyanide poisoning from any source (see page 6.32). Artificial respiration and oxygen are given and the stomach washed, and left filled with 5 per cent aqueous sodium thiosulphate solution. Sodium nitrite and thiosulphate may be injected intravenously, but intravenous dicobalt edetate is now the treatment of choice.

Toxicity to the liver. Composite plants of the genera *Crotalaria* and *Senecio* (ragwort) contain families of alkaloids related to jacobine which are cumulative poisons, causing liver cirrhosis. They are a frequent cause of fatalities in domestic stock. Liver cirrhosis is common in drinkers of 'bush tea' prepared from these plants in the West Indies.

Liver toxicity of a different kind is caused in Jamaica by the unripe fruit of *Blighia sapida* (akee) which contains hypoglycins, alkaloids that cause a fall in blood sugar and severe depletion of liver glycogen. Vomiting occurs 6–24 hours after ingestion, followed by a period of remission of 8–10 hours; then further vomiting, convulsions, coma, and death within four days. Sometimes convulsions and coma occur at the outset.

Treatment. Glucose should be given intravenously at once and electrolyte balance monitored and restored.

Fungi

Mushrooms and toadstools have been used as sources of poison from the earliest times. They contain active substances in great variety, with effects that range through simple alimentary tract irritation, stimulation of the autonomic or central nervous systems, or almost certain death from their toxic action on the liver and kidneys. In recent years, attention has been directed to the widespread effects of mycotoxins generated in stored foodstuffs as a result of fungal contamination.

Mushrooms and toadstools. Poisoning is usually the result of mistaking the identity of toxic species for edible ones. Individuals vary greatly in their susceptibility to poisoning, and fungi that grow in different localities may vary in the amounts of toxic substances they contain.

Many species produce transient nausea, vomiting, and diarrhoea which begin within an hour or two of ingestion, especially if they are eaten raw.

Species of *Clitocybe* and *Inocybe* contain muscarine and produce the characteristic 'muscarinic' actions of acetylcholine. *Amanita muscaria*, the toadstool from which muscarine was originally isolated, contains it in only small amounts; the excitement, hallucinations, elation, and the fly-killing properties for which this fungus is renowned, are now known to be caused by the isoxazole derivatives, ibotenic acid and muscimol.

Species of *Conocybe* and *Psilocybe*, fresh or dried, produce pleasant hallucinations and a state of hilarity as a result of the central nervous effects of psilocin and psilocybin; they are used for self-intoxication.

Most fatal mushroom intoxications are caused by *Amanita phalloides*, gathered and eaten in mistake for field mushrooms. This fungus contains phallotoxins and amatoxins, cyclic peptides that interfere with ribonucleic acid synthesis. The cyclic octapeptide,

---

Table 4   Plants with atropine-like effects

Plant species	Toxic agents	Symptoms and signs	Treatment
Atropa (deadly nightshade) *Datura* (thornapple) *Hyoscyamus* (henbane) *Cestrum* (jessamine)	atropine, hyoscyamine, scopolamine	photophobia and visual disturbance due to mydriasis and loss of accommodation, dryness of the mouth, and intense thirst; hot, dry, flushed skin, sometimes erythematous rash; tachycardia; fever, headache, confusion, delirium, hallucinations; urinary retention, and constipation; convulsions, stupor, coma, and respiratory failure	prompt gastric lavage; slow intravenous infusion of physostigmine; diazepam for sedation and to control convulsions; external cooling; pilocarpine drops to reduce eye discomfort

Table 5 Plants that affect the central nervous system

	Plant species	Toxic agents	Symptoms and signs	Treatment
Convulsants	*Cicuta* (cowbane) *Oenanthe* (water drop-wort)	cicutoxin oenanthetoxin	nausea, salivation, vomiting; tremors, followed by severe intermittent seizures, exhaustion, and respiratory failure	control convulsions with barbiturates or diazepam and support respiration
	Strychnos (nux vomica)	strychnine and brucine	stiffness of face and neck muscles, reflex excitability, severe tetanic convulsions, and medullary paralysis	gastric lavage when convulsions are controlled
	Thuja (arbor vitae) *Cupressus* (cypress) *Juniperus* (juniper) *Tanacetum* (tansy)	thujone and other terpenes	diarrhoea and vomiting; personality change, renal damage, and convulsions after repeated doses.	monitor and adjust fluid and electrolyte balance; control convulsions.
Hallucinogens	*Cannabis* (Indian hemp)	tetrahydrocannabinols	nausea, thirst, euphoria, ataxia, tremor, drowsiness and hallucinations	do not leave alone; reassurance and support may be needed to control panic reactions
	Ipomoea and *Rivea* (morning glory) *Lophophora* (peyote) *Myristica* (nutmeg)	lysergic acid and ethylamides mescaline myristicin	also mydriasis and other sympathomimetic effects	
	Vinca (periwinkle)	vincristine and vinblastine	also alopecia and paraesthesias	

α-amanitin is a potent and selective inhibitor of RNA polymerase B.

Treatment. This is outlined in Table 6. The prognosis of poisoning by *A. phalloides* is grave and, until recently, death resulting from profound degeneration of the alimentary mucosa, hepatic atrophy, and severe renal damage was almost inevitable within a week of eating the fungus. There is no specific antidote but lives have been saved by haemodialysis, initiated within 24–36 hours of ingestion. Intermittent peritoneal dialysis is of value if facilities for haemodialysis are not available. Thioctic (lipoic) acid or its amide, given by slow intravenous infusion (100–300 mg daily, with 100 g dextrose) has been reported to assist recovery of liver function in *A. phalloides* intoxication.

Contaminants of foodstuffs. The potential hazard of fungal toxins in foodstuffs was recognized in the eighteenth century, when it was realized that the ingestion of rye contaminated with the sclerotia of *Claviceps purpurea* was associated with ergotism in man and

Table 6 Poisonous mushrooms

Species	Toxic agents	Symptoms and signs	Treatment
Boletus luridus *B. satanas* *Lactarius* *Rhodophyllus* *Russula* *Scleroderma* *Tricholoma*	unknown	onset rapid, within two hours of ingestion; severe, but usually transient nausea, vomiting, and diarrhoea	gastric lavage
Clitocybe *Inocybe*	muscarine	frequently within 15 minutes of ingestion; nausea, visual disturbance, perspiration, salivation, lachrymation, colic, and muscular weakness	gastric lavage; atropine
Amanita muscaria *A. pantherina*	ibotenic acid and muscimol	frequently within 15 minutes of ingestion; drowsiness, nausea, and sometimes vomiting; elation, hyperkinesis, compulsive shouting, and visual hallucinations	gastric lavage; tranquillizers if agitation or hallucinations are severe (atropine aggravates the symptoms)
Conocybe *Psilocybe*	psilocin and psilocybin	within 3 hours of ingestion; drowsiness, dizziness, ataxia, skin paraesthesias, hallucinations, and hilarity	recovery usually uneventful in 3–6 hours; restrict destructive behaviour during hallucinations; tranquillizers if agitation is severe
Amanita phalloides *A. verna* *A. virosa* *Galerina*	phallotoxins and amatoxins	onset delayed for 6–12 hours; vomiting, abdominal cramps, and continuous diarrhoea; thirst, albuminuria, haematuria, anuria; jaundice in 2–3 days; prostration, peripheral circulatory collapse, hepatic coma, and death in 3–8 days	gastric and colonic lavage; immediate haemodialysis; thioctic acid with electrolytes and dextrose by slow intravenous infusion
Helvella (uncooked)	gyromitrin		

domestic animals. Outbreaks of 'St Anthony's fire', resulting from the vasoconstrictor properties of the ergot alkaloids frequently followed wet, rainy summers favourable to the growth of the fungus in the ears of grain.

Almost all plant products can serve as substrates for the growth of moulds. When contamination is heavy as a result of a damp growing season or insect damage, and when grain is gathered and stored before it is dry, moulds grow and some species produce mycotoxins (Table 7). Ingestion of grain infected with *Fusarium* or *Stachybotris* is associated with alimentary toxic aleukia (ATA), probably caused by toxic trichothecenes. Some strains of *Aspergillus flavus* and *A. parasiticus* produce aflatoxins, which are toxic to the liver and are carcinogenic. The common occurrence of liver cancer in some regions of Africa and Asia has been correlated with a high dietary intake of aflatoxins in contaminated groundnuts, maize, or cassava.

Ochratoxins, produced by species of *Aspergillus* and *Penicillium*, give rise to chronic renal illness, and a specific nephrotoxin has been extracted from *Penicillium verrucosum* var. *cyclopium*, isolated from contaminated maize in a Bulgarian village where endemic Balkan nephropathy occurs.

Inhalation of fungal spores during the handling of contaminated grain, flour, or animal feeding stuffs can give rise to respiratory disease. This may result from direct invasion of respiratory tissue by the growing fungus (histoplasmosis, actinomycosis) from the toxic effects of fungal metabolites (stachybotryotoxicosis) or from aller-gic responses that cause asthma, rhinitis, or 'farmers' lung' (*Aspergillus* and actinomycetes).

In order to protect health from the hazards of myotoxins, contamination of foods by moulds must be reduced to a minimum, and attention given to storage and quality control.

References

Arena, J. M. (1974). *Poisoning.* C. C. Thomas, Springfield, Illinois.
Austwick, P. C. K. (1981). Fungi and Actinimycetes. In *Scientific foundations of respiratory medicine* (eds. J. G. Scadding, G. Cumming, and W. M. Thurlbeck). Heinemann, London.
Chopra, R. N., Badhwar, R. L., and Ghosh, S. (1940). *Poisonous plants of India.* Govt. of India Press, Calcutta.
Dalziel, J. M. (1937). *The useful plants of west tropical Africa.* Crown Agents for the Colonies, London.
Forsyth, A. A. (1954). *British poisonous plants.* Bull. 161, MAFF, HMSO, London.
Lampe, K. F. and Fagerstrom, R. (1968). *Plant toxicity and dermatitis.* Williams and Wilkins, Baltimore.
Morton, J. S. (1977). Poisonous and injurious higher plants and fungi. In *Forensic medicine* (eds. C. P. Tedeschi, W. G. Eckert, and L. G. Tedeschi), Vol. 3, ch. 71, W. B. Saunders, Philadelphia.
Pammel, L. H. (1911). *A manual of poisonous plants.* Torch Press, Cedar Rapids, Iowa.
Ramsbottom, J. (1923). *A handbook of the larger British fungi.* British Museum (Natural History), London.
World Health Organization (1979). *Environmental health criteria II. Mycotoxins.* WHO, Geneva.

Table 7   Moulds

Fungus	Toxic agents	Toxic effects in man
Claviceps purpurea	ergot alkaloids	nausea, vomiting, diarrhoea, pruritus, numbness, and tingling of the extremities, confusion, and unconciousness; chronic poisoning causes vasoconstriction and thrombosis, resulting in muscle pain, dry peripheral gangrene, or epilepsy
Aspergillus flavus *A. parasiticus*	aflatoxins	liver necrosis; hepatic and renal cancers
Fusarium poae *F. sporotrichioides*	tricothecenes (probably)	alimentary toxic aleukia (ATA); leucopenia, with necrotic lesions of the mouth, oesophagus, and stomach
Aspergillus ochraceus *Penicillium viridicatum*	ochratoxins	renal tubular degeneration, interstitial fibrosis, and glomerular hyalinization
Penicillium verrucosum var. *cyclopium*	unidentified nephrotoxin	

Environmental extremes

HEAT, COLD, AND DROWNING

W. R. Keatinge

Heat

Effects of heat on the body. In a hot environment thermal receptors in the skin initiate reflex vasodilatation and sweating through cholinergic sympathetic nerves. At a later stage, as body temperature rises, deep receptors in the heat-loss centre in the preoptic region of the base of the brain reinforce these responses. Vasodilatation is also directly produced by warming of the blood vessels of the skin. The vasodilatation alone is able to dissipate resting metabolic heat production of the body as long as skin temperature is about 1 °C or more below body core temperature. Conduction and convection in the air can keep skin temperature low enough to allow this in slowly moving air up to about 32 °C, but in warmer air, or in cooler air during exercise, the heat produced can only be lost if sweat is formed and can evaporate to cool the skin. Sweat can be formed in larger amounts and with a lower salt content in heat-acclimatized than in unacclimatized people. If heat loss is insufficient, the consequent rise in body temperature leads to hyperventilation, to cerebral dysfunction involving irritability and confusion, and ultimately to cardiovascular collapse and cessation of sweating with rapid rise in body temperature and death. As body temperature rises above 41 °C, heat denaturation of proteins causes damage first to large cells of the cerebellum and cerebral cortex, and later to vascular endothelium, hepatic and renal cells, and striated muscle. Almost all cells of the body are killed if their temperature rises to 50 °C for a few minutes. Surface burns represent heat necrosis of this kind from brief localized surface heating, but are not often associated with general overheating of the body core.

Heat stroke. Heat stroke describes the clinical syndrome produced by overheating of the body core. It can be produced in normal people by several hours' physical exercise in a hot, humid environment close to or above body temperature. Exercise in hot, dry air can cause it if sweating is limited, either by lack of acclimatization to heat, by the rare condition of congenital absence of sweat glands, by dehydration, or by a failure of sweating known as tropical anhydrosis which can follow prolonged exposure to hot climates. Tropical anhydrosis is usually preceded by the common tropical complaint of prickly heat, which represents an inflammation of the sweat glands. After the inflammation subsides, the sweat glands may become functionless to produce tropical anhydrosis; the glands then form papules surmounted by vesicles. The face and axillae are not affected; sweating continues normally there. People with prickly heat recover rapidly, and people with tropical anhydrosis slowly, on return to cool surroundings, but both conditions are liable to recur on subsequent exposure to heat.

In hot, humid air above body temperature, heat stroke can develop even if sweating is normal, and in the absence of exercise. Many hours are normally required for a dangerous degree of overheating, but in hyperbaric gas at high temperature uptake of heat by the body can be rapid, both at the body surface and from respiratory gas. Rapid deaths from heat stroke have accordingly occurred among divers in pressure chambers after chamber temperature has risen as a result of difficulties with equipment.

Otherwise, heat stroke in sedentary people is usually associated with impairment of sweating and vasodilatation, either by drugs or disease. In industrial countries, heat stroke in hot weather is most commonly seen in psychiatric patients receiving drugs such as barbiturates or phenothiazines which depress reflex regulation of body temperature generally, or anticholinergic drugs which specifically suppress sweating and vasodilatation. General autonomic hypofunction due to diabetes is also a common cause of heat stroke in hot weather. Old age without other obvious disability is also sometimes associated with liability to heat stroke. A rare cause of a dangerous rise in body temperature is damage to the heat-loss centre in the preoptic region of the brain, usually by a tumour or by surgical interference with one. Shivering and vasoconstriction due to unrestrained action of the heat-gain centre in the hypothalamus can then cause a rapid and often fatal increase in body temperature even in temperate surroundings.

Diagnosis of heat stroke is generally easy, particularly in otherwise healthy people, from the history and the presence of irritability, confusion, headache, a hot, dry skin, and a deep body temperature (oral or rectal) close to or above 41 °C. Blood pressure is normal in heat stroke until it falls in the terminal stage of cardiovascular collapse. There is initially respiratory alkalosis due to hyperventilation, often followed by metabolic acidosis due to accumulation of lactic acid as hepatic failure develops. Serum calcium may be low in severe cases due to calcium binding by proteins of damaged cells.

Treatment consists of immediate cooling. Mild cooling by sponging with tepid water, which is allowed to evaporate on the skin, is often as effective as intense surface cooling by very cold water or refrigerated rubber blankets; mild cooling allows high blood flow in the skin to continue and to facilitate heat loss to the body surface. Rapidity of treatment is more important than the precise method used. In mild cases, recovery is generally rapid and complete, except in the ill or elderly when mortality is often due to other coexisting conditions. Severe cases of heat stroke may die suddenly, or, if they recover, may show lasting cerebellar or cerebral signs.

Post mortem may show little abnormality in cases of rapid death from heat stroke apart from degeneration of Purkinje cells and other large cells of the cerebellar and cerebral cortex. Less rapid deaths show oedema and petechial haemorrhages in the brain, and sometimes in other tissues.

Water-depletion heat exhaustion. Severe cases generally result from deprivation of water in hot environments. They are often complicated by heat stroke. Unlike other forms of heat illness, water depletion can develop more rapidly in heat acclimatized than in unacclimatized people because of their increased ability to sweat. The diagnosis is usually obvious from the history and from the

presence of thirst, dehydration with sunken face and eyes, and elevated serum sodium and chlorine. Haematocrit is normal since the water loss involves cell fluid and extracellular fluid equally. Death occurs when weight loss is 15–25 per cent bodyweight, and is due to excess concentration of salts in the body fluids. Contrary to some earlier views, present evidence indicates that shipwreck victims without fresh water cannot prolong survival by drinking seawater. Since seawater contains salt in higher concentration than can be excreted by the kidney, drinking of seawater accelerates death in victims of simple water depletion.

Treatment consists of giving up to 8 l of water by mouth during the first 24 hours, if the patient can swallow. In more severe cases, up to 5 l of 5 per cent glucose should be given by intravenous drip.

Salt-depletion heat exhaustion. Salt depletion usually develops insidiously in people working in hot environments, particularly in unacclimatized people in whom loss of salt in sweat is relatively high. Sodium chloride intake of up to 20 g per day, in food and by salt tablets, may be needed to prevent it. The sodium chloride must be accompanied by an adequate intake of water and should not be given to people threatened by dehydration due to restricted supply of water.

Early cases show fatigue, weakness, headache, nausea, and sometimes vomiting. One characteristic symptom is the appearance of sudden, very painful muscle cramps (e.g. 'miner's cramp'), but these only develop if the salt depletion is associated with muscular exercise.

There are a few signs of salt depletion apart from those of dehydration of the face and the skin generally, and often low blood pressure with marked postural hypotension. It is important to realize that serum sodium and chlorine are normal in mild cases of salt deficiency since osmotic pressure is initially regulated at normal levels at the expense of falling blood volume. However, haematocrit is raised and so are plasma protein concentrations. Blood urea is elevated. In severe cases, water is retained at the expense of osmotic pressure, and serum sodium and chlorine fall.

Treatment consists of giving 25 g sodium chloride in 5 l of water by mouth, and then ensuring adequate daily salt intake. In severe cases, immediate intravenous infusion of 500 ml isotonic saline may be needed.

Cold

Effects of cold on the body. In a cold environment cutaneous thermal receptors and later the deep receptors in the preoptic region of the brain bring about reflex vasoconstriction in the skin through noradrenergic sympathetic nerves. With moderate cooling of the skin, this is assisted by direct constrictor action of cold on the arterioles in the skin, so that even after sympathectomy there is marked local vasoconstriction when a limb is cooled in water or moving air at 15 °C. Aided by reflex noradrenergic drive to the heart, the vasoconstriction can result in large increases in arterial pressure on sudden exposure to cold. If cold exposure is severe enough to reduce the mean skin temperature of an adult below 33 °C, there are also reflex increases in muscle tone and shivering, brought about by ordinary somatic motor nerves, which can increase heat production by as much as fivefold for many hours at a time. The newborn infant does not shiver, but in a cold environment can increase heat production by metabolizing specialized brown fat, much of which is over the upper part of the back of the rib cage. This metabolism of brown fat is induced by noradrenergic sympathetic nerves which innervate the fat. That response, like reflex vasoconstriction in the skin, and muscular heat production brought about in response to cold in the adult, is mediated by the so-called heat-gain centre located in the posterior hypothalamus. Acclimatization by brief periods of exposure to cold generally reduces the degree of vasoconstrictor and of other responses to cold, leading to higher peripheral temperatures but greater tendency to lose central body heat. However, different patterns of acclimatization can produce other patterns of change in thermo-regulatory responses.

Although a mean skin temperature below 33 °C causes discomfort, these responses to cold enable most healthy and well-fed adults to maintain body temperature for long periods with skin temperatures as low as 12 °C if the individual is fat, but only as low as 25–30 °C if the individual is thin and so has little internal insulation when vasoconstricted. Children are also at a disadvantage because of a high surface area in relation to body mass. Most adults can maintain body temperature when lightly clothed in still air at about 5 °C, but not in much colder air, or in much less cold surroundings if external insulation is reduced by immersion in water or by wind and rain. Even fat people are liable to cool in water below 12 °C, since cold paralysis of the peripheral blood vessels then results in cold vasodilatation with rapid loss of heat.

Hypothermia. Hypothermia is usually defined by the presence of a deep body temperature, measured by reliable means, of less than 35 °C. Reliable measurement of this may be made sublingually in air warmer than 24 °C, in the external auditory meatus with servo-controlled external heating (zero gradient aural probe) in air warmer than 18 °C, rectally or from flowing urine in any environment if body temperature is reasonably stable, or oesophageally if the patient is not swallowing cold saliva. Rectal temperature is usually 0.2–0.5 °C higher than the others and both it and urine temperature lag behind the others if deep body temperature is changing rapidly.

Increasing disturbances of cerebral and cardiac function appear as the temperatures of the heart and brain fall below 35 °C. There is first listlessness and confusion, often with subsequent amnesia for events at the time of low body temperature. Consciousness is lost at a lower but variable temperature of 26–33 °C. After an initial rise in cardiac output associated with shivering, cardiac output falls with slowed heart rate due to direct effects of cold on the cardiac muscle, and at a temperature of 17–26 °C the cardiac output becomes insufficient to supply even the reduced oxygen requirements of the cold tissues, so that death ultimately ensues unless the patient is rewarmed. Failure of haemoglobin to release normal amounts of oxygen, due to a shift of the dissociation curve to higher values of P_{O_2}, contributes to tissue anoxia. One consequence in man and other large animals is that oxygenation of the cardiac muscle itself is impaired and the likelihood of arrhythmia increased. Atrial fibrillation is common at temperatures of 28–35 °C. Ventricular fibrillation may occur at temperatures below 28 °C, but otherwise, slow cardiac activity may be maintained for a time by a normal or ectopic pacemaker at temperatures as low as 11 °C. Respiration is depressed in hypothermia, but generally almost in proportion to metabolic needs, so that there is only slight respiratory acidosis. Accumulation of lactic acid from shivering in the early stages of cooling often produces some metabolic acidosis, but generally of mild degree unless very prolonged, severe hypothermia has resulted in anoxic liver damage. Glucose metabolism is depressed during hypothermia, and blood glucose and serum K rise as body temperature falls, and return to or below normal during recovery. Blood volume falls a little at the start of exposure to cold due to cold diuresis, which involves loss of both salt and water. This diuresis ceases after a while provided that deep body temperature remains near normal, but if hypothermia develops it returns, due to inability of renal tubular cells to reabsorb sodium chloride and water at low temperature. Loss of fluid from the circulation to the extravascular tissue space during hypothermia also contribute to a fall in blood volume. Hypotension is therefore liable to develop when a victim of prolonged hypothermia is warmed and vasodilatation takes place. Gastric erosions and haemorrhage, and pancreatitis occasionally follow severe hypothermia.

Immersion injuries and frostbite. Local cooling of the limbs can induce either non-freezing 'immersion' injury, or frostbite due to freezing of the tissues. Local cooling for many minutes below 12 °C, without freezing, causes sensory and motor paralysis. This is due to

blockage by low temperature of the sodium pump across cell membranes, with consequent net entry of sodium ions and ultimate inexcitability of nerve and muscle fibres. After short periods of cooling this recovers completely on warming, but after several hours at low temperatures nerve and muscle undergo lasting damage and subsequently degenerate when normal temperature and blood flow are restored. Local cooling below −0.54 °C can freeze human tissues, though they often supercool initially and only freeze when rather lower temperatures are reached. Unless the temperature is very low, only part of the tissue water freezes, leaving the remainder with an increased concentration of salts which denatures proteins. Endothelial cells of blood vessels are particularly vulnerable to such damage, and when the tissue thaws, the capillaries leak plasma and the red cells left behind may sludge, block the vessel, and then clot. Ischaemic necrosis produced in this way is responsible for most of the tissue damage in frostbite.

Prevention and management of hypothermia and cold injury
Immersion hypothermia and immersion injury. These usually result from shipwrecks. Most people without protection develop a dangerous degree of hypothermia after several hours' immersion in water at 15–20 °C. People who survive immersion in water below 12 °C are in addition liable to suffer non-freezing immersion injury of the limbs, particularly if they subsequently spend many hours on a lifeboat or raft, where body heat loss is reduced but the limbs remain cold. The other cause of non-freezing cold injuries on a large scale has been 'trench foot' caused by prolonged standing in flooded trenches in wartime. Body tissues cannot, of course, freeze in fresh water. They can freeze in seawater, which itself freezes at −1.9 °C, but once they do freeze in this situation survival is unusual, and few cases of frostbite from general body immersion in seawater have required medical attention.

The most important measures are preventive. Body cooling during immersion and the risk of immersion injury can both be reduced, and the risk of frostbite in the water virtually eliminated, by advising survivors abandoning ship to put on thick conventional clothing including gloves and footwear. Body cooling in the water can also, surprisingly, be reduced by advising survivors to float still in lifejackets rather than exercising; exercise in cold water generally increases heat loss substantially more than heat production. Wet suits of foam rubber, or waterproof suits, of course provide excellent protection if they are available.

After an immersion victim is rescued, the immediate treatment is what matters most. It must first be decided whether the patient is suffering mainly from hypothermia or from inhalation of water. A fully conscious person can say whether or not he has inhaled water. With a semi-conscious or unconscious person, someone still alive after immersion in cold water for many hours with an adequate lifejacket is likely to be hypothermic, while someone unconscious after a few minutes' immersion without one would have drowned. However, in rough water mixed conditions are not uncommon, and an immediate measure of body temperature is always useful. Rectal temperature by a low-reading thermometer is the most reliable and practical method in this situation, though it must be remembered that rectal temperature can lag as much as 1–2 °C behind cardiac temperature when the latter is falling very rapidly, as it may be in someone just removed from very cold water.

People who have a body temperature below about 31 °C at the time of rescue, and who have not inhaled water, are liable to die suddenly from cardiac arrest or fibrillation during the next 30 minutes, since deep body temperature continues to fall for a time. This can often be prevented, or cardiac action restored after it has failed, if the victim is rewarmed by immediate immersion of the trunk in a bath no hotter than the observer can tolerate with his own hand, or 42–44 °C. Conscious victims of hypothermia demand a rather lower bath temperature. External cardiac massage and artificial ventilation, at slower rates than usual, may be useful if cardiac action and respiration are definitely absent, but can be dangerous if spontaneous heartbeat and respiration are present, as they may precipitate ventricular fibrillation. P_{CO_2} is not normally high enough, or P_{O_2} low enough, to require artificial ventilation in simple hypothermia. Adrenaline usually precipitates ventricular fibrillation in hypothermia and should not be given. In order to minimize hypotension during rewarming, the patient should be removed from the hot bath when body temperature has risen to 33 °C or when general condition is clearly returning to normal, and placed recumbent in warm air on under blankets to continue rewarming more slowly. When no hot bath is available initial warming in warm air or under blankets with mild heat input, for example from hot-water bottles at 44 °C, is usually effective.

Victims of immersion hypothermia who are still alive 30 minutes after rescue almost always recover, and as long as improvement continues, no further active treatment should generally be given at that stage. Admission to hospital is desirable for chest X-ray, in case water has been inhaled. It is advisable to monitor arterial pressure and ECG, and to keep a defibrillator available. Atrial fibrillation and ventricular ectopic beats, if present, usually cease as temperature rises and do not require treatment. Antifibrillatory agents should generally be avoided as they are liable to produce arrest or even induce fibrillation in deep hypothermia. Blood glucose, pH, and serum K may be measured once a good bloodflow is restored to the limbs so that a venous sample can give meaningful information. However, attempts to correct apparent abnormalities of pH and K are rarely needed and should not be made unless the abnormalities are large and the patient is in poor general condition in spite of rising body temperature. They should never be made unless the validity of the blood sample itself, and of the assay and any temperature corrections made to it, are known without doubt to be dependable.

The limbs of people rescued from water below 12 °C are initially often anaesthetic and paralysed. If the duration of cooling was prolonged, they will, on warming, develop signs of immersion injury, becoming bright red, hot, oedematous, and painful. They should then be elevated to reduce oedema, and analgesics given for the pain. During the next few weeks, muscles and nerves may degenerate, and physiotherapy is needed to prevent contractures. Partial denervation of blood vessels due to degeneration of their motor nerves often leads to vascular instability with excessive vasoconstriction in the cold and dilatation in the heat. Some improvement in the disabilities is usual over the course of months as nerves regenerate, but weakness due to muscular damage often persists.

Exposure without severe frostbite. Hillwalkers, climbers, and skiers who are inadequately clothed in air colder than 0 °C are liable to both hypothermia and frostbite, and in air above 0 °C to hypothermia alone. These generally develop after people become lost, or immobilized by bad weather or injury, and have to spend one or more nights without shelter. However, hypothermia can develop during even mild exposure to cold if people take ethanol after exercise and without food, as inexperienced hillwalkers sometimes do. Two hours' exercise depletes the body's reserve of carbohydrate, and metabolism of ethanol leads to reduction of the pyruvate needed for gluconeogenesis, so that less than 30 ml of ethanol can then produce hypoglycaemia. This not only causes mental confusion but virtually eliminates the normal reflex vasoconstrictor and metabolic responses to cold, so that body temperature can fall to 33 °C in as little as 80 minutes in slowly moving air at 14–22 °C. Hypothermia due to ethanol hypoglycaemia should be considered when people who have taken insufficient ethanol to cause drunkenness are found confused, unconscious, or dead after relatively mild exposure to cold.

Since apathy and confusion can be produced by exhaustion as well as by hypothermia, an immediate measurement of body temperature is important when people are found in this state in open country. Urine temperature provides a convenient way of excluding hypothermia in conscious people in field conditons, if a low-reading thermometer and funnel needed for it are carried by the rescue party; otherwise, rectal temperature should be measured.

Table 1 Hypoglycaemia and hypothermia induced by ethanol after exercise. All groups had taken 28 ml ethanol by mouth and then sat in air at 14–22 °C for 80 minutes. Some had also taken approximately 60 g glucose, and some had previously exercised for approximately two hours, as indicated. Means ± SE, seven experiments

	Exercise No glucose	No exercise No glucose	Exercise Glucose
Blood glucose (mmol)	1.77 ± 0.20	2.82 ± 0.61	4.96 ± 0.61
Rectal temperature (°C)	34.49 ± 0.34	26.82 ± 0.14	36.94 ± 0.14
Metabolic rate (kcal/m²/hour)	45.00 ± 2.90	76.10 ± 7.70	91.00 ± 10.40
Blood ethanol (mmol)	5.11 ± 0.29	5.12 ± 0.18	5.80 ± 0.74

From Haight, J. S. J. and Keatinge, W. R. (1973). *J. Physiol.* **229**, 87

In cases of exposure on land, unlike immersion hypothermia, body temperature has usually fallen slowly, so that it has been low for many hours and is relatively stable at the time of rescue. In such cases, provided that there is no serious injury or extensive frostbite, recovery is almost invariable if the victim is placed recumbent in a well-insulated sleeping bag. Although respiratory heat loss is relatively small, it is helpful in very cold air to control it by a simple heat exchanger or heater, until the patient can be moved into warm surroundings. Small amounts or extra heat from hot water bottles at 44 °C or an electric blanket are important if hypothermia is severe, but since loss of blood volume has often been substantial in the prolonged exposure that such cases have usually experienced in open country, more rapid rewarming in hot water can be dangerous to them. Even with slow rewarming, their arterial pressure often falls considerably as body temperature rises. This can almost invariably be controlled by recumbent posture and raising the legs, but 500 ml of saline or dextran intravenously is often helpful. Body temperature is most conveniently monitored, during slow rewarming, by a zero gradient aural thermometer. Depletion of body carbohydrate by prior exercise is common in cases of exposure, and sugary drinks should be given during recovery, once body temperature is above 31 °C so that glucose can be metabolized. As in immersion hypothermia, ECG may be monitored and blood glucose, pH, and serum K may be measured in severe cases, once peripheral circulation is restored to allow valid samples of circulating blood, but they rarely call for further treatment.

Frostbite is obvious as hard, white areas of skin on the extremities. As long as it involves only parts of the fingers, toes, hands, or feet, it is best treated by sudden thawing in water no hotter than the observer can stand without discomfort. This allows optimal tissue recovery, probably because return of bloodflow is so rapid that blood flowing through damaged capillaries has too little time to lose all its plasma and to block the vessels with sludged red cells. Subsequently, analgesics should be given for pain and the part elevated to reduce oedema. The skin may subsequently turn black, but then often sloughs off to leave almost normal tissue beneath. Surgery should be considered only after the necrotic region is fully delineated.

Exposure with massive frostbite. Exposure in very cold climates can result in massive freezing of most of the tissue of the limbs, together with general hypothermia. People in this condition have sometimes survived slow rewarming in warm air without early medical help, but the best results seem to have been obtained by transporting them at once to hospital and rewarming them there at moderate speed under full biochemical control. Such people have extensive tissue damage comparable to massive crush injury. Rapid thawing leads to massive release of toxic substances, particularly potassium, into the circulation. These can cause ventricular fibrillation, so that treatment in an intensive care unit with full biochemical control, haemodialysis, and even extracorporeal circulation in cases of persistent ventricular fibrillation, may be needed for recovery. Subsequent necrosis of tissue in the damaged limbs is often extensive in those who survive.

Hypothermia complicating poisoning, disease, injury, undernutrition, old age, and infancy. Approximately 3 per cent of patients admitted to British hospitals in winter have rectal temperatures below 35 °C, the recognized level for hypothermia. The great majority of these have cooled as a result of the effects of drugs or disease in cold surroundings. Ethanol, barbiturates, and other drugs which depress the central temperature regulatory centres are commonly responsible; in most cases anaesthetic or near-anaesthetic quantities have been taken. Malnutrition, insulin hypoglycaemia, myxoedema, and anoxia due to carbon monoxide poisoning, also reduce heat production in cold conditions and are important causes of hypothermia. Other patients cool after collapsing and being immobilized as result of injuries, strokes, heart attacks, or pneumonia. Provided that rewarming is carried out at a moderate rate in warm air or with a low wattage electric blanket, it has been found that the hypothermia has little effect on the outcome, and mortality is essentially that of the underlying condition. In cases of carbon monoxide poisoning or hypoglycaemia, the hypothermia can even be beneficial before help is available, by protecting the brain from damage until the treatment can be started. No specific treatment of hypothermia, other than moderate application of surface heat, is generally required. The depressant effect of hypothermia on respiration can make artificial ventilation necessary during poisoning by quantities of depressant drugs which would be insufficient to stop respiration on their own. Otherwise, the main importance of hypothermia resulting from poisoning, disease, or injury is that it often complicates diagnosis of the underlying disease.

Rare cases of hypothermia are due to defective responses to cold, so that in cool surroundings body temperature drops to the point of mental confusion and coma without the patient shivering or feeling cold. The defect is rarely complete and the patients, who are not always elderly, may continue to work and lead normal lives provided they spend most of the day in warm surroundings. They usually show no other defect in function, and no obvious abnormality on brain scan. Malnutrition must always be excluded, but in its absence, and in the absence of hypothalamic tumour or disease, degeneration of thermoregulatory neurones in the hypothalamus must be assumed to be responsible.

In even rarer cases, hypothermia is induced actively by epileptic discharge in the preoptic heat-loss centre. The attacks involve a sensation of warmth with sweating, vasodilatation, and rapid fall in body temperature below 35 °C. When the discharge ends, there is a sensation of cold, with shivering, vasoconstriction, and rise of body temperature to normal. The attacks may be prevented by anticonvulsant drugs, or failing that controlled by sympathectomy.

There has been uncertainty over whether old people who are not suffering from one of these rare major defects of temperature regulation or from poisoning, malnutrition, or disease are particularly prone to hypothermia in cool surroundings. Old people's ability to discriminate small rises or falls in skin temperature is often less than that of younger adults. Present evidence suggests that general tendency to hypothermia associated with this exists but is mild in degree. A British survey of over 1000 elderly people at home during a winter in which all heating was stopped from time to time as a result of a miners' strike revealed nobody with a temperature below 35 °C in the evening, and only four with both mouth and urine temperatures a little below 35 °C in the early morning at the bottom of the normal diurnal temperature fluctuation. There was no correlation between body temperature and age, which varied from 65 to 85 years. As we have seen, very few people of any age admitted to hospital have hypothermia except as an occasional secondary consequence of their main disease. Excess mortality occurs in cold weather but is due mainly to deaths from coronary insufficiency and other cardiovascular disease, usually apparently precipitated not by hypothermia but by the reflex effects of sudden

exposures to cold. The case for special care with home heating for the elderly rests mainly on maintaining the comfort and general health of a group whose physical activitiy, and therefore heat production, tend to be less than those of younger adults.

Infants are liable to hypothermia in cool surroundings which would present no threat to an adult. Their high surface area to mass ratio and their lack of subcutaneous fat, particularly in premature infants, are mainly responsible. Once the store of brown fat is exhausted, body temperature of lightly clothed infants can fall rapidly in a cold room. The diagnosis is often not obvious since the face is often red due to engorgement of capillaries with stagnant but oxygenated blood. Drowsiness, oedema, and coldness of the skin to the touch suggest hypothermia, which can be confirmed by low-reading rectal thermometer. The oedema may later be followed by a hardening of the tissues called sclerema. Severe cases carry a high mortality. Rewarming is generally carried out at a moderate speed by exposure in an incubator kept just warmer than the infant's own temperature. Hypoglycaemia often develops when body temperature rises above 31 °C. It can be treated by 60 ml/kg of 10 per cent glucose intravenously per day, with further glucose by mouth when the infant can suck and swallow.

Cold allergy. Cold allergy is a rare condition in which local exposure to cold is followed by vasodilatation and oedema of the region involved. The symptoms usually develop only after the exposure to cold, and consequent local vasoconstriction, has ended. The severest consequences are seen after susceptible people have swum in cold water. On coming ashore, they may develop a reaction over the entire body, with widespread vasodilatation, headache, hypotension, and sometimes loss of consciousness. Even the severest cases usually recover spontaneously. The cause is not understood in detail, and the most effective treatment is preventive; repeated exposures to progressively more severe cold generally produce desensitization. Antihistamines can be given before cold exposure, though they are only moderately effective. In the acute phase, little treatment is usually needed apart from placing the patient recumbent in a comfortably warm environment, elevating the legs if necessary, and giving antihistamines and mild analgesics if needed for headache.

Drowning

Classical drowning. Total submersion is usually followed by breath-holding for about five minutes and then massive inhalation of water into the lungs. In seawater drowning, calcium and magnesium ions in the water are then rapidly absorbed into the blood and cause cardiac arrest. In freshwater drowning, absorption of the inhaled water causes haemolysis, with consequent increase in serum K, and ventricular fibrillation. In either case, the immediate treatment of a victim without pulse or respiration is to clear the airway and start external cardiac massage and artificial ventilation. As soon as a gastric tube can be obtained, the stomach should be emptied, as it is often distended with water swallowed during the submersion, which is liable to be vomited. The trachea should be intubated before passing the gastric tube if the gag reflex is absent. Victims of seawater drowning frequently recover rapidly if treatment is given within five minutes of the drowning; artificial restoration of the circulation allows the high levels of calcium and magnesium in the blood to be dissipated by diffusion into the tissues, and spontaneous heartbeat and respiration to return. The ventricular fibrillation and haemolysis produced by freshwater drowning are less easily treated, and recovery is rare after freshwater drownings in summer in water above about 20 °C. However, when people drown in colder water, cooling of the brain and other body tissues protects them from rapid anoxic damage during circulatory arrest so that more time is available for resuscitation. This is particularly true of water near 0 °C, and of children, whose smaller size allows more rapid tissue cooling. Resuscitation has then been successfully carried out without serious brain damage after more than 30 minutes under water. When facilities are available, positive pressure ventilation to reduce pulmonary collapse and oedema and, exchange transfusion and electrical defibrillation may all be needed as soon as the victim, receiving continuous cardiac massage and mouth-to-mouth ventilation, can be brought to hospital.

Many cases involving inhalation of small amounts of water do not progress to cardiac arrest or fibrillation, but require treatment for respiratory failure. Inhalation of relatively small amounts of water can cause respiratory failure within minutes by obstructing bronchioles or inducing laryngeal spasm, or after periods up to several hours by pulmonary collapse and oedema. Animal experiments show that inhalation of as little as 3 ml/kg body weight, representing a little over 200 ml for a human adult, can sometimes cause death in these ways. If the heart is still beating after sudden obstruction, rapid recovery may follow clearing of the airways and mouth-to-mouth resuscitation. However, removal of pulmonary surfactant and local irritation and obstruction by the inhaled fluid can lead to delayed pulmonary collapse and oedema, causing secondary respiratory failure hours after rescue. Anyone who has inhaled significant amounts of water should therefore be admitted to hospital for at least 24 hours for chest X-ray and observation. Artificial ventilation with positive end expiratory pressure can then be given if it becomes necessary. A broad spectrum antibiotic is often given to prevent infection.

'Dry drowning' and sudden death in water. Dry drowning is essentially a post-mortem description of death due to submersion but without water in the lungs at post mortem; in classical drowning the lungs are partially flooded with water and partially ballooned with air as a result of obstruction of bronchioles by water. Most cases of rapid death in water with dry lungs at post mortem are due to inhalation of water which has been absorbed into the blood from the lungs before the circulation stopped. Evidence of this can often be found in a higher chloride content and specific gravity in the left than the right side of the heart in seawater drownings, and the reverse in freshwater drownings. The most reliable indication that water has been inhaled during life can be obtained by the demonstration, in body tissues remote from the lungs, of large numbers of diatoms of types which match species present in the water in which the victim died.

There are also occasional rapid deaths due to immersion, but in which there is no inhalation of water into the lungs. People sometimes hyperventilate before swimming underwater, to increase the time that they can hold their breath and stay submerged. The hyperventilation reduces the CO_2 content of the body without adding to its oxygen content, so that the increased duration of breath-holding allowed by the reduced CO_2 is accompanied by fall of arterial P_{O_2} to low levels. In these circumstances cold water on the face or upper airway can cause marked reflex bradycardia. These people are accordingly liable to lose consciousness, and to die if not rescued rapidly and ventilated. Another rare group involves reflex cardiac death within the first few minutes of immersion, induced by sudden cooling of the body surface in water. These deaths are probably due in most cases to ventricular fibrillation, resulting from intense noradrenergic reflex drive to the ventricular muscle and peripheral vasoconstriction, and sometimes assisted by cooling of the face which causes vagal slowing of the normal pacemaker. Such deaths may occur just after a brief swim, as in a recent case in which a young man dived into a pool, swam fifteen yards across it, climbed out, and then fell to the ground unconscious. He was breathing but was blue and no pulse could be felt, and he died in spite of immediate attempts at external cardiac massage and artificial ventilation. Such cases are rarely resuscitated successfully, and revival is likely to require continuation of effective cardiac massage and artificial ventilation until the patient can be transported to a hospital with facilities for defibrillation. Peripheral vasoconstriction can bring about pulmonary oedema during more prolonged cold swims or dives, but no deaths from this seem to have been recorded in healthy people.

References

Daly, M. de B. and Taton, A. (1979). Interactions of cardio-respiratory reflexes elicited from the carotid bodies and upper airways receptors in the conscious rabbit. *J. Physiol.* **291**, 34.

Fox, R. M., Woodward, P. M., Exton-Smith, A. N., Green, M. F., Donnison, D. V., and Wicks, M. H. (1973). Body temperatures in the elderly: a national study of physiological, social and environmental conditions. *Br. med. J.* **i**, 200.

Golden, F. St. C. and Rivers, J. F. (1975). Thoughts on immediate care: the immersion incident. *Anaesthesia* **30**, 364.

Haight, J. S. J. and Keatinge, W. R. (1973). Failure of thermoregulation in the cold during hypoglycaemia induced by exercise and ethanol. *J. Physiol.* **229**, 87.

Keatinge, W. R. (1969). *Survival in cold water. The physiology and treatment of immersion hypothermia and drowning.* Blackwell Scientific Publications, Oxford.

Ledingham, I. McA. and Mons, J. G. (1980). Treatment of accidental hypothermia: a prospective clinical study. *Br. med. J.* **i**, 1102.

Maclean, D. and Emslie-Smith, D. (1977). *Accidental hypothermia.* Blackwell Scientific Publications, Oxford.

Sprung, C. L., Portocarrero, C. J., Fernaine, A. V., and Weinberg, P. F. (1980). The metabolic and respiratory alterations of heat stroke. *Archs intern. Med.* **140**, 665.

DISEASES OF HIGH TERRESTRIAL ALTITUDES

D. Rennie

High altitude terrain and populations. Until the late nineteenth century, mountains were viewed by Europeans as dangerous, mysterious, hostile, and remote. Yet there is evidence that mountainous regions have, for many thousands of years, been the home of large and elaborate civilizations such as that of the Incas, which in the fifteenth century included Ecuador to the north and much of northern Chile and Argentina some 5000 km to the south, an empire of at least 12 million people. The Altiplano or high plateau of the Andes is still home to millions of descendants of these Incas, many of whom have never been below altitudes around 4000 m above sea level.

Temperature tends to determine the fauna and flora. Since, other things being equal, temperature falls with increasing altitude, the high altitude climate tends to be an arctic one. The snow line and tree line become lower with increasing distance from the equator and to live, work, hunt, and cultivate at altitudes above 3000 m is possible only within about 40 degrees of the equator. This includes the Andes of Ecuador, Bolivia, Peru, and northern Chile, the Rocky Mountains in the United States, the high lands of east Africa, the Caucasus, the Pamirs, and the Himalayas, but does not include, for example, the European Alps.

The fall in temperature of some 1 °C for every 150 m rise in altitude, irrespective of latitude, and the high winds increase the danger of cold injury. The low humidity contributes greatly to fluid loss and dehydration, as does the increased solar radiation which may be very much exaggerated by reflection from the snow. These factors are, however, common to most arctic environments and will be discussed elsewhere (see page 6.55).

The fact that so many people of diverse races have been born and have lived at such altitudes, and the fact that, excluding Antarctica, about 2.5 per cent of the land lies above 3000 m, gives high altitude physiology and medicine an economic, political, and cultural relevance. As modern transport brings the highest mountains within range of the meanest purse, tourists, hikers, mountaineers, and downhill and crosscountry skiers, as well as mining engineers, geologists, and surveyors, are flocking up into the hills. Every day in July and August about 3600 people visit the summit of Pike's Peak in Colorado (4300 m) and there is now even a 42 km marathon race up and down that mountain. In 1950, three expert Western climbers first reached the base of the ice fall below Mount Everest's Western Cwm, at 5300 m. Twenty-five years later, in a mere four weeks, well over 500 inexpert tourists did so.

The vast majority of mankind lives below 1000 m altitude and, though there is this exponential rise in the numbers of lowlanders going to high altitude, they cannot assume that they can make the ascent with impunity.

Hypoxia. Though the proportion of oxygen in the air (20.93 per cent) is the same at every altitude, the atmospheric pressure, as was shown by Blaise Pascal on the Puy de Dome in his 'Great Experiment' of 1648, decreases with increasing altitude. The total atmospheric pressure at sea level (barometric pressure, P_B) varies but is usually around 760 torr (mmHg) (101 kPa) and that due to oxygen (the partial pressure of oxygen) is 20.93 per cent of this, i.e. 159 torr (21.2 kPa). In the lung, the air is rapidly saturated with water vapour at body temperature. At any altitude this is 47 torr (6.25 kPa) at 37 °C. The actual combined pressures of gas taken into the lungs is therefore $(P_B - 47)$ torr and the inspired oxygen tension (P_{IO_2}) is 20.93 per cent of this: $0.2093 \times (P_B - 47)$. At sea level this is $0.2093 \times (760 - 47) = 149$ torr (19.8 kPa). At about 5500 m the atmospheric pressure is about half that at sea level and at the summit of Everest (8848 m), allowing for the fact that the earth's atmosphere is an oblate spheroid—flattened at the poles—the atmospheric pressure is about 250 torr (33 kPa; one third that at sea level) and the partial pressure of oxygen is $0.2093 \times 250 = 52.3$ torr (7 kPa). The partial pressure of water, however, reduces the P_{IO_2} from 52.5 torr to $0.2093 \times (250 - 47) = 42.5$ torr (5.7 kPa). It is clear that the fraction of total inspired gas pressure due to water vapour, which at sea level is 6 per cent, increases with altitude. At the summit of Everest it will be nearly 19 per cent and at 19 200 m (63 000 feet), the total pressure of inspired gases would be a fatal 47 torr—fatal because all of it would be water vapour. Conversely, the proportion of inspired gas due to oxygen, which is 19.6 per cent at sea level, is reduced to 17 per cent at the summit of Everest and is, of course, zero at 19 200 m.

Following a plane's sudden decompression or a rapid balloon ascent, for example, a resting man, just up from sea level, would lose consciousness in a matter of minutes at altitudes between 6400 m and 7300 m ($P_{AO_2} = 24$–15 torr; 3.2–2 kPa) and in seconds above 7300 m (P_{AO_2} below 15 torr; 2 kPa), yet during one year (1978–9) a total of 14 men, on the three highest peaks in the world (Everest, K2, and Kanchenjunga) were not only fully conscious at rest more than 1000 m higher than this but were able to climb over difficult terrain in bad weather to their respective summits (8848 m, 8611 m, and 8598 m) all without the benefit of supplemental oxygen.

Acclimatization. These are obviously extreme examples, but anyone who has driven by car in a few hours from the coast up to mining towns of the Peruvian Andes at between 4000 m and 4900 m, is immediately struck by the contrast between their own discomfort and helplessness and the energy with which the locals after a hard shift in the mines, set about playing soccer. The difference consists of a myriad of physiological adjustments which collectively we call 'acclimatization'. As far as we can tell, it depends solely upon the length of exposure and the age when first exposed and has little if anything to do with genetic factors. It is not, therefore, an adaptation in the Darwinian sense and the physiologist has yet to demonstrate any discrete long term adjustment that cannot be made by, say, Caucasians born at high altitude.

The processes of acclimatization, which affect every system in the body, proceed at different speeds but though changes may continue for many years thereafter, the time of greatest adjustment is in the hours and days after arrival at a higher altitude. During this early process, when the most marked changes are occurring, the newcomer to high altitude is not only comparatively weak and ineffectual but may suffer the signs and symptoms of acute mountain sickness (AMS), a disease which may itself be caused by the rapid physiological responses to the new and oxygen-deficient environment.

There are huge numbers of people who have ascended to high altitudes and, having had a measurable deficit in performance on arrival, but no signs or symptoms, have gradually acclimatized until their performance is identical with that of natives. The presence of AMS, therefore, indicates that the early and most dramatic adjustments are not merely incomplete but distorted or deranged.

The changes that occur within the body, in response to hypoxia, affect every tissue and it is inappropriate to detail them here: I refer to excellent reviews of this subject at the end of this chapter. In general they may be briefly summarized as a series of adjustments which boost oxygen supply to the mitochondria by keeping the partial pressure of oxygen in the tissue capillaries as high as possible, by decreasing the distance oxygen has to diffuse in the tissues, and by increasing the concentrations of respiratory enzymes.

A few of the principal steps involved may be summarized thus:

Ventilation. When P_{AO_2} has fallen to 55–60 torr (7.3–7.9 kPa) at an altitude of about 2000–3000 m, the peripheral chemoreceptors are stimulated by hypoxia and ventilation is increased. This initial reaction is amplified over the next three or four days so that P_{AO_2} levels which are only very slightly lower than normal (as one would find at, say, 1000 m altitude) now begin to stimulate ventilation. After a few weeks of sojourn, however, ventilation slowly decreases and this process continues for years, though ventilation is always higher in sojourners than in people who were born and have lived all their lives at altitude. With exercise, ventilation increases more at high altitude than at sea level and more in sojourners than in natives.

Driving respiration by hypoxia implies, from the point of view of carbon dioxide (CO_2), 'hyperventilation', since CO_2 is blown off, and a respiratory alkalosis develops. The P_{CO_2} falls in a linear manner with altitude, and the alkalosis is only partly compensated by a rise in urinary excretion of bicarbonate. The effect of this hypocarbia and alkalosis would normally be to inhibit respiration, as well as, for example, to diminish cerebral blood flow, but a heightened sensitivity of the respiratory centre to CO_2 tends to counteract this. The exact mechanisms by which changes in brain stem extracellular $[H^+]$ are produced during early and late exposure to high altitude and how they affect respiration are at present a matter of vigorous controversy.

The *effect* of the increased ventilation is rapidly to increase the alveolar oxygen pressure by reducing the oxygen gradient between ambient and alveolar air and by reducing P_{ACO_2}.

Pulmonary diffusion. Though no increase in pulmonary diffusing capacity occurs in sojourners at high altitude, natives have increased pulmonary diffusing capacity with a lowered alveolar–arterial oxygen gradient, associated with an increased capillary surface for diffusion. This is due to an opening up of pulmonary capillaries, and to polycythaemia which decreases the distance necessary for gaseous diffusion. There is no increase in pulmonary blood flow so the increase in lung capillary volume is equivalent to allowing the blood longer for gaseous equilibration.

In the newcomer to high altitude, exercise is accompanied by a marked fall in arterial oxygen saturation, in contrast to the unchanged values on exercise at sea level and this may be partly due to a limitation in diffusion. Pulmonary blood flow is unchanged and though ventilation increases in the newcomer at high altitude, there still seems to be an odd mismatch between ventilation and perfusion, possibly due to increased lung water or obstruction to some of the airways by oedema.

Circulation. Though there is an abrupt increase in cardiac output on ascent to high altitude, there follows a progressive decrease in stroke volume and maximal cardiac output is reduced at all levels of exercise including maximal exercise. There is no evidence for insufficient myocardial oxygenation and there is argument about whether or not the myocardium is actually depressed by the hyoxia. There is an immediate alteration in the distribution of blood flow. For example, coronary and cutaneous flow both fall, cerebral and retinal flow increase, renal flow temporarily decreases, and then, with acclimatization, returns to normal.

The oxygen-carrying ability of the blood is considerably increased by the massive increase in red cell production, in total red cell mass and, more importantly, in tissue capillarity. It is somewhat offset by the higher haematocrit which increases the blood viscosity and decreases the rate of flow. The shift in the oxyhaemoglobin dissociation curve to the right, which occurs on ascent and is due to an increase in red cell 2,3-diphosphoglycerate (2,3-DPG), favours unloading of oxygen to the tissues, but this particular adjustment is not now thought to be of much practical importance.

Tissue adaptations. Apart from the very major role of increased tissue capillarity which reduces the average capillary-mitochondrial distance and so dramatically reduces the distance for diffusion, increased myoglobin facilitates oxygen diffusion and there is an increase both in mitochondrial density and in many enzymes of the respiratory pathway (e.g. in cytochrome oxidase).

Many alterations in the body that follow ascent are quite unexplained and it may be that these changes are not coping mechanisms at all but direct and deleterious results of the effect of hypoxia—or of other alterations such as alkalosis—upon the body. As a trivial example, one may quote the minimal increase in urine protein excretion of high altitudes, and, more importantly, the shifts of fluid from the extracellular to the intracellular compartments, or the failure of coronary artery blood flow to increase following ascent.

Oxygen uptake. Though the oxygen uptake at rest is not diminished even at very high altitudes, above an altitude of 1500 m the maximal oxygen uptake ($\dot{V}_{O_2 \text{(max)}}$) falls about 10 per cent for each gain in altitude of 1000 m between 1500 m and 6700 m and though it is improved by administration of pure oxygen, it does not return to normal until several days after descent. The *cause* of this drop in $\dot{V}_{O_2 \text{(max)}}$ has been debated. If, at any one altitude, the work load is increased, $\dot{V}_{O_2}$ may reach a maximum but ventilation, already increased at high altitude, is still able to increase further and so does not seem to be the factor limiting $\dot{V}_{O_2 \text{(max)}}$.

At altitude, as opposed to at sea level, arterial oxygen saturation falls with increasing exertion, but, at moderate altitudes, rises again near maximal exertion. There is probably no increase in alveolar–arterial oxygen gradient and because of the rise in haemoglobin, the amount of oxygen carried is kept up. Diffusion may be a little limited—this is controversial—but diffusion and the blood's oxygen carrying capacity are probably not factors limiting $\dot{V}_{O_2 \text{(max)}}$ either. After a few days at high altitude, however, maximal heart rate and particularly maximal cardiac stroke volume are reduced, the cause (a defect in myocardial contractility, for example) being unclear, and so the inability of the heart to go on increasing cardiac output seems to be the reason for the fact that $\dot{V}_{O_2 \text{(max)}}$ declines progressively with increases in altitude.

Extreme altitudes. Only serious climbers venture above altitudes of around 5800 m, where the atmospheric pressure is well below half that at sea level, but elaborate physiologic measurements have been made at altitudes of 7500 m ($P_B = 300$ torr; 40 kPa).

At these extreme values, where every increment in height results in a precipitous fall in $\dot{V}_{O_2 \text{(max)}}$, the oxygen cost of the work of ventilation rises considerably and it assumes an even greater proportion of total oxygen cost when $\dot{V}_{O_2 \text{(max)}}$ is reduced to really low levels. Moreover, the maximal ventilation itself is reduced at such altitudes and in addition, there undoubtedly is a diffusion defect within the lungs which becomes very marked on exercise. This, together with the steady decline in maximal cardiac output causes *maximal* oxygen uptake to fall very precipitously when P_B is below 300 torr, reaching, at around 8000 m altitude, resting or basal levels of oxygen uptake, a figure of about 350 m/kg per min. The state of a climber at 8000 m who is comfortable resting in his tent but whose $\dot{V}_{O_2 \text{(max)}}$ is reached when he puts on his boots, for example, is interesting physiologically but is also, practically speaking, perilous.

As others have noted, it is an extraordinary coincidence that the highest point on earth, the summit of Everest—where the atmospheric pressure is 250 torr or 33 kPa; the arterial P_{aO_2} about 25 torr (3.33 kPa) at rest and barely 20 torr (2.67 kPa) on exercise, and the P_{aCO_2} about 10 torr (1.3 kPa)—is the point where the best acclimatized and fittest athletes finally reach their physiological limit and find their $\dot{V}_{O_2 \text{(max)}}$ levels reduced to levels necessary to sustain life at rest.

ILLNESS DUE TO ALTITUDE

Acute mountain sickness

For centuries it has been known that when lowland dwellers climb mountains, some of them become ill. The illness, usually called acute mountain sickness (AMS), generally begins after a few hours, and is characterized by non-specific symptoms such as headache and vomiting. In the vast majority of people it is transient and trivial but in a few becomes progressive, severe, and may be fatal. It is to some extent relieved by breathing oxygen and it is cured by descent to sea level. Its cause is unknown.

AMS itself may be a miserable condition, but it is of concern to the physician practising in mountainous areas only because it may progress to one or both of two very serious conditions, *high altitude pulmonary oedema* and *high altitude cerebral oedema*, which are part of the syndrome of AMS but which are often discussed separately from it. Reasons for classifying them together include the fact that pulmonary oedema never occurs without symptoms and signs of AMS; that cerebral oedema seems clinically to be an exaggeration of AMS; that they may coexist, and that all have the same predisposing and relieving factors: in particular, they only occur at high altitudes or in low pressure chambers, and they are relieved by descent.

Symptoms and signs. Symptoms usually begin 24–48 hours after ascent to a higher altitude, but sometimes begin in as little as 8 hours or as many as 96 hours. On arrival, the sufferer may have been aware of a curiously disordered breathing and some light headedness but frequently feels well and even euphoric. Within the passage of a few hours, an unaccustomed lethargy assails him but sleep is fitful, disturbed by dreams, little bouts of breathlessness, and frequent arousals. On waking, he has a headache, often severe and occipital, which tends to diminish a little with activity but which may be unaffected by aspirin and codeine. He may vomit quite suddenly and nausea compounds his anorexia. Trying to keep up on his feet and active is made harder by dizziness and he may even lose his balance and fall. While the others organize the camp, he lies groaning in his sleeping bag, refusing food and dozing but the increasing periodicity of his respirations leads to frequent arousals and complaints of insomnia. After a day or two of rest, the symptoms disappear and are soon forgotten yet they may recur on further ascent to a greater altitude.

The signs are few: an irritable, depressed, but usually fit person, often, because he is starved, smelling of ketones and vomit, and holding his aching head. The most useful diagnostic sign is ataxia, best demonstrated by getting the patient to walk heel-toe (remembering that this may be awkward in boots and on snow) and then to turn around rapidly without staggering. Occasionally the patient, if he has been vomiting a great deal and especially if he has been taking diuretics, may be too dehydrated and hypotensive to stand up.

In a few, the symptoms rapidly worsen with the onset of *pulmonary oedema*. Soon the breathlessness, even at rest, is extreme and may be accompanied by a dry cough. The patient, anxious and sometimes incoherent, becomes progressively more dyspnoeic and sometimes orthopnoeic. He is very cyanosed, though this is hard to judge in tents of differing colours. He may have a mild pyrexia (38.3 °C). There is a pronounced tachycardia and sometimes mild hypotension. There are no signs of cardiac failure, but loud crackles can easily be heard all over the chest and frothy sputum, sometimes tinged with blood, wells out of the mouth and nose. At this point the patient, like anyone with severe acute pulmonary oedema, of whatever cause, is near death.

Pulmonary oedema, if very severe, tends to be accompanied by high altitude *cerebral oedema* but each syndrome may occur independently as features of AMS. In cerebral oedema without pulmonary manifestations, the patient, having had progressively worsening symptoms of AMS for three or four days (the range seems to vary from one day to as many as 21 days) becomes incoherent, hallucinated, and too ataxic and drowsy to stand up or look after himself. He may be unable to get out of his tent, or he may do so and then fall into a snow drift and lie there. Soon he is stuporose and snoring stertorously. His sleeping bag may be wet with urine and in a few hours he is in deepening coma. There are rarely any localizing signs—merely a generalized flaccid paralysis and pupillary reactions depending upon the depth of coma, though mild bilateral papilloedema is characteristic. In addition, the bladder may be palpable.

Predisposing factors. Though males and females are equally likely to develop the AMS syndrome, there are a number of factors which broadly predispose to AMS (including pulmonary oedema and cerebral oedema), though it is important to remember the large differences in susceptibility between individuals.

1. Age. The incidence and severity of AMS are inversely related to age and there is some evidence that young children are particularly susceptible to pulmonary oedema.

2. Previous AMS. Most investigators have the strong impression that AMS, and in particular pulmonary oedema, are more common in those who have in the past suffered badly from these conditions.

3. Re-ascent. Workers in Colorado and Peru have both produced evidence that healthy high altitude dwellers are at unusually high risk from high altitude pulmonary oedema after brief descent to lower altitudes followed by re-ascent. Once again we lack the large epidemiological surveys necessary to test the truth of this assertion.

4. Speed of ascent. Whether on foot, or horseback, by train, or by air, the faster the ascent, the more likely and the worse the AMS. In particular, the more *nights* spent on acclimatizing en route, the less the AMS. There is good evidence for the wisdom of the climber's maxim: 'Climb high, sleep low'.

5. Altitude. The incidence and severity of AMS following a 2000 m ascent to 5000 m from 3000 m are both much greater than from, say, 1000 m to 3000 m in the same amount of time.

6. Exertion. Independent of speed of ascent, severe exertion involved in the ascent (coping with snow; carrying loads) predisposes to AMS.

7. Physiological functions measured at sea level. There is no good evidence that the incidence of AMS relates to prior physical fitness as expressed by, say, maximal oxygen consumption, and much anecdotal evidence from many experienced observers that there is no such relationship. We now know, however, that statistically-speaking, the higher the vital capacity, the less the chance of AMS. Many other physiological functions have been measured at sea level but none usefully predict whether any one individual will develop AMS.

There is no evidence that the presence of upper respiratory tract infection predisposes to AMS, though pulmonary oedema must be distinguished from pneumonia. Nor is there evidence that the heat or cold at high altitudes influences AMS, though once again such factors may complicate diagnosis. For example, the symptoms and signs of AMS are identical with most of those found in hypothermia.

Pathophysiology. The initiating cause of AMS is hypoxia but it is probable that the disease is due to a combination of failed and exaggerated physiological adjustments to that hypoxia. We do not know why some people respond poorly to ascent. Reports of rare cases of patients with congenitally absent hypoxic ventilatory response who develop high altitude pulmonary oedema below 2000 m suggest that the respiratory centre might be primarily at fault. The individual's hypoxic ventilatory response at sea level fails to predict AMS, but people who have AMS do, as a group, have lower arterial oxygen pressures and saturations at high altitudes than those who feel well. The extent of the lowering correlates well with the severity of AMS, and this inadequate oxygenation is associated with high blood P_{CO_2} levels (and lower arterial pH), due to poorer ventilation. Whether as cause or result of the AMS, they are therefore more hypoxic. Clearly, if they develop pulmonary oedema they will become yet more hypoxic and get into a vicious cycle of deepening hypoxia.

Perhaps as a result of the hypoxia (or relative hypercarbia), people with AMS retain fluid and gain weight. Typically they have a prounounced antidiuresis on ascent which contrasts with the diuresis and the unchanged or even lowered weights of those who feel well. This antidiuresis is independent of the anorexia and vomiting of AMS. On ascent, in people who feel well, as well as in those with AMS, there is a movement of fluid into the cells from the plasma and interstitial fluid compartments. No one knows whether this movement is more pronounced in the brain, or in general greater in those people who will develop AMS. At the same time there is a considerable hypoxic cerebral vasodilatation in people ascending to high altitude.

A reasonable but not fully tested hypothesis to account for AMS proposes that all the symptoms and signs and all the physiological abnormalities of the disease can be explained as being due to brain stem and cerebral malfunction, itself due to minimal oedema of the respiratory and cardiovascular centres consequent upon the fluid shifts and the vasodilatation. In other words, in even mild AMS, there is very mild (and transient) oedema within the brain and that, as the cerebral oedema increases, so do the symptoms from headache and anorexia to coma. Autopsies in people who have died from cerebral oedema have shown, besides oedema, numerous tiny haemorrhages from the capillaries. They have also shown arterial, capillary, and venous sludging and clotting. It is unlikely that these are primary events but more probably that the clotting system has been activated by the oedematous process which, by increasing intracranial pressure, has closed the cerebral capillaries.

The pathophysiology of high altitude pulmonary oedema is yet more obscure. Pulmonary oedema at sea level is known to follow numerous intracranial lesions including cerebral oedema, but the relationship at high altitude is unclear.

It is known that on ascent to high altitude, there is a shift in blood from the systemic 'capacitance vessels' (veins) to the pulmonary circuit. In addition, there is a brisk hypoxic pulmonary arterial vasoconstriction with a rise in pulmonary artery pressure. Neither of these processes cause the oedema but both contribute to it.

The oedema fluid at high altitude has a high protein content, suggesting that there is a breakdown in the blood/alveolar junction and that it is not 'high pressure' cardiogenic pulmonary oedema. The fact that minor degrees of such breakdown occur early and frequently is suggested by the finding, in large studies at altitude, of a high incidence of pulmonary crackles in the asymptomatic newcomers, as well as by the finding in newcomers of an increased pulmonary liquid content.

The weight of evidence suggests that cardiac function is not really impaired. Pulmonary wedge pressures, reflecting average pulmonary venous pressures, are normal and so are atrial pressures when they have been measured. At autopsy, cuffs of oedema have been found around pulmonary arteries, as well as blebs of oedema within arteries and these may be associated with the thromboses that may be found at autopsy.

Four cases of high altitude pulmonary oedema have recently been described which are instructive. They all occurred after minimal exertion at modest altitudes and in each case the exceedingly rare anomaly of congenital absence of one pulmonary artery was revealed, suggesting that pulmonary hypertension and shearing forces due to a massively increased circulation (in these cases through one lung) might together contribute to high altitude pulmonary oedema. Experimentally, whether in dogs or sheep, this is very hard to reproduce, oedema occurring only when almost all but one upper lung lobe has been removed and the heart is assisted by pumps to force all the circulating blood through this tiny remnant of the pulmonary circulation. Nevertheless, most physiologists believe that in high altitude pulmonary oedema some lung capillary beds are closed off, whether by hypoxic vasoconstriction or by capillary wall oedema and thrombosis. There is, therefore, diversion of the whole circulation through the remaining widely patent capillaries which are damaged both by the increased pressure and the shear-stress of the large flow. As a consequence, they leak: pulmonary oedema.

Incidence. Both the incidence and severity of AMS depend upon the altitude and the terrain where they are assessed and upon the method of ascent used. Since there is wide individual variation in susceptibility, there is a wide variation in altitudes at which it has been reported. Also, as all the symptoms (which are found commonly in all sorts of maladies at sea level) and most of the signs are not specific to AMS, and since there is variability in the criteria investigators use for diagnosing AMS, it is impossible to give an exact value for the altitude at which AMS occurs. The difference in access and terrain has undoubtedly contributed to the belief once held that AMS was a peculiarity of some mountain regions, particularly the Andes, and that AMS might be due to some local abnormality in the air. Eighty years ago the Andean mining towns could be reached in a few hours from the coast by railway, but to get the same altitudes of around 4500 m in the Himalayas required weeks of gradual trekking, riding, and travelling on foot. The Peruvians have had names for AMS ('soroche', 'puna') for hundreds of years simply because one can go from coast to Altiplano in a very few days, even on foot, and very large numbers of people had to do so, going up to around 4000 m in the process. In contrast, the main trade route between Tibet and India, through central Nepal, passes through the Himalayas, squeezed between two mountains over 8000 m high but is itself at an altitude of only about 2400 m.

We now know that the atmosphere is less dense towards the poles so that the 250 mmHg isobar (which cuts through the summit of Everest (8848 m) at 27° 59′ N) is at a much lower altitude at the poles and much higher at the equator. All this implies that AMS might tend to occur at lower altitudes towards the poles, but this has yet to be tested, and other moderating factors such as mode of access and speed of ascent are likely to be far more important.

A fundamental problem in studying this problem is that though there are very many resorts and touring, climbing, and skiing areas at high altitudes, we do not have any really large-scale studies of AMS and its complications which give us both the numbers affected (the numerator) and the population at risk (the denominator) so that true incidence may be calculated.

Suffice it to say that AMS has been reported below 1550 m; that it is uncommon below 3000 m, and that the higher the altitude, the faster the ascent, and the greater the exertion (in load-carrying, dealing with difficult terrain, and so on), the higher the incidence and the worse the illness.

Because of difference in terrain, access, height, and criteria for diagnosis, and lack of both numerators and denominators, the incidence of AMS has been reported variously as from fewer than 10 per cent to 60 per cent. Most large studies suggest that some symptoms, for example, a bad headache that is not relieved by 600 mg of aspirin, occur in over half of those lowlanders going to above 4000 m and that over 10 per cent of climbers have more than one severe symptom at that altitude. High altitude pulmonary oedema occurs in about 5 per cent of people at that altitude, but symptomless crackles in the lung in almost a quarter. Cerebral oedema is less common: occurring in perhaps 0.5 to 2 per cent. Since it usually takes several days to develop, it is unlikely to occur on mountains climbed in a day or two.

Diagnosis. The differential diagnosis is small. For mild AMS the non-specific symptoms mean that hypothermia, exhaustion, and dehydration should be considered. The effects of alcohol and marijuana may duplicate those of AMS. The absence of diarrhoea speaks against, for example, dysentery or giardiasis. For pulmonary and cerebral oedema, only infectious diseases (pneumonia, or meningo-encephalitis) are likely possibilities. It must be remembered that periodic breathing with apnoeic phases is normal at high altitude and not by itself a cause for alarm, though it may be very marked indeed and associated with very severe oxygen desaturation in cerebral oedema. In most high mountain settlements it is impossible to get chest X-rays or electrocardiographs or examine specimens of cerebrospinal fluid, even if such fluid could be obtained. Though high altitude pulmonary oedema may be accompanied by a slight fever, this is moderate, and the extreme tachycardia and tachypnoea and the absence of purulent sputum and of signs or symptoms of pleurisy are characteristic, as is gross cyanosis. Sometimes the pulmonary oedema is one-sided or there may have been an upper respiratory infection, both of which confuse the diagnosis. In cerebral oedema there is no meningism and little if any pyrexia, nor evidence of ear infection or of localizing signs. There is a striking absence of any signs of cardiac decompensation (cardiac enlargement; raised neck veins). Giving oxygen—which is expensive, often not available, and has to be given in 4–5 l/min amounts—frequently produces equivocal results as everyone at high altitude, with almost any illness or none at all, feels temporarily better on oxygen.

Whilst it is true that *all* illnesses, from laryngitis to haemorrhoids, which develop at high altitude, tend to improve much more rapidly at sea level, the very dramatic recovery in AMS, and particularly in pulmonary and cerebral oedema on going down is so striking as to be diagnostic in itself. Numerous cases have been described of people unconscious and worsening at 4000 m who were fully conscious at 3000 m.

The physician who sees the patient on descent is, however, usually obliged to perform a battery of tests on the patient who, except in the case of very prolonged cerebral oedema, is recovering fast. The chest X-ray will show scattered fluffy patches of oedema; the electrocardiogram shows simple right ventricular hypertrophy and 'strain', and the cerebrospinal fluid will be normal.

Prophylaxis. AMS and its complications are the consequence of ascent that for any one individual is too high or too fast and are therefore easily and completely preventable by going up slowly. It is essential for the physician to remember and stress the vast individual differences in susceptibility when advising people who are to take part in one of the many thousands of high altitude treks organized each year. These often have strict, cramped, and too optimistic schedules, and there is frequently great pressure on those who feel unwell to keep up with the rest of the party. It is essential that everyone should realize that AMS, unless it is very mild, has ruined many an idyllic and expensive holiday and that it cannot be cured except by rest or temporary descent. They must be told very emphatically that high altitude pulmonary or cerebral oedema may be rapidly fatal, that they have a responsibility to keep an eye on their fellows, for the natural tendency is to leave people with headache and drowsiness to sleep it off, unwatched as they drift into coma. Everyone must know that to help a sick person down on his own feet is quick, easy, and safe, while a few hours later, when he is unconscious, 20 or 30 expert climbers may spend days in risking their lives trying to carry down that same patient. They should know that even in the 1980s, communications are frequently very faulty, planes and helicopters may not exist or may crash, or because of terrain and bad weather, may be unable to get near. They must know, therefore, that any rescue is chancy and dangerous to others.

Everyone, especially those who have flown to high altitude, has a personal duty to rest on arrival, to be sure to ascend at a pace that is personally comfortable (about 300 m per day above 3000 m with days of rest every 1000 m is usually a good pace), to spend nights as low down as possible and to climb less far each day as higher altitudes are reached. Time spent in acclimatizing to be able physically to work harder is also time spent in avoiding the miseries and dangers of AMS. Since insensible water loss is increased due to the increased exertion, the extra ventilation and the dry air, every effort must be made to avoid dehydration, by drinking enough to urinate clear, dilute urine. The climber should also eat plenty, especially carbohydrates.

The drug acetazolamide (Diamox), which is a carbonic anhydrase inhibitor, and was introduced in order, by its action in increasing urinary bicarbonate excretion, to counteract the respiratory alkalosis, reduces the incidence and severity of AMS when taken before and during ascent. It probably works by decreasing cerebrospinal fluid formation and, more importantly, stimulating nocturnal respiration so that periodic episodes of apnoea, which are very common at altitude, are abolished and blood oxygen saturation is never allowed to fall. Its principal side effect is tingling in the hands, feet, and around the mouth. It is poor advice to recommend drugs such as acetazolamide except in the case of an emergency ascent, say for rescue, since slow ascent allowing time for acclimatization is so effective.

Energetic propaganda advising slow ascent and rest days and nights has been shown to lower the incidence of AMS. There is evidence that sleeping tablets, which further lower the already lowered oxygen saturation during sleep should be avoided.

Treatment. In mild AMS, aspirin for the headache and rest are usually adequate. If not, the sufferer should descend 300–500 m and rest for a couple of nights. Occasionally an anti-emetic should be given, and even intravenous fluids for dehydration. If there is ataxia or mild cerebral or pulmonary oedema, the patient should at once be assisted down 700 m to 1000 m, rested, and watched carefully. If pulmonary oedema is severe or the patient is comatose, he must be immediately carried down at least 1000 m and further if recovery is not evident. While helicopters, etc., may be sent for at the same time and while oxygen, if available, should be administered (if the patient is comatose, tracheal intubation and sucking out of the airways must be performed, and the oxygen should be delivered at 5–6 l/min), it is *essential* to begin evacuation immediately because communications may be defective, helicopters are not always available or crash, oxygen may run out and is often ineffective, changes in weather can prevent evacuation, and people with pulmonary or cerebral oedema are in extreme danger of dying in a matter of hours, while quite a small decrease in altitude may improve them dramatically.

In pulmonary oedema, sit the patient up if this makes him comfortable. Give frusemide 20–40 mg orally and morphine 15 mg intravenously. Both these drugs divert blood from the pulmonary to the systemic circuit. Frusemide causes a diuresis and morphine decreases anxiety and respiration rate.

In cerebral oedema, intravenous dexamethazone in large doses (e.g. 16 mg) should be given to reduce the oedema. Intravenous infusion of hypertonic agents such as glycerol and mannitol have been used. They are logical and appropriate but are hard to set up in the mountains. A cuffed endotracheal tube should be passed, the lungs kept inflated and the bladder kept empty with a Foley catheter (all these devices should form part of the kit of any responsible physician travelling at high altitudes).

Prognosis. This depends not merely on the altitude and terrain but on the speed with which early signs are noticed by the patient's colleagues and their determination and skill in evacuating him to lower altitudes immediately. There are numerous reports of death due to pulmonary oedema and to the rarer but more dangerous cerebral oedema. Once either of these have developed the patient probably has about a one-third chance of dying. If he recovers fully, it is probable that he will have no demonstrable physical after-

effects and also likely that he will be able to ascend to high altitudes again, but using great caution.

Retinal haemorrhage of high altitude

Twelve years ago it was noticed that some people flown to altitudes of around 5600 m developed flame-shaped retinal haemorrhages. Retinal pathology occurring at between 4000 m and 8000 m altitude has now been confirmed by numerous studies.

On ascent, there is not merely a considerable increase in cerebral blood flow but in retinal blood flow also. Ophthalmoscopy at around 5000–6000 m shows a 20–25 per cent increase in diameter of both arteries and veins, and striking increase in the tortuosity of these vessels (Fig. 1). The optic disc takes on a pink tinge as it becomes suffused with blood due to capillary dilatation. This can delude the examiner into diagnosing papilloedemea, a condition which may, as shown above, occur in very ill subjects and be diagnostic of cerebral oedema. This vasodilatation is accompanied by a brisk increase in retinal blood flow.

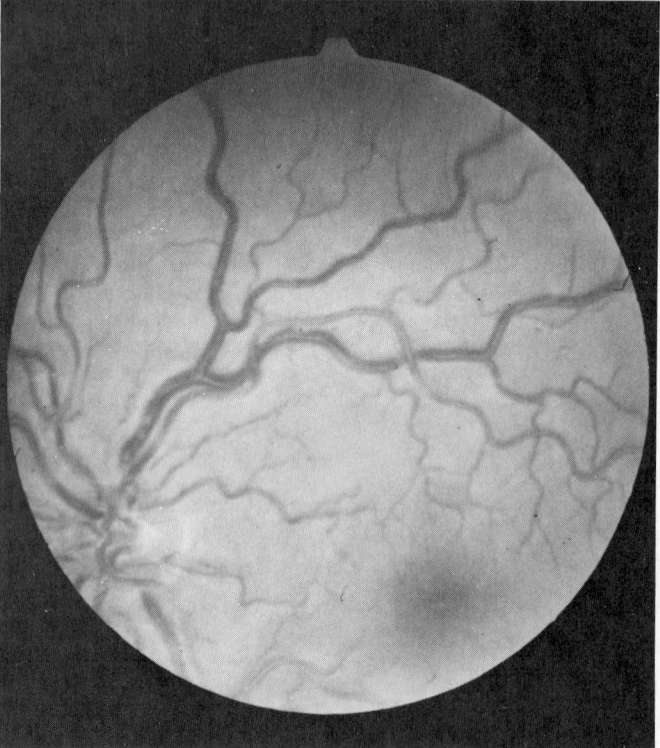

Fig. 1   The left optic fundus of a 26-year-old male climber photographed at 5900 m altitude. Both the veins and arteries are dilated and tortuous and there is hyperaemia of the optic disc as well as mild papilloedema. This climber had severe headache, nausea, and vomiting.

At 5600 m studies have shown that one-third to one-half of people develop flame-shaped retinal haemorrhages (Fig. 2) and further studies, carried out at 5900 m have confirmed this figure in fit, symptomless climbers descending from 7000–8000 m altitude. Clearly the exact figure depends upon whether pupillary dilators and retinal photography were used in the surveys. The haemorrhages are usually near the optic disc and may be of any size and number. Since they tend to occur adjacent to the disc and since the macula constitutes a tiny proportion of the area of the retina, it is not surprising that they are rarely noticed by those who develop them. Though their presence bears a statistical relation to ASM, they also occur in people who feel very well.

It is not known whether the occurrence of haemorrhages relates to the unusual sheer stresses associated with an increased flow through dilated vessels. It may be that they are caused by transmittal of high thoracic pressures developed during straining or

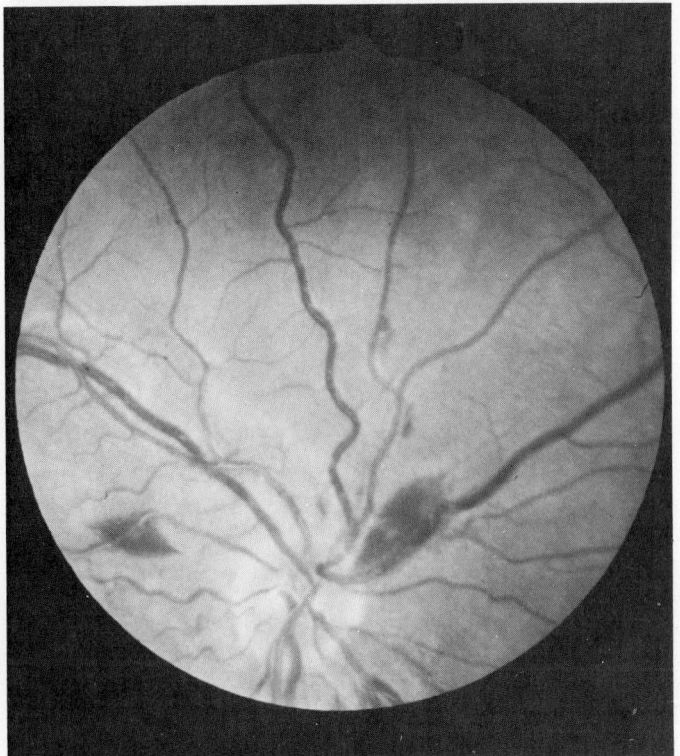

Fig. 2 The right optic fundus of a fit and symptomless 28-year-old male climber photographed at 5900 m altitude. The vessels are dilated, as in Fig. 1, but less tortuous. There are numerous, scattered retinal haemorrhages.

prolonged coughing, and transmitted through a vasculature dilated because of hypoxia. Their presence is reminiscent of the small haemorrhages found over the brain in high altitude cerebral oedema.

On descent, retinal blood flow, vascular diameter, and tortuosity all rapidly return to normal and the haemorrhages resolve, though when they impinge on the fovea, despite the fact that an observer can no longer see them, the victim may have a permanent blind spot. It is probable that the finding of retinal haemorrhages in someone at high altitude is not by itself a reason to counsel descent.

Peripheral oedema

Swelling of hands, face, and ankles may occur in climbers on ascent to high altitude and rarely there may be gross anasarca. The oedema is commoner in women than men though no association with menses has been found. It is associated with AMS and pulmonary oedema but may occur by itself, and it is relieved by the diuresis that accompanies descent. Levels of antidiuretic hormone (ADH) are raised in severe AMS but the relationship between ADH and peripheral oedema at high altitude is obscure. Treatment with a mild oral diuretic is easy. It should be noted that peripheral oedema may also follow long-continued daily hiking at sea level.

Other illnesses of high altitudes

On theoretical grounds (and occasionally this has been borne out by practical experience), people with diseases which limit ventilation (e.g. kyphoscoliosis, alveolar hypoventilation syndrome), diffusion (e.g. pulmonary fibrosis), circulation (e.g. general, as in heart failure or anaemia; specific as in vascular disease), and tissue adaptation, fare badly at high altitudes. Often, however, there is little evidence that any particular patient will succumb to the hypoxia. Doctors should remember that spas such as St Moritz, in Switzerland, have been receiving the sick for many centuries and that tuberculosis sanatoria at, say, Davos (1529 m) were places where people with lung disease were sent, and they should be

cautious about the constraints they place on a patient's activities and frank about our ignorance.

On the other end of the spectrum, there are not enough people with abnormal haemoglobins shifting the oxy-haemoglobin dissociation curves to the left (e.g. Hb Andrew–Minneapolis) who can take on more oxygen and who do well at high altitude, for this sort of abnormality to make much difference to the average physician's practice.

In addition, some acclimatizing features may in themselves cause problems: the erythropoietic stimulus, to take an example, never shuts off above an altitude of about 5500 m: the consequent high viscosity of the blood makes it hard to pump and easy to clot and it is probably that, as in severe cyanotic congenital heart disease and chronic mountain sickness (see below), venesection is beneficial.

Chronic mountain sickness (Monge's disease). This is a clinical syndrome affecting a few very long-term residents at altitudes. It is to be distinguished from the persistent failure of a newcomer to adjust to the altitude which results in weeks or even months of acute mountain sickness. It usually occurs in men between the ages of 20 and 50, and the symptoms are of headache, dizziness, depression, irritability and, most strikingly, drowsiness and even episodes of coma. The signs are those of severe polycythaemia and cyanosis with suffused, congested conjunctiva, ear lobes, cheeks, and lips, as well as clubbed finger nails. Signs of congestive heart failure may be present. The right heart may be enlarged on chest X-ray and there is evidence of right ventricular hypertrophy on ECG, itself a reflection of marked pulmonary hypertension.

These patients have a polycythaemia that is inappropriately high for the altitude, the haematocrit usually being in the high 70s. The total circulating red cell volume is increased, probably due to the arterial oxygen saturation which is very low, itself a reflection of inadequate ventilation as shown by the arterial P_{CO_2} which is high. All the symptoms, signs, and physiological abnormalities are cured by descent to sea level, and sufferers should move there permanently.

Where there is, for example, gross kyphoscoliosis, massive obesity, or a pneumoconiosis, it is possible to blame a specific defect for the excessive hypoxia and therefore the body's natural adjustments (for example, the great polycythaemia and pulmonary vasoconstriction) which themselves produce the syndrome. Where no such cause is found, it is probable that the cause lies in alveolar hypoventilation, similar to the alveolar hypoventilation syndrome that may occur at sea level, and due to a sluggish response to oxygen on the part of the peripheral chemoreceptors or to carbon dioxide on the part of the respiratory centre.

Myocardial infarction. There is a low rate of coronary arterial disease in all indigenous populations studied at high altitudes, whether in the Andes, the Himalayas, or the Pamirs. This might be unexpected since most workers find a reduction of cardiac output and of coronary arterial flow in such residents.

It may be that as such indigenous populations tend to be more active physically, to eat differently and less (especially salt), when compared with people in the West, and to have lower serum lipids and less systemic hypertension, the reasons for the low prevalence of coronary disease and infarction has little to do with the altitude. However, it may have little to do with racial differences and to the factors listed above because most epidemiologic evidence suggests that mortality from arteriosclerotic disease in the United States declines with increasing altitude of residence. Whether this is because mild arterial hypoxia 'trains' the myocardium to open more capillaries and thus make it less vulnerable to occlusions is not known.

The physician at sea level is often asked by people whether it is safe for them to go up to 3000 m or 4000 m altitude to ski or to climb. Logic dictates that as the myocardium has no oxygen reserves; that as myocardial oxygen extraction even at sea level leaves no room for improvement, and as coronary flow is decreased, people who have poor coronary circulation will be at great risk when they ascend from sea level and start hard exercise. There are, however, no credible studies to guide the physician. The few anecdotal reports suffer from the absence of a denominator, so we have no idea if such people are more or less likely to have suffered their infarct than when exercising at sea level. Morover, age, state of training, cold, and a host of other variables confound the issue. A prudent physician might tell the patient not to go until they are fit to take exercise at sea level, but unless the patient has had a previous myocardial infarction, we have no evidence that an electrocardiogram, with or without exertion or breathing low oxygen mixtures simultaneously, has any predictive value at all, and the patients' previous history of fitness and of illness is likely to be far more useful. Since the predictive value of tests is critically dependent upon the prevalence of the condition, the utility of doing large numbers of such tests in the absence of symptoms is likely to be very low.

Pulmonary emboli. Deep vein thrombosis tends to occur in climbers at very high altitudes partly because of the extreme polycythaemia and partly because of enforced inactivity due to storms. Pulmonary emboli, sometimes fatal, occur. Evacuation to lower altitudes and the administration of aspirin as an anticoagulant should be tried. More powerful anticoagulants require careful supervision of, say, prothrombin times, and this is impossible under the circumstances.

Sickle cell anaemia. Since cells containing HbS sickle, when hypoxic, becoming sticky and rigid, it is not surprising that homozygous cases of HbS (sickle cell anaemia) are at great danger from high altitude. In Denver, at 1609 m, people who are heterozygotes (sickle cell trait) apparently lead normal lives, but cases of splenic infarction in people with sickle cell trait have been described in men at between 3500 m and 4500 m. The effect here of exercise is unclear. Clearly one should be cautious in advising anyone with sickle cell trait to exercise at altitudes above about 2000 m.

References

Health, D. and Williams, D. R. (1977). *Man at high altitude*. Churchill Livingstone, Edinburgh.
Lenfant, C. and Sullivan, K. (1971). Adaptation to high altitude. *New Engl. J. Med.* **284**, 1298.
Rennie, I. D. (1976). See Nuptse and die. *Lancet* **ii**, 1177.
Ward, M. (1975). *Mountain medicine*. Crosby Lockwood Staples, London.

Aviation medicine

F. S. Preston and D. M. Denison

Aviation medicine, or more correctly aerospace medicine, concerns the welfare of man in the upper atmosphere and outer space. Air and space travel expose people to many risks that are usually avoided and pass unnoticed. Some are associated with the high speeds needed to get the vehicles off the ground, others concern the dangers of sitting in a structure travelling fast through very cold low-pressure surroundings, and others again relate to the hazards that are encountered getting the vehicle, or failing that its occupants, back to ground safely. As the altitude, range, and speed of aircraft have increased and rockets have been developed, these risks have become more severe (Fig. 1).

Some of the problems created by these stresses are common to other aspects of occupational medicine and will not be considered here. These include, for example, keeping people cool or warm, protecting them against crash injury, providing them with instruments that give essential information in an unequivocal manner, designing warning systems that sense crucial events swiftly but do not go off inadvertently, and making sure that all controls can be reached from a comfortable seat and operated smoothly and efficiently. Other problems, such as mild-prolonged and brief-profound hypoxia, sustained accelerations, rapid decompressions, and certain spatial disorientations, are not experienced elsewhere. They, and the problems of aircrew selection and medical care, form the substance of this chapter and will be discussed after the physical features of the aviator's environment have been described.

Physical features of the atmosphere. The atmosphere is a uniformly mixed oxygen-enriched gas which shields the ground below from thermal and other high-energy radiations above. Because it is held to the Earth by gravity and compresses under its own weight it is denser close to the ground than further away. The long waves of infrared sunlight travel easily through the atmosphere, warming it very little but heating the ground below. The hot ground re-radiates some of this heat at other wavelengths which are absorbed by

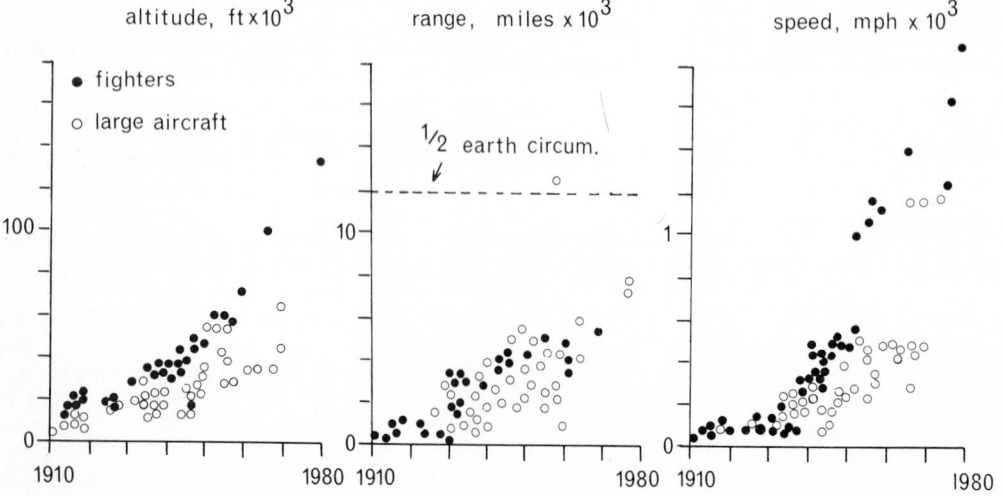

Fig. 1 Improvements in the altitude, range, and speed of aircraft over the years 1910 to 1980.

carbon dioxide and water vapour, making the air close to the ground much warmer than that elsewhere. By contrast, the short waves of ultraviolet sunlight entering the upper atmosphere, are absorbed by oxygen molecules early in their journey, creating a belt of warm ozone at high altitudes. Most of the other high-energy rays are also intercepted in the same region but generate secondary rays that extend lower down. Very few of these reach the ground. At sea-level, air exerts a pressure of about 1 atmosphere (760 mmHg), is variably moist, has a temperature that ranges from $-60\ °C$ to $+60\ °C$ and moves at wind speeds from 0–160 km/h. With increasing altitude its temperature, pressure, and water-content fall and wind-speeds increase. Some of these features are summarized in Fig. 2. In general, on ascent, conditions become more severe and more uniform.

Atmospheric pressure. Although the Earth is almost perfectly spherical its atmosphere is not, being more extensive over the Equator than the Poles. On average the total gas pressure falls with altitude in a regular, almost exponential, way, halving every 18 000 ft. Thus it is easy to sketch a reasonable model of atmospheric pressure (i.e. half an atmosphere at 18 000 ft, a quarter at 36 000 ft, an eighth at 54 000 ft, a sixteenth at 72 000 ft, etc., as in Fig. 3). Since the oxygen content of the atmosphere (20.93 per cent) is constant to very high altitudes indeed, the same curve can be used to obtain the ambient oxygen pressure at any altitude, by re-scaling the ordinate as shown in Fig. 3. The values obtained in this manner are slight overestimates since they make no allowance for the atmosphere's water-vapour content. Its water-vapour pressure is largely determined by temperature and introduces errors that are just significant at low altitudes where the air is warm. However, the oxygen pressure of physiological importance, is that which exists in ambient air when it is warmed and wetted on entering the bronchial tree. This process necessarily raises water-vapour pressure to about 47 mmHg, regardless of the total gas pressure outside. Thus the oxygen pressure in moist inspired gas (P_{IO_2}) fully saturated with water vapour at 37 °C, is given by the relationship:

$$P_{IO_2} = F_{IO_2}(PB - 47) \qquad (1)$$

where F_{IO_2}, the fractional concentration of oxygen in the inspirate, is 0.2093 when the air is inspired.

Atmospheric temperature drops more or less linearly with altitude, at about 2 °C/1000 ft, to the tropopause (40 000 ft), is stable at

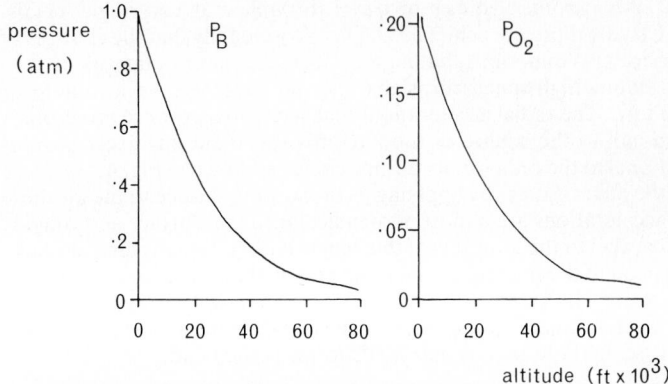

Fig. 3 The variations of barometric pressure and ambient oxygen pressure with altitude.

$-56\ °C$ up to about 80 000 ft and then rises to almost body temperature at about 150 000 ft, but by then air density is so low that its temperature is unimportant (cf. the dense cold air below).

Atmospheric ozone (O_3) is formed by irradiation of diatomic oxygen molecules which dissociate into atoms. At very high altitudes the ultraviolet irradiation is so intense that all oxygen exists in the monatomic form. Lower down those that are produced combine with oxygen molecules to form the triatomic gas O_3 (ozone) at concentrations from 1 to 10 p.p.m. The ozonosphere normally exists between 40 000 and 140 000 ft, i.e. from one-fifth to one-thirtieth of an atmosphere. Below 40 000 ft the irradiation is normally too weak for significant amounts of ozone to form. Concentrations of 1 p.p.m. at sea-level pressures cause lung irritation. Ten times that concentration can cause fatal lung oedema. Although the ozonosphere is at much lower pressure, aircraft ventilation systems can take it in and compress it to pressures at which pulmonary irritation is a real threat.

Mechanical aspects. Propeller-driven aircraft need sufficient air to 'bite' on but not enough to slow them down. They fly best at altitudes below 30 000 ft. Jet aircraft are propelled by throwing a stream of hot gas behind them but they need atmospheric oxygen to ignite the fuel that does this. They fly best at altitudes below 65 000 ft. Rockets take an oxygen supply with them, and fly best in a vacuum.

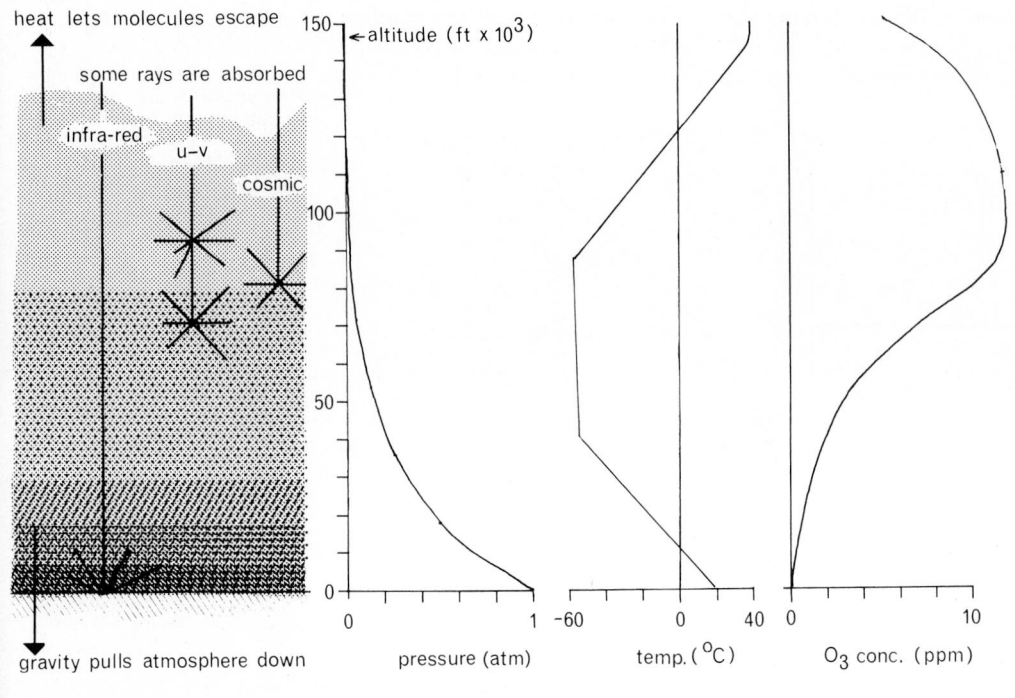

Fig. 2 Some physical features of the Earth's atmosphere, showing the variations in barometric pressure, air temperature, and ozone concentration with altitude. (NB There is an international aviation safety convention that all altitudes are given in feet.)

Air permits vehicles to travel through it at very high speeds. Usually these are achieved and lost so gradually that the changes of pace pass unnoticed, but high-performance aircraft may make continuous high-speed turns that can be sustained for a minute or more. The radial accelerations that such turns produce are proportional to the square of the aircraft's speed and inversely proportional to the radius of its turning circle (as shown in Fig. 4). Because the aircraft turns by applying its broad wing surface to the air these accelerations are almost perpendicular to that surface and roughly parallel to the long axis of the people within. Usually aircraft make 'head to the middle' turns causing tissue fluids and loosely tethered organs like the liver and heart to fall footwards (positive 'g' or $+Gz$ accelerations). Occasionally the aircraft makes 'head-out' turns forcing these organs and fluids towards the head.

Summary. In brief, the important features of the atmosphere are that its temperature and pressure fall and radiation intensities rise with altitude. In addition there is a poisonous belt of ozone at high altitude. The atmosphere also permits vehicles to travel at high speeds and make sustained severe accelerations.

The physiological problems posed by these stresses are extremely challenging but on the whole they only affect professional aircrew. One risk that is shared by all who fly, impinges on everyday life in many ways, and is a common feature of several diseases. It will be discussed first.

Hypoxia

Oxygen has a dual role in most animal cells, since it is life-giving and extremely poisonous at the same time. In the form in which it exists in the air or dissolved in simple solution it is benign and only ionized with difficulty. However, once an electron is successfully attached to an oxygen molecule it becomes a highly corrosive *superoxide ion*, capable of pulling the (electron) lynch-pins from neighbouring molecules of all sorts. This is an essential feature of oxygen toxicity which is discussed on page 6.80. Superoxide dismutase and various peroxidases have evolved to protect most cells from the effects of the spontaneous superoxide ion formation that occurs, by quenching the ions as rapidly as they appear.

More recently in evolution, other enzymes have developed that can harness this property of oxygen molecules in a controlled way. There are three sorts. Firstly, there are the oxidases which take oxygen and free-electrons attracting hydrogen, to make water. Quantitatively, cytochrome a3 oxidase is the most important

because, using oxygen as the ultimate electron sink, it allows many metabolic processes to proceed and at the same time unlocks and traps most of the energy the body needs (oxidative phosphorylation). However, there are several other oxidases that release the power but are unable to trap it. They are used to denature various unwanted products of metabolism.

Secondly, there are oxygenases which take the oxygen molecule and introduce it into an organic molecule creating a new compound. Although these enzymes, of which there are many, only consume a small fraction of the body's total oxygen need, they are particularly important, because they are responsible for production and dismemberment of many critical compounds such as the amine transmitters of the brain.

The third group of enzymes that handle oxygen have the attributes of both the other groups and so are called mixed function oxidases. They take one atom of an oxygen molecule and use it to make water as would an oxidase, but with another hand take the other atom of the oxygen molecule and put it into an organic moleculer as would an oxygenase. That atom takes hydrogen with it, so these enzymes are also known as hydroxylases. They too are responsible for many critical metabolic processes and for the denaturation of many drugs in the liver, kidney, and elsewhere.

These three groups of enzymes, which handle virtually all the oxygen uptake measured at the lips in man, differ from each other in a crucial respect, which is in their affinity for oxygen. That property can be described by a commonly-used term in enzyme kinetics, the Michaelis constant (for oxygen). This constant (K_{mO_2}) is that partial pressure of oxygen which, when all other factors are equal, just allows an oxygen-consuming reaction to proceed at half its maximum velocity. The major oxidase (cytochrome a3), which is the co-catalyst of oxidative phosphorylation, has a very high oxygen affinity and thus a very low K_{mO_2}, of 1 mmHg or less. That means this particular type of oxygen consumption, representing 80–90 per cent of the whole, can proceed full-tilt down to very low levels of oxygen supply indeed. By contrast (Fig. 5), the other enzymes which are qualitatively less important but qualitatively critical, have Michaelis constants for oxygen that vary from 5 to 250 mmHg. A fall in oxygen supply will influence these processes long before oxidative phosphorylation is affected and at times when overall oxygen consumption is diminished little if at all.

Although Fig. 3 describes how ambient oxygen pressure is related to altitude, it does not convey the measure of oxygen supply which is critical to man, namely the pressure of oxygen to be found in the lungs. That pressure is determined by two equations (Fig. 6). The *alveolar ventilation equation* states that alveolar CO_2 pressure

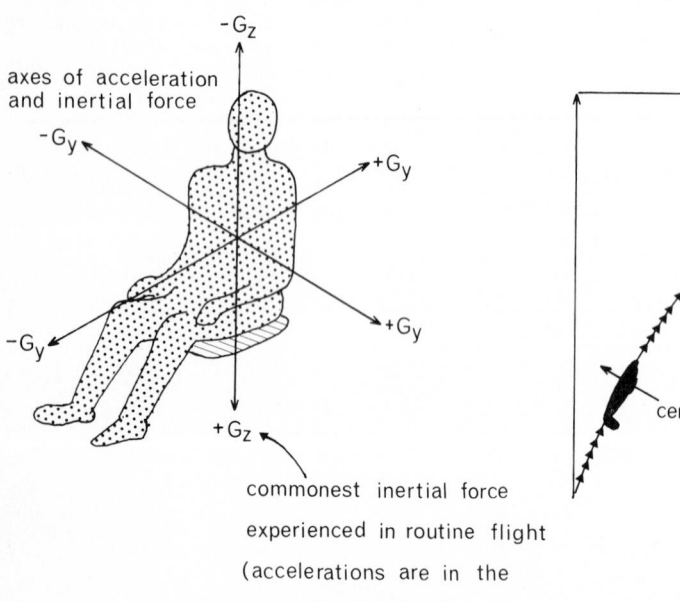

axes of acceleration and inertial force

$-Gz$
$-Gy$
$+Gy$
$+Gy$
$-Gy$
$+Gz$

commonest inertial force experienced in routine flight (accelerations are in the opposite direction)

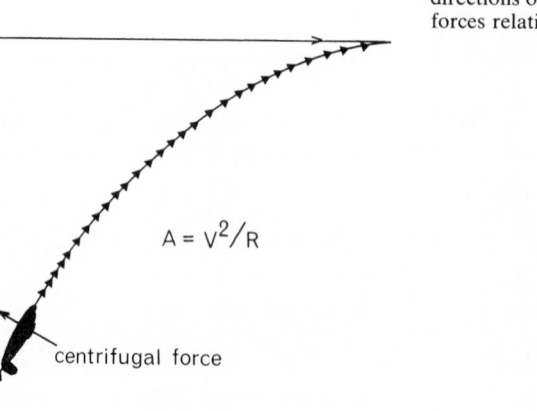

$A = V^2/R$

centrifugal force

the commonest cause is a banked turn in rapid flight

Fig. 4   The axes used to express the directions of accelerative and inertial forces relative to the body.

The Michaelis–Menten equation when the substrate is oxygen:

$$\dot{M}_{O_2}/\dot{M}_{O_2}max = P_{O_2}/(P_{O_2}+Km_{O_2})$$

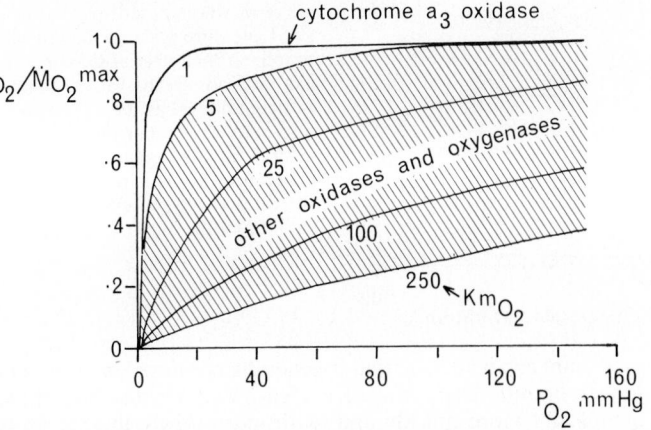

Fig. 5 Curves of oxygen uptake (M_{O_2}) as a fraction of the theoretical maximum (M_{O_2} max) against the partial pressure of oxygen (P_{O_2}) for a family of oxygen-handling enzymes with Michaelis constants for oxygen (K_{mO_2}) from 1 to 250 mmHg.

(P_{ACO_2}) depends only on CO_2 excretion ($\dot{M}_{CO_2}$) and alveolar ventilation ($\dot{V}_A$), so:

$$P_{ACO_2} = k(\dot{M}_{CO_2}/V_A).$$

The *alveolar air equation* states that since at any one time there is a fixed trading ratio between oxygen uptake and CO_2 excretion ($R = \dot{M}_{CO_2}/\dot{M}_{O_2}$), alveolar oxygen pressure (P_{AO_2}) can be calculated from the moist inspired oxygen pressure ($P_{IO_2}*$) and alveolar P_{CO_2}, so:

$$P_{AO_2} = P_{IO_2}*/R.$$

Progressive hypoxia leads to a mild hyperventilation (i.e. rise in $\dot{V}_A$ and fall in P_{ACO_2}). Knowing this it is possible to sketch a graph of alveolar oxygen pressure against altitude as in Fig. 7(a).

When arterialized blood leaves a healthy lung it has an oxygen pressure some 10 mmHg less than that in the alveoli, due to uneven matching of ventilation to perfusion, some anatomical shunting, and an almost nominal obstacle to diffusion. In resting people, this alveolar–arterial oxygen gradient does not change much with altitude, although the relative importance of the factors contributing to

it alter considerably; so, subtracting a further 10–15 mmHg describes the relation between arterial oxygen pressure and altitude (also shown in Fig. 7).

The most important change is the loss of the head of pressure driving oxygen from the alveoli to blood, since the fall in alveolar P_{O_2} is much greater than that in mixed venous P_{O_2}, (because of the shape of the oxygen dissociation curve). As a result the aveolar–venous gradient for oxygen diffusion is smaller and equilibration slower than at ground level.

During the early part of the Second World War many rear-gunners who were quite alert breathing air while sitting in their turrets at 18 000 ft, lost consciousness when they attempted to crawl back into the body of the plane, at the same altitude. That occurred because exertion speeds up blood flow through individual capillaries in the lung, leaving even less time for oxygen equilibration. Since the obstacle to diffusion, that is nominal at ground level, is dominant at altitude, exertion leads to arterial desaturation that is not present at rest. The same phenomenon is seen at ground level in patients with fibrotic lung disease.

When sytemic blood leaves the central arterial tree it loses a surprising amount of oxygen through the thin arteriolar walls. Some areas of the central nervous system, such as the part of the optic nerve around the central retinal artery and parts of the retina immediately adjacent to some of its branches, depend upon this diffusion for their supply of oxygen. The fall in this driving head (of arterial P_{O_2}) may explain some of the visual impairment experienced on ascent to altitude. Most tissues do not get their oxygen in this way but receive it from the blood as it travels through the systemic capillaries. Until a few years ago it was supposed that there was a fairly even fall of P_{O_2} along the length of any capillary with the oxygen diffusing radially, leaving a most deprived area (the 'lethal corner') at the outer limit of that part served by the venous end of the capillary. Nowadays it is believed that most of the oxygen floods out of the vessel very early in its course, to diffuse parallel to the capillary, holding the great bulk of the tissue at much the same P_{O_2} as in the blood leaving the servant venule. The arteriovenous oxygen content and partial-pressure differences are fixed by the ratio of metabolism to perfusion. In any respiratory steady-state local blood flow is the prime determinant of tissue P_{O_2}.

People suddenly exposed to altitude make two adaptive responses to hypoxia, (an increase in blood flow and the modest hyperventilation mentioned previously). These limit but do not abolish the effects of oxygen lack. The consequences (Fig. 8) include loss of night vision, impairment of the ability to learn complex and then simple tasks, a deterioration in the performance of already

The ALVEOLAR VENTILATION EQUATION ignores dead-space, and supposes there is a stream of oxygen-rich CO_2-free gas, $\dot{V}_A$

and says, for practical purposes,

$$P_{ACO_2} \propto \dot{M}_{CO_2}/\dot{V}_A$$

The ALVEOLAR AIR EQUATION pictures $\dot{V}_A$ trapped in a bag, and notes there must be a link between the rise in P_{CO_2} and the fall in P_{O_2}, so that, for most practical purposes:

$$P_{AO_2} = P_{IO_2} - P_{ACO_2}/R$$

Fig. 6 Graphical representations of the alveolar ventilation and alveolar air equations.

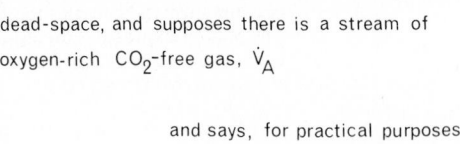

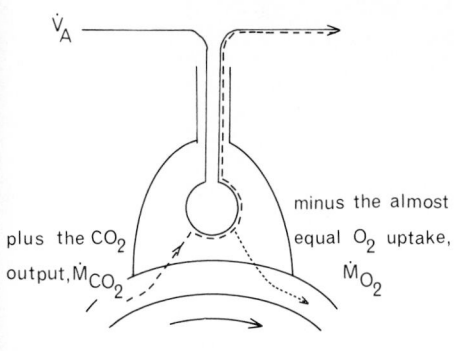

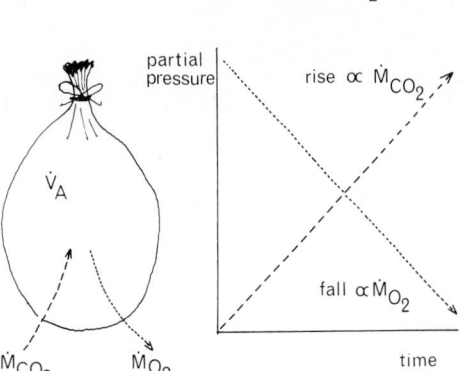

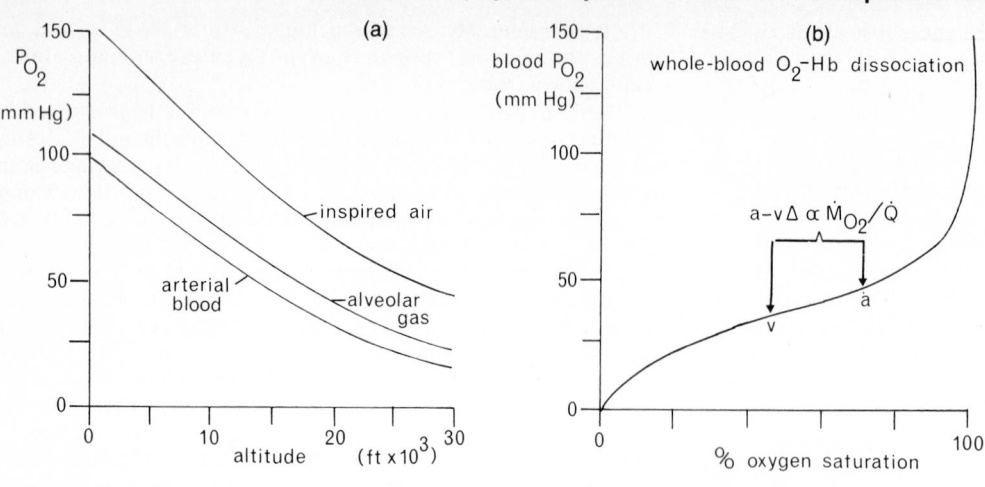

Fig. 7 (a) Variations in moist-inspired, alveolar, and arterial oxygen pressures (P_{O_2}) with altitude, in normal men. (b) The conventional oxygen–haemoglobin dissociation curve of whole blood, plotted to the same pressure scale as the left hand graph, so that arterial O_2 content can be read directly (at the same horizontal level as the P_{O_2} curve). It also emphasizes that the arterio-venous oxygen content difference (a-v∆) is proportional to the ratio of oxygen uptake (M_{O_2}) to local blood flow (Q).

learnt skills, a progressive loss of muscular power (aerobic capacity), and eventually loss of consciousness, convulsions, and death.

As Fig. 8 shows, people suddenly exposed to an altitude of 10 000 ft and above are unreliable and physically weak. This altitude is taken as the ceiling above which it is mandatory to provide aviators with oxygen. To be safe, the ceiling that is actually used is almost always 8 000 ft, at which barometric pressure is 565 mmHg, arterial oxygen pressure is around 55 mmHg (i.e. sitting just at the top of the sloping part of the oxyhaemoglobin dissociation curve; and venous oxygen pressures have only fallen by 1–2 mmHg. It is the

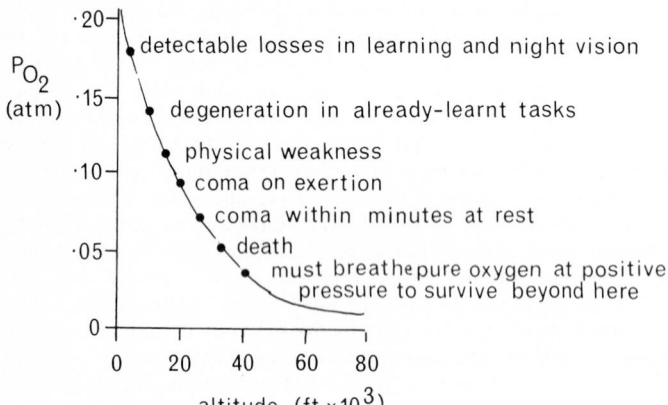

Fig. 8 A summary of the functional consequences of altitude hypoxia.

maximum cabin altitude that is generally permitted in civilian passenger aircraft. There is some evidence that, even at this altitude, people tire more quickly and learn more slowly than at ground level. Some aircraft have a lower maximum to cabin altitude, but this requires a stronger and thus heavier cabin to contain the higher pressure, which makes the aircraft less economical to run and more difficult to get off the ground.

Two physiological features of altitude hypoxia are especially important in aviation. The first is a total lack of awareness that the mind is breaking down. This means that an affected man cannot be relied on to take corrective action himself, however well trained. It follows that protective equipment has to be designed to sense his hypoxia and come into operation automatically. The second feature, known as the time of useful consciousness describes how rapidly consciousness is lost and thus dictates how quickly this equipment must respond.

The time of useful consciousness is the interval after the onset of hypoxia during which an aviator can be relied on to act sensibly. This is a difficult characteristic to test, since sophisticated abilities need to be sampled in an adequate and time-consuming way at moments when the level of consciousness may be changing rapidly.

Many studies have confirmed the general relationship between this time-interval and the altitude of sudden exposure, which is shown in Fig. 9(a). The time of useful consciousness diminishes from about four minutes at 25 000 ft to a minimum of roughly 15 seconds which is reached at 35 000 to 40 000 ft. This asymptote represents the sum of the seven seconds or so required for blood to

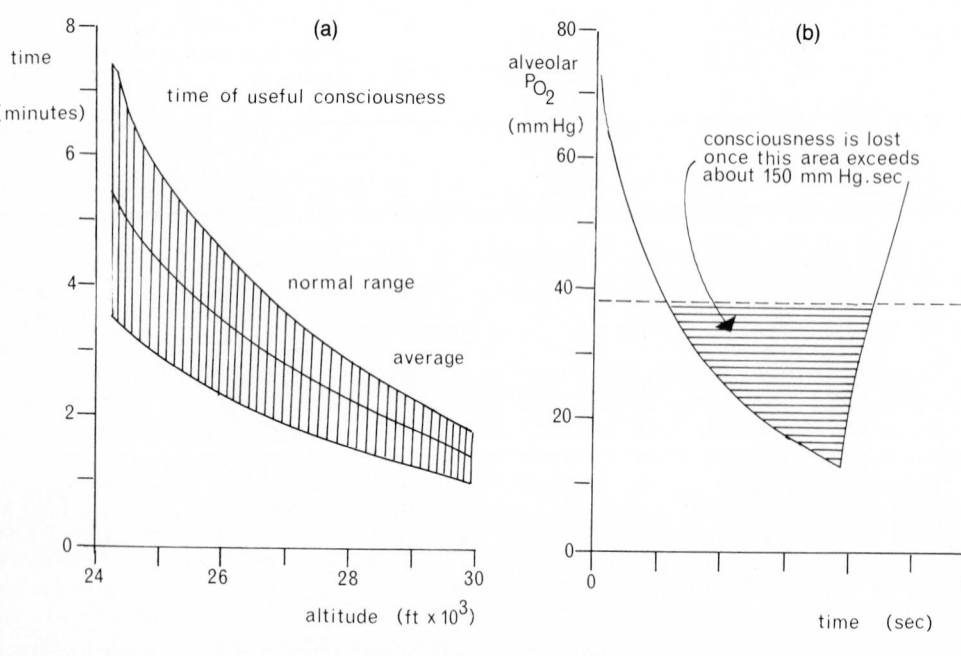

Fig. 9 (a) Variations in the time of useful consciousness with altitude. (b) One way of expressing the dose of hypoxia needed to bring about the loss of consciousness.

travel from the lungs to the brain and the equal time needed for the brain to consume the oxygen that is already dissolved in its substance.

Some recent studies have defined the dose of hypoxia which can be suffered before useful consciousness is lost. In trained and healthy men breathing normally (i.e. with an alveolar P_{CO_2} of 35–40 mmHg), it is equivalent on a curve of alveolar P_{O_2} against time, to an area of 150 'millimetre of mercury seconds', where P_{O_2} is less than 38 mmHg (Fig. 9(b)). However, this is sensitive to many other factors of which the most important are the degree of hyperventilation and the acceleration that the person is exposed to at the time. Hyperventilation causes cerebral vasoconstriction, and 'positive g' opposes the upward flow of blood to the brain (see below). Sometimes deterioration in consciousness is quickened by vasovagal syncope, but more often the heart is beating quite rapidly as consciousness is lost. Exertion also quickens loss of consciousness, as mentioned previously, because it forces blood to rush through the lungs, leaving insufficient time for oxygen equilibration.

It is quite remarkable that resting unadapted men suddenly exposed to the pressure which exists at the top of Mount Everest will lose consciousness in about two minutes, but after a few weeks of gradual exposure they are able to climb strenuously to the top without benefit of oxygen (see p. 6.58). All the available evidence suggests that exposure of at least 15 hours a day is needed to produce sustained adaptation. No useful responses of this sort are ever seen in aviation. It is interesting that a very similar time per day is needed if chronic bronchitic and emphysematous patients are to benefit from long-term oxygen therapy.

The minimum cabin pressure of 565 mmHg (8000 ft), is sufficiently low to bring a normal person's arterial P_{O_2} along the plateau of the oxyhaemoglobin dissociation curve until it is sitting just at the top of the steep part (Fig. 7). Because their blood is still fully saturated with oxygen they will not be cyanosed at this altitude. At ground level, many people with chest diseases have arterial oxygen pressures that are as low as 55–60 mmHg (or even lower, in which case they become cyanosed). As they ascend to 8000 ft their arterial P_{O_2} will fall further. If their hypoxaemia at ground level is due to a mismatch of ventilation to perfusion, as is usually the case, the drop in arterial P_{O_2} will not be as extensive as in normal people (about 40 mmHg), but if it is due to diffusion defect associated with desaturation on exertion, as in some fibrotic conditions, it may be greater. However, in either event, it can be reversed completely by the administration of oxygen, since 30 per cent oxygen at 8000 ft is equivalent to breathing air at ground level. The medical services of all the major airlines can provide a personal oxygen supply for any passenger if they are given notice beforehand. (It is worth checking the altitudes of the patient's destination and of any stopping-point en route at the same time.)

Oxygen equipment and pressure cabins

Aircraft that fly below 10 000 ft do not need any oxygen equipment at all. Most of those that fly higher have reinforced cabins capable of holding a higher pressure inside them than out. These are of two sorts, the high-differential type, seen in passenger and transport aircraft generally, and the low-differential variety found in military high-performance aircraft. The former, holding a high transmural pressure, usually prevent pressure falling below 565 mmHg (8000 ft). They provide an environment in which oxygen equipment is not needed routinely and the occupants breathe cabin air. However, it is always possible that the pressure-cabin system can fail, allowing the pressure within to fall to the level of that outside. This fall can be limited by descent to a lower altitude, but it is not always practical to put the aircraft into a very steep dive, for structural reasons. Similarly, it is not always practical to descend below 10 000 ft because, in mid-Atlantic for example, there may not be sufficient fuel for the vehicle to reach the nearest land through dense air. For these reasons, if there is a cabin-pressure failure, people can be exposed to dangerously hypoxic environment for some time.

A high-differential cabin limits the vehicle's range and manoeuvrability. It also increases the risk of catastrophic damage if the fuselage is punctured. For these reasons military high-performance aircraft are fitted with low differential cabins. These usually prevent cabin pressure falling below 280 mmHg (equivalent to a pressure altitude of 25 000 ft). That is the level at which decompression sickness becomes a serious hazard (see below). In such aircraft oxygen equipment is needed routinely.

The requirements such equipment must meet are demanding, and much ingenuity has gone into its design. In principle, it must

1. conserve oxygen, which itself is heavy to carry;
2. not allow the inspired oxygen pressure to rise above half an atmosphere (this avoids pulmonary oxygen toxicity and absorbtion atelectasis);
3. not allow the inspired oxygen pressure to fall below about 100 mmHg, equivalent to breathing air at 8000 ft;
4. therefore it must mix cabin air and stored oxygen in proportions that vary with cabin altitude and have to be regulated automatically.
5. routinely, it must provide the air-oxygen mix at a slight positive pressure (safety pressure) to ensure that any leaks in the breathing system are outboard, since inward leaks of air cannot be detected but are dangerous;
6. in the event of pressure-cabin failure at altitudes above 40 000 ft, it must deliver oxygen to the lung at pressures substantially greater than ambient air in such a way that the man can remain conscious and breath easily until the aircraft is brought below 40 000 ft, where pressure-breathing is not required.

Devices the size of a match box can perform all these functions automatically, sensing the altitude, regulating the airmix, providing the safety pressure and when necessary much greater over-pressures, and at the same time constantly matching the volume demanded, in response to respiratory pressure swings of at most a few mmHg. They usually deliver gas to an oronasal mask with a reflected edge seal, that is held onto the face by a harness capable of withstanding the greatest over-pressure likely to be encountered.

Sometimes occupants have to escape from aircraft in flight. The faster the aircraft is travelling the more difficult this is to do. All modern fighters are equipped with ejector seats to launch the man into the high-speed airstream and get him clear of the tail. Usually the man free-falls in the seat until he is below 10 000 ft. This gets him through the cold hypoxic upper air as quickly as possible. A small seat- or man-mounted emergency oxygen supply sees him safely through this stage.

Mechanical effects of pressure change

When any rigid gas-filled cavity (e.g. an aircraft cavity or a paranasal sinus) is exposed to an abrupt fall of external pressure, it tends to vent in an exponential manner, with a time-constant (i.e. time taken to follow 62 per cent of the external pressure change) that depends upon the volume of the cavity and the resistence of the pathway to the outside world (i.e. to the product RC in Fig. 10). If the external pressure change is gradual (i.e. if its time-constant is much longer than that of the cavity in question), the pressure in the cavity will almost exactly follow that outside, and the transmural pressure developed during the decompression will be slight. If the time-constant of the external pressure change is substantially shorter than that of the cavity, the transmural pressure will approach the magnitude of the decompression outside. This may be sufficient to rupture the cavity. If the wall of the cavity is pliable (as in the lung, gut, and middle ear), then part of the decompression is accommodated by expansion of the gas within, stretching the walls but limiting the maximum transmural pressures that can develop.

In civilian passenger and transport aircraft the climb from take-off to cruise altitude takes about 30 minutes and involves a fall of about 200 mmHg in cabin pressure (to 8000 ft). The descent to ground, which involves an equivalent rise in cabin pressure, takes much the same time. Body fluids and tissues generally are virtually

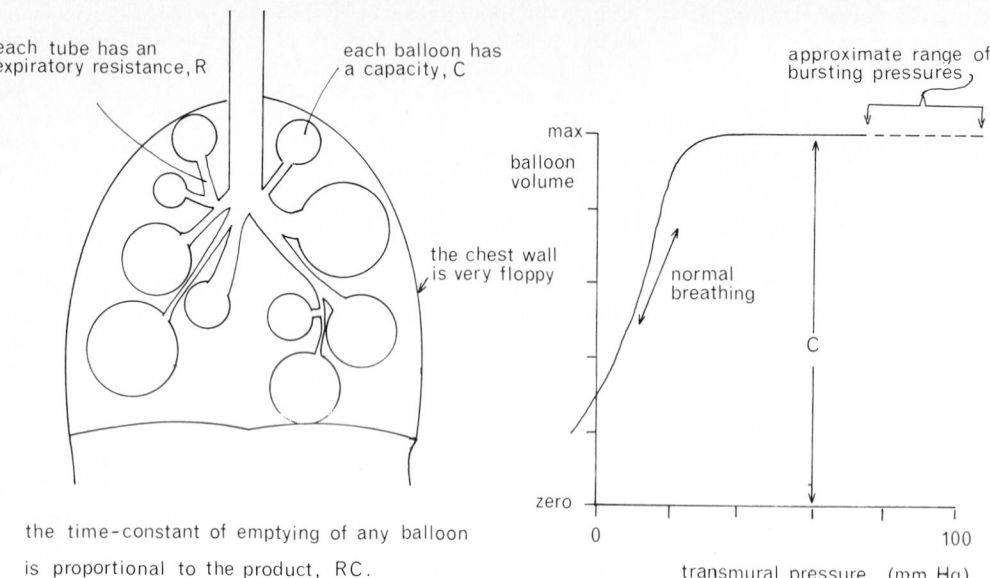

each tube has an expiratory resistance, R

each balloon has a capacity, C

the chest wall is very floppy

the time-constant of emptying of any balloon

is proportional to the product, RC.

Fig. 10   A graphical summary of the factors determining lung rupture.

incompressible and do not alter shape to any important extent when these pressures are applied (cf. diving), but cavities such as the lungs, gut, middle-ear, and facial sinuses, which do contain air, behave differently.

The thoraco-abdominal wall is a floppy structure that can develop an internal pressure of 100 mmHg or so briefly but is normally flaccid and has a transmural pressure of a few millimetres of mercury. Thus, any gas inside the wall must be at a pressure very close to that outside, and must also follow Boyle's law. Ascent from ground level (760 mmHg) to 8000 ft (565 mmHg) will expand a given volume of gas in a completely pliable container by about 35 per cent, which is equivalent to a radial increase of 10 per cent if it were in a sphere or 18 per cent in a cylinder of fixed length. In the abdomen this may cause slightly uncomfortable gut distension in healthy people but it is not an important problem.

Expansion of gas in the chest is a different matter. The lungs can be thought of as a cluster of tubes and balloons of different sizes. A small balloon served by a wide-bore tube can empty freely and poses no threat, but the air in any space served by an inappropriately small airway will empty slowly and behave as 'trapped gas'. Since most spaces in the lung are only about half full during quiet breathing, they can accommodate the 35 per cent increase in volume that would accompany complete obstruction, without bursting. If there is a large obstructed space, e.g. a pneumothorax, this expansion can be functionally embarrassing. However, if any of the 'trapped gas' is already in a fairly tense container at ground level, there is a risk of lung rupture, since it has a bursting pressure of about 100 mmHg (cf. the 200 mmHg that are available on ascent to 8000 ft). The time-constant of emptying is about 1 s in the healthy lung (witness the normal FEV1/FVC ratio) and even very diseased lungs can vent themselves over a minute or so. Most patients with obstructive chest disease are able to fly quite safely and should not be prevented from doing so, but those with very severe asthma, obviously tense cysts or a pneumothorax, should not fly. In this regard, flying in small helicopters and small private planes at low altitudes is perfectly acceptable.

The pressure cabins of civilian passenger aircraft are designed so that the failure of any single element (e.g. a window, an air-intake, or a pressure-relief valve) will lead to a decompression that takes place over many seconds. In military aircraft, especially in high-performance fighters, decompressions are more likely and more rapid, perhaps taking a second or less, (as in 'through-canopy ejection). To meet these circumstances aircrew are trained to breath-out throughout the decompression. Many experiments have shown that, if they are correctly trained, healthy people can survive quite wide-range decompressions over such short times, but it is quite clear that anyone with obstructive lung disease would not. For

this reason, aircrew medical examination set stringent spirometric requirements (see below).

The cavity of the middle ear poses a separate problem because it vents easily but sometimes fails to fill since the lower part of the Eustachian tube behaves as a non-return valve, especially when it is inflamed. As a result, the cavity equilibrates quite easily on ascent but does not refill on descent, and the ear-drum bows inwards causing pain that can be severe. Patients with colds or a history of middle-ear infection should take a decongestant spray with them and use it before descent. In general, people who really cannot move their ear-drums outwards on performing a Valsalva manoeuvre are best advised to delay their flight.

The facial sinuses present a different hazard because their walls are rigid. If the sinus is obstructed before ascent, it will fail to vent and ultimately will hold a positive pressure of up to 200 mmHg. This is sufficient to obstruct the blood flow to the mucosa and may rupture the sinus. Occasionally, as with the thin roof of the ethmoid sinuses, this can force infected material through the floor of the skull, leading to cerebral abscess. If a sinus that was patent on ascent obstructed during descent, its cavity would contain a relative vacuum that could reach −200 mmHg. This is sufficient to cause gross mural oedema and to rupture some vessels, filling the cavity with blood. Occasionally, air-filled spaces in the teeth and jaw may behave in the same way (aerodontalgia).

Decompression sickness

One unexpected hazard that passengers in civil aircraft can experience is decompression sickness (see pp. 6.81–82). In principle, if the pressure around the person quickly falls to less than half its original value, the gas dissolved in blood and tissue fluids may come out of solution precipitously, forming bubbles and obstructing flow in small blood vessels. Although this cannot develop on simple ascents from ground level to 8000 ft, it may arise if the person has been scuba-diving immediately before their flight. It is a particular hazard for holiday-makers on package tours who often fly back home at night and have all day to swim beforehand. It is customary to advise people not to scuba-dive to a depth greater than 30 feet in the 12 hours before take-off. This condition should be kept in mind when looking at anyone who has developed neurological signs or symptoms during or soon after a flight. The correct treatment is immediate descent and ideally transfer to the nearest compression chamber, giving oxygen and other non-specific support meantime.

In aircraft with low-differential pressure cabins, the risk of developing decompression sickness is greater and people flying in them should not dive at all in the preceding 12 hours. The time symptoms take to develop varies widely between individuals and

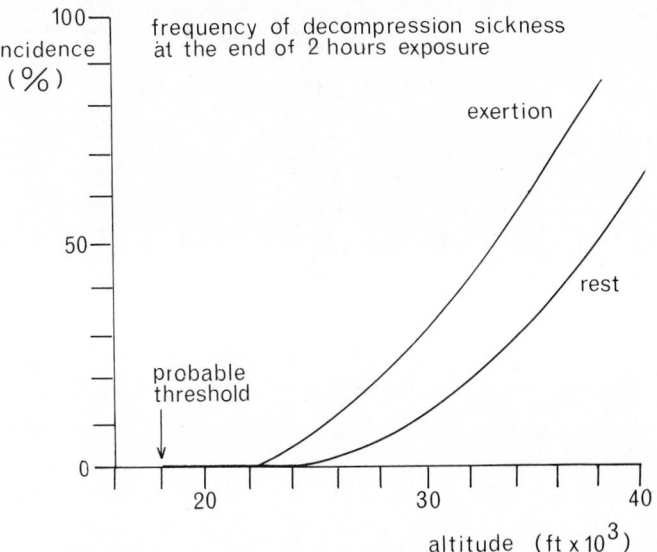

Fig. 11 The incidence of decompression sickness (percentage) at the end of 2 hour exposure to various altitudes in men at rest, or exerting themselves.

shortens markedly as the altitude of exposure rises. A guide to these times and variability is given in Fig. 11.

Acceleration

The human body is continuously acted upon by the force of earth's gravity and is well adapted to a force of 1 G. Modern aircraft, particularly in the military role, are capable of high speed and may be subjected to violent and sustained manoeuvres which may expose the occupants to accelerative forces of high magnitude. In addition, man in space faces a new phenomenon in that the pull of the earth's gravitational field is lost, exposing the individual to a so-called weightless condition.

There are three main types of duration when describing acceleration: firstly, short duration when the forces acting on the body act for less than one second. Secondly, long duration when the forces act for more than one second and may last for minutes, and thirdly, intermediate duration when the force acts from one-half to two seconds. In flight prolonged changes in velocity lasting longer than one second can result from changes in speed or direction of flight.

Linear acceleration. We refer to a linear acceleration as a change in speed without a change in direction. These are generally of low magnitude in that even supersonic aircraft accelerating in a straight line do not produce profound changes on the body. However significant linear accelerations can be experienced in the accelerated launch of an aircraft from an aircraft carrier or the use of re-heat in a supersonic fighter.

Radial acceleration. This is described as a change of direction without a change of speed when for example the line of flight is changed or the aircraft goes into a steep and prolonged turn. Accelerations of 6–8 Gz can be reached in high-performance military aircraft or in centrifuge studies on man in the laboratory. On the other hand linear or radial accelerations are of a low order in the operation of civil transport aircraft and have little effect on the crew or passengers.

Long-duration positive acceleration. The pilots and aircrew of high speed combat aircraft can be exposed to long-duration positive accelerations in normal training and in combat flying in the range of 5–7 Gz for 10 seconds and even 8–10 Gz for up to 60 seconds. In civil aviation, even in supersonic transport operations, these loadings are never experienced.

The general effects of long-duration positive accelerations have profound effects on the body and on human performance, and crews have to be trained in exposure to these levels and positive means of protecting them provided.

At +2 Gz the facial soft tissues begin to sag and the weight of the trunk and limbs increases, creating difficulty in standing up from a sitting position which becomes an impossibility at +3 Gz and could preclude unassisted escape from an aircraft. At +8 Gz upward movement of the arms is impossible, and, if the head has been allowed to flex before this level, raising of the head is impossible. Because of these limitations, unassisted escape is impossible, and hence the development of the ejector seat became necessary over 25 years ago to ensure that aircrew could escape under such G loadings.

Vision. As exposure to positive acceleration increases so does progressive loss of visual acuity and loss of peripheral vision—the so-called 'grey-out'. At +4.5 Gz there is usually a complete loss of vision or 'black-out', whilst hearing and mental activity remain. There are, of course, wide variations in the levels of acceleration required to produce loss of peripheral vision in individuals, and this loss also varies with the intensity of the illumination of the visual field, for instance, in the dark peripheral vision seems to be lost more rapidly. At +5.0 Gz 'black-out' may occur at 6 seconds, but vision may be restored some 6 seconds later and normal vision 3–5 seconds after the manoeuvre ceases.

Unconsciousness. Positive accelerations above the levels producing black-out produce loss of consciousness, but with higher rates of onset, loss of consciousness may occur first with loss of muscle tone and slumping of head, trunk, and limbs. Convulsions of varying degree may be seen in the subject during such periods with slow recovery and confusion lasting from 30 seconds to one minute. These changes are due to changes in the pressures of the cardio-vascular system under the effects of positive accelerations, resulting in shift of blood to the more dependant parts of the body which in turn result in reflex changes compensating, to some extent, the initial effects. These changes are partly due to initial hydrostatic effects and accentuation of the pressure gradients which normally exist due to gravity. The magnitude of the changes of pressure in the circulation produced by positive acceleration are proportional to the point at which the pressure is measured and the heart, and the degree of acceleration.

Vibration. Vibration in aircraft may arise from the engines, propellers in propeller-driven aircraft, and from helicopter propeller blades in helicopters in the range of 10–1000 Hz. In multi-engined aircraft, for instance, a lack of precise synchronization of engine speeds may result in 'beats' of very low frequencies (1–10 Hz) which may be more intense and disturbing than the primary vibration of the power-plants.

Helicopters have peculiar characteristics in that they vibrate in all major axes, particularly at frequencies related to the rotational speed of the main rotor blades. In addition, vibrations of different frequencies emanate from the engines, gearbox, and tail rotor blades to a considerable degree generating both internal and external noise fields in the infrasonic frequency range below 10 Hz. Low frequency structure-borne vibration may be of considerable concern and effect during changes of flight profile, e.g. from hovering to straight and level, etc.

In civil aircraft, particularly in supersonic aircraft at high speed and high altitude, there may be major modes of structural vibration at 10 Hz or below at crew stations and at certain passenger positions. In addition, because of the long extended nose with the crew position well forward of the nose-wheel, small oscillations during taxying and take-off may be amplified, resulting in considerable vertical motion of the cockpit and difficulty in reading instruments during these critical phases of flight.

High speed, low-level flight also produces problems, particularly in military aircraft flying perhaps in excess of 400 knots at 90 m altitude to avoid radar detection. Very severe vibrations may be set up in the aircraft structure and its crew particularly during the penetration of turbulent air. This may be compounded by manoeuvres by the pilot to avoid terrain or by automatic terrain-following systems which direct the autopilot. In such conditions the aircraft may pitch and yaw unpleasantly, and with irregular random vibrations the body can be excited into a mass/spring type of resonance.

Physiological effects of vibration. The vibration ranges of concern in flight are those in the low frequencies (1–50 Hz). They give rise to effects related to the resonance of the body, its contained organs and tissues. Other factors affecting resonance are the type of aircraft, the effects of external turbulence, position in the aircraft, type of seating, and the provision of protective anti-G clothing.

Whole body vibration in the range of 1–10 Hz may cause severe hyperventilation if the amplitude exceeds 0.5 G. The aetiology of this hyperventilation is not clear but may partly be due to the upward piston-like thrust of the viscera transmitted via the diaphragm, plus widespread stimulation of somatic mechanoreceptors in the lungs and respiratory passages. Hyperventilation, which may also be associated by anxiety, apprehension or fear, results in a vicious circle since the hypocapnia induced by the hyperventilation produces anxiety and anxiety in turn aggravates the hyperventilation. This can result in collapse and unconsciousness, but well before that, there are well-defined decrements of performance in psychomotor tasks, mental tasks, and the ability to perform manual tasks due to muscle spasm.

Spatial disorientation. This term is used in aviation to describe a variety of incidents when a pilot fails to sense correctly the position, motion, or attitude of his aircraft in flight within the bounds of the surface of the earth and the gravitational vertical.

Generally speaking, all aircrew at one time or another experience illusory sensations of aircraft attitude and motion or fail to appreciate the attitude of the aircraft in flight. These illusions are caused by the physiological limitations of the sensory mechanisms in the body. The most important result of such sensory illusions is of course loss of control of the aircraft resulting in a subsequent accident.

Although the incidence of such accidents is small (about 5–10 per cent in military aviation in the UK and USA), they nevertheless account for up to 20 per cent of all fatal accidents. In civil air transport the figures are smaller (about 12 per cent of all UK civil air transport causes to UK aircraft had a disorientation implication). Nevertheless, approach and landing accidents still account for some 62 per cent of all civil transport hull losses over the last fifteen years and 25 per cent of these 'visual misjudgement of distance, altitude, or speed'—in other words disorientation—played quite a major part.

Mechanisms of orientation. Man's ability to preserve his true orientation in flight comes from a number of sensory receptors. Some of these are grouped together to form special sense organs like the eye or the vestibular apparatus, others are distributed throughout the body in the skin, muscles, joints, and viscera.

Pilots often refer to the 'seat of the pants' sensation. What they really mean is sensory messages coming from skin, muscle, joints, and viscera—in other words all non-visual sensory mechanisms involved in maintaining orientation in flight.

In our natural environment when standing, sitting, or walking about we receive very accurate information regarding our spatial orientation via visual cues. The eyes in fact are the most important organs in providing information about the orientation of the body with respect to the immediate environment. They also inform the pilot about the position and altitude of the aircraft relative to the surface of the earth.

In the dark, or in cloud or poor visibility, the pilot must determine the aircraft's orientation from his instruments, a skill he acquires from training in instrument flying and by experience.

In addition to visual cues the pilot obtains further information from his vestibular organs and other kinaesthetic receptors elsewhere in the body such as muscle, capsules of joints, etc. The vestibular apparatus can sense linear and angular accelerations and

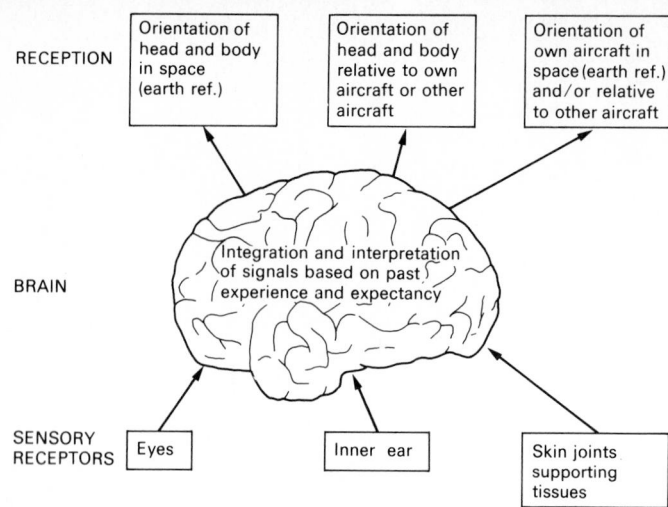

Fig. 12 Sense organs used by man to determine his spatial orientation in flight (after Benson (1978), by permission).

movements of the head, and under certain conditions can give erroneous information regarding orientations, particularly where well-defined external visual cues are lost.

Types of disorientation. The ability to maintain control of an aircraft without adequate visual cues is quite short—about 60 seconds even in straight and level flight, but much shorter in a turn. Loss of control will quickly follow if the pilot does not go over immediately to his instrument panel. In addition, his vestibular apparatus may well give him false cues during such conditions and these may be so overwhelming that he may be tempted, if insufficiently trained, to ignore the information being presented to him on the instrument panel.

There are certain well-known types of disorientation experienced by pilots in flying. These can be classified as 'the leans', somatogravic and oculogravic illusions, and the coriolis effect. One could also add to these pressure vertigo, flicker vertigo, dissociative sensations, and disorientation during approach and landing.

'The leans'. This is a false sensation of bank when the aircraft is in a straight and level condition. It is caused when the pilot allows one wing to drop at a rate below the threshold for the detection of a change in angular velocity. There is, as a result, no stimulation of the vestibular otoliths or his kinaesthetic receptors by linear accelerations.

The pilot, however, usually becomes aware of the situation by reference to his artificial horizon and thus initiates recovery to level flight. If the recovery is rapid, and as he felt his wings were level before the recovery, the angular velocity in roll so perceived may be above the sensory threshold so that he rolls the other way, causing a further erroneous perception of his true position.

Quite apart from this, 'the leans' can also be induced from external visual cues in that the pilot can line up his aircraft to correspond with sloping streets of cloud assuming them to be horizontal. Only by reference to his instruments will he perceive his mistake.

Somatogravic and oculogravic illusions. Disorientation can occur when a pilot is exposed to accelerations he is not exposed to normally on the face of the earth where gravity is stable and assumed to be vertical.

For instance, in a prolonged co-ordinated turn the pilot may be unable to sense—apart from outside visual reference— the angle of bank. In a flat prolonged turn he may feel he has rolled out of the turn and in a prolonged co-ordinated turn has no sensation of being in a banked attitude—he feels his wings are straight and level. Even more dangerous in flight are somatogravic illusions connected with pitch attitudes. In an aircraft which accelerates rapidly, the initial force due to the increase in forward speed produces a resultant force which is inclined backwards. In such a case and, in particular, if there are no external visual cues, such as in cloud or night flying, the pilot feels that he and the aircraft are in a marked nose-up attitude. If he does not refer to his instruments, he experiences the sensation of falling backwards as the nose of the aircraft continues to give the illusion of pitching-up. The great temptation then is to push the nose of the aircraft down with—if the aircraft is near the ground—nearly always fatal results. This is the classic night take-off accident and can also be seen during an overshoot in conditions of fog or poor visibility.

If head movements are made in a turning or banking aircraft—for instance to look for some object or at some instrument or switch in an inaccessible area of the cockpit—erroneous sensations of angular motion can be evoked. These can be most powerful, particularly if the head is moved quickly, resulting in complete loss of control of the aircraft. Forward head movement in pitch during a +6 Gz pull-up from a dive will result in the sensation of tumbling forward in pitch.

Oculogravic illusions are regarded as being part of a situation where linear acceleration stimulate the otoliths and other receptors resulting in displacement of the visual scene. They are rarely a problem when good external cues are available, as the illusory movement affects all objects in the visual field, including the interior of the aircraft and the instruments.

At night however, with inadequate external visual references and few stars, the oculogravic illusion can cause disorientation and the apparent movement of external lights can lead the pilot to assume a change in altitude of the aircraft. In addition, isolated single lights which apparently move can be regarded as being the light of another aircraft.

Somatogyral illusions are induced during prolonged turning manoeuvres when the receptors only give correct information during the first few seconds of the manoeuvre. Once a steady speed of rotation has been achieved the signals from the semicircular canals die away. For instance, in a spinning aircraft most pilots are unable to perceive spinning from vestibular stimulation after 15–30 seconds. However, with external visual cues and by checking cockpit instruments, they can usually appreciate the true situation.

Coming out of the spin results in angular acceleration in the opposite direction so that the pilot has the sensation of turning in the opposite direction—this may be overwhelming, particularly if he does not pay complete attention to his instruments. In addition, because of nystagmus which may take several seconds to decay, visual reference from external sources may be completely unreliable.

Pressure vertigo. Pressure changes within the middle ear can, in susceptible subjects, produce quite powerful vertigo effects and may be of sudden onset, for example, on descent when the pilot 'clears his ears' by performing a 'Valsalva manoeuvre'. There may be very intense vertigo with blurring of vision and possible movement of the visual scene which usually lasts 15–20 seconds, but in some cases may persist.

The mechanism of stimulating the semicircular canals by pressure changes in the middle ear is not fully understood, but Eustachian catarrh can be a contributory factor in this condition, and for this reason aircrew should not fly whilst suffering from upper respiratory tract infections or any condition impairing ventilation of the middle ear.

Flicker vertigo. Some pilots experience vertigo, particularly in helicopters where the shadow of the rotor blades passes across the cockpit probably several times a second, but also from the flashing of aircraft anti-collision lights, particularly when the lights are reflected into the cockpit by cloud or snow. In one case a pilot under training in a helicopter developed an epileptiform fit and became unconscious. In such cases the photic stimulus may flicker at a frequency close to a dominant rhythm of the electroencephalogram (8–10 Hz of the α waves). Fortunately this is a very rare occurrence in aviation experience.

Motion sickness. Motion sickness is a generic term applied to sea sickness, car sickness, swing sickness, simulator sickness, air sickness, and space sickness, and its existence is probably as old as man himself. The condition was well-known to the early Greeks and the word nausea is derived from the word *nauxia* meaning sea sickness, itself derived from *naus* meaning ship. The condition has plagued travellers through the ages: Julius Caesar, Lord Nelson, Charles Darwin, and Lawrence of Arabia being a few sufferers of note. Little seemed to be done until the Second World War when it became necessary to transport large numbers of troops by land, sea, and air, and to ensure that they arrived in a suitable physical condition to go straight into combat. In addition, due to the large number of survivors from air crashes and shipwrecks, it was necessary to provide some sort of preventive treatment for those who were faced with survival, adrift on the sea.

The condition is characterized by nausea, followed by vomiting, pallor, and cold sweating when man is exposed to real or apparent motion stimuli with which he is unfamiliar and unadapted. Generally the first symptom is epigastric discomfort followed by nausea of increasing severity. At the same time circum-oral or facial pallor may be noted, and sweating of the face and hands may be seen. There is increased salivation at this stage with swallowing of the saliva, lightness of the head, and a feeling of apathy or depression, followed by vomiting. This sequence has been termed the 'avalanche effect'. Some individuals on the other hand do not proceed as far as vomiting and others report that only induced vomiting will relieve the preceding symptoms.

Continued exposure to the causitive motion results in a cyclical pattern of waxing and waning symptoms with recurrent vomiting and retching, which may last for several days. In such cases the victim becomes severely anorexic, depressed, apathetic, and unable to carry out his normal duties. The mental symptoms may be so severe that personal safety and safety of the group in general may be completely abandoned.

Operational aspects. Motion sickness can have a very adverse effect on performance in that the loss of a sense of well-being in the air or on the sea results in distraction from the task in hand with mistakes in navigation, aircraft handling, operating radar equipment, and arithmetical calculations involving, say, fuel reserves.

Air sickness in pilots is frequently seen during flying training and this may be so severe as to result in the individual's complete withdrawal from training.

In the case of airline passengers this may be also a problem if they have to carry out business appointments immediately on arrival where there is no time for recuperation.

Fortunately with the advent of the turbo-prop and turbo-jet transport aircraft which have the capability of climbing through and flying above adverse weather conditions, motion sickness amongst crew and passengers has been reduced to a very low incidence indeed. The only areas where motion sickness occurs in passengers is where the aircraft is held by air traffic control for operational reasons in areas of high turbulence or during penetration during climb or descent of rough air.

Prevention of motion sickness. The best method of prevention of motion sickness is to avoid the causative motion altogether, but this is perhaps not helpful. The exact causes of the condition are still unknown but it is necessary to have an intact vestibular mechanism to experience the disease. In animals or humans where these organs have been destroyed by disease or surgically extirpated, motion sickness is not experienced.

The visual mechanism plays a large part in the occurrence of the disease. In ships it is important to remain on deck, keeping eyes focused on distant horizons and the same applies to rail or car travel. The individual should not attempt to focus on objects passing nearby. Below decks or in aircraft the eyes should be kept closed and the head kept fixed to, say, the seat back. In addition, many individuals subject to the condition will become less prone when given a task to perform, thus occupying the mind.

The use of drugs. Many drugs have been tried over the years to deal with, or better, to prevent the condition developing. The exact mechanism by which they work is unknown and as a result many and varied drugs have been tried with mixed success over the years. All drugs have side effects and most appear to act on the central nervous system and have included the antihistamines, belladonna derivatives, belladonna itself, phenathiazones, and the barbiturates either separately or in combination.

In selecting a drug particular care should be taken in ascertaining the duties of the individual. For instance, to give an antihistamine to a driver or pilot with its known side effects of drowsiness and disorientation is to invite disaster. Secondly, it would be pointless to give an oral drug to a victim already vomiting. For instance, in life-raft survivors it was found that the best method of giving drugs, e.g. 1-hyoscine hydrobromide, was by intramuscular injection (0.2 mg).

Others have found that 1-hyoscine hydrobromide by mouth (0.6 mg) is still the best prophylactic for the bad risk case undergoing short exposure. Less effective drugs are meclozine hydrochloride (50 mg twice daily) or cyclizine hydrochloride (50 mg twice daily). The latter should not be given to expectant mothers. Dimenhydrinate (50 mg twice daily) is also effective but drowsiness is a side effect.

Work carried out by Wood and Graybiel in the United States has shown that combining promethazine hydrochloride (25 mg) with dexamphetamine (10 mg) gives consistently good results, as good as 1-hyoscine hydrochloride, but further studies has shown that the best results can be obtained by combining promethazine hydrochloride (25 mg) with ephedrine hydrochloride (25 mg). 1-hyoscine hydrobromide should not be used in elderly men with incipient urinary retention, in cases of glaucoma, or where impairment of visual accommodation may be a problem. In addition, dry mouth may be unpleasant to some people.

Dexamphetamine should not be given in cases of high blood pressure, and, as it is a known drug of addiction and closely controlled in many countries it may not be available without a prescription.

Whatever drug is employed it is essential that it is taken at least 30 minutes to one hour before exposure to the motion. In the case of children positive steps should be taken to prevent overdosage, particularly in long journeys, and repeated doses.

Advances in the stability of modern transport vehicles, such as the use of stabilizers in ships, improved railway rolling stock, hydro-elastic suspension in road vehicles, and jet transport aircraft which can quickly penetrate and ride above the weather, has done much to reduce the incidence of motion sickness, but much still depends on the susceptibility of the individual and the duration and the severity of the motion imparted to them.

In long-established vomiting dehydration and loss of electrolytes results with consequent loss of interest in surroundings and the will to survive or co-operate in rescue attempts. Drugs in this situation must be given parenterally, either by intramuscular injection or by suppository. In addition fluids, electrolytes, and calories may need to be given intravenously.

Selection of aircrew and medical maintenance

As a result of the very high cost of training pilots, military forces and airlines demand the highest physical and mental standards on entry, for if a pilot has to retire on medical grounds before the age of 55 in a civil airline or even earlier in the military role, there is considerable economic loss not only to the individual but also to his employer. As far as airlines are concerned aircrew require to be in possession of a current licence to fly which is granted by the statutory licensing authority of the country concerned and in accordance with the recommendations of the International Civil Aviation Organization (ICAO) publication *Personnel Licensing*. These re-

commendations are amended every ten years or so and were last revised in 1970 (Amendment 156). Most countries adhering to the United Nations adopt these recommended medical standards. In formulating medical standards ICAO has to take note of the fact that general medical facilities and practices vary from country to country, and, while advanced standards of biochemical analysis may be highly desirable, many developing countries do not have the medical expertise to meet these.

For this reason, the standards set by certain countries may in fact be higher than expected by ICAO. To enable all signatories to agree, any changes in ICAO practices are therefore deliberately cautious and slow to appear in print.

Medical standards for civil aircrew. In the United Kingdom the Civil Aviation Authority (CAA) is the responsible mandatory authority for issuing licences to the various categories of aircrew. The regulations are contained in an Air Navigation Order issued under the authority of the Minister of Trade & Industry. The CAA issues a handbook for Authorized Medical Examiners which details the standards which are to be met in granting licences to airmen—pilots, flight engineers, flight radio officers, and air traffic control officers. In addition, pilots are divided into several groups, i.e. airline transport pilots, senior commercial pilots, commercial pilots, private pilots, and student pilots.

The CAA divide airmen into three main classes, medically speaking:

Class I includes: airline transport pilot (ALTP); senior commercial pilot (SCPL); commercial pilot (CPL); and air traffic control officer (ATCO).

Class II includes: flight navigator (F/N); flight engineer (F/E); and flight radio officer (FRO).

Class III includes: private pilot (PPL) and Student Pilot (S/PPL).

The holder of a class III licence would not be eligible for licences whose minimal requirements were a class II or a class I certificate. The standards applied in the UK by CAA are in fact those recommended by ICAO and are summarized in Table 1.

Table 1　Medical standards for aircrew

Type of licence	Physical standard	Visual standard	Colour vision standard	Hearing standard
S/PPL	3	3	1	2
PPL	3	3	1	2
F/N	2	2	1	1
F/E	2	3	1	1
FRO	2	3	1	1
CPL	1	1	1	1
SCPL	1	1	1	1
ALTP	1	1	1	1
ATCO	4	1	1	1

Physical standards. Generally speaking candidates should be free from (*a*) any abnormality, congenital or acquired; (*b*) any active, latent, acute or chronic disability; or (*c*) any injury or sequelae from operation such as would entail a degree of functional incapacity likely to interfere with his safe handling of an aircraft at any altitude throughout a prolonged or difficult flight.

Abnormality or absence of limbs or fingers may interfere with the safe handling of an aircraft and special orthopaedic problems may need evaluation by a special flight test and/or orthopaedic opinion.

With reference to the special systems the following limitations apply to applicants for any form of airman's licence.

The cardiovascular system. The history of a proven myocardial infarction or definite evidence of myocardial ischaemia or any significant ECG changes even in the absence of clinical symptoms are causes for rejection. The frequency of ECG examination varies with type of licence and age. At the moment resting ECGs are routine and post-stress ECGs would only be used for diagnostic purposes. An applicant with congenital disease would be rejected; but if a right bundle branch block is shown to be congenital rather than acquired, the licence may be granted.

Blood pressure 'shall be within acceptable limits' states the regulations, but previous recordings, body build, state of the urine, weight and height should all be taken into account when assessing blood pressure. The CAA give some figures (Table 2) purely for guidance.

Table 2   CAA guidelines on blood pressure

| Age | Pressure (mmHg) | |
	Systolic	Diastolic
20–29	140	82
30–39	145	92
40–49	155	96
50+	160	98

Generally speaking for airmen under the contol of their own physicians or company medical advisers, the CAA will only allow the use of simple diuretic type anti-hypertension drugs, which are thought to be compatible with the safe performance of flying duties. At present very limited use of β-blockers have been allowed in selected and carefully supervised cases.

It is not proposed to go into great detail about the medical standards for military and civil aircrew on entry as this would entail a complete chapter in itself. The enquiring reader is referred however to the standard mandatory regulations previously referred to and also to *Aviation Medicine* (vol. 2, 1978).

Medical care and maintenance of aircrew. Only military air forces and the larger airlines maintain medical departments with fulltime medical officers who are specially qualified in aerospace medicine.

It has long been the tradition in the Armed Forces that doctors concerned with aircrew should live, fly, and work closely with their patients and develop a close rapport with them. In this way individual aircrew will bring their worries and anxieties to the doctor at an early stage. The civilian doctor, if he is to be accepted by aircrew, who tend to be suspicious, as a group, of outsiders, must strive hard to establish a good relationship if he is to be accepted.

In addition, it is essential that the aircrew medical centre is not only close to the centre of flight operations, but that it is also available at all times and a round-the-clock service is available. Nursing staff and other staff must be dedicated in their approach to good relations as, if this mutual trust is lost, it may take many years to correct a misunderstanding made by some unfortunate remark.

It is important to maintain the best relationships with pilots' general practitioners, and where necessary hospital consultants, as the former may have little insight into the problems facing aircrew and resultant medication given with good intention may have serious effects on pilots' performance.

Medication, drugs, and flying. Generally speaking no aircrew member should undertake flying duties while on medication as a drug or combination of drugs can have adverse, serious, or even dangerous effects on flying skill which may result in disaster. In addition, the exposure of the individual to hypoxia even in the safer confines of a pressurized cabin can heighten the effects of many drugs. It is essential that doctors dealing with aircrew whether they be hospital consultants, general practitioners, or flight medical officers are thoroughly familiar with the effects of the drugs they prescribe for aircrew, and that the latter should inform the doctor of their profession and in addition adopt a critical and responsible attitude to drug-taking of any sort.

The CAA recommend that a pilot should ask himself three questions if he is on medication and intends to fly: (a) Do I really feel fit to fly? (b) Do I really need any medication at all? (c) Have I given this particular medication a trial on the ground for at least 24 hours before flight to ensure that it will not have any adverse effects whatever on my ability to fly?

Generally speaking the nature and the degree of the medical condition will determine the final decision to fly or not rather than the medication, but, with the increasing complexity of drugs and their possible interaction, unwanted effects on performance and skill may result.

Drug groups and flying. The following are only a few of the drug groups where serious thought should be given to their possible effects on pilot or aircrew performance in the air.

Hypnotics and sedatives. Aircrew should not normally fly whilst under medication by these drugs. In addition, the antihistamines must be included here due to their secondary-effects of sedation. Sleep loss is usually incurred in aircrew crossing time zones with increased fatigue at the end of flight resulting in heightened effects from these drugs. Abuse of hypnotic drugs overseas is common and many drugs of this category, normally on prescription in the West, can be obtained by direct over-the-counter purchase in several overseas countries. Abuse of hypnotics by aircrew, often potentiated by the injudicious use of alcohol, can lead to bizarre effects.

Hypnotics also affect the quality of sleep in that REM (rapid eye movement sleep) which occurs in the latter part of the night may be diminished.

It is known that many hypnotics may have measurable effects on performance up to 30–36 hours after the ingestion of a therapeutic dose. Generally speaking the routine use of hypnotics in aircrew is not to be recommended, and flight schedules should be so designed as to allow the aircrew adequate time for sleep and recovery.

Tranquillizers and antidepressants. There is no place for the use of these drugs in aircrew who fly, and doctors must be made aware of their very severe effects on performance and judgement. If it is neccessary to prescribe such drugs to aircrew, they should be removed from the active flying roster during the period of treatment and for several days after the cessation of therapy.

Antihistamine drugs. Nearly all this group produce side effects such as drowsiness, fatigue, gastro-intestinal disturbances, and a dry mouth. Coupled with hypoxia the combination may be lethal to any airman. Many of these drugs are prescribed for 'cold-cures', motion sickness, hay-fever, urticaria, etc. Their use in active flying personnel must be discouraged at all times.

Analgesics. Whilst aircrew suffering severe pain would not normally report for flying duties, nevertheless, some analgesics could be self-administered. Salicylates can and do cause gastric erosion and haemorrhage, as do indomethacin and phenylbutazone.

Antibiotics. Generally speaking if an airman requires antibiotics then he should be removed from the flying roster as the condition being treated usually means that he is unfit anyway.

Streptomycin should never be given to aircrew in case of possible vestibular damage. Other broad-spectrum antibiotics may cause gastrointestinal upsets and diarrhoea, but tetracycline taken in small doses as long-term treatment for acne can probably be taken safely. Penicillin can give rise to hypersensitivities and its use should be avoided in those who fly.

Steroids. Generally speaking any crew member requiring steroids should be grounded, but the conditions requiring such therapy usually means the individual is unfit to fly anyway.

Motion sickness cures. These are usually of the belladonna or antihistamine groups and may cause drowsiness, diplopia, dry mouth, and tinnitus. Air-sickness in professional aircrew is of such a low incidence that it is rarely seen except amongst new trainee pilots submitted to extreme aerobatic manoeuvres. It is rarely necessary to submit these categories to prolonged therapy unless the case is severe, when termination of flying training may have to be considered as the final cure.

Antimalarial drugs. Most authorities in the UK recommend the daily use of 100 mg of proguanil continued for 28 days after leaving an infected area. However some areas of the world have become resistant to proguanil and in these high risk areas a weekly tablet of

Maloprim (dapsone 100 mg, pyrimethamine 12.5 mg) or Fanisdar (sulphadoxine 500 mg, pyrimethamine 25 mg) should be taken in addition. Chloroquine should not be used for prophylaxis but rather for treatment of an attack, for ocular complications, such as corneal deposits and a typical retinopathy, can be seen on occasions.

Gastric and intestinal remedies. Simple antacids are perfectly safe to use but mixtures containing belladonna alkaloids or anticholinergics are not. Some preparations in addition may contain barbiturates or other sedatives. In the case of anti-diarrhoea drugs, careful administration is necessary in the case of aircrew because opiates and belladonna derivatives often are added, causing drowsiness or visual disturbances. Overdosage of Lomotil can be particularly prone to produce visual upsets—in one case a Captain was unable to read his flight-check list due to visual side-effects of an excessive dose of Lomotil prescribed to him before take-off.

Treatment of hypertension. Generally speaking, if a hypertensive pilot needs drug therapy to control his blood pressure, then serious questions should be asked about his continued flying.

At present most licensing authorities will only allow the use of a simple thiazide diuretic or spironalactone, or both together, as these very rarely produce side-effects. Other hypotensive drugs can produce serious side-effects which could be disastrous when flying. Recently it has been suggested and agreed by the ICAO Aviation Medical Division that in some cases of hypertension in aircrew treatment by beta adrenegic blocking agents or by hydrallazine can be allowed in carefully controlled cases. It is likely that state licensing authorities will follow this advice.

Drugs and alcohol abuse. Fortunately, drug abuse is not common amongst professional aircrew, but has been seen from time to time amongst cabin crew who can be exposed to the dangers of drug abuse in some parts of the world. Another problem commonly seen amongst the latter group of staff is the tendency to experiment with hypnotic-type drugs which can be freely obtained by over-the-counter purchase in some countries. These combined with alcohol can be lethal on occasions. Careful and frequent education of these categories of staff is essential.

Alcohol and its abuse is of course, another problem. With its widespread availability throughout the world, it can be abused by those who fly professionally. In fact the very nature of long-distance commercial flying with extended stays at hotels in uninteresting areas of the world can and does lead to over-indulgence in alcohol. Most airlines and air forces have very strict rules about the use of alcohol, and many insist on complete abstinence from 8–12 hours before rostered duties. Some countries insist on 24 hours but this may be unrealistic in practice and frequently abused.

Education of aircrew in the use and abuse of alcohol is essential, as is the provision of a clearly stated policy on alcoholism and the provision of specialist facilities for treatment. Air crew tend to be very protective to the alcoholic in their midst and must be educated to advise the victim to seek early professional advice and treatment.

In summary, aircrew should not take any medication whilst on flying duties. If it is absolutely necessary that they do fly under medication, then they should fly only under the strict control of a physician trained in aviation medicine.

Table 3 Adult dosages for anti-motion sickness drugs

Drug	Dose (mg)	Time of onset (hours)	Duration of effect (hours)
1-hyoscine hydrobromide (Kwells)	0.3–0.6	$\frac{1}{2}$–1	4–6
Cyclizine hydrochloride (Marzine, Valoid)	50	1–2	4–6
Dimenhydrinate (Dramamine, Gravol)	50–100	1–2	6–8
Promethazine hydrochloride (Phenergan)	25	1½–2	24–30
Promethazine theoclate (Avomine)			
Meclozine hydrochloride (Ancolan)	50	1–2	12–24

References

Benson, A. (1978) In *Aviation medicine*, Vol. 2 (ed. G. Dhenin, T. C. D. Whiteside, T. J. G. Price, J. G. Taylor, and J. Ernsting) 19. Tri-med, London.

Denison, D. M. (1981*a*). High altitudes and hypoxia. In *Principles and practice of human physiology* (ed. O. G. Edholm and J. S. Weiner) 241. Academic Press, London.

—— (1981) The distribution and use of oxygen in tissues. In *Scientific foundations of respiratory medicine* (ed. G. Cumming, G. Scadding and W. Thurlbeck) 221. Heinemann Medical, London.

Dhenin, G., Sharp, G. R., and Ernsting, J. (eds.) (1978) *Aviation medicine*, Vol. 1. *Physiology and human factors*. Tri-med, London.

—— Whiteside, T. C. D., Price, T. J. G., Taylor, J. G., and Ernsting, J. (eds.) (1978) *Aviation medicine*, Vol 2. *Health and clinical aspects*. Tri-med, London.

Department of Trade and Industry (1970) *Air navigation orders*. HMSO, London.

Department of Trade and Industry (Civil Aviation Medical Branch) (1972) *Authorized Examiners Handbook*. HMSO, London.

Glaister, D. H. (1970) *The effects of gravity and acceleration on the lung*. Technivision Services, Slough.

Howard, P. (1981) Acceleration. In *Principles and practice of human physiology* (ed. O. G. Edholm and J. S. Weiner) 191. Academic Press, London.

ICAO (1970) Medical requirements. In *Personnel licensing*, annexe ch. 6. ICAO, Montreal, Canada.

ICAO (1973) Amendment 156. ICAO, Montreal, Canada.

Wood, D. C. and Graybiel, A. (1968) Evaluation of 16 anti-motion sickness drugs. *Aerospace Med.* **39**, 1341.

—— —— (1970) Evaluation of motion sickness drugs. A new effective remedy revealed. *Aerospace Med.* **41**, 932.

Diving medicine

D. M. Denison

We often think of man as an able creature that has conquered the globe, but almost three-quarters of the Earth's surface is covered by sea which he invades with very little success indeed. Other mammals, such as dolphins, explore it with much greater mastery because they have various features, such as a highly streamlined shape, a much thicker layer of subcutaneous fat, a more mobile chest wall, and bronchioles reinforced all the way to the alveoli, which men are unable to engineer or match for themselves except by very cumbersome means.

Because this is so, human divers are exposed to many hazards that marine mammals avoid. Frequently it is too late or too impractical to give divers specific help once they are in trouble, so Diving

Medicine is largely concerned with prevention. It depends upon a thorough understanding of the job a diver must do and the risks he runs in completing it. In this sense, almost every diving accident is a failure of education or equipment design. However, many well-trained and well-equipped divers come to grief when they are driven or drive themselves beyond limits that are clearly understood but expensive to maintain.

The section begins with a description of the environment, which is usually dark, cold, and too deep to stay in without risk for much time. After discussing some features of the sea, and the basic but minor problems of vision, hearing, dexterity, and mobility, it concentrates on the major hazards of air embolism, inert-gas narcosis, oxygen toxicity, decompression sickness, the high-pressure syndrome, and the difficulty of keeping warm. It finishes with a note on the selection and general medical care of divers.

The shape of the sea. Most people have a hazy idea of the shape of the sea (Fig. 1). Leaving a typical shore, the sea bed falls away gently, with a slope of about 1:50 until it is 200 to 300 metres deep. This shallow stretch is the Continental Shelf. It then angles more steeply (roughly 1:15), the Continental Slope, to descend to vast flat expanses of soft mud, known as the Abyssal Plains, which lie at depths of 3 to 6 kilometres. These are interrupted by occasional mountain peaks and deep chasms. One of the mountains is slightly taller than Mount Everest. The deepest point is just over 11 kilometres below the surface.

Various deep currents, arising from differences in water temperature and salinity, take regular courses across the Abyssal Plains, welling up the sides of the Continental Shelves as mineral-rich streams. These supply the vegetable life that exists in the sunlit upper zone. The animals that feed on these plants, or each other, become concentrated in these waters so that 80 per cent of the biological wealth of the sea lies in the top 0.2 km, mainly close to the Continental Shelves. Put together, these sites form an area equal to that of Africa, infinitely more fertile, and, as yet, unfarmed.

At the surface, regular tidal currents vary widely in velocity from point to point as they are accelerated or slowed down by features of the shore. They often exceed the speed at which a man can swim (Fig. 2a), so that it may only be practical to dive in slack water, i.e. for an hour or two each day. Similarly, waves are often sufficiently tall to prevent a diver being launched into the sea or recovered with safety (Fig. 2b). These surface phenomena rarely penetrate below 100 m or so, but tidal currents can be tunnelled along marine canyons, and springs of fresh water, or falls of cold ocean water, can carry divers in unexpected directions without them necessarily being aware that they are moving at all.

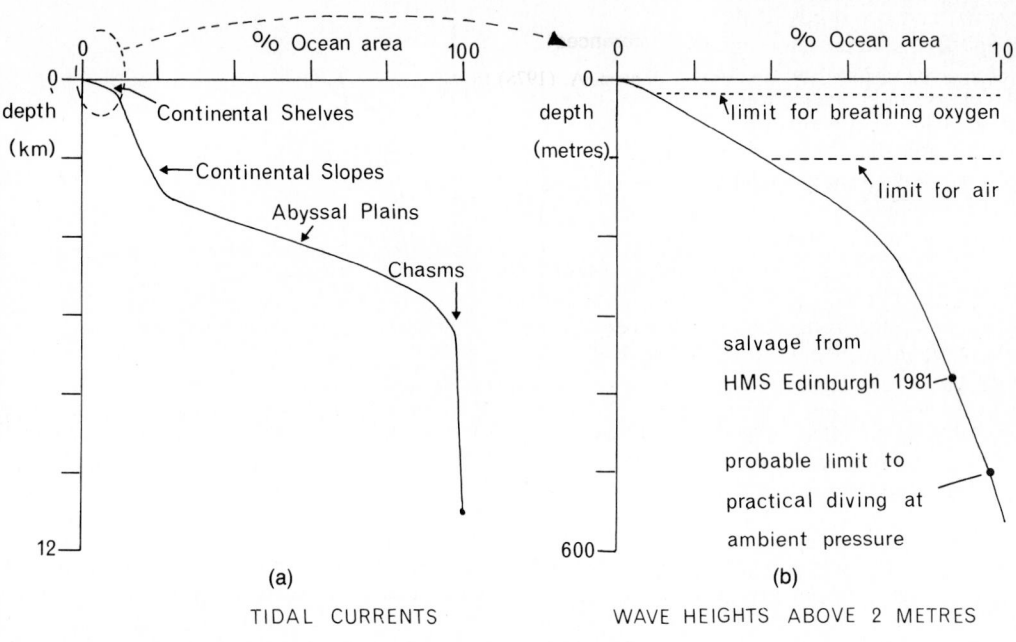

Fig. 1 (a) A cumulative depth versus area plot of the oceans. (b) a similar plot of the top 600 metres, including the Continental Shelves.

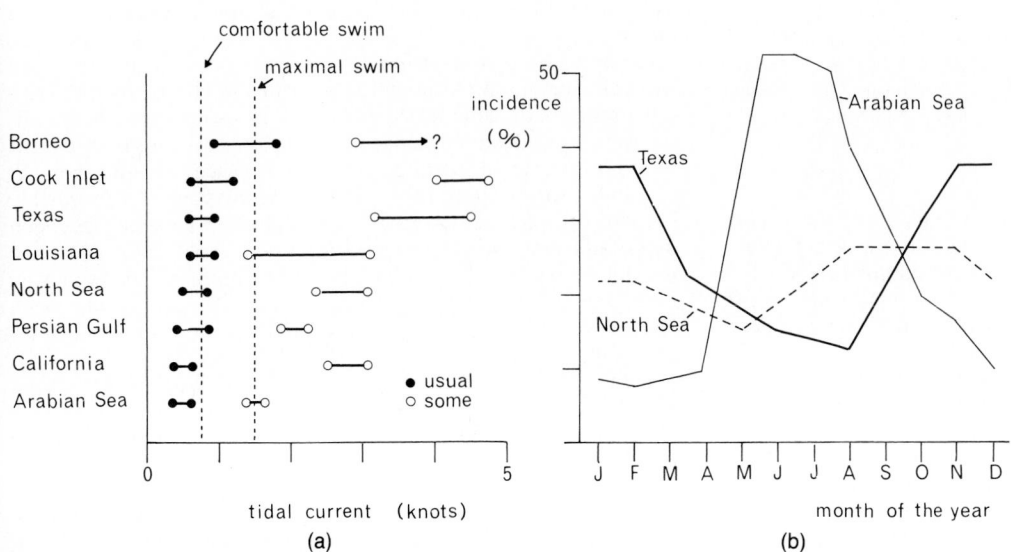

Fig. 2 (a) A plot of the usual and the not uncommonly seen tidal currents in eight diving sites around the world. (b) A plot of the percentage incidence of waves exceeding a height of 2 metres at different times of the year in three of the diving sites.

Vision

Most recreational diving takes place in clear warm waters at placid times of the year, but many tasks in professional diving, e.g. harbour work, hull inspections and repairs, pipe-line surveys, oil-rig work, and wreck salvage, occur throughout the year, alongside or beneath large obstructions, in waters where simply finding the task, let alone completing it properly, may be very demanding indeed.

There are many reasons why this should be so. During the middle of the day about 5 per cent of the light falling on the surface of the sea is reflected back to the sky, but, whenever the sun is lower, much more is reflected, so dawn arrives late and dusk comes early to the sea. The light that does penetrate the surface is quickly altered by absorption and scattering. On average, intensity halves with every one or two metres of descent. In consequence, even in very clear water, it is effectively 'night' below 80 metres. However, even in shallow water, e.g. in harbours, near estuaries, close to wrecks, and after storms, sea-water can be very turbid, blurring the boundaries of objects to such an extent that the diver may have to be within a foot or two of the objects to see them at all. In these circumstances, artificial illumination is often ineffective because of back-scattering.

Normally, some 65 dioptres of refracting power are needed to focus parallel rays of light on the retina, and two-thirds of this refraction occurs at the air–cornea interface. Underwater, this boundary is lost unless some form of gas-filled goggles or mask are worn. If they are worn, the additional glass–water boundary makes objects seem 30 per cent bigger and nearer than they actually are. This distortion is easily adjusted to but very often the margins of the goggles or mask restrict the visual fields severely giving the diver a blinkered, as well as blurred, view of his surroundings.

Hearing and blast injury

Underwater, localization of sound is poor because binaural cues disappear. They are lost because sounds are transmitted almost five times as fast and many times more efficiently through water than air. So there is very little alteration or delay as sound passes from ear to ear. Localization is also affected by echoes bouncing from the air–water interface above and the water–ground boundary below. The loss of air-conduction alone, raises auditory thresholds by 30–60 dB. The neoprene-foam hoods that keep the head warm raise them by a further 30 dB or so.

The superior transmission of sound in water also increases susceptibility to blast injury. This is important, even in civilian fields, because plastic explosives are often used to free propellers from shafts or to ease buried objects from marine concretions, and the sort of detonation that would leave a man unharmed at 5 metres range in air, would be sufficient to kill him at the same range under water. Damage is mainly due to abrupt decompression and recompression of the lungs, gut, and sinuses (see later). Gas-free tissues, such as the liver and spleen, are usually undamaged. The air-filled foam of some wet suits provides some protection

Dexterity and mobility

Except for the surface-waters of tropical seas, all of the oceans are too cold for men to stay long without insulation (Fig. 3). In air, men maintain body temperature at 37 °C with minimal effort when the air temperature is 18–24 °C, the zone of thermal neutrality. In water, this zone is higher and very narrow (35 to 35.5 °C). Loss of tactile discrimination and manual dexterity are major problems for divers working in cold water. In general, there is a steep loss of discrimination once finger-skin temperature drops below 8 °C, and there is a substantial loss of dexterity and grip-strength whenever the effective cold exposure of the forearm exceeds that of 20 °C water for 30 minutes. Re-examination of Fig. 3 indicates how easily such conditions are realized.

The most serious, and least treatable, problems of diving occur from working in a dense and viscous medium. Water is some 1300 times denser than air. Since it is virtually incompressible (the water at the deepest part of the ocean is 4 per cent denser than at the surface), ambient pressure rises linearly with depth. It does so, at very nearly 1 atmosphere for every 10 m descent. Thus at 10 metres depth, the surrounding pressure is 2 atm (one of water plus one of air), at 20 m it is 3 atm, and so on. Immersion in a fluid of this density makes the diver weightless and vertically unstable, it opposes any movement generating turbulent flow and exposes him to much higher pressures than on land. Since water is also many times more viscous than air, it is useless as a ventilating fluid and opposes any body motion generating streamline flow.

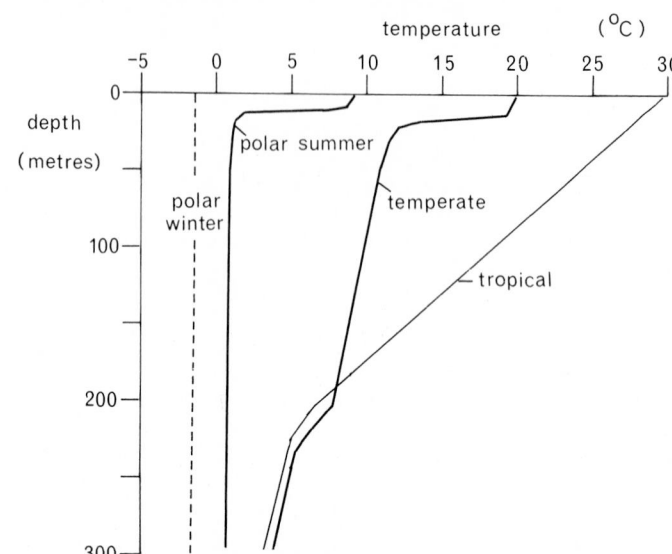

Fig. 3 Variations in sea temperature with site and depth. Note that water temperatures less than 20 °C are too cold for unclothed men to stay in for very long.

When a diver enters water his body becomes 'weightless' because the density of sea-water, blood, tissue-fluids, and the body as a whole, are very nearly the same. As a result, his tissues are rehung on the skeleton, and blood and other fluids are displaced upwards, some 500 ml entering the chest, distending the large veins and the right atrium. Stretch-receptors in the chest interpret this signal as an excess circulating volume and promote diuresis until the central distension is reduced to its normal value. When the man emerges from the water the normal hydrostatic gradient of body materials is unopposed and blood drops away from the chest, leaving the man hypovolaemic. Any negative pressure-breathing exaggerates this effect (see later).

Because the immersed body is weightless it can be displaced vertically with ease. Although this permits the diver to poise himself anywhere or examine the full height of a submerged rig at will, it is a great disadvantage, since he can no longer use his body weight to apply leverage or torque, or to stay in place when a current is running. More importantly, any vertical movement can quickly become uncontrolled because of the positive feedback between depth and buoyancy. The deeper a breath-hold diver goes, the heavier he becomes and the more rapidly he falls. The higher he rises, the lighter he becomes and the faster he ascends. Such changes should be seen in the context of the man's actual buoyancy and swimming power.

Although the rises of cardiac output and alveolar ventilation, with effort, are the same in air and water, much of the effort is dissipated in simply moving the limbs through the medium, making most tasks more tiring, and much less efficient below the surface than above (Fig. 4). The maximum sustained thrust that a swimmer can develop underwater is about 5 kg, which is just enough to propel him at about 1½ miles an hour. An opposing force of 5 kg,

CONSTANT SPEED

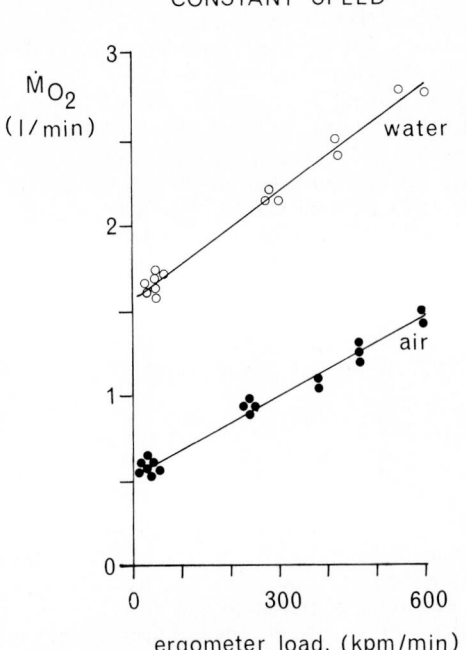

CONSTANT LOAD

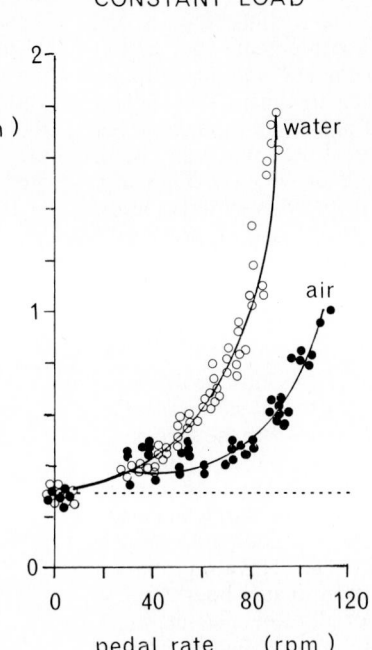

Fig. 4 A comparison of oxygen consumption ($\dot{M}_{O_2}$) when pedalling a cycle ergometer in air and underwater (a) at a constant speed (60 r.p.m.) and at a constant light load. Note the high cost of moving the limbs through water. Most people's aerobic capacity is about 2.5 litres O_2/min.

i.e. that weight on a string over a pully, would immobilize him. If a normally built man takes a full inspiration he is about 2.5 kg positively buoyant and so requires half of his maximum swim-power to descend. If he breathes out to residual volume he is about 2.4 kg negatively buoyant and needs half his maximum swim-power to ascend. Since the chest wall is a floppy structure that can only maintain a pressure-difference equivalent to 1 or 2 metres of sea water, the gas in the lungs is at virtually the same pressure as the water surrounding the chest. Thus a breath-hold diver leaving the surface with a full lung and diving 30 metres (4 atmospheres absolute) will compress his lung from total lung capacity to residual volume, forcing the man to use half his aerobic capacity to overcome positive buoyancy at the start of the dive and the same amount of effort to ascend. If he is wearing insulating clothing (e.g. a foam 'wet suit', normal buoyancy about 8 kg) the total changes in buoyancy are very close to maximum swimming capacity leaving little margin for controlling unexpected ascent or descent.

Mechanical effects of compression and decompression

When a breath-hold diver descends the gas in his lungs is compressed by the surrounding water, according to Boyle's law, as just instanced. On return to the surface the gas will re-expand to its original volume, with no risk of lung rupture. However, if a diver has access to fresh gas at any time after leaving the surface, he can fill his lungs with enough gas to burst them on ascent, unless they are adequately vented. The principles that determine whether the lung will rupture have been mentioned in detail elsewhere: the lung can be considered as a cluster of tubes and balloons with bursting pressure of about 75 mmHg (1 metre of sea-water) and time-constants of emptying that are normally close to 1 second. The latter may be grossly prolonged by injury, inhalation of water, or by disease. Divers are taught to exhale continuously whenever they ascend, and to ascend no faster than the bubbles they exhale. If people with healthy lungs ascend in this manner, the alveoli have time to empty sufficiently and the risk of lung rupture is very low. Occasionally, apparently healthy people do tear a lung during a normal ascent but they are found to have abnormal lungs subsequently.

Lung rupture usually occurs in divers breath-holding while making emergency ascents after losing their gas supply. Central tears of lung tissue lead to mediastinal emphysema. Peripheral tears cause

pneumothoraces. In both cases, but more commonly the former, gas may also enter the circulation as air emboli. Whether it is in the tissue, pleural space, or bloodstream, the escaped gas expands as the ascent continues, making matters worse. The victim usually notes dyspnoea, cough, of haemophysis during the ascent, or no more than a few minutes later. If the tear is central he may also note dysphasia, voice change, or a sense of fullness in the throat or behind the sternum. On examination there may be surgical emphysema of the neck and upper chest, subcutaneous crepitus, increased cardiac dullness, or cardiac crepitus. If a pneumothorax has developed it is often accompanied by one-sided pleuritic pain, diminished respiratory movement, deviation of the trachea and apex-beat, hyper-resonance, and distant breath sounds. If air embolism has occurred, there will be additional neurological signs. Patients with uncomplicated mediastinal and/or superficial emphysema are treated by giving them pure oxygen to breath, but they must never be positive-pressure ventilated. The oxygen accelerates bubble absorbtion by emptying the blood or inert gas so it is a more efficient sink for the gas in the bubble. After two or three days the emphysema will have subsided and the patient will be fit for release. Small pneumothoraces can be treated in the same way. If the pneumothorax is large it can be relieved in the ordinary way with a chest drain, however, if it is critically large the patient should be recompressed immediately to reduce its size. This is rarely necessary for uncomplicated pneumothoraces. The chest drain must be clamped on compression and must be exposed to continuous suction at depth and during recompression.

If there is *any* evidence of air embolus, or any doubt about the diagnosis, the patient should immediately be laid semi-prone, on his left side, with the head down and the buttocks up. He should be given oxygen, without positive-pressure ventilation, and be recompressed as soon as possible (details of recompression therapy are discussed below).

Lung rupture is the most worrying form of barotrauma (pressure damage) but others are more common. On descent, the diver may have difficulty in 'clearing his ears' because the mounting pressure on the outside of the drum is not balanced by an equal rise on the inner side, due to the valvular nature of the Eustachian tube. This can be very painful, and may lead to drum-rupture, but the strain on the drum usually resolves immediately on stopping the descent and ascending slightly. Sometimes the sinuses are affected on ascent or descent, in the same way. Pain on descent is always relieved by ascent. However, pain due to gas trapped in an obstructed space, gets worse on ascent. Sometimes blood that has filled a sinus, and partly clotted during descent, is expelled in this manner as the diver returns to the surface. Occasionally, an ethmoid sinus may rupture into the cranial cavity. Usually, no specific treatment is needed for these injuries, but the diver is laid-off diving until the cause has been established and he is fit to return. Pressure-injuries also occur if the gas pressure inside the goggles, mask, or helmet does not keep pace with that outside. Sometimes, reversed-ear injury occurs because on descent the soft foam wet-suit helmet prevents a matching build-up of pressure in the external auditory canal, and the drum blows outwards.

Inert-gas narcosis

Because the chest wall is a floppy structure, gas must be delivered to the diver at the same pressure as the water that surrounds him. This may be sent to him via an umbilical pipe from the surface, in which case it can flush through his helmet or face-mask continuously, which is wasteful of gas, but easily engineered, or it can supply a regulating valve that provides gas on demand only (surface-demand systems). Alternatively, the diver can take a self-contained underwater breathing apparatus (SCUBA) with him. This always feeds a demand regulator and rarely lasts for more than 1 hour. Professional divers often use a combination of all three systems, i.e. a surface-demand supply for routine use, with a helmet-flushing capability for occasional comfort or emergency use, and a small back-mounted gas supply ready in case the surface supply fails.

Nowadays demand-regulators and compensated outlet-valves are well-designed and there are few practical obstacles to providing the diver with gas at the right pressure. The composition of the gas to be breathed is a much more complex decision. Air can be breathed quite safely down to depths of 50 metres although tests of sophisticated cerebral function show there is already some impairment at 20 metres. Below 50 metres mental deterioration becomes increasingly obvious, manifested by such actions as the diver offering his mouthpiece to neighbouring fish.

This condition is described as nitrogen-narcosis or '*l'ivresse des profondeurs*'. It is a specific example of the more general condition of *inert gas narcosis* related to inhalation anaesthesia. An extension of the Meyer–Overton lipid solubiltity theory of anaesthesia supposes that the size or thickness of the nerve membrane, or some part of it, is dependent upon the size and number of gas molecules dissolved in it, and once the size or thickness of the membrane exceeds critical limits it cannot conduct an impulse. On descent breathing air, ambient and arterial nitrogen pressures rise, and more nitrogen dissolves in nerve membranes, making them thicker, until at a depth of about 50 metres, interference in neural transmission becomes obvious functionally. Replacing the nitrogen molecules with smaller and less numerous helium molecules allows the membrane to shrink to an acceptable size and the impairment of function regresses (cf. replacing nitrogen molecules by bulkier xenon molecules, which is sufficient to cause anaesthesia at sea level). As would be expected, these changes in function develop within a few minutes and are rapidly reversible, because they depend purely on the process of passive chemical solution.

If men breath an oxygen–helium mix, rather than air, they can descend to the lowermost parts of the Continental Shelves (730 m) without narcosis. Thus, nitrogen narcosis is a wholly preventable hazard in diving which if it occurs by accident can be completely reversed within minutes, by ascent, and therefore needs no treatment. Unfortunately, helium is an expensive gas and there is an understandable reluctance for diving operators to use it. Medical advisers must oppose this and emphasize that it is dangerous for men to breath air below a depth of 50 metres or so.

High-pressure nervous syndrome

At great depths, breathing oxygen ± helium mixtures, men show various neurological disturbances which are apparently not narcotic but are due to the direct effect of pressures on nerve tissues. This is thought to be so because very similar states can be induced in animals who are ventilated on fluorocarbon liquids containing normal sea-level quantities of oxygen and nitrogen or helium. It is also known that many organic and inorganic processes are disturbed by the applications of high barometric pressures *in vitro*. The high pressures are believed to alter the natural aggregations of water molecules to increase the ionization of salts, oppose ionic bonding, liquify gels, and cause various enzymes to fail. It appears to be the major obstacle to ambient-pressure diving much below the edges of the Continental Shelves. At present, men are able to make experimental dives to about 700 metres. Various drugs have been investigated as modifiers of the syndrome, but its fundamental cause and protean manifestations suggest this depth will be close to the absolute limit to ambient-pressure diving.

Oxygen toxicity

The hazards of inert-gas narcosis, and of decompression sickness (see below) could be avoided completely if people breathed pure oxygen when they dived. Unfortunately it becomes toxic to the lungs when the alveolar oxygen pressure exceeds half an atmosphere (5 metres of sea water) and it becomes toxic to the nervous system when the alveolar, and the arterial, oxygen pressure exceed 2 atmospheres (10 metres of sea water). These effects are due to complex chemical interactions, rather than physical solution, and so take time to develop and reverse.

As mentioned elsewhere respired oxygen is handled by a large number of enzymes and used in very many ways. Some, such as the production and destruction of neurotransmitters and the synthesis of some steroid hormones, are critical. Increasing the amount of oxygen in simple solution not only affects the balance of some of these processes but also increases the risk of randomly forming the destructive superoxide ion. So, high-pressure oxygen affects body tissues in many ways.

It has two principal actions on the lung. Firstly, it promotes simple absorbtion atelectasis by replacing the relatively insoluble nitrogen in alveolar spaces. As their servant airways shut off due to transient obstructions, pulmonary blood flow rapidly removes the highly soluble oxygen and CO_2 causing the alveolar spaces to collapse, leading to linear regions of atelectasis that are most obvious in the well-perfused and more readily collapsed basal regions of the lung. Paradoxically, blood leaving the lung is then hypoxic due to admixture with blood perfusing the collapsed spaces.

Secondly, oxygen damages the lung by irritating its endothelial and epithelial surfaces. Some people suggest this is due to the extrapulmonary generation of a noxious agent because the endothelial damage appears first, but it is much more likely to be a direct action of alveolar oxygen on these surfaces. At first there is an exudation of fluid and proliferation of macrophages and an interference with surfactant production. This damage is reversible. If the exposure is prolonged, fibrosis occurs and the lung is permanently scarred.

The time taken for symptoms to appear depends upon the dose. It varies from several hours at half an atmosphere Po_2 to a few hours at 2 atmospheres. Above that pressure, the neurological sequelae overshadow the pulmonary damage that still occurs (Fig. 5).

Oxygen interferes with nervous tissue in a manner that is not yet understood, perhaps because it disrupts many processes rather than one. It manifests itself by epileptiform convulsions that are sometimes, but not always, preceded by aura such as twitching of the face and hands. Any convulsion underwater is potentially fatal and must be avoided. There is a safe latent period, during which oxygen can be breathed without any detectable harm to the CNS. This time is inversely proportional to depth (i.e. to Po_2). However, the time and threshold level can vary widely in the same individual from day to day. CO_2 retention and exertion lower the threshold and shorten the latent period. Like nitrogen narcosis, oxygen toxicity is a preventable hazard in diving. Divers should not breathe oxygen at

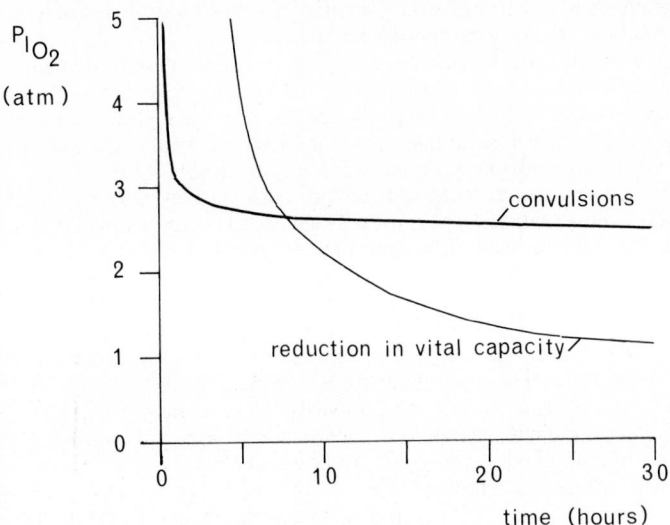

Fig. 5 The pulmonary and CNS O_2-toxicity versus time curves that are commonly observed (constructed from the data of many workers).

partial pressures greater than two atmospheres except under observation in the decompression chamber. Diving mixtures that are to be breathed for several hours should maintain inspired Po_2 between 0.5 and 1.0 atmospheres. Those that are to be breathed for longer periods should maintain inspired Po_2 between 0.2 and 0.5 atmospheres.

Decompression sickness

Oxygen toxicity, nitrogen narcosis, and the high-pressure nervous syndrome set depth-limits to diving of 10, 50, and 500 metres respectively, and so are physicochemical obstacles to *invading* the sea. By contrast, the major medical hazard to diving, decompression sickness, is a physicochemical obstacle on *returning* from the sea. It occurs because, during any dive, extra inert gas, usually nitrogen or helium, goes into passive solution in the body. On ascent, as the ambient pressure falls, this gas can come out of solution in an uncontrolled way, forming bubbles in the circulation and within tissues. As the ascent continues, these bubbles increase in size and number, blocking blood vessels, and distorting or rupturing cells. On re-descent the bubbles contract and are eventually resorbed. If the first or the subsequent ascent is slow enough, few if any bubbles are formed, the extra gas diffuses into the bloodstream and out of the lungs easily, and the diver reaches the surface unharmed.

Experiments by Haldane at the turn of the century, which have been confirmed subsequently many times, suggest bubble formation occurs whenever ambient pressure falls below half the total pressure of inert gas in solution. It follows that it is normally safe to ascend from dives to 10 metres or less, without hesitation, however long they have endured, and to ascend without stopping, from any deeper dive which has been too brief to take this critical mass of gas on board. For any other dive, return to the surface must be delayed so the ratio of pressure of gas remaining in solution: ambient pressure, never exceeds the critical value of 2.

A vast amount of experimental work has been done to determine the safe limits to 'no-stop' diving and the depth–time profiles that have to be followed on returning to the surface after any longer dive. The time-limiting curve for 'no-stop' diving is shown in Fig. 6. It represents the time taken to accumulate 2 atmospheres of dissolved gas in the tissues at the depths shown. The rate of gas accumulation in tissues is determined by the ratio of the solubility of the gas in that tissue to the speed of its blood flow. Because the tissues vary widely in these respects, the body behaves as if it were made up of a series of compartments, the 'fast' ones having short time-constants of inert gas uptake, and the 'slow' ones having long

time-constants. The fast tissues such as working muscle dominate the time course of safe short dives. The slow tissues such as body fat determine the safe ascent rate from long dives. Knowledge of safe practice is tabulated in a series of lengthy decompression schedules, that vary somewhat from one country to another, and are to be found in any textbook of diving medicine. After long (saturation) dives, the ascent is very slow and can take several days.

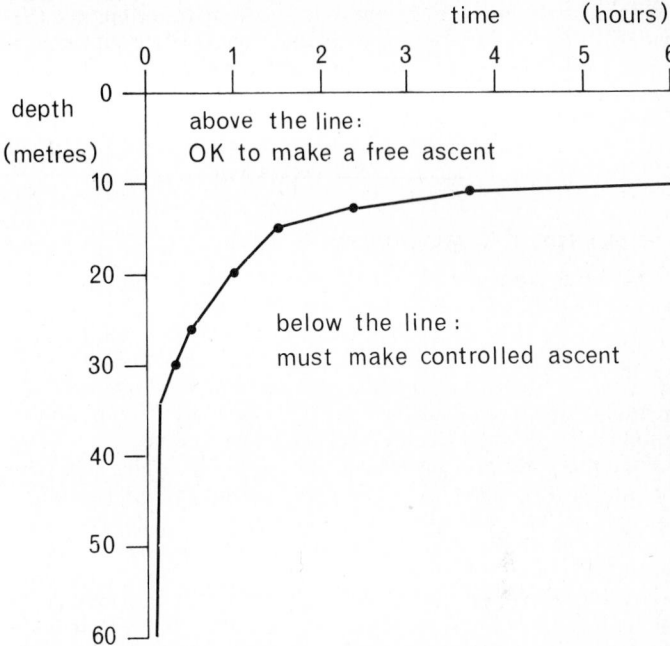

Fig. 6 The 'no-stop' diving curve which determines whether a dive has been shallow and brief enough for the diver to make a free ascent to the surface.

After relatively brief, shallow descents, divers can return to the surface slowly, stopping for a few minutes at scheduled depths. To do this they normally ascend up a marked shot-line. It is not practical or safe to ascend from deeper or longer dives in this manner so a submersible recompression chamber is sent to the bottom to collect the diver and return him to the surface in warmth and comfort, or the divers make a limited number of stops in the water and then quickly ascend to the surface and immediately enter a deck-mounted chamber to be recompressed and then decompressed slowly and safely. Usually they are recompressed to 20 metres and then given oxygen to breathe intermittently, to accelerate inert-gas excretion.

About 1 per cent of dives conducted to authorized schedules, and many badly conducted dives, lead to decompression sickness. This can take two forms, skin irritation or limb pain only (type 1 'bends'), or any other serious manifestation (type 2 'bends'). Skin irritation and mottling alone is treated by oxygen inhalation at the surface and does not require recompression. It is the mildest form of decompression sickness. All other cases should be recompressed as soon as possible. This is the only effective treatment. The object is to reduce the size of existing bubbles and prevent the formation of new ones, before irreversible infarction and oedema have occurred.

About half of all cases involve the CNS, most often the lower cervical, the thoracic or the upper lumber segments of the spinal cord. Visual disturbances and other cerebral signs are seen often also. Many others involve limb pain, commonly of the shoulders or elbows in divers and of the knees and hips in tunnel workers. A minority of victims experience sudden chest pain, dyspnoea, and cough, believed to be due to bubbles in the pulmonary circulation. Symptoms appear minutes to hours after the end of a dive. Some of them are due to bubble formation directly—others are believed to be secondary to clumping of red cells.

If the symptoms are of limb pain only, the patients are recompressed to 20 metres on oxygen. Providing the pain disappears within 10 minutes of recompression, they are then decompressed over a period of 2¼ hours. If the pain persists, the decompression time is doubled. If there is any evidence of CNS or chest involvement, at the time of initial diagnosis or subsequently, the patient is immediately put semi-prone on the left side, with the buttocks raised, recompressed to 20 metres on oxygen and decompressed over at least 4½ hours. Sometimes it is necessary to recompress the patient briefly to 50 metres or so to relieve persistent symptoms or signs. Some people give low molecular weight dextran to combat the clumping of red cells and heparin to reduce any lipaemia from tissue disruption. It is important to emphasize that the only effective treatment is recompression, and that this may still be beneficial even if it can not be achieved for several hours.

The problem of keeping warm

The general problems of survival in cold water are described on pages 6.54–55. However, some difficulties are peculiar to divers. They insulate themselves in one of three ways: by cramming as much clothing as possible beneath a supposedly impermeable layer of rubber or canvas sealed at the neck and wrists (a 'dry' suit); by wearing an open-cell foam 'wet' suit that contains air at the surface but immobilizes water freely percolating in; or by wearing a closed-cell suit that consists of gas-filled plastic bubbles. All three suits rely on some air for insulation and thus are buoyant and compressible. Typically a wet suit will provide some 8 kg of buoyancy—i.e. contain some 8 litres of air. As the diver descends, this gas compresses, making him heavier and colder. The loss of insulation is very noticeable. At depths greater than 50 metres it is compounded by the need to breath helium, which has a high thermal conductivity especially when it is compressed. In fact, the conductivity of helium is so high that gas-filled habitats for saturation diving have to be kept at temperatures close to 30 °C to achieve thermal neutrality. When divers emerge from the habitat they lose heat rapidly through the respiratory tract and through the 'air' filled insulation which now contains helium. It is often necessary to provide them with personal heating systems (e.g. piped hot water).

Atmospheric pressure diving

In classical diving, men invade the sea breathing gas at ambient pressures which rise linearly with depth. These men are able to deploy most of their sensory and motor skills but are very seriously limited by cold and the chemical consequences of breathing gases at high pressures. Two of these, oxygen toxicity and inert-gas narcosis, restrict the choice of breathing mixtures. A third, decompression sickness, greatly reduces the maximum permissible rate of ascent. Divers cannot be launched or recovered when wave-heights exceed a few feet, are unable to swim against currents greater than 1½ knots and are usually too cold to work for longer than 1½ hours. The long times spent in controlled ascent cannot usually be employed profitably, but detain expensive equipment, sometimes in the face of worsening weather. At present, it is difficult to imagine that classical divers will be able to descend much lower than 500 metres. This gives them access to the whole of the Continental Shelves but not to the Continental Slopes or the Abyssal Plains beyond.

There are three other ways in which one can explore the sea.

Firstly and most safely, one can send down unmanned sensors and manipulators. Almost all of our present knowledge has been obtained in this way. Many of the exploratory devices are dropped at one point as spot samplers to measure local values of particular variables which they record and transmit from the bottom or on return to the surface. Others can be towed with a fair degree of vertical and lateral control relaying similar information along a cable. Some can be envoyed remotely under sonar or an internally programmed control, storing or transmitting information as they go. As investment pressure rises, more of these will be fitted with manipulators to perform specific tasks.

Unmanned devices do not imperil human life, may be designed to work without a bulky pressure protection, should be able to move freely to and from great depths, and have the important advantage that in need they can be instructed to wait at the bottom indefinitely until surface conditions are favourable for their recovery. Their serious disadvantages are cost, lack of dexterity, and inflexibility of mission purpose. (To get these in perspective, it may be helpful to consider as a parallel the problems of exploring and redeveloping a dry continent, if it could only be done with towed or remote robots operated from night-flying helicopters.) There are bound to be considerable technical improvements in manipulators, sensors, power sources, and programme controls. Similarly more marine engineering and mining plants will be designed to be built and maintained by telechiric devices. Nevertheless, at present, no-one can envisage a time when submarine robots with anything like human capabilities could be constructed for sums less than several thousand pounds.

Secondly, men can enter the sea in pressure resistant vessels that can be towed, powered via a cable, or moved under their own steam. All of the present submersibles are fitted with porthole transparencies, most have additional sensors and some have primitive manipulators. They can search large areas and some can perform simple tasks. Their present disadvantages are weight, restricted vision and manoeuvreability, bulk, poor manipulator performance, limited operability (most cannot be launched or recovered when wave heights exceed 3–4 feet), high capital and operating costs, and the need for a large and specially equipped surface support vessel.

Thirdly, men can invade the sea in armoured diving suits, i.e. a relatively cheap weightless but warm second skin capable of resisting high ambient pressures but putting less restriction on touch, vision, and dexterity than the larger devices. These leave the diver with many of his sensorimotor skills and gives him vertical freedom, greater depth range, and very reduced ascent times.

Although such suits were tried and found wanting in the 1930s, they are now easier to make and the need for them has risen greatly. At present they have a working depth limit of about 500 metres and are able to ascend and descend freely. The inhabitant remains dry and warm, breathing air at atmospheric pressure throughout. When he surfaces, someone else can descend immediately using the same suit. It is likely that, in the future, much deep-sea diving will be conducted in this way.

The selection and medical care of divers

Divers have a physically demanding job and often must work in sites remote from any medical aid. They must have a high exercise tolerance and be free of any active or latent condition that could erupt while they were away from medical help. In addition, specifically, they must not have any condition that could imperil their own lives or those of their would-be rescuers when they are underwater.

In Britain all divers have to pass an annual medical examination conducted by a doctor competent in diving medicine. If the diver is found to be unfit to dive and disagrees with the decision of the examiner he has the right of appeal to an independent tribunal set up by the Health and Safety Executive. The codes of safe diving practice have been summarized recently in the British 'Health and Safety—Diving Operations at Work Regulations' which took effect in July 1981. These regulations have been nationally and internationally accepted.

In principle, all divers are expected to be physically able and mentally stable people, free of conditions such as epilepsy and ill-controlled diabetes or asthma. They should not be addicted to alcohol or any other drug and they should not have a history, or any other evidence, of obstructive lung disease, ruptured ear-drums, or aural surgery. Divers who are generally fit to dive should not be allowed to do so when they have chest, upper airway or ear infections, or when they are overweight (since obesity predisposes to decompression sickness). Neither should they dive while taking any medication that could impair their ability to think clearly or orientate themselves in space correctly.

References

Bennet, P. B. and Elliott, D. H. (1975). *The Physiology and medicine of diving and compressed air work.* Baillière Tindall, London.
Elliott, D. H. (1981). Underwater physiology. In *The principles and practice of human physiology* (ed. O. G. Edholm and J. S. Weiner) p. 309. Academic Press, London.
Kooyman, G. L., Castellini, M. A., and Davis, R. W. (1981). Physiology of diving in marine mammals. *A. Rev. Physiol.* **43**, 343.
Shilling, C. W., Werts, M. F., and Schandelmeier, N. R. (1976). *The underwater handbook.* Wiley, London.
Statutory Instrument 1981 No. 399. Health and Safety Diving Operations at Work Regulations 1981. HMSO. London.
Strauss, R. H. (1976). *Diving medicine.* Grune and Stratton, London.

ELECTRIC SHOCK AND LIGHTNING

B. A. Pruitt, Jr and A. D. Mason, Jr

Electric injury is a phenomenon of modern society. Its frequency, though not precisely known, roughly parallels the per capita use of electric power. In burn centres, the reported frequency of admission for electric injury ranges from 2 to 8 per cent of total admissions, a variation which depends partly upon whether patients with flame injury due to electric ignition of clothing, with minimal electric injury *per se*, are included or excluded.

Pathophysiology of electric injury. The accidental insertion of part of a living body into an electric circuit may produce injury in two ways. The first, which has been called electric shock, may occur at low or high voltage while the second, thermal injury, occurs principally with higher voltage.

The known determinants of electric injury include voltage, amperage, type of current, frequency of alternating current, duration of current passage, physical size and configuration of the part involved, and specific points of contact. Unfortunately, the frequencies which are ideal for electric power transmission are within the most dangerous part of the frequency spectrum for the production of both electric shock and thermal injury. Lightning injury is most easily viewed as contact with a direct current source at very high voltage and amperage and does not differ in principle from other forms of electric injury.

Electric shock produces disruption of cyclic bio-electric rhythms in affected organs, e.g. ventricular fibrillation; or induces membrane depolarization, e.g. muscular contraction. The power required to produce such effects is determined by the nature of the current involved and by the precise path of current through the body; the effects are strongly dependent upon the contact site as well as upon the voltage, power, and frequency of the source.

Thermal injury may be induced either by electric arcing outside the body or by power dissipation in tissue. High voltage electric arcs develop very high temperatures which are directly injurious to skin and may cause more extensive thermal injury by producing ignition of clothing. Power dissipation in any element of an electric circuit is determined by the voltage gradient (*V*) and current flow (*I*) within that element:

$$I = V/R \text{ (Ohm's Law)}$$
$$P = VI = V^2/R = I^2R$$

When part of the body becomes included in a circuit, power dissipation within the part produces heat and an increase in temperature. Skin exhibits moderate resistance, especially when dry, but like any insulator, breaks down at sufficient voltage gradient. When this occurs at a contact point, current density and power dissipation

reach high levels, producing severe local injury (Fig. 1). In the deeper tissues, current flow is not isotropic, because individual tissues differ in resistance; except for bone, which has relatively high resistance, these differences are not great. For any specific voltage gradient, power dissipation is greater in tissues of lower resistance, and it is a common clinical observation that deep tissues having low resistance are more susceptible to electric injury than those having high resistance. The heat generated within any particular tissue is not confined to that tissue; it is, instead, distributed within the affected part according to the laws of heat flow. Thus the low resistance soft tissues, contained between an inner core of high resistance bone and an outer shell of high resistance skin, behave as a nearly isotropic volume electric conductor and in any cross section are nearly uniformly heated by the passage of current. Soft tissue heating parallels current density, which may be reasonably approximated as an inverse function of the square of the radius of the body segment in question. In such a system, heat production per unit volume and rate of temperature increase are greatest in segments of small diameter. The actual temperature achieved is, in turn, a complex function whose principal determinants are current density and the duration of current passage.

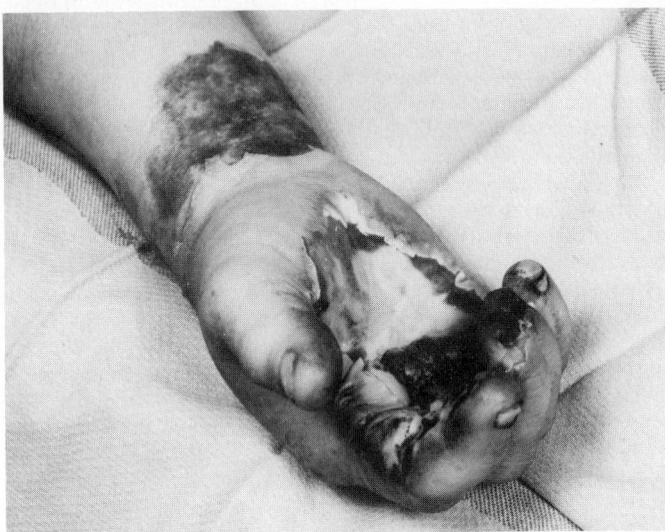

Fig. 1 The right hand of this patient illustrates charring at a high voltage contact site on the palm, a flexion deformity of digits indicative of severe deep tissue injury, and a typical skin injury at the site of the wrist-watch band.

Thermal injury to tissue is a function not only of temperature but also of duration of exposure to that temperature. At the threshold for injury, which probably lies between 45–50 °C, injury occurs when exposure is of the order of 100 seconds; at higher temperatures the requisite time decreases exponentially. A block of tissue heated in such a way as to make its temperature uniform throughout and then exposed to a cooler environment cools more rapidly at its periphery than at its core. This suggests that central segments of body parts sustain longer thermal exposure times and are more liable to injury following contact with a source of electric power; the studies of Hunt *et al.* appear to verify this expectation. Those studies also suggest that duration of current flow is, in a sense, self-limiting, since desiccation and carbonization of the points of contact greatly increase the resistance at those points and effectively interrupt current flow at a time inversely proportional to voltage.

Following such deep tissue injury, occlusion of small nutrient vessels occurs rapidly and tissue ischaemia ensues. In such areas, the patency of larger vessels is often maintained, and the observation of bleeding at the time of early debridement does not necessarily define vascular integrity.

These pathophysiological elements allow certain predictions about electric injury.

1. Maximal tissue destruction may be expected at points of arcing or of maximal current density, i.e. at contact points and in segments of small diameter.

2. Extremities are more liable to injury than the trunk, and the distal portions of extremities are more vulnerable than the proximal because of current density relationships.

3. Low resistance soft tissues are most liable to thermal injury by power dissipation; one may expect injured muscle to underlie intact skin.

4. Core tissues in the current path are more liable to injury than more peripheral tissues; one may anticipate the occurrence of injured periosseous muscle overlain by uninjured muscle.

5. The true extent of injury is unlikely to be well correlated with the extent of cutaneous burn.

Diagnosis and treatment. These physiological characteristics of high voltage electric injury are responsible for the differences in clinical presentation and treatment needs between patients sustaining such injury and patients sustaining conventional thermal injury. Significant differences include a high occurrence rate of cardiopulmonary arrest, greater susceptibility to acute renal failure, frequent need for fasciotomy and early debridement of damaged subfascial tissues, and the occurrence of organ dysfunction of delayed onset.

Cardiopulmonary arrest is much more common in the immediate post-injury period in patients with high voltage electric or lightning injury than in patients with conventional burns. The arrest may be due to either asystole or fibrillation and must be treated by immediate cardiopulmonary resuscitation. Cardiac arrhythmias can also occur following resuscitation, and patients with such injuries should undergo ECG monitoring for at least 48 hours following injury even in the absence of arrhythmias, and for 48 hours beyond the last electrocardiographic evidence of dysrhythmias if such occur. Hyperkalaemia, which may occur as a consequence of massive tissue destruction, is yet another reason for early post-injury electrocardiographic monitoring in patients with high voltage electric injury, since the serum potassium concentration may reach levels which affect the cardiac conduction system. Hyperkalaemia, depending upon its severity and persistance, should be treated by administration of hypertonic glucose combined with insulin and calcium gluceptate, administration of an ion exchange resin, or performance of haemodialysis.

Two factors conspire to increase the incidence of acute renal failure in patients with high voltage electric injury. Fluid needs may be underestimated as a result of there being little cutaneous injury, coupled with extensive but inapparent deep tissue injury. Accordingly, inadequate volumes of resuscitation fluids may be administered so that oliguria results. Moreover, myoglobin may be liberated from injured muscle and may precipitate in the renal tubules in the presence of oliguria. Resuscitation fluids should, accordingly, be infused in sufficient volume to obtain a 75–100 ml hourly urinary output in patients who exhibit elevated levels of urinary haemochromogens. If oliguria persists or the haemochromogen level does not promptly diminish despite otherwise adequate resuscitation, a diuretic should be administered to prevent the development of acute renal failure. Although some clinicians advocate the use of a loop diuretic, we prefer the use of mannitol as an osmotic diuretic and administer 12.5 g (one ampule) in each litre of intravenous fluid given until the pigment has cleared from the urine. It is important to remember that diuretic administration invalidates the hourly urinary output as a reliable guide to the adequacy of resuscitation; under these conditions one must rely upon other haemodynamic indices to assess the adequacy of resuscitation.

If the electric current has caused injury to tissues beneath the investing fascia of a limb, sufficient oedema may be produced in a muscle compartment to impair nutrient blood flow further or interrupt flow to distal unburned tissue. Fasciotomy is required in such a situation (Fig. 2) to prevent further ischaemic damage of unburned tissue by relieving intracompartmental pressure and improving nutrient blood flow. The clinical signs indicating a need for fas-

ciotomy include stony hardness of muscle compartments upon palpation, cyanosis of distal unburned skin, impaired capillary refilling of distal unburned skin or nail beds, and absent or diminished pulsatile flow in distal vessels as assessed by ultrasonic flowmeter examination. Although direct intracompartmental pressure measurements have been used in other types of patients to determine the need for fasciotomy, the risk of infection secondary to placing the pressure measurement cannula in burned tissue is great and prevents the use of such devices in the burn patient. If the indications are present, fasciotomy should be performed under general anaesthesia as soon as resuscitation has restored haemodynamic stability.

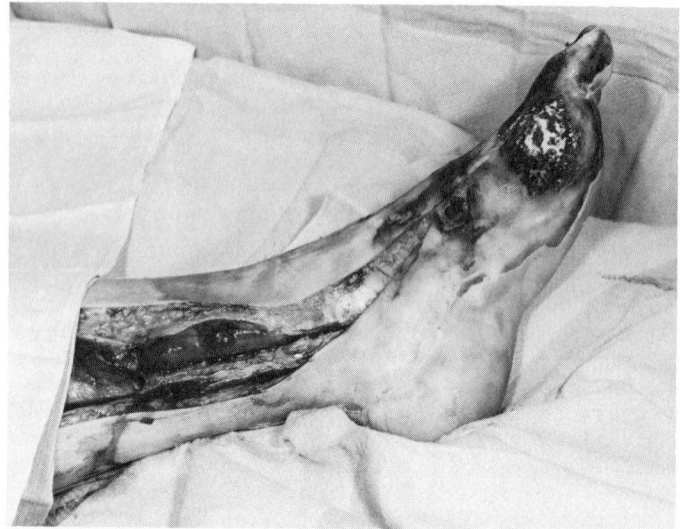

Fig. 2 Note severe tissue injury at the level of first metacarpophalangeal joint contact point. Fasciotomy revealed ischaemic oedematous muscle which is seen bulging above the cut edge of the fascia. Above-knee amputation was required in this patient because of the extent of muscle damage.

If significant deep tissue injury is suggested by clinical signs but large vessel pulses are intact, arteriography may be helpful in determining the need for operative debridement. Arteriographic evidence of large vessel occlusion secondary to thrombosis may merely confirm clinical findings, but when the arteriogram is performed in the immediate post-injury period, luminal narrowing, irregularity, or 'beading' may be observed in severely injured vessels which will subsequently be occluded by thrombosis. Regional muscle injury of variable extent may be indicated by a decrease in the density or 'pruning' of muscular nutrient vessels in a limb, and the identification of such changes helps define the level of amputation which is required to remove muscle which is irreversibly damaged in the absence of other clinical signs of such injury. Some investigators have used a ^{133}Xenon wash-out technique or technetium ^{99}Tc^m pyrophosphate scanning to assess muscle viability following electric injury. Muscle blood flow of less than 1 ml per minute per 100 g of tissue as measured by the ^{133}Xenon wash-out technique has been taken to indicate non-viable muscle. Both the absence of technetium uptake, interpreted as reflecting avascularity, and increased uptake, interpreted as indicating impairment of blood flow, are considered positive indications for excision of muscle. But since these diagnostic procedures have been evaluated in such a small number of patients their reliability, accuracy, and clinical usefulness are not yet established. Arteriography, ^{133}Xenon wash-out studies, and technetium ^{99}Tc^m pyrophosphate muscle scanning should only be carried out when resuscitation has averted or corrected hypovolaemia and hypotension.

Exploration of tissues damaged by high voltage electrical injury should be carried out under general anaesthesia as soon as the patient is haemodynamically stable. The affected muscle is thoroughly explored, bearing in mind that non-viable deep periosseous muscle can be present beneath more superficial viable muscle. All necrotic tissue is debrided to reduce the risk of infection and to remove a source of potassium contributing to post-injury hyperkalaemia. Destruction of nerves, tendons, and vessels, and muscle necrosis so extensive as to render a limb useless are indications for amputation, which is frequently required in patients with high voltage electric injury (Table 1). Oedema of the pectoral muscles in such patients with upper limb injury suggests the need for exploration of that area and excision of any non-viable muscle found. All wounds are packed and left open, and are re-examined 24–48 hours later, when any residual necrotic tissue is debrided, the wound again packed and left open, and the patient scheduled for further re-exploration 48–72 hours later. Since the morphological changes used as an index of cell damage due to high voltage electricity are seldom evident within 24 hours following injury, frozen section microscopy is generally of little help if operation is carried out during the first day after injury.

Table 1 Amputations required in 28 patients with electrical injury of the upper limb

Level of amputation	Number of amputations	Mean post-burn time of amputation (days)
Shoulder disarticulation	5	2
Above elbow	6	6
Below elbow	9	8
Wrist	5	19
Digit	8	21

In patients whose injuries are confined to skin and subcutaneous tissue, and those with full-thickness burns due to electrical ignition of clothing, bacterial control is best achieved by the use of Sulphamylon burn cream. The active ingredient, mafenide acetate, can diffuse into the non-viable tissue in effective concentrations.

Other injuries. The physical characteristics of electrical injury make visceral damage uncommon, but intestinal perforation, focal necrosis of gall bladder or pancreas, and direct liver injury have been reported. In the case of at least one patient with high voltage electric injury of the liver, hepatic damage was associated with a coagulopathy. In one series, three-quarters of patients with high voltage electric injury developed symptoms of gastrointestinal dysfunction within 12 to 18 months of the injury, and 13 of 45 patients developed cholelithiasis within two years.

Neurological abnormalities indicating either peripheral nerve or spinal cord injury may be evident immediately after injury or may be delayed. A complete neurological examination must be performed on admission and at defined intervals thereafter in order to detect these abnormalities. Motor nerves are more commonly affected than sensory nerves. If peripheral nerve damage is apparent immediately after injury, recovery is rare. Delayed neuropathies may involve nerves far removed from the points of electrical contact and may occur as part of a polyneuritic syndrome with highly variable recovery of function. Immediate post-injury spinal cord deficits are considered to reflect direct neuronal injury, but return of function is more common than in the case of spinal cord deficits of delayed onset, which tend to be permanent. The latter include localized nerve deficits with signs of ascending paralysis, transverse myelitis, an amyotrophic lateral sclerosis-like syndrome, and hemiplegia and quadriplegia.

Significant haemorrhage and even exsanguination have been reported to occur from large blood vessels in patients with high voltage electric injury. Although this complication has been attributed to an 'arteritis' caused by the electric injury *per se*, our experience suggests that it is usually the result of inadequate initial debridement or exposure of the vessel following debridement leading to desiccation and necrosis of the vessel wall.

Tetanic contractions of the paraspinous muscles due to the electric injury may produce compression fractures of the vertebral bodies as in patients with tetanus and those receiving electro-convulsive therapy. Vertebral injuries and long bone fractures are not uncommon in linemen who fall from a height following electric shock. Radiographs should be obtained as indicated by clinical signs and symptoms to exclude such fractures.

Cataracts may occur in any patient who has sustained high voltage electric injury but particularly those when the contact point is the head or neck (Fig. 3). Such cataracts may form during the initial hospital period or may develop as late as three or more years after the injury. An ophthalmological examination should be obtained prior to discharge from the hospital, and the patient should be informed of the possibility of such sequelae.

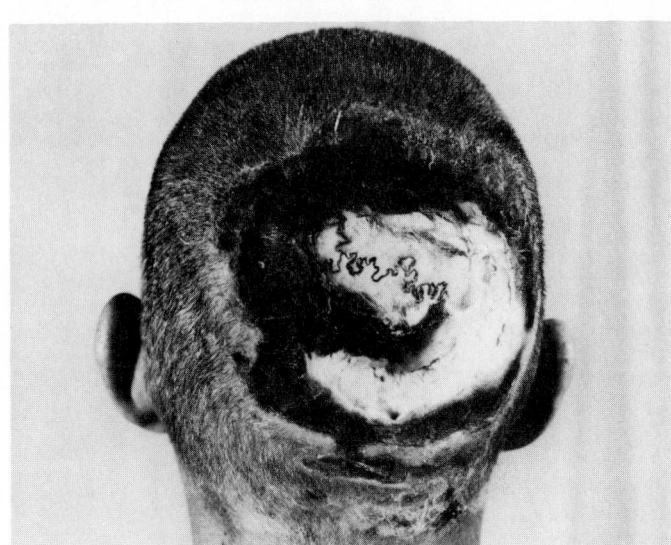

Fig. 3 Contact with a high voltage source produced extensive full-thickness destruction of scalp and calvarium in this patient. Note charred scalp at the margin of the defect and an exposed cranial suture line. The patient slowly regained consciousness, and no long-term neurological sequelae occurred. Bone grafting was needed to repair the calvarial defect, several months after the defect was initially closed by split-thickness skin grafting. Bilateral cataracts developed after discharge from hospital.

Lightning injury. Cardiopulmonary arrest is particularly common in patients who have been struck by lightning and immediate cardiopulmonary resuscitation is life-saving in such patients. Patients who have been reported to be without signs of life for 15 or more minutes after being struck have recovered, so cardiopulmonary resuscitation must be instituted when such patients are received in the emergency room. Although a few patients struck by lightning may later develop acute myocardial damage, persistent or recurrent ECG abnormalities are infrequent.

Neurological sequelae are common: they range from coma to isolated nerve deficits and even lower limb paraplegia. These abnormalities commonly resolve within hours or days.

The cutaneous burns present in patients with lightning injury are characteristically superficial and often exhibit a branching, spidery, or 'splashed-on' appearance. Myoglobinuria in such patients is surprisingly uncommon in view of the current flow which occurs during lightning injury. Adequate resuscitation will prevent vasoconstriction and mottling of the skin, which were previously considered to be changes uniquely characteristic of lightning injury. Today, two-thirds of patients who have sustained lightning injuries survive as a result of prompt cardiopulmonary resuscitation and treatment of the other pathophysiological consequences.

References

Apfelberg, D. B., Masters, F. W., and Robinson, D. W. (1974). Pathophysiology and treatment of lightning injuries. *J. Trauma* **14**, 453.
Baxter, C. R. (1970). Present concepts in the management of major electrical injury. *Surg. Clin. N. Am.* **50**, 1401.

Burke, J. F., Quinby, W. C., Jr, Bondoc, C., McLaughlin, E., and Trel-stad, R. L. (1977). Patterns of high tension electrical injury in children and adolescents and their management. *Am. J. Surg.* **133**, 492.

Clayton, J. M., Hayes, A. C., Hammel, J., Boyd, W. C., Hartford, C. E., and Barnes, R. W. (1977). Xenon-133 determination of muscle blood flow in electrical injury. *J. Trauma* **17**, 293.

DiVincenti, F. C., Moncrief, J. A., and Pruitt, B. A., Jr (1969). Electrical injuries: A review of 65 cases. *J. Trauma* **9**, 497.

Hunt, J. L., Mason, A. D., Jr, Masterson, T. S., and Pruitt, B. A., Jr (1976). The pathophysiology of acute electric injuries. *J. Trauma* **16**, 335.

Hunt, J. L., McManus, W. F., Haney, W. P., and Pruitt, B. A., Jr (1974). Vascular lesions in acute electric injuries. *J. Trauma* **14**, 461.

Hunt, J. L., Sato, R. M., and Baxter, C. R. (1980). Acute electric burns: Current diagnostic and therapeutic approaches to management. *Archs Surg.* **115**, 434.

Kleiner, J. P. and Wilkin, J. H. (1978). Cardiac effects of lightning stroke. *J. Am. Med. Ass.* **240**, 2757.

Lancet (1977). Death by lightning *Lancet* **i**, 230

Levin, N. S., Atkins, A., McKeel, D. W., Jr, Peck, S. D., and Pruitt, B. A., Jr (1975). Spinal cord injury following electrical accidents: case reports. *J. Trauma* **15**, 459.

Newsome, T. W., Curreri, P. W., and Eurenius, K. (1972). Visceral injuries: an unusual complication of an electrical burn. *Archs Surg.* **105**, 494.

Pontén B., Erikson, U., Johansson, S. H., and Olding, L. (1970). New observations on tissue changes along the pathway of the current in an electrical injury: case report. *Scand. J. plast. reconstr. Surg.* **4**, 75.

Pruitt, B. A. Jr (1979). The burn patient: I. Initial care. *Curr. Probl. Surg.* **16**, 1.

Ugland, O. M. (1967). Electrical burns. *Scand. J. plast. reconstr. Surg.* (Suppl. 2), 1.

Valdes, R. R., Torres, V. C., de Castro, A. B., and Toribio, J. A. (1974–5). Electric cataract. *Burns* **1**, 317.

RADIATION

R. J. Berry

What kind of radiation? Radiations are either *ionizing* or *non-ionizing*. Ionization involves the forcible ejection of an orbital electron from an atom of matter, hence creating an ion. When this takes place in a molecule of biological importance, it may lead to biological damage. Non-ionizing radiations may be capable of *excitation*, but cannot convey sufficient energy to the target molecules to produce this gross structural change.

Ionizing radiations

X-rays. These are electromagnetic waves in the continuous spectrum which includes light and radio waves, but of very short wavelength. They have no mass and no charge, and are produced in machines by the bombardment of a positively charged anode with a stream of electrons from a heated filament. The energy of the X-rays is determined by the voltage through which they are accelerated, and their penetration increases with increasing acceleration voltage. They were first discovered by Roentgen in 1895.

Gamma-rays. These are identical in properties to X-rays but are produced by the spontaneous disintegration of radioactive atoms (see below).

Particle radiations. Unlike the above these have mass, and are produced by the composite parts of atoms such as electrons (β-particles), protons, or neutrons, or by the nuclei of larger atoms, e.g. helium nuclei (α-particles). They may be charged or uncharged. Particulate radiations may come either from the spontaneous disintegration of radioactive atoms or from electrical accelerators, where beams of a wide variety of subatomic particles have been produced.

Sources of radiation

Natural.Cosmic rays. Throughout his evolution man has been exposed to cosmic radiation emanating from the sun, which can be regarded as a large thermonuclear reactor. The majority of cosmic rays are high energy particles, protons, and electrons, and their intensity at the surface of the earth is now reduced compared to that in prehistoric times due to the development of a stable belt of charged particles, the van Allen belt, thickest at the equator and thinnest at the poles, but encircling the globe. This belt of particles interacts with and attenuates incoming cosmic rays. In addition, the ionized ozone layer of the atmosphere decreases the total cosmic radiation reaching the earth's surface. Cosmic rays are energetic and can not only irradiate man on the earth's surface but can also pass through many metres of earth.

Radioactivity. Many of the earth's minerals are naturally radioactive. Atoms are stable only if their nuclei contain an approximately equal number of protons and neutrons, and unstable atomic nuclei may undergo spontaneous disintegration. *Isotopes*, atoms with the same number of protons but different numbers of neutrons in their nuclei, may be stable or radioactive. In body fluids, the naturally occurring radioactive isotope ^{40}K forms the largest contribution to the internal radiation background. In the environment, building materials such as granite may have significant levels of natural radioactivity.

Man-made. Amongst man-made radiations, all the types listed above can be produced by machines: X-rays used by doctors are the greatest single man-made source of irradiation of the general population. Nuclear reactors are not only sources of direct radiations (usually absorbed in appropriate shielding) but also are copious producers of radio-isotopes. Finally, and it is hoped never to be used, nuclear weapons are intense sources of man-made radiation. However, except for 'radiation-enhanced' weapons, the so-called 'neutron bomb', potential lethal effects of blast and heat occur at greater distances from the point of detonation than do lethal effects from direct radiation.

For both natural and man-made substances, the qualities of importance are the type of disintegration, the particles or non-particulate radiation produced by the disintegration, the half-life (the time for one half of the initial activity to have disappeared, half of the remaining activity taking the same time to disappear, etc.), and the initial activity. This is specified in units of disintegrations per second, given the eponym becquerel, after the discoverer of radioactivity. The unit which has been used in the past related the number of radioactive disintegrations to the number of disintegrations taking place in 1 g of pure radium, 3.7×10^{10} per second = 1 curie (1 Ci = 3.7×10^{10} Bq, 1 Bq = 2.7×10^{-11} Ci).

Radiation effects

Ionization density. Radiations differ in their effects both qualitatively and quantitatively. X-rays and gamma-rays produce their damage by ejecting orbital electrons from atoms of matter with which they interact. These radiations are sparsely ionizing because the ejected particle is of low mass and limited in its capability for producing damage, so that interactions of many particles are needed to cause major chemical and biological damage. These sparsely ionizing radiations are described as being of low linear energy transfer (low LET) and their effects are dependent upon the rate at which the radiation dose is accumulated, whether protracted in time or fractionated in multiple short bursts. The chemical state of the target molecule can also affect the damage produced by low LET radiations, chemical interactions causing either potentiation of the radiation damage or protection against it.

Protons, neutrons which eject protons from atoms of matter, and other larger particles are more densely ionizing, and are said to be of high linear energy transfer (high LET). These radiations are less dependent for their effects on the accumulation of multiple damaging events within one target molecule, so that their action is often 'all or none'. They are also less dependent upon the dose rate, dose fractionation, or the chemical state of the target molecule.

Radiation dose. All effects of radiation depend upon the magnitude of the accumulated radiation dose. After a chequered history, beginning with the definition of the Roentgen in 1928 (that quantity

Radiation

6.87

of radiation which produces in 1 cm³ of air 1 unit of charge of either sign), absorbed radiation dose is now cited in SI units which have the dimensions of joules (energy) per kilogram (mass of absorbing material). The older radiation units are due to disappear from use in 1985. Throughout this section the new units will be given, followed by the old units in brackets. The basic unit of absorbed radiation dose, 1 J/kg has been given the eponym 1 gray (1 Gy = 100 rad). Conventional SI prefixes are used for multiples and submultiples of this unit. To compare the effects of different radiations with the reference standard which is the effect of sparsely ionizing radiations such as X-rays, a unit of *dose equivalent* is used. Absorbed radiation dose is multiplied by Quality Factor, a measure of the maximum Relative Biological Effectiveness of the particular radiation. The values of Quality Factor are determined by the International Commission on Radiation Protection and are intended to represent the highest value of the effectiveness of that particular radiation which has been encountered. The unit of dose equivalent is the sievert (1 Sv = 100 rem).

Table 1 lists a thousand millionfold range of radiation doses, and their effects upon biological systems.

Table 1   Effects of total-body irradiation

Dose equivalent		Effect
Sv*	(rem)	
Sublethal for man		
0.0001	0.01	*circa* 1 month's natural background radiation, no detectable effect
0.001 (1 mSv)	0.1	*circa* 1 year's natural background radiation, no detectable effect
0.01	1	no detectable effect
0.1	10	minimal decrease in peripheral lymphocyte count, no clinical effect
1	100	mild acute radiation sickness in some individuals (nausea, possible vomiting), *no acute deaths*, early decrease in peripheral lymphocyte count, decrease in all WBC and platelets at 2–3 weeks, increase in late risk of leukaemia, solid tumours
Lethal for man		
10	1000	severe acute radiation sickness, severe vomiting, diarrhoea, *death within* circa *30 days* of all exposed individuals. Severe depression of blood cell and platelet production, damage to gastrointestinal mucosa
100	10 000	immediate severe vomiting, disorientation, coma, *death within hours*
1000	100 000	death of some microorganisms, some insects
10 000	1 000 000	death of most bacteria, some viruses
100 000	10 000 000	death of all living organisms, denaturation of proteins

* for X-rays and γ-radiation dose equivalent in Sv is equal to absorbed dose (Gy)

Total body irradiation of man. As seen in Table 1, the major consequence of radiation exposure is life-shortening, either acutely for doses in excess of 5–10 Gy, or due to late effects which may be seen 1–40 years after radiation exposure for smaller doses. Clinically important radiation syndromes are as follows:

Central nervous system. Above acute exposures of 30–100 Gy (3000–10 000 rad) there is a rapid onset of nausea, vomiting which may be severe and repeated, anxiety, disorientation, and within hours, coma and death due to direct radiation effects on central nervous system conduction and to cerebral oedema. There are no definite pathological signs of damage at autopsy of such individuals.

Gastrointestinal syndrome. Individuals who have received doses in excess of 10 Gy (1000 rad) will also show early onset of nausea and vomiting, usually starting 1–2 hours after radiation exposure, but often recovering from this in 4–6 hours. However, they are doomed to die within 4–14 days because of radiation damage to the gastrointestinal tract. The convoluted epithelial lining of the small intestine is perhaps the most rapidly renewed tissue in the body; cells born in the intestinal crypts are shed from the tips of villi to the intestinal contents at the end of their normal life span approximately 4 days later. Radiation inhibition of cell division, followed by the reproductive death of the intestinal stem cells results in first a shortening of the intestinal villi until the lining of the intestine is as flat as a garden hose. This drastically reduces the surface area available for nutrient and electrolyte diffusion, and results in intractable diarrhoea. Failure of survival of sufficient intestinal stem cells and their proliferation to yield intestinal epithelial cells leads to denudation of areas of the bowel, with consequent free access of bowel contents and infection to the blood, and leakage of body fluids into the intestinal contents. Dehydration, overwhelming infection, and death follow.

Haemopoietic syndrome. At doses between 1 and 10 Gy (100–1000 rad) although transient nausea and occasional vomiting may be seen in some individuals, the frequency increasing with increasing dose, these early prodromal symptoms disappear rapidly, followed by a period of relative well-being. However, second only to the small bowel, the haemopoietic system is the body tissue which has the most rapid cell turnover. Mature lymphocytes, unlike the majority of body cells, do not need to attempt division before being killed by radiation damage, and undergo rapid interphase cell death within a period of hours. In fact, the change in peripheral lymphocyte count over the first 24 hours after acute radiation exposure can be used as a rough dosemeter for the magnitude of the exposure. As the majority of differentiated peripheral blood cellular elements have normal lifetimes of two to three weeks for most white cells and platelets, and around 100 days for red cells, no other immediate alterations in blood count are seen. However, haemopoietic stem cells are damaged by radiation, as are cells of other tissues, primarily by the loss of their ability to divide and by their subsequent death on attempting division. Hence, when the normal division stimuli occur there is an initial abortive repopulation of the peripheral blood achieved by 'short-cutting' the normal differentiation steps, which further depletes the already damaged haemopoietic stem cell population. By two to three weeks, there is no new input of differentiated, functional white cells and platelets, and the clinical syndrome develops of easy and overwhelming infection due to lack of white cells, and bleeding starting with petechial haemorrhage due to shortage of platelets.

Therapy of acute radiation exposure. It is unlikely that prior warning of radiation exposure would have allowed the ingestion or injection of a radioprotective substance. The only effective, potentially usable radioprotectors so far evolved depend on the production of intracellular hypoxia and/or increasing intracellular-SH concentration. Agents such as cysteine, cysteamine, aminoethylisothiouronium (AET) and mercaptoethyl guanidine (MEG) used in near-toxic concentrations have been shown in animal experiments to increase the LD$_{50}$ radiation dose by up to 20 per cent. A thiophosphate compound, S-2-(3-aminopropylamino) ethyl phosphorothioic acid, numbered WR 2721, has been evaluated by the US Army and has achieved similar or greater effectiveness with lower toxicity. However, a more likely scenario is that radiation exposure will occur without prior warning. If large populations have been irradiated even crude estimation of the radiation dose received will be of importance. Scarce medical resources will have to be devoted only to those patients who have received doses in the LD$_{10}$–LD$_{50}$ range; the most ill will have been irretrievably lethally irradiated, and those who have received less than an LD$_{10}$ radiation dose will recover spontaneously. As the haemopoietic syndrome is life-limiting, those patients at highest risk of haemopoietic death will have to be identified by initial peripheral blood lymphocyte count. A better biological dosemeter but useable for only small numbers of exposed individuals is the number of chromosome aberrations in peripheral blood cells cultured *in vitro* with phyto-haemagglutinin. If facilities exist, venesection and the storing of white cells and platelets against future need is considered by many to be a useful step, as well as providing a major early stimulus to proliferation of surviving haemopoietic stem cells. Another useful haemopoietic stimulation is challenge with a strong antigen such as TAB/tetanus toxoid. This is a good public health measure in a disaster, and has the advantage of a useful degree of early haemopoietic stimulation. If only a small number of radiation casualties are expected, a programme of isolation, gastrointestinal tract sterilization by non-absorbable antibiotics, the provision of a 'soft' environment to minimize chances of injury and bleeding, and the provision of sterile foods may tide the patients through the critical period of the nadir in peripheral white blood cell and platelet count. A number of such sterile units exist in the UK, established in the 1960s under the NAIR scheme following the incident in which the core of a nuclear reactor at Windscale in Cumbria was severely damaged, resulting in the release to the environment of gaseous and particulate radioactive contamination, but fortunately without acute hazard to man.

If a major radiation exposure results not from external irradiation but from contamination by radioactive isotopes, e.g. from nuclear weapon fallout, information from health physics personnel as to the nature of the hazard expected and determination of the initial amount of radioactivity in contaminated casualties will be vital—to assess danger to staff as well as patients. If exposure to fallout is expected a major amount of skin contamination can be avoided by wearing all possible clothing and removing this contaminated clothing once the fallout danger has passed.

First treatment of exposure to radioactive materials by wounding (skin penetration), ingestion, or inhalation may be directed towards removing the radioactive material from the body. Dangerously radioactive material in a wound is treated initially by washing and mechanical scrubbing, and if necessary by adequate surgical excision of the contaminated tissue. Ingestion of radioiodine is treated by the ingestion of a single 200 mg dose of stable sodium iodide/iodate so that the amount of the radioisotope which is fixed in the thyroid is minimized. This is most effective if taken *before* exposure and is only of use within a few hours of exposure. Ingestion of bone-seeking radionuclides such as ^{90}Sr and ^{137}Cs may be treated by the administration of chelating agents such as ethylene diamine tetraacetic acid (EDTA) to minimize their deposition in bone. Massive oral doses of stable calcium and parathyroid hormone have also been used with limited success. Particulate radioactive contamination which has been inhaled may, when the material has particular long-term hazards (e.g. ^{239}Pu), be removed in part by bronchial lavage carried out in centres with appropriate skills, but this technique is still largely experimental.

Late effects of radiation exposure

Leukaemogenesis. Over the period between 3 to 10 years after acute radiation exposure there is increased risk of the development of leukaemia, predominantly acute myeloid leukaemia. The magnitude of risk is proportional to the total radiation dose received. The male preponderance is in a ratio of 3 to 1. Other types of leukaemia are less likely to be increased by radiation exposure. Larger scale human experience is based on early radiation workers who were exposed unwittingly to large cumulative radiation doses, and the survivors of the Hiroshima and Nagasaki nuclear weapon detonations. From such data the dose to double the natural incidence of leukaemia is estimated to lie in the region 30–50 cGy (30–50 rad). However, leukaemia represents only about 3 per cent of all new malignancies in the UK, and even a relatively large increase in

leukaemia incidence may represent a small change in the overall numbers of patients presenting with malignant disease.

Carcinogenesis. Solid tumours are also induced by ionizing radiation exposure, once again increasing in risk as a function of increasing dose, but over periods up to 40 and more years after radiation exposure. The commonest sites of radiation-induced tumours are related to the sites in which the cancer is most prevalent in the general population. Skin cancer is inevitably high in incidence; other cancers in which increased incidence following radiation exposure has been demonstrated include lung, breast, bone, and lymphomas. A large pool of human experience exists, once again in the early radiation workers, the Hiroshima and Nagasaki survivors, and in specific groups exposed to either inhalation or ingestion of radioactive materials (e.g. uranium miners, radium dial painters) or to the medical use of ionizing radiation for diagnostic or therapeutic purposes (breast cancer in women TB patients, given a therapeutic artificial pneumothorax; skin and other cancers in patients treated by radiation for ankylosing spondylitis, etc.). For establishment of permissible population and occupational exposure limits, it is assumed that there is no threshold radiation dose below which no harm is caused, and the risk of inducing malignancy is assumed to be proportional to accumulated radiation dose. Animal and human studies suggest, however, that as the radiation dose increases there is a departure from this inexorable increase in induced malignancy due to the killing by the additional radiation dose of the transformed cells which presumably would have evolved into a malignant clone. As a guide, on best human data it is suggested that total body exposure of 1 cGy (1 rad) gives at most a 1 in 6000 risk of the development of fatal malignant disease in a particular individual. Thus, uniform exposure of a population of 1 million people to 1 cGy may result in the eventual development of about 165 fatal cancers against a background of 200–250 000 'spontaneous' cancer deaths.

Radiation damage to the fetus. Damage to the fetus by ionizing radiation is a special case of somatic damage. In the UK, accidental irradiation of early pregnancies is minimized by the application of a '10 day rule' that women of child-bearing age will only be subjected to radiographic examination including the abdomen on the first ten days after the start of last menses, unless there is some vital overriding medical reason. The developing fetus is particularly susceptible to damage during the period of organogenesis when the loss of reproductive capacity of a cell rest due to evolve into a particular organ may be catastrophic. The fetus, like the adult, is also subject to an increased risk of the development of leukaemia and solid tumours which is related to the total accumulated radiation dose.

Genetic damage. Radiation can produce both dominant lethal events and recessive changes not evinced in the first generation. However, with increasing radiation dose, an increasing proportion of those cells in which such transformations have taken place are rendered reproductively inert and cannot pass on their genetic misinformation. Hence, somatic rather than genetic damage is the limiting factor in determining permissible radiation exposure to populations.

Estimation of radiation hazards

Dose limits to the general population. Since the institution of maximum permissible annual radiation exposure levels, pioneered by the International Congress of Radiology in 1928 and intended for radiation workers, progressively more restrictive limits have been imposed for maximum exposure to ionizing radiation among members of the general public. The present average exposure to the general public from all sources of radiation in the UK and USA is shown in Table 2. Note that by far the greatest source of man-made radiation exposure to the general population is from the medical use of diagnostic X-rays. Following the recommendations of the International Commission on Radiological Protection, the maximum permissible total body exposure per annum to a member of the general public in the UK is now 5 mSv (0.5 rem). However, in its most recent recommendations, the Commission declares that 'all exposures shall be kept as low as reasonably achievable, economic and social factors being taken into account,. This dose limit is designed to keep at an acceptably low level the stochastic harmful effects of radiation exposure (those which occur with increasing frequency with increasing dose) and to prevent the occurrence of non-stochastic harmful effects (all-or-none effects for which there is a dose threshold). If only part of the body is irradiated, proportionally higher doses are allowed. Limits for the inhalation or ingestion of radioactive material depend on the concentration of those materials in limiting target organs. Thus, the limit for ingestion of radioactive iodine is set by the maximum radiation dose to the thyroid in which it would be concentrated; in fact the limit is set by the concentration in the thyroid of the most susceptible member of the population, a young child. Maximum permissible concentrations of other important isotopes such as ^{60}Co are set by the exposure of the bone marrow or of ^{90}Sr or ^{137}Cs by the dose to bone.

Table 2 Annual radiation exposure of the general public

Source	Average dose equivalent, mSv (rem)/year	
	UK 1978	USA 1970
Environmental		
Natural	1.10 (0.11)	1.02 (0.10)
Fallout from atmospheric testing of nuclear weapons	0.01 (0.001)	0.04 (0.004)
Nuclear power	0.002 (0.0002)	0.00003 (−)
Medical		
Diagnostic radiology	0.50 (0.05)	0.72 (0.072)
Radiopharmaceuticals		0.010 (0.001)
Occupational	0.008 (0.0008)	0.008 (0.0008)
Miscellaneous	0.008 (0.0008)	0.02 (0.0002)
Total	1.63 (0.16)	1.82 (0.18)

Data from Taylor and Webb (1978), National Academy of Sciences (1972)

Dose limits to radiation workers. As for the general public, recommendations of the International Commission on Radiological Protection set the dose limits for permissible annual exposure for radiation workers. This is now 50 mSv (5 rem) per year to the whole body, once again with specific exposure limits to individual organs when less than the whole body is irradiated. These limits are based on the assumption that the radiation worker will not be so employed for more than 40 years. Present regulations of the EEC require that persons be designated radiation workers if there is a likelihood that their annual radiation exposure will exceed three-tenths of the current maximum permissible exposure levels. Volunteers giving informed consent to participate in medical experiments in which radiation is used may not receive a dose greater than the annual maximum permissible dose to radiation workers, except in very special circumstances. Current dose limits to the general population and to radiation workers are summarized in Table 3.

Table 3 United Kingdom dose limits for radiation exposure

	General public annual exposure mSv (rem)	Radiation workers annual exposure mSv (rem)
Whole body	5.0 (0.5)	50 (5.0)*
Bone marrow/gonads	5.0 (0.5)	50 (5.0)
Eye (lens)	30.0 (3.0)	300 (30.0)
Extremities	50 (5.0)	500 (50.0)
Other organs	50 (5.0)	500 (50.0)

* Subject to maximum of 30 mSv (3 rem)/quarter; 13 mSv (1.3 rem)/quarter to the abdomen of women of reproductive age
Data from Council of the European Communities (1980)

Emergency reference levels. In the event of an unscheduled release of radioactive material into the environment, from the detonation of a nuclear weapon, from a fault in a plant handling radioactive material, or in the unlikely event of uncontrollable malfunction of a nuclear reactor, it is necessary to assess the potential radiation dose to the population at risk and then to decide whether appropriate counter-measures should be taken. There are some radiation levels low enough that the risks inherent in taking *any* action, be it the distribution of stable iodine tablets after a nuclear weapon detonation or a reactor burn-out, or the evacuation of population, may be greater than the risks from the radiation exposure. For this reason it is necessary to have Emergency Reference Levels (ERL) as a planning guide. ERLs of dose can be translated into initial activities in the air, on pasturage, in the water, which would lead to a total body commitment to a dose equal to the emergency reference levels. An incident which produced population doses lower than the ERL would not require specific action, but above this level consideration would be given to intervention such as the destruction of milk, the removal of animals from contaminated pasture, evacuation of populations, etc. Thus, above a lower bound, there will be a range of action levels up to an upper dose bound above which the introduction of countermeasures is virtually certain. For taking shelter this dose range has been set in the UK as 5–50 mSv (0.5–5 rem), for taking stable iodine tablets 50–250 mSv (5–25 rem), while for more disruptive countermeasures such as evacuation the range is 100–500 mSv (10–50 rem).

Partial body exposure—local radiation effects. When less than the whole body is irradiated, the effects will once again depend on radiation dose, and critically upon what parts of the body are irradiated. Radiation therapy, limited to appropriate parts of the body, has been used to treat malignant diseases since the 1880s, and there is a considerable literature of the effects of such local irradiation on limiting normal tissues. The radiation effect will also be determined by the fractionation or protraction of the dose in time, the longer the overall time or the larger number of individual radiation exposures, the greater the total dose which can be accumulated before damage is produced. On the skin a single radiation dose in excess of around 8 Gy (800 rad) will cause a transient reddening within a few hours, followed by a more vigorous erythema at 7–10 days, its intensity once again depending on total dose accumulated. With increasing radiation dose to the skin, dry or moist desquamation will result, healing by repopulation of the denuded epithelium from surviving basal epithelial cells. For the majority of body tissues the major effect of irradiation is the cessation of division in the stem cells which replenish the differentiated population of the particular tissue. Therefore, radiation effects will be most severe in those tissues in which cell turnover is most rapid. In many organs, although the turnover of parenchymal cells is slow, irradiation damage is produced because of damage to blood vessels resulting in focal ischaemia and often leading to fibrosis. Limiting normal tissues for the clinical radiotherapist in the treatment of cancer include lungs, gastrointestinal tract, kidneys, and central nervous system. Modern radiation therapy uses supervoltage (greater than 1 MV) X-rays or the gamma-rays from ^{60}Co which physically spare the skin. The skin is therefore no longer the limiting normal tissue. Normal tissue tolerance is determined by the induction of fibrosis in subcutaneous connective tissues and in limiting organs within the irradiation volume.

Effects on non-ionizing radiations
Ultraviolet light. Although non-ionizing, ultraviolet light is capable of penetration to at least the basal layer of the skin epithelium, and is specifically absorbed in nucleic acid, including DNA. Because of this it is capable of causing both chromosomal damage and cell killing. In the less pigmented races the incidence of skin cancer is highly correlated with exposure to solar ultraviolet. The intensity of solar ultraviolet radiation increases rapidly with increasing altitude due to the reduced atmospheric scattering and absorption of these

light wavelengths. The mechanism of ultraviolet light damage has been relatively well studied. Much of the damage is repaired, and individuals deficient in such repair systems, such as patients with xeroderma pigmentosum, are exquisitely sensitive to ultraviolet light because of their inability to excise thymine dimers formed by this irradiation in their DNA. Protection against ultraviolet light can be achieved by ingestion of para-aminobenzoic acid and a number of sulphonamide antibiotics, and by the use of suitable UV absorbing barrier creams such as Uvistat or Eversun 7.

Radio frequency electromagnetic waves. Much less is known about the hazard to man of exposure to high intensity radio frequency electromagnetic waves, but individuals chronically exposed to such radiations in high intensity have been reported as developing anaemia, alopecia, psychological disorders, etc. In animal studies, changes in the high spontaneous rate of cancer in particular strains has been reported. The widespread use of radio frequency 'microwave' ovens for home and restaurant cookery has made their safety a more important question. With the exception of the danger from induction heating, with consequent thermal burn damage, there is no evidence that there is significant risk of danger to the general public from the use of such appliances. Further studies are, however, in progress to determine the effects of acute and chronic exposure to high intensity radio frequency waves.

Ultrasound. As with radio frequency waves, ultrasound can produce local tissue damage by heating or by the production of minute bubbles due to cavitation within individual cells. The effects are critically dependent upon the sound frequency, the duty cycle, and the overall length of exposure. For the power levels used conventionally in diagnostic ultrasonography, no significant damage to mammalian cells has been demonstrated, although sophisticated studies of the effect of low power ultrasound on chromosomes suggests that the margin may not be very wide. The widespread use of medical ultrasound as a non-invasive imagining technique makes it essential that such studies are repeated or disproved, but the clinical experience of more than 25 years without significant suspicion of induction of fetal abnormalities by diagnostic ultrasound gives reassurance.

References

Bond, V. P., Fliedner, T. M., and Archambeau, J. O. (1965). *Mammalian radiation lethality: a disturbance in cellular kinetics*. Academic Press, London.

Council of the European Communities (1980). Council directive of 15 July 1980 amending the Directives laying down basic safety standards for the health protection of the general public and workers against the dangers of ionizing radiation. *Off. J. Eur. Communit.* no. L246, 1, 17 September 1980, available from HMSO, London.

Dainton, F. and McLean, A. (1981). *Living with radiation*, 2nd edn. National Radiological Protection Board, Harwell, Oxfordshire.

Hall, E. J. (1973). *Radiobiology for the radiologist*. Harper and Row, Hagerstown, Maryland.

ICRP Publication 26 (1977). Recommendations of the International Commission on Radiological Protection. *Annals of the IRCP* **1**, no. 3.

National Academy of Sciences (1972). *The effects on populations of exposure to low levels of ionizing radiation (BEIR Report)*. National Academy of Sciences/National Research Council, Washington, DC.

National Radiological Protection Board (1981). *Emergency reference levels: criteria for limiting doses to the public in the event of accidental exposure to radiation*. ERL 2, HMSO, London.

Taylor, F. E. and Webb, G. A. M. (1978). *Radiation exposure of the UK population*. National Radiological Protection Board, Harwell, Oxfordshire.

NOISE

D. H. Glaister

'Sound is of great value to man. It warns him of danger and appropriately arouses and activates him. It allows him the immeasurable advantage of speech and language. It can be beautiful. It can calm, excite, and it can elicit joy or sorrow' (Miller 1974). Unwanted sound, however, constitutes noise, though the distinction is frequently blurred. Noise can cause masking of wanted sounds, interference with speech and communication, pain and injury, and temporary or permanent loss of hearing. With few exceptions, loud noises are the product of modern man, and evolution has had insufficient time to develop adequate protection against extreme exposures. It is the permanent noise induced hearing loss (NIHL, noise deafness, or acoustic trauma) which is of most concern to the clinician.

Measurement of sound. The range of sound level from that which is just audible to that which is deafening is so great that normal units (of energy, or pressure) are unwieldy and recourse is made to a logarithmic scale based on the bel (named from Alexander Graham Bell, of telephone fame). One bel represents a tenfold increase in sound intensity, and is divided into ten decibels (dB). A decibel is, therefore, a ratio, and must be referred to an appropriate standard. Accepted values are 10^{-12} W for sound energy and 2×10^{-5} N/m² for sound pressure. The logarithm of two is 0.3 and an increase in sound pressure of 3 dB indicates a two-fold rise. For example, when two 80 dB sources of sound are added together, their sum is 83 dB. In contrast, a subjective doubling of noise results from an increase of around 10 dB in intensity.

Sounds are built up from various frequency components in the audible range (30 Hz to 18 kHz in a young person). Noises tend to be of broad spectrum, but often contain particularly energetic components. For example, Fig. 1 shows spectra recorded in two different types of aircraft. The upper curve shows the cockpit noise in an aircraft flying at high-speed and at low-level. Sound energy of all frequencies is present at more or less equal amplitude. Such noise is known as broad band and contrasts with the lower curve.

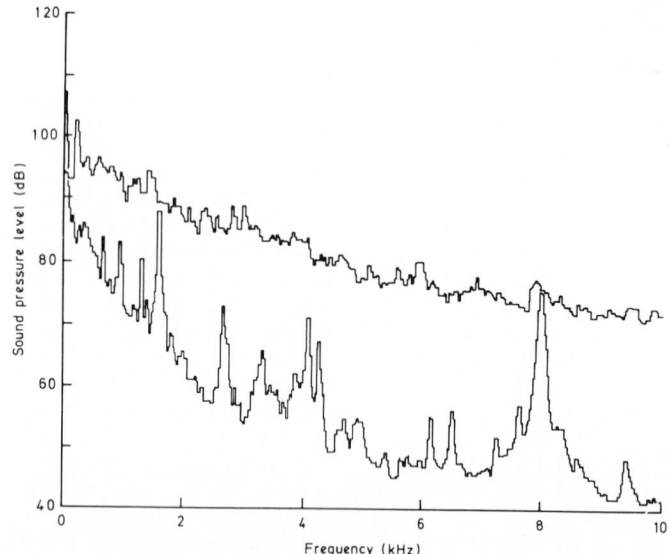

Fig. 1 Narrow band analyses of noise recorded in a fighter aircraft (upper curve) and helicopter (lower curve).

This shows the cockpit noise in a helicopter. It contains components related to rotor r.p.m. and the number of rotor blades, to the meshing of gears and to the rotational speed of various engine components, and to jet eflux. The overall noise level can be obtained by summing each frequency component, but since the ear does not have a flat frequency response, an estimate of the overall perceived noise is obtained by using an appropriate weighting, referred to as dB(A). The curves of Fig. 1 are dominated by low frequency components (especially in the helicopter example) and the overall levels were 114 dB(A) and 104 dB(A) respectively.

On the equal energy principle, confirmed for steady state noise on a large industrial population (Burns and Robinson 1970), equal quantities of A-weighted sound energy cause equal amounts of hearing loss. Thus, a sound intensity of 90 dB(A) for eight hours would have the same effect as one of 93 dB(A) for four hours, or 102 dB(A) for 30 minutes. Occupational exposures may be assessed over a working week by noting times spent at differing noise levels and then making use of tables set out in the International Organization for Standardization (ISO) Recommendation R 1999. The outcome is an equivalent continuous sound level (L_{eq}) from which the risk of hearing damage may be obtained. Alternatively, a personal noise dose meter may be worn, calibrated in L_{eq}, or as a percentage of the maximum permitted daily dose. It must be noted, however, that these relationships apply to populations on a statistical basis and can only give a rough indication of the risk of injury in individual cases.

The sensitivity of hearing is determined by finding, in a quiet room, the level of a pure tone which can just be detected, the process being repeated for a number of frequencies from, usually, 250 Hz to 8kHz (standard intervals are 250 and 500 Hz and 1, 2, 3, 4, 6, and 8 kHz). The level of hearing for each ear can be assessed using manual or automatic pure tone audiometry. The resulting plot of threshold versus frequency is referred to as an audiogram, and any hearing loss can be assessed by reference to normal values, or by comparing it with a previous audiogram from the same subject. In either case the effect of age must be taken into account. As the test uses pure tones based on octave spacing, the discrimination tends to diminish with increasing frequency. It is, however, found to be sufficiently sensitive for clinical use.

Noise-induced hearing loss

Aetiology. A temporary shift in the threshold of hearing may follow any exposure to noise in excess of 60–80 dB(A), though there is great individual variation. The effect is most marked in the 2–6 kHz frequency range and, in effect, the louder the noise and the longer its duration (up to 24 hours or so), the more profound and longer lasting the temporary shift. It may be associated with tinnitus and, by definition, complete recovery occurs after a few hours to two weeks or more (depending on the degree of hearing loss and individual susceptibility). Threshold shifts of up to 40 dB may occur, but above this level the loss becomes compound with complete recovery unlikely. Any residual effect then constitutes a permanent hearing loss.

A permanent threshold shift may follow a single exposure to intense noise, for example, the firing of a heavy gun, but the noise level required is so great that it is seldom tolerated voluntarily. More usually the permanent loss of hearing follows repeated exposures on a daily basis over a period of many years. Whilst these exposures are usually occupational, field studies have shown the very significant contribution of household sources—domestic appliances, power tools etc.—and of leisure activities—hi-fi, motor sport, pop concerts and discos, where noise levels of up to 122 dB(A) have been recorded. Occupational noise exposures occur predominantly in heavy industry, especially ship-building and re-pairing, and in aerospace activities. Particularly damaging sources are drop-forging and the use of percussive tools. An example of noise induced permanent threshold shifts for jute workers with up to 40 years exposures to a working noise level of about 98 dB(A) is illustrated in Fig. 2.

Pathology. The primary site of damage is the organ of Corti in the inner ear. The outer ear, eardrum, and middle ear are virtually never damaged by exposure to noise though the eardrum may be ruptured by the blast of an explosion (impulsive noise), or by extremely intense noise (150 dB or more). Excessive chronic exposure leads to gradual destruction of hair cells and to collapse and eventual destruction of parts of the organ of Corti. Auditory neurones may also degenerate. This sequence of changes is illustrated in Fig. 3, and loss of auditory function will be virtually complete by the stage illustrated in panel (c).

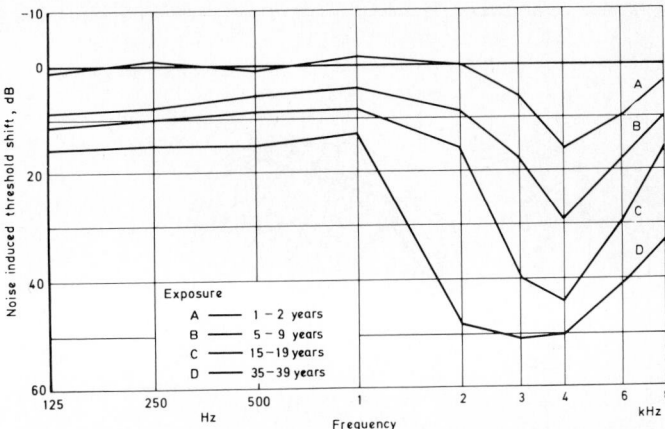

Fig. 2 Estimated noise-induced threshold shift as a function of frequency, for various durations of exposure of jute weavers to sound levels of about 98 dB(A). (Redrawn from Taylor *et al.* (1965), by permission of the authors and the American Institute of Physics.)

The organ of Corti contains some 500 hair cells per millimetre of its 34 mm length and the loss of 1–2 mm may not lead to a measurable change in function. Damage is, however, more critical in the lower part of the cochlea responsible for the perception of high-frequency sound.

The mechanism of damage is unclear, but very intense sounds can cause direct mechanical disruption, the relevant portion of the organ of Corti being simply torn apart. It is also possible that constant over-exposure causes the organ's cells to work at an excessive rate so leading to a local metabolic disturbance with a developing loss of function and eventual cell death. These cells are highly specialized and once destroyed cannot regenerate. Thus there can be no recovery from noise induced cochlear damage and the resulting hearing loss is permanent.

Symptoms and signs. The clinical picture is one of gradually increasing difficulty in hearing, usually in men of late-middle to elderly age and leading, in severe cases, to considerable social handicap. In moderate cases there may be difficulty in speaking with groups of people against background noises, whilst there is no problem in conversing with an individual at home. Words may be confused and wrong answers given to questions. A typical audiogram would show bilateral hearing loss of 40 dB or more at frequencies above 2 kHz (for example, Fig. 2, curves C or D). With a more severe loss difficulty is experienced even with loud speech and conversation becomes difficult even at home. Simply turning up the radio or television volume is of little help as sounds are distorted, the problem being one of speech discrimination rather than of sound perception. The distance and direction of sounds may also be misjudged, so putting the subject at risk from accidents at home and on the roads.

Tinnitus is common (30 per cent incidence in one series) and may be the only symptom, the subject being unaware of any deafness. In these cases the hearing loss may be confined to a dip in the audiogram at 4 kHz (Fig. 2, curves A and B). A disturbance of balance may also occur though caloric tests usually give normal reactions.

Differential diagnosis. This depends upon the presence of the symptoms referred to above together with a characteristic audiogram, a history of noise exposure over many years, and the absence of any other cause for the deafness. The picture may be complicated by other factors such as age, old middle and/or inner-ear infection, head injury, or the effect of drugs. It must be remembered that the possibility of compensation for industrial injury may cloud the issue, but a well-conducted audiogram should provide clear objective evidence.

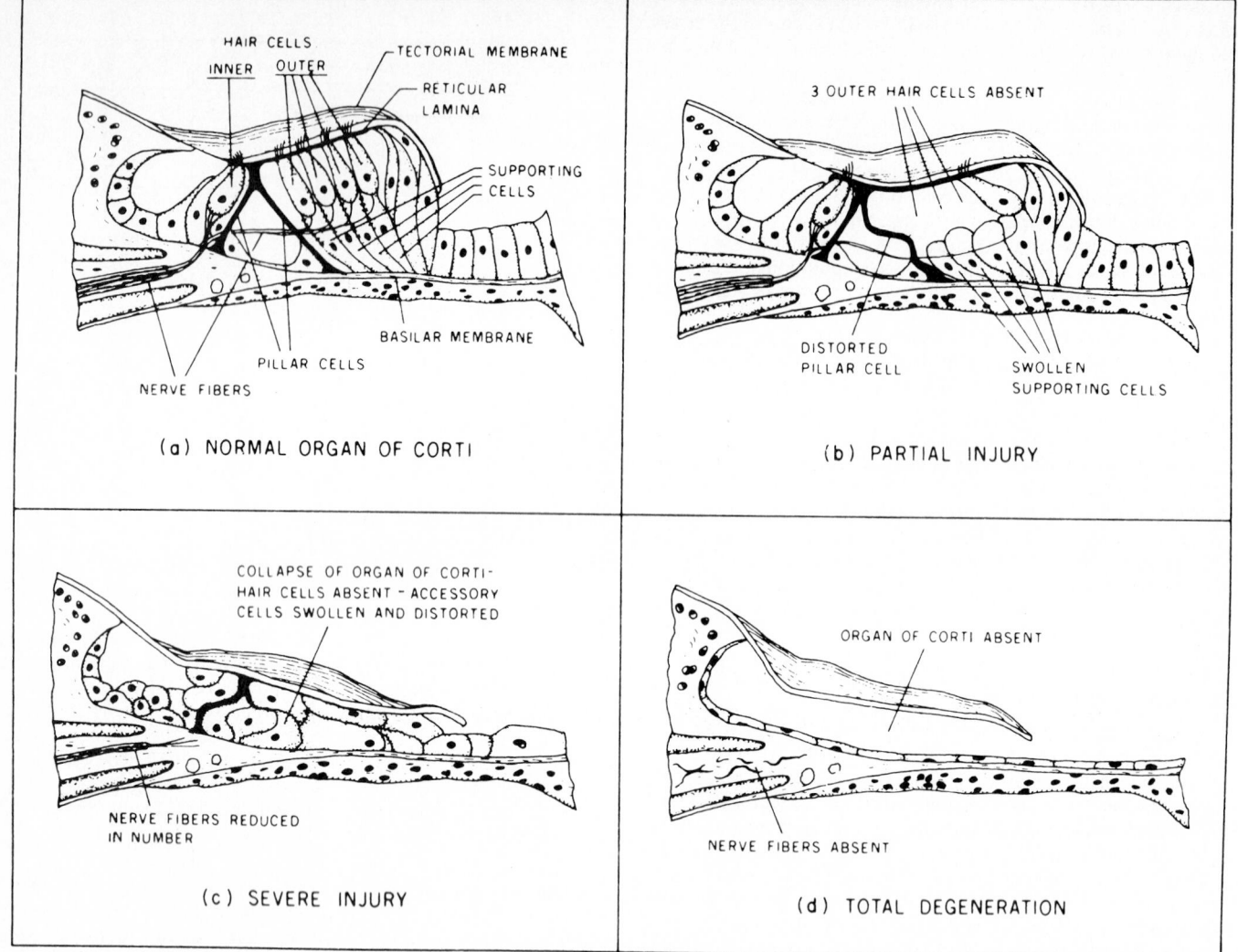

Fig. 3 Drawings of the human organ of Corti to illustrate (a) the normal state, and (b), (c), and (d) increasing degrees of noise induced permanent injury. (From Miller (1974), by permission of the author and the American Institute of Physics.)

Management. 'There are few more depressing or unrewarding patients than those with permanent occupational hearing loss. In the present state of medical knowledge, once the diagnosis is established, little can be done to alleviate matters. The answer lies in the realms of preventive medicine' (Chadwick 1971). Thus, this section is entitled management, not treatment. Withdrawal from further noise exposure will preclude any worsening of the condition, but will not prevent further loss of hearing due to the normal effect of ageing. The condition is frequency selective so that mere amplification of the incoming sound is usually of little value as the sound distortion is unaffected and amplified to the same degree. However, when symptoms are disabling, a hearing aid should be given an adequate trial.

If early signs of noise induced hearing loss appear on routine audiometry, for example notching at 4 kHz, it should be sufficient to warn the individual of the likely outcome and to institute protective measures. Hearing should subsequently be checked at three to six-monthly intervals and, if there is no further deterioration, the individual can continue at work. However, an individual appearing in middle-age with hearing loss attributable to noise presents a greater problem. Age is certain to exacerbate his symptoms, but withdrawal from his place of work is likely to cause difficulties, as by then he will be skilled and may find alternative employment in quiet surroundings difficult. It is, however, essential to isolate him from the noise environment for a period of at least two months so that an accurate estimate of his permanent threshold shift may be made.

His work environment and use of personal protection should be checked. Return to work under supervision could then be allowed, but his hearing must be checked three-monthly. Should there be further deterioration it is essential that he should move to a quieter environment, whatever the personal consequences.

Prevention. The other side of the coin is that noise induced hearing loss is an almost wholly preventable disease and adequate preventative measures are available. Hearing conservation measures include the identification of hazardous noise sources and a detailed investigation of their frequency characteristics, the control of exposure, the provision (and wearing) of protective devices, and the use of routine audiometry. Furthermore, although initial exposures to high noise levels may be unpleasant to the novice, familiarity breeds contempt and at least temporary threshold shift. Recent anecdotal support of this was provided by a mechanic at a drag-race meeting who commented 'you get used to the noise after a while'. Presumably for the same reason, disc jockeys gradually turn up the volume to maintain a 'good atmosphere'!

Initially, a hazardous source may be defined as one with an overall sound pressure level of at least 90 dB(A), but lower values may still be hazardous if they contain discrete energetic frequency components. The noise reaching the individual may be reduced by diminishing the sound energy at source (the change from straight jet to fan jet engines on commercial aircraft for example), by attenuating the sound by use of appropriate building construction and insulating materials, and by use of personal protection. Soft synthetic rubber ear plugs can give up to 30 dB protection at higher frequencies whilst an ear muff can give up to 40 dB protection over the critical 2–4 kHz frequency range. However, both devices must be closely fitted and worn consistently to be of benefit.

References

Burns, W. and Robinson, D. W. (1970). *Hearing and noise in industry.* HMSO, London.

Chadwick, D. L. (1971). Occupational hearing loss and the otologist. In *Occupational hearing loss* (ed. D. W. Robinson), 217. Academic Press, London and New York.

ISO (1971). *Recommendation R 1999.* Acoustics: assessment of occupational noise exposure for hearing conservation purposes. International Organization for Standardization.

King, P. J. (1978). Otorhinolaryngology in aviation. In *Aviation Medicine,* vol. 2 (eds. G. Dhenin and T. C. D. Whiteside), 232, Tri-Med Books, London.

Kryter, K. D. (1970). *The effects of noise on man.* Academic Press, New York and London.

Miller, J. D. (1974). Effects of noise on people. *J. acoust. Soc. Am.* **56**. 729.

Taylor, W., Pearson, J., Mair, A., and Burns, W. (1965). Study of noise and hearing in jute weaving. *J. acoust. Soc. Am.* **38**, 113.

AIR POLLUTION

P. J. Lawther

Sources and varieties of pollutants. In the absence of a definition of pure air, pollution is difficult to define. Among the natural sources of pollution which have caused injury or death are emissions from volcanoes, other subterranean emissions such as hydrogen sulphide and carbon dioxide, and the products of rotting vegetation. Dusts from the land can cause damage; recently the occurrence of endemic mesothelioma in Turkey has been attributed to the presence of fibres in the local volcanic tuff; pollens, spores, and moulds pollute the air. But most air pollution is man-made. The most important source is the burning of fossil fuels for the generation of heat and power. The source may be stationary or mobile; combustion may be complete or incomplete. Industry may pollute the communal air by emitting by-products or by the loss of prime products. The concentration of a pollutant will obviously depend on the strength of the source, factors which influence dilution or removal from the air, and the site at which samples are taken. Weather and climate are of obvious importance as determinants of the concentration of a pollutant. After emission many pollutants undergo physical and chemical changes in the air which may enhance or lessen their potential toxicity. Because these reactions may occur and since ground level concentrations may vary widely both in time and in space, much caution must be exercised when selecting sites for sampling and in choosing analytical methods; the dangerous tendency to confuse the relevance of emission rates and ground level concentrations must be avoided when assessing the possible effects of suspect pollutants.

In this necessarily brief account the nature and possible effects of three main groups of pollutants will be discussed: those from the burning of coal, oil, wood, and gas; those emitted by motor vehicles; and some (the list must be short and consist merely of examples of this class) from industry which might affect the general population. Pollution within workplaces will not be discussed, nor will pollution by radioactive species (see page 6.86).

Pollution from combustion of coal, oil, wood, and gas

Nature. When hydrocarbon compounds are burnt completely, water and carbon dioxide, plus traces of nitrogen oxides derived from the fixation of atmospheric nitrogen, are produced. Less complete burning produces carbon monoxide in addition. Some combustion processes allow pyrolysis and destructive distillation of the fuels which result in the formation of complex organic compounds among which may be irritants or carcinogens, including the polycyclic aromatic hydrocarbons. Impurities present in the fuel may be emitted to air or retained in ash. The commonest impurities in coal and heavy fuel oil are compounds, organic and inorganic, of sulphur: the sulphur content of these fuels varies widely. Light distillate oils used for domestic heating contain much less sulphur. Other impurities include fluoride in some coals, vanadium in some heavy oils, and many trace elements.

When coal is burned in large furnaces, such as those in power stations and big industrial installations, combustion is usually very nearly complete (it must be for economic considerations) and the pollutants emitted, apart from water, carbon dioxide, and some oxides of nitrogen, are sulphur oxides and the fine ash particles which escape retention by precipitators. When coal is burned in domestic open grates and other small appliances, tars, soot, and carbon monoxide may also be emitted. This complex mixture of pollutants was common in many towns in temperate zones before legislation led to its reduction in some. The tarry component contains the potentially carcinogenic polycyclic hydrocarbons of which class of compounds benzo(a)pyrene is commonly used as an indicator. Sulphur dioxide may be oxidized to sulphuric acid in the chimney or in the air; the reaction is catalysed by several compounds; fog droplets in polluted town air may be very acidic. Atmospheric ammonia tends to neutralize these acids. Because of their height, tall stacks ensure relatively good dispersion whereas emissions from low domestic chimneys are often trapped under temperature inversion conditions. Oil is more easily burnt efficiently than coal; soot may result from inadequate combustion but tar is uncommon. Wood contains no sulphur though incomplete combustion may produce irritant smoke. Coal gas contains carbon monoxide and is poisonous in itself; liquid petroleum gas and other 'natural' gases contain no carbon monoxide but this pollutant may be produced in dangerous amounts by faulty heaters or stoves in the home. Attention is currently being directed to pollution of the indoor environment by several compounds including oxides of nitrogen from unflued heaters and cookers. Faulty flues may allow the accumulation of lethal amounts of pollutants indoors. The use of free-standing kerosene heaters in poorly ventilated rooms can also lead to asphyxiation.

Acute effects. The acute effects have been seen most clearly in the so-called 'smogs' (smoke-polluted fogs) when pollution, derived mainly from coal smoke and its attendant gases, had reached high concentrations in the still, calm, cold weather associated with winter anticyclones. Temperature inversions favour the accumulation of pollutants which disperse only gradually by a process of diffusion. Many such incidents have been described; the London 'smog' in December 1952 was associated with the occurrence of 4000 deaths in excess of those expected during the week in Greater London. The deaths were among the elderly, the very young, and the sick. The clinical picture was consistent with irritation of the respiratory tract. No specific disease pattern was recognized, nor any specific toxic substance identified. Whilst an immense amount of subsequent work has failed to identify with certainty the causal agent, it would seem reasonable to attribute the effects seen to irritation of the respiratory tract by sulphur dioxide, sulphuric acid, and acid particles present in the fog which accompanied the stagnation of the air. The role of more subtle reactions and components is not known. Whereas subjects with normal lungs and hearts felt little more than discomfort, the likely increase in resistance to air-flow caused by bronchospasm and/or the hypersecretion of bronchial mucus could have produced serious and often fatal disturbances of ventilation/perfusion ratios in susceptible subjects, and an intolerable stress to those persons already suffering from other chest diseases and cardiovascular disorders. The increases in mortality derived from vital statistics in such incidents give little idea of the number of deaths occurring after the fumigation, and good indices of morbidity are difficult to obtain. Although it is now of historic interest only in the United Kingdom, the account of the 1952 London episode (Ministry of Health 1954) is still relevant; the type of pollution which caused such a dramatic increase in mortality and morbidity still occurs in many parts of the world.

Treatment should aim to alleviate bronchospasm and to protect the cardiovascular system by orthodox therapy. Some protection might be afforded against acid particles by the use of ammonia dispensers in which a mixture of equal parts of 0.880 ammonia solution and industrial methylated spirit is allowed to evaporate on a wick protruding from a bottle. Masks have been tried; they must be tolerable, of low resistance to airflow, and have a high filtration efficiency. Susceptible patients should be advised strongly to remain at rest indoors during episodes of high pollution. Air conditioners, which filter the air and absorb sulphur dioxide, are obviously desirable. They may be in the form of large commercial installations or can be free-standing appliances which recirculate cleaned air in the sick room. Some air filters use electrostatic precipitators which, whilst having the advantages of high efficiency and low resistance to airflow, might emit undesirable amounts of ozone which may be irritant.

Acute pollution from the burning of heavy fuel oil gives a picture similar to that caused by burning coal. Though tarry matter is uncommon, pollution by sulphur oxides might be more severe depending on the sulphur content of the oil used. In many towns the sources will be mixed. Fortunately techniques exist for ensuring the efficient combustion of coal and oil so that smoke need not be a problem; means of reducing the emissions of sulphur dioxide are expensive and are the subject of much debate in terms of cost–benefit.

Exposure to concentrations of pollutants much lower than those found in 'smogs' may affect patients with chronic disease of the lungs or heart. The threshold concentrations supposed to have perceptible effects are the basis of much argument in the formulation of air quality criteria and standards. It had been hoped that observation of the responses of groups of sick patients to varying concentrations of sulphur dioxide and smoke, would have allowed discrimination between the effects of the two classes of pollutants since smoke control measures were not expected to reduce sulphur dioxide concentrations. In fact the concentrations of both pollutants fell; the most that can be said is that groups of patients with chronic bronchitis and other chronic chest complaints appear not to react (subjectively) when 24-hour average concentrations of smoke and sulphur dioxide are less than $250\ \mu g/m^3$ and $500\ \mu g/m^3$ respectively. There is some evidence that the reported effects are related more to short term peaks rather than to average levels. There is no convincing evidence that sulphur dioxide and particulate matter act synergistically.

Acute effects of wood burning are not well described; they are being studied now because wood is an attractive alternative to coal and oil in some parts of the world. The negligible sulphur content may be an advantage but some wood smoke is highly irritant.

The acute effects of carbon monoxide, derived from any fuel which is poorly burned, are well documented (see page 6.31). Pollution of indoor spaces by leaky flues or maladjusted gas burners may be lethal or may result in malaise and headache. When carbon monoxide, which is odourless, produces saturations of more than 40 per cent exposed subjects are likely to become unconscious; the subsequent prognosis depends on the concentration of carbon monoxide and the duration of exposure. Immediate removal from the foul room is essential; the expulsion of the carbon monoxide from the blood is hastened by the administration of oxygen and stimulation of pulmonary ventilation, but the use of oxygen containing carbon dioxide may cause further damage to the respiratory centre.

Chronic effects. Chronic bronchitis is more prevalent in towns than in rural areas and is especially common in the United Kingdom. There are good reasons for blaming irritant air pollutants for playing a prominent part in its aetiology. But simple chemical irritation might not be enough to explain the later infective stage and it is clear that many other factors play a part in the development of the disease. There is good evidence that air pollution by coal smoke favoured infection of the lower respiratory tract in childhood and appeared to lay the foundation for the later development of chronic bronchitis. As air pollution by this source has declined in the United Kingdom, it is abundantly clear that smoking, especially of cigarettes, has supplanted air pollution as the main cause. Pollution of indoor air by parental tobacco smoke and by heating and cooking apparatus has been shown recently to be associated with the later development of bronchitis in children.

The tarry fractions of coal smoke which are capable of producing skin cancer have been blamed for the observed excess of carcinoma of the bronchus seen in towns compared with rural areas. Whilst tobacco smoking is almost universally accepted as being the overwhelmingly important cause of the disease, attention must be paid to arguments in favour and against air pollution as another aetiological factor. Carcinogenic polycyclic aromatic hydrocarbons are undoubtedly present in town air polluted by coal smoke (other sources, including vehicle exhausts, contribute). There is an excess of bronchial carcinoma in gas works retort-house operatives and those who work on coke ovens, where exposure to these compounds exceeds that experienced in towns by two or three orders of magnitude. British towns have been heavily polluted by coal smoke for very many years until the comparatively sudden decline in the last 25 years, yet the increase in incidence of bronchial carcinoma was seen to start soon after the First World War. Men were affected before women; the rate of increase in men is falling yet it continues to rise among women. The prevalence of the disease has increased as pollution by coal smoke has decreased. An urban excess over that observed in rural areas occurs in countries, such as Norway, in which there is little urban/rural difference in pollution by carcinogenic hydrocarbons. Despite these observations which diminish the argument for the contribution of air pollution, an explanation is still required for the excess of cases of carcinoma of the bronchus in town dwellers who do not smoke. Carcinogens other than the polycyclic hydrocarbons might be involved and the easier access to diagnostic facilities in the larger towns could have influenced the figures.

There are tars in wood smoke and it is likely that there will be concern about their possible carcinogenic properties as the use of wood as a fuel increases.

Chronic effects of exposure to the combustion products of gas may cause disease: the oxides of nitrogen produced by burning it in high temperature flames in unflued appliances are regarded with suspicion as an indoor pollutant which might favour the development of chronic bronchitis. There is no evidence that repeated exposure to low concentrations of carbon monoxide has chronic effects though the sequelae of acute poisoning, which include damage to the extrapyramidal system, may be chronic. Exposure to concentrations of carbon monoxide indoors too low to cause acute signs and symptoms may produce lassitude, fatigue, and vague headache. Should no other cause be found for such a picture, diligent enquiry and subsequent analyses of the air in the home may reveal pollution from a faulty appliance. Modern heating and building techniques designed to conserve energy, are leading to decreased ventilation rates in homes so that pollutants produced indoors now reach levels higher than formerly. This trend will continue.

Pollution from motor vehicles

Nature. Private cars are usually driven by petrol (gasoline) engines and heavier commercial vehicles are commonly diesel-powered, but there is a trend for diesel engines to be used in lighter vehicles, including private motor cars. There are important differences between the two types of engine which determine the nature of their exhaust products. In the petrol engine (spark ignition) fuel is burned in a stoichiometrically inadequate supply of air (it 'runs rich') and consequently its exhaust gases include carbon monoxide in addition to carbon dioxide and water. In contrast, the diesel engine (compression ignition) 'runs lean'; the fuel is burned in a considerable excess of air. The exhaust of a well-adjusted diesel engine ought to contain little more than a trace of carbon monoxide. Both engines emit oxides of nitrogen derived from fixation of atmospheric nitrogen and oxygen in the combustion chamber at high temperature and pressure. Nitric oxide predominates which, contrary to popular belief, oxidizes only slowly in the ambient air since it is, after emission, rapidly diluted. If a diesel engine is maladjusted, worn, or overloaded it may emit soot which consists of aggregates of very small particles of carbon (less than 1 μm diameter). These may be associated with small amounts of polycyclic aromatic hydrocarbons. Even a well-maintained diesel engine might emit a small puff of smoke on moving from a stationary position.

Although in crowded streets in calm weather carbon monoxide has been found in concentrations well in excess of those allowed in industry for continuous exposure for eight hours (50 parts per million by volume), kerbside concentrations in daytime are more usually about 20 parts per million which, if breathed indefinitely would produce a carboxyhaemoglobin saturation of about 3 per cent. In tunnels and car parks much higher ambient CO levels may occur. The absorption of carbon monoxide and the ultimate effect on the blood is dependent on the Haldane equation:

$$\text{COHb/HbO}_2 = \text{M} \, (P_{CO}/P_{O_2})$$

where M is the affinity constant (about 210 to 245) and P_{CO} and P_{O_2} are the ambient partial pressures of oxygen and carbon monoxide. The amount of carboxyhaemoglobin found in the blood will also depend on the duration of exposure and on pulmonary ventilation, as well as on the initial content before exposure to the polluted atmosphere. Table 1 gives examples of the relationship between ambient gas concentrations, exposure time, and COHb levels.

Table 1   Relation between ambient CO concentrations, exposure time, and levels of carboxyhaemoglobin*

Ambient CO		Carboxyhaemoglobin level (%) at		
mg/m³	p.p.m.	1 hour	8 hours	Equilibrium
117	100	3.6	12.9	16.0
70	60	2.5	8.7	10.0
35	30	1.3	4.0	5.0
23	20	0.8	2.8	3.3
12	10	0.4	1.4	1.7

* Assumes an average individual engaging in light activity and with an initial 'basal' value
From Lawther (1975)

In the non-smoker saturations of more than 3 per cent are rarely found as a result of exposure to traffic. Smokers who inhale the smoke commonly have levels of between 5 and 15 per cent COHb. The effects of smoking and exposure to air containing carbon monoxide are not simply additive; if at the beginning of exposure a subject's COHb is higher than that which would be in equilibrium with ambient carbon monoxide concentration, he will exhale the gas until equilibrium is achieved. The half-life of COHb at rest in a CO-free atmosphere is about four-and-a-half hours.

Modern petrol engines are designed to have a high compression ratio by which means performance and efficiency are increased, requiring fuel which has a high octane number. Should such engines be driven on petrol with low octane rating, performance falls and there is premature detonation of the fuel/air mixture (pinking); efficiency is decreased and damage may occur. In order to adjust the effective octane rating of petrols having a different hydrocarbon content, alkyl lead compounds (commonly tetraethyl lead) are added as antidetonants. At present in the United Kingdom petrol might contain as much as 0.4 g/l; this is to be reduced to 0.15 g/l by 1986. Other compounds, known as scavengers, are added in order to ensure that some of the lead compounds produced during combustion are retained, as the chlorobromo compounds, in the lubri-

cating oil. The remainder are emitted mostly as very small particles associated with complex aggregates of sub-micron size carbon particles. The 'bio-availability' of the lead on inhalation of these particles is the subject of current research. Diesel engines do not emit lead.

The relationship between the concentrations of lead in air and those in blood has been the subject of much research. There are good reasons for the assumption that 1 μg/m³ in air may contribute about 2 μg/dl to the blood lead. The relationship is curvilinear at higher concentrations but there appears to be rough linearity over the range encountered in non-industrial conditions. In places where pollution from traffic is high, such as on central reservations on motorways and in narrow crowded streets, the air might contain more than 6 μg/m³; more commonly, town air might contain between 2 and 3 μg/m³ near busy streets; the value falls to about 0.5 μg/m³ in suburban areas and to 0.1 μg/m³ in rural districts. Surveys of blood lead concentrations show mean differences between values found in inner city and outer suburban areas which are consistent with a relationship to air concentrations (the alpha value) of about 2 mentioned above. Mean blood lead values are usually less than 20 μg/dl. Much of the lead emitted by motor vehicles eventually settles and contributes to the lead content of deposited dust, and it can contaminate leafy crops growing by busy roads. Translocation of lead compounds from contaminated soil to the plant substance is less important when considering the total contribution made to the body burden by pollution by motor cars. Dust may be eaten by children. While the contribution made by the motor car is minor compared to that from food and drink, it can be proportionately high if these other sources are low. Similarly, if lead in food and drink has produced an unacceptably high burden, then any contribution from the air is potentially dangerous. Of the total lead in the air fouled by traffic, up to 10 per cent may be in the organic form, and comes mainly from spillages and evaporation of petrol.

Both types of engine emit hydrocarbons; these may be derived from feeding excess fuel or they may be new compounds derived from chemical reactions which have taken place in the engine. When a diesel engine is started from the cold state it may emit an aerosol of partly burned fuel together with other 'cracked' compounds which together form an intensely lachrymatory mixture; exhaust from operating diesel engines has a characteristic odour which many people find disagreeable. Some hydrocarbons, especially the olefines, may take part in complex secondary reactions in the presence of strong sunlight, ozone, and oxides of nitrogen forming the 'photochemical smog' which was first seen and studied in Los Angeles. Among the lachrymatory compounds formed as a result of these reactions are the peroxyacyl nitrates. Many regulations have been applied to motor vehicle exhausts in order to avoid the production of these secondary pollutants; these include the fitting of catalytic devices in which the hydrocarbons are oxidized. The catalysts used are poisoned by lead. Petrol engines also emit small amounts of polycyclic hydrocarbons, but emissions of this class of potentially carcinogenic hydrocarbons are small and localized when compared with the contribution from coal smoke which was common some years ago.

Usually the concentration of pollutants from motor vehicles falls away rapidly as distance from the source increases. Dilution is rapid and is aided by the turbulence caused by the movement of the vehicles. There are obvious exceptions to this general statement: dispersion is impaired in still weather, and canyon-like streets favour the accumulation of pollutants. Tunnels and car parks merit special attention.

Faulty exhaust systems may lead to serious pollution within a vehicle; the fumes caused by leaking fuel oil dripping on to a hot exhaust manifold have caused the death of at least one driver of a diesel van.

Effects. Of the pollutants emitted by motor vehicles, carbon monoxide is potentially the most toxic. It causes tissue hypoxia not merely by the formation of carboxyhaemoglobin but also because the presence of COHb shifts the dissociation curve of oxyhaemoglobin to the left. There are good reasons to suspect that exposure to the gas might, by causing hypoxia of the central nervous system, impair perception and the performance of fine tasks; the relevance of such effects on driving are obvious. However, as a result of carefully controlled trials and observations, no sound evidence has been produced which links such impairment with concentrations of COHb in the region of 5 to 8 per cent saturation. Lower concentrations have been shown to have an effect on the rate of onset of angina of effort and on ECG patterns in patients with ischaemic heart disease and it is reasonable to expect that pollution by carbon monoxide could affect unfavourably any patient whose tissues are hypoxic by virtue of disease of the cardiovascular or respiratory systems. Ambient concentrations which could lead to COHb levels of 2.5 per cent are held to be undesirable in such patients. Again, one must remember that exposure to high concentrations of carbon monoxide which might be found in tunnels and cark parks where ventilation is deficient, might have undesirable effects in special cases, though the time usually spent in such atmospheres by susceptible subjects is usually too short to allow the absorption of dangerous amounts of carbon monoxide. There have been notable exceptions.

The dominant contribution made by smoking must not be forgotten, but carbon monoxide derived from tobacco smoke produced by other persons is of little importance to the non-smoker.

The possible effects of lead absorbed from the air or from food polluted by motor exhausts have been the subject of much work and many review articles. Polluted air is but one source of lead and cannot be studied in isolation. Acute lead poisoning in children, almost always as a result of pica, may be followed by impairment of intelligence and certain behavioural disturbances; this fact has led many to suspect that the presence in the body of amounts of lead well below those seen to be associated with symptoms might be the cause of 'subclinical' impairment of intelligence, disturbances of behaviour and learning ability. The literature on this topic is vast and of grossly uneven quality; strong emotions are aroused. Careful assessment of the evidence by the British Department of Health and Social Security Working Party indicated that there was little doubt that blood lead levels in children of over 80 µg/dl were associated with impairment. There was some evidence that within the range of 35 µg/dl and 80 µg/dl deficits of intelligence quotients of up to 5 points could occur, but no such association had yet been demonstrated in children with blood levels below 35 µg/dl (which has been regarded as the 'paediatric upper limit of normal' in clinical practice). Whilst it is obvious that much work is needed in this important field, it must be borne in mind that airborne lead is but one source of the potentially toxic element. If body burdens from other sources are high, then any further contribution from the air could be undoubtedly most undesirable.

The DHSS Working Party made strong recommendations that lead in food, water, air, and paint be reduced and that attention be paid to adventitious sources. Any child whose blood lead levels exceeds 35 µg/dl ought to be investigated in order to identify the source leading to this high figure.

The soot emitted by faulty diesel motors is noisome and unnecessary. By causing offence to the nose and eye and by soiling it can cause stress, but there is no evidence that the polyclyclic hydrocarbons sometimes associated with the soot are a cause of lung cancer. The most important source of information on this vexed topic is the study of populations who are exposed in their occupation to high concentrations of exhaust products. The same comments apply to the polycyclic compounds emitted by petrol engines. Likewise there is no evidence that the oxides of nitrogen emitted by both types of vehicle cause ill effects, but they may take part in photochemical reactions which produce lachrymation and impair vision. Despite much work on the question there is little convincing evidence that the products of these complex reactions affect the lung although by the indirect effects of stress, they may cause

symptoms. Many people find the smell of the exhaust products of either type of vehicle objectionable enough to provoke stress. Ozone is involved in many secondary reactions and may sometimes reach concentrations (in the ambient air) which exceed the upper limit accepted in industrial atmospheres (0.1 parts per million by volume). In high concentrations this gas is a powerful irritant but no sound evidence has been put forward to support claims that concentrations found in the ambient air on occasion (usually in hot weather) have any demonstrable effects on health.

Adventitious sources of pollution. The pollutants of the ambient air which might come from industrial plants are legion. They may be prime products, intermediate compounds, or by-products. Useful information about the possible effects they may have on the general population may be derived from the study of the effects on healthy people exposed in the plant. But the general population includes those who are very young, elderly, or sick. Although the concentrations to which the general population might be exposed are almost always much less than those which the work force may experience, the duration of exposure might be greater outdoors and pollutants might include waste products to which the worker might not be exposed. The common practice of dividing the industrial maximum allowable concentration of a pollutant for workers by a factor (usually 40) to arrive at a concentration which might be acceptable to the general public is to be deplored. Results of sound epidemiological surveys and clinical observation ought to be studied. Extrapolation of experimental work on animals is of limited value in view of the different reactions of various species and the non-linear relation between dose and response. Ideally one would like to be able to forecast the effects of various pollutants from industry by knowing the mechanisms by which certain classes of compounds exert their effects. Hope that this sort of predictive toxicology might prevent exposure of the public to harmful compounds is dashed when minute concentrations of substances such as crocidolite asbestos are seen to produce such rare tumours as mesotheliomata among people in the neighbourhood of industrial sources after many years of exposure. Similarly there was no reason to suppose that a molecule as simple as vinyl chloride used in the plastics industry could cause angiosarcoma of the liver. Beryllium in minute amounts has been found to cause illness in people living near factories in which it is used. Lead has been mentioned at some length as a pollutant from motor cars; much higher amounts may be found in the neighbourhood of lead smelters and other works using the metal. Casual trades such as scrap metal dealing and the burning of old car batteries have produced dangerous amounts of lead in the communal air.

When considering the possible effects of the emission of a pollutant from an industrial source, attention must be paid to its physical and chemical nature as well as to the amount evolved. The emission of fluorine compounds is an example of the importance of this; fluoride from brickworks and aluminium smelters falls out rapidly and affects grazing animals rather than humans living in the area. Dioxin, which is extremely toxic, can be produced accidentally if the reaction producing the herbicide 2,4,5T overheats. There has been catastrophic dissemination of this compound in industrial accidents. The seriousness of such events is due to the persistence of this very stable compound on surfaces and soil. It exerts its effects through skin contact and ingestion. Some pollutants, such as cement dust, are too coarse to enter the lung and cause pneumoconioses but they ought not to be dismissed as a mere nuisance since they may be hazardous in relation to the sequelae of the stress they may cause. The same caution must be exercised when tempted to dismiss odours as being merely a nuisance.

There is a common tendency to dismiss the effects of cigarette smoking as being harmless to persons other than the smoker. Mention has been made of the possible role of parental smoke on the development of bronchitis in children, and the contribution to non-smokers' body burden of carbon monoxide has been dismissed, but the irritant effects of the smoke may be intolerable to a patient with chronic bronchitis and may indeed lead to irreversible effects in a seriously ill patient by virtue of the coughing and bronchospasm it might provoke.

The list of air pollutants is virtually endless: the effects of many are unknown; the vast amount of published work reflects the complexity of the subject as well as our ignorance. The variety of pollutants will increase as industrial processes diversify. Dramatic trends have been seen in many places as a result of the implementation of preventive legislation and these changes must be taken into account in studies of mortality and morbidity. The references quoted below contain more detailed accounts and extensive bibliographies of the commoner problems met with in clinical medicine.

References

Department of Health and Social Security Working Party (1980). *Lead and health* HMSO, London.
Ellison, J. McK. and Waller, R. E. (1978). A review of sulphur oxides and particulate matter as air pollutants with particular reference to effects on health in the United Kingdom. *Env. Res.* **16**, 302.
Hobson, W. (ed.) (1979). *Theory and practice of public health*, 5th edn. Oxford University Press, Oxford.
Lawther, P. J. and Waller, R. E. (1978). Trends in urban air pollution in the United Kingdom in relation to lung cancer mortality. *Env. Hlth Perspectives* **22**, 71.
Ministry of Health (1954). *Mortality and morbidity during the London fog of December 1952.* HMSO, London.
Royal College of Physicians (1970). *Air pollution and health.* Pitman, London.
World Health Organization (1972). *Air quality criteria and guides for urban air pollutants.* World Health Organization, Geneva.
— (1979). *Sulfur oxides and suspended particulate matter.* Environmental Health Criteria no. 8. World Health Organization, Geneva.

NON-FILARIAL ENDEMIC ELEPHANTIASIS OF THE LOWER LEGS

E. W. Price

A non-filarial but endemic form of elephantiasis limited to the lower legs has been described in Africa and Central and South America under a variety of names: pseudo-lepra, verrucosis lymphostatica, lymphoedema, chronic sclerosing lymphangitis, Robles–Lowenthal disease. The clinical entity is characterized by bilateral but asymmetrical swelling of the feet and lower legs as a result of obstructive lymphopathy of the distal superficial lymphatics.

Aetiology. The disease is found in tropical or subtropical areas at an altitude between 1000 and 2000 m, with certain recognizable features. Affected areas are usually notably fertile with seasons alternately wet and dry. The underlying rocks are volcanic and produce a slippery, reddish-brown adhesive clay which is characteristic of an endemic area. The disease has also been noted at the mouths of some rivers draining affected highlands.

It occurs in both sexes in a barefooted population engaged in arable farming, and may affect as many as 60 per 1000 adults in a hyperendemic area. The recognition of a familial tendency is reflected in various objections to marrying into an 'elephantiasic' family. This tendency has led to speculations of a possible congenital inadequacy of the lymphatic system of the lower legs as a contributory factor.

The occurrence in some cases of episodes of acute lymphangitis, when a streptococci may sometimes be found in the lymph, has suggested 'repeated erysipelas' as a cause, but the disease may develop in the absence of acute attacks.

More recently the presence of microparticles of silica and alumino-silicates has been noted in the macrophages of the femoral lymph-nodes (Fig. 1). An associated fibrosis of the afferent lymphatics has raised the possibility that the disease is a silicosis of the

peripheral lymphatics following absorption of these substances from the soil through the feet. The colloid size typical of clay particles facilitates any passage through skin or up sweat ducts.

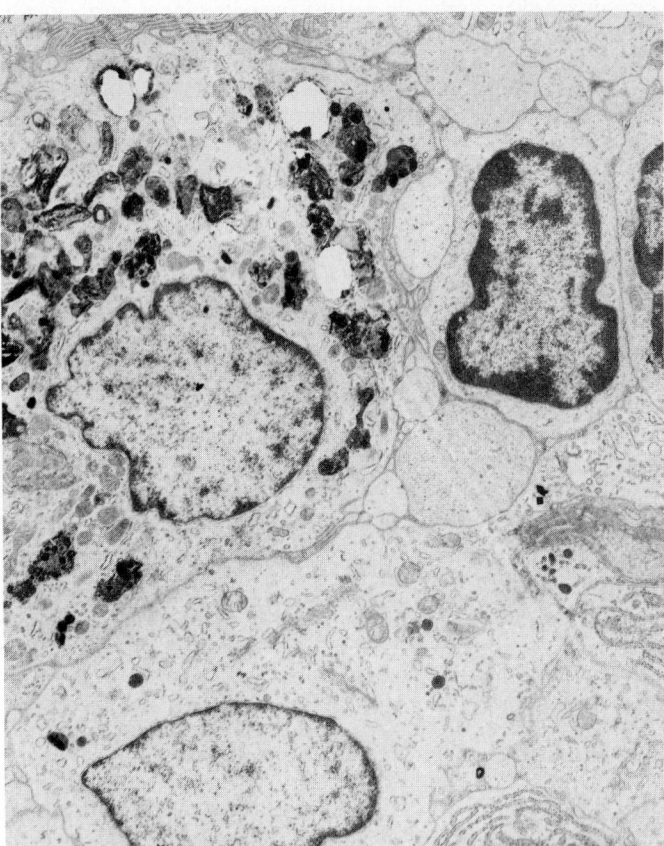

Fig. 1 Micrograph of femoral lymph-node of an elephantiasic. Note two macrophages on the left, the upper of which contains a number of clumps of microparticles. On analysis, most of these were silica with varying amounts of aluminium, iron, and titanium (× 7200).

Pathology. In the early stages of the disease, the peripheral lymphatics may be found by lymphography to be dilated or irregular in number and diameter. Multiple microgranulomata may be seen in relation to the sinuses of the node, and eventually macrophages appear which contain electron-dense particles of less than two microns within their phagolysosomes. On analysis these consist of silica, mainly amorphous, with varying amounts of aluminium, iron, and titanium. Some larger particles are crystalline and may be bi-refringent.

As the disease develops, there is evidence of loss of lymph-flow through the node, with fibrous thickening of the capsule. Histological evidence implies that the block to lymph-flow is in the peripheral lymphatics, which in a late stage are fibrotic and even indistinguishable in the fibrotic subcutaneous tissues. Lymphography is not easily accomplished because of the pathology of the peripheral lymphatics.

Clinical appearances. These vary with the type of disease and may be described as 'water-bag', 'rubbery', and 'wooden'. The type is usually established in the early stages of the disease, and remains a feature unless repeated infective episodes produce induration of the skin and superficial tissues. The recognition of the type is important for planning effective treatment.

The *'water-bag'* type is bulky and soft with smooth, relatively healthy oedematous skin which can be picked up between the fingers, sometimes with pitting oedema (Fig. 2(a)). There may be large horizontal folds in front of the ankle. On elevation of the limb, the size diminishes considerably during four or five days, but, except in the early stages, never entirely.

At the other extreme, the 'wooden' type is hard, the skin cannot be picked between the fingers, and is fibrous, with marked hyperkeratosis, especially distally and in front of the ankle; local globular swellings of 0.5–2 cm diameter may occur, notably at the base of the toe–clefts and on the transverse folds in front of the ankle (Fig. 2(b)). Dermatologically, it is known as 'nodular subepidermal fibrosis of Michelson' and ascribed to microtraumata; but it occurs also in other conditions. Bacterial infection at the base of these nodules is common and produces an unpleasant odour which is a characteristic of the disease.

Between these two are the common or 'rubbery' types, with features of both 'water-bag' and 'wooden'.

Natural history. The disease progresses through a prodromal to a progressive and finally permanent stage. The prodromal symptoms include a burning sensation with or without itching over the track of the main lymphatic channels of the lower legs; discomfort of the femoral lymph nodes is sometimes experienced. The symptoms occur commonly at night in bed and are alleviated by uncovering the leg. Unaccustomed use of the legs, sitting before a fire, the drinking of alcohol, or the occurrence of the monthly menses may initiate symptoms. These are confined initially to one or other leg.

In the absence of treatment, the progressive stage supervenes. Itching with slight thickening of the skin of the dorsum of the foot around the base of the first toe cleft on one or other side appears, at first intermittently, but finally permanently, and spreads with or without acute episodes, proximally on the dorsum of the foot as far as the ankle. The skin is thickened and loses its hair and sweat glands. The oozing of lymph commonly attracts flies. Hyperkeratosis is common. Both legs may be affected together but one side is always more advanced than the other. The second foot may not be affected for some time, or may show plantar oedema only, leading to statements that one-sided disease has been observed.

The progressive stage is sometimes interrupted by acute episodes of infective or non-effective lymphangitis with tender swelling of the femoral nodes, but suppuration is rare. The episode, often induced by long exertion, may begin with rigor a few hours after the exertion and incapacitates the patient for several days. There is tense and reddened swelling of the lower limb which, when the episode subsides, leaves an increase in size and extent for the swelling. An acute episode rarely affects both legs at the same time.

The permanent stage is reached either spontaneously or as a result of treatment. Elderly patients commonly report the cessation of acute episodes or of progression with age.

Treatment. The efficacy of active treatment depends on the clinical type of disease, the 'water-bag' type responding best and the 'wooden', least. The oedema can be reduced either by elevation of the limb or by intermittent compression. The 'water-bag' type decreases in size within 48–72 hours, and may then be controlled by compressive stockings; these reduce the frequency of acute attacks but are usually insufficient to prevent swelling recurring. In this event, long leather boots, reaching up to the knee, have proved to be the only effective measure; plastic or other substitutes do not sustain the pressure for long.

More rapid reduction of swelling can be achieved by intermittent compression machines, providing repeated pressures of 90 mmHg for periods of 50 seconds, followed by 10 seconds relaxation. Details are given by Price (1975). The surgical removal of nodules is facilitated by their lack of sensory nerves.

Only minimal reduction in size can be achieved in the 'wooden' types, and treatment is limited to the protection of the hard skin from traumata and secondary infection.

In all cases, the condition can be alleviated or its progression arrested by the transfer of the patient to live in a non-endemic area, as has been long recognized by the local people.

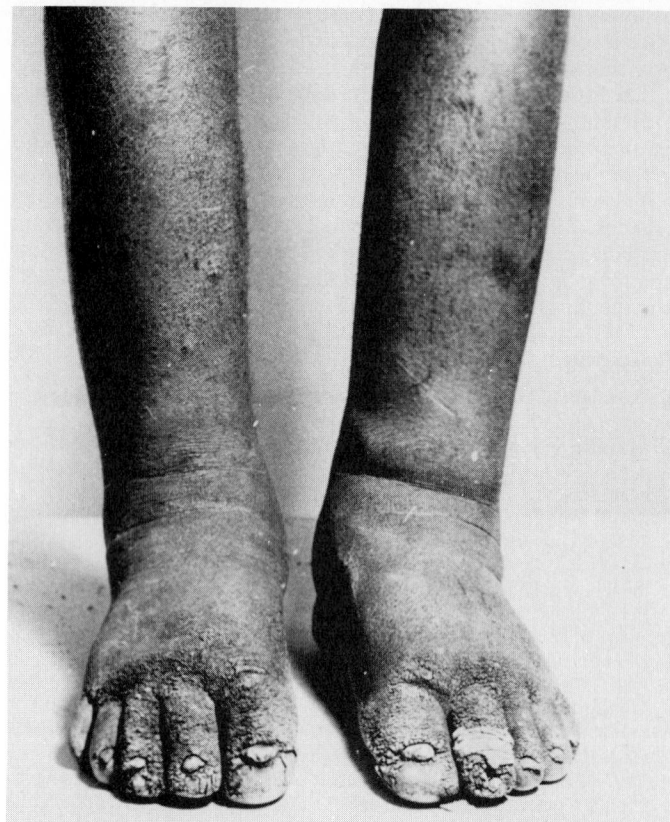

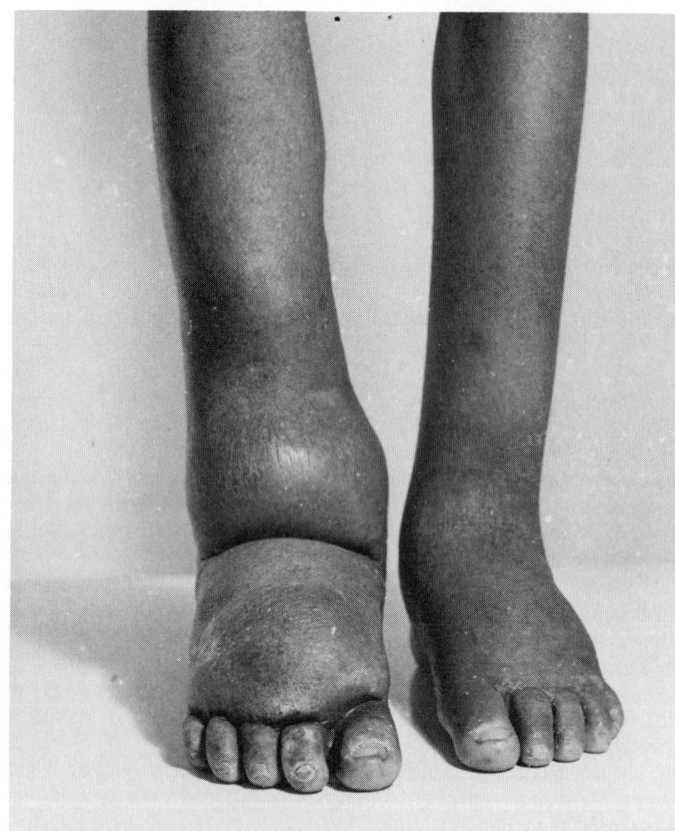

Fig. 2 Clinical types of elephantiasis: (a) the wet or 'water-bag' type. Swelling readily reduced by compression or elevation. Skin soft and can be pinched off the bones; (b) the dry or 'wooden' type. Swelling irreducible by compression or elevation. Note prominence of hyperkeratosis of toes with trauma to one toe. Nodulation is frequent.

Prophylactically, and in the present state of knowledge, children of elephantiasic families are well-advised to use footwear as far as possible, and to keep the feet clean; but the economic situation of many of these families make some type of subsidy desirable if this is to be practicable.

References

Price E. W. (1972). The pathology of endemic elephantiasis of the lower legs. *Trans. R. Soc. trop. Med. Hyg.* **66**. 150.
— (1974). Endemic elephantiasis—natural history and clinical study. *Trans. R. Soc. trop. Med. Hyg.* **68**. 44.
— (1975). Management of endemic elephantiasis. *Tropical Doctor* **5**. 70.

Occupational diseases

OCCUPATIONAL EXPOSURE TO NOXIOUS AGENTS

G. Kazantzis

From industrial disease to occupational health. Occupational medicine is a broad discipline concerned with the interaction between health and work. That certain occupations were injurious to health was known since ancient times, for Hippocrates recognized lead colic and Pliny described mercurialism in the slaves who worked the mercury mines at Almaden in Spain. Agricola (1494–1555) gave a classic description of metalliferous mining in Central Europe and observed the harmful effects on the lungs of the inhalation of dry dust. However, it was Ramazzini (1633–1714) professor of medicine in Padua, who first systematized industrial diseases and taught on the importance of enquiring about a patient's occupation in history taking.

In the United Kingdom the industrial revolution brought its attendant evils of overcrowding, environmental pollution, insanitary conditions, and infectious and industrial disease. The Leeds physician, Charles Thackrah (1795–1833) wrote of the miners who 'rarely work for more than six hours a day, yet they seldom attain the age of forty' and of the price paid for Sheffield cutlery: 'the fork-grinders, who use a dry grindstone, die at the age of 28 or 32, while the table-knife grinders who work on wet stones, survive to between 40 and 50'. In 1900, over 1000 cases of lead poisoning were notified to the statutory authority, compared with 23 cases in 1978. During the present century industrial technology has expanded at an ever increasing rate, a great number of new chemical compounds have been synthesized and used in industry, ionizing radiation has found increasing uses, and gas and oil are being recovered from beneath the sea. However, despite increasing hazards, industrial disease, with the exception of injury, is becoming progressively less prominent in the United Kingdom and other industrial communities. This control has been brought about by what may be summarized as a conceptual change from the acceptance of industrial disease to the promotion of occupational health. Thus occupational medicine has now become in large part a discipline in the prevention of disease. However, there is a danger that many developing countries today, through a combination of failure to recognize needs and inadequate resources to meet them, may repeat the unfortunate experiences of Britain and other pioneer countries in the industrial revolution.

From the Factory Act, 1833, which appointed inspectors and regulated the labour of children in the mills and factories of Britain, legislation has been progressively introduced aimed at the protection of the worker, culminating in replacement of the cumbrous legal edifice which had evolved, by the Health and Safety at Work Act, 1974. This was an enabling act covering all aspects of health and safety at work including the use, storage and transport of potentially noxious agents, control of processes which may affect the health and safety of the general public, emissions into the atmosphere, and the disposal of waste. The Health and Safety Executive is responsible for enforcing the statutory provisions through its inspectorates and Employment Medical Advisory Service (EMAS). They have a right of entry into work places and powers to issue improvement or prohibition notices to require action to be taken against dangerous processes. The main functions of the medical arm, EMAS, are helping to prevent ill health caused by work and advising people with health problems on suitable or inappropriate work on health grounds. It will advise the inspectors on medical matters; and employers, unions, workers, and medical practitioners on the risks from dangerous substances and other problems. The Act places the onus on employers and the employed to ensure that safe systems of work are maintained. Thus employers have to prepare safety policies and establish safety committees, and employees have a duty to co-operate with employers in meeting the statutory requirements.

Notifiable and prescribed diseases. Certain industrial diseases have for long been compulsorily notifiable, now to the Chief Employment Medical Adviser, where the diagnosis is suspected by the medical practitioner. Such notification serves a useful purpose in control and prevention, by enabling EMAS to investigate the circumstances under which the disease had arisen and to take appropriate action. The notifiable diseases are shown in Table 1.

Table 1 Industrial diseases statutorily notifiable to the Chief Employment Medical Adviser

Lead poisoning, including organic lead compounds
Arsenic poisoning, including organic arsenic compounds
Mercury poisoning, including organic mercury compounds
Phosphorus poisoning, including organic phosphorus compounds and their anticholinesterase action
Manganese poisoning
Beryllium disease
Cadmium poisoning
Chrome ulceration
Carbon bisulphide poisoning
Aniline poisoning
Chronic benzene poisoning
Toxic jaundice
Toxic anaemia
Epitheliomatous ulceration due to tar, pitch, bitumen, mineral oil, or paraffin or products containing these
Anthrax
Compressed air illness

Certain processes which involve health risks, for example in the lead industry, are governed by regulations which require workers to be examined at regular intervals. Such examinations are performed by EMAS or by other doctors specially appointed for the purpose.

Persons who have contracted certain industrial diseases are entitled to financial benefit under the Social Security Act, 1975. These are known as the Prescribed Diseases and Part I of the schedule is shown in Table 2. Part 2 is concerned with pneumoconiosis and byssinosis. A claimant has to show that he has worked in a scheduled occupation, that is, one recognized as offering a risk of

Table 2   The Prescribed Diseases (Part I) with abridged notes on the nature of the occupations which may give rise to them

PD
no. Description of disease or injury

Poisoning by:
1 Lead or a compound of lead
2 Manganese or a compound of manganese
3 Phosphorus, phosphine, or poisoning due to the anticholinesterase action of organic phosphorus compounds
4 Arsenic or a compound of arsenic
5 Mercury or a compound of mercury
6 Carbon disulphide
7 Benzene or a homologue
8 A nitro- or amino- or chloro-derivative of benzene or of a homologue of benzene, or poisoning by nitrochlorbenzene
9 Dinitrophenol or a homologue or by substituted dinitrophenols or by the salts of such substances
10 Tetrachlorethane
11 Tricresyl phosphate
12 Triphenyl phosphate
13 Diethylene dioxide (dioxan)
14 Methyl bromide
15 Chlorinated naphthalene
16 Nickel carbonyl
17 Nitrous fumes
18 *Gonioma kamassi* (African boxwood)
19 Anthrax
20 Glanders
21 (a) Infection by *Leptospira iterohaemorrhagiae*
   (b) Infection by *Leptospira canicola*
22 Ancylostomiasis in work in or about a mine
23 (a) Dystrophy of the cornea (including ulceration of the corneal surface)
   (b) Localized new growth of the skin, papillomatous, or keratotic
   (c) Squamous-cell carcinoma of the skin due to arsenic, tar, pitch, bitumen, mineral oil (including paraffin), or any compound, product, or residue, including quinone or hydroquinone
25 Inflammation, ulceration, or malignant disease of the skin, subcutaneous tissues, or of the bones; blood dyscrasia, or cataract due to electromagnetic radiations (other than radiant heat) or to ionizing particles
26 Heat cataract following exposure to rays from molten or red hot material
27 Decompression sickness
28 Cramp of the hand or forearm due to repetitive movements
31 Subcutaneous cellulitis of the hand (beat hand)
32 Bursitis or subcutaneous cellulitis of the knee (beat knee)
33 Bursitis or subcutaneous cellulitis of elbow (beat elbow)
34 Traumatic inflammation of tendons of hand or forearm or of their tendon sheaths
35 Miners' nystagmus
36 Poisoning by beryllium or compound of beryllium
37 Carcinoma of mucous membrane of nose or associated air sinuses and primary carcinoma of bronchus or lung following exposure to nickel by decomposition of a gaseous nickel compound
38 Tuberculosis in a health care worker or in a research or laboratory worker exposed to infected material
39 Primary neoplasm of epithelial lining of bladder, renal pelvis, or ureter associated with work in a building in which one of a group of specified aromatic amines is produced, or any occupation involving the handling, or contamination by these substances
40 Poisoning by cadmium
41 Inflammation or ulceration of the mucosae of the upper respiratory tract or mouth produced by dust, liquid, or vapour
42 Non-infective dermatitis, including chrome ulceration following exposure to dust, liquid, or vapour or other external agent capable of irritating the skin
43 Farmers' lung
44 Primary malignant neoplasm of the mesothelium of the pleura or peritoneum in relation to asbestos exposure
45 Adenocarcinoma of the nasal cavity or associated air sinuses in work in a building where wooden furniture is manufactured
46 Infection by *Brucella abortus* in farm workers and others occupationally exposed to infected material
47 Poisoning by acrylamide monomer
48 Permanent sensorineural hearing loss due to occupational noise amounting to at least 50 dB in the better ear
49 Viral hepatitis following close and frequent contact with blood or blood products or with a source of viral hepatitis in health care personnel
50a Angio sarcoma of the liver following work in or about a plant for the polymerization of vinyl chloride monomer
50b Osteolysis of the terminal phalanges of the fingers, as in PD 50
51 Carcinoma of the nasal cavity or associated air sinuses in work in a building used for the manufacture or repair of footwear made wholly or partly of leather or fibreboard
52 Occupational vitiligo
53 Occupational asthma

developing the disease. The table shows the wide range of disorders which can be clearly identified as capable of being occupational in origin.

Occupational health services. Occupational health services in the United Kingdom are outside the jurisdiction of the National Health Service and are provided voluntarily by the larger private and nationalized industries. In some parts of the country, where there is a concentration of small and medium-sized industry, occupational health services have been set up on a group basis. However, much of the workforce employed in small industrial undertakings remains without adequate occupational health cover. This system, in which the state plays a supervisory and advisory role within a statutory framework requiring the employer to provide certain services has in general been adopted by the countries of the European Economic Community and the USA. In the latter, the National Institute of Occupational Safety and Health is responsible for recommending hygiene standards which have received a measure of international acceptance. In Eastern Europe the state is responsible for the provision of occupational health services. At an international level, the World Health Organization and the International Labour Office are actively engaged in the setting of standards for occupational safety and health, with emphasis on the needs of developing countries.

Prevention of occupational disease. Health risks are commonly identified by observing adverse effects on people at work, and clinical observation has more often provided the first indication of such a risk. This may require confirmation by epidemiological investigation, which provides the only method for detecting an excess risk in an occupational group of a disease which is also common in the general population. The risk can be quantified where data are available to establish an exposure–effect (or dose–response) relationship. However, the setting of standards for safe working conditions presents considerable problems. The earliest effect may be difficult to detect, may be behavioural rather than physical, or may consist of a change in a biochemical parameter of uncertain significance. Again the exposure, or dose received, may be difficult to determine, especially where this is culmulative over a long period and where a latent interval of years exists between initial exposure and the recognition of an adverse effect or disease. All human activity involves a degree of risk. Scientific enquiry at its best can establish an exposure–effect relationship in terms of risk, but it is for society to decide on an acceptable level of risk in relation to standard setting.

A health risk may also be predicted and thus an adverse effect prevented from occurring. In a number of countries new substances which are intended for industrial use are screened for hazard evaluation, taking account of their physical, chemical, and biological properties, utilizing tests for toxicity, carcinogenicity, mutagenicity, teratogenicity, and assessing their behaviour in the environment. In the United Kingdom, new substances to be used in quantities greater than 1 tonne per annum are to be screened in this way.

Environmental monitoring. Noxious agents in the working environment may take the form of gases, vapours, fumes, dusts, and both ionizing and non-ionizing radiation. Other physical factors are extremes of temperature and pressure, high intensity noise, and vibration. The measurement of exposure to these various agents requires specialized equipment and methodology and is best performed by trained industrial hygienists. Environmental monitoring is necessary to maintain exposures below those associated with adverse effects. Airborne contaminants are monitored by air sampling techniques. In the USA and Western Europe, permissible levels of exposure are expressed in terms of Threshold Limit Values (TLVs). These represent conditions under which it is believed that nearly all workers may be repeatedly exposed day after day without adverse effect. Because of wide variation in individual susceptibility, however, a small percentage of workers may experience discomfort from some substances at concentrations at or below the threshold limit; a smaller percentage may be affected more seriously by aggravation of a pre-existing condition or by development of an occupational illness. Thus, adherence to a TLV does not ensure worker safety, and in practice exposure levels should be kept well below this value. TLVs are expressed as time weighted average concentrations for a normal eight-hour work day or 40-hour week, in parts per million and mg/m^3.

Biological monitoring. A measure of absorption via respiratory, gastrointestinal, and dermal routes may be obtained by estimating the concentration of an environmental chemical agent in blood or its excretion in the urine, or by estimating a metabolite, enzyme, or other altered biochemical parameter. Such estimations may be more reliable indicators of health risks than environmental measurements, but they require the active participation of the worker. Biological monitoring should be regarded as complementary to environmental monitoring and in practice both procedures are often employed. Biological monitoring for absorption of toxic agents forms one part of more general health monitoring, including periodic medical examinations.

Control measures. *Substitution.* A health hazard can be eliminated by substituting a noxious material or a hazardous process by a safer alternative. Thus silica grindstones which gave rise to silicosis in the Sheffield cutlery industry have been replaced by carborundum, aromatic amines causing bladder cancer used as anti-oxidants in the rubber industry have been replaced by other compounds and crocidolite or blue asbestos responsible for mesothelioma is no longer imported into the United Kingdom. However, the substitute could turn out to be even more hazardous, especially if inadequately tested for long-term effects.

Segregation. Where a hazardous process has to be performed, it is good practice to isolate this in order to limit those exposed to essential workers who can be more readily kept under close surveillance. A potential environmental hazard can be more effectively contained in this way. Nuclear power stations, for example, are built in isolated sites.

Enclosure. The fume cupboard in a chemistry laboratory is a familiar example of an enclosure where toxic chemicals can be handled in relative safety. Hazardous materials can be handled in totally enclosed cabinets through gloved inlets and radioactive sources can be appropriately shielded and handled with mechanical devices or by automation.

Exhaust ventilation. A fume cupboard functions under a small negative pressure so that air is drawn in from the laboratory to prevent the emission of toxic chemicals. Many industrial processes use exhaust ventilation at the site of origin of a toxic fume or dust, which may be applied to a small source on the work bench or to a series of furnaces in a foundry. Exhaust ventilation systems to be effective have to be correctly designed and are expensive. The exhausted material may have to be recovered, for its emission into the atmosphere may give rise to widespread environmental pollution.

Dust suppression. It may be possible to suppress dust at its site of origin thus preventing its dissemination into the atmosphere of the workplace. This simple method has been successfully used in the miners' drill where a jet of water wets the dust as it is generated. Many processes can be carried out in wet stages thus minimizing the handling of chemicals in powder form.

Good housekeeping. This evocative term implies a well-ordered, clean and tidy system of work practice. Work places may require frequent hosing with water or vacuum cleaning and adequate provision has to be made for the disposal of waste, which is often controlled by legislation for the protection of the environment.

Personal protection. The workers may require protection with a complete set of appropriate clothing, boots, gloves, and head gear. Contaminated clothing is removed at the end of the work shift, the worker passing through a shower to gain access to his outdoor clothes. The miner's hat, metal toe caps in boots, and the radiologist's lead apron are examples of specialized protective equipment. The eyes may require protection with goggles, the ears with ear muffs or plugs, and the hands with barrier creams. Respiratory protection is afforded with a variety of masks, ranging from simple dust filters to helmets with external airlines. Protection against infection acquired through work may require immunization. The problem with all personal protective measures is the reliance on the individual worker in their use. Familiarity with work processes breeds contempt for their hazards. Medical research workers take short cuts in the handling of pathogens and chemical carcinogens and construction workers on building sites often do not wear their hard hats.

Worker education. Good housekeeping, safe work procedures, and compliance with procedures for personal protection can be fostered by providing information on the nature of the hazard and the methods for its containment. Health and safety representatives and committees help to ensure active worker participation in all measures directed to health and safety.

The diagnosis of industrial disease. All clinical history taking should include some information on the patient's present occupation. This is important not only in the diagnosis of industrial disease, but also for assessing the patient's suitability for his job in relation to his illness. Unhelpful descriptive terms such as 'maintenance worker', 'process' worker, or 'fitter' should be avoided, for all may be exposed to noxious agents at work. Where an industrial disease may be suspected, it is necessary to take a full occupational history, starting with the first job after leaving school and proceeding in chronological order, with approximate dates, to include an adequate description of what each job entailed. Spare-time occupations and even hobbies may be relevant. It should be borne in mind that the present, or the last job may not be the relevant one with respect to the patient's illness. An asbestos worker or a miner with reduced effort tolerance will seek a less demanding job and a cancer may be related to an exposure at work more than forty years previously. Where the patient is unable to provide information on the nature of his work exposure, this may often be obtained, in confidence, from the occupational physician, the regional employment medical adviser, the company management, or the manufacturer of a material used at work.

The occupational history may be of importance in assessing the contribution of the work environment to pre-existing, non-occupational disease. This may be exacerbated not only by physical but also by psychosocial factors encountered at work. Finally, the effect of health and capacity for work is of relevance not only to the patient but also to the health and safety of the public. Airline pilots, drivers of public service and heavy goods vehicles, other railway workers, health care staff, food handlers, administrators, and senior government officials are examples of categories of workers whose health is of great relevance to the society in which they function and whose health requires appropriate surveillance.

Classification of occupational noxious agents. An adverse reaction to an occupational exposure may be immediate, as following the inhalation of a chemical or a simple asphyxiant gas, may occur within a few hours, as with occupational asthma or allergic alveolitis, or within days, months, or years following initial exposure. Many chemical agents absorbed in trace quantities while at work accumulate in critical organs to give rise to subacute and to chronic poisoning. Thus the heavy metals such as lead, mercury, and cadmium although excreted in part, accumulate in the body and may cause chronic intoxication. Some exposures cause cancer after a latent interval ranging from a few to more than 40 years. Physical, chemical, and biological agents may affect the embryo to be responsible for abortion, stillbirth, or teratogenic effects, and exposure of both male and female germ cells may give rise to adverse mutagenic effects. The more important categories of occupational agents which cause adverse health effects are shown in Table 3, and some of these are discussed below while others are referred to elsewhere in this work.

PRINCIPAL ADVERSE HEALTH EFFECTS OF OCCUPATION

Respiratory system

The respiratory tract and the skin are readily accessible to noxious agents in the working environment and not surprisingly they manifest a high proportion of all occupational disease. The more important noxious agents which are absorbed through the lung with the main types of pulmonary reaction to these are shown in Table 4.

Table 3 Classification of principle occupational factors giving rise to adverse health effects

Category	Agent	Examples of principal effects
Physical	trauma	head and skeletal injury; backache; tenosynovitis; beat disorders
	heat and cold	heat cramps; heat exhaustion and stroke; hypothermia; cold tissue injury
	atmospheric pressure	decompression sickness; aseptic necrosis of bone
	noise	occupational deafness; psychoneurosis
	vibration	Raynaud syndrome; gangrene of fingers
	radiation	
	ionizing	acute radiation syndrome; depression of haemopoiesis; radiation dermatitis; malignant disease, teratogenic, and mutagenic effects
	non-ionizing	thermal effects; cataract; skin cancer; miners' nystagmas
Chemical	industrial e.g., metals, solvents, plastics, dyes and paints	acute and chronic poisoning; teratogenic and mutagenic effects; hypersensitivity reactions; irritant dermatitis; behavioural effects
	fibrogenic dusts (in part physical)	coalworkers' pneumoconiosis; silicosis; asbestosis; other pneumoconioses
	pharmaceutical	steroid, hormone, and antineoplastic drug effects
	agricultural pesticides	orgenophospherous and carbonate poisoning; paraquat; arsenicals; thallium
Biological	plants, woods and venomous predators	hypersensitivity reactions; acute poisoning
	parasites	anclyostomiasis; schistosomiasis; malaria
	bacteria	anthrax; brucellosis; glanders; leptospirosis; tetanus; tuberculosis
	rickettsial and viruses	Q fever; ornithosis; yellow fever; rabies; hepatitis; lassa fever; Marburg disease
	fungi	histoplasmosis; allergic alveolitis, e.g., farmers' lung
Psychosocial	physical inactivity cigarette smoking stress	} coronary heart disease
	shift work	disruption of circadian rhythms; sleep disorders; peptic ulcer
	job dissatisfaction alcoholism stress over- or underwork	} work absence, psychoneurosis, low morale, industrial unrest

Table 4 Principal inhalational hazards of occupational origin with pulmonary reactions to these

Acute reactions
  Systemic intoxication
    Carbon monoxide; cyanides; hydrogen sulphide; solvents; toxic metals
  Asphyxiants
    Carbon dioxide; nitrogen; methane
  Irritants
    Ozone; phosgene; oxides of nitrogen and sulphur; ammonia; chlorine; some metallic compounds
  Specific infections
    Tuberculosis; anthrax; Q fever; ornithosis; coccidiomycosis; histoplasmosis
  Asthma
    See Table 5
  Extrinsic allergic alveolitis
    See Table 6

Chronic reactions
  Pulmonary fibrosis
    Silica; coal dust; asbestos; talc; kaolin; fuller's earth; mica; haematite; 'hard metal', graphite
  Cancer
    Asbestos; ionizing radiation; chromium and nickel ore processing; arsenic; polycyclic hydrocarbons in coal gas manufacture; ?cadmium; ?beryllium
  Other effects
    Cadmium oxide (emphysema); aluminium oxide (emphysema and fibrosis); beryllium (granuloma and fibrosis)

Acute reactions. Acute reactions may manifest with asphyxia, irritative, inflammatory, or asthmatic symptoms. A number of highly toxic substances are absorbed through the respiratory tract but have systemic rather than local effects. Carbon monoxide, hydrogen cyanide, hydrogen sulphide, many organic solvents, and metal fumes and dusts and their compounds act in this way. The asphyxiants, carbon dioxide, nitrogen, and methane act by excluding oxygen. They are dangerous because they are colourless, odourless, and non-irritant so that workmen may meet them unawares and be overcome before rescue is possible. These gases are found principally in wells, tunnels, pits, and mines, although carbon dioxide is also encountered in cellars, boiler rooms, and silos. Nitrogen with carbon dioxide is known as 'black damp' and methane as 'fire damp' by miners.

Of the irritant gases, nitrous fumes, ozone, and phosgene may produce minor effects at the time of inhalation but delayed pulmonary oedema may have a fatal outcome some hours later. Nitrous fumes are evolved in many chemical processes, in electric arc welding, in silos at certain stages of fermentation, in explosions, and in fires. Phosgene is evolved when certain halogenated hydrocarbons are overheated. Sulphur dioxide, ammonia, and chlorine are more intensely irritant when inhaled, producing cough, irritation of the eyes and nose, laryngeal spasm, tracheobronchitis, bronchopneumonia, and sometimes delayed pulmonary oedema. These gases are encountered in mining, agriculture, fire fighting, and in the chemical and metal industries.

Inhalation of beryllium dust or fume or of cadmium fume may give rise to a delayed chemical pneumonitis (see below). Transient systemic and respiratory symptoms with fever and rigors may follow some hours after the inhalation of freshly formed zinc oxide fume, a condition known as metal fume fever or brass founders' ague.

Asthma and extrinsic allergic alveolitis may follow the inhalation of a variety of organic products of animal, vegetable, or microbial origin or certain groups of chemicals, in particular isocyanates, epoxy resin curing agents, certain complex platinum salts, and formaldehyde. Many occupations are involved, especially farming, and in the food, textile, pharmaceutical, and detergent industries, where the chemical compounds are encountered in the manufacture of foam rubber, paints, and plastics, in metal refining, and in health care services. Whereas most occupational diseases reflect both toxicity and dose of the aetiological agent, in the asthma/alveolitis group of disorders, susceptibility appears related to a state of hypersensitivity which develops after a variable latent interval and is not dose related. Further consideration of these acute reactions is given in the section on occupational allergies. Respiratory infectious disease occurs in persons whose work brings them into close contact with human or animal sources. Tuberculosis remains an increased risk in health service personnel. Q fever and ornithosis are widespread infections in such groups as farmers and poultry keepers, and pulmonary anthrax, now virtually unknown in industrialized countries, still occurs in slaughterhouse men, hide and wool workers in less developed parts of the world. Soil infected with *Histoplasma capsulatum* and other pathogenic fungi causes acute pulmonary reaction in farmers, migrant workers, and construction workers over wide geographical areas. Infectious diseases exotic in industrialized countries may, however, be seen in health service personnel, in particular in medical laboratory workers.

Chronic reactions

Pulmonary fibrosis. (See also Section 15.) Chronic industrial respiratory diseases are sometimes loosely referred to as pneumoconioses. This term has a precise meaning in the United Kingdom for the purpose of industrial injury benefit, where it is defined as 'fibrosis of the lungs due to silica dust, asbestos dust, or other dust, and including the condition of the lungs known as dust reticulation'. This latter term describes only a radiological abnormality. Within this definition are included silicosis; coal workers' pneumoconiosis; asbestosis; other silicate pneumoconioses such as those caused by talc, kaolin, Fullers' earth, and mica; and pulmonary fibrosis caused by beryllium, haematite, hard metal dust (tungsten carbide with cobalt), and graphite.

In Britain, a little under 1000 new cases of pneumoconiosis are diagnosed annually by the statutory medical panels. More than one half of these are cases of coal workers' pneumoconiosis, the next commonest being asbestosis, while the remainder are mainly cases of silicosis in mining (other than coal) and quarrying, in foundry work, pottery manufacture, steel dressing, refractories, and other industries. In recent years, only a handful of cases have been diagnosed below the age of 40 years, an indication of the present time scale for the development of pneumoconiosis in occupations initially taken up by young men.

Data from pneumoconiosis panels can give only an approximate guide to incidence rates, which can only be obtained by epidemiological studies. These are of course necessary to evaluate the effectiveness of preventive measures in use. Such studies rely on regular screening of the work force using standardized methods for clinical evaluation, assessment of radiological abnormality, and of respiratory function.

The Medical Research Council's questionnaire on respiratory symptoms is a validated and useful tool for clinical evaluation. For radiological assessment, full size, good quality films are required. Because the interpretation of these films is subject to both inter- and intra-observer variation, their reading should be incorporated in a design which can be subjected to statistical analysis. The International Classification of Radiographs of Pneumoconioses uses standard films for limits of normality, classifies opacities in the lung fields in terms of size, shape, profusion, and situation, and enables the extent of pleural involvement to be recorded. Sets of standard films issued by the International Labour Organization are now used on an international basis. Respiratory function tests also require careful standardization of instruments and technique. The simplest tests which can be performed in the field are estimation of peak flow rate and forced vital capacity with timed subdivisions, but more elaborate tests such as sub-divisions of lung volume and transfer factor have been performed in mobile physiological laboratories.

Biological investigation needs to be accompanied by environmental measurement of dust concentration or of chemical contaminants. Personal samplers worn by the workers measure the dust concentration in the breathing zone and static sampling devices give information on its evolution and distribution through the work place. The dust particles can then be identified, sized, and counted, so that estimates can be made of exposure levels and of cumulative exposures over time for the calculation of exposure effect relationships.

The pneumoconioses are all preventable provided the inhalation of respirable particles over a working lifetime is kept below the minimum required to give rise to the disease. A set of Threshold Limit Values (TLVs) act as guidelines for exposure, but these are not sharp dividing lines between safe and dangerous concentrations of inhaled dust. While exposure should in any case be kept within the TLV by the application of suitable engineering controls, this should also be kept as low as reasonably practical below the TLV. Where necessary suitable respiratory equipment should be provided as a backup for other techniques that aim to control the risk at source rather than as a first line of defence. For dusts, TLVs are expressed in terms of millions of particles per cubic foot or as a respirable or a total mass in mg/m³. The clinical features of the pneumoconioses are described elsewhere (see Section 15), but some epidemiological aspects are considered in the following paragraphs.

Silicosis. Silicosis is caused by the inhalation of free silica (SiO_2) in a respirable size range. This is released into the atmosphere whenever silica-containing minerals are worked either by hand or by mechanical processes. Thus miners, including gold, tin, and haematite miners as well as coal miners who drill through siliceous rock strata, are high-risk groups, others are stone masons who fashion sandstone or granite, potters who handle powdered flint, slate quarriers, metal grinders, iron and steel foundry workers, sand blasters, and boiler scalers. Foundry workers clean their castings of adherent sand in the process of fettling, which fractures the sand particles into a respirable size range. Sand blasters are exposed in a similar way and normally require protection with a helmet and external air line.

In industrialized countries, with progressive control of dust exposure and tuberculous infection, most cases of silicosis are now diagnosed over the age of 50 years and run a chronic course. However, silicosis or silico-tuberculosis can still occur as a rapidly fatal disease in younger age groups, as was evidenced in a group of sand blasters in New Orleans in the previous decade. In a cohort of South Dakota gold miners employed for 21 years or more, there was a large excess mortality from silicosis and silico-tuberculosis, which was shown to be linearly related to estimated dust concentration. Progression of silicosis may occur even after cessation of exposure, when massive fibrosis may develop, probably as a result of an immunological reaction.

Coal workers' pneumoconiosis. This form of pulmonary fibrosis follows the inhalation of respirable coal dust which may contain a variable proportion of free silica and other minerals. While by far the most common form of industrial pulmonary fibrosis in the United Kingdom, the numbers must be interpreted in relation to the size of the population at risk, of the order of a quarter of a million men. Incidence rates, from the National Coal Board's surveys were, in the 1970s, between 2.2 and 2.8 per 1000 men employed. In the mid 1970s the average age at diagnosis was 61 years compared with 53 years in 1951. Prevalence, expressed as a diagnosis of pneumoconiosis on the chest radiograph as a percentage of all men examined has fallen from 13.4 per cent in 1959–60 to 7.6 per cent in the mid 1970s. Large regional differences have been consistently maintained, with a low of 2.8 per cent in the Scottish coal fields contrasted with a high of 20.0 per cent in South Wales over the latter period. These differences between collieries in the risk of pneumoconiosis hold for equivalent levels of exposure and are probably dependent on 'coal-rank', a classification of coal based on its mineral content. For coal dust of constant composition, the development of simple pneumoconiosis is determined by the accumulated dust exposure, which is better expressed in terms of respirable mass concentration rather than the number of respirable particles.

The natural history of coal workers' pneumoconiosis is clearly separable into 'simple pneumoconiosis', a prolonged and essentially benign phase determined by accumulated dust exposure, and 'complicated' or progressive massive fibrosis which may be rapidly progressive in a proportion of men with heavy exposure and in part determined by immunological factors. Coal workers with rheumatoid arthritis and even those with no more than a rheumatoid diathesis have a higher prevalence of massive fibrosis than others. The massive opacities, appearing unusually distinct and rounded on the chest X-ray may develop on a background of minimal simple pneumoconiosis and may progress rapidly. First recognized in Welsh miners as Caplan's syndrome, the condition, which represents a state of enhanced tissue response has since been observed following exposure to other fibrogenic dusts. A long-term mortality study of South Wales miners and ex-miners showed that those with simple pneumoconiosis survived as well as those without the disorder, a finding supported by observations elsewhere. However, with advanced massive fibrosis, clinical deterioration is often rapid.

The essential requirement for a diagnosis of pneumoconiosis is evidence of pulmonary fibrosis, and this, for purposes of certification in Britain is assessed on the presence of parenchymal opacities on the chest radiograph. Indeed, the chest X-ray is seen before a claim for benefit can be considered by the pneumoconiosis medical panels. Where these opacities amount to no more than a simple pneumoconiosis, or even the earliest grade of progressive massive fibrosis, there are no associated symptoms, signs, or abnormalities on respiratory function tests. However, chronic bronchitis and emphysema are common amongst miners and other workers exposed to fibrogenic dusts. Most are cigarette smokers and experience other adverse factors associated with social class and general environment, such as atmospheric pollution. Epidemiological studies have sought to disentangle this complex aetiological maze, but so far without complete success. Some studies have shown cigarette smoking and social factors to be more important determinants than dust exposure in giving rise to respiratory symptoms. However, long-term prospective studies in miners have also shown a progressive reduction in ventilatory function with increasing cumulative exposure to airborne dust. In British and American coal miners, cough, phlegm, and ventilatory impairment appears now to be related both to cigarette smoking and to dust exposure, with evidence that the effects are additive. What is much less certain is whether dust exposure, in the absence of cigarette smoking or pulmonary fibrosis can lead to emphysema with its more serious effects on health and life expectancy.

Asbestosis. Asbestos is a generic term for a group of fibrous silicates which differ physically, clinically and in their biological activity although all can cause pulmonary fibrosis.

Chrysotile is a hydrous magnesium silicate forming the bulk of commercial asbestos and mined principally in Canada, Russia, and South Africa. The fibres are made up of bundles of fine, flexible, wavy fibrils in parallel array.

Crocidolite is a hydrous sodium iron silicate known also as South African blue asbestos because of its colour and origin. These are generally short, sharp, straight fibres.

Amosite, a hydrous magnesium iron silicate is brown and long fibred, and also comes from South Africa.

Anthophyllite, Tremolite, and Actinolite, are commercially less important forms. All except chrysotile belong to the amphibole group.

The longer fibres can be corded and spun to make yarns and fire-proofing fabrics and equipment. The shorter fibres are mixed with paper, rubber, cement, plastics, and paints to make a variety of products from brake-linings and clutch plates to floor coverings, roofing, water pipes, and thermal and electrical insulating equipment. Increasing quantities are being mined and used annually, and, as asbestos is virtually indestructible, being fireproof and chemically indissoluble, the increasing total quantity in use presents a problem in general environmental contamination. Workers in many industries have been exposed to asbestos especially in asbestos processing plants, and amongst workers engaged on the stripping of old lagging from boilers and heating systems. Casual exposure may occur in many trades in people who are not specifically asbestos workers, as for example in transport or in the building industry. A code of practice for the safe handling of asbestos has been delineated and there are also legal requirements. Crocidolite has not been imported into the United Kingdom since 1970, but it had been widely used in the past in lagging and fireproofing of buildings.

Asbestos exposure causes pulmonary fibrosis, pleural plaque formation, bronchogenic carcinoma, and mesothelioma. The malignant conditions are considered elsewhere (see page 6.112, and Section 15). The fibrosis in asbestosis is interstitial and often accompanied by pleural thickening, in contrast to the more focal distribution seen with silica and coal dust. As a result, functional impairment in relation to radiological abnormality occurs at an earlier stage, and sometimes precedes X-ray change. Because of this, the preliminary scrutiny of the chest X-ray by the pneumoconiosis medical panels does not apply and all claimants for benefit are examined. As with the other pneumoconioses, asbestosis is a disease of the later years of life, but with a rather higher proportion in the 40–49 age group. Prevalence surveys, using chest radiography and respiratory function tests have shown that some degree of asbestosis is present in a high proportion of workers exposed for long periods in poorly controlled conditions of asbestos production, manufacture, and application. Fibre concentration and duration of exposure seem to be the principal determinants, while fibre type is not an important variable for fibrosis. Progression is usually slow and insidious, increasing fibrosis leading to increasing breathlessness terminating in cardiorespiratory failure. Progression also occurs after withdrawal from exposure.

A few large-scale cohort studies have attempted to elucidate the dose–response relationship for asbestos exposure. The evidence suggests that there is no apparent threshold limit below which exposure to asbestos dust entails no risk to health, but this includes consideration of carcinogenicity too. The Advisory Committee on Asbestos of the Health and Safety Executive in the United Kingdom proposed, in 1979, the abolition of the hygiene standard for asbestos on the grounds that this implied a level below which exposure is safe. The Committee proposed a control limit, with legal backing, for chrysotile of 1 fibre/ml; for amosite of 0.5 fibre/ml, and for crocidolite of 0.2 fibre/ml over a four-hour sampling period. This, it is proposed, would replace the existing standard of 2 fibres/cm³ for all forms of asbestos.

Other pneumoconioses. Other fibrous silicates, talc and mica, and some non-fibrous silicates such as kaolin or china clay and Fuller's earth also produce pulmonary fibrosis, talc pneumoconiosis having features resembling those of asbestosis. Exposure has occurred in mining and milling and in the use of talc as a dusting powder for rubber. China clay, mined in Cornwall, is used in the ceramics industry and has given rise to pulmonary fibrosis. However, most cases of silicosis in the bone china industry have been caused by flint dust, used in the past to support the article in the process of firing. Haematite mining has been responsible for a mixed dust fibrosis from exposure to free silica together with iron oxide. Another mixed dust fibrosis is seen in boiler scalers, exposed to dusts containing soot, iron oxide, vanadium oxides, and probably free silica as well. The fibrogenic factor in the mining of mica and of slate has again probably been the free silica content of the dust.

Pulmonary fibrosis in the absence of free silica or of silicates has occurred in the 'hard-metal' industry, where cobalt, which is probably the fibrogenic agent, is used as a binder for powdered tungsten carbide. The inhalation of a large quantity of carbon dust, as has occurred in the manufacture of carbon electrodes or in the grinding of graphite, has also been followed by simple pneumoconiosis and progressive massive fibrosis.

Other chronic pulmonary reactions to inhaled dust

Beryllium. When inhaled in sufficient concentration, beryllium causes acute tracheobronchitis and a chemical pneumonitis. Lower exposures give rise to a non-caseating granulomatous reaction in the lung and other tissues. The condition resembles sarcoidosis but with a more chronic course and more serious prognosis, for the inflammatory reaction is followed by interstitial fibrosis often terminating in cardiorespiratory failure. Beryllium, alloyed with copper and other metals, is used in precision instruments, electronic equipment, space vehicles, and nuclear energy installations. In the past, beryllium phosphors were used in fluorescent lamps, but these have now been replaced by materials which are safer to handle. In addition to the workers, wives of beryllium employees and other neighbourhood contacts have developed the disease, which has some features of a hypersensitivity disorder.

Cadmium. The inhalation of freshly formed cadmium fumes as may happen inadvertently with the use of low melting point cadmium containing solders or the flame-cutting of cadmium-plated steel also produces an acute inflammatory reaction of the airway with a pneumonitis followed by alveolar cell proliferation. The longer term inhalation of lower concentrations of cadmium oxide fume or dust gives rise to progressive obstructive airways disease and there is some evidence which suggests it may cause emphysema without an associated chronic bronchitis. Exposure to the fume occurs in alloy manufacture, cadmium plating, and soldering; to the dust in the cadmium nickel battery industry and in the manufacture of cadmium based pigments and plastics stabilizers.

Aluminium. Pulmonary fibrosis has also been observed following the inhalation of aluminium oxide and of aluminium powder. The affected workers developed recurrent spontaneous pneumothorax and were found to have interstitial fibrosis with emphysematous blebs on the pleural surface (Shaver's disease). Exposure to the oxide occurred in the manufacture of corundum, an abrasive material, and the powdered metal was used in explosives.

Inert dusts. A number of inhaled dusts at work produce radiological opacities over the lung fields which are not associated with any adverse effect or with underlying pulmonary fibrosis or evidence of inflammatory reaction. Most striking is the chest radiograph in workers exposed to barium sulphate, with multiple, dense rounded opacities. These opacities represent barium, a metal of high atomic number, deposited in the lung. Antimony, tin, titanium, and iron oxide in its pure form also produce focal opacities which may be indistinguishable from the appearances of simple pneumoconiosis. Freshly formed ferric oxide is inhaled in oxyacetylene cutting and arc welding and these workers frequently develop respiratory abnormalities. However, irritant gases, such as ozone and oxides of

nitrogen, free silica and other biologically active metals inhaled simultaneously may be responsible for the adverse effects.

Nervous system

Occupational factors are associated with a broad spectrum of disorders affecting peripheral nerves and the central nervous system, with both organic and behavioural manifestations.

Central effects. The commonest occupational factors are mechanical and acoustic trauma, the former occurring predominantly in mining, transport, and construction and the latter throughout heavy industry. The construction industry in Britain accounts for about 300 deaths per million workers per year, mainly through head injury. The effects of noise exposure are considered elsewhere (see page 6.90).

Carbon monoxide remains the most frequent cause of death from poisoning because of its ubiquitous nature. Survivors may be left with permanent damage to the cerebral cortex and the extrapyramidal system. Inhaled in lower concentration, as may occur in blast furnace workers, traffic policemen and others, it may give rise to impaired performance of tasks requiring perceptual and motor skills.

A number of metals, in particular lead, mercury, and manganese, have specific central effects. Acute encephalopathy may be the presenting feature in *lead poisoning*, but this is now more likely to be seen in childhood than in industrial lead poisoning. *Tetraethyl lead* when inhaled causes a toxic organic psychosis seen in workers handling leaded petrol, but again, because of preventive measures cases are rare in industrialized countries. Workers in *manganese* mines and mills have developed psychotic symptoms followed by extra-pyramidal involvement with akinesia, rigidity, and tremor.

The inhalation of *mercury vapour* has been followed by acute psychosis and rarely by a Parkinsonian syndrome, but, more commonly, by a milder mental disturbance known as erethism, so frequently seen in the past in the felt hat industry that 'mad as a hatter' and 'hatter's shakes' passed into everyday speech. The latter term refers to the irregular tremor of chronic mercurialism. The short chain *aliphatic mercury* compounds synthesized primarily as seed dressings produce a specific disorder characterized by selective cerebrocortical and cerebellar damage, affecting primarily the granular layer in the cerebellum and the visual cortex with neuronal loss and glial proliferation. The condition is characterized by paresthesia, ataxia, dysarthria, and concentric constriction of the visual fields with blindness in more severe cases. While initially described in formulators of seed dressings, methyl mercury poisoning gained notoriety in more recent years as an environmental pollutant from an industrial source in Minamata disease and as a large-scale epidemic in Iraq following the ingestion of contaminated bread. Aluminium, bismuth, and organo tin compounds have also given rise to encephalopathy, in isolated cases in industry but again in epidemic proportions in other population groups.

Certain aliphatic and aromatic organic compounds, volatile and frequently used as solvents have a narcotic effect when inhaled and in lower concentration depress the level of consciousness, affecting initially higher mental functions. Subjective changes in mood and some slowing of reaction time has been observed in studies of behavioural effects in exposed workers, and it is possible that lasting brain damage may occur. Some solvents have other toxic effects too, such as carbon tetrachloride on liver and kidneys, trichloroethylene on cranial nerves, and methyl alcohol causing optic atrophy.

Peripheral effects. Organophosphorus compounds, used as pesticides the world over, are readily absorbed by inhalation or skin contact to interfere with nerve transmission through the inhibition of cholinesterase. Some of the triaryl phosphates, in particular triorthocresyl phosphate, used in the plastics industry, in addition cause demyelination. The carbamate pesticides are also inhibitors of cholinesterase. Agricultural workers in developing countries are particularly at risk, mainly through spraying without adequate protection, but also from the combined effects of pesticide with heat exposure and malnutrition.

Toxic neuropathies account for only a small proportion of all peripheral neuropathy, most of which has an obscure aetiology. In evaluating the possible role of an occupational exposure as a cause of peripheral neuropathy, a careful history is essential, with special reference to drug intake, alcohol ingestion, and the presence of pre-existing disease. Of the metals, lead produces a motor neuropathy affecting principally the extensors of the wrist and fingers, the classical lead palsy. Lower exposures have caused subclinical dysfunction of peripheral nerve detectable on electromyography. Arsenic and thallium give a mixed motor and sensory neuropathy, the former sometimes after a single large exposure and the latter delayed in onset, progressive, and accompanied by central effects.

A number of organic compounds encountered at work have also caused neuropathy. Workers preparing acrylamide polymer have been affected and a mixed neuropathy has followed exposure to carbon disulphide. N-hexane is a commonly used solvent which was responsible for a symmetrical, largely motor neuropathy affecting a group of Japanese workers responsible for cementing sandals. An outbreak of symmetrical, mainly motor neuropathy involved a large group of workers at a plastic-coated, printed fabrics plant in the USA, where no previously known neurotoxic agent had been used. The cause of the outbreak was traced to the substitution of the apparently innocuous methyl N-butyl ketone for methyl *iso*-butyl ketone used previously in a solvent mixture. Workers, and others, have also developed neuropathy following the practice of glue-sniffing.

Cardiovascular system

Although heart disease is the major cause of death in industrial communities today, occupational factors in its causation have been little explored. That coronary arteriosclerotic heart disease is commoner in some occupational groups than others does not necessarily imply a causal relationship to occupation, for risk factors such as cigarette smoking, physical inactivity, obesity, and stress are often features of the life style of employees in certain occupations. However, the lifestyle itself may be determined by the occupation. The hypothesis that physical activity at work affords protection against ischaemic heart disease was first found to hold in a study of bus drivers and bus conductors, and later in government clerks, postmen, and American longshoremen, with a remarkably consistent relationship between mortality and inactivity, within the same social class. The large social class differential in coronary heart disease with its higher mortality in professional and managerial groups in the earlier part of the century is no longer evident, perhaps as a result of the reduction in the physical effort of work and modern transportation.

A randomized controlled trial performed in industry to assess the effectiveness of a programme aimed at preventing heart disease by the control of risk factors showed that these can be changed in a working population, but the changes obtained were small and not sustained. Advice was given on dietary reduction of plasma cholesterol, on stopping or reducing smoking, weight reduction, daily exercise, and treatment of hypertension.

There is evidence for a causal association between certain toxic agents in the working environment and coronary arteriosclerotic heart disease. Workers exposed to carbon disulphide, as in the manufacture of rayon and carbon tetrachloride, have experienced a significantly increased mortality associated with hypertension and hyperlipidaemia. Carbon monoxide, which is atherogenic in rabbits and monkeys, is believed to be a causal factor in arteriosclerotic heart disease in cigarette smokers. In a prevalence study of angina in Finnish foundry workers, the highest rate was found in smokers with industrial carbon monoxide exposure and the lowest rate in

non-smokers without such exposure. Munitions workers exposed to glyceryl trinitrate and other organic nitrates have been shown to have an increased mortality, believed to result from coronary artery spasm after a short period of absence from work. Exposure to a number of halogenated hydrocarbons has been associated with sudden death from cardiac arrhythmia, in particular trichloro-ethane, trichloroethylene, and fluorocarbon aerosol propellants.

Of the metals, cobalt used as a foaming agent in beer has caused an epidemic of cardiomyopathy with a high mortality, including some cases among the brewery employees. An increased mortality from cerebrovascular disease has been observed in a group of lead battery workers in Britain, but this has not been confirmed elsewhere.

Alimentary system and liver

Acute gastroenteritis has followed the ingestion of soluble salts of a number of metals, in particular arsenic, antimony, cadmium, copper, iron, mercury, thallium, and zinc. Where this is followed by neuropathy and skin pigmentation arsenic poisoning is a possibility, whilst gastroenteritis followed by neuropathy and alopecia is the classic presentation of thallium poisoning. Lead poisoning may present with attacks of intestinal colic with constipation.

During the present century, duodenal ulceration increased in prevalence until the 1940s and then progressively declined. It has been considered to be related to stress and an increased prevalence has been observed in occupations thought to be stressful, although an objective measure of stress is difficult to obtain.

Occupational exposures are more likely to affect the liver than the gastrointestinal tract. Type B hepatitis is an important hazard in health care personnel, especially in those working in hospital laboratories, and dialysis and oncology units. A survey of doctors showed high levels of seropositivity in pathologists and surgeons, but low levels were found in those without patient contact. Infection with *L. icterohaemorrhagiae* (Weil's disease) or with other leptospiral serotypes may cause liver cell damage with jaundice. The condition is endemic worldwide but occurs with greater frequency in those whose occupation brings them into contact with water contaminated by urine from infected rats or other animals. It is thus most frequently seen in sewer workers, miners, agricultural workers, canal workers, and fish workers.

A number of chemicals, in particular organic solvents, may give rise to liver cell damage with jaundice. Toxic jaundice has followed occupational exposure to certain aliphatic hydrocarbons, such as carbon tetrachloride, chloroform, and tetrachlorethane, and in the aromatic series to the nitrobenzenes, trinitrotoluene, the chlorinated naphthalenes, and less commonly to other compounds.

Hepatic fibrosis or cirrhosis may follow liver cell damage from these infective or chemical agents. Cirrhosis is most commonly associated with excessive consumption of alcohol, although multiple risk factors have been proposed to explain variation in susceptibility. In Britain, where alcohol has been relatively expensive, professional groups have experienced the highest cirrhosis rates, whilst in the USA, where alcohol has been cheap, unskilled workers have the highest rates. Among the occupations with the highest mortality from cirrhosis are publicans and barmen, seamen, and medical practitioners.

Chronic arsenic poisoning has been followed by cirrhosis among vintners using arsenical pesticide sprays in the Moselle Valley. Non-cirrhotic perisinusoidal fibrosis has been observed in some instances, both in workers exposed to arsenic compounds and in vinyl chloride workers. In the latter, cases have come to light following haematemesis from an associated portal hypertension, the discovery of thrombocytopenia associated with splenomegaly or the development of angiosarcoma. In all cases, previous exposure to vinyl chloride monomer had been heavy, and occurred mainly in the cleaning of the pressure vessels used in the polymerization process.

As a general principle, workers who are unavoidably exposed to a potentially hepatotoxic chemical should avoid exposure to a second such agent and should therefore avoid alcohol and any drug which is potentially injurious to the liver. The converse also applies, for those who are taking drugs capable of liver injury or enzyme induction should avoid occupational exposure to potentially hepatotoxic agents.

Urinary system

Toxic chemicals encountered in the workplace may cause glomerular or tubular damage, or, after a latent interval to cancer of the urinary tract or bladder, considered elsewhere (see Section 18). Acute tubular necrosis has followed the absorption of certain inorganic salts of mercury, in particular mercuric chloride, and also of bismuth, ethylene glycol, tetrachlorethane, and carbon tetrachloride. In France this latter, because of its widespread useage, was considered to be the most common cause of acute renal failure. Workers exposed to inorganic mercury vapour have been shown to have an increased prevalence of proteinuria compared with controls. In a few cases more severe glomerular damage following exposure to metallic mercury and mercurials led to the nephrotic syndrome with a likely immune complex pathogenesis.

Following occupational or environmental exposure, cadmium accumulates in the renal cortex giving rise to tubular proteinuria and other defects of both proximal and distal tubular function, including aminoaciduria, renal glycosuria, high clearance rates of phosphate and uric acid, and defects in acidification and water concentration. Hypercalciuria and renal stone formation have been described in cadmium workers and in a few instances osteomalacia. Widespread renal tubular dysfunction with a high prevalence of osteomalacia in multiparous postmenopausal women (itai-itai disease) in Japan has been associated with environmental cadmium pollution from an industrial source. Excessive lead absorption from occupational exposure has also given rise to tubular dysfunction and also to interstitial nephropathy, progressing to renal failure sometimes associated with gout. Uranium salts too will give rise to renal tubular dysfunction. Animal studies have shown damage to the lower two-thirds of the proximal convoluted tubule together with the glomerular basement membrane. Gold nephropathy has followed therapeutic administration rather than occupational exposure.

Exposure to a number of organic compounds had been associated with the development of chronic glomerulonephritis. Carbon tetrachloride has been implicated, also solvents found in glue and certain cleaning fluids, and the pesticides 2,4-D and paraquat. There is some evidence that sniffing toluene in high doses has been followed by the development of renal stones.

Haemopoietic system

Ionizing radiation and many chemical substances encountered at work may cause disorders of the formed elements of the blood and of their precursors. However, commoner on a global scale, especially in the tropics, than blood dyscrasia caused by chemical exposure is chronic anaemia as a result of parasitic infestation. Hookworm infestation has also been known as miners' or tunnel workers' anaemia because of its frequency in the past in such working groups and the severe anaemia produced. Hookworm infestation is especially common in Southeast Asia where it affects agricultural workers, in particular labourers in rice fields in contact with damp soil. Schistosomiasis giving rise to anaemia through chronic blood loss can also be considered an occupational disease in certain situations.

With regard to chemical exposure, host sensitivity may play an important part in determining outcome. A haemoglobinopathy or glucose 6-phosphate dehydrogenase deficiency may be responsible for a haemolytic crisis following exposure to concentrations quite harmless to normal persons. It has been suggested that racial groups with a high prevalence of this condition should be screened before exposure to haemolytic chemicals or welding fumes.

Of chemicals which give rise to haemolysis, arsine is probably the most insidious, for it is formed whenever arsenic, often present in traces in scrap metal, flue dusts, or refinery residues, comes into contact with nascent hydrogen. Thus arsenic contamination in the reaction of metals with acids, or arsenides of alkali metals coming into contact with water will liberate arsine; which if unsuspected and inhaled, may cause massive haemolysis with jaundice and secondary renal failure. Naphthalene also gives rise to severe haemolysis. A number of industrial chemicals, some of which are readily absorbed through the skin, cause severe methaemoglobinaemia with a degree of haemolysis, imparting a lilac colour and inhibiting oxygen transport. These are the nitrobenzenes, trinitrotoluene and aniline. Sodium chlorate, commonly used as a weed killer, will also give rise to methaemoglobinaemia.

Excessive inorganic lead absorption produces a mild to moderate anaemia as a result of both haemolysis and inhibition of haem synthesis. The earliest effect of lead is inhibition of red cell δ-amino laevulinic acid (ALA) dehydratase activity, which occurs with blood lead concentrations common in urban populations, and whose significance is unknown. With higher degrees of lead absorption, as may occur in those occupationally exposed to lead, erythrocyte zinc protoporphyrin and serum ALA concentration is raised, as is the urinary excretion of ALA and of coproporphyrin. These parameters are useful for monitoring workers exposed to lead.

Both reduced and increased haemopoietic activity have been observed following industrial exposure to benzene either in pure form or as a component of many solvent mixtures, glues, and paint removers. Over the past 50 years many reports have associated benzene exposure with the subsequent development of non-lymphocytic leukaemia. Epidemiological studies suggest such an association, but a causal relationship has yet to be convincingly demonstrated.

Exposure to high doses of ionizing radiation produces an immediate fall in lymphocyte count, followed by a diminution in granulocytes and platelets with a more gradual fall in erythrocytes. Aplastic anaemia or pancytopenia may supervene, or alternatively proliferation of cellular elements may occur, in particular to give rise to acute or chronic myelogenous leukaemia. In the case of leukaemia, a linear dose–response curve has been shown, although in the very low dose range quantitative data are insufficient to determine whether this relationship still holds. In the luminizing industry the ingestion of traces of radioactive substances resulted in aplastic anaemia and osteogenic sarcoma. Secondary myelofibrosis with hypoplasia has followed the diagnostic administration of thorium dioxide. Lower doses of radiation and exposure to radiomimetic chemicals such as benzene have produced chromosome abnormalities in circulating lymphocytes.

Locomotor system

The extent to which occupation gives rise to disorders of the skeletal system has been little investigated in population-based studies. In addition to the extensive and varied effects of accidental trauma, low back pain and osteoarthrosis are common conditions and a major cause of lost working time. Back pain is very common in both manual and sedentary workers, but in the former, such as miners, dockers, and nurses, it is an important cause of disability. Osteoarthrosis of the spine, hips, or knees is particularly common in heavy manual workers, and the interphalengeal joints were said to be affected in tailors, in whom Heberden's nodes produced a characteristic deformity. Disabling osteoarthrosis of hip, knee or shoulder also occurs as a sequel to aseptic necrosis of bone in compressed air workers, where the infarcted area is in proximity to the joint and involves the articular cartilage. In a study of decompression sickness and aseptic necrosis of the bone in tunnellers, a quarter of the men who were radiographed showed evidence of damage to one or more bones, although most of the lesions were symptomless. Osteoarthrosis, in particular of the elbow and wrist joints, is seen in workers who handle vibrating tools, both with and without associated Raynaud syndrome. These and other heavy manual workers may have multiple small areas of decalcification in the carpal bones.

Acro-osteolysis has occurred in workers engaged on the polymerization of vinyl chloride, in particular in those whose work entailed cleaning of the pressure vessels, where intermittent exposure to the monomer fume used to be high. Cystic lesions in the terminal phalanges of the fingers and toes and sometimes in the patella and sacroiliac bones together with a Raynaud's syndrome and sclerodermatous change of the hands have been found.

Housemaid's knee, or prepatellar bursitis, is a descriptive term for one of a number of conditions characterized by a collection of synovial fluid in bursae subjected to repeated friction or pressure. The most important of these are the beat disorders of miners, involving the elbow or the knee, where the bursae are liable to become infected and where subcutaneous cellulitis may occur. Such a cellulitis may involve the hand in boilermen as well as in miners. Although declining in frequency, these conditions continue to be important causes of sickness absence.

Repetitive movement of the hands is required in many occupations, for example, carpenters, braiders, and typists. The tendon sheath or the musculotendinous junction of the most used muscles may become inflamed, with fluid exudation, giving rise to an incapacitating tenosynovitis. The most commonly affected are the radial extensors and the abductors of the wrist and thumb. In a study in a motor vehicle assembly plant the main aetiological factors were occupational change necessitating unaccustomed movement, resumption of work after absence, and repetitive, stereotyped movement. In Britain in 1978, tenosynovitis was the second most frequent cause of certified incapacity after occupational dermatitis.

Reproductive effects

Certain physical and chemical exposures at work may affect either sex to give rise to adverse reproductive effects. Ionizing radiation and many chemicals, both organic, such as benzene, and inorganic, for example salts of some heavy metals, can produce genetic alterations in somatic cells. In some instances such changes have been demonstrated following occupational exposures, but in others, only in cultured mammalian cells. If such effects can also occur in human germ cells, deleterious mutations are likely to occur. The present average population exposure to ionizing radiation from all sources has been estimated to increase the spontaneous mutation rate by about 2 to 15 per cent. However, evaluation of the mutagenic effects of occupational exposures is difficult to obtain.

Reproductive effects in the male may manifest with diminished libido or infertility with abnormal sperm production, but again objective data is at present scanty and difficult to acquire. Infertility and a high abortion rate have been reported in the wives of lead workers and an increased risk of spontaneous abortion and congenital abnormality has been observed in the wives of vinyl chloride workers and of male anaesthetists. Loss of libido and impotence have been reported in pharmaceutical workers in manufacturing oestrogens and in the manufacture of kepone and dibromochloropropane, both pesticides.

In women menstrual disorders, in particular amenorrhea, are common in nurses and airline stewardesses, and menstrual, breast, and genital changes have been observed in those who manufacture oral contraceptives.

Occupational exposure to noxious chemicals during pregnancy may result in enhanced maternal toxicity, or in fetal toxicity with little evidence of maternal effect, as has occurred following absorption of alkyl mercury used as a seed dressing. The effects on the fetus may be incompatible with life to give rise to spontaneous abortion or still birth, or if less severe to prematurity, low birthweight, congenital malformation, or abnormal postnatal development. A toxic chemical absorbed at work may be secreted into breast milk to cause poisoning in the baby. Transplacental carcinogenesis has been observed following prenatal exposure to diethyl-

stilboestrol, and this possibility has been raised but not confirmed with regard to exposure during pregnancy to anaesthetic gases.

Certain infective agents, in particular rubella, toxoplasma, and cytomegalovirus cause specific teratological effects: teachers, animal minders, and others may thus be at increased risk in pregnancy from these infections.

At the present time there is little reliable information on the effects of noxious agents encountered at work on reproductive capacity or outcome of pregnancy. A system of data collection is required to enable records of work exposure to be related to the occurrence of congenital malformation and other measures of the outcome of pregnancy.

Occupational allergies

Occupational asthma. (See also Section 15). *Definition.* Occupational asthma is defined for the purpose of prescription for disablement benefit in the United Kingdom as asthma which develops after a variable period of symptomless exposure to a sensitizing agent encountered at work. The initial symptom-free period of exposure may vary from weeks to years, and usually only a minority of those exposed develop asthma. Once sensitization has developed, asthmatic reactions recur following exposure to concentrations, often minute, which do not affect other workers similarly exposed. Other allergic effects, such as conjunctivitis, rhinitis, or skin sensitization may or may not be present. Byssinosis may be regarded as a form of occupational asthma, but because of differences in the pattern of symptoms, it is usually considered as a separate entity.

Aetiology. Over 200 agents encountered at work have now been reported as causing asthma, and with the ever increasing introduction of new industrial processes, this list of causal agents is likely to grow. Seven groups which have been most clearly identified have been proposed for prescription in the United Kingdom, and these, together with other likely sensitizing materials are shown in Table 5. Bakers' asthma was known since ancient times, and Ramazzini in 1700 described shortness of breath and urticaria in grain workers. Grain and flour dust contain many potential allergens, from the flour itself to wheat hairs, fungi, and mites. The condition is not uncommon, for in one survey 20 per cent of bakers had rhinitis and most had asthma as well. Workers engaged in harvesting, transporting, and storing grain are also at risk.

Refinery workers exposed to platinum compounds containing reactive halogen ligands may become sensitized after as little as 10

Table 5   Clearly established agents causing occupational asthma (P = proposed for prescription in the United Kingdom)

Complex salts of platinum (P)
  Ammonium hexachloroplatinate
Isocyanates (P)
  Toluene di-isocyanate; hexamethylene di-isocyanate;
  naphthalene di-isocyanate
Epoxy resin curing agents (P)
  Phthalic acid anhydride; trimellitic acid anhydride;
  triethylene tetramine
Colophony fumes (P)
Proteolytic enzymes (P)
  Bacillus subtiis (alkalase)
Laboratory animal urine (P)
  Rats, mice, guinea pigs, rabbits, locusts
Flour and grain dusts (P)
  Barley, oats, rye, wheat
Formaldehyde
Antibiotics
  Penicillin
Wood dusts
  South African boxwood (*Gonioma kammassi*); Canadian red cedar
  (*Thuja plicata*); Mansonia (*Sterculiacea altissima*)
Natural gums
  Gum acacia, gum arabic, tragacanth

days or as long as 20 years' exposure, developing asthma, rhinitis, conjunctivitis, or urticaria. A large proportion of the workforce can become sensitized, with reactions developing after minute subsequent exposures. While few workers are likely to be exposed to platinum salts, many are exposed to di-isocyanates, used extensively in the manufacture of polyurethane foams, paints, inks, and adhesives. Again, sensitization may occur at a variable period of exposure and attacks may follow not only re-exposure but also non-specific irritants such as cigarette smoke or physical exertion. Several chemicals used with epoxy resins in curing processes have caused asthma in a high proportion of those exposed in the plastics and electronics industries. Colophony is the natural resin from pine trees which is a constituent of most of the fluxes used in hard soldering, mainly in electronics. The fumes given off when colophony is heated during soldering have given rise to asthma in those engaged in the process and to neighbourhood workers, with many experiencing symptoms even after removal from exposure. Biological washing powders containing derivatives of *B. subtilis* produce in sensitized subjects asthma, rhinitis, urticaria, blistering of the skin, and malaise. Laboratory animal handlers, in particular those working with rats, mice, guinea pigs, and rabbits, and those handling certain insects, expecially locusts, have developed asthma and other allergic manifestations. Investigation has shown that with rats and mice the sensitizing agents are low molecular weight urinary proteins rather than blood or animal dander. Health care workers have become sensitized to formalin used, for example, in the sterilization of artificial kidney machines and also to antibiotics, in particular to the penicillins.

Diagnosis. A detailed clinical and occupational history is essential in the diagnosis of occupational asthma and in many cases this alone will suffice. Symptoms often increase in severity during the working week and remit at weekends, to recur on return to work. However, the relationship to occupational exposure is not always clear, for symptoms may persist for days or weeks in some cases, although improvement usually occurs after a holiday or other period away from work. The relationship can be further clouded by attacks triggered by non-specific stimuli such as repiratory infection or even exercise. A marked diurnal variation in airway resistance may even give rise to symptomatic improvement while exposed to the allergen in the mornings, with the most severe effects experienced while at home at night. Again, the symptoms do not always suggest allergic asthma, for episodic breathlessness and wheezing may be accompanied by dry cough or by mucopurulent expectoration or in some cases by an additional extrinsic allergic alveolitis.

Objective evidence of a causal relationship between exposure and the development of asthma should be sought where this is not clear or where the implication would be a loss of employment. Such evidence can be obtained from (a) skin-prick tests, (b) respiratory function tests, and (c) bronchial provocation tests. In addition, serological tests are being developed for demonstrating allergen specific IgE and IgG antibodies by means of the radioallergosorbent test (RAST). Skin-prick tests giving an immediate reaction are of value with platinum salts and rat urine allergens. With other allergens they may lack sensitivity and specificity or they may not have been sufficiently evaluated. Assessment of ventilatory function in relation to exposure is most conveniently performed by the subject using a peak flow meter at regular intervals before, during, and after exposure at work on different days of the week. Isolated readings may be misleading, because of the marked diurnal variation in airway resistance which occurs in some subjects.

Bronchial provocation tests involve admission to hospital and giving graded exposures under carefully controlled conditions employing adequate controls. The test is potentially hazardous and should only be performed where the necessary expertise is available. Such testing may be indicated where doubt remains about the diagnosis after other investigations have been performed, where the symptoms are so severe that further work exposure, even

for testing, is unjustified, and where complex exposures occur or a hitherto unrecognized allergen is being investigated.

Course and prognosis. Bronchial provocation testing with soluble antigens has shown three distinct patterns of reaction. An asthmatic reaction may develop (a) within one hour of testing—an immediate reaction; (b) within 12 hours of testing—a late reaction; or (c) during the night following challenge—a nocturnal dip. In addition, a febrile reaction with malaise, leucocytosis, crepitations, and a fall in transfer factor within 24 hours signifies an associated alveolar reaction.

Many cases of occupational asthma clear following permanent removal from exposure to the sensitizing agent. However, in others disability may persist for years or a state of bronchial hyperreactivity may develop with reactions to common allergens, exercise or upper respiratory infection.

Prevention. In the absence of a safe substitute, the concentration of potent allergens in the working environment must be kept below a level where the majority of those exposed are unlikely to develop an adverse effect. This requires a high standard of industrial hygiene and ventilation engineering. In the platinum refining industry in the United Kingdom, persons with a history of respiratory disorder, allergy, or asthma are not employed, and an atopic state or sensitivity to platinum confirmed by a skin-prick test precludes employment where contact with platinum salts is possible. During employment workers are monitored with repeated skin-prick testing and tests of ventilatory function.

Byssinosis. Workers exposed to cotton, hemp, flax, and sisal dusts for a number of years develop a condition characterized by attacks of breathlessness, wheezing, tightness of the chest, and an irritating cough which occurs initially on the first day of return to work after a weekend or after absence (Monday fever). Over a period of years the symptoms progress to involve successive days of the week, until eventually complete and permanent incapacity may result. At this stage the condition is indistinguisable from chronic obstructive bronchitis.

The condition is seen wherever the above fibres are processed, in some countries significant exposure occurring in homes and farms, with a high prevalence in rural populations. The prevalence of byssinosis is related to the concentration of dust inhaled irrespective of whether or not the particles are respirable. Bronchoconstriction appears to be caused by a histamine releasing agent found, for example, in the pericarp of the seed present as a contaminant in raw cotton fibre rather than by an immune response as in occupational asthma which in some ways it resembles.

The diagnosis of byssinosis is made from the occupational and medical history. The episodes of chest tightness are initially associated with a fall in ventilatory capacity with an increase in airway resistance on the first day at work, respiratory function being normal on other days of the week. As the condition progresses, the fall in ventilatory capacity becomes permanent, but again, with a more marked fall on the first day back at work. The maximum expiratory flow rate at 50 per cent has been found to be more sensitive than the FEV_1 in detecting acute ventilatory changes from cotton dust.

Provided the concentration of raw cotton dust is kept below the threshold limit value of 200 $\mu g/m^3$, byssinosis is unlikely to occur in the majority of exposed workers.

Extrinsic allergic alveolitis. Allergens in organic dusts encountered in a variety of occupations give rise to the syndrome of extrinsic allergic alveolitis usually associated with the presence of precipitating antibody in the blood (Table 6).

The most common of these conditions seen in Britain is farmers' lung which follows the inhalation of dust from mouldy hay or other vegetable produce. Farmers' lung is seen more frequently after the harvesting of crops in rainy weather, which favours the growth of a variety of moulds, the most important being *Micropolyspora faeni* (*Thermopolyspora polyspora*) of the group of thermophilic acti-

Table 6 Occupational causes of extrinsic allergic alveolitis

Condition	Source of allergen	Precipitins against
Farmers' lung	mouldy hay	*Micropolyspora faeni*
Pigeon breeders' lung	pigeon droppings	serum proteins and
Bird fanciers' lung	budgerigar droppings	droppings
Mushroom pickers' lung	mushroom compost	*M. faeni; T. vulgaris*
Malt workers' lung	mouldy barley/malt	*Aspergillus clavatus*
Wheat weavil disease	infested wheat flour	*Sitophilus granarius*
Cheese washers' lung	mouldy cheese	*Penicillium casei*
Bagassosis	mouldy bagasse	*T. vulgaris*
Suberosis	mouldy cork dust	
Maple bark strippers' lung	mouldy maple-bark	*Cryptostroma corticale*
Woodpulp workers' lung	woodpulp	*Alternaria* spp.
Sequoisis	mouldy sawdust	*Aureobasidium pullulans*
New Guinea lung	mouldy dust from thatched roof	

nomycetes. This mould acts as an antigen giving rise to precipitating antibodies in the serum.

The clinical features of extrinsic allergic alveolitis are given in Section 15. The diagnosis is made on the occupational and medical history, the clinical findings, the chest radiograph, respiratory function tests which show a fall in transfer factor and possibly a restrictive defect, and on the presence of precipitating antibody. The diagnosis may easily be missed if an occupational history is not taken, for the condition has been mistaken for influenza, acute bronchitis, pneumonia, or asthma, for there may be an associated immediate or late asthmatic reaction. Repeated exposure is followed by recurrent attacks until eventually pulmonary fibrosis may develop with its sequel of cor pulmonale. Farmers' lung is not uncommon. A survey in Wales based on a combination of relevant symptoms with positive serology found a prevalence rate of 54 per 1000 in random samples of the farming population.

Inhaled avian protein acts as an antigen in pigeon breeders' and birdfanciers' lung, with features resembling farmers' lung seen even in owners of a single budgerigar or other bird. Precipitins have been demonstrated against feathers and droppings and against serum proteins from the birds.

Thermoactinomyces vulgaris has been incriminated as an allergen both in bagassosis and in mushroom pickers' lung. The former follows the inhalation of dust from the crushing and processing of the residue of sugar cane, while the latter condition may develop after exposure to spores present in the compost of horse manure and straw on which the mushrooms are grown. Maple logs may be infected with the fungus of *Cryptostroma corticale* which grows beneath the bark. Stripping the bark or sawing logs can produce a very high spore count to which sensitization has occurred. A similar disorder has been described in malt workers heavily exposed to the spores of *Aspergillus clavatus* and *A. fumigatus* which may contaminate the grain to give rise to malt workers' lung. There are other similar disorders where the allergen has yet to be identified.

Occupational skin disease. (See also Section 20.) Occupationally related skin disorders are common. In Britain in 1978, 61 per cent of all new spells of certified incapacity for which injury benefit was payable were due to occupational skin diseases, and these accounted for more than twice the number of working days lost by all the other prescribed occupational diseases together.

Skin disorders of occupational origin, especially if involving the hands have to be differentiated from endogenous eczema, pimpholyx, psoriasis', and fungal infections which they may closely resemble. A wide range of agents in the working environment may be involved, which may be classified into: (*a*) mechanical: e.g., trauma, friction or pressure; (*b*) physical: climate or radiation; (*c*) biological: plant or animal contact, insects, or micro-organisms; or (*d*) chemical: inorganic and organic compounds.

Whether a disorder of the skin develops is dependent not only on the pattern and intensity of exposure but also on individual susceptibility, in part related to skin pigmentation and to atopy. For example, fair skinned and poorly pigmented mariners, farmers, and other workers exposed to high intensity sunlight have an increased incidence of skin cancer in comparison with pigmented races. Atopy has a complex relationship to industrial skin disease. Thus a nurse with a history of eczema has a greater risk of developing not only an allergic but also an irritant contact dermatitis.

Mechanical. Repeated friction or mechanical pressure on the skin causes the beat disorders and cellulitis commonly seen in miners. Gangrene of the finger tips may accompany the Raynaud syndrome associated with the handling of vibrating tools.

Physical. Workers exposed to climatic extremes develop skin disorders ranging from chapped and dessicated skin, chilblains, and frostbite on cold exposure to prickly heat and other sweat disturbances on exposure to high temperatures. Ultraviolet light causes sunburn and skin cancer. The effects of exposure to ionizing radiation were dramatically demonstrated by the pioneer radiologists early this century who developed chronic X-ray dermatitis, post-irradiation telangiectasis, and eventually skin cancer.

Biological. Grain itch in grocers and men unloading grain from ships is caused by infestation with *Pediculoides ventricosus*, Dogger Bank itch is an eczematous eruption in North Sea fishermen caused by contact with the sea-chevril, *Alcyonidium gelatinosum*, and erysipeloid, seen in fishworkers, cooks, housewives, butchers, and veterinary surgeons follows infection with *Erysipelothrix rhusiopathiae*. Anthrax is a potential hazard to all who come into contact with animals or animal products including hides and wool. Many plants, fruits, and vegetables cause irritant or allergic contact dermatitis seen in numerous occupations. Amongst the most potent sensitizers are the *Anardiacae*, the *Primulaceae*, and certain woods, such as South African boxwood.

Chemical. The skin can be damaged in a variety of ways by many chemical products. Thus mineral oils and chlorinated hydrocarbons can cause acne, while hydroquinone derivatives give rise to leukoderma, and soot, tar, pitch, and shale oils are precursors of papilloma and skin cancer. Chromates can cause chronic skin ulceration (chrome holes) and nasal septum perforation. However, the commonest occupational skin disorder is a contact dermatitis. This can take one of two forms, an irritant, or an allergic contact dermatitis.

Irritant contact dermatitis. Primary irritant contact dermatitis, which is the most common form, may be acute or chronic, and is caused by a multitude of agents which damage the skin directly. Such damage is caused by acids and alkalis, by solvents which defat the skin, by certain metal salts which precipitate cellular proteins, by detergents and even by dryness of the air. The cutaneous response depends on the strength of the irritant and the length of time it is in contact with the skin. Lesions occur on exposed areas of skin and clear on removal from exposure.

Chronic irritant contact dermatitis is seen most commonly in bricklayers, nurses, car mechanics, lathe workers, and housewives. Multiple environmental factors are often responsible. Contact with cement may cause acute or chronic irritant contact dermatitis due to its alkaline, hygroscopic nature, or allergic contact dermatitis from its chromium content.

Allergic contact dermatitis. Allergic contact dermatitis may not differ in appearance from non-occupational eczema and diagnosis is dependent on careful history taking with knowledge of the materials to which exposure occurs and their sensitizing properties. Sensitization may occur after a variable and sometimes long period of exposure without ill effects, and is usually permanent, with an inflammatory reaction occurring on each re-exposure.

Allergic contact dermatitis is an example of delayed cell mediated hypersensitivity (type IV immune response) which may be detected by patch testing. However, misinterpretation of results can easily occur. Irritant contact dermatitis may develop if the test solutions are too strong, and both false positive and false negative reactions are not uncommon. Prick testing is used to demonstrate immediate hypersensitivity reactions (type I). Atopy is the state where multiple sensitivities of this type occur to common allergens.

A large number of biological and chemical agents can sensitize the skin. On the former, some have been mentioned above, while the commoner chemical sensitizers are shown in Table 7. Positive patch tests to nickel sulphate, potassium dichromate, thiomersal, p-phenylene diamine, ethylenediamine, neomycin sulphate, colophony, balsam of Peru, and wood alcohols are common in the general population. Hexavalent chromium allergy is commoner in males and is more likely to be occupational in origin, due to the opportunities for exposure in cement, paints, printing, tanning, and coal mining. In women, nickel sensitivity predominates, much of it being non-occupational, originating from cheap jewellery and metal fastenings on clothing. p-Phenylene diamine, a constituent of hair dyes, is also a more common skin sensitizer in women. In the industrial setting, dermatitis is seen most frequently, in descending order of importance, in coal mining, metal working, leather, chemical, and textile manufacture.

Table 7 Examples of potent chemical sensitizing agents in industry giving rise to allergic contact dermatitis (type IV immune response)

Metals
  Salts of nickel,* chromium,* cobalt; arsenicals; complex platinum salts; inorganic and organic mercury* compounds
Resins
  Epoxy resin monomers and accelerators; colophony
Rubber additives
  Vulcanization agents, antitoxidents, accelerators, etc. e.g. thiuram derivatives; mercaptobenzothiazole; Isopropyl-phenyl-phenylene diamine
Dyes
  p-phenylene diamine;* inks and paints
Antibiotics
  Penicillins; neomycin*
Miscellaneous
  Ethylene diamine;* turpentine;* benzocaine; formalin; balsam of Peru; wood alcohols; parabens; vioform

* Sensitizers common in the general population.

Occupational cancer

Since the observation by Percivall Pott in 1775 on the role of soot in the causation of cancer of the scrotum, many substances, both man-made and naturally occurring, encountered in the working or the general environment, have been found to give rise to cancer. Estimates of the influence of environmental factors on the expression or induction of cancer have ranged as high as 90 per cent. Observations on cancer in relation to occupational exposures are of particular value in the study of aetiology, for exposures tend to be higher than in the general population, levels can be more readily estimated, and exposed groups more easily defined. However, confounding factors are still plentiful. Occupational groups are exposed to environmental carcinogens common to the population as a whole; for example, most industrial workers are also cigarette smokers, and many smoke heavily. Occupational exposures are often complex with more than a single suspect agent, they change over time both qualitatively and quantitatively, and the long latent interval between initial exposure and clinical presentation of cancer makes it difficult to obtain adequate data in retrospective studies. It may only be possible to conclude that a certain occupation or process runs an increased cancer risk without defining the responsible carcinogen, a situation analogous to cigarette smoking, where one can only speculate on the nature of the active agent.

Information on occupational cancer can be obtained in the following ways:

1. Clinical observation. Astute observation by clinicians has been of greater value than epidemiological study in suspecting a relationship between an environmental exposure and the subsequent development of cancer. Percivall Pott made his observations and wrote his monograph on scrotal cancer in chimney sweeps while practising as a highly successful surgeon.

2. Epidemiological enquiry. Well-designed cohort studies require identification of exposed workers, accurate information on mortality or morbidity, qualitative and quantitative information on exposure over time, sufficient exposure, and an adequate follow-up period to allow for the long latency of many carcinogens. Such studies are expensive and time-consuming but nevertheless provide the only way by which an increased human cancer risk in relation to a particular exposure can be identified.

3. Animal experimentation. Life-time studies in animals of more than one species are performed for the estimation of carcinogenic potential. Species, dose, route, and pattern of administration, chemical and physical form of the test agent, and its metabolism in the species selected have to be taken into account. The results of animal experimental studies cannot be directly extrapolated to man. Nevertheless, a WHO task group concluded that if a substance has been shown to be carcinogenic in animals, it should be considered carcinogenic for man, unless adequate epidemiological evidence exists to the contrary. Animals studies also are expensive and time-consuming.

4. Short-term tests. Over the last decade a battery of laboratory tests have been developed which either seek evidence of genetic toxicity or of alterations in the behaviour of cells in culture. These tests are rapid and inexpensive, but although there appears to be a relationship between mutagens and carcinogens, effects in bacteria, in cell cultures, and in cell-free systems cannot be extrapolated to complex organisms, let alone man. Cytogenetic studies, in which a search is made for chromosome aberrations or sister chromatid exchanges in somatic cells may be performed *in vivo* in occupationally exposed groups or again *in vitro*, in cultured mammalian cells. Ionizing radiation produces both chromosome abnormality and cancer, and chemicals which have the former effect are said to be radiomimetic, and suspect as carcinogenic.

Principal occupational carcinogens. Chemicals which are undoubted human carcinogens and processes associated with an increased cancer risk are shown in Table 8. Ionizing radiation and

Table 8 Substances, and substances associated with industrial processes, classified as human carcinogens by the American Conference of Governmental Industrial Hygienists

Carcinogen	Target organ
Aromatic amines	
B-naphthylamine	bladder
Benzidine	bladder
4-amino diphenyl	bladder
4-nitro diphenyl	bladder
Asbestos	
Chrysotile	bronchus
Crocidolite	bronchus; pleura; peritoneum
Amosite	bronchus; pleura; peritoneum
Other forms	bronchus
Arsenic trioxide production	bronchus; skin; liver
Chloromethylmethyl ether	bronchus
Chromite ore processing	bronchus
Nickel sulphide roasting	bronchus; nasal sinuses
Bis(chloromethyl)ether	bronchus
Chromium (VI), certain water insoluable compounds	bronchus
Vinyl chloride	angiosarcoma of liver
Coal tar pitch volatiles	bronchus; skin
Acrylonitrile	bronchus
Ethylene dibromide	uncertain

ultraviolet light can be included in the same category, as physical agents. In addition, a number of other chemical compounds, for example benzene, certain hydrazines and nitrosamines, beryllium and cadmium have been suspected as human occupational carcinogens. Some of the more important occupational cancers will be considered in more detail.

Polycyclic aromatic hydrocarbons. Percivall Pott's observation on scrotal cancer in chimney sweeps was followed by Butlin more than a century later who showed that pitch, tar, and mineral oil similarly affected the same site. Skin cancer was later produced experimentally with coal tar and Scottish shale oil. In the 1920s Kennaway, using fluorescence spectroscopy identified the first chemical carcinogen, 1,2,5,6-dibenzanthracene and then isolated 3,4-benzopyrene from pitch. In the early years of this century skin cancer was not uncommon in workers handling tar, pitch, creosote, asphalt, and anthracene. Cotton mule spinners used Scottish shale oil for lubricating their machines. Constant friction with oil soaked clothing gave rise to skin cancer in particular affecting the scrotum. While this risk has been removed from the cotton industry by the substitution of noncarcinogenic oils, an excess incidence of epithelioma of the skin is still seen in the engineering industry. Here mineral oils are used as lubricants, coolants, and quenching agents, in particular in automatic machine tool processes. Gross contamination of the skin has occurred in the past, giving rise to oil folliculitis, multiple hyperkeratosis, and epithelioma. Fine droplets of mineral oil in the breathing zone are believed to be responsible for an excess mortality from lung cancer. In the process of coal carbonization, the mortality from lung cancer in retort house workers was higher than that in other gas workers, and this has been attributed to the very high levels of polycyclic hydrocarbons to which these workers were exposed in the past.

Aromatic amines. Bladder cancer in the synthetic dyestuff industry was first recorded in 1895, some thirty years after the process had been established in Germany. Subsequently, cases were associated with the manufacture of synthetic dyes, in the rubber cable making, and chemical industries in the United Kingdom and other countries. These workers were exposed to a large number of chemicals, but from epidemiological studies and animal experiments, the principal carcinogens were identified as B-naphthylamine and benzidine. 4-amino diphenyl was used as a rubber anti-oxidant in the USA, where it gave rise to a number of cases of bladder cancer, and workers in the British rubber industry showed a large excess of bladder cancer in cohort studies performed in the 1950s. Routine occupational mortality statistics failed to reveal the problem because of the small total number of workers involved, but in one plant, fifteen distillers of B-naphthylamine all developed bladder cancer. In 1967, importation and use of the four aromatic amines listed in Table 8 was statutorily prohibited. Alternative anti-oxidants were found in the rubber industry, but as no alternative to benzidine has been devised for manufacturing dyes, it continues to be used, but in totally enclosed processes. A recent survey in which over 40 000 men employed for at least one year in the rubber and cable-making industries have now been observed for eight years has shown a significant excess of deaths from bladder cancer throughout the industry, including firms where exposure to acknowledged bladder carcinogens had not occurred. Occupational bladder cancer is, therefore, a continuing problem. The tumours are frequently multifocal in origin and involve the epithelium of the renal pelvis and ureters as well as the bladder. They tend to arise as multiple papillomata which may be initially benign or malignant. Characteristically, the presentation is one of painless haematuria, occurring at a rather younger average age than non-occupational bladder cancer, with a latent interval from first exposure of between four and over 40 years. Workers with known past exposure to these aromatic amines are regularly followed up with exfoliative cytology and in some cases cystoscopy. The active carcinogens are not the parent amines, but hydroxylated metabolic products of these excreted in the urine.

Asbestos. The different forms of asbestos and their principal uses are considered on page 6.104. The initial observations were made in cases of asbestosis, in which an increased frequency was found of carcinoma of the bronchus. Subsequently, many well designed cohort studies have shown a substantial excess mortality from bronchial carcinoma with all types of asbestos fibre in a variety of industries where it is produced, manufactured, and applied. However, the amphibole group, mainly crocidolite and amosite, appears to have a higher risk of bronchial carcinoma than chrysotile. Estimates of total, cumulative exposure have shown an exposure–response relationship which appears linear, without a no-effect threshold. Large-scale cohort studies on North American insulation workers and Quebec chrysotile miners and millers have shown an important interaction between asbestos exposure and cigarette smoking, an interaction which is at least additive and which may even be multiplicative. Most asbestos related lung cancers have occurred in smokers, but non-smokers are also at risk.

Mesothelioma of the pleura was a rare tumour until twenty years ago, when it was first associated with asbestos exposure amongst the inhabitants of the small townships which had grown around the crocidolite, or blue asbestos workings in South Africa. Since then the association has been amply confirmed in several countries in miners, process workers, shipyard and insulation workers, and in a few instances in the families of asbestos workers and in people living in the vicinity of asbestos factories. Most of the cases have been related to crocidolite or amosite exposure, the risk of mesothelioma following chrysotile exposure appears to be very small. However, it is probable that carcinogenic activity is determined by the size and shape of the fibre rather than its actual type. Mesothelioma develops clinically up to 50 years after exposure to asbestos dust, which has made it difficult to identify the nature or the intensity of past exposure. Where tissue is available, it is now possible to identify and count the mineral fibre content of the lung, adding to the accuracy of exposure data in epidemiological studies. The risk of mesothelioma also appears to increase with dose, but in contrast to bronchial carcinoma, asbestosis has only been identified in a minority of cases, and more cases have occurred following short exposures.

The mortality from mesothelioma has increased over the past decade in industrial countries, mainly in older men. The increasing uses of asbestos with opportunities for exposure to the dust over recent years makes it likely that the number of new cases will continue to rise to reach a peak during the final decade of the century. The geographical distribution of the cases is remarkable, showing clustering in cities with shipyards. In the United Kingdom the concentration in areas with naval shipyards is likely to be related to the past use of crocidolite in marine insulation with high exposure in confined spaces over many years.

About half of the total number of cases of asbestos-related mesothelioma have arisen from the peritoneal rather than the pleural surface. This may perhaps be due to the ingestion of fibres at work, or their translocation from the respiratory to the gastrointestinal tract. In amosite factory workers in the USA, and in insulation workers in Belfast, an increased risk has been demonstrated of cancer of the gastrointestinal tract. However, other studies have not shown such an effect. A similar situation exists with cancer of the larynx, although here the increased risk appears to be small.

Other naturally occurring and synthetic mineral fibres. Experimental work suggests that both natural non-asbestos mineral and synthetic fibres less than 0.5 μm diameter and more than 8 μm in length may be hazardous. Some fibrous clays have been shown to cause mesothelioma experimentally, and epidemiological evidence suggests that fibrous erionite, a zeolite found in deposits of volcanic ash, may well have been responsible for a high incidence of mesothelioma in man. It will be some years yet before the effects of exposure to synthetic mineral fibres of equally fine diameter are known.

Arsenic. An increased mortality from bronchial carcinoma has been found in chemical process workers engaged in the production of inorganic arsenicals, in sheep dip workers, in vineyard workers using arsenical pesticide sprays, and in copper smelter workers. Exposure had in the past been heavy, and while predominantly to arsenic trioxide, in smelter workers exposure patterns are mixed, with other suspected carcinogens frequently present. In a group of copper smelters a linear relationship was shown between lifetime exposure to arsenic and excess mortality from lung cancer.

Data from other than occupational sources support the carcinogenic role of arsenic. For long, inorganic arsenicals, in particular Fowler's solution, have been used medicinally for the treatment of psoriasis and other chronic ailments. Arsenic pigmentation of the skin and hyperkeratosis have been followed by epithelioma, often multifocal in origin, and in some cases by basal cell carcinoma. Similar lesions have been described in some parts of the world with a high arsenic content in drinking water. Finally, angiosarcoma of the liver has followed chronic arsenic poisoning both following medication and in vintners in the Moselle valley using arsenical sprays. It is of interest, though not necessarily of relevance, that arsenic is the only example of a human carcinogen which has not given rise to experimental tumours despite many attempts.

Chromium. Since the 1930s workers engaged in the production of chromates from the raw material, chromite, or chrome iron ore by roasting with soda ash and lime have been known to have an increased mortality from bronchial carcinoma. The highest incidence of the disease was in people in their early 50s, that is, about five years earlier than the peak incidence in heavy smokers. The mean time interval between first exposure to the dusts and the development of cancer is of the order of 15–17 years. An increased mortality from lung cancer has also been shown in the chromate pigment industry, but not in chromium plating or other industries using chromium. The increased risk appears to be related to exposure to partly soluble hexavalent compounds but the precise nature of the carcinogen is not known.

A number of chromium compounds, in particular calcium chromate, are carcinogenic in the rat; they show mutagenic activity in bacterial test systems and will induce transformation in cell culture. Of the metals, chromium fits best the hypothesis that carcinogenesis entails mutagenic initiation of somatic cells as a result of direct interaction with DNA.

Nickel. A highly significant excess of both bronchial and nasal sinus cancer has been found in nickel refinery workers in several countries. In the Mond nickel works in South Wales where exposure occurred to, amongst other agents, nickel carbonyl gas, a 10-fold increase in mortality from lung cancer and a 900-fold increase in nasal cancer was found in men who had worked there in the early years. At first it was thought that highly poisonous nickel carbonyl gas was the specific carcinogen, but this supposition was discarded when a similar risk was found in nickel refinery workers in Canada, where an electrolytic process had been used. As with chromium, no excess mortality has yet been demonstrated in nickel plating or alloy production, although adequate epidemiological studies are lacking. Under the old nickel refinery conditions exposure had been heavy and from the fall in cancer mortality as exposure was progressively reduced, it seems unlikely that the much lower levels encountered in nickel plating would constitute a hazard. The time interval between initial exposure to nickel and the diagnosis of cancer is long, about 25 years, with a range of 10–40 years. Epithelial tumours of the lung have been most frequent but anaplastic and pleomorphic growths have also been seen.

In animal studies tumours have been produced with several nickel compounds in more than once species, and nickel subsulphide is probably the most potent metal carcinogen tested in animals. Cell transformation in culture has been shown, but not mutation in bacterial test systems.

Other metals. The evidence for a carcinogenic effect by metals other than arsenic, chromium, and nickel is much less conclusive. A small excess of lung cancer has been found in beryllium workers, some of whom had very short exposures. A small excess of carcinoma of the prostate has been found in cadmium workers, and both metals have shown a carcinogenic potential in animals. The excess lung cancer mortality observed in haematite miners is probably not related to iron oxide but to radioactivity present in the atmosphere of the mines.

Vinyl chloride. Angiosarcoma of the liver, a rare and highly malignant tumour was first observed in 1974 in a group of workers exposed to vinyl chloride monomer engaged in the polymerization process for the production of polyvinyl chloride. Exposure to the gaseous monomer in over 40 years preceding recognition of the hazard had been high in men engaged in the cleaning of the reactor vessels. Cases have since come to light in similar plants in several countries and exposure has now been drastically reduced. Angiosarcoma, as already described, has followed exposure to arsenic compounds and also the diagnostic use of thorium dioxide.

Ionizing radiation. The biological properties of ionizing radiation and its effects at population level are discussed elsewhere. In the sixteenth century, Paracelsus referred to the fatal disease of workers in the metal mines of Schneeberg and Joachimsthal as the *mala metallorum*. An excess lung cancer risk has been shown in these miners, exposed not only to metallic ores, but to ionizing radiation from the inhalation of radon and daughter products. An increased lung cancer mortality has now been found in the uranium miners of the Colorado plateau, where an exposure–response relationship with airborne radiation could be demonstrated. While the strength of the association was not great, compared with that between lung cancer and asbestos exposure, it is consistent, for a similar increase in lung cancer mortality has been found in fluorspar miners in Newfoundland and in the zinc-lead miners of northern Sweden. The excess lung cancer in the haematite miners of Cumberland in relation to the amount of airborne radiation there is in keeping with the above. There is some evidence too of a synergistic interaction with cigarette smoking.

In the luminizing industry, oral absorption of trace quantities of radium and related products in luminous paint by girls who tipped paint brushes in their mouths led to aplastic anaemia, radiation osteitis, and osteosarcoma from continuous exposure to α- and β-emissions from these bone-seeking elements. Plutonium 239, styled the deadliest poison known, radioactive products of uranium fission, and especially radio-isotopes of strontium are selectively retained and act in a similar way. Carcinoma of the nasal and mastoid sinuses has also developed in workers in the luminizing industry.

A number of physicists and pioneer radiologists working with X-rays from unshielded sources developed chronic X-ray dermatitis followed by squamous cell carcinoma, and occasionally basal cell carcinoma of the skin. At a later date American radiologists experienced an increased mortality from myeloid leukaemia. The leukaemogenic potential of X-irradiation is further demonstrated from the therapeutic field, for an increased mortality from myeloid leukaemia was found in patients irradiated in the treatment of ankylosing spondylitis. Thyroid carcinoma also developed in patients who had received irradiation of the thymus gland in infancy.

The use of thorium dioxide as a radiological contrast medium in diagnosis was abandoned after the discovery of angiosarcoma of the liver, an otherwise rare malignant tumour, in a number of patients between two and 25 years after administration. An increased mortality from leukaemia and from other forms of malignant disease was experienced by the population irradiated by the atomic bombs in Hiroshima and Nagasaki. The problems of general environmental contamination from fission products of atomic explosions are considered on page 6.86. Nuclear reactor workers are a high risk group in the event of a criticality accident, which has occurred from time to time.

Vibration injuries

Noise and mechanical vibrations are frequently encountered at work and both are responsible for adverse health effects.

Noise. See page 6.90 for a detailed discussion.

To prevent occupational deafness, it is necessary to limit noise exposure above 90 decibels. Where this level is exceeded, the exposure pattern and total dose over time should be determined, and where this is excessive, the following options considered. It may be possible to modify the machine or other noise source, to segregate it or to enclose it. This is often impracticable, in which case exposure time may have to be reduced and personal ear protection provided. Ear plugs or muffs have to be carefully fitted and may not be readily acceptable. The effectiveness of control measures instituted can be ascertained with regular audiometry.

Mechanical vibration. Vibration can be transferred to the body as a whole, or to a limb, as for example, when a vibrating tool is held in the hand. It can be described in terms of vibratory frequency, displacement, velocity, and acceleration. Vibratory frequency is made up of a fundamental oscillation with a series of harmonics to produce a vibration spectrum, and furthermore at certain frequencies resonance effects in the body may actually amplify the vibration.

Whole body vibration is experienced in both surface and air transport. Motion sickness must undoubtedly be the most familiar effect. Some studies have shown an increase in oxygen consumption and a decrease in performance levels. Various other adverse effects have been claimed which require substantiation, including loss of visual acuity. Vertical oscillations of about 0.25 Hz appear to be most effective in producing motion sickness.

Extensive use of vibratory hand tools may lead to the development of Raynaud's syndrome, known as vibration white finger (VWF). The condition is seen frequently in chain sawing, in both hand and pedestal grinding, in chipping with pneumatic tools, and in swaging. The power-driven chain saw is used extensively in forestry and timber operations, while grinding involves the cleaning of castings with the use of air drills on hard, resisting material. Quarrymen, miners, and others handling pneumatic drills, hammers, and chisels are also affected. In one study, 89 per cent of chain sawyers were affected, but prevalence rates in different groups have varied widely. The latent interval from initial exposure to vibration to the development of VWF has ranged from a few months to more than 20 years. Following withdrawal from exposure, a proportion of affected workers improve, the majority show no change, and a small number, mainly the more advanced cases, continue to deteriorate.

VWF develops with an initial complaint of intermittent tingling or numbness of the fingers. This is followed by blanching of one or more fingertips, with or without tingling or numbness (stage 1) usually first noticed in cold weather; progressing to frequent episodes of extensive blanching with all fingers involved, occurring in summer or winter, interfering with work and social activities and necessitating a change of occupation (stage 4). In a minority of cases trophic changes have occurred in the skin with gangrene of the terminal digits. Arteriography has shown subintimal fibrosis, medial hypertrophy, and digital artery occlusion with thrombus formation. Bone cysts in the hand are frequently seen, but these appear to be related more to heavy manual work than to vibration.

In the prevention of VWF, those who have experienced Raynaud's phenomenon should be excluded from work with vibrating tools. Cold exposure should be avoided, and gloves to maintain adequate warmth of the hands and wind-resistant clothing should be worn where appropriate. The main factors leading to the more advanced stages of VWF are exposure time, high energy vibration, the tightness of the grip, and susceptibility of the subject. Exposure time should be kept as short as possible with frequent breaks, avoiding long periods of continuous use of the vibrating tool. The characteristics of the vibration can be determined with the aid of a piezoelectric accelerometer. It appears that low frequency vibration is the most injurious, but tools should be designed to reduce transmission from the source to the handle as far as possible.

References

Advisory Committee on Asbestos (1979) Vol. I. *Final report of the Advisory Committee*; Vol. II. *Papers commissioned by the Committee.* HMSO, London.

Cronin, E. (1980). Contact dermatitis. Churchill Livingstone, Edinburgh.

Environmental health Perspectives (1981). Proceedings of a workshop conference on the role of metals in carcinogenesis. *Env. Hlth Perspec.* **40**, 1.

Friberg, L., Nordberg, G. F., and Vouk, V. B. (eds.) (1979). *Handbook on the toxicology of metals.* Elsevier/North-Holland, Amsterdam.

Hollstein, M., McCann, J., Angelosanto, F. A., and Nichols, W. W. (1979). Short-term tests for carcinogens and mutagens. *Mutation Res.* **65**, 133.

Hunter, D. (1978). *The diseases of occupations.* Hodder and Stoughton, London.

International Agency for Research on Cancer (1979): *Monographs on the evaluation of the carcinogenic risk of chemicals to humans.* Supplement 1, World Health Organization, Lyon.

International Labour Office (1980). Guidelines for the use of ILO International Classification of radiographs of pneumoconioses, revised edn. *Occupational Safety and Health Series* 22 (rev. 80) International Labour Office, Geneva.

Kazantzis, G. (1978). The role of hypersensitivity and the immune response in influencing susceptibility to metal toxicity. *Env. Hlth Perspec.* **25**, 111.

McDonald, J. C. (ed.) (1981). *Recent advances in occupational health.* Churchill Livingstone, Edinburgh.

Parkes, W. R. (1981). *Occupational lung disorders*, 2nd edn., Butterworth, London.

Rosenman, K. D. (1979). Cardiovascular disease and environmental exposure. *Br. J. ind. Med.* **36**, 85.

Royal Society (1979). *Long-term hazards from environmental chemicals.* A Royal Society discussion organized by Sir Richard Doll and A. E. M. McLean. Royal Society, London.

Schilling, R. S. F. (ed.) (1981). *Occupational health practice.* Butterworth, London.

Taylor, W. and Pelmear, P. L. (eds.) (1975). *Vibration white finger in industry.* Academic Press, London.

Waldron, H. A. (ed.) (1980). *Metals in the environment.* Academic Press, London.

ACCIDENT PREVENTION

R. T. Booth

The prevention of accidents at work demands the contribution of many disciplines and the coalition of several interests. The objectives of the chapter are to review the development of the conflicting approaches to the control of danger, and to suggest the most fruitful directions for future efforts. Similar measures are necessary to prevent occupational diseases. The approach is epitomized by the British Health and Safety at Work Act 1974. It is a duty of all employers of five or more persons to prepare a written statement of their policy on the health and safety of their employees and to describe how it is to be implemented.

Accidents at work occur in diverse circumstances and settings. A small number of accidents result from component or structural failures or from maloperations (*contingent* dangers); but the majority of accidents are associated with the dangers which form an everyday element of working life: contact with moving machinery, falls, cuts from material being handled, slipping on or striking against objects, injuries from hand tools, and so on. The weakness of many efforts to prevent accidents associated with component or other failures is that they are considered to be purely technical matters, exclusively the responsibility of engineers. The control of ever present dangers is seen either as a problem capable of solution only with physical safeguards, or as a behavioural issue relating only to the personnel directly exposed to risk. In fact to achieve high safety standards it is necessary to employ competent personnel at all levels and to create a coherent safety organization within which they can work.

Accident statistics. Table 1 shows the number of fatal accidents at work reported to the Health and Safety Commission (HSC) and

Table 1 Fatal accidents at work, with incidence rates where available, 1973–7 (UK)

Sector	Number of deaths *(deaths per 100 000 at risk)*				
	1973	1974	1975	1976	1977
Reported to HSC enforcement authorities under:					
1. Factories Act					
Manufacturing industries	236	254	196	175	179
	(4.2)	*(4.5)*	*(3.7)*	*(3.4)*	*(3.4)*p
Construction industry	231	166	182	156	130
	(21.6)	*(16.0)*	*(17.7)*	*(15.3)*	*(13.1)*p
Other industries	82	59	49	51	49
Total Factories Act	549	479	427	382	358
2. Offices, Shops, and Railway Premises Act	15	20	16	20	34
3. Explosives Act	8	3	6	4	—
4. Regulation of Railways and Railway Employment (Prevention of Accidents) Acts	42	38	46	46	35
	(18.3)	*(14.8)*	*(18.7)*	*(18.8)*	*(16.8)*
5. Mines and Quarries Act					
Coal mines	80	48	64	50	40
	(29.6)	*(18.7)*	*(24.7)*	*(19.6)*	*(15.8)*
Other mines	8	2	2	8	2
Quarries	14	16	15	16	12
	(29.0)	*(31.2)*	*(29.0)*	*(32.6)*	*(24.2)*
Total Mines and Quarries Act	102	66	81	74	54
6. Agriculture (Safety, Health, and Welfare Provisions) Act	46	33	34	41	32
	(14.7)	*(10.9)*	*(11.7)*	*(14.1)*	*(10.7)*
7. Mineral Workings (Offshore Installations) Act	3	12	10	17	11
Total reported to HSC enforcement authorities	765	651	620	584	524
Reported to other authorities under:					
8. Merchant Shipping (Returns of Births and Deaths) Regulations:					
Seamen	71	58	77	58	52
Fishermen:					
Deep sea trawlers	20	46	16	14	9
Other fishing vessels	8	27	13	16	19
Total Merchant Shipping etc. Regulations	99	131	106	88	80
9. Civil aviation (various legislation)	9	4	3	10	10
Total reported to other authorities	108	135	109	98	90
Total reported to all authorities	873	786	729	682	614

From Health and Safety Executive (1980). *Health and safety statistics 1977.* HMSO, London

other relevant authorities for the years 1973–7. Table 2 presents the total numbers of accidents at work reported to the same authorities over the same period. It may be seen that the number of fatalities at 614 in 1977 represented a reduction of about 30 per cent from the 1973 figure. The reduction in reported accidents has been much less dramatic. Reported accident statistics are notoriously unreliable. The figures may be affected by under-reporting; moreover the period of absence from work is likely to be affected by factors other than the actual severity of the injury. In any case it must be acknowledged that a proportion (about 80 per cent on the basis of factory accident data only) of the reported accidents involve either relatively minor injuries, or injuries of uncertain relationship to work (e.g. strains and sprains). Thus Table 2 is included only to show the general magnitude of the problem. The fatalities and the reduction in fatalities, shown in Table 1, are probably a better guide to the trend of safety performance.

Table 3 shows the fatal accident rates in manufacturing industry for selected countries. Bearing in mind that the average number of hours worked in a year will be about 2000 so that incidence rates (per 10^5 man-years) will tend to be about double the frequency rates (per 10^8 man-hours), the UK record compares well with that of the other countries. Such statistics need to be viewed with caution because of the complexities of comparing data based on different criteria. For example the German figures may include occupational diseases as well as accidents.

Review of approaches to accident prevention. Research effort has, at first sight, been concentrated in the right area: namely the study of causation. An understanding of causation is obviously a prerequisite to the choice of preventive measures. Unfortunately researchers have tended to pursue causation in narrow behavioural terms, with an emphasis on the circumstances immediately before, and directly leading to, an accident. The more distant causes (in time) which may be crucial for prevention have been largely neglected. Hale and Hale state: '. . . researchers have not paid enough attention to the part played by the work and the social and physical environment in accident causation. They have concentrated on the factors associated with the people who have suffered the accidents.' '. . . research has concentrated on the search for causes of accidents. The effectiveness of preventive measures has received little attention . . . .'

The emphasis of behavioural factors in accident causation—in scientific papers factors such as accident proneness, fatigue, and intelligence, and in other sources, recklessness, carelessness, and ignorance—is associated with the widespread (though controversial) presumption that most accidents are caused by human failings,

Table 2   Accidents at work, with incident rates where available, 1973–7 (UK)

Sector	Number of accidents (accidents per 100 000 at risk)				
	1973	1974	1975	1976	1977
Reported to HSC enforcement authorities under:					
1. Factories Act					
Manufacturing industries	209 699	199 090	184 324	181 065	187 261
	(3 710)	(3 520)	(3 490)	(3 480)	(3 590)
Construction industry	37 920	34 598	35 579	36 139	32 815
	(3 540)	(3 330)	(3 460)	(3 530)	(3 330)
Other industries	24 899	23 242	23 237	24 481	24 324
Total Factories Act	272 518	256 930	243 140	241 685	244 400
2. Offices, Shops, and Railway Premises Act	17 742	16 669	17 198	18 359	19 159
3. Explosives Act	54	24	32	51	50
4. Regulation of Railways and Railway Employment (Prevention of Accidents) Acts	5 912	5 592	5 781	5 620	6 001
	(3 010)	(2 770)	(2 920)	(2 920)	(2 980)
5. Mines and Quarries Act					
Coal mines	66 074	49 642	54 071	50 788	49 315
	(24 610)	(19 340)	(20 860)	(19 960)	(19 520)
Other mines	569	539	583	870	807
	(–)	(12 450)	(11 580)	(16 490)	(13 920)
Quarries	2 265	2 003	1 889	1 672	1 891
	(4 690)	(3 900)	(3 730)	(3 400)	(3 810)
Total Mines and Quarries Act	68 908	52 184	56 543	53 330	52 013
6. Agriculture (Safety, Health, and Welfare Provisions) Act	6 172	5 742	5 230	5 247	4 818
	(1 970)	(1 890)	(1 800)	(1 800)	(1 600)
7. Mineral Workings (Offshore Installations) Act	190	449	591	718	868
Total reported to HSC enforcement authorities	371 496	337 590	328 515	325 010	327 309
Reported to other authorities:					
8. Merchant seamen (non-fatal accidents only)	–	1 347	1 390	1 255	1 426
9. Fishermen—deep sea trawlers	825	781	624	827	618

From Health and Safety Executive (1980). *Health and safety statistics 1977*. HMSO, London

Table 3   Fatal accident rates in manufacturing industry for selected countries, 1973–7

Country	Incidence (I) or frequency (F) rate*	Accidents reported (R) or compensated (C)	1973	1974	1975	1976	1977
Great Britain	I	R	4	5	4	3	3¶
France†	I	C	10	10	10	8	–
Federal Republic of Germany	I‡	C	17	16	16	14	13
Irish Republic	I‖	R	10	8	9	5	–
Italy	I‡	C	8	8	8	–	–
Netherlands	I‡	R	4	4	4	3	–
Sweden	F	C	3	3	3	–	–
Canada	I	R	15	21	15	10¶	9¶
United States of America¶	F	R	3	3	3	3	–
Japan**	F	R	3	2	2	1	2

* Incident rates: deaths per 100 000 employees
   Frequency rates: deaths per 100 million man-hours
 † Including mining and quarrying
 ‡ Based on standard man-years of 300 working days. With a 5-day week accidents per actual man-year are likely to be some 20 per cent fewer
 ‖ Rate per 100 000 wage earners
 ¶ Based on sample surveys
 ** Establishment employing 100 or more workers
 Sources: Health and Safety Executive, International Labour Office
 From Health and Safety Executive (1980). *Health and safety statistics 1977*. HMSO, London

not by shortcomings in the physical environment and laid-down methods of work. Heinrich in an influential book first published in 1931 stated that about 90 per cent of preventable accidents were caused by 'unsafe acts' and the remainder by 'unsafe conditions'. Many participants in the increasingly sterile causation debate have overlooked Heinrich's further observation: '. . . although man failure *causes* the most accidents, mechanical guarding and engin-

eering revision are nevertheless important factors in *preventing* the most accidents'.

Kletz has summarized the way opinion has developed: 'Searching my company's old files, I found a report . . . in which one of our first safety officers announced a new discovery: most accidents are due to human failing. . . . The remedy was obvious: we must persuade men to take more care. For 50 years our sites have been adorned with posters urging us to do just this—though no one has ever produced evidence that they have any effect. . . . It took nearly 50 years for the next breakthrough in thought: the realization that well-trained, well-motivated men . . . make occasional mistakes, have their moments of aberration . . . and that punishment, reprimand, or exhortation will not prevent these occasional errors. . . . We came to realize that to say "Accidents are caused by human failing" is not untrue, but not very helpful. It encourages us to tell people to be more careful, instead of looking for ways of reducing opportunities for error.'

In marked contrast to the attitudes described above Her Majesty's Factory Inspectorate has for the last 140 years argued for, and enforced, legal provisions narrowly demanding absolute standards of physical safeguards. For example, it is no defence in law for occupiers of factories to argue that their obligation to fence securely dangerous parts of machinery is waived when an employee wilfully removes a machinery guard. Notwithstanding this stringency many accidents continued to occur in circumstances where the law was rigorous (and yet more occurred in circumstances where no legal provisions existed, or the law was not relevant).

In parallel with the general failure to reduce accidents associated with continuous dangers, the early 1970s saw a growing concern about the potential for catastrophe from the increasing scale, complexity, and potential for harm of technological development in 'high-risk' industries. Her Majesty's Chief Inspector of Factories stated in his report for 1972: 'Some risks are now so great that a major failure is unacceptable and the possibility must be eliminated at the very outset. . . . We are faced increasingly with the risk of failures which could result in multiple deaths and injuries of near disaster proportions.'

These forebodings were justified shortly afterwards by the Flixborough explosion in 1974. Moreover in the same time period a substantial number of serious accidents occurred as a result of *contingent* dangers in traditional industries, for example the collapse of falsework at Loddon Bridge in 1972, the eruption of molten metal at the Appleby-Frodingham Steelworks in 1975, and the cage winding system brake failure at Markham Colliery in 1973. The initial investigations of most of these accidents concentrated on the immediate, technical causes of the accidents. The Report of the Inquiry into the Flixborough Disaster suggested that attention to certain technical details should prevent a recurrence. This approach was attacked amongst others by Atherley and Booth. Incidentally the explosion at Flixborough occurred without any breach of the Factories Act 1961. No legal provisions applied to the pressure vessels which contained highly flammable cyclohexane. Paradoxically if the vessels had contained more innocuous air or steam there would have been several breaches of law. However, the committees established to look more deeply into these accidents, for example the Advisory Committee on Falsework (1978) and the Advisory Committee on Major Hazards (1976 and 1979), considered the underlying (non-technical) *pre-conditions* for the accidents. The Final report on the Advisory Committee on Falsework stated: 'Our studies showed that failures arise from many different causes. Each one has two elements: the technical cause which led to the collapse; and the procedural errors which allowed the faults to occur and to go undetected and uncorrected. . . . In hardly any case did we find that failure was the result of a problem beyond the scope of current technology.'

Legal developments. The preceding sections have described how accident prevention effort has been less than fully effective where there has been a compartmentalized concentration on behavioural or technical measures, aided and abetted by legal provisions which were out-of-date both in terms of the scope of dangers covered and the range of preventive measures.

All the developing forces referred to led to a watershed in approaches to the control of dangers at work, and to the Report of the Committee on Safety and Health at Work —the Robens' Report.

The Report stated: 'It is not to underrate the importance of physical safeguards to say that the preoccupation with the physical environment has tended to dominate this field, to the neglect of the equally important human and organizational factors such as the role of training . . . the arrangements for monitoring safety performance, or the influence of work systems on attitudes and behaviour.'

The Robens' Report led directly to the Health and Safety at Work Act 1974. The crucial point about the more recent legislation is that it is not a substitute for the old; the absolute duties remain extant. But the new law provides the basis for a broadening of the scope of the old law together with the basis for better compliance with the old. The new law does not replace the duty to fence securely dangerous parts of machinery; rather, in its general duties, it requires consideration of the factors which determine standards of compliance: obligations on all parties concerned with safety; the requirements to devise safe systems of work, training, and supervision to be used in conjunction with, and in support of the requirements for physical safeguards.

Safety organization and expertise. The Health and Safety at Work Act 1974 places unrestricted obligations on employers to control workplace dangers. Whereas previous enactments could be complied with by rote (the law identified the dangers and specified the preventive action) the 1974 Act obliges employers to identify *for themselves* the dangers within their undertaking and to devise an implement their own solutions. The new legislation quite properly allows much greater discretion to companies to select countermeasures of their choice (although there is now scope for argument in circumstances where the new general duties apparently conflict with the old specified duties, as is the case with machinery guarding standards). But the new law also allows much greater scope for making expensive mistakes.

Industrial managements have not appreciated fully the significance of the change in the character of health and safety legislation. Many managers still request and require detailed guidance from the enforcement agencies concerning their specific duties. The philosophy of earlier legislation—'do it this way'—remains. Managers sometimes appear to labour under two inter-related misapprehensions. Firstly, a belief, encouraged by the old law, that the control of danger is essentially a straightforward, even a trivial, subject which could be dealt with with a minimum of expertise. Secondly, the presumption that safety can be achieved by the combination of good intentions and exhortation. The Health and Safety Executive (HSE) report *Success and Failure in Accident Prevention* states: 'in many (companies) the . . . understanding of the problem weakened successively the higher up the management chain the subject was followed'. It is not surprising that some managers are woefully ignorant of this subject if no attempts have been made to teach them and convince them that skill in health and safety is an essential part of their professional make up. 'The Report identifies an almost total absence of any form of safety training or knowledge enlargement at the more senior management levels'.

Typical consequences of weaknesses in safety management appear to be:

1. Failures to identify certain workplace dangers, for example relatively straightforward dangers which are 'hidden' in the details of a complex machine or process.

2. Delays in recognizing dangers, e.g. a failure to identify a hazard at the design stage (the costs of control are likely to be substantially greater once a machine is installed).

3. Failure to respond to identified dangers because of a 'lack of closure' in the safety procedures: 'important safety issues are . . . raised and may be studied to some degree of depth, but are not carried through to resolution; and the lessons learned from these studies do not reach those individuals . . . that most need to know about them' (Kemeny 1979).

4. Inappropriate allocation of safety resources, typically undue

attention to the prevention of accidents with a relatively trivial potential for harm.

5. Failure, primarily involving shortcomings in safety methods, to select optimal control measures, and the adoption of control measures which simply do not work.

6. Failure to provide long-term control of dangers because, for example, monitoring arrangements are not thought to be necessary. Examples include checks on the use of machinery guards, protective clothing, and safe systems of work.

7. Failure to persuade employees or the HSE of the efficiency of safety arrangements leading to the possibility of production losses associated with safety-related industrial action, or prohibition orders.

The deficiencies in safety management referred to in the previous section appear to be attributable to:

1. Shortcomings in health and safety skills (the consequence may be wrong decisions but could also include a reluctance of managers to take decisions because of a lack of confidence in their own knowledge).

2. The absence of adequate procedures for the systematic evaluation of dangers and their control.

3. The absence of adequate arrangements for monitoring compliance with safety procedures and working methods.

There appear to be four crucial ingredients in an effective safety organization designed to cope with the identification and long-term control of dangers. The list represents a summary of the arrangements which have been found to work well in companies that have adopted them:

1. Competent staff at all levels, and in particular management and technical staff who are appropriately trained in the execution of their safety duties.

2. The availability from within or outside the organization of specialist advisers on health and safety matters.

3. An effective safety organization including an appropriate and balanced use of detailed safety procedures, and arrangements for consultation with employees at all levels.

4. The provision of sufficient funds to ensure that the policy objectives are met.

The employer's policy statement and arrangements for carrying out this policy required under Section 2 (3) of the 1974 Act should manifestly give specific detail of its provisions under each of the four headings.

The fundamental responsibility of all managements must be to employ competent staff and to organize them sensibly to deal with health and safety matters. Two crucial questions should be asked at a senior level within the organization:

1. How much safety skill is required within the organization?

2. How should (a) safety skill, and (b) safety responsibilities and duties be 'allocated' and shared between line and functional staff, for example engineers, occupational physicians, and between specialist safety advisers within and outside the Company?

The Chief Inspector of Factories has drawn particular attention to the shortcomings of safety policy statements in providing coherent answers to the above questions: 'The majority of policies suffered from similar defects and these were . . . (a) a failure to identify adequately the organization for implementing the general policy statement; (b) a complete lack of detail about the arrangements for ensuring that the policy statement was observed; (c) no laid-down information about basic or specific hazards and no written procedures for hazardous routine jobs; and (d) an over-emphasis on the responsibilities of employees for their own safety.'

It is clear that safety arrangements generally lack depth and detail. The adequacy of the detail of safety arrangements should be tested in relation to a particular danger. For example, with re-ference to the problems associated with mechanical dangers from (new) machinery, the following questions might be asked:

Whose job is it to:

Identify the dangers and determine risk?

Select and implement the appropriate safeguarding measures?

Devise a planned maintenance schedule for the safety devices?

Devise the safe work systems, and written procedures where judged necessary?

Instruct operators and maintenance staff of their duties?

Monitor compliance with the safe systems of work?

For each task, what are the training needs involved?

I believe that safety arrangements should, in general, deal with safety matters at this level of detail. The fundamental point is that unless safety issues are pursued in detail it is impossible to draw up a coherent training programme. The starting point for safety training must be instruction for senior managers to ensure that the formulation of safety policy and arrangements ceases to be the vacuous exercise that it is so often at present.

References

Atherley, G. R. C. (1975). Strategies in health and safety at work. *Production Engineer* **54**, 49.

— and Booth, R. T. (1975). Could there be another Flixborough? *Sunday Times* 14 September.

Booth R. T. (1979). *Safety: too important a matter to be left to the engineers?* University of Aston in Birmingham.

— (1980). Safety training for management. Management responsibilities and the development of suitable training methods. *National Health and Safety Conference.* Victor Green Publications, London.

Committee on Safety and Health at Work (1972). *Safety and health at work. Report of the committee.* HMSO, London.

Department of Employment (1974). *Accidents in factories.* HMSO, London.

— (1975). *The Flixborough disaster. Report of the court of inquiry.* HMSO, London.

Department of Energy (1974). *Accident at Markham Colliery Derbyshire.* HMSO, London.

Hale, A. R. and Hale, M. (1972). A review of the industrial accident research literature. *Committee on Safety and Health at Work research paper.* HMSO, London.

Health and Safety Commission (1976). *Advisory Committee on Major Hazards: first report.* HMSO, London.

— (1979). *Advisory Committee on Major Hazards: second report.* HMSO, London.

Health and Safety Executive (1976). *The explosion at Appleby-Frodingham steelworks Scunthorpe 4 November 1975.* HMSO, London.

— (1976). *Final Report of the Advisory Committee on Falsework.* HMSO, London.

— (1976). *Success and failure in accident prevention.* HMSO, London.

— (1979). *Health and safety in manufacturing and service industries 1976.* HMSO, London.

— (1980). *Effective policies for health and safety.* HMSO, London.

— (1980). *Health and safety statistics 1977.* HMSO, London.

Heinrich, H. W. (1959). *Industrial accident prevention.* McGraw-Hill, New York.

HM Chief Inspector of Factories (1972). *Annual report.* Comnd 5398, HMSO, London.

— (1974). *Annual report.* Comnd 6322, HMSO, London.

HM Factory Inspectorate (1973). *Report on the collapse of falsework for the viaduct over the River Loddon on 24 October 1972.* HMSO, London.

Kemeny, J. G. (1979). *Report on the Presidents Commission on the accident at Three Mile Island.* Pergamon Press, Oxford.

Kletz, T. A. (1979). *Industrial safety: the shaking of the foundations.* Loughborough University.

Powell, P. I., Hale, M., Martin, J., and Simon, M. (1971). *2000 accidents.* National Institute of Industrial Psychology, London.

Surry, J. (1969). *Industrial accident research.* University of Toronto, Canada.

Section 7
Principles of clinical pharmacology and therapeutics

Principles of clinical pharmacology and therapeutics

A. Breckenridge and M. L' E. Orme

Introduction. The rational use of drugs dates from the latter part of the nineteenth century and may be attributed to three distinct developments. First was the birth of synthetic organic chemistry and the question whether some new compounds might have medicinal value. Among the earliest chemicals recognized to be of therapeutic importance were the general anaesthetics and chemotherapeutic agents such as salvarsan. The second pillar of modern therapeutics was the elucidation of the mode of action of these chemicals by means of experiments in animals and in man. Third has been the development in the understanding of the basis of human disease expressed in terms of perturbation of underlying physiological control mechanisms and morbid anatomical changes.

From these disparate origins, clinical pharmacology has emerged as a discipline whose aim is, broadly speaking, the scientific study of drugs in man. There are many aspects of clinical pharmacology. Pharmacokinetics, the mathematical description of the fate of drugs in the body, including the processes of drug absorption, distribution, metabolism, and excretion, has probably attracted attention disproportionate to its importance because of the ability to make precise measurements of drug concentrations in biological fluids using refined analytical technology. Pharmacodynamics encompasses studies of the effects of drugs on the body and of the underlying modes of drug action; this still remains the main challenge in clinical pharmacology since available techniques are either invasive and thus generally inapplicable or are non-invasive and tend to be crude and imprecise. Toxicology is that aspect of pharmacology dealing with the adverse effects of drugs used in therapy and of chemical substances used in the household, in industry, or found in the environment. For political reasons this is the face of clinical pharmacology most frequently shown to the public and is one reason for current trends away from allopathic medicine. A separate facet of clinical pharmacology is the testing of new drugs in man by means of the clinical trial. Such studies are only as good as the methods used to assess drug effects, and the statistical methods to evaluate the results.

The principles underlying drug therapy are fundamentally similar for any condition in which drugs are used. Obvious variables include the nature and stage of the disease, the chemical nature and dose of the drug used. The aim of all therapy is to administer the appropriate drug in the correct dose to produce the desired therapeutic effect with the minimum of adverse side-effects. This chapter outlines the principles on which the achievement of this aim rests.

Basic concepts of drug action

Physicochemical characteristics of drugs. The three most important physicochemical properties of a drug are lipid solubility, degree of ionization, and molecular size.

Lipid solubility is the principal determinant of the ability of a drug to cross the membranes of cell walls be they of the gastrointestinal tract, renal tubule, or blood–brain barrier. The relevance of lipid solubility can best be appreciated by considering the fate of drugs in the nephron. Filtered at the glomerulus, a lipid soluble drug is completely reabsorbed in the renal tubular system to remain in the body for an indefinite time. Drug metabolism can thus be viewed as a mechanism to change lipid soluble compounds into those with a higher degree of water solubility, i.e. greater polarity. The behaviour of water soluble metabolites in the renal tubules is quite different from the parent compound. By virtue of their new found polarity, metabolites tend not to be reabsorbed in the renal tubules and will be eliminated in the urine. Lipid solubility can be measured by *in vitro* methods using partition of a drug between an organic and an aqueous solvent. Table 1 shows the partition coefficients of a series of beta adrenoceptor blocking agents between octanol and water. This has clinical relevance since those beta blockers with a high degree of lipid solubility, e.g. propranolol and oxprenolol, tend to be well absorbed from the gut, to show a high first pass effect in the gut and the liver, and to have a relatively short half-life. They also gain easy access to the cerebral cortex and thus have the propensity to produce central side-effects. On the other hand less lipid soluble beta adrenoceptor blocking drugs such as atenolol and sotolol are not so readily absorbed, are not extensively metabolized in the liver, and tend to be eliminated unchanged via the kidney. Further, they do not gain such easy access to the brain as more lipid soluble counterparts.

Table 1 Principal pharmacological properties of some beta-adrenoceptor blocking drugs

Drug	Cardio-selectivity	Intrinsic sympatho-mimetic activity	Membrane stabilizing activity	Log partition coefficient octanol/water
acebutolol	±	+	+	1.87
alprenolol	−	+	+	2.61
atenolol	+	−	−	0.23
metoprolol	+	−	±	2.15
nadolol	−	−	−	0.71
oxprenolol	−	+	+	2.18
pindolol	−	+ +	+	1.75
practolol	+	+	−	0.79
propranolol	−	−	+	3.65
sotalol	−	−	−	0.79
timolol	−	−	+	2.10

The extent to which a drug is ionized depends on the pKa of the drug and the pH of the medium in which the drug is dissolved. pKa is defined as the pH at which 50 per cent of the drug is ionized. If a weakly acidic drug is represented as HA, then:

$$HA \rightleftharpoons H^+ + A^- \qquad (1)$$

and therefore $\quad Ka = \dfrac{H^+ + A^-}{HA} \qquad (2)$

where Ka is the dissociation constant. pKa is the negative logarithm of Ka.

Logarithmic transformation of equation (2) gives:

$$pH = pKa + \log_{10} \frac{(A^-)}{(HA)} \qquad (3)$$

From this, it can be seen that changes in pH near the pKa of a drug such as phenobarbitone (pKa 7.4) will give rise to considerable changes in extent of its ionization. This is put to clinical use in patients overdosed with phenobarbitone in whom the urine can be made alkaline by sodium bicarbonate administration to facilitate its excretion. At urine pH of 8.0, over 95 per cent of phenobarbitone will be ionized and thus will not be reabsorbed in the kidney. For a basic drug, e.g. amphetamine or quinidine, (represented as BH), equation (3) is rearranged so that:

$$pH = pKa + \log_{10} \frac{BH}{B^+} \qquad (4)$$

By the same arguments as above, acidification of the urine will promote the elimination of basic drugs and this may also be made use of in treating an overdose.

The degree of drug ionization has implications for drug absorption from the gastrointestinal tract. Under the acid conditions in the stomach, it can be appreciated from equation (3) that acidic drugs such as salicylate or warfarin will exist preferentially in the non-ionized lipid soluble form. Basic drugs such as chlorpromazine and tricyclic antidepressants will tend to be ionized and relatively lipid insoluble in the stomach on this pH partition hypothesis. However, the larger surface area of the small intestine dictates that both types of drug, pH and pKa notwithstanding, will tend to be maximally absorbed lower in the gastrointestinal tract than the stomach. The basis that only non-ionized drugs will preferentially cross the gastrointestinal tract is illustrated in Fig. 1.

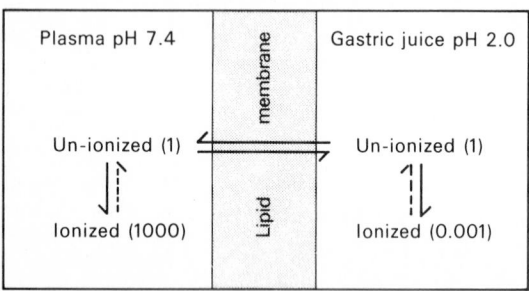

Fig. 1 Distribution of weakly acidic drug (e.g. warfarin) between plasma and gastric juice. The figures in brackets refer to the relative concentrations of warfarin in arbitrary units.

Molecular size is probably the least important of the three physical properties of a drug. Biliary excretion is largely determined by molecular size; in man, compounds of molecular weight of greater than 400 are excreted in the bile. This molecular weight shows considerable species variation and applies to drug conjugates too. This property can also be used therapeutically. Ampicillin is excreted in the bile and use is made of this in the treatment of biliary tract infections. Once drug conjugates have reached the gut via the bile, they may be broken down by the enzymes of gut bacteria, liberating free drug for reabsorption. This process of enterohepatic recirculation is described below.

Pharmacokinetic considerations. Pharmacokinetics is the mathematical description of the processes of drug absorption, distribution, and elimination. The body can be considered for mathematical purposes as either a single compartment or a series of interconnected compartments each of a finite volume containing a drug at a definite concentration and whose ingress into and egress from the compartment is described by a series of rate constants.

Figure 2 represents the body as a single compartment. This has a volume V which is also referred to as the apparent volume of drug distribution. In Fig. 2 K_{ab} is the rate constant of absorption and K_{el} the rate constant of elimination. Most kinetic processes can be described by first order kinetics, that is the rate at which a drug enters or leaves a compartment is proportional to the concentration therein. This is illustrated in Fig. 3 where the plasma concentration of warfarin versus time is plotted over 100 hours after adminis-

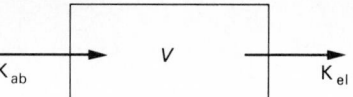

Fig. 2 Schematic diagram of the body as a one-compartment model.

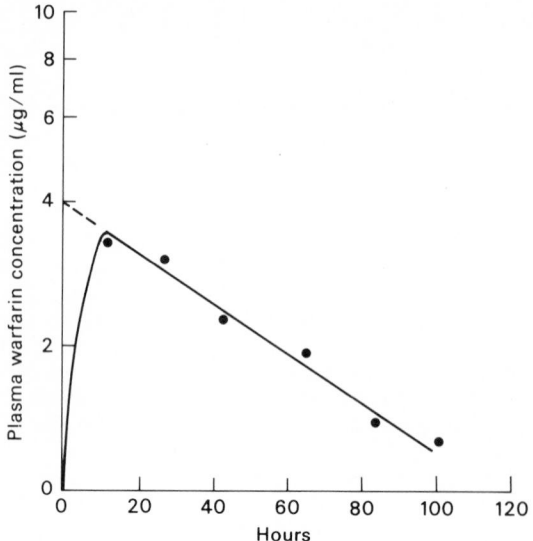

Fig. 3 Plasma concentrations of warfarin over a 100 hour period in a man given a single oral dose of 35 mg. The vertical axis is on a logarithmic scale.

tration of a single dose of 35 mg. The vertical axis (warfarin concentration) is logarithmic, thus converting the exponential decay slope seen on an arithmetical scale into a straight line; the slope of this line gives the rate constant for elimination (K_{el}). The half-life of the drug in plasma is the time it takes for any concentration to fall by 50 per cent.

In a one-compartment model, the plasma concentration (C_p) at any time is proportional to the amount of drug in the compartment. Thus

$$\frac{d}{dt} C_p = K.C_p \qquad (5)$$

On integration with respect to time,

$$C_p = C_{p_0} e^{K_t} \qquad (6)$$

where C_{p_0} is the concentration at time zero. To calculate the plasma half-life of warfarin (i.e. the time to take C_p to decline by 50 per cent):

$$C_p = C_{p_0}/2$$

$$\text{or} \quad C_{p_0} = C_{p_0} e^{-K_t_\frac{1}{2}}$$

$$\therefore t_\frac{1}{2} = 0.693/K \qquad (7)$$

If, in Fig. 3, the decay slope of warfarin in plasma is extrapolated back to time zero, the plasma concentration at time zero is 4 µg/ml. The elimination plasma half-life of warfarin is approximately 50 hours.

The apparent volume of distribution (see below) of warfarin using the one-compartment model system is calculated by dividing the dose (35 mg or 35 000 µg) by the value for C_0 (4 µg/ml). The result is 8750 ml or 8.75 l. This, it should be noted, is of the same order as the plasma volume.

Two-compartment model. When the plasma concentration of a drug versus time is plotted, the result may not be a linear decay as in Fig. 3 but may yield two linear portions as in Fig. 4, which shows the decline in plasma ethinyloestradiol after oral administration. The

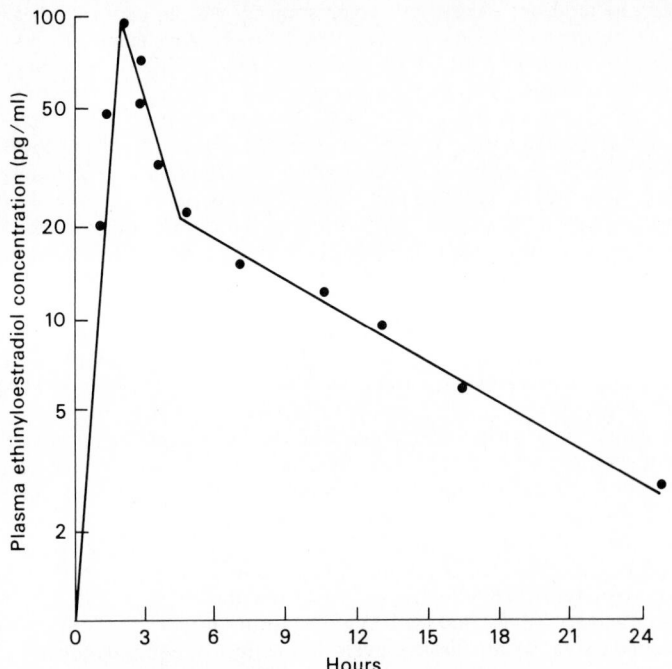

Fig. 4 Plasma concentrations of ethinyloestradiol over 24 hours in a woman given a single oral dose of 30 μg. The vertical axis is on a logarithmic scale.

first phase can broadly be equated with the distribution of drug into the tissues of the body and the second phase represents elimination from the body. Rate constants for these two phases can be calculated as described above. The body can thus be considered as comprising two compartments, a central and a peripheral compartment which are connected as shown in Fig. 5. It is customary but not essential to consider absorption and elimination as occurring into and from the central compartment.

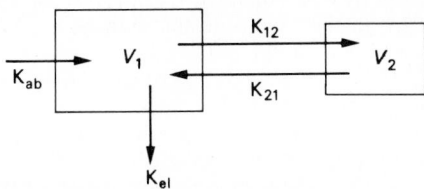

Fig. 5 Schematic diagram of the body as a two-compartment model. K_{12} and K_{21} are the transfer rate constants between the two compartments.

Apparent volume of distribution. The apparent volume of distribution is the sum of the volumes of the compartments defined above. Irrespective of the model chosen, the apparent volume of distribution is merely a proportionality constant which describes the amount of drug in the body relative to that in the plasma at any one time. Thus the total amount of drug in the body is equal to its apparent volume of distribution multiplied by the plasma concentration. The apparent volume of distribution is a notional volume rather than one with anatomical significance. Drugs (such as warfarin) which have a low apparent volume of distribution tend to be located within the plasma, by virtue of their high affinity to plasma albumin. Drugs such as tricyclic antidepressants have a large apparent volume of distribution, i.e. their concentration in tissues relative to plasma is high. Table 2 gives the apparent volume of distribution for some commonly used drugs. One important therapeutic implication of the size of the apparent volume of distribution is the assessment of the ease by which drugs may be removed from the body by haemodialysis after overdosage. A drug with a low volume of distribution located primarily in the plasma may be dialysed more readily than a drug with a high volume of distribution

which is located primarily in the tissues. Thus aspirin (apparent volume of distribution 0.15 l/kg) may be dialysed but nortriptyline (apparent volume of distribution 20 l/kg) may not, and any attempt to do so is automatically doomed to failure.

The apparent volume of distribution may be calculated in several ways. As described already for warfarin, if one assumes rapid absorption after oral dosage, or more properly after intravenous dosage, the logarithmic decay in drugs in plasma versus time is linear. Then the dose of drug administered, divided by the plasma concentration at zero time gives the apparent volume of distribution.

Table 2   Apparent volumes of distribution of various commonly used drugs

Drug	V_D l/kg
frusemide	0.1
warfarin	0.1
phenylbutazone	0.1
aspirin	0.15
sulphafurozole	0.2
nalidixic acid	0.3
penicillin G	0.3
diphenylhydantoin	0.6
diazepam	0.7
indomethacin	0.9
lignocaine	1.3
procainamide	2.0
digoxin	6.0
propranolol	15.0
nortriptyline	20.0

A more general approach is to measure the total area under the plasma concentration time curve (AUC). Then:

$$V_D = \text{Dose}/(AUC \times K_{el}) \qquad (8)$$

where V_D is the apparent volume of distribution and K_{el} is the rate of elimination. This formula is model independent.

Plasma clearance of drugs. Clearance of a drug is a better index of the efficiency of its elimination than the more commonly used term half-life, described above. Clearance is defined as the volume of biological fluid totally cleared of drug per unit of time. A fundamental expression for clearance is:

$$CL = \text{Rate of elimination/Concentration} \qquad (9)$$

Where the rate of elimination is equal to the rate at which drug is removed from the body and the term concentration is the concentration of drug in the biological fluid that defines the clearance. This expression can be applied to whole body, renal, or hepatic clearance. If the liver is the sole organ of elimination of the drug, then systemic and hepatic clearance are equal. If the disposition of a drug can be described by a one compartment model, clearance (CL) can be defined as:

$$CL = V_D \times K_{el} \qquad (10)$$

From equation (8) another expression for clearance is:

$$CL = \text{Dose}/AUC \qquad (11)$$

Bioavailability. The amount of a drug reaching the systemic circulation irrespective of route of administration is termed its bioavailability. By definition, the bioavailability of a drug after intravenous administration is 100 per cent. If the same drug is given intravenously, and then orally in the same dose in the same individual, the bioavailability is the ratio between:

AUC after oral dosing/*AUC* after intravenous dosing

Figure 6 shows such data for ethinyloestradiol, which can be seen to have a low bioavailability—on average only 40 per cent of the drug

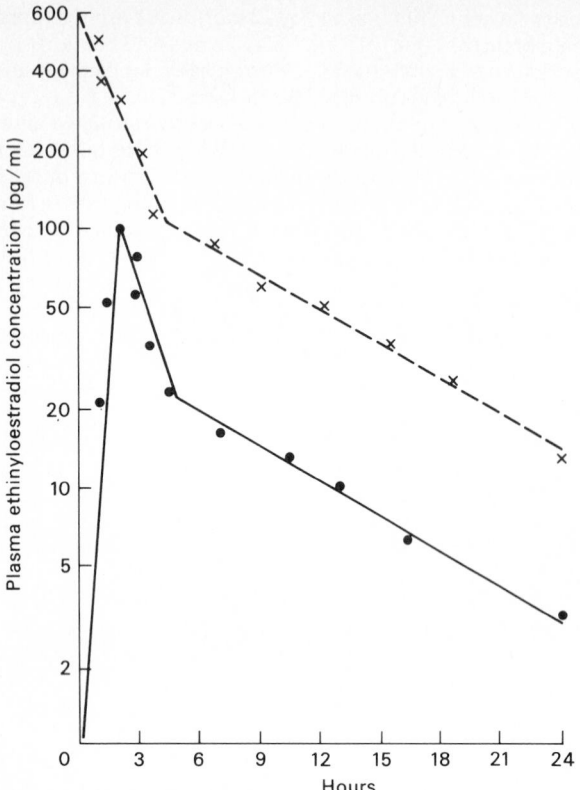

Fig. 6   Plasma concentrations of ethinyloestradiol over a 24 hour period in a woman given 30 μg by the intravenous (......) and oral (————) routes. The vertical axis is on a logarithmic scale.

reaches the systemic circulation. Other evidence shows that ethinyloestradiol is well absorbed from the gastrointestinal tract, but it is extensively metabolized in both gut wall and liver, thus accounting for its low bioavailability. This metabolic breakdown in gut wall and liver is termed the first pass effect.

Steady state plasma concentration. Most therapeutic agents are not given as single doses but on a regular basis. If a drug has a plasma half-life of 36 hours, irrespective of its route of elimination, and is administered twice daily, the drug will accumulate. However, if the elimination of the drug obeys first order kinetics, as the concentration in the plasma increases, then the amount eliminated per unit of time will increase too. Thus a balance will eventually be reached when the amount of drug absorbed will equal the amount eliminated, i.e. a steady state will be reached, around which the plasma concentration will fluctuate, depending on dosing. The rate at which the steady state will be reached may be calculated from a knowledge of the plasma half-life of the drug. As seen from Table 3 50 per cent of the steady state concentration will be reached in one half-life, 75 per cent in two half-lives and so on. It takes approximately five half-lives of continuous administration (i.e. intravenous

Table 3   The plasma concentration at different time points as a percentage of the steady-state concentration

Number of $t_{1/2}$	Plasma concentration as % of steady state concentration
1	50
2	75
3	87.5
4	94
5	97
6	98
7	99

or repeated oral dosing) to reach some 97–98 per cent of steady state plasma levels. As a consequence, the shorter the half-life of a drug the sooner the steady state will be achieved. For a drug such as phenobarbitone with a plasma half-life of some 60 hours, it will take some 12–24 days for steady state kinetics to be achieved. The shorter the half-life, the greater the fluctuation in plasma level between doses unless the drug is given very frequently. For example, heparin has a plasma half-life of one to two hours. If the drug were given six-hourly by bolus injections, there would be marked fluctuations in plasma levels and in therapeutic effect. Thus a continuous infusion of heparin is the preferred route of administration. If a drug given orally has a short half-life (e.g. propranolol or procainamide) then consideration of the manufacture of a slow release formulation is appropriate. If, however, a drug has a plasma half-life of some 24–36 hours, as is the case for tricyclic antidepressants, it makes no sense to consider slow release formulations. Further, if the drug is eliminated by the kidney and renal failure supervenes, either the dose of the drug or the frequency of administration, or both, should be decreased if the same steady state plasma concentration is required as when the renal function was normal. This applies particularly to drugs such as aminoglycoside antibiotics where high plasma concentrations are associated with ototoxicity. In renal failure, prolongation of the plasma half-life of gentamicin means that with regular dosing it will take longer to achieve steady state plasma levels. If an effect is required quickly, a loading dose may be administered.

Inter-individual differences in drug response

Drugs are, in general, organic molecules with varying degrees of lipid solubility. To aid elimination, as described above, they must be converted from lipid to water soluble compounds in the body, and this is performed by the process of metabolism. There are four main processes determining the fate of administered drugs: absorption, distribution, metabolism, and excretion.

Drug absorption. Drugs are frequently given by mouth. After a drug has been swallowed as a tablet or capsule it must disintegrate and dissolve in the gastrointestinal fluids prior to absorption. Most drugs are absorbed in the small intestine but some acidic drugs, which will be unionized in the acid stomach contents, will be absorbed from the stomach itself as described above. The balance between lipid and water solubility is an important determinant of a drug's absorption, since only unionized (and lipid soluble) drugs can cross the cell membrane from the gastrointestinal contents into the body itself. There are four possible mechanisms of drug absorption.

Passive diffusion. This is the process by which most drugs are absorbed and involves the transfer of a drug down a concentration gradient from the gut to the blood stream with no expenditure of energy; the net transfer of the drug is directly proportional to the concentration gradient of the drug. The drug must initially achieve an aqueous solution at the surface of the cell, must then dissolve in the lipid of the cell membrane in order finally to pass into the aqueous phase on the other side of the membrane. There is no competition for absorption between drugs even of similar structure.

Active transport. Only drugs with a structure similar to a naturally occurring compound that undergoes active transport are absorbed by this method. The mechanism is highly specific for compounds such as sugars, amino acids, and some vitamins. Alpha methyldopa and levodopa are two drugs that are probably absorbed by an active transport mechanism because of the similarity to the naturally occurring amino acid tyrosine.

Filtration through pores. Pores are present between cells, but they are so small that only compounds with a molecular weight of less than 100 may be absorbed in this way, and very few commonly used drugs are so small.

Pinocytosis. The process whereby microscopic particles are engulfed by cells is not of major importance for drug absorption. An interesting development of pinocytosis is the preparation of drugs enclosed in a membrane as a liposome which may than be directly engulfed by the target cell. Liposomes, however, usually need to be administered systemically.

Factors affecting oral absorption. Factors affecting the absorption of drugs from the gastrointestinal tract are listed in Table 4. The formulation of a drug may have dramatic effects on its absorption; for example, when the excipient contained in phenytoin capsules in Australia was changed, its bioavailability increased and this resulted in an epidemic of phenytoin intoxication. The presence of other drugs in the gut may also modify drug absorption. It is well known that the absorption of tetracycline is impaired by the presence of iron salts as well as other cations such as calcium or magnesium. Anion exchange resins such as cholestyramine may impair the absorption of drugs given at the same time, e.g. warfarin. It is often stated that food in the stomach has a deleterious effect on the absorption of drugs, but there is no consistent pattern in this effect. The absorption of some drugs (e.g. propranolol) is improved if taken with food. Perhaps the most important patient factor affecting drug absorption is the gastric emptying time. If gastric emptying is slow, then the absorption of acidic drugs from the stomach may be enhanced (see below). In general, factors slowing gastric emptying will tend to slow the *rate* at which a drug is absorbed but will not normally reduce the *amount* of drug absorbed.

Table 4   Factors affecting the absorption of drugs from the gastrointestinal tract

1 Formulation of drug
   Disintegration time
   Dissolution time
   Presence of excipient
2 Patient characteristics
   pH of lumen
   Gastric emptying time
   Intestinal transit time
   Surface area of gastrointestinal tract
   Presence of gastrointestinal disease
3 Presence of other substances in the gastrointestinal tract
   Interaction with other drugs or ions
   Food
4 Pharmacokinetic characteristics of drug
   Drug metabolism by gut bacteria
   Drug metabolism by gut wall

Alternative routes of drug administration

Intramuscular or intravenous administration. Drugs may be given by intramuscular injection because they are destroyed in the stomach (e.g. benzylpenicillin), because they are subject to extensive first pass effect (e.g lignocaine) to aid compliance with therapy, or to speed up the rate of onset of the therapeutic effect. However, problems can arise if the drug is not soluble in water and may precipitate out of solution before absorption can occur (e.g. diazepam). Absorption after intramuscular administration may be delayed if the blood flow to skeletal muscle is reduced, e.g. in shocked patients given intramuscular morphine after myocardial infarction.

Buccal administration. This is used to ensure both a rapid onset of action (e.g. glyceryl trinitrate) by virtue of direct absorption into the systemic circulation and absorption of a drug which would be destroyed by gastric acidity or by an extensive first pass metabolism (buprenorphine or glyceryl trinitrate).

Rectal administration. Drugs may be given as a suppository for the same reaons as for the buccal route, but in general with less efficacy. A first pass effect is not completely avoided due to the dual venous drainage of the rectum into the portal and systemic systems. Since the surface area of the rectum is small, absorption may be slow. However, this can be put to advantage when asthmatic patients are given aminophylline suppositories at night to ensure a prolonged effect.

Percutaneous administration. Many drugs are well absorbed across the skin especially if diseased or inflamed. An ointment containing glyceryl trinitrate can be applied on to the skin to relieve angina; motion sickness can be relieved by applying a disc impregnated with hyosine to a suitable site, e.g. the skin behind the ear from which drug absorption is rapid. This route has a further advantage that drug administration can be terminated by removing the application from the skin.

Pulmonary adminstration. Anaesthetic gases are typically absorbed in this way. The beta stimulants, salbutamol or terbutaline given by inhaler produce more rapid benefit and in a smaller dose than when given by the oral route. Sodium cromoglycate is not well absorbed from the gastrointestinal tract and it is only active in preventing asthma when the powder is inhaled. Patients need to be trained in the use of inhalers and even then, over 90 per cent of the drug will be swallowed. Inhaled particles need to be 2–5 µm in size to reach the smallest bronchioles.

Other routes of drug administration can be used, e.g. conjunctival, vaginal, and nasal, but they tend to be for specialist indications.

Binding and distribution of drugs. Following absorption, drugs are distributed via the blood stream to sites of action, e.g. receptors, to sites of storage in plasma or in tissues, and to sites of metabolism and excretion. The process of distribution largely depends on the physicochemical characteristics of the drug and on the blood flow to the various organs.

In the blood, drugs are often carried bound to plasma proteins, especially albumin. Basic drugs may also bind to acute phase proteins such as α_1-glycoprotein. Forces involved in protein binding include ionic and hydrogen bonding. It is now recognized that there are at least two independent types of binding site on human serum albumin and each site will bind a variety of drugs. As Table 5 shows, some drugs, e.g. tolbutamide, naproxen, or indomethacin, will bind to both sites, while other drugs will only bind to one of the sites.

Table 5   Protein binding sites of highly bound acidic drugs on human serum albumin

Site 1 ('warfarin site')		Site 2 ('diazepam site')	
Drug	% bound	Drug	% bound
warfarin	99	diazepam	98
frusemide	91–99	ethacrynic acid	85
nalidixic acid	93–97	cloxacillin	95
phenytoin	87–93	probenecid	85–95
tolbutamide	95–97	tolbutamide	95–97
naproxen	98–99	naproxen	98–99
indomethacin	92–99	indomethacin	92–99

The interaction between protein and drug is usually reversible and obeys the law of mass action:

$$\text{Drug} + \text{Protein} \rightleftharpoons \text{Drug–Protein complex}$$

The rate at which a drug–protein complex can dissociate is rapid with half-life of only a few milliseconds. As stated earlier, only an unbound drug can diffuse into tissues according to current theory, and only an unbound drug can interact with a receptor to produce a pharmacological effect. The drug–protein complex thus acts as a store for the drug. For drugs which are rapidly cleared from the blood stream by the liver (e.g. propranolol), increased protein binding may increase the delivery of drug to the liver and hasten its elimination.

Displacement of protein bound drugs. In theory, if two drugs that can bind to the same sites on human serum albumin are given together, they will compete for those sites. Thus, if a patient taking warfarin is given a non-steroidal anti-inflammatory drug such as indomethacin the non-steroid anti-imflammatory drug will tend to displace warfarin from its binding sites to form a new equilibrium. This type of interaction is discussed in more detail on page 7.13.

Drug metabolism. Drugs are, in general, lipid soluble compounds that cannot be excreted as such by the kidney. The process of drug metabolism renders them more water soluble thus allowing excretion from the body. The main site of drug metabolism is the liver, but other tissues including skin, lung, blood, and intestinal wall may also contribute. The gut wall is an important site of drug metabolism during the process of absorption, and drugs such as isoprenaline, ethinyl oestradiol, and morphine are, in part, converted there to inactive compounds by metabolism.

The rate of metabolism of a drug in any individual is usually determined genetically, but can be changed by environmental factors (see below). The rate of metabolism of any one drug varies widely from individual to individual, and a ten-fold variation in the rate of drug metabolism is not unusual. Metabolites formed are usually less pharmacologically active than the parent compound but some drugs (e.g. cyclophosphamide) are only active through the production of a metabolite. Other drugs are active themselves but, in addition, produce metabolites that are also pharmacologically active. In some of these cases the metabolite of the drug has a similar spectrum of activity to the parent drug (e.g. propranolol, procainamide, or diazepam). However, the metabolite produced may differ in its pharmacological effects from the parent drug (e.g. pethidine), whose metabolite norpethidine causes no analgesia but muscular twitching, or may have specific toxic effects (e.g. paracetamol, one of whose metabolites is responsible for causing liver necrosis).

Pathways of drug metabolism. A variety of biochemical reactions can take place during the metabolism of a drug to more water soluble compounds. They are of two types; phase I reactions are those whereby polar groups are introduced into the molecule by oxidation, reduction, or hydrolysis; phase II reactions are synthetic and involve conjugation of the drug with glucuronic acid, glycine, sulphate, or other groups. Some drugs may only undergo phase II reactions whilst others may first have to undergo a phase I reaction before a phase II reaction can take place. The enzymes that metabolize drugs in the liver are non-specific compared with the enzymes in intermediary metabolism. Oxidation is the most frequent metabolic pathway and involves the transfer of molecular oxygen through the agency of cytochrome P450. At one time it was thought that there was only one moiety of cytochrome P450, but it now appears that there are may subtypes of the cytochrome in the liver, each responsible for the metabolism of different groups of drugs.

Factors affecting drug metabolism. Many factors can affect the rate of drug metabolism. Pharmacogenetic variations are dealt with in a later section. Important environmental factors that may affect drug metabolism are listed in Table 6. The maximal rate of drug metabolism is not fully developed at birth. Certain enzyme systems, particularly those involved in drug conjugation rather than those dealing with oxidation develop slowly in the newborn. The ability to metabolize drugs may diminish with age, but this is a gradual process and the changes seen are small compared to the overall inter-individual differences in drug metabolism that are known to occur.

Heavy cigarette smoking increases the rate of drug metabolism. It is known that smokers require higher doses of theophylline and pentazocine than non-smoking patients to produce a similar pharmacological effect. Prolonged occupational exposure to insecticides such as lindane or DDT will enhance drug metabolism. Diet may affect drug metabolism in a number of ways. High protein, low carbohydrate content diets will enhance the rate of drug metab-

Table 6   Factors affecting drug metabolism

Factor	Response
Age	
Neonates	reduced rate of drug metabolism
Elderly	
Environment	enhanced rate of drug metabolism with occupational exposure to insecticides
Smoking	enhanced rate of drug metabolism
Diet	increased rate of drug metabolism by high protein/low carbohydrate diet
	reduced rate of drug metabolism in malnutrition
Alcohol	
Acute ingestion	inhibition of drug metabolism
Chronic ingestion	increased rate of drug metabolism
Drugs	may increase or decrease rate of metabolism (enzyme induction or inhibition)

olism and low protein/high carbohydrate diets may inhibit drug metabolism. In extreme malnutrition the rate of drug metabolism is reduced. Alcohol, in excess on a single occasion, will tend to inhibit drug metabolism, but in chronic alcoholics, at least until liver damage ensues, the rate of drug metabolism is increased. Liver damage may result in diminished rates of drug metabolism. Co-administration of other drugs influences the rate of drug metabolism and this is probably the most important environmental factor in clinical practice. A number of drugs are known to enhance the rate of drug metabolism in man (enzyme inducers) and these, together with drugs that inhibit drug metabolism, are listed in Table 7. This subject is considered further in the drug interaction section (page 7.12).

Table 7   Drugs that are known to inhibit or induce drug metabolism in man

Inhibitors	Inducers
allopurinol	barbiturates
cimetidine	carbamazepine
chloramphenicol	glutethimide
phenylbutazone	phenytoin
sulthiame	rifampicin

Excretion of drugs

Renal excretion of drugs. There are relatively few drugs (e.g. digoxin and gentamicin) in regular clinical use that are excreted unchanged by the kidney. Most tend to be, at least in part, metabolized and their metabolites are excreted in the urine. Active tubular secretion does occur for a few drugs. Bases such as mecamylamine and acids such as penicillin, probenecid, and salicylate are carried across the renal tubular cell by an active transport mechanism against a concentration gradient. Probenecid will compete for the carrier mechanism with penicillin, thus inhibiting the renal clearance of penicillin and causing its plasma concentrations to increase.

The renal clearance of some drugs is affected by the pH of the urine. The pH partition hypothesis has been described in an earlier section. Weak acids such as phenobarbitone and salicylates are ionized at alkaline urine. Only unionized drugs can be reabsorbed into the body across the renal tubular epithelium. Similarly basic drugs such as amphetamine are excreted more rapidly in an acid urine. The urine can be made alkaline by the use of sodium bicarbonate and acid with ammonium chloride, and these principles can be helpful in the treatment of drug overdoses.

Biliary excretion of drugs. Drugs may be excreted by hepatic cells into the bile. They are occasionally excreted unchanged but more usually as conjugates (e.g. with glucuronic acid, sulphate, or glycine). Polar metabolites are likely to be excreted in bile if their molecular weight exceeds 400. Biliary excretion may serve as an alternative to renal excretion in patients whose kidney function is impaired, but it is unlikely that excretion in the bile will entirely compensate for deficiencies in renal excretion.

Some drugs are excreted in the bile and then undergo an enterohepatic circulation. For example, the contraceptive steroid ethinyloestradiol is absorbed from the small intestine forming sulphate and glucuronide conjugates in the gut wall and liver. A high proportion of these metabolites are excreted via the bile into the intestine. Bacterial flora hydrolyse then conjugates to liberate free ethinylestradiol which is then available for reabsorption; thus the enterohepatic recirculation can be seen as a mechanism to prolong the action of the drug.

Pharmacogenetics. Pharmacogenetics (see also Section 4) deals with the modification of drug responses by hereditary influences. Table 8 shows that some examples involve drug metabolism while others involve a variation in response to the drug. The interplay between genetic and environmental influences on response is one of increasing interest. It has been calculated that for phenylbutazone at least two-thirds of the variation in rates of metabolism is due to genetic influences and the remainder to environmental effects. Another interesting example is that about 5 per cent of people in the United Kingdom are poor hydroxylators of debrisoquine and this inability to metabolize the drug has a genetic basis. Whether the same applies to other drugs which are oxidized is a matter of continuing interest.

The importance to therapy can be seen in a number of examples shown in Table 8. A number of drugs such as isoniazid, procainamide, and hydralazine are metabolized by acetylation. This process is performed by the enzyme N-acetyl transferase in the liver. The ability to acetylate isoniazid is inherited as an autosomal recessive trait and distribution histograms show a bimodal pattern. In a Caucasian population about 60 per cent of the population are slow acetylators, but in Japan the incidence falls to 10 per cent. However, in the Canadian Eskimo races nearly 100 per cent of the population are fast acetylators; the reason for this geographical variation is unknown. It is now clear that slow acetylators of isoniazid are more likely to develop toxic effects such as peripheral neuropathy than are fast acetylators. On the other hand, patients with tuberculosis, who are fast acetylators, may respond less well to isoniazid if the drug is given on a twice weekly basis. Fast acetylators seem to be more likely to develop liver damage following the use of isoniazid because this toxicity is caused by a metabolite

acetylhydrazine; rapid acetylators will produce higher concentrations of this substance. Slow acetylators of procainamide and hydralazine are more prone to develop systemic lupus erythematosus than are fast acetylators.

Acute intermittent porphyria may be precipitated by drugs such as phenobarbitone. This disease is inherited as an autosomal dominant and is due to an abnormal inducibility of the enzyme δ-amino laevulinic acid synthetase.

About 100 million people in the world are at risk of developing drug induced haemolysis due to lack of glucose 6-phosphate dehydrogenase in the red cell. Haemolysis may be precipitated by a variety of drugs such as primaquine, nitrofurantoin, and sulphonamides (see Table 9). This condition is considered in detail in Section 19. Malignant hyperthermia is a recently recognized condition that occurs approximately 1 in 20 000 anaesthetics and may be due to an abnormality of calcium binding by the muscular sarcolemma. Following the use of anaesthetic drugs such as halothane, suxamethonium, or nitrous oxide, the body temperature may rise by 2 °C or more per hour.

Table 9 Some drugs causing haemolysis in patients with glucose 6-phosphate dehydrogenase deficiency

primaquine	sulphonamides
quinine	dapsone
chloroquine	nalidixic acid
quinidine	nitrofurantoin
probenecid	chloramphenicol
aspirin	

The therapeutic use of measuring plasma concentrations of drugs

A fundamental premise in pharmacology is that the intensity and duration of drug response is determined by the concentration of drug at the sites of action, i.e. receptors. Since the concentration of drug in plasma can usually be measured, it is important to know whether changes in this reflect changes in concentration at receptors. For drugs that act reversibly, the formation of drug receptor complexes obeys the law of mass action. Thus:

$$\text{Drug} + \text{Receptor} \rightleftharpoons \text{Drug–Receptor complex}$$

At equilibrium, the rates of formation and dissociation of drug–receptor complexes are equal. There are, however, many instances when pharmacological effects are not related to the plasma level of the drug. There are several possible reasons for this. First, a thera-

Table 8 Genetically determined abnormal drug responses

Condition	Response	Inheritance	Drugs involved
Slow and fast acetylators	slow acetylators may show toxicity; fast acetylators show diminished response	autosomal recessive	isoniazid hydralazine procainamide dapsone
Suxamethonium sensitivity	prolonged apnoea	autosomal recessive	suxamethonium (succinylcholine)
Porphyria	abdominal pain paralysis	autosomal dominant	barbiturates
Favism	haemolysis on exposure to certain drugs	sex-linked incomplete dominant	e.g. primaquine nitrofurantoin sulphonamides
Malignant hyperthermia	uncontrolled rise in body temperature	autosomal dominant	certain anaesthetic agents, e.g. halothane suxamethonium
Glaucoma steroids	glaucoma due to abnormal response to intraocular steroids	autosomal recessive	topical corticosteroids, systemic corticosteroids

peutic substance may act at least in part through a metabolite, e.g. the activity of cyclophosphamide, the cytoxic agent, resides in one or more metabolites formed from the parent substance by the hepatic microsomal enzyme system. α-Methyldopa, the anti-hypertensive agent acts via α-methylnoradrenaline which is two steps removed from the parent drug. Procainamide, the anti-arrhythmic agent, has an active metabolite N-acetyl procainamide. Second, drugs may act irreversibly, i.e. the quantity of active drug attached to receptors is not related to steady state plasma concentrations. Such drugs often attach to their receptors and then bind covalently with them. A small amount of drug remains attached to these sites long after the rest of the drug has vanished from the body. Certain drugs act non-reversibly without bonding covalently, but they are attached so tightly to receptors that they remain fixed to their sites after the concentration of unbound drug has declined to levels which are unmeasurable by our present analytical techniques. Non-reversible drugs are inherently dangerous since their effects tend to accumulate even though the drug may not. Third, the assay method for plasma drug concentrations may be too insensitive to reflect an important pool of the drug, such as that for guanethidine stored in adrenergic neurones. In such instances it may be useful to foresake kinetic analyses based on plasma drug concentrations and examine urine excretion as it reflects the kinetics of the drug in plasma.

Thus there are several prerequisites for using the plasma concentration of a drug to monitor clinical effects.

1. The drug should act by a reversible mechanism.

2. The drug should not have active metabolites.

3. The concentration of unbound drug in plasma should reflect the concentration of unbound drug at receptor sites. For drugs with a small aparent volume of distribution it is reasonable to picture the plasma concentration representing the amount of drug in the body. For drugs with a large apparent volume of distribution, the relationship between plasma level and total drug may be more tenuous and difficult to ascertain. Tissue levels of the drug may be of more importance as a determinant of effect.

4. The development of tolerance at receptor sites should not be an important problem as with barbiturates and ethyl alcohol.

5. The pharmacological effects of the drug should be recorded in an accurate way. While the measurement of drug levels may pose certain technical problems, these are usually soluble. The question of measurement of drug effects is much more challenging. For psychotropic drugs, 'rating' scales employing both subjective and objective assessment may have to be used. Visual analogue scales for analgesic drugs are popular (see Fig. 7). Even the measurement

No pain   Very severe pain

Fig. 7   Visual analogue scale for use in the assessment of pain.

of a physiological end point such as blood pressure may pose problems. Should lying or standing blood pressure be used, systolic or diastolic and if the latter, phase 4 or phase 5 Korotkoff sounds?

What to measure—total plasma concentration or free concentration? In principle, it is free (unbound) drug which is in equilibrium with receptor sites. There are variations in plasma protein binding of drugs, although these are usually small in comparison with the differences which occur in rates of drug metabolism, suggesting that in most instances total drug concentration measurements are adequate. There are, however, several limitations to this.

When more than one drug is administered. Displacement of one drug by another leads to an increase (albeit transitory) in free drug concentration and when this is monitored, a better correlation is obtained between free concentration than total concentration and effect.

In patients with diseases which perturb plasma protein binding. The unbound fraction of diphenylhydantoin is markedly increased

in uraemia. It has been found that epileptics with uraemia respond both therapeutically and in terms of adverse effects at much lower total plasma concentrations of diphenylhydantoin than epileptics with no renal disease.

Certain drugs tend to localize within the red cell. Propranolol and chlorthalidone have concentrations within the red blood cell considerably higher than in plasma. Whether the effect for drugs such as these are related more to total blood level than to plasma level remains to be explored in most instances.

Indications for monitoring drugs in plasma

Therapeutic monitoring. For several drugs it is more difficult to assess the clinical effect of the drug than to monitor the plasma concentration. This is not true for drugs such as antihypertensive agents, anticoagulants, and hypoglycaemic agents where clinical observation (blood pressure) or simple laboratory tests (prothrombin time or blood sugar) must always form the basis of dose adjustment. For drugs which have a narrow therapeutic ratio (e.g. lithium) or show dose dependent kinetics (e.g. diphenylhydantoin), plasma concentrations are a better guide to both efficacy and potential toxicity than pure clinical observation although this must always play an extremely important role in dose adjustment.

Patient compliance. One of the most difficult problems in therapeutics is to decide whether a patient is taking his medication as prescribed. While certain dosage regimes (e.g. three or four times daily dosing) and certain patient characteristics (the old, those with poor doctor/patient relationship) predispose to poor compliance, many aspects of this important area have not been explored. If a patient responds poorly to a drug, it is useful to monitor its concentration in a biological fluid, e.g. plasma or urine. If a drug has a relatively long half-life and a low volume of distribution and no drug can be detected in plasma a few hours after alleged dosing, it is difficult to escape the conclusion that the patient has not taken the drug.

Measurement of drug (or metabolite) in the urine helps to distinguish between the patient who metabolizes a drug rapidly and a non-complier. In the former, the urine metabolite concentration in a specified time (e.g. 24 hours) should account for a defined and predictable amount of the ingested drug. In some situations attention is now being focused on the measurement of drug concentrations in saliva as a 'non-invasive' procedure. In general, salivary concentrations of drugs reflect their unbound concentration in plasma, and salivary levels have been successfully used in the monitoring of therapy with diphenylhydantoin, phenobarbitone, theophylline, and isoniazid. One drawback to this method is that if the drug has an effect on salivary flow the interpretation of salivary concentrations may be difficult. Salivary concentrations may, of course, also be used in therapeutic monitoring although it may be in the area of drug compliance that this technique may be most widely used.

Patients with renal or liver dysfunction. In patients with increasing renal dysfunction but who require drug therapy, drugs which are excreted predominantly by the kidney may pose toxicological problems. Examples are the aminoglycoside antibiotics (causing inner ear disease and also further renal dysfunction) and digoxin (causing nausea, vomiting, and arrhythmias).

The handling of many drugs in patients with hepatitis or cirrhosis may be altered by the disease, especially if these drugs undergo phase 1 metabolism. Thus the clearance of theophylline and phenytoin (drugs with a low therapeutic index) are diminished in cirrhosis and monitoring is mandatory.

Drug overdosage. If a definitive procedure such as haemodialysis or peritoneal dialysis is to be instituted for intoxication with drugs such as phenobarbitone or salicylate, it is wise to check the efficacy of the manoeuvre, e.g. monitoring plasma concentrations. In the case of intoxication with paracetamol, plasma concentrations above 200 µg/ml at four hours or 50 µg/ml at 12 hours after ingestion of the overdose are indications for administration of a specific antagonist such as *n*-acetyl cysteine (Fig. 8).

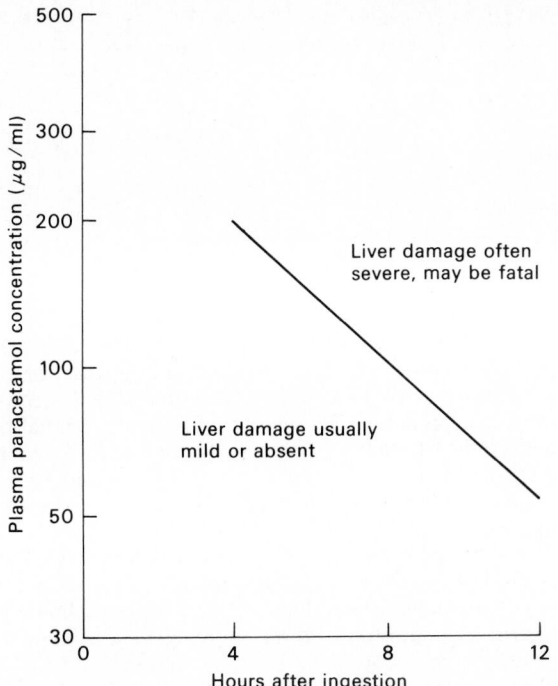

Fig. 8 Relationship between plasma paracetamol concentrations and time after ingestion to liver damage following an overdose of paracetamol. Treatment with sulphydryl compounds such as *n*-acetyl cysteine is indicated with values above the solid line. (After Prescott, L. F. (1981). Drug overdosage and poisoning, in *Drug therapy*, 2nd edn. (ed. G. S. Avery), p. 263. Adis Press, Sydney.)

Drugs whose plasma concentrations should be monitored

Anticonvulsants. Phenytoin is a difficult drug to use because of its capacity limited metabolism, i.e. if one doubles the dose, plasma concentrations may rise six-fold. It is now well established that monitoring the plasma concentration of phenytoin is helpful clinically and adjusting the dose to bring the plasma concentration into the range 10–20 µg/ml will reduce fit frequency in most patients and will diminish drug toxicity. Some epileptic patients will have good epileptic control at plasma concentrations outside this range (e.g. patients in renal failure, see above). The main problem with phenytoin is probably underdosing. Workers in Sweden showed in a series of epileptic patients on phenytoin that more than 50 per cent had plasma concentrations below the therapeutic range, either because of poor compliance or rapid metabolism.

There is no persuasive evidence that monitoring plasma levels of phenobarbitone is of clinical value. A case can be made for monitoring carbamazepine levels in plasma (therapeutic range 2–6 µg/ml, toxic effects seen above 8 µg/ml), although the presence of an active metabolite may render such data more difficult to interpret. Ethosuximide (therapeutic plasma concentration 40–80 µg/ml, toxic effects above 100 µg/ml) is also being monitored although wider experience is necessary to confirm its value (Table 10).

Cardiovascular drugs. To check compliance and to adjust the dose in patients with renal failure, monitoring of plasma concentra-

Table 10 Drugs for which therapeutic and toxic plasma ranges have been defined

Drug	Therapeutic range	Toxic effects
digoxin	1–2 ng/ml	3 ng/ml
digitoxin	10–25 ng/ml	40 ng/ml
theophylline	10–20 µg/ml	25 µg/ml
phenytoin	10–20 µg/ml	25 µg/ml
lithium	0.5–1.5 mmol/l	1.5 mmol/l
nortriptyline	50–140 ng/ml	200 ng/ml

tions of digoxin has been shown to be of value. Considerable controversy exists as to how far plasma digoxin concentrations should be measured in routine clinical practice. Digitoxin, unlike digoxin, is metabolized by the liver rather than excreted by the kidney. In some centres this is used as an alternative to digoxin in patients with renal failure. The role of digitalis glycosides in the long-term management of congestive heart failure is the source of continuing debate; in patients with atrial fibrillation there is no question as to its value but when the patient is in sinus rhythm, diuretic therapy may be more appropriate long-term monotherapy.

Procainamide is less used as an anti-arrhythmic drug than previously. Although therapeutic plasma concentrations have been suggested, the presence of an active metabolite N-acetyl procainamide in plasma calls into question the value of measuring only unchanged drug. A similar reservation pertains with lignocaine. The importance of active metabolites remains to be clarified in routine therapeutic monitoring.

Bronchodilators. Many studies have confirmed the value of monitoring plasma theophylline concentrations in asthmatic patients, especially in children. With attention to maintaining plasma concentrations within the prescribed range, theophylline is increasingly shown to be a most valuable first lime drug in asthma therapy. The therapeutic range is between 10 and 20 µg/ml.

Central nervous system drugs. Lithium, used in the management of mania and manic-depressive psychoses, has a low therapeutic index. Handled by the body in a similar manner to sodium, monitoring of plasma concentrations has been shown to be mandatory for its optimal use. (The therapeutic range is 0.5–1.5 mmol/l). Coadministration of diuretics has been shown to cause perturbation of plasma concentrations. There is the further strong possibility that long-term therapy with lithium may cause renal dysfunction making plasma level monitoring even more important.

Although several high quality research investigations have demonstrated the value of measuring plasma concentrations of nortriptyline, this has not yet achieved routine status. The problems with antidepressant administration are the wide inter-individual range of rates of metabolism, the difficulty in monitoring their clinical effect, the long duration (sometimes three to four weeks) before an optimum response is obtained after starting therapy, and the relatively narrow 'therapeutic window' in which maximum benefit is seen.

Antibiotics. As mentioned above, aminoglycoside antibiotics, e.g. gentamicin, are excreted by the kidney. In renal failure accumulation may result in ototoxicity and further renal damage unless appropriate dosage adjustment is made.

Drugs taken in overdosage. Paracetamol causes liver damage when taken in overdosage. A nomogram has been constructed (Fig. 8) using plasma concentrations relative to time after dosing as a basis for deciding whether administration of an antagonist, e.g. *n*-acetyl cysteine or methionine, should be administered to avert hepatotoxicity.

Effect of disease on drug response

Most initial studies of new drugs are performed in volunteers and the results are then applied to patients who may have a variety of diseases often quite distinct from the one for which the drug was designed. In some cases the presence of disease may alter the responsiveness of tissues to the drug; for example, hypokalaemia enhances the toxicity of digitalis, morphine-like drugs have greater CNS depressant effects in patients with cirrhosis of the liver. Most reliable information in this area, however, relates to the effects of disease on the pharmacokinetics of drugs.

Drug absorption in disease. Drug absorptive processes are usually so efficient that it rare for disease to have much effect. If gastric emptying is delayed, then the rate of drug absorption will be slowed but the amount of drug absorbed will not change. This may mean a delay in the peak effect of the drug, but little overall change in effect. Delayed gastric emptying may produce therapeutic failure with levodopa partly because the drug is metabolized in the stomach wall leaving less to be absorbed by active transport in the small intestine. In patients with malabsorption syndromes drug absorption may be delayed, but it appears that the disease has to be very severe before clinically significant changes in overall absorption will occur.

Drug distribution in disease. As described above, the distribution of drugs to their sites of action, storage, or elimination are mainly influenced by physicochemical characteristics of the drug and regional blood flow. Changes in plasma pH may, on occasion, result in a change in drug ionization sufficient to alter distribution of a drug whose pKa approximates to that of plasma. This may contribute to the reduced effect and myocardial uptake of lignocaine in acidotic states. Reduction in blood flow in heart failure or following a myocardial infarction may also affect drug distribution.

Protein binding is also affected by disease. In severe hypoalbuminaemia, such as may occur in patients with the nephrotic syndrome, or with cirrhosis, the binding of acidic drugs in plasma will be reduced. The protein binding of acidic drugs is also reduced in patients with impaired renal function. As this becomes reduced, a number of endogenous compounds are retained in the plasma and compete with drugs for the binding sites on plasma albumin. Drugs such as phenytoin, warfarin, phenylbutazone, sulphonamides, and salicylates, show reduced binding to albumin in patients with renal impairment. One implication of this finding is in the interpretation of plasma concentration data. Phenytoin is measured in plasma as the total concentration (i.e. free + bound) of which the free concentration is the pharmacologically active moiety. If under normal conditions a total plasma concentration of 15 µg/ml is desired, then the free concentration will be about 1 µg/ml. However, in a patient with impaired renal function a free concentration of 1 µg may be achieved at a total plasma concentration of only 7.5 µg/ml or less. Under these circumstances it is obviously important to reduce the dose given.

Protein binding of basic drugs is not disturbed in renal failure. However, in inflammatory states, basic drugs (e.g. propranolol, chlorpromazine, quinidine, or imipramine) will become more extensively bound because of the increased plasma concentrations of α_1-glycoprotein.

Drug metabolism in disease. Since the liver is the main organ of metabolism, it would not be too surprising to find that disease of the liver causes impaired drug metabolism. In general, liver disease needs to be fairly extensive before the metabolism of drugs is affected because of its large reserve capacity. It is now recognized that the metabolism of drugs in disease states will depend largely on the pharmacokinetic characteristics of the drugs. In terms of their hepatic clearance, drugs can have either high clearance or low clearance characteristics. The extraction ratio across the liver of high clearance drugs is large and the ability of the liver to eliminate them after intravenous administration is dependent more on liver blood flow than on the intrinsic ability of the liver to metabolize them. Thus, reduction in hepatic blood flow, as may occur in heart failure, will lead to reduced clearance of drugs such as lignocaine and propranolol given intravenously. In contrast, low clearance drugs are more dependent upon the intrinsic metabolizing ability of the liver and will be more affected by disease of the liver parenchyma than by changes in liver blood flow. Some examples of these changes are shown in Table 11.

Drug excretion in disease. (See also Section 18.) Those drugs which are primarily cleared from the body by renal excretion show a prolonged half-life in patients with impaired function. Renal function may be reduced not only by disease but also in increasing age. With increasing degree of renal failure such drugs may progressively accumulate in the body. It is generally assumed that drugs which are metabolized can safely be given in normal doses to

Table 11   Drugs whose clearance may be reduced in liver disease

High clearance drugs	Low clearance drugs
lignocaine	diazepam
labetalol	prednisolone
chlormethiazole	ampicillin
propranolol	theophylline
pethidine	

patients in renal failure. This is true only if the metabolites have no pharmacological effect. In some cases polar metabolites will not be excreted readily by the patient in renal failure and any activity of the metabolite will be seen as increased therapeutic and toxic effects. The main active metabolite of procainamide, N-acetyl procainamide, accumulates in the plasma of patients in renal failure and has been the cause of arrhythmias. Norpethidine is a metabolite of pethidine that is not readily excreted in patients with renal function impairment. Norpethidine has little analgesic effect but may cause muscular irritability and twitching.

It is obviously of prime importance for safe therapy in patients with renal disease to know the fate and metabolism of administered drugs. In order to achieve a defined steady state plasma concentration in these circumstances three main points need to be understood.

1. If a loading dose is given, this dose will not need to be changed provided that the distribution volume is unaltered in the disease state.

2. The maintenance dose of the drug should be smaller and/or the dose should be given less frequently.

3. The time taken to achieve steady state plasma concentrations, and therefore the optimum therapeutic effect, will be longer.

Several nomograms have been introduced into clinical practice to guide the physician in his choice of drug dosage in patients with renal failure, but in general these have not been shown to be of great clinical value. Table 12 shows the changes in plasma half-life of some drugs that may be seen in anuric patients.

Table 12   Elimination half-lives (hours) of some drugs in normal and impaired renal function

Drug	Normal	Anuria
penicillin G	0.5	23
cephaloridine	1.7	23
gentamicin	2.5	35
vancomycin	5.8	230
tetracycline	8.5	90
doxycycline	23	23
digoxin	30	100
digitoxin	170	170

Drug interactions

The likelihood of adverse reactions occurring increases with the number of drugs prescribed. It has been calculated that if five drugs are given simultaneously, there is a 75 per cent chance of causing an adverse reaction due to the interactions perpetrated. In many respects, drug interactions have attracted an attention disproportionate to their clinical significance, but on the other hand, they may give clear insights into underlying pharmacological mechanisms. However, the important clinical examples are drawn from a relatively short list of groups of drugs with a narrow therapeutic ratio, i.e. whose dose must be adjusted within a small range and whose adverse effects are pronounced when this range is either exceeded or not attained. Such drug groups include oral anticoagulants, anticonvulsants, antidepressants, and antihypertensive agents. Some interactions may be beneficial and are deliberately perpetrated. Examples of drugs used in combination to achieve a therapeutic effect or minimize an adverse reaction in a way which could not be done with a single drug regimen include L-dopa and decarboxylase inhibitors used for Parkinson's disease, diuretics and beta-adrenoceptor blockers for hypertension, oestrogen–progestogen combinations for contraception, and trimethoprim with a sulphonamide for infections.

Mechanisms of interactions. In broad terms, the basis of underlying drug interactions may either be pharmacokinetic or pharmacodynamic. Pharmacokinetic interactions depend either on a change in free drug concentrations in plasma, or at the sites of drug action in the tissues. Pharmacodynamic interactions result from a modification of drug occupancy of a receptor or a modification of an underlying physiological control mechanism. The additive effects of drugs with a similar action are often cited as a type of drug interaction, but strictly speaking an interaction should result in either an enhancement or diminution of the combined separate effects of the drugs.

Sites of interactions. Interactions may be classified according to their sites. Table 13 shows one such classification.

Table 13 Sites of drug interaction

1 Prior to administration
2 Drug absorption
    Within the gut lumen
    By altering gut motility
    By altering gut flora
    Within the gut wall
3 Protein binding
4 Drug metabolism
    Stimulation
    Inhibition
5 Drug excretion
    Changes in urine pH
    Competition for active renal tubular excretion
    Fluid and electrolyte changes
6 Interactions at receptors

Prior to administration. If drugs such as heparin or benzyl penicillin are mixed with infusion fluids of low pH (e.g. certain dextrose solutions), appreciable loss of drug activity may occur due to chemical inactivation. Further, since drugs may interact in the infusion bottle (e.g. carbenecillin is inactivated by gentamicin), administration of more than one drug in the same infusion should be avoided wherever possible. If it is essential that this should be done, the therapeutic consequences should always be considered.

A further example of a pharmaceutical interaction is when the excipients in the formulation of a tablet may alter the release characteristics of an active drug. A recent example of this is the change in the formulation of digoxin (resulting in altered efficacy by changing its bioavailability).

Drug absorption. *Within the gut lumen.* Calcium, magnesium, and aluminium interact with tetracycline to form a non-absorbable chelate and thus antacids containing these cations(or even milk) should not be taken with tetracycline or they should be given as far apart in time as possible. Cholestyramine, an ion exchange resin, will bind acidic drugs such as warfarin and digitoxin, preventing their absorption.

By altering gut motility. If a drug which either enhances gastric emptying (e.g. metoclopramide) or diminishes it (e.g. propantheline, tricyclic antidepressants, or opiates) is given with a drug that is mainly absorbed in the small intestine, the rate of absorption of the second drug may be altered. This has been illustrated very clearly with paracetamol (Fig. 9). Metoclopramide increases gastric emptying and therefore the rate of paracetamol absorption. (This combination is widely used in migraine.) Conversely, propantheline

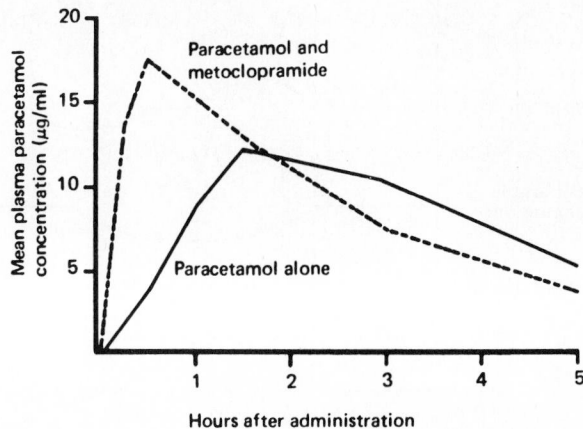

Fig. 9 Increased rate of absorption of paracetamol following the use of metoclopramide. (After Nimmo *et al.* (1973). *Br. med. J.* **i**, 587.)

decreases the rate of paracetamol absorption and thus, presumably, the onset of effective analgesia.

By altering gut flora. In the past few years several reports have appeared of an increased incidence of intermenstrual bleeding and unwanted pregnancy in women given broad spectrum antibiotics and oral contraceptives. The putative mechanism of this effect is that conjugates of the contraceptive steroid ethinyloestradiol, are excreted in bile; under control conditions these conjugates are hydrolysed by gut bacteria and unchanged ethinyloestradiol is then reabsorbed (enterohepatic circulation). In the presence of antibiotics which either kill or alter gut flora, this hydrolysis will not occur, the enterohepatic circulation is interrupted, and conjugated ethinyloestradiol excreted in the faeces. This mechanism has been clearly demonstrated in animals but its therapeutic importance awaits clarification.

Within the gut wall. The gut wall is an important organ for phase II metabolism (conjugation). For example, over 40 per cent of ethinyloestradiol is metabolized to a sulphate conjugate within the gut wall in man, and if vitamin C, which competes for available sulphate, is administered with the steroid, plasma ethinyloestradiol concentrations are increased significantly. A similar mechanism underlies the interaction between isoprenaline (which forms a sulphate conjugate in the gut wall) and salicylamide (which competes for available sulphate). Under those circumstances, the amount of unchanged, and therefore active, isoprenaline that is absorbed increases.

Protein binding. As discussed on page 7.7, many drugs are transported in the blood bound to either albumin or specialized globulins. The significance of displacement of drugs from binding sites as a cause of drug interaction has probably been exaggerated. There are several reasons for this. If a drug is 90 per cent bound to plasma proteins, and if, in the presence of a displacing agent this percentage falls to 80 per cent, there is a doubling of the concentration of the free drug. This free drug will then leave the plasma and be cleared by normal processes. Thus the total plasma concentration will fall until equilibrium is re-established, i.e. 90 per cent of the new total plasma concentration is bound (Fig. 10). As a result any effect of displacement will be transient and the final result may be an overall diminution in therapeutic effect. A second consideration is the relative distribution of the drug between plasma and the tissues. A drug must be both highly bound (e.g. 90 per cent) and have a low apparent volume of distribution (i.e. be predominantly localized to the plasma) for displacement to have any therapeutic significance. Displacement of warfarin (99 per cent bound, V_D 9 l) by 1 per cent leads to a doubling of the free concentration. Displacement of digoxin (20 per cent bound V_D 300 l) by 5 per cent leads to a very small increase in free concentration both because of the high initial percentage free and its large apparent volume of

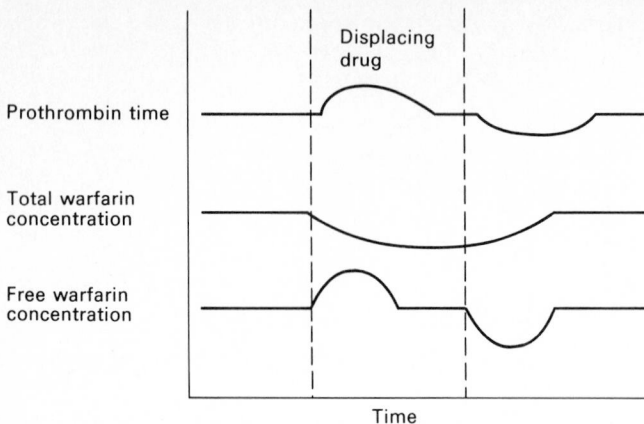

Fig. 10 Theoretical effect of protein binding displacement. (After Koch-Weser, J. and Sellers, A. M. (1971). *New Engl. J. Med.* **294**, 311.)

distribution. There are instances, however, when displacement of one drug by another could be dangerous. When the displacing drug is injected intravenously, the concentration of unbound drug could be increased instantaneously and thus highly perfused organs such as brain, heart, and liver may be exposed to high free concentrations during redistribution. In other instances, if drug–protein complexes serve as transport carriers rather than drug depots (e.g. propranolol) displacement of the drug from binding sites in plasma could retard drug elimination and thus alter the steady state drug concentration of the unbound drug. Not only may drugs be displaced from binding sites by other drugs with a higher affinity for the site, but endogenous substances which may accumulate in disease may also compete for these sites. Bilirubin in liver failure, and various endogenous metabolites in renal failure, will displace drugs from albumin binding. Toxic effects from sulphonamides, phenytoin, and warfarin have been documented in these instances.

Finally, it should be mentioned that several interactions, whose basis is alleged to be displacement, may have an entirely different mechanism. The enhancement of the pharmacological effect of warfarin by phenylbutazone (frequently cited as being due to displacement, since this can be demonstrated *in vitro*) is, in fact, more likely to be attributed to a stereo-selective alteration in the metabolic degradation of warfarin by phenylbutazone. Warfarin is a racemic mixture and phenylbutazone inhibits the metabolism of S-warfarin (the more potent isomer) while increasing the elimination of R-warfarin (the less potent isomer).

Drug metabolism

Stimulation. Many lipid soluble drugs cause non specific stimulation of drug metabolism in both man and experimental animals. The number of drugs shown to be inducing agents in man is relatively small (see Table 7). The administration of an inducing agent stimulates not only the metabolism of many drugs and physiological compounds which are substrates for microsomal enzymes but also the metabolism of the inducing agent itself. Microsomal enzyme induction occurs in many tissues—gut wall, lung, kidney, skin, as well as the liver. Depending on the dose and drug, induction usually develops over a period of several days or weeks and persists for a similar period following withdrawal of the inducing agent. The effect of some inducing agents such as chlorinated hydrocarbon insecticides is more persistent since these compounds are stored in body fat and remain for long periods within the body. Induction is often considered to equate with drug inactivation, but if drug metabolites have a greater pharmacological activity or a different spectrum of action from the parent substances, then drug effects may be enhanced by induction. For example, hepatic necrosis following paracetamol overdosage is more severe in patients previously given inducing agents due to increased production of toxic metabolites of paracetamol. Similarly, prior use of inducing agents increases the risk of nephrotoxicity after methoxyflurane.

Many of the important parameters of enzyme induction were worked out using barbiturates (e.g. time course of induction, dose dependence, structure activity relationships).

If barbiturates are given to a patient taking (for example) warfarin or an oral contraceptive steroid, then over a period of two to three weeks the clinical effect of the drug will be reduced because plasma concentrations of the relevant drug will fall due to the increased rate of metabolism. When the barbiturate is stopped, the rate of drug metabolism slowly returns to its previous level, but this may take several weeks. Figure 11 shows an example of the interaction between amylobarbitone and warfarin.

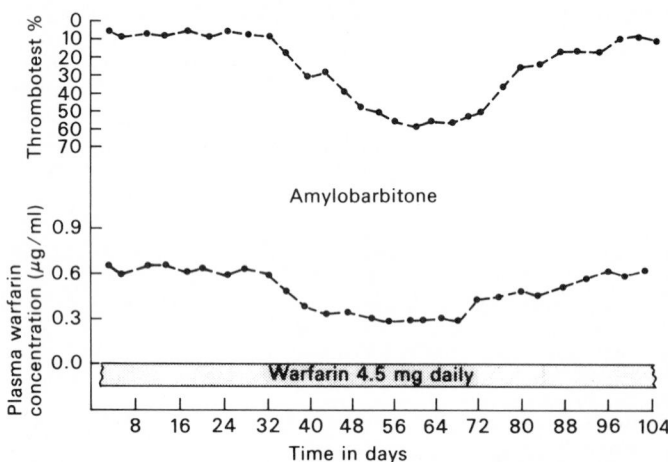

Fig. 11 The effect of amylobarbitone on the plasma warfarin concentration and anticoagulant control (measured as thrombotest) in a patient taking 4.5 mg warfarin daily).

With the decrease in use of barbiturates (except in epilepsy), rifampicin is probably more important nowadays as an inducing agent. Rifampicin, in particular, has been shown to diminish the efficacy of oral contraceptive and oral anticoagulant therapy and to alter the rate of metabolism of various natural substrates such as vitamin D and cortisol.

An interesting facet of enzyme induction is the increase in liver blood flow which it produces, and this is due to an increase in portal venous flow rather than hepatic arterial flow. For drugs which are highly cleared by the liver, e.g. propranolol, the increase in liver blood flow is a more important determinant of their increased elimination than increase in liver microsomal enzyme activity when an inducing agent is given.

Not all increases in rates of metabolism are due to induction. There is some evidence of activation of drug metabolizing enzymes in certain experimental situations, e.g. with certain steroids. Activation implies a more rapid effect and is probably due to structural alteration in the drug metabolizing enzyme without necessarily increased *de novo* protein synthesis as occurs in enzyme induction.

Inhibition. Inhibition of drug metabolism may result in prolonged and exaggerated drug responses and an increased risk of toxicity. The time course of changes is quite different from that seen with induction, depending on the rate of elimination of the drug whose metabolism has been inhibited. This potentially rapid effect is of greater clinical significance than induction. Inhibition of drug metabolism may be competitive or non-competitive; an example of the latter type is the destruction of cytochrome P450 by quinalbarbitone. Azathioprine is converted in the body to 6-mercapto-purine which is metabolized by xanthine oxidase. Allopurinol inhibits this enzyme and, if azathioprine and allopurinol are prescribed together, the dose of the former must be reduced two- to three-fold to minimize bone marrow toxicity. Monoamine oxidase inhibitors (MAOI) are weak inhibitors of drug oxidation but are the source of an important drug interaction with noradrenaline. In the presence of MAOI noradrenaline accumulates in all adrenergic nerve endings including those in the gut wall. When an indirectly acting catecholamine (i.e. one which releases catecholamines such as phenylpropanolamine, which is a common constituent of many cold cures, or tyramine, present in many foods) is taken, noradrenaline is released into the circulation and the blood pressure may rise abruptly. A recent example of interest is the effect of the H_2 receptor antagonist, cimetidine, shown to be a potent inhibitor of the metabolism of warfarin (Fig. 12), diazepam, and other drugs. This effect is probably due to its imidazole structure, since other H_2 antagonists with different chemical structures do not show this effect. As mentioned in the drug metabolism section, inhibition of metabolism may have a stereospecific basis, e.g. phenylbutazone and S-warfarin.

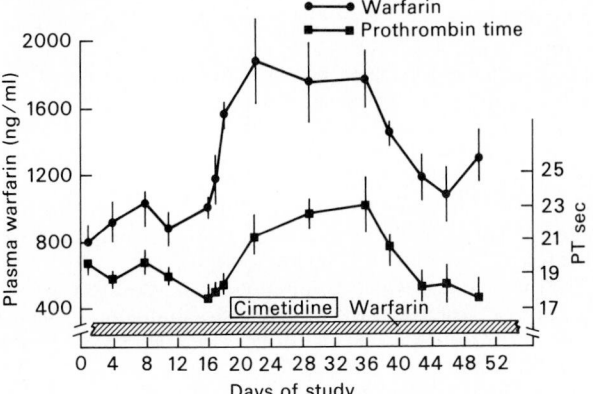

Fig. 12 The effect of cimetidine on the plasma warfarin concentrations and prothrombin times in seven volunteers. (After Serlin *et al.*, (1979). *Lancet* **ii**, 317.

Interactions at the level of the kidney (See also Section 18.)
Changes in urine pH. The renal clearance of weak acids (i.e. pKa 4.0–7.5) is increased in alkaline urine, and renal clearance of weak bases (pKa 7.5–10.0) increased in acid urine due to the impermeability of renal tubules to ionized molecules and the permeability to non-ionized molecules. These facts are used in the treatment of overdosage with phenobarbitone (pKa 7.4) and aspirin (pKa 3.5); alkalinization of urine increases their elimination. Amphetamine overdosage (pKa 9.9) is treated by urine acidification. The half-life of the antifilarial drug diethylcarbamazine (pKa 7.8) can be increased up to three-fold in alkaline urine after therapeutic dosing.

Of course, if drugs are eliminated by hepatic metabolism rather than renal excretion, change in urine pH in the normal clinical situation is irrelevant, irrespective of the pKa.

Competition for active renal tubular excretion. The proximal part of the renal tubule has an active transport mechanism which is used by many drugs. There is probably one system for acidic drugs and one for basic compounds. Examples of acidic drugs using this transport mechanism include penicillin, probenecid, thiazide diuretics, methotrexate, and some sulphonamides. Probenecid is sometimes given to block the renal tubular secretion of penicillin to augment its activity. Another interaction currently causing great interest is the augmentation of digoxin toxicity by quinidine. Quinidine (a weak base) blocks the renal tubular secretion of digoxin, but this interaction may have another component, which is not clearly defined, at the level of digoxin distribution.

Fluid and electrolyte changes. Changes in electrolyte balance may have profound effects on therapeutic effect of drugs acting on the myocardium, CNS, and the kidney. Hypokalaemia (caused by steroids or carbenoxolone) for example, markedly enhances the toxicity of digoxin, prolongs the paralysis produced by non-depolarizing muscle relaxants, and may antagonize the action of acetylcholine by producing hyperpolarization of the motor end-plate. Fluid retention caused by phenylbutazone antagonizes antihypertensive drug effects. (Interestingly, other non-steroidal anti-inflammatory drugs, which act by inhibiting prostaglandin synthesis, may

antagonize the antihypertensive effect of the beta blocker, propranolol.) Certain prostaglandins have vasodilator properties and this may be the basis of this interaction.

Interactions at receptors. There are many examples of pharmacodynamic interactions where one drug alters the effect of another by virtue of its greater affinity for a receptor site. The antagonism of warfarin by vitamin K_1, of morphine by naloxone, of acetylcholine by tubocurarine or atropine, and of dopamine by chlorpromazine are all such examples. The 'receptors' concerned are better defined in some instances than others. In some instances the underlying mechanism is slightly more complicated. The muscle relaxation produced by tubocurarine can be reversed by neostigmine which inhibits cholinesterase and thus increases the concentration of acetylcholine at nerve endings.

Interference with intracellular transport mechanisms constitute a further type of receptor interaction. The adrenergic neurone blocking drugs guanethidine, bethanidine, and debrisoquine lower blood pressure by being actively taken up into sympathetic nerve endings where they replace the neurotransmitter noradrenaline. Several drugs will inhibit their uptake and thus antagonize their antihypertensive effect. Best known antagonists of these adrenergic neurone blockers are the tricyclic antidepressants, although chlorpromazine and amphetamine have a similar attenuating action.

Some interactions are said to occur 'by altering receptor sensitivity', e.g. clofibrate and warfarin, or anabolic steroids and warfarin. This is not an especially valuable concept and the mechanism is frequently postulated when no obvious kinetic or dynamic explanation is quickly forthcoming. As pharmacological knowledge advances, the underlying basis of many of these interactions may become obvious and will fit into the schemes suggested above.

Adverse drug reactions

Incidence. The reported incidence of adverse drug reactions varies depending on the method of data collection used. If trained personnel ask each patient specific questions, higher prevalence figures are reported than if reliance is placed solely on patients volunteering the information. In various series, therefore, the incidence of adverse reactions ranges between 1 and 30 per cent. It has been estimated that between 1 and 3 per cent of all hospital admissions are due to adverse drug reactions. The number of reactions leading to death is also difficult to quantitate since studies are, by definition, carried out in hospital on patients who are seriously ill; the contribution of the adverse drug reaction to the fatal outcome is frequently impossible to quantify.

In spite of the very large number of prescribed drugs, most adverse reactions are attributed to a relatively small group. In most series some 6–10 drugs are most commonly implicated (Table 14).

Table 14   Drugs most commonly implicated as the cause of adverse drug reactions

antibiotics	heparin
aspirin	insulin
digoxin	prednisone
diuretics	warfarin

Epidemiology. Some important determinants of adverse drug reactions are given below.

Age and sex. Adverse effects are more likely to occur in the very young and the elderly, probably because of their relative inability to eliminate drugs. More adverse reactions are recorded in women than men in the ratio of 2:1, and a similar ratio applies to the incidence of fatal drug reactions. This may, in part, be attributable to the use of contraceptive steroids, but there is a greater tendency for women to seek medical attention and thus receive drugs, although this may change as society and employment patterns evolve.

Previous allergic history. Adverse reactions to drugs are more likely to ocur in patients with a history of previous abreaction to other drugs. In some surveys of adverse reactions, up to 25 per cent of patients had previously demonstrated an adverse reaction to drug therapy.

Effect of disease. The disease for which the drug is given may alter the patient's response. A potentially toxic drug whose use may be acceptable in the management of a life threatening situation, should not be used for a relatively trivial indication (e.g. chloramphenicol in typhoid fever versus its use in urinary tract infection).

Pregnancy. Pregnancy alters the response of the mother to certain drugs as well as exposing the fetus to potentially harmful agents. For example, tetracycline in large doses has been implicated as a cause of hepatic damage in pregnancy, but not at other times; it also damages bone and teeth in the fetus. Further, the normal pattern of drug handling may be distorted in pregnancy when both the rate of gastric emptying (leading to delay in drug absorption) and the rate of drug metabolism are slower. Most drugs given to the mother are readily transferred via the placenta to the fetus; this depends largely on the relative lipid solubility of the drug. Once drugs have reached the fetus, they may accumulate there because of its poorly developed ability to eliminate them by metabolism. Special problems of toxicity thus arise when drugs are given in early stages of pregnancy and may cause developmental defects. For this reason drug administration in pregnancy should be kept to a minimum.

Two other aspects of pregnancy merit special mention. During labour, sedatives and analgesics that are given to the mother may pass to the fetus and may interfere with the onset of spontaneous respiration after birth. After birth, drugs may be excreted in breast milk in sufficient concentrations to cause toxic effects in the neonate. Such drugs include thiouracil, phenobarbitone, diazepam, and some laxatives. Interestingly, the oral anticoagulant, warfarin, is not excreted in breast milk and may be used safely in mothers who are breast feeding.

Drug dose. Idiosyncratic drug reactions are not related to dose, but many others, which are related to alteration in drug handling by the body, clearly are.

Timing of reactions. Adverse reactions to drug therapy can occur at any stage during a course of treatment or after its completion. Anaphylactoid reactions characteristically occur with the first administration of a drug course when the patient had been previously exposed, while others may not be observed for months after the drug has been withdrawn (e.g. peritonitis with practolol).

Multiple drug therapy. The greater the number of drugs administered, the higher the incidence of adverse reactions since the number of drug interactions will be greater. The topic of drug interactions is dealt with on page 7.12.

Types of adverse drug reactions. Adverse reactions to drugs can be divided into two main types. First, there are those which arise from an exaggerated but otherwise normal pharmacological action of the drug concerned. In most studies about 80 per cent of adverse drug reactions noted have been of this type. Examples include bleeding on anticoagulant therapy, postural hypotension on antihypertensive therapy, and drowsiness on sedatives. These are termed type A adverse effects and are usually predictable and dose-dependent. Although their incidence is high, the resulting mortality is usually low. Since most of these reactions are merely an extension of the pharmacological action of the drug, it follows that factors affecting these reactions are those that modify the therapeutic effect of the drug. These are conventionally divided into pharmocokinetic factors and pharmacodynamic factors. The responsible pharmacokinetic and pharmacodynamic factors are described on page 7.4 *et seq.*

In contrast to type A reactions, type B adverse effects represent a totally aberrant, novel, and unpredictable action of the drug. Examples of this type of reaction include agranulocytosis due to drugs such as chloramphenicol and phenylbutazone, and malignant hyperthermia from anaesthetic agents. Although these are less common than type A reactions, they carry a higher mortality.

The cause of type B reactions may be within the drug or within the patient. For example, out-of-date tetracycline may degenerate to anhydrotetracycline and epiandrotetracycline particularly in warmer climates and may produce a Fanconi-like syndrome in the patient. Old paraldehyde (more than six months old) may contain acetaldehyde, and the acetic acid which is then formed is highly toxic when injected. Drug preparations contain many other substances than the drug itself, e.g. stabilizers, colouring and wetting agents, and other excipients designed to produce an identifiable tablet of suitable size. Sensitivity to tartrazine, an orange-yellow dye used to colour drugs and soft drinks has been reported frequently. The prevalence may be as high as 1 in 10 000 and the most usual manifestations are urticaria, acute asthma, and non-thrombocytopenic purpura, but anaphylactic shock has also occurred. Cross-reaction to tartrazine occurs with aspirin; probably 10 per cent of patients with aspirin sensitivity are also sensitive to tartrazine.

A novel metabolite of a commonly given drug may produce a type B adverse effect. This was seen in two members of a Swiss family who developed methaemoglobinaemia when phenacetin was given, due to the idiosyncratic formation of a minor metabolite (2-hydroxyphenetedin). Glucose 6-phosphate dehydrogenase (G6PD) deficiency, which is inherited as a sex-linked dominant characteristic, leads to lack of reduced glutathione in red cells, which, on exposure to certain drugs (see Table 9), haemolyse. Males and homozygous females are particularly at risk of developing haemolysis because the deficiency of G6PD is likely to be greater (see Section 19). Other genetic traits carrying with them an increased likelihood of developing adverse drug reactions have been discussed in the section on pharmacogenetics.

Type B adverse drug reactions are sometimes described as being 'allergic' in nature, but this word is often not used in its proper sense denoting an altered reactivity. An allergic mechanism depends on an interaction between the drug (or drug–protein complex) and host antibodies or sensitized lymphocytes. Frequently it is not the native drug which acts as an allergen but a metabolite which becomes tightly bound to larger macromolecules which act as the antigen. The antigen reacts with T lymphocytes to initiate the immune response, and this is followed by activation of B lymphocytes to form anti-drug antibodies. The antigen must have the capability of forming a bridge between cell bound antibody molecules thus producing conformation changes in the cell membrane. Reaction with complement and release of various vasoactive peptides ensue. Two manifestations of type B adverse reactions are of special importance.

Anaphylactic reactions. These are mediated by IgE antibodies and occur very quickly after drug administration. The reaction may be in the skin (acute urticaria), in the respiratory tract (asthma), or in the gastrointestinal tract (abdominal pain and vomiting). A generalized anaphylactic reaction may be life threatening. It usually occurs at the start of a treatment to which the patient has previously been exposed. Penicillin is a common cause of this type of reaction which tends to occur more frequently in atopic individuals.

Serum sickness. This is a less acute form of reaction and results from damage by circulating immune complexes. Current theory is that it results when antigen remains in the circulation for a long period; when antibody (usually IgG or IgM) is first formed, circulating antigen reacts with it forming antigen–antibody complexes. If antibody is in relative excess, the complexes are small and may lodge in blood vessels causing local inflammation and a general systemic response.

Allergic drug reactions may take many forms and may involve other mechanisms than the two detailed above. The formed elements of the blood are frequently involved probably because the antigen (drug) antibody complex is absorbed on to the cell surface, complement is activated, and haemolysis or cell damage occurs.

Why platelets should be damaged in one patient and red cells in another, is currently uncertain (see Section 19).

Clinical trials of new drugs

The aim of an early clinical study of a new compound is to see if the effects seen in animals may also be seen in man, and if the way in which the drug is handled by man corresponds to that in animals. Toxicology studies must also be performed to examine the effect of the drug on standard haematological and biochemical indices. Such early studies will usually be performed in volunteers but with some agents such as cytotoxic drugs it will be necessary to do these studies in patients with the disease for which the drug was designed.

Once the initial studies have been performed in man, it will be necessary to conduct more formal clinical trials. The formal clinical trial is a most powerful tool for the investigation of new drugs, but in some situations this type of study may be too rigid and unsuitable (e.g. if the rate of onset of a drug's effect is being studied). Before a clinical trial is mounted, it is important to establish its real purpose. The aim should be to answer *one* precisely framed question. It is all too easy to attempt to design a trial which asks a number of questions, such as 'is the drug effective?', 'in what patients should it be used?', 'what is the most appropriate dosage?', and 'how does it compare with other drugs?'. Such a trial will fail because it will become too complicated to perform. The comparative clinical trial should be carried out in equivalent groups of patients who are as closely matched for important variables (e.g. age, sex, severity of disease, etc.) as possible. Although in initial clinical trials, controls may not be needed (i.e. the study is an open one), it is important to introduce control observations as soon as possible in the study programme. Thus patients receiving the new drug under test may be compared with patients receiving no treatment, or receiving a matching placebo. However, most commonly the new compound will be compared with a drug that is considered to be the standard treatment for the disease under study at the time. Thus, for example, a new beta-adrenoceptor blocking drug may be compared with placebo to show that it lowers blood pressure in hypertensive patients, or with an existing beta blocker to see if it is more (or less) effective than that drug. Historical retrospective controls are rarely satisfactory. In some situations it may be unethical to withhold active treatment from the control group of patients and in this situation placebo should not be given. Usually the two treatments are studied in comparable patients over the same period of time. It will be necessary to ensure that enough patients are included to minimize any inter-patient variability. When the variability between individuals is a cause for concern, it is often useful to use each patient as his own control, but this can only be done if the disease is stable. Here all patients are exposed to each treatment in a cross-over design and it is important to ensure that each treatment both precedes and follows each other treatment the same number of times. This will minimize any 'carry-over' effect from one treatment to the next. In a crossover design if 'carry over' is a problem, it may be useful to include a placebo 'washout' period between two active periods. It is important to realize that placebo treatment is not synonymous with no therapy. Although the placebo will not contain a pharmacologically active agent, it may have measurable effects. About 30 per cent of patients develop side-effects on placebo therapy, and in many clinical situations the placebo may have therapeutic effects too.

Double blind studies. The information given forms the basis for randomized double blind studies. Patients will be selected for the study on the basis of criteria that have been written down and they will be allocated to control or active treatment groups in a random manner. Since both doctors and patients are capable of bias due to previously held beliefs, by the use of matching placebo capsules both patient and doctor will be made unaware of the precise nature of any patient's therapy. A third party (e.g. a pharmacist) will hold the code which can be broken if it becomes clinically necessary to identify the treatment of an individual patient. If two active treatments (A and B) are compared, the 'double dummy' technique can be used. Here a patient receives either active A and placebo B or active B tablets and placebo A tablets. In this way the study remains double blind. In some instances it may be impossible to preserve the 'blindness' of the doctor. If, for example, a beta-adrenoceptor blocking drug is being studied, as low heart rate may indicate which patient is having active therapy. In these circumstances it may be better to compare one beta-adrenoceptor blocking drug with another similar drug.

Clinical assessment of drugs. When clinical trials of drugs are performed, it is very important to obtain an accurate assessment of their therapeutic effect. This is easy if a hypotensive or anticoagulant drug is being studied. The fall in blood pressure is a fairly objective measure although even here appropriate steps are needed to reduce observer bias (e.g. to use a muddled zero sphygmomanometer). In certain areas a drug has effects which can only be assessed by subjective measures and clinical assessment is less reliable. In the assessment of CNS active drugs such as antidepressants and tranquillizers, 'rating scales' have been developed which require skilled personnel to undertake them. Visual analogue scales can be very useful to assess many subjective sensations such as pain and sleepiness. The patient places a mark on the line corresponding to the assessment of pain suffered, and this is repeated at each examination, the 'score' being measured. This method of assessment is remarkably accurate, repeatable, and relatively free of observer error. The same method can be applied to the assessment of adverse effects. An example is shown in Fig. 7.

Statistical and ethical considerations. In designing a clinical trial the initial hypothesis is that there is no difference between the two treatments. It then has to be decided if the results obtained could have been due to chance or if there is a real probability of difference between the two treatments. The statistical aspects of clinical trials can be complicated and the interested reader is referred elsewhere for more detailed information (Hill, A. B., 1971, *Principles of medical statistics*). In most cases it can be assumed that the data is normally distributed but this is not always the case and simple statistical methods will then not be applicable. Before the start of a trial it is usual to assume that a given level of probability (p) will be accepted. Thus, with a p value of less than 0.05, a difference would be found by chance less than 5 in 100 times. It is important to realize that even if a p value of 0.01 is chosen there is still a risk, albeit small, that any difference found in the trial may not be real but due to chance alone.

Statistical considerations will often help in the design of a trial, particularly in knowing how many patients to include. The smaller the expected difference between two treatments the more patients will be required to show a significant result. Many trials are rendered invalid by a failure to include enough patients.

In the conduct of any clinical trial the ethical aspects are of great importance. Nowadays all trial protocols should be scrutinized by an independent review body. Each participant in the study should have the details of the trial explained to them and they should give their written informed consent to take part in the study. This consent should be witnessed by a third party. Any patient entering a clinical study must, of course, be free to leave the study at any time.

References

Breckenridge, A. (1975). *Advanced medicine symposia: topics in therapeutics 1*. Pitman Medical, London.

Ciba Foundation Symposia (1980). *Symposium 76. Environmental chemical enzyme function and human disease*. Exerpta Medica, Amsterdam.

Davies, D. M. (ed.) (1981). *Textbook of adverse drug reactions*, 2nd edn. Oxford University Press, Oxford.

Davies, D. S. and Prichard, B. N. C. (eds.) (1973). *Biological effects of drugs in relation to their plasma concentrations*. Macmillan, London.

Goodman, L. S. and Gilman, A. (1980). *Pharmacological basis of therapeutics*, 6th edn. Macmillan, London.

Hill, A. B. (1960). *Controlled clinical trials*, Blackwell Scientific Publications, Oxford.

Prescott, L. F. and Nimmo, W. S. (1980). *Drug absorption*. Adis Press, Sydney.

Rowland, M. (1978). In *Clinical pharmacology, basic principles in therapeutics*, 2nd ed. (eds. K. Melmon and H. Morelli), p. 25. Macmillan, London.

Sjöqvist, F., Borga, O., and Orme, M. L'E. (1980). Fundamentals of clinical pharmacology. In *Drug treatment*, 2nd edn. (ed. G. S. Avery), p. 1. Adis Press, Sydney.

Vesell, E. S. (ed.) (1971). Drug metabolism in man. *Ann. N. Y. Acad. Sci.* **179**.

Williams, R. T. (1959). *Detoxication mechanisms*. Wiley, New York.

World Health Organization (1972). Clinical pharmacology: scope, organization, training. *Tech. Rep. Ser. Wld Hlth Org.* **446**.

Section 8
Nutrition

Introduction

R. Smith and W. P. T. James

Adequate nutrition is essential to life, and many of the conditions mentioned in this book are partly nutritional in origin. The nutritional aspects of some diseases, such as those of the liver, kidney, and pancreas, and of inherited metabolic diseases, are best dealt within the context of the diseases themselves. This introduction deals particularly with nutrition of the hospital and surgical patient, and with the problems of obesity and starvation.

It is widely considered that nutrition is badly taught and that the student is ignorant of its theory and practice. This is partly because the effects of malnutrition are not so striking in temperate climates as in the tropics, and also because the average student regards nutrition merely as a branch of dietetics. Where it has been a practical necessity to understand nutrition, as in starvation and in the post-operative care of surgical patients, there has fortunately been more interest and research.

Much of our understanding of nutrition is based on biochemical advances which the following pages will take into account. This does not imply that disturbances of nutrition are primarily biochemical in origin nor that they are treated mainly by biochemical means.

The basis for many nutritional diseases is multifactorial and involves the cultural aspects of food preparation and social and economic influences, all of which may contribute to an inappropriate diet. These aspects are particularly emphasized in the account of protein energy malnutrition (pages 8.12–21). Similarly obesity has many causes, with an interplay between environmental factors and individual constitutional variations in susceptibility to weight gain.

In many nutritional diseases the patient may be the individual most susceptible to the prevailing pattern of food intake within the community. Only now are we beginning to disentangle the biochemical basis for the individual susceptibility to such conditions as ischaemic heart disease, hypertension, and obesity. This biochemical progress is matched by a recognition that particular items in the diet are being ingested in excessive or insufficient amounts. This is a very different view of nutrition from the traditional one which considered nutritional disorders simply as due to protein deficiency or the result of mineral or vitamin lack.

The last few decades have seen little advance in our knowledge of vitamins, except for vitamin D, but the clinical effects of their deficiencies can be striking. In contrast clinical syndromes due to trace element deficiencies continue to be recognized, and are often precipitated by the artificial effects of prolonged intravenous nutrition.

Amongst those conditions in which malnutrition is only one aspect of the clinical picture anorexia nervosa is an example; here protein energy lack is associated with complex endocrine and psychological disturbances. Other conditions such as ischaemic heart disease and colonic diverticulosis, where nutrition is of undoubted importance, but where the clues are elusive and the findings controversial, are considered on pages 8.55–8.

A very important aspect of nutrition concerns different types of food, their structure, composition, and preparation. These are dealt with generally under the heading of dietetics and details will be found in the bibliography; however, there are certain important points which should now be considered.

Man is an omnivore, but by necessity many millions of people eat a virtually vegetarian diet. Many forms of edible matter are not used as food; the decision to do so or not depends on many social, religious, and economic factors and may bear no relation to nutritive value. There is usually one food which is the staple diet of a particular culture and this is nearly always vegetable in origin (for instance wheat, rice, maize, cassava); another form may be labelled as a prestige food, since it is expensive and is, therefore, reserved for special occasions; this is usually meat.

When attempts are made to find out what individuals or communities actually eat, it is usual to enquire about the types of food ingested or to estimate in more detail the amount of each item of food. By reference to tables for the average composition of these foods it is then possible to calculate the nutrient intake. Despite their demonstrated usefulness, food composition tables are available only in developed countries; they require continuous revision because of the wide variety of new products; and they can give only an approximate estimate of food actually consumed by individuals. Intake can be assessed retrospectively or prospectively. To ask an individual about the types or quantities of food he has consumed over the previous days, weeks, or months gives results which are of little use. Prospective methods can be divided into those where individuals record the type and approximate amounts of food which they consume over a period of a week or so, and those which involve weighing the diet. The last method requires some explanation by the investigator, and co-operation, some intelligence, and literacy on the part of the individual, and time to analyse the results. Many studies which have shown the importance of diet in relation to disease have been carried out in this way. An important aspect of the food consumed is its physical characteristics and its method of preparation. With advances in technology many foods, particularly cereals, rice, and bread, are partly deprived of their nutritive value during preparation, which can lead to specific vitamin deficiencies. The importance of retaining the fibrous element of food has received much recent emphasis.

Although obesity is a major nutritional disease in the western world, international organizations such as the Food and Agriculture Organization (FAO) and the World Health Organization (WHO) have rightly concerned themselves more with the worldwide problems of starvation, and have made recommendations for food requirements with particular emphasis on protein. The general principles of nutrient requirements have been summarized by Waterlow and Eddy. Although it is possible to make an approximation of the average food requirement for a group, based on data of variable validity, the difficulty is to specify an intake which will meet the needs of all or nearly all individuals within the group.

Statistically a level of intake two standard deviations above the average should cover the needs of 97.5 per cent of the group, and this has been called the safe level or safe intake; but in fact the standard error is often not known and the individual variation is very wide.

Energy requirements clearly differ considerably from one person to another and one of the main causes of this variation is occupational physical work (Table 1). In addition there is considerable variation in individuals' metabolic rate. The safe protein intake can be estimated by adding two standard deviations to the average requirement derived from studies on nitrogen balance, and a correction is made for the quality of the protein, using milk or eggs as 100 per cent. With energy, however, this manipulation of data to derive a safe value for nearly all the population cannot be made

Table 1   Estimate of energy expenditure of a normal adult

	Time	kcal*	kJ	Total range kcal (kJ)
Male				
Bed	8 h	500	2100	
Non-occupational activities	8 h	700–1500	3000–6300	
Work	8 h			
Light		1100	4600	2300–3100 (9660–13 000)
Very heavy		2400	10 100	3600–4400 (15 100–18 500)
Female				
Bed	8 h	420	1760	
Non-occupational activities	8 h	580–980	2430–4120	
Work	8 h			
Light		800	3360	1800–2200 (7560–9240)
Heavy		1400	5880	2400–2700 (10 100–11 340)

These figures refer to a 'reference' man of 65 kg and woman of 55 kg. Energy expenditure decreases with age and these figures should probably be reduced by at least 10 per cent over the age of 50 years. The main difficulty in calculation arises from the variation in 'non-occupational' or 'leisure' activities.

* kcal = Cal

Adapted from Waterlow and Eddy (1978)

since a surfeit of energy can only be metabolized by a proportion of the population, the rest then showing varying degrees of obesity. As will be emphasized in subsequent chapters, and particularly with

regard to parenteral nutrition, protein intake cannot be considered on its own independent of energy intake; nitrogen balance depends on the intake both of protein and energy since insufficient non-protein energy will lead to protein itself being used as an energy source. The approximate daily requirements for energy and the safe intakes of protein at different ages are summarized in Table 2.

Table 2   Daily requirements for energy and safe intakes of protein at different ages

	Age	Energy kcal/kg	Energy kJ/kg	Safe intake of protein (g/kg)
Infant	3 months	120	500	2.40
Child	4–6 years	90	380	1.30
Adolescent				
Male	13–15 years	57	240	0.90
Female	13–15 years	50	210	0.80
Adult				
Male		46	190	0.70
Female		40	170	0.65

The figures refer to an individual of moderate activity, and the protein intake for milk protein

Adapted from Waterlow and Eddy (1978)

References

Davidson, S., Passmore, R., Brock, J. F., and Truswell, A. S. (1979). *Human nutrition and dietetics*, 7th edn. Churchill Livingstone, Edinburgh.

McLaren, D. S. (1980). *Nutrition and its disorders*, 3rd edn. Churchill Livingstone, Edinburgh.

Waterlow, J. C. (1981). Nutrition of man. *Br. med. Bull.* **37**, 1.

— and Eddy, T. P. (1978). Nutrition and nutritional disorders. In *Price's Textbook of medicine*, 12th edn. (ed. R. Bodley Scott). Oxford University Press, Oxford.

Biochemical background

R. Smith and D. H. Williamson

Such is the ease with which nutrition usually occurs that it is taken for granted; and only when it is disturbed does this complex physiological process become of clinical interest. At such times it is essential for the physician or surgeon to have some knowledge of the fundamental biochemical processes which underlie normal nutrition, such as the supply and utilization of energy-containing nutrients (upon which life depends), the control of the metabolism of protein, fat, and carbohydrate, and results of imbalance between fuel supply and demand. It is necessary to know, for example, how metabolic fuels are provided to the tissues; which biochemical changes occur in a patient deprived of food; how an injured person survives; and what are the principles and problems of parenteral feeding. This section aims to summarize the relevant biochemical facts of normal human nutrition. It will concern itself exclusively with the metabolism of protein, fat, and carbohydrate and their intermediates. Since much recent knowledge on energy exchange has been derived from studies on obese patients undergoing short or long periods of starvation; the effects of this will also be considered. Further relevant biochemical information will be found in the sections on diabetes mellitus and on vitamin deficiencies.

Production of energy from metabolic fuels. The body requires energy for many functions. These include the synthesis of new

tissues, the maintenance of ionic gradients, the processes of secretion and detoxification, the generation of heat, and the performance of exercise and locomotion. To provide this energy the tissues oxidize glucose (from carbohydrate) non-esterified fatty acids and ketone bodies (from fat), and amino acids (from protein). These energy-containing substrates or metabolic fuels are provided as a mixture to the tissues in the blood stream, and their proportional utilization depends on many factors. The oxidation of these fuels is linked to the generation of the high energy phosphate of adenosine triphosphate (ATP) (Fig. 1) through the tricarboxylic acid (TCA), or citric acid, cycle. A high proportion of the ATP is generated in the mitochondria, where the energy released by the oxidation of reducing equivalents, in the form of $NADH_2$ and $FADH_2$, by O_2 is coupled to the formation of ATP in oxidative phosphorylation. Although most of the reducing equivalents are generated in the TCA cycle, some are also produced by the partial oxidation of glucose, fatty acids, and amino acids. ATP can additionally be formed anaerobically during glycolysis but the amount is insignificant compared with total energy production.

Details of oxidative phosphorylation can be obtained from the references listed at the end of this section. Figure 1 demonstrates the central position of acetyl-CoA whose acetyl group is derived from glucose, fatty acids, and many amino acids. This carrier

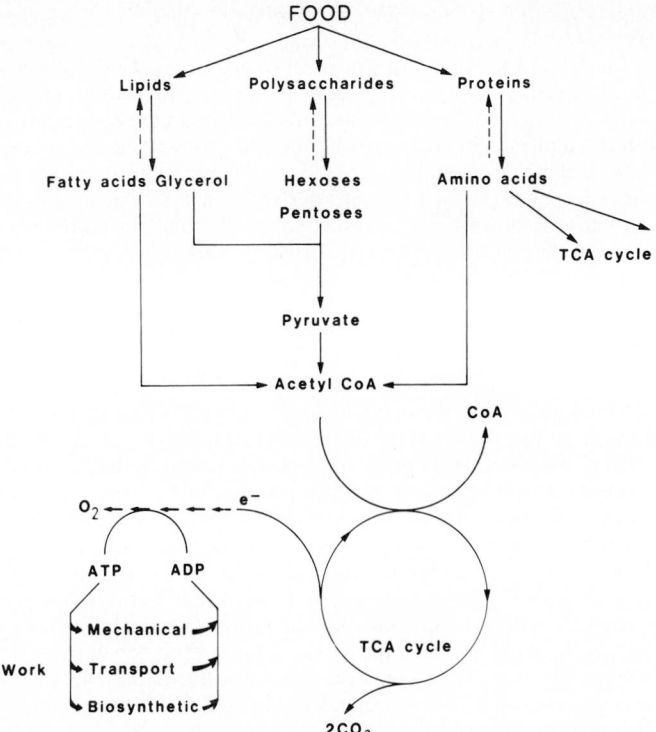

FOOD

Fig. 1 The source, production, and utilization of energy from food. The lipids, polysaccharides, and proteins are degraded into their constituents by digestive enzymes. After transport to the tissue cells they are either used for resynthesis (dotted arrows) or mainly converted to acetyl-CoA. The TCA cycle is located in the mitochondria. For further explanation see text.

molecule brings acetyl units into the TCA or citric acid cycle. The cyclical oxidation of acetyl-CoA produces 3 moles of $NADH_2$, 1 mole of $FADH_2$, and 2 moles of CO_2 for each mole of acetyl-CoA oxidized. These reducing equivalents are the substrates utilized by the electron transport chain (represented by e^-) to form ATP. Oxidation of a single glucose molecule can result in the formation of 36 molecules of ATP.

Energy requirements. The normal energy requirements in the adult (which are equal to the energy expenditure) are shown in Tables 1 and 2, on page 8.4. In the healthy person, energy consumption increases considerably with exercise; fever, surgery, burns, and neoplasms also increase energy demand. Of the total oxygen consumption (which is a convenient measure of aerobic metabolism), more than 90 per cent in the basal state is accounted for by the major organs; approximate figures are skeletal muscle 30 per cent, abdominal organs 25 per cent, brain 20 per cent, and heart about 11 per cent. During exercise the energy requirements of muscle may increase 10–15 fold compared with insignificant changes in other organs. Other physiological circumstances increase the energy requirements of other tissues; for instance that of abdominal organs is increased by eating; and that of a large number of tissues is increased by growth, particularly during infancy or fetal life. In contrast, energy expenditure decreases after middle age.

Some clues about the fuels used to provide this energy may be provided by a comparison between CO_2 production and O_2 consumption (the respiratory quotient), which is 1.0 when carbohydrate is used exclusively as a fuel, and 0.7 for fat. The use of the respiratory quotient to predict the type of fuel being burnt is valid only with certain assumptions and does not provide any information about the proportion of fuel used by different organs.

Body composition and metabolic fuels. The available metabolic fuels are related to body composition (Table 1). There are two main protein sites within the body. One of these is extracellular (col-

Table 1   The approximate normal composition of a 70 kg man

	kg	% body weight
Water	42	60
Intracellular	28	40
Extracellular	14	20
Solids		
Fat	12.6	18
Protein*	11.2	16
Intracellular (muscle)	8.4	12
Extracellular (collagen)	2.8	4
Minerals	3.8	5.4
Carbohydrate	0.4	0.6

* The figures for intracellular and extracellular protein are estimates only and the fat content is less than in Fig. 2

lagen), located particularly in the bone matrix and skin, and this does not appear to be readily available as a source of fuel. The other is intracellular (striated muscle) which in man is the main protein source of fuel. The amount of adipose tissue may alter very considerably, and an obese person may have between 50 and 100 kg above normal. The significance of the differences between muscle and adipose tissue as potential energy sources becomes obvious when it is recalled that muscle protein is associated with about three times its own weight of water and provides 4 kcal/g (about 17 kJ/g) whereas adipose tissue fat is virtually anhydrous, and provides 9 kcal/g (about 38 kJ/g). Thus 100 g of skeletal muscle will yield 100 kcal whereas 100 g of adipose tissue will yield about 900 kcal (3780 kJ). This means that for a given utilization of energy the weight loss is far less rapid when fat is consumed than muscle; that fat is by far the most efficient way of storing energy; and that an obese person with an extra 55 kg of adipose tissue has half a million kcal 'in store'. The prime importance of adipose tissue triglyceride as a fuel 'store' is emphasized in Fig. 2. Apart from fat, the only

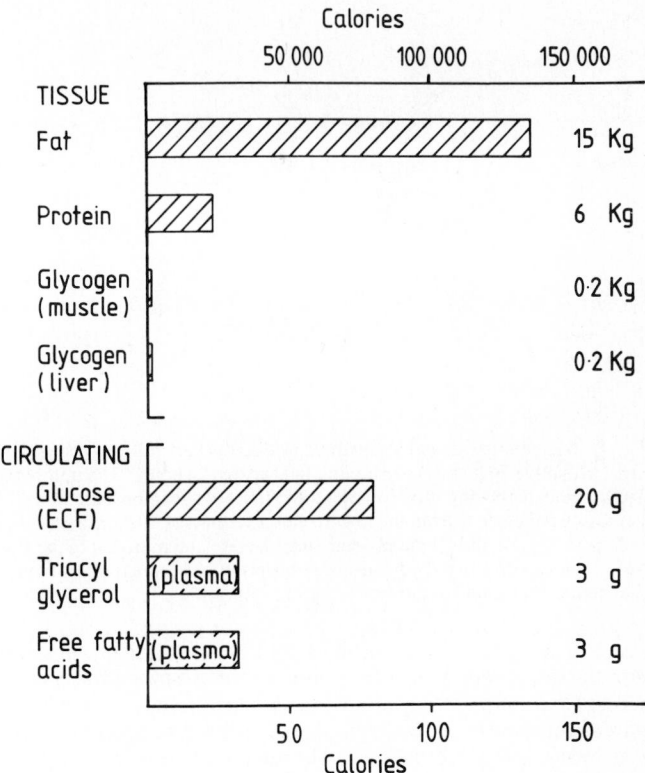

Fig. 2 To demonstrate the available metabolic fuels in the normal adult. After the rapid utilization of glycogen, protein and fat are the main fuel 'stores' in fasting. In comparison the energy to be derived from circulating metabolites is insignificant. Note that the scale for the circulating metabolites is 1000 less than for the tissue stores.

other significant body store of fuel which can be used on a relatively long-term basis is protein, particularly that of skeletal muscle. In starvation, degradation of this tissue for energy purposes is reduced by the selective utilization of fat. In the non-fasting person there are also a number of minor short-term body stores of fuel. These include glycogen, the circulating body pools of free glucose, free fatty acids, and amino acids, which are readily used in an overnight fast.

The main metabolic fuels circulate in the plasma as their constituents; protein in the form of amino acids, particularly alanine and glutamine from skeletal muscle; carbohydrate, predominantly as glucose but also (as in exercise) lactate and pyruvate produced in the Cori cycle; and fats as non-esterified fatty acids (NEFA) and glycerol. Ketone bodies are formed by partial oxidation of NEFA in the liver.

Fuel supply, utilization, and balance. The supply and utilization of energy-containing substrates is most simply considered in the way represented by Cahill and his colleagues where the liver occupies a central position as the transformer between the fuel supply and those tissues which utilize it. An outline of this is shown in Fig. 3. This shows the main metabolic exchanges, determined by direct cannulation of appropriate vessels, by measurement of isotopically labelled substrate turnover, and by indirect calorimetry in post-absorptive man. After the rapid utilization of short-term fuel stores such as glycogen, the main suppliers of further fuel are fat (in adipose tissue) and protein (in skeletal muscle), and the main utilizers the brain and central nervous system, the muscles, the abdominal organs, and the circulating blood cells. The proportional utilization of fat and protein by tissues will depend on such factors as their availability, and on the changes in concentration of hormones and other metabolites discussed below.

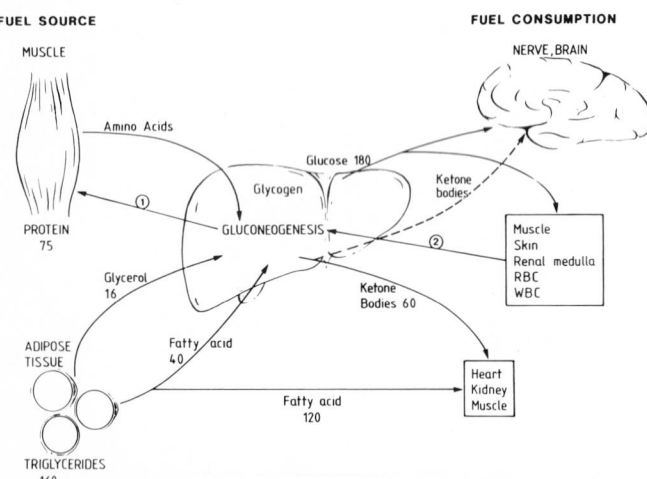

FUEL SOURCE   FUEL CONSUMPTION

Fig. 3   To demonstrate daily substrate production and utilization (in g) in a post-absorptive 70 kg man consuming 1800 kcal in 24 hours. The numbered arrows indicate the direction (but not the extent) of two important cycles:① the transfer of glucose from the liver to muscle as part of the glucose-alanine cycle (see Fig. 9); and② the production of lactate and pyruvate in the Cori cycle. The dotted arrow indicates the utilization of ketone bodies by nervous tissue (particularly the brain) during starvation.

In a 24-hour period the tissues of a normal fasting man will utilize approximately 1800 kcal derived from about 75 g of protein (mainly muscle) and 160 g of triglyceride from adipose tissue. Of the 180 g of glucose released from the liver, about 144 g will be totally oxidized by nervous tissue, mainly brain. The remaining 36 g is converted by glycolytic tissues—for example, bone marrow, renal medulla, peripheral nerve, erythrocytes and to a lesser extent skeletal muscle—to lactate and pyruvate. These metabolites are carried to the liver and kidney and are there resynthesized into glucose. This cycle, the Cori cycle (② in Fig. 3), provides a shuttle of carbon which spares

gluconeogenesis from protein by limiting the complete oxidation of glucose to carbon dioxide.

In addition to complete oxidation of glucose (in the brain) and glycolysis (in red cells), the remaining tissues, heart, kidney cortex, skeletal muscle and other organs, in fasting man use fatty acids or ketone bodies. The liver, which efficiently converts lactate, pyruvate, and the glucogenic amino acids to glucose, requires energy for these processes; again it is mainly derived from fatty acid oxidation.

Figure 3 shows how energy is supplied from the body's own tissues; clearly where there is an exogenous source of fuel the picture will be more complex, but the mechanisms which control the metabolic pathways will be the same. However, where the food intake either exceeds or is less than the energy requirements, there may be considerable changes in the fuel stores with subsequent alteration in body composition.

The regulation of the overall balance between fuel supply and its consumption is poorly understood. In the normal person the intake and utilization of food appear to be closely linked so that at least in some adults body weight and composition may remain virtually constant for years. Intake is influenced by appetite and hunger and probably by other unidentified endocrine or intestinal signals. Many studies on fuel intake which have been done on rats are not directly applicable to man, whose larger brain imposes complex controls on eating behaviour and also utilizes a larger proportion of energy. In man the role of the hypothalamus is still debated and the factors which control short and long-term fluctuations in weight remain obscure. These are further considered in relation to obesity (see pages 8.34–6).

Regulation of substrate metabolism. Before the specific pathways of carbohydrate, fat, and protein are considered further it is important to outline the basic principles which regulate substrate metabolism. The utilization of a given energy-containing substrate by a tissue depends on many factors; amongst these are its circulating concentration, the blood flow to the tissue, the permeability of the cells and their compartments to the substrate, the mechanism of the entry into the metabolic pathway, subsequent intracellular metabolism, and the effects of other substrates and hormones.

Availability of substrate. The concentration of a particular substrate in the circulation must represent the balance between its utilization and production (either from endogenous or dietary sources). Most metabolites are utilized in proportion to their concentration. Changes in concentration are important not only for energy supply, but they may also act as signals to regulate the utilization or production of other substrates; their regulation can be direct, or indirect by altering hormone concentrations (for instance the increase in insulin produced by an elevation of blood sugar decreases lipolysis, the release of non-esterified fatty acids, and the production of ketone bodies). The total amount of substrate (calculated as oxidizable fuels) in the blood is remarkably constant in various physiological states but the proportion of glucose, non-esterified fatty acids (NEFA), ketone bodies, triglycerides, and amino acids may vary considerably (compare for instance the fed with the starved state). Since all tissues of the body necessarily receive the same prevailing substrate 'mixture', the question arises as to how the removal of these substrates by particular tissues is controlled.

The role of blood flow in controlling tissue metabolism is often underestimated. A clear example is the depression of blood flow to the splanchnic area during prolonged exercise and its reciprocal increase to the peripheral tissues which leads to the provision of more substrates, in particular NEFA, to working muscle. Further it is now appreciated that the increased metabolism and concomitant heat production by brown adipose tissue is partly regulated by a large increase in blood supply.

Permeability to substrate. For a substrate which is available in the circulation the next potential site of regulation is entry into the cell through the plasma membrane, or into the particular cellular compartment such as the mitochondrion, where its metabolism is initiated. The substrate can enter the cell by simple diffusion or by a specific transport system, whose activity may be altered by hormones. There is, for instance, a carrier system for transport of glucose into muscle and adipose tissue which is stimulated by insulin: and pyruvate enters the matrix of hepatic mitochondria via a carrier which may be activated by glucagon.

There are different systems in different tissues; for instance, in the rat, the rate of diffusion of ketone bodies into skeletal muscle does not limit their utilization, whereas in the brain there is evidence of a transport system for these metabolites. Triglycerides occupy a special position, since they are not transported as such into cells, and the initial enzyme involved in their metabolism is located at an extracellular site on the capillary endothelium.

Entry into metabolic pathway. Inside the cell the next factor involved in utilization of the substrate is the concentration (activity) of the first or 'initiating' enzyme in its metabolic pathway. Although the majority of substrates eventually yield acetyl-CoA which can enter the tricarboxylic acid cycle for oxidation (see Fig. 1), each substrate has its own initiating enzyme, examples of which are given in Table 2. The activity of these enzymes may be regulated either by acute changes in the concentration of effector metabolites (for instance the inhibition of hexokinase by glucose 6-phosphate limits further glucose utilization) or by longer-term alteration in the amount of enzyme (for example a decrease in hepatic glucokinase concentration in starvation and insulin-deficiency limits hepatic extraction of glucose).

Such changes in the amounts of the initiating enzyme in various tissues mean that the metabolism of substrates may be partitioned to particular tissues. This tissue-specific metabolism does not imply that a substrate is solely removed by a single tissue of the body but rather that a particular tissue predominates in its removal. The differences in the amounts of initiating enzymes between tissues may be constitutive and not alter with change in the physiological state, or be adaptive and therefore changeable; for example, the reciprocal alteration in the lipoprotein lipase activity in adipose tissue and mammary gland during lactation results in a re-direction of the available plasma triglycerides from adipose tissue to the lactating gland for milk fat production. An important question is what signals bring about such changes in the activity of initiating enzymes? As an example it appears that during lactation prolactin plays a role in suppressing lipoprotein lipase activity in adipose tissue.

Intracellular regulation. Although the first enzyme involved in the metabolism of a substrate is often a site of regulation, other regulatory sites exist within the metabolic pathway. These other regulatory enzymes are usually situated at branch-points in the pathway, and are low activity enzymes whose reactions are far from equilibrium. The regulation of the activity of these enzymes is of two main types: short-term (or fine) and long-term (or coarse). Long-term regulation requires a period of time (usually hours) to take place and involves a change in the amount (concentration) of active enzyme, brought about by alterations in the rate of synthesis and/or degradation of the protein. In contrast, fine control of metabolism is exerted on a minute-to-minute basis and involves changes in the activity of existing enzymes. Such rapid changes can be produced in a number of ways. For instance, if the enzyme is not saturated with substrate then an increase in substrate concentration will increase its activity. Alternatively the enzyme may be susceptible to inhibition or activation by effector metabolites (e.g. inhibition of phosphofructokinase by citrate: activation of liver-type pyruvate kinase by fructose 1,6-bisphosphate). It is now well established that many regulatory enzymes, in particular those concerned with storage or mobilization of stored fuels (fat or glycogen) exist in active and inactive forms which can be rapidly inter-converted. Phosphorylation or dephosphorylation of the protein brings about the change in activity and is catalysed by two types of enzyme; a kinase for phosphorylation and a phosphatase for dephosphorylation (Fig. 4). Pairs of interconvertible enzymes (such as phosphorylase and glycogen synthetase) which bring about opposite effects on storage depots (such as glycogen) have their active and inactive forms in opposing states of phosphorylation, so that a hormonal signal can affect both enzymes simultaneously and bring about a uni-directional change in flux rate. The obvious advantage of this type of regulation is that within seconds the concentration of active enzyme can be increased without the need to stimulate protein synthesis, a process which takes the order of one-half to two hours. In addition effector molecules can regulate the activity of the active

Table 2 Initiating enzymes

Substrate	Initiating enzyme	Product	Intracellular site
A. Carbohydrate			
Glucose	hexokinase glucokinase	glucose 6-phosphate	cytosol
Lactate	lactate dehydrogenase	pyruvate	cytosol
Pyruvate	1. pyruvate dehydrogenase	acetyl-CoA	mitochondrial inner membrane
	2. pyruvate carboxylase	oxaloacetate	mitochondrial matrix
Glycerol	glycerol kinase	glycerol 3-phosphate	cytosol
B. Lipid			
Triacylglycerols	lipoprotein lipase	fatty acids plus glycerol	extracellular
Non-esterified fatty acids	fatty acyl-CoA synthetase	fatty acyl-CoA	1. microsomes 2. mitochondrial outer membrane
Hydroxybutyrate	hydroxybutyrate dehydrogenase	acetoacetate	mitochondrial matrix
Acetoacetate	1. 3-oxoacid CoA transferase	acetoacetyl-CoA	1. mitochondrial matrix
	2. acetoacetyl-CoA synthetase	acetoacetyl-CoA	2. cytosol
Acetate	acetyl-CoA synthetase	acetyl-CoA	1. cytosol 2. mitochondrial matrix
C. Amino acids			
Alanine	alanine amino-transferase	pyruvate	1. cytosol 2. mitochondrial matrix
Glutamine	glutaminase	glutamate	mitochondrial matrix
Branched-chain amino acids (leucine, isoleucine and valine)	corresponding amino-transferases	corresponding ketoacids	1. cytosol 2. mitochondrial matrix

The initiating enzymes are grouped according to the main metabolic fuels. Apart from lipoprotein lipase they are all intracellular and may be found in different locations within the cell

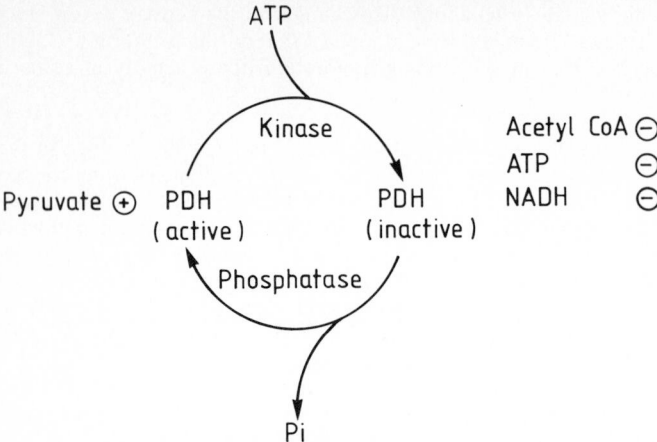

Fig. 4 An example of interconversion between active and inactive forms of an enzyme. Pyruvate dehydrogenase (PDH) is converted to an inactive phosphorylated form by a kinase and to an active dephosphorylated form by a phosphatase. The activity of PDH is decreased by acetyl CoA, ATP, and NADH; and increased by pyruvate.

enzyme and of the two interconverting enzymes (kinase and phosphatase).

Another method of controlling flux through a metabolic pathway utilizes a 'substrate cycle'. A reaction in a pathway may be catalysed by a regulatory enzyme in the forward direction and opposed by another regulatory enzyme in the reverse direction (Fig. 5). If the two enzymes are simultaneously active, a substrate cycle is created and the rate of the overall flux through the reaction step will depend on the relative activity of the two opposing enzymes. These enzymes themselves may be controlled by effectors or by interconversion cycles. Examples of enzymes catalysing substrate cycles are: (a) glucokinase versus glucose 6-phosphatase in liver and (b) phosphofructokinase and fructose 1,6-bisphosphatase in muscle. These substrate cycles dissipate chemical energy and it is the conversion of this energy into heat which may be a major limitation to the rate of cycling. For further information on the role of substrate cycles in regulation the reader should consult Newsholme.

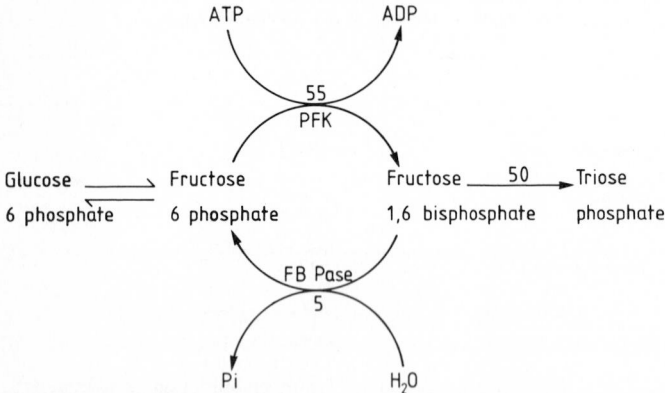

Fig. 5 An example of a substrate cycle between fructose 6-phosphate and fructose 1, 6-bisphosphate. This cycle is considered important in the control of glycolysis, which provides energy for muscle under anaerobic or hypoxic conditions. The figures represent the hypothetical reaction rates of the forward (phosphofructokinase; PFK) and reverse (fructose 1, 6-bisphosphatase; FBPase) reactions at rest. The glycolytic flux is the difference between these two. (Modified from Newsholme, 1980).

Substrate interactions. Changes in substrate concentration in the blood can in certain situations regulate the utilization or production of another substrate. For example, the increased availability of NEFA and/or ketone bodies in starvation inhibits glucose utilization by muscle. The accepted mechanism for this inhibition is shown in Fig. 6. The increased production of acetyl-CoA within the

mitochondria from fatty acids or ketone bodies results in increased availability of citrate which is transported to the cytosol where it inhibits phosphofructokinase. Consequently, the concentrations of fructose 6-phosphate and glucose 6-phosphate rise; the latter is an inhibitor of hexokinase. The net result is that less glucose is utilized and that which still undergoes glycolysis to pyruvate is not oxidized because acetyl-CoA is an inhibitor of pyruvate dehydrogenase. The pyruvate and lactate which accumulate can be returned to the liver to be reconverted to glucose (see Fig. 9).

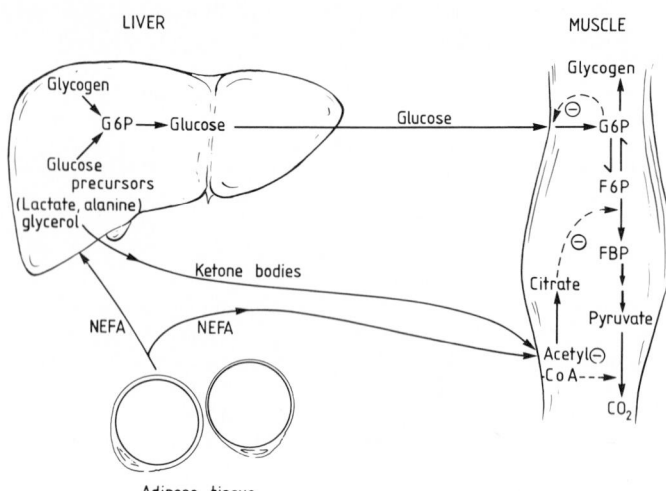

Fig. 6 To show how one substrate may regulate the use of another. The increasing concentration and availability of non-esterified fatty acids (NEFA) and ketone bodies in starvation decreases the utilization of glucose by muscle. For explanation see text and Randle *et al.* (1966). ⊖ signifies inhibition.

Regulation of substrate concentrations in the blood can also be exerted via a 'feed-back' loop. Ketone bodies stimulate the secretion of insulin by the pancreatic ß-cells and this in turn decreases the release of NEFA, the major precursors of ketone bodies, from adipose tissue. In addition, ketone bodies exert a direct antilipolytic effect on adipose tissue. The advantage of this 'feed-back' control is that it assists in maintaining the circulating concentrations of ketone bodies at a level which is optimum for their utilization by peripheral tissues, but which causes the minimum disturbance of the acid–base balance and little loss of ketone bodies in the urine. Further, this method of regulation also allows ketone bodies to control the availability of glycerol (released on mobilization of adipose tissue triglycerides) to form glucose in the liver.

Hormones and metabolism. (See also Section 10.) As discussed above, alterations in available substrate play a key role in fuel supply and the intracellular control of metabolism. In the postabsorptive state, changes in concentration of circulating substrates mainly represent the direct response to changes in the hormonal milieu. Thus, following a carbohydrate meal, the rise in blood glucose and in various enteric hormones increases insulin secretion. This in turn decreases hepatic glucose release, promotes glycogen synthesis and inhibits lipolysis in adipose tissue. Consequently, blood glucose remains within a relatively narrow range (avoiding renal loss of substrate) and the concentrations of the alternative substrates, fatty acids, and ketone bodies, decrease.

The way in which hormones alter substrate supply are mainly rapid (short-term regulation), but longer-term changes do occur. Insulin, glucagon and the 'stress' hormones (catecholamines, growth hormone, vasopressin) usually have acute effects, although they can also bring about long-term changes in enzyme concentration. The effects of corticosteroids and thyroxine appear to be confined to long-term regulation. The rapid effects of hormones involve either changes in the rate of transport of substrates into the cell or particular cellular compartment or alterations in the activity of key regulatory enzymes. The accepted mechanisms for their action involve: (*a*) binding of the hormone to its receptor (usually located on or within the plasma membrane); (*b*) generation of a change in concentration of the 'second messenger' (cyclic AMP, cyclic GMP, Ca^{2+} ions); and (*c*) interaction of the second messenger with the target enzyme (or transport system). The target enzyme may not directly be involved in the metabolic process which the particular hormone regulates. In many cases it acts to change the activity of an enzyme (e.g. protein kinase and/or phosphatase) which controls the interconversion of a regulatory enzyme in the metabolic pathway. In this way very small amounts of hormone can bring about large changes in the rate of a metabolic process by a form of enzyme cascade (Fig. 7). Impairment of hormone action can occur at any of these stages, by alteration in the number and affinity of the cell-surface receptors, by defects in the generation of the second messenger, or by a deficiency in some other post-receptor event.

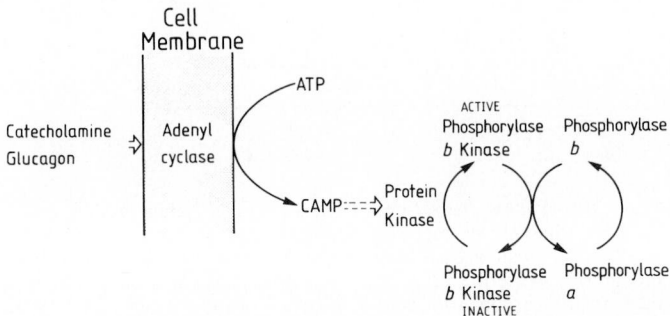

Fig. 7   To demonstrate how a hormone such as adrenaline or glucagon activates a metabolic process in the cell through the adenyl cyclase mechanism and may initiate an enzyme 'cascade'. In this way the eventual metabolic effects of a hormone may be far removed from the initial ones and can be considerably augmented. (Diagram redrawn from Newsholme and Start, 1977).

By such mechanisms hormones regulate the supply and utilization of metabolic fuels both in health and disease. There is no need to describe their individual effects in detail since much is dealt with in Section 10, but the short-term effects of insulin, glucagon, and catecholamines (Table 3) require mention.

All the actions of insulin are anabolic; protein, glycogen, and fat synthesis are stimulated, and lipolysis and gluconeogenesis inhibited. In contrast those of catecholamines and glucagon are catabolic. Glucagon exerts its major effect through the liver, increasing glycogen breakdown, gluconeogenesis, and ketogenesis from fatty acids; it also stimulates lipolysis in adipose tissue but has no important effect on muscle. The catecholamines have similar catabolic effects, with muscle as an additional target tissue.

Cortisol is often included as a 'catabolic' hormone, and it may be that its 'permissive' role has been overstressed. It appears to inhibit glucose uptake by peripheral tissues and to increase proteolysis. However, its effects (which are still debated) are delayed rather than immediate.

Finally it is unwise to deal with the effects of particular hormones in isolation. Just as there are interactions between metabolites there are also hormone–hormone interactions; for instance glucagon appears to stimulate the production of insulin and growth hormone, whereas catecholamines have the opposite effect.

Carbohydrate metabolism. Although the relative importance of the different metabolic fuels may alter in starvation and other conditions, it is accepted that glucose occupies a central role in whole body metabolism. This is because it serves as an optimal fuel for so many tissues and an obligatory fuel for brain (except during prolonged starvation), red blood cells, and the renal medulla.

Glycogen is the storage form of glucose in many tissues, and

Table 3   Summary of the short-term metabolic effects of some hormones

Hormone	Target tissues	Effects	Changes in substrate concentration
Insulin	liver muscle adipose tissue mammary gland	increases glucose transport (not liver) increases glycogen synthesis protein synthesis lipogenesis esterification decreases lipolysis gluconeogenesis	lowers glucose, fatty acids, ketone bodies, and amino acids
Glucagon	liver adipose tissue	increases glycogen breakdown gluconeogenesis alanine transport (liver) lipolysis ketogenesis decreases esterification lipogenesis	increases glucose, fatty acids, and ketone bodies
Catecholamines	liver muscle adipose tissue	increases glycogen breakdown gluconeogenesis glycolysis lipolysis ketogenesis decreases esterification lipogenesis	increases glucose, fatty acids, ketone bodies, and lactate

glucose can be liberated from the liver by the action of glucose 6-phosphatase, which is absent in muscle. After an overnight fast about 25 per cent of the 180 g of glucose required daily by a 70 kg man is produced from glycogen. The remainder is formed from lactate and pyruvate, alanine (the main gluconeogenic amino acid), and glycerol (from fat). In post-absorptive man the formation of glucose from lactate represents one part of the Cori cycle (see Fig. 3). Glucose from the liver is converted to pyruvate and lactate in muscle and any which is not oxidized re-enters the liver to form glucose. Alanine is the other major precursor of glucose and its release from the muscle is an important part of the glucose–alanine cycle (see Fig. 9). Finally glycerol released during lipolysis contributes a minor proportion of the circulating glucose.

In the fed state the concentration of glucose remains very constant. This implies that ingested glucose is very rapidly disposed of. The main organ for its disposal is the liver, where glucose is rapidly converted to glycogen and fatty acids (for triglyceride secretion). The details of glucose metabolism are discussed in the section on diabetes (see Section 9).

Protein metabolism. The subject is a very large one. Particularly relevant are a knowledge of turnover rate, of the metabolism of different amino acids, and of the glucose–alanine cycle.

Protein turnover. Body protein is being continuously broken down and resynthesized. The rate at which this occurs will of course differ widely from one patient to another, and a significant contribution to this turnover is provided by skeletal muscle. Isotope measurements suggest that the whole body protein breakdown rate (equivalent to the protein synthetic rate) in a young adult is between 3.0 and 3.5 g/kg per day. Measurements of 3-methylhistidine (see below) also suggest that the myofibrillar breakdown rate is about 25 per cent of this. Striated muscle contains sarcoplasmic and myofibrillar protein in approximately equal amounts, and the rate of muscle protein turnover derived from measurements of 3-methylhistidine refers only to that of myofibrillar protein. Even if we disregard the sarcoplasmic contribution to protein turnover, it is important to realize that the measurements imply a daily breakdown of at least 250 g of muscle tissue, since muscle protein is associated with three times its weight of water; if this is not restored by equivalent synthesis, as may occur after operation, the rapid loss of muscle bulk at such a time is readily explained.

Urine nitrogen and 3-methylhistidine. The amino groups derived from the metabolism of amino acids in the liver are excreted largely as urea but a significant proportion is also excreted as ammonium ions (Fig. 8). The total amount of nitrogen excreted in the urine represents the balance between protein breakdown and synthesis and reflects the reincorporation of amino acids, liberated into the amino acid pool, into newly formed protein. However, not all amino acids can be re-utilized for synthesis and these include amino acids which have been modified after their incorporation into the peptide chain (i.e. post-translationally modified amino acids). 3-Methylhistidine and hydroxyproline provide examples of these; hydroxyproline excretion gives an indication of collagen breakdown rate and 3-methylhistidine that of myofibrillar protein. Both actin and myosin contain 3-methylhistidine derived from post-translational methylation of some histidine residues. In contrast the sarcoplasmic proteins, which comprise about 50 per cent of the striated muscle, do not contain 3-methylhistidine. 3-Methylhistidine is quantitatively excreted in the urine and under certain circumstances its rate of excretion can provide an indicator of endogenous muscle protein breakdown, provided that dietary protein is reduced. Since creatinine excretion is an approximate biochemical indicator of muscle mass the ratio of 3-methylhistidine excretion to that of creatinine can be used to indicate the fractional catabolic rate of skeletal muscle. Measurements have been made in starvation, injury, and various clinical states.

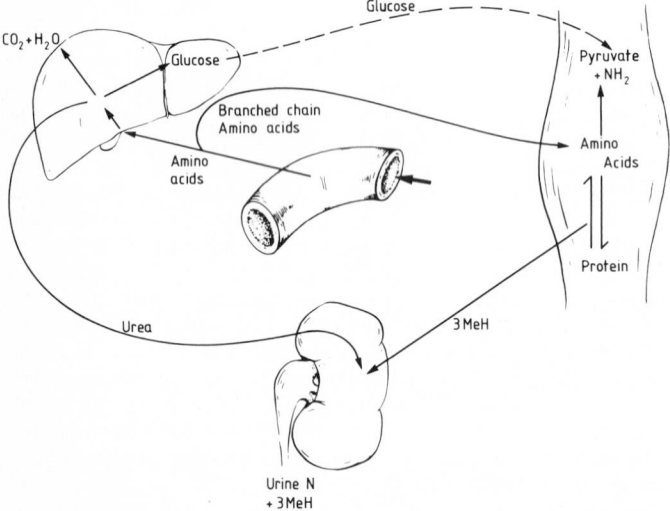

Fig. 8   A diagram to distinguish the differing metabolic pathways of amino acids and the origin of 3-methylhistidine (3MeH). The glucose–alanine cycle is dealt with in Fig. 9.

The branched chain amino acids. These are leucine, isoleucine, and valine: both their initial and subsequent metabolism is different from those without branched chains (Fig. 8). Thus when they are ingested they largely bypass the liver and are initially metabolized in muscle. This localization in muscle is presumed to have functional significance, and it has been suggested that leucine in particular can stimulate the synthesis of protein. The way in which it does this is not known, but forms the basis for the attempted therapeutic use of these particular amino acids in nitrogen-losing states.

The glucose–alanine cycle. One pathway that is of particular importance in the exchange of energy is the so-called 'glucose–alanine' cycle (Fig. 9) whereby glucose from the liver is supplied to the peripheral tissues such as muscle and alanine is supplied to the liver for deamination. In this way amino groups derived from various

amino acids by transamination are transported to the liver in the form of alanine and subsequently disposed of as urea; and the carbon skeletons are used as a source of glucose. Since the proportion of alanine in the amino acids released from muscle is considerably more than that in the amino acids of muscle, it is clear that the released alanine is not entirely derived from muscle protein breakdown. The other major precursors of alanine appear to be glutamate and the branched chain amino acids. The quantitative importance of this cycle in different conditions and the relative contributions to alanine from different sources remain controversial.

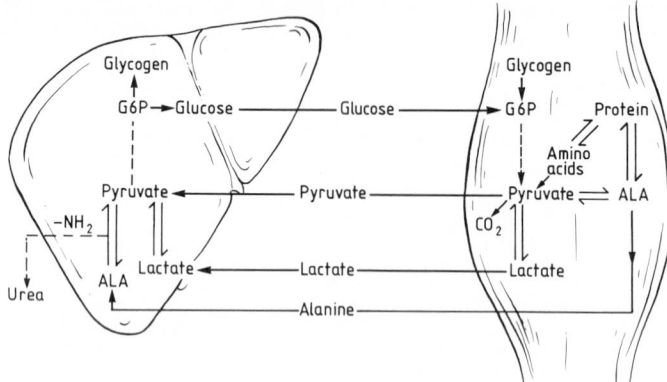

Fig. 9   The glucose–alanine cycle. The sources of alanine within muscle differ according to the state of nutrition. In post-absorptive man alanine (ALA) comes mainly from the transamination of pyruvate derived from glucose. In short-term starvation, alanine is also derived from proteolysis, and pyruvate carbon from partial oxidation of other amino acids. With prolonged starvation less alanine comes from glucose-derived pyruvate and proteolysis is reduced.

Fat metabolism

Lipolysis. In the adipose tissue cell (the adipocyte) stored triglyceride is continually broken down to glycerol and non-esterified fatty acids by the action of a hormone sensitive lipase; the glycerol is eventually used for gluconeogenesis in the liver, and fatty acid may be re-esterified by glycerol-3-phosphate derived from glucose. In the fed state metabolism is directed towards fat storage. During food deprivation or insulin deficiency non-esterified fatty acids are released into the circulation, where they may be used directly as fuel, or converted in the liver to ketone bodies. Most tissues, apart from red cells and nervous tissue, are capable of using non-esterified fatty acids and some, such as resting muscle, prefer them to glucose.

Ketogenesis. There is increasing evidence of the importance of the ketone bodies, acetoacetate and 3-hydroxybutyrate, as tissue fuels, and there are a number of conditions in which their concentration is increased. The control of their production depends on two main steps; the hydrolysis of adipose tissue fat by a hormone-sensitive lipase into glycerol and fatty acids; and the metabolism of the long chain fatty acids into ketone bodies. The former system appears to be largely under the control of insulin, lack of which increases lipolysis. The latter occurs within the liver and is more complex (Fig. 10). Fatty acids entering the liver may either be re-esterified into triglycerides or oxidized. If the rate of fatty acid oxidation is high, there is an increase in the production of ketone bodies; this does not passively follow an increase in the supply of fatty acids but is critically dependent on the activation of the carnitine acyl transferase reaction, itself influenced by the amount of carnitine present, which provides a mechansim to transport long chain fatty acids into the mitochondria. This process appears to be stimulated by an excess of glucagon relative to that of insulin.

The utilization of ketone bodies as a tissue fuel is particularly important in starvation (see below), where the circulating concentration increases to between 2 and 5 mmol/l, since in this way the

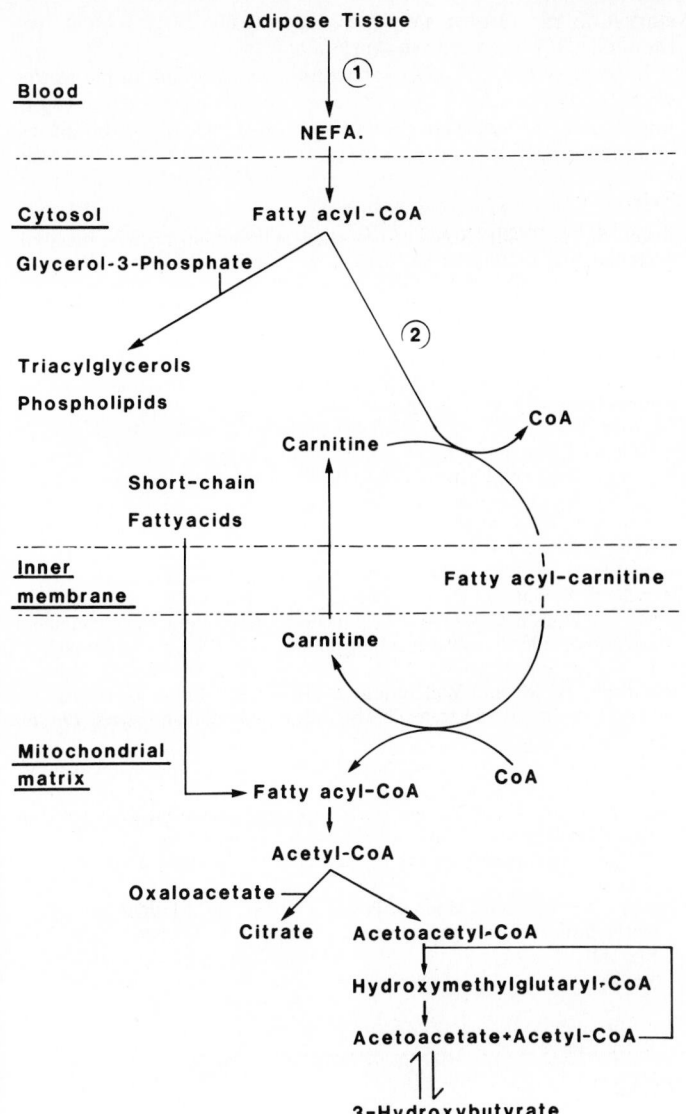

Fig. 10 To show the pathway of fatty acid metabolism in the liver (from Williamson 1979). Step ①, lipolysis, is particularly stimulated by insulin deficiency (absolute or relative to glucagon), and by an increase in catecholamines: Step ② by glucagon excess in relation to insulin. These hormones may also have their effects by modulation of the malonyl-CoA concentration (see text and Fig. 11).

breakdown of protein for gluconeogenesis is minimized. So far as the brain and central nervous system (which are normally the main consumers of glucose) are concerned, the degree to which ketone bodies are utilized probably depends more on their circulating concentration than on any form of adaptation to starvation, since these tissues already appear to have the necessary enzymes for their metabolism.

Glucose–lipid interactions. The relationships between the utilization of glucose, hepatic carbohydrate status and lipid metabolism are of considerable nutritional importance. Figure 6 demonstrates one way in which increased availability of ketone bodies may reduce the utilization of glucose. Figure 11 illustrates another link between carbohydrate and lipid metabolism. In order to enter the mitochondrion for subsequent metabolism fatty acyl CoA must be converted to the carnitine derivative via the enzyme carnitine acyl transferase I (CAT I) located on the outer surface of its inner membrane.

On the inner surface carnitine acyl transferase II(CAT II) then reforms fatty acyl-CoA from the fatty acyl carnitine with liberation

of carnitine. It has long been known that the hepatic carbohydrate state, i.e. glycogen content and predominance of glycolysis or gluconeogenesis, has a major influence on the rate of ketogenesis. For instance if ample hepatic glycogen is available there is no need to produce large amounts of ketone bodies, even if the flux of NEFA to the liver increases. What has not been clear is the nature of the regulatory signal which links hepatic carbohydrate status and the rate of ketogenesis. It has now been shown that malonyl CoA, an intermediate in the pathway of lipogenesis, itself inhibits CAT I. Glucose derived from glycogen is a major source of carbon for lipogenesis in the liver, and the concentration of malonyl-CoA is directly related to this rate of lipogenesis. Thus an increase in malonyl-CoA will inhibit the further metabolism of fatty acyl-CoA by CAT I and encourage its esterification thus reducing the formation of ketone bodies. This explains the reciprocal relationship between lipogenesis and ketogenesis, (Fig. 11). The hormonal regulation of ketogenesis may also involve this system, since current evidence suggests that insulin and glucagon alter the rate of ketogenesis in liver cells by modulation of malonyl-CoA concentration. Recently it has also been shown that vasopressin has important antiketogenic effects, which may be relevant in the body's biochemical response to stress.

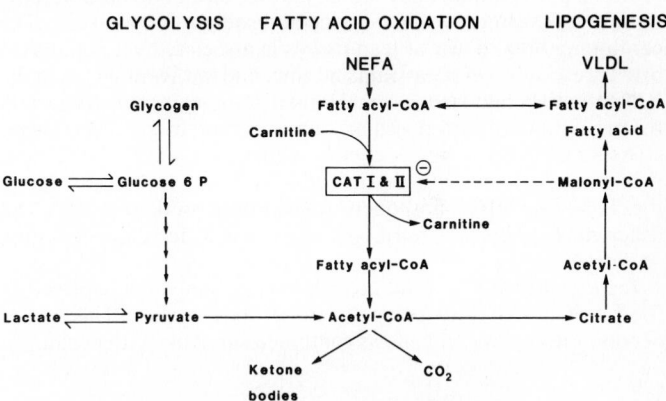

Fig. 11 A scheme of the regulatory links between hepatic carbohydrate status, lipogenesis and ketogenesis. ⊖ indicates site of inhibition; CAT I and II indicate carnitine acyl transferase I and II respectively. For explanation see text.

The biochemical effects of starvation. Experimental study of short- and long-term fasting, usually in obese subjects, has shed considerable light on normal metabolic processes and on the way in which the body can adapt to food deprivation. The results obtained from brief fasts have been incorporated in the previous account; in effect they deal with the post-absorptive phase where the small carbohydrate stores, particularly glycogen, have been utilized and energy is provided from protein and fat alone. If the pathways demonstrated during brief fasting persisted during prolonged food deprivation, the loss of protein to provide glucose would be very rapid indeed. However, as we have mentioned, the brain can substitute a fat-derived product, namely ketone bodies, for glucose, and with prolonged starvation this progressively occurs. The reduction of protein breakdown is reflected in a fall in urinary nitrogen. As the brain increasingly uses ketone bodies and the liver reduces gluconeogenesis, the kidney produces increased amounts of glucose. This last alteration appears to make the kidney the chief gluconeogenetic tissue in prolonged starvation; the glucose is made from deaminated amino acids (mainly glutamine), whilst the amino groups provide ammonia required to neutralize the keto-acids lost in the urine.

The progressive reduction in gluconeogenesis and protein breakdown does not result from the accompanying fall in insulin levels which would, in contrast, increase gluconeogenesis. It seems likely that proteolysis is reduced by the hyperketonaemia of starvation in two independent ways; first the increasing utilization of ketone bodies, as an alternative fuel to glucose, decreases the requirement of the brain for glucose (derived from protein); and second the direct effect of ketone bodies reduces glucose utilization and alanine release from muscle. This effect can be demonstrated in starving man where the infusion of ketone bodies further reduces the already low nitrogen excretion.

In starvation there are only minor changes in the excretion of 3-methylhistidine and hydroxyproline. At the beginning of food deprivation urine 3-methylhistidine falls to a constant low level as the effect of exogenous protein declines, but the subsequent changes are small. The reported changes in urinary hydroxyproline are variable, but they do suggest that prolonged food deprivation leads to an increase in collagen breakdown rate. How much this breakdown reflects the use of collagen as a protein source for gluconeogenesis, and how much comes from the skeleton as the result of immobility (especially after surgery, see below) is impossible to say. It does not appear to be due to the effect of acidosis on the skeleton, since it is not affected by the administration of alkali. The combined effects of loss of protein and fat produce considerable changes in body composition, with a reduction of lean body mass in relation to body water. In initial starvation the rapid weight loss is largely due to loss of sodium and water; however, with prolonged starvation body water and extracellular fluid volume decline less than that of lean tissue and sodium is conserved. The continuing breakdown of lean tissues is associated with increased urinary excretion of potassium and zinc, and the eventual fall in the K/N ratio to below 3 (the normal ratio in muscle) is compatible with the breakdown of non-muscular sources of protein such as collagen.

As starvation continues energy requirements also fall. This is partly due to decreasing physical activity; but there is also a fall in the T_3 levels with a subsequent reduction in metabolic rate. The other most important hormonal change is a decrease in insulin secretion.

In summary the fat (and the normal) person when deprived of food switches over to being a ketone body burner. This spares protein breakdown and allows continued survival. With prolonged starvation the rate of weight loss decreases, fluid is selectively retained, and the metabolic rate falls.

In practice the effects of starvation are rarely as simple as this, since food deprivation usually occurs against a background of injury or infection, or as part of a complex picture of protein energy malnutrition.

References

Adibi, S. A. (1980). Roles of branched-chain amino acids in metabolic regulations. *J. lab. clin. Med.* **95**, 475.
Cahill, G. F. (1976). Starvation in man. *Clins Endocr. Metab.* **5**, 397.
Dickerson, J. W. T. and Lee, H. A. (1978). *Nutrition in the clinical management of disease.* Arnold, London.
Elia, M., Carter, A., Bacon, S., Winearls, C. G., and Smith, R. (1981). Clinical usefulness of 3-methylhistidine in indicating muscle protein breakdown. *Br. med. J.* **282**, 351.
Garrow, J. S. (1978). *Energy balance and obesity in man.* Elsevier/North Holland Biochemical Press, Amsterdam.
McGarry, J. D. and Foster, D. W. (1977). Hormonal control of ketogenesis. *Archs intern. Med.* **137**, 495.
Newsholme, E. A. (1980). A possible mechanism for the control of body weight. *New Engl. J. Med.* **302**, 400.
— and Start, C. (1977). *Regulation in metabolism.* Wiley, London.
Randle, P. J., Garland, P. B., Hales, C. N., Newsholme, E. A., Denton, R. M., and Pogson, C. I. (1966). Protein hormones. Interactions of metabolism and the physiological role of insulin. *Recent Prog. Hormone Res.* **22**, 1.
Robinson, A. M. and Williamson, D. H. (1980). Physiological roles of ketone bodies as substrates and signals in mammalian tissues. *Physiol. Rev.* **60**, 143.
Snell, K. (1980). Muscle alanine synthesis and hepatic gluconeogenesis. *Biochem. Soc. Trans.* **8**, 205.
Williamson, D. H. (1979). Recent developments in ketone body metabolism. *Biochem. Soc. Trans.* **7**, 1313.
— (1981). Mechanisms for the regulation of ketogenesis. *Proc. Nutrition Soc.* **40**, 93.
Young, V. R. and Munro, H. N. (1978). N^T-Methylhistidine (3-methylhistidine) and muscle protein turnover: an overview. *Fed. Proc.* **37**, 2291.

Undernutrition

PROTEIN ENERGY MALNUTRITION

A. A. Jackson and M. H. N. Golden

The term protein energy malnutrition (PEM) covers a wide spectrum of clinical conditions in both adults and children. It encompasses the syndromes known as kwashiorkor, nutritional or famine oedema and marasmus, cachexia, and phthisis. The large number of terms that have been used often reflect differences in a single clinical feature. Notwithstanding the differences, most of the physiological, biochemical, and body compositional features are common, and the principles of classification, investigation, and treatment are the same for both adults and children.

Apart from famine conditions, the development of PEM in adults is usually secondary to a specific illness (Table 1). This illness may be physical or psychiatric, e.g. anorexia nervosa (see page 8.51), and in the elderly includes conditions such as slight dementia, grief, physical frailty, or social isolation. In temperate countries children with PEM are often labelled 'failure to thrive' which carries the connotation of an underlying primary disorder. PEM, however, is usually associated with developing countries, where it is estimated that over 100 000 000 children under five years of age are affected.

Natural history. In demographic terms childhood PEM is the product of an environment which is characterized by material, social, and cultural poverty. In this respect PEM can be seen as a common expression of illiteracy, inadequate sanitation, poor personal hygiene, insufficient access to medical services, poor earning capacity, poor crop management and agricultural practices, overpopulation, and inefficient or inappropriate use of resources. These factors act at a national, regional, and village level, as well as at the level of the individual family. The developing world is in a position of technological and economic dependency, lacking the infrastructure of adequate medical, educational, and managerial skills that are needed to effect a change in the country's condition. A similar situation prevailed in the industrialized nations until the recent past, and was associated with high prevalence rates for malnutrition. PEM has always accompanied social upheaval, oppression, and war wherever they have occurred.

Table 1 Common causes for the reduced dietary intake leading to PEM

1 Infection
2 Imbalanced diet, or a specific nutrient deficiency
3 Psychological problems
4 Starvation and famine
5 Malabsorption syndromes and diseases leading to loss of nutrient
6 Metabolic disease including specific renal, hepatic, or cardiac disease, and inborn errors of metabolism
7 Malignancy

In clinical terms identification of how poverty and disruption affects the individual is required. Normal growth and development is a continuous ordered process with consecutive and predictable changes in body composition, physiological maturation, and mental development. Any insult may cause a cessation or stuttering of this process, necessitating an acceleration following the insult, to make up the deficit. A faltering in growth can be caused by increased frequency or severity of insults, or by a failure to catch up between insults, or by a combination of both these causes. In childhood intercurrent infections form the commonest insults.

All children suffer from infections from time to time. In advantaged societies infections are infrequent because of improved sanitation, lack of overcrowding, vaccination, and eradication of many serious diseases. Infections are treated quickly and adequately. The child receives a varied, balanced and wholesome diet. The child from a disadvantaged society contracts infections frequently. The infections are inadequately treated, tending to become more severe and long lasting. Even when the child recovers from the infection, the monotonous diet is inadequate in quantity and quality, so that he fails to catch up. The more the child falls behind, the more vulnerable he becomes, so that the episodes of infection become more frequent and severe. His opportunities for catch-up growth become fewer and of shorter duration. Trauma or psychological stress can take the place of infection in this cycle of insult/malnutrition that leads to PEM.

The clearest picture of the natural history of PEM in a poor rural community has been provided through a detailed longitudinal study, from conception to puberty, by workers in Guatemala. Many studies from different parts of the world provide corroborative evidence that the overall pattern is similar wherever PEM is widespread.

Pregnancy. The adult height of mothers is short, a result of their own malnutrition during growth. Therefore, they are liable to give birth to relatively small infants. In addition, during pregnancy the mother has a poor dietary intake, usually has hard manual work to perform, and a large family to cater for. She has a low weight gain during pregnancy. The mother has multiple infections whilst pregnant and studies on the levels of IgM and IgA in cord blood show that one-fifth of fetuses have an intra-uterine infection. The mother has little access to medical care and obstetric management is poor. These factors combine to give an increased frequency of low birthweight infants, both pre-term and small for gestational age, with an increased risk of neonatal disease. The insanitary environment determines the flora with which the umbilicus, skin, gut, and respiratory tract are colonized.

Lactation. In all societies infants who are not breast fed, but weaned at a young age, have an increased risk of developing infections, particularly in the intestine and respiratory system. In some very poor communities those infants who are never breast fed invariably die. Human milk contains a number of substances which give protection against infection: lysozyme, leucocytes, lactoferrin, interferon, complement, and secretory IgA. In particular antibodies to specific pathogens in the environment are secreted in the milk. Moreover, human milk has a composition that is generally inhibitory to bacterial growth. In gross composition the biochemical and physiological differences between human and cow's milk are enormous, most components differing by a factor of up to ten. The two milks have evolved to fulfil completely different functions with respect to bacteria: human milk is inhibitory to bacterial growth; cow's milk facilitates the development of a rumen, and readily supports bacterial growth. Feeding human infants with cow's milk predisposes to the overgrowth of bacteria in the small intestine. Substitutes for human milk not only lack its anti-infective properties, but are also all nutritionally inferior in quality, and usually in quantity as well.

Weaning. All weaning foods used in poor communities tend to have a very high level of contamination with faecal organisms. This is a result of the mode of preparation and so applies equally to a locally produced traditional pap as to an expensive commercial product. Commercial products are less satisfactory than traditional weaning foods because the cost of the commercial formulae results in them being given in inadequate quantities. Furthermore, the commercial product is often reconstituted incorrectly. The instructions have to be read by a hardly literate mother who lacks the facilities needed to carry them out.

The infant's ability to resist the pathogens in the weaning food depends upon the adequacy and duration of breast feeding. The infant requires sufficient nourishment and time to develop his own immune resistance. As weaning progresses the passive protection afforded by breast milk is withdrawn and the infant is exposed to the full brunt of the contaminated environment. The usual age of developing PEM varies in different communities and is largely determined by the traditional age of weaning.

The common feature of all causes of PEM, whether in the adult or child, is a reduced dietary intake. The pattern and amount of the actual nutrient intakes in relation to the metabolic demands probably determines the balance of clinical signs in any one patient. Normally food is used for tissue maintenance, to make good physiological losses, for activity, and for growth. In the face of an inadequate intake there is a hierarchy in which these functions can be sacrificed. Initially growth and then activity are curtailed to maintain the integrity of the organism. Further saving is brought about by reductive metabolic adaptations in every tissue and organ of the body.

In the well-fed individual the metabolic capacity greatly exceeds that usually demanded. Energy is used to maintain this excess capacity for metabolic work. It allows the individual to cope easily with rapid changes in metabolic function, activity, or environmental stress: running at 30 km/h, achieving a cardiac output of 20 l/min; or eating 950 kcal (4 MJ) of energy with 70 g protein at one sitting, then fasting for several days, without any untoward effects. In health the digestive, absorptive, and hepatic capacity to deal with the meal are maintained without upsetting the *milieu interieur*. There is considerable physiological redundancy in all organs. This is why unphysiological stress tests have to be used to diagnose the disordered function of an organ, measuring the maximum capacity before determining if there is impairment of function. The reserves of tissue and of functional capacity are energetically very expensive to synthesize, replace, and maintain. This is the basis for the reduction in functional capacity of all the organs in PEM. However, the cost of this reduction is that the patient with PEM can no longer respond as appropriately to metabolic or environmental stresses as a healthy individual. As the adaptation becomes more and more complete, there is a loss of homeostasis and the patient becomes extremely sensitive to any perturbation.

Clinical features. The classical childhood syndrome of kwashiorkor (from a Ghanaian word meaning the disease suffered by a child displaced from the breast) was described by Williams in 1933. A child of 18–24 months is weaned abruptly and develops a desquamating skin rash, oedema, fine friable discoloured hair, and hepatomegaly. Psychologically he is apathetic when undisturbed and irritable when disturbed. The marasmic child is classically younger, with normal skin, short, wasted with an anxious 'old man' expression. All gradations between these extremes have been described and occur at all ages. Each clinical sign must have a metabolic basis: the inconsistency with which signs appear between individuals, and the changing pattern from country to country suggests that each sign probably has a different metabolic basis, although they are often associated to form the recognized syndromes.

Linear growth failure. Skeletal growth failure is usually present to some degree, but varies from mild to very severe, and is assessed by measuring the height/length. Severe linear growth failure is usually the result of chronic PEM, often starting in the first six months of life.

Anorexia. Loss of appetite is a common feature of all forms of severe PEM and can be caused by any of the conditions listed in

Table 1. In the child infections, especially diarrhoea, and specific nutrient deficiencies are the most common causes.

Oedema. Pitting oedema is an indispensable condition for the diagnosis of kwashiorkor. The extent of sodium and water retention in the extracellular fluid is variable. It is commonly 10–30 per cent of body weight but may reach 50 per cent in very severe cases. The oedema is usually both dependent and periorbital. Small accumulations of fluid may be found at post mortem in the peritoneal, pleural, or pericardial spaces. In severe cases the entire body and internal organs may be oedematous.

The retained sodium and water is not evenly distributed throughout the compartments of the extracellular fluid. Thus depletion of the intravascular volume can coexist with enormous expansion of the interstitial fluid space. This is because the patients have difficulty controlling the distribution of fluid across membranes. The maldistribution gives rise to the paradoxical statement that an oedematous child is dehydrated.

Cheeks. Fullness of the cheeks is commonly associated with oedematous malnutrition but may occur in marasmics or in malnourished adults. The cause is unknown. It is not due to parotid enlargement.

Skin changes. The dermatosis progresses from hyperpigmentation to peeling and cracking of the superficial skin to hypopigmentation, where the skin is extremely thin and eventually ulcerates. These changes are most marked in areas subject to trauma and maceration, the perineum, flexures, and behind the ear. The ulcerated skin is notable for the absence of a local inflammatory response.

Hair and nails. There is atrophy of the hair roots of the scalp. The hair may be plucked out easily and painlessly and in severe cases the patient may be bald. The hair itself becomes thin and straight. The colour changes to red, brown, grey, or blond. If there are successive periods of PEM interspersed with periods of normal growth, the hair may become banded, giving a flag sign. The morphological changes of the hair are so constant that they have been used to identify and classify patients with PEM.

The eyebrows may be lost but the eyelashes grow long. The whole body may become covered with fine lanugo hair. In adults axillary and pubic hair is lost.

The rate of growth of the nails is impaired and they may show colour changes.

Hepatomegaly. In some areas hepatomegaly is frequently encountered. The liver may extend to the iliac brim and is smooth, regular, and often tender. The increase in size is usually due to fat accumulation, mainly as triglyceride. Hepatomegaly may also be associated with endemic infections such as malaria or kala azar. Signs of liver dysfunction, such as petechiae or slight hyperbilirubinaemia, are serious prognostic indicators.

Brain function. Children are apathetic when undisturbed but cry when picked up. Adults become introspective and lethargic with a shuffling gait, downcast eyes, and a dejected demeanour. The higher cerebral functions are most severely affected. A variety of abnormal neurological signs, such as spasticity, hypotonia, hypo- and hyper-reflexia, and abnormal movements have been described. They are relatively uncommon and may be caused by specific limiting nutrient deficiencies or an underlying disease process. The peripheral nervous system is relatively well-preserved.

Specific nutrient deficiencies. In addition to the general signs of PEM, other signs more easily associated with recognized specific nutrient deficiencies may be present. Most commonly these are eye signs with vitamin A deficiency; anaemia, from folic acid, iron, or copper deficiency; and bone disease from vitamin C or D, phosphate, or copper deficiency. These signs have regional differences in prevalence.

Infection. In well-nourished people infection produces hyperaemia, swelling, and an inflammatory cell infiltrate locally, with fever, tachycardia, and malaise. Metabolically, the liver produces acute phase proteins and there is stimulation of the immune system, resulting in an immune response. It is principally this response by the patient that leads to the diagnosis of the presence of infection. Malnutrition dampens or abolishes all the responses to infection. Consequently the malnourished patient has a reduced resistance to infection. A diligent search will reveal an infection in nearly every case.

The thymolymphatic system is atrophied with severe depression of the cell-mediated immune response. Those diseases which the body deals with primarily through the cell-mediated immune system (tuberculosis and measles, for example) are devastating in malnourished populations.

The normal diagnostic criteria for infection are inappropriate for malnourished patients. Pneumonia can be overlooked because radiological shadowing reflects an inflammatory response. Pyuria rarely accompanies a significant urinary tract infection. Septicaemia is not commonly associated with the usual systemic manifestations, rather the malnourished patient has hypothermia, hypoglycaemia, or a severely depressed sensorium.

The relationship between the patient and his normal resident flora is altered, so that organisms which are usually non-pathogenic overgrow body surfaces and invade the tissues. The upper small intestine and stomach become overgrown with bacteria, in particular anaerobes, facultative anaerobes, and often yeasts. Gas produced from fermentation by these organisms gives rises to the distended abdomen, so typical of malnutrition. The overgrowth leads to a functional 'blind loop syndrome' and hence to chronic diarrhoea. It is unusual to find specific pathogens in the stools because the small intestine is overgrown with normal faecal organisms. The chronic diarrhoea, which most malnourished children have, has to be differentiated from episodes of acute diarrhoea which are usually caused by a specific organism and are a short-lived, self-limiting disorder, although they may so deplete the host that they predispose to bacterial overgrowth.

Infection in general, and diarrhoea in particular, lead to an unbalanced loss of nutrients from the body. Even if the patient is receiving a balanced intake, the unbalanced losses can lead to specific deficiencies, particularly of minerals, which in turn lead to loss of appetite and rapid progression of PEM.

Pathophysiology

Body composition. Although there is some wasting of most tissues the loss is not even, so that the composition of the body changes. Fat and muscle are most severely affected. In severely malnourished individuals subcutaneous fat may disappear and the muscle mass may be reduced by half. Cadaver analyses show that muscle wasting is due to loss of soluble and contractile proteins with a relative preservation of collagen protein; histologically there is a decrease in both fibre diameter and fibre number.

Total body water as a proportion of body weight is clearly increased in all oedematous patients. Although it has been stated that marasmic children have an increase in body water, this is not so. However, the total body water in marasmic children increases rapidly once catch-up growth starts.

An increase of total body sodium is invariably present in all forms of PEM, with a loss of total body potassium. In part this loss of potassium is due to a loss of potassium-rich tissue leading to a reduction of the potassium capacity of the body. However, the fall in intracellular potassium and the accumulation of intracellular sodium is principally due to a decrease in the activity of the sodium–potassium pump in the cell membrane. It has been estimated that up to one-third of the basal metabolic rate is consumed by the sodium–potassium pump, and, therefore, by allowing intracellular sodium to rise and relinquishing potassium, the body can save a considerable proportion of its energy expenditure. One of the main difficulties in treatment is the correction of this abnormal distribution of the body's major electrolytes.

There are nearly always total body deficits of other intracellular ions even though plasma concentrations may be maintained. Balance studies have shown avid retention of magnesium, zinc, and phosphorus. Iron and copper are often deficient. There is evidence for depletion of chromium, selenium, manganese, and vanadium. Each mineral has specific metabolic roles which are compromised in the malnourished patient.

Whole body metabolism. *Basal oxygen consumption.* This is decreased whether expressed per unit height, weight, surface area, or lean body mass. In children the basal metabolic rate (BMR) is reduced from 79 kcal/kg/day (332 kJ/kg/day) to 66 kcal/kg/day (280 kJ/kg/day), a reduction of about 15 per cent. A demonstration of the effect of this adaptation is that a diet which contains sufficient energy to maintain the body weight of a malnourished child results in a loss of body weight in the same child after he has recovered.

Protein turnover. The wasting and loss of body protein is the result of a change in the balance of the rate of protein synthesis and the rate of protein degradation. Protein synthesis and breakdown are continually occurring in normal individuals. The intensity of this turnover is about 7 g/kg/day in children and 4 g/kg/day in adults accounting for about one-quarter of the BMR. Measurements in malnourished children show that the turnover is reduced by almost 40 per cent. This represents a considerable saving in energy expenditure. The main changes that occur are in the rate of protein synthesis so that, as the dietary intake is reduced, the rate of synthesis falls below that of breakdown resulting in a negative nitrogen balance and a net loss of protein from the body. It is important to realize that a loss of protein from the body is often due to a deficiency of energy or of the minerals and vitamins needed as building blocks for protoplasm; loss of body protein cannot be equated with dietary deficiency of protein.

Thermoregulation. The malnourished patient becomes poikilothermic with an abnormal response to variations in environmental temperature. In the face of a cold stress there is a reduction in oxygen consumption whereas the normal response is an increased consumption. Thus, even a modest reduction in room temperature may lead to hypothermia (rectal temperature < 35 °C). Hypothermia is frequently seen in severe PEM in the tropics. In temperate climates it is common in malnourished elderly patients. Hypoglycaemia is often found in association with hypothermia. Both these features may be related to low catecholamine output because there seems to be impairment of both gluconeogenesis and the ability for non-shivering thermogenesis in brown fat.

Malnourished patients are also sensitive to mild heat stress. They do not have a normal sweating response and so may develop daytime pyrexia. In malnourished patients heat stress is probably a more frequent cause of pyrexia than an endogenous response to infection.

Organ function. The reduction in the whole body responses is reflected in the capacity of the individual organs. No physiological system has been found to be normal in the malnourished patient.

The kidney has a decreased capacity to concentrate or dilute the urine, or to excrete an acid load.

The heart has a decreased rate and stroke volume. There is prolongation of the circulation time.

The intestine has a thin atrophic wall with a reduction in villous height and mitotic index. There is a marked reduction in the functional capacity of all the digestive enzymes and the transport systems for nutrient absorption.

The extent of hepatic dysfunction is closely related to the overall prognosis. The synthesis of transport proteins such as transferrin and albumin are sensitive to the nutritional state and are reduced before many of the other features of PEM supervene. Fatty liver is probably a result of difficulty in mobilizing triglyceride, possibly due to a limitation in synthesis of the lipoprotein or to a deficiency of carnitine.

There are marked changes in the hormonal balance in PEM. Growth hormone levels are usually elevated in association with low insulin concentrations and a reduced insulin response to a test meal. Somatomedin, catecholamine, and glucagon levels are low. The cortisol concentration tends to be high. Thyroid status is unclear,

but injected radioactive thyroxine is degraded more rapidly than normal. The hormonal changes are difficult to interpret in functional terms as the differences in hormonal profile and metabolic state between individuals provide no clear pattern in terms of our present understanding of the action of these hormones. This is probably partly due to variability in the immediately antecedent diet, and to the variable effects of specific nutrient deficiencies and adaptations of the endocrine organs themselves.

Aetiology. The understanding of the aetiology of malnutrition has been hampered because undue emphasis has been placed on one or other clinical sign. For many years the kwashiorkor syndrome has been described as a disease caused by a dietary deficiency of protein. The basis for this supposedly causal association was not direct and was largely based on theoretical considerations. The hypothesis has become increasingly untenable as knowledge has advanced.

Field studies have failed to show any differences in the protein content or quality of the diets of children who developed kwashiorkor from those that developed marasmus. Virtually all the diets in which protein intake was insufficient have had even greater deficiencies of energy and other nutrients. For example, examination of modern food composition tables shows that if the recommended dietary allowances are correct, it is not possible to have protein deficiency without an even more profound zinc deficiency. Malnourished children and adults can gain or lose oedema in a way that bears no relationship to the ingestion of protein. Furthermore, during treatment of severe kwashiorkor syndrome, oedema may be lost on a diet supplying considerably less protein than the recommended dietary protein allowance, with no change in the plasma albumin concentration. Excessive emphasis on this one feature of a complex disease had blunted appreciation of many other features which have important implications for the management of individual patients as well as for public health programmes. Some features have been identified with specific nutrient deficiencies, thus zinc deficiency has been associated with severe skin lesions and a depressed cell-mediated immune response. The metabolic basis of most of the features is probably complex; the resultant of an inadequate intake, unbalanced losses of nutrients, and infection.

Classification. Any system of classification should have a practical use, either in identifying the individuals who require intervention or to indicate the extent of malnutrition so that preventative measures can be taken. Ideally the system chosen should identify those individuals at most risk of death, should be simple to apply, and should have international acceptance.

Children. During childhood a sensitive indicator of malnutrition is a failure of growth, in that the individual falls behind with time. Of the many systems of classification three have gained general acceptance. Each has its uses and drawbacks.

Gomez. The Gomez classification characterizes the child according to the weight of the child in relation to the weight of a normal child of the same *age*. In this system the 'normal child' used as the reference is the 50th centile of the Boston standard. The grades are shown in Table 2. This system is useful in public health screening. It also defines epidemiologically the extent of PEM in a population, and can thus be used to evaluate the impact of public health programmes. It suffers from limitations. Thus, in areas where

Table 2 Gomez classification

Weight for age (% of reference)	$\dfrac{\text{weight of subject}}{\text{weight of normal child of the same age}} \times 100$
90–110	normal
75–89	grade I mild malnutrition
60–74	grade II moderate malnutrition
less than 60	grade III severe malnutrition

oedematous malnutrition is common, the oedema itself leads to an increase in body weight, so that oedematous children may be misclassified into less severe grades.

Wellcome. In order to overcome this difficulty the Wellcome classification was introduced. This system groups children according to two criteria; one qualitative, the presence or absence of oedema and the other, similar to the Gomez system, the weight deficit of the children for their age. This system is shown in Table 3. Each child is assessed for each feature independently so that four possible diagnoses are obtained. One result of the introduction of this system has been the restriction of the definition of kwashiorkor to patients with nutritional oedema, and the term has now become synonymous with the term 'oedematous malnutrition'. It is no longer generally restricted to the clinical syndrome described by Williams, where the skin and hair changes were of importance in the definition. A weight for age of less than 60 per cent is now used as the definition of marasmus. In reading the literature one has to be clear about the changing use of the terms marasmus and kwashiorkor.

Table 3 Wellcome system of classification

Weight for age	With oedema	Without oedema
60–80%	kwashiorkor	undernutrition
less than 60%	marasmic-kwashiorkor	marasmus

Both the Gomez and the Wellcome classifications, by using the deficit in weight for age, fail to differentiate between long standing failure of growth and an acute loss of weight.

Waterlow. Normal growth is a continuous process of balanced accretion of tissue resulting in a steady increase in both height and weight. Even a relatively mild insult which continues for a period of time will result in slowing or cessation of growth. The child is normally proportioned but as time passes he falls further behind the child who is actively growing, and will eventually fulfil the criteria for severe malnutrition because he is diminutive. Because of the shape of the normal growth curve, the younger the child the more rapidly will he fall behind the normal child. In the older age groups growth has to cease for many months or years if a child is to fall below 60 per cent of the standard weight. A child who is exposed to a more severe insult will not only stop growing in height but will also lose weight. He will become underweight for his age much more rapidly, and when he is malnourished he will not be normally proportioned: his tissues will be wasted. Thus, within the group of children underweight for age (Gomez and Wellcome) these two conditions will represent the extremes of a spectrum: (*a*) stunted but normally proportioned; and (*b*) normal height but wasted. The two separate groups can be differentiated by measuring the weight for height (wasting) and height for age (stunting). These are shown in Table 4.

The wasted child presents an immediate clinical problem where rehabilitation can lead to restoration of the lost tissue. Correction of stunting on the other hand is more likely to depend upon public

Table 4 Waterlow classification

	Stunting (ht/age)	Wasting (wt/ht)
Normal	> 95	> 90
Mild	87.5–95	80–90
Moderate	80–87.5	70–80
Severe	< 80	< 70

$$\text{Weight for height (\%)} = \frac{\text{weight of subject}}{\text{weight of a normal child of the same height}} \times 100$$

$$\text{Height for age (\%)} = \frac{\text{height of subject}}{\text{height of normal child of same age}} \times 100$$

health measures aimed at environmental improvement. This system, together with the presence or absence of oedema, is the most useful for deciding which individuals require intensive treatment.

The Gomez and Wellcome classifications are limited because the age of the child has to be known. The Waterlow system has the advantage that measuring wasting is more or less age independent. However, height (or length) is not an easy measurement to make under field conditions, or in mass screening programmes. For these purposes a simple measurement is required which will identify those individuals who require to be brought to a centre where weight and height can be measured.

Upper arm circumference. Between the ages of 1 and 5 years there is very little change in the normal child's arm circumference. This measurement therefore gives a simple anthropometric measure of wasting which is almost age independent. Table 5 gives an indication of the degree of severity of PEM in children with various upper arm circumferences. Simple tools and standards have been devised to measure arm circumference in the field.

Table 5 Mid upper arm circumference in children aged 1–5 years

Circumference	Level of nutrition
> 14 cm	normal
12.5–14 cm	mild/moderate malnutrition
< 12.5 cm	severe malnutrition

Adults. The assessment of malnutrition in adults is similar to the Waterlow classification for children, and is based upon weight for height usually using the Metropolitan Life Assurance tables of ideal weight for height. Less than 80 per cent of expected weight or the presence of nutritional oedema represents severe malnutrition. Stunting in adults often represents childhood malnutrition.

Diagnostic investigations. A careful history and examination usually provide most of the information required to treat these patients. The laboratory has a relatively minor role to play and is mainly used for the identification and characterization of infection.

Urine should always be cultured if the facilities are available. If there are perineal lesions, urine should be obtained by suprapubic tap. Although pyuria can be looked for, its absence should not alter the diagnosis of urinary tract infection in the presence of significant bacteriuria in a urethral specimen or any growth at all in a suprapubic specimen.

Tuberculosis is common, and its diagnosis presents especial difficulties as the Mantoux test is usually negative irrespective of the presence or absence of active disease. The chest X-ray is particularly important in diagnosing TB. Acid-fast bacillae can sometimes be recovered from gastric washings or from a laryngeal aspirate using a neonatal mucous extractor. Tuberculosis can sometimes be diagnosed by observing a tubercle on the retina. About 50 per cent of cases of miliary TB have retinal tubercles, so that careful examination of the fundus, in the dark, with mydriasis should be carried out if this diagnosis is expected. The blood should be examined for malarial parasites and a fresh specimen of stool for ova, cysts, and specific pathogens.

Haematocrit or haemoglobin may be helpful, although anaemia is usually clinically obvious. Changes in haematocrit often give clues to changes in the distribution of fluid between the interstitial and vascular compartments. This may be of importance during early treatment when, for instance, the causes for increasing hepatomegaly have to be differentiated.

Measuring the concentration of plasma constituents is often unhelpful. Plasma concentrations bear no relationship necessarily to total body content. This is particularly true for intracellular constituents, such as potassium; but applies equally well with respect to sodium. If oedema is present, there is a greatly increased sodium content in the extracellular fluid, and even in marasmus the total body sodium is invariably increased because of an increase in intracellular sodium. However, hyponatraemia is frequently found, and is a severe prognostic sign. Making this measurement can trap the unwary into fatal therapeutic decisions.

Therapy. The hospital treatment of malnutrition is relatively expensive, and has been associated with mortality rates of up to 50 per cent or more. This has led to the suggestion that in the tropics PEM should not be treated in hospital, but is more appropriately managed at home or in some form of nutrition rehabilitation centre. However, these alternative approaches have been no more successful for the severe forms of the disease. We consider that each approach has a role to play, and that the choice as to which is most appropriate should be based upon an adequate understanding of the cause of the disease.

We feel justified in stating that there are two criteria for admission to residential care for active intervention where the child should be under continuous observation and treated by someone skilled in the management of PEM.

1. The presence of anorexia of more than a few days duration for which no immediately obvious cause can be identified.
2. Any child with severe malnutrition who does not respond immediately to outpatient therapy, that is a child with oedematous malnutrition, regardless of weight, or < 75 per cent weight for height and < 60 per cent weight for age, or < 70 per cent weight for height.

This recommendation is based upon the premise that simple food deficiency is seldom the cause of severe malnutrition, except at times of famine. Malnutrition is usually secondary to or accompanied by some other disorder. The mere provision of an abundance of food with instructions to force the child to eat excessive amounts will rarely be successful and is often the cause of death.

The approach to therapy must be holistic. All the various abnormalities have to be attended to in a balanced way; relatively slowly at first so that the child is enabled to correct his own disordered metabolism, and to synthesize the metabolic machinery necessary to utilize the building blocks required for growth. All this has to be done within the child's homeostatic capacity. This principle may be best illustrated with an example. All children with PEM have deficiencies of lactase, sucrase, and maltase when compared with normal individuals. If a *small* amount of isotonic disaccharide is given to a malnourished patient, it will be absorbed at the same rate as in a normal patient. However, as either the absolute amount or the tonicity of the disaccharide is increased, the absorption rate falls further and further behind that of the normal subject. The actual level at which the capacity is exceeded in either amount or tonicity depends upon the severity of the individual case. The same considerations apply to the amount of other nutrients in the diet, the loads presented to the liver for metabolic conversion, the heart for circulation, or to the kidney for excretion. When the effects of infection, specific nutrient deficiencies, small bowel bacterial overgrowth, and gross changes in body composition are superimposed on this lack of homeostasis, it is apparent that the successful treatment of these patients can be extremely complex.

Attention to simple details is much more important than the actual physical surroundings where they are carried out. Sophisticated equipment is not required and so treatment in hospital need not be expensive. It should be possible to achieve the same results in a small village hospital as in a modern teaching hospital.

The residential management of PEM can be divided into five phases: (a) resuscitation; (b) preparation for high energy feeding; (c) rehabilitation; (d) preparation for discharge; and (e) follow up and outpatient support. At each stage attention should be paid both to the physical and mental well-being of the child. Education of the mother and the rest of the family forms an essential part of treatment.

Resuscitation. As we have seen in the first part of this section all the physiological, biochemical, and behavioural measurements

that have been made in malnourished patients are abnormal. To single out a particular abnormality, usually because there is a laboratory that can perform the measurement, and to concentrate on treating that abnormality is fraught with danger. For example in the past, we have attempted to correct abnormal plasma sodium concentrations using standard therapeutic procedures that have been formulated from experience in well-nourished populations, only to find the response of the malnourished patient is opposite to that anticipated. Often there is conflict between the specific treatments for different aspects of the child's condition. Thus, oedema is associated with sodium retention yet diarrhoea is known to be associated with sodium depletion. Which should take precedence in the oedematous child with diarrhoea? The attempts to resolve this therapeutic dilemma by giving conventional treatment to one facet, while ignoring the other face of the illness lead to the death of many of these patients. We are still ignorant of the relative importance of the factors involved in deranged homeostasis. Many of the 'abnormalities' are in fact appropriate adaptations in response to the metabolic state. Hence, rather than attempting to correct the abnormality, it is better to remedy the basis for the adaptation. Reversal of the abnormality will follow. This is particularly true of the abnormal distribution of fluid and electrolytes between body compartments.

The guiding principles of the resuscitation period are (a) to give supportive therapy to allow repair to proceed; (b) to keep within the functional capacity of the patient; and (c) to think in terms of balance of nutrients in the whole child and not in terms of concentrations. These guidelines can be viewed from the various aspects of treatment:

1. Control of infection and overgrowth of bowel flora.
2. Repletion of specific nutrient deficiencies.
3. Control of metabolic state through dietary energy and protein.

Control of infection and overgrowth of bowel flora. Patients with PEM should be presumed to have an infection until proven otherwise. Diligence and care should be exercised to identify the location and nature of the infection. In sick patients in whom a specific infection has not been identified it is reasonable to introduce therapy blindly using powerful broad spectrum antibiotics active against anaerobic, Gram-negative and Gram-positive organisms. The combination of penicillin and gentamicin is particularly effective. When supplies of gentamicin are limited, chloramphenicol and tetracycline are relatively cheap alternatives.

In areas where malaria is prevalent all children should receive antimalarials unless a laboratory can confirm the absence of malarial parasites. Tuberculosis must be sought diligently, and if there is any doubt, tuberculosis should be assumed to be present and active.

A clinical diagnosis of small bowel overgrowth can be made on the basis of gaseous abdominal distension, often obvious on plain X-ray of the abdomen, or the lower parts of the chest X-ray. These patients usually have a history of chronic diarrhoea with offensive or watery stools. Metronidazole has a dramatic effect and should be continued until the patient has reached a stage of recovery where he can resist recolonization of his small intestine. In most situations it is wise to give metronidazole to all children with PEM.

Intestinal parasites are extremely common, and, if facilities are available, stools should be examined for ova and cysts, if not, antihelminthics should be given routinely. Mebendazole (100 mg, twice daily for three days) is currently the best antihelminthic to use. Thiabendazole can be used, but as it often gives rise to nausea and vomiting, routine treatment is better delayed until after the acute phase of the illness is controlled. Piperazine is not adequate for all the common worms. Giardiasis is treated with metronidazole.

Our knowledge of pharmokinetics in PEM is very poor. Drugs like gentamicin which are distributed in the extracellular fluid will have a larger volume of distribution in malnutrition, while others which are fat soluble or which bind to albumin may have a smaller volume of distribution. Intestinal absorption of drugs may be impaired as may the mechanisms of elimination. It is advisable to use standard therapeutic doses, until more information becomes available.

Repletion of specific nutrient deficiencies. In normal clinical practice one is almost entirely dependent upon the identification of clinical signs to recognize the presence of specific nutrient deficiencies. There are nutrient deficiencies in three senses.

1. Loss of tissue leads to a balanced deficiency of all the normal constituents of that tissue. Repletion is accomplished by stimulating regrowth of the whole tissue.

2. Within the tissue unbalanced losses lead to some constituents being much more depleted than others. The normal balance of nutrients has to be redressed before new tissue synthesis can take place.

3. For many micronutrients there is an absolute deficiency relative to the demands of the body, despite the metabolic adaptations that have taken place.

The nutrient which becomes limiting first for the function of a particular tissue, will determine the pattern of deranged function displayed by that tissue.

Minerals (cations). Potassium and magnesium are invariably deficient in all tissues, and this may account for a wide range of the metabolic disturbances. Potassium should be given orally as potassium chloride, between 2 to 4 mmol/kg/day, once the patient has been seen to pass urine. The potassium can only be effectively retained if magnesium deficiency is corrected. Magnesium should be given as a soluble salt (chloride or acetate) 0.5–1.0 mmol/kg/day. Magnesium hydroxide is cheap, but it is relatively insoluble and because of the presence of achlorhydria is unlikely to be efficiently utilized by malnourished patients. Correction of the deficiency of these two minerals may take several weeks.

Zinc deficiency is always present with chronic diarrhoea, skin atrophy or ulceration, or oedema, and is a potent cause of anorexia. Zinc plays an important role in maintaining the cell-mediated immune response and in protein synthesis. Zinc (2 mg/kg/day) should be given as the acetate. Zinc sulphate can be used but is not as efficacious.

Copper tends to be dificient in diets based on cow's milk and so a clinical deficiency is common. This is indicated by osteoporosis, with splaying of the ends of the ribs, associated with a hypochromic anaemia that is unresponsive to iron, and an inappropriately low neutrophil count. Copper (0.2 mg/kg/day) can be given as the acetate, chloride, or sulphate.

Iron deficiency anaemia is frequently present. However, early supplementation is to be discouraged as the levels of iron binding proteins are particularly depressed and easily saturated. Free transferrin exerts bacteriostatic effects which are lost when the molecule is bound with iron. Parenteral iron should never be given to malnourished patients and a severe deficiency is better treated with a blood transfusion. Otherwise, as soon as the resuscitation phase is completed, iron (2–4 mg/kg/day) is given as ferrous sulphate.

Most milk based diets contain adequate calcium but supplementation may be required with diets formulated entirely from local produce.

The situation is unclear for other cations at the present time. There is evidence that chromium, vanadium, and manganese may be important.

Minerals (anions). Phosphate depletion contributes to the limited ability of the kidney to excrete an acid load. Intracellular levels of phosphate are deficient, which is of importance for energy production. The phosphate content of milk is adequate for phosphate repletion.

Selenium deficiency is common, except in areas where the soil contains large amounts of selenium. It is an integral part of the enzyme glutathione peroxidase. Cell membranes are susceptible to peroxide and other oxidant damage in the absence of selenium. A

supplement of 20 µg/day should be given where a deficiency is suspected.

Iodine should be given in areas where endemic goitre is encountered.

Vitamins. Deficiency of nearly all the vitamins has been described. A vitamin mix should be given routinely to all malnourished children. In some instances the quantities of vitamins in commercial supplements are insufficient and additional specific therapy is required. In rice-eating areas additional thiamine should be given parenterally on admission. In most malnourished populations oral folic acid (5 mg/day) should be given. In many countries vitamin A deficiency is very common. The early manifestations are very slight loss of reflectivity of the conjunctiva or cornea and perhaps a conjunctivitis. Bitot's spots are uncommon in young children and the other eye signs are late manifestations of deficiency. Vitamin A, 150 000 units intramuscularly, should be given routinely in affected areas.

Supplementation with the first limiting nutrient may unmask deficiencies in other nutrients. This is particularly likely to happen if more than maintenance energy and protein is given so that the child attempts to synthesize new tissue before the imbalances are corrected.

Control of energy and protein intake. The recommended dietary allowance for energy has a narrow range. The energy required for maintenance varies with age and weight, and in a child between six and 24 months is about 95 kcal/kg/day (400 kJ/kg/day). A relatively small increase or decrease in energy intake leads to marked metabolic changes, and affects the requirements for other nutrients.

A patient remains in a steady state when he takes exactly enough energy to cover his needs. A small increase in energy intake leads to synthesis of new tissue, requiring all the essential building blocks (vitamins, minerals, and amino acids) for building new tissue. In the absence of one essential nutrient protoplasm cannot be made and the extra energy, protein, and minerals have to be disposed of harmlessly. If the excess is large, it may overwhelm the existing metabolic machinery. Fortunately, the child develops anorexia, which functions as a protective mechanism in this respect. Conversely the other nutrients cannot be utilized if the energy intake is insufficient, and weight loss will continue. The adaptive mechanisms will not be reversed, and the functional capacity will not be restored.

The requirement for protein is relatively small at this time and 0.6 g/kg/day of milk protein covers all the needs. On this intake oedema is lost.

In an oedematous child, an estimate of the contribution of oedema fluid to the measured body weight has to be made, otherwise the child will receive an excess intake relative to his metabolic body mass. In an anorectic child a maintenance intake must be given by nasogastric tube. It is very dangerous to force feed a patient in *excess* of his requirements. Strict attention to detail is needed, with accurate recording and precise formulation of the feeds. Anorexia may be the response to excessive feeding, to an unfulfilled need for a specific nutrient, or to an undiagnosed or inadequately treated infection. A cup should always be used for feeding.

Intravenous therapy. The use of intravenous therapy is to be avoided, and is only indicated where there is actual circulatory collapse. The loss of homeostasis makes the child very vulnerable to error, furthermore the risks of septicaemia are increased and the intestine is not stimulated to regrow.

The same fluids can be given cheaply, effectively, and with greater safety with a nasogastric drip. Even the catastrophic watery diarrhoea of cholera can be successfully treated with oral fluids.

Blood transfusion. In particularly ill patients who fail to respond to therapy, a blood transfusion may result in dramatic improvement (Table 6). The blood is given as a non-specific source of nutrients or for the anti-infective proteins and cells it contains, and not as a rule for anaemia. Whenever possible it is advisable to give whole fresh blood rather than packed cells or plasma. A volume of 10 ml/kg usually suffices, but may have to be repeated after a period of time in the most severely ill patients. It should be given slowly to minimize the risk of precipitating low output cardiac failure and special care has to be taken with patients who have received more than a maintenance intake of energy.

Table 6 Indications for a transfusion of fresh whole blood (10 ml/kg) before energy intake exceeds maintenance

1 Severe infection	4 Persistent anorexia
2 Loss of sensorium	5 Unresponsive oedema
3 Liver failure	6 Anaemia

Diarrhoea. The intestine has taken part in the process of reductive adaptation as well as being damaged by bacterial overgrowth. Treatment of the overgrowth will relieve much of the diarrhoea. Parenteral rather than oral feeding leads to rapid atrophy of the intestine (up to 50 per cent of intestinal weight in one week). The concept of 'resting the intestine to allow it to repair itself' is pernicious and only leads to more profound malnutrition. The intestine must be stimulated, within its absorptive capacity, to allow it to recover.

Undue emphasis has been placed upon acquired lactase deficiency as a cause for malnutrition: even though all these children will fail to meet the standards of normal lactase absorption set by severe stress tests, they can absorb lactose if given in small amounts and frequently. Many thousands of children have been successfully treated for severe malnutrition with cow's milk based diets. In PEM all the digestive enzymes are reduced in amount. Any food which is presented in a bolus that is too large or too concentrated will cause diarrhoea, by exceeding the capacity for absorption. When the intestine is stimulated by food, and has its own infections and nutrient deficiencies treated, it is able to synthesize new enzymes and transport proteins. As its capacity for digestion and absorption returns, the quantity and strength of each bolus of food can be increased. The principle is to give *little, often, isotonically*. It may be necessary to start with 4.3 per cent dextrose and 0.18 per cent sodium chloride into which the other mineral supplements have been incorporated during the formulation. The feed intakes are increased until maintenance requirements are being given.

Vomiting. Vomiting is seldom a major problem when small volumes of isosmotic feed are given and bacterial overgrowth treated. Occasionally stale curds in the stomach need to be removed by washing with isotonic clear fluid. Persistent vomiting may be due to regurgitation and rumination. This difficult problem is best managed by loving firmness administered by a single, persistent experienced nurse. If the child is very sick, then a nasojejunal tube or the judicious use of small doses of metoclopramide may be indicated.

Hypothermia and hypoglycaemia. These conditions often occur together and are hallmarks of severe infection. Hourly feeds night and day are often effective, although radiant heat from a lamp may be required. Each child needs a blanket at night. Occasionally unresponsive children require intravenous therapy with 50 per cent dextrose.

Conclusion of resuscitation period. Using this regimen we have found that most metabolic derangements correct themselves within a week. In the sickest patients a longer period is required. This is often due to our failure to recognize a specific nutrient deficiency or infection.

The successfully treated child manifests his improvement with a return of appetite. The disappearance of anorexia and the development of a voracious appetite marks the successful end of the resuscitation phase.

Preparation for high energy feeding. The transition from a maintenance diet to an intake that allows for catch-up growth should be made gradually. If large energy intakes are introduced abruptly,

some children develop a syndrome which frequently results in death. The children who are intolerant to excess energy rapidly develop congestive cardiac failure followed by profuse diarrhoea and circulatory collapse, some time during the first four days of high energy feeding. At post mortem the condition can be recognized by the quantities of straw coloured clear fluid in the intestinal lumen. This condition is similar to the sudden death which may occur on refeeding patients released from concentration camps, and following starvation for morbid obesity. The patients at risk can be identified on admission because the sodium pump of their leucocytes responds *in vitro* to provision of energy with a rapid extrusion of sodium. The exact mechanism of the salt and water shifts is not clear, but the syndrome can be prevented by the gradual introduction of high energy feeds. An increasing pulse and respiratory rate at this time are danger signals which should lead to a reduction in food intake.

Rapid catch-up weight gain
(Rehabilitation). In 1961 Waterlow demonstrated that the rate of weight gain during rehabilitation is directly proportional to the dietary *energy* intake, and not related to the protein intake once sufficient protein is given. Once maintenance energy requirements have been met the extra energy is available for tissue synthesis and deposition. Approximately 5–6 kcal (20–25 kJ) are utilized to lay down one gram of new tissue. The theoretical implication that this has for the time taken for recovery is shown in Table 7. Relatively small increments in energy intake can have a marked effect on the rate of weight gain.

Table 7 Predicted effect of calorie intake on recovery from malnutrition

Example: a 7 kg child who should, according to his height weigh 10 kg
Assumptions: (*a*) maintenance requirements = 100 kcal/kg/day
(*b*) weight gain (g/day) = excess (kcal) / 6

Total intake (kcal/day)*	Excess (kcal/day)*	Weight gain (g/day)	Days to gain 3000 g
700	0	0	∞
760	60	10	300
820	120	20	150
940	240	40	75
1180	480	80	38
1660	960	160	19

* 1 kcal = 4.2 kJ
From Kerr, D., Ashworth, A., Picou, D., Poulter, N., Seakins, A., Spady, D., Wheeler, E. (1973). Accelerated recovery from infant malnutrition with high calorie feeding. In *Endocrine aspects of malnutrition* (ed. L. I. Gardner and P. Amacher). Kroc Foundation Symposia, no. 1

During rehabilitation maximum weight gain is achieved in the shortest possible time by increasing the energy intake. The energy density of the feed is increased by adding a concentrated source of calories to the diet. Oil is particularly effective as it has over twice the energy density of carbohydrate, but does not increase the osmolality of the diet. Milk based examples are given in Table 8. The patient must be fed not less than four hourly throughout the whole 24-hour period. The volume of the feed offered is increased progressively during the early phase of rehabilitation.

When the patient is growing rapidly he should be fed *ad libitum*. The only way to ensure that the patient is fed to appetite is to make certain that something is left uneaten at each feed. At this stage as much as 240–310 kcal/kg/day (1000–1300 kJ/kg/day) may be taken with the patient gaining weight at over 20 times the normal rate.

Supplements of minerals and vitamins must be continued throughout this period. The requirements for these nutrients are much higher in the rapidly growing child than in the child growing at a normal rate. The child must retain all the constituents of lean tissue; they must be provided in the diet. During rapid weight gain any lack in the diet is quickly translated into clinical deficiency.

Table 8 Composition of high energy formulae suitable for use in the rehabilitation of patients with kwashiorkor

Type of milk	Amounts to weigh			
	Milk (g)	Sugar (g)	Oil (g)	Volume of water (cm³)
Dried skim milk	86	67	86	811
Evaporated milk	443	67	52	488
Semilko	98	66	74	812
Pelargon	190	—	55	805
Nespray	118	65	54	813
Lactogen	183	14	43	810
Ostermilk (⅔ cream)	111	70	66	803
Olac	135	42	61	812
Cow and Gate	115	57	66	812
Ostermilk (½ cream)	100	69	73	808
Complan	100	67	71	812
Sustagen	132	23	84	811
Klim	116	67	55	812
Lactogen 'full protein'	163	26	56	805
Cow's milk (fresh)	885	67	56	42

From Picou et al. (1978)

Progress is most easily followed if weights are regularly plotted on a chart. The standard growth chart is unsatisfactory for this as the intense changes that take place over a short period cannot be demonstrated on the compressed axes. We have constructed a weight chart suitable for use in 6 month to 2-year-old children, which is target-seeking. In general the weight gain should be 2–3 kg in a period of less than 10 weeks. The axes are filled in on admission for a particular child. Any child who fails to reach the target requires further investigation. A list of the common causes of failure to gain weight are as follows:
1. Unrecognized infection or infestation.
2. Unrecognized specific nutrient deficiency.
3. Feed incorrectly prepared.
4. Child not offered enough feed.
5. Unrecognized underlying disorder, e.g. congenital heart disease.
6. Psychological causes.

Residential treatment aims to correct oedema and wasting. Once a child has achieved his appropriate weight for height his appetite decreases to an intake that can be met easily on an ordinary diet. Rapid catch-up growth can be achieved on diets that are not milk based, provided the principles of energy density, *ad libitum* feeding, and supplementation are adhered to.

Hospital treatment is usually necessary for resuscitation. It may be advantageous to carry out rehabilitation in a centre where the involvement of the family is increased, and the setting is similar to that in their own home. The family should be encouraged to visit and assist actively in the care of their child.

One of the most serious effects of malnutrition is the delay it causes in mental development. This can be minimized with suitable programmes of educational play and other forms of stimulation. This aspect of treatment, despite its importance, is the one area most neglected in centres managing malnutrition. In order to sustain any benefit gained in the institution it is essential to include the mother and older siblings so as to maintain the level of stimulation once the child returns home. One of the most cogent arguments against hospitalization is the additional psychological trauma for a child who is severed from his family and environment. Every effort should be made to minimize this effect.

Preparation for discharge. It is desirable to do everything possible to prevent a child relapsing with a further episode of PEM after discharge. A number of simple steps may help.

Most malnourished children have only received a fluid diet. It is important to ensure that all children are established on the type of

mixed feeding that is recommended for the region. The transition from formula feed to solid food is more difficult the older the child gets. During the first day or so of the transition period, food is often refused and some weight loss takes place. The mother must be given practice in preparing the feed and giving the food to the child, so that she sees precisely the type, consistency, and way that the child takes the food.

Education of the mother as to feeding the child, what to do in case of intercurrent infection, and how to stimulate the child mentally is an integral part of treatment.

A full course of immunization should be initiated before discharge.

After discharge the patient should be followed up at regular intervals. At each visit the education given to the mother must be reinforced, she must be encouraged and supported, the child should be weighed and measured and the results recorded on a graph. Any faltering in the normal growth pattern is then recognized early and appropriate remedial measures taken.

Prognosis. Using the approach outlined above the mortality from severe PEM can be reduced to less than 1 per cent.

The long-term effect on intellectual and physical functioning is a matter of great concern. In experimental animals a severe nutritional insult at a time when tissues are growing rapidly may result in irreversible damage and limitation of function. The exact timing of the sensitive period varies for each tissue; the severity of the damage depends upon the intensity and period of exposure to the insult. It is difficult to determine the extent to which a single severe nutritional insult exerts a lasting effect in the human. Firstly there is a large reserve of functional capacity in all organs and tissues. Secondly the lifelong experience of malnourished children is of an environment that is deprived and hostile to optimal development.

The human brain is growing rapidly from the last trimester of pregnancy up to the second year of life. This covers the period during which PEM is most prevalent. Clinical studies show that malnutrition during this period is associated with stunted brain growth, in terms of the number of cells and the sophistication of their intercellular connections. Childhood PEM is associated with retarded psychomotor development. Attempts to tease out the different factors contributing to this delay suggests that malnourished children are more seriously handicapped than other children from the same environment. With a programme of increased stimulation children who have been malnourished can catch up or even surpass their unstimulated peers. Children who have recovered from PEM show an increased frequency of behavioural disorders in later childhood, with antisocial traits which increase their alienation and accentuate their learning disabilities.

Long-term follow up of physical growth shows that children tend to remain stunted in height and head circumference. The longer growing period brought about by delayed puberty alleviates this effect somewhat.

The body composition at the end of the resuscitation period is not normal, in that there is increased adiposity and muscle tissue has not been fully repleted. These abnormalities seem to correct themselves after discharge from hospital, and may be related to specific deficiencies in the high energy diet, so that it is not optimal for lean tissue growth. The small bowel histology returns to the normal for the community from which the child comes. There is no evidence that there are any sequelae to the severe fatty liver.

Malnourished children who are subsequently fostered into wealthy homes may become entirely normal physically, and go on to high intellectual achievement. This illustrates that the long term prognosis is closely related to the quality of the environment into which the child is discharged. The reserves that he builds up in hospital may help to carry him over several critical periods of his development.

Preventive programmes. Bitter and very expensive experience has shown that PEM is not caused simply by a deficiency of food or even a particular nutrient in food. Food production and distribution do have a role to play, but must be seen as one factor in a complex situation. Prevention or alleviation of the long term effects of the condition requires a whole series of related environmental and social developments. Clearly there is a close relationship between malnutrition and poverty, but the pure possession of wealth by a nation does not necessarily alleviate PEM. In the last analysis major political decisions have to be made and carried through, concerning the mobilization of a nation's resources. Malnutrition is a preventable disease and appropriate measures can be introduced at a number of levels to minimize its effects.

Surveillance. The principle of surveillance is that PEM is the end result of a process. Identification of individuals at an early stage of this process should lead to the institution of appropriate curative measures at a personal level. To be effective this approach requires that young children are seen and assessed at regular intervals. Invariably those most at risk are the very individuals with whom it is difficult to maintain correct contact. The expense of tracing these people can be minimized if the surveillance is carried out by a member of the community who knows all the families personally. A respected member of the community can be trained with skills to an appropriate level.

It is easiest to follow progress, and pick up faltering early if regular weights are taken, and plotted accurately on a growth chart. A Gomez classification chart is useful in this respect, although there are a number of other types in use. A smooth procedure for referral is required for patients who are identified as faltering. If a system is really effective the community will use it; most systems fail because of administrative ineptitude or medical incompetence to deal with the problems that are set by the surveillance agent, who thereby loses respect in the community.

Supplementation and fortification. Fortification programmes are designed on the premise that the basic diet is deficient in one or more essential nutrients. An appropriate vehicle is identified to ensure that the nutrient reaches the target population in the ordinary diet. Where the premise is in fact true these programmes have been successful, for example fortification of table salt with iodide and margarine with vitamin D have reduced the prevalence of goitre and rickets considerably. These techniques are much less effective in populations of subsistence farmers who may not purchase manufactured food items. Fortification programmes have not had any effect on PEM.

Supplementation involves the provision of additional food items, either free or at low cost, to 'at risk' groups. The effectiveness of these programmes is limited by our inadequate understanding of the aetiology of PEM. Provision of protein supplements has generally been without demonstrable effect. In areas where vitamin A deficiency is prevalent, distribution of supplemental vitamin A has been effective in reducing the prevalence of vitamin A associated eye disease.

Maternal nutrition during pregnancy and lactation. The effects of maternal undernutrition are most marked in groups with low socio-economic status. Calorie supplements during pregnancy have been shown to increase the birth weight of the offspring. During lactation it is much better to supplement the mother's diet to ensure efficient milk production. Supplementation of the infant leads to early weaning.

The families of children with PEM are large. It is an arguable point whether large families cause poverty or whether poverty leads to large families. Nevertheless, multiple pregnancies in rapid succession quickly affects the nutritional state of the mother so that subsequent pregnancies are likely to be of poorer quality. A rational family planning policy and programme is part of any strategy to prevent PEM.

Nutrition rehabilitation centres. Nutrition rehabilitation centres can have a valuable educational effect in teaching mothers appropriate ways to wean and feed young children. The experience with these centres is that they have not been as successful as originally hoped. Part of this failure is due to unrealistic expecta-

tions from the centres and part due to failure to appreciate the nature of the illness itself, with undue emphasis being placed upon the provision of a high protein diet. Children are only likely to benefit if all the underlying disease problems are recognized and adequately treated. In particular the anorectic child is unlikely to benefit from simply being offered more food, regardless of how appetisingly it has been made.

Health centres. Local clinics where minor ailments, infections, cuts, and diarrhoea can be seen and treated have an important role to play in the prevention of malnutrition.

National food and nutrition policies. Many countries, recognizing the important role that adequate nutrition and good health play in national development, have formulated some form of national food and nutrition policy. By their very nature these policies involve many different sectors of the society and therefore it is essential that decisions be taken at the highest level of government, and they need to enjoy the support of the political will and administrative skill, if they are to be successful. Furthermore most policies require considerable cooperation at an international level.

Conclusion. The problems raised by PEM cover the whole spectrum of human experience, from that of the individual to that of society. Childhood PEM is the most common serious illness in the world today. Lessons learnt from the study and management of these children have relevance for malnourished individuals of all ages and for those whose malnutrition is secondary to a wide spectrum of disorders. A clear understanding of the aetiology and pathogenesis of this disorder is a prerequisite for designing effective intervention and prevention at an early age.

References

Alleyne, G. A. O., Hay, R. W., Picou, D. I., and Whitehead, R. G. (1977). *Protein-energy malnutrition.* Arnold, London.

Beaton, G. H. and Bengoa, J. M. (1976). *Nutrition in preventive medicine.* Monograph Series, No. 62. World Health Organization, Geneva.

Gardner, L. I. and Amacher, P. (eds.) (1973). *Endocrine aspects of malnutrition.* Kroc Foundation Symposia, no. 1.

Golden, M. H. N. and Jackson, A. A. (1981). Chronic severe undernutrition. In *Present knowledge in nutrition,* 5th edn. (ed. R. E. Olsen) in press.

Landman, J. P. and Jackson, A. A. (1981). The role of protein deficiency in the aetiology of kwashiorkor. *W. Indian Med. J.* **29**, 229.

Mata, L. J. (1978). *The children of Santa Maria Cauque.* Massachusetts Institute of Technology Press, Cambridge, Mass.

McLaren, D. S. and Burman, D. (1976). *Textbook of paediatric nutrition.* Churchill Livingstone, Edinburgh.

Olsen, R. E. (1975). *Protein-calorie malnutrition.* Academic Press, New York.

Picou, D., Alleyne, G. A. O., Brooke, O., Kerr, D. S., Miller, C., Jackson, A. A., Hill, A., Bogues, J., and Patrick, J. (1978). *Malnutrition and gastroenteritis in children: a manual for hospital treatment and management.* Caribbean Food and Nutrition Institute, Kingston, Jamaica.

United Nations University (1979). *Protein-energy requirements under conditions prevailing in developing countries.* Tokyo.

Waterlow, J. C. (1981). Nutrition of man. *Br. Med. Bull.* **37**.

VITAMINS AND TRACE ELEMENTS

D. S. McLaren

Vitamins

There are three kinds of disorders of vitamin nutrition and metabolism: deficiency, toxicity, and dependency. Deficiency arises from inadequate intake and is common in developing countries. It also occurs secondary to diseases that impair intake, absorption, transport, or cellular metabolism of vitamins. Toxicity results from excessively high or prolonged dosage, especially of fat-soluble vitamins. Dependency arises from apoenzyme defects affecting some of the vitamins and in which the co-enzyme pool is normal.

This section does not consider vitamin D (see Sections 17 and 10), vitamin B$_{12}$ (see Section 19), and folic acid (see Section 19).

Vitamin A

Deficiency (night blindness, xerophthalmia, keratomalacia). Dietary deficiency is usually accompanied by protein energy malnutrition (PEM, see page 8.12) in young children, and is common in parts of South and East Asia, the Middle East, Africa, and Latin America. Secondary deficiency occurs sporadically, accompanying malabsorption and liver disease.

Symptoms and signs. Growth retardation, increased susceptibility to infections and impaired cell-mediated immunity, anaemia, and perifollicular hyperkeratosis are frequent signs, but they are not specifically related to deficiency of vitamin A. Characteristic changes resulting from deficiency affect the eye, the first sign being impaired dark adaptation proceeding to night blindness. This is difficult to detect in the very young but a carefully elicited history from the mother and observation of the child's ability to grasp objects and avoid obstacles in a poorly illuminated room is a useful indication.

With advancing deficiency, dryness or xerosis of the conjunctiva occurs, the exposed parts of the bulbar aspect being most affected. This results from diminished mucin production and keratinization of the epithelial cells. Bitot's spots (Fig. 1) are part of this process. They consist of one or more areas of foamy or cheesy material made up of keratinized exfoliated epithelial cells, and commonly occupy the temporal aspect of the conjunctiva in the inter-palpebral fissure. Only in pre-school age children are they commonly associated with active vitamin A deficiency, while in older children and adults they are usually stigmata of prior deficiency or caused by exposure.

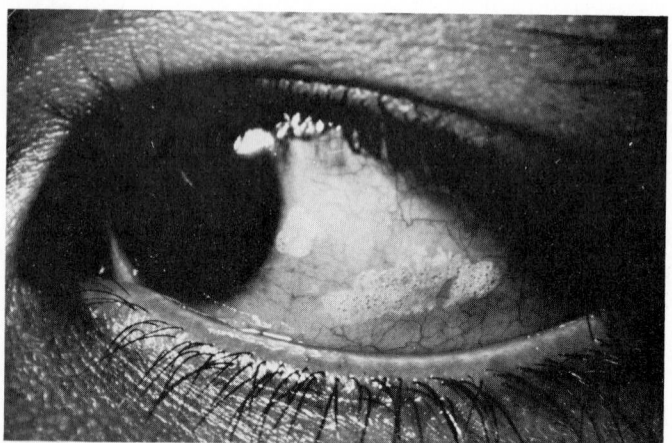

Fig. 1   Bitot's spots, a sign of advancing vitamin A deficiency.

Xerosis of the cornea, preceded by a punctate keratopathy visible only under the slit-lamp, proceeds rapidly to liquefaction and dissolution of part or all of the corneal substance resulting in keratomalacia (Fig. 2). This results inevitably in some degree of impairment of vision. Fortunately the two corneae are often affected to different degrees and some useful vision can sometimes be preserved with prompt treatment (Fig. 3). In advanced deficiency there is complete disorganization of the globe, often accompanied by secondary infection, resulting in panophthalmitis leading to phthisis bulbi or corneal ectasia. It has been estimated that at least 250 000 children go blind annually from corneal xerophthalmia. In these severe cases the mortality is very high, at least 50 per cent.

Diagnosis and laboratory tests. In making a diagnosis other causes of night blindness, e.g. retinitis pigmentosa, must be excluded. Also secondary eye infections may mask deficiency. The response of the patient to vitamin A will aid diagnosis. On testing, plasma retinol will be low (less than 10 μg/100 ml) and plasma retinol-binding protein will usually be less than 30 μg/ml.

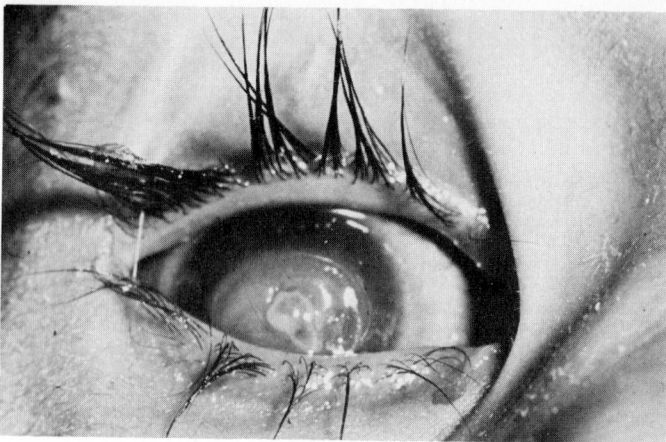

Fig. 2   Keratomalacia resulting from vitamin A deficiency.

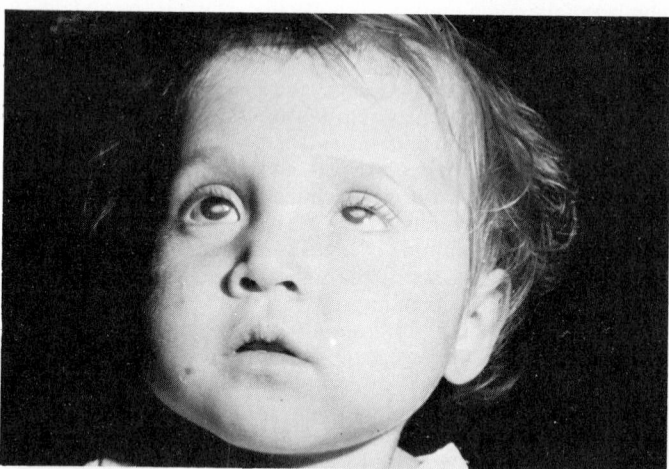

Fig. 3   Some useful vision was preserved in this child suffering from keratomalacia as a result of prompt treatment.

Treatment. The effective treatment is vitamin A palmitate oil capsules, 200 000 units (66 000 μg) immediately, repeated on the second day. If the patient is suffering from severe vomiting or diarrhoea, water-miscible vitamin A (100 000 units) should be given intramuscularly. Oil injection should *not* be used as it is not absorbed from the injection site.

Prophylaxis. Dark green leafy vegetables are a rich and readily available source of carotenoid precursors of vitamin A and should be incorporated into the diet of all young children. In some countries bread, sugar, or monosodium glutamate are fortified with vitamin A, and capsule distribution programmes (200 000 units six-monthly) are also used.

Hypervitaminosis A. Acute toxicity occasionally occurs in children after a large dose of vitamin A, and it has also been reported in Arctic explorers who have consumed large quantities of polar bear or seal liver. Symptoms include headache, drowsiness, vomiting, and peeling of skin. This non-fatal condition subsides rapidly with cessation of intake.

Chronic toxicity in children and adults results from the prolonged intake of large doses of vitamin A. A bizarre syndrome of generalized weakness, headache, dry skin, bone hyperostosis and hepatosplenomegaly results. Fasting plasma retinol exceeds 100 μg/100 ml. Symptoms subside slowly when vitamin A ingestion is stopped.

Hypercarotenosis. This benign condition results from prolonged, excessive intake of carrots and other rich sources or is caused by a defect in carotene metabolism in diabetes mellitus, myxoedema, and anorexia nervosa. The palms, soles, and other areas rich in sebaceous glands are stained yellow-orange, but the sclerae are clear. Plasma carotenoids exceed 250 μg/100 ml.

Thiamin (vitamin B₁). Primary deficiency occurs in those subsisting on a diet of highly polished, non-parboiled rice, resulting in *beriberi*. Deficiency is not uncommon secondary to low intake, poor absorption and impaired liver function in chronic alcoholism. It may also occur in patients given prolonged dextrose infusion without consideration of nutritional requirements (see page 8.45).

Symptoms and signs. The nervous and cardiovascular systems are especially affected. Polyneuropathy (dry beriberi) affects symmetrically mainly the legs and is ushered in by paraesthesiae, calf muscle cramps, and diminution of vibration sense. Continual deficiency leads to loss of tendon reflexes, muscle atrophy, and foot and toe drop. Cerebral beriberi (*Wernicke–Korsakoff syndrome*) manifests as mental confusion, aphonia, ataxia, and nystagmus in the early stage of Korsakoff psychosis, leading on in untreated cases to Wernicke's encephalopathy with total ophthalmoplegia, coma, and death. It has recently been shown that patients with the Wernicke–Korsakoff syndrome have an inborn defect of the thiamin-requiring enzyme transketolase which impairs the binding of thiamin pyrophosphate and predisposes them to develop thiamin deficiency. Rarely there is amblyopia (see Section 21). Cardiovascular beriberi (wet beriberi) consists of biventricular congestive failure and pulmonary congestion with oedema, anasarca, and dyspnoea. Infantile beriberi occurs in infants breast fed by thiamin-deficient mothers, usually between the second and fourth months of life. Cardiac failure, aphonia, and absent deep tendon reflexes are characteristic of this potentially fatal condition.

Diagnosis and laboratory tests. Polyneuropathy from diabetes and other causes has to be distinguished. A response to thiamin is specific to the heart disease of vitamin B₁ deficiency. Elevated blood pyruvate and changes in urinary thiamin excretion are late phenomena. More sensitive is erythrocyte transketolase activity, measured before and after addition of thiamin pyrophosphate (TPP effect). Variations in apoenzyme levels in some diseases may complicate interpretation.

Treatment. In mild polyneuropathy 10–20 mg thiamin hydrochloride is given orally per day. In cardiovascular and cerebral beriberi 50–100 mg subcutaneously or intravenously is usually given daily and continued until response or a strong odour of thiamin occurs. Rarely, fatal anaphylactic reactions have followed intravenous injection.

Riboflavin (vitamin B₂). Dietary deficiency, although widespread, is usually mild and sympatomatology is trivial.

Symptoms and signs. Lesions consist of mucous membrane and cutaneous changes. Angular stomatitis and fissuring of the vermilion surfaces of the lips (cheilosis) are the most common (Fig. 4). Dyssebacea (shark skin) is a heaping up of sebaceous material in the nasolabial folds and ear roots. A dermatosis may affect the scrotum or labia majora. There may rarely be neovascularization of the cornea and some cases of nutritional amblyopia respond to riboflavin.

Diagnosis and laboratory tests. These changes often accompany pellagra (see below) and may be related to deficiency of iron or of other B group vitamins. Urinary riboflavin excretion is low but an earlier change is increased activation of erythrocyte glutathione reductase by riboflavin.

Treatment. Riboflavin 10–30 mg/day orally in divided doses is given until response is evident.

Niacin (nicotinic acid). *Pellagra* usually occurs in populations subsisting on a maize diet of porridge or gruel. The lime treatment used in producing tortillas makes niacin unavailable for absorption. It is also seen secondary to malabsorption in diarrhoeal and liver diseases, and in alcoholism. It may complicate prolonged isoniazid therapy (the drug replaces niacinamide in NAD), phaeochromocytoma (tryptophan is diverted to form 5-hydroxytryptamine), and Hartnup disease (failure in tryptophan absorption).

Symptoms and signs. Pellagra dermatosis is characteristically symmetrical and on the exposed parts of the body. Erythema is followed by chronic hypertrophy and then atrophy. Pressure points may also be affected. Casal's necklace (the skin lesion whose distribution in the neck is limited by clothing) is pathognomonic (Fig. 5). The tongue is usually scarlet and painful, there is generalized gastrointestinal hyperaemia, and ulceration may occur.

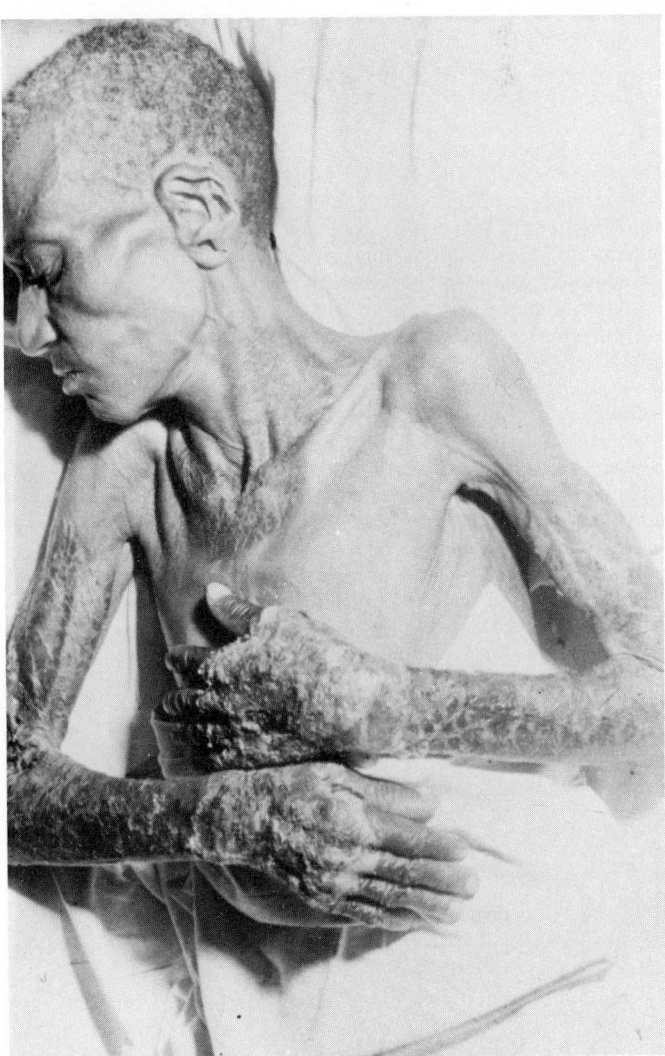

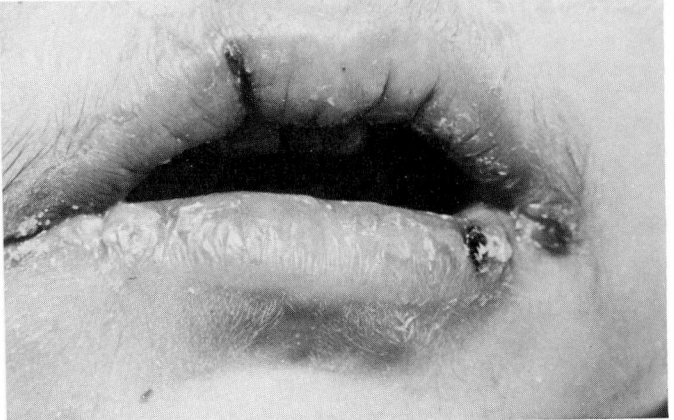

Fig. 4 Angular stomatitis and fissuring of the vermilion surfaces of the lips are the most common signs of riboflavin deficiency.

Fig. 5 Pellagra dermatosis affecting exposed parts of the body.

Diarrhoea and dementia are common and an encephalopathy indistinguishable from Wernicke–Korsakoff syndrome (see above) may rarely be seen.

Diagnosis and laboratory tests. Other causes of dermatosis (the lesions in kwashiorkor are not photosensitive), diarrhoea, and dementia have to be distinguished. There is decreased excretion of N-methylnicotinamide and its pyridones in urine.

Treatment. Deficiencies of other vitamins and protein are commonly present and should be corrected. Nicotinamide 300–500 mg per day orally in divided doses is recommended for severe cases. This may be reduced to 50 mg for maintenance and for milder cases.

Vitamin B₆ (pyridoxine)

Vitamin B₆ deficiency. Dietary deficiency is rare but it may complicate malabsorption and result from drug inactivation (e.g. isoniazid, hydralazine, DL-penicillamine). In some patients with homocystinuria the biochemical lesion can be corrected by pyridoxine (see Sections 9 and 17).

Symptoms and signs. Seborrhoeic dermatosis, glossitis, cheilosis, peripheral neuropathy, and lymphopenia have been produced experimentally. Anaemia, usually normoblastic but occasionally megaloblastic, and convulsions in infants have been reported.

Laboratory tests. The tryptophan load test (2 g) shows increased excretion of xanthurenic acid (greater than 50 mg/day) and other intermediates on the niacin pathway. Plasma pyridoxine falls (less than 25 ng/ml) as does urinary excretion of pyridoxine (less than 20 µg/g creatinine) and 4-pyridoxic acid (less than 0.5 mg/day). Glutamic-oxaloacetic transaminase (GOT) and glutamic-pyruvic transaminase (GPT) determinations on the various blood components are insufficient to detect deficiency.

Treatment. Underlying causes should be treated. Pyridoxine 50–100 mg/day orally results in cure.

Vitamin B₆ dependency

Symptoms and signs. Several recessive or X-linked states have been described, affecting different apoenzymes and producing convulsions, mental deficiency, and cystathioninuria; iron overload anaemia, urticaria and asthma; and xanthurenicaciduria.

Treatment. In the infant the daily requirement (normally 0.4 mg) is increased many times (up to 10 mg) and as much as 200–600 mg daily may be required for the treatment of older children and adults.

Biotin

Deficiency. This is very rare and has only occurred in patients consuming large quantities of raw egg white which contains avidin, an antagonist of biotin. A dermatosis, painful tongue, and cracked lips have responded to 150–300 µg biotin daily.

Dependency. Retarded physical and mental development, alopecia, keratoconjunctivitis, and defects in T-cell and B-cell immunity have been reported in children with deficiencies of biotin-dependent carboxylases. Urinary excretion of various organic acids assists diagnosis and response has been complete to large doses (10 mg) of biotin daily.

Pantothenic acid. As its name suggests, this vitamin is widely distributed in foods and deficiency, well-substantiated in experimental animals, is of doubtful occurrence in man. Claims have been made for its efficiency in relieving the painful condition known as 'burning feet' syndrome seen in prisoners of war and some patients.

Vitamin C (ascorbic acid). Scurvy commonly affects infants fed boiled milk without vitamin supplements and the elderly, especially those living alone (so-called 'bachelor's' or 'workhouse' scurvy).

Symptoms and signs. Infantile scurvy. Supplies of vitamin C are usually adequate at birth and the majority of cases present in the second half of the first year of life. The triad of irritability, tenderness of the legs, and failure to use them (pseudoparalysis) is charac-

teristic. Bleeding manifestations are uncommon at this age and are usually confined to the site of erupting teeth when they do occur.

The infant characteristically lies in the 'pithed frog' position with the legs flexed at the knees and the hips partially flexed and externally rotated. This is due to pain resulting from subperiosteal haemorrhages which can often be palpated at the distal end of the femur and proximal end of the tibia, and can be seen on X-ray. Costochondral beading or scorbutic rosary is usually palpable, can sometimes be seen clinically, and is always evident on X-ray when present (see Section 17). Anaemia is commonly present, usually microcytic and hypochromic in type, but may present megaloblastic features relating to accompanying folic acid deficiency which results from lack of protection of folate co-enzymes due to vitamin C deficiency. There is often fever, leucocytosis, and an accompanying infection, and rickets may occasionally co-exist.

X-ray appearances are characteristic but rather late in appearance, involving first the sites of rapid bone growth: sternal ends of ribs, distal end of femur, proximal end of humerus, both ends of tibia and fibula, and distal ends of radius and ulna. The corner sign appears early and consists of a defect at the corners of the ends of the long bones due to the pulling away of the abnormal scorbutic lattice. Fraenkel's line is an area of radiotranslucency in the metaphysis due to debris of broken down bone trabeculae and connective tissue. Atrophy of trabecular substance and blurring of trabecular markings cause a ground glass appearance of the shafts and the epiphyses show a similar change with the denser unaffected cortical bone giving rise to what is known as pencil outlining.

Pathology of infantile scurvy. Mesenchymal tissues are chiefly affected, with failure of deposition of intercellular substances by fibroblasts, osteoblasts, and odontoblasts. There is widespread rupture of capillaries and haemorrhage. Cessation of osteoid deposition in bone causes the thinning of the cortex, diminution in the size of trabeculae, and haemorrhage under the periosteum.

Adult scurvy. Elderly bachelors and widowers who live alone are especially prone, but food faddists are also at risk. Early symptoms are weakness and aching in bones, joints, and muscles, especially at night. Keratosis of the hair follicles occurs with surrounding haemorrhage. In advanced deficiency ecchymoses are common and haemorrhage may occur deep in muscles, into joints, and under the nails. Gum changes occur in relation to natural teeth or hidden roots and consist of swelling, congestion, and spongy degeneration with bleeding. Secondary infection, gangrene, and loosening of the teeth eventually supervene. In the skin old scars break down and new wounds fail to heal.

Diagnosis and laboratory tests. Rickets in children and various diseases with haemorrhagic manifestations have to be distinguished. On X-ray zones of rarefaction are visible at the sites of most active bone growth. The anaemia is microcytic and hypochromic. Plasma vitamin C is nearly zero in manifest scurvy but the range in healthy subjects is too great to be of value for early diagnosis. Vitamin C of less than 0.1 mg/100 ml in the leucocyte–platelet layer is indicative of deficiency and very little of a large dose will be excreted in the urine in a saturation test.

Treatment. Ascorbic acid 50 mg four times daily should be given for one week in infantile scurvy followed by 50 mg twice daily for one month. The total amount of ascorbic acid may be given as 110–225 ml orange juice or 340–680 ml tomato juice per day and reduced thereafter for prophylaxis. In adult scurvy 250 mg four times daily is recommended until signs have disappeared. Haemorrhage ceases and blood regeneration begins almost immediately. Bone changes take several weeks to disappear and skin pigmentation may linger for months.

Prophylaxis. Artificially fed infants should receive supplements and excessive destruction of vitamin C by prolonged and high temperature cooking should be avoided at all times. There is no convincing evidence for the claims that large doses of vitamin C (4 g or more daily) prevent or decrease severity of the common cold; the evidence for protection against cancer is stronger, but not conclusive.

Vitamin E (tocopherols). Primary deficiency may occur in low birth weight infants and those fed a formula rich in polyunsaturated fatty acids. Children with protein energy malnutrition (PEM) often have low plasma vitamin E levels. Adult subjects show increased fragility of erythrocytes only after many months on a deficient diet. Secondary deficiency may occur in malabsorption, especially with steatorrhoea from any cause and in abeta-lipoproteinaemia due to transport dysfunction.

Symptoms and signs. These are confined to increased erythrocyte fragility and a haemolytic anaemia in infants.

Diagnosis and laboratory tests. Deficiency is considered to be present when plasma tocopherol is less than 0.8 mg/100 ml in the adult. Below 0.5 mg/100 ml erythrocyte fragility in the presence of hydrogen peroxide is increased. On a creatine-free diet excessive creatinuria and increased plasma creatine phosphokinase can be demonstrated.

Treatment. If there is malabsorption, DL-α-tocopheryl acetate 30–100 mg daily should be given intramuscularly. Infants should receive the recommended daily allowance of 0.5 mg/kg (the amount usually obtained from breast milk).

Vitamin K

Vitamin K deficiency. Low birth weight infants may synthesize inadequate amounts of the vitamin K-dependent clotting factors in the liver. Breast-fed infants are susceptible as human milk is a poor source of the vitamin. Non-absorbable sulphonamides or other antimicrobials given by mouth may interfere with intestinal synthesis. Coumarin anticoagulants are antagonistic to vitamin K. Secondary deficiency may result from impaired absorption due to lack of bile salts in patients with external biliary fistulae or obstructive jaundice, and in malabsorption states. Severe liver disease may inhibit prothrombin synthesis, a condition unresponsive to vitamin K.

Symptoms and signs. These are of hypoprothrombinaemia superimposed upon the underlying disease. Haemorrhage may occur almost anywhere but is common from surgical wounds, the gums, nose, or into the gastrointestinal tract. Some intracranial haemorrhages at birth are due to vitamin K deficiency.

Diagnosis and laboratory tests. Many haemorrhagic diseases without hypoprothrombinaemia have to be distinguished by laboratory tests. All vitamin K-dependent coagulation factors are depressed in plasma. Reduction of quantitive prothrombin below 80 per cent of normal requires treatment and reduction to less than 20 per cent is associated with active bleeding, and bleeding and coagulation times are altered at this level.

Treatment. Phytonadione (vitamin K_1) is the preparation of choice and the usual dose is 10 mg intramuscularly. In emergencies 10–50 mg dissolved in 5 per cent dextrose or 0.9 per cent sodium chloride should be given intravenously at a rate not more than 1/mg/minute. This may be repeated in six to eight hours.

Phytonadione 1–2 mg intramuscularly should be given prophylactically to all newborn infants. Alternatively 2–5 mg orally may be given to the mother daily for one week prior to expected confinement or 2–5 mg intramuscularly 6–24 hours before delivery.

Vitamin K toxicity. Menadione and its water-soluble analogues may cause haemolysis in persons with G6PD deficiency and in others when large doses are used. In the newborn large doses have produced anaemia, hyperbilirubinaemia, and kernicterus, especially in low birth weight infants with erythroblastosis. The dose should be limited; 2–5 mg for women in labour, 1–2 mg for newborn babies.

Essential fatty acids.

Essential fatty acids. There is a dietary requirement of about 10 g per day for arachidonic, linolenic, and linoleic acids mostly in the form of the latter. Deficiency has been produced experimentally in infants and has occurred in patients receiving long-term total parenteral nutrition using fat-free solutions (see page 8.48). A dermatosis results and early deficiency may be diagnosed by low plasma levels of linoleic and arachidonic acids and the abnormal presence of 5,8,11-eicosatrienoic acid from lack of inhibition of its synthesis from oleic acid.

A 10 per cent soyabean emulsion contains 56 g/l linoleic acid and is a safe way of administering it intravenously.

Trace elements

By convention these are elements that are present in amounts less than 0.005 per cent of body weight. At present 15 have been accepted as essential for animals: iron (see Section 19), iodine (see Section 10), copper, zinc, cobalt, selenium, chromium, manganese, fluorine, molybdenum, nickel, silicon, tin, vanadium, and arsenic. The last six have not hitherto been shown to be of special significance in man. Preliminary work in the rat suggests that cadmium may also be essential.

Another group of trace elements, notably lead and mercury, are not known to have biological significance apart from their toxicity. Many other elements such as barium, bromine, gold, silver, and rubidium occur in the body in trace amounts and have no known toxic or functional significance.

Copper

Copper deficiency. Breast and cow's milk are low in copper and infants exclusively so fed have occasionally developed hypocupraemia accompanied by hypoproteinaemia, hypoferraemia, and anaemia. The latter respond to iron but copper alone corrects the hypocupraemia. Children with protein energy malnutrition (PEM) rehabilitated with milk diets may develop anaemia, neutropenia, and bone changes which respond rapidly to copper.

Menkes' kinky hair syndrome is a sex-linked abnormality caused by a defect in absorption of copper (see Section 17). Plasma levels of copper and caeruloplasmin are low, leading to progressive cerebral degeneration, retarded growth, abnormally sparse and brittle hair, arterial lesions, and scurvy-like bone changes. Surprisingly, anaemia has not been reported. Copper given intravenously (200 μg/kg/day) in early infancy has resulted in some improvement.

Copper toxicity. Primary toxicity is known only to occur as an industrial hazard but it results from disorders of metabolism.

Wilson's disease (hepatolenticular degeneration) (see Section 9) is an autosomal recessive disease in which there is excessive accumulation of copper in many tissues. Hepatic insufficiency is followed by cirrhosis and liver failure. Accumulation in nerve cells, especially in the putamen and caudate nuclei, the dentate nuclei, and cerebral cortex results in tremors, choreoathetoid movements, rigidity, dysarthria, and eventually dementia. Haemolytic anaemia, renal tubular dysfunction, corneal Kayser–Fleischer rings, and sunflower cataracts are characteristic.

Plasma copper and caeruloplasmin are low but urinary excretion of copper is increased. Heterozygous carriers show these changes to some degree and siblings should be screened and may require treatment. The cause is not known but there is evidence that the binding power of the protein metallothionein in lysosomes, where copper is mainly concentrated, is increased fourfold in Wilson's disease.

Foods high in copper should be avoided. D-penicillamine treatment is indicated for symptomatic or apparently healthy subjects in whom the disease has been diagnosed. A dose of 250 mg daily by mouth is increased weekly to a maintenance dose of 1–2 g daily in divided doses on an empty stomach. After several months the dose may be reduced to 1.5 g per day after clinical and biochemical improvement. Pyridoxine 25–50 mg daily has been recommended and serum iron, platelet, and white counts should be monitored. These measures may be necessary throughout life.

Indian childhood cirrhosis is a rapidly progressive disorder and an important cause of death in the Asian subcontinent. Recent reports have demonstrated prolific deposition of orcein-staining material in hepatocytes and renal tubules, suggesting accumulation of copper-binding protein.

Zinc. A diet in young children rich in milk products, of low zinc content, has been reported to result in retarded growth, poor appetite, and impaired taste (hypogeusia). Zinc content of plasma and hair was low and zinc therapy resulted in catch-up growth and disappearance of symptoms.

A syndrome of dwarfism and hypogonadism, with low zinc status, seen in the Middle East, has been shown to respond to zinc supplementation. Geophagia or chelation of zinc by dietary phytate or fibre may be responsible.

Zinc status is low in many diseases resulting in malabsorption or impaired liver function, and some instances of impaired dark adaptation and night blindness have responded to zinc and not to vitamin A.

Acrodermatitis enteropathica, an inherited, previously fatal disorder has been shown to result from malabsorption of zinc. It is characterized by psoriasiform dermatitis, hair loss, paronychia, growth retardation, and diarrhoea. The frequency of monilial and bacterial infections may be related to a zinc-responsive defect in chemotaxis of neutrophils and monocytes. The precise cause of the malabsorption is uncertain but it has been suggested that it may be due to lack of an oligopeptidase, normally secreted by the enterocyte, thus allowing an oligopeptide presumed to be present in all diets except human milk (for babies thus fed do not develop the disease) to chelate zinc. Zinc sulphate 30–150 mg per day results in complete remission.

Cobalt. The significance of cobalt in human nutrition is confined, as far as is known, to its presence in the cobalamin (vitamin B_{12}) molecule and dietary deficiency is not known. Cobaltous chloride in large doses (20–30 mg/day) has been advocated in the treatment of the chronic renal failure, but should be used cautiously as it is potentially toxic. Overdosing in infants has caused hypothyroidism and congestive heart failure.

Selenium. Low selenium plasma levels and depressed activity of erythrocyte glutathione peroxidase have recently been reported in patients on prolonged total parenteral nutrition (see page 8.48). In one case muscle pain and tenderness responded to selenium therapy. An endemic cardiomyopathy in parts of China, called Keshan disease, has been attributed to selenium deficiency, and protection has been claimed from sodium selenite 0.5 mg/week for children 1–5 years old and 1 mg/week for those six to nine years old.

Livestock may be affected by excessive intake (selenosis) and oral ingestion of selenium salts is highly toxic.

Chromium. Glucose tolerance is usually impaired in protein energy malnutrition and some cases have shown response to trivalent chromium, a cofactor of a glucose tolerance factor (GTF). Brewer's yeast, rich in the cofactor, has been shown to improve glucose tolerance and lower serum cholesterol and triglycerides in some elderly subjects and reduce insulin requirements in some diabetics. Deficiency has been reported in one patient on prolonged total parenteral nutrition. Hexavalent chromium is much more toxic than trivalent chromium and its excessive use in industry necessitates protection of workers.

Manganese. It is a component of several enzyme systems and is

essential for normal bone structure. Human deficiency has not been reported. Poisoning is usually limited to those who mine and refine ore. Prolonged exposure causes neurological symptoms resembling Parkinson's or Wilson's disease.

Fluorine. Predisposition to dental caries occurs in communities where the level of fluorine in drinking water is less than 1 p.p.m. Fluoridation of the water supply to about this level significantly reduces the incidence of dental caries, as does the topical application.

Fluorosis affects most members of communities where the level in drinking water is excessively high (greater than 10 p.p.m.). Permanent teeth are usually affected, with chalky-white patches on the enamel which eventually become infiltrated with yellow or brown pigment, giving rise to the characteristic mottled appearance (Fig. 6). Severe and prolonged fluorosis results in pitting due to weakened enamel and osteosclerosis and exostoses of the spinal vertebrae and may cause genu valgum and genu varum (see Section 17).

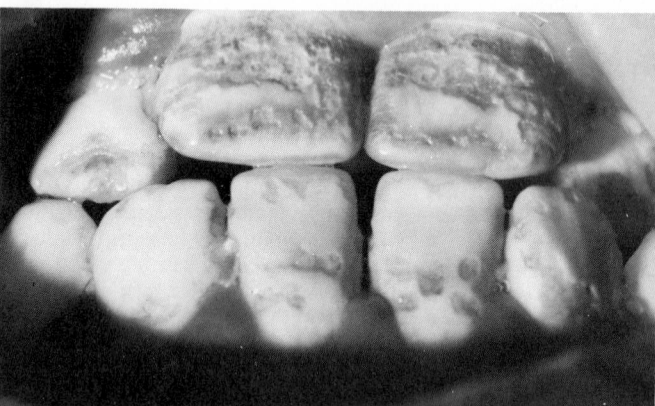

Fig. 6   The characteristic mottled experience of permanent teeth as a result of fluorosis.

Cadmium. Cadmium poisoning is known to be an industrial hazard, and in Japan many cases of severe and often fatal osteomalacia with amino-aciduria resulted from the consumption of rice contaminated by the effluent from a zinc mine.

Cadmium accumulates throughout life, much of it coming from cigarette smoke. The renal concentration may be especially high and has been considered as a factor contributing to hypertension.

Vanadium. Recent work suggests that high dietary intake of vanadium interferes with the sodium pump in susceptible individuals and induces manic-depressive symptoms which are relieved by the vanadium inhibitors vitamin C or EDTA.

References

McLaren, D. S. (1980). *Nutrition and its disorders*, 3rd edn. Churchill Livingstone, Edinburgh.
Underwood, E. J. (1977). *Trace elements in human and animal nutrition*, 4th ed. Academic Press, New York.

Obesity

W. P. T. James

Most of the body's fat is stored in adipose tissue but some is also stored in liver, muscle and other cellular structures, e.g. bone marrow. The 'fat-free' mass refers to the mass of all tissues once the fat content has been subtracted. Fat stored in non-adipose tissue sites as well as the fat component (i.e. the ether soluble fraction) of the adipose tissue itself is excluded so that the fat-free mass includes the water and protein fractions of adipose tissue. The term 'lean body' mass is different and is usually taken to include the weight of all tissues other than adipose tissue. This difference is the source of some confusion but attempts to measure total body fat includes fat in all tissues and does not simply involve measuring the mass of adipose tissue.

Measuring body fat content. A series of methods for estimating the fat content of the body is available, but all are indirect and depend on the physical and compositional differences between fat and lean tissue. Methods which estimate the amount of a fat-soluble gas taken up by the body have proved too difficult for widespread use. Current methods depend on several simple properties of body fat: fat contains no water, no potassium, and has a density of about 0.9 g/cm³. Measurements of total body water, total body potassium, and body density have therefore been used to estimate the fat-free mass. The fat-free mass is taken to have a density of 1.1 g/cm³, a water content of 72 per cent and a potassium content of 66 mmol/kg in men and 60 mmol/kg in women. The calculation of body fat from any of these measurements assumes that the figures for water and potassium content and density are constant in all individuals; the values certainly do not apply to infants nor to the elderly and individual variability in the values must also be recognized. For example, the water content of cadavers varies from 67.4 to 77.5 per cent of the lean tissue so the use of an average figure of 72 per cent in the individual patient can give only an estimate for total body fat.

Body water. The volume of body water is readily found by measuring the dilution of a standard dose of either the radioactive or stable isotopes of water once the isotope has equilibrated with the total body water pool: the degree of isotope dilution is proportional to the volume of body water. An accuracy of 1 per cent may be expected by careful techniques but this does not overcome the variability between individuals in the true water content of the body. The measurement is also in error if conducted in patients who have oedema or are dehydrated.

Total body potassium. About 99 per cent of total body potassium exists within cells and naturally contains 0.0118 per cent of the natural ^{40}K isotope, a gamma ray emitter of high energy. Thus sensitive machines which measure the ^{40}K content of the body can be used to estimate the total amount of body potassium. An isotope dilution technique with the short half-life isotope ^{42}K can also be used but the development of low background and highly sensitive whole body counters means that repeated measurements of the ^{40}K content of an individual can readily be obtained, with an accuracy of about 3 per cent. This statistical error in counting is small but there may be just as great a variability in the potassium content of tissues as in its water content. States of diarrhoea, malnutrition, or the use of diuretics with low potassium intakes also lead to tissue potassium depletion and can lead to erroneous estimates of fat-free mass.

Total body density. This is the technique most favoured by experts attempting to measure body fat accurately. The principle involved is that of Archimedes; the body displaces a weight of water equivalent to its own volume and this displacement is reflected in the change in weight of individuals when weighed under water rather than in air. Unfortunately, allowances in the figure for body volume must include the large residual volume of air in the lung and this is normally measured directly by nitrogen or helium dilution in the subject at the same time. Intestinal gas is neglected in these calculations and the subjects need to be trained to control their breathing while being weighed under water. New methods which automatically measure residual lung volume and body density are being developed and can provide reproducible measurements within 1 per cent of each other.

Skinfold thickness and body fat. Body density has been used as the primary measure to derive equations which relate the thickness of subcutaneous skinfolds to the body fat content. By use of a pair of Harpenden calipers (see Figs. 1a and b) it is possible to measure the thickness of subcutaneous fat at standard sites. By reference to Table 1, the amount of body fat can then be estimated. The table, taken from measurement on Glaswegian adults, shows that women have more of their fat distributed subcutaneously than internally and the internal fat expands disproportionately with advancing years, particularly in men who tend to develop a paunch.

Healthy young men and women have a body fat content of less than 20 and 25 per cent respectively. In affluent societies there is on average a progressive increase in total body fat in middle-aged men and women. There is no evidence that this is a fundamental feature of ageing since in developing communities where food patterns are different and physical activity high, there is no increase in body fat with advancing years.

The determination of optimal body fat content. Whilst an excess of fat may be clinically obvious in an individual patient, there is a need to define obesity more precisely by relating the excess body fat to some agreed standard of normality. Some populations are fatter than others, so if one classified the average fat content of adults in every country as the specific standard for that population, then the standard would vary from country to country. On this basis patients might be considered obese in one country but normal in another.

Table 1   The equivalent fat content, as a percentage of body weight, for a range of values for the sum of four skinfolds (biceps, triceps, subscapular, and suprailiac) of males and females of different ages

Skinfolds (mm)	Percentage fat							
	Males (age in years)				Females (age in years)			
	17–29	30–39	40–49	50+	16–29	30–39	40–49	50+
15	4.8				10.5			
20	8.1	12.2	12.2	12.6	14.1	17.0	19.8	21.4
25	10.5	14.2	15.0	15.6	16.8	19.4	22.2	24.0
30	12.9	16.2	17.7	18.6	19.5	21.8	24.5	26.6
35	14.7	17.7	19.6	20.8	21.5	23.7	26.4	28.5
40	16.4	19.2	21.4	22.9	23.4	25.5	28.2	30.3
45	17.7	20.4	23.0	24.7	25.0	26.9	29.6	31.9
50	19.0	21.5	24.6	26.5	26.5	28.2	31.0	33.4
55	20.1	22.5	25.9	27.9	27.8	29.4	32.1	34.6
60	21.2	23.5	27.1	29.2	29.1	30.6	33.2	35.7
65	22.2	24.3	28.2	30.4	30.2	31.6	34.1	36.7
70	23.1	25.1	29.3	31.6	31.2	32.5	35.0	37.7
75	24.0	25.9	30.3	32.7	32.2	33.4	35.9	38.7
80	24.8	26.6	31.2	33.8	33.1	34.3	36.7	39.6
85	25.5	27.2	32.1	34.8	34.0	35.1	37.5	40.4
90	26.2	27.8	33.0	35.8	34.8	35.8	38.3	41.2
95	26.9	28.4	33.7	36.6	35.6	36.5	39.0	41.9
100	27.6	29.0	34.4	37.4	36.4	37.2	39.7	42.6
105	28.2	29.6	35.1	38.2	37.1	37.9	40.4	43.3
110	28.8	30.1	35.8	39.0	37.8	38.6	41.0	43.9
115	29.4	30.6	36.4	39.7	38.4	39.1	41.5	44.5
120	30.0	31.1	37.0	40.4	39.0	39.6	42.0	45.1
125	30.5	31.5	37.6	41.1	39.6	40.1	42.5	45.7
130	31.0	31.9	38.2	41.8	40.2	40.6	43.0	46.2
135	31.5	32.3	38.7	42.4	40.8	41.1	43.5	46.7
140	32.0	32.7	39.2	43.0	41.3	41.6	44.0	47.2
145	32.5	33.1	39.7	43.6	41.8	42.1	44.5	47.7
150	32.9	33.5	40.2	44.1	42.3	42.6	45.0	48.2
155	33.3	33.9	40.7	44.6	42.8	43.1	45.4	48.7
160	33.7	34.3	41.2	45.1	43.3	43.6	45.8	49.2
165	34.1	34.6	41.6	45.6	43.7	44.0	46.2	49.6
170	34.5	34.8	42.0	46.1	44.1	44.4	46.6	50.0
175	34.9					44.8	47.0	50.4
180	35.3					45.2	47.4	50.8
185	35.6					45.6	47.8	51.2
190	35.9					45.9	48.2	51.6
195						46.2	48.5	52.0
200						46.5	48.8	52.4
205							49.1	52.7
210							49.4	53.0

From Durnin, J. V. G. A. and Womersley, J. (1974). *Br. J. Nutr.* **32**, 77

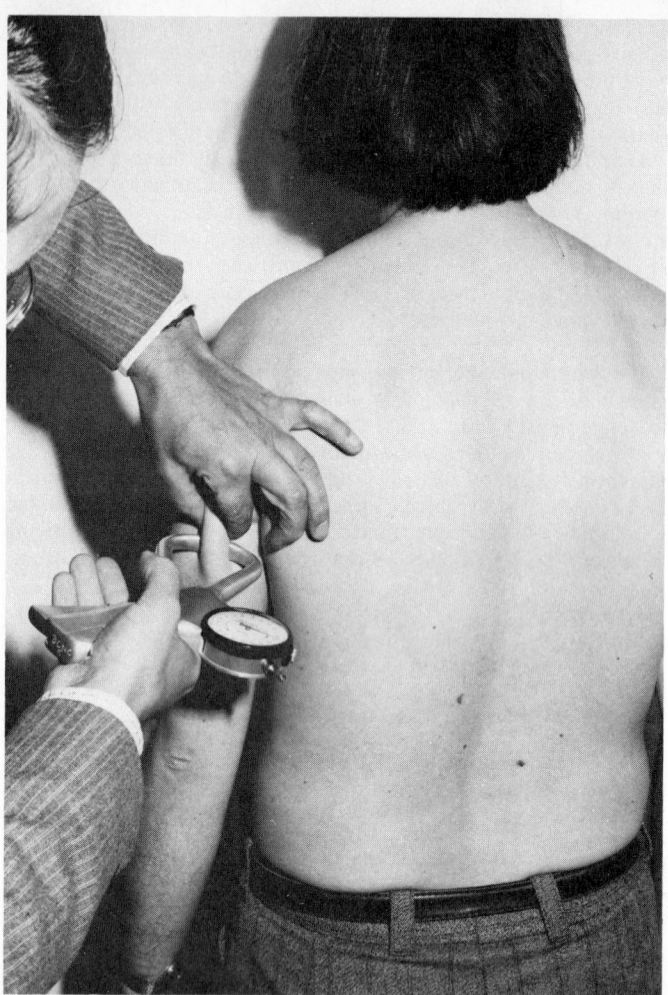 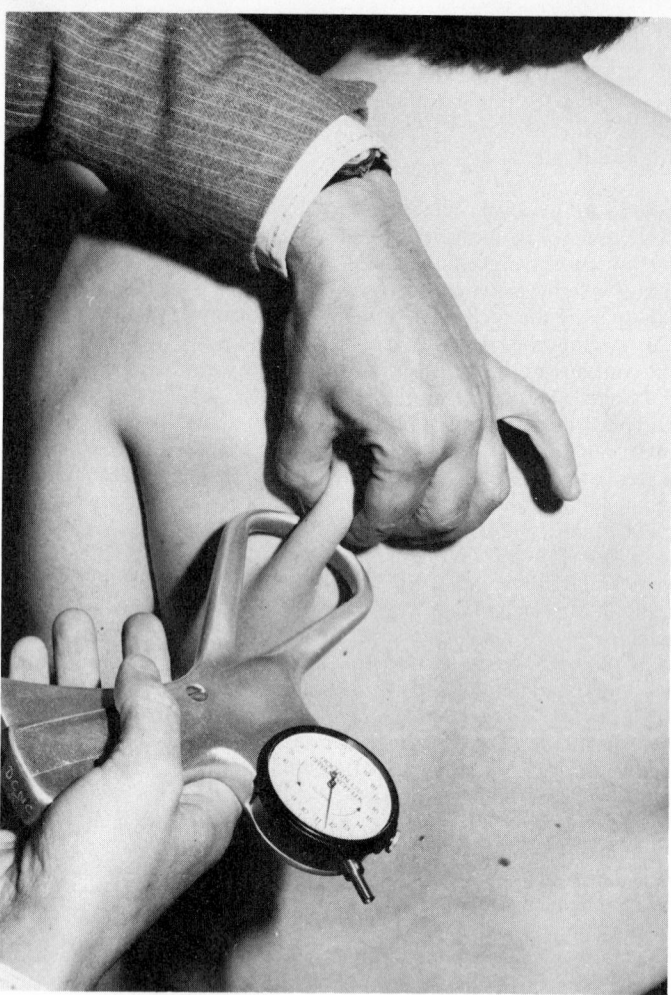

Fig. 1 *The measurement of skinfold thicknesses.* The point at which the skinfold is taken on the arm is measured as half the distance between the acromial and the olecranon processes. A fold of skin and subcutaneous tissue is taken by pinching the tissue between thumb and forefinger as shown and initially placed 2 cm apart. It is essential to maintain the grip with the left hand as shown while the right hand relaxes pressure completely on the handle of the calipers. Above a reading of 20 mm the measurement may decrease despite a firm hold with the left hand. In this case the reading should be taken 2 seconds after the caliper is applied. The biceps reading is taken in the same plane but at the front of the arm with the hand supinated. The suprailiac measurement is also taken on the left side in the mid-axillary line just above the iliac crest. (Photographs by permission of J. M. Tanner and R. H. Whitehouse, from *Growth and development chart SEB 45*, Castlemead Publications, Hertford, UK. Calipers are obtainable from Holrain Ltd, Crosswell, Crymmych, Dyfed, UK)

This approach is unsatisfactory and it is better to have a universal standard which also has some practical usefulness.

An excess body fat is associated with medical complications and an increased risk of early death and a very low body fat content, e.g. in anorexia nervosa, is also dangerous. It is therefore sensible to work out a range of body fat where the risks are minimized and regard this as optimal or desirable. The most detailed attempts to do this have been based on mortality statistics collected by Life Insurance Companies. Those wishing to take out a policy provide details of themselves and are medically examined; subsequent analyses of their age of death is used to define those groups with the lowest risk of an early death. Unfortunately, these studies have not included measurement of body fat content and have relied simply on measuring body weight. Extreme degrees of overweight are taken to indicate obesity.

Table 2 lists the new values published in 1979 by the United States Fogarty Conference and originally derived by the Metropolitan Life Insurance Company which presented the analysis of the mortality rates of nearly five million policy holders taking out insurance policies in the United States between 1935 and 1953. These tables have been adjusted since heights were actually reported in shoes and weights in indoor clothing! The original tables listed values for three frame sizes but no definition of frame size has

ever been specified and the practice of specifying frame size is now being discarded. The new tables encompass values for all frame sizes and therefore provide very generous allowances. The tables had no adjustment for age despite the usual tendency for adults in affluent societies to gain weight. The appropriateness of the choice of these limits in terms of mortality risk has been confirmed by the recent 1979 Build Study in the USA, which finds that the risk of being overweight is less than it was 20 years earlier. The latest study dealt with nearly 4 200 000 men and women issued with an ordinary insurance policy between 1950 and 1971, these policies being traced through to 1972. The upper limit of optimal weights suggested are almost identical to those given in Table 2. The risk associated with being underweight in adults in affluent societies appears to be less than it was and the new Insurance Statistics suggest that values of 7 kg less in men and 5.7 kg less in women than the lower limits given in Table 2 are still appropriate and not associated with a significantly increased risk.

Overweight is defined when weight is 110 per cent or more of the upper limit of these standards and obesity when weight is 120 per cent or more. Greater precision in estimating excess fat in the individual patient can come from measuring skinfold thickness. Weight for height values for men and women within the acceptable range shown in Table 2 are equivalent to an upper normal limit for

Table 2 Appropriate body weight and the lower limits for defining overweight and obesity

Height (cm)	Men				Women			
	Average (kg)	Acceptable range (kg)	Overweight (kg)	Obese (kg)	Average (kg)	Acceptable range (kg)	Overweight (kg)	Obese (kg)
145					46.0	37–53	58	64
148					46.5	37–54	59	65
150					47.0	38–55	61	66
152					48.5	39–57	63	68
156					49.5	39–58	64	70
158	55.8	44–64	70	77	50.4	40–58	64	70
160	57.6	44–65	72	78	51.3	41–59	65	71
162	58.6	46–66	73	79	52.6	42–61	67	73
164	59.6	47–67	74	80	54.0	43–62	68	74
166	60.6	48–69	76	83	55.4	44–64	70	77
168	61.7	49–71	78	85	56.8	45–65	72	78
170	63.5	51–73	80	88	58.1	45–66	73	79
172	65.0	52–74	81	89	60.0	46–67	74	80
174	66.5	53–75	83	90	61.3	48–69	76	83
176	68.0	54–77	85	92	62.6	49–70	77	84
178	69.4	55–79	87	95	64.0	51–72	79	86
180	71.0	58–80	88	96	65.3	52–74	81	89
182	72.6	59–82	90	98				
184	74.2	60–84	92	101				
186	75.8	62–86	95	103				
188	77.6	64–88	97	106				
190	79.3	66–90	99	108				
192	81.0	68–93	102	112				

Figures taken from the Fogarty table but adjusted to take account of extended lower range suggested by 1979 Build study. Limits of overweight taken to be 110–119 per cent of upper limit, with obesity present when weight is 120 per cent or more

the sum of the four skinfolds of 40 mm in both men and women. A total value of 60 mm is equivalent to a substantial excess of fat, i.e. 'overweight', and 80 mm is equivalent to the weight for height values used to define obesity.

Reference weights for children. Traditionally the practice followed in defining the lower limits of overweight and obesity in children is similar to that in adults and is taken as 110 per cent and 120 per cent of the standard weight. The standard in children is not, however, based on morbidity or mortality risk but on average weight of children in a well-nourished society. Recently new reference standards for weight, height, and weight for height of children have been agreed by the World Health Organization and are presented in Table 3 both as the median and the limits for two standard deviations from the median value. Unlike the system for defining obesity in adults by referring excess weight to the upper limit of the range of weights, the tradition in children is to define obesity when weight exceeds 120 per cent of the median weight for height. On this basis it must be recognized that the 110 per cent limit of weight for height for defining overweight corresponds to approximately the 80th percentile and that a 'normal' population would therefore be expected to have about 20 per cent of the children classified incorrectly as 'overweight'.

Few attempts have been made to define adiposity in children by first documenting the normal limits for skinfold thickness but a suggested set of standards is presented in Fig. 2. Figure 3 shows that the fat content of the child's body increases rapidly in the last trimester of pregnancy and in the first year of life. Thereafter the body's fat falls steadily until the onset of puberty. At this stage girls put on much more fat than boys and the increase is usually apparent earlier because of the earlier onset of puberty in girls than boys. These changes in body fat are also apparent in the changes in the skinfold thicknesses. The triceps skinfold thickness measurement, although widely used on its own, is unreliable since there are ethnic differences in the distribution of subcutaneous fat, and children of Black, Malaysian, and Chinese extraction tend to have less fat distributed on their limbs than on their trunk: the use of a combina-

tion of trunkal and limb measurements of skinfold thickness is therefore important.

Assessing overweight and obesity in adolescents is more difficult because of the marked variability between children in the time of their growth spurt. Measurements of weight and height are therefore less useful and it is more appropriate to measure skinfold thickness. There are no internationally agreed standards for these but the normal range derived from British studies is shown in Fig. 2. These values include measurements at the triceps and subscapular sites only rather than the four skinfold measurements used in adults. The upper limit of normal may therefore be taken as 20 mm for the combination of the two with 30 mm and 40 mm being equivalent to the adult classifications of 'overweight' and 'obesity'

The hazards of overweight and obesity. In affluent societies increases in body weight are associated with hazards to health (see page 8.55). Table 2 lists the optimal weights for the insured American population. These figures are very similar to those derived from the uninsured general population studied by the American Cancer Society. Three questions immediately arise from these figures: why do overweight people die early, do mild degrees of overweight matter, and are there a number of debilitating effects of weight gain which are not life-threatening but which nevertheless make weight gain unwise?

Causes of early death in obesity. Table 4 lists the causes of death from which overweight men are likely to die early. In the last 20 years the risk of operative deaths in obesity is less because of the advances in anaesthetic techniques, but the increased risk of death is nevertheless appreciable in patients who are frankly obese. The time needed for other risks to become evident may be 15–20 years so overweight and obesity are particularly disadvantageous in young adults, who tend to remain with their condition throughout life. This is illustrated in Fig. 4 which shows the different mortality rates by weight of young and middle-aged men. In the young men there is a clear relationship between weight and risk, whereas later in life

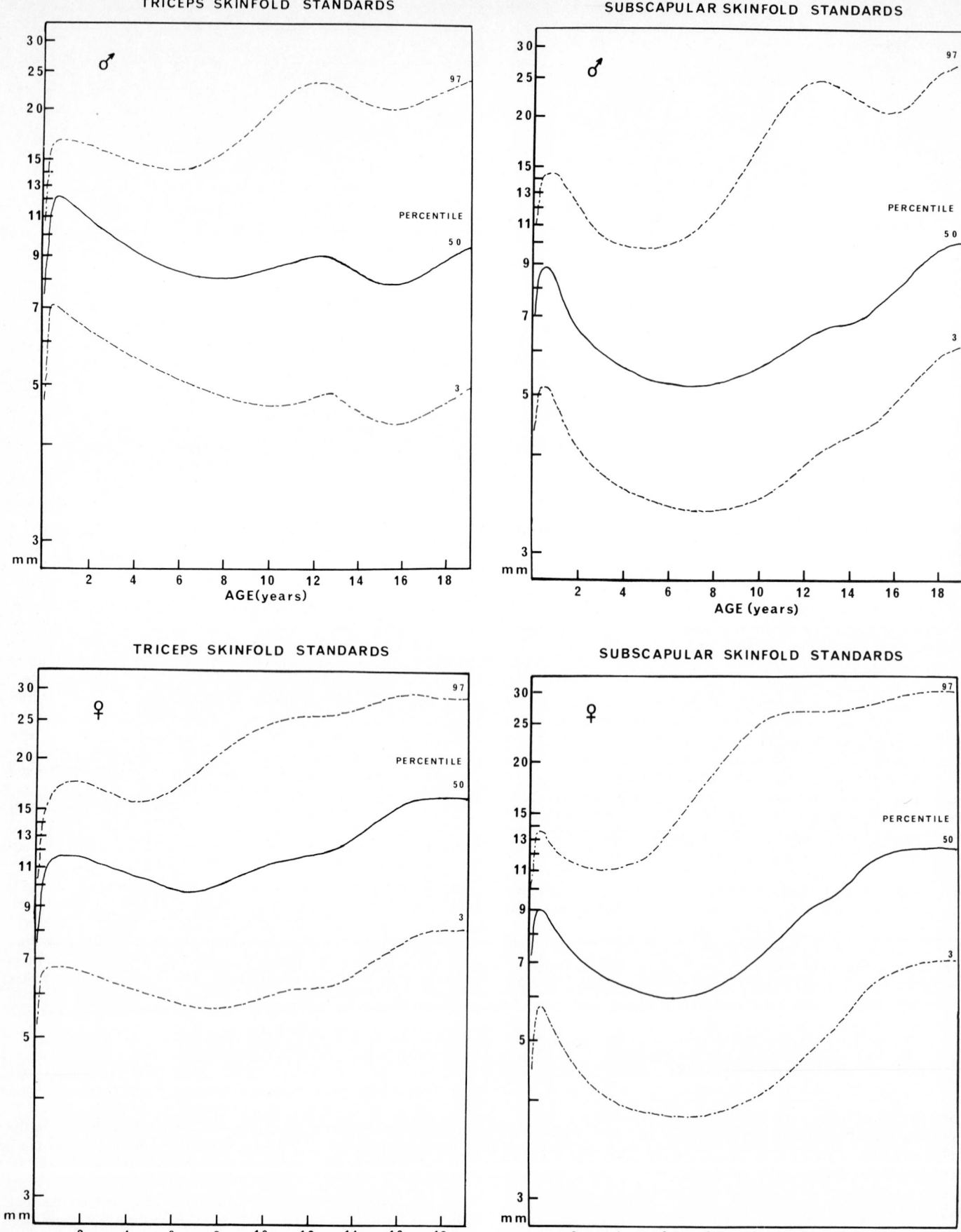

Fig. 2   Standards for triceps and subscapular skinfold thickness in boys and girls.

the excess risk of being overweight is less obvious in a population which has gained on average 3 kg in men and 6 kg in women between the ages of 25 and 55 years.

Table 3(a) The median and range (± 2 s.d.) of standard values for weight for length or height of boys

Length (cm)	Weight (kg) Median	Weight (kg) Range	Height (cm)	Weight (kg) Median	Weight (kg) Range
50	3.3	2.5–4.4	102	16.3	13.4–19.6
52	3.7	2.8–4.8	104	16.8	13.9–20.2
54	4.1	3.1–5.3	106	17.4	14.4–20.8
56	4.6	3.4–5.9	108	18.1	14.9–21.5
58	5.1	3.9–6.4	110	18.7	15.5–22.2
60	5.7	4.4–7.1	112	19.4	16.1–23.0
62	6.2	4.9–7.7	114	20.0	16.7–23.9
64	6.8	5.4–8.7	116	20.7	17.3–24.8
66	7.4	6.0–9.0	118	21.5	17.9–25.8
68	8.0	6.5–9.6	120	22.2	18.6–26.9
70	8.5	7.0–10.2	122	23.0	19.3–28.2
72	9.1	7.5–10.8	124	23.9	20.0–29.5
74	9.6	8.0–11.4	126	24.8	20.7–30.9
76	10.0	8.4–11.9	128	25.7	21.5–32.3
78	10.5	8.8–12.4	130	26.7	22.3–33.9
80	10.9	9.2–12.9	132	27.8	23.1–35.6
82	11.3	9.6–13.3	134	29.0	23.9–37.4
84	11.7	9.9–13.8	136	30.2	24.8–39.3
86	12.1	10.3–14.2	138	31.5	25.7–41.3
88	12.5	10.6–14.7	140	33.0	26.6–43.4
90	13.0	11.0–15.1	142	34.5	27.5–45.5
92	13.4	11.4–15.6	144	36.1	28.4–47.8
94	13.9	11.9–16.1			
96	14.4	12.3–16.6			
98	14.9	12.8–17.1			
100	15.5	13.3–17.7			

From World Health Organization (1979). Monograph (WHO/FAP/79.1).

Table 3(b) The median and range (± 2 s.d.) of standard values for weight for length or height of girls

Length (cm)	Weight (kg) Median	Weight (kg) Range	Height (cm)	Weight (kg) Median	Weight (kg) Range
50	3.4	2.6–4.2	100	15.4	12.7–18.8
52	3.7	2.8–4.7	102	15.9	13.1–19.4
54	4.1	3.1–5.2	104	16.5	13.6–20.0
56	4.5	3.5–5.7	106	17.0	14.0–20.6
58	5.0	3.9–6.3	108	17.6	14.5–21.3
60	5.5	4.3–6.9	110	18.2	15.0–22.0
62	6.1	4.8–7.5	112	18.9	15.6–22.8
64	6.7	5.3–8.1	114	19.6	16.2–23.7
66	7.3	5.8–8.7	116	20.3	16.8–24.7
68	7.8	6.3–9.3	118	21.0	17.4–25.8
70	8.4	6.8–9.9	120	21.8	18.1–27.0
72	8.9	7.2–10.5	122	22.7	18.8–28.3
74	9.4	7.7–11.0	124	23.6	19.5–29.8
76	9.8	8.1–11.4	126	24.6	20.3–31.4
78	10.2	8.5–11.9	128	25.7	21.0–33.2
80	10.6	8.8–12.3	130	26.8	21.9–35.1
82	11.1	9.3–12.9	132	28.0	22.7–37.3
84	11.4	9.6–13.2	134	29.4	23.6–39.6
86	11.8	9.9–13.6	136	30.8	24.5–42.2
88	12.2	10.3–14.1			
90	12.6	10.7–14.5			
92	13.0	11.1–15.0			
94	13.5	11.5–15.6			
96	14.0	12.0–16.1			
98	14.6	12.5–16.8			
100	15.2	13.1–17.4			

From World Health Organization (1979). Monograph (WHO/FAP/79.1).

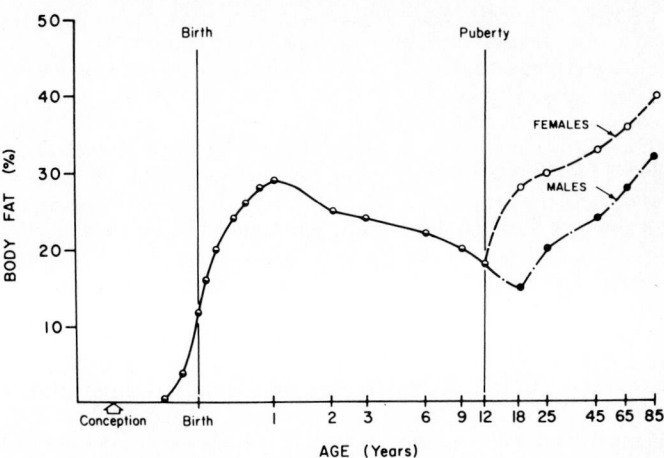

Fig. 3 The changes in body fat with age. (From Bray 1976, by permission)

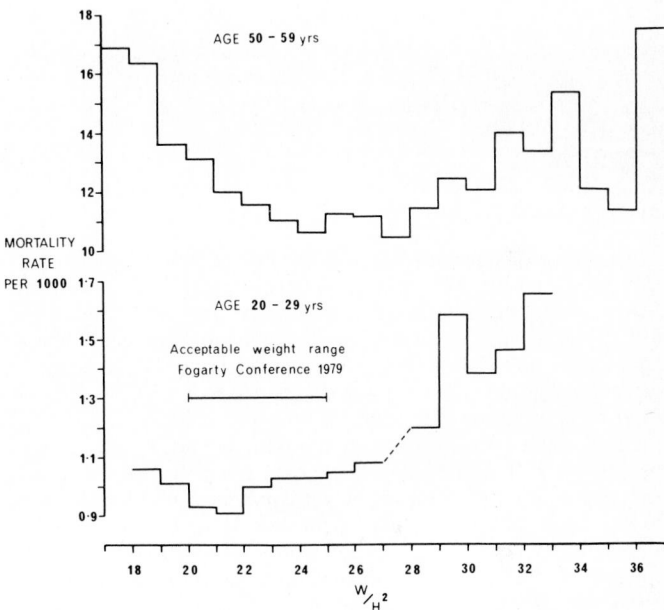

Fig. 4 The mortality rate of men of different ages, recalculated in relation to the body mass index. (From the Build study, 1979)

Table 4 Causes of increased mortality with excess weight in men

	Degree of overweight (%)	Mortality ratio (%)
Diabetes mellitus	5–15	125
	15–25	200
	>25	>500
Coronary artery disease	15–25	130
	25–55	160
	60	180
Hypertensive heart disease	5–15	170
	>15	250
Vascular lesions of CNS, e.g. strokes	>25	130
Digestive diseases, e.g. gall-bladder and colonic disease	15–35	140
	>25	250

Mortality ratios refer to the excess risk compared with the 100 per cent 'normal' risk for the population as a whole in the 1979 Build study

Obesity and cardiovascular disease. The major long-term health hazards of obesity are those affecting the cardiovascular system, e.g. hypertension and coronary artery disease. The effect of obesity on coronary artery disease has remained controversial with some experts considering that when the contributions of hyper-cholesterolaemia and hypertension have been assessed, then obes-ity has little influence. Since an increase in weight leads to an increase in plasma cholesterol and blood pressure, and slimming on an appropriate diet reduces both, the argument becomes academic: obesity's effects on cardiovascular disease are, to a substantial degree, mediated through a series of mechanisms as illustrated in Fig. 5. Physical activity may have its own protective effects on coronary artery disease by improving coronary circulation and the cardiorespiratory reflex responses to exercise, but it is also known to enhance HDL cholesterol concentrations and reduce circulating triglyceride levels. The HDL cholesterol concentration is now being recognized as a good predictor of coronary artery disease and in some studies high triglycerides are also a risk factor (see Section 13).

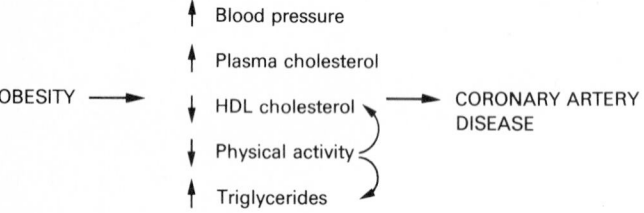

Fig. 5 The mechanisms whereby obesity increases the risk of coronary artery disease.

Smoking, weight, and disease. One major contributor to coronary artery disease which interacts with both obesity and coronary artery disease is smoking. Smoking is associated with a lower body weight, and many young women seem to recognize this and smoke cigarettes as an aid in slimming. On giving up smoking men gain on average 8 kg and a similar weight gain is observed in women. Figure 6 shows, however, that for both men and women the risk associated with smoking is far greater than that incurred by gaining weight and the risk of being 140 per cent above the average weight for all ages, i.e. frankly obese, only just matches the risk of smoking 20 cigarettes a day at a normal weight. It is clearly better, therefore, to encourage normal or overweight adolescents and adults to give up smoking first rather than being concerned with being a few kg above the optimal weights shown in Table 2.

Much of the confusion over whether obesity is important in the development of coronary artery disease has come from analysing statistics where no distinction is made between smokers and non-smokers. A group of thin or normal weight individuals are more likely to have a higher proportion of heavy smokers who are there-fore at greater risk than the moderately overweight non-smoker.

The progressive increase in risk of coronary artery disease in young men of increasing weight is illustrated in Fig. 7. This figure also displays the optimal weight range suggested in Table 2. Clearly the risk does increase with even moderate increases beyond the optimal range and there is no suggestion that it does not matter if weight gain does occur in middle age. It is therefore sensible to maintain weight within the range indicated and maintain this weight throughout life.

Obesity and hypertension. Both obesity and hypertension are fami-lial conditions with obesity enhancing the rise in blood pressure in those who are susceptible to hypertension (see Section 13). Popula-tion statistics have shown that a 10 per cent gain in body fat leads to an average rise of 6 mm and 4 mm in systolic and diastolic blood pressures, and there is a progressive increase in risk of hypertension with increasing age and weight.

Additional support for the interaction of excess weight and high blood pressure comes from the effects of weight reduction on blood pressure. Successful treatment of overweight hypertensives is much

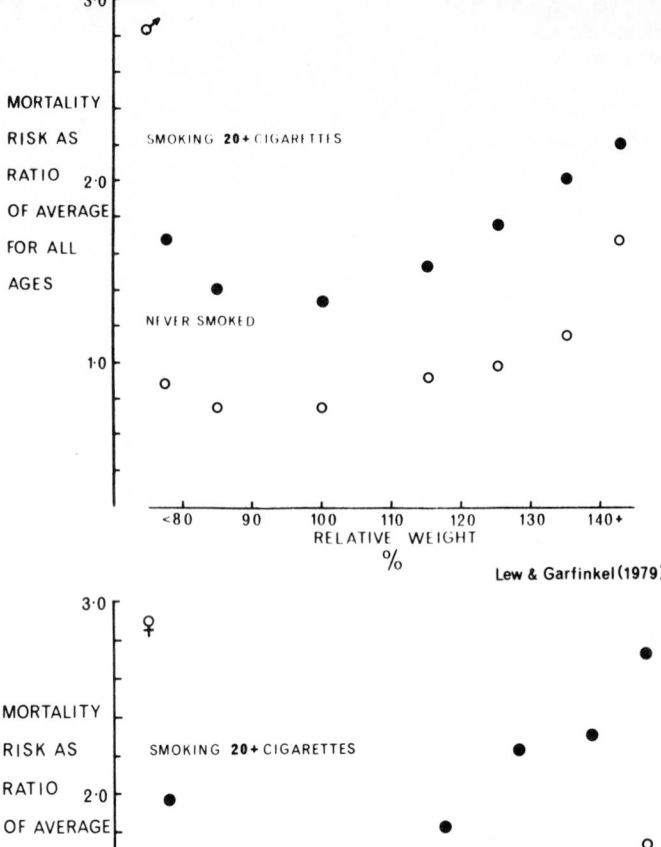

Fig. 6 The relationship between weight, smoking, and mortality in men and women. (Data recalculated from Lew and Garfinkel, 1979)

easier if they lose weight. Comparatively small weight losses may be effective in both sexes and at all ages. This effect of weight reduc-tion on blood pressure is independent of sodium intake in both normotensive and hypertensive obese patients. The mechanisms seems to depend not only on weight reduction as such but on changes in energy and perhaps carbohydrate intake which, in ani-mal studies, affect the sympathetic control of the cardiovascular system.

The evidence that a reduction in weight reduces blood pressure in moderately overweight individuals has now been applied to a population in a coronary prevention programme. Of 519 middle-aged men living in Chicago, 333 managed to maintain a weight loss of 5 kg for 10 years; systolic blood pressure fell by 7–16 mm de-pending on the degree of weight loss and diastolic pressures by 4–10 mm. Decreases of this order may lead to a fall in morbidity and a reduced need for pharmacological treatment with its poten-tial side-effects. The beneficial effect of quite modest reductions in weight make this a particularly appealing approach to dealing with hypertensive patients, some of whom may be only marginally over-weight.

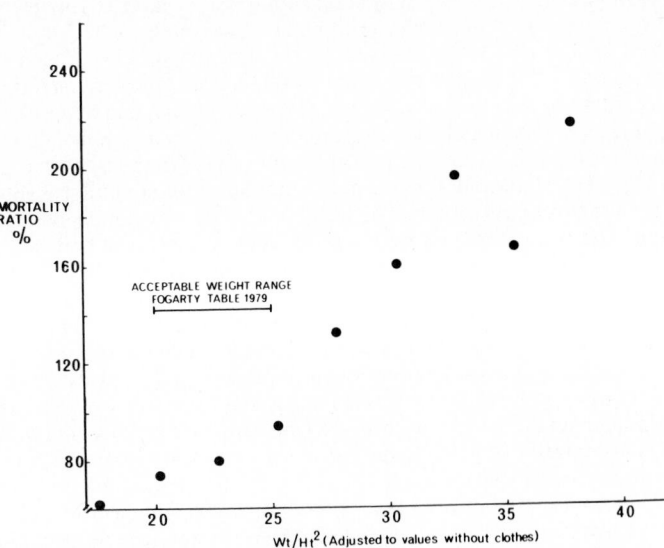

Fig. 7 The risk of coronary artery disease in relation to weight of young men. (Recalculated from the Build study, 1979)

are closely related epidemiologically and physiologically. With the development of obesity the endogenous synthesis of cholesterol by the liver and other tissues increases, and although there may be only a modest rise in circulating cholesterol concentrations, the body pool of cholesterol expands and there is a marked increase in the rate at which cholesterol is excreted in the bile. Since the development of gallstones depends on the precipitation of cholesterol from a supersaturated bile, any factor which increases cholesterol excretion will enhance the likelihood of gallstones. There is a remarkable increase in gall-bladder disease with increasing obesity (Fig. 9). The predominance of gallstone disease in women, and the increase in the problem with an increasing number of pregnancies, probably reflects the important stimulating effect of oestrogens on biliary cholesterol secretion. The use of oestrogen-containing contraceptives also enhances the cholesterol saturation of bile and there is increased production of endogenous oestrogens in obesity.

Obesity and diabetes. The effect of obesity in precipitating biochemical and clinical evidence of diabetes mellitus is well known (see Section 9). The risk of diabetes increases with age and with the degree of obesity (Fig. 8). The development of overt diabetes depends on a decline in the pancreatic capacity for insulin production with age and a need to increase markedly the output of insulin to compensate for the insulin resistance which develops in obesity.

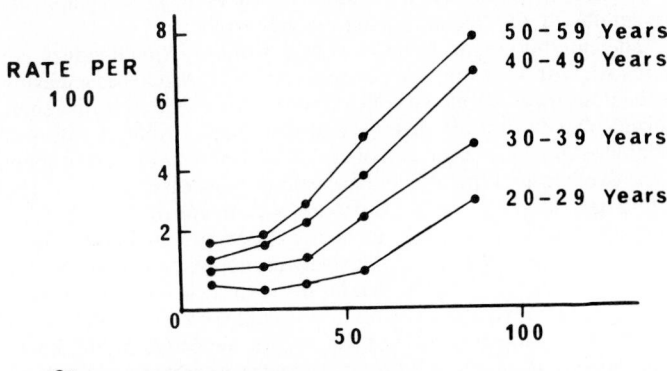

Fig. 8 The increasing prevalence of diabetes with age and overweight. (Redrawn from Rimm et al. 1975)

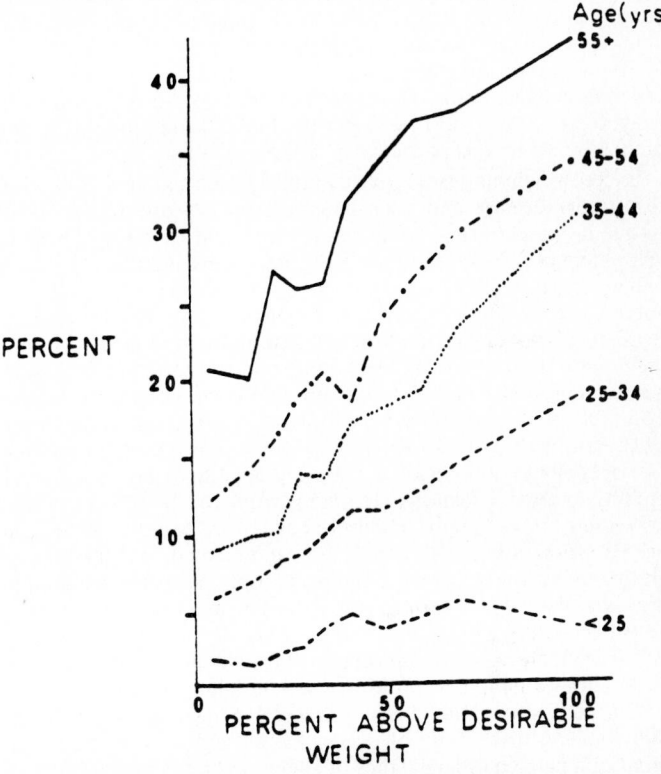

Fig. 9 The percentage of women with gall-bladder disease in relation to age and overweight. (Redrawn from Rimm et al. 1975)

The problem of individual susceptibility to diabetes has been well recognized in type I (juvenile onset) diabetes with its associations with HLA antigenic markers. What is less well recognized is the familial aggregation of type II (maturity onset) diabetes and its interaction with obesity. If a diabetic patient is not obese, his brothers and sisters are much more likely to develop diabetes if they are obese. This would be in keeping with the patient case having type I diabetes which is known to be familial. Obesity in a sibling will, therefore, more readily precipitate the development of diabetes because in these individuals the genetic predisposition to diabetes and obesity are additive in their effects. If the patient is obese and more likely, therefore, to have type II diabetes, the risk of diabetes developing in his siblings is still more than double if they too become obese. Particular care is therefore needed in diabetic families to prevent the development of obesity. Reducing weight places less demand on the pancreas and may often be the key to resolving the clinical and biochemical manifestations of diabetes.

Obesity and gall-bladder disease. Obesity and gallstone formation

Another factor in obese patients which may exacerbate the tendency to gallstone formation is the choice of inappropriate slimming diets. One of the common slimming regimens, the low carbohydrate diet, leads to a fall in cereal fibre intake. Cereal fibre normally aids laxation and thereby reduces the reabsorption of the secondary bile salt, deoxycholate, which acts on the hepatic-biliary system to reduce chenodeoxycholate concentrations and the solubility of cholesterol. Thus a low fibre diet will not only lead to constipation in the obese patient but may well accentuate the risk of gallstone formation.

Other problems in obesity. Table 5 lists many of the other conditions which have now been linked to obesity. The deranged hormonal status of obese women leads to menstrual irregularities and menorrhagia. The oestrogenic stimulus may also explain the increased risk of endometrial cancer but this stimulus has not been linked to the excess number of obese women who develop cancer of the breast.

Osteoarthritis is a very common condition in obese individuals.

Table 5 The morbid effects of moderate obesity

Both sexes	
Psychological disturbances	Hyperlipidaemia
Breathlessness	Coronary artery disease
Ankle swelling	Hypertension
Arthritis	Diabetes mellitus
Skin irritation	Cerebrovascular accident
Varicose veins	Post-operative infections, poor
Gallstones and gall-bladder disease	wound healing
Hiatus hernia	Renal disease
Constipation	

In women	
Menstrual irregularities and	Endometrial cancer
menorrhagia	Breast cancer
Hirsutism	

The two conditions may well be frequently associated by chance in elderly people but arthritis leading to reduced physical activity would appear to be one ready explanation for an interaction. Gout is a less common complication of obesity and only occurs in susceptible individuals. Patients become well aware of the advantages of weight loss if they do have arthritis, but reducing weight in the physically inactive is particularly difficult.

Excess weight imposes a considerable burden on individuals with respiratory disease and even in simple obesity one of the most frequent complaints is breathlessness on mild exertion. The development of obesity leads to a deterioration in a number of indices of lung function, including the vital capacity, maximum ventilatory volume, and compliance of the lung. The heavy chest wall impedes respiratory movements and the increase in internal fat also limits the range of movement of the diaphragm so that a marked improvement in well-being and exercise tolerance occurs with weight reduction. The more extreme syndromes with hypoxia and respiratory failure are usually only seen in those who are markedly obese but the overweight individual can be an operative risk with postoperative chest infections stemming from the poor respiratory movement. Overweight children have also been reported to become susceptible to chest infection and many excessively heavy infants recover more slowly from pneumonia. Severely obese children may also develop the hypoventilation syndrome, but this is unusual.

The frequency of varicose veins in obese subjects has been found to be about double that of normal-weight adults of the same age. Backache is also common and is induced by ligamentous strain in individuals whose centre of gravity has shifted with the development of a paunch or large folds of abdominal fat. These folds also lead to perspiration and intertrigo in the flexures.

Many of these consequences of obesity are reversible with weight loss and this is particularly true of insulin resistance and hyperlipoproteinaemia. Cholesterol deposited in gallstones is less likely to be dissolved.

Causes of obesity

Genetic. Obesity may be recognized in childhood as part of a number of genetic abnormalities which are usually accompanied by hypogonadism and have been classified as follows: (a) syndromes with primary hypogonadism and no polydactyly: (i) Prader–Willi; (ii) Alström; (iii) Edwards; (iv) Vasquez; (b) syndromes with secondary hypogonadism: (i) with polydactyly: Lawrence–Moon; Biemond type II; (ii) without polydactyly: Bardet–Biedl; and (c) obesity without hypogonadism: (i) early onset: triglyceride storage disease; (ii) late onset: Morgagni–Stewart–Monel syndrome.

All these syndromes are extremely unusual and those with obesity and hypogonadism are characteristically short in stature for their age, and often mentally retarded. In contrast, those with simple obesity of childhood onset are often taller than their peers and within the normal range of intelligence. Assessing a child's height is therefore important in the preliminary assessment. The Prader–Willi syndrome is by far the commonest of the conditions, occurring at an estimated frequency of 1 in 20 000 births. Hypotonia, mental retardation, obesity, short stature, hypogenitalism, and hyperphagia are characteristic, the syndrome arising from a genetic abnormality based on a translocation at chromosome J in the q-11 or q-12 locus. The condition does cluster in families, although the parents are not necessarily obese. The onset of obesity may not be evident until the age of three to five years and there is a delay in bone age. Many cases become exceptionally obese and are very difficult to manage because of their poor intelligence and hyperphagia.

The Alström syndrome is inherited as an autosomal recessive condition with early retinal degeneration, nerve deafness, and later diabetes mellitus as additional complications. The Edwards' syndrome is very similar but shows pigmented retinopathy whereas the Vasquez syndrome is a recently recognized X-linked syndrome with gynaecomastia as well as hypogonadism, mental retardation, short stature, and obesity.

The obesity syndrome associated with hypogonadism includes the Lawrence–Moon and Bardet–Biedl syndromes (see Section 23) which have five principle features: retinal degeneration, obesity, mental deficiency, polydactyly, and hypogonadism. These conditions are usually autosomally recessive in their inheritance and the Bardet–Biedl group have now been separated off because of the absence of polydactyly. Consanguinity of parents is common and the decreased visual acuity becomes apparent at school age as the first sign of the disease, most with the disease becoming blind by the age of 30. Most subjects are of subnormal intelligence but the hypogonadism only becomes apparent in adult life, some of the women having had children. Small testes, a feminine hair distribution, and occasional gynaecomastia is evident in the men. Obesity appears in childhood and becomes progressively worse.

The childhood syndromes of obesity without hypogonadism are unusual, with very few cases of triglyceride storage disease having been described. Localized collections of fat are evident with generalized obesity in most members of the family. Abnormalities of adenyl cyclase activation and of cyclic AMP activation of hormone-sensitive lipase in the affected areas have been distinguished. The Morgagni–Stewart–Morel syndrome is characterized by virilism, obesity, and hyperostosis, but does not become obvious in childhood, being found almost exclusively in older women who have a variety of neuropsychiatric symptoms with headache, irritability, and poor memory. Epileptic fits occasionally occur, the skull X-ray showing a diffuse shrinking of the inner table of the orbital bone. This appearance has given the syndrome another name of hyperostosis frontalis interna, but the condition is very unusual.

Hormonal. Hypothyroidism (see Section 10) is frequently but not always associated with obesity. In cretinism obesity is commonly found but this condition is rare. Many obese patients and their doctors hope to find biochemical evidence of hypothyroidism, but this is relatively uncommon occurring in only about 1 per cent or less of patients presenting to a specialized obesity clinic.

Cushing's syndrome (see Section 10) is less frequent a condition than hypothyroidism. It is suspected clinically in patients who show a combination of truncal accumulation of fat with poor muscular development of the arms and legs, skin thinning with striae, and hypertension. It is occasionally necessary to use laboratory investigation to distinguish obesity from Cushing's syndrome.

There is accelerated turnover of cortisol in obesity, mediated by a small increase in plasma ACTH and reflected by a rise in urinary 17-hydroxycorticosteroid excretion. The primary change in cortisol metabolism in obesity may be its increased metabolic degradation. Other tests for abnormalities of cortisol metabolism are, however, normal in obesity, e.g. urinary free cortisol, plasma unbound cortisol concentration, and total plasma cortisol. The diurnal variation in plasma cortisol is usually preserved in obesity, but suppression by dexamethasone may be less than in normal subjects.

Obesity and abnormalities of sex-hormone metabolism. There are a number of syndromes in which obesity seems to be associated with primary abnormalities in sex-hormone secretion. The hormones responsible for inducing obesity have not been identified but the association is nevertheless strong. The Stein–Leventhal syndrome of polycystic ovaries, menstrual abnormalities, and hirsutism is frequently associated with obesity. Patients who have had their ovaries removed also seem to gain weight readily but the basis of the weight gain is unknown. Secondary amenorrhoea in association with obesity suggests the possibility of hyperprolactinaemia. Obesity often slowly remits once the prolactin concentrations return to normal, suggesting that prolactin may contribute to increases in body fat.

A major change in body fat is found in pregnancy. There is a progressive increase with a maternal retention of approximately 36 000 kcal) (150 MJ) in the 4 kg of extra triglyceride stores as part of the total weight gain of 12.5 kg in a well-nourished woman. This is an average figure and many obese patients with a family history of obesity put on much more weight and fat at this stage. The basis for the weight gain seems to involve changes in metabolism as well as in food intake. Hormones in the progesterone class are known to increase body fat content by both increasing appetite and by altering the efficiency of metabolism; oestrogens antagonize these effects. In pregnancy the hormonal control of metabolism is modified by placentally derived sex-hormones which may also be responsible for the increased amount of fat stored. It seems likely that the development of obesity in adolescent girls depends on similar effects of sex-hormones on metabolism.

Drug-induced obesity. The contraceptive pill is probably the drug which is most widely recognized by the public as inducing weight gain. Yet formal trials often suggest that any gain is usually small, most of it being accounted for by water retention alone. About 10 per cent of women give up using the contraceptive pill because of weight gain which often exceeds the 2–3 kg ascribable to water retention. Doctors tend to avoid the pill in patients who are already overweight or from a fat family. A physiological basis for the pill's capacity to increase weight is readily established. Ovulation normally initiates an increase in metabolic rate of about 10 per cent for the second half of the menstrual cycle and this change is readily documented by the rise in body temperature at ovulation. The oral contraceptive, by inhibiting ovulation, prevents the increase in metabolism and body temperature; less energy is therefore dissipated and unless compensatory changes in metabolism or food intake occur, body fat will slowly accumulate. Additional direct effects of the oestrogen and progestogen in oral contraceptives on metabolism and appetite may occur but no definite advantages in terms of limiting weight gain have been linked to specific hormone preparations. Although similar changes in metabolism are to be expected at the menopause, no direct link has been established between the time of the menopause and the well-recognized tendency of women to gain weight at this stage of life.

Other drugs have been linked with weight gain. Those used for the treatment of thyrotoxicosis have a well-recognized mechanism of action. Corticosteroid analogues, lead to serious weight-gain in many patients but the mechanism underlying steroidal obesity is unknown (see Section 10).

Cyproheptadine is a drug introduced for its effects in stimulating the appetite as well as for use in allergic disorders. More commonly used drugs leading to weight gain, however, are the phenothiazine series which can lead to very large increases in body fat in susceptible patients. A large number of drugs developed for use as anti-depressants increase body weight either by improving the appetite of a depressed patient who cannot be bothered to eat, or by altering metabolism.

Other specific causes of obesity. Unusual cases of obesity occur in patients who have brain damage or who have a brain tumour in the hypothalamic area responsible for controlling appetite and meta-

bolism. Often it is difficult to disentangle the mechanism underlying the obesity because patients, in addition to having pituitary or hypothalamic abnormalities, may be immobilized by their injury or disease, bored by their limited range of opportunity, or stressed by their condition.

The cause of 'simple' obesity

Familial obesity: is it genetic? A number of studies have shown that in 60–80 per cent of obese children, one or both parents are obese, usually the mother rather than the father. This has been taken in the past to indicate that the maternal influence on a child's obesity is exerted through an effect on eating patterns rather than through any genetic mechanism. Table 6 shows an analysis of the weight of children of fathers and mothers of different weights. Thin parents did not have fat children and obese parents never had thin children.

Table 6 The relationship between various degrees of under- and overweight in parents and their offspring

Parental size	Parental body mass index	% Children				
		Thin	Under-weight	Normal	Over-weight	Obese
Thin	14.0–18.0	20	60	10	10	–
Underweight	18.1–21.4	10	69	21	–	–
Normal	21.5–25.6	1	12	61	25	21
Overweight	25.7–30.5	–	9	39	39	13
Obese	30.6–45.0	–	–	40	27	33

Recalculated by Bray (1981) from Davenport (1923) *Body build and its inheritance*. Publication no. 329, Carnegie Institute, Washington

This familial aggregation, however, does not help in distinguishing the genetic from the environmental factors. When adopted or fostered children are compared with the biologically related children within a family, the association between body weight of the parents and children is far greater for the biologically related children even when the adopted or fostered children enter the family within a few weeks of birth. Twin studies also suggest the importance of genetics since the heights and weights of monozygotic twins are closer to each other in adult life than of dizygotic twins, even if the monozygotic twins are raised apart. Similar findings have been obtained by looking at the skinfold thickness of twins as a more specific measure of body fatness, the similarity in skinfold measurements becoming more obvious in older children who presumably are less likely to be influenced by the environmental pressures on feeding behaviour within the home.

This evidence all points to the important contribution which genetics can make in determining body fat, but environmental factors can also be of great importance. The environment can have a long-term effect if it acts sufficiently early in a child's life. Obese mothers tend to have much larger placentae and bear children who may weigh about 10 per cent more than children of lean mothers. These differences in weight persist until at least seven years of age. Obese mothers who have small placentae, e.g. in association with pre-eclampsia, have smaller babies who are still smaller at seven years old, and about half the difference in weight of children appears to be accounted for by the environmental effect of placental weight. That intra-uterine nutrition may be the key to this effect is suggested by the finding that if differences in weight of monozygotic twins are found in later life, this can usually be traced back to marked differences in birth weight and in the relative dominance of the twins *in utero*.

The work on identical twins of widely differing weight and on placental weight in relation to a child's stature at the age of seven, all seems to indicate that long-term programming of body size can occur in the early phase of life. This concept has received considerable support from animal experiments which show that there appear to be critical periods when restricting food has a long-term effect on body size and adiposity. From this developed a very popular theory that over-feeding in infancy could programme the body to lay down fat preferentially. The theory was developed by suggesting that infants who became obese, e.g. as a result of an excess energy intake from bottle feeding, laid down the excess fat by multiplying the number of fat cells which then remained stable in number, sequestering fat and altering the body's energy economy for the rest of the individual's life.

There is very little evidence for these propositions. Fat infants are more likely to become fat children at the age of four to five years and weight gain in infancy has been linked with the degree of adiposity in boys (but not girls) at the age of 10. By the age of 10 years, only half an obese population of children can date their obesity to early childhood. That children are fat later in life because they were induced to be fat in infancy is doubtful and the link may merely mean that those individuals with a propensity to fatness are those displaying rapid weight gain under the adverse effects of inappropriate bottle feeding in infancy. These children are also more likely to be the group displaying obesity in adult life. In one group of infants who exceeded the 90th percentile of weight, 36 per cent were overweight 20–30 years later, compared with 14 per cent of average and light-weight infants. Thus permanent obesity is far from inevitable in the overweight infant but there is an increased risk, and once obesity is found in older children, the risk of persisting obesity should not be underestimated: 80 per cent of overweight young teenagers may be expected to be markedly overweight 30–35 years later compared with 20 per cent of young teenagers of normal weight.

Environmental factors. Although the interaction of genetic factors and early perinatal influences may have a permanent effect on the susceptibility to obesity, a variety of environmental factors are needed to display this susceptibility. The old adage that no obese subject came out of a concentration camp is frequently mentioned by unhelpful doctors seeking to cope with patients struggling to lose weight. This truth is not particularly illuminating.

Energy balance and obesity. Figure 10 shows the various factors which need to be considered when assessing the metabolic basis of obesity. Body fat only accumulates slowly in the obese individual and it has always seemed to be difficult to understand how some people can remain almost the same weight throughout their lives with a body energy content of about 191 000 kcal (800 MJ) while ingesting on average 2400 kcal (10 MJ) every day for over 60 years. Only a small discrepancy between intake and output will therefore lead to a rapid change in the stores of body energy. On this basis it used to be thought that the amount of food energy ingested was controlled by an exquisitely sensitive system which in some way monitored body fat. In practice food intake is not so finely regulated but varies considerably from day to day in a manner which does not seem to bear any relation to changes in body energy. However, big discrepancies between energy intake and expenditure are recognized by some physiological system which then adjusts appetite appropriately. Thus strenuous exercise after a few days leads to an increase in food intake. A disguised dilution of the food of both infants and adults is also followed by a compensatory

Table 7   Calculating excess body energy stores in obesity

1. Measure all 4 skinfold thicknesses and calculate body fat content a percentage of weight (see Table 1).
2. Weigh patient and calculate absolute fat content in kg.
3. Obtain optimal weight from average optimal weight (see Table 2).
4. Assume optimal fat content 15 per cent for men and 25 per cent for women and calculate optimal fat content in kg.
5. Subtract optimal weight from actual weight of fat.
6. Multiply excess fat content by (a) 37 to obtain excess energy deposited in MJ; or (b) 9000 to express in kcal.

increase in food intake after a few days so that the energy deficit is minimized.

A further component of energy regulation is the fluctuation in energy output in response to changing energy intakes. Physical activity is reduced in semi-starvation and increases with refeeding: these changes affect an important fraction of energy output. A variety of metabolic processes demanding energy also vary in relation to the energy content of the diet and minimize changes in the body fat content. Thus both the rate of input and output is modulated to help preserve energy balance and these combined regulatory processes ensure that only slow changes in body weight and fat content occur.

Energy expenditure. Figure 10 shows the normal components of energy output in man. Women have, at an equivalent height, an energy output which is almost 15 per cent less than a man's; this relates to their lower basal metabolic rate which in turn relates to their smaller lean body mass. Since women are also usually shorter and lighter than men, there is a further reduction in energy requirements which on average amounts to 20 per cent.

All components of energy expenditure fluctuate in response to changes in food intake, but the mechanisms controlling the body's responses are unknown; thyroid hormone activity influences a number of metabolic processes, including those which contribute to the basal metabolic rate, e.g. protein turnover, fatty acid and glucose turnover, and sodium pumping; in addition, the sympathetic nervous system affects metabolism, increasing its activity on overfeeding and reducing its activity during semi-starvation. In babies the sympathetic system appears to have a major effect on non-shivering thermogenic processes in brown adipose tissue, an organ specifically developed biologically to maintain body temperature when the environmental temperature falls. As the size of the lean body mass increases during growth, the need for additional heat production to maintain body temperature diminishes. Brown adipose tissue atrophies during childhood and cold-induced thermogenesis plays only a minor role in adult life. Brown adipose tissue can still be demonstrated, however, around the internal organs and along the intercostal nerves in the elderly. In animals the tissue responds to overfeeding by increasing its activity and this minimizes weight gain. In adult man histological evidence of brown adipose tissue activity remains and indirect evidence suggests that it may still retain its capacity to change its activity and affect energy balance. However, its quantitative contribution remains uncertain.

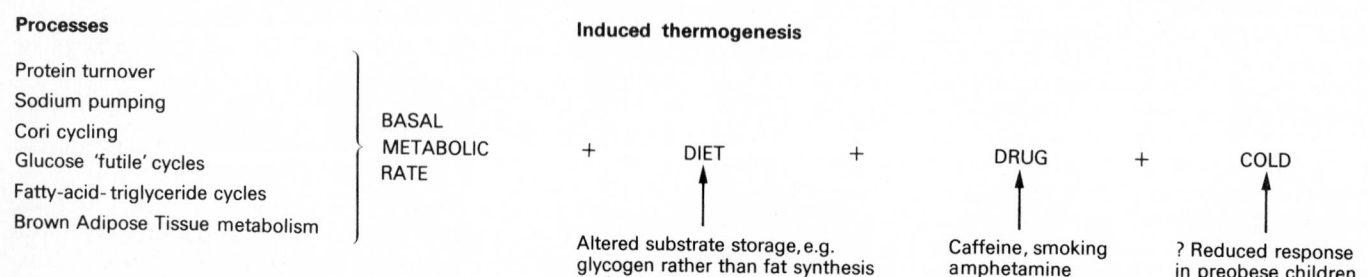

Fig. 10   Some of the metabolic factors potentially contributing to the metabolic basis of obesity.

The basal metabolic rate (BMR), i.e. the rate measured in the morning at rest and when relaxing in the fasting state, was often measured as a way of assessing changes in metabolism. However, even in sedentary individuals it contributes only about 50–60 per cent of the total energy expenditure. Expressing BMR as total energy output per day and not relating it to surface area in the traditional manner, shows that few adults have a BMR below 1000 kcal (4.2 MJ) per day. In adult life BMR declines with age and this decline is often considered to represent part of the ageing process. In Western societies, however, the fat free mass also declines with age, perhaps because of reduced physical activity. When the BMR is related to the mass of lean tissue, then no decline in the energetics of the tissues is apparent.

A very sedentary individual increases his energy output to 1.5 times his BMR by a range of processes costing a small amount of energy, e.g. increased muscle tone, fidgeting, and by the termogenic response to meals, smoking, and caffeine. The physical activity of a moderately active person, e.g. a carpenter, plumber, or docker, increases his energy expenditure by about 20 per cent and few individuals in societies geared to the use of machines are involved in the heavy manual work normally associated with coalminers and lumberjacks. These individuals may in unusual circumstances expend twice as much energy as the sedentary person. The comparatively low cost of physical exercise is often emphasized but it is still important since increases in body fat may develop insidiously from small discrepancies in energy balance. Reduced physical activity also tends to be accompanied by a slow fall in BMR as muscle tissue with its own basal energy requirements slowly atrophies with inactivity.

Food intake and obesity. Formal studies of food intake support the common view of obese subjects that they do not eat more than their slim counterparts. This has been found not only in adults but also in adolescents and even infants. In one study 63 obese women were found to have an intake of 1184 ± 534 kcal/day (7.85 ± 2.23 MJ/day; mean ± s.d.), whereas the intake of 26 normal weight controls was 1978 ± 479 kcal/day (8.24 ± 2.0 MJ/day). Even when care is taken to match obese and lean women for age, similar intakes are found. There tend to be more obese individuals in working-class homes but social class does not affect the comparison of intakes since consistently lower energy intakes have been observed in obese adolescent girls of similar age and background.

These studies deal with the findings in groups of obese infants, adolescents, and adults and not in individuals. It would therefore be wrong to assume that food intake is never increased in obesity. The reasons for the large quantities of food eaten by some obese patients are many. One obese subject may have been accustomed to consuming such quantities when very active physically. Young men and women who are injured at sport or are unable to compete for other reasons may continue to eat at their previous level or fail to reduce their intake sufficiently when giving up sport; others find that eating helps them to cope with boredom, stress, or unhappiness. One of the most difficult groups of obese patients with whom to deal are the compulsive eaters who find it difficult to explain their behaviour, some women finding this compulsion a particular problem in the pre-menstrual phase.

The cultural environment is also important in determining the amount of energy ingested. Many children are reared in an environment of poverty where food is not only linked with communication within the family and between friends, but is a visible demonstration of affluence. The constant availability of a variety of snacks, sweets, and drinks on display in several areas of the home, and the cultural links which establish food as a symbol of affection all lead to a tendency to eat more than that warranted by the physiological drives of hunger.

The variety of food available in affluent societies also contributes since it is well recognized that a subject satisfied after a large meal may still find a new variety of food appetizing and start eating once more. Given these social and psychological pressures, it would not be surprising if most children and adults in affluent societies tend to eat much more: an increase in weight and the development of obesity is then displayed by those most susceptible to adiposity for psychological or metabolic reasons.

Nutritional factors may also be involved in the development of obesity but their exact role is still debated. Foods which are dense in energy can be ingested easily and physiological signals may then be too slow to respond in producing satiety to limit further consumption. Energy-dense foods are characteristically those which are rich in sugar and fat but poor in dietary fibre. Fibre-rich foods tend to contain much more water and are therefore low in energy density. The remarkable difference in the energy density of foods in different cultures is illustrated by the finding that one to three year old children in Uganda subsisting on a matoke diet have to ingest 500 g of food to meet their energy needs, whereas a European child living in the same area on a British diet needed to eat only 210 g to obtain 40 per cent more energy. Gastric distension appears to be one of the short-term satiety signals, so a meal of low energy density is likely to provide a lower energy intake than meals which are rich in sugar and fat. The satiety value of different nutrients is difficult to test but some studies suggest that protein-rich foods have a high satiety value. The type of diet also has different effects on energy output. If carbohydrate is ingested, about 5 per cent of the energy is dissipated in the cost of storing glycogen; when converted to triacyl glycerol, however, the energy cost increases and about 18–20 per cent of the dietary carbohydrate energy is lost. The cost of storing ingested dietary fat is very small and amounts to only 3–5 per cent of the energy ingested. Thus energy absorbed as fat will lead to more triglyceride being deposited than if the same amount of energy is ingested as carbohydrates and then converted to triglyceride.

Physical inactivity may be a precipitant of obesity in an individual patient but a comparison of groups of lean and obese subjects provides little evidence that physical inactivity is a major factor in the development of obesity. Once a substantial increase in weight has occurred, there is, however, a fall in the time devoted to strenuous exercise. This can most readily be explained as a secondary effect of weight gain rather than an aetiological factor.

The metabolic basis of obesity: thermogenesis. Table 8 shows that normal-weight children of obese parents ingest 20 per cent less energy than similar-weight children of non-obese parents. Their metabolic rates are also lower and their calculated total energy expenditure matches the low food intake. These children therefore appear to be genetically predisposed to obesity by virtue of having a lower energy requirement than normal. Given the social pressure to eat the same as their peers, these children will tend to gain weight; it is therefore not surprising that obese children are found to remain obese on a normal intake of food.

Table 8   The physical characteristics and energy turnover of 4-year-old children of obese and normal-weight parents

	Normal-weight parents	Obese parents
Height (cm)	111.3±7.4	110.7±7.5
Weight (kg)	19.1±3.5	19.5±3.5
Body fat (%)	14.3±5.2	16.8±3.7
Daily energy intake (kJ) (kcal)	5996±787 (1433±188)	4665±1255(1115±300)
Daily resting expenditure	4950±770 (1183±184)	4180±611 (999±146)
Daily energy expenditure	6309±1473(1508±352)	4912±1243(1174±297)

Data are mean ± s.d. with 12 children of normal weight parents and 8 of obese parents

From Griffiths and Payne (1976)

One of the metabolic factors involved in the development of obesity relates to the metabolic response to fat. A normal-weight subject adjusts his thermogenic response to dietary fat depending on whether the extra fat is ingested as an excess above his normal energy requirements or as part of a slimming diet. Fat in excess of requirements is more readily metabolized whereas fat added to a low energy diet is stored with only a small loss of energy. This change illustrates the normal metabolic flexibility to ingested nutrients. If thin young men without a family history of obesity and normally requiring about 3000 kcal (12.6 MJ) per day to maintain weight are then overfed a high fat diet for many months, only a small weight gain results even if they are persuaded to reduce their activity. Studies on prisoners in Vermont, USA showed that they could ingest daily about 6000–8000 kcal (25–34 MJ) and yet stabilize their weight. After months an intake below 5750 kcal (24 MJ) led to weight loss! These classic studies conducted by Sims and his colleagues on volunteer prisoners agree with the personal accounts early this century of scientists who deliberately manipulated their own energy intake over a wide range without gaining or losing weight. This is in striking contrast to the problem of obese patients who often feel the need to restrict their intake to prevent even further weight gain. Obese individuals have a subnormal response to dietary fat, expending only 3 per cent of the fat's energy even when overfed. The obese are therefore very susceptible to further weight gain if consuming a high fat diet.

One biochemical and physiological explanation suggested for this flexibility in metabolic response to changes in dietary energy is that brown adipose tissue is modulated in its activity by the sympathetic nervous system and that dietary fat provides an appropriate and readily available substrate for this tissue. Inactive or absent brown adipose tissue in pre-obese or obese patients may then predispose them to obesity when faced with a high energy and fat-enriched diet. These susceptible individuals become obese and in doing so accumulate not only extra fat but additional lean tissue. This lean tissue increases the basal metabolic rate and thereby limits further weight gain. The higher basal metabolic rate in obese patients relates directly to their greater lean body mass and this should be considered a consequence of obesity and not a cause. Figure 10 shows that the high BMR compensates for the lower thermogenic response to food in the obese individual. The figure also illustrates a fundamental problem faced by the obese individual wishing to slim. As the excess fat is lost there is also a loss of lean tissue and the BMR falls back to the normal range. This means that the obese individual has to re-educate himself so that he learns to eat less than normal permanently if he is to maintain his reduced weight. This integration of input and output in constitutionally thin and obese individuals is set out in Fig. 11, but these must be regarded as only one possible explanation for the observations in obesity. In some individuals the key factor appears to be obesity developing during pregnancy and in others there may be a major psychologically based hyperphagia with no family history of obesity. In yet others there may be an unusually low BMR as a primary predisposing factor. This multiplicity of causes must be recognized

so that the management of the patient can be linked to the cause of their obesity whenever possible.

Treatment

Assessing the patient. The success of treatment depends on assessing the principal factors responsible for the development of obesity. Drugs may need to be changed, and a detailed analysis of a patient's life style is essential. This helps both the patient and doctor to appreciate the problems to be tackled. A simple method of assessment is to ask the subject to write down a detailed record of his normal eating and exercise pattern for a month *while maintaining a constant weight*. A period of four weeks is needed to overcome the patient's claim that the pattern of a few days eating is particularly unusual and may make him realize that 'unusual' events occur frequently. The need to maintain weight is essential if an estimate of current energy requirements is to be made. Occasionally patients attempt to convince their doctors (and often themselves) that they are able to manage on very few calories, deluding themselves while eating larger amounts of food than those recorded, or eating secretly. A 24-hour collection of urine will then reveal a high potassium and urea output at variance with the dietary record. All too often doctors rely on a series of simple questions to elicit an obese individual's eating pattern. These questionnaires are extremely unreliable (in both thin and obese patients) and to ask a dietician to conduct a dietary history may improve the reliability of the data a little but indicate to the patient that the doctor will only deal with his 'medical' problems and not his pattern of living. The use of questionnaires also neglects the value of the individual reassessing his own behaviour.

Patients weighing in excess of 120 kg usually have a metabolic rate of over 1900 kcal (8 MJ) and are often hyperphagic. Only the exceptional patient has a basal metabolic rate below 1000 kcal (4.2 MJ) per day. Nevertheless, patients claim not to lose weight on an 800 kcal (3.4 MJ) diet or complain that the benefits of the diet were only short lived. Detailed enquiries often reveal that patients weighed themselves daily for only two to three weeks or followed only the principles of the 800 kcal diet. The patient is also confused by popular accounts of spectacular weight losses on low energy diets and by the poor correlation between their own monitoring of the foods ingested and their daily fluctuations in weight. Few patients realize that a 1 kg weight loss corresponds to the loss of 7700 kcal (32 MJ) from adipose tissue but a low carbohydrate diet can induce a weight loss of 3–4 kg once muscle glycogen has been mobilized and muscle protein begins to be broken down to provide aminoacids for gluconeogenesis. Both glycogen and protein are stored with four times their weight of water. The combination of glycogen and protein breakdown therefore leads to spectacular early weight losses which boost the confidence of the patient only to depress him when in the third and fourth weeks weight loss seems negligible. When depressed, the patient may then ingest comparatively small amounts of carbohydrate which promptly lead to glycogen storage, and renal sodium retention. Both these effects are accompanied by water retention and a weight gain of as much as 4 kg, which then masks the loss of up to 30 000 kcal (132 MJ) from adipose tissue! The individual is thereby convinced that the simple principles of energetics do not apply to him and that weight loss is impossible. The examination of the patient is often neglected and can be difficult. Obese patients tend to have all their complaints ascribed to their excess weight and pathological conditions, e.g. abdominal masses, may remain undiagnosed. Examination may reveal additional problems requiring treatment, e.g. severe varicose veins with incipient ulceration of the leg, xanthelasma, or the presence of coexisting hypertension. Urinary testing may suggest a urinary infection or undiagnosed diabetes. The unusual case of hypothyroidism or Cushing's disease is usually readily diagnosed clinically. Measuring weight, height, and skinfold thickness also allows a simple calculation of the excess amount of fat and energy to be lost over a period of weeks or months, as shown in Table 8.

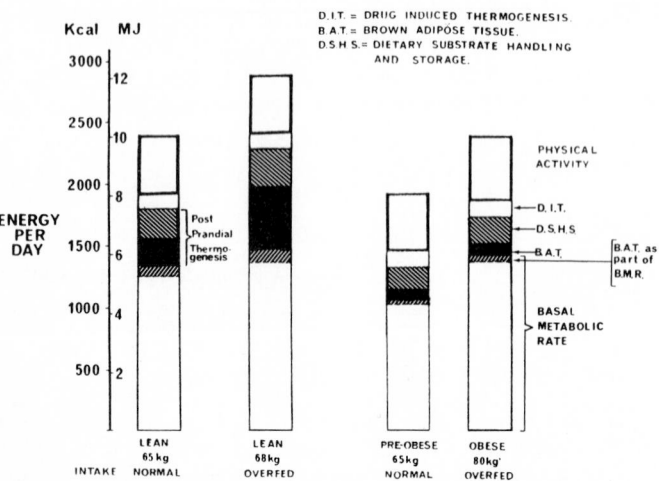

Fig. 11   An integrated view of the possible metabolic basis of obesity.

Dietary management. Many diets have been devised and continue to be produced for the weight conscious individuals in affluent societies. It has been estimated that in any one year about a third of adults in Britain are attempting to reduce their weight. Since this proportion of slimmers remains constant, it is evident that few, if any, of the many diets advocated are particularly successful. Much of this failure stems from the frequent failure to recognize the prolonged dieting necessary for any substantial loss of body fat. The common but incorrect view that slimming is a temporary need and that once slim the subjects can return to their former life-style also explains the poor long-term results of slimming. The problem is one of changing individuals' behaviour permanently so that they end up either expending more energy or ingesting less energy. This is true whether a patient has a predominantly psychological basis for obesity or metabolic 'simple' obesity.

Most weight-reducing schemes are based on the choice of a suitable diet. Two diets, the low carbohydrate diet and a calorie counting diet, have been the traditional approaches, but neither has

been shown to be particularly effective. The low carbohydrate diet has many disadvantages, including hypotension in susceptible individuals. With Government Departments of Health now advocating as part of their Health Education programme a reduction in fat intake and an increase in complex carbohydrates, it is irrational to advocate a reduction in bread and potato intakes in the overweight; permanent reduction in sugar and fat intake is both logical for preventive health and is appropriate in view of the obese subject's propensity to weight gain on fat-enriched diets. Those dietary schemes which advocate 'eat as much fat as you like while slimming' are based on the finding that in practice a protein and fat diet given *ad libitum* with an avoidance of sugar and starch intake leads to a reduction in total energy intake. These schemes do, however, increase total plasma cholesterol and are not in the long-term interest of the patient who may attempt to continue slimming unsuccessfully for years on a diet which may be conducive to atherosclerosis and many other diseases.

Tables 9 and 10 list a variety of diets based on the two underlying

Table 9   Principal items in diets of different energy content

Addenbrooke's 7	Addenbrooke's 8
Daily allowance Wholemeal bread 3 × 25 g slices 1 pint skimmed milk Potatoes 100 g boiled or 1 large potato, baked, or 60 g rice	*Daily allowance* Wholemeal bread 3 × 50 g slices 1 pint skimmed milk Potatoes 100 g boiled or 1 large potato, baked, or 60 g rice Low fat spread 12 g, i.e. one 250 g pack of butter/margarine substitute to last 3 weeks
Breakfast ½ grapefruit without sugar or 1 orange or 1 apple or 100 g fresh orange juice	*Breakfast* ½ grapefruit without sugar or 1 orange or 1 apple or 100 g fresh orange juice
Two main meals	*Two main meals* Vegetable soup (home-made without fat)

Either   60 g poultry or game: chicken, duck, turkey (with skin removed), hare, rabbit, venison, pheasant, or pigeon
or   90 g white fish: cod, flounder, halibut, John Dory, lemon sole, ling, monkfish, plaice, pollak, skate, sole, turbot, whiting, or haddock (if smoked. use only once weekly)
or   60 g fatty fish: eel, herring, bloater, kipper, mackerel, pilchards (in tomato sauce), salmon, sardines (in tomato sauce or with oil discarded), or trout
or   60 g meat: heart, liver, kidney, tongue, lean beef, lean minced beef, lean steak, lean lamb or pork (including chops if fat discarded)
or   90 g shellfish: crab, lobster, mussels, oysters, prawns, shrimps, whelks, winkles
or 100 g cottage cheese
or   50 g cheese: camembert, cheddar, Danish blue, stilton (use no more than 5 times weekly)
or   2 eggs: (use only 3 times weekly)

| *Vegetables*
Unlimited: cabbage (savoy, red, or Dutch), cauliflower, lettuce, cucumber, beans (runner, French, dwarf, or baked), broccoli, tomatoes, brussels sprouts, winter and spring greens, marrow, celery, mushrooms, mustard and cress, spinach, asparagus, artichokes, onions | *Vegetables* (two portions per day allowed) |

or   and
50 g peas, beans (butter, haricot, or red kidney), carrots, leeks, parsnips, swedes, turnip (peas should be fresh, frozen, or canned *garden* peas only)

| *Fruit*
One piece of fruit: orange, apple, half a grapefruit without sugar, pears, plums, peaches, and all soft fruit or 100 g melon (canteloupe, honeydew, or water). No bananas | *Fruit* |
| *Unlimited*
Water, tea, coffee | *Unlimited*
Water, tea, coffee |

Approximate nutrient content		*Approximate nutrient content*	
Energy (kcal)	721	Energy (kcal)	1116
(kJ)	3075	(kJ)	4741
Protein (g)	62.7	Protein (g)	77.9
Fat (g)	6.1	Fat (g)	18.2
Carbohydrate (g)	111.4	Carbohydrate (g)	171.4
Fibre (g)	19.6	Fibre (g)	35.9
Minerals (mg)		Minerals (mg)	
Na	954	Na	1706
K	3003	K	4269
Ca	915	Ca	995
Mg	249	Mg	377
P	1190	P	1514
Fe	5.56	Fe	9.37
Zn	6.00	Zn	8.65

Table 10 Principal items in slimming diets of higher energy content

	Addenbrooke's 6	Addenbrooke's 9
Allowed freely:	Herbs, spices, mustard, pepper, vinegar, salt in cooking, dietetic (low 'calorie') squashes and fizzy drinks, soda water, clear soups, yeast and yeast extracts, stock cubes, all vegetables (for special comments on potatoes, peas, and beans, see below), saccharin, and saccharin sweeteners.	
Carbohydrate		
A. Sugars	4 pieces of fruit allowed per day. This includes natural fruit juice.	Fruit should be raw or stewed/baked without sugar.
B. Starches	6 portions from list below:	8 portions from list below:
	30 g home-made, sugar-free muesli, 2 Weetabix, 30 g wholemeal bread, 90 g potatoes (boiled or baked in skins), 60 g boiled rice or 20 g cornflour or custard powder	50 g home-made, sugar-free muesli, 2 Weetabix, 50 g wholemeal bread, 90 g potatoes (boiled or baked in skins), 60 g boiled rice or 20 g cornflour or custard powder
Protein	2 portions from list below:	2 portions from list below:
	up to 100 g lean meat, up to 150 g white fish, up to 90 g fatty fish (tuna, mackerel, etc.) or shellfish, up to 150 g cooked pulses (dried peas, beans, lentils, baked beans), 120 g cottage cheese, 60 g hard cheese, 2 eggs (not more than 4 eggs per week)	up to 75 g lean meat, up to 90 g fish, up to 150 g cooked pulses (dried peas, beans, lentils, baked beans), 90 g cottage cheese, 40 g hard cheese, 2 eggs (not more than 4 eggs per week)
Fat	20 g butter or margarine daily 300 ml (½ pint) whole milk or preferably 600 ml (1 pint) skimmed milk	20 g butter or margarine daily 300 ml (½ pint) whole milk or preferably 600 ml (1 pint) skimmed milk
Alcohol	None	Single measure of spirits with low calorie soft drink or ½ pint beer per day

Approximate nutrient content					*Approximate nutrient content*				
Energy (kcal)	1313	Minerals (mg)			Energy (kcal)	1657	Minerals (mg)		
(kJ)	5540	Na		894	(kJ)	6996	Na		1284
Protein (g)	80.0	K		3737	Protein (g)	76.0	K		4372
Fat (g)	38.1	Ca		646	Fat (g)	40.1	Ca		731
Carbohydrate (g)	173.0	Mg		319	Carbohydrate (g)	247.7	Mg		432
Fibre (g)	27.3	P		1292	Fibre (g)	36.7	P		1452
		Fe		9.59			Fe		12.53
		Zn		6.76			Zn		8.35

principles that starch and fibre intakes should be maintained while sugar and fat intakes are reduced during slimming. A number of studies have shown that if these (or any other diets) are simply issued to patients without considering their individual energy needs, their personal idiosyncrasies and their home circumstances, then early failure is usual.

A number of dietary principles are commonly enunciated by nutritionists without any demonstrable scientific basis. These include the requirement that all slimmers should have breakfast, that food should be taken in numerous small meals rather than as larger, fewer meals per day, and that specific items of food be taken at particular times during the day. These 'rules' help those individuals who delight in mystical rituals, but detract from the development of an educated view of sensible eating.

Commercial slimming organizations. There are several of these in most Western countries. They provide a reasonable service, usually at a modest cost. Research has shown that overweight and obese subjects often do better when helped by individuals in similar circumstances and there is a need for constant support during the dieting period which can often be supplied by groups. Personal and regular supervision, e.g. at two-weekly intervals for overweight and moderately obese patients, does not necessarily require a doctor who unfortunately rarely learns the skills needed to re-educate his patient's eating and activity patterns.

Despite the apparent advantages of making use of specially trained individuals for supervising slimming groups, and with most attenders not severely obese, the success of these groups is limited; about 15–20 per cent finally achieve a weight within the range shown in Table 2. Reasons for failure include the dogmatic insistence that all attenders follow the same scheme whatever their individual needs, and the failure to change the diet of the whole family rather than of the individual alone: if family food patterns do not alter then it is highly unlikely that the slimming individual can maintain a different and more appropriate diet long-term. A further reason for failure is the choice by most commercial organizations of diets relatively high in energy value, e.g. 1500 kcal (5–

6 MJ), while still expecting most subjects to have a progressive rapid weight loss on this scheme. If a patient's energy requirements are 1900 kcal (8 MJ) when obese, and these fall during slimming to perhaps 1550 kcal (6.5 MJ), it is not surprising that weight loss will be slow given that 1 kg of adipose tissue represents a loss of 7700 kcal (32 MJ). Patients, particularly those short and elderly women with a small lean body mass who are relatively inactive, may show no discernible weight loss on these diets.

Behavioural modification programmes. These have become very popular, particularly in the USA. They are based on an attempt to produce permanent changes in behaviour by involving the patient in his own management. Subjects are encouraged to examine their current pattern of living, including eating habits. Systems are then devised to give the individual greater awareness of his own behaviour and control of his activities. If eating is precipitated by the ready availability of unsuitable foods, steps are taken to ensure that these items are not purchased or are stored out of sight. Meals are organized carefully and the subject must sit down to all meals, which are then made into a ritual to ensure that the food being provided is seen as a full meal and not a minute and restricted diet. Few, if any, subjects who 'nibble' between meals while standing on their feet ever succeed in reducing their weight on a long-term basis, so the principle of sitting while eating and drinking is a key feature of this scheme.

Similarly, the obsession which patients have with weighing themselves is often best met by removing the scales completely from the home and concentrating on modifying behaviour rather than just considering weight changes. Positive encouragement is also needed: subjects learn to give themselves a bonus, e.g. a holiday with money saved on food when their reorganization has progressed through a number of steps. Displacement activity is also important to cope with times when boredom, depression, or stress are common. Too many doctors consider these approaches as mundane, but the use of simple dietary advice in association with behavioural modification programmes is proving to be the most effective medical approach for long-term success. Several of the commercial slimming clubs are beginning to adopt the behavioural modification approach.

Extreme measures. Total starvation used to be used for the inpatient treatment of severe obesity. It is rarely justified, does nothing to re-educate the patient, and may be dangerous since it induces electrolyte imbalance, particularly potassium deficiency, and a marked loss of body protein. It is almost always associated with a rapid return to the pre-starvation weight and should only be considered in exceptional circumstances. Protein-sparing modified fasts are becoming increasingly popular with the underlying principle that the provision of protein, e.g. about 70–80 g, with no carbohydrate or fat will lead to a selective loss of body fat and a preservation of body protein. Few reports have documented adequately the preservation of body protein, although there is undoubtedly far less loss of protein than that observed in starvation. Unfortunately a variety of nitrogen-containing preparations were introduced into the USA, some of which contained inadequate minerals and vitamins and several contained predominantly non-available nitrogen rather than the full range of essential and non-essential aminoacids. At least 17 patients died of cardiac arrhythmia of unknown cause and it is now suggested that these very low energy protein-based diets should only be used in research until satisfactory explanations for these observations are found. Even the use of a variety of mixed animal proteins providing only 300–400 kcal (1.3–1.7 MJ) daily has been shown to lead to cardiac irregularity when 24 hour heart recordings are used.

Surgical procedures used to combat obesity have included jaw wiring, plastic surgery, jejuno-ileal bypass, gastric bypass, gastric plication, and truncal vagotomy.

Jaw wiring has been recently introduced as a temporary measure to limit food intake. It is not suitable for edentulous patients, and must be used only in selected patients, e.g. those who must lose weight before essential surgery. Careful dental hygiene is needed while the wires are in place, the patient having to rely on liquid nutrients, e.g. 2 pints of milk with vitamin supplements while slimming. Some still manage to retain weight by ingesting large volumes of energy-rich fluid: this indicates a failure to select the appropriate patient for the procedure. Weight gain is usual once the wires have been removed and the procedure is not widely used.

Plastic surgery, e.g. an apronectomy to remove a huge fold of abdominal fat, may help the patient who is very embarrassed by his appearance, but further weight gain in other areas is then likely. Plastic surgery is usually reserved for those patients who are left with large folds of loose skin after substantial weight loss.

Jejuno-ileal by-pass (Fig. 12) has been performed on many thousand patients, particularly in the USA. The operation is not now viewed with favour because of its long-term complications. It involves the anastomosis of 35 cm of jejunum to 10 cm of ileum, the bypassed small intestine being left *in situ* in case re-anastomosis is necessary when complications develop. The operative mortality in the very obese patient varies from 1 per cent in specialist centres to 5 per cent in hospitals with little experience of this procedure. Post-operatively severe diarrhoea may develop, with profound electrolyte losses. Food is malabsorbed and hepatic enlargement with fatty infiltration of the liver is exacerbated by protein malabsorption in the early stages and a failure to mobilize triglyceride from the liver because of limited apoprotein synthesis. Hepatic damage may become evident and liver failure in the first few months may require high protein feeding or an immediate reversal of the by-pass. After 6–12 months the intestine adapts with improved absorption of protein, water, and electrolytes; faecal losses diminish but malabsorption persists. Gut overgrowth syndromes, electrolyte disturbances, renal oxalate stones, osteomalacia, and hepatic abnormalities are particularly common in the long term.

Despite the frequency of these complications, about half of the patients are very satisfied with the operation and consider it far superior to any medical therapy; the others, however, remain unwell or may be worse after surgery than before. Weight loss is almost universal provided care is taken with measuring the length of small intestine left in continuity. Few patients return to normal weight and commonly weight loss stops after one to two years at about 130–140 per cent of the optimal weights. The loss in weight depends not only on malabsorption but also on a marked reduction in food intake, the reason for which is unclear; patients learn that eating too much leads to profound diarrhoea and extremely unpleasant flatus; some feel too ill to eat too much, while others have a genuine reduction in appetite which may relate to the altered gut and changes in reflex and hormonal responses.

Gastric bypass (Fig. 12) has the advantage that it does not lead to such severe complications as the jejuno-ileal bypass. It is tending to replace the jejuno-ileal bypass. The operation in very obese individuals is still hazardous and technically difficult, but the weight loss is approximately the same as that achieved by jejuno-ileal bypass. The effect seems to depend predominantly on reducing food intake, and this may be achieved mainly by limiting the volume of food which can be eaten at a single meal.

Gastric plication is increasingly popular because stapling machines are available which facilitate the formation of a small gastric pouch. For success considerable care must be taken to preserve the lesser and greater gastric blood supply to the upper pouch which otherwise becomes ischaemic and tends to perforate; the upper pouch needs to be measured to contain only 50–60 ml and a 12 mm ring round the aperture from the upper pouch needs to be reinforced to prevent later dilatation. This operation has not been assessed in such detail as the other two procedures.

Truncal vagotomy is experimental and too few subjects have been studied to warrant its general use.

Drugs in the treatment of obesity. Drugs may be used either to limit food intake or to increase energy expenditure. Anorectic drugs have fallen into disrepute because one of the most effective agents, amphetamine, proved to be addictive. The later development of non-addictive analogues and other drugs allow a reassessment of their role.

Anorectic drugs. Figure 13 shows the small differences in the structure from amphetamine of the anorectic drugs currently in use. Most act on the central nervous system and stimulate catecholaminergic receptors. Behavioural changes are evident in addition to anorexia and the relative potency of cerebral activation and anorexia varies. Diethylpropion is one of the most widely tested agents which improves weight loss when given in conjunction with a diet. Some cerebral activation also occurs so that it may interfere with sleep. This agitation becomes obvious at higher doses but there is wide individual variability in response. Mazindol tends to lead to greater cerebral activation and all these compounds may have a thermogenic effect by acting on some peripheral catecholaminergic

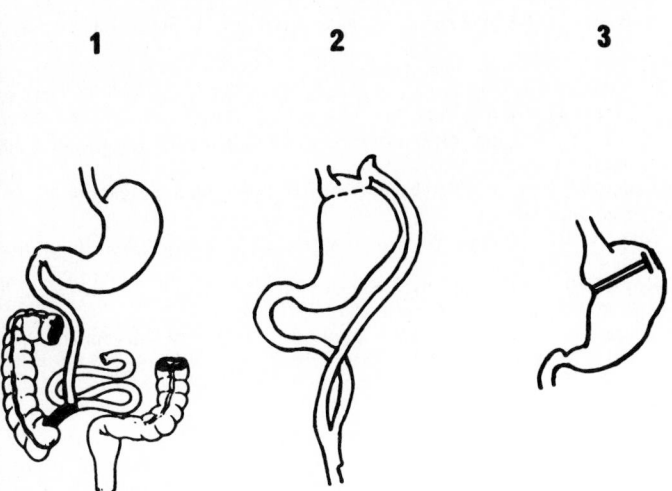

1 2 3

Fig. 12 Three of the operative techniques used in the surgical management of obesity.

receptors as well as centrally. It is often claimed that these drugs lead to habituation but there is little evidence for this; suggestions that 'tolerance' to the drug occurs has also led to inappropriate intermittent therapy. Individual adjustment of doses is necessary, and the rapidly available form of tablet preparation rather than the slow-release forms are preferable in allowing flexibility of therapy so that patients with a specific pattern of hunger at one time in the day (usually the early evening) can be treated with a single tablet at this time. The amphetamine-like drugs are rapidly metabolized so that therapy geared to dealing with hunger at specific times of the day is appropriate.

Fenfluramine differs from the other agents in not acting through the catecholaminergic system and being more slowly metabolized.

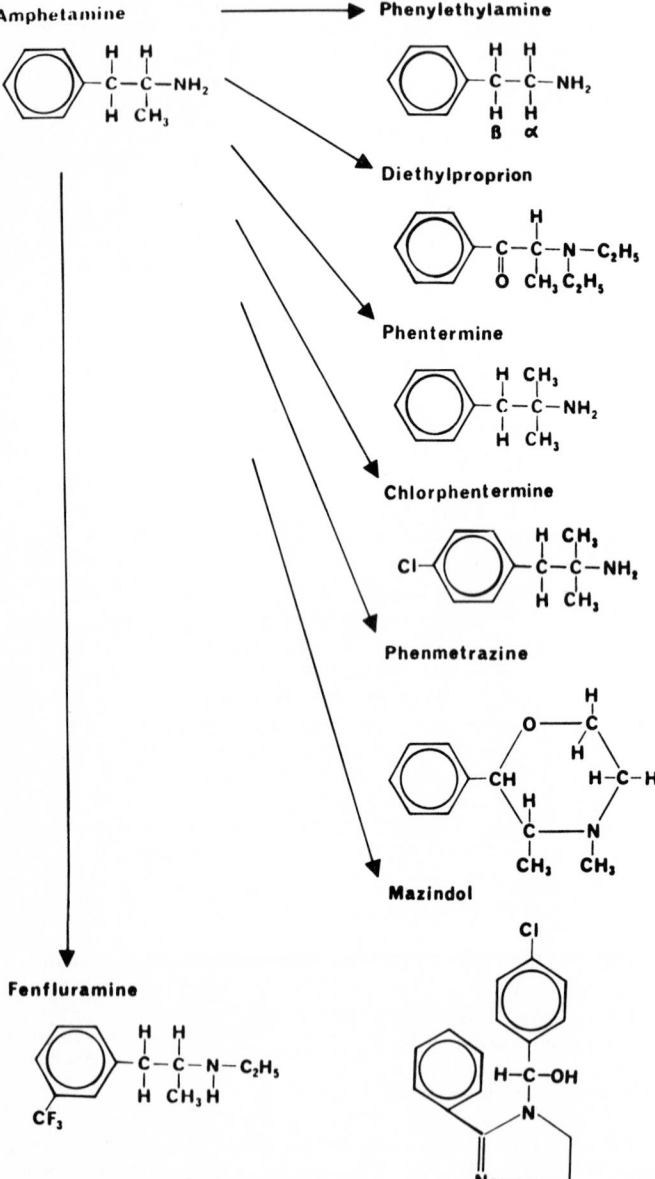

Fig. 13 The derivatives of amphetamine used commercially for their anorectic properties. Compounds on the right act via catecholaminergic systems whereas fenfluramine acts through a serotoninergic mechanism.

Fenfluramine is effective as an anorectic agent once it has been converted to norfenfluramine, but this conversion is variable and the metabolite acts on the serotoninergic rather than the catecholaminergic system. The efficiency of the drug has been shown to relate to its blood concentration and therefore to its rate of metabolism. Drug metabolism is much slower than with the amphetamine-like derivatives so therapy aimed at counteracting hunger only at specific times of the day is inappropriate. Intermittent therapy is also unwise since depression may occur if the drug is suddenly stopped.

Anorectic drugs should not be used as the sole method for treating obesity since they can only act by changing energy balance temporarily and their role should be to support appropriate dietary therapy. Continuous therapy for the duration of slimming is appropriate but should be reserved for those individuals who are persistently hungry once converted on to a slimming regimen. Diethylpropion is a cheap, short-acting drug, and is an appropriate first choice, but if it fails occasional patients may respond to another of the amphetamine-like group. Otherwise fenfluramine may be tried to combat hunger. Whichever drug is used it should be continued until weight loss no longer occurs or until a satisfactory weight is achieved.

Weight loss may stop despite both dietary advice and drug treatment. If this occurs, the drug may be withdrawn slowly to test its continued efficacy in suppressing hunger. Subsequent weight increase, despite no change in hunger or apparent food intake, may signify the usefulness of the drug in its thermogenic effects, but long-term treatment should only be contemplated if the patient is regularly assessed and care is taken to ensure that dietary advice is being followed rigorously.

Thermogenic drugs. Caffeine is regularly consumed in tea and coffee and increases metabolism. It may also suppress hunger. Other commonly consumed thermogenic agents include ephedrine taken in some herbal remedies, but unwanted side-effects, e.g. cardiac stimulation, limit its general usefulness. Other thermogenic agents acting on selective catecholamine receptors may prove more effective in the future.

Thyroid hormones have been widely used in the management of obesity but the high doses commonly used lead to protein loss as well as a reduction in body fat. Since the conversion of thyroxine (T_4) to triiodothyronine (T_3) is slowed by slimming, it is more appropriate to give high physiological daily doses of 60 μg T_3 to combat the reduction in circulating T_3 concentrations, but the usefulness and safety of this therapy is still in considerable doubt.

References

Bray, G. A. (1976). *The obese patient* (ed. L. H. Smith Jr). Saunders, Philadelphia.
— (ed.) (1979). *Obesity in America.* Proceedings of the 2nd Fogarty International Center Conference on Obesity. Washington DC. USDHEW, NIH Publication No. 79.
Garrow, J. S. (1981). *Treat obesity seriously.* Churchill Livingstone, Edinburgh.
James, W. P. T. and Trayhurn, P. (1981) Thermogenesis and obesity. *Br. med. Bull.* **37**, 43.
Jung, R. T. and James, W. P. T. (1980). Is obesity metabolic? *Br. J. Hosp. Med.* **24**, 503.
Royal College of Physicians (1982). Working Party on Obesity Report. *J. R. Coll. Physns*, in press.
Symposium on Surgical Treatment of Morbid Obesity. Hirschman, G. H. and Barton, B. T. (eds.) (1980). *Am. J. clin. Nutr.* suppl. **33**.

Special nutritional problems

R. Smith

Many clinical conditions pose special nutritional problems. Some are best dealt with under the appropriate disease headings, for example, renal disease, liver disease, diabetes mellitus, and inborn errors of metabolism. Others, particularly those associated with various forms of injury, are considered here.

Many advances in clinical nutrition have come directly from the need to understand and to treat the effects of surgery, accidental injury, and burns. Such matters are conventionally dealt with in surgical texts, but the nutrition of the hospital patient (surgical or not) is of importance to all concerned with their care.

Accidental injury and burns most often occur in well-nourished subjects (especially in times of war) whereas in contrast surgery is often carried out on patients whose body composition and response to stress has been modified by malnutrition begun outside hospital and worsened by a hospital diet; and the effect of malnutrition may be further complicated by sepsis, cancer, and prolonged immobility. These factors combine to produce a clinical picture far more complex than that resulting from simple food deprivation, but this complexity may go unrecognized. Since it is the injured and post-operative patient who most often requires specialized means of nutrition, it is important first to summarize the biochemical effects of injury on the body; the account which follows should be compared with that of normal metabolism (see page 8.4).

Surgery and accidental injury. The effects of elective surgery and of mild to severe accidental injury produce a continuous spectrum of biochemical change directed towards survival. Modern elective surgery is often so small an insult to the body that the metabolic changes it produces are insignificant; in contrast multiple injuries, such as those produced by road traffic accidents, lead to considerable biochemical disturbances proportional to their severity. The so-called 'metabolic response' to injury is the result of many factors which can only be outlined here; recent detailed reviews are available (see references).

First and most important is the effect of the injury itself, which produces powerful afferent stimuli of pain, blood loss, volume depletion, and tissue damage. Second is the response to these stimuli, with important hormonal and biochemical changes which lead to the provision of readily utilizable metabolic fuels such as glucose, fatty acids, and ketone bodies. These changes are often less in the elderly and the malnourished, and the endocrine response appears to be smaller in women than men. Third is the effect of variable food deprivation, leading to a reduction in the intake of nitrogen and energy-providing substrates; and fourth is the effect of immobility which causes loss of muscle and skeletal mass and which may be prolonged. To these may be added the complications of sepsis (see page 8.44) or burns (see page 8.45).

The biochemical effects of injury are not those of starvation, despite some similarities between them (Table 1). In particular injury is characterized by an increase in circulating catecholamines and cortisol, by initial hyperglycaemia, and by a greater eventual loss of nitrogen than in starvation alone. The amount of weight subsequently lost will vary according to the degree of starvation and the severity of the injury. Weight loss will be more rapid in total starvation than in uncomplicated injury, but will be most where injury and starvation are combined.

In general the biochemical effects of an injury are related both to its severity and nature. Thus after accidental injury the amount of nitrogen lost is proportional to an injury severity score (see page 8.44); and it increases in the following order—elective surgery, multiple injuries, sepsis, and burns.

Table 1 Similarities and differences between the effects of injury and starvation

	Total starvation	Injury	Starvation and injury
Weight loss	++	+	+++
Nitrogen loss	+	++	+++
Blood glucose	↓	↑	↑
Blood alanine	↓	↓	↓
Blood BCAA*	↑	↑	↑
Endocrine response			
Catecholamine	↓	↑	↑
Cortisol	↓	↑	↑
Insulin	↓	↓ (early)	↓
Metabolic rate	↓	↑	↑↑
Ketonaemia	++	variable	variable
Water and sodium	early loss	retention	retention
Potassium loss	+	++	+++

* Branched chain amino acids—leucine, isoleucine, and valine

Clearly the weight loss resulting from injury and starvation will be more than that from either alone. Nitrogen loss is a reflection of the gluconeogenesis which occurs early in all these conditions; in the starving subject this falls with increasing utilization of fat

It is useful to divide the time after injury into the phases originally proposed by Cuthbertson (Fig. 1). In the immediate 'ebb' phase the body is reacting to the injury; there is a fall in temperature and in energy production and expenditure; and rapid hormonal changes occur appropriate to survival. During this phase necrobiosis and death may occur. In survivors this is followed by a 'flow' phase in which metabolic processes accelerate and energy production, metabolic rate, and temperature increase, leading to eventual recovery with catabolic giving way to anabolic processes. These processes have been better defined in animals than in man; their duration differs with many factors, and particularly the severity of the injury. Many metabolic studies have been done in the initial ebb phase, and some attempt has been made to relate the biochemical changes in this phase to the subsequent outcome.

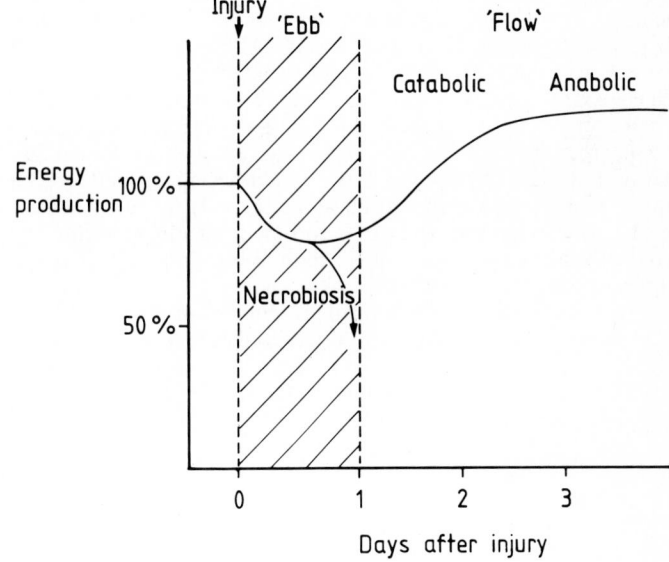

Fig. 1 A diagram of the phases after injury. The time scale is variable and the phases merge into each other.

Metabolic changes in injury. The best known biochemical changes after injury are an increase in blood sugar and in urinary nitrogen, both reflections of net protein breakdown and increased gluconeogenesis. There may also be an increase in lipolysis and in ketone body production. Considerable changes also occur in fluid and electrolytes which are particularly relevant where intravenous nutrition (see page 8.48) becomes necessary.

Water and electrolytes. Following injury there is a retention of water in excess of sodium and a dilutional hyponatremia. This is partly due to an increase in secretion of antidiuretic hormone and may be associated with potassium deficiency. However, this relatively simple picture is likely to be confused by loss of fluid and blood and by their intravenous replacement. If the effects of injury are prolonged and recovery is delayed the composition of the body may alter considerably, with an increase in water relative to both lean body mass and body weight, and a continuing loss of intracellular electrolytes such as magnesium, potassium, and zinc. The causes of these changes are not fully understood; but in practice it is important to remember that after surgery or injury hyponatremia rarely means sodium deficiency and that during recovery from such trauma the composition of the patient can no longer be regarded as normal.

Protein and amino acids. Urinary nitrogen excretion, which reflects net protein loss (see Fig. 8, page 8.10), is greatest on the second and third day after injury. Nitrogen loss is most marked after severe injury in a previously fit young adult; it is exaggerated by infection and reduced in the elderly and by an increase in the external temperature to the thermoneutral zone (28–32 °C). Its extent is not always appreciated; the loss of 15 g of nitrogen per day (which is not unusual, especially where surgery and semi-starvation are combined) is equivalent to nearly 100 g of protein, much of which will come from skeletal muscle. Theoretically such a loss may be due either to increased protein catabolism or to decreased synthesis. Current isotopic measurements of protein turnover and of 3-methylhistidine excretion (see page 8.10) suggest that after elective surgery the main early change is a decrease in synthesis of protein without any significant increase in its breakdown. Severe injury, in contrast, also increases protein catabolism, if only from damaged tissues, and produces a significant increase in the excretion of 3-methylhistidine. The relationship between protein synthesis and catabolism presumably alters during recovery.

Important changes occur in the circulating concentration of amino acids. That of alanine, the main precursor for gluconeogenesis (see page 8.10) tends to fall after the first day; in contrast the concentration of the branched chain amino acids may remain considerably increased. The concentration of both of these amino acids is highest after the most severe injuries and when ketone body levels are not increased. Although the changes in circulating amino acid levels are similar to those in starvation, their cause is probably different. The increase in circulating branched chain amino acid concentration after surgery and injury is related to the degrees of protein loss and appears to reflect net protein breakdown. Recent work has concentrated on the changes which occur in the protein of muscle and of the whole body. However, there are also well documented increases in specific circulating proteins, the so-called 'acute phase reactants', soon after injury, but their significance is not known.

The consequences of prolonged protein loss are deleterious but difficult to define. Apart from loss of weight and muscle tissue, there is often an impairment of immunity with increased susceptibility to infection, delayed wound healing, generalized weakness, and hypoproteinaemic oedema. Importantly, continuing loss of nitrogen appears to increase mortality rate.

Fat and ketone bodies. The effects of injury on triglyceride metabolism and ketone body production are not fully understood. It seems that some subjects produce ketone bodies in response to injury or surgery whilst others do not. Whether this represents an inbuilt or acquired difference is unknown. However, protein loss appears to be less in hyperketonaemic subjects than in others. This could be due to a possible inhibitory effect of ketone bodies on proteolysis.

The main immediate stimulus to lipolysis after injury is an increase in catecholamine concentration, associated with a deficiency of insulin relative to that of glucagon. Recent work suggests that hepatic ketogenesis may also be reduced by an increase in the circulating levels of vasopressin. It is important to know what factors control the production and utilization of ketone bodies after surgery and injury since the survival of a patient could depend on the use of adipose tissue fat rather than muscle protein as an energy source. Interestingly there is now evidence that in some circumstances 'hypermetabolic' patients with sepsis and injury may utilize endogenous fat despite a continuing supply of intravenous glucose.

Hormones. After injury, and less markedly after elective surgery, the combined effect of changes in hormones is to stimulate the breakdown of protein, fat, and carbohydrate and to increase the production of metabolic fuels, in particular glucose. There are early increases in circulating concentrations of catecholamines, cortisol, and vasopressin and a similar rise in glucagon. A temporary lack of insulin in relation to glucagon contributes towards lipolysis and hyperglycaemia; there is also an apparent resistance to the effect of insulin with a reduction in the insulin–glucose ratio. The extent of these hormonal changes, particularly in cortisol, is roughly proportional to the degree of injury. There are alterations in other hormones but their significance is not clear; these include growth hormone, thyroxine, and probably endorphins. The increase in growth hormone may have an anabolic effect and that of cortisol a catabolic one; but the main hormonal determinants of the metabolic changes after injury appear to be catecholamines, insulin, and glucagon. Damage to the tissues will also stimulate the production of locally acting substances such as prostaglandins.

The severity of injury. The biochemical changes are related to the type and severity of injury whose effects are in part due to the afferent stimuli they produce. Thus the relatively minor metabolic effects of elective surgery may be due to the partial removal of pain. Extensive epidural anaesthesia, and possibly some synthetic opiates, considerably reduce the biochemical effects of surgery. It is difficult to measure accurately the severity of an injury, although quantitative methods have been devised by summating the severity of injuries from different defined parts of the body to produce an 'injury-severity score'. When such scores are compared with biochemical and hormonal changes, injury-severity is related directly to the initial circulating concentration of cortisol, pyruvate, and alanine, and inversely to concentration of ketone bodies. Subsequent nitrogen loss is also significantly related to injury-severity.

Immobility. The mass of both the skeleton and of voluntary muscle appears to depend on the mechanical stress to which they are subjected, although the underlying mechanisms are unknown. Most patients lose mobility for a variable time after injury. After a minor operation such as hernia repair, this may be of no significance, but after the multiple fractures of a road traffic accident immobility produces widespread effects. Those on the skeleton have been mentioned elsewhere (see Section 17); there is a fall in the rate of new bone formation relative to that of resorption, with a negative calcium balance and hypercalciuria. Muscles of immobilized limbs rapidly waste, but it is not clear whether this is due to a failure of synthesis or to an increase in breakdown. Neither the skeletal nor muscular wasting can be satisfactorily reversed or prevented until mobility is restored, and for this reason it is very difficult to maintain muscle mass, whatever form of nutrition is used, in the immobile patient. Other effects of immobility, such as venous thrombosis, urinary and pulmonary infections are well known.

Sepsis. Infection is a common complication of injury. It is known to increase the negative nitrogen balance and to worsen the prognosis, but knowledge of its other biochemical effects is fragmentary. The few measurements of 3-methylhistidine excretion suggest that myofibrillar breakdown is increased, and of respiratory quotient that endogenous fat may sometimes be utilized as a fuel source in preference to exogenous glucose.

Burns. The most extreme biochemical and hormonal changes are found in patients who have been burned. This represents a severe form of injury to which is added the important feature of excessive fluid loss. Protein losses are also large, and the increase in basal metabolic rate is prolonged and proportional to the area of surface burnt. Infection is common. Energy requirements are so high that they may be very difficult to supply.

Nutrition of the hospital patient. The nutrition of medical and surgical patients is an everyday hospital problem. Like so much else in nutrition it is taken for granted until particular problems or gross disturbances occur. It is becoming increasingly clear that the nutritional status of patients admitted to hospital is often poor and that subsequent treatment may accentuate this. Therefore the nutritional problems of the hospital patient, especially the surgical one, start before admission and continue until after discharge. Treatment before and after surgery often calls for the provision of additional fuel which may be provided through the gastrointestinal tract (enteral nutrition) or by partial or total intravenous feeding (parental nutrition). Recent studies have suggested that a significant percentage of patients are undernourished before admission to hospital and that more than 50 per cent of them have signs of malnutrition before they leave it. Observations have been made mainly on patients with gastrointestinal disease and those with cancer, before or during treatment, but malnutrition does occur in other groups. Starvation in hospital can be attributed to reduction in food intake due to a combination of fear, apprehension, and gastrointestinal symptoms. Additionally the diet provided in hospital may be unbalanced, and deficient in calories, protein, and vitamins. For the patient unable to tolerate solid food this is commonly in the form of jellies, soups, and similar preparations. Intake may also be considerably reduced during periods of investigation, and by the prolonged hypocaloric infusions which often follow surgery.

Even very simple measurements of the nutritional state of hospital patients are often not done; as an example, surveys have suggested that patients are only occasionally weighed. It is especially important to assess the nutritional state of surgical patients in order to estimate their likely nutritional needs and to prevent further malnutrition. Nutrition may be clinically assessed (Table 2)

Table 2   Measurements used as evidence of protein energy malnutrition

Weight loss	more than 10%
Mid-triceps skinfold thickness	less than 10 mm (men)
	less than 13 mm (women)
*Arm muscle circumference	less than 23 cm (men)
	less than 22 cm (women)
Serum albumin	less than 35 g/l
Serum transferrin	less than 2 g/l
Lymphocyte count	less than 1500/μl
Impaired cell-mediated immunity (delayed hypersensitivity)	negative skin tests to candida, PPD, mumps, streptodornase, streptokinase

* For derivation see text

by the measurement of body weight, triceps skinfold thickness (an indication of fat stores), and mid-arm muscle circumference. This last indicates muscle mass; it is equal to the arm circumference (measured at the same level as the triceps fold thickness) minus the product of π and the triceps skinfold thickness. Although it is widely used, it can only be an approximation, since muscle mass must be affected by many factors other than nutritional ones, including age, body size (particularly height), and physical activity.

Likewise to use an isolated measure of triceps skinfold thickness as an index of nutritional status would be unwise. More useful is the information derived from skinfold thicknesses in various parts of the body (see page 8.28).

Biochemical measurements commonly used to indicate protein energy malnutrition include plasma albumin and transferrin. Undernutrition is also said to alter the immune response, to depress the lymphocyte count, and to produce a reversible suppression of delayed hypersensitivity reactions but these changes have little clinical usefulness.

The nutritional significance of different anthropomorphic and biochemical measurements is not fully agreed upon. For example, in a recent study of surgical patients in an American hospital there was a close correlation between arm muscle circumference and serum albumin; but weight–height ratio was not found to be a useful index of malnutrition. Superficially, overall weight or the ratio of weight to height might be expected to be related to nutritional status. In practice weight is not often recorded; and the changes in it have so many causes that it is difficult to separate them. It is also possible for an overweight person to have a reduced lean body mass. However, in a United Kingdom study of surgical patients low body weight, arm muscle circumference, and plasma albumin tended to occur together with a high frequency. Measurements of the urine creatinine–height ratio can also provide a useful index of muscle mass. The serum albumin concentration is a valid indicator of severe protein energy malnutrition but its intravascular concentration may be maintained during short periods of malnutrition and it may also be reduced for non-nutritional reasons by gastrointestinal loss, liver and kidney disease. Short-term reduction of energy and protein intake may thus be better detected by measurement of rapid turnover transport proteins such as thyroxine-binding prealbumin and retinol-binding protein. Jeejeebhoy has recently pointed out the usefulness of measurements of total body nitrogen, which may not necessarily be closely related to total body potassium, as an additional more sophisticated nutritional index. All these measurements are designed to detect protein energy malnutrition, but it is also important to look for anaemia and specific vitamin deficiencies. This is particularly so in the elderly patient who is often housebound, and in whom lack of vitamin D, iron and less often vitamin C may occur.

Nutritional requirements. The nutritional requirements of a patient are both quantitative and qualitative. Normal energy requirements, the effect upon them of activity, and the safe intake of protein have been summarized (see Tables 1 and 2, page 8.4). Of the 40 or so essential nutrients all must be supplied regularly and where possible on a daily basis; and tissue maintenance, repletion, and nitrogen balance will be defective if any of them is lacking. The correct amount of an essential nutrient may not be known, even for a normal subject, but if the minimal requirement is known, this should be given.

In the group of micronutrients (which contrasts with the macronutrients carbohydrate, proteins, and fat), particular attention should be paid to the vitamins, trace elements, and essential fatty acids. The recommended daily intake of vitamins (Table 3), and minerals and trace elements (Table 4) are taken from a variety of sources. The stated requirements for vitamins are often approximate, and few preparations contain them all. In the trace elements, zinc, copper, chromium, and manganese are all essential, and zinc deficiency often occurs in patients with gastrointestinal disease. Lack of trace element is of particular importance in patients on prolonged parenteral nutrition (see page 8.48); it should also be remembered that trace elements given in excess can be toxic. When zinc or copper are being given intravenously, their circulating concentrations should be regularly measured; and since zinc and chromium are excreted via the kidneys and copper and manganese through the biliary tract it is important to take malfunction of these organs into account. Lack of the essential fatty acids, linoleic and arachidonic, has often been reported in patients who are fed paren-

Table 3　Recommended daily intake of vitamins for a 70 kg adult

	Water Soluble									Fat Soluble			
	Thiamin* B_1 (mg)	Riboflavin* B_2 (mg)	Niacin* (nicotinic acid) (mg)	Pyridoxin B_6 (mg)	Folate (mg)	Vitamin B_{12} (µg)	Pantothenic acid (mg)	Biotin (mg)	Ascorbic acid (mg)	Vitamin A (µg)	Vitamin D (µg)	Vitamin K (µg/kg)	Tocopherol (mg)
Oral†	1.4	1.6	18	2.2	0.4	3			60	1000	5		10
Intravenous‡	3.0	3.6	40	4.0	0.4	5	15	60	100	1000	5	0.03–1.5	10

* The requirements increase according to energy intake
† From National Academy of Sciences (1980)
‡ From American Medical Association (1975)
Modified from Grant and Todd (1982)

Table 4　Recommended daily intake of mineral and trace elements for a 70 kg adult

	Calcium (mmol)	Phosphorus (mmol)	Iron (µmol)	Magnesium (mmol)	Zinc (µmol)	Manganese (µmol)	Copper (µmol)	Chromium (µmol)	Fluorine (µmol)	Iodine (µmol)	Selenium (µmol)	Molybdenum (µmol)
Oral*	12		180	12	82–165	54	31–84	95–190				
Intravenous† ‡	7–14	14–70	21–70	7–28	49–210 38–90	7–35 2.7–14.4	5–70 7.5–22.5	1 0.19–0.29	49	1–7	0.4	0.2

* From Department of Health and Social Security (1979) and World Health Organization
† From Shenkin and Wretlind (1977)
‡ From American Medical Association (1979)
In general the UK recommendations are less than those from the USA
Modified from Grant and Todd (1982)

terally. Only the first is normally provided by the diet, but it is converted to arachidonic acid which is essential for membrane function and is a precursor of the prostaglandins.

Provided that specific deficiencies of micronutrients can be avoided, the most important aspect of nutrition is to provide the correct amount of nitrogen and energy-containing metabolic fuels in the form of protein, carbohydrate, and fat. Although there are various ways in which this can be done it should be noted that a complex relationship exists between nitrogen and energy balance which is altered by nutritional depletion and trauma. In normal subjects nitrogen balance will be increased by an increase in energy balance, provided that the nitrogen intake is adequate; and in the normal adult in a steady state increasing nitrogen intake will not increase nitrogen balance if the energy balance is zero. In contrast a nutritionally depleted subject can achieve a positive nitrogen balance if given sufficient nitrogen even though the energy balance is zero. Such relationships between nitrogen balance and fuel supply are dealt with by Elwyn. In assessing the nutritional needs of surgical patients the requirements differ according to the degree of nutritional depletion, and to the resting energy expenditure. In nutritionally depleted patients, often with considerable and recent weight loss, the main aim is restoration of lean body mass, with or without fat. In the patient who has an increased resting energy expenditure (hypermetabolism) and considerable nitrogen loss (hypercatabolism), for instance after severe accidental injury, the situation is by no means clear. Although it appears logical to provide both a high nitrogen and high energy intake, to compensate for protein depletion and for the increased energy expenditure, there is some evidence that such patients may continue to utilize fat. It is suggested that under such circumstances the overenthusiastic administration of glucose which is not utilized may lead to excessive glycogen deposition, increased glucose oxidation, and increased resting energy expenditure.

Thus the guidelines to treatment are not so simple as might be expected. In the post-operative patient the main aim is to prevent the loss of lean tissue; and if the patient is unable to eat properly in five to seven days after operation, total parenteral nutrition should be started. Amino acids should be given at a rate of 200–300 mg of nitrogen per kg body weight daily, with glucose and fat in roughly isocaloric amounts to provide a total energy intake equal to expenditure. The nutritionally depleted patient should be given more nitrogen (300–400 mg of nitrogen per kg daily) and more energy-containing fuel (50 per cent above estimated resting energy expenditure) again in the form of equal amounts of fat and glucose. Such a regimen should restore tissue mass in the ratio of lean body mass to fat of approximately 2:1. The severely injured hypermetabolic patient who is also hypercatabolic clearly requires an increased intake of both nitrogen and energy. Intake of the former is suggested at 400–500 mg of nitrogen per kg per day; in view of the possible deleterious effects of excessive glucose, the recommended energy intake is moderate, at about 25 per cent above the resting energy expenditure.

Enteral and parenteral nutrition. Since most evidence shows that protein energy malnutrition reduces immunological competence, increases the incidence of sepsis, delays wound healing, and reduces patient survival, its detection and correction is important. This is particularly so in surgical patients and in those with cancer and gastrointestinal disease. Protein and energy-providing substrates may be given by mouth or by tube feeding (enteral nutrition), or, when enteral feeding is impossible, by the intravenous route (parenteral nutrition). In the practical decision whether or not to feed parenterally there are situations where an inadequate nutritional intake for a short period only (as after operation) is preferable to complicated attempts to feed. In all patients it is important to consider: (*a*) the previous food intake, both over the last 24 hours and the previous few weeks; (*b*) the need for more nutrition; (*c*) the possibility of enteral feeding; and (*d*) the need for parenteral nutrition.

Enteral nutrition. Where the gastrointestinal tract is available, enteral feeding is always preferable to parenteral nutrition. Enteral feeding includes feeding by mouth, by tube, and through a gastrostomy, duodenostomy, or jejunostomy. Many of the indications for enteral feeding (Table 5) are the same as those for parenteral nutrition, but the enteral route should be used wherever possible since it requires less attention, is less costly, and has fewer complications—particulary sepsis. Enteral feeding may be useful in patients with inflammatory bowel disease, and to provide supplemental nitrogen and energy after burns. Nutritional alternatives available are food by mouth (liquidized where necessary), standard hospital tube feeds, and proprietary enteric feeds. The latter in-

Table 5   Indications for enteral feeding*

In gastrointestinal disease
Short bowel syndrome
Malabsorption syndrome
Gastrointestinal fistulae
Granulomatous disease of the gastrointestinal tract
As a supplemental source of nitrogen and energy in several catabolic states, particularly burns
As an adjunct to cancer therapy

* Where it is not possible to use the gastrointestinal tract these are also indications for parenteral feeding

Table 7   Examples of daily energy and nitrogen requirements in the adult

	Starving (non-catabolic)	Catabolic	Hypercatabolic
Nitrogen (g)	7.5	15	25
Total kcal	2000	3000	4000
Approximate ratio of non-protein kcal/nitrogen	250	200	135

These figures are approximate and based on those necessary to maintain nitrogen equilibrium. Hypercatabolic patients include injured patients with sepsis, and those with extensive burns

clude whole protein preparations and elemental diets. Elemental diets have chemically defined constituents and originate from diets developed for use in the American aerospace programme (hence 'space diets'); they are not palatable enough for oral use without modification. They are also hypertonic and tend to cause diarrhoea so that if given at all they should be sufficiently diluted and preceded by a 'starter' regimen. The use of elemental diets, rather than whole protein enteric feeds, is declining; they are considered only when hydrolysis within the gut lumen is severely reduced, as in pancreatic failure, or where the absorptive capacity of the small intestine is very defective, as in the short bowel syndrome. Early commercial (non-elemental) feeds were high in protein and also produced diarrhoea because of their hypertonicity. More acceptable preparations which are virtually isosmotic, contain soya protein isolates, corn or soya oil or MCT (medium chain triglyceride) oil, corn syrup solids, and caseinates.

For enteral feeding it is important that the preparations should be easily prepared and economical; that the requirements, particularly of nitrogen, should be previously assessed; that attention be paid to water and electrolyte balance; and that the essential biological elements and water-soluble vitamins are included. In practice the use of proprietary enteric feeds is often preferable to their manufacture within the hospital pharmacy or preparation in the hospital diet kitchen. Table 6 gives examples of some commercially available solutions. Of those available, Isocal, Clinefeed, and Ensure are good general purpose tube feeds; the last is the most palatable but also the most hypertonic. Flexical and Vivonex are both elemental feeds but of different composition; the place of elemental diets in enteral nutrition is currently being reassessed. The nitrogen requirement for a moderately catabolic patient may be estimated at 15 g or more daily, and the regimen for enteral (or parenteral) feeding can be devised on this basis (Table 7). Nitrogen will normally be given as protein, with the exception of elemental diets which contain mixtures of amino acids. Some amino acids are now known to be better absorbed in peptide form so that pure amino acids preparations may offer no nutritional advantage. Energy must always be given with nitrogen and the usual recommended ratio between the two is about 200 non-protein kcal to 1 g of nitrogen.

With enteral feeding the provision of energy may depend more on carbohydrate and less on fat than for parenteral nutrition. To increase the fuel provided by carbohydrate without increasing tonicity the glucose polymer Caloreen may be used which has an average chain length of 5 molecules. When fats are used, at least some can be given in the form of medium chain triglycerides (MCT). These are hydrolysed in the lumen of the gut and directly absorbed into the portal blood via the small intestinal mucosa; in contrast long-chain fatty acids are reesterified in the intestine to form chylomicrons which are then transported via the lymphatic system and thoracic duct into the circulation. Medium chain fatty acids are also relatively water soluble. For the differences in hepatic metabolism between fatty acids with long chains, and those with medium or short chains, see Fig. 10, page 8.11. In practice provided that tube feeding is introduced slowly (over two to three days) and that the constituents are given sufficiently diluted at room temperature through narrow tubes, it is possible (although rarely necessary) to give up to 4000 kcal and 200 g of protein in about 4 litres of water daily. Some complications of enteral feeding are given in Table 8.

Table 8   Some complications of enteral nutrition

Mechanical
Tube insertion: Misplacement and oesophageal problems (inflammation, erosions, stricture)
Regurgitation and aspiration
Gastrointestinal
Diarrhoea and vomiting
Abdominal pain and distention
Metabolic
Hyperglycaemia
Low circulating levels of K, P, and Zn
Low red cell folate
Hypoprothrombinaemia
Deficiency of essential fatty acids

The mechanical problems of tube insertion are particularly prominent if a wide inflexible tube is used, and diarrhoea is most troublesome with hypertonic elemental feeds. For these reasons protein solutions given through narrow bore tubes are to be preferred

Table 6   Examples of some solutions available for enteral feeding (approximate composition per 2000 kcal in 2 litres)

	Isocal	Clinifeed 1S0	Ensure	Flexical	Vivonex
Protein (g)	65	56	70	45	42
Fat (g)	84	82	70	68	2.9
Carbohydrate (g)	250	260	274	305	260
Approximate osmolality (mosmol/kg water)	300	270	380	550	550
Protein source	Na caseinate soya protein isolate	milk whey protein	casein soya protein isolate	casein hydrolysate plus amino acids	synthetic amino acids
Fat source	MCT oil, soya oil	vegetable oil butter fat	corn oil	MCT oil, soya oil	safflower oil
Carbohydrate source	glucose, oligo-saccharides	malto-dextrin	corn syrup solids sucrose	corn syrup solids tapioca starch	glucose

MCT = medium chain triglycerides
For electrolytes, trace elements and vitamin composition see Philips and Odgers (1980) and Grant and Todd (1982)

In patients who are unconscious, or cannot protect their airway if they vomit, a tube large enough to allow aspiration of gastric contents is essential. In others a fine bore silastic tube is more comfortable and less likely to lead to oesophagitis.

Parenteral nutrition. Parenteral nutrition may vary from short periods of intravenous therapy given, for instance, after surgery, to more prolonged provision of nitrogen and energy either as a supplement to other forms of nutrition or on its own (complete or total parenteral nutrition). In the former the need is mainly for fluid and electrolytes and it is traditional to provide energy in the form of glucose; however, there is a vogue for the use of amino acids (see below). More prolonged total parenteral nutrition has proved its usefulness in many clinical situations but it should be given only with specific indications when enteral nutrition is impracticable. Predictably the indications for parenteral nutrition are very similar to those for enteral feeding (see Table 5), with the addition of temporary post-operative feeding when the gastrointestinal tract is not available. Parenteral nutrition has proved particularly useful in upper gastrointestinal fistulae, in patients with cancer, and in improving resistance to infection. Long-term parenteral nutrition has been used especially in patients with severe granulomatous disease of the bowel, and in the short gut syndrome. In specialized units total parenteral nutrition may be given successfully to outpatients. Parenteral feeding should not be regarded merely as the provision of an intravenous meal; it should not be undertaken lightly, and it has many complications. Since it bypasses the gut and the nutrients are not modified by digestion, it is easy to produce side-effects. The important constituents provided by parenteral nutrition are protein, readily utilizable energy containing substrates, water, electrolytes, and essential biological or trace elements.

Protein. Nitrogen is given in the form of amino acids, either as protein hydrolysates or more frequently as mixtures of synthetic L-amino acids. Hydrolysates of protein such as casein (Aminosol) have a significant amount of their total nitrogen in the form of small peptides; synthetic amino acid solutions are therefore preferable but are more expensive. Plasma, or protein fractions derived from it, should not be given primarily to provide nitrogen and energy but as a temporary measure to maintain the circulating fluid volume. Amino acids given on their own produce a more positive nitrogen balance than glucose alone. It has been suggested that this relative advantage of amino acids arises from the lower insulin concentrations and greater availability of ketone bodies than with glucose alone, but the evidence for this is not convincing. The addition of glucose to an amino acid regimen certainly does not reduce its protein sparing effect and it is common practice to give the nitrogen and non-protein energy sources together.

The amount of nitrogen required can be decided arbitrarily or from measurement of nitrogen losses, assuming that the urinary urea nitrogen accounts for about 80 per cent of the total urine nitrogen. As with enteral nutrition, a moderately catabolic patient can be considered to require 15 g of nitrogen daily or 0.20 to 0.24 g of nitrogen per kg body weight. Table 9 gives some help in calculating intravenous nutritional requirements; further details can be found in the reference list. The choice of an appropriate amino acid solution may be difficult since of those available none has particular advantages. Trials of the effectiveness of different amino acid mixtures have shown that the nitrogen balance obtained depends more on the nitrogen and energy input than on the composition of the infused solution. Some amino acid solutions are incomplete, lacking aspartic or glutamic acid, or cystine, or serine or tyrosine. One complete formulation is Vamin N (Nutramin N); in this preparation the essential amino acids form 41 per cent of the total, and the branched chain amino acids 19 per cent. It has been suggested that essential amino acids should constitute about 30 per cent of the total amino acids in adults and about 40 per cent in children. There is certainly little evidence that giving an excessive proportion of essential amino acids, branched chain amino acids, or ketoacids, is therapeutically advantageous. However there are occasions in

Table 9   The calculation of intravenous nutrient requirements

Nitrogen	0.20–0.24 gN/kg body weight
Energy	40–50 kcal/kg body weight
Energy/nitrogen ratio	about 200:1
Energy source	glucose and fat emulsion equally
Sodium	8 mmol/gN
Potassium	5 mmol/gN
Magnesium	1 mmol/gN
Calcium	0.5 mmol/gN
Phosphorus	0.5–0.75 mmol/kg body weight
Other requirements	water-soluble vitamins
	vitamin A, D, and K
	essential trace elements; Zn, Cu, Mn, etc

This table gives the approximate nutritional requirements of a moderately catabolic adult who requires about 15 gN daily. Fluid requirements vary widely. In practice 2–3 l daily are infused in most patients. The electrolyte requirements are also considerably dependent on daily losses. The concentration of electrolytes may not be sufficient in commercially available solutions such as those containing synthetic amino acids. More magnesium is required where gastrointestinal fluid loss is considerable, and more phosphate where the daily energy input is more than 3000 kcal

renal and hepatic disease and in paediatric practice when solutions of particular amino acid composition are required. Finally in selecting an amino acid solution it is important to take note of the electrolyte composition; for instance many such solutions do not contain phosphate.

Energy sources. The ideal intravenous energy source should be rapidly utilized and have no abnormal side-effects. A number have been tried and a mixture of glucose and fat is probably the best. Since glucose provides about 4 kcal/g it is necessary to administer a hypertonic solution to achieve an acceptable intake of energy. Patients will tolerate 300–400 g of glucose a day but at this intake some will require exogenous insulin. Fat is most often given as an emulsion of 10 or 20 per cent soya bean oil (containing 2–5 per cent glycerol and egg yolk phosphatides as an emulsifier) in a preparation called Intralipid. Most of the early objections to fat emulsions have now been removed, but they are contra-indicated in patients with hyperlipidaemia. Their advantages are a high energy content (1000 kcal per 500 ml of a 20 per cent solution), low osmolality and the prevention of essential fatty acid deficiency. Intralipid can be given in amounts up to 2 g/kg body weight daily, or approximately one third of the non-protein energy intake, over 6–8 hours; it should not be stored frozen or mixed with other solutions.

In patients receiving parenteral nutrition it is important to monitor whether the glucose or fat is being properly utilized. Four-hour urine testing and daily blood sugar measurement are necessary to detect glycosuria and hyperglycaemia. If the plasma glucose consistently exceeds 10 mmol/l, insulin is probably required; and if the plasma is lipaemic six hours after the fat infusion has been discontinued this suggests that the lipid is not being properly metabolized. A fat overload syndrome with hyperlipidaemia, gastrointestinal disturbance, hepatosplenomegaly, and haematological abnormality with spontaneous bleeding can occur. Previously a number of other non-protein energy-providing substrates used as alternatives to glucose produced troublesome side-effects; examples of these include the lactic acidosis of fructose sorbitol ethanol combinations; and the hyperuricaemia, oxaluria, and hyperbilirubinaemia which may follow xylitol. As in enteral nutrition, energy-containing substrates and nitrogen should be given together.

Differences of opinion remain about the best way to provide non-protein fuel. Most centres in the United Kingdom give fat as well as glucose but elsewhere glucose alone is still widely used. In view of the reported hepatic and respiratory problems produced by the administration of excessive amounts of glucose in hypermetabolic patients and in those with poor respiratory reserve, this metabolic fuel may need to be used with more caution in future.

Water and electrolytes. The amount of fluid required varies considerably with losses, especially from the intestine which may be difficult to estimate. Whilst 2–3 l per day is normal, up to 6 l may be needed where losses are excessive. Nutritional requirements and the need for some drugs to be given by separate infusion, or for fluids to maintain a central venous line impose an obligatory minimum input which can cause difficulty in the presence of heart disease or renal failure.

Other constituents. These include minerals such as calcium and phosphate, the essential biological or trace elements such as zinc and copper, and vitamins. The requirements for phosphate are often underestimated, and hypophosphataemia may impair white cell function, contribute to muscle weakness and produce osteomalacia. The trace elements which have been proven to be essential for man are zinc, copper, manganese, iodine, chromium, iron, and cobalt. Selenium deficiency syndromes have been described in man. During long-term parenteral nutrition, especially in patients with gastrointestinal disease, deficiency of these elements is likely to occur, and is not adequately replaced by intravenous preparations. Trace element solutions are available to correct these deficiencies, and if given in the correct formula and amounts, they are without side-effects. Unless supplemented, the most frequent deficiency is that of zinc; it is not commonly recognized that the requirements for zinc are quantitatively of the same order as those for iron.

Many, but not all, vitamins are provided in parenteral nutrition solutions. The majority contain the B group (thiamine, riboflavin, nicotinic acid, and pyridoxine), pantothenic acid, and ascorbic acid, but no other water-soluble or fat-soluble vitamins. In short-term parenteral nutrition deficiencies of vitamins A or D and of E or of B_{12} are unlikely to develop. In contrast folic acid deficiency can develop rapidly. Care needs to be taken in the administration of vitamins because of their probable instability in parenteral nutrition solutions. Thus vitamin K, folic acid, and vitamin B_{12} are often given by weekly intramuscular injection; and if water-soluble vitamins are given in parenteral solutions they should be added immediately before use.

Administration and monitoring. The number of solutions for parenteral nutrition need not be large. They can be administered by different routes. The two main alternatives are peripheral and central venous lines. A central venous line is unnecessary for short periods of intravenous therapy with electrolyte, glucose, and amino acid solutions, but is needed for longer periods of complete parenteral nutrition. The percutaneous infraclavicular approach is often preferred and a subcutaneous tunnel may be made for the catheter so that the site of entry through the skin is some distance from that into the vein; strict asepsis, radiography to check that the catheter tip is in the superior vena cava and to exclude a pneumothorax, and subsequent monitoring, are important. There should be regular measurements of infusion rate and fluid balance; daily measurement of body weight and of plasma urea, creatinine, electrolyte, and glucose concentrations; and less frequent plasma measurements of such elements as calcium, phosphorus, and magnesium. Other measurements in such patients should include tests of hepatocellular function, blood counts, urine urea and electrolytes, urine and serum osmolality, and of acid–base balance. Most parenteral nutrition teams have a basic formula made in the hospital pharmacy from commercially available solutions. The standard regimen used for adults in Oxford provides 2350 kcal and and 3.0 l of fluid per day; 0.5 l of 20 per cent intralipid is given over six to eight hours, and the non-fat constituents, containing 250 g glucose and 14 g nitrogen in 2.5 l from a single separate container continuously over 24 hours. Folic acid and water-soluble vitamins of the B complex in the form of parenterovite, are given daily with the non-fat constituents. Electrolytes, trace elements, and fat soluble vitamins are given according to requirements.

Effectiveness. On the whole parenteral nutrition works well, may prevent continuing weight loss, and can produce significant clinical improvement. An increase in well being, an increase in weight without oedema, correction of the reduced levels of short half-life proteins such as transferrin, production of a positive nitrogen balance, improvement in wound healing with reduction of infection, and an improvement in skin fold thicknesses are all reported

beneficial therapeutic effects. In contrast some studies suggest that in severely catabolic patients parenteral feeding merely prevents further nutritional deterioration. It may be that parenteral nutrition is more beneficial when given before surgery than after it, but this has been difficult to prove. Undoubtedly it can be life saving when correctly administered; but because of the attention it requires, which may not be available in the wards of a general hospital, there are good reasons for it to be carried out by a parenteral nutrition team which should include a physician and/or surgeon, a dietitian, a trained nurse, and a pharmacist. With such an approach complications can be reduced to a minimum. This particularly applies to long-term parenteral nutrition and parenteral nutrition at home, where complete metabolic homeostasis may be maintained for years.

Complications. The complications of parenteral feeding are mechanical, septic and metabolic (Table 10). Mechanical complications depend on which intravenous route is used, and sepsis limits the length of time parenteral nutrition can be continued. The metabolic complications arise from a number of causes. These are mistakes in water and electrolyte balance, giving rise to over or underhydration, to hyponatraemia or hypernatraemia, and to changes in osmolality. Others include the incorrect use of energy-providing substrates, giving too much glucose without insulin, or excessive amounts of fat; the use of inappropriate substrates such as fructose and xylitol; the failure to provide adequate amounts of basic constituents, particularly phosphorus; the failure to balance the components in a parenteral nutrition regimen; and deficiency of essential biological elements such as copper, zinc, and essential fatty acids.

Table 10   Some complications of parenteral nutrition

Mechanical
Pneumothorax; catheter embolus; air embolus
Septic
Thrombophlebitis; septicaemia
Metabolic
Errors in water and electrolyte balance
Inappropriate use of energy substrates: excess glucose; excess fat
Use of inappropriate substrates
Fructose, xylitol, sorbitol, ethanol
Failure to provide individual constituents
Failure to balance constituents
Absolute deficiency syndromes: for example, copper; zinc; essential fatty acids
Other: metabolic bone disease

Of the specific deficiencies following parenteral nutrition that of copper is seen most often in paediatric practice; leucopaenia, anaemia, and bone disease may occur. Deficiency of zinc may occur in patients with copious diarrhoea or large intestinal losses from fistulae. Zinc is important in protein synthesis and nucleic acid metabolism. To correct severe deficiency up to 80 mg of zinc sulphate daily intravenously has been suggested. Zinc deficiency may be associated with apathy, depression, and alopecia. A nasolabial rash and bullous or pustular lesions on other parts of the face, hands, feet, and the groins is described. A form of bone disease whose exact cause is unknown can also occur in patients on parenteral nutrition (see Section 17) and the effects of phosphate deficiency have been mentioned. Deficiencies of chromium, manganese, selenium, vitamin D, and biotin have also been described. The importance of zinc and other trace elements is fully discussed by Golden and Golden.

In summary although patenteral nutrition is widely used, problems of its safe administration and effectiveness still remain. The provision of large amounts of energy containing fuels does not ensure therapeutic success; the relative use of glucose and fat as fuel sources remains controversial; the overadministration of glucose may lead to hyperglycaemia, to excessive glycogen and fat deposits in the liver, and to the overproduction of CO_2 which may be troublesome in patients with a poor respiratory reserve; and electrolyte and trace element deficiency remains a constant hazard where gastrointestinal losses are considerable.

Nutrition and cancer. The nutritional management of cancer patients may often be difficult. Cancer can be associated with rapid weight loss, loss of muscle bulk and of subcutaneous fat, weakness and tiredness, and sometimes an increase in the basal metabolic rate, features which are generally considered to be those of 'neoplastic cachexia'. It should come as no surprise that there is a high incidence of protein energy malnutrition in patients with advanced cancer, even though its cause is not fully understood. This has been assessed by methods used for surgical and other patients (see Table 2) including the urine creatinine–height ratio. The ability to withstand anticancer therapy, and the overall prognosis, appears to lessen in proportion to weight loss, and to be increased by adequate nutrition.

Neoplastic cachexia is often associated with anorexia and can be largely attributed to reduced energy and protein intake. However, the loss of weight in cancer may be more complex than this. It is stated that the resting metabolic rate of patients with solid tumours is usually within the normal range, but that there is a discrepancy between the reduced energy intake and continuing energy utilization. It is not established whether utilization of the endogenous sources of fuel is altered, or whether such fuel is derived mainly from muscle (which could lead to weakness and wasting) or from fat.

Many biochemical studies done on tumour-bearing animals show abnormalities not found in man. In the human neoplastic cachexia, with an inappropriately high energy expenditure in the presence of a reduced energy intake, is associated with a tendency to hyperglycaemia and insulin resistance, and a two to three fold increase in Cori cycle activity, and according to some, increased lipolysis. Protein loss has been attributed to both decreased synthesis and increased breakdown. The commonest change in mineral metabolism is hyponatremia, probably dilutional in origin. The cause of these changes is unknown, but at least some may be due to the production of hormonally active peptides by the tumour.

Descriptions of the effects of parenteral nutrition in neoplastic patients vary in their enthusiasm. It has been suggested that to provide energy and protein to the patient with a neoplasm merely feeds the tumour, but there is little evidence to support this. In contrast parenteral nutrition often improves the physical and psychological well being of the cancer patient, improves the immune response (which is often impaired), and facilitates anticancer therapy. Whilst it seems self-evident that the cancer patient will do better (with or without antineoplastic treatment) if properly fed, prospective controlled trials on the effects of parenteral nutrition in patients with cancer are now being done. Some early results in children show that weight may be maintained during treatment but falls as soon as parenteral nutrition is stopped; so that three months after the end of a course of radiotherapy there is no detectable difference between those children given or not given parenteral nutrition. Not least of the nutritional problems in neoplastic disease is to decide how vigorous should be attempts to provide protein and energy for the patient with advanced cancer.

Nutrition and burns. Adequate nutritional treatment of the burned patient is very difficult. Burns may double the metabolic rate and considerably increase the loss of protein until the burnt surface is healed. The degree of hypermetabolism is related to the type and extent of the burn; it is most with full thickness skin loss and increases with burn size up to about 40 per cent of the body surface area. Without adequate nutritional support such a severely burnt patient will lose about 30 per cent of his body weight in three weeks and almost certainly die. As in other forms of stress the outcome is affected both by the previous nutritional state and the occurrence of complications, particularly infection and renal failure. The severity of the nitrogen loss may also be somewhat reduced by minimizing afferent stimuli such as pain and hypovo-

laemia, and by nursing at an ambient temperature of 30 °C with high humidity. Large amounts of nitrogen and energy need to be given; a simple formula for protein which takes into account the age of the patient and extent of the burn is 1 g/kg body weight plus 3 g for each percentage burn for adults and up to 3 g/kg plus 1 g/percentage burn for children. There are technical and metabolic difficulties in following this advice in young children. Energy should be supplied in the normal approximate ratio of 200 non-protein kcal/g of nitrogen. In badly burned patients this represents a considerable bulk of food which cannot be taken orally but can often be given (at least in part) by a narrow nasogastric tube. In this situation parenteral feeding is restricted to those with disturbed gastrointestinal function, with severe facial or nasal burns, and in those who require nutritional supplementation in addition to that provided orally. In severe burns intravenous therapy is also necessary in the immediate period of resuscitation and for several days afterwards. It is particularly in the severe catabolic state produced by burns that the administration of insulin in addition to glucose reduces nitrogen loss and corrects hyponatremia.

Nutrition and pregnancy. Pregnancy can produce specific nutritional problems, of which those of iron, folate, glucose and carbohydrate are considered briefly elsewhere (see Section 11). There are also important changes in overall energy requirements and in fat and protein metabolism. The metabolic changes which occur during pregnancy have nutritional implications; for a full review the reader is referred to Hytten and Chamberlain.

A previously held view of the nutritional effect of pregnancy was to regard it as a form of stress, in which the fetus behaved as an intra-uterine parasite imposing its metabolic requirements on those of an otherwise normal adult. This oversimplified approach ignores the fact that the metabolic changes induced by pregnancy occur long before the conceptus is large enough to make significant demands on maternal resources. It has also been pointed out that these changes are too widespread, complex, and fundamental to be produced by stress alone; and the evidence is that (at least until the last weeks of the pregnancy) maternal and fetal tissues are both in an anabolic state.

During pregnancy additional maternal and fetal tissues are laid down, and there are also energy requirements for the extra metabolism of pregnancy. Together these account for the extra nutritional costs of pregnancy. The increase in maternal tissues begins early and the cumulative total of protein and fat deposited in the fetus and maternal body during pregnancy has been estimated at 925 and 3825 g respectively. The increase in maternal fat (some 3.5 kg) is particularly striking, and has an animal equivalent in hibernation or before migration.

The daily increment of protein during late pregnancy which is required for structural purposes, is some 6 g, corresponding to an additional daily requirement of some 8.5 g in the diet. During the third quarter of pregnancy the main demands for energy come from the deposition of maternal fat; the rate of this deposition declines in the last quarter, but the increase in fetal tissues continues. The energy needs are greatest in the middle of pregnancy, when relatively large amounts of maternal fat are being laid down. In late pregnancy the average estimated additional daily requirement of energy of 250 kcal may be largely compensated by a reduction in physical activity, without any increase in dietary intake. Physiological measurements provide a background for the recommended dietary allowances during pregnancy. Although these are variable, it is generally true that the recommendations for energy and nutrients have become smaller as knowledge of the physiological effects of pregnancy has increased.

Of the widespread hormonal changes which occur during pregnancy, those which affect calcium metabolism are of particular importance. In the last ten weeks of pregnancy the fetus obtains approximately 18 g of calcium from maternal sources. This additional calcium appears to come from an increase in the intestinal absorption of calcium, associated with an approximate doubling of the circulating concentration of 1,25-dihydroxycholecalciferol, rather than from the maternal skeleton. The maternal skeleton is presumably also protected by the observed increase in calcitonin levels during pregnancy. Supplementation of the maternal diet with vitamin D is only indicated in those populations known to be at risk of vitamin D deficiency; thus pregnant Asian immigrants should be given 500 i.u. (12.5 μg) of vitamin D daily.

Osteoporosis can occur during or after pregnancy (see Section 17); whether there are significant abnormalities in calcium-controlling hormones in such patients is unknown.

References

American Medical Association. Department of Foods and Nutrition (1975). Multivitamin preparations for parenteral use. *J. enteral parenteral Nutr.* 3, 258.

American Medical Association. Department of Foods and Nutrition (1979). Guidelines for essential trace element preparations for parenteral use. *J. Am. med. Ass.* 241, 2051.

Askenazi, J., Rosenbaum, S. H., Hyman, A. I., Silverberg, P. A., Milic-Emili, J., and Kinney, J. M. (1980). Respiratory changes induced by the large glucose loads of total parenteral nutrition. *J. Am. med. Ass.* 243, 1444.

Bistrian, B. R., Blackburn, G. L., Hallowell, E., and Heddle, R. (1974). Protein status of general surgical patients. *J. Am. med. Ass.* 230, 858.

Cancer (1979). *Cancer* 43, May suppl.

Department of Health and Social Security (1979). Recommended daily amounts of food energy and nutrients for groups of people in the United Kingdom. *Report on Health and Social Subjects*, 15.

Elwyn, D. H. (1980). Nutritional requirements of adult surgical patients. *Critical Care Med.* 8, 9.

Grant. A. M. and Todd. E. (1982). *Enteral and parenteral nutrition: a clinical handbook*. Blackwell Scientific Publications, Oxford.

Grant, J. P. (1980). *Handbook of total parenteral nutrition*. W. B. Saunders, Philadelphia.

Golden, M. H. N. and Golden, B. (1981). Trace elements. Potential importance in human nutrition with particular reference to zinc and vanadium. *Br. med. Bull.* 37, 31.

Hill, G. L., Blackett, R. L., Pickford, I., Burkinshaw, L., Young, G. A., Warren, J. V., Schorach, C. J., and Morgan, D. B. (1977). Malnutrition in surgical patients. An unrecognised problem. *Lancet* i, 689.

Hytten, F. E. and Chamberlain G. (1980). *Clinical physiology in obstetrics*. Blackwell Scientific Publications, Oxford.

Jeejeebhoy, K. N. (1981). Protein nutrition in clinical practice. *Br. med. Bull.* 37, 11.

Johnston, I. D. A. and Lee, H. A. (1978). *Developments in clinical nutrition*. Proceedings of a Symposium at the Royal College of Physicians, London, October 1978. MCS Consultants.

Karren, S. J. and Alberti, K. G. M. M. (1980). *Practical nutritional support*. Pitman, London.

Koretz, R. L. and Meyer, J. H. (1980). Elemental diets—facts and fantasies. *Gastroent.* 78, 393.

Lancet (1980). Nutritional management of enterocutaneous fistulas. *Lancet* i, 507.

Lee, H. A. (1974). *Parenteral nutrition in acute metabolic illness*. Academic Press, London and New York.

Munro, H. N. (1979). Hormones and the metabolic response to injury. *New Engl. J. Med.* 300, 41.

National Academy of Sciences (1980). *Recommended dietary allowances*, 9th edn. Committee on Dietary Allowances, Food and Nutrition Board, National Academy of Sciences, Washington, D.C.

Nixon, D. W., Heymsfield, S. B. Cohen, A. E. Kutner, M. H., Ansley, J., Lawson, D. H., and Rudman, D. (1980). Protein calorie undernutrition in hospitalized cancer patients. *Am. J. Med.* 68, 683.

Phillips, G. D. and Odgers, C. L. (1980). *Parenteral and enteral nutrition. A practical guide*. New Zealand.

Richards, J. R. and Kinney, J. M. (eds.) (1977). *Nutritional aspects of care in the critically ill*. Churchill Livingstone, Edinburgh.

Shenkin, A. and Wretlind, A. (1977). In *Nutritional aspects of care in the critically ill* (eds. J. J. Richards and J. M. Kinney), 345. Churchill Livingstone, Edinburgh.

Shetty, P. S., Jung, R. T., Watrasiewkz, K. E., and James, W. P. T. (1979). Rapid turnover transport proteins: An index of subclinical protein-energy malnutrition. *Lancet* ii, 230.

World Health Organization (1973). *Trace elements in human nutrition*. Technical Report Series no. 532, WHO, Geneva.

Anorexia nervosa

G. F. M. Russell

The most obvious clinical manifestation of anorexia nervosa is general undernutrition associated with marked weight loss. Since the earliest descriptions of anorexia nervosa there has been much interest in its possible relationship to endocrine disorders. At one time confusion reigned because it was thought that destruction of the anterior pituitary caused loss of weight and emaciation, so-called Simmond's cachexia. This mistaken view still lingers today and may give rise to unnecessary investigations of endocrine function when the diagnosis of anorexia nervosa should be obvious. The illness does include an endocrine disturbance, but it is specific and confined to the hypothalamic–anterior pituitary–gonadal axis. It is also essential to recognize that the loss of weight is self-induced and that there is a characteristic psychological disorder.

Typical anorexia nervosa in the female

Aetiology, psychopathology, and pathogenesis. Although the fundamental cause of anorexia nervosa is unknown, the psychopathology underlying the illness and the hypothalamic disorder associated with the amenorrhoea have become more clearly understood. It has been proposed that anorexia nervosa is a self-protective device employed by a vulnerable young girl who dreads the prospect of growing up, leaving home, becoming independent, or coming to terms with her sexuality. These conflicts may be caused by and are certainly aggravated by tensions within the family, especially disturbances between the parents. These ideas are rendered plausible by the common setting of the illness in young girls soon after puberty, for whom changing expectations from modern society might appear particularly bewildering. They are consistent with the increase in the incidence of anorexia nervosa within western cultures during the past thirty years. Theander has reported a five-fold increase in Malmö, Sweden, from the 1930s to the 1950s. Kendell and his associates found a higher incidence in Britain in recent years, which they estimated as 0.6 to 1.6 per 100 000 of the entire population per year. Anorexia nervosa is now commonly recognized among certain groups at special risk: 1 in 250 among schoolgirls in England aged 16 and over (Crisp *et al.* 1976), 6 per cent of ballet students in Canada (Garner and Garfinkel 1978). These findings suggest that culturally determined attitudes contribute to the genesis of anorexia nervosa. The illness is commoner among upper social classes, but no social class is exempt.

The nutritional disorder in anorexia nervosa reflects mainly a prolonged insufficient intake of carbohydrate foods. The tissue lost from the body is composed of over three times as much adipose tissue as other cellular (non-fatty) tissue. In a study of refeeding anorectic patients the surplus calories required to restore lost weight amounted to 7500 calories per kilogram. The relative preservation of protein in the body is probably due to the initial large adipose stores in the female. Levels of plasma amino acids are normal and vitamin deficiencies are surprisingly uncommon. Serum cholesterol may be raised, possibly for dietary reasons (e.g. a high intake of cheese).

The psychological disturbances in anorexia nervosa are much in evidence, and a psychogenesis for at least part of the illness is undoubtedly present. Patients will often give strongly held reasons for curtailing their food intake. They may feel guilty after eating. More often they express a fear that they will lose control over their eating and become odiously fat. Associated with this fear is a disturbance of body image causing the patient to feel and see herself as fat, in spite of her painfully obvious thinness. The disturbance is also demonstrable experimentally as a tendency for the patient to overestimate the width of her body. This distorted perception of fatness leads the patient to starve herself further in an attempt to gain more acceptable proportions. Paradoxically the faulty perception of body size increases as she loses weight, hence a self-perpetuation of the starvation and a further preoccupation with body size.

The endocrine disturbance in anorexia nervosa which results in amenorrhoea is specifically a disorder affecting the hypothalamic-anterior pituitary-gonadal axis. When the patient presents in an undernourished state, blood levels of luteinizing hormone (LH), follicle-stimulating hormone (FSH), and oestradiol are found to be abnormally low. The primary site of the disturbance is in the hypothalamus, since the administration of synthetic gonadotrophin-releasing hormone (LHRH) results in a rise in plasma LH and FSH, indicating that the anterior pituitary remains responsive. Recovery occurs slowly in the course of treatment leading to weight gain. First plasma FSH and LH levels rise. Next the hypothalamus begins to respond to the negative feedback effects of oestrogens and progesterone secreted by the ovaries. This can be shown by a rise in plasma LH following the administration of clomiphene, a drug which blocks the negative feedback action of the gonadal hormones on the hypothalamus. Finally there occurs a positive feedback effect of oestrogens on the hypothalamus; this can be shown by administering a high dose of oestradiol over three days and observing a peak rise in plasma LH. It is at this stage, usually when normal nutrition has been restored for some weeks, that cyclical menstruation and ovulation are resumed.

There is a complex relationship between the psychological, nutritional, and endocrine disorders in anorexia nervosa. The most likely chain of events is that the patient's abnormal attitude to her body size leads to the avoidance of food and the loss of weight, which in turn causes amenorrhoea. But poor nutrition is not the only explanation for amenorrhoea, for in a substantial proportion of patients this symptom precedes the loss of weight. An additional factor may be an interference of hypothalamic function mediated through the psychological disturbance at the onset of the illness. Self-perpetuating mechanisms are also at play: for example, the psychological symptoms are themselves aggravated by the undernutrition. In spite of much research it is still not clear to what extent the eating disorder in anorexia nervosa can be attributed to a disturbance of hypothalamic function. It is clear, however, that the psychological and physical disorders are closely interwoven, and that it is a crude over-simplification to interpret the illness as having either a purely psychological or physical basis.

Clinical features. The patient is usually a girl aged 14–17 years who has only recently gone through her puberty. The illness may occasionally precede puberty, or occur at a later age up to the menopause. The patient begins to follow a 'slimming diet', avoiding foods such as bread, pastries, potatoes, or sugar. She exercises excessively and walks in preference to travelling by public transport. These alterations of habit may initially be mistaken for healthy pursuits. When questioned about them the girl will persuasively argue that she wishes to look like a friend or sister whose figure appears more slender and desirable. She may say that an acquaintance has teased her about fatness. More searching questions will often reveal that she has recently suffered an emotional upset such as a family bereavement, an acute illness, or the stress of

school examinations. The emotional difficulties may be of longer standing and the result of serious tensions within the family. The patient's initial weight would probably be within the normal range (50–60 kg). The parents may not have been aware of any problems until they observe that their daughter's weight has fallen to 45 kg and that her menses have ceased. In a minority of patients amenorrhoea may coincide with the initial loss of weight or even precede it. Over the course of the next three to six months there may be a further loss of weight down to 35 kg or less. The patient may still fail to understand the concern of others though restlessness, irritability, and preoccupation with school studies will have become apparent. If the girl had a boyfriend, she is likely to have lost interest in him and withdrawn from other social contacts. When pressed she may admit to symptoms of depression, insomnia, difficulty in concentration, and sensitivity to cold. It may be only at this late stage that she will reluctantly acquiesce to entreaties from her parents to seek medical advice.

Mental state. The patient is likely to minimize her problems and question the need for treatment. She attempts to justify her wish to become thin and her need to exert a precise control over her eating in order to avoid becoming fat. She expresses a dread of fatness, not only for aesthetic reasons but also because she would feel ashamed of herself. For example, she may feel that to be fat is incompatible with social success. She may also express sensitivity about the appearance of a particular part of her body, e.g., her stomach, hips, thighs, legs, or, less often, her breasts. The patient may deny that she looks thin and may even assert that her wasted limbs look fat to her. An assessment of her over-valuation of thinness can be made by asking her what weight would be 'right' for her. Her answer will be expressed as a precise threshold which she would be unwilling to exceed and this level will fall markedly below her previously healthy weight. It is commonly found that the patient is anxious about her sense of individuality, often expressed as a wish to become independent from her parents and to leave home, but with a fear of the consequences. Depressive symptoms are common and may be severe. Obsessional ideas are often concerned with the food eaten and a precise count of calories may be kept.

Physical examination. The patient's weight will be markedly below normal. Physical examination will reveal severe or gross wasting involving mainly subcutaneous fat with resulting hollowness of the cheeks, stick-like limbs, shrunken breasts, a flat belly, and wasted thighs and buttocks. Bony points stand out sharply. The hands and feet are blue and cold to the touch, especially at times of cool weather. The skin is dry with an excess of downy hair (lanugo) over the nape of the neck, cheeks, forearms, and legs. The heart rate is slow (50–60 per min) and the blood pressure low (e.g. 90/60 mm Hg)

Investigations. Plasma levels of LH, FSH, and oestrogens are low or undetectable. It is worthwhile estimating plasma electrolytes, especially if self-induced vomiting or purging is suspected, when the potassium level in particular may be found to be low. A blood count is also advisable, since a normochromic anaemia may coincide with refeeding, but the initial haemoglobin level is likely to be normal. Other laboratory investigations are unnecessary. A slight reduction in thyroid activity, or elevations in plasma growth hormone or cortisol may be recorded, but these changes rapidly disappear as soon as the undernutrition becomes corrected.

Typical anorexia nervosa in the male. Anorexia nervosa is relatively uncommon in the male with an incidence one-tenth to one-twentieth that in the female. There is a close similarity in the age of onset, the psychopathology, and other clinical features. The main difference is in the mode of expression of the endocrine disorder in the male: recently acquired sexual interest and potency will have declined or disappeared. Plasma LH and testosterone levels are low.

With an early age of onset there is a greater risk of undernutrition causing a delayed puberty and a retardation of growth, the age of normal physical maturation being later in the male than in the female. The undernutrition is more likely to be a combination of calorie and protein deficiency in view of the smaller stores of adipose tissue in the male.

Diagnosis of typical anorexia nervosa. The regular association of a triad of clinical disturbances provides the essential criteria for the diagnosis of anorexia nervosa in its typical form.

1. There is *considerable weight loss* resulting mainly from the patient depriving herself of foods she considers 'fattening' (i.e. rich in carbohydrate content). Weight loss may be accentuated by additional devices such as self-induced vomiting or purging or excessive exercise.

2. There is a *specific psychopathology*: the patient clings tenaciously to the idea that fatness is a dreadful state to be avoided at all costs. Her definition of fatness is uncommonly harsh and she sets herself a weight threshold which she will not exceed.

3. *The endocrine disorder* differs according to sex. In the female amenorrhoea occurs at an early stage of the illness. In the male there is a loss of sexual interest and potency.

Treatment of typical anorexia nervosa. There are three main aims in the treatment of anorexia nervosa: (*a*) to obtain the patient's confidence and some measure of cooperation; (*b*) to restore the patient's weight to its previously healthy level; and (*c*) to shorten the duration of the illness and reduce residual disability. Although there is no specific treatment available the results of a general management are highly rewarding.

As a rule better results are obtained by admitting the patient to a psychiatric unit, but many patients seek to avoid a psychiatric referral as part of a denial of their emotional problems. General physicians are of course capable of supervising the necessary regime, but should resist the common temptation of prolonged and useless searches for endocrine or intracranial disease. In most patients the diagnosis is straightforward. Most patients will require in-patient treatment for at least six weeks and the therapeutic effort should be concentrated on refeeding the patient. There is no simple drug treatment to achieve the desired result, and the admitting physician must accept responsibility jointly with his nursing staff for a carefully structured and diligently applied regime.

During the initial stage of treatment the doctor uses his skills to establish a good relationship with the patient and her family. It is often clear from the outset that the patient requires treatment in hospital, but two or three outpatient interviews may be needed to persuade her to accept admission voluntarily. In this way a compulsory admission can usually be avoided, but in a small proportion of cases it is justified to invoke the powers of the Mental Health Act, if the patient's life and health are to be safeguarded.

During the phase of in-patient treatment the principal aim is to restore the patient's weight to its previously healthy level. The patient's food requirements are often underestimated. It has already been seen that a surplus calorie balance of 7500 cal (31.5 kJ), is needed for each kg of weight gain. For the first 7 to 10 days only a moderate food intake of 1500–2000 cal (6.3–8.4 kJ) daily is provided in order to avoid the rare but dangerous complication of gastric dilatation. Thereafter the patient is asked to consume approximately twice the intake of a normal adult (3000–5000 cal, 12.6–21 kJ, daily). The resulting positive energy balance should amount to 1500–3000 calories daily, which will lead to a daily gain in weight of 200 to 400 g, with a steeper initial rise due to selective water retention. Figure 1 shows a typical response of a 19-year old patient whose weight over the course of seven weeks rose from 36 to 53.5 kg. The photographs in the colour plate section show the patient before and after treatment.

The refeeding regime naturally requires more than the physician prescribing a high calorie intake. He should train his nursing staff to become skilful in persuading the patient to accept a healthy

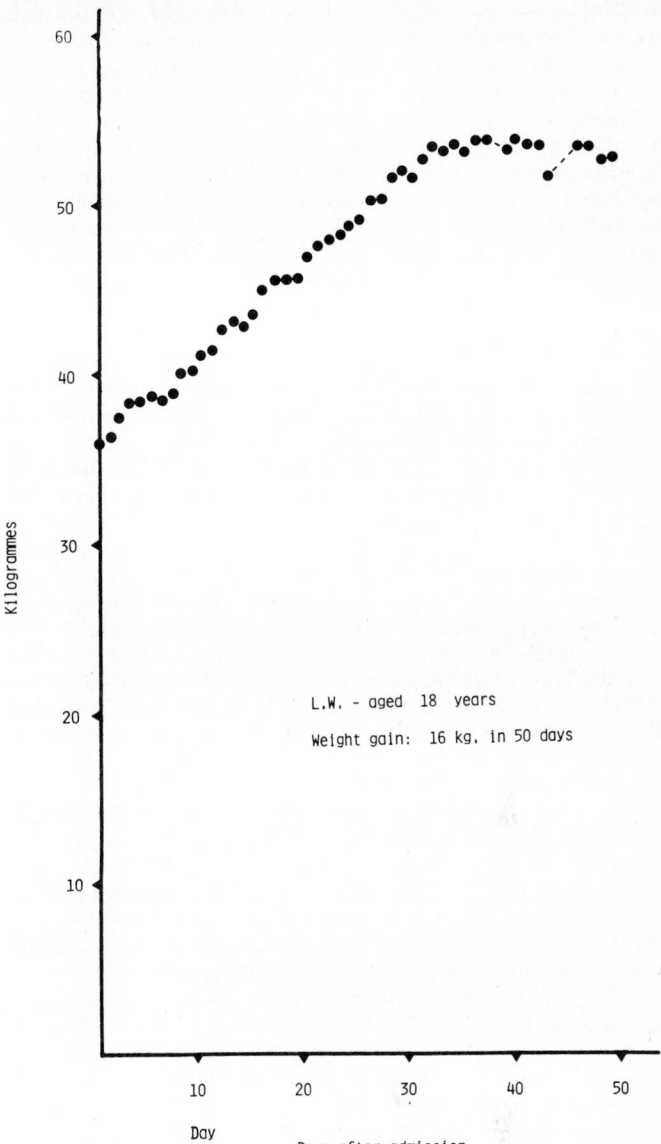

Fig. 1 Weight chart of a 19-year old patient showing weight gain during seven weeks of treatment.

weight. The nurse needs to become familiar with the psychopathology of anorexia nervosa, including the conflicts and distress experienced by the patient, and the risk that she may avoid weight gain by concealing food, inducing vomiting, or exercising. The nurse's main task is to establish a relationship of trust with the patient. She will express sympathy with her preoccupations about her weight, and offer to become responsible for the choice of food and its amount. She will promise that the refeeding will fall short of inducing 'fatness', but avoid the trap of committing herself to any limit in weight that the patient may stipulate. No false bargains may be entered into. As the patient gains weight and expresses sensitivity about 'acquiring a fat stomach', the nurse reassures her that the weight will later become generally distributed. The patient is complimented on regaining her good looks as soon as her emaciation is corrected, and is encouraged to care for her hair and use cosmetics. The patients are asked to buy new clothing to fit the healthier figure. The nursing care should concentrate on friendly support rather than inquisitorial supervision. The patient will give up attempts to discard food when she becomes aware that the nurses will discover such deceptions. The basic supervision needed to discourage subterfuges is to confine the patient to the ward and for the nurse to remain present at meal times, chatting amiably to her, until the whole meal has been consumed. Body weight is the best index of progress and should be recorded each morning before breakfast. Within five to eight weeks it should be restored to its former level. A moderate normochromic anaemia may develop during refeeding but becomes corrected spontaneously. The characteristic psychological symptoms diminish or disappear in most patients including the preoccupation with body size. This paradoxical psychological improvement may be due partly to the correction of the debilitating effects of undernutrition and partly to the exposure of the patient to her former body size and convincing her of its acceptability. During the inpatient stay it is important to initiate appropriate psychotherapeutic support which will become the mainstay of treatment after leaving hospital.

The long-term phase of treatment is aimed at preventing relapses and reducing morbidity. At the least the patient must be followed up and weighed at two-weekly intervals; she is strongly urged to maintain regular eating habits and a healthy weight. If possible, she should receive supportive psychotherapy and an attempt should be made to resolve any psychological conflicts which may have led to her illness. An important area to explore is the young girl's hesitations about achieving independence from her family, a theme well discussed by Bruch. The frequency of disturbed relationships within the families of anorexic patients has led some therapists to treat the family as a whole, with the aim of promoting more healthy patterns of family interaction and reducing the patient's need to solve the family's problems by starving herself. This method has had some success in the early stages of treatment but so far there is no proof that this or any other form of long-term treatment is effective in modifying the course of anorexia nervosa and its eventual outcome.

Endocrine treatment is indicated only occasionally. The patient who maintains her weight will usually menstruate spontaneously within two to twelve months. In the case of delays one or two courses of clomiphene (50–100 mg daily for 7 days) may be effective. The administration of hypothalamic gonadotrophin-releasing hormone (LHRH) is effective in inducing menstruation and ovulation even in patients of low weight but fails to produce any overall benefits. It is therefore indicated only in cases of amenorrhoea persisting in spite of weight gain.

Prognosis. The course of the illness is variable but often lasts two or three years or even longer. Relapses may occur after successful weight gain in hospital. Nevertheless the eventual prognosis is reasonably good with some two-thirds of patients recovering or making a fairly good adjustment. There is a small but definite mortality rate (about 5 per cent), mainly due to suicide. A proportion of patients who fare badly enter a chronic phase of bulimia nervosa.

Bulimia nervosa

A minority of patients with anorexia nervosa do not recover but enter a chronic phase of the illness with an altered clinical picture. This is called bulimia nervosa because one of its main features is the recurrence of gross overeating.

Pathogenesis and psychopathology. It is uncertain why the bulimic patient should crave for food and suffer bouts of overeating. It is postulated that this represents a response of the hypothalamus to a suboptimal body weight which has been maintained by the patient over several years as a result of her morbid concern with slimness. It is this essentially unchanged concern which leads the patient to avoid fattening effects of the food ingested by inducing vomiting, purging, or both. The resulting loss of body fluids causes a depletion of potassium and an alkalosis which in turn may lead to urinary infections, renal impairment, epileptic seizures, and tetany.

Clinical features. The patient is plagued with almost constant thoughts of food. Much of the time she attempts to avoid eating fattening foods, but then succumbs to bouts of overeating. She may consume enormous amounts at one sitting such as a whole loaf of bread, packets of biscuits, several bars of chocolate, or whole cartons of cottage cheese. The total food and drink ingested may weigh 3 kg and contain 15–20 kcal (63–84 kJ). The frequency of these bouts may vary from once weekly to several times daily. The episode is usually terminated by the induction of vomiting, either by pushing the fingers in the mouth and throat, or by using an instrument such as a toothbrush. With continued practice some patients need no longer stimulate the pharynx but induce vomiting almost effortlessly by bending forward and exerting pressure over the abdomen. Purgative abuse is often combined with vomiting or may be used as an alternative, less efficient method of preventing the absorption of food. Senokot is a favourite preparation with 12 to 20 or more tablets being taken daily. The overeating and consequent vomiting and purging are conducted in secret, and may become so habitual that they fill much of the patient's day. The patient becomes depressed and her personal and social relationships suffer. She is seldom as thin as during the preceding anorexic phase. Indeed she may not appear unduly thin or may even be mildly obese. However, her weight will probably be several kilograms less than before the onset of her illness. Menstruation and fertility may be retained.

Mental state. The patient is very distressed by her preoccupation with food and her irresistible urges to overeat. Depressive symptoms include feelings of gloom, irritability, impaired concentration, and suicidal ideas. The bulimic patient shares with the anorexic patient the overvalued idea that it is odious to be fat and that her weight must not exceed a certain self-determined threshold.

Physical examination. Physical appearance may be unremarkable. An unusual sign is the presence of calluses or ulcers over the dorsum of the hand which result from abrasions of the skin against the upper incisors while inducing vomiting (Fig. 2). Occasionally there is swelling of the salivary glands. Signs of latent tetany may be elicited.

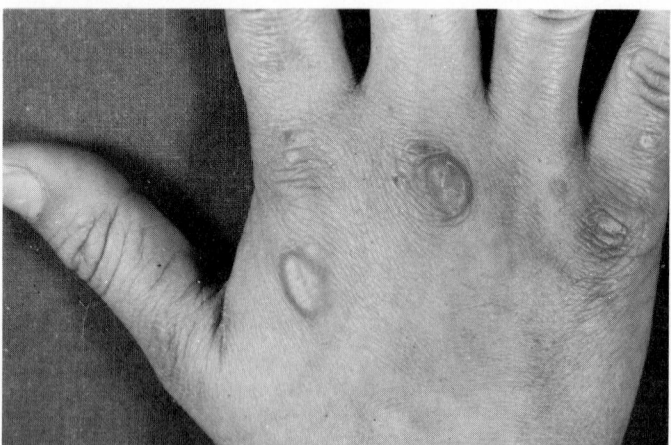

Fig. 2   Calluses on the back of the hand of a patient who habitually pushed her fingers down her throat to induce vomiting.

Investigations. Serum potassium levels may be low and bicarbonate levels elevated. Renal function may be impaired as shown by a reduced creatinine clearance. The EEG may show small sharp waves or epileptiform discharges.

Diagnosis. The essential diagnostic criteria are:
1. Severe cravings for food and recurrent bouts of gross overeating
2. Self-induced vomiting or purging, or both
3. An exaggerated dread of becoming fat with a self-imposed weight threshold

Treatment. In contrast with anorexia nervosa, treatment is difficult and its results often disappointing. Admission to hospital is indicated when depression is severe, physical complications are serious, or the patient's habitual overeating and vomiting are out of control. The first aim is to help the patient to control the bouts of overeating. The structured nursing regime described above is most effective in helping the patient to eat regular meals and the supervision prevents the acquisition of food which acts as a source of temptation. Vomiting soon ceases, and serum potassium levels rapidly return to normal. The benefits are short-lived, however, unless the patient's attitudes and way of life change. In particular it is desirable to attempt to persuade her to accept a higher weight which hopefully will reduce her cravings for food. The same arguments hold for the provision of individual psychotherapy or family therapy as in the case of typical anorexia nervosa. Antidepressants may relieve depressive symptoms but are unlikely to help the eating disorder.

Prognosis. Follow-up studies of bulimic patients have not been undertaken but the impression is that the prognosis is much less favourable than in typical anorexia nervosa, and that the risk of suicide is greater.

References

Bruch, H. (1978). *The golden cage: the enigma of anorexia nervosa.* Open Books, London.

Crisp, A. H., Palmer, R. L., and Kalucy, R. S. (1976). How common is anorexia nervosa? A prevalence study. *Br. J. Psychiat.* **128**, 549.

Garner, D. M. and Garfinkel, P. E. (1978). Socio-cultural factors in the development of anorexia nervosa. *Lancet* **ii**, 674.

Kendell, R. E., Hall, D. J., Hailey, A., and Babigian, H. M. (1973). The epidemiology of anorexia nervosa. *Psychol. Med.* **3**, 200.

Minuchin, S., Rosman, B., and Baker, L. (1978). *Psychosomatic families: anorexia nervosa in context.* Harvard University Press, Cambridge, Mass.

Morgan, H. G. and Russell, G. F. M. (1975). Value of family background and clinical features as predictors of long-term outcome in anorexia nervosa: four-year follow-up study of 41 patients. *Psychol. Med.* **5**, 355.

Nillius, S. J. and Wide, L. (1977). The pituitary responsiveness to acute and chronic administration of gonadotrophin-releasing hormone in acute and recovery stages of anorexia nervosa. In *Anorexia nervosa* (ed. R. Vigersky), 225. Raven Press, New York.

Russell, G. F. M. (1979). Bulimia nervosa: an ominous variant of anorexia nervosa. *Psychol. Med.* **9**, 429.

— and Mezey, A. G. (1962). An analysis of weight gain in patients with anorexia nervosa treated with high calorie diets. *Clin. Sci.* **23**, 449.

Slade, P. D. and Russell, G. F. M. (1973). Awareness of body dimensions in anorexia nervosa: cross-sectional and longitudinal studies. *Psychol. Med.* **3**, 188.

Theander, S. (1970). Anorexia nervosa. A psychiatric investigation of 94 female cases. *Acta psychiat. scand.* suppl. 214.

Wakeling, A., de Souza, V. A., and Beardwood, C. J. (1977). Assessment of the negative and positive feedback effects of administered oestrogen on gonadotrophin release in patients with anorexia nervosa. *Psychol. Med.* **7**, 397.

Diseases of overnourished societies and the need for dietary change

J. I. Mann

A wide range of diseases, which are common in affluent societies and occur rarely in developing countries, has been ascribed in part to aspects of the Western diet. Ischaemic heart disease, diabetes, gall stones, constipation (and irritable bowel syndrome), diverticular disease of the colon, cancer of the large bowel, dental caries, appendicitis, haemorrhoids, varicose veins, and obesity are probably the most important of these conditions. The features of the Western diet which have been incriminated are an excessive quantity of total and saturated fat (or perhaps a deficiency of certain polyunsaturated fatty acids), excessive amounts of sucrose and other refined carbohydrate, a deficiency of dietary fibre, and energy intake in excess of requirements.

The following paragraphs will summarize the evidence in favour of regarding these conditions as manifestations of malnutrition in affluent societies and consider the arguments for and against recommending dietary change.

Ischaemic heart disease. The suggestion that certain dietary practices may be associated with an increased risk of ischaemic heart disease (IHD) is based principally upon epidemiological and animal studies. The epidemiological studies are reviewed in detail in Section 13. Animal studies have yielded some confirmatory data: several research groups have shown that in monkeys it is possible to induce atheromatous lesions by feeding a diet high in saturated fat. The experimental lesions can be reversed by lipid-lowering measures. The process in animals may differ considerably from that in humans, but such findings do provide additional evidence of the role of diet in atherosclerotic disease.

Diabetes mellitus. Diet undoubtedly plays an important aetiological role in non-insulin dependent diabetes. As early as 1920 Himsworth suggested that excessive energy intake, deficiency of dietary carbohydrate, and possibly an excessive intake of fat might increase the risk of diabetes. His conclusions were based on the following observations: in non-diabetics blood glucose levels following an oral glucose load were lower when eating a high carbohydrate as compared with a high fat (low carbohydrate) diet. When examining mortality rates from diabetes, he found that in countries with high death rates, the diets contained a relatively low proportion of carbohydrate and a high proportion of fat. During the First World War, when death rates from diabetes fell, the main dietary change was a reduction in the proportion of fat and an increase in the proportion of carbohydrate. Finally, when taking diet histories (concerning diet before the onset of symptoms) from newly presenting diabetics, it was found that diabetics ate more in general than non-diabetic controls and fat intake appeared to be especially high.

Controversy has raged subsequently between those who have argued the case for excessive intakes of sugar and others who have suggested a deficiency of dietary fibre as being particularly relevant. The most helpful study involved careful survey techniques in 12 countries for the determination of both diabetes frequency and dietary histories (rather than much less reliable mortality statistics and population food consumption figures) in an attempt to discover the most important environmental factors in the aetiology of non-insulin dependent diabetes. Both sugar and fat intake correlated with diabetes frequency but the most striking association ($r = 0.9$) was with energy intake. More detailed analysis of these data suggested that correlations with individual foods were occurring simply as a consequence of the most important factor—energy intake in excess of requirements.

Whilst excessive energy intake seems likely to explain the

previously observed correlations between sugar and fat, a protective role for dietary fibre should not be dismissed since there is considerable circumstantial evidence. In Pakistan diabetes is less common among those who eat chapatti (wholewheat unleavened bread) than those using white flour. In India the disease occurs less frequently in those areas where unpolished rice is eaten as compared with the urbanized areas where rice is polished. Diets high in fibre-rich carbohydrate are associated with an improvement in several measures of diabetic control when compared with the standard low carbohydrate diet still in use in most British diabetic clinics. More research is needed to determine whether any single dietary factor is as important as excessive energy intake in a genetically predisposed individual in determining the risk of developing diabetes. Although diet is important in the management of insulin-dependent diabetes, nutritional factors have not been incriminated as a cause of the disease. Here, genetic and other environmental influences appear to be particularly important.

Obesity. Of all the conditions associated with overnutrition, obesity is the most obvious and perhaps at the same time one of the least understoood. There is little consensus with regard to definition and, consequently, epidemiological data are scanty. There is, however, no doubt about the increased risk of morbidity and mortality associated with marked obesity, and it has been suggested that during the past 40 years the average body fat content of the adult population of the United Kingdom has increased by about 10 per cent. Consequently the prevalence of obesity must also have increased. The precise role of nutritional factors is unclear and is discussed in more detail on page 8.26. However, in the long term only a reduction in energy intake or a substantial increase in output will reduce the proportion of overweight people in the population. It is possible that a diet in which carbohydrates are taken in fibre-rich forms will help to reduce obesity by encouraging satiety at a lower level of energy intake.

Diverticular disease of the colon. The first suggestion that deficiency of dietary fibre might be implicated in the aetiology of diverticular disease of the colon came from the striking geographic variations and the documented increase in disease rates in several European countries since the 1920s. The variation and trends in rates are certainly compatible with fibre deficiency but could be explained by several alternative dietary and other environmental factors. The best documented evidence comes from studies of patients with diverticular disease and controls, animal experiments, and the effects of treatment with bran. Diet histories taken from patients with diverticular disease and from controls have shown that before the onset of symptoms the patients reported a lower intake of crude fibre than the controls, but symptoms could have modified eating habits and influenced the memory of what was eaten before the onset of symptoms. Another study involved barium follow-through investigations on 220 asymptomatic volunteers (including 56 vegetarians) which identified 95 individuals with asymptomatic diverticular disease. Careful dietary histories were obtained from all participants. The vegetarians, with a substantially higher fibre intake than non-vegetarians, were less prone to diverticular disease (12 per cent versus 33 per cent). In non-vegetarians over the age of 60 dietary fibre intake was 19 g/day in those with diverticular disease and 23 g/day in those without. The difference was more striking in vegetarians with (28 g/day) and without (43 g/day) diverticular disease. Differences in total dietary fibre were principally due to differences in intake of cereal fibre. No other dietary constituents differed significantly in subjects with and without diverticular disease. Vegetarians with diverticular disease ate more fibre than non-vegetarians without it. This study provides strong evidence for a protective role of cereal fibre in diverticular disease but also suggest that factors other than fibre are involved. Animal experiments provide confirmation. An increase in dietary fibre is widely recommended to patients with symptomatic diverticular disease, a treatment justified by at least one double-blind crossover trial and numerous uncontrolled studies.

Plausible theories concerning pathogenesis have been suggested: small hard faeces, undoubtedly features of a fibre deficient diet, are associated with narrowing of the colon and the formation of closed segments in which pressure increases. Additional work is needed by colonic muscles to provide the pressure to move the more solid faeces, producing muscular hypertrophy in addition to the diverticula at sites of weakness where blood vessels penetrate the muscular coat.

Although no formally conducted intervention study in humans has ever shown dietary fibre to be protective against diverticular disease, the indirect evidence seems strong.

Constipation and the irritable colon syndrome. Ninety-nine per cent of a large population sample studied in Britain reported that their bowels functioned at least three times per week. Yet perceived constipation is a frequent complaint. In 1976 3 per cent of all prescriptions written in the National Health Service (in the United Kingdom) were for purgatives and laxatives, at a cost of around £4 million, and many times this amount was bought over the counter. In another survey 6 per cent of people aged 18–80 described straining when passing stools. No data are available concerning the frequency of passing small stools. There seems little doubt that constipation is uncommon in populations eating a high fibre diet. In rural Africa stool weights are frequently around 500 g daily and bowel transit times around 40 hours. In Britain stool weights in non-vegetarians are more usually around 100 g (with a very wide range), whereas in vegetarians the average stool weight is over 200 g. Factors other than fibre might be involved but the fact that British vegetarians and non-vegetarians with average daily intakes of dietary fibre greater than 30 g have transit times of less than 75 hours whereas those with small fibre intake have transit times ranging from 20 to 124 hours suggest that fibre must be particularly relevant. There is no doubt that increasing the fibre (in particular cereal fibre) content of the diet relieves the symptoms of constipation, an observation now confirmed by controlled clinical trials. On average the addition of about 10 g of dietary fibre to the usual daily diet is required. There is no direct evidence of a causal link between a fibre-depleted diet and the irritable colon syndrome but high fibre diets are widely recommended in treatment and are believed to be of value even in the absence of formal clinical trials.

Dental caries. Dental caries was exceptionally rare among young people in ancient Britain. In 1975 80 per cent of five-year-olds required treatment for dental caries and about 10 per cent of all children enter school with more than half their teeth seriously decayed. Some 5 per cent of the adult population in England and Wales and 15 per cent of that in Scotland are edentulous by the age of 30 years. Careful oral hygiene, fluoridation of the water supply, and perhaps in the future a vaccine to raise resistance against cariogenic organisms will decrease the frequency of dental caries, but there are impressive data to suggest a nutritional cause. Amongst the indigenous population of many countries where unrefined foods used to form the bulk of the diet (e.g. China, Uganda), dental caries had a very low prevalence. Within a few years of the addition of sugar and other refined foods the frequency showed a rapid increase. In a classical experiment carried out in a Swedish mental hospital, volunteers given toffee apples, chocolate, and caramel in addition to their control diet had a 13-fold greater number of tooth surfaces becoming carious each year, as compared with those eating the control diet alone.

Other diseases. Cancer of the large bowel, gall stones, appendicitis, haemorrhoids, varicose veins, and hiatus hernia all occur frequently in developed countries and rarely in developing countries, but the evidence linking these conditions to a nutritional cause is more tenuous. Gall stones are undoubtedly associated with obesity and in the case of both gall stones and appendicitis there are some rather indirect data suggesting an association with fibre deficiency or excessive quantities of refined carbohydrate. The addition of bran to the diet can make bile less saturated, and experimentally induced gall stones in animals tend to be reduced if fibre-rich food is given. Data from the United Kingdom and South Africa taken together provide interesting information concerning appendicitis: appendicitis rates were compared in two matched South African Caucasian groups, the privileged group living in University halls of residence and the other living in establishments for the more indigent where the diets contained more fibre. Annual rates were 7.8 and 1.8 per 1000 respectively. Of course factors other than diet might explain this but the similarity in rates to those found in an almost identical study in Bristol (7.6/1000 in a public school and 0.8/1000 in an orphanage) are very striking.

The case for dietary change. Ischaemic heart disease, non-insulin dependent diabetes, diverticular disease, constipation, dental caries, and obesity are conditions in which malnutrition plays a definite role in aetiology. It is of some interest to consider the frequency of these diseases. The first three accounted for approximately 10 per cent of all hospital admissions to acute hospitals in the Oxford Region in 1978. Ischaemic heart disease and diabetes accounted for 40 per cent of all deaths in men aged 45–54 years in England and Wales in the same year.

The case for recommending dietary change hinges on (a) the importance of these conditions in affluent societies; (b) the strong evidence for a nutritional aetiology in a substantial number of the diseases; (c) the evidence from clinical trials that lowering of cholesterol (of the order of magnitude that can be achieved by dietary means) reduces the risk of non-fatal IHD; and (d) the evidence from animal experiments which suggest that atheroma, and perhaps other diseases of disordered nutrition, might be reversible. Numerous official and semi-official bodies have suggested dietary change. The great majority have been aimed at reducing the frequency of IHD and have centred around increasing the proportion of fat coming from polyunsaturated sources, with or without a reduction in total fat. More recently advice has been offered concerning a more generally 'prudent diet' than the typical British diet which comprises 45 per cent energy from carbohydrate (substantially refined and low in fibre), 44 per cent from fat, and 11 per cent from protein. Criticisms of this approach have been (a) lack of conclusive evidence concerning the beneficial effects of such change; (b) possible harmful effects of dietary change; (c) infringement of personal liberties; and (d) the fact that dietary modification would not be compatible with traditional dietary practices in many affluent societies. The two latter objections are of less relevance to scientific arguments since recommendations themselves do not affect individual rights—certainly no more than present national policies determined by political considerations (e.g. the subsidy of butter and other dairy products). The most difficult issue when recommending dietary change is the lack of conclusive evidence, i.e. from adequately conducted clinical trials. It is necessary to point out that in view of the very considerable costs such trials will probably never be conducted and the evidence will perhaps only come from natural experiments—observations of disease rates in populations or sections of populations who do change their dietary practices. A little of this kind of evidence is already available from the fall in IHD mortality rate in the USA which appears to be at least to some extent associated with the dietary change which has occurred in that country.

Despite this there would appear to be a few general recommendations which are likely to be reasonably free of controversy and may be beneficial to the health of affluent societies. The importance of maintaining ideal body weight is perhaps the only entirely non-controversial suggestion. There does in addition seem to be a quite strong case to recommend an increase in complex fibre-rich carbohydrate, especially whole grain cereals, dried beans, and unprocessed fruit and vegetables at the expense of fats, simple sugars, and refined carbohydrate. This represents, for many affluent societies, a trend towards past eating habits and certainly a trend towards the diet of populations where the diseases of affluence occur very infrequently. It should be stressed that there is no single clinical trial which has confirmed the benefits of such modifications and consequently it is impossible to give a precise proportion of total daily energy which might be derived from carbohydrate but 55 per cent rather than 45 per cent as at present is the most frequently quoted suggestion, together of course with a radical change in the type of carbohydrate. Dietary fibre intake in the UK is currently 20 g/day and at least as far as gastrointestinal function is concerned it would seem from the data on bowel transit times that intake ought to be increased to at least 30 g/day. Possible adverse effects of increasing dietary fibre do need to be considered. Calcium, iron, and zinc absorption could be impaired chiefly as a result of the cation-binding effect of phytate in cereal fibre. In vulnerable groups such as the elderly and Asian immigrants supplementation of the diet with calcium rich foods might be necessary. In vegetarians there is at least a theoretical possibility of iron and zinc deficiency (since meat is a particularly good source of both) but this has not been evident in a recent study of vegetarians. Such deficiencies if they do exist must be uncommon and probably need not act as a deterrent from recommending a general increase in fibre-rich carbohydrate.

An increase in complex carbohydrate will need to be associated with a reduction in total fat in order to avoid obesity. If carbohydrate is increased to 55 per cent of total energy, fat will need to be reduced from the current level of 44 per cent of total energy to 30–35 per cent. Controversy surrounds any recommendations relating to the nature of the dietary fat. Currently the ratio of polyunsaturated to saturated fatty acids (p/s) is 0.3. The early studies of IHD prevention (and also the earliest recommendations) suggested increasing this ratio to 2 in the context of an overall 40 per cent fat diet. This change increased the risk of gall stones and it is now known that a p/s ratio of about 0.8 (in a diet where fat provides 30–35 per cent of total energy) can produce a long-term reduction in plasma cholesterol of about 10 per cent in well-motivated adults. For this reason a p/s ratio of 0.8 to 1.0 is suggested in more recent recommendations for a 'prudent diet'. It is, however, criticized on the one hand by those who claim that this proportion of polyunsaturated fat has not been tested in any clinical trial, and on the other by enthusiasts for the hypothesis that polyunsaturated fatty acids may have an antithrombotic effect who feel that, while this ratio may be adequate to lower cholesterol, it may not be sufficient to exert the antithrombotic effect. Clearly the situation is unresolved. It would seem that a ratio of 0.8 is a reasonable compromise; it would certainly reduce cholesterol levels, might be sufficient to produce some antithrombotic effect (though the addition of eicosopentanoate, may be necessary) and is unlikely to be harmful.

Dietary change along these lines is possible, but represents a fairly substantial change from the 'typical' British diet. It could not be achieved without a substantial reduction of meat and dairy products (which account for the present relatively high fat intake) and an increase in vegetable protein and fibre-rich cereals. Furthermore, major changes would be required in agricultural policy which in the United Kingdom and many other countries favours the dairy industry.

Dietary recommendations made by various official bodies have ranged from a 'no change' policy to far more wide-ranging recommendations than offered here (e.g. to include reduction in salt intake in the hope of reducing frequency of hypertension; and concerning fluoridation, breast feeding, alcohol, food-additives, and measures to reduce the incidence of iron deficiency anaemia, rickets, and oesteomalacia). All these recommendations have been criticized. There is, therefore, considerable advantage in suggesting simple changes which are likely to have the greatest effect on the health of entire populations. These suggestions imply a trend back towards an eating pattern which was prevalent in the United Kingdom and other European countries earlier in the century.

References

Ahrens, E. H. (1979). Dietary fats and coronary heart disease: unfinished business. *Lancet* **ii**, 1345.

Gear, J., Ware, A., Fursdon, P., Mann, J. I., Nolan, D. J., Brodribb, A., and Vessey, M. P. (1979). Symptomless diverticular disease and intake of dietary fibre. *Lancet* **i**, 511

—, Brodribb, A. J. M., Ware, A., and Mann, J. I. (1981). Fibre and bowel transit times. *Br. J. Nutrition* **45**, 77.

Mann, J. I. (1979). A prudent diet for the nation. *J. hum. Nutrition* **33**, 57.

— (1980). Diet and diabetes. *Diabetologia* **18**, 89.

— and Marr, J. W. (1981). In *Lipoproteins, atherosclerosis and coronary heart disease* (eds. W. E. Miller and B. Lewis), ch. 12. Elsevier/North Holland Biomedical Press, Amsterdam.

Royal College of Physicians of London (1980). *Medical aspects of dietary fibre*. Pitman Medical, London.

US Senate (1977). *Select Committee on Nutrition and Human Needs*. US Government Printing Office, December, stock no. 052–070–03913–2.

Section 9
Metabolic disorders

The inborn errors of metabolism: general aspects

R. W. E. Watts

There are about 180 diseases due to an inherited single enzyme defect. These are the inborn errors of metabolism. In most cases, the change in the structure of the enzyme reduces its catalytic activity. This causes a block on the relevant metabolic pathway and the phenotype arises from lack of a metabolic product, or the accumulation of intermediary metabolites, or the opening up of alternative metabolic pathways. There are a few examples in which the mutation alters the structure of the enzyme in such a way as to increase its activity. In another group of diseases, the underlying abnormality is a defect in an active transport mechanism, and these disorders manifest themselves by a failure to transport specific low molecular weight compounds across the intestinal and proximal renal tubule epithelial cells. Lysosomal enzyme defects cause the lysosomal storage diseases in which the undegraded substrates distend the lysosomes and distort the subcellular anatomy. Some inborn errors of metabolism are of no clinical significance, others produce more or less serious degrees of morbidity, and some may be incompatible with an independent existence.

Heterogeneity in the inborn errors of metabolism. The individual inborn errors of metabolism are defined on the basis of specific constellations of clinical and biochemical features including the demonstration of a specific enzyme lesion. Such a basis for identification might be expected to delineate the individual diseases very precisely. The study of a series of cases of any particular inborn error of metabolism reveals unexpected heterogeneity, and this can be ascribed to one or more of the following factors:

1. Multiple allelism.
2. Mutations at different gene loci affecting the structure of different polypeptide chains in a single enzyme protein.
3. Mutations at different gene loci affecting different proteins with similar catalytic functions.
4. The overall genetic background against which the specific gene acts.
5. Environmental factors.

Clinical pointers towards a diagnosis of an inborn error of metabolism. The detailed symptomatology of the different inborn errors of metabolism spreads across all of the medical subspecialties. There are, however, certain clinical findings, which in the absence of an acquired cause, suggest the presence of an inherited metabolic disorder (Table 1).

The inborn errors of metabolism are inherited in a unifactorial manner, that is, they behave as simple Mendalian characters so that a carefully taken family history is essential. Special inquiries should be made about affected siblings, possible parental consanguinity, paternity, miscarriages, perinatal deaths, abortions, and about the sexes of possibly affected relatives as well as their placement on the maternal or paternal side of the family.

General approaches to the treatment of inborn errors of metabolism. The fundamental cause of the inborn errors of metabolism, namely the abnormal gene, cannot be corrected so that all treatments are in a sense palliative. The main general approaches which are available are summarized in Table. 2.

Treating inborn errors of metabolism by various types of enzyme replacement therapy (for example: enzyme infusion, leucocyte infusion, fibroblast transplantation, bone marrow transplantation)

is still of unproven value. These approaches are being evaluated in some diseases, and it is clear that different types of disease will require different therapeutic approaches.

Table 1 Clinical presentations, which in the absence of acquired or other congenital causes, suggest an inborn error of metabolism

---

Unexplained acute neonatal illness and/or failure to thrive in early infancy. (Marked muscle hypotonia, recurrent fits, comas, acidosis and vomiting, especially if withholding milk feeds causes temporary improvement, are especially suggestive)
Developmental slowing and arrest followed by retrogression
Developmental slowing and arrest leading to unexplained mental handicap
Unusual physiognomy, multiple skeletal deformities with developmental delay and retrogression
Multiple skeletal deformities alone
Gross visceromegaly
Specific dietary intolerances
Haemolytic anaemia
Unusual body odour*
Recurrent urolithiasis
Cataracts in early life
Persistent jaundice and hepatic cirrhosis in infancy
Abnormal cutaneous photosensitivity
Abnormal drug sensitivity
A history of recurrent perinatal deaths and/or stillbirths

---

* Examples are: phenylketonuria (mousy, musty), branched chain keto acidaemia (maple syrup), methionine malabsorption (oast house, dry celery), isovaleric acidaemia (sweaty feet), methylaminuria (stale fish)

Screening for inborn errors of metabolism. The realization that very early diagnosis is essential in order to achieve good results in some of the inborn errors of metabolism such as phenylketonuria and galactosaemia has stimulated interest in the possibility of examining either whole populations or selected groups of predisposed individuals for the biochemical differences which characterize particular inherited metabolic diseases. Diagnosis is needed at a stage which is not only presymptomatic but which precedes the onset of self-perpetuating secondary pathological changes.

Screening programmes should only be established for treatable or preventable diseases and the consistency of the association of the proposed biochemical marker and the serious clinical phenotype must have been proved beyond any doubt. The possibility that metabolic screening will bring to light previously unrecognized variants, which are either mild and do not require treatment, or which by virtue of a fundamentally different biochemical lesion will resist the currently established therapies has to be borne in mind. Phenylketonuria illustrates these problems. Here, beside classical phenylketonuria, whole population screening identified the clinically unimportant, so-called essential (mild) hyperphenylalaninaemia, and the abnormalities of the dihydrobiopterin part of the phenylalanine hydroxylase system, in which correction of the hyperphenylalaninaemia by dietary phenylalanine restriction does not cause clinical improvement.

Metabolic screening may be either non-selective and aim to cover the whole population or be selective and aim to cover a part of the population which may be defined on clinical, genetic, ethnic, or geographical grounds. Selective screening includes carrier detection studies within the family of the propositus. Screening for

Table 2 General approaches to the treatment of the inborn errors of metabolism

Method	Example
1 Restriction of a dietary substrate which cannot be metabolized	phenylalanine restriction in phenylketonuria; protein restriction in the hyperammonaemias; elimination of galactose in galactosaemia
2 Avoidance of specific hazards	ultra-violet radiation (congenital erythropoetic and variegate porphyrias, and in albinism); ionizing radiation in the DNA repair enzyme defects (xeroderma pigmentosum, ataxia telangiectasia) infections (agammaglobulinaemia); medications (oestrogens, barbiturates, etc. in acute intermittent porphyria)
3 Replacement of a missing metabolic product	orotic aciduria: treatment by uridine which is metabolized to uridylic acid; Hartnup disease: nicotinic acid to control skin manifestations
4 Removal of a toxic metabolite	haemodialysis and peritoneal dialysis as temporary treatment of an acute metabolic crisis due to a diffusible toxic metabolite, and to correct certain secondary biochemical abnormalities quickly; specific chemical detoxication or solubilization: penicillamine in Wilson's disease and cystinuria
5 Pharmacological doses of a cofactor (only some cases of each disease respond)	propionic acidaemia: biotin; homocystinuria: pyridoxine; primary hyperoxaluria: pyridoxine; methylmalonic acidaemia: vitamin B_{12}
6 Replacement of a missing gene product	haemophilia: factor VIII

phenylketonuria (incidence between about 1:6000 and 1:12 000 in Caucasian populations) is the only generally accepted example of non-selective (whole population) screening which is currently practised, although there is widespread agreement that screening for congenital hypothyroidism (incidence about 1:6000 in Europe) should also be introduced.

Attempts are being made to develop screening methods for the simultaneous detection and differentiation of large classes of clinically and chemically related diseases. Recent work in relation to the non-amino organic acidurias and to the inborn errors of glycoconjugate metabolism has shown this to be feasible, but it may require high level technology. The amino acidopathies are exceptional in that relatively simple, although labour intensive, chromatographic methods can be used for preliminary broad screening.

Prenatal diagnosis. The state of the fetus can now be directly assessed from an anatomical viewpoint by ultrasonography, and at the cellular level by examining the amniotic fluid and the cells which it contains by biochemical and cytological techniques. Amniocentesis for the diagnosis of chromosomal and inherited biochemical abnormalities should be undertaken at the sixteenth week of pregnancy (determined by ultrasonography) because the volume of fluid is then sufficiently large to reduce the risk of inducing the miscarriage of a normal fetus to about 1 per cent, and there is sufficient time for cell culture and detailed biochemistry so that an elective abortion can be undertaken by about the twenty-first week of the pregnancy. Amniocentesis for prenatal diagnosis should not be recommended unless the mother wishes to have an abnormal fetus aborted. Amniotic fluid taken for the diagnosis of an inborn error of metabolism should be routinely examined for alpha-

fetoprotein in order to diagnose an unsuspected open neural tube defect, as well as for chromosomal abnormalities. Only a proportion of the known inborn errors of metabolism can be diagnosed prenatally because the relevant enzyme is not expressed in cultured amniotic cells. The fact that the relevant enzyme activity can be demonstrated in cultured fibroblasts does not prove that it will be found in cultured amniotic cells and a prenatal diagnosis should not be attempted unless this is known to be the case. The examination of the DNA of amniotic cells by restriction endonuclease analysis may have considerable potential in prenatal diagnosis; it has already been applied successfully to sickle cell disease and β-thalassaemia.

Carrier state diagnosis. The incidence of carriers of autosomal recessive disorders can be calculated approximately by halving the square root of the denominator of the vulgar fraction describing the incidence of the disease. For example, the incidence of cystic fibrosis in Caucasian populations is approximately 1 in 2000; the square root of 2000 is 44.72 so the incidence of heterozygous carriers of the abnormal gene causing cystic fibrosis is about 1 in 22.

The accuracy of genetic counselling is greatly improved if the carriers of abnormal recessive genes can be positively identified. The general approaches to this in the case of the inborn errors of metabolism are:

1. The detection of minor clinical abnormalities.

2. The demonstration of levels of enzyme activity in tissue (e.g. leucocytes, hair follicles, or cultured fibroblasts) which are intermediate between those observed in individuals homozygous for the abnormal and the normal forms of the enzyme respectively (the observed level of activity may not be exactly 50 per cent of the normal value).

3. The demonstration of intermediate levels of a characteristic metabolite in an accessible body fluid.

4. The demonstration of mosaicism with respect to the product of the mutant X-linked gene in the case of sex-linked recessive disorders using, for example, hair follicles or cultured fibroblasts.

It is particularly important to determine the carrier status of the female siblings and other female blood relations on the maternal side of the family of the propositus in the case of sex-linked disorders.

References

Bickel, H., Guthrie, R., and Hammersen, G. (eds.) (1980). *Neonatal screening for inborn errors of metabolism.* Springer-Verlag, Berlin.

Burton, B. K. and Nadler, H. L. (1978). Clinical diagnosis of the inborn errors of metabolism in the neonatal period. *Paediatrics* **61**, 398.

Crawford, M. d'A., Gibbs, D. A., and Watts, R. W. E. (eds.) (1982). *Advances in the treatment of inborn errors of metabolism.* Wiley, Chichester.

Gibbs, D. A. (1977). Enzyme measurements of hair follicles in the study of some inborn errors of metabolism, with particular reference to Hunter's disease. *Ann. Clin. Biochem.* **14**, 757.

Kyrieckos, A. A. and Shapiro, L. J. (1978). Genetic metabolic considerations in the sick neonate. *Pediat. Clin. N. Am.* **25**, 431.

Little, P. J. R. (1981). DNA analysis and the antenatal diagnosis of hemoglobinopathies. In *Genetic engineering 1* (ed. R. Williamson), 61. Academic Press, London.

Raine, D. N. (1979). Inborn errors of metabolism. In *Chemical diagnosis of disease* (eds. S. S. Brown, F. L. Mitchell, and D. S. Young), 927, Elsevier/North-Holland Biomedical Press, Amsterdam.

Watts, R. W. E. (1978). Progress in screening for inborn errors of metabolism. *Experientia* **34**, 143.

—, Gibbs, D. A., and McKeran, R. O. (1975). Some aspects of the use of hair follicles for the biochemical study of inborn errors of metabolism. In *Inborn errors of skin hair and connective tissue* (eds. J. Holton and J. T. Ireland), 27. MTP Press, Lancaster.

Diabetes mellitus

K. G. M. M. Alberti and T. D. R. Hockaday

Definition, diagnosis, and classification

Definition. Diabetes is generally defined by a particular degree of hyperglycaemia. This is certainly current usage, but can be thought a limited approach to a complex metabolic disorder with various long-term sequelae. It is, however, difficult to produce a single binding definition because of the heterogeneous aetiologies of diabetes. In many ways there are parallels with jaundice, where the manifold causes are unified in a raised bilirubin concentration.

In diabetes, the fundamental defect is in insulin secretion and/or action. In the classical young-onset form of the disorder, there is near-total insulin deficiency, with inevitable widespread metabolic changes. In the older-age onset form, there is diminished and/or delayed insulin secretion in response to glucose, combined with varying degrees of diminished effectiveness of circulating insulin, whilst when diabetes is associated with obesity insulin resistance predominates. Diabetes can therefore be defined as a state of diminished insulin action, due to its decreased availability or effectiveness, in varying combinations.

It is arguable whether tissue damage should be included in the definition. To one well-known Danish diabetologist, 'diabetes is a dot in the eye in 20 years' time'. Certainly, the likelihood of developing tissue damage, or the particular complications of microangiopathy and neuropathy, have influenced diagnostic criteria, but this is not true of macroangiopathy. This is largely an academic argument, in that the glycaemic diagnosis is usually clearcut when tissue damage is clinically evident, but one may add to the earlier definition 'and associated with the development in the long term of retinopathy, nephropathy, neuropathy, and macrovascular disease'. Whether these sequelae are inevitable is discussed below.

Diagnosis. Much heat, and little light, has been generated in the last five years over the diagnostic criteria for diabetes mellitus. It must be stressed that usually the diagnosis is obvious: thus, if a patient presents with weight loss, fatigue, polyuria and polydipsia, and 2 per cent glycosuria, all that is required is an elevated random blood glucose estimation to make the diagnosis. Similarly, with patients presenting in diabetic ketoacidosis; or being referred to the clinic with classical retinopathy, or gangrene, or having recurrent candidiasis with glycosuria: all these need little in the way of rigorous chemical testing. In some, however, glycosuria is detected during routine medical examinations or as part of a general screen in hospital. It is here that more clearcut guidelines for diagnosis are required. One important practical point is that many members of the general public are aware that diabetics should avoid eating free sugar. If the general practitioner tells the patient that he may have diabetes before measuring blood glucose, dietary treatment may be self-imposed, and the patient be normoglycaemic and aglycosuric when seen later. It is better, therefore, if the GP immediately takes a blood sample for blood glucose estimation.

Recently, both the American Diabetes Association (ADA) and the World Health Organization (WHO) have suggested new criteria for the chemical diagnosis of diabetes. These are important, particularly for occasional asymptomatic patients and for epidemiological surveys. It is suggested that in the symptomatic patient a random plasma glucose value of 11.1 mmol/l (200 mg/dl) or more is diagnostic. This is certainly adequate for the asymptomatic patient as well, if found on more than one occasion (and not due to an obvious hyperglycaemic stimulus such as glucose infusion in a surgical patient). If hyperglycaemia is not marked, then two further

measures may be employed: (i) estimation of fasting glucose levels; and (ii) an oral glucose tolerance test.

The generally ignored differences between plasma and whole blood glucose levels, and between capillary and venous levels, should be stressed. Whole blood values are some 10–15 per cent lower than plasma values. Similarly, capillary values are 7 per cent higher than venous values in the fasting state and 8 per cent higher after a glucose load. This has become more important, since clinical laboratories may use venous plasma whilst bedside monitoring techniques use whole blood or plasma capillary blood.

Fasting venous or capillary whole blood values equal or greater than 7 mmol/l (WHO) or 120 mg/dl (6.7 mmol/l) (ADA), or fasting venous plasma levels of 8 mmol/l (WHO) or 140 mg/dl (7.8 mmol/l) (ADA) are considered diagnostic of diabetes mellitus. Absolute dependence should not, however, be placed on a single value for a life-time diagnosis, and a second abnormal fasting value or a diagnostic post-glucose load value should also be obtained. It is now generally agreed that a 75-g oral glucose load should be used in adults (in a minimum of 250 ml of water) with loads of 1.75 g/kg ideal body weight in children, to a maximum of 75 g. Table 1 shows suggested diagnostic values, with greatest reliance placed on the two-hour post-glucose value (≥ 10 mmol/l; 180 mg/dl for venous whole blood and ≥ 11.0 mmol/l; 200 mg/dl for capillary or venous whole blood). A normal value is cited as a fasting venous blood glucose and two-hour post-load value both of < 7.0 mmol/l (WHO) or 120 mg/dl (ADA). Any intermediate values or combination of intermediate values has been put in a new class: 'impaired glucose tolerance'.

Table 1 Diagnostic glucose values for oral glucose tolerance tests

Diabetes mellitus	Fasting(mM)	and/or	2 h post-glucose(mM)
Venous whole blood	≥ 7		≥ 10
Capillary whole blood	≥ 7		≥ 11
Venous plasma	≥ 8		≥ 11
Impaired glucose tolerance	Fasting	*and*	2 h post-glucose
Venous whole blood	< 7		$\geq 7 - < 10$
Capillary whole blood	< 7		$\geq 8 - < 11$
Venous plasma	< 8		$\geq 8 - < 11$
Normal	Fasting	*and*	2 h post-glucose
Venous whole blood	< 7		< 7
Capillary whole blood	< 7		< 8
Venous plasma	< 8		< 8

All for 75-g oral glucose load in 250–350 ml water, or 1.75 g/kg ideal body weight for children to a maximum of 75 g. Values are for a *specific enzymatic* glucose assay. Table adapted from Second Report of WHO Expert Committee on Diabetes Mellitus, Technical Report Series 646.

The choice of particular values rests on epidemiological data: thus, patients with two-hour values diagnostic of diabetes are the main risk group for development of diabetic retinopathy, while those in the impaired glucose tolerance bracket carry an increased risk of (i) worsening to diabetes (2–4 per cent per year); and (ii) developing macrovascular disease but not specific microangiopathic lesions. There are certain defects in these criteria, for they may apply neither to all races nor all ages. However, they emphasize a 'grey' area between normality and clinical diabetes, and are a useful working basis for the present. However, the importance of GTT diagnosis of diabetes should *not* be over-emphasized. Its main use in clinical practice is in the diagnosis of abnormal glucose tolerance in pregnancy, and in that situation change of nomenclature should not alter *clinical practice*. Such patients require therapy—just as the non-pregnant with 'impaired glucose tolerance' require following from the cardiovascular point of view.

Presenting features. Diabetes may be diagnosed when a patient consults his doctor because of certain symptoms which lead to measurement of glucose levels, while both diabetes and impaired glucose tolerance may be diagnosed through the finding of high glucose levels on screening asymptomatic patients or those without specific symptoms. Pathognomonic types of tissue damage (e.g. background diabetic retinopathy) or associated clinical findings (cardiac infarction) may also lead to detection of high glucose levels. This applies only to more elderly diabetics, but 4 per cent of type II patients have retinopathy visible when they are diagnosed.

The classic symptoms of hyperglycaemia are polyuria, thirst, and weight loss. While thirst and polyuria can have other explanations (Table 2), diabetes mellitus is one of the commonest, and either of these features should always lead at least to a urine test for glucose. In type I diabetes weight loss may be severe, while in type II it has often been substantial even though the patient is still obese. However, in type II there may be no significant weight loss at diagnosis. Nocturnal frequency is often two to four times, and the thirst severe enough for patients to take a drink after passing urine.

Table 2   Causes of combined thirst and polyuria

1. Diabetes mellitus
2. Hypercalcaemia
3. Some forms of renal failure, including those due to cardiac insufficiency
4. Habitual water drinking
5. Diabetes insipidus

In women, pruritis vulvae is a frequent symptom, even without development of a full-blown monilial rash in the perineum. Balanitis (sometimes causing a paraphimosis) is much less common, but equally can be severe. Other common but non-specific symptoms are cramps, particularly at night, in the calves or feet and tingling in the fingers (rare in the feet). Some patients complain of loss of appetite, but others develop a craving, particularly for sweet foods. Occasionally glycosuria causes crystallization of glucose, as on the shoes of elderly males. Patients are often relatively constipated, while in a minority a mild (though occasionally severe) change in lens refraction causes visual blurring.

Classification. This is also an area of change and conflict. The only certainty is that the age-old terms of 'juvenile onset' and 'maturity onset' diabetes have outlived their usefulness. It is now obvious that the term diabetes mellitus covers a heterogeneous group of disorders with widely varying aetiologies. Two main classifications have appeared in the past few years. The first refers to type I and type II diabetes, with subcategorization of type I into types Ia and Ib. The second refers to 'insulin-dependent' (IDDM), 'non-insulin-dependent' (NIDDM), and 'others', although this is logically unappealing. It is probably preferable to use the type I, type II scheme, in that considerable confusion arises from the term 'insulin-dependent', which is often equated in practice with insulin-*treated*, which will depend on clinical practice and the state of the patient at a particular time; neither is it clearly stated that the dependence refers to avoidance of ketoacidosis.

Table 3 shows a simplified classification, which is based in part on the monumental document produced by the ADA in 1979.

Type I diabetes. We prefer this term because it is often difficult to classify a patient as 'insulin-dependent' or not. Thus, a classical type I diabetic may present in childhood with ketoacidosis without measurable insulin secretion. Shortly afterwards, the patient may go through a period of remission, at which time he is not strictly insulin-dependent. Similarly, a type II diabetic may be adequately treated by diet alone but develop ketoacidosis during a severe infection and be insulin-dependent for a period.

The classic type I Caucasian diabetic develops the disorder before age 30 years, with peaks of onset at age five and in early adolescence. The prevalence is approximately two per 1000 in the United Kingdom under 20 years old, with somewhat higher rates in Scandinavia, but lower in Asian countries. Males and females are affected almost equally. However, patients can present at any age. Such patients classically have demonstrable insulin secretory function (as assessed by C-peptide secretion) for the first 1–5 years. They may develop ketoacidosis at any time, secondary to well-recognized precipitating factors (see below).

There is a major association with HLA antigens on chromosome 6: particularly B8, B15, DR3, and DR4, although these associations are different for other racial groups. There is also an association with the presence in the circulation of cytoplasmic and complement-fixing islet-cell antibodies. The aetiological role of these factors is discussed below. Type Ib is a subgroup of type I, characterized by the persistent presence of islet-cell antibodies, and a close personal and familial association with other autoimmune endocrinopathies. Biochemically the metabolic disorder is indistinguishable from the commoner type Ia. Type Ib patients are typically older (e.g. onset in their thirties), and females outnumber males.

Type II diabetes. This is a heterogeneous group of disorders characterized by hyperglycaemia; appreciable insulin secretory capacity, although it may be decreased or delayed; and varying degrees of insulin resistance. It is probably wise on aetiological grounds to distinguish between non-obese and obese forms, but there is no clearcut dividing line for this. There is an association between prevalence and Gross National Product world-wide. In the United Kingdom the prevalence is probably between 0.5 and 1.0 per cent. The non-obese type II diabetic tends to be relatively insulinopenic, whilst the obese patient has absolutely hyperinsulinaemia, although levels are lower than in non-diabetic obese subjects. In the obese form, peripheral insulin resistance plays a major role, with both insulin receptor down-regulation and post-receptor defects. These defects, and the glucose intolerance, may return to normal with weight loss.

Strong familial aggregation is characteristic of the type II diabetic. Studies of identical twins show 100 per cent concordance three years after the first twin is diagnosed, compared with less than 60 per cent concordance in identical twins where one has type I diabetes. Even in apparently unaffected siblings of type II diabetics, metabolic abnormalities may be present, and indeed glucose intolerance may be found even though the apparently unaffected twin is asymptomatic.

In most cases the age of onset is delayed to middle or old age. There are, however, many examples of younger onset. One group has been described as MODY (maturity-onset diabetes of the young). This type tends to be strongly familial, but it remains to be proven whether it is a separate entity.

Recently it was suggested that type II diabetics could be divided usefully by presence or absence of flushing when given alcohol after preloading with the oral sulphonylurea, chlorpropamide. It was said that 'flushers' were relatively protected against the development of diabetic complications; this has not been substantiated, and indeed much criticized, and further information is required.

Almost by definition, type II diabetics are not 'ketosis-prone'. This does not mean, however, that they may not present with ketoacidosis or develop diabetic ketoacidosis when severely ill. This is generally due to the excess secretion of the anti-insulin hormones associated with infection, trauma, or illness.

Other types. There are many other causes of diabetes. Some are listed in Table 3. One group has recently been described as 'periodic' insulin dependence' or PID (perhaps more consistently called type III). Others include some of the forms of pancreatic diabetes: the J, K, and Z types (see below). Many other rare forms of diabetes are found. These include hormone and drug-induced

Table 3 Simplified classification of diabetes mellitus

	Other names	Aetiological features	Clinical characteristics
Type Ia	Insulin-dependent diabetes Juvenile onset diabetes Ketosis-prone diabetes	(i) Association with HLA types (e.g. DR3, DR4) (ii) Generally cytoplasmic and complement-fixing islet-cell-antibody positive at diagnosis but later become negative	In early phase retain some endogenous insulin secretion, and may have honeymoon phase. Later have no endogenous insulin. Develop ketosis when insulin withdrawn or with stress. May present with weight loss. Mostly young.
Type Ib	Same as type Ia	(i) Close association with other autoimmune endocrinopathies (ii) Persistent islet-cell antibodies (iii) Presumed autoimmune aetiology	Same as type Ia
Type II (non-obese)	Non-insulin-dependent diabetes (NIDDH) Maturity-onset diabetes Maturity-onset diabetes of the young (MOD)	(i) Heterogeneous aetiologies (ii) Familial aggregation (iii) Environmental factors?	Always measurable insulin present Tendency to insulin resistance Ketosis not provoked by insulin withdrawal but may become ketoacidotic with severe illness. Onset usually above age of 40
Type II (obese)	As for type II (non-obese)	(i) Related to obesity (ii) Glucose tolerance often normal after weight loss (iii) Probably different aetiology from type II (non-obese)	Hyperinsulinaemic and insulin resistant. Rarely if ever ketotic
Other types A. Pancreatic disease	Secondary diabetes J type K type Type III Z type	Chronic pancreatitis. Pancreatic calcification. Alcohol may be important (K type). Malnutrition and cassava consumption also implicated (Z type). Pancreatecomy). Haemochromatosis.	Often underweight with history of malnutrition. Mostly restricted to tropical countries and non-caucasians. May have severe insulin resistance although pancreatectomized subjects are insulin sensitive
B. Hormonal		(i) Corticosteroid excess (exogenous or endogenous) (ii) Glucagonoma (iii) Acromegaly (iv) Thyrotoxicosis (v) Phaeochromocytoma (vi) ?Hypothalamic lesions	Obvious signs of steroid excess Associated with skin rash Diabetes mild Obvious signs and symptoms of excess of particular hormone
C. Drug-induced		(i) Diuretics (ii) Psychoactive agents (iii) Catecholaminergic agents (iv) Analgesics	
D. Insulin receptor abnormalities		(i) Congenital lipodystrophy (ii) Associated with acanthosis nigricans (iii) Autoimmune insulin receptor antibodies	
E. Genetic syndromes		Examples: glycogen-storage disease; ataxia telangiectasia; DIDMOAD syndrome; Huntington's chorea; Laurence–Moon–Biedl syndrome; Werner's syndrome; Prader–Willi syndrome	
Impaired glucose tolerance (IGT)	Asymptomatic diabetes Chemical diabetes Borderline diabetes Latent diabetes Subclinical diabetes	Mild glucose intolerance from any cause (see Table 1)	Increased risk of macrovascular disease. Likely to be obese
Gestational diabetes		Pregnancy. Normal GTT beforehand	Diagnosis as for IGT or more severe forms of glucose intolerance

Adapted from National Diabetes Data Group, *Diabetes* **28**: 1039–1057, 1979, from where further details may be obtained. It should also be noted that the term *Prediabetes* has been replaced by 'Potential Abnormality of Glucose Tolerance' (PotAGT) types, as well as the interesting varieties caused by abnormalities of the insulin receptor. Several genetic syndromes also include diabetes, such as DIDMOAD syndrome (diabetes insipidus, diabetes mellitus, and optic atrophy), hypothalamic disorders, and lipodystrophic diseases.

Pathogenesis—genetic and environmental

For clinical diabetes to develop, those with genetic predisposition must encounter undefined environmental influences (Table 4). Type I and type II diabetes will be discussed separately, though these headings imply a sharper division between the two major types of preliminary diabetes than exists clinically, even if the classification proves to be justified aetiologically, at least in Western societies. Present knowledge certainly cannot exclude unrecognized patterns of disease that will in future distinguish patients now allocated between these two groups.

Table 4 Pathogenic factors of diabetes

Type I diabetes
  Predisposing
    HLA type: DR3, DR4, B8, B15 (Caucasian)
    Chromosome 6 markers: properdin factor B (Bf), glyoxalase-1, Kidd blood group locus

  Precipitating factors
    Viral infection: Coxsackie B4, mumps
    'Stress'?
    Trauma?
    Emotional upset?
    Islet cell antibodies?
    Autoimmune (type Ib)

Type II diabetes
    Family history
    Obesity

The genetics of diabetes is far from resolved. Among the difficulties is that most of those carrying the identifying markers (among the leucocyte histocompatibility antigens) of increased risk of type I diabetes do not develop clinical disease. Also, there is no agreed marker of type II diabetes, although from identical twin studies there is a much stronger genetic contribution (at least for those living in affluent societies) in this than in type I.

Type I diabetes. The two crucial clues to the pathogenesis of this condition are its association with circulating islet cell antibodies and an increased risk of developing type I diabetes in those with certain HLA (human leucocyte A) antigenic markers.

The islet-cell antibodies first recognized reacted with all the components of the pancreatic islets, but now cell-surface antibodies have been identified which react specifically with the β-cells. Two main groups of antibodies have been identified, one reacting directly but the other requiring complement for its fixation. One or other type of antibody has been detected in over 90 per cent of type I diabetics when sought within a month of diagnosis. Complement-fixing antibodies are particularly liable to be present close to diagnosis and disappear earlier than the other. Most diabetics positive for the cell-surface antibody show β-cell specificity. Five years after diagnosis some 15–20 per cent of diabetics still show positive plasma antibody tests. This proportion declines only slowly thereafter, so even 20 years after diagnosis 10 per cent may still show circulating islet cell antibodies. This is the type Ib (Table 3), in which autoimmunity is a prime factor in development of the disease. Such patients are particularly liable to have circulating antibodies to other endocrine tissue or to have frank disease of other endocrine organs, e.g. thyroid or adrenal, or relatives with one or other such feature. Islet-cell antibodies have been detected in non-diabetics but are more likely to be found in non-diabetic first-degree relatives of type I diabetics than in the general

population. In prospective studies their presence (and again particularly that of the complement-fixing antibody) increases the likelihood of imminent development of clinical diabetes, but as the numbers of those developing diabetes in these studies are still small, this is still a tentative conclusion.

Islet-cell antibodies can be present for several years without development of clinical disease, as is also true of thyroid or intrinsic-factor antibodies and their respective associated disease.

These type Ib patients show on average a different pattern from the larger group of type Ia diabetics. Females predominate over males, the patients are older at presentation, 30–50 years rather than under 25, and they are more likely to retain for several years after diagnosis some endogenous insulin secretion.

The exciting discovery of increased liability to type I diabetes in those with certain alleles at the B HLA locus has led to further work which has defined the D3 and D4 loci as the most useful markers of liability to this condition. The two markers would seem to be associated with different risks, for when both are present there is a synergistic effect. Other genetic factors in this part of chromosome 6 have been implicated, e.g. properdin factor B, glyoxylase, and the Kidd blood group locus. Particular genetic constellations, e.g. rare allotypes such as HLA C4–B2 or -B4, may indicate especially high risk of diabetes. A child carrying the same HLA markers as a sib already diabetic, has a 90-fold increased risk of developing clinical type I diabetes. It must be emphasized, though, that this means an absolute risk of only 5–10 per cent, so low is the incidence of type I diabetes in the population. This reinforces the importance of the environmental factor.

It is unknown whether the HLA antigens are mechanistically involved in disease development, or whether they serve purely as markers for neighbouring genes associated via linkage disequilibrium; and that it is these neighbours that carry the risk of diabetes. The association with circulating islet-cell antibodies and the possible link with preceding infection have been used to support the mechanistic involvement of the loci, while geographical differences in the associated risk, with members of the B group at least, have been used against it. This latter would not seem a strong objection if different B alleles have different functional significance in different parts of the world, quite apart from the likelihood that the B relationship is secondary to that of the D alleles.

Although certain viral illnesses, such as mumps and Coxsackie B infections, have sometimes been followed by a spate of cases of type I diabetes, it has been impossible to fix any particular viral agent or group of agents as regular forerunners of the disease. It is also uncertain whether the mononuclear cell infiltration of pancreatic islets found at post-mortem examination of patients dying soon after onset of type I diabetes indicates defence against a viral infection or, as is perhaps more likely, some immune response. The suggestion that such a response can be triggered by particular infections, or perhaps particular viruses after necessary passage through pancreatic tissue of previous hosts, is unsubstantiated, just as it is arguable that the probable link between viral infection and subsequent development of type I diabetes is non-specific through the generalized 'stress' of infection rather than a more direct effect of the infective agent. The increased incidence of type I diabetes during the winter months in both the northern and southern hemispheres has been attributed to such infections.

Type II diabetes. The generalization that there is a greater genetic influence in type II than in type I diabetes is based on the study of identical twins by Tattersall and Pyke, despite the selective elements doubtless affecting their case collection. Thus, they report many more identical twin pairs with type I than with type II diabetes, though the former is much less common. Again, 40 per cent of the type II propositi had another first-degree relative with diabetes, an unusually high prevalence. However, with 90 per cent concordance among their type II diabetics, and no pairs discordant for longer than three years, a substantial genetic component seems established.

It is uncertain whether the new WHO and ADA class of 'impaired glucose tolerance' should be considered together with 'true' diabetes in assessing the type II condition, but results in selected populations (Pima Indians, Nauru Micronesians) with a very high (e.g. 50 per cent) prevalence of type II diabetes seems to justify their inclusion. These populations show a bimodal distribution of glucose tolerance, and this deteriorates with age only in the 'higher glucose' groups. In the United Kingdom about 3 per cent of those with impaired tolerance annually reach the chemical criteria for the diagnosis of diabetes; this is different from, and precedes, clinical symptoms, apart from those caused by macrovascular tissue damage. A careful community survey is needed, but meanwhile genetic influences are best analysed from family studies. Fajan's results from such observations also argue strongly for a larger genetic component in type II than in type I diabetes. He first drew attention to the clinical pattern of maturity-type onset diabetes in relatively young patients, even during adolescence, often with a strong family history of diabetes, even through three generations. However, such MODY patients are now generally thought to be merely extreme examples of type II, and not qualitatively different.

Defective insulin secretion. There is little understanding of the defect in islet-cell function in type II diabetes. In perhaps a quarter, the failure of insulin production is purely relative to excessive needs imposed by the development of insulin resistance. This is obviously so in diabetic acromegalics. It is questionable whether grossly obese diabetics with marked hyperinsulinaemia, both fasting and in response to glucose loads, should be thought of as primary type II diabetics, or be classified as having diabetes secondary to obesity. They may return to virtually normal glucose and insulin relationships after substantial weight loss, but many do progress later to definite failure in insulin production. There is also the problem that their insulin secretion, though greater than normal, is still less than that in equally obese but euglycaemic subjects.

From the results of a strong, sustained stimulation of insulin secretion with intravenous glucose, Cerasi and Luft characterized normal subjects as having 'lower' or 'higher' insulin responses. The importance of this awaits long-term observations on the incidence of clinical diabetes in the two groups. The characteristics of insulin secretion they recognized were at least partially familial.

With the remaining three-quarters of type II diabetics, impaired insulin secretion to a hyperglycaemic stimulus at least partially underlies the hyperglycaemia. It is uncertain how much this impairment derives from loss of functioning β cells, how much from 'fatigue' by hyperglycaemia of 'weak' β cells, and how much from inhibition of potentially normally functioning cells. Post-mortem studies show a destructive process in this condition, with reduction of the β cell mass to somewhere between 10 and 50 per cent of normal through hyalinization of islets, often with intracellular deposition of an amyloid-like material. These changes do not appear secondary to primary vascular disease. Impairment through over-stimulation, or disordered function secondary to hyperglycaemia is indicated by the improved insulin secretion often seen if near normal glycaemic levels are maintained for hours or days. However, this is neither a large nor a sustained recovery. It is less easy to assess whether the β cells are inhibited. This could occur, for example, through a paracrine influence of somatostatin from neighbouring D-cells, or sympathetic (α-adrenergic) neurogentic inhibition.

The nature of the destructive process in type II diabetes is unknown, as is the extent to which it is linked to present or prior obesity. Patients have often followed a 'weight trajectory' that carries them into marked obesity, from which they decline then to be diagnosed diabetic after loss of 10–20 kg but still obese. The reason for this positive energy balance over several years is unknown, as is the mechanism of the reversal to negative balance before gross glycosuria develops.

The common deterioration of glucose tolerance with age is also not understood, though a decreasing muscle mass and increasing percentage of adipose tissue may be partly responsible. Such mechanisms would hardly explain the tendency to increasing fasting blood glucose concentration. It is more likely that the wide range of rate of deterioration of glucose control with time reflects differences in rates of 'aging'. The argument is made more complicated by the possibility that diabetes leads to (or is associated with) accelerated 'aging'. Features common both to diabetics and to aging are increased arteriosclerosis, increased thickening of capillary basement membranes, and increasing rigidity of collagen.

Increased insulin resistance. Insulin resistance has been categorized by Olefsky as occurring either at the level of the insulin receptor, or at a post-receptor stage. The former site predominates in the obese diabetic, and the latter in the non-obese, as well as in secondary diabetes, e.g. Cushing's. Resistance may be assessed in any insulin-sensitive tissue, and indeed may differ from one to the other. Early studies concentrated on the forearm (mainly muscle), while recently whole-body sensitivity has been examined with the 'glucose-clamp' technique, or hepatic metabolism has been tested. In the human forearm, sensitivity to insulin-stimulated glucose uptake correlates well with skinfold thickness, i.e. obesity, but most studies to date (including the glucose–insulin infusion studies with adrenaline and propanolol-blocked islets) neglect the numerical association between resistance and the initial plasma insulin concentration. This has been suggested as a prime determinant of insulin resistance, through a negative feedback effect on insulin receptors (see below). Alternatively, the resistance associated with obesity may depend simply upon the energy stored within cells. When these contain much lipid they may become less avid for further glucose uptake, e.g. from stretching of the cell membrane.

Insuling sensitivity may also be increased by exercise: again, the mechanism is unknown. Some insulin resistance certainly depends upon the catabolic hormones, as discussed later (page 9.13). Apart from obesity, the overall importance of insulin resistance in the pathogenesis of usual type II diabetes is probably small, with oversecretion of catabolic hormones contributing even less. However, in established type II diabetics with poor glycaemic control there will be the insulin resistance associated with hyperglycaemia, even in the non-obese.

Other types of diabetes. Secondary diabetes has already been discussed (page 9.6). The different forms of pancreatic diabetes deserve special mention because of their widespread distribution in tropical countries. These include J, K, and Z types.

J-type diabetes was first described in Jamaica but has since been widely described in Africa and Asia. It is associated with a history of childhood malnutrition, although patients may be normally nourished at presentation. There tends to be severe insulin resistance, although no ketosis even if insulin treatment is withdrawn. The Z type is associated with pancreatic calcification, malnutrition, and cassava consumption. The latter, when unripe, contains cyanide, which is normally counteracted by sulphur-containing amino-acids. If these are lacking, as in protein malnutrition, pancreatic damage ensues. These patients too may be insulin-resistant. The third type, K diabetes, is associated with consumption by males of strong local liquors and is mainly restricted to Africa. Pancreatic fibrosis, with or without calcification, is found, but patients are insulin-sensitive.

Metabolic basis of diabetes

Normal metabolic homeostasis. There is normally a fine balance between anabolic and catabolic processes, so that weight is steady about a healthy level and an adequate supply of fuel is maintained to the body tissues. The organism has become adapted to periods of feasting interspersed with times of fasting.

During feasting there is a large positive fuel surplus absorbed from the gastrointestinal tract. Excess carbohydrates and amino acids pass first to the liver via the portal system. The liver is particularly well designed to dispose of carbohydrate loads. It can be calculated that if 100 g of glucose were ingested, and distributed instantaneously around the extracellular fluid, glucose concentration would rise by 37 mmol/l, with a large osmotic imbalance. Instead the rise is only 2–3 mmol/l. The liver takes up approximately 60–80 per cent of such a load, storing some as glycogen for later use, and converting the rest to fatty acids and triglycerides which are then secreted as very-low-density lipoproteins (VLDL), whose fatty acids are subsequently stored in adipose tissue. The rest of the glucose enters the peripheral tissues where it is stored as glycogen or oxidized. Amino acids are not stored as such but protein synthesis from them is increased after feeding while excess amino acids are oxidized in the liver, apart from those of branched chain structure (BCAA) which tend to be broken down in extrahepatic tissues. Fats, after digestion and absorption, are reassembled in gastrointestinal mucosal cells as chylomicra, which traverse the thoracic duct and deposit their fatty acids again into adipose tissue stores.

In fasting, the body depends on supplies of fuels from the stores built up during feeding. In short-term fasting the brain, nervous tissue, red blood cells, and renal medulla have an obligatory requirement for glucose amounting to 180 g per day. This is produced in the main (90 per cent) by the liver from glycogen (80 per cent after an overnight fast) and gluconeogenesis from recycling lactate, pyruvate, gluconeogenic amino acids (mainly alanine and indirectly glutamine) and glycerol. As fasting progresses, so the brain increasingly uses ketone bodies and thus spares glucose from oxidation, with consequent saving of vital amino acids. The kidney also contributes to gluconeogenesis in this state, but total glucose requirements are halved. It is crucial that alternative fuels to protein should be used and adipose tissue provides this need.

In adipose tissue there is a continuous recycling of fatty acids from the free state to triglycerides and back through re-esterification and lipolysis. The latter generates glycerol which cannot be reutilized for re-esterification as the enzyme glycerokinase is not present in adipose tissue. Instead new glycerol 3-phosphate must be produced from glucose. In fasting, such production is decreased with net release of fatty acids, which may be used directly as oxidative fuels. Muscle in the resting state, for example, derives 80–90 per cent of its energy from fatty-acid oxidation. In addition approximately 30 per cent of the fatty acid is taken up by the liver, enters the mitochondria via the carnitine shuttle and is oxidized to acetyl-CoA. Most of this acetyl-CoA is then converted to the ketone bodies acetoacetate and 3-hydroxybutyrate through the 3-hydroxymethyl-glutaryl-CoA pathway. The ketone bodies cannot normally be used in the liver owing to the lack of the enzyme thiolase but diffuse into the circulation for use elsewhere. Most tissues of the body are adapted to use several alternative fuels, and their metabolism is determined by the amounts of these that reach them. Heart muscle, for example, can use glucose, fatty acids, lactate, or 'ketone bodies', in amounts depending primarily on availability.

There is thus a highly adaptable series of metabolic processes which are designed to ensure continuation of fuel supply at all times, and storage of appropriate substrates at times of excess. The whole system is finely integrated and is regulated by a group of hormones. Insulin is the prime anabolic hormone designed for fuel storage and with an anticatabolic role in fasting. The catabolic hormones comprise glucogen, cortisol, and catecholamines, which ensure fuel supplies during fasting and stress. Growth hormone is designed primarily to preserve protein, and has mixed anabolic and catabolic functions.

In diabetes insulin is lacking or is present but acts ineffectively. In the rest of this section the normal synthesis, secretion, and actions of insulin, together with the biochemical actions of the opposing catabolic hormones are reviewed, after which the biochemical effects of insulin deficiency are described.

Insulin biosynthesis. Insulin is found in the β cells of the islets of Langerhans in the pancreas. The islets comprise 1–3 per cent of the pancreatic mass and are probably derived from the ectoderm. Estimates of the numbers of islets vary from 100 000 to 2.5 million. They contain not only β cells which secrete insulin, but α cells (glucagon), D cells (somatostatin), PP cells (pancreatic polypeptide), and other less well-defined neuroendocrine cells. Approximately half the cells are β cells. The islets have a rich sympathetic and parasympathetic nerve suppy.

Insulin is synthesized initially on the rough endoplasmic reticulum as a large precursor, preproinsulin, of molecular weight 11 500 daltons. This has a very short half-life, being cleaved almost immediately to yield a long polypeptide chain, proinsulin, of molecular weight 9000, which is joined in an overlapping circle by two disulphide bridges. The proinsulin is packed into granules surrounded by a single membrane layer at the Golgi apparatus. Part of the molecule is then removed—the connecting or C-peptide—leaving the characteristic double chain of insulin plus C-peptide in the granule. The A-chain comprises 21 amino acids and the B-chain 30 amino acids, with the two chains linked at the A7–B7 and A20–B19 positions by cystine disulphide bridges. The A-chain contains a further disulphide link between the 6 and 11 positions.

The structure of insulins of different species are remarkably similar. Thus human and porcine insulin differ only in the B30 amino acid (threonine in man, alanine in the pig) while beef insulin is different only at the A8, A9, and B30 positions. In the β-cell, insulin exists as a hexamer bound to zinc, but is almost certainly monomeric after release into the circulation.

Insulin secretion. Insulin is formed from proinsulin in the β-cell granules. These migrate to the cell surface where the granule membrane fuses with the cell membrane and the contents of the granule are discharged. The microtubular–microfilamentous system is involved in the passage of the granules from the Golgi apparatus to the cell surface.

The mechanism of action of the different insulin secretagogues has not been clearly established. Glucose is the prime stimulus, but it remains controversial as to whether it acts through a glucoreceptor on the β-cell surface or through metabolism to an active intermediate. Both glyceraldehyde phosphate and fructose 2,6-biphosphate have been suggested for the latter role, and both may indeed by involved. Glucose, unlike most other stimuli to insulin secretion, also increases insulin synthesis.

There are several further crucial components to the insulin release system even if no clinical link is yet recognized. Extracellular calcium is required for glucose to act and calcium may be needed for the microtubules to function normally. Cyclic AMP also acts as a trigger to insulin release but is ineffective in the total absence of glucose. Many factors act through cyclic AMP system, such as glucagon, to increase insulin secretion, while α-adrenergic stimulation by adrenaline or noradrenaline decreases cyclic AMP and so inhibits secretion. β-stimulation acts in an opposite sense but normally the α-inhibitory effect predominates. It was once thought that the sulphonylurea drugs acted through the cyclic AMP system. This is now less certain although they do enhance glucose-stimulated insulin secretion.

Several metabolic fuels also affect insulin secretion (Table 5). Thus amino acids increase insulin release. Leucine may act via a separate mechanism and is effective in the absence of glucose, unlike other amino acids such as arginine. Fatty acids and ketone bodies may also increase insulin secretion. Gut hormones almost certainly modulate insulin secretion. Insulin secretion is much greater in response to an oral than an equivalent intravenous glucose load. Many hormones have been suggested to be responsible, but only GIP remains as a reasonable candidate and even then all the changes cannot be explained. Glucagon is also a potent stimulus to insulin secretion. The physiological importance of this is unknown, although the anatomical juxtaposition of the α and β cells should be remembered; glucagon may prove to have a local regulatory function. This may also be true for somatostatin (from the islet D cell), a potent inhibitor of insulin and of glucagon secretion.

Neural regulation of insulin secretion is also important *in vivo*. The vagus, through acetylcholine release, stimulates insulin secretion, while sympathetic discharge predominantly inhibits it. It is very likely that other neurotransmitters, such as somatostatin, dopamine, serotonin, and VIP also have effects. Recently there has been considerable interest in the central regulation of insulin secretion by the hypothalamus, with the ventrolateral nucleus controlling vagal drive to the islets and the ventromedial nucleus stimulating the sympathetic innervation.

Table 5 Stimulators and inhibitors of insulin secretion

	Mechanism	Glucose required
Stimulator		
Glucose	? glucoreceptor	
	? metabolite	
	± Ca^{2+} shifts	
Glucagon	↑ cyclic AMP	+
Gut hormones (GIP)	↑ cyclic AMP	+
β-Adrenergic agents	↑ cyclic AMP	+
Prostaglandins	↑ cyclic AMP	+
Leucine	? membrane effect	−
	? metabolite	
Other amino acids		
(arginine)	?	+
Fatty acids	?	−
Ketone bodies	?	−
Acetylcholine	? Ca^{2+} shifts	−
vagal stimulation		
Inhibitors		
α-Adrenergic agents	↓ cyclic AMP	−
Sympathetic nerve		
stimulation		
Dopamine	? Ca^{2+} shifts	−
Serotonin	? Ca^{2+} shifts	−
Somatostatin	?	

Secretion occurs in two phases, a fast first phase, probably from secretion of already formed granules situated near the cell surface. If the stimulus is sustained there is then a slower second phase of secretion, in which much of the insulin is newly synthesized. Attempts have been made to relate the two phases of insulin secretion to morphological compartments with small and large storage pools but their exact identity remains uncertain. In man the two phases are not seen clearly unless a constant stimulus is applied, as with a constant glucose infusion. There is some diminution in the first-phase and slight delay in the second in mild type II diabetics, but the response to a non-glucose stimulus such as arginine may be normal. In type I and severe type II diabetes, the first phase is generally entirely absent, and in type I the second phase is greatly diminished, and eventually disappears altogether.

Insulin secretion *in vivo* is controlled by a finely integrated combination of metabolic, hormonal, and neural mechanisms. For example, there is a rise in insulin secretion on eating a mixed meal. First there is the 'cephalic' phase due to vagal secretion. This is followed by release of gut hormones and absorption of glucose, which together cause a steady rise in insulin levels to peak at 45–60 min. Absorbed amino acids have a synergistic effect with glucose. There may be an added effect from amino-acid-stimulated glucagon secretion, although this will be counteracted by the action of glucose on the α cell and will only be of real importance with a pure protein meal. As food absorption is completed the stimulus to insulin secretion falls and plasma levels return to baseline after 2–3 h.

In the fasting state, basal insulin secretion is maintained in part by glucose and in part by neuroregulation. In addition, as levels of fatty acids and 'ketone bodies' rise, so there will be a slight increase in insulin secretion which serves to damp down lipolysis. Basal insulin secretion is crucial in the restraint of catabolism.

Insulin physiology. Insulin is secreted into the portal vein and immediately reaches its main target organ—the liver, which takes up to 20–70 per cent of the insulin reaching it, the exact amount depending on nutritional state, with greater uptake in the fed state. The combination of hepatic extraction and subsequent dilution in the circulation results in a considerable portal: peripheral insulin gradient, varying between 3 and 10:1, which has implications both with respect to insulin action and to the therapeutic use of insulin given into the peripheral circulation. Insulin degradation by the liver follows its action there. Insulin is also degraded to some extent by the kidney, apart from the substantial urinary excretion; about 40 per cent is extracted in a single passage. Other tissues, e.g. lung and muscle, extract small amounts of insulin. The half-life of insulin in the circulation is 4–5 min, with a metabolic clearance rate of 1.2 to 1.4 l/min and an apparent distribution space of approximately 10 to 13 l.

C-peptide is secreted in equimolar amounts with insulin. Its practical importance is twofold. First, it is not metabolized by the liver so that its peripheral blood measurement gives a better index of pancreatic β-cell function than peripheral insulin measurement. Second, C-peptide measurement can be used to assess endogenous insulin secretions in insulin-treated diabetics, in whom both exogenous and endogenous insulin cross-react with the antibody, or insulin antibodies prevent the assay being used at all. C-peptide is degraded by the kidney and has a half-life in the circulation of 20–35 min.

Mechanism of action of insulin. Controversy still surrounds the mechanism of the metabolic actions of insulin. The first step, however, now seems clear. Insulin binds to specific cell surface receptors in insulin-sensitive tissues, including fat, muscle, liver, and brain; binding to circulating white cells and red blood cells can also be demonstrated. The receptor is postulated to be a glycoprotein of molecular weight approximately 350 000. It comprises two α subunits of 125 000 daltons and two smaller subunits of 90 000 with disulphide linkages between subunits. There is still argument about subunit size, particularly in different tissues. The receptor, both in the intact cell and isolated, displays the property of 'negative co-operativity', a form of negative feedback control in which the affinity of unoccupied receptors for insulin falls the greater the number of receptors that have been occupied. Another feature of the receptor is that maximal insulin action on the fat cell for example can be obtained with only 10 per cent of the receptors occupied, giving rise to the concept of 'spare' receptors. It is possible that *in vivo* these are either buried within the cell membrane or inaccessible to insulin because of shielding by neighbouring cells.

Insulin receptors also appear to be regulated by the amount of insulin that they are exposed to. Thus in chronic hyperinsulinaemia the number of receptors decreases—so-called 'down-regulation'. Conversely in hypoinsulinaemic states such as untreated insulin-deficient diabetes the number of receptors increases. The classical example of down-regulation is obesity. If obese patients diet there is an immediate increase in affinity and then a slower increase in receptor number. This regulation of receptor number may be a protective mechanism. Thus in obesity with hyperphagia cells become less responsive to insulin to limit, for example, triglyceride synthesis and deposition. A vicious circle can, however, result with more and more insulin secreted to overcome the fall in receptor number and activity, a sequence of events which can lead to diabetes in a susceptible individual when insulin secretion has reached a maximum.

The physiology of insulin receptors has therapeutic importance. The sulphonylureas not only promote insulin secretion, but also increase insulin receptor number, thereby increasing the effectiveness of insulin action.

The insulin–receptor complex is internalized as a vesicle. The vesicle probably fuses with lysosomes resulting in degradation of both insulin and the receptor. It is possible that internalized receptors are recycled to the cell membrane although it is more likely that new receptors are synthesized within the cell and then inserted into the cell membrane.

Although the process of insulin binding to the receptor is now well characterized there is much less information on the subsequent steps in the action of insulin. It is uncertain whether insulin acts solely through cell-membrane interactions or whether the internalized insulin–receptor complex may have an active biological role. The evidence would support the former view at present. Any hypothesis must encompass the intermediate and delayed actions of the hormone, and the modification of the effect of insulin on glucose transport by several agents. After the discovery of cyclic AMP it was assumed that insulin acted through inhibition of adenyl cyclase. This cannot be the sole mechanism, although insulin may act to decrease intracellular cyclic AMP concentration. It has been suggested that the insulin–receptor interaction activates a cell membrane protease, which is arginine specific and releases a small peptide (2000 to 10 000 daltons) from a membrane protein precursor. This peptide then has several effects within the cell, such as activating the phosphatase in the pyruvate dehydrogenase complex and inhibiting cyclic AMP activation of protein kinases.

The overall effect would be to decrease phosphorylation of particular enzymes. This hypothesis still needs to be substantiated and other postulated mechanisms such as changes in the intracellular distribution of Ca^{2+}, or changes in membrane structure must still be considered.

It is possible that the slow actions of insulin are due to effects on protein synthesis by the putative peptide, but it is unlikely that such a mechanism explains the effects of insulin on membrane transport of substrates such as glucose and amino acids, or electrolytes. These could be due to changes in membrane configuration induced by the insulin–receptor interaction. Recently it has been shown that whole segments of membrane-glucose transport units are mobilized from within the cell from the Golgi apparatus, suggesting a different mechanism for glucose transport stimulated by insulin.

Much remains to be discovered about the actions of insulin on cells; new data may allow more effective use of insulin or its substitutes in diabetic patients.

Effects of insulin *in vivo*. The overall effects of insulin are summarized in Table 6. Many tissues are responsive to insulin, including liver, muscle, adipose tissue, brain, peripheral nerve, smooth muscle, large arteries, skin, cartilage, bone, fibroblasts, leucocytes, and seminal vesicles, but in terms of whole-body homeostasis, only the first three are important.

Table 6 Metabolic effects of insulin in major metabolic tissues

	Tissue	Mechanism
Carbohydrate metabolism		
Increase		
Glucose transport	Muscle, adipose tissue	Mobilization of glucose transport units
Glucose phosphorylation	Liver	Induction of glucokinase; activation of hexokinase
	Muscle, adipose tissue, etc.	Activation of hexokinase
Glycogenesis	Liver, muscle	Activation of glycogen synthase
Glycolysis	Liver, muscle, adipose tissue	Activation of phosphofructokinase, pyruvate kinase, pyruvate dehydrogenase
Pentose phosphate pathway	Liver, adipose tissue	Activation of glucose 6-phosphate dehydrogenase and 6-phosphogluconate dehydrogenase
Decrease		
Glycogenolysis	Liver, muscle	Decreased phosphorylase; ? decreased cyclic AMP
Gluconeogenesis	Liver	Decreased pyruvate carboxylase, phosphoenol-pyruvate carboxykinase, Fructose 1,6-bisphosphatase Decreased precursor availability
Lipid metabolism		
Increase		
Fatty acid synthesis	Liver	Activation (dephosphorylation of PDH, acetyl-CoA caboxylase)
Triglyceride synthesis	Liver, adipose tissue	Increased glycerol 3-phosphate. ? Increased esterase
VLDL formation	Liver	?
Lipoprotein degradation	Adipose tissue	Increased lipoprotein lipase activity
Decrease		
Lipolysis	Adipose tissue, ? liver ? muscle ? heart	Inhibition of hormone sensitive lipase activity ? Decrease cyclic AMP
Fatty acid oxidation	Liver, muscle	Decreased mitochondrial fatty acid entry
Ketogenesis	Liver	Increased malonyl-CoA
Lipoprotein degradation	Muscle	Increased lipoprotein lipase
Protein metabolism		
Increase		
Amino acid transport	Liver, muscle, etc.	?
Protein synthesis	Liver, muscle, etc.	Increased nucleic acid synthesis, monoribosome attachment, polyribosome formation
Decrease		
Protein degradation	Liver, muscle, etc.	?
Ureagenesis	Liver	?
Electrolyte metabolism		
Increase		
Potassium transport	Muscle, liver, etc.	Membrane effect
Phosphate entry	Muscle, liver, etc.	?
Decrease		
Sodium uptake	Muscle, liver, etc.	Membrane effect

Liver. Insulin has a key role in maintenance of glucose supplies to tissues. In the basal, or fasting, state insulin modulates hepatic glucose production by restraining glycogenolysis and gluconeogenesis. In the fed state insulin levels rise and there is virtual total inhibition of these processes, so that hepatic glucose production drops to zero. This is achieved by inhibition of phosphorylase and the key gluconeogenic enzymes pyruvate carboxylase, phosphoenolpyruvate carboxykinase, and fructose 1,6-diphosphatase, probably through inhibition of protein kinases. At the same time insulin is crucial in the hepatic disposal of incoming glucose. This it does by enhancing glucokinase activity and hence glucose phosphorylation. Glucose 6-phosphate then follows any of three routes. First is to glycogen with activation of glycogen synthase, but glycogen storage capacity is limited and further excess glucose is diverted to lipid synthesis. Thus increased glycolysis (at first sight a catabolic effect), through activation of phosphofructokinase and pyruvate kinase, increases pyruvate availability; this through increased activation of pyruvate dehydrogenase and acetyl-CoA carboxylase is then diverted into fatty acid synthesis. Secondly, increased flux of glucose 6-phosphate into the pentose phosphate shunt, which increases NADPH (diphosphopyridine nucleotide) availability for fatty acid synthesis. The fatty acids are esterified with glycerol 3-phosphate, also formed during glycolysis. The resultant triglycerides are incorporated into VLDL (very-low-density lipoproteins) and secreted by the liver, so that newly formed lipid is transported to extrahepatic sites for storage. Fatty acids absorbed from the gut will follow the same route, although short-chain fatty acids will first be elongated.

While fatty acid synthesis is promoted, fatty acid oxidation and ketogenesis are inhibited. Malonyl-CoA is formed as the first committed step of fatty acid synthesis. This is the major factor regulating entry of fatty acids into mitochondria. Increased levels inhibit carnitine acyltransferase I, the key first step in transport. If fatty acids, or at least fatty acylCoA, do not enter mitochondria, they cannot be oxidized and so are not available for esterification. Similarly lack of oxidation of fatty acids prevents ketogenesis through lack of acetyl-CoA as precursor.

Net hepatic synthesis is also promoted by insulin, partly through increased DNA polymerase and RNA polymerase activity and also through effects on ribosomal aggregation. There is also increased amino-acid uptake, and decreased amino-acid and protein breakdown.

Overall the hepatic actions of insulin lead to preservation of fuels. There is decreased production of substrates for immediate use, i.e. ketone bodies and glucose, and fuel storage with dispersal of newly synthesized high-energy substrates for storage in other tissues.

Muscle. The effects of insulin in muscle are directed mainly towards local metabolism. Glucose transport is enhanced, and glucose 6-phosphate formation and glycogen synthesis are increased. Muscle, unlike liver, cannot release glucose into the circulation as it lacks glucose 6-phosphatase; but it can contribute glucose indirectly by breaking down glycogen to lactate and pyruvate, which pass into the circulation and are used for gluconeogenesis by the liver (Cori cycle).

Lipoprotein lipase in muscle capillary endothelium is inhibited by insulin so that less fatty acid is delivered to muscle when insulin levels are raised; although triglyceride synthesis is increased, this is a much smaller effect than in adipose tissue or liver, owing to shortage of available fatty acid. In the fasting state, muscle derives 80–90 per cent of its energy from fatty acid and ketone body oxidation. In the fed state, owing to the comparative unavailability of these substrates, and the actions of insulin, fuel utilization is switched more to glucose. All these effects are less sensitive to insulin than are the anticatabolic effects in the liver.

Insulin also has a major effect on muscle protein metabolism. Amino-acid transport is increased (mainly the two neutral amino-acid transport systems) and protein synthesis enhanced

through effects at several points in the synthetic pathway. Simultaneously protein degradation is decreased. One further point of clinical importance is the effect of insulin on electrolyte transport. This is probably a direct effect on the membrane, the net result being an increase in intracellular potassium and phosphate.

Adipose tissue. Lipolysis is extremely sensitive to insulin with considerable inhibition evident even at normal basal insulin concentrations. In the fed state lipolysis decreases further. This is a major controlling factor, not just on fatty acid supply for oxidation, but on ketogenesis as the lack of substrate supply to the liver will sharply decrease ketogenesis. After food the higher insulin levels have several additional effects on adipose tissue. Glucose transport is stimulated and this provides glycerol 3-phosphate, for re-esterification of fatty acid released by lipolysis or entering the adipocyte *de novo*. Re-esterification is also stimulated. In contrast to muscle, lipoprotein lipase in the capillary endothelium is activated with release of fatty acids from circulating chlyomicrons and VLDL. The fatty acids enter the adipocyte where they are esterified for storage as triglyceride. There are smaller effects of insulin on protein synthesis.

Whole-body effects. Several studies have been performed to examine the overall effects of different doses of insulin on metabolic processes. Infusion of small amounts of insulin to give increments of 10–20 μU/ml over the fasting levels of 5–10 μU/ml causes inhibition of glucose production and a sharp fall in circulating fatty acid, glycerol, and ketone body levels. Two- to threefold greater increments are required to increase glucose utilization and to cause significant effects on amino acid and potassium transport and on lipid synthesis.

Actions of catabolic hormones. The actions of insulin cannot be isolated from the effects of the catabolic or anti-insulin hormones which balance and oppose it. As insulin levels fall in fasting, for example, the actions of these other hormones become more important, while in the fed states the effects of insulin predominate.

Table 7 summarizes the actions of glucagon, cortisol, catecholamines and growth hormone. Glucagon is predominantly an hepatic hormone with most, if not all, of its effects mediated by cyclic AMP. It has a long-term tonic effect on gluconeogenesis, inhibiting the glycolytic enzymes phosphofructokinase (through fructose 2,6-bisphosphate) and pyruvate kinase. At the same time it causes the activation of phosphoenolpyruvate carboxykinase and fructose 1,6-biphosphatase. Glucagon also causes glycogenolysis via the phosphorylase reaction, but this is short-lived. Gluconeogenesis is also enhanced by a glucogen-mediated increase in hepatic uptake of gluconeogenic amino acids, particularly alanine.

Glucagon also has important effects on hepatic lipid metabolism. The enzyme acetyl-CoA carboxylase is inhibited, with a fall in fatty acid synthesis, and a decrease in malonyl-CoA formation. This latter stimulates the carnitine-mediated transport of fatty acids into mitochondria with consequent increased fatty acid oxidation, acetyl-CoA formation, and ketogenesis. The secretion of VLDL and triglycerides is also inhibited. All these effects of glucagon are antagonized by insulin, and much has been made of the 'glucagon:insulin ratio' in the regulation of hepatic metabolism. Certainly both hormones are important in determining the anabolic or catabolic direction of metabolism, but to view them out of context of the other catabolic hormones is inappropriate. Glucagon may also increase lipolysis, but this effect is not seen with physiological excursions of glucagon concentration in the presence of even basal amounts of insulin. Similarly the ketogenic effects of glucagon on the liver will be irrelevant if there is insulin suppression of lipolysis, and thereby few fatty acids arriving at the liver.

The *catecholamines*, adrenaline and noradrenaline, act chiefly on adipose tissue and liver. Both hormones stimulate adipose tissue lipolysis even in the presence of insulin, through activation of hormone-sensitive lipase. This and other effects are mediated both

Table 7   Some metabolic actions of the catabolic hormones

	Glucagon		Catecholamines		Cortisol		Growth hormone	
	Increase	Decrease	Increase	Decrease	Increase	Decrease	Increase	Decrease
Liver	Glycogenoly-sis Gluconeo-genesis Fatty acid oxidation Ketogenesis Alanine uptake Ureagenesis	Glycolysis Fatty acid synthesis Triglyceride formation VLDL secre-tion Protein secre-tion	Glycogenoly-sis (adrena-line) Gluconeo-genesis Ketogenesis†	Glycolysis	Gluconeo-genesis Amino acid uptake Amino acid degradation Protein syn-thesis Ketogenesis† Lipid syn-thesis‡		Gluconeo-genesis Protein synthesis Amino acid transport Ketogenesis†	
Adipose tissue	Lipolysis*		Lipolysis*		Lipolysis*	Re-esterifica-tion Glucose uptake	Lipolysis* (long-term)	
Muscle	–	–	Glycogenoly-sis (adrena-line) Glycolysis Lactate release	–	Proteolysis Alanine release Lactate release	Glucose uptake	Glucose up-take (short term) Amino acid transport Protein synthesis Fatty acid uptake (short-term)	Glucose uptake (long-term)

* In the absence of insulin.
†Probably secondary to increased fatty acid supply from adipose tissue.
‡ In the presence of insulin.

by cyclic AMP effects on protein kinases and cyclic-AMP-independent effects, probably involving calcium. In the liver both hormones increase gluconeogenesis but adrenaline alone causes glycogenolysis. Intrahepatic lipolysis may be stimulated but there are few other effects on hepatic lipid metabolism. The increase in ketogenesis seen *in vivo* is primarily due to increased fatty acid delivery to the liver. Adrenaline also increases glycogenolysis in muscle. This causes increased lactate production which is available for gluconeogenesis in the liver.

Cortisol has widespread metabolic effects. It inhibits glucose uptake in many tissues. In adipose tissue this decreases re-esterification and so increases fatty acid mobilization. The sensitivity of lipolysis to other catabolic hormones is also increased. Perhaps the most important effect of cortisol is to increase protein degradation, particularly in muscle. Amino acids are released into the circulation, mainly as alanine and glutamine, major substrates for the main effect of cortisol, an increase in hepatic gluconeogenesis through induction of transaminases and gluconeogenic enzymes. Fatty acid synthesis and triglyceride formation are also enhanced by cortisol in the presence of insulin, but ketogenesis occurs if insulin is absent. Protein synthesis is also increased in the liver.

Growth hormone has many effects which may differ in the short and long term, and some are mediated by somatomedins. Glucose uptake by muscle is increased acutely but impaired chronically. At the same time lipolysis is stimulated and ketogenesis may thereby be increased indirectly in the absence of insulin. The main effects, however, are to increase amino acid uptake and protein synthesis by most tissues.

Altogether the actions of the catabolic hormones oppose the various effects of insulin described earlier. An important considera-tion for diabetics is that some of the effects of catabolic hormones, particularly on ketogenesis, are of importance early in insulin deficiency.

Insulin deficiency. The metabolic effects of insulin deficiency may be predicted from the known actions of insulin and of the counter-regulatory hormones described above.

Partial deficiency. In some forms of type II diabetes there is partial insulin deficiency (in others there is primary insulin resistance, as described below) in which the anticatabolic effects persist, as they require only small (normal basal) amounts of insulin. In this situation lipolysis and ketogenesis are not increased, and glyco-genolysis and gluconeogenesis are at most slightly increased. In contrast ingested foods are handled inadequately. A glucose load is disposed of slowly; glycogen deposition is impaired; and protein synthesis may be decreased.

Hyperlipidaemia is a further concomitant of partial as well as total insulin deficiency. Newly diagnosed diabetics commonly present with hypertriglyceridaemia and hypercholesterolaemia. There is no single characteristic defect in lipoproteins and many different abnormalities are seen. There is a clear association between glycaemic control and raised plasma triglyceride, total cholesterol and LDL-cholesterol levels, and an inverse relation to HDL-cholesterol. A major cause is impaired clearance of chylo-microns and VLDL, owing to inadequate activation by insulin of adipose tissue lipoprotein lipase.

There are also associated endocrine changes. Basal glucagon secretion is increased, and may increase further on feeding, in contrast to the normal fall, tending to increase gluconeogenesis. In addition growth hormone levels may be increased, but the effect of this is uncertain.

Total deficiency. In total, or near-total insulin deficiency there are much more profound metabolic changes. Many type I diabetics retain some endogenous insulin secretion, particularly early on. This is normally sufficient to prevent unrestrained lipolysis and gluconeogenesis unless there is an increase in the catabolic hormones due to stress or illness. Initially the changes will be as in partial insulin deficiency, but later these will be followed by loss of inhibition of gluconeogenesis, glycogenolysis, lipolysis and hence fatty acid mobilization, and ketogenesis. It is rare for total insulin deficiency to be isolated from changes in other hormones. This has been shown experimentally by treating C-peptide-negative (totally insulin-deficient) type I diabetics subcutaneously only with short-acting insulins for 48 h, and then infusing insulin intravenously for a further 12 h before stopping insulin altogether. Blood glucose levels then rise from near normal to plateau at 10–12 mmol/l after three or four hours. Plasma fatty acids, blood glycerol, and ketone bodies rise less abruptly but continue to increase so that ketone body levels are 6–8 mmol/l after 12 h, compared with normal overnight fasting values of 0.05–0.4 mmol/l. These changes are consistent with a stepwise increase in glucose production rate, but a steady increase in ketone body production. In parallel, plasma glucagon levels rise throughout the deprivation period and correlate closely with the rises in lipid metabolites in particular. Alanine levels fall due to glucagon enhanced hepatic extraction. The role of glucagon has been illustrated by the much slower rises in glucose than in ketone bodies found in insulin-deprived pancreatectomized subjects who, obviously, lack pancreatic glucagon. If insulin deprivation is continued, cortisol secretion also increases, which will potentiate both gluconeogenesis and ketogenesis. Later growth hormone levels also rise. It is probable that catecholamine secretion only rises significantly if substantial circulatory changes occur because of dehydration and desalination induced by hyperglycaemic osmotic diuresis. Acidaemia from hyperketonaemia will also affect both blood pressure and catecholamine levels. Once this occurs, the metabolic state will further deteriorate, in particular from the marked effects of catecholamines on lipolysis, and hence further enhanced ketogenesis.

These are the results of 'pure' insulin deprivation. However, similar changes may occur in relative insulin deficiency. In this state insulin levels may be unchanged or at least equivalent to normal fasting levels, but the levels of the catabolic hormones have increased greatly. For example half the patients presenting in ketoacidosis do so because of infection, during which glucagon and cortisol secretions increase markedly. Unless extra insulin is given there will be an imbalance in favour of the catabolic hormones, with increase in lipolysis and hepatic metabolism set in favour of gluconeogenesis and ketogenesis. Other stress states will have similar effects. Thus, myocardial infarction or trauma are associated with increases not only in cortisol and glucagon, but also catecholamines. The metabolic derangements of either mild diabetes or ketoacidosis can therefore be understood on the basis of the known actions of insulin and the catabolic hormones.

Insulin resistance. Considerable interest has centred on insulin resistance, particularly with respect to the mildly or grossly obese type II diabetic, where insulin levels may appear to be normal, and metabolic changes are not attributable solely or even partly, in some cases, to impaired insulin secretion.

Possible causes of insulin resistance are listed in Table 8. There is down-regulation of insulin receptors in obesity but in view of the large number of 'spare' receptors there would have to be a very large decrease in receptor number to cause a decrease in sensitivity, i.e. the dose–response curve is shifted to the right but the maximum effect remains the same. This phenomenon has been shown both

Table 8 Causes of insulin resistance

1. Target tissue defects
    (a) Insulin receptor defects
    (b) Post-receptor defects

2. Circulating antagonists
    (a) Increased concentrations of catabolic hormones: glucagon, cortisol, growth hormone, catecholamines
    (b) Anti-insulin antibodies
    (c) Anti-insulin receptor antibodies

Adapted from Olefsky and Kolterman (1981) *Am. J. Med.* **70**, 151.

for adipose tissue and for hepatic functions, but in some obese type II diabetics the maximum effect is also decreased, perhaps implying an as yet unidentified post-receptor disturbance. Decreased insulin sensitivity in both obese and non-obese type II diabetics can be demonstratated using the glucose clamp technique where euglycaemia is maintained by variable glucose infusion, while insulin is infused at a constant rate. Very large doses of insulin may be needed in the extremely obese diabetic; indeed it is often impossible to achieve good glycaemic control in such patients until weight loss has been obtained. Insulin therapy in them may only worsen control by increasing down-regulation.

Other possible causes of insulin resistance are listed in Table 8. The insulin-dependent diabetic often shows mild insulin resistance, most likely through insulin antibodies (see below) which bind insulin and prevent its access to receptors. It is also possible that increased concentrations of the catabolic hormones cause some insulin resistance with regard to carbohydrate, although not lipid, metabolism. Certainly, inhibition of glucagon secretion decreases insulin requirements but this occurs in normal man too, and it is uncertain whether the small elevations in circulating glucagon levels found in the average type I diabetic cause significant resistance. The same is true for the raised growth hormone levels of poorly controlled type I diabetics.

Insulin resistance is also found in patients with severe diabetic ketoacidosis. This is due partly to acidaemia, partly to high levels of the catabolic hormones, and sometimes to hypothermia. This resistance rarely lasts for long after appropriate fluid and insulin therapy has been instituted (see below).

Importance of metabolic control

The two main aims of therapy in diabetes are to prevent day-to-day symptoms secondary to hyperglycaemia or hypoglycaemia and to prevent the long-term tissue damage of diabetes: macroangiopathy, microangiopathy (retinopathy and nephropathy), and neuropathy. The latter is much the more difficult to achieve, and even now there is no unanimous view on how best to approach the problem, although a reasonable consensus is forming.

One strong view is that good control of glycaemia will prevent or delay the onset of tissue damage. Before discussing the evidence, it should be stressed that the aetiologies of tissue damage are different for different 'complications' (Table 9). Thus, macroangiopathy has been suggested to be related to hyperinsulinaemia and lipid disorders; small blood vessel disease to hyperglycaemia through protein glycosylation, insulin deficiency, and other metabolic disturbances; and neuropathy could be associated with

Table 9 The chronic complications of diabetes

		Possible causes
A.	Macroangiopathy (atherosclerosis, myocardial disease)	Hyperlipidaemia Hyperinsulinaemia ? Hyperglycaemia ? Increased growth hormone levels ? Platelets and other vascular factors
B.	Microangiopathy (retinopathy, neuropathy, capillary basement membrane thickening)	Hyperglycaemia Protein (basement membrane) glycosylation Hormonal factors, e.g. growth hormone Insulin deficiency
C.	Neuropathy	Sorbitol accumulation Deficient myoinositol Myelin glycosylation Hyperglycaemia
D.	Diabetic cataract	Hyperglycaemia Protein glycosylation
E.	Collagen change	

hyperglycaemia, sorbitol accumulation and abnormalities in myoinositol metabolism. It is not unlikely, therefore, that different aspects of metabolism may need to be controlled to prevent the individual complications.

The term 'diabetic control' is confusing. To most clinicians this now implies normoglycaemia, but in the past it has even been used synonymously with aglycosuria or near normal blood glucose levels when assessed randomly at the diabetic clinic. It is not possible to monitor blood glucose levels continuously, but in the last five years, developments have allowed assessment of glycaemic control more easily than before (see below).

Hyperglycaemia is but one facet of diabetes mellitus. Insulin has effects on many different metabolic pathways, which in sum involve virtually the whole of metabolism. It may not be possible, therefore, by monitoring glucose alone, to establish whether diabetes is or is not 'well controlled'. Strictly the terms 'glycaemic' or 'blood glucose' control should be used. It is still uncertain whether glucose is the best metabolite to measure and to correct in relation to the prevention of chronic complications, but the evidence increasingly favours this. It remains also one of the few metabolites which is easy to monitor, and so will be used for the time being, in combination with attempts to achieve normal physiological patterns of circulating insulin.

Short of absolute certainty, there is extremely strong suggestive evidence that the physician should approach as closely as possible a normal metabolic pattern in his patients. This stems from three lines of evidence: epidemiological work, animal experiments, and a few prospective studies in patients.

Studies in Oxford, Massachusetts, in Bedford, in Athens and in Pima Amerindians have shown a close association between the two-hour post-glucose blood glucose levels and the risk of developing retinopathy. There appeared to be a cut-off point of approximately 11 mmol/l (200 mg/dl) below which retinopathy developed infrequently. The studies in Bedford and Oxford also showed an association between risk of cardiovascular disease and blood glucose, with the degree of risk much lower than for retinopathy.

There is other clinical evidence. There was a lower rate of complication in patients treated with multiple injections than in patients treated with once-daily injections in Malmö, Sweden, in the 1930s, the inference being that 'control' was better in the former group. Many further studies were published in the 1950s and 1960s which cannot be considered seriously because the criteria for control were inadequate. Of 14 prospective studies at this time, four showed no relation of glucose to complications, whilst the other ten each provided some evidence that improved control slows the development of retinal or glomerular changes. In a Belgian study, 4398 subjects entered a 25-year period prospective observation. The authors summed up that 'the duration and severity of hyperglycaemia seem to be the only factors which can be definitely linked with the development, at whatever age, of diabetic retinopathy . . .'. Many criticisms may be levelled at this work, not least that no biochemical parameters other than glucose were followed in a systematic way. It is also pertinent to ask why 20–30 per cent of the poor-control group did *not* develop retinopathy after 20–25 years. None the less, the association with glycosuria and intermittently measured hyperglycaemia was strong. Other factors must, however, also be involved. This is most evident in type II diabetics, where severe retinopathy in one study was found despite persistent near-normoglycaemia. In these patients hypoinsulinaemia and raised growth hormone levels were also found.

Animal work supports the view that long-term tissue damage results from the metabolic disturbance. Dogs, rats, and mice with uncontrolled experimental diabetes all develop tissue damage which has many features in common with the human syndromes. Transplantation of the pancreas can both prevent lesions developing and reverse some of the early changes. Little success has been gained in man or animals in the reversal of late renal or retinopathic changes by achievement of normoglycaemia, but this is perhaps not surprising when major morphological changes, including fibrosis, have occurred. It certainly emphasizes the need for prevention.

If there is a strong association between poor glycaemic control and the different chronic complications of diabetes, the exact relationship to macrovascular disease is uncertain. It is also unknown whether glucose *per se* is the toxic agent or whether other metabolic consequences of diabetes are responsible. None the less, the onus now is on the physician to attempt to produce normoglycaemia and, at best, good overall metabolic control, in the belief that chronic tissue damage will not then occur.

Treatment of diabetes mellitus

Diet. Dietary treatment is a difficult issue in diabetes. Obesity so commonly contributes to the relative pancreatic failure in type II diabetes, through the associated increase in insulin resistance, that successful management depends most importantly on weight loss. It is difficult to impose a negative energy balance on these patients, perhaps because a tendency to a positive energy balance is one component inherent in the basic abnormality. This view is strengthened by the even greater weights previously reached by many of these patients years before they present as diabetic (and still fat). Indeed, such a vague measure as their highest remembered weight is a useful guide to the likely need for sulphonylurea treatment (in addition to diet) in the first year after diagnosis.

With type I diabetes less fundamental ignorance has been cloaked with excessive attention to the wrong type of detail, and two heresies have become widespread. The first arose from the controversy, particularly active around 1920, as to whether diabetes was a disorder of total, or just of carbohydrate metabolism. Allen's arguments for the former view were swept aside with the increased concentration on glucose levels that followed the discovery of insulin, and emphasis on a low carbohydrate diet became widespread in the 1930s. There were two theoretical reasons to doubt its validity; first, that diabetics in Africa or India often showed sustained good control of glucose levels despite following the high carbohydrate diet traditional there, and second that, since a low carbohydrate diet was likely to be high in fat, it might contribute to the hyperlipidaemia seen in some diabetics, particularly with only moderately controlled glucose levels, with the further argument that such hyperlipidaemia could contribute to macroangiopathy. Although good clinical studies around 1930 had indicated that even in the West high carbohydrate diets worked well, it was only with the renewed interest in natural or 'high-fibre' diets that arose in Africa and from the American 'green revolution' that the argument was re-opened. Direct experiment in America and separately in Oxford have shown that a high carbohydrate diet (avoiding its quickly absorbed forms) achieves at least as good glycaemic control in diabetics as the traditional 'low carbohydrate' regime. Indeed slightly better results were often obtained, providing the overall level of control was close to normal.

The second fallacy came from the emphasis on chemical analysis of foods 'on the shelf', without any thought as to how they were dealt with in the body. The content of carbohydrate, fat, and protein was categorized and any form of carbohydrate thought equivalent to any other, so that diets were based on building blocks of 10-g portions of carbohydrate. Many patients (and their advisers) had more sense in practice than to believe 10 g of carbohydrate as table sugar really to be equivalent in a diabetic diet to 10 g of carbohydrate taken as potato, but that was the theoretical position in much dietary instruction. Mainland Europe showed a more logical approach than Britain and America, listing separately 'bread portions', 'milk portions', 'fruit portions', etc.

Eventually, it was realized that what mattered was the effect of the food on the blood glucose of the recipient, and that this would be greatly influenced by the speed of its passage through the gut and its rate of digestion, all determining the rate at which the nutrients reached the blood. Two main lines of experiment have contributed to this understanding. First, Kinsell showed around 1970 that diabetic patients showed a smaller rise in blood glucose when a 50 g glucose load was taken together with a liquid fat and protein meal than when it was taken alone. Further, he showed that this was not a simple phenomenon, as in different patients the lower glucose levels with more nutrient were accompanied by either higher or lower plasma insulin concentrations. The important consideration then is the effect on the blood glucose of a food when it is taken as part of a meal, and not when it is ingested alone. The variables include the effect on the absorption of the food of the other foods with which it is taken, and its own effect in speeding or slowing the absorption of those other foods. The way in which a particular food is cooked may affect its rate of absorption, clearly illustrated by Haber and colleagues (amplifying previous work by Campbell) who observed that the blood glucose increases more when the juice from a particular weight of apples is drunk than when the apples are taken as a purée, with the least rise if the apples are eaten raw.

Secondly, studies in which suitable dietary fibre was added to meals have shown lesser rises of blood glucose and of insulin concentrations both in normal and in diabetic subjects. Jenkins established that this was due to *delayed*, but not *decreased*, absorption. This effect may be useful both in preventing hypoglycaemia in insulin-treated diabetics as well as reactive hypoglycaemia in non-diabetics. The delayed absorption may be because of slower gastric emptying, slower enzymatic digestion of these foods, or directly from the more viscous alimentary contents. There may also be changes in the response to the different meals of the gastrointestinal hormones.

When different fibres are examined, the viscosity of their standard solutions in water correlate strongly with the reduction in hyperglycaemia. Consequently it is the 'viscous fibres' (e.g. pectin or guar) rather than the 'fibrous fibres' (e.g. bran) which are effective in this way. No association can be shown relating the reduction in hyperglycaemia produced by a fibre, and its effect on a stool bulk.

The delayed absorption is accompanied by earlier satiety, increased feelings of epigastric fullness and abdominal distention with borborygmi together with increase rectal flatus and looser, bulkier stools. As when a European eats rural African food, such abdominal symptoms lessen greatly within three months, but those subjects who find 'viscous fibres' repugnant in the mouth from their 'slimy' or 'gummy' feel do not lose this with time. Unfortunately, 'mouth feel' is closely associated with viscosity.

Increase in the viscous fibre content of the diet may be achieved by either of two methods. Natural foods, rich in these substances, may be made predominant constituents of the diet, and in practice this means a high legume content. The storage polysaccharides (galactomannans) of the legumes are a major source of viscous fibre. The pectins of cell walls (especially fruits) form another major group, and to some extent galactomannans and pectins have additive qualities. The other approach is to use gums rich in viscous fibre, such as the guar gum (or flour) from the cluster bean of India as a pharmacological additive. While soups or crispbreads containing such a compound are acceptable to many, perhaps a quarter of subjects are unable to take an adequate quantity because of the unacceptable mouth feel. Such addition of viscous fibre is of most effect in improving postprandial glycaemia, while the increased carbohydrate in the diet is effective primarily in reducing overnight glucose levels and those well away from a meal. To obtain the best results from these two dietary changes, quickly absorbed simple sugars should be avoided, and the overall level of glycaemia should be fairly strictly controlled.

There is still much scope for improved understanding of the inter-reactions between different foods, and for observation on which foods, combined in a meal, give the lowest glucose response (Fig. 1). This can no doubt be predicted to an extent from studies on single foods (Table 10), but only direct observations can give the required knowledge.

As a generalization, foods taken in a more natural state are likely

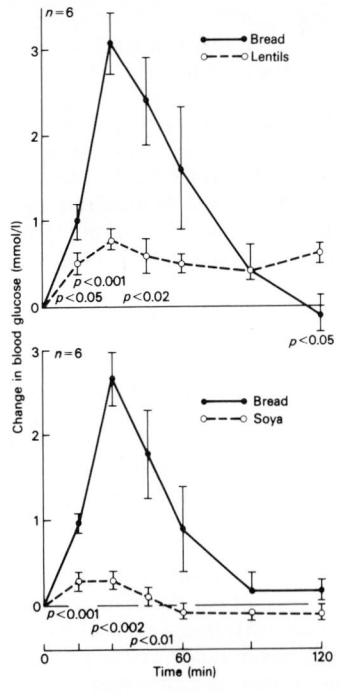

Fig. 1   Rise in blood glucose concentrations in six healthy volunteers after meals containing 50 g carbohydrate as wholemeal bread or lentils (top) or wholemeal bread and soya beans (bottom). From Jenkins, D. J. A. (1980). *Br. med. J.* **281**, 16.

Table 10   Areas of blood glucose increase after ingestion by non-diabetics of food portions of equal carbohydrate content, as a percentage of area of increase after 50 g of glucose in aqueous solution

	$\% \pm SD$
Apples	62 ± 9
Orange juice	46 ± 6
Bananas	62 ± 9
Soya beans	15 ± 5
Lentils	29 ± 3
Kidney beans	29 ± 8
Haricot beans	31 ± 6
Peas (black-eye)	33 ± 4
Peas (marrowfat)	47 ± 3
Porridge oats	49 ± 8
All-bran® (high-fibre breakfast cereal)	51 ± 5
Cornflakes	80 ± 6
Oatmeal biscuits	54 ± 4
Ryvita	69 ± 10

to be more slowly absorbed, for digestion has to break down containing cell walls and other natural 'wrappings'. To obtain 'lente' carbohydrate (to match long-acting insulins), one needs it in 'spansuled' form, and nature often provides such 'spansule' coatings. However, preparation of food for the table in lightly cooked form is often more time-consuming than using the convenience foods widely marketed today. Of course, raw food may be the easiest to serve, even if it takes longer to chew.

Timing, indeed, is important. Slowly taken meals will be advantageous in avoiding peaks of glucose, just as small, frequent meals are more suitable for any type of diabetic (but particularly those treated with insulin) than a few large ones.

High carbohydrate diets are likely to prove less satisfactory in grossly glycosuric patients. When blood glucose is elevated implying increased hepatic gluconeogenesis, absorbed carbohydrate will produce sharper rises in glucose levels than would equicaloric absorption of other nutrients. This will increase the heavy glycosuria already present, and the extra loss of fluid and electrolytes may further impair metabolism. The benefit of improved lipaemic and glycaemic control of diabetics through high carbohydrate diets (containing 50–55 per cent of the calories as carbohydrate) is therefore to be sought only together with tight control of glucose levels.

Practical advice. The important aspects are:

1. To provide the correct calorie intake that will both support necessary activity and, where appropriate, normal growth, and bring the patient's weight to the correct value. For many type II diabetics this means weight loss. Any particular activity has very different energy demands in different people, and so each insulin-taking diabetic must work out the right balance between extra food intake and extra energy output. As a general rule one may expect walking for one hour to need some 20 g carbohydrate extra, while more active exercise such as playing tennis or football may require at least 40 g/h. This is best taken as extra food at a preceding meal, but small amounts of it may be taken as quickly absorbed carbohydrate just before the exercise or half way through it.

2. The food should be well spread out throughout the day, and those taking insulin reckon on three main meals and three snacks, the latter because of the relatively slow absorption of insulin from subcutaneous sites. Older patients who wake regularly during the night can be advised on a small intake then (e.g. a digestive biscuit, etc.).

3. Meals should consist of foods that are slowly digested and absorbed, with particular reference to slowly absorbed carbohydrate and increased fibre content, especially of the more viscous type. Simple sugars (e.g. glucose, sucrose) should be avoided as completely as possible, and certainly never added by the patient. The only exceptions are treatment of hypoglycaemia and illness, especially gastrointestinal, when simple sugars may be added to drinks to supplement a grossly reduced total food intake.

4. The total carbohydrate content of the diet should provide 50–55 per cent of the total calories, though in individual meals this can vary widely, e.g. from 30 to 60 per cent.

5. The patients should be thoroughly instructed in the caloric as well as the carbohydrate content of their food, with particular emphasis on the high caloric content of fatty foods. They should also aim at a ratio of polyunsaturated to other dietary fatty acids of 0.9 or above and be advised to restrict intake of eggs to a maximum of eight a week, with only modest intake of the rarer high cholesterol foods such as shellfish.

6. The need for a regular pattern of feeding should be stressed in insulin-dependent diabetics who are on fixed insulin regimes. In some patients appropriate advice can be given on varying the timing of insulin injection to match altered meal times. This is socially important for young diabetics.

Three specimen diets are given in Table 11 with calorie content of 1000, 1500, and 2500 respectively, with the carbohydrate content of each meal also given.

Sulphonylureas. Although they are the most widely used and completely accepted oral hypoglycaemic agents, the role of sulphonylureas in diabetic treatment is far from settled and may vary considerably from place to place, or doctor to doctor. They act in two different ways. First, they sensitize the β-cell to the stimulatory effect of glucose (and perhaps other agents) on insulin secretion. This causes a left-shift in the dose–response curve of insulin secretion against glucose concentration, an effect which sometimes persists for years. There are also clearly defined 'extrapancreatic' actions; sulphonylureas do not affect glucose levels in the depancreatectomized animal but appear to 'up-regulate' the insulin receptors, increasing their number and so magnifying the effect of the available insulin. Some members of the group have other actions, e.g. chlorpropamide both potentiates the antidiuretic effect of vasopressin and enhances the flush after drinking alcohol.

There is argument about the extent to which these drugs can be replaced by proper dieting, or indeed may interfere with this. Dieting alone can be remarkably successful in reducing glucose levels quickly, and long-term weight loss (in absence of gross glycosuria) often renders sulphonylureas, initially necessary for glucose control, superfluous. But dietary treatment on its own has limitations, especially in the more hyperglycaemic type II diabetic, and sulphonylureas can be a real aid in glucose control. They probably interfere with dietary effort only when used in excess.

The University Group Diabetes Program in the USA reported data which implied an excessive risk of cardiovascular deaths in diabetics capable of control by diet alone, if they were treated with a fixed dose of tolbutamide (500 mg t.d.s.) together with their diet. The concern which this report aroused has been largely dissipated with greater understanding of this work and lack of confirmation of risks from tolbutamide (and by implication all sulphonylureas) in a number of other, albeit smaller, studies.

Toxic effects. As with most drugs, the sulphonylureas can cause a wide range of allergic reactions, especially on the skin. Some compounds are particularly associated with rare but severe bone marrow depression, but most of those developing this during chlorpropamide treatment were on more than 500 mg daily, a dose that would rarely be exceeded today. All can produce hypoglycaemia, but this is rarely severe enough to cause unconsciousness. This may happen spontaneously but occurs particularly under special circumstances, as in synergy with β-adrenergic blocking agents, monoamine oxidase inhibitors, when displaced from binding plasma proteins by another drug, or in the neonate if the agent was unwisely still administered to the mother within a few days of delivery. This risk is generally greater the longer acting the agent, and will be enhanced by hepatic or renal disease, affecting the usual elimination of the drug. This increases its plasma concentration, probably one mechanism for the increased risk of nocturnal hypoglycaemia in some elderly persons on chlorpropamide.

Plasma concentrations of the sulphonylureas are rarely measured. They should be taken at least 30–45 min before the relevant meal, though this can increase the risk of mild hypoglycaemic symptoms, particularly with the rapidly acting forms, such as glibenclamide or glipizide or after extra physical exertion.

Administration. The commonly used sulphonylureas are listed in Table 12, grouped according to high, medium, or low dose levels. Many patients prefer a long-acting agent such as chlorpropamide, or sometimes glibornuride, even though more effective glucose control and higher insulin levels may be achieved by shorter-acting, frequently administered drugs such as tolbutamide or glipizide. While there is no advantage in adding a second sulphonylurea when a maximum dose of one has already been prescribed, it is reasonable to supplement a small dose of long-acting agent with a quick-acting one, e.g. before a large evening meal, or regularly before breakfast in those with a marked morning hyperglycaemic surge.

Particular agents may have special advantages. Thus, gliquidone may be relatively more suitable in presence of renal impairment, as it is mostly metabolized in the liver with excretion of its metabolites in the bile. Again, glymidine is chemically a sulphapyrimidine rather than a sulphonylurea and so may be acceptable when sensitivity to a sulphonylurea proves a group phenomenon (as occasionally happens) rather than a more specific response.

Indications for sulphonylurea prescription will depend mostly on the ability of a type II diabetic to initiate and sustain dietary effort, and in the physician's aim in glucose control. Although neither the mechanism nor time course of continuing β-cell deterioration in type II diabetes is understood, this will be a major cause of secondary failure of these agents. They are relatively contraindicated in the younger, thinner, and more ketonuric patients. While some slow-onset type I diabetics can achieve adequate glucose control on sulphonylureas for months or years, recognition of the type (e.g. by a positive islet-cell antibody test) should increase the readiness to transfer to insulin should glucose control become borderline.

Most diabetics requiring sulphonylureas are prescribed them within a year of diagnosis, but there is a continuing tail of 'secondary' dietary failures. Somewhere around 30 per cent of

Table 11 Menus for three specimen diets

Meal	1000 kcal	approx CHO(g)	1500 kcal	approx CHO(g)	2500 kcal	approx CHO(g)
Breakfast	Fresh orange segments 1 Weetabix® with skimmed milk (130 ml) Wholemeal toast—one slice with margarine Tea with skimmed milk (20 ml)	40	Fresh grapefruit: half Small bowl All Bran® with skimmed milk (150 ml) Wholemeal toast—one slice with margarine Tea with skimmed milk (20 ml)	38	Large bowl Puffed Wheat® with milk (150 ml) (or medium helping Puffed Wheat® + one banana) wholemeal toast—one slice with baked beans One glass of milk (150 ml)	73
Mid-morning	Tea with skimmed milk (20) ml	1	Tea with skimmed milk (20 ml) One apple	12	Tuna and cucumber sandwiches from two slices wholemeal bread Tea with milk (20 ml)	30
Lunch	Butter beans, sweetcorn, and ham salad Lemon juice dressing One apple Tea with skimmed milk (20 ml)	37	Tuna and cucumber sandwiches from two slices wholemeal bread One small banana and a small carton of natural yoghurt Tea with skimmed milk (20 ml)	53	Beef and bean hot pot Rice and pineapple condé Low-calorie squash	81
Mid-afternoon	Coffee with skimmed milk (40 ml)	2	Coffee with skimmed milk (40 ml) One wholewheat cracker biscuit	10	One wholewheat fruit scone Coffee with milk (40 ml) One apple	29
Evening meal	Lean roast lamb—two slices Sugar-free mint sauce Garden peas and carrots One large jacket potato Stewed pear with cinnamon Low-calorie squash	42	Red bean and lamb casserole One large jacket potato Runner beans Fresh fruit jelly Diabetic squash	86	Vegetable and pasta soup Red bean and cheese flan Red cabbage salad with yoghurt dressing Orange fruit jelly Coffee with milk (40 ml)	90
Bedtime	Skimmed milk as tea/hot milk/ coffee (40 ml) Two rye crispbreads (Ryvita®)	15	Skimmed milk as coffee/hot milk (50 ml) One digestive biscuit	13	One tall glass unsweetened fruit juice (or one glass milk) Two digestive biscuits	39
		137		212		342

Table 12 Major oral hypoglycaemic agents available in the United Kingdom

	Trade names	Daily dose range (mg)	t_{max} (h)	$t_{\frac{1}{2}}$ (h)	Number of daily doses	Site of metabolism
Sulphonylureas						
Acetohexamide	Dimelor	250–1500	1–2	1.3–4.5	1–3	Liver
Chlorpropamide	Diabinese Melitase	100–500	1–7	33–43	1	Mostly excreted unchanged in urine
Glibenclamide	Daonil	2.5–20	1–2	6–10	1–3	Liver
Glibornuride	Glutril	12.5–75	2–4	8–9	1–2	Liver
Gliclazide	Diamicron	80–240	4–8	10–12	1–3	95% liver
Glipizide	Glibenese	2.5–30	0.5–2	3–7	2–3	90–95% excreted unchanged
Gliquidone	Glurenorm	30–180	2–3	—	1–3	95% liver—metabolites excreted in bile
Glymidine	Gondaphon	500–2000	1–2	5–8	1–2	?
Tolazamide	Tolanase	100–1000		7	1–3	Liver
Tolbutamide	Pramidex	1000–3000	3–4	7	2–3	Liver
Biguanides						
Metformin	Glucophage	500–1500	2–4	12–20	1–2	Excreted unchanged in urine

those on sulphonylureas will be transferred to insulin treatment within four years. There is no recognized benefit from combining insulin and sulphonylurea therapy.

Although the issue is not clear cut, the sulphonylureas seem to have no appreciable effect in reducing deterioration of blood glucose homeostasis with time in mild type II diabetics.

The choice between sulphonylurea and insulin treatment has been made easier in some centres by measuring the maximal C-peptide secretory response to a stimulus such as glucagon, or even the response to a sulphonylurea itself, but glucose levels, especially if combined with a simultaneous insulin concentration (in a relatively steady state), may be as useful.

Biguanides. These compounds act by reducing the efficiency of ion exchange across membranes with resulting decreased cellular efficiency, so that both hepatic gluconeogenesis, and the efficiency of obtaining chemical energy from peripheral utilization of a glucose, are decreased, with resulting fall in blood glucose. The same properties no doubt underlie the toxic effects that these agents may cause, ranging from generalized lassitude and vague muscular discomfort via increased intestinal motor activity (and occasionally malabsorption of vitamin B_{12}) to the serious complica-tion of lactic acidosis.

Lactic acidosis, though rare, is particularly liable to occur with phenformin (phenethylbiguanide) therapy. Hence, this agent has been proscribed in some countries and recently has been withdrawn from use in the United Kingdom. Lactic acidosis is particularly likely to occur when there is impaired liver function, commonly from acute reduction in hepatic blood flow (e.g. cardiac infarct, pulmonary embolus, Gram-negative septicaemia), but is also predisposed to by excess alcohol intake or certain systemic illnesses, e.g. leukaemia. Since the biguanides are largely elimin-ated via the kidney, renal impairment is another contraindication to their use.

The risk of lactic acidosis is least with metformin (Table 12) but the dose of this drug should probably not exceed 500 mg t.d.s. or 850 mg b.d. It is best taken during meals, to reduce the risk of dyspepsia.

The biguanide's principal role in treatment is as a synergist to a sulphonylurea when this, together with dietary advice, has failed to produce satisfactory glucose control. That is often an indication for transfer to insulin, but in 'class I' (see below) patients combined sulphonylurea–biguanide therapy is a useful method of attempting continued adequate oral treatment. The biguanides remain active after months or years of therapy, and their efficacy is little dependent on the residual effective β-cell mass. However, it is rarely advantageous to combine them with insulin treatment.

Their special renown in the treatment of obese diabetics is perhaps little justified despite some observations to the contrary. Their use may favour weight loss because of anorexia rather than minimal malabsorption, but there is little evidence that sulphony-lureas are often fattening, though any agent improving glucose control may be associated with weight gain in a diabetic. It is reasonable, however, to use a biguanide in the occasional obese diabetic refractory to dietary therapy who gains weight on sulphonylureas.

Other oral hypoglycaemic agents. None are widely used in Europe or North America in the treatment of diabetes. Certain herbal preparations, e.g. *kerala*, are widely used in India, and are weakly hypoglycaemic, as is onion extract. Other agents may be grouped as:

1. Specific hypoglycaemic agents, of no practical advantage, e.g. dichloroacetate, dimethylpyrazole.

2. Widely used pharmaceuticals with a weak hypoglycaemic action. The salicylates are a special case, for they have a variety of potential actions, including a direct metabolic hypoglycaemic effect, impaired insulin production from their antiprostaglandin action, and their interaction with sulphonylureas in displacing them from binding proteins.

3. Hypoglycaemic effect purely from enhancing sulphonylurea activity, e.g. phenylbutazone or dicoumarols displace sulphony-lureas from their plasma binding proteins; monoamine oxidase inhibitors potentiate sulphonylureas, especially in depressives.

Insulin

Aims. In order to define the aims of insulin therapy it is necessary first to distinguish those patients for whom insulin is to be prescribed. Three main groups of diabetics are best treated with insulin.

1. The first is of type I or II diabetics with relatively limited life expectancy (usually from age) in whom insulin is necessary to prevent symptomatic hyperglycaemia, or even ketoacidosis, and in whom maximum doses of oral hypoglycaemic agents have failed. The principal concern is to keep the patient symptom free and free from hypoglycaemia rather than to achieve perfect metabolic control. There may also be social reasons to simplify management, e.g. the avoidance of twice-daily injections. The aim therefore is to use the simplest therapy to minimize symptoms.

2. The second group is of younger type II diabetics where excellent control is desired. Treatment may be prompted by amyotrophy, chronic infection, painful neuropathy or foot lesions, but it may be best to attempt to achieve normoglycaemia from the time of diagnosis and before tissue damage has evolved, for at least some forms of tissue damage may have an inherent momentum for deterioration irrespective of later glycaemic control.

3. The third and largest group are type I (insulin-dependent) diabetics, in whom the same considerations apply as in 2 above. These can be divided into two subgroups: those with and those without some remaining endogenous insulin secretion. Good control of blood glucose is more difficult in the latter, but every effort must be made in both these subgroups to achieve normoglycaemia, although however well an insulin regime may be designed, it is only part of the overall strategy for good metabolic control. If dietary advice is not followed, and education of the patient about the effects of everyday life on insulin requirements is not given, precise insulin therapy is pointless. The overall aim in patients in the second and third groups is to mimic normal metabolism including plasma insulin profiles, even if only in the systemic circulation. In the average patient taking three main meals per day, this implies three peaks in circulating insulin levels with basal levels maintained at all times between.

Types of insulin available. The various insulin preparations have three main characteristics, in respect of species of origin, purity, and duration of action (Table 13); to this may be added concentration: presently 40 and 80 i.u./ml but shortly to change to 100 i.u./ml.

Table 13   Main types of therapeutic insulins

Species	Bovine
	Porcine
	Human
Purity	Conventional
	Single peak
	Highly purified
Duration of action	Short
	Intermediate
	Long

Species. Insulin was first isolated from beef pancreas in 1921. Shortly afterwards it was extracted also from porcine pancreas. Since then beef and pork insulins have been the mainstays of therapy, with the majority of bovine origin. Recently, synthetic human insulin has been available for extensive clinical trials, and will be available commercially in 1983. The three insulins are naturally similar. Human insulin differs from porcine only at the amino acid in position 30 of the β-chain where the former has threonine and the latter alanine. Bovine insulin differs at two other sites, aminoacids 8 and 10 of the A-chain, where alanine and valine have been substituted for threonine and isoleucine respectively. Commercial human insulin is currently produced by two methods. The first is chemical substitution of the B30 amino acid of pork insulin. The second involves DNA coding of *E.coli* to produce separately the A- and B-chains of human insulin, and then combining the chains *in vitro*. This method will shortly be replaced by coding for the whole proinsulin sequence.

The potency of the three insulins is remarkably similar. So far no convincing difference has been shown between human and porcine insulins *in vivo*. There is a small but so far therapeutically unimportant difference in solubility. Acute experiments with beef insulin also show it to be similar to human and pork insulin, but it is probably less desirable than pork or human insulin because of its greater antigenicity (see below). In this respect, purity is probably more important than the species of origin of the preparation. Other insulins have been prepared, e.g. fish insulin, but in general they have not found therapeutic use.

Purity. Insulin was prepared for many years by acid-ethanol extraction of porcine or bovine pancreas followed by a series of isoelectric precipitations and recrystallizations. The resulting aqueous solution or suspension was mainly insulin, but also contained small amounts of other pancreatic hormones, such as glucagon, pancreatic polypeptide, and VIP, as well as insulin dimers and degradation products, and significant amounts of proinsulin (10 000–40 000 p.p.m.). The standard British insulins listed in Table 14 are of this type. In the last 20 years, purer preparations have become available. Thus gel-filtration chromatography can be used to remove most of these contaminants, reducing the proinsulin content to less than 50 p.p.m. Significant amounts of desamido-insulin, arginyl insulins, and insulin ethylesters still remain. These insulins are the so-called 'single peak' or purified insulins as available now from Weddell (Hypurin insulins) and Wellcome (Neusulin and Neuphane). Further purification has been achieved by ion-exchange chromatography of the single-peak. This yields 'highly-purified' (so called 'monocomponent') or 'rarely immunogenic') insulins as marketed by the Danish insulin manufacturers which contain <10 p.p.m. proinsulin and insignificant amounts of other contaminants. The significance of the purity of the insulin preparations will be discussed below (see complications of insulin therapy) but the less pure the preparation, the more antigenic it is. Antibodies to insulin have been recognized in the circulation of insulin-treated diabetics for nearly 30 years. The bulk

of the antigenicity lies in the contaminants, particularly proinsulin, with the added factor that substances used to prolong the action of insulin (e.g. protamine and zinc) appear to increase antigenicity, acting perhaps as adjuvants. Originally, species was suggested as a major factor but highly purified beef and pork insulins are much less antigenic than less pure preparations, although even in the highly purified preparations beef is slightly more antigenic than pork insulin. Human preparations appear to be not dissimilar in antigenicity from porcine insulin, suggesting strongly that purity or local change after injection are the important determinants.

It is debated whether insulin antibodies are of clinical significance. One of their possible effects is to delay the onset of action of short-acting insulins with a later, sustained, release of insulin at times when high concentrations are not required. These effects may be detrimental if precise therapy is required but will be irrelevant if *only* background treatment is necessary. Insulin doses are on average less in patients with low antibody titres—an economical rather than clinical argument. Development of insulin antibodies may shorten the phase of low insulin requirement often seen in the early stages of type I diabetes. The antibodies cross the placenta, and may increase the risk of hypoglycaemia in the neonates of diabetic mothers. One suggestion that enjoyed a brief vogue was that insulin antibodies were implicated in the development of diabetic tissue damage, particularly retinopathy and nephropathy. This was deduced from animal but not human experiments and has not been substantiated; indeed type II diabetics, never treated with insulin, develop tissue damage which is qualitatively indistinguishable from that in insulin-treated diabetics.

It is questionable whether there is clinical significance in the antibodies formed to the non-insulin components of conventional

Table 14 Insulin preparations available in the United Kingdom

Type of insulin*	pH Acid	pH Neutral	Species	Purity†	Retarding agent	Action (h) Initial	Maximum	Total
Short-acting								
Soluble	+	–	Beef	3	–	$\frac{1}{2}$	2–4	6–8
Neutral soluble	–	+	Beef	3	–	$\frac{1}{2}$	2–4	6–8
Neusulin (Wellcome)	–	+	Beef	2	–	$\frac{1}{2}$–1	2–4	6–8
Hypurin Neutral (Weddell)	–	+	Beef	2	–	$\frac{1}{2}$	2–4	6–8
Actrapid (Novo)	–	+	Pork	1	–	$\frac{1}{4}$–$\frac{1}{2}$	2$\frac{1}{2}$–5	6–8
Velosulin (Nordisk)	–	+	Pork	1	–	$\frac{1}{4}$–$\frac{1}{2}$	2–4	6–8
Semilente	–	+	Beef	3	Zinc	1	4–6	14
Semitard (Novo)		+	Pork	1	Zinc	1–2	4–8	10–16
Intermediate								
Isophane	–	+	Beef	3	Protamine	1–2	5–8	18
Hypurin isophane (Weddell)	–	+	Beef	2	Protamine	1–2	5–8	18
Neuphane (Wellcome)	–	+	Beef	2	Protamine	1–2	5–8	18
Insulatard (Nordisk)	–	+	Pork	1	Protamine	1–2	5–7	16–18
Lente	–	+	Pork and beef	3	Zinc	1–2	3–12	20–30
Lentard (Novo)	–	+	Pork and beef	1	Zinc	1–3	7–15	18–24
Neulente (Wellcome)	–	+	Beef	2	Zinc	1–2	6–10	20–26
Hypurin Lente (Weddell)	–	+	Beef	2	Zinc	1–2	6–10	20–26
Monotard (Novo)	–	+	Pork	1	Zinc	1–3	7–15	16–22
Long-acting								
Protamine zinc	–	+	Beef	3	Protamine and zinc	3	8–12	30–40
Hypurin protamine zinc (Weddell)	–	+	Beef	2	Protamine and zinc	3	8–12	30–40
Ultralente	–	+	Beef	3	Zinc	3	8–12	60–80
Ultratard (Novo)	–	+	Beef	1	Zinc	3	10–30	60–80

Mixed preparations
Initard (Nordisk): 50% Velosulin + 50% Inulatard
Mixtard (Nordisk): 30% Velosulin + 70% Insulatard
Rapitard (Novo): 25% highly purified pork neutral + 75% highly purified crystalline

*Unspecified insulins are available from British Insulin Manufacturers. All are available at 40 and 80 i.u./ml (100 i.u./ml from 1983).
†3: Conventional insulin; 2: purified insulin; 1: highly purified insulin.

insulin preparations. Antibodies to glucagon, VIP, and somato-statin have been detected, but to date they have not been found deleterious.

In summary, insulins of various grades of purity are now available and in clinical use. It seems wise to use the purest preparations which have the least antigenic potential, i.e. highly purified porcine or pork-derived human insulins, in those patients where excellent control is sought and where long-term use is probable. It is also desirable to use the pure preparations in patients receiving insulin intermittently for short periods, e.g. pregnancy and surgery, so as to decrease the possibility of sensitization.

Duration of action and pharmacokinetics. The other main properties of available insulins are speed and duration of action, and time of peak action (Table 14). Broadly, when given subcutaneously the insulins can be divided into short-acting, intermediate, and long-acting preparations (Tables 13 and 14).

The duration of action depends on where the insulin is administered. Insulin injected intravenously has a half-life in the circulation of 4–5 min, and an effective half-life of 20 min. Thus if i.v. insulin is used, it must be given by continuous infusion to produce a sustained effect. This is pertinent to the therapy of diabetic ketoacidosis and of diabetics undergoing surgery. Only the short-acting insulins should be used intravenously. The longer-acting insulins are particulate and carry a theoretical risk of embolism. Insulin may also be given intramuscularly, when the half-life of crystalline (short-acting) insulin is approximately 2 h. In therapeutic use insulin is commonly given subcutaneously, when the half-life in the circulation of the quick-acting preparations is longer: 3–4 h in diabetics already treated with insulin, although much shorter in normal subjects. The time to onset of action varies between 15 and 60 min, with peak effects at 2–6 h and some activity for up to 8 h, although this may exceed 12 h in patients with high antibody levels. It is probably correct to include the semilente insulins as short-acting insulins. They are crystalline zinc insulins which are popular as twice daily preparations in children, but are unsuitable in totally insulin deficient patients as they rarely last for the required 12–14 h.

Absorption of insulin from subcutaneous sites is variable both within and between subjects (Table 15). This makes it necessary to

Table 15 Factors influencing the rate of absorption of insulin

---

Type of insulin
? pH
Species
Concentration
Anatomical site (abdomen>arm>thigh)
Depth of injection
Massage
Exercise
Interaction with antibodies
? Local degradation

---

individualize therapy but even then the same dose of insulin may have quite different effects on different days in the same patient. Some of the main factors affecting absorption are shown in Table 14. The type of insulin has been referred to already. The pH of the preparation may also have an effect: the older insulins are acid rather than neutral preparations, and the former may be absorbed slightly more slowly than the neutral insulins. Species of origin may also have an effect: it has been claimed, for example, that human insulin is absorbed more rapidly than pork insulin, which in turn is absorbed more quickly than beef insulin. This may reflect differences in solubility of the insulins, but even if true the changes are small and of dubious clinical significance. More concentrated insulin is also absorbed more quickly than dilute preparations. Patients should therefore not change to and fro between 40 i.u./ml and 80 i.u./ml insulin.

Tissue blood flow is an important factor influencing rates of absorption and this is influenced by temperature and by the site of injection. Absorption is significantly more rapid from the abdomen than from the arm, which is in turn more rapid than from the thigh. A consistent approach should be taught to the patient. Depth of injection is also important—more shallow injections are absorbed more rapidly than deeper injections, providing of course that the former are not intradermal and the latter not intramuscular. Exercise of the injected part, as well as massage, can also speed absorption to a clinically important degree. Insulin may also be sequestered locally by antibodies, with slowed absorption.

Many of these considerations influencing variation in absorption rate also apply to the intermediate and long-acting insulins listed in Table 14. Indeed the variability between and within patients is even greater with these insulins. Several intermediate insulins are available. Either protamine or zinc are used as retarding agents. The lente insulins (which are mixtures of amorphous and crystalline zinc insulin) depend on zinc whilst protamine is used for the isophane insulins. Both of these agents may increase the antigenicity of insulin. The duration of action varies from 16–30 h with peak actions at 5–12 h. In most cases the duration of action is less than 24 h and these preparations must therefore be used twice daily if total insulin replacement is sought.

The long-acting (bovine) insulins, protamine zinc insulin and ultralente insulins, have a broad peak of maximum effect and a duration of action up to three days. There is a vogue for using ultralente insulins to give a constant background of insulin but they require familiarity for easy use. Because of the long half-life it can take several days to reach a stable dose; and, more important, if too much is given the patient may remain at risk of hypoglycaemia for several days.

Mixed insulin preparations are also available (Table 14). These are useful for our first class of patient (see page 9.20), but prevent the patient from flexibly altering his insulin regimen according to glucose levels. Rapitard is often used in children, where precise control may be difficult but there really seems little need to use it even here.

Routine use of insulins. The aims of insulin therapy differ between different patient groups. If the patient is simply to be kept asymptomatic, then a once-daily regimen may be used. Commonly this would be achieved with a single dose of an intermediate insulin such as lente or Monotard insulin. The latter in particular bears little risk of nocturnal hypoglycaemia, an important consideration in the elderly (Table 16). It may be necessary to add a short-acting insulin if there is severe post-breakfast hyperglycaemia.

Once daily therapy may also be successful in type II diabetics not controlled satisfactorily by oral agents, using, for example, Actrapid plus Monotard. Fasting blood glucose is here the best index of the adequacy of glycaemic control. If there is persistent fasting hyperglycaemia, an additional evening injection is required. Ultratard or Ultralente insulin injected once daily has also been suggested as an alternative (or adjuvant) to sulphonylurea therapy in type II diabetics. The need for it probably depends primarily on the success of the sulphonylurea in controlling hyperglycaemia.

In most type I diabetics two (or even three) injections of insulin are required as one aim of precise therapy is to reproduce peak levels of insulin at meal times with basal concentrations in between. From the above discussion of the pharmacokinetic behaviour of insulin this is difficult—if not impossible—to achieve when patients lack endogenous insulin secretion. The absorption of even short-acting insulin from subcutaneous tissue is slower than the physiological pancreatic response to a meal. More important, circulating levels do not return to baseline sufficiently quickly. However, some of these disadvantages can be countered by appropriate dietary adjustments. Thus a smaller breakfast with more slowly absorbed carbohydrate followed by an equivalent carbohydrate load two hours later as a snack can match the profile of a short-acting insulin injection in the morning. Similar dietary adjustments can be made at other times of the day.

Table 16 Regimens for insulin therapy in diabetic patients

	Patient group
1. Once daily	
Monotard or Lente	Elderly patients requiring symptomatic relief
Monotard or Actrapid plus Monotard	Non-obese type II diabetics, uncontrolled on oral agents. Older type I patients with significant residual insulin secretion*
Ultratard or Ultralente	Type II diabetes uncontrolled by diet
2. Twice daily	
Intermediate insulin, e.g. Isophane, Insulatard, or Monotard	New type I diabetics
Short- and intermediate-acting insulin, e.g. Actrapid or Velosulin + Monotard or Insulatard Soluble + isophane	Type I diabetics Pregnant diabetics
3. Three times daily	
Short + intermediate with breakfast, short before evening meal, intermediate at bedtime, e.g. Actrapid + Insulatard, Actrapid, Insulatard	Type I diabetics with morning hyperglycaemia and/or nocturnal hypoglycaemia
Short-acting t.i.d. plus intermediate or long-acting before evening meal, e.g. Actrapid t.i.d. + Monotard (or Ultratard)	Labile diabetics. Diabetics requiring near perfect glycaemic control

*Continue until there is persistent fasting morning hyperglycaemia.

In the new diabetic who retains endogenous secretion, a twice daily regimen of intermediate insulin (e.g. Insulatard, Monotard, or Isophane) can give excellent control; endogenous secretion is then adequate to deal with meal-time insulin requirements. Later the majority of patients can be dealt with satisfactorily using a twice-daily mixture of short- and intermediate-action insulins (e.g. soluble and isophane, Velosulin or Actrapid with Insulatard, etc.). This does not produce a clear insulin peak at lunchtime, and is best matched by a small lunch and a small mid-afternoon snack. Guidelines for modifying b.d. insulin therapy are shown in Table 17.

The day is generally divided into unequal portions with respect to insulin injections. Thus the morning injection may be taken at 8 a.m. and the pre-evening meal injections at 6.00 or 6.30 p.m. This leaves a larger night-time fraction of the 24 hours. It has been found recently that many patients on twice-daily therapy have morning hyperglycaemia, which correlates with low levels of circulating insulin at that time. If more intermediate insulin is given in the early evening, there may be nocturnal hypoglycaemia. Either a longer-acting insulin is required in the evening, or the evening meal should be later, or a different insulin regimen is required. One successful manoeuvre is to give short-acting insulin alone before the evening meal and then an intermediate-acting insulin at bedtime.

Another version of twice-daily therapy is the use of twice-daily short-acting insulin against a background of long-acting insulin (Ultratard or Ultralente). Thrice-daily insulin may be necessary or desirable in some patients. These include labile diabetics, the diabetic with rapidly advancing tissue damage, the pregnant diabetic who is not 'perfectly' controlled on twice-daily therapy, or the diabetic requiring maximum flexibility in life-style. In these patients, therapy can be altered frequently depending on glucose levels and approaching events. The most popular versions of t.i.d. therapy are thrice-daily quick-acting highly purified insulin before each meal with additional intermediate insulin or long-acting insulin before the evening meal.

Practical aspects of insulin therapy. Particular emphasis should be placed on teaching correct injection technique at the start of insulin therapy. Simple problems such as air bubbles in the syringe can make a large difference to the amount of insulin injected. Neutral short-acting and intermediate insulins can be mixed in the same syringe providing that the injection is given immediately. The insulin used in smaller dose should be drawn up first, unless protamine zinc insulin is used when it should always be drawn up second as its admixture changes the characteristics of short-acting insulins. Injections are considerably less traumatic if finer rather than blunter needles are used. Indeed, wherever possible plastic syringes with fixed needles should be used as these can safely be reused many times, at least up to a week; they do not require special sterilization (insulin solutions contain a preservative), and have a small dead space. Children in particular should be issued with these

Table 17 Guide to modification of b.d. (short- and intermediate-acting) insulin regimen

	Fasting	Pre-lunch	Pre-evening meal	Bedtime
Persistent hyperglycaemia (>10 mmol/l) or glycosuria (>½%)	↑ Evening* Intermediate 2–4 units	↑ Morning short-acting 2–4 units	↑ Morning intermediate 2–4 units	↑ Evening short-acting 2–4 units
		or	or	or
		Decrease breakfast or mid-morning carbohydrate	Decrease afternoon carbohydrate	Decrease evening carbohydrate
Persistent hypoglycaemia —symptomatic or BG <4 mmol/l	↓ Evening Intermediate 2–4 units	↓ Morning short-acting 2–4 units	↓ Morning intermediate 2–4 units	↓ Evening short-acting 2–4 units
		or	or	or
		↑ Mid-morning carbohydrate	↑ Afternoon carbohydrate	↑ Evening meal carbohydrate

*NB this may result in nocturnal hypoglycaemia in which case the evening intermediate-acting insulin should be moved to bedtime.
Intermediate acting insulin, e.g. Isophane, Monotard, Insulatard.
Short-acting insulin, e.g. soluble, Nuso, Actrapid, Velosulin.
†Carbohydrate should be increased or decreased in approximately 10 g amounts.

syringes, which unfortunately cannot yet be prescribed by general practitioners in the United Kingdom.

Rotation of injection sites should also be taught. This can be advantageous if rapidly absorbing sites (abdomen and arm) are used in the morning and more slowly absorbing sites (thigh, buttocks) in the evening when a longer action is required. The initial delay in absorption of s.c. administered insulin should also be allowed for. If the insulin is given 30 min before food, the upstroke of the resulting plasma insulin profile closely matches the physiological rise.

Complications of insulin therapy. The complications of insulin therapy are listed in Table 18. Hypoglycaemia is far the commonest and results from inadequate matching of insulin against diet and activity, or the use of inappropriate insulin therapy. These should be avoidable but intermittently patients can be surprised, often through failure of concentration on the hypoglycaemic risk. If hypoglycaemia does occur, it is generally recognized as such by patients and can then be counteracted by consumption of rapidly absorbed carbohydrate (biscuits, barley sugar, Dextrosol). Long-standing and/or older diabetics may lose their typical warning symptoms of hypoglycaemia, and so become vulnerable to catastrophic attacks, even when driving. The timing of 'hypos' is often predictable, e.g. late morning or late afternoon in patients taking twice-daily mixed insulins, and if repeated should lead to modification of therapy and/or diet. A major disadvantage of frequent hypoglycaemia is weight gain due to the extra carbohydrate ingested. The family of a diabetic should be instructed about the symptoms and signs of hypoglycaemia, which may be bizarre, as well as the action to be taken (see below). It is a mistake to assume that all short-lived recurrent attacks in diabetics are due to hypoglycaemia; other causes must always be considered.

Table 18   Complications of insulin therapy

Hypoglycaemia
Antibody formation–? impaired control, transplacental transfer
Lipoatrophy
Lipohypertrophy
Local allergy
Generalized allergy
Insulin resistance
Insulin oedema
Sepsis

The second commonest complication of insulin therapy is the lipodystrophies: atrophy and hypertrophy. Lipoatrophy is the loss of fat at the sites of insulin injection. From 25–75 per cent of patients treated with conventional insulins may show signs of lipoatrophy, and this can be quite disfiguring. It is commonest in countries where less pure insulins are used. It may be due to immunogenic components of conventional insulin preparations which lead to the formation of either immune complexes or IgE antibody, which binds locally and so stimulates lipolysis. Lipoatrophy is rare in patients using highly purified insulins, confirming that it is caused by impurities in the older insulin preparations. It is treated by injecting a purer insulin into the centre or edge of the atrophic area, until this fills. In patients who also have local allergy (see below) the latter may need to be treated before the lipoatrophy responds to therapy.

Lipohypertrophy is commoner than lipoatrophy in countries where most patients are treated with highly purified insulins. It is due to repeated injection at the same site, which is particularly common in children. It presumably results from continued lipid synthesis in response to a high local concentration of insulin. It is prevented by proper rotation of injection sites, and disappears in time if the patient stops injecting into the affected area.

Insulin therapy is affected by the formation of insulin antibodies. High titres of circulating antibodies are commoner with conven-

tional insulins, but may still occur even with highly purified biosynthetic human insulin lacking proinsulin contamination. The possible significance of insulin antibodies has been discussed previously (page 9.21). There is a greater tendency to develop antibodies in Aryans who are HLA B15 or HLAA2 + BW44 than in those who are, for example, B8 or DRW3.

Insulin allergy, either local or general, is a rare complication of insulin therapy. The local form comprises pruritic, erythematous indurated lesions subsequent to insulin injection, which are occasionally also painful. There are three distinct types. The commonest is a biphasic IgE-dependent reaction called the 'late-phase reaction'. Arthus-type or delayed reactions also occur. Insulin impurities, and the retarding agents zinc and protamine, have all been implicated as causative agents. The incidence is much decreased in populations using predominantly highly purified insulins. The first step in treatment is to ensure that the lesions are not due to faulty technique, e.g. intradermal injection. Skin testing with different insulins, including zinc-free insulins, can then be used to find a non-reactive insulin preparation. Oral antihistamines may also be useful. Local steroid therapy may be necessary, and this can be mixed with the insulin before injection, e.g. 1 mg/ml prednisolone. Generalized allergy is extremely rare and presents classically. The antigen is usually insulin itself, and the B-chain of all commonly used insulins induces the response. The allergy responds to conventional desensitization regimens.

Occasionally septic lesions are due to insulin injection. If recurrent, they are usually a result of faulty injection technique and some special state of the patient, e.g. staphylococcal carriage or impaired antibacterial defences (gross hyperglycaemia can contribute to the latter).

Insulin resistance is a relatively uncommon complication of insulin therapy in type I diabetics in the United Kingdom. It may or may not depend upon altered immunity. Before purer insulins were available, it was much commoner, and most cases were due to high levels of antibodies. At the time it was indicated by a daily insulin dose of more than 200 units. It would be more accurate to define insulin resistance now as present in any patient taking more than 1.5 units insulin/kg body weight per day. Obesity is its commonest non-immunological cause. Treatment is obvious but difficult. With immunologically-based resistance, the insulin preparation should be changed to highly purified versions, preferably from a different species. If this is unsuccessful, the porcine desala-insulin or human insulin may be tried. Failing this, systemic prednisolone may be useful, but only when the resistance is severe, because of its own diabetogenic and other side-effects. Other forms of insulin resistance, antireceptor antibodies, elevated levels of counter-regulatory hormones, have been discussed above.

'Pseudo-insulin resistance' has been characterized among those patients who are overtreated with insulin, become hypoglycaemic, eat excessively in response, become hyperglycaemic, and then have their insulin dose increased. The Somogyi phenomenon is a version of this. A dramatic improvement in glycaemic level and stability can be obtained by drastic reduction of the insulin dose, and appropriate dietary advice.

Insulin oedema is the last complication to mention. It also is rare, but extremely troublesome when encountered. It occurs when proper glycaemic control is achieved in poorly controlled, often previously undiagnosed, diabetics. Marked pitting oedema can develop quickly, to resolve spontaneously, usually in 5–10 days. Its cause is unknown.

Alternative methods of insulin delivery. In view of the moderate glycaemic control that is achieved in most insulin-dependent diabetics, better methods of insulin therapy have been sought over the past decade (Table 19). This has involved (a) improving upon the slow insulin absorption that occurs with conventional injection, and (b) devising a system which will respond to ambient blood glucose by automatic provision of insulin. One of the earliest attempts was to deliver insulin subcutaneously by jet injection, in which an insulin is driven through the cutis by compressed air as a microdispersion. Absorption is significantly more rapid than with injected insulin, which may be partly due to intramuscular delivery. There are problems with size, cost, and delayed pain, but the approach is perhaps worth pursuing to obtain more natural insulin profiles.

Table 19 Alternative methods of insulin delivery in the treatment of diabetes

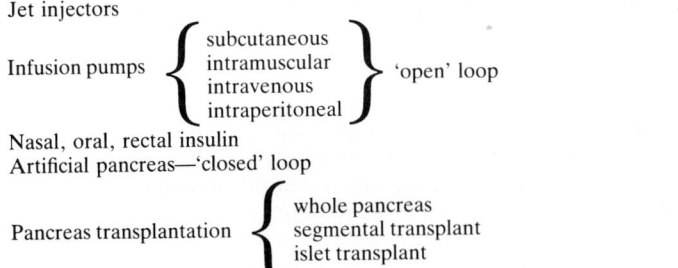

Jet injectors

Infusion pumps   { subcutaneous / intramuscular / intravenous / intraperitoneal } 'open' loop

Nasal, oral, rectal insulin
Artificial pancreas—'closed' loop

Pancreas transplantation { whole pancreas / segmental transplant / islet transplant }

In the last four years most attention has been paid to insulin infusion pumps. These have been widely used to deliver insulin subcutaneously using a fine cannula—inserted under the skin—most commonly with a 25-gauge butterfly. A background infusion is given at a predetermined rate (0.5 to 1.2 units/h on average). Extra boluses are delivered as desired at mealtimes, using an override switch or a manual drive. Most systems are simple syringe pumps, and the newer generation are reasonably small. Much more sophisticated programable pumps with long-lasting insulin reservoirs are also available, but seem unnecessary for extracorporeal use. Pumps or 'open-loop' devices should only be used in conjunction with appropriate patient education and self-monitoring (see below). Already their over-liberal use has resulted in several hypoglycaemic deaths in the United States.

Results so far show that near-normal glycaemic control can be obtained using continuous subcutaneous insulin infusion (CSII), and that this can be achieved more easily than with conventional (i.e. twice daily) multiple injections. The indications for use of such devices are not yet established. They have been suggested in pregnancy, but in most pregnant diabetics excellent control can be obtained by conventional means. It may be more useful to use pumps in patients with rapidly developing early tissue damage or in patients with labile diabetes. This latter group, however, may remain labile even with pump therapy, as the lability may have causes unrelated to the insulin therapy. The other use of pumps is to test the hypothesis that 'good control' delays or prevents tissue damage.

Pumps can also be used to deliver insulin intramuscularly, intravenously, or intraperitoneally. Intramuscular delivery has been used in the treatment of that subgroup of brittle diabetics who have defective absorption of insulin from subcutaneous sites. The technique is, however, difficult and rarely suitable for prolonged use. The intravenous route has also been used in these patients, and is now being used experimentally in uncomplicated juvenile type I diabetics in Canada, Germany, and Austria. The risks of septicaemia and thrombosis are considerable, even though the technique works well and is the only insulin delivery route whereby normal plasma insulin profiles can be reproduced accurately. If the i.v. route is to be used for pumped insulin, it is logical to implant the pump to reduce the possibility of infection, and then operate the pump externally by radio control. This is perhaps a prelude to development of a fully autonomous artificial pancreas but as yet has little practical application.

A more interesting and potentially more practical route for insulin delivery is via the peritoneal cavity. Endogenously secreted insulin is delivered into the portal venous system, whence it passes immediately to the liver where a large fraction of the insulin is extracted. This produces a marked portal: peripheral insulin gradient, with the liver constantly exposed to much higher insulin levels than extrahepatic tissues such as fat and muscle. Therapeutically insulin always enters the circulation *peripherally*, so either the peripheral tissues receive the correct amount of insulin and less than usual reaches the liver, or the liver receives the correct amount and there is peripheral hyperinsulinaemia. Current data indicate raised peripheral insulin levels in insulin-treated diabetics with, for example, constant reduction in lipolysis as well as other biochemical abnormalities; these are not corrected even if the patient is made normoglycaemic. More important is the possibility that hyperinsulinaemia increases the deposition and synthesis of lipid in arterial walls, potentially worsening macrovascular disease.

Delivery of the insulin into the peritoneum, which at least partly drains via the portal venous system, could resolve this difficulty. Peritoneal insulin is used routinely in diabetics undergoing chronic ambulatory peritoneal dialysis, but it is as yet impossible to judge whether this will show long-term benefits. Intraperitoneal infusion from either external or implanted pumps results in good glycaemic control with less hyperinsulinaemia peripherally, suggesting that at least some insulin is going intraportally.

Other attempts to deliver insulin intraportally have used the gastrointestinal tract. 'Oral' insulin has been protected from proteolytic degradation by inclusion within liposomes, but unfortunately only a variable, small number of these are absorbed. Rectal insulin suppositories give greater absorption, but again it is very fickle, and they have little aesthetic appeal. Also, it is uncertain what fraction of that absorbed passes into the portal circulation. Recently insulin has been given intranasally. A hypoglycaemic effect may be found, but it has no practical importance as yet, again because of a variable and very small percentage absorption.

Two major developments are already underway. The first aims at an artificial endocrine pancreas. This comprises a glucose sensor, a small computer, programed to respond both to absolute levels of, and changes in, glucose concentration, and an insulin infusion pump directed by the computer. At present effective systems are available, but they are large, expensive and extracorporeal. Miniaturization is feasible, but the outstanding problem is the lack of a glucose sensor which is reliable and can function for lengthy period *in vivo*. Its lack has blocked development.

Finally comes pancreatic transplantation, which has been technically successful, particularly with segmental grafts, but unsuccessful in terms of long-term endocrine function. Most grafted patients have received simultaneous pancreas and renal transplants, which probably does not assess the technique fairly. Autologous islet transplants have been used in patients after total pancreatectomy for chronic pancreatitis. Several have been independent of insulin for up to three years, although there is always the problem that there may be functioning islets in small amounts of remaining pancreas. The results from pancreatic and islet transplantation indicate much more work to be necessary. Rejection problems are considerable, although cyclosporin A looks hopeful as an immunosuppressive agent. Eventually pancreatic or islet transplantation may have a significant role to play in the treatment of insulin dependent diabetes, particularly because normoglycaemia should be possible, with insulin possibly delivered into the portal system, and with normal insulin: glucagon relationships. There are formidable problems still to be overcome, not the least the provision of sufficient pancreatic tissue for widespread use.

Exercise. The role of exercise in the treatment of diabetes remains controversial. Exercise, however, is well recognized as a major factor influencing day-to-day food and insulin requirements, and hence diabetic control. This is particularly so in children and adolescents whose unpredictable and intermittent activity may be intense.

In normals, the requirements for glucose and other fuel increase rapidly on exercise. Muscle glucose utilization increases independently of variations in insulin levels, providing basal amounts of insulin are present. There is a parallel increase in hepatic glucose production, probably resulting from associated increases in glucagon and catecholamine secretion, and often a slight drop in insulin levels. Consequently, plasma glucose levels alter little.

Several of these responses are lacking in type I diabetics, so that in the well-controlled diabetic glucose levels fall and hypoglycaemia may result unless treatment is modified. This is particularly true in the diabetic given too much insulin. Paradoxically, in the poorly controlled diabetic (blood glucose >12mmol/l) blood glucose rises with exercise, because of insulinopenia. Muscle glucose uptake increases but less than usual while hepatic glucose production shows a normal or excessive rise. In this situation there may also be a marked increase in ketonaemia—a magnification of the normal post-exercise ketosis.

Increased insulin absorption from a subcutaneous injection site also occurs in exercise, particularly if the injection has been made into an exercising limb. This alone can lead to a hypoglycaemic response.

Treatment will vary with the individual. In the mildly overweight subject it is probably wisest to decrease insulin before planned exercise. Thus, less morning intermediate insulin should be given if afternoon exercise is anticipated. In the lean diabetic extra carbohydrate should be taken before exercise begins, and more may be necessary during prolonged exercise. It is also sensible to inject insulin into a non-exercising part on the day of exercise, e.g. the abdomen or upper arm in a runner. Hypoglycaemia may occur several hours after excercise; and patients with autonomic neuropathy may have both diminished exercise capacity and a highly metabolic response.

A fall in blood glucose with exercise also occurs in type II diabetics. This is thought to be due to failure of the catecholamine response to lower insulin levels, particularly in the obese. This prevents the normal compensatory increase in hepatic glucose production.

Exercise as part of treatment is more arguable. In the obese type II diabetic, contrary to popular belief, little weight is usually lost even with intense exercise, but this will depend on how zealously dietary advice is followed; and indeed whether exercise affects appetite and food intake. However, insulin sensitivity is increased by regular physical training, through up-regulation of insulin receptors. This obviously benefits glucose tolerance even without any weight loss, but training must be sustained and the benefits are relatively small. Exercise may be more important in diminishing risk factors for cardiovascular disease. This is probably true in the non-diabetic population, but information is not available for diabetics.

Education. It is self evident that diabetics who know little or nothing about their disease are unlikely to be able to maintain good day-to-day control. There is an increasing trend towards self-management in both type I and type II patients. Education should be directed not only at patients and their families but also at their physicians, general practitioners and nurses and dieticians.

A good knowledge of dietary needs and food composition is important for all diabetics. They should know too of the effects of exercise, alcohol, and the means of self-monitoring. The insulin-treated patient should be taught injection techniques and dose adjustment and should understand the principles of balancing insulin dose and diet to meet changes in health and life-style. In the elderly or long-standing diabetic education in foot care is mandatory. All diabetics should be advised how the risks of cardiovascular disease can be reduced.

There are many possible ways in which to inform diabetics. Least satisfactory is a personal interview with a physician if this is hurried or unduly brief. Simple booklets, film strips, and audiovisual aids are likely to be helpful, but frequent reinforcement is necessary. A team of teaching nurses and dieticians may well make the greatest impact, and group teaching is often successful. A phone-in service is also useful. Crucial factors are kindness and patience from the instructors, and repetition of material which must be suitably expressed for the particular audience. There is little concrete guidance or information available on the best means to educate patients, although it is well established that *any* system will cut down both acute admissions and chronic foot problems. What is essential is that each group responsible for diabetic care has a positive commitment to teach self-care to diabetic patients.

Monitoring of therapy. Urine testing for glucose has for well over 50 years been the cornerstone in assessing metabolic control to monitor therapy biochemically. With the recent emphasis on much closer control of diabetes, several new methods have been introduced, most of which concern blood glucose measurement. Body weight should be added as another index of progress. Table 20 lists the available means of monitoring control, and adds some which may prove useful in the future. The indices measured may change when the causes of diabetic tissue damage are clarified, but those listed are appropriate to present knowledge.

Table 20 Biochemical methods for monitoring effectiveness of therapy and metabolic control in diabetes

A. Clinical methods	
Urine glucose	(a) Clinitest, Diastix, Diabur
	(b) 24-h collection
Urine ketones	(a) Acetest, Ketostix, Ketodiastix
Blood glucose	(a) Random clinic measurement
	(b) Timed post-prandial
	(c) Fasting
	(d) In-hospital profile
	(e) Home blood glucose monitoring
Glycosylated protein	(a) Haemoglobin
	(b) Albumin
Blood lipids	(a) Cholesterol
	(b) Triglyceride
B. Experimental methods	
Blood metabolites	(a) Lactate, pyruvate
	(b) Ketone bodies, glycerol, fatty acids
Free insulin	(a) Diurnal profiles
Flux measurements	(a) Glucose turnover and recycling
	(b) Ketone bodies

Urine glucose measurement gives only limited information. The renal threshold for glucose varies between 7 and 12 mmol/l but may rise much higher in renal disease. In general, glycosuria implies blood glucose values at least twice normal. A negative test does not discriminate between a blood glucose of 2 or 10 mmol/l. However, unlike a spot blood glucose test, the urine sugar excretion reflects blood glucose concentrations over several hours. If short-term information is needed, a 'second void' speciment is tested, a technique too troublesome for routine use, and dependant on the basic assumption that the volume of residual urine is very small.

Passing the analytic strip through the stream of urine is the quickest and easiest of all glucose tests. The commonest method used, Clinitest, measures reducing substances and is subject to interference from non-glucose compounds, e.g. ascorbic acid. The glucose-specific methods such as Diastix and Diabur are preferable. Despite the disadvantages of urine testing, a patient persistently aglycosuric and free of hypoglycaemic symptoms, is probably in good control.

In children, where control is highly erratic, use of a method (two-drop Clinitest, Diabur test strips), which measures up to 5 g/100 ml glucose in urine is useful in indicating how bad glycaemic control is. There is also some benefit from periodic 24-h urine quantiative glucose measurement. These are more useful than spot testing since the confounding effects of change in the rate of urine flow on concentration are reduced by a longer collection period.

Urine ketones need not be measured routinely in the majority of type I nor in any type II diabetics. This test is useful for home-monitoring in labile ketosis-prone diabetics, where it can serve as a guide to increased insulin need or a call for medical assistance. The available tests measure only acetone and aceto-acetate and not the quantitatively major 'ketone body', 3-hydroxybutyrate. The tests are insensitive, and blood levels may be 10- to 20-fold elevated before positive response is found. A high urinary ketone concentration interferes to a practically important extent with the detection of glucose by Diastix, which should therefore never be relied on in a sick patient suspected of ketoacidosis (ketodiastix should then be used).

Blood glucose measurement is the obvious test to assess glycaemic control, but a spot sample gives only momentary information. There are many different approaches to blood-glucose measure-ment. In many centres it is only measured routinely at the diabetic clinic, generally at a random time. This means that in most patients blood glucose is measured two to four times per year, which is quite inadequate if any attempt at good control is sought in type I patients; although this frequency may be acceptable in stable type II patients. Moreover patients may live very differently near clinic appointments, be stricter with dietary compliance for the few preceding days, or indeed miss meals in order to lower their blood glucose. Conversely, irritation at waiting for one to two hours may cause an adrenergic hyperglycaemic response.

Timed post-prandial glucose measurements may be more useful, again in the type II diabetic, but the same strictures apply with regard to unnatural behaviour on clinic days. There is an arguable case for not measuring blood glucose routinely in diabetic clinics, but only if arrangements are made to obtain more useful information elsewhere.

Fasting blood glucose estimation is enjoying a vogue in assessing control in type II diabetics. It appears to reflect overall glycaemic control accurately but is limited in usefulness if done only two or three times a year. It may be difficult in some individuals, e.g. those who start work at unusual hours. A monthly measurement reasonably close to home, e.g. in a health centre, can give very useful information for the management of type II disease.

A single blood glucose level may give a totally misleading impression of glycaemic control even on that day in insulin-treated type I diabetics. There may be a two- to fourfold difference between blood glucose levels measured two hours after breakfast and those measured in the late morning or late afternoon. The only way to assess control in such patients is to perform a blood glucose profile with measurements before and one to two hours after each main meal. This can be done in day clinics and is useful in the investigation of problem patients, with the reservation that the results may provide a poor reflection of normal life.

Home blood glucose monitoring (HBGM) has revolutionized assess-ment of blood glucose fluctuations, particularly in insulin-dependent diabetics. It has also enabled self-adjustment of insulin and dietary therapy to be achieved more safely and accurately, as well as providing a useful educational guide. It has become practicable through the development of simple methods for the quantitative assessment of blood glucose.

There are two main forms of HBGM. In one, fingerprick blood is taken on to impregnated filter paper or test-strips, which are delivered to the hospital laboratory or health centre for later measurement. This is useful for assessing control, but is not immediate enough for true self-management. The second, and more commonly employed method uses test-strips whose colour can be read visually or with a meter. Adequate accuracy can normally be achieved visually, but meters may be useful if greater accuracy is required during initial education, or for the colour-blind. The various methods available are shown in Table 21.

Patients use small lances (Monolets) with or without an additional spring-loaded device (Autolets) to draw blood, and it is surprising how many are prepared to do this repetitively. Indeed, approx-imately two-thirds of patients prefer HBGM to routine four-times-daily urine testing. But these comparisons have usually been with Clinitest, the most complicated form of urine testing. The frequency of HBGM varies between centres and patients. One common protocol is for the patient to measure blood glucose before and after each main meal and at bedtime on one weekday and one weekend day each week, with fasting and bedtime samples on the other days. Alternatively, four-times-daily testing is used on two or three days per week with intermittent urine testing. Such frequent testing is unnecessary in type II diabetics, where periodic fasting and post-prandial sampling is adequate. If the renal threshold for glucose is known to be approximately normal, there is little need for blood testing so long as there is sustained substantial (e.g. ½ per cent or more) glycosuria, except in brittle patients.

Table 21 Methods of home blood glucose monitoring

1. Methods not giving immediate results
    Blood collection into containers
    Blood collection on to filter paper
    Reflotest strips (strips read later with Reflomat at health centre or clinic

2. Methods giving immediate results
(a) Visual methods
    BM-Glycemie 20–800 test strips
    Visidex test strips (previously Dextrostix)

(b) Methods using meter read strips

Test strip	Meter (in United Kingdom)
BM-Glycemie	Hypocount B
Reflotest	Reflomat†
Dextrostix*	Glucometer
	Hypocount
	Glucochek
	Eyetone†

†Expensive and cumbersome.
*Shortly to be replaced by Accudex.

The accuracy of patients' measurements has been questioned. Provided that initial instructions are adequate, patients' results are at least as accurate as tests performed by hospital staff, and are certainly accurate enough for clinical purposes. Undoubtedly HBGM provides much more information on the glycaemic control of patients. The educational benefits derived may also lead to improved overall control; and most patients are satisfied by having more precise information about control. However, not all patients are prepared to self-monitor blood glucose. Present indications are shown in Table 22. The more cautious have objected that more vigorous attempts to achieve good glycaemic control could lead to a catastrophic increase in hypoglycaemia. HBGM has shown this not to be the case and has given patients reassurance that they are not on the verge of hypoglycaemia. HBGM is a *sine qua non* when intensive therapy is contemplated, as, for example, with subcu-taneous infusion, and allows all hypoglycaemic therapies to be used to their maximum potential.

Table 22 Indications for home blood glucose monitoring

1. Labile and brittle diabetics
2. Pregnant diabetics
3. Renal threshold abnormalities
4. Problem solving, e.g. nocturnal hypoclycaemia
5. In association with intensive therapy, e.g. pumps, multiple injection regimens
6. When normoglycaemia is sought
7. Patient preference
8. Educational aid

Glycosylated protein measurements may provide a better answer to assessment of overall glycaemic control. Haemoglobin A is glycosylated post-translationally at the terminal valine of the β-chain. This produces HbA_{1c}. There are two further minor glycosylated fractions HbA_{1b} and HbA_{1a}. Together they are referred to as glycosylated haemoglobin. The percentage of haemoglobin A glycosylated is directly proportional to the time the red cell has been exposed to glucose, and the height of the glucose levels. If the whole glycosylated haemoglobin fraction is measured, it gives an integrated picture of the mean blood glucose level during the average lifespan of the red blood cell, i.e. 120 days, providing that the stable, irreversibly glycosylated form is separated from an unstable intermediate. The result will be unduly low for a given blood glucose level if the lifespan of the red blood cell is appreciably shortened.

Measurement of glycosylated haemoglobin therefore gives a useful assessment of mean blood glucose control over a period of several weeks. It does not indicate sudden changes in control nor give any indication of daily variation, but is useful in assessing control in patients who do not consistently perform any type of home monitoring; in detecting patients who are not providing honest records of self-assessment, and in directing attention to patients who require more intensive education and/or care. It is reasonable to measure HbA_{1c} monthly in all clinic patients, and this has replaced routine glucose measurement in many centres.

The best method for measuring glycosylated haemoglobin is still debated. Dialysis or incubation in saline is needed to remove the unstable fraction before measurement. Column chromatography is popular, but labour-intensive and temperature-sensitive; the colorimetric method, which measures derived 5-hydroxymethylfurfural, is lengthy but can be automated, although it is not an easy routine method; electroendosmosis is simple and rapid, but the available kits are expensive. As yet, despite early promise, there is no immunoassay.

The glycosylation of haemoglobin is an example of the much wider process of glycosylation of many proteins, both intra- and extracellular, which have appropriate amino acids. Albumin is one such, and glycosylated albumin may prove easier to assay than glycosylated haemoglobin. However, albumin has a shorter half-life than haemoglobin, so glycosylated albumin will reflect the integral of glycaemic levels over a shorter time than glycosylated haemoglobin. This could sometimes be advantageous, particularly when therapy is being changed or after intercurrent illness.

It is important to recognize limitations in interpreting these techniques. For instance, a normal or minimally raised glycosylated HbA level may depend upon frequent and dangerous episodes of hypoglycaemia. Measurement of glycosylated haemoglobin or other proteins is a parallel estimation to HBGM, and of equal importance in assessing the efficacy of therapy.

Blood lipid concentrations do not assess carbohydrate metabolism directly through glucose control. They are not a particularly sensitive index of insulin status but, if abnormal, should be corrected either by changes in the hypoglycaemic agent (type or dose) or, often more usefully, by dietary modification. Cholesterol can be assessed at any time of day, but triglycerides and lipoproteins should only be measured after an overnight fast, perhaps annually unless abnormalities are known. Fractioned cholesterol estimations, i.e. HDL and LDL cholesterol, are considerably more helpful than measurement of total cholesterol, but the methods are considerably more sophisticated technically. If hyperlipaemia persists despite satisfactory blood sugar control and suitable dieting, hypolipidaemic agents may be required.

Experimental methods of assessing therapy are also listed in Table 20, to emphasize the simple nature of current metabolic monitoring, despite the major analytic advances of recent years. Blood metabolite measurement has been used experimentally to assess intermediary metabolism during different therapies. Blood lactate levels, for example, are raised during biguanide therapy, and to a lesser degree may be increased during conventional insulin therapy, even when blood glucose is kept normal with the artificial pancreas. In this instance, it almost certainly indicates a peripheral insulin excess relative to portal venous concentrations. Similarly, measurement of lipid metabolites has shown that their diurnal patterns are abnormal in all treated type I diabetics, because of excessive suppression of lipolysis. Such measurements may become useful in the future for fine-tuning of therapy. New methods (e.g. strip-tests) for many such metabolites are under active development. Home monitoring may be extended in the future but there is as yet no reason to believe raised blood levels of metabolites such as lactate or 'ketone bodies', which oscillate widely in health, contribute directly to diabetic tissue damage.

If one aim of therapy is to produce normal circulating insulin profiles, it is logical to measure plasma insulin. This is technically difficult in insulin-treated patients if insulin antibodies are present. An approximation can be achieved, using pre-precipitation of antibody–insulin complexes, and this has proved invaluable in the investigation of insulin pharmacokinetics. It has also confirmed the supposition that there is peripheral hyperinsulinaemia in conventionally treated diabetics, but probably unduly low portal vein insulin levels.

Even these methods are biochemically naive. Measurement of appearance and disappearance rates of glucose, ketone bodies and other substances have shown abnormalities of flux despite normal concentrations of circulating substrates. The relevance of such findings to the future clinical management of diabetic patients is unknown, but they emphasize the possibilities for continuing progress in our methods for assessing therapy.

Diabetic tissue damage

Introduction. This section lists the many varieties of tissue damage to which diabetics are particularly prone. Their prevalence is increased in those with less controlled glucose levels, although it is increasingly apparent that the extent of the damage depends upon the interaction with hyperglycaemia of other factors (both environmental and inherited). The biochemical processes causing damage are probably different with different lesions. Understanding of these processes is necessary for the design of correct treatment. It is also important to identify patients whose constitutions predispose them to such deterioration, so that protective measures, e.g. rigid glycaemic control, can be concentrated upon them rather than imposed on all.

One useful generalization is that development of the more specific microangiopathic lesions requires higher sustained glucose levels than those that give an increased risk of macroangiopathy. None the less, blood glucose control has to be extremely good by the standards pertaining even a few years ago if an appreciable increased risk of microangiopathy is to be avoided. The necessary target would appear to be blood glucose values below 7 mM fasting and to avoid increases above 10–11 mM throughout the day, though evidence of the need for such precision is slight and the variation between individual patients likely to be substantial.

Tissue damage tends to occur according to certain clinical patterns; if diabetic nephropathy develops severely enough to cause renal failure, the patient is most likely to be under 50 years old and to have had diabetes diagnosed less than 35 years previously. Severe diabetic retinopathy and neuropathy are also likely to be present. On the other hand, foot ulceration, particularly if mainly ischaemic in origin, is rare under 45 years of age and increasingly common thereafter, up to 70 years; this is predominantly a lesion of type II diabetics. Visual disturbance in this group is more likely to be due to cataract or exudative retinopathy than to proliferative retinopathy, found mainly in type I diabetics, often together with nephropathy.

Such divisions may underlie the trough in age-corrected diabetic mortality seen between 45 and 55 years old, at which stage the more vulnerable type I diabetics have died, while type II diabetics have not had time for much damage to develop.

Type I diabetes is associated with a mortality rate increased about five times over that of the general population, the relative risk being greater the younger the patient. It is difficult to state an exact rate for type II diabetes. It depends on accurate detection, particularly so in studies undertaken before the new definition of 'impaired glucose tolerance' came into use. Values range upwards from the increased mortality of around 40 per cent in the most widely based study, that in Birmingham in the United Kingdom. This relatively low excess mortality was probably because more older patients were included than in other studies. Insurance company figures indicate values nearer to 300 per cent, but these are not unbiased. Whatever the precise figures, the risk is larger the younger the patient. The relative risk of macroangiopathic disease is also always greater than that of mortality with foot ulceration a particular cause of morbidity.

A recent study of deaths of diabetics under 50 years old showed the great majority of these to occur in those above 40, mostly from cardiac infarction but also from renal failure in the long-term type I diabetic. However, some 15 per cent of these deaths are still the result of acute metabolic derangement, whether hyperglycaemic or hypoglycaemic (Table 23), which also gives the experience of the Joslin Clinic with mostly type I diabetics, but without age restrictions.

Table 23   Principal causes of death in diabetics

	Joslin Clinic 1966–1968 (%)	United Kingdom survey of deaths in diabetics under 50 years old (via death certificate) (%)
Cardiovascular		
Cardiac causes	54.6	35
Cerebral	10.0	7
Other	1.6	—
Renal	8.0	17
Diabetic nephropathy	(6.0)	
Infections	5.9	2
Cancer	12.8	7
Hepatic cirrhosis	1.5	2
Hyperglycaemic comas	1.0	16
Hypoglycaemia	0.7	4
Suicide	0.3	—
Others	3.6	10
Respiratory		5
Chronic neurological		3

It is difficult to give accurate quantitative expression to the ill effects of diabetes, because there have been no conclusive cohort studies yet reported which assess both prevalance and incidence, and because the results are influenced by many interacting factors, e.g. whatever determines the much greater frequency of peripheral vascular disease in European or North American diabetics than among the Japanese, who have the relatively greater liability to severe retinopathy. Some generalizations may be advanced as a guide. The average expectation of life of type I diabetics diagnosed below 30 years old has been 29 years, with only half reaching 50 years of age. A third of such patients have severe renal failure before death, which comes from cardiac disease in at least half. The risks of this, and of peripheral vascular disease of leg and brain, are greatly increased by hypertension, which is commoner among diabetics than others (especially after more than 10 years of type I). Amputative operation on the leg (at any level) is uncommon below 60 years, but then affects about 10 per cent of all diabetics, with marked deterioration in prognosis. After even as relatively mild an operation as a unilateral transmetatarsal amputation, only 60 per cent are alive five years later, while after a second operation at knee

level on the remaining leg, only 50 per cent survive more than two years.

Among type I patients, one-third will be 'legally blind' in at least one eye before death; and they show most clearly the increased relative risk in females of severe or fatal cardiac disease, up to five times that of non-diabetics, even if the absolute risk of such trouble does not exceed that in males.

The 10–15 per cent of type I patients who live more than 40 years with the disease disclose a more cheerful prospect, for they are relatively free from serious morbidity, with under 10 per cent legally blind (even if another 10 per cent have proliferative retinopathy), and uraemia a rare ending. Somehow, and probably constitutionally, hyperglycaemia is not for them the harbinger of serious tissue damage that it is to so many.

Nephropathy. The kidneys of a diabetic are at risk from a specific lesion, typified by the nodular glomerulosclerosis described by Kimmelstiel and Wilson, as well as from a more generalized arteriolar lesion. They may also be affected by pathological processes dependent upon some other form of diabetic tissue damage, e.g. recurrent pyelitis or pyelonephritis dependent upon incomplete bladder emptying because of autonomic neuropathy. Thirdly, they may be affected by diseases unconnected with diabetes.

The specific microangiopathic renal lesion has four main structural facets. These are:

1. Hyaline tissue, particularly near the glomerular hilum. This change is associated with capillary basement membrane thickening and perhaps impaired ability to remove mesangial debris.

2. Diffuse lesions of the glomeruli, approximately twice as common as the nodular lesions, with thickening of the whole circumference of the peripheral capillary walls in the tufts, and narrowed lumens. By light microscopy this lesion may be confused with amyloidosis or membranous glomerulonephritis, but can be distinguished by electron microscopy.

3. Less specific is an exudative lesion, a relatively late change, with rounded or concentric deposits of intensely acidophilic material either as a cap over a glomerular loop or attached to the inside of Bowman's space. It contains fibrinoid.

4. All these lesions can result in complete hyalinization of glomeruli. While these changes are not uniform they are widely scattered and show no clustering. This specific glomerular degeneration is complicated by the liability to diffuse intimal fibrosis in the large renal vessels and even more by hyalinization of the efferent arterioles. Functionally, diabetic nephropathy does not affect the tubule specifically, for the proteinuria is 'non-selective'. Similarly, there are no specific tubular lesions, for light microscopy reports of thickening of the tubular basement membranes have not been confirmed by electron microscopy.

Early in diabetes there is renal hypertrophy with enlargement of the glomeruli, both generally and in the amount of basement membrane substance. This is associated with increased glomerular filtration and microproteinuria. Such a change could possibly occur with any prolonged osmotic diuresis. An excess of glycogen is often also found in diabetic kidneys, but it is not known to contribute to the nephropathy. In experimental animals most of these changes are reversible by restoration of normoglycaemia.

Symptoms and signs. These are remarkably few and although terminal renal failure is one of the important causes of death of type I diabetics, patients may be unaware of progressive renal disease until insidious symptoms of uraemia develop with those of the accompanying anaemia. There may be increasing lassitude, breathlessness on effort, nocturia unexplained by glycosuria, or gastrointestinal disturbance unexplained by autonomic neuropathy (all too likely, though, to be present at the same time). An increasing instability of glucose control in insulin-treated patients, and particularly a decreasing insulin requirement, suggests developing uraemia.

Perhaps a quarter of those doomed to terminal renal failure pass through a nephrotic phase, with gross albuminuria and ankle swelling. There may be hypoalbuminaemia but, perhaps because of a special liability to increased capillary permeability, ankle oedema may occur without severe hypoalbuminaemia. As with other forms of the nephrotic syndrome, its disappearance often heralds increasing uraemia.

Proteinuria is therefore the major clincal index of developing diabetic nephropathy. It is present in perhaps 10 per cent of those attending a typical hospital diabetic clinic, but there can be great variability in the interval between its first appearance and the development of heavy proteinuria, or between the first finding of proteinuria and developing uraemia. Even after exclusion of urinary tract infection, or the orthostatic proteinuria of the young, proteinuria may be transiently present at diagnosis, then to disappear for many years. Excluding these, perhaps a fifth of patients have intermittent proteinuria, which typically becomes constant three years later. Should it remain intermittent for six years, the clinical course is considerably more benign.

In typical type I diabetics of young onset, proteinuria develops about 15 years from diagnosis. In the small number of proteinurics among diabetics treated by oral agents or diet alone, the average interval is as short as four years between diagnosis and appearance of constant proteinuria. The interval between developing proteinuria and a significant increase in plasma creatinine may vary from one to ten or more years, but as a generalization this interval is shorter the greater the age at which proteinuria appears. Once hypercreatininaemia has developed, its time course is remarkably predictable, with a linear relationship between the reciprocal of the plasma creatinine concentration and time in any individual, though the gradient of deterioration can vary considerably between patients. Reasonably reliable predictions can therefore be made as to when terminal renal failure may need treatment.

Investigation of proteinuria. A search for urinary infection is obviously indicated, as is measurement of the plasma creatinine. The kidneys are not palpable in this condition, which is painless (in the absence of infection). Proteinuria is non-selective. Diagnosis can only be reliably achieved by biopsy, after intravenous urography. Undue dehydration must be avoided during the pyelogram, and glycosuria must be well controlled. Other specialized examination of the kidneys may be necessary, as by ultrasound or renal angiography, but this is to detect lesions other than diabetic nephropathy.

In the absence of any feature suggestive of a non-diabetic renal lesion, it is a moot question (or when) one should recommend renal biopsy for a diabetic with sustained proteinuria. This is likely to be done more frequently, and earlier in the course of the disease, if increased opportunities arise for renal transplantation of diabetics, and it proves beneficial to transplant earlier than later in the course of the disease (particularly if this retards the evolution of cardiac or ocular disease). Further, if near normalization of glucose levels were to prevent (or retard) the evolution of serious diabetic nephropathy, it would become important to detect developing nephropathy early, so that such patients could be offered optimal methods of blood glucose control. At present biopsy is usually recommended only when plasma creatinine rises beyond 300 μm/l.

Differential diagnosis. Biopsy may be performed to clarify diagnosis and is particularly indicated if the developing nephropathy is unaccompanied by retinopathy, or if in a relatively young (say, under 40 years) patient proteinuria develops within a short time of diagnosis (say, four years). Proteinuria present at diagnosis, and persisting for six months after start of effective hypoglycaemic treatment, indicates biopsy particularly in those under 50 years. Sudden development of heavy proteinuria is another indication.

Associated factors. There is general belief that the more hyperglycaemic a diabetic the greater the chance of nephropathy, and this is illustrated in Pirart's series, although only a small percentage of his patients were followed long-term. Perhaps one-fifth of patients remain free of any important degree of nephropathy, even after 40 or more years of type I diabetes, but some post-mortem lesion will be found in over 90 per cent of diabetics of all types. Type II diabetics develop typical renal lesions, but the arterial and arteriolar changes are the more likely to predominate. Typical glomerular lesions may be seen in secondary diabetes.

No reliable marker of increased risk has been seriously suspected apart from hyperglycaemia. Hypertension is present in perhaps 10 per cent of patients with proteinuria, but there is no evidence that diabetics with hypertension are more liable to serious nephropathy than others. However, Mogensen showed that effective hypotensive treatment retarded the progression of uraemia in diabetics, but only over the relatively short period of a year; the results of more prolonged treatment are yet to be announced. However, proper hypotensive treatment, promptly started, is part of the correct management of these patients, as with other forms of renal disease. The extent to which the hypertension results from the diabetic kidney lesion is unknown.

Diabetics with severe renal disease are particularly liable to proliferative retinopathy as well as to cardiac lesions. They may die from myocardial infarction before or after treatment for renal failure is begun, rather than from the consequences of renal failure itself.

Diet. A low-protein diet with a low carbohydrate content tends to lead to hyperlipaemia (hypertriglyceridaemia sometimes with hypercholesterolaemia). Adequate calories can always be provided by slowly absorbed carbohydrate, which should supply at least 50–60 per cent of the total calories. The liability to hyperlipaemia may well increase the likelihood of myocardial infarction, and the biochemical lesion at least can be reversed substantially by proper dietary advice.

Other renal lesions. In any disease with gross polyuria, especially if it starts young, there can be gross dilation of the bladder and even ureters. However, diabetes mellitus is nearly always adequately treated early enough for this to be no more than a curiosity, especially when it is part of the rare syndrome of deafness with diabetes insipidus as well as diabetes mellitus (Didmoad syndrome). However, if diabetic autonomic neuropathy develops, urinary retention may develop in a low-pressure bladder. Thus, even though the residual bladder volume may be considerable, it is much less painful and less readily palpable than the high-pressure bladder of an obstructed overflow (e.g. prostatic hypertrophy). Percussion is particularly helpful clinically, but the enlarged bladder is often best detected by IVP or ultrasound. Treatment may be conservative or surgical. Bladder neck resection can give great relief, but may produce an unpleasant degree of urinary incontinence. Slight relief may come from cholinergic agents such as ambostigmine or anticholinesterases.

Ascending urinary tract infection, or blood-borne infection may develop into the rare complication of renal carbuncle or perinephric abcess. The former must be treated surgically, and operation will usually be required for the latter. Palpable enlargement of the renal (or perirenal) tissues as well as marked tenderness and guarding occur in both conditions, but gross pyuria is more characteristic of renal carbuncle.

Renal failure: treatment. This may be by regular dialysis, or by renal transplantation. Haemodialysis often proves unsatisfactory in diabetics. In the past it has probably been started too late, and there are features of the treatment (e.g. anticoagulation, fluid shifts, etc.) that are particularly unhealthy for the diabetic. Certainly retinopathy and cardiac disease seem to proceed apace in these patients, quite apart from the technical problems of inserting a shunt in those whose arm arteries, even at the wrist, are liable to medial thickening and calcification.

Recent trends favour continuous ambulatory peritoneal dialysis. This can work well in diabetics; it allows excellent control of glucose levels through insulin introduced into the peritoneal cavity with the dialysate. The limiting factor is peritoneal infection but evidence that this is a greater risk for diabetics than for patients with other causes of renal failure is lacking to date.

Transplantation. The main problem is the stage at which a diabetic is most suitable for such treatment. Once an inexorable progression of renal failure can be predicted, the benefits of transplantation in likely improvement in general health, and perhaps removal of factors accelerating progression of diabetic tissue damage, must be weighed against possible involvement of a transplanted kidney by diabetic nephropathy, and the hazards of the surgical procedure, as well as the liability to infection associated with immunosuppression.

The results of transplantation using first-degree relatives as living donors have been as good with non-diabetic recipients. Graft survival of cadaver kidneys is less than in non-diabetic recipients but the gap between the two has narrowed. Transplantation is probably the treatment of choice for diabetics who are otherwise reasonably healthy. If graft rejection occurs, patients can be transferred (or returned) to a dialysis programme to await a further suitable graft. Different centres take different precautions to exclude unsuitable recipients. Some do not exclude the blind, while others regard proliferative retinopathy as a barrier. Some centres carry out pre-transplant coronary angiopathy, while others would be guided more by the ECG, cardiac function, and a history of ischaemic pain.

Diabetic eye disease. This is the main cause of blindness in the United Kingdom between the ages of 20 and 65 years. It is mainly due to diabetic retinopathy or to cataract. Much less frequently, glaucoma associated with rubeosis iridis is the mechanism, while occlusion of the retinal vein or artery is also unduly frequent in diabetics. Although there are abnormalities of the intraocular pressure in diabetics, open-angle glaucoma is not established as increased.

Diabetic retinopathy. This almost certainly has a multifactorial pathogenesis, with contributions from sex and other genetic factors, in addition to the metabolic abnormalities of diabetes. Increased retinal blood flow, with widening of the smaller retinal vessels, is suspected to be an important early abnormality, but the stimulus to it is unknown. There are also, perhaps later, changes in the endothelial cells, thickening of the capillary basement membrane, and a decreased number of intramural pericytes. These changes are accompanied by increased permeability of the blood–retinal barrier (measurable by fluorescein leakage).

Somehow these changes lead to blockage of retinal capillaries and arterioles with reduced blood flow, and non-perfusion of certain retinal areas. The veins draining such areas may become abnormally variable in diameter, as well as showing increased tortuosity, while vessels close to the non-perfused area become abnormally permeable, with risk of development of surrounding oedema and fatty deposits which are the basis of retinal exudates. At the margins of such areas, too, new blood vessels develop. There is little risk of serious visual loss from peripheral neovascularization, or from small degrees of neovascularization unassociated with previous haemorrhage, but marked neovascularization, particularly when it occurs on or very close to the optic disc, is associated with rapidly advancing retinopathy. The stimulus to such neovascularization, perhaps a vascular growth factor, is thought to arise from ischaemic retina, and presumably reaches the affected vessels by diffusion. Alternatively, neovascularization could be the response to a deficiency.

Retinopathy may be divided into three types:
1. Simple, 'background', harmless in itself and often present without substantial alteration for many years, but nearly always observed before either of the two other vision-threatening types of retinopathy.
2. *Proliferative*, associated with neovascularization, vitreous haemorrhage, fibrous overgrowth and retinitis proliferans, and retinal detachment.
3. *Exudative*, only threatening vision severely when involving the macula by either oedema or exudates.

1. Simple retinopathy. This has a number of ophthalmoscopic features ranging from small red dots (microaneurysms or dot haemorrhages) to much larger, though still usually regular, red 'blot haemorrhages'. There may also be small areas of exudate, either cottonwool spots (prognostically worrying, as these indicate areas of retinal ischaemia) or small 'fatty' exudates, either circular or crescentic, and usually slightly yellow in colour. There may be increase in the size and tortuosity of the veins.

2. Proliferative retinopathy is dominated by neovascularization and evidence of pre-retinal, usually vitreous, haemorrhage. Neovascularization is recognized by an increased density of fine arteriolar elements arranged in a disorganized fashion, as a crazy lattice. Such areas are often smaller than quarter of the optic disc, but sometimes they are widespread throughout the retina. They are particularly likely to be seen close to the disc or even on it. Vitreous haemorrhages vary in size but are rarely as small as a typical sub-hyaloid haemorrhage as seen in subarachnoid haemorrhage. They usually resolve over two to four months, with complete remission or even if the initial loss of vision was complete. However, any single haemorrhage, and particularly repeated haemorrhages, may be organized with forward spread of fibrous elements, often as a sheet running at right angles to the retina. This is liable to cause a retinal detachment and to be a source of further vitreous haemorrhage, as the vessels growing forward over these fibrous sheets are particularly fragile.

No single feature of diabetic proliferative retinopathy is unique to it, but the evolution of retinal change is characteristic. Similar features are seen in hypertensive retinopathy and in the reaction to ischaemic areas of retina, as after fat embolus, in sickle cell disease, after venous occlusion, and in the hyperviscosity syndromes.

Smoking and hypertension exacerbate proliferative retinopathy and, while there are claims that increased intraocular tension may retard its development, this is unproven. There are much data which associate an increased risk of retinopathy with higher blood glucose values, but there is no proof of a causal relationship in man. However, Engerman and Bloodworth have shown, in dogs with experimental diabetes that those with the higher glucose values (who had received less insulin) had marked retinopathy after five years, while those with better control showed little or no abnormality.

Exudative retinopathy may present as macular oedema or macular exudates or, much less seriously for vision, with exudates away from the macula. Of the serious forms of retinopathy, macular oedema is much the most difficult to recognize ophthalmoscopically, so any deterioration of visual acuity in a diabetic should be taken seriously until the cause is determined. The retina shows a glazed appearance, with some diminution of vascular calibre and number, but there are none of the obvious focal features, seen with either haemorrhage or exudate. Oedema is often accompanied by such features, but not necessarily. Exudates are particularly liable to occur as crescents just lateral to the macula, but they may be sited anywhere in the retina. They should be distinguished from the usually smaller, highly refractile, cholesterol deposits in the walls of vessels, particularly where they bifurcate. These indicate vascular change but are usually less directly related to visual disturbance. Fluorescein angiography may be particularly helpful in assessing the likely course of oedema or exudates by indicating the nature of the vascular pattern close to them, and whether there is markedly increased permeability. This can be particularly helpful in deciding whether to coagulate vessels thought responsible for the formation of perimacular exudates.

Management. The corrected visual acuity should be assessed in each eye separately in every diabetic one to three months from diagnosis, to allow for the not uncommon, but temporary, refractile disturbance of rapid onset hyperglycaemia to settle. The fundi should be examined after pupillary dilatation. Examination through undilated pupils misses about a third of abnormalities. In patients under 40, an interval of two years may separate successive checks until 10 years after diagnosis, when annual checks should start. Annual review is wise in all those diagnosed above 40 years. Some 4 per cent of diabetics have retinopathy at diagnosis, and nearly all these are type II patients, at least 50 years old. Younger patients are more prone to develop proliferative retinopathy, and the older to show exudative changes, with insidious visual disturbance from macular exudate or oedema. A minority of patients can be diabetic for 40 or 50 years without any ophthalmoscopic sign of retinopathy, while others may develop background retinopathy 10–20 years after the disease is recognized, but this never progresses to threaten vision. Minor ophthalmoscopic features (such as microaneurysms) may disappear, but this does not always indicate improvement, in that fluorescein angiography may show that the area is less well perfused than before. However, even by fluorescein, retinopathy is often observed spontaneously to stop deteriorating. Proliferative retinopathy may worsen substantially during pregnancy, but the deterioration tends to regress after delivery.

The mechanism by which background retinopathy evolves into a vision-threatening form is unknown and, while the chances of this are related to blood glucose levels, these are far from the whole story. This deterioration must involve individual constitution (as indicated by identical twin studies), while physical (e.g. infection) or emotional stress may be related to it in time.

Treatment. Blood sugar must be controlled as well as possible.

1. The fasting blood glucose may need to be consistently below 7 mM and the two-hour blood glucose value in the artificial oral glucose tolerance test to be below 11 mM if the chance of evolving retinopathy is to be reduced substantially. These values are extremely difficult to achieve in type I diabetics and are obtained in only a minority of type II diabetics.

2. Attention must be paid to contributory factors such as smoking, blood pressure, and hyperlipidaemia. High lipid levels are likely to increase the liability to retinal exudates, though this has not been directly shown, but they will certainly affect both viscosity and liability to blood coagulation or aggregation.

3. Photocoagulation can be achieved by either the xenon or argon arcs. The former gives a larger lesion and is absorbed deeper in the retina than the argon beam, which is absorbed by intravascular haemoglobin. Hence, the xenon arc may be preferable for widespread peripheral ablation, while the argon beam is certainly better for accurate coagulation of small vessels near the optic disc. The treatment has two aims: to close friable vessels likely to be the source of vitreous haemorrhage, and to destroy retina that may serve as the source of the vasoproliferative factor discussed above. The treatment is paradoxical, in that it mimics the disease, by reducing retinal blood flow by blocking vessels; but its specific aims are to attack selectively particularly dangerous vessels and to preserve the function of the crucial retinal areas, even if this involves destruction of less important peripheral parts.

Photocoagulation has been shown to be effective by randomized control trials in both America and Britain. Its use is associated with a decrease over three (or even five) years in the incidence of blindness by some 60 per cent, both in proliferative retinopathy and when perimacular lesions threaten function. In the untreated of this second group, loss of vision was not always associated with progression of the macular lesion, but sometimes with proliferative complications.

Once retinitis proliferans has become established, or retinal detachment is present, or large exudates are well established close to the macula, treatment has no effect. Similarly, as with heavy proteinuria in diabetic nephropathy, it is probable that at a severe level of retinopathy improved glycaemic control will no longer retard deterioration.

4. Pituitary ablation was used in the past, to prevent growth hormone and perhaps also prolactin production, though the exact role of diminished gonadotrophin secretion was never fully elucidated. Hypophysectomy is followed by a decrease in capillary fragility which may be secondary to changes in catecholamine levels. In two small studies hypophysectomy was shown to be beneficial in severe proliferative retinopathy, but it is unsuitable in patients over 40 years old. It also requires an intelligent patient to cope thereafter with the increased lability of the blood glucose and can only be done when there is unusually well preserved renal function despite severe retinopathy. Nowadays photocoagulation is virtually always the treatment of choice, as hypophysectomy produces so much endocrine disturbance. However, the very few patients with florid diabetic proliferative retinopathy in whom photocoagulation alone is ineffective should be recognized early and referred for consideration of hypophysectomy within weeks of the photocoagulation treatment.

Recently, vitrectomy has developed as a treatment for blindness from unresolved vitreous haemorrhage and as a treatment of retinal detachment subsequent to vitreous haemorrhage. Specialist opinion may well be required, therefore, before diabetics even blind in an eye for five years are considered to have irreversible loss of sight.

Ocular cataract. As with some other types of tissue damage, there is both a specific 'diabetic' lesion and an increased incidence of a severe, common, but non-specific lesion.

The metabolic or 'snowflake' cataract of poorly controlled juvenile diabetics happily is much less common than in the past. It may be seen at first diagnosis of type I diabetes, but more often after a few years of poor glycaemic control. It may be very severe, causing blindness within a few days but, in contrast, early successful control of blood glucose may reverse it. If the cataract progresses, it can be extracted, but this is now very rarely necessary.

Quite different is the common accelerated 'senile' cataract that leads to a disproportionate number of diabetics among those operated on for cataract. While some doubt must remain, the development of cataract seems no commoner among diabetics than non-diabetics but, should a cataract start, it extends more rapidly and interferes more with vision among diabetics. Around 50 per cent of diabetics diagnosed more than 20 years previously have some lens opacity visible on examination, while the frequency of cataract extraction among diabetics is perhaps six times that in the general population. Nowadays there is no increased risk of rupture of the lens capsule at operation, and results in diabetics are almost as good as in non-diabetics, although there is still an increased risk of severe infection. Lens opacities are commoner in diabetic women than in men, and women show a faster progression of cataract. On average diabetics coming to cataract extraction are five years younger than non-diabetics.

Again, mild lens opacities may disappear during periods of tight glucose control, but usually develop slowly until extraction is required. With a dense cataract it is always difficult to know whether diabetic retinopathy may have developed during its maturation. However, retinopathy accounts for blindness after extraction in only one-third of retinopaths from whom a lens is removed.

Although there are hopes of development of a medical treatment of cataract, surgery still remains the only effective method. The planned medical treatment is based on the hypothesis that the sugar alcohol sorbitol, formed by reactions of the hexose 6-phosphate pathway, accumulates within the lens and damages it. Thus, an inhibitor of aldose reductase could be effective by preventing the accumulation of sorbitol. In animals the inhibitor has been found to reduce lens opacities in experimental galactosaemia in which dulcitol, the corresponding sugar alcohol, accumulates. Development of a suitable enzyme inhibitor for man is still experimental.

Diabetic macroangiopathy. In all diabetics, and among those with impaired glucose tolerance, there is a greatly increased liability to develop arteriosclerosis in large- and medium-sized arteries throughout the body. It is clinically important, particularly in the coronary vessels and those supplying the legs. Arteriosclerosis of vessels near the wrist makes installation of access sites difficult to fashion in renal failure and narrowing of renal vessels can be a substantial component of ailing renal function in elderly diabetics. The neck and cerebral vessels are also involved.

It is debatable whether the lesion is merely an acceleration of the disease of non-diabetics, or whether it has specific features. If the latter, these are relatively minor, but clinically there is a distortion of the pattern typical of the non-diabetic. The lesions are more widespread and more peripheral particularly in the legs, and fewer are amenable to vascular surgery which is less practicable in long or multiple vascular obstructions, and is still almost confined to lesions above the knee. Medial calcification is also commoner in diabetics, though present in non-diabetics as Monckeberg's sclerosis. This calcification, causing a tramline appearance on X-ray, can extend even to the small plantar arteries running between the metatarsals. Calcification alone is rarely a cause of major vascular occlusion, but in diabetics is associated with poor tissue prognosis, particularly when distal.

The clinical effects may be summarized as:

1. Coronary vessels. Coronary artery disease is not the only cause of diabetic cardiomyopathy, but is of major importance and has an increased incidence among diabetics. Heart disease is the main cause of death among diabetics, increasing the mortality of all types. The relative risk is particularly increased in women. Diabetics with advanced renal disease often die of cardiac disease, perhaps because hyperlipidaemia has been aggravated by hitherto ill-judged dietary treatment.

The coronary artery disease usually presents as it does in non-diabetics, but there is an increased likelihood of painless cardiac infarction, perhaps twice as common among diabetics. Whether or not this is due to cardiac autonomic neuropathy, it is a possible cause of insidious cardiac failure or dysrhythmia, or even sudden onset of poor glucose control. It is most uncommon for an infarct in known diabetics not to be followed by at least a few days of heavy glycosuria, or blood glucose values rising to 15 mM or higher.

2. Aortic, pelvic, and leg vessels. Marked narrowing near the aortic bifurcation may contribute to Leriche's syndrome of impotence and intermittent claudication with pain in the buttocks or thighs. Much more commonly the major lesions are distal even to the iliac vessels and are seen mostly in the femoral or profunda femoris arteries or below the knee. Delineation of the lesion may be necessary in patients with intermittent claudication, with troublesome foot lesions, and always before any major amputation, in case vascular repair could either push the chosen amputation site distally or just improve its healing. Proper attention must be given to interacting factors, such as smoking, hypertension, and hyperlipidaemia.

3. Arm and neck vessels. More commonly than in non-diabetics, but still rarely, pain on exercise of the arm is due to vascular block at the subclavian or closely proximate level. There may be an accompanying vascular bruit and in some cases vascular repair may improve symptoms. Subclavian 'steal' may occur, as may carotid narrowing or obstruction. There is some evidence of a small increase in liability to cerebrovascular accidents among diabetics, but this is not so pronounced as the increased risk of heart disease, and to date no increase in damage to the distal cerebral arteries has been established.

Any damaged vessel may be the source of emboli, whether of platelets or other material. This should always be considered to explain lesions in the foot, the retina, the kidney, or the brain.

Diabetic heart disease. As well as macroangiopathy diabetics have a separate risk of cardiac disease, particularly of the left ventricle. This results from microangiopathy in the heart and from altered structure of diabetic collagen, whether or not these are interdependent. Clinically, this has been recognized by: (a) the increased incidence of left ventricular failure, inexplicable after investigation by ECG or coronary angiography in epidemiological studies, as in Framingham; (b) the high percentage of diabetics among those investigated by coronary angiography because of left ventricular failure who prove to have normal vessels; (c) pathological studies. Non-invasive investigation of cardiac function indicates a stiffer muscular wall. The likelihood of associated alcoholic cardiomyopathy must always be considered in type II diabetics, particularly if there is hyperlipidaemia.

Management of hyperlipidaemia. The most important steps to decrease the raised concentrations of plasma lipids not uncommonly found in diabetics are: (a) achieve excellent control of blood sugar; (b) an increase in the ratio of polyunsaturated to other fatty acids in the diet, with limitation of extremely cholesterol-rich foods such as eggs or shellfish; and (c) to consider the use of hypolipaemic agents such as cholestyramine, long-acting nicotinic acid preparations, and other newer agents whose role is still to be evaluated. Weight loss in the obese and increased exercise in all is likely to be important.

Coagulative or thrombotic abnormalities. Although no severe disturbance in the clumping of the formed elements of the blood has been attributed to diabetes, the associated increase in macroangiopathy has been linked with various indices of an increased liability to thrombosis. These include increased mean fibrinogen concentrations with duration of diabetes and/or the prevalence of tissue damage increase; and an increased concentration of von Willebrand's factor. There are also indices of increased platelet aggregation, such as raised plasma β-thromboglobulin in man, and experimental evidence *in vivo* in animals of increased platelet aggregation at sites of damage to vascular endothelium when ADP (adenosine diphosphate) is applied. Suspicions have been raised of abnormalities of endothelial function, particularly in respect of the prostaglandins, but no abnormality has been definitely established.

It is more debatable whether such abnormalities contribute to microangiopathy for instance in the retina, where the reduced deformability of the red cells, and their increased tendency to aggregate, may disturb the microcirculation. Increased viscosity may also be important, caused by either an increased packed-cell volume, as in uncontrolled diabetes, or an increased tendency to hyperlipidaemia or other changes in plasma constitution, such as an increase in α_2-macroglobulins.

Neuropathy. Diabetic peripheral neuropathy affects somatic and autonomic neurones in their axonal processes. It is debatable whether there is primary neuropathy within the central nervous system, especially of the neuronal bodies themselves. All accept an increased liability to cerebral and presumably spinal arterial disease, and its consequences for neuronal health, as well as the possibility of damage from hypoglycaemia, particularly to certain layers of the cerebral cortex. Specific changes among cerebral neurones have been reported but this work has not yet been confirmed.

Peripheral neuropathy is both common and symptomatic, although more often annoying than life-threatening. Neuropathy also contributes to much of the foot ulceration of diabetes, and is the cause of the uncommon Charcot's neuro-arthropathy. Autonomic neuropathy, initially only a nuisance, later causes major morbidity and may result in fatal complications. Severe postural hypotension is uncommon but disorders in motility of stomach, large bowel, or urinary bladder can all be distressing, and predispose to infection or malnutrition. Impotence may be the straw that makes a relatively young type I diabetic cynically adopt self-destructive behaviour, particularly if his marriage has already ended through this lesion.

The most important factor in the prevalence of neuropathy is the time from diagnosis of diabetes. In diabetics of 20 years' duration, aged 40 years or more (for age also contributes), there is usually clinical evidence of peripheral neuropathy, even though this affects the patient little. The frequency of excruciating dysaesthesiae has been estimated at 3 per cent, of incapacitating proximal motor neuropathy in at least one leg at 7 per cent, of feet so numb that they are at real risk of traumatic ulceration at 24 per cent, of diabetic bowel disturbance at 28 per cent, and of impotence (males only) at 40 per cent. By contrast, each clinic will usually, at one time, contain only two or three patients with severe postural hypotension, and urinary retention severe enough for operation is rare.

It has long been known that various electrical properties of peripheral nerves are altered by diabetes, e.g. delayed conduction velocity in motor and sensory nerves, and that treatment at least of newly diagnosed type I diabetics can improve this substantially within three to four weeks, though failing to restore it to normal. Further, a recent study of vibration sense in the feet of newly diagnosed, mainly type II, diabetics has shown a positive correlation between the mean fasting blood glucose concentration and the degree of deterioration in the sensory threshold during the first three or five years from diagnosis, and this applies across the whole range of fasting blood glucose concentrations (from under 5 to over 12 mM). Glucose levels are not the only factor contributing to the deterioration in vibratory threshold, e.g. women are less affected than men. Multifactorial influences on diabetic neuropathy, at least in large sensory fibres, accord with clinical experience, where the degree of glucose control seems far from an exclusive determinant. The impairment of vibratory threshold at diagnosis is strongly correlated with that three or five years later. Two factors linked with this initial value are age (the worse the older) and the patient's maximum remembered weight (allowing for height), which is a stronger correlate than the degree of obesity at diagnosis.

The pathology of diabetic neuropathy is multiple. In addition to vascular lesions and segmental demyelination there are abnormalities both of axoplasmic transport and of the mechanism generating the action current and perhaps of the nodal membranes. One hypothesis to explain the Schwann cell and myelin abnormalities is an excessive entry of glucose during hyperglycaemia into the glucose 6-phosphate pathway of insulin-dependent cells with resulting increase in sorbitol. This sugar alcohol remains largely within those tissues in which it forms, e.g. ocular lens and Schwann cell. There is no doubt of the high sorbitol contents of diabetic peripheral nerve, and one argument for the involvement of sorbitol is improved peripheral nerve conduction in animals with experimental diabetes given an inhibitor of the relevant enzyme, aldose reductase. There is a further analogy from the effects of galactitol on peripheral nerve and ocular lens in hereditary galactosaemia or after excessive galactose feeding of animals. These features can be partially reversed in animals by an aldose reductase inhibitor. Other possible pathogenetic possibilities include myoinositol deficiency with consequent disturbance of phospholipid metabolism and direct glycosylation of myelin.

Classification (Table 24) I. *Somatic sensory* neuropathy involves large fibres, such as serve joint position and vibration sense, and contribute to touch and small fibres, such as serve pain and temperature sensation, as well as contributing to touch.

This type of neuropathy is nearly always virtually symmetrical and affects the arms as well as the legs, but the latter predominantly. It is also responsible for loss of tendon jerks, first at the ankles, via failure on the afferent side of the two-neurone arc.

II. *Motor neuropathy*. Affects proximal nerves asymmetrically and usually involves some of the femoral plexus. Some believe this to be a special example of type III.

III. *Mononeuropathy* (mononeuritis) can result from pressure or from a vascular accident to a nerve. Motor and sensory nerves are unduly vulnerable in diabetics to pressure as in the carpal tunnel, from cervical spondylitis, or in relation to a thoracic rib. Occasionally, clinical episodes occur that suggest a 'stroke' of a peripheral nerve, with excruciating, short-lived pain followed by interrupted nerve function; but more commonly the onset is insidious. Obstruction of the vasa nervorum is common in this condition, particularly with femoral neuropathy or third cranial nerve palsy. External ophthalmoplegia is not uncommon in diabetics and, if an elderly man develops a painless sixth nerve palsy, diabetes is as likely a diagnosis as any.

Mononeuropathy may be multiple to give the striking clinical picture of 'mononeuritis multiplex', with interruption of more than one peripheral nerve trunk, otherwise seen in other disorders, such as polyarteritis nodosa or sarcoidosis.

IV. *Autonomic neuropathy*. Small afferent and efferent unmedullated fibres may be affected as early as somatic nerves, as shown by impaired sweat tests on the legs. The defect is often more obviously patchy in distribution than with somatic sensory nerves.

Table 24　Diabetic neuropathies

Type	Structure involved	Main parts affected
Radiculopathy	Nerve root	
Mononeuro-pathy	Mixed spinal or cranial nerve	Single dermatome
	Nerve terminal	Arm, leg, third and sixth cranial nerve
Polyneuropathy	? Nerve terminal ?Muscle	Feet
		Quadriceps, gluteals, hamstrings
Autonomic neuropathy	Sympathetic ganglia	Cardiovascular
		Gastrointestinal
		Bladder
		Impotence

Clinical features I. *Peripheral sensory*. Large-fibre disease is clinically demonstrable as decreased appreciation of vibration (at frequency of 128 c.p.s.). More importantly to the patient, it underlies loss of joint position sense. This may affect the toes and contribute to the 'hammer toe' deformity often seen in long-term diabetes. It is uncommon for postural loss to be severe enough to interfere with walking, but rarely it produces a pseudotabetic picture. Loss of ankle jerks even after reinforcement is an early feature of this type of neuropathy.

Loss of postural sense also contributes to the gross disorganization of the small joints of the foot in Charcot's neuroarthropathy, but loss of pain is probably even more important. Large-fibre neuropathy also contributes to numb feet, with the feeling first that the subject is walking on a bed of feathers or a thick pile of carpets, and later a total loss of appreciation of the underlying surface, so that vision becomes unusually important in walking.

Small-fibre damage causes loss of normal sensibility to pain, in stocking distribution, clinically examined by pinprick. Curiously some patients will show impairment of pain sensation with little evidence of large-fibre neuropathy, while others show the reverse, although commonly both modalities are affected. Small-fibre neuropathy probably underlies the troublesome dysaesthesiae of diabetics, which range from feelings of numbness or compression via bizarre sensations of warmth or cold to the common tingling, pricking or diffuse irritability. In a few the discomfort is excruciating and they are totally incapacitated, spending hours sitting with their feet either in bowls of cold water or raised high against a wall.

Most dysaesthesiae become more obtrusive as the patient settles for sleep or later in the night, so interfering with rest. Management consists of a combination of simple sedation or analgesia with identification of exacerbating physical factors. These probably involve an interaction between the neuropathy and the peripheral circulation. Many find relief by sleeping with their feet exposed but others are helped by bedsocks. Again, several are helped by raising the foot of the bed on blocks, while in others raising the head is more successful. There is no fixed relationship between which manoeuvre will be successful and the presence or absence of foot pulses except that an erythromelalgic picture with retained and even bounding peripheral pulses, and a reddish-blue, but often cool, foot is most likely helped by cool surroundings and elevation. It is important to prevent the patient becoming unduly attentive to the sensation. Any successful distraction may be helpful, at least in part.

One comforting aspect of the prognosis is that as the neuropathy worsens and the foot becomes more numb, so the dysaesthesiae lessen. However, the need for good care of the feet then becomes critically important; well-fitting shoes and avoidance of trauma to the feet are essential but even more important otherwise invisible parts of the foot must be inspected each evening to ensure absence of any break in the skin or consequent infection. Advice on foot care is often given to young diabetics at diagnosis only to be forgotten or disregarded by the time it is really needed.

The hands are only rarely seriously involved clinically, although, curiously, paraesthesiae of recent onset are commoner at diagnosis in the hands than the feet. Diabetics are possibly more liable than others to nocturnal or early morning tingling of the fingers but otherwise dysaesthesiae in the hands are rare apart from their vulnerability to pressure in 'entrapment' syndromes, e.g. carpal tunnel. A failure of full extension of the fingers, particularly at the metacarpophalangeal joint, is not rare after ten or more years of diabetes, and is quite separate from the increased liability to Dupuytren's contracture. While this may be due to change in collagen, it may also reflect peripheral neuropathy and an imbalance of postural muscle tone at the joint. Uncommonly diabetics may develop a painful swollen hand with discoloured clammy skin, suggestive of rheumatoid arthritis. However, the typical joint deformities are absent, while muscle wasting is more localized than the generalized involvement characteristic of rheumatoid. This lesion, although it usually involves both hands may suggest the causalgic syndrome and is presumably due to neuropathy, not least of vasomotor nerves. Sympathectomy is not a successful treatment of this or other forms of diabetic dysaesthesia, but may give temporary relief to predominantly ischaemic 'rest' pain.

Proximal motor neuropathy, typically of rapid onset, and very rare in the young type I diabetics, usually causes sudden weakness at the hip and knee of a diabetic over 50 years old, and seldom on insulin treatment. Within weeks or months the other leg is often affected, but one is usually substantially the worse. The thighs may sometimes feel uncomfortable or painful. There may or may not be accompanying peripheral sensory neuropathy. The lesion can be severe enough to prevent walking, even with a supporting frame. Rising from a chair or climbing stairs are often difficult. The one benign aspect is the excellent long-term prognosis so that within 12–24 months the patient will be walking again, albeit with one or two sticks, because a substantial but usually incomplete recovery is the rule. In the same way external ophthalmoplegia usually recovers substantially, so that one can promise loss of diplopia in 3–9 months.

The affected muscles waste and uncommonly fasciculate. The tendon jerk is lost or retained as a flicker. There is no reason to believe that forced or excessive exercise speeds recovery, but passive movement is essential to maintain health of the neighbouring joints, and some practice in voluntary effort is almost certainly a help. The lesion can make movement in bed very difficult. It is very rare for it to affect the proximal shoulder muscles and when these are involved in a diabetic it may well be a coincidence of diabetes with 'neuralgic amyotrophy'.

Diabetic mononeuropathy. The typical pressure mononeuropathies are (a) carpal tunnel, (b) lateral popliteal nerve just below the knee, (c) cervical spinal roots as they pass through the spinal foramina, and (d) the first thoracic root if a cervical rib (or corresponding fibrous structure) is present.

Autonomic neuropathy probably affects nerves anywhere in the body. It is uncertain whether it most affects the longest nerves, as do somatic sensory lesions. The degree of automatic neuropathy of vasomotor nerves, e.g. in the feet, is uncertain.

Postural hypotension is rare but dramatic with, at its worst, syncope and collapse on standing. The effect of a given degree of autonomic failure will vary with circumstances. If there has been a spell of heavy glycosuria with loss of sodium and water, the circulating blood volume may have dropped, and postural hypotension be more likely. A similar exacerbation may occur a half to two hours after subcutaneous injection of insulin, due to increased transcapillary passage of albumin, again with reduction in circulating blood volume, though by no more than 5 per cent. This is asymptomatic when autonomic function is normal. The vasodilation of hot weather or a febrile illness may exacerbate the symptoms similarly, as may the temporary disturbance caused by spinal herpes zoster. Treatment is by simple management; for example, by careful change from a lying or sitting position, on rising in the morning, e.g. by sitting on the edge of the bed and exercising the legs for a minute before standing. This is particularly necessary if patients wake at night to micturate, when they should also act to avoid associated syncope, by sitting on the lavatory during and after micturition. Glycosuric natriuresis must be avoided. 9-α-fluorohydrocortisone can expand the extracellular volume and in a minority of patients is very useful, even at the relatively low dose of 0.05 or 0.1 mg daily. More than 0.1 mg b.d. is rarely needed. Its use may be accompanied by mild ankle oedema, but it is rare for it to cause significant hypertension in the lying position, if there was not already a tendency to this. Elastic bandages to the legs or better full-length elastic stockings can be helpful, but these must be applied with caution if there is impairment of the arterial supply to the feet. In most severely affected patients use of an anti-gravity suit (G-suit) may be considered.

Diabetics may become *impotent* insidiously or suddenly through failure of the autonomic functions controlling erection. Libido is normal and there is often other evidence of autonomic neuropathy. Again, there is often accompanying somatic sensory neuropathy, but autonomic neuropathy may be present without clinical evidence. The cremasteric or bulbocavernous reflexes may be tested, and their absence certainly supports the diagnosis or organic neuropathic impotence, but their presence by no means excludes it. The differential diagnosis includes the rare Leriche's syndrome from macroangiopathy of the aortic bifurcation or the smaller arteries carrying blood to the pelvis, where impotence is accompanied by intermittent claudication, classically involving the thighs as much as the calves.

Impotence of higher central nervous origin is much commoner than organic impotence. This may stem from emotional disturbance from the diagnosis of diabetes itself, either because this has diminished self-image or because the patient has heard that the disease may produce impotence. Onset of type I diabetes of any severity may cause a temporary organic impotence because of the general weakness and catabolic state, and this may be confused with a long-term disability. Balanitis at the time of diagnosis or later may also lead to undue anxiety over erection and intercourse, not unknown too, in the husbands of diabetics with puritus vulvae. Later in the disease a temporary period of impotence, either from intercurrent disease, exacerbation of hyperglycaemia or from functional causes may be made permanent by overwhelming anxiety. Impotence occasionally arises from a fear that children may develop diabetes.

Management requires careful history both as to erections other than with the spouse, and as to possible causes of emotional upset in either the marriage or the patient. Much depends upon the attitude of the partner, and it is important that she should not confuse a temporary, or even long-lasting period of impotence with loss of affection. Marriage guidance counselling should be freely recommended, but to help clarify the situation the plasma prolactin concentration should first be determined to exclude hyperprolactinaemia as a rare cause, and other endocrine tests performed if there are suggestive features.

Nocturnal penile plethysmography records expansion of the base of the penis during sleep, as normally happens during the recurrent phases of REM (rapid eye movement) sleep. If a normal tracing is seen, this both gives good evidence of an adequate neurovascular mechanism and allows substantial reassurance, particularly by showing the tracing. As with most investigations, the more difficult clinical problems may be associated with an indeterminate result, for instance from partial erections, with expansion of the base without full erection of the shaft.

If a fixed neuropathy seems the cause, then apart from counselling on other methods of gratification, consideration may be given to artefactual erections, either by an attached inflatable rubber prosthesis or by implantation into the corpora cavernosa of silastic rods sufficiently ductile to mimic an erection. The wisdom of such manoeuvres greatly depends upon the individuals concerned, and careful understanding of their needs is essential. All too little is known as to the extent of any comparable abnormalities in female diabetics.

Diabetic diarrhoea is usually intermittent, occuring for a few days and then possibly disappearing for weeks or months, but gradually increasing in frequency as the condition worsens. The motions are typically watery with mucus and only small amounts of faecal material, but the first one or two motions of a cluster may be fairly normal. Typically, diarrhoea begins in the early morning with up to ten further motions during the day, and it often settles by evening. However, a burst of diarrhoea may begin at any time and in some there is undue frequency of defecation soon after meals. There doubtless can be an emotional contribution and sometimes the condition mimics the irritable bowel syndrome. However, there is rarely pain, but there may be abdominal distension.

Differential diagnosis includes the irritable bowel syndrome or other more serious organic causes of diarrhoea, but particularly pancreatic steatorrhoea. Diabetes may always be the presenting feature of chronic pancreatitis. Also, many patients with type I diabetes in time show deficient pancreatic exocrine function and though it is rare for this to progress severely enough to produce clinical steatorrhoea, it may cause some malabsorption

The pathogenesis may depend upon incomplete digestion in an abnormal upper alimentary tract, altered bowel flora or motor disturbance of the gut. There is no clear evidence of altered neurotransmitter production in any diabetic neuropathy but it cannot be excluded. Nor can the possibility of disturbance in gastrointestinal hormonal production and response.

Codein is the most effective treatment but this should become the main approach only if there is no good response to a five-day course of a broad-spectrum antibiotic such as neomycin, tetracycline, or a cephalosporin. If there is marked gastroparesis (see below) treatment for this should be proffered. Increased dietary bulk is usually helpful. Diabetic gastroparesis can produce at its worst a gastric stagnation almost as severe as pyloric stenosis, and can cause intermittent vomiting or a succussion splash on examination, but it is usually asymptomatic except for feelings of upper abdominal distension after meals. It probably conduces to diabetic diarrhoea from production of irritant compounds in the sluggishly moving contents of the dilated viscera. Breath hydrogen studies may indicate abnormal flora of colonic origin in the small bowel. Glucose control is erratic because the absorption rate of meals becomes unpredictable.

Sever gastroparesis has a grave prognosis with 50 per cent dead within two years if there is marked stasis on the barium meal. Treatment is either with ambostigmine 10 mg b.d. or t.d.s. a.c. or, metoclopramide; but in some patients neither helps.

Sluggish motility of the gall-bladder in long-standing diabetes may contribute to either gallstone formation or to impaired digestion. Any hint of pancreatic steatorrhoea should produce a trial of pancreatic enzymes given with meals, and sometimes this also considerably improves the hyperlgycaemic state.

Urinary retention may result from impaired urinary bladder motility. Treatment is, by trial of anticholinesterase or cholinergic agents, with only secondary consideration of surgery. This carries a risk of subsequent dribbling incontinence to set against the liability of the incontinent to chronic urinary tract infection.

Rarely, on starting a meal, a diabetic has diffuse sweating and reddening of the face and blush area (*gustatory sweating*). The sweating may be so profuse that it is both uncomfortable and embarrassing, and this condition may make a patient into a recluse. In some, particular foods, e.g. cheese, precipitate attacks.

Cardiac autonomic disturbance may occur but it is difficult to know how serious this is. ECG studies show frequent failure of the normal cardiac acceleration with deep breathing, standing, or mental arithmetic, and a plethora of manoeuvres have been used to illustrate this. Simple clinical tests include measurement of the R-R interval on an ECC during sleep, slow breathing, or determining the ratio of the R-R interval on standing to that when lying down. More severe degrees of the condition are more likely to present when there is evidence of other forms of autonomic neuropathy. A moderate resting tachycardia is presumably due to vagal neuropathy but this phenomenon is not rare in elderly non-diabetics, particularly if there is cardiomyopathy.

This condition may contribute to postural hypotension, via impaired function of cardiac and venoconstrictor fibres, as well as via those to adrenal medullary and renin-producing cells.

It is unknown whether autonomic neuropathy contributes to sudden death from cardiac dysrhythmia either independently of, or following, cardiac infarction, but there is strong circumstantial evidence that patients with marked cardioneuropathy are at risk of sudden death from cardiorespiratory arrest following anaesthesia. Such patients should therefore be watched particularly carefully in the post-anaesthetic period, with the necessary equipment for resuscitation at hand until they have regained normal alertness.

Collagen disturbance. This is a relatively recently recognized form of diabetic tissue damage. It may result from increased glycosylation of collagen, with consequent change in its physical properties. Biopsy of skin collagen has shown it to be abnormal in diabetics, and it has long been suspected that Dupuytren's contracture is more frequently found in diabetics than others. This is truer of men than women but in women (or hypogonadal males) surprisingly soft fibrous cords may be felt causing deformity of the metacarpophalangeal joints. It is uncertain whether the tendency to slight flexion of the hand seen even in quite young diabetics of several years' standing is also due to a change in collagen or is a result of muscular imbalance from sensory neuropathy. Certainly failure to press one palm completely against another, or, better, closely to oppose the palmar surfaces of the fifth digits is not uncommon in young type I diabetics. It is uncertain whether it indicates an increased liability to retinopathy.

Collagen disturbance may contribute to diabetic dermopathy, which presents mainly as trivial pigmented macules found particularly on the shins and usually regarded as the result of past trauma. These areas neither ulcerate nor cause discomfort, and may indeed be an abnormal response to old trauma. They are sometimes called 'hockey stick marks'. Secondly, there is the curious blistering that can occur in diabetics through accumulation of serous fluid in a split in the epidermis, similar to that which may occur in non-diabetics after deep coma from self-intoxication. In diabetics the blisters may be precipitated by exposure to cold or wet, but equally sometimes occur without obvious cause. The sterile fluid within them may be mildly bloodstained. The lesions are best treated conservatively, but if the blister is large, the fluid may be aspirated with a thin needle. Even then the pierced overlying skin is best left in place, at least until some repair of the base of the blister has occurred, when the overlying and then dead skin should be removed with scissors. Dressings are subsequently applied as necessary. The only indication to remove the overlying skin straightaway is an infection of the contained fluid, but this is rare.

A third type of diabetic skin lesion is necrobiosis lipoidica diabeticorum. This presents as larger painless lesions, usually on the anterior aspects of the lower leg. They are yellowish in colour, often with slightly raised edges. Rarely they become infected, and then they are slow to heal. They persist for many years, typically in type I diabetics between 15 and 40 years old. Microangiopathy is nearly always found in the underlying dermis on skin biopsy. Similar lesions may occur in non-diabetics in whom the pathogenesis is not known.

Diabetic foot disease. Different types of diabetic tissue damage interact and summate in the feet, to give a wide variety of lesions ranging from the minor dysaesthiae to fulminating infections and widespread ulceration. Ulcers of ischaemic death of tissue can occur without appreciable neuropathy, but never without some circulatory disturbance. However, this may be slight, and neuropathy and subsequent infection the prime cause of the lesion. Certainly the circulatory disturbance may be confined to small vessels distal to two palpable ankle pulses.

Infections of painless traumatic abrasions of neuropathic feet hold the best prognosis (Plate 3(c),(d)). They occur particularly with trauma to the sole, which becomes progressively infected before the patient realizes what is happening, to an extent that would be impossible if there were normal sensation. The poor eyesight of elderly diabetics may exaggerate this tendency. The spreading infection may, through local endarteritis obliterans, cause acute local vascular damage that leads to cell death and faster spread of the infection, resulting in wet gangrene. This contrasts with the dry gangrene that occurs with ischaemia of uninfected tissue (Plate 3(d)) though such dead tissue may be secondarily infected to produce a common 'wet' state. Infarction of toes may be due to thrombosis, often of the deep plantar arch or its prime branches. Less commonly it is due to an embolus, either of thrombus from the atrium of a fibrillating heart or of grumous material discharged from an arteriosclerotic ulcer of the abdominal aorta or more distal large vessel.

Another serious lesion is the Charcot neuro-arthroporotic foot, grossly distorted usually at the tarsal level, but remarkably painless, though sometimes there is discomfort as the distorted foot causes traumatic ulceration of the skin. Much more benign are the curious blisters that can form rapidly in a cleft in the epidermis, which may occur anywhere from the heel to the toe.

The rules of treatment are the same for every type of ulcer, even if different aspects become more important with some than with others. They are based on (*a*) the elimination of infection (by draining pus or removing infected bone, by removing dead tissue likely to provide a focus for infection, and by using antibiotics if necessary); and (*b*) speeding healing, by encouraging the greatest possible blood flow, and resting the foot from traumas that will interfere with healing. Treatment may be summarized as:

(i) *Debridement*. This must be thorough, extensive, and readily repeated when dealing with diabetic feet. The aim is to remove all dead tissue and any excessive healing by primary intention. Easy drainage of infection must be ensured by opening out narrow sinuses into deep-lying pus, as well as 'saucerizing' more superficial lesions. X-ray evidence of bony infection is an immediate indication for amputation of such tissue, for however successful conservative management of osteomyelitis may be in the young and healthy, antibiotics do not succeed in diabetic feet. The bony infection will always persist, to break out again later, whatever resolution of the soft-tissue infection may have occurred. It may be difficult radiologically to distinguish a vascular necrosis from early osteomyelitis, so another X-ray a few days later may be needed for certainty. There is rarely need for instant decision, and once bone is removed it cannot be replaced. The debrided tissue should be packed with ribbon gauze soaked in a solution such as half-strength Eusol-saline, and only when primary healing is well established should drier dressings be contemplated. As healing proceeds it is wise to test its integrity by gentle probing, e.g. with a throat swab. This may reveal that granulation tissue from secondary healing conceals remaining and spreading infection.

(ii) *Antibiotics*. Local antibiotic application is avoided, in general, as in time it is too liable to cause local skin sensitivity and further reduce the health of the skin already compromised by vascular and neuropathic damage. Culture of pathogens from the surface of otherwise well-healing lesions is not an indication for systematic antibiotics. However, they should be used if the infection invades surrounding tissue, and particularly if there is systemic upset, such as fever or deterioration in glucose control. The choice of agent should be guided by culture, either of the local lesion or of blood when infection is widespread. If a staphylococcus has been found, then it is best to prescribe both cloxacillin and fucidic acid, as the latter seems useful in preventing emergence of resistant strains of staphylococci. Often a more broad-based antibiotic may be required, such as one of the cephalosporins or amoxycillin. The most difficult organisms to treat are *Pseudomonas* or *Proteus*, and their elimination usually depends upon successful local therapy, which may include antiseptics such as iodine soaks, or acriflavin. If there is excessive granulation tissue, and while awaiting debridement, lotions such as acerbin may help. Care should be taken to prevent the lesion becoming either too dry or excessively wet from unduly wet dressings.

(iii) *Pain relief*. This should be effective and repeated, as pain is vasoconstrictive.

(iv) *Adequate rest*. The use of this in healing is long established and has been well defended.

(v) *Assessment of vascular supply*. Before any substantial amputation of tissue, vascular repair to improve the blood supply should be considered. This does not apply if at least one of the two ankle pulses is palpable, and as yet vascular surgery does not tackle blocks distal to the arterial trifurcation just below the knee. Hence, a palpable popliteal artery also contra-indicates likely successful vascular repair, though this may well change in the coming years. With evidence of higher obstruction, assessment by Doppler measurements or angiography should always be considered. In perhaps 10–15 per cent of patients likely to undergo a mid-tarsal or more severe amputation, there may be a substantial obstruction local enough for worthwhile vascular surgery. The disappointment is that often lesions in the diabetic iliac and more distal arteries are so widespread that they are beyond the scope of effective vascular surgery.

(vi) *Smoking*. The patient should not smoke, because of its ill effects on the peripheral circulation.

(vii) *Glycaemic control*. The control of glucose levels should be as strict as possible, and certainly blood glucose levels above 15 mM should be avoided, as this impairs the functions of the leucocytes, both polymorphonuclear and mononuclear. Good glucose control should never be achieved by excessive restriction of food intake in someone with tissues to heal and an infection to combat. Insulin will often be required in those not previously receiving it, even if only for a few weeks while the lesion heals. The anabolic effect of the insulin may well be an advantage, but there is no evidence that it is helpful as a local dressing.

The indications for amputation are: (i) *Life threatening infection*. This is now rare because of antibiotics, but is still occasionally necessary, particularly if there is surgical crepitus or gas within the tissues on X-ray, indicating a gas-forming organism. The three likely to be found are (*a*) anaerobic streptococci, (*b*) gas-forming coliforms, and (*c*) clostridia. With all there must be extensive debridement to allow good access of aerial oxygen to the tissues; effective antibiotics are required certainly including penicillins for the first and third organisms, and clostridial antitoxin if it should be considered that organism is the culprit.

(ii) *Removal of dead tissue.* The only exception is in the very ill or very old when, if a single toe has undergone dry gangrene, it may be best to leave it to wither and slowly separate spontaneously, when the bare area exposed to possible infection will be much smaller than after surgery. This indication includes removal of osteomyelitic bone.

(iii) *Intractable pain.* This is rarely a problem with infections, but sometimes results from dry gangrene, or severe ischaemia short of that.

(iv) *Social reasons.* These range from inability of a wage-earner to spend the long period of rest necessary for conservative management, to undue boredom and deterioration of personality in an old person excessively confined, whether in hospital or the home, through the immobility necessary to attempt healing.

Nibbling amputations should be avoided wherever possible. The strain of successive anaesthetics in an elderly and infected patient may be lethal, as removal of a toe is followed successively by amputation of a metatarsal, a mid-tarsal operation, and finally a below-knee amputation. It is much better to go to the latter first, if it really seems likely that things will end so.

While amputation is under consideration, care should be taken that the blood supply to the foot is of as good quality as possible, as well as maximizing its quantity. Thus, anaemia should be treated; if necessary by a transfusion of packed cells. Again, oedema is inimical to healing, so heart failure should be treated, if present, and the limb elevated to reduce the swelling. Such elevation, however, must not be excessive if there is real limitation of the arterial supply.

It may not be in the patient's best interest to choose definitely between perfect healing by long drawn-out conservative measures on the one hand and a major amputation on the other. The patient may be more mobile and happier to return home with a low-grade infection discharging via a sinus, even with the realization that this may persist for months if not years. Much depends upon the required degree of activity and general prognosis. Occasionally such a 'draw' between the host and the organisms may be best, even where there is osteomyelitis, perhaps particularly of the calcaneum, because removal of even the posterior third of that bone rarely eradicates infection, even when on X-ray this seems confined to the posterior margin. A low-grade infection controlled by long-term antibiotics may seem preferable to the patient to amputation at knee level.

Special problems

Pregnancy (see Section 11)
Infection. Poorly controlled diabetics are particularly prone to develop bacterial or fungal infections. Indeed one of the classical presentations of diabetes is with recurrent infections, such as boils or abscesses or fungal infections such as candida; and more than half of the cases of ketoacidosis in known diabetics are precipitated by infection. In the 1920s 20 per cent of deaths in diabetics were due to infection; with the development of chemotherapy and antibiotics this figure had already dropped to 5 per cent by the 1960s. There are three aspects of the problem: first, the effect of infection on metabolism; secondly, the increased liability to serious infections in poorly controlled diabetics; and thirdly, those infections which occur with much increased frequency in diabetics, and might almost be termed diabetes-specific.

Metabolic effects of infection. Infections, particularly bacterial, lead to a clearly defined stress response, marked particularly by increased ACTH (and cortisol) and glucagon secretion. There is

also activation of the adrenergic system with increased secretion of catecholamines. These effects combine to produce hyperglycaemia and, in the absence of normal insulin response to both hyperglycaemia and reticuloendothelial system activity, increased ketogenesis. In the type II diabetic there may be a need temporarily for exogenous insulin, and in the type I diabetic insulin requirements may rise dramatically. Infected patients often stop eating and may mistakenly be advised to, or spontaneously, decrease their insulin, though at least as much or even more insulin is usually needed. Home glucose monitoring, either of blood or urine, can be used to guide insulin therapy during such illness. Patients (and general practitioners) should receive clear appropriate instructions for the action to be taken, particularly in type I diabetics, in such situations.

The two basic principles are, first, that even when no food is being taken (e.g. in a vomiting illness) the daily dose of insulin is likely to be very much as usual; and, secondly, that if the diabetic is too ill to do his own urine or blood tests it is more important than ever that they are done by someone else. Every effort should be made to maintain a reasonable calorie intake, if necessary purely as liquids, e.g. lemon squash with 20 g of sucrose, glucose, or honey every 2 h, or Ribena or Lucozade, or milk with added sucrose. If food intake is likely to be erratic it may be easier to rely upon several injections a day of quick-acting soluble insulins, but this is to deny the increase in the basal, 'round-the-clock' insulin requirement. Those on Ultratard and Actrapid should increase the Ultratard dose by some 20 per cent and decrease the Actrapid by about the same number of units (initially), but divide this between three injections instead of the usual one or two. Patients on twice-daily mixtures of medium and short-acting insulins may do well to move 10 per cent of their medium morning insulin to the evening injection and split their total quick-acting dose into three, as with the Ultralente patients. Glucose testing will then indicate whether small adjustments, up or down, are necessary in the total daily dose. As the infection clears, insulin doses will probably need reduction once satisfactory glucose levels are seen, for otherwise they are likely to suffer hypoglycaemia.

Host defences against infection in diabetes. In normal man the response to infection is complex, including immunological responses as well as the mobilization and action of phagocytic cells, particularly polymorphonuclear leucocytes (PMN). The four steps in the normal functioning of PMN are: chemotaxis in response to bacterial products; adherence of the PMN to endothelium at the site of invasion; phagocytosis involving opsonins; and microbicidal activity. Components of the complement system are involved in the first three steps.

Chemotaxis and phagocytosis have long been known to be defective in hyperglycaemic as well as ketotic diabetics, whilst more recently it has been shown that PMN microbicidal activity may also be impaired. On the other hand there is no evidence to suggest any defect in the response to infection in well-controlled diabetics. Similarly no defect has been found in the complement system or in opsonin production and function even in ketoacidotic diabetics. This suggests strongly that intrinsic properties of the PMN are altered and function is impaired by poor diabetic control. Abnormalities are consistently found when fasting blood glucose levels exceed 10 mmol/l.

It is probable that the abnormalities are secondary to impaired energy metabolism in the PMN. Sustained energy production is required for normal PMN function. The PMN is freely permeable to glucose but thereafter there are several insulin-dependent steps including glucose phosphorylation, glycogen synthesis, and pyruvate formation. Diabetic granulocytes have diminished glycogen content which proves critical in limiting energy production when activity is required. Many *in vitro* studies show that high glucose levels and acidaemia impair PMN function, in addition to the obvious defects found in PMN taken from hyperglycaemic patients.

There is thus good *in vivo* and *in vitro* evidence for impaired host resistance to infection in the poorly controlled diabetic. This should be taken as a strong indication for rigorous glycaemic control in any diabetic patient with an infection.

Specific infections in diabetes. Some of the proven and suggested infections associated with diabetes are shown in Table 25. The commonest are urinary tract infections, particularly in females. The prevalence of bacteriuria has been found three times higher in diabetic than non-diabetic women. Poor control was not the only factor: for instance, abnormal bladder function from autonomic neuropathy can be another major factor. Pyelonephritis, perinephric abscesses, and papillary necrosis are also associated with diabetes, particularly when there has been poor glycaemic control.

For many years there has been a presumptive association between tuberculosis and diabetes mellitus. Again the incidence has been said to be greater in poorly controlled diabetics. Prior to good antituberculous therapy and the emphasis on good control of diabetes, 5 per cent of diabetic deaths were due to tuberculosis and the combined diagnosis was almost invariably fatal. One underlying factor may be impaired metabolism of the lymphocyte which is found in poorly controlled diabetes. Other pulmonary infections are shown in Table 25.

Table 25 Infections associated with diabetes mellitus

Urinary tract infections (females):* cystitis, pyelonephritis, perinephric abscess*, acute papillary necrosis*, fungal UTI*, emphysematous pyelonephritis*
Mucocutaneous candidiasis
Furunculosis (staphylococcus)
Gram-negative pneumonia*, staphylococcal pneumonia
Tuberculosis*
Foot-ulcer related infections*
Cryptococcosis, histoplasmosis, blastomycosis, coccidioidomycosis
Rhinocerebral mucormycosis*, malignant otitis externa*
Emphysematous cholecystitis*
Influenza*

*Proven association. The rest are possible or suggested associations.

Fungal infections are also commonly associated with poorly controlled diabetes. *Candida albicans* is the commonest agent, particularly in females who present with vaginal or vulval moniliasis. Candidial infections of the bladder and skin are also found. Other fungal infections are rarer but can be catastrophic, as with rhinocerebral mucormycosis. Most of the fungal infections are directly related to both impaired host defences and increased fungal growth in high-glucose media.

Cutaneous infections are commoner in poorly controlled diabetics than in either non-diabetics or well-controlled diabetics. Staphylococcal infections are the commonest, but respond well to therapy if the diabetes is brought under control. The rare but severe malignant otitis externa due to *Pseudomonas aeruginosa* should probably be included in this group.

Infected foot lesions are only too common in diabetes. These are due not only to poor control, but also impaired circulation. They may lead to local osteomyelitis and often require surgical debridement to allow adequate healing.

Treatment. In most cases, infections in diabetics respond to standard therapy providing that the glucose levels are simultaneously brought under good control. As glycaemic control is often poor because of the infection, type II diabetics may need to be treated with insulin for a period, possibly of several months with chronic infections such as foot ulcers or tuberculosis. Type I diabetics will generally require increased doses of insulin. Infections which respond less well to therapy are those in which there are added complicating factors, such as bladder dysfunction with some urinary tract infections or circulatory impairment with foot ulcers.

In many of these cases, however, effective preventative medicine can be practised.

Special problems

Anaesthesia and surgery. A diabetic has a one in two risk of requiring surgery any time after diagnosis. Though there are no recent comprehensive figures there is probably both increased morbidity and mortality compared with non-diabetics. Many of the diabetics are older, of type II, and have increased cardiovascular disease, which will increase per- and postoperative morbidity; similarly many are obese, which also carries a less favourable prognosis for surgery. Neurological impairment, particularly autonomic neuropathy, also adds to morbidity. This suggests particular care with both elective and emergency surgery. Although many of the factors cannot be modified it is possible to avoid metabolic disaster by clear knowledge of the usual metabolic response to surgery and its control with insulin. There is need for straightforward therapeutic guidelines. Examples are outlined below.

Metabolic response to anaesthesia and surgery. Anaesthesia provokes a stress response. This was greater with the older anaesthetics such as ether, but even with modern inhalational anaesthetics there is in general an increase in ACTH, and hence cortisol, and also catecholamine secretion (although halothane does not increase catecholamines). These effects are only avoided by spinal anaesthesia. There will therefore be an initial decrease in insulin secretion (in those patients with endogenous insulin secretion) and an increase in insulin resistance. These effects are small, however, when compared with the stress of surgery itself.

Surgery has long been known to cause a major catabolic response. There is an immediate neuroendocrine response with release of ACTH, cortisol, catecholamines, and growth hormone. Noradrenaline increases, particularly peroperatively, with adrenaline rising later. Glucagon secretion also increases, primarily as a result of the rise in noradrenaline secretion. Insulin levels may fall due to inhibition by catecholamines and other factors, with a loss of responsiveness to glucose. Hyperglycaemia is the end result of these endocrine changes, with the rise in blood glucose proportional to the severity of surgery. This is primarily due to increased gluconeogenesis. During and after surgery the mobilization of lipid fuels is less than would be expected, particularly in fasting patients. This is probably because postoperatively insulin levels rise in response to the hyperglycaemia and suppress lipolysis, despite levels inadequate to control the hyperglycaemia. There is then dependency on glucose for oxidative metabolism, and there is increased utilization of amino acid for gluconeogensis. The increase in cortisol also increases protein catabolism, which is the main cause of postoperative morbidity in the non-diabetic.

These changes will be exaggerated in the non-insulin-treated (type II) diabetic, where insulin secretion is already compromised and insulin resistance is present. Thus severe hyperglycaemia and increased protein losses are likely. In the untreated type I diabetic the increases in cortisol, catecholamines, glucagon, and growth hormone will lead to severe hyperglycaemia and ketoacidosis, as well as disturbances of electrolyte metabolism and large-scale protein losses. Hyperosmolarity will also ensue. The rise in blood glucose levels may not be very large if glucose solutions are not infused, but this may just mask impending severe ketoacidosis (see below).

Aims of treatment during surgery of the diabetic. The main aim of therapy is to avoid excess mortality and morbidity. More specifically hypoglycaemia, excessive hyperglycaemia and protein catabolism, and electrolyte disturbances are to be avoided. There is no need to achieve absolute normoglycaemia, but the patient should be given adequate insulin which is essential for adequate healing and response to infection. Regimens should be designed which are robust in use, because they are simple to follow and have a large margin of safety.

Surgical management of type I (insulin-dependent) diabetics. All elective surgery requiring general anaesthesia, be it minor or major, may be managed in a similar fashion in insulin-treated patients, with few exceptions. A guideline to pre-, per-, and postoperative management is shown in Table 26.

Table 26   The management of type I (insulin-dependent) diabetics during surgery

A. Preoperative
1. Admit to hospital 2–3 days before operation
2. Stop long-acting insulins and stabilize on *either* twice daily short- and intermediate-acting insulins *or* thrice daily short-acting insulin with intermediate insulin in the evening
3. Monitor blood glucose (bedside methods) before and after each main meal and at bedtime
4. Aim to maintain fasting blood glucose <8 mmol/1, and other values between 4 and 10 mmol/1
5. Check urea; electrolytes; and renal, cardiovascular, and neurological systems

B. Peroperative
1. Schedule operation for early in day
2. Check fasting glucose. If >10 mmol/1, delay operation
3. Omit morning insulin and breakfast
4. Start infusion of glucose–insulin–potassium (see Table 27), as early as possible and at least one hour preoperatively
5. If operation delayed more than 2 h from onset of infusion, recheck blood glucose; adjust infusion if necessary
6. Recheck blood glucose at end of operation (and during lengthy operations). Modify regimen if necessary
7. Check K^+

C. Postoperative
1. Check glucose 2–4 hourly, and K^+ six-hourly then b.d.
2. Continue infusion until first meal. Restart s.c. insulin at preoperative dose 1 h before infusion stopped
3. Consider total parenteral nutrition if oral refeeding not recommenced within 48 h

For major procedures particularly patients should be admitted to hospital two or three days preoperatively. This allows full assessment and facilitates good glycaemic control. Long-acting insulins should be stopped and the patient stabilized on twice daily mixtures of short- and intermediate-acting insulins; alternatively a thrice daily regimen can be used if glycaemic control is initially very poor. Blood glucose should be monitored frequently at the bedside (using test-strips with or without meters, Table 21) so that dose adjustments can be made rapidly.

The anaesthetist should be contacted and details of peroperative management agreed. On the morning of operation insulin and food should be omitted regardless of the time of operation, and blood taken for bedside glucose analysis, and laboratory potassium measurement. The operation should, whenever possible, be scheduled for early in the day. An intravenous infusion of glucose, insulin, and potassium should be begun (Table 27). If the operation is delayed for more than two hours blood glucose should again be measured and the insulin content of the infusate adjusted accordingly (Table 27). If blood glucose level is high (<13 mmol/l) the operation should be postponed or at least delayed until late in the day. During lengthy operations (>1½ hours) a further blood glucose should again be measured in theatre, and it should always be checked in the recovery room. These measurements can well be made with test-strips, which give immediate results, and prevent undue strain on the laboratory.

Postoperatively plasma potassium should be re-checked, and blood glucose measured by test-strip two to four hourly, with appropriate changes in the infusion regimen. In practice few

changes are necessary if the defined aim is to maintain blood glucose between 5 and 10 mmol/l. The infusion should be continued until the first meal is taken, when the preoperative subcutaneous insulin regimen may be reinstituted. The s.c. insulin should be given at least one hour before the infusion is discontinued, owing to the relatively slow absorption of s.c. insulin and the rapid decay of plasma insulin once i.v. infusion is stopped.

Table 27   Insulin infusion regimen for per- and postoperative management of diabetes during surgery

1. Add 16 units short-acting insulin (soluble, Actrapid) + 10 mmol KCl to 500 ml 10% glucose (dextrose)
2. Run 25–50 ml through infusion tubing before attaching to patient
3. Infuse at 100 ml/h
   If there is need to limit fluids, use double amounts of insulin and KCl in 20% glucose and infuse at 50 ml/h

If blood glucose >10 mmol/l increase insulin by 4 units/500 ml; check blood glucose 2 h later; increase by further 4 unit increments as necessary. If blood glucose <5 mmol/l decrease insulin by 6 units/ 500 ml; check blood glucose 2 h later; decrease by further 4 unit decrements as necessary.

There are several ways in which the insulin can be given. The safest is to put the insulin directly into the bag or bottle of dextrose (glucose). In this case variations in infusion rate will effect all components equally, and hypoglycaemic or hyperglycaemic disasters are less likely. Some advocate insulin administration via a pump, because absorptive problems are less from concentrated solutions of insulin, but in practice, this is not a problem with combined glucose–insulin infusions.

Several situations are associated with insulin resistance, and so increased insulin requirement per gram of glucose. These are predictable and listed in Table 28, together with approximate insulin requirements. The most severe insulin resistance is found during and following cardiopulmonary bypass surgery. In this case, the standard glucose–insulin–potassium infusion should be used preoperatively, but the insulin alone should be infused during surgery when as much as 20 units per hour may be needed. A combined glucose–insulin infusion should be restarted at the end of the operation, but insulin requirements will continue high for the next 24 h.

Table 28   Insulin requirements during surgery in insulin-resistant states

	i.v. insulin requirement	
	units/g glucose	units/500 ml 10% glucose
1. Normal	0.32	16
2. Obesity	0.4–0.6	20–30
3. Liver disease	0.5–0.6	25–30
4. Severe infection	0.5–0.8	25–40
5. Steroid therapy	0.5–0.8	25–40
6. Cardiopulmonary bypass	0.8–1.2	40–60

Other infusions are often required during surgery; these should be infused through separate lines, in amounts dictated by clinical need. If too much fluid is being given with the glucose–insulin–potassium then half the volume of 20 per cent dextrose can be used in place of 10 per cent dextrose.

Some authorities prefer subcutaneous to intravenous insulin in the surgical management of type I diabetics. One regimen is to give the usual s.c. short- and intermediate-acting insulins morning and evening. The usual oral carbohydrate intake is then substituted with an equivalent amount of i.v. glucose given as 5 or 10 per cent dextrose. Thus if 50 g carbohydrate is normally consumed at breakfast and the midmorning snack, 500 ml of 10 per cent glucose is given between 8 a.m. and noon. Blood glucose is monitored as for the i.v. regimen, and if blood glucose equals or exceeds 20 mmol/l additional i.m. insulin (6–20 units) is given two hourly until the blood glucose <12 mmol/l. The regimen is continued until the patient is eating normally again. This is a reasonable alternative but is more complex than the totally intravenous regimen, depends on adequate subcutaneous perfusion and requires more care and attention on the parts of the anaesthetist, surgeon, and physician.

One further problem concerns day admission for minor procedures. This should not be encouraged for type I diabetics, but may be tolerated because of lack of beds. There are two approaches. In both cases patients should come to the hospital early in the day, omitting their usual insulin and breakfast. Blood glucose should then be checked. If it is less than 13 mmol/l the patient can go immediately to theatre, have the procedure, then return to the day ward and be given insulin plus breakfast as usual. Blood glucose should be checked once more and the patient can return home in the late afternoon. If the procedure becomes a lengthy one a glucose–insulin–potassium intravenous infusion should be commenced. The alternative is to start an infusion on admission, and this will apply also to all patients with FBG ⩾13 mmol/l. The infusion is then continued until the first meal (i.e. lunch) when short-acting insulin is given, and usual therapy reinstituted with the evening meal, after which the patient may return home. It must be stressed that it is always more satisfactory to have the patient in hospital both pre- and postoperatively.

Surgical management in type II diabetics (Table 29). The general principles of management are as for type I diabetics. However, treatment is simpler for well-controlled patients undergoing minor procedures.

Table 29 The management of type II diabetes during surgery

A. Minor operations	
Diet-treated	If FBG ⩽ 8 mmol/l treat as non-diabetic
	If FBG >8 mmol/l treat with insulin infusion regimen during operation
Oral agent treated	1. Stop biguanides and long-acting sulphonylureas 2–3 days preoperatively. Stabilize on diet alone or short-acting sulphonylureas
	2. If FBG ⩽ 8 mmol/l on day of operation treat as non-diabetic. If FBG >8 mmol/l treat with insulin infusion regimen during operation
B. Major operations	
Diet-treated	1. If FBG ⩽ 7 mmol/l, treat as type I diabetic on day of surgery
	2. If FBG >7 mmol/l stabilize on short-acting insulin t.i.d. for two days preoperatively. Treat as type I diabetic on day of surgery
Oral agent treated	1. Stop all oral agents 2–3 days preoperatively
	2. Stabilize on t.i.d. short-acting insulin
	3. Treat as type I diabetic on day of surgery
C. Postoperative management	
	1. *Minor surgery*: recommence usual therapy with first meal
	2. *Major surgery*: convert to t.i.d. s.c. insulin with first oral feeding. Recommence oral agent or diet-alone therapy 24–48 hours later

In diet-treated patients who are well controlled (fasting blood glucose concentration <8 mmol/l) the patient may be treated as a non-diabetic. Similarly in well-controlled patients taking short-acting oral hypoglycaemic agents, therapy should be omitted on the day of operation and the patient treated as a non-diabetic. Oral therapy should then be reinstituted, if necessary, with feeding.

In general, particularly for major procedures, biguanides and long-acting sulphonylureas should be stopped a minimum of three days before surgery and the patient restabilized on short-acting sulphonylureas. Patients undergoing minor surgery who are poorly controlled should be treated like type I diabetics, i.e. with a glucose–insulin–potassium infusion on the day of surgery. The infusion can be stopped at the time of the first meal and sulphonylurea therapy recommended.

Patients undergoing major surgery can be left on sulphonylurea therapy if fasting glucose is less than 7 mmol/l, until the morning of surgery, when sulphonylureas should be omitted and infusion therapy commenced as for type I diabetics. If patients are poorly controlled preoperatively (fasting glucose levels >7 mmol/l; interval blood glucoses >10 mmol/l), they should be stabilized on insulin, best given as highly purified porcine short-acting insulin before each meal. They should then be treated as type I diabetics preoperatively.

Blood glucose monitoring both pre- and postoperatively should be two to four hourly, as for type I diabetics. After major surgery, when refeeding begins, it is probably safest to use t.i.d. insulin therapy for one or two days before attempting reconversion to sulphonylureas or therapy with diet alone. It is in these patients that there is particular risk of cardiovascular illness and meticulous attention should be paid to potassium and fluid balance, and myocardial function.

Emergency surgery in diabetes. Diabetics are as likely as non-diabetics to require surgery: 2–5 per cent of operations in diabetics fall into this category, with infection the main cause. In nearly all there is some metabolic decompensation, with frank ketoacidosis in some cases. The trap of apparent abdominal emergencies in younger patients must be emphasized (see page 9.44), with abdominal pain consequent on the ketoacidosis and disappearing rapidly with rehydration and insulin therapy. One important guide is that if vomiting precedes abdominal pain, the latter is more likely to be due to ketoacidosis, whilst the converse also holds true.

The first priority is to assess glycaemic and acid/base status. While results are awaited a saline infusion should be started and nasogastric suction applied where appropriate. If moderate or severe ketoacidosis is confirmed, operation should be delayed if at all possible for 4–5 h whilst standard rehydration and ketoacidosis therapy is applied (see below). After reasonable metabolic correction has been achieved, surgery can be performed safely using the glucose–insulin–potassium regimen. Similarly with less severe hypoglycaemia and ketosis the glucose–insulin infusion can be used throughout. In all such cases hourly blood glucose monitoring is desirable. It must be stressed that both metabolic decomposition and infection will cause insulin resistance and a higher insulin infusion rate will be required (0.5–0.8 units/g glucose compared with the usual 0.3 units/g). If extra fluids are required these should be given through a separate line. Good glycaemic control should be sought postoperatively to aid healing, particularly if infection was a precipitating factor.

'Brittle' diabetes. A small proportion of type I diabetics are unstable and difficult to control. These are referred to variously as 'labile' or 'brittle'. The terms are used loosely, and indeed some paediatricians claim that all children with diabetes are 'brittle'. In practice, 5 per cent of diabetics at most fall into this category. A useful working definition of a brittle diabetic is a 'patient whose life is constantly disrupted by episodes of hypoglycaemia or hyperglycaemia, whatever their cause' (Tattersall 1977). Such patients have frequent admissions to hospital for hypoglycaemia or ketoacidosis, and one or two such patients can provide a significant proportion of the total workload of a diabetic unit.

Broadly, the causes of brittle diabetes fall into four main groups. These are: therapeutic errors, intercurrent illness, emotional causes, and brittle diabetes of unknown aetiology.

The commonest causes are therapeutic errors either on the part of the physician or the patient. Inappropriate insulin therapy can create unstable diabetes. Thus, attempts to achieve morning normoglycaemia in a totally insulin-deficient patient by once-daily therapy can cause repeated severe hypoglycaemia in the late afternoon. Similarly, nocturnal hypoglycaemia can be produced by over-enthusiastic increases in intermediate insulin in the late afternoon. The rare so-called Somoygi phenomenon fits into this category. This occurs when an undetected period of hypoglycaemia (e.g. during the night) triggers a counter-regulatory response, with subsequent hyperglycaemia, glycosuria, and ketonuria. These latter findings suggest insulin lack, so that the insulin may easily be increased, thereby worsening the situation. Proof comes when a *decrease* in insulin dose improves control. The existence of this phenomenon has been questioned, but it is a clinical entity, although rare, and not easy to prove. Improper or imperfect dietary advice can also result in wide day-to-day glycaemic fluctuations. Equally, the patient can 'generate' the brittle state by erratic insulin dosage, erratic exercise, and total lack of dietary compliance.

The second main cause of brittle diabetes is intercurrent illness. This can be subdivided broadly into infections, endocrine disorders, and pancreatic disease. The most common occult infective cause is tuberculosis, generally 'atypical', but other infections can have equally severe effects on diabetic stability. The brittle diabetes always resolves with cure of the infection. Endocrine causes include hyperthyroidism, Addison's disease, and hypopituitarism. Again, treatment resolves the diabetic problem. Amongst pancreatic causes are pancreatectomy, which is predictable and due to lack of pancreatic glucagon, and chronic pancreatitis, which is a not uncommon cause and may present insidiously.

The third and fourth groups of causes may well be linked. Home disturbances and family conflict may cause glycaemic instability. It is not certain how much of this is due to a neuroendocrine disturbance of metabolism and how much to manipulative behaviour. Whatever the cause, this type of brittle diabetes is not uncommon in adolescence, may disappear spontaneously when the psychosocial problems resolve, or may occasionally respond dramatically to psychotherapy or family group therapy. The liability to premenstrual hyperglycaemia, most marked in adolescence and, indeed, sometimes episodic before menarche, could be allocated anywhere among the last three groups.

The fourth group, i.e. those of unproven aetiology, is the most difficult to deal with. We would estimate a prevalence of 1 per 1000 type I diabetics in the United Kingdom. It is perhaps not as heterogeneous a group as originally thought. The majority of such patients are female, between the ages of 14 and 26, with onset soon after menarche. They are all mildly overweight, which may be secondary to overeating in response to intermittent hypoglycaemia. Their brittle state is reflected, however, more in recurrent ketoacidosis. The majority require large doses of insulin s.c. with considerable day-to-day variations in requirement. Many, indeed, have impaired subcutaneous insulin absorption, which is often an intermittent defect. They respond well to intravenous insulin, but still have slightly higher than normal i.v. insulin requirements. They also show persistent metabolic abnormalities which are consistent with adrenergic overactivity, although circulating catecholamine levels are normal. They show an accelerated response to insulin withdrawal. Few psychiatric abnormalities have been found and, although there is often a disturbed home background, psychotherapy or improvement in the background may not improve glycaemic control. As yet, no good long-term treatment has been discovered, apart from chronic intramuscular insulin therapy, which is technically difficult, and chronic intravenous insulin infusion, with considerable risks of septicaemia. However, with home monitoring and rigorous self-management, many can at least limit the number of hospital admissions. The real nature of this severely brittle form of diabetes remains elusive.

Adolescence. There are probably only two features of diabetes particular to adolescence. Otherwise, the problems are no more than an intensification of many factors that contribute to unstable diabetes at any age: unusually large daily variations in energy output and routine, especially in the nature and timing of meals, with a generally increased inner emotional (and so hormonal and neutral) turmoil. Much of this expresses the difficulties in self-discipline of this age group, as they seek self-determination.

One of the particular problems is that of a minority of girls around menarche. Either during the first few menstrual cycles, or at approximately monthly intervals before these have begun (negating a total explanation through emotional 'shock' at menstruation), rapid deterioration in glycaemic control may occur, sometimes even into ketoacidosis. So far no convincing hormonal explanation has been forthcoming, nor has the absorbability of subcutaneously injected insulin at these times been examined. It remains a clinically important, but usually relatively short-lived conundrum. Prescription of oral contraceptives (low oestrogen) for a few months sometimes helps rapid response to incipient loss of control with extra insulin is also very important.

The other special problem is that posed by cessation of growth in height. If the large energy intake necessary for growth continues after it, a correspondingly large dose of insulin may become customary. This then sustains the food intake at a time when it would have fallen in the healthy, self-regulating adolescent. Obesity then develops and a conflict of interests and guilt may develop if good advice is not given as to coincident reduction of food intake and insulin dose.

Coma in diabetics

Comas in diabetics may be grouped as in Table 30.

Table 30   Coma in diabetics

---

1. Abnormal glycaemia
   (a) Hypoglycaemic
   (b) Hyperglycaemic: (i) ketoacidotic (ii) non-ketoacidotic
2. Other metabolic, consequent upon the diabetic state
   (a) Uraemic coma, with or without glycaemic upset
   (b) Lactic acidosis, with or without glycaemic upset
   (c) Alcoholic coma, with possible upset in 'ketones', lactate, or glucose
3. Non-metabolic coma
      e.g. subarachnoid haemorrhage

Hypoglycaemia. Hypoglycaemia in diabetics is rare except in those treated with insulin. Symptomatic hypoglycaemia is well recognized, although relatively uncommon, in those treated with sulphonylureas. True coma is uncommon except when there is some synergistic action between the sulphonylureas and another agent (e.g. monoamine oxidase inhibitors), or when a long-acting sulphonylurea accumulates, e.g. gross chlorpropamide overdosage, or in a newborn baby whose diabetic mother has been unwisely treated with chlorpropamide.

Usually there are three important points in the history, should this be available from a friend or bystander: (*a*) the patient is a known diabetic, probably on insulin; (*b*) the patient was in normal health as little as 15 or 30 min before the onset of the stupor; and (*c*) there may have been a phase of typical symptomatic hypoglycaemia or of abnormal behaviour. This third phase is not a constant feature, as hypoglycaemia may occur with remarkable rapidity, particularly when the patient is no longer aware of any premonitary symptom. This is more likely the longer a patient has been on insulin treatment and may be because of developing autonomic neuropathy, with failure to secret catecholamines normally.

On examination of the stuporose or comatose patient, the diagnostically important points in the known diabetic are negative ones: namely, that the patient is not dehydrated, nor hyperventilating, nor ketotic. The most important positive evidence is of insulin injection sites, whether from needle marks or local change in subcutaneous fat. There may be non-specific helpful physical signs, such as symmetrically dilated pupils, which react normally to light, and tachycardia, but a drenching sweat is often the most useful sign. The body temperature tends to be low. The condition clearly has to be distinguished from non-metabolic comas; the neck is not stiff, but the plantar reflexes may be upgoing. A rapid assessment of the blood glucose (by bedside glucose oxidase sticks) is essential in any undiagnosed comatose patient.

Hypoglycaemic episodes are more likely to occur several hours after the last meal or after unusual physical exertion without compensating intake of extra food, but attacks do not always occur classically. Sometimes they happen inexplicably within one to two hours of an insulin injection, and it is probable that occasionally subcutaneous insulin is absorbed more rapidly than usual into the circulation, perhaps through damage to local blood vessels at the time of injection.

Self-willed insulin overdosage must always be remembered as a further possibility, as must simple errors in the preparation of the insulin injections, or confusion between 'units' and 'marks' of insulin when others take on responsibility for the injection, as in hospital.

Symptoms. Each individual usually maintains a fairly constant pattern in the evolution and occurrence of the many possible symptoms of hypoglycaemia. They may be divided into two categories: one is consequent on neuroglycopaenia, with defective function of the central nervous system. It includes visual blurring, a feeling of uncertainty as to what is happening and then increasing ignorance of this, intense hunger, and a throbbing headache. The second group probably stems from increased catecholamine release as a counter-regulation against impending hypoglycaemia. It includes palpitation, paraesthesiae in the fingers or lips, a feeling of impending doom, a fine muscular tremor and excessive sweating, which is due to cholinergic fibres, albeit of the sympathetic system.

Onlookers may note increasing pallor, as well as curious mannerisms such as stroking the back of the head or yawning. Some patients wake during the night feeling unduly warm when mildly hypoglycaemic. As hypoglycaemia develops, diabetics are very likely to resist advice to take sugar from onlookers who feel the patient is becoming 'hypo' and great firmness may be needed by relatives or friends to achieve intake of quickly absorbed carbohydrate by the patient.

Treatment. Prevention is better than cure. It is easy for a diabetic to take some oral sucrose or glucose, in solid or liquid form, at a time when there are early symptoms or signs of hypoglycaemia, but once the mental state has altered significantly this may be difficult. It is vital, though, that no quantity of fluid be put into the mouth of a patient so comatose that he cannot swallow properly. In that state medical help is urgently required so that an i.v. injection of concentrated glucose solution is given, usually 20 ml of 50 per cent glucose initially. Only when arrangements for this are under way, e.g. by telephone, should other means be considered, e.g. intramuscular glucagon (1 mg) which can be injected by relatives. This may increase the blood glucose sufficiently to allow oral glucose to be given. However, there are some patients in whom it does not help, and many in whom it is much less effective than i.v. glucose.

After i.v. glucose the patient commonly opens his eyes, and takes notice within 90 s, but then often lapses back into stupor or sleep. If there has been no substantial response at all to the first injection within 5 min, a further intravenous injection of 30 ml of 50 per cent glucose should be given. There is no point in further increasing the dose but if again the patient has not responded a continuous intravenous infusion of 5 per cent glucose in water (or 4 per cent glucose in saline) should be started. The blood glucose should be checked by glucose oxidase strips and confirmed in the laboratory.

If the patient has not returned to near normal consciousness, even if sleepy and somewhat vague, within an hour further treatment should be considered. There is no objective evidence that high-dose glucocorticoid treatment, or any other measure against cerebral oedema, is beneficial but equally none that they do harm, though the steroids will increase the insulin required in management over the next 24–48 h. Many physicians use such agents.

Immediately after a severe hypoglycaemic attack a patient may be best managed either by continuous intravenous insulin (if an intravenous drip is running for other reasons) or by frequent injections of small doses of quick-acting insulin. The routine daily dose of insulin should be decreased by at least 4 units when it is resumed, unless there is some obvious explanation for the hypoglycaemic episode.

Hyperglycaemic comas. The majority of patients ill from hyperglycaemia are not comatose as a neurologist would define it, but confused or stuporose. Type I diabetics mostly suffer ketoacidotic hyperglycaemia; type II may present with or without ketosis. In the United Kingdom as many as 70 deaths occur annually from hyperglycaemic comas even in those under 50 years old, and the mortality increases with age to approximately 50 per cent in the over-70s. These emergencies occur at a rate of perhaps one per 200 patients per annum, but as particular patients may contribute several of these emergencies, somewhat fewer individual patients are affected annually. Ketoacidosis is relatively common in girls around menarche who may suffer repeated attacks at monthly or two monthly intervals.

A clinic can monitor its education of insulin-taking diabetics from the ratio of previously unknown to treated diabetics admitted in ketoacidosis coma. The total number of admissions per year is also an index of the general state of education throughout a community and its health service.

The mortality from ketoacidosis remains as high as between 3 and 10 per cent in hospitals that admit all the emergencies from particular localities. If individual factors are examined for their correlation with high mortality, age is the most important. However, when the interaction between factors is considered, associated illnesses (such as overwhelming infection, cardiac infarction, pulmonary embolism, etc.) are dominant; it is just that the elderly are more likely to present with coma accompanied by, and very likely precipitated by, such associated conditions. The depth and duration of coma are also prognostic factors, but as a general guide to therapy the clinical state of the patient is of greater prognostic influence than plasma biochemistry. Indeed the blood urea concentration is a more important guide than the blood glucose, the blood 'ketones', the plasma bicarbonate or the arterial pH; presumably the blood urea mainly reflects the adequacy of the renal circulation.

The plasma osmolality is the biochemical feature most related to the depth of unconsciousness, which correlates poorly with either the height of the blood glucose, or the degree of acidosis or ketosis. In experimental diabetes the fall in cerebral oxygen uptake also correlates with depth of coma.

The cause of ketoacidotic coma is uncertain and only increased knowledge and the application of catastrophe theory seem likely to explain it. Certainly patients can walk about with equally high blood glucose values. The onset of severe symptomatic ketoacidosis is linked indirectly to depletion of total body water, sodium, and potassium, and no doubt major changes in the intracellular electrolyte state. The final catastrophe may depend upon a switch from fat to protein to provide the alternative fuel to carbohydrate, or may depend upon the steadily increasing loss of total body water and electrolytes. Because of either the circulatory or metabolic disturbance, or through one of the common precipitating causes, e.g. infection or sterile inflammation as in myocardial infarction, the levels of the anti-insulin, catabolic, hyperglycaemic hormones increase markedly to magnify the crisis.

There is probably no fundamental difference between the ketoacidotic and non-ketotic varieties of coma. The latter occur in older patients and there tends to be less severe insulin deficiency. The crucial differences may be defective renal function in the older patients, so that more water and electrolytes are lost together with severe persistent glycosuria. There may also be differences in the size and effectiveness of the counter-regulatory hormonal and autonomic nervous responses.

Ketoacidotic hyperglycaemia coma. The three cardinal clinical features on examination are:

(a) dehydration, affecting the whole body and not just a dry tongue, as from excessive mouth breathing; (b) air hunger with an increased depth and rate of breathing; (c) ketosis. The latter is recognizable by many clinicians from the typical sickly sweet smell on the breath. However, about 20 per cent of medical attendants cannot detect this usefully, and the sensitivity of the remaining 80 per cent varies greatly. Hence during training every student should learn to appreciate how sensitive they are to it. The degree of ketosis can also be readily assessed, either by testing the urine (often not available in dehydrated and comatose patients), or by centrifuging heparinized blood and dipping Ketostix into the clear supernatent. Acetest tablets can also be used.

When a history is available, this varies from several weeks to a few days, particularly in those previously undiagnosed. There may be weight loss, fatigue, excessive thirst and polydipsia with polyuria. Other typical symptoms of developing hyperglycaemia may also be present. However, even in previously unrecognized patients the history may be as short as three or four days, while excessive physical activity may precipitate ketoacidosis (e.g. one youth ran a mile race in an only slightly slower time than usual 36 hours before his admission). Other cardinal features are of anorexia or vomiting with or without diarrhoea. The onset of vomiting is always a threatening symptom, particularly useful as a warning in those already known to be diabetic. An uncommon but well recognized complicating symptom is of abdominal pain, particularly likely to occur in younger patients as a dull persistent discomfort often affecting the whole abdomen but usually centred on the umbilicus. It may cause unjustified suspicions of an abdominal emergency.

On examination, as well as the three cardinal clinical features mentioned above, the patient is likely to show signs of weight loss, with rapid pulse of low volume, and low systolic pressure. There may be postural hypotension, certainly because of dehydration and decreased total body sodium, but perhaps also because of temporary autonomic neuropathy which may contribute to the vomiting and diarrhoea. Significant postural hypotension in a young patient, however alert and physically active, should always be a pointer to the need for immediate parenteral fluid treatment. In newly diagnosed patients it is most unusual to find evidence pathognomic of tissue damage but in any there may be symptoms and signs of a precipitating condition, e.g. infection (broncho-pneumonia, or an infected foot ulcer in a known diabetic). Evidence of infection of the urinary tract or other inaccessible sites, e.g. ischiorectal or perinephric abscess, should be sought.

Differential diagnosis. Table 31 gives pointers towards this. The main problems are:

Any other illness with over-ventilation, usually due to acidosis, e.g. uraemia or lactic acidosis, whether or not they complicate hyperglycaemia. Hyperventilation from salicylate overdosage is a potential problem but the most confusing clinical picture is Claude Bernard's 'piqure' diabetes, a short-lived hyperglycaemia from a lesion in the region of the fourth ventricle or the *iter*, leading to it from the third ventricle. It probably results from massive discharge of the sympathetic division of the autonomic nervous system. The accompanying hyperventilation is due to irritation of pathways involved in respiration, and such overbreathing produces a respiratory alkalosis rather than the usual metabolic acidosis. Determination of the arterial pH is decisive, as the plasma venous bicarbonate concentration will be low in both instances. Patients with such fourth ventricle lesions (e.g. subarachnoid haemorrhage) may have mild ketonaemia because of reduced food intake and a degree of hypermetabolism, possibly with fever, and their conscious state will also be disturbed. The hyperglycaemia settles spontaneously in 6–12 h, and unless the glucose concentration is watched carefully, insulin treatment can cause a rapid swing to hypoglycaemia. The initial fall in glucose is unaccompanied by any improvement in consciousness unlike the course in true diabetes, and so insulin can be persisted with mistakenly. Hypoglycaemia then further worsens central nervous function.

Fourth ventricle lesions are often accompanied by neck stiffness but a degree of meningism (rather than true meningitis) may be present as a facet of a general irritability which is present in about 5 per cent of stuporose ketoacidotic patients. If there is doubt, a lumbar puncture (having checked the absence of papilloedema) will differentiate, or a small intravenous injection of diazepam (e.g. 2 mg) may be given to see if this relaxes the neck.

Certain physical signs expected in ketoacidotic coma may not be present. Even if there is a pyrogenic infection there is usually no fever until treatment has been given for 6–12 h. Again, perhaps due to gross dehydration, classical signs of consolidation in patients with lobar pneumonia may not be elicited even though the X-ray shows lung shadows.

Non-ketotic hyperglycaemia states. Of the previously mentioned cardinal features, only dehydration is present. The condition is not uncommon in elderly patients, so glucose levels should be checked urgently in any stuporose patient, particularly if old. Unilateral signs of central nervous system abnormality do not exclude the diagnosis, for if a metabolic disturbance coincides with asymmetry of cerebral blood flow focal neurological signs may result.

Investigation. The pretreatment state must be determined both for diagnosis and to allow a later measure of the progress of recovery. Treatment can be started on clinical grounds when blood samples have been obtained for urea, sodium, potassium, and arterial pH as well as glucose and 'ketones'. The arterial P_{O_2} in perhaps 20 per cent of patients is surprisingly low initially, even below 60 mmHg; the hypoxia is not associated with the usual degree of cyanosis because of a shift of the dissociation curve of oxyhaemoglobin to the left (i.e. oxyhaemoglobin dissociates less

Table 31 Differential diagnosis of the diabetic comas

	Blood glucose* (mmol/l)	Plasma ketones†	Dehydration	Hyperventilation	BP
Hypoglycaemic coma	≤ 2	0	0	0	Normal
Severe diabetic ketoacidosis	>13	+ to +++	+++	+++	Normal or low
Hyperglycaemic hyperosmolar non-ketotic coma	>13	0 to 0	+++	0	Normal or low
Lactic acidosis	Variable	0 to +	0 to +	+++	Low
Non-metabolic comas	Normal to high	0 to +	0 to +	0 to +	Variable

*Assessed with Dextrostix or BM-Glycemie 20–800.
†Assessed with Ketostix or Acetest.

readily to release oxygen to the tissue). The haematocrit may provide a guide to dehydration but chronic infection or uraemia will affect the premorbid value. The clinical state of the patient must be assessed initially and regularly with records of heart rate, blood pressure, respiratory rate, and level of consciousness. It is also useful to note the discrepancy between warmth of the centre (e.g. abdominal wall temperature) and the periphery (big toe or tip of nose).

Blood glucose and potassium levels should be reassessed one hour after start of insulin treatment and, unless the clinical course is convincingly satisfactory, arterial pH and blood urea should be remeasured three hours after start of treatment, together with glucose and potassium. These latter two should anyhow be measured after five hours. Crucial targets are that plasma potassium remains normal, and that the level of blood glucose at which it may be necessary to add glucose to the i.v. infusion be detected.

Treatment (Tables 32 and 33)

Metabolic   *(a) Fluid.* The bases of treatment are provision of water, sodium, insulin, and potassium. The two former are the most important as restoration of an adequate circulation is the single most important need. Despite a greater loss (usually) of water than of sodium, the correct replacement fluid is 'physiologi-

Table 32 Management of diabetic hyperglycaemic comas

Initial assessment	
Clinical examination	Hydration, respiration, pulse, BP, consciousness, signs of infection
Biochemical	(a) Bedside. Glucose, ketone body test strips (b) Laboratory. Glucose, Na+, K+, urea, arterial pH, pO$_2$
Treatment	
Fluid	1 l 0.15 M saline in 15–30 min, 2 l in 2 h, 3 l in 4 h, then 500 ml 2–4-hourly. Change to 10% dextrose, 500 ml four-hourly, when blood glucose 10–16 mM. If plasma Na+ >150 mM use hypotonic saline. Consider use of CVP
Insulin	(a) i.v. regimen. 6 unit i.v. bolus, then 6 units/h continuous i.v.; change to 2–4 units/h continuous i.v. when dextrose infusion commenced. Change to s.c. with first meal (b) i.m. regimen. 20 units i.m. (or 10i.m./10i.v.) initially, then 6 units every h. Change to 6u two-hourly or 12u s.c. four-hourly when dextrose infusion commenced
Potassium	Start at 13–20 mM/h in saline from time of first insulin. Adjust rate according to plasma values (26 mM/h if plasma K+ 3–4 mM; 39 mM/h if K+ < 3 mM; 10 mM/h if K+ 5–6 mM; stop i.v. potassium if plasma K+ > 6 mM)
Bicarbonate	(a) Give 100 mM + 13 mM KCl in 20–40 min if pH < 7.0; repeat after 60–90 min if pH still < 7.0 (b) Give 50 mM + 10 mM KCl if patient distressed by hyperventilation

Table 33 General measures in the treatment of diabetic hyperglycaemic comas

1. Nasogastric tube in unconscious patients
2. CVP line in patients with cardiovascular disease
3. Low dose s.c. heparin in comatose, obese, or severely hyperosmolar patients, provided that there are no contraindications
4. Antibiotics if infection detected or suspected
5. ECG. Cardiac monitor as guide to K+ therapy
6. Bladder catheterization if prolonged failure to pass urine
7. Frequent monitoring of pulse, BP, respiration, conscious state

cally normal' saline (0.9 per cent) and this should be given fast, e.g. 500 ml in the first quarter of an hour, a litre in the next three quarters of an hour, and another in the next hour, with infusion of 500 ml hourly thereafter to a total of about 5 l (or until a normal circulation is present and obvious clinical features of dehydration have disappeared). The use of hypotonic sodium chloride is indicated only when there is marked hypernatraemia, e.g. an initial plasma sodium concentration of 145 mM or higher (see below).

Once insulin has been administered, the plasma sodium rises because water moves intracellularly together with glucose and potassium. There is abnormal water balance of the central nervous system in ketoacidosis, with undue liability to oedema. Hence the osmolarity of the extracellular fluid should be kept relatively high, another benefit of physiologically normal saline. Most patients with ketoacidosis have a low plasma sodium on admission as an osmolar compensation for hyperglycaemia, so a sodium concentration of 145 mM, still within the normal range, represents a marked excess loss of water over sodium. This may be an indication to infuse half-normal physiological saline after two litres of normal saline, to prevent undue hypernatraemia. The mechanisms that can underlie this are poorly understood but hypernatraemia is particularly liable to occur in non-ketotic patients.

Insulin. The necessary actions of insulin in diabetic ketoacidosis are to inhibit inappropriate gluconeogenesis and excessive lipolysis. Relatively low concentrations of insulin are adequate for this, e.g. 30–40 mU/l, half the normal maximum peripheral insulin concentration during an oral glucose tolerance test, and less than half the insulin concentration necessary to achieve maximum glucose uptake in the forearm, at normal blood glucose levels. However, during treatment of ketoacidosic hyperglycaemic coma the aim is to decrease blood glucose by 5–10 mmol/l. Insulin can be administered either by hourly intramuscular injection or by continuous i.v. infusion. Every institute should choose the method which suits its facilities best. The aim is continuous entry into the blood of small but adequate amounts of insulin.

(a) *Intramuscular regime.* An initial injection of 20 i.u. crystalline insulin (e.g. soluble, actrapid, velosulin) should be followed by a further 5 i.u. hourly. It is important that the injections are intramuscular and not subcutaneous, for absorption of insulin from the poorly infused subcutaneous site is slow. If blood glucose has not dropped by 5 mM after two hours a change to the i.v. route is indicated.

(b) *Intravenous.* After an initial bolus of 6 i.u. of crystalline insulin the same amount (6 i.u.) is infused hourly. In children the loading dose is 0.1 units/kg with 0.1 units/kg per hour subsequently. This is best given by an automatic pump with insulin joining the giving set from a separate line. If this facility is unavailable, insulin can be added to an ordinary giving set (or Metriset). Again a Y-connection is best, so that the rate of insulin administration is independent of that of the volume of intravenous fluid. Absorption of insulin to the walls of syringes or tubing can be prevented by addition of purified human albumen, or more easily by drawing back 1 ml of the patient's blood into a syringe containing between 0 and 60 ml of the saline carrier for the insulin, but this precaution is not necessary clinically. When i.v. infusion of insulin was evaluated, the differences between individual patients in the clearance and distribution space of insulin were greater than the variation with or without added albumen. It is always vital to check that insulin is given in an amount adequate to produce the expected rate of fall of blood glucose of between 3 and 5 mM/h. The recommended rate of infusion should be doubled if glucose falls less than 5mm/l the first two hours. The rate of fall is remarkably constant in individual patients, and allows a rough and ready prediction of when i.v. glucose should be infused, i.e. at a blood glucose between 16 and 12 mM. This serves both to provide necessary fuel to a starving patient, and further to reduce the chances of cerebral oedema. The i.v. glucose is best given as 125 ml/h of 10 per cent dextrose.

Insulin can be continued by infusion of 2–4 i.u./h. If the

intramuscular route has been used, the injections may be changed to 6 i.u. two hourly or to four-hourly injections of about 12 i.u. subcutaneous insulin. The i.v. route should be used only as long as it is necessary to give the i.v. fluids on other grounds. Ingestion of nourishing fluids should be encouraged as soon as possible, beginning with small quantities of simple fluids.

(c) *Potassium.* The details of potassium replacement treatment remain surprisingly contentious. Many regard the greater attention given to this during the last ten years as one of the more important developments in the treatment of diabetic ketoacidosis, but one recent authority wrote: 'I prefer to delay the start of (potassium) treatment until the (plasma) level has fallen to about 4.5 mM or less'. The reasons for more active potassium infusion, advanced at least ten years ago, are still valid. Patients in diabetic ketoacidosis have a total body deficit of potassium averaging 500 mM and sometimes more than twice this. A major action of insulin is to increase tissue potassium uptake. Once insulin treatment has been started, therefore, it is safe to infuse potassium, providing both the potassium and the insulin will reach their target tissues. The only contraindication to early potassium supplementation is a grossly inadequate circulation, such that potassium added to a small circulating blood volume does not reach enough cells for its uptake to be increased effectively by insulin, with an equally limited distribution. It is also perhaps only in patients with such an inadequate circulation that there is real risk of acute renal tubular necrosis, with a risk of 10 days or so of anuria or gross oliguria. Previously, the risk of renal failure made potassium administration potentially dangerous, but this problem has been reduced by the development of peritoneal and haemodialysis.

Even though a quarter of the patients admitted with diabetic ketoacidosis have a plasma potassium above the normal range, potassium should be given once saline infusion and insulin treatment have started; i.e. within a few minutes of intravenous insulin and about ten minutes after intramuscular insulin, with the exceptions noted above. Blood for plasma potassium assay will have been sent before insulin was given. In the first hour 13–20 mM potassium chloride can be safely given, by which time the initial potassium concentration should be available. At this stage another sample should be sent for potassium assay, for the change over the first hour helps greatly in predicting future doses, which can be altered accordingly. With resalination and insulin treatment, plasma potassium may fall fast, perhaps particularly from high values. Thus, a drop from 6.4 to 5.2 mM may occur in the first hour, even though 13 mM potassium were given. If plasma potassium is between 3 and 4 mM, the rate of intravenous infusion can be increased to 26 mM/h, while if it is below 3.0 at least 39 mM/h should be given.

Patients particularly liable to have a low initial plasma potassium concentration in diabetic ketoacidosis are both the newly diagnosed when the period of kaliuresis is likely to have been considerably longer than those already on insulin, and patients treated with a thiazide or similar diuretic, as the usual urinary potassium loss caused by these agents will be magnified by the osmotic diuresis of heavy glycosuria. Such patients may require 400–600 mM potassium in the first 12 hours of treatment.

Plasma potassium should certainly be measured one and five hours after the start of treatment, as well as initially, and if there is any doubt, three hours after treatment started also. The ECG is a useful albeit indirect guide to potassium states, with particular reference to the .T waves, whose inversion implies a low plasma potassium (page 8.28). However, the T waves can also be influenced by acidosis, so they are an uncertain guide to absolute potassium levels, though a useful index of change. Potassium is usually given intravenously as the chloride, but may also be administered as a hydrogen phosphate salt.

Potassium should be started orally as soon as fluids are taken, initially as potassium-rich fluids, such as meat soups, fruit juice, or even milk, and later as more definite supplements, when solid food is being taken.

Observations on diabetics in Oxford under treatment with old high-dose insulin regimens showed that the decrease in plasma potassium correlated inversely with the amount of potassium infused over the first five hours; plasma levels would drop an average of 2.0 mM if no potassium at all was given, while, to prevent any fall from initial values some 110 mM potassium was needed over that time. Urinary potassium losses may continue large during the first 12–24 hours, despite the deficit of total potassium, perhaps because of intracellular deficits in renal tubular cells. As expected, it is the patients with lower initial potassium concentrations who both conserve most added potassium and lose the least in the urine. There is a smaller drop in plasma potassium concentration on the low-dose insulin regime described here, an advantage over older high-dose regimes.

Particular attention must also be paid to potassium replacement when intravenous bicarbonate is given (see below).

(d) *Bicarbonate.* There is good reason for this to be a contentious aspect of treatment. The advantages of bicarbonate infusion are reduction in the metabolic acidosis and consequent relief in a conscious patient of distressing hyperventilation. If acidaemia is severe (pH < 7.0) tissue function may be impaired, with a negative ionotropic effect on the heart, peripheral vasodilation, and central nervous system depression. The disadvantages of bicarbonate infusion are first, hypokalaemia with possible consequent cardiac dysrhythmia and a leftwards shift in the dissociation curve of oxyhaemoglobin, so that oxygen reaches the tissues less readily. The dissociation curve is approximately normal before treatment of ketoacidotic patients, despite the marked acidosis which by the Bohr effect would be expected to have moved the curve to the right. However, that right shift is approximately balanced by decreased red cell 2,3-diphosphoglycerate. If the metabolic acidosis is rapidly corrected, the curve will shift to the left as the 2,3-diphosphoglycerate deficit is not corrected until 24–72 h after treatment starts. Another consideration is that, after bicarbonate a metabolic alkalosis often appears as ketonaemia disappears. This is rarely severe enough to disturb health, but it shows that less bicarbonate is needed than is often given.

Ketosis disappears through oxidation of the 'ketone bodies' in the periphery, coincident with inhibition of their further formation in the liver, once insulin has checked the typical excessive lipolysis. The drop in concentration of these organic acids is faster than the rise in bicarbonate concentration of the plasma, and usually a mild hyperchloraemic acidosis occurs for a short while during replacement therapy.

Bicarbonate should not be given so long as the peripheral circulation is grossly restricted, for it will almost certainly reduce oxygen delivery to the periphery; but once sufficient saline has been given to restore a reasonable circulation, if arterial pH is still below 7.0, sodium bicarbonate 100 mmol should be given over 20 min, and 50 mmol in that time if it is between 7.1 and 7.0. Such bicarbonate should be accompanied by an extra 13 mM of potassium chloride per 100 mM of bicarbonate. Arterial pH should be measured 60–90 min after bicarbonate, to decide whether more is needed.

(e) *Oxygen.* Approximately one-fifth of patients have an initial arterial p_{O_2} below 8 torr. If this is coincident with any leftward shift of the dissociation curve of oxyhaemoglobin, it may help to administer oxygen via a facemask. Initially 100 per cent can be given but this should be stopped for 10 minutes before arterial blood is taken and pH and p_{O_2} determination. If p_{O_2} is low, oxygen is continued at at least 28 per cent until the peripheral circulation has improved substantially.

General management. The hyperosmolar, hyperglycaemic, non-ketotic patient should be treated in similar fashion to the more classical ketoacidotic case. There are, however, some special points of note.

1. Approximately half of such patients are normo- or hypernatraemic, so that hypotonic fluid replacement will be necessary.

2. There is an increased likelihood of thrombotic events, so that anticoagulation should be seriously considered.

3. Bicarbonate replacement is obviously unnecessary, and smaller amounts of potassium are required than in ketoacidotic patients: a replacement rate of 10 mM/h is probably adequate.

4. Blood glucose levels are likely to be extremely high, so that restoration of normoglycaemia will take many hours but, as with ketoacidotic patients, too great a fall of glucose levels could be harmful because of the effects of osmotic disequilibrium on the CNS.

An unconscious patient should be nursed semiprone until a thin (Ryle's type) nasogastric tube has been passed and any gastric content aspirated. Frequently this is of large volume and if vomited by an unconscious patient, aspiration of the acid liquid will produce a severe chemical pneumonitis, possibly with a fatal outcome. If aspiration occurs, anti-inflammatory doses of glucocorticoids should be given, even though this will probably mean an increased need for insulin. Thus the nasogastric tube should be passed as soon as possible after admission in the unconscious patient.

Urethral catheterization is sometimes recommended early in management, for instance if no urine has been passed after 4–6 h of treatment: but it is not surprising if an hypotensive and severely dehydrated patient does not void urine in this time, and catheterization of devitalized tissues readily introduces infection. It may therefore be an advantage to delay catheterization unless there is clinical evidence of distressing bladder distention. Such delay is more permissible now than in the past, in that fewer patients are admitted in such severe circulatory collapse that acute tubular necrosis of the kidneys is likely. At the same time, even should eight or ten days' anuria follow resolution of the diabetic metabolic emergency, excess potassium is readily removed by dialysis, so it is less urgent now to recognize early the onset of oliguria. If oliguria persists 6–8 h after the start of i.v. fluids, 80 mg frusemide may be helpful.

Central venous catheterization. Although some advocate this for the majority, it is probably better confined to those in whom there is real suspicion of cardiac embarrassment, as when intravenous fluid is rapidly administered to those with known cardiac disease, or in the aged. If there is any suspicion of cardiac dysfunction from this, a central line should be installed but it should equally be removed as soon as it becomes unnecessary, to reduce the risk of infection. Failure of the heart rate to decrease during treatment can indicate cardiac insufficiency, but another cause may be the uncommon deterioration in pulmonary function that can occur 4–8 h after treatment starts. This is associated with X-ray appearances of pulmonary oedema; there is a marked drop in arterial P_{O_2}, while medium or coarse crepitations are heard over the lung fields, quite unlike the fine, moist crepitations of left sided failure. If the condition is severe enough to warrant artificial ventilation, pulmonary compliance is found to be very low. The cause of such stiff lungs is uncertain, but possibly they result from interstitial pulmonary oedema, or alternatively from a disseminated intravascular coagulation affecting particularly the lung circulation.

ECG. This should always be recorded early in management, in case an acute, and possibly painless, cardiac infarction has precipitated the metabolic emergency. It is an advantage to repeat the recording frequently or, ideally, for the patient to be on an ECG monitor to detect extremes of hyper- or hypokalaemia.

It is rare for ketoacidosis to be associated with *disseminated intravascular coagulation* of clinical significance. Clinically, evidence of vascular occlusion and/or excessive bruising or spontaneous bleeding should suggest this possibility, diagnosed by the conjunction of low platelet count, reduced plasma fibrinogen and increased amounts of fibrin degradation products. If there is spontaneous bruising some advocate the use of heparin treatment.

Routine anticoagulation has been suggested for diabetics with metabolic emergencies. It is probably wiser to confine prophylaxis to high-risk patients, such as those in deep coma, those with a known history of venous thrombosis, the very obese and the very

hyperosmolar. Subcutaneous heparin injections should not be started until 8 h after admission, to allow time for clinical assessment of any predisposing or precipitating factors, some of which might contraindicate anticoagulation.

Antibiotics. While 'routine' use has been suggested, prescription on more positive grounds is preferable. When hitherto undiagnosed diabetes presents as a metabolic emergency, and there is a history of steadily increasing severity, infection is rarely a precipitating cause. Also, bacterial infection is rarely present in known diabetics who present after two or three days of vomiting with or without accompanying diarrhoea, particularly if admission has been precipitated by marked reduction in their usual insulin dose. But in any patient and particularly in known diabetics, infection must be sought avidly, e.g. an ischiorectal abscess, or relatively small foot ulcer at the mouth of a sinus leading to a deeper collection of pus. The white blood cell count, certain physical signs, and especially abdominal pain and guarding, may all be potentially misleading in ketoacidosis. With a suspected 'acute abdomen', the management is perhaps not so difficult as the differential diagnosis in the early state. Whether or not there is intraperitoneal infection, conservative treatment by intravenous fluids and insulin, together with gastric aspiration, is best for at least the first 4–6 h. If the illness is purely metabolic, there should then be substantial improvement in the signs in the abdomen while, if peritonitis is indeed present, a fever is likely to have appeared, and the patient's condition to have worsened rather than improved as expected. Surgery, for however good a cause, is dangerous in the presence of severe ketoacidosis, which should be combated first. With antibiotics, intravenous fluids, and gastric aspiration little will be lost on the surgical side by such delay, but a great deal gained medically.

If antibiotics are to be given, blood, urine, and throat swabs should first be taken for culture.

Routine observations include the usual nursing records of pulse and respiration rate, level of consciousness and temperature, together with blood pressure. These are the most important guides to the success of treatment in that they report the patient's condition directly; metabolic measurements only predict what that condition is likely to be in the coming minutes or hours.

Occasionally the metabolic reports give strange results, such as a plasma sodium under 110 mM, and this should raise suspicion of gross lipaemia, which may be missed if the plasma is not looked at after centrifugation (the blood should not stand on the bench long enough for chylomicra to separate). A clinical clue to this may be the uncommon lipaemia retinalis, in which the small retinal vessels are yellow and highly reflective. The high chylomicra count may occupy even 30 per cent of the plasma volume and so distort the biochemical results.

Organization of therapy

Perhaps half the diagnosed diabetics in the United Kingdom regularly attend hospital clinics. This proportion varies from region to region and is higher among the insulin treated. Clinic care is often far from ideal and alternative methods include general practitioner 'mini-clinics' and 'shared care' between health centre and hospital. Increased participation of medical ancillary workers and increased education of patients have also been used to improve care for the diabetic. Whichever system is used the key should be increased self-care by well-informed and well-monitored patients.

The diabetic clinic. In Britain care has centred on the hospital-based diabetic clinic, all too often under-staffed. Individual doctors may see 20–30 patients in a single clinic (one every 5–6 minutes). The patient may see six different junior doctors, often without particular training in diabetes, at six successive visits, which may be spaced at 4–12-month intervals. If clinic care is wrongly over-emphasized, general practitioners become alienated and restrict themselves to issuing repeat prescriptions. A dietician may be attached to the clinic, but often gives different advice to that offered by the doctor (if indeed he offers any), and is unlikely to have sufficient time to see an adequate number of patients.

Hospital clinics should be staffed by doctors of at least registrar (resident) status in sufficient numbers to allow at least 15 minutes per patient. Each patient should see the same doctor at successive visits. Each visit should include educational reinforcement. Patients should be screened for complications at appropriate intervals by adequately trained medical staff. A dietician should be in attendance and should have her own clinic on a separate occasion when she can reinforce and extend advice given at the diabetic clinic. A chiropodist should also be present for foot care and preventive foot education. A teaching nurse as an integral part of the clinic is a major advantage. She can both teach practical aspects of therapy—home blood-glucose monitoring, injection technique, urine testing—and provide general advice on self-management. The provision of simple brochures and videofilms may also be helpful. The major requirement, however, is for consistent continued care, which requires a lot of time.

In centres responsible for many diabetics it is advantageous to have separate clinics for separate functions: a pregnancy clinic shared with an obstetrician, a pre-pregnancy clinic for 'super-control', an adolescent clinic (with perhaps a psychologist in attendance) and, should they prove necessary, infusion pump clinics. Even separating clinics into 'routine' and 'problem' sessions may be helpful. Use of a day unit for more detailed investigations, and for further education, is another advantage, as are clinics held at special times, e.g. evening.

These ideal aims are unlikely to be provided against the background of increasing costs of health care in all countries.

'Shared-care'. In the conventional diabetic clinic the general practitioner plays at most a small role, possibly involved only when emergencies occur. One approach to the staffing problem is for general practitioners to involve themselves more in day-to-day care of diabetic patients. Hospital clinics can be restricted to particular problem patients plus an annual biochemical and clinical review for chronic complications. The patient carries a shared-care card and is seen routinely and regularly by the practitioner. The latter sends blood samples for glucose or HbA_1 to the hospital and, with appropriate organization, this can serve as a check on the frequency of the general practitioner's contact with the patient. This system is theoretically sensible, but requires real and sustained interest from both hospital and family doctors.

'Mini-clinics'. An alternative to 'shared-care' is the establishment of small clinics outside the main centre. This can be done in cottage hospitals or health centres. The clinics are staffed by general practitioners with periodic visits from the consultant diabetologist. If a prevalence of diabetes of 1–2 per cent is accepted, then a group practice of 10 000 patients will have 100 to 200 diabetics, more than enough to have a monthly diabetic clinic. The general practitioners who run the clinic will require initial training, and there must be a strong local organization for continuing education. Open access to hospital investigations, to an ophthalmologist, to the dietician, and to the chiropody services is essential, plus provision of appropriate educational materials. The advantage of this system is the increased attention given to the individual patient, continuity of care, and knowledge of family background. The disadvantage is the more limited access to specialized facilities.

'Diabetes nurse'. Over the years there has been a slow increase in the number of nurses with a special responsibility for diabetes in the United Kingdom. They are variously labelled diabetes health liaison officers, community nurses, sisters, health visitors, etc. Whatever their title, they have an essential role to play in total diabetic care. The 'diabetes nurse' is generally attached to a specific clinic and has several distinct roles. These may include: (*a*) teaching practical and theoretical aspects of diabetes in the clinic; (*b*)

co-ordinating the care of diabetic patients in different parts of the hospital, advising on their therapy, and teaching them and their families where necessary; (*c*) following new patients, into their homes, and patients with specific problems (compliance, feet, labile diabetes) in liaison with district nurses. This last task is particularly important in that problems may be unravelled which have their roots in home circumstances, which might not be revealed during a busy diabetic clinic. It is also almost axiomatic that patients communicate more freely with nurses than with doctors.

'Teaching units' (diabetes education centres). There are few formal education centres in the United Kingdom, the concept being more fully developed in the United States and continental Europe. The centre may be headed by the diabetes physician and staffed with diabetes nurses and a dietician. Coherent teaching programmes can be organized for new patients and their families and, as reinforcement, for old patients, with different programmes for type I and type II diabetics, and the young and old patients. Both group and individual teaching can be useful. There is much scope for tape-slide programmes and films. Such a scheme should include evaluation and audit, to ensure the objectives initially established are met.

The exact structure of such centres and their relation to the diabetic clinic will depend on local circumstances and resources. At the simplest level, one teaching nurse in a single room can have a great effect. For a large health district, three or four staff who also serve as diabetic nurses in the clinic and community is probably the minimum requirement. The centre should include a 'phone-in' service for patients, and families, which can have a dramatic effect on both patient health and clinic work-load.

'The diabetic record'. In most clinics, the notes of diabetic patients form part of the overall medical records system, are disorganized, and offer little help to the physician doing a busy clinic. There are three possible solutions to this problem. The first is to have separate diabetic records. This has the disadvantages that the records though less voluminous may still be disorganized, and problems arise when patients are admitted or seen with non-diabetic problems. The second solution is to have a flow sheet at the front of the notes, which records all major events, inpatient admissions, the dose of antidiabetic and other therapeutic agents, diet, weight, indices of control, and indicates when appropriate physical examinations and interviews were performed (i.e. eyes, feet, blood pressure, neurological, visits to chiropodist, and dietician). This is certainly preferable to the usual 'random notes'.

The final possibility is to introduce a computerized records system. In the past most such schemes have been unduly complicated, and required main-frame computers, and a computer programmer. At best they have been used to run appointments systems, to identify defaulters, and to provide research information. Nowadays clinic microcomputers can provide a summary of each patient seen, ask appropriate questions of the clinician, and receive new information typed in directly. Such interactive systems are being developed; they should be relatively simple and inexpensive, and could prove a major advance in patient care.

References

Brownlee, M. (ed.) (1981). *Diabetes mellitus*, Vols. 1–5. Garland STPM Press, New York.

Ireland, J. T., Thomson, W. S. T., and Williamson, J. (1980). *Diabetes today*. HM + M Publishers, Aylesbury.

Johnston, D. G. and Alberti, K. G. M. M. (1980). Diabetic emergencies: practical aspects of the management of diabetic ketoacidosis and diabetes during surgery. *Clins Endocr. Metab.* **9**, 437.

———— (eds.) (1982). Diabeties mellitus. *Clins Endocr. Metab.* **11**, No. 2.

Keen, H. and Jarrett, J. (eds.) (1982). *Complications of diabetes*, 2nd edn. Edward Arnold, London.

Porte, D. Jr and Halter, J. B. (1981). The endocrine pancreas and diabetes mellitus. In *Textbook of endocrinology*, 6th edn (ed. R. H. Williams) p. 715. Saunders, Philadelphia.

Reaven, G. M. and Steiner, G. (eds.) (1981). Diabetes and atherosclerosis. *Diabetes* **30**, Suppl. 2.

Skyler, J. S. and Cahill, G. F. (eds.) (1981). *Diabetes mellitus*. Yorke Medical Books, New York.

Tattersall, R. B. (1977). Diabetes. *Clins Endocr. Metab.* **6**, 283.

Volk, B. W. and Wellmann, K. F. (eds.) (1977). *The diabetic pancreas*. Plenum Press, New York.

West, K. M. (1978). *Epidemiology of diabetes and its vascular lesions*. Elsevier North Holland, New York.

HYPOGLYCAEMIA

R. C. Turner

Hypoglycaemia is an unusual symptom in adults, except in diabetic patients treated with insulin. Spontaneous hypoglycaemia usually can be divided into two categories. *Fasting hypoglycaemia* is precipitated by lack of food for several hours with symptoms during the night or on walking. *Reactive* or *post-prandial hypoglycaemia* occurs two to five hours after meals. Patients with reactive hypoglycaemia never have symptoms during a fast, although occasionally some patients with fasting hypoglycaemia may have a reactive component, e.g. in some with insulinomas. Fasting hypoglycaemia indicates an identifiable underlying disease, while reactive hypoglycaemia usually occurs in the absence of organic disease.

Clinical features. Hypoglycaemic symptoms are unusual unless the plasma glucose falls to less than 2.5 mmol/l. However, patients with prolonged hypoglycaemia often have a lower threshold for symptoms. Patients with an insulinoma, or diabetic patients chronically overtreated with insulin, can have a plasma glucose of 1 mmol/l for several hours without overt symptoms.

Adrenergic symptoms usually predominate, particularly when the plasma glucose falls rapidly as in reactive hypoglycaemia. Adrenaline is secreted (together with other counter-regulatory hormones including glucagon, growth hormone, and cortisol) and induces pallor, sweating, tremor, and palpitation. These early, premonitory adrenergic symptoms can be lost in insulin-dependent diabetics with a long duration of diabetes who have developed an autonomic neuropathy. They then find it less easy to detect hypoglycaemia and can have more severe attacks. Diabetics with prolonged hyperglycaemia, abruptly corrected with insulin therapy, sometimes have an adrenergic response although the blood glucose has only been reduced to 5–7 mmol/l.

Neuroglycopenic symptoms occur because of the lack of glucose substrate required for normal CNS function. The brain, unlike most other tissues, is primarily dependent on glucose for its energy supply. It can utilize ketone bodies, but the development of significant ketosis requires several hours in man, and cannot protect against acute hypoglycaemia. If excess insulin has induced hypoglycaemia, it will have inhibited ketogenesis, and thus have removed both the glucose and ketone body substrate of the brain. The ketosis of starvation may help to prevent symptoms in the presence of marked hypoglycaemia.

Neurological symptoms include poor concentration, sluggishness, dysarthria, incoordination, diplopia, tingling around the mouth, transient strokes, epileptic attacks, and coma. Each patient may have a characteristic group of symptoms which he can recognize. Patients may have features resembling ethanol intoxication, and poor judgement and incoordination can be dangerous if they are driving a car, swimming or near to dangerous machinery.

Fasting hypoglycaemia. In the fasting state, the liver maintains a normal plasma glucose level initially by the breakdown of stored glycogen. When glycogen stores are depleted after 12–36 hours, glucose production by the liver depends on gluconeogenesis. Any disease or drug that inhibits glycogenolysis or gluconeogenesis may lead to fasting hypoglycaemia (Table 1).

Table 1 The differential diagnoses and investigations appropriate to either fasting hypoglycaemia or post-prandial hypoglycaemia

Fasting attacks	Post-prandial attacks

Exclude clinically
  Hypopituitarism
  Addison's disease
  Cirrhosis or liver failure
  Sarcoma (including chest X-ray, plain abdomen X-ray)
  Ethanol after a fast
  Availability of insulin/sulphonylurea for self-administration
	Exclude clinically
	  Gastric surgery
	  Mild diabetes

Investigation
  Sarcoma: spontaneous hypoglycaemia with low plasma insulin and no ketosis
  Self-administration of insulin: insulin antibodies; during 'spontaneous' hypoglycaemia, low plasma C-peptide with high plasma insulin
	Investigation
	  Extended oral glucose tolerance test

Insulinoma
  Inordinately raised plasma insulin during hypoglycaemia: during spontaneous episode; after an overnight fast; fish insulin suppression test with human insulin assay, or insulin suppression test with C-peptide assay; during a prolonged fast
  High fasting plasma pro-insulin (if assay available)	

Insulinomas, although rare, are one of the most common causes of fasting hypoglycaemia in adults. The tumours are semi-autonomous and maintain insulin secretion in the presence of hypoglycaemia, which normally would suppress beta cell secretion. The persistent basal insulin secretion of insulimonas inhibits hepatic glucose efflux and causes hypoglycaemia. Patients characteristically present with drowsiness on waking, relieved by a sweet drink or breakfast. They may have specific symptoms such as diplopia or parasthesiae, or become confused or have epileptic fits. Symptoms can also occur during the day, particularly after exercise, e.g. prior to lunch after digging the garden. It is unusual for patients to notice specifically that the symptoms can be prevented by frequent meals, and thus eat more and develop obesity.

Ethanol-induced hypoglycaemia occurs because ethanol is oxidized in the liver, and hence NAD^+ is reduced to NADH. This alteration in redox state inhibits gluconeogenesis, e.g. by preventing lactate to pyruvate conversion. In rats, this effect is at its maximum at an ethanol concentration of 10 mmol/l, a level less than the legal limit for car driving in the United Kingdom of 18 mmol/l. After a fast of approximately 36 hours the liver glycogen reserves are depleted and drinking ethanol will induce hypoglycaemia. Alcohol-induced hypoglycaemia is thus usually only seen in alcoholics who drink and do not eat. Children, with their greater turnover of fuel supply, occasionally get ethanol-induced hypoglycaemia after a few hours without food, e.g. at wedding receptions. Starvation is probably the commonest, and ethanol the second commonest, cause of fasting hypoglycaemia in the world.

Cortisol deficiency from *pituitary* or *adrenal insufficiency* inhibits gluconeogenesis. Whilst cortisol deficient patients have a slightly low fasting plasma glucose, frank hypoglycaemia is rare and only occurs after a fast of about one day.

Liver disease has to be severe to diminish gluconeogenesis and glycogenolysis sufficiently to produce hypoglycaemia. Thus symptoms only occur in patients with acute hepatic failure, gross cirrhosis, or marked hepatic congestion secondary to heart failure.

Factitious hypoglycaemia can occur when a patient surreptitiously takes either insulin or a sulphonylurea drug. If a doctor, nurse, or other hospital worker has hypoglycaemia, it is often self-induced. These patients often do not appear to have a psychiatric disorder and will usually deny self-administration. They are often remarkably plausible.

Extra-pancreatic sarcomas, e.g. retroperitoneal fibrosarcoma or mesothelioma, occasionally cause hypoglycaemia by secreting a pro-insulin-related peptide (i.e. NSILA, non-suppressible insulin-like activity, so-called because insulin antibodies do not inhibit the peptide's action, or IGF, insulin-like growth factor). The tumours are usually large, and can be either easily palpated in the abdomen or become apparent on the chest or abdomen X-ray.

Diagnosis of fasting hypoglycaemia. Anybody with a 'funny turn' or transient stroke should probably immediately have a blood glucose measurement with a glucose-oxidase strip to exclude hypoglycaemia. If that result is low, a blood sample for laboratory glucose (and insulin) assay should be taken.

A fasting plasma glucose of less than 3.5 mmol/l is likely to be pathological. Women have a slightly lower fasting plasma glucose than men; thus after a three-day fast the lower limit of normal for women is 2 mmol/l compared with 3 mmol/l for men.

If a patient with fasting hypoglycaemia has raised plasma ketone levels or ketonuria, this excludes an insulinoma, mesothelioma, or self-administration of insulin or of sulphonylurea, as endogenous or exogenous insulin or NSILA inhibit ketogenesis as well as gluconeogenesis. Other causes of decreased hepatic glucose production, e.g. ethanol-induced hypoglycaemia, are associated with increased ketone body production.

In adults most of the causes of fasting hypoglycaemia, other than an insulinoma, can be easily recognized clinically. Thus the hormone deficiencies or liver disease have to be gross and easily clinically apparent before hypoglycaemia is induced. The extra-pancreatic tumours are usually large and either palpable or easily seen on an X-ray. Ethanol hypoglycaemia only occurs in people who have had a prolonged fast, and can often be excluded from the history. Thus, an adult with a definite fasting hypoglycaemia, who is otherwise well and has no large tumour on palpation or chest abdomen X-ray, will either have an insulinoma or be self-administering insulin or a sulphonylurea.

Insulinomas usually can be diagnosed easily by means of a blood sample taken during a spontaneous attack or after an overnight fast, when 90 per cent of patients have fasting hypoglycaemia. Normally hypoglycaemia inhibits insulin secretion, the plasma insulin being less than 1.5 mU/l for a fasting plasma glucose of less than 2 mmol/l (normal range 3–13 mU/l at normal fasting plasma glucose concentrations). The semi-autonomous insulinomas continue to secrete insulin, and can be diagnosed by inordinately high fasting plasma insulin levels during spontaneous hypoglycaemia (Fig. 1). Most endocrine tumours are diagnosed by a suppression test, and patients with insulinomas in effect do their own suppression test. The 10 per cent of patients with insulinoma who have normal fasting plasma glucose concentrations need to be distinguished from the more common situation of a patient with a 'funny turn' in whom an insulinoma needs to be excluded. Those patients used to be admitted for a two-day fast, in which it was important to maintain exercise to try to provoke hypoglycaemia. If at any time the fasting plasma glucose fell below the normal range, a blood sample would be taken for plasma insulin assay to demonstrate excess secretion. However, this test is uncomfortable for patients, and is expensive, requiring hospital admission. Two alternative *dynamic suppression tests* are available:

1. *Fish insulin* can be administered over a two-hour period to induce hypoglycaemia, with measurement of the *endogenous plasma human insulin concentration* with an antibody which does not detect fish insulin. Hypoglycaemia can be induced in all subjects, and one can determine if insulin secretion has been appropriately suppressed, or inappropriately remains elevated.

2. Fish insulin is not widely available, and the alternative is to induce hypoglycaemia with any insulin, and then measure the *plasma C-peptide* which is secreted on an equimolar basis with each insulin molecule. The greater C-peptide than insulin differences

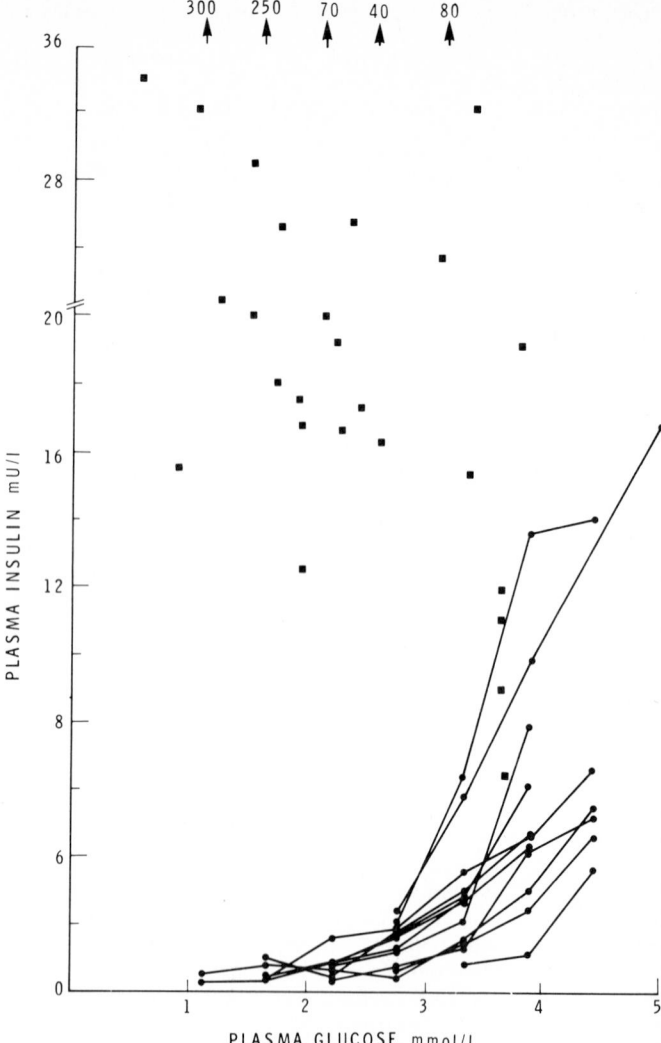

Fig. 1   Inordinately raised fasting plasma insulin concentrations after an overnight fast in 30 patients with *insulinomas* (each shown as a black square). The lines show suppression of plasma human insulin by hypoglycaemia induced by a fish insulin suppression test in 12 normal subjects. The majority of patients with insulinomas have a diagnostic high plasma insulin during their spontaneous hypoglycaemia. Those with normal fasting plasma glucose fail to suppress their plasma insulin to < 1.5 mU/l during a hypoglycaemic suppression test. (Adapted from Turner, R. C. (1976). Hypoglycaemia: Proceedings of European Symposium, Rome. *Horm. Metab. Res.* **6**, 40)

between species means that endogenous beta cell secretion can be monitored by a specific human C-peptide immunoassay.

A simple method of diagnosing insulinomas is to measure the *fasting plasma pro-insulin*. The tumours are always moderately undifferentiated. and secrete a high proportion of pro-insulin. There is an apparent complete distinction between normal subjects and those with insulinomas, even with normal fasting plasma glucose levels. In theory, therefore, a single fasting plasma pro-insulin assay would be an ideal way to diagnose an insulinoma. However, pro-insulin assays are not yet widely available. In their absence the basis of the diagnosis rests on (*a*) documentation of a spontaneous hypoglycaemic episode, and (*b*) inordinately high insulin secretion during hypoglycaemia.

Self-administration of insulin until now has usually been easily detected, because impure insulin preparations have induced insulin antibodies, which can be detected with a suitable modification of the insulin immunoassay. The development of pure pork and human insulins, which are rarely immunogenic, will make detection of self-administration more difficult. If a blood sample is taken when the patient has a hypoglycaemic episode, the presence of immunoreactive insulin, in the absence of immunoreactive C-peptide or pro-insulin, confirms the exogenous origin of the insulin.

Self-medication with sulphonylurea presents exactly like an insulinoma. These patients can usually only be detected because of clinical suspicion which leads to discovery of sulphonylurea tablets in a patient's possession. The wide variety of sulphonylurea drugs makes detection of sulphonylurea compounds in urine or plasma very difficult.

Localization of insulinoma. Coeliac axis angiography localizes an adenoma in 60–70 per cent of patients, but additional superior mesenteric artery angiography may be needed for an adenoma in the uncinate lobe of the head or of the pancreas. Extra-pancreatic insulinomas are exceedingly rare, with three poorly documented cases of insulinoma from an abdominal carcinoid, and one from a bronchial carcinoid. If arteriography fails to show an insulinoma, it can still be assumed to be in the pancreas, but is also usually too small to be detected either by computerized tomography or ultrasonography.

Treatment of insulinoma. If a tumour is seen on angiography, it can usually be enucleated at laparotomy without need for resection of the pancreas. If not apparent on angiography, a tumour can often be palpated at operation after mobilization of the pancreas. In those cases in which a tumour cannot be found, distal pancreatectomy should *not* be undertaken as the tumour is most likely to be hidden in the head of the pancreas. The abdomen should then be closed, and the patient later referred to a centre which undertakes percutaneous trans-hepatic cannulation of the portal vein for multiple blood sampling of effluent from the pancreas in the portal, splenic, and superior mesenteric veins. High localized plasma insulin concentrations indicate the position of the tumour. If this technique is readily available, it is reasonable to use it prior to laparotomy in a patient in whom the tumour cannot be seen on angiography. If the tumour is in the body or tail of the pancreas, it can subsequently be removed by distal pancreatectomy. If the tumour is localized to the head of the pancreas, operation is technically more difficult, and medical therapy with *diazoxide* is usually preferable. This approach only relieves symptoms in about 50 per cent of patients, and may induce nausea or, in women, hirsutes. Sodium retention can be counteracted with a diuretic. Despite its limitations, medical, rather than surgical, treatment can be the therapy of choice in elderly, or other patients in whom surgery is undesirable.

Malignant insulinomas occur in about 5 per cent of patients, and often hepatic metastases have developed by the time of presentation. Diazoxide is usually of little benefit. Streptozotocin, particularly combined with fluorouracil, can dramatically decrease the size of the tumour and its deposits and relieve persistent hypoglycaemia. Relapse usually occurs within a year, but some patients are symptom free for two or three years. Death may ensue from uncontrollable hypoglycaemia or from metastases.

Tumours of the islets may secrete more than one hormone, and patients with insulinomas, particularly when malignant, may have symptoms from hypersecretion of gastrin or somatostatin.

Multiple endocrine adenoma syndrome. Insulinomas can be multiple, or associated with other peptide secreting tumours, e.g. parathyroid tumours and acromegaly as part of the type I multiple endocrine adenoma (MEA) syndrome. All these tumours are characterized by similar histological staining revealing amine precursor uptake and decarboxylation (apud), a property which may be related to a common embryological origin from neural crest cells. This syndrome may be familial, with other members of the family also harbouring endocrine tumours. Insulinomas are not associated with the MEA type II syndrome, including hyperparathyroid, phaeochromocytoma, and various neuro-ectodermal defects.

Reactive post-prandial hypoglycaemia

Alimentary hypoglycaemia. Several abnormalities of the gastrointestinal tract can give rise to rapid gastric emptying, with brisk absorption of glucose and prompt release of enteric insulin-stimulating hormones which induce excessive insulin release and hypoglycaemia 90 minutes to three hours after a meal. These phenomena can occur following partial gastrectomy, gastrojejunostomy or pyloroplasty, and are particularly provoked by a meal with a high refined carbohydrate content. The symptoms are distinct from the 'dumping' syndrome of light headedness, sweating, and fullness of the abdomen which occurs about 30 minutes after a meal.

Diabetes. Patients with mild diabetes and near-normal fasting plasma glucose levels occasionally present with post-prandial hypoglycaemia two to four hours after a meal. An initial subnormal insulin response to a meal leads to hyperglycaemia which may stimulate sufficient late insulin release to produce reactive hypoglycaemia. The symptoms disappear as diabetes progresses and fasting hyperglycaemia ensues.

Idiopathic reactive hypoglycaemia is the most frequently diagnosed form of post-prandial hypoglycaemia in the USA. The diagnosis is usually made because of attacks of tiredness, loss of concentration, faintness, perspiration, or palpitation a few hours after a meal, and an oral glucose tolerance test shows a rebound 'hypoglycaemia'. However, many of these patients do not have symptoms at the same time. It is normal for plasma glucose to fall to 2.5–3 mmol/l 90–150 minutes after a glucose tolerance test, and similar hypoglycaemia is often not seen after a normal meal. It is probable that many of these patients have adrenergic symptoms secondary to stress and anxiety, rather than to hypoglycaemia. Patients with symptomatic reactive hypoglycaemia can most easily be treated by appropriately timed snacks between meals.

Treatment of hypoglycaemia. If a patient is semi-conscious and unable to take glucose by mouth, 20–30 ml of 50 per cent glucose is given intravenously, repeated as necessary. The administering needle should not be withdrawn from the vein immediately, as the pressure on the vein to secure haemostasis maintains the glucose in the vein and can cause venous thrombosis. There should either be a pause before withdrawing the needle, or the glucose followed by an intravenous injection of saline.

Hypoglycaemia of short duration does not produce obvious permanent neurological sequelae, but the longer the hypoglycaemia the longer it takes for normal cerebral function to recover. If the patient remains unconscious for longer than 30 minutes, it is possible that secondary cerebral oedema may occur; mannitol or dexamethasone therapy sometimes appear to expedite recovery.

Hypoglycaemia in childhood. A completely separate differential diagnosis applies to hypoglycaemia in children compared with adults. In the neonatal period, hypoglycaemia is found in small-for-dates babies with poor liver glycogen reserves, and in babies of diabetic mothers who have excess insulin secretion.

Nesidioblastosis is a rare condition causing persistent hypoglycaemia in the neonatal period. A developmental abnormality of the pancreas includes a large number of duct overgrowths associated with beta cells which are not distributed as normally in islets, but in 'nests', the pathological feature which provides the name of the disorder. The beta cells in this condition, as in insulinomas, are semi-autonomous, and their excess insulin secretion causes hypoglycaemia. A defect of somatostatin cells and secretion of somatostatin has been suggested to be a cause of the increased insulin secretion. The infants seldom respond to glucagon or diazoxide, and usually require 95 or even 100 per cent pancreatectomy. It is very important to monitor closely and maintain the baby's plasma glucose concentration during diagnosis, to prevent long-term brain damage and mental retardation. An infusion of somatostatin, in addition to glucose, can be a useful temporary measure whilst surgery is being planned.

Several rare hepatic enzyme defects present in childhood. These include type I glycogen storage disease, galactosaemia, and fructose intolerance. 'Leucine-sensitive hypoglycaemia' probably relates to patients with either nesidioblastosis or an insulinoma, and may not be a separate entity.

Ketotic hypoglycaemia is the common form of hypoglycaemia in infancy, usually presenting at the age of one to eight in boys, who have often been small-for-dates when born. A defect in hepatic glucose efflux can be due to several causes, including hepatic glycogen synthetase deficiency, decreased release of glucogenic aminoacids from muscles, or decreased adrenergic stimulation. Symptoms of drowsiness or fits usually present after a period without food, often induced by an intercurrent illness, or after exercise. A low plasma glucose reduces plasma insulin, so leading to the ketosis which is a feature of the disease. Frequent feeding prevents attacks, which disappear in adult life.

References

Fajans, S. S., Floyd, J. C., Jr, and Vij, S. K. (1975). Differential diagnosis of spontaneous hypoglycaemia. In *Endocrinology and diabetes* (eds. L. Kryston and S. Shaw), 453. Grune and Stratton, New York.

Gorden, P., Hendricks, C. M., Kahn, C. R., Megyesi, K., and Roth, J. (1981). Hyperglycaemia associated with non-islet-cell tumour and insulin-like growth factors. *New Engl. J. Med.* **305**, 1452.

Moertel, C. G., Hanley, J. A., and Johnson, L. A. (1980). Streptozotocin alone compared with streptozotocin plus fluorouracil in the treatment of advanced islet-cell carcinoma. *New Engl. J. Med.* **303**, 1189.

Service, F. J., Dale, A. J. D., Elveback, L. R., and Tiang, N-S. (1976). Insulinoma: Clinical and diagnostic features in 60 consective cases. *Mayo Clin. Proc.* **51**, 417.

Turner, R. C., Lee, E. C. G., Morris, P. J., Harris, E. A., and Dick, R. (1978). Localisation of insulinomas. *Lancet* **i**, 515.

INBORN ERRORS OF CARBOHYDRATE METABOLISM

R. W. E. Watts

Glycogen storage diseases

Glycogen is a high molecular weight glucose polymer with a branched structure and about 12 glucose residues between the branch points. All mammalian cells have the capacity to make glycogen, but the extent of this depends on their function. Glycogen is abundant in the liver, where it is used predominantly to form blood glucose, and in muscle where it is the fuel for muscle contraction. The brain contains very little glycogen although it uses glucose preferentially as a source of energy.

Glycogen synthetase catalyses the addition of single glucose residues to the ends of the polysaccharide chains, and branching enzyme catalyses the intramolecular rearrangement which produces the branches. Phosphorylase mobilizes glucose from the ends of the chains until a branch point is reached, debranching enzyme catalyses the degradation of this region of the molecule after which phosphorylase catalyses further chain shortening. Some glycogen is also synthesized by the reversed action of phosphorylase acting with branching enzyme, and producing the same overall effect as that of glycogen synthetase and branching enzyme. This process of glucose storage and mobilization occurs in the cytosol. Glycogen, which becomes incorporated into lysosomes by either autophagy or endocytosis, is hydrolized directly to glucose within the lysosome under the catalytic influence of α-glucosidase. The amylases also break down glycogen directly to glucose. Fig. 1 shows the metabolic inter-relationships of glycogen and glucose and the sites of the metabolic lesions in the main types of the glycogen storage diseases.

Table 1 summarizes the classification and biochemistry of the glycogen storage diseases. The glycogen is in the cytosol fraction of the cells in all except Type II which is a lysosomal storage disease. Their combined incidence is about 1 in 60 000 and, except for type IXB they are all inherited as autosomal recessives. Precise diagnosis requires direct tissue assay of the enzymes concerned,

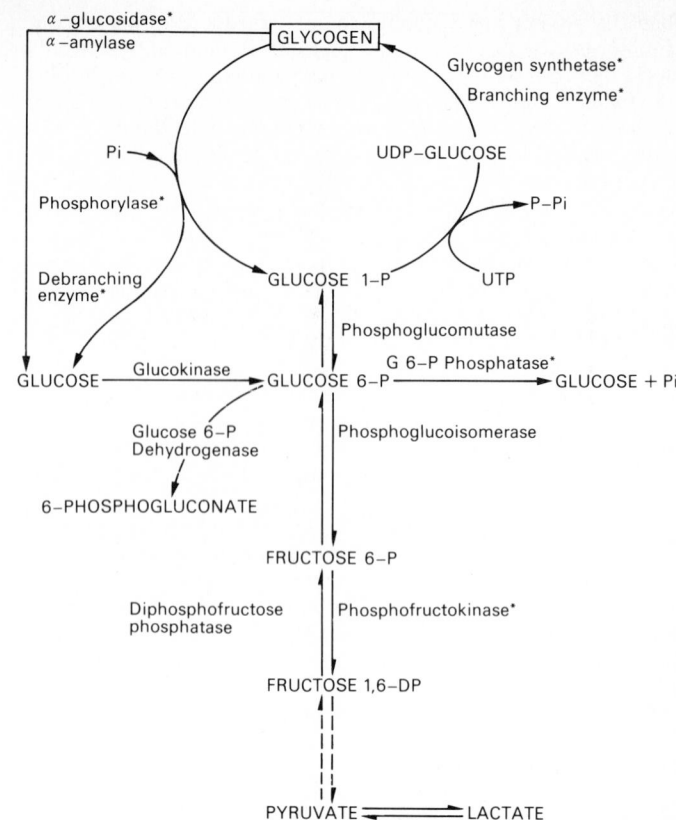

Fig. 1   The metabolic pathways leading to and from glycogen. Deficiency of each of the enzymes marked * cause a different glycogen storage disease. See Table 1. Glucose 1-P = glucose 1-phosphate; glucose 6-P = glucose 6-phosphate; UDP-glucose = uridine diphosphate glucose; fructose 1,6-DP = fructose 1,6-diphosphate; UTP = uridine triphosphate; P-Pi = inorganic pyrophosphate; Pi = inorganic orthophosphate.

measurement of the tissue glycogen content, and studies of its structure. Open liver biopsy is recommended. The tissue should be frozen immediately, wrapped in aluminium foil, kept in the deep frozen state in a sealed container until it is to be analysed, and the surgeon should not use starch-containing glove powder. Histochemical and electron microscopic examination of biopsy tissues may provide ancillary information on the distribution of glycogen and of some of the enzyme activities.

Studies of the response of the blood glucose and lactate to glucagon, adrenalin, and different sugars may give some preliminary diagnostic help, but they do not provide definitive information. Failure of the lactate content of the venous return from an ischaemic exercising limb to rise suggests a diagnosis of one of the muscle glycogenoses.

Type I (Von Gierke's disease, glucose 6-phosphatase deficiency)

Clinical aspects. Hepatic enlargement is present at birth, and abdominal distension may be the presenting symptom. These children rapidly become hypoglycaemic on fasting and the stress of an intercurrent infection or surgical operation may precipitate fatal hypoglycaemia and lactic acidosis. They are otherwise resistant to the effects of hypoglycaemia because the brain adapts to using the ketone bodies as a source of energy instead of glucose. Growth is stunted but there is no mental handicap. Obesity and a round florid 'doll-like' facies are characteristic. The skeletal musculature is hypotonic and poorly developed, the bones are osteoporotic, the kidneys are enlarged, and the optic fundi show discrete yellow paramacular lesions. Xanthomata develop on the extensor aspects of the limbs and have to be distinguished from the gouty tophi which appear in early adult life. Impaired platelet function causes an abnormal bleeding tendency.

Table 1 Glycogen storage diseases

Type	Name	Main site of glycogen storage	Glycogen structure	Enzyme defect	Tissue for diagnostic enzymology
I	Von Gierke	liver, kidney, intestine	normal	glucose 6-phosphatase	liver, jejunal mucosa
II	Pompé	liver, myocardium, muscle	normal	lysosomal α-glucosidase (acid maltase)	liver, muscle, leucocytes, fibroblasts, amniotic cells
III	Forbes (Cori's limit dextrinosis)	(a) liver and muscle (b) liver	short outer branches	amylo 1,6-glucosidase (debranching enzyme)	liver, muscle, leucocytes, fibroblasts, amniotic cells
IV	Andersen (amylopectinosis)	liver	long outer branches	1,4-α-glucan branching enzyme	liver, fibroblasts, leucocytes, amniotic cells
V	McArdle	muscle	normal	phosphorylase (muscle)	muscle
VI	Hers	liver	normal	phosphorylase (liver)	liver, muscle
VII	Tauri	muscle	normal	phosphofructokinase	muscle, erythrocytes
VIII	—	liver and brain	normal	phosphorylase (mainly in inactive form in spite of normal phosphorylase kinase)	liver
IX	—	(a) liver and muscle	normal	phosphorylase kinase (autosomal recessive)	liver
		(b) liver and muscle		phosphorylase kinase (sex-linked recessive)	
X	—	liver and muscle	normal	phosphorylase kinase (partial deficiency loss of 3′,5′-cAMP dependent kinase activity)	liver, muscle
XI	—	liver and kidney	normal	none suggested	
O	—	gross deficiency of liver glycogen	normal	glycogen synthetase	liver

Biochemical aspects. The hypoglycaemia is unresponsive to adrenaline, glucagon, or to the intravenous administration of galactose or fructose. Infusion of these sugars may precipitate acidosis. There is a marked hyperlipidaemia (involving triglycerides, phospholipids, and cholesterol), hyperlactic acidaemia, and sometimes acidosis. Ketosis is not a feature. There is both abnormal retention and increased endogenous synthesis of urate, causing tophaceous gout and gouty arthritis in later childhood and early adult life. Impaired renal tubular transport functions, due to glucose 6-phosphate toxicity and glycogen accumulation, may be associated with a generalized amino aciduria and some other components of the Fanconi syndrome although glycosuria is unlikely because of the low blood sugar levels. An increased incidence of hepatoma has been reported in Type I patients who survive into adult life.

Types I, III, VI, and IX are the most frequently confused of the glycogen storage diseased, and their differentiation requires the detailed study of liver tissue. Some cases are encountered with all the stigmata of Type I but no identifiable enzyme abnormality *in vitro*. This may reflect an abnormality of the membrane binding of the enzyme in the cells which prevents it working normally *in vivo* but not *in vitro*.

Treatment. Treatment aims to maintain normoglycaemia throughout the whole 24-hour period. This has usually been done by 2-hourly feeds of glucose and starch, the latter as a slow release source of glucose. Nasogastric drip feeding with glucose at night is a major advance in the management of these children. Provided that normoglycaemia is achieved and maintained, the other biochemical parameters also improve. There is catch-up growth and normal somatic development, the liver becomes smaller and the decreased platelet adhesiveness is corrected. It should be emphasized that the successfully treated patients lose their ability to withstand hypoglycaemia.

The crises associated with intercurrent infections and other stressful situations require intravenous glucose and sodium bicarbonate with close biochemical monitoring as well as vigorous treatment of the precipitating cause.

Prognosis. Type I glycogen storage disease carries a high mortality and morbidity in the early years of life unless the risk of acute episodes of hypoglycaemia and lactic acidosis is recognized and

unless an efficient regimen to maintain normoglycaemia throughout the 24-hour period is instituted. The patients who survive into adult life are mainly troubled by the complications of their hyperuricaemia and this can be satisfactorily controlled with allopurinol. The increased incidence of hepatoma is disturbing.

Type II (α-glucosidase deficiency). All tissues of the body, including the motor nuclei of the brain stem and spinal cord and the Schwann cells are involved. There are infantile, juvenile, and adult variants.

Patients with the classical infantile form (Pompé's disease) present during the first months of life with cardiac enlargement and failure, and with generalized muscle hypotonia without muscle wasting. The QRS complexes are large and the PR interval is short. The blood sugar, lipids, and ketones and the responses to adrenaline and glucagon are normal. Treatment is symptomatic and few patients survive beyond the first six months of life. The differential diagnoses are those of congestive cardiac failure due to congenital heart disease and the other causes of gross muscle hypotonia in infancy such as the inherited neuromuscular diseases.

The juvenile variant presents in infancy or early childhood and progresses more slowly than the infantile form. Muscle involvement is the only constant feature. The patients die in the second or third decade.

The adult type presents as a slowly developing adult onset myopathy.

Type III (Forbes' disease; debrancher enzyme deficiency). This is a relatively mild disease resembling Type I. There is a variable degree of hypoglycaemia, massive hepatomegaly, slowly progressive myopathy, and some asymptomatic cardiac enlargement in older patients. Mild hyperlipidaemia and hyperuricaemia are inconstant features. Glucagon and adrenaline raise the blood sugar in the fed but not in the fasting state, and galactose and fructose infusions also raise the blood sugar.

Treatment involves the effective correction of hypoglycaemia. Extra dietary protein has also been recommended on the grounds that gluconeogenesis is enhanced. The prognosis appears to be good from the viewpoint of both life expectancy and morbidity.

Type IV (Andersen's disease; branching enzyme deficiency). Hepatomegaly and failure to thrive appear during the first months of life. There is cirrhosis with portal hypertension, ascites and splenomegaly, muscle hypotonia, and death during the first three years of life. Only symptomatic treatments for the liver failure and ascites are available.

Type V (McArdle's disease, muscle phosphorylase deficiency). These patients usually present in adult life with muscle cramps after exertion which may be associated with myoglobinuria. They may give a history of undue fatiguability in childhood and adolescence, and they develop increasingly severe proximal muscle wasting and weakness as they grow older. The disease is compatible with a normal life span and little morbidity. It is not associated with hypoglycaemia. Lactate dehydrogenase, creatine phosphokinase and aldolase leak out of the muscles on exertion. The lactate content of blood draining a muscle which is exercising under ischaemic conditions does not increase as is normally the case.

Histologically, the muscles show central migration of the nuclei, and subsarcolemmal glycogen deposits. The latter changes are more marked in Type I fibres and the Type II fibres may be a little hypertrophied.

Type VI (Hers disease, liver phosphorylase deficiency). Some authorities have grouped all cases of glycogen storage disease which do not belong to Types I–V under this heading. This is unsatisfactory and the term Type VI glycogen storage disease should be reserved for patients with biochemically proven virtually complete deficiency of liver phosphorylase. There is marked hepatomegaly, no splenomegaly, no hypoglycaemia, no acidosis, no hyperlipidaemia, and no rise in blood sugar after glucagon administration. Mental development is normal and the overall prognosis is good. These patients are sometimes confused with mild cases of Type I.

Type VII (Tauri disease; muscle phosphofructokinase deficiency). These patients resemble Type V.

Type IX (phosphorylase kinase deficiency). Patients with this disorder were formerly included in Type VI which they resemble clinically. Autosomal recessive and sex-linked recessive variants exist. There is marked hepatomegaly, no splenomegaly, no hypoglycaemia or acidosis and, unlike Type VI, a normal rise in blood sugar after glucagon. The prognosis is good and no treatment may be needed. The liver size may decrease in adulthood although the enzyme defect persists.

Types VIII, X, XI, and O. Type VIII patients present in early childhood with hepatomegaly, increased hepatic glycogen, increased catechol amine excretion and progressive degenerative brain disease with death in mid-childhood. Axon cylinders and synapses in the brain contain abnormal glycogen deposits.

Type X is a very rare liver and muscle glycogenosis presenting in childhood with mild muscle cramps and hepatomegaly.

Type XI are children in whom renal tubule dysfunction is especially prominent. They show stunted growth and hepatomegaly, but mental development is normal. Their response to glucagon is impaired but the metabolic lesion has not been identified.

Patients with liver glycogen synthetase deficiency (Type O) have fasting hypoglycaemia, prolonged hyperglycaemia after glucose administration, and mental handicap. Frequent protein-rich feeds prevent the hypoglycaemic attacks and can promote normal psychomotor development. Their muscle glycogen synthetase activity is normal.

Inborn errors of galactose metabolism

Galactose is converted to glucose by four sequential metabolic reactions (Fig. 2) and metabolic lesions affecting the first three of these are known. They all produce a measurable level of circulating galactose and are detected by the recently developed bacterial inhibition screening test for galactose in blood. The term galactosaemia is customarily used for the galactose 1-phosphate uridyl transferase deficiency which is the commonest of the group. The clinical manifestations in galactosaemia are due to the toxic actions of galactose 1-phosphate which accumulates behind the metabolic block. The cataracts which are a feature of both galactosaemia and galactokinase deficiency result from the action of galactitol which is formed via alternative metabolic pathways which become operative at high galactose concentrations.

$$\text{Galactose} + \text{ATP} \xrightarrow{\text{Galactokinase}} \text{Galactose 1-phosphate} + \text{ADP}$$
$$\text{Galactose 1-phosphate} + \text{UDP glucose} \longrightarrow \text{UDP galactose} + \text{glucose 1-phosphate}$$

$$\text{UDP galactose} \longrightarrow \text{UDP glucose}$$
$$\text{UDP glucose} + \text{P-Pi} \longrightarrow \text{UTP} + \text{glucose 1-phosphate}$$

Fig. 2 The galactose–glucose interconversion pathway. ATP = adenosine triphosphate; ADP = adenosine diphosphate; UDP = uridine diphosphate; UTP = uridine triphosphate; P-Pi = pyrophosphate.

Galactosaemia (galactose 1-phosphate uridyl transferase deficiency)

Clinical aspects. The incidence of galactosaemia is about 1:60 000 births and it is inherited in an autosomal recessive manner. The symptoms classically begin a few days after birth. The infant rejects its feeds, develops diarrhoea and becomes hypoglycaemic, acidotic, and dehydrated. The liver enlarges, jaundice, ascites, proteinuria, and a generalized amino aciduria develop, and in the absence of treatment, the child dies within a few weeks. Cataracts may be detectable with a slit lamp at birth and they usually become obvious if the baby survives beyond a few weeks. Older children who have survived without treatment show marked psychomotor retardation, hepatic cirrhosis, and a Fanconi syndrome. Some cases develop a Gram-negative septicaemia immediately after birth and die during the first day or two of life. These patients remain undetected unless a specimen of umbilical cord blood (erythrocytes) is examined for galactose 1-phosphate uridyl transferase activity. The diagnosis should always be confirmed enzymologically; blood galactose or galactose 1-phosphate, and urine galactose levels should not be the sole criteria for diagnosis. Prenatal and carrier state diagnosis are both possible.

Genetic variants. There are two well recognized genetic variants of galactosaemia: the Duarte and Negro variants. Patients with the Duarte variant have about half the normal erythrocyte galactose 1-phosphate uridyl transferase activity and are asymptomatic; they may be confused with individuals who are heterozygous, the classical type of galactosaemia. Electrophoretic analysis differentiates the two abnormal enzymes. Double heterozygotes for classical galactosaemia and the Duarte variant have been described. Patients with the Negro variant have no detectable galactose 1-phosphate uridyl transferase activity in their erythrocytes, but retain about 10 per cent of the normal level of activity in their liver and small intestine. They may show galactose toxicity in infancy. Other galactose 1-phosphate uridyl transferase polymorphisms have been described, including one, the Los Angeles variant, with supernormal catalytic activity.

Treatment. A diet containing as little galactose as possible is essential, and a milk substitute such as Nutramigen must be used in infancy. It has been customary to relax the diet when the child is 7–10 years of age, although there is increasing evidence to suggest that dietary restriction of galactose intake should be life long. Treatment is controlled by measuring the erythrocyte galactose 1-phosphate concentration, blood and urine galactose measurements being too insensitive for this purpose. The galactose restricted diet should certainly be reintroduced before galactosaemic women conceive in order to avoid the heterozygous fetus being damaged by the mother's galactose 1-phosphate and galactitol.

Prognosis. Untreated infants with classical galactosaemia rarely survive more than a few months. Treatment starting at birth prevents the acute manifestations of galactose 1-phosphate intoxication, the liver and ocular damage. The long-term outlook from the viewpoint of intellectual development is less certain. Many early and conscientiously treated children develop normally but a minority are left with some degree of handicap. Any delay in starting the dietary treatment and any relaxation of it in early childhood worsens the prognosis. Furthermore, the possibility of some prenatal brain damage cannot be excluded. The patients should be followed up throughout childhood and adolescence and preferably into adult life, with particular reference to their psychological and emotional development, liver function, and possible cataract formation.

Galactokinase deficiency. The incidence of galactokinase deficiency is about 1:100 000 births, and it is inherited as an autosomal recessive.

Cataracts are the only clinical manifestation and the diagnosis should be considered in any child with this presentation. They are prevented but not cured by a galactose restricted diet.

Galactokinase is assayed on erythrocytes. Heterozygotes can be detected by this means, and screening the cord blood of siblings of known cases for galactokinase will permit early treatment. Galactokinase deficiency can be diagnosed prenatally.

Uridine diphosphate 4'-epimerase deficiency. The reported examples of this metabolic lesion have been asymptomatic. Its incidence is about 1:50 000 and the pattern of inheritance is autosomal recessive.

The enzyme is assayed on red blood cells and both the homozygous and heterozygous individuals can be identified.

Pentosuria

Pentosuria is due to an inherited deficiency of L-xylulose reductase which causes a metabolic block in the glucuronic acid cycle with the excretion of several grams of L-xylulose daily. This is increased by feeding glucuronolactone or drugs which are excreted as glucuronides and which therefore stimulate glucuronic acid synthesis. Pentosuria is of no clinical significance except that L-xylulose reduces the alkaline copper reagents (e.g. Clinitest) which are used to detect glycosuria, and so may lead to an erroneous provisional diagnosis of diabetes mellitus. It does not react with the glucose oxidase based reagents (e.g. Clinistix). The incidence of pentosuria among Ashkenazi Jews is between about 1:2000 and 1:5000. It rarely, if ever occurs in non-Askenazi Jewish subjects and is inherited in an autosomal recessive manner. The specific enzyme defect can be demonstrated in erythrocytes. Individuals who are heterozygous for the abnormal gene concerned have enzyme levels intermediate between normal subjects and those who are homozygous for the abnormal gene. The heterozygous individuals also have some impairment of the ability to metabolize a glucuronolactone load.

Inborn errors of pyruvate metabolism

Pyruvate dehydrogenase deficiency. The pyruvate dehydrogenase complex catalyses the oxidative decarboxylation of pyruvate, and a deficiency of the decarboxylase part of the complex has been recognized. Pyruvate accumulates and is either transaminated to alanine or reduced to lactate so that the patients have hyperalaninaemia and hyperalaninuria with increased levels of lactate and pyruvate in the body fluids. The latter may only be intermittent and may not always produce an acidosis. The patients usually present with intermittent cerebellar ataxia, torsion dystonia, and involuntary eye movements beginning in early childhood, and follow a progressive downhill course. More acute presentations with neonatal acidosis and muscular hypotonia, and cases presenting as hereditary spinocerebellar degeneration in early adult life, have also been described.

The enzyme defect can be demonstrated in leucocytes and fibroblasts and the less severe syndromes are associated with more residual enzyme activity. Thiamine and lipoate responsive and non-responsive variants are described. Autosomal recessive inheritance appears to be usual. The extent to which the hereditary spinocerebellar ataxias can be regarded as inborn errors of the pyruvate dehydrogenase complex is uncertain.

Pyruvate carboxylase. Pyruvate carboxylase is a biotin dependent enzyme which catalyses the production of oxaloacetate for gluconeogenesis, lipogenesis, and the supply of tricarboxylic acid cycle intermediates. The patients either present in the neonatal period with collapse, hypoglycaemia, and acidosis, or they survive for a few years with mental handicap and brain damage. Others present the picture of Leigh's encephalomyelopathy in which there is hypotonia, ocular palsies, and progressive psychomotor retardation, and retrogression beginning in infancy. The body fluids contain increased concentrations of pyruvate, lactate, and alanine. The metabolic lesion can be demonstrated in liver tissue. Thiamine and lipoic acid, both of which are cofactors in the pyruvate dehydrogenase system have been reported to modify the biochemical changes. Another approach to treatment has been to give large doses of L-glutamate or aspartate with pyridoxine in order to increase the supply of tricarboxylic acid cycle intermediates and thereby improve the supply of oxaloacetate.

Inherited carbohydrate intolerance

The enzymes which complete the hydrolysis of starch and glycogen to glucose, and lactase and sucrase which cleave lactose and sucrose to their respective constituent monosaccharides are situated in the brush border of the small intestine epithelium. Glucose and galactose are absorbed by an energy and sodium ion requiring active transport process and fructose is absorbed by facilitated diffusion.

There are three inherited carbohydrate malabsorption syndromes. They have non-specific symptomatology due to the osmotic action of unabsorbed carbohydrate and the results of its bacterial degradation in the intestine. Other absorptive processes are inhibited and there is secondary malabsorption of fat in about 30 per cent of patients.

An isolated deficiency of lactase with lactose intolerance occurs in such a large proportion of some non-Europeans (acquired isolated lactase deficiency) who have been fed milk in infancy without any problems that a decrease in intestinal lactase activity should probably be regarded as physiological, at least in these individuals. It may be that the non-development of acquired isolated lactase deficiency in other races who have practised dairying for millennia results from natural selection.

The inherited carbohydrate intolerance syndromes are summarized in Table 2, p. 9.56. They have to be distinguished from carbohydrate intolerance due to diffuse intestinal disease and surgical resections. This subject is dealt with in Section 12.

References

Blass, J. P. (1980). Pyruvate dehydrogenase deficiencies. In *Inherited disorders of carbohydrate metabolism* (eds. D. Burman, J. B. Holton, and C. A. Pennock), 239. MTP Press, Lancaster.

Fernandes, J. (1980). Hepatic glycogenoses: diagnosis and management. In *Inherited disorders of carbohydrate metabolism* (eds. D. Burman, J. B. Holton, and C. A. Pennock), 297. MTP Press, Lancaster.

Gitzelmann, R. and Hansen, R. G. (1980). Galactose metabolism hereditary defects and their clinical significance. In *Inherited disorders of carbohydrate metabolism* (eds. D. Burman, J. B. Holton, and C. A. Pannock), 61. MTP Press, Lancaster.

Hug, C. (1980). Pre- and postnatal diagnosis of glycogen storage disease. In *Inherited disorders of carbohydrate metabolism* (eds. D. Burman, J. B. Holton, and C. A. Pennock), 327. MTP Press, Lancaster.

Hommes, F. H., Schriver, J., and Dias, Th. (1980). Pyruvate carboxylase deficiency, studies on patients and on an animal model system. In *Inher-*

Table 2 Inherited carbohydrate intolerance syndromes

Disorder	Pathophysiology	Treatment

1 Lactose intolerance
  Lactase deficient
    Congenital and permanent in infants and children
	autosomal recessively inherited abnormality of intestinal lactase (β-galactosidase)	lactose-free diet

Temporary, especially in premature infants	delayed enzyme maturation	
Acquired isolated lactase deficiency	physiological loss of enzyme activity in some racial groups	
Non-lactase deficient	? toxic effect of lactose which is unrelated to an enzyme deficiency	
2 Sucrose intolerance	autosomal recessively inherited abnormality of intestinal sucrase (β-fructose furanosidase)	sucrose-free diet
3 Trehalose intolerance	autosomal dominantly inherited deficiency of trehalase	exclude dietary trehalase (present in young mushrooms)
4 Glucose–galactose malabsorption	autosomal recessively inherited abnormality of the energy mediated carrier system for glucose and galactose. Associated glycosuria due to renal tubular reabsorption defect	fructose as sole source of carbohydrate

ited disorders of carbohydrate metabolism (eds. D. Burman, J. B. Holton, and C. A. Pennock), 269. MTP Press, Lancaster.

Ryman, B. E. (1974). The glycogen storage diseases. *J. clin. Path.* **27**, Suppl. **8**, 106.

— (1975). The glycogen storage diseases. In *The principles and practice of diagnostic enzymology* (ed. J. H. Wilkinson), 503. Arnold, London.

Stacey, T. E., Macnab, A., and Strang, L. B. (1980). Recent work on treatment of Type I glycogen storage disease. In *Inherited disorders of carbohydrate metabolism* (eds. D. Burman, J. B. Holton, and C. A. Pennock), 315. MTP Press, Lancaster.

Inborn errors of fructose metabolism

H. F. Woods

D-Fructose is a normal dietary constituent being widely distributed among fruits and vegetables, in honey, and as a constituent of the disaccharide sucrose. The average Western diet provides 50–100 g of fructose per day.

Three metabolic defects in fructose metabolism have been described in man: (*a*) essential fructosuria (EF); (*b*) hereditary fructose intolerance (HFI); and (*c*) fructose 1, 6-diphosphatase deficiency (FDD). All are due to either a total or partial lack of an enzyme involved in fructose metabolism together with secondary enzyme inhibitions in HFI and FDD. The defects are best discussed in the light of normal fructose metabolism.

Normal fructose metabolism (Fig. 1). Fructose is absorbed from the gut lumen via a specific transport mechanism. Once absorbed, the main site of fructose metabolism is in the liver, the small intestine and kidney having a small capacity to metabolize fructose.

The first step is the phosphorylation to fructose 1-phosphate a reaction catalysed by the enzyme fructokinase. In the mammalian liver this enzyme has a high maximal rate and a low Km so that this organ has a large capacity to metabolize fructose. The fructose 1-phosphate is then split via the adolase reaction to form dihydroxyacetone phosphate and D-glyceraldehyde. Aldolase can also split fructose 1, 6-diphosphate into the triose phosphates, dihydroxyacetone phosphate and D-glyceraldehyde 3-phosphate. This is a reversible reaction, the two triose phosphates reacting to give fructose 1, 6-diphosphate.

Once formed from fructose the D-glyceraldehyde can follow three pathways (Fig. 1):

1. Phosphorylation to D-glyceraldehyde 3-phosphate.

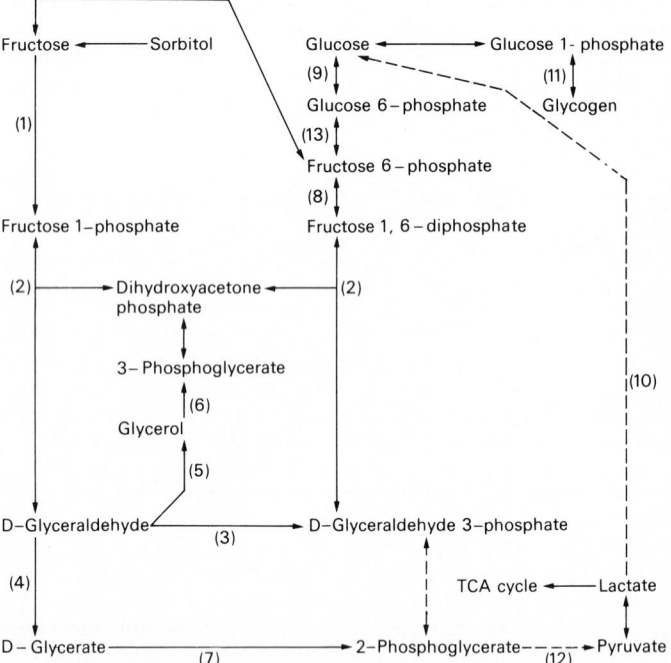

Fig. 1 The pathways of fructose metabolism—enzyme defects in inherited disorders of fructose metabolism. The enzymes and enzyme sequences are numbered as follows: (1) Fructokinase; (2) aldolase; (3) triokinase; (4) aldehyde dehydrogenase; (5) alcohol dehydrogenase; (6) glycerol kinase; (7) glycerate kinase; (8) fructose 1,6-diphosphatase; (9) hexokinase; (10) the gluconeogenic pathway; (11) the glycogenolytic pathway; (12) the glycolytic pathway; (13) phosphohexose isomerase. The enzyme defects in the inborn errors of metabolism are as follows:

Primary enzyme defect		Secondary enzyme defect
EF	(1)	nil
HFI	(2)	(1), (11), (2), (13)
FDD	(8)	(11)

2. Oxidation to glycerate and subsequent metabolism to 2-phosphoglycerate.

3. Reduction to form glycerol followed by phosphorylation to glycerol 3-phosphate which can then be oxidized to dihydroxyacetone phosphate.

The first of these pathways is the main route for D-glyceraldehyde in mammalian tissues, and thus the overall reaction for the initial stages of fructose utilization can be represented as:

$$\text{fructose} + 2\text{ATP} \rightleftharpoons \text{D-glyceraldehyde 3-phosphate} + \text{dihydroxyacetone phosphate} + 2\text{ADP}$$

The triose phosphates can either be metabolized through the glycolytic chain to lactic acid or can act as a substrate for glucose synthesis. In man about 20 per cent of splanchnic fructose metabolism is to lactic acid, the remainder forming glucose or being deposited as glycogen in the liver. During this process there is an accumulation of fructose 1-phosphate in those tissues with fructokinase activity, namely liver and kidney. These pathways account for more than half of the ingested fructose in man and are present in intestine, liver, and kidney. Alternatively fructose can be directly phosphorylated to fructose 6-phosphate by the enzyme hexokinase present in adipose tissue and muscle. This is normally a minor pathway.

Essential fructosuria. Essential fructosuria (EF) is a condition in which one of the pathways of fructose metabolism is blocked and is best considered as a harmless metabolic abnormality and not as a disease. It is rare having an estimated incidence of 1 in 130 000 of the general population and is inherited as an autosomal recessive trait.

In affected individuals 10–20 per cent of ingested fructose appears in the urine and, if fructose is given orally, the blood fructose concentration rises to very high levels and the subsequent clearance from the blood is slower than in normal individuals, a large portion of fructose being metabolized in adipose tissue and muscle via the hexokinase pathway. The block is due to a deficiency of hepatic fructokinase.

Essential fructosuria is usually diagnosed as a result of finding a reducing sugar in the urine which is not glucose. Occasionally diabetes mellitus has been diagnosed in error when the reducing sugar present in urine has not been chemically identified.

Hereditary fructose intolerance. Hereditary fructose intolerance (HFI) was first described in 1956 and is characterized by the de-velopment of hypoglycaemia and vomiting soon (20 minutes) after fructose ingestion. In affected children a syndrome develops characterized by vomiting, hepatomegally, jaundice, proteinuria, aminoaciduria, and failure to thrive. Older patients develop an aversion to fructose-containing foods and have a low incidence of dental caries.

The condition is inherited as an autosomal recessive trait. Some affected children die in early life, but among those who survive, the intelligence is normal and the hepatic and renal lesions are completely reversible on withdrawal of fructose from the diet; adults do not show any pathological effects. Treatment is by adherence to a diet completely free of fructose.

When fructose is ingested, the blood fructose concentration rises and this is accompanied by a profound fall in blood glucose concentration. The plasma inorganic phosphate concentration also falls while that of magnesium rises and some fructose appears in the urine. The hypoglycaemia provoked by fructose administration can be prevented by galactose infusion, but glucagon injection, and glycerol or dihydroxyacetone infusion do not have any beneficial effect.

The diagnosis is established by an intravenous fructose tolerance test which produces the symptoms, with the exception of the vomiting which accompanies oral fructose administration. The blood glucose and inorganic phosphate concentrations fall while that of lactic acid is unchanged.

The enzyme defects are of two types. The primary defect is a lowered activity of fructose 1-phosphate aldolase. The amount of enzyme protein in liver is usually lowered to 20 per cent of normal and in some cases its activity may be as low as 2 per cent of normal.

The secondary enzyme defects are probably due to the large accumulation of fructose 1-phosphate in those tissues possessing the fructokinase pathway of fructose degradation. These are:

1. An inhibition of fructokinase.
2. An inhibition of glycogen breakdown.
3. An inhibition of fructose 1,6-diphosphate synthesis via the aldolase reaction.
4. Inhibition of the conversion of fructose 6-phosphate to glucose 6-phosphate via phosphohexoisomerase.

The biochemical mechanisms involved in the pathogenesis of the acute effect of fructose loading in HFI are partially unclear but

Table 1 Disorders of fructose metabolism: a summary

	Essential fructosuria (fructokinase deficiency)	Hereditary fructose intolerance (fructose-aldolase deficiency)	Fructose 1,6-diphosphatase deficiency
Incidence	1:130 000	1:20 000	?
Inheritance	autosomal recessive	autosomal recessive	autosomal recessive
Appearance of symptoms	after exposure (fructose sucrose, sorbitol)	after exposure to fructose	after prolonged fasting, especially in neonatal period and during infections after exposure to fructose
Symptoms and signs	none	acute: vomiting, sweating, tremor, coma, convulsions chronic: failure to thrive, vomiting, hepatomegaly, jaundice ascites, oedema, hypoglycaemic convulsions, aversion to sweets	hyperventilation, apathy, unconsciousness, convulsions, hepatomegaly, hypotonia
Laboratory findings	fructosaemia, fructosuria	fructosaemia, fructosuria, hypoglycaemia, liver dysfunction, renal tubular syndrome	hypoglycaemia, lactic acidosis, ketonaemia, hyperalaninuria
Diagnosis	fructose in blood or urine after ingestion	fructose-tolerance test (0.2–0.3 g/kg body weight i.v. in adults or 3 g/m² surface area in children): enzyme activity	prolonged fasting; loading tests (fructose, glycerol); enzyme activity in liver or intestine
Treatment	none	fructose-free diet	fructose-restricted diet
Course without treatment	harmless	episodic, possibly fatal	episodic, possibly fatal
With treatment	—	benign	benign

many result from an exaggeration of the events which follow fructose loading in a normal subject, namely fructose 1-phosphate accumulation and adenosine triphosphate (ATP) depletion in those tissues possessing the fructokinase pathway. A transient form has been described in newborn infants.

Fructose 1,6-diphosphatase deficiency. This rare disorder was first described in 1970. Patients usually present before the age of six months with severe lactic acidosis, hypoglycaemia, and hepatomegaly often precipitated by infections. The reaction to fructose ingestion is less severe than in HFI. The defect is a complete lack of hepatic fructose 1,6-diphosphatase which means that gluconeogenesis from lactic acid, glycerol, and amino acids cannot take place. Thus, when hepatic glycogen stores are depleted, fasting hypoglycaemia develops.

The diagnosis is difficult to make, the least harmful procedure being a fast with frequent blood glucose determinations. After some 12–16 hours of fasting, the blood sugar concentration falls and is not restored by glucagon administration. Loading tests with fructose, glycerol, or dihydroxyacetone are dangerous because they lead to hypoglycaemia and lactic acidosis.

The mechanism of the hypoglycaemia is unclear but, like HFI, it may result from a secondary enzyme defect. Glycogenolysis is inhibited by the hepatic accumulation of the phosphorylated intermediates fructose 1-phosphate, fructose 1,6-diphosphate and 3-phosphoglycerate, the hepatic concentrations of which rise if fructose is administered in the absence of fructose 1,6-diphosphatase activity.

Clinical and biochemical features of the three inherited disorders of fructose metabolism are summarized in Table 1.

References

Baker, L. and Winegrad, A. I. (1970). Fasting hypoglycemia and metabolic acidosis associated with deficiency of hepatic fructose 1,6-diphosphatase activity. *Lancet* **ii**, 13.

Chambers, R. A. and Pratt, R. T. C. (1956). Idiosyncrasy to fructose. *Lancet* **ii**, 340.

Froesch, E. R. (1978). Essential fructosuria, hereditary fructose intolerance, and fructose 1,6-diphosphatase deficiency. In *The metabolic basis of inherited disease*, 4th edn (eds. J. B. Stanbury, J. B. Wyngaarden, and D. S. Fredrickson), 121. McGraw Hill, New York.

Sachs, B., Sternfeld, L., and Kraus, G. (1942). Essential fructosuria: its pathophysiology. *Am. J. Dis. Child.* **63**, 252.

Woods, H. F. (1972). Hepatic accumulation of metabolites after fructose loading. *Acta med. scand.* (Suppl. 542), 87.

Disorders of lipid transport

B. Lewis

Abnormalities of plasma lipid transport are associated with a wide clinical spectrum, from silent aberrations of plasma lipoprotein concentration to grave disorders in which life-limiting cardiovascular, abdominal, or neurological manifestations are part of the natural history. Of particular clinical significance is the evidence that certain plasma lipoprotein abnormalities are risk factors for atherosclerotic heart disease.

The physiology of lipid transport in plasma

Lipids are by definition poorly soluble in water. Their transport in plasma is dependent upon the existence of a system of complex soluble proteins, the lipoproteins; these contain nine specific polypeptides, the apolipoproteins A-I, A-II, B, C-I, C-II, C-III, D, E, and F, together with triglyceride, cholesteryl ester, cholesterol, and phospholipid in varying proportion. The major classes of plasma lipoprotein are illustrated in Fig. 1. From their compositions it is clear that increased levels of chylomicrons or very-low density lipoprotein (VLDL) lead to hypertriglyceridaemia with relatively little increase in cholesterol concentration; an elevated level of low density lipoprotein (LDL) is the usual cause of hypercholesterolaemia with relatively normal plasma triglyceride concentration, though mild hypercholesterolaemia can also occur as a result of elevated concentrations of high density lipoprotein (HDL). Increased levels of intermediate density lipoprotein (IDL) leads to a rise in concentration of both cholesterol and triglyceride, i.e. combined hyperlipidaemia.

Chylomicrons are synthesized in the small intestinal mucosa during fat absorption. They are the main form in which dietary fat is transported, and also carry fat-soluble vitamins. Being of large particle size (80–500 nm), they impart lactescence to plasma. Normally present 1–10 hours after a fatty meal, their presence in the fasted state is pathological. VLDL (30–80 nm) are synthesized chiefly in the liver and are also large triglyceride-rich particles, but much of their lipid is of endogenous origin; most of the triglyceride is derived from plasma-free fatty acid which has its origin in adipose tissue. Chylomicrons and VLDL are initially metabolized in peripheral tissues, chiefly muscle and adipose tissue (Fig. 2). The triglyceride of these particles is hydrolysed by the enzyme lipoprotein lipase, situated in the capillary endothelium of most

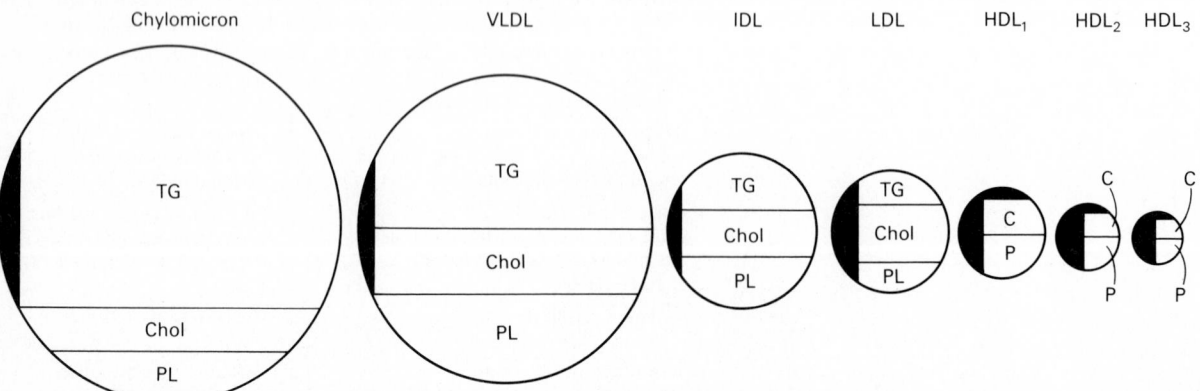

Fig. 1 the plasma lipoproteins, to indicate relative size, physical properties, and composition (not to scale). TG = triglyceride; PL = phospholipid.

peripheral tissues; the fatty acids so produced largely enter the parenchymal cells and are either oxidized, an important energy source in the post-absorptive state, or reconverted to triglyceride and stored. One of the apolipoproteins of chylomicrons and VLDL, apo-CII is an obligatory activator of the lipoprotein lipase system. Hence the presence of apo-CII in these particles determines their sites of catabolism, i.e. those tissues rich in lipoprotein lipase.

All plasma lipoproteins are influenced, directly or indirectly, by lipoprotein lipase. Activity of the enzyme in adipose tissue rises in the fed state, and is increased by insulin. The rate of catabolism of triglyceride-rich lipoproteins appears to be regulated by activity of lipoprotein lipase. These particles are catabolized within the circulation, yielding a series of particles which are progressively depleted of triglyceride and are consequently denser, smaller in diameter, and proportionally enriched in cholesteryl ester. These have been termed 'remnant' particles; physically they comprise the denser subclass of VLDL, and IDL. As their diameter decreases some of the more polar components which comprise the surface of the particles become redundant. These include phospholipid, unesterified cholesterol, and the apo-C group of polypeptides, which transfer to HDL. The apo-A peptides of HDL appear to be largely derived in this way, being synthesized in the small intestine, incorporated into and released as chylomicrons, and finally transferred to HDL to become its major apoproteins.

The remnant particles, particularly IDL, are normally of low concentration in plasma because they are avidly taken up and metabolized in the splanchnic bed, probably in the liver. Hepatocytes have high affinity receptors for these particles, evidently 'recognizing' the apo-E which is one of their major polypeptides. There is evidence in man that about 50 per cent are catabolized, the remainder being converted to LDL by further remodelling of their composition. The enzyme hepatic endothelial lipase possibly plays

a role in this conversion and/or in IDL catabolism. Hence a series of reactions takes place in which VLDL is initially catabolized intravascularly in peripheral tissues, yielding denser VLDL and ultimately IDL; these products are further catabolized in the liver, LDL being a major end-product. One LDL particle is derived from one IDL and ultimately from one VLDL particle, and during the cascade the apo-B moiety is conserved, i.e. it remains a constant component of each particle as its lipids and other proteins are progressively depleted.

LDL is more slowly catabolized than its precursors, thus its plasma concentration is considerably greater. It is catabolized to a large extent in peripheral cells including fibroblasts, adipocytes, smooth muscle, endothelium, and mononuclear cells, but the liver is also an important site of catabolism. LDL is metabolized intracellularly. It is internalized via cell surface receptors. At least one-third is bound by high-affinity receptors in the coated pit regions of the cell surface, which recognize the apo-B of LDL and also the apo-E of other lipoproteins; the coated pits, with bound LDL, invaginate and fuse with lysosomes where LDL is degraded by acid hydrolases. This appears to be a further instance of direction of a lipoprotein class to its catabolic site by its apoprotein moiety. The number of receptors is regulated by intracellular cholesterol levels; this and other homeostatic processes stabilize the cell's cholesterol content. There is also a low-affinity receptor pathway (or 'scavenger' pathway), which is not known to be regulated but which becomes proportionately more important at higher LDL concentrations. The activity of the high affinity receptors is a major determinant of plasma LDL and cholesterol levels, of cholesterol synthesis in peripheral cells, and perhaps of the homeostatic response to a high cholesterol diet. It permits an adequate supply of cholesterol (as LDL) to these cells even at very low LDL levels in plasma and tissue fluid. Peripheral cells acquire most of their cholesterol from the LDL of tissue fluid, at least at the

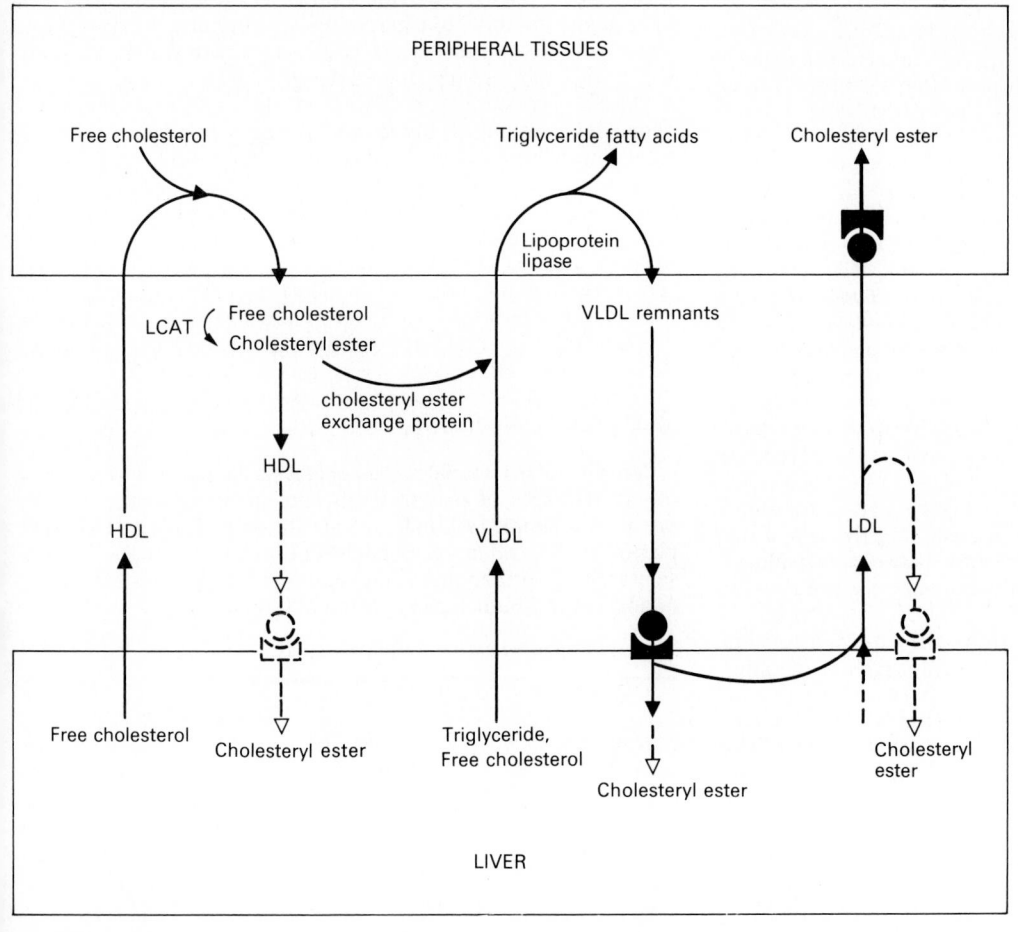

Fig. 2 Classes of lipoprotein molecules involved in lipid transport between the liver and peripheral tissues (postulated model). Dotted lines indicate receptor-mediated uptake.

relatively high plasma LDL concentrations typical of man consuming a high fat, high cholesterol 'westernized' diet.

In summary, the chylomicron–VLDL–LDL system probably serves to transport fat and cholesterol of both dietary and endogenous origin from liver and intestine centrifugally to peripheral tissues.

HDL is secreted by the liver and small intestine (Fig. 3). The nascent form is a discoidal particle comprising phospholipid, unesterified cholesterol, and apoproteins. In the circulation the cholesterol is converted to cholesteryl ester by the plasma enzyme lecithin-cholesterol acyltransferase (LCAT). The conformation of the HDL changes, the cholesteryl ester forming the core of a spherical particle with the other components forming its surface. Further, it is probable that HDL acquires unesterified cholesterol from peripheral cells, the first stage in the reverse (centripetal) transport of cholesterol from the periphery to the liver. Compatible with this is the finding that the mass of tissue cholesterol pools is inversely related to plasma HDL-cholesterol concentration. As indicated above, HDL acquires apo-A, cholesterol, and phospholipid from chylomicrons and VLDL during catabolism of the latter; HDL-cholesterol levels are directly related to lipoprotein lipase activity in adipose tissue. Clearly the plasma levels of the components of HDL are determined by several metabolic processes.

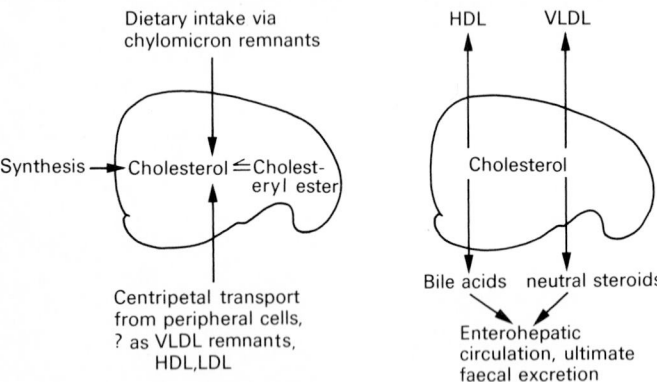

Fig. 3   Sources of metabolic fates of hepatic cholesterol.

The lipoprotein system serves to transport triglyceride as an energy source of high caloric yield, readily stored. Its role in cholesterol transport permits the supply of cholesterol to many tissues which normally depend on uptake of sterol derived from diet or hepatic synthesis. Cholesterol is an essential cell membrane constituent, the phospholipid:cholesterol ratio influencing membrane fluidity and hence permeability and cell division. Cholesterol is also required for steroid synthesis, and as a vitamin D precursor. Almost all cells possess the enzyme system for cholesterol synthesis, the rate of which is determined by the activity of hydroxymethyl glutaryl coenzyme A reductase (HMA CoA reductase). While the pathway is probably largely repressed in most peripheral cells *in situ*, active synthesis occurs in the liver at a rate which varies inversely with the intake and absorption of dietary cholesterol (which reaches it as 'remnant' particles). The effectiveness of this homeostatic process shows wide variation between individuals, leading to differing sensitivity of plasma and tissue levels of cholesterol to dietary intake.

In the steady state, cells must lose cholesterol at a rate equal to the uptake and synthesis of this sterol. A role for HDL in initiating the centripetal transport of cholesterol has been alluded to, and there is evidence that unesterified cholesterol transfers from cells to HDL *in vitro* (Fig. 2). Ultimately most cholesterol is excreted by the liver, or is converted to bile acids which are excreted. Some cholesterol is probably transported to the liver by HDL. It is likely that a major proportion of centripetal transport of cholesterol follows a more indirect route. Conversion to cholesteryl ester takes place in HDL (the LCAT reaction); this transfers via a plasma cholesteryl ester exchange protein to VLDL and enters the cascade

of conversion via IDL to LDL. It seems plausible that IDL and LDL play a major role in the transport of cholesterol to the liver.

Determinants of plasma lipid levels. Plasma lipoprotein levels are to some extent genetically determined, by polygenic inheritance; some have estimated that up to 40 per cent of the variance between individuals is genetic. Sex hormones, catecholamines, thyroxine, and insulin influence lipid metabolism. Regular aerobic physical activity increases HDL-cholesterol, particularly that of the HDL$_2$ subclass, decreases VLDL and total triglyceride levels, and, in some studies, slightly reduces LDL-cholesterol.

Nutritional factors are profoundly important determinants of lipid metabolism. VLDL and LDL levels are directly related, and HDL-cholesterol inversely related to relative body weight. During or after weight reduction of obese subjects, VLDL and LDL levels usually decrease and HDL-cholesterol concentrations rise. Several nutrients influence plasma and LDL cholesterol levels. Fats rich in saturated fatty acids of chain length 12–16, predominant in dairy products and meat, increase LDL levels and intake of such fats to a large extent accounts for the wide variation of plasma cholesterol levels between populations. Due to dietary homogeneity, nutritional factors play a much smaller role in accounting for within-population variation in lipid levels, though some reports indicate significant correlations with total fat intake. Mono-unsaturated fatty acids, as in olive oil, have little influence on plasma lipid levels; polyunsaturated fatty acids, e.g. linoleic acid obtained from many seed oils have a moderate effect in reducing LDL and VLDL concentrations. Some forms of fibre, notably the mucilaginous types present in fruit, vegetables, and oat bran, decrease plasma cholesterol and LDL levels, and a similar relatively small effect is seen when dietary proteins of animal origin are replaced by vegetable proteins such as soy-protein. Dietary cholesterol increases plasma cholesterol levels (influencing LDL and to a lesser extent IDL and HDL concentration); though the average effect is a modest one, there is a wide individual variation in the plasma cholesterol response to this, and indeed most nutrients. Alcohol has a consistent effect in increasing HDL levels, and elevates VLDL-triglyceride to a varying, sometimes gross extent.

Plasma cholesterol and triglyceride levels increase from low neonatal values until about six years of age, then remain stable—sometimes with a dip at the time of puberty—until adult life. In some populations there is little subsequent trend with age, but in affluent western countries levels increase during adult life to reach a peak in the sixth decade. The inconsistency of this adult increase makes it unlikely that these changes are physiological; they may reflect trends in life style, and an increasing prevalence of obesity. Plasma cholesterol and LDL levels are higher in men than in premenopausal women; after the menopause female levels exceed those in men. HDL levels are higher in women than in men throughout adult life, and the converse is true of triglyceride and VLDL concentration.

Concepts of the normal ranges of plasma lipid concentration. The observed ranges of plasma lipids and lipoproteins in a healthy population sample of Londoners are shown in Table 1. The mean plasma cholesterol in young adults in London, 5.8 mmol/l, is considerably higher than that in the same age group in South Italy, 4.7 mmol/l, or in South Japan, 3.9 mmol/l.

Table 1   Reference ranges for plasma lipids*

	mmol/l	mg/dl
Cholesterol	4.0–6.7	160–260
Triglyceride: male	0.70–2.1	60–185
female	0.60–1.5	55–135

* Based on apparently healthy adult population sample in London, age range 20–39 years; in fasted state. Enzymatic methods

Note: to convert cholesterol concentrations from SI units (mmol/l) to mg/dl, multiply by 39; to convert triglyceride levels, multiply by 89

These differences have prompted some authorities to seek other criteria than simple population data to identify optimal, as opposed to observed 'normal' ranges. Such considerations have suggested an optimal population mean plasma cholesterol level in adults of about 4.9 mmol/l (190 mg/ml) with a desirable upper limit of 5.7 mmol/l (220 mg/ml). If such definitions are accepted, it follows that a large proportion of many affluent populations are hyperlipidaemic; this carries the implication that mass hyperlipidaemia of dietary origin is to a large extent a public health problem. Clinical care is chiefly appropriate for patients with the more florid disorders of plasma lipoprotein metabolism, and for those with a strong family history of early-onset ischaemic heart disease.

Investigation of hyperlipidaemic states

The extent of the investigation of hyperlipidaemia depends upon its purpose, and upon the severity of the hyperlipidaemia. If the goal is to assess the extent of lipoprotein-mediated risk of atherosclerosis and its complications, the minimum investigation is the measurement of total plasma cholesterol and of HDL-cholesterol in a random, i.e. non-fasted, specimen. Necessary preconditions are that the subject has been following his or her habitual diet for at least two weeks, that there has been no major illness, operation, or injury for at least two to four weeks and no minor febrile illness in the preceding week. Lipid-active drugs should be withdrawn at least three weeks prior to sampling. The blood should be drawn without venous stasis, with the subject recumbent or seated.

The preferred baseline investigation of plasma lipoprotein abnormalities is more comprehensive. It is performed on plasma (EDTA, 1 mg/ml, is used as anticoagulant), obtained after a 14 hour overnight fast; water or fat-free fluids are permitted. Cholesterol, triglyceride, and HDL-cholesterol concentrations are measured. The lipoproteins(s) responsible for any substantial degree of hypertriglyceridaemia are qualitatively identified by the stored plasma test: the tube of plasma is stored vertically for 18 hours at 4 °C and inspected for lactescence. Diffuse lactescence usually indicates an excess of VLDL or IDL, while floating lactescence with a clear subnatant is characteristic of chylomicronaemia. Although less dependence is placed on lipoprotein electrophoresis than formerly, the method may suggest the presence of the broad beta band of remnant hyperlipoproteinaemia, and helps to recognize high HDL levels as a cause of mild hypercholesterolaemia. A diagnosis of hyperlipidaemia should be based upon at least two samples obtained at an interval of about one week.

Other investigations relevant to particular lipoprotein disorders are discussed in the clinical section below. In addition, hyperlipidaemic patients should be investigated for underlying causes of lipid abnormalities and common accompaniments of hypertriglyceridaemia such as elevated urate levels and glucose intolerance. A full history and examination most often reveal such causes of secondary hyperlipidaemia; it is usual to obtain a biochemical 'profile' including plasma levels of creatinine, urate, albumin, globulins, γ-glutamyl transpeptidase, alkaline phosphatase, and alanine transaminase. Plasma thyroxine levels and a free thyroxine index may reveal unsuspected hypothyroidism but more often confirm a clinical diagnosis. It is necessary to seek evidence of cardiovascular disease, and to assess risk factors for ischaemic heart disease as part of a comprehensive evaluation of risk, notably family history, blood pressure, cigarette consumption, and relative body weight. Lastly, the use of drugs which can influence plasma lipid levels, particularly thiazides, chlorthalidone, corticosteroids, contraceptives, oestrogens, and microsomal inducing agents should be noted.

Severe hypertriglyceridaemia can interefere with certain biochemical measurements, by displacement of plasma water, or by preventing accurate colorimetric analysis. Of practical importance is the masking of elevated serum amylase levels in pancreatitis complicating hypertiglyceridaemia. Apparent hyponatraemia is another source of confusion, occurring despite the presence of a normal sodium concentration in plasma water. In many laboratories, most of the interfering lipoprotein can be removed by brief ultracentrifugation or by ultrafiltration, permitting reliable analyses. Measurement of urinary amylase may be helpful.

Lastly, plasma cholesterol and triglyceride levels should be measured in the first-degree relatives of patients with substantial hyperlipidaemia. This may lead to diagnosis of hyperlipidaemia at an asymptomatic stage, and permits identification of the pattern of inheritance.

Secondary hyperlipidaemia. Depending on the pattern of referral and the extent of the investigation, some 10 to 20 per cent of hyperlipidaemic patients are found to have an underlying cause. Hence the hyperlipidaemia may provide the lead to a full diagnosis and often to a therapeutic opportunity. Not infrequently primary and secondary hyperlipidaemias coexist, correction of the cause for the latter (e.g. diabetes, alcohol overindulgence) uncovering the former. Not surprisingly this situation is often associated with gross hyperlipidaemia. While the causes of secondary hyperlipidaemia are numerous, two are strikingly common: hypothyroidism as a cause of predominant hypercholesterolaemia and alcohol abuse as a cause of hypertriglyceridaemia.

Hypothyroidism. In hypothyroidism, hypercholesterolaemia is the rule and it is often gross. Typical levels are 9–20 mmol/l. Xanthomas are unusual. The severity of the lipid abnormality does not appear to parallel the degree of hypothyroidism, pronounced hypercholesterolaemia sometimes resulting from a modest reduction of thyroxine levels. Not infrequently moderate hypertriglyceridaemia is also seen. Genetically-predisposed patients may show remnant (type III) hyperlipoproteinaemia with the typical skin lesions (see page 9.66). The hypercholesterolaemia is associated with reduction of the rate of catabolism of LDL mediated by the high-affinity LDL receptors, leading to decreased excretion of cholesterol and reduced conversion of cholesterol to bile acids. An occasional diagnostic pitfall is the occurrence of hypothyroidism in two or more members of a family, which may be confused with a genetic hyperlipidaemia.

Alcohol. The relationship between alcohol consumption and hyperlipidaemia is complex. Experimentally, moderate doses of alcohol consistently produce a slight hypertriglyceridaemia, an effect which may wane with ongoing intake. Probably only a minority of alcoholics have hyperlipidaemia, either because of individual differences in susceptibility or because of coexisting liver disease and/or malnutrition. Gross hypertriglyceridaemia due to increased VLDL levels with or without chylomicronaemia (type IV or V) is the typical alcoholic lipaemia; in some patients withdrawal of alcohol is followed within 10–14 days by completely normal plasma lipid levels, but more often a mild or moderate primary hypertriglyceridaemia is revealed. Another pattern is of moderate hypertriglyceridaemia in patients consuming quite modest amounts of alcohol which is corrected or ameliorated by reduction of intake or abstention. The effect of alcohol in increasing HDL-cholesterol levels has been mentioned. In a hypertriglyceridaemic patient concealed alcohol abuse may be suspected from the presence of hepatomegaly, parotid enlargement, macrocytosis and elevated serum γ-glutamyl transpeptidase activity. In most hypertriglyceridaemic states HDL-cholesterol levels tend to be low; the coexistence of increased levels of triglyceride and HDL-cholesterol is strongly suggestive of alcohol lipaemia, but is also seen as an oestrogen effect. Alcohol lipaemia may result in part from reduced hepatic NAD levels, the consequence of oxidation of alcohol by the alcohol dehydrogenase pathway; the consequent impairment of free fatty acid oxidation leads to increased fatty acid esterification to triglyceride and is followed by development of a fatty liver and increased secretion of VLDL-triglyceride.

In addition alcohol, in common with other microsomal inducing agents, may directly enhance hepatic synthesis and secretion of

VLDL and HDL. Zieve's triad of alcoholic lipaemia, jaundice, and haemolytic anaemia is rarely seen.

Diabetes mellitus. About 40 per cent of uncontrolled diabetics have elevated VLDL levels, and when hypertriglyceridaemia is severe there is usually also chylomicronaemia. Mean LDL-cholesterol levels are increased, but normal levels are present in many diabetics. Raised VLDL levels contribute to the hypercholesterolaemia. HDL–cholesterol is often low. With good diabetic control and correction of obesity, these changes usually revert to normal and treated diabetics sometimes have relatively high HDL levels. However, persisting hyperlipidaemia is sometimes seen. Frequently this is related to imperfect control; but the coexistence of diabetes or impaired glucose tolerance and primary endogenous hypertriglyceridaemia is remarkably common. The relationship is incompletely understood but may reflect a common predisposing factor such as obesity and/or insulin resistance. Often treatment has to be directed empirically to both abnormalities in patients with diabetes and severe or resistant hypertriglyceridaemia. Diabetic hypertriglyceridaemia is most commonly moderate but can be gross leading to eruptive xanthomas and abdominal pain. Severe hyperlipidaemia may be due to the coexistence of a primary lipid disorder, but can occur in insulin-dependent diabetes alone, usually without ketoacidosis but with a history of severe weight loss. Diabetic hypertriglyceridaemia is associated with reduced fractional removal of VLDL-triglyceride from plasma. Adipose tissue lipoprotein lipase activity is often but not always subnormal, and the defect in VLDL catabolism is possibly due in part to impairment of other steps in triglyceride removal. Most studies of VLDL metabolism in experimental insulin deficiency reveal low rates of synthesis. However, there is good evidence of VLDL overproduction in some diabetics. This may the result of very high plasma levels of free fatty acids due to insulin deficiency. Hyperinsulinism and hypertriglyceridaemia often coexist, but it is not clearly established that elevated insulin levels, as seen in some non-insulin-dependent diabetics and some patients with endogenous hypertriglyceridaemia, is a cause of increased VLDL synthesis in man.

Cholestasis. The hypercholesterolaemia of cholestatic jaundice is due to the secretion of abnormal discoidal LDL particles ('LP–X') rich in unesterified cholesterol and phospholipid. Plasma LCAT activity is frequently decreased. This accounts for the elevated ratio of free-to-esterified cholesterol in plasma. LP–X may be demonstrated in plasma in many but not all patients with obstructive jaundice using immunochemical methods or electrophoresis; the majority view is that tests for LP–X are not reliable predictors of cholestasis. Xanthomatosis develops if the cholestasis is unrelieved as in long-standing primary biliary cirrhosis. Pain in the hands and feet are usually ascribed to a hyperlipidaemic peripheral neuropathy; this sometimes-incapacitating symptom has been relieved following reduction of the hyperlipidaemia by plasma exchange or drug treatment.

Other causes. Hypertriglyceridaemia is seen in about one-third of patients with *gout*. Excessive intake of alcohol contributes to this association in some but seemingly not all, aggravating the hyperuricaemia and the lipid abnormality.

Chronic renal failure is commonly accompanied by hypertriglyceridaemia or combined hyperlipidaemia with low levels of HDL-cholesterol. Low lipoprotein lipase activity in adipose tissue may contribute to these changes and a circulating inhibitor of the enzyme has been postulated. Hepatic endothelial lipase activity is also low, and there is commonly insulin resistance. After renal transplantation these lipoprotein abnormalities are ameliorated but mild combined hyperlipidaemia may persist; a role of corticosteroid therapy is possible. The *nephrotic syndrome* is a familiar cause of lipoprotein abnormalities; when plasma albumin levels are moderately reduced, hypercholesterolaemia due to increased LDL concentration is the rule, while severe hypoalbuminaemia is often accompanied by gross elevation of VLDL-triglyceride. HDL-cholesterol is sometimes very low; with non-selective proteinuria substantial urinary losses of HDL occur. Overproduction of VLDL and probably LDL occurs in the nephrotic syndrome. One explanation of this is that it is part of a generalized increase in hepatic protein synthesis in response to the proteinuria. Alternatively or additionally, it has been attributed more directly to the hypoalbuminaemia. Albumin has two high-affinity binding sites per molecule for free fatty acid; with marked reduction in plasma albumin, free fatty acids become bound to weaker sites. This would favour uptake of fatty acids by tissues including the liver, promoting VLDL-triglyceride synthesis.

Marked hyperlipidaemia is an occasional complication of *myelomatosis* and also *polyclonal hypergammaglobulinaemias*, and a role of auto-antibodies that inactivate lipoprotein lipase or bind lipoproteins has been demonstrated. Increased LDL and IDL levels due to reduced catabolism, with tendon xanthomas, have been observed in *primary amyloidosis*.

In children, noteworthy causes of secondary hyperlipidaemia include *diabetes, glycogen storage diseases Types I, III, and VI, Werner's syndrome, progeria, hypothyroidism,* and *idiopathic hypercalcaemia.*

Drugs which can lead to hypertriglyceridaemia include oral contraceptive formulations and oestrogens. The effect is modest except in a minority of susceptible individuals, particularly patients with primary endogenous hypertriglyceridaemia in whom pancreatitis has been so induced. Oestrogens reduce LDL levels in postmenopausal women; they ameliorate remnant hyperlipoproteinaemia, and increase HDL levels. Thiazide diuretics tend to increase plasma triglyceride, usually mildly, and cholesterol levels also are elevated; chlorthalidone has been reported to increase LDL-cholesterol substantially. High-dosage corticosteroids may elevate cholesterol and triglyceride levels.

Secondary hyperlipidaemia and ischaemic heart disease. The impact of risk factors for ischaemic heart disease may be taken to be a function of their duration as well as their severity. As secondary hyperlipidaemia is usually of shorter duration than genetic lipoprotein disorders, its effects on the atherosclerotic process must be presumed to be smaller.

This may explain the variability of the published reports on myocardial infarction mortality in patients with secondary hyperlipidaemia. Nevertheless, the majority of accounts indicate an excess risk of ischaemic heart disease in chronic renal failure, the nephrotic syndrome, and hypothyroidism. There is an undoubted increase in the frequency of ischaemic heart disease, peripheral vascular disease, and stroke in diabetes, though asymptomatic hyperglycaemia is not a risk factor except, perhaps, when very pronounced (the upper 5 per cent of the distribution). LDL levels are normal or mildly elevated in untreated diabetes. These lipoprotein changes are cardiovascular risk factors. The common hypertriglyceridaemia of diabetes is less certainly a risk factor (see below). There is also an unexplained increase in frequency of hypertension in diabetes which contributes to cardiovascular disease. In addition, abnormalities of platelet function and composition in untreated diabetes may well contribute to the atherogenic process and thrombosis.

There is a J-shaped relationship between alcohol consumption and ischaemic heart disease. Mortality is higher in total abstainers than in modest drinkers (up to about two alchoholic drinks per day). This protection may be mediated by the consistently higher levels of plasma HDL-cholesterol in the latter. However, heavier alcohol intake, in problem drinkers, is an independent risk factor for fatal ischaemic heart disease.

Primary hyperlipidaemic states

Classification. While the last word has yet to be said on classifying hyperlipidaemia, two approaches have proved helpful in describing

Type	I	IIa	IIb	III	IV	V
Chylomicrons	++	−	−	+	−	++
VLDL	N	N	++	+	++	++
Remnants	N	N	N,+	++	N	N
LDL	low	++	++	low	N	low
Plasma cholesterol	+	++	++	++	+	+
Plasma triglyceride	+++	N	++	++	++	++
Stored plasma appearance						

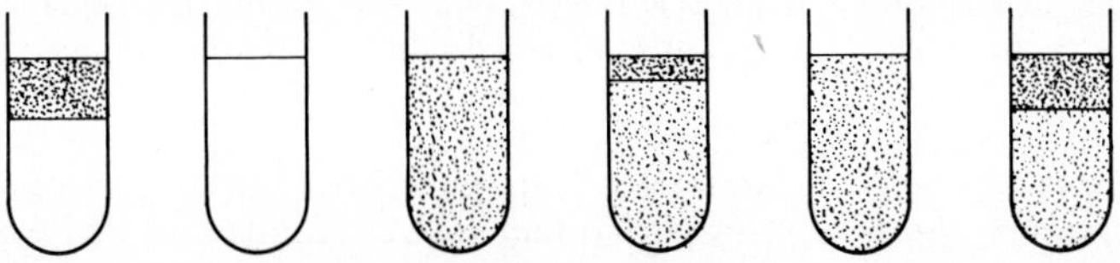

Fig. 4 Frederickson/WHO classification of hyperlipoproteinaemias.

the several clinical, genetic, and metabolic entities. In practical terms a classification should aid in deciding upon optimal therapy and in estimating prognosis. Diagnosis of a major lipoprotein disorder may bear the implication of lifelong dietary and drug therapy, insurance problems, and considerations of genetic counselling. The classification of Fredrickson, Levy, and Lees, extended by a World Health Organization committee, defines six types of hyperlipoproteinaemia on the basis of the pattern of lipoprotein abnormality (Fig. 4), without dependence upon clinical, genetic, or metabolic considerations. It provides a convenient and widely-used terminology for these lipoprotein patterns. The classification introduced by Goldstein, Hazzard, Motulsky, and their colleagues, on the other hand, distinguished several patterns of familial distribution of hyperlipidaemia in the relatives of patients with ischaemic heart disease, providing a genetic classification. Studies of the underlying disorders of lipoprotein metabolism in genetically defined patients by Janus, Nicoll, and Lewis indicate that this genetic classification separate metabolically distinct disorders. The genetic-metabolic classification, slightly extended, is given in Table 2.

Familial hypercholesterolaemia. Hypercholesterolaemia due to elevation of LDL levels, of autosomal dominant inheritance, is a relatively common disorder comprising of the order of 20 per cent of referrals to the St Thomas' Hospital lipid clinic. The usual heterozygous form affects between 1 in 300 and 1 in 500 individuals in the United Kingdom and USA (but appears to be considerably commoner in the Lebanon and South Africa). Unless detected by the screening of affected families or other screening approaches, its commonest mode of presentation is with early-onset ischaemic heart disease. Fifty per cent of male heterozygotes develop

ischaemic heart disease due to typical atherosclerosis by age 50, and presentation in the thirties or twenties is not unusual. It has been suggested that 5 per cent of ischaemic heart disease is primarily due to this genetic disorder. Affected men show a tenfold excess risk of cardiac ischaemia. Women are also at substantially increased risk. The unique vascular hazard in familial hypercholesterolaemia is ascribed to the relatively severe elevation of LDL levels, and to its early age of onset; cord blood LDL concentration is increased.

The increase in LDL concentration is due to a decreased rate of fractional removal of this lipoprotein from plasma. There is also overproduction of LDL in many heterozygotes. The defect in catabolism is due to a reduction in the number of high-affinity cell-surface LDL receptors which mediate one of the pathways for internalization of the lipoprotein and its lysosomal catabolism.

In heterozygotes the receptor number is reduced by about 50 per cent while high-affinity receptors are absent in the commonest form of the homozygous disease. Several lesions of the LDL pathway have been described, including functionally defective receptors. Overproduction of LDL is less readily explained. It occurs by an abnormal pathway not involving VLDL, and can contribute up to 50 per cent of LDL entering plasma. In adult patients increased cholesterol synthesis or impaired excretion or catabolism have not been demonstrated but increased cholesterol synthesis is seen in younger children homozygous for the disease. As plasma LDL levels increase, internalization and intracellular catabolism of the lipoprotein via low-affinity receptors become quantitatively more important. This 'scavenger' pathway, though it permits a normal absolute rate of LDL removal at the expense of an elevated plasma LDL concentration, must be presumed to mediate the accelerated development of atheromatous plaques and xanthomas. Abnormalities of LDL composition have been reported; these may well be

Table 2 Genetic metabolic classification of major primary hyperlipidaemias

	Plasma cholesterol	Plasma triglyceride	Lipoprotein in excess	WHO type	Relative prevalence	Inheritance	Xanthomas	Athero-sclerosis risk
Familial hypercholesterolaemia	+++	normal, +	LDL	IIa, IIb	++	autosomal dominant	tendon planar	+++
Familial combined hyperlipidaemia	+	+	LDL, VLDL	IIa, IIb, IV	+++	undetermined, ? dominant	—	++
Familial hypertriglyceridaemia	+	+++	VLDL, CM	V, IV	+	autosomal dominant	eruptive	?−
Lipoprotein lipase deficiency; apo-CII deficiency	+	+++	CM, VLDL	I, V	+	autosomal recessive	eruptive	−
Remnant hyperlipoproteinaemia	++	++	(IDL) CM, remnants,	III	+	apo-E₃ deficiency coincident with other factors	tuberous, planar	++
Common hypercholesterolaemia	+	normal	LDL	IIa	++++	polygenic	—	+

Cm = chylomicrons   VLDL = very low density lipoproteins   IDL = intermediate density lipoprotein   LDL = low density lipoprotein the consequence of the prolonged mean survival of these particles in the circulation.

In the heterozygotes, xanthomas are unusual in childhood, but are present in at least 50 per cent of patients in early adult life and in about 75 per cent by middle age. They occur typically in the Achilles tendons and the extensor tendons on the dorsum of the hand, especially over the heads of the metacarpals, and may occur at the insertion of the patella tendon, and in the flexor tendons in the feet. The fusiform or irregular swellings range from a few millimetres to several centimetres in size. The only common cutaneous lesions in heterozygotes are xanthelasmas, papular or plaque-like orange-coloured lesions in the eyelids. Corneal arcus may appear in adolescence (and usually indicates hypercholesterolaemia when it develops in the first three decades of life). Absent peripheral pulses and bruits over major arteries are often noted. Rheumatological manifestations include episodes of pain and tenderness in xanthomatous Achilles tendons, and an acute large-joint migrating polyarthritis chiefly affecting the knees and ankles and most often occurring in adolescence. It closely resembles rheumatic fever; the ESR is elevated and xanthomas could be mistaken for rheumatic nodules though the sites of predilection differ.

In the homozygous state the natural history is shortened and qualitatively somewhat different. At least until recently the average life span was about 20 years. The typical xanthomas are cutaneous, appearing in the first decade. They are planar orange-coloured lesions, commonly on the buttocks, the backs of the thighs, in the interdigital clefts, and over the knees and elbows. Supravalvar aortic stenosis, often with a substantial pressure gradient, results from massive xanthomatous deposits in the ascending aorta; involvement of the coronary ostia is frequently seen. Angina pectoris and other manifestations of cardiac involvement develop in the first or second decade. Stature is often short. The acute polyarthritis described above is common in homozygotes.

Diagnosis of heterozygous familial hypercholesterolaemia requires the presence of hypercholesterolaemia (typically about 10 mmol/l and ranging from 7.5 to 15 mmol/l), due to increased LDL concentration. Triglyceride and VLDL levels may be normal or mildly elevated. HDL-cholesterol concentration tends to be low. The lipoprotein pattern is type IIa, less often type IIb. The presence of tendon xanthomas renders the diagnosis almost certain but they are also seen in cerebrotendinous xanthomatosis and rarely, in remnant hyperlipoproteinaemia. Screening of relatives reveals an autosomal dominant distribution of hypercholesterolaemia. There is usually a family history of early-onset ischaemic heart disease. In children of an affected family, a plasma cholesterol concentration of 7 mmol/l or more is likely to be due to familial hypercholesterolaemia. Cord blood LDL-cholesterol levels are increased, permitting neonatal diagnosis in affected families. It is of interest that the extent of the excess risk of ischaemic heart disease varies from family to family and it has been reported that HDL-cholesterol levels are particularly low in those especially prone to cardiovascular disease.

The homozygous state is recognized by more severe hypercholesterolaemia (15–30 mmol/l), the presence of cutaneous xanthomas before 20 years of age, and the presence of hypercholesterolaemia in both parents. A definitive diagnosis may be made using cultured skin fibroblasts or blood mononuclear cells in the homozygote. Absence of high-affinity LDL receptors, or other receptor defects is demonstrable. Though receptor studies have been claimed to discriminate between hypercholesterolaemia due to heterozygous familial hypercholesterolaemia and other conditions, their clinical value has yet to be confirmed.

Familial combined hyperlipidaemia (multiple-type hyperlipidaemia). This strongly-familial form of hyperlipidaemia was first described in 1973 in the relatives of ischaemic heart disease patients. Its characteristics include mildly to moderately elevated plasma levels of both cholesterol and triglyceride, or of cholesterol or triglyceride alone. The form of hyperlipidaemia differs in the affected members of the family, and may vary from time to time even in the individual patient; it reflects increased concentrations of VLDL, LDL, or of both lipoproteins. HDL-cholesterol levels tend to be low. Not all authorities accept that this description defines a specific metabolic disorder, and the original view that it is due to a single mutant gene, with autosomal dominant transmission, has also been debated. Nevertheless several accounts correspond in indicating that a strongly familial variable pattern of hyperlipidaemia is relatively common and that ischaemic heart disease is frequent in affected patients. Studies of lipoprotein kinetics indicate that overproduction of VLDL and LDL is the mechanism of the combined hyperlipidaemia, fractional catabolism of these lipoproteins being normal. Thus it appears to be metabolically distinct from other heritable forms of hyperlipidaemia. Lipoprotein composition is not abnormal. Its association with ischaemic heart disease seems well established. The disorder is seldom detectable until adult life. Hypertriglyceridaemic patients have increased turnover of cholesterol and increased faecal bile acid excretion, though this has not as yet been related to the various genetic types of hyperlipidaemia.

The variable expression in terms of the pattern of hyperlipoproteinaemia is likely to represent interactions between the genetic disorder and environmental factors such as diet. Elevated VLDL levels are usually seen in obese patients, and with weight reduction they rapidly revert to normal.

Typical plasma cholesterol concentrations range from normal to about 9 mmol/l, and the triglyceride levels from normal to about 6 mmol/l. The lipoprotein pattern may be type IIb, IIa, or IV. Pronounced hyperlipidaemia may result from the coexistence of familial combined hyperlipidaemia with a cause of secondary hyperlipidaemia such as diabetes. Xanthomas are not a feature. Early-onset corneal arcus and xanthelasmas may be noted. Family studies show the presence of differing patterns of hyperlipidaemia in the affected relatives. Although autosomal dominant inheritance has not been rigorously established, vertical transmission is common and roughly half of each sibship is hyperlipidaemic.

Familial hypertriglyceridaemia. This is an uncommon disorder characterized by pronounced hypertriglyceridaemia, typical levels ranging from 6 to more than 50 mmol/l. There is a marked increase in VLDL concentration, and most often there is chylomicronaemia even in the fasted state (type IV or V). Plasma cholesterol levels are more modestly increased; LDL and HDL levels are low. The VLDL includes a high proportion of the least dense, most triglyceride-rich subclass. Unlike familial combined hyperlipidaemia, affected relatives show a consistent pattern of increased VLDL levels with or without chylomicronaemia. Common associated features include impaired glucose tolerance or overt diabetes, hyperinsulinism, and obesity. The causal links between these findings and the hypertriglyceridaemia have not been identified with certainty; weight reduction rapidly lessens the hypertriglyceridaemia.

Unlike hypertriglyceridaemia consequent upon lipoprotein lipase deficiency (see below), the hyperlipidaemia of this disorder is not consistently ameliorated by a fat-free diet. When a low-fat isocaloric diet (which is necessarily rich in carbohydrate) is fed, the total plasma triglyceride may increase, remain unchanged, or slightly decrease; the chylomicronaemia usually abates. Hence the excess circulating triglyceride is largely of endogenous origin.

Relatively little information is available as to the mechanism of the hyperlipidaemia. Overproduction of VLDL triglyceride was reported in one study; however, there is no consistent evidence of overproduction of VLDL particles, as reflected by VLDL–apo-B kinetic studies which reveal subnormal fractional catabolism. If increased triglyceride synthesis is an important mechanism, it may be speculated that this is consequent upon the hyperinsulinism, but such an effect of insulin has not been firmly established in man.

The low LDL levels are due to increased catabolism, and there is decreased synthesis of apo-AI, the major peptide of HDL. The chylomicronaemia probably reflects competition between chylomicrons and VLDL for catabolism by lipoprotein lipase, the removal mechanism being saturated at high triglyceride concentration.

The few family studies have been interpreted to indicate autosomal dominant inheritance. While the disorder may present at any age, most cases have been diagnosed during adult life.

Two major clinical manifestations are seen. Eruptive xanthomas, which may appear acutely, occur as multiple macular or vesicular lesions on extensor surfaces—the back, buttocks, elbows, and knees. Occasionally they appear in other sites including the mouth. They are unusual when triglyceride levels are less than 6–8 mmol/l, but above this value differences in the severity of the hypertriglyceridaemia do not appear to correlate with the presence or number of xanthomas. The lesions regress and disappear within several weeks of successful treatment of the hyperlipidaemia.

Several acute abdominal pain is the other major mode of presentation of pronounced hypertriglyceridaemia (i.e. levels exceeding 6–8 mmol/l). The common basis for this is acute pancreatitis. The pain is epigastric or diffuse, often radiates to the back and is accompanied by tenderness and guarding, sometimes by vomiting, fever, and leucocytosis. Pancreatic calcification is unusual. If laparotomy is inadvertently performed, there may be clear evidence of pancreatitis, or the only abnormality may be the presence of a little turbid free fluid in the peritoneal cavity. It is not clear whether other bases than pancreatitis exist for the abdominal pain of hypertriglyceridaemia. Reports of normal serum amylase in this situation may be misleading as discussed earlier; urinary amylase, or enzyme measurement on the clear subnatant of plasma after ultracentrifugation may establish the diagnosis of pancreatic disease. The mechanism of the pancreatitis is uncertain. If it is assumed that small amounts of amylase normally enter the pancreatic capillary bed, then a reasonable hypothesis is that in the presence of high triglyceride concentration lipolysis may give rise to fatty acid soaps at a concentration sufficient to damage parenchymal cells. This would promote further enzyme release and a vicious circle of pancreatic damage.

Other signs of severe hypertriglyceridaemia include retinal lipaemia and hepatosplenomegaly. An uncommon neurological syndrome of peripheral neuropathy with or without dementia has been well documented; the manifestations were reversible within 6–12 weeks in the reported cases.

Based on the stated definition, diagnosis depends on the presence of substantial hypertriglyceridaemia (6–100 mmol/l) due to elevated levels of VLDL with or without chylomicronaemia, and milder hypercholesterolaemia (8–20 mmol/l), with evidence of familial distribution compatible with autosomal dominant transmission of a similar lipoprotein pattern. The disorder is not substantially ameliorated by an isocaloric low fat diet. Triglyceride levels remain elevated due to high VLDL levels, though chylomicronaemia may abate. If assay of adipose tissue lipoprotein lipase and plasma apo-CII levels are available results lie within the normal range. The disorder most often presents in adult life.

Defects of the lipoprotein lipase system. At least two defects, deficiency of lipoprotein lipase or of its circulating activator apo-CII, occur as familial disorders leading to severe hypertriglyceridaemia. The elevation of triglyceride levels is largely dependent on the accumulation in plasma of triglyceride of dietary origin. The excess lipid is transported entirely or chiefly in chylomicrons, and the presence of a high concentration of these particles in the fasted state is the hallmark of this condition (type I hyperlipoproteinaemia). There may also be a moderate excess of VLDL; hence lipoprotein lipase deficiency can lead to the type I or type V pattern. Plasma triglyceride concentration is grossly elevated, probably from birth; the diagnosis is possible within the first days of neonatal life though it may not be recognized until early adult life. Typical triglyceride levels are 20–100 mmol/l: reflecting the composition of chylomicrons, the elevation of cholesterol levels is

comparatively slight, 7–10 mmol/l. LDL and HDL levels are often strikingly low.

The clinical manifestations are those of gross hypertriglyceridaemia of any cause. As described for familial hypertriglyceridaemia these include eruptive xanthomatosis, acute pancreatitis, hepatic and splenic enlargement, and retinal lipaemia. There is no evidence of excess risk of ischaemic heart disease. A characteristic feature of lipoprotein lipase deficiency is the grave aggravation of the hyperlipidaemia during pregnancy plausibly due to increased VLDL-triglyceride production. Intractable pancreatitis may ensue, leading to spontaneous or induced termination of pregnancy. It is of interest that one woman with apo-CII deficiency has undergone an entirely uncomplicated pregnancy.

Absence or severe deficiency of the extrahepatic lipoprotein lipase was until recently the only known basis for primary chylomicronaemia due to exogenous hypertriglyceridaemia. It is now clear that the identical lipoprotein pattern can also result from absence or grossly subnormal levels of apo-CII, a component of chylomicrons, VLDL, and HDL which potently activates lipoprotein lipase. Both disorders are transmitted by autosomal recessive inheritance. As assessed by referral patterns they are amongst the rarest forms of heritable hyperlipidaemia; twelve families have attended the St. Thomas' Hospital lipid clinic.

Clearance of circulating triglyceride of dietary origin is severely impaired by lipoprotein lipase deficiency or failure of activation of the enzyme, leading to the pronounced hypertriglyceridaemia. Removal of triglyceride-rich particles appears to be carried out by the reticulo-endothelial system, presumably the basis of the hepatosplenomegaly. While lipoprotein lipase undoubtedly plays a major role in catabolism of circulating triglyceride of dietary and of endogenous origins (transported chiefly by chylomicrons and VLDL respectively) defective functioning of the lipoprotein lipase system consistently leads to accumulation of chylomicrons with normal levels or only moderate increase of VLDL. This is best explained by considering the preferred substrates of lipoprotein lipase and of the hepatic endothelial triglyceride lipase. Lipoprotein lipase hydrolyses the triglyceride of chylomicrons far more rapidly than that of VLDL; by contrast the hepatic lipase splits chylomicron triglyceride very slowly, and has increasing activity against the denser triglyceride-rich remnant particles, particularly against IDL. In deficiency of lipoprotein lipase or of apo-CII, activity of the hepatic enzyme is normal or somewhat increased. In this clinical situation, and possibly physiologically, hepatic endothelial lipase may account for catabolism of VLDL and the denser remnant particles. The fractional catabolism of VLDL particles, as assessed by VLDL–apo-B metabolism, and its fractional conversion to LDL proceeds at a normal rate in lipoprotein lipase and apo-CII deficiencies.

Study of apo-CII deficiency has provided further physiological insights. Temporary replacement of the activator by fresh-frozen plasma infusion strikingly demonstrates the influence of lipoprotein lipase on every lipoprotein class: chylomicron concentrations fall steeply, and to a lesser extent VLDL levels decrease; concentrations of IDL, LDL, HDL$_2$, and HDL$_3$ increase, reflecting the direct or indirect role of the enzyme in their formation.

Differential diagnosis of severe hypertriglyceridaemia. In the differential diagnosis of severe hypertriglyceridaemia the first step is recognition of underlying causes, notably diabetes mellitus, alcohol abuse, nephrosis, glycogen storage disease, or myelomatosis. If familial, the distinction between endogenous and diet-related hyperlipidaemia must be made and is crucial in offering effective therapy. Lipoprotein patterns are helpful but type V may result from either mechanism. Lipoprotein lipase deficiency is characterized by predominant chylomicronaemia and by autosomal recessive inheritance. It is confirmed by assay of the enzyme in adipose tissue at a specialized centre, or in plasma obtained ten minutes after injection of heparin 40 units/kg i.v. to release endothelium-bound lipases into the blood stream. Post-heparin plasma contains more than one lipase, hence a lipoprotein-lipase-specific assay is required. The differential diagnosis may also be made by serial measurement of plasma triglyceride and assessment of chylomicronaemia quantitatively or by the stored plasma test at baseline and at 24-hour intervals after instituting an isocaloric fat-free diet (< 5 g fat/24 hours). Triglyceride levels fall to < 5 mmol/l and chylomicrons virtually disappear within 72 hours. Apo-CII deficiency is recognized by immunoassay and may be strongly suspected if hyperlipidaemia is greatly ameliorated within 24 hours of infusing 500 ml of normal fresh-frozen plasma.

Remnant hyperlipoproteinaemia (type III hyperlipoproteinaemia, broad-beta disease). Recognition of this uncommon variety of familial hyperlipidaemia provides an important therapeutic opportunity. Untreated, it is associated with increased risk of early-onset atherosclerosis, and with xanthomas and, occasionally, pancreatitis; it is however extremely responsive to appropriate treatment. Most often it is diagnosed during adult life but some case reports describe presentation during childhood.

Though the majority of patients have cutaneous xanthomas, which can be very florid, such lesions can be quite inconspicuous. Tuberous xanthomas are most often seen on the elbows though they can appear at almost any site. They are elevated sessile or hemispherical pink or orange-pink lesions often occurring in clusters, 0.5–3 cm in diameter, and are commonly surrounded by several eruptive xanthomas. The other skin lesion, almost diagnostic of remnant hyperlipoproteinaemia is the linear planar xanthomas which are seen in the palmar creases, orange-coloured usually-impalpable streaks. They range from pronounced bands 5–6 mm in diameter to easily-missed lesions best detected in daylight. Tendon xanthomas have also been reported in this condition. Clinical observation suggests that the distribution of atherosclerosis is somewhat different from that in other hyperlipidaemic states, lower-limb ischaemia being commoner than heart disease; three personal cases have had thrombotic strokes in middle age, in the absence of other known risk factors. Other clinical features, less often observed, are hepatosplenomegaly and episodes of pancreatitis. Glucose intolerance and hyperuricaemia may be present.

Marked combined hyperlipidaemia is the rule, with typical cholesterol levels of 10–15 mmol/l and triglyceride concentration 5–12 mmol/l. This is chiefly due to accumulation in plasma of IDL and of the denser subclasses of VLDL. There may also be mild chylomicronaemia. LDL and HDL levels are usually low. VLDL in this disorder has several atypical features: slow electrophoretic mobility (to the β or fast-β position instead of pre-β or α_2), a high ratio of cholesterol to triglyceride (a molar ratio exceeding 1:1 being virtually diagnostic), and an abnormally high content of apo-E. The less-dense VLDL, and chylomicrons too, are cholesterol-rich. These findings have been interpreted as indicating an increase within each lipoprotein class in the proportion of the later products of intravascular catabolism of VLDL and chylomicrons, i.e. an accumulation of remnant particles. During normal catabolism triglyceride, phospholipid, and apo-C are selectively lost, resulting in a relative enrichment in cholesteryl ester and apo-E. Kinetic studies of lipoprotein metabolism indicate decreased catabolism of IDL and denser VLDL. The uptake of such particles in the splanchnic bed was reduced, and the fraction converted to LDL was 10–15 per cent (normal 30–70 per cent) in two patients studied in the author's laboratory.

The key to the complex genetics of type III was the demonstration by Utermann that apo-E (a major apoprotein of remnant particles) shows genetic polymorphism with at least four isoproteins. A consistent finding in such patients is the low ratio of apo-E$_3$ to apo-E$_2$ (the apo-E–D phenotype). This phenotype is common, being present in about 1 per cent of a healthy population; hence it is a necessary but not a sufficient cause of type III, and in fact most individuals bearing this phenotype are mildly hypocholesterolaemic. It may be transmitted as an autosomal recessive. Studies of type III kindreds by Utermann and by Hazzard suggest that other heritable hyperlipidaemias are often present. These investigators proposed that type III hyperlipoproteinaemia arises as a result of the coexistence in the affected individual of apo-E deficiency and either familial combined hyperlipidaemia or, less often, familial hypercholesterolaemia. Possibly hypothyroidism or diabetes mellitus can also interact with apo-E$_3$ deficiency to cause type III. Thus several variants of type III are possible. There is evidence suggesting that hepatic 'recognition' and the consequent avid uptake and catabolism of remnant particles is dependent upon their high proportion of apo-E, and that such recognition is impaired when the ratio of apo-E$_3$ to apo-E$_2$ is low. Occurring alone, this leads to subnormal LDL production and hypocholesterolaemia, but in the presence of other disorders of lipid metabolism the rare type III hyperlipoproteinaemia develops.

Recent investigations have shown more extensive polymorphism of apo-E. This is determined by alleles coding for three major isoproteins; in the heterozygous state these produce the α pattern of apo-E proteins, and in the homozygous state the β pattern. These patterns are rendered more complex by post-transitional changes in E proteins which determine their number of sialic acid groups, yielding a multiplicity of proteins. Six patterns of apo-E isoproteins result from these genetic and post-transatational determinants. One of these, βIV is uniquely present in remnant (Type III) hyperlipoproteinaemia. The presence of βIV rather than the absence of a specific protein may prove to be a necessary factor in the causation of Type III; but if, as has been estimated, βIV occurs in about 3 per cent of people, it follows that an additional abnormality must be present for remnant hyperlipoproteinaemia to develop.

The diagnosis of type III or remnant hyperlipoproteinaemia requires the presence of combined hyperlipidaemia, usually but not always severe, due to 'atypical' VLDL. Combined hyperlipidaemia occurring in a patient with the classical physical signs is relatively specific for this disorder, but confirmation depends upon the demonstration of a cholesterol:triglyceride molar ratio > 1.0 in isolated VLDL, or of definite β mobility of VLDL on agarose or polyacrylamide gel electrophoresis. At specialized centres the abnormal apo-E isoprotein pattern may be confirmed.

Lecithin-cholesterol acyltransferase deficiency. This is an extremely rare recessively inherited disorder. The enzyme deficiency leads to very low levels of cholesteryl ester in plasma; there is marked hyperlipidaemia, with high concentrations of unesterified cholesterol and of triglyceride. The clinical manifestations include ocular and renal lesions. Corneal opacities due to lipid deposits are common. Foam cells are present in the renal glomeruli, due to deposition of grossly abnormal plasma lipoproteins. Proteinuria is a consistent feature and renal failure is the major cause of death. There is anaemia with target cells, and the erythrocyte membrane is abnormal.

All plasma lipoproteins show striking chemical and structural abnormalities including the presence of LP-X, underlining the role of lecithin-cholesterol acyltransferase in intravascular lipoprotein metabolism. The condition should be suspected when chronic renal disease is accompanied by corneal opacities and marked hyperlipidaemia. The diagnosis is confirmed by the very low ratio of esterified to free cholesterol in plasma (< 0.1) and by assay of the transferase. There is no specific treatment at present; medical treatment of renal failure is required and renal transplantation has been performed. A familial distribution must be sought.

Fish-eye disease. This is a familial disorder so far recognized only in northern Sweden, in which hypertriglyceridaemia is accompanied by visual impairment due to dense corneal opacities. VLDL levels are increased, LDL is abnormally enriched in triglyceride, and HDL levels are very low. Lecithin-cholesterol acyltransferase activity is normal.

Common hyperlipidaemia. As discussed in an earlier section, selection of an upper limit for a 'normal' or 'desirable' range of plasma cholesterol concentration may be based on varying criteria. Whatever limit is chosen, a proportion of the population is thereby assigned to a hypercholesterolaemic range. The frequency distribution of plasma cholesterol levels is skewed to the right. For this reason, too, the prevalence of hypercholesterolaemia is very considerable, e.g. 10 per cent of adult Londoners have cholesterol levels exceeding 6.5 mmol/l. The majority of hypercholesterolaemic subjects by this definition do not have any of the major primary or secondary hyperlipidaemias described in the foregoing sections, but their lipoprotein status is a cause for concern in that their lipoprotein-mediated risk of ischaemic heart disease is substantially greater than that of normolipidaemic people (see below).

The term common hypercholesterolaemia may be applied to this state. It is not a disease, but rather a risk factor for disease. Genetic factors play a role in determining the level of plasma cholesterol, the pattern of transmission being polygenic.

Expression of the genetic make-up is powerfully influenced by diet, notably the intake and saturation of fatty acids, energy balance, intake of fibre, and of cholesterol. Correspondingly, reduction of plasma cholesterol in this portion of the population should chiefly be based upon dietary modification.

Hyperalphalipoproteinaemia. Population surveys have revealed that remarkably high levels of HDL-cholesterol (α-lipoprotein) are not infrequent. This may only be evident on lipoprotein analysis, but in some subjects total plasma cholesterol is mildly elevated. High levels of HDL-cholesterol are seen physiologically in highly-trained athletes. They may also result from alcohol abuse, exogenous oestrogen treatment and the use of or exposure to microsomal enzyme inducers such as phenobarbitone, phenytoin, and halogenated insecticides, effects which are very slowly reversible.

A familial elevation of HDL concentration has been well described. The lipoprotein is of normal composition and the mechanism is unknown. Xanthomas do not occur, and the exchangeable mass of cholesterol in the non-plasma compartments of the body tends to be low. It has been claimed that such families enjoy unusual longevity and that ischaemic heart disease is conspicuously infrequent. No treatment is known or indicated. Recognition of elevation of HDL levels as a cause of mild hypercholesterolaemia is within the competence of almost every laboratory. It will prevent committing a patient to inappropriate dietary or pharmacological treatment.

Management of the hyperlipidaemic states

Before embarking on potentially life-long dietary or drug treatment of hyperlipidaemia, the objectives must be clearly defined. Prevention of relapsing pancreatitis justifies the correction of severe hypertriglyceridaemia, and the excess risk of ischaemic heart disease in familial hypercholesterolaemia is so great as to call for adequate intervention by drugs, diet, and if necessary surgical or other procedures. Regression or non-progression of disfiguring cutaneous and tendon xanthomas can be achieved. More generally, however, judgement must be used in deciding whether to treat, and how intensively, in an attempt to reduce ischaemic heart disease risk. The younger the patient, the more pronounced the lipoprotein abnormality, and the worse the family history, the more assiduously should one attempt to reduce plasma lipid levels towards the desirable range. A further indication is the presence of multiple risk factors, especially hyperlipidaemia with hypertension or diabetes; a corollary is that attempted reduction of cardiovascular risk requires intervention against all known risk factors, the cigarette habit deserving the same attention as hyperlipidaemia for example.

There is strong evidence that hypercholesterolaemia due to elevated LDL levels is causally associated with a high risk of atherosclerotic heart disease (see page 13.151), hence judicious treatment is justified despite the current lack of rigorous proof of benefit. The treatment of mild to moderate hypertriglyceridaemia is more controversial, chiefly because it is not yet clear whether its status as a cardiovascular risk factor is direct or due to the often-associated low levels of HDL-cholesterol. Hypertriglyceridaemia can be a marker for the presence of familial combined hyperlipidaemia, a disorder which is clearly over-represented in ischaemic heart disease patients. Interventions designed to increase plasma HDL-cholesterol levels, seemingly desirable on epidemiological grounds, are currently unsupported by evidence from clinical trial or laboratory experimentation. On the other hand, reduction of moderate hypertriglyceridaemia and increased levels of HDL-cholesterol can usually be achieved by an appropriate programme of physical exercise and by correction or partial correction of obesity; and the correction of even modest over-use of alcohol in hypertriglyceridaemia is most effective. It is difficult to take exception to such interventions.

The following is a brief account of the better-authenticated measures for treating primary hyperlipidaemia. Few if any are specific for individual disorders. Wherever possible secondary hyperlipidaemia is dealt with by management of the underlying condition.

Weight reduction. Weight reduction of the obese hyperlipidaemic patient decreases endogenous hypertriglyceridaemia (due to elevated levels of VLDL or IDL) often to a striking extent, the improvement usually persisting when an isocaloric diet is resumed. Common hypercholesterolaemia is also usually ameliorated. During weight reduction HDL-cholesterol shows little change or decrease but there is evidence that levels gradually increase to above baseline values after the weight loss is completed. Hence correction or even partial correction of obesity is a valuable first step in hyperlipidaemia management, requiring calorie restriction preferably together with a suitable exercise programme.

Isocaloric dietary modification. This is the mainstay of treatment of most hyperlipidaemic patients, alone or together with lipid-active drugs. Satisfactory results can be achieved with a single set of dietary modifications in many hypercholesterolaemic and endogenously-hypertriglyceridaemic states; but a distinct diet is required in the exogenous hypertriglyceridaemia due to defects of the lipoprotein lipase system. Reduction of saturated fatty acid intake is the most important component of the generally applicable diet, typically to 8–10 per cent of energy requirements compared with 20 per cent in the normal British diet. The intake of carbohydrate, specifically of complex carbohydrates as in cereal products and vegetables is increased. Total fat intake becomes 25–30 per cent and polyunsaturated fatty acids, particularly linoleic acid, provide 7–10 per cent of food energy (cf. 3–4 per cent normally). This chiefly requires reduction of the intake of fat from dairy products, meat, and baked foods, with a moderate increase in linoleic acid sources, i.e. edible oils and polyunsaturate-rich margarines. Such a diet is necessarily low in cholesterol because of restriction in foods of animal origin, and the cholesterol intake may be specified as 200–250 mg/day (cf. about 500 mg normally). The expected mean fall in plasma cholesterol concentration is about 20 per cent though incomplete compliance usually reduces this in practice to nearer 15 per cent. Other dietary measures which reduce plasma cholesterol concentration include supplementation with fruit, vegetables, and oat bran. Other sources of dietary fibre such as wheat bran are not effective. Reduction of saturated fatty acid and cholesterol intake, modest supplementation with linoleic acid and with fruit and vegetable fibre have an additive and potent cholesterol-lowering effect.

In hyperlipidaemia due to deficiency of lipoprotein lipase or apo-CII the treatment is severe restriction of all long-chain fatty acids, i.e. all fat-rich foods. Treatment is commenced with a very low fat intake, which is progressively increased under close observation; most adult patients maintain acceptable plasma triglyceride levels (< 6 mmol/l) when consuming 20–30 g fat per day. Medium chain triglyceride is not transported in chylomicrons and can be added to the diet if liver function is normal.

Physical activity. Physical activity of the aerobic type, undertaken for periods of at least 20 minutes, at least on alternate days, reduces triglyceride levels, increases HDL-cholesterol, and in some studies has been shown to reduce plasma cholesterol. Institution of an exercise programme should not be undertaken lightly. In a sedentary middle-aged patient the initial stages must be gentle, with progressive increments as fitness develops; suitable limits for the exercising pulse rate are 60 per cent of calculated maximum heart rate initially, and rising to 75 per cent. The programme should take into account cardiorespiratory capacity, age, musculoskeletal problems, and, especially, effort-induced symptoms. A baseline exercise ECG is often recommended.

Bile-acid sequestrants. Cholestyramine and colestipol are valuable in the treatment of severe or resistant hypercholesterolaemia. They are non-absorbable anion exchange resins which bind bile acids, reduce their enterohepatic circulation, and enhance the catabolism of cholesterol to bile acids and receptor-mediated catabolism of LDL. Cholestyramine is effective in heterozygous familial hypercholesterolaemia at a dosage of 8–12 g twice daily, with meals. Xanthomas commonly show partial regression over a period of 1–3 years. A controlled trial of colestipol suggests that ischaemic heart disease incidence and mortality may be reduced in hypercholesterolaemic men, but female patients were not significantly benefited. The bulk of sequestrant drugs is somewhat inconvenient. Many patients develop mild constipation which can be offset by increased fibre intake. Dyspepsia is sometimes a problem. The most serious difficulties arise from malabsorption of other drugs taken within 1–2 hours of these resins, including warfarin and digoxin. Folate deficiency is a potential problem, especially in children and pregnant women who require a supplement of 5 mg daily taken at a time well separated from sequestrant ingestion.

Nicotinic acid. Taken in pharmacological doses nicotinic acid effectively reduces triglyceride levels, and plasma cholesterol decreases to a smaller but valuable extent. HDL-cholesterol increases. It reduces free fatty acid release from adipose tissue, limiting the supply of substrate for hepatic VLDL-triglyceride synthesis; cholesterol synthesis is probably also reduced. The drug is of use in severe endogenous hypertriglyceridaemia; in familial hypercholesterolaemia its effect is usefully additive with bile acid sequestrants. With many preparations initial flushing is a problem, requiring a gradually increasing dosage schedule. Other side-effects are dyspepsia, cholestatic jaundice, and hyperuricaemia. Diabetes may be aggravated but the drug can sometimes be successfully used in the presence of diabetes. Inositol nicotinate 1–1.5 g three times daily with meals (adult dose) appears to cause flushing and dyspepsia less often than other preparations.

Clofibrate. This was used for all forms of hyperlipidaemia, and is the drug of choice for remnant (type III) hyperlipidaemia. It can be effective in severe diet-resistant hypertriglyceridaemia, where there is a risk of acute pancreatitis. It is the only drug which has unequivocally been shown to reduce myocardial infarction morbidity in previously healthy men. It decreases endogenous hypertriglyceridaemia, has a smaller effect on elevated plasma cholesterol levels, and increases HDL-cholesterol. Its effect is additive with that of cholestyramine in reducing plasma cholesterol. The modes of action include an increased activity of lipoprotein lipase and increased biliary excretion of cholesterol. The latter effect leads to an increased risk of cholesterol gallstones. It is appropriate to deal effectively with obesity whenever possible, before prescribing lipid-lowering drugs such as clofibrate and nicotinic acid. This may offset the increase in lithogenicity of bile. Other untoward effects are potentiation of coumarin anticoagulants, an acute myopathy causing pain and stiffness in large muscle groups, impotence, leucopenia, and ventricular bigeminy. In one extensive controlled trial there was an increase in non-cardiovascular mortality, not confirmed in another large trial. Clofibrate must be used with great caution, and in low dosage, if used for the hyperlipidaemia of renal failure; there is a particular risk of acute myopathy, and deterioration in renal function has been reported. Several fibric acid analogues are now becoming available in many countries. None has been shown to protect against myocardial infarction, and their appearance is too recent to compare their risk–benefit ratios with that of clofibrate, but in their favour there is a several fold increase in potency.

Probucol. This drug introduced relatively recently, is used for treatment of hypercholesterolaemia and does not significantly alter triglyceride levels. Its effect is additive with that of diet. In diet-resistant hypercholesterolaemia due to familial combined hyperlipidaemia, or to common hypercholesterolaemia, LDL-cholesterol levels decrease by about 20 per cent. Some patients with heterozygous familial hypercholesterolaemia respond to probucol. Mild diarrhoea may occur. Gallstone risk is not increased. The drug reduces HDL-cholesterol levels, probably by depressing the HDL_3 subclass; this effect requires further evaluation.

Ileal bypass surgery. This has proved successful in the treatment of heterozygous familial hypercholesterolaemia, interrupting the enterohepatic circulation of bile acids with consequent effects similar to but more pronounced than those of bile-acid sequestrant drugs. A greater increase in faecal bile acid excretion occurs. Cramping and diarrhoea are the major side-effects, and malabsorption of vitamin B_{12} necessitates monthly injections of the vitamin. The operation is worthy of consideration for patients with heterozygous familial hypercholesterolaemia who respond inadequately to, or do not comply with a two-drug regimen such as cholestyramine with nicotinic acid. There is limited evidence that atherosclerotic plaques show partial regression following the operation.

Plasma exchange. At intervals of 7–14 days, together with drug therapy, plasma exchange now appears to be the treatment of choice for the extremely rare homozygous familial hypercholesterolaemia. Extensive reduction of plasma cholesterol is attainable, with regression of xanthomas and suggestive evidence of retardation of atherogenesis. HDL-cholesterol levels fall to a lesser extent than LDL. The use of selective LDL-absorbing columns is likely to supersede this technique.

Hyperlipidaemia, other risk factors, and the pathogenesis of ischaemic heart disease

The pathogenesis of coronary atherosclerosis (see also page 13.151) may well have been the subject of greater research effort in the past quarter century than any other single disease. Though this permits many conclusions with a high degree of probability, wide areas of uncertainty remain. Atherosclerotic plaques vary in composition, their major components including smooth muscle cells, evidently monoclonal or oligoclonal in a single plaque, cholesteryl esters and other lipids, collagen, and glycosaminoglycans. According to Baroldi about 50 per cent of myocardial infarctions are associated with thrombosis in the coronary artery branch supplying that region; the more consistent finding, with rare exceptions, is extensive coronary atherosclerosis, and increasing evidence indicates a role of localized coronary spasm in precipitating at least some acute occlusions. Early events in the pathogenesis of the atheromatous plaque are not well understood. A plausible hypothesis envisages a sequence of events commencing with localized endothelial injury, platelet aggregation, release of a platelet polypeptide which is mitogenic for arterial smooth muscle cells, and local increase in permeability to plasma proteins including lipoproteins; smooth muscle hyperplasia and lipid accumulation ensue, followed by fibrosis and ulceration.

While fatty streaks are seen in the major arteries of young adults from many parts of the world, the International Atherosclerosis Project has shown marked regional differences in the frequency of raised atheromatous plaques. The rank order of coronary plaque frequency is similar to that of mean plasma cholesterol in population samples from the corresponding regions. Evolution of early plaques into raised occlusive lesions may therefore be a function of high plasma cholesterol levels and of the several other risk factors defined by prospective epidemiological studies: risk increases directly with cholesterol and LDL-cholesterol levels and inversely with HDL-cholesterol; the HDL effect is probably mediated by its HDL_2 subclass. Risk increases with blood pressure and the number of cigarettes smoked. The behaviour pattern described as type A personality is an independent risk factor, as is diabetes. While moderate asymptomatic hyperglycaemia is unassociated with excess risk of heart disease, glucose levels exceeding 5.3 mmol/l two hours after 50 g oral glucose, are predictive of ischaemic heart disease mortality. Other risk factors include insulin and fibrinogen levels and factor VII and VIII activity.

The association between hypercholesterolaemia and atherosclerotic heart disease is beyond dispute and is evident from a variety of epidemiological approaches. The probability that this association is one of cause and effect is suggested by several sources of evidence. Coronary lesions closely resembling human atherosclerosis are inducible in primates and other animals in which hyperlipidaemia is induced by high fat, high cholesterol diets. Such lesions show considerable regression in primates when cholesterol levels are reduced by dietary change or medication, regression being demonstrable at plasma cholesterol levels below 5 mmol/l. In man severe, typical atherosclerosis consistently develops in patients with elevated LDL levels due to heterozygous familial hypercholesterolaemia. The results of the many controlled trials of plasma cholesterol reduction in reducing ischaemic heart disease incidence have been variously interpreted. Few have been large enough, and few have achieved sufficient change in plasma cholesterol to test the causal hypothesis. Comparison of 14 major trials indicates that those studies which demonstrated a fall in incidence were most often the ones in which the reduction in plasma cholesterol was greatest, i.e. 13–20 per cent.

Other studies with bearing on the causal hypothesis have provided plausible mechanisms by which certain plasma lipoprotein abnormalities would favour growth of the atheromatous plaque. LDL is present in plaques and normal intima, and LDL influx provides a mechanism for transfer of cholesteryl ester into the intima; its net rate of transfer from plasma into the arterial wall is directly related to its plasma concentration. LDL has also been shown to induce smooth muscle cell proliferation. Conversely HDL appears to play a role in transfer of tissue cholesterol into plasma, initiating its centripetal transport and ultimately its excretion. High plasma HDL levels are associated with low tissue cholesterol content, a relationship which may be reflected in the amount of cholesterol present in the arterial wall.

In assessing the lipoprotein-mediated risk of cardiovascular disease, total plasma cholesterol level has stood the test of time as a useful predictor. It is usually a good index of the concentration of LDL-cholesterol, though the latter is a better measure of risk in that it remains predictive in the seventh decade of life while the total plasma cholesterol is not informative beyond age 60. From the viewpoint of risk of ischaemic heart disease an optimal plasma cholesterol level may well be 4.7 mmol/l, with an upper acceptable limit of 5.7 mmol/l; corresponding levels of LDL-cholesterol would be about 2.8 and 3.6 mmol/l. In clinical practice such levels are often difficult to attain by available methods of treatment of hypercholesterolaemia. In many prospective studies a progressive increase in ischaemic heart disease risk with rising cholesterol level is seen, from the lowest to the highest extremes of the distribution.

The inverse relationship between HDL-cholesterol level and risk is independent of that of total or LDL cholesterol. The probability of developing ischaemic heart disease is greatest in men with HDL-cholesterol levels of 1 mmol/l or less, and is least when levels of 1.6–1.8 mmol/l or more are present. There are insufficient data to define optimal levels at present. Corresponding values in women are 1.2 and 2 mmol/l.

It is by no means proven that a knowledge of plasma triglyceride or VLDL levels will provide additional knowledge of cardiovascular risk if plasma cholesterol and HDL-cholesterol levels are known. This by no means excludes a possible role of IDL or VLDL in atherogenesis, for which there is circumstantial evidence from clinical and experimental sources. Nor does it detract from the necessity for measuring plasma triglyceride as part of the characterization of disorders of lipoprotein metabolism.

The hypolipidaemias

Hypocholesterolaemia may be secondary to end-stage parenchymal liver disease, the distal malabsorption syndrome, severe intestinal protein loss, and sideroblastic anaemia. Very low cholesterol and triglyceride levels are a feature of malnutrition, particularly protein-energy deficiency in infants (kwashiorkor).

Abetalipoproteinaemia. This leads to severe clinical manifestations and most patients do not survive beyond 40 years of age. It is inherited as an autosomal recessive, and there appears to be failure to synthesize apolipoprotein B. Not only LDL, but also VLDL and chylomicrons, which contain this protein, are absent from serum. Because of this there is mild impairment of fat absorption, and the condition may present in infancy as failure to thrive often with diarrhoea and anorexia. By the second decade, neurological and visual abnormalities appear. Nystagmus, ataxia, dysarthria, and motor and sensory deficits develop, often with kyphoscoliosis, and sight becomes impaired due to a pigmentary retinopathy. Night blindness and colour blindness may occur, but visual impairment is seldom gross. The circulating red cells show acanthocytosis. Jejunal biopsy reveals normal villi with vacuolated mucosal cells; lipid is normally absorbed into these cells and fat droplets accumulate because of the failure of chylomicron synthesis. Malabsorption is not reversed by short-term infusions of LDL. It has been suggested that the neurological and retinal lesions may result from impaired transport of vitamins E and A.

The features described are distinctive, and the diagnosis is supported by the finding of marked hypolipidaemia. Serum cholesterol levels of 1–2 mmol/l are characteristic, and triglyceride is barely detectable in plasma. Electrophoresis reveals that only α-lipoprotein (HDL) is present. The absence of apolipoprotein B is confirmed by immuno-electrophoresis. Treatment of the malabsorption is by restriction of ordinary fat with partial substitution by medium chain triglyceride. Fat-soluble vitamin supplements have been given; it has been suggested that vitamins A and E may arrest progress of the retinal and neurological lesions. Supplements of these vitamins should certainly be given if their plasma concentrations are low.

Familial hypobetalipoproteinaemia. This is a separately inherited condition, an autosomal dominant. Hypocholesterolaemia is less pronounced with levels of 1–4 mmol/l. LDL is present in low concentration as shown on electrophoresis or ultracentrifugation. VLDL and HDL are present. Chylomicrons are formed after a fatty meal and malabsorption is uncommon. The disorder is often unassociated with clinical abnormalities; but some patients show features similar to those of abetalipoproteinaemia, including neurological changes developing in middle age, distorted red cell morphology, and fat-engorged intestinal mocosal cells. The synthetic rates of both VLDL and its product LDL are subnormal. In the homozygous state, this disorder may be indistinguishable from abetalipoproteinaemia but family studies reveal the distinct genetic basis.

Familial alphalipoprotein deficiency (Tangier disease). Another rare but clinically well-defined disorder, HDL deficiency occurs in patients homozygous for an autosomal recessive gene. One of the two major HDL apoproteins, apo-AI, is deficient and the trace of HDL detectable in plasma is abnormal in its protein and lipid composition. Serum cholesterol levels are low (1–3 mmol/l) and triglyceride concentration is moderately high or normal (1.5–3 mmol/l); this combination of abnormal lipid concentrations is highly suggestive of the diagnosis. On electrophoresis α-lipoprotein (HDL) is undetectable, and the β-and pre-β-regions are occupied by a broad band similar to that seen in type III hyperlipoproteinaemia. More detailed analysis shows an accumulation in plasma of IDL and the denser components of VLDL, accounting for the hypertriglyceridaemia. The diagnosis is confirmed by the faintness of the line of precipitation on immuno-electrophoresis against anti-HDL serum.

Accumulation of cholesteryl esters in reticulo-endothelial tissues accounts for most clinical manifestations. The tonsils and adenoids are enlarged and orange in colour; after tonsillectomy the tonsillar tags and adenoids retain the characteristic colour. The spleen, and sometimes the liver are enlarged. Corneal opacities are common, and a motor and sensory neuropathy is frequently present. There is no definite evidence of predisposition to ischaemic heart disease despite the absence of normal HDL. It may be relevant that LDL concentration is also low in Tangier disease. The pathogenesis of the lipid storage is uncertain. The activity of lecithin-cholesterol acyltransferase is somewhat low, but this is unlikely to be of functional significance. The deficiency of HDL may limit the rate of centripetal transport of cholesterol. The metabolic basis for the HDL deficiency is unknown. Normal HDL shows rapid fractional disappearance in Tangier patients but it cannot be concluded that increased catabolism explains the laboratory findings. The reasons for accumulation in plasma of triglyceride-rich intermediate density lipoproteins is unclear. There is no known treatment.

References

Blackburn, H., Lewis, B., Stamler, J., Wissler, R. W., and Wynder, E. L. (1979). Conference on the health effects of blood lipids: optimal distributions for populations. *Preventive Medicine* **8**, 609.
Brown, M. S. and Goldstein, J. L. (1976). Receptor-mediated control of cholesterol metabolism. *Science* **191**, 150.
Dietschy, J. M. and Wilson, J. D. (1970). Regulation of cholesterol metabolism. *New Engl. J. Med.* **282**, 1128.
Eisenberg, S. and Levy, R. I. (1975). Lipoprotein metabolism. *Adv. Lipid. Res.* **13**, 1.
Goldstein, J. L., Schrott, H. G., Hazzard, W. R., Bierman, E. L., and Motulsky, A. G. (1973). Hyperlipidaemia in coronary heart disease: genetic analysis. *J. clin. Invest.* **52**, 1544.
Janus, E. D., Nicholl, A. M., Turner, P. R., Magill, P., and Lewis, B. (1980). Kinetic bases of the primary hyperlipidaemias. *Eur. J. clin. Invest.* **10**, 161.
Lewis, B. (1976). *The hyperlipidaemias: clinical and laboratory practice.* Blackwell Scientific Publications, Oxford.
Miller, N. E. (1979). Plasma lipoproteins, lipid transport and atherosclerosis. *J. Clin. Path.* **32**, 639.

DISORDERS OF PURINE METABOLISM

G. Nuki

Gout

Gout is a name given to a group of metabolic diseases in which symptoms and signs result from tissue deposition of crystals of *monosodium urate monohydrate* from hyperuricaemic body fluids. Major clinical manifestations include: (a) acute inflammatory arthritis, tenosynovitis, bursitis, or cellulitis; (b) chronic, erosive, deforming arthritis associated with periarticular and subcutaneous urate deposits (tophi); (c) nephrolithiasis and urolithiasis due to deposition of crystals of *uric acid* from urine at acid pH; (d) chronic renal disease and hypertension.

The biochemical hallmark of the disorder is hyperuricaemia. Prolonged elevation of serum urate is a necessary, but not sufficient, prerequisite for the development of clinical gout. Hyperuricaemia may result from increased purine intake, turnover, and production; decreased urate elimination; or a combination of genetic and environmental factors.

Serum urate levels. Serum urate concentrations are distributed in the community as a continuous variable (Fig. 1). Mean values are higher in men than in women and the sex-specific distribution curve is broader for males than females with skewing to the higher end of the scale in both sexes. Serum urate levels rise in boys at puberty and then remain virtually unchanged throughout adult life. In girls the pubertal rise is smaller and the serum urate level only approaches that of the males after the menopause (Fig. 2).

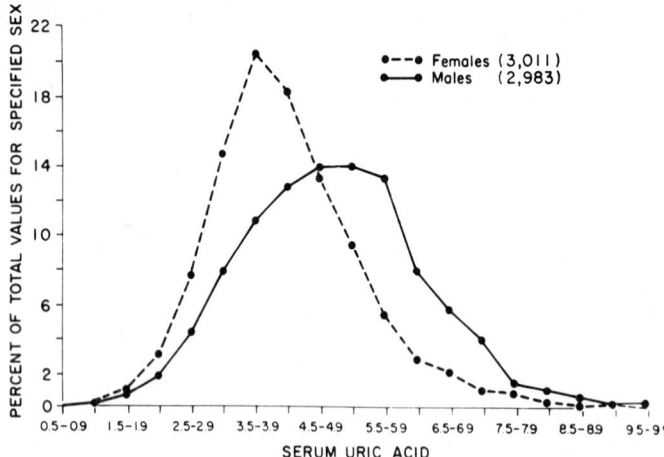

Fig. 1 Distribution of serum urate (mg%) values in male and female populations of Tecumseh, Michigan, 1959/60 (from Mikkleson *et. al.: Am. J. Med.* **39**, 242 (1965), permission of the *American Journal of Medicine*).

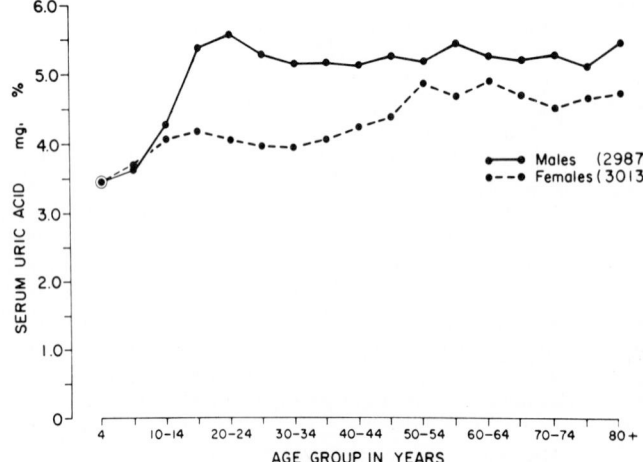

Fig. 2 Sex and age specific mean serum urate values in the population of Tecumseh, Michigan, 1959/60 (from Mikkleson *et. al.: Am. J. Med.* **39**, 242 (1965), with permission of the *American Journal of Medicine*).

Epidemiological studies demonstrate significant variations of serum urate in different ethnic groups. The Maoris of New Zealand and the Polynesians of the Western Pacific, for example, have very high levels. Although some polygenic control of serum urate levels is well established, environmental factors are also important. The Chinese community in Taiwan have lower serum urate levels than those in Malaysia or British Columbia; Philippinos resident in the United States have higher serum urate levels than those in the Philippine Islands and urban South African negroes have significantly higher levels than those in rural communities. There is some evidence to suggest that these differences within ethnic groups result from a less than average capacity to increase the renal excretion of urate when the purine load is increased. These data, and positive correlations between high serum urate levels and protein intake, alcohol consumption, weight, body bulk, social class, and intelligence have led to the understanding that in most communities environmental factors are the major determinants of the level of serum urate—'the associates of hyperuricaemia are the associates of plenty'.

Hyperuricaemia. Serum is saturated with monosodium urate at a concentration of 7 mg per 100 ml (0.42 mmol/l) but much higher concentrations of urate may remain in stable supersaturated solution for long periods. The majority of subjects with hyperuricaemia are asymptomatic. Nevertheless, epidemiological studies suggest that risks of clinical manifestations of gout gradually increased with rising values of serum urate without any evidence of a critical threshold level (Table 1). The age of onset of gouty arthritis is also inversely related to the level of serum urate, rising from a mean of 39 years in men with serum urate levels greater than 9 mg/100 ml (0.52 mmol/l) to 55 years in those with levels between 6 and 7 mg/100 ml (0.35–0.42 mmol/l).

Hyperuricaemia is usually arbitrarily defined as a serum urate level greater than two standard deviations from the mean. Using a specific enzymatic (uricase) spectrophotometric assay, upper limits of normal are 7 mg/100 ml (0.42 mmol/l) for adult males and 6 mg/100 ml (0.36 mmol/l) for females in UK and US communities. Automated colorimetric assays used in most clinical laboratories may give results which are 1 mg/100 ml (0.06 mmol/l) higher, and hospital populations have higher levels, largely attributable to diuretic drug therapy.

Uric acid metabolism. Uric acid is the end-product of purine metabolism in man and some higher apes. These species lack the enzyme uricase which degrades uric acid to allantoin in the majority of mammals.

Plasma and tissue urates are derived from the catabolism of preformed dietary purines and purine nucleotides synthesized *de novo*. The miscible body pool of urate in normal individuals ranges from 0.9–1.6 g, of which about 60 per cent is replenished daily from the catabolism of newly synthesized purines. Two-thirds of the urate formed each day is eliminated by the kidney and one-third via the gastrointestinal tract.

Purine synthesis. Purine nucleotide synthesis in mammalian cells is regulated by a balanced interaction of a number of biochemical pathways (Fig. 3). The *de novo* pathway of purine biosynthesis consists of a series of ten enzymatic reactions in which glutamine, glycine, carbon dioxide, aspartate, and one-carbon formyl derivatives of folate are added to the ribose phosphate moiety of phosphoribosyl pyrophosphate (PRPP) to form inosinic acid (IMP). Adenosine monophosphate (AMP) and guanosine monophosphate (GMP) are each formed from IMP by two enzymatic steps before phosphorylation to their respective di- and triphosphates. Alternatively the nucleotide monophosphates can also be synthesized by phosphorylation of purine bases by phosphoribosyl transferase enzymes reacting with PRPP, and AMP can be formed by phosphorylation of adenosine by adenosine kinase. *In vitro* studies of PRPP amidophosphoribosyl transferase (PAT), the first enzyme in the *de novo* pathway of purine synthesis, show it to have allosteric properties that one might associate with a

rate-limiting enzyme, and have provided a molecular model for the mechanism whereby the rate of purine synthesis is regulated. The enzyme exists in two forms; a catalytically inactive dimer and an active monomer. PRPP converts the larger form of the enzyme to the active monomer while purine nucleotide monophosphates have the opposite effect. A good deal of evidence suggests that PRPP, which is present in cells at limiting concentrations, is the major regulator of the rate of *de novo* purine synthesis in clinical situations associated with increased or decreased purine production.

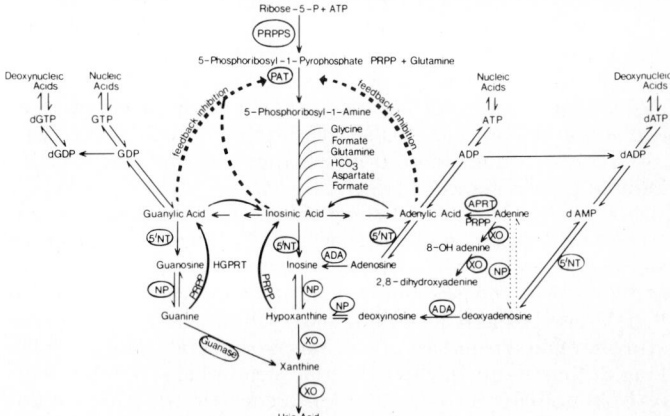

Fig. 3 Pathways of purine metabolism in man.
ADA = Adenosine deaminase
APRT = Adenine phosphoribosyl transferase
HGPRT = Hypoxanthine–guanine phosphoribosyl transferase
NP = Nucleoside phosphorylase
5′NT = 5′-nucleotidase
PAT = Phosphoribosyl pyrophosphate amidotransferase
PRPPS = Phosphoribosyl pyrophosphate synthetase
XO = Xanthine oxidase
(From Nuki: *Advanced Medicine* **15**, 138 (1979), with permission of the publishers, Pitman Medical, London.)

The purine nucleotide monophosphates are degraded to nucleosides by 5′ nucleotidase. Adenosine is deaminated by the enzyme adenosine deaminase and inosine and guanosine dephosphorylated to purine bases by nucleoside phosphorylase. Guanine and hypoxanthine are converted to xanthine by guanase and xanthine oxidase and this latter enzyme is also responsible for the final oxidation of xanthine to uric acid.

Uric acid excretion. Uric acid excreted in the urine is derived from both endogenous purine production and exogenous dietary purines. On an unrestricted diet, urine uric acid excretion can be as much as 1000 mg/day, each gram of dietary nucleic acid contributing 115–150 mg of urinary uric acid. Although 100–200 mg of uric acid are secreted daily into the gastrointestinal tract prior to degradation by bacterial uricolysis, an approximate estimate of uric acid synthesis can be made by measuring urine uric acid excretion

Table 1 Prevalence of gouty arthritis and urinary stones in relation to maximal serum uric acid over twelve years

Serum uric acid level (mg/100 ml)	Men			Women		
	Total number examined	% Gout	% Stones	Total number examined	% Gout	% Stones
< 6	1281	0.6		2665	0.08	
> 6	1002	6.1		179	5.0	
> 7	212	21.7	12.7	28	14.3	7.1
> 8	50	38.0	22.0	5	0	0
> 9	10	90.0	40.0	1	0	0
Totals	2283	2.8	1.4	2844	0.4	0.07

From the Framingham study (Hall *et al.* (1967), by permission).

on an isocaloric purine-free diet. Twenty-four-hour excretion of more than 600 mg (3.6 mmol) of uric acid on a 2600-calorie, 70-g protein, purine-free diet strongly suggests an increase in *de novo* purine synthesis or increased turnover of cellular purine nucleotides. Accurate assessment of the rate of *de novo* purine synthesis requires measurement of incorporation of ^{14}C-isotopically-labelled glycine into urine uric acid with simultaneous administration of ^{15}N-labelled uric acid to allow for extrarenal disposal of urate.

Renal handling of uric acid follows a four-component system: glomerular filtration, proximal tubular reabsorption, tubular secretion, and post-secretory reabsorption. Glomerular ultrafiltration is complete as there is no significant protein binding of urate *in vivo*. Proximal tubular reabsorption occurs by an active-transport mechanism closely linked or identical with the transport mechanism responsible for the tubular reabsorption of sodium. Evidence for active secretion comes from inherited and pharmacologically induced tubular defects in which urate clearance can exceed inulin clearance. The paradoxical effect of high- and low-dosage aspirin on uric acid excretion can be explained by differential effects on active secretion and reabsorption. Low-dosage aspirin blocks urate secretion with consequent hyperuricaemia while high-dosage therapy also blocks reabsorption and results in a net increase in uric acid excretion. Post-secretory reabsorption of urate is suggested by the fact that pretreatment with probenecid, which inhibits tubular reabsorption of urate, prevents the decrement in uric acid excretion that normally follows administration of low-dosage aspirin or pyrazinamide.

Renal clearance of urate in normal subjects ranges from 6–9 ml/min which is less than one-tenth of inulin or creatinine clearance. Decreased fractional clearance of urate is the cause of hyperuricaemia in 75 per cent or more of gouty patients. In up to 25 per cent there may be some evidence of primary purine overproduction.

Pathogenesis of hyperuricaemia. The concentration of urate in body fluids depends on a balance between purine synthesis plus ingestion and uric acid elimination. Hyperuricaemia may be the result of increased urate production, decreased renal excretion, or a combination of both mechanisms. Decrease in extrarenal elimination of uric acid in the gut has not been shown to be a cause of hyperuricaemia. Dietary ingestion of purines can be an important contributing factor and there is evidence to suggest that gout and hyperuricaemia are much more frequent in affluent than malnourished populations. To a large extent, however, the normal kidney is able to increase uric acid excretion in response to a dietary purine load.

In 75–90 per cent of patients with gout, hyperuricaemia is associated with impairment of fractional excretion of uric acid (Fig. 4). In the presence of normal creatinine clearance, uric acid clearance is significantly reduced (mean 3.6 ml/min).

Secondary hyperuricaemia, and gout, may, however, be a consequence of a variety of factors that influence renal blood flow, tubular reabsorption, and secretion of uric acid (Table 2).

Increased uric acid production and excretion are found in 10–15 per cent of patients with gout. In the majority of these patients the basis for increased synthesis of purines *de novo* is unknown, but in a few there is evidence of a specific inherited purine enzyme defect. In approximately 10 per cent of patients with gout, hyperuricaemia results from increased turnover of preformed purines and in a few accelerated *de novo* purine synthesis may be a secondary subordinate manifestation of an inherited enzyme defect (Table 2).

Pathogenesis of crystal inflammation. The factors leading to the precipitation of monosodium urate crystals from supersaturated solution in connective tissues are complex and poorly understood. A good deal of evidence suggests that symptomatic gout is always preceded by a long period of asymptomatic hyperuricaemia. Silent deposition of urate crystals in relatively avascular articular cartilage

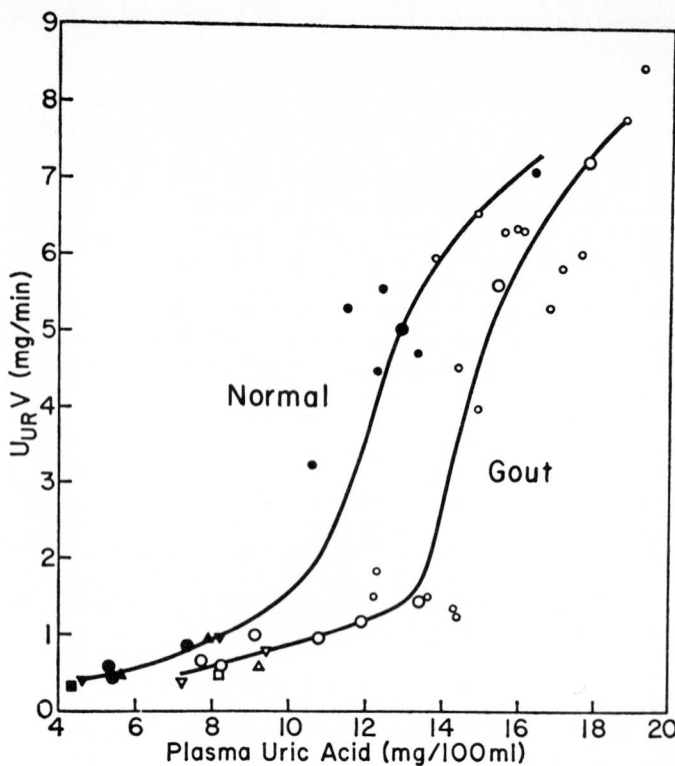

Fig. 4 Rate of uric acid excretion at various plasma urate levels in non-gouty (solid symbols) and gouty (open symbols) subjects. Large symbols represent mean values; small symbols represent individual data of some mean values to illustrate scatter within groups. Data obtained under basal conditions, after RNA feeding and after infusions of lithium urate.
▲△ Nugent and Tyler: *J. clin Invest.* **38**, 1890 (1959).
▼▽ Seegmiller *et. al.*: *J. clin Invest.* **41**, 1094 (1962).
● ○ Yu *et. al.*: *Am. J. Med.* **33**, 829 (1962).
■ □ Latham and Rodnan: *J. clin Invest.* **41**, 1955 (1962).
(From Wyngaarden: *Adv. metab. Dis.* **2**, 2 (1965), with permission of Academic Press.)

and tendons may well be a prelude to the induction of acute crystal synovitis by a process of crystal shedding. Direct trauma, or local metabolic changes leading to loosening of crystals from their connective tissue mould can predispose to crystal synovitis and may explain why it is possible to develop acute gouty arthritis at a time when the plasma uric acid level is not raised. Sudden lowering of plasma urate levels following initiation of uricosuric or allopurinol drug therapy may provoke acute gout by a similar mechanism but other factors which precipitate acute attacks, such as alcohol, dietary excess, severe dieting, diuretic drug therapy, or severe physical exercise do so by suddenly elevating the plasma urate.

Microcrystals of monosodium urate preferentially absorb IgG to their surface. This facilitates phagocytosis by Fc receptor-bearing polymorphonuclear leucocytes. Crystal-induced membranolysis follows phagocytosis and degradation of the adsorbed protein. Although the molecular mechanisms underlying crystals membranolysis are incompletely understood the physicochemical interaction is accompanied by complement activation and a release of a wide variety of inflammatory mediators, chemotactic factors, and lysosomal and cytoplasmic enzymes.

Clinical features. There are four stages in the natural history of gout: asymptomatic hyperuricaemia, acute gouty arthritis, inter-critical gout, and chronic tophaceous gout. Symptomatic gout is usually preceded by many years of asymptomatic hyperuricaemia. Nineteen out of 20 hyperuricaemic subjects remain asymptomatic throughout life, but up to 25 per cent of those who do go on to get symptoms have one or more attacks of renal colic before their first attack of crystal synovitis.

Table 2 Causes of hyperuricaemia and gout

Decreased uric acid excretion		Increased uric acid production	
Primary	Secondary	Primary	Secondary

Decrease in fractional urate excretion
  Idiopathic
	1. Reduction in functional renal mass
	    Chronic renal disease
	2. Reduction in glomerular filtration
	    Volume depletion
	    Nephrogenic diabetes
	      insipidus
	3. Reduction in fractional urate clearance
	    Hypertension
	    Hyperparathyroidism
	    Sickle cell anaemia
	    Myxoedema
	    Bartter's syndrome
	    Down's syndrome
	    Chronic beryllium
	      poisoning
	    Lead nephropathy
	    Sarcoidosis
	    Increased levels of
	      organic acids (e.g.
	      exercise, starvation,
	      alcohol, ketoacidosis)
	    Drug administration
	      (e.g. diuretics, low-dose
	      salicylates, pyrazinamide,
	      ethambutol, angiotensin)
		Increased purine synthesis *de novo*
		  Idiopathic
		  Specific enzyme defects
		    HGPRT deficiency
		    (partial)
		    PRPP synthetase over-
		      activity
		    Ribose 5-phosphate
		      overproduction
			1. Increased purine synthesis *de novo*
			   Specific enzyme defects
			   a. HGPRT deficiency (complete)
			     Lesch–Nyhan syndrome
			   b. Glucose 6-phosphatase
			     deficiency—Type 1
			     glycogen storage disease
			2. Increased turnover of preformed purines
			   Myeloproliferative disorders,
			     e.g. polycythaemia rubra vera
			     granulocytic leukaemia
			   Lymphoproliferative disorders,
			     e.g. lymphomas
			     myeloma
			     lymphocytic leukaemia
			     Waldenström's
			      macroglobulinaemia
			     Infectious mononucleosis
			   Carcinomatosis
			   Chronic haemolytic anaemia
			   Secondary polycythaemia
			   Gaucher's disease
			   Severe exfoliative psoriasis

Acute gouty arthritis is eight times more common in men than women and seldom occurs in boys before puberty or women before the menopause. The first attack occurs commonly in men between the ages of 30 and 60. It is almost always monoarticular and the metatarso-phalangeal joint of the great toe is the first joint affected in 20 per cent of cases. Other sites of attack in decreasing order of frequency include the ankle, knee, wrists, elbows, and small joints of the hands and feet. The axial skeleton and large central joints such as the hip and shoulder are seldom involved but acute gout may present as tenosynovitis, bursitis, or cellulitis.

The initial attack may be sudden, waking the patient from sleep. The affected joint becomes hot, red, and swollen with shiny overlying skin, and is extremely painful and tender. Very acute attacks may be accompanied by fever, leucocytosis, and a raised erythrocyte sedimentation rate, and are occasionally preceded by prodromal symptoms, such as anorexia, nausea, or a change in mood. Untreated, the attack lasts days or weeks before subsiding spontaneously, but mild episodes may resolve in a few hours. Resolution of the acute arthritis can be accompanied by pruritus and desquamation of the overlying skin.

Some patients have just one attack or suffer another only after many months or years. Others have recurrent attacks with progressive shortening of the intercritical period between each episode. At this stage polyarticular attacks of acute gouty arthritis are not uncommon and can give rise to diagnostic confusion. Eventually, the recurrent acute attacks of gouty arthritis may become less severe but so prolonged that they merge into one another. First attacks are seldom associated with residual disability but recurrent acute attacks are followed by progressive cartilage and bone erosion (Fig. 5), deposition of tophi, secondary degenerative arthritis, and more permanent restriction of joint function.

Chronic tophaceous gouty arthritis inevitably follows recurrent acute attacks and is characterized by asymmetrical joint swelling (Fig. 6). Tophi are found typically in the periarticular tissues, the cartilagenous helix of the ear, bursae, and tendon sheaths. Rarely tophi may form in the eye, the tongue, the larynx, and the heart and have been recorded as interfering with cardiac conduction and

valvular function. Before the advent of uric-acid-lowering drugs, 60 per cent of patients with untreated gout developed tophi after 10 years. Tophus formation is related to the serum urate concentration as well as to local factors but is not seen in persons with asymptomatic hyperuricaemia. In those with recurrent gouty arthritis, the higher the serum urate level, the earlier and more extensive is the development of tophaceous deposits.

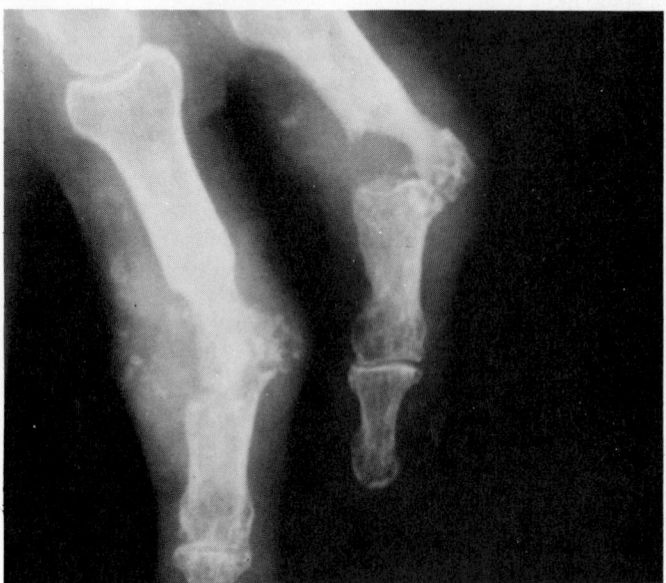

Fig. 5 Radiographic appearances of fingers in chronic gouty arthritis. Note soft tissue swelling with patchy calcification; lucent pockets with cortical erosions of shafts of phalanges as well as punched-out erosion, destructive and secondary hypertrophic changes.

Urolithiasis (see page 18.81). In the UK uric acid stones account for 5 per cent of all renal calculi and 10 per cent of patients with gout have a history of renal colic. In Israel, uric acid calculi are

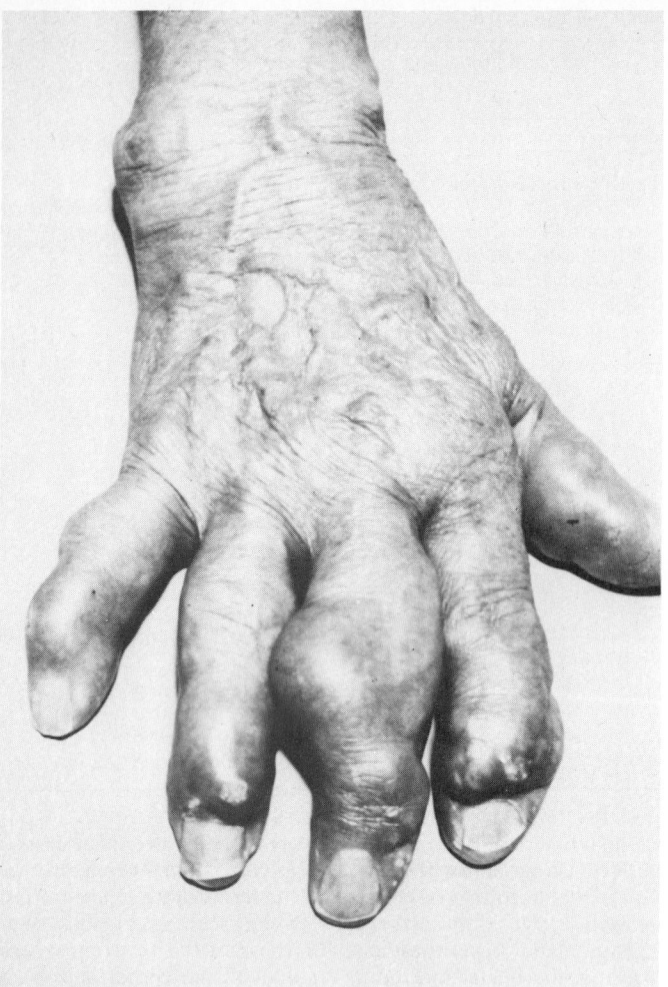

Fig. 6 Chronic tophaceous gouty arthritis. Note irregular asymmetrical joint involvement and massive subcutaneous tophi.

responsible for 40 per cent of cases of nephrolithiasis and 75 per cent of patients with primary gout get renal calculus disease. Urine uric acid concentration is the most important aetiological factor and in temperate climates this is mainly determined by urate production and purine ingestion. The prevalence of renal stones in patients with primary gout is 20 per cent in patients excreting up to 200 mg of uric acid per 24 hours and 50 per cent in those excreting more than 1100 mg/day. In addition to dehydration, primary purine overproduction, increased turnover of purines, and excessive purine ingestion, uric acid calculi may be associated with defects in tubular reabsorption of uric acid, uricosuric drug therapy, chronic diarrhoeal diseases, and ileostomy; the latter as a result of lowered urine pH.

Acute uric acid mephropathy. Acute renal failure may result from sudden precipitation of unionized crystals of uric acid in the renal collecting ducts and ureters. This dramatic form of acute obstructive uropathy occurs most often when ill, dehydrated, acidotic patients with leukaemia or lymphoma are treated with cytotoxic drugs, but has also been recorded following epilepsy, severe muscular exercise, and in patients with gout and grossly accelerated primary purine synthesis. The diagnosis is suggested by finding crystals of uric acid and a uric acid: creatinine ratio > 1.0 in the residual urine of an oliguric patient with renal failure. The problem is entirely preventable by careful attention to a high fluid intake and alkalinization of the urine, and/or the prophylatic administration of allopurinol to prevent the sudden rise in uric acid which follows the breakdown of cellular nucleoproteins during chemotherapy.

Chronic urate nephropathy. Clinically significant, progressive, chronic renal disease is an important complication of untreated chronic tophaceous gout and renal failure accounts for 20–25 per cent of deaths in these patients. There is evidence to suggest, however, that this form of progressive renal failure may be largely limited to one or more poorly defined subgroups of patients with familial or acquired disorders that include hyperuricaemia, urate nephropathy, hypertension, and gouty arthritis; but which differ significantly from the bulk of the gouty population. Recent studies have particularly implicated low-grade lead poisoning as an important environmental determinant of renal insufficiency in patients with gout.

Mild intermittent proteinuria is found in 20–30 per cent of patients with gout but the minor progression of renal insufficiency that occurs in the majority of subjects with gout is largely age-related and overall life expectancy is not reduced. Significant renal disease is a very rare complication of hyperuricaemia in the absence of recurrent gouty arthritis. When faced with a patient with renal insufficiency and hyperuricaemia it can, however, be extremely difficult to ascertain whether the raised serum urate is a cause or consequence of the renal failure.

The pathogenesis of chronic urate nephropathy is complex and poorly defined. It seems likely that the initial lesion may be crystal-induced damage to the tubular epithelium of the loop of Henle and adjacent interstitial tissue, and this is later complicated by tubular obstruction, tophus formation, hypertensive damage, glomerulosclerosis, and secondary pyelonephritis.

Other clinical associations. Gout and hyperuricaemia are often associated with obesity, type IV hyperlipoproteinaemia, impaired glucose tolerance, and ischaemic heart disease.

Obesity may be the major linking factor. Patients with gout are on average 15–20 per cent overweight and the prevalence of hyperuricaemia in the community rises from 3 per cent in those whose weight is in the 20th percentile to 11 per cent in those above the 80th percentile.

Hypertriglyceridaemia occurs in more than 75 per cent of patients with gout and hyperuricaemia in a similar proportion of individuals with hypertriglyceridaemia. The pattern is most commonly one of type IV hyperlipoproteinaemia with elevated very-low-density lipoproteins and normal levels of serum cholesterol. Heavy alcohol intake and obesity are both predisposing factors.

Hypertension occurs in 25–50 per cent of patients with gout, and hyperuricaemia is a feature in one-third of untreated hypertensives and two-thirds of those receiving antihypertensive drug therapy.

Impaired glucose tolerance and ischaemic heart disease are associated with gout and obesity rather than with asymptomatic hyperuricaemia and there is no good evidence to suggest that hyperuricaemia alone is a risk factor for diabetes mellitus or myocardial infarction.

Diagnosis. The diagnosis of gout can be reasonably regarded as being established if a young man or postmenopausal woman develops spontaneous excruciating pain, redness and swelling in the metatarsophalangeal joint of the great toe in association with a raised plasma uric acid level. Suspicion can be strengthened by a history of a previous episode which resolved completely especially when this was in response to treatment with colchicine, a personal history of renal colic or a family history of hyperuricaemia, gout, or renal calculi. Gout should always be considered in patients with acute monoarticular arthritis, tenosynovitis, or bursitis but it should be remembered that 10 per cent of cases may present with acute polyarticular gout with sparing of the great toe. It is also important to remember that asymptomatic hyperuricaemia is relatively common and that a raised serum uric acid level alone does not prove a diagnosis of gouty arthritis. Conversely although the serum uric acid is usually raised at the time of an acute attack of gout, and must be documented at some time to sustain the diagnosis, acute attacks can occur when serum levels are normal. Whenever possible synovial fluid should be examined under polarizing-light microscopy for crystals of monosodium urate and where appropriate possible causes of secondary hyperuricaemia (Table 2) should be considered. Patients should always be examined for evidence of tophi and an asymmetrical chronic arthritis.

Compensated polarized-light microscopy. Using a microscope fitted with polarizing filters and a first-order red compensator, monosodium urate crystals can be distinguished from crystals of calcium pyrophosphate dihydrate which occur in patients with chondrocalcinosis and pseudogout. Monosodium urate crystals are 3–20 μm in length, needle-shaped, and strongly negatively birefringent (yellow in colour when the crystal axis is parallel to the slow ray of the compensator). Calcium pyrophosphate crystals are shorter, rhomboidal, and weakly positively birefringent (blue when the crystal axis is parallel to the compensator).

Radiology. Early in the disease X-rays show no abnormality. After repeated attacks joint radiographs may show characteristic erosive changes (Fig. 5). Typical lesions are punched-out erosions, described as 'sharply marginated lucent pockets with overhanging margins', but the erosions may be indistinguishable from those seen in other types of inflammatory arthritis. Secondary degenerative changes are common and adjacent tophi may be detected as periarticular soft-tissue swelling with partial calcification.

Differential diagnosis. Acute gouty arthritis must be distinguished from other causes of acute monoarthritis; notably infective arthritis, traumatic arthritis, haemarthrosis, sarcoid arthritis, rheumatoid arthritis with 'palindromic' onset, acute seronegative inflammatory arthritides such as psoriatic arthropathy, or a spondarthritis presenting with peripheral joint involvement. Chronic tophaceous gout can be confused with nodular rheumatoid arthritis, osteoarthritis with Heberden and Bouchard nodes, xanthomatosis with joint involvement or reticulohistiocytosis. The pattern of arthritis in gout is usually less symmetrical.

Treatment. No other form of arthritis can be managed as well with drugs as gout.
Treatment is directed towards:
1. Prompt termination of the acute attack.
2. Prevention of subsequent acute attacks.
3. Dissolution of tophaceous deposits and preventing the formation of tophi and renal calculi.
4. Management of associated disorders such as hypertension, obesity, and hyperlipoproteinaemia.

Acute attack. The first line of treatment is to rest the affected joint and administer an adequate dose of a non-steroidal analgesic anti-inflammatory drug (NSAID). Oral indomethacin can be given in a dose of 50 mg 4–6 hourly until the symptoms of the acute attack subside and should then be tailed off gradually over 5–10 days. Any NSAID can be used in full dosage as an alternative but aspirin and other salicylates are best avoided. Phenylbutazone and oxyphenbutazone can be very effective but carry a small risk of inducing serious bone-marrow depression.

Colchicine has more specificity than NSAI drugs in gout and can therefore have some diagnostic as well as therapeutic value. Dramatic remission of symptoms within a few hours of the administration of colchicine is characteristic of gout but may occasionally also occur in patients with pseudogout or sarcoid arthritis. The use of colchicine for the routine management of acute gouty arthritis has been largely superseded by the use of NSAID because the margin between therapeutic and toxic doses is very

small. An initial dose of 1 mg of oral colchicine is followed by 0.5 mg every two hours until the acute attack subsides or nausea, diarrhoea, and abdominal cramps preclude further therapy. If the acute attack of arthritis does not show signs of resolution 12–48 hours after administration of adequate doses of colchicine or an NSAID, an alternative diagnosis, especially infection, should be considered.

If oral therapy is precluded a single i.v. dose of 2–3 mg of colchicine can be effective but care must be taken to avoid extravenous extravasation. Indomethacin suppositories, intramuscular hydrocortisone, or corticotrophin are further alternatives.

It is important not to administer allopurinol or uricosuric drugs until the symptoms have completely settled as these agents may prolong the acute attack. Salicylates and diuretics should also be avoided if at all possible.

Long-term management and prevention. Life-long therapy to lower the serum uric acid level should be considered carefully several weeks after resolution of an acute attack if:
1. Acute attacks have been recurrent and troublesome.
2. There is evidence of tophi or chronic joint damage.
3. There is renal disease.
4. The patient is young, the uric acid level is high and there is a family history of renal or heart disease.
5. There is evidence of primary purine overproduction and hyperexcretion.

Allopurinol is the drug of choice. It lowers the uric acid level by inhibiting the enzyme xanthine oxidase (Fig. 3) and in most patients also depresses the rate of de novo purine synthesis. The dose must be adjusted carefully according to individual needs. In most patients therapy is commenced with 300 mg OD adjusting the dose up or down within the range 100–900 mg daily in order to keep the serum uric-acid level normal. In patients with renal insufficiency excretion of the active metabolite oxypurinol is delayed and therapy should be commenced with smaller doses of 100 mg/day. In most patients uricosuric drug therapy with probenecid 0.5–1.0 g b.d. or sulphinpyrazone 100 mg 3–4 times daily is an acceptable alternative for lowering the uric acid but uricosuric drugs are generally contraindicated in patients with primary overproduction of uric acid and gross hyperuricosuria, those with evidence of urolithiasis and patients with renal insufficiency. Salicylates interfere with the action of uricosuric drugs and must be avoided.

Patients beginning treatment with allopurinol or uricosuric drugs are prone to develop 'breakthrough' attacks of acute gouty arthritis during the early phases of treatment. These can be largely prevented by the administration of prophylatic colchicine 0.5 mg b.d. or a standard dose of an NSAID during the first three months of therapy. It is important not to start hypouricaemic drugs until the acute attack has resolved completely.

Serious side-effects are unusual with allopurinol or uricosuric agents. Only about 5 per cent of patients have to discontinue one or other of these drugs usually on account of minor skin rashes or dyspepsia. Very rare, but serious toxic reactions include toxic epidermal necrolysis and vasculitis (allopurinol), nephrotic syndrome (probenecid), and hepatitis and bone-marrow suppression with both types of hypouricaemic drugs. Uricosuric agents interfere with the excretion of lactam antibiotics and many other drugs. Allopurinol is associated with an increased prevalence of ampicillin drug rashes and has important interactions with coumarin anticoagulants owing to inhibition of hepatic microsomal enzymes and purine analogues such as azathioprine which are normally inactivated by xanthine oxidase.

With modern drug therapy there is no need for stringent dietary restriction but patients should be advised to avoid gross excesses of alcohol and purine containing foods. Correction of obesity by mild caloric restriction is associated with a gradual fall in serum uric acid but severe dietary restriction may precipitate lactic acidosis, hyperuricaemia, and acute gouty arthritis. Any associated hypertension should be treated but it should always be remembered that diuretic drugs will raise the serum urate and may precipitate attacks of acute gout in patients who have not been stabilized on allopurinol.

Asymptomatic hyperuricaemia. Although hyperuricaemia may be associated with hypertension, atherosclerosis, ischaemic heart disease, and renal insufficiency there is no evidence to suggest that the raised serum urate itself is a risk factor. Since the majority of hyperuricaemic individuals never develop gout or renal complications, there is no indication to treat asymptomatic hyperuricaemia unless the serum urate is very high (> 0.8 mmol/l) and the urine uric-acid excretion very great (> 7.2 mmol/24 h). In the majority of persons with asymptomatic hyperuricaemia it is reasonable to exclude a history, family history, and clinical evidence of gout; search for a secondary cause of the hyperuricaemia, and monitor the blood pressure and renal function annually.

Inborn errors of purine metabolism

Lesch-Nyhan syndrome. Severe cellular deficiency of the purine-salvage enzyme *hypoxanthine–guanine phosphoribosyl transferase* (HGPRT see below) is associated with primary purine overproduction, hyperuricaemia, and gout together with a neurological syndrome comprising choreoathetosis, spasticity, a variable degree of mental deficiency, and a striking behavioural disturbance characterized by self-mutilation (Fig. 7).

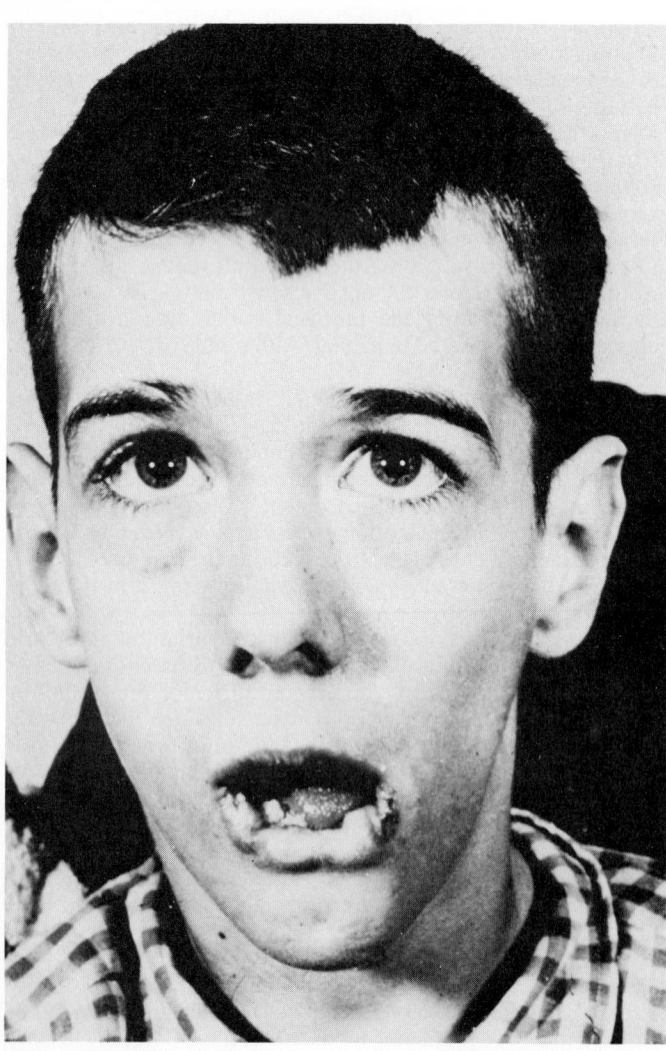

Fig. 7 Boy with Lesch–Nyhan syndrome showing evidence of self mutilation of lips (courtesy of Dr J. E. Seegmiller).

Hypoxanthine–guanine phosphoribosyl transferase

$$\text{Hypoxanthine} + \text{PP-ribose-P} \xrightarrow{Mg^{2+}} \text{inosine } 5' - \text{phosphate} + \text{PPi}$$
$$\text{Guanine} + \text{PP-ribose-P} \xrightarrow{Mg^{2+}} \text{inosine } 5' - \text{phosphate} + \text{PPi}$$

Clinical features. Clinical expression of disease is limited to males. Babies appear normal at birth but mothers may observe the presence of orange crystals in the diapers. Occasional vomiting and hypotonia is followed by delay in motor development at the age of 3–4 months. The characteristic pyramidal and extrapyramidal signs which eventually progress to severe spasticity and choreoathetosis are seldom apparent before one year and the compulsive behavioural disturbance may start at any time between the ages of 2 and 16 years. Episodes of involuntary and occasionally unilateral self-mutilation come and go without any clear relationship to endogenous or environmental factors. These episodes are often associated with agitation and anxiety which can be partially relieved by physical restraint to prevent finger biting. In some cases self-mutilation of the lips can only be prevented by extraction of teeth. Aggression towards others may take the form of hitting, spitting, biting, and abusive language typically accompanied by a smile and an apology. The majority of boys affected are mentally retarded with an IQ in the range 40–65 but the severity of the behavioural disturbance is unrelated to the degree of mental deficiency.

Haematuria and renal colic may occur during the first decade of life but gouty arthritis and tophi seldom develop before puberty. A macrocytic or frankly megaloblastic anaemia is an occasional feature. Recurrent bacterial infections may be associated with B lymphocyte immunodeficiency as well as self-inflicted wounds and obstructive uropathy. Death from infection or renal failure commonly occurs between the ages of 20 and 30.

Biochemical findings. Grossly accelerated production of uric acid results in greatly increased urine uric acid excretion (0.15–0.75 mmol/kg per 24 hours) and a characteristically high urine uric acid:creatinine ratio (Fig. 8). The serum urate is usually, but not invariably, raised in the range 0.42–0.9 mmol/l.

Lesch–Nyhan syndrome is characterized by raised concentrations of phosphoribosyl pyrophosphate (PP-ribose-P) and severe

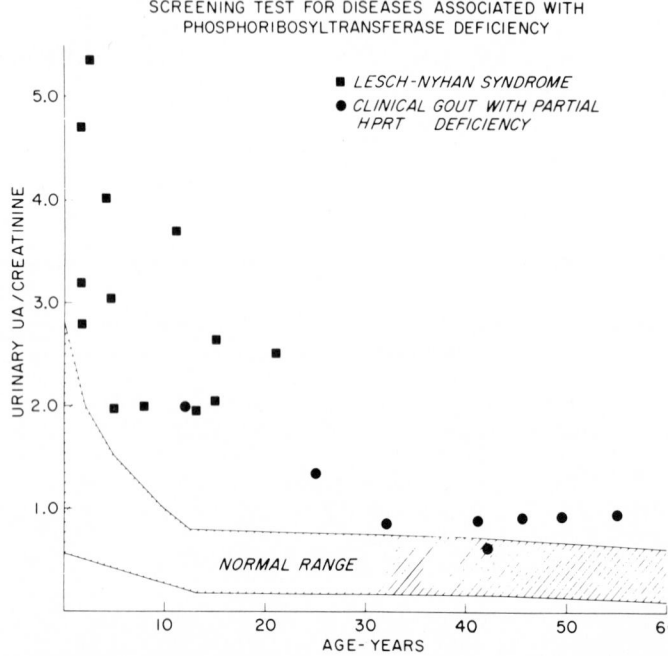

Fig. 8 Ratio of uric acid to creatinine concentrations (expressed as mg/100 ml) in urine samples from patients with Lesch–Nyhan syndrome and gout with partial HGPRT deficiency (from Kaufman *et. al.*: *J. Paediatr.* **73**, 583 (1968), with permission of the *Journal of Pediatrics*).

deficiency of HGPRT in red-cell lysates. Complete or nearly complete deficiency of the enzyme is also found in leucocytes, cultured fibroblasts, amniotic fluid cells, and other tissues such as liver and brain. Associated biochemical abnormalities include increased activity of adenine phosphoribosyl transferase (APRT), inosine monophosphate dehydrogenase (IMPD), and the pyrimidine enzymes orotate phosphoribosyl transferase (OPRT) and orotidine 5'-phosphate decarboxylase (ODC). Concentrations of the pyrimidine nucleotides UDP, UTP, and CTP are increased in HGPRT-deficient lymphoblasts and fibroblasts but steady-state purine nucleotide concentrations are not reduced as might be expected. It seems probable that the acceleration of *de novo* purine biosynthesis *in vivo* is primarily due to the effect of increased availability of PP-ribose-P on the rate-limiting amidophosphoribosyl transferase (PAT) enzyme rather than decreased feedback inhibition by purine nucleotides.

The biochemical basis for the neurological dysfunction in Lesch–Nyhan syndrome remains uncertain. Morphological abnormalities have not been detected in post-mortem studies of the brain. As neuronal cells are able to synthesize purine nucleotides *de novo* it seems reasonable to assume that accumulation of purine metabolites, rather than deficiency of purine nucleotides, interferes in some way with neurotransmitter function in the brain stem. The recent demonstration of decreases in dopamine, homovanillic acid, dopa decarboxylase, and tyrosine hydroxylase activity in the dopamine-terminal-rich regions of the putamen and caudate nucleus suggest that there may be secondary abnormalities of terminal arborization of dopaminergic neurones.

The biochemical bases for the putative immunological dysfunction and the megaloblastic anaemia are also unclear. In isolated cases the anaemia has been shown to respond to adenine rather than folic acid.

Genetics, prenatal detection, and prevention. Lesch–Nyhan syndrome is an X-linked disorder which is only fully expressed in males. Asymptomatic carrier females can be detected by hair-root analysis or by finding HGPRT-positive and HGPRT-negative populations of cells in fibroblast cultures from skin biopsies using an autoradiographic technique; incidentally providing confirmation of the Lyon hypothesis of random inactivation of the X-chromosome. Using these techniques only four out of 47 mothers were homozygous normal, suggesting a lower than expected ratio of new to established mutations. Culture of amniotic fluid cells following amniocentesis allows the detection of affected males *in utero* and preventive therapeutic abortion.

Biochemical studies of normal human HGPRT have revealed a variety of electrophoretic HGPRT variants. Although much of this electrophoretic heterogeneity appears to be the result of post-transcriptional modification there is evidence of true genetic heterogeneity in cells from patients with the disease. In the majority of cases of Lesch–Nyhan syndrome complete absence of catalytic enzyme activity is associated with absence of protein cross-reacting with antibody to normal enzyme (CRM-negative mutants), but CRM-positive mutants with absent catalytic activity have also been detected providing good evidence of structural gene mutations. Amino-acid sequencing has recently been accomplished in three such mutations. It is now clear that there is a whole spectrum of mutations at the HGPRT locus which result in cells with varying amounts of residual enzyme activity and HGPRT with altered substrate affinities. Indeed the level of HGPRT activity in red cells from some patients with Lesch–Nyhan syndrome overlaps the range of activity seen in some families with gout and overproduction of purines alone. Heterozygote carriers can have subtle sub-clinical alterations in purine metabolism with modest increases in the rates of *de novo* purine biosynthesis, increase in urine uric acid excretion and occasional asymptomatic hyperuricaemia.

Treatment. Treatment with allopurinol is mandatory in all affected subjects. Serum and urine uric acid levels are effectively lowered by inhibition of xanthine oxidase but total purine excretion is not reduced when allopurinol is given to patients with Lesch–Nyhan syndrome as it is in other patients with gout and purine overproduction. Nevertheless, gouty arthritis, urate stone formation, and urate nephropathy can be prevented effectively and the possibility of xanthine stone formation is minimized by ensuring adequate hydration and urine flow. Hypouricaemic drug therapy does not, however, influence the neurological manifestations nor the behavioural disturbance. Diazepam, haloperidol, and barbiturates can be helpful in managing the extrapyramidal movements but tooth extraction and physical restraint with splints and bandages are often required to control the compulsive self-mutilation.

Partial HGPRT deficiency. Severe familial X-linked gout with minor or absent neurological features may be associated with 'partial' deficiency of HGPRT.

Clinical features. These patients usually present with uric acid calculi or gouty arthritis in adolescence or adult life. In about 25 per cent there is a mild neurological disturbance. In some families this resembles a *forme fruste* of Lesch–Nyhan syndrome with disorders of movement and compulsive behaviour. In others there has been a history of convulsions, mental retardation, and a spinocerebellar syndrome. As in the Lesch–Nyhan syndrome, macrocytosis and megaloblastic marrow changes may be observed.

Biochemical findings and genetics. Serum uric acid levels are high and there is evidence of primary purine overproduction with urine uric acid excretion usually in excess of 5 mmol/24 h and a uric acid:creatinine ratio greater than 0.75 unless renal insufficiency has already supervened. HGPRT activity in erythrocyte lysates is usually in the range of 0.01–30 per cent of normal activity with similar levels of residual enzyme activity in individuals from the same family. Identical phenotypes have, however, been reported in which red blood cell HGPRT was undetectable or apparently normal. In the latter instances, structural gene mutations had led to subtle abnormalities of the HGPRT protein with an altered K_m for PP-ribose-P in one case and abnormal sensitivity to feedback inhibition by purine nucleotides in the other. These cases illustrate how the clinical features of disease associated with HGPRT deficiency cannot be reliably predicted from simple assays of erythrocyte HGPRT alone. Phenotypic expression is, however, always similar within each family; typical Lesch–Nyhan syndrome and X-linked gout without neurological features never occurring in related patients.

As in Lesch–Nyhan syndrome intracellular concentrations of PP-ribose-P and pyrimidine nucleotides are increased and there is increased activity of APRT, IMPD, OPRT, and ODC in erythrocyte lysates.

Carrier detection of heterozygotes is the same as for Lesch–Nyhan syndrome but amniocentesis, prenatal detection, and preventive abortion are not justified.

Treatment is with allopurinol.

Adenine phosphoribosyl transferase (APRT). This enzyme catalyses the reaction:

$$\text{Adenine} + \text{PP-ribose-P} \xrightarrow{Mg^{2+}} \text{Adenosine } 5'\text{- phosphate} + \text{PPi}.$$

Severe homozygous deficiency is associated with the formation of renal calculi of 2,8-dihydroxyadenine from early childhood. This rare autosomal recessive disorder is not associated with primary purine overproduction, hyperuricaemia, or gout although the renal calculi may be mistaken for uric acid stones if only standard laboratory methods of analysis are used. Their true identity can be established by X-ray diffraction, infrared, and ultraviolet spectroscopy. Homozygous APRT deficiency is characterized by increased urinary excretion of adenine and its metabolites 8-hydroxyadenine and 2,8-dihydroxyadenine, formed by the action of xanthine oxidase. Renal stone formation in this condition can be successfully prevented by administration of the xanthine oxidase inhibitor allopurinol.

Heterozygous APRT deficiency is a rather common trait. As many as 1 per cent of the normal population may be heterozygotes with partial APRT deficiency and 8–45 per cent of normal enzyme activity in erythrocyte lysates. Partial APRT deficiency does not appear to be associated with clinical metabolic disease.

Phosphoribosyl pyrophosphate synthetase (PRPPS). This enzyme catalyses the reaction:

Ribose 5-phosphate + ATP$\xrightarrow{\text{Mg}^{2+}\ \text{Pi}}$ PP-ribose-P + AMP.

A number of families have been described in which X-linked gout and severe primary purine overproduction are associated with structural enzyme mutations resulting in *superactive* PP-ribose-P synthetase. In some, increased enzyme activity is associated with abnormal resistance to feedback inhibitors while in others superactive PRPPS appears to be associated with an increased V_{max} or affinity for ribose 5-phosphate.

Affected males develop uric acid lithiasis or gouty arthritis in childhood or early adult life. Hyperuricaemia is often severe and in the range 0.5–1.0 mmol/l with urine uric acid excretion of 5–15 mmol/24 h. Heterozygotes remain asymptomatic although clinical investigation shows them to have evidence of increased purine synthesis *de novo*. Deafness may be an associated clinical feature in both affected males and their heterozygous mothers.

Heterozygotes can be identified by studies of cultured skin fibroblasts but amniocentesis, prenatal diagnosis, and preventive abortion are not justified in this condition.

The hyperuricaemia, primary purine overproduction, and uricosuria can be well controlled with allopurinol.

Glucose 6-Phosphatase. This enzyme catalyses the reaction: the reaction:

Glucose 6-phosphate + H$_2$O $\longrightarrow$ glucose + Pi.

Severe deficiency of glucose 6-phosphatase (glycogen storage disease type I, Von Gierke's disease) is associated with marked hyperuricaemia from infancy. Gouty arthritis may become a problem before the age of ten and chronic tophaceous gout with renal involvement can be a major cause of morbidity in those lucky enough to survive to adult life, unless preventive measures are taken.

Clinical features. Children with this condition have a characteristic appearance. They are pale, with chubby cheeks, stunted growth, and a large protruberant abdomen due to massive hepatomegaly. Severe and recurrent hypoglycaemia may result in convulsions or insidious and progressive mental retardation. Epistaxes and other bleeding phenomena may be a consequence of abnormal platelet function. Xanthomata frequently develop over the buttocks and extensor surfaces of the extremities and need to be distinguished from tophi.

Biochemical findings and diagnosis. In the absence of glucose 6-phosphatase the liver is unable to generate glucose from glycogen stores or glycogenic precursors. Glycogen accumulates in the liver and kidneys but not the heart or skeletal muscle. Maintenance of blood sugar in these patients is entirely dependent on regular feeding and absorption of glucose from the gut. Recurrent hypoglycaemia is accompanied by increased lipolysis, glycogenolysis, and gluconeogenesis with elevation of serum levels of lactate, pyruvate, free fatty acids, glycerol, cholesterol, triglycerides, phospholipids, and urate.

Renal clearance of uric acid is decreased but urine uric acid: creatinine ratios are frequently greater than 0.75 and glycine incorporation into urine uric acid is increased. Thus hyperuricaemia is a consequence of both decreased urate excretion

secondary to competitive inhibition of renal tubular urate secretion by lactate and excessive purine synthesis *de novo*. It has been suggested that the accelerated purine synthesis which occurs in these patients may result from increased availability of phosphoribosyl pyrophosphate following shunting of metabolites through the pentose phosphate pathway (Fig. 9).

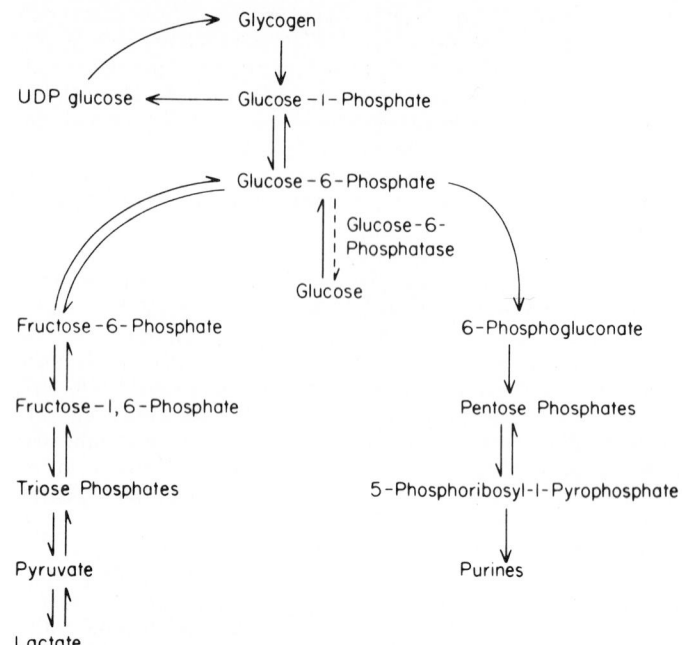

Fig. 9 Metabolic pathways of glucose 6-phosphatase showing postulated mechanism for purine overproduction (after Howell: *Arthritis Rheum.* **8**, 780 (1965), with permission of *Arthritis and Rheumatism*).

Glucose 6-phosphatase deficiency can usually be distinguished from glycogen storage disease type III (Debrancher enzyme deficiency) by an exaggerated increase in lactic acid and a failure to mount a glucose response to injections of glucagon or galactose. Definitive diagnosis is made by direct assay of the enzyme which is confined to liver, intestinal mucosa, and renal tissue. Patients have been described with clinical and biochemical features identical to those of classical Von Gierke's disease in whom glucose 6-phosphatase levels are normal in the liver biopsy (glycogen storage disease type 1b). A less severe form of the disease characterized by absence of hypoglycaemia and partial deficiency of glucose 6-phosphatase has also recently been described.

Treatment. Dramatic reversal of metabolic abnormalities and increases in growth often follow continuous intragastric feeding. This may be followed by portocaval shunting in severely affected cases. Nevertheless, it is advisable to administer allopurinol to all patients in order to prevent the consequences of severe and prolonged hyperuricaemia.

Xanthine oxidase. This enzyme catalyses the reactions:

Hypoxanthine + H$_2$O + O$_2$ $\longrightarrow$ Xanthine + H$_2$O$_2$.
Xanthine + H$_2$O + O$_2$ $\longrightarrow$ Uric acid + H$_2$O$_2$.

Hereditary xanthinuria is a rare autosomal recessive disorder in which severe deficiency of xanthine oxidase is associated with hypouricaemia and excessive urinary excretion of xanthine and hypoxanthine.

Some persons affected appear to remain free from symptoms throughout life, the condition being detected only by finding a low serum urate on routine biochemical testing. In others the formation of xanthine calculi has been associated with renal colic, a mild myopathy, and crystal synovitis.

Plasma uric acid levels are usually less than 1 mg/100 ml and urinary uric acid excretion is less than 50 mg/24 h. Plasma oxypurines are correspondingly raised in the range 0.1–1.0 mg/100 ml and urine oxypurine excretion may be as high as 500 mg/24 h. Assays of hepatic or intestinal xanthine oxidase usually show no detectable activity but cases with as much as 10 per cent (liver) and 25 per cent (intestine) residual activity have been recorded.

Not all patients with xanthine stones have xanthine oxidase deficiency or even increased oxypurine excretion.

Treatment is usually restricted to maintaining a high fluid intake. Since xanthine solubility increases at higher pH, oral administration of alkali can be considered in recurrent stone formers, but care must be taken. Allopurinol should be considered in those patients with residual enzyme activity as hypoxanthine is significantly more soluble than xanthine.

Other causes of hypouricaemia (Table 3). Hypouricaemia may be associated with reduction in uric acid formation in patients with deficiencies of PP-ribose-P synthetase and purine nucleoside phosphorylase as well as in hereditary xanthinuria, allopurinol therapy, and severe hepatic disease. More commonly, however, hypouricaemia results from increased excretion which may be associated with isolated or more generalized defects of renal tubular transport and particularly with drug therapy of various kinds.

Table 3   Causes of hypouricaemia

Decreased production of uric acid	Increased excretion of uric acid
Purine enzyme defects	Isolated defects in renal tubular handling
xanthine oxidase	idiopathic (Dalmatian dog
PP-ribose-P synthetase	mutation)
purine nucleoside phosphorylase	malignant diseases
Severe hepatic disease	hepatic diseases
Metastatic carcinoma	Generalized defects in renal tubular transport (Fanconi syndrome)
Acute intermittent porphyria	idiopathic
	Wilson's disease
	carcinoma of bronchus
	multiple myeloma
	lymphomas
	hepatic disease and alcoholism
	hyperparathyroidism
	heavy metal poisoning
	cystinosis
	galactosaemia
	Drugs
	allopurinol
	uricosuric agents
	radiographic contrast agents
	NSAID with uricosuric properties
	(e.g. phenylbutazone,
	azapropazone
	High-dose aspirin)
	oestrogens
	glyceryl guaicholate

Inborn errors of purine metabolism in immunodeficiency

A number of immunodeficiency disorders appear to be a direct consequence of inherited defects in purine metabolism.

Adenosine deaminase (ADA). This enzyme catalyses the reaction:

$$\text{Adenosine} \longrightarrow \text{Inosine} + \text{NH}_3.$$

In about half the patients with the autosomal recessive form of severe combined immunodeficiency (SCID) the enzyme adenosine deaminase is absent.

Affected babies usually come to medical attention soon after birth, with diarrhoea, chest infections, and failure to thrive. Some infants present with lymphopaenia and hypogammaglobulinaemia with low or absent T and B lymphocytes, while others initially have normal immunoglobulins and a normal or increased percentage of B lymphocytes. T lymphocytes and especially T suppressor cells appear to be particularly vulnerable, possibly because these cells require expansion of their effector population for functional expression. In about a third of cases there are multiple radiological abnormalities including fraying of the long bones, abnormally thick growth arrest lines and chondro-osseous dysplasia affecting the costochondral junctions. In a few there are additional abnormalities such as renal tubular acidosis, choreoathetosis, spasticity, and the development of fine sparse hair.

Biochemical findings. ADA deficiency is associated with the accumulation and excretion of deoxyadenosine as well as adenosine. Intracellular dATP, a potent inhibitor of ribonucleotide reductase, is markedly elevated in erythrocytes and T lymphoid cells but not B cells. Initially, this differential toxicity for T and B cells was attributed to the relative deficiency of ecto-5′-nucleotidase in T cells but it now seems intrinsically unlikely that this ecto-enzyme can be serving such an important regulatory role. Deoxyadenosine is also a 'suicide' inactivator of S-adenosylhomocysteine hydrolase which catalyses the synthesis of S-adenosyl homocysteine from adenosine and L-homocysteine and is a key enzyme for numerous methylation reactions.

The prognosis in ADA deficiency SCID is very poor, death due to infection usually occurring in the first year of life.

Treatment. Following the demonstration that addition of ADA to lymphocyte cultures *in vitro* resulted in restoration of mitogenic responsiveness in cells from ADA deficient patients, attempts have been made to treat these children with red-cell infusions rather than marrow transplants.

Purine nucleoside phosphorylase (PNP). This enzyme catalyses the reaction:

$$\text{Inosine} + \text{Pi} \longrightarrow \text{hypoxanthine} + \text{ribose 1-P.}$$

Inherited PNP deficiency is associated with isolated T cell immune deficiency. These children present with recurrent upper and lower respiratory tract infections, usually during the first year of life. Susceptibility is particularly to virus infections such as varicella, vaccinia, or cytomegalovirus. The tonsils are small or absent and lymph nodes are deficient in thymic-dependent areas. Circulating lymphocyte counts are usually very low with a low percentage of T lymphocytes and depressed or absent responsiveness to phyto-haemagglutinin (PHA) transformation. Serum immunoglobulin levels and antibody responses to pneumococcal polysaccharide and keyhole limpet haemocyanin are typically increased in these children and the occasional finding of a monoclonal IgG paraprotein strongly suggests that the changes in antibody production are secondary to T-cell defects. Autoimmune haemolytic anaemia, megaloblastic bone marrow, and spastic tetraplegia have been occasional associations.

Biochemical findings. PNP deficiency is associated with the accumulation and excretion of deoxyguanosine and deoxyinosine as well as guanosine and inosine. Paradoxically there is massive purine overproduction and excretion, although all patients are severely hypouricaemic. Erythrocyte concentrations of dGTP are markedly raised in PNP deficient cells. T cells but not B cells appear to be susceptible to deoxyguanosine toxicity probably as a result of accumulation of dGTP, inhibition of ribonucleotide reductase, impairment of DNA synthesis, and eventually cell death.

Treatment. The prognosis in children with PNP deficiency is often much better than that in SCID with ADA deficiency. Since some children have remained healthy and free from viral infection until the age of six years, high-risk procedures such as marrow transplantation are currently thought not to be justified in all cases. Conservative treatment with gammaglobulin replacement with later attempts at enzyme replacement with red cell transfusions in children with recurrent infections are the current approach to management.

5'-Nucleotidase. This enzyme catalyses the reaction:

Adenylic acid $\longrightarrow$ Adenosine + Pi.

Deficiency of the ectoenzyme 5'-nucleotidase is found in some patients with X-linked and 'acquired' adult onset hypogamma-globulinaemia. There is no evidence that the enzyme deficiency causes the immunodeficiency in either case. It is currently thought to be much more likely to reflect simply an arrested stage of lymphocyte development in these patients.

References

Gout

Becker, M. A. and Seegmiller, J. E. (1974). Genetic aspects of gout. *Ann. Rev. Med.* **25**, 15.

Diamond, H. S., Meisel, A., and Kaplan, D. (1977). Renal tubular transport of urate in man. *Bull. Rheum. Dis.* **27**, 876.

Emmerson, B. T. (1980). Uricosuric diuretics. *Kidney Internat.* **18**, 677.

Fox, I. H. and Kelley, W. N. (1971). Phosphoribosyl pyrophosphate in man: Biochemical and clinical significance. *Ann. Int. Med.* **74**, 424.

Halla, J. T. and Ball, G. V. (1982). Saturnine gout: a review of 42 patients. *Seminars Arthr. Rheum.* **11**, 307.

Healey, L. A. and Hall, A. P. (1970). The epidemiology of gout and hyperuricaemia. *Bull. Rheum. Dis.* **20**, 600.

Hershfield, M. S. and Seegmiller, J. E. (1976). Gout and the regulation of purine biosynthesis. In *Horizons in biochemistry and biophysics*, Vol. 2, p. 132. (ed. E. Quagliariello). Addison–Wesley, Reading, Mass.

Holmes, E. W., Kelley, W. N., and Wyngaarden, J. B. (1976). Control of purine biosynthesis in normal and pathologic states. *Bull. Rheum. Dis.* **26**, 838.

Kelley, W. N. (ed.) (1977). Crystal induced arthropathies. *Clin. Rheum. Dis.* **3**, 1.

Klinenberg, J. R. (ed.) (1975). Proceedings of the second conference on gout and purine metabolism. *Arthritis Rheum.* (Suppl.) **18**, 659.

Nuki, G. (1971). The significance of hyperuricaemia. In *Advanced medicine*, Vol. 11, (ed. A. F. Lant), p. 334. Pitman Medical, London.

— (1979). Crystals, arthritis and connective tissue. In *Advanced medicine*, Vol. 15 (ed. P. S. Harper and J. R. Muir), p. 138. Pitman Medical, London.

Purine and pyrimidine metabolism (1977). Ciba Foundation symposium No. 48. Elsevier/Excerpta Medica, Amsterdam.

Reif, M. C., Coustantiner, A., and Levitt, M. F. (1981). Chronic gouty nephropathy: a vanishing syndrome? *New Eng. J. Med.* **304**, 535.

Rieselbach, R. E. and Steele, T. H. (eds) (1975). Symposium on influence of the kidney on urate homeostasis in man. *Nephron* **14**, 5.

Scott, J. T. (1980). Long-term management of gout and hyperuricaemia. *Br. med. J.* **281**, 1164.

Seegmiller, J. E. (1980). Human aberrations of purine metabolism and their significance for rheumatology. *Ann. Rheum. Dis.* **39**, 103.

— (1980). Diseases of purine and pyrimidine and metabolism. In *Metabolic control and disease*, 8th ed. (by P. K. Bondy and L. E. Rosenberg), pp. 777 and 937. W. B. Saunders, Philadelphia.

Talbott, J. H. and Yu, T. F. (eds) (1976). *Gout and uric acid metabolism.* Stratton, New York.

Weiner, I. M. and Kelley, W. N. (eds) (1977). *Uric acid, handbook of experimental pharmacology.* Springer-Verlag, Berlin–New York.

Wyngaarden, J. B. and Kelley, W. N. (1976). *Gout and hyperuricaemia.* Grune and Statton, New York.

— and — (1978). Gout. In *The metabolic basis of inherited disease* (eds J. B. Stanbury, J. B. Wyngaarden, and D. S. Fredrickson, p. 916. McGraw-Hill, New York.

Hypoxanthine–guanine phosphoribosyl transferase

De Bruyn, C. H. M. M. (1976). Hypoxanthine–guanine phosphoribosyl transferase deficiency. *Hum. Genet.* **31**, 127.

Emmerson, B. T. and Thompson, L. (1973). The spectrum of hypoxanthine guanine phosphoribosyl transferase deficiency. *Q. J. Med.* **42**, 423.

— and Wyngaarden, J. B. (1978). The Lesch–Nyhan syndrome. In *The metabolic basis of inherited diseases*, 4th ed. (eds J. B. Stanbury, J. B. Wyngaarden, and D. S. Fredrickson), p. 1011. (1980). McGraw-Hill, New York.

Kelley, W. N., Green, M. L., Rosenbloom, R. M., Henderson, J. F. and Seegmiller, J. E. (1969). Hypoxanthine–guanine phosphoribosyl transferase deficiency in gout. A review. *Ann. int. Med.* **70**, 155.

Seegmiller, J. E. (1980). Diseases of purine and pyrimidine metabolism. In *Metabolic control and disease*, 8th Ed. (eds P. Bandry and L. E. Rosenberg), p. 777. W. B. Saunders, Philadelphia.

Sorenson, L. F. and Pepe, P. (1970). Hypoxanthine–guanine phosphoribosyl transferase deficiency. *Bull. rheum. Dis.* **21**, 621.

Adenine phosphoribosyl transferase

Fox, I. H., Lacroix, S., Planet, G., and Moore, M. (1977). Partial deficiency of adenine phosphoribosyl transferase in man. *Medicine* **56**, 515.

Simmonds, H. S., Barratt, T. M., Webster, D. R., Sahota, A., Van Acker, K. J., Cameron, J. S., and Dillon, M. (1980). Spectrum of 2,8-dihydroxyadenine urolithiasis in complete APRT deficiency. In *Purine metabolism in man III* (ed. A. Rapado, R. W. E. Watts, and C. H. M. M. De Bruyn, *Adv. exp. Med. Biol.* **122A**, 337.

Phosphoribosyl pyrophosphate synthetase

Becker, M. A. (1978). Abnormalities of PRPP metabolism leading to an overproduction of uric acid in *Handbook of experimental pharmacology* (eds W. N. Kelley, and I. M. Weiner), p. 155. Springer-Verlag, Berlin.

Becker, M. A., Raivio, K. O. and Seegmiller, J. E. (1979). Synthesis of phosphoribosyl pyrophosphate in mammalian cells. In *Adv. Enzymol.* **49**, (ed. A. Meister), p. 281. John Wiley, New York.

Sperling, O., Boer, P., Brosh, S., Sonef, E. and De Vries, A. (1977). Superactivity of phosphoribosyl pyrophosphate synthetase due to feedback resistance causing purine overproduction and gout. In *Purine and Pyrimidine metabolism*, Ciba Foundation Symposium no. 48, p. 143. Elsevier/Excerpta Medica, Amsterdam.

Glucose 6-phosphatase

Alepa, F. P., Howell, R. R., Klinenberg, J. R., and Seegmiller, J. E. (1967). Relationships between glycogen storage disease and tophaceous gout. *Am. J. Med.* **42**, 58.

Greene, H. L., Wilson, F. A., Hefferan, P., Terry, A. B., Moran, J. S., Slonim, A. E., Claus, T. H., and Burr, I. M. (1978). ATP depletion, a possible role in the pathogenesis of hyperuricaemia in glycogen storage disease Type I. *J. clin. invest.* **62**, 321.

Howell, R. R. (1965). The interrelationship of glycogen storage disease and gout. *Arth. Rheum.* **8**, 780.

Xanthine oxidase

Wyngaarden, J. B. (1978). Hereditary xanthinuria. In *The metabolic basis of inherited disease*, 4th ed (eds J. B. Stanbury, J. B. Wyngaarden, and D. S. Fredrickson, p. 1037. McGraw-Hill, New York.

Hypouricaemia

Dwosh, I. L., Roncari, D. A. K., Marliss, E., and Fox, I. H. (1977). Hypouricaemia in disease: a study of different mechanisms. *J. Lab. clin Med.* **90**, 153.

Kelley, W. N. (1975). Hypouricaemia. *Arthr. Rheum.* (Suppl.) **18**, 731.

Disorders of purine metabolism associated with immunodeficiency (ADA, NP, 5'NT)

Asherson, G. L. and Webster, A. D. B. (1980). Purine metabolic defects in immunodeficiency. In *Diagnosis and treatment of immunodeficiency diseases*, p. 202. Blackwell Scientific Publications, Oxford.

Giblett, E. R. (1981). Inherited biochemical defects in lymphocytes causing immunodeficiency diseases. *Prog. clin. Biol. Res.* **58**, 123.

Hirschhorn, R. (1977). Defects of purine metabolism in immunodeficiency diseases. *Prog. clin. Immunol.* **3**, 67.

Martin, D. W. Jr. and Gelfand, E. W. (1981). Biochemistry of diseases of immunodevelopment. *Ann. Rev. Biochem.* **50**, 845.

Thompson, L. F. and Seegmiller, J. E. (1980). Adenosine deaminase deficiency and severe combined immunodeficiency disease. *Adv. Enzymol.* **58**, 167.

Porphyrin metabolism and the porphyrias

A. Goldberg, M. R. Moore, K. E. L. McColl, and M. J. Brodie

The porphyrias are metabolic disorders, hereditary in origin, which, though comparatively rare, may mimic many other common conditions. They are disorders of the porphyrin chemistry of the body of which the striking clinical expression is often the passage of dark urine. They belong to that larger family of diseases called by Garrod 'inborn errors of metabolism'. The metabolism of the body is regulated by an intricate mosaic of enzymes, the synthesis of which is under genetic control. A defect in this control may result in the defective formation of one or more specific enzymes and thus lead to an 'inborn error of metabolism'. The porphyrias are an example of such a group of diseases in which specific enzyme defects relating directly or indirectly to porphyrin biosynthesis may cause generalized clinical abnormalities.

The tetrapyrrolic porphyrin ring is a unique and intriguing biological structure ubiquitously distributed in nature. By virtue of its ring structure and available ligand bonding, it is capable of binding many metals, but reaches its true apotheosis when binding either iron or magnesium. As the ferrous iron-containing complex, haem. it is central in all biological oxidation reactions. Chlorophylls, the magnesium-porphyrin compounds, are the basis of biological solar energy utilization and carbohydrate synthesis. In all biological systems the biosynthetic intermediates of haem and chlorophyll synthesis are the porphyrinogens, the hexahydro-porphyrins, which are chemically quite distinct from the porphyrins. Porphyrinogens are non-conjugated colourless compounds which may easily be oxidized to the totally conjugated and highly coloured porphyrins. Porphyrins typically absorb radiation about 400 nm, the so-called 'Soret' maximum and re-emit it as the characteristic red porphyrin fluorescence around 600 nm. The structures of biologically important porphyrins and porphyrinogens are shown in Fig. 1.

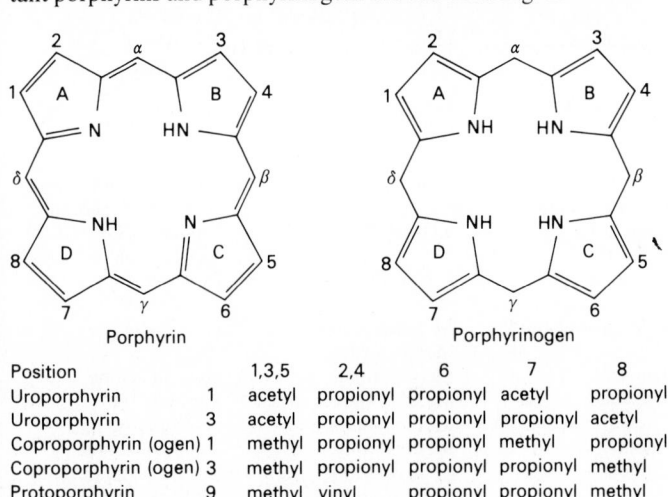

Position		1,3,5	2,4	6	7	8
Uroporphyrin	1	acetyl	propionyl	propionyl	acetyl	propionyl
Uroporphyrin	3	acetyl	propionyl	propionyl	propionyl	acetyl
Coproporphyrin (ogen)	1	methyl	propionyl	propionyl	methyl	propionyl
Coproporphyrin (ogen)	3	methyl	propionyl	propionyl	propionyl	methyl
Protoporphyrin	9	methyl	vinyl	propionyl	propionyl	methyl

Fig. 1 The structures of porphyrins showing the positioning of the different substituents round the porphyrin nucleus.

Biochemistry. In man the principal respiratory pigment, haem, is synthesized from the simple precursors, glycine and succinyl CoA by the pathway shown in Fig. 2. This pathway is now well understood and developing knowledge has linked the specific biochemical lesions to the clinical manifestations of the porphyrias. The initial stage is the rate-limiting one, that is the condensation of glycine and succinyl CoA through the aegis of the mitochondrial enzyme delta-aminolaevulinic acid synthase to form delta-aminolaevulinic acid (ALA). Control of this enzyme takes place both through feedback repression and inhibition by haem. The next step occurs in the cytoplasm where ALA dehydratase condenses two molecules of ALA and cyclizes them to form the monopyrrole porphobilinogen. Still within the cytoplasm, uroporphyrinogen I synthase and uroporphyrinogen cosynthetase act concertedly, to cyclize and isomerize four molecules of porphobilinogen to form the first of the reduced tetrapyrroles, the hexahydro octacarboxylic porphyrin, uroporphyrinogen III. In circumstances where there is a deficiency of the enzyme uroporphyrinogen cosynthetase or isomerase there is an excessive production of uroporphyrinogen I and coproporphyrinogen I which cannot be used further and are therefore excreted, mainly in the urine, as the I isomer porphyrins. Coproporphyrinogen III is produced by a stepwise decarboxylation from uroporphyrinogen III by uroporphyrinogen decarboxylase and thence by oxidation and decarboxylation, once more within the mitochondrion; coproporphyrinogen oxidase forms protoporphyrinogen IX which is oxidized by protoporphyrinogen oxidase to protoporphyrin IX, into which ferrous iron is inserted by ferrochelatase to form haem.

Classification. The classification of the porphyrias is dependent upon three features. Firstly, the principal site of porphyrin biosynthesis, secondly, whether the disease shows an acute presentation, and finally the pattern of production of the porphyrin precursors and formed porphyrins. A classification of the porphyrias is shown in Table 1. The porphyrias, as mainly inborn errors of metabolism, involve aberrations of specific enzymes in the haem biosynthetic pathway. The major sites of abnormal porphyrin production are liver and bone marrow, although porphyrin biosynthesis is a function of every cell in the body. These determine one classification, the hepatic (see below) and the erythropoietic porphyrias. The other, the acute and non-acute porphyrias, is based upon the clinical presentation of these diseases. The activity of the rate-limiting enzyme delta-aminolaevulinic acid synthase is elevated in all porphyrias. The prevalence of the various forms of porphyria varies widely from country to country. In the United Kingdom this has not been definitively established. In Scotland 1 person in 50 000 has some form of porphyria with a predominance of acute intermittent porphyria and cutaneous hepatic porphyria. In South Africa the prevalent form of the disease is variegate porphyria with an incidence of 1 in 9000 in the white population, whilst the Bantu suffer mainly from cutaneous hepatic porphyria.

Table 1

Hepatic porphyrias	
Acute intermittent porphyria	
Variegate porphyria	Acute porphyrias
Hereditary coproporphyria	
Cutaneous hepatic porphyria	
genetically predisposed	
toxic	
neoplastic	Non-acute porphyrias
Erythropoietic porphyrias	
Congenital porphyria	
Erythropoietic protoporphyria	

Solar photosensitivity. The production of solar photosensitivity of the skin by formed porphyrins is a characteristic feature of all the porphyrias excluding acute intermittent porphyria. This skin photosensitivity is brought about by deposition of free porphyrin

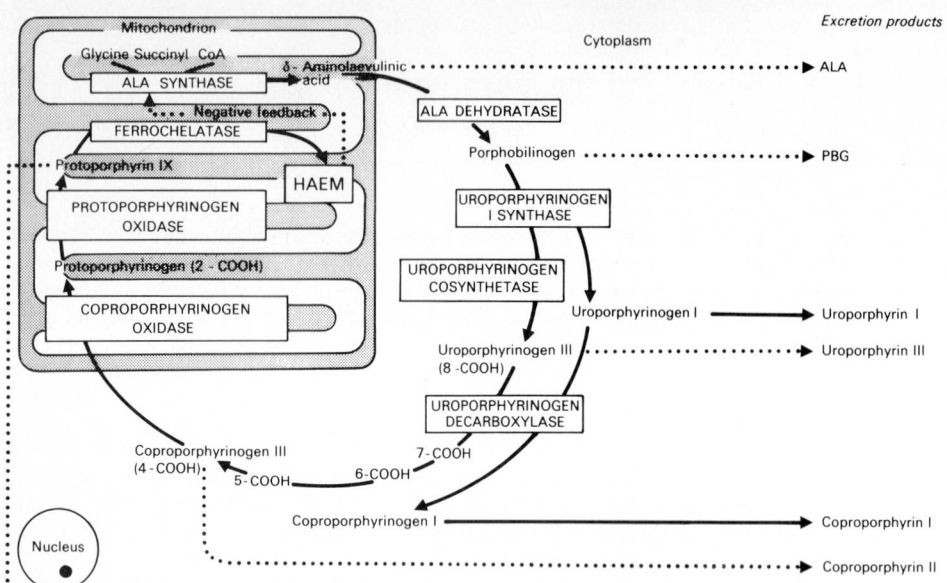

Fig. 2   Haem biosynthesis within the cell. This figure shows how haem is synthesized from the precursors glycine and succinyl CoA and the different compartmentation of the stages of the pathway in the mitochondrion and in the cytoplasm. Control of the pathway is maintained by haem acting by negative feedback on ALA synthase. Any of the series I isomer porphyrins synthesized will be excreted.

within the upper epidermal layers, after photo-oxidation of the non-photosensitizing porphyrinogens to porphyrins. This deposition is facilitated by the decreased availability of porphyrin binding by proteins such as haemopexin caused by the associated hepato-cellular insufficiency, as well as the massive increase of porphyrins.

The photochemistry of porphyrins is, in general, complex but it is on the basis of this photochemistry that many of the adverse reactions may be explained. It is generally accepted that the most prominent electronic transition is that from the π electron state to the π^* activated state, the lifetime of which is wholly dependent on the porphyrin concerned. Some metallo-porphyrins show phosphorescence, some fluorescence, and some both of these. Activated porphyrins have been shown to participate in photo-reductive and photo-oxidative procedures. By virtue of these photodynamic properties, that is the sensitization of biomolecules and cells such that they may be damaged by visible light, porphyrins will exhibit their damaging properties on skin cells in porphyria. Cancer cells will accumulate porphyrins more avidly than normal cells, a feature which has been used in the phototherapy of cancer. This property has been shown to continue throughout the cell cycle when a haematoporphyrin derivative is used as the photodynamic agent in cultured human cells.

Hepatic porphyrias

The acute porphyrias. These comprise acute intermittent porphyria (AIP), variegate porphyria (VP), and hereditary coproporphyria (HC), which have several features in common. They are all transmitted by Mendelian autosomal dominant modes of inheritance. Acute attacks are followed in most cases by complete remission, but death may be the outcome especially in AIP. Latent cases can occur. In attacks they can all display similar abdominal and neuropsychiatric disturbances, although VP and HC may also present with photosensitivity. All can be precipitated by some sex hormones, alcohol, and especially by certain drugs (Table 2), often hepatic microsomal enzyme inducers but which also have the characteristic of being lipid soluble. All patients excrete the porphyrin precursors ALA and PBG in excess in the urine in attack. Finally the management of the acute porphyric attack is similar in each of these porphyrias.

Acute intermittent porphyria. This is the most severe of the acute porphyrias. The abnormality lies at the level of uroporphyrinogen I synthase in the haem biosynthetic pathway and may be detected in

Table 2   Drugs unsafe in the acute porphyrias

Alphaxolone	Flufenamic acid	Oral contraceptives
Aluminium	Flunitrazepam	Oxyzolidinediones
preparations	Fluroxine	(Paramethadione
Aminoglutethimide		and Trimethadione)
Amitriptyline	Glutethimide	Oestrogens
Amphetamines	Gold preparations	Oxazepam
Apronalide	(Myocrisin)	
Azapropazone	Griseofulvin	Pancuronium
		Pargyline
Barbituvates	Halothane	Pentazocine
Bemegride	Hydantoins	Pentylenetetrazol
Busulphan	(Phenytoin, Ethotoin,	Phenoxybenzamine
	Mephenytoin)	Phenylbutazone
Carbromal	Hydrallazine	Phenylhydrazine
Carbamazepine	Hydrochlorthiazide	Primidone
Chlorambucil	Hydrocine butyl	Probenecid
Chloramphenicol	bromide	Progesterone
Chlordiazepoxide		Pyrazinamide
Chlormezanone	Imniprime	Pyrazolones
Chloroform	Isoniazid	(amidopyrine,
Chloroquine	Isopropyl	antipyrine,
Chlormethiazole	meprobamate	isopropylantipyrine,
Chlorpropamide		dipyrone, sodium
Cimetidine	Ketoprofen	phenyl dimethyl
Clonidine		pyrazolone)
Cocaine	Lignocaine	Pyrimethamine
Colistin		
Cyclophosphamide	Mefenamic acid	Rifampicin
	Mephenezine	
Danazol	Meprobamate	Spironolactone
Dapsone	Mercury preparations	Steroids
Dichloralphenazone	Methoxyflurane	Succinimides
Diethylpropion	Methyldopa	(ethosuximide,
Dimenhydrinate	Methylprylone	methsuximide,
	Metoclopramide	phensuximide)
Enflurane	Metyrapone	Sulphonamides
Ergot preparations	Metronidazole	Sulphonylureas
Erythromycin		Sulthiame
Ethanol	Nalidixic acid	
Ethchlorvynol	Nikethamide	Tetracyclines
Ethinamate	Nitrazepam	Theophylline
Etomidate	Nitrofurantoin	Tolazamide
	Novobiocin	Tolbutamide
		Tranylcypromine
		Troxidone
		Xylocaine

the erythrocyte even when porphyrin precursor excretion is normal. Women are affected more often than men in a ratio of 3:2. The disease occurs mainly in young adults; the mean age of onset of symptoms is 27 years in women and about 35 years in men. Only a few cases have been described in children and first attacks are unusual in people over 50 years.

Clinical features. The gastrointestinal and neuropsychiatric symptoms and signs are common to attacks of all the acute porphyrias and are summarized in Fig. 3. Gastrointestinal symptoms are commonest occurring in 95 per cent of cases. Most patients present acutely with colicky central abdominal pain. On examination there is tenderness but not much rigidity. There may be limb pain or generalized muscular aches. Vomiting may be troublesome and severe; constipation is usual, although diarrhoea has been noted in about 10 per cent of patients. Where vomiting is severe or prolonged, the patient may become dehydrated with associated electrolyte abnormalities. Hyponatraemia may rarely be associated with inappropriate secretion of antidiuretic hormone, in which case one finds low plasma osmolality, high urine osmolality, and diminished water clearance.

A peripheral neuropathy may be the presenting feature and it complicates two-thirds of porphyric attacks. This begins most commonly with cramp-like pain and stiffness progressing to muscular weakness. The motor signs are usually symmetrical, involving limb and girdle muscles more frequently than trunk muscles. Upper limbs are most affected, proximal muscles before distal ones. Involvement of the wrists, ankles, and small muscles of the hand are important as permanent deformity can be produced. Weakness of trunk muscles has serious consequences as it is frequently associated with respiratory embarrassment. Upper motor lesions may develop and rarely the cerebellum and basal ganglia may be involved. Sensory signs and symptoms may occur, e.g. paraesthesiae, numbness, and objective evidence of sensory impairment (usually loss of pin prick sensation) most marked around the shoulder and hip areas. Urinary retention and cranial nerve palsies have also been described but are less common. Grand mal epileptic seizures

and non-specific abnormalities of the electroencephalogram sometimes occur during attacks but the EEG reverts to normal in remission.

The cardiovascular system is involved in about 70 per cent of attacks of acute intermittent porphyria. Sinus tachycardia with a rate of up to 160 per minute and systemic hypertension are the usual findings. Blood pressure usually reverts to normal as the attacks subside but during the attack there may be associated left ventricular failure and fundal changes including papilloedema. Permanent hypertension may be a long-term sequel. Hypotension, sometimes postural, with syncope has also been described.

Depression, anxiety, hysteria, and frank psychosis are important and sometimes presenting manifestations but rarely extend beyond the duration of the somatic illness.

Pathogenesis of symptoms. Histopathological changes have been found in the peripheral and autonomic nerves and in the central nervous system, which can explain all of the acute clinical manifestations of the porphyrias. The relationship between the biochemical aberrations and the neuropathology of the porphyrias is still unclear.

Diagnosis. Although acute porphyria is an uncommon disorder, its characteristic symptoms and signs are shared by many other diseases. Abdominal pain, a common cause of hospital admission, is only rarely associated with a primary porphyrin abnormality. However, if abdominal pain occurs in a patient with some neuropsychiatric presentation, the diagnosis of acute porphyria should be considered. This suspicion is increased if there is a positive family history, if the urine turns dark brown or red on standing, or if one observes an association of onset of attack with certain drugs (Table 2).

The acute attack can be diagnosed at the bedside by one of the chemical tests for the presence of excess porphobilinogen. One volume of urine (i.e. 2 ml) is mixed with one volume of Ehrlich's aldehyde reagent (p-dimethyl amino benzaldehyde in acid solution) in a test-tube. If a pink colour is produced, either excess porphobilinogen or urobilinogen is present. Porphobilinogen can

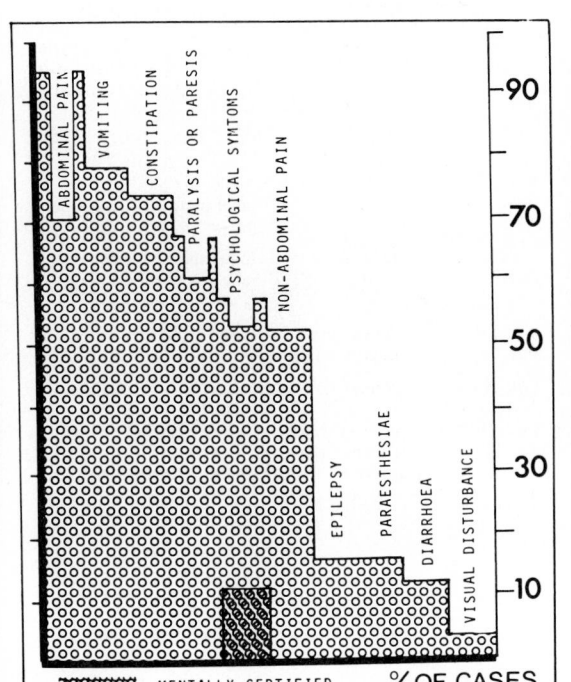

INCIDENCE OF SYMPTOMS IN 50 CASES OF ACUTE INTERMITTENT PORPHYRIA

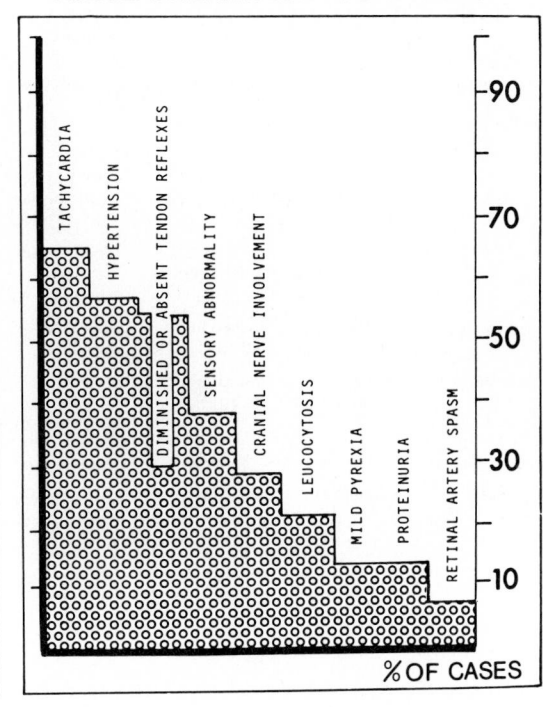

INCIDENCE OF PHYSICAL SIGNS, BLOOD & URINE FINDINGS IN 50 CASES OF ACUTE INTERMITTENT PORPHYRIA

Fig. 3 Incidence of symptoms and signs of acute intermittent porphyria in attack.

be identified by adding two volumes of chloroform (i.e. 4 ml), shaking and observing that the pink colouration remains in the upper part of the test-tube, i.e. is insoluble in chloroform. The pattern of abnormality in porphyrin and porphyrin precursor excretion is outlined in Table 3. The peripheral blood picture is normal apart from an occasional modest neutrophil leucocytosis. Liver function tests may be abnormal with elevated transaminases and bilirubin being the most common findings. The serum cholesterol and protein-bound iodine may be elevated together with total thyroxine and triiodothronine concentrations, and moderate proteinuria is found in about 10 per cent of patients. The blood urea is often raised during and for some months after the acute attack.

Precipitating factors. The porphyrias have been described as pharmaco-genetic diseases, that is a group of genetically defined diseases which show an idiosyncratic reaction to many common drugs. Patients at risk may develop an attack after taking certain drugs, especially those which are lipid soluble and which are known to be inducers of monooxygenases. The most important of these are listed in Table 2. Great care must be taken to ensure that patients with porphyria are not prescribed any of these drugs. Barbiturates and, more recently, oral contraceptive preparations are most frequently involved. Attacks sometimes occur in the later stages of pregnancy and in the early puerperium. In some young women, there is an association with menstruation. Infection at any site may provoke symptoms and starvation has been associated with an acute attack. In about 40 per cent of patients there is no evident provoking factor. There is evidence of endogenous hormonal precipitating agents. Women show much greater monthly fluctuation in porphyrin production and steroid hormone levels. Urinary excretion of individual 17-oxosteroids are elevated both in attack and remission and one of these steroids (dehydroepiandrosterone) has been shown to induce the production of hepatic ALA synthase, the rate-limiting enzyme of haem biosynthesis, when injected into rats. This observation could explain the rarity of childhood cases, the female preponderance and the association with pregnancy and menstruation.

Variegate porphyria. This form of porphyria, also known as mixed porphyria or porphyria variegata, combines the clinical features of an acute porphyria with those of a cutaneous porphyria. The abnormality has been shown to lie at the level of protoporphyrinogen oxidase with consequently increased production of protoporphyrin in the haem biosynthetic pathway. A number of large family trees have been compiled, but by far the biggest is that of a South African pedigree in which over a 1000 patients with variegate porphyria were traced to a Dutch Cape settler who married an orphan girl in 1688.

Variegate porphyria affects young adults and is very rare in childhood. There is no sex preponderance, but, for reasons which are poorly understood, acute systemic symptoms are commoner in women, while cutaneous symptoms are found more often in men. An acute attack may present with gastrointestinal and neuropsychiatric features together with bullous dermatosis identical to that seen in cutaneous hepatic porphyria. The skin lesion often persists when the acute attack has passed and indeed may be the only manifestation of the disease. Systemic attacks are nearly always precipitated by a drug; barbiturates and the contraceptive pill have hitherto been the most commonly implicated.

Hereditary coproporphyria. This is the least common of the acute porphyrias. Since the disease was first named in 1955 by Berger and Goldberg, about 100 further cases have been reported. Coproporphyrinogen oxidase is the enzyme in the haem biosynthetic pathway which is the site of the biochemical lesion. The disease has no sex preponderance and affects people from 7 to 75 years old, with a peak at 30 years. The condition is often latent.

As in variegate porphyria there are systemic and cutaneous manifestations. Abdominal pain, vomiting, and constipation are the usual presenting features. Psychiatric symptoms, particularly depression, have been recorded in about a third of active cases. Epileptic seizures have also been reported. Photosensitive bullous eruptions may occur and often such cases have been associated with disordered hepatic function. The skin lesion does not occur in isolation in contrast to variegate porphyria. Once again attacks may be precipitated by drugs. Diagnosis depends on demonstrating the specific abnormal pattern of porphyrin excretion (Table 3).

Another acute porphyria. A further type of porphyria has recently been described, but as yet is unnamed, in which the biochemical

Table 3 Normal values and abnormal porphyrin and precursor patterns in the porphyrias

	Erythrocyte proto-porphyrin	Erythrocyte copro-porphyrin	Urinary ALA	Urinary PBG	Urinary uro-porphyrin	Urinary copro-porphyrin	Faecal X porphyrin	Faecal proto-porphyrin	Faecal copro-porphyrin
Normal levels	0–50 µg/dl cells	0–4.2 µg/dl cells	0–5.3 mg per day	0–3.6 mg per day	0–41 µg per day	0–280 µg per day	0–15 µg per g dry wt	0–113 µg per g dry wt	0–50 µg per g dry wt
SI units	0–900 nmol/l	0–64 nmol/l	0–40 µmol per day	0–16 µmol per day	0–49 nmol per day	0–432 nmol per day	—	0–200 nmol per g dry wt	0–76 nmol per g dry wt
Acute intermittent porphyria	normal	normal	raised—very high in attack	raised—very high in attack	usually raised	sometimes raised	normal	sometimes raised	sometimes raised
Variegate porphyria	normal	normal	raised in attack	raised in attack	sometimes raised	sometimes raised	raised very high in attack	raised	raised
Hereditary coproporphyria	normal	sometimes raised in attack	raised only in attack	raised only in attack	sometimes raised in attack	usually raised —always raised in attack	sometimes raised normal	usually normal	raised
Cutaneous hepatic porphyria	normal	normal	normal	normal	raised—very high in attack	slightly raised	raised	raised in remission	raised in remission
Congenital porphyria	usually raised	usually raised	usually normal	usually normal	raised	sometimes raised	normal	sometimes raised	raised
Erythropoietic proto-porphyria	raised—usually very high	sometimes slightly raised	normal	normal	normal	normal	normal	usually raised	normal

presentation is analogous to that found in lead poisoning. In this disease, inherited as a Mendelian autosomal dominant, the activity of ALA dehydratase is depressed. In the few cases described to date in Germany and in the USA, there are acute features together with excess urinary excretion of delta-aminolaevulinic acid. Latent cases have been found.

Management of the acute porphyrias. In remission and in the latent cases, prophylaxis is important. Blood relatives of patients should be tested for latency. The drugs listed in Table 2 are contra-indicated. Alcohol should also be avoided as should severe dietary restriction. No dogmatic statement can be made about the possible effect of pregnancy on acute porphyria. A patient in the midst of attacks should certainly avoid pregnancy, but must avoid the contraceptive pill. After a suitable period of remission, e.g. one year, she may reasonably contemplate pregnancy. The danger does not stop at labour, for the early part of the puerperium may be treacherous. Pregnancy appears to be less dangerous in variegate porphyria than in acute intermittent porphyria. When a patient needs an anaesthetic, nitrous oxide, ether, and cyclopropane have been safely used while suxamethonium appears to be a safe muscle relaxant. The opiates and belladona derivatives can be used for premedication. Infection should be sought and treated since this can precipitate or aggravate an acute attack.

The more important points in the management of a patient in an attack of acute porphyria are to identify and remove any precipitating factors and provide effective supportive therapy until the attack spontaneously resolves. A high carbohydrate intake should be maintained throughout the attacks as this represses hepatic ALA synthase and reduces the overproduction of porphyrins and precursors. In attack the carbohydrate may be given orally or via a naso-gastric tube in the form of high calorie drinks. If nausea or vomiting is a problem, then glucose or laevulose should be administered intravenously through a central venous line. About 1500–2000 kcal carbohydrate should be given every 24 hours.

During the attack, patients are often difficult to nurse and to treat. Their constant requests for analgesia for intractable abdominal pain may even give a false impression that they are drug addicts. Pethidine and dihydrocodeine may control the pain but stronger analgesics such as morphine or its analogues may be required. Vomiting can be controlled through the use of promazine, and the hypertension and tachycardia may be treated with propranolol or other beta-blockers. Guanethidine, reserpine, and diazoxide may also be used without exacerbating the attack. The commonly observed neurosis and psychosis can be controlled with chlorpromazine, promazine, or trifluoroperazine while epileptiform seizures may be treated with diazepam, or chlormethiazole. Constipation, when it occurs, is severe to the point of obstipation and neostigmine (7.5–15 mg orally) is helpful in these circumstances. Weakness and paralysis—consequences of the neurological features of these diseases—require early physiotherapy and assisted respiration. Respiratory paralysis may develop and progressive weakening of the voice is an important premonitory sign. Artificial respiration with tracheostomy and intermittent positive pressure respiration may be required. Full recovery has occurred following such ventilation for some months. The treatment of fluid imbalance is important. Hypochloraemia and hyponatraemia may complicate an acute attack, associated with excessive vomiting and inadequate fluid intake. In these cases one should ensure that there is adequate fluid and salt replacement. Where there is evidence of inappropriate secretion of antidiuretic hormone rather than sodium depletion, the water excess should be treated by fluid restriction, with 24 hour intake limited to 700 ml. Infection which can precipitate or aggravate an acute attack, should be sought and treated.

Intravenous haematin therapy has been shown consistently to reduce the over production of porphyrin and precursors in patients in an attack of acute porphyria. The haematin is administered once or twice daily for several days. The most commonly used dose has been 4 mg/kg body weight/24 hours and this is infused slowly over 30 minutes. The haematin is mainly taken up by the liver and results in repression of ALA synthase (Fig. 4). The clinical response unfortunately has not been as consistent as the biochemical response, since improvement has occurred in only about 50 per cent of patients treated. The haematin may cause localized phlebitis if injected in a small peripheral vein and should be given into a large vein or via a central venous line. No other side-effects have been reported with haematin, when given at the recommended dosage. Experience is still limited and fuller clinical assessment is required. Some centres have found high doses of propranolol to result in some clinical and biochemical improvement; others recommended the use of folic acid.

There is no specific treatment for the skin photosensitivity occurring in variegate porphyria and hereditary coproporphyria, although β-carotene treatment has been suggested as useful (see Erythropoietic protoporphyria below). Barrier creams may be used and avoidance of excess sunlight advised. The dermatological features often subside with the acute attack as the amount of formed porphyrin in the serum is reduced.

Cutaneous hepatic porphyria. There is a genetic predisposition to this disease, also known as porphyria cutanea tarda or symptomatic porphyria, although there is rarely more than one member of the family affected. The biochemical abnormality lies in hepatic uroporphyrinogen decarboxylase. Diagnosis, once again, is by the analysis of the porphyrin excretion pattern in which the dominant finding is an increased urinary uroporphyrin excretion. The urinary porphyrin precursors ALA and PBG are never elevated. The changes in porphyrin excretion in attacks, remission and in the treated case are outlined in Fig. 5.

The most striking and consistent clinical feature of cutaneous hepatic porphyria is bullous dermatosis on exposure to sunlight. The lesions are encountered on exposed areas such as the scalp, face, neck, and backs of the forearms and hands. They usually start with erythema progressing to vesicles that become confluent to form bullae. Haemorrhage may occur into the bullae which heal, leaving scars. Pruritus is often troublesome. There may be local pitting oedema at the site of the skin lesion. Increased fragility of the skin is an important feature and in less severe cases may be the only clinical sign. Hyperpigmentation is common and women often complain of hirsutes. Histological examination of the skin shows gross hyaline swelling in the walls of the capillaries in the upper corium of the bullae. Monochromator studies demonstrate that light of about the same wavelength as that absorbed by the porphyrin molecule (400 nm) will cause skin lesions in the porphyric patient.

In addition to the cutaneous signs there may be evidence of hepatic disease both clinically and biochemically. Hepatomegaly is particularly common where alcohol has an aetiological role. Severe abdominal pain with vomiting is rare but there may be mild abdominal pain. The deranged porphyrin biochemistry is considered in Table 3, and several other laboratory tests may be helpful. In nearly all cases liver function tests are abnormal including elevated bilirubin, alkaline phosphatase, and serum transaminase levels. Serum iron and transferrin saturation are often increased and there may be an increased plasma iron turnover with early uptake of radioactive iron by the liver. Histological examination of the liver usually reveals features which reflect the whole spectrum of alcoholic liver disease, although occasionally liver damage is minimal and non-specific. Siderosis invariably occurs and an underlying active chronic hepatitis may rarely be present. There is a 25 per cent incidence of diabetes mellitus.

Alcohol is the most important precipitating agent in cutaneous hepatic porphyria. More than 90 per cent of patients admit to excessive alcohol consumption. Oestrogenic steroids are also implicated in some cases. An outbreak of cutaneous hepatic porphyria occurred in Southeast Turkey in 1956 and this was traced to seed wheat dressed with the fungicide hexachlorobenzene. There was

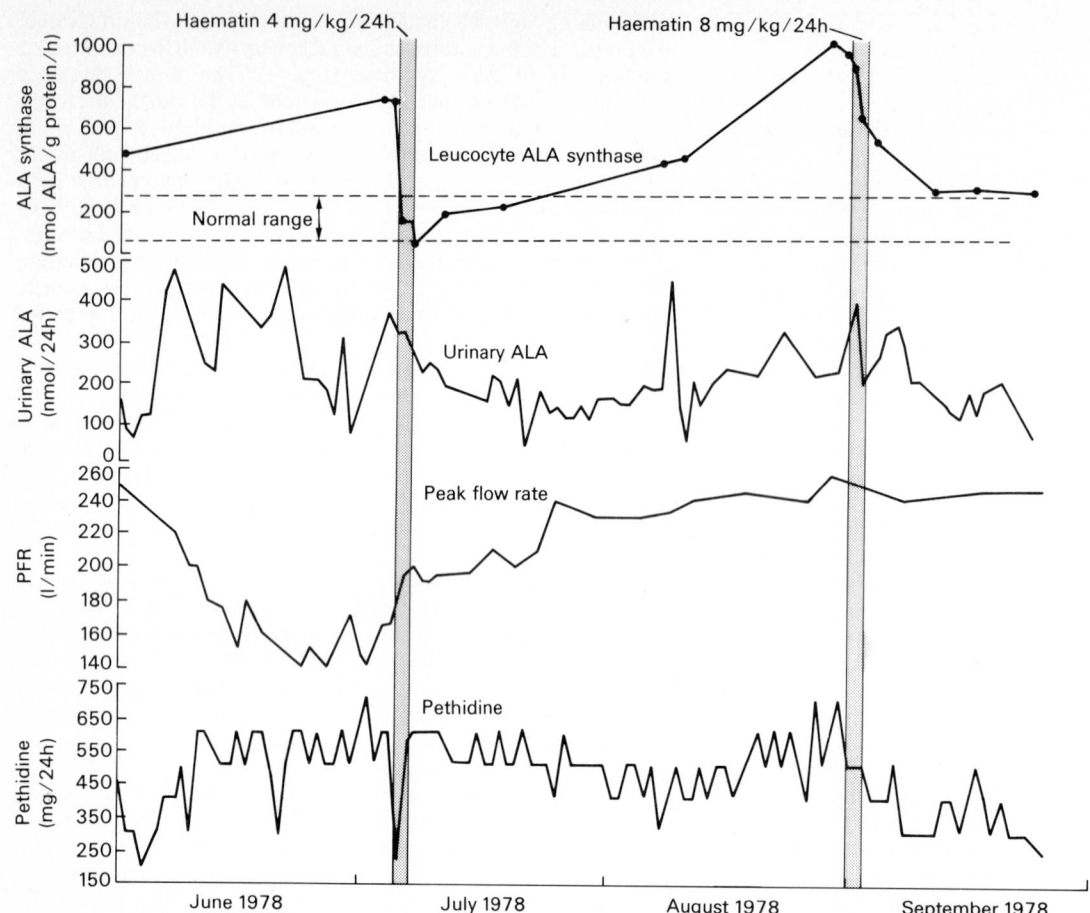

Fig. 4 Biochemical and clinical response to three course of haematin therapy in a 29-year-old woman in prolonged attack of acute intermittent porphyria. The haematin repressed the activity of ALA synthase which was monitored in peripheral leucocytes and reduced the urinary excretion of ALA. There was associated improvement as reflected in rise in respiratory peak flow rate and drop in analgesic requirement.

evidence of organic liver disease as well as photosensitivity and a number of patients died. Abnormal porphyrin excretion has been shown in animals given dietary hexachlorobenzene. More recently other polychlorinated hydrocarbons have been implicated in production of this toxic form of cutaneous hepatic porphyria. A neoplastic subgroup includes a similar condition secondary to benign or malignant primary liver tumour.

The clinical features are reduced and even reversed by withdrawal of the offending agent. Alcohol, in particular, should be avoided. Venesection of about 2–4 litres of blood in total may bring about clinical remission. Regular venesection of 500 ml is carried out until clinical remission occurs or until the haemoglobin level

falls below 12 g/dl. A rising urinary uroporphyrin level is a useful index of the requirement for further venesection before clinical symptoms become manifest. Treatment may be required for the underlying liver disease, e.g. active chronic hepatitis. Chloroquine has recently been found to be of value in the treatment of cutaneous hepatic porphyria. It is taken in the small dose of 125 mg twice per week and results in increased urinary excretion of uroporphyrin with an associated fall in plasma and tissue levels and symptomatic improvement. The precise mechanism of its action is not clear but it probably forms complexes of uroporphyrin which are more readily cleared by the kidney. There is also evidence that it modifies hepatic iron and porphyrin metabolism.

DEVIATION OF PORPHYRINS IN CUTANEOUS HEPATIC PORPHYRIA

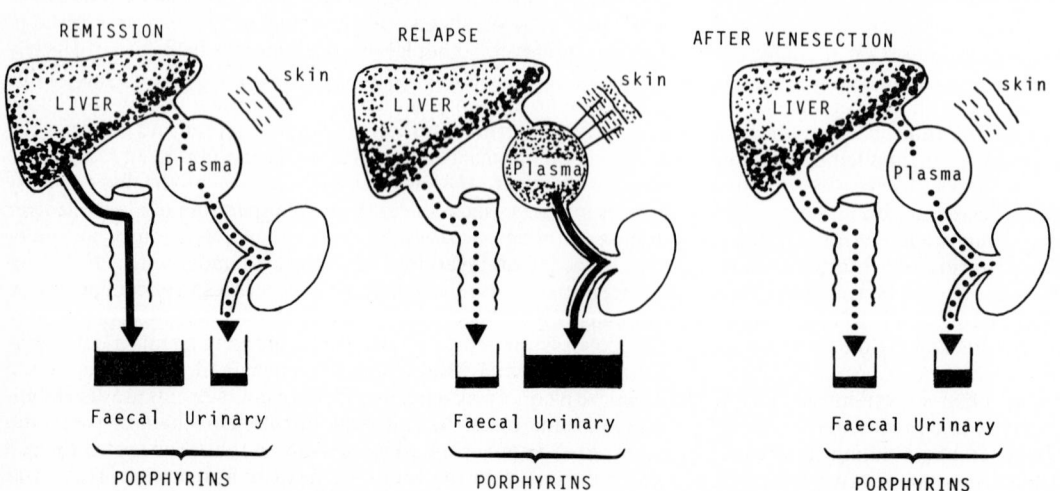

Fig. 5 In cutaneous hepatic porphyria in remission, porphyrins pass from the liver to the bile and are excreted in the faeces. As the disease relapses and the liver disease progresses, this route of excretion becomes less available and porphyrins are deviated to the systemic circulation to be excreted in the urine. Some porphyrins, in addition, pass to the skin to cause solar photosensitivity. After venesection the disease goes into remission with relatively less porphyrin synthesized by the liver and consequent depression of both urinary and faecal excretion of porphyrins. There is complete remission of cutaneous signs.

Erythropoietic porphyrias

Congenital porphyria. Although extremely rare, this congenital porphyria, also known as erythropoietic porphyria or Gunther's porphyria, was probably the first porphyria to be described, in 1874. Since then, less than 100 cases have been reported. Solar sensitivity is the most striking symptom but systemic effects may also be severe. The disorder is inherited in a Mendelian autosomal recessive manner. There is evidence that the defect lies at the level of uroporphyrinogen cosynthetase in the biosynthetic pathway. Boys and girls are equally affected and symptoms usually begin during the first few years of life, although the disease can rarely present in middle age.

The skin reaction to sunlight is more severe than that of cutaneous hepatic porphyria. Pruritus and erythema are the initial features followed by vesicle and bullous formation. The bullae rupture leaving ulcers that frequently harbour secondary infection. Eventually the ulcers heal leaving scars. The severity of the lesions varies considerably but the result in most cases is devastating. Dystrophic changes in the nails may cause them to curl and drop off. Scarring of the skin on the hand may produce a claw-shaped deformity; lenticular scarring may lead to blindness. Hypertrichosis may be seen on the face, arms, and legs. Eyebrows and eyelashes become thick and long. Pigmentation may be marked. The teeth become brownish-pink (erythrodontia) due to their high porphyrin content.

In addition to these integumentary lesions, a number of cases also develop anaemia and splenomegaly. The anaemia is caused by ineffective erythropoiesis with shortened red cell survival. The bone marrow reveals normoblastic hyperplasia and the peripheral blood film shows a normocytic normochromic anaemia with polychromasia. There is usually a moderate reticulocytosis with Howell–Jolly bodies; leucopenia and thrombocytopenia may occur when the spleen is large. Splenectomy may improve the anaemia and can reduce the degree of photosensitization. Treatment with chloroquine has been shown to be helpful in this disease, as it may be in cutaneous hepatic porphyria, reducing erythrocyte fragility and diminishing the photosensitization lesions. Patients with congenital porphyria have a much shortened life expectancy.

Erythropoietic protoporphyria. Although not described until 1961, this form of erythropoietic porphyria, also known as erythrohepatic protoporphyria, is much commoner than congenital porphyria. It is inherited as an autosomal dominant character and symptoms may occur at any age including infancy and childhood. Ferrochelatase activity is reduced in peripheral blood, liver, bone marrow, and skin. The clinical features are mainly cutaneous with pruritic urticarial swelling and redness of the skin on exposure to sunlight. The most distressing symptom is a burning sensation of the affected parts which may be unbearable. There may also be an eczematous skin reaction with scarring.

Systemic manifestations are not usually severe, but hepatic involvement occurs. There is evidence that protoporphyrin is hepatotoxic and that its deposition in the liver can lead to fatal liver failure from an active chronic hepatitis with cirrhosis. Histological assessment of liver damage is essential. There is also a tendency to the formation of protoporphyrin-containing gallstones, which may be the clinically presenting feature.

Diagnosis can be made by demonstrating fluorescence in a proportion of red cells (fluorocytes) in the peripheral blood and confirmed by measurement of greatly increased protoporphyrin content of erythrocytes and stool. β-carotene taken orally is an effective protective measure against solar sensitivity. There is the side-effect of some yellowing of the skin after prolonged treatment which may be controlled by concurrent ingestion of canthaxanthin. The mode of action of β-carotene may be by quenching of activated porphyrin triplet states, but it does not affect the biochemical presentation of the disease. Treatment of the liver lesion is more problematical. Interruption of the enterohepatic circulation of pro-

toporphyrin by bile salt sequestering agents such as cholestyramine reduces plasma protoporphyrin levels and retards the activity of the liver disease.

Pathogenesis of the porphyrias

The principal linking feature in this group of diseases is an elevation of the initial and rate limiting enzyme ALA synthase which explains the primary overproduction of porphyrins and their precursors. Control of this enzyme has been shown to take place both by feed-back repression and inhibition by haem at both transcriptional and translational cellular levels. In the liver a major portion of the haem is required for the maintenance of microsomal cytochromes which have a rapid turnover. This is the primary control point of the pathway; but changes in ALA synthase activity cannot alone fully explain the differences in porphyrin production and excretion and differences in clinical manifestations of the acute and non-acute porphyrias. One may then postulate the existence of some secondary control mechanisms. The acute porphyrias are characterized by acute generalized neuropathies which are absent in the non-acute porphyrias. In each of the three acute diseases there is excessive production and urinary excretion of ALA and PBG but in the other non-acute porphyrias no such excess of porphyrin precursors is found. This may be of importance since ALA has been shown to have pharmacological, biochemical, and possible behavioural effects in experimental animals, but such effects can only take place at concentrations of ALA greater than those found in the human diseases. The monopyrrole porphobilinogen may have similar properties although this is less likely, but other monopyrroles have been found to be elevated in the urine of patients with acute porphyria.

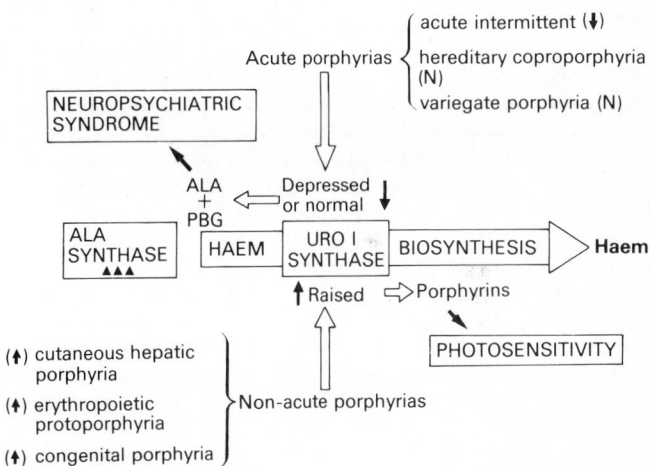

Fig. 6 Control of the biosynthetic pathway. The principal control of the pathway takes place by the action of haem by negative feedback on ALA synthase. Secondary control takes place at the level of uroporphyrinogen I synthase. In the acute porphyrias where uroporphyrinogen I synthase activity is either normal or depressed, excessive concentrations of circulating porphyrin precursors delta-aminolaevulinic acid and porphobilinogen are produced thus potentially resulting in the proven neuro-psychiatric syndrome in these diseases. In the non-acute porphyrias uroporphyrinogen I synthase activity is raised. No precursors accumulate and only porphyrins are elaborated in excess giving the typical photosensitization lesions found in the cutaneous porphyrias.

If one then considers the pattern of activities for the enzymes of the haem biosynthetic pathway in each of the porphyrias, one feature becomes immediately clear; that uroporphyrinogen I synthase activity is either normal or depressed in the acute porphyrias but raised in all of the non-acute porphyrias. The importance of this finding is that since the activity of the initial enzyme is always raised, greater quantities of substrate than normal enter the pathway. It is essential that some of this excess substrate be excreted, either as porphyrin precursor or as formed porphyrin, since the quantities produced are in excess of the biological requirement for haem. In the acute porphyrias the activity of uroporphyrinogen I synthase is low (acute intermittent porphyria), or normal (hereditary coproporphyria and variegate porphyria) and, the excessive production of both ALA and PBG accumulates and is subsequently excreted. It is possible that during the period of raised circulating concentrations of these compounds, the various abnormal effects may become manifest. In hereditary coproporphyria and variegate porphyria enough free porphyrins will be formed and accumulate (because of the depressed activity of coproporphyrinogen oxidase and protoporphyrinogen oxidase respectively) to allow photosensitization lesions to occur. In each of the non-acute porphyrias uroporphyrinogen I synthase activity is raised. There is no accumulation of porphyrin precursors and the subsequent formation of free porphyrins will cause solar photosensitive lesions in the skin (Fig. 6). This view of control does not exclude the possibility that other means might come into play to alter the characteristics of the pathway such as biological oxidation changes or changes in the concentration of mononucleotides or indeed of partition differences across cellular membranes. The exact relation of these biochemical aberrations to the neuropathological abnormalities and clinical features of the acute porphyrias is still speculative.

Other diseases associated with abnormal porphyrin metabolism

Increased excretion of circulating porphyrins is found in a number of other diseases either because the synthesis of haem is disturbed or because the mechanism of excretion is abnormal. The most important of these are lead poisoning, iron deficiency anaemia, and alcohol ingestion, although there is a heterogenous group of other diseases in which porphyrin metabolism is deranged.

Lead poisoning. It has been known for some time that in patients suffering from lead poisoning, there is accumulation of protoporphyrin in erythrocytes and increased urinary excretion of delta-aminolaevulinic acid and coproporphyrin. This accumulation of porphyrins and precursors is due to the inhibition by lead of several enzymes of haem biosynthesis; ALA dehydratase, coproporphyrinogen oxidase, and ferrochelatase. An increase in the activity of the rate-controlling enzyme ALA synthase results.

Many of the clinical manifestations of lead poisoning may be the result of altered haem biosynthesis. The anaemia of lead poisoning is due in part to the depressant effect of the lead on haem biosynthesis though haemolysis and depression of globin synthesis are also important. The abdominal pain, constipation, and peripheral neuropathy which occur in lead poisoning are also seen in acute attacks of hepatic porphyria. These manifestations can be explained at least in part by circulating concentrations of delta-aminolaevulinic acid, which may be high enough to cause neurological dysfunction. There may also be a contribution from disordered haem biosynthesis in nervous tissue.

Alterations in porphyrin metabolism have provided a useful means of detecting and assessing the severity of lead exposure and poisoning. The diminution in activity of erythrocyte ALA dehydratase and elevated erythrocyte protoporphyrin levels are the most sensitive measures although others, such as raised urinary ALA and coproporphyrin are more frequently used. For screening purposes portable front-surface fluorimeters have been developed for the rapid determination of protoporphyrin mainly as its zinc chelate in an untreated drop of blood.

Iron deficiency anaemia. It has been recognized for some time that in iron deficiency anaemia there is a marked accumulation of protoporphyrin in erythrocytes where insufficient iron is available for incorporation into haem. This rarely reaches the level seen in erythropoietic protoporphyria. There have been a number of conflicting reports regarding alterations of other porphyrins and precursors. The measurement of erythrocyte protoporphyrin is a useful diagnostic procedure in the investigation of anaemia. It may be raised in latent iron deficiency before changes appear in peripheral blood. It is also helpful when serum iron and ferritin levels are misleading after patients have started iron therapy. Protoporphyrin concentration is also different in the small red cells of iron deficiency and those of beta-thalassaemia in which levels are normal.

Alcohol. The association between ethanol ingestion and alterations in porphyrin metabolism was first noted in 1935 when it was found that after drinking one litre of beer or 90 ml of Cognac, a subject generally doubled his urinary coproporphyrin excretion. Chronic alcoholics have an increased urinary excretion of coproporphyrin, mainly isomer III, but normal urinary excretion of uroporphyrin, ALA, and PBG. The ratio of urinary excretion of coproporphyrin isomer I to III varies with drinking habit. More recently ethanol has been noted to cause marked alteration in activity of several of the enzymes of haem biosynthesis. In rats, acute ethanol dosage results in depression of activity of ALA dehydratase and ferrochelatase and increased activity of the rate-controlling enzyme of the pathway, ALA synthase in hepatic tissue: and in humans acute and chronic ethanol ingestion markedly depresses the activity of ALA dehydratase in peripheral blood. Ethanol administration to normal subjects results in increased activity of leucocyte ALA synthase and erythrocyte uroporphyrinogen-I-synthase, the two rate-controlling enzymes of the pathway. The activity of each of the other four enzymes is depressed. Ferrochelatase, the enzyme which inserts iron into protoporphyrin to form haem, shows the most marked depression, and in alcoholism there is prolonged depression of uroporphyrinogen decarboxylase. These ethanol-related alterations in haem biosynthesis may be relevant to ethanol-related sideroblastic anaemia. In this condition, there is accumulation of non-haem iron in the mitochondrion of blood cell precursors and accumulation of protoporphyrin and coproporphyrin in erythrocytes. The alcohol-related and marked depression of ferrochelatase activity may explain both of these findings. Patients with ethanol-related sideroblastic anaemia have been noted to have increased activity of ALA synthase in bone marrow. The depression of ferrochelatase activity may also be relevant to ethanol-related siderosis. The depression of uroporphyrinogen decarboxylase in alcoholism provides a rationale for the importance of ethanol in the aetiology of cutaneous hepatic porphyria.

Other conditions. Abnormalities of haem biosynthesis have been reported in a variety of other haematological conditions including several forms of sideroblastic anaemia, megaloblastic anaemia, the anaemia of chronic renal failure, haemolytic anaemias, sickle cell anaemia, leukaemia, and polycythaemia. In hereditary tyrosinaemia excess urinary ALA is excreted and, like the acute porphyrias and lead poisoning, this disease is associated with neurobehavioural disturbance. In liver disease there may be increased urinary excretion of coproporphyrin predominantly the isomer I type. In the Dubin–Johnson syndrome there is increased urinary excretion of coproporphyrin isomer I and reduced excretion of coproporphyrin isomer III possibly as a result of deficiency of hepatic uroporphyrinogen III cosynthase. In Rotor syndrome urinary excretion of coproporphyrin I is increased with normal coproporphyrin III excretion and in Gilbert's disease there is increased urinary excretion of coproporphyrin I and III isomers. A slight alteration of faecal porphyrin excretion may be seen in patients with malabsorption. Increased urinary excretion of porphyrin-like substances has been found in a varying proportion of psychiatric patients not having porphyria. The association between this biochemical finding and the psychiatric disorder is not known although the monopyrrole, haemopyrrole lactam, is excreted in excess in urine in both acute intermittent porphyria and schizophrenia.

References

Brodie, M. J., Moore, M. R., and Goldberg, A. (1977). Enzyme abnormalities in the porphyrias. *Lancet* **ii**, 699.

De Matteis, F. and Aldridge, W. N. (eds.) (1978). *Heme and hemoproteins.* Springer-Verlag, Berlin.

Doss, M. (1978). *Diagnosis and therapy of porphyrias and lead intoxication.* Springer-Verlag, Berlin.

Goldberg, A. and Moore, M. R. (eds.) (1980). The porphyrias. *Clinics Haemat.* **9**.

— and Rimington, C. (1962). *Diseases of porphyrin metabolism.* Thomas Springfield, Illinois.

McColl, K. E. L., Moore, M. R., and Goldberg, A. (1982). Porphyrin metabolism—The porphyrias. In *Blood and its disorders*, 2nd edn. (eds. R. N. Hardisty and D. J. Weatherall). Blackwell Scientific Publications, Oxford.

—, —, Thompson G. G., and Goldberg, A. (1981). Treatment with haematin in acute hepatic porphyria. *Q. Jl Med.* **50**, 161.

Moore, M. R. (1980). International survey of drugs in acute porphyria. *Int. J. Biochem.* (in press).

—, McColl, K. E. L., and Goldberg, A. (1979). The porphyrias. *Diabetes and Metabolism* **5**, 323.

Pimstone, N. R. (1975). The hepatic aspects of the porphyrias. In *Modern trends in gastroenterology* (ed. A. E. Read). Butterworth, London.

Ridley, A. (1969). The neuropathy of acute intermittent porphyria. *Q. Jl Med.* **38**, 307.

Smith, K. M. (ed.) (1975). *Porphyrins and metalloporphyrins.* Elsevier, Amsterdam.

Inborn errors of amino acid and organic acid metabolism

R. W. E. Watts

Removal of the amino group is an early step in the intermediary metabolism of amino acids after which the metabolic pathways followed by their carbon skeletons are progressively less distinguishable from those of similar molecules derived from other sources. The amino acids can be detected and measured relatively easily in biological fluids, and they are important biochemical markers of inborn errors of metabolism. In some cases a non-amino organic acid provides the biochemical hallmark. Inborn errors of amino acid and organic acid metabolism together account for between one third and one half of all the inborn errors of metabolism. The main biochemical and clinical features of the more important of these disorders are summarized in Table 1.

Table 1 Inborn errors of amino and organic acid metabolism. (The most commonly used and succinct names have been used as far as possible and prefixes indicating quantity have been omitted.)

Disease	Inheritance	Urinary metabolites	Enzyme defect	Comments
β-Alaninaemia (hyper β-alaninaemia)	?	β-alanine, taurine, β-amino-*iso*-butyric acid	β-alanine-pyruvate aminotransferase presumed	somnolence, seizures, hypotonia microcephaly
Alkaptonuria	autosomal recessive	homogentisic acid	homogentisic acid oxidase	urine darkens on exposure to air and stains nappies; connective tissues, especially cartilages become blue-grey or black (ochronosis); premature cartilage degeneration, arthropathy, spondylosis with intervertebral disc calcification in later life
β-Amino-*iso*-butyric aciduria	autosomal recessive	β-amino-*iso*-butyric acid	unknown	harmless trait present in 5–10% of Caucasians but with greater prevalence (up to 95%) in Southeast Asia
Ammonaemia (hyperammonaemia)				suggestive evidence only; blood ammonia measurement gives the definitive diagnosis
Type I	autosomal recessive	glutamine and glycine	carbamoylphosphate synthetase	
Type II	sex-linked dominant	glutamine and orotic acid	ornithine carbamoyltransferase	
Argininaemia (hyperargininaemia)	autosomal recessive	arginine with relatively smaller amounts of cystine, lysine, and ornithine	arginase	spastic diplegia, fits and severe mental handicap in childhood; associated hyperammonaemia, especially postprandially
Argininosuccinic aciduria	autosomal recessive	argininosuccinic acid	argininosuccinate lyase	most cases present with psychomotor delay in later childhood; at least some of the brain damage is thought to be due to intermittent hyperammonaemia; trichorrhexis nodosa is characteristic
Carnosinaemia	?	carnosine	aminoacyl-histidine dipeptidase	psychomotor retardation, epilepsy, myoclonus, spasticity; one clinically normal case (female) reported
Citrullinaemia (hypercitrullinaemia)	autosomal recessive	citrulline, homocitrulline, N-acetylcitrulline, glutamine, orotic acid, and uracil	argininosuccinate synthetase	associated hyperammonaemia, especially postprandially; some cases run a subacute course, others are atypical in that they have only minor neurological abnormalities

Table 1 cont.

Disease	Inheritance	Urinary metabolites	Enzyme defect	Comments
Cystathioninuria	autosomal recessive	cystathionine	cystathionine γ-lyase	some cases associated with mental handicap
Cystinuria	autosomal recessive and incompletely recessive pedigrees	cystine, lysine, ornithine, arginine homocysteine–cysteine, homoarginine	defective common transport mechanism	only individuals who are homozygous for a trait causing classical cystinuria excrete all of the abnormal amino acids; heterozygotes for incompletely recessive cystinuria excrete abnormally large amounts of cystine and lysine
Fanconi syndrome	—	generalized amino aciduria	renal tubule transport defect	a complication of both inherited and acquired renal tubule damage
Glutathionaemia	autosomal recessive	glutathione	γ-glutamyltranspeptidase	associated with mental handicap
Glycinaemia (hyperglycinaemia: non-ketotic)	autosomal recessive	glycine	serine hydroxymethyl-transferase	psychomotor retardation; mental handicap; some die in neonatal period
Hartnup disease	autosomal recessive	indole-3-acetic acid, indole-3-lactic acid indole-3-acetylglutamine neutral monoamino monocarboxylic acids except glycine and the iminoacids indican	neutral amino acid transport system	intermittent psychiatric and neurological symptoms; pellagra-like rash; some patients are mentally handicapped
Histidinaemia	autosomal recessive	imidazole pyruvic, imidazole acetic, and imidazole lactic acids	histidine ammonialyase	the previously suggested causal relationship between specific speech defect and/or mental handicap has not been confirmed in prospectively studied cases
Homocystinuria				
Type I	autosomal recessive	homocystine	cystathionine β-synthase	mental handicap inconstant Marfan-like syndrome and thrombotic tendency in some cases
Type II	autosomal recessive	homocystine	5,10-methylenetetra-hydrofolate reductase	mental handicap inconstant
Hydroxyprolinaemia	autosomal recessive	hydroxyproline	hydroxyproline oxidase	mental handicap inconstant
Iminoglycinuria	autosomal recessive	proline, hydroxyproline, glycine	iminoacid-glycine transport system	no clinical significance; genetic heterogeneity; the obligate heterozygotes have isolated hyperglycinuria in some pedigrees only
Isovaleric acidaemia	autosomal recessive	iso-valeric and 3-hydroxy-iso-valeric acids and iso-valerylglycine	iso-valeryl-CoA dehydrogenase (not proven)	older patients show psychomotor delay; leucopenia, anaemia, and thrombocytopenia with the acute acidotic episodes; smell of sweaty feet
Lysinaemia (hyperlysinaemia)				
Type I	autosomal recessive	lysine	L-lysine: NAD+ oxidoreductase (not proven)	periodic hyperlysinaemia with hyperammonaemia; neonatal vomiting, fits, intermittent coma
Type II	autosomal recessive	lysine	lysine: 2-oxoglutarate (NADPH) oxidoreductase	persistent hyperlysinaemia without hyperammonaemia; no data on clinical presentation in infancy; mental handicap in some cases
Type III	autosomal recessive	lysine, citrulline, saccharopine, homocitrulline, and 2-amino adipic acids	aminoadipic semialdehyde reductase	psychomotor retardation
Maple syrup urine disease (branched chain keto-aciduria)	autosomal recessive	leucine, iso-leucine, valine, 2-oxo-iso-caproic 2-oxo-3-methylvaleric and 2-oxo-iso-valeric acids, and hydroxyacid derivatives	branched chain keto acid decarboxylase	neonatal acidosis, fits, failure to thrive; psychomotor retardation; milder intermittent forms of later onset known
β-Mercaptolactate-cysteine disulphiduria	?	β-mercaptolactatecysteine	?	no specific clinical phenotype; originally described in association with severe mental handicap

Table 1 cont.

Disease	Inheritance	Urinary metabolites	Enzyme defect	Comments
β-Methylcrotonyl-glycinuria	autosomal recessive	3-methylcrotonic and 3-hydroxy*iso*valeric acids and 3-methylcrotonylglycine	3-methylcrotonyl-CoA carboxylase	biotin responsive and non-responsive types; Gompertz *et al.* (1973) reported a case with tiglylglycinuria (1,2-methylacroylglycinuria); this is now considered to have been an example of the holocarboxylase-synthetase deficiency which produces an organic aciduria with the features of both β-methylcrotonyl-glycinuria and propionic acidaemia
Methylmalonic acidaemia*				
Type I	autosomal recessive	methylmalonic, methylcitric, propionic, and 3-hydroxypropionic acids	methylmalonyl CoA mutase	death from neonatal acidosis; survivors physically and mentally handicapped; leucopenia, thrombocytopenia, osteoporosis
Type II	autosomal recessive	methylmalonic acid, homocystine, cystathionine	failure of cellular cobalamin accumulation and/or retention with secondary failure of both methylcobalamin and 5'-adenosylcobalamin production	mental handicap in surviving cases; often associated with megaloblastic anaemia
Type III	autosomal recessive	methylmalonic, methylcitric and 3-hydroxypropionic acids	primary failure of 5'-adenosylcobalamin synthesis	death from neonatal acidosis; survivors physically and mentally handicapped
Type IV	autosomal recessive	methylmalonic acid	methylmalonyl CoA racemase	the true existence of this type is uncertain
Oast house urine disease (methionine malabsorption syndrome)	autosomal recessive	methionine, 2-hydroxybutyric, phenylpyruvic, and branched chain ketoacids especially 2-oxo-*iso*-valeric	methionine malabsorption (amino acid transport defect)	diarrhoea, seizures, psychomotor retardation, oast house smell
Ornithinaemia (hyperornithinaemia)				
Type I	autosomal recessive	homocitrulline	ornithine decarboxylase	protein intolerance, vomiting; seizures, lethargy, psychomotor retardation
Type II	autosomal recessive	generalized amino aciduria	ornithine-oxoacid aminotransferase	impaired hepatic and renal tubular function; psychomotor retardation
Type III	autosomal recessive	ornithine	—	gyrate atrophy of choroid and retina, mentally normal
5-Oxoprolinuria	autosomal recessive	5-oxoproline	glutathione synthetase (generalized)	neonatal acidosis; mental handicap in some cases
Phenylalaninaemia				
Type I (phenylketonuria)	autosomal recessive	phenylpyruvic, phenyllactic, phenylacetic, and 2-hydroxyphenylacetic acids; phenylacetylglutamine, phenylalanine	phenylalanine-4-hydroxylase	severe psychomotor retardation, variant forms with less or no brain damage also occur; dietary phenylalanine restriction prevents brain damage; a benign transient neonatal hyperphenylalaninaemia exists and is attributed to delayed enzyme maturation
Type II	autosomal recessive	phenylalanine	dihydrobiopterin reductase	severe psychomotor retardation which is not prevented by dietary phenylalanine restriction
Type III	autosomal recessive	phenylalanine	dihydrobiopterin synthetase	severe psychomotor retardation which is not prevented by dietary phenylalanine restriction
Prolinaemia (hyperprolinaemia)				
Type I	autosomal recessive	proline hydroxyproline glycine	pyrolline-5-carboxylate reductase (proline oxidase)	no specific clinical phenotype; originally described in association with congenital renal disease
Type II	autosomal recessive	proline hydroxyproline glycine	1-pyrolline-5-carboxylate dehydrogenase	no specific clinical phenotype; originally described in association with mental handicap
Propionic acidaemia (ketotic hyperglycinaemia)	autosomal recessive	propionic, 3-hydroxypropionic, methylcitric, 3-hydroxy-*n*-valeric acids and glycine	propionyl-CoA carboxylase (ATP-hydrolysing)	episodes of acidosis and leucopenia; death in infancy or survival with psychomotor retardation; biotin responsive and non-responsive types

* Types I and IV refer to methylmalonic aciduria produced by mutations which alter the structure of the individual apoenzymes. Type III methylmalonic aciduria includes metabolic lesions affecting the reduction of cobalamin, its combination with adenosine, and the linking of adenosyl cobalamin to the apoenzyme

Table 1 cont.

Disease	Inheritance	Urinary metabolites	Enzyme defect	Comments
Sarcosinaemia (hypersarcosinaemia)	autosomal recessive	sarcosine	sarcosine dehydrogenase	no consistent clinical abnormality; originally described in association with mental handicap
Sulphite oxidase deficiency				
Type I (simple sulphite oxidase deficiency)	?	S-sulpho-L-cysteine, sulphite, thiosulphate	sulphite oxidase	psychomotor delay and retrogression; dislocated lenses
Type II	?	S-sulpho-L-cysteine, sulphite, thiosulphate, hypoxanthine, xanthine	sulphite oxidase and xanthine oxidase	increased hypoxanthine and xanthine levels in blood and urine, hypouricaemia, hypouric aciduria; the postulated fundamental abnormality is a disorder of molybdenum metabolism or transport
Tyrosinaemia				
Type I (hepatorenal type)	autosomal recessive	4-hydroxyphenyllactic, 4-hydroxyphenylpyruvic, and 4-hydroxyphenylacetic acids; generalized amino aciduria with prominent tyrosine, methionine δ-aminolaevulinic acid	4-hydroxyphenylpyruvate dioxygenase (not proven); fumarylacetoacetase deficiency suggested in some patients	acute or chronic course; renal tubule reabsorption defects and nodular cirrhosis; raised plasma tyrosine and methionine
Type II (oculo-cutaneous tyrosinosis)	autosomal recessive	tyrosine, 4-hydroxyphenyllactate, 4-hydroxyphenylpyruvate, 4-hydroxyphenylacetate N-acetyl tyrosine	tyrosine aminotransferase (cytosol isoenzyme only)	psychomotor retardation; microcephaly; ocular and skin lesions; no renal or hepatic damage
Tyrosyluria	—	4-hydroxyphenylpyruvic, 4-hydroxyphenyllactic, and 4-hydroxyphenylacetic acids	delayed maturation of 4-hydroxyphenylpyruvate dioxygenase	a harmless anomaly responsive to ascorbic acid; occurs transiently in the neonatal period, especially in premature infants
Valinaemia (hypervalinaemia)	autosomal recessive	valine	valine-isoleucine aminotransferase	failure to thrive and psychomotor retardation

Disorders of aromatic amino acid metabolism

The hyperphenylalaninaemias

Biochemistry. The hydroxylation of phenylalanine to form tyrosine is an oxidative process linked to the simultaneous oxidation of tetrahydrobiopterin (Fig. 1).

Infants are normally screened for hyperphenylalaninaemia when they are six days old, and on a full protein diet for their age. The plasma phenylalanine concentration is normally less than 0.12 mmol/l (2 mg/dl) at this age. Screening tests which depend on detecting an abnormal urinary excretion of aromatic acidic metabolites (e.g. Phenistix) are unreliable for this purpose.

Metabolic lesions affecting either phenylalanine mono-oxygenase or the production of the tetrahydrobiopterin cofactor produce hyperphenylalaninaemia. The latter may be either reduced activity of dihydropteridine reductase or of dihydrobiopterin synthetase (Fig. 1). Classical phenylketonuria is due to a complete phenylalanine mono-oxygenase deficiency, incomplete deficiencies causing less severe clinical manifestations which fall into two groups, namely atypical (variant) phenylketonuria and essential hyperphenylalaninaemia. As judged clinically and by the usual biochemical criteria (plasma phenylalanine levels and the abnormal excretion of phenylalanine metabolites) these three disorders form a continuum and they cannot be absolutely delineated from one another without recourse to direct measurement of the residual enzyme activity in liver tissue. This is rarely undertaken and they are normally defined on the basis of fasting blood phenylalanine concentrations, the plasma phenylalanine response to oral phenylalanine loading, the aromatic amino acid excretion pattern, and the clinical course of untreated members in a sibship. Delayed matura-

tion of phenylalanine mono-oxygenase causes transient neonatal hyperphenylalaninaemia. This is seen most frequently in premature infants.

The patients with dihydropteridine reductase and dihydrobiopterin synthetase defects account for about 3 per cent of all apparent phenylketonuric patients, and they are sometimes described as having malignant phenylketonuria because there is progressive neurological degeneration in spite of good dietary control of the plasma phenylalanine concentration. Tetrahydrobiopterin is a cofactor for 5-hydroxytryptamine, dopamine, and noradrenaline synthesis, and this may account for the poor results of dietary phenylalanine restriction. Tetrahydrobiopterin may be of use therapeutically in these cases. Precise diagnosis of the defects in tetrahydrobiopterin production require enzymological studies on liver tissue, although measurement of blood and urine neurotransmitter substances and pterins may give some diagnostic help.

Clinical aspects. Patients with all of the hyperphenylalaninaemia syndromes appear superficially normal at birth, and unless they are detected by routine screening, usually present with psychomotor delay in early childhood. There is some evidence suggesting that as a group they have slightly (about 0.5 kg) lower birth weights than normal children in the same population and have a higher than normal incidence of prematurity and perinatal difficulties. The incidence of positive Guthrie screening tests for hyperphenylalaninaemia is between 1:6000 and 1:12 000 in Great Britain and Ireland. It is highest in the groups with strong Celtic genetic admixture and about half of the positive reactors require long-term treatment for phenylketonuria.

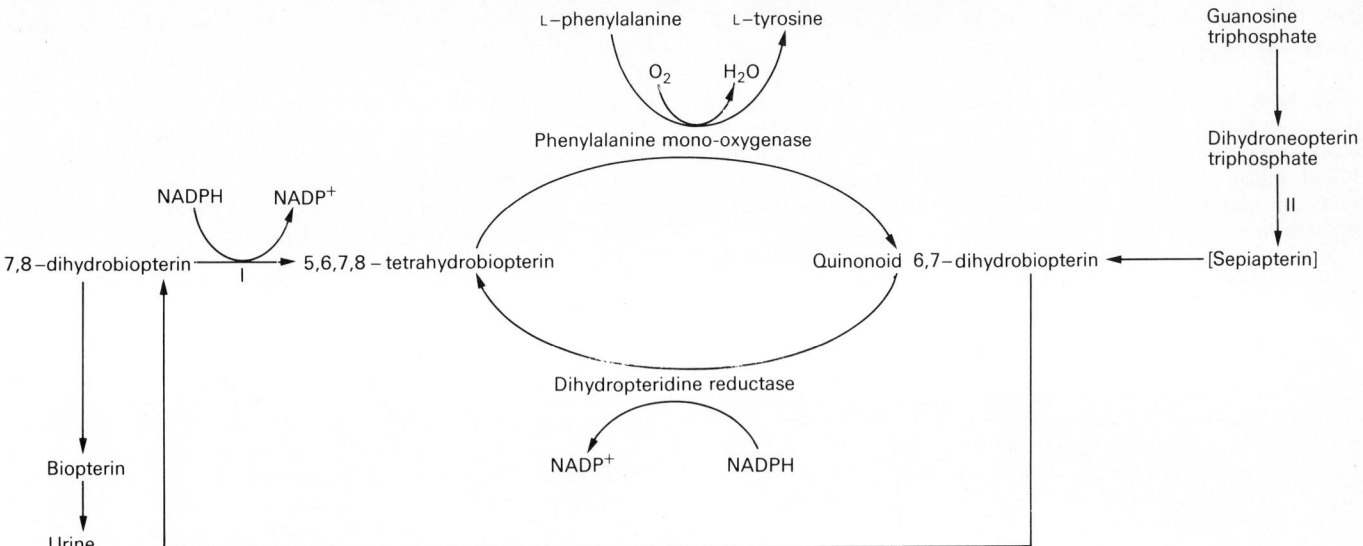

Fig. 1 The phenylalanine hydroxylase system.
I = tetrahydrofolate dehydrogenase (dihydrofolate reductase) catalyses the reduction of (7,8)-dihydrobiopterin to (5,6,7,8,)-tetrahydrobiopterin.
II = Dihydrobiopterin synthetase.
The conversion of quinonoid (6,7)-dihydrobiopterin to (7,8)-dihydrobiopterin is non-enzymatic.

Cases of classical phenylketonuria have hyperphenylalaninuria and excrete abnormal phenylalanine metabolites (Table 1) in their urine, and have plasma phenylalanine concentrations above 1.2 mmol/l (20 mg/dl). Their phenylalanine tolerance varies with age and may only be sufficient to meet their estimated minimum requirement of 70–90 mg/kg bodyweight at one month although the situation may be somewhat easier by age two years when the estimated minimum requirement of phenylalanine has decreased to about 35 mg/kg.

The term atypical phenylketonuria embraces patients with plasma phenylalanine concentrations in the range 0.61–1.21 mmol/l (10–20 mg/dl), who excrete abnormal phenylalanine metabolites and phenylalanine. There is some disagreement as to the extent to which these patients are at risk from mental handicap and therefore of the need to institute treatment. The risk does not parallel the plasma phenylalanine concentration exactly, but it is generally accepted that infants in whom this exceeds 0.85 mmol/l (14 mg/dl) should be treated although some authorities now recommend treatment at a lower level, e.g. 0.61 mmol/l (10 mg/dl).

Patients with plasma phenylalanine concentrations consistently in the range 0.12–0.61 mmol/l (2–10 mg/dl) are described as having persistent (essential) hyperphenylalaninaemia; they excrete no phenylalanine metabolites and do not appear to be at risk for the development of mental handicap. They can tolerate a normal diet without their plasma phenylalanine concentration moving into the atypical phenylketonuria range.

The degree of mental impairment is variable although it is usually profound in the untreated classical cases, with Intelligence Quotients (IQ) varying from immeasurably low values to about 50. Adult untreated phenylketonurics are occasionally encountered with IQ values of 70–80, living in the general population, and it is in this group that cases of severe oligophrenia and other developmental defects (e.g. cardiac and ocular) in children, who are not themselves homozygotes for classical phenylketonuria, arise due to the effect of untreated material phenylketonuria on the developing fetal brain. This also occurs in women who were successfully treated in childhood and who are taking a normal diet when they conceive. The damaged fetus is referred to as having the 'maternal phenylketonuria (PKU) syndrome'.

Apart from oligophrenia, patients with classical phenylketonuria show dilution of skin, hair and iris pigmentation, microcephaly, seizures in about 50 per cent, and cerebral dysrhythmia on electroencephalography in about 90 per cent. They tend to be hyper-

kinetic and have irascible personalities. Tendon reflexes are generally increased and they may have eczematous skin eruptions particularly on the exposed surfaces. The excreted aromatic acids have a mousy or musty odour.

Heterozygous phenylketonuria carriers are asymptomatic. Some show reduced phenylalanine tolerance on acute loading with the amino acid. Minor reductions in verbal IQ have also been reported.

Treatment. Treatment aims to keep the plasma level of phenylalanine in the range 0.18 to 0.49 mmol/l (3–8 mg/dl) by means of a diet of reduced phenylalanine content. The plasma phenylalanine is monitored twice weekly while treatment is being initiated, weekly in infants, every two or three weeks in toddlers, and monthly thereafter until it is discontinued. The diet is based on a synthetic substitute for most of the dietary protein and its continued use until the child has passed the period when brain damage is most likely to occur can put a great strain on the family; skilled social as well as medical and dietetic support is necessary. The diet must include sufficient calories, essential amino acids, vitamins, and trace elements. Overtreatment causing phenylalanine deficiency leads to mental impairment, eczematous rashes, hair loss, failure to thrive and gain weight, hypoproteinaemia, diarrhoea, and increased susceptibility to intercurrent infections. The degree of phenylalanine intolerance may change as the child grows older, and it may be necessary to challenge the patient with a test dose of phenylalanine (100 mg/kg bodyweight) and observe the time course of the change in the blood phenylalanine concentration several times during childhood.

It is customary to relax the diet when the child is about eight years old, the perinatal and subsequent burst of brain myelination being complete by age about five years. In the present state of knowledge the intake of first-class protein should be restricted sufficiently to keep the plasma phenylalanine concentration at least below about 1.82 mmol/l (30 mg/dl) after the main dietary restriction has been lifted, because of the behaviour problems and seizures which are sometimes associated with hyperphenylalaninaemia even in the treated patient, and the possibility of some effect on the later stages of brain development. There is increasing evidence that a completely free diet after the main period of treatment is associated with a failure to develop full IQ potential. Some authorities recommend that phenylketonuric women should remain on a phenylalanine restricted diet until they are past the childbearing years. They should certainly resume the diet before conception in order to protect the fetus.

Prognosis. Conscientious and well controlled treatment beginning in the first weeks of life gives development with IQ values in the normal range. However, in some cases these are a little less than those predicted from the intelligence of the unaffected members of the family. Poor control with episodes of hyper- or hypophenylalaninaemia worsens the prognosis.

Successfully treated children with atypical (variant) phenylketonuria have IQ values consistent with those of the unaffected family members, but untreated children with atypical phenylketonuria have lower IQ values.

Inborn errors in tyrosine metabolism. Tyrosine is either derived from the diet or from the hydroxylation of phenylalanine, and its metabolism follows the sequence shown in Fig. 2.

Four disorders have been claimed to involve the steps between tyrosine and homogentisic acid: tyrosinosis, tyrosinaemia types I and II, and tyrosyluria.

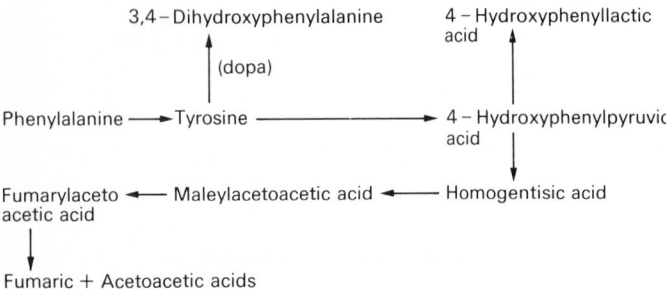

Fig. 2   The metabolism of tyrosine.

Tyrosinosis. The description of tyrosinosis dates from a single case report. The patient was a 49-year-old man with coincidental myasthenia gravis who excreted large amounts of 4-hydroxyphenylacetic acid in the urine. This continued during fasting, and was increased by dietary tyrosine supplements, which also led to the excretion of 4-hydroxyphenyl-lactic acid and 2,4-dihydroxyphenylalanine (dopa). A metabolic block between 4-hydroxyphenylpyruvic acid and homogentisic acid was suggested. However, this suggestion could not be proved at the time and the patient had none of the features observed in the more recently reported cases of Type I tyrosinaemia (hepatorenal tyrosinaemia) in which the same metabolic lesion has been proposed (Table 1). The term tyrosinosis should be reserved to describe this still unique case until further examples are encountered and studied by modern methods.

Tyrosinaemia: Type I
Clinical aspects. The main biochemical and clinical features of this disorder are summarized in Table 1. A single metabolic lesion to explain all the findings has not yet been identified, and it has been argued that Type I tyrosinaemia is not in fact primarily a disorder of tyrosine metabolism. Some cases have been reported in association with perinatal cytomegalovirus infection and neonatal hepatitis, but it is uncertain if they are the cause. There is considerable geographical variation in incidence, and a particularly high incidence has been reported in some genetic isolates in French Canada. This supports the view that in at least some cases the disease is inherited, and that it may follow either an acute or chronic course in different members of the same family.

Patients with the acute variant present with failure to thrive during the first six months of life, and 90 per cent die from liver failure before they are a year old. Chronic active hepatitis with fatty infiltration and cirrhosis with some evidence of lobular regeneration and hepatomas have been recorded. The patients have hepatosplenomegaly, a haemolytic tendency, oedema, and sometimes develop a cabbage-like odour due to the excretion of abnormal

methionine metabolites. Damage to the renal tubules causes the Fanconi syndrome to develop and hypophosphataemic rickets is a prominent feature. There is also hyperplasia of the islets of Langerhans with hypoglycaemia. Cases with the chronic phenotype (Baber's syndrome) present with similar but more slowly evolving manifestations in later childhood. The main differential diagnoses are Type II tyrosinaemia, and tyrosyluria. However, hereditary fructose intolerance and galactosaemia can both cause combined hepatic cirrhosis and renal tubule damage.

Treatment. Restriction of dietary tyrosine, phenylalanine, and methionine, with careful control of the plasma amino acid concentrations to ensure that normal levels are being maintained, correction of hypoglycaemia and electrolyte imbalance, and sufficiently large doses of vitamin D (for example 10 000–50 000 units per day) or 1α-hydroxycholecalciferol (1–2 μg daily) to heal the rickets.

Prognosis. Although treatment corrects the abnormal biochemical findings, most cases die in infancy or early childhood. The hepatic cirrhosis becomes self-perpetuating and leads to death from liver failure. It is not known if treatment from birth can lead to completely normal growth and development.

Tyrosinaemia: Type II. The main biochemical and clinical features of these patients are presented in Table 1. The excretion of the metabolites derived from the activity of enzymes distal to the metabolic block has been explained by the action of mitochondrial tyrosine transaminase and the lack of 4-hydroxyphenylpyruvic acid oxidase in that location. Drastic restriction of tyrosine intake reduces the excretion of aromatic amino acid metabolites to normal, but the possible benefit of dietary treatment of presymptomatic cases has not been assessed.

Tyrosyluria. Neonatal tyrosyluria (Table 1) occurs in about 30 per cent of premature infants and 10 per cent of full term infants. It is believed to be associated with delayed enzyme maturation. Males are more often affected than females. The highest levels of hypertyrosinaemia occur towards the end of the first week of life and persist for several weeks. Neonatal tyrosyluria is abolished by administering ascorbic acid (50–100 mg per day), and this distinguishes it from the tyrosinaemias.

Albinism
Biochemistry. Melanocytes are specialized cells which synthesize melanin in cytoplasmic vesicles called melanosomes. These vesicles contain tyrosinase which catalyses the oxidation of tyrosine to 3,4-dihydroxyphenylalanine (dopa) and then to the corresponding quinone. The later stages of melanin formation occur nonenzymatically in the melanosomes and specifically require zinc ions.

The term albinism covers a group of diseases due to mutations of the gene directing the synthesis of tyrosinase.

Oculocutaneous albinism. Oculocutaneous albinism is the classical form of the disease. It exists in two forms, tyrosinase negative and tyrosinase positive, which are due to non-allelic mutations, and are distinguished by testing the patient's hair bulbs for tyrosinase. Both forms are autosomal recessives so that individuals who are heterozygous for both of the abnormal genes (double heterozygotes) will be normally pigmented, and this explains the observation that two albino parents do not necessarily have albino children.

The tyrosinase negative patients have snow white hair, pink-white photo-sensitive skin, grey or grey blue irides, and a prominent red reflex from the unpigmented fundus oculi. Nystagmus, photophobia, and loss of visual acuity are severe, and 90 per cent of the patients also have a strabismus. There are no brown pigmented naevi and accumulations of naevus cells produce small red or purple spots on the skin. Prolonged exposure to sunlight may produce a yellow tinge in the hair tips due to a change in the keratin configuration.

Tyrosinase positive albinism is a less severe phenotype. The affected infants are indistinguishable from those with the tyrosinase negative variant at birth but they develop some light pigmentation of the hair, skin, and eyes later. The ocular complications, although present are usually less severe than in the tyrosinase negative type. Tyrosinase positive albinism is also a feature of the Chediak–Higashi syndrome (oculocutaneous albinism, reduced resistance to infection and hepatosplenomegaly) and the Hermansky–Pudlak syndrome (oculocutaneous albinism and haemorrhagic diathesis with abnormal platelets and ceroid-like pigment in reticulo-endothelial cells).

'Yellow mutant oculocutaneous albinism' is due to a separate mutation which produces a phenotype resembling tyrosinase positive oculocutaneous albinism, except that the hair bulb test for tyrosinase gives an equivocal or negative result, and a yellow pigment develops if cysteine is added to the incubation medium. The metabolic lesion is thought to be a failure of the final polymerization step in melanin-formation.

Ocular albinism. In the usual X-linked type, the affected male hemizygotes have depigmented fundi, translucent irides, and nystagmus, and the female heterozygous carriers have patchy depigmentation of the fundi with partial pigmentation of the iris. There have been claims for autosomal recessive ocular albinism and for X-linked pedigrees with no expression in the females (the Åland variant).

Cutaneous albinism. This type shows patchy failure of pigmentation involving the skin and hair, and is inherited in an autosomal dominant manner. The white forelock is a common finding and the skin may show various degrees of a piebald appearance. The eyes are not involved.

Abnormalities of the optic neuronal pathways in albinism. Albinos, both animal and human, have anatomically abnormal visual pathways in that all the nerve fibres from the lateral half of the retina decussate in the optic chiasma, and there are associated anatomical and histological abnormalities in the lateral geniculate nuclei. Grossly, the lateral geniculate bodies are buried in the adjacent brain tissue and microscopically the nuclei lack their normal organization into six layers of cells. These abnormalities deprive albinos of binocular vision although they have normal visual fields. They are found in association with all of the genetic defects which cause hypopigmentation of the fundus oculi.

Treatment of albinism. The major problems encountered by albino patients are their sensitivity to sunlight with an increased susceptibility to skin cancers, and their poor visual acuity. They should avoid direct sunlight wherever possible and apply sun screen preparations (e.g. 5 per cent para aminobenzoic acid) to exposed areas of skin. The skin of older patients should be inspected annually for pre-malignant or malignant lesions. The use of tinted spectacles may be helpful in reducing photophobia. Operations for strabismus are appropriate for cosmetic reasons but because of abnormalities in the visual pathways binocular vision will not improve. Near vision is substantially better than far vision in most cases.

Patients with Hermanski–Pudlak syndrome should avoid aspirin and related drugs because of their platelet abnormalities, and platelet transfusions may be necessary to arrest massive haemorrhage.

Alkaptonuria
Biochemistry and pathology. Alkaptonuria is due to deficiency of homogentisic acid oxidase which catalyses the oxidation of homogentisic acid to maleylacetoacetic acid. Homogentisic acid slowly polymerizes *in vivo*. The brown-black product is deposited most intensively in cartilages and the fibrous tissues of tendons and ligaments. These structures are stained black at post mortem in long-standing cases. The endocardium and tunica interna of the main blood vessels and the epidermis are also involved. The pigment is both inter- and intracellular. The urine darkens on exposure to air, but this process may occur so slowly at acid pH values and in the presence of normal urinary vitamin C levels that the phenomenon may not be noticed until it is specifically sought for, the patient having presented with other clinical manifestations. Homogentisic acid reduces the alkaline copper reagents (e.g. Clinitest) which are used to detect glycosuria, producing an orange precipitate in a muddy brown supernatant. It also reduces photographic emulsions and produces a purple-black reaction with aqueous ferric chloride solution.

Clinical aspects. The patients may present in early life because of dark urine and brown staining of the urine soiled underclothes. Other cases remain undetected until revealed by either a false positive test for glycosuria or by the development of ochronotic arthritis. The confusion of homogentisic aciduria with glycosuria does not arise with the glucose oxidase based tests for glycosuria (e.g. Clinistix). The term ochronosis refers to the fact that the pigment appears blue-black or grey grossly but ochre microscopically.

The pigmentation of the affected subcutaneous structures such as the aural and nasal cartilages and the subcutaneous tendons is visible through the skin. The cartilages feel abnormally stiff. The sclerae develop brown pigmentation beginning at the points of attachment of the medial and lateral rectus tendons. Pigmented perspiration stains the patients' clothes and the skin of the axillae and genital regions. Ochronotic arthritis is a degenerative arthritis associated with ochronitic pigmentation of, and damage to, cartilages. It affects mainly the large joints and can be severe and incapacitating. The intervertebral joints degenerate, and the intervertebral discs are characteristically densely calcified. The suggestion that alkaptonuria predisposed to heart valve calcification and to myocardial infarction is unproven. An acquired form of ochronosis was formerly encountered in patients in whom phenol dressings were applied to chronic cutaneous ulcers.

Alkaptonuria is inherited as an autosomal recessive. The heterozygous carriers cannot be identified on either clinical or biochemical grounds.

There is no curative or prophylactic treatment for alkaptonuric arthritis.

Inborn errors of thyroid hormone synthesis. Each stage in the process of thyroid hormone biosynthesis and release can be the site of an inherited metabolic lesion. A series of inherited abnormalities of thyroid gland regulation are known and end-organ resistance to the action of thyroid hormone has also been described. The metabolic blocks in thyroid hormone synthesis produce hereditary goitres and hypothyroidism, although the latter may be compensated to a variable degree. Table 2 summarizes the inherited disorders of the thyroid gland. The regulation of thyroid function and the pathophysiology of the gland are dealt with in detail in Section 10.

Urea cycle disorders

General aspects. The urea cycle (Fig. 3) is the biochemical mechanism whereby α-amino nitrogen derived from the deamination or transamination of the amino acids is converted to urea. An inborn error of metabolism is associated with a metabolic block at each stage of the cycle. The individual diseases with their specific enzyme deficiency, inheritance, and main biochemical and clinical features are included in Table 1.

The normal venous blood ammonia concentration in neonates is about twice the adult value of 10–50 mmol/l (17–85 mg/dl); arterial samples are about 20 per cent lower than venous samples. All of the urea cycle disorders have some degree of hyperammonaemia, but

Table 2 Inherited disorders of thyroid function

Thyroid hormone synthesis (congenital hypothyroidism with goitre, data compatible with autosomal recessive inheritance in each case)
1 Iodide transport failure (gland cannot concentrate iodide)
2 Failure to iodinate tyrosyl residues (peroxidase deficiency)
   (a) without nerve deafness
   (b) with nerve deafness (Pendred's syndrome)
3 Oxidative coupling defect
4 De-iodinase defect (loss of iodine from the gland as MIT and DIT)
5 Reduced thyroglobulin synthesis

Thyroid gland regulation
1 Familial pituitary hypothyroidism
   (a) Isolated deficiency of thyroid stimulating hormone (autosomal recessive)
   (b) Familial panhypopituitrism (autosomal recessive and sex-linked variants)
   (c) Familial pituitary agenesis
   (d) Familial absence of sella turcica
2 Impaired response to thyrotropic hormone

Thyroid hormone transport (data compatible with sex-linked inheritance in each case)
1 Familial lack of thyroid hormone binding globulin (TBG) with complete deficiency in the affected males and half normal TBG levels in the female carriers
2 Familial partial deficiency of TBG with residual TBG in the affected males and higher sub-normal levels in carrier females
3 Familial increase TBG concentration

Target organ resistance to thyroid hormones

---

this is most severe in carbamoylphosphate synthetase (CPS) deficiency and ornithine carbamoyltransferase (OCT) deficiency. Apart from its occurrence in patients with hepatic failure due to both acquired and congenital causes, hyperammonaemia is associated with some inborn errors of metabolism, which are not primarily related to the urea cycle. These include the hyperornithinaemias, some of the hyperlysinaemic syndromes and some of the non amino organic acidurias of which methylmalonic, propionic, and *iso*valeric acidurias are the best known.

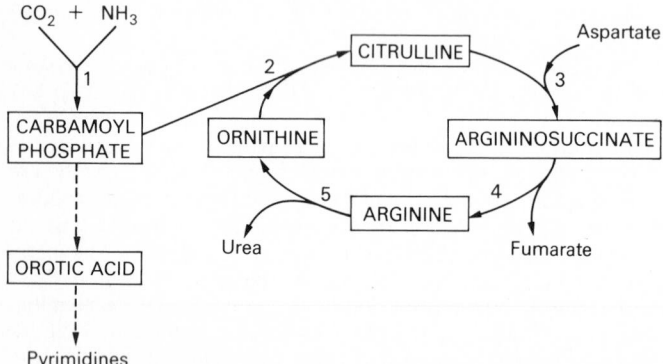

Fig. 3 The urea cycle. The enzymes are as follows: (1) carbamoyl phosphate synthetase; (2) ornithine carbamoyltransferase; (3) argininosuccinate synthetase; (4) argininosuccinate lyase; and (5) arginase.

The urea cycle disorders have the following common features: (*a*) vomiting in infancy and dislike of protein foods in later life; (*b*) episodes of ataxia, disordered behaviour, irritability, confusion, ketoacidoses, seizures, lethargy, and coma; and (*c*) mental handicap. Presentation with life-threatening symptoms during the first day of life has been recorded in all of this group of disorders exept for arginase deficiency which has not so far been recognized before about 18 months of age.

Most patients with urea cycle disorders have normal blood urea levels and exrete urea in their urine. It is generally thought that this is due to the metabolic lesion being incomplete, and that a total absence of one of the urea cycle enzymes would be incompatible

with life. The urea cycle enzymes are all expressed in leucocytes as well as in liver tissue.

Hyperammonaemia is the common pathophysiological basis for the brain damage in the urea cycle disorders. Dietary protein restriction beginning immediately after birth should therefore be the basis of their treatment. The protein requirement is highest during the first months of life and a balance has to be struck between providing sufficient protein for growth (at least 1.0–1.5 g/kg body weight/day in infancy) and control of hyperammonaemia. The diet must also supply sufficient essential amino acids, vitamins, trace elements, and energy. Arginine supplements may be needed because of reduced synthesis of this amino acid via the urea cycle. A short period of protein-free feeding may be necessary while the diagnosis is being established. Protein is then introduced at a level of 0.5 g/kg body weight and subsequently increased. Peritoneal dialysis and exchange blood transfusion may be needed in order to gain time for the diagnosis to be made, and for the institution of treatment when severe brain damage *may* be preventable. These measures are also appropriate if a deterioration has been precipitated by hypercatabolism due to an intercurrent illness. The possibility of replacing essential dietary amino acids by their α-keto analogues in order to further reduce the need for urea cycle activity in situations where dietary protein restriction does not control the hyperammonaemia, and as an adjunct to peritoneal dialysis in the severely ill patient, has been recommended.

The neuropathological findings, which roughly parallel the clinical severity, are similar in all of the urea cycle disorders and are ascribed to chronic ammonia intoxication. They comprise: loss of cortical neurones, demyelination, abnormal astrocytoses, and ventricular dilatation.

Carbamoyl phosphate synthetase (CPS) deficiency. Hyperammonaemia Type I. These patients present with severe symptoms of hyperammonaemia and usually die. If they survive, there is extensive brain damage with mental handicap and focal neurological signs. The pattern of inheritance appears to be autosomal recessive. The urinary excretion of orotic acid is normal or low; this is in contradistinction to the findings in ornithine carbamoyl transferase (OCT) deficiency (Fig. 3). The definitive enzymological diagnosis is made on liver tissue or leucocytes. Prenatal diagnosis and carrier state diagnosis have not yet been reported.

Ornithine carbamoyltransferase (OCT) deficiency. Hyperammonaemia Type II. Ornithine carbamoyltransferase deficiency is inherited in a sex-linked dominant manner. The hemizygous males are more severely affected than the female heterozygous carriers in whom random chromosome inactivation leaves more overall residual activity. Two populations of cells, one lacking OCT activity and the other with normal OCT activity have been demonstrated histochemically in the liver of an obligate heterozygous female carrier. The affected boys, although normal at birth, present with milk intolerance and manifestations of gross hyperammonaemia during the first day or two of life and usually die within a few days. Occasional males survive into early childhood with severe brain damage. The clinical manifestations in the females vary from dislike of protein foods to recurrent episodes of hyperammonaemia with death in childhood and some are mentally handicapped. The symptoms are aggravated by pregnancy, intercurrent illness, and surgical procedures. Some cases of migraine and cyclic vomiting have proved to be carriers of the abnormal gene for OCT deficiency.

Measurement of the blood ammonia level establishes the diagnosis and the orotic aciduria may be a useful diagnostic pointer. Liver tissue, leucocytes and jejunal mucosa can all be used for diagnostic enzymology.

The blood ammonia level in the carrier rises 60–90 minutes after a protein meal and this response is not seen in normal subjects. Orotic aciduria has also been reported after protein loading in the carriers. Prenatal diagnosis is not currently possible. Patients with OTC deficiency have to be distinguished from cases in whom the activity of both CPS and OTC are secondarily depressed by exogenous factors as in Reye's syndrome.

Citrullinaemia (argininosuccinate synthetase deficiency). These patients have usually presented with manifestations of severe neonatal hyperammonaemia and have died almost immediately. Others have presented later with psychomotor retardation, a history of early feeding difficulties, and episodic neurological disturbances. Asymptomatic cases are also recognized. The enzyme defect can be demonstrated in leucocytes, skin fibroblasts and liver tissue. Carrier state diagnosis and prenatal diagnosis appear to be possible although the available experience is insufficient for an assessment of their reliability.

Argininosuccinic aciduria (argininosuccinate lyase deficiency). There are neonatal, subacute, and late-onset types. The neonatal group develop serious hyperammonaemia and die in the perinatal period. The subacute type present in infancy with a history of feeding difficulties, failure to thrive, seizures, psychomotor delay, and hepatomegaly. The late onset group have similar manifestations but present in later childhood and their episodes of neurological dysfunction may be more clearly related to either protein ingestion or intercurrent infection. The degree of mental handicap is variable in the late-onset type and variants without brain damage may exist. Abnormally short friable hair due to trichorrhexis nodosa is characteristic.

The biochemical diagnosis depends on the demonstration of argininosuccinic acid in the urine, and on the measurement of erythrocyte argininosuccinate lyase activity. Prenatal diagnosis based on the argininosuccinate lyase activity of cultured amniotic fluid cells has been reported.

Hyperargininaemia (argininaemia). The known cases of this disorder have presented in early childhood with marked psychomotor retardation, seizures, ataxias, pareses, and tremors. They had postprandial hyperammonaemia with increased plasma and urinary arginine levels. The large filtered load of arginine impairs the renal tubule reabsorption of cystine, lysine, and arginine. The specific enzyme defect can be demonstrated in erythrocytes and in liver tissue.

Branched chain amino acid disorders

General aspects. Leucine, isoleucine, and valine are essential amino acids which contain a non-terminal methyl group so that the carbon chain branches. They are all metabolized by a similar series of enzymatic reactions and at some points the specificity of the enzyme includes the analogous derivatives of all three acids. They are first transaminated to the corresponding α-oxoacids and although the same enzyme can catalyse the transamination of all three acids, valine appears to have a separate transaminase and a second transaminase appears to act on leucine and isoleucine. Defective oxidative decarboxylation of the α-oxo derivates causes maple syrup urine disease (branched chain ketoaciduria). There are five further steps on the metabolic pathway between the α-oxo derivatives and the metabolic products which can enter the tricarboxylic acid cycle.

Branched chain amino acid transaminase deficiencies. Hypervalinaemia is a very rare disorder presenting in the neonatal period with rejection of feeds and failure to thrive, followed by hyperkinesia and psychomotor retardation. A specific valine transamination defect has been demonstrated in leucocytes. An analogous transamination defect has also been reported for leucine and isoleucine.

Maple syrup urine disease (branched chain keto aciduria). Although the existence of maple syrup urine disease is well known and it has been included in several surveys to detect inborn errors of metabolism, it remains one of the rarer diseases of this group, with an incidence of about 1:120 000 live births in Europe. The characteristic maple syrup or burnt sugar odour of the patients and their urine is due to the branched chain keto acids which they excrete in the urine and sweat.

There are four clinically distinguishable genetic variants of maple syrup urine disease: classical, intermittent, mild, and thiamine responsive. The classical form presents in the perinatal period with a severe metabolic acidosis, feeding difficulties, lethargy, and convulsions. The smell of maple syrup may be detectable as early as the fifth day of life, although it is usually first noticed much later. About half of the patients die at this stage of the illness and the survivors have severe brain damage. The high circulating levels of leucine induce a variable degree of hypoglycaemia. The plasma and urine levels of the branched chain amino acids are very high and there is a heavy ketoaciduria.

Patients with the intermittent type of maple syrup urine disease have episodes resembling those of the classical type but only in association with an intercurrent infection. They are well between the attacks although some have a mild degree of psychomotor retardation. The metabolic abnormalities are also only present during the acute episodes.

The term 'mild maple syrup urine disease' refers to a group of patients with continuous but less marked biochemical changes than in the classical type. They show some degree of psychomotor retardation and the severity of the clinical and biochemical phenotypes has been correlated with the amount of residual enzyme activity in leucocytes and cultured fibroblasts.

The biochemical abnormalities are relatively small and can be abolished by pharmacological doses of thiamine (10 mg/day), in the thiamine-responsive variant of maple syrup urine disease. These patients show some psychomotor retardation which may be preventable by thiamine treatment. The partial enzyme deficiency in these cases can also be corrected *in vitro* by raising the thiamine concentration.

Maple syrup urine disease is diagnosed biochemically by the abnormal pattern of amino acids and organic acids in the blood and urine, and confirmed in leucocytes or cultured fibroblasts. Prenatal diagnosis is possible by demonstrating the specific enzyme defect in cultured amniotic fluid cells.

Maple syrup urine disease is treated by restricting the intake of branched chain amino acids to an extent which keeps the plasma concentrations of these compounds at or a little above the normal values. The diet must provide adequate calories, essential amino acids, vitamins, and trace elements. Treatment along these lines beginning immediately after birth has proved to be successful but there is at present no experience as to when, if ever, the dietary restrictions may be relaxed. Acute episodes with acidosis, dehydration, hyperglycaemia and electrolyte imbalance are readily induced by hypercatabolic situations such as acute infections. Peritoneal dialysis or exchange blood transfusion and a period of protein-free feeding may be necessary, both in the presenting neonatal illness and in the acute exacerbation. Intermittent infections should be treated vigorously.

Isovaleric acidaemia. Isovaleric acidaemia is due to a block in the metabolism of leucine one step after the reaction which is defective in maple syrup urine disease. Patients present with feeding difficulties, failure to thrive, and severe metabolic acidosis in the neonatal period. There is a high mortality at this time and survivors have psychomotor retardation and acute episodes with vomiting, acidosis, focal neurological signs, and comas. The isovaleric acid imparts a smell resembling sweaty feet to the child and its surroundings. The acute episodes are associated with leucopenia and thrombocytopenia. Except for the odour, the clinical picture is a non-specific one and the diagnosis is established by identifying isovaleric acid in the blood and/or urine, and by inability of the patient's leucocytes to catabolize radioactively labelled leucine normally.

The treatment is on the same lines as for maple syrup urine disease except that only the leucine intake is restricted.

β-methylcrotonylglycinuria. β-methylcrotonylglycinuria is due to a metabolic block involving the biotin dependent carboxylase step on the leucine metabolic pathway beyond the one which is deficient in isovalericacidaemia. The patients present with severe acidosis and failure to thrive in the early months of life and a rash. Biotin (10 mg per day) causes clinical and biochemical improvement in some cases. The other aspects of treatment are as outlined for isovaleric acidaemia.

Propionic acidaemia. The coenzyme-A activated form of propionic acid (propionyl-CoA) is formed by the catabolism of *iso*-leucine, valine, methionine, threonine, the odd-numbered chain fatty acids, and cholesterol, and is carboxylated to methylmalonyl-CoA (see below). The spectrum of excreted metabolites in propionyl-CoA carboxylase deficiency (Table 1) includes glycine and acylglycines, so that the condition was formerly called ketotic hyperglycinaemia. Most patients present in the neonatal period with a very severe metabolic acidosis, vomiting, dehydration, and lethargy, and pass rapidly into coma. Some cases present later with episodic ketoacidosis and/or psychomotor retardation. Acute episodes may be precipitated by infection and by protein ingestion. Thrombocytopenia, neutropenia and some degree of hyperammonaemia are additional features.

A specific enzymological diagnosis is possible on leucocytes or cultured fibroblasts. Prenatal and carrier state diagnoses are also possible.

Acute episodes of ketoacidosis require vigorous treatment with intravenous sodium bicarbonate and a period of protein-free feeding. A low protein diet (0.5–1.5 g/kg body weight per day) should be given between the acute episodes. Some of the clinically milder cases are improved, at least biochemically, by biotin supplements (5 mg twice daily).

Methylmalonic acidaemia (methylmalonic aciduria) and cobalamin metabolism

Biochemistry. Methylmalonic acid may accumulate because of several metabolic lesions, and has to be considered in relation to some aspects of vitamin B_{12} metabolism. Figure 4 summarizes the intracellular metabolism of the cobalamin coenzymes.

Propionyl-CoA (the coenzyme-A activated form of propionic acid) is metabolized via methylmalonyl-CoA to succinyl-CoA as shown in Fig. 5.

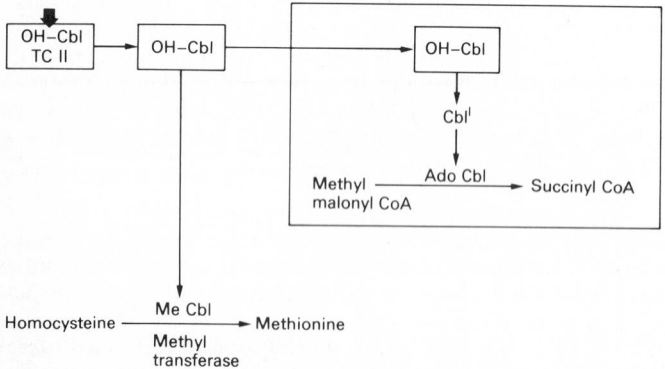

Fig. 4 The intracellular utilization of hydroxycobalamin. The formation and utilization of methylcobalamin (Me Cbl) takes place in the cytosol. The production and utilization of adenosylcobalamine (Ado Cbl) are mitochondrial functions. OH—Cbl = hydroxycobalamin. OH—Cbl TC II = transcobalamin II linked hydroxycobalamin. Cbl^I = cobalamine in which the cobalt has been reduced from the III to the I valency state. The top right rectangle represents the mitochondrial membrane.

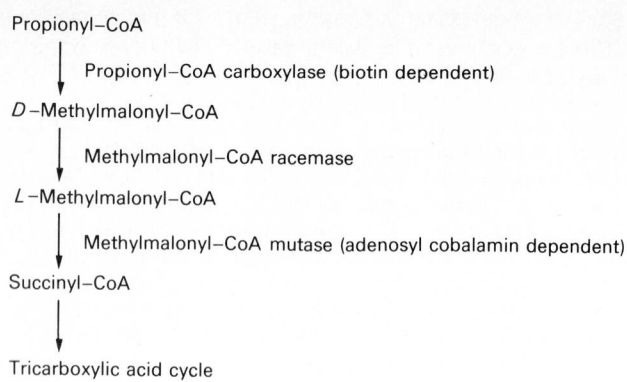

Fig. 5 The metabolism of propionyl-CoA.

Abnormalities of the methylmalonyl-CoA racemase and mutase apoenzymes cause Type I and Type IV methylmalonic acidaemia respectively (Table 1).

Hydroxycobalamin is bound to the carrier protein transcobalamin II and this complex is taken into the cells which require cobalamin coenzymes. The cobalt is reduced from the III to the I valency state before the cobalamine combines with adenosine to form adenosylcobalamine (Fig. 4). Methylmalonic aciduria due to a block in adenosylcobalamin synthesis from hydroxycobalamin is termed Type III methylmalonic aciduria (Table 1). The metabolic abnormality may be either a failure to reduce the cobalt from the III to the I valency state or a failure of the mechanism linking the adenosylcobalamin to the apoenzyme.

Homocysteine-N^5-methyltetrahydrofolate methyltransferase which catalyses one of the reactions converting homocysteine to methionine (Fig. 4) requires methylcobalamin. A metabolic lesion affecting simultaneously the production of adenysylcobalamin and methylcobalamin produces Type II methylmalonic aciduria in which there is also homocystinuria and cystathioninuria (Table 1). Failure of the cellular uptake of transcobalamin II linked hydroxycobalamin would produce such a combined biochemical abnormality (Fig. 4).

Clinical aspects. The defects of methylmalonic acid metabolism present with severe life-threatening neonatal ketoacidosis. The survivors are physically and mentally retarded, leucopenic, thrombocytopenic, and osteoporotic. Hypoglycaemia has been observed in the acute episodes and the urinary excretion of glycine may be increased. The latter is derived from the breakdown of the conjugate methylmalonylglycine. Megaloblastic anaemia is not a feature of Types I, III, and IV.

Patients with methylmalonic aciduria associated with defective methylcobalamin as well as adenosylcobalamin synthesis (Type II), and therefore impaired conversion of homocysteine to methionine, have severe megaloblastic anaemia, seizures, psychomotor delay, and fail to thrive from birth onwards. Signs of cerebellar and long tract involvement in the spinal cord appear in the older children. The reported patients who have survived the crises of infancy died in later childhood or adolescence.

Vitamin B_{12}-responsive and vitamin B_{12}-resistant variants of methylmalonic aciduria are recognized clinically. Impaired methylmalonyl-CoA mutase activity due to primary failure of adenosylcobalamin synthesis may respond to pharmacological doses of hydroxycobalamin (1 mg daily).

The metabolic crises which occur in the neonatal period and which are precipitated later by intercurrent infection are treated by the temporary withdrawal of protein feeds, the provision of calories from carbohydrate sources, the correction of fluid electrolyte and pH abnormalities, and vigorous treatment of any infection. Hydroxycobalamin (1 mg daily intramuscularly) is given to the vitamin B_{12}-responsive cases and when vitamin B_{12} responsiveness has not been established. Urinary methylmalonate excretion and blood pH are closely monitored. In the long term, the intake of dietary protein has to be restricted to levels which minimize the excretion of methylmalonic acid and its metabolites, and prevent ketonuria and acidosis.

Methylmalonic aciduria can be diagnosed prenatally but the analytical methods have not yet been refined sufficiently to allow the detection of carriers with certainty.

Methylmalonic aciduria due to an inborn error of metabolism has to be distinguished from transient neonatal methylmalonic aciduria which may be due to either immaturity of the enzyme systems responsible for converting propionate and methylmalonate to succinate or to temporary vitamin B_{12} deficiency.

Inborn errors of the metabolism of the sulphur-containing amino acids

The homocystinurias. (See also Section 17.) The term homocystinuria is usually used for the disease due to cystathionine synthase deficiency in which homocysteine accumulates proximal to the metabolic block and is oxidized to homocystine in the extracellular environment. The urinary excretion of homocystine is also increased in: (a) Type II methylmalonic aciduria (Table 1); (b) vitamin B_{12} deficiency; and (c) decreased activity of N^5, N^{10}-methylenetetrahydrofolate reductase.

The clinical manifestations of classical homocystinuria (cystathionine synthase deficiency) are neurological, ocular, skeletal, and vascular. About half of the patients are mentally handicapped and between 10 and 15 per cent of cases have seizures with corresponding electroencephalographic abnormalities. Dislocation of the lens of the eye, usually downwards, and due to weakening of the suspensory ligaments, is the commonest clinical abnormality. This develops in childhood and is complicated by glaucoma, myopia, iridodonesis, and cataracts. Optic atrophy and retinal detachment also occur. Multiple venous and arterial thrombo-embolic lesions may be recurrent major problems in these patients; the malar flush and livedo reticularis are characteristic concomitants. The patients are unusually tall, with arachnodactyly, high arched palate, kyphoscoliosis, flat feet, pectus excavatum, abnormally lax ligaments, and poor muscle development. There is generalized osteoporosis which is probably due to occlusion of the small nutrient blood vessels of the bones. These patients have to be distinguished from cases of Marfan's syndrome (see page 17.27). Homocystine gives a positive reaction with the cyanide nitroprusside reagent which is sometimes used to screen for cystinuria. The two conditions are easily distinguished by chromatographic or electrophoretic methods of urinary amino acid analysis. The associated hypermethioninaemia and hypermethioninuria are more reliable diagnostic criteria than measurements of homocystine excretion in the early weeks of life. They also distinguish cystathionine synthase deficiency from the defects of homocysteine remethylation, the methionine excretion being reduced in the latter group.

Dietary restriction of methionine with cystine supplementation and the administration of pharmacological doses of pyridoxine have been proposed as treatments for homocystinuria. Treatment needs to be given immediately after birth. Although the biochemical abnormalities can be modified by dietary restriction and in some cases by pyridoxine, the extent to which the natural history of the disease and its complications can be modified in the long term is uncertain. Homocystinuric women should not take oestrogen containing oral contraceptives, and elective surgical procedures should be undertaken after a period of pyridoxine treatment in the pyridoxine sensitive patient and low methionine diet in the pyridoxine resistant cases.

Cystathioninuria (cystathionase deficiency). The metabolic lesion in cystathioninuria involves the next reaction on the transsulphuration pathway after cystathionine synthase. It was originally identified in association with severe mental handicap, but intellectually normal individuals with the same metabolic anomaly have

also been identified. Pharmacological doses of pyridoxine reduced the cystathionine excretion markedly in some patients but this effect does not appear to be specifically related to the presence or absence of mental handicap. There have been conflicting claims as to the value of pyridoxine in controlling fits in patients with cystathioninuria.

Cystinosis. Cystinosis is a lysosomal storage disease in which cystine accumulates primarily in the cells of the reticulo-endothelial system. Cystinosis is not related to cystinuria; confusion has arisen in the past because the generalized amino aciduria, which is a component of the Fanconi syndrome induced by cystinosis, includes cystine and this amino acid was more easily detectable than most others before chromatographic methods became available. The underlying metabolic lesion remains to be identified. The cysteine–cystine couple is almost entirely in the reduced form (cysteine) inside cells and almost wholly in the oxidized (cystine) form in the extra-cellular enviroment. Some authorities suggest that the mechanism which maintains the position of the equilibrium in the lysosomes is defective in cystinosis so that cystine/cysteine liberated by intralysosomal proteolysis remains as cystine which cannot cross the lysosomal membrane.

There are three clinically definable types of cystinosis: infantile (nephropathic), juvenile (intermediate), and adult (benign). These types are also distinct genetically and are inherited as autosomal recessives.

Infantile (nephropathic) cystinosis. Children with infantile cystinosis appear normal at birth but develop signs of nephrogenic diabetes insipidus and fail to thrive from about six months of age. Some patients have recurrent episodes of prostration and cardiovascular collapse which may prove fatal. Growth retardation, rickets, and acidosis are apparent by age one year, progressive renal failure develops and the patients die during the first decade. Intellectual development is normal and there is no special liability to intercurrent infection. Most of the patients are less pigmented than their parents or siblings. Photophobia associated with refractile corneal opacities usually develops in childhood. Cystine crystals also accumulate under the conjuctiva. The peripheral part of the retina shows pigmentary degeneration most marked in the temporal quadrants, and these changes may antedate the other manifestations of cystinosis. The diagnosis is usually confirmed by demonstrating cystine crystals in a bone marrow aspirate, in leucocytes, or a conjunctival biopsy. Renal tubule damage produces a Fanconi syndrome (see page 9.101), acidosis, and tubular proteinuria with an excess of gamma-globulin light chains.

Treatment has to be directed at the individual facets of the disease: namely, correction of the dehydration, hypokalaemia, and acidosis in the acute episodes, sufficient vitamin D and phosphate to heal the rickets, and management of the overall renal failure. Cystinosis is not a contra-indication to renal transplantation. The transplanted kidney does not develop the renal tubule and progressive glomerular failure of cystinosis, although cystine containing interstitial and mesangial cells migrate into the graft. Attempts to treat cystinosis by dietary restriction or by drugs (penicillamine) which solubilize cystine and by large doses of vitamin C (a reducing agent) have been unsuccessful.

Juvenile (intermediate) cystinosis. These patients have presented at between 18 months and 17 years of age. They are less stunted than the infantile type, and have an incomplete Fanconi syndrome with less rapidly developing glomerular failure than the infantile variety. Cystine deposits are present in the cornea, conjunctiva, and in the bone marrow.

Adult (benign) cystinosis. These patients are asymptomatic and are usually detected when corneal deposits of cystine are observed during a routine slit-lamp examination. The bone marrow and leucocytes contain cystine crystals. The kidneys and retina are unaffected.

Histidinaemia

Histidinaemia (Table 1) was originally recognized because one of the abnormal excretion products, imidazole pyruvic acid, reacts with ferric chloride and gives a false positive test in colorimetric screening tests (Phenistix) for phenylketonuria. The original cases were associated with speech defects and a moderate degree of mental handicap. The elevated level of histidine and histidine metabolites in the body fluids can be corrected by restricting the dietary intake of histidine and practicable regimens for dietary treatment have been evolved. However, the association of brain damage and histidinaemia has proved to be an inconstant one, and it is unclear whether the original observations were due to chance association, which then appeared to be confirmed because screening programmes to detect histidinaemia were initiated among mentally handicapped populations, or due to heterogeneity in the histidinaemia phenotype. Most authorities would not now recommend dietary restriction of histidine.

Hyperlysinaemias and lysinuric protein intolerance

The main features of the three inborn errors of lysine metabolism with hyperlysinaemia are summarized in Table 1.

Lysinuric protein intolerance is an autosomal recessive inborn error of dibasic amino acid transport. It presents in infancy with protein intolerance and failure to thrive. There is severe growth failure, osteoporosis, neutropenia, and mental handicap in about one quarter of the cases. Blood urea values are low and hyperammonaemia develops postprandially. There is impaired dibasic amino acid transport involving intestinal absorption, renal tubule reabsorption, and uptake of these amino acids by the liver. It is proposed that this combination starves the urea cycle of two of its essential intermediates, arginine and ornithine, causing inefficient urea synthesis and hyperammonaemia. Lysine is an essential amino acid, deficiency of which causes growth failure. Dietary supplementation with arginine or with its precursor citrulline plus lysine has been reported to prevent hyperammonaemia and to promote growth.

The hyperprolinaemias

Types I and II hyperprolinaemia (Table 1) were originally reported as being associated with inherited renal disease and mental handicap respectively. Further experience has shown these to have been chance associations.

The increased filtered load of proline saturates the renal tubular common transport mechanism for proline, hydroxyproline, and glycine, so that the excretions of hydroxyproline and glycine are also increased. This has to be distinguished from familial iminoglycinuria in which the common transport system is itself deficient (see page 9.103).

5-oxoprolinuria (pyroglutamic aciduria)

5-oxoproline is an intermediate of the cyclic mechanism, the γ-glutamyl cycle whereby glutathione is synthesized. A generalized deficiency of glutathione synthetase causes a massive accumulation and excretion of 5-oxoproline. The patients present with severe metabolic acidosis in infancy followed by mental handicap in some cases. They also show low-grade spontaneous haemolysis. Patients with glutathione synthetase deficiency affecting the erythrocyte have haemolytic disease but no 5-oxoprolinuria. These disorders appear to be inherited as autosomal recessives.

Carnosinaemia and β-alaninaemia

The main clinical and biochemical feature of these rare disorders are presented in Table 1.

The occurrence of β-aminoisobutyric aciduria and hypertaurinuria in β-alaninuria is attributed to the large filtered load of β-alanine saturating the transport system for the β-amino acids in the renal tubule.

Non-ketotic hyperglycinaemia

This condition is due to serine hydroxymethyltransferase deficiency. This blocks the serine–glycine interconversion pathway, which is a major route for the metabolism of these two amino acids. Glycine utilization is impaired but serine can still be converted to glycine. The original description included hypo-oxaluria in the biochemical phenotype but this has not been substantiated. Profound psychomotor retardation, spasticity, and seizures are consistent clinical findings if the child survives the neonatal period. There is no treatment, although transient decreases in the plasma glycine have been claimed after large doses of N^5,N^{10}-methylene-tetrahydrofolate and after methionine supplementation.

References

Bachmann, C. (1974). Urea cycle. In *Heritable disorders of amino acid metabolism: patterns of clinical expression and genetic variation* (ed. W. L. Nyhan), 361. Wiley, New York.

Berry, H. K., O'Grady, D. J., Perlmutter, L. J., and Bofinger, M. K. (1979). Intellectual development and academic achievement of children treated early for phenylketonuria. *Dev. Med. Child Neurol.* **21**, 311.

Bremer, H. J., Duran, M., Kamerling, J. P., Przyrembel, H., and Wadman, S. K. (1981). *Disturbances of amino acid metabolism: clinical chemistry and diagnosis.* Urban and Schwarzenburg, Baltimore and Munich.

Bickel, H. and Schmidt, H. (1982). Dietary and coenzyme therapy. In *Advances in the treatment of inborn errors of metabolism* (eds. M. d'A. Crawford, D. A. Gibbs, and R. W. E. Watts). Wiley, Chichester.

Clayton, B. E. (1975). The principles of treatment by dietary restriction as illustrated by phenylketonuria. In *The treatment of inherited metabolic disease* (ed. D. N. Raine), 1. MTP Press, Lancaster.

Ghadimi, H. (1978). The hyperlysinemias. In *The metabolic basis of inherited disease* (eds. J. B. Stanbury, J. B. Wyngaarden, and D. S. Fredrickson), 387. McGraw-Hill, New York.

La Du, B. N. (1978). Histidinemia. In *The metabolic basis of inherited disease* (eds. J. B. Stanbury, J. B. Wyngaarden, and D. S. Fredrickson), 317. McGraw-Hill, New York.

— and Gjessing, L. R. (1978). Tyrosinosis and tyrosinemia. In *The metabolic basis of inherited disease* (eds. J. B. Stanbury, J. B. Wyngaarden, and D. S. Fredrickson), 256. McGraw-Hill, New York.

The Lancet (1979). New varieties of PKU. *Lancet* i, 304.

Meister, A. (1978). 5-Oxoprolinuria (pyroglutamic aciduria) and other disorders of glutathione biosynthesis. In *The metabolic basis of inherited disease* (eds. J. B. Stanbury, J. B. Wyngaarden, and D. S. Fredrickson), 328. McGraw-Hill, New York.

Mudd, H. S. and Levy, H. L. (1978). Disorders of transulphuration. In *The metabolic basis of inherited disease* (eds. J. B. Stanbury, J. B. Wyngaarden, and D. S. Fredrickson), 458–503. McGraw-Hill, New York.

Nyhan, W. L. (1978). Non-ketotic hyperglycinemia. In *The metabolic basis of inherited disease* (eds. J. B. Stanbury, J. B. Wyngaarden, and D. S. Fredrickson), 518–27. McGraw-Hill, New York.

Rosenberg, L. E. (1978). Disorders of propionate, methylmalonate, and cobalamin metabolism. In *The metabolic basis of inherited disease* (eds. J. B. Stanbury, J. B. Wyngaarden, and D. S. Fredrickson), 411. McGraw-Hill, New York.

Schneider, J. A. and Schulman, J. D. (1977). Cystinosis: a review. *Metabolism* **26**, 817.

Scriver, C. R., Nutzenadel, W., and Perry, T. L. (1978). Disorders of β-alanine and carnosine metabolism. In *The metabolic basis of inherited disease* (eds. J. B. Stanbury, J. B. Wyngaarden, and D. S. Fredrickson), 528. McGraw-Hill, New York.

— and Rosenberg, L. E. (1973). Imino acids. In *Amino acid metabolism and its disorders*, vol. 10 of *Major problems in pediatrics* (ed. A. L. Schaffer). W. B. Saunders, Philadelphia.

Shih, V. E. (1978). Urea cycle disorders and other congenital hyperammonemia syndromes. In *The metabolic basis of inherited disease* (eds. J. B. Stanbury, J. B. Wyngaarden, and D. S. Fredrickson), 362. McGraw-Hill, New York.

Snyderman, S. E. (1975). Maple syrup urine disease. In *The treatment of inherited metabolic disease* (ed. D. N. Raine), 71–90. MTP Press, Lancaster.

Thalhammer, O., Havelic, L., Knoll, E., and Wehle, E. (1977). Intellectual level (IQ) in heterozygotes for phenylketonuria (PKU). *Human Genet.* **38**, 285.

Witkop, C. J., Quevedo, W. C., and Fitzpatrick, T. B. (1978). Albinism. In *The metabolic basis of inherited disease* (eds. J. B. Stanbury, J. B. Wyngaarden, and D. S. Fredrickson), 283. McGraw-Hill, New York.

Amino acid transport defects

R. W. E. Watts

General pathophysiology. This discussion concerns the transport of amino acids across plasma (cell) membranes, with particular reference to the epithelial cells lining the renal tubule. Solutes cross cell membranes by passive diffusion along concentration and electrochemical gradients, by facilitated diffusion, and by energy requiring active transport mechanisms. These processes, and in particular, the energy requiring active transport processes regulate the internal composition of all cells. In certain specialized situations, active transport mechanisms affect the transfer of specific solutes across a sheet of cells at rates which are optimum for maintaining the composition of the internal environment and the nutritional state of the whole organism.

This situation involves transport across two cell surfaces as in the gut and the renal tubule. Active transport processes confer a specificity in relation to the organism's requirements as well as individual cell composition, which non-energy requiring passive and facilitated diffusion processes lack. They provide a barrier as well as a portal of entry.

Active transport systems show specificity and saturability as well as competitive and non-competitive inhibition. The terms permease, carrier protein, and pump have been used to describe the concept of a specialized region of the cell membrane which effects the active transport of specific substances across the membrane. Structurally, such a region could be a catalytic protein inserted through the lipid bilayer.

The active transport of amino acids across cell membranes is linked to the activity of the membrane bound, ouabain inhibitable, enzyme sodium–potassium adenosine triphosphatase (Na–K ATPase). It is, therefore, sodium-dependent and can be inhibited by ouabain.

Although unidirectional flow predominates, transport across the whole renal tubule cell as well as across the luminal and antiluminal borders is always at least potentially bi-directional. Transport from the peritubular capillary (tubule or tubular secretion) and movement from the tubule lumen (tubule or tubular reabsorption) can be active processes. The distinction should be drawn between renal tubule reabsorption and secretion considered separately, and the algebraic sum of their effects when they occur simultaneously, namely net reabsorption and net secretion.

The study of disorders of amino acid transport has shown some parallelism between the intestinal mucosa and the renal tubule from this viewpoint. The extent to which similar mechanisms operate in cells generally is unknown. It is noteworthy that most of the products of protein digestion are absorbed from the gut as low molecular weight peptides and not as free amino acids.

Some transport systems are shared by groups of related compounds, and in the kidney such transport mechanisms have been identified for the dibasic amino acids, the dicarboxylic amino acids, glycine and the imino acids (proline and hydroxyproline), neutral aliphatic and aromatic α-amino acids, and β-amino acids. The same compound may be transported by more than one carrier mechanism, for example, cystine which shares the dibasic amino acid system and also has a separate carrier mechanism.

Although there is a considerable measure of localization of function to different regions of the nephron, individual transport functions are located in the same epithelial cell and in adjacent cells. Thus, disease of a specific part of the renal tubule commonly affects more than one transport function.

Amino acids are fully filterable at the glomerulus and more than 95 per cent of the filtered load is reabsorbed in the proximal convoluted tubule. The pattern of renal amino acid clearance matures postnatally and an adult pattern is achieved by the age of two years. Abnormal amino-acidurias are due to: (a) saturation of the reabsorptive mechanism due to an abnormally large filtered load, which may be generalized as in hepatic failure or isolated as in phenylketonuria; (b) competition by one of a group of amino acids, which share a common transport system, for all of the available carrier sites, as in prolinaemia; (c) renal tubule abnormalities which may produce either a generalized amino-aciduria, as in the Fanconi syndrome, or an amino-aciduria confined to those amino acids which are transported by a single carrier system as the primary pathophysiological phenomenon as in Hartnup disease.

Identifiable clinical syndromes of renal tubule dysfunction are associated with disordered transport of amino acids, glucose, phosphate ions, sodium ions, potassium ions, bicarbonate ions, hydrogen ions, uric acid, and water. Renal tubule lesions will clearly impair the transport of other physiologically important substances, for example, peptides and vitamins, but the results of such losses are not apparent clinically.

The generalized amino-acidurias

The Fanconi syndrome

Pathophysiology. The Fanconi syndrome comprises osteomalacia (or rickets), renal glycosuria, generalized amino-aciduria, and phosphaturia. Juvenile and adult variants are known. The juvenile Fanconi syndrome is sometimes referred to as the de Toni–Fanconi syndrome or the de Toni–Fanconi–Debré syndrome. The following features have been added to the original syndrome: hyperchloraemic acidosis (renal tubular acidosis) due to failure to reabsorb bicarbonate and transport hydrogen ions normally, hypokalaemia, polyuria, hypouricaemia, the excretion of immunoglobulin light chains and other low molecular weight proteins with the electrophoretic properties of α_2-, β_2-, and γ-globulins. It is caused by damage to the proximal convoluted tubule of the kidney (Table 1). Cystinosis (cystine storage disease, page 9.99) was the first recognized cause of the syndrome and the situation was confused by the early failure to differentiate juvenile cystinosis (nephropathic cystinosis) from cystinuria. The increased excretion of cystine observed in cystinosis is part of a generalized amino aciduria. The amounts excreted are similar to those of the other amino acids, and less than in cystinuria. Nephropathic cystinosis is sometimes referred to as Lignac's disease, or the Lignac–Fanconi syndrome. This is not a synonym for the juvenile Fanconi syndrome. Similarly adult, or benign, cystinosis in which there is no renal damage is a distinct entity from the adult Fanconi syndrome as well as from juvenile cystinosis.

The proximal convoluted tubules are short with epithelial cell atrophy ('swan neck' deformity of the nephron). The bones show the histological appearances of osteomalacia due to phosphate-depletion. Potassium depletion may be caused by a primary renal tubule reabsorption defect or be secondary to the disturbance of acid–base regulation, and polyuria with isosthenuria is characteristic of the nephropathy of potassium depletion.

The individual components of the Fanconi syndrome may occur separately or together in different combinations (Table 2).

Clinical aspects. Symptoms of the juvenile form of the Fanconi syndrome usually begin when the child is about six months old. Failure to thrive and grow is accompanied by bouts of vomiting, and unexplained fever. Severe rickets develops and is resistant to the usual replacement doses of vitamin D. Chronic systemic acidosis,

Table 1 Causes of generalized renal amino-aciduria

Inherited
  Cystinosis
  Galactosaemia
  Hereditary fructose intolerance
  Glycogen storage disease Type 1
  Tyrosinosis
  Wilson's disease
  Osteogenesis imperfecta
  Congenital renal tubular acidosis
  Congenital haemolytic anaemias (sickle cell disease, thalassaemia, spherocytosis)
  Adult Fanconi syndrome (idiopathic)
  Busby syndrome (familial growth retardation, cor pulmonale, amino aciduria)
  Luder–Sheldon syndrome (glycosuria and amino-aciduria)
  Paine's syndrome (microcephaly, spastic diplegia amino-aciduria)

Acquired
  Poisons
    cadmium, zinc, uranium, mercury, lead, nitrobenzine, lysol, salicylate, maleic acid (in experimental animals), methyl-3-chromone, 5α, 6-anhydro-4-epi-tetracycline (a tetracycline degradation product)
  Nutritional deficiencies
    vitamin B_{12} deficiency, vitamin C deficiency, vitamin D deficiency, kwashiorkor,
  Endocrine disorders
    primary hyperparathyroidism
  Renal disease:
    acute tubular necrosis, nephrotic syndrome, multiple myelomatosis, renal transplant rejection, potassium depletion nephropathy
  Malignant disease
  Thermal burns

Table 2 The renal tubule reabsorption deficiency syndromes

Renal glycosuria
Hypophosphataemic (vitamin-D resistant) rickets and/or osteomalacia
Generalized amino-aciduria
Renal glycosuria with hypophosphataemic rickets
Generalized amino-aciduria with vitamin D resistant rickets and/or osteomalacia
Renal glycosuria with generalized amino-aciduria
Glycosuria with generalized amino-aciduria and hypophosphataemic rickets
  and/or osteomalacia (the Fanconi syndrome)
Renal tubular acidosis
Renal hypouricaemia

polyuria, and dehydration are prominent features. The urine is alkaline with a high ammonium content in spite of the systemic acidosis. The classical generalized amino aciduria, glycosuria, and phosphaturia are accompanied by hypophosphataemia, hypokalaemia with increased kaliuresis, and hypo-uricaemia with hyperuricaciduria.

The adult cases of the Fanconi syndrome show essentially the same clinical and biochemical features as the juvenile cases, except that osteomalacia with fractures and pseudo-fractures (Looser's zones) of the demineralized tender bones is the dominant clinical feature, and the symptoms of hypokalaemic myasthenia are more readily elicited. Common sites for Looser's zones are the ischiopubic rami, lateral border of the scapula, subtrochanteric region of the femur, upper third of the tibia and humerus, and the ribs.

Many cases of the adult Fanconi syndrome lack a demonstrable cause and familial cases have been described. Some cases are due to multiple myelomatosis, and the renal abnormalities may antedate the appearance of other manifestations of the primary disorder by several years. It is suggested that, like other peptides, the immunoglobulin light chains are absorbed into the epithelial cells of the proximal convoluted tubules where they form crystalline structures and damage the functional integrity of the cells. Conversely, it has been claimed that all patients with the Fanconi syndrome excrete immunoglobulin light chains as part of their characteristic low molecular weight proteinuria.

The bone disease usually dominates the clinical picture so that the main differential diagnoses are rickets and osteomalacia. In children, the earlier cases need to be distinguished from other causes of failure to thrive. If skeletal deformities are not prominent, the main differential diagnoses will be renal tubular acidosis and other causes of hypokalaemia with muscle weakness. The latter include familial hypokalaemic periodic paralysis, and potassium depletion nephropathy.

Treatment. Large (milligram) doses of vitamin D (50 000–400 000 units daily) or physiological (1–2 µg) doses of 1,25-dihydroxy-D_3 or 1,α-hydroxy-D_3 heal the bone lesions. The serum calcium should be checked every few days until it has been confirmed that the patient is in fact resistant to the vitamin. Thereafter it should be checked at longer intervals. Acidosis and potassium depletion are corrected. These replacement therapies do not prevent renal failure.

Lowe's syndrome (the oculocerebral syndrome, the Lowe–Terry–McLachlan syndrome). The combination of generalized amino aciduria, mental handicap, congenital cataracts, and muscular hypotonia define the syndrome which is inherited in a sex-linked recessive manner. The heterozygous female carriers develop cataracts which may be of only minor severity. The patients are also physically retarded with dolichocephaly, saddle nose, prominent forehead, shield chest, cryptorchidism, umbilical herniae, and high arched palate. More extensive ocular abnormalities include glaucoma, myopic pupils, posterior synaechiae, and pigmentary degeneration of the macula. Hypophosphataemic rickets and hyperchloraemic acidosis complicate the clinical picture, and impaired transport of amino acids across the small intestine mucosa has been claimed. The cataracts, dysmorphic features, and hypotonia are present at birth, and the amino aciduria becomes apparent during the first weeks or months of life. Most patients die from renal disease in infancy. Some cases, however, evolve more slowly, with psychomotor retardation, blindness, and chronic renal insufficiency, and occasionally survive into early adulthood.

The pathological changes are non-specific and Lowe's syndrome has to be distinguished from other examples of multiple developmental abnormalities, including the results of intrauterine infections. It cannot be diagnosed prenatally or in the carrier state.

The metabolic acidosis and hypophosphataemic rickets respond to alkali and large doses of vitamin D (or small doses of active metabolites) respectively.

Specific amino-acidurias

Hartnup disease (Harts disease, H-disease)

Pathophysiology. Hartnup disease is an autosomal recessively inherited disorder in which increased renal clearance of the neutral amino acids (alanine, serine, threonine, valine, leucine, *iso*leucine, phenylalanine, tyrosine, tryptophan, histidine, glutamine, and asparagine), is associated with photosensitive skin eruptions and neuropsychiatric manifestations. The transport defect is expressed in the small intestine epithelium as well as in the epithelium lining the proximal convoluted tubules of the kidney. The estimated prevalence of Hartnup disease is about 1:16 000 live births.

Tryptophan malabsorption causes nicotinamide deficiency and a pellagra-like picture. The unabsorbed tryptophan is metabolized by the intestinal flora to a series of indolic compounds including indican which are absorbed and excreted into the urine.

The abnormal amino aciduria is the only constant feature amounting to an increase of 5 to 10 times the normal excretion, and the extent of the renal tubule reabsorption defect varies for the different amino acids. The abnormal amino-aciduria is of no clinical significance except in so far as the tryptophanuria contributes to the state of tryptophan deficiency.

Clinical picture. Some patients are asymptomatic and are only detected during urine screening for abnormal amino-aciduria. About 20 per cent of patients have a mild to moderate degree of mental retardation. The psychiatric symptoms vary from a mild increase in emotional lability to a major psychotic illness with delirium. Intermittent cerebellar ataxia with nystagmus, intention tremor, as well as hyper-reflexia, impaired consciousness, and convulsions may occur. The neuro-psychiatric manifestations vary in their occurrence in different patients and at different times in the same case, but when present are associated with some cutaneous involvement. The skin lesions occur on the exposed surfaces, the face, neck, hands, wrists, knees, and legs in children. They may be dry and scaly or inflamed and moist, and tend to heal in the winter. Fever, psychiatric stress, sunlight, and sulphonamide therapy may all precipitate clinical signs and symptoms in these patients.

The amino-aciduria differentiates Hartnup disease from nutritional pellagra, and from other causes of abnormal photosensitivity in normally pigmented subjects. These include the DNA repair enzyme defects (ataxia telangectasia, xeroderma pigmentosum, and Cockayne's syndrome) and the cutaneous porphyrias. Hartnup disease has not been diagnosed prenatally or in the carrier state. Oral nicotinamide (40–200 mg daily) improves the cutaneous and neurological manifestations. Some patients improve spontaneously, especially as they grow older. There is no decrease in life expectancy.

Blue diaper syndrome (tryptophan malabsorption syndrome). The patients have an isolated transport defect for tryptophan. They excrete tryptophan metabolites including indican, which is oxidized to indigo blue and this stains the child's underclothes. There are no neurological or cutaneous manifestations, and no abnormal amino aciduria. The male patients have presented in infancy with recurrent fever, growth retardation, irritability, and hypercalcaemia. A female sibling with increased indican excretion as the only abnormality has been reported. The available data are too scanty to permit assessment of the long-term prognosis and the pattern of inheritance.

Familial iminoglycinuria
Pathophysiology. Familial iminoglycinuria is due to dysfunction of the mechanism which transports glycine, proline, and hydroxyproline across the renal tubule epithelial cell membrane, and which is shared by these three amino acids only. It is inherited as an autosomal recessive, its incidence being quoted as 1:20 000 in the north eastern region of the United States. There are no structural or anatomical abnormalities specifically associated with iminoglycinuria. Glycine normally accounts for about 30 per cent of the total excretion of unconjugated urinary amino acids. Premature infants and neonates excrete free proline and hydroxyproline, but these disappear from the urine during the first year of life.

Clinical aspects. Familial iminoglycinuria appears to be a harmless autosomal recessive biochemical anomaly. Cases have been described in association with mental retardation, ocular abnormalities, and congenital nerve deafness. These associations are inconstant and reflect the practice of screening selected populations with these abnormalities without comparative screening of strictly identical normal control populations. Iminoglycinuria has also been described fortuitously associated with cystathioninuria and with cystinosis. These associations presumably reflect the identical methods used for the study of all the amino acidopathies. The differential diagnoses are: (a) physiological prolinuria and hydroxyprolinuria occuring during the first year of life; (b) the hyperprolinaemias; (c) hydroxyprolinuria; and (d) isolated hyperglycinuria.

In some families, the heterozygous individuals have isolated renal hyperglycinuria and this accounts for reports of dominantly inherited isolated hyperglycinuria. Iminoglycinuria is unrelated to glucoglycinuria in which the dominantly inherited metabolic lesion specifically affects the transport of glucose and glycine. Hyperglycinuria without other amino aciduria also occurs in the ketotic and non-ketotic hyperglycinaemia syndromes (see page 9.100).

Cystinuria
Pathophysiology. The synthesis of the group-specific carrier protein for cystine and the dibasic amino acids (lysine, ornithine, and arginine) is directed by a single pair of allelic genes, and there are three possible mutant alleles which cause cystinuria when present in the homozygous state. Individuals who are homozygous for one of the mutant alleles or heterozygous for two of them have the classical cystinuria phenotype. The detailed classification of patients requires study of the transport of the individual amino acids in the small intestine as well as consideration of their renal handling.

A simpler but clinically useful classification, which depends only on the study of urinary amino acid excretion divides the families into: (a) the completely recessive genotype, in which the heterozygotes for the abnormal gene causing cystinuria have no abnormal amino aciduria; and (b) the incompletely recessive genotype in which the heterozygotes show only increased excretions of cystine and lysine. On this basis hyperlysinuria may be the only abnormality in the heterozygotes and hyperargininaemia usually indicates that the individual is homozygous for an abnormal gene causing cystinuria or a double heterozygote for two different abnormal genes.

Cystine is also reabsorbed from the renal tubule lumen by a cystine-specific mechanism. The intracellular concentration of cystine is negligible, the disulphide amino acid being reduced to the free thiol form (cysteine). The active tubular secretion of cystine has also been proposed to explain the observation that the renal clearance of cystine exceeds the glomerular filtration rate in some cases of cystinuria. This would involve a specific carrier mechanism for cysteine. The dibasic amino acids are also reabsorbed by a carrier system, which does not handle cystine, as well as by the shared mechanism. Isolated cystinuria is presumably due to a lesion of the cystine specific system, and several syndromes of hyperdibasic amino aciduria with normal cystine excretion are known. In classical cystinuria, the degree of amino acid transport defect does not affect the individual amino acids to the same extent in a particular patient, as judged by renal clearance studies.

Bacterial action in the colon converts some of the unabsorbed lysine to cadaverine (1,5-pentane diamine) and piperidine. Arginine and ornithine are similarly converted to putrescine (1,4-butane diamine) and pyrrolidine. These compounds are absorbed and excreted in the urine, in amounts which vary between different patients and at different times in the same patient. Cystinuric patients have normal absorption of cysteine and oligopeptides containing the amino acids, which they are unable to absorb in the free state. This presumably protects them from growth retardation due to malabsorption of the essential amino acids lysine and arginine.

There are no morbid anatomical or histopathological changes which are peculiar to cystinuria. The findings in cystine stone-formers are the same as in other types of urolithiasis without nephrocalcinosis. The stones may be multiple, small and faceted, or single and sometimes of the 'stag-horn' type. Their yellow-brown colour with small glistening crystals on their surface is characteristic. Phosphatic stones or stones containing both cystine and phosphate occur in patients whose primary disorder has been complicated by urinary tract infections.

Clinical aspects. In Europe between 1 and 4 per cent of urinary stones are due to cystinuria. The risk of stone formation depends only on the extent and length of time for which the urinary cystine concentration exceeds the solubility of the amino acid in the urine. Urinary stones and the passage of cystine gravel or sand are the only manifestations of cystinuria. The stones tend to recur after surgical removal, and bacterial infections often complicate the clinical picture. The clinical history sometimes dates from childhood although the third decade is the peak for the onset of symptoms. The pattern of amino aciduria observed in heterozygotes of incompletely recessive cystinuria has been observed in association with hereditary pancreatitis sufficiently frequently to suggest that the two conditions may sometimes be specifically associated with one another. Other reported clinical associations, for example with facioscapulohumeral muscular dystrophy, retinitis pigmentosa, mental retardation, and hyperuricaemia appear to be coincidental. The production of a cystinuria type of amino acid excretion pattern in hyperargininaemia which itself causes mental handicap is noteworthy. Cystine stones are radio-opaque, and although they are often less dense than calcium-containing stones, the difference is not sufficiently marked or sufficiently consistant to be of material diagnostic help.

Treatment. Patients with cystinuria who have never had stones should be advised to maintain a urine volume of about three litres per 24 hours as a prophylactic against stone formation. In temperate climates, this involves drinking about the same volume of fluid with special attention to taking extra drinks at bed time.

Cystine stone formers are treated either by maintaining a vigorous water diuresis throughout the 24-hour period, or with penicillamine. Treatment by hydration is cheap and free from side-effects. α-Mercaptopropionylglycine (Thiola) can also be used but it is not generally available in the United Kingdom. The patient needs to drink sufficient fluid, about 600 ml every four hours to maintain a urine volume of at least 500 ml in each four hours throughout the day *and night*. The solubility of cystine in urine is about 400 mg per l (1.66 mmol per at pH 7.0 and 37°C). Increasing the urine pH up to this value has little effect on the solubility of cystine. However, increasing the pH to about 7.8 doubles the solubility. Large doses of sodium bicarbonate are needed to keep the urine pH in this high range and are not recommended as a routine because of the increased risk of urinary infection and the possibility of favouring the formation of phosphatic stones. At least one third of cystine stones will become smaller if the hydration regimen is followed conscientiously. It is not possible to assess whether the failures are genuine therapeutic failures or due to the patients' inability to follow the regimen.

In clinical practice in the United Kingdom, the term 'penicillamine' refers to D(−)penicillamine; the L(+) stereoisomer is much more toxic than D(−) penicillamine; neither D, L(−), nor L(+) penicillamine should be given to human subjects. D(−) penicillamine is available as tablets (50 mg, 125 mg or 250 mg). Penicillamine reacts *in vivo* with cystine to form penicillamine-cysteine which is excreted in the urine in place of cystine. This makes the urine unsaturated with respect to cystine so that cystine stones dissolve and further stone formation is prevented. Penicillamine-cysteine is 50 times more soluble than cystine. α-Mercaptopropionylglycine also acts by forming a mixed disulphide with cysteine. Patients with cystinuria usually excrete 4.25–8.50 mmol (1–2 g) cystine per 24 hours, so that their urine is often oversaturated with amino acid.

The urinary cystine concentration should be kept below 0.83 mmol (200 mg) per g creatinine (approximately 100 μmol cystine per mmol creatinine) or about 0.83 mmol per litre when measured on a 24-hour urine collection, the total cystine excretion being about 1.45 mmol (300 mg) per 24-hours. An alternative way of controlling treatment is to measure the urinary cystine concentration in timed six-hour urine collections throughout several 24-hour periods with the patient drinking an accustomed volume of fluids. The cystine concentration of all the specimen should be less than 1.66 mmol (400 mg) per litre, particular attention being paid to the urine voided between 02.00 and 08.00 hours. Most patients require a total dose of 1–2 g of penicillamine per 24 hours. This is usually given in three equal and approximately equally spaced doses. However, if the drug is being given to prevent a recurrence of stones rather than to dissolve stones which are already present, it may be possible to use a smaller dose (for example, 750 mg per 24 hours) given at about 22.00 hours and thereby prevent the cystine

concentration of the night time urine exceeding the solubility limit.

The effect of penicillamine on the urinary cystine excretion is not lost with time, although the dose may need adjusting especially in children. Calculi are usually visibly smaller after 6–12 months of penicillamine treatment, provided that they are in a region of the pelvicalcyceal system which is perfused with urine and they usually dissolve silently. The stone matrix remains, and may cause renal colic or form the basis of a calcium containing stone. The drug crosses the placental barrier and penicillamine administration (about 1 g per day) has been continued throughout pregnancy without any adverse effect on the fetus or growth of the baby. Larger doses (2 g per day) have been reported to cause a generalized connective tissue dysplasia in the fetus with a picture resembling the Ehlers–Danlos syndrome in the neonate. It is therefore wise to discontinue penicillamine administration if possible during pregnancy. About half of the cystinuric patients treated with penicillamine develop morbilliform or urticarial rashes with or without fever on about the tenth day of treatment. Prednisolone (initial dose 15 mg followed by 10 mg every eight hours) controls the manifestations of acute hypersensitivity. Penicillamine is introduced under this prednisolone cover, and when the urinary cystine excretion has been lowered sufficiently, the steroid dose is reduced to zero over the course of about one week. Abnormal sensitivity to penicillamine is sometimes accompanied by allergy to penicillin.

Proteinuria occurs less frequently and usually develops insidiously after at least several months of treatment. Clinically, there appear to be two groups of patients, those who progress rapidly to a nephrotic syndrome and those in whom the proteinuria does not increase, even if the drug is continued. Recovery occurs in all cases if the drug is withdrawn; steroids have been used to hasten recovery in the most severe cases but their contribution to this is difficult to evaluate. Penicillamine should be stopped as soon as proteinuria is detected, unless there are particularly strong reasons for continuing.

There is no evidence that pyridoxine deficiency induced by penicillamine is responsible for any of the adverse side effects of penicillamine treatment and it is not necessary to give this vitamin routinely during penicillamine therapy.

The surgical treatment of cystine stones does not differ from the approach to urolithiasis in general. Stones in a region of the pelvicalyceal system which is perfused with urine can be treated medically provided that they are not obstructing the flow of urine. Complicating urinary tract infections should be treated vigorously under strict bacteriological surveillance, and prolonged antibiotic treatment may be needed to eradicate active pyelonephritis.

Methionine malabsorption syndrome

Pathophysiology. Failure to transport methionine normally across the intestinal epithelium leaves an abnormal amount of the amino acid in the bowel lumen where it is metabolized by bacteria to yield α-hydroxybutyric acid. This is absorbed and excreted in the urine, faeces, and sweat to which it imparts the characteristic oast house, or dry celery-like odour. The urine also contains the branched chain ketoacids (α-ketoisocaproic, α-keto-β-methylvaleric and α-keto-isovaleric acid), which are derived from the branched chain amino acids leucine, isoleucine, and valine respectively. This is attributed to inhibition of the absorption of the amino acids by unabsorbed methionine and their metabolism by the colonic flora. Methionine is the predominant urinary amino acid presumably because the proximal convoluted tubule has the same transport defect as the intestinal epithelium; there is also increased excretion of phenylalaline and tyrosine.

Clinical aspects. Methionine malabsorption syndrome presents in early childhood with psychomotor delay, epilepsy, and acute episodes of vomiting, diarrhoea, and ketoacidosis. The patients die from the severe metabolic acidosis unless dietary methionine is restricted. The possible effect on mental development of instituting this regimen from birth has not been assessed. The diet abolishes the convulsions, diarrhoea, and α-hydroxybutyric aciduria, and normalizes the EEG pattern.

Dicarboxylic amino-acidurias. Two groups of patients with a specific renal tubule transport defect for the dicarboxylic acids (aspartic and glutamic acids) have been described. In one, the only abnormality is a high renal clearance of these amino acids which exceeds the glomerular filtration rate. This was an incidental finding in a 38-month old baby. The metabolic lesion may involve excessive renal production of these amino acids with a failure to transfer them into the blood stream so that they accumulate and are excreted into the urine. The second type of dicarboxylic aciduria is associated with impaired intestinal absorption of these compounds, oligophrenia, and fasting hypoglycaemia. This patient was also athyreotic. The extent to which this contributed to the oligophrenia and the specificity of the association between impaired renal and intestinal transport of the dicarboxylic acids is not known.

References

Bremer, H. J., Duran, M., Kamerling, J. P., Przyrembel, H., and Wadman, S. K. (1981). *Disturbances of amino acid metabolism: clinical chemistry and diagnosis.* Urban and Schwarzenburg, Baltimore and Munich.
Crawhall, J. C. (1974a). Cystinuria—diagnosis and treatment. In *Heritable disorders of amino acid metabolism: patterns of clinical expression and genetic variation* (ed. W. L. Nyhan). Wiley, New York.
— (1974b). The uncommon disorders of sulphur amino acid metabolism. In *Heritable disorders of amino acid metabolism: patterns of clinical expression and genetic variation* (ed. W. L. Nyhan). Wiley, New York.
—, Purkiss, P., Watts, R. W. E., and Young, E. P. (1969). The excretion of amino acids by cystinuric patients and their relatives. *Ann. human Genet., Lon.* **33**, 149.
Scriver, C. R. and Rosenberg, L. E. (1973a) Amino acid metabolism and its disorders. In *Major problems in clinical pediatrics* (ed. A. L. Schaffer), vol. 10. W. B. Saunders, Philadelphia.
—, — (1973b). Nature and disorders of cystine and dibasic amino acid transport. In *Amino acid metabolism and its disorders.* W. B. Saunders, London and Toronto.
Stephens, A. D. and Watts, R. W. E. (1971). The treatment of cystinuria with N-acetyl-D-penicillamine, a comparison with the results of D-penicillamine treatment. *Q. Jl Med.* **40**, 355.
Watts, R. W. E. (1982). Cystinuria and xanthinuria. In *Scientific foundations of urology*, 2nd edn.(eds. D. I. Williams and G. D. Chisholm). Heinemann, London.

Lysosomal storage diseases

R. W. E. Watts

Lysosomes are subcellular cytoplasmic particles which contain hydrolytic enzymes. These enzymes catalyse the intralysosomal breakdown of complex molecules derived either from macromolecules entering the cell by endocytosis, or from the internal structural components of the cell itself. The lysosomal storage diseases are due to inborn errors of metabolism affecting specific lysosomal enzymes so that either undegraded or partially degraded macromolecules accumulate in the lysosomes. The engorged lysosomes distort the internal architecture of the cell and disturb its function, and there are secondary abnormalities of other lysosomal enzyme activities which are unrelated to the primary enzyme deficiency.

It has recently been shown that lysosomal enzymes are discharged from cells during exocytosis and taken up again by either the same or a different cell during endocytosis. The re-uptake depends on the carbohydrate recognition markers which are attached to the enzyme protein, and the corresponding recognition marker on the cell surface.

Sphingolipidoses

The sphingolipid molecule contains a hydrophobic portion, ceramide (N-acylsphingosine) and a hydrophylic portion which is a carbohydrate in the case of the gangliosides and phosphorylcholine in the case of sphingomyelin. The galactose residues are sulphated in the sulphatides. The sphingolipids are degraded by a series of lysosomal hydrolases and deficiencies of the individual enzymes cause the degradation products, which are characteristic of each disease (Fig. 1, Table 1), to accumulate intralysosomally. The different diseases and different variants of the same disease have characteristic organ distribution patterns of the abnormal storage products. The diseases in which there is an abnormal sphingolipid accumulation in the neuronal cells of the central nervous system, and, therefore, in the ganglion cells of the retina also, show retinal degeneration, which is particularly apparent at the macula causing pallor of this part of the retina with a central red area (the cherry red spot); pigmentary retinal changes are also found in some cases. The cherry red spot is a useful general pointer to the sphingolipidoses with neuronal involvement.

Except for Fabry disease which is inherited in a sex-linked recessive manner, the sphingolipidoses are all autosomal recessive disorders.

Farber's disease (ceramidase deficiency). A hoarse cry, painful swollen joints with peri-articular nodules, and pulmonary infiltrations developing in a previously healthy infant between two and four months of age suggest this diagnosis. The retina in the macular region appears grey with a cherry red centre. The disease exists in severe and mild forms and death is usually due to pulmonary involvement. Most cases have developed severe mental handicap. Thickening of the heart valves is usual, but hepatosplenomegaly and generalized lymphadenopathy are inconstant features.

Niemann–Pick disease (sphingomyelin lipidosis; sphingomyelinase deficiency). There are five phenotypic variants: type A, the acute neuronopathic form; type B, the chronic form without neurological involvement; type C, the chronic neuronopathic form; type D, the Nova Scotia variant; type E, the adult non-neuronopathic form. They all show abnormal lipid storage in the reticulo-endothelial macrophages and this is demonstrable in the sternal marrow and sometimes in circulating monocytes. The abnormal cells are large (50–90 μm in diameter) and look foamy.

Type A is the most common variety: hepatosplenomegaly, lymphadenopathy, and neurological retrogression with epileptic attacks begin during the first 6–12 months of life, and most patients die before the age of two years. About half the cases have the cherry red spot appearance at the macula. The type B patients develop hepatosplenomegaly and pulmonary infiltration with sphingomyelin laden histiocytes, but there is no neurological involvement. Type C patients show psychomotor delay and retrogression during early childhood and die in later childhood or adolescence. Hepatosplenomegaly is less marked in this variant than in types A and B. Type D patients resemble those with the chronic neuronopathic variant but they have been shown to share a common ancestry arising in western Nova Scotia. Type E patients present in adult life with moderate hepatosplenomegaly, but no neurological involvement. Some late presenting cases have shown mild cerebellar ataxia and the cherry red spot at the macula.

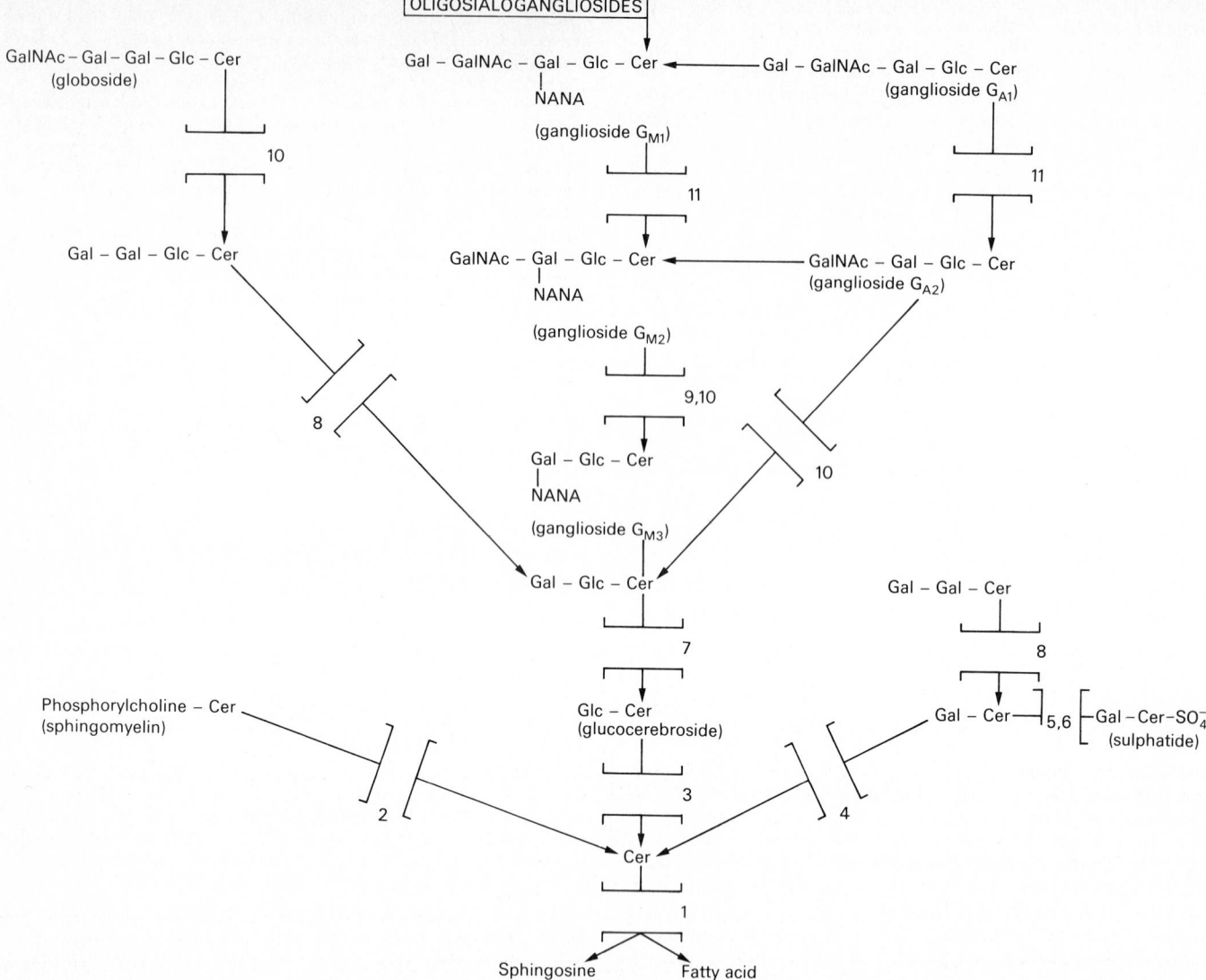

Fig. 1   Sphingolipid catabolism and the abbreviated structures of the sphingolipids which accumulate in the sphingolipidoses. The numerals indicate the metabolic blocks in the individual sphingolipidoses and correspond to those used in Table 1. Oligosialogangliosides are gangliosides with either 2, or 3, N-acetylneuraminic acid (NANA) residues per molecule as opposed to the monosialogangliosides (G_M series) and the asialogangliosides (G_A series). Cer = ceramide; Glc = glucose.004 galactose; GalNAc = N-acetylgalactosamine; NANA = N-acetylneuraminic acid (sialic acid). There are no known diseases due to lack of the enzyme which catalyses the cleavage of NANA from the sialogangliosides. G_{M3} gangliosidosis is due to reduced activity of the transferase which converts the G_M series gangliosides to the more highly sialylated G_D and G_T series (oligosialogangliosides).

Gaucher disease (glucocerebrosidosis, glucocerebrosidase deficiency). There are three clinical types of Gaucher disease: type 1, chronic non-neuronopathic (adult); type 2, acute neuronopathic (infantile); type 3, subacute neuronopathic (juvenile). All types of patients have hepatosplenomegaly and large (20–80 μm diameter) glucocerebroside-containing reticulo-endothelial histiocytes (Gaucher cells) in the bone marrow. These cells have a crumpled-silk appearance in the usual stained preparations. Increased amounts of glucocerebroside occur in the plasma and erythrocytes.

Type 1 is the commonest and has an especially high incidence in Ashkenazi Jews (1:2500 births). It may present with hepatosplenomegaly in childhood although the main disabilities occur later. The spleen becomes very large and attacks of left upper abdominal pain due to splenic infarction occur. Grey-brown pigmentation of the forehead, hands, and pretibial region is characteristic. Wedge-shaped yellow brown subconjuctival plaques (pingueculae) develop in the region of the corneoscleral junction. Bone marrow infiltration interferes with bone growth and mineralization; pathological fractures, bone pain and deformities including the classical

Ehrlenmeyer flask-like expansion of the lower end of the femur, and avascular necrosis of the femoral head are major complications in older patients. Anaemia is common, due to bone marrow replacement and to hypersplenism. Haemorrhages due to thrombocytopenia are a major complication. The serum level of non-prostatic acid phosphatase is increased. The hepatic involvement is not usually reflected in the results of biochemical tests of liver function.

Thrombocytopenia, hypersplenism, recurrent painful splenic infarction, and abdominal discomfort due to a greatly enlarged spleen are indications for splenectomy. Attempts at treatment by enzyme replacement are still being evaluated.

Patients with acute neuronopathic (type 2) Gaucher disease have hepatosplenomegaly, and show developmental delay and retrogression by the age of six months. There are fits, focal neurological signs, and pulmonary infections due to infiltration of the lung parenchyma by Gaucher cells. These patients die during the first year of life.

The subacute neuronopathic (type 3) cases present in later child-

Table 1 The sphingolipidoses. The materials listed under biochemical diagnosis are those which have been most frequently used for this purpose. The enzyme defect is usually more generally demonstrable. Prenatal diagnosis is only recorded as being possible if a correct predictive result has been obtained. The presence of the enzyme in normal fibroblasts or amniotic cells does not guarantee that prenatal diagnosis will be possible

Number in Fig. 1	Systematic name	Eponymous and/or other generally used name	Main storage compound	Enzyme deficiency	Biochemical diagnosis	Prenatal diagnosis	Carrier state diagnosis
1	Ceramidosis	Farber disease	ceramide	ceramidase	ceramide in skin nodules; enzyme in leucocytes, fibroblasts	no	no
2	Sphingomyelinosis	Niemann–Pick disease	sphingomyelin	sphingomyelinase	enzyme in leucocytes, fibroblasts	yes	yes
3	Glucocerebrosidosis	Gaucher disease	glucocerebroside	glucocerebroside β-glucosidase	glucocerebroside in liver, erythrocytes; enzyme in leucocytes, fibroblasts	yes	yes
4	Galactocerebrosidosis	Krabbé disease globoid cell leucodystrophy	galactocerebroside	galactocerebroside β-galactosidase	enzyme in serum, leucocytes, fibroblasts	no	yes
5	Sulphatidosis	metachromatic leucodystrophy	cerebroside sulphates	arylsulphatase A (cerebroside sulphatase)	enzyme in leucocytes, fibroblasts, hair bulbs, urine	yes	yes
6	Mucosulphatidosis	multiple sulphatase deficiency syndrome	cerebroside sulphates steroid sulphates	arylsulphatase A, B, C and steroid sulphatase	enzymes in leucocytes, fibroblasts, urine; dermatan and heparan sulphates in urine	no	no
7	Lactosylceramidosis	—	lactosylceramide	lactosylceramide β-galactosidase	enzyme in fibroblasts; lactosyl ceramide in erythrocytes, plasma, bone marrow, urine sediment	no	yes
8	α-galactosyl-lactosyl-ceramidosis	Fabry disease, Anderson–Fabry disease, angiokeratoma corporis diffusum	α-galactosyl-lactosyl-ceramide	α-galactosidase	enzyme in leucocytes, hair bulbs, fibroblasts, tissue biopsies, trihexoside in urine deposit	no	yes
9	G_{M2}-gangliosidosis type $A_O B_H$	Tay–Sachs disease	ganglioside G_{M2}	N-acetyl-β-D-hexosaminidases	enzymes in leucocytes, fibroblasts, plasma	yes	yes
10	G_{M2}-gangliosidosis type $A_O B_O$	Sandhoff disease	ganglioside G_{M2} globoside	N-acetyl-β-D-hexosaminidases A and B	enzymes in leucocytes, fibroblasts, plasma	yes	yes
11	G_{M1}-gangliosidosis	—	ganglioside G_{M1}	β-galactosidase	enzymes in leucocytes, fibroblasts, urine	yes	yes

hood and may survive into adult life with a variable degree of intellectual impairment, focal neurological manifestations, and seizures as well as the systemic manifestations of the disease.

Krabbé's disease (globoid cell leukodystrophy: galactosyl ceramide lipidosis). Most of these patients present with signs of progressive neurological degeneration between three and nine months of age and die before three years. Apart from the developmental delay and retrogression, optic atrophy, deafness, and progressive long tract signs are prominent features. A few cases presenting later in childhood and running a slower but equally fatal course have been reported. The main pathological changes are in the white matter of the central nervous system which contains large PAS-positive cells some of which are multinucleate, the globoid cells. These are rich in galactosylceramide, which accumulates behind the metabolic block (Fig. 1). The globoid cells are mesodermal and not modified neuroglia as was formerly thought; and they are a specific histiocytic response to galactosylceramide as opposed to the sphingolipids which accumlate in the other sphingolipidoses. The white matter shows very extensive demyelination and astrocytic gliosis.

Metachromatic leucodystrophy (sulphatidosis). The three clinical types of metachromatic leucodystrophy are defined by the age of onset of symptoms and their evolution. The late infantile type (incidence about 1:40 000) usually presents with increasing flaccid paresis and inco-ordination between ages of one and four years, although a few patients have a phase of spastic paraplegia or diplegia; the deep reflexes are usually reduced. There is psycho-motor retrogression until the patient reaches a bedridden vegetative state having lost all contact with his surroundings. Optic atrophy, and a grey discoloration with a cherry red spot at the macula are characteristic ophthalmoscopic findings. The juvenile form (incidence about 1:160 000) presents in later childhood and adolescence with a greater emphasis on intellectual deterioration and emotional disorders as early symptoms, and locomotor disturbances including dystonia beginning somewhat later. Adult patients present with psychosis and dementia, followed by progressive loss of motor functions and seizures, and die in early middle life. The enzyme deficiency can be shown in leucocytes, cultured fibroblasts, hair bulbs, and plasma. Metachromatic deposits are demonstrable in sural nerve biopsy specimens, and the conduction velocity in peripheral nerves is reduced.

Multiple sulphatase deficiency (mucosulphatidosis). The clinical course of these patients resembles that of late infantile metachromatic leucodystrophy except that features reminiscent of the muco-polysaccharidoses are added. Thus, the facies is coarse and Hurler-like, the liver and spleen are enlarged, and the skeleton shows dysostosis multiplex. The urine contains dermatan and heparan sulphates.

Lactosylceramidosis. The few reported cases of this rare condition have shown psychomotor delay and retrogression beginning at about the age of two years. There is marked muscle hypotonia, ataxia, and tremor with optic atrophy. Progressive neurological damage leads to death within a year or so of presentation. The liver, spleen, and lymph nodes are enlarged. There are no skeletal abnormalities but the cells of the reticulo-endothelial system contain fine lipid droplets and these can be demonstrated in a bone marrow aspirate.

Fabry disease (Anderson–Fabry disease; glycosphingolipid lipidosis, ceramide trihexosidosis). Fabry disease is inherited in an X-linked recessive manner. The male hemizygotes, therefore, show the full syndrome and the heterozygous female carriers either show the disease in a mild form or are asymptomatic.

The clinical manifestations are mainly due to intralysosomal deposits of α-galactosyl-lactosyl-ceramide (trihexoside) in the endothelial, perithelial, and smooth muscle cells of the blood vessels and in the histiocytic cells of the reticulo-endothelial system. The crystalline trihexoside is birefringent with a characteristic Maltese cross apearance. Deposits are prominent in the epithelial cells of the cornea, the glomeruli, and tubules of the kidney, myocardium, ganglion cells of the autonomic nervous system and Schwann cells of peripheral nerves. The abnormal cells in the kidney look foamy. Intra and extracellular trihexoside is present in the urinary centrifuge deposit.

Attacks of severe burning pain and paraesthesiae in the extremities may be the presenting feature in childhood and adolescence. Heat, cold, and physical exertion may precipitate the attacks, which may be accompanied by fever. Episodes of nausea, vomiting, abdominal pain, Raynaud phenomenon, and musculoarticular pains may also occur. The cutaneous lesions (*angiokeratoma corporis diffusum*) usually appear in childhood or around puberty and their number increases with the passage of time. They are bright red to blue-black telangiectases, which may be flat or slightly raised and scaly, and are most numerous on the lower trunk and thighs. Small numbers of these lesions are usually present elsewhere, including the buccal mucosa and conjuctiva.

The eyes show corneal and lens opacities, the aneurysmal dilatation of small thin-walled retinal venules. The trihexoside deposits in the walls of the coronary arteries predispose to ischaemic heart disease, and heart valves are distorted by infiltration with trihexoside laden histiocytes and secondary fibrosis. Pulmonary infiltration and avascular necrosis of bone are other complications.

The hemizygous males die in the fourth or fifth decade from renal failure, cerebrovascular disease, myocardial infarction or cardiac failure. The heterozygous carrier females may have any of the manifestations which occur in the affected males but to a lesser degree. The characteristic renal histological appearances are seen in the carrier females, and they may die of renal or cardiovascular disease due to the abnormal trihexoside deposition. Careful examination of the eyes often shows corneal changes in otherwise unaffected female carriers.

The angiokeratomas have to be distinguished from Campbell de Morgan spots (senile angiomas) which are usually brighter red in colour, on the upper trunk, and less numerous; and angiokeratomas of the scrotum (Fordyce) which are common in older men. The lesions of Osler–Weber–Rendu disease (congenital haemorrhagic telangiectasia) are brighter red, less grouped, and occur chiefly around the mouth, nose, lips and on the fingers. Angiomas identical to those of Fabry's disease have been reported in fucosidosis.

Renal transplantation, performed because of renal failure, has been shown to provide a source of the missing enzyme.

The G_{M2}-gangliosidoses. There are two isoenzymes (A and B) of the hexosaminidase which catalyses the coversion of the G_{M2}- and G_{A2}-gangliosides to G_{M3}-gangliosides and of globoside to α-galactosyl-lactosyl-ceramide (Fig. 1). Severe deficiency of both isoenzymes causes Sandhoff's disease, and a severe deficiency of isoenzyme-A causes Tay–Sachs disease. Less severe deficiencies of hexosaminidase-A are associated with the juvenile and adult variants of G_{M2}-gangliosidosis. These four disorders are genetically distinct and no clinical phenotype has as yet been associated with a specific deficiency of hexosaminidase B.

Tay–Sachs disease (infantile G_{M2}-gangliosidosis). This has a particularly high incidence (1:2000) among Ashkenazi Jews. Progressive generalized motor weakness begins at about six months of age, and there is rapid psychomotor regression with seizures, blindness, and deafness between 12 and 18 months. The child lapses into a vegetative state with decerebrate rigidity, increasingly severe fits, and dies before it is three years old. The cherry red spot appearance of the macula is often present early in the evolution of the disease, and the head enlarges abnormally rapidly due to neuronal ganglioside accumulation and cerebral gliosis. A doll-like facies, pale skin, and the startle reaction (a flexion of the arms and extension of the legs in response to a sudden sound) are classical although non-specific features of patients in the late stages of the disease. Microscopically, the neuronal cells of the central and autonomic nervous systems contain large amounts of ganglioside G_{M2} which is arranged as laminated masses within engorged lysosomes. These appearances in the autonomic nervous sytem can be demonstrated by a rectal biopsy.

Sandhoff's disease. This cannot be distinguished from very rapidly evolving Tay–Sachs disease clinically or on histopathological grounds. There are, however, minor differences in the proportion of the different gangliosides in the brain and other tissues.

Juvenile G_{M2}-gangliosidosis. This presents between two and six years of age usually with ataxia. There is loss of speech, progressive spasticity, dystonic posturing, and seizures. Blindness occurs late although optic atrophy, retinitis pigmentosa, and the macula cherry red spot have been reported. The patients die in later childhood or in their teens.

Adult G_{M2}-gangliosidosis. This presents with slowly progressive difficulty in walking, muscular atrophy, inco-ordination, dystonia, and dysarthria. Intellect and vision are not affected.

The G_{M1}-gangliosidoses (generalized gangliosidoses). Undegraded gangliosides (G_{M1} and G_{A1}) accumulate in the viscera as well as in the nervous tissues in this group of disorders, and some of the phenotypic features resemble the dysmorphism of Hurler disease. The term *generalized gangliosidoses* emphasizes the more extensive changes in the composition of the visceral gangliosides in contradistinction to the situation which prevails in the G_{M2}-gangliosidoses, where the changes are mainly neuronal.

Infantile G_{M1}-gangliosidosis. Symptoms begin at birth or shortly thereafter; there is oedema of the extremities, and psychomotor retardation is obvious from the first weeks of life. Sucking and swallowing are poor and there are frequent seizures. The patient passes into a state of decerebrate rigidity with blindness, deafness, spastic quadriplegia, and dies before the age of two years. There is marked muscle hypotonia. The facial features are coarse, with frontal bossing, depressed nasal bridge, low set ears, gum hypertrophy, and macroglossia. The corneae are usually clear and the cherry red spot appearance of the macula is often present. Head size increases abnormally rapidly but to a lesser degree than in Tay–Sachs disease. Hepatosplenomegaly is usually evident by the time the child is a few months old, and dysostosis multiplex develops. The undegraded gangliosides accumulate in neuronal cells, parenchymal cells of the viscera, and in reticulo-endothelial macrophages. The abnormal ganglioside storage impairs the degradation of the mucopolysaccharides so that some tissues also contain a keratan sulphate-like glycosaminoglycan. The cells look foamy in the visceral organs.

Juvenile G_{M1}-gangliosidosis. Symptoms begin between the ages of 6 and 20 months but these patients rarely survive beyond 10 years. Psychomotor delay is often apparent by the end of the first year and is followed by retrogression. Ataxias, squints, generalized muscle weakness, inco-ordination and progressive spasticity, and sometimes blindness develop. The facial features are not coarsened, the retina and macula appear normal, and the liver and spleen are not usually enlarged. The dysostosis multiplex is minimal. The appearances of the neurones with stored gangliosides are identical with those seen in the infantile type. Some visceral histiocytosis is usually present, and the bone marrow contains foamy-looking histiocytes.

G_{M3}-gangliosidosis. No clinical phenotype has so far been identified which is associated with a failure to convert G_{M3}-ganglioside to glucocerebroside (Fig. 1) due to ganglioside neuraminidase deficiency. This enzyme is distinct from the sialyloligosaccharide neuraminidase, deficiency of which causes sialidosis (mucolipidosis I).

G_{M3}-gangliosidosis is due to biosynthetic failure whereby G_{M2}-ganglioside cannot be converted to G_{M2}-ganglioside by the addition of N-acetylgalactosamine. The deficient enzyme is G_{M3}-UDP-GalNAc transferase. There is progressive failure of neurological functions with fits from birth, macroglossia, and coarse facies but no visceromegaly or mucopolysacchariduria. There are no gross intraneuronal deposits of gangliosides but the proportion of G_{M3}

relative to the longer chain gangliosides and the more highly sialy-
ated homologues is abnormally high.

Mucopolysaccharidoses

The mucopolysaccharidoses are a group of seven inborn errors of
metabolism in which the activity of one of the exoglycosidases
which catalyse the sequential removal of individual carbohydrate
groups from the mucopolysaccharides (glycosaminoglycans) is deficient. Their combined incidence is about 1:10 000. These diseases
were originally classified on the basis of the clinical features and the
pattern of mucopolysacchariduria. Their eponymous names are
still widely used although McKusick and his colleagues have prepared a numerical classification. The terminology, biochemistry,
genetics and main clinical features are summarized in Table 2.
Hurler and Hunter diseases were formerly called gargoylism
because of their characteristic facies. Maroteaux–Lamy disease,
some of the mucolipidoses, α-fucosidosis, and mannosidosis have
similar Hurler-like features.

The term dysostosis multiplex is now used specifically for the
skeletal changes demonstrated radiologically in this group of disorders. The term lipochondrodystrophy, which was formerly used
because it was thought that the stored material was a lipid, has been
abandoned. The primary abnormal storage products are carbohydrate polymers. These produce secondary changes in lysosomal
function, including some impairment of ganglioside turnover. The
tissue deposits of highly sulphated mucopolysaccharides stain
metachromatically.

Mucopolysaccharide deposits in relation to the meninges can
cause hydrocephalus, spinal cord compression, arachnoid cysts,
and radiculopathies. These complications arise in all of the mucopolysaccharidoses irrespective of whether the functions of the
neuronal and glial cells are primarily impaired by intracellular
mucopolysaccharide deposits or not.

The presence of mucopolysaccharide inclusion bodies (Alder–
Reilly bodies) in the white blood cells is another feature which is
common to all of the mucopolysaccharidoses. Except in Morquio
disease (mucopolysaccharidosis IV) their accumulation in cultured
fibroblasts can be demonstrated by studying the uptake and release
of $^{35}SO_4$ by the cells *in vitro*. The cross correction of the enzyme-
deficient cells can also be demonstrated by growing them in tissue
culture medium in which normal cells or cells from a patient with
another lysosomal storage disease have been grown. The precise
enzymological diagnosis is made on either leucocytes or cultured
fibroblasts and prenatal diagnosis on cultured amniotic cells.

Hurler disease (mucopolysaccharidosis I H). The classical Hurler
facies (Fig. 2) comprises thickenend, stiff, soft tissues of the lips,
nares, and face generally, depressed nasal bridge, wide bony ridge
in the centre of the forehead, bushy eyebrows, and some degree of
macrocephaly. There is upper respiratory obstruction with mouth
breathing and chronic upper respiratory tract infection. The gums
are hyperplastic and the teeth widely spaced and poorly formed.
Corneal clouding, deafness of multifactorial origin, and generalized thickening and stiffening of the skin are other features.

The diagnosis is usually suggested at age 6–12 months by the
association of psychomotor delay and the developing facial
appearance. Corneal clouding and loss of the normal lumbar lordo-
sis are other early signs. Dwarfing is usually evident by age two or
three years and the children die before they are 10 years old having
shown profound psychomotor regression. Other prominent clinical
features are hepatosplenomegaly, progressive joint stiffness and
contractures; the latter affect the terminal interphalangeal joints
and radioulnar joints early and there is a dorsolumbar kyphosis.
Figures 3–7 show the bone changes, some of which are visible
radiologically during the first weeks of life.

A complicating hydrocephalus due to mucopolysaccharide de-

Table 2 The mucopolysaccharidoses

McKusick's classification	Eponymous name	Enzyme deficiency	Excreted glycosaminoglycans	Inheritance	Organs mainly affected	Facial appearance
I H	Hurler	α-L-iduronidase	dermatan sulphate heparan sulphate	autosomal recessive	central nervous system skeleton viscera	classical Hurler appearance
I S	Scheie	α-L-iduronidase	dermatan sulphate heparan sulphate	autosomal recessive	skeleton (mild relative to Hurler) viscera (mild relative to Hurler)	coarse features ± (not specifically Hurler like)
I H/S	Hurler/Scheie	α-L-iduronidase	dermatan sulphate heparan sulphate	autosomal recessive	phenotype intermediate between Hurler and Scheie diseases	coarse features ± (not specifically Hurler-like); micrognathism
II	Hunter	iduronate sulphate sulphatase	dermatan sulphate heparan sulphate	sex-linked recessive	central nervous system skeleton viscera mild and severe phenotypes reported	Hurler-like
III A	Sanfilippo A	heparan N-sulphatase	heparan sulphate	autosomal recessive	central nervous system	not characteristic
III B	Sanfilippo B	N-acetyl-α-D-gluco-saminidase	heparan sulphate	autosomal recessive	central nervous system	not characteristic
III C	Sanfilippo C	α-glucosamine-N-acetyl transferase	heparan sulphate	autosomal recessive	central nervous system	not characteristic
III D	Sanfilippo D	N-acetyl-glucosamine-6-sulphate sulphatase	heparan sulphate	autosomal recessive	central nervous system	not characteristic
IV	Morquio	galactosamine 6-sulphatase	keratan sulphate	autosomal recessive	skeleton	not characteristic
V*						
VI	Maroteaux–Lamy	N-acetylgalactosamine 4-sulphatase (aryl sulphatase B)	dermatan sulphate	autosomal recessive	skeleton mild and severe phenotypes reported	Hurler-like
VII		β-glucuronidase	dermatan sulphate heparan sulphate	autosomal recessive	central nervous system skeleton viscera	Hurler-like

* Originally Scheie disease which was re-classified as mucopolysaccharidosis I S when the enzyme defect was shown to be the same as that in Hurler disease. The possibility that Hurler and Scheie diseases are due to allelic mutations and that the intermediate Hurler/Scheie phenotype (mucopolysaccharidoses I H/S) is due to double heterozygosity for the allelic mutations concerned has been widely proposed. The Hurler/Scheie phenotype could also be due to homozygosity for a third allelic mutation at the same gene locus

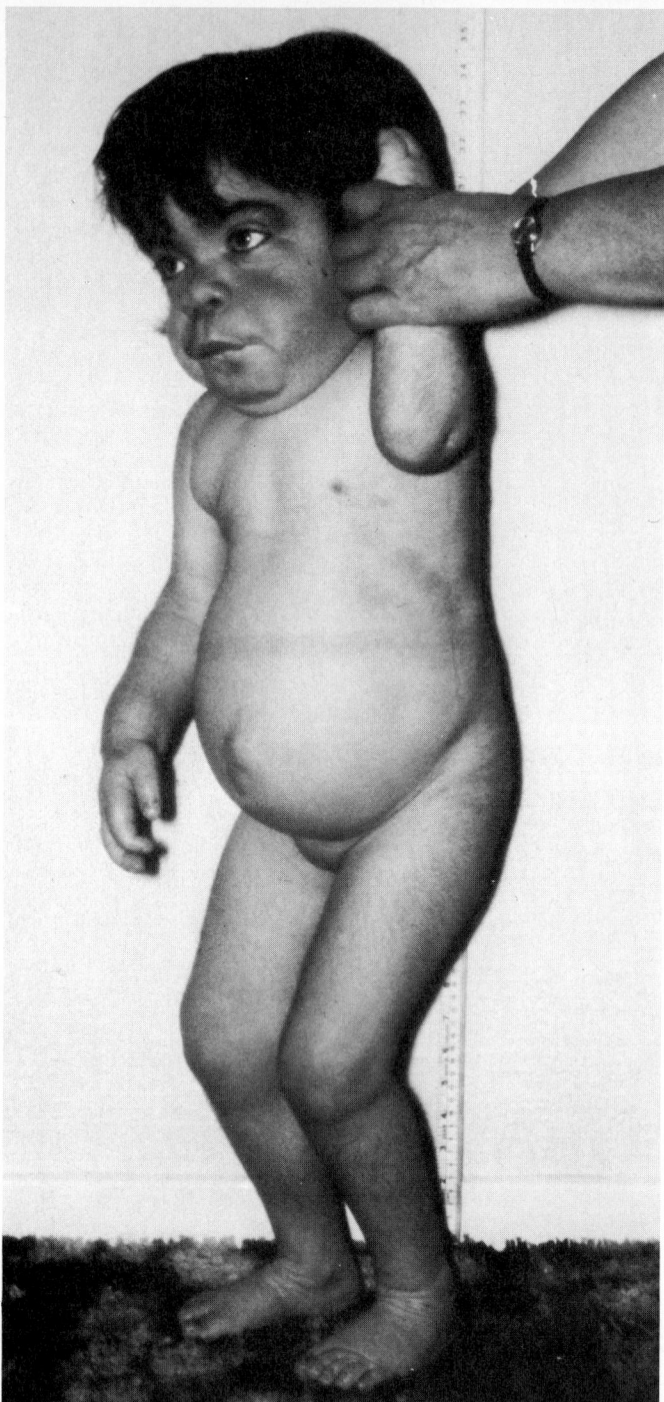

Fig. 2 The typical facies of a patient with Hurler disease.

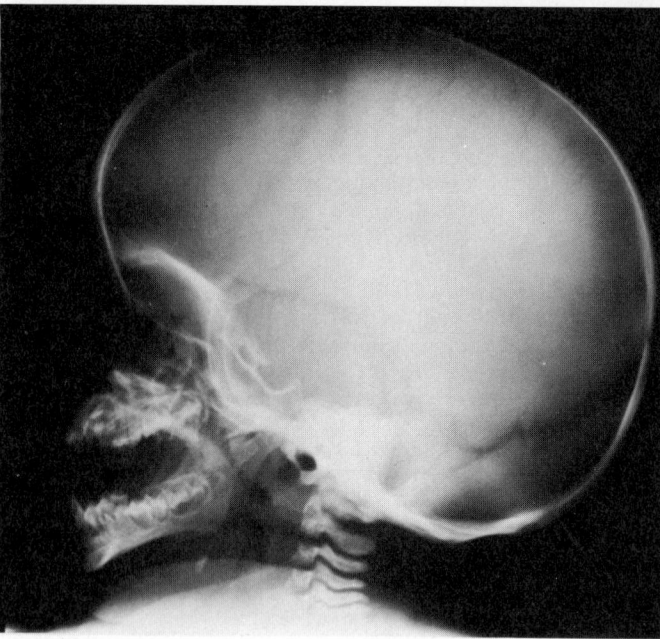

Fig. 3 Dysostosis multiplex. The skull in a case of Hurler disease (female age 13 months). Premature fusion of the sagital suture produces dolichocephaly. The pituitary fossa is J-shaped or shoe-shaped, with a large recess extending under the anterior clinoid processes. The normal markings on the skull vault are reduced due to thickening of the meninges. The occipital suture is widened, other radiological signs of hydrocephalus may occur as the disease progresses. The teeth are irregularly placed.

posits at the base of the brain or interference with the function of the arachnoid granulations may accelerate the neurological deterioration. Blindness is due to the combined effects of corneal clouding, retinal degeneration, damage to the visual pathways, cerebral infiltration, hydrocephalus, and glaucoma. The latter may develop acutely due to mucopolysaccharide deposits in the cells lining the trabecular meshwork of the iridocorneal angle.

Hunter disease (mucopolysaccharidosis II). Although this disease usually follows a slower course than Hurler disease, cases of the severe variant cannot be distinguished from Hurler disease on clinical grounds except for the almost universal absence of corneal clouding. Patients with the genetically distinct mild variant may survive beyond the age of 30 and have either low or near normal intelligence. Most cases die in childhood or in their teens.

Sanfilippo disease (mucopolysaccharidosis III). The four biochemically distinct types are indistinguishable from one another clinically. There is severe mental deterioration with hyperkinetic behaviour but relatively mild somatic features. The patients usually die before the end of the second decade. Physical growth tends to be accelerated, and there is abundant coarse scalp hair which may be a useful diagnostic pointer. The routine qualitative tests for abnormal mucopolysacchariduria sometimes becomes negative in older children with Sanfilippo disease.

Morquio disease (mucopolysaccharidosis IV). The severe skeletal deformities dominate the clinical picture and growth virtually stops after about six years of age. The development of the vertebral bodies is grossly disordered producing flat anteriorly beaked vertebrae, kyphoscoliosis, a lumbordorsal gibbus, and hypoplasia of the odontoid process. Spinal cord compression is a frequent complication. Other features are: deafness, pectus carinatum with flaring of the lower ribs, fine corneal opacities, a broad mouth with widely spaced teeth, cardiac valvular lesions especially aortic incompetence, a moderate hepatosplenomegaly, and hypermobility of the joints. Intellect is normal and the facies is not Hurler-like.

The metabolic lesion prevents the normal degradation of keratan sulphate, which is a constituent of cartilage, the nucleus pulposus, and cornea. There are mild and severe variants of Morquio disease. Cardiorespiratory complications and cervical cord compression can be fatal.

Maroteaux–Lamy disease (mucopolysaccharidosis VI). Skeletal, corneal, and cardiac involvement, and hepatosplenomegaly are prominent features. The facies resembles that in Hurler disease but the intellect is unimpaired. Phenotypically mild, intermediate and severe variants have been described.

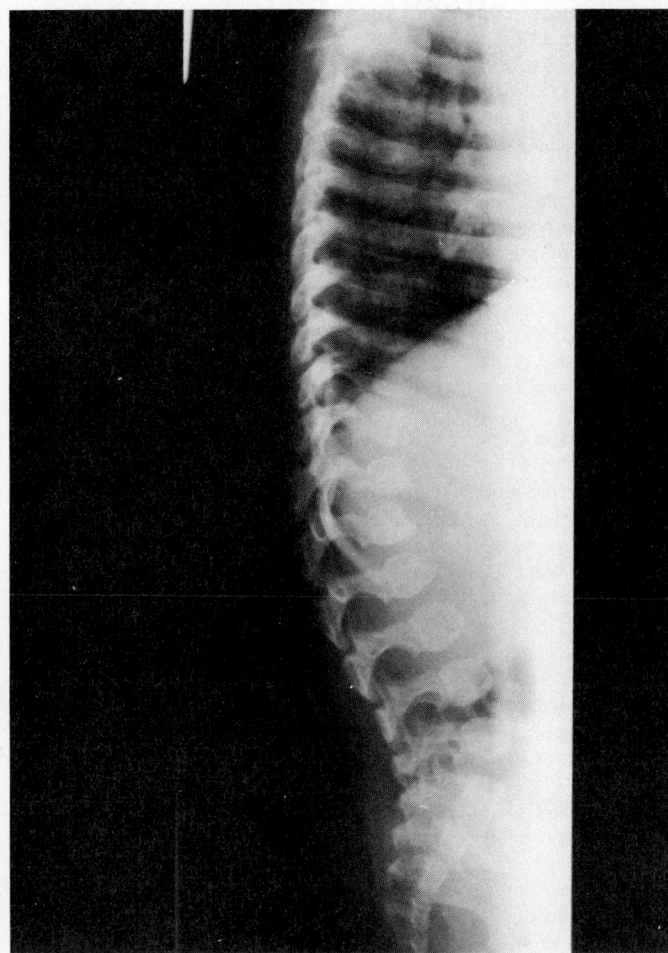

Fig. 4 Dysostosis multiplex. The spine in a case of Hurler disease (female age 13 months) showing oval vertebral bodies, anterior inferior beaking of the lumbar vertebrae and elongation of the vertebral pedicles. The loss of the normal lumbar curvature is noteworthy.

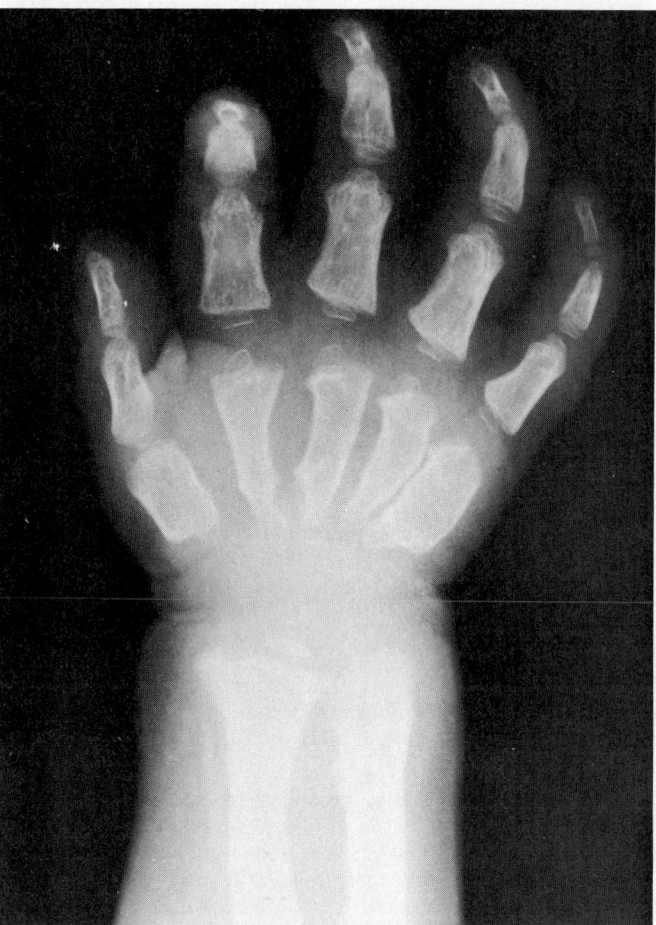

Fig. 6 Dysostotis multiplex. The hands in the case of Hurler disease (female age eight years). Bone remodelling is very abnormal with marked under-tubulation. The proximal phalanges show the bullet-shaped appearance, proximal tapering of the metacarpals is marked and the fingers are curved radially. Ossification is delayed and disordered, the lower end of the radius is expanded, and the radial and ulnar metaphyses are slanted and tilt towards each other.

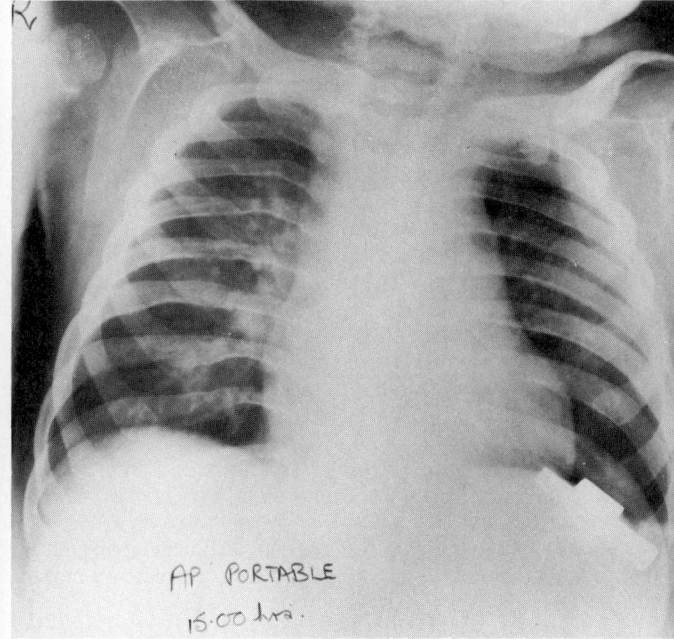

Fig. 5 Dysostotis multiplex. The chest in a case of Hurler disease (male age seven years). The ribs appear to lie more horizontally than normal, their anterior ends are expanded, and they are constricted posteriorly so that they assume a paddle shape. The clavicles are hypoplastic.

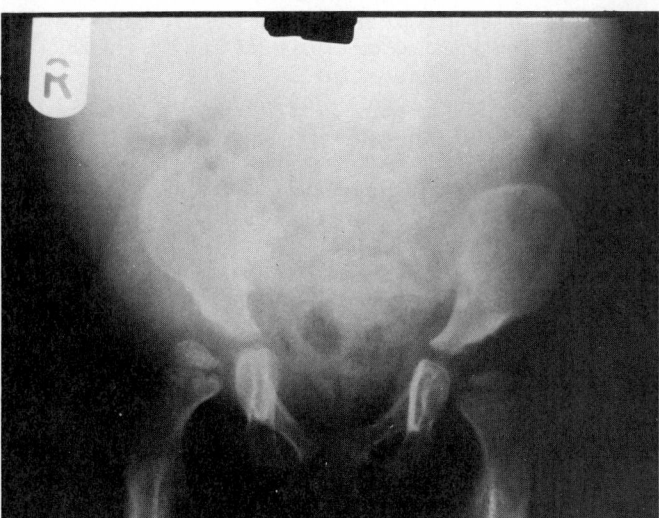

Fig. 7 Dysostosis multiplex. The pelvis in a case of Hurler disease (female age seven years). The triradiate cartilage and ischiopubic synchondroses are widened. The femoral heads are hypoplastic and uncovered due to hypopla-sia of the supra-acetabular part of the ilium. The wings of the ilia are flared and there is a marked coxa valga deformity.

Scheie disease (mucopolysaccharidosis I S). Scheie disease is a clinically mild phenotype due to a mutation at the α-iduronidase locus allelic with that which causes Hurler disease. The patients are mainly incapacitated by the arthropathy but they may develop cardiac valvular lesions and glaucoma. Mucopolysaccharide deposits in the meninges cause hydrocephalus, cervical myelopathy, radiculopathy, and arachnoid cysts. Carpal tunnel syndrome is also a well-recognized neurological complication. Mental handicap is not a feature.

Hurler–Scheie disease (mucopolysaccharidosis I H/S). This phenotype is intermediate in severity between Hurler and Scheie diseases. The patients may be homozygous for a third allelic mutation or they may be heterozygous for both Hurler disease and Scheie disease. They usually present in childhood with joint involvement, the degree of mental handicap, if any, is variable, and they are liable to have the same neurological, cardiac, and ocular complications as patients with both Hurler and Scheie diseases.

β-glucuronidase deficiency (mucopolysaccharidosis VII). These patients have the clinical features of Hurler disease but the degree of mucopolysacchariduria is relatively slight.

Mucolipidoses

The mucolipidoses were originally delineated as a group of disorders resembling the mucopolysaccharidoses clinically but in which there was no abnormal mucopolysacchariduria.

Mucolipidosis I (sialidosis: the cherry red spot/myoclonus syndrome). Mucolipidosis I is due to the deficiency of the N-acetyl-neuraminic hydrolase which cleaves sialic acid from oligosaccharides, glycoproteins, and glycolipids. The urine contains large amounts of sialic acid rich oligosaccharides. The patients are divided into Type 1 and Type 2 according to the absence or presence respectively of dysmorphic features and mental deterioration. Infantile (onset at or below one year of age) and juvenile (onset at 8–15 years) variants of Type 2 are recognized. The Type 1 patients present at 8–15 years with visual failure and action myoclonus, and have the cherry-red spot at the macula. They appear normal, and have normal or near normal intelligence. The features and skeletal abnormalities in the Type 2 patients resemble those of Hurler disease, these patients also having spasticity and ataxia, as well as cherry red spots and myoclonus. Seizures may occur in both types. Visceromegaly is rare except in the infantile variant of Type 2. Vacuolated mononuclear cells (foam cells) are seen in the blood and/or bone marrow in most cases.

Mucolipidoses II (I cell disease, inclusion cell disease) and III (pseudo-Hurler polydystrophy). Mucolipidoses II and III are due to an abnormality of multiple lysosomal enzymes whereby their carbohydrate recognition markers are defective. The basic biochemical abnormality in mucolipidoses II and III interferes with the re-uptake of exocytosed lysosomal enzymes. The levels of multiple lysosomal enzymes are greatly elevated in the body fluids, but deficient in the tissues and cultured fibroblasts. Patients with mucolipidosis II resemble cases of Hurler disease (mucopolysaccharidosis IH) clinically, and those with mucolipidosis III resemble Scheie disease (mucopolysaccharidosis IS). They may also be confused with mild variants of the Maroteaux–Lamy syndrome (mucopolysaccharidosis VI) clinically. Cultured fibroblasts from both mucolipidosis II and III patients contain highly refractile inclusions. Hence the synonym I (inclusion) cell disease for Type II.

Mucolipidosis IV. This is a recently recognized lysosomal storage disease in which there are corneal opacities, full (but not Hurler-like) facial features, and psychomotor retardation. Abnormal inclusions have been demonstrated by electron-microscopy in amniotic cells, brain, and other tissues. These patients have no dysostosis multiplex and this differentiates them from other types of mucolipidoses.

Fucosidosis and mannosidosis

α-Fucosidase and α-mannosidase are lysosomal enzymes which cleave terminal fucose and mannose residues respectively from the carbohydrate moieties of glycoproteins and glycolipids. Inherited deficiency of one of the enzymes causes oligosaccharide-containing fragments rich in the corresponding sugar to accumulate in the cells of the brain, viscera, and connective tissues and to be excreted into the urine. These enzyme deficiencies can be demonstrated in leucocytes, plasma, and cultured fibroblasts during life and prenatally in cultured amniotic cells.

Fucosidosis. The external appearances, visceromegaly, and skeletal changes resemble those of Hurler disease but there is no abnormal mucopolysacchariduria. Phenotypically mild and severe genetic variants are recognized. There is extensive and rapidly evolving neurological damage with psychomotor regression and increased sweat sodium and chloride in the former group, who die in early or mid-childhood. The mild cases have angiokeratomas resembling those seen in Fabry disease, there is less neurological damage, normal sweat salinity, and they survive longer. The erythrocyte and saliva Lewis blood group antigen (Le[a] and Le[b]) titres are raised, and the abnormal tissue glycoconjugates have Le blood group activity. These findings reflect the failure to cleave fucose residues from glycoproteins.

Mannosidosis. These patients also resemble Hurler disease clinically but have no abnormal mucopolysacchariduria. Mild and severe variants exist. The sweat electrolytes are normal. There are no angiokeratomata although a bullous hyperkeratotic condition of the skin (ichthyosiform erythroderma bullosa) has been reported.

Acid cholesteryl ester hydrolase deficiency

There are at least two allelic mutations of the gene directing the synthesis of the lysosomal acid esterase which catalyses the hydrolysis of both cholesteryl esters and triglycerides. The corresponding phenotypes are *Wolman's disease* and *cholesteryl ester storage disease*. Foamy-looking bone marrow histiocytes and lipid droplet inclusions in the circulating leucocytes occur, and the enzyme defect can be demonstrated in leucocytes, and cultured fibroblasts during life, and prenatally in cultured amniotic fluid cells.

Wolman's disease. This is the clinically more severe phenotype presenting in the first weeks of life with vomiting, diarrhoea, failure to thrive, hepatosplenomegaly, and intestinal malabsorption with adrenal gland enlargement and calcification. Symptoms specifically related to the nervous system are unusual and psychomotor delay occurring later in the disease seems to be related to the systemic illness. The infants usually die before the age of six months. Lysosomes distended with tryglycerides and cholesteryl esters are found in the parenchymal, reticulo-endothelial, and vascular endothelial cells of most organs including the central and autonomic nervous systems.

Cholesteryl ester storage disease. This follows a more benign course and may not be detected until adult life. There are widespread intralysosomal cholesteryl ester and trigyceride deposits although hepatomegaly may be the only clinical abnormality. Hypercholesterolaemia is common there may be severe premature atherosclerosis. No specific treatment is available.

The main differential diagnoses of cholesteryl ester storage disease are: (*a*) Tangier disease (familial high density lipoprotein deficiency; (*b*) familial lecithin cholesterol acyl transferase deficiency; (*c*) neutral lipid storage disease; (*d*) type I glycogen storage disease.

Other lysosomal storage diseases

Cystinosis (cystine storage disease) and Pompé's disease (type II glycogen storage disease, α-glucosidase deficiency) are reviewed on page 000 and page 000 respectively.

Lysosomal acid phosphatase deficiency is a rare cause of failure to thrive and death in the first weeks or months of life. It is inherited as an autosomal recessive.

Aspartylglycosaminuria is an autosomal recessive disorder, which has been mainly recognized in Finland. The patients have coarse features and a severe degree of mental handicap.

The results of ultrastructural studies suggest that the ceroid-lipofuscinoses are lysosomal storage diseases but their enzymological basis is unknown.

Familial diseases with storage of sterols additional to cholesterol

Cerebrotendinous xanthomatosis and β-sitosterolaemia are two apparently inherited disorders in which tendon xanthomata appear to be initiated by a metabolic lesion which primarily affects the metabolism of cholesterol in the case of cerebrotendinous xanthomatosis, and a group of plant sterols in the case of β-sitosterolaemia. In spite of this aetiology, cholesterol is quantitatively the main chemical component of the xanthomata. The specific enzyme defects have not been identified. Table 3 summarizes the main features of these two disorders.

The relationship between cerebrotendinous xanthomatosis and spinal cholesterosis (progressive spastic paraplegia with cholesterol and possibly other lipid deposits in the medulla oblongata and spinal cord) is uncertain.

Refsum's disease

Refsum's disease (see also Section 21) is an autosomal recessively inherited disease in which the long chain aliphatic alcohol phytol, which is a component of chlorophyll, cannot be degraded beyond the stage of the corresponding acid, phytanic acid, because of phytanic acid α-hydroxylase deficiency. This compound accumulates in the plasma, blood cells, and tissues generally. The peripheral nerves show segmental demyelination with hypertrophy due to concentric Schwann cell proliferation. Symptoms begin in the second decade and the course may be relapsing or steadily progressive. The main abnormalities are mixed motor and sensory polyneuropathy, cerebellar ataxia, pigmentary degeneration of the retina with failing night vision, pupillary abnormalities, nerve deafness, anosmia, ichthyosis, and cardiomyopathy.

The cerebrospinal fluid protein level is raised without a pleocytosis. A chlorophyll-free diet may produce clinical improvement and it should be begun as early in life as possible.

References

Bhattacharya, A. K. and Conmor, W. E. (1978). Familial diseases with storage of sterols other than cholesterol. In *The metabolic basis of inherited disease* (eds. J. B. Stanbury, J. B. Wyngaarden, and D. S. Fredrickson), 656. McGraw-Hill, New York.

Brady, R. O. (1978). Sphingolipidoses. *Ann. Rev. Biochem.* **47**, 687.

Cantz, M. and Gebber, J. (1976). The mucopolysaccharidoses: inborn errors of glycosaminoglycan catabolism. *Human Genet.* **32**, 233.

Desnick, R. J., Thorpe, S. R., and Fiddler, M. B. (1976). Toward enzyme therapy for lysosomal storage diseases. *Physiol. Rev.* **56**, 57.

Hers, H. G. and Van Hoof, F. (eds.) (1973). *Lysosomes and storage diseases*. Academic Press, New York.

Neufeld, E. F., Lim, T. W., and Shapiro, L. J. (1973). Inherited disorders of lysosomal metabolism. *Ann. Rev. Biochem.* **44**, 357.

Sandhoff, K. (1979). Biochemistry and genetics of gangliosidoses. *Human Genet.* **50**, 107.

Steinberg, D. (1978). Phytanic acid storage disease syndrome: Refsum's syndrome. In *The metabolic basis of inherited disease* (eds. J. B. Stanbury, J. B. Wyngaarden, and D. S. Fredrickson), 688. McGraw-Hill, New York.

Watts, R. W. E., Spellacy, E., Kendall, B. E., du Boulay, G., and Gibbs, D. A. (1981). Computed tomography studies on patients with mucopolysaccharidoses. *Neurocardiology* **9**, 23.

Table 3 Xanthomatosis with sterols additional to cholesterol

	Cerebrotendinous xanthomatosis	β-sitosterolaemia
Age at presentation	childhood or early adulthood	childhood or early adulthood
Inheritance	autosomal recessive	? autosomal recessive
Storage products	free and esterified cholestanol (dihydrocholesterol) and cholesterol	mainly unesterified cholesterol unesterified plant sterols (mainly β-sitosterol, with some campesterol and stigmasterol)
Blood chemistry	plasma lipids usually normal; no other characteristic findings	β-sitosterol, campesterol, stigmasterol; no other characteristic findings
Pathology	granulomas (xanthomas) in most tissues, especially brain, tendons, lungs, bones; ? premature atherosclerosis	granulomas (xanthomas) in tendons
Clinical features	tendon xanthomas progressive mental handicap and neurological dysfunction (ataxia, spasticity, dysarthria, focal signs) cataracts	tendon xanthomas, no neurological deficits
Treatment	none	diet low in plant sterols
Prognosis	death in middle age	? compatible with normal life-span
Metabolic lesion	? failure to degrade cholestanol ? transport defect	hyperabsorption of plant sterols which may impair stability of lipoprotein complexes and cause cholesterol deposition

Wilson's disease

A. G. Bearn

Wilson's disease is a rare autosomal, recessively inherited abnormality in the hepatic excretion of copper that results in excessive and toxic accumulations of the metal in the brain, liver, kidneys, and certain other organs. A golden brown pigmented ring at the corneal margin, the Kayser–Fleischer ring, although not an invariable finding, is virtually pathognomonic of the disease.

Clinical manifestations. Wilson's disease has an insidious onset and alertness to the possibility of the diagnosis is unusually important since, if recognized early and treated appropriately with penicillamine, the patient's condition will nearly always improve. Without treatment, the disease is relentless and leads to progressive disability and death.

Although the disease, if not suspected, is notoriously easy to misdiagnose, the clinical manifestations, although frequently protean, usually fall under two principal categories: those due to disturbances of neurological function and those of hepatic origin.

Neurological manifestations usually begin with tremor or, less commonly, rigidity. The tremors are usually apparent in the second or third decade of life and, while minimal at rest, are made markedly worse when purposive movements are attempted. Very rarely, symptoms occur as early as four years of age or, more commonly, may be delayed until the fourth decade of life. In childhood and adolescence, the untreated disease may run an accelerated course with fever, spasticity, rigidity, wild choreiform movements, drooling, dysphagia, and dysarthria. The sensory system is characteristically spared, and pyramidal signs are usually absent. In the terminal stages, the often febrile patient is emaciated and unable to swallow or care for himself. Completely bedridden, mentally impaired, and physically distorted by severe contractures, patients with the disease usually succumb to intercurrent infections. Since the introduction of penicillamine, this tragic neurological picture is rarely seen.

Cirrhosis of the liver is an essential pathological feature of Wilson's disease and can be diagnosed by liver biopsy. Clinical evidence of hepatic insufficiency is less common in adults and in those with predominantly neurological manifestations of the disease. In children and young adults, however, signs of hepatic dysfunction are frequent and may be the first evidence of Wilsons disease. The presenting symptoms and signs maybe those of acute hepatitis, or cirrhosis of the liver. A mistaken diagnosis of juvenile cirrhosis of uncertain aetiology may be made. Portal hypertension can usually be demonstrated and ascites and hepatic coma may supervene in the terminal stages of the disease. Mild, transient jaundice may be an early symptom and may be followed by several years of normal health. Wilson's disease should always be considered in the differential diagnosis of asymptomatic hepatosplenomegaly and cirrhosis of the liver, particularly in adolescents and young adults. Although mild tremor may occasionally be seen in patients who present with a hepatic features neurological symptoms are frequently absent and the neurological examination may be quite normal.

Psychiatric symptoms are common and may be the first sign of the disease. Syndromes indistinguishable from classic schizophrenia or manic depression are seen. Behavioural and personality changes, including aggressive outbursts, may be early signs.

The disease may also present with a variety of unusual signs and symptoms that obscure the diagnosis until the disease is far advanced. An acute unexplained Coombs-negative haemolytic anaemia is a not an uncommon feature and may be a presenting symptom. It usually occurs in young adults with the hepatic form of the disease, and is presumed to be due to the sudden and massive release of copper from the overladen hepatic cells of the liver. Unusual melanotic pigmentation of the lower extremities, azure lunulae, and bone lesions, including spontaneous fractures, occur.

The Kayser–Fleischer ring deserves special comment. The brownish gold, occasionally green, discoloration of the cornea is due to the deposition of copper in Descemet's membrane (Plate 4). It is virtually diagnostic and, although it may not be seen in the early stages of the disease, by the time neurological symptoms are manifest it is invariably present. However, in young patients, particularly those with the hepatic form of the disease, the ring is not always detectable. Most Kayser–Fleischer rings are visible to the naked eye and are best observed by standing behind the patient's head and shining a light on the cornea from above as the patient looks downward. The ring is most marked superiorly. It can, however, also be seen with decreasing ease inferiorly, laterally, and medially; a complete ring is not unusual. Rarely, sunflower cataracts, due to the intraocular accumulation of copper, may accompany the Kayser-Fleischer ring. The presence of a Kayser–Fleischer ring cannot be excluded with confidence without a slit lamp examination.

Genetics. (See Section 4.) The disease is found all over the world, and is particularly common in relatively isolated populations with a high inbreeding coefficient. As anticipated in rare autosomal recessive disorders, the parents of those affected are frequently first cousins. The disease has an estimated frequency of 1 in 200 000 with a carrier frequency of 1 in 500. The age of onset and clinical manifestations tend to be similar within single sibships.

Pathogenesis. A decrease in the normal biliary excretion of copper leads to a disturbance in the near-normal zero copper balance of the body. The excess copper first accumulates in the hepatocytes. As the disease progresses, the capacity of the hepatocytes to store the copper is exceeded. The copper leaks from the damaged hepatocytes and accumulates in lysozomes. Subsequently the excess copper is distributed and deposited in various organs and tissues of the body, where it causes cellular and organ damage.

In normal persons, approximately 95 per cent of the serum copper is tightly bound to caeruloplasmin. The remainder is loosely bound to serum albumin. In Wilson's disease, the total serum copper and serum caeruloplasmin decreases and the loosely bound, easily dissociable, albumin-bound copper increases. The urinary excretion of copper is usually increased. Exceptionally, but particularly in young women with chronic active hepatitis or cirrhosis, the serum copper and caeruloplasmin levels may be normal. Accumulation of copper in the kidney predominantly damages the renal tubule resulting in Fanconi's syndrome. Aminoaciduria, glycosuria, phosphaturia, uricosuria, and calciuria occur. Proteinuria may be present. A markedly increased excretion of beta microglobulin is common and may be an early sign of tubular disease. A decreased glomerular filtration rate and effective renal blood flow, as well as inadequate acidification of the urine, can often be demonstrated but are clinically unimportant.

Pathology. Although it is evident that accumulation of copper in the tissues is responsible for the symptomatology, the brain may appear surprisingly normal at autopsy. Slight cerebral atrophy is common, particularly in the basal ganglia. A non-diagnostic accumulation of large astrocytes is found throughout the central nervous system and is most marked in the region of the basal ganglia. In the increasingly rare acute form of the disease with rapidly deteriorating cerebral function, cavitation in the putamen, globus pallidus, caudate nucleus, and cerebal cortex may be evident. Abnormal fat and glycogen deposits are early findings that can be observed by light microscopy. As the disease progresses, liver damage occurs and the characteristic features of chronic active hepatitis or post-necrotic cirrhosis are evident. Mitochrondrial abnormalities are seen early in the disease by electron microscopy and are considered moderately specific. In the asymptomatic stage of the disease, the liver is grossly and histologically normal, despite an increase in the concentration of copper.

Diagnosis. The diagnosis should be suspected in all cases of unexplained tremor and rigidity, particularly in early adult life. Indeed, in any patient under the age of 40, unexplained neurological, psychiatric, or hepatic symptoms should raise the suspicion of Wilson's disease. Patients with signs or symptoms of chronic active hepatitis, or of liver disease of unknown origin should be suspected of having the disease. Although the presence of a Kayser–Fleischer ring is diagnostic and invariable in patients with neurological manifestations of the disease, the ring may be absent in children and in patients with predominantly hepatic disease. A careful slit-lamp examination should be undertaken when the diagnosis is in doubt, and in all siblings of patients with the disease.

In the absence of gross malnutrition, protein losing enteropathy, sprue, or the nephrotic syndrome, the disease is diagnostically confirmed by the finding of a reduced serum caeruloplasmin—less than 20 mg/100 ml (approximately 1.25 µmol/l). Additionally, an increased urinary excretion of copper, greater than 1.6 µmol (100 µg) per day, is usually found in the untreated patient but is not diagnostic since it can also occur in biliary cirrhosis and in liver disease due to a variety of causes.

Unless specifically contra-indicated, a needle biopsy of the liver should be undertaken in all those patients in whom the disease is strongly suspected, but in whom the serum caeruloplasmin is normal. In most patients the concentration of copper in the liver is greater than 200 mg per gram of dry weight. Many patients with liver disease have a moderate increase in the liver copper but, in contrast to patients with Wilson's disease, the serum caeruloplasmin in such patients is usually normal or elevated. However, since 5 per cent of patients with Wilson's disease have a normal caeruloplasmin (and will also have an increased liver copper), diagnostic uncertainty may exist. A firm diagnosis can still be made, however, since patients with Wilson's disease with a normal caeruloplasmin concentration, unlike patients with liver disease, will fail to incorporate radiolabelled copper into caeruloplasmin normally.

Treatment. Treatment should be instituted in both symptomatic and asymptomatic patients as soon as the diagnosis is secure. The goal of treatment is to return the copper content of the body to normal and to prevent its reaccumulation. A low-copper diet is impractical but it is probably wise for patients to avoid foods high in copper such as nuts, chocolate, shellfish, and liver.

The oral administration of D-penicillamine, 1–2 g a day, depending on body weight, is the treatment of choice, and should be continued indefinitely. Chemical effectiveness of therapy can be monitored by measuring the 24-hour urinary copper excretion. After the institution of penicillamine therapy, a daily excretion of 30–60 µmol (2–4 mg) of copper is not unusual; as the total body stores decrease the urinary excretion of copper will slowly diminish. A modest decrease in the serum caeruloplasmin level accompanies therapy. Because pyridoxine deficiency has been noted following penicillamine therapy in animals, it is customary to supplement the diet by the addition of 25 mg pyridoxine daily. Although clinical improvement is frequently rapid, in some patients several weeks may elapse before improvement is evident.

Penicillamine is a toxic drug and care must be exercised in its administration. An acute sensitivity reaction to the drug, which may be IgE mediated, is not uncommon. Sensitivity manifests itself within one to three weeks and occurs in about 10–20 per cent of patients. The acute reaction is characterized by any or all of the following: fever, urticaria, morbilliform rashes, arthralgia, lymphadenopathy, leucopenia, thrombocytopenia, and proteinuria. If these reactions occur, the drug should be temporarily discontinued; it should be restarted slowly with a smaller dose and, if the reactions are severe, under an umbrella of prednisone 20 mg/day for 10 days, after which the steroid should be slowly discontinued.

Among many additional untoward effects, penicillamine may provoke systemic lupus erythematosus, dermatomyositis, Goodpasture's syndrome, the nephrotic syndrome, and pemphigus. These reactions are probably mediated by penicillamine antibodies. DNA antibodies can be detected in penicillamine-induced lupus, and epithelial antibodies have been reported in pemphigus. If any of these serious complications arise, temporary discontinuation of penicillamine is imperative, but cautious resumption at a lower dosage with steroid cover should be undertaken in most cases. Additional complications include optic neuritis and, particularly in patients who have been on treatment for many years, structural alterations in skin collagen may occur and may be reflected clinically in the syndrome of elastosis serpiginosa perforans, or cutis hyperelastica.

On the exceptionally rare occasions when penicillamine therapy must be permanently discontinued, the experimental drug triethylene tetramine may be tried. Liver transplantation has been suggested as a logical form of therapy. Although dramatic improvement has been occasionally reported, it remains, at the present time, the treatment of last resort for those patients in whom liver disease is progressive and alternate forms of therapy are contra-indicated. Because of the frequency of toxic reactions, it is prudent to follow the patients closely, particularly during the early months of treatment. Thereafter, regular examination of the urine for protein, and white blood cell and platelet counts should be carried out at intervals of 8–10 weeks.

After many years of treatment, the urinary excretion of copper falls below 24 µmol (1.5 mg) per day, the Kayser–Fleischer ring fades and ultimately disappears. Liver function abnormalities, particularly the transaminase, slowly return to normal. Despite clinical and biochemical normality, however, it is necessary to continue penicillamine indefinitely at a lower dosage, 500 mg/day.

Because it is now apparent that asymptomatic homozygotes will not develop the disease if treated, it is important, without exception, to examine all siblings of patients and institute therapy in those in whom the diagnosis can be confirmed. Heterozygotes do not develop the disease and treatment for them is not indicated.

References

Sass–Kortsak, A. and Bearn, A. G. (1978). Hereditary disorders of copper metabolism; Wilson's disease (hepatolenticular degeneration) and Menkes' disease (kinky-hair or steely-hair syndrome). In *The metabolic basis of inherited disease*, 4th edn (eds. J. B. Stanbury, J. B. Wyngaarden, and D. S. Fredrickson), 1090. McGraw-Hill, New York.

Schaffner, F., Sternlieb, I., Barka, T., and Popper, H. (1962). Hepatocellular changes in Wilson's disease; histochemical and electron microscopic studies. *Am. J. Path.* **41**, 315.

Strickland, G. T., Frommer, D., Leu, M.-L., Pollard, R., Sherlock, S., and Cumings, J. N. (1973). Wilson's disease in the United Kingdom and Taiwan. I. General characteristics of 142 cases and prognosis. II. A genetic analysis of 88 cases. *Q. Jl Med.* **42**, 619.

Walshe, J. M. (1973). Copper chelation in patients with Wilson's disease; a comparison of penicillamine and triethylene tetramine dihydrochloride. *Q. Jl Med.* **42**, 441.

Disturbances of acid–base homeostasis

R. D. Cohen and H. F. Woods

The hydrogen ion is critically involved in numerous fundamental aspects of biochemical and physiological organization and control. The need for close homeostasis of extra- and intracellular pH becomes immediately obvious when the role of hydrogen ion activity in determining the rates of many metabolic pathways, the conformations of proteins, and the distribution of many substances across biological membranes is considered. This section deals firstly with the general mechanisms by which acid–base homeostasis may be disrupted and the clinical consequences of such disruption. An account then follows of specific acid–base disorders and their therapy.

The normal acid burden. In resting man arterial blood pH (pH_a) is normally tightly maintained between 7.36 and 7.42, as a result of control of arterial P_{CO_2} (P_{a,CO_2}) and plasma bicarbonate between the limits 4.7–5.7 kPa and 24–30 mmol/l respectively. Intracellular pH is also controlled and varies between tissues within the range 6.5–7.35 depending on prevailing physiological circumstances. Most physiological and clinical disturbances shift, or tend to shift, pH in the acid direction, and are due to the accumulation in the body fluids of H^+ derived from metabolism. Table 1 shows the approximate order of magnitude of the various sources of endogenous acid in moles H^+ per day in a resting normal man. The many extra- and intracellular buffers, notably haemoglobin, other proteins, bicarbonate, and phosphate, play a transient role in counteracting pH changes but normally the acid burdens listed in Table 1 are quantitatively eliminated in the middle or long term. They have been grouped into three classes according to the mode of elimination. It may be seen that CO_2 derived from cellular respiration is much the largest component, the burden from lactic and other organic acid production being approximately ten times less and that derived from the metabolism of sulphur and phosphorus-containing compounds is a further order of magnitude lower. The modes of elimination of these three types of acid are also shown in Table 1. Disposal of CO_2 is, of course, dependent on adequate lung function. The metabolism of sulphur-containing amino acids in the diet eventually results in the production of sulphuric acid, and phosphoric acid may be derived from many sources. Both these acids are non-volatile and not disposable in the present context by metabolism; excretion of H^+ from these sources must, therefore,

occur in the urine, mainly as ammonium and dihydrogen phosphate ions.

The organic acids (Table 1) have pK values much less than blood pH and are, therefore, present in blood as the organic acid anions rather than as the undissociated acid, the equivalent H^+ which was formed at the site of production of these acids having titrated blood bicarbonate and other buffers. The organic acid anions (lactate, 3-hydroxybutyrate, acetoacetate, and fatty acids) are non-volatile but may be eliminated by metabolism. Figure 1 shows an example of the general principle that when these organic acid anions are metabolized to electroneutral products (e.g. glucose, or carbon dioxide and water), H^+ is consumed and the bicarbonate is regenerated. H^+ from organic acids can also be eliminated by the usual urinary route referred to above, but this is under normal circumstances a much slower process than the metabolic route. In the case of the ketone bodies for which the renal threshold is quite low, substantial amounts can be lost in the urine. Although maximally acid urine (pH 4.5) results in about half of the urinary ketone body excretion being as the undissociated acid, the remaining free anion moiety in fact represents loss of potential alkali from the body, since by escaping into the urine it eludes eventual metabolism to bicarbonate. In the case of lactate the renal threshold is high (approximately 5–10 mmol/l—normal blood lactate ≈ 1 mmol/l) and its pK is so low that lactate is not lost in the urine until blood

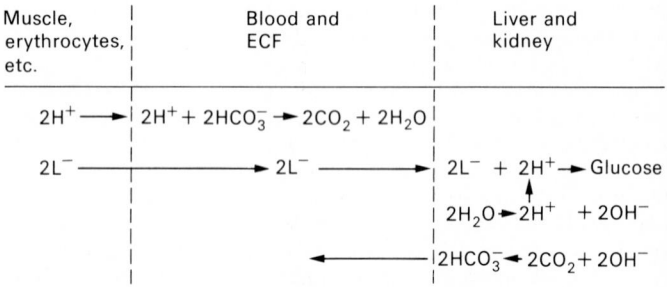

Fig. 1 A scheme, using lactate conversion to glucose as an example, showing how the conversion of an organic acid of low pK to an electroneutral substance consumes H^+ and regenerates HCO_3^-. The lactate ion is shown as L^-.

Table 1   Production and elimination of hydrogen ions

Class		Daily production (moles)	Source	Respirable	Metabolic removal possible	Organ of elimination
I	CO_2	15	tissue respiration	+	−	lungs
II	Organic acids					
	Lactic	1.2	muscle, brain, erythrocytes, skin, etc.	−	+	liver (≈50%) kidneys, heart
	Hydroxybutyric and acetoacetic	0.6*	liver	−	+	many tissues (not liver)
	Free fatty acids (FFA)	0.7*	adipose tissue	−	+	most tissues
III	'Fixed' acids					
	Sulphuric	⎫ 0.1	dietary sulphur-containing aminoacids	−	−	urinary excretion
	Phosphoric	⎭	organic phosphate metabolism	−	−	urinary excretion

The daily production rates for the organic acids are calculated from results obtained in resting 70 kg man after an overnight fast, and are proportioned up to 24-hour values.
*Because of ingestion of food during daytime and consequent suppression of FFA and ketone body production, the values for these acids may be considerable over-estimates.

lactate is grossly elevated; most of any lactate so lost represents loss of potential alkali.

In spite of the large quantitative differences in the burden due to the three classes of acid in Table 1, their correct elimination is in a sense equally important, for no class is able substantially to use a disposal route normally associated with another class. The distinction lies in the potential rate at which the clinical state may become critical when a disposal route is deranged. Thus it has been calculated that total failure of elimination of CO_2 would result in critically severe acidosis in 30 minutes. Observations in clinical lactic acidosis suggest that elimination of the lactate removal mechanisms would take several hours to produce a lethal acidosis; in acute renal failure several days may elapse before acidosis becomes a major problem. Normally production and elimination of each class of acid are balanced. The homeostasis of pH_a that this balance provides is given quantitative expression in the classical Henderson–Hasselbalch equation:

$$pH_a = 6 \cdot 1 + \log_{10} \frac{[HCO_3^-]}{(0 \cdot 255 \times P_{a,CO_2})}$$

Where P_{a,CO_2} is the partial pressure of artificial carbon dioxide exposed in kP_a the constancy of $[HCO_3^-]$ is maintained by the elimination of class II and III acids and that of P_{CO_2} by the lungs, thereby fixing pH_a within a narrow normal range.

The genesis of acid–base disturbances. The terminology of acid–base disturbances has always been confused. Here we use the terms *acidaemia* and *alkalaemia* simply to indicate that the pH_a is lower or higher than the normal range respectively. The term *acidosis* is used to encompass both the situation where pH_a is low, and also that in which pH_a is normal, but the nature of the responsible disturbance is such that if compensatory mechanisms had not operated, pH_a would be low. An equivalent definition applies to *alkalosis*

Most acid–base disturbances are due to imbalance of production and elimination of hydrogen ions derived from the endogenous sources classified in Table 1. However, some are due to ingestion or infusion of excessive amounts of acids or bases (particularly bicarbonate). When the *primary* disturbance is related to abnormal CO_2 elimination, the acidosis or alkalosis is termed 'respiratory'. All other primary disturbances (i.e. those due to difficulties with class II and III acid metabolism or elimination) are termed 'metabolic' or 'non-respiratory'. The term 'primary' is used in contradistinction to 'secondary' disturbances which are compensatory in nature. Thus metabolic acidosis is compensated for by hyperventilation due to stimulation of the respiratory centre and consequently P_{a,CO_2} is lowered; respiratory acidosis is compensated for by increased renal secretion of H^+ into the urine and concomitant 'reabsorption' of bicarbonate.

Two points must be made about the compensatory mechanisms. Firstly, respiratory compensation for metabolic acidosis is much more rapid than metabolic compensation for respiratory acidosis. Secondly, compensation for metabolic alkalosis by hypoventilation often, but by no means invariably, poor.

The diagnosis of acid–base disturbances. The clinical manifestations of acid–base disturbances are described later. They are rather non-specific and may not be evident until the disturbance is quite severe. Thus although clinical features may provide the first indication of a disturbance of acid–base homeostasis, accurate characterization, both qualitatively and quantitatively, requires laboratory investigation. Measurement of pH and P_{CO_2} on arterial, or arterialized venous blood is the most definitive procedure. Additional valuable information may be obtained from measurement of plasma sodium, potassium, chloride, and bicarbonate and subsequent calculation of the anion gap.

Measurement of pH_a and P_{a,CO_2}. A variety of apparatus is available for this purpose. Usually bicarbonate is automatically calculated

from the Henderson–Hasselbalch equation. Despite the automated nature of the equipment, the first response to a clinically unexpected set of results should be to request another after restandardization.

Interpretation of the results is best achieved by the use of an acid–base diagram which has pH_a on one axis and P_{a,CO_2} on the other. Diagrams which use $[HCO_3^-]$ instead of either pH_a or P_{a,CO_2} are less suitable, since $[HCO_3^-]$ is calculated from pH_a and P_{CO_2} and is not only affected by the errors in both the latter measurements, but also by the fact that pK_a in the Henderson-Hasselbalch equation is subject to some unexplained variations in blood from severely ill patients.

The acid–base diagram shown in Fig. 2 has bands drawn in to show the range of expected response to *uncomplicated* acid–base disorders. The shaded square represents the approximate limits of pH_a and P_{a,CO_2} in normal individuals. Thus a patient with uncomplicated metabolic acidosis will have values lying in the band marked '*metabolic*' in the region to the left and above the shaded area; the metabolic band is in fact the envelope of measurements of pH_a and P_{a,CO_2} from patients in the literature with completely uncomplicated metabolic acidosis or alkalosis. The band marked *acute respiratory* is the 95 per cent confidence range of values obtained in normal man voluntarily hyperventilating or breathing air/CO_2 mixtures for short periods of time. Since after a few days of CO_2 retention in respiratory acidosis, renal reabsorption of bicarbonate has produced substantial or complete compensation, the response expected in chronic respiratory acidosis is different from the acute response, the presence of the extra bicarbonate reducing the fall in pH for a given rise in P_{a,CO_2}. Figure 2. shows the uncomplicated response to *chronic respiratory acidosis*. It may be seen that the band for *metabolic alkalosis* (to the right of and below the shaded region) is rather restricted, extending only a short distance along the P_{a,CO_2} axis. This is because compensation by hypoventilation for metabolic alkalosis is variable and poor, perhaps because hypoxia sets a limit to compensating hypoventilation and also possibly because a number of conditions in which metabolic alkalosis is a feature may be associated with intracellular acidosis affecting the respiratory centre. Masked hypercapnia is, however, occasionally seen in metabolic alkalosis.

The pH_a and P_{a,CO_2} measurements in some patients will not fall within any of the defined bands shown in Fig. 2. Such patients have a mixture of acid–base disorders. Thus a patient whose pH_a and

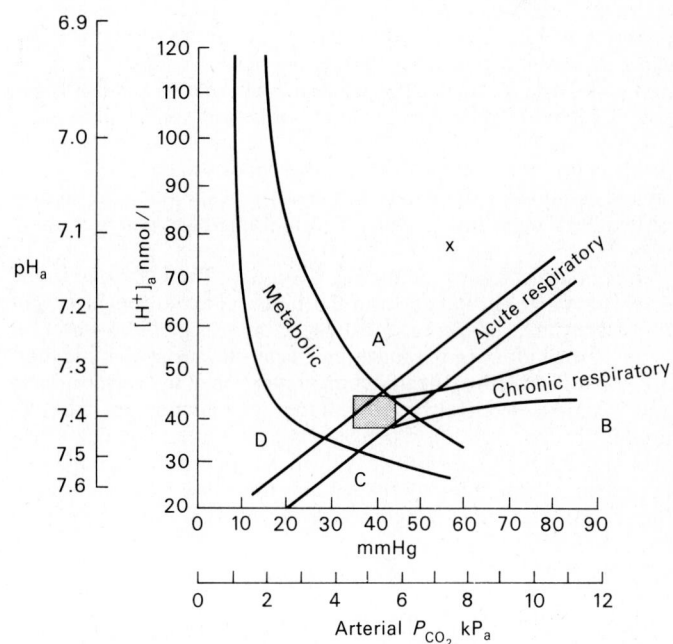

Fig. 2 For explanation see text.

P_{CO_2} are represented by the point x has mixed respiratory and metabolic acidosis (e.g. a patient with an exacerbation of chronic bronchitis and coexistent diabetic ketoacidosis). It may be noted that a disturbance lying in sectors A or C results from the combination of two primary acid–base conditions; in sector B and D one of the two disturbances could be compensatory for the other. The diagram not only permits the diagnosis of acid–base disorders, but by serially plotting results the course of an individual patient's disturbance and its response to treatment may be closely followed.

Contemporary acid–base analytical equipment usually also provides at least two further acid–base variables if the haemoglobin concentration is also known. These are the 'standard bicarbonate' and the 'base excess' or 'base deficit'. The standard bicarbonate represents what the plasma bicarbonate would be if the blood had a normal P_{a,CO_2} (5.33 kPa, 40 mmHg) rather than its actual value. Standard bicarbonate was introduced in an attempt to provide a measurement which was independent of respiratory disturbance and thus to provide an estimate of pure metabolic disturbance. 'Base deficit' represents the amount of alkali in mmol required to restore the pH of 1 litre of the patient's blood *in vitro* to normal at P_{CO_2} of 5.33 kPa and might at first sight be considered a quantitative measure of metabolic acidosis. Unfortunately the titration curve of blood *in vitro* is different from that when it is circulating *in vivo*, since in the latter situation the interstitial and intracellular fluids are in equilibrium with blood and may gain or lose bicarbonate from it; in addition their buffering capacity differs from that of blood. These considerations detract from the usefulness of standard bicarbonate and base excess or deficit as a guide either to diagnosis or therapy. Further difficulties arise from ambiguities in the interpretation of base excess or deficit. Thus a patient with chronic respiratory acidosis will certainly have a base excess due to compensatory renal retention of bicarbonate. It could be said, therefore, that this patient has simultaneously a respiratory acidosis *and* a metabolic alkalosis, since base excess indicates the latter. This way of regarding the situation, which is quite widely adopted, seems to us confusing, and is not compatible with the definitions of acidosis and alkalosis we have given, which are intended to indicate the direction of the *primary* disturbance.

For these reasons we prefer the use of the acid–base diagram shown in Fig. 2 which is based entirely on directly measured variables and is not subject to the difficulties associated with the derived variables described above.

Use of the anion gap. Normally the main electrolytes measured in plasma are Na^+, Cl^-, K^+, and HCO_3^-. The sum of the measured cations $(Na^+ + K^+)$ exceeds that of the measured anions by 10–18 mmol/l. This difference is known as the 'anion gap' and is attributable largely to negatively charged proteins but also to phosphate, sulphate, and some organic acids. Calculation of the anion gap is principally of value in the differential diagnosis of metabolic acidosis and in following the progress of therapy. Metabolic acidosis may be divided broadly into those with normal and those with high anion gap.

Metabolic acidoses with normal anion gap. These are due to the direct loss of bicarbonate from the body, either through the gut (e.g. diarrhoea, pancreatic fistulae, ureterosigmoidostomy) or through the kidney (e.g. renal tubule acidosis, acetazolamide therapy) or very rarely, to the ingestion or infusion of hydrochloric acid or substances effectively giving rise to it (e.g. ammonium chloride, arginine hydrochloride). When bicarbonate is lost, more chloride is retained by the renal tubules; thus low plasma bicarbonate is accompanied by hyperchloraemia and the anion gap remains unaltered. In the case of hydrochloric acid intake bicarbonate is titrated and replaced by chloride.

Metabolic acidoses with high anion gap. These are due to the ingestion or endogenous generation of acids, usually organic, whose anions are not routinely measured. Plasma bicarbonate is titrated and the anion gap is now widened by the presence of these unmeasured anions. The principal causes are ketoacidosis, lactic

acidosis, uraemic acidosis and poisoning by salicylates. In uraemic acidosis the anion gap seldom exceeds 28 mmol/l, but considerably higher values may be found in severe lactic acidosis and ketoacidosis. It should be noted that there are causes of raised anion gap other than metabolic acidosis—namely therapy with sodium salts of relatively strong acids (e.g. lactate, acetate), high-dose sodium carbenicillin therapy, and respiratory or metabolic alkalosis. The infusion of sodium lactate or acetate only gives rise to a raised anion gap if metabolism to bicarbonate is delayed, and the raised anion gap in alkalosis is usually trivial, being at least partly due to stimulation of lactate production.

Causes of acid–base disturbance. In surveying the spectrum of causation of acid–base disorders, by far the most diverse problems of aetiology and classification arise in *metabolic acidosis*. Table 2 classifies those conditions associated with high anion gap metabolic acidosis and attempts to divide them into those in which the predominant unmeasured anion is lactate, ketoacids or other often less well-defined acid anions. The term 'ketoacid' is loosely used to refer both to a ketoacid itself (e.g. acetoacetic) and its reduced (hydroxy) derivative (e.g. 3-hydroxybutyrate). It may be seen from Table 2 that high anion-gap acidosis is often due to a mixture of acids, but where possible the predominant acid has been indicated in italic type. It is often the case that the acid anions actually identified in plasma can only account for a part, often minor, of the acidosis and this has been shown by an asterisk. The common form of uraemic acidosis is the best example of this.

It is not possible reliably to ascertain the contribution of an individual organic acid to the acidosis by determination of its urinary excretion; a good example of this is methylmalonic aciduria, where, in spite of major elevation in urinary methylmalonate excretion, the blood levels although elevated can only account for a very minor part of the severe acidosis which may be seen. Conversely, lactic acidosis may be quite severe before any substantial amount of lactate appears in the urine. In Table 3 metabolic acidoses with normal anion gap are classified according to whether they are due to gut or renal bicarbonate loss, or to ingestion or infusion of acidifying agents.

Metabolic alkalosis (Table 4) is due either to ingestion or infusion of excessive alkali in circumstances (e.g. poor renal function) when it cannot be excreted, or to loss of acid, either from the stomach as in pyloric stenosis, or in secretion of an inappropriately acid urine. Most of the causes of the latter occurrence are related to the complex disturbances occurring in potassium and chloride deficiency (see page 18.28).

Respiratory acidoses, presented in Table 5, are due to problems at one or more of three levels, namely the lungs and airways, the neuromuscular and mechanical aspects of respiration, and the central nervous system. *Respiratory alkalosis* (Table 6) is nearly always due to some form of stimulus to the respiratory centre, whether it be psychogenic, reflex, chemically induced, or due to local lesion; the exception is deliberate or inadvertent hyperventilation during anaesthesia or other occasions when assisted ventilation is used.

Tables 2–5 illustrate both the wide range of aetiology and the major causes of acid-base disturbances; they are not intended to be totally comprehensive.

The consequences of acid–base disturbances. The effect of acid base disturbances on physiological and biochemical mechanisms are widespread. We limit ourselves here to a brief description of those currently known, or thought probably to have clinical relevance.

Respiratory effects. Both metabolic acidosis and acute respiratory acidosis induced by breathing high P_{CO_2} gas mixtures result in hyperventilation. Deep sighing respiration (Kussmaul breathing) is a familiar sign of metabolic acidosis. The degree of hyperventilation achieved in given clinical circumstances is dependent on complex factors which are related both to the magnitude and the rate of

Table 2   High anion gap metabolic acidoses

	Associated serum acid anions*
Predominant ketoacidosis	
Diabetic ketoacidosis	*3-hydroxybutyrate*, acetoacetate, lactate
Starvation ketoacidosis	*3-hydroxybutyrate*, acetoacetate, lactate
Alcoholic ketoacidosis	*3-hydroxybutyrate*, acetoacetate, lactate
Ketotic hypoglycaemia of childhood	*3-hydroxybutyrate*, acetoacetate, lactate
Predominant lactic acidosis	
Type A lactic acidosis	
Exercise	*lactate*
Post-epileptic	*lactate*
Shock (traumatic, haemorrhagic cardiogenic, septic)	*lactate*
Severe hypoxia	*lactate*
Type B lactic acidosis	
Biguanide associated (phenformin, buformin, metformin)	*lactate*, 3-hydroxybutyrate
Ethanol associated	*lactate*, 3-hydroxybutyrate
Fructose, sorbitol, or xylitol infusion	*lactate*
Other poorly characterized acquired lactic acidoses	lactate
Severe liver disease	*lactate*
Leukaemia and reticulosis	*lactate*
Paracetamol poisoning	*lactate*
Thiamine deficiency	†*lactate*
Type I glycogenosis	*lactate*
Hepatic fructose 1,6–, diphosphatase deficiency	*lactate*
Lactic acidosis associated with metabolic myopathies	*lactate*
Pyruvate carboxylase deficiency	†*lactate*
Other poorly characterized hereditary lactic acidoses	†*lactate*
D(−) lactic acidosis due to lactabacillus ingestion	*lactate*
Conditions with imperfectly defined source of acidosis	
Uraemic acidosis	†phosphate, sulphate, etc.
Salicylate poisoning (acidotic phase)	salicylate, lactate, ketoacids
Methanol poisoning	*lactate*, formate
Ethylene glycol poisoning	†*lactate*, oxalate
Paraldehyde poisoning	?
Reye's syndrome	†*lactate*
Jamaican vomiting sickness (ackee poisoning)	?
Glutaric aciduria type II	†lactate, free fatty acids
Ethylmalonic-adipic aciduria	?
Propionyl CoA carboxylase deficiency	†higher ketoacids, propionic acid
Methylmalonic aciduria	†ketoacids (including higher ones, lactate, methylmalonate)
β-Ketothiolase deficiency	†methyl—hydroxybutyrate, methylacetoacetate

* The predominant acid anion is shown in italics
† Indicates that the named acids may only partly account for the acidosis

Table 3   Metabolic acidoses with normal anion gap

Gastrointestinal bicarbonate loss
  Diarrhoea
  Pancreatic fistula

Ureteroenterostomy

Renal causes
  Renal tubular acidosis
  (a) Gradient (distal type)
    Primary
      Transient, in infancy
      Permanent (childhood or adult)
    Secondary
      In hypergammaglobulinaemic states
      Amphotericin B therapy
      Vitamin D intoxication
      Hyperthyroidism
      Obstructive uropathy (pre- and post-treatment)
  (b) Bicarbonate wastage (proximal type)
    Primary
      Isolated
      As part of idiopathic Fanconi syndrome
    Secondary
      Hyperparathyroidism
      Hypoaldosteronism
      Uraemia (occasionally)
      Dysproteinaemic states (myeloma, Sjögren's syndrome)
      Heavy metal poisoning (cadmium, mercury)
      Outdated tetracycline
      Renal transplant rejection
      Hereditary disorders (e.g. cystinosis, Wilson's disease, hereditary fructose intolerance, galactosaemia, Lowe's sydrome)
  (c) Acetazolamide

Ingestion or infusion of acidifying agents
  Ammonium chloride
  Arginine hydrochloride
  Intravenous feeding with solutions containing excess cationic aminoacids

Rapid intravenous hydration (dilutional acidosis)

Table 4   Causes of metabolic alkalosis

Ingestion or infusion of alkali in excess of excretory ability
  Milk-alkali syndrome
  'Alkaline overshoot' during therapy of high anion-gap acidoses
  Forced alkaline diuresis therapy of salicylate and barbiturate poisoning

Loss of acid inappropriately (gastric or renal routes)
  Pyloric stenosis
  Potassium depletion
  Chloride depletion   } frequently
  Hyperaldosteronism   } associated

'Contraction alkalosis'
  Rapid diuresis

development of the acid–base disturbance. pH control of ventilation is determined both by the pH perceived by the carotid and aortic body chemoreceptors and also by chemoreceptors in the medulla which appear to monitor the pH of brain extracellular fluid (ECF). In the steady state brain ECF pH is closely similar to that of cerebrospinal fluid (CSF). Sudden development of metabolic acidosis, resulting in low pH_a and plasma bicarbonate, induces hyper-

ventilation by stimulating the carotid and aortic body chemoreceptors and P_{a,CO_2} is thus lowered. However, the first effect on brain ECF pH is to raise it. This is because brain ECF P_{CO_2} is lowered since CO_2 is rapidly equilibrated across the blood–brain barrier. In contrast, it takes many hours for the brain ECF bicarbonate concentration to fall in response to the lowering of plasma bicarbonate since active and passive movement of bicarbonate across the barrier is very much slower than that of CO_2. The temporary alkalinization of brain ECF pH in the presence of systemic metabolic acidosis somewhat offsets the ventilatory drive provided by the peripheral chemoreceptors. In the long-term brain ECF and CSF pH are rather tightly controlled, and their initial high pH in acute metabolic acidosis is eventually restored to normal or slightly below normal. This removes the partial inhibition of ventilatory response and the degree of hyperventilation increases. Though clinical circum-

Table 5 Causes of respiratory acidosis

Structural and mechanical pulmonary disease
Chronic obstructive airways disease
Severe asthma (uncommonly)
Large airway obstruction

Neuromuscular and mechanical problems
Acute ascending polyneuritis
Poliomyelitis
Acute porphyria
Myasthenia gravis
Motor neurone disease
Muscular dystrophies
Traumatic 'flail chest'
Ankylosing spondylosis
Severe kyphoscoliosis
Gross obesity
Muscle relaxant drugs

Respiratory centre disorders
Organic disease affecting respiratory centre
Numerous respiratory centre depressant drugs
    e.g. opiates, barbiturates, benzodiazepines, anaesthetic agents
Respiratory arrest

Table 6 Causes of respiratory alkalosis

Spontaneous or psychogenic hyperventilation

Reflex hyperventilation (e.g. in pulmonary disease)

Other stimuli to respiratory centre
Via chemoreceptors: low inspired oxygen concentration (e.g. high
    altitude); alveolar-capillary diffusion block; right-to-left shunt;
    carbon monoxide poisoning
Via drugs or metabolites: salicylate poisoning; acute liver failure
After recovery from metabolic acidosis
Local lesion affecting centre

Overventilation during anaesthesia or other assisted ventilation

stances usually prevent the observation of this sequence of events, the opposite effect, namely the persistence of hyperventilation after restoration of normal arterial pH during the therapy of metabolic acidosis is very commonly seen. In this situation systemic alkalinization has suppressed the peripheral chemoreceptors, raising P_{CO_2} and thus causing paradoxical acidification of brain ECF and CSF. Over 24 hours may elapse before the resulting persisting hyperventilation ceases. In acute and chronic respiratory acidosis the ventilatory manifestations of phased events equivalent to those seen in metabolic acid base disorders are seldom given full expression, because the respiratory disease usually prevents this. However, the ventilatory drive in response to acute respiratory acidosis should fall with time as the initial rapid fall of brain ECF and CSF pH is gradually eliminated. In the presence of chronic hypercapnia a further effect, namely direct depression of the respiratory centre, occurs, and the respiratory response to increments of P_{a,CO_2} becomes progressively lost, ventilation becoming increasingly dependent upon hypoxic drive.

A further effect of acute metabolic acidosis on the respiratory system is its role in the development of 'shock lung'. This syndrome, consisting of pulmonary congestion, oedema, capillary endothelial swelling, shunting, and high pulmonary vascular resistance is a common complication of severe shock and is to a considerable extent preventable in animals subjected to experimental shock if the metabolic acidosis of shock is not allowed to occur.

Cardiovascular effects. *On the heart.* It is generally agreed that acidosis has adverse effects on cardiac contractility (negative inotropism) and alkalosis smaller but opposite effects. The negative inotropic effects are particularly related to changes in cardiac intracellular pH and are experimentally found to be rather greater in

acute respiratory than in acute metabolic acidosis in the presence of the same extracellular pH. The negative inotropic effect of acidosis is due to a combination of mechanisms connected with excitation–contraction coupling and energy supply; amongst other effects, acidosis inhibits the inward slow calcium current during the action potential and the release of calcium from sarcoplasmic reticulum, possibly inhibits the binding of calcium to troponins and depresses glycolysis. In the rat progressive metabolic acidosis induced by oral feeding of ammonium chloride results in fall of cardiac output due to both bradycardia and to negative inotropy, with consequent hypotension and decreased renal and hepatic blood flow. This sequence of events may provide a model for the circulatory collapse which is often seen to occur in patients after some hours of severe metabolic acidosis not primarily due to shock.

Although mild to moderate acidosis has often not been associated with negative inotropic effects in intact animal studies this appears to be due to the protective effect of catecholamine release, which is increased in acidosis. The beta-adrenergic stimulation of contractility is sufficient to overcome the negative effects of mild to moderate acidosis, but in more severe acidosis this protection breaks down. Patients receiving beta-blocking drugs are thus potentially more susceptible to the negative inotropic effects of acidosis.

Other effects of acidosis are also important in cardiac arrest. It has been found experimentally that correction of the metabolic acidosis greatly facilitates defibrillation, and in cardiac arrest it is usual to infuse bicarbonate immediately prior to defibrillation attempts.

On the peripheral vasculature. The simplest effects of acid–base disturbance on the peripheral vasculature are observed in the cerebral circulation, where these effects are relatively little obscured by changes in circulating catecholamines. Cerebral arterioles are very sensitive to the pH of brain ECF, being dilated when this falls and constricted by increases. The cerebrovascular resistance is therefore subject to similar phased responses to different types of acute acid–base disturbances as is ventilation, due to the differential time response of brain ECF pH, P_{CO_2} and bicarbonate to acute systemic changes. Dilatation is also the response of most systemic arterioles to acidosis, although this response may be modified or offset completely by catecholamine effects. The peripheral veins, however, constrict in acidosis, resulting in a shift of blood from the peripheral capacitance vessels to the central circulation. This effect has been demonstrated during treatment of the dehydration and acidosis associated with cholera. It might, therefore, be expected that administration of fluids would have a greater risk of precipitating pulmonary oedema in acidotic subjects. In animals, acidosis raises pulmonary vascular resistance, but the extent of this effect in man is uncertain.

Effects on intermediary carbohydrate metabolism. In all tissues in which observations have been made, glycolysis is inhibited by acidosis and stimulated by alkalosis, due to effects of intracellular pH on phosphofructokinase, the rate-limiting step of glycolysis. Respiratory alkalosis might, therefore, be expected to raise blood lactate, but in normal man the effect is very small, no doubt due to removal of lactate by the liver. However, in the presence of severe liver disease gross elevation of blood lactate may be seen in association with respiratory alkalosis and the increased production of lactic acid may partially compensate for the alkalosis.

In animal experiments, hepatic gluconeogenesis from lactate is inhibited by severe acidosis due to an effect on the step between pyruvate and oxaloacetate. This phenomenon may be responsible for perpetuating and worsening lactic acidosis. It may be partially offset by the effects of the increased catecholamine levels seen in lactic acidosis due to shock. Acidosis has a stimulatory effect on lactate removal by the kidney but this may not be sufficient in magnitude to compensate for the opposite hepatic effects.

Effects on blood oxygen uptake and delivery. One of the major factors determining pulmonary oxygen uptake and tissue oxygen delivery is the position of the blood oxygen dissociation curve with respect to the ordinate (the oxygen saturation) and abscissa (the partial pressure of oxygen, P_{O_2}). Right shifts of this curve improve unloading of oxygen in the tissues, but, in the presence of low inspired O_2 concentration or pulmonary disease, impair oxygen uptake in the lungs; left shifts have the opposite effect. The position of the curve is determined by three ligands capable of interacting with the haemoglobin molecule, namely H^+, CO_2, and 2,3-diphosphoglycerate (2,3-DPG). Increases in the concentration of any of these result in a shift to the right. The effects of changes in extracellular H^+ (Bohr effect) and CO_2 are immediate and operate through changes in intraerythrocytic H^+ and CO_2. In addition, an increase in intra-erythrocytic H^+ (i.e. fall in pH) inhibits the synthesis of 2,3-DPG and encourages its breakdown. 2,3-DPG is a by-product of the glycolytic pathway unique to erythrocytes and the acidotic inhibition of the pathway at phosphofructokinase referred to above, together with inhibition of DPG-mutase and stimulation of 2,3-DPG phosphatase result in a fall in its concentration. Opposite effects occur in alkalosis. These reactions are, however, very slow in comparison with the immediate Bohr effect.

The effect of these differences in time scale on oxygen delivery during the course of acid–base disturbances may be exemplified by the changes occurring during the development (over a few hours) and treatment of acute metabolic acidosis. Initially the acute acidosis causes a right shift and hence improved oxygen delivery. After several hours the 2,3-DPG level falls, thus restoring the position of the curve approximately to normal. If the patient is now rapidly treated with alkalinizing solutions, the Bohr effect results in an immediate shift to the left; it may be many hours, even up two to three days, before 2,3-DPG concentrations are restored. The sudden deterioration in oxygen delivery caused by alkalinization may have adverse clinical effects unless the shift in the curve is counteracted by other factors, such as increase in blood flow through the tissues. A further example is acute metabolic alkalosis which in certain circumstances could jeopardize the cerebral cortex, both because of the Bohr effect and because of cerebral vasoconstriction due to alkalosis.

Effects on the nervous system. The effects of acid–base disturbances on the central nervous system are a resultant of many factors, including changes in cerebral blood flow and oxygen dissociation (see above) and other mechanisms less well characterized.

Severe acidosis is frequently associated with a variety of degrees of impairment of consciousness, varying from mild drowsiness to coma. The degree of disturbance is not closely related to systemic pH, and the mechanism is not understood. Attempts to relate this effect of acidosis to CSF pH have proved unsuccessful.

The excitability of neuromuscular tissues is in general increased by alkalosis and decreased by acidosis. Tetany is a common feature of respiratory alkalosis, and may also be seen when a chronic metabolic acidosis is corrected in a patient with low plasma calcium, a combination of events which may occur in renal failure. The effect has been attributed to increased protein binding of plasma calcium but it is very doubtful whether this is sufficient quantitatively to account for the phenomenon. Epileptic attacks in those prone are precipitated by alkalosis and suppressed by acidosis.

Effects on potassium homeostasis. (See also page 18.28.) Acute acidosis results on a shift of potassium out of the intracellular compartment into the extracellular fluid. Hyperkalaemia is thus often seen in the acidosis of renal failure, untreated diabetic ketoacidosis, and in acute respiratory failure. The mechanism is unclear, possibly related to proton binding, in response to a fall in intracellular pH, by acidic groups of intracellular proteins which normally act as counter-ions for potassium. Alkali therapy in such patients causes shift of potassium back into cells. Since substantial amounts of potassium may be lost through the kidneys during the period of hyperkalaemia, the body may be potassium depleted even in the presence of hyperkalaemia, and alkali therapy may result in serious hypokalaemia. This is a well known hazard in the treatment of diabetic ketoacidosis and is even more dangerous in renal tubular acidosis, when, because of prior potassium depletion, plasma potassium may be low even in the severely acidotic patient. Such patients should be treated with potassium salts *before* alkalinization, or at least concomitantly. Treating the acidosis first may result in cardiac arrest due to further fall of plasma potassium.

Chronic metabolic alkalosis is frequently accompanied by potassium depletion, due to distal tubular potassium secretion uninhibited by competition for secretion with hydrogen ions and associated with high intracellular potassium concentrations. The increased tubular potassium secretion is further enhanced by the chloride depletion which is frequently present in chronic metabolic alkalosis (see below).

Effects on the kidney. Since the kidney is a major organ of acid–base control, most of its responses to acid–base disturbances are geared to their correction. Acidosis causes a marked increase in renal gluconeogenesis, primarily due to increased activity of the relevant rate-limiting enzyme, phosphoenolpyruvate carboxykinase. The increased gluconeogenesis is thought to be causally linked with the increase of renal ammoniagenesis which is a crucial part of the renal response to acidosis. The mechanism of this link is still under debate. The ammoniagenic response to acidosis also depends on adequate supply of ammonia precursors to the kidney, and an intact ammonia production mechanism within the distal tubular cells. The main precursor of renal ammonia is glutamine and substantial changes take place in glutamine metabolism in acidosis. Glutamine release from skeletal muscle is increased and disposal of glutamine nitrogen is shifted away from urea production in the liver to ammoniagenesis in the kidney. This is due not only to the stimulatory effects of acidosis on renal ammoniagenesis, but also to direct inhibition of urea production; this switch in the route of nitrogen disposal can be shown to result in the loss of hydrogen ions from the body. In addition to the above mechanisms for increasing ammoniagenesis, chronic acidosis also results in the increased activity of renal glutaminase, the critical enzyme of ammoniagenesis.

The detailed mechanisms by which urinary acid excretion is increased in acidosis is discussed extensively in physiology textbooks and will be referred to again in the section on renal acidosis. Here it will suffice to note that the kidneys are capable of increasing their acid secretion from a typical normal value of 100 mmol/day to about 500 mmol/day. Their capacity to do so depends on (*a*) the ability to lower the urine pH (normal range of *minimum* urine pH 5.3–4.3); (*b*) the urinary buffer excretion; and (*c*) ammonium excretion. In alkalosis other than that due to potassium, chloride, and extracellular volume depletion, large quantities of bicarbonate are excreted in the urine, the maximum pH of which is about 8.

In respiratory acidosis, high P_{a,CO_2} acts as a direct stimulus to tubular H^+ secretion and concomitant bicarbonate secretion in the opposite direction, i.e. into the peritubular capillaries. This results in a rise in plasma bicarbonate over a few days and restoration of pH_a to normal or near normal. Respiratory alkalosis has opposite effects, and loss of bicarbonate in the urine helps minimize the change in pH_a.

Effects on bone. It has been shown that bone acts as a buffer in chronic metabolic acidosis, in that leaching out of a calcium carbonate phase in bone and exchange of extracellular phosphate for carbonate within the apatite crystal result in the neutralization of H^+. The first of these mechanisms gives rise to a negative calcium balance in chronic metabolic acidosis, and in chronic uraemic acidotic subjects it has been shown that calcium balance can be restored by treatment with sodium bicarbonate. Although chronic experimental metabolic acidosis in rats leads to osteoporosis, renal tubular acidosis and the acidosis of ureterosigmoidostomy in man lead to osteomalacia, which can be corrected by alkali therapy alone. Osteomalacia is usually related to vitamin D deficiency or inappropriate metabolism, or to phosphate deficiency; its mechanism in the context of acidosis is unknown.

Effect on leucocytes. Severe acidosis is often associated with marked leucocytosis, unrelated to the presence of infection. Blood leucocyte counts of up to 60 000 mm³ have been recorded in lactic acidosis. It has been suggested that this phenomenon may be partly specifically related to the acidosis and not merely an indication of stress.

Effects on the distribution of metabolites and drugs. When weak acids and bases are distributed between body compartments by non-ionic diffusion, pH differences between two compartments will determine their relative concentration in these compartments. Weak bases are concentrated in the more acid and weak acids in the more alkaline compartments. Examples of physiological metabolites thus affected are ammonia (weak base) and urobilinogen (weak acid). The urinary excretion of ammonia is thus markedly increased in acid urine and that of urobilinogen decreased. The distribution of ammonia between blood and CSF is partly determined by the blood–CSF pH difference. Examples of drugs exhibiting this behaviour are salicylates and phenobarbitone which are both weak acids; use of the pH dependence of distribution is made in the therapy of salicylate and phenobarbitone poisoning by forced alkaline diuresis.

Principles of treatment of acid–base disorders. In general the mainstay of treatment is to eliminate the primary cause of the disorder, the acid–base control mechanisms then restoring the normal situation in due course. However, it is frequently necessary to make a direct attempt to restore normality and this is far more often the case in respiratory and metabolic acidosis than in the alkaloses. The treatment of respiratory failure is dealt with elsewhere.

In deciding whether to treat acute metabolic acidosis the main difficulty is in assessing the relative risks of treatment against the advantages. The main advantages are improvement in cardiac performance, redistribution of blood volume away from the central circulation, correction of hyperkalaemia and restoration of hepatic lactate removal, and reduction of distressing hyperventilation. Disadvantages lie in adverse effects on the oxygen dissociation curve, and, in the case of lactic and ketoacidosis, the production of 'alkaline overshoot' due to metabolism of the organic acids after pH_a has been normalized. A certain amount of empirical guidance is available. Thus in diabetic ketoacidosis it is generally accepted that provided pH_a is not below 7.05, alkalinization is unnecessary, rehydration and insulin therapy being sufficient. In type B lactic acidosis due to biguanides there is evidence to suggest that a more vigorous approach is indicated, pH being restored to normal by bicarbonate infusion over about six hours. The most difficult decisions are in shocked patients where the acidosis may, through its negative inotropic effects, be a major contributor to circulatory failure. Yet it is in these patients who are unable to raise the cardiac output that the theoretical disadvantage effects of alkalinization on the O_2 dissociation curve might have most serious consequences. In these patients alkalinization should be combined with other essential means of restoring the circulation (e.g. fluids and pharmacological intervention). The dangers of 'alkaline overshoot' have perhaps been over-emphasized, but should be borne in mind particularly if there is reason to suppose that the cerebral circulation is in jeopardy.

The alkalinizing agent most generally used is sodium bicarbonate, usually administered intravenously in acute metabolic acidosis and orally in the chronic forms. Sodium lactate has the disadvantage that lactate has to be metabolized before the alkalinizing effect occurs and in many patients lactate metabolism is impaired. THAM (trishydroxyaminomethane) may be indicated when the patient has sodium and water overload and cannot tolerate sodium bicarbonate. However, a rise in P_{a,CO_2}, hypoglycaemia and adverse effects on

the renal tubules are possible complications of its use. Sodium bicarbonate is given either as hypertonic (1 mol/l) or isotonic (0.163 mol/l) solution.

In general it is best to alkalinize by slow infusion of isotonic bicarbonate rather than by boluses of hypertonic bicarbonate, in order to minimize deleterious effects on oxygen dissociation. Hypertonic bicarbonate obviously also carries the danger of inducing a severe hypertonic state. In shocked patients who are volume depleted it is more appropriate to treat the acidosis with isotonic sodium bicarbonate. Nevertheless in some patients the acidosis, through the effect on the heart, may be the major contributor to the circulatory failure. In these patients more rapid alkalinization may be indicated together with oxygen therapy, and hypertonic bicarbonate is also standard treatment for the acidosis of cardiac arrest. Central venous pressure is a helpful guide to the rate and type of alkali therapy. The amount of alkali therapy should be determined by an iterative process of administration of a relatively small quantity (e.g. 80 mmol), followed by reassessment of the clinical condition and pH_a and P_{a,CO_2} before repeating the cycle. Attempts to calculate the amount of alkali needed from the 'base deficit' have little validity both for reasons outlined earlier and because the primary cause of proton accumulation may still be operative; such estimates can in no way replace the need for repeated clinical and biochemical monitoring.

It is seldom necessary to treat metabolic alkalosis by direct attempts at acidification. However, occasions arise when a severe metabolic alkalosis unrelated to potassium and chloride deficiency may need treating because of tetany or suspected effects on the central circulation. In such rare instances oral ammonium chloride or intravenous infusion of arginine hydrochloride may be indicated.

Major syndromes of metabolic acidosis

The causes of metabolic acidosis can be divided into two groups, one with a high anion gap and one with a normal anion gap (Tables 2 and 3). In this section some of the important causes of metabolic acidosis of both types will be discussed in some detail.

High anion gap metabolic acidosis
Uraemic acidosis. An important function of the kidneys is to excrete the 'fixed' acid produced during the course of normal metabolism which amounts to 60–100 mmol/day on a diet containing a normal amount of protein. When the number of normally functioning nephrons is lowered in renal disease, the production of this metabolic acid will continue unchanged if the protein intake is not restricted, and a metabolic acidosis will occur. In uraemic acidosis the unmeasured anions are those which accumulate as a result of tubular and glomerular dysfunction, such as sulphate and phosphate. In most of the conditions listed in Table 2 the increased anion gap is due to the accumulation of unmeasured anions produced by increased endogenous acid synthesis. In uraemic acidosis this is not the case; the unmeasured anions are produced in normal quantities but are not excreted to a normal extent.

The acidosis of renal failure often gives a plasma bicarbonate concentration of 12–15 mmol/l but this may be lower in advanced failure. In this type of metabolic acidosis the total excretion of ammonia is lowered although there may be an adaptive increase in total ammonia production per nephron, and the amount of titratable acid in the urine is normal unless either the dietary intake or intestinal absorption of phosphate are lowered. The total renal bicarbonate production and hydrogen ion excretion may fall below the total rate of hydrogen production.

Logically this imbalance between acid production and removal should result in a progressive acidosis and yet the patient usually has a relatively stable acidosis whose extent is defined above. There must therefore be a further method of removing or buffering hydrogen ions which involve buffers outside the extracellular fluid in addition to the buffering provided by plasma proteins. It is probable that the large reserves of carbonate and bicarbonate within bone are the source of this buffering capacity. With the exception of renal disease causing renal tubular acidosis, the urine pH in uraemia is usually below 5.5. At this pH the loss of bicarbonate into the urine is minimal but if bicarbonate is administered to a patient it tends to leak into the urine as the plasma bicarbonate concentration rises. It is thus difficult to sustain a normal plasma bicarbonate concentration by the administration of alkali.

Acidosis of hyperglycaemic diabetic coma (diabetic ketoacidosis). The pathogenesis of hyperglycaemic ketotic diabetic coma is described in detail elsewhere (see page 9.43); only the acid–base disturbances will be discussed here.

Diabetic ketoacidosis is a classical high anion gap metabolic acidosis due to the accumulation of organic acids as a result of their increased production and decreased peripheral utilization. The acids responsible are acetoacetic acid and 3-hydroxybutyric acid which are interconvertible through the enzyme 3-hydroxybutyrate dehydrogenase, and which are produced in large amounts when there is a lack of insulin. If the ketones are the only acids present in excess, the extent of the acidosis as measured by the decrease in plasma bicarbonate concentration and the increase in the anion gap above the normal value can be fully accounted for by the increased ketone concentration in blood. The total ketone body concentration in blood in the well-controlled fed diabetic patient attending a diabetic clinic is about 0.1 mmol/l. In diabetic ketoacidosis the concentration is often above 10 mmol/l and can rise as high as 30 mmol/l. The acidaemia produces both respiratory and renal responses. The rate and depth of respiration are increased (Kussmaul breathing) and the decreased P_{CO_2} and carbonic acid tend to return the blood pH to normal although the respiratory responses are slow to achieve maximum effect, and cases where the arterial blood pH is less than 7 are quite often seen. The renal response is to conserve base through the tubular re-absorption of bicarbonate resulting in an acid urine. Large amounts of acid are excreted through the titration of the urinary buffers ammonia and phosphate and as undissociated ketoacids themselves which are approximately half ionized at the minimum pH of urine. Thus the amounts of urinary titratable acid in ketoacidosis may be as high as ten times that normally excreted.

After insulin and fluid therapy the tissue metabolism of the ketones via oxidation generates alkali which results in a return of the blood and tissue pH to normal over the course of several hours. Another mechanism works to correct the pH although its contribution is quantitatively small. This is the non-enzymic conversion of aceto-acetate to acetone which is then excreted.

However, this is a simplistic view of diabetic coma and the clinical picture may be complicated in two ways, firstly by the contribution of underlying disease or other factors to the pathogenesis of the acidosis and secondly by the occurrence of mixed acid–base abnormalities one part only of which is ketone accumulation. In the first case the presence of renal disease with impairment of renal function may blunt the normal renal response to an acidosis and the occurrence of volume depletion caused by fluid loss via an osmotic diuresis or vomiting may compromise renal function. Secondly complex acid–base changes can occur during treatment.

A metabolic alkalosis can follow ketoacidosis when vomiting has been severe and when excessive amounts of bicarbonate have been infused to treat the acidaemia. In such a case, although pH_a may initially be returned to normal, the quantity of acid anions in the form of ketones remains high as does the anion gap. When the ketones are metabolized during treatment metabolic alkalosis ensues.

When the acutely ill diabetic patient has an underlying infective disease such as pneumonia, the hyperventilation accompanying this may effectively increase the usual compensation of the acidosis. In such a case the pH may be normal with a low plasma bicarbonate concentration. A similar abnormality can occur during the therapy of ketoacidosis when, as the ketones are metabolized to produce base, the respiratory compensation returns to normal more slowly and thus the P_{a,CO_2} remains low when the plasma bicarbonate is normal or near normal and the pH_a may then become alkaline. A third mixed abnormality is that of lactic acidosis either developing during therapy or playing a major role in the pathogenesis of the presenting acidosis. During the therapy of diabetic ketoacidosis, if the blood sugar is falling satisfactorily and the blood ketone concentration is also decreasing, the persistence of a severe metabolic acidosis should alert the clinician to the possibility of a supervening lactic acidosis. In addition there is a significant contribution to the metabolic acidosis by the accumulation of lactic acid to concentrations of 5 mmol/l or above in 5 to 10 per cent of cases of ketoacidosis. In most cases these concentrations fall with successful treatment of ketoacidosis but may, on occasions, rise further late in the progress of the disease. This occurs particularly when there is shock or hypoxia or infection as an underlying condition. A mixed acidosis of this type has also been described during phenformin therapy.

Lactic acidosis. *Nature and classification.* In a normal, healthy human the concentration of lactate in the venous blood varies within the narrow limits of 0.6–1.2 mmol/l. It is low after fasting and rises after meals, but the homeostatic mechanisms are such as to maintain the concentration within the limits defined above. The main exception to this is severe physical exercise where the concentration may rise to 10 mmol/l or above. In this case however the concentration rapidly returns to normal on cessation of exercise.

Lactic acid has a pK of 3.86 and thus over a wide range of pH will be completely dissociated so that the accumulation of the lactate ion in body fluids and tissues is accompanied by a similar amount of hydrogen ion.

There are conditions under which the regulation of lactate metabolism is disturbed in such a way as to cause the accumulation of lactic acid. These conditions can be divided into two groups: firstly hyperlactataemia where there is a raised lactate concentration without changes in blood pH, and secondly lactic acidosis when the rise in lactate concentration and the accompanying hydrogen ion accumulation is sufficient to lower the blood pH. Many definitions of lactic acidosis exist, and for practical purposes a working definition is that lactic acidosis is characterized by a persistently raised blood lactate concentration together with a lowered blood pH. Clinical experience has shown that the blood lactate concentration has to be 5 mmol/l or above in such cases irrespective of the concentration of other anions; below this concentration the homeostatic mechanisms described earlier in this chapter are able to keep the pH within normal limits. Cases of lactic acidosis fall into two groups (A and B). In type A lactic acidosis, which is the most common the patients have signs of poor tissue perfusion with or without hypoxia. Patients with haemorrhagic shock or a severe myocardial infarct and left ventricular failure provide good examples of this type. Here the accumulation of lactic acid can mostly be explained by its overproduction in those tissues having a high glycolytic capacity. The type B patients, however, do not have signs of tissue hypoxia or underperfusion except as a secondary and late event and thus to explain lactate accumulation in such cases there must be occult overproduction or underutilization or a combination of these two mechanisms. The type B cases can be further sub-classified into those occurring as a result of the administration of certain drugs, chemicals, and toxic compounds and those in which the patient has an inherited metabolic defect which results in lactate accumulation (a detailed classification is given in Table 2). Many of the causes listed in this Table are rare, being the subject of single case reports. The vast majority of information has been collected from the study of either patients with shock (type A) or those associated with phenformin therapy (type B). The condition has been almost exclusively confined to the accumulation of the natural L(+) isomer of lactic acid. Although man has the capacity to metabolize the D-isomer, it is not a product of normal metabolism, but a small amount is ingested in food and produced by bacterial metabolism in the gut. One case of D-lactic acidosis in man has been described due to excessive D-lactic acid production in the gut.

The clinical presentation in type B lactic acidosis is fairly uniform, the patients having the following collection of symptoms listed in order of frequency: vomiting, coma or impairment of consciousness, nausea, epigastric pain, loss of appetite, overbreathing, lethargy, diarrhoea, and thirst. This list was compiled from the presenting symptoms of a large collected series of phenformin-associated cases and may in part reflect underlying or accompanying disease together with the more specific symptoms of an acidosis such as impairment of consciousness and overbreathing. The onset of symptoms and signs is usually rapid with development of the acidosis over the course of a few hours accompanied by a deterioration in the level of consciousness which varies from mild confusion to coma and may, in the early stages, be accompanied by profound lethargy.

Although these symptoms and signs are not specific, some indication that lactic acidosis may be present can be obtained from general clinical assessment and biochemical tests. Lactic acidosis has been described in association with many disorders but most frequently with diabetes mellitus (especially in association with biguanide therapy), liver disease, renal impairment, acute pancreatitis, bacterial infections, septicaemia, leukaemia, and lymphoma. Although the reported cases may reflect the experience and speciality of the reporting author rather than the true incidence, the associations listed above may alert the clinician to the possibility of lactic acid accumulation as a cause of a metabolic acidosis. Determination of the plasma electrolytes can indicate that a metabolic acidosis is due to the accumulation of organic acids. In such cases the plasma bicarbonate concentration is lowered and the anion gap is increased.

The definitive diagnosis depends on the identification of lactate as the organic anion causing the acidosis. The measurement of lactate in plasma, urine, and other body fluids is simple, rapid, and specific through the use of enzymic spectrophotometric micromethods. The concentrations of several other blood constituents are altered in lactic acidosis such as inorganic phosphate, uric acid, and some amino acids, but these changes are not universal and are thus of limited diagnostic use. In patients with hyperglycaemic ketotic diabetic coma a substantial contribution to the metabolic acidosis is made by lactate, and occasionally, while the patient may not have a very raised blood lactate concentration at presentation, lactic acidosis may develop during the course of treatment (see above).

Pathogenesis. Disturbances of lactate homeostasis sufficient to cause an acidosis must be due to either (*a*) an increased lactate production, or (*b*) impaired lactate utilization or a combination of these two processes.

Catheter studies have shown that between 30 and 50 per cent of the total daily lactate production of about 1.2 mol/24 hours/70 kg body weight in man is taken up by the liver. Many patients with liver disease have an elevated resting blood lactate concentration and their ability to dispose of an exogenous lactate load is impaired. Some 30–40 per cent of patients with lactate acidosis have evidence of liver disease and thus many explanations of the pathogenesis of lactic acidosis have centred upon the liver.

Although hyperlactataemia is a common finding in patients with liver disease only a few develop lactic acidosis. The hyperlactataemia in liver disease can be explained by impaired utilization but before lactic acidosis can develop the extent of impairment must be severe or increased production must be present.

The weight of evidence leads to the conclusion that phenformin therapy and lactic acidosis are causally related. The drug has been shown to both increase lactate production in the splanchnic bed and decrease hepatic lactate uptake. Increased peripheral production of lactic acid may also be involved.

Increased lactate production is probably the main contributing factor in type A lactic acidosis but impaired utilization is also involved. This latter factor may be a result of impaired energy supply in those tissues usually removing lactate and both animal and human experimental data show that organs which usually

remove lactate may produce lactate in the presence of shock. Infusion of fructose, sorbitol, or xylitol have all been associated with lactic acidosis in man and during fructose infusion the liver becomes a site of net lactate production because a major portion of the infused substrate is metabolized to lactate at a rate which is greater than the removal capacity of the extrahepatic tissues. In the cases described in association with cancer the increased lactate production consequent upon the high glycolytic capacity of malignant tissue is probably important.

Skeletal muscle is another potential site of lactate uptake but the evidence proving uptake and removal in this tissue in man is incomplete. A final factor which deserves mention is the possibility that a defect in hydrogen ion buffering capacity and renal hydrogen ion excretion may contribute. Moderate hyperlactataemia is not usually accompanied by acid–base changes apart from an alkalosis in some patients with liver disease and thus, if buffering ability or renal excretion of hydrogen ion were impaired, they could help to initiate lactic acidosis. Cases of lactic acidosis have been described where previous unexplained episodes of metabolic acidosis preceded the lactic acidosis and an impaired capacity to excrete an acid load has been demonstrated in some patients treated with phenformin.

Treatment and prognosis. There are two main objectives of treatment, firstly, to identify the precipitating factors and treat them particularly in patients with type A acidosis where reversal of hypoxia and treatment of circulatory collapse are vital, and secondly, the correction of the acidosis with the aim of restoring the arterial hydrogen ion concentration to normal. In addition, where a drug or toxin has been identified attempts can be made to accelerate its elimination from the body. There is evidence that strenuous early treatment of hypoxia and circulatory collapse with oxygen, plasma volume expanders and other drugs may lead to a favourable response in type A cases. Some caution, however, should be exercised in the use of vasoconstrictor drugs as these, while raising blood pressure, may decrease the perfusion of already anoxic tissues and can in the case of sympathomimetic agents have the effect of increasing tissue glycolysis and thus lactic acid production.

The negative inotropic effect of a systemic acidosis on left ventricular output makes correction of the acidosis vital. The infusion of isotonic sodium bicarbonate solution is the method of choice and large amounts (over 1000 mmol of base in some cases) may be needed, reflecting probably the continuing production of an acid load. The effects of bicarbonate infusion are complex because in addition to restoring the pH of the plasma to normal it also expands the plasma volume and alters the activity of key enzymes in lactate metabolizing and producing pathways. The efficacy of bicarbonate treatment is difficult to assess. The amounts given to survivors and non-survivors have been similar but there is some evidence that the mortality is lower in patients whose plasma hydrogen ion concentration has been restored to normal with bicarbonate. There has been no controlled trial and the information is largely anecdotal, a successful outcome being more likely to be reported.

Other agents have been used. The use of sodium lactate is contra-indicated as the production of alkali from this compound depends upon its metabolism which may be impaired in lactic acidosis. The amine buffer THAM (trishydroxymethyl-aminomethane) has been used to avoid the sodium load accompanying bicarbonate infusion and attempts have been made to increase lactate removal by giving the hydrogen acceptor methylene blue or using peritoneal or haemodialysis against acetate-containing dialysis fluids. Dialysis against a hypertonic fluid may be useful if large volumes of sodium bicarbonate need to be administered to correct the acidosis. In cases of drug-induced lactic acidosis it may increase clearance of the causative drug. Again the evidence of benefit is slender and anecdotal in nature.

An alternative approach is to accelerate lactate removal by stimulating the activity of pyruvate dehydrogenase and hence lower the concentrations of pyruvate and lactate in blood. The administration of insulin together with a glucose infusion has been tried on these grounds, but it can deepen the acidosis through a stimulation of tissue glycolysis. More recently the compound dichloroacetate has been suggested as a specific form of treatment. This compound stimulates pyruvate dehydrogenase activity but its usage has been limited and no proper assessment of its value can be made. Overall the prognosis of lactic acidosis is poor, the mortality being very high in type A cases where their survival is clearly related to the blood lactate concentration on presentation. A blood lactate concentration of 9 mmol/l or greater is accompanied by a mortality of 80 per cent or greater. In the type B cases, the mortality is about 50 per cent, still high but lower than in type A. In part this may be due to earlier diagnosis in phenformin-related cases because of widespread knowledge of the association. There is some evidence that since the withdrawal of phenformin in some countries and the restrictions placed upon its use in others the incidence of type B cases has fallen.

Conditions with imperfectly defined source of acidosis. In Table 2, (part 3) there is a list of high anion gap metabolic acidoses where the source of the acidosis has not been well defined. These are, with certain exceptions, rarely seen in clinical practice but deserve some discussion here.

Alcoholic (ethanol) acidosis. A high anion gap metabolic acidosis can occur after heavy ethanol intake, usually in premenopausal women. The acidosis is due to the accumulation of 3-hydroxybutyrate predominantly together with a small excess of acetoacetate. In some cases the blood lactate concentration is normal but lactic acidosis has also been described following ethanol abuse. In this case the lactic acid accumulation is most probably due to the inhibition of gluconeogenesis from lactate by ethanol.

Methanol-induced acidosis. When large outbreaks of methanol poisoning have been well documented a metabolic acidosis of rapid onset has frequently been described. The acids responsible for the acidosis are lactic acid and formic acid. The latter is formed as a result of the metabolism of methanol via formaldehyde and has been shown to accumulate in blood but the extent of accumulation is not usually sufficient to account for the whole of the increase in anion gap in poisoned patients. Recent observations have shown lactic acid to be the major organic acid in such cases. This may accumulate because of the inhibition of gluconeogenesis from lactate by methanol or the effect of formaldehyde in uncoupling oxidative phosphorylation. The onset of such an acidosis after methanol ingestion requires treatment with bicarbonate to correct the blood pH because there is some evidence that this will decrease the retinal toxicity of methanol and decrease the overall mortality. In some cases dialysis to remove the methanol and the administration of ethanol to inhibit the metabolism of methanol have been used.

Paraldehyde-induced acidosis. The prolonged administration or ingestion of paraldehyde can be followed by a profound metabolic acidosis. The cause for the acidosis is unknown. One suggestion has been acetic acid which is a decomposition product of paraldehyde which is stored for long periods particularly when exposed to sunlight. However, the acidosis occurs after the administration of fresh paraldehyde and there have been no cases where sufficient acetate has been detected in the blood to explain the degree of acidosis recorded.

Ethylene glycol poisoning. The ingestion of ethylene glycol can cause a metabolic acidosis. This compound is metabolized to oxalic acid but, although this acid and lactate have both been shown to accumulate in the blood of patients after ethylene glycol ingestion, the quantities involved are not sufficient to account for the acidosis.

Salicylate poisoning. The initial acid–base abnormality in cases of salicylate poisoning is a respiratory alkalosis secondary to hyperventilation. In some cases, however, in both child and adult, a metabolic acidosis can occur as a later event. This is thought to be secondary to the effects of salicylate upon intermediary metabolism, particularly its action in uncoupling oxidative phosphorylation and inhibitionary lactate disposal via gluconeogenesis. The acids

responsible are the salicylate itself, the keto acids acetoacetate and 3-hydroxybutyrate, and lactate. This response to salicylate overdose is most often seen in childhood.

Normal anion gap metabolic acidosis
Renal tubular acidosis. Renal tubular acidosis is a syndrome consisting of a persistent or episodic acidosis with a low serum bicarbonate concentration and an elevated serum chloride concentration occurring in patients who are unable to excrete a normal quantity of acid into the urine. The hyperchloraemic acidosis may be accompanied by other abnormalities of electrolyte metabolism, and their consequences. Thus large urinary potassium losses can result in hypokalaemia and its symptoms and signs such as muscle weakness and paralysis. Excessive urinary calcium losses may contribute to the pathogenesis of osteomalacia, nephrocalcinosis, and renal stones found in some types of the disorder. Renal damage consequent upon the nephrocalcinosis and potassium deficiency can result in loss of urine concentrating ability and polyuria.

Two distinct types of defect have been described. In the first, the so called 'classical' or gradient renal tubular acidosis the patient cannot lower the urinary pH below 6 however severe the systemic acidosis. Such patients, however, have a near normal capacity to reabsorb bicarbonate from the glomerular filtrate.

In the second type of disorder, while the biochemical features can be similar to those in the classical type, the patients have a decreased capacity to reabsorb bicarbonate from the glomerular filtrate. This variant has been named the 'bicarbonate wastage' (proximal) form.

Classical renal tubular acidosis. This condition can present with a number of clinical features. The systemic acidosis is of the hyperchloraemic type and the serum concentrations of sodium, potassium, calcium, and phosphate may all be lowered. The serum alkaline phosphatase activity may be increased. Polyuria may occur. The urine is inappropriately alkaline in relation to the systemic acidosis. It contains lowered quantities of ammonia and titratable acid but increased amounts of potassium, calcium, and phosphate. Osteomalacia, renal stones, and nephrocalcinosis can occur and the patient may experience bone pain and muscle weakness. In some cases, the muscle weakness may be periodic and periodic paralysis may be a clinical feature.

All these abnormalities are consequent upon a single defect of urinary acidification. The capacity to secrete hydrogen ions in the proximal tubule is normal as shown by the complete reabsorption of bicarbonate from the glomerular filtrate; bicarbonate does not leak out of the proximal tubule. In addition the excretion of ammonia, corrected for the glomerular filtration rate and urine pH, is normal and thus the key abnormality is the loss of the power of the distal tubule to maintain a steep pH gradient between the blood and the urine within the tubule. This may be due to an increased permeability of the distal tubular cells to hydrogen ions which can thus diffuse back into the blood from the tubular urine. The electrolyte disturbances are corrected by treatment with sodium and potassium and bicarbonate. However, where permanent renal damage has occurred, the response to therapy may be incomplete.

Classical renal tubular acidosis may have several causes and classifications have usually subdivided these into primary and secondary types. In cases of the primary type there is no history of previous disease and the disorder is not part of another disease. This form of renal tubular acidosis may occur as a transient disorder in infancy and as a permanent disorder starting in childhood or adult life. Both types can be familial but this is rare in the transient variety and common in the permanent variety and this latter type can also be sporadic in nature. In families with the permanent type of primary renal tubular acidosis a dominant transmission has been described, although expression may vary within the members of an affected family. The genetics of the primary type starting in infancy are unclear.

In the secondary type of classical renal tubular acidosis the disorder accompanies existing systemic disease or some types of poisoning. One group consists of patients having raised gamma globulins from various causes. Thus secondary classical renal tubular acidosis has been described in idiopathic hypergammaglobulinaemia, lupus hepatitis, and coccidioidomycosis where raised concentrations of 7S gamma globulin occur in the blood. Waldenström's macroglobulinaemia can also be accompanied by this type of renal tubular acidosis as can cryoglobulinaemia. The mechanism through which these abnormal proteins produce renal tubular damage is not known.

The secondary type of the classical disorder has also been described with hyperparathyroidism, hyperthyroidism, vitamin D toxicity, amphotericin B toxicity, and a number of other rare disorders.

Bicarbonate wastage (proximal) renal tubular acidosis. This type of renal tubular acidosis is due to a defect in the proximal tubular reabsorption of bicarbonate. The patients excrete a large amount of bicarbonate which results in a reduction in plasma bicarbonate concentration. The concentration falls until the filtered load reaches that level at which proximal tubular function is able to reabsorb the filtered load, a threshold at which bicarbonate disappears from the urine, the urine pH falls sharply and the urinary content of ammonia and titratable acidity rise. In these patients, therefore, the urine may have a low pH at presentation, in contrast to the findings in classical distal renal tubular acidosis.

There are two types of this disorder, primary and secondary. The primary type can occur as an isolated renal tubular defect or as a part of the idiopathic Fanconi syndrome. The secondary type has been described as a complication of many disorders which are accompanied by an increased urinary lysozyme content, resulting either from renal damage or systemic overproduction. This enzyme is bound to the proximal tubule and has been implicated as a causative factor. Thus the defect has been described in dysproteinaemic states, heavy metal poisoning, and rejection after renal transplantation.

The broad diagnosis of renal tubular acidosis can be established by using the ammonium chloride load test. After an overnight fast but with ample water intake ammonium chloride is given by mouth, in a dose of 100 mg per kg body weight. After discarding the urine passed in the first two hours after dosage the urine is collected at hourly intervals between three and eight hours after dosing and its pH immediately measured. The diagnosis is established if the patient is unable to lower the urinary pH below 6. The ability to acidify the urine as shown by a lower urinary pH rules out the diagnosis and the test can then be stopped.

It is difficult to distinguish between the types of renal tubular acidosis because they may both give positive results in the ammonium chloride load test. The presence of the bicarbonate wastage (proximal) type may have to be confirmed by the determination of the Tm for bicarbonate during bicarbonate infusion. There are other clinical features which can help to classify a particular case. In the classical type with a gradient defect nephrocalcinosis is common, being rare in the bicarbonate wastage type. Also in the gradient type the urine is always relatively alkaline however profound the systemic acidosis and thus if the urine pH is low the defect cannot be of this type. The classical gradient type of defect is easily corrected with bicarbonate therapy while the bicarbonate wastage type is not, the patients in these cases being very resistant to alkali therapy. In the bicarbonate wastage type the reabsorption of bicarbonate is always impaired while it is not altered in the classical type. The main clinical and other features of the two types of defect are summarized in Table 7.

Table 7   A summary of the main features of the types of renal tubular acidosis

	Classical or gradient type	Bicarbonate wastage (proximal) type
Site of defect	distal tubule	proximal tubule
Nephrocalcinosis	common ($> 70\%$)	rare
Aminoaciduria + glycosuria	rare	common
Ammonia excretion	normal	normal
Maximum lowering of urine pH		
(a) when serum bicarbonate is greater than 18 mmol/l	>6.0	>6.0
(b) when serum bicarbonate is less than 13 mmol/l	>6.0	<5.4
Response to alkali therapy	sensitive	resistant

References

Campbell, E. J. M. (1974). Hydrogen ion (acid–base) regulation. In *Clinical physiology,* 4th edn (eds. E. J. M. Campbell, C. J. Dickinson, and J. D. H. Slater). Blackwell Scientific Publications, Oxford.

Cohen, R. D. and Iles, R. A. (1980). Lactic acidosis: diagnosis and treatment. *Clins Endocr. Metab.* **9**, 513.

— and Woods, H. F. (1976). *Clinical and biochemical aspects of lactic acidosis.* Blackwell Scientific Publications, Oxford.

Emmett, M. and Narins, R. G. (1977). Clinical use of the anion gap. *Medicine, Baltimore* **56**, 38.

Huehns, E. R. (1976). Disorders of carbohydrate metabolism in the red blood corpuscle. *Clins Endocr. Metab.* **5**, 651.

Mitchell, J. H., Wildenthal, K., and Johnson, R. C. (1972). The effects of acid–base disturbances on cardiovascular and pulmonary function. *Kidney Int.* **1**, 375.

Muldowney, F. P. (1979). Renal acidosis. In *Renal disease* (eds. D. Black and N. F. Jones), 588. Blackwell Scientific Publications, Oxford.

Poole-Wilson, P. A. (1978). Measurement of myocardial intracellular pH in pathological states. *J. Molec. Cell. Cardiol.* **10**, 511.

Seldin, D. W. and Wilson, J. D. (1978). Renal tubular acidosis. In *The metabolic basis of inherited disease* (eds. J. B. Stanbury, J. B. Wyngaarden, and D. S. Fredrickson). McGraw-Hill, New York.

Section 10
Endocrine disorders

Introduction to endocrinology

Pamela C. B. MacKinnon

Historical perspectives. The first recorded experiment in the field of endocrinology appears to have been that of Berthold (1849) who, having removed the testicles of a cock, observed the subsequent regression of its wattle and its loss of interest in the opposite sex. Transplantation of the testes to the abdominal cavity of the deprived animal led not only to the revival of its appendages but a renewed attention to the local hens. Towards the end of the century, further observations were made along these lines when Brown-Séquard, a well-respected physician, suggested that all animal tissues produced specific chemical substances which were required for full healthy vigour. But his objectivity in the matter was open to question when he reported a certain invigoration which followed a course of subcutaneous self-injections of testicular extracts obtained from dogs and guinea-pigs. Albeit, a little later, Dr George Murray (1891) injected extracts of thyroid tissue into a patient with myxoedema and reported a cure, while Oliver and Schäfer (1894) published a report on the vasopressor effect of adrenal medullary extract. When, in 1904, Bayliss and Starling demonstrated that acidification of the intestinal mucosa caused 'secretin' to enter the circulation and regulate the flow of pancreatic juices, the disciplined study of the 'internal secretions' had started. A further important landmark was the isolation of insulin by Banting and Best (1922), who first ligated the pancreatic duct to ensure enzymatic digestion of the acinar portion of the gland before extracting the tissue. Over the next two decades new chemical techniques were developed and isolation and purification of most of the protein and steroid hormones derived from the pituitary gland and its target organs were achieved. Furthermore, P. E. Smith (1929) developed a technique for the removal of the pituitary gland in the rat which enabled meaningful experiments to be designed with respect to the influence of pituitary hormones on their target organs.

Following the collation of evidence by F. H. A. Marshall (1942) of environmental influences on pituitary gland activity and the description of a portal system between the hypothalamus and the anterior pituitary gland in humans (Popa and Fielding 1930), G. W. Harris (1955) produced a monograph in which he emphasized the functional significance of this unique vascular connection. Harris promoted the concept that neurohumours, secreted in the brain and released into the portal vessels, caused either an increase or an inhibition of the release of anterior pituitary hormones. Complementing Harris' investigations were those of the Scharrers; they shocked conventional neurophysiological notions by demonstrating that neurones of the central nervous system could secrete appreciable quantities of what was then called neurosecretory material into blood sinusoids of the posterior lobe of the pituitary. Subsequent work has substantiated the claims of both sets of workers. Hypothalamic 'releasing' and/or 'inhibitory' factors have been isolated for each of the anterior pituitary hormones, and at least three of these factors have been characterized and synthesized by Guillemin (1969) and by Schally (1971); while the posterior lobe octapeptides, oxytocin and vasopressin, are now well recognized.

Almost invariably scientific knowledge expands very rapidly in the wake of new technical advances and at no time has this been more apparent than in the late 1960s when Berson and Yalow developed and promoted the sensitive methods of competitive protein binding and radioimmunoassay which superceded bioassays and enabled minute amounts of circulating hormones to be measured reliably and at a relatively low cost. Since then considerable knowledge has been acquired, not only with respect to the physiology of individual endocrine glands but to the neural control of the pituitary gland and the reciprocal effects of target gland hormones on the hypothalamus and the pituitary.

The most recent chapter in this brief history has been written by Kosterlitz and Hughes (1975) who reported the presence, in the forebrain, of a peptide (encephalin) possessing many of the properties of exogenously administered morphine. A number of different peptides, largely related to specific neuronal pathways, have been found in many parts of the central nervous system (e.g. neurotensin, VIP, substance P). Moreover, peptides with similar immunoreactive properties have been discovered in the pituitary gland, the mucosa of the gut and in certain organs derived from it. The molecular structure of these peptides suggests that many are enzymatically cleaved from certain common parent molecules, some of which may have their origins in primitive phyla. Although the functions of this somewhat ubiquitous peptidergic system are only beginning to be recognized, it would seem that certain peptide producing cells have endocrine-like activity, others have neurotransmitter or neuromodulatory activity, and yet others possess a morphology and apparent function that defies a strict classification along these lines. Clearly, however, no study of endocrinology will now be complete without a consideration of these peptides.

Homeostasis. Any organism, if it is to achieve optimal performance or to survive when exposed to potentially lethal fluctuations of its external environment, must possess homeostatic mechanisms which control the quantity and quality of its body fluids. For instance, the rates at which various nutrients enter and leave the extracellular space must be controlled. If the flux of glucose into the extracellular space was permitted to fall below its flux out of the space, then glucose deficiency would ensue and the proper function of the glucose-dependent central nervous system would be endangered. Homeostasis is effected by the interaction of the endocrine and neural systems and failure within either is a threat to survival.

Endocrine contribution to homeostasis is achieved by the production of a variety of different chemical messengers or hormones which are synthesized either by endocrine or by neurosecretory cells. *Endocrine cells* exert their effects by secreting hormones which act either locally on neighbouring cells (paracrine activity), or at a distance by virtue of having been secreted into the lumen of the gut (lumocrine activity) or into the blood stream (classical endocrine activity). *Endocrine neurones* on the other hand synthesize hormones within their perikarya and transport the material along axons for release into blood vessels at their terminations (Fig. 1). Before proceeding to the study of functions of individual glands and cells of the endocrine system, it is well worth while considering the basic principles of hormone synthesis and release, of plasma transport and cellular action and of integration within this diffuse and seemingly complex system.

Principles of hormone synthesis and release. The understanding of hormone production has been achieved by collation of data from microscopic studies of peripheral endocrine glands and from electrophysiological and electronmicroscopic studies of the hypothalamo-neurohypophysial system. All the available evidence suggests

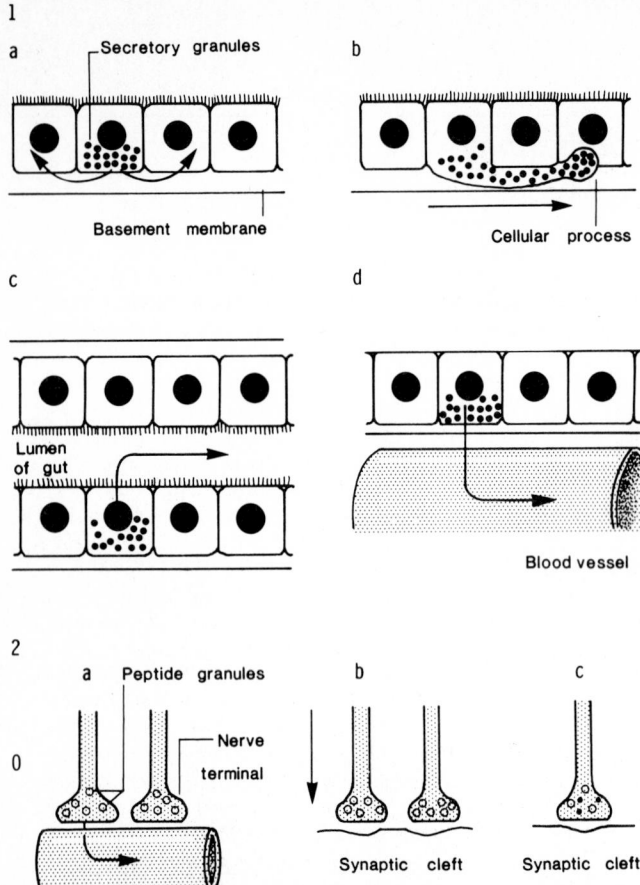

Fig. 1 Schematic representation of methods by which endocrine cells achieve their hormonal effects. 1a. local diffusion or paracrine effect; somatostatin cell within a pancreatic island. 1b. modified paracrine effect; cholecystokinin cell in intestinal mucosa. 1c. lumocrine effect; gastrin cell having effect at distal site within lumen of gut. 1d. classical endocrine effect; adrenocortical cell secreting into blood vessel. 2a. neuroendocrine effect; hypothalamic releasing hormone secreting into blood vessel. 2b and c. peptides having possible neurotransmitter or neuromodulatory effects respectively.

that neural or circulatory stimuli appropriate to protein-producing endocrine cells or endocrine neurons stimulate DNA and RNA mechanisms and that this leads to enlargement of both the cell nucleus and the cytoplasm. With the augmented production of RNA, protein synthesis increases, and this is associated with a multiplication of rough endoplasmic reticulum (RER), and the formation of cisternae. The Golgi apparatus also enlarges since it receives vacuoles containing secretory products from the RER which are packaged into granules (Fig. 2); some of these may contain precursor molecules (which are not necessarily biologically active), while others contain active hormones. These granules, which are frequently of varying electron density, are subsequently transported to their site of release at the membrane.

The release of secretions from protein-producing endocrine cells or endocrine neurones depends on neural and/or hormonal stimuli. As an example the release of neurosecretory material into the blood sinusoids of the posterior pituitary is determined by volleys of action potentials passing down the axons. This activity causes depolarization of the terminals and an influx of Ca^{2+} upon which the discharge of hormones depends. An acute neural stimulus causes a fast but transient release of hormone which represents only a fraction of the total content, yet chronic stimulation will result in a steady basal secretion. These findings imply the presence of two hormonal pools, one of which is 'readily releasable' and the other which is not as easily available. If newly synthesized hormone is

labelled by an intravenous injection of a radioactive marker and release is then stimulated, the specific radioactivity of the released hormone is far higher than that of the gland as a whole. This observation suggests that the readily releasable pool contains newly formed granules; moreover, autoradiographic studies have shown that such granules are the first to be transported to the nerve terminals. If new granules are not quickly released from neurosecretory axons, they move to storage swellings. Release from the nerve endings is primarily by exocytosis but the precise mechanism by which the neurosecretory granules fuse with the terminal membrane to release their contents into the bloodstream is not known. The membrane surrounding the granule is not extruded but is retrieved, forming a vacuole in the terminal cytoplasm, the membrane of which is either recycled or broken down by lysosomal action. These general principles do not apply to steroid hormones which may after synthesis diffuse across the cell membrane or to the synthesis and release of thyroxines.

Plasma transport. When considering the transport of many hormones to their cellular site of action, it is useful to classify them into two groups: those which act at the cell surface, generally without broaching the plasma membrane; and those which enter the cell before effecting a response. The catecholamines and protein hormones belong to the first group and circulate in relatively low concentrations in a free or unbound state in the plasma. The second group consists of thyroid and steroid hormones which circulate in somewhat higher concentrations but are largely adherent to macromolecules. Active thyroid hormones (T_3 and T_4) bind to thyroid binding globulin (TBG), prealbumin, and to a lesser extent, albumin. The affinity of binding to these large plasma proteins depends on the character of the amino side-chains and the number of iodine substituents that the thyronines possess, T_4 binding better than T_3. However, only the free or unbound fraction of these hormones is available to the tissues and capable of action.

From a functional point of view such binding alters the metabolism of the thyroid hormones in that filtration through the kidney glomeruli is lowered, the rate of turnover is slowed, and the distribution volume is affected. This metabolically inert reservoir represents an important homeostatic mechanism in that it prevents the rapid breakdown of the thyroid molecules, and minimizes the effects of any fluctuations in hormonal output.

The major transport mechanism for cortisol or corticosterone and also progesterone is an α globulin known as corticosteroid binding globulin (CBG). If the binding sites on this macromolecule become saturated, then the spillover of hormone adheres loosely to albumin. Transport macromolecules for oestrogens and androgens also exist in the circulation as sex binding globulin (SBG).

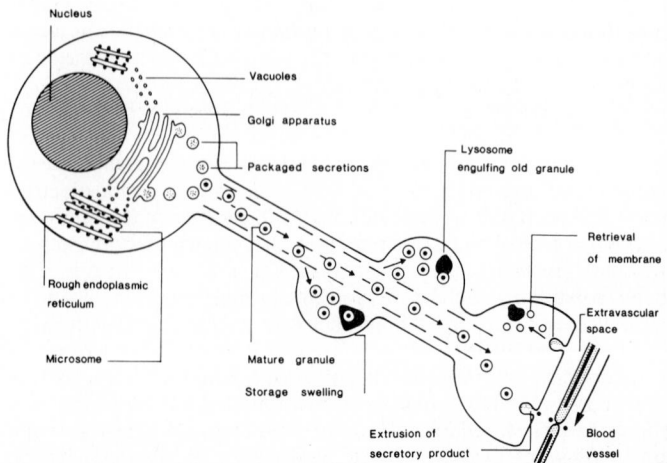

Fig. 2 Schematic summary of a neurosecretory cell indicating processes of synthesis, packaging of granules, transport, and release of secretory products.

Alterations of hormone binding interactions may be caused by variations in the appropriate endocrine organs which can lead to either excessive or subnormal concentrations of hormones in the blood, or alternatively they may be caused by alterations in the concentration or affinity of the binding mechanisms.

Action. Hormones which act at the cell surface (Fig. 3a). The low concentrations at which catecholamines or protein and peptide hormones are known to circulate are commensurate with the high affinity of their respective receptor sites and their marked specificities which permit recognition of the relevant hormone amid an excess of protein molecules in the circulation. As the hormone binds to the cell surface receptor, it is coupled by a regulatory protein to adenylate cyclase which in many cases (though not invariably) catalyses the formation of cyclic adenosine monophosphate (cAMP) from adenosine triphosphate (ATP). This so-called 'second messenger' triggers a cascade of biochemical events which leads either to a rapid response such as ion transport, carbohydrate metabolism or steroidogenesis, or to a slow response such as DNA, RNA, and protein synthesis, with a resultant cell growth or cell division. Although RNA mechanisms appear to be stimulated by many hormone activities, this is not invariably the case, and there are many instances in which hormonal activities are expressed in the presence of inhibitors of nucleoprotein synthesis.

The ability of peptide hormones to regulate the concentrations of their specific receptor sites has been demonstrated in numerous tissues. Generally speaking, after activation the receptor population becomes de-sensitized or 'down regulated' which is thought to be attributable to depletion or a decreased availability of a proportion of the receptor population. Recent studies, however, indicate that the process of down regulation may in addition involve an alteration of transmembrane events.

Hormones which act within the cell. Steroids (Fig. 3b). Our present understanding of steroid binding and its action on DNA and RNA mechanisms in promoting target tissue growth and metabolism is derived largely from studies of oestrogen binding in the rat uterus. This steroid enters most cells of the body where it may be loosely bound in the cytoplasm. On entering the cells of its well-recognized target tissues, however, it is bound by a cytoplasmic molecule with a low capacity but high affinity for the steroid. This receptor-hormone complex is immediately translocated to the nucleus. A second receptor protein (type II) has recently been found in the cytoplasm with a high capacity and low affinity for the steroid. Although the function of the type II receptor is not clear, it has been suggested that it may help to concentrate hormone in the cytoplasm. Oestrogen, once it has been translocated to the nucleus, is retained by its nuclear type I receptor for a period of four to six hours and its presence apparently causes an increase in a further nuclear receptor (nuclear type II), the levels of which remain elevated for 4–48 hours. The subsequent uterine growth which takes place over 24–48 hours can be correlated with the increased levels of nuclear type II receptors.

Thyroid hormones (Fig. 3b). Thyroid hormone receptors have been found in almost all mammalian cells and are only absent in tissues obtained from lower forms (e.g. *Drosophila*) which do not respond to these hormones. Unlike steroid receptors which are in cytoplasm and bind to chromatin only in the presence of the hormone, thyroid receptors are not in the cytoplasm. They are permanently associated with non-histone proteins within the chromatin. On entering the cell, T_4 converts largely to T_3 which binds immediately and with high affinity to the nuclear core-receptor.

Degradation. Degradation of *protein and peptide hormones* occurs in all tissues as a result of general proteolytic action. However, the glycoproteins TSH, LH, FSH, and human chorionic gonadotrophin are worth special mention in that they are formed from two subunit chains of amino acids to which carbohydrates are attached. Sialic acid forms part of the carbohydrate moiety and it appears to be an important factor in the biological potency of the molecule: if it is

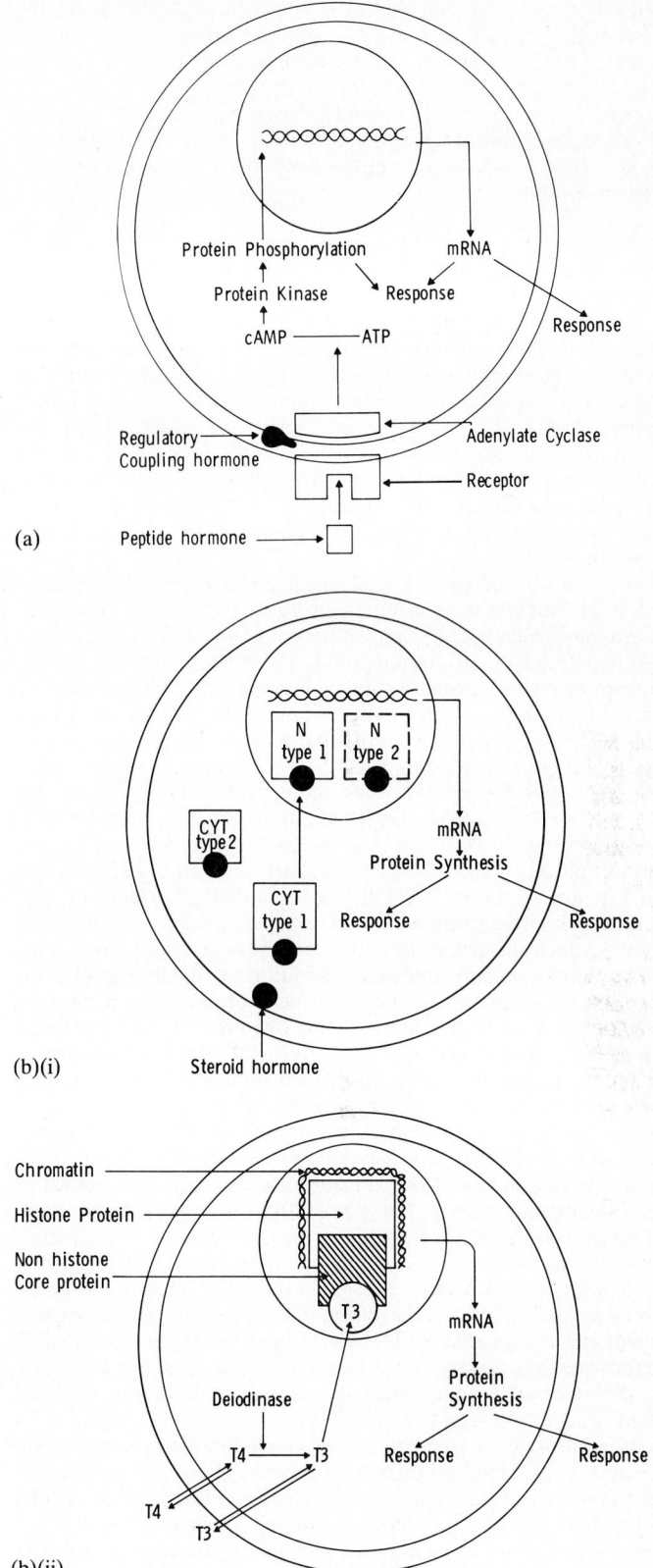

Fig. 3 Diagrams of hormones acting (a) at the cell surface; protein hormones. (b) within the cell: (i) steroid hormones; (ii) thyroid hormones.

cleaved off and degraded in the bloodstream there is a loss of hormonal activity. *Steroids*, on the other hand, are metabolized by enzymes in the liver and conjugated either with glucuronate or sulphate moieties. The resultant esters are water soluble and are therefore easily excreted in the urine and to a lesser extent in the bile. The rate at which this process occurs will depend on the binding affinities of the respective plasma binding proteins and the integrity of the liver. Thus, in cases of liver dysfunction, a decrease in the rate of degradation will lead to an increase in plasma steroid concentrations. Although *thyroid hormones* also undergo conjugation with glucuronate and sulphate moieties in the liver and kidney, they are first deiodinated by enzyme action in the tissues in order to conserve iodine.

Principles of integration between the endocrine and nervous system

Feedback mechanisms. Integration between certain systems of endocrine organs and their target tissues, or between endocrine and central nervous mechanisms, is brought about by a series of what systems engineers term 'feedback loops'. These are of two main types: 'long-loop' feedback mechanisms in which effects are exerted either directly between the parent gland and its distant target organ, or indirectly through the inclusion of other agents within the circuit, and 'short-loop' feedback mechanisms whereby secretions from a parent gland can influence its own output directly or indirectly.

Long-loop feedback. It is well recognized that control of anterior pituitary function is greatly influenced by releasing or inhibitory hormones which are secreted by neurones situated somewhere in the hypothalamus or preoptic area. These peptide hormones are transported along axons to the median eminence where they are stored until electrical or chemical stimuli reach the nerve terminals and dictate their release into capillaries of the pituitary portal system. On reaching the appropriate receptors on the plasma membranes of anterior pituitary cells, the peptides stimulate or inhibit the release of their specific trophic hormones. Certain of these hormones, e.g. growth hormone and prolactin have a direct action on peripheral tissues while luteinizing hormone (LH), follicle stimulation hormone (FSH), thyroid stimulating hormone (TSH), and adrenocorticotrophin (ACTH) exert their effects on peripheral glands which in turn secrete their own (target organ) hormones. These target organ hormones, in addition to affecting specific tissues in the periphery of the body and brain, exert a *negative feedback action* at the level of the hypothalamus and anterior pituitary, effecting in this way control over output of the corresponding trophic hormones. Evidence obtained from studies of primates suggests that feedback effects at pituitary level are of greater importance than those which may be taking place at the level of the hypothalamus. Nevertheless, anterior pituitary cells, at least the gonadotrophs, are unable to secrete normal amounts of gonadotrophins unless the gonadotrophin releasing hormone (GnRH) is released in a pulsatile fashion and at a specific frequency from the appropriate nerve terminals. If the frequency is reduced, then gonadotrophin levels in the plasma fall to minimal or undetectable values. Clearly, therefore, plasma concentrations of these hormones can be affected by two factors: the frequency of GnRH pulses which is controlled by neural influences; and the sensitivity of the anterior pituitary which depends on its hormonal environment.

In contrast to the negative feedback action on gonadotrophin release occasioned by low plasma concentrations of oestrogen, is the massive surge output of this trophic hormone which is the immediate stimulus to ovulation. This so-called *positive feedback* occurs as a result of a sustained increase in the secretion of oestrogen from developing ovarian follicles. That this effect of oestrogen is mediated at the pituitary level in primates was demonstrated by Knobil and his colleagues. Rhesus monkeys with regular menstrual cycles were subjected to an operation designed to destroy GnRH synthesizing neurones and to remove any influence of endogenous GnRH on the pituitary gonadotrophs. This led to minimal or undetectable levels of gonadotrophins in the plasma although concentrations of GH, prolactin, and TSH remained normal. A subsequent infusion of GnRH into the systemic circulation

at a specific pulse frequency led to restoration of normal gonadotrophin levels and normal menstrual cycles with pre-ovulatory oestrogen-stimulated LH surges. These elegant experiments demonstrate that, although proper functioning of the anterior pituitary is undoubtedly dependent upon a pulsatile release of GnRH, the ovarian oestrogen stimulus which triggers the pre-ovulatory LH surge (positive feedback) is directed at pituitary level. The significance of a pulsatile release of GnRH is not fully understood, but it may be associated with stimulation of receptors on the gonadotrophs which, after occupancy, are inhibited or 'down-regulated' and require a period of time for functional recovery. That these mechanisms can be altered at different times of life is clearly demonstrated by the marked fluctuations of LH which occur at night in pubertal boys and girls and which change when adulthood is reached to pulses of smaller amplitude and greater frequency throughout the day and night. It is of considerable interest that patients with anorexia nervosa show pubertal-like fluctuations in LH release during the stage of marked weight-loss and that on recovery there is a return to an adult-like pattern of LH release. Further investigations of neural mechanisms underlying the control of pituitary hormone output are obviously essential.

Short-loop feedback. There are many examples of short-loop feedback effects, perhaps the most familiar being the reciprocal effects between insulin and blood sugar levels. The trophic hormones of the pituitary also appear to be regulated to some degree by a feedback action at the level of their releasing factors. This type of control mechanism can be found in nearly all systems of the body and it is not surprising that 'ultra short-loop feedback' has also been described.

Synergistic action. An aspect of endocrine integration to which more attention should be paid is the synergistic activities of different hormones. One clear cut instance of this can be seen when pituitary tumour cells are incubated in an artificial serum with the addition of either T_3 or dexamethasone (Dx). Whereas each drug acting alone exerts only a minor effect on the output of GH, the addition of both T_3 and Dx at the same time leads to a highly significant increase in GH.

The peptidergic system. A potentially important set of integrating mechanisms, and one which acts on both the endocrine and nervous systems, can be found in the peptides of the nervous system, the gut, and certain endocrine glands. Their similar structures raise the intriguing question of their evolutionary origin. It has been suggested that since many of the peptide-producing cells share certain features, such as the ability to take up amine precursors and decarboxylate them, they may have a common origin in ectodermal stem cells. This became known as the APUD (amine precursor uptake and decarboxylation) theory and tumours of such cells are now termed 'apudomas'. Experimental embryological studies have not entirely supported this idea. A more recent suggestion has been that since all somatic cells have the capacity to produce a particular peptide or protein by virtue of possessing identical genomes, changes in the pattern of gene expression could account for the presence of similar molecules in both endocrine cells and neurones. It seems possible that during the course of evolution, duplication and the mutation of relatively few genes could have resulted in the formation of certain peptides which, favoured by the processes of natural selection, have been used by different cells for different purposes. Utilization of the same active molecule at different sites appears to reflect a biological economy, but it also necessitates the development of mechanisms to ensure specificity. Such mechanisms could include the blood–brain barrier and the existence of specific metabolic enzymes which ensure that activity is strictly localized.

The varied functions of these ubiquitous peptides are only just beginning to be recognized but current research indicates that although some—for example, calcitonin, secretin, and angiotensin—are transported via the blood stream to their sites of action and have undoubted endocrine function, others such as somatostatin or gastrin may have local effects on neighbouring cells or may act on distal parts of the gut. Yet others may have a classical neurotransmitter function or exert modulatory effects on both endocrine and neural units (Fig. 1). A strict classification of this peptidergic complex based on either their endocrine or their neural activities is therefore not tenable. But it is becoming abundantly clear that any consideration of integrated endocrine-neural activities should now take account of the possible modulatory role of these peptides. Especially challenging in this respect is the influence they might exert on neural pathways concerned with emotional control and mood swing.

Conclusion. The broad outline of the principles of endocrinology and some of the advances which have taken place in the field over the past century have been presented. Recently, an explosive increase in research has taken place; moreover its rate of advance does not appear to be slackening. A far reaching future can therefore be predicted which should lead not only to a deeper understanding of the actions of individual hormones within the cell but also of their interactions. Furthermore, when neurohormonal mechanisms which underlie the output of pituitary hormones are better understood, it may well provide us with a long awaited insight into psychosomatic and perhaps psychiatric dysfunctions.

References

Barrington, E. J. W. (1979). Introduction. In *Hormones and evolution* (ed. E. J. W. Barrington) Vol. 1. Academic Press, London.
Dockray, G. J. and Gregory, R. A. (1980). Relations between neuropeptides and gut hormones. *Proc. R. Soc. Lond. B* **210**, 151.
Krieger, D. T. and Hughes, J. C. (ed.) (1980). *Neuroendocrinology. A hospital practice book.* Sinauer, Mass.
Medvei, V. C. (ed.) (1982). *A history of endocrinology*. MTP, Lancaster.
Williams, R. G. (ed.) (1981). *Textbook of endocrinology*. W. B. Saunders, Philadelphia.

PITUITARY AND HYPOTHALAMIC DISORDERS

R. Hall

ANTERIOR PITUITARY

Anatomy and embryology

The pituitary gland is divided into an anterior lobe, a pars intermedia (intermediate lobe), and a neural lobe (posterior pituitary) which is a downward extension from the hypothalamus. The pars intermedia is poorly developed in man, making up less than 0.8 per cent of the total weight of the gland but in addition other cells of intermediate lobe origin are distributed diffusely through the anterior and posterior lobes.

The anterior and posterior lobes have distinct embryological origins and function largely independently of one another. The anterior lobe is formed from an upward extension of the stomodaeum of ectodermal origin known as Rathke's pouch. This loses its attachment to the pharyngeal roof and forms the anterior pituitary which is in contact with a downgrowth of the floor of the diencephalon, the infundibulum which forms the posterior pituitary. The pars tuberalis of the anterior lobe is derived from cells in its upper part which partly surround the pituitary stalk.

In man the pituitary weighs about 0.6 g being about 6 mm in depth, 15 mm across, and 9 mm anteroposteriorly. It is larger in women especially the parous when it may weigh up to 1 g and smaller in the elderly. The anterior lobe makes up about three-quarters of the weight of the whole gland.

The pituitary lies within the sella turcica, a depression in the sphenoid covered by the diaphragma sellae, a layer of dura, through which the pituitary stalk passes. The position of the diaphragm is variable but it can usually be located on a lateral X-ray of the skull by the line joining the tuberculum sellae and the anterior convexity of the posterior clinoid processes (Fig. 1).

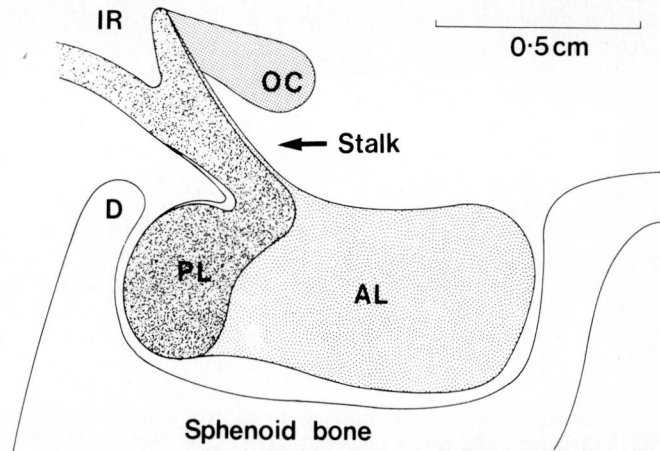

Fig. 1   Anatomy of the pituitary. AL, anterior lobe; PL, posterior lobe; D, dorsum sellae; OC, optic chiasm; and IR, infundibular recess

Radiology of the normal pituitary. This can be observed on plain radiographs of the skull and pituitary fossa, only a lateral view being required in most cases. If this shows any abnormality, additional films may be required including a coned lateral centred on the sella and an anteroposterior view taken with the patient's head slightly extended. This radiograph should identify the floor of the sella seen through the sphenoid and ethmoidal sinuses. The major errors in radiological technique are angulation or rotation of the patient's head—a good lateral skull X-ray should show accurate superimposition of the anterior clinoid processes. Another error is to compare fossae in skull X-rays taken at different tube distances though this should be apparent by the difference in size of the skull. There is much debate about the need for tomography of the sella. In the writer's opinion this procedure adds little to the diagnosis but leads to significant radiation exposure.

The sellar dimensions and area vary widely in both children and adults and their measurement is of little help. Where the normal dimensions are exceeded there is usually ample other evidence of sellar abnormality. The normal sella varies widely in shape and a double floor can be a normal variant or can signify asymmetrical fossa enlargement or poor positioning of the patient.

Relations of the pituitary. Anteriorly and below lies the sphenoid sinus and laterally are the cavernous sinuses containing the third, fourth, and sixth cranial nerves and the carotid siphon. Superiorly the diaphragma sellae is related to the optic chiasm and optic nerves and above this to the hypothalamus and third ventricle behind which are the mamillary bodies. These relationships explain the well-known local effects caused by expansion of pituitary tumours.

Blood supply of the pituitary. The pituitary receives its blood supply from superior and inferior hypophyseal arteries. The superior hypophyseal arteries arise from each internal carotid and divide into anastomosing branches supplying the pituitary stalk and the distal part of the gland via the 'artery of the trabecula'. Capillaries from the arteries to the stalk ramify into the median eminence and around the various hypothalamic nuclei and tracts where they come in contact with a variety of neuro-regulatory peptides and dopamine. These are transported down the pituitary stalk to the anterior lobe sinusoids by a portal venous system. The surrounding venous sinuses receive the drainage of the pituitary veins. In some instances a large intercavernous sinus can pose problems during the trans-sphenoidal approach to the gland.

Cytology of the anterior pituitary. The earlier classification of anterior lobe cell types into chromophobe, acidophil, and basophil based on the tinctorial properties of the cytoplasm is now largely outmoded. Five distinct cell types can be recognized at present based on more specific staining procedures, immunocytology, and electron microscopy.

Somatotrophs. These growth hormone secreting cells which stain with acid dyes make up half of the cells in the anterior lobe. They are usually densely granulated with a granule size measuring 250–500 nm.

Lactotrophs. These are also acidophilic cells comprising 10–20 per cent of the cell population. The cells increase in number during pregnancy and in response to oestrogens. They can be separated from somatotrophs by immunoperoxidase staining and by electron microscopy which reveal the characteristic large (up to 1200 nm, average about 600 nm) variably shaped granules.

Corticotrophs. These cells produce corticotrophin (ACTH) and the lipotrophins and comprise about 20 per cent of the cells. They are PAS positive and contain granules measuring 250–400 nm, a similar size to growth hormone-containing granules but other ultrastructural and immunoperoxidase features differentiate the cell types.

Thyrotrophs. Thyrotrophs producing thryotrophin (TSH) make up only 5 per cent of the cell population. They stain with the PAS method and contain secretory granules ranging in size from 150–300 nm. Thyrotrophs are found predominantly in the anteromedial portion of the gland.

Gonadotrophs. These cells also make up about 5 per cent of the anterior lobe cells. It is still uncertain whether one cell type secretes both luteinizing hormone (LH) and follicle stimulating hormone (FSH). The cells are PAS positive and it has been suggested that the average granule size of putative LH-containing cells is somewhat smaller than those secreting FSH.

Pituitary hormones

There are at present six recognized anterior lobe hormones (Table 1). The role of the lipotrophins is still uncertain.

Table 1 Anterior lobe hormones

Hormone	Abbreviation
Growth hormone	GH
Prolactin	PRL
Thyrotrophin	TSH
Luteinizing hormone	LH
Follicle-stimulating hormone	FSH
Corticotrophin	ACTH
Beta-lipotrophin	β-LPH
Gamma-lipotrophin	γ-LPH

Growth hormone. Growth hormone (GH) is present in large amounts making up between 5 and 10 per cent of the dry weight of the human pituitary (10 mg per gland). It is derived from a pre-GH which is converted to GH by proteolysis. GH is made up of 191 amino acids with two intramolecular S—S bonds. Its structure differs in different species but it shows considerable similarities in structure to both prolactin and placental lactogen suggesting that the three hormones have evolved from a single progenitor. Despite many attempts it has not yet been possible to isolate a biologically active core from the GH molecule.

Secretion. The regulation of GH secretion is complex and Fig. 2 shows some of the factors and pathways involved in determining the set point of GH release. A growth hormone releasing hormone (not yet identified) and somatostatin, a growth hormone release inhibiting hormone (GHRIH) are likely to be involved. There is some evidence that GH may regulate its own secretion, acting via a short loop feedback on hypothalamic somatostatin. Dopamine enhances growth hormone release in normal man but suppresses secretion in acromegaly. Alpha-noradrenergic pathways via noradrenaline are involved in GH release in response to hypoglycaemia and also possibly to glucagon, vasopressin, and arginine. Somatomedins (see below) may also be involved in the negative feedback inhibitory control of GH secretion. Evidence for this view is seen in the syndrome of Laron dwarfism in which there is defective somatomedin production in the liver, and GH levels are high.

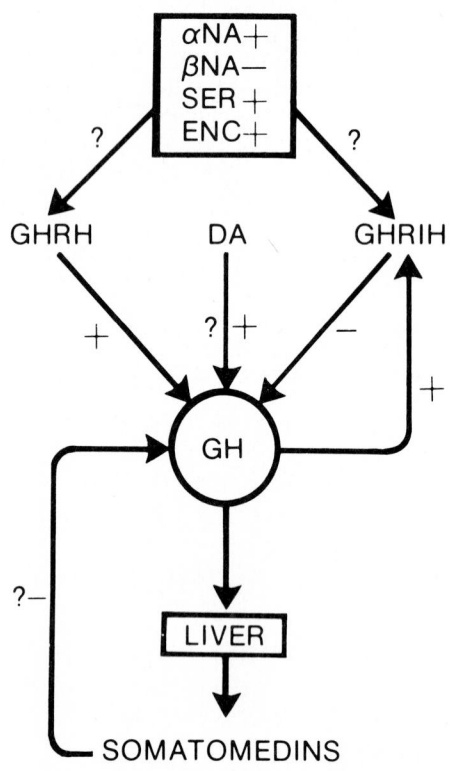

Fig. 2 Control of GH secretion

Growth hormone is normally secreted in short bursts lasting one to two hours, especially in the first half of the night during rapid eye movement (REM) sleep. Secretion is greater in children and adolescents in whom more frequent secretory bursts occur. Normal GH levels are usually less than 5 mU/l except during secretory bursts. The half-life of endogenous growth hormone is about 20–25 minutes but its metabolic effects are of longer duration since GH deficient children can be treated effectively by twice weekly injections of GH.

Metabolic effects. Most, if not all, of the metabolic effects of GH are mediated by the somatomedins, a family of small peptides which circulate bound to larger carrier proteins. They resemble proinsulin in amino acid sequence and tertiary structure but show little cross-reactivity with insulin in binding to receptors in the tissues. They have an anabolic insulin-like action on muscle and fat and promote growth by enhancing cell multiplication and by stimulating proliferation of cartilage. Circulating inhibitors counteract these effects and form part of the regulatory process. Somatomedins are produced in the liver in response to the action of GH, insulin, and nutritional factors, particularly dietary protein.

GH may also have a direct action on protein synthesis by increasing amino acid transport into cells.

Prolactin. Unlike GH there are only small amounts of prolactin (PRL) present in the normal pituitary, about 100–200 µg per gland, though *in vivo* levels may be higher since the hormone is labile during extraction. The structure of human PRL has been established to be a single chain polypeptide of 198 amino acids, molecular weight 22 550, containing three loops formed by disulphide bridges.

Like GH it circulates in several molecular forms, at least two being of larger molecular weight. Their pathophysiological relevance is not yet understood.

Secretion. An outline of some of the factors involved in the control of PRL secretion is shown in Fig. 3. There is general agreement that prolactin secretion is under a dominant inhibitory control by dopamine synthesized in the hypothalamus, stored in the median eminence, and transported to the lactotrophs by the portal capillaries. Thyrotrophin releasing hormone (TRH) releases prolactin as well as TSH but it is likely that there is another PRL–RH independent of TRH. There is no known peripheral negative feedback control of PRL secretion but there is evidence that PRL may regulate its own release by a short loop positive feedback by inducing hypothalamic dopamine production.

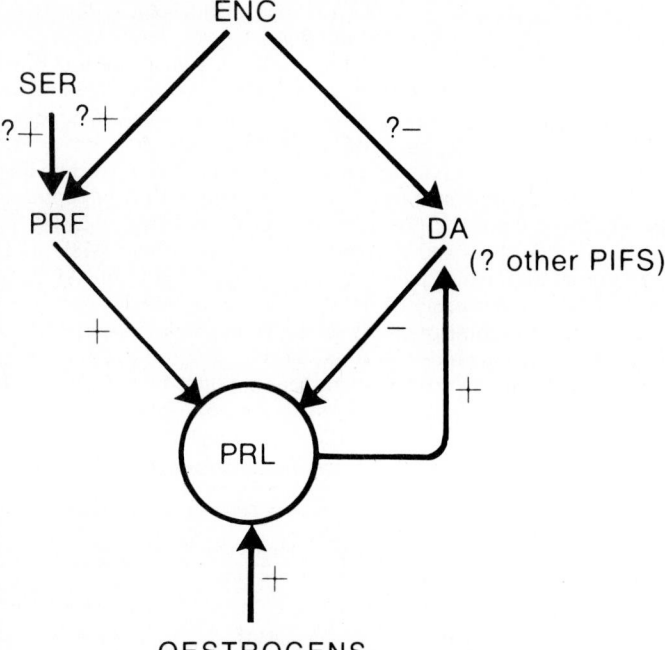

Fig. 3 Control of PRL secretion

Serum PRL levels are generally less than 400 mU/l (20 ng/ml) in the morning, levels being slightly higher in women. It is secreted intermittently in pulses lasting about 90 minutes. Secretion is highest at night after the onset of sleep and falls during the morning. Although stress may lead to a rise in PRL levels, it is probable that this effect has been overestimated in clinical practice.

Lactotrophs multiply in number and become more active in response to oestrogens, hence serum PRL levels are higher during pregnancy and in women receiving oestrogen-containing oral contraceptives. The physiological causes of hyperprolactinaemia, relative to normal adult daily values are shown in Table 2.

Prolactin levels rise from the twentieth week of fetal life but fall rapidly after birth to reach the adult range at four to six weeks. At puberty in girls there is a slight rise and levels later decline after the menopause. Only minor changes occur during the menstrual cycle.

Table 2 Physiological causes of hyperprolactinaemia

Sleep
Pregnancy
Suckling
Coitus and orgasm
Nipple stimulation
Neonatal period
Puberty in girls
Stress

A late follicular rise culminates in a mid-cycle peak and is followed by luteal levels marginally higher than those in the follicular part of the cycle.

Actions. PRL has remarkably diverse actions throughout the animal kingdom but great caution should be exercised in extrapolating functions in one species to those in another.

PRL together with oestrogens and adrenal steroids is essential for normal breast development, though raised levels of PRL do not themselves cause enlargement of the breast. Levels of PRL are slightly raised in boys with puberty gynaecomastia but probably result from the increased oestrogen/androgen ratio which is responsible for the breast enlargement. During pregnancy, PRL, along with placental lactogen, oestrogens, and progesterone, is responsible for breast growth and for milk secretion. When suckling is maintained for several months, prolactin levels fall into the normal range.

Prolactin has not been shown to have a definite luteotrophic action in women. Raised levels of PRL do interfere with gonadal function both directly and indirectly at the hypothalamic level.

Thyrotrophin. Thyrotrophin (TSH) is the principal regulator of thyroid function. It is a glycoprotein containing 15 per cent carbohydrate with a molecular weight of 28 300. It is composed of two dissimilar subunits, an α-subunit (96 residues) which is common to LH, follicle-stimulating hormone (FSH), and human chorionic gonadotrophin (hCG) and a hormone specific β-subunit (110 residues). The individual subunits are not biologically active.

Secretion (Fig. 4). Thyroid hormones exert a powerful negative feedback control on TSH secretion, acting at hypothalamic and pituitary levels. Other inhibitory influences include dopamine and somatostatin although their physiological role remains to be determined. The tripeptide thyrotrophin-releasing hormone derived from hypothalamic sources is also involved.

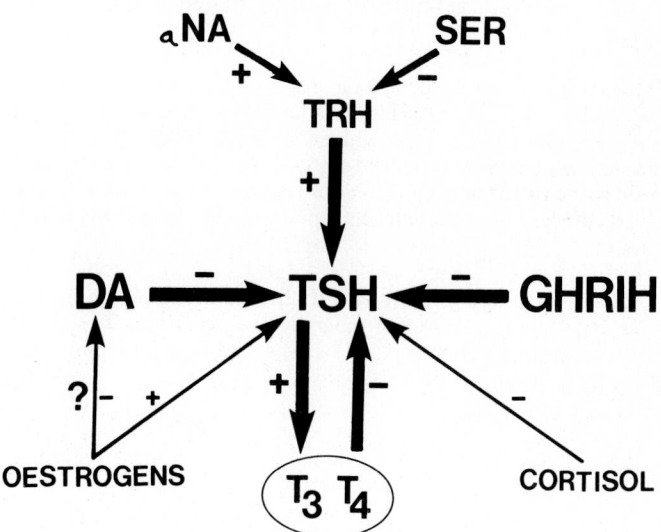

Fig. 4 Control of TSH secretion

There is a circadian rhythm of TSH secretion which is not entirely sleep-related since TSH levels begin to rise during the evening before the onset of sleep, reaching a peak at about 2300 hours, when the TSH response to TRH is also enhanced. Levels remain elevated overnight and gradually decline over the ensuing morning to reach a nadir at 1100 hours. The neuro-endocrine mechanisms responsible for this circadian rhythm are not known.

The normal serum TSH level is in the region of 1 mU/l. There is a transient surge for a few hours in the newborn but apart from this TSH levels remain remarkably constant throughout life in the absence of thyroid disease. Free α-subunit can be detected comprising 3–7 per cent of the total circulating TSH. A larger form of TSH is also present in the circulation possibly representing a pro-TSH molecule.

Actions. The physiological role of TSH is to control thyroid hormone secretion. In common with other polypeptide hormones it first binds to a specific receptor on the thyroid plasma membrane leading to an activation of adenylate cyclase. The increased cAMP then mediates the effect of TSH by interaction with protein kinases which phosphorylate certain key enzymes. In experimental situations TSH can also be shown to stimulate lipolysis and to interact with the joint synovium but it is unlikely that these effects have any physiological relevance.

Luteinizing hormone. The peptide portion of luteinizing hormone (LH) has a molecular weight of about 28 000 and, like TSH and FSH, is composed of a common α-subunit and a hormone specific β-subunit. LH differs from hCG largely in the β-subunit structure, lacking the 30 amino acid carboxyl fragment of hCG.

Secretion. LH secretion is modulated by the action of a single gonadotrophin releasing hormone (GnRH) modified by the effects of oestrogens, progesterone, and androgens. Blood concentrations of LH alter with 5–20 minute pulsations. GnRH normally causes a greater rise in LH than FSH but this pattern of response may be reversed before puberty, in the early follicular phase of the cycle, and after castration. The mid-cycle surge of gonadotrophins is preceded by a rise in oestradiol and is accompanied by a rise in progesterone and other steroids. It is an example of the positive feedback effect of oestradiol on gonadotrophin secretion which contrasts with an earlier negative feedback effect.

There is no circadian rhythm of LH secretion except in early puberty when sleep-related surges can be detected. LH values show a gradual rise in men over the age of 50 years and a sharp rise which commences just before the menopause in women. Secretion of gonadotrophins can normally be stimulated by the anti-oestrogen clomiphene which is bound to gonadal steroid receptors in the hypothalamus.

Actions. LH binds to specific receptors on the Leydig cells of the testis in the presence of FSH to stimulate testosterone secretion and is also involved in FSH-determined spermatogenesis possibly via the action of locally produced testosterone. In women the mid-cycle surge of LH is responsible for rupture of the ovarian follicle and the lower luteal phase levels support the function of the corpus luteum.

Follicle-stimulating hormone. Follicle-stimulating hormone (FSH) has a molecular weight and basic structure similar to LH with a 96 amino acid α-chain and a 115 amino acid β-subunit. Sialic acid is an important part of the carbohydrate portion of the molecule.

Secretion. FSH secretion is controlled by similar factors to LH with the addition of inhibin. Inhibin is an as yet uncharacterized peptide secreted by the testis during the process of spermatogenesis. Early tubular failure with azoospermia as in Klinefelter's syndrome is associated with deficient production of inhibin and a secondary rise in FSH. Hence elevation of FSH levels are a poor

prognostic sign in testicular disease so far as fertility is concerned. It is likely that inhibin is also produced by the ovary during the process of oogenesis although its role in the control of FSH release in women is uncertain. Fluctuations of blood FSH are less than for LH. Factors involved in the mid-cycle surge of FSH are similar to those affecting LH.

Serum FSH levels are higher in the follicular part of the cycle, decline before the LH peak, rise transiently along with LH, and then gradually rise during the luteal phase. In post-menopausal women FSH levels show a striking rise but in men there is only a gradual increase with age. FSH levels rise before LH during early puberty. There is no clear circadian rhythm of FSH secretion.

Actions. FSH stimulates the development of LH receptors in the Leydig cells and induces responsiveness to LH. FSH is the major factor involved in spermatogenesis acting along with LH-induced testosterone. FSH appears to enhance the synthesis of a testicular androgen-binding protein by the Sertoli cells and to increase tubular permeability to testosterone. In the female FSH stimulates follicular development along with locally produced oestrogens and androgens. The elevation of FSH is a major component of the ovulatory surge.

Corticotrophin and the lipotrophins. Corticotrophin (ACTH) is a single chain 39 amino acid polypeptide with a molecular weight of about 4500. The amino-terminal 24 amino acids are needed for its biological activity (the production of cortisol and some corticosterone and to increase adrenal blood flow).

Pro-γ-MSH, ACTH, and β-LPH originate from a common precursor molecule pro-opiocortin which comprises some 239 amino acids (Fig. 5). In the anterior lobe pro-opiocortin is broken down to its three constituent peptides and further processing does not occur. Pro-opiocortin is also synthesized in the melanotrophs which make up the bulk of the pars intermedia. Here a wide variety of peptides are produced from the precursor molecules including γ-LPH, β-MSH, β-endorphin, and α-endorphin from β-LPH; α-MSH and corticotrophin-like intermediate lobe peptide (CLIP) from ACTH, and γ-MSH from pro-γ-MSH. While the breakdown of pro-opiocortin in the anterior lobe is similar from species to species, the products of the pars intermedia are more variable, e.g. the human fetal pars intermedia produces only four peptides from ACTH and β-LPH whereas in the rat 11 peptides can be recognized.

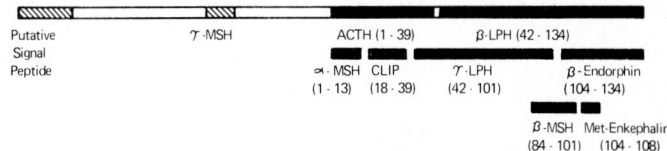

Fig. 5　Synthesis of ACTH and related peptides

Secretion. ACTH, β-LPH, and pro-γ-MSH appear to be secreted concomitantly in response to a corticotrophin-releasing factor. Distinct hypothalamic sites are responsible for the response to low and high cortisol levels as part of the negative feedback system and also to stress such as hypoglycaemia, fever, and trauma.

There is a striking circadian rhythm of ACTH secretion determined by the hypothalamus which is mirrored by plasma cortisol levels. ACTH secretion peaks at about 0900 hours and is lowest at midnight. Loss of this rhythm is seen in Cushing's syndrome, depression, heart failure, and stress of any sort. Stress can overcome the other control mechanisms of negative feedback and circadian rhythm.

Normal ACTH levels between 0800 and 1000 hours range from 10–80 pg/ml with lower values being recorded at midnight. The half life of ACTH is short ranging from 5–20 minutes.

Actions. ACTH binds to receptors on the adrenocortical cell membrane, activates adenylate cyclase, and the cAMP produced effects the resultant increase in steroid biosynthesis. The rate limiting step between cholesterol and pregnenolone is particularly affected but other sequences in the pathway may also be stimulated. Physiological levels of ACTH have little effect on aldosterone biosynthesis, but many adrenal steroids other than cortisol can also be affected by ACTH.

ACTH also has a variety of extra-adrenal actions, the most important of which is to stimulate melanin production by melanocytes, an effect responsible for the increased pigmentation seen in any variety of ACTH-induced Cushing's syndrome and in Nelson's syndrome. The physiological relevance of its actions on fat and carbohydrate metabolism is uncertain. It increases free fatty acid release from adipose tissue, increases fat concentration in the liver and induces ketosis.

Pituitary disease

A wide variety of diseases can affect the pituitary. These include local disorders of the pituitary and/or hypothalamus or local manifestations of primary disease elsewhere. Pituitary disease may become manifest as a local lesion, as hormone deficiency, as hormone excess, and often as a variable combination of all three. The major causes of hypopituitarism are shown in Table 3.

Table 3   Causes of hypopituitarism

---

1 Congenital
    Deficiency of growth hormone either isolated or combined with other deficiencies, e.g. of LH, FSH, TSH, ACTH
    Other isolated hormone deficiency, e.g. of TSH, ACTH
    Deficiency of LH, FSH with anosmia (Kallman's syndrome), or without anosmia
2 Pituitary tumours
    Secretory or non-secretory pituitary tumours, craniopharyngiomas, infarction of a pituitary tumour
3 Malignant disease
    Secondary deposits particularly from breast or lung, reticuloses (rarely), local tumours, e.g. meningiomas, optic nerve gliomas
4 Infectious diseases
    Tuberculous basal meningitis, encephalitis, syphilis
5 Granulomatous diseases
    Sarcoidosis, Hand–Schuller–Christian disease, eosinophilic granuloma, multi-system granulomas
6 Vascular disease
    Post-partum hypopituitarism or following other causes of severe blood loss, diabetes mellitus, cranial arteritis, carotid aneurysms, pituitary apoplexy, vascular malformations
7 Iatrogenic
    Surgical or radiotherapeutic intervention, selective trophic hormone deficiency after prolonged exposure to target organ hormones, e.g. ACTH deficiency after steroid medication, TSH deficiency after thyroid hormone therapy
8 Trauma
    After head injury usually with a fracture of the base of the skull
9 Secondary to hypothalamic disease (usually associated with diabetes insipidus, hypogonadism and field defects)
    Craniopharyngiomas, aqueduct stenosis due to neurofibromatosis, other causes of internal hydrocephalus, other brain tumours
10 Functional
    Anorexia nervosa, emotional deprivation syndromes, malnutrition from any cause

---

The patterns of hormone deficiency and the clinical features of these will be discussed under the appropriate pituitary hormones (see below). The commonest cause of hypopituitarism is now a pituitary tumour, especially a prolactin-secreting tumour in adults or a craniopharyngioma in children. Iatrogenic hypopituitarism may result from surgical or radiotherapeutic interference with the hypothalamus or pituitary or from hormone therapy, e.g. corticosteroid medication causing functional ACTH deficiency. Isolated GH or GH and gonadotrophin deficiencies are the commonest

congenital lesions. Post-partum hypopituitarism is now rare in developed countries but still makes a significant contribution to the disease in Africa and Asia.

Deficiency of posterior lobe hormones does not usually occur with lesions confined to the pituitary fossa except as a transient phenomenon, e.g. after trans-sphenoidal hypophysectomy. Permanent posterior lobe deficiency is commonly a sign of hypothalamic disease or of suprasellar extension of a pituitary tumour.

Growth hormone deficiency. GH deficiency occurs early in the presentation of most pituitary diseases. In children GH deficiency is manifest as shortness of stature whereas in adults few clinical features result other than fine wrinkling of the skin and a tendency to hypoglycaemia. The common causes of GH deficiency are shown in Table 4. GH deficiency is often partial even in the congenital variety. GH does not affect growth *in utero* and growth is usually normal for the first few months of life which is useful in separating GH deficiency from intra-uterine growth retardation and neonatal hypothyroidism where growth failure occurs earlier. Usually the condition remains unrecognized until the child starts school. Apart from growth failure the only other clinical manifestations at this stage may be occasional hypoglycaemic episodes. After three years of age the annual increment in growth is usually less than 3 cm and the height is below the third percentile. Some increase in growth rate may occur at puberty although puberty is usually delayed. The children are often plump with immature facies and small hands, feet, and genitalia. One-third of boys with isolated GH deficiency have a micropenis. Muscular development is poor and dentition delayed. The possibility of a pituitary tumour should always be considered and the fundi and visual fields examined.

Table 4   Congenital and acquired causes of growth hormone deficiency

Congenital	Acquired
Genetic, usually autosomal recessive, occasionally X-linked or dominant	Tumours of the pituitary, hypothalamus (especially craniopharyngiomas) and pineal
Midline embryonic defects, e.g. septo-optic dysplasia, cleft lip and palate; absence or hypoplasia of the pituitary; Laron type dwarfism	Head injury or surgery to the region
Pygmies	Granulomas, e.g. sarcoidosis, eosinophilic granuloma
Haemorrhagic infarction at birth, e.g. with breech delivery	Postmeningitis, especially after tuberculous meningitis
	Postradiation to the head, e.g. for nasopharyngeal tumours
	Temporary failure due to emotional deprivation or hypothyroidism

Diagnosis. Most children with short stature are not suffering from GH deficiency. Unless there are suspicious signs such as anaemia or pyuria, it is only necessary to carry out full investigation of a short child if the height is more than 3 s.d. below the mean or the growth rate is slow. Particular points to be considered include the patient's birth weight and length, the pattern of growth in height and development, facial features, bone and dental development, body weight, appetite and nutrition, infections, previous diseases, and intelligence. Examination should include measuring the height and span, lower segment, weight, skull circumference, and assessing body configuration, e.g. fat distribution, webbing of the neck, carrying angle, sexual maturation, particularly penile and testicular size, vulval development, and body hair distribution.

Investigations should include urinalysis for sugar and albumin, blood count, sedimentation rate, and urea and electrolytes. X-rays should include lateral skull X-ray, left hand and wrist for bone age (Greulich and Pyle), and left knee for state of epiphyseal fusion. Further investigations, e.g. chromosomal karyotype and jejunal biopsy will depend on the clinical findings and initial tests.

Tests for GH deficiency. The GH response to exercise or Bovril may be used as screening tests to exclude GH deficiency. The standard test used to confirm GH deficiency is the insulin tolerance test. In children the GH response to soluble insulin (0.1 U/kg intravenously) is assessed at half-hourly intervals for two hours in the fasting patient. If hypoglycaemia is adequate—lowest blood glucose less than 2.2 mmol/l (40 mg/100 ml)—and there are symptoms of hypoglycaemia, the GH level should rise to greater than 20 mU/l (10 ng/l). The patient should not be left unattended during the test and if severe symptoms, e.g. convulsions or loss of consciousness occur, the test should be terminated by intravenous glucose and hydrocortisone after removal of blood for glucose and hormone estimations. The patient should be given a meal at the end of the test and kept under observation for several hours.

In adults who are obese 0.15 U/kg or 0.2 U/kg of insulin may be required to produce adequate hypoglycaemia and in untreated acromegalics 0.3 U/kg may be necessary. In the elderly (over the age of 65 years) the test should rarely be performed and clinical or electrocardiographic evidence of ischaemic heart disease or of epilepsy is ordinarily a contra-indication.

In some prepubertal normal children a partial GH response may be observed and it is now customary to repeat the test after the administration of androgens or oestrogens for a few days. If the hypoglycaemic stimulus is inadequate and an impaired response is obtained, the test should be repeated on a separate occasion using a larger dose of insulin (an increment of 0.05 U/kg). If the hypoglycaemia was adequate yet an absent or impaired GH response observed and GH therapy is to be considered, it is usually wise to measure the GH response to intravenous arginine or subcutaneous glucagon.

Tests should always be carried out to assess the adequacy of secretion of the other pituitary hormones (see below).

Differential diagnosis. Other endocrine causes of short stature include hypothyroidism, Cushing's syndrome, congenital adrenal hyperplasia, and sexual precocity. The differential diagnosis of some important causes of short stature is considered in Table 5. Coeliac disease may cause diagnostic difficulties since many of the investigations may be within the normal range including full blood count. The plasma or red cell folate estimation can be helpful but a jejunal biopsy should be considered in a short child without a family history or other causes of shortness.

Treatment. Once a diagnosis of GH deficiency is established and X-rays of the epiphyses at the knee indicate growth potential, treatment should be commenced with human growth hormone in a dose of 5–10 mg three times weekly. The response to treatment is monitored by height and growth velocity charts. Treatment is usually continued for several years until an acceptable adult height is achieved and/or the epiphyses have fused. If there is concomitant deficiency of gonadotrophins, sex hormone replacement is delayed as long as possible to prevent epiphyseal fusion. Similarly in the presence of TSH or ACTH deficiency replacement therapy is kept to the minimum acceptable level. With the newer growth hormone preparations antibody formation is less common and the effects of treatment are usually maintained. It is sometimes justifiable to withhold therapy in patients who are unco-operative or in those with a progressive lesion and a poor prognosis.

Prolactin deficiency. Prolactin deficiency is a cause of failure of lactation in Sheehan's syndrome or other varieties of hypopituitarism but does not otherwise lead to any clinical problem.

Thyrotrophin deficiency. Isolated deficiency of TSH is a rare and often familial condition. Hypothyroidism due to TSH deficiency is often mild and easily overlooked. It is uncommon, but not unknown, for the patient to develop a full blown myxoedematous appearance. Loss of energy, cold intolerance, and some dryness of the skin may be apparent but only rarely are the tendon reflexes prolonged. Clinical TSH deficiency is usually a late manifestation of pituitary disease though abnormalities are more commonly revealed by sophisticated tests.

Diagnosis. The great majority of patients who present with thyroid failure of any degree of severity are suffering from some form of primary thyroid disease. A pituitary cause of hypothyroidism is only suspected if there are additional features suggestive of pituitary disease, e.g. amenorrhoea or impotence, loss of body hair, or undue pallor of the skin, although all of these findings may be seen in primary thyroid disease. The presence of a goitre, particularly if it is firm and finely nodular as in auto-immune thyroid disease suggests a thyroid cause but does not necessarily exclude hypopituitarism since goitre is so common in the female population. Obviously a pituitary cause is most likely in patients with pituitary tumours, particularly after destructive therapy. The presence of a

Table 5 Diagnosis of important varieties of short stature

	Constitutional delay in growth and adolescence	Familial short stature	Pituitary dwarfism	Hypothyroid dwarfism	Turner's syndrome	Coeliac disease
Family history	positive	positive	usually negative	negative	usually negative	may be positive
Birth weight and height	normal	reduced	normal	normal	slightly reduced	normal
Pattern of growth	rather slow from birth	slow from birth	slow from few months after birth	slow from birth	slow from birth	slow from birth
Epiphyseal development	moderate but not progressive retardation	almost normal	progressive retardation	marked retardation	within normal but wide variation	retarded
Features	immature but later normal	mature	immature	infantile	often characteristic	immature
Puberty	late but eventually normal	normal	usually delayed even with solitary growth hormone deficiency	delayed	usually no signs except in mosaics	delayed
Serum cholesterol	normal	normal	raised	raised	normal	normal or low
Growth hormone level	normal	normal	low	normal	normal	normal
Gonadotrophin level (after puberty)	normal	normal	low unless solitary growth hormone deficiency	normal or may be raised	raised	normal

scar at or above the hair line in the frontal region is easily over-looked.

Tests for TSH deficiency. Patients with any variety of symptomatic hypothyroidism usually have a low serum thyroxine (T_4) level though this may be in the lower part of the normal range. Patients with hypopituitarism and treated gonadotrophin deficiency can cause diagnostic problems since androgens lower the thyroxine-binding globulin (TBG) level and cause a low serum T_4, and oestrogens raise TBG and produce a high T_4 value. It is better to defer gonadal hormone replacement till a T_4 estimation has been carried out. In patients receiving gonadal steroids the changes in TBG can be corrected by a thyroid hormone binding test, calculating from this and the T_4, a free thyroxine index. Conversely a measurement of true free T_4 can now be performed and this is unaffected by changes in TBG level.

Most patients with TSH deficiency have an impaired or absent TSH response to thyrotrophin releasing hormone (TRH) but normal responses are not uncommon. A delayed response, where the 20 minute TSH level after TRH is less than the 60 minute value is frequently seen in disease of the pituitary or hypothalamus.

Some patients with pituitary disease and hypothyroidism have a TSH level which is at the upper limit of normal or actually raised. In these cases it is important to exclude concomitant primary thyroid disease by estimating levels of circulating thyroid auto-antibodies and measuring the thyroidal radio-iodine response to exogenous TSH. Once primary thyroid disease has been excluded it is likely that the patient is secreting an abnormal form of TSH with reduced biological activity which retains some of its immunoreactivity.

Treatment. As in primary thyroid failure, pituitary TSH deficiency is treated with thyroxine in a dose ranging from 0.1–0.2 mg daily, building up to this dose gradually in patients over 50 years of age. The final dose is assessed by the patient's response and by the establishment of a serum thyroxine level in the mid-normal range, i.e. about 100 nmol/l. It is obviously not possible to monitor TSH levels as a guide to therapy in hypopituitarism. In patients with ACTH deficiency it is important to treat the cortisol lack first lest an adrenal crisis be produced.

Gonadotrophin deficiency. Gonadotrophin deficiency may involve both LH and FSH or more rarely either alone. Congenital deficiency of gonadotrophin secretion, presumably on the basis of a defect in production of the gonadotrophin releasing hormone, may occur alone or in combination with deficiency of GH or other pituitary hormones. The association of gonadotrophin deficiency and anosmia is termed Kallman's syndrome (see also page 10.76). This familial, recessively inherited condition may affect either sex. The defect in the sensation of smell may be partial or complete and may occur independently of the hormone deficiency. There may be other associated mid-line defects such as hare lip or a cleft palate. One form of hypogonadotrophic hypogonadism not associated with anosmia may resolve either spontaneously or after a prolonged course (one year) of human chorionic gonadotrophin (hCG) therapy.

In children gonadotrophin deficiency is silent and only becomes manifest when the onset of puberty is delayed. The separation of the gonadotrophin deficiency from constitutional or familial delay in the onset of puberty can be difficult before the age of 16 years though, in the latter, some testicular development or breast formation is usually apparent.

In the adult gonadotrophin deficiency causes thin skin, which is particularly fine and wrinkled at the corners of the mouth. This loss of skin thickness is due to a decrease in skin collagen. Body hair is absent or reduced. In isolated gonadotrophin deficiency the body proportions become eunuchoid (span 5 cm greater than height, lower segment greater than upper segment). Penile growth is lacking and the testes are small (less than 8 ml volume in an adult) and soft. Reduced potency and libido are associated with loss of fertil-ity. Primary or secondary amenorrhoea and infertility occurs with a variable loss of libido.

Diagnosis. Gonadotrophin deficiency occurs early in the course of pituitary disease and normal gonadal function as assessed clinically and normal LH and FSH levels should always cast some doubt upon a diagnosis of pituitary disease. Low or normal serum levels of LH and FSH are found (depending on the sensitivity of the assay) but the response of these to gonadotrophin-releasing hormone is sometimes normal despite clear evidence of hypogonadism. Measurements of plasma testosterone or oestradiol should be performed to confirm the diagnosis of hypogonadism. If LH and FSH levels are within the normal range in a patient with pituitary disease and evidence of hypogonadism, the LH and FSH response to the anti-oestrogen clomiphene provides a useful stress test.

The major differential diagnostic problem is to determine whether a patient presenting with hypogonadism has pituitary or primary gonadal disease. In the latter gonadotrophin levels, particularly of FSH, are invariably elevated. Occasionally gonadotrophin levels are elevated in patients with prolactinomas because prolactin blocks the action of the gonadotrophins on the gonads.

Treatment. In adolescents or adults with pituitary/hypothalamic hypogonadism the secondary sexual characteristics may be restored using gonadal steroids. In men sublingual testosterone in the form of Testoral, 10–20 mg four times daily is usually adequate. If potency or beard growth are inadequate on this regimen an intra-muscular preparation, e.g. Sustanon, 250 mg alternate weeks, can be used. Again if intramuscular therapy is inadequate subcu-taneous implants of testosterone, e.g. 600 mg can be given into the abdominal wall. In women substitution therapy can be given with a low oestrogen (20–30 μg daily) oral contraceptive or with a cyclical regimen consisting of ethinyl oestradiol 10 μg twice daily for 24 days (commencing after menstruation) along with norethisterone 5 mg twice daily from days 14 to 24 of the cycle. Withdrawal bleeding occurs a few days after cessation of therapy and the next course of treatment is commenced after this stops.

In some women with secondary anemorrhoea and infertility where a functional disturbance of gonadotrophin release is postulated, clomiphene therapy may restore ovulation, menstruation, and fertility. It is given in a dose of 50–200 mg daily for five days early in the cycle, i.e. after menstruation if bleeding is occurring. Administration of hCG five days after the clomiphene may facilitate ovulation. Ovarian enlargement may occur, particularly in women with the polycystic ovary syndrome, and other minor side-effects include hot flushes, nausea and vomiting, and blurring of vision. The role of clomiphene in male fertility is uncertain.

Gonadotrophin therapy should be reserved for men or women with organic hypopituitarism in whom hyperprolactinaemia, treatable by bromocriptine, has been excluded and who wish to have children. Treatment is expensive and in men may need to be continued for up to 18 months. Human menopausal gonado-trophin—Pergonal—is used, largely as a source of FSH. When treating women, the total dose is divided into three equal injections over five days followed by 5000 i.u. of hCG of the eighth day. The total dose of Pergonal is increased at monthly intervals till ovulation occurs, as indicated by plasma and/or urinary oestrogen and progesterone measurements. It is important to start with a low dose of Pergonal and to check the oestrogen response to this before giving hCG. Such therapy is best performed in specialized centres to reduce the risk of multiple ovulation and the hyperstimulation syndrome. The latter consists of massive ovarian enlargement, abdominal pain, ascites, pleural effusions, thrombo-embolism, and sometimes death. In men a standard dose of Pergonal and hCG is given, monitoring the response by semen analysis.

Corticotrophin deficiency. Isolated ACTH deficiency may be congenital or acquired and is a very rare condition. ACTH deficiency *per se* is responsible for the pallor of the skin which is a feature of hypopituitarism due to lack of its stimulating action on the melanocytes. Secondary hypoadrenalism causes a wide variety of non-specific clinical features such as anorexia, nausea, vomiting, loss of energy, and muscle weakness leading to prostration, coma, and death. Body hair may be reduced in females due to lack of adrenal androgens. Hypotension is a late event. Hypoglycaemia results from lack of cortisol action on gluconeogenesis and hyponatraemia may be more marked than in primary hypoadrenalism due to water retention. Acute hypoadrenalism, e.g. after hypophysectomy may present with weakness, fever, and general aches and pains including headaches.

Diagnosis. In an acute situation where the diagnosis of pituitary disease has been established blood should be removed for measurement of plasma cortisol prior to initiating therapy. In a more stable situation the investigation of choice is the insulin tolerance test, using a low dose, 0.05 U/kg of insulin intravenously if the diagnosis is very likely see page 10.12). Before assuming that an impaired cortisol reponse is due to ACTH deficiency it is important to ensure that adequate clinical and biochemical hypoglycaemia was produced. A normal response is indicated by a rise in plasma cortisol to greater than 550 nmol/l. In long-standing hypopituitarism or after corticosteroid medication secondary adrenal atrophy will impair the response. Under these circumstances it is important to correct adrenal atrophy with tetracosactrin depot, giving 1 mg intramuscularly and measuring plasma cortisol levels 8 and 24 hours later when a value greater than 750 nmol/l indicates adequate adrenocortical reserve. If the response is inadequate, the patient should be given twice weekly tetracosactrin depot for two weeks and the response confirmed before proceeding to an insulin tolerance test.

The urinary 17-hydroxycorticosteroid (17-OHCS) response to the 11-hydroxylase blocking agent metyrapone (750 mg four-hourly for 24 hours) can also be used to monitor pituitary ACTH reserve. In normal subjects there is a doubling of 17-OHCS output after metyrapone.

Primary hypoadrenalism is usually easily differentiated from ACTH deficiency by the presence of pigmentation of the skin and mucous membranes caused by the high ACTH levels. Patients with Addison's disease show an impaired or absent response to ACTH stimulation in the tetracosactrin depot test.

Treatment. Acute hypoadrenalism warrants treatment with hydrocortisone hemisuccinate in an initial dose of 100 mg intravenously followed by 50 mg intramuscularly eight-hourly till the situation improves. Saline infusions may be required if the patient is hypotensive or acutely ill. It should be noted that intravenous hydrocortisone is only effective for two to four hours and an intramuscular dose for six to eight hours. Standard oral therapy consists of hydrocortisone 10 mg twice or three times daily. A mineralocorticoid is not required since aldosterone secretion continues in the absence of ACTH. A Steroid Card and Medic Alert bracelet or pendant should always be provided.

Pituitary tumours

Pathology. Based on histological, immunocytological and electron microscopic criteria eight different types of pituitary adenoma can be recognized (Table 6).

Growth hormone, prolactin, and corticotroph cell adenomas can be divided into densely and sparsely granulated varieties. Undifferentiated cell adenomas include the oncocytomas detected by electron microscopy.

GH cell adenomas. Densely granulated GH cell adenomas are acidophil adenomas by light microscopy and contain numerous secretory granules 300–600 nm in diameter. Sparsely granulated GH cell adenomas are chromophobic by light microscopy and contain smaller granules.

Prolactin cell adenomas. Densely granulated PRL cell adenomas are acidophilic by light microscopy with granules 400–1200 nm in

Table 6   Types of pituitary adenoma

	Frequency (%)
Growth hormone cell	21
Prolactin cell	32
Mixed growth hormone cell–prolactin cell	6
Acidophil stem cell	3.5
Corticotroph cell	13
Thyrotroph cell	0.5
Gonadotroph cell	1.0
Undifferentiated cell	23

From Kovacs and Horvath (1979)

diameter. Sparsely granulated adenomas are chromophobic by light microscopy again with smaller granules but characteristic ultrastructural features.

Mixed growth hormone cell-prolactin cell adenomas. These adenomas are associated with acromegaly and occasionally with the amenorrhoea, galactorrhoea syndrome. They consist of two cell types—producing either GH or PRL. They are acidophilic–chromophobe adenomas by light microscopy, and densely or sparsely granulated GH cells can be mixed with similar varieties of PRL cells.

Acidophil stem cell adenomas. These adenomas are not accompanied by acromegaly or increased GH levels but sometimes cause hyperprolactinaemia. They consist of immature cells derived from a common precursor of the two acidophil cell types. They are chromophobic on light microscopy and both GH and PRL may be detected in their cytoplasmic granules.

Corticotroph cell adenomas. These tumours may result in Cushing's disease or Nelson's syndrome or they may be non-secretory. By light microscopy they are basophilic or chromophobic adenomas which contain ACTH, β-lipotrophin, and endorphin in their cytoplasmic granules.

Thyrotroph cell adenomas. These rare tumours may be secondary to long-standing hypothyroidism or, because of inappropriate TSH secretion, may cause hyperthyroidism. They are chromophobic on light microscopy and contain 100–200 nm diameter granules on electron microscopy.

Gonadotroph cell adenomas. These rare tumours may be feedback or primary in origin. They are chromophobic in type and contain 100–250 nm diameter granules.

Undifferentiated cell adenomas. These non-secretory chromophobic cell tumours cause their effects by local compression and do not secrete any known hormones. Some tumours show a striking increase in mitochondria and are termed oncocytomas.

Craniopharyngiomas. These are the commonest tumours in the pituitary region in children and adolescents although they can present at any age. They are derived from elements of Rathke's pouch and have a variable histological appearance from squamous cells with cornified areas and calcification to groups of columnar cells.

Other tumours in the pituitary region. Tumours of the third ventricle, optic chiasm gliomas, pinealomas of varying types, and tumours of the hypothalamus and mid brain may all affect the pituitary–hypothalamic region. Secondary tumours arise most often from breast or lung and reticuloses may rarely affect this area.

Associations of pituitary adenomas. Pituitary adenomas may occasionally form part of the multiple endocrine adenoma type I syndrome when they are associated with tumours of the parathyroid, adrenal cortex, or pancreas. Rarely an acidophil adenoma is associated with a phaeochromocytoma. Feedback tumours may arise as a result of long-standing target organ deficiency, e.g. in hypothyroidism, Addison's disease, or primary gonadal failure. Such feedback tumours usually remain responsive to target organ hormones, e.g. TSH hypersecretion can be suppressed by thyroxine.

Clinical features. Pituitary tumours can produce their effects in three ways—as a result of hormone hypersecretion by the tumour cells, from damage to the normal pituitary causing hypopituitarism, or from local pressure effects in the region. The clinical and laboratory features of hypopituitarism have already been described (see pages 10.11–14) and in this section the effects of the local lesion and of hormonal oversecretion will be discussed.

Effects of the local lesion. Lesions confined to the pituitary fossa are usually asymptomatic but may cause headache because of local extension with pressure on the dura or blood vessels. The headaches are variable in location and may be retro-orbital, frontal, vertical, or temporal. Their severity is also very variable but they are not usually disabling in nature.

Inferior extensions into the sphenoid sinus can lead to cerebrospinal fluid (CSF) rhinorrhoea and this complication should be suspected after yttrium implantation or trans-sphenoidal hypophysectomy if clear fluid drips down the nose. Meningitis is a frequent and dangerous sequel of CSF rhinorrhoea. The fluid has a higher sugar content than normal nasal secretions and a fluid level is sometimes seen in the sphenoid sinus on lateral skull X-rays.

Lateral extension into the cavernous sinus characteristically causes palsies of the third cranial nerve which are often partial and usually unilateral. The fourth and sixth cranial nerves and the internal carotid may also be affected by lateral spread.

Superior extensions cause compression of the optic pathways or their vascular supply, hypothalamic syndromes (see page 10.23), or internal hydrocephalus. A bitemporal hemianopia, commencing in the upper quadrants is the result of pressure on the optic chiasm. The optic nerves or tracts are sometimes affected depending on the route of extension of the tumour and whether the chiasm is pre- or post-fixed. In any patient suspected to have a supra sellar extension it is important to test the visual fields to confrontation and also to obtain an expert field assessment by perimetric techniques. Corrected near vision should be tested using the Jaeger test type and distance acuity using the Snellen test chart at 6 m. Colour vision defects are tested by the Ishihara plates and are useful indicators of optic nerve compression. Papilloedema is rare in patients with pituitary tumours unless extension into the third ventricle has caused internal hydrocephalus. Optic atrophy may follow chiasmal or optic nerve compression and can progress after the lesion has been removed. The pupillary reaction to light may also be abnormal if there is optic nerve compression.

The hypothalamic syndromes are considered further on page 10.23.

Radiology of pituitary tumours. The radiology of the normal pituitary has been considered on page 10.7. Lateral and anteroposterior views of the fossa usually suffice to demonstrate the size and extent of intrasellar lesions. An intrasellar tumour causes sellar enlargement and deformity, thinning and erosion of its bony outline, and sometimes expansion of the tumour into the sphenoid sinus. Uneven downward extension may produce a second contour of the sellar floor but this appearance can be due to poor radiological technique or to a normal variation in shape of the fossa. As mentioned earlier there is still debate as to the value of tomography of the sella and the writer is sceptical of the need for the procedure except in unusual circumstances.

Pneumoencephalography is of value in demonstrating the extent of the suprasellar extension of a pituitary tumour but is often a painful procedure even with careful pre-medication. The complication of infarction of a pituitary tumour should be suspected if headache, vomiting, and prostration is severe and persist for more than a day or two.

Computerized tomography (CT scanning) has now revolutionized the neuroradiological investigation of pituitary lesions. Axial (horizontal) plane scans can usually demonstrate a suprasellar extension which may show enhancement after intravenous contrast medium (Conray). Coronal or semi-coronal scans give an even better demonstration of the extent of the lesion. A water-soluble contrast medium, metrizamide, can be run into the basal subarachnoid cisterns and around the brain after introduction by the lumbar route. The suprasellar cistern can be easily specified and lateral radiographs of this area demonstrate all the structures shown by pneumo-encephalography. The technique is simpler and the side-effects fewer and less severe, so that serial examinations can be made. An empty sella is clearly shown by this technique. A metrizamide cisternogram can be combined with a CT scan—a metrizamide CT cisternogram—in both the axial and coronal planes which provides a three-dimensional appreciation of the extent of the lesion.

Angiographic procedures are not usually required in the investigation of pituitary tumours although some surgeons prefer to know the precise location of the carotid arteries before embarking on pituitary surgery.

Acromegaly and gigantism

Increased GH secretion from a pituitary adenoma leads to overgrowth of the skeleton and soft tissues. Before the epipyses have fused there is an increase in linear growth resulting in gigantism but there are always concomitant features of acromegaly. Acromegaly occurs in about 40 per million of the general population in the United Kingdom but gigantism is much rarer probably representing only about one per cent of all cases of GH oversecretion. About one-third of patients present because of a change in their features, one-third because of associated disturbances such as field defects, carpal tunnel syndrome, and headaches, and the rest are recognized to have acromegalic features when seeking medical attention for an unrelated complaint. There is a significantly higher mortality in both sexes, in males from malignancy, respiratory, cardiovascular, and cerebrovascular disease and in females from cerebrovascular disease. There is a slight preponderance of the disease in females.

The clinical manifestations of acromegaly are shown in Table 7. Local effects of the tumour are not listed since they have been considered earlier.

Diagnosis. In patients with florid clinical features it is necessary to confirm GH oversecretion by measurements of the GH response during a standard glucose tolerance test. GH levels should normally suppress to less than 4 mU/l (2 ng/ml). A skull X-ray is performed to assess the size of the tumour. If surgical or yttrium–90 therapy is contemplated, it is necessary to determine the upper level of the tumour by CT scanning (see above) or pneumoencephalography. In patients in whom active therapy is not contemplated, and who have normal visual fields, invasive neuroradiological procedures may not be justified, although any patient with a visual field defect should be fully investigated. Evidence of hypopituitarism should be sought by appropriate tests (see pages 10.11–14) including an insulin-tolerance test, bearing in mind the insulin resistance of active acromegaly. Oversecretion of PRL should be sought by measurements of basal hormone levels.

The common diagnostic problem at present is to decide which patients with rugged features and large hands and feet justify further investigation. Patients who complain of a change in their appearance, especially if this is confirmed by inspection of previous photographs, are worthy of investigation. Other causes of enlargement of the hands include manual work, obesity, hypothyroidism, and primary amyloidosis. Enlargement of the feet usually affects their width rather than their length. Enlargement of the tongue may also be complained of in hypochondriasis, hypothyroidism, and primary amyloidosis. A lateral skull X-ray is the most rapid screening test since 90 per cent of acromegalics show enlargement of the pituitary fossa. Conversely the pituitary fossa is normal in 10 per cent of acromegalics so a normal fossa does not exclude the diagnosis, particularly in early cases. Measurement of the GH response to glucose is then necessary to confirm or refute the diagnosis.

Table 7 Clinical manifestations of acromegaly

1 Endocrine
  (a) Effects of excess GH on tissue growth and metabolism
     Overgrowth of skin, soft tissues, and skeleton
     Visceromegaly, e.g. of liver, spleen, kidneys, lungs
     Increased metabolic rate, sweating and heat intolerance
     Impaired carbohydrate tolerance, diabetes mellitus
     Hypercalciuria and hypercalcaemia
     Hyperphosphataemia
  (b) Alterations in other pituitary hormone secretion
     Hyperprolactinaemia
     Hyperthyroidism and goitre—TSH oversecretion
     Hypopituitarism
     Diabetes insipidus (only if there is a suprasellar extension or
       after surgical or radiation therapy)
  (c) Thyroid abnormalities
     Nodular goitre (no change in TSH secretion) either non-toxic
       (common) or toxic (less common)
     Hypothyroidism as part of hypopituitarism
     Alterations in levels of thyroid hormone binding proteins
  (d) Association with multiple endocrine adenoma
     Hyperparathyroidism, pancreatic, adrenocortical tumours
     Phaeochromocytoma
     Carcinoid syndrome (? ectopic production of a GH-releasing
       factor)
2 Neuromuscular
  (a) Related to tumour growth (see page 10.15)
  (b) Related to GH oversecretion
     Carpal tunnel syndrome
     Tarsal and other nerve entrapment syndromes
     Hypertrophic neuropathy
     Neurological syndromes complicating diabetes mellitus
     Brachial neuritis, lumbago, and sciatica
     Proximal myopathy
3 Respiratory
     Voice changes
     Upper respiratory tract obstruction
     Increased lung volume
4 Skeletal
     Bone and soft tissue changes
     Arthropathy
     Cervical, dorsal, and lumbar spondylosis
5 Cardiovascular
     Hypertension and its complications
     Diabetes mellitus complications
     Cardiomyopathy
6 Dermatological
     Thickened coarse, greasy skin with increased sebum production
     Skin papillomas and lipomas
     Hirsutes
     Pigmentation
     Raynaud's phenomenon

Treatment. The objectives of therapy are to restore GH levels to normal and to prevent further tumour growth without causing hypopituitarism or other local complications. As yet no form of treatment fulfills these objectives in all patients. For patients up to the age of 60 years or so with active disease and a tumour confined to the fossa, or with only a small suprasellar extension, the treatment of choice is now trans-sphenoidal hypophysectomy. Most surgeons attempt to 'clear the fossa' but hypopituitarism is only produced in about one-quarter of the patients so it is assumed that enough normal tissue is usually left around the stalk. Cure rates (as defined by return to normal GH levels) of about 80 per cent are achieved in the best centres. If GH levels remain high, post-operatively residual tumour growth can usually be prevented by external radiation in a total dose of up to 4500 rad. Treatment with bromocriptine can be used to lower GH levels and cause symptomatic improvement during the interval, which may be several years before radiation becomes effective.

In experienced hands yttrium-90 implantation is effective using 50 000 rad if the GH level is less than 100 mU/l and 150 000 rad if the level exceeds 100 mU/l. If GH levels are not lowered satisfactorily, a further dose can be given. Field defects from small suprasellar extensions can also be relieved.

In patients with large suprasellar extensions, inaccessible from the trans-sphenoidal route, trans-frontal decompression of the chiasm is performed followed by external radiation to the residual tumour. Again bromocriptine can be used to cause further symptomatic improvement.

In patients in whom invasive therapy is thought inappropriate because of their wishes, their age, or concomitant disease, medical treatment with bromocriptine, a long-acting dopamine agonist, produces a worthwhile clinical response in about 75 per cent of cases. Treatment is built up gradually to an average dose of 5 mg four times daily (for details of therapy and its complications, see page 10.17). GH levels fall although not usually into the normal range and there is some evidence for the preferential reduction of biologically active GH secretion.

There is now convincing evidence that bromocriptine reduces the size of some GH-secreting tumours though its effects on prolactinoma size is more dramatic.

Plastic surgery may be used to improve the patient's appearance once GH levels have been low and static for some time.

Hypopituitarism can complicate untreated acromegaly or be an early or late effect of treatment. All patients with acromegaly should be kept under long-term review by an endocrinologist.

Prolactinomas

A wide variety of drugs and diseases may cause hyperprolactinaemia (Table 8). The physiological causes have been considered in Table 2. Before carrying out detailed investigation for pituitary–hypothalmic disease it is important to exclude physiological causes and hypothyroidism, and to take a careful drug history. Elevated PRL levels may be due to stress or, before 1100 hours, to settling of the physiological nocturnal surge. Prolactin-secreting pituitary adenomas are being recognized more often although it remains uncertain whether this is due to a true increase in frequency, an increased index of suspicion, the ready availability of PRL immunoassays, the advent of an effective therapy (bromocriptine), or to a combination of these factors. Certainly in animals PRL-secreting adenomas can be induced by oestrogen medication.

Table 8 Non-physiological causes of hyperprolactinaemia

1 Drugs
     Dopamine receptor blocking agents:
       Phenothiazines, e.g. chlorpromazine
       Haloperidol
       Metoclopramide, sulpiride, pimozide, domperidone
     CNS-dopamine-depleting agents:
       Reserpine
       Methyldopa
     Others:
       Oestrogens
       TRH
2 Hypothalamic or pituitary stalk lesions
     Craniopharyngiomas, gliomas, pinealomas
     Granulomas—sarcoidosis, eosinophilic granuloma, TB meningitis
     Stalk section following trauma, pituitary surgery, or pressure from a
       tumour
3 Pituitary tumours (see page 10.14)
     Prolactin cell
     Mixed growth hormone cell prolactin cell
     Acidophil stem cell
     Mixed corticotrophin cell prolactin cell
4 Miscellaneous
     Idiopathic/functional
     Hypothyroidism
     Chronic renal failure
     Ectopic, e.g. from bronchogenic carcinoma or hypernephroma

There is still no clear evidence that oral contraceptive medication induces prolactinomas although this possibility remains open.

The clinical features associated with hyperprolactinaemia are shown in Table 9. Hyperprolactinaemia is commoner in women and should be suspected if any of the clinical features shown in Table 9 are present. It is a common finding in post-oral contraceptive amenorrhoea, and PRL levels should always be checked if this persists for more than six months. Oral contraceptives should not be used to regularize menstruation since this treatment is often followed by 'post-pill' amenorrhoea in such patients.

Table 9 Clinical features associated with hyperprolactinaemia

Women
  Amenorrhoea or oligomenorrhoea
  Galactorrhoea
  Infertility
  Hirsutes

Men
  Impotence
  Galactorrhoea
  Oligospermia
  Reduced size of prostate
  Reduced semen volume
  Infertility
  Female distribution of body fat

It is important to realize that hyperprolactinaemia with or without galactorrhoea is not a cause of gynaecomastia. Gynaecomastia is due to an oestrogen effect on the breast due either to excessive oestrogens or reduced androgens.

The hypogonadism that frequently accompanies hyperprolactinaemia may be due to hypopituitarism or to a direct action of PRL on the gonads where it interferes with the action of the gonadotrophins. PRL may also act on the adrenal cortex to divert normal corticosteroid biosynthesis to androgenic pathways, a factor which may be responsible for hirsutes, secondary amenorrhoea, and the polycystic ovary syndrome in some cases. Raised levels of PRL may also interfere with the positive feedback mechanism whereby oestrogens trigger the ovulatory surge of LH.

Diagnosis. In the appropriate clinical context PRL levels should be taken after 1100 in the unstressed patient. If the PRL levels are raised (greater than 400 mU/l) and drugs and hypothyroidism excluded as possible causes, the problem is to decide whether the hyperprolactinaemia is due to stress, functional hyperprolactinaemia, or a pituitary tumour. In general the higher the PRL level the more likely is the patient to have a pituitary tumour although tumours may sometimes be found in patients with only a modest increase in PRL levels. A lateral skull X-ray should be performed, and if this shows a definitely enlarged fossa, the diagnosis is established and the extent of the tumour and secretion of other pituitary hormones must be determined.

If the PRL level is raised and the pituitary fossa normal or only 'suspicious query normal', one is faced with what has been termed 'the prolactinoma problem'. Is the hyperprolactinaemia functional or does the pituitary fossa harbour a micro-adenoma? It has been shown that patients with prolactinomas have an impaired PRL response to both TRH and to dopamine receptor blockade with metoclopramide or domperidone. Patients with functional hyperprolactinaemia show a normal, i.e. several hundred per cent increase in PRL in response to these stimuli.

Treatment. Prolactinomas can be treated by trans-sphenoidal hypophysectomy, by external radiation, or by bromocriptine. At present the optimal therapy is still undecided.

If the tumour is large, the pituitary fossa grossly enlarged, and PRL levels very high (e.g. greater than 2000 mU/l) it is unlikely that the tumour can be completely removed by any surgical procedure.

In this situation bromocriptine is the treatment of choice. In some centres this treatment is complemented by external radiation.

If the tumour is large enough to cause clear but not massive enlargement of the fossa, trans-sphenoidal hypophysectomy is performed in some centres, again complemented by radiation and bromocriptine if PRL levels remain high post-operatively.

If the pituitary fossa is not enlarged, some centres prefer to use bromocriptine alone, particularly if the patient's complaint is primarily of infertility. In other centres, if the neuro-endocrine tests indicate the presence of a micro-adenoma, an attempt is made to remove the lesion trans-sphenoidally.

In patients with suprasellar extensions of the tumour or recurrence after previous surgery and/or external radiation, bromocriptine is the treatment of choice and there is now unequivocal evidence of shrinkage of the tumour with this drug. At present the duration of therapy required is uncertain but probably the hormonal activity and extent of the tumour should be checked every year.

Bromocriptine therapy has revolutionized the management of prolactinomas, and there is much to be said for treating all patients with this drug alone. Its side-effects, which are shown in Table 10, can be divided into early and late. It is usual to work up to a dose of 2.5 mg eight hourly over a week or two. Half a tablet (1.25 mg) is given in bed at night after a meal for a few nights and the dose gradually increased after meals with the patient sitting or lying at first. Once a dose of 7.5 mg daily is established, the initial side-effects usually resolve and the later ones are rarely troublesome at this dose. Occasional patients require doses up to 20 mg daily, but in general patients with hyperprolactinaemia are more sensitive to bromocriptine than those with acromegaly.

Table 10 Side-effects of bromocriptine

Early
  Nausea, vomiting
  Postural hypotension, syncope

Late
  Raynaud's phenomenon
  Nasal stuffiness
  Constipation
  Flickering of vision
  Dyspepsia
  Dyskinesia (at doses > 20 mg/day)

If the patient becomes pregnant as a result of bromocriptine therapy, it is usual to discontinue the drug. There is no evidence that bromocriptine causes any ill effect in the fetus. Because of the small risk, probably about 5 per cent, of tumour extension during the pregnancy, the patient should be seen at monthly intervals for review and visual field testing and warned to report immediately if she develops headaches or nausea. If tumour expansion does occur during pregnancy, it is rarely necessary to resort to surgery and tumour shrinkage can be effectively and safely produced by recommencing bromocriptine.

If functional hyperprolactinaemia is associated with galactorrhoea or infertility, bromocriptine can be a most effective treatment.

Cushing's disease

Cushing's syndrome is considered in detail on page 10.58. Cushing's disease is the term applied to Cushing's syndrome of pituitary origin. There is still debate as to whether ACTH-secreting adenomas represent a primary pituitary disease or whether they arise from long continued hypothalamic stimulation from a corticotrophin-releasing factor. The recent 'cures' obtained by selective removal of the adenoma would support the former view.

The clinical features of Cushing's disease include facial plethora, hirsutism, hypertension, thin skin, easy bruising, proximal muscle weakness, and truncal obesity. The most discriminating signs are the thin skin and proximal myopathy which are absent in simple obesity and the polycystic ovary syndrome, the two conditions which tend to mimic Cushing's syndrome.

Diagnosis. Cortisol overproduction must first be confirmed by measurement of the urinary free 11-hydroxycorticosteroids on at least three occasions. In Cushing's disease the normal circadian rhythm of ACTH and hence the cortisol secretion is lost and this should be confirmed by measurements of 0900 and 12 midnight cortisol levels over 48 hours.

Once cortisol overproduction is confirmed, the cause for this must be ascertained. If ACTH levels are undetectable, the cause is an adrenal adenoma or carcinoma and the least invasive procedure available is performed to determine the side of the lesion. Whole body CT scanning is the best procedure, if available, and ultrasound can also be valuable. Adrenal arteriography and venography with selective venous catheterization should be kept in reserve for use if the non-invasive procedures are equivocal.

If ACTH levels are raised, the problem is to decide if the lesion is a pituitary adenoma or an ectopic source of ACTH. An enlarged pituitary fossa and modest ACTH elevation supports the former diagnosis as does suppression of adrenal steroid output by dexamethasone and a rise in response to metyrapone. An abnormal chest X-ray, marked elevation of ACTH levels, skin pigmentation, oedema, and hypokalaemic alkalosis support the latter diagnosis. Again in the ectopic ACTH syndrome there is usually no response in adrenal steroid excretion to either dexamethasone or metyrapone.

Treatment. Adrenal tumours obviously require removal although the prognosis is poor in the case of carcinomas. Recurrence of Cushing's syndrome after removal of a carcinoma can be treated by adrenal blockade or by aggressive chemotherapy in a specialized centre. Ectopic ACTH syndromes, if due to an inoperable tumour, can also be treated by blockade although it is often possible to remove a bronchial carcinoid completely. There is still disagreement as to the optimal therapy for Cushing's disease and this will largely depend on the local facilities. External radiation to the pituitary cures about one-third of patients (rather more in children) after a delay of several years and adrenal blockade can be used to render the patient euadrenal over this period. For small tumours the treatment of choice is selective removal of the adenoma by the trans-sphenoidal route. Yttrium implantation can be very effective in experienced hands.

It should be stressed that the investigation and management of patients with Cushing's disease are best carried out by an endocrinologist in a specialized centre.

Thyrotroph adenomas

Raised TSH levels are usually the result of primary thyroid failure. Rarely, if thyroid failure is prolonged, a thyrotrophin-secreting adenoma may arise and cause enlargement of the pituitary fossa. Mild long-standing thyroid failure associated with an ectopic thyroid is a common cause of such feedback tumours.

In some patients hyperthyroidism, with increased circulating thyroid hormone levels is associated with a raised serum TSH level. In the majority of these patients the pituitary fossa is enlarged and the disease can be cured by removal of the tumour. A characteristic finding is the presence of circulating α-subunits, presumably of TSH, but neither these nor the TSH level usually rise after TRH.

In the less frequent non-tumour TSH-induced hyperthyroidism α-subunit cannot be detected in the circulation. Most of these patients have had previous destructive therapy to the thyroid. They show a partial TSH response to TRH and some suppression of TSH thyroidal radioiodine uptake by triiodothyronine. They may be familial and due to selective pituitary resistance to thyroxine. Cases have been described where the TSH level is lowered by giving

triiodothyronine and clinical remission of the hyperthyroidism induced.

Gonadotroph adenomas

As for TSH, these tumours can also arise from long-standing gonadal failure as occurs in Klinefelter's syndrome or Turner's syndrome. Here low levels of sex steroids are associated with raised FSH and either raised, normal, or low LH levels and enlargement of the pituitary fossa. The tumours are normally responsive to gonadal steroid replacement therapy.

Rarely gonadotrophin-secreting tumours, usually secreting FSH, may arise *de novo*. Here sexual function is often well maintained and the presence of normal sized testes in a patient with an apparently non-functioning pituitary tumour should lead to measurement of gonadotrophin levels. Some patients may have reduced libido, potency, and sexual function and this may on occasion result from concomitant hyperprolactinaemia. An attempt should be made to remove the tumour whenever possible.

POSTERIOR PITUITARY

The posterior lobe of the pituitary consists of the median eminence, the infundibular stem, and the posterior lobe. It is made up of nerve cells and fibres, neuroglia, connective tissue, and blood vessels. Its two hormones, vasopressin or antidiuretic hormone (ADH) and oxytocin, are synthesized in the hypothalamus in the supra-optic (SON) and paraventricular (PVN) nuclei along with their carrier proteins, the neurophysins. All of the cells of the SON and many in the PVN secrete ADH. The PVN is probably the main source of oxytocin. Vasopressin is combined with neurophysin II, a protein with a molecular weight of about 10 000, and is transported by axonal streaming to the posterior lobe. Here it reaches the bulbous expansions of the axons which rest on the basement membrane of the posterior lobe capillaries to be secreted into the systemic circulation. Oxytocin, combined with neurophysin I, follows a similar path from the PVN to the posterior lobe.

Vasopressin

Vasopressin is a nonapeptide with a molecular weight of about 1000, consisting of an S—S bonded ring of five amino acids and a three amino acid tail (Fig. 6). Arginine vasopressin (AVP) is the

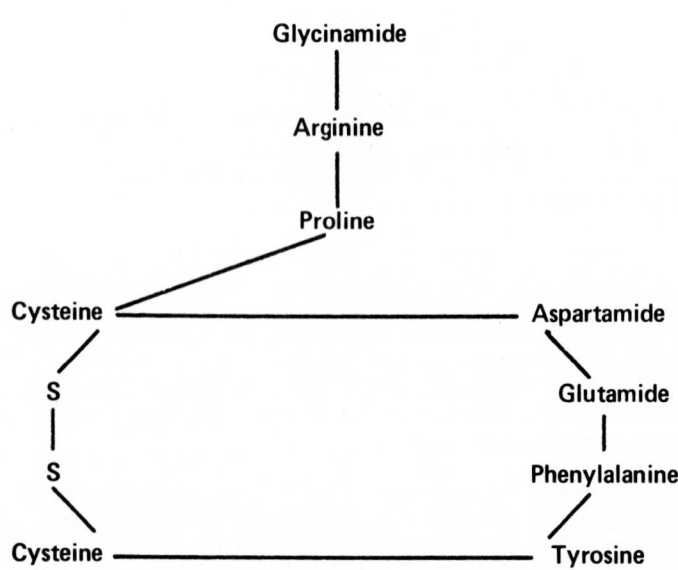

Fig. 6 Structure of arginine vasopressin.

natural ADH in man and mammals other than the pig, hippopotamus, and peccary in which lysine vasopressin is the ADH. Lysine vasopressin is more stable than AVP and a synthetic LVP is still used in the treatment of mild diabetes insipidus, although it has now largely been replaced by the long acting analogue 1-deamino-8-D-arginine vasopressin (DDAVP).

Factors affecting ADH secretion are shown in Table 11. Alterations in tonicity of the body fluids and volume contraction are likely to be the major physiological factors, the former being more important.

Table 11   Factors affecting ADH secretion

Stimuli	Inhibitors
Osmolar	
increased body fluid tonicity	decreased body fluid tonicity
Cardiovascular	
volume contraction	volume expansion
decreased blood pressure	increased blood pressure
Hormonal	
beta-adrenergic stimulation	alpha-adrenergic stimulation
angiotensin II	
hypothyroidism	
hypoadrenalism	
Environmental factors	
heat	cold
stress	
Drugs	
nicotine	ethanol
barbiturates	
clofibrate	
vincristine	

Metabolism of ADH. Vasopressin is dissociated from its carrier protein as it is released from the posterior lobe and levels of neurophysin II alter in parallel with those of ADH in response to a variety of stimuli. The half-life of ADH is between seven and 20 minutes. Radioimmunoassays of ADH have been developed for research purposes but are not yet widely available for clinical practice.

Actions of ADH. ADH increases the permeability of the distal convoluted tubular and collecting ducts to water by a cAMP-dependent mechanism. This leads to the production of more concentrated urine as a result of water extraction. In pharmacological doses it causes smooth muscle contraction with resultant pallor, coronary vasoconstriction, and constriction of the smooth muscle of the gut. The various factors reducing the renal action of ADH are shown in Table 12.

Table 12   Factors reducing the renal action of ADH

Increased solute excretion
Decreased glomerular filtration rate
Decreased protein intake
Increased water intake
Decreased salt intake
Hypercalcaemia
Hypokalaemia
Amyloidosis
Sickle cell disease
Drugs
    Frusemide, ethacrynic acid
    Lithium salts
    Demethylchlorotetracycline

Demethylchlorotetracycline is useful in the treatment of the syndrome of inappropriate secretion of ADH.

Chlorpropamide and carbamazepine appear to potentiate the action of ADH on the kidney and have been used clinically in mild cases of diabetes insipidus.

Vasopressin deficiency (diabetes insipidus). This condition is dealt with fully in Section 18 and only a brief outline will be given here.

Vasopressin deficiency causes polyuria and secondary polydipsia, the syndrome of cranial diabetes insipidus. This condition is due to a variety of hypothalamic diseases and to pituitary tumours which have extended upwards beyond the pituitary fossa. It occurs transiently after damage to the pituitary stalk by head injury, usually when there has been a fracture of the base of the skull, and sometimes after trans-sphenoidal hypophysectomy or yttrium implantation. Sometimes there is no apparent cause for the diabetes insipidus and such cases may be familial. The syndrome of diabetes insipidus, diabetes mellitus, optic atrophy, and deafness (DIDMOAD) is inherited on an autosomal recessive basis.

Nephrogenic diabetes insipidus is a sex-linked recessive disorder which is due to lack of ADH action on the nephron, a similar syndrome being produced by the various diseases or drugs listed in Table 12.

Diagnosis. It is first necessary to demonstrate that the patient has polyuria and polydipsia by recording fluid intake and urine volume. Diabetes insipidus usually occurs with other evidence of hypothalamic–pituitary disease so the clinical context of the symptoms is important. Renal disease should be excluded by urinalysis and measurement of urea and electrolytes which will also reveal evidence of hypokalaemia. Hypercalcaemia is tested for and diabetes mellitus ruled out by urinalysis and blood glucose estimation.

The major diagnostic problem is then to differentiate between diabetes insipidus and compulsive water drinking. In both the urine osmolality is usually low and in compulsive water drinking the plasma osmolality is reduced (less than 285 mosmol/kg.). A fluid deprivation test may be required to confirm the diagnosis. In normal subjects from whom fluid is withdrawn for eight hours the plasma osmolality remains unchanged and the urine osmolality at the end of the test exceeds twice the plasma value. In diabetes insipidus the plasma osmolality rises and the test should be discontinued if the patient loses more than 3 per cent of body weight. By the end of the test the urine osmolality remains less than twice that of the plasma. In compulsive water drinking the initial plasma and urine osmolalities are low and the plasma level rises into the normal range (285–95 mosmol/kg) by the end of the test. The urine osmolality rises during the test but does not always exceed twice that of the plasma since the excessive water intake leads to a renal concentrating defect. Once a diagnosis of diabetes insipidus is established, it is usual to confirm the response to vasopressin (DDAVP) which excludes a nephrogenic cause.

Treatment. Although there is a variety of vasopressin preparations and drugs enhancing the effect of endogenous vasopressin, the treatment of choice in virtually all cases of cranial diabetes insipidus is DDAVP given intranasally in a dose of 10–20 µg once or twice daily. It can be given intramuscularly in a dose of 2–4 µg once or twice daily if the need arises.

Nephrogenic diabetes insipidus can be treated with thiazide diuretics, e.g. polythiazide (1 mg daily for a child). Hypokalaemia is prevented by potassium supplements and sometimes a potassium-sparing diuretic, e.g. triamterene 25–50 mg twice daily can be added. The mechanism of action of the diuretics in this situation is not known.

Vasopressin excess. Vasopressin excess may be derived from the pituitary or from an ectopic tumour source (Table 13) (see also page 18.20).

The feature of vasopressin excess is urine hyperosmolality in the

Table 13   Cause of vasopressin excess

1 Increased pituitary ADH
   Hypothyroidism
   Hypoadrenalism
   Stress
   Drugs:
      Nicotine, barbiturates, clofibrate, vincristine
   Lung disease:
      Pneumonia, abscess, tuberculosis, pleural effusion
   Intracranial disease:
      Head injury, cerebrovascular disease, cerebral tumours, encephalitis, TB meningitis
   Other neurological disorders:
      Guillain–Barré syndrome, Poliomyelitis
   Systemic diseases
      Acute intermittent porphyria
2 Increased sensitivity to ADH
   Chlorpropamide
   Carbamazepine
3 Ectopic source of ADH
   Bronchogenic carcinoma

face of plasma hypo-osmolality, hence the secretion of ADH is inappropriate.

The clinical features of vasopressin excess are those of water intoxication and hyponatraemia. They depend on the nature of the underlying disease and the rate of development and severity of the hyponatraemia. Symptoms are almost invariable at plasma sodium levels of less than 120 mmol/l. The major clinical features are shown in Table 14.

Table 14   Clinical features of vasopressin excess

Symptoms	Signs
Loss of energy	Clouded consciousness
Drowsiness	Drowsiness, coma
Disorientation	Depressed reflexes
	Extensor plantar responses
Agitation	Cheyne–Stokes respiration
Muscle cramps	Hypothermia
Anorexia, nausea	Convulsions
	Pseudobulbar palsy
	Absence of oedema

The patient may have few complaints. The neurological signs may suggest cerebral secondary deposits which can of course co-exist with this syndrome.

Diagnosis. The plasma sodium is usually less than 120 mmol/l and sometimes values as low as 100 mmol/l are recorded although the total body sodium is normal. The urine osmolality is greater than twice that of the plasma.

The plasma chloride, bicarbonate, urea, and creatinine are also lowered because of the haemodilution.

Other causes of hyponatraemia are often obvious from the clinical context although inappropriate ADH secretion may contribute to their evolution in some cases (Table 15).

A low plasma sodium may be recorded in hyperglycaemia,

Table 15   Other causes of hyponatraemia

Congestive heart failure
Cirrhosis of the liver
Chronic renal failure
Nephrotic syndrome
Decreased intravascular or extracellular fluid volume
Diuretics
Pseudohyponatraemia

hyperlipidaemia, hyperproteinaemia, and in patients receiving mannitol therapy. High blood glucose or mannitol levels lead to withdrawal of intracellular water with a dilution phenomenon. High protein and lipid levels reduce the sodium concentration by virtue of the volume they occupy.

Treatment. The underlying cause should be treated when possible, e.g. hypothyroidism, withdrawal of chlorpropamide or resection of a bronchogenic carcinoma. Symptomatic improvement is produced by limiting the fluid intake to rather less than the urine output, usually to about 500 ml per day. Renal potassium loss may necessitate replacement therapy but it is rarely necessary to give additional sodium. If coma supervenes, a single infusion of 500 ml of 3 per cent saline may be justified. The patient should be weighed daily to confirm water loss. If water restriction is unacceptable on a long term basis, demethylchlortetracyline can be given to antagonize the action of ADH on the nephron.

Oxytocin

Oxytocin, like vasopressin, is an nonapeptide (Fig. 7). Its actions overlap with those of vasopressin but in a physiological situation are confined to the breast and uterus. Its role in men is unknown.

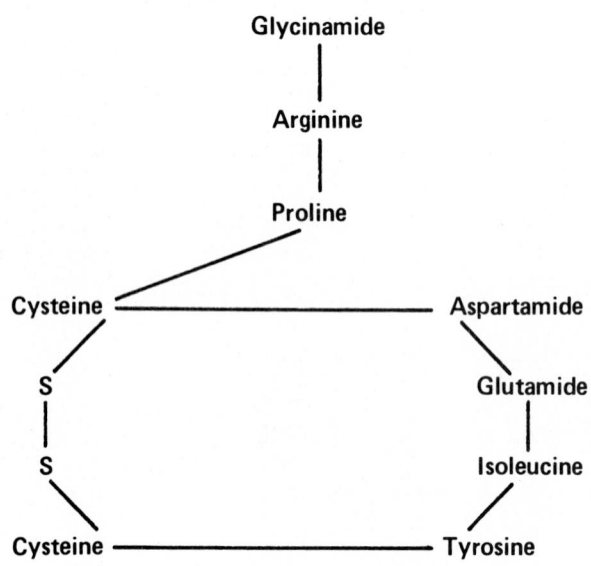

Fig. 7   Structure of oxytocin

It is synthesized largely in the PVN and to a lesser extent in the SON. Along with its carrier protein neurophysin I, it is transported by axonal flow to the posterior lobe for storage and release in response to nervous impulses transmitted from the hypothalamus.

During suckling afferent stimuli from the nipples and areolae are transmitted via spinothalamic fibres to the brainstem. Here the impulses relay via collaterals to the midbrain reticular formation to reach the hypothalamic neurosecretory nuclei via the tegmento-hypothalamic pathways.

Oxytocin causes contraction of the myoepithelial cells of the breast leading to milk ejection. After hypophysectomy, when the action of oxytocin is lost, women may fail to lactate.

Oxytocin stimulates myometrial contraction but its role in the onset and maintenance of labour is still uncertain. The uterus becomes more sensitive to oxytocin as pregnancy advances and there is a rise in levels of the enzyme oxytocinase during pregnancy, an observation of unknown significance.

Other than failure of suckling there are no obvious clinical sequelae of oxytocin deficiency, or excess. Oxytocin and neurophysin have been extracted from some tumours secreting vasopressin but do not appear to contribute to the syndrome of inappropriate ADH secretion.

HYPOTHALAMUS

The hypothalamus fulfills an integrating role between the central nervous, autonomic nervous, and endocrine systems, co-ordinating short-term neurological and longer-term endocrine responses. It also plays a major part in the control of body temperature, appetite, water balance, and sexual function.

Anatomy

Relations. The hypothalamus, as its name implies, lies below the thalamus and above the pituitary to which it is connected by the pituitary stalk. It also includes the lateral walls of the lower part of the third ventricle. Laterally it is related to the optic tracts, the ansa lenticularis, the globus pallidus, the internal capsule, and the lower part of the thalamus. In front it extends to just beyond the optic chiasm and behind to the posterior aspect of the mamillary bodies.

Blood supply. The anterior hypothalamus receives its blood supply from the anterior cerebral and anterior communicating arteries; the middle hypothalamus from the posterior communicating arteries; and the posterior hypothalamus from the bifurcation of the basilar artery and posterior cerebral arteries. Hence the occurrence of hypothalamic dysfunction from aneurysms of vessels of the circle of Willis, from subarachnoid haemorrhage from these vessels and from neurosurgical intervention. The supra-optic and paraventricular nuclei receive their blood supply from several sources—the anterior cerebral, internal carotid, posterior cerebral, and posterior communicating arteries. The capillaries of a portal system are located between the median eminence and pituitary stalk. Portal veins drain this region, passing down the pituitary stalk to the sinusoids of the anterior lobe and providing a route whereby neurotransmitters reach the pituitary from the hypothalamus. Other veins leave the hypothalamus to enter the veins above the circle of Willis to reach the basal vein and the vein of Galen.

Structure. The neurons of the hypothalamus can be divided into two categories relating to their connection to the anterior or posterior lobe respectively.

The hypothalamic parvicellular-adenohypophyseal system is made up both of well-defined nuclei and diffusely scattered neurons. The nuclei are responsible for synthesis of the various hypothalamic regulatory hormones.

The hypothalamic magnocellular-neurohypophyseal system comprises the SON located above the lateral edge of the optic chiasm and the PVN situated more dorsally on both sides of the third ventricle. The cells of these nuclei are larger than those of other hypothalamic nuclei and have characteristic staining properties.

Afferent pathways. The hypothalamus receives a wide variety of afferent fibres, the most important of which originate in limbic structures, particularly the amygdala and hippocampus. The extent of the control of these afferent pathways on the pituitary gland remains to be defined.

Hypothalamic control of the anterior pituitary. If the pituitary stalk is transected, serum prolactin levels rise whilst the levels of other anterior pituitary hormones fall. This indicates dominant inhibitory hypothalamic control of PRL secretion and dominant stimulation of the other anterior pituitary hormones by the hypothalamus. The anterior pituitary receives blood via the hypophyseal portal system which originates at the median eminence of the hypothalamus from the hypophyseal artery and direct arterial connections have not

been demonstrated. However, the sustained hyperprolactinemia which follows complete stalk section indicates the presence of alternate sources of blood supply to the anterior pituitary perhaps by diffusion from the posterior pituitary which does not possess a direct arterial supply.

The hypothalamic effects on anterior pituitary function are mediated by chemical messengers which are transported from the median eminence of the hypothalamus to the anterior pituitary via the hypophyseal portal vessel system. The hypothalamic regulatory hormones are small peptides which are synthesized and secreted by so called 'peptidergic' neurons whose cell bodies lie in different hypothalamic nuclei. Functional control of these neurons by higher brain centres is mediated by conventional neurotransmitters such as the catecholamines, dopamine (DA) and noradrenaline (NA), and serotonin (SER).

So far three such peptides have been characterized and synthesized. Thyrotrophin releasing hormone (TRH), somatostatin [growth hormone release inhibiting hormone (GHRIH)] and gonadotrophin releasing hormone (GnRH) are found in highest concentrations in the hypothalamus although TRH and somatostatin are also widely distributed throughout the central nervous system. They have been shown to alter the release of anterior pituitary hormones *in vitro* although the precise receptor mechanisms and intracellular events involved are incompletely understood.

The pentapeptides methionine (met) and leucine (leu) encephalin (which again have a wide CNS distribution but are found in highest concentrations in the hypothalamus), their synthetic analogues, β-endorphin and the undecapeptide substance P, have also been shown to affect anterior pituitary gland function.

Because of the wide CNS distribution and very short half-life (less than four minutes) of all these peptides, it has been suggested that they may have a central neurotransmitter role in addition to their known effects on anterior pituitary function. High concentrations of vasoactive intestinal peptide (VIP) have also been detected in portal blood, although the significance of this is unknown at present. There is good bioassay evidence for the existence of a separate GH releasing factor (GHRF), PRL releasing factor (PRF), and corticotropin (ACTH) releasing factor (CRF) although their structure remains unknown.

In addition to the hypothalamic 'peptidergic' neurons another pathway has now been described which is known as the tuberoinfundibular dopaminergic system whose terminal axons lie in juxtaposition to the perivascular spaces of the portal capillaries in the median eminence. Thus DA itself is secreted directly into hypophyseal portal blood and transported to the anterior pituitary gland. DA can be measured in portal blood where its concentration (10^{-9}–10^{-8} M) is much greater than in arterial blood from the same animal. By contrast NA concentrations in portal and arterial blood are similar. DA infusion *in vivo* effects the release of several anterior pituitary hormones and since catecholamines do not cross the blood–brain barrier to any appreciable extent, these effects reflect a direct action of DA on either the anterior pituitary or median eminence, tissues which lie outside the blood–brain barrier.

In this way the hypothalamic regulatory hormones interact with central neurotransmitters in the control of anterior pituitary gland function. The trophic hormones, thyroid stimulating hormone, follicle stimulating hormone, luteinizing hormone, and ACTH are subject to inhibitory peripheral negative feedback control by target gland hormones. GH may also be subject to negative feedback control by circulating somatomedins but additionally and in common with PRL may regulate its own secretion through a short loop positive feedback on specific hypothalamic inhibiting factors. In a recent study it was demonstrated that retrograde blood flow occurred in the pituitary stalk and was responsible for the delivery of high concentrations of TSH, PRL, LH, ACTH, and vasopressin to the median eminence. It was proposed that this might constitute an anatomical basis for such short loop positive feedback effects.

Hypothalamic regulatory hormones and factors

The hypothalamic substances affecting the synthesis and release of the anterior lobe hormones are termed hormones if their structure has been defined and their synthesis achieved. If merely a biological action has been described in a hypothalamic extract, the term factor is applied. These regulating hormones and factors are shown in Table 16.

Table 16 The hypothalamic regulatory hormones (RH) and releasing factors (RF)

Anterior lobe hormone	Release	Inhibition of release
Growth hormone	GHRF	GHRIH (somatostatin)
Prolactin	TRH	dopamine
	? PRF	? PIF
Thyrotrophin	TRH	?
Gonadotrophins	GnRH	?
Corticotrophin	CRF	?

Growth hormone release inhibiting hormone (somatostatin). The structure of this substance is:

H-Ala-Gly-Cys-Lys-Asn-Phe-Phe-Trp-Lys-Thr-Phe-Thr-Ser-Cys-OH

GHRIH is a cyclic tetradecapeptide with a short half-life of less than four minutes. In common with other hypothalamic regulatory hormones it lacks phylogenetic specificity in its actions. Somatostatin has a wide distribution throughout the CNS, although its concentrations are highest in the hypothalamus. It is also found in several other tissues in cells of APUD origin, particularly in the gut and the D cells of the pancreas.

Actions. Somatostatin has a wide variety of inhibitory actions on the pituitary and other tissues (Table 17).

Table 17 Inhibitory actions of somatostatin

1 Anterior pituitary	
TSH	
ACTH (in Nelson's syndrome)	
GH	
PRL (weak effect)	
2 Other tissues	
Endocrine	
Insulin	GIP
Pancreatic and gut glucagon	VIP
Gastrin	Cholecystokinin
Motilin	Renin
Exocrine	
Gastric acid	Pancreatic juice and enzymes
Pepsin	Salivary amylase

It is as yet uncertain which of the actions are physiological and which pharmacological. It inhibits GH secretion both basally and in response to stimuli in normal subjects and in acromegaly. Administration of antibodies to somatostatin to animals causes a rise in GH suggesting a physiological role for GHRIH.

Somatostatin also inhibits TSH secretion both basally and in response to TRH in normal subjects and in hypothyroidism. As for GH, administration of antibodies to somatostatin to rats is followed by a rise in basal TSH and the TSH response to a cold stimulus again suggesting a physiological role.

Somatostatin's location in the D cells of the islets adjoining the insulin and glucagon secreting cells indicates that it may have a local paracrine role in adjusting the balance of insulin and glucagon secretion.

The importance of locally mediated (paracrine) and blood-borne (endocrine) effects of somatostatin is uncertain. It can be detected in the systemic circulation at levels of 10–80 pg/ml. The source of this circulating material remains to be determined though the rise in response to glucose, protein, and fat ingestion suggests a gut origin.

Clinical applications. As yet the short half-life, the need for intravenous administration, and the wide variety of actions have precluded any clinical use of GHRIH. Search has gone on for analogues with selective actions capable of being given by mouth, so far without real success. Recently a 28 amino acid prosomatostatin has been isolated which has a greater and more prolonged action on GH release than GHRIH on an equimolar basis; and is more effective in inhibiting PRL.

Thyrotrophin releasing hormone. TRH is a tripeptide with the following structure:

pyro-Glu-His-Pro-NH$_2$

It has been isolated from the hypothalamus, and from other parts of the brain though in lesser amounts. It is also found in many other tissues including the spinal cord and pancreas.

Actions. TRH releases both TSH and PRL from the anterior pituitary. The hypothyroidism which results from pituitary stalk section suggests a physiological role for TRH as does the fall in TSH in response to certain stimuli following the administration of antibodies to TRH in animals. The role of TRH in sites other than the hypothalamus and pituitary is uncertain though it could function as some sort of neurotransmitter.

TRH also releases small amounts of FSH in men and LH in women around mid-cycle. In certain diseases such as acromegaly and chronic renal failure it causes GH release.

The nature and origin of the TRH-like material detected in the circulation and in the urine remains uncertain since assays of the hormone are prone to many methodological artefacts.

Clinical applications. TRH causes a rise in serum TSH levels which peak 20–30 minutes after intravenous injection. This observation has formed the basis of the TRH test which is widely used in clinical practice. The major value of the test is to exclude hyperthyroidism in borderline cases or where equivocal results have been obtained in serum T$_4$ and T$_3$ estimations. All patients with hyperthyroidism have an absent response to 200 μg of TRH given intravenously though there are other reasons than hyperthyroidism for an absent or impaired response (see below). A normal TSH response to TRH (value rising to outside the normal basal range for TSH) excludes hyperthyroidism. An impaired or absent response is seen in opthalmic Graves' disease, in some euthyroid multinodular goitres, in subclinical toxic adenomas, in de Quervain's thyroiditis, in acromegaly and hypopituitarism, and in Cushing's syndrome. A delayed TSH response to TRH when the 60 minute level is greater than that at 20 minutes is seen in hypothalamic and sometimes in pituitary disease.

Gonadotrophin releasing hormone. GnRH is a decapeptide with the following structure:

pyro-Glu-His-Trp-Ser-Tyr-Gly-Leu-Arg-Pro-Gly-NH$_2$

It is present in highest concentrations in the hypothalamus. So far only one GnRH has been isolated and this releases both LH and FSH. In adults more LH than FSH is released, but before puberty the reverse is true.

Actions. Since apparently one GnRH releases different amounts of LH and FSH under different conditions it seems likely that the effect of GnRH on the pituitary is modulated by the hormonal milieu at the time. In mid-cycle the positive feedback of oestrogens sensitizes the gonadotrophs to GnRH and also increases the amount of GnRH produced. Further sustained secretion of oestradiol-17β and progesterone in the luteal phase of the cycle reduces GnRH release and its action on the pituitary.

In men the negative feedback mechanism involving testosterone lowers the pituitary response to GnRH and hence lowers LH levels. The interaction of gonadally produced inhibin with GnRH in both sexes is poorly understood.

In children there is little LH and FSH response to GnRH but as puberty approaches the FSH response becomes greater. Once puberty is established the adult pattern of a greater LH response than FSH develops.

Clinical applications. GnRH can be used as a test of pituitary gonadotrophin reserve, measuring the LH and FSH levels before and at 20 and 60 minutes after 100 µg of GnRH given intravenously. An absent response in a patient with pituitary disease confirms lack of gonadotroph function. However, a normal response is often seen in patients with clear clinical evidence of pituitary–gonadal failure. An exaggerated LH response is seen in some patients with hyperprolactinaemia and in the polycystic ovary syndrome.

Initially it was considered that GnRH would have an important role in the treatment of some patients with hypogonadotrophic hypogonadism in whom the primary defect is believed to be a lack of GnRH. Some such patients treated with 500 µg of GnRH eight-hourly for several months do have restoration of gonadal function.

In normal adults and in patients with functional secondary amenorrhoea or oligomenorrhoea the gonadotrophin response to GnRH falls off after repeated administration and it has been suggested that GnRH may have a role as a contraceptive. Analogues with a D-amino acid at the 6 position of GnRH have a greater and more prolonged action and some are effective intranasally. They may find a place in the treatment of undescended testes or as a safe and reversible contraceptive agent.

Hypothalamic disease

A wide variety of diseases may affect the hypothalamus either directly, by spread from the pituitary or from disease elsewhere. The major disorders affecting the hypothalamus are shown in Table 18. As in pituitary disease, hypothalamic disease may present as a result of the local lesion, from hormone deficiency, from hormone excess, or from varying combinations of the three.

Headaches and visual field defects are commoner than in pituitary disease. A striking group of disorders make up the hypothalamic syndromes comprising disorders of:

Appetite
Sleep
Sexual behaviour and puberty
Thirst
Temperature control
Emotional behaviour
Motor activity
Cyclical hormonal activity

Obesity is a characteristic feature of hypothalamic disease although it should be stressed that there is no evidence for any hypothalamic abnormality in the vast majority of obese patients. The underlying cause for the obesity of hypothalamic disease is dysfunction of the ventromedial satiety centre. It is likely that the Prader Willi syndrome with gross obesity, hyperphagia, diabetes mellitus, mental retardation, hypogonadism, and small hands and feet, results from hypothalamic dysfunction.

Rarely damage to the lateral feeding centre results in aphagia with profound weight loss.

Disturbances of the normal pattern of sleep are another feature of hypothalamic disease particularly somnolence during the day which may be associated with insomnia at night.

Sexual behaviour may be grossly disturbed with embarassing promiscuity or with loss of libido. Puberty may be delayed or precocious. The latter disorder is seen particularly in lesions in the

region of the pineal. In girls true precocious puberty is more often functional whereas in boys an organic lesion is commonly responsible.

Table 18 Diseases of the hypothalamus

1 Congenital
  Deficiency of GH with or without other deficiencies
  Deficiency of LH and FSH with anosmia (Kallman's syndrome) or without anosmia
  Isolated hormone deficiencies, e.g. of TSH or ACTH
  Laurence–Moon–Biedl syndrome (mental retardation, polydactyly, retinitis pigmentosa and hypogonadism)
2 Tumours
  Hypothalamic
    Craniopharyngiomas
    Pinealomas (germinomas)
    Sphenoidal ridge meningiomas
    Gliomas of the optic chiasm
    Other cerebral tumours
    Secondary deposits
  Pituitary
    Suprasellar extension of pituitary tumours
3 Infectious diseases
  Encephalitis
  Tuberculosis
  Syphilis
4 Granulomatous diseases
  Sarcoidosis
  Hand–Schuller–Christian disease
  Eosinophilic granuloma
  Multi-system granulomas
5 Vascular disease
  Post-partum hypopituitarism
  Carotid and other aneurysms
  Subarachnoid haemorrhage
  Pituitary apoplexy
6 Structural
  Secondary to internal hydrocephalus from any cause, e.g. aqueduct stenosis in neurofibromatosis
7 Iatrogenic
  Radiation or neurosurgical treatment of pituitary lesions
  After prolonged steroid or thyroid hormone medication
8 Trauma
  After head injury
9 Functional
  Anorexia nervosa, starvation, emotional deprivation syndromes

Damage to the thirst centre in the hypothalamus can lead to dangerous dehydration and gross hypernatraemia, particularly if this lesion has also affected the SON and produced diabetes insipidus.

Alterations in the normal control of body temperature more often cause hypothermia than hyperthermia. It is likely that the anterior hypothalamus and adjacent pre-optic area are involved in body temperature regulation. In hypothalamic disease the body temperature may vary independently of the environment or may fall precipitately in response to cold due to lack of the normal compensatory mechanisms.

Behaviour may be immature, inappropriate, or psychopathic in patients with hypothalamic disease but the underlying mechanism for these effects is not known.

Motor activity can be strikingly reduced so that the patient is content to sit in a chair all day. No hormonal factors appear to be responsible and the condition persists even after full correction of all hormonal deficiencies.

Cyclical hormonal activity may be lost in some hypothalamic diseases, e.g. the nocturnal surge of GH, PRL, and ACTH. Likewise monthly rhythms may be affected, e.g. the mid-cycle elevation of LH and FSH.

Deficiency of any pituitary hormone other than PRL may be seen with hypothalamic disturbances. Characteristically diabetes insipidus and hypogonadism may be associated with hyperprolactinaemia.

The possibility exists that the syndromes of pituitary hormone excess may sometimes result from a primary disorder of the hypothalamus. For example acromegaly could result from excess GHRF, Cushing's syndrome from excess CRF, or pituitary hyperthyroidism from excess TRH, although there is as yet no firm evidence to support this view. In Albright's syndrome of polyostotic fibrous dysplasia which may be associated with precocious puberty, acromegaly, Cushing's syndrome, or hyperthyroidism, structural hypothalamic abnormalities can be demonstrated. It is possible that inappropriate secretion of various hypothalamic regulatory hormones could be involved in the development of these endocrine sequelae. Certainly hyperprolactinaemia is a common and characteristic feature of hypothalamic disease as a result of decreased formation of dopamine which now appears to be the major prolactin inhibitory factor.

References

DeGroot, L. J., Cahill, G. F., Odell, W. D., Martini, L., Potts, J. T., Nelson, D. H., Steinberger, E., and Winegrad, A. I. (1979). *Endocrinology*, vols. 1–3. Grune and Stratton, London.

Doyles, F. and McLachlan, M. (1977). Radiological aspects of Pituitary-Hypothalamic Disease. *Clin. Endocr. Metab.* **6**, 53.

Hall, R., Anderson, J., Smart, G. A., and Besser, M. (1980). *Fundamentals of clinical endocrinology*, 3rd edn. Pitman Medical, London.

—, Evered, D. C., and Greene, R. (1979). *A colour atlas of endocrinology*. Wolfe Medical Publications, London.

Kovacs, K. and Hovath, E. (1979). Pituitary adenomas. In *Pathologic aspects in clinical neuroendocrinology: a patho-physiological approach* (ed. G. Tolis, F. Labrie, J. B. Martin, and F. Naftolin), 367. Raven Press, New York.

Martini, L. and Ganong, W. F. (1980). *Frontiers of neuroendocrinology*, vol. 6. Raven Press, New York.

Nakanishi, S., Inoue, A., Kita, T., Nakamura, M., Chang, A. C. Y., Cohen, S. N., and Numa, S. (1979). Nucleotide sequence of cloned cDNA for bovine corticotropin-β-lipotropin precursor. *Nature, Lond.* **278**, 423.

Phillips, L. S. and Vassilopoulou-Sellin, R. (1980). Somatomedins, parts 1 and 2. *New Engl. J. Med.* **302**, 371, 438.

Post, K. D., Jackson, I. M. D., and Reichlin, S. (1980). *The pituitary adenoma*. Plenum Medical, New York and London.

Scanlon, M. F., Pourmand, M., McGregor, A. M., Rodriguez-Arnao, M. D., Hall, K., Gomez-Pan, A., and Hall, R. (1979). Some current aspects of clinical and experimental neuroendocrinology with particular reference to growth hormone, thyrotropin and prolactin. *J. endocr. Invest.* **2**, 307.

Tolis, G., Labrie, F., Martin, J. B., and Naftolin, F. (1979). *Clinical neuroendocrinology: a pathophysiological approach*. Raven Press, New York.

Thyroid disorders

R. Hoffenberg

According to Rolleston, the thyroid gland was first described by Galen (AD 130–200) but Vesalius (1514–64) furnished a fuller account. The name 'thyroid' was applied by Thomas Wharton (1614–73) and derived from its shield-like shape (θυρεος, an oblong shield); in German it is the *schilddrüse* or shield-gland. T. W. King, writing in *The Structure and Function of the Thyroid Gland* (1836), prophetically said '. . . We may one day be able to show that a particular material is slowly formed and partially kept in reserve, and that this principle is also supplementary, when poured into the descending cava, to important functions in the course of the circulation'. We now know that the thyroid gland slowly forms the protein, thyroglobulin, some tyrosine residues of which become iodinated to constitute the active thyroid hormones, thyroxine (T_4) and triiodothyronine (T_3), which are partially kept in reserve and released into the circulation to fulfil important functions.

Embryology and anatomy

The thyroid gland develops as an endodermal downgrowth from the tongue and can be identified in the human embryo by the end of the third week. Lateral extensions are joined by ultimobranchial cells that are the origin of calcitonin-secreting C cells. Colloid spaces may be seen in the gland by the end of the ninth week; follicular elements form and can be shown to contain colloid, to accumulate iodide, and synthesize hormone by the eleventh to twelfth week. These follicles extend in size and number and demonstrate increasing capacity to concentrate iodide and synthesize hormone. By the fourteenth week the thyroid of the fetus is essentially an adult gland in miniature. But fetal plasma hormone concentrations remain low until the second half of pregnancy, partly due to low circulating levels of thyroxine-binding globulin (TBG). Increased synthesis of TBG and maturation of the hypothalamic–pituitary axis to produce high fetal serum TSH (thyroid-stimulating hormone) concentration are associated with gradually-increasing levels of fetal T_4 and T_3 in the last trimester of pregnancy.

In the adult, the thyroid gland consists of two lobes connected by an isthmus; the upper poles of the lateral lobes reach up as far as the thyroid cartilage. Each lateral lobe measures approximately 40 mm tall by 15–20 mm broad by 20–40 mm deep, and the weight of the whole gland in a normal non-goitrous adult is 15–20 g, which makes it the largest single endocrine gland in the body. It consists of innumerable small follicles, like a bag of berries; Vercelloni (1711) could not be blamed for considering it a receptacle for worms which released their ova into the circulation. The lobes lie laterally close to the trachea and the isthmus crosses the trachea just below the cricoid cartilage. Important neighbouring structures include the oesophagus, parathyroid glands, recurrent laryngeal nerves, and carotid arteries; all of these may be affected by an enlarging thyroid gland.

Each thyroid follicle functions separately, the surrounding cells as the site of hormone formation, the lumen as a storage depot. Follicles are roughly spherical with diameters ranging from 50–500 μm. The activity of the thyroid gland is reflected directly by the height of the epithelial cells lining the follicle and indirectly by the diameter of the lumen. In the resting gland the cells are flat with a large colloid-filled lumen; in a more active phase, cell-height increases ('columnar' epithelium) and the lumen is smaller. In general, cell-height and luminar volume are inversely proportional.

Physiology of the thyroid gland

Hormone synthesis and secretion. The follicular cells of the thyroid gland produce two powerful metabolically active modified amino-acids, thyroxine (T_4) and 3,3′,5-triiodothyronine (T_3) (Fig. 1). Their synthesis depends on the availability of iodine which is absorbed from the diet via the small intestine. The average daily intake of iodine is 100–150 μg per day but this figure has increased

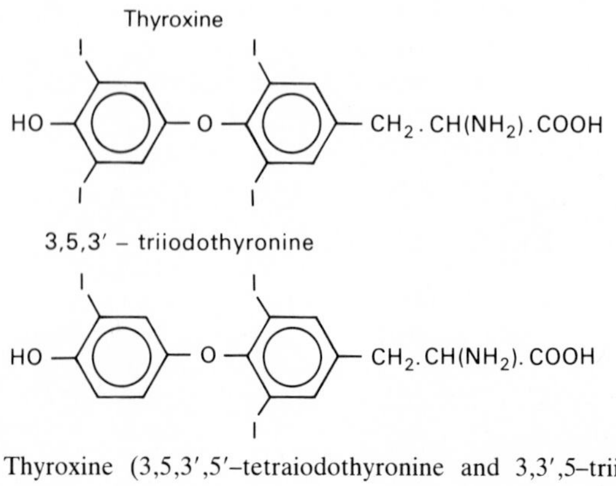

Fig. 1 Thyroxine (3,5,3′,5′–tetraiodothyronine and 3,3′,5–triiodothyronine).

recently in many parts of the world due to iodide supplementation of salt, milk products, and bread. Dietary iodine is reduced to iodide before absorption and is effectively removed from plasma by competition between the kidneys and the thyroid gland. The uptake of iodide by the thyroid cell involves both an active transport process and passive diffusion. Once inside the cell, iodide is rapidly metabolized and bound to tyrosyl residues of thyroglobulin; this step ('organification') depends on oxidation of iodide, probably through a peroxidase-H_2O_2 system. Thyroglobulin is the major protein constituent of the thyroid gland, a glycoprotein (molecular weight 660 000) formed on polyribosomes in the endoplasmic reticulum of the follicle cell. Each thyroglobulin molecule has about 110–125 tyrosyl residues, only a fraction of which are accessible for iodination which gives rise to monoiodotyrosines (MIT) and diiodotyrosines (DIT), still part of the large parent molecule. Coupling of suitably-placed iodotyrosines then takes place to form T_4 (from two DIT molecules) or T_3 (from a DIT and a MIT molecule); extrusion of an alanine side-chain accompanies this process. The ratio of T_4/T_3 formed depends largely on the relative abundance of DIT and MIT precursors. The MIT/DIT ratio within the thyroid is increased in thyrotoxicosis and some nodular goitres; the ratio of T_3/T_4 formed is therefore increased. In iodine-deficiency DIT is less abundant than MIT and relatively less T_4 is formed than T_3, presumably because of the greater chance of coupling of an MIT and a DIT molecule than of two DITs. Iodinated thyroglobulin is promptly extruded into the follicular lumen where it is stored. About 1 per cent of this organic iodide colloid pool is used each day in normal euthyroid man, but the rate of turnover is greatly increased in hyperthyroid states and the luminar pool diminishes rapidly.

Secretion of thyroid hormones is initiated by recovery by the cell of the stored iodoprotein and cleavage of T_4 and T_3 from it. The first step is the appearance of microvilli at the apical membrane of the cell which envelop a small piece of colloid and pinch it off to form an intracellular 'colloid droplet'. This process is greatly influenced by thyroid-stimulating hormone (TSH) and intracellular colloid droplet counting has been used as a bioassay for TSH. The colloid droplets fuse with intracellular lysosomes which contain proteolytic enzymes that completely degrade the thyroglobulin into its constituent amino acids, releasing T_4 and T_3 into the cell and then into the bloodstream. Uncoupled iodotyrosines within thyroglobulin are also released and rapidly de-iodinated; the iodide arising from this reaction is recycled within the same cell by incorporation into iodotyrosines and iodothyronines in newly-formed thyroglobulin, thus completing the cycle.

It is clear from this description that secretion from the thyroid gland consists almost exclusively of T_4 and T_3. But small amounts of MIT, DIT, iodide, and thyroglobulin may also leak into the circulation, as well as other metabolites of T_4 such as $3,3',5'$-T_3 (reverse T_3).

Hormone transport and action. T_4 and T_3 are poorly soluble in water and are transported in plasma in close linkage to plasma proteins. At physiological pH, 75–80 per cent of both serum T_4 and T_3 is bound to a specific thyroxine-binding globulin (TBG), which migrates electrophoretically between α_1- and α_2-globulin. It is a glycoprotein with a molecular weight of about 64 000 and is present in plasma at a concentration of 6–16 mg/l. This may be affected by a number of factors, hereditary and acquired (see page 10.27). A second important T_4 binding protein, thyroxine-binding prealbumin (TBPA), has a concentration in plasma of about 200–300 mg/l and normally binds 10–15 per cent of circulating T_4 and approximately 10 per cent of circulating T_3. TBPA is a tetrameric protein consisting of four symmetrical subunits so placed as to form a channel into which the thyronines are inserted. Each tetramer has two binding sites for T_4 but binding to the second site is inhibited once the first is occupied so that each is capable of binding a single T_4 molecule. TBPA circulates in close linkage to retinol-binding protein and its metabolically important ligand, retinol. TBPA is an

acute phase reactant and its concentration may be greatly reduced after various forms of medical or surgical stress.

TBG has a high binding affinity for T_4 and is capable of binding up to about 400 nmol/l of the hormone, but the normal circulating T_4 concentration is only 60–150 nmol/l, i.e. only about one-third of the binding sites of the protein are occupied. TBPA has a far greater capacity for binding T_4 and T_3 but a lower binding affinity. Albumin acts as a third binding protein and has a very large capacity but low affinity for both hormones. Small fractions of T_4 (± 0.03 per cent of the total or 4×10^{-11} mol) and T_3 (0.3 per cent or 1×10^{-11} mol) are thought to circulate 'free' or not bound to a plasma protein. The free fraction is thought to cross cell membranes to evoke the intracellular action of thyroid hormones and thus constitutes the important biologically active moiety of the circulating hormones. The concentration of free T_4 and T_3 must clearly depend on the concentration of total hormone in plasma as well as that of the binding proteins and their affinity for the hormones. This aspect will be considered later (see page 10.27).

Because of their lipid solubility T_4 and T_3 can enter the cell by diffusion across the cell membrane. There is a little evidence to suggest the existence of specific binding sites for T_3 on the plasma membrane of some cells and of an active transport system. The main intracellular binding protein for T_4 and T_3 is within the cytosol and this appears to act simply as a transport protein, allowing passage of the hormones to the specific nuclear binding site where action takes place. Cytosol binding proteins would thus serve the same functions within the cell as the main binding proteins within the plasma: to transport T_4 and T_3 from one site to another and perhaps to serve as a reservoir of hormone. The presence of high affinity binding proteins in the plasma and in the cell would modulate the movement of free T_4 and T_3 across the cell membrane and prevent their excessive and uncontrolled access to the nuclear site of action. Mitochondria also appear to possess specific binding sites for T_3, the significance of which remains to be determined.

There is abundant evidence that T_3 is the most active form of the thyroid hormones and specific nuclear binding receptors have been found in cells of the liver, anterior pituitary, kidney, lymphocytes, and heart—all known target-sites of thyroid hormone action. At the nuclear site T_3 is thought to produce its effects by activation of protein kinases and stimulation of protein synthesis. Other theories exist to explain the actions of thyroid hormones; one of the oldest suggests that they uncouple oxidative phosphorylation which would result in uneconomic oxygen and substrate utilization for energy production. This theory has lost support in recent years although the demonstration of mitochondrial binding sites for T_3 has provided some indirect evidence in its favour. Another possible mode of action of T_3 would be via stimulation of adenosine triphosphatase (ATPase).

The metabolism of thyroid hormones. The thyroid gland normally secretes about 80 µg of T_4 (100 nmol) and about 5 µg of T_3 (7–8 nmol) per day. Both hormones are subject to three main metabolic transformations: de-iodination, conjugation, and side-chain modification (Fig. 2). De-iodination is the most important route of

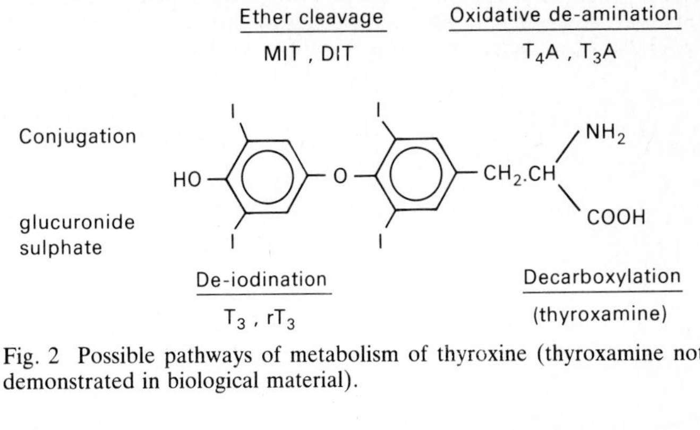

Fig. 2 Possible pathways of metabolism of thyroxine (thyroxamine not demonstrated in biological material).

metabolism of T_4 and is thought to proceed by serial removal of iodine atoms finally to produce thyronine, the fully de-iodinated skeleton of T_4 (Fig. 3). The first-line products of T_4 are $3,3',5-T_3$ (T_3) and $3,3',5'-T_3$ (reverse T_3 or rT_3). The former is produced by removal of an iodine atom in the $5'$-position through the action of an enzyme known as $5'$-monodeiodinase, the regulation of which has been the focus of attention in recent years. T_3 possesses three to five times the metabolic activity of T_4 (depending on the end-point used), and specific high-affinity binding sites for it have been found in the nuclei of those tissues that are most responsive to the actions of thyroid hormones. It is generally accepted, therefore, that T_3 is the active form of thyroid hormone and T_4 has assumed the role of a prohormone. Whether T_4 has any intrinsic action or whether it needs first to be converted to T_3 in order to achieve an effect remains a matter of controversy. Removal of the 5-position iodine atom of T_4 produces rT_3, considered under physiological conditions to be inert. The concentration of rT_3 may also be modulated by $5'$-monodeiodinase since its clearance by further de-iodination depends on the activity of this enzyme.

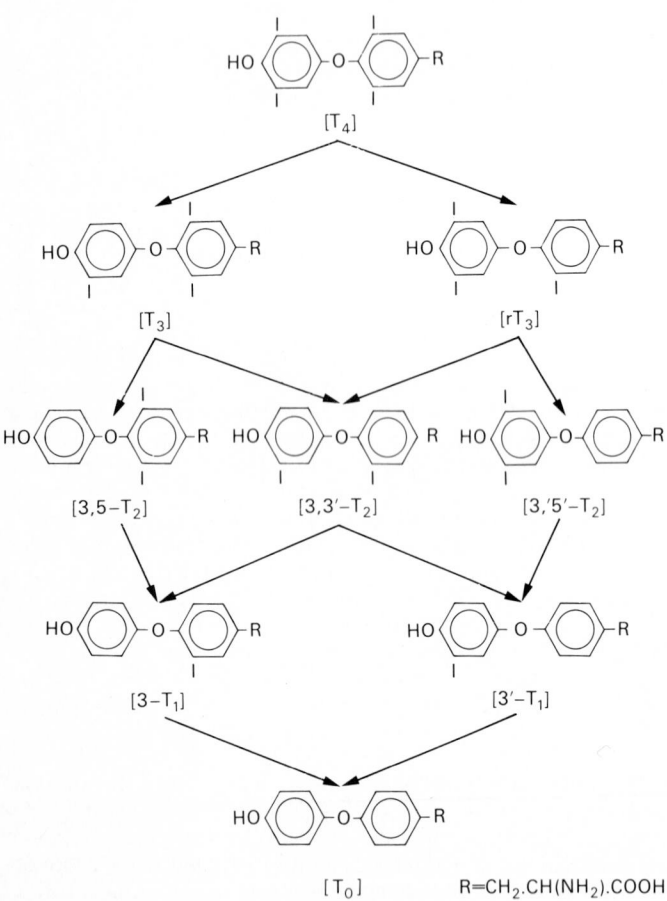

Fig. 3 Serial de-iodination of thyroxine to yield two triiodothyronines, three diiodothyronines, two monoiodothyronines and thyronine. All metabolites have been demonstrated in biological fluid.

The conversion of T_4 to T_3 may be inhibited by a large number of factors: acute medical or surgical stress; chronic illness; dietary intake; and a number of conditions have now been recognized in which plasma T_4 remains within the normal range but plasma T_3 is reduced. Generally this is linked to an increase in rT_3 concentration. It is not yet clear whether functional hypothyroidism accompanies this fall in T_3 production. Most of the metabolites that result from sequential de-iodination of T_3 and rT_3 have now been identified in biological fluids but their role is probably unimportant as they seem to possess no significant metabolic activity.

Side-chain modification may produce the acetic acid analogues of T_4 and T_3, tetraiodothyroacetic acid (tetrac) and triiodothyroacetic acid (triac). The latter has been shown to possess quite marked biological activity in certain systems, and the nuclear thyroid hormone receptors bind triac with an affinity 3 to 4 times that of T_3. There is at present little evidence to support an important role for these acetic acid analogues in health or disease.

Conjugation of T_4 or T_3 takes place at the phenolic hydroxyl group, mainly to glucuronic and sulphuric acids. The former enter the usual biliary/enteric pathway of glucuronides and hydrolysis in the gut may release thyroid hormones and iodine for recycling; the fate of sulpho-conjugates is less clear.

The control of thyroid function. The primary regulator of the thyroid gland is thyroid-stimulating hormone (TSH) produced by the pituitary gland. Regulation is achieved by a negative feedback system (Fig. 4) in which the pituitary responds to low circulating thyroid hormone concentrations by secretion of TSH, which accelerates the production and release of thyroid hormones by the thyroid gland until circulating concentrations are restored to normal. Conversely, a high concentration of thyroid hormone inhibits secretion of TSH. The pituitary gland itself is under the control of thyrotrophin-releasing hormone (TRH) produced in the median eminence region of the hypothalamus. Several questions about feedback control of thyroid function have not finally been answered: is control exerted through T_4 or T_3 or both? Is the negative feedback exerted at hypothalamic as well as pituitary level? Are there 'short-loop' feedbacks between, say, the pituitary and hypothalamus?

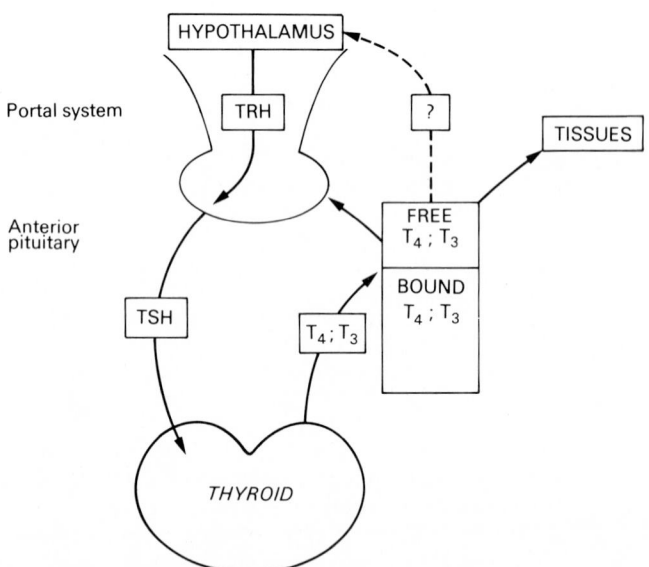

Fig. 4 Simple negative feedback system controlling thyroid hormone secretion. Suppression of anterior pituitary response has been demonstrated but direct action on the hypothalamus is still uncertain.

TSH is a glycoprotein (molecular weight 14 000) consisting of two subunits, alpha and beta, linked by disulphide bridges. The alpha chain is common to other trophic hormones of the pituitary gland, luteinizing hormone (LH), follicle stimulating hormone (FSH), and to chorionic gonadotrophin, but the beta chain is characteristic of TSH and confers specificity of action on the thyroid cell. TSH can be measured in several bio-assay systems and with greater sensitivity in a radio-immunoassay. In primary hypothyroidism (of thyroidal origin) plasma TSH is elevated, in hyperthyroidism it is generally undetectable. TSH binds to receptors on the membrane of thyroid cells and activates the adenylate cyclase system to increase intracellular cAMP. Within minutes changes can be detected within the thyroid cell, in particular the appearance of pseudopods which engulf intraluminal colloid as described on page 10.25. The production and secretion of T_4 and T_3 is stimulated by TSH.

TSH secretion is inhibited by both T_3 and T_4 and is stimulated by TRH, a tripeptide (Fig. 5) which is carried directly to the anterior pituitary gland by the hypophysial-portal system. TRH binds to the membrane of anterior pituitary cells and also acts via activation of the adenylate cyclase–cyclic AMP system. TRH also stimulates secretion of prolactin. The availability of synthetic TRH allowed the recognition of a dose-responsive secretion of TSH and the development of a TRH-test in the investigation of pituitary and thyroid disease. In primary hypopituitarism the TSH response to TRH is blunted or absent. In hypothyroidism there is a prolonged and exaggerated response to TRH, but in hyperthyroidism it is absent or greatly attenuated. The reason for the enhanced response to TRH in hypothyroidism and the attenuated response in hyperthyroidism is not completely understood. TRH is rapidly degraded *in vitro* in the presence of blood plasma. This degradation proceeds slowly in the absence of thyroid hormones and is greatly accelerated in their presence. In hyperthyroidism rapid degradation of TRH by high concentrations of thyroid hormones could explain its lack of effect; in hypothyroidism the low thyroid hormone concentrations could explain the prolonged and exaggerated response.

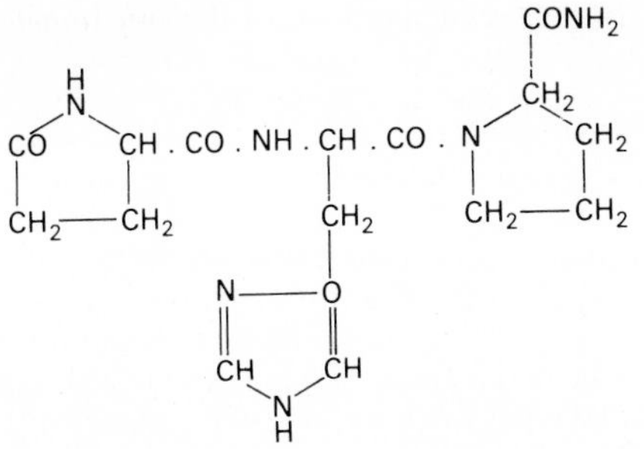

Fig. 5 Structure of thyrotrophin releasing hormone (pyroglutamyl-histidyl-prolineamide).

Many other factors, intrinsic and extrinsic, enter into the control of TSH and thyroid function. Of great importance is the availability of iodide, mainly through dietary source. This affects the total amount of thyroid hormone formed as well as the ratio of T_4 to T_3, and thus determines the output of TSH. In iodide-deficient areas the output of thyroid hormone is low and TSH secretion is high; goitre results from this prolonged stimulation. In addition, large doses of iodide have direct inhibitory effects on the thyroid gland, on the binding of the element within the gland and, most marked, on the pinocytic processes that lead to enhanced engulfment of colloid and secretion of T_4 and T_3. This effect is exploited in the treatment of thyrotoxic storm or crisis (see page 10.35).

Thyroid gland function in the fetus and in infancy. (See also pages 10.24 and 11.14.) In general the placenta is impermeable to the passage of peptide hormones such as TSH. Development of the fetal thyroid gland is thus independent of maternal control and wholly dependent on the maturation of its own hypothalamic-pituitary function. TSH is detectable in the fetal pituitary by the eleventh week of pregnancy and at about this time colloid formation and small follicular precursors are identifiable. Iodide-concentration and thyroglobulin synthesis are evident and the fetal thyroid gland gradually assumes full 'adult' function over the remainder of pregnancy. Plasma thyroxine-binding proteins (TBG and TBPA) are synthesized by the fetus through the second half of pregnancy and reach adult levels by term, so that cord blood thyroxine levels are similar to those of the adult. Thyroid hormones cross the placenta poorly if at all, so the fetus is dependent on its own thyroid secretions. Iodide crosses readily as do most antithyroid drugs, a point to be remembered in the treatment of pregnant thyrotoxic patients. Gamma-globulins are transported from mother to fetus and neonatal hyper-

thyroidism may follow the transplacental passage of maternal immunoglobulin thyroid stimulators (see page 11.14).

At birth rapid changes take place in thyroid hormone metabolism and control. There is a surge of TSH secretion which reaches a peak value of 80–100 µg/l about 30 minutes after birth and remains elevated for about 48 hours when it reaches normal adult values. At birth serum T_3 is low and rT_3 high due apparently to inhibition of 5'-deiodinase activity during the final stages of pregnancy and in parturition; in normal infants this returns to adult values within 24 hours. Perhaps as a result of the TSH surge, serum T_4 values are high in the newborn infant but return to normal in two to three weeks. Deviation from this pattern of hormonal change in the newborn has allowed the early recognition of neonatal hypothyroidism and the development of screening programmes for its detection (see page 10.40).

Thyroid function tests

Thyroid function tests are most commonly used to determine whether too much or too little thyroid hormone is being produced, i.e. whether the patient is hyper-, hypo-, or eu-thyroid.

Serum T_4, TBG, T_3 uptake tests and 'free T_4'. The most widely-used first-line test is measurement of the concentration of circulating T_4, usually by a specific radio-immunoassay. The normal range in most laboratories is 40–110 µg/l (50–150 nmol/l). The concentration is increased in hyperthyroidism, decreased in hypothyroidism.

Assay of serum T_4 is an assay of all circulating T_4, 99.96 per cent or more of which is bound to TBG, prealbumin, or albumin. Only about 0.2–0.04 per cent is not bound to protein or 'free', and this moiety is thought to cross from the plasma into cells to effect a biological action. Because of variable concentration of the major T_4-binding protein, TBG, in health and disease and under the influence of many drugs (Table 1), allowance must be made for the

Table 1 Alterations in serum TBG

Increased
Pregnancy, oestrogens, oral contraceptive pill
Phenothiazines, perphenazine, clofibrate
Viral hepatitis, acute intermittent porphyria
Myxoedema
Hereditary
Decreased
Androgens, asparaginase
Corticosteroids, anabolic steroids
Active acromegaly
Nephrotic syndrome
Malnutrition
Major illness, surgery
Thyrotoxicosis
Hereditary

concentration of serum TBG in evaluating the result of a T_4 assay. If TBG concentration is increased, total T_4 will increase; if TBG concentration is decreased, total T_4 will decrease. In both instances, although the percentage of free hormone will change, homeostatic adjustment will keep the absolute concentration stable. The same reduction of total T_4 with normal free T_4 concentration is seen with some drugs that displace T_4 from TBG. In hyperthyroidism the circulating pool of T_4 is increased by excessive secretion from the thyroid gland; total T_4 *and* free T_4 concentrations are elevated. In hypothyroidism the opposite obtains. These different situations are illustrated diagrammatically in Fig. 6. It is clear that a raised concentration of serum total T_4 may be due either to hyperthyroidism or to an increase in the concentration of TBG; in the former the free T_4 concentration is also raised, in the latter it is normal. Some means must be found to distinguish these two causes of a high serum T_4. It would be advantageous to measure free T_4 concentrations directly and there are techniques that do so; but they are not

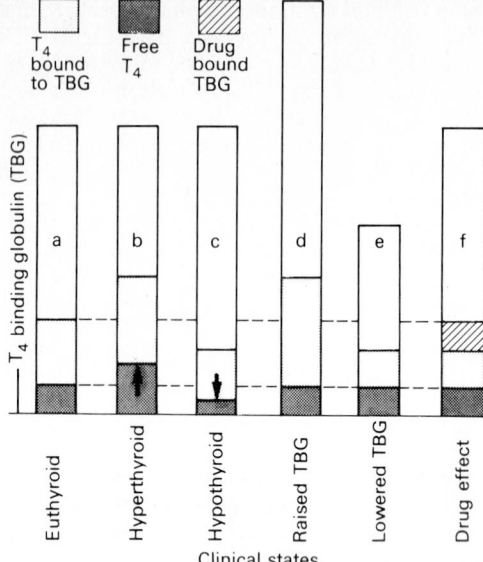

T₄ bound to TBG · Free T₄ · Drug bound TBG

Fig. 6 Diagrammatic representation of the relation between serum T₄ and the 'occupancy' of binding sites on serum proteins in different clinical states: (a) euthyroid; (b) hyperthyroid, serum T₄ and free T₄ raised; (c) hypothyroid, serum T₄ and free T₄ lowered; (d) raised T₄ binding globulin, serum T₄ raised, but free T₄ normal; (e) lowered T₄ binding globulin, serum T₄ lowered, but free T₄ normal; (f) drugs occupying binding sites on T₄ binding globulin but free T₄ normal.
(Reproduced from Hoffenberg, 1978. The thyroid. *Medicine* 3rd series no. 8, 392, by kind permission of Medical Education International Ltd.)

available in many centres, so some form of indirect assessment of free T₄ concentration is usually made.

The relationship between total T₄ concentration, its binding protein, and free T₄ may be expressed by the formula:

$$(\text{T}_4) = \frac{K \times (\text{T}_4 \cdot \text{TBP})}{(\text{TBP})}$$

where (T₄) = concentration of free T₄; (T₄. TBP) = T₄ bound to protein; and (TBP) = T₄ protein binding sites not occupied by T₄. This equation shows that the free T₄ concentration is directly related to the concentration of T₄ bound to protein and inversely to the unoccupied binding sites on that protein. Since 99.96 per cent or more of T₄ is bound to protein, simple assay of total serum T₄ will suffice to give (T₄. TBP). The problem is to measure (TBP), the unoccupied T₄ binding sites; this is achieved by so-called T₃ uptake tests, in which radioactive T₃ is added to the patient's serum and allowed to partition between the endogenous unoccupied protein binding sites and added T₃-binding substrates (resins or gels). From such tests it is possible to derive a figure that reflects the unoccupied binding sites and thus an 'index' of the free T₄ concentration. Recognition of this important relationship and the derivation of various types of free T₄ 'index' allows proper interpretation of serum T₄ assays even when TBG concentrations are grossly abnormal. In recent years several direct assays of TBG concentration have become available. One can thus express circulating T₄ concentration in terms of TBG concentration (T₄/TBG ratio) which gives a different but equally valid indication of free T₄ concentration.

Serum T₃ concentration; discrepancies between T₄ and T₃. Not to be confused with T₃ uptake tests, the concentration of serum T₃ may also be measured by a specific radio-immunoassay (normal range usually 0.7–2.0 µg or 1.0–3.0 nmol/l). High values are almost always found in hyperthyroidism, low values in hypothyroidism. Generally serum T₃ changes in the direction of serum T₄, but there are several circumstances in which the two hormones are discrepant:

T₃-toxicosis (see page 10.36). This syndrome must be thought of in cases of clinical hyperthyroidism with normal total or free serum T₄ values;

'T₄-toxicosis'. A rare condition of hyperthyroidism with high serum T₄ but normal or low circulating T₃. This may reflect a combination of hyperthyroidism with impaired de-iodination of T₄;

Low T₃ syndrome. Mono-iodination of T₄ to T₃ is impaired in a variety of clinical states: acute and chronic illness, acute stress, starvation or low-calorie intakes, liver disease, and drug effects (propylthiouracil, propranolol, glucocorticoids). The clinical significance of this finding is uncertain but it may cause functional hypothyroidism if sustained for long periods of time in chronically ill patients.

High T₃–low T₄ syndrome with clinical euthyroidism. This is seen particularly after treatment of hyperthyroidism by surgery or ¹³¹I or during treatment with antithyroid drugs. In these patients serum T₄ is low and serum TSH high, a combination that should suggest hypothyroidism, but serum T₃ is high or high-normal, and clinical euthyroidism is apparently achieved through its action. Some of these patients advance to develop overt hypothyroidism with failure of T₃ secretion as well as T₄; others show the discrepancy for years without evidence of progression.

In all of these circumstances measurement of both hormones is desirable for proper understanding of the functional state of the individual.

Serum TSH and the TRH test. TSH in serum is usually measured by a specific radio-immunoassay. In most laboratories the normal range is 0–4 mU/l, with 10–30 per cent of normal subjects having immeasurably low concentrations; this reflects the relative insensitivity of the assay. In primary hypothyroidism serum TSH concentration is elevated; in hyperthyroidism it is depressed (but not distinguishable from the normal range). Serum TSH concentration within the normal range in a clinically or biochemically hypothyroid patient exludes a primary thyroidal cause and points to hypopituitarism or a mistaken diagnosis. Conversely, a high serum TSH excludes the diagnosis of hyperthyroidism with the exception of rare cases due to excessive pituitary stimulation. It is not necessary to perform a TRH test if the basal TSH concentration is high as it adds nothing to the diagnosis.

Unfortunately, these responses are not specific and other conditions may produce similar effects so that the TRH test is best used in the negative sense: a positive response of TSH secretion excludes hyperthyroidism, failure of response excludes primary hypothyroidism. In the TRH test 200 µg is usually administered intravenously and blood samples are taken immediately before injection and 30 minutes later. It is no longer thought necessary to measure the response at two time-points after injection.

DISEASES OF THE THYROID GLAND

Diseases of the thyroid gland cause enlargement (goitre) and/or disturbance of function (hyper- or hypothyroidism).

Goitre

Goitre is the term applied to enlargement of the thyroid gland. The normal gland is barely visible, usually only in females with thin necks; visibility, therefore, implies that the gland is enlarged.

Palpation of the thyroid. Confirmation of enlargement is achieved through palpation. In orthodox surgical teaching this is carried out with the patient seated and the examiner standing behind using the fingers of both hands to define the gland; some examiners prefer to sit face to face with the patient, mainly using the thumbs to dislodge the trachea laterally, thus bringing each lobe in turn into greater prominence; my own preference is to stand at the side of the patient using the index and third fingers of the right hand to palpate the gland, with my left hand placed on top of the patient's head to move it into the position that most easily exposes each lobe to the examining fingers. The choice of method is personal but students are advised to select the method they find easiest and to persevere with it to gain efficiency. It is most important to achieve relaxation of the sternocleidomastoid muscles so the examining fingers can explore deeply into the paratracheal region normally covered by them. Manoeuvres such as extension, flexion, or lateral movement of the head help to secure relaxation and facilitate palpation of each lobe and the isthmus separately. Because of his adherence to the trachea, the thyroid gland generally moves up and down on swallowing. A sip of water often helps to confirm the presence of a goitre or a nodule within it. 'Fixation' or failure to move on swallowing suggests the presence of carcinoma, thyroiditis, or scarring but may be found if the gland is extremely large.

The examiner should attempt to define the gland's outline, symmetry, and overall consistency. The normal thyroid gland is usually palpable only in young people with thin necks and relaxed muscles; in older people or those with thick or short necks palpation may be extremely difficult. The gland usually enlarges symmetrically but one lobe may be more prominent and more easily palpated even in diffuse disorders. Asymmetry with displacement of the trachea implies nodularity of the gland. When the patient swallows the lower borders of the enlarged thyroid gland can usually be felt; if one cannot get 'below' the gland it may be assumed to extend retrosternally.

The normal thyroid gland has the consistency of soft rubber or meat; it is often described as 'fleshy'. Undue hardness may be found in chronic thyroiditis, in which the gland is usually diffusely enlarged and its borders very easy to delineate; in carcinoma an asymmetrical area of hardness is often present. One or more nodules or lumps within the thyroid gland may be felt as smooth rounded cystic swellings or poorly defined irregularities or variations in consistency. Occasionally a nodule on one side of the trachea may be the only palpable thyroid tissue. The distinction between 'diffuse' and 'nodular' enlargements of the thyroid gland, is of importance aetiologically and therapeutically, but even experts find it difficult to make this distinction with accuracy on palpation in all cases.

Palpation of the thyroid gland should always include a search for enlargement of neighbouring lymph nodes, most commonly found in cancer but often present in thyroiditis. The anterior cervical chain is most commonly involved but enlarged glands may also be found more laterally in the supraclavicular fossa, or just above the isthmus (Delphian nodes).

Local examination of the thyroid gland is incomplete without enquiry about and search for involvement of other neighbouring neck structures. Compression or deviation of the trachea may give rise to dyspnoea, stridor, and cough; hoarseness or loss of voice may suggest involvement of a recurrent laryngeal nerve, perhaps by carcinoma; Horner's syndrome may result from sympathetic nerve damage; and signs of venous obstruction may indicate local pressure often in the mediastinum.

Diffuse goitre. This term refers to enlargement of both lobes (and the isthmus) of the thyroid gland; it is usually but not always symmetrical, and may contain nodules especially if it has been present for a long time. This section will not consider the diffuse hyperplastic goitre of Graves's disease, only 'simple' or 'non-toxic' diffuse enlargement of the thyroid gland. Theoretically, this type of goitre can be looked on as compensatory to decreased secretion of thyroid hormones. Loss of negative feedback inhibition would lead to increased stimulation of the gland by TSH with resultant hypertrophy and hyperplasia. This simple explanation may obtain in some cases but fails to take into account three common observations: (*a*) plasma TSH concentration is not elevated in most cases of non-endemic simple goitre; this may reflect the insensitivity of our assay methods to distinguish normal from slightly elevated levels; (*b*) failure or diminution of thyroid hormone synthesis or secretion is not demonstrable in most cases of non-endemic goitre; (*c*) administration of thyroid hormones in full and prolonged dos-

age to suppress TSH does not often lead to regression of the goitre. While it is clear that some other explanation needs to be found to account for most cases of simple goitre, failure of hormone production, for whatever cause, may give rise to diffuse enlargement of the thyroid gland.

Iodine lack and endemic goitre. Endemic goitre is one of the most common diseases known and has been estimated to affect 200 million people. The term 'endemic' is applied when goitre is present in a significantly large proportion of a population but the definition is arbitrary since neither thyroid size nor the required proportion of an affected population is universally agreed. Endemic goitre is generally attributed to insufficiency of iodine in the diet and is found in most mountainous areas of the world, e.g. the Himalayas, the Andes, the Alps, Greece, New Guinea. It also occurs in non-mountainous areas which have a low concentration of environmental iodine. It is important to realize that sporadic goitre indistinguishable from endemic is found in areas that are not deficient in iodine, and that the prevalence of goitre varies greatly within endemic regions, from district to district, and within and between families. These differences are generally ascribed to an inability of some individuals, perhaps for genetic reasons or at times of increased demand, to adapt to relatively low iodine intakes.

The minimum daily requirement for iodine is probably 50–70 μg and dietary intake is reflected by the urinary excretion of iodine. In endemic goitre regions urine output of iodine is low (40 μg per day or less) and the thyroid gland shows marked avidity for the element, demonstrable by a high thyroidal uptake of radioactive iodine. An inverse relationship thus exists in endemic areas between thyroidal uptake and urinary excretion of iodine. If the deficiency is not too severe, compensation may be found with normal or low-normal values of plasma T_4 and a normal or slightly raised concentration of TSH. There is often a relative increase in serum T_3, reflecting the less complete iodination of tyrosines by the thyroid gland and the higher intrathyroidal MIT/DIT and T_3/T_4 ratios; this may be sufficient to maintain the subject in a euthyroid state despite the presence of a goitre. If the deficiency of iodine is severe, however, hypothyroidism will ensue with low plasma T_4 and T_3 and elevated TSH.

Clinically, the picture is one of goitre with or without hypothyroidism. Thyroid enlargement becomes apparent in early childhood and affects both sexes equally; after puberty females tend to be affected more than males in a ratio as high as six or seven females to one male. In early stages the goitre is diffuse but it tends to become nodular in older subjects. There is no satisfactory explanation for this nodule formation but repeated cycles of hyperplasia and involution have been incriminated (see page 10.31). If these large multinodular glands are scanned with radioactive isotopes, uptake is shown to be patchy, some nodules appearing hyperactive, others inactive. Endemic goitres may reach an immense size, extend retrosternally and give rise to pressure symptoms particularly venous obstruction.

The most important clinical consequence of iodine deficiency is cretinism (see page 10.39), but mention must be made here of a related but separate syndrome in which neurological features predominate. In this form of cretinism deaf-mutism is almost always present associated with spastic paralysis, squint, and ataxia. These patients do not show the characteristics of myxoedemic cretinism such as coarseness of features, thick dry skin or sluggish movement but share the intellectual retardation. The existence of these two syndromes and the fact that goitres are not present in all cases of endemic cretinism have caused some controversy about their aetiology and the relationship of dietary iodine deficiency to their development. The role of ingested goitrogenic substances has been postulated for many years based on early demonstrations of development of goitre in experimental animals fed naturally-occurring foodstuffs (cabbage and plants of the *Brassica* species, such as rape, kale, and turnip). This observation led to the identification, isolation, and synthesis of the commonly used thionamide antithyroid drugs. Evidence for the existence of a naturally-occurring goitrogenic substance in food as a cause of endemic goitre in man is not convincing.

Endemic goitre is not usually associated with hyperthyroidism, but this has been induced in epidemic form after introduction of iodide as a prophylaxis for iodine-deficient goitre (Iod Basedow); it is probable that the increase of iodine available for hormone synthesis unmasks in some people a pre-existing tendency to hyperthyroidism previously kept in abeyance by lack of iodine substrate. In the later multinodular stage of endemic goitre one or more nodules may appear more active on scanning but hyperthyroidism is rarely seen. Although the evidence is confusing, it is probably true that endemic goitre does not predispose to thyroid malignancy.

Eradication of goitre by iodine supplementation in some parts of the world has been one of the successes of modern medicine. Goitre-prevention programmes in the mid-western states of North America, Switzerland, Austria, and Central and some parts of South America have reduced the prevalence of cretinism and deafmutism as well as goitre, and are being extended to many other countries. Addition of iodine to salt or to flour used for breadmaking is most commonly practised but these techniques may fail to reach some regions of severe endemicity. A remarkably successful method is the injection of iodized oil, as used in radiographic contrast media, from which iodine is slowly released, the effects of a single injection lasting three to five years. Pioneered in New Guinea this method has now been applied with striking benefit in other parts of the world. Iodine-supplementation prevents the appearance of goitre in children and may induce a decrease in size or disappearance of existing goitres. As large glands begin to involute, pre-existing nodules may become easier to feel. The induction of hyperthyroidism referred to above is rare and is thought predominantly to affect older women with nodular goitres in whom slightly smaller doses of iodine may need to be used.

Treatment of large goitres is more effectively achieved by administration of thyroxine (150–200 µg per day). Diffuse hyperplastic goitres may shrink rapidly but many do not alter in size. In addition, thyroxine treats existing or incipient hypothyroidism, often with impressive clinical improvement even when biochemical evidence of the disorder is unconvincing. Surgery may be needed if the gland is very large and features of local compression are present, e.g. stridor or venous congestion, but a trial of thyroxine therapy is first justified in all but the most urgent cases.

Hereditary defects in hormone synthesis. This group of conditions is rare and of limited clinical importance but they help to elucidate the processes by which thyroid hormones are normally formed. As in most other inherited metabolic disorders, the degree of completeness of the defect is variable. As a result, some children present with goitre and severe cretinism, some with only mild hypothyroidism, and others with goitre alone. Even within a single family the clinical picture can be variable. Because of the comparative rarity of these disorders, patterns of inheritance have often not been worked out. The existence of a defect in thyroid hormone synthesis may be suspected when familial goitre with or without hypothyroidism is encountered in a non-endemic region. Characterization of the defect is exceedingly difficult and usually requires *in vitro* study of excised abnormal thyroid tissue. Most clinicians would be content to suspect the existence of a synthetic block and to treat the patient without detailed confirmatory investigation. The main categories of defect include:

Inability to concentrate iodide in the thyroid gland. The mechanism underlying this disorder of transport is unexplained but salivary glands also lose their iodide-concentrating ability. It is possible to overcome the disability by administering large amounts of iodine to the subject to take advantage of simple diffusion processes, but, as with all synthetic defects, thyroxine administration is the preferred form of treatment.

Inability to iodinate thyroglobulin. Iodide trapped by the thyroid gland is normally oxidized to iodine before it can displace hydrogen from the tyrosine residues of thyroglobulin (organification). Various defects have been described that affect the generation of peroxidase activity or of hydrogen peroxide, on which oxidation of iodide depends. The most commonly recognized form is Pendred's syndrome in which the defective iodination is incomplete and there is an associated nerve-deafness; hypothyroidism, if present at all, is usually mild. This defect is the easiest to detect: non-protein bound (non-organified) iodide which is present in the thyroid gland may be displaced or discharged by perchlorate ions. Radioactive iodine is therefore given to suspect patients, time allowed for its accumulation by the thyroid gland, and its loss from the gland then observed after oral administration of potassium perchlorate (perchlorate discharge test).

Deficiency of iodotyrosine dehalogenase. When thyroglobulin is hydrolysed by a normal thyroid cell, MIT and DIT are released in addition to T_4 and T_3. These tyrosines are then de-iodinated by an intrathyroidal dehalogenase enzyme and the iodide released is taken up for new hormone formation. A defect in the activity of this enzyme leads to loss of this extra iodide (which is excreted in the urine as MIT or DIT) and to a relative state of iodine deficiency. The diagnosis may be confirmed by demonstration of MIT or DIT in the urine after administration of radioactive iodine or labelled DIT. In theory the disorder may be treated by giving iodine supplements sufficient to balance the loss; in practice, thyroxine replacement therapy is advised.

Abnormality of thyroglobulin synthesis and of iodothyronine synthesis. Coupling of iodotyrosines is a necessary step in the synthesis of T_3 and T_4. A specific coupling enzyme has been postulated but not demonstrated, and defective coupling may simply be due to abnormalites of thyroglobulin structure or conformation that fail to provide the steric relationship of iodotyrosines that favours this step. A number of patients have been studied who showed an abnormality or absence of thyroglobulin synthethis; unusual iodoproteins such as iodoalbumin are found in their thyroid glands and plasma. No defect of coupling of iodotyrosines has been demonstrated that could not be explained by synthesis of abnormal thyroidal proteins.

Target organ unresponsiveness to thyroid hormones. A few cases have been described in whom variable degrees and forms of peripheral resistance to T_4 or T_3 have been demonstrated. The clinical picture is one of euthyroidism or even hypothyroidism in the face of elevated plasma concentrations of T_4 and T_3. In one form the unresponsiveness is thought to be confined to the pituitary gland; in these subjects hyperthyroidism is present with elevation of plasma TSH due to failure of feedback inhibition.

In all cases of hereditary goitre due to enzyme blocks, with or without hypothyroidism, treatment with T_4 is advisable. In some, the extent of TSH-drive is extreme with plasma TSH values often in excess of 1000 mU/l. This is reflected by intense hyperplasia of the thyroid gland and a notable tendency to recur after surgery. In this group as a whole there is thought to be an enhanced tendency to develop malignancy and it is hoped that adequate T_4 replacement therapy may eradicate this risk.

Interference by antithyroid agents (goitrogens). A large number of chemical substances can impair the synthesis of T_4 at a variety of points in the pathway. Thiocyanate, once used extensively in the treatment of hypertension, and perchlorate block transport of iodide into the thyroid cell, perhaps by direct competition resulting from a similarity of molecular volume and charge.

Most goitrogens act by blocking the iodination of thyroglobulin, perhaps competing as substrate for the enzyme, peroxidase. This is the basis for the successful application of thionamide and thiourylene drugs to the treatment of hyperthyroidism. Other drugs share this mechanism of antithyroid action: paraaminosalicylic acid (PAS), phenylbutazone, resorcinol, some sulphonylureas and sulphonamides, cobalt, and aminoglutethamide are examples.

Secretion of thyroid hormones is strongly inhibited by iodide, an observation that is exploited in the management of thyrotoxic crisis or storm (see page 10.36). It is paradoxical that iodine excess as well as iodine deficiency can give rise to goitre. This is seen in areas of Japan were milligram amounts of iodine are consumed each day in the form of seaweed. Individual susceptibility to iodine ingestion is apparent even in areas of endemic high intake, and goitre is more commonly seen in glands that have previously been damaged by thyroiditis or irradiation. Chronic ingestion of iodine-containing asthma remedies or vitamin preparations is occasionally associated with goitre. Lithium acts by a similar mechanism and may cause goitre or even hypothyroidism.

Many drugs are known to affect the peripheral metabolism, transport, or action of T_4. Propylthiouracil, for instance, in addition to its action on organification, inhibits the conversion of T_4 to T_3; propranolol shares this property but also blocks the beta-adrenergic-mediated effects of hyperthyroidism; many compounds are capable of displacing T_4 or T_3 from plasma binding proteins. But there is no suggestion of goitre-production except through mechanisms directly related to function of the thyroid gland.

In treating drug-induced goitre, withdrawal of the drug is advisable. This may not always be desirable, e.g. with the use of lithium for manic depressive psychosis. In such cases, thyroxine may be employed in normal replacement doses.

Thyroiditis. This term covers a variety of disorders of an inflammatory nature that will be dealt with separately (see page 10.40). Although goitre is partly explained by the aggregation within the gland of cellular infiltrates and fibrosis, there is commonly compensatory hyperplasia of residual intact parenchymal cells presumably as a response to deficient thyroid hormone production and enhanced thyrotrophic stimulation. Thyroxine administration frequently achieves diminution in the size of the gland.

Colloid goitre. In the variety of diffuse goitres discussed above, I have suggested that TSH-stimulated hyperplasia resulting from deficient hormone production might be an important component of the mechanism by which the glands enlarge. The hyperplasia is reflected histologically by the presence of tall columnar epithelium with small follicles containing scanty colloid. Another form of diffuse goitre exists in which follicles are normal-sized or even larger than normal, filled with colloid, and lined by flat epithelium. This 'colloid goitre' may represent a stage of involution as proposed by Marine many years ago. In his theory the initial response to iodine deficiency is one of hyperplasia, but later the gland becomes 'exhausted' and enters a resting phase characterized by histological appearances of the colloid goitre. Marine extended this theory to suggest that nodules developed in such glands if they were subjected to repeated cycles of hyperplasia and involution, perhaps through an erratic supply of dietary iodine or an intermittent increase in the demand for thyroid hormone, as might occur during pregnancies. Marine's hypothesis has gained support from clinical and experimental observations.

Colloid goitre is most commonly found in young females, often at adolescence. The gland enlarges symmetrically and feels characteristically soft and spongy. Because of its soft consistency it rarely gives rise to symptoms of compression. Within a few years the gland may disappear or it may persist and evolve into a multinodular gland. Some of these nodules can enlarge to cause compression of surrounding tissues and may extend retrosternally. The commonest form of goitre in young females is that of chronic thyroiditis which usually feels firmer and is more clearly defined; colloid goitre can only be diagnosed with certainty by histology.

Surgery is not necessary for colloid goitre unless it is very large, unsightly, or causing pressure symptoms, and reassurance about the nature of the enlargement is often all that is necessary. Thyroxine may be given in standard replacement doses to reduce the size of the gland, but is seldom of dramatic benefit.

Nodular enlargement of the thyroid gland
Multinodular goitre. The term 'nodule' as applied to the thyroid

gland means a lump. This is usually palpated but the term applies equally well to 'lumps' found by any imaging technique, at surgery or autopsy. Nodules of the thyroid gland can vary in size from 1–2 mm to 10–15–20 cm in diameter, can be single or multiple, hyper-functioning or hypofunctioning. Pathologically, they may consist of true tumours (adenoma, carcinoma, lymphoma) or simple aggregates of colloid-filled follicles. Within a nodule there may be cystic degeneration, haemorrhage, fibrosis, calcification, or papillary changes that suggest microcarcinomas.

Various terms are used to describe these goitres: 'multinodular' or 'non-toxic nodular' gland are clinical descriptions based usually on palpation; 'nodular colloid', 'cystic colloid', or 'adenomatous' goitre are sometimes loosely applied to the feel of a gland without pathological justification.

The prevalence of nodules within the thyroid gland varies from country to country and depends on the means of ascertainment. By careful palpation, nodules may be felt in 4–5 per cent of a normal female population over the age of 50 years. At autopsy even in non-goitrous areas nodules of the thyroid may be found in 40–50 per cent of subjects. Women are more commonly affected than men and nodules are particularly common in areas of high goitre endemicity. Perhaps because of various interventions, it is generally felt that the incidence of nodular goitres is declining.

There is no completely satisfactory explanation of nodule formation, but Marine's theory of cyclic hyperplasia and involution is widely accepted. Nodule formation seems likely to occur in any longstanding hyperplastic gland whether this is due to iodine deficiency, goitrogens, or a hereditary enzyme defect. With thyroxine treatment of a gland of this sort, shrinkage of surrounding hyperplastic tissue may bring a pre-existing nodule into prominence so that it may be felt more easily. With practice one should be able to palpate nodules of 1 cm diameter provided they are not too deeply placed.

Nodules of the thyroid gland may present because of pressure symptoms (dysphagia, cough, hoarseness of voice, dyspnoea) but more commonly the patient (or her doctor) notices a lump in the neck which is painless and symptomless. Once aware of the lump, the patient may develop symptoms of discomfort, dyspnoea, dysphagia, or a dry cough because of anxiety. Occasionally haemorrhage into a nodule may give rise to acute pain and swelling which usually subsides partially within two to three days and fully within two to three weeks. Large multinodular goitres tend to shelve retrosternally and may cause the syndrome of superior vena caval obstruction.

Older patients may present with hyperthyroidism (Plummer's disease or secondary hyperthyroidism), the features of which are often less typical than those associated with toxic diffuse goitre (Graves's disease); these aspects will be discussed later (see page 10.37). Why some nodules should become hyperthyroid is not at all clear. As time passes one or more nodules in a multinodular gland may show greater activity than the surrounding tissue on a thyroid scan (a 'hot' nodule). This activity may increase to the extent that it suppresses the function of all other thyroid tissues and it may then independently produce enough thyroid hormone to cause clinical and biochemical hyperthyroidism (a 'toxic' nodule). The presence of hyperthyroidism in a patient with nodular goitre does not neccesarily imply that it is a nodule that is responsible for the hyperfunction: Graves's disease can affect the internodular tissue of such glands and non-toxic nodules may be present in the diffuse hyperplastic gland of Graves's disease. It is rare for patients with multinodular goitre to be hypothyroid and the combination of an apparently nodular thyroid gland with hypothyroidism should raise the possibility of Hashimoto's (auto-immune) thyroiditis.

Various types of imaging technique may be used to detect nodules of the thyroid gland. A straight X-ray of the neck may show deviation of the trachea, retrosternal extension, or calcification; barium or other contrast media may show nodular indentation of the oesophagus; ultrasound may additionally reflect whether a nodule is solid or cystic; and scanning with radioactive isotopes adds information about the relative activity or inactivity of the nodule.

The most difficult decision facing the clinician who feels one or more nodules in a thyroid gland is whether these are benign or malignant. This aspect will be discussed in the section on *thyroid cancer* but one or two points should be made at this stage: by careful examination pathologists may find papillary carcinoma in 5–15 per cent of all thyroid glands, whether these are nodular or not. The problem is whether these are 'significant', i.e. if left alone would they enlarge to invade locally or spread to other parts of the body? In the case of multinodular goitre the presence of carcinomatous elements seems to confer no or extremely little risk of spread: in a Framingham study Vander *et al.* were able to follow 218 patients with non-toxic nodular glands for more than 15 years and found no clinical suspicion of malignancy in any patient. The case of the single nodule of the thyroid may be slightly different (see below).

The treatment of multinodular goitre depends to a large extent on one's willingness to accept that the risk of malignancy is insignificant. Thyroxine replacement (200–300 μg per day) is the treatment of choice and should be tried first in almost all cases. Response rates differ from centre to centre but generally do not support the earlier enthusiasm for this mode of treatment; at best 10–20 per cent of multinodular goitres will regress with continued thyroxine replacement therapy. A little care must be exercised as the function of some autonomous nodules may not be suppressed by exogenously administered hormone and the effect may be additive thus precipitating hyperthyroidism; this is an uncommon finding.

Unless the goitre is very large or producing compressive features, nothing needs to be done about it, and reassurance about its benign nature often dispels symptoms of anxiety. Cosmetic considerations, especially in a young girl, might sway one toward surgery, as might the supervention of features that are accepted as evidence of malignancy, such as rapid increase in size. If surgery is undertaken, as much nodular tissue as possible should be removed without putting the parathyroid glands or recurrent laryngeal nerves at risk, and thyroxine replacement therapy is subsequently advisable.

Radioactive iodine is excellent treatment for toxic nodular goitre, especially if there is a single hyperactive nodule. Since the surrounding thyroid tissue is suppressed, uptake of radioactivity is confined to the hyperactive nodule and large doses of ^{131}I may be used without fear. Hypothyroidism is most unlikely to follow as the suppressed tissue should soon regain its normal function.

Single nodules of the thyroid. One of the most difficult and controversial aspects of thyroid disease is the approach to the single nodule. The majority are true benign adenomas but some, especially those containing papillary elements, are thought to be potentially malignant, and clinically the distinction is not easy. Because of this some clinicians advocate surgery for all single nodules of the thyroid gland, despite evidence to show that at least half the nodules diagnosed as single prove to be multiple at surgery, with a far lower incidence of malignancy. Others would not advocate surgery unless there was clear suggestions of malignancy on clinical or investigational grounds: recent rapid increase in size; the presence of a nodule in a young person, especially a male; past history of exposure of the thyroid region of the neck to irradiation, especially in childhood; irregularity of the nodule; the presence of enlarged regional lymph nodes; or involvement of laryngeal nerves. Scanning of the thyroid with radioactive isotopes may provide further information. A nodule that is 'hot' is most unlikely to be malignant, some would say never. The reported incidence of carcinoma in 'cold' nodules varies widely, 10 per cent being a generally accepted figure. Recently ultrasound examination with or without needle-aspiration has been used for cold nodules that are thought to be cystic, as they show a very low incidence of carcinomas and surgery may be obviated if a cyst is found. There is little firm data to reconcile these opposing views, which reflect a lack of agreement about the histopathological criteria for the diagnosis of cancer in single nodules, uncertainty about their natural history, and geo-graphic differences in the prevalence of goitre and cancer. Whatever approach is adopted, consideration must always be given to the skill and experience of the available surgical team.

Thyroid carcinoma

The reported prevalence of carcinoma of the thyroid gland varies with the effort made by the pathologist to identify small 'occult' neoplasms usually regarded as non-significant. Routine autopsies usually reveal cancer in 4–5 per cent of thyroid glands, but in some parts of the world, e.g. Japan, this figure rises to about 25 per cent on careful serial sectioning. It has been estimated that 0.8 per cent of the population could have clinical carcinoma, and about 30 new cases are diagnosed annually per million people but only about 6 per million die each year from the disease. The discrepancy between pathology, clinical diagnosis, and mortality reflects the benign nature of the disease as well as the lack of uniformity about diagnostic criteria, and makes it difficult to offer firm recommendations about treatment.

Little is known about the aetiology of thyroid cancer in humans. Exposure of the upper mediastinum or neck to irradiation during childhood has been identified as an important factor, and many cases of thyroid tumour have been reported 10 to 30 years after X-ray therapy for cervical tuberculous adenitis, thymic or tonsillar enlargement, and acne. In one series a 7 per cent incidence was found 30 years after irradiation, but doubts must be expressed about the clinical significance of this finding and the need to take active therapeutic steps. It is reassuring that there appears to be no increased risk of cancer in adult patients who have been treated with ^{131}I for hyperthyroidism.

It is customary to consider primary malignancy of the thyroid gland under specific headings:

1. Papillary carcinoma
2. Follicular carcinoma
3. Medullary carcinoma
4. Anaplastic carcinoma
5. Miscellaneous, e.g. sarcoma, lymphoma.

Papillary carcinoma. This shows papillae around a fibrovascular stalk and usually contains elements of follicular differentiation. These tumours tend to infiltrate locally to involve lymph nodes, the strap muscles of the neck, and perhaps the trachea, but may metastasize to the lungs or bone. They tend to be very slow-growing and may be present for decades without causing symptoms. The prognosis is especially good in children and young adults. Of all thyroid cancers 60–80 per cent are classified as papillary, and about 20 per cent are said to be multicentric, although it is not clear whether this is intrathyroidal spread or true multicentricity.

Follicular carcinoma. This tends to occur slightly later in life (peaking in the fifth decade), affects females three times as commonly as males, and accounts for 20–25 per cent of all thyroid cancers. Many are resectable with a good prognosis but they tend to metastasize by bloodspread to the lungs and bone rather than to infiltrate locally. Their differentiation into relatively normal-looking follicles reflects a greater degree of TSH-responsiveness and they often take up iodine and even form thyroid hormones; rarely hyperthyroidism ensues.

Medullary carcinoma. This arises from the parafollicular or C cells of the thyroid of ultimobranchial origin, and constitutes about 3–5 per cent of all thyroid cancers. Histology is characterized by sheets of cells with large nuclei, amyloid deposits, and extensive fibrosis. They tend to infiltrate locally and also to metastasize to the lungs and other soft tissues. These tumours secrete calcitonin which provides a useful diagnostic criterion and a marker to monitor response or relapse after treatment. In cases of doubt, calcitonin secretion may be enhanced by infusion of calcium, pentagastrin or ingestion of alcohol. This manoeuvre may be particularly valuable in screening families as the disease may be transmitted as a dominant trait. Medullary carcinoma of the thyroid gland forms part of the multiple endocrine syndrome in conjunction with phaeochromocytoma (see page 13.278), parathyroid adnomas (see page 10.56), and multiple mucosal and cutaneous neurofibromata; diarrhoea is often present but is not explained. The prognosis is poor.

Anaplastic carcinoma. This occurs most commonly in women and is associated with a poor prognosis. Spread takes place locally and may involve the trachea to cause dyspnoea, or the oesophagus giving rise to dysphagia. Most patients with this disease die within a year of diagnosis.

The diagnosis of thyroid carcinoma. Thyroid nodules are common, thyroid carcinoma rare. The investigation of multinodular goitres for suspect cancer is only justified if there are strong indications; solitary nodules would be investigated by most clinicians. The ultimate diagnosis depends on demonstration of tumour tissue on biopsy, which may be carried out at open surgery, by use of a cutting needle, or aspiration using a small needle. I prefer open biopsy from which sufficient tissue may be taken to allow a reliable diagnosis to be made. The distinction between benign and malignant lesions is often difficult, especially with well-differentiated papillary or follicular tumours. Secretion of abnormal tumour products does not help to distinguish carcinomas (apart from calcitonin in medullary tumours). Thyroglobulin may be detected in the serum of patients with benign or malignant lesions of all kinds and is therefore of no diagnostic value; its assay may be useful in monitoring patients after surgery or other forms of treatment.

Thyroid scanning with radioactive iodine or technetium is widely used. A hot nodule is very rarely malignant; cold nodules are usually benign, but have a greater chance of being malignant. Ultrasound may help to distinguish cystic from solid lesions; the former are almost always benign. These imaging techniques are helpful but never entirely reliable in the identification of malignant thyroid swellings.

Before embarking on treatment, especially surgery, it is customary to X-ray the chest for lung secondaries. A skeletal X-ray survey or scan is probably not justified without some hint of bone involvement.

Treatment of thyroid cancer. With the exception of medullary and anaplastic variants, thyroid carcinomas are generally slow-growing and relatively benign. A trial of TSH suppression with oral thyroxine (200–300 µg daily) is usually worthwhile in the case of both multinodular goitres and solitary nodules in which the diagnosis is suspected but not proved; even 'cold' nodules occasionally regress. Once the diagnosis of cancer is established by histology, surgery is usually undertaken. In principle a lobectomy is performed on the affected side, with a subtotal lobectomy on the other. The amount removed depends on the surgeon's assessment of the risks to the parathyroid glands and, perhaps, the laryngeal nerves. Lymph glands which are readily accessible may be removed but radical neck dissection is seldom undertaken as it probably does not alter life expectancy. Post-operatively the patient must be closely observed for hypoparathyroidism and appropriate treatment instituted if clinical or biochemical features are present. Once again, there are differing views about how to proceed after surgery.Some authorities would simply give the patient suppressive doses of thyroxine and observe, arguing that a recurrence or metastasis could be treated on its merits if and when it appeared; serial measurement of plasma thyroglobulin may be valuable in this circumstance. Others would favour ablation of all functioning thyroid tissue and would arrange a schedule of regular (6–12 monthly) [131]I whole body scans in the hope of showing sufficient uptake for a therapeutic ablative dose of this isotope to be effective; in between scans, the patient would be maintained on thyroxine therapy. Large doses of ^{131}I are usually needed (50–150 mCi) and this may uncommonly cause radiation sickness with nausea or parotitis; rarely

acute radiation thyroiditis may be seen. Various methods to stimulate tumour uptake of ^{131}I have been tried but are of limited value. Because of the slow progression of thyroid cancer and its variable natural history, it is difficult to offer dogmatic advice about the best course of treatment.

Medullary and anaplastic tumours in general do not concentrate radioactive iodine; surgery may be followed by X-ray therapy to the neck, but the clinical course of established disease is seldom mitigated. Chemotherapy has been tried without much success, adriamycin having received most attention.

In the case of lymphoma or lymphosarcoma excellent responses to X-ray therapy may be seen.

Hyperthyroidism

Hyperthyroidism or thyrotoxicosis is the syndrome that results from an excess of circulating thyroid hormones (T_4 and/or T_3). Although this may be derived from extrathyroidal sources (Table 2), the syndrome results in 99 per cent of cases from hyperfunction of the thyroid gland that falls into two broad groups: diffuse hyperplasia and hypertrophy (Graves's disease); hyperactive or 'toxic' single or multiple nodules of the thyroid (Plummer's disease). Very rarely a well-differentiated cancer of the thyroid may cause hyperthyroidism. In this section Graves's disease will be considered in detail.

Table 2 Causes of hyperthyroidism

1 Graves's disease (diffuse toxic goitre)	

2 Toxic nodular goitre
    Multinodular (Plummer's disease)
    Single toxic adenoma
	99% of cases

3 Nodular goitre with Graves's disease	
4 Well-differentiated thyroid carcinoma	

5 Excess thyroid stimulating hormone
    Inappropriate secretion of TSH by pituitary tumour
    Non-tumorous
    Choriocarcinoma and hydatidiform mole
    Embryonal testicular carcinoma	

6 Extraneous thyroid hormone
    Intentional (factitious)
    Overenthusiastic therapy
    During T_3 suppression test
	exogenous

Metastatic thyroid cancer Struma ovarii	endogenous
7 Transient thyroiditis following irradiation	

Graves's disease

Aetiology. This syndrome affects females more than males in a ratio of 5–7 to one, and occurs at all ages with a peak in the third and fourth decades. Its geographical distribution is uncertain but it seems more common in developed and affluent nations; no community is immune. Psychological stress has frequently been postulated as a precipitating factor but the evidence for this is unconvincing.

It is possible by a variety of *in vivo* and *in vitro* techniques to demonstrate the presence of thyroid-stimulating immunoglobulins in the plasma of almost all patients with Graves's disease. The first of these to be described was initially called long-acting thyroid stimulator (LATS) because of its prolonged stimulatory action in test animals, but a number of other terms are applied depending on the system used to detect the presence of what appear to be different types of stimulating immunoglobulins. Although their exact nature remains to be clarified, these immunoglobulins appear to be auto-antibodies directed against the TSH-receptor or a closely associated protein on the plasma membrane of the thyroid cell. Graves's disease is thus generally accepted as another example of auto-immune disease. This concept is supported by the histological appearance of the gland and by frequent association with other auto-immune diseases, such as rheumatoid arthritis, pernicious anaemia, and myasthenia gravis.

It has long been known that thyrotoxicosis tends to run in families. Indeed, other disorders of thyroid function (goitre and hypothyroidism) are also commonly seen in the relatives of patients with Graves's disease. Other auto-immune diseases and even thyroid stimulating immunoglobulins have been found in non-thyrotoxic family-members. This genetic predisposition to Graves's disease conforms to the usual pattern of auto-immune disturbances but, in common with them, the precise precipitating mechanism in Graves's disease is not explained.

Pathology. The thyroid gland is usually markedly enlarged due to hypertrophy and hyperplasia. The enhanced activity of the gland is shown by the change of epithelium from cuboidal to columnar with papillary infoldings of redundant cells and reduction in the size of the follicular lumen, which contains sparse colloid with increased vacuolization (Fig. 7). There is often infiltration with lymphocytes and plasma cells, and the stroma is very vascular. This appearance is characteristic of a thyroid gland that is under intense stimulation as may be seen as a result of TSH stimulation after prolonged and excessive administration of antithyroid drugs.

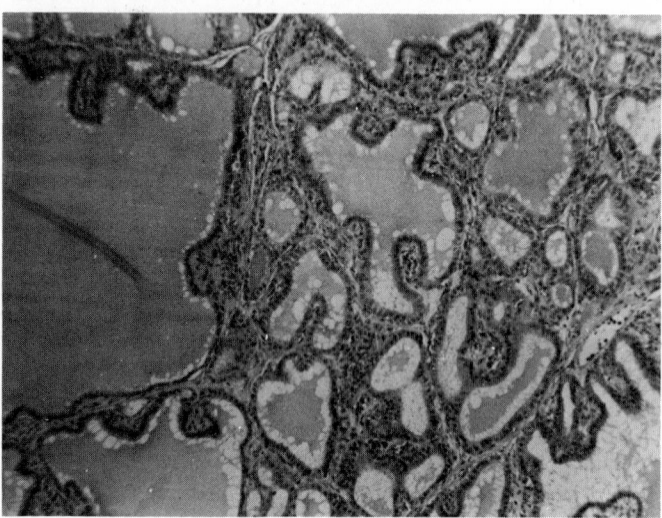

a

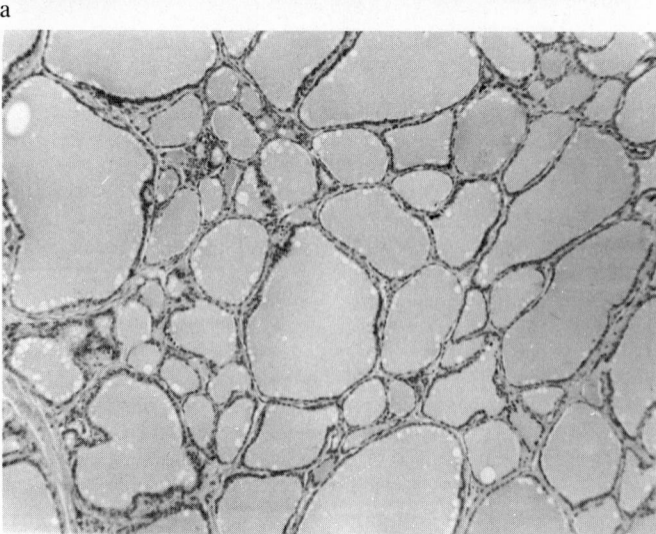

b

Fig. 7 Contrast between appearance of hyperthyroid (a) and inactive thyroid (b) glands. In the former note the cellularity, infoldings, and relative paucity of colloid; in the latter the flat epithelium and distended colloid spaces.

Onset and course. The onset of the disease is characteristically gradual, often insidious, but it may be quite dramatic with florid manifestations appearing in the course of a few days. These more rapid developments are occasionally attributed to psychic or other stress, but careful questioning after such episodes usually reveals evidence of pre-existing disease. Iod Basedow refers to hyperthyroidism that may follow rapidly after the ingestion of iodide, especially in elderly patients.

The natural history is no longer easy to observe as treatment is usually started as soon as the diagnosis is made. It is important to appreciate that the disease may be self-limited, as was frequently observed in the days before specific therapy was available. This forms the rationale on which medical treatment is based (see page 10.36). Once adequate treatment is established, the disease abates and will remain quiescent so long as treatment is maintained. In patients who receive no or too little treatment, acute exacerbations may occur at any time, rarely constituting the serious exaggerated form of the disease known as 'thyroid storm' or 'crisis' (see page 10.35).

Clinical picture. Almost all systems of the body may be affected in hyperthyroidism but the emphasis often falls more strikingly on one, e.g. the cardiovascular or neuropsychiatric. In a classic case the diagnosis should be suggested by the appearance and general demeanour of the patient (Fig. 8): wide-eyed, hollow-cheeked, agitated, restless, shaky and tremulous with rapid bounding carotid pulsations, and a visible goitre. More difficult to diagnose are cases of 'masked' or 'apathetic' hyperthyroidism in which the classical manifestations are subdued and the clinical picture may consist

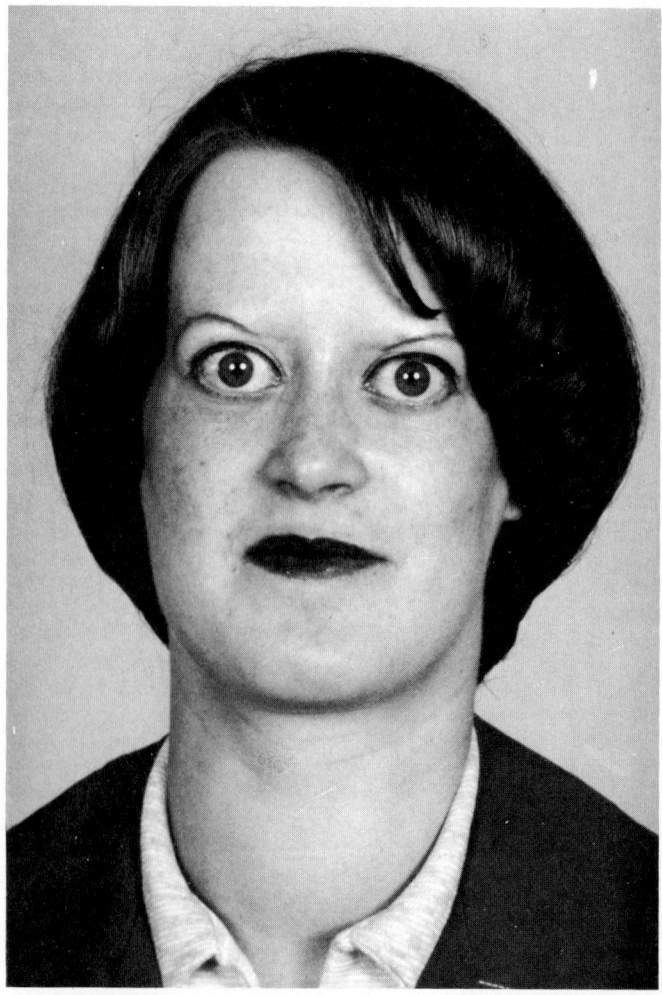

Fig. 8 Typical appearance of patient with Graves's disease.

solely of cardiac features such as atrial fibrillation or cardiac failure, profound muscle weakness, or apathy and asthenia.

Important *symptoms* of hyperthyroidism include loss of weight, often with maintenance of a good appetitie, fatigue, nervousness, increased sweating and intolerance of heat, palpitation, dyspnoea, weakness, diarrhoea, or simply an increased frequency of bowel movement. The patient may complain that the eyes have become more prominent or painful ('grittiness'), of double vision, or lacrimation.

Objectively, a *goitre* is felt in the vast majority of cases; it is diffusely enlarged but may be asymmetrical with one lobe larger than the other; occasionally it is extremely large displacing the carotid arteries posteriorly. The gland is usually vascular with an easily-audible systolic bruit. The absence of a goitre makes the diagnosis of hyperthyroidism less likely and should lead one to consider other conditions or thyrotoxicosis factitia.

A fine *tremor* is usually present, the *skin* feels hot and damp, palmar erythema and spider naevi may be seen; vitiligo may be present (often indicating an auto-immune background) or occasionally hyperpigmentation. *Alopecia* of the scalp occurs in severe cases. The *nails* may show onycholysis, a lifting up of the nailbed distally with accumulation of dirt beneath it (Plummer's nails).

The common *eye signs* include a stare, lid-retraction with visible sclera above the iris, and lidlag, seen as the patient moves the eyeball downwards. Only a mild degree of proptosis is found in most cases of Graves's disease but more severe forms of ophthalmopathy may occur (see below).

Cardiovascular features are often prominent. Almost all patients show a rapid pulse which may be due to sinus tachycardia or atrial fibrillation. A high-output state is shown by bounding peripheral pulses often with a clear collapsing impulse; expansile pulsation of the terminal digits may be felt. In some patients angina pectoris may be experienced and cardiac failure is not uncommon. It is important to stress that cardiac features may dominate the clinical picture and thyroid function tests must be done in all unexplained cases of atrial fibrillation or cardiac failure.

Neuropsychiatric manifestations include nervousness, hyperactivity, and tremor; choreoathetosis may be seen and a Parkinsonian tremor is occasionally associated. Emotional lability is very common, giving rise to short-temper and easy crying. Occasionally frank psychosis is seen, or a picture of encephalopathy.

Muscular weakness is frequent, often affecting the proximal muscles, occasionally profuse and profound. Fatiguability may mimic myasthenia gravis which may indeed be independently associated with Graves's disease. In chronic thyrotoxic myopathy, the course may be insidious and slowly progressive, simulating motor neurone disease. The tendon reflexes are maintained and sensory loss does not occur. In the Far East a form of hypokalaemic periodic paralysis is often seen, particularly in men; this syndrome is rare in the West (see page 18.29).

Gastrointestinal features may include anorexia, nausea, and vomiting (although the appetite is usually maintained). Hyperemesis may be a presenting feature of hyperthyroidism. Increased frequency of bowel action is common, occasionally amounting to frank diarrhoea. Steatorrhoea may occur. The liver and spleen rarely enlarge and jaundice is unusual.

Less common or specific features of hyperthyroidism include oligomenorrhoea or amenorrhoea in the female, gynaecomastia and loss of libido in the male. In children exaggerated growth is seen and behavioural disturbances tend to dominate the picture.

A high serum calcium may rarely be found in hyperthyroidism. More often than not this is due to the concomitant presence of hyperparathyroidism. Very rarely a high serum calcium level is found which responds to treatment of the hyperthyroidism; this is usually attributed to exaggerated bone metabolism with mildly impaired renal clearance of calcium.

Hyperophthalmopathic Graves's disease. Mild ocular involve-ment is an integral part of the clinical syndrome of Graves's disease. Occasionally more severe involvement is found with marked proptosis, ophthalmoplegia, chemosis, and increasing retro-orbital pressure that might lead to papilloedema or optic atrophy and loss of vision (malignant exophthalmos). The disease may start with puffiness and itching of the eyelids and redness of the conjunctivae which may be diagnosed erroneously as allergic conjunctivitis. The condition is usually bilateral but is often asymmetrical and may be unilateral; in this case it may be confused with a retro-orbital tumour or other space-occupying lesion. These severe eye signs usually accompany the general constitutional picture of hyperthyroidism but occasionally occur in the absence of overt hyperthyroidism or even after its successful treatment. In some cases exophthalmos may be associated with pretibial myxoedema or clubbing of the fingers. *Pretibial myxoedema* is due to deposition of mucopolysaccharides in the subcutaneous tissue of the legs, anteriorly or posteriorly. Small plaques of thickened skin gradually coalesce and may extend to involve the lower half of the legs and feet. Rarely the same lesions may affect the arms, face, or pectoral regions. Pretibial myxoedema is usually pink or reddish-brown with a *peau d'orange* appearance, and its borders are well demarcated from normal skin. The deposits are difficult to treat but may respond to topical applications of steroids such as triamcinolone. It is important to appreciate that pretibial myxoedema is not usually a feature of myxoedema; nor should it be confused with the accumulation of oedema fluid in the legs that is quite commonly seen in hyper- and hypothyroidism.

The cause of the hyperophthalmopathic form of hyperthyroidism is not understood. Excess secretion of TSH is not responsible. Pathologically there is retro-orbital deposition of mucopolysaccharides with oedema and round-cell infiltration; the extraocular muscles are greatly thickened as may be demonstrated on computerized axial tomography of the orbit.

If systemic hyperthyroidism is present, it should be treated by conventional means and the eye signs often improve. If the patient is euthyroid or the hyperthyroidism has been brought under control and the ocular features are severe or progressive, oral adrenocortical steroids may be needed. It is usually necessary to give massive doses initially to achieve an effect, e.g. prednisolone 120–150 mg daily in divided doses, but a reduced dose may sustain the improvement. Orbital irradiation has been recommended and success has been claimed for plasmapheresis, provided the disease is not long-standing. Decompressive surgery may be needed in unresponsive or threatening disease. It is of particular value where retro-orbital tension builds up to the point that papilloedema and visual failure occur or the eyeball threatens to protrude excessively. At all times local palliative measures may help: eyedrops such as methylcellulose to protect the cornea, an eyepad, diuretics, or elevation of the head during sleep. Lateral tarsorrhaphy may be needed to ensure adequate closure of the lids to prevent damage to the cornea by debris with consequent ulceration and infection; this operation often improves the appearance of the eyes.

Fortunately severe life- or vision-threatening exophthalmos is not common. Since it is a disease of spontaneous remissions and relapses, it has been difficult to evaluate properly the many forms of treatment that have been tried. In my own experience adrenal steroids or surgery offer the best chance of quick relief when the condition is severe and progressive.

Thyroid crisis or storm. This is a life-threatening augmentation of the hyperthyroid state, usually but not always abrupt in onset and related to a precipitating factor in many cases. Inadequate preparation for thyroidectomy remains an important and completely avoidable cause, but a thyroid storm may follow any non-thyroidal surgery in patients whose hyperthyroidism has not been recognized or adequately controlled. Infection, especially of the upper respiratory tract, may be important. In about half the cases a precipitant is not identified.

In most instances hyperthyroidism is known to exist and the

condition suddenly worsens. Fever is almost invariable and the main clinical features are:

1. *Cardiovascular*: tachycardia, arrhythmia, congestive cardiac failure, and shock;
2. *Central nervous*: agitation, tremor, restlessness, mania, delirium, stupor, or coma;
3. *Abdominal*: pain, jaundice, diarrhoea, vomiting, and hepatomegaly.

Thyroid storm is an emergency, requiring prompt and energetic treatment. Antithyroid drugs may begin to act within an hour of administration and it is customary to give 600–1200 mg of propylthiouracil or 60–120 mg of carbimazole orally or by intragastric tube.

Iodide is a powerful and prompt inhibitor of release of thyroid hormones by the gland; lithium salts have a similar action.

Beta-blocking agents are most effective; 1–5 mg of propranolol should be given intravenously, or 20–80 mg six-hourly by mouth. Tachycardia, fever, tremor, and restlessness usually respond promptly.

General measures are also needed, e.g. parenteral fluids, anti-cardiac failure treatment, antipyretics and antibiotics if infection is present. Adrenal steroids are usually given without clearcut evidence of benefit.

Plasmapheresis, exchange transfusion, and dialysis have all been tried but should perhaps be reserved for patients who fail to respond to more conservative measures.

The diagnosis of hyperthyroidism. Essentially the diagnosis is clinical but the condition must be excluded in unexplained atrial fibrillation, cardiac failure, myopathy or weight-loss, despite the absence of classical features of hyperthyroidism. Even where the clinical diagnosis is reasonably certain, a confirmatory test is advisable as a hyperthyroid state may be mimicked by conditions such as anxiety, occult infections like tuberculosis, carcinoma, phaeochromocytoma, or diabetes mellitus.

The diagnosis is best established by the demonstration of a high circulating concentration of thyroid hormones, T_4 and T_3, after allowance has been made for the influence of their binding proteins in the plasma (see page 10.27). A free thyroxine index may be derived or the concentration of free thyroxine in plasma assayed directly. T_3-toxicosis is a term applied to hyperthyroidism resulting from excessive circulating T_3 without an increase in total or free T_4. This condition is reported in up to 5–10 per cent of all thyrotoxics in some parts of the world but selection of cases introduces a bias and the figure for the United Kingdom is probably around 1 per cent T_3-toxicosis is reported more commonly with toxic nodular goitre, especially single toxic nodules, in recurrent hyperthyroidism after any form of treatment, and often in the early phase of the disease before both T_4 and T_3 become elevated, but it is not certain that it differs in any way from conventional forms of hyperthyroidism. The syndrome is important as it must be considered in patients with a clinical picture suggestive of hyperthyroidism without elevation of serum T_4. In T_3-toxicosis the thyroidal uptake of ^{131}I is elevated and a TRH test demonstrates the typical hyperthyroid picture of diminished or absent TSH response.

Measurement of plasma total or free T_4 or T_3 is usually all that is needed to diagnose or exclude hyperthyroidism. There is little or no place for a thyroid uptake test except to detect 'silent' thyroiditis (see below), or to exclude the rare condition of struma ovarii or thyrotoxicosis factitia.

In hyperthyroidism the gland is under intense stimulation by a thyroid stimulating immunoglobulin. The resulting high serum concentration of T_4 and T_3 causes suppression of pituitary TSH secretion. In hyperthyroid states of all types, therefore, serum TSH concentration should be low (within the normal range allowing for insensitivity of the assay). Inappropriate elevation of TSH in a case of hyperthyroidism suggests a pituitary tumour or the rare condition of excessive TSH production due to a postulated receptor defect of the pituitary gland.

A TRH test is only of value in the exclusive sense. Other non-hyperthyroid conditions may produce an attenuated response of TSH, e.g. non-toxic nodular goitre. But a clear-cut TSH response after injection of TRH rules out the diagnosis of hyperthyroidism, which is valuable information in some difficult cases.

It is seldom necessary to scan the thyroid gland in hyperthyroidism, but a single toxic nodule may be picked up by this procedure, a finding that might influence choice of treatment.

The treatment of hyperthyroidism. There are three forms of treatment for hyperthyroidism: medical, radioactive iodine, and surgical.

Medical treatment. This includes the use of antithyroid drugs and beta-adrenergic blocking agents. The use of antithyroid drugs is based on the observation that in a proportion of patients with hyperthyroidism, the course is self-limited, allowing suppression of the disease to tide them over until a spontaneous natural remission has occurred. It is customary to give medical treatment for 12 to 18 months and to start with a loading dose of the drug (30–60 mg of carbimazole per day or 300–600 mg of propylthiouracil). This is rapidly reduced as the hyperthyroidism is brought under control; within a week or two the patient may experience symptomatic improvement but an objective clinical response is not usually seen before three to six weeks; slowing of the pulse and weight-gain are the most reliable signs of response. Maintenance doses are usually about 5–15 mg of carbimazole per day and 50–150 mg of propylthiouracil. (In the United Kingdom carbimazole is the most commonly-used antithyroid drug; it is converted in the body to its active metabolite, methimazole. In North America and other parts of the world methimazole is, more logically, the drug of choice.)

The major drawback of medical treatment is the high relapse rate after a full course of treatment, certainly over 50 per cent; this should be considered and explained to the patient before treatment is decided upon. Side-effects of carbimazole and propylthiouracil drugs are similar and include skin rashes, arthralgia, jaundice, lymphadenopathy, nausea, vomiting, and fever; these are often transient and may respond to antihistamines. Sensitivity to one drug may be managed by changing to the other. The only dangerous toxic effect is agranulocytosis, fortunately rare, affecting perhaps 1 in 1000 patients; an early warning feature is often a sore throat, which should always lead to an immediate white blood count and smear. Agranulocytosis, although serious, is always temporary and, if one can tide the patient over, granulocytes reappear in the peripheral blood within a few days of stopping the drug. If side- and toxic effects of the antithyroid drugs are not seen within two months they are unlikely to occur, and these drugs are then extremely safe. This very occasionally justifies their use indefinitely in older patients with hyperthyroidism.

Beta-adrenergic receptor blocking drugs such as propranolol achieve prompt but short-lived control of many of the features of hyperthyroidism. Within 12–48 hours propranolol 40 mg three or four times daily produces a fall in pulse-rate, diminution of tremor, anxiety, restlessness, heat intolerance, and sweating in most thyrotoxics; if a response is not seen within 48 hours the dose may be increased to 80 mg or even 160 mg four times daily. In addition to blocking the peripheral adrenergic features of hyperthyroidism, propranolol partially inhibits the conversion of T_4 to T_3 which may contribute to its clinical effectiveness. It is important to realize that propranolol does not reduce the output of hormone by the thyroid gland nor reduce the circulating pool of T_4 and 40 mg orally is effective for only about six hours; this is of particular importance before or after surgery for hyperthyroidism as omission of a single dose may be followed by the reappearance of severe hyperthyroidism or even crisis.

Beta-adrenergic blocking drugs are most valuable where rapid control of hyperthyroidism is needed. Standard antithyroid drugs do not achieve a response in less than two to three weeks as a rule; propranolol will do so within 12–24 hours. These drugs are therefore of use while awaiting confirmation of the diagnosis as they do not interfere with the usual tests of diagnosis; they may be used during the two to four weeks needed for the standard antithyroid drugs to bring the patient under control, or for the two to three months that ^{131}I takes to achieve the same result. They may occasionally be used in the immediate pre-operative period for patients considered still to be mildly hyperthyroid, if there are good reasons for wishing to proceed rapidly with surgery. In general, despite the practice of several excellent centres, beta-adrenergic blockers are not recommended for routine pre-operative preparation, nor would I recommend them for long-term medical treatment as the degree of control of hyperthyroidism is not usually as satisfactory as with standard antithyroid drugs.

Radioactive iodine. This cures hyperthyroidism by destroying the functioning cells of the thyroid gland. It is not possible to predict with confidence whether a given dose will destroy too much, leading to hypothyroidism, or too little, leaving the patient hyperthyroid. Probably 10–15 per cent of ^{131}I-treated thyrotoxics become hypothyroid within two years, and this figure is added to slowly year by year to reach perhaps 50–60 per cent after 20 years. Failure of response to ^{131}I is seen in about 30 per cent of patients who may then need second, third, or even fourth doses. To some extent the outcome of ^{131}I treatment is dose-related: A very large dose cures more patients but leads to a higher incidence of hypothyroidism; a small dose cures fewer patients but causes less hypothyroidism. Many authorities today select an arbitrary dose of ^{131}I, say, 3–4 mCi for hyperthyroidism with a small goitre, 6–8 mCi for a large gland.

^{131}I takes 6–10 weeks to achieve a clinical response, and cover with an antithyroid drug or propranolol is often required during this time. If the patient has not improved within about four months, a repeat dose may be given.

One can be reassuring about the risks of cancer or leukaemia after ^{131}I therapy; after almost 40 years there is no evidence that either of these conditions is induced by ^{131}I. There remains a theoretical risk of genetic damage which usually limits its use to women beyond the child-bearing age in the United Kingdom.

Surgery. This aims to cure hyperthyroidism by removing the bulk of functioning thyroid tissue. In good hands it offers prompt and effective control with little or no risk of complications. Hypoparathyroidism and damage to the recurrent laryngeal nerves should hardly ever be seen. There is a small recurrence rate after surgery but the incidence of hypothyroidism is substantial (perhaps 30 per cent over a 10-year period).

It is most important that surgery is not carried out until the hyperthyroidism is brought under control. A common schedule would include the use of antithyroid drugs for 4–8 weeks followed by iodine for 7–10 days; most surgeons have personal preferences about dosage and timing. In some units propranolol is used as the sole means of controlling hyperthyroidism before surgery; in less experienced centres thyroid storm, occasionally fatal, has been reported due to omission of one or more doses post-operatively.

The choice of treatment. For a particular patient this is often made on arbitrary grounds. The skill and experience of the available surgeon is a most important factor, and one should take into account the preference and convenience of the patient, including factors such as loss of time from work or separation of a mother from young children. Antithyroid drugs are always worth trying in children and young adults especially if the thyroid gland is not very large and the disease not too severe. They may be valuable in the very old as definitive treatment in preference to surgery or ^{131}I. Surgery is probably best if the gland is large or if there is compression of neighbouring structures. Radioactive iodine is especially valuable where surgery is contra-indicated or for recurrent disease.

Toxic nodular goitre. Hyperthyroidism may be due to autonomous hyperfunction of a single thyroid nodule or of one or more nodules in a multinodular gland. These nodules appear 'hot' on a thyroid scan. It is important to realize that one or more non-toxic nodules may be present in a diffusely overactive gland of Graves's disease.

Toxic multinodular glands produce the same picture of hyperthyroidism as Graves's disease but since they arise in previously enlarged glands of long standing, the patients tend to be older. The clinical presentation may be dominated by cardiovascular or neuromuscular features. In this group eye signs are rare.

The treatment of toxic nodular goitre follows the same lines as for diffuse Graves's disease. Because local compressive features are more commonly found with nodular goitre, there may be a bias towards surgery. On the other hand, patients with nodular glands are often older and more likely to have disorders of cardiac rhythm or function that might argue in favour of long-term medical treatment or ^{131}I.

The single toxic nodule (adenoma) is most simple to treat. Medical treatment is not recommended as recurrence is the rule when it is stopped. After surgery (simple excision) or ^{131}I recurrence is most unlikely and there is little or no danger of post-treatment hypothyroidism. Very large doses of ^{131}I may be given as the isotope is concentrated in the hyperactive nodule, and, after its ablation, function should be restored to the remaining suppressed part of the gland.

Hyperthyroidism due to thyroiditis. Acute or subacute thyroiditis generally presents as a painful enlargement of the thyroid gland, tender to the touch and associated with systemic manifestations such as fever and sweating. It has long been known that patients with this disease could pass through a transient phase of hyperthyroidism. It has recently been suggested that a 'silent' form of thyroiditis might occur, without pain, tenderness or fever, but producing the clinical and biochemical picture of hyperthyroidism. Such patients may be distinguished by a low or absent uptake of radioactive iodine by the thyroid gland (typical of thyroiditis) and a rapid return—within a month or two—to euthyroidism or even hypothyroidism. In some parts of North America this disorder is thought to account for up to 15 per cent of all hyperthyroid subjects. In the United Kingdom it appears to be far less common; in a personal series of 100 successive hyperthyroid patients, elevated thyroidal uptake tests were shown in all. The declining use of thyroid uptake tests will make it harder to diagnose 'silent thyroiditis' as a cause of hyperthyroidism. Other causes of hyperthyroidism with low or absent thyroid uptakes would include iodine-induced thyrotoxicosis, thyrotoxicosis factitia, struma ovarii (ectopic hyperfunctioning thyroid tissue present in an ovarian dermoid tumour).

Hyperthyroidism due to excess secretion of TSH. Very rarely a TSH-producing tumour of the anterior pituitary gland may cause hyperthyroidism. This would normally only be diagnosed by the finding of an inappropriately high circulating TSH concentration. The condition responds to treatment of the primary tumour.

Even more rarely hyperthyroidism has been described with choriocarcinoma, certain embryonal tumours of the testis, or hydatidiform mole. This is thought to result from non-specific responsiveness of thyroidal TSH receptors to high concentrations of chorionic gonadotrophin.

Recently a third type of TSH-induced hyperthyroidism has been described, also due to pituitary hypersecretion but without a demonstrable tumour. This form of disease is postulated to result from an abnormality of T_3 nuclear receptors confined to the anterior pituitary gland which fails to respond to a high concentration of T_3 by suppression of TSH.

Neonatal hyperthyroidism. Thyroid stimulating immunoglobulins, like other immunoglobulins, may pass from the mother to the infant via the placenta (see also page 11.14). If a newborn infant has a high concentration of these stimulators, hyperthyroidism may ensue. These babies show goitre, exophthalmos, feeding problems, fever, and usually develop marked tachycardia with cardiac failure unless treatment is instituted promptly. The condition is serious and demands the immediate use of antithyroid agents and iodine in addition to the usual supportive and anti-cardiac failure treatment. Fortunately the disease is transient, lasting not more than a few months, reflecting the rate of degradation of the acquired maternal immunoglobulin. Although Graves's disease is not too uncommon in pregnancy, neonatal hyperthyroidism is rare. It occurs only when the maternal concentration of circulating thyroid stimulating immunoglobulin is extremely high. Since pretibial myxoedema is a good marker for high concentrations of these thyroid stimulators, pregnant women with this disorder, and their offspring, need very close observation.

Hypothyroidism

The term denotes the slowing down of all body functions that results from a deficiency of circulating thyroid hormones; myxoedema is usually applied to more severe forms of the disease in which deposition of mucinous substances leads to thickening of the skin and subcutaneous tissues.

The causes of hypothyroidism. (Table 3). The syndrome may be secondary to disorders of the hypothalmus or pituitary gland with deficient secretion of TSH, such as craniopharyngiomas, functioning or non-functioning tumours of the pituitary, and infarction of the pituitary gland as seen in post-partum necrosis (Sheehan's syndrome). Hypothyroidism in these cases is usually part of a syndrome of panhypopituitarism with deficiency of other hypophysial hormones, but isolated TSH deficiency is occasionally seen.

Table 3   Causes of hypothyroidism

Secondary to hypothalamic-pituitary disease
   Panhypopituitarism
   Isolated deficiency of TSH

Primary thyroidal
   Agenesis
   Idiopathic atrophy (? auto-immune)
   Impaired synthesis or release of T_4, T_3
      Iodine deficiency
      Antithyroid drugs
      Inherited enzyme defects
   Destruction of gland
      Post-surgery
      Post-irradiation (usually therapeutic ^{131}I)
      Auto-immune disease (Hashimoto's)
      Post-thyroiditis
      Replacement by tumour
   Peripheral resistance to thyroid hormones
   ? Inhibition of T_3 production from T_4
      (Functional hypothyroidism not clearly documented)

Transient hypothyroidism
   Post-pregnancy (in auto-immune subjects)
   Post- ^{131}I-therapy

Primary failure of the thyroid gland may be due to idiopathic agenesis or atrophy. It may result from reduction or inhibition of the synthesis of thyroid hormones, as with dietary iodine deficiency, inherited enzyme defects, or the ingestion or administration of antithyroid drugs or other inhibiting compounds. It may follow widespread destruction of the gland, e.g. after acute or subacute thyroiditis or irradiation, especially with therapeutic ^{131}I; excessive removal by surgery; replacement by non-functioning nodules, cancer, or other disease. But most cases probably arise as an end stage of auto-immune thyroiditis; in many a firm goitre is present which shows the characteristic histological features, and tests for thyroid auto-antibodies are positive. Similar positive tests are found in many

cases of idiopathic atrophy of the gland with hypothyroidism, presumably reflecting more profound destruction of the gland by the autoimmune process.

Transient hypothyroidism, both clinical and biochemical, has been reported in a high proportion of patients who have received ^{131}I treatment for hyperthyroidism, and also after pregnancy in women who show evidence of auto-immune thyroiditis.

The clinical picture of hypothyroidism. This is one of the most insidious of all diseases. The symptoms are often present for years before the diagnosis is made and, because of their non-specific and vague nature, are often attributed to non-organic causes. Even severe myxoedema can be missed by those who fail to appreciate the slow inexorable progress of the disease; minor or more subtle manifestations may cause the patient to present to almost any specialist in any department.

Like hyperthyroidism, this is a disease that predominantly affects women (females to males about 5 to 1). It occurs in a slightly older age group as a rule, peaking in the fifth or sixth decades, but no age is immune and juvenile hypothyroidism is a common and important entity.

Typically the patient has no complaints and the diagnosis is made almost accidentally. Fatigue, lethargy, and physical and mental slowness are common symptoms but patients may present with aches and pains in the muscles and joints, menorrhagia, alopecia, deafness, paraesthesiae, angina pectoris, cardiac failure, constipation, anaemia, or goitre. In other words, almost every organ or tissue of the body may be affected and the presentation is so variable that all clinicians must constantly be alert to the diagnosis (Fig. 9). The gruff voice, puffy eyes, gross features, and slowness of

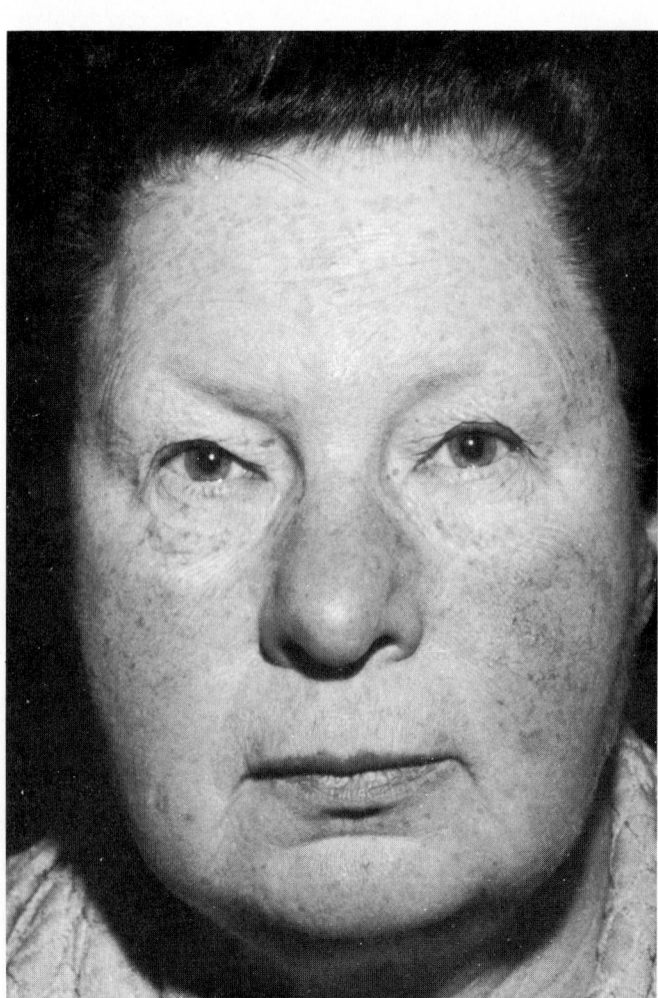

Fig. 9   Typical appearance of patient with hypothyroidism.

expression and movement are often give-away features but signs may be found in all systems.

The skin is characteristically dry and scaly, cold and thickened; a malar flush may be seen against a generally pale facial appearance ('strawberries and cream'); the lips are often thick and tinted mauve; halitosis is common. The hair of the scalp may be coarse and brittle, lack-lustre and balding.

The pulse rate is slowed, often quite markedly; the apex beat may be hard to locate or auscultate often due to the presence of pericardial effusion. An ECG shows low voltage complexes with flattening or inversion of T waves. The blood pressure may be slightly low but is more often normal or even elevated.

Many neurological disturbances are reported in myxoedema: Carpal tunnel syndrome; polyneuritis; cerebellar syndrome with slurred speech and ataxia; muscle cramps and stiffness; myopathy and myotonia. A delay in the relaxation phase of the ankle jerk is characteristic. Bizarre psychiatric features are recognized as 'myxoedema madness'.

Anaemia is common. This may be microcytic and hypochromic due to blood loss from menorrhagia, or macrocytic due to associated B_{12} deficiency from pernicious anaemia. Normocytic, normochromic anaemia is most common and may respond to treatment with thyroxine.

Myxoedema coma. A number of more acute crises requiring emergency treatment may affect the patient with myxoedema, such as cardiac failure or intestinal obstruction. The most important by far is coma, which even today has a mortality of about 50 per cent.

A patient with myxoedema may present for the first time in coma; more commonly the desease progresses insidiously and somnolence and torpor gradually merge into coma. Exposure to cold is an important precipitant, the complication being far more common in winter months especially among old people who live alone in poorly-heated houses. Various drugs (phenothiazines, narcotics, and anaesthetics) as well as infections may precipitate the onset of coma (see also *hypothermia*, pages 6.54 and 26.10).

The pathogenesis of coma is obscure but hypothermia, respiratory acidosis, and hyponatraemia with inappropriate secretion of antidiuretic hormone may all play a part.

In myxoedema coma, bradycardia and bradypnoea may be profound. About 80 per cent of patients are hypothermic with body temperatures as low as 24 °C, requiring special low-reading thermometers and rectal measurement. The body feels cold and dry—cadaveric—and shivering is notably absent. It must be emphasized that not all cases of hypothermia are due to myxoedema, and not all myxoedemics in coma are hypothermic. In a series of 88 hypothermic patients, 70 were thought to be euthyroid, 18 myxoedemic.

Coma may develop within hours in a known case of myxoedema and treatment should never be delayed unnecessarily once the diagnosis has been made. Treatment of established myxoedema coma will be discussed below.

The diagnosis of hypothyroidism. Essentially the diagnosis is clinical and must be kept in mind at all times in view of the protean manifestations of the disease. Confirmation is usually provided by the demonstration of low concentrations of T_4 and T_3 after appropriate correction for the level of binding proteins. The most useful single test is probably estimation of plasma TSH which is elevated in all cases of primary thyroidal myxoedema; in hypopituitarism, of course, plasma TSH will not be high. Other tests of thyroid function, e.g. thyroidal uptake tests, BMR, or serum cholesterol are of little or no value in the diagnosis. A TRH test may be used in a negative way: patients with primary myxoedema demonstrate a prolonged and exaggerated response of TSH to TRH injection; failure of TSH response excludes hypothyroidism unless it is due to pituitary disease.

The treatment of hypothyroidism. Replacement of the deficient thyroid hormones is the basis of treatment. This is most satisfac-

torily achieved by using l-thyroxine sodium 100–200µg per day taken as a single oral dose. The response may be monitored clinically and biochemically; return of an elevated concentration of TSH to normal is probably the best indication of satisfactory response. In the elderly or those with heart disease (angina pectoris, cardiac failure) it is probably wise to start cautiously using 25–50 µg of T_4 daily and increasing the dose by 25 to 50 µg per day every two or three weeks until a full maintenance dose is reached. This schedule is normally well-tolerated but may rarely exacerbate ischaemia or precipitate psychosis; an even more gradual build-up of T_4 dosage is then indicated. Some authorities prefer to use T_3 in these circumstances because of its shorter duration of action.

There is no need to give mixed tablets of T_4 and T_3, as peripheral mono-deiodination of administered T_4 to T_3 occurs in myxoedematous patients. There is no place for T_3 alone in the usual management of myxoedema.

The treatment of myxoedema coma is a medical emergency, the essential part of which is replacement of the body's stores of thyroid hormone. A gradual build-up of the dose is no longer thought necessary and the modern approach would be to give 400–500 µg of T_4 as a bolus intravenous injection. If an intravenous preparation is not available, the same dose may be given by intragastric tube. It is not clear at present whether T_3 has any advantage over T_4. After bolus injection, no further dose of T_4 is needed for about a week as the therapeutic effect is maintained. It is customary also to administer cortisol but the benefits are unproved; intravenous fluids, usually glucose, are given; respiratory acidosis may respond to oxygen administration; tracheostomy and assisted ventilation may be needed. Controversy surrounds the question of rewarming; most authorities would simply expose patients to normal ambient room temperatures without taking special measures. In successful cases, recovery takes place in about 24 hours, and lifelong T_4 therapy will then be needed.

Hypothyroidism in the newborn and during childhood. The diagnosis of neonatal hypothyroidism is now most commonly made on the basis of screening programmes. It is well-recognized that a clinical diagnosis of the disease is difficult and many cases are not diagnosed or treated in time to avoid the permanent consequences of thyroid hormone lack. It is for this reason that universal adoption of screening programmes is advocated.

As a result of the information that has accrued from such programmes and the detailed investigation of cases exposed by their adoption, it is now possible more accurately to define the causes of neonatal hypothyroidism. Agenesis (non-development) of the thyroid gland accounts for between 25–40 per cent of cases. Ectopic thyroid tissue is reported in about 25–40 per cent in the USA, in up to 60 per cent in Europe; it is usually at the base of the tongue, sometimes between this site and the usual location of the thyroid gland. About 30 per cent of cases are associated with goitre, for which the same reasons apply as for adult goitrous hypothyroidism; genetic defects in hormone synthesis probably predominate in this group but the role of availability of iodide needs final assessment. In about 10 per cent of cases the hypothyroidism is transient, perhaps reflecting maternal ingestion of drugs that have passed across the placental barrier or other transmitted abnormalities of maternal thyroid function. Pituitary failure of TSH production accounts for 3–5 per cent of all cases of neonatal hypothyroidism.

The hallmark of neonatal hypothyroidism is retardation of physical and mental development. Early symptoms are non-specific, vague, and difficult to detect; they include feeding problems, torpor, constipation, jaundice, and respiratory distress. The diagnosis may suggest itself within three weeks of life but is not usually made before six weeks, by which time deficiency of thyroid hormones may have produced irreversible damage. The classical objective manifestations of cretinism—large tongue, distended abdomen, umbilical hernia, and dry skin and hair—are not usually found before three of four months of age. Later still, one may find delay in growth, bone maturation, or motor development.

Biochemical tests, especially the finding of high circulating TSH, provide confirmation of the diagnosis, and it is probably no longer necessary to carry out other investigations such as X-rays. Precise delineation of an inborn defect in thyroid hormone synthesis adds nothing to the prognosis or management of a particular case.

Treatment is carried out with oral thyroxine in the standard way. Overtreatment is thought to cause accelerated bone development. It is usually recommended that the dose of T_4 should be adjusted to keep the serum T_4 concentration at the upper end of the normal range.

Hypothyroidism may appear at any stage of childhood or adolescence and is most frequently due to auto-immune chronic thyroiditis. Goitre and hypothyroidism due to an inherited defect of hormone synthesis may also appear at this stage. The clinical picture of juvenile hypothyroidism is not much different from that of adult disease, but may additionally show evidence of delayed skeletal growth and maturation or delayed dental development. The picture of delayed growth and development, including perhaps sexual immaturity, may suggest a diagnosis of hypopituitarism which should be easy to distinguish on biochemical grounds. Sexual precocity and hirsutes are rare manifestations of juvenile hypothyroidism. Treatment at this stage of life is the same as it is for adults.

Neonatal hypothyroidism: screening programmes. Increasing availability of reliable and sensitive radio-immunoassay techniques has led to the widespread introduction of screening programmes to detect neonatal hypothyroidism. In all reports so far about 1 in 3500–4000 infants shows biochemical evidence of hypothyroidism and, since the effects of the disease should be avoidable with prompt administration of T_4, there is justification for the view that all newborn infants should be screened.

The ideal test would be one that identifies all abnormal infants with very few false positive results. Assay of serum TSH from five to seven days after birth has proved more satisfactory than assay of T_4 for this purpose; the rare case of secondary hypothyroidism (due to hypopituitarism) would be missed by this procedure, but the unnecessary recall rate is very low. TSH can be assayed without elution from the same filter paper discs that are used for screening for phenylketonuria. If neonatal hypothyroidism is diagnosed, treatment with T_4 should be instituted promptly. Careful follow-up is needed to ensure adequacy of therapy and to assess the benefits of screening programmes in the long run.

Thyroiditis

Acute thyroiditis. This term should be reserved for an extremely rare form of thyroid disease caused by invasion by micro-organisms; various cocci, yeasts, and anaerobes have been incriminated. The patient presents with pain and tenderness over the thyroid gland, often with systemic features such as fever; signs of an acute abscess of the thyroid gland may be present. Surgical drainage or antibiotics are indicated.

Subacute thyroiditis. Also known as de Quervain's, granulomatous, giant-cell, or acute non-suppurative thyroiditis, this is a disease of unknown aetiology, possibly viral, associated with an acutely tender painful thyroid enlargement with constitutional features (fever, sweating, high ESR). It most commonly affects young women and may start insidiously with features of an upper respiratory infection. Tenderness is usually bilateral but only one lobe may be affected. Painful dysphagia is common.

Symptoms and signs of hyperthyroidism may be present, and the condition is characterized by a low or absent thyroidal uptake of radioactive iodine. A painless form of thyroiditis has recently been recognized that gives rise to transient hyperthyroidism without the high thyroidal uptake of ^{131}I seen in Graves's disease. The reported prevalence of thyroiditis as a cause of hyperthyroidism ranges from less than 1 to 15 per cent and may be dictated by geographical factors. Very rarely the destructive process of subacute thyroiditis may progress leading to permanent hypothyroidism. In the vast majority of cases, the disease is self-limited, settling down within a few months to leave the patient euthyroid.

In some cases the severity of symptoms justifies treatment. Simple analgesia with salicylates may suffice in mild cases. If this is not immediately effective, response to adrenal steroids is generally impressive. Prednisone 10–20 mg three times daily is usually given and may need to be continued for several weeks, or even months in a reduced dosage.

Chronic thyroiditis

Riedel's thyroiditis. This is an extremely rare, sclerosing disease of the thyroid gland, sometimes called ligneous or woody. Dense fibrous tissue involves the gland and extends into the surrounding tissue so that the edges of the gland may be difficult to define on palpation or even at surgery. It is related to and may be associated with other idiopathic fibrosing conditions such as retroperitoneal fibrosis, sclerosing cholangitis, and fibrous mediastinitis.

Lymphocytic (Hashimoto's) thyroiditis. Also called struma lymphomatosa, this is an extremely common and most important condition. Its aetiology is still uncertain but it is associated with the presence in the serum of affected persons of antibodies to thyroglobulin and the microsomal fraction of thyroid homogenates; anti-

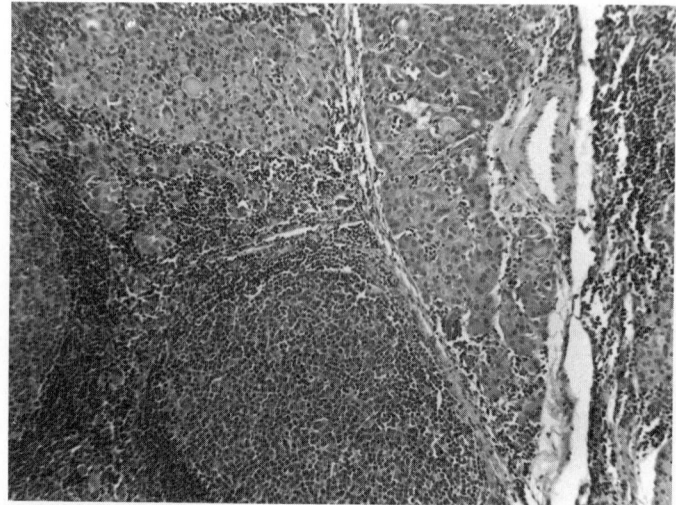

a

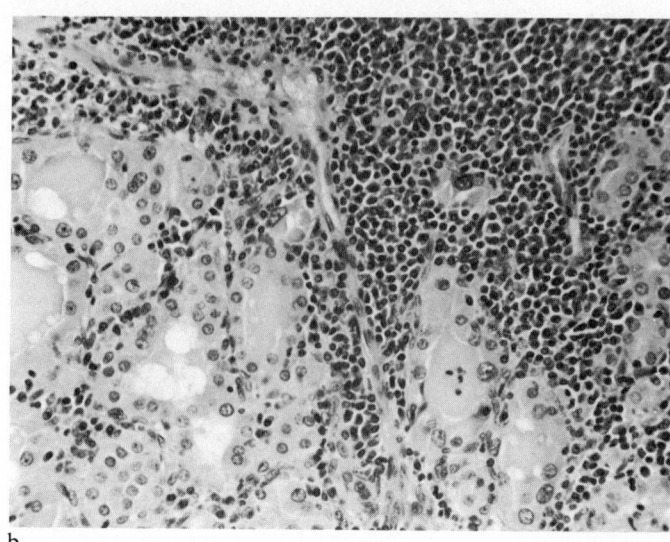

b

Fig. 10 Low (a) and high power (b) views of typical Hashimoto's thyroiditis showing cellular infiltration and lymphoid follicles.

bodies to other thyroidal cytosolic antigens may be demonstrated. It is not clear why similar antibodies are so commonly found in subjects who do not have chronic thyroiditis or, for that matter, any evidence of thyroid disease or dysfunction; it is suggested that suppressor T cells help to prevent manifestations of disease in these individuals.

Lymphocytic thyroiditis is usually regarded as the prototype of autoimmune disease. It is often familial and other autoimmune diseases are commonly present in the patient or the family; other forms of thyroid disease may also be present.

Pathologically, the thyroid gland is usually enlarged with varying degrees of lymphocytic infiltration, cell destruction, and fibrosis (Fig. 10); some cells may show the tall columnar appearance of hyperplasia; extensive atrophy may be present in parts or may affect the whole gland.

Clinically, lymphocytic thyroiditis may present as a case of goitre or hypothyroidism or both. The goitre results from a mixture of cellular and fibrous tissue infiltration and hyperplasia. If the destructive process outweighs the capacity of unaffected parts of the gland to hyperplase, hypothyroidism will ensue; very rarely, this form of thyroiditis may be associated with clinical hyperthyroidism. The goitre in Hashimoto's disease characteristically feels firm and very well-defined; the pyramidal lobe may be enlarged and neighbouring lymph nodes may be palpable.

The diagnosis of Hashimoto's thyroiditis may be suspected clinically because of the nature of the goitre with or without hypothyroidism. Confirmation is provided by the finding of high titres of antibodies against thyroglobulin or complement fixing antibodies against microsomes but neither is specific to this form of thyroiditis.

The gland occasionally feels lumpy or irregular and biopsy may be needed to distinguish it from carcinoma of the thyroid. At surgery incision of a typical Hashimoto's gland feels like cutting through an unripe pear, and the cut surface of the gland may show the same uniformly pale and granular appearance.

As the disease progresses, further destruction of the gland ensues with increased fibrosis; atrophy may follow and clinical hypothyroidism. Treatment consists of oral thyroxine, usually in a dosage of 200 µg per day. This will keep the patient euthyroid and may lead to resolution of a goitre. In a small number of cases thyroid carcinoma or lymphoma may supervene.

References

Devisscher, M. (ed.) (1980). *Thyroid gland*. Raven Press, New York.

Degroot, L. J. and Stanbury, J. B. (1975). *The thyroid and its diseases*. John Wiley, New York.

Fisher, D. A. and Burrow, G. N. (1975). *Perinatal thyroid physiology and disease*. Kroc Foundation Symposia Series vol. 3. Raven Press, New York.

Kidd, A., Okita, N., Row, V. V., and Volpe, R. (1980). Immunologic aspects of Graves's and Hashimoto's diseases. *Metabolism* **29**, 80.

Oppenheimer, J. H. (1979). Thyroid hormone action at the cellular level. *Science* **203**, 971.

Werner, S. C. and Ingbar, S. H. (eds.) (1971). *The thyroid*. Harper and Row, New York.

Disorders of calcium metabolism

J. A. Kanis

Introduction. There has been a rapid growth in our understanding of the biochemistry, metabolism, and actions of the calcium regulating hormones which has clarified the pathophysiology of several disorders and led to the identification of several new syndromes. There are still large gaps in our understanding of hormone action, particularly on the skeleton, and very little is known about the local control of skeletal growth and remodelling.

This contribution reviews the common disorders of plasma calcium homeostasis, but there are inevitably overlaps with disorders of skeletal metabolism since the skeleton is the major reservoir of extracellular calcium. Detailed discussion of disorders of the skeleton are discussed in Section 17. Reference should be made to page 18.83 for details of renal stone disease.

Distribution and function of calcium

Function of calcium. Calcium and phosphate are widely distributed throughout living tissue. The great majority is found in bone, and the ability of the skeleton to turn over calcium and phosphate is essential for growth, the prevention and healing of fractures, and skeletal remodelling in response to physiological and pathological stresses. During skeletal growth and remodelling of bone, there is a bidirectional flux of calcium between bone and the extracellular fluid compartment. The skeleton can also provide substantial amounts of buffers, such as phosphate and carbonate, to the extracellular fluid, for example in acidosis, but at the risk of inducing metabolic bone disease.

The extracellular fluid concentration of calcium is critical to maintain normal neuromuscular activity, and a fall in plasma calcium concentration results in tetany and convulsions. Also a rise in extracellular fluid calcium levels has many adverse effects including delayed neuromuscular conduction and muscle paralysis.

The maintenance of the skeleton and the maintenance of extracellular fluid calcium concentrations are closely related and disorders of the one may induce disorders of the other. This is commonly but not invariably the case. For example, in primary hyperparathyroidism, skeletal disease and disturbed plasma calcium homeostasis, commonly coexist. On the other hand, in Paget's disease, where bone turnover is characteristically increased, plasma calcium is usually normal.

The total amount of calcium within soft tissues is similar to that found in the extracellular fluid (approximately 25 mmol). However, cytosol calcium *concentrations* are thought to be 100 to 1000 times lower than extracellular. Within cells, mitochondria are capable of accumulating large amounts of calcium against electrochemical gradients, to an extent that mitochondrial deposits of insoluble calcium phosphate can form. The activation of many different types of cells by hormones or pharmacological agents is now thought to be accompanied by increases in intracellular calcium concentration, derived from the extracellular fluid or from mitochondria. Hormonal activation, enzyme activity, membrane function, and cell division are all important roles for intracellular calcium. Calcium is also essential for neurotransmitter release as well as for the release of hormones and other secretory products. This is true for every endocrine system that has been thus far studied. Hormonal activation is often associated with the stimulation of an adenylate cyclase specific to the target tissues. Changes in cyclic AMP and intracellular calcium can produce further responses within the cells. The ability of parathyroid hormone (PTH) to stimulate adenylate cyclase in the kidney can be used clinically to distinguish various types of hypoparathyroidism and in the investigation of hypercalcaemia.

Plasma calcium. The concentration of plasma calcium in health is maintained within a very narrow range, varying by less than 5–10 per cent, despite the large movements of calcium across gut, bone, kidney, and cells. Several hormones, including parathyroid hormone and 1,25-dihydroxy vitamin D_3 ($1,25(OH)_2D_3$) appear to regulate the ionized fraction of plasma calcium (approximately 50 per cent of total plasma calcium; Table 1) by modulating calcium fluxes to and from the extracellular fluid. In turn the secretion rates for these hormones are regulated in part by the calcium concentration of the extracellular fluid thereby completing a negative feedback loop.

Changes in plasma calcium are usually due to changes in the total amount of calcium in the extracellular fluid, since there is a passive

Table 1   Distribution of plasma calcium

Ultrafilterable calcium		
Ionized calcium	47%	
Complexed calcium		
Phosphate	1.5%	⎫
Citrate	1.5%	⎬ 53%
HCO₃, etc.	3%	⎭
Protein bound calcium		
To albumin	37%	⎫ 47%
To globulin	10%	⎭
Total plasma calcium (2.12–2.6 mmol/l)	100%	

distribution of ionized calcium throughout the extracellular fluid compartment. Within the plasma compartment, however, approximately half of the calcium is bound to proteins, mainly albumin, and the binding is pH dependent. Major changes in plasma protein concentrations, the presence of abnormal proteins, and large shifts in extracellular hydrogen ion concentration can therefore affect the proportion of total plasma calcium that is bound so that the estimation of total plasma calcium may not accurately reflect the ionized calcium concentration. These changes in protein binding have some important clinical consequences. Thus, the paraesthesiae seen in patients with hyperventilation syndrome are associated with a decreased ionized calcium concentration due to alkalosis, but total plasma calcium is normal. Also, the infusion of alkalis into patients with long-standing metabolic acidosis (e.g. chronic renal failure) may precipitate hypocalcaemic convulsions due to a decrease in ionized calcium, without changing the total plasma calcium.

In the absence of severe acidosis or alkalosis, the major factor influencing total plasma calcium to concentration is the quantity of albumin present, since the proportion of calcium which is bound varies little. Failure to account for protein binding may result in the erroneous diagnosis of hypercalcaemia in conditions where increased levels or abnormal plasma proteins are found, e.g. dehydration, prolonged venostasis, myeloma, and sarcoidosis. Also, in hypoproteinaemic states such as disseminated carcinoma or chronic renal failure, total plasma calcium may be low, though ionized calcium is normal. Similarly, in such disorders total plasma calcium may be normal and mask true hypercalcaemia.

Since the ionized plasma calcium is the physiologically relevant fraction, it is this fraction which should be measured, but the available methods are often unreliable and not widely available. Many formulae have been proposed for predicting the ionized calcium from the total plasma calcium, or 'correcting' the total plasma calcium to a normal protein value. These methods depend on the concurrent measurement of total proteins, albumin, or specific gravity of plasma. None are entirely satisfactory but a simple correction factor for plasma calcium which is widely used is to subtract from the total plasma calcium 0.02 mmol per litre for every 1 gram per litre that the plasma albumin exceeds 40 g/l, provided the sample is withdrawn without venostasis. A similar addition is made when the plasma albumin is less than 40 g/l. Many laboratories now report 'corrected' plasma calcium or 'ionized' plasma calcium, but it should be realized that these are at best a guide as to the true ionized calcium concentration.

A small proportion of total plasma calcium is complexed with cations such as phosphate, citrate, and bicarbonate (see Table 1). The calcium which is normally filtered by the kidney includes this complexed calcium as well as ionized calcium. In several disorders the proportion of ultrafilterable calcium which is complexed is increased (i.e. disorders of acid–base, phosphate and citrate metabolism).

Distribution of calcium and phosphate. Most of the total body calcium and phosphate resides in bone (99 and 88 per cent respectively). The concentration of calcium is low in most soft tissues, but 12–15 per cent of phosphorus lies outside the skeleton as organic phosphate compounds such as nucleic acids, nucleotides, phospholipids,

and phosphorylated metabolites. Extracellular concentrations, and probably intracellular concentrations of phosphate vary much more than levels of calcium, particularly in response to circadian rhythms, growth, and meals. The measurement of plasma phosphate is a valuable adjunct in the diagnosis of disturbances of plasma calcium homeostasis but it is important to recognize that high levels occur after food and that plasma phosphate in childhood is commonly higher than in adults.

Principles of regulation of plasma calcium. The total amount of calcium in the extracellular fluid, and hence its concentration, is dependent upon movements of calcium to and from the extracellular fluid. The major fluxes occur across the gut, bone, and kidney. The relative sizes of these fluxes determine their potential in plasma calcium homeostasis (Fig. 1).

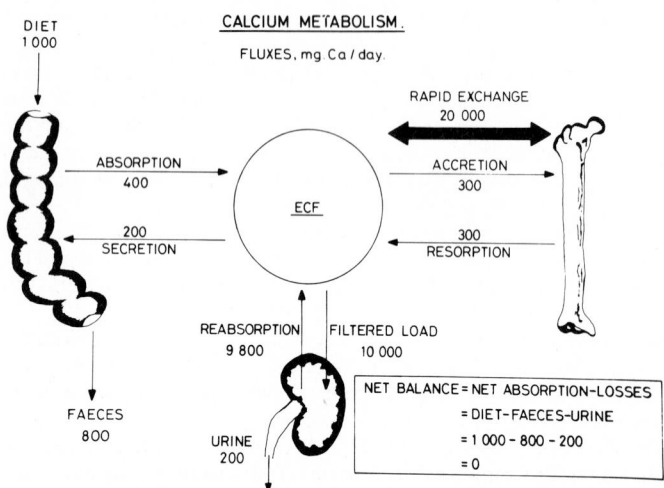

Fig. 1   Major fluxes of calcium (mg/day) in a healthy adult. Exchange of calcium in the extracellular fluid occurs with bone, gut, and kidney. The net balance for calcium equals the net absorption minus the losses of calcium in faeces and urine, which in a healthy adult is zero. The major fluxes of calcium are regulated by the regulating hormones. PTH increases renal tubular reabsorption of calcium and bone resorption, calcitonin inhibits bone resorption, and vitamin D augments intestinal absorption of calcium. The precise role of vitamin D in augmenting bone resorption and mineralization *in vivo* is unclear.

There is a significant exchange of calcium between extracellular fluid and bone. Studies with radioisotopes in normal human adults show that between 1 and 2 per cent of total body calcium is exchanged over a few days. This represents 1000 or 2000 mmol, which is a substantial amount considering that the extracellular fluid contains somewhat less than 20 mmol as ionized calcium. This exchangeable pool may therefore be very important in plasma calcium homeostasis, although the extent to which the large movements of calcium between body fluids, cells, and surfaces of bone are subject to metabolic regulation is controversial.

These large and rapid fluxes should be distinguished from the movements of calcium which occur in bone as a result of mineralization and bone resorption. Bone resorption is defined as the complete removal of bone mineral and matrix which occurs during physiological remodelling and is a result of osteoclast activity. This accounts for only a fraction of the total calcium exchange between bone and extracellular fluid, the remainder occurring across the large surface area of osteocytes and their canaliculi without synthesis or destruction of bone matrix. Between 1 and 4 per cent of the adult skeleton is thought to be renewed each year, although this is not uniformly distributed throughout the skeleton, since trabecular bone has a faster turnover than cortical bone. This means that disturbances of bone turnover commonly have greater and more dramatic effects at trabecular than cortical sites.

The body is not a closed system with respect to calcium, in the sense that calcium is lost by urinary and intestinal excretion and to a lesser extent in sweat, and enters by intestinal absorption and renal tubular reabsorption of glomerular filtrate. The true intestinal absorption of calcium is greater that the net absorption because some calcium is returned to the gut lumen in biliary, pancreatic, and intestinal secretion. Thus, from an average daily dietary intake of 25 mmol, approximately 10 mmol is absorbed. This is offset by intestinal secretion amounting to approximately 5 mmol daily, leaving a net transport into the extracellular fluid pool of 5 mmol. Apparent and real fluxes across the gut can be measured by tracer and balance studies, some of which are used in specialized clinical practice.

The kidney is a major site for calcium excretion. A large amount is filtered (see Fig. 1), but most is reabsorbed leaving only 5 mmol for urinary excretion. Several hormones, particularly parathyroid hormone alter renal tubular reabsorption and, since the fluxes to and from the extracellular fluid compartment are large, this means that small changes in tubular reabsorption have profound effects on the extracellular fluid concentrations. This has led to the view that the kidney is a major site for plasma calcium regulation. Calcium is also lost from the body in sweat, but these losses are usually small. However, losses may be as high as 8 mmol daily under extreme conditions where sweat production is increased, e.g. fever and in tropical climates.

In mature adults who are neither gaining nor losing calcium, bone and soft tissue contribute neither a net gain nor loss of calcium to the extracellular fluid; the amount of bone resorbed exactly matches the amount formed. Also, the total amount of calcium absorbed by the gut matches the urinary excretion. Because plasma and intracellular calcium levels are controlled within a narrow range, changes in bone mass are reflected as changes in the external balance for calcium. For example, during growth where there is a net daily gain of calcium which is incorporated into the skeleton, plasma and intracellular concentrations of calcium are normal. In the long term, therefore, the total body balance of calcium reflects exactly the skeletal balance for calcium (in this case positive calcium balance). Mineral losses begin at middle age (negative balance). Between the age of 25 and 45 the body should be neither gaining nor losing calcium so that inflow and outflow of calcium are matched.

The transport of calcium between the extracellular fluid and bone, gut, and kidney is continually changing and is regulated by a variety of factors including several hormones (see Fig. 1). These can be subdivided into 'controlling hormones' and 'influencing hormones'. The controlling group are the major regulating hormones of plasma calcium which include PTH, calcitonin, and vitamin D metabolites, the secretion of each of which is altered in response to changes in ionized calcium levels. The influencing group are those other hormones such as thyroid hormone, growth hormone, adrenal and gonadal steroids which have effects on calcium metabolism, but whose secretion is determined primarily by factors other than changes in plasma calcium.

Major regulating hormones

Parathyroid hormone (PTH). In the circulation PTH consists of several polypeptide fragments which are degraded in the liver, kidney, and skeleton. The major stimulus to the secretion of PTH is a fall in the ionized fraction of plasma calcium. The biological actions of PTH at a variety of target organs serve to increase plasma calcium and thus there exists an efficient negative feedback hormonal loop.

In man there are usually four parathyroid glands, two embedded in the superior poles of the thyroid and two in the inferior poles. There is considerable individual variation both in the site and the number of parathyroid glands. Parathyroid tissue is occasionally found in the mediastinum. Each gland, approximately the size of a match head, comprises chief cells, with clear cytoplasm, and larger oxyphil cells.

PTH is released as a single peptide chain containing 84 amino acids (molecular weight 5500). In common with several other peptide hormones, PTH is synthesized as a prohormone which contains an additional six amino acids on its amino-terminal end. A further precursor form, pre-pro-PTH containing a total of 150 amino acids has been identified in studies *in vitro*. The site of synthesis of the precursor hormone is the rough endoplasmic reticulum of the chief cells. The function of the oxyphil cells is unknown. The precursor forms of PTH are probably converted to the 84 amino acid polypeptide before secretion from the gland in secretory granules.

Only the first 32–34 amino acids, reading from the amino-terminal end, are necessary for biological activity. There is evidence that cleavage occurs naturally, partly in the liver, to produce a short amino-terminal fragment with biological activity and a larger inactive carboxy-terminal fragment. This cleavage may be necessary for PTH to act on bone. There are also many less well characterized circulating fragments of PTH. The liver and kidney are important sites for degradation. For example, the C-terminal fragment normally cleared by the kidney may be increased in chronic renal failure, although the circulating levels of biologically active PTH may be normal. This causes some problems in the interpretation of radioimmunoassay results, particularly in patients with renal impairment since the C-terminal fragment is the major component measured in many assay systems. Sensitive biological assays for PTH have been developed but are not yet available in clinical practice.

Secretion of PTH. The major physiological stimulus to the secretion of PTH is a fall in the plasma ionized calcium concentration. A rise suppresses PTH secretion. Many other factors are known to influence PTH secretion including beta-adrenergic agonists, vitamin D metabolites, growth hormone and somatostatin, vitamin A, prostaglandins, prolactin, and other divalent cations such as magnesium and strontium. With the exception of magnesium, the physiological or clinical relevance of these factors is uncertain. In the presence of very low levels of magnesium, the release of PTH from parathyroid tissue is impaired, and this, together with an impaired target organ response to PTH probably accounts for the hypocalcaemia occasionally observed in magnesium deficiency.

Actions of PTH. The target actions of PTH include effects on bone, kidney, and indirectly on the gut. PTH acts on the proximal and distal tubules of the kidney to increase the renal tubular reabsorption of calcium and to depress the tubular reabsorption of phosphate. This leads to a rise in plasma calcium and fall in plasma phosphate. Inhibition of proximal tubular reabsorption of phosphate appears to be mediated by cyclic AMP as a result of activation of adenylate cyclase in the renal cortex. PTH also decreases the proximal renal tubular reabsorption of bicarbonate which leads to increased excretion of bicarbonate ions and to a hyperchloraemic acidosis. A mild metabolic acidosis is commonly seen in primary and secondary hyperparathyroidism whereas in hypoparathyroidism a metabolic alkalosis is observed. Alkalosis may also occur when the secretion of PTH is suppressed, for example by hypercalcaemia due to malignant disease affecting the skeleton. In this example the alkalosis is also partly due to the release of buffer from bone. It is possible that the acidosis induced by PTH augments the resorption of bone.

PTH has a further important effect on the kidney to stimulate the 1α-hydroxylase enzyme responsible for the production of 1,25-dihydroxyvitamin D_3 $(1,25(OH)_2 D_3)$ from 25-OHD$_3$. This potent metabolite of vitamin D increases calcium absorption from the gut and possibly releases calcium from bone. Thus, the various effects PTH on the kidney appear either directly or indirectly to increase the extracellular fluid concentration of calcium. Other actions of PTH on the kidney include decreased proximal tubular reabsorption of sodium and increased amino-acid excretion.

The major effect of PTH on bone is to increase bone resorption, by increasing the activity and numbers of osteoclasts. This is associated with activation of cyclic AMP. Both primary and secondary hyperparathyroidism can be associated with obvious radiographic and histological evidence of increased bone resorption. There is increasing evidence, however, that PTH also increases bone formation. In kinetic studies, the rate of mineral accretion often matches the rate of bone resorption in primary hyperparathyroidism, suggesting that a major effect of PTH on the skeleton is to increase bone turnover.

There is controversy as to whether PTH (and indeed calcitonin) can affect the rapid exchange of calcium that occurs between the extracellular fluid and bone and soft tissue. This rapid transfer may be very important in the minute to minute maintenance of plasma calcium if subject to control, though it is difficult to envisage its importance in long-term regulation, since the net unidirectional flux of calcium must be close to zero.

Calcitonin (CT). Calcitonin is a peptide hormone containing 32 amino acid residues with a disulphide bond between cystine residues in positions 1 and 7. The major stimulus to its secretion is an increase in the plasma level of calcium. Many of its actions serve to lower plasma calcium.

Calcitonin is produced from the parafollicular (C cells) of the thyroid in man, but is related embryologically to the ultimobranchial body of lower vertebrate species. The entire amino-acid sequence is essential for biological activity. There are several differences in amino-acid composition of the calcitonins from different species and this is associated with different potencies. Surprisingly, the salmon hormone resembles the human more than other mammalian calcitonins and it is interesting that it is more potent in man than the human hormone. The site of calcitonin secretion is not exclusively in thyroid tissue. C cells are derived embryologically from the APUD cell series of the neural crest. Extrathyroidal sites for calcitonin production have been demonstrated in the thymus and adrenal, and recently it has been suggested that calcitonin-like material is synthesized in the pars intermedia of the pituitary gland.

Many agents are known to affect the secretion of calcitonin in addition to calcium. These include gastrointestinal hormones such as glucagon, gastrin, beta-adrenergic agents, and whisky. Since an obvious action of calcitonin is to inhibit osteoclast numbers and activity and thereby lower plasma calcium, it is widely believed that calcitonin is a calcium-regulating hormone with a negative feedback loop provided by plasma calcium. Thus, calcitonin can be seen to have actions opposite to those of parathyroid hormone with respect to the maintenance of plasma calcium.

The physiological role for calcitonin is, however, unclear. In addition to inhibiting bone resorption it decreases renal tubular reabsorption of calcium, sodium, phosphate, magnesium, potassium, and some other ions. Calcitonin also inhibits the secretion of several gastrointestinal hormones including gastrin, cholecystokinin, insulin, and glucagon. Whether or not these multiple effects are physiological or pharmacological is still uncertain. One difficulty of ascribing any physiological role to calcitonin is that calcitonin deficiency (total thyroidectomy) or excess (medullary carcinoma of the thyroid) are associated with only minor disturbances in skeletal or calcium homeostasis.

A further difficulty in assessing the role of calcitonin arises from conflicting radioimmunoassay data. As in the case of PTH, calcitonin circulates in heterogeneous forms and many of the fragments measured do not have biological activity. The assay for calcitonin is important in the diagnosis of medullary carcinoma of the thyroid, and for the detection of family members with the disease in a presymptomatic form. Interest has recently been shown in the use of calcitonin as a tumour marker since a variety of non-thyroidal cancers appear to be associated with raised plasma levels of calcitonin. Once again, there are considerable qualitative difference in results between centres, so that its value for this purpose is unclear.

The major clinical interest in calcitonin is its use as an inhibitor of bone resorption and turnover for the treatment of Paget's disease and of hypercalcaemia associated with increased bone resorption.

Vitamin D. Man derives his vitamin D_3 (cholecalciferol) from the diet and from the skin by ultraviolet irradiation of 7-dehydrocholesterol. Vitamin D_2 (calciferol) is a product originally derived from the ultraviolet irradation of plant sterols and is used to supplement the diet, particularly in margarine. In most respects these vitamin Ds are comparable in their metabolism and their actions.

Following the photochemical conversion of 7-dehydrocholesterol to vitamin D, it is transported in plasma bound to a specific alpha-globulin (vitamin D-binding protein). Vitamin D is fat soluble and absorbed primarily from the duodenum and jejunum into the lymphatic circulation. A large amount of the vitamin may be stored in adipose and muscle tissues.

Before exerting biological effects, vitamin D undergoes a series of further metabolic conversions (Fig. 2). The first step involves its conversion in liver to a 25-hydroxylated derivative. The 25-OHD so formed is the major circulating vitamin D metabolite and is commonly measured to provide an index of vitamin D nutrition. There are marked seasonal variations in plasma 25-OHD levels with a peak in late summer and a trough in late winter reflecting exposure to ultraviolet irradiation. In northern Europe, plasma levels in winter commonly approach those associated with vitamin D-deficiency states suggesting that both sunlight and dietary intake may be of crucial importance in maintaining vitamin D nutrition. A proportion of the 25-OHD formed is secreted into the intestinal lumen, some of which is probably available for reabsorption. The physiological importance of this enterohepatic circulation is not known but it could be responsible for loss of vitamin D in malabsorption syndromes and liver disease. Plasma levels of 25-hydroxy vitamin D less than 5 ng/ml (12.5 nmol/l) occur in vitamin D-deficiency.

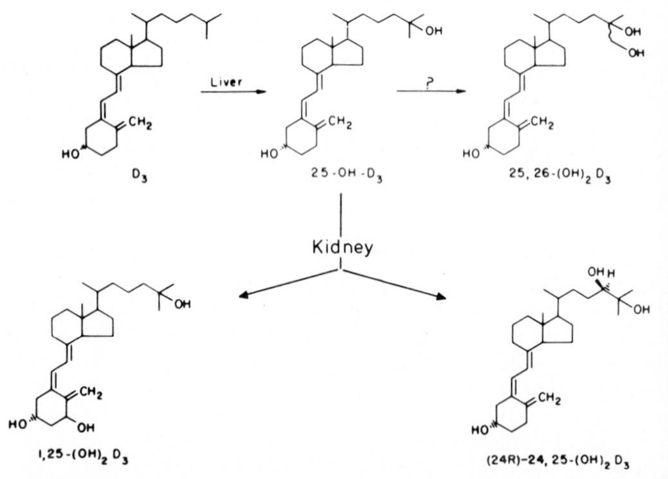

Fig. 2 Steps in the metabolism of vitamin D. The site of synthesis of 25-hydroxy-vitamin D_3 is in the liver. The active form of vitamin D [$1,25(OH)_2D_3$] is made in the kidney and placenta. $24,25(OH)_2D_3$ is synthesized in several tissues, but the kidney is probably the major site. The site of synthesis and function of $25,26(OH)_2D_3$ is unknown.

The next step in the metabolism of vitamin D is its further hydroxylation, mainly in the kidney to 1,25-dihydroxy-vitamin D_3, $24,25(OH)_2D_3$ or $25,26(OH)_2D_3$. Apart from the placenta and decidua, the kidney is the sole site for 1α-hydroxylation, a factor which is of considerable importance in the pathogenesis of vitamin D resistance in renal failure. The renal metabolism of $1,25(OH)_2D_3$ is closely regulated, and its production is favoured under conditions of vitamin D, calcium, or phosphate deficiency. Production of $1,25(OH)_2D_3$ is also augmented by a variety of hormones including PTH, oestradiol, prolactin, and growth hormone, but it is unclear whether or not all these are direct effects.

The kidney is a major site for production of $24,25(OH)_2D_3$. In many experimental systems its production is favoured under conditions which inhibit synthesis of $1,25(OH)_2D_3$ such that a reciprocal relationship is commonly observed between their respective production rates. Thus, under conditions of vitamin D, calcium, or phosphate repletion, it is the major circulating dihydroxy-metabolite. A variety of observations suggest that this metabolite once considered a 'waste' product, may prove to have a physiological role in cartilage, bone, or parathyroid homeostasis. Several other vitamin D metabolites have been isolated from plasma and identified, such as 25,26-dihydroxycholecalciferol. Some of these metabolites appear to have some biological activity but their tissue of origin and metabolic function is unclear.

$1,25(OH)_2D_3$ has a biological half-life measured in hours and a normal plasma concentration of approximately 30 pg/ml in adults. Higher concentrations are observed in growing children and during late pregnancy and lactation. Plasma levels of 25-OHD_3 and $24,25(OH)_2D_3$ are 1000-fold and 100-fold greater than those of $1,25(OH)_2D_3$ and both metabolites have a long biological half-life in the circulation, perhaps related to their greater affinity for the vitamin D-binding protein. Despite these differences in plasma levels, $1,25(OH)_2D_3$ is considered the active form of vitamin D because it is so much more potent than other derivatives in exerting actions on the target organs.

Actions of vitamin D. The principal effects of $1,25(OH)_2D_3$ are to increase intestinal absorption of calcium and phosphate and to increase resorption of bone mineral and matrix. Although lack of vitamin D in man is associated with defective mineralization of cartilage and bone, the question whether or not vitamin D and its metabolites directly increase mineralization of bone is unsettled. There is also surprisingly little evidence that *physiological* amounts of $1,25(OH)_2D_3$ or of any other vitamin D metabolite increase bone resorption although increased resorption is well documented in vitamin D toxicity. From a teleological viewpoint, the action of $1,25(OH)_2D_3$ can be thought of as a mechanism for increasing the availability of calcium and phosphate for mineralization. Alternatively, its function may be to maintain plasma levels of calcium and phosphate in concert with PTH. $1,25(OH)_2D_3$ can be considered to be a hormone in the sense that its secretion from endocrine tissue (the kidney) is controlled by the calcium and phosphate status of the individual, and that its action reverses the stimulus to its secretion.

Receptors for $1,25(OH)_2D_3$ have been found in many other tissues apart from bone and gut. These include skin, breast, salivary, and parathyroid tissue. Their physiological significance is unclear but in the case of parathyroid tissue there is some evidence that $1,25(OH)_2D_3$ and probably some of the other metabolites of vitamin D may also influence parathyroid hormone secretion.

A striking weakness of skeletal muscles, particularly of the pelvic and shoulder girdles are well described features of vitamin D-deficiency. Moreover, myopathy improves rapidly following treatment with vitamin D or one of its metabolites. The mechanisms whereby vitamin D produces an effect on muscle function is unknown but it may involve calcium transfer across the sarcoplasmic reticulum or modifications in the metabolism of troponin C. It is notable that severe phosphate deficiency induced by dietary deprivation or by hyperparathyroidism is associated with muscle weakness, suggesting that the effects of vitamin D deficiency could be due to hypophosphataemia. However, in the inherited tubular disorder, hypophosphataemic osteomalacia, muscle weakness is characteristically absent even though profound hypophosphataemia is found. There are several other poorly understood trophic effects of vitamin D, particularly on growth, the maintenance of intestinal mucosa, and on the maturation of collagen and cartilage.

Other hormones. The hormones PTH, calcitonin, and $1,25(OH)_2D_3$ are all detectable under physiological conditions, and their secretion might be expected to exert continuous influences on bone. But, since they are regulated by changes in plasma levels of calcium or phosphate, the physiological role of these hormones seems less important for skeletal homeostasis itself than for plasma

calcium homeostasis. Other factors must maintain the integrity of the skeleton in health and under various conditions of stress. Many of these factors are reviewed in Section 17 but a summary of their effects are important in the consideration of plasma calcium homeostasis, since disorders of their metabolism commonly induce changes in plasma calcium.

Growth hormone. Growth hormone is best known for its effects on the growth of cartilage, which is probably brought about indirectly by growth hormone-dependent production of somatomedins. There may be several somatomedins not all of which are dependent on growth hormone. Growth hormone also causes a rise of plasma phosphate by increasing its renal tubular reabsorption. Growth hormone excess or deficiency is associated with obvious abnormalities in skeletal growth. In acromegaly there is increased periosteal apposition of bone, but there is no convincing evidence for the widely expressed view that acromegaly causes osteoporosis. Changes in growth hormone secretion have very little effect on plasma calcium and the occasional finding of hypercalcaemia in acrogmegalic patients should alert one to the possibility of coexistent primary hyperparathyroidism (pluriglandular syndrome).

Thyroid hormones. Deficiency of thyroid hormones early in life produce the well-known skeletal abnormalities of cretinism. Before skeletal maturity, thyrotoxicosis may increase skeletal growth. In the adult, thyrotoxicosis is associated with hypercalciuria, hypophosphataemia, augmented bone turnover, and occasionally hypercalcaemia, probably due to direct effects of thyroid hormones on bone.

Adrenal steroids. The most important effect of glucocorticoids on the skeleton is to regulate growth. Their action on calcium metabolism is complex and probably involves effects on many target tissues in addition to effects on the metabolism and action of other hormones including $1,25(OH)_2D_3$. In the adult, adrenal insufficiency is not associated with skeletal abnormalities but is occasionally accompanied by hypercalcaemia. This is probably due to haemoconcentration and to increased renal tubular reabsorption of calcium because of volume depletion. Chronic glucocorticoid excess can induce osteoporosis, but the mechanisms are far from clear. The ability of corticosteroids to decrease plasma calcium in hypercalcaemia other than that due to primary hyperparathyroidism has been used for many years as a diagnostic aid (see page 10.51), but once again the mechanism of action is uncertain. One effect of corticosteroids is to suppress the secretion of osteoclast activating factors and prostaglandins, both of which may have direct effects on bone to increase bone resorption.

Sex steroids. Characteristic growth abnormalities are associated with deficiencies of either male or female sex hormones which appear to play a crucial role in epiphyseal closure and in the growth spurts seen before this event. They may also influence the amount of calcium present in the skeleton at the time of maturity. In adults, the effects of oestrogens are of particular interest because of the loss of bone that occurs in women after the menopause (see Section 17). Administration of exogenous oestrogen may slow down this loss. Oestrogen administration also lowers plasma calcium slightly, an effect more noticeable in post-menopausal women with hyperparathyroidism or hypercalcaemia from carcinoma of the breast. Hypercalcaemia is also occasionally seen with the use of tamoxiphen, an oestrogen inhibitor, when used in carcinoma of the breast. This probably reflects the effects of oestrogen on tumour growth, and it is notable that normal breast as well as malignant breast tissues do have receptors for $1,25(OH)_2D_3$.

Gastrointestinal hormones. There are many interactions between calcium regulating and gastrointestinal hormones. The relationships between gastrin and calcitonin secretion have been described earlier. Calcium and parathyroid hormone also influence gastrin levels which are increased in hyperparathyroidism, due to the stimulation of gastrin secretion by calcium. Large doses of glucagon may induce hypocalcaemia by inhibiting bone resorption, either directly or by stimulating the secretion of calcitonin. Secretin may cause hypercalcaemia perhaps by stimulating parathyroid hormone release. Insulin is important for skeletal growth and diabetics often have diminished skeletal mass; it is one of the few hormones shown to stimulate bone collagen synthesis.

Osteoclast activating factor. Osteoclast activating factor (OAF) is a potent bone resorbing substance derived from mononuclear leucocytes. The factor has not been fully identified chemically, but unlike PTH it is inhibited by corticosteroids. The physiological importance of OAF is unknown but its production is increased in haematological neoplasia and may be responsible for the hypercalcaemia and bone loss seen in myeloma, which is characteristically sensitive to treatment with corticosteroids.

Sites of calcium regulation

With the exception of the pregnant or lactating female, the major fluxes of calcium to and from the extracellular fluid occur across the intestinal mucosa, bone, and kidney. The following pages describe the extent to which these fluxes are controlled by hormonal agents and the influence they have on plasma calcium.

Intestine. Unlike the fluxes of calcium between the extracellular fluid, bone, and kidney, intestinal absorption of calcium is episodic and is dependent on an adequate supply of calcium delivered in an available form to the intestinal mucosa. The availability of calcium for absorption depends on many dietary factors. For example, the presence of excess phosphorus, lipids, and phytates bind calcium and render it unavailable for absorption. The influx of calcium depends both on active transport and diffusion processes. Absorption occurs throughout the length of the small intestine and to a lesser extent in the colon. The major site for active transport is the duodenum and upper part of the jejunum. However, because the duodenum is relatively short compared to the entire length of the gastrointestinal tract, more calcium is probably absorbed at the sites distal to the duodenum at normal dietary intakes than within the duodenum itself.

At very low intakes of calcium, net absorption may be negative since endogenous faecal calcium secretion may exceed the amount absorbed. In malabsorption syndromes the endogenous faecal calcium may appear to rise, but this does not necessarily mean that calcium secreted in the digestive juices is increased, since the rise is probably due to malabsorption of this digestive juice calcium.

Man is able to adapt to variations in dietary intake of calcium so that net absorption remains relatively constant over a fairly wide range of intake, possibly regulated by $1,25(OH)_2D_3$. The biochemical mechanisms involved in active calcium transport have been partially identified. $1,25(OH)_2D_3$ stimulates the synthesis of a calcium binding protein in addition to an intestinal alkaline phosphatase, by a mechanism similar to that described for many other steroid hormones. This involves the translocation of this vitamin D metabolite plus its receptor protein to the nucleus to stimulate the synthesis of messenger RNA and new protein.

There is good evidence that calcium and phosphate can be absorbed separately from each other, though $1,25(OH)_2D_3$ has independent effects to enhance the absorption of each. Unlike the absorption of calcium which appears to be closely regulated, the proportion of the dietary phosphate absorbed does not decrease with increasing intake but remains relatively constant at approximately 80 per cent of the dietary intake over a wide range. This explains in part the fluctuations in plasma phosphate that can occur following a meal and underlines the need for studying phosphate metabolism under controlled conditions.

A variety of tests are available to study calcium and phosphate absorption, including metabolic balance and the use of tracer techniques. These are generally available only to a few centres. A 24-hour urine collection for calcium or phosphate provides an indirect index of absorption provided it is assumed or known that the net flux of calcium across bone is zero. The expression of excretion as a ratio of creatinine excretion standardizes somewhat for variations in body weight and for incomplete urine collections.

Increased intestinal absorption of calcium is found in pregnancy,

during lactation, and in several disease states including hyperparathyroidism, sarcoidosis, and idiopathic hypercalciuria; it is thought to be due to increased production of $1,25(OH)_2D_3$. Conversely, malabsorption of calcium is often associated with low levels of $1,25(OH)_2D_3$, for example in hypoparathyroidism, vitamin D-deficiency states, and in chronic renal failure. Calcium malabsorption is also seen in untreated coeliac disease where a target tissue for $1,25(OH)_2D_3$ has been destroyed.

Kidney. The fluxes of calcium across the kidney are much greater than those of the gut. Renal tubular reabsorption of calcium in the kidney is a complex process involving several mechanisms in various parts of the nephron. The total amount of calcium reabsorbed can be estimated by subtracting the amount of calcium excreted by the kidneys from the filtered load. The filterable calcium is approximately 60 per cent of total plasma calcium, and the filtered load represents the product of the glomerular filtration rate and the filterable calcium (approximately 200–250 mmol/day).

In health there is a curvilinear relationship between plasma calcium (an index of filtered load) and renal excretion. The renal excretion may be expressed per unit of GFR to take account of variations in glomerular filtration rate (Fig. 3). Any value below the

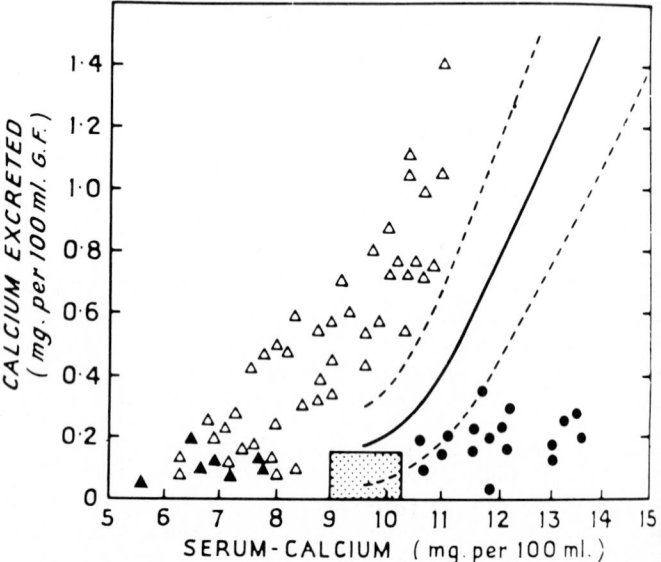

Fig. 3   Relationship between urinary calcium excretion (expressed as milligrams per 100 ml of glomerular filtrate) and serum calcium in health and disorders of parathyroid function. The solid and dashed lines denote the mean values (± 2SD) obtained in normal subjects during calcium infusions. The shaded area represents the normal basal range. Patients with primary hyperparathyroidism (●) lie to the right of the line describing normal subjects, indicating increased renal tubular reabsorption of calcium. In contrast, patients with hypoparathyroidism (▲ untreated; △ during calcium infusion) lie to the left of the normal line indicating decreased renal tubular reabsorption of calcium. Note that the determination of calcium excretion alone (without concurrent measurement of serum calcium) does not give information concerning renal tubular reabsorption of calcium. Note also that hypoparathyroid patients, not infused with calcium, and many hyperparathyroid patients have calcium excretion values which are normal. (From Nordin, B. E. C. and Peacock, M., 1969. *Lancet* ii, 1280).

line depicting the normal relationship would indicate an increase in the net tubular reabsorption of calcium, and values above the lines denote decreased tubular reabsorption. A high value for renal calcium excretion indicates an increase in the filtered load (gut or bone derived) or a low glomerular filtration rate. When calcium excretion is measured in the fasting state, this will reflect more closely calcium derived from skeletal sources. An important corollary is that the estimation of urinary calcium excretion does not give information concerning renal tubular reabsorption unless the filtered load is also known. Some normal ranges for these values are shown in Table 2.

The assessment of renal tubular reabsorption in this way has several limitations in clinical practice since ultrafilterable calcium is rarely measured, and its derivation from total plasma calcium may be difficult in the presence of disorders of acid–base metabolism, dysproteinaemia, or renal damage.

Table 2 Typical normal adult ranges for some simple biochemical measurements used in the investigation of patients with disorders of calcium homeostasis (M or F denotes sex)

Measurement	Units	Normal range	
Plasma			
Total calcium	mmol/l	2.12–2.60	
Ionized calcium	mmol/l	1.10–1.35	
Fasting inorganic phosphate	mmol/l	0.6 –1.5	
Urine			
Calcium	mmol/24h	2.5–10	(M)
	mmol/24h	2.5–9.0	(F)
Phosphate	mmol/24h	16–32	
Total hydroxyproline	μmol/24h	55–250	(M)
	μmol/24h	75–430	(F)
Fasting urine			
Calcium/creatinine ratio	mmol/mmol	0.10–0.32	
Calcium excretion	mmol/1 GF	<0.04	
TmP/GFR	mmol/l	0.8–1.35	
Total hydroxyproline/creatinine	μmol/mmol	<40	

In health approximately 97 per cent of the calcium filtered by the kidney is reabsorbed. Many hormones influence renal tubular reabsorption of which PTH is probably the most important. In mild primary hyperparathyroidism the hypercalcaemia is due mainly to increased renal tubular reabsorption. Conversely, in hypoparathyroidism the fasting renal excretion per unit of GFR is commonly normal. The low plasma calcium is therefore due to decreased renal tubular reabsorption for calcium.

Plasma phosphate varies more than plasma calcium and its level is set mainly by the kidney. The measurement of renal tubular reabsorption of phosphate may be used in clinical investigation, for example in the diagnosis of hyperparathyroidism. There are several methods available to calculate phosphate reabsorption; the best is probably an estimation of TmP/GFR (tubular maximum for phosphate reabsorption). This examines the relationship between filtered load and renal excretion which, like that for calcium reabsorption, is curvilinear. A nomogram has been produced for deriving this measurement (Fig. 4). Phosphate reabsorption is increased by growth hormone, in hypoparathyroidism, and in phosphate deprivation. It is low in several inherited or acquired renal tubular disorders and may also be influenced by drugs, e.g. corticosteroids.

Both calcium and phosphate excretion are influenced by other factors, notably sodium excretion, extracellular fluid volume expansion, and by the administration of diuretics. Infusion of sodium chloride increases the excretion of both calcium and phosphate, an effect which contributes to its value in the treatment of hypercalcaemia.

The biochemical mechanisms of transport of calcium and phosphate are not elucidated, but the action of PTH on the kidney is known to produce an increase in cortical adenylate cyclase activity which increases tubular cell and urine concentrations of cyclic AMP. It is not known whether this increase in cyclic AMP is the cause of the subsequent changes in phosphate and calcium transport.

Bone. The major organic component of bone matrix is type I collagen, but other constituents may have considerable importance. The metabolism of the organic component of bone is reviewed in Section 17. Mineral turnover and the indirect indices of bone turnover are considered here. The processes of bone formation, its mineralization, and subsequent resorption are closely coupled but do not occur in the same anatomical site at the same time. These processes are governed by bone cells which include osteoblasts which form bone matrix and are rich in alkaline phosphatase, and osteoclasts which are multinucleate giant cells responsible for bone destruction. Alkaline phosphatase may function in calcification as a component of a membrane pump for calcium and phosphate, or it may be involved in the metabolism of potential inhibitors of calcification such as inorganic pyrophosphate. The possible importance of alkaline phosphatase in mineralization is illustrated in hypophosphatasia (a rare and recessively inherited disorder of mineralization, see Section 17). This is characterized by low or absent levels of bone-derived alkaline phosphatase.

Plasma alkaline phosphatase provides a useful and readily measured index of osteoblast activity. It is important to note that plasma alkaline phosphatase is also partly derived from liver and gut sources, and that diseases of these organs may also result in hyperphosphatasia. This can be resolved by the concurrent measurement of liver enzymes (e.g. 5′-nucleotidase) or isoenzyme studies.

Bone resorption is accompanied by a release of enzymes such as collagenase and lysosomal enzymes capable of degrading bone matrix. Proline is a major constituent of the bone collagen molecule which is hydroxylated to hydroxyproline in the post-translational stage of collagen formation. The liberation of hydroxyproline by osteoclasts is therefore an index of collagen degradation and bone resorption which can be used clinically in the assessment of metabolic bone disease. Other sources of hydroxyproline include the diet (meats and gelatin), non-skeletal collagen, and the first component of complement. There is, however, a surprisingly good correlation

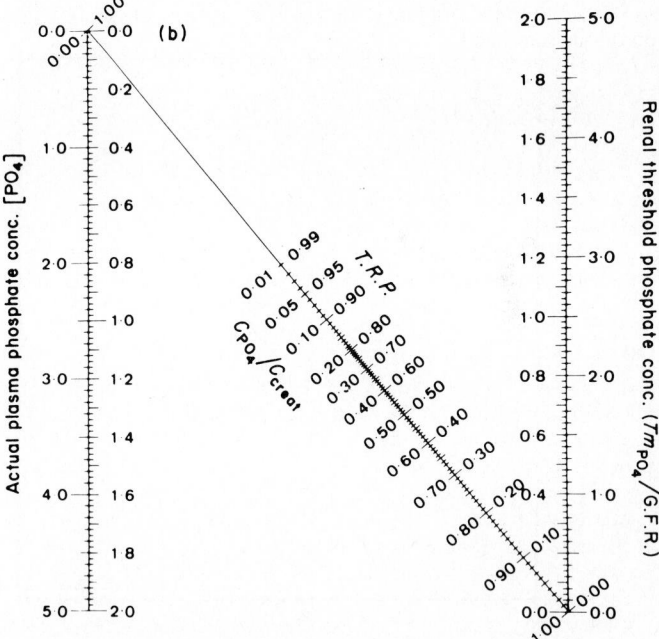

Fig. 4 Nomogram for the derivation of TmP/GFR (estimate of phosphate reabsorption) from simultaneous measurements of tubular reabsorption (TRP) or the ratio of clearance of phosphate to clearance of creatinine (C_{PO_4}/C_{creat}) and plasma phosphate (PO$_4$). TRP can be calculated from the concentrations of phosphate and creatinine in plasma and urine. The urine volume is not required:

$$\frac{\text{Phosphate clearance}}{\text{Creatinine clearance}} = \frac{\text{urine phosphate} \times \text{plasma creatinine}}{\text{plasma phosphate} \times \text{urine creatinine}}$$

A straight line through the appropriate values of plasma phosphate and TRP or phosphate/creatinine clearance passes through the corresponding value of TmP/GFR. TmP/GFR and phosphate are expressed in the same units. The scale in units of the figure are arbitrary. (From Walton R. J. and Bijvoet, O. L. M., 1975. *Lancet* ii, 309.)

between hydroxyproline excretion and other indices of bone resorption. The use of the fasting urinary calcium excretion as an index of bone resorption has been discussed previously.

The factors affecting bone formation and mineralization are ill-understood and more is known of the agents which affect bone resorption, possibly because this is easier to study *in vitro*. $1,25(OH)_2D_3$ and PTH are potent bone resorbing agents but probably act by different mechanisms. A number of agents are known to inhibit the rate of bone resorption. Administration of calcitonin inhibits bone resorption and decreases the activity and numbers of osteoclasts. Oestrogens also inhibit the rate of bone resorption, though receptors for oestrogen have not yet been demonstrated in bone cells. Other inhibitors of bone resorption include mithramycin, corticosteroids, and the diphosphonates which have become useful therapeutic agents in the treatment of disorders of bone turnover and of hypercalcaemia associated with increased bone resorption.

In a variety of physiological and pathological states, there is a remarkably close correlation between the rates of mineral deposition in bone and mineral resorption (Fig. 5). Even though these individual rates may be altered many fold (e.g. Paget's disease) the net gains or losses of the skeletal mass are minimized by the tight coupling between these rates. Dissociations do, however, occur in response to immobilization, and in the loss of bone mineral that occurs in malignant disorders, particularly myeloma. In osteoporosis, where there is a gradual diminution of bone mass, there is clearly an imbalance in the rate of bone formation and that of bone resorption in favour of net mineral losses. However, there still appears to be a coupling mechanism in the sense that attempts to alter bone resorption, e.g. by calcitonin, result not only in the inhibition of bone resorption but also the inhibition of bone formation. Thus, changes in bone turnover alone have only transient effects on plasma calcium.

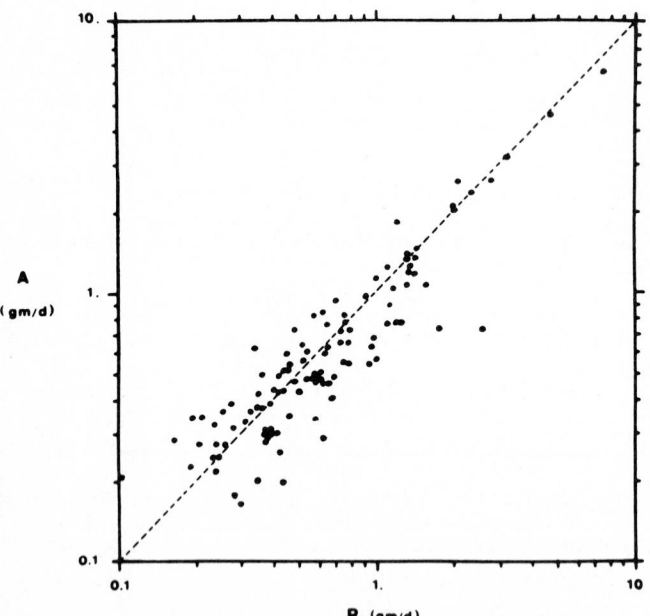

Fig. 5 The relationship between the rate of mineral accretion (A) and resorption (R) in patients with a variety of metabolic bone disorders. Note the logarithmic scales for accretion and resorption and the close relationship of these measurements. The dotted line represents the state in which resorption of bone matches its accretion. (From Harris, W. H. and Heaney, R. P., 1969. *New Engl. J. Med.* **280**, 193.)

A variety of techniques exist for the assessment of skeletal turnover other than the measurement of alkaline phosphatase and the urinary excretion of hydroxyproline. These include metabolic balance studies with concurrent tracer kinetic studies and quantita-

tive histology of bone. These are useful in the understanding of pathophysiology of skeletal disorders and their response to treatment but are not generally critical in the assessment and treatment of most patients. Techniques are also available for measuring bone mass. These include density and cortical width measurements on X-rays, photon absorption to measure bone density, *in vivo* neutron activation analysis, and computerized axial tomography. The quality of bone itself can be more directly estimated by the use of bone biopsy. Some of these techniques are discussed in greater detail in Section 17.

Integrated responses. In considering plasma calcium homeostasis, it is useful to separate acute changes from chronic changes. When the system is disturbed a steady state no longer exists. A response occurs which adjusts the system to produce a new steady state. Deviations of plasma calcium away from its normal value are rapidly corrected by alterations in the secretion of the regulating hormones. PTH can be considered the fast-acting component of the regulatory system, whereas vitamin D is responsible for adaptation over a longer time. The rapid control of plasma calcium by PTH is mainly due to its ability to regulate renal tubular reabsorption and possibly by effects on rapid exchange of calcium in bone. After parathyroidectomy, the fall in plasma calcium can be largely accounted for by the continued loss of calcium into urine until a new steady state is achieved in which calcium exretion is the same as its starting value but takes place at a much reduced filtered load of calcium. During the transient state, when plasma calcium is falling, urinary excretion of calcium will increase. In contrast, when a new steady state is established, urinary calcium excretion will fall to normal despite a lower level of plasma calcium.

A further example of the difference between the steady and transient state is seen during the infusion of calcium. During a calcium infusion (or, for example, increased absorption of calcium from the gut or increases in bone resorption not mediated by PTH) plasma calcium rises. If the rate of calcium entry into the extracellular fluid is constant, levels of plasma calcium will not rise indefinitely but only until the rate of efflux of calcium from the ECF pool (from bone, gut, and other tissues but mainly from the kidney) matches the rate of influx. At this point, extracellular calcium levels will rise no further despite continuing the infusion, and a new steady state prevails. In practice, the infusion of calcium would result in the suppression of secretion of parathyroid hormone and a decrease in the renal tubular reabsorption of calcium. This increases the rate at which a new steady state is achieved, and also decreases the final level of plasma calcium obtained. It is notable that the rate of rise of plasma calcium during a calcium infusion is to some extent buffered by the exchange of calcium in bone. Thus, rises or falls in plasma calcium are partially compensated by increased net movements of calcium in or out of bone.

Hyperparathyroidism

Definitions. The term hyperparathyroidism is applied to those clinical disorders characterized by an increase in circulating concentrations of parathyroid hormone. These can be arbitrarily classified into primary, secondary, tertiary, and ectopic (pseudo) hyperparathyroidism.

Secondary hyperparathyroidism is due to hypocalcaemia, such as is seen in vitamin D-deficiency or chronic renal failure, which results in increased secretion of parathyroid hormone and leads to hyperplasia of the parathyroid glands. In general, all four parathyroid glands are enlarged. The biochemical and skeletal lesions which result are a reflection of the underlying disorder, as well as hypocalcaemia and high circulating levels of parathyroid hormone. The skeletal abnormalities seen, for example in vitamin D-deficiency, represent a combination of hyperparathyroidism, calcium deficiency, and varying degrees of osteomalacia. Secondary hyperparathyroidism can be cured by treatment which restores the plasma calcium to normal (for example, vitamin D in simple nutritional deficiency of vitamin D). This removes the stimulus to parathyroid overactivity. Levels of parathyroid hormone fall quickly but the involution of parathyroid hyperplasia may take many months. More detailed considerations of secondary hyperparathyroidism are found in the sections on disorders of vitamin D metabolism (see page 10.54), on renal bone disease (see page 18.137), and on osteomalacia (see page 10.55).

Tertiary hyperparathyroidism is a term used to denote those patients with long-standing secondary hyperparathyroidism who develop autonomous gland function and hypercalcaemia. Nowadays this is most commonly seen after renal transplantation, but may also be observed in patients with long-standing malabsorption or chronic renal failure. As in the case of many endocrine disorders, the term 'autonomous secretion' is probably a misnomer since parathyroid hormone can be suppressed by calcium infusion, or further augmented by lowering plasma calcium. Tertiary hyperparathyroidism therefore implies a change in the set point with respect to the calcium control of PTH secretion. In this disorder, plasma calcium and PTH are both raised and treatment includes parathyroidectomy and the management of the cause.

Primary hyperparathyroidism implies autonomous hyperfunction of one or more parathyroid glands which results in a change in the set point for the control of plasma calcium such that plasma calcium levels are higher than normal. Pseudohyperparathyroidism is the elaboration of PTH-like material in association with certain malignancies, particularly of the lung. This gives rise to biochemical abnormalities not unlike those of primary hyperparathyroidism.

Primary hyperparathyroidism. Primary hyperparathyroidism is usually due to a single parathyroid adenoma of the chief or clear cells of the parathyroid gland. More rarely it is due to diffuse hyperplasia or multiple adenomata (Table 3). Hyperplasia and adenoma may be difficult to differentiate histologically. Carcinoma is very rare. Since the widespread use of multiple channel autoanalysers in clinical practice, the most common presentation (50–70 per cent of cases) is hypercalcaemia which is asymptomatic. This has also resulted in revised estimates of the disease prevalence which is now estimated as between 2 and 10 per 10 000 of the population. It occurs with greatest frequency between the fourth and sixth decades of life when it is twice as common in females as in males. At other age groups the sex incidence is roughly equal. The cause of primary hyperparathyroidism is unknown. An increased risk occurs some years following irradiation of the head and neck.

Table 3   Causes of primary hyperparathyroidism. Chief cell hyperplasia is associated with multiple endocrine abnormalities

Single adenoma	83.0%
Multiple adenoma	4.3%
Carcinoma	1.7%
Hyperplasia: clear cell	7.6%
Hyperplasia: chief cell	3.6%

Since the major effect of PTH is to raise plasma calcium, the main biochemical abnormality is an increase in the circulating concentration of both PTH and calcium. There are, however, instances where patients with proven adenoma have normal total serum calcium levels or intermittent hypercalcaemia. Thus, primary hyperparathyoidism can be defined as a circulating level of PTH that is inappropriately high for the prevailing plasma calcium (Fig. 6). In some instances, the patient with primary hyperparathyroidism may be normocalcaemic because of co-existent vitamin D-deficiency.

In primary hyperparathyroidism, the hypercalcaemia is mainly maintained by resetting of the renal tubular reabsorption for calcium, so that reabsorption is enhanced at any given filtered load (see Fig. 3). There is often also increased bone resorption reflected by increased hydroxyprolinuria and increased intestinal absorption of calcium due to the stimulation of production of $1,25(OH)_2D_3$. These factors will tend to increase the 24-hour urinary excretion of

calcium. In contrast, in secondary hyperparathyroidism, calcium malabsorption is common since $1,25(OH)_2D_3$ is generally low and plasma and urine calcium are very low despite high levels of PTH. Although resorption of bone is commonly enhanced in primary hyperparathyroidism, so too is bone formation, reflected as an increase in alkaline phosphatase. Thus the balance for calcium is usually normal, but at the expense of an increased bone turnover. Calcium balance may, however, be negative, particularly in patients with severe bone disease and in female patients with coexisting post-menopausal osteoporosis. Renal stones are also a feature of primary hyperparathyroidism. The aetiology of renal stones in hyperparathyroidism is discussed elsewhere (see page 18.83) but is related in part to an increase in the filtered load of calcium and the passage of an alkaline urine.

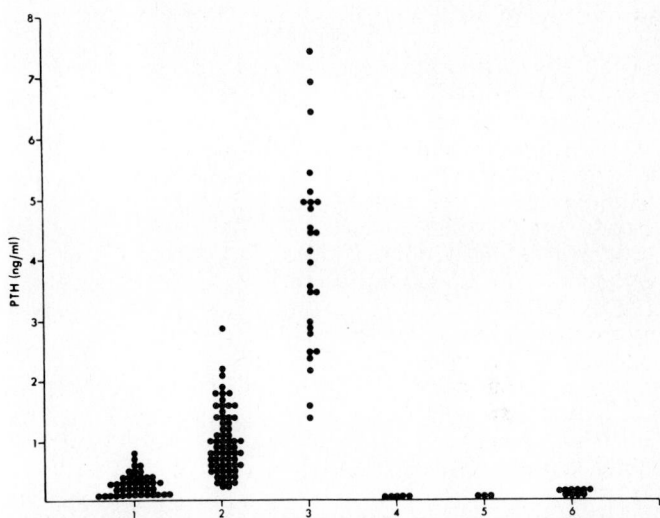

Fig. 6   Plasma levels of parathyroid hormone in normal subjects (group 1) and patients with hypercalcaemia (2–6). Patients with surgically proven hyperparathyroidism (groups 2 and 3) have higher levels of PTH but there is an overlap with the normal range. However, these patients were hypercalcaemic indicating that levels of PTH were inappropriately high for the level of plasma calcium. Thus, patients with vitamin D intoxication (group 4), idiopathic hypercalcaemia of infancy (group 5), and patients with skeletal metastases and hypercalcaemia (group 6) have very low or undetectable levels of PTH. (From Woodhead, J. S. and Walker, D. A., 1976. *Ann. clin. Biochem.* **13**, 549.)

Clinical features. The manifestations of primary hyperparathyroidism largely reflect the result of parathyroid hormone actions and hypercalcaemia itself. Approximately 50 per cent of patients present with renal stone disease and primary hyperparathyroidism accounts for approximately 5 per cent of patients with renal stone disease.

Bone disease is a common feature of primary hyperparathyroidism. It is usually apparent on quantitative histology of bone but it is rarely overt. Biochemical indices of increased bone turnover (raised alkaline phosphatase and increased urinary hydroxyproline excretion) occur in up to 50 per cent of patients. Radiographic manifestations of primary hyperparathyroidism occur in less than 2 per cent of patients and in them hyperparathyroidism is severe and sometimes due to parathyroid carcinoma; renal calculi are uncommon in this group. The characteristic radiographic feature of hyperparathyroidism is subperiosteal erosion of bone (Fig. 7). The skeleton may also be diffusely osteoporotic or osteosclerotic though the latter findings are usually confined to patients with severe and long-standing secondary hyperparathyroidism. Hyperparathyroidism in growing children causes appearances which are radiographically similar though histologically quite different from rickets. This is due to resorption of metaphyseal bone which may give rise to crippling skeletal deformities. Cystic lesions may also be found in primary hyperparathyroidism, 'brown tumours' which may result in pathological fracture. In the skull extensive bone resorption may give a mottled 'salt and pepper' appearance on X-rays. Subperiosteal erosion is most frequently noted in the hands with resorption of the phalangeal tufts and the radial borders of the middle phalanges. The distal ends of the clavicles are also commonly involved by resorption but are more difficult sites to X-ray. The loss of the lamina dura and the appearance of brown tumours in the mandible are late complications of primary hyperparathyroidism and the radiographic appearances are not specific.

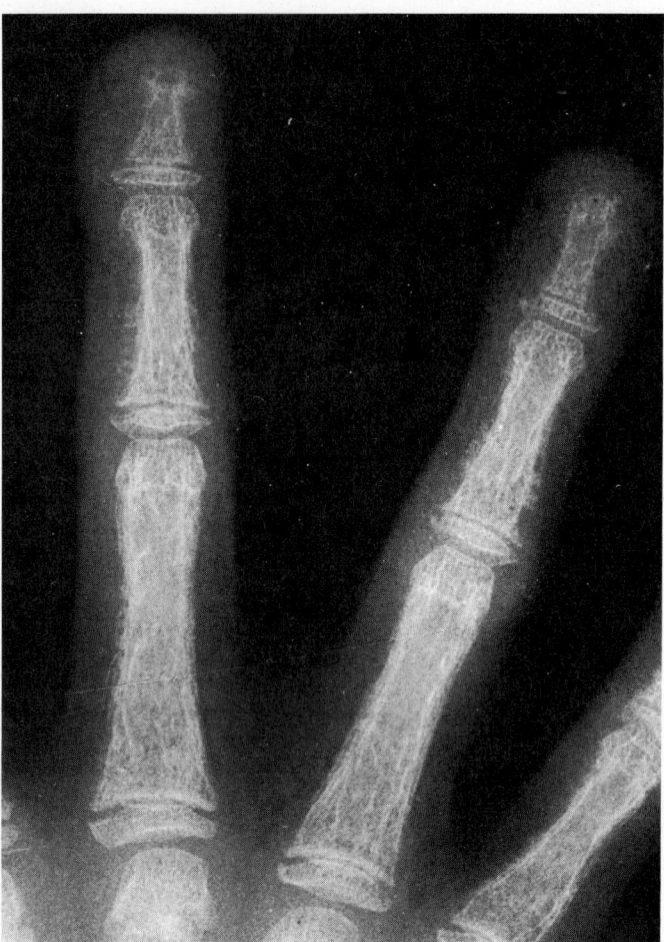

Fig. 7 Radiographic features of hyperparathyroid bone disease. Note the marked subperiosteal bone resorption involving the terminal phalanges. Note also the cortical porosity.

There are many other features of primary hyperparathyroidism, many of which are due to hypercalcaemia. It is important to realize that in a third of patients hypercalcaemia will have been an incidental finding and many patients are asymptomatic. However, the symptoms of hypercalcaemia are often very vague and include nausea, vomiting, fatigue, constipation, and hypotonicity of the muscles and ligaments. Bone pain and tenderness is seen in primary hyperparathyroidism but is more common in secondary hyperparathyroidism. Hypercalcaemia induces polyuria, and this may lead to dehydration or polydipsia. The raised plasma calcium and dehydration may also lead to renal abnormalities in addition to renal stone disease such as nephrocalcinosis and progressive chronic renal failure. Calcification may also occur in other sites such as cartilage (pseudogout) and blood vessels. Periarticular soft tissue calcification is more commonly seen in hyperparathyroidism due to renal failure. Calcification in the eye is reflected as a band keratopathy of the cornea or as conjunctival deposits which are seen with the use of a slit lamp. Proximal myopathy is an unusual

feature and may be due to concurrent phosphate depletion. Gastrointestinal symptoms may be an early clue to the diagnosis of hyperparathyroidism since peptic ulceration is seen in 5–10 per cent of patients, possibly related to hypercalcaemia-induced secretion of gastrin. Acute or chronic pancreatitis is also associated with hyperparathyroidism and calcification of the pancreas may be evident on X-ray or on radionuclide scanning. Pancreatic symptoms often precede the diagnosis of hyperparathyroidism and the failure of serum calcium levels to fall during acute pancreatitis raises the suspicion of coexisting primary hyperparathyroidism.

Mental disturbances attributable to hypercalcaemia are very varied and often subtle. They range from behavioural disorders and mood variation to organic psychosis and dementia. They are associated with abnormalities in the EEG which disappear with treatment.

Less common laboratory findings in hyperparathyroidism include aminoaciduria, hypomagnesaemia, elevated ESR, and a shortening of the QT interval on the electrocardiogram. A monoclonal increase immunoglobulins has been described in primary hyperparathyroidism and does not necessarily indicate myeloma.

A number of other disorders have been associated with primary hyperparathyroidism including gout, hypothyroidism, Paget's disease, and diabetes mellitus. These are relatively common disorders and it is unclear whether or not the association is causal. Hypercalcaemia is occasionally seen in Paget's disease, particularly during immobilization of the patient, and is commonly associated with primary hyperparathyroidism. There is a familial form of hyperparathyroidism and suspicion should be alerted when hyperparathyroidism is found in young adults or children. It has an autosomal dominant mode of transmission. It may occur without other abnormalities but is frequently part of the pluriglandular syndrome. It may be associated with pituitary or pancreatic tumours with peptic ulceration and gastric hypersecretion, or tumours of the adrenal cortex (multiple endocrine neoplasia type I). Combinations of hyperparathyroidism, medullary carcinoma of the thyroid, phaeochromocytoma, Cushing's disease, and carcinoid tumours also occur (multiple endocrine neoplasia type II).

Diagnosis. The characteristic feature of primary hyperparathyroidism is the raised level of plasma calcium in the presence of high or normal circulating levels of PTH. Both plasma calcium and PTH should be interpreted with caution. Account should be taken of possible abnormalities in the protein concentration or in protein binding of calcium. The kidney is an important site of degradation of PTH and a degree of renal impairment is found in approximately 10–15 per cent of patients with primary hyperparathyroidism. Depending on the characteristics of the immunoassay, the increased levels of PTH in the presence of renal failure may not reflect an increase in the biologically active fraction of PTH. The majority of patients with primary hyperparathyroidism also have low levels of plasma phosphate due to decreased renal tubular reabsorption for phosphate. The estimation of TmP/GFR (see Fig. 4), however, does not always discriminate various groups of patients with hypercalcaemia. In the majority of patients, the diagnosis is quite straightforward and rests on the finding of an increase in plasma calcium, increase in plasma PTH, reduction in tubular reabsorption of phosphate, and an increase in renal tubular reabsorption of calcium. The finding of augmented calcium absorption and high levels of $1,25(OH)_2D_3$, hyperphosphatasia or increased urinary excretion of hydroxyproline support the diagnosis. It is important to recognize that renal failure makes the interpretation of these tests difficult.

Most patients with primary hyperparathyroidism present with hypercalcaemia alone or with renal stone disease. The greatest diagnostic difficulties among patients with renal calculi are encountered in distinguishing between hyperparathyroidism and idiopathic hypercalciuria. In the case of idiopathic hypercalciuria, plasma calcium is always normal but there are well documented cases of patients with parathyroid adenoma in whom plasma calciums lie within the normal range. The administration of a thiazide diuretic such as bendrofluazide which increases renal tubular reabsorption of calcium, will induce persistent hypercalcaemia in patients with primary hyperparathyroidism but not in the case of idiopathic hypercalciuria.

Hypercalcaemia is commonly seen in patients with malignant disease. This is usually due to increased calcium release from bone, but in some instances may be due to the production of PTH-like material by the tumour itself. This latter syndrome has been variously described as ectopic hyperparathyroidism or pseudo-hyperparathyroidism and, although once thought common, is probably a rare cause of hypercalcaemia in patients with carcinoma. The majority of patients with carcinoma and hypercalcaemia have overt radiographic or scintigraphic evidence of bone metastases. Patients with myelomatosis and other haematological tumours associated with hypercalcaemia may show diffuse osteoporosis rather than the more characteristic punched-out lesions. Other causes for hypercalcaemia are discussed on page 10.57. A variety of tests have been advocated to distinguish these disorders, partly because of the lack of easy access to PTH assays. The hydrocortisone suppression test has been widely used. Hydrocortisone (usually 40 mg thrice daily for 10 days) fails to lower plasma calcium in the majority of patients with primary hyperparathyroidism but usually does so in hypercalcaemia due to other causes. False positive and false negatives are encountered and with the advent of radioimmunoassay for PTH (see Fig. 6), this test is somewhat outdated.

Other tests have been devised to distinguish the hypercalcaemia of hyperparathyroidism from that due to other causes. Discriminate function analysis depends on the simultaneous measurement of several biochemical variables including albumin, phosphate, alkaline phosphatase, chloride, bicarbonate, urea, and ESR. One of the major drawbacks of this approach is that the measurements need to be calculated independently in each laboratory. Their discriminating power in prospective studies is often disappointing. In the absence of renal impairment, a plasma bicarbonate may be useful. Thus, in hyperparathyroidism a metabolic acidosis is commonly found which is reflected by a low plasma bicarbonate and a high plasma chloride, whereas in disorders where PTH secretion is depressed a metabolic alkalosis is to be expected. Moreover, in hypercalcaemia due to rapid bone destruction, alkalosis may be accentuated by the release of bicarbonate from bone. Patients with carcinoma frequently have low levels of plasma albumin and low levels of plasma phosphate due to malnutrition.

More recently, the urinary excretion of cyclic AMP has been used as a test of parathyroid function. Considerable overlap occurs between patients with hyperparathyroidism and normal subjects, but expression of the excretion of cyclic AMP as a ratio to that of creatinine improves discrimination. A proportion of patients with malignant disease and hypercalcaemia excrete increased amounts of cyclic AMP in the urine, in the absence of evidence for ectopic hyperparathyroidism. This may be due to the secretion of humoral substances other than PTH.

Treatment. A moderate elevation of plasma calcium may lead to progressive renal impairment and severe hypercalcaemia may cause an immediate threat to life. At the other extreme, many patients with primary hyperparathyroidism have mild hypercalcaemia (plasma calcium < 3.0 mmol/l) without symptoms and it is probable that many patients with adenomas of the parathyroid glands die of unrelated causes. Opinion varies as to whether such patients should undergo parathyroidectomy but it is probably wise to err in the favour of surgery since many of the signs of hypercalcaemia are subtle and not always appreciated until after removal of excess parathyroid tissue. The aims of surgery are to remove the adenoma or to resect sufficient hyperplastic parathyroid tissue to render the patient euparathyroid.

The surgical management of patients with primary and tertiary hyperparathyroidism is controversial because of the variable anatomy of the parathyroids, problems of differentiation between multiple gland hyperplasia and single gland adenoma, and the incidence of post-surgical hyper- and hypoparathyroidism. The approach of many centres is to identify all cervical parathyroid tissue since more than one parathyroid gland is affected in an appreciable minority of patients (Table 3). On the other hand, the majority of patients with primary hyperparathyroidism have a single adenoma and some surgeons, on finding an adenoma, undertake no further exploration, particularly if other glands already identified have been shown to be normal or atrophic. In cases of diffuse hyperplasia the tendency is to remove three and a half glands. This has become a standard treatment of the secondary hyperparathyroidism of renal disease requiring resection. It has recently been suggested that total parathyroidectomy may be undertaken followed by transplantation of parathyroid tissue into the forearm muscles. This is not without technical difficulties and is, at present, experimental. Whatever the strategy employed, the operative implantation of radio-opaque markers at sites of remaining parathyroid tissue is helpful if re-exploration is required. Multiple operations carry greater risk and cause difficulty for the surgeon because of distorted anatomy and local fibrosis.

Arteriography or venography with radioimmunoassay for PTH in the thyroid effluent can be used as a pre-operative localizing procedure for abnormal parathyroid tissue. Venous sampling is most useful in localizing parathyroid tissue after failed surgery, although there may be difficulties in interpretation because of variations in venous drainage from the parathyroids particularly after previous surgery. The technique is particularly useful for detecting mediastinal tumours. Other approaches to localization include scanning (e.g. ^{75}Se), computerized axial tomography, and selective injection of a contrast dye such as methylene blue to discolour the parathyroids. Unfortunately, the yield of all these techniques is better in patients not previously explored than at re-exploration.

After operation, plasma calcium should be monitored at least daily for the first few days. Post-operative tetany is common in patients who have significant bone disease. They should be treated with intravenous calcium (10 per cent calcium gluconate, 10–30 ml in 1 litre of saline), and at the same time vitamin D should be begun. The 1,α-hydroxylated derivatives of vitamin D[(1,25(OH)$_2$D$_3$) and its synthetic analogues 1,α-OHD$_3$ and dihydrotachysterol] act quickly and are preferable in acute management. Hypocalcaemia usually persists for several days but occasionally it may take weeks of even months to reverse. Permanent hypoparathyroidism is rare when surgery has been undertaken by experienced surgeons.

Medical treatment can be considered in some asymptomatic or high-risk individuals with borderline or mild hypercalcaemia. Oestrogens have been shown to be effective in post-menopausal women with mild hypercalcaemia and oral cellulose phosphate and calcium restriction may transiently lower plasma calcium in other patients, but other features of the disease may progress. The use of neutral phosphate has been advocated in doses between 1 and 2.5 grams daily. Significant falls in plasma calcium have been shown but these have been associated with increases in serum creatinine. Specific inhibitors of bone resorption such as calcitonin and the diphosphonates may have transient effects on hypercalcaemia. There has been recent interest in the use of cimetidine and propranolol as a means for suppressing hyperparathyroidism but these approaches are experimental and there is to date little evidence to suggest that these drugs might be widely suitable. There is no ideal long-term medical treatment for primary hyperparathyroidism and surgery should be undertaken wherever this is feasible.

Hypoparathyroidism

Definitions. Decreased secretion of PTH may arise in hypercalcaemic conditions which suppress the secretion of PTH. The term hypoparathyroidism is, however, usually confined to those disorders associated with defective secretion or action of PTH (the latter is termed pseudohypoparathyroidism). These disorders, irrespective of their aetiology, are characterized by hypocalcaemia, hyperphosphataemia, and the clinical manifestations of hypocalcaemia.

Many of the biochemical and metabolic abnormalities seen in hypoparathyroidism can be understood by an appreciation of the physiological effects of PTH. Plasma phosphate is raised due to an increase in the TmP/GFR. Hypocalcaemia is due, in part, to a decrease in tubular reabsorption of calcium (Fig. 3). PTH directly or indirectly stimulates the synthesis of $1,25(OH)_2D_3$ from its precursor 25-OHD_3; and hypoparathyroidism is associated with decreased circulating concentrations of 1,25-dihydroxy-vitamin D_3. Hyperphosphataemia may be another reason for low levels of $1,25(OH)_2D_3$. It is a commonly held view that hypocalcaemia in hypoparathyroidism is also due to an inhibition of osteocytic calcium transfer from bone due to deficiency of PTH or $1,25(OH)_2D_3$ or both. Hypoparathyroidism is also characterized by decreased urinary excretion of cyclic AMP.

Hypoparathyroidism is characterized by absent or low levels of plasma PTH, but it is important to interpret PTH levels according to the plasma calcium, and the presence of low but detectable levels of PTH with hypocalcaemia is abnormal. Indeed plasma levels of PTH commonly fall to undetectable levels in such cases when plasma calcium is raised during treatment. A further characteristic is that hypoparathyroid patients have normal target tissue responses to parathyroid hormone. This can be examined by the administration of exogenous PTH in the Chase–Auerbach test (Ellsworth Howard test). The infusion of PTH normally elicits phosphaturia and an increase in plasma and urinary cyclic AMP. This contrasts with pseudohypoparathyroidism (sometimes termed PTH-resistant hypoparathyroidism) characterized by resistance of one or more target tissues to the action of PTH.

General clinical features. The symptoms and signs of most forms of hypoparathyroidism are attributable to hypocalcaemia and hyperphosphataemia. Hypocalcaemia is responsible for neuromuscular irritability which may cause carpopedal spasm, paraesthaesiae of the face, fingers, and toes, and occasionally abdominal cramps. Latent tetany may be detected by tapping the facial nerve to induce contraction of the facial muscles (Chvostek's sign) or by inducing carpal spasm following occlusion of the arterial circulation of the forearm (Trousseau's sign). Chvostek's sign has limited clinical usefulness since approximately 5 per cent of the normal population have a positive response. The neurological changes which accompany profound hypocalcaemia include irritability, emotional lability, impairment of memory, generalized lethargy, and convulsions which are usually of the grand mal type. Occasionally petit mal is a presenting feature. Abnormal EEG patterns are observed which disappear with effective treatment. Papilloedema occasionally associated with increased intracranial pressure may also accompany the hypocalcaemia of hypoparathyroidism. Both return to normal with adequate treatment. Hypocalcaemia in early life causes mental retardation which is not reversible. Cataracts are common consequences of chronic hypocalcaemia. Soft tissue calcification is not infrequent and has a curious predilection for the basal ganglia or subcutaneous tissue. If hypocalcaemia occurs in early life and is sustained, dental abnormalities such as blunting of the roots of the teeth and enamel dysplasia occur. Nails may be malformed, brittle, and have transverse grooves. Other ectodermal changes which may be found include a dry rough skin. A prolonged QT interval in the ECG may be found in hypocalcaemia and a partial insensitivity to digoxin has been reported. There are certain clinical presentations and features that are specific for particular forms of hypoparathyroidism which are discussed subsequently since they aid the differential diagnosis.

Causes (Table 4). Simple (PTH-deficient) hypoparathyroidism most commonly results from damage to the parathyroid glands during thyroid, parathyroid, or laryngeal surgery. The incidence of hypoparathyroidism after thyroidectomy varies enormously depending on the surgeon, the length of the follow-up, and the criteria used for diagnosis. Surgical hypoparathyroidism may be latent for many years, sometimes becoming manifest in association with increased calcium demands such as pregnancy and lactation.

Table 4   Major causes of hypoparathyroidism

1. Inadequate secretion of PTH
   Surgical—thyroid, parathyroid, and radical neck surgery
   Familial
   Sporadic
   DiGeorge syndrome
2. Suppression of PTH secretion from normal parathyroid glands
   Neonatal—from maternal hypercalcaemia
   Severe magnesium depletion
3. Defective end-organ response to PTH
   Pseudohypoparathyroidism Types I and II

Idiopathic hypoparathyroidism. This is a relatively rare condition associated with absence, fatty replacement, or atrophy of parathyroid glands. In the familial form it may be inherited as a sex-linked recessive, autosomal recessive, or autosomal dominant with variable penetrance. The sporadic form, occurring at any age, may be associated with pernicious anaemia, Addison's disease, or moniliasis. Addison's disease and moniliasis may also occur in the familial form although less commonly than in the sporadic form. These observations together with the presence of antibodies to parathyroid tissue suggest that these are autoimmune endocrine disorders. There is no evidence, however, that the antibodies to endocrine tissues are cytotoxic and they are not proven to be important in pathogenesis.

Children with idiopathic hypoparathyroidism have impaired growth and malformations of the nails and teeth. X-ray examination is usually normal although bone density may be increased and calvarial width increased. Idiopathic hypoparathyroidism is also associated with intestinal malabsorption, steatorrhoea, and osteomalacia. Moniliasis, a recognized feature of this form of hypoparathyroidism, does not complicate the surgically induced disease.

Other causes of hypoparathyroidism. Rarely hypoparathyroidism may result from infiltration of parathyroid glands by iron in haemochromatosis or from the invasion of parathyroid tissue by malignant metastases. In DiGeorge's syndrome there is a congenital absence of the parathyroid glands. It is associated with immunological deficiencies (thymic aplasia) and is a consequence of failure of development of the third and fourth branchial pouches from which the parathyroids and thymus arise. Thymic agenesis leads to a severe immunodeficiency state of the cellular type. Delayed hypersensitivity and allograft rejection may be suppressed or absent, and chronic mucocutaneous candidiasis is common. Patients with this syndrome usually die in early childhood from hypocalcaemia, severe infections, or both.

Neonatal tetany may arise because of maternal hypercalcaemia which causes the fetal parathyroid glands to become suppressed. Hypocalcaemia may become overt when infants are stressed with a high phosphate diet (cows' milk). The presence of neonatal tetany should alert one to investigate the mother for primary hyperparathyroidism. Hypoparathyroidism has also been reported following I^{131} treatment for hyperthyroidism, but radiation of the neck with X-rays appears to be one of the factors predisposing to hyperparathyroidism. Severe magnesium depletion impairs the release of PTH.

Pseudohypoparathyroidism. Pseudohypoparathyroidism results from the resistance of one or more target tissues to the actions of PTH. The physiological control of PTH secretion is partially intact in the sense that PTH levels are appropriate to the degree of hypocalcaemia. However, the administration of PTH does not produce the normal response of an increase in the renal excretion of phosphate and cyclic AMP. This is somewhat analogous to the failure of patients with nephrogenic diabetes insipidus to respond to antidiuretic hormone. There is an association between pseudo-hypoparathyroidism and somatic abnormalities. These include short stature, round face, short neck, shortening of the metacarpals and metatarsals. Characteristic radiographic findings include shortening of the fourth, fifth, or all metacarpals and metatarsal bones (Fig. 8). These features are not invariably found in pseudohypoparathyroidism and may be rarely present in idiopathic hypoparathyroidism. An X-linked dominant inheritance has been postulated for pseudohypoparathyroidism, but reports of male-to-male transmission suggest that a recessive inheritance pattern may also occur. In contrast to idiopathic hypoparathyroidism, pseudohypoparathyroidism is associated with hypothyroidism. The defect appears to be a selective deficiency of TSH. Other associated disorders include diabetes mellitus, amenorrhea, and gonadal dysgenesis so that there appears to be a striking overlap in the disorders associated with Turner's syndrome and pseudohypoparathyroidism.

The resistance to PTH may be partial or complete. In many patients neither phosphaturia nor increased urinary cyclic AMP production is stimulated during the infusion of PTH (type I); in others a marked rise in urinary cyclic AMP occurs without a phosphaturic response (pseudohypoparathyroidism type II). In yet other patients, the responsiveness to PTH may be restored by calcium infusion. Not all target tissues need be affected and occasionally pseudohypoparathyroidism may be associated with radiographically obvious osteitis fibrosa, suggesting that the skeleton is sensitive to PTH.

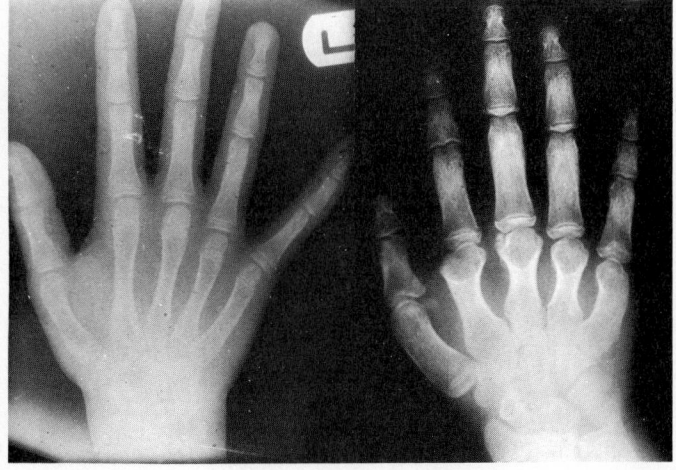
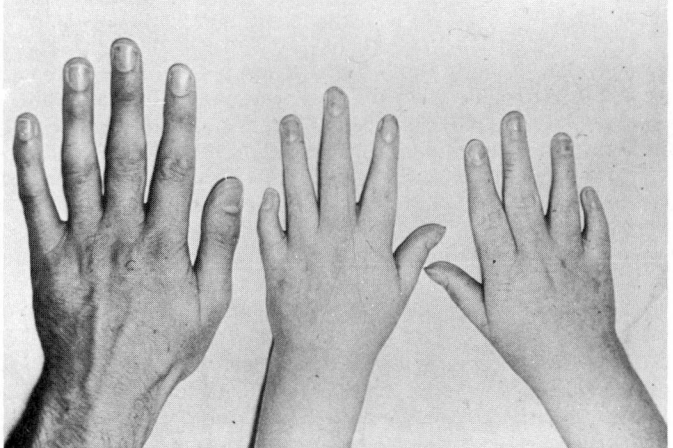

Fig. 8 Brachydactyly in a patient with pseudohypoparathyroidism. The photograph and radiograph on the left hand side show a normal hand for comparison.

Pseudopseudohypoparathyroidism. Rarely the somatic features of pseudohypoparathyroidism may be found in patients with normal plasma levels of calcium and phosphate. This condition is termed pseudopseudohypoparathyroidism. PTH levels are usually normal but may be raised. There are patients with pseudopseudohypoparathyroidism who are relatives of patients with pseudohypoparathyroidism and who indeed may undergo transitions from hypocalcaemia to normocalcaemia or vice versa. It is notable that cataracts may develop in patients with pseudopseudohypoparathyroidism who have been demonstrated to have consistently normal plasma calcium, suggesting that mechanisms other than hypocalcaemia are responsible for this feature.

Diagnosis. The diagnosis of hypoparathyroidism does not present any difficulty and is based on the finding of hypocalcaemia and hyperphosphataemia in the absence of renal failure, osteomalacia, or malabsorption. The clinician should be aware of the association of hypocalcaemia secondary to magnesium deficiency. A careful history, including one of previous neck surgery and physical examination usually indicates the underlying cause. The finding of Addison's disease, pernicious anaemia, moniliasis, atypical epilepsy, or bizarre mental symptoms raises the possibility of hypoparathyroidism. Apart from extremely rare forms of vitamin D-deficiency, the only other disorder commonly associated with hyperphosphataemia and hypocalcaemia is chronic renal failure. Measurement of plasma creatinine easily resolves this possibility. Since many patients with the more unusual forms of hypoparathyroidism are children, it is important to be aware that both plasma levels of alkaline phosphatase and phosphate are commonly higher in children than in adults. The differential diagnosis and investigation of hypocalcaemia is discussed subsequently (see page 10.57). The 24-hour excretion of urinary calcium is commonly low but the fasting urinary calcium excretion is usually normal. In order to distinguish the various forms of idiopathic and pseudohypoparathyroidism, more detailed investigation including the measurement of PTH and the responses to exogenous PTH are required. The principles of treatment, however, are similar for all forms of hypoparathyroidism although the doses required of the vitamin D-like agents used may vary.

Treatment. The priorities of treatment are to restore normal circulating levels of calcium and phosphate. This is rarely attainable by the use of calcium supplements alone but they are commonly used (1–1.5 g daily) in conjuction with vitamin D or its metabolites. The use of intravenous calcium (10–30 ml of 10 per cent calcium gluconate in 500 ml or 1 litre of saline) may be required in patients with tetany. In the past, the most commonly prescribed vitamin D preparation has been calciferol (vitamin D_2) in doses from 0.25 to 20 mg daily (10 000–800 000 units). One of the disadvantages of vitamin D_2 or 25-hydroxylated derivatives such as 25-hydroxy vitamin D_3 is that the onset and reversal of action of these preparations are very slow (Fig. 9). It is very difficult to titrate the dose quickly according to requirements and inadvertent hypercalcaemia may take weeks or months to resolve. The 1α-hydroxylated derivatives of vitamin D ($1,25(OH)_2D_3$, 1α-hydroxy-vitamin D_3, and dihydrotachysterol) all have a more rapid onset and offset of action. The daily maintenance dose required of these agents is 1–2 μg in the case of 1α-OHD$_3$ and $1,25(OH)_2D_3$ and 0.25–2 mg of DHT. Occasionally higher doses are required. High doses may also be used in the initiation of treatment, since the rise in plasma calcium is then more rapid. It is mandatory to follow plasma calcium closely to avoid toxicity in the first two to three weeks of treatment and at least six-monthly in patients on stable doses. The requirements for vitamin D and its metabolites may vary, particularly when the defect in PTH secretion is incomplete. Treatment may be required for concurrent hypomagnesaemia and other endocrinopathies when present.

Medical treatment such as phosphate depletion with the use of antacids, thiazide duretics, ammonium chloride, and acetazolamide are experimental and cannot be recommended, but their use for other reasons may alter the requirements for vitamin D.

Many patients who are hypocalcaemic may take anticonvulsant drugs. The requirements for vitamin D are probably increased when patients are taking anticonvulsants. These may be withdrawn when normocalcaemia is attained, bearing in mind that requirements for vitamin D treatment may alter at the same time.

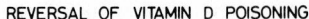

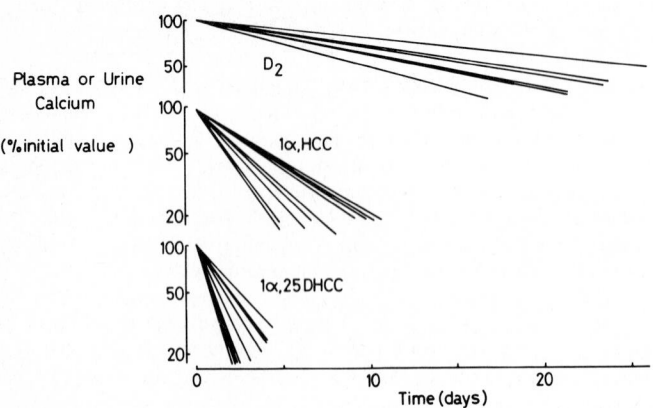

Fig. 9 The rate of reversal of biological effects after stopping treatment with vitamin D compounds. The fall in plasma or urine calcium is shown on a logarithmic scale. Note that the reversal of vitamin D toxicity is more rapid in the case of 1,25-hydroxy-vitamin D (1α, 25-DHCC) and its synthetic analogue 1α-hydroxy-vitamin D (1,α-HCC) than with vitamin D$_2$. (From Kanis, J. A. and Russell, R. G. G., 1977. *Br. med. J.* **i**, 78.)

The prognosis of adequately treated hypoparathyroidism is excellent. It is, however, unclear whether or not cataracts can be prevented. Major difficulties with long-term vitamin D treatment include prolonged hypercalcaemia which may lead to renal stone formation and progressive renal failure. Further details of treatment with vitamin D and its metabolites are discussed in the section on renal bone disease (see page 18.137) and in Section 17.

Disorders of vitamin D metabolism

The unravelling of the metabolism and actions of vitamin D has been one of the most rapid developments in endocrinology. An ever-increasing number of disorders has been associated with disturbances in the metabolism of vitamin D. It is, however, not yet clear in many instances to what extent changes in plasma levels of vitamin D metabolites reflect aetiological factors or adaptive responses to the disorder.

Hypervitaminosis D. Vitamin D toxicity is a common finding in clinical practice and is usually iatrogenic. Since vitamin D increases calcium absorption, and in high doses augments bone resorption, these patients develop hypercalcaemia. Plasma phosphate is commonly also elevated due to similar effects on phosphate transport. If over-dosage is prolonged, increased bone resorption is reflected by progressive loss of bone. The effects of prolonged hypercalcaemia are discussed in the section on hypercalcaemia (page 10.56), but the effects on renal function and structure are clinically the most important. Vitamin D toxicity is still an important cause of morbidity, and it should be a responsibility of the physician initiating treatment to ensure that adequate monitoring is undertaken. Vitamin D preparations should be stopped when hypercalcaemia is confirmed or suspected. The rate of fall of plasma calcium depends upon the agent used. The biological half-life of vitamins D$_2$ or D$_3$ may be months or even years, particularly when pharmacological amounts have been used over prolonged periods, resulting in high body stores. A long half-life of several weeks is also seen with 25-hydroxy-vitamin D$_3$. In disorders which require very high doses of vitamin D, the current fashion is to use 1α-hydroxylated metabolites of vitamin D such as 1,25(OH)$_2$D$_3$, 1α-hydroxy-vitamin D$_3$, or dihydrotachysterol. These have the theoretical advantage of bypassing the metabolic block in vitamin D metabolism; but they also have the practical advantage of having a much more rapid offset of action. The half-life of reversal of hypercalcaemia is measured in days rather than weeks or months (see Fig. 9).

The principles of treatment include the general management of hypercalcaemia (see page 10.57). Protracted hypercalcaemia can be additionally treated with the use of corticosteroids or a specific inhibitor of bone resorption such as calcitonin. In life-threatening situations, particularly in the face of renal impairment, patients may require treatment with haemodialysis or peritoneal dialysis.

Increased production of 1,25(OH)$_2$D$_3$. The production of 1,25(OH)$_2$D$_3$ is under metabolic control. The factors which augment its synthesis include hypophosphataemia, hypocalcaemia, and excessive secretion of PTH. Abnormally high levels of 1,25(OH)$_2$D$_3$ have been reported in patients with primary hyperparathyroidism and may account for the increased calcium absorption in this disorder. Increased calcium absorption is also seen in acromegaly, which may be due to high levels of 1,25(OH)$_2$D$_3$. Many patients with calcium-containing stones are classified as having idiopathic hypercalciuria because of a normal plasma calcium, a low plasma phosphate, and increased gastrointestinal absorption of calcium. Approximately one-third of these patients have increased levels of 1,25(OH)$_2$D$_3$, perhaps related to the hypophosphataemia. Sarcoidosis is occasionally associated with hypercalcaemia and more commonly with hypercalciuria, and increased bone turnover: increased intestinal absorption of calcium may be associated with high circulating levels of 1,25(OH)$_2$D$_3$. Hypercalcaemia in sarcoidosis may be aggravated by relatively low doses of vitamin D$_3$ and is more common in the summer months. Plasma levels of 25-hydroxy-vitamin D$_3$ are normal suggesting that the vitamin D sensitivity seen in this disorder is due to abnormal metabolism of 25-OHD$_3$ to 1,25(OH)$_2$D$_3$.

Defective production of vitamin D metabolites (Table 5). The hallmarks of vitamin D-deficiency include defective mineralization of bone and retardation of growth. Simple vitamin D-deficiency is associated with hypocalcaemia, hypophosphataemia, and high plasma levels of bone derived alkaline phosphatase, but in the early stages of vitamin D-deficiency, plasma calcium may be normal. The hypocalcaemia is caused by malabsorption of calcium from the gut and a decrease in the calcium efflux from bone. Hypocalcaemia stimulates PTH secretion and the hypophosphataemia is due to secondary hyperparathyroidism (decreased TmP/GFR) as well as malabsorption of phosphate. Indeed, it is possible that defective mineralization of bone is due, in part, to phosphate depletion.

Not all cases of osteomalacia or rickets result from deficiency of vitamin D or its metabolites. For instance, in X-linked or sporadic hypophosphataemia (vitamin D-resistant rickets) defective mineralization of bone is probably due to abnormalities in phosphate transport rather than to impaired metabolism of vitamin D. Conversely, deficiency of 1,25(OH)$_2$D$_3$ does not invariably lead to osteomalacia. Thus, osteomalacia is an unusual finding in hypoparathyroidism and is not invariably seen in end-stage chronic renal failure even though plasma levels of 1,25(OH)$_2$D$_3$ are reduced in both these disorders.

The clinical manifestations of osteomalacia, its investigation and differential diagnosis are discussed elsewhere (see Section 17). The purpose of this section is to review the manner by which disorders associated with defective production of vitamin D metabolites arise, rather than to discuss in detail the disorders themselves.

Simple vitamin D-deficiency. Simple vitamin D-deficiency may be due to dietary deficiency or inadequate exposure of the skin to sunlight. In northern Europe it commonly occurs in young children, particularly at the time of adolescence, in the immigrant Asian population, and in the very old. It is probable that the high phytate content of Eastern diets which binds calcium in the gut, aggravates vitamin D-deficiency.

The characteristic biochemical findings are hypophosphataemia, a raised level of plasma alkaline phosphatase and a low level of plasma calcium. In young children, plasma calcium may be sufficiently low to cause tetanic symptoms, but in the elderly may lie within the normal range. Levels of 25-hydroxy-vitamin D_3 in plasma are below 5 ng/ml where there are clinical signs of rickets, but these low values may also be found in asymptomatic individuals.

The term rickets is confined to vitamin D-deficiency occurring before epiphyseal closure. The characteristic features of rickets are expanded epiphyseal cartilage plates and deformity of the long bone. In adults, vitamin D-deficiency results in osteomalacia. The main symptoms are skeletal pain and proximal muscular weakness. There may be infolding of the chest to produce an hour-glass shaped thorax. Radiographically there may be diminished bone density. Characteristic radiographic signs are pseudofractures or Looser zones appearing as translucent bands of decalcification, usually at right-angles to the bone surface. They are most commonly found in the pubic rami, ribs, and on the neck of femur and humerus. X-rays may show evidence of secondary hyperparathyroidism, for example subperiosteal bone resorption.

The clinical, biochemical, and radiographic abnormalities show complete recovery with the oral administration of between 50 and 150 µg of cholecalciferol or ergocalciferol (vitamin D_2) daily. It is important to ensure that adequate supplies of calcium are available from the diet since severe deprivation of dietary calcium may delay healing or make a patient refractory to treatment. The failure of the patients to respond to small doses of vitamin D in the presence of adequate amounts of dietary calcium suggests that causes other than simple vitamin D-deficiency have given rise to the disorder.

The use of the 1α-hydroxylated derivatives of vitamin D in simple deficiency of vitamin D is unnecessary and presents certain risks to the patient since the ratio between effective and toxic dose is much less in the case of the 1α-hydroxylated metabolites than with the use of the parent vitamin D. These derivatives of vitamin D have a

Table 5   Vitamin D-deficiency states

Reduced availability of vitamin D
  Inadequate sunlight or diet
  Intestinal malabsorption of vitamin D, e.g. malabsorption syndromes, subtotal gastrectomy, ileal bypass surgery
Reduced availability of 25-OHD$_3$
  Liver disease
  Drugs, e.g. phenobarbitone, phenytoin, glutethimide
  Decreased enterohepatic circulation, e.g. malabsorption syndromes and liver disease
  Nephrotic syndrome
Reduced availability of 1,25(OH)$_2$D$_3$
  Enzyme deficiency (1α-hydroxylase), e.g. vitamin D-dependent rickets (type I)
  Enzyme destruction, e.g. chronic renal failure
  Enzyme suppression, e.g. hypoparathyroidism, pseudohypoparathyroidism
  Fanconi syndrome and acidosis
  Tumour associated osteomalacia (Mesenchymal tumours)
  Itai–Itai disease (cadmium toxicity)
Reduced end organ response
  Vitamin D-dependent rickets type II
  Anticonvulsants
  ?Steroid induced osteoporosis
  Coeliac disease and chronic renal failure (tissue damage to gut)
Uncertain relationship to vitamin D
  X-linked hypophosphataemia
  Diabetes mellitus
  Neonatal hypocalcaemia
  Treatment with corticosteroids
  Osteoporosis

more crucial role in the treatment of those disorders refractory to physiological amounts of vitamin D (Table 5).

The occurrence of a vitamin D-deficiency state despite adequate supplies of vitamin D and calcium is termed vitamin D-resistance in the sense that doses of vitamin D necessary to achieve therapeutic effects are greater than the normal physiological requirement. Not all vitamin D-resistant disorders are due to defective metabolism of vitamin D. Defective action or production of vitamin D metabolites may arise in a number of ways (see Table 4), by impaired conversion of vitamin D to its natural metabolites, or by impaired target organ responses. In many disorders where vitamin D resistance is a feature, there is evidence for more than one abnormality.

Malabsorption syndromes. Patients with long-standing malabsorption due to diseases such as cystic fibrosis or gluten-sensitive enteropathy (coeliac disease) are likely to develop osteomalacia. Not all such patients have symptomatic steatorrhoea and further investigation, such as intestinal biopsy or the determination of faecal fat excretion, may be necessary. The pathophysiology of the disorder is related in part to malabsorption of vitamin D which is fat soluble, but in patients with active disease, the intestinal cells themselves have been destroyed and hence the vitamin D-deficiency is partly related to the destruction of one of the target organs for vitamin D. The absorption of 25-hydroxy-vitamin D_3 is also decreased in patients with intestinal disease, including those with small bowel resection and it is possible that vitamin D deficiency also results from a defect in the enterohepatic circulation of 25-hydroxy-vitamin D_3. A high prevalence of osteomalacia is also seen in patients with liver disease and those with partial gastrectomy. Malabsorption of vitamin D may contribute to the former but the causes of osteomalacia after partial gastrectomy remains somewhat of a mystery and may be more related to malabsorption of calcium.

Reduced availability of 25-hydroxy-vitamin D. Vitamin D is hydroxylated in the liver to form 25-hydroxy-vitamin D. It might be expected that severe liver disease would impair this hydroxylation and there is some evidence that the prevalence of osteomalacia is higher in patients with liver disease than in normal subjects. There is, however, little direct evidence for defective 25-hydroxylation: low levels of 25-hydroxy-vitamin D, when found, may be due to losses of 25-hydroxy-vitamin D by interruption of the enterohepatic circulation, or to a poor dietary intake of vitamins D_3.

Osteomalacia has been associated with the administration of anticonvulsant drugs such as phenobarbitone and phenytoin. These drugs are potent inducers of hepatic microsomal enzymes and it has been claimed that there is an increased metabolic degradation of vitamin D to inactive metabolites. This is unlikely to be the sole explanation and there is increasing evidence that drug-induced target organ resistance is a major feature.

A convincing role for impaired 25-OHD metabolism is seen in the nephrotic syndrome. Certain features of vitamin D deficiency are common, such as reduced plasma calcium, hypocalciuria, and decreased intestinal absorption of calcium, even when the glomerular filtration rate is normal or increased. The hypocalcaemia is partly related to the low levels of plasma albumin which occur as a consequence of protein losses in the urine, but ionized calcium is also low as are levels of 25-hydroxy-vitamin D due to losses of vitamin D-binding protein in the urine.

Reduced availability of 1,25(OH)$_2$D$_3$. Chronic renal failure, pseudo-hypoparathyroidism, and hypoparathyroidism are disorders in which conversion of 25-hydroxy-vitamin D_3 to 1,25(OH)$_2$D$_3$ is probably impaired. Plasma levels of 1,25(OH)$_2$D$_3$ are low, and physiological quantities of 1,25(OH)$_2$D$_3$ may reverse some of the biochemical abnormalities, whereas pharmacological amounts of vitamin D_3 are required to achieve the same response. Not all these disorders are associated with osteomalacia. In the case of parathyroid disorders, the low levels of 1,25(OH)$_2$D$_3$ are probably due to raised levels of plasma phosphate as well as low levels of PTH, or, in the case of pseudohypoparathyroidism a resistance in response of renal tissue to PTH. In chronic renal failure, low levels of $1,25(OH)_2D_3$ are probably a reflection of destruction of the renal tissue which converts $25\text{-}OHD_3$ to $1,25(OH)_2D_3$.

Vitamin D-dependency rickets (pseudodeficiency rickets) is a rare disorder inherited as an autosomal dominant. These patients have all the features of vitamin D-deficiency except that vitamin D must be given in very large doses to correct the biochemical and skeletal abnormalities (10 000–50 000 units daily). Pharmacological doses of 25-hydroxy-vitamin D are also needed. Whereas physiological doses of $1,25(OH)_2D_3$ (1 μg daily) cure the disorder. It is thought that some of these patients have a deficient $1,\alpha$-hydroxylase enzyme system. There are, however, patients with similar biochemical characteristics who have normal or even high levels of $1,25(OH)_2D_3$—the vitamin D equivalent of pseudohypoparathyroidism. This rare condition, sometimes associated with alopecia, has been described as vitamin D-dependent rickets type II. It reflects presumably an inherited defect associated with target tissue resistance to $1,25(OH)_2D_3$.

Target tissue resistance to $1,25(OH)_2D_3$. Aside from vitamin D-dependency type II, it is probable that target tissue resistance to the action of vitamin D metabolites is an important component of the osteomalacia associated with anticonvulsant treatment and with intestinal disorders.

It is thought that the osteomalacia associated with phosphate deficiency, due, for example, to antacid abuse or to the genetically determined disorder of hypophosphataemic rickets, is unrelated to defects in the metabolism of vitamin D. Some of the renal tubular disorders, e.g. the Fanconi syndrome, are associated with a profound metabolic acidosis which might impair the activity of renal 1α-hydroxylase. In some cases correction of the acidosis alone without phosphate supplements may lead to healing. Sporadic cases of acquired hypophosphataemic rickets or osteomalacia have been found in association with various mesenchymal tumours and in many cases this is also associated with a defect in the synthesis of $1,25(OH)_2D_3$. Excision of the tumour results in cure.

Low levels of $1,25(OH)_2D_3$ have also been described in postmenopausal osteoporosis. It is unclear whether this contributes to the pathophysiology of osteoporosis, or whether the low levels of $1,25(OH)_2D_3$ reflect the chronic efflux of calcium into the extracellular fluid by the osteoporotic process, which in turn suppresses the production of $1,25(OH)_2D_3$.

Wider availability of the assays for vitamin D and its metabolites will aid in the precise diagnosis of patients with and without vitamin D-related disorders. Treatment should, wherever possible, be directed at the underlying cause, which in many cases may be reversible. The choice of whether to use large doses of vitamin D or lower doses of the metabolites of vitamin D is often a matter of personal preference and familiarity with the use of the particular agents available. It is probable that the use of 1α-hydroxy-vitamin D, $1,25(OH)_2D_3$ and dihydrotachysterol offer significant advantages in the treatment of hypoparathyroidism, pseudohypoparathyroidism, vitamin D-dependency rickets, and renal bone disease.

Disorders of calcitonin secretion

Medullary carcinoma of the thyroid. Increased secretion of calcitonin occurs in medullary carcinoma of the thyroid, a malignant disorder of the C cells. It may be inherited in a number of distinct syndromes. Where direct evidence of inheritance is found, it is termed familial, and the term sporadic medullary carcinoma is otherwise used. Medullary carcinoma accounts for between 3 and 10 per cent of thyroid carcinomas but there is a considerable geographic variation in the incidence. The majority of patients present with a thyroid mass, often with palpable cervical lymph nodes. The tumour may spread to the mediastinum but spread beyond the neck and mediastinum usually occurs late with the lungs, liver, adrenal,

and bones being the most common sites. Metastases to bones are sometimes osteoblastic. The tumour may be associated with other endocrine abnormalities such as phaeochromocytoma and hyperparathyroidism—the so-called multiple endocrine adenoma syndrome (MEAS). Medullary carcinoma may become clinically evident by the expression of these endocrinopathies. Severe diarrhoea may occur which is probably related to the synthesis of prostaglandins or serotonin. Hypocalcaemia is very rare. Calcitonin is consistently produced by medullary carcinoma of the thyroid, and the measurement of serum calcitonin is of value in establishing the diagnosis, the presence of metastases, and in following the effects of treatment. It is also of value in family studies for tracing asymptomatic cases. A number of other humoral agents may be synthesized by the tumour including prostaglandins, 5-hydroxytryptamine, and ACTH. The latter may give rise to Cushing's syndrome. Other genetically related disorders include multiple mucosal neuromas, ganglio-neuromatosis of the gastrointestinal tract, Marfanoid features, muscular weakness, and a high arch palate. A feature of associated phaeochromocytoma is the large amounts of adrenalin secreted which usually forms more than 70 per cent of the total catecholamine excretion.

Treatment is surgical. In view of the high incidence of a phaeochromocytoma, it is advisable to screen for this preoperatively and if present this should be dealt with first (see page 13.278). Because of the high proportion of adrenaline produced by these tumours, beta-adrenergic blockade should be used in addition to alpha-adrenergic blockade during surgery. The extent of surgery depends, in part, on the spread of disease and the associated symptoms. In the presence of distant spread it may still be worth resecting a large tumour mass to control severe diarrhoea or Cushing's syndrome.

It is important to screen members of the family who may be submitted to partial or total thyroidectomy if raised basal plasma levels of calcitonin are demonstrated or if exaggerated responses to provocative tests of calcitonin secretion (whisky, pentagastrin, or calcium infusion) are demonstrated. The majority of patients with medullary carcinoma have basal calcitonin levels which are clearly distinguishable from normal. In those in whom there is doubt, provocative tests of calcitonin secretion are used.

Until recently an elevated plasma calcitonin was considered diagnostic of medullary carcinoma of the thyroid, but high levels have also been demonstrated in patients with hypercalcaemia and a variety of non-thyroidal tumours such as oat-cell carcinoma of the lung and carcinoma of the breast. There is, however, a wide variability in the reported prevalence of high levels of calcitonin in these disorders, probably because of the difficulties of radioimmunoassay. High levels have also been described in chronic renal failure, in part related to delayed metabolism of some of the circulating fragments. Defective secretion of calcitonin has been implicated in the pathophysiology of hyperparathyroid bone disease in chronic renal failure. Athyroidal patients may have detectable levels of calcitonin and when these patients are given thyroid supplements, calcium metabolism is not markedly disturbed. This observation and the apparent lack of effect of excessive amounts of calcitonin on skeletal metabolism in medullary carcinoma of the thyroid illustrate the difficulty in elucidating the normal physiological role of calcitonin.

Hypercalcaemia

Differential diagnosis. Many of the causes of hypercalcaemia have been reviewed previously and are summarized in Table 6. The most common in hospitalized patients is malignant disease. The hypercalcaemia is complex and arises by several mechanisms. Most commonly it is due to the widespread destruction of bone by metastases. In such cases the secretion of PTH may be suppressed. In addition, hypercalcaemia may cause intrinsic renal damage due to the deposition of calcium phosphate which decreases the renal sensitivity to antidiuretic hormone resulting in dehydration. Decreased renal tubular delivery of sodium increases reabsorption of calcium and aggravates hypercalcaemia.

The investigation and diagnosis of primary hyperparathyroidism has been discussed previously (see page 10.48). The majority of other causes may be accurately detected by a good history (including a full drug history) and the simple measurement of plasma calcium, phosphate, and creatinine, and an estimate of tubular reabsorption for phosphate. X-rays or bone scans are helpful in detecting malignant disease not otherwise clinically apparent. The investigation of the rarer forms of hypercalcaemia (Table 6) is commonly straightforward and they are easily excluded by the appropriate investigations or history.

Table 6 Causes of hypercalcaemia

Common
  Artefactual: hyperproteinaemia due to venous stasis, hyperalbuminaemia (dehydration, i.v. nutrition), hypergammaglobulinaemia (myeloma, sarcoidosis)
  Neoplasia: carcinoma with skeletal metastases (e.g. breast, lung), carcinoma without skeletal metastases (? ectopic secretion of humoral agent), haematological disorders (myeloma, lymphoma)
  Primary hyperparathyroidism
Rare
  'Tertiary' hyperparathyroidism: transplantation, chronic renal failure, malabsorption
  Vitamin D toxicity
  Vitamin D 'sensitivity': sarcoidosis, ? hypercalcaemia of infancy
  Immobility: Paget's disease
  Milk alkali syndrome
  Thyrotoxicosis
  Thiazide diuretics
  Adrenal failure
  Phaeochromocytoma
  Familial hypocalciuric hypercalcaemia
  Haemodialysis: high dialysate calcium

The major difficulties arise in those patients without overt skeletal disease and hypercalcaemia. Mention has been made previously of the use of PTH assays (see Fig. 6), discriminant function analysis, and the hydrocortisone suppression test. These investigations together with a search for sarcoidosis or myeloma usually resolve further diagnostic difficulties. Hypercalcaemia and malignancy may occur in the absence of any obvious bone involvement by the tumour. In such patients there is presumed to be a humoral mechanism and the terms ectopic and pseudohyperparathyroidism have been used to describe such patients with raised levels of PTH. Some patients also have an increased excretion rate of nephrogenous cyclic AMP. In some this could be due to ectopic hyperparathyroidism but in others there is probably an additional (non-PTH) circulating factor which stimulates both renal tubular reabsorption of calcium, and the production of cyclic AMP.

Demonstrable bone involvement with metastases occurs in approximately 20 per cent of all patients with advanced cancer. Bone lesions and hypercalcaemia are most frequently seen in patients with tumour of the breast, lung, and kidney. Carcinoma of the prostate commonly involves bone but induces osteoblastic lesions in 90 per cent of patients. In patients with carcinoma of the breast, hypercalcaemia may be precipitated by factors which influence the tumour growth, such as the administration of oestrogen or oestrogen antagonists such as tamoxiphen.

Hypercalcaemia can develop rapidly in patients with malignancy and initiate a vicious cycle of increasing nausea, vomiting, dehydration, and impaired renal function. These patients often have a hypochloraemic metabolic alkalosis, whilst hyperchloraemic acidosis is more common in primary hyperparathyroidism. Serum phosphate concentrations are variable, depending on the presence or absence of malnutrition, disturbed renal function, and increased bone resorption. Plasma levels of PTH are usually low in malignant disease but raised in primary hyperparathyroidism.

Treatment. The aims of treatment should be to reduce the high serum calcium values and to remove the underlying cause. Severe hypercalcaemia should be treated as an emergency but chronic management is required in some patients because of difficulties in identifying or controlling the underlying disorder. Therapeutic strategy should be based on the mechanism of the hypercalcaemia, particularly the contributions of dehydration, increased renal tubular reabsorption of calcium, and decreased renal function.

Hypercalcaemia that is neither symptomatic nor progressive requires treatment only of the underlying disorder. The hypercalcaemia associated with myeloma commonly responds to adequate chemotherapy alone. On the other hand, progressive and severe hypercalcaemia may be life-threatening. Patients with serum calcium concentrations greater than 3 mmol/l are commonly dehydrated and it is important to restore the extracellular fluid volume by the use of intravenous saline. Care should be taken in patients with very low plasma proteins, or impaired cardiac or renal function. Frusemide and other loop diuretics increase urinary calcium excretion and can accelerate the effects of rehydration, but the use of diuretics without adequate rehydration may aggravate hypercalcaemia. Thiazide diuretics should be avoided since these increase renal tubular reabsorption of calcium. Only a small minority of patients, mainly those with impaired renal function, do not show an adequate response to the combination of adequate rehydration and loop diuretics.

Additional agents which may help in the acute management of hypercalcaemia include calcitonin (100–200U intravenously or intramuscularly) which consistently induces a decrease in serum calcium, but this may be of short duration. The cytotoxic agent, mithramycin (15 μg/kg i.v.), and the diphosphonates can also be used. Corticosteroids have been widely advocated in the acute management of hypercalcaemia but their efficacy has not been adequately demonstrated except in patients with myeloma, vitamin D intoxication and sarcoidosis. If more prolonged treatment of hypercalcaemia is indicated, a number of agents may be considered. Oral phosphate has been widely employed and is particularly indicated in patients with a low serum phosphate concentration and normal renal function. It frequently causes dose-dependent diarrhoea and is contra-indicated in patients with high plasma levels of phosphate or impaired renal function since this may lead to soft tissue calcification of kidney, lungs, and blood vessels. Intravenous phosphate therapy is particularly likely to cause this and should be avoided.

There may be a reluctance to treat mild hypercalcaemia complicating malignant disease, but the symptoms of hypercalcaemia can be subtle and may include a decrease in the pain threshold. This suggests that a more aggressive approach may have worthwhile clinical dividends. Intestinal hyperabsorption of calcium (e.g. vitamin D toxicity or sarcoidosis) can be controlled with the use of corticosteroids (5–20 mg prednisone daily). Additional approaches include a low calcium diet and the use of cellulose phosphate which is non-absorbable but binds calcium in the gut.

There is increasing evidence that some tumours induce osteolysis by the production of prostaglandins. The use of indomethacin or aspirin in long-term treatment has been disappointing but it is nevertheless worthy of trial in appropriate patients.

Hypocalcaemia and tetany

The more common causes of hypocalcaemia are shown in Table 7; most of them have been discussed earlier in this chapter. The measurement of plasma calcium, phosphate and creatinine, together with plasma albumin distinguishes patients with artifactual hypocalcaemia, vitamin D-deficiency, chronic renal failure, and hypoparathyroidism.

The symptoms and signs of hypocalcaemia have been discussed under parathyroid disorders. The most important of these is tetany. Tetany may develop in the presence of alkalosis, potassium and magnesium deficiency as well as in hypocalcaemia. Hyperventila-

Table 7   Causes of hypocalcaemia

Low plasma albumin: malnutrition, liver disease, etc.
Vitamin D-deficiency or resistance
Chronic renal disease
Hypoparathyroidism, pseudohypoparathyroidism
Acute pancreatitis
Drugs, e.g. calcitonin, phosphate, diphosphonates
Carcinoma, particularly of the prostate

tion alters the protein binding of calcium such that the ionized fraction is decreased and may therefore cause hypocalcaemic tetany in the face of a normal plasma calcium. Hypocalcaemic tetany may also occur during the administration of alkalis. This is particularly prone to occur during the treatment of acidotic patients with bicarbonate, particularly those with chronic renal failure in whom total plasma calcium may be low. Alkalosis may also occur in intestinal disorders where excess alkalis are ingested or there is excessive loss of gastric acid. Alkalotic tetany is diagnosed by an increase in plasma bicarbonate and an alkaline urine. Hypochloraemic alkalosis may be a feature of primary aldosteronism or the administration of corticosteroids.

The principles of treatment are those of the underlying disorder.

Emergency treatment for hypocalcaemia has been described under parathyroid disorders and the use of the 1α-hydroxylated derivatives of vitamin D on page 10.51.

References

Avioli, L. V. and Krane, S. M. (eds.) (1977). *Metabolic bone disease* (2 volumes). Academic Press, New York.

DeGroot, L. J., Cahill, G. F., Jr, Odell, W. W., Martini, L., Potts, J. T., Jr, Nelson, D. M., Steinberger, E., and Winegard, A. I. (eds.) (1979). Section on disorders of the bone and bone mineral metabolism: relation to parathyroid hormone, calcitonin, and vitamin D. In *Endocrinology*, vol. 2, 551. Grune and Stratton, New York.

Kanis, J. A. (ed.) (1980). Etiology and medical management of hypercalcaemia. *Metab. Bone Dis. related Res.* **2**, 141.

Lawson, D. E. M. (ed.) (1978). *Vitamin D*. Academic Press, London.

Nordin, B. E. C. (ed.) (1976). *Calcium, phosphate and magnesium metabolism. Clinical physiology and diagnostic procedures*. Churchill Livingstone, Edinburgh.

Peacock, M. (ed.) (1977). The clinical uses of 1-alpha-hydroxy-vitamin D_3. *Clin. Endocr.* **7**, suppl.

Potts, J. T., Jr and Deftos, L. J. (1974). Parathyroid hormone, calcitonin, vitamin D, bone, and bone mineral metabolism. In *Duncan's diseases of metabolism—endocrinology*, 7th edn (ed. P. K. Bondy and L. E. Rosenberg), 1225. W. B. Saunders, Philadelphia.

Adrenocortical diseases

C. W. Burke

Adrenocortical diseases are not common. Their clinical importance lies in the threat they pose to life and health, and in the success with which they can be treated, while their clinical and laboratory diagnosis are typical lessons in endocrine methods.

As with other endocrine glands, the pathogenesis of adrenal disease is of four types. These are: destruction or reduction of function by auto-immunity, primary tumour of the gland with or without hyperfunction, inborn errors of hormone synthesis, and overproduction of the trophic hormone (ACTH). ACTH overproduction is the commonest cause of clinical adrenocortical disease, the cortex itself being generally a remarkably 'reliable' organ. Usually the ACTH source is a tumour, whether of the pituitary or of a non-endocrine organ (ectopic ACTH production).

Cushing's syndrome: the syndromes of cortisol excess

The disease described by Harvey Cushing in 1932 as 'pituitary basophilism' is often referred to as *Cushing's disease*, which is a shorthand for 'Cushing's syndrome due to pituitary-dependent adrenal hyperplasia'. The term 'Cushing's syndrome' is a wider one, including a group of disorders which have essentially the same symptoms and signs due to overproduction of cortisol. The varieties of Cushing's syndrome, however, differ in other associated features (Table 1). The differential diagnosis is often possible on clinical features, and the treatment of Cushing's syndrome varies according to the cause.

Aetiology of Cushing's syndrome. Views on the pathogenesis of Cushing's disease have evolved considerably in recent years. Cushing himself thought that the pituitary was the primary cause of the adrenal hyperplasia which had been described many years before; but it was not until the 1960s that inappropriately high ACTH levels were shown in blood. In the following decade it was increasingly accepted that the pituitary hyperactivity was itself secondary to excess of a putative corticotrophin-releasing factor (CRF) from the hypothalamus; pituitary adenomas were not always found by the methods then available, and when they were

shown, it was presumed that they were themselves secondary to hypothalamic CRF activity.

The evidence for excess of CRF activity was, however, indirect and circumstantial, and it now seems probable that Cushing's original view was correct. Radiological or clinical evidence of pituitary enlargement is absent in 90–95 per cent of cases, but microsurgery and improved pathological techniques show the pituitary is in fact abnormal in all patients. The majority show a more or less localized

Table 1   Varieties of Cushing's syndrome

Clinical syndrome	Incidence	Causation
Clinically typical features mainly of cortisol overproduction	80–90% of cases	pituitary microadenoma secreting ACTH ('Cushing's disease')
	5–10% of cases	primary adrenal adenoma
	5–10% of cases	ectopic ACTH production by benign tumours
	very rare	micronodular adrenal dysplasia
Features mainly of cortisol overproduction but with other disease present	very common	iatrogenic Cushing's syndrome—due to glucocorticoid medication
	common	alcoholic pseudo-Cushing's syndrome
	uncommon	severe depressive psychosis
Severe cortisol overproduction with features other than those of Cushing's syndrome (e.g. hypokalaemic alkalosis)	common	ectopic ACTH production by malignant tumours
Variable and mixed steroid overproduction by adrenal often including androgens and cortisol	rare (1% of cases)	primary adrenal carcinoma

microadenoma, with suppression of the normal corticotroph cells in the rest of the gland. Removal of the microadenoma cures the ACTH excess, and after a variable period of ACTH insufficiency, the suppressed corticotrophs recover in a successful case, and completely normal ACTH function is restored. This normal ACTH function includes the normal physiological changes such as the day–night rhythm, and appropriate responses to stimulation and suppression tests. Restoration of function by extirpation of a small pituitary lesion shows that in most cases hypothalamic activity was not the primary abnormality. However, the question is not finally settled; the microadenomas are not completely autonomous, and they retain, for instance, some suppressibility by dexamethasone. Moreover, in some patients the pituitary abnormality is rather more diffuse than localized, and may resemble pituitary hyperplasia rather than adenoma.

In some patients with Cushing's disease, there may be adrenal nodules up to 2 cm diameter which resemble adenomata ('nodular adrenal hyperplasia'). The distinction from primary adrenal adenoma is clear in two ways, however. First, such patients have detectable ACTH in plasma, unlike those with primary adrenal adenoma; secondly, in primary adenoma the non-adenomatous adrenal tissue is atrophic, and not hyperplastic as it is in nodular adrenal hyperplasia.

A rare cause of Cushing's syndrome in children is micronodular adrenal dysplasia. The enlarged adrenals show disorganization of architecture, with multiple tiny (millimetre) nodules. Plasma ACTH is undetectable, and the aetiology is unknown.

The aetiology of primary adrenal adenomas and carcinomas is also unknown.

Ectopic ACTH-secreting tumours outside the pituitary are embryologically of neuro-ectodermal origin (Table 2). The ACTH they produce is immunologically indistinguishable from natural $^{1-39}$ACTH. The tumours also secrete other peptide sequences contained in the normal pituitary precursor pro-opiocortin, whose fission releases a molecule of ACTH and a molecule of β-lipotrophin in the normal pituitary.

Table 2   Tumours associated with ectopic ACTH production

	Approximate incidence
Oatcell lung carcinoma	50%
Other lung carcinomas	10%
Pancreatic malignant tumours (including carcinoids)	10%
Thymoma, benign or malignant	10%
Benign carcinoids of lung	5%
Benign carcinoids elsewhere (e.g. appendix)	2%
Medullary carcinoma of thyroid	2%
Phaechromocytoma	2%
Ganglioneuromas	1%
Primary carcinomas of: ovary, prostate, liver, other chromaffin tissue, breast, parotid	isolated cases only

After Liddle (1974) and Rees and Ratcliffe (1974)

These sequences secreted by tumours include 'big' ACTH, corticotrophin-like intermediate lobe peptide (CLIP), and others not normally secreted by the pituitary. Such tumours may also secrete other peptide hormones (e.g. gastrin, vasopressin) or amines (e.g. serotonin), depending on the tissue of origin. Factors controlling ectopic hormone production are not well understood.

Excess cortisol production in association with alcoholism or severe depressive psychosis is certainly ACTH-dependent, but whether the mechanism is cerebral or pituitary in site is uncertain.

General clinical features of cortisol overproduction. While the familiar picture of the patient exposed to excess cortisol as gross, plethoric, and obese is often accurate, some of the most diagnostically important clinical features are due to tissue destruction.

In the skin, atrophy can be found by pinching the skin on the back of the hand and the thickness may be measured as subnormal with calipers. In obesity, and in such disorders as acromegaly or hypothyroidism, skin thickness is increased, but in Cushing's syndrome of any severity the skin is palpably thin. The atrophy of the elastic lamina allows disruption of the dermis along lines of stretch so that capillaries can be seen below. This causes the typical purple striae on abdomen, breasts, and thighs: but abrupt weight gain especially in the young or old can also cause striae without cortisol excess, so that they are common in simple obesity. Weakening of the capillaries in the skin leads to purpura or bruising, but the greatest significance should be given to bruises that are spontaneous and not due to trauma. The same capillary fragility commonly gives rise to dependent oedema, which is seen in over 70 per cent of cases and is not primarily due to the sodium-retaining effects of adrenal steroids. This oedema sometimes affects the conjunctiva.

These effects may be due to the protein-catabolic effects of cortisol, as are some other features. Muscle wasting is common, and like other endocrine myopathies, it affects the proximal (especially girdle) muscles more than peripheral ones. But proximal myopathy without wasting may often be demonstrated by asking the patient to sit up from the lying position without the use of the hands, to rise from the squatting position unaided, or to get out of the bath without hands. Most patients with simple obesity will pass these tests. This muscle weakness in Cushing's syndrome is aggravated by potassium depletion in many cases. The skeleton is also wasted: osteoporosis, especially of the axial skeleton, is common and in severe cases will result in spontaneous vertebral and rib fractures. Again this is due to protein loss, in this case from the skeletal matrix. Poor healing of wounds is also seen (Fig. 1).

Most patients with Cushing's syndrome are obese, and typically (but not at all always) this obesity is central, affecting the trunk. The classical 'buffalo hump' of fat across the shoulders is neither characteristic nor invariable, but in the well-developed case of Cushing's syndrome the patient may present an 'orange-on-matchsticks', appearance, the central obesity contrasting with leg wasting. The degree of facial plethora is variable, though facial rounding is common. Hirsuties and pigmentation are not signs of cortisol overproduction, and are referred to below.

Over half the patients are hypertensive at the time of diagnosis, but malignant hypertension is not common. About 30 per cent are frankly diabetic and another 20 per cent have chemical diabetes. The associated complications thus include ischaemic heart disease, peripheral vascular insufficiency, and strokes. The well-known tendency of excess steroids to promote infection is evident mainly in relation to urinary tract infection. Sometimes the combination of cortisol and androgen excess is associated with acne. The ESR and often the white cell count are commonly suppressed, eosinophils in particular being absent from peripheral blood.

Psychiatric complications are common, around 20 per cent of patients having some degree of depressive psychosis while a similar number of other patients experience mood lability and insomnia, sometimes with inversion of the normal sleep rhythm.

As well as diabetes and hypertension, there are metabolic complications. The increased skeletal turnover is associated with hypercalciuria in about half the patients (more show increased hydroxyproline excretion), and urinary tract stones occur in as many as 10 per cent of patients in some series. Elevated triglycerides in plasma are found in patients with the disorder even if they are not diabetic. Total body potassium is reduced by 100–500 mmol, but serum K is not usually reduced except in the malignant forms of the disease (see below). Polycythaemia is unusual, though as a group the patients show an increase in red cell mass.

Features of hypopituitarism are seldom present even in pituitary-dependent Cushing's disease. Oligomenorrhoea, impotence, and infertility, however, are common. In children, Cushing's syndrome causes growth arrest regardless of the variety of the syndrome. Some childhood cases present solely with growth arrest and obesity. Table 3 gives an assessment of the relative value of some of these symptoms and signs.

Special features of some varieties of Cushing's syndrome. When due to *adrenal carcinoma*, Cushing's syndrome may be associated with hypokalaemia (due to the enormous cortisol overproduction),

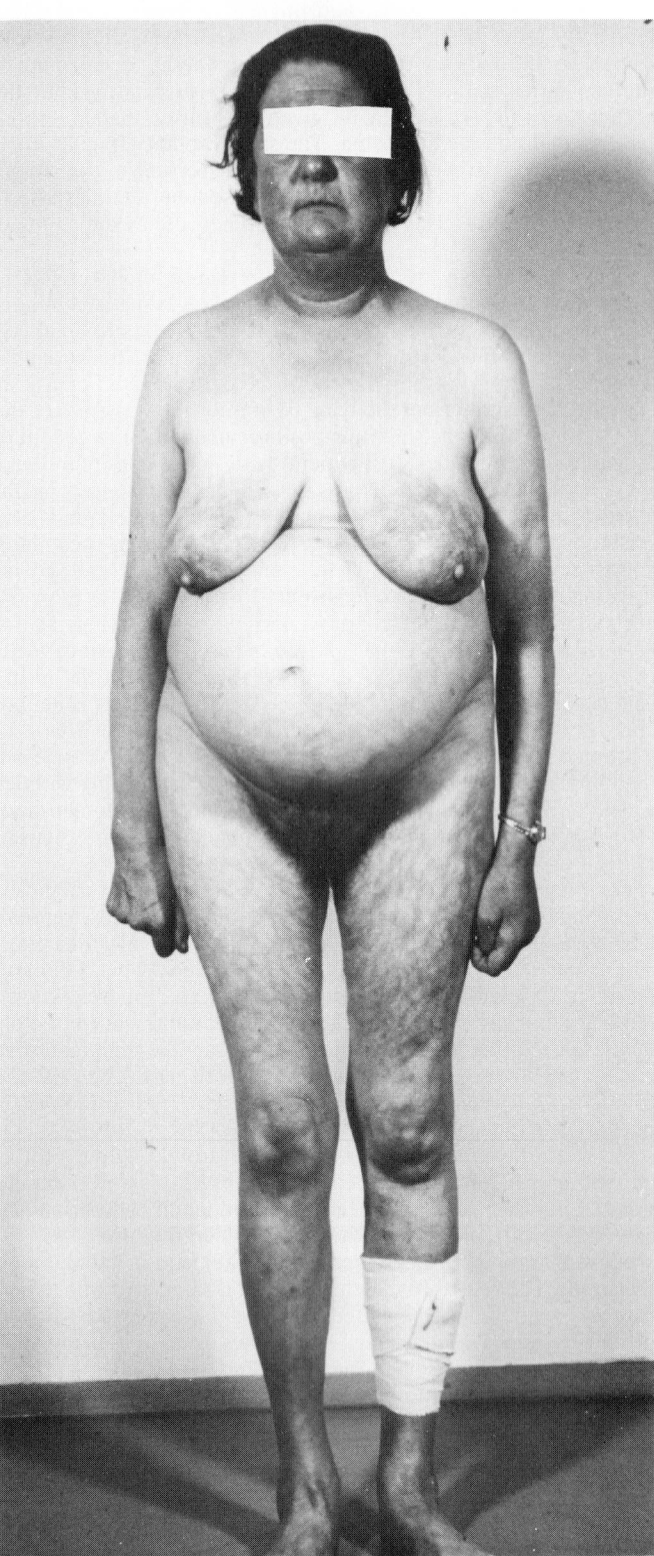

Fig. 1 Cushing's syndrome, showing wasting of quadriceps and deltoids, plethora, some obesity, and a dog bite on the shin unhealed after nine months.

Table 3 Clinical value of some symptoms and signs in Cushing's syndrome

Regularly occurring and of high diagnostic value
   Skin atrophy
   Myopathy and proximal wasting
   Spontaneous purpura
   Growth arrest in children
   Osteoporosis and fractures

Regularly occurring and of value in generating suspicion
   Oedema
   Livid striae, paper-thin scars, poor healing
   Facial mooning
   Facial hirsuties and scalp hair loss
   Mood lability with inverted sleep rhythm

Non-specific and of makeweight value only
   Central obesity, 'buffalo hump'
   Pale striae
   Hypertension
   Diabetes
   Oligomenorrhoea
   Plethora
   Acne

with weight loss due to the tumour, and with virilization due to androgen excess. If the androgen excess predominates, there may be fewer of the 'atrophic' features described above. This variety of Cushing's syndrome is disproportionately rather commoner than the others in childhood, and is a cause of precocious puberty in the male.

With *primary adrenal adenoma*, there are often no specific clinical features other than a slight tendency to excess androgen production. In general, benign tumours of the adrenal cortex tend to retain specialist production of either glucocorticoids, androgens, or mineralocorticoids; while carcinomas characteristically secrete various biologically active and inactive steroids in large amounts.

In cases of *ectopic ACTH production*, the clinical picture is particularly variable. At one end of the scale small benign tumours, such as lung carcinoids with a fairly modest output of ACTH and cortisol, may produce the typical features of classical Cushing's syndrome. At the other end larger and rapidly-growing cancers, such as oat-cell carcinoma of the bronchus, produce much greater amounts of ACTH and cortisol: the metabolic features of cortisol excess then appear before there is time for 'Cushingoid' symptoms and signs to develop. The most usual of these metabolic features are profound muscle weakness, hypokalaemic alkalosis (which no doubt contributes to the weakness), and sudden diabetes or hypertension. The very high ACTH levels may be associated with pigmentation, unlike the more modest levels in Cushing's disease. ACTH itself is not a pigmentary hormone, as shown by lack of pigmentation in ACTH-treated patients. The β-MSH sequence, which is contained in pro-opiocortin, may be responsible for ACTH-associated pigmentation.

Clinical differential diagnosis of Cushing's syndrome. The main clinical problem is to distinguish between patients who are obese, diabetic, hypertensive, hyperlipidaemic, and perhaps plethoric on the one hand, and patients with Cushing's syndrome on the other. Sometimes patients with polycystic ovary syndrome may look Cushingoid, but their increased skin thickness contrasts with the atrophy in Cushing's syndrome. The two, however, may occur together. A special problem is the obese plethoric alcoholic, who may show elevated cortisol excretion ('alcohol-induced pseudo-Cushing's syndrome') and details of the patient's habits should always be sought. Severe depressive psychosis with secondary raised cortisol excretion can only be distinguished from Cushing's syndrome with secondary psychosis by an insulin hypoglycaemia test (see below).

Investigation of patients with Cushing's syndrome. *Is Cushing's* *syndrome present or not? Screening tests.* Virtually all patients with Cushing's syndrome show elevated *urinary unconjugated cortisol* excretion (Fig. 2). This is a better discriminator than 17-hydroxysteroid or 17-oxogenic steroid excretion, which reflect cortisol metabolism rather than prevailing blood levels, and hence depend on nutrition, liver function, and so forth. In principle, the amount of cortisol excreted in 24 hours represents an integrated plasma sample for unbound cortisol. It does, however, depend on renal function and may be affected by proteinuria. Non-specific increases in urinary cortisol may be due to stress, oral contraceptives, and pregnancy.

24-HOUR URINARY STEROID EXCRETION

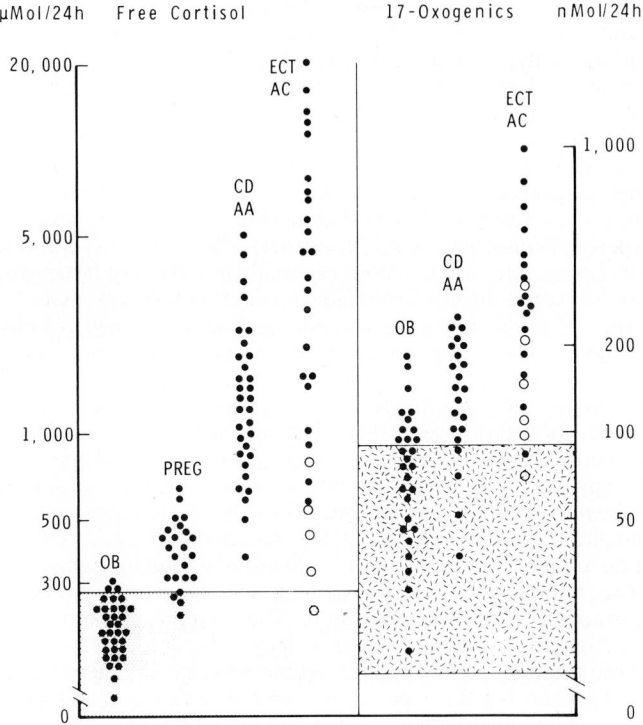

Fig. 2 Urinary cortisol (left) and 17-oxogenic steroid (right) excretion in normal subjects (hatched area), women in the third trimester of pregnancy (PREG), obese persons suspected of Cushing's syndrome, in whom that was disproved (OB); Cushing's disease (CD), and in Cushing's syndrome due to adrenal adenoma (AA) or carcinoma (AC) and ectopic ACTH production (ECT) (log scale). The open circles are for patients with adrenal carcinoma but no overt features of Cushing's syndrome.

Plasma cortisol concentration varies so much under normal circumstances that it should only be measured under defined conditions. In Cushing's syndrome, the only constant finding is failure of the normal fall in plasma cortisol at night, when it is normally less than 250–300 nmol/l. Samples should therefore be drawn around midnight, with the patient rested beforehand. Morning samples are of less value (Fig. 3), for many patients with Cushing's syndrome have normal morning cortisol concentrations. Elevated values for midnight cortisol may, however, be found in stress, pregnancy, and in oral contraceptive users.

In Cushing's syndrome there is a variable degree of resistance to suppression by exogenous steroids. *Dexamethasone* does not interfere in cortisol assays, which enables its inhibition of the pituitary adrenal control of endogenous cortisol to be tested. The normal pituitary is most susceptible to suppression at midnight, and a popular outpatient test is to give 2 mg of dexamethasone at midnight, and measure plasma cortisol at 9 a.m. the following morning. A normal value is less than 250–300 nmol/l.

At this stage pituitary fossa X-ray does not help to decide if the

PLASMA CORTISOL CONCENTRATION

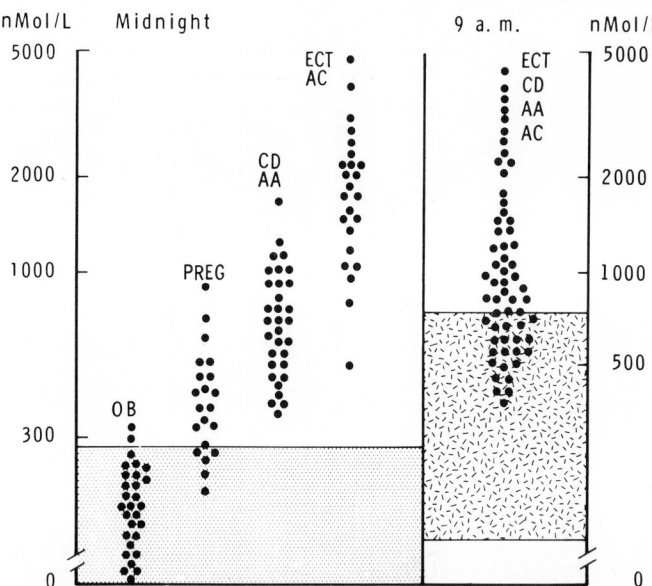

Fig. 3 Plasma cortisol at nine a.m. and midnight in normal subjects (hatched area), patients with Cushing's syndrome (same groups as Fig. 2) (log scale).

syndrome is present, as even if it is, the appearances are likely to be normal. X-rays of the spine and chest may be taken to show osteoporosis and fractures.

None of these tests is completely specific, and the interpretation depends on the level of clinical suspicion. The occasional occurrence of cyclical Cushing's disease has to be borne in mind.

What is the aetiology of the Cushing's syndrome which has now been shown to be present? Although it is of no help as a screening test, immunoassay of *plasma ACTH* is of the greatest value in determining the cause. Levels are undetectable when Cushing's syndrome is due to primary adrenal adenoma or carcinoma (Fig. 4), but normal or elevated levels are seen in cases due to pituitary or ectopic ACTH production. Since the main value is to show undetectable levels in primary adrenal disease, it is most logical to take the sample in the morning, as ACTH is often undetectable in normal persons at night. The sample has to be drawn with special precautions. The ACTH level is not always capable of differentiating between pituitary and ectopic ACTH production, although values above 500 ng/l are almost always due to ectopic production in untreated Cushing's syndrome.

The *metyrapone* test is also useful. This drug inhibits adrenal 11β-hydroxylase, causing a fall in cortisol secretion which normally stimulates a rise of ACTH. This can be measured in several ways; by measuring ACTH itself, by measuring the ACTH-mediated rise in the precursor 11-deoxycortisol, or by measuring the general production of precursors as 17-oxogenic steroids. In theory, in primary adrenal adenoma or carcinoma the pituitary is suppressed and there is no rise, while ectopic ACTH-producing tumours should also be unresponsive; in Cushing's disease the pituitary will respond. This is true in 90 per cent of cases but not all. The method is to give 750 mg metyrapone four-hourly, measuring urine 17-oxogenic steroids the day before, the day of, and the day after metyrapone. The highest excretion is often seen on the day after, and in Cushing's disease is, on average, three times basal.

The *height of the steroid overproduction* is helpful in that urinary cortisol excretion over 5000 nmol/day is almost always associated with adrenal carcinoma or ectopic ACTH (Fig. 2). Such cases are the most likely to show a hypokalaemic alkalosis. In adrenal carcinoma a disproportionate rise in androgen metabolites may be measured as 17-oxosteroid excretion. More specific assays such as

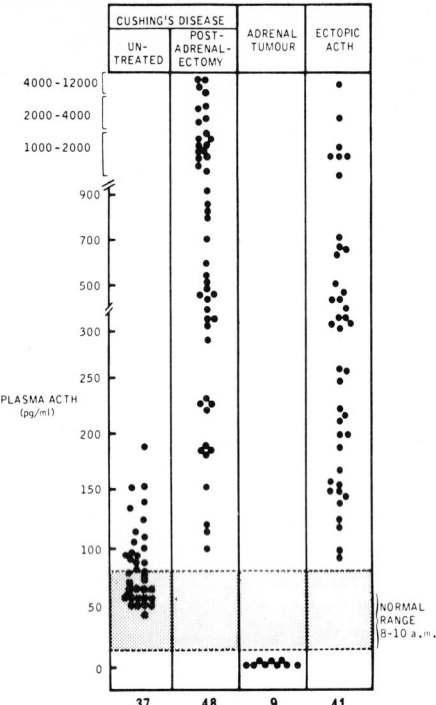

PLASMA IMMUNOREACTIVE ACTH LEVELS IN CUSHING'S SYNDROME

Fig. 4 Nine a.m. immunoreactive N-terminal ACTH concentrations in plasma of normal subjects (hatched area), and patients with Cushing's disease (pituitary-dependent adrenal hyperplasia), Cushing's syndrome due to primary adrenal tumour, and the ectopic ACTH syndrome. (Reproduced by courtesy of Professor L. H. Rees).

dehydroepiandrosterone (DHEA) are helpful in carcinoma if available.

Suppression tests with *dexamethasone* have been largely superseded as 30–40 per cent of patients give false positive or negative results. It used to be held that patients with any form of Cushing's syndrome would show resistance to suppression with 0.5 mg of dexamethasone six-hourly, while those with obesity suppressed normally. Plasma or urinary steroid assays were used as the index. If 2 mg six-hourly was given, patients with Cushing's disease would suppress, but patients with primary adrenal disease or ectopic ACTH production would not. However, suppressibility is a matter of degree, and there are so many exceptions that more modern methods of testing should take precedence.

In Cushing's disease, *pituitary fossa X-ray* should form part of the assessment. Only 5–10 per cent will show fossa enlargement, and in these cases a CT scan is necessary to determine the presence of upward extension of the tumour. In other cases, a small blister on the pituitary fossa may suggest the site of a microadenoma, but interpretation is often clouded by osteoporosis of the sella turcica. If plasma ACTH is detectable, a careful search for tumours elsewhere is required; small bronchial carcinoids secreting ACTH may be overlooked, for example.

If primary adrenal disease is suspected on the basis of low ACTH levels and the clinical features, pyelography to detect renal displacement and ultrasound examination of the adrenal areas should be performed, and followed by adrenal ateriography or venography to localize the lesion. At venography, adrenal vein cortisol samples are useful to confirm the lateralization. ^{125}I-cholesterol is taken up by the adrenals; in adenoma or carcinoma unilateral uptake on cholesterol scanning demonstrates the side of the lesion for the surgeon.

Where an ectopic source of ACTH is suspected but is not easy to locate, cannulation of the great veins with venous sampling for ACTH is a good method of localization, in practised hands.

Where cortisol excess is shown and is ACTH-dependent but there is confusion as to whether it is alcohol-induced, due to depressive psychosis, or due to Cushing's disease, an *insulin hypoglycaemia test* may help. Patients with Cushing's disease are insulin-resistant, and require 0.3 u/kg of insulin to generate an adequate hypoglycaemia (less than 2 mmol/l glucose) for 20 minutes, but they show no plasma cortisol rise in response. Patients with alcoholism or depression commonly respond normally, with a rise in plasma cortisol.

The treatment of Cushing's disease and the prognosis. The prognosis of untreated Cushing's syndrome has been compared in the past to that of breast cancer: 50 per cent dead in five years. Deaths are due to various combinations of hypertension, stroke, ischaemic heart disease or heart failure, and pyelonephritis. A few cases of spontaneous remission of Cushing's disease have been reported. Uncommonly, but regularly, cases of cyclical Cushing's disease are encountered, the disease running a fluctuant course with a periodicity of weeks, months, or occasionally years.

The treatment of Cushing's disease used to be by bilateral total adrenalectomy, subtotal adrenalectomy having fallen into disrepute because either adrenal failure or relapse of the hypercorticolism usually resulted. Total adrenalectomy of course relieves the hypercorticolism permanently, restores relative health, and does not destroy pituitary function, especially fertility. But it has great disadvantages. In the Cushingoid patient with fragile tissues, it carries morbidity and a mortality in some centres as high as 5 or 10 per cent. Deaths are due to infection, potassium disturbances, haemorrhage, pulmonary complications (the pleura often being entered by the posterior surgical approach), and damage to the spleen and inferior vena cava. The operation implies endocrine mutilation by engendering life-long dependence on replacement therapy. Further, 20–30 per cent of patients go on to develop *Nelson's syndrome* (very high ACTH levels with deep pigmentation and pituitary enlargement) (see Fig. 4). This may be due to release of the pituitary adenoma from feedback inhibition by high cortisol levels, but it means that many patients need some form of pituitary destruction after adrenalectomy. The current place of adrenalectomy is in treating patients with the ectopic ACTH syndrome whose tumour cannot be removed but who, nevertheless, have a good prognosis if the hypercorticolism can be relieved; and for the occasional patient in whom treatment by the pituitary route fails. But nowadays treatment is usually directed at the primary lesion, i.e. the pituitary.

What this pituitary treatment should be is less certain. The options are surgical removal of the microadenoma if present, or irradiation. Methods for the latter include external X-ray therapy, heavy particle irradiation with a proton beam, or interstitial implantation of radioactive sources, usually ^{90}Y. Total surgical hypophysectomy is no more indicated than is total adrenalectomy, unless it is the only means of dealing with an invasive pituitary adenoma as happens on occasion. Where the fossa is enlarged, surgical treatment of the pituitary would usually be advised and pituitary destruction should be anticipated. Irradiation should be carried out as well in these cases. At present, the objective of treatment in cases without pituitary enlargement should be to remove the hyperfunction without endocrine deficit. Where a truly selective, transphenoidal removal of a localized microadenoma can be performed (and it requires considerable technical expertise), this optimal result will be achieved; after a year or so of ACTH insufficiency, the patient will recover normal function and replacement therapy can be withdrawn. When the lesion is found to be more diffuse (as happens in about 30 per cent of cases), then cure is not to be expected unless the pituitary is extirpated. There is a risk of pituitary damage even with selective microsurgery, but this may be as low as 5 per cent depending on the skill available. Similar results have been claimed for ^{90}Y implantation and proton beam irradiation; again the cure rate, extent of endocrine deficit, and complications of the procedure vary with the skill and experience of the centre. All these methods, however, may be considered broadly similar in their results: a failure to cure 10–30 per cent, and induction of endocrine deficit in about the same number if enthusiasm to cure promotes more invasive treatment.

The results of these methods do contrast, however, with those of external X-ray therapy; the best large series reported shows only a 25 per cent cure rate by external irradiation alone, and the response is slow, taking up to four years and requiring adrenolytic therapy meantime. This approach is more popular in the USA, perhaps because there is little risk of pituitary damage using conventional doses of about 4000 rad.

If treatment either by the pituitary or adrenal routes is satisfactory in Cushing's disease, most patients will lose their diabetes and after two years the mean blood pressure of such patients is reduced into the normal range. About three-quarters of patients will lose their hypertension. Osteoporosis does not heal in middle or late life after treatment of Cushing's disease, but the occurrence of fresh fractures is prevented. Any osteoporosis in children, however, tends to heal well. Muscle strength is always improved, and the oedema diminishes. The skin atrophy and muscle wasting reverse, except in the elderly where tissue repair is impaired. In children, normal growth and development is resumed.

Survival data are relatively limited, but indicate that after the first year after treatment (when excess deaths still occur though in small numbers), the survival of successfully treated patients with Cushing's disease is near-normal.

Removal of a primary *adrenal adenoma* will effect a cure, but the surgeon must take care to examine the non-adenomatous adrenal tissue for atrophy to confirm the diagnosis. Replacement steroids are required for 6 to 24 months after adrenal adenomectomy; the pituitary is profoundly suppressed and the only way of reactivating its ACTH production is by persistent attempts to wean the patient from replacement. With patience, by about two years the patient should have regained a good cortisol response to hypoglycaemia as well as to ACTH administration.

The results of removal of a primary adrenal adenoma are equivalent to those in successfully treated Cushing's disease.

The treatment of *adrenal carcinoma* is much less satisfactory, and is discussed in the section on adrenal tumours below. Most patients are dead in two years.

The management of the *ectopic ACTH syndrome* depends on whether the ACTH-secreting tumour can be found and removed. Many patients have been surgically cured of Cushing's syndrome due to benign appendicular or bronchial carcinoids or thymomas. At the opposite end of the scale the patient who presents with florid cortisol overproduction and widespread cancer is beyond much help, although his welfare may be improved by adrenolytic therapy (see below). It is almost always possible to control the cortisol overproduction with adrenolytic drugs, which greatly helps the patient. Quite startling improvements in muscle weakness, and relief of diabetes and hypertension occur very rapidly and may be maintained for long periods if the tumour itself permits continued life. In any patient in whom the tumour cannot be removed but appears to be going to run a benign course of more than six months, bilateral total adrenalectomy after a period of adrenolytic drugs to improve surgical fitness should be considered to improve the quality of the patient's life.

Adrenolytic drug therapy. The 11β-hydroxylase inhibitor *metyrapone* in a daily dose of 3–4.5 g is capable of curtailing cortisol production to acceptable levels in many cases of Cushing's syndrome. It has the disadvantages of causing nausea (which is improved by taking it with milk) and of having a short action so that it must be given four-hourly. Very high ACTH levels as in some ectopic cases often override the 11β-hydroxylase inhibition after some weeks or months; the response in adrenal carcinoma is very variable, but often useful. The main use of this drug alone is in Cushing's disease, either to improve the fitness of frail patients for operation or while awaiting remission after pituitary irradiation.

Aminoglutethimide inhibits the conversion of cholesterol to Δ5-pregnenolone, thus interfering with production of mineralocorticoids and androgens as well as cortisol. It is effective in a daily dose of 1.5–3 g, but this tends to produce unacceptable side-effects such as ataxia, profound lethargy or sedation, and rashes. Some groups have claimed good results from combinations of lower doses of both drugs, e.g. aminoglutethimide 250 mg eight-hourly plus metyrapone 500 mg four-hourly, with few side-effects. Indeed, so potent is this combination that it is usually necessary to give replacement fludrocortisone and dexamethasone (the latter chosen so that steroid assays may be followed). Such therapy is most useful in cortisol overproduction due to malignant lesions.

More recently the 3β-steroid dehydrogenase inhibitor trilostane has been introduced. This also inhibits all three major pathways of steroid biosynthesis. There are few side effects, but its effectiveness in Cushing's syndrome is quite unknown. Personal experience suggests it is very ineffective, if cortisol overproduction is more than mild.

o, p'-DDD is a selective adrenal poison, and unlike the reversible enzyme inhibitors described above, can cause adrenal atrophy or necrosis. Rather than in Cushing's disease, its main use has been in adrenal carcinoma. In daily doses up to 8 g, control of steroid overproduction and even regression of tumour metastases have been achieved. Improvement is usually not permanent, however, and fatigue, gastrointestinal side-effects, and rashes are prominent.

Adrenal tumours

Adrenocortical carcinoma. As well as causing Cushing's syndrome, this rare disease may present with virilization, associated or unassociated with features of cortisol excess. Hirsuties, clitoromegaly and loss of libido, deepening of the voice, and increased skin thickness are typical. There may be weight gain. Alternatively, and especially in the male, there may be malaise, weight loss, or even the appearance of metastases as presenting features without endocrine symptoms or signs. These tumours may be found as a symptomless mass in the abdomen.

As noted above, the hallmark of adrenal carcinoma is disordered steroid synthesis in large amounts, whether the products are biologically active or not. Elevated levels, in plasma or urine, of such steroids as dehydroepiandrosterone (DHEA), 11-deoxycortisol, testosterone, or cortisol may be sought. However the bulk of steroid synthesis is usually revealed by massive excretion of 17-oxo or 17-oxogenic steroids. The diagnosis is essentially radiological; the tumour mass may displace a kidney, as shown by pyelography, and will usually be evident on ultrasound examination, but selective arteriography will show the nature and site of the lesion (Fig. 5).

At surgery such tumours frequently show invasion of the renal veins, diaphragm, or liver. Metastases are commonly to the lung or spine. The tumours present late and are often large, weighing several kg. Even if complete removal is possible, metastases often become evident later. They are not very radiosensitive, although irradiation is useful for metastases in locations such as spine. The use of *o, p'*-DDD to control this disease is described above. The prognosis of adrenocortical carcinoma is very poor. Very few patients are alive at 5 years after diagnosis, and most are dead within 2 years.

Adrenocortical adenomas. Five per cent of routine necropsies show adrenal adenoma, presumably functionless in life. As well as the cortisol-secreting adenomas described above, mineralocorticoid-secreting adenomas occur. They give rise to primary hyperaldosterism (Conn's syndrome), which is described elsewhere (see page 13.278). Androgen-secreting adenomas are very uncommon. They present with hirsuties, clitoromegaly, voice deepening, some skin thickness increase, and (usually) menstrual disturbance. Urinary 17-oxosteroid excretion is increased and does not suppress normally with dexamethasone. The androgens produced are variable: weak androgens such as DHEA may be present in excess, but usually testosterone and androstenedione are elevated.

The differential diagnosis from ovarian tumour is difficult biochemically, but may be made on ultrasound or laparoscopy. Polycystic ovary disease usually causes less severe clinical abnormalities. Virilizing adrenal carcinoma tends to run a more aggressive course. The definitive pre-operative diagnosis is made by arteriography or venography; such adenomas may be as small as 2 cm. The prognosis after surgical removal is, of course, excellent.

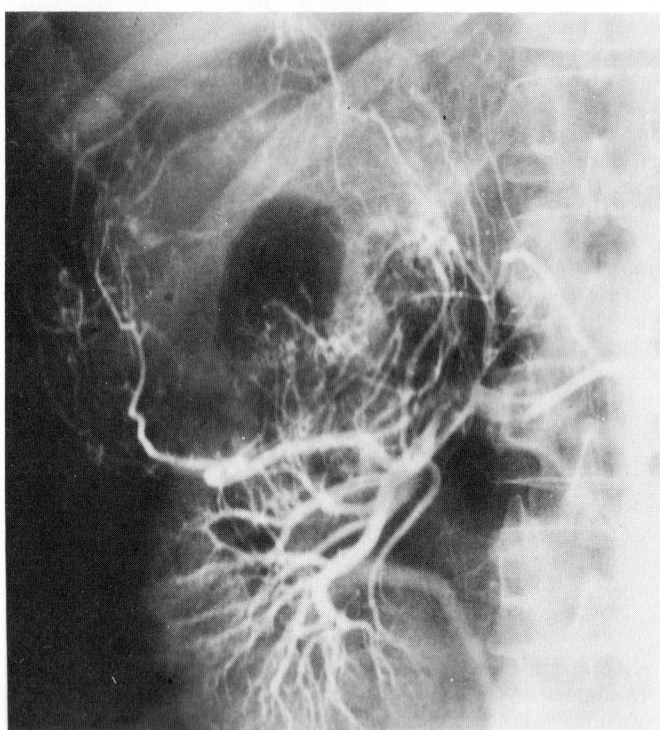

Fig. 5 Adrenal arteriogram in a patient with a right-sided adrenal carcinoma who presented with weakness and a mass in the flank thought clinically to be kidney. Note the ring of capsular vessels and the tumour 'blush'.

Adrenal medullary tumours. These are described elsewhere (see page 13.278).

Cortisol deficiency syndromes: Addison's disease

Aetiology

Primary hypoadrenalism (Addison's disease). This may be due to adrenal destruction by tuberculosis (formerly the commonest cause), metastatic carcinoma, infarction, amyloidosis, or auto-immune adrenalitis. As tuberculosis has become less common, auto-immune Addison's disease has emerged as the most usual cause of an uncommon condition. Unlike the total adrenal destruction (both medulla and cortex) formerly seen, auto-immune adrenal disease affects the cortex alone. The cortex shows atrophy with lymphocytic infiltration, and abnormal T-cell action against it has been shown. Circulating auto-antibodies against adrenal cortex are present in the great majority of women with Addison's disease, and over half the men. The antibodies are not present in tuberculous cases.

Infarction of the adrenal cortex is a not uncommon agonal event in dying patients. It has characteristically been identified in meningococcal septicaemia (the Waterhouse–Friedrichsen syndrome, 'adrenal apoplexy'). When cortisol levels have been measured in such patients in life, they have usually been appropriately elevated, and it is now thought that 'adrenal apoplexy' is no different in nature from other terminal adrenal infarction.

Although adrenal metastases are not uncommon at necropsy in cancer cases, it is uncommon for steroid deficiency to be recognized

in them before death. Rare causes of primary hypoadrenalism include Schilder's disease (hereditary leucodystrophy and adrenocortical atrophy) and Wolman's disease (adrenal insufficiency, hepatosplenomegaly and steatorrhoea with lipid storage) see Goldstein and Motulsky 1974, for further details).

Secondary hypoadrenalism (ACTH deficiency). This is most usually due to pharmacological steroid therapy, which is discussed on page 10.94. Otherwise it sometimes occurs in pituitary disease, especially after unselective pituitary destruction (see page 10.13). Spontaneous isolated ACTH deficiency is very rare.

Clinical features of adrenal insufficiency. The only clinical feature which distinguishes primary from secondary hypoadrenalism is pigmentation: in primary hypoadrenalism ACTH levels are very high with associated pigmentation possibly due to β-MSH, as described above. Unfortunately Addisonian pigmentation is often absent in auto-immune Addison's disease, being commoner in tuberculous cases. When present it is a very helpful sign. Characteristically it is seen in the palmar creases, other skin creases, exposed areas, scars, and inside the lips and cheeks. Just as commonly seen in Addison's disease (as in other auto-immune endocrinopathies) is patchy depigmentation (vitiligo), and if this is widespread, the remaining islands of normally-pigmented skin may give the impression of patches of pigmentation (see Section 20).

Other symptoms and signs are common to both primary and secondary hypoadrenalism. The commonest symptom of chronic cortisol insufficiency is weight loss. This is often associated with episodes of vomiting and diarrhoea. Non-specific abdominal pain, often severe and colicky, is a feature of these attacks, which may occur over a period of many months at intervals. Although the patient may be able to maintain work between attacks, malaise and loss of energy are typical complaints. Eventually these unexplained symptoms may lead to hospital admission, often with the patient shocked, hypotensive, and hyponatraemic (Addisonian crisis). Such crises are sometimes provoked by intercurrent disease or infections. Acute cortisol insufficiency is often associated with muscle cramps or myalgia, and with unexplained fever. Cortisol deficiency is a cause of spontaneous hypoglycaemia, though this is more likely to occur when ACTH deficiency is associated with growth hormone deficiency in hypopituitarism. Acute steroid insufficiency is marked by hypotension and shock; chronic insufficiency tends to cause postural hypotension with a fall in blood pressure on standing of 20 mmHg or more after a couple of minutes.

In secondary hypoadrenalism not due to exogenous steroid treatment there are usually associated features of failure of other pituitary hormones. Usually there is reproductive failure (whether due to hyperprolactinaemia or gonadotrophin failure) and loss of body hair, though this last does sometimes occur in post-menopausal females with Addison's disease due to a failure of adrenal androgens. If growth hormone deficiency is present, there may be skin thinning and the tendency to hypoglycaemia is accentuated. Secondary hypothyroidism is often a late feature of pituitary disease, in which reproductive failure (which is not a feature of Addison's disease) is the paramount early symptom.

Associations of Addison's disease. Organ-specific auto-immune disease seems to have a predilection for the endocrine system (Table 4). The commonest of these disorders is primary hypothyroidism with thyroid auto-antibodies (see page 10.40), and hypothyroidism is present in up to 10 per cent of patients with auto-immune Addison's disease. A word of caution is necessary, however, since it has recently been shown that low thyroxine in plasma with elevated TSH occurs frequently in Addison's disease and these changes reverse with treatment after some months: the mechanism is unknown. This makes it unwise to assume an Addisonian patient also has primary hypothyroidism until steroid replacement is complete and the presence of thyroid antibodies has been shown.

Other auto-immune associations are striking, and include insulin-dependent diabetes, premature menopause with ovarian

Table 4 Epidemiology of Addison's disease

Incidence*
    Tuberculous M:F 1.5:1   Prevalence 12/million
                        Death rate 0.7/million
    Auto-immune F:M 2.5:1   Prevalence 27/million
                        Death rate 0.7/million

Non-tuberculous presumed autoimmune
    Clinical associations
        Diabetes about 15%
        Hypothyroid about 10%
        Pernicious anaemia about 10%
        Atrophic gastritis about 10%
        Hypoparathyroidism about 5%
        Cutaneous moniliasis about 5%
        Premature menopause about 5%
    Antibodies present to (approximately)
        Adrenal: female   80%; male 10–20%
        Thyroid tanned rbc   25%
        Thyroid microsomal   45%   } some will be present in
        Parietal cell   30%   } two-thirds of all patients
        Intrinsic factor   10%
    Adrenal antibodies also found in absence of Addison's disease
        Mainly in Hashimoto's disease, but even then < 5%
        Very rare in diabetes, pernicious anaemia, etc.

* In 1960; tuberculous probably since declined
From Burke (1973)

auto-antibodies, primary hypoparathyroidism, gastric parietal cell antibodies and pernicious anaemia, vitiligo (already referred to), alopecia, and less commonly mucocutaneous candidiasis (Table 4).

Laboratory investigations in hypoadrenalism. A clue to the presence of hypoadrenalism may be found from plasma electrolyte estimations, the characteristic abnormalities being hyponatraemia, hyperkalaemia, and elevation of the blood urea. Of these, the most constant is the last, reaching perhaps 8–15 mmol/l, the sodium and potassium abnormalities being more marked in the patient with hypoadrenal crisis. These changes are found both in primary hypoadrenalism, where aldosterone deficiency and cortisol deficiency may coexist, and also in secondary hypoadrenalism with pure cortisol insufficiency. Anaemia, eosinophilia, and a raised ESR may be present as non-specific abnormalities.

Cortisol measurements give variable results and must be carried out under defined conditions. Urinary cortisol assays are of no help in diagnosis as a rule, since the lower normal limit of urinary cortisol excretion approaches the detection limit of standard assays and some urinary cortisol is often detectable in hypoadrenalism. Resting plasma cortisol levels are also often in the low-normal range in hypoadrenalism, especially at night when the normal range approaches the limit of detection by routine methods. The main application of an isolated plasma cortisol estimation in hypoadrenalism is in the acutely ill patient in whom hypoadrenalism appears possible. A sample for cortisol should always be drawn from such patients before any treatment is given. This is for later analysis which need not delay therapy based on clinical judgment, but a subsequent result from the laboratory over 600 nmol/l disproves hypoadrenalism and indicates a pituitary-adrenal response that is appropriate to acute illness. A low or normal result does not prove or disprove adrenal insufficiency.

The proof of primary adrenal insufficiency is by two principal methods. The more elegant is to show that an estimation of plasma ACTH (which requires special precautions and facilities) gives an elevated result which is disproportionately high compared with a simultaneous plasma cortisol result which is low or normal. Typical ACTH values in Addisonian patients are shown in Fig. 6. The second and usually more convenient method is to simulate the adrenal: the synthetic 1-24 N-terminal (bioactive) sequence of ACTH is used (tetracosactrin). Intramuscular injection of 250 µg of tetracosactrin in normal subjects results in plasma cortisol concen-

tration rising 45 minutes later to 600 nmol/l, and values less than this are consistent with primary or secondary hypoadrenalism. The test may be carried out in patients who are already under treatment with steroids for suspected hypoadrenalism, provided such treatment has been given for three weeks or less and the patient is changed to dexamethasone treatment 48 hours in advance of the stimulation test. A more sensitive variant of this test is to give 2 mg of depot tetracosactrin intramuscularly and draw samples for plasma cortisol at four hours and 24 hours. Patients with normal adrenal function reach a plasma cortisol concentration of 1000 nmol/l by four hours; patients with secondary hypoadrenalism show a higher value at 24 hours than at four hours, due to recruitment of adrenal function by the continued supply of tetracosactrin; patients with primary hypoadrenalism show no response at either time, nor do they respond to further injections which in secondary hypoadrenalism produce progressive increments in plasma cortisol over several days.

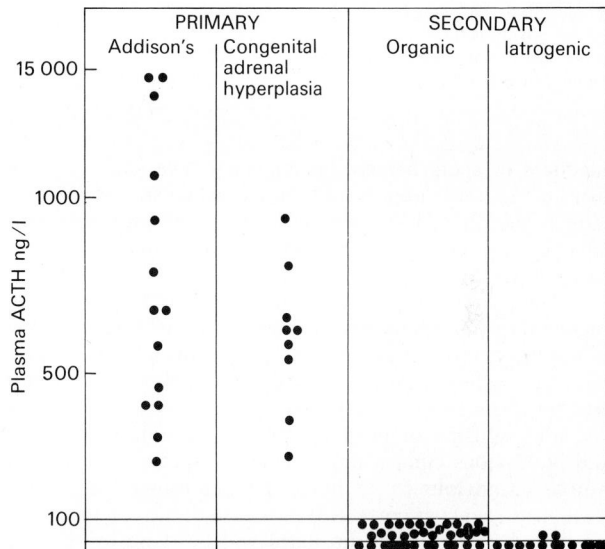

Fig. 6 Morning N-terminal immunoreactive ACTH values in patients with hypoadrenalism. The normal range is indicated by the horizontal lines. (Reproduced by courtesy of Professor L. H. Rees.)

In auto-immune Addison's disease adrenal auto-antibodies are usually demonstrable, especially in females. In tuberculous Addison's disease adrenal calcification may be seen on X-ray. A useful test in the acutely ill patient suspected of adrenal insufficiency is the ECG. This often shows S–T segment flattening or low voltage; the changes are non-specific (for example being seen also in hypothyroidism) but in hypoadrenalism they specifically revert to normal within a few hours of cortisol adminstration. As already emphasized, such patients should have blood drawn for later cortisol assay.

Hypoadrenalism: differential diagnosis (Table 5). Weight loss, hypotension, and some pigmentation are common in terminal illness and in debilitating diseases such as cancer, tuberculosis, salt-losing chronic renal failure, anorexia nervosa, and malnutrition, and in severe gastrointestinal disease and malabsorption. If the primary diagnosis is unrecognized, such patients may be suspected of adrenal failure. Only a proper test, e.g. stimulation with tetracosactrin, can distinguish the normal adrenal reserve such patients possess, since resting urinary and plasma hormone assays may be subnormal or otherwise disturbed in those conditions. The differential diagnosis from pituitary failure is mentioned above. Confusion with congenital enzyme defects of cortisol synthesis (congenital adrenal hyperplasia) is unlikely, since, if these result in cortisol insufficiency, they usually do so in infancy when Addison's disease is rare.

Table 5 Differential diagnosis of Addison's disease

Pigmentation and/or gastrointestinal symptoms; especially weight loss
   Steatorrhoea and malabsorption
   Crohn's disease
   Intestinal polyposis
   Cirrhosis of liver
   Anorexia nervosa
   Thyrotoxicosis
   Malnutrition
Other wasting disorders with or without pigmentation and often with
hyponatraemia
   Tuberculosis
   Chronic renal failure, especially salt-losing
   Aleukaemic leukaemia
   Tumours with ectopic vasopressin production
Skin disorders
   Dermatomyositis
   Acanthosis nigricans
   Scleroderma
Other diseases
   Haemochromatosis
   Heavy metal poisoning (e.g. silver)
   Drugs: atabrine, busulphan

Treatment of acute adrenal insufficiency. The shocked patient requires circulatory support and normal saline should be infused initially at the rate of 1 litre within the first hour, and thereafter as dictated by the patient's condition. Blood should be drawn for glucose analysis and for later plasma cortisol assay. Hypoglycaemia should be corrected by glucose infusion. Cortisol hemisuccinate or cortisol sodium phosphate 100 mg should be given intravenously, or intramuscularly if the intravenous route is impracticable. Insoluble steroid acetates, especially cortisone acetate, should not be used. Thereafter 200 mg of cortisol should be given in the next 24 hours by intravenous infusion or in divided doses intramuscularly. There should be obvious clinical improvement, especially in the blood pressure, within four to six hours if the presumed diagnosis of cortisol insufficiency is correct. If the cause of the collapse is other than adrenal insufficiency, no harm will be done by the above treatment, provided that no delay in recognition of septicaemia, haemorrhage, or other causes has occurred.

In acute adrenal insufficiency treated as above, 100 mg cortisol in divided doses orally, intramuscularly, or intravenously should suffice in each of the second and third 24 hours. Thereafter the patient should be maintained on replacement therapy (see below). If no other cause for the collapse is found, the diagnosis of acute insufficiency is at this stage still uncertain, and steps must be taken to confirm it during convalescence for it implies lifelong therapy. At a convenient point, the patient's treatment should be changed to dexamethasone 0.5 mg twice daily for 48 hours; on the second day any previously administered cortisol will have been metabolized and the dexamethasone does not register in plasma cortisol assays so that a tetracosactrin stimulation test should then be carried out. Positive proof of primary adrenal insufficiency is afforded by a failure of plasma cortisol to respond to prolonged tetracosactrin stimulation over four to six days, by injection of 2 mg depot tetracosactrin on alternate days with daily plasma cortisol samples.

Replacement steroid therapy. There is a difference in need between patients with primary hypoadrenalism (Addison's disease or adrenalectomy) who lack both cortisol and aldosterone, and patients with secondary hypoadrenalism (ACTH lack) who are cortisol deficient but maintain normal mineralocorticoid function.

In primary hypoadrenalism both cortisol and aldosterone replacement must therefore be provided. The usual daily dose of glucocorticoid required is 30 mg of cortisol by mouth (more or less equal to daily normal production), and it is traditional (though not necessary) to mimic the normal daily cortisol rhythm by giving 20 mg in the morning and 10 mg in the evening. Few patients require

more or less cortisol than this; occasionally patients with a small requirement appear Cushingoid unless the dose is reduced to 20 mg daily, and in some patients pigmentation persists unless 40 mg daily is given. If more than this appears to be needed, then either the diagnosis is wrong or there is a problem with steroid absorption. Cortisone acetate is insoluble and has to be converted to cortisol to become active; its use is now of historic interest. Some physicians use prednisone or prednisolone (which bear the same molecular relationships to each other as cortisone and cortisol); the lack of mineralocorticoid effect of these synthetic steroids is a slight disadvantage in primary hypoadrenalism. Similar clinical effects can be expected from the following doses of these various steroids: cortisone acetate 25 mg, cortisol 20 mg, prednisolone 5 mg, dexamethasone 0.5 mg. Mineralocorticoid replacement with aldosterone itself is impracticable as it is not absorbed; instead 9α-fluorocortisol (fludrocortisone) is used. An average daily need is 0.1 mg, but this varies: the dose may be adjusted on the lying and standing blood pressures, or with greater sophistication by measuring plasma renin which should be suppressed into the normal range. Formerly treatment was by periodic injection of deoxycorticosterone acetate (DOCA); this is now of historical interest only.

Patients on such replacement should be advised to double the daily dose of glucocorticoid in the event of fever of 38 °C or more, intercurrent infection, accident and so forth. They should carry a steroid-dependency card or bracelet. In the event of vomiting for 24 hours, they should receive their cortisol parenterally. There is no need to alter the dose of replacement in pregnancy, although it is traditional to increase the dose temporarily during parturition. For surgical operations, such patients should be treated as for acute adrenal insufficiency described above.

Patients with secondary hypoadrenalism requiring only glucocorticoid replacement may be treated with cortisol alone (20 mg morning, 10 mg evening) or with equivalent doses of prednisolone (5 mg morning, 2.5 mg evening). The same precautions for vomiting, intercurrent illness, and surgery apply. Higher doses than these are virtually never needed, and if they appear to be required some other explanation for the symptoms should be sought.

Congenital adrenal hyperplasia ('adrenogenital syndrome')

The out-of-date term 'adrenogenital syndrome' will not be referred to further, as it was an umbrella term which included congenital adrenal hyperplasia and other abnormalities of the adrenal affecting the genitalia.

Congenital adrenal hyperplasia (CAH) is a complex family of congenital disorders of adrenal steroid-synthesizing enzymes, with a wide spectrum of clinical presentation varying from neonatal collapse through intersex, to presentation in the adult with sex-hormone disorder. The essential features common to all varieties of CAH are defects (often partial) in cortisol biosynthesis with resulting elevated ACTH levels and consequent disorders in production of other adrenal steroids, notably androgens and mineralocorticoids. A few cases, however, have a defect on the aldosterone pathway alone, with resulting high renin levels.

Aetiology. Congenital adrenal hyperplasias are due to inheritance of a recessive gene. The prevalence of this gene in the population has been estimated to be as high as 1 per cent, and if this is so, the rarity of the resulting disease (variously estimated between 1 in 5000 and 1 in 50 000 live births) must mean that the gene has poor penetrance, although it appears to be reinforced by consanguinity. It may bear a relationship to polycystic ovary syndrome or idiopathic hirsuties, as it has been proposed that adults with these conditions suffer from a partial form of one or more of the enzyme defects. Firm proof of this relationship is not available.

The commoner enzyme defects responsible for CAH are shown in Fig. 7. The most frequent is the *21-hydroxylase defect*. This causes impairment of both cortisol and aldosterone biosynthesis.

The cortisol deficiency results in elevated ACTH levels, which in turn cause excess androgen production by stimulation of the left-hand pathways. In mild cases, with a partial defect, resting cortisol production may be compensated back to normal by the elevated ACTH; and aldosterone may also be normal or even raised. Clinically, the androgen excess is the predominant feature and the presentation ranges from virilization at birth or later on (even into adult life) to isosexual precocity in the male. In some infants with a mild 21-hydroxylase defect there is also a temporary tendency to salt loss and hyponatraemia which may require fludrocortisone and salt treatment for the first year of life. The obvious explanation for this, that such children are aldosterone-deficient, proves to be incorrect. Among a number of possible explanations for it, the one currently favoured is that elevated levels of progesterone and 17α-hydroxyprogesterone (17α-OHP), which are aldosterone antagonists, are responsible for the salt loss.

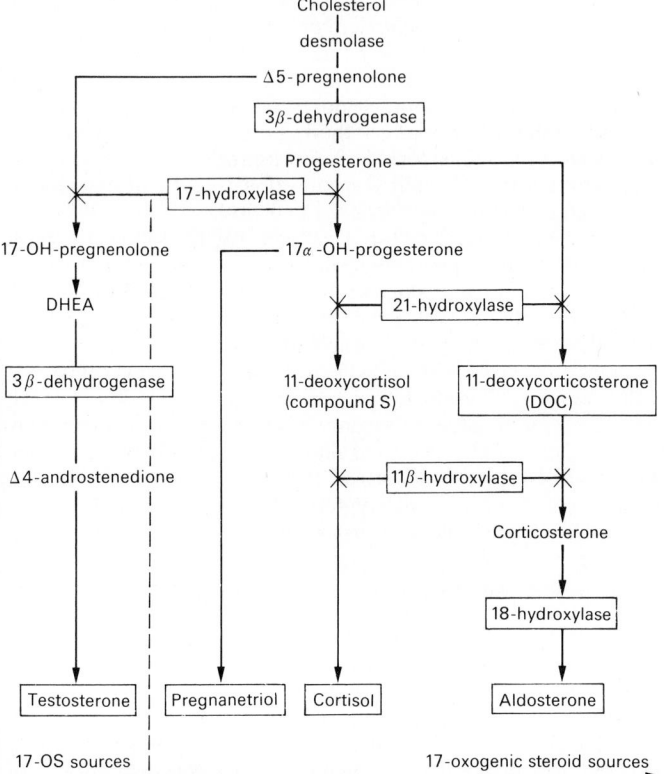

Fig. 7 The principal steroid biosynthetic pathways affected by enzyme defects in congenital adrenal hyperplasia.

In severer cases of 21-hydroxylase defect, there is salt loss in neonatal life. In some this is due to aldosterone deficiency, but in others aldosterone levels are normal or raised. Cortisol-deficient adrenal crisis is unusual, but acute hyponatraemic collapse may be provoked by ACTH administration, perhaps again because of the resulting increased 17α-OHP. Clearly the biochemistry of a 21-hydroxylase defect is variable, but the hallmarks are over-production of progesterone, 17α-OHP and its metabolite pregnantriol and various 17-oxosteroids such as DHEA. Usually therefore both 17-oxosteroid and 17-oxogenic steroid excretions are raised.

A less common defect affecting the same steroid pathways is an *11β-hydroxylase defect*. The same overproduction of 17α-OHP and of androgens occurs, so that these patients posses the genital abnormalities of 21-hydroxylase defect; but in addition they are hypertensive (see page 13.278). The hypertension is ascribed to accumulation of the precursor 11-deoxycorticosterone (DOC) which has mineralocorticoid and hypertensive activity. The enzyme defect causes accumulation of 11-deoxycortisol and the excretion of

this steroid is raised; as it is a 17-oxogenic steroid, the excretion of both 17-OGS and 17-OS is raised.

A rare defect is that of *18-hydroxylase*; in this cortisol production is unimpaired so that neither ACTH levels nor androgens are elevated. Aldosterone production is impaired, and so the essential features are salt loss, elevated plasma renin, and the absence of genital abnormality. 17-OS and 17-OGS may be normal.

17-hydroxylase deficiency has been described; it affects several steroid pathways (Fig. 7) and it is also present in the ovary. In the male, androgen synthesis does not proceed to the fully biologically-effective androgens, and there may be ambiguous genitalia. In the female, these features are not apparent until puberty when the presentation is with primary amenorrhoea and lack of sexual development. In both sexes, hypokalaemia and hypertension are probably due to excess mineralocorticoid production. 17α-OHP is not elevated.

A few cases of *3β-hydroxysteroid dehydrogenase defect* have been reported. Cortisol synthesis is defective and ACTH levels high, resulting in the production of DHEA and other adrenal androgens behind the block. There are weak androgens which do not produce full biological effect, but are measurable as urinary 17-oxosteroids. The patients are severely cortisol and aldosterone-deficient and hence are salt losers, prone to death in infancy. The lack of effective androgens leads to pseudohermaphroditism in affected male infants. Expected urinary steroid results are elevated 17-oxosteroids and normal 17-oxogenic steroids.

Desmolase deficiency, which also affects the ovary and testis, is rarely compatible with life and is a rare cause of neonatal death. The steroid deficiency affects all pathways. All appear phenotypic females, due to androgen lack in affected male fetuses. At necropsy the adrenal cortex is stuffed with accumulated cholesterol ('lipoid hyperplasia').

A number of cases with other or partial defects have been reported, and it is clear that 'congenital adrenal hyperplasia' is very heterogenous. Most patients, however, if treated have a normal life expectancy, and so it is very important to be able to recognize the presence of an adrenal enzyme defect.

Clinical features. Certain categories of infants can be regarded as more liable to have enzyme defects than others, and these should be observed carefully after birth. Included are those with a family history of abnormal genitalia, including cryptorchidism and hypospadias; those with a family history of neonatal deaths; perhaps those with a parental or sibling history of hirsuties who might be heterozygotes; and of course those infants with siblings affected by CAH. Infants born with the slightest ambiguity of genitalia or with cryptorchidism or hypospadias should be carefully followed and tested: most cases of CAH which are diagnosed late show such abnormalities which were overlooked in infancy.

As seen above the incidence of CAH is a matter of dispute but it may be estimated at perhaps 1 in 10 000 live births. This is half as common as phenylketonuria, which is considered worth screening for. Certainly at the least, infants with ambiguous genitalia or cryptorchidism should have the appropriate steroid assays performed in the second week of life, and the chromosomal sex should be determined. 46 XX chromosome constitution, or the presence of a Barr body in a buccal smear, make congenital adrenal hyperplasia likely in such cases.

In the neonatal period, symptoms to alert the paediatrician to think of this group of conditions include failure to gain weight, and lack of feeding enthusiasm. Urinary salt loss can usually be shown before the plasma sodium falls. By the time hyponatraemia has occurred, the infant may well be vomiting, have diarrhoea, acidosis, hyperkalaemia, and elevated blood urea. Severe mineralo-corticoid or cortisol deficiency may present as neonatal hypoglycaemia.

In later life the diagnosis usually presents with less urgency. In childhood it may be with cryptorchidism, especially if hypospadias is present; or with clitoromegaly and pubic hair development in the female, or isosexual precocity in the male. In virilized infants or children the bone age will be advanced. In the absence of such features presentation with salt loss after the first year of life is unusual. Later still, presentation may be with primary amenorrhoea with or without hirsuties or even frankly masculinizing features such as clitoromegaly. To the adult endocrinologist cases sometimes present with hirsuties or later masculinizing features, and the diagnosis has been substantiated in patients as old as 65 years; these are partial enzyme defects and often can be proved only on biochemical findings.

Finally, the hypertensive types should be remembered as presenting at any age (though usually in childhood) with hypertension and hypokalaemia, and either some degree of intersex or failure of sexual development, depending on the defect. Some features of the differential diagnosis are shown in Table 6.

Table 6 Differential diagnosis of congenital adrenal hyperplasia

Presentation	Differential diagnosis
Neonatal salt-losing state	pyloric stenosis gastroenteritis
Female infants	maternal ingestion of androgens, or progestogens which can be converted to androgens genetic causes of intersex male pseudohermaphroditism testicular feminization
Female children	adrenal tumours ovarian tumours
Male children	any cause of precocious puberty and rapid growth
Adults: with amenorrhoea with hirsuties, etc. with cortisol deficiency	any cause of primary amenorrhoea polycystic ovaries adrenal tumours ovarian tumours Cushing's syndrome Addison's disease hypopituitarism

From Burke (1973)

Laboratory diagnosis. In infancy the first biochemical information obtained may be a urinary sodium excretion which is inappropriate in that it exceeds intake; urinary sodium concentrations over 50 mmol/l in the first days of life are consistent with urinary salt loss. Salt-losing or hyponatraemic infants should have their 24-hour excretion of 17-oxogenic steroids measured, and time for this can be bought by salt therapy. Interpretation of urinary steroids in the first four to seven days of life is difficult as considerable physiological changes occur in the first week of life. A plasma cortisol assay is useful in some types, though a normal result is unhelpful; it must, however, be measured in hypoglycaemic infants. Where suspicion of an enzyme defect is high, plasma ACTH assay is most valuable, for it is likely to be inappropriately elevated compared with a normal or low result for a simultaneous determination of plasma cortisol. In certain types 17α-hydroxyprogesterone assay will give an abnormally high result.

These tests are generally available but may not identify the exact enzyme defect. To do this it may be necessary later to identify the concentrations of individual steroids and precursors by gas-liquid chromatography or specific radio-immunoassays. The important measures in the infant, however, are to identify salt loss and cortisol insufficiency if present. The investigation of androgen excess or deficiency is a little less urgent, although advanced bone age with its implications for future development makes early diagnosis and complete therapy highly desirable. The need for determination of chromosomal sex has already been referred to.

In older children and in adults the same principles apply. Suitable screening tests are measurement of urinary 17-oxo and 17-oxogenic steroids and pregnantriol, plasma testosterone, plasma 17α-hydroxyprogesterone, and the plasma cortisol response to tetracosactrin. Abnormalities in these tests suggest the need for determination of individual steroids (for example deoxycorticosterone, 11-deoxycortisol, DHEA) appropriate to the suspected defect. Information on the interpretation of different patterns in relation to the clinical features is given in the references listed below.

Treatment. Treatment of salt loss in infancy requires appropriate saline infusion or addition of salt to the feed, and fludrocortisone 0.05 mg daily. If vomiting prevents the latter, deoxycorticosterone acetate 0.5–1.0 mg may be injected intramuscularly. Cortisol, in doses as high as 20–30 mg/day for a few days, is usually only needed in babies who have hypoglycaemia or do not respond quickly to saline and mineralocorticoid therapy. It will, however, be introduced when the results of the initial steroid assays are available, if they show cortisol deficiency either directly or indirectly by elevated 17-oxosteroid excretion (implying high ACTH levels). As with Addison's disease, cortisone replacement is out of date and cortisol should be used; suitable doses for different ages are given in paediatric reference works. Synthetic glucocorticoids such as dexamethasone or prednisolone are not appropriate in infancy and childhood because of their disproportionately greater effects on growth and bone development than cortisol.

After the first weeks of life, treatment has the following objectives: replacement of cortisol insufficiency; replacement of mineralocorticoid to prevent salt loss; suppression of ACTH to relieve androgen overproduction and so prevent overadvancement of bone age with its implication of eventual growth stunting, and to prevent progression of virilization or male precocity; suppression of ACTH with excess DOC production in certain cases, to allow reversal of the hypertension; allow emergence of normal gonadotrophin function at puberty; and above all to allow normal growth, which will be suppressed by excessive cortisol therapy. In addition, intersex, genital abnormalities, and cryptorchidism require surgical treatment. This formidable task list requires considerable skill and experience to accomplish. Accurate measurement of growth at frequent intervals is necessary, with repeated bone age assessments. Mineralocorticoid replacement is adjusted on blood pressure and urinary salt excretion, and in some centres plasma renin assays are used to test adequacy of replacement. Cortisol replacement is given in sufficient quantity, but no more, to suppress ACTH excess. As the suppressive effect of each dose is transient, isolated ACTH assays are of limited help, and the dose is adjusted to bring elevated 17-oxosteroid excretion toward the upper limit of normal; no attempt should be made to suppress 17-OS completely, as the dose will then be too high with resulting growth impairment. The best suppression of ACTH is achieved by spreading the daily dose throughout the 24 hours, and the last dose at night should be given as late as possible.

In the adult female, a good guide to cortisol replacement is to give the minimum dose which will maintain menstruation with ovulation. Otherwise, adults of both sexes require replacement as for Addison's disease if they are salt-losers, cortisol alone if not, and fludrocortisone alone in the case of 18-hydroxylase defect. Precautions for surgery and stress are as in other forms of hypoadrenalism.

Surgical correction of genital abnormalities often requires more than one stage. Clitoral reduction is deferred until genital growth allows determination of the correct eventual size, but correction of hypospadias or labial fusion is performed earlier; vaginoplasty may be required. Occasionally a severely affected female with unrecognized CAH may be reared as a boy, and there may be real difficulty in deciding which phenotypic sex it is appropriate to achieve. But if the case is diagnosed early and treated correctly, normal growth, reproductive function, and life span should be realized.

References

Brook, C. G. D., Zachmann, M., Prader, A., and Mürset, G. (1974). Experience with longterm therapy in congenital adrenal hyperplasia. *J. Pediat.* **85**, 12.

Burke, C. W. (1978). Disorders of cortisol production: diagnostic and therapeutic progress. In *Recent advances in endocrinology and metabolism* (ed. J. L. H. O'Riordan), 61. Churchill Livingstone, Edinburgh.

Goldstein, J. L. and Motulsky, A. G. (1974). Genetics and endocrinology. In *Textbook of endocrinology*, 5th edn. (ed. R. H. Williams), 1017. W. B. Saunders, Philadelphia.

Hughes, I. A. and Davies, P. A. (1980). Neonatal endocrine and metabolic emergencies. *Clins Endocr. Metab.* **9**, 595.

Hung, W., August, G. P., and Glasgow, A. M. (1978). *Paediatric endocrinology*. Henry Kimpton Publishers, London.

Hutter, A. M. and Kayhoe, D. E. (1966). Adrenal cortical carcinoma. *Am. J. Med.* **41**, 572, 581.

Irvine, W. J. and Barnes, E. W. (1972). *Clins Endocr. Metab.* **1**, 549.

Janne, O., Perheentupa, J., Vinikka, L., and Vinko, R. (1975). Plasma pregnenolone, progesterone, 17-hydroxyprogesterone, testosterone and 5α-dihydrotestosterone in different types of congenital adrenal hyperplasia. *Clin. Endocr.* **4**, 39.

Liddle, G. W. (1974). The adrenals. In *Textbook of endocrinology*, 5th edn. (ed. R. H. Williams), 254. W. B. Saunders, Philadelphia.

Lipsett, M. B., Hertz, R., and Ross, G. T. (1963). Adrenocortical carcinoma. *Am. J. Med.* **35**, 374.

Rees, L. H. and Radcliffe, J. G. (1974). Ectopic hormone production by non-endocrine tumours. *Clin. Endocr.* **3**, 263.

Salassa, R. M., Kearns, T. P., Kernohan, J. W., Sprague, R. F., and MacCarty, C. S. (1959). Pituitary tumours in patients with Cushing's syndrome. *J. clin. Endocr. Metab.* **19**, 1523.

Disorders of the reproductive systems

D. R. London

THE MALE

Introduction. The testis has two functions, the production of spermatozoa and the elaboration of hormones (Fig. 1). The former happens in the seminiferous tubules while the latter are synthesized principally by the Leydig cells. It takes approximately 70 days for the stem cells to develop into mature spermatozoa. This process is controlled by follicle stimulating hormone (FSH) and testosterone formed both by the Leydig cells and by the Sertoli cells, which are non-germinal cells within the seminiferous tubules and which probably have a nutrient function for spermatogenesis. FSH is under feedback control from the testis possibly via a non-steroidal substance produced by the Sertoli cells, termed 'inhibin'. Luteinizing hormone (LH) from the pituitary gland regulates the secretion of testosterone and other steroids and itself forms part of a negative feedback loop with the endocrine products of the Leydig cells. The synthesis and secretion of both gonadotrophins are controlled by gonadotrophin releasing hormone (GnRH, or LHRH or FSH/LHRH) produced within the hypothalamus and secreted into the hypothalamic–hypophyseal portal system. The mature sperms pass via the epididymis and vas deferens to the seminal vesicles where they are stored. The production of the seminal fluid in which the sperms are bathed occurs in the seminal vesicles and is controlled by androgens.

The principal androgen secreted by the testis is testosterone. This circulates in the blood stream largely bound to a protein, sex hormone binding globulin (SHBG), as an inactive complex, which is in equilibrium with an active, unbound fraction. The concentration of SHBG is controlled by the androgen/oestrogen ratio with the former lowering and the latter raising SHBG levels. The unbound (or 'free') hormone is taken up by target tissue where it can be enzymatically converted to dihydrotestosterone (DHT) which in turn binds to an intracellular receptor protein. This intracellular protein also binds testosterone. The steroid protein complex is then translocated into the nucleus where it exerts its biological effects; these are set out in Table 1.

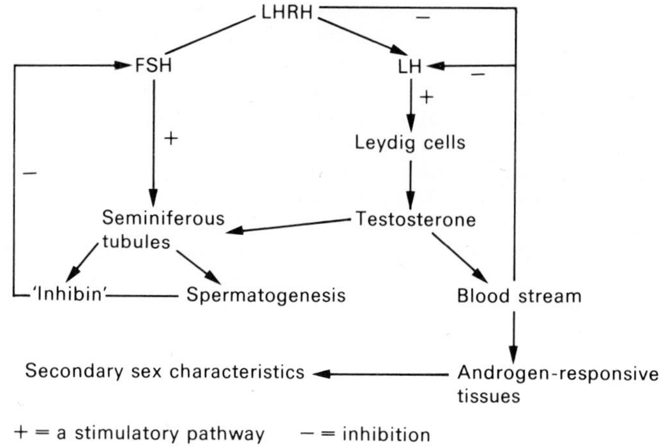

Table 1 Physiological effects of androgens

Growth and development of skeleton
Development of muscle
Growth of beard, pubic, axillary, body, and limb hair
Deepening of the voice
Frontotemporal balding
Enlargement of the phallus and (in the male), testes and scrotum with rugosity of the scrotum

Infertility

An abnormality in the male can be defined in a third of couples presenting with infertility. Often a seminal analysis with abnormal results is the reason for referral, since it is now common practice for gynaecologists to obtain a specimen of semen from the male partner during the initial assessment of a sterility problem. Indeed it cannot be stressed too strongly that it is the couple and not the individual that presents the problem, although on full investigation, it may be either the male or the female wherein an abnormality is found. Not infrequently, however, it is in both.

Once the male has been shown to be abnormal, he should be clinically assessed by history and examination with further investigations performed only when necessary.

Spermatogenesis. The formation of the male gamete from germ cell to mature spermatozoon takes approximately 70 days and procedes within the confines of the seminiferous tubules. These comprise more than 90 per cent of the bulk of the normal testis. Maturation of the sperm is controlled by hormones as well as by cytogenetic activities. Of the former, FSH and testosterone are of particular importance to the clinician. FSH acts mainly on the seminiferous tubules. These secrete 'inhibin' which controls FSH secretion through a negative feedback loop, so that severe deficiencies of spermatogenesis are reflected in elevated blood levels of FSH. Testosterone is also required for spermatogenesis, although small amounts may be sufficient since states of partial androgen

Fig. 1 The pathways for the hormonal control of reproductive function in the male together with the tissues involved.

deficiency can in some very rare instances—'the fertile eunuch syndrome' (see below)—be associated with relatively adequate spermatogenesis.

Genetic factors also control spermatogenesis, so that translocations of autosomal and sex chromosomes in the germinal tissue, abnormal association of sex chromosomes during meiosis, and probably, meiotic mutation can also be responsible for otherwise inexplicable oligo- or azoospermia. Additionally, the easily identifiable abnormalities of the sex chromosomes in somatic cells, as described in the relevant sections below, can also give rise to infertility.

History. Specific questions additional to those normally listed in a general enquiry should be asked. These are listed in Table 2. Enquiry

Table 2 Clinical assessment of the infertile man

History
  Frequency and success of intercourse
  Use of lubricants
  Urethral discharge and frequency of micturition
  Present or past pain or swelling of testes
  Trauma (including surgery) to testes or inguinal region
  Sense of smell
  Result of investigation of female partner

Examination
  Position, size, and consistency of testes and epididymis
  Penis and external urethral meatus
  Secondary sexual characteristics
  Spermatic cords (with patient standing and performing a Valsalva
    manoeuvre)
  Prostatic and seminal vesicles (if suspicion of genital infection)

about the details of intercourse will reveal if insemination is satisfactory, whether orgasm is achieved, and whether there is an ejaculate. Very infrequent intercourse reduces the chances of conception. Orgasm without emission may indicate retrograde ejaculation into the bladder. Use of lubricants to facilitate penetration may provide a clue to the cause of infertility since some jellies are spermicidal. The other questions will help in assigning one or other of the listed causes (Table 3) affecting the testes or the passage of sperms into the ejaculate. An absent or diminished sense of smell suggests a diagnosis of Kallman's syndrome with its associated gonadotrophin deficiency. Query about the female partner will reveal whether she also requires help and whether her problems are

Table 3 Causes of male infertility

Abnormalities of the generative organs
  Commoner
    Idiopathic
    Varicocele
    Obstruction to epididymis or vas
    Local infection
    Cryptorchidism
    Testicular trauma or torsion
  Rarer
    Chronic disease
    Immunological
    Drugs
    Irradiation
    Industrial hazards
    Kartagener's syndrome
    Dystrophia myotonica
Abnormalities of intercourse
  Infrequency of intercourse
  Use of spermicidal lubricants
  Retrograde ejaculation
  Hypospadias

such as to make diagnostic and therapeutic pursuit of the male an unnecessary interference.

Examination. Particular features relevant to this problem are given in Table 2. Attention should be paid to the development of the secondary sexual characteristics, the size of the penis, whether or not hypospadias is present, and the position, consistency and volume of the testes, the latter measured with the Prader orchidometer. Since so much of the bulk of the testes is made up of germinal tissue, small soft gonads are an index of defective spermatogenesis. The spermatic cords should be carefully palpated with the patient lying down and again standing while performing a Valsalva manoeuvre in order to detect the presence of a varicocele, or less commonly, absence of the vas.

Investigations. Seminal analysis is the principle test for assessing the 'male factor' in infertility. This should be performed on at least three occasions with an interval of at least one week between each specimen and following at least three days abstinence from sexual activity. The semen should be obtained by masturbation into a warm clean glass receptacle and examined by the laboratory within two hours of production. The important indices are volume of ejaculate, sperm density, motility, morphology, and continued viability. The semen can be graded as to likelihood of fertility. If it appears completely normal by stringent criteria—i.e. a volume of greater than 2 ml with a sperm density greater than 40 million of which 60 per cent are normally formed and are motile—post-coital testing and mucus penetration can be assessed, and sperm antibodies measured.

Should there be any suspicion of an endocrinopathy, the appropriate hormonal measurements should be performed (see below). Other specific tests may be done as indicated in subsequent paragraphs.

Causes. Unfortunately, it is most unusual to find a remediable cause of infertility in the male. The largest single group consists of patients in whom no clear diagnosis can be found despite careful history, clinical examination, and investigation. Even when pathology can be identified, it is the exception to find something amenable to treatment. The conditions listed in Table 3 should all be considered as, occasionally, a simple measure like the abandoning of a spermicidal lubricant or the eradication of a prostatitis can have a gratifying outcome. On the other hand, the identification of, say, Kartagener's syndrome (see Section 15) or congenital absence of the vas is of academic interest only since there is no treatment for either. Moreover, when treatment is undertaken its effectiveness must be judged against the fact that the partners of 20 per cent or so of patients with oligospermia will become pregnant within a year even without treatment. The more important causes are discussed in detail below.

Varicocele. The commonest identifiable condition is varicocele. It is found in a third of infertile men compared with an incidence of one in ten in an apparently normal population. However, in half of the latter some seminal abnormality may be apparent. The mechanisms by which spermatogenesis is affected remain unclear. Two theories, based on observation, prevail. The first is that there is a reflux of 'toxins' down the spermatic vein into the testes, the second that the increased scrotal temperature which has been noted is harmful. Usually, the varicocele is left-sided and affects the right as well as the left testis through the rich venous anastomoses that link the two sides of the scrotum. Occasionally, a varicocele can occur on the right side. The diagnosis is made by palpating the spermatic cords with the patient performing a Valsalva manoeuvre while standing upright. The varicocele is detected as a 'bag of worms' that usually disappears when the examination is repeated with the patient recumbent. Although its efficacy is not universally accepted, treatment is by ligation of the spermatic vein at the level of the internal inguinal ring. A scrotal approach is contra-indicated.

Semen quality improves in over half those who have had surgery and pregnancy results in 30–50 per cent of the wives, usually within a year.

Endocrine. The majority of infertile males with endocrine deficiency present with eunuchoidism rather than infertility. These abnormalities are discussed in detail in the section on androgen deficiency but it is necessary to stress a number of points here.

Klinefelter's syndrome. Patients with this condition can be normally virilized and present with infertility due to oligospermia or azoospermia. Thus, if plasma FSH levels are high, particularly in a patient with small but firm testes, chromosome studies should be performed. An XXY sex chromosome pattern is most common in Klinefelter's syndrome, with mosaicism and other variants being found occasionally. No treatment is available for the infertility.

Hyperprolactinaemia. High plasma concentrations of prolactin have been reported in approximately 3 per cent of men attending infertility clinics. Occasionally, slightly elevated (500–900 mU/l) levels are found in men with oligospermia. Usually, there is no obvious cause either for this observation or the seminal deficiency. In this situation no benefit is gained by giving bromocriptine or other dopamine agonists. When hyperprolactinaemia is gross and due to an identifiable condition such as a pituitary tumour specific treatment can lead to an increase in spermatogenesis, but there is no proven case of fertility being restored.

Gonadotrophin deficiency. The loss of gonadotrophin secretion normally affects spermatogenesis as well as Leydig cell function. The former can be restored by giving FSH prepared either from human pituitary glands or, more usually, extracted from post-menopausal urine.

Acute febrile illness. There is good evidence that fever can depress the sperm count. While infertility is not a complaint of patients with infection, the observation is relevant to the interpretation of apparent oligospermia: it is important to enquire about any significant fever within the previous three months in patients found to be oligospermic.

Chronic illness. Chronic disease can also inhibit spermatogenesis. In some conditions such as chronic renal failure the endocrine mechanisms have been established. In others, the causal relationship is not known.

Drugs. The list of drugs inhibiting spermatogenesis is impressive, and is displayed in Table 4. The mechanisms are varied and include

Table 4 Drugs inhibiting spermatogenesis

Alcohol, cannabis, and barbiturates
Oestrogens, progestogens, anabolic steroids, danazol, and androgens (high doses)
Anti-androgens, alkylating agents, and antimetabolites
Phenothiazines, butyrophenones, and other psychotropics
Monoamine oxidase inhibitors
Nitrofurantoin and sulphasalazine
Bis-diamine amoebicides
Phenytoin

endocrine as well as purely biochemical effects. From the clinical point of view it is important to emphasize the need to stop a drug if possible whenever a new problem develops. There is always the chance that the drug and the problem are causally related.

Radiation to the testes may also induce infertility.

Industrial hazards. Chronic exposure to lead results in low sperm counts, and arsenic and zinc may also be harmful. It is possible that other chemicals, such as some chlorinated pesticides and herbicides have similar effects. Since excessive heat has been shown by experiment to inhibit spermatogenesis, foundry workers and others who are exposed to high temperature for prolonged periods could be at risk of sub-fertility, there is no firm evidence that this is so.

Infection. Mumps orchitis occurring in adults may produce infertility if both testes are affected. Corticosteroid treatment and even incision of the tunica albuginea to reduce pressure, have been recommended. Smallpox is still an important cause of infertility in those regions in which it was endemic.

Tuberculosis can involve the testis, epididymis, and vas and should be considered in patients with a history of the condition and complaining of infertility. Treatment, *vis-à-vis* sterility, is seldom effective. Leprosy also produces infertility. Gonorrhoea may cause an epididymitis that can scar and obstruct the outward passage of sperms from the testes. Non-specific epididymitis and prostatitis can have the same consequences as gonorrhoea. Sub-clinical low grade infection can be suspected if the semen contains pus cells and can be confirmed by examination of the urethral discharge following prostatic massage. Oxytetracycline or metronidazole should be given, as indicated, to both partners.

Immunological. Antisperm antibodies of the IgA and IgG classes have been identified in the sera and on the sperms of sub-fertile men. They have also been found in the cervical mucus and sera of their consorts. In the former case, it has been postulated that there may be an immune orchitis, and corticosteroids have been prescribed with some benefit having been claimed. In the latter instance, the use of a condom for several weeks to allow the antibody titre to fall, or the direct insemination of husband's sperm into the uterine cavity to avoid the cervical mucus, have been advocated and employed, but with little success.

Trauma and torsion of the testis. Trauma to the gonad may interfere with spermatogenesis. This may be relatively minor and clinically apparently inconsequential. However, it is relatively easy to damage vessels in operations for testicular maldescent or inguinal hernia for instance. Torsion, clinically a more dramatic condition, is well recognized as a cause of testicular atrophy.

Obstructive aspermia. Blockage of both epididymes or both vasa deferentia can cause infertility. Obstruction can be suspected if the patient has normal testes but no sperms in the ejaculate. Blockage of the vas may be found by surgical exploration with a fine nylon wire. Pathology of the vas can be congenital, post-infective, traumatic, or deliberate in the case of vasectomy. In the latter situation, reconstructive surgery may be curative. Males with cystic fibrosis are infertile because of lack of development of the vas deferens or of deficiencies in the seminal vesicles or epididymis. In Kartagener's syndrome it has been proposed that there is a lack of ciliary function in the genital as well as the respiratory tract.

Idiopathic oligospermia. In at least a third of males with oligo- or azoospermia, there is no obvious pathological mechanism. Abnormalities of the seminiferous tubules may range from a complete lack of germinal tissue (known as the Sertoli cell-only syndrome) to varying degrees of arrest of the maturation of spermatogenesis. An elevated serum FSH concentration indicates a more severe defect. There is very rarely an indication for testicular biopsy, particularly when sperms are present in the ejaculate. The procedure is uncomfortable as well as being unhelpful as a guide to therapy, since there is no reliably effective treatment for this condition. In the situation where some sperms are present, partial coitus interruptus with insemination of the first part of the ejaculate has been proposed; however, there is no clear evidence that this works. Other treatments, such as artificial insemination with the husband's semen (AIH) or various hormonal regimes, are useless.

Retrograde ejaculation. This is found in some patients with a diabetic neuropathy and occasionally after surgery to the prostate. Attempts have been made to treat the infertility by removing the semen from the bladder after masturbation and inseminating it into the wife.

Treatment. As indicated above, the treatment is wherever possible that of the cause. However, this can be achieved in only a minority of instances. There is no sound evidence to prove that the various non-specific therapies that have been employed such as testosterone rebound, mesterolone, or cooling the scrotum do anything more for the patient than put off the time when he must learn that he is infertile. In the absence of cure, there are two 'therapeutic' avenues, adoption and artificial insemination by donor (AID). The choice of one or other, or neither, can only be made by considered discussion between the doctor and the couple.

Cryptorchidism

Testes bilaterally undescended by the time puberty is reached are almost invariably associated with infertility. This may be due to the destructive effect of heat on spermatogenesis while the testes are intra-abdominal, or it may be that the testes themselves are abnormal thus contributing to their own maldescent. Indeed, both primary testicular disease, such as Klinefelter's syndrome, and gonadal disease secondary to gonadotrophin deficiency are found in patients with cryptorchidism.

The patient, often a child, should be examined with warm hands one of which should be over the internal inguinal ring to prevent a retractile gonad being missed while the other is used to palpate gently from the scrotum up to the inguinal canal. If this manoeuvre fails to reveal a testis, the little finger should be delicately invaginated into the inguinal canal. The identification of a small swelling or a discreet tenderness may indicate the presence of a hitherto undiscovered gonad. Additionally, the superficial inguinal pouch should be palpated as this may harbour a maldescended gland.

By five years of age, the normal male will have scrotal testes. After that age, there is an increasing risk of damage to the germinal epithelium and investigation and treatment is indicated as early as possible. A six-week course of chorionic gonadotrophin 3000 units once a week intramuscularly may on occasions produce descent and is worth trying. Intranasal LHRH may also be used but currently is much more expensive. The testes may enlarge with this treatment, making surgical exploration and discovery easier, and a rise in serum testosterone may reassure that exploration is worthwhile in that there is evidence of testicular tissue to be found. CT scanning is an alternative, non-invasive way of finding the organ, but the resolving power of this technique must be taken into consideration if no testis is identified. Since intra-abdominal testes have an increased risk of developing a malignancy, orchidectomy and scrotal prostheses with androgen replacement therapy are recommended when the condition presents after puberty.

Androgen deficiency

This is most often due to lack of testosterone but it can also be caused by absent or diminished cytosolic androgen receptors, or by a deficiency of the 5α-reductase which converts testosterone to dihydrotestosterone (DHT). Testosterone deficiency can result from primary gonadal disease or from a disorder of the hypothalamus or pituitary with diminished gonadotrophin secretion. In either instance, the patient will manifest the clinical features of hypogonadism (see Tables 5 and 6). Sometimes, androgen deficiency may present with infertility, and has already been discussed. Most often,

Table 5 Symptoms of androgen deficiency

Absent or diminished
  Beard growth
  Pubic, axillary, and limb hair
  Libido, erections, and ejaculations
Voice remains high pitched

Table 6 Signs of androgen deficiency

Small or impalpable testes
Infantile or poorly developed penis and scrotum
Diminished facial, pubic, and axillary hair
Unbroken voice with unnotched thyroid cartilage
Smooth, feminine skin
Lack of muscular development
Long limbs

though, the clinical problem is dominated by the somatic consequences of the hormonal pathology.

History. The symptoms encountered in the androgen-deficient patient are set out in Table 5. The man, or if a boy, his parental spokesman, may encapsulate all these with a complaint of failing to achieve manhood or failing to grow normally, since the puberty growth spurt is a feature of sexual maturation. He may also present with 'delayed puberty'.

Examination. The physical findings that may be encountered on examination are listed in Table 6. The teenager may be shorter than normal whereas the adult may have long limbs with a sitting height at least 5 cm less than half the standing height. In the former instance, the increase in growth that comes with sexual maturation will not have taken place, whereas in the latter there will have been delayed epiphyseal fusion of the long bones: growth has continued well into adulthood, giving the classical proportions of the eunuch.

Investigation. The causes of androgen deficiency can be distinguished from each other on clinical grounds with the aid of the investigations set out in Table 7. Serum testosterone levels will indicate whether there is indeed an endocrine abnormality at all; FSH and LH measurements will point either to a primary or a secondary testicular abnormality. Elevated gonadotrophins indicate primary testicular disease. Secondary disease is diagnosed when gonadotrophin levels are low or low normal in the presence of low serum testosterone concentrations.

Table 7 Investigations of androgen deficiency

To ascertain the cause
  Essential (with normal ranges)
    FSH (1–8 u/l), LH (2–14 u/l), and testosterone (15–50 nmol/l)
  Often indicated
    Prolactin, FSH, and LH responses to LHRH
    Stimulation tests for other pituitary hormones
    Radiology of skull and pituitary fossa
    Chromosome analysis
  Occasionally indicated
    Precursors and metabolites of testosterone
    Nocturnal FSH and LH at 30 minute intervals
    Tests of smell

To evaluate consequences of androgen deficiency
  Radiological bone age
  Semen analysis

The cause of gonadotrophin deficiency can be ascertained by dynamic tests of gonadotrophin secretion together with other investigations of hypothalamic pituitary function including prolactin measurements. In some cases of delayed puberty, estimations of night-time gonadotrophin concentrations are done in order to detect the earliest signs of episodic release that indicate impending puberty. However, this procedure is prodigal with resources and provides no more clinical information than an LHRH test, since gonadotrophin release after LHRH can be observed whenever nocturnal surges in these hormones occur spontaneously. Chromosome studies should be performed whenever Klinefelter's syndrome or one of its variants is suspected. Tests of smell assist in the diagnosis of Kallman's syndrome. Radiological bone age is helpful in assessing the degree of sexual immaturity and seminal analysis gives information on reproductive capacity. Height and weight measurements are also informative in the initial evaluation of the problem and also when the effects of treatment are being monitored.

Causes. The disorders causing lack of normal male secondary sex characteristics are tabulated in Table 8. The classification is, as far as is possible, based on physiological principles. Each condition is described in detail below.

Table 8 Causes of androgen deficiency

Lack of androgen receptors	
Incomplete male pseudohermaphroditism	
Lack of 5α-reductase	
Pseudovaginal perineoscrotal hypospadias	
Diminished gonadal testosterone	
Congenital	Acquired
Testosterone biosynthetic enzyme	Castration
deficiencies	Protein malnutrition
Leydig cell agenesis	Sickle cell disease
Anorchia	Cirrhosis
Chromosome abnormalities	Renal failure
(including Klinefelter's syndrome)	Leprosy
Bonnevie–Ullrich syndrome	Alcohol
Noonan's syndrome	Cancer chemotherapy
Miscellaneous (see text)	
Diminished gonadotrophins	
Panhypopituitarism	
Fertile eunuch syndrome	
Haemochromatosis	
Lead poisoning	
Diminished LHRH	
Selective gonadotrophin deficiency	
Hyperprolactinaemia	

Congenital abnormalities. *Incomplete male pseudohermaphroditism.* In this condition, transmitted through the X chromosome, there is a relative deficiency of the intracellular androgen receptor. The clinical picture, which has a number of eponymous attributions—Gilbert–Dreyfus, Lubs, Rosewater or Reifenstein—covers a spectrum of hypogonadism ranging in severity from azoospermia and gynaecomastia to gross perineoscrotal hypospadias and cryptorchidism with deficient chest and facial hair and an unbroken voice. The psychological orientation is male. The chomosomal pattern is XY with normal, or even elevated, levels of testosterone and LH. The treatment is surgical, to correct the perineal abnormalities and to perform mammoplasty. If orchidectomy is carried out for undescended testes, testosterone replacement is required.

Although the pathophysiological basis of this disorder is somewhat similar to that of the testicular feminization syndrome where there is complete deficiency of the androgen receptor, the latter condition is described in the section on the female reproductive system (see page 10.82) since the clinical problem is that of an abnormal female rather than of an abnormal male.

Pseudovaginal perineoscrotal hypospadias. This is an autosomal recessive abnormality of XY males where there is a lack of enzyme responsible for the conversion of testosterone to dihydrotestosterone. This results clinically in apparently female external genitalia and an internal Wolffian (male) system. At puberty, the external genitalia virilize with enlargement of the phallus and the development of pubic hair. Facial, axillary, body, and limb hair also appear and the voice deepens. There is no gynaecomastia, but in severe cases hypospadias, with a pseudovagina, remains. Untreated, there is male orientation at puberty, but if castration has been carried out in childhood and oestrogen given, the sexual attitude may be female. Homozygous XX and heterozygous XY individuals are normal. The diagnosis is made by noting the clinical

picture and family history and by finding high testosterone and low dihydrotestosterone levels in plasma. In addition, there is low 5α-reductase activity in fibroblasts taken from the genital skin. Plastic surgery to the perineal structures is indicated in those who go through a male puberty. If castration has been performed prior to this time, oestrogens will produce feminization.

Defects in androgen biosynthesis. A number of very rare syndromes have been recognized as being due to a deficiency of one or other steps in the biosynthetic pathway of testosterone synthesis. The pathways involved together with the various abnormalities and their biochemical markers are shown in Table 9.

Table 9 Defects in testosterone biosynthesis

Cholesterol
  ↓ 1   2
Pregnenolone ───────→Progesterone
  ↓ 3   2   ↓ 3
17OH-pregnenolone ───→17OH-progesterone
  ↓ 4   2   ↓ 4
  DHA ──────→Δ⁴androstenedione ───→Oestrone
  ↓ 5   2   ↓ 5   ↓ 5
Δ⁵androstenediol ─────→Testosterone ───────→Oestradiol

Deficiency	Biochemical markers*	
	Increased	Decreased
20,22-desmolase	†	†
3β-hydroxysteroid dehydrogenase	DHA	testosterone cortisol
17α-hydroxylase	corticosterone	testosterone cortisol
17,20-desmolase	pregnanetriolone	testosterone androstenedione
17-oxosteroid reductase	androstenedione pregnanetriol	testosterone

* Steroids, measurement of which can be used to identify the enzyme defect
† This is a rapidly fatal condition and therefore does not present a problem in adult life

Adapted from Givens J. R., et al. (1974), *New Engl. J. Med.* **291**, 938 and reproduced from London D. R. (1975), *Clin. Endocr. Metab.* **4**, 597.

The clinical picture is variable. In 20,22-desmolase, 3β-hydroxysteroid dehydrogenase isomerase, and 17α-hydroxylase deficiencies, the synthesis of cortisol in the adrenal cortex is also affected. The genitalia of these subjects, karyotypically male, are phenotypically female. Those suffering from 17,20-desmolase and 17-oxosteroid reductase deficiencies have ambiguous genitalia, and the latter may additionally suffer from gynaecomastia. All these conditions, with the exception of the 17,20-desmolase abnormality, which is X linked, are transmitted via an autosomal recessive gene. 17,20-desmolase deficiency is distinguished from partial androgen receptor deficiency by the latter feminizing at puberty. The distinction of partial androgen insensitivity from the 17-oxosteroid reductase deficiency must be made biochemically.

Persistent Mullerian tract. The patient is a phenotypic male with cryptorchidism and with an inguinal hernia containing uterus and fallopian tubes. The diagnosis is usually made at herniorrhaphy. Puberty is normal and in the best documented cases, oligospermia or azoospermia is found. The mode of inheritance is unclear.

Klinefelter's syndrome. This is the commonest cause of testicular disease involving both seminiferous tubules and Leydig cells. It has a genetic aetiology. Classically, the patients have an XXY chromosomal pattern but many karyotypic variations have been described. The testes show hyalinization of the basement membranes of the seminiferous tubules together with defective spermatogenesis, and there are usually clumps or even sheets of Leydig cells. Clinically, the patients present with defective sexual maturation, infertility, or maldescended testes, and are usually found to be hypogonad with small firm testes. They may also have gynaecomastia and be mentally retarded. In the variant where there is a 49 XXXXY karyotype there is a high incidence of skeletal deformities including short neck, kyphosis and scoliosis, radio-ulnar synostosis, clinodactyly of the fifth finger, coxa valga, genu valgum, and pes planus. There is also a tendency to wide-set eyes and epicanthic folds, strabismus, malformed ears, and prognathism. The cytogenetic basis of this is obscure. Patients with Klinefelter's syndrome have an increased incidence of breast cancer compared with other males and they may also have a slight predisposition to germ cell tumours.

The combination of hypogonadism, small but firm testes, and gynaecomastia is neither universal in, nor diagnostic of, Klinefelter's syndrome. Some patients may be normally developed and only have small testes and oligospermia or azoospermia, while hypogonadism and gynaecomastia together are found in a number of other conditions. The final diagnosis can only be made by detecting the appropriate chromosome abnormality and a high FSH concentration. Treatment of the endocrine deficiency is with androgen replacement, although caution must be exercised in this regard, if the patient is mentally subnormal and manifests any antisocial tendency. The infertility is irremediable.

Sex reversal. These patients are clinically identical to those with Klinefelter's syndrome. The distinction from that condition is made by observing that in sex reversal there is no Y chromosome, only a 46 XX karyotype. The aetiology of the condition is unknown but it may be due to a translocation of the testicular determinants of the Y chromosome either to an X or to an autosome, or the Y material may be lost after the initiation of testicular development during embryogenesis.

True hermaphroditism. Usually, these patients are raised as males since the external genitalia appear more male than female although a urogenital sinus is usually present. Ovotestes may be found or alternatively there may be separate ovarian and testicular tissue on one or both sides. A uterus is usually present together with Wolffian and Mullerian systems. Menstruation may present as cyclical haematuria. Both ovulation and spermatogenesis have been recorded. The chromosome pattern is 46 XX or 46 XY but various mosaics have been reported. The reconstructive and ablative surgery, on which treatment is based, should attempt to preserve the gender assigned at birth. Gonadal tumours are rare in these patients and gonadectomy is therefore not usually necessary.

Anorchia. The condition can present in childhood, when the problem is of cryptorchidism, in adolescence with delayed puberty, or in adult life with a clinical picture of eunuchoidism.

The aetiology is usually obscure. Rarely there may be a history of accidental trauma, surgery, or infection, and a chromosomal disturbance has on occasion been reported, but most frequently there is no apparent cause. Since the external genitalia are male and the Wolffian system is present testosterone must have been produced by an embryonic organizer, presumably the testes. Thus, the condition is sometimes called the 'vanishing testes syndrome'.

The diagnosis is made by failing to find testes after surgical exploration of the scrotum and abdomen in an XY eunuchoid male. Gonadotrophin levels are high and there is no rise in serum testosterone concentrations after prolonged stimulation with HCG. Treatment is with testosterone and the implantation of testicular prostheses into the scrotum.

Bonnevie–Ullrich and Noonan's syndromes. These are also referred to as 'male Turner's syndrome'. In both there is primary testicular deficiency with hypogonadism. Chromosomes may be normal but sometimes an abnormal karyotype is noted. Familial as well as sporadic forms occur.

In the Bonnevie–Ullrich syndrome, the somatic abnormalities include short stature, neck webbing, cubitus valgus, short fourth metacarpal, arched palate, chest deformity, hyperteleorism, ptosis, low set ears, naevi, lymphoedema, and malformations of the urinary tract. An auto-immune thyroiditis has been reported in association. There may also be congenital deformity of the left-sided outflow tract of the heart with aortic stenosis or coarctation. This is in contrast to Noonan's syndrome where right-sided cardiac abnormalities are found as well as a higher incidence of mental subnormality and a hyperplasticity of the skin that can be confused with the Ehlers–Danlos syndrome. In both Noonan's and Bonnevie–Ullrich syndromes, gonadotrophin levels are high. The hypogonadism is treated with testosterone.

Miscellaneous. A large number of inherited diseases have primary gonadal failure as part of the condition. These are listed in Table 10.

Table 10 Syndromes in the male that include primary gonadal failure

Condition	Abnormalities involving gonads	Somatic features	Mode of inheritance
Alström syndrome	Germinal cell aplasia with varying degrees of tubular sclerosis and slight immaturity; normal sexual development Elevated gonadotrophin levels	Obesity beginning in infancy, nystagmus, sensitivity to light, progressive visual impairment with blindness by age 7, retinal degeneration, cataracts, neurosensory hearing loss, diabetes mellitus with onset after puberty	Autosomal recessive
Ataxia-telangiectasia	Absence of hypoplasia of gonads, cryptorchidism Elevated gonadotrophin levels	Cerebellar ataxia, choreoathetosis, nystagmus, recurrent sinopulmonary infections, telangiectasias of skin and bulbar conjunctiva, IgA deficiency, defects in cellular immunity, chromosome breakage	Autosomal recessive
Borjeson syndrome	Cryptorchidism, micropenis, sexual infantilism, germinal aplasia, interstitial fibrosis Decreased gonadotrophin levels	Mental retardation, obesity, grotesque facies, dwarfism, seizures	X-linked recessive
Fanconi syndrome	Small, firm testes, tubular hypoplasia, decreased spermatogenesis	Pancytopenia, bone marrow hypoplasia, skin hyperpigmentation, short stature, upper limb malformations, chromosome damage	Autosomal recessive
Fraser syndrome	Cryptorchidism, hypospadias, micropenis	Cryptophthalmus, hypoplastic eyebrows, coloboma of alae nasi, midfacial cleft, cleft lip and palate, ankyloglossia, small ears, hearing loss, syndactyly, umbilical hernia, laryngeal stenosis, nipple displacement, renal malformations	Autosomal recessive
Geominne syndrome	Seminiferous tubule failure, normal Leydig cell function, cryptorchidism	Congenital torticollis, keloids, renal dysplasia, cutaneous naevi, varicose veins	X-linked recessive

Table 10 Syndromes in the male that include primary gonadal failure—*cont.*

Condition	Abnormalities involving gonads	Somatic features	Mode of inheritance
Multiple lentigines syndrome	Small or absent testes, hypospadias	Multiple lentigines, pulmonary stenosis, short stature, hypertelorism, sensorineural deafness, ECG changes	Autosomal dominant
Myotonic dystrophy	Normal gonadal function until young adult life, with later testicular atrophy, involving primarily the seminiferous tubules; germinal aplasia or tubular fibrosis Elevated basal FSH level with exaggerated LHRH response. Normal LH level with exaggerated LHRH response	Muscle atrophy, myotonia, cataracts, frontal balding, diabetes mellitus	Autosomal dominant
Noonan syndrome	Complete absence of testicles, cryptorchidism, germinal aplasia: Gonadal function may be normal	Short stature, mental retardation, cardiac defect, ear abnormalities, epicanthal folds, ptosis, downward slanting palpebral fissures, anterior open bite, micrognathia, webbed neck, pectus excavatum, cubitus valgus, vertebral anomalies, renal anomalies, lymphoedema	? Autosomal dominant
Osteochondritis dissecans syndrome	Eunuchoid habitus, high-pitched voice, sparse facial and axillary hair	Osteochondritis dissecans in multiple joints, hypertelorism, ptosis, pectus excavatum	Uncertain
Prader–Willi syndrome	Sterility, sexual infantilism, testicular atrophy, deficient spermatogenesis, cryptorchidism, hypoplastic scrotum, small penis Variable basal LH and FSH levels, variable response to LHRH	Mental retardation, obesity, short stature, infantile hypotonia, delicate facial features	Uncertain
Ruthmund–Thomsen syndrome	Cryptorchidism, delayed puberty and/or deficient masculinization	Erythema, telangiectasia, skin atrophy and irregular pigmentation, short stature, juvenile cataracts, saddle nose, small hands and feet, sparse hair, mental retardation	Autosomal recessive
Russell–Silver syndrome	Cryptorchidism, hypospadias Variable gonadotrophin levels	Low birthweight, dwarfism, triangular face, asymmetry, macrocephaly (relative)	Uncertain
Sohval–Soffer syndrome	Small, soft testes, small penis, defective secondary sex development, azoospermia, gynaecomastia, germinal aplasia, tubular fibrosis Elevated gonadotrophin levels	Mental retardation, multiple skeletal anomalies involving cervical spine and ribs	Uncertain
Van Benthem syndrome	Cryptorchidism, testicular agenesis	Chest deformities, muscle hypoplasia, deficient subcutaneous fat, dolichocephaly, mental retardation	Autosomal or X-linked recessive?
Weinstein syndrome	Small, soft testes, small hyalinized tubules, germinal hypoplasia, normal Leydig cell function, normal virilization, thick lamina propria Low plasma testosterone levels unresponsive to HCG	Blindness, neurosensory deafness, cataract, retinal degeneration, hyperuricaemia, hypertriglyceridaemia, obesity, short stature	Uncertain
Werner syndrome	Small testes and penis, decreased pubic hair, diminished libido, sterility, testicular atrophy, hyalinized tubules, absent spermatogenesis	Premature aging, short stature, cataracts, sclerodermatous skin changes, mild diabetes mellitus	Autosomal recessive
Xerodermic idiocy syndrome	Small testes, cryptorchidism	Xeroderma pigmentosa, cutaneous malignancy, progressive mental retardation, microcephaly, dwarfism, ataxia, athetosis, retarded bone age, sensorineural deafness Defective DNA repair	Autosomal recessive

Adapted from Summitt, R. L. (1980), Genetic forms of hypogonadism. In *Progress in medical genetics* (ed. A. G. Steinberg et al.), vol. 3. W. B. Saunders, Philadelphia

Acquired abnormalities. *Castration*. If this has been done pre-pubertally, the boy will continue to grow and develop eunuchoid proportions and there will be no development of male secondary sex characteristics and no libido. If the operation is performed after puberty, various androgenic characteristics may persist with the occasional patient maintaining erections and continuing to shave. For full sexual activity, testosterone replacement is required.

Protein malnutrition. In this situation, there may be loss of libido and potency as well as a decrease in facial and body hair. The finding of high gonadotrophins with a low testosterone points to a primary gonadal effect.

Cirrhosis of the liver. Gonadal pathophysiology and its clinical consequences in cirrhosis are very similar to the pattern found in alcoholism (see below).

Alcohol. Acutely, alcohol can increase the libido but, frustrating-ly, diminish the ability to perform sexually. In large amounts it may induce stupor and hence remove desire. Taken to excess over a long period, the libido is reduced and there may be gynaecomastia with testicular atrophy as well as loss of pubic, facial, and axillary hair. Usually, this is associated with gross disturbances of liver function, but not necessarily so. Leydig cell function can be depressed by alcohol and what testosterone is produced undergoes increased metabolism in the alcoholic. An important product of metabolism in this context is oestradiol, leading to an abnormal testosterone/oestradiol ratio, with concentrations of free testosterone further reduced by the high SHBG levels found in the condition. Spermatogenesis may also be impaired.

Renal failure. Decreased libido, impotence, and infertility are all found in males with chronic renal failure. Testosterone levels may be normal or low and gonadotrophin concentrations may be normal or elevated, but the responses of the latter to LHRH may be impaired. In addition, prolactin levels may be high. Haemodialysis does not produce clinical improvement but transplantation may.

Leprosy. Approximately 15 per cent of men with lepromatous leprosy have testicular atrophy and gynaecomastia with acid-fast bacilli present in the gonads. This contrasts with the tuberculoid form of the disease where the testes are spared.

Cancer chemotherapy. While the Leydig cells are usually not harmed, administration of these drugs to adolescent boys can cause gynaecomastia and gonadal dysfunction with low levels of testosterone and high LH concentrations (see also page 18.53 and Section 19).

Diminished gonadotrophin secretion. *Panhypopituitarism*. This is discussed on page 10.11. In the context of the current section it must be stressed that this condition may present as a problem of hypogonadism, so any patient found to be deficient of gonadotrophins should have all other aspects of pituitary function carefully evaluated.

LH deficiency. The 'fertile eunuch' syndrome is a rare condition where there may be normal or absent spermatogenesis in a clinic-ally eunuchoid man. It is associated with normal FSH but low LH levels. Testosterone concentrations are also low but respond to HCG injections. The 'fertile eunuch' syndrome may occur sporadi-cally, or in association with Kallman's syndrome (see below) or in men with intra- or suprasellar tumours. The treatment is to give HCG which promotes the development of secondary male charac-teristics and spermatogenesis where the latter is abnormal. Isolated FSH deficiency has not been convincingly described in men.

Haemochromatosis and lead poisoning. These may both cause hypogonadism. Haemochromatosis can do so, independent of an effect on the liver, through iron deposition in the pituitary gland. Lead may have the same effect, although it is possible that in this case lead accumulates in Leydig cells as well.

Selective gonadotrophin deficiency. This condition which is secondary to LHRH deficiency, or to selective loss of gonadotrophes, may present as delayed puberty or as adult hypogonadism. The disorder may occur with or without gynaecomastia and may be due to generalized disease of the hypothalamus or pituitary. Alter-

natively, there may be no obvious pathology as in Kallman's syndrome, where the gonadotrophin deficiency is associated most commonly with hyposmia or anosmia and, more rarely, with other abnormalities such as colour blindness, renal and midline facial deformities, syndactyly, short fourth metacarpals and mental retardation. Kallman's syndrome may be familial but the mode of genetic transmission is unclear. Treatment is ordinarily with testosterone to induce sexual maturation but human menopausal gonadotrophin (HMG) and human chorionic gonadotrophin (HCG) are necessary to induce fertility and recently, LHRH has been used successfully.

Ataxia-hypogonadism. Gonadotrophin deficiency has been reported in males with cerebellar ataxia, including that of the Friedreich type. In association with this may be pes cavus, pectus excavatum, spina bifida, and disturbance of the electrical activity of the heart. The mode of transmission is genetically heterogeneous.

Nevoid basal cell carcinoma. This occurs with hypogonadism and also with anosmia, as in Kallman's syndrome. Transmission is via an autosomal dominant gene.

All other causes of gonadotrophin deficiency, as listed in Table 10, are considered elsewhere.

Delayed puberty. It may be important to distinguish a physiological retardation in the onset of puberty from the foregoing pathological causes of sexual infantilism and also from other conditions such as growth hormone deficiency and a malabsorption syndrome. The distinction may be difficult on clinical grounds although clues to prospective normality may be gleaned from noting the appearance of various milestones of sexual maturation in the patient in relation to those recorded for a normal population. Also, there is often a history of later development in the father and siblings. A testicular volume of more than 5 ml makes pathology unlikely and an appropriate serum testosterone level or gonadotrophin response to LHRH, or a radiological bone age within two years of the chronological age are also findings that may be used to encourage the child and his parents. A poor rise in GH after stimulation should, unless clinically appropriate, be rechecked after androgen therapy, since an apparently abnormal pattern can simply be a manifestation of the pre-pubertal state. Where possible, a temporizing approach should be adopted and the patient followed at three monthly intervals for at least one year with recording of height, weight, and the relevant milestones. If treatment is forced by psychological pressures, a normal future is not compromised by the administration of testosterone to hasten growth and sexual maturation. However, a careful check should be kept to ensure that the epiphyses are not fused prematurely, and any treatment should be withdrawn as soon as the boy has developed in line with his peers.

Ageing

There is a progressive loss in sexual function after the age of 40 with a reduction in the frequency and ability to perform sexual intercourse. Nocturnal emissions and morning erections also become less and fertility is reduced. The age of onset of this decline varies from individual to individual but there is no such thing in normals as the 'male climacteric'. Testicular volume diminishes relative to the reduction in spermatogenesis and testosterone secretion decreases with a fall in serum levels and a resultant gradual loss in secondary sexual hair. Gonadotrophin levels rise, indicating that the failure originates in the gonad and not in the hypothalamus or pituitary.

Tumours

Introduction. Testicular neoplasms account for 1–2 per cent of all malignancies and are therefore rare. There are two main types, seminoma and teratoma, of which the histogenesis is debated. The seminoma is undoubtedly of germinal origin but there is no agreement as to the line of stem cells from which teratomas are derived. Choriocarcinoma is a term applied particularly in the USA to some teratomas. These two tumours make up the majority of testicular cancers. Other pathological entities are: combined seminoma and teratoma, Sertoli cell tumour, interstitial cell tumour and orchioblastoma.

Clinical features. These tumours can occur at any age but particularly affect men in their prime between the ages of 20 and 50. Predisposing factors are maldescended testes and the testicular feminization syndrome 10.82. They may present with pain or as a hard mass accidentally discovered in the testis, or with the symptoms and signs of distant spread. Metastases can be to regional lymph nodes, particularly the para-aortic chain, or to distant sites such as liver, lung, mediastinum, and left supra-clavicular nodes. The author has seen one case and knows of another where the tumour was growing as a core in the right atrium, right ventricle and within the pulmonary artery which it finally obstructed. Gynaecomastia is an occasional feature.

Investigation. Diagnosis is by orchidectomy which should be always carried out if a hard mass develops in the testis. This enables the cell type to be identified as a prelude to treatment. About 90 per cent of patients with non-seminomatous tumours have elevated blood levels of HCG and alpha-fetoprotein (AFP) which can be used as tumour markers for following the progress of the disease and the success of treatment. Occasionally, a seminoma can secrete HCG, in which case there should be a hard search for choriocarcinomatous elements. If AFP is found with a seminoma, teratomatous tissue may co-exist.

Other investigations may include chest X-ray, inferior vena cava angiography, lymphangiography via the foot, intravenous urography, and CT scanning of abdomen and mediastinum. Using a combination of these, the severity of the disease can be graded by whether it is local (Stage 1), involving the retroperitoneal lymphatics (Stage 2), or spread distally (Stage 3). There are sub-divisions for each of these.

Treatment is selected according to cell type and clinical stage as assessed by clinical findings, radiology, and measurement of biochemical markers. Seminomas, which have a relatively good prognosis, are radiosensitive. The other tumours may need node dissections and combination chemotherapy of which there are a number of permutations.

Agents currently in use include actinomycin-D, adriamycin, bleomycin, chlorambucil, cyclophosphamide, 5-fluoro-uracil, methotrexate, phenylalanine mustard, vinblastine, and vincristine. The management of these patients requires careful monitoring and should be carried out in specialized centres.

Disorders of sexual performance

Normal sexual activity can be divided into three phases: desire, excitement, and orgasm. The physiology of desire is complex involving psychological as well as hormonal factors. Testosterone is necessary for a normal libido in the male and is said to play a facultative role in the female. The endocrine control of sexual desire in the female remains a mystery; however, it is known that oestrogens are necessary for adequate vaginal lubrication. During the stage of excitement the penis becomes erect and the vagina balloons. These changes are due to increased local blood flow which is controlled via the sacral parasympathetic outflow. Psychological factors as well as hormones, at least in the male, play a part in maintaining excitement and engorgement. Orgasm is dependent on hormones in the male and the psyche in both sexes. Orgasm in the male is accompanied by emission which involves contraction of the smooth muscle of the vas deferens, seminal vesicles, prostate, and prostatic urethra, and ejaculation which is seen as the rhythmic contraction of the striated muscle of the perineum and penis. The female orgasm is analogous with contraction of the perineal and vaginal muscles. The nervous pathways for this are centred on the lumbar sympathetic. In the male there is a refractory period after orgasm. The duration of this increases with age with a decrease in the desire for, or the possibility of, frequent ejaculations. Erection, however, is not affected.

Clinical aspects. Sexual performance can be impaired by a loss of libido, by an inability for the male to have an erection, or through failure of orgasm. Analogous abnormalities in the female have in the past been grouped together and termed 'frigidity' but at least in part are capable of being split into their component parts and diagnosed and treated accordingly. Nevertheless, sexual function is much more vulnerable to disturbance in the male and so emphasis will be given to problems in men.

Lack of desire, or a diminished libido, may occur in psychiatric or any general medical illness as well as in endocrine disease or following drug therapy. Erectile difficulty or ejaculatory failure may be endocrine in origin, neurogenic, psychological, or due to drugs. Among the latter which are in common use are alcohol and cannabis. Of those used therapeutically, antihypertensive agents and psychotropics are associated with copulatory failure. Autonomic neuropathy, of which the most important cause is diabetes mellitus is the commonest disease leading to the problem. Unfortunately, there is no satisfactory treatment for diabetic impotence. Various mechanical devices are available but they are a poor substitute for the real thing. Drug therapy whenever thought to be a cause of sexual dysfunction should be altered. Surgery within the lower abdomen and pelvis can produce impotence by interruption of the parasympathetic nerves to the genitalia and the Leriche syndrome of narrowing of the common iliac arteries produces similar symptoms through a reduction in blood flow through the penis and accessory tissues.

A history should include questions about drug therapy, social habits, and marital attitudes. The presence of nocturnal emissions and morning erections excludes an endocrinopathy. The physical examination necessitates assessment of endocrine status as well as neurological testing and palpation of the arteries of the lower limbs. If there is any doubt as to the cause, a serum testosterone level should be estimated.

In the majority of cases, no organic cause is found and the patient should therefore receive psychosexual counselling. Sometimes, the problem can be resolved by talking to the patient alone, but more often both partners should be seen and advised together. Treatment is usually given by specialists in the field, either psychiatrists or marriage guidance councillors working together or individually. Premature ejaculation, a common problem, can also be treated psychosexually.

References

Amelar, R. D., Dubin, L., and Walsh, P. C. (1977). *Male infertility*. W. B. Saunders, Philadelphia.

Blatt, J., Poplack, D. G., and Sherins, R. J. (1981). Testicular function in boys after chemotherapy for acute lymphoblastic leukaemia. *New Engl. J. Med.* **304**, 1121.

Cancer (1980). Supplement. *Cancer* **45**, 1735.

de Kretser, D. M. (1979). The effects of systemic disease on the function of the testis. *Clin. Endocr. Metab.* **8**, 487.

Griffin, J. E. and Wilson, J. D. (1980). The syndromes of androgen resistance, *New Engl. J. Med.* **302**, 198.

Grumbach, M. M., Grave, G. D., and Mayer, F. E. (1974). *Control of the onset of puberty*. Wiley, New York.

Javadpour, N. and Bergman, S. (1978). Recent advances in testicular cancer. *Cur. Prob. Surg.* **15**, 1.

Kaplan, H. S. (1974). *The new sex therapy*. Baillière Tindall, London.

— (1979). *Disorders of sexual desire*. Brunner Mazel, New York.

Kurohara, S. S., Webster, J. H., Badib, A., Doctor, Z., and Woodruff, M. W. (1969). The clinical features of the common testicular cancers. *J. Urol.* **101**, 587.

Lipsett, M. B. (1980). Physiology and pathology of the Leydig cell. *New Engl. J. Med.* **303**, 682.

Odell, W. D. and Swerfloff, R. S. (1978). Abnormalities of gonadal function in men. *Clin. Endocr.* **8**, 149.

Pepperell, R. N., Hudson, B., and Wood, C. (1980). *The infertile couple*. Churchill Livingstone, Edinburgh.

Summitt, R. L. (1979). Genetic forms of hypogonadism in the male. In *Progress in medical genetics* (eds. A. G. Steinberg, A. G. Bearn, A. G. Motulsky, and B. Childs) vol. 3, 1. W. B. Saunders, Philadelphia.

Wilson, J. D. and Walsh, P. C. (1979). Disorders of sexual differentiation. In *Campbell's Urology* (eds. J. H. Harrison, R. F. Gittes, A. D. Permutter, T. A. Stamey, and P. C. Walsh). W. B. Saunders, Philadelphia.

Yen, S. S. C. and Jaffe, R. (1978). *Reproductive endocrinology*. W. B. Saunders, Philadelphia.

THE FEMALE

Introduction. Disorders of the female reproductive system may occur through disease of the hypothalamus, pituitary, ovary, or of the lower genital tract. Although the physician more commonly encounters hypothalamic, pituitary or ovarian pathology, occasionally abnormalities of fallopian tubes, uterus, or vagina can masquerade as a medical problem.

There may be problems of sexual differentiation and development, menstrual disturbances, infertility and states of masculinization. Advice may also be sought on contraception and the management of menopausal symptoms. Each of these will be considered in separate sections in this chapter. Central to all is an understanding of the endocrine function of the ovary and its control.

Physiology

Ovarian steroidogenesis. The adult ovary serves two inter-related purposes, to secrete hormones and to provide germ cells. As is described in the next section, the endocrine products (Fig. 1) of the ovary are secreted in varying amounts according to the phase of the menstrual cycle (Fig. 2). The main hormones of the ovary are oestradiol (E) and progesterone (P). Oestradiol together with another oestrogen, oestrone, is responsible for the feminization of the adult. Oestrogens are also produced by extra-ovarian sites from precursors such as androstenedione and dehydroepiandrosterone (DHA) secreted by ovary and adrenal; this extra-ovarian production becomes clinically significant when the ovary is abnormal, as in the polycystic ovary syndrome, or when it is non-functioning, as after the menopause. The precursors can also be metabolized to androgens, as can be clinically manifest in ovarian or adrenal disease. The normal ovary secretes insignificantly small amounts of testosterone, but twice as much androstenedione as oestradiol.

As with oestradiol, output of progesterone alters with the stage of the cycle, with secretion in the luteal phase approximately 15 times that of the follicular phase. Progesterone acts mainly on the uterus to produce a secretory endometrium and on the uterine cervical glands increasing the viscosity of their secretion.

These steroids act on their target tissues first by binding with a specific cytosolic receptor and then being translocated to the nucleus in a manner analogous with androgens. The physiological effects of oestrogens are set out in Table 1.

Cholesterol

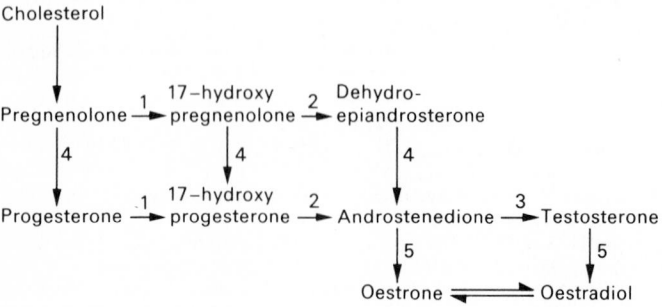

1 = 17α-hydroxylase   2 = 17,20-desmolase   3 = 17β-hydroxylase

4 = 3β-ol-dehydrogenase   5 = 'Aromatase'

Fig. 1   The biosynthetic pathways in the ovary leading to oestrogen and progesterone formation. The numbers refer to the enzymic steps involved. This figure should also be considered in conjunction with Table 1 and Fig. 2 in the section on intersex (page 10.88).

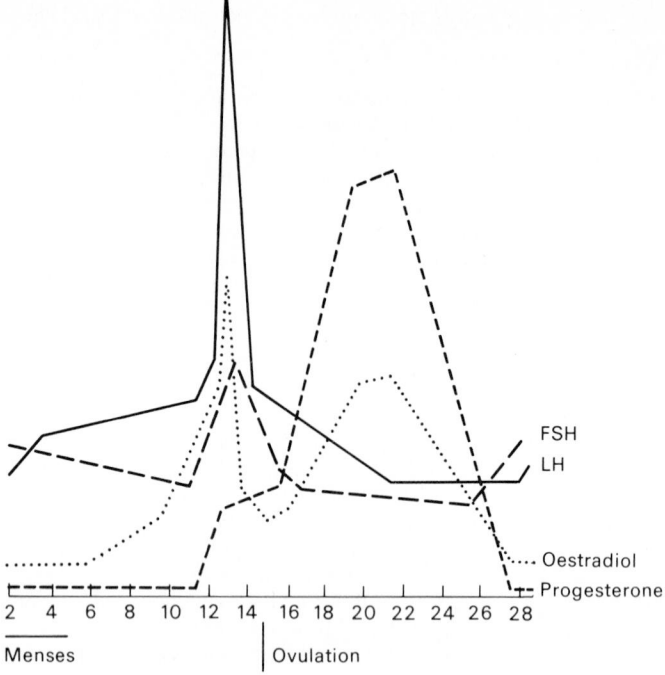

Fig. 2 Diagrammatic representation of the hormonal changes in the menstrual cycle. The concentration of the hormones at the various phases of the normal cycle are given in Table 4. (Adapted from Speroff L. *et al.*, 1978. *Clinical gynaecologic endocrinology and infertility*, 2nd edn., 31. Williams and Wilkins, Baltimore).

Table 1 Physiological effects of oestrogens

Uterine
  Myometrial hypertrophy
  Endometrial proliferation
  Cervical gland proliferation and secretion
Tubal
  Muscular hypertrophy and contractility
  Epithelial proliferation
Vaginal
  Epithelial proliferation
  Glandular proliferation and secretion
  Vulval growth
Breast
  Development of connective tissue
  Enlargement of nipple
  Areolar pigmentation
  Ductal proliferation
Pubic hair development
Epiphyseal fusion
Control of hypothalamus-pituitary function (see text)

Control of the menstrual cycle. As in the male, the endocrine and germinal functions of the ovary are controlled by the hypothalamic pituitary unit, but in the female the modulation of hormone secretion is more complex, involving positive as well as negative feedback loops (Fig. 3). Hypothalamic LHRH (gonadotrophin releasing hormone) initiates synthesis and secretion of follicle stimulating hormone (FSH) and luteinizing hormone (LH). Oestradiol can inhibit gonadotrophin secretion or can promote it depending on the level of steroid perfusing the hypothalamus and pituitary. In the presence of high concentrations of progesterone, oestradiol does not have a stimulatory effect.

Hormonal changes of the menstrual cycle. These interactions form the basis of the control of the normal menstrual cycle (Fig. 2). The most important biological event of this cycle is ovulation although

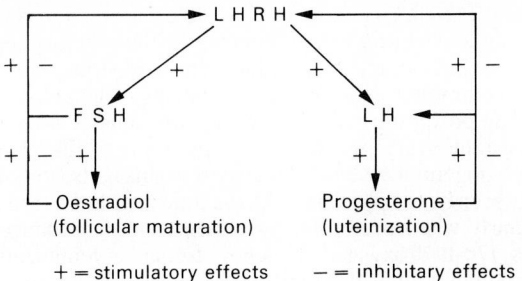

+ = stimulatory effects   − = inhibitory effects

Fig. 3 The control of gonadal function in the female. Where both + and − are shown there is both negative and positive feedback (see text for full description).

that most obvious to the woman and her medical attendant is menstruation.

Ovulation follows soon after the mid-cycle surge in gonadotrophin levels. These result from the positive feedback effect of oestradiol, and to a lesser extent, progesterone. The pre-ovulatory increase in oestradiol levels comes from the follicle that has developed through the influence of FSH. The slight decrease in the concentration of this hormone during the late follicular phase is a manifestation of the negative feedback of oestradiol. The initiation of follicular development, and hence of the menstrual cycle, is a result of increasing FSH secretion. The hormonal pattern of the luteal phase which follows ovulation is characterized by progesterone secretion and a secondary rise in oestradiol. Menstruation follows the shedding of the endometrium which occurs when progesterone and oestradiol levels fall. In anovular cycles, there is no luteal elevation of progesterone but the changes in oestradiol are enough to produce endometrial proliferation followed by a loss sufficient to give menstrual bleeding.

The control of LHRH secretion is regulated by neural mechanisms as well as by feedback from the gonadal hormones. Nerve pathways terminating in the hypothalamus play a part in controlling LHRH release. For example, dopaminergic neurons and opiate pathways of the tubero-infundibular system inhibit LHRH as do 5-hydroxytryptamine and melatonin, a pineal hormone. Noradrenergic pathways stimulate gonadotrophin release probably via LHRH.

Abnormalities of the menstrual cycle

Amenorrhoea. Lack of menses can be due to structural abnormalities of the hypothalamopituitary unit or ovary or to various functional disorders where the anatomy is apparently normal but the control of hormonal secretion is faulty. Additional to these general causes, primary amenorrhoea may result from anatomical problems of the lower genital tract such as an absent uterus or imperforate hymen.

Clinical aspects. The important points to establish in the history of a patient with amenorrhoea are set out in Table 2.

Any adult woman who is not pregnant, lactating, or menopausal has pathological amenorrhoea if she has not menstruated for six months. The same is true of an otherwise normal girl who has had no period by the age of 16. A younger person with amenorrhoea and stigmata of congenital disease also warrants a clinical review.

While amenorrhoea may be a symptom of general, or non-gonadal, endocrine disease, Table 2 emphasizes those features that would draw the attention of the clinician specifically to disease of the hypothalamopituitary-ovarian axis. The reasons why these are important are made apparent in subsequent paragraphs.

Investigation. The investigations that should be performed in the amenorrhoeic patient in whom gross anatomical abnormality of the lower genital tract has been excluded are shown in Table 3. Rep-

Table 2 Clinical assessment of amenorrhoea

History
  Age of onset of symptoms
  Sudden or gradual menstrual disturbance
  Age of menarche (if any)
  Possibility of pregnancy
  Change in weight
  Change in location, occupation, or life style
  Headache
  Hot flushes
  Medication
Examination
  Height
  Weight
  Breast development
  Amount and distribution of body hair
  Presence of galactorrhoea
  Abdominal and pelvic examinations
  Evidence of virilism (q.v.)
  Evidence of other endocrine disease (q.v.)

resentative normal values are quoted, but each laboratory should establish its own normal range.

All females of reproductive age with amenorrhoea should have a pregnancy test performed before they are assessed further. The results of the initial tests narrow the diagnostic field and act as a guide for further more detailed investigation. If pregnancy can be excluded, FSH and prolactin measurements are helpful. The former will be elevated if there is gonadal failure and high levels of the latter will set the investigator off on the appropriate diagnostic trail (see Table 5). LH concentrations may parallel changes in FSH, but a monotropic rise in LH suggests, in the absence of pregnancy, a diagnosis of the polycystic ovary syndrome (PCO). Low gonadotrophin concentrations are difficult to define as many normal subjects have basal levels that are at the limit of sensitivity for the assay. It is generally considered that basal oestradiol measurements are not very useful.

Progesterone estimates between days 18 and 22 of the cycle are used to follow the effects of therapy and to detect ovulation. Androgens must be measured when virilization accompanies amenorrhoea and are also useful in the PCO syndrome as a guide to treatment. Thyroid disease is detected by abnormal concentrations of thyroxine. Measurement of serum gonadotrophins after an injection of LHRH, is useful in distinguishing low normal levels from

Table 3 The investigation of amenorrhoea due to anovulation

Essential
  Measure FSH (follicular phase 1–9 u/l, ovulatory phase 6–26 u/l, luteal phase 1–9 u/l)
  Measure LH (follicular phase 1–12 u/l, ovulatory phase 16–104 u/l, luteal phase 1–12 u/l)
  Prolactin (follicular phase 70–460 mu/l)
  (Pregnancy test)

Often useful
  Measure oestradiol (follicular phase 160–1310 pmol/l, ovulatory phase 900–2290 pmol/l, luteal phase 220–1480 pmol/l)
  Measure progesterone (luteal phase 16–60 nmol/l)
  Measure testosterone (0.8–3.0 nmol/l)
  Measure thyroxine (60–135 nmol/l)
  LHRH test
  Chromosome analysis
  Pituitary fossa radiology
  Ultrasound and/or CT scanning of pelvis

Occasionally helpful
  Pelvic examination under anaesthesia (EUA)
  Dilatation and curettage (D&C)
  Progestogen administration
  Oestrogen amplification

true gonadotrophin deficiency. Cytogenetic disorders are detected by chromosome analysis. X-rays of the pituitary fossa are indicated if a tumour is suspected for clinical reasons or if prolactin levels are high, or there is evidence of unexplained gonadotrophin deficiency. Computerized tomography with or without enhancement by metrizamide is required if a hypothalamic or pituitary space-occupying lesion poses a surgical problem. Imaging of the pelvis is useful in defining an ovarian tumour or absence of the uterus.

Other investigations that may occasionally be called for include an EUA and D and C to define further the pelvic anatomy and establish uterine pathology. An endometrial biopsy is still occasionally used to confirm ovulation. Progestogen may be administered as a biological test of oestrogen activity since bleeding after progesterone will only occur in a woman whose endometrium has been primed by oestrogen. This test is also used as a guide to the likely outcome of clomiphene therapy; a positive result makes it more probable that clomiphene will induce ovulation. Lack of a bleed indicates the need for gonadotrophin treatment in addition. Oestrogen amplification provides similar information; an LHRH test is followed by oestrogen, usually given by injection. The LHRH test is then repeated after 48 and 92 hours. The normal will show amplification of the LHRH effect—hence the name of the test.

Patients with this normal response will ovulate with clomiphene.

The causes of amenorrhoea with their functional diagnosis are listed in Table 4. The further investigation depends in part on whether there is evidence of virilism (see page 10.85).

Table 4 Pathological amenorrhoea

Cause	Primary	Secondary	Pattern of laboratory findings (see Table 5)
Hypothalamic/pituitary			
Tumour	+	+	3,4
Empty sella syndrome	±	+	3,4
Trauma	+	+	3,4
Granuloma	±	+	3,4
Infarction	−	+	4,5
Weight loss	+	+	4,5
Weight gain	+	+	4,5
Psychogenic/idiopathic	+	+	4,5
Kallman's syndrome	+	−	4
Hyperprolactinaemia	±	+	3
Gonadal			
Dysgenesis	±	±	1,2
17α-hydroxylase deficiency	+	−	1,2
Resistant ovary	±	+	1,2
Iatrogenic	±	±	1,2
Galactosaemia	+	+	1,2
Autoimmune	+	±	1,2
Tumour	±	+	5
Polycystic ovary	±	+	2
Testicular feminization	+	−	1
Uterine/vaginal			
Malformed vagina	+	−	
Imperforate hymen	+	−	
Mullerian agenesis	+	−	
Loss of endometrium	−	+	
Adrenal			
Congenital hyperplasia	+	±	5
Cushing's syndrome	±	+	3,4,5
Virilizing tumour	±	+	4,5
Thyroid			
Hypothyroidism	±	+	3
Hyperthyroidism	±	+	?5
Severe generalized disease (chronic infection, neoplasms, etc.)	+	+	

+ = commonly   ± = uncommonly   − = not found

Causes. The classification used in Table 4 is based on anatomical and physiological principles. Tumours of the pituitary region, including prolactinomas, weight loss, and idiopathic amenorrhoea are the commoner causes of abnormalities of gonadotrophin release. The polycystic ovary syndrome and gonadal dysgenesis and the 'resistant ovary' are the most important of the ovarian disorders. Congenital absence of uterus or vagina is also important but is rarely seen by the physician. All the other conditions are unusual, particularly when presenting as a menstrual disturbance. Some, such as 17α-hydroxylase deficiency, testicular feminization, and auto-immune oophoritis are very rare indeed. These are discussed because they illustrate important physiological or pathological principles. In the majority of instances the diagnosis will be straightforward and the tests purely confirmatory. Occasionally, the cause of the illness will not be obvious, in which case the ancillary investigations are needed.

Hypothalamic/pituitary disorders. Many of these conditions have already been considered (see pages 10.7–24). Only those aspects germane to ovarian disorders, or of special significance in reproductive endocrinology, will be considered here.

Many tumours in the region of the third ventricle, the hypothalamus, and pituitary can present with disturbances of reproductive function. In the absence of information leading to a definitive diagnosis either from the clinical picture or from the result of the preliminary investigations, an X-ray of the skull and pituitary fossa should be obtained. A double floor or rarefaction in the wall of the pituitary fossa or erosion of the posterior clinoid processes may raise suspicion of a tumour. Visual fields should be charted as they may reveal an unexpected loss. CT scanning may show an empty sella or a large suprasellar extension but current techniques do not allow the non-invasive demonstration of small projections of tumour above the diaphragma sellae, or of distortions to the anatomy of the third ventricle. For these to be shown, procedures such as pneumo-encephalography or metrizamide cisternography, or even carotid angiography, are necessary, but should only be done when surgery or radiotherapy are contemplated. Visual field disturbances and the effects of raised intracranial pressure, but not amenorrhoea or infertility, are indications for surgery; even with modern microsurgical techniques, the results vis-à-vis fertility are less satisfactory than with drugs.

A woman with a pituitary tumour who becomes pregnant should be managed conservatively with monthly checks of her visual fields and instructions to report immediately if she should develop severe headache or disturbance of vision. While the pituitary gland, and thus the tumour, tends to enlarge during pregnancy, only in a minority of instances is an emergency hypophysectomy required. There is no evidence that prophylactic radiotherapy reduces the risk and indeed the long-term effects of such treatment might be harmful.

A condition specifically related to reproduction is Sheehan's syndrome where there is hypothalamic and pituitary dysfunction following an obstetric catastrophe, usually a severe post-partum haemorrhage. The diagnosis is clinched by the history of subsequent failure to establish lactation or menstruation. However, an occasional pituitary tumour may present in this way, with an incidental severe blood loss post-partum, and anorexia nervosa likewise can superficially mimic the condition.

Weight loss. The greater the percentage decrease from ideal body weight, the more the chance of amenorrhoea. When weight falls below 90 per cent of ideal body weight there is a chance of amenorrhoea; below 75 per cent amenorrhoea is inevitable. Some patients diet in order to model clothes, or to become ballet dancers, but more often the weight loss and amenorrhoea form part of the picture of anorexia nervosa (see page 8.51). The endocrine disturbance in mild cases of this disease is associated with a loss of oestrogen positive feedback and in severe forms to a lack of gonadotrophin secretion even in response to acutely administered

Table 5 Pattern of laboratory findings

	1	2	3	4	5
Finding	raised FSH	raised LH	raised prolactin	low FSH and oestradiol; no LH release	normal hormone levels
Functional diagnosis	ovarian failure	ovarian failure (FSH raised, E lowered) PCO (FSH lowered or normal, E raised or normal) pregnancy (FSH normal, E raised)	hyperprolactinaemia	gonadotrophin deficiency	defect of cycle initiation and/or disorder of positive feedback
Further investigation	karyotype laparoscopy and ovarian biopsy	pregnancy test measure androgens laparoscopy	find cause (q.v.)	X-ray pit fossa LHRH test	measure androgens laparoscopy progesterone administration oestrogen amplification

LHRH. Experimental evidence points to a deficiency of LHRH since it has been reported that replacement doses given in pulses over a period of weeks will restore the cycle to normal. The diagnosis of anorexia nervosa is usually easy. Cortisol and growth hormone levels are often high and distinguish the disease from hypopituitarism. Management is difficult and prolonged. Fashions for therapy change. Ovulation is restored in the majority of those who regain their weight.

Weight gain. Obesity may also be associated with amenorrhoea. The reason for this is not clear but it may be due to the conversion of inactive steroid precursors to oestrogens and to androgens by fat, thereby disturbing the normal cyclical changes in oestradiol levels that modulate gonadotrophin release.

Polycystic ovarian disease (see below) may occur in obese women, presumably as a consequence of the abnormal acyclic gonadotrophin secretion. Reduction in weight towards normal usually results in restitution of ovulatory cycles. It is most important to bear in mind that a combination of amenorrhoea and increase in weight is most commonly due to pregnancy.

Psychogenic/idiopathic. Minor psychological factors as well as severe mental disturbance can cause amenorrhoea, but the ascribed precipitating event may be so minor that it turns out to be the invention of the physician looking for a cause, rather than the true reason. Change of status, job, locale, or hours of working can all upset the normal cycle but usually not for more than two or three months. Should the amenorrhoea exceed six months, further investigation is warranted. If no abnormality is found, then the diagnosis is by definition 'idiopathic'. In idiopathic secondary amenorrhoea, there may be an abnormality of cycle initiation or of mid-cycle feedback. Recent experimental data suggest that this may be due to activation of opiate pathways since naloxone can restore the hormonal pattern to normal. The amenorrhoea of this condition is not of itself harmful but may be very worrying to the sufferer who will be aware that fertility will be impaired. Periods can be restored by giving oral contraceptives but these are rarely necessary since the amenorrhoea *per se* is not damaging. Strong reassurance that the periods will return spontaneously may be all that is required, with the added rider that ovulation can usually be induced by medical means (see below) to facilitate pregnancy.

Kallman's syndrome. Kallman's syndrome (see page 10.13) may occur in the female, but is much commoner in the male. The somatic features are the same, namely anosmia, colour blindness, midline facial deformities, and renal abnormalities. There may also be a family history. Investigation will show low gonadotrophin levels that are unresponsive to acute administration of LHRH. Treatment with cyclical oestrogen and progesterone will induce sexual maturation and menstrual periods but LHRH given in a pulsatile manner over a prolonged period or gonadotrophin therapy is necessary for ovulation.

Hyperprolactinaemia (see page 10.16). Elevated prolactin levels are found in approximately 20 per cent of women of reproductive age presenting with amenorrhoea. In one half of these a pituitary tumour will be found. In all but a few of the remainder no definite aetiology is apparent but occasionally there may be one of the other of the causes listed in Table 6. The cause of the ovulatory defect leading to the amenorrhoea is complex. There is a hypersensitive and prolonged negative feedback by oestradiol on FSH and defective positive feedback on LH. The disordered gonadotrophin dynamics result in a poorly stimulated ovary and hence oestrogen deficiency. The level at which hyperprolactinaemia acts is not known for certain; the pattern of gonadotrophin secretion suggests the hypothalamus with faulty secretion of LHRH. Apart from some data showing that prolactin inhibits luteinization of the ovary, there is no support for the theory that prolactin has an antigonadotrophic effect.

Besides amenorrhoea, the clinical consequences of hyperprolactinaemia are galactorrhoea and dyspareunia, the latter being due to the lack of vaginal secretion consequent to the oestrogen deficiency. Recent studies have revealed osteoporosis as an additional consequence of low oestrogen concentration. Only a half to two-thirds of patients with hyperprolactinaemia suffer from galactorrhoea.

The management of hyperprolactinaemia depends on the cause. In the majority of cases there will be either a tumour or there will be no obvious pathology. Unless urgent treatment is required for a rapidly expanding space-occupying lesion, the therapy of choice is bromocriptine (see page 10.17) which reduces prolactin levels into the normal range in almost all patients and shrinks some tumours.

Table 6 Causes of hyperprolactinaemia

Physiological
  Midcycle
  Pregnancy
  Lactation
  Stress
  Sleep
Pathological
  Disease in region of hypothalamus and pituitary
  Hypothyroidism
  Chest wall injury
  Ectopic production by non-endocrine tumours
  Renal failure
  Drugs
  Idiopathic

Gonadal disease

Gonadal dysgenesis. In its classical form it is known as Turner's syndrome. The patients present with primary amenorrhoea, although 10 per cent give a history of having had at least one vaginal bleed independent of any oestrogen therapy. Typically, the patients are short with a large number of skeletal abnormalities including cubitus valgus, arched palate, short fourth metacarpals, and shield chest with widely spaced nipples. Radiologically, other osseous abnormalities such as osteoporosis, 'beaked' vertebral bodies, fused cervical vertebrae, and abnormal carpal angles may be detected. Coarctation of the aorta or renal anomalies such as horseshoe kidney may occur, as may hypertension. The high frequency of kidney anomalies makes intravenous urography mandatory. Lymphoedema is also a feature together with a low hairline and multiple naevi. The patients are sexually infantile with poorly developed breasts and external genitalia and scanty axillary and pubic hair. Auto-immune thyroiditis and diabetes mellitus are commoner in these patients than in the general population.

The diagnosis is made by the detection of elevated FSH concentrations and, in the classical case, a 45 XO karyotype with chromatin-negative buccal squames. Laparoscopy may reveal streak ovaries. There are many chromosomal variants of the condition, for details of which the reader should refer to a text on cytogenetics. Some of them are associated with a tall eunuchoid stature and secondary, rather than primary amenorrhoea. Other variants are considered below (see Swyer syndrome).

Management requires great sensitivity since the chance of conception is vanishingly small and the news of sterility comes hard. The oestrogen deficiency is best treated with cyclical ethinyl oestradiol 100 µg a day for three weeks in the month for 6–12 months and then an oral contraceptive preparation containing oestrogen and progesterone. Hypertension, if present, is controlled by appropriate drugs. If a Y chromosome is found, gonadectomy should be performed, because of an increased risk of dysgerminoma.

Pure gonadal dysgenesis. This differs from Turner's syndrome in that the stigmata of that condition are absent and the chromosome pattern is that of a normal female. There may be an associated neurosensory deafness. Familial studies suggest that the condition is inherited via an autosomal recessive gene.

Swyer syndrome. This eponym has been given to the co-existence of an XY karyotype and gonadal dysgenesis. The condition, inherited either as an X-linked recessive or male limited autosomal dominant, is notable for a 20–30 per cent incidence of dysgerminomas or gonadoblastomas usually in the first two decades of life. Gonadectomy should therefore be carried out in any patient with this syndrome.

17α-hydroxylase deficiency. This is a very rare congenital enzyme deficiency affecting the ovary and adrenal. Oestradiol levels are low so the patient does not develop secondary sex characteristics. There is also hypertension and hypokalaemia since deoxycorticosterone and corticosterone are produced to excess by the adrenal (see page 10.67). Treatment is with cyclic gonadal steroids and continuous glucocorticoids.

The resistant ovary. A minority of women may develop ovarian failure before the age of 40 with menopausal flushing, secondary amenorrhoea, and elevated gonadotrophin levels. In the absence of an obvious cause, such as iatrogenic or auto-immune reactions, the terms 'resistant ovary' or 'premature menopause' are used. The latter is incorrect since a proportion of these women may spontaneously resume normal ovarian function, ovulate and even conceive. Thus, a guarded prognosis should be given. The treatment is that of menopausal symptoms (see below) when they occur.

Iatrogenic ovarian failure. Irradiation and cytotoxic drugs used in the treatment of malignant disease can affect the ovary. In this instance, infertility and menopausal symptoms may result. However, spontaneous recovery can occur once chemotherapy is finished.

Galactosaemia. Females with this inborn error of metabolism may have ovarian failure as a feature. This may be due to a toxic effect of galactose or its metabolites. While some patients have had successful pregnancies, a recent series reported over half had either primary or secondary amenorrhoea.

Auto-immune oophoritis. Auto-antibodies to ovarian tissue have been described and may be responsible for ovarian failure. They may occur in association with pernicious anaemia, auto-immune hypophysitis, hypoparathyroidism. Addison's disease, hypothyroidism, and diabetes mellitus.

Ovarian tumours. Androgen-producing tumours of the ovary, in particular, may cause amenorrhoea. In the presence of elevated androgen levels hirsutism and virilism will develop; this cause of amenorrhoea is discussed in the section on virilism (see page 10.85).

Polycystic ovary syndrome. This usually presents in early adulthood when typically, after a year or two of regular menstruation, the periods become grossly irregular with the intermenstrual interval ranging from a few days to many months and the loss varying from sparse to very heavy. This pattern may be described as menstrual chaos. Fertility is impaired, but not absolutely. In approximately half the women there may be hirsutism, and, in a few, more obvious features of virilism. Some degree of obesity is found in 50 per cent of patients. The typical hormonal pattern is of low FSH and high LH levels. There is also a tendency to high oestradiol and androgen concentrations. The anovulation may be due to an abnormality in cycle initiation with, in some instances, a loss of positive feed-back for the mid-cycle surge of gonadotrophins. There is a defective ovarian biosynthesis of oestradiol with the overproduction of precursors that may be metabolized in extraglandular tissue to oestrone and testosterone. This in turn maintains the abnormality of gonadotrophin release. The diagnosis may be made on the clinical picture and confirmed by laparoscopy of the ovaries which appear large and have multiple cysts under a glistening white capsule. Biopsy clinches the diagnosis but often a cyst is not sampled so the histology is not then diagnostic. Furthermore, thecal hyperplasia of the ovary without cysts may mimic the clinical features of the polycystic ovary syndrome. The diagnosis is usually straightforward but it is important to bear in mind that hyperandrogenic states such as congenital adrenal hyperplasia, virilizing adrenal tumours, Cushing's syndrome, arrhenoblastoma, and hilus cell tumour of the ovary can co-exist with, and possibly predispose to, the polycystic ovary syndrome. Ovarian hyperthecosis has also been reported in association with hypertension, hyperuricaemia, hyperlipidaemia, insulin-resistant diabetes mellitus, and acanthosis nigricans. The clinical problems of the polycystic ovary syndrome are anovulation and hirsutism and there is an increased incidence of endometrial carcinoma presumably due to the prolonged effect of oestrogen unopposed by post-ovulatory, luteal progesterone.

The ovulatory deficiency may be treated with clomiphene with or without added human chorionic gonadotrophin (HCG) or with corticosteroids. Wedge resection of the ovary is now almost never recommended. The management of the hirsutism is discussed on pages 10.85–87.

Testicular feminization. This term is a misnomer since the testis does not feminize the patient. It is that the affected male is resistant to the action of testosterone and dihydrotestosterone and so a female phenotype is found. In testicular feminization, binding of androgen to receptors on target tissues is deficient with the result that androgens cannot act normally at the cellular level. This results in a patient who is phenotypically female with well-developed breasts at puberty and female external genitalia including a normal clitoris. However, the vagina is short and there may be inguinal herniae, which sometimes contain testes. Pubic and axillary hair are absent or scanty. The testes, if not in hernial sacs, may be intra-abdominal or scrotal. The diagnosis is usually easy. In the adult the presentation is with primary amenorrhoea. In childhood, it is with inguinal herniae. The chromosome karyotype is 46 XY. Serum testosterone and luteinizing hormone levels tend to be high due to diminished receptors in the pituitary, thus preventing the operation of normal feedback. The hyperactivity of the testes is responsible for the high oestrogen levels that are found. These cause the development of the female secondary sex characteristics at puberty. The sex orientation is also female.

The metabolic abnormality is transmitted genetically although the mode of inheritance is not absolutely clear. The alternatives that have been proposed are via an X-linked recessive or a sex-limited autosomal dominant gene.

Treatment is to castrate the patient soon after puberty since there is a high risk of the testes undergoing malignant change. Unfortunately, a frequent consequence of this is disabling hot flushes, which are often, but not always, responsive to treatment with oestrogens. Plastic surgery to the genitalia may also be necessary to increase the size of the vagina to allow satisfactory sexual intercourse. Many of the patients marry and have entirely satisfactory sexual relationships.

Partial receptor deficiency usually manifests as an abnormally virilized male, and so has been discussed in the section on the male reproductive system (see page 10.73).

Adrenal disease. disorders of the adrenal cortex are commonly associated with menstrual disturbances. Usually, this is due to excess androgen production so the clinical picture, pathophysiology, and diagnosis are detailed in the section on hirsutism and virilism (page 10.85). However, patients with Addison's disease can also become amenorrhoeic. 17α-hydroxylase deficiency occurs in the adrenal as well as the ovary.

Thyroid disease. Both hypo- and hyperthyroidism may be associated with amenorrhoea as part of the symptom complex. In hypothyroidism this may be associated with hyperprolactinaemia. The mechanism for the menstrual disturbance of thyrotoxicosis is not clear. Nevertheless, both abnormalities should be born in mind in the obscure case.

Generalized illness. Any disease significant enough to cause constitutional disturbances can produce amenorrhoea. Usually this symptom is merely one of a more complex number but occasionally, as for example, in secondary deposits in the ovary or in tuberculosis, it may provide an important clue to diagnosis and indicate focal involvement of the genital tract.

Delayed puberty

The chronological age of onset of breast development and menses often follows a familial pattern, so the timing of these landmarks in mother and sisters should be ascertained. Usually breast development has begun by the age of 13 and, in the United Kingdom, 95 per cent of normal girls have menstruated by the time they are 15 years old. Delay beyond these ages merits investigation in an analogous manner to the male. A bone age within two years of chronological is grounds for reassurance as is a gonadotrophin response to LHRH. Otherwise an investigation should be undertaken for evidence of hypothalamic pituitary or gonadal disease, with a high FSH pointing to the latter.

Anatomical abnormalities of the lower genital tract

There may be developmental disorders of the Mullerian tract any of which may cause primary amenorrhoea. The conditions that are found may be: (a) an imperforate hymen, with haematocolpos,

presenting with a mass arising out of the pelvis; (b) a 'blocked' vagina, that will have the same physical signs as imperforate hymen; and (c) the Mayer–Rokitansky–Kuster–Hauser syndrome, i.e. lack of Mullerian development. In (c) there may be a complete absence of uterus, or malformation of that organ, in addition to vaginal abnormality. Sometimes, cyclical abdominal pain may occur in those patients who have partial canalization of the endometrial cavity. This is due to retained menstrual loss. In a high proportion of cases, skeletal abnormalities occur. These include scoliosis, spina bifida, and malformations of limbs and ribs. Likewise, disorders of the renal tract such as absent or ectopic kidneys or abnormalities of the pelvis or ureters are common. Occasionally, congenital heart disease, cleft palate, and situs inversus have been reported in association. There are instances of one or more manifestations of the syndrome occurring in families, but the mode of transmission remains undefined. The defect involves a maldevelopment of mesoderm. While the condition will present only rarely to the physician, it is important to appreciate that it lies second only to gonadal dysgenesis as a cause of primary amenorrhoea. The diagnosis can usually be made on clinical grounds but a chromosome karyotype may be necessary to distinguish it from some patients with male pseudohermaphroditism. Normal cyclical function can be proved with serum progesterone measurements; abdominal ultrasonography or CT scanning can assist where abdominal or rectal examinations fail. If the sole genital problem is an uncanalized vagina, then surgery is the treatment of choice.

A cause of secondary amenorrhoea found more frequently in the United States than elsewhere is Asherman's syndrome where over-enthusiastic curettage has completely denuded the uterus of endometrium and caused the cavity to scar. Treatment consists of hysteroscopy with reforming of the uterine cavity and maintenance of patency with a small urinary catheter.

Infertility

The management of this problem in the female falls usually within the province of the gynaecologist or the specialist reproductive endocrinologist. However, the principles involved are of interest to the general physician who will then be able to refer the patient as appropriate.

It is first necessary to locate the nature of the problem. In approximately a third of cases there is an abnormality in the male. This can be identified by seminal analysis, which is mandatory in the investigation of the infertile couple. An abnormality here is dealt with in the manner described on page 10.70. In approximately a fifth of the couples there is disease of the Fallopian tubes. This may be suspected from a past history or pelvic inflammation or may be found at laparoscopic examination or by hysterosalpingography. This requires the expertise of the gynaecologist. In a small proportion there may be an abnormality of the cervical mucus making it 'hostile', or at least not friendly, to the sperms. In 20 per cent there is no apparent reason for infertility. The remaining sixth have a failure of ovulation. The causes of this together with the differential diagnosis have already been discussed in the section on amenorrhoea see page 10.79). The treatment is that of the cause whenever possible, but in many instances the cause is functional and in some cases the ovulatory failure can be treated despite an inability to remedy the primary condition.

The aim of treatment is to reproduce as closely as possible the hormonal changes of the normal cycle by stimulating the ovary to produce a mature follicle, ovulation, and luteinization.

If the defect is solely one of the cycle initiation, an oral anti-oestrogen is used, usually clomiphene, but others are available. This will result in a rise in gonadotrophins, follicular maturation, increasing oestradiol secretion, and the oestrogen-stimulated gonadotrophin surge in those women with intact positive feedback. This mid-cycle surge results in ovulation. In those women who have an abnormality of positive feedback in addition to a failure of cycle initiation, HCG, which is rich in LH activity, is injected after the clomiphene at a time when the mid-cycle surge would normally occur.

In the absence of gonadotrophins, or in those instances when clomiphene fails, human FSH is given by injection to produce maturation of the Graafian follicle followed by HCG to induce ovulation. FSH is obtained from post-menopausal urine.

Many of the clomiphene failures are among the patients with hyperprolactinaemia. The specific treatment here is bromocriptine, a drug which produces ovulation in over 95 per cent of women treated, with a resulting pregnancy in 70–90 per cent.

Any woman being treated with gonadotrophins for anovulation requires monitoring by a specialized unit. Serum or urinary oestrogen measurements with rapid reporting of results are necessary to monitor the follicular development. Ovulation can be implied from the fall and then rise in basal body temperature, but is more accurately assessed by measurement of serum progesterone levels. In hyperprolactinaemia the response of serum prolactin concentrations to treatment should also be checked.

The main hazard of treatment with clomiphene or gonadotrophins is massive painful ovarian enlargement, particularly when clomiphene is given to women with polycystic ovary syndrome. Fortunately, this is very rare and subsides with masterly inactivity. Very rarely, haematoperitoneum and dehydration may occur; these are managed symptomatically. Ovarian cystectomy, or ovarectomy, should not be performed. Minor side effects of clomiphene are hot flushes, breast discomfort, nausea, headache, or vomiting.

The menopause

Introduction. Reproductive capacity starts to fail in women in the Western world from their mid-forties to mid-fifties with a mean age of approximately 50.

During this time there is a steady disorganization of the hormonal changes associated with the menstrual cycle. There are episodic rises in FSH concentrations much higher than those found during early adult life with a loss of cyclicity. At the same time oestradiol levels gradually fall and the luteal increase of progesterone diminishes. Ultimately, the mid-cycle gonadotrophin peak disappears and the hormonal pattern of the menopause becomes established. This results from ovarian failure and consists of low oestradiol and high gonadotrophin concentrations, with FSH being the more markedly raised. There is also a fall in the concentration of oestrone, although this is not decreased to the same extent as oestradiol since the latter comes mainly from the follicle whereas the former is produced not only by this source but also by the ovarian stroma, which does not atrophy in the menopause. Peripheral conversion of androstenedione to oestrogens from the stroma and from the adrenal gland is also decreased. This reduction in the circulating levels of oestrogens produces the clinical manifestations of the menopause.

Clinical aspects. These are shown in Table 7. The menopause is heralded in the majority of women by the menses becoming irregular and scanty and then finally ceasing. In some, it presents suddenly with the amenorrhoea coming 'out of the blue' while in others there may be excessive and prolonged vaginal bleeding before the periods stop. The majority of women, but not all, develop hot flushes during the menopausal transition. These consist of attacks of flushing of the face and trunk associated with sweating and a

Table 7   Clinical features of the menopause

Amenorrhoea
Hot flushes
Mammary atrophy
Atrophic vaginitis
Pelvic floor weakness
Osteoporosis

sensation of heat. They may range in severity from the infrequent, mild, and inconsequential, to repeated long-lasting and disabling episodes significantly interfering with the conduct of a normal life. The mechanism of the flush is unclear although it is known to be related to the fall in oestrogen secretion and is associated with rapid surges in LH secretion. Recent work has indicated an involvement of opiate receptors since naloxone, a specific opiate antagonist, can be shown by experiment to reduce the frequency and severity of the flushes.

The atrophy of the breasts and genitalia associated with the menopause is a clear consequence of the reduction in oestrogen secretion. There is now also abundant evidence that the osteoporosis that appears in the post-menopausal years and is associated with the high incidence of Colles' fractures, and fractures of the femoral neck in the elderly is related to oestrogen deficiency.

There is an increased frequency of ischaemic heart disease following the menopause. This too might be a result of the biochemical changes at the menopause.

The lay term for the menopausal years, 'the change of life' encapsulates not only the physical alterations that occur but also the altered psychology. The decrease in libido that may occur can be due to pain in intercourse as a result of an atrophic vaginitis. Alternatively, it may be the consequence of a sense of loss of femininity. This change in self-perception can predispose to other depressive symptoms such as headache, non-specific aches and pains, insomnia, loss of concentration, and irritability. These latter symptoms together with the more clearly defined consequences of oestrogen deficiency comprise the menopausal syndrome that makes life so wearisome for some women.

Treatment. Treatment is based on the assumption that the majority of symptoms are due to the decline in oestrogen levels. Treatment is now usually given cyclically with oestrogens in combination with progestogen except when a hysterectomy has been carried out, when the progestogen may be omitted. The oestrogens may be either synthetic or naturally occurring products. Although there are proponents of both types, there is probably nothing to choose between them. In the former category fall oestradiol valerate and mestranol, while in the latter are conjugated equine oestrogens and oestrone sulphate. The benefits, disadvantages, hazards and contra-indications are set out in Table 8. Most women tolerate therapy well and derive improvement from it but the precautions listed in the Table must be noted and oestrogen-only pills should not be given because of the risk of endometrial carcinoma, protection from which is afforded by adding a progestogen and giving the therapy cyclically.

Other hormonal approaches are used from time to time. Progestogen alone can decrease flushing but not as effectively as oestrogens, and androgens are said to increase libido and reduce the rate of bone loss. However, they also induce virilization and cholestasis and so are not generally recommended. Clonidine in

Table 8   Oestrogen therapy

Benefits	Contra-indications
Reduction in	Absolute
Hot flushes	Liver disease
Vaginal atrophy	Cerebrovascular disease
Rate of bone loss	Venous thrombosis
Hazards	Hormone-dependent tumours of
Gall bladder disease	Breast
? Thrombo-embolic disease	Uterus
Endometrial cancer	Kidney
Disadvantages	Malignant melanoma
Tender breasts	Relative
Breakthrough bleeding	Hypertension
Nausea and vomiting	Gall bladder disease
Cramps	Cardiac failure
	Nephrogenic oedema

small doses (0.025–0.075 mg twice daily) may reduce the flushes but has no effect on oestrogen deficiency *per se*. The controversy still rages as to how long therapy should be continued. The large majority hold the view that it should only be given to tide the patient over the period when symptoms are at their worst. Unfortunately, there is no evidence that oestrogens are the Elixir of Youth for women.

Hormonal contraception

The most popular and effective method of contraception in the developed world is the oral contraceptive pill (see also page 11.1). In its usual form this consists of a combination of oestrogen and progestogen, although progestogen-only pills are available and depot progestogen injections are also used.

Mechanism of action. The combined pill suppresses gonadotrophin release and hence follicular maturation, ovulation, and luteinization. Thus endogenous oestrogen levels are low and there is no luteal rise in progesterone secretion. The consequence of this is an atrophic endometrium together with a progestogen-stimulated cervical mucus that is hostile to spermatoza.

Hazards. The chief adverse effect is of thrombo-embolic disease with myocardial infarction, cerebrovascular disease, and pulmonary emboli being the clinical manifestations. All these are rare but their incidence is increased by obesity and smoking. Moreover, age is also a factor with the reactions being more frequent in women over 35. Thus, women with these risk factors should be advised to seek alternative means of contraception such as intra-uterine contraceptive devices, mechanical measures, or sterilization of one or other partner. Furthermore, women with a previous episode of venous thrombosis due to one of the common causes rather than the 'pill' should stop oral contraception for one month before and two after surgery. Other side-effects which may be encountered are hypertension, depression, gall bladder disease, and weight gain. Although there may be an initial impairment in glucose tolerance, there is not a significant increase in the incidence of diabetes mellitus in pill users compared with women not on the pill. Breakthrough bleeding may be a problem with some women, particularly when the product contains small amounts of oestrogen. *Breakthrough bleeding as well as contraceptive failure can occur in women on rifampicin or enzyme-inducing anticonvulsants such as phenytoin and carbamazepine.*

Reproductive function returns to normal in two or three months in the majority of women after they stop the pill. If amenorrhoea should persist for six months or more, the patient should be fully investigated for this symptom rather than be labelled 'post-pill amenorrhoea' and the problem cast aside. A small proportion will be found to have prolactinomas but there is no evidence to support the view that these have been caused by the pill. Indeed, there are no firm grounds for incriminating the pill as a cause of long-term reproductive failure since many of the women with this problem give a history of menstrual disturbances before starting with the contraception.

Contra-indications. The effect of age, particularly in smokers and the obese, on the incidence of side-effects make it wise clinical practice to recommend changing the pill in the mid-thirties for some other contraceptive method. Patients with hypertension and diabetes should avoid the pill, as should patients with recurrent venous thromboses. Liver disease can be worsened in pill-users so this too is a contra-indication. Women taking enzyme-inducing drugs may take the pill providing they are aware of the risks and providing they do not use a preparation with a low oestrogen content.

Hirsutism and virilism

Introduction. Excessive hair growth is among the commoner endocrine afflictions of women. The complaint may exist in isolation or it may be one of a constellation of abnormalities found in the virilized state.

The ultimate cause of this group of disorders is an increase in the amount of androgen to which the target issue is exposed or an increased responsiveness of the target tissue to normal amounts of androgen.

Androgenic hormones may be secreted in excess by diseased adrenals (see page 10.60) or ovaries (see Fig. 1). They may also be produced by non-endocrine tissue from precursors secreted by these glands. The strong androgen that circulates in the highest concentration is testosterone. This is thought to contribute half the circulating androgenicity in the normal female.

The serum concentration of these and other hormones with similar action is given in Table 9. Androstenedione is very weak when tested in bioassay. However, it is important as a precursor for conversion in non-endocrine tissue to testosterone as well as to oestrone. Another weak androgen is dehydroepiandrosterone (DHA). As with androstenedione, this substance is secreted by both adrenal and ovary. Present in much higher concentrations than either of these is DHA-sulphate (DHA-S). This steroid is secreted by the adrenal but not by the gonad. The reason for the high serum concentrations is a metabolic clearance rate approximately 100 times lower than DHA. The production rate is similar.

Table 9 Concentrations of androgens and precursors in the serum of normal women of reproductive age

Testosterone   1–3 nmol/l
Dihydrotestosterone (DHT)   1–2 nmol/l
Androstenedione   4–10 nmol/l
Dehydroepiandrosterone (DHA)   10–40 nmol/l
DHA-sulphate (DHA-S)   3–7μmol/l
17-OH progesterone (17-OHP)   2–7 nmol/l
Sex hormone binding globulin (SHBG) capacity 70–90 nmol/l

A scheme showing the pathways for androgen synthesis and breakdown is set out in Fig. 4. DHA, androstenedione, and testosterone can all be transformed to dihydrotestosterone (DHT) in androgen sensitive tissue. The final step in this pathway is dependent on a 5α-reductase, unique to cells that respond to androgens. The DHT interacts with an intracellular receptor protein prior to manifesting its biological effect as an androgen. DHT is metabolized to androstanediol and thereby inactivated. This takes place in various tissues such as liver and skin and other sites that respond to androgens. Excretion of androgens usually takes place after conjugation with glucuronide or sulphate in the liver. These products are measured in the urine as '17-oxosteroids (17-OS)'. The hormone which contributes most to the 17-OS is DHA-S. Testosterone is a relatively minor contributor. In order to assess the androgenic state of the female, it is best to measure serum concentrations of testosterone and DHA-S. 17-OS estimations in urine may be substituted if DHA-S determinations are unavailable. There are in-

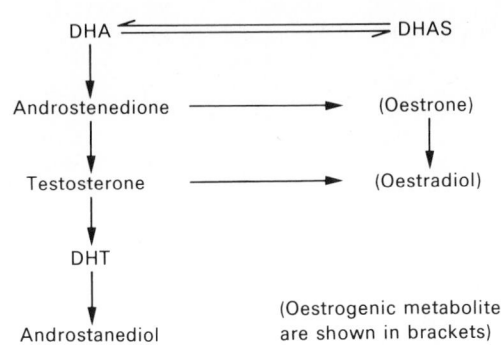

Fig. 4 Pathways of androgen metabolism. The oestrogens, oestradiol, and oestrone are inserted to emphasize that increased oestrogen formation can be a by-product of androgen excess.

stances when all the usual indices of androgen production are normal despite the woman being abnormal. This may be due to an increased intradermal conversion of precursors to DHT which is then further metabolized within the skin. Androstanediol measurements would show this, but the assay is still a research procedure.

Another marker of androgenicity is a low serum concentration of sex hormone binding globulin (SHBG). This is a hepatic protein, secreted into the bloodstream, which binds both androgen and oestrogen. The affinity for androgen is higher than that for oestrogen. The latter increases the concentration of the protein whereas it falls in response to the former. Since it is the free rather than the bound hormone that is physiologically active, it has been proposed that SHBG may act as an amplifier for sex steroid action with high levels of oestrogen producing increased androgen binding and thus low circulating free androgens, and vice versa when androgen levels are elevated.

Clinical consequences of excess androgen production or action. The effects of androgens on women are shown in Table 10. The most common of these is hirsutism. However, it is possible to have the other features of masculinization with little or no increase in hair growth.

Table 10   Effects on androgens in the female

Growth of hair on face, lip, chin, abdomen, and thighs
Fronto-temporal balding
Seborrhoea and acne
Deepening of voice
Clitoral hypertrophy
Skeletal muscular development
Oligomenorrhoea or amenorrhoea
Mammary atrophy

Causes. Hirsutism, having many causes as listed in Table 11, presents the greatest difficulty in differential diagnosis. The type and distribution of hair helps with ascertaining the underlying disorder. Soft downy hair on the limb extremities is not hormone dependent in contrast to a coarse hair on the face, trunk and thighs. Although excess hair may indeed be found in conditions such as anorexia nervosa, acromegaly, and porphyria, it is not a salient

Table 11   Causes of hirsutism

Adrenal
  Congenital adrenal hyperplasia
  Tumours
  Cushing's disease
Ovarian
  Tumours
  Polycystic ovary syndrome
Pituitary
  Acromegaly
Thyroid
  Juvenile myxoedema
Iatrogenic
  Phenytoin
  Diazoxide
  Minoxidil
  Corticosteroids
  Anabolic steroids
  Androgens
  19 nortestosterone progestogens
  Psoralens
'Idiopathic'
  Porphyria
  Anorexia nervosa
  Familial
  Racial
  Menopausal

symptom of these diseases which invariably present in other ways, so they will be considered no further in the differential diagnosis.

Women from the Indian subcontinent tend to have darker thicker hair than Caucasian women so minor deviations from the norm may appear more obvious, certainly when viewed through European eyes. Hairgrowth in dark Caucasians is more apparent than in those with a lighter skin. Thus, a familial or racial tendency to hirsutes should be noted when taking a history and examining a woman with this complaint.

A wide variety of drugs can produce hirsutism. Some such as anabolic steroids and androgens for obvious reasons, others such as corticosteroids because of an induced fall in SHBG. The antihypertensive agents, diazoxide and minoxidil, may act by increasing cutaneous blood flow. It is therefore important to enquire of the patient whether she is on any medicament.

In the majority of instances the cause is not one of the above and so the differential diagnosis lies between an adrenal or ovarian aetiology, or the hirsutism is idiopathic. The clinical features which help in distinguishing one pathology from another are shown in Table 12.

Table 12   Differential diagnosis of hirsutism

	Frequency	Age of onset	History	Menses
Adrenal				
Congenital hyperplasia	rare	infancy to early adulthood	short	variable (absent or normal)
Carcinoma	rare	any age	short	usually absent
Cushing's syndrome	unusual	any age	short	usually absent
Ovarian				
Polycystic ovary syndrome	common	near menarche	long	chaotic
Arrhenoblastoma	rare	menarche onwards	short	absent
Hilar cell tumour	rare	perimenopause	short	absent
Krukenberg tumour	rare	adulthood onwards	short	absent
Luteoma of pregnancy	very rare	pregnancy	short	absent
'Idiopathic'	common	near menarche	long	normal

The important factors to note in the history are the age of onset and duration of the presenting symptoms and whether there is an associated menstrual disturbance. If the periods are normal, it is most unlikely that there is serious underlying organic disease, particularly if the history is a long one. On the other hand, a short history with associated features of masculinization makes the existence of a significant adrenal or ovarian disorder more probable.

The initial investigations of a patient with hirsutism should include serum testosterone and DHA-S estimations. If there is a possibility of congenital adrenal hyperplasia measurement of 17-hydroxyprogesterone (17-OHP) and of the urinary 11-oxygenation index should be added.

A diagnosis of the polycystic ovary syndrome is supported by the finding of a high serum LH. In most cases of adrenal disease causing hirsutism the plasma DHA-S level and the urinary 17-OS are grossly elevated, with only a moderately high testosterone. In ovarian tumours, testosterone is very high and DHA-S concentrations are normal. Stimulation and suppression tests with corticosteroids, oestrogens, ACTH, or HCG are only of limited value and can indeed be misleading since tumours can respond in a physiologically inappropriate manner because of altered specificity of their receptors. In many instances, hormone measurements require supplementation with morphological studies to make a final diagnosis. Non-invasive investigations that are employed are CT, or less usefully, ultrasound scanning for either ovarian or adrenal lesions or adrenal scintiscanning with Se-cholesterol. On rare occasions, adrenal venography may help or the adrenal or ovarian veins may be catheterized to obtain samples for the determination of hormone levels in the effluent blood.

Endocrine causes

Adrenal. Disease of this gland are considered in detail elsewhere (page 10.58). Suffice it to say here that congenital adrenal hyperplasia can present in adult life with hirsutism, virilism, and often disturbed menstrual cycles as well as at the commoner times of early in life. The diagnosis is made by finding high serum 17-OHP levels that rise further when ACTH is given. Alternatively, a urinary 11-oxygenation index, which measures the ratio of cortisol precursors to cortisol may be used. Other diagnostic tests are the serum DHA-S or the urinary 17-OS and a plasma ACTH concentration which will all be elevated. Adrenal tumours are usually rapidly growing so that the development of symptoms may be dramatic. Often a tumour is palpable or there are hepatic or osseous metastases present when the patient is first seen. If not, diagnosis can be made by finding a high DHA-S and an adrenal mass on imaging. ACTH levels are low. The treatment for congenital hyperplasia is corticosteroid suppression. For a tumour a surgical approach should be adopted wherever possible. Palliation may be achieved with ortho-para DDD, metyrapone, or aminoglutethimide, all of which inhibit steroid biosynthesis in the adrenals.

Ovary. The polycystic ovary syndrome (PCO) is the commonest ovarian cause of hirsutism. Usually, there is a history of the typical menstrual disturbance but very occasionally the periods can be regular. Other features of virilization in addition to the hirsutes are encountered from time to time in women with this disorder. The diagnosis is supported by the finding of high LH levels and confirmed laparoscopically. Sometimes, the polycystic ovaries co-exist with another condition giving rise to excessive androgens, such as congenital adrenal hyperplasia or a virilizing adrenal or ovarian tumour. The latter may be so small as to escape notice on laparoscopy. There is increased incidence of endometrial carcinoma in women suffering from the PCO. This is due to the continued exposure to high levels of oestrogen, infrequent menstrual shedding of endometrium, and relatively low progesterone concentrations.

Ovarian tumours secreting androgens are rare. They may occur at any age, but are usually found in the reproductive years and shortly after. The endocrine features appear rapidly and are often responsible for the clinical presentation when the tumour is small. The diagnosis is suggested by a high serum testosterone and a normal or minimally elevated DHA-S. CT scanning and laparoscopy may provide further evidence but sometimes surgical exploration is required to clinch the diagnosis.

Idiopathic hirsutism. This ailment usually presents two or three years after the menarche with increasing hair growth on the face, trunk, and thighs. Menses are normal. Often the more usual endocrine measurements reveal no disturbance but specialized testing such as for SHBG or 'free' testosterone concentrations in serum reveals an abnormality. Androstanediol levels may be high, indicating that the skin itself is the site of increased androgen formation.

Treatment. The therapy available for the treatment of hirsutism is listed in Table 13. If the underlying cause is known and is amenable to treatment this should be done. Even when endocrine cure can be achieved in this way, the hirsutism will respond slowly, over several months, and indeed does not always disappear. However, in almost all instances, there will be clear amelioration of symptoms with a slowing of the rate of growth and the hair becoming finer. Signs of masculinization, if present, may diminish, but not disappear.

Periods may normalize and breasts may grow but a deep voice will not become high pitched nor will clitoromegaly atrophy.

Two types of treatment are available for idiopathic hirsutism, local and endocrine. The former includes bleaching, plucking, waxing, and shaving hair, or using electrolysis or depilatory creams. Plucking and electrolysis may suffice, if the hairs are few and coarse. Both may cause scarring and the latter is expensive. Shaving is cosmetically and psychologically unacceptable to many women, and the belief persists, albeit unsupported by evidence, that shaving stimulates hair growth. Waxing can be painful and, together with creams, may lead to inflammation and secondary infection of the skin.

Table 13   Treatment of hirsutism

Local	Endocrine
Plucking	Corticosteroids
Shaving	Oral contraceptives
Waxing	Cyproterone acetate
Electrolysis	
Depilatory creams	

Thus, endocrine treatment is indicated for the more severe cases. Corticosteroids suppress adrenal function and may also influence ovarian activity. They can be given in small doses in the late evening to suppress the rise in ACTH secretion that begins in the latter part of the night. Unfortunately, this form of treatment is not often effective and may indeed occasionally cause the hirsutes to worsen. Oral contraceptives work by suppressing hypothalmic/pituitary and hence ovarian activity. The oestrogenic component stimulates a rise in SHBG concentrations and thereby lowers the free circulating fraction of testosterone. This approach is moderately beneficial but only occasionally dramatically so. The choice of agent is important since the progestogenic component of some of the combinations is mildly androgenic and hence could worsen rather than ameliorate the complaint. The most effective treatment is with the anti-androgen, cyproterone acetate. This is given cyclically in a dose of 100 mg daily from days 5–14 of the cycle together with ethinyl oestradiol 50 µg daily on days 5–25. It is important that this cyclical regimen with the oestrogen is used since contraception must be effective during therapy. This is because of the risk of femininization of a male fetus by the anti-androgen.

Occasionally cyproterone produces lethargy and loss of libido and the long-term effects of anti-androgen treatment are unknown and could potentially be disadvantageous. Thus, this regime should be prescribed with caution. However, it is currently the best treatment available and is indicated when the complaint is having a profound effect on psyche and social life. As with all the endocrine treatments, the response may be slow so the patient should be warned that there may be no amelioration in hair growth before three months and that it may indeed be six or even nine months before a change is noticed. However, acne and seborrhoea may improve dramatically. Recently cimetidine and spironactone have been used experimentally to control hirsutism. The rationale behind both is apparent anti-androgenicity but there is as yet insufficient experience with either to recommend their use for this indication.

Gynaecological oncology

Only those aspects of the subject that the physician could encounter in practice are dealt with here.

Ovarian tumours. This group, of which three-quarters are benign, comprises one-third of tumours of the female genital tract. The symptoms are more commonly those of a pelvic space-occupying lesion, so will therefore usually present to the gynaecologist or surgeon. Only those with endocrine features are likely to be referred to the physician.

The hormonally active tumours are listed in Table 14 together with their respective secretions. All are rare, but need to be considered in unusual cases of diagnostic difficulty. The presentation and diagnosis of those secreting androgens has already been discussed. Oestrogen-producing tumours may cause precocious puberty, inter-menstrual, or post-menopausal bleeding and may be associated with endometrial carcinoma. The diagnosis is often made clinically but may be supplemented with hormonal measurements as well as CT scanning and ultrasound.

Table 14 Ovarian tumours

Type	Hormone
Arrhenoblastoma	androgen
Hilar cell	androgen
Gynandroblastoma	androgen, oestrogen
Granulosa cell	oestrogen
Thecoma	oestrogen
Choriocarcinoma	HCG
Struma ovarii	thyroxine
Carcinoid	serotonin

Substances such as placental lactogen (HPL), carcino-embryonic antigen (CEA), alpha-fetoprotein (AFP), and chorionic gonadotrophin (β-HCG), as well as the steroid hormones, which produced the clinical symptoms, can be used as tumour markers for diagnosis and following the effects of treatment.

As with other malignancies there is a vogue for staging laparotomies and radiology. Treatment may be surgical, radiotherapeutic, or chemotherapeutic or a combination of all three. A variety of drugs are employed in ovarian cancer including the usual antimetabolites. Among the more promising is the recently introduced *cis*-platinum.

Familial aspects. About 40 per cent of patients with ovarian cancer give a history of malignancy in other members of the family. Occasionally, more than two members of the family have an ovarian tumour and there may also be a clustering with breast cancer. Other familial associations are the concurrence of granulosa cell tumours with the Peutz–Jeghers syndrome and ovarian fibromas with the basal cell naevus syndrome of skin tumours, face cysts, and skeletal abnormalities.

Another genetic factor predisposing to ovarian neoplasia is gonadal dysgenesis with an inactive Y chromosome where there is an increased risk of dysgerminoma.

Choriocarcinoma. This has been described in the section on the testis (page 10.76). In addition to its spontaneous appearance in gonadal tissue of either sex, it can also arise as a product of conception either as a hydatidiform mole or following a miscarriage or a normal delivery. Rapid uterine enlargement or irregular menstrual bleeding may be the presenting features but the disease can manifest with the clinical consequences of disseminated disease. The management in the female is the same as in the male.

Endometrial cancer. This is a relatively benign condition that presents either with intermenstrual or post-menopausal bleeding. It is commoner in women exposed to long periods of hyperoestrogenization 'unopposed' by progestogen. Thus, it occurs with increased frequency in women with the polycystic ovary syndrome, oestrogen secreting tumours, and menopausal therapy where oestrogen alone is given. It is also twice as common in patients with diabetes mellitus compared with a normal population.

References

Andrews, W. C. (1979). Oral contraception. *Clins Obstet. Gynaec.* **6**, 3.
Gold, J. J. and Josimovich, J. B. (1980). *Gynaecologic endocrinology.* Harper and Row, Hagerstown.
Govan, A. D. T. (1976). Ovarian tumours: clinical and pathological features. *Clins Obstet. Gynaec.* **3**, 89.
Grumbach, M. M., Grave, G. D. J., and Mayer, F. E. (1974). *Control of the onset of puberty.* Wiley, New York.
Greenblatt, R. B. and Studd, J. (1977). The menopause. *Clins Obstet. Gynaec.* **4**, 1.
James, V. H. T., Serio, M., and Giusti, G. (1976). *The endocrine function of the human ovary.* Academic Press, London.
Lurain, J. R. and Piver, M. S. (1979). Familial ovarian cancer. *Gynaec. Oncol.* **8**, 185.
Mauvais-Jarvis, P., Kuttenn, F., and Mowszowicz, I. (1981). *Hirsutism.* Springer, Berlin.
Speroff, L., Glass, R. H., and Kase, N. G. (1978). *Clinical gynaecologic endocrinology and infertility.* Williams and Wilkins, Baltimore.
Yen, S. S. C. and Jaffe, R. (1978). *Reproductive endocrinology.* W. B. Saunders, Philadelphia.

Intersex

Disorders of sexual differentiation can present with an abnormal male, an abnormal female, or with a person whose sex is indeterminate. The details of the various clinical conditions are described in the sections on the male and female reproductive systems. Here the principles governing the pathogenesis of these disorders together with their differential diagnosis are discussed.

Sexual ontogenesis. The 'social' sex, or gender, of an individual depends on the appearances of the external genitalia. In the normal person these are a reflection of gonadal function evident, at least in the male, by the secretion of a gonadal factor, or factors, controlling sex differentiation. Thus, phenotypic sex is a manifestation of gonadal sex. Gonadal sex, in turn is determined by chromosomal sex. In the human, the Y chromosome controls maleness by initiating differentiation to a gonad which secretes testosterone. This stimulates the development of the Wolffian (male system of epididymis, vas deferens, seminal vesicle, and prostrate. Testosterone is responsible for the development of the undifferentiated external genitalia of early embryonic life into penis and scrotum of which the critical steps are enlargement of the genital tubercle and midline fusion of the urogenital sinus to form the penis; the latter change is also involved in the development of the scrotum. There is also an inhibitor which induces atrophy of the Mullerian (female) system of Fallopian tubes, uterus, and vagina. Dihydrotestosterone is the hormone responsible for midline fusion, and so 5α-reductase, which catalyses its formation from testosterone, is necessary for the complete defferentiation of that male external genitalia. Differentiation of the human female is largely a negative phenomenon; that is, in the absence of the male factors, feminization will take place.

Clinical aspects. It is possible thus to have three types of clinical abnormality, chromosomal, gonadal and phenotypic (Table 1).

The majority of these disorders tend towards either a male or a female phenotype and therefore are considered in the differential diagnosis of the abnormal male or female respectively. Nevertheless, on occasion there is some overlap and doubt, and some patients may be of indeterminate sex. The particular features which should be sought on examination and the investigations that may be useful are shown in Table 2. Usually, the diagnosis can be made on clinical grounds together with chromosome analysis. Occasionally, however, steroid measurements will be necessary to identify both virilizing and non-virilizing adrenal and ovarian biosynthetic defects in the female and abnormalities of testosterone synthesis and action producing hypogonadism with or without feminization in the male. Schemes for the differential diagnosis of the abnormalities are shown for the 'male' in Fig. 1 and the 'female' in Fig. 2.

Table 1 Disorders of sexual differentiation

	Female	Indeterminate	Male
Chromosomal	Turner's syndrome	True hermaphroditism	Klinefelter's syndrome Mixed gonadal dysgenesis Sex reversal syndrome
Gonadal	Pure gonadal dysgenesis Swyer syndrome		Anorchia Bonnevie–Ullrich syndrome
Phenotypic	Congenital adrenal hyperplasia (21-and 11-hydroxylase deficiencies) 17 α-hydroxylase deficiency Administration to mother of testosterone progestogens Virilizing tumours Congenitally absent vagina		Biosynthetic defects testosterone 20,21,22-desmolase 3β-hydroxysteroid dehydrogenase 17α-hydroxylase 17,20-desmolase 17β-hydroxysteroid dehydrogenase Receptor defect complete testicular feminization incomplete male pseudohermaphroditism 5α-reductase deficiency pseudovaginal perineoscrotal hypospadias persistent Mullerian system administration to mother of anti-androgens

Table 2 Diagnosis of intersex

Clinical features
  External genitalia
  Breasts
  Pubic and axillary hair
  Hernial orifices
  Stigmata of Turner's syndrome, etc.

Pelvic examination under anaesthesia

Laparoscopy

Chromosome analysis

Steroid measurements

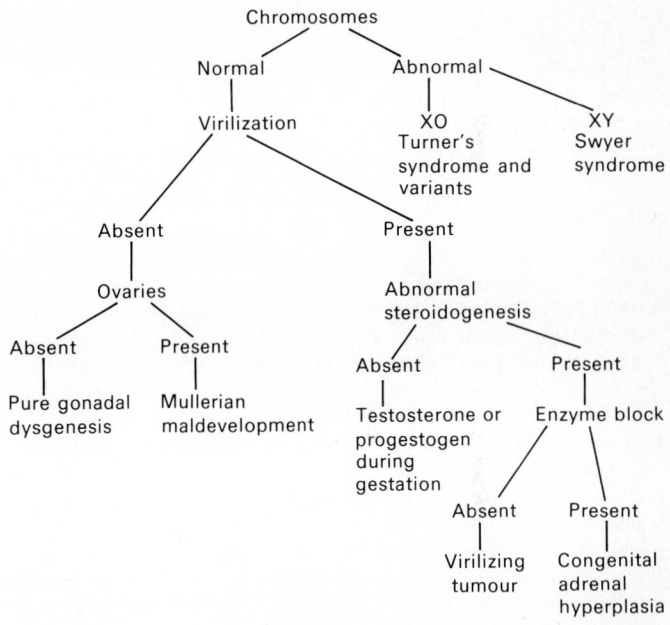

Fig. 2 The format is the same as Fig. 1. The individual abnormalities are described in the section on the female reproductive system (page 10.78).

References

Gold, J. J. and Josimovich, J. B. (1980). *Gynaecologic endocrinology.* Harper and Row, Hagerstown.

Griffin, J. E. and Wilson, J. D. (1980). The syndromes of androgen resistance. *New Engl. J. Med.* **302**, 198.

Wilson, J. D. and Walsh, P. C. (1979). Disorders of sexual differentiation. In *Campbell's Urology* (eds. J. H. Harrison, R. F. Gittes, A. D. Perlmutter, T. A. Stamey, and P. C. Walsh). W. B. Saunders, Philadelphia.

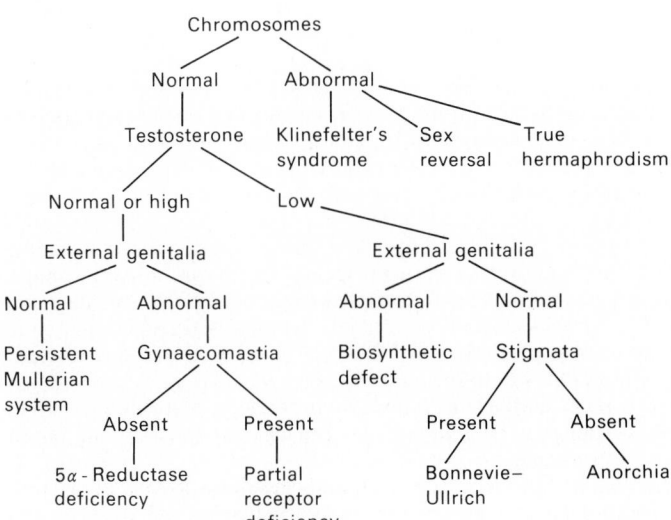

Fig. 1 An approach to the differential diagnosis of intersexual states looking superficially more male than female. The important points in the assessment are underlined. Details of each condition are given in the section on the male reproductive system (page 10.69).

Puberty

Introduction. The precise mechanisms responsible for the onset of puberty have not been fully defined. Ultimately, the hormonal changes that distinguish the adult from the child are an increase in testosterone in the male, and the cyclical changes in the secretion of gonadotrophins and sex steroids in the female. It has been postulated that the trigger setting off those processes is a change in sensitivity of the various feedback loops which operate between the gonadotrophin releasing hormone (LHRH), the gonadotrophins, and the gonadal steroids. The somatic, but not the reproductive, changes of puberty can be induced by administration of testosterone or oestradiol, as appropriate. LH given in the form of chorionic gonadotrophin (HCG) will produce sexual maturation in the male, but will not allow normal spermatogenesis. For this, FSH also is required. In the female it is possible to induce normal reproductive activity by cyclical administration of FSH and LH, and in both sexes LHRH given in a pulsatile manner may induce puberty. Thus, ultimately, it would seem that the critical site of control is at the level of LHRH release. Influencing this are factors such as the physical and psychological environments as well as an intrinsic 'clock'. The hypothalamic–pituitary–gonadal axis is also affected by melatonin, a pineal hormone which inhibits gonadotrophin release, and adrenal androgens, of which the most important in the context of puberty is dehydroepiandrosterone (DHA).

The hormonal changes of puberty are first a rise in DHA, then an increase in FSH followed by a rise in LH, first in nocturnal pulses and then during the day. This is associated with, in the male, a steady increase in testosterone levels. The cyclical changes in the female do not appear until late in puberty. Seminal fluid is secreted moderately early in sexual development but mature spermatogenesis is a late phenomenon. The same is true of analogous changes in the female—the first cycles are anovulatory, with regular ovulation being the final event marking sexual maturity.

The physical and psychological features on which puberty is judged start to appear at the age of 9 or 10 in the average European child and are completed by 16 or 17. It is however important to recognize that the age ranges of normal puberty vary widely from individual to individual, family to family, and race to race. Menarche usually appears by the age of 13 in Europe but for example, may be as late as 18 in the New Guinea highlands. Although reproductive maturity signals the end of puberty, other events such as somatic growth and psychological adaptation also take place.

It is useful to stage puberty for clinical purposes using pubic hair and changes in the penis and scrotum in the male, and pubic hair and breasts in the female as criteria. These stages have been defined both in words and pictures. For details the reader is referred to the bibliography. Other features occur at the same time, notably facial, axillary, limb, and body hair in the male, and axillary hair and an increase in the panniculus adiposus in the female. Linear growth accelerates at puberty with peak velocity occurring two years earlier in girls than in boys. The former manifest peak growth rate before the menarche whereas the maximum speed of growth occurs later in puberty in boys and lasts longer. Thus men tend to be taller than women.

The hormonal and physical changes of puberty are accompanied by alteration in the bones with the appearance and fusion of new epiphyses. This phenomenon is used as a basis to estimate the radiological age of the child which, by using a reference atlas, can be compared with the chronological age. Thus the stage of puberty can be assessed by a combination of physical, radiological, and hormonal measurements which can be then used as objective criteria for the evaluation of clinical problems.

Delayed puberty. This has already been discussed in the sections on the individual reproductive systems. Constitutional delay occurs in girls as well as boys, but because of current social attitudes, it is the male rather than the female who is brought to the clinic. This is not to say that the undeveloped girl is not equally distressed, merely that her parents' generation consider the sexual immaturity more socially acceptable.

Precocious puberty. The causes of this condition are shown in Table 1. By convention menstruation before the age of 9 is considered abnormal as is secondary sexual development in boys.

Table 1 Cause of precocious puberty

Complete
  Idiopathic
  Obesity
  'Cerebral'
  Weil–Albright–McCune–Sternberg syndrome
  Silver syndrome
  Juvenile hypothyroidism
  Gonadotrophin-secreting tumours
  HCG administration

Incomplete
  Premature thelarche
  Premature adrenarche
  Adrenocortical congenital hyperplasia, Cushing's disease, tumour
  Leydig cell hyperplasia, tumour
  Ovarian tumour
  Androgen or oestrogen consumption

Usually, the precocity is isosexual but occasionally it may be heterosexual. The cause of the condition is established by considering the features listed in Table 2. A full clinical examination should be performed in all cases but the further investigations will depend on clinical indications and should not be performed in a blanket manner. The details of what should be done will be described for each individual disease. It must, however, be stressed that the results of stimulation with ACTH or HCG for adrenal and gonad respectively, or suppression with dexamethasone or synthetic sex hormones, may be diagnostically misleading since tumours of the adrenal or the gonad can have inappropriate receptors and thereby respond paradoxically.

Table 2 Diagnosis of the cause of precocious puberty

Presenting symptoms
Family history
Examination of breasts, sex organs, and secondary sexual characters
Abdominal and rectal examination
Measurement of gonadal and adrenal steroids and gonadotrophins
Radiology of the skull, long bones, and bone age
Imaging of pelvis and skull

Causes.
Isosexual idiopathic precocity. This is the commonest condition comprising two-thirds of cases. The condition affects girls approximately eight times more frequently than boys. The diagnosis is usually made by exclusion. The clinical problems are of sexual maturation inappropriate for the child's years and of an early growth spurt which, with premature epiphyseal fusion, eventually results in short adult stature. Treatment is with danazol, a mildly anti-androgenic progestational agent, or with cyproterone acetate, a stronger anti-androgen also with progestogenic activity. There is a risk of adrenal suppression when the latter is used in children, so the parents should be warned of the hazards and a steroid card carried.

Obesity may be associated with an advance in pubertal development, particularly in the female. In the male, if anything, it seems to retard puberty. The pathological mechanisms underlying either effect are unclear.

Cerebral. The next most frequent cause of isosexual precocious puberty is the 'cerebral' group. The particular associated conditions are those involving the hypothalamus and its connections. Thus neoplasms and hamartomas of the region, which includes the tuber cinereum and mammillary bodies, the pineal, and the optic chiasm, together with infections of the basal meninges of the brain or developmental abnormalities that disturb the anatomy in the region of the third ventricle or trauma can all produce precocious puberty. The diagnosis can often be made clinically, but sometimes brain imaging is necessary before the true nature of the disease is revealed. The causal relationship between the symptoms and the disease is ill-understood. One possibility is that pathways from the pineal to hypothalamus through which melatonin normally inhibits gonadotrophin release are interrupted.

Weil–Albright–McCune–Sternberg syndrome. This condition, more usually called Albright's syndrome, occurs much more commonly in girls than in boys and consists of sexual precocity, segmental patches of pigmentation of the skin, and polyostotic fibrous dysplasia. The vaginal bleeding occurs earlier than would be expected from the other aspects of sexual maturation, and the child has a tendency to suffer pathological fractures before puberty, but less so afterwards. An association with hyperthyroidism, hypersecretion of growth hormone, or Cushing's syndrome have also been described. There is no treatment for the underlying condition but danazol may be symptomatically useful.

Juvenile hypothyroidism. The clinical picture is of accelerated sexual development but with stunted growth, hypothyroidism, and sometimes galactorrhoea. The diagnosis is made by the findings of a low thyroxine and high TSH level in the blood. Treatment is of the hypothyroidism.

Silver's syndrome. In this disorder there is an association of precocious puberty with low birth weight, small stature, craniofacial disproportion, clinodactyly, and inappropriately high gonadotrophin levels, which presumably cause the early sexual maturation.

Gonadotrophin secreting tumours. These arise in ovary or testes, although they have also been described in hepatoblastomas. In addition to an elevation of FSH and LH levels, β-HCG sub-unit is found.

HCG used in treatment of maldescended testes if given for long enough and in large enough doses can cause premature sexual maturation. LHRH given for this purpose is less likely to do so.

Premature thelarche. Development of the breast in the absence of other pubertal changes usually occurs in affected children between the ages of two and four and disappears spontaneously over several months. The differential diagnosis is easily made since the breast development is the only abnormality.

Premature adrenarche. This is found in girls more often than boys when pubic and axillary hair appear prematurely. The other changes of puberty are, however, minimal. DHAS and urinary 17-osoxteroid levels are slightly increased. This is a slight exaggeration of the hormonal changes that accompany a normal puberty. Ultimately, development is normal.

Hyperplasia and tumours of adrenals or gonads. The clinical features of these together with the differential diagnosis are described in the relevant sections.

Iatrogenic. Oestrogens given to fuse the epiphyses of tall girls or a child surreptitiously eating the mother's oral contraceptive pills can result in feminization. Virilization can occur with consumption of androgens or anabolic steroids.

References

Bierich J. R. (ed.). (1975). Disorders of puberty. *Clin. Endocr. Metab.* **4**, 1.
Brook, C. G. D. (ed.) (1981). *Clinical paediatric endocrinology.* Blackwell Scientific Publications, Oxford.
Grumbach, M. M., Grave, G. D., and Mayer, F. E. (1974). *Control of the onset of puberty.* Wiley, New York.
Ojeda, S. R., Andrews, W. W., Advis, J. P., and Smith White, S. (1980). Recent advances in the endocrinology of puberty. *Endocr. Rev.* **1**, 228.

Disorders of the breast

D. R. London

The development and function of this gland is influenced by a large variety of endocrine factors, most important of which are prolactin and oestrogens. However, other hormones such as growth hormone, thyroxine, and progesterone also play a role, and insulin and cortisol are required for lactation. Androgens have an inhibitory effect on breast development and lactation. The clinical conditions most likely to be encountered by the physician are gynaecomastia, galactorrhoea, and carcinoma.

Gynaecomastia. This is the breast abnormality most frequently seen by the physician. The causes are listed in Table 1.

Often the cause of the breast enlargement is apparent from the clinical picture as in pubertal gynaecomastia or when it appears in the course of an already diagnosed condition, but sometimes the aetiology is obscure. In this instance a full history and physical examination are necessary to establish the nature of the underlying process. Special attention should be paid to the symptoms and signs suggestive of androgen deficiency or oestrogen excess with a particular search for evidence of hypogonadism or feminization. The testes should be palpated carefully for a tumour and signs of liver disease or hyperthyroidism should be sought. A history of drug ingestion or excessive alcohol intake is important. The diagnosis is often obvious and requires no laboratory investigation, but measurements of testosterone, oestradiol, prolactin, and gonadotrophin may be required. In obscure cases, tests for adrenal neoplasia should be done and if gonadotrophin levels in the presence of normal testes are high, an ectopic source may be revealed by the appropriate biochemical and radiological procedures.

Important individual causes are considered below.

Table 1 Causes of gynaecomastia

Physiological	Prolactinoma
Neonatal	Hyperthyroidism
Pubertal	Liver disease
Senescent	Starvation and refeeding
Pathological	Drugs
Deficient testosterone secretion	Oestrogenic
or action	Oestrogens
Increased oestrogen secretion	Digitalis
True hermaphroditism	Marijuana
Tumours of testis	Heroin
adrenal	Anti-androgens
liver	Cyproterone
Increased HCG secretion	Spironolactone
Tumours of testis	Cimetidine
lung	Testosterone
GI tract	Gonadotrophins
pancreas	Prolactinogenic
liver	Cytotoxics
breast	Trauma
	Malignancy

Pubertal. The commonest breast problem in the male undoubtedly is puberty gynaecomastia. Some breast development is found in most boys as they begin to mature sexually. Usually this is of no consequence and soon disappears spontaneously. But in a few, breast enlargement continues so that it becomes unsightly and embarrassing. The mechanism is probably of breast stimulation by unopposed oestrogens at the beginning of puberty. This happens before androgen levels rise. The breast responds to the abnormal oestrogen/testosterone ratio.

The diagnosis is made by noting that the secondary sex characteristics are appearing normally and that FSH and testosterone levels are appropriate for age. Wherever possible a temporizing policy should be pursued as mild gynaecomastia usually subsides as puberty advances. However, when the breasts become very large or painful, or when the boy's psyche is severely affected, treatment is indicated. Testosterone may be given and anti-oestrogens such as clomiphene and tamoxifen are also used, but their effectiveness has not been scientifically evaluated. Mammoplasty may be necessary in extreme cases.

Androgen deficiency. Any cause of impaired secretion or action of androgens can lead to gynaecomastia. This is as true of Kallman's syndrome (see page 10.13) as of Klinefelter's syndrome (see page 10.73). The clinical clue to aetiology is a lack of male secondary sexual development and on investigation, a lower serum testosterone level than would be predicted by the age of the patient.

A high FSH and LH indicates a primary gonadal disorder, and demonstration of abnormal chromosomes leads to a diagnosis of Klinefelter's syndrome or one of its variants. The details of the differential diagnosis of this group of disorders is more fully discussed in section on the male reproductive system (see page 10.72).

Increased oestrogen secretion. This occurs in states of true hermaphroditism when ovarian and testicular tissues co-exist. The differential diagnosis is discussed in the section on intersex. Tumours of endocrine elements in the testis may secrete abnormal amounts of oestradiol and thus produce gynaecomastia, and liver tumours may transform steroid precursors to active oestrogens.

Increased gonadotrophin secretion. Testicular tumours of the germinal tissue can produce HCG, or an active sub-unit of the hormone, that can stimulate the normal interstitial cells or Sertoli cells to secrete amounts of oestradiol in large quantities. HCG from ectopic sites such as the lung, gastrointestinal tract, pancreas, liver, and breast can have a similar effect. Thus, in cases of gynaecomastia it is most important to search carefully for a hard testicular mass and to review the general health of the patient. Elevated HCG levels provide the diagnostic clue.

Adrenal tumours. These can cause gynaecomastia by secreting oestrogenic precursors such as androstenedione and dehydroepiandrosterone sulphate (DHA-S) which are converted peripherally to oestrone.

Prolactinoma. A high plasma prolactin *per se* is not responsible for gynaecomastia but combined with the associated androgen deficiency secondary to low gonadotrophins, can result in breast development.

Hyperthyroidism. The gynaecomastia of this condition is due to three factors. The first is increased peripheral conversion of androstenedione to oestrogens. The second is increased production of androstenedione, and the third is a high sex hormone binding globulin (SHBG) concentration which will amplify the effects of the altered androgen/oestrogen ratio. Usually there is no difficulty in diagnosis as hyperthyroidism will have presented with features other than the gynaecomastia.

Liver disease. The mechanisms for the breast development in this disorder have already been discussed. Clearly it is necessary to look for features of hepatic dysfunction in unexplained breast development.

Malnutrition. The pathogenesis here is thought to be similar to that in liver disease. The gynaecomastia which occurs on refeeding is due to the recurrence of sexual activity after the hypogonadism of malnutrition so the pathophysiology is the same as for the pubertal variety.

Drugs. *Oestrogen-like activity*. Oestrogens given for prostatic carcinoma commonly cause gynaecomastia. Digitalis derivatives, which have oestrogenic effects can do likewise; marijuana depresses androgen levels and its metabolite, tetrahydrocannabinol, is oestrogenic. Heroin depresses androgen levels and opiates also increase prolactin secretion.

Anti-androgens. Cyproterone acetate given to male sexual deviants with criminal tendencies may by its anti-androgenic action cause gynaecomastia. Other drugs with similar action are cimetidine and spironolactone. The latter also acts as progestogen, which may be another reason for gynaecomastia.

Testosterone. Paradoxically, testosterone given as replacement therapy occasionally produces gynaecomastia. The reason for this is unclear but it could be because some is converted to oestrogen.

Gonadotrophins. The therapeutic administration of HCG in gonadotrophin deficiency or delayed puberty may result in gynaecomastia by mechanisms similar to those described for the physiological condition arising at puberty. However, here the gynaecomastia is more likely to be painful owing to its rapid appearance.

Prolactinogenic drugs. There is some controversy in the literature as to the incidence of gynaecomastia in men receiving drugs known to raise prolactin levels. While the symptom is very rare in clinical practice, it has been reported during experimental administration. As with all symptoms that might be drug induced, it is wise to stop or reduce the drug wherever possible.

Trauma. Damage to the breast may produce a swelling that is usually unilateral. These patients present to surgeons.

Malignancy. Carcinoma of the male breast manifests as unilateral swelling. It is discussed further below.

Galactorrhoea. This is found in the majority of women with hyperprolactinaemia but is very rare in men with the condition. Any cause of sustained elevation of prolactin levels (q.v.) can produce the symptom. The galactorrhoea may be gross and spontaneous, with staining of the brassiere and excoriation of the areola and nipple, or it may be so slight that the finding can only be produced by manual expression. If the galactorrhoea is caused by hyperprolactinaemia, there will also be a reproductive abnormality almost invariably manifested in the women as a gross disturbance of the menstrual cycle. The diagnostic protocol is as for any patient with elevated prolactins (q.v.). However, galactorrhoea can also occur, for unknown reasons, in women with normal prolactin concentrations. In this instance, the menses are normal.

The treatment is wherever possible that of the cause. When this is not possible or desirable, bromocriptine or another dopamine agonist should be prescribed.

Carcinoma. Breast cancer is the commonest tumour in women, but it may also occur in the male, particularly if suffering from Klinefelter's syndrome. It is commoner in North America, where it accounts for one quarter of all cancers in women, and in northern Europe than in the Far East, for environmental rather than racial reasons. The risk increases with age.

Tumour initiation probably precedes clinical presentation by two to three decades. Since the breast is under endocrine control, many studies have been carried out to implicate hormonal mechanisms in the genesis of the carcinoma. Unfortunately, however, nothing clearcut has yet emerged. Prolactin does not seem to be an aetiological agent, nor is there general agreement that, as has been suggested, metabolism of adrenal androgens is different in women with breast cancer compared with normal women. Likewise, there is no consistently described ovarian or thyroid disturbance. Nevertheless, reproductive and ovarian function may be involved in some way since there is a striking correlation between relative risk for developing breast cancer and the age of the woman at first birth of an offspring. Moreover, bilateral removal of the ovaries reduces the incidence of breast cancer, and the disease is, of course, much commoner in women than men.

Viruses have been implicated as aetiological agents but there are no firm grounds for considering these crucial in human disease. There may be a genetic factor since familial clusters are found, but it is not clear whether an environmental agent may be to blame. Ionizing radiation in large doses, as with repeated chest fluoroscopy is associated with carcinoma of the breast, but this is not of a sufficient scale to be of epidemiological importance. Fibrocystic disease probably does predispose to cancer, but in an unknown manner. The clinical details will be considered only in outline since management falls more within the province of the surgeon than the physician.

Diagnosis. A solitary lump in the breast must be regarded with suspicion until proved benign. Hardness, tethering to skin or deep tissues, skin ulceration, nipple retraction, or the presence of enlarged axillary nodes are all features pointing towards malignancy. Mammography using radiological methods, thermography, and needle biopsy are used in establishing diagnosis.

Various systems of staging have been devised. They all grade the extent on criteria such as localization within the breast, extension to adjacent groups of lymph nodes, involvement of skin and deep structures, and metastases to distant sites. The aim of each classification is to indicate prognosis principally to provide an objective way of comparing methods of treatment. Histology of the tumour is of prognostic significance. Recently there has been considerable interest in tumour oestrogen receptors as a guide to the suitability of oestrogen of anti-oestrogen therapy. Tumours that lack these receptors are unlikely to respond to hormone treatment.

Treatment. Radical breast surgery is less widely used than formerly. Now endocrine and chemotherapy are increasing in popularity as adjuvants to the basic treatment.

Schedules are continually evolving and there are no strict guidelines apart from reserving oophorectomy for premenopausal patients. The presence of oestrogen receptors in the tumour increases the likelihood of response to castration and indeed to adrenalectomy. This latter manoeuvre is of greatest benefit to the perimenopausal group who have responded to oophorectomy and then relapsed.

Hypophysectomy is also practised but less so than the other endocrine ablations possibly owing to the more restricted availability of the necessary surgical expertise.

Oestrogens are the most commonly used hormonal agents and are particularly effective in post-menopausal women with oestrogen receptors in the tumour cell. Androgens have been employed but are currently unpopular because of their virilizing effects. Progestogens and corticosteroids have also been used but are generally thought to be of only minor value. Anti-oestrogens, of which the most used in tamoxifen, induce remissions in the majority of oestrogen receptor-positive patients both pre- and post-menopausal.

Cytotoxic therapy is usually reserved for advanced cases. The view that micrometastases are already present in many patients who on clinical grounds had been thought to have early local disease has widened the indications for chemotherapy, so that some centres are giving drugs with the primary excision whether or not there is distant spread. The list of agents employed is ever-increasing and includes alkylating agents, antitumour antibiotics, antimetabolites, and the vinca alkaloids. These drugs may be given in various combinations, and may be combined with hormones as well as with surgery and radiotherapy.

References

Calson, H. E. (1980). Gynecomastia. *New Engl. J. Med.* **303**, 795.

Donegan, W. L. and Spratt, J. S. (1979). *Cancer of the breast*. W. B. Saunders, Philadelphia.

Wilson, J. D., Aiman, J., and MacDonald, P. C. (1980). The pathogenesis of gynecomastia. *Adv. intern. Med.* **25**, 1.

Corticosteroid and corticotrophin treatment in non-endocrine disease

R. I. S. Bayliss

In addition to their use as physiological replacement therapy in acute and chronic adrenal insufficiency, hypopituitarism, and congenital adrenal hyperplasia, corticosteroids are used systemically and topically in the treatment of a wide variety of non-endocrine conditions. In these the therapeutic rationale largely depends upon the suppression of an inflammatory response that usually stems from a cell-mediated delayed hypersensitive immune reaction. The corticosteroid dosage necessary often exceeds normal physiological requirements and is therefore termed pharmacological. Systemic corticosteroid treatment may be given by mouth or be induced endogenously by stimulation of the patient's own adrenal glands by the injection of corticotrophin (ACTH) or one of its analogues.

Corticosteroids. In non-endocrine disorders synthetic compounds are used in preference to the naturally occurring substance cortisol (hydrocortisone) or its closely related analogue cortisone because they have less potential for causing sodium retention, oedema, hypertension, and potassium loss. These synthetic substances are usually marketed in tablets containing an amount of the compound that has an anti-inflammatory action approximately equivalent to that of 20 mg cortisol or 25 mg cortisone (Table 1). The differences

Table 1 Comparative anti-inflammatory potency of corticosteroids given orally

		Tablet strengths commonly available (mg)
Cortisone	25 mg	5, 25
Cortisol (hydrocortisone)	20 mg	10, 20
Prednisone	5 mg	1, 5
Prednisolone	5 mg	1, 2.5, 5
Methylprednisolone	4 mg	2, 4, 16
Triamcinolone	4 mg	1, 2, 4
Paramethasone	2 mg	2
Dexamethasone	0.75 mg	0.5, 0.75
Betamethasone	0.75 mg	0.5

in biological potency depend upon stereochemical molecular changes which influence adherence to receptor sites on the cell membrane, intestinal absorption, protein binding, and the rates of degradation and excretion. The more potent analogues seldom show any therapeutic superiority over prednisone or prednisolone although sometimes one preparation may suit a particular patient better than another. Certain compounds are used in special situations, for example dexamethasone in the treatment of cerebral oedema.

Corticotrophins. Therapeutic uses of ACTH and its analogues include adrenocortical insufficiency secondary to deficient endogenous corticotrophin secretion and non-endocrine diseases that respond to corticosteroids. The ACTH used is usually rendered long-acting with a gelatin or zinc adjuvant. Synthetic analogues, containing the biologically active first 24 amino acids of the total 39 and rendered long-acting in a zinc adjuvant, are in common use as tetracosactrin depot.

The material must be injected intramuscularly. The degree of stimulation of the adrenal cortex is unpredictable because absorption from the injection site may vary, the trophic hormone may be destroyed locally or in the blood stream by proteolytic enzymes, and the responsiveness of the adrenal cortex may vary, often becoming greater as the stimulus is repeated and the adrenal cortex hypertrophies.

The fact that corticotrophins stimulate the adrenal cortex to secrete increased amounts of androgens should theoretically reduce the liability to such side-effects as osteoporosis but this remains unproven.

Because they have to be given by injection, because of the unpredictability of the adrenal response, and because of no substantiated therapeutic superiority over corticosteroids, ACTH and its analogues have a limited role; their main application is in diagnostic tests of adrenocortical function.

Indications. Except in adrenocortical insufficiency and as a life-saving measure in certain non-endocrine diseases corticosteroids are seldom the treatment of first choice because of inevitable and potentially dangerous side-effects and because their action is palliative rather than curative. Table 2 summarizes the more important disorders in which corticosteroids given systemically may play a therapeutic role: reference to the appropriate sections elsewhere in this textbook will define more precisely the circumstances in each disease which merit such therapy. In an emergency, such as status asthmaticus or an anaphylactic reaction, the compound should be given intravenously; suitable preparations are 100–200 mg hydrocortisone sodium succinate or 4–8 mg dexamethasone sodium phosphate.

Principles of treatment. Some conditions may respond to a short sharp course of corticosteroids and these should be treated with an initially large dose of corticosteroid, e.g. 40–60 mg prednisone daily in divided dosage, which over 10–21 days is rapidly reduced. Others require prolonged treatment for months, years, or for life; in these it is often best to start with a smaller dose (e.g. 10–15 mg prednisone) and increase this, if necessary, to the minimal dose that suppresses adequately but not completely the symptoms or clinical manifestations of the disease. In every patient the therapeutically effective dose can only be found by trial and error. It is important to remember that the disease being treated may fluctuate in its severity without discernible reason and the patient's responsiveness to treatment may vary from time to time. Hence, in prolonged illnesses requiring prolonged corticosteroid treatment, frequent manipulation of the dose is often required, and the golden rule is to use the acceptable minimum. Treatment with systemic corticosteroids should never be undertaken without first balancing the possible benefits against the potentially dangerous side-effects. The larger the dose and the more prolonged the treatment, the greater is the liability to side-effects. Although these may be reduced by

Table 2 Non-endocrine diseases responding to systemic corticosteroid treatment

Collagen diseases	systemic lupus erythematosus* cranial arteritis* polymyalgia rheumatica* polyarteritis nodosa* Wegener's granulomatosis* rheumatoid arthritis
Cardiac diseases	acute rheumatic fever* benign (viral) pericarditis Dressler's syndrome*
Pulmonary diseases	status asthmaticus* asthma* sarcoidosis with pulmonary infiltration* allergic alveolitis*
Renal diseases	nephrotic syndrome*
Gastrointestinal diseases	ulcerative colitis Crohn's disease malabsorption syndromes
Haematological diseases	idiopathic thrombocytopenia* haemolytic anaemias lymphatic leukaemia and lymphomas*
Hepatic diseases	chronic active hepatitis
Allergic diseases	angio-neurotic oedema anaphylaxis* serum sickness
Dermatological diseases	pemphigus* exfoliative dermatitis* erythema nodosum
Miscellaneous disorders	mammary carcinoma organ transplantation* cerebral oedema

* Conditions in which systemic corticosteroid may be especially indicated or may be life-saving

alternate day therapy, such a frequency of dosage may fail to control the symptoms of the underlying disease and cannot be relied upon to reduce suppression of the hypothalamo-pituitary-adrenal (HPA) axis.

Contra-indications. Unless necessary to save life, ACTH or corticosteroids in pharmacological dosage should be avoided in patients with a peptic ulcer or a previous history of peptic ulcer, haematemesis, or melaena, in those with past or present mental instability and, unless antibacterial treatment is given concurrently, when an acute or chronic bacterial infection, including tuberculosis, is present.

Side-effects and complications. The consequences of treatment with corticosteroids or ACTH can be divided into two major categories—those that arise from continued use of large doses and those that, on stopping treatment, occur as a result of a suppressed hypothalamo-pituitary-adrenal axis.

The prevalence, severity, and importance of side-effects depend mainly on the duration of treatment and the size of the dosage used as well as on the individual patient's responsiveness. Table 3 shows the most common; those contributing to, or responsible for, death in patients subjected to prolonged treatment are marked with an asterisk.

Gastrointestinal complications are common. About 25 per cent of patients complain of dyspepsia and of these 5 per cent have proven peptic ulceration. Perforation of a peptic ulcer may be difficult to recognize because high corticosteroid dosage may mask the usual symptoms and signs. Similarly the manifestations of an acute opportunistic infection may be obscured with little rise in temperature or white cell count. Uncontrolled, often unrecog-

Table 3 Side-effects and complications of corticosteroid or ACTH treatment

Gastrointestinal	oesophageal candidiasis dyspepsia proven peptic ulcer perforation of peptic ulcer* haemorrhage* acute pancreatitis (especially in children)
Endocrinological	weight gain with Cushingoid distribution moon facies hirsutism amenorrhoea diabetes mellitus suppression of hypothalamo-pituitary-adrenal axis* impaired growth in children
Musculo-skeletal	osteoporosis with crush fracture of vertebrae aseptic necrosis of femoral head myopathy with wasting and weakness
Dermatological	thinning of the skin striae acne
Cardiovascular and renal	sodium retention with hypertension oedema and heart failure potassium depletion thrombosis (venous, coronary, cerebral)*
Neuro-psychiatric	euphoria, insomnia, restlessness hypomania depression corticosteroid addiction pseudotumour cerebri in children
Ocular	posterior subcapsular cataracts
General	liability to opportunistic infection* rekindling of dormant tuberculosis

* Side effects contributing to or responsible for death in patients subjected to prolonged treatment

nized, infection is the most common complication to cause death and is found in 25 per cent of those who die while having corticosteroid or ACTH therapy. Diabetes mellitus develops in some 5 per cent of patients on corticosteroids particularly when the dosage is high, and in those with latent glucose intolerance who might be expected to develop diabetes later in life.

Side-effects peculiar to children are acute pancreatitis, pseudotumour cerebri, and retardation of growth. Pseudotumour cerebri is a syndrome characterized by headache, vomiting, raised intracranial pressure, and papilloedema which may lead to blindness. Usually this condition develops when the dosage of corticosteroids is reduced and is relieved by increasing the dose again to be followed by a very gradual weaning process.

Retardation of growth, which may result in permanent dwarfism, may occur in children on prolonged corticosteroid therapy for control of asthma or the nephrotic syndrome. In asthmatic patients this may be obviated by using corticosteroid inhalations (beclomethasone dipropionate or betamethasone valerate) in place of systemic steroids. Growth retardation may be avoided in children with conditions that can only be controlled with systemic corticosteroids by alternate day treatment or by switching them to the less convenient and less acceptable injections of ACTH or tetracosactrin.

ACTH and tetracosactrin. Painful local reactions at the site of injection are more frequent after tetracosactrin than ACTH although generalized allergic reactions are more common after the latter.

Such reactions may, however, occur with both types of compound, and for this reason it is recommended that patients should not inject themselves and should remain under observation for an hour after the injection has been given by a doctor or nurse.

Patients on such treatment are particularly prone to increased bruising, acne, pigmentation, sodium retention, and hypertension.

Suppression of the hypothalamo-pituitary-adrenal axis. Systemic corticosteroids by increasing the plasma steroid level suppress the secretion of corticotrophin releasing factor (CRF) from the hypothalamus and the output of ACTH from the anterior pituitary. The degree of this suppression depends upon the dosage and duration of corticosteroid administration. Over a prolonged time little or no secretion of ACTH causes physiological and eventually anatomical atrophy of the adrenal cortex. Similar consequences may follow the too liberal application of topical corticosteroids particularly to the skin or as enemas.

ACTH and its analogues increase cortisol secretion from the cortex of the adrenal glands. This and the ACTH suppress the release of CRF from the hypothalamus and of corticotrophin from the pituitary. Thus, in response to stress the corticosteroid-treated patient may fail to respond because of adrenocortical atrophy, and the ACTH-treated patient may also fail to respond because of hypothalamo-pituitary suppression.

The consequence of HPA suppression is the development of hypotensive, potentially fatal, collapse of patients subjected to stress (infective, traumatic, or occasionally psychological) who are having or have had in the recent past treatment with corticosteroids, ACTH, or their analogues. About 10 per cent of deaths in patients receiving such treatment can be ascribed to this cause, which emphasizes the need to give additional corticosteroid treatment to these patients when they are under stress and to withdraw treatment slowly to allow the HPA axis to resume normal responsiveness.

Resumption of normal HPA activity. On stopping corticosteroid or corticotrophin treatment there may be a delay of several months before the atrophic adrenal glands, suppressed by steroid therapy, or the hypothalamo-pituitary secretion of CRF and ACTH, suppressed by high cortisol levels and injected corticotrophin or its analogues, respond normally to stress. The recovery process follows a sequential pattern:

1. The suppressed plasma level of ACTH returns to normal.
2. The circadian variation in ACTH level is resumed with higher levels in the early morning and low levels at midnight.
3. The plasma cortisol concentration returns to normal and shows a circadian rhythm.
4. Finally, the HPA system responds normally to a neurogenic stimulus, such as insulin-induced hypoglycaemia.

Some resumption of cortisol secretion may be observed when the dosage of prednisone is reduced to 7.5–12.5 mg daily. A normal functioning HPA axis may be evident on testing when the prednisone dosage is reduced to 2.5–5.0 mg daily. Less suppression occurs when the corticosteroid treatment is given in a single dose during the first part of the day or in divided doses that diminish during the course of the day.

Mitigation of HPA suppression. Although HPA suppression cannot be avoided when prolonged treatment in high dosage is given, the consequences can largely be circumvented by withdrawing treatment gradually, particularly when the treatment in the past has been prolonged. Except when a short sharp course over 7–10 days has been given, a reduction in steps of 2.5 mg prednisone (or the equivalent of other corticosteroids) every two to four weeks is recommended until the total daily is 10–12.5 mg. Thereafter the weaning process should continue at the rate of 1.0 mg every two to four weeks.

Prevention of adrenocortical insufficiency. Patients currently receiving corticosteroids or ACTH or tetracosactrin will require an increased dosage during a surgical operation, labour, or any other severe stress. Minor surgical procedures and stresses, physical and psychological, can usually be countered by temporarily doubling the daily dose of corticosteroid or giving an extra injection of ACTH or its analogue depending on which type of therapy the patient is having. Greater coverage will be required for more major stresses, particularly in patients who are currently on corticosteroid treatment or have ceased prolonged high-dosage therapy within the last 12 months. Patients who have been off treatment for 12 months usually respond normally to stress. When practically possible an insulin tolerance test should be done to assess the responsiveness of the HPA axis in these patients.

Coverage for a major operation is given with 100–200 mg hydrocortisone sodium succinate by intramuscular injection at the same time as the premedication and thereafter 50–100 mg six-hourly until the patient is able to take prednisone or hydrocortisone orally. Thereafter, if the operation is unassociated with complications, the dosage can rapidly be reduced from 100–200 mg hydrocortisone (or 25–50 mg prednisone) in divided dosages daily to a maintenance dose. The same coverage is necessary for patients who have been adrenalectomized, have Addison's disease, or congenital adrenal hyperplasia, hypopituitarism, or are undergoing adrenal exploration for Cushing's syndrome. A major surgical operation normally stimulates the adrenal cortex to secrete 200–400 mg cortisol, and it is safer to give too much coverage than too little.

Patients who stopped having corticosteroid or corticotrophin therapy for longer than a year should be watched carefully during the operative and post-operative period. If hypotension develops, 200 mg hydrocortisone sodium succinate should be injected intravenously, followed by intramuscular and then by oral hydrocortisone beginning with 100–150 mg daily, and then in diminishing amounts.

Identification of patients at risk. All patients taking corticosteroids or ACTH compounds or analogues either for substitutional therapy (Addison's disease or hypopituitarism) or for pharmacological effect should carry a card in their wallet or handbag stating the diagnosis and the precise medication being taken.

Alternatively, or preferably in addition, a stainless steel bracelet or necklace, as supplied by Medic Alert Foundation of 9 Hanover Street, London W.1. (telephone 01 499 2261) should be worn stating the underlying diagnosis. Full details of the patient's condition can be readily obtained from this source which has worldwide connections.

References

Ackerman, G. L. and Nolan, C. M. (1968). Adrenocortical responsiveness after alternate-day corticosteroid therapy. *N. Engl. J. Med.* **278**, 405.

Axelrod, L. (1976). Glucocorticoid therapy. *Medicine, Baltimore* **55**, 39.

British Thoracic and Tuberculosis Association. (1975). Inhaled corticosteroids compared with oral prednisone in patients starting long-term corticosteroid therapy for asthma. *Lancet.* **ii**, 469.

Byyny, R. L. (1976). Withdrawal from glucocorticoid therapy. *N. Engl. J. Med.* **295**, 30.

Daly, J. R., Fletcher, M. R., Glass, D., Chambers, D. J., Bitensky, L., and Chayen, J. (1974). Comparison of effects of long-term corticotrophin and corticosteroid treatment on responses of plasma growth hormone, ACTH, and corticosteroid to hypoglycaemia. *Br. med. J.* **ii**, 521.

Graber, A. L., Ney, R. E., Nicholson, W. E., Island, D. P., and Liddle, G. W. (1965). Natural history of pituitary-adrenal recovery following long term suppression with corticosteroids. *J. clin. Endocr. Metab.* **25**, 11.

Jasani, M. K., Boyle, J. A., Greig, W. R., Dalakos, T. G., Browning, M. C. K., Thompson, A., and Buchanan, W. W. (1967). Corticosteroid-induced suppression of the hypothalamo-pituitary-adrenal axis: Observations on patients given oral corticosteroids for rheumatoid arthritis. *Q. Jl Med.* **36**, 261.

Kehlet, H. and Binder, C. (1973). Value of ACTH test in assessing hypothalmic, pituitary-adrenocortical function in glucocorticoid treated patients. *Br. med. J.* **ii**, 147.

Levine, S. B. and Leopold, I. H. (1973). Advances in ocular corticosteroid therapy. *Med. Clins N. Am.* **57**, 1167.

Melby, J. C. (1974). Systemic corticosteroid therapy: pharmacology and endocrinologic considerations. *Ann. intern. Med.* **81**, 505.

Westerhof, L., van Ditmars, M. J., der Kinderen, P. J., Thijssen, J. H. H., and Schwarz, F. (1970). Recovery of adrenocortical function during long-term treatment with corticosteroids. *Br. med. J.* **iv**, 534.

Section 11
Reproductive medicine

BENEFITS AND RISKS OF ORAL CONTRACEPTIVES

M. P. Vessey

Introduction. Oral contraceptives were first approved for use in the United States in 1959. Just 20 years later, it was estimated that about 55 million women around the world were taking them. Although sales are levelling off, or even declining a little, in Western Europe and North America (where use rates are now mostly in the range of 20–30 per cent of women aged 15–44 years), increasing numbers of women in Asia and Latin America are 'going on the pill'.

There are several different types of oral contraceptive regimen, but by far the most important is the combined preparation, in which both an oestrogen and a progestogen are administered daily for three weeks out of every four. This chapter is entirely concerned with preparations of this type. In the United Kingdom, only two oestrogens have been used, ethinyl-oestradiol and mestranol, but four progestogens are currently available (norethisterone, norethisterone acetate, ethynodiol diacetate, and levonorgestrel), while many others have been used in the past (e.g. norethynodrel, chlormadinone acetate, and megestrol acetate). Since the dosage of the constituent steroids may be varied (the trend has generally been downwards over the years both for the oestrogen and for the progestogen component), it is not surprising that the number of different combined oral contraceptive formulations marketed currently or in the past is very large—approaching 100 in the United Kingdom. This adds greatly to the difficulties confronting those trying to assess the safety of the pill.

Oral contraceptives have many metabolic effects. Indeed, Briggs, has stated 'almost every metabolic parameter that is capable of laboratory investigation has been reported to be altered in one way or another by some contraceptive steroid'. This implies that the results of many routine laboratory tests are altered by the pill, a point of considerable practical importance. In this chapter, however, most attention will be concentrated on its effects on morbidity and mortality as revealed by epidemiological studies, although a brief reference will be made to laboratory findings where they appear to provide a clue to underlying mechanisms.

Until the mid-1970s, most of the available data about the benefits and risks of the pill had been derived from uncontrolled clinical trials and from case-control studies. Since then, an enormous amount of information has been obtained from two large British cohort studies, the Royal College of General Practitioners Oral Contraceptive Study and the Oxford Family Planning Association Contraceptive Study. Between them, these investigations recruited 63 000 women of childbearing age (about half of whom were users of the pill and half users of other methods or no method of contraception) who have now been carefully followed up for an average of over seven years. Many of the findings described in this chapter are derived from these two cohort studies.

Information about the benefits and risks of oral contraception in developing countries is extremely sparse although a number of agencies, such as the World Health Organization, are trying to mount appropriate studies. In the meantime, the reader is cautioned *not* to extrapolate the date summarized here to parts of the world to which they clearly do not apply.

Benefits of oral contraception
High efficacy. By far the most important beneficial effect of the pill is its remarkable efficacy which, coupled with a high degree of acceptability (at least among the young), has given many women a new freedom from anxiety about pregnancy. If taken conscientiously, no more than about two to four women in every thousand using a combined preparation should become accidentally pregnant each year. In practice, pills are often missed and much less satisfactory results are then obtained.

Suppression of menstrual disorders. It has long been known that oral contraceptives suppress some menstrual disorders, notably menorrhagia and dysmenorrhoea, leading to a reduction in hospital admissions for dilatation and curettage and for hysterectomy, and to a lessened risk of iron-deficiency anaemia.

Suppression of benign breast disease. Epidemiological studies have consistently shown that use of the pill is negatively associated with the occurrence of benign lumps in the breast (chronic cystic disease and fibroadenoma), thus reducing the need for surgical biopsies by up to 50 per cent. The effect is most pronounced in long-term users, appears to wear off after discontinuation of use, and is probably attributable to the progestogen component of the pill. Taken together with the known positive association between chronic cystic disease and cancer of the breast, these results have led some to suggest that the pill might protect against malignant disease of the breast. This point of view is supported by those studies which have shown no histological differences between lumps excised from pill users and those excised from non-users. A recent study has, however, suggested that oral contraceptives protect against only those forms of chronic cystic disease in which epithelial atypia are minimal or absent and which are little, if at all, associated with an increased risk of breast cancer.

Suppression of functional ovarian cysts. Since oral contraceptives act principally by inhibiting ovulation, it is not surprising that follicular cysts and corpus luteum cysts are relatively uncommon in pill users. Such cysts usually pass undetected and are of no consequence, but from time to time they rupture and precipitate an acute abdominal emergency or give rise to a mass demanding investigation.

Other possible beneficial effects. While the beneficial effects already described may be considered established, a number of others which have been reported in some studies also deserve mention. These include a lessened risk of cancer of the ovary, cancer of the uterine body, thyroid disease, rheumatoid arthritis, peptic ulceration, and pelvic inflammatory disease. Further work is necessary before the significance of these observations can be assessed. It should be stressed, however, that if substantiated these effects could have a profound influence on our present thinking about the balance of benefits and risks associated with pill use.

Risks of oral contraception.
Oral contraceptives are well known to cause minor side-effects such as nausea, headache, and breast tenderness. Although such symptoms are common enough and unpleasant enough to lead to the discontinuation of the pill by up to 25 per cent of women, they disappear immediately medication is stopped and need not be considered a hazard. More important are adverse effects of the pill of sufficient severity to require hospital investigation or treatment (and which may, occasionally, prove fatal) and influence on fertility and the unborn child.

Cardiovascular effects. The best known adverse effects of oral contraceptive use are the cardiovascular ones; thus, it is now clear that the pill is a cause of venous thrombosis and embolism, thrombotic stroke, and acute myocardial infarction. The evidence concerning haemorrhagic stroke is rather less convincing. Some features of the association between oral contraceptive use and these conditions are summarized in Table 1.

Little work has been done on the interrelationship between oral contraceptives and other risk factors in the production of venous thrombo-embolism and stroke. There is, however, appreciable evidence that, as far as myocardial infarction is concerned, the risks associated with pill use, cigarette smoking, and increasing age multiply together. The same may also be true of other risk factors such as hypertension, hyperlipidaemia, and diabetes.

The mechanisms underlying adverse cardiovascular reactions to the pill are uncertain. The following findings may, however, be relevant:

Haematological studies. Poller has concluded 'the consensus of findings . . . on the effects of oral contraceptives indicates some acceleration of the clotting of the procoagulants in the extrinsic and intrinsic clotting systems as well as reduction of antithrombin III levels. There is also evidence of increased fibrinogen levels, depression of fibrinolytic activator activity, and associated changes of antiproteases.'

Serum lipids. On average, oral contraceptives stimulate an increase in fasting serum triglyceride levels of around 30–70 per cent and in cholesterol levels of around 10–30 per cent. The changes in serum cholesterol appear to be a result of steroid induced alterations in the concentrations of VLDL and HDL. There is strong evidence that HDL cholesterol is increased by oestrogen and depressed by progestogen. It follows that the net effect of a combination oral contraceptive on HDL cholesterol depends on its formulation.

Carbohydrate metabolism. Many women treated with oral contraceptives show a modest deterioration in glucose tolerance, especially after an oral test. An exaggerated plasma insulin response is also frequently seen. Fasting blood glucose concentrations are rarely altered by the pill.

Blood pressure. A modest rise in blood pressure (say 2–5 mmHg in systolic pressure and rather less in diastolic) is common in pill users. An occasional subject develops frank hypertension while taking oral contraceptives. These effects appear to be reversible in most cases (see Section 18).

Other findings. A handful of studies have indicated that oral contraceptives may reduce the rate of venous blood flow in the limbs and may have adverse effects on the structure of vessel walls. Beaumont has suggested that immunological mechanisms may be involved in the aetiology of adverse cardiovascular events in pill users.

Gall bladder disease. Surgically proven gall bladder disease is increased about 25–30 per cent among users of oral contraceptives. One careful study has shown that gall bladder bile is significantly more saturated with cholesterol during oral contraceptive treatment than during the normal menstrual cycle. Gall bladder emptying does not, however, seem to be altered by the pill.

Hepatocellular adenoma. Hepatocellular adenoma is an extremely rare (but serious) condition in women of childbearing age. In those without exposure to the pill, the incidence is around one per million per annum. Oral contraceptive users suffer a much higher incidence than this, the risk being very strongly correlated with the steroidal content and duration of use of the preparations on the one hand and with the age of the user on the other.

Some workers suspect that oral contraceptives may also increase the risk of hepatocellular carcinoma. The evidence is, however, inconclusive.

Cervical erosion. Cervical erosion (in which a zone of columnar epithelium develops on the vaginal portion of the cervix in place of the stratified squamous epithelium normally found there) occurs about twice as often in pill users as in others. Although a trivial condition in itself, a diagnosis of cervical erosion may lead to hospital admission for cautery under general anaesthesia.

Impairment of fertility. Despite a vast literature, prior use of oral contraceptives has not been conclusively incriminated either as a cause of prolonged secondary amenorrhoea or of prolactinoma of the pituitary which is sometimes associated with this condition (see Section 10). Many women do, however, experience some temporary impairment of fertility after stopping the pill. In the majority this lasts only a month or so, but in some recovery may be much slower. It seems unlikely that oral contraceptives are a cause of permanent infertility.

Other possible adverse effects. Not surprisingly, many epidemiological studies have been concerned with the possible relationship between oral contraceptive use and malignant disease. On balance, the results so far have been fairly reassuring; indeed, as already mentioned, there is mounting evidence that the pill may offer some protection against endometrial and ovarian cancer. It should be noted, however, that a few studies have suggested that oral contraceptives may increase the risk of breast cancer and pre-invasive cervical cancer in certain subgroups of women already predisposed to these diseases. A particularly worrying finding in one recent investigation was an association between the occurrence of breast cancer and use of oral contraceptives for prolonged periods prior to the first pregnancy. A Californian study has also hinted that the pill might slightly increase the risk of malignant melanoma. Work on

Table 1 Some features of the association between oral contraceptives and cardiovascular disease

Adverse effect	Approximate relative risk, users: non-users	Relation of risk to steroidal content of pill	Relation of risk to duration of use of pill	Relation of risk to current or past usage
Venous thrombosis and embolism	6:1	positive association with oestrogen dose; progestogen probably unimportant	increase in risk independent of duration of use	increased risk in current users only
Thrombotic stroke	6:1	weak evidence for a positive association with both oestrogen and progestogen dose	data inadequate	increased risk in current users; data for past users inadequate
Haemorrhagic stroke	2:1	data inadequate	data inadequate	increased risk in current users; some evidence of increased risk in past users also
Myocardial infarction	3:1	weak evidence for a positive association with both oestrogen and progestogen dose	increase in risk independent of duration of use	increased risk in current users; little evidence of increased risk in past users

the relationship, if any, between oral contraceptives and cancer will have to continue since few of the women in the investigations reported to date have had prolonged exposure to the pill (say for 10 years or more).

A number of reports have suggested that oral contraceptives taken inadvertently during (or even just before) pregnancy might increase the risk of malformation of the fetus (especially cardiac defects, neural tube defects, and limb reduction defects). The evidence is, however, uneven and difficult to interpret and the risk certainly cannot be regarded as substantiated.

Finally many other disorders including migraine, depression, and urinary tract infection have been reported in some studies, but not in others, as possible adverse effects of oral contraception.

Balance of benefits and risks. In Table 2, an attempt has been made to draw together information about the morbidity associated with the use of the pill. For comparative purposes, data are also provided about women using the diaphragm, a simple contraceptive device which (unlike the pill) has not been conclusively demonstrated to have any 'medical' effects (although occlusive methods of contraception may protect against cervical neoplasia). The medical audit in Table 2 is largely based on data derived from the Oxford Family Planning Association Contraceptive Study and is limited to a consideration of hospital admissions.

Table 3 presents the best available data on mortality associated with use of the pill obtained from the Royal College of General Practitioners Oral Contraceptive Study. The rates shown are subdivided according to age and cigarette smoking habits.

Simple analyses of the sort shown in Tables 2–3, while of value in providing a sense of proportion when comparing contraceptive methods, should not be taken too seriously. Thus, many of the estimates (especially of the risk of death) are based on small numbers of events, while no allowance has been made for variations in risk with different oral contraceptive formulations, different durations of use, and so on.

The pill has been studied extremely intensively over the last two decades. On the whole it has stood up well to close scrutiny. It remains an excellent method of contraception for younger women. Those over 35, especially if they smoke or have other cardiovascular disease risk factors would, however, be well advised to use some other method if at all possible.

Table 2 Morbidity experienced by women aged 25–44 using either oral contraceptives or the diaphragm to try to prevent pregnancy for one year

Reason for hospital admission	Numbers of hospital admissions in one year among 100 000 women using	
	Oral contraceptives	diaphragm
Beneficial effects of pill:		
menstrual disorders	450	575
anaemia	40	60
benign breast disease	120	280
functional ovarian cysts	85	120
Adverse effects of pill:		
venous thromboembolism	90	20
stroke	45	10
acute myocardial infarction	10	3
gall bladder disease	170	130
hepatocellular adenoma	3	0
cervical erosion	540	250
Accidental pregnancy:		
term birth	90	3040
spontaneous abortion	19	640
ectopic gestation	1	20
termination	40	1300

It has been assumed that the accidental pregnancy rate for pill users is 1.5/1000/year and for diaphragm users is 50/1000/year

References

Briggs, M. H. (1978). Steroid contraception: metabolic and endocrine effects. In *Risks, benefits and controversies in fertility control* (eds. J. J. Sciarra, G. I. Zatuchni, and J. J. Speidel), 214. Harper and Row, Hagerstown.

Laragh, J. H. (1976). Oral contraceptive-induced hypertension—nine years later. *Am. J. Obstet. Gynec.* **126**, 141.

Poller, L. (1978). Oral contraceptives, blood clotting and thrombosis. *Br. med. Bull.* **34**, 151.

Rooks, J. B., Ory, H. W., Ishak, K. G., Strauss, L. T., Greenspan, J. R., Paganini-Hill, A., and Tyler, C. W. (1979). The epidemiology of hepatocellular adenoma. The role of oral contraceptive use. *J. Am. med. Ass.* **242**, 644.

Royal College of General Practitioners (1974). *Oral contraceptives and health.* Pitman Medical, London.

Scientific Group (1978). *Steroid contraception and the risk of neoplasia.* Technical Report Series no. 619. World Health Organization, Geneva.

— (1981). *The effect of female sex hormones on total development and infant health.* Technical Report Series no. 657. World Health Organization, Geneva.

Vessey, M. P. (1979). Results of epidemiological studies of the return of fertility in ex-users of the pill. In *The regulation of fertility— evaluation and perspectives*, p. 185. Institut National de la Sante et de la Recherche Médicale. Paris.

— (1980). Female hormones and vascular disease—an epidemiological overview. *Br. J. Fam. Plan.* **6**, Suppl., 1.

—, Doll, R., Peto, R., Johnson, B., and Wiggins, P. (1976). A long-term follow-up study of women using different methods of contraception—an interim report. *J. Biosoc. Sci.* **8**, 373.

Table 3 Mortality experienced by women aged (a) 25–34 and (b) 35–44 using either oral contraceptives or the diaphragm to try to prevent pregnancy for one year

Age group and cause of death	Numbers of deaths in one year among 100 000 women			
	Using oral contraceptives and smoking	Using oral contraceptives but not smoking	Using diaphragm and smoking	Using diaphragm but not smoking
Ages 25–34				
cardiovascular disease	14.2	4.4	4.2	2.7
pregnancy	0.0	0.0	0.7	0.7
Total	14.2	4.4	4.9	3.4
Ages 35–44				
cardiovascular disease	63.4	21.5	15.2	6.4
pregnancy	0.1	0.1	2.3	2.3
Total	63.5	21.6	17.5	8.7

It has been assumed that the accidental pregnancy rate for pill users is 1.5/1000/year and for diaphragm users is 50/1000/year. The numbers of deaths attributable to pregnancy are based on the maternal mortality rates for England and Wales for the year 1977

HYPERTENSION IN PREGNANCY

C. W. G. Redman

The cardiovascular system in pregnancy. Cardiac output increases during the first trimester to about 1.5 l/minute above non-pregnant levels. No further increase occurs in the second and third trimesters. Towards term it declines in the supine but not lateral recumbent positions. This is the result of pressure from the gravid uterus on the inferior vena cava which reduces the total venous return. In the third trimester about two-thirds of the additional cardiac output is distributed either to the placental circulation or to augment renal plasma flow. The increased output is a product of both a greater stroke volume and a higher pulse rate.

Arterial pressure falls in the second half of the first trimester at about the same time as the cardiac output is increasing. Thus peripheral resistance must decrease proportionately more than the cardiac output has increased. This cannot be caused by the development of the uteroplacental circulation which is small at this time and must therefore result from a generalized arteriolar dilatation. During the second and third trimesters this relaxation of arterial tone is associated with a marked insensitivity to the constrictor action of angiotensin II.

In the later weeks of pregnancy there is a tendency for the diastolic pressure to rise slowly towards its non-pregnant level whereas the systolic pressure remains constant. At this time measurement of the arterial pressure in the recumbent position may be atypically low because of the pressure effects of the enlarged uterus—the 'supine hypotension' syndrome which affects about 10 per cent of women in the third trimester.

Definition. The definitions for arterial hypertension used in general medical practice are not applicable to pregnant women who are both young and healthy and have lower blood pressures than when they are not pregnant. The mean blood pressure at the first visit before 20 weeks will be about 120/70 supine: two and three standard deviations above this will be about 145/85 and 160/95 respectively. The actual reading will depend on many factors, particularly body weight. Women weighing 80 kg or more have blood pressures about 15 mmHg more than women weighing less than 50 kg.

Obstetric hypertension is conventionally diagnosed at the arbitrary cut-off point of 140/90 which is a low threshold by general medical standards. This is appropriate for the first half of pregnancy. In the second half of pregnancy about one-quarter of all women will be hypertensive by this criterion, meaning that the limits are set too low to define an unusually hypertensive section of the population. About 2.5 per cent have a maximum arterial pressure of 160/105 or more and 1 per cent of 170/110 or more and these are more realistic limits; but note that the maximum blood pressure is a biased statistic and women whose highest blood pressures peak to 170/110 for example will tend to have a lower basal blood pressure.

Aetiology. Hypertension in pregnancy has three possible aetiologies: it may be caused by the pregnancy itself; it may represent a long-term problem, present before the pregnancy began; or, much more rarely, it may be a new medical problem by chance coinciding with pregnancy.

Hypertension caused by pregnancy has previously been thought of as a quite separate problem from other forms of hypertension. For this reason it has in the past been managed by obstetricians who developed modes of treatment which largely ignored the developments of treatment of hypertension in other fields. At the same time physicians have remained ignorant of the specifically different features of pre-eclampsia.

Hypertension caused by pregnancy. Pre-eclampsia, pre-eclamptic toxaemia, gestosis, pregnancy-induced hypertension, or gestational hypertension are all terms which have been used to describe the same syndrome. The most precise is pre-eclampsia which identifies the end-point of the problem namely eclampsia. Toxaemia is an obsolete term which was used previously to refer to any hypertension or proteinuria in pregnancy whether pregnancy-induced or not. Eclampsia can occur rarely before the twentieth week of pregnancy but is confined ordinarily to the second half of pregnancy. It is a brief and violent illness characterized by generalized convulsions, hypertension which may be extreme, and renal impairment with proteinuria. It is similar but not identical to malignant hypertension (Table 1). In England and Wales pre-eclampsia/eclampsia remains one of the most significant causes of maternal death. Cerebral pathology is the dominant feature at autopsy (Table 2) especially cerebral haemorrhages which in distribution and histological features are indistinguishable from hypertensive cerebral haemorrhage seen in non-pregnant individuals. Thus hypertension is not only a defining feature of pre-eclampsia but must be considered the cause of its most dangerous terminal complications.

Table 1   The similarities and differences between malignant hypertension and eclampsia

	Malignant hypertension	Eclampsia
Convulsion	+	+
Cerebral haemorrhage	+	+
Retinal haemorrhage	+	rarely
Heart failure	+	+
Proteinuria	+	+
Renal failure	+	+
Disseminated intravascular coagulation	+	+
Microangiopathic haemolysis	+	+
Hepatic pathology	0	+
Renal artery intimal proliferation	+	0

The main difference between eclampsia and malignant hypertension is that even if the precise cause of eclampsia is unknown, it is at least localized to the gravid uterus and the simple expedient of delivery always terminates the illness. Thus with normal obstetric care severe pre-eclampsia or eclampsia are brief episodes. This is probably why renal artery intimal proliferation (a feature of malignant hypertension) is not seen; this is a secondary response to arterial injury which takes more time to develop than the usual duration of an eclamptic illness.

Table 2   The causes of maternal death (39 cases) from pre-eclampsia and eclampsia in England and Wales, 1973–5

Complications	
Cerebral	23
Anaesthetic	5
Hepatic	4
Cardiopulmonary	3
Haemorrhage	1
Renal	1
Hepato-renal	1
Sickle cell crisis	1

A further difference is found in the hepatic pathology of eclampsia which comprises periportal haemorrhages and infarcts. These are not a feature of malignant hypertension and cannot be explained by any process of hypertensive injury. Hepatic pathology is a more significant cause of maternal death than renal pathology (Table 2). This underlines the fact that pre-eclampsia is not *only* a hypertensive disorder and that hypertension is but one component of a generalized systemic maternal disorder caused by pregnancy.

Pre-eclampsia, the forerunner of eclampsia, begins and progresses with much the same sequence of changes in different patients, but varies in the speed with which it evolves. It may last only a few days or extend over several months. The patient is asymptomatic until the terminal stages. The onset of symptoms—headaches, vomiting, and epigastric pain—indicates that convulsions are imminent. The diagnosis of pre-eclampsia is thus made in the asymptomatic woman by screening.

Conventionally, medical practitioners have been taught to recognize pre-eclampsia by the triad of hypertension, oedema, and proteinuria. However, this is both inadequate and inaccurate.

Hypertension is an early feature. It is caused by vasoconstriction of unknown aetiology associated with reduced circulating plasma volume and a normal or reduced cardiac output. Vascular reactivity is altered so that the normal insensitivity of the pregnant arterial system to angiotensin II is lost. Basal blood pressure becomes characteristically unstable with sudden spikes unrelated to any external stimuli. The nocturnal fall of the blood pressure is attenuated, and in advanced pre-eclampsia the highest blood pressures may be recorded during sleep at night, a reversal of the usual circadian pattern.

Eighty-five per cent of women with proteinuric pre-eclampsia have generalized fluid retention which may extend to the serous cavities, for example as ascites, or it may involve the lungs—pulmonary oedema being a rare life-threatening complication of the disorder. This pathological oedema which is associated with abnormally low plasma protein concentrations is easily and frequently confused with the physiological oedema of pregnancy. Nearly nine out of 10 normal pregnant women have some oedema by term and in some this may be gross. But this normal fluid retention is almost certainly not in any way related to pre-eclamptic oedema. Oedema is not an essential part of pre-eclampsia or eclampsia: the 'dry' variants have long been recognized as particularly dangerous forms. Because of the confusion between physiological and pathological oedema in pregnancy and because oedema is not consistently present in pre-eclampsia, it is now no longer included as a basic diagnostic feature.

Proteinuria is a late sign of pre-eclampsia and once present indicates a poorer prognosis for both mother and baby than when it is absent. It may be heavy (more than 5 g/day) and is moderately selective in terms of the molecular size of the filtered proteins. Overall, pre-eclampsia is the commonest cause of nephrotic syndrome in pregnancy. The proteinuria is but one manifestation of involvement of the kidney as a principal target organ of the pre-eclamptic process. Renal biopsy (for research purposes only) has shown a characteristic, non-inflammatory lesion, primarily a swelling of the glomerular endothelial cells which occlude the capillary lumina. The epithelial foot processes and the glomerular basement membrane are intact. There may be deposits of IgM and C3 demonstrable by immunofluorescence. It should be noted that renal biopsy is never indicated for the diagnosis or management of pre-eclampsia.

Renal function is also impaired. The changes are biphasic involving first tubular function and later glomerular function. An early feature of pre-eclampsia is a reduced uric acid clearance whilst glomerular filtration continues to be normal. Later, at about the time that proteinuria develops, glomerular filtration becomes impaired. A rising plasma urate is thus an early feature of pre-eclampsia, and precedes a later rising plasma creatinine or urea. It is also the biochemical change which best correlates with the renal biopsy appearances of the disorder.

In pregnancy there is an increased turnover of the clotting system indicating an activation which is probably needed for haemostasis at delivery. This process is exaggerated in pre-eclampsia and in the severe disorder may progress to a pathological disseminated intravascular coagulation with widespread small vessel occlusion, depletion of clotting factors, and even a micro-angiopathic haemolytic anaemia. The features of this terminal stage are the same as in other medical situations. The early activation of the coagulation system is not easy to detect except by research techniques, but it can be shown that it begins at about the same time as the blood pressure and plasma urate are rising. Later there is severe thrombocytopenia, raised fibrin/fibrinogen degradation products, and prolonged bleeding times. If there is haemolysis haemoglobin concentration may suddenly fall with haemoglobinaemia, schistocytes, and an increased reticulocyte count.

The fundamental pathology of pre-eclampsia lies within the uterine spiral and basal arteries which supply the placental intervillous space and the uterine decidua respectively. In pre-eclampsia these are partially or completely blocked by intimal aggregates of fibrin, thrombi, and large lipid-laden cells. Although termed acute atherosis, this lesion has no histological relation to degenerative arterial disease of middle and old age. Nor is it the sort of lesion associated with direct hypertensive injury. Furthermore its presence has been documented with maternal arterial pressures so low as to make direct pressure injury a very unlikely primary cause. We can therefore conclude that hypertension is probably a secondary feature of pre-eclampsia consequent on the processes which cause the spiral artery changes. The spiral artery lesions account for the reduction of placental blood flow characteristic of pre-eclampsia and hence the increased incidence of placental infarction and failure. The fetal consequences of the disease—intra-uterine asphyxia and nutritional deprivation—are also clearly explained.

Diagnosis of pre-eclampsia. None of the features of pre-eclampsia is specific; even convulsions in pregnancy are, in modern practice, more likely to have causes other than eclampsia. Diagnosis therefore depends on the demonstration of a coincidence of several pre-eclamptic features together. The final proof is their regression after delivery. An abnormal rise in maternal arterial pressure combined with a rising plasma urate are early signs which are easy to detect. The diagnosis of pre-eclamptic hypertension depends more on showing a change from a baseline than finding a blood pressure level at or above an arbitrary limit. Whether or not an increase is clinically significant depends on the reliability of the measurements, the magnitude of the change, and the time in pregnancy when it occurs. The errors of indirect blood pressure readings are well known; to detect small changes at different times in the same individuals therefore requires standardization particularly with respect to posture. In pregnant women the Korotkoff sounds are occasionally audible at zero cuff pressure; for this reason phase IV (the point of muffling) has to be used to define diastolic pressure. Between weeks 20 and 30 the blood pressure is normally steady so that even a small consistent rise is clinically significant. Between weeks 30 and term the diastolic will normally rise 10 mmHg. Overall, therefore, a sustained rise of 30/15–20 mmHg from the first reading taken in the first half of pregnancy is an accepted diagnostic criterion. There is as yet no consensus about what changes in plasma urate are diagnostic of pre-eclampsia. As a rough guide abnormal levels can be said to be present if they exceed 0.35 mmol/l at 32 weeks or earlier and 0.40 mmol/l after this time. If a baseline reading is available in early pregnancy then rises of 0.1, 0.15, and 0.2 mmol/l at 28, 32, and 36 weeks respectively are typical of the pre-eclamptic process.

Proteinuria and evidence of a reduced glomerular filtration rate are later signs. The changes in the measurements of renal function are usually within the normal range for non-pregnant individuals. As a rough guide abnormal levels for plasma creatinine and urea are at or above 100 µmol/l and 6.0 mmol/l respectively. Pre-eclamptic proteinuria is usually in excess of 1 g/24 hours but the exact amount will depend at what stage in the evolution of proteinuria the measurements are made.

Gross thrombocytopenia, raised fibrin degradation products, and evidence of hepatic impairment are preterminal developments immediately preceding or coinciding with the onset of symptoms.

The absence of all these signs can refute the diagnosis. The presence of hypertension and the *de novo* occurrence of at least one other sign allows the diagnosis to be made with reasonable certainty. But a raised blood pressure on its own, without any other sign, can never justify a confident diagnosis of pre-eclampsia. On occasions, although a raised blood pressure may be the first indication of the onset of the disorder, spontaneous or induced delivery terminates its further evolution so that a final certain diagnosis cannot be made.

Complications of pre-eclampsia. Obstetric complications include primarily the consequences of placental ischaemia and infarction, namely fetal growth failure and asphyxia, and abruptio placentae. Medical complications include cerebral haemorrhages which are the commonest cause of maternal death. Cerebral oedema, on the other hand, only rarely occurs. Retinal haemorrhages are seen infrequently (about 1–2 per cent of all women with proteinuric pre-eclampsia). Retinal detachment has been reported resulting from retinal oedema. Loss of vision is one of the symptoms which may precede eclamptic fits. Heart failure and pulmonary oedema are uncommon antenatal complications, but constitute an indication for immediate delivery after reversal by treatment. Circulatory collapse within the first 24 hours after delivery used to be seen in pre-eclamptic women treated by vigorous salt restriction, but is not seen in modern practice. Pre-eclampsia/eclampsia has been one of the prime obstetric causes of renal failure through partial or complete renal cortical necrosis. The combination of severe pre-eclampsia and abruptio placentae is particularly dangerous in this respect. Jaundice is a rare but dangerous presentation of pre-eclampsia. It is associated with signs of hepatocellular damage without evidence of biliary obstruction. Both hypertension and proteinuria are present and the patient usually complains of vomiting and abdominal pain. Immediate delivery is the right management and the condition completely regresses thereafter. This form of jaundice must be distinguished from cholestasis of pregnancy where there is a mild obstructive jaundice which presents with itching. A rare and potentially lethal complication of liver involvement is spontaneous rupture of the liver capsule. Severe disseminated intravascular coagulation has in the past caused presentations which have been confused with thrombotic thrombocytopenic purpura.

Management of pre-eclamptic hypertension. Pre-eclampsia is not merely a hypertensive disease but a profound disturbance of pregnancy involving many maternal systems and the fetus as well. Therefore, control of the blood pressure is only part of patient management. The definitive management of the established disorder is always delivery, which, if expedited before irreversible damage has occurred (e.g. cerebral haemorrhage), guarantees a complete and rapid cure. No medical regimen has ever been shown to alter in any significant way the relentlessly progressive course of pre-eclampsia. Until such specific treatment is available, the purpose of medical management is to protect the mother from the dangers of her illness during that relatively brief period after the disease is diagnosed and before elective delivery.

The main objective is to prevent extreme hypertension. The threshold at which hypotensive therapy should be given is disputed. The evidence is that the risk of acute arteriolar damage begins at a mean arterial pressure of about 140 mmHg. For this reason it is our custom to begin treatment if maximum readings (systolic or diastolic) are repeatedly reaching or exceeding a pressure of 170 mmHg or 110 mmHg respectively.

Parenteral diazoxide and hydralazine are employed for the acute reduction of blood pressure. Diazoxide has been used mainly for intrapartum hypertensive emergencies. It reduces the blood pressure within minutes but the standard dose of 300 mg by rapid intravenous injection is excessive and can cause serious hypotension. The tendency to hypotension is aggravated by the plasma volume depletion of pre-eclampsia and is more likely if the patient is already on drugs that inhibit the sympathetic nervous system. Titration, by intermittent administration of small intravenous boluses of 30–60 mg is preferable and effective. Apart from hypotension the side-effects of diazoxide include the inhibition

of labour and the possibility of hyperglycaemia in both mother and fetus. Hydralazine can be given by continuous intravenous infusion (5–10 mg per hour) or intermittently (10–20 mg intramuscularly or subcutaneously). Its action takes 30–50 minutes to develop and lasts for the relatively brief time of one to three hours. Side-effects are common and include reflex tachycardia, headaches, vomiting, and hyper-reflexia. These mimic the symptoms of impending eclampsia, which complicates the further assessment of the pre-eclamptic patient.

It is not known if the rapid reduction of maternal blood pressure affects placental blood flow and hence fetal well-being. In pre-eclampsia, placental perfusion is already compromised and there is circumstantial evidence that fetal problems may be precipitated by acute hypotensive treatment. However, if perfusion of a pre-eclamptic placenta can only be maintained by a blood pressure that directly threatens maternal well-being, then urgent delivery is the first priority for both mother and baby. The potential dangers of a sudden (and possibly excessive) drop in the blood pressure should, therefore, be recognized and parenteral therapy avoided if possible. Short-term blood pressure control can usually be achieved over about 12 hours by an adequate oral loading dose of methyl dopa (0.5–1.0 g) followed by 2–3 g/day in divided doses. If there is vomiting, intravenous methyl dopa can be substituted. Its hypotensive action can be augmented by oral hydralazine limited to less than 300 mg/day. Methyl dopa is used because there is extensive evidence indicating its safety for the fetus. Beta-adrenergic blocking agents are avoided because their possible fetal side-effects in these circumstances have yet to be defined. Diuretics are not given because they exacerbate the often severe hypovolaemia of pre-eclampsia.

Good blood pressure control in pre-eclampsia does not ameliorate its other features. The disease persists and remains relentlessly progressive until delivery. Therefore 'escape' from control is common. Nor does adequate treatment prevent other complications such as placental abruption or progressive fetal asphyxia.

A persisting inability to control maternal arterial pressure is one of several indications for immediate delivery.

The second objective of medical management is to prevent eclamptic fits if these are thought to be imminent. This will always be for a brief period before delivery because if a patient is ill enough to require anticonvulsant therapy, she is ill enough to need immediate delivery. Intravenous diazepam or chlormethiazole are the preferred agents in the United Kingdom; parenteral magnesium sulphate is used in the USA. Claims that one regime is superior to the other are meaningless because they have never been formally compared.

Numerous regimens have been advocated for the prevention of pre-eclampsia. None has been shown to be effective. They include bed-rest, restriction of maternal weight gain, salt restriction, diuretic administration, and the use of non-specific sedatives.

Diuretics have been considered to be useful because of the oedema and salt retention of pre-eclampsia. However, controlled trials have shown that their use neither prevents nor ameliorates pre-eclampsia and has no impact on the eventual perinatal mortality. They aggravate the hypovolaemia of established pre-eclampsia which can adversely affect renal function. They cause hyperuricaemia and so obscure one of the more useful diagnostic signs of the disorder. They are, however, clearly indicated for the management of left ventricular failure, which is a rare complication of severe pre-eclampsia.

Chronic hypertension complicating pregnancy. Women with chronic hypertension coinciding with pregnancy tend to be older, fatter, and slightly taller. Frequently they have clear family histories of hypertension. Because of the physiological changes of pregnancy, their hypertension may be ameliorated or masked by the beginning of the second trimester and therefore not necessarily diagnosable unless pre-pregnancy blood pressure readings are available.

Chronic hypertension is one of the major predisposing factors to pre-eclampsia so that the two conditions, which in their pure forms are easily separable, may commonly occur together. Pre-eclampsia superimposed on chronic hypertension tends to be more severe, to occur at earlier stages of pregnancy, to cause more fetal growth retardation, and to be recurrent in later pregnancies. Pre-eclampsia occurring in a normotensive individual tends not to recur in second and later pregnancies. If a blood pressure of 140/90 in the first half of pregnancy is taken as evidence of chronic hypertension, then the affected individuals have an approximately fivefold increased risk of later pre-eclampsia compared to normotensive individuals. This close link between the two conditions led earlier clinicians to conclude that chronic hypertension is extremely dangerous when combined with pregnancy. It is now clear that the particular risks of chronic hypertension in pregnancy are entirely attributable to the increased chance of developing superimposed pre-eclampsia, and that the majority of chronically hypertensive women who do not get pre-eclampsia can expect a normal and uncomplicated perinatal outcome.

Hypertension in pregnancy can only be diagnosed with certainty as being non-gestational if it is detected in the first half of pregnancy, preferably before the sixteenth week. In the second half of pregnancy the possibility that mild hypertension could be pre-eclamptic in origin can never be entirely excluded unless the readings can be related to early or pre-pregnancy levels. The signs of pre-eclampsia in chronically hypertensive women are the same as in other women except that the blood pressure levels start from a higher baseline. Thus the demonstration of a rise in the blood pressure (+ 30/+ 20 mmHg from baseline), of a progressive hyperuricaemia, or abnormal activation of the clotting system is evidence of superimposed pre-eclampsia which will progress to proteinuria unless pre-empted by delivery. When proteinuria develops, intrauterine growth retardation is almost the rule.

The easiest diagnostic guide is a maternal plasma urate level. Values below 0.3 mmol/l are not in favour of pre-eclampsia and in a hypertensive woman would suggest the diagnosis of a chronic problem. Values above 0.35 mmol/l before 32 weeks and above 0.40 mmol/l after this time are more characteristic of pre-eclamptic hypertension. Thus the differential diagnosis of chronic hypertension from pre-eclamptic hypertension rests on the demonstration of the absence of pre-eclamptic features such as a change of the blood pressure from baseline, a rise in maternal plasma urate levels, and absence of proteinuria and activation of the clotting system.

Treatment of chronic hypertension in pregnancy. If antihypertensive treatment has been started before conception, the patient may seek advice about the possible effects of her medication on the growth and development of her fetus. None of the commonly used antihypertensive drugs is known to be teratogenic. This does not preclude the possibility of subtle problems which are as yet unknown. For this reason it is appropriate that women with no more than moderate hypertension stop treatment before conception so that only those whose hypertension constitutes an immediate health hazard continue taking treatment through the first trimester. By the twelfth week the normal fall in blood pressure is such that the need for treatment is either temporarily diminished or no longer present.

If chronic hypertension is diagnosed for the first time in pregnancy, it is then necessary to treat those in whom it presents an immediate (as opposed to a long-term) hazard to the patient. The precise levels at which this is necessary have not been agreed upon; we take a cut-off point at or above 170/110.

The problem of less severe chronic hypertension (i.e. 140–170/90–110 mmHg) needs to be considered. In general medical practice the purpose of treating this degree of hypertension is to prevent long-term complications such as heart failure, aortic dissection, and coronary or cerebral vascular disease. Although these problems do present in pregnant women, and are associated with hypertension, they are so rare that in themselves they cannot justify treatment for the brief period of gestation. Thus moderate hypertension *per se* carries no intrinsic maternal risk in pregnancy except in so far as it

may be the precursor of more severe hypertension. However, the higher the arterial pressure the greater is the eventual perinatal mortality. If the mild hypertension indicates early pre-eclampsia, the risks evolve through simple progression. If the mild hypertension indicates a pre-existing problem, then the risk is of later superimposition of pre-eclampsia which is, as we have seen, several times more likely to develop in hypertensive than in normotensive women. If antihypertensive treatment is indicated for moderate hypertension in pregnancy, it must either be because it can *retard* the progression of mild pre-eclampsia or because it can *prevent* the superimposition of pre-eclampsia in chronically hypertensive women.

There is no evidence that the early control of pre-eclamptic hypertension retards its progression. There is also clear evidence based on randomized controlled trials that the early control of moderate chronic hypertension does not lessen the eventual incidence of superimposed pre-eclampsia. Thus there is no clear fetal indication for the control of moderate hypertension in pregnancy, and consequently the medical management hinges entirely around considerations of maternal welfare.

Oral antihypertensive agents that are used in pregnancy. The choice of drugs is dictated by fetal considerations. Methyl dopa is the preferred agent because its fetal effects have been defined much more clearly than those of any other agent. Its antihypertensive action and side-effects are the same as in non-pregnant individuals. It does not cause any discernible fetal problem although fetuses exposed *in utero* to methyl dopa for the time between 16 and 20 weeks gestation may have slightly reduced head circumferences. However, developmental follow-ups to the age of four years confirm the absence of any adverse drug reaction. The usual treatment schedule is 1–4 g/day in divided doses. The effect of methyl dopa can be supplemented by low doses of oral hydralazine as for the treatment of pre-eclamptic hypertension. Beta-adrenergic blocking agents have been used less extensively in pregnancy and their possible fetal effects have not been completely evaluated. The fetus depends on an intact adrenergic nervous system to compensate for periods of hypoxaemia so there is a theoretical risk that beta-adrenergic blockade could impair survival in certain vulnerable fetuses. This has not been confirmed in practice nor have other predicted side-effects been observed, namely a stimulant action on the gravid uterus which could precipitate pre-term labour, or neonatal hypoglycaemia. Nevertheless, these agents should be used with caution in pregnancy until the results of current controlled trials are fully evaluated and reported.

If diuretics are essential for good blood pressure control, they can be continued throughout pregnancy, but their use carries certain disadvantages if pre-eclampsia should supervene, as already discussed. Bethanidine, clonidine, and prazosin have all been used in pregnancy but their effects on the fetus are not defined. Reserpine and the angiotensin-converting enzyme inhibitor, captopril, both have adverse effects on the fetus and therefore should not be used.

Long-term sequelae of hypertension in pregnancy. Severe pre-eclampsia and eclampsia can cause irreversible maternal damage, particularly acute renal cortical necrosis or cerebral haemorrhage. In the absence of these complications there is no evidence at the present time that long-term health is impaired by a pre-eclamptic illness. However, in terms of life expectancy, pre-eclamptic women fall into two groups. Those who have an episode in the first pregnancy only and become normotensive soon after delivery have a normal life expectancy. The second group have recurrent pre-eclampsia in several pregnancies, or blood pressures which remain elevated in the puerperium. They have a higher incidence of later cardiovascular disorders and a reduced life expectancy compatible with the diagnosis that the initial episode of pre-eclampsia was superimposed on pre-existing hypertension.

Conclusions. Extreme hypertension in pregnancy is as dangerous as it is in any other medical situation and demands urgent treatment. The perinatal risks of chronic hypertension in pregnancy are mediated through the increased incidence of pre-eclampsia. The treatment of mild chronic hypertension in pregnancy does not prevent the later superimposition of pre-eclampsia. Methyl dopa is the most thoroughly tested hypotensive agent in pregnancy. Apart from a possible effect on fetal head growth, if treatment is started between 16 and 20 weeks gestation, no significant adverse reactions have been observed. Beta-adrenoceptor antagonists may be safe to use in pregnancy but there are as yet inadequate trial data. Diuretics should primarily be reserved for the treatment of heart failure complicating pre-eclampsia.

References

Chesley, L. C. (1978). *Hypertensive disorders in pregnancy*. Appleton-Century-Crofts, New York.

Redman, C. W. G. (1980). Treatment of hypertension in pregnancy. *Kidney Int.* **18**, 267.

RENAL DISEASE IN PREGNANCY

C. W. G. Redman and J. G. G. Ledingham

Renal function in pregnancy. Renal function changes during the first trimester of human pregnancy. Effective renal plasma flow increases by about 60 per cent and glomerular filtration rate by about 50 per cent. In late pregnancy, renal function may become dependent on posture (although this point is disputed by several investigators). In particular, supine recumbency may reduce renal perfusion and glomerular filtration because of pressure from the gravid uterus. These physiological changes alter the criteria for diagnosing abnormal renal function clinically. As a rough guide, abnormal values for plasma urea, creatinine, and uric acid are above 6.0 mmol/l, 100 μmol/l, and 0.40 mmol/l respectively.

The renal collecting systems dilate during pregnancy. The volume of the ureters may increase as much as 25 times. The changes are more marked on the right side and in primigravida. They begin to regress soon after delivery but have not completely returned to more normal dimensions until about two months after delivery; indeed the right ureter above the pelvic brim may remain a little dilated chronically. This point is of importance when interpreting postpartum intravenous pyelograms.

Infection. About one in 20 pregnant women have asymptomatic bacilluria. If left untreated, one quarter of those affected will progress to an acute attack of pyelonephritis, which can be prevented in more than half by adequate treatment at the symptomless stage. Asymptomatic bacilluria in pregnancy is associated with an increase in incidence of premature delivery. This need not be a direct cause and effect but may be mediated through a third common factor, such as a poor socio-economic status. Nevertheless it is well known that an attack of acute pyelonephritis can precipitate premature labour and that the endotoxin of *Escherichia coli* (the commonest offending organism) can be toxic to the fetus.

Bacilluria is commoner in gravida with major renal abnormalities. The more persistent the infection, the higher the likelihood of finding significant pathology. It is, therefore, a sensible routine that all pregnant women are screened once for bacilluria, that all confirmed infections are treated, and that women with persistent or recurrent infections are investigated postpartum with full evaluation of the renal system including intravenous pyelography. More than half the women in whom bacilluria persists, despite treatment, will be shown to have radiographic abnormalities of the urinary tract or kidneys.

Acute pyelonephritis is the most common serious medical complication of pregnancy affecting 1–2 per cent of all gravid women. It may cause septic shock, and, before the availability of antibiotics, caused maternal deaths. It usually presents in the second or third trimesters with the typical symptoms and signs of loin pain, fever,

headache, nausea, vomiting, frequency, and dysuria. Transient renal dysfunction is not uncommon. A prompt response to treatment with intravenous fluids and antimicrobial agents can be expected. Nearly one-quarter of the affected women will have recurrent attacks during pregnancy and the incidence of persisting bacilluria is equally high. The marked tendency to recurrences distinguishes acute pyelonephritis complicating pregnancy from its presentation in non-pregnant subjects. The effect of the acute illness on the pregnancy is hard to assess but most investigators find an increased incidence of pre-term labour, fetal growth retardation, and perinatal deaths. The drugs that are commonly used for the treatment of renal infection in non-pregnant patients can be used during pregnancy. These include the broad-spectrum antimicrobials including ampicillin, cephalosporin derivatives, and the aminoglycosides such as gentamicin or amikacin.

Acute renal failure in pregnancy. Acute renal failure complicates about 1 in 6000 pregnancies. Previously, there was a bimodal pattern of occurrence with two peaks in incidence occurring respectively in early and late pregnancy. The commonest presentation was with septic abortion at 12 to 18 weeks' gestation. Recently the incidence of septic abortion has declined so that acute renal failure in late pregnancy (i.e. the third trimester) is now more important. The underlying pathology includes a high incidence of acute cortical necrosis which develops in 5–30 per cent of all cases of obstetric renal failure. Both partial and complete necrosis occur. Pregnant women are so much more susceptible than others to acute cortical necrosis that they comprise the greater part of any series of cases. The reason for this is not known. Disseminated intravascular coagulation is common to all the obstetric conditions which pre-dispose to acute cortical necrosis: septic abortions, pre-eclampsia/eclampsia, antepartum haemorrhage, prolonged intra-uterine death, amniotic fluid embolism, and acute yellow atrophy of the liver. So it is possible that coagulation disorders mediate its occurrence. The commonest causes of acute renal failure in pregnancy are abruptio placenti and severe pre-eclampsia. The affected women tend to be older than the average and parous. Full recovery is anticipated if there is acute tubular necrosis. Recovery occurs more slowly (extended over several months) and less completely after partial cortical necrosis and is not expected after complete cortical necrosis. Both peritoneal dialysis and haemodialysis can be used to prevent the complications of acute renal failure whilst recovery is awaited. Antenatal peritoneal dialysis is both feasible and safe, but which technique is chosen will depend on both circumstances and clinical facilities. In the interests of fetal health, early dialysis of undelivered mothers is to be preferred.

Despite improvements in management, maternal mortality remains high at 10–15 per cent. The perinatal mortality is also extremely high, but this reflects the conditions precipitating the renal failure as much as the renal failure itself.

Idiopathic postpartum renal failure. This is a rare and frequently fatal complication of the first weeks of the puerperium usually after an uncomplicated pregnancy. It is characterized by acute renal failure with severe hypertension and disseminated intravascular coagulation. The clotting problems may be severe enough to cause micro-angiopathic haemolysis and may mimic thrombotic thrombocytopenic purpura. The principal renal pathology is of 'mucinous' subendothelial thickening of the small muscular arteries producing changes which resemble those of scleroderma. The condition may remit after bilateral nephrectomy but spontaneous recovery has also been reported occasionally. No definitive treatment for this condition has been established.

Chronic renal failure. Women in chronic renal failure are usually amenorrhoeic and infertile so that pregnancy is not likely to complicate their condition. However, there are a few cases of successful pregnancy in patients dependent on maintenance haemodialysis. Nearly all the infants have survived but most have weighed less than

2000 g, indicating a high incidence of prematurity and fetal growth retardation.

The situation is transformed by successful renal transplantation. Ovulation and menstruation are restored in about six months. The experience of more than 200 pregnancies following renal transplantation has been reported. Most of those which have progressed to viability have ended successfully in that a normal and surviving infant has been delivered.

It is not known if pregnancy alters the natural history of the transplanted kidney. A decline in transplant function is relatively common during or after pregnancy, affecting 10–20 per cent of women with renal allografts. About one-third of the episodes of deterioration occur in the puerperium. In the majority of instances, the loss of function has been small, but in some it has been total. The incidence of pre-eclampsia is high (25 per cent), and this may contribute to reversible impairment of function. Urinary tract infections are common (20 per cent) despite the careful supervision that these patients receive. The transplanted kidney is not at risk of damage by vaginal delivery.

The use of immunosuppressive therapy during pregnancy is discussed more fully on page 11.15. One-quarter of mothers with renal transplants will also need hypotensive agents. The incidence of congenital abnormalities has not been strikingly increased, but there may be problems relating to immunosuppression of the baby at delivery, including lymphopenia, adrenocortical insufficiency, cytomegalovirus, or bacterial infection. Nearly half the infants are born prematurely, which further complicates the neonatal period.

Glomerulonephritis. Acute post-streptococcal glomerulonephritis is extremely rare in pregnancy, whereas the group of disorders encompassed by chronic glomerulonephritis occurs more commonly. Systemic lupus erythematosus is discussed separately on page 11.14. In most women pregnancy seems to have no effect on the natural history of chronic glomerular disease. In some, there is a coincidental worsening of the disorder, but it is impossible to tell whether or not it was caused by, rather than just associated with, pregnancy.

Even if there is renal impairment, the outcome of the pregnancy should be good, provided the non-pregnant blood pressure is normal. However, if there is pre-existing hypertension, then a high incidence of superimposed pre-eclampsia (30–50 per cent) with its associated effects on perinatal survival can be expected. Furthermore, the superimposition of pre-eclampsia will cause further impairment of renal function and can itself precipitate permanent renal damage by cortical necrosis. Thus, two clinical features determine the advisability of pregnancy in patients with chronic glomerulonephritis: concurrent hypertension and, where available, the previous obstetric history.

Patients with previously undiagnosed chronic glomerular disease may present with proteinuric hypertension in pregnancy, and the differential diagnosis from pre-eclampsia is extremely difficult. The only certain discriminant is provided by renal biopsy. This presents no additional hazards to the gravid patient, provided her blood pressure is controlled and her coagulation status is known to be normal. However, it should only very rarely be an antepartum procedure, because the best test for pre-eclampsia is to observe what happens after delivery. Only if the proteinuria persists, for example, at six weeks after delivery should renal biopsy be considered.

Nephrotic syndrome. The commonest cause of heavy proteinuria in late pregnancy is pre-eclampsia. More rarely it will result from a glomerulonephritis, lupus nephropathy, or diabetic nephropathy. Causes such as renal vein thrombosis or amyloidosis are extremely rare. Certain women may present with heavy proteinuria which remits at the end of pregnancy, only to recur cyclically with further pregnancies. The nature of this disorder has not been elucidated. In the absence of hypertension, the pregnancy is not likely to be complicated.

Other renal problems. In general, the pregnancy is likely to be complicated by superimposed pre-eclampsia if there is pre-existing hypertension. Otherwise few problems need to be anticipated. Women with chronic interstitial nephritis ('chronic pyelonephritis') are particularly prone to acute renal tract infection. Women with polycystic renal disease need genetic counselling so that they understand the chances of their children inheriting this autosomal dominant disorder. Women with single kidneys tolerate pregnancy well, provided the remaining kidney is not scarred nor has poor function for other reasons. Congenital abnormalities of the renal tract are associated with uterine abnormalities which can affect fertility and the success of gestation. Urolithiasis, being more a disease of men, is not commonly a complication of pregnancy. However, both renal colic and acute obstruction due to a calculus can occur in gravid women, and must be managed as in other circumstances.

References

Lindheimer, M. D. and Katz, A. L. (1977). *Kidney function and disease in pregnancy*. Lea and Febiger, Philadelphia.
Katz, A. L., Davidson, J. M., Hayslett, J. P., Singson, E., and Lindheimer, M. D. (1980). Pregnancy in women with kidney disease. *Kidney Int.* **18**, 192.

HEART DISEASE IN PREGNANCY

C. W. G. Redman and P. Sleight

Introduction. During the first trimester, cardiac output increases to about 40 per cent above non-pregnant levels and thereafter during the second and third trimesters there is little further change. During the third trimester there may be transient falls in the venous return and cardiac output which result from pressure on the inferior vena cava by the gravid uterus in the supine position. The majority of pregnant women develop a loud third sound and a minority a soft fourth sound. Almost all have a soft ejection systolic murmur best heard at the left sternal edge. About half of these seem to originate in the pulmonary artery and the remainder are left-sided in origin. The change in heart position causes a leftward deviation in the axis of the electrocardiogram associated with a flattening or inversion of the T wave in lead III. The heart size on X-ray increases by about 10 per cent. These normal changes may sometimes lead to a false diagnosis of organic heart disease and thus cause unnecessary anxiety.

Pregnancy may predispose to additional morbidity and mortality in women with heart disease in four ways. First, it imposes additional burdens on the heart antenatally. Secondly, during labour and delivery, the cardiovascular system has to adapt rapidly to the effects of the 'bearing down' or Valsalva manoeuvres of the second stage, to the sudden extinction of the uteroplacental circulation in the third stage, to blood loss, and to the haemodynamic changes of regional and general anaesthesia. Thirdly, the clotting system changes to increase the risk of thrombo-embolic complications of cardiac disorders. Fourthly, sepsis is an obstetric hazard, particularly at delivery, and exposes susceptible individuals to the risk of infective endocarditis.

In England and Wales just under 10 per cent of all maternal deaths are caused by heart disease comprising nearly equal proportions of congenital heart disease, rheumatic valvular disease, infective endocarditis, coronary artery disease, and 'other' problems. Overall, the death rate has dropped more than threefold since 1960.

Amongst women who become pregnant with known heart disease, the lower the initial cardiac reserve, the more likely there are to be complications. At the most extreme, a patient with cardiac decompensation at rest is unlikely to survive pregnancy. On the other hand, absence of symptoms is no guarantee of absence of complications. For example, a woman with symptom-free mitral stenosis before pregnancy may suddenly develop life-threatening pulmonary oedema during pregnancy. In other patients, the cardiovascular demands of pregnancy may suddenly reveal, for the first time, previously undiagnosed cardiac disorders.

Finally, the pregnancy itself may produce new circulatory disease. The most obvious example is pre-eclamptic toxaemia. Peripartum cardiomyopathy is less clearly defined.

Rheumatic heart disease. Acute rheumatic carditis is now very rare in technically advanced countries but previously was a grave complication of pregnancy with a high maternal mortality. Chronic rheumatic heart disease now complicates less than 1 per cent of all pregnancies in the United Kingdom and over the last 40 years has comprised a diminishing proportion of all cardiac disease in pregnancy (now about two-thirds of the total). Mitral stenosis is the commonest lesion encountered. The complications of rheumatic heart disease in pregnancy are, in order of their importance, pulmonary oedema, heart failure, atrial fibrillation, and thrombo-embolism—either systemic or pulmonary. Heart failure can occur at any stage but most commonly during the third trimester. It is particularly precipitated by atrial tachycardia, flutter or fibrillation. Chest infection and pre-eclampsia are other predisposing factors. Its treatment is the same as in the non-pregnant individual. The aim of medical supervision is, by the appropriate use of digoxin and diuretics, to pre-empt the life-threatening emergency of acute pulmonary oedema.

The onset of atrial fibrillation in pregnancy is often a medical emergency with a high risk of heart failure and thrombo-embolism. The risks are less if atrial fibrillation presents and is controlled before pregnancy begins. Electroconversion to sinus rhythm is safe in pregnancy and may be used for the management of the atrial disorders of rhythm. Systemic and pulmonary thrombo-embolism complicates about 1.5 per cent of all pregnancies in patients with rheumatic heart disease, increasing to 25 per cent if there is an acute episode of atrial fibrillation. Anticoagulant therapy may be necessary and presents special hazards in pregnancy (see below).

Infective endocarditis is a rare but well recognized hazard of labour. Antibiotic prophylaxis is usually used to cover delivery in women with susceptible lesions, although the effectiveness of this prophylaxis has never been proven; various combinations of bactericidal agents have been recommended, but usually a broad spectrum antibiotic is used to cover the Gram-negative organisms of the genital tract.

Cardiac surgery and pregnancy. Closed mitral valvotomy has been carried out at all stages of pregnancy for mitral stenosis sufficiently severe to cause acute pulmonary oedema or uncontrolled haemoptysis. The maternal mortality of the procedure is about 1.5 per cent and the fetal mortality 5–10 per cent. Open heart procedures seem to carry the same operative risks for pregnant women as for non-pregnant patients. However, as many as one in three fetuses die, probably as a result of the cardio-pulmonary bypass procedures. Previous mitral valvotomy is not in itself a contra-indication to pregnancy but does not preclude the possibility of pregnancy-induced pulmonary oedema.

Valve prosthesis. Successful pregnancies have been reported in women with single, double, and triple valve prostheses. However, fetal wastage is high, particularly if oral anticoagulants have to be used (see below). With non-biological valves the risk of thrombosis in the valve when anticoagulants are reversed during labour poses a major hazard for the mother, which should be clearly understood. In this respect, there are particular advantages for young women who have valvular homografts rather than prosthetic valves.

Congenital heart disease. The decline in the incidence of rheumatic heart disease means that congenital heart lesions form an increasing proportion (between one-quarter and one-third) of all forms of cardiovascular disorder in pregnancy. The risks both for mother and fetus are increased if there is a right to left shunt. The highest risk group is among those in whom the shunt is associated with severe pulmonary hypertension—Eisenmenger's syndrome (see Section 13). Between 1961 and 1975, Eisenmenger's syndrome constituted the major cause of maternal death from congenital heart disease in England and Wales. Death particularly occurs during labour or with sudden circulatory collapse in the immediate puerperium. Blood loss or coincident pre-eclampsia seem to be predisposing factors.

There is no consensus about the management of this rare condition in pregnancy. Early delivery to pre-empt progressive pre-eclampsia, obsessive management of blood loss, and postpartum anticoagulation to prevent pulmonary thrombo-emboli are advocated. Sudden increases in right to left shunting are managed by increasing systemic arterial resistance by giving phenylephrine, methoxamine, or noradrenaline.

There is a similarly high maternal mortality with the rarer condition of primary pulmonary hypertension. It is clear that a high pulmonary arterial resistance predisposes to severe maternal problems in pregnancy.

A high fetal loss, and an increased incidence of prematurity or growth retardation, are complications of maternal cyanosis of all causes. Thus, the outlook with corrected Fallot's tetralogy is much better than with the untreated condition, which is associated with losses of up to one-third of all fetuses.

Patients with acyanotic heart disease usually tolerate pregnancy well. The commonest lesion encountered is atrial septal defect. If not corrected this may predispose to heart failure and disorders of rhythm arising in the atria. Uncorrected coarctation of the aorta in pregnancy is associated with an increased risk of aortic rupture or dissection as well as bacterial infection of the lesion itself. After correction, uncomplicated pregnancies are the rule. Mild to moderate aortic stenosis causes no problems during gestation. If severe, episodes of left ventricular failure or syncope may develop. Infective endocarditis is the other major complication.

Cardiomyopathy in pregnancy (See also Section 13.)
Hypertrophic obstructive cardiomyopathy (HOCM). Women with this inherited condition tolerate pregnancy well. Beta-adrenergic antagonists may need to be administered throughout pregnancy as part of medical management. This is compatible with a normal outcome, and to date no teratogenic effects have been recorded. The possibility that beta-adrenergic blockade may adversely affect the neonate is still disputed and has been raised in relation to the treatment of hypertensive pregnancies where the condition itself can cause fetal and neonatal compromise (see page 11.9). If there is a fetal disadvantage in the use of beta-adrenergic antagonists, it is a relative one. Patients with HOCM may be allowed a vaginal delivery and ergometrine is not contra-indicated. Factors which increase left ventricular outflow gradients should be avoided. These include vasodilatation from epidural anaesthesia, hypotension caused by blood loss and the physical effort of the second stage of labour.

Peripartum cardiomyopathy. This is a syndrome of unexplained heart failure and cardiomegaly occurring at the end of pregnancy and in the puerperium. It has usually been reported in women of African origin. It is very rare in the United Kingdom but in central Nigeria is one of the commonest medical problems amongst female patients. It responds rapidly to conventional management with digoxin and diuretics but is frequently recurrent in further pregnancies. Persistent cardiomegaly or associated hypertension are associated with a shortened life expectancy. It seems likely that pregnancy is the final extra load in a heart already burdened with other adverse factors such as hypertension, anaemia, malnutrition, and perhaps some toxic factor.

Myocardial infarction. This is rare, complicating about 0.01 per cent of pregnancies, but carrying a high maternal mortality of around 25 per cent. Women who have had previous cardiac infarction or known myocardial ischaemia should probably not embark upon a pregnancy although there are no data to give an exact estimate of the risks involved.

Paradoxical embolism. The increased risk of deep vein thrombosis in pregnancy may, in association with an atrial septal defect, give rise to a systemic embolus, particularly after Valsalva-like manoeuvres in labour.

Labour and delivery in the cardiac patient. Caesarean section should be performed for obstetric reasons only. The physical effort of labour should be reduced to a minimum by adequate pain relief and assisted delivery in the second stage. Epidural analgesia may be appropriate where a fall in systemic resistance is not likely to create problems as with Eisenmenger's syndrome. Blood loss should be minimized and promptly but carefully replaced. Prophylactic antibiotics should be used where the lesion places the patient at risk for infective endocarditis.

Advice about pregnancy to patients with heart disease. If a woman with heart disease is relatively free of symptoms, is able to exercise without undue dyspnoea, and does not have orthopnoea, she will usually be able to tolerate pregnancy and labour well. Advice about the number of pregnancies and their timing should be based on the following considerations.

1. The long-term prognosis of the heart disease is probably the biggest single factor. Rheumatic heart disease is usually progressive so it is better to advise limitation in numbers of children and to have them early in life.

2. The need to cope with other small children imposes a major physical strain on a pregnant woman.

3. With valvular heart disease it is better to have children before the necessity for prosthetic valve replacement arises, with anticoagulant complications. It should be borne in mind that valve replacement in non-pregnant patients carries a mortality risk of 1–10 per cent.

Drugs for heart disease in pregnancy

Digoxin. Digoxin crosses the placenta and maternal and umbilical venous blood concentrations are similar. Women taking digoxin in late pregnancy have blood concentrations which are reduced to about half of their non-pregnant levels whilst remaining on the same drug regimen. This implies increased clearance of the drug by mechanisms which remain undefined. However, it should not be necessary to alter treatment schedules during pregnancy. Digoxin is not known to be teratogenic and seems to be well tolerated by the fetus although one case of transplacental digitalis intoxication has been reported.

Diuretics. There are some relative disadvantages in the widespread use of diuretics for the treatment of pre-eclampsia (see page 11.8). These do not form an absolute contra-indication to their administration in pregnancy. Where there is a clear indication for their use, such as cardiac failure, ordinary medical regimens using 'loop' diuretics or the thiazide preparations can be administered without any special restriction. All the side-effects that occur in non-obstetric patients can be anticipated. Major fetal side-effects have not been reported. The thiazide diuretics are not known to be teratogenic.

Anticoagulants. Of the coumarin derivatives, warfarin has been used most commonly in pregnancy. Its administration is associated with potentially major maternal and fetal side-effects. Haemorrhage is the single most significant maternal factor particularly during the delivery period. The fetal problems are all derived from the transplacental passage of warfarin. Exposure between the sixth and ninth weeks of gestation leads to a characteristic syndrome of nasal hypoplasia and abnormal calcification of the epiphyses which is radiologically evident as 'stippling'. This so-called warfarin embryopathy is frequently associated with further abnormalities of

the central nervous system which can cause mental retardation and blindness. They include congenital abnormalities of the cerebral structures and lesions which have been attributed to cerebral haemorrhage. There is no specific time of pregnancy when warfarin therapy is particularly associated with this problem, which can be more debilitating than that of warfarin embryopathy itself. Intrauterine fetal haemorrhage has also been the cause of death, contributing to a high overall rate of fetal loss from both spontaneous abortion and stillbirths.

Heparin has the advantage that it does not cross the placenta. Like warfarin, its use in pregnancy can predispose to maternal bleeding. It has been given during pregnancy for prolonged periods of time both prophylactically in low doses and therapeutically, by the subcutaneous or intravenous routes. A high perinatal mortality has also been a feature of the reported cases of heparin use. Whether this reflects the treatment, or the conditions for which the treatment is used, is not clear. Apart from haemorrhage and the discomfort of administration, there are other problems. Osteoporosis is rare, but potentially serious, in that it has been associated (in one case) with vertebral crush fractures.

There is no ideal anticoagulant in pregnancy. What is used must depend on individual assessment of the patient and her problems. The fact that heparin does not cross the placenta is an advantage in the first trimester and the peripartum period. Warfarin needs to be used with caution. It is probably appropriate to restrict its use to the second trimester and the first half of the third trimester. To avoid neonatal haemorrhage it should be replaced by heparin well before delivery.

Breast-feeding. Except in the case of premature infants the amount of warfarin which is excreted in the milk is insufficient to cause any alteration in the infant's prothrombin time.

Sterilization. This is not advisable in the puerperium because of the special risks of thrombo-embolism.

Conclusion. We are now much less cautious about the risks of pregnancy in women with heart disease, but advice is necessary with regard to the timing and number of pregnancies. It is particularly important not to induce a cardiac neurosis in patients with physiological murmurs caused by the hyperkinetic circulation in pregnancy.

References

Szekely, P. and Snaith, L. (1974). In *Heart disease and pregnancy*. Churchill Livingstone, London.

Gleicher, N., Midwall, J., Hochberger, D., and Jaffin, H. (1979). Eisenmenger's Syndrome and Pregnancy. *Obstet. Gynaec. Surv.* **34**, 721.

THYROID DISEASE IN PREGNANCY

C. W. G. Redman

Normal changes. During normal human pregnancy renal clearance of iodide increases and plasma iodide falls. Thyroidal clearance of circulating iodide shows a compensatory increase to maintain absolute levels of iodide uptake. The resulting increase in thyroid activity may be reflected by visible enlargement of the thyroid gland particularly when dietary intake of iodide is low. The increasing levels of placental oestrogen stimulate hepatic synthesis of thyroxine binding globulin (TBG). In consequence the total concentrations of circulating thyroxine (T_4) and triiodothyronine (T_3) are increased to levels which would indicate hyperthyroidism in non-pregnant individuals. However, the levels of unbound, or free, T_4 and T_3 remain unchanged. The binding capacity of TBG remains unsaturated so that its measurement in pregnancy (for example by T_3 resin uptake) gives values which would indicate hypothyroidism in non-pregnant individuals. The free thyroxine index, which is calculated from the measurement of total circulating T_4 (bound and unbound) and T_3 resin uptake, therefore remains at the upper end of the normal range. The responsiveness of the thyroid to thyroid-stimulating hormone continues to be normal during pregnancy. It is thought that maternal T_3 and T_4 do not cross the placenta to a significant extent. Human chorionic gonadatrophin is structurally related to thyrotrophin (TSH) and has a weak stimulatory action on the thyroid. Normally this is of no consequence but when HCG is unusually high, as for example with hydatidiform mole or choriocarcinoma, maternal hyperthyroidism may ensue.

Maternal hyperthyroidism. This complicates about one in 500 pregnancies. It is usually associated with diffuse thyroidal enlargement (Graves' disease) rather than a toxic nodular goitre. Some of the clinical features of hyperthyroidism—small diffuse goitre, tachycardia, heat intolerance, and weight loss—may be either mimicked or masked by normal pregnancy. A high sleeping pulse, a fine tremor, persistent weight loss, eye signs (lid lag, proptosis) or pretibial myxoedema may all indicate the diagnosis. Frequently there is a positive family history of thyroid disease. Confirmation is sought by measurement of either the free thyroxine index or the circulating levels of free T_3 or T_4, which should be elevated.

The impact of untreated hyperthyroidism on the outcome of pregnancy has to be assessed from older reports which indicate a high perinatal mortality and possibly an increased incidence of toxaemia. The treated condition is associated with a tendency for smaller and lighter babies and a perinatal mortality which may be slightly above average. Current or previous maternal Graves' disease is the principal cause of neonatal thyrotoxicosis which results from placental transmission of the maternal immunoglobulins—long-acting thyroid stimulator (LATS) or LATS-protector (LATS-P). The neonatal condition, being passively acquired, is self-limiting after delivery. The other auto-antibodies associated with Graves' disease are thought to be secondary signs of the disorder and are not known to affect the fetus or neonate adversely. Pregnancy may induce temporary remission of Graves' disease, and exacerbations may occur in the puerperium.

Pregnancy is not the ideal time to embark upon surgical treatment of thyrotoxicosis. On the other hand there is no evidence that subtotal thyroidectomy in pregnancy is any more difficult or less successful than at any other time. Conventionally medical treatment is preferred using the thiourea drugs carbimazole or propylthiouracil. Both readily cross the placenta and inhibit fetal thyroid iodination of tyrosine. In consequence neonatal hypothyroidism is likely and about 10 per cent of fetuses exposed to treatment will be born with a goitre resulting from increased fetal TSH. In certain circumstances this fetal action of the drugs may be desirable, notably when fetal and neonatal thyrotoxicosis occur. This is predictable from a knowledge of maternal LATS and LATS-P levels. In certain cases fetal thyrotoxicosis may be provisionally diagnosed *in utero* if there is persistent fetal tachycardia. More commonly this complication is neither anticipated nor diagnosed and maternal treatment must be adjusted to minimize fetal side-effects. In the past it has been claimed that antithyroid treatment combined with supplementary thyroxine achieves this objective. Now that it is known that maternally administered thyroxine does not enter the fetal compartment to any significant extent, this approach seems unnecessary. Rather, the aim should be simply to reduce maternal treatment to a minimum.

Mild hyperthyroidism is well tolerated in pregnancy; but the risks of undertreating thyrotoxicosis must be borne in mind, in particular that pregnancy does not preclude the possibility of a thyrotoxic crisis. Given this approach, mild and transient hypothyroidism will occur in most neonates. The present evidence is that this is unlikely to have long-term effects on growth and development. Thiourea drugs are secreted in breast milk so breast-feeding is not recommended. Investigation or treatment of hyperthyroidism in pregnancy with radio-isotopes is contra-indicated.

Maternal hypothyroidism. Severe hypothyroidism impairs ovulation and hence pregnancy rarely complicates this condition. However, patients with normal full-term pregnancies have been reported. Mild hypothyroidism in pregnancy may frequently not be recognized. The diagnosis may be suggested by a history of cold intolerance and tiredness, a puffy face, slow pulse, and delayed relaxation of the ankle jerks. A low free thyroxine index or free T_4 will give confirmation. Frequently thyroglobulin or thyroid microsomal auto-antibodies will be present. The treatment should be straightforward. Replacement therapy does not have to be modified because of pregnancy and its adequacy can be monitored by the patient's well-being and free thyroxine index. Women who are already on thyroxine when they become pregnant present few problems. It is unlikely that their therapy will need to be changed with advancing pregnancy.

Postpartum thyroiditis. This presents in the first six months after delivery with the development of a painless goitre and symptoms and signs of hypothyroidism or, more rarely, hyperthyroidism. The patient may already have a history of thyroid disease but more commonly does not. Very high titres of thyroglobulin and thyroid microsomal auto-antibodies are observed. When the goitre has been biopsied lymphocytic thyroiditis has been confirmed. Frequently the episode is transient and only a relatively short period of treatment is required. The condition is thought to appear in the postpartum period as a consequence of the release of the maternal immunoregulatory mechanisms from the suppressive influences of pregnancy.

Thyroid carcinoma. Pregnancy seems to have no adverse effects on current or previously treated carcinoma of the thyroid. Conversely the tumour does not affect the outcome of pregnancy. Treatment needs to be modified only in so far as radioactive iodine cannot be used.

References

Burrow, G. N. (1975). Thyroid diseases. In *Medical complications during pregnancy* (eds. G. N. Burrow and T. F. Ferris), 196. W. B. Saunders, Philadelphia.

Ramsay, I. D. (1980). The thyroid gland. In *Clinical physiology in obstetrics* (eds. F. Hitton and G. Chamberlain), 400. Blackwell Scientific Publications, Oxford.

SYSTEMIC LUPUS ERYTHEMATOSUS AND RELATED DISORDERS IN PREGNANCY

C. W. G. Redman

Systemic lupus erythematosus (SLE) and rheumatoid arthritis are the most common of the collagen diseases to present in pregnancy. Polyarteritis nodosa, scleroderma, dermatomyositis, and Wegener's granulomatosis are all very much rarer and most clinicians will see at most one or two cases complicating pregnancy in a lifetime.

Systemic lupus erythematosus mainly affects women and its peak incidence is during the child-bearing years. It may, therefore, not uncommonly complicate pregnancy. Whether or not pregnancy has any effect on the severity of the disease is disputed. Exacerbations affect about 10 per cent of women who, at the start of pregnancy, are in remission compared to about 50 per cent of women who enter pregnancy with active disease. Older reports emphasized the likelihood of relapses either in the first half of pregnancy or in the puerperium. When maternal deaths have been described, they have tended to occur after, rather than during, pregnancy.

Patients with SLE, amongst other problems, may have renal impairment, the nephrotic syndrome, and/or hypertension. Thus, if the disease starts during pregnancy, it may be easily confused with pre-eclampsia. Furthermore, during the third trimester, pre-eclampsia can be superimposed on SLE so that the differential diagnosis may be difficult. Pre-eclampsia does not cause the skin, joint, or pleuritic symptoms of SLE. It is not associated with signs of active glomerular disease, i.e. granular and red cell casts in the urinary sediment. SLE will not remit at the end of pregnancy, whereas pre-eclampsia will. Raised levels of antinuclear factor (ANF) or DNA binding antibody confirm the diagnosis of SLE or a closely related collagen disorder. These investigations should always be done in women presenting with features ascribable to severe or atypical pre-eclampsia to elucidate the differential diagnosis.

There is no question that SLE adversely affects the outcome of pregnancy. Spontaneous abortions, premature labour, and perinatal deaths all occur more commonly than expected. The likelihood of these complications is increased if the disease is active at the start of pregnancy or there is a relapse during pregnancy. Recurrent spontaneous abortions are particularly associated with the presence of the lupus anticoagulant which prolongs the partial thromboplastin and kaolin–cephalin clotting times. The outcome of pregnancy is not adversely affected further if there is an associated nephrotic syndrome, but is compromised if there is renal impairment (plasma creatinine greater than 150 μmol/l).

Neonatal SLE is a rare complication of maternal SLE presumably caused by the transplacental passage of maternal IgG autoantibodies. The baby manifests three categories of problem. First, there are cardiac disorders particularly heart block. Secondly, there may be haematological complications which include auto-immune haemolysis or thrombocytopenia. Finally, classical discoid skin lesions may occur. Some of these problems may impair perinatal survival, for example heart block may lead to heart failure and fetal hydrops. The problems result from passively acquired antibodies. They are naturally self-limited. However, the presence of ANF in cord blood does not correlate with the signs of neonatal auto-immune disease. Occasionally neonatal disorders of this sort may be the first indication of a previously unsuspected maternal problem.

Patients with active SLE should therefore be advised to defer pregnancy until in remission. The management during pregnancy depends, as in other circumstances, on the use of immunosuppressive drugs, the problems of which are discussed below. The postpartum period is a time when dangerous exacerbations have been reported, so close clinical supervision should continue after delivery.

Polyarteritis nodosa. Very few cases have been described in pregnancy. The majority have resulted in maternal death after delivery. The condition may easily be confused with pre-eclampsia/eclampsia in that it may present with hypertension, proteinuria, and convulsions. However, it does not remit after delivery. The diagnosis may be further confirmed by biopsy demonstration of the arterial lesion. The fetus seems not to be adversely affected by the disease process, which is a further difference from pre-eclampsia or eclampsia.

Systemic scleroderma. The association of pregnancy and scleroderma is rare. If there is renal involvement, the outcomes of the pregnancies have been poor, with a high incidence of spontaneous abortion, stillbirth, and pre-term delivery. The maternal presentation has mimicked both pre-eclampsia and eclampsia and maternal mortality has been high. Pregnancy is less hazardous in women without renal involvement and the course of the disease is unaffected by concurrent pregnancy. There is no evidence of transmission of auto-immune problems to the fetus. Patients with active systemic sclerosis with renal involvement should be advised against pregnancy.

Wegener's granulomatosis. This condition affects an older age group. There is only one case report of its occurrence in pregnancy. There was apparently no renal involvement and the pregnancy was uncomplicated. Prognosis in pregnancy probably depends most on renal function and arterial pressure.

Dermatomyositis. Of the small number of cases reported, the majority were unaffected by pregnancy. However, nearly half the women had no surviving child so the fetal mortality was exceptionally high.

Rheumatoid arthritis. During pregnancy, symptoms of rheumatoid arthritis characteristically ameliorate although exacerbation or even onset of the disease can occur more rarely. However, relapses are common within the first six months after delivery. If the disease begins during pregnancy, it is important that it is distinguished from rheumatic fever, which has a grave prognosis in the gravid women if there is active carditis.

There is no evidence that the disease itself adversely affects the growth and development of the fetus, although the drugs used for treatment may do so (see below). Rheumatoid factor is an IgM and is therefore not transmitted by the placenta to the fetus.

Severe joint disease may complicate the delivery process if it involves the hips, with impairment of abduction or flexion. Involvement of the cervical spine may impede hyper-extension of the neck, and thus make administration of a general anaesthetic more difficult or more dangerous.

Drugs used for the treatment of the collagen diseases. Chloroquine, corticosteroids, azathioprine, soluble gold salts, and prostaglandin synthetase inhibitors may all be administered for the treatment of the auto-immune connective tissue disorders which coincide with pregnancy.

Chloroquine should not be used in gravid women because it is concentrated in the fetal uveal tract and may cause retinal damage. There is also evidence that it may cause chromosomal damage. Large doses of corticosteroids may cause cleft palates in both experimental animals and humans. However, congenital abnormalities are not prominent if administration is limited to conventional therapeutic doses. If corticosteroids are given throughout pregnancy, fetal growth may be retarded, which may be an effect analogous to the stunting of growth in corticosteroid-treated children. Fetal adrenal cortical activity may be suppressed, which manifests itself as reduced maternal urinary oestriol excretion antenatally and adrenal cortical insufficiency in the neonatal period. The latter complication is, however, rare. Although it is orthodox advice that a mother on corticosteroids should not breast feed, the only study available indicates slow excretion of prednisolone into breast milk at low concentrations.

Azathioprine is teratogenic if given to mice early in pregnancy, being associated with a high incidence of skeletal and central nervous system malformations. However, with normal therapeutic regimens the incidence of malformations in babies of treated women is not markedly increased. Azathioprine may cause neonatal leucopenia and thereby an increased susceptibility to infection. The long-term consequences of intra-uterine exposure to this drug have not yet been defined. Breast feeding is inadvisable in treated patients, mainly because there is no information about how much azathioprine is secreted into breast milk. Soluble gold salts, used for the treatment of rheumatoid arthritis, have been administered rarely to pregnant women. Because of their high toxicity this cannot be considered advisable. Small quantities are transmitted in breast milk and may cause neonatal rashes.

Prostaglandin synthetase inhibitors (e.g. aspirin or indomethacin) used for the treatment of joint pain may prolong pregnancy by inhibiting the onset of labour. Aspirin given in large doses to animals may be teratogenic, but this has not been observed in human pregnancy. Aspirin may also inhibit platelet function and haemorrhagic problems have been reported in neonates exposed to the drug *in utero*. Indomethacin is used in neonatal medicine to stimulate closure of a patent ductus arteriosus. There is evidence that fetuses exposed to this drug or mefenamic acid may undergo premature closure of the ductus arteriosus *in utero* and develop pulmonary hypertension in consequence. For these reasons, these drugs should be used sparingly in pregnancy.

References

Gifford, R. H. (1975). Rheumatic diseases. In *Medical complications during pregnancy* (eds. G. M. Burrow and T. F. Ferris), 773. W. B. Saunders, Philadelphia.

Hayslett, J. P. and Lynn, R. I. (1980). Effects of pregnancy in patients with lupus nephropathy. *Kidney Int.* **18**, 207.

DIABETES IN PREGNANCY

C. W. G. Redman and T. D. R. Hockaday

In this section, we will consider the metabolic changes in normal pregnancy; the management and outcome of pregnancy in insulin-dependent and type II diabetic women; and the problems of chemical diabetes during gestation. The term 'chemical diabetes' will be used to mean asymptomatic changes in carbohydrate metabolism detectable and defined by glucose tolerance tests. The term 'gestational diabetes' will be used to mean either symptomatic or chemical diabetes induced by pregnancy but resolving at the end of pregnancy.

Metabolic changes in normal pregnancy. The disposition of every major class of nutrient is altered in normal late gestation, reflecting the way in which maternal metabolism adapts to meet the energy needs of the rapidly growing conceptus. The circulating levels of glucose and amino- acids decline, whereas free acids, ketones, triglycerides, and lipoproteins all increase. In particular there is an accelerated maternal response to food deprivation. Thus, after a brief overnight fast, a pregnant woman will demonstrate raised plasma ketones and free fatty acids at levels which are characteristic of prolonged starvation in non-pregnant individuals. This tendency has been called 'acceleration starvation'. It is thought that these responses are needed to 'spare' circulating maternal glucose for the demands of the fetus.

A well-grown term baby *in utero* may drain as much as 25–30 g of glucose per day from its mother. The removal of maternal glucose by the placenta probably accounts, at least in part, for the small but progressive decline in maternal plasma glucose which reaches a nadir at about 36 weeks gestation. Early in pregnancy plasma insulin decreases in line with the changes in plasma glucose. The second half of pregnancy is marked by a progressive development of peripheral insulin resistance leading to raised plasma insulin levels despite normal carbohydrate tolerance. Responses to all known insulogenic stimuli are also markedly exaggerated. The peripheral resistance to insulin disappears suddenly at delivery. It may in part be caused by utilization of insulin in the placenta which is not only rich in insulin receptors but has insulinase activity. But the greater part of the insulin resistance of pregnancy is thought to depend on hormones secreted by the placenta of which the most important is human placental lactogen (HPL).

Human placental lactogen is a polypeptide hormone comprising 191 amino acids with a similar but not identical structure to human growth hormone and human prolactin. HPL is a major placental product accounting for 10 per cent of all placental protein production at term. The rise of HPL in the maternal circulation begins at the fifth week after the last menstrual period and reaches a plateau at 34 to 36 weeks of pregnancy when on average its concentration is about 5–6 μg/ml. The concentration in the fetal circulation is about 100 times less. HPL is thought to induce some of the metabolic changes characteristic of pregnancy including the tendency to lipolysis and the reduced sensitivity to insulin. However, successful pregnancies have been reported where the placenta is apparently producing almost undetectable amounts of HPL; its possible role in the maintenance of normal pregnancy is therefore not clear.

The other main hormones elaborated by the placenta are oestrogens and progesterone. Oestrogens are thought to cause pancreatic islet cell hyperplasia and in combination with progesterone to promote an exaggerated insulin response to standard stimuli. Oestrogen and progesterone combinations also stimulate hypertriglyceridaemia and an augmented tendency to ketosis.

Glycosuria. Between 10 and 90 per cent of gravid women can be shown to have glycosuria depending on the frequency of testing and the timing of urine samples in relation to food intake. This is because glucose excretion in the urine increases about fivefold in pregnancy, on average to 350 mg per day. This tendency to glycosuria is already apparent in the first trimester. Typically the same pregnant individual excretes very variable quantities of glucose from day to day. Glycosuria develops because renal absorption of filtered glucose is less effective than in the non-pregnant state. It is even less effective in gravid women who have marked glycosuria but this group also has a reduced capacity for reabsorption even when they are not pregnant. These observations on renal handling of glucose do not explain the characteristic intermittency of gestational glycosuria, the reason for which remains obscure.

Transport of nutrients to the fetus. Neither maternal nor fetal insulin traverses the placenta so each individual has separate insulin compartments. Glucose crosses the placenta by a system of facilitated diffusion which is stereospecific with more rapid transport of D-glucose than L-glucose and of glucose than of other hexoses. Changes in fetal blood glucose lag about 10 minutes behind maternal changes. The transfer system becomes saturated when maternal levels reach about 15 mmol/l. Fetal blood glucose has to be lower than maternal levels to maintain this system of diffusion. Part of the gradient is accounted for by the metabolism of glucose by the placenta.

Amino acids are transferred by an active process. For every amino acid, fetal plasma levels are higher than maternal. Lipid traffic across the placenta is restricted to the transfer of maternal free fatty acids at a rate determined by maternal plasma levels. The fatty acid profiles of umbilical and maternal plasma are similar and there is no evidence for selective transfer of particular fatty acids. Ketones also freely diffuse from the maternal to the fetal compartments.

Fetal insulin. Insulin is present in the human pancreas from about the 11th week of fetal life and its concentration increases as development progresses. Plasma insulin can be detected from about the same stage of development but up to the end of the second trimester does not correlate with fetal body weight. Sensitivity of human fetal pancreatic beta cells to glucose stimuli develops during the first part of the third trimester. *In vitro* studies suggest that fetal insulin responsiveness to arginine or agents that increase intracellular concentrations of cAMP (glucagon, theophylline) is present at rather earlier stages of gestation. Even at term, the fetal insulin responses to changes in plasma glucose are relatively sluggish so that at all stages of pregnancy the main determinant of circulating fetal glucose is the circulating maternal glucose. This is an important factor when the fetal consequences of maternal diabetes are examined.

Human and experimental observations demonstrate that fetal insulin has a key role in promoting intra-uterine growth. Its absence is associated with abnormally small fetuses. Its presence in excess causes abnormally fast fetal growth, particularly affecting body fat and fetal organs such as the heart, liver, adrenals, spleen, and thymus. Brain weight, however, is not affected.

A mature human fetus has about 35 g of glycogen and more than 500 g of fat. Hepatic glycogen reserves are utilized very quickly after birth and thereafter energy is supplied by rapidly increased lipolysis until neonatal feeding is established.

Insulin-dependent diabetes in pregnancy. Pregnancy adversely affects diabetes and vice versa. The likelihood and magnitude of the problems increase with the severity of the diabetic state. Thus it is useful for clinical purposes, and essential for comparative studies, to have some method of grading the severity of the diabetes. The system devised by Dr Priscilla White (Table 1) has been widely adopted in the USA but is not used so much in the UK. Despite its drawbacks it does provide a simple identification of women most at risk, i.e. those with complicated diabetes, or diabetes of longstanding (particularly classes D, F, and R).

Table 1   Classification of diabetes in pregnant women

Class A Chemical diabetes
Class B Aged 20 years or more at onset
     and duration less than 10 years
     and no vascular or renal complications
Class C Aged 10–19 years at onset
     or duration 10–19 years
     and no vascular or renal complications
Class D Under 10 years at onset
     or duration of more than 20 years
     or calcification in leg arteries
     or hypertension
     or non-proliferative retinopathy
Class E Calcification of pelvic arteries
Class F Nephropathy
Class R Proliferative retinopathy

The true incidence of diabetes in pregnant populations is not known. Women with insulin dependent diabetes form a tiny fraction of the total (0.1–0.3 per cent). The incidence of chemical diabetes depends on both the definitions of the abnormality and the screening procedures used. An estimate of 0.5–1.0 per cent would fit the available data.

Effect of pregnancy on insulin-dependent diabetes. In patients with pre-existing diabetes the first few weeks of pregnancy are sometimes marked by reduced insulin requirements and hypoglycaemia. These have two causes. First, the physiological decline in maternal blood glucose begins at this time. Secondly, pregnancy-induced sickness and changes in appetite can reduce overall carbohydrate and calorie intake.

From about 16 weeks onwards peripheral insulin resistance develops gradually but progressively, as do the physiological changes promoting 'accelerated starvation'. It is not difficult to see how these demands of normal pregnancy specifically aggravate a condition characterized by a relative or absolute deficiency of insulin and a tendency to ketoacidosis. Between 16 and 36 weeks on average about two-thirds more insulin will be needed, but in some women insulin requirements will increase two- or threefold. The increased dietary requirements of pregnancy will need to be met and even short periods of food deprivation (for example with a mild intercurrent illness) may rapidly lead to ketosis and acidosis. At the same time, for reasons already discussed, urine testing for glucose ceases to be a reliable screen for hyperglycaemia. Thus diabetic women who are accustomed to regulating their condition according to the presence or absence of glycosuria have to reorientate themselves to control by direct measurement of blood glucose.

At the moment of delivery the insulin resistance induced by pregnancy is abruptly curtailed; a brief transitional period of enhanced insulin sensitivity is then followed by a rapid return to pre-pregnancy conditions.

Despite great improvements in management, the mortality of diabetic pregnant women is still about 10 times higher than average. The principal causes of death are metabolic factors (both ketoacidosis and severe hypoglycaemia) and infection. For this reason alone, the management of the diabetic gravida demands great care and attention to detail. There is, however, no evidence that pregnancy alters the long-term health of diabetic women. This is particularly important with respect to nephropathy and proliferative retinopathy. Both may progress in relation to gestation, but what information is available indicates that this is likely to be a temporary rather than a permanent deterioration.

Effect of insulin-dependent diabetes on the pregnancy. Diabetes has many adverse affects on the outcome of pregnancy. In general, the incidence of obstetric complications increases with the severity of the diabetes as listed in Table 1. The complications that may develop are summarized in Table 2.

Table 2   Obstetric complications of insulin-dependent diabetes

Polyhydramnios
Pre-eclampsia
Maternal infection

Fetal macrosomia
Intra-uterine death
Neonatal hypoglycaemia
Other neonatal factors
    Hypocalcaemia
    Hyperbilirubinaemia
    Polycythaemia
    Renal vein thrombosis
    Cardiomyopathy

Congenital malformations

Polyhydramnios. Polyhydramnios is a rare complication of pregnancy affecting about 0.5 per cent of all women. However, it occurs 40 to 50 times more commonly in diabetic women, so that about one quarter of all cases of polyhydramnios are associated with this condition. The likelihood of polyhydramnios is increased with complicated or poorly controlled diabetes. Conversely, if polyhydramnios is present the perinatal outcome is worse. In insulin-dependent diabetic women it presents typically at 32 to 36 weeks gestation; with chemical diabetes somewhat later at 37 to 40 weeks. It is not known why diabetes should predispose to polyhydramnios. The amniotic fluid itself has a slightly increased osmolality but normal glucose content. Where fetal urine output has been estimated, it has not been found to be increased. The management of this complication is its prevention by good diabetic control.

Pre-eclampsia. Vascular disease combined with renal disease is a major predisposing factor to the development of pre-eclampsia (see pages 11.6 and 11.10). It is therefore not surprising that women with complicated diabetes, particularly with renal involvement, have a two to threefold increase in susceptibility to pre-eclampsia. In contrast, uncomplicated diabetes enhances the risk of pre-eclampsia by negligible amounts.

Pre-eclampsia is associated with placental ischaemia and infarction, which in turn causes fetal compromise in terms of nourishment, and respiratory function. Thus, pre-eclampsia contributes significantly to the perinatal morbidity and mortality of diabetic pregnancies.

Infection. Both diabetes and pregnancy predispose to urinary tract infection. In some series the incidence has been high with as many as one in 20 diabetic pregnant women developing symptomatic pyelonephritis. Acute pyelonephritis has an adverse effect on pregnancy outcome (see pages 11.10 and 11.11). More recent experience is that, with adequate control and attentive management, the incidence of this complication can be greatly reduced.

Macrosomia. The maternal hyperglycaemia of diabetic pregnancies results in fetal hyperglycaemia, which in turn causes fetal hyperinsulinism when the fetal pancreatic beta cells become responsive to the higher circulating glucose at the start of the third trimester. The fetal islets of Langerhans become larger, more numerous, and richer in stored insulin.

This easily understood disturbance of the metabolic relationship between the diabetic mother and her fetus—of an excessive transplacental flux of glucose, and of a responding fetal hyperinsulinism—underlies much of the perinatal morbidity and mortality which is now to be summarized.

Fetal growth is stimulated by fetal insulin. At the same time the metabolic disturbances of poorly controlled maternal diabetes make available to the fetus, and increase the supply, not only of glucose but other nutrients such as ketones, free fatty acids, and amino acids. The final outcome is of overgrowth of the fetus caused by 'forced feeding'. Thus fetal gigantism or macrosomia is characteristic of the neonate born to a diabetic woman. Such infants have typical round, fat faces with sunken eyes, a short neck, a red skin and a lot of head hair. Although most of the excessive weight is due to fat, the babies are not only heavier but longer. These features only become apparent, however, if the baby is born after pancreatic beta cell responsiveness has begun to develop, that is after 28 weeks gestation. Not all babies of diabetic women are 'large for dates'. If pre-eclampsia supervenes, a second pathology impairing fetal growth by placental ischaemia begins to operate and may become dominant. Thus, typically, the babies of women with more complicated diabetes (classes D, F, and R) tend to show less macrosomia.

Two other causes of human fetal giganticism—nesidioblastosis and Beckwith–Wiedmann syndrome—are also characterized by hyperinsulinaemia, resulting from islet-cell pathology.

Perinatal mortality. At the Joslin Clinic (Boston, USA) records of the outcomes of diabetic pregnancies date from 1898. At that time perinatal mortality was 60 per cent in the very few pregnancies that were seen. For the first fifteen years after the introduction of insulin the perinatal mortality remained extremely high at slightly less than 50 per cent, but since 1938 it has progressively improved to its current level of less than 3 per cent.

Three phases in this sequence of gradual progress can be discerned. In earlier years the problem of sudden intra-uterine death in mature and well-grown fetuses was defined. In order to pre-empt this disaster clinical management changed in favour of preterm delivery, especially by Caesarean section. During the second phase neonatal death, particularly from hyaline membrane disease, a disorder of prematurity, became a major problem. Currently better timing of delivery has reduced the complications of prematurity so that a third problem has emerged, namely a high incidence of congenital malformations which are now the commonest cause of perinatal death.

The many factors that contribute to the high perinatal mortality of diabetic pregnancies demonstrate the complexity of the derangements to which the fetus is exposed.

Intra-uterine deaths. Typically these occur suddenly after 36–38 weeks in macrosomic but otherwise normal fetuses. The cause of death is not known but, because of the absence of gross placental pathology, it is thought to result from fetal metabolic problems caused by poor control of the maternal diabetes. One theory postulates that the fetus dies with a lactic acidosis which develops when the influx of maternal glucose exceeds the fetal capacity for its oxidative metabolism. This pathology can be demonstrated in animal models. An alternative is that inappropriate fetal hyperinsulinism causes fatal hypoglycaemia. However, the clinical evidence is that the fetus survives periods of maternal hypoglycaemia remarkably well. Both explanations imply the corollary that the risk of fetal death will be reduced by meticulous control of the maternal diabetes, a postulate that can explain the great improvement in perinatal outcome with modern management.

Intra-uterine death can also occur secondary to the placental pathology of pre-eclampsia. Unlike the 'metabolic' deaths discussed above, these problems are mirrored by easily detectable changes in the maternal condition (see page 11.7) and are not in any sense sudden or unpredictable.

In England and Wales the stillbirth rate of diabetic women is still about five times more than normal. The proportion of stillbirths ascribed to diabetes increases with birthweight so that as many as a quarter of stillborn infants weighing more than 4750g are born to diabetic gravidae.

Hyaline membrane disease. Hyaline membrane disease (HMD) affects premature neonates who cannot synthesize and release enough pulmonary surfactant, the phospholipids which are necessary to maintain alveolar aeration. Infants born to diabetic women seem to be about five times more susceptible to this complication than normal infants of the same gestational maturity. As many as one quarter of all infants of diabetic mothers have been affected in some series, and overall it has been a major cause of neonatal mortality and morbidity. The total size of the problem depends primarily on the pattern of preterm delivery, either spontaneous or induced. Elective preterm delivery has been practised so as to avoid the risk of intra-uterine death in the last few weeks of gestation. In consequence at least part of the high incidence of HMD has been iatrogenic. Furthermore the babies have been frequently delivered by Caesarean section, which itself augments the risks of developing HMD. Apart from these considerations hyperglycaemia and hyper-insulinaemia seem to impair lecithin synthesis in the fetal lung so that the greater risk of HMD might be offset by better maternal management. This possibility has not been tested in formal controlled trials but would explain some of the improvement in perinatal outcome in recent years. HMD can be anticipated by measuring the lecithin-sphingomyelin ratio (L/S ratio) in amniotic fluid. A ratio greater than two would normally indicate a low risk of HMD. Diabetic pregnancies have frequently been associated with an unacceptable number of false positive results. Whether this has resulted from technical problems in measuring the true L/S ratio or whether the synthesis of surfactant lecithin is deficient in some respect has not been determined. Many clinicians demand a ratio of 3 at which level even in diabetic pregnancies the incidence of HMD is low.

Neonatal hypoglycaemia. The insulin status of the human fetus can only be studied in umbilical blood samples at birth. Conventional measurements of plasma insulin are not possible because maternal antibodies to exogenous insulin cross the placenta and their presence in fetal blood interferes with the assay. However, appropriate measures of insulin C peptide demonstrate increased levels compatible with hyperinsulinism, and which correlate with infant size. At birth the transplacental supply of glucose ends abruptly and this, combined with the continuing hyperinsulinism, leads to an abnormal fall in the blood glucose. In addition the neonates of diabetic women seem to have impaired mechanisms for compensating for hypoglycaemia; in particular secretion of catecholamines and glucagon remains inappropriately low. Thus, although the infant has increased hepatic glycogen stores as well as quantities of fat he or she is unable to draw on these reserves.

Hypoglycaemia is therefore the commonest neonatal problem of diabetic pregnancies. Its incidence should be less if the maternal condition is well treated. Since its occurrence is now well established its detection and treatment should not present problems.

Other neonatal problems. These include hypocalcaemia, jaundice, polycythaemia, renal vein thrombosis, and cardiomyopathy. Polycythaemia seems to result from increased erythropoiesis in the liver; it causes increased blood viscosity and poor peripheral perfusion and predisposes to multiple organ thrombosis of which renal vein thrombosis is the most important. Cardiac septal hypertrophy may cause neonatal congestive heart failure which resolves spontaneously during the first few months of life. It is possible that this may be induced by fetal hyperinsulinism.

Congenital malformations. The factors contributing to perinatal mortality and morbidity which have been discussed so far are all in some way or another related to events in the third trimester of pregnancy, and, being the consequences of maternal metabolic disturbances at this time, are therefore ameliorated by better management. Congenital malformations present a different problem in that they arise during the first trimester.

With the decline in the overall perinatal mortality of diabetic pregnancies, congenital malformations have emerged as the single most important cause of perinatal death. They now account for 10–45 per cent of all deaths in this group. They occur two to four times more commonly in the offspring of diabetic mothers but not in the offspring of diabetic fathers. This demonstrates that they are not primarily genetic in origin.

All organ systems are involved but lesions of the skeleton, and of the cardiovascular and central nervous systems, predominate. Multiple malformations are common (about a threefold increase in incidence above normal) but usually cannot be categorized to any specific syndrome. The exception is the rare caudal dysplasia syndrome which includes bony abnormalities of the sacrum (including sacral agenesis), coccyx, and lower limbs. This occurs about 600 times more frequently in diabetic than in normal women.

Abnormalities of the central nervous system occur about three times more commonly than expected. Neural tube defects are frequent. Cardiovascular anomalies are noted about five times more than expected; the commonest lesions reported have been ventricular septal defects, aortic anomalies, and situs inversus. The likelihood of all lesions is increased the more complicated and severe is the maternal diabetes, and the highest incidence occurs in women with diabetic renal disease or proliferative retinopathy.

It is not known what is the teratogenic factor, or whether it operates before or after conception. Whether or not better medical control during the first trimester will lessen the number of malformations is also not known. The present evidence indicates that severe hypoglycaemia including hypoglycaemic coma is not the contributory factor.

Organization of antenatal care. Women with insulin-dependent diabetes comprise a tiny fraction of the total obstetric population. Their care demands co-ordination between physician, obstetrician, general practitioner, dietitian, and midwife as well as the services of biochemistry and pathology laboratories. Good care cannot be well organized except from a combined obstetric diabetic clinic. Such clinics are only justified if they serve obstetric populations of 15 000 to 20 000 deliveries per annum or more. Small units will not see enough of the disorder to generate and maintain the necessary clinical skills. Therefore, wherever possible, obstetric care of the diabetic woman should be concentrated at tertiary or referral centres.

Prepregnancy assessment. It is desirable that the diabetic services for medical and obstetric patients are properly unified so that women who become pregnant are seen in advance by the physician and obstetrician who will care for them in pregnancy; that the risks and special demands of pregnancy are fully explained; and that the patient is evaluated with special respect to factors that are relevant to the success of pregnancy. A full prepregnancy assessment should no longer be considered an unanticipated bonus but an ordinary requirement of good care.

Three aspects should be examined before pregnancy begins: the success of current schedules of treatment, because it is desirable that pregnancy starts with as good control as possible; the presence and degree of diabetic complications to allow a grading such as in Table 1 to assess the likelihood of perinatal complication; and the details of any previous pregnancies. If there has been a child with a neural tube defect the capabilities of antenatal diagnosis must be discussed. If there has been severe pre-eclampsia the possibility of recurrence is more likely if there is persisting hypertension or nephropathy. Baseline measurements of blood pressure and renal function will be useful in allowing later changes due to pregnancy to be separated from changes due to the diabetic condition.

Management in pregnancy. The third trimester is the critical time in the management of diabetes in pregnancy. Maternal insulin requirements reach their peak. Concurrently, the fetal beta cells become responsive to hyperglycaemia, fetal hyperinsulinism can develop, and the stage is set for all the perinatal problems already discussed. These difficulties are largely resolved by very stringent control of the maternal diabetes. The objective is to keep all maternal blood glucose measurements below 7 mmol/l during the final 12–14 weeks of pregnancy. The preceding or middle trimester must be used to create the most favourable conditions for these final critical months.

Insulin. Good control in the third trimester will not be achieved with a once-a-day regimen. Furthermore, rapid responses to day to day fluctuations in the blood glucose cannot be made with long-acting preparations. Instead it is usual to employ twice daily combinations of highly purified porcine short and medium acting insulins. Insulin requirements for each 12 hours are met almost entirely by what is given at the start of each period. The change to a twice-a-day regimen should be completed before the start of the second half of pregnancy. If good control in the first trimester is shown to minimize the incidence of congenital abnormalities, a prepregnancy adjustment of insulin schedules along these lines will also become necessary.

Diet. The best control of the maternal blood glucose will not be achieved if food intake is erratic in terms either of its calorie and carbohydrate content or of the timing of meals and snacks. The pregnant patient must be carefully educated as to how and why she can help herself in this respect, so that early in pregnancy she learns the disciplines necessary for the third trimester.

The objectives of dietary control are not primarily caloric restriction nor weight restriction but a precise titration of diet against administered insulin. A normal woman gains on average 12.5 kg during pregnancy. Many studies indicate no benefit and potential harm in attempting to restrict this physiological weight gain. There is further no purpose in arbitrary rules which attempt to stereotype the calorie intake of a diabetic gravida. Instead her normal diet should be reviewed and then adjusted in terms of the balance of calories between carbohydrate and other constituents and of the content and timing of individual meals and snacks. Approximately 45–50 per cent of the total calories will come from carbohydrate, but quickly-absorbed carbohydrate should be used sparingly. Once a pattern has been settled which is right for an individual patient, control of blood glucose levels can thereafter often be more readily achieved by moving portions of diet from one part of the day to another rather than by changing insulin doses.Thus an experienced dietician plays a vital part in the patient's management.

Monitoring of blood glucose. The need for precise blood glucose control and the altered relationship between glycosuria and glycaemia mean that the monitoring of management depends on blood glucose measurements. In the past this demanded the patient's presence in hospital so that much of the third trimester was spent as an inpatient. Measurement of blood glucose using glucose oxidase reagent strips supplemented, if necessary, by reflectance colorimeters, now allows the patient to monitor her own blood glucose levels at home. This is far more satisfactory, not only because it avoids prolonged periods in hospital but because the patient is a more active participant in her care. She quickly learns how her diet, insulin regimen, and daily activities interact and what she needs to do to achieve good control. It is simple to review blood glucose levels at least once a week. Blood is sampled fasting in the morning, two hours after breakfast, before and two hours after lunch, before the main evening meal and before going to bed. The results are recorded on a specific chart along with insulin doses used, results of urine testing, and untoward events such as hypoglycaemic symptoms.

Under the most ideal conditions, the best diabetic control never exactly simulates the physiological state. The blood glucose level is always likely to fluctuate over a wider range than normal. Hyperglycaemia is most common during the middle of the morning. If enough soluble insulin is administered in the morning to control this, its action becomes excessive before lunch and hypoglycaemia develops. Increasing the mid-morning snack or reducing breakfast or inceasing the interval between the insulin injection and breakfast are all moves that may help here. The tendency to morning hyperglycaemia is aggravated by the next most common aberration, which is nocturnal hypoglycaemia. If this is undetected, it may only become apparent in the morning with its hyperglycaemic rebound (the Somoygi effect). The right therapeutic response to a high fasting morning blood sugar is not immediately to increase the evening dose of medium-acting insulin but first to check the blood glucose at about 0200 hours. This can easily be done by the patient herself at home. If the measurement is low, correction of the morning hyperglycaemia depends on reducing, not increasing, the evening medium-acting insulin.

The patient should learn to monitor her own blood glucose in the second trimester and hence assess her daily increasing insulin requirements. At this stage, because fetal hyperinsulinism is not a potential problem, control need not be over-stringent: the aim should be to keep all blood glucose measurements at less than 8.0 mmol/l. Hypoglycaemic reactions are the main problem. Fortunately, because of the insulin resistance of pregnancy the extreme 'brittleness' of some non-pregnant diabetics is usually not encountered. The insulin needs of the pregnant patient can usually be titrated up or down without violent swings in her own blood glucose levels. Hypoglycaemic attacks in the final weeks of pregnancy may herald a decline in insulin needs which, if marked, may be a reflection of placental failure and impending fetal problems. At the moment of delivery insulin requirements suddenly fall and dangerous hypoglycaemia will occur if insulin doses are not markedly reduced. Nearly all pregnant women have hypoglycaemic symptoms during pregnancy and in some these will be severe. There is little evidence that any fetal damage results from these episodes.

Even with home blood glucose measurements, frequent outpatient review at the combined antenatal diabetic clinic is necessary. A minimum schedule is once every two weeks until the third trimester, at which time weekly visits become necessary.

Other problems and complications. Monitoring and care will be needed for problems other than blood glucose control. Proliferative retinopathy may need to be managed concurrently as discussed in Section 9. Fluorescein angiography can be undertaken if necessary. Changes ascribable to pre-eclampsia must be detected, and because these may be superimposed on pre-existing vascular and renal disease the techniques outlined on pages 11.7 and 11.8 should be used. Fetal growth and well-being require continual assessment; and all the other components of antenatal preparation, education and clinical care should be given their due importance.

Timing of delivery, delivery, and puerperium. Pre-term delivery is indicated if problems in management arise or there is a poor obstetric history. Uncomplicated, well controlled diabetic patients can be allowed to go to term provided fetal size is normal. Vaginal delivery is preferable. On the day of delivery blood glucose is controlled by an intravenous regimen comprising 5 g of dextrose and 2 units of soluble insulin per hour. The blood glucose is measured frequently using glucose oxidase reagent strips. At delivery the insulin infusion rate is immediately halved to one unit per hour. During the first 24 hours after delivery food intake is frequently restricted (particularly after a Caesarean section), the maternal system is very sensitive to insulin, and there is no longer the absolute need for tight control of blood glucose. During this time the insulin requirements will be considerably less than those before pregnancy in marked contrast to the situation just before delivery. Insulin dosage will then be increased as normal eating resumes to approximately the pre-pregnancy level. There is no contra-indication to breast-feeding.

Gestational diabetes. Diabetes may be diagnosed for the first time in pregnancy. If it remits afterwards, it can correctly be called gestational or pregnancy induced. If it does not, then it is simply a diagnosis made concurrently with pregnancy. Gestational diabetes cannot be diagnosed with certainty, therefore, until a postpartum assessment has been made to demonstrate a return to normal.

Almost all gestational diabetes is asymptomatic and detected biochemically. It is a subset of the category of chemical diabetes and perhaps should be more correctly called 'chemical diabetes of pregnancy'. The diagnosis depends on a glucose tolerance test (GTT), usually with an oral glucose load, although some investigators use intravenous glucose. The criteria for an abnormal GTT are arbitrary but usually are defined so as to identify between 1 and 2 per cent of the population.

Chemical diabetes causes fetal problems similar to but less severe than those encountered in insulin-dependent disease. Fetal macrosomia and neonatal hypoglycaemia are the most significant. The incidence of congenital malformation is, however, not increased. These perinatal disadvantages can be ameliorated by appropriate management, and therefore the problem of how to screen for the affected individuals is an important one.

Screening for chemical diabetes. The diagnosis is made by the oral GTT and the problem is to know which women to select for this procedure. All the cases of chemical diabetes would only be detected if all gravid women were given a GTT, an expensive approach which would be unacceptable to the great majority of unaffected women. Significant numbers of women with chemical diabetes will not show glycosuria, and conversely the majority of women with glycosuria will not have chemical diabetes. The value of a urine test can be enhanced if the second fasting specimen in the morning is tested ('fasting glycosuria'). Fasting glycosuria is found in 0.8 per cent of all pregnant women and about 15 per cent of these will have chemical diabetes, but many cases will be missed using this as the primary screening system.

A different approach is to reserve the GTT for women with features which make them potentially diabetic (see Table 3). More than a quarter of all pregnant women will have one or more of these features and hence will need to be tested. Moreover, about one third of those with chemical diabetes will show none of these features and will remain undetected. This is clearly both wasteful and inefficient. A simplified GTT can also be used in which a one-hour blood sugar is estimated after a 50–100 g glucose load given to all women (unfasted) attending their routine antenatal clinics. Those above a specific limit (e.g. plasma glucose greater than or equal to 7.7 mmol/l at 60 minutes after 50 g glucose by mouth) are then tested with a full oral GTT. In this way a full GTT is done on 8 per cent of the gravid population of whom about one-fifth will eventually be shown to have chemical diabetes. This is still a relatively expensive and time-consuming approach.

Table 3   Risk factors for chemical diabetes in pregnancy

Family history of diabetes (parent or sibling)
'Fasting glycosuria'
Polyhydramnios
Previous obstetric history
   Chemical diabetes
   Large baby (> 4500 g)
   Unexplained stillbirth

A simpler technique is based on random blood glucose sampling at a defined gestation, for example 28 weeks. The results are assessed according to the interval from the last meal before the blood was taken. If the upper limit of normality is defined as a blood glucose of 6.4 mmol/l within two hours of eating, or 5.8 mmol/l if not, about 1 per cent of a pregnant population exceed these limits and go on to a full GTT. In this small group nearly all the cases of chemical diabetes will be identified. This method seems to offer the best compromise between convenience and efficiency.

Metabolic status of women with chemical diabetes in pregnancy. In chemical diabetes of pregnancy the insulin response to a glucose load is sluggish so that post-prandial hyperglycaemia persists for longer. Overall the mean circadian plasma glucose is raised and there is a greater variability between minimum and maximum values over a 24-hour period. Fasting plasma free fatty acids are raised and decrease less after a meal. Plasma triglycerides tend to be higher at most times. The maternal plasma levels of certain amino acids are also higher either in the fasting state or post-prandially. The effects are those of a relative deficiency of maternal insulin. This does not cause abnormalities only of maternal plasma glucose but of other circulating maternal fuels, all of which can traverse the placenta to be utilized by the fetus. The effect of chemical diabetes upon the fetus is to increase the supply of many classes of nutrients and to provoke a relative degree of hyperinsu-linism which causes macrosomia.

Management of chemical diabetes in pregnancy. Management is straightforward and depends on control of blood glucose by diet alone or supplemented by insulin. The milder abnormalities nearly always respond to diet alone, the intake being spread throughout the day and providing a proper balance of different nutrients. If insulin is needed, it may be at surprisingly high doses, because of the insulin resistance of pregnancy which may frequently be combined with that caused by obesity. Management of patients requiring insulin proceeds as for Class B diabetic patients, except that in mild cases once-daily injections of long-lasting insulin may be adequate. After delivery insulin can be stopped.

Chlorpropamide has been used in pregnancy without causing specific problems. However, it does cross the placenta and, with its long half-life, particularly in the new-born, causes severe and protracted hypoglycaemia. It must therefore never be given within five days of a possible delivery, which means it cannot be given entirely safely after the 26th week. For this reason insulin is considered preferable. The problem of chemical diabetes will tend to recur in future pregnancies. Using current definitions more than half the patients will develop maturity onset diabetes within 15 years of pregnancy.

Contraceptive advice for patients with diabetes in pregnancy. The use of contraceptive steroids carries a potential risk of exacerbating the metabolic disorders of diabetes. There is also the further possibility that the development of complications, particularly vascular disease, may be accelerated. Both oestrogens and progestogens increase carbohydrate intolerance. Oestrogenic oral contraceptives increase fasting triglyceride and blood cholesterol whereas progestogens on their own have no effect.

Women who have had gestational diabetes and who are likely to become permanently diabetic in later life may therefore significantly aggravate their metabolic problems by taking oestrogen–progestogen combination. If mechanical methods of contraception are not acceptable, a progestogen-only preparation should be used. Insulin-dependent diabetics need not be excluded from taking oestrogen-containing agents. However, the possible advantages in limiting the duration of their use should be emphasized. In particular, once a diabetic woman's family is complete, the medical advantages of sterilization should be discussed.

References

Pregnancy Metabolism, Diabetes and the Fetus (1979). CIBA Foundation Symposium 63. Excerpta Medica, Amsterdam.
Symposium on Gestational Diabetes (1980). *Diabetes Care* **3**, 399.
Clinical Obstetrics and Gynecology (1981). *Clin. Obstet. Gynec.* **24**, 3.

BLOOD DISORDERS IN PREGNANCY

C. W. G. Redman and D. J. Weatherall

Plasma volume increases progressively during pregnancy, reaching a peak during the third trimester which is about 45 per cent or 1250 ml above non-pregnant values. The change is greater in multiple pregnancy. The total red cell mass increases proportionately less, that is by about 20–30 per cent. The net result is haemodilution and hence a decline in haemoglobin concentration, packed cell volume, and red cell count. In the absence of iron deficiency, the mean cell haemoglobin concentration and mean cell volume remain at non-pregnant values. As a result of these changes anaemia cannot be diagnosed in pregnancy using criteria applied to non-pregnant individuals.

Iron-deficiency anaemia. The expansion of red cell mass represents a net gain of iron of about 500–600 mg and a further 250–350 mg is required for transfer to the fetus. These additional requirements are met, at least in part, by an increased rate of absorption of dietary iron from the gut. The mean serum iron concentration of healthy pregnant women is about two-thirds of the levels for non-pregnant individuals. Total iron-binding capacity (TIBC) is increased because transferrin levels more than double as pregnancy advances. In consequence, the saturation of iron binding capacity is, in healthy pregnancy, lower (at about 25 per cent) than is normal for other situations. Serum ferritin (reflecting iron stores) declines markedly during the first half of pregnancy to a nadir of about 15–20 μg/l where it remains until delivery. In an antenatal population routinely given iron supplements, about 0.5 and 3.0 per cent of women have a haemoglobin of less than 9.0 g/dl and 10.0 g/dl respectively. However, 18 per cent have a haemoglobin of 11.0 g/dl or less at some stage in their pregnancy. Thus, the conventional limit of 11.0 g/dl for diagnosing anaemia in gravid women is probably too high—a more practical limit would be 10.0 g/dl or less. A low haemoglobin concentration combined with hypochromia and microcytosis in the peripheral blood film suggests iron deficiency. This is further confirmed if the serum iron is less than 10 μmol/l, the saturation of iron binding capacity is less than 15 per cent or the serum ferritin less than 15 μg/l. It should be necessary to assess iron stores directly in a bone-marrow aspirate only if there is a failure to respond to iron replacement.

It is now routine to provide all pregnant women with iron supplements. The justification for this is still being debated. The main point to consider is that if iron deficiency develops in the third trimester there will not be time to correct it by oral supplements. Thus blood transfusions may be needed with their associated hazards.

Folic acid deficiency. The pregnant woman needs approximately twice as much folic acid—800 μg daily—compared with non-pregnant individuals. This meets the needs of the growing uterus and conceptus and the expanded maternal red cell mass. As pregnancy advances serum folate falls to about half the non-pregnant value at term. The red cell folate content shows a slight decline over the same period.

Megaloblastic anaemia in pregnancy is usually the result of dietary folate deficiency (see Section 19). Its incidence is therefore very variable, dependent upon the socio-economic status of the parturient population and whether or not folic acid supplements are given routinely as part of antenatal care. It occurs more frequently in multiple pregnancies. About half the cases present in the third trimester and the remainder after delivery. Commonly, deficiencies of iron and folate are combined; folate deficiency may then be revealed by the failure of a patient to respond to iron supplements. The peripheral blood film shows macrocytosis (which may be mixed with microcytosis if there is also iron deficiency) and hypersegmentation of the neutrophils. The diagnosis is confirmed by examination of a bone marrow aspirate. Diagnosis, using other tests, may be difficult because the results need to be related to the normal range that is expected for healthy pregnant women and not those derived from non-pregnant subjects. This applies to measurements of serum and red cell folate concentrations, as well as the excretion of formimino-glutamic acid after a histidine load (which is increased in normal pregnancy).

It is still argued to what extent folate deficiency may alter the outcome of pregnancy. It has been suggested that it can predispose to congenital malformation, particularly neural tube defects, prematurity, and antepartum haemorrhage. These associations however are still not proven.

Vitamin B_{12} deficiency is rarely seen in pregnancy.

Haemoglobinopathies
Sickle cell trait and disease. The sickling disorders are described in detail in Section 19. It is essential to carry out a sickling test on all pregnant women of the appropriate racial background, and if the test is positive, to determine whether they are heterozygous or homozygous.

Women with the *sickle cell trait* have no difficulties in pregnancy, but it is important to warn the anaesthetists if an anaesthetic is required during labour. Tissue infarction can occur even in the sickle cell trait if an adequate oxygen level is not maintained or if there is severe dehydration or shock. It is also necessary to check the husbands of all women with a positive sickling test. At the present time, some centres are starting programmes for antenatal diagnosis of sickle cell anaemia using fetal blood sampling, although this is not yet widely applied. However, it is important to identify homozygous infants of all mothers at risk of giving birth to an infant with sickle cell anaemia. The infant's blood should be examined by agar gel electrophoresis immediately after birth. The first two years of life are particularly hazardous for an infant with sickle cell anaemia because of the high incidence of death due to infection and splenic sequestration. Hence the mothers must be advised to present the infants early with any unusual symptoms.

It is difficult to evaluate the reported effects of *sickle cell anaemia* on women who are pregnant. Early studies indicated a relatively high maternal morbidity and mortality due to a marked increase in sickle cell crises and a high incidence of severe anaemia. These studies also stressed the high perinatal mortality, as great as 50 per cent in some series. However, it is clear that many of these reports dealt with populations in which antenatal care was either inadequate or totally lacking. There have been very few good studies of series of pregnant women with this disorder who have received adequate antenatal care with regular folate supplementation and early treatment of infection. The little information that is available indicates that women with sickle cell anaemia have a greater incidence of crises during pregnancy and that there is an increased likelihood of fetal loss, prematurity, or growth retardation.

For these reasons there is an increasing tendency to carry out prophylactic exchange transfusion starting between 24 and 28 weeks of pregnancy. The object is to increase the packed cell volume to at least 30 per cent and to reduce the level of haemoglobin S to below 40 per cent. Women treated in this way seem to have uneventful pregnancies and the incidence of fetal loss seems to be reduced. However, these regimens are expensive and time-consuming and may not be applicable in developing countries with a massive sickle cell population. Furthermore, studies of this type have not been carried out in a controlled way and there is still relatively little information about the course of pregnancy in sickle cell anaemia when there is careful antenatal care.

Against this background of uncertainty, a reasonable compromise, particularly where blood transfusion facilities are limited, is to follow pregnant women with sickle cell anaemia extremely carefully throughout the pregnancy and to administer regular folate supplements. If they are becoming severely anaemic, or if they have crises during the second half of pregnancy, then it is appropriate to proceed to an exchange transfusion. Alternatively, if they present with haemoglobin values of less than 7 g/dl it is also acceptable to transfuse them up to a level of 12–14 g/dl since this will reduce the level of haemoglobin S to a safe value without the need for exchange transfusion. During labour, management is directed towards preventing dehydration and acidosis. Regional rather than general anaesthesia should be used wherever possible.

Special mention should be made of the problems of *haemoglobin SC disease* (see Section 19) in pregnancy. Many women with this disorder go through pregnancy with no complications. However, occasionally there may be severe thrombotic episodes either late in pregnancy or early in the puerperium, which may lead to maternal death due to pulmonary thrombotic crises. Any women with this disorder who develop a painful crisis late in pregnancy, or who develop symptoms and signs suggestive of a chest infection or small pulmonary embolus, require urgent exchange transfusion; the dangerous thrombotic complications of this disorder are nearly always heralded by symptoms or signs of a thrombotic crisis; the lungs seem particularly vulnerable.

Thalassaemia. The clinical and haematological manifestations of the α and β thalassaemias are described in Section 19. The homozygous state for α° thalassaemia produces the haemoglobin Bart's hydrops syndrome. The obstetric complications of this condition are described on page 19.47.

Any woman of an appropriate racial background should be screened for β thalassaemia early in pregnancy. Since antenatal diagnosis for homozygous β thalassaemia is now available in the United Kingdom, the USA, and many parts of Europe, it is important to check the husband of women who are known to be carriers and to offer these women this possibility if the husband is also found to carry the disease.

Heterozygous β thalassaemia may be associated with anaemia in pregnancy. Although this is not usually severe, occasionally it requires transfusion late in pregnancy. Heterozygous thalassaemic women should have adequate folic acid supplementation; iron deficiency may occasionally complicate this disorder, and when in doubt it is important to determine the serum iron or serum ferritin level. Although non-pregnant heterozygous β thalassaemic women should not receive iron, there is no harm in giving iron supplementation during pregnancy.

Pregnancy is extremely rare in transfusion-dependent homozygous β thalassaemics but is now being seen with increasing frequency in women with β thalassaemia intermedia (see Section 19). These patients may become profoundly anaemic and require regular transfusion during pregnancy.

Genetic counselling and identification of the different carrier states for α and β thalassaemia are described in detail in Section 19.

Disorders of haemostasis. During normal pregnancy the concentrations of factors VII, VIII, X, and fibrinogen in the blood increase. Fibrinolytic activity is inhibited. Some of these changes are thought to be oestrogen-induced. They become detectable by the end of the first trimester and predispose to a more rapid and larger response to coagulant stimuli.

Haemophilia A and haemophilia B are deficiencies of factor VIII and IX respectively and are the commonest inherited disorders of coagulation. But because they are sex-linked recessive diseases, pregnant women may present only as carriers. The affected women usually have lower than average levels of the relevant clotting factor but remain clinically normal. Rarely, carriers may have bleeding tendencies, but these are not usually a problem during pregnancy because of the pregnancy-induced increases in the concentrations of the involved factors. Half the sons of known carriers will have the disorder. Antenatal diagnosis has previously been limited to identifying the sex of the fetus and offering the option of termination if it is a male. Currently, techniques of sampling fetal blood at fetoscopy are being developed, and the ability to identify affected males may become more generally available.

Von Willebrand's disease is the commonest abnormality of blood coagulation in women, and therefore the most likely to affect pregnancy. The diagnosis is suggested by a history of excessive bleeding and an appropriate family history; and confirmed by a prolonged bleeding time associated with abnormally low levels of both factor VIII procoagulant and factor VIII related antigen. Diagnosis in pregnancy is made more difficult because of the pregnancy-induced increases in both these factors. The only known complication is postpartum haemorrhage. The likelihood of this is increased if factor VIII levels fall below 50 per cent and prevented by an infusion of fresh frozen plasma or cryoprecipitate when delivery is anticipated, and continuing for three to five days postpartum. Thus, the management hinges around careful monitoring of the factor VIII levels.

Platelet disorders. The platelet count is slightly reduced in normal pregnancy. Pre-eclampsia causes further decrements mediated by a process of low-grade intravascular coagulation. However, except in extreme circumstances, the platelet count rarely falls below 50×10^9/l and bleeding problems do not ensue. Acute intravascular coagulation severe enough to cause defibrination associated with marked thrombocytopenia occurs with eclampsia, abruptio placentae, retained dead fetus, amniotic fluid embolism, and septic abortion. The treatment in these situations is primarily of the underlying disorder.

Idiopathic thrombocytopenic purpura is rare in gravid women. Its course is not made worse by pregnancy, but it can cause complications for both mother and baby. The fetus may acquire the condition passively by transplacental passage of the antiplatelet auto-antibodies (see page 19.121). Approximately half the neonates are significantly affected; their thrombocytopenia tends to worsen in the first week of life before spontaneous improvement occurs; there may be bleeding problems if the count at birth is less than $50 \times 10^9/l$.

Since corticosteroids are relatively ineffective in chronic idiopathic thrombocytopenic purpura, women of reproductive age who wish to have children should undergo splenectomy before they are allowed to become pregnant. If a woman with this disorder presents early in pregnancy, she requires extremely careful assessment and management. It is important to treat the patient and not the platelet count. On the whole, bleeding is likely to occur during either pregnancy or labour if the platelet count is persistently less than $20 \times 10^9/l$. Levels higher than this in an asymptomatic woman can probably be observed and the pregnancy allowed to continue. If the platelet count is extremely low, it is reasonable to proceed to splenectomy, certainly during the first 20 weeks. In women with symptomatic thrombocytopenic purpura, who present later in pregnancy, corticosteroids should be tried although they are frequently ineffective. If so, and if there is dangerous bleeding (see page 19.121), the pregnancy may have to be terminated and splenectomy carried out. The major hazard of sending a woman to term with an extremely low platelet count and bleeding is intracranial haemorrhage during labour. Unfortunately, platelet infusions are of little value, and severe and uncontrollable maternal bleeding is an indication for termination of the pregnancy.

Aplastic anaemia in pregnancy. Women with aplastic anaemia which is associated with recurrent infection or bleeding should not be allowed to become pregnant. If they do, treatment should follow the lines described on page 19.145 for patients with bone marrow failure. There is a rare but extremely interesting form of aplastic anaemia which occurs for the first time in pregnancy, remits after delivery, and then recurs again in subsequent pregnancies. The mechanism of this condition has not been worked out. It does not respond to any form of bone marrow stimulant or corticosteroid therapy and the management is symptomatic.

Leukaemia and lymphoma. These neoplastic conditions occasionally coincide with pregnancy. There is no evidence that their course is adversely affected by pregnancy. However, pregnancy becomes complicated because of the need for treatment with either radiotherapy or cytotoxic agents. Termination of pregnancy is necessary if radiotherapy needs to be started without delay. Successful pregnancies have been reported where cytotoxic therapy has been administered for the treatment of leukaemia. Teratogenic effects may occur with the use of folate antagonists (aminopterin or methotrexate), chlorambucil, cyclophosphamide, and vincristine. Prematurity and growth retardation seem to be the main problems in later gestation.

References

Horger, E. O. (ed.) (1979). Obstetric hematology. *Clin. Obstet. Gynec.* **22**, 783.

Letsky, E. (1980). The haematological system. In *Clinical physiology in obstetrics* (eds. F. Hytten and G. Chamberlain), 43. Blackwell Scientific Publications, Oxford.

Section 12
Gastroenterology

Introduction

This section describes the major disorders of the gastrointestinal tract, liver, and pancreas. Where possible these conditions are described in groups which have a common form of pathophysiology, i.e. disorders of motility, or vascular disorders, rather than by the more conventional approach of considering the different pathologies of one particular part of the gastrointestinal tract together. This approach seems particularly appropriate because of the increasing evidence regarding the functional interdependence of the various sections of the gastrointestinal tract and its related organs.

Methods for investigation of gastrointestinal and related diseases

ENDOSCOPY

D. P. Jewell

The advent of fibre-optic endoscopy has made a major impact on the practice of gastroenterology both with respect to diagnosis and, more recently, therapy. Basically, light from a cold light source passes down a bundle of quartz fibres to illuminate the lumen of the gastrointestinal tract. The reflected light is returned to the observer's eye via the image bundle which may contain up to 20 000 fibres and is 'coherent', i.e. the alignment of fibres is strictly maintained throughout the bundle in order to prevent distortion of the image.

The tip of all modern instruments can be angulated in both directions which usually allows a deflection of about 180°. Fingertip controls are provided for suction, air insufflation, and for water injection to clean the lens or mucosa.

Indications

Oesophageal disease. Endoscopy with a forward-viewing instrument is essential for the diagnosis of oesophagitis and for obtaining biopsies of strictures and neoplasms. Barium studies are still required, however, since motor disorders of the oesophagus are frequently difficult to appreciate by the endoscopist, and oesophageal reflux is much better assessed by the radiologist. Interpretation of oesophageal biopsies from patients with endoscopic evidence of oesophagitis is difficult and the macroscopic appearances are usually more reliable. Endoscopic dilatation of benign strictures with Eder–Puestow dilators is now a well-established form of therapy. Oesophageal tubes (e.g. the Celestin tube) can also be inserted through malignant strictures using the endoscope and this has now become the method of choice.

Stomach and duodenum. If facilities are available, endoscopy should be the first-line investigation. In the hands of a good endoscopist, the investigation provides maximal diagnostic information. Gastritis (acute, chronic, superficial, and atrophic), the presence of erosions, and mucosal tears are readily recognized by an experienced endoscopist and their presence can be confirmed by biopsy. Even with the best air-contrast barium studies, these lesions can be difficult to detect. Endoscopy is also essential for gastric lesions in order that cytological specimens and biopsy specimens can be obtained. Patients who present with dyspeptic symptoms following gastric surgery should also proceed to endoscopy as the radiological assessment of the post-operative stomach is notoriously difficult. However, radiological studies can be more useful in the assessment of gastric disease in certain situations. Motor disorders are better appreciated radiologically and this also applies to infiltrative diseases (e.g. linitis plastica, lymphoma) and to extrinsic compression of the stomach. Duodenal disease is always better assessed endoscopically than radiologically although ulcers in the roof of the duodenum immediately distal to the pylorus can be missed as this is a difficult area to examine.

Colonic disease. In general, patients presenting with suspected colonic disease should have a barium enema performed as the initial procedure. Colonoscopy is indicated in the following situations:

1. To biopsy polyps or suspected carcinomas for histological confirmation.

2. To examine and biopsy strictures.

3. To perform polypectomy.

4. If the barium enema is negative and the patient is still suspected of having organic disease, e.g. patients with persistent occult blood in the stools.

5. In the investigation and treatment of patients with severe colonic bleeding with a negative barium enema, i.e. those suspected of having angiodysplasia.

6. In the assessment of patients with ulcerative colitis or Crohn's disease.

7. Patients with radiological evidence of diverticulosis in whom there is a high index of suspicion that another lesion may be present, e.g. a polyp, a carcinoma, or Crohn's disease.

Pancreatic disease. Visualization of the pancreatic duct by direct endoscopic cannulation should be performed in all cases of suspected pancreatic disease. This procedure coupled with a functional test of pancreatic function (see page 12.162) will give maximal diagnostic information.

Biliary disease. Visualization of the bile duct may be obtained either by endoscopic cannulation or by radiology. If oral cholecystography or cholangiography fail, then the choice lies between endoscopic visualization and percutaneous trans-hepatic cholangiography. The latter procedure is usually best done in patients who have dilated bile ducts seen on an ultrasound scan, but in patients with normal ducts endoscopic cannulation is the procedure of choice. Some patients may require both investigations. The advent of endoscopic sphincterotomy has been a major advance in the management of bile duct stones.

Premedication. This varies according to the preference of the endoscopist. For upper gastrointestinal endoscopy and endoscopic retrograde cholangiopancreatography (ERCP), a lignocaine spray is often applied to the patient's throat and is followed by intravenous sedation. Diazepam and pethidine in combination provides a satisfactory regimen. However, many endoscopists prefer not to use pharyngeal anaesthesia, for the reason that it may predispose to inhalation, and some use minimal sedation, if any. Intravenous atropine can also be used, but there is little objective evidence that it decreases secretions sufficiently to make a notable difference.

Preparation for colonoscopy. Many regimens exist. Most involve a low residue or a fluid diet for 24–48 hours prior to the examination together with purgation with senna or castor oil. It is usual to combine this with a colonic washout. Osmotic purgation with mannitol with a high fluid intake is an effective preparation. However, the presence of a disaccharide in the colon may lead to fermentation with the production of hydrogen and explosions have been reported when diathermy has been used.

Complications. Trivial complications include a sore throat, peripheral thrombophlebitis from diazepam injection, and some abdominal discomfort if insufflated air has not been aspirated at the end of the procedure. These are fairly common and can be ameliorated by good endoscopic practice.

Major complications are rare and the mortality rate is extremely low. When deaths do occur, they are usually due to apnoeic attacks in the elderly patients who have been given too much sedation. Perforation of the oesophagus and of the colon can also occur but the frequency of these complications is low and may be decreasing with increased endoscopic skill and improved design of instruments.

Following ERCP, a rise in serum amylase is a frequent finding but clinical attacks of pancreatitis are much less common. They tend to occur in patients with pancreatic calculi or in those cases where there has been over-filling of the duct with contrast medium. The presence of a pancreatic pseudocyst is a contraindication to ECRP as pancreatitis usually occurs and the cyst may become infected. Ascending cholangitis may follow cannulation of the bile duct, especially when organic disease is present, e.g. stones or strictures. In these patients, antibiotics such as gentamicin and metronidazole should be given for 48 hours following the procedure.

Cross-infection from endoscopes has occasionally been reported—salmonella and pseudomonas are the commonest organisms involved. Although there is concern about hepatitis B virus, no convincingly documented case has so far been reported. Good cleaning schedules should prevent these complications.

Haemorrhage may occur following polypectomy.

Care of instruments. Fibre-optic endoscopes are expensive to purchase and to repair. Their care should be the responsibility of a specially trained nurse or technician—this is especially important in busy units where the instruments are handled by many different endoscopists. Each endoscopist should also be taught the cleaning procedures.

Bacteriological studies have shown that the first patient on the morning's list is particularly at risk from cross-infection since organisms remaining in the instrument from the previous day have multiplied during the night. All instruments should therefore be thoroughly cleaned before and after a list and a 20 minute contact with glutaraldehyde is recommended. A five minute cleaning schedule between examinations is also recommended. Regular microbiological sampling from the tip, the channels, and the biopsy valve should be made. The wash bottle should also be checked as this is an important reservoir of potential infection.

References

Morrissey, J. F., Browning, T. H., and Reichelderfer, M. (1980). Endoscopy. In *Current gastroenterology* (ed. G. L. Gitnick), vol. 1, 353. Houghton Mifflin, Boston.

Williams, C. B. and Hunt, R. (1980). In *Practical gastrointestinal endoscopy* (eds. P. B. Cotton and C. B. Williams). Blackwell Scientific Publications, Oxford.

RADIOLOGICAL INVESTIGATION OF THE DIGESTIVE SYSTEM

D. J. Nolan and E. W. L Fletcher

Radiological and imaging techniques play a role in the diagnosis and management of diseases of the digestive system. Plain radiographs may provide some help, but to obtain the required information in the majority of cases it is necessary to outline the upper gastrointestinal tract, small intestine, colon, or biliary tract with positive contrast medium. The newer imaging techniques of ultrasound, computerized tomography, and radionuclide scanning are valuable for investigating the hepatobiliary system and the pancreas.

The gastrointestinal tract

Plain abdominal radiographs. Plain radiographs of the chest and abdomen are important in patients who present with symptoms or signs of an 'acute abdomen'. Perforation or obstruction of the gastrointestinal tract may be evident on plain radiographs.

Barium studies of the upper gastrointestinal tract. The barium examination remains the procedure of choice for the routine examination of the upper gastrointestinal tract which from the radiological viewpoint consists of the oesophagus, stomach, and duodenum as far as the ligament of Treitz. The double-contrast barium meal is now used routinely in most centres as it gives much better results than the conventional single-contrast examination. The technique allows the stomach to be distended with gas while a thin coating of barium enables its inner surface to be visualized (Fig. 1). The gas,

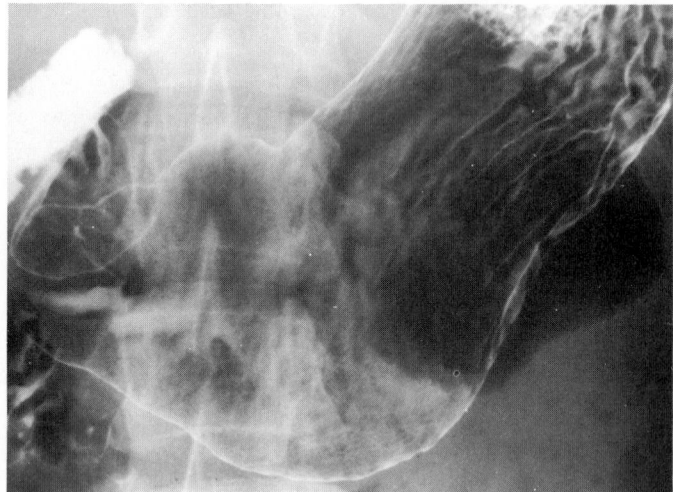

Fig. 1 Normal double-contrast view of the lower body and antrum of the stomach as well as the duodenal cap.

introduced as an effervescent agent, puts the gastric mucosa under slight tension and lesions causing lack of distensibility result in a clearly visible series of converging folds. Carcinomas, ulcers, and ulcer scars that have a converging fold pattern are easily detected. Small lesions and slight irregularity of the mucosa can be identified. It is possible with this examination to detect small carcinomas that have not spread beyond the mucosa and the prognosis for such patients has improved as a result. The lesions are shown *en face* and the mucosal relief pattern closely resembles the endoscopic and macroscopic appearances. Lesions most frequently seen in the upper gastrointestinal tract include carcinomas and benign strictures of the oesophagus, oesophageal varices (Fig. 2), hiatal

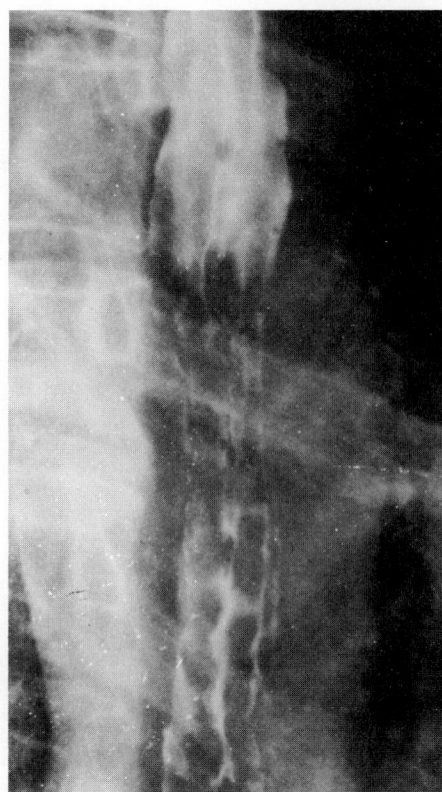

Fig. 2 Oesophageal varices shown on a barium swallow.

hernias, gastric ulceration (Fig. 3), gastric carcinomas, and duodenal ulceration (Fig. 4).

Special barium studies are sometimes indicated, such as cine radiography which is performed to demonstrate functional abnormalities of the oesophagus. Patients who have had a previous Billroth I or Polya-type partial gastrectomy are examined by a modified double-contrast examination. If the prime interest is the duodenal loop, hypotonic duodenography should be performed as a separate study. When perforation is suspected in the upper gastrointestinal tract and plain films are inconclusive, water-soluble contrast agents are used instead of barium.

Fibre-optic endoscopy is widely used to visualize lesions and to obtain aimed biopsy and cytology specimens. It has been claimed

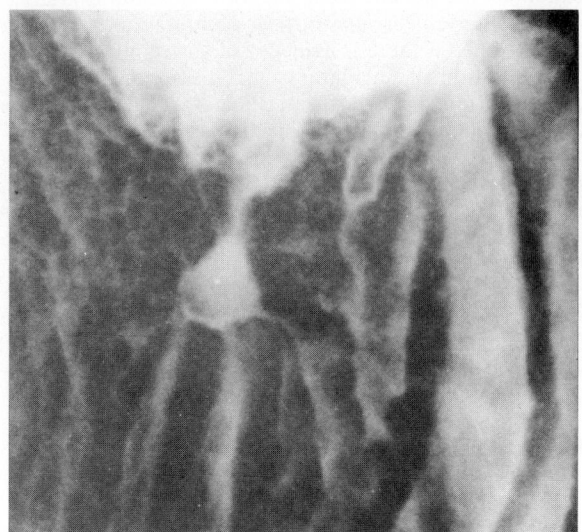

Fig. 3 Gastric ulcer. A shallow ulcer crater is seen on the posterior wall of the upper body of the stomach with distortion of the adjacent mucosal pattern. The patient presented with acute gastrointestinal bleeding.

that endoscopy is more accurate in detecting lesions of the upper gastrointestinal tract than the barium meal. This was true with the single-contrast barium examination, but the argument no longer holds when proper double-contrast barium studies are performed. The accuracy of both double-contrast barium studies and endoscopy depends on the experience and skill of the person performing the examination. The main advantages of the double-contrast barium examination are that it is safer and more comfortable for the patient and can be performed quickly. Each radiograph obtained provides an image of a large area of the oesophagus, stomach, or duodenum which can be retained as a permanent record and is available at any time for detailed review.

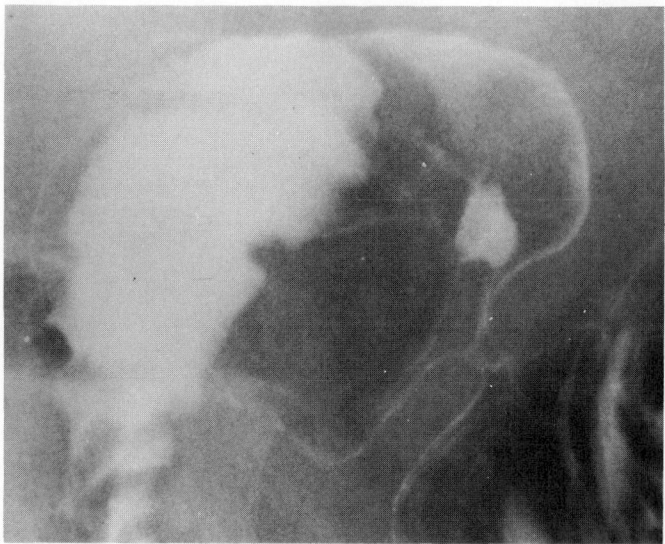

Fig. 4 Duodenal ulcer. A moderate-sized ulcer crater is seen in the base of the duodenal cap.

Barium examination of the small intestine. The follow-through is the most widely used procedure for examining the small intestine with barium. The examination is normally performed following a barium meal examination of the oesophagus, stomach, and duodenum. Large films of the abdomen are taken at half-hourly intervals as the barium progresses through the small intestine.

Many investigators are dissatisfied with the accuracy of the barium follow-through and at the present time more and more centres are adopting the barium infusion technique (small bowel enema, enteroclysis) instead. A large volume of dilute barium suspension is infused directly into the small intestine through a duodenal tube (Fig. 5). The examination, including duodenal intubation, normally takes 20–25 minutes. The infusion examination gives excellent visualization of the small intestine, delineating clearly between healthy and diseased segments. It is indicated when diseases causing morphological changes in the small intestine such as Crohn's disease, tuberculosis, tumours, radiation damage, or ischaemia are suspected. If coeliac disease is suspected, a jejunal biopsy should be the initial diagnostic procedure and the barium study should be reserved for patients in whom the jejunal biopsy is normal or for detecting suspected complications of coeliac disease such as lymphomas.

Reflux of barium through the ileocaecal valve may occur during barium enema examinations and this barium can be used to visualize the terminal ileum. Diseases affecting the small intestine often involve the distal ileum and the diagnostic value of refluxed barium should not be overlooked.

Barium enema. Digital examination of the rectum and sigmoidoscopy should have been carried out before the barium enema is requested. Indications for performing a barium enema are to detect colorectal cancer and polyps, and in the diagnosis and management of inflammatory bowel disease. There is evidence to show that cancers of the colon develop from previously benign adenomas. If cancer of the colon is diagnosed at an early stage, the survival rate of patients is much higher than if lesions are extensive at the time of diagnosis. The barium examination of the colon is therefore a most important diagnostic procedure; it should be sensitive enough to detect small polyps of the colon as well as cancers. The double-contrast barium enema fulfils this requirement and it should be used routinely.

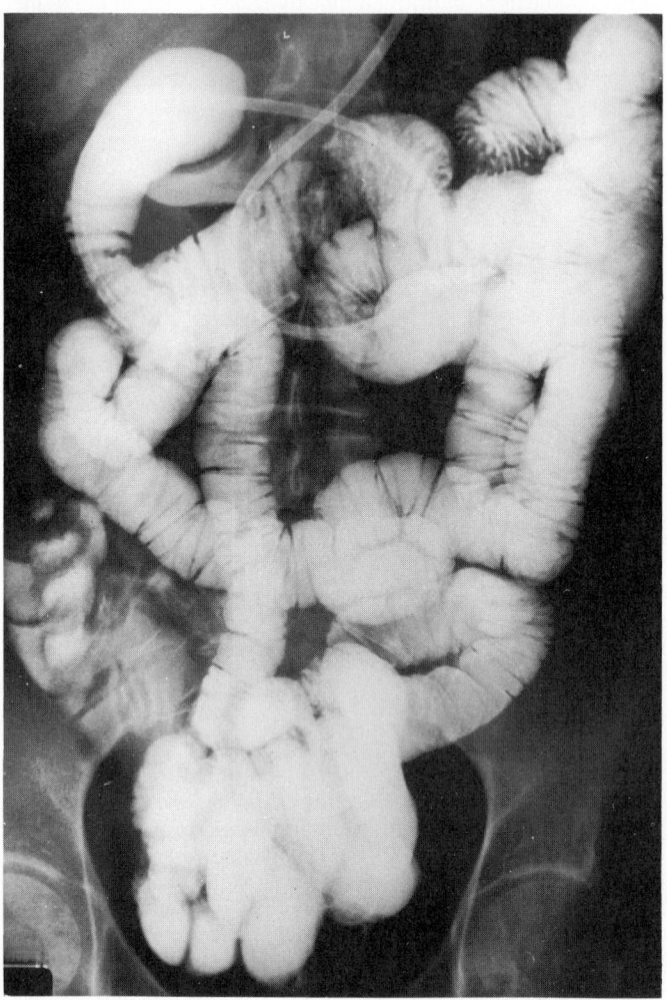

Fig. 5   A normal barium infusion examination of the small intestine.

A clean colon, a suitable barium suspension, air insufflation, and the routine use of smooth muscle relaxant drugs together with a good radiographic technique are essential for consistently good results. Barium is introduced into the rectum and it is allowed to flow in a column as far as the hepatic flexure before being drained off. A smooth muscle relaxant such as 20 mg of hyoscine butyl-bromide (Buscopan) is injected intravenously and air is introduced into the rectum. Radiographs are obtained following air insufflation. Cancers and polyps of the colon are shown either as infiltrating (Fig. 6) or polypoid lesions. The changes of inflammatory bowel disease are shown as mucosal ulceration seen *en face* and in profile and as alterations in the normal mucosal pattern.

Barium enemas should not be performed in patients with suspected perforation of the colon or with toxic megacolon. A single-contrast barium enema is indicated in patients with obstruction.

Fibre-optic colonoscopy can be accurate in the diagnosis of colonic lesions, but digital examination, sigmoidoscopy, and the barium enema remain the initial diagnostic procedures in patients with suspected colonic disease. At colonoscopy lesions may be missed at the flexures because of sharp angulation and the colonoscopist fails to reach the caecum in at least 10 per cent of cases. Good endoscopy

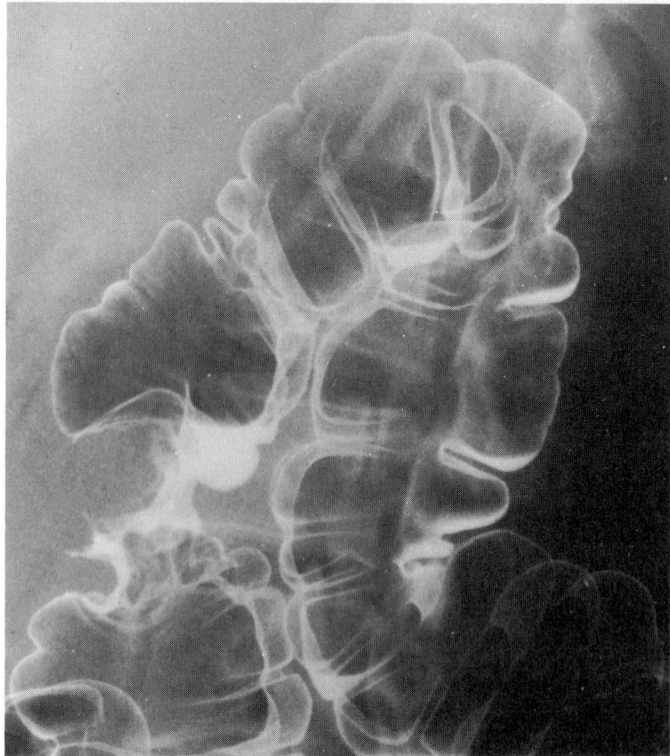

Fig. 6   An infiltrating carcinoma of the ascending limb of the splenic flexure shown on a double-contrast barium enema examination.

and double-contrast barium radiology are complementary and their combined diagnostic accuracy exceeds that of either technique.

Gastrointestinal angiography. Selective visceral angiography is indicated in certain patients who present with bleeding from the gastrointestinal tract. In patients with acute bleeding angiography is performed for two reasons—to locate the source of bleeding when it is unknown (Fig. 7) and to stop the bleeding by selective infusion of drugs or embolic material into the bleeding territory. Angiography can also yield valuable diagnostic information in patients with obscure gastrointestinal bleeding when barium studies and fibre-optic endoscopy are negative. Lesions that are likely to cause obscure bleeding include angiomatous malformations, small tumours, Meckel's diverticulum, and small ulcers. Selective catheterization of the coeliac axis, superior mesenteric artery, and inferior mesenteric artery may be necessary. Barium studies should not be performed if there is evidence of gastrointestinal bleeding until the question of angiography has been considered, as the presence of barium in the gastrointestinal tract makes it impossible to carry out adequate angiographic studies.

Radionuclide studies. Meckel's diverticulum can be detected using $^{99}Tc^M$ pertechnate and it should be the initial radiological procedure if this condition is suspected. Meckel's diverticulum is identified as an area of increased radionuclide activity in the lower abdomen, usually on the right side. Radionuclide studies can also be used to locate the site of obscure bleeding from the gastrointestinal tract. The general anatomical location of bleeding can be identified in many patients and further investigations such as barium studies or angiography can then be performed to define the site of bleeding more precisely.

The liver. Enlargement of the liver may be identified on plain films, but adds little to clinical examination. Inflammatory masses such as subphrenic abscess under the right diaphragm may cause elevation and impairment of movement of the diaphragm together with a pleural effusion. Calcification is occasionally seen in the liver and the commonest causes are old granulomatous disease and hydatid cyst.

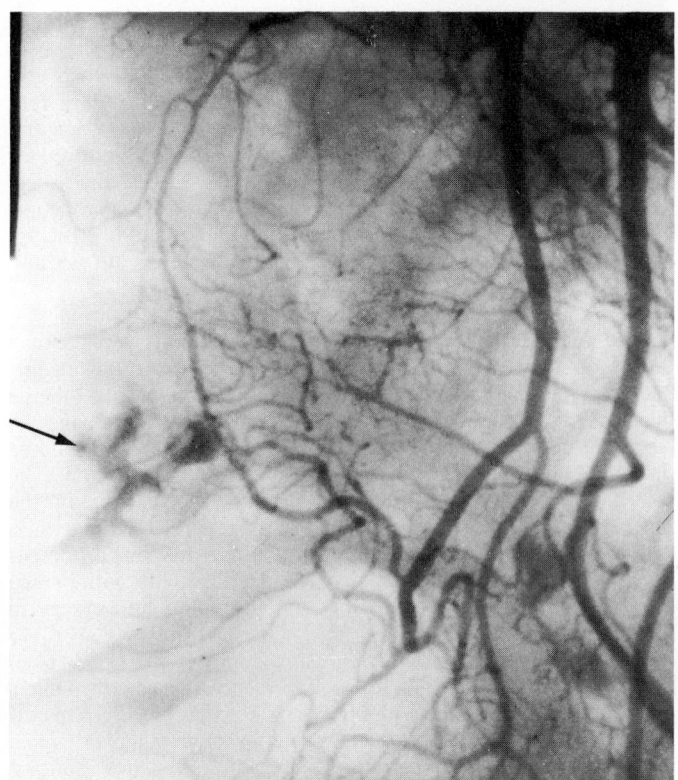

Fig. 7   Subtraction film of a superior mesenteric arteriogram showing contrast leaking into a diverticulum of the caecum (arrow). This was successfully treated by colonoscopic diathermy.

Ultrasound. Ultrasound of the liver is safe, cheap, and accurate in experienced hands. Abscesses appear as black transonic areas surrounded by high intensity echoes whilst cysts have black transonic areas surrounded by a thin echogenic rim. Neoplasia produces areas of discontinuity in the homogeneous pattern of the liver. Most commonly, the echo amplitude is less than that of the surrounding liver, but some metastases, particularly from the colon, produce high intensity echoes. Cirrhosis produces a higher amplitude of echoes than does the normal liver and a large portal vein may be demonstrated. In heart failure the hepatic veins may be dilated. Diagnostic biopsy of liver tumours is greatly facilitated by ultrasound control.

Radionuclide studies. Radio-isotope imaging is a relatively inexpensive and accurate method of identifying metastases in the liver as they produce defects in the uptake of isotope by the Kupffer cells of the normal liver. Abscesses, cysts, haematomas, arteriovenous malformations, and ischaemia produce defects and additional ultrasound may increase diagnostic accuracy. Diffuse liver disease such as cirrhosis can be identified by poor uptake of radio-isotope in the liver whilst the use of gallium will often identify an infective process. Hepatic isotope imaging can be combined with lung scintigraphy to localize a right subphrenic abscess.

Computerized tomography (see page 12.9). Computerized tomography is of use in demonstrating metastatic disease and primary neoplasia of the liver. Cysts and abscesses also show well on computerized tomography, but cirrhosis may be difficult to identify with certainty.

Nuclear magnetic resonance. This technique is reported to be excellent for differentiating malignant tumours from benign cysts, and for providing useful information in patients with cirrhosis and with metastatic deposits.

Angiography. Coeliac axis angiography is useful in identifying haemangiomas as they have feeding vessels of normal size, but with a slow flow of contrast through the lesion. Angiography will help to differentiate hepatic tumours, but is more commonly used

to identify the exact site and blood supply of tumours before partial hepatectomy. If a tumour is inoperable, the hepatic artery can be embolized to alleviate symptoms, which is partially effective in secondary carcinoid.

The late films of a coeliac angiogram usually give a good picture of the portal vein which is invaluable if portocaval shunting is contemplated.

The biliary system. Plain radiographs are normally the initial diagnostic procedure in patients with symptoms of disease of the biliary tract. The plain film may show pathological calcification of the gall-bladder, opaque calculi, gas in the biliary tree, or radio-opaque bile in the gall-bladder.

Oral cholecystography. About 80–85 per cent of gallstones are not radio-opaque and oral cholecystography remains the method of choice for examining the gall-bladder with contrast medium to detect calculi and to demonstrate abnormalities causing a change in the outline of the gall-bladder such as adenomyomatosis. The contrast medium used for oral cholecystography is lipid-soluble and contains iodine. It is absorbed from the intestine and transferred through the liver to the bile, the majority of it reaching the gall-bladder where it becomes concentrated.

Ultrasound. High definition sector scanners provide an excellent real-time image of the gall-bladder, and the intrahepatic and extra-hepatic bile ducts. The small probe can be used between the ribs and allows scanning with the patient erect. The accuracy in detecting gallstones (Fig. 8) is similar to that of oral cholecystography with the added advantage that the bile ducts may be examined at the same time. A thickened gall-bladder wall is sometimes seen in acute cholecystitis. Dilated hepatic and common bile ducts may be identified and, if the bowel is relatively free from gas, intraductal calculi or an enlarged head of pancreas may be identified. Ultrasound is the initial method of imaging in the jaundiced patient.

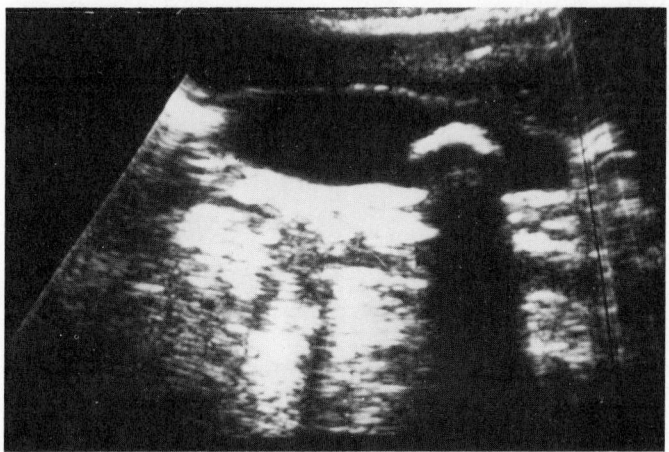

Fig. 8   Ultrasound of the gall-bladder showing a gallstone reflecting the sound and casting a black shadow.

Intravenous cholangiography. Intravenous cholangiography is the method used if examination of the bile ducts is required. The gall-bladder is also opacified unless patients have had a previous cholecystectomy or have cystic duct occlusion. The contrast agents used are water-soluble and are preferentially excreted in the bile.

Intravenous cholangiography is indicated to investigate patients who have had a previous cholecystectomy that present with symptoms suggestive of biliary tract disease or patients who present with episodes of biliary colic and transient jaundice. Combined severe liver and renal disease and monoclonal IgM paraproteinaemia (Waldenström's macroglobulinaemia) must be regarded as absolute contra-indications to the use of intravenous biliary contrast media. Relative contra-indications include a history of asthma or allergy to contrast media or drugs. Normal or near-normal liver function is essential for a satisfactory examination. Intravenous cholangiography should not be carried out within 48 hours of oral cholecystography. When the examination is properly carried out, it is an accurate method for detecting calculi in the bile ducts, assessing the degree of obstruction and the calibre of the bile ducts in patients with chronic pancreatitis, and demonstrating choledochal cysts. Until recently intravenous cholangiography was often performed to assess the gall-bladder and bile ducts in patients whose gall-bladder had failed to opacify at oral cholecystography. Now ultrasound is being used as an alternative procedure for these patients. Likewise, radionuclide scanning is now replacing intravenous cholangiography in the diagnosis of acute cholecystitis.

Radionuclide studies. ^{99}Tc^M HIDA cholescintigraphy is the procedure of choice for investigating suspected acute cholecystitis. It can accurately detect functional obstruction or patency of the cystic duct.

Percutaneous trans-hepatic cholangiography. Percutaneous trans-hepatic cholangiography has been used for some time to demonstrate the bile ducts in obstructive jaundice, but in recent years the introduction of the fine Chiba needle has led to a more widespread use of the technique. The examination is carried out in the X-ray department on a fluoroscopic table with an image intensifier and television monitor. The lateral approach is used as this allows the fine needle to pass through the wide right lobe of the liver before encountering a bile duct and as a result the risk of bile and blood leakage is lessened. Following adequate premedication and with the use of local anaesthesia the needle and stylet are passed through the liver. The stylet is removed and the needle is connected to a syringe containing contrast medium. The needle is slowly withdrawn under fluoroscopic control while contrast medium is gently injected. When contrast medium enters an intrahepatic bile duct withdrawal is halted and the contrast medium is injected to outline the biliary tract. It may be necessary to repeat the procedure a number of times before an intrahepatic bile duct is entered.

Common bile duct calculi (Fig. 9), carcinoma of the head of the pancreas, cholangiocarcinoma, and benign bile duct strictures are the most common causes of extrahepatic bile duct obstruction. The

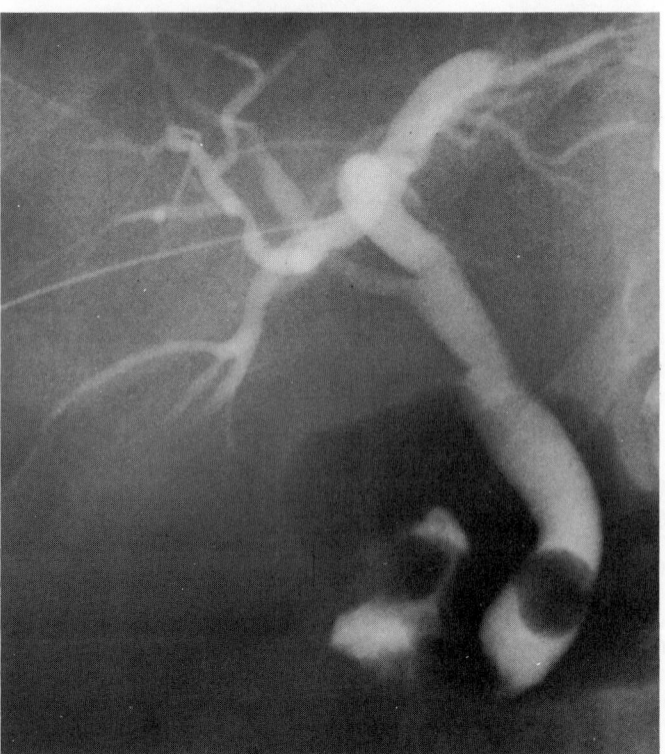

Fig. 9 A calculus is shown in the common bile duct at percutaneous transhepatic cholangiography. The patient presented with obstructive jaundice.

success rate of visualizing the biliary tract is 95–100 per cent in patients with extrahepatic bile duct obstruction and 60–80 per cent in patients with non-dilated ducts. Contra-indications to percutaneous trans-hepatic cholangiography include a bleeding tendency, cholangitis, ascites, and a history of allergy to contrast media.

Patients with normal bile ducts should be carefully monitored for evidence of bleeding or other complications following the procedure. Biliary peritonitis, cholangitis, and septicaemia are most likely to occur in patients with extrahepatic bile duct obstruction and when surgery is indicated it should be carried out without delay.

Percutaneous trans-hepatic catheterization of the bile ducts is now being used as a therapeutic procedure in patients with bile duct obstruction due to inoperable lesions. It is performed following fine needle percutaneous trans-hepatic cholangiography whilst the bile ducts are still outlined with contrast medium. Internal drainage can be performed by passing a catheter through the liver and the bile ducts and through the obstructive lesion to the duodenum. The side-holes in the catheter are positioned above and below the obstructive lesion, allowing the bile to pass from the proximal ducts to the duodenum. Insertion of an endoprosthesis via the percutaneous trans-hepatic route is also possible in patients with benign or malignant biliary strictures as an alternative to surgery in selected cases.

Endoscopic retrograde cholangiopancreatography (ERCP). Cannulation of the papilla of Vater under direct vision through a duodenoscope combined with injection of contrast medium to outline the bile and pancreatic ducts is a very useful diagnostic procedure. It is used to demonstrate the ducts in obstructive jaundice when a satisfactory percutaneous cholangiogram is unlikely because of the size of the ducts, and in the investigation of patients with suspected bile duct disease when the findings at intravenous cholangiography are equivocal. It is also possible to carry out endoscopic papillotomy during the procedure and thus relieve obstructive jaundice by releasing bile duct calculi.

The pancreas. The plain radiograph of the upper abdomen is an important investigation in patients presenting with symptoms of acute or chronic disease of the pancreas. In acute pancreatitis it may show the colon 'cut-off' sign, a sentinel loop, evidence of displacement of the stomach, or of a pancreatic abscess. Pancreatic calcification may be seen in patients with chronic pancreatitis.

Barium studies. Displacement of the stomach may be caused by a pseudocyst of the pancreas and in such cases the barium examination can be a useful diagnostic procedure. Hypotonic duodenography often shows a double contour or reversed 3 sign of Frostberg which is characteristic of carcinoma of the head of the pancreas. Barium studies have been replaced by the newer imaging techniques in most centres, mainly because barium remains in the gastrointestinal tract for some time and obscures detail if other investigations are required.

Ultrasound. Ultrasound allows the measurement of size and the visualization of parenchyma of the pancreas. Acute pancreatitis, tumours, and pseudocysts may be identified and, if a neoplasm is diagnosed, it may be biopsied using a Chiba needle guided by ultrasound. Ultrasound is often used to investigate epigastric masses with the advantage that other organs in the region of the pancreas including the aorta, para-aortic lymph nodes, and adrenal glands may be seen.

Computerized tomography (see page 12.9). The ability of high-resolution computerized tomography (CT) to detect small intra-pancreatic pseudocysts, pseudocysts containing gas or solid contents, pancreatic calcification, and peripancreatic fascial thickening make it the most accurate method for evaluating pancreatitis. Accurate assessment of carcinoma of the pancreas is also possible with CT, particularly when combined with ERCP.

Retrograde pancreatography. Endoscopic retrograde cholangiopancreatography (ERCP) is an extremely useful procedure in the diagnosis of carcinoma of the pancreas and chronic pancreatitis. It is an accurate technique for detecting carcinoma of the pancreas; tapered strictures or occlusions of the main pancreatic duct are seen (Fig. 10). The signs of chronic pancreatitis include stricturing and irregular dilatation of the pancreatic duct, retention cyst formation, and duct concrements.

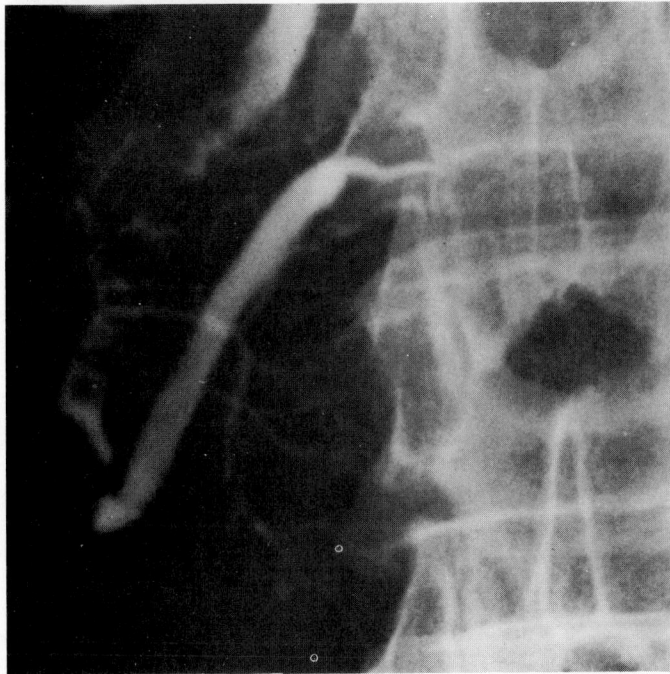

Fig. 10   Carcinoma of the body of the pancreas is shown at endoscopic pancreatography. A tapered occlusion of the main duct has produced a 'rat-tail' appearance. (Reproduced from Baddeley, Nolan, and Salmon (1978), by permission.)

Angiography. Coeliac angiography will usually show insulinomas of the pancreas (Fig. 11), but trans-hepatic portal catheterization will allow samples of blood to be taken from the splenic vein to localize insulinomas if angiography is unsuccessful.

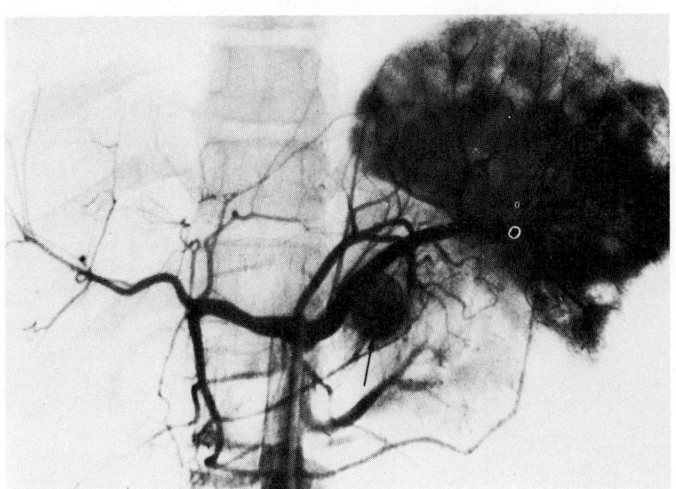

Fig. 11   Subtraction film of a coeliac angiogram of a ten-year-old girl with an insulinoma of the pancreas (arrow).

The spleen (See Section 19.) A plain radiograph will usually show an enlarged spleen as is found in blood disorders, disorders of the reticulo-endothelial system, infection, hepatic cirrhosis, and trauma. A single area of calcification may be seen in atherosclerosis or aneurysm of the splenic artery. Multiple calcifications occur in healed tuberculosis, phleboliths, haemangiomas, and histoplasmosis.

The spleen can be examined by radio-isotopes and this may be particularly useful in trauma or where a small splenunculus is suspected. Ultrasound may be employed to measure splenic size and in identifying splenic cysts whilst computerized tomography shows the spleen well and is useful following trauma.

Portal phlebography may be performed by injecting contrast medium directly into the spleen in order to show that the portal vein is patent and to identify oesophageal or other varices. The anatomical information provided is helpful to a surgeon contemplating a porto-caval shunt.

Trans-hepatic portal phlebography is performed by inserting a catheter through the liver into the portal vein. This technique allows obliteration of oesophageal varices to be undertaken.

References

Alavi, A. (1980). Scintigraphic demonstration of acute gastrointestinal bleeding. *Gastroint. Radiol.* **5**, 205.

Allison, D. J. (1980). Gastrointestinal bleeding—radiological diagnosis. *Br. J. hosp. Med.* **23**, 358.

Baddeley, H., Nolan, D. J., and Salmon, P. R. (1978). *Radiological atlas of biliary and pancreatic disease.* HM.+M, Aylesbury.

Dooley, J. S., Dick, R., Irving, D., Olney, J., and Sherlock, S. (1981). Relief of bile duct obstruction by the percutaneous transhepatic insertion of an endoprosthesis. *Clin. Radiol.* **32**, 163.

Foley, W. D., Stewart, E. T., Lawson, T. L., Geenan, J., Loguidice, J., Maher, L., and Unger, G. F. (1980). Computed tomography, ultrasonography and endoscopic retrograde cholangio pancreatography in the diagnosis of pancreatic disease: a comparative study. *Gastroint. Radiol.* **5**, 29.

Gelfand, D. W. (1975). The double-contrast upper gastrointestinal examination in the Japanese style. *Am. J. Gastroent.* **63**, 216.

Lunderquist, A. and Vang, J. (1974). Transhepatic catheterization and obliteration of the coronary vein in patients with portal hypertension and oesophageal varices. *New Engl. J. Med.* **291**, 646.

Miller, R. E. and Lehman, G. (1978). Polypoid colonic lesions undetected by endoscopy. *Radiology* **129**, 295.

Muto, T., Bussey, H. J. R., and Morson, B. C. (1975). The evolution of cancer of the colon and rectum. *Cancer* **36**, 2251.

Nolan, D. J. (1980). *The double-contrast barium meal. A radiological atlas.* HM.+M, Aylesbury.

— (1981). Barium examination of the small intestine. Progress report. *Gut* **22**, 682.

Sellink, J. L. (1976). *Radiological atlas of common diseases of the small bowel.* Stenfert Kroese, Leiden.

Smith, F. W., Mallard, J. R., Read, A., and Hutchison, J. M. S. (1981). Nuclear magnetic resonance. Tomographic imaging in liver disease. *Lancet* **i**, 963.

Weissmann, H. S., Frank, M. S., Bernstein, L. H., and Freeman, L. M. (1979). Rapid and accurate diagnosis of acute cholecystitis with [99]TcM HIDA cholescintigraphy. *Am. J. Roent.* **132**, 523.

COMPUTERIZED TOMOGRAPHY

R. Dick

Computerized tomography (CT) in the investigation of gastroenterological disorders is mainly used for the diagnosis of liver and pancreatic disease. It may also be useful in detecting retroperitoneal tumours, abdominal lymph node enlargement, and intra-abdominal abscesses.

Computerized tomography of the liver and biliary system. Due to its bulk and relationships the liver is well suited for examination by CT (Fig. 1). Abnormalities of size and shape are well demonstrated. It is particularly effective in focal lesions, the attenuation number giving an accurate indication as to the nature of the abnormal tissue (cyst, abscess, neoplasm). Most primary and secondary neoplasms show diminished attenuation, compared with the normal tissue (Fig. 2). CT shows calcification, not visible on routine X-rays or standard tomography. Occasionally, neoplasms are

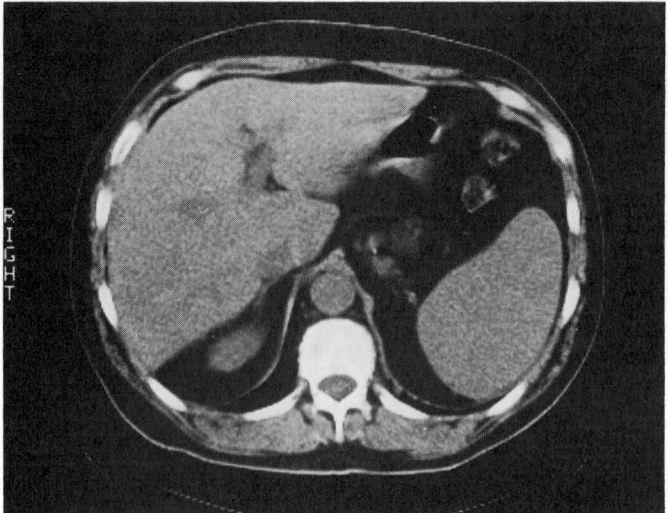

Fig. 1   CT scan of the normal liver: the portal vein is seen at the hilum, the linear branching structure within the right lobe of the liver being portal vein tributaries. Anterior to the inferior vena cava lies the caudate lobe.

isodense and only an alteration in liver contour can be seen. Intravenous contrast media may be given to highlight the difference between normal and abnormal tissue.

Cysts are well shown down to a diameter of 1.5 cm, their attenuation value being 0–20 Hounsfield units.

Infiltration of liver by fat or iron causes a dramatic change in liver density which can be well shown on CT. As yet, however, CT is not of great help in demonstrating the cirrhotic liver.

The gall-bladder and biliary ducts are not as reliably shown as by ultrasound. Faster scanners, with an improved image quality, should result in better quality CT of the liver and biliary system.

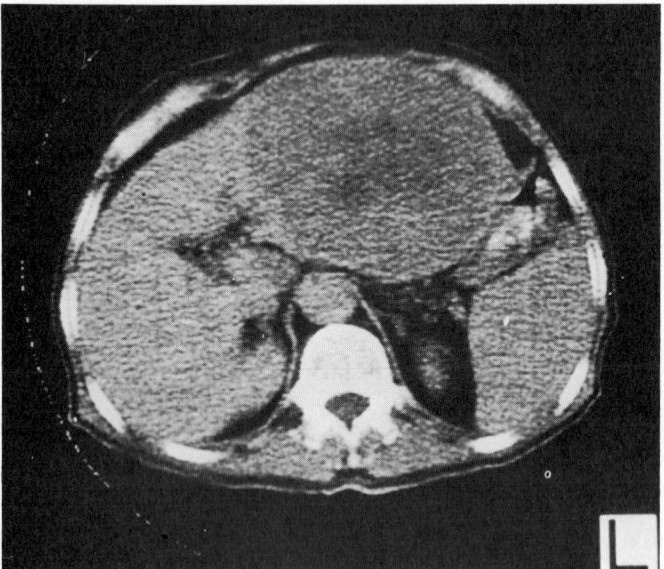

Fig. 2   CT scan of the liver: enlarged left lobe with deformed anterior border, due to primary liver cancer (decreased attenuation).

Computerized tomography of the pancreas. As the pancreas lies in the transverse axial plane, it is an organ well suited to CT. It is the best current technique for showing pancreatic morphology, being especially good for lesions in the pancreatic head, an area where ultrasound may have difficulty because of surrounding gas.

CT scanning of pancreas is performed with the patient supine. The organ is well seen in most patients as it is surrounded by a layer of retroperitoneal fat. The head, neck, body, and tail may be seen

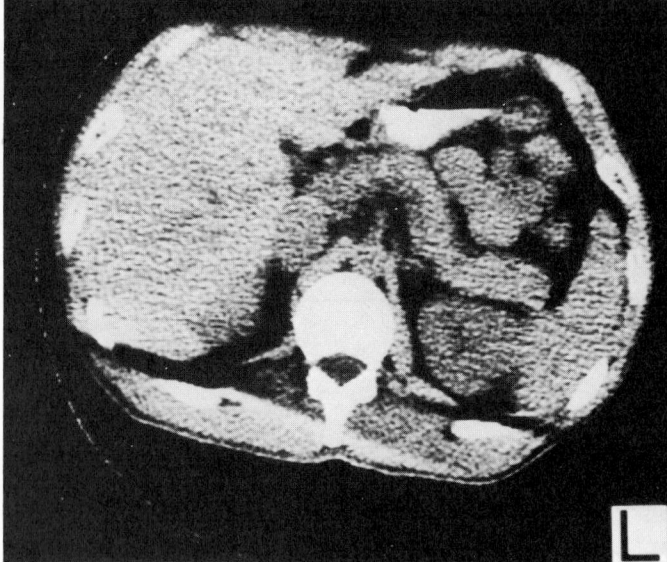

Fig. 3   CT scan of the normal pancreas: the head, neck, body, and tail are well demonstrated on one slice.

on one cut (Fig. 3) or on 1-cm sequential cuts. If the head is not well seen, CT may be repeated with the patient lying on the right side to allow gastrograffin to gravitate into the duodenal loop.

Abnormalities seen include local enlargement, suggesting neoplasm (Fig. 4), general enlargement with loss of peripancreatic fat planes (acute pancreatitis), and calcification, cyst formation, or dilatation of the pancreatic duct (chronic pancreatitis). Fine needle aspiration biopsy may be readily performed under CT control.

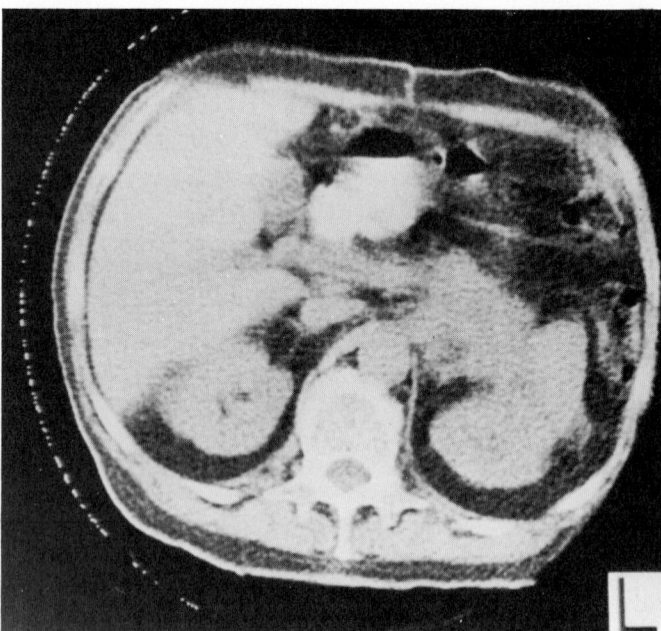

Fig. 4   Irregular mass affecting the tail of the pancreas with an attachment to the left kidney and spleen. Carcinoma.

References

Hounsfield, G. N. (1976). Computerized tomography. In *Topics in gastro-enterology*, vol. 4 (eds. S. C. Truelove and J. A. Ritchie), 299. Blackwell Scientific Publications, Oxford.

Stephens, D. H., Hattery, R. R., and Sheedy, P. F. (1976). CT of the abdomen; early experience with the EMI body scanner. *Radiology* **119**, 331.

LIVER BIOPSY

J. M. Trowell

Percutaneous liver biopsy is a useful investigation in many patients with liver disease. However, it is not without risks and should never be performed by inexperienced clinicians or without appropriate indications.

Indications. 1. Patients with acute liver dysfunction, where the aetiology of the liver damage is not clear. It is rarely necessary in patients with extrahepatic obstruction as there are other techniques which are usually available and which demonstrate the bile ducts and localize the lesion more precisely.

2. After two to three months in patients with acute hepatitis. This is to discover if progression to chronic active hepatitis has occurred.

3. If chronic liver disease is suspected, to determine the aetiology and to see whether irreversible changes have occurred.

4. In patients with unexplained hepatosplenomegaly to establish a diagnosis.

5. Assessment of treatment in patients with chronic liver disease, for example, patients with haemochromatosis treated with venesection or chronic active hepatitis treated with corticosteroids.

6. In various systemic diseases to determine whether there is hepatic involvement and to make a histological diagnosis, e.g. lymphoma, tuberculosis, storage disease.

7. To determine tissue iron levels such as in patients with primary haemochromatosis or iron loading anaemias (see Section 19).

8. Tumours, either primary or secondary, in the liver can be diagnosed histologically by needle biopsy, although if they are localized and predominantly in the left lobe of the liver, it may be difficult to do this safely without laparoscopic visualization of the tumour.

Contra-indications. All contra-indications are a measure of the relative risk of the procedure and in many instances experienced physicians may decide that the specific risks can be overcome and that the value to be obtained by liver biopsy outweighs the additional risks of the procedure.

1. Lack of co-operation of the patient greatly increases the risk attached to the biopsy which is done with the patient conscious and holding his or her breath in expiration. Lack of co-operation may be the result of confusion or coma, or because of a language or other communication problem. A patient who for any reason is reluctant to have a liver biopsy may not be entirely compliant, and children are usually not able to co-operate and require a general anaesthetic.

2. Patients must be able to lie flat and hold their breath for a few seconds and it is therefore not possible to carry out a biopsy in those with cardiorespiratory failure. The classical route for needle biopsy is transpleural with a slight risk of pneumothorax and this is an additional reason for avoiding the procedure in any patient with reduced respiratory reserve.

3. Any bleeding tendency is a relative contra-indication and

before the procedure clotting and haemostatic function, normally assessed by the prothrombin time and platelet count, should be measured. It is frequently possible to correct a bleeding tendency if the biopsy is thought to be essential, and appropriate platelet concentrates or clotting factors can be infused prior to biopsy.

4. Ascites and a right pleural effusion add greatly to the technical problems of the biopsy, and if it is essential, it may be necessary to drain some fluid before the procedure is undertaken. For similar reasons subphrenic abscess or empyema may make the technique difficult, with the added problem of dissemination of infection.

5. Biopsy should be avoided in patients suspected of having intrahepatic abscesses or cysts. Although they may be treated by needling, liver tissue may not be obtained for histological examination, and there are technical problems for the inexperienced. If hydatid disease of the liver is suspected percutaneous liver biopsy should *not* be undertaken.

6. Obstruction to the large bile ducts increases the pressure within the biliary system, and needling with the relatively large needles required to obtain a liver biopsy may precipitate a bile leak and biliary peritonitis. If the bile ducts are dilated, any needling should be restricted to the small needle used for trans-hepatic cholangiography which has the advantage of visualizing the bile ducts and demonstrating the anatomy prior to surgical correction.

7. Hepatic angiomas may bleed profusely even after a well-performed liver biopsy.

Complications. Pleuritic pain, sometimes referred to the shoulder, occurs quite often and requires mild analgesia. The most serious complications are bleeding, so that procedure should always be followed by a period of close observation for 24 hours, and biliary peritonitis which was considered earlier. The incidence of serious complications from this procedure is in the region of one per 1000 biopsies, or less.

References

Mendhini, G. (1970). One second biopsy of the liver—problem of its clinical application. *New Engl. J. Med.* **283**, 582.

Scheuer, P. J. (1980). *Liver biopsy interpretation*, 3rd edn. Baillière Tindall. London.

Sherlock, S. (1981). *Diseases of the liver and biliary system*, 6th edn., 44. Blackwell Scientific Publications, Oxford.

OTHER DIAGNOSTIC METHODS USED IN GASTROINTESTINAL AND HEPATIC DISEASES

Other diagnostic methods are described in the sections which follow; these include small intestinal biopsy (page 12.89), liver function tests (page 12.177), pancreatic function tests (page 12.162), and motility tests (page 12.38).

Symptomatology of gastrointestinal disease

D. P. Jewell

Gastrointestinal diseases frequently occur in the absence of symptoms, e.g. peptic ulcers, carcinomas, and Crohn's disease. When symptoms occur, they are protean. The following account is selective for the major symptoms, namely: vomiting, abdominal pain, diarrhoea, constipation, gastrointestinal bleeding, and dysphagia.

Vomiting

Vomiting is a common symptom associated with many gastrointestinal disorders—functional, inflammatory, and obstructive. In addition it may be a symptom of many other non-gastroenterological conditions which include: infections, metabolic disturbances, migraine, travel sickness, pregnancy, myocardial infarction, drug toxicity, raised intracranial pressure, and psychogenic syndromes.

The act of vomiting consists of three stages. The first stage is that of nausea during which there is reduced motor activity of the stomach but an increase in the activity of the duodenum and jejunum. This allows reflux of duodenal contents into the stomach. Retching is the next stage during which there are a series of contractions of the chest muscles and diaphragm associated with the simultaneous contraction of the abdominal muscles, the glottis remaining closed. During these spasms, gastric contents reflux freely into the lower oesophagus. Finally, there is a powerful and sustained contraction of the abdominal muscles with descent of the diaphragm causing a large rise in intra-abdominal pressure and emesis occurs.

The neurophysiology of vomiting has been worked out mainly in the cat. The pathways are probably similar for man but obviously this has not been completely proven. The vomiting centre is situated in the reticular formation of the medulla and is excited directly by visceral impulses from the gastrointestinal tract. It is closely associated with the centres for salivation and respiration which probably explains the hypersalivation and respiratory disturbances which are usually associated with vomiting. In addition, there is a chemoreceptor trigger zone in the floor of the fourth ventricle which is stimulated by drugs such as morphine, digoxin, and anaesthetics, but this only initiates vomiting if the vomiting centre is intact. Nausea and vomiting due to travel sickness, uraemia, and diabetic ketoacidosis are also mediated by prior stimulation of the chemoreceptor trigger zone. Other receptors and areas of the medulla may also be involved in causing vomiting but, whatever the trigger, all the emetic responses are mediated via reflex arcs which pass through the vomiting centre.

Clinical features. Vomiting in the morning soon after waking is characteristic of pregnancy, alcoholism, and metabolic disturbances such as uraemia. It may also occur following gastric surgery. Vomiting associated with psychological disorders usually occurs during or soon after a meal. Pyloric canal ulcers may also cause vomiting immediately after a meal. Delayed vomiting (more than one hour after a meal) is the usual pattern associated with peptic ulcer, gastric carcinoma, gall-bladder disease, and intestinal obstruction. Projectile vomiting, which is the forceful ejection of vomitus without retching, is often seen in pyloric stenosis and is said to occur in patients with raised intracranial pressure.

The content of the vomitus may provide some diagnostic clues. Vomiting of undigested food suggests that it is regurgitation secondary to achalasia, an oesophageal stricture, or a pharyngeal diverticulum. Intestinal contents in the vomitus suggest intestinal obstruction or ileus and the vomit usually has a faecal odour. Bilious vomiting characteristically occurs following gastric surgery. Altered blood ('coffee-grounds') is of obvious significance.

Patients who are vomiting because of delayed gastric emptying (whether due to outlet obstruction or to gastric atony) may show gastric distension on physical examination and a succussion splash may be present. Visible peristalsis may be seen in patients with gastric outlet or intestinal obstruction.

Metabolic consequences. Prolonged vomiting causes a metabolic alkalosis and hypokalaemia. Potassium deficiency results from a reduced intake, potassium loss in the vomit, and renal loss. The renal loss is due to hyperaldosteronism secondary to salt and water deficiency with contraction of the plasma volume. Alkalosis occurs because of the loss of H^+ in the vomit and also because there is a shift of H^+ into cells in response to potassium depletion.

Treatment. Treatment partly depends on the cause of the vomiting. For nausea and vomiting associated with vestibular disorders (Ménière's disease, middle-ear diseases), hyoscine, antihistamines, and phenothiazines may be useful. However, phenothiazines are ineffective for travel sickness; hyoscine or an anticholinergic (e.g.

cinnarizine, cyclizine, or dimenhydrate) should be used. Nausea and vomiting of pregnancy should not be treated if at all possible. If therapy is required, an antihistamine should be given. Phenothiazines, metoclopramide, and dicyclomine should be avoided. Phenothiazines are particularly beneficial when vomiting is caused by agents acting on the chemoreceptor trigger zone (e.g. drugs, metabolic disturbances). For nausea and vomiting secondary to gastrointestinal disease, metoclopramide is the drug of choice. As well as acting centrally, it also acts locally to increase the peristaltic activity of the stomach and to increase the lower oesophageal sphincter pressure.

Specific syndromes. Psychogenic vomiting. Chronic and recurrent vomiting due to psychological causes is not uncommon and mainly affects women. There is often a long history of vomiting (e.g. vomiting associated with school examinations) and there may be a family history. Vomiting normally occurs after a meal but can usually be suppressed until the patient reaches a bathroom or lavatory. Vomiting is frequently a feature of patients with anorexia nervosa (see Section 8) and then it is often initiated by inserting a finger into the pharynx. Although organic disease must be excluded, the diagnosis should be recognized quickly and extensive investigation avoided. Treatment is difficult since anti-emetics are not usually beneficial. Psychiatric assessment and psychotherapy may be helpful (see also page 12.46).

Cyclical vomiting. This is a syndrome that occurs in children and is characterized by recurrent attacks of severe vomiting, which may last for several days. The onset is sudden and may be associated with headache, abdominal pain, and, occasionally, fever. Vomiting may be severe enough to cause profound dehydration and alkalosis. The syndrome usually starts before the age of six and the frequency of the attacks varies from more than one a month to one or two each year. The cause is unknown but the many hypotheses that have been put forward include: epilepsy, migraine, psychogenic, peri- and post-natal brain damage. Organic disease, especially intracranial pathology, must be excluded. Most children gradually improve with increasing age and the attacks usually stop by the end of puberty.

Abdominal pain

Table 1 summarizes the main causes of abdominal pain.

The abdominal viscera are insensitive to cutting, tearing, and crushing, but they are sensitive to distension or tension. The nerve endings of the hollow organs are found in the muscle layers of the wall, whereas for solid organs (liver, kidneys, spleen), they are found in the capsule. The sensory nerves may also be stimulated by inflammation, ischaemia, or direct involvement by neoplasms.

Since the viscera mostly receive afferents from both sides of the spinal cord, the pain is usually midline, dull, and poorly localized to the epigastrium, peri-umbilical area, or hypogastrium. It may be described as colicy, burning, or the gnawing sensation of hunger pains.

Parietal pain arises from the parietal peritoneum as a result of inflammation. The pain is usually sharp and can be precisely located. It is usually exacerbated by movement or coughing.

Referred pain is felt in skin or muscles remote from the affected organ and is due to the sharing of central pathways by the peripheral neurones. Examples of referred pain are the back and leg pain associated with intestinal distension.

Nerve pathways. Although 90 per cent of the nerve fibres in the vagus are sensory, none of them transmit pain. The ability to feel abdominal pain is therefore unaltered by vagotomy. The main pathways by which painful stimuli are relayed to the spinal cord are shown in Table 2. Following relay in the dorsal root ganglion, fibres are transmitted in the posterior horn and the tract of Lissauer to synapse in the reticular formation and thalamus. From there, pain

Table 1 Causes of abdominal pain

Intra-abdominal
Generalized peritonitis
Perforated viscus; primary infective peritonitis; rupture of cyst
Localized peritonitis
Appendicitis; cholecystitis; pancreatitis; abscesses; salpingitis
Motility disorders
Intestinal obstruction; biliary obstruction; ureteric
obstruction; irritable colon; diverticulosis; uterine contraction
Ischaemia
Mesenteric angina/infarction; splenic infarction; torsion—
ovarian cyst, testicle, omentum; tumour necrosis—hepatoma,
fibroid
Other
Peptic ulcer; inflammatory diseases; retroperitoneal tumours

Extra-abdominal
Thoracic
Lung disease; ischaemic heart disease; oesophageal disease
Neurological
Herpes zoster; spinal arthritis; radiculopathy from tumours;
tabes dorsalis; abdominal epilepsy
Metabolic
Diabetes mellitus; chronic renal failure; porphyria; acute
adrenal insufficiency
Toxins
Snake and insect bites; lead poisoning; strychnine

Table 2 Nerve pathways from the abdominal viscera to the spinal cord

Oesophagus	Un-named sympathetic nerves
Liver, spleen	Phrenic nerve (C3–C5)
Gall-bladder Pancreas, stomach Small intestine	Coeliac plexus, greater splanchnic nerves (T6–T9)
Appendix, colon Pelvic viscera	Mesenteric plexus, lesser splanchnic nerves (T11–L1)
Kidneys, bladder Rectum	Pelvic nerve (S2–S4)

impulses are relayed to the post-central gyrus at which point pain is experienced.

Pain from specific viscera. Pain from the *oesophagus* is felt retrosternally and is usually felt at the site of disease. It may occasionally radiate and can mimic cardiac pain. The Bernstein acid infusion test may be useful clinically in reproducing the pain of oesophagitis. Severe oesophageal pain is referred into the back. Pain from the *stomach* and *duodenum* is usually mid-line in the epigastrium or in the right upper quadrant. Again, it may be felt in the back. *Small intestinal* pain is central and mid-line, usually colicy and radiating into the back. *Colonic* pain can be felt centrally, along the line of the colon, or in the hypogastrium. It is often poorly localized but frequently radiates into the back or into the thighs. Pain from the *gallbladder* and *bile duct* is colicy and is felt in the right upper quadrant. Characteristically it is also felt in the back, between the scapulae or in the right shoulder tip. *Pancreatic* pain is epigastric and mid-line, and radiates into the back. As with *retroperitoneal* pain, pancreatic pain is often made better by curling up and is aggravated by lying flat.

Diagnosis. The major features of the pain to be determined are: site, intensity, character, timing, and aggravating and relieving factors. Associated symptoms, such as bowel disturbance, vomiting, heartburn, and urinary and gynaecological symptoms must be

elicited. Physical examination will reveal areas of abdominal tenderness, rebound tenderness, and rigidity. Abdominal distension or visible peristalsis must be looked for. Organ enlargement and the presence of masses must be excluded. A rectal examination is essential. The hernial orifices should be carefully examined and the abdomen should be auscultated for bruits. General examination may reveal the presence of fever, tachycardia, jaundice, weight loss, or anaemia.

Investigation of abdominal pain will be directed by the clinical findings. However, in cases of chronic pain it is not usually possible to make a firm clinical diagnosis as the symptom complexes of many diseases overlap, e.g. gastric ulcer, gastric carcinoma, duodenal ulcer, gallstones, or irritable colon syndrome. Radiological and endoscopic investigations will therefore be necessary. The diagnosis of specific disorders is dealt with in the appropriate sections.

The acute abdomen. Acute inflammation of any of the abdominal viscera, perforation of a hollow organ, rupture of a cyst, intestinal or ureteric obstruction, strangulation of an intestinal loop, or an aortic dissection can all present as an acute abdomen. Diagnosis rests on the history, the exact site and nature of the pain, the findings on physical examination, and the results of emergency investigations: white blood cell count, plain abdominal X-rays and, if necessary, an intravenous pyelogram (see page 12.148).

Diarrhoea

Diarrhoea is one of the commonest symptoms encountered in medical practice. The major mechanisms in the production of diarrhoea are: an increased osmotic load, increased secretion into the intestinal lumen, the failure of electrolyte absorption, and an altered intestinal motility (Table 3). Obviously the diarrhoea associated with any one disease may involve more than one of these mechanisms, e.g. the diarrhoea of ulcerative colitis may be due to failure to absorb ions from the colon, increased salt and water secretion, and a disturbance in colon motility.

Table 3 Mechanisms of diarrhoea

Osmotic
Disaccharidase deficiency
Magnesium salts
Secretory
1. Associated with activation of adenylate cyclase
Bacterial enterotoxin (*Vibrio cholerae*, *Escherichia coli*); prostaglandins; vasoactive intestinal polypeptide (VIP); dihydroxy bile acids; theophylline, caffeine
2. Not proven to be associated with adenylate cyclate activation
Serotonin; cholecystokinin; laxatives (phenolphthalein, oxyphenisatin); bacterial enterotoxins (*Clostridium difficile*, *Staphylococcus aureus*, *Shigella dysenteriae*); villous adenoma
Failure of ion absorption
Congenital chloridorrhoea
Bile acids in the colon (following ileal resection)
Hydroxy fatty acids in the colon (steatorrhoea)
Inflammatory diseases
Deranged intestinal motility
Irritable colon syndrome
Diverticulosis
Tumours
Inflammatory diseases

Clinical assessment. The following points must be determined:
1. Is the diarrhoea acute or chronic?
2. What is the consistency of stool—watery, loose, or fatty?
3. What is the volume or weight of stool?
4. Is there a non-gastrointestinal cause—thyrotoxicosis,

medullary carcinoma of the thyroid, neurogenic diarrhoea (e.g. diabetes mellitus)?

5. Is steatorrhoea present or absent?

6. Are pathogenic bacteria and parasites (e.g. giardiasis, helminthic infestations) present or absent?

7. Is inflammatory or neoplastic disease of the intestine present or absent?

8. Can cholestasis and chronic pancreatitis be excluded?

In patients who have chronic diarrhoea with no adequate explanation, it is particularly important to measure stool volume. Secretory diarrhoea nearly always produces an output of at least 1.5 l/24 hours. It may also be useful to give the patient intravenous fluids and nothing by mouth. Osmotic diarrhoeas stop under these conditions, but a secretory diarrhoea usually persists. There are exceptions, however. For example, secretory diarrhoea caused by unabsorbed fatty acids and bile salts usually lessens with fasting. Nevertheless, this simple test can be useful if a vipoma or laxative abuse is suspected. *Laxative abuse* is notoriously difficult to diagnose. The presence of melanosis coli (see page 12.155) on sigmoidoscopy and in the rectal biopsy suggests prolonged ingestion of senna. The stools should always be tested with alkali for the presence of phenolphthalein and measurement of the magnesium content is useful in the rare patient who is purging himself with magnesium salts. Locker searches are an essential part of the investigations. Drugs should always be considered as a cause of diarrhoea and this includes alcohol. *Chronic alcoholism* may present as diarrhoea and may be misdiagnosed as an irritable colon syndrome. The mechanism of the diarrhoea is unclear although alcohol is known to cause abnormalities in enterocyte function and there may be disturbances of villous architecture. *Food allergy* as a cause of diarrhoea is a controversial issue. Patients with an eosinophilic gastroenteritis, many of whom appear to be sensitive to milk proteins, have diarrhoea or even steatorrhoea. However, the majority of patients who claim an association between individual foods and diarrhoea have a histologically normal intestine. Once *hypolactasia* has been eliminated, then the majority are probably examples of the *irritable colon syndrome*. Nevertheless, when patients are strongly atopic, it is worth attempting to treat with elimination diets.

Treatment. The primary aim is to treat the underlying cause of the diarrhoea. Symptomatic treatments for diarrhoea are grossly oversubscribed and their only major indication is in the control of infective diarrhoeas once the specific antibiotic therapy (if indicated) has been given and also in the management of antibiotic-induced diarrhoea. Patients with ulcerative colitis or Crohn's disease rarely need antidiarrhoeal agents and, indeed, the opiate derivatives may be dangerous. Patients with the irritable colon syndrome should be treated as described on page 12.46.

The major antidiarrhoeal agents are codeine phosphate, lomotil (diphenoxylate hydrochloride and atropine), loperamide, and the bulking agents which also act as absorbants (e.g. methyl cellulose, ispaghula, fybogel). If patients have associated pain, opiates usually increase the pain and should be avoided. Loperamide is probably the most effective agent but it is also the most expensive.

Constipation (see also page 12.46)

There is no universally accepted definition of constipation but it usually implies a diminished stool frequency and the passage of hard small stools (see also page 12.46). Some patients complain of constipation when they have the feeling of incomplete evacuation.

Diet plays a major role in stool frequency and consistency. High fibre diets decrease the colonic transit time, increase faecal weight, and lead to a softer, bulkier stool.

Constipation may be a symptom of colonic or anal disease but may also be caused by a wide variety of non-gastrointestinal disorders (Table 4). Investigation of constipation will depend upon which group of disorders is thought to be present. A history, clinical

Table 4 Causes of constipation

Motility disorders
  Irritable colon syndrome; diverticulosis; megacolon from laxative abuse

Intestinal obstruction

Anal and rectal disease
  Proctitis; anal fissure; mucosal prolapse

Drugs
  Analgesics; antacids (aluminium compounds); anticholinergics; iron tablets; tricyclic antidepressants; lead poisoning

Metabolic and endocrine disorders
  Diabetes; hypokalaemia; hypothyroidism; hypercalcaemia; phaeochromocytoma; pregnancy; porphyria

Neurological disorders
  Aganglionosis (Hirschsprung's disease); pseudo-obstruction; Chagas' disease; spinal cord lesions—paraplegia, cauda equina tumour, meningocoele, tabes dorsalis; cerebral lesions—Parkinson's disease, cerebrovascular disease

examination, and some simple laboratory investigations are usually sufficient to decide whether the constipation is due to a gastrointestinal cause in which case a barium enema is indicated. Hypothyroidism, hypercalcaemia, and drugs are fairly frequent causes of constipation in patients presenting to a gastroenterological clinic and the true diagnosis can easily be missed. Assessment of colonic transit time by radiopaque markers, for example, or measurement of intra-colonic pressures is rarely necessary for standard clinical practice.

Treatment. Treatment will depend on the underlying cause of the constipation. The following account assumes that no underlying metabolic, endocrine, or structural abnormality has been found (see page 12.47).

Therapeutic agents

Hydrophilic bulking agents. These include dietary fibre and the hemicelluloses which are polysaccharides of plant origin. Patients should be advised to take a high fibre diet which includes wholemeal bread and plenty of fresh vegetables and fruit. However, it is often necessary to supplement the diet with either bran itself or a pharmaceutical preparation such as methylcellulose, an ispaghula husk preparation (Isogel, Metamucil, Fybogel), or a sterculia gum (Normacol).

Chemical laxatives. These agents include the anthraquinone glycosides, bisacodyl (Dulcolax), antispasmodics, lactulose, castor oil, and local treatment in the form of suppositories or enemas.

The anthraquinone glycosides are mainly senna, cascara, frangula, and rhubarb. The precise mode of action is unknown but they stimulate peristalsis in the colon with very little effect on the small intestine. Free anthraquinone (e.g. Danthron) is probably less effective and more toxic than senna. Prolonged usage of these agents causes melanosis coli, which is probably of no clinical significance, and a cathartic megacolon. The aetiology of the megacolon may in fact be due to a direct toxic effect on the myenteric plexuses of the colonic wall. Hypokalaemia from excessive purgation may be a contributing factor.

Antispasmodic agents include anticholinergic agents (e.g. propantheline), dicyclomine, and mebeverine. Mebeverine (Colofac) is a phenylethylamine derivative of reserpine and is more specific in its action on the colon than the other two. It has fewer side-effects, such as dry mouth and urinary retention, and is the drug of choice in first-line management.

Lactulose is a non-absorbable disaccharide (one molecule of fructose and one of galactose). It is useful in patients whose colons are full of hard scybala as it softens the stool partly by an osmotic effect and partly by the production of lactic acid and other organic acids caused by the fermenting effect of bacteria. Large doses may have to be given and the laxative effect is often accompanied by abdominal distension and flatus which may be unacceptable to the patient.

Castor oil is hydrolysed in the small intestine with the release of ricinoleic acid. This is a potent irritant to both the small and large intestine. It is only successful as a preparative agent prior to a colonic examination, e.g. barium enema or colonoscopy. It is dangerous for prolonged use as it induces water and electrolyte losses.

Local preparations include large volume washouts with warm normal saline, oil retention enemas (olive oil, arachis oil), and disposable hypertonic saline enemas and suppositories (glycerin, bisacodyl). These agents are frequently useful in the management of constipation in the elderly, in patients with neurological deficits, and in the transient constipation that follows abdominal surgery or bed rest.

Other therapeutic agents. Liquid paraffin is a traditional and widely used laxative but it has many adverse effects and its use should be strongly discouraged. The side-effects include: deficiencies of fat-soluble vitamins as liquid paraffin is a solvent for them, a lipoid pneumonia from aspiration, paraffinomas in mesenteric nodes, liver, spleen, and mucosa due to absorption, and an association with gastrointestinal cancer. Oxyphenisatin has now been withdrawn from the British Pharmacopoeia due to its effect on the liver—chronic administration causes jaundice, hepatomegaly, and a rise in the aspartate transaminase. Histologically, oxyphenisatin produces a lesion resembling chronic active hepatitis.

Dioctyl sodium sulphosuccinate is another widely used laxative. It is an emollient and is thought to act by reducing surface tension and allowing water to penetrate more readily the faecal mass. Its detergent effect may be potentially damaging to the gastrointestinal tract and it must not be used in combination with liquid paraffin as it increases the absorption of the mineral oil.

Gastrointestinal bleeding

The major causes of bleeding from the gastrointestinal tract are listed in Table 5. In terms of diagnosis and management, they are best considered as acute bleeding from either the upper or lower gastrointestinal tract and as chronic bleeding.

Table 5   Causes of gastrointestinal bleeding

Inflammatory
  Oesophagitis; gastritis; peptic ulcer; Crohn's disease; ulcerative colitis; enterocolitis—infective, ischaemic, radiation

Mechanical
  Hiatus hernia; Mallory–Weiss tears; Meckel's diverticulum; diverticulosis coli

Neoplasms
  Carcinoma; polyps—single, multiple; leiomyoma; carcinoid

Vascular
  Varices; hereditary telangiectasia; angioma; aorto-intestinal fistula; mesenteric thrombosis or embolus; arteritis

Systemic
  Chronic renal failure; thrombocytopenia; coagulation defects; connective tissue disorders; dysproteinaemia

Acute upper gastrointestinal bleeding. (See also page 12.62.) This presents as haematemesis and/or melaena. It is very rare for lesions distal to the ligament of Treitz to cause a haematemesis. Brisk bleeding may, however, occur from a proximal lesion, e.g. oeso-phageal varices, without haematemesis and present as melaena. Upper gastrointestinal bleeding can be severe enough to cause the passage of dark red blood per rectum which may cause diagnostic confusion. Table 6 shows the approximate frequency of lesions causing upper gastrointestinal bleeding and has been compiled from a number of recent British series. Bleeding from oesophageal varices is a common cause in those countries where the incidence of

Table 6   Causes of upper gastrointestinal bleeding and their frequency

Duodenal ulcer	35%
Gastric ulcer	20%
Acute gastric erosions	
Haemorrhagic gastritis	18%
Gastric carcinoma	6%
Oesophageal varices	5%
Other	16%

alcoholic cirrhosis is high and is being seen more frequently in Britain. It should be noted that acute bleeding from a gastric carcinoma is relatively uncommon. Bleeding from *Mallory–Weiss tears* usually follows an episode of violent retching. This is particularly common following large volumes of alcohol. The degree of bleeding ranges from a cupful of blood to torrential bleeding. The majority of patients stop bleeding spontaneously and, indeed, the tears may heal within 24 hours. However, occasionally blood loss can be sufficiently prolonged and severe to require emergency surgery. Rare causes of acute bleeding include vascular abnormalities (telangiectasia, angiomata), leiomyoma, haemophilia, thrombocytopenia, Ehlers–Danlos syndrome, pseudoxanthoma elasticum, and rupture of the aorta into the duodenum.

The role of aspirin in initiating bleeding from whatever cause is still controversial. Certainly up to one-third of patients presenting with acute bleeding may have ingested aspirin within the previous 24–48 hours. However, some series have shown a similar proportion of aspirin-takers amongst patients presenting with other acute medical emergencies. All the anti-inflammatory drugs may be associated with bleeding.

Assessment. A rapid clinical assessment must be made before resuscitation is begun. Except in severely shocked patients, the patient should be questioned with regard to dyspepsia, vomiting, alcohol and drugs, previous episodes of bleeding, and jaundice. Pulse, respiratory rate, blood pressure, and the state of the peripheral circulation must be noted and recorded. Specific signs to look for are those of chronic liver disease, iron deficiency, telangiectasia (these may only be present on the under surface of the tongue), and signs of malignancy.

Blood should be taken for cross-matching and for determination of haemoglobin, haematocrit, platelet count, and prothrombin time. A plain X-ray of the abdomen is also useful but can be delayed until resuscitation has begun.

Assessment must be made by the physician and surgeon working as a team so that joint decisions on management can be made.

Management. An intravenous line is set up immediately. Patients who are shocked or who are elderly should have central lines so that central venous pressure can be monitored during subsequent transfusion. Saline should be given initially but, occasionally, uncross-matched blood (blood group O, Rhesus negative), albumin, or plasma expanders may be required if bleeding is severe. Half-hourly observations of pulse, respiratory rate, and blood pressure are instituted although these can be reduced to an hourly pulse, and a two-hourly blood pressure once bleeding has stopped. The use of a nasogastric tube is controversial but it adds to the discomfort of the patient and may cause fresh bleeding. Repeated nasogastric aspiration as a means of detecting a recurrent bleed is less sensitive than observing the pulse rate. Nasogastric tubes can be used for gastric lavage with ice-cold water but there is no good evidence that this is an effective procedure for stopping bleeding and it can no longer be recommended. The use of intravenous cimetidine in the acute stage is common practice but there is little evidence to support this. Small trials have variously reported some benefit in patients bleeding from oesophageal varices, in elderly women bleeding from gastric ulcers, and in patients with upper gastrointestinal bleeding following renal transplantation. However, most studies have shown disappointing results for intravenous cimetidine when used either during a bleeding episode or prophylactically to prevent acute bleeding in patients undergoing intensive care for burns, major trauma, or septicaemia. Continuous intragastric instillation of antacids may be a more beneficial prophylactic measure.

For patients bleeding from oesophageal varices, further procedures may be necessary. Intravenous pitressin (20 units/hr) may be helpful—the arterial route confers no greater advantage. A Sengstaken–Blackemore tube is indicated if bleeding is severe and prolonged and the decision has been made to subsequently obliterate the varices. Percutaneous trans-hepatic or endoscopic sclerosis of the varices or a surgical operation may be considered (see page 12.189). Many patients with chronic liver disease will become encephalopathic during a gastrointestinal bleed and will require the appropriate treatment (see page 12.188).

Endoscopic laser therapy for bleeding peptic ulcers and erosions is currently being evaluated. So far, however, the results are not encouraging for either the argon or the NdYAG laser. Endoscopic diathermy has successfully treated angiomata of the stomach but these are a rare cause of bleeding. Bleeding peptic ulcer is discussed in detail on page 12.62.

Diagnostic procedures. Initially, the management of acute upper gastrointestinal bleeding must consist of restoring the circulation. Once bleeding has stopped, and the patient is in a good haemodynamic state, the diagnosis of the cause of bleeding can begin. Emergency endoscopy or barium meals while the patient is still bleeding and in a state of shock are usually hazardous and often reveal little more than the fact that the stomach is full of blood. However, diagnostic procedures must be done within 12 hours of bleeding since erosions and tears can heal rapidly.

The diagnostic procedure of choice is fibre-optic endoscopy as this will reveal tears and acute erosions of the stomach or duodenum which may frequently be missed radiologically even when air contrast studies are performed. Furthermore, endoscopy allows biopsies to be taken of a gastric ulcer or a tumour if found. If varices are found at endoscopy, it is safe to pass the endoscope through into the oesophagus (especially if a small diameter endoscope is used) and, indeed, it is essential to make a full examination of the stomach and duodenum in order to exclude other causes of bleeding. Even if endoscopy, or radiology, is delayed until bleeding has stopped, the stomach may still be full of clots. If they are troublesome, they can be washed out with a large stomach tube. However, as this procedure can damage the gastric mucosa and the lesions produced may be confusing to the endoscopist, gastric washouts are best avoided.

Angiography should be reserved for patients with continuing bleeding and in whom no cause of bleeding has been found at upper gastrointestinal endoscopy. It is especially useful in detecting angiomata, the presence of duodenal or ileal varices, bleeding from Meckel's diverticulum or non-specific ulcers of the ileum, and small bowel tumours. Small lesions, however, can only be visualized when active bleeding is occurring; this usually means a bleeding rate of at least 0.5 ml/min.

Indications for surgery. As previously stated, all patients presenting with acute upper gastrointestinal bleeding must be assessed by a physician and surgeon working as a team. The precise indications for surgery will partly depend on the cause of bleeding. For bleeding peptic ulcers, the indications are discussed on page 12.62. If bleeding is occurring from a haemorrhagic erosive gastritis, surgery should be avoided if possible as the surgeon may have to perform a total gastrectomy. Bleeding from a carcinoma is rarely severe and continuous enough to require emergency surgery. Mallory–Weiss tears or isolated erosions may require emergency surgery. The managment of bleeding varices is considered elsewhere (see page 12.189).

In general, early surgery can be recommended for elderly pa-

tients once initial resuscitation has been achieved. Continuous bleeding which results in transfusion in excess of eight pints or bleeding to the point at which the central venous pressure cannot be maintained are obvious indications. Patients with recurrent bleeds should also be recommended for early surgery.

Course and progress. This again depends on the cause of bleeding. Patients bleeding from varices and malignant tumours are discussed on pages 12.189 and 12.117. The majority of patients with ulcers and erosions will stop bleeding within a few hours and, if rebleeding does not occur within 48 hours, they can be considered for early discharge from hospital.

The overall mortality of upper gastrointestinal bleeding is about 10–15 per cent and has remained constant over the last 15–20 years. The major mortality, of course, is in the elderly. However, bleeding from a haemorrhagic gastritis also has a high mortality. It is disappointing that early diagnosis or early recourse to surgery have failed to influence the mortality rate or, indeed, the length of hospital stay. Nevertheless, mortality can be reduced considerably if patients are managed in specialized gastroenterological units, where a policy of managment of acute bleeding exists.

Acute colonic bleeding. This usually presents with the passage of fresh blood and clots per rectum. Diverticular disease and tumours of the rectum and colon are the commonest causes. However, ulcerative colitis, Crohn's disease, and ischaemic colitis must be considered. Infectious causes include shigella dysentery, campylobacter, amoebiasis, schistosomiasis. Elderly patients presenting with massive bleeding of sudden onset, especially if they have had a previous episode, are likely to have *angiodysplasia*. This vascular lesion occurs mainly in the caecum and ascending colon but may occur elsewhere in the colon. It is said to be more common in patients with aortic valve disease (see page 12.126).

Management of these patients is similar to that described for upper gastrointestinal bleeding. After initial assessment, intravenous infusion and subsequent transfusion of blood should begin with monitoring of pulse, blood pressure, and central venous pressure if indicated.

Abdominal and rectal examination with sigmoidoscopy may diagnose the cause of bleeding. In general, emergency barium enema or colonoscopy is not practicable while active bleeding exists. An urgent barium enema should be obtained as soon as the colon can be adequately prepared. If negative, then colonscopy is indicated.

Angiodysplasia may be visualized at colonoscopy or, if performed while the patient is bleeding, by angiography. If angiodysplasia is seen endoscopically, it may be treated using the 'hot' biopsy technique, i.e. the passage of a diathermy current while taking a biopsy. An alternative treatment involves injecting thrombosing agents (e.g. thrombin, gel foam) at angiography.

Chronic gastrointestinal bleeding. Chronic gastrointestinal bleeding may present one of the most difficult diagnostic problems in gastroenterology. Upper gastrointestinal endoscopy, colonoscopy, and angiography have greatly increased the diagnostic rate. Nevertheless, there is a significant proportion of patients who continue to bleed and in whom these investigations, as well as barium studies, have failed to reveal a cause. In this situation, all X-rays should first be reviewed. Then the possibility of a vascular lesion in the stomach or colon should be considered and it may be worthwhile repeating the endoscopic procedures specifically to look for these abnormalities. Angiography should also be repeated if the patient starts to bleed rapidly and it is essential to selectively catheterize each of the major vessels.

If bleeding is occurring in patients with chronic liver disease and no apparent cause has been found, ileal varices must be considered. Selective angiography may reveal them but a splenoportogram is usually preferable. Angiography usually demonstrates small bowel tumours. These may also be seen on a small bowel enema which should also pick up lymphomas, the early lesions of Crohn's disease, and strictures. Meckel's diverticulum may be detected by a careful small bowel enema but a negative examination does not exclude it. A $^{99}Tc^m$ scan may be useful since the technetium is concentrated in gastric mucosa and gastric heterotopes are found in about 30 per cent of Meckel's diverticula. Ulcers of the ileum are notoriously difficult. There may be a history of potassium ingestion but this is often absent. A small bowel enema may reveal them. Ulcerating jejuno-ileitis is also best diagnosed with barium studies. Finally, the possibility of factitious bleeding should never be forgotten.

Many patients with chronic or recurrent acute bleeds from the gastrointestinal tract are brought to laparotomy when all the above tests have proved negative. The surgeon may find the cause (e.g. a Meckel's diverticulum or an ileal ulcer) but about 30 per cent of these patients will still remain undiagnosed.

Disorders of swallowing

The act of swallowing is divided into three phases; oral, pharyngeal, and oesophageal. During the first phase the tongue is pressed against the hard palate so propelling the food bolus into the back of the pharynx. Aspiration into the trachea is prevented by closure of the soft palate, glottis, and epiglottis. As the pharyngeal muscles contract, the upper oesophageal constrictor muscles relax, so establishing a gradient which propels the bolus into the upper oesophagus. A wave of peristalsis then moves the material down the oesophagus and, following relaxation of the lower oesophageal sphincter, the food enters the stomach. The reflexes involved in these functions are mediated through the fifth, seventh, ninth, tenth, and eleventh cranial nerves.

Dysphagia. Dysphagia describes difficulty in swallowing. True dysphagia must be distinguished from *globus hystericus* which is described as a feeling of a lump or obstruction in the throat. Dysphagia may result from motor disorders or obstructive lesions. In the former case it is characterized by difficulty in swallowing liquids and solids whereas the latter occurs typically with solid foods. Common neurological causes of dysphagia include cerebrovascular accidents, motor neurone disease, poliomyelitis, and any form of progressive bulbar palsy. Mechanical causes include neoplasms of the pharynx or oesophagus, inflammatory strictures of the oesophagus, cricopharyngeal webs, diverticular of the upper or lower oesophagus, and external pressure on the oesophagus due to a variety of lesions in the mediastinum (see page 12.41).

Heartburn. Heartburn consists of a retrosternal burning sensation which may be referred to the neck or back. It usually results from reflex oesophagitis (see page 12.40).

Belching. Belching is caused by the retropulsion of air from the oesophagus or from the stomach through the oesophagus. It frequently results from air swallowing which occurs in anxious individuals.

Rumination. This is an unusual symptom in man. It is characterized by the regurgitation of food into the mouth which is then swallowed again. The symptoms usually occur shortly after meals although occasional patients are encountered who can ruminate at will. Although this symptom is sometimes associated with anxious or neurotic individuals, this is not always the case and the cause of the condition is unknown (see page 12.45).

References

Avery Jones, F., and Godding, E. W. (eds.) (1972). *The management of constipation.* Blackwell Scientific Publications, Oxford.

Bernuau, J., Nouel, O., Belghiti, J., and Rueff, B. (1981). Severe gastrointestinal bleeding Part II: guidelines for treatment. *Clins Gastroent.* **10**, 17.

Protell, R. L., Silverstein, F. E., Gilbert, D. A., and Feld, A. D. (1981). Severe gastrointestinal bleeding. Part I: causes, pathogenesis and methods of diagnosis. *Clins Gastroent.* **10**, 38.

Schiller, K. F. R., Truelove, S. C., and Gwyn Williams, D. (1970). Haematemesis and melaena with special reference to factors influencing the outcome. *Br. med. J.* **iv**, 7.

The mouth and salivary glands

T. Lehner

Stomatology is a branch of medicine which deals with oral diseases. Due to historical reasons and the rather technical aspects of treatment of teeth, dentistry has been separated from the main body of teaching of medicine. This has created a curious anomaly in the training of doctors, in that oral diseases receive the lowest priority in the medical curriculum. The aims of this chapter are to present briefly some aspects of stomatology of particular concern to the physician, with special reference to the differential diagnosis of the soft tissue lesions of the mouth.

Dental caries and sequelae

Aetiology. Dental decay or caries is probably the most common disease in man and is responsible for a great deal of pain and discomfort. The prevalence of caries is greatest in children and young adults. Intensive investigations during the past two decades have shown that caries is an infection caused by aggregations of bacteria on the tooth surface, usually referred to as dental plaque. The development of dental caries requires: (*a*) the presence of cariogenic bacteria that are capable of rapidly producing acid below the critical pH required for dissolving enamel; and (*b*) sugar in the diet that favours colonization of these bacteria and that can be metabolized by the bacteria to form acid. Germ-free studies have clearly shown that *Streptococcus mutans* can induce caries rapidly in the absence of other organisms. *Strep. mutans* is a facultative anaerobic, non-haemolytic, acidogenic organism, producing extracellular and intracellular polysaccharides. The organism fulfils Koch's postulates as a cause of dental caries.

In addition to micro-organisms a sugar substrate is essential for caries formation. The most common carbohydrates in our diet are starches and sucrose, with smaller amounts of glucose, fructose, and lactose. Quantitatively and functionally the most important substrate in man is sucrose. Addition of glucose to this diet makes little difference, but sucrose gives rise to heavy plaque formation, with considerable amounts of extracellular polysaccharide around the bacterial plaques. The most important polysaccharide is dextran (glucan) which is synthesized in large amounts by the constitutive enzyme glucosyltransferase (dextran-sucrase). Dextran may give plaque the necessary quality of stickiness to the enamel surface.

Streptococci do not possess a cytochrome system but contain the Embden–Meyerhof glycolytic enzymes which will convert glucose to lactic and other organic acids. The pH inside the plaque may fall within two to three minutes of rinsing the mouth with glucose or sucrose from a level of about 6.5 to 5; the critical pH below which decalcification of enamel occurs is thought to be about 5.5. Caries is the end-result of a complex sequence of microbial and biochemical processes terminating in acid formation.

Pathology. Caries develops as a result of acid formed by the bacterial plaque acting on sucrose. The enamel becomes demineralized and plaque bacteria penetrate along the enamel prisms. This process progresses slowly through the enamel layer, but once the dentine is reached destruction by decalcification and proteolysis of the dentine is rapid. The pulp reacts by an acute inflammatory response and results in necrosis, as the pulp is enclosed within the rigid walls of the tooth and the exudate cannot expand to adjacent tissues. Eventually spread of infection and toxic materials occurs from the root canal opening to the tissues around the apex of the tooth and induces peri-apical inflammatory changes which may terminate in an acute or chronic abscess, or chronic granuloma. If epithelial proliferation takes place within the granuloma or abscess then a cyst may develop which will increase in size over many years before it may be revealed clinically. A dental abscess shows a mixed bacterial infection with a variety of streptococci, staphylococci, and other organisms.

Clinical features. The patient complains of toothache which is made worse with any hot or cold drinks or food. The throbbing pain becomes progressively worse, affects the patient especially at night-time, and may radiate to the face and ear. If relief is not sought the pain becomes excruciating in intensity, and the tooth becomes tender to bite on. This will be followed by death of the dental pulp and the development of an acute swelling due to an abscess or cellulitis. With an acute abscess the inflammatory exudate may penetrate through the bone to the soft tissues. Whilst the pain is reduced the facial oedematous swelling increases and if the upper canine is involved the swelling spreads to the eyelid and may present an alarming appearance. The regional lymph nodes are tender and enlarged, there may be fever and some malaise. Much less commonly a cellulitis or infection by β-haemolytic streptococci may give rise to a spreading infection along the fascial planes, especially of the submaxillary and sublingual spaces. The inflammatory exudate may occasionally spread along the parapharyngeal spaces into the loose connective tissue of the glottis causing oedema of the glottis and respiratory obstruction. The attendant brawny swelling of the neck and floor and the mouth, difficulty in swallowing, trismus, fever, and malaise is referred to as *Ludwig's angina*. An alternative chronic course is the development of a chronic pulpitis, granuloma, abscess, and eventually cyst around the apex of the offending tooth and these may proceed without symptoms or only slight discomfort.

Although the patient may point out the painful tooth, this can be misleading, because the pain often radiates to adjacent teeth. The offending tooth is located by finding the caries, most commonly in the pits and fissures of the occlusal surfaces or the approximal surfaces of adjacent teeth. The tooth responds with pain on application of a hot or cold stimulus and later is tender to percussion and may be discoloured. If in doubt, a dental X-ray may confirm the carious tooth and at a later stage the periapical pathological changes.

Treatment. The principles of treatment are to remove the caries, apply a non-irritant material, such as zinc oxide and eugenol dressing, to protect the pulp and then restore the tooth with a filling. If the pulp is damaged irreversibly it will have to be extirpated and root canal therapy instituted. The alternative to conservative treatment is extraction of the offending tooth. A dental abscess is effectively dealt with by extraction of the diseased tooth, for this removes the source of infection and drains the pus.

If the tooth is to be saved, the pus is drained by an intra-oral incision and/or establishing drainage through the root canal. Antibiotics are usually given in acute abscesses and oral penicillin, such as phenoxymethylpenicillin, 250 mg four times a day for about seven days is adequate. Cellulitis should first be treated by intramuscular penicillin, in the form of benzylpenicillin, 1 mega unit four times a day. The swelling should then be incised, to relieve the pressure and provide drainage; extraction of the tooth under general anaesthesia should take place as soon as the patient's condition permits it.

Prevention of dental caries is best practised by careful plaque removal by the individual. The type of toothpaste used matters less than the method of tooth brushing, though fluoride in toothpaste may decrease the incidence of caries in children by up to 40 per cent. Water fluoridation, however, is the only effective public health preventive measure. One part per million of fluoride in the drinking water will decrease the incidence of caries in children by up to 60 per cent. There is no evidence of toxicity from water fluoridation. The ethical and scientific issues of water fluoridation are complex and have been the subject of a report by the Royal College of Physicians.

Differential diagnosis. Toothache has a characteristic quality but occasionally needs to be carefully differentiated from sinusitis and neuralgia. The throbbing pain which is exacerbated by thermal stimuli and is more severe at night are important diagnostic features. An abscess or cellulitis caused by dental caries has been on a few occasions confused with mumps though the latter is confined predominantly to the parotid fascia, earache may be a prominent feature and pain is elicited by pulling on the ear lobe. A chronic granuloma or a dental cyst are usually diagnosed radiologically, unless the cyst becomes large and a swelling becomes clinically evident.

Course and prognosis. The acute sequence of events from dental caries are acute pulpitis, periodontitis, resulting in an abscess or cellulitis. If treated promptly the sequelae can be prevented, but if not treated the patient will loose the tooth and may also develop some facial scarring due to a discharging sinus. With slow progression of caries or incomplete removal of decay, a chronic pulpitis may supervene, followed by chronic periadentitis which may result in a periapical granuloma, abscess, or cyst. Dental caries is in most instances a progressive condition and can be halted only by the dental surgeon.

Gingival and periodontal disease

Aetiology. A mild inflammation of the gingiva (gum) and slight destruction of the collagen fibres of the periodontal membrane are found in most adults. Advanced destruction of the periodontal membrane, including the supporting bone, is found in about half of the middle-aged or older population. Gingivitis is caused by dental plaque, and both Gram-positive and negative organisms are involved. However, *Actinomyces viscosus*, *Bacteroides asaccharolyticus*, and other anaerobes seem to be of particular significance. The organisms do not penetrate the gingival epithelium and damage is thought to be caused by toxic and antigenic products, particularly endotoxins from the Gram-negative organisms. Dental plaque may calcify, especially in adults and the elderly, to produce calculus. This is often found above the gingival margin, especially on the lingual surface of the lower incisors and the buccal surface of the upper molars, i.e. opposite the orifices of the major salivary glands. Dental plaque is the primary cause of gingivitis, but if not removed some of it becomes calcified and the resulting calculus may exacerbate the gingivitis.

Chronic gingival inflammation may persist for many years and breakdown of the periodontal membrane, with loss of the supporting bone, may follow and increase in severity over the years. This is referred to as periodontitis, or 'pyorrhoea', as it used to be called, and is the most important cause of loss of teeth after the age of 40, when the incidence of dental caries has greatly diminished. An important feature of periodontitis is that it affects many and often all the teeth, resulting in a complete loss of the dentition. A very rare type of rapid destruction of the supporting dental tissues is found in children or young adults and is referred to as *juvenile periodontitis*; one or more teeth may become mobile and may be lost before 21 years of age.

Pathology. The initial change is a chronic inflammatory response of the gingival epithelium, with ulceration, followed by hyperplasia of the crevicular epithelium. The adjacent connective tissue is infiltrated by a large number of neutrophils and mononuclear cells; lymphocytes and monocytes appear in the early stage and may persist, though the plasma cell infiltration becomes more prominent as the lesion becomes chronic. Extension of the infiltration into deeper tissues is associated with breakdown of the periodontal fibres, bone resorption, and proliferation of the crevicular epithelium towards the root apex. Repair, with collagen formation and destruction of the tissues, eventually leads to loss of support of the teeth.

Clinical features. The symptoms of chronic gingivitis or periodontitis are usually so mild that they go unnoticed by the patient. They may, however, complain of discomfort from their teeth, bleeding of gums, difficulty on eating, looseness of teeth, and occasionally abscess formation. A lack of severe symptoms permits the disease to progress to an irreversible stage before help is sought, so that the loss of teeth from 'pyorrhoea' was often considered in the past as a process of ageing.

Differential diagnosis. Chronic gingivitis can be differentiated from acute ulcerative gingivitis by the sudden onset, malaise, halitosis, pain, and ulceration of the gingiva in the latter (see page 12.21). Herpetic gingivostomatitis occurs predominantly in children and again the onset is acute, with fever, malaise, pain and ulceration of the gingiva and oral mucosa (see below). Desquamative gingivitis may cause difficulties in differential diagnosis and the points to bear in mind are that the attached gingiva shows diffuse erosive areas and evidence of bullous lesions may be found in the oral mucosa.

Treatment. The aims in the management of gingivitis and mild periodontitis are to remove dental plaque and calculus by scaling the teeth and this can be done only by the dentist, or where available, by a dental hygienist. Prevention is, however, much more effective by plaque control which involves careful tooth brushing, with the aid of plaque disclosing solutions. However, once deep periodontal pockets have been formed, these will have to be eradicated surgically by gingivectomy or a variety of other procedures. It should be appreciated that the management of periodontal disease is in the hands of the patient, for any type of treatment is dependent on meticulous plaque control.

Course and prognosis. If the bacterial plaque is not removed, the gingivitis will progress to periodontitis and after many years will result in increased mobility and loss of teeth. This process, however, is reversible by plaque control and, if necessary, eradication of pockets, as long as there is sufficient bone to support the teeth.

Herpes simplex infection

Synonym. Herpesvirus hominis type 1 infection. (See also Section 5.)

Primary herpetic gingivostomatitis
Aetiology. Clinical or subclinical primary infections by herpesvirus type 1 is acquired in early childhood, probably in the second and third years of life. Primary herpetic infection in the first year is rare, because most mothers have neutralizing antibodies to the virus which are transferred through the placenta to the fetus. Serum virus complement-fixing and neutralizing antibodies are found in about 50 per cent of children at 5 years of age. The disease is common in children, but is also seen, less frequently, in adults.

Pathology. Infection starts with the herpes virus gaining entry into epithelial cells. Virus replication takes place inside the nucleus and this is associated with formation of intranuclear inclusion bodies and giant cells. As more epithelial cells become infected, degenerative and oedematous changes give rise to vesicle formation. The intra-epithelial vesicles contain oedematous fluid, with giant cells and degenerating cells with intra-nuclear inclusion bodies. The vesicles rupture early resulting in ulcers that heal without scarring.

Clinical features. The disease is recognized by an acute onset of a sore mouth and often sore throat, fever, and extensive inflammation of the gum, followed by formation of vesicles and ulcers of the oral mucosa, and regional lymphadenitis. Infants display considerable fretfulness, sleeplessness, and refusal to eat. Initially there are crops of small ulcers but these coalesce to produce large, shallow, irregular ulcers with surrounding inflammation. Herpetic keratitis is not often associated with herpetic stomatitis, and herpetic encephalitis is extremely rare but may occasionally complicate herpetic stomatitis.

Diagnosis. The early phase of infection can be confused with a cold but the development of vesicles and ulcers makes the latter diagnosis unlikely. Recurrent aphthous ulcers may occasionally be misdiagnosed in the adult, though the important differentiating points are the acute onset, sore throat, fever, and lymphadenitis in herpetic infection. Laboratory tests can be useful in confirming the diagnosis. Direct examination of a smear from the lesion can be helpful if intranuclear inclusion bodies or giant cells are found. Culture of the virus may assist in the diagnosis, but the herpesvirus is also found in carriers. A rise in antibody titre to the virus during an infection is a useful aid to diagnosis.

Treatment. Patients are advised to rest for two to four days; a soft diet is indicated and an adequate fluid intake is emphasized. The mouth is cleansed by thorough rinsing with hot salt water six times daily and the teeth are cleaned with a wet flannel. Special attention must be paid to infants with regards to the fluid intake and sleep. A useful sedative to use is promethazine elixir given in doses of 1 teaspoonful (5 mg/5 ml) at night-time.
Until recently the only agent found to be helpful was tetracycline mouthwash; in infants the elixir is applied to the ulcers. This produces considerable symptomatic improvement, possibly due to control of secondary infection. However, idoxuridine is an anti-DNA agent which inhibits growth of herpesvirus and can be helpful. It is usually used as a solution containing 0.1 per cent of idoxuridine and is applied to the lesions with a brush or cotton wool hourly if possible on the first day, and then six times daily for the next four days.

Course and prognosis. The natural course of this infection is seven to 14 days, during the initial days of which eating is usually difficult, but healing of the ulcers occurs spontaneously. Recurrence of herpetic lesions intra-orally is extremely rare, though a type of recurrent oral ulceration due to herpes virus has now been recognized.

Recurrent herpetic infection

Synonyms. Recurrent herpes labialis; cold-sores.

Aetiology. The lesion is caused by herpes simplex virus (HSV) and is commonly found from childhood to past middle age and affects both sexes. A variety of factors may precipitate the lesions: fever, exposure to sunlight, local trauma, emotional stress, menstruation, and section of the sensory root of the trigeminal ganglion are among the best-known ones. Severe herpetic infections, affecting the lips, peri-oral skin and mouth are seen in patients receiving immunosuppressive drugs for transplantation.

Pathology. Primary herpes simplex infection is followed by the virus becoming latent in the trigeminal ganglion. The relation between primary infection, latency, and recurrent infection by HSV has not been completely elucidated but the following immunological hypothesis is supported by current evidence.

Primary infection induces immune responses to the virus, and antibody and cell-dependent cytotoxic mechanisms kill most of the virus and virus-infected cells which are accessible to killer cells. HSV will be sequestered to the nerves and will migrate centripetally along the axons to the trigeminal ganglia. Latency in the trigeminal ganglion may be mediated by antibodies. Some alteration in the surface charge of neurons, triggered off by the various clinical precipitating factors, may induce derepression of the viral genome and virus replication which will then migrate centifugally along the axon, to be shed at the nerve endings. In the presence of some defect in cell-mediated immunity, acting at the neuroepithelial junction, a recurrent herpetic lesion will be precipitated.

Clinical features. The lesions are usually limited to the vermilion border of the lips and adjacent skin. A single blister or a crop of blisters may develop a day after the prodromal phase of a burning sensation. The duration of the lesion varies usually between three and 10 days, but secondary infection by *Staphylococcus pyogenes* occurs commonly. The lesion recurs at various intervals, for many years, and the rate of recurrence may be related to the type of precipitating factor involved.

Diagnosis. Localization to the vermilion border of the lips and the history of recurrences make this a readily recognizable condition. Laboratory assistance is rarely required but the findings are similar to those described for primary herpetic infection, except that there is an elevated initial antibody titre which does not usually increase during recurrent infection. Staphylococcal infection from the anterior nares should be excluded.

Treatment. Idoxuridine solution (0.1 per cent) or an ointment of 5 per cent idoxuridine in dimethyl sulphoxide applied four times daily can be effective, especially if applied during the prodromal phase. Staphylococcal infection responds readily to tetracycline (1 per cent) or neomycin (1 per cent) ointment, applied four times daily. In the severe type of muco-cutaneous herpetic infection in immunosuppressed patients it has been recently found that Acyclovir (acycloguanosine) given intravenously in doses of 5 mg/kg, every eight hours, for five days, can be effective in clearing the lesions.

Course and prognosis. The lesions heal usually within about seven days but recurrences are difficult to prevent. If the precipitating factors are known, some preventive measures can be taken, as by applying a barrier cream to the lips before exposure to the sun.

Herpes zoster infection. Herpes zoster infection of the skin of the face, innervated by the second or third branches of the trigeminal nerve, may be associated with unilateral oral vesicles. These break down early to produce ulcers along the oral distribution of the maxillary or mandibular branches.

Herpangina. This is a rare infection by the Coxsackie group A viruses, usually affecting the soft palate and the oropharyngeal region. Children tend to be affected more often than adults and the mode of presentation of the disease is similar to that in primary herpetic stomatitis. The diagnosis can be firmly established only by isolating the virus from a lesion or by showing an increase in antibody titre. The disease appears to be self-limiting and specific treatment is not necessary.

Hand, foot, and mouth disease. This is another virus infection caused by Coxsackie A5, 10 and 16 (see Section 5). The mouth is sore due to multiple small vesicles or ulcers which affect most commonly the hard palate, tongue, and buccal mucosa. There are associated vesicular lesions on the hands and feet. The diagnosis is confirmed by isolating the virus from the lesion. The disease is self-limiting within about two weeks and no specific treatment is necessary.

Measles. This is an acute exanthematous virus infection of children (see Section 5). Whitish macules on the buccal mucosa, known as Koplik's spots, may precede the development of the red macular rash by two to three days.

Fungal infections (see Section 5)

Candidiasis
Synonyms. Moniliasis; thrush.

Aetiology. Species of candida are found as commensal organisms in the mouth of 20 to 40 per cent of the normal population. Most normal subjects show serum-agglutinating antibodies and skin delayed hypersensitivity reaction to candida. It is not clear whether candida infection of the oral mucosa is endogenous or exogenous, but as the organism is ubiquitous, a suitable environment and impaired immune responses are the most important conditions conducive to infection by candida. Although most species of candida can become pathogenic, *Candida albicans* is most frequently found in oral infections.

Pathology. The different varieties of candidiasis have in common a superficial invasion of epithelium by hyphae of candida and it is unusual for the hyphae to penetrate the basement membrane. However, occasionally candida may spread by the vascular route particularly to the heart, kidneys, and brain. Raised titres of antibodies to candida are found in serum and secretory IgA antibodies in saliva of patients with oral candidiasis. A spectrum of increasing cell-mediated immunodeficiencies is found in chronic mucocutaneous candidiasis affecting the skin delayed hypersensitivity, lymphocyte transformation, and macrophage migration inhibition to *C. albicans*.

Clinical features. There are four varieties of oral candidiasis.
Acute pseudomembranous candidiasis (thrush). This disease is commonly seen in infants as well as in debilitated adults, particularly in diabetes mellitus and malignant diseases, especially leukaemia and lymphoma. Iatrogenic agents are also important predisposing factors; systemic antibiotics, corticosteroids, and immunosuppressive drugs seem to enhance candida infection. Local antibiotic and corticosteroid treatment can enhance oral candidiasis. Clinical manifestations of thrush are usually symptomless white papules or cotton-wool like exudates which can be rubbed off leaving an erythematous mucosa.
Acute atrophic candidiasis. This may follow acute pseudomembranous candidiasis and is usually associated with broad-spectrum antibiotic therapy, hence referred to as 'antibiotic sore tongue'. It is the only type of oral candidiasis that is consistently painful, showing a smooth erythematous tongue, with angular cheilitis and less often inflamed lips and cheeks.
Chronic atrophic candidiasis. This type of candida infection is better known as 'denture stomatitis', for it presents as a diffuse erythema of the palate, limited to the denture-bearing mucosa. The denture covering the palatal mucosa predisposes to proliferation of candida. The lesion is usually symptomless but is often associated with angular cheilitis.
Chronic hyperplastic candidiasis. This lesion presents as a firm, diffuse, white patch, or as numerous white papules with intervening erythema on the tongue, cheeks, or lips. The lesion may persist for many years or for life and should be separated from leucoplakia. This variety of candidiasis can be associated with skin lesions and there are three clinical types of mucocutaneous candidiasis.
Chronic localized mucocutaneous candidiasis. This starts in childhood as an intractable oral candida infection, with involvement of nails and sometimes the adjacent skin of hands and feet. A number of other skin sites may show persistent candida infection.
Chronic localized mucocutaneous candidiasis with granuloma. The onset of this condition is in infancy and the clinical manifestations are similar to those in the previous type of candidiasis, with

the important additional feature of granulomatous masses affecting the face and scalp. Recurrent respiratory tract infection was recorded in a quarter of these children.

Chronic localized mucocutaneous candidiasis with endocrine disorder. This used to be found in children only, as the mortality was particularly high in the presence of Addison's disease, but nowadays the disease is also seen in young adults. A strong familial incidence is often found and candidiasis commonly precedes the endocrine abnormalities. The clinical features of candida infection are similar to those seen in the localized mucocutaneous variety and the association with hypoparathyroidism and Addison's disease, and less often pernicious anaemia and hypothyroidism, illustrates the relationship beteeen cell-mediated immunodeficiencies and auto-immune endocrine disorders.

Differential diagnosis. Chronic hyperplastic candidiasis can cause some difficulties in differentiation from leucoplakia and the laboratory tests are useful in this, as well as in the other types of candidiasis, in establishing the diagnosis. A culture from the lesion yields candida, usually *C. albicans*, and direct examination of scrapings shows Gram-positive hyphae and yeast cells of candida. Biopsy of the lesion in chronic mucocutaneous candidiasis is helpful, as in addition to the superficial invasion of epithelium by candida hyphae, there is usually extensive epithelial hyperplasia. The dermis shows an intense mononuclear cell infiltration with a large proportion of plasma cells.

A rise in convalescent serum antibody titre to candida may assist in the diagnosis of the acute types of candidiasis, but there may be an impaired antibody titre in the chronic type of candidiasis. Chronic mucocutaneous candidiasis usually shows some defect in cell-mediated immunity and these should be defined, especially with reference to the skin delayed hypersensitivity, lymphocyte transformation, and macrophage migration inhibition tests to candida. It is essential that the endocrine function should be tested in children with chronic candidiasis of the mouth and nails.

Treatment. All varieties of oral candidiasis except the chronic hyperplastic type respond readily to topical oral treatment with antifungal drugs; sucking tablets of nystatin 500 000 units four times a day or amphotericin B 100 mg four times a day, for one to two weeks are very effective. Chronic mucocutaneous candidiasis, however, usually does not respond to tropical oral treatment and necessitates intravenous administration of amphotericin B. Although almost complete eradication of the lesions can be accomplished, amphotericin B is nephrotoxic and the disease tends to return after the drug is discontinued. Some of the more recent antifungal agents (e.g. clotrimazole and miconazole) suffer from the same disadvantage, that the disease recurs if treatment is stopped. This is comprehensible on the basis of an underlying immunological defect which, if it is not rectified, will lead to reinfection with candida. Transfer factor and levamisole have been used as immunopotentiating agents with some success, in patients lacking delayed hypersensitivity, migration inhibition factor, or lymphocyte transformation to candida, resulting in clinical remission and a restored capacity of cell-mediated immunity.

Bacterial infections

Acute ulcerative gingivitis

Synonyms. Vincent's gingivitis; acute fusospirochaetal gingivitis.

Aetiology. An infective cause of acute ulcerative gingivitis has been widely accepted, though the organisms thought to be responsible are greatly disputed. *Fusobacterium fusiformis* and *Borrelia vincenti* have been favoured on account of their presence in large numbers in direct examination of smears from the lesions. *Bacteroides melaninogenicus* has been later implicated as the causative organism, but evidence is accumulating in favour of a mixed, bacterial pathogenesis of Gram-negative organisms (fusobacteria, veil-

lonella, bacteroides, leptotrichia) which may be responsible for the lesions by their endotoxin activity.

Whatever role micro-organisms may play, a number of predisposing factors are recognized. Of the local factors, poor oral hygiene, with accumulation of dental bacterial plaque, defective restorations, and pericoronitis are most important. The prevalence of acute ulcerative gingivitis is rather high and it is seen more commonly in young adults and smokers. A lowered general resistance may also predispose to the disease, as was commonly seen during trench warfare during the First World War.

Pathology. The gum undergoes an acute inflammatory reaction, with an intense polymorphonuclear response and fibrinous exudate. This leads soon to necrosis of the epithelium and thrombosis of the small blood vessels.

Clinical features. Acute ulcerative gingivitis is readily recognized by the sudden onset of painful, bleeding gums and a characteristic foul breath. Except for primary herpetic stomatitis, this is the only other oral mucosal infection in which there is a rise in temperature which may reach 39 °C, regional lymphadenitis, anorexia, and significant malaise. Oral examination reveals necrotic, punched out ulcers, affecting predominantly the interdental gingiva. At times there are shallow necrotic ulcers affecting the oropharyngeal mucosa which shows diffuse erythema; this has been referred to as Vincent's angina. In the presence of erupting wisdom teeth, the overlying gum can show ulceration and oedema causing partial trismus of the jaws.

Diagnosis. This disease is often confused with primary herpetic stomatitis, because of the acute onset. However, these patients are usually younger, their breath is stale and lacks the distinct foul quality of that found in ulcerative gingivitis. First vesicles, and then numerous well-defined ulcers are scattered over the oral mucosa, unlike the tendency to localization of necrotic sites to the gingiva in ulcerative gingivitis. Direct examination of a smear from the lesion reveals a large number of spirochaetal and fusiform organisms, with a decrease in the mixed bacterial flora.

Treatment. Phenoxymethl penicillin, 250 mg taken four times daily for a week is effective in clearing the symptoms within 24 hours of start of treatment. Metronidazole is as effective as penicillin: the dosage is 200 mg taken by mouth three times daily for four days. Oxidizing agents, hydrogen peroxide mouthwash, and a variety of peroxyborate preparations are also useful. During the acute phase patients are advised to use a soft toothbrush or a soft cloth to clean their teeth, and they are encouraged to rinse their mouths forcibly with warm saline every three hours.

Although treatment by drugs is effective in clearing up the acute phase, recurrences can be prevented only by careful attention to oral hygiene. The teeth have to be scaled and polished, and the patient is instructed as to the best method of toothbrushing and dental plaque control. Frequent examinations by the dental surgeon are advisable.

Course and prognosis. In the absence of treatment the acute phase may gradually disappear leaving behind a partially necrosed gingiva and chronic inflammation. Inadequate treatment commonly leads to recurrent ulcerative gingivitis over many years, with halitosis, gingival bleeding, and recession.

Cancrum oris (noma). This is a rapidly spreading gangrene of the lips and cheeks, mostly confined to children in parts of tropical Africa. It is thought to be an extension of acute ulcerative gingivitis when associated with other diseases, especially measles. Cancrum oris is rare in the United Kingdom, but can be seen during the terminal stages in patients with leukaemia, especially when treated by a variety of cytotoxic, anti-inflammatory, and immunosuppressive drugs.

Tuberculosis. Oral tuberculosis is rare and usually secondary to pulmonary tuberculosis. Commonly the presenting feature is a painful ulcer or a firm small swelling. Ulcers may be single or multiple, but they are usually large, with a depressed and granulomatous floor and some induration of the base. The tongue, lips, and cheeks may be affected. Diagnosis is based on microscopical and cultural demonstration of *Mycobacterium tuberculosis* and a biopsy of the lesion which will show a tuberculous granuloma. Oral tuberculosis responds readily to specific chemotherapy.

Syphilis. *Treponema pallidum* may affect the mouth in all stages of syphilis (see also Section 5).

Primary stage. A chancre appears within two to four weeks of infection. The lesion presents on the lip or tongue as a painless, small, firm nodule which breaks down and forms an ulcer with raised indurated edges. The regional lymph nodes show discrete rubbery enlargement. The diagnosis depends on direct observation of *Treponema pallidum* by dark-ground illumination. This stage is highly infective, but serological tests are usually negative during the initial three to four weeks.

Secondary stage. This develops one to four months after infection and presents as a generalized maculopapular rash and lymphadenitis. Shallow, snail-track ulcers affect the tonsils, tongue, or lips, and the saliva is highly infective. The serological tests for syphilis are positive.

Tertiary stage. This is delayed by three to 15 years after infection. Gumma and leucoplakia are the typical oral manifestations at this stage. A gumma starts as a swelling of the palate, tongue, or tonsils; it undergoes necrosis and results in a painless, punched-out, deep ulcer, with a 'wash-leather' floor. The lesion may heal by scarring, or give rise to perforation. Leucoplakia usually affects the dorsum of the tongue as an irregular, diffuse white patch which cannot be rubbed off.

The treatment of oral syphilis is the same as that administered to other sites, but the response in the tertiary stage is rather poor.

Oral ulceration

In view of the great variety of oral ulcers a classification will be given first. Only recurrent oral ulcers will be dealt with fully and the other types of ulcers will be considered predominantly under differential diagnosis.

Recurrent oral ulcers

Synonyms. Three types of ulcers will be described; minor aphthous ulcers, also known as Mikulicz's aphthae; major aphthous ulcers, often referred to in the literature as periadenitis mucosa necrotica recurrens; and herpetiform ulcers.

Aetiology. These are the most common lesions affecting the oral mucosa and the prevalence varies between 10 and 34 per cent. Although a large variety of causes have been suggested, the aetiology of recurrent aphthous ulcers has not been fully established. Trauma is unlikely to play an essential role, though it might precipitate ulceration. There is no evidence that vitamin deficiency or food allergy are involved. Infection by the herpes virus has been excluded as a cause of this type of ulceration. Whilst emotional stress may often influence the pattern of the disease, it is unlikely to be the direct cause. A family history of recurrent aphthous ulcers is often present and the highest incidence of ulcers is recorded in siblings in whom both parents have recurrent aphthous ulcers. A hormonal disturbance may play a part, as in some female patients there is a relationship between the ulcers and menstrual period; the onset of ulceration may coincide with puberty, and the ulcers often disappear during pregnancy. The part that auto-immunity may play in the pathogenesis of this disease has not been fully elucidated, but the *in vitro* response of lymphocytes to epithelial antigens has been related to the clinical features, and lymphocytes are cytotoxic to oral epithelium. The possibility that oral mucosa shares common antigens with some microorganisms has not been fully explored.

Table 1 Classification of oral ulcers

1 Recurrent oral ulcers	(a) Minor, major aphthous, and herpetiform
	(b) Behçet's syndrome
2 Microbial infection	(a) Primary and recurrent herpes simplex infection
	(b) Herpes zoster infection
	(c) Acute ulcerative gingivo-stomatitis
	(d) Tuberculosis
	(e) Syphilis
3 Neoplastic ulcers	(a) Carcinoma
	(b) Leukaemia
4 Haematological disorders	(a) Anaemia
	(b) Neutropenia, agranulocytosis
5 Dermatological disorders	(a) Erosive lichen planus
	(b) Pemphigus
	(c) Benign mucous membrane pemphigoid
	(d) Erythema multiforme and Stevens-Johnson syndrome
	(e) Reiter's syndrome
6 Granulomatous disorders	(a) Histiocytosis X
	(b) Wegener's granulomatosis
7 Iatrogenic agents	(a) Drug allergy
	(b) Drug-induced agranulocytosis
	(c) Cytotoxic drugs
	(d) Radiotherapy
8 Trauma	(a) Denture, teeth, or foreign body
	(b) Chemical

Pathology. An early intense lympho-monocytic infiltration, especially with a perivascular distribution, is a constant histological finding suggesting a delayed hypersensitivity reaction. This is followed by a polymorphonuclear infiltration.

Clinical features. *Minor aphthous ulcers.* About 80 per cent of recurrent oral ulcers are of this type; they are extremely common, especially in the 10–40 year group, and they are found more frequently in females than males.

A prodromal phase is recognized by most patients, one to two days before the onset of ulceration, as a soreness or burning sensation. With the breakdown of epithelium and associated inflammatory reaction the pain increases in severity, particularly on eating. The ulcers are round or oval, up to five in number, and enlarge in size, although they remain well under 10 mm. They have a yellow floor with a slightly raised margin and often marked surrounding erythema and oedema. The most common sites of involvement are the mucosa of lips and cheeks and margin of the tongue, and the ulcers last four to 14 days. The rate of recurrences varies from one to four months and is usually irregular, though in some females ulcers may precede the menstrual period. Enlargement of lymph nodes is uncommon and the patients do not have a raised temperature.

Major aphthous ulcers. These are severe variants of minor aphthous ulcers and less than 10 per cent of patients with recurrent oral ulcers have this type of ulcers. The pain which develops after the prodromal symptoms can be severe and persistent, so that patients find it difficult to eat and swallow food and often lose weight. Examination may reveal one to 10 ulcers at a time and some of these may enlarge to about 30 mm. The ulcers are necrotic with a raised margin and inflammation of the adjacent tissue, so that they occasionally mimic a carcinomatous ulcer. In addition to the lips, cheeks and tongue, the soft palate and tonsillar region are commonly involved. Healing of an ulcer may take 10–40 days and recurrences are so frequent that the patient suffers from continuous ulceration. Multiple small scars may result from the large ulcers and these may assist in the diagnosis of major aphthous ulcers. It is probable that the incidence of major aphthous ulcers is significantly raised in ulcerative colitis.

Herpetiform ulcers. These are recurrent crops of small ulcers, up to 100 in number, affecting any part of the mouth, including the gum, palate, and dorsum of the tongue. They account for less than 10 per cent of recurrent oral ulcers and are much more common in females than males. Patients present with pain on eating and talking, and often with dysphagia; malaise and loss of weight can be prominent features. The lesions persist for seven to 14 days and commonly new ulcers appear before the previous crop has healed so that ulceration becomes continuous.

Diagnosis. The differential diagnosis of the three types of recurrent oral ulcers are given in Table 2. It is important to differentiate these ulcers from pseudoaphthous and pseudoherpetiform ulcers which account for less than 5 per cent of recurrent oral ulcers; the diagnosis is established here predominantly on haematological grounds. These ulcers may also be found in coeliac disease and occasionally may be the only feature of this disease. The diagnosis is based on a flat jejunal biopsy, and a gluten-free diet may prevent the ulcers.

Agranulocytosis or neutropenia may manifest themselves as shallow necrotic ulcers, affecting predominantly the oropharyngeal region. The ulcers tend to persist, unlike the major aphthous type which recur at different sites. However, cyclical neutropenia can mimic minor aphthous ulcers and the diagnosis depends on serial weekly white blood counts.

One of the commonest diagnostic errors is to confuse the results of denture trauma and aphthous ulcers, although the former are usually localized to the mucosa covering the mandibular and maxillary alveolus and the buccal and lingual sulci. The relationship between denture trauma and ulceration is usually simple to find and requires the attention of a dentist.

The differential diagnosis from pemphigus, benign mucous membrane pemphigoid, and erythema multiforme will be stressed below.

Not infrequently patients with major aphthous ulcers are suspected of having a carcinoma, though a careful history will make it evident that these ulcers have been recurring at different sites in the mouth. Although major aphthous ulcers may have a raised margin, this is due to inflammation and not invasion, so that palpation fails to elicit induration usually detected in carcinomatous ulcers.

Treatment. Topical corticosteroids are at present the most helpful agents in alleviating aphthous ulcers. They are most effective if application is started during the prodromal phase, when the mucosa has not ulcerated yet, and the intensity of lymphocyte transformation is reaching peak values. If steroids are applied early, an ulcer may not appear, but application at a later stage may reduce the severity and duration of ulceration. The most useful preparations are triamcinolone in orabase, containing 0.1 mg triamcinolone per 100 g of an adhesive base; hydrocortisone sodium succinate, having 2.5 mg of the steroid per tablet; and betamethasone,

containing 0.5 mg steroid per tablet. The tablets are kept in the mouth, or the ointment is applied to the ulcers, three times daily until the ulcer disappears. Systemic prednisolone or tetracosactrin has to be resorted to rarely in patients with major aphthous ulcers, when topical corticosteroids fail to control the ulcers.

Topical tetracycline is the drug of choice in suppressing herpetiform ulcers, but is also useful in controlling some major aphthous ulcers, particularly when there is excessive amount of inflammation. Its mode of action is not clear and an effective preparation which does not induce acute atrophic candidiasis is Mysteclin; a capsule contains 250 mg tetracycline and 250 000 units of nystatin and is used by dissolving the powder from a capsule in water and keeping this in the mouth four times daily.

Course and prognosis. Minor aphthous ulcers may recur from early childhood for many years, and often these ulcers may cause only transient discomfort to which the patient becomes accustomed. However, major aphthous and herpetiform ulcers usually cause a great deal of discomfort, difficulty in eating, and loss of weight. In children major aphthous ulcers are particularly troublesome and need careful management. In the majority of patients with recurrent oral ulceration the disease burns itself out and this may vary from one year to 20 or more years. In some patients the ulcers recur to old age and may become more severe. In a very small proportion of patients extra-oral sites may become involved, of which the vulvovaginal region is most common, to form part of *Behçet's syndrome*. There is no way of predicting the development of Behçet's syndrome in patients with recurrent oral ulcers (see Sections 20 and 21).

Bullous lesions

These are diseases which often affect the skin and oral mucosa, but sometimes involve only one type of epithelium. Three conditions will be discussed in this section; pemphigus vulgaris, benign mucous membrane pemphigoid, and erythema multiforme (see Section 20).

Pemphigus vulgaris

Aetiology. It is a rare disease which presents in the mouth in half the patients, but the mouth is involved at some stage of the disease in all patients. There is considerable evidence in favour of auto-immunity playing a part in this disease, as serum antibodies are found against interepithelial antigens of mucous membrane and skin.

Pathology. This shows intra-epithelial bullae and acantholytic cells, with a diffuse leucocytic infiltration of the lamina propria.

Clinical features. The disease affects males and females, usually over the age of 30 years. Painful fluid-filled blisters or bullae may appear in the mouth and burst within a few hours, resulting in shallow ulcers. These persist for weeks or months, but new lesions recur throughout the disease process. Oral manifestations of the

Table 2 Differentiating features of the three varieties of recurrent oral ulcers

	Minor aphthous ulcers	Major aphthous ulcers	Herpetiform ulcers
Sex ratio F:M	1.3:1	0.8:1	2.6:1
Age of onset (peak incidence)	10–19 years	10–19 years	20–29 years
Number of ulcers	1–5	1–10	10–100
Size	< 10 mm	> 10 mm	1–2 mm
Duration	4–14 days	10–30 days	7–10 days
Healing with scars	8 per cent	64 per cent	32 per cent
Recurrence	1–4 months	< monthly	< monthly
Sites	lips, cheeks, tongue	lips, cheeks, tongue, pharynx, palate	lips, cheeks, tongue, pharynx, palate, floor, gum
Total duration	< 5 years	> 15 years	> 5 years
Associated oral lesions	—	erythema migrans	—
Treatment (local)	corticosteroids	corticosteroids	tetracycline

disease may persist for many months, without overt ill-health but skin lesions, malaise, and loss of weight may occur later.

Differential diagnosis. Clinically the lesions can be differentiated from recurrent aphthous ulcers by the presence of bullae and when these ulcerate the edges lack the well-defined character of aphthous ulcers. Only occasionally is the Nikolsky sign helpful, that is rubbing the mucosa induces a bulla. The most important diagnostic test is the presence of acantholytic cells on microscopic examination of direct scrapings from the lesion and a biopsy must always be taken. Antibodies to interepithelial antigens also assist in the diagnosis.

A less severe and rather rare variant of pemphigus vulgaris is *pemphigus vegetans*. Vegetations may be found on the oral mucosa and lips and histological examination shows intra-epithelial abscesses containing numerous eosinophils.

Treatment. Systemic corticosteroids such as prednisolone are administered initially in doses of 40–60 mg a day and this is gradually reduced to the minimal dose that will prevent formation of new lesions. In order to keep the steroid dose to a minimum azathioprine can also be used with a starting dose of 200 mg a day.

Course and prognosis. Treatment with corticosteroids has completely changed the prognosis of the disease. Patients rarely die now from the disease but they develop the side-effects of steroid therapy which must be maintained for the rest of life.

Benign mucous membrane pemphigoid

Aetiology. This is a rare disease, affecting women twice as often as men, usually over the age of 40 years. The aetiology is ill-understood but there is some evidence that auto-antibodies to the basement membrane of epithelium may play a part in this disease.

Pathology. This shows subepithelial bullae, and the epithelium tends to detach itself from the underlying lamina propria.

Clinical features. Bullous lesions involve the oral mucosa, conjunctiva, and skin around the genitals and orifices, but in some patients only the mouth is involved. The bullae rupture within a day or two leaving large erosive areas and ulcers. The gingiva is commonly involved, giving rise to persist pain, bleeding, and a diffuse raw fiery red lesion. Other mucous membranes can be involved, such as the nose, larynx, pharynx, oesophagus, vulva, vagina, penis, and anus.

Differential diagnosis. Benign mucous membrane pemphigoid can be differentiated from pemphigus vulgaris on clinical grounds but only a biopsy examination will establish the diagnosis. There are no acantholytic cells and the bullae are subepithelial and not suprabasilar. Furthermore, fluorescent antibodies can be detected, probably in less than half the patients, binding to the basement membrane of epithelium and not to the interepithelial substance.

Treatment. If the disease is confined to the mouth, topical corticosteroids are often adequate to control the lesions. However, with involvement of other sites systemic corticosteroids are indicated, as in pemphigus.

Course and prognosis. This is a chronic disease which persists, often with exacerbations and remissions, over many years. The conjunctivitis may result in adhesions, corneal opacity and blindness.

Erythema multiforme

Aetiology. Erythema multiforme may develop at any age but often occurs in young males. There are many agents which have been associated with this disease; drugs, such as sulphonamides and barbiturates, microbial infections, especially with herpes simplex virus, but a large proportion appear to be idiopathic.

Pathology. There is intracellular oedema with a zone of liquefaction degeneration of the upper layers of the epithelium. Often subepithelial bullae are present and the lamina propria is infiltrated with leucocytes, especially lympho-monocytic cells, neutrophils, and eosinophils.

Clinical features. The disease involves most prominently the skin, and oral manifestations may not be a significant feature. However, the mouth can be affected without skin involvement and the diagnosis then is more difficult. The patient develops painful, extensive erosions and ulcers with a predilection for the palate, tongue, and cheeks. The gum may show extensive erosions which tend to bleed. Haemorrhagic crusting of the lips is often seen. A severe variant of erythema multiforme, which affects the eyes and genitalia, in addition to the skin and mouth, is referred to as *Stevens–Johnson syndrome*.

Differential diagnosis. The diagnosis of oral lesions without the typical skin manifestation can be very difficult. The clinical features to note are the very extensive erosions affecting the palate, tongue, cheeks, and gingiva and the haemorrhagic crusting of the lips. These features should avoid confusion with aphthous ulcers. An association with drugs or microbial infection is helpful. The age and sex prevalence differs from those in benign mucous membrane pemphigoid. A biopsy examination can definitely exclude pemphigus and erosive lichen planus. The differential diagnosis of Stevens–Johnson from Behçet's syndrome has been discussed (see page 12.23) and the points noted about Reiter's syndrome also apply here.

Treatment. Whenever possible the offending drug or infection should be eliminated. The oral lesions often respond to topical tetracycline and Mysteclin capsules dissolved in water and applied four times daily are often used. With extra-oral manifestations treatment with systemic corticosteroids may be indicated.

Course and prognosis. If the offending agent is not found, the lesions may recur over many years and cause a great deal of discomfort. In Stevens–Johnson syndrome, blindness may result from intercurrent bacterial infection.

Lichen planus. This is a disease which may affect the skin, or the mouth or both muco-cutaneous surfaces (see Section 20).

Aetiology. Although the prevalence of oral lichen planus is not known it is surprisingly common in adults. Very little is known about its aetiology, except that the lesions may appear after taking some drugs (e.g. mepacrine) and seems to be associated with emotional or psychiatric stress. However, in most patients no cause can be determined.

Pathology. The pathological changes are hyperkeratosis, hyperplasia, and a characteristic liquefaction degeneration of the basal cell layers of epithelium. The lamina propria shows a well-defined lympho-monocytic cell infiltration.

Clinical features. In the mouth the lesions may remain symptomless for years and not infrequently they are first noticed by the dentist during routine examination. Some patients notice a furry thickening of the mucosa and others complain of pain or bleeding of the gums on eating. There are three types of oral lichen planus: hypertrophic, erosive, and bullous types. The hypertrophic variety is most common and is usually seen in all three types. There are white striae and minute papules, most commonly affecting the posterior part of the buccal mucosa, lips, and dorsum of tongue, though the palate, gum, and floor of the mouth are also involved. The striae criss-cross giving rise to a fine lacey or fern-like pattern, and less commonly a honeycomb or annular pattern. At times the striae may fuse together and result in a diffuse, somewhat smooth, shiny white plaque which may be difficult to differentiate from leucoplakia. Indeed, the dorsum of the tongue usually manifests diffuse white patches instead of the striated pattern.

Bullous lichen planus is rarely seen presumably because the bullae burst to produce ulcers. Erosive lichen planus however, is common and patients complain of pain and discomfort on eating. There may be large shallow ulcers up to 30 mm in size surrounded by white striae and papules. The sites of predilection are the same as in the hypertrophic variety, and whilst the latter may break down to result in erosive lichen planus, it is remarkable how often the hypertrophic variety remains unchanged. Except for discomfort and occasionally loss of weight, there are no general manifestations and the regional lymph nodes are not enlarged, except with secondary infection. Not infrequently lichen planus may affect only the gum, inducing a diffuse fiery red gingivitis and scattered erosions. This is a particularly troublesome type of lichen planus, with pain and bleeding, and tends to be resistant to treatment. It should be stressed that many patients with oral lichen planus do not have skin lesions.

Differential diagnosis. The striae and papules of lichen planus are sufficiently distinctive features in the mouth to differentiate lichen planus from other lesions, without the necessity of a biopsy examination. However, the diffuse hypertrophic variety can be confused with leucoplakia and then a biopsy is helpful. Erosive lichen planus may very occasionally lack the distinctive striae, and then erythema multiforme and benign mucous membrane pemphigoid should be excluded. Both systemic and discoid lupus erythematosus can present in the mouth as central erosions, surrounded by a keratinized margin.

Treatment. In the absence of symptoms hypertrophic lichen planus does not require any treatment. The patient, however, needs to be reassured as to the nature of the disease. Topical corticosteroids are usually effective in the treatment of erosive lichen planus but also suppress the striae and papules of the hypertrophic variety. Triamcinolone in orabase ointment applied four times a day is useful in localized lesions, but betamethasone is more effective and is usually used in the form of 0.5 mg tablets kept in the mouth three times daily. For these drugs to be helpful, they must be applied for a minimum of a month and sometimes for several months. The lesions recur almost invariably, though the length of remissions vary greatly and corticosteroids may have to be applied with every remission.

Cleaning the teeth tends to be painful and the accumulation of a large amount of dental plaque aggravates the gingivitis. The patient should use a camel-hair toothbrush and needs to have the teeth scaled every three to six months.

Course and prognosis. The disease is chronic and tends to persist for decades, with natural remissions and exacerbations. Topical corticosteroids prolong the remissions, and the erosions and discomfort are kept under control. In a very small number of patients carcinomatous transformation, especially of erosive lichen planus can take place. In view of this possibility patients should be followed up regularly on stomatological clinics.

Leucoplakia

White patches of the oral mucosa which cannot be removed by scraping are referred to as leucoplakia. By convention lichen planus and lupus erythematosus are excluded from this group.

Aetiology. The prevalence of leucoplakia has not been established but it seems that during the past two decades it has become less frequent. There are many causes of leucoplakia and as these may have distinctive features they will be classified below. It should be however, noted that in about half the leucoplakias a cause cannot be found. Syphilitic and candidal leucoplakias will not be consid-

ered as these have been discussed elsewhere (see pages 12.22 and 12.20). There is some immunological evidence to support herpes simplex virus as another aetiological agent in the pathogenesis of some leucoplakias. Causes include:
1. Physical and chemical agents: frictional keratosis, smoker's keratosis.
2. Microbial infection: chronic hyperplastic candidiasis, tertiary syphilis.
3. Congenital and hereditary leucokeratosis.
4. Idiopathic.

Pathology. The microscopical features of leucoplakia show a spectrum of changes; at the benign end is epithelial keratosis alone, followed by hyperplasia and then epithelial atypia at the pre-malignant end of the spectrum. The lamina propria shows in parallel an increase in mononuclear cells, especially plasma cells. Carcinoma in situ is the least common histological finding.

Clinical features. The white patches vary from a soft, slightly thickened mucosa, involving a small or very large mucosal surface, to hard, irregular white plaques, with intervening normal, erosive, or ulcerated sites. The latter is often referred to as speckled leucoplakia and must be recognized clinically because of its greater propensity to carcinomatous transformation. Any part of the oral mucosa or gum may be involved but the cheeks and tongue are most often affected.
Frictional keratosis is usually found along the occlusal line of the buccal mucosa and presents as a linear white patch of even consistency.
Smoker's keratosis shows a characteristic distribution of the soft and adjacent hard palate, as keratinized papules with central red dots. The distribution is due to involvement of the palatal mucous glands and the red dots are the openings of the ducts. It is usually caused by pipe smoking, but cigarette smoking may also lead to keratosis of a diffuse type, affecting most commonly the cheeks.
Congenital and hereditary leucokeratosis can be distinguished by the presence of diffuse soft white plaques, often with a folded surface. The lesions tend to be symmetrical; they affect the floor of the mouth. Other members of the family may have similar lesions.

Differential diagnosis. All leucoplakias should be biopsied, except smoker's keratosis of the palate, as even small white patches have at times proved to be early carcinomas. It is, furthermore, essential to find out the degree, if any, of epithelial atypia as this affects the prognosis of leucoplakia. Direct examination of scrapings can be helpful in the presence of hyphae of candida; cultures should also be set up for candida. Serological tests can further aid in the diagnosis of candidiasis but are essential in the diagnosis of syphilitic leucoplakia.

Treatment. Smoker's keratosis is reversible in many instances, if the patient gives up smoking. Frictional keratosis can also be cleared, if some local cause of irritation is removed. Candidal leucoplakia, however should be treated with topical antifungal drugs (see page 12.20), though this rarely results in permanent clearance of the lesion. Syphilis should be managed by a course of penicillin and stringent follow-up, so as to detect early any carcinomatous transformation. Leucoplakia showing evidence of epithelial atypia should be excised and if the lesion is large a skin graft may be required. However, in many cases the lesion recurs, even after repeated excision. There is no satisfactory treatment of leucoplakia and the most important point is long-term follow-up, so as to detect in time the development of an incipient carcinoma.

Course and prognosis. Leucoplakia may persist for life, without any discomfort or change. However, about 5 per cent of all leucoplakias undergo malignant changes and this figure increases to about 30 per cent in leucoplakias showing histological evidence of epithelial atypia. It seems that epithelial atypia is more commonly

associated with speckled leucoplakia and the latter as well as syphilitic leucoplakia have a worse prognosis. In contrast smoker's keratosis and frictional keratosis have a very good prognosis if the
offending cause is removed. Congenital or hereditary leucokeratosis were thought to be free of malignant changes, though recently a
few cases with carcinomatous transformation have been reported.
Long-term follow-up is indicated in all leucoplakias in order that an
incipient carcinoma can be diagnosed in time.

Benign neoplasms, cysts, and developmental and inflammatory lesions of the soft tissues

There are numerous benign neoplasms and soft-tissue lesions of the
mouth. The section will be restricted to some essential features of
the following lesions: papilloma, fibroma, lipoma, neurofibroma,
hamartoma, pigmented naevus, lymphangioma, denture granuloma, giant-cell reparative granuloma, fibrous polyp, pregnancy
tumour, mucous retention, and extravasation cysts.

Aetiology. The cause of benign neoplasms is unknown and the
parts that physical or chemical irritation and microbial infection
may play are ill-understood. Mucous retention or extravasation
cysts are caused by trauma or obstruction of the duct orifice of the
minor salivary glands. Whereas true benign neoplasms are rare,
inflammatory lesions and cysts are commonly found in the mouth.

Clinical features. The soft tissue tumours present as painless, slow-
growing swellings affecting any part of the mouth but if they originate from the gum they are referred to as epulides. Fibrous polyps
are the most common inflammatory lesions of the oral mucosa and
result from trauma or irritation from rough edges of carious teeth.
Most of the tumours are sessile, some are pedunculated as with
some fibromas, and others are flat and pigmented as with the naevi.
They are usually symptomless except for bleeding from hamartomas and giant-cell reparative granulomas.

Differential diagnosis. There are some distinguishing clinical features but the definitive diagnosis will depend on the histological
examination of the excised specimen. A papilloma can be recognized by its firm, small, keratinized, finger-like processes. Lym-
phangiomas are soft swellings which may cause considerable enlargement of the lip or tongue. Hamartomas are flat or nodular red
lesions which may blanch when compressed; they are occasionally
confused with pregnancy tumours which are rather vascular granulomatous swellings of the gingiva found during pregnancy. Giant-
cell reparative granulomas are also very vascular maroon-coloured
lesions originating from the gingiva. Denture granuloma can be
readily recognized from their relationship to the flange of a denture; the lesion is often elongated, can be indented or ulcerated by
the denture. Mucous retention or extravasation cysts are small,
often bluish swellings affecting the lips or cheeks.

Treatment. Surgical excision, with a margin of normal tissue at the
base of the lesion, is usually indicated. Pregnancy tumours, however, commonly regress spontaneously.

Course and prognosis. The soft-tissue neoplasms will enlarge over
the years and interfere with the normal functions of the mouth.
Bleeding from any of the lesions is rarely profuse. Only the giant-
cell reparative granuloma has a tendency to recur after excision.

Oral carcinoma

Aetiology. Carcinoma of the mouth accounts for about 2 per cent
of all cancers of the body. The prevalence increases significantly
after the age of 45 years and more than twice as many men as
women are affected. The incidence of oral cancer has been decreasing over the last four decades, unlike that of lung cancer. As in
other carcinomas the causes are not known, but smoking and
alcohol have been implicated. There is some epidemiological evidence to support this, but unlike lung cancer it is pipe or cigar,
rather than cigarette smoking that have been associated with oral
cancer. The relationships with chronic oral sepsis and irritation
have not been critically examined. There is some evidence that
microbial agents, particularly *Treponema pallidum*, *Candida albicans*, and possibly herpes simplex virus, may directly or indirectly
influence the development of carcinoma by affecting the immune
system.

Among the predisposing lesions leucoplakia is the best-known
one; in 5 per cent of all patients and in about 30 per cent of those
showing evidence of epithelial atypia the leucoplakia may undergo
carcinomatous transformation. Submucous fibrosis is another precancerous condition and is found predominantly in India and Sri
Lanka. It seems to be related to eating chillis and affects the palate,
buccal mucosa, and tongue.

Pathology. Squamous-cell carcinoma in the mouth is usually a
well-differentiated keratinizing neoplasm invading the surrounding
tissue. Poorly differentiated and anaplastic oral carcinomas are
much less frequent and especially rare with carcinoma of the lip.
Spread occurs by local invasion and lymph node metastasis is less
common than is generally thought, and then at a late stage.

Clinical features. The presenting features of carcinoma vary with
the site of involvement but there are two types, a lump or an ulcer.
The patient complains of a swelling or ulcer which is resistant to
healing and is gradually enlarging in size. There may be little pain
initially, but at a later stage discomfort and occasional bleeding may
occur. Cancer of the tongue may give rise to local pain and earache.
Whereas some patients complain of excess of saliva, especially with
the larger tumours, a dry mouth may be found during the early
stages of malignant change and should be noted as another feature
favouring malignancy. A small lump may enlarge to a hard swelling
before the covering mucosa breaks down. A malignant ulcer shows
a raised and often everted edge and the most important feature is
induration at the base of the lesion. Any part of the mouth can be
involved but the lips (usually the lower lip) and tongue are most
common, each accounting for about 25 per cent of oral carcinomas.
The floor of the mouth, gingiva, cheek, hard and soft palate, and
oropharynx may account for about 10 per cent of the carcinomas. In
most patients there is only one lesion but some patients may have
two or even multiple carcinomas. Metastasis may occur at a late
stage to the submandibular or upper cervical lymph nodes, and
occasionally to the submental nodes.

Differential diagnosis. Any long-standing or indurated lesion in the
mouth, especially of elderly or middle-aged patients, should be
queried for malignancy and biopsy examination is essential. A
traumatic ulcer caused by a denture can be confused with a malignant ulcer, but it may lack induration, the offending part of the
denture may fit into the ulcer, and removing the denture for about a
week may bring about healing of the lesion. Major aphthous ulcers
have been mentioned elsewhere (see page 12.22), but the salient
differentiating features are a history of recurrent ulcers at different
sites of the mouth, over many years.

Adenocarcinoma of the small salivary glands may present as a
lump of the soft palate, lips, or cheeks and only a biopsy will
establish the diagnosis firmly. Carcinoma *in situ* is rare in the
mouth, but it may present as a diffuse, erythematous, somewhat
velvety lesion, affecting the mucosa of one half of the soft palate or
cheek. Again a biopsy examination must be carried out for diagnosis.

Treatment. The principles of treatment of oral carcinomas are
those applied to other carcinomas of the body. Surgical excision of
the lesion and a margin of adjacent tissue is the most common
practice and this may be extended if necessary to a block dissection
of the regional lymph nodes. Radiotherapy is an alternative approach and is commonly used in primary treatment of cancer of the

lip. However, it is most often used in inoperable cases, or with recurrent carcinoma following surgery. Remarkable results have been claimed recently with 'fast neutron' therapy. Cytotoxic drugs have also been used in the management of cancer of the mouth with variable results. Management of oral cancer is a complex subject outside the scope of this section. It should be emphasized that oral hygiene is particularly important with any treatment so as to avoid ascending parotitis. A dry mouth usually follows radiotherapy and again meticulous oral hygiene should be advised, so as to prevent rampant caries and candida infection.

Course and prognosis. The five-year survival rates differ considerably with the anatomical site of the cancer. Carcinoma of the lip has by far the best prognosis, irrespective of whether treatment is by surgery or radiotherapy, and the five-year survival rate is about 80 per cent. In contrast the figures for carcinoma of the tongue range from 25 to 35 per cent, floor of the mouth 20–40 per cent, cheek 30–50 per cent and oropharynx, palate, and gingiva at about 25 per cent. The prognosis is significantly better in the absence of lymph node involvement.

Salivary gland diseases

Xerostomia. Xerostomia is a term describing dryness of the mouth and can be due to a variety of conditions.

Aetiology. Dry mouth is a common manifestation especially in middle-aged women and can be caused by anxiety, emotional, and mental stress. Iatrogenic xerostomia is secondary to a number of drugs, the most common of which are antihistamines, tranquillizers, hypotensive agents, diuretics, and preparations, containing atropine. Another common cause is secondary to radiotherapy, but the salivary flow tends to recover, though it may take many months. Some diseases affect the salivary glands directly and cause dryness of the mouth, e.g. Sjögren's syndrome and sialadenitis. Another large group of agents cause xerostomia by inducing changes in fluid balance; diabetes, anaemia, dehydration, and oedema are common examples.

Pathology. Diseases affecting the salivary glands cause a destruction of the secretory components by a mononuclear cell infiltration and fibrosis of the salivary acini.

Clinical features. The patient complains of dryness of the mouth and sometimes the eyes, soreness of the mouth, especially the tongue and throat, and discomfort on swallowing of solids and at times difficulty in speaking. The best clinical evidence of xerostomia is an atrophic dry oral mucosa, often fiery red, due to infection by candida. Inspection of the duct orifice of the major salivary glands will fail to reveal salivary flow and in severe cases even stimulation by lemon juice applied to the tongue may not induce a flow of saliva. The patient may develop rampant caries, or if he wears dentures these may cause difficulties with retention.

Differential diagnosis. A thorough history may establish psychogenic or iatrogenic causes, and diseases affecting fluid balance. Sialography and labial gland biopsy may be necessary in the diagnosis of Sjögren's syndrome, though a raised erythrocyte sedimentation rate, rheumatoid factor, ANF, auto-antibodies, and HLA-typing may assist in the diagnosis. Nevertheless there will be a large proportion of patients in whom a specific cause cannot be found.

Treatment. Management of the patient is clearly directed to eliminate the cause of xerostomia but this may be difficult or at times impossible to achieve. In such cases palliative measures are helpful and these include frequent sips of water, meticulous oral hygiene, early treatment or preferably prevention of candidiasis by topical nystatin or amphotericin B. Each patient responds differently; some prefer glycerin, other carboxy methylcellulose as a lubricant, and many find both unacceptable.

Sialadenitis. Bacterial or viral infections and rarely allergic reactions may cause inflammation of the salivary glands. These agents may give rise to acute, chronic, and allergic sialadenitis, and recurrent parotitis.

Aetiology. Ascending infection of the parotid gland used to be a common complication in the past, in elderly post-operative patients who were predisposed by dehydration, reduced salivary flow, and lack of oral hygiene. Acute parotitis may also follow the use of drugs causing xerostomia. The most common micro-organisms involved are Staphylococcus aureus, Streptococcus viridans, and pneumococcus. The most common acute parotitis is mumps (see Section 5). Chronic sialadenitis is usually associated with duct obstruction and therefore affects usually the submandibular gland. Recurrent sialadenitis is a disease of unknown aetiology and may be associated with a decreased salivary flow causing retrograde infection. The disease may affect both adults and children.

Pathology. Acute sialadenitis shows an acute inflammatory reaction of the salivary tissue, with a predominantly neutrophil infiltration, except in mumps which shows an infiltration by mononuclear cells. In both chronic and recurrent sialadenitis there is a marked periductal and acinar infiltration by mononuclear cells, with some duct epithelial hyperplasia, accompanied by acinar atrophy and fibrosis.

Clinical features. The presenting symptoms in acute sialadenitis are a painful swelling in one of the parotid glands of an elderly patient. Commonly the patient has a low-grade fever, oedema of the cheek, and some trismus, and a purulent discharge may be expressed from the duct opening. In contrast mumps affects healthy children and young adults.

In chronic sialadenitis there are usually clinical features of duct obstruction of one of the submandibular glands. There is pain and swelling in the submandibular or retromandibular region, with a reddened duct orifice discharging pus. Recurrent parotitis presents as an acute pain and swelling of one or both parotid glands, with erythema of the duct orifices and pus discharging from them. There may be an associated fever and malaise. Recurrences vary from weeks to months and after repeated attacks the affected gland may remain enlarged.

Differential diagnosis. There is little clinical difficulty in the differential diagnosis between acute sialadenitis of the parotid gland in the elderly patient due to ascending infection and mumps in the healthy young subject. Any discharging pus should be cultured for the organism and its antibiotic sensitivity should be determined. Recurrent parotitis however, can cause difficulties, for in addition to a history of recurrent painful swelling the discharging pus may show a 'snow storm' appearance. Sialography may help and show sialectasis and duct dilatation. In chronic sialadenitis there is usually clinical or radiological evidence of a calculus and sialography may show duct dilatation.

A variety of granulomatous diseases may very occasionally affect the salivary glands, such as sarcoidosis, tuberculosis, syphilis, and actinomycosis. When there is bilateral salivary and lacrimal enlargement this is often referred to as Mikulicz's syndrome. Allergic sialadenitis is also rare and to determine the allergic agent can be difficult as drugs, foods, pollen, and other agents have been implicated.

Treatment. In acute, chronic, or recurrent sialadenitis the relevant antibiotics should be used to control the infection but occasionally surgical drainage may also be necessary. Careful oral hygiene measures are important in all types of sialadenitis. There is no special treatment for mumps, but rest and isolation for about a week are indicated. In chronic sialadenitis the cause of obstruction, such as a calculus should be removed. The treatment of recurrent parotitis is more difficult and if antibiotics do not control the disease, surgical intervention should be considered.

Course and prognosis. Acute sialadenitis will resolve with the aid of antibiotics and general management of the patient. Mumps will resolve spontaneously and second attacks are very rare. Chronic sialadenitis may persist for many years and may lead to destruction of the gland, unless the cause of duct obstruction is removed early. Recurrent parotitis in childhood may show spontaneous recovery after puberty.

Salivary duct obstruction due to calculus
Aetiology. The submandibular salivary ducts and, to a less extent, glands are the most common sites for the development of stones. Calcium phosphates and carbonates are deposited from the saliva round a nidus of desquamated cells or micro-organisms.

Clinical features. Salivary calculus is usually found in adults and the presenting symptoms are a sudden unilateral swelling and pain of the gland related to eating. The swelling may take minutes to appear and hours to subside. Examination reveals a soft swelling of the affected gland and careful digital palpation along the course of the salivary duct will localize the calculus. This may vary in size from a small grain to a concretion 10–20 mm in length. The presence and localization of a stone in a duct should be confirmed by radiographs and the presence of calculi in the gland itself can be diagnosed only by radiography.

Differential diagnosis. Recurrent unilateral swelling associated with eating is characteristic of salivary gland obstruction but occasionally this may be caused by external agents. Trauma from a denture or sharp tooth may cause obstruction of the orifice of the parotid duct.

Treatment. If the calculus is near the orifice of the duct it can occasionally be teased out, otherwise surgical removal is indicated.

Course and prognosis. Single calculi do not tend to recur, but if treatment has been delayed numerous calculi may have formed inside the gland which may occasionally have to be excised.

Salivary gland tumours.
A variety of epithelial tumours affect the major and minor salivary glands of which the most common is the pleomorphic adenoma, or mixed salivary tumour (74 per cent), followed by adenocarcinoma (12 per cent), adenoma (8 per cent), muco-epidermoid tumour (3 per cent), and acinic cell tumour (2 per cent); the percentages give the prevalence in the parotid glands. Only pleomorphic adenoma will be considered in any detail and the references should be consulted for other tumours.

Pleomorphic adenoma
Aetiology. The cause of this tumour is unknown, though salivary gland tumours can be produced in animals by carcinogenic hydrocarbons, polyoma virus, and other agents. The tumour originates from epithelial cells of the ducts, acini, or myoepithelial cells; the latter are thought to be capable of producing the stromal mucins of this tumour.

Pathology. The epithelial cells proliferate in duct-like structures, sheets, and cords, within a connective tissue stroma which may show mucous, cartilagenous, or hyaline appearance. The tumour is encapsulated, though satellite tumours are often found outside the capsule.

Clinical features. The tumour is usually found in adults and the parotid salivary gland is most commonly affected, followed by the submandibular gland and rarely the sublingual gland. The minor salivary glands, however, are also affected and the most frequent sites are the glands of the palate, lips, and cheeks. The tumour presents as a small, painless swelling which may take years to enlarge and is not attached to the overlying skin or mucosa.

Differential diagnosis. As the tumour is slow growing it needs to be differentiated only from other tumours. Adenocarcinoma, mucoepidermoid carcinoma, and adenoid cystic carcinoma may mimic pleomorphic adenoma in its slow growth, but some may grow more rapidly, invade the adjacent skin or mucosa, and metastasize. These tumours can often be differentiated only on histopathological examination, and wherever possible an excision biopsy should be carried out.

Treatment. Surgical excision with a margin of normal tissue is always practised, as the tumour is radioresistant.

Course and prognosis. If left untreated the tumour may enlarge to a grotesque size. A small proportion of pleomorphic adenomas may undergo carcinomatous transformation. The tumour has a bad record for recurrences after excision and this is thought to be due to leaving behind satellite tumours outside the capsule.

Neoplasms, cysts, developmental lesions, and dystrophies of the bones and teeth

This section covers a very large number of lesions found in the jaws. Only essential features, especially of differential diagnosis, will be covered in the following disorders: (*a*) benign neoplasms: osteoma, chondroma, fibroma, ossifying fibroma, and giant-cell tumour; (*b*) malignant neoplasms: osteosarcoma, and chondrosarcoma; (*c*) cysts and tumours of dental origin: periodontal and dentigenous cysts, keratocysts, and ameloblastoma; (*d*) dental malformations or odontomes; (*e*) osteodystrophies: giant-cell reparative granuloma, brown tumour of hyperparathyroidism, fibrous dysplasia, and Paget's disease.

Aetiology. The cause of the neoplasms and osteodystrophies is not known. Periodontal cysts, which are the most common lesions in this group, develop as a consequence of chronic periapical infection.

Clinical features. The bony tumours and cysts are commonly symptomless, unless they have reached a large size and the patient notices a swelling, or a denture ceases to fit. Often pathological changes are noticed by the dentist through movement of teeth or on routine X-ray examination of the teeth. Hyperparathyroidism should be excluded, in case a giant-cell granuloma is suspected. Cysts can be found at any age, but giant-cell reparative granulomas, ossifying fibroma, and fibrous dysplasia are often seen in young people, unlike Paget's disease of bone which is seen only in old people. There is a predilection for the mandible to be involved more commonly with ossifying fibroma and giant-cell reparative granuloma. Odontomes are developmental malformations of dental tissue which become calcified. This is a diverse group of disorders and vary from a simple enamel pearl, consisting of a nodule of ectopic enamel attached to a tooth, to a complex composite odontome which is an irregular mass of calcified dental tissues. Ameloblastoma is a rare but important epithelial neoplasm of the jaws. Young adults are most often affected, the tumour is slow-growing and affects the mandible more often than the maxilla. The neoplasm is locally invasive but does not metastasize. Osteosarcoma and chondrosarcoma are found in children or young adults but may develop in the elderly with Paget's disease. They present as fast growing, painful, and firm swellings and they may metastasize to the lungs early.

Differential diagnosis. The diagnosis of bony lesions of the jaws is made on the basis of a characteristic radiological picture, coupled with the histological features of the biopsy. Periodontal cysts are very frequent and show a radiolucent rounded area with a sharply defined outline. If the crown of a tooth is enclosed within the cyst, it is referred to as a dentigerous cyst. The latter and keratocysts are usually found in the young, but with some keratocysts a tooth may be missing. Dental cysts must be differentiated from ameloblastomas which tend to show on X-rays multilocular and sometimes a honeycomb pattern. These radiolucent lesions should also be differentiated from secondary carcinoma and myelomatosis. Giant-cell reparative granuloma and tumour (osteoclastoma) show a radiolucent area, sometimes loculated, and the outline is not as well-defined as a dental cyst. Hyperparathyroidism can be excluded by radiological appearance of other bones and by the calcium and phosphate levels in blood. Ossifying fibromas are more common than fibromas and the X-rays show a well-defined radiolucent area with speckled calcification. This can usually be distinguished from the 'ground-glass' appearance, without a distinct border, found in fibrous dysplasia. In Paget's disease there is a distinctive 'cotton-wool' appearance on X-ray examination and the alkaline phosphatase levels are high. Odontomes can be readily recognized on clinical examination, but those that are unerupted, particularly the compound and complex composite odontomes show on X-rays a mass of overlapping denticles and an irregular radio-opaque mass, respectively. Osteosarcoma and chondrosarcoma show patchy areas of bone resorption and deposition.

Treatment. The treatment of dental cysts is by enucleation of the cyst lining and usually extracting the involved tooth. The tumours and malformations are usually excised but some, such as giant cell reparative granuloma can be curettaged. Brown tumours will recur unless the underlying hyperparathyroidism has been dealt with. Fibrous dysplasia may require removal of excessive tissue for cosmetic or functional reasons, but this should be delayed until normal bone growth has ceased. Bony changes in Paget's disease are best not interfered with, except if there are functional reasons, such as inability to fit a denture. Composite odontomes should be removed surgically. The treatment of ameloblastoma is by local excision, with a generous margin of normal bone, or by hemimandibulectomy. Sarcoma of the jaw must be dealt with by early radical excision.

Course and prognosis. If the cysts and benign tumours are removed surgically, they do not recur, except with keratocysts and the reparative granulomas. Ameloblastomas may recur after several excisions, without metastases, and this is why some surgeons prefer to perform a hemimandibulectomy. The prognosis of the jaw sarcomas is very poor and the five-year survival rate is between 25 and 40 per cent. Fibrous dysplasia tends to be self-limiting, but in Paget's disease there may be progressive enlargement, especially of the maxilla.

Miscellaneous

In this section a brief discussion will be given on the following three topics: (a) oral manifestations of blood disorders, (b) halitosis, and (c) disorders of the temporo-mandibular joint.

Oral manifestations of blood disorders. Mild anaemias or deficiencies of iron, folate, or vitamin B_{12} may manifest themselves as *glossitis* with a sore tongue or mouth, angular cheilitis, or recurrent ulceration (see Section 19). The tongue is commonly depapillated, the corners of the mouth may be inflamed and fissured, and occasionally there may be small shallow ulcers affecting the lips, tongue, and cheeks. The cause of any haematological deficiency, should be investigated and, especially with folate deficiency, coeliac disease should be excluded. Replacement therapy usually deals with the clinical features effectively. It should, however, be emphasized that the complaint of a sore tongue can be associated with many other causes, such as erythema migrans, candidiasis,

lichen planus, recurrent aphthous ulceration, and black hairy tongue. *Erythema migrans (geographical tongue)* is particularly common and is characterized by oval-shaped red areas with a well-defined edge affecting the dorsum of the tongue. The lesions move from one site to another. The aetiology of erythema migrans is unknown and treatment is rather unsatisfactory. A sore tongue is a frequent complaint in middle-aged women, often without any demonstrable aetiological factor.

Acute leukaemia, particularly the myelo-monocytic form, may occasionally present in the young in the form of sore, bleeding gums. This may vary from slight inflammation to that showing bulbous enlargement of the gingiva. There are usually inadequate local causes for such a gingivitis and anaemia may be evident; blood tests should be requested to exclude leukaemia.

Leucopenia and agranulocytosis, especially that due to drugs, may become clinically evident by ulceration of the throat or the mouth. Purpura may be associated with a deficiency of platelets, so that bleeding from the gum may also be a feature.

Many haemorrhagic disorders may become evident after extraction of a tooth, because bleeding does not stop. Less commonly gingival bleeding may attract attention to the blood disorders.

Halitosis. Bad breath is usually a trivial complaint, though it seems to be heightened by the attention drawn to it by advertising. There are four possible sources of halitosis: the mouth, nasopharynx, lungs, and the gastrointestinal tract. Altered blood round the gum may be the most important oral cause and this may be associated with debris or pus from gingivitis and periodontal pockets. A characteristic halitosis is found in acute ulcerative gingivitis. It should be noted that bad taste and bad breath are subjective sensations which are often confused. Excessive bacterial plaque on the teeth is not a principal cause of halitosis, but meticulous oral care should be advised.

Chronic tonsillitis may be responsible for halitosis but atrophic rhinitis causing ozena is probably the most important cause to be excluded. Occasionally respiratory tract infections may cause halitosis and a variety of gastrointestinal disorders have been associated with bad breath but there is little evidence to substantiate this. Frequently all these sources of halitosis may be excluded without finding a cause and these patients may have a fixation about bad breath related to emotional or sexual problems.

Temporo-mandibular joint disorders. Temporo-mandibular arthrosis is the commonest disorder of this joint and the patient complains of pain, clicking, or limitation of movement. It is found in young women more often than men. Examination may reveal limitations in jaw movement, tenderness of the joint, and crepitus on movement, discovered by palpating the head of the condyle through the overlying skin. The cause is difficult to establish but malocclusion might be one of several factors. The condition may clear spontaneously, but in some patients the occlusion should be checked and a bite-raising appliance is usually helpful. Rheumatoid and osteo-arthritis of this joint are occasionally seen clinically. Dislocation of the joint which becomes fixed in the open position may be caused by a blow on the jaw or during dental extractions under general anaesthesia. Ankylosis of the joint is nowadays extremely rare and used to be secondary to osteomyelitis.

References

Bahn, S. L. (1972). Drug related dental destruction. *Oral Surg. Med. Path.* **33**, 49.

Binnie, W. B., Cawson, R. A., and Soaper, A. E. (1972). *Oral cancer in England and Wales*. Studies on medical and population subjects, no. 23. HMSO, London.

British Medical Journal (1974). Recurrent oral ulceration. *Br. med. J.* **ii**, 757.

Cawson, R. A. (1975). Premalignant lesions in the mouth. *Br. med. Bull.* **31**, 164.

Cooke, B. E. D. (1960). The diagnosis of bullous lesions affecting the oral mucosa. *Br. Dent. J.* **109**, 83.

Farmer, E. D. and Lawton, F. E. (eds.) (1966). *Stone's oral and dental diseases.* Churchill Livingstone, Edinburgh.

Hartles, R. L. and Leach, S. A. (1975). *Effect of diet on dental caries. Br. med. Bull.* **31**, 137.

Juel–Jensen, B. E. and MacCallum, F. O. (1972). *Herpes simplex, varicella and zoster.* Heinemann, London.

Lehner, T. (1966). Classification and clinico-pathological features of candida infections in the mouth. In *Symposium on candida infections* (eds. H. I. Winner and R. E. Hurley). Churchill Livingstone, Edinburgh.

— (1975). Immunological aspects of oral diseases. In *Clinical aspects of immunology* (eds. P. G. H. Gell, R. R. A. Coombs, and P. J. Lachmann), 1409. Blackwell Scientific Publications, Oxford.

—, Wilton, J. M. A., and Ivanyi, L. (1972). Immuno-deficiencies in chronic mucocutaneous candidosis. *Immunology* **22**, 775.

—, —, and Shillitoe, E. J. (1975). Immunological basis for latency, recurrences and putative oncogenicity of herpes simplex virus. *Lancet* **ii**, 60.

Luna, M. A., Stimson, P. G., and Bardwell, J. M. (1968). Minor salivary glands of the oral cavity. *Oral Surg. Med. Path.* **25**, 71.

MacPhee, T. and Cowley, G. (1973). *Essentials of periodonotology and periodontics.* Blackwell Scientific Publications, Oxford.

Mason, D. K. and Chisholm, D. M. (1975). *Salivary glands in health and disease.* W. B. Saunders, Philadelphia.

Maynard, J. D. (1965). Recurrent parotid enlargement. *Br. J. Surg.*, **52**, 784.

Mitchel, C. D., Gentry, S. R., Boen, J. R., Bean, B., Groth, K. E., and Balfour, H. H. (1981). Acyclovir therapy for mucocutaneous herpes simplex infections in immunocompromised patients. *Lancet* i, 1389.

Morgan, M. N. and MacKenzie, D. H. (1968). Tumours of salivary glands, a review of 204 cases with 5-year follow-up. *Br. J. Surg.* **55**, 284.

Royal College of Physicians (1976). *Fluoride, teeth and mouth.* Report, Royal College of Physicians, London.

Seward, G. R. (1968). Anatomic surgery for salivary calculi: symptoms, signs and differential diagnosis. *Oral Surg. Med. Path.* **25**, 150.

Shklar, G. (1972). Lichen planus as an oral ulcerative disease. *Oral Surg. oral Med. oral Path.* **33**, 376.

Sircus, W., Church, R., and Kelleher, J. (1957). Recurrent aphthous ulceration of the mouth. A study of the natural history, aetiology, and treatment. *Q. Jl Med.* **26**, 235.

Thackray, A. C. and Lucas, R. B. (1974). *Tumours of the major salivary glands.* Washington.

The tonsils and pharynx

R. F. McNab Jones

Acute tonsillitis

Aetiology. This common disease principally affects children and young adults. Children are particularly subject to the condition during their early school years. The infecting organism is usually a haemolytic streptococcus of Lancefield's group A. The mode of spread is by droplet or dust infection and the disease flourishes in conditions of overcrowding and poor ventilation. Occasional outbreaks can be traced to infected milk supplies. The disease also occurs in scarlet fever, measles, and many acute infections of the upper respiratory tract.

Symptoms. There is severe soreness of the throat and a marked general reaction. Children occasionally do not complain that their throat is sore but swallowing is obviously difficult for them and examination of the throat reveals the condition. The temperature may rise to 39.5 °C or more and there is a variable degree of malaise with headache and muscle and joint pains. The throat symptoms are made worse by swallowing, even liquids and saliva causing acute discomfort in many cases. The voice becomes thick and the breath foul, and there is tender adenitis in the submandibular and upper deep cervical glands. Earache during the course of the disease is often a referred pain but it may be due to the development of acute otitis media as a complication so that inspection of the eardrums is a wise precaution.

The tonsils are swollen and inflamed often with pus exuding from the crypts. This exudate may coalesce to cover most of the tonsil, and is soft and may be readily wiped away. The tongue is coated; the fauces, soft palate, and uvula are inflamed and may be covered with sticky mucus.

Acute suppurative otitis media is the most frequent complication. Occasionally peritonsillar abscess or lung infection occurs and rarely acute nephritis or acute rheumatism may follow.

Diagnosis. Many conditions begin with a sore throat and fever and the differential diagnosis is important and may be difficult. Diphtheria, although rarely seen nowadays, should not be forgotten. This disease begins more insidiously than acute tonsillitis and the symptoms and general reaction are less marked while the adenitis is often very considerable. The diphtheritic membrane may cover the

fauces and soft palate as well as the tonsil. It can only be removed with difficulty and leaves a raw bleeding surface. There is a characteristic musty odour easily recognized by those with previous experience of the disease. If there is any suspicion of diphtheria, a throat swab should be taken and antitoxin given immediately.

Nowadays the most common alternative diagnosis is the anginal type of glandular fever (see also Section 5). Superficial ulceration may affect the tonsils and pharynx, but is not always present, while the cervical adenitis is more generalized than in acute tonsillitis and there may be lymphadenitis elsewhere, splenomegaly, and hepatomegaly. Blood examination and a Paul–Bunnell reaction will confirm the diagnosis.

Agranulocytosis and acute leukaemia may also simulate acute tonsillitis, though in these conditions ulceration in the pharynx is usually a marked feature. With adequate treatment acute tonsillitis should resolve within a week. If this does not occur, suspicions of one of these alternative diagnoses should be investigated by means of a throat swab, full blood investigation. Paul–Bunnell test, and a chest X-ray.

Treatment. With bed rest, most cases quickly recover. The appetite is poor and the patient should be encouraged to take ample bland fluids and can usually manage a semi-solid diet. Swallowing is made easier if a tablespoonful of aspirin mucilage is taken just before meals. A mild purgative may be required. Many types of lozenges are available but probably have very little beneficial effect, and penicillin lozenges are contra-indicated because of the severe stomatitis that they cause in susceptible subjects.

Although antibiotics are almost always prescribed for this condition, it is doubtful if they speed recovery in many cases. Ideally their use should be reserved for severe cases with marked general reaction and adenitis and for those in whom a complication is suspected. Penicillin is still the first choice and should be given in adequate dosage for at least one week.

Peritonsillar abscess or quinsy

Aetiology and pathology. The abscess develops between the capsule of the tonsil and the muscular bed of its fossa. The usual situation is above and lateral to the tonsil but in rare cases it develops behind it.

Previous tonsillitis or peritonsillar abscess are predisposing causes. If untreated the abscess usually bursts and discharges through the supratonsillar cleft. Resolution of the infection and fibrosis of the abscess cavity then follows in most cases, but occasionally a chronic abscess develops which discharges imtermittently.

Symptoms. The affection is almost always unilateral and develops during an attack of acute tonsillitis. The patient's condition suddenly worsens with increased pain radiating to the ear and enlarged tender glands on the affected side. Marked trismus develops and there is a sharp rise in temperature. Examination of the throat is difficult, but if a good view is obtained, the affected side shows a large red swelling of the soft palate with the tonsil pushed downwards and medially. Pus forms in two to four days, and if spontaneous rupture occurs, there is immediate relief of symptoms.

Diagnosis. Mixed salivary tumours developing in the soft palate adjacent to the tonsil produce similar physical appearances, but there is no acute illness, pain, or trismus.

Complications. These are rare. If the abscess ruptures during sleep, the pus may be inspirated and cause lung infections. Severe haemorrhage from the internal carotid artery has been reported. Suppuration in the cervical glands, pneumonia, and blood infection may occur. Spreading inflammation in the pharynx may lead to laryngeal oedema and necessitate tracheostomy.

Treatment. The general treatment is the same as that for acute tonsillitis and antibiotics should be administered to reduce the risk of complications. Pus is probably present after four days and as soon as the swelling has assumed a well-defined rounded form, still more so if there is a boggy area in the centre. The abscess should be opened without delay, for this cuts short the attack and relieves the worst of the symptoms. The swelling should be incised at a point halfway between the last upper molar tooth on the affected side and the base of the uvula. This area is painted with 20 per cent cocaine solution and the abscess incised with a special quinsy forceps or a scalpel with a half centimetre unguarded blade. Pus usually gushes forth and should be expectorated into a bowl; the patient should then use a hot mouthwash. Further hot mouthwashes used four times daily for the next few days aid drainage of the abscess. After the disease has subsided, removal of the tonsils is indicated in order to prevent recurrence.

Recurrent tonsillitis in children

Symptoms. Some children are subject to frequent attacks of acute tonsillitis. These may start before the child begins school but the first few years of school life are the commonest period for these recurrent infections. They may occur without much evidence of infection elsewhere in the upper respiratory tract but more usually there is associated nasal and sometimes chest infection. The attacks are particularly frequent following one of the exanthemas.

The tonsils hypertrophy in most cases and may reach a very large size so that swallowing food becomes mechanically difficult and the child eats slowly. Associated adenoid hypertrophy and nasal infection is common and the child then presents the classical picture with a perpetually open mouth, nasal discharge, and a history of snoring and nocturnal cough. Recurrent earache and suppurative otitis media often complicate this condition. Cervical adenitis accompanies the acute attack and enlargement of the glands often persists between the acute episodes. If this enlargement seems out of proportion to the throat symptoms, the glands may be tuberculous. Simple hypertrophy may occur without severe recurrent infection while in a few cases the tonsils become fibrosed at an early age, and although the seat of severe recurrent infection, do not enlarge. Children with an allergic diathesis who have suffered from infantile eczema often develop considerable hypertophy of the tonsils and adenoids and suffer from nasal obstruction and discharge.

Treatment. Each acute episode is treated as described already for acute tonsillitis. The problem is to decide when the condition warrants surgical removal of the tonsils which is combined in most cases with curretage of the adenoids.

If four or more attacks of severe tonsillitis have occurred during the preceding 12 months without the predisposing cause of an acute exanthem, and especially if there has been associated acute otitis media, the tonsils should be removed. They should also be removed if there is suspected tuberculous cervical adenitis or if it is considered that recurrent tonsillar infection is the cause of repeated attacks of rheumatic fever or acute nephritis. The operation should be avoided in an allergic child unless there is much infection associated with the hypertrophy of the tonsils and adenoids. The operation is also contra-indicated if the child has a bleeding diathesis and during an epidemic of poliomyelitis. Details of the operation may be found in surgical textbooks.

Chronic tonsillitis

Symptoms. Young adults are the usual sufferers. There may be a history of frequent attacks of acute tonsillitis, often dating from childhood or the condition may have developed recently. In others there are no severe acute exacerbations but a more or less constant discomfort and soreness in the throat without much general reaction, and sometimes accompanied by laryngeal infection. Chronic tonsillitis may be secondary to chronic sinusitis or dental sepsis.

Treatment. Any dental or sinus infection must be treated appropriately. Mandl's paint applied with a soft brush to the fauces and tonsils twice daily for two weeks may help, and smoking, alcohol, and dusty atmospheres should all be avoided. If the symptoms are severe, tonsillectomy is indicated.

Vincent's angina

Aetiology. This affection (see also Section 5) is generally believed to be due to two organisms, the fusiform bacillus and *Borrelia vincenti* which are commonly found together in many ulcerative lesions of the mouth or throat, as well as in tropical ulcer, pulmonary spirochaetosis, and certain ulcerative lesions of the genitalia. It has never been established beyond doubt that these two organisms are the cause of these lesions: it is quite possible that they are only secondary invaders. Affection of the throat is frequently secondary to periodontal infection. It occurs especially in debilitated persons and under insanitary conditions and was common during both World Wars.

Symptoms. The attack begins insidiously with malaise, general pains, and a temperature of 38–38.5 °C. The pain in the throat is often slight, but in some cases may be severe; the glands on the affected side become enlarged and tender, and the breath is characteristically offensive.

There is superficial ulceration which commonly involves the tonsils and fauces but may affect the inner surface of the cheek, pharyngeal wall, or larynx. The ulcers vary in size; their base is covered with a yellowish-grey pseudomembrane which is not easily detached, and there is marked hyperaemia around the edges. By the end of a week the membranes cease to form, and the ulcers begin to heal. If dental hygiene is poor, there may be recurrent attacks of ulceration.

Diagnosis. The disease may imitate diphtheria in its early stage, and syphilitic ulceration later. In both cases the discovery of numerous spirilla and fusiform bacilli in smear preparations—they are difficult to cultivate—will help to confirm the diagnosis. However, these organisms can be found in syphilitic ulcers and the Wassermann reaction is sometimes positive in Vincent's angina. The subacute onset, the raised temperature, and the tenderness of the glands aid the differentiation from syphilis; and from diphtheria the milder constitutional symptoms, the soft pliable character of the membrane, and the absence of the diphtheria bacillus. Ulceration of the fauces and tonsils also occurs in glandular fever, agranulocytosis, and leukaemia, and in the elderly it may be a tuberculous infection secondary to phthisis. Recurrent non-specific ulceration of the mouth, palate, fauces, and tonsils is not uncommon. In most cases the cause is unknown, but some are due to herpes simplex while in rare instances it is a manifestation of Behçet's syndrome, pemphigus vulgaris, or pemphigoid.

Treatment. The lesions respond to parenteral penicillin in full dosage. Alternatively, administer metronidazole, 200 mg thrice daily for three days.

A paint of 5 per cent neoarsphenamine in equal quantities of glycerin and water may be applied to the ulcers.

Attention to dental hygiene and a course of ascorbic acid and vitamin B complex will prevent recurrent attacks.

Acute catarrhal pharyngitis

This is not a well-defined affection, and is usually accompanied by acute rhinitis on the one hand, and by laryngitis on the other; the tonsils also often participate in the inflammation.

Aetiology. The affection is generally the result of coryza, and it is a feature of various acute infectious fevers, such as measles, German measles, scarlet fever, influenza, and typhoid.

Symptoms. The discomfort varies from a tickling sensation, or the feeling of a lump in the throat, to severe dysphagia. The voice is husky and thick, and the cervical glands tender and somewhat enlarged. There is slight fever and general malaise.

The pharynx is to a varying degree red and swollen, especially at the sides behind the posterior faucial pillars, where the swelling forms the so-called 'lateral bands'. The palate is swollen and relaxed, and the uvula elongated. The posterior wall is often covered by a film of tenacious mucus.

Treatment. The patient should stay in a warm room and avoid the irritation of smoking, talking, alcohol, or irritating foods. Aspirin, or sodium salicylate, is helpful and it is important to treat any primary cause.

Acute septic pharyngitis

This term includes a series of severe infective inflammations: oedematous, phlegmonous, and gangrenous pharyngitis and laryngitis, and Ludwig's angina. Any classification must necessarily be a clinical one, based on the severity of the symptoms and their localization, for they can be produced by a variety of micro-organisms, though they are usually caused by a streptococcus. These severe inflammations are fortunately uncommon, and most often, though by no means invariably, occur in debilitated or alcoholic persons.

Symptoms. These vary greatly with the severity of the infection, which ranges from a mild inflammation to the most severe septic intoxication. They include malaise, sore throat, dysphagia, hoarseness, and dyspnoea. The temperature in some cases rises to 40.5–41 °C, but in many of the worst cases it is hardly raised at all, and may be subnormal. Pleurisy, pneumonia, and pericarditis may ensue, or death may result from asphyxia; but the worst cases die from general toxaemia and heart failure, even within 24 hours of the onset of the disease.

The objective appearances, also, are very variable. The pharynx and palate are of a deep purplish-red, and there may be sloughy pseudomembranous patches. The entire mucosa may be enormously swollen, and the oedema may involve the upper aperture of the larynx and produce asphyxia. The sublingual region is sometimes occupied by a peculiar brawny swelling, of a hardness like wood, which spreads downwards into the neck to a variable extent, and is known as Ludwig's angina.

Treatment. The patient must be in bed and well nursed, and every care must be used to ensure that he takes as much nourishment as possible. Antibiotics must be administered in full dosage and a high fluid intake be assured. Oedema of the glottis may call for emergency tracheostomy. For Ludwig's angina it is now only rarely necessary to make an incision deeply into the neck in the hope of striking pus; the swelling will either subside or a fluctuating abscess will become apparent.

Retropharyngeal abscess

There are two forms: acute, and chronic.

The acute form occurs in children up to the age of three or four years, but is far more frequently met with in the first 12 months. It is due to suppuration in the prevertebral glands situated behind the posterior pharyngeal wall; these glands disappear in later life. The abscess is secondary to nasal, nasopharyngeal, or tonsillar infection and may occur during the course of an infectious fever.

Though rare the condition is an important one for it may easily remain unrecognized in a young infant and could then cause death either by rupturing with inspiration of the pus, or by spread to the mediastinum, or by general toxaemia and septicaemia. The symptoms are fever and restlessness, a hoarse cry, and croupy cough, with difficulty in swallowing and dyspnoea. Such symptoms should arouse a suspicion of retropharyngeal abscess, which may be seen on inspection as a rounded swelling of the posterior pharyngeal wall.

As soon as the condition is recognized a broad-spectrum antibiotic should be administered in high dosage. Intramuscular penicillin is the first choice unless specifically contra-indicated. The abscess must then be incised and, as it is often large, care is needed to avoid aspiration of pus and blood. It should be opened widely over the most prominent and inferior part of the bulge. In a child under one year old this can be done without anaesthesia if the child is firmly held lying on its back with the head hanging almost vertically. Over one year old general anaesthesia with a cuffed endotracheal tube is used and suction should be availabe in all cases. A specimen of the pus should be sent for bacteriological examination and if the sensitivity reports indicate it the antibiotic must be changed. Antibiotic therapy should continue for at least one week after incision of the abscess. Recovery is usually rapid unless the child was severely debilitated before treatment commenced.

The chronic form also is found most frequently in children but generally after the third year. This is a tuberculous abscess forming behind the prevertebral fascia and is secondary to caries of the cervical spine. X-rays of the spine usually demonstrate the lesion well. It should not be opened through the mouth as this may lead to secondary infection of the diseased bone but is best drained via a vertical incision along the posterior border of the sternomastoid. General antituberculous chemotherapy is indicated and temporary support for the cervical spine may be necessary.

Chronic pharyngitis (pharyngeal hyperaesthesia)

Aetiology. Chronic pharyngitis is usually secondary to chronic infection in the nasal sinuses, tonsils, or teeth. It is aggravated by mouth breathing, smoking, and over-indulgence in alcohol. Excessive use or misuse of the voice perpetuates the condition which may be initiated by an acute pharyngitis which fails to resolve satisfactorily.

Symptoms. Discomfort may take the form of aching, fullness, or feeling of a lump, a hair, or a pricking. The voice has a dead tone, and there is usually much hawking and frequent swallowing. The sufferer often becomes depressed, and fears that he has cancer of the throat. The unpleasant sensations are markedly lessened after a meal.

The mucosa of the pharynx and palate is thickened, and there is a loss of the finer modelling of the faucial pillars; the uvula is elongated, often slightly oedematous at its edges and tip, and fails to retract on phonation. The posterior wall is covered by a film of mucus, which puckers up and becomes more obvious on touching it with a probe or swab. The wall of the pharynx is traversed by enlarged venules, and sometimes it is set with slightly raised pink lenticular nodules of lymphoid tissue, constituting a variety known as 'granular pharyngitis'. In other cases two elongated masses of lymphoid tissue appear behind and parallel to the posterior pillars; these are the 'lateral bands', and this form is called 'lateral pharyngitis'. Patients suffering from atrophic rhinitis may complain of dryness of the throat; the posterior pharyngeal wall presents a glazed desiccated appearance, sometimes alluded to as pharyngitis sicca.

Treatment. Any focus of infection elsewhere in the nose or mouth should be eradicated. Tobacco, alcohol, spiced foods, and excessive use of the voice must be avoided. A warm alkaline saline nasal douche and throat spray may help, but local medication should be avoided when possible as it concentrates the patient's attention on his throat. In cases of chronic granular pharyngitis and those with enlarged 'lateral bands' of lymphoid tissue the hypertrophied lymph follicles may be reduced by painting them at weekly intervals for one month with a 5 per cent solution of silver nitrate. Alternatively they may be ablated by superficial cryosurgery. It is most important to reassure these patients that there is no growth in their throat as many of them have an underlying cancer phobia and this reassurance will often cause their symptoms to abate.

Keratosis pharyngis

In this condition a number of sharply defined white or yellow spikes project from the surface of the tonsils; they also occur, though less profusely, scattered over the lingual and nasopharyngeal tonsils and on any lymphoid granules in the pharynx. They occur at any age after childhood and the causation is unknown. The projections consist of heaped-up epithelium and detritis containing numerous micro-organisms of the kind ordinarily present in the mouth. On microscopical examination branching fungus mycelium can usually be demonstrated. They sometimes disappear quickly, in other cases they remain for many months, or they may recur. They produce no symptoms, or at most a slight discomfort, and are of interest chiefly because they are frequently mistaken for the exudation of chronic follicular tonsillitis. Once seen they can, however, be recognized at a glance, for they are hard and adherent, discrete and prominent, and occur beyond the limits of the tonsils, on the pharynx and base of the tongue. They are usually discovered accidentally by the patient, who is naturally alarmed at their appearance. They are quite harmless, and local treatment is useless, for they are removed with difficulty and usually recur; it is wise to reassure the patient by telling him these facts and, if any treatment be required, to trust to attention to the general health, a holiday and change of air. In rare cases when the condition is confined to the tonsils, marked symptoms and persistence of the condition may justify tonsillectomy.

References

Ludman, H. (1981). Throat infections. *Br. med. J.* **282**, 628.
Lund, W. (1981). The pharynx and larynx. In *Scientific foundations of surgery*, 3rd edn. (eds. J. Kyle and J. D. Hardy), 271. Heinemann, London.
Ransome, J., Holden, H., and Bull, T. R. (1973). *Recent advances in otolaryngology*, vol 4. Churchill Livingstone, Edinburgh.
Valman, H. B. (1981). Tonsillitis and otitis media. *Br. med. J.* **283**, 119.

Disorders of motility

D. L. Wingate

The principal function of the digestive tract is the assimilation of nutrients; of the major processes contributing to this, two—exocrine secretion and intestinal absorption—are well understood, but the third, motility, is not. In the absence of any clear understanding of 'normal' motility, it is not surprising that most problems of 'abnormal' motility are ill-defined.

It is important to appreciate the dimensions of the problem, and to have a clear understanding of the few established facts. The absence of well-defined syndromes dictates a measure of improvisation in the investigation and treatment of presumed abnormal motility, and this approach can be clinically valuable only if the physician has some understanding of normal function and, hence, how it might be disorganized.

To the layman (and to not a few doctors), the digestive tract is thought of as something akin to a slot-machine, in which food is inserted in the upper orifice with the consequent emergence of faeces at the lower end. According to this model, the ingesta are assumed to travel under the influence of gravity through a maze of tubes offering a varying degree of resistance to flow. Nothing could be further from the truth; gravity plays little or no part in the normal transit of ingesta. The digestive tract is indeed a hollow tube invested by smooth muscle, but the transit of ingesta through the tract is regulated not only by the intrinsic characteristics of the muscle, but also by complex neurohumoral controls. The purpose of these controls appears to be to regulate flow so that each stage of physicochemical transformation occurs at the appropriate region of the tract. Thus, the mechanical breakdown of large particles must be accomplished before the ingesta are subjected to chemical breakdown in order to permit penetration of digestive enzymes to the nutrient molecules; it is the function of the stomach to achieve this breakdown and also to ensure, if possible, that ingesta do not proceed beyond the stomach until dispersed into fine particles.

The obstacles to progress in this field have been the difficulties of defining normal patterns of activity. This requires the simultaneous observation and correlation of muscular activity in the wall, and the passage of material in the lumen; in practice, this is surprisingly difficult. Conventionally, three types of investigation have been pursued:

1. *Imaging of ingesta during transit.* This can be accomplished using radio-opaque substances with fluoroscopy, or radionuclide labels with scanning. Radio-opaque substances are non-nutrient; replacement of nutrient with barium sulphate undoubtedly alters the motor response of the digestive tract and gives a false picture of the transit of normal ingesta. Radionuclides can be incorporated into a normal meal but give a poorer image, and tend to be confined to a single phase (solid, lipid, aqueous) of the meal which may become separated from other phases.

2. *Measurement of intraluminal pressure.* This can be performed in a number of ways in the proximal digestive tract, and in the rectosigmoid region. It gives an approximate picture of muscle activity patterns, but little information on transit. Since the pressure change at any point in the lumen is not only a function of muscle activity at that point, but also the contractile activity proximally and distally, it does not always serve as an accurate guide to local muscle activity.

3. *Measurement of contractile activity.* Sensors may be attached to the wall of the digestive tract to give information on tension changes or electromyographic changes at the recording site. Such

techniques have been used extensively in experimental animals, but only limited studies are possible in man. Again, the correlations between contractile activity and the propulsion of ingesta are not always clear.

If such techniques have failed to provide a complete picture of 'normal' motility, they do provide limited information. In clinical practice, where the likelihood of dysfunction may be comparatively circumscribed, these methods may give useful diagnostic or therapeutic information, but, overall, the diagnosis of motility disorders in the present state of knowledge depends upon the ability of the physician to select, or even devise, a diagnostic manoeuvre to answer specific questions. Both for the selection and the interpretation of such procedures, an understanding of 'normal motility'—in so far as it is understood at all—is essential.

Normal motility

Motor anatomy of the digestive tract. While the detailed anatomy of the gastrointestinal motor system is complex, a simple knowledge of the groups of components of the system is sufficient basis for the appreciation of function. Muscles and nerves comprise the essentials of the system.

With the exception of the proximal third of the oesophagus, which is composed of voluntary muscle, the *musculature* of the digestive tract is composed of smooth, or non-striated muscle, largely orientated in two planes, *circular* and *longitudinal*. The configuration of these two muscle layers varies between a simple arrangement of two groups of fibres at right angles to each other which completely invest a hollow tube, as in the small intestine, to the more complex arrangements of muscle groups in specialized organs, as exemplified by the stomach and colon. Essentially, the muscle fibres are arranged so that contraction will result in both circular constriction and longitudinal shortening; relaxation will have the converse effect. It should be appreciated that these movements alone, arranged in complex spatial and temporal patterns, confer an almost infinite variety of possible movements to the gut.

A third muscle group is the muscle layer of the mucous membrane, the *muscularis mucosae*. The function of this layer is unknown, but the penetration of fibres into the intestinal villi suggests that it is involved in villous contraction and lengthening, and thereby in the modulation of epithelial function.

Morphologically, the most important characteristic of gastrointestinal smooth muscle is the arrangement of cells within layers in a syncytium, as in the myocardium. Adjacent cells are connected by *nexuses*, or gap junctions, permitting the spread of electrical activity from one cell to another to allow co-ordinated movement of the muscle mass, which is potentially independent of neural control.

The *sphincters* of the gastrointestinal tract are specialized muscular structures; each end of the digestive tract is protected by a pair of sphincters, one of each pair being composed of smooth muscle, and the other of striated muscle under voluntary control. At the proximal end, the pair of sphincters (upper and lower oesophageal sphincters) are widely separated, whereas the distal pair (internal and external anal sphincters) are closely approximated. But, while the passage of material in and out of the gastrointestinal tract is under voluntary control, there is considerable controversy concerning the exact role of the smooth muscle sphincters within the tract. For example, there is reasonable agreement that the pyloric sphincter is, in health, more important in the prevention of reflux of duodenal contents than in the control of gastric emptying; it is only the pylorus which is fibrotic, or even stenotic, as a result of chronic ulceration, which obstructs gastric emptying. The lower oesophageal sphincter does appear to have a true sphincter action, but this action is considerably impaired when the sphincter is anatomically displaced as in hiatus hernia, even though the intrinsic neuromuscular apparatus is undamaged.

The *innervation* of the digestive tract is intrinsic and extrinsic.

The *intrinsic* nerves are arranged in plexuses which lie along the wall of the digestive tract. The principal plexus is the myenteric plexus, containing fibres interconnecting ganglia; the myenteric plexus lies between the longitudinal and circular muscle coats. Subsidiary plexuses lie within the myenteric plexus itself, including plexuses of fine fibres that penetrate the muscle coats. The submucosal plexus is located submucosally, and is both less dense and morphologically simpler than the myenteric plexus; it is also probably absent in the oesophagus.

The *extrinsic* nerves connect the enteric plexuses to the central nervous system through sympathetic nerve trunks, each containing both sensory and motor fibres. The sympathetic nerves are connected to the gut through perivascular plexuses connected to the retroperitoneal ganglia associated with major arteries (coeliac, superior mesenteric, and inferior mesenteric); splanchnic nerves link the ganglia to the central nervous system. The parasympathetic nerves travel to the gut through the pelvic nerves and the vagus nerves; the latter are mixed motor and sensory nerves, with the sensory fibres being in the majority.

It is now apparent that the nerves of the gut may be classified into three functional groups; probably further groups or subgroups remain to be identified. This classification is based on histochemical evidence and on the response of nerve and muscle to neurotransmitter substances. *Cholinergic* parasympathetic receptors are either muscarinic and blocked by atropine, or nicotinic and blocked by hexamethonium and D-tubocurarine. *Adrenergic* sympathetic receptors are of both alpha and beta classes, blocked by phentolamine and propranolol respectively. The third group of receptors are *non-adrenergic*, *non-cholinergic* receptors. Controversy exists concerning the transmitter or transmitters in the latter group. At the time of writing, opinion is polarized between two possibilities, which are not mutually exclusive. The 'purinergic' hypothesis embodies the concept that the transmitters are cyclic nucleotides, and ATP (adenosine triphosphate) in particular, based on responses of nerve-muscle preparations to ATP in the presence of adrenergic and cholinergic inhibition. The 'peptidergic' hypothesis is based principally on the immunohistochemical identification of 'gut hormone' peptides, such as vasoactive intestinal peptide, within the enteric plexuses, and also the identification of such peptides, including gastrin, cholecystokinin, neurotensin, and somatostatin, in both the enteric nervous system and the central nervous system.

The complexity of the myenteric plexuses, and certain morphological features, have led to the concept that they may function as a type of primitive brain—networks capable of initiating co-ordinated muscular activity without reference to the central nervous system.

Motor physiology of the digestive tract

Characteristics of gastrointestinal smooth muscle. The cardinal characteristic of gastrointestinal smooth muscle is its spontaneous electrical rhythmicity, in which it resembles myocardial smooth muscle. Smooth muscle cells exhibit an endless cycle of depolarization and repolarization, and because of the syncytial arrangement of the cells and their intercommunication through nexuses, this electrical change tends to spread rapidly to adjacent cells, producing an almost synchronous change in the muscle mass. This electrical change can be recorded by an electrode on the surface of the muscle mass as an electric slow wave, and the electrogastrogram, or electro-enterogram, first described in 1921, is analogous to the electro-cardiogram. Unfortunately for diagnosticians, the electrical signal cannot be reliably picked up at remote points on the body surface, as can the electro-cardiogram, because of the differing electrical geometry of the respective viscera.

The fundamental difference between gastrointestinal smooth muscle and cardiac smooth muscle is that, in the digestive tract, the electrical cycle resulting in the slow wave does not represent contraction; one, or many, cycles of depolarization may occur in a gut smooth muscle cell without any tension change (Fig. 1). Contraction *may* occur, and if it does, it will occur during the depolarization phase. In general, at the intercellular level, contraction is marked by action potentials during the plateau phase, and thus, in a muscle mass, these action potentials will be synchronous, and in a fixed temporal relationship to the slow wave; the term 'phase-locked' is sometimes employed. The electrical cycle of the smooth muscle cell determines when a contraction may occur in each cycle, but not *whether* it will occur.

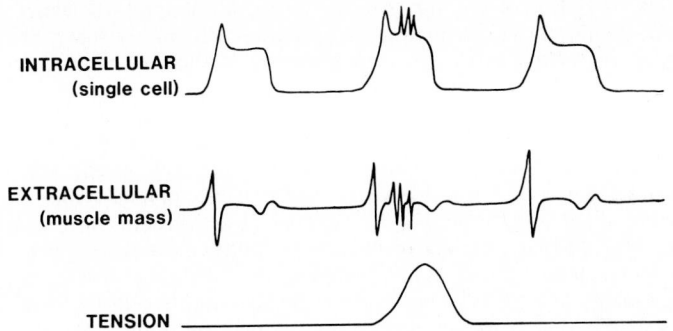

INTRACELLULAR
(single cell)

EXTRACELLULAR
(muscle mass)

TENSION

Fig. 1 Schematic comparison of intracellular activity of smooth muscle (upper trace), electrical activity as recorded by serosal electromyography (middle trace), and tension change in the muscle (lower trace). Intracellular depolarization is represented extracellularly as a QRS-type complex, the slow wave. Tension change does not occur with the slow wave, but with the associated action potentials, if present; summated action potentials are detected extracellularly as spike bursts.

The slow wave frequency varies from region to region. In the stomach, the cycle duration is 20 seconds, whereas in the small intestine, it is about six seconds. Thus the maximum number of contractions that can occur in the stomach is three per minute, and in the small intestine, 10–12 per minute. Whether or not a contraction will occur is, presumably, a function of the neurohumoral control systems which are modulating the release of acetylcholine (and other transmitters) within the muscle. Pursuing the analogy with the myocardium, the activity of the myocardial cell is altered by altering the period of the electrical cycle, since each cycle is accompanied by contraction; by contrast, the electrical cycle of the gut smooth muscle cell is remarkably constant, varying within less than 10 per cent, and the activity of the cell is altered by external controls which determine whether each slow wave cycle will or will not be accompanied by contraction.

It is possible, although difficult, to detect gastric and intestinal smooth wave cycles—but not spike bursts—on the body surface. From the foregoing it should be obvious that this is not helpful as a diagnostic procedure, since the regularity of the slow wave cycle gives no indication of the contractile events.

Again as in the myocardium, pacemakers are found. These are areas with the highest slow wave cycle rate and they are sited proximally in the viscera. These pacemaking sites over-ride adjacent and more distant cells with slower intrinsic frequencies; consequently the electrical slow waves are determined by these pacemakers and travel through the longitudinal muscle layers. For the stomach, the pacemaker site lies in the fundus, and electrical slow waves pass down as far as the pylorus. In the small intestine, the pacemaker is just distal to the pylorus, and slow waves radiate from it caudally as far as the ileocaecal junction. Pacemaking activity as such is not seen in the oesophagus, and considerable uncertainty exists about the number and location of pacemakers in the large intestine. Transection of the small bowel interrupts the caudal propagation of slow waves from the duodenal pacemaker, and the muscle immediately distal to the transection then assumes the role of pacemaker for the remaining length of bowel.

The practical consequence of proximal pacemaker sites transmitting slow waves which propagate distally is that the trend of contraction should always be aboral. Slow waves in the small intestine travel several centimetres in one second. Consider a (hypothetical) situation where several centimetres of bowel are simultaneously subjected to cholinergic stimulation to produce contractile activity

in the first available slow wave cycle. The effect of slow wave propagation is to ensure that this contraction will occur proximally at first, and then travel rapidly through the stimulated segment. In fact, such a rapid contraction wave would probably be of little value in the propulsion and transit of ingesta, and such waves probably occur rarely, although animal experiments suggest that they may occur in infective diarrhoea.

Movements of gastrointestinal smooth muscle. Conventionally, three characteristic movements of gastrointestinal smooth muscle have been described. These are *peristalsis, segmentation,* and *pendular movements.* The first two movements are predominantly circular muscle contractions, while the third movement is assumed to be contraction and relaxation of longitudinal muscle. This terminology is not altogether helpful, although it finds a place in radiological practice. The terms *ring contraction* and *longitudinal contraction* are better; *moving* ring contractions are the equivalent of peristalsis, while multiple *standing* ring contractions are the equivalent of segmentation (or, in the colon, haustration). Moving ring contractions are essentially propulsive, while standing ring contractions serve to mix intraluminal content. Description of these movements gives little clue to organ function; while such contractions are the bricks from which the edifice of integrated organ movement is constructed, the complexity of organ function arises from the organization of these movements in time and space. Similarly, pharmacological studies in which muscle strips are induced *in vitro* to exhibit contraction or relaxation may not easily relate to *in situ* organ function. Muscle movement in the gastrointestinal tract appears to be *organ-specific*, related to the function of the viscus and the disposition of the muscle layers, and *time-specific* according to temporal patterns of activity.

Spatial and temporal organization of muscle activity. Since the digestive tract is a tube consisting of two layers of muscle orientated at right angles, and since each muscle layer consists of a syncitium of individual cells, the possible permutations of movements that might occur are almost infinite. In fact, specific patterns of movement recur, and these patterns may be characterized in three ways.
1. *Spatial organization.* Contractile activity occurs at specific sites, and in a specific temporal sequence so that a specified operation on ingesta (i.e. swallowing) can be accomplished.
2. *Temporal organization.* As well as contraction being organized into specific movements, patterns of activity occur that are specific to the physiological state of the individual; as will be seen, movements of the stomach and small intestine have a marked pattern during fasting which is abolished on feeding.
3. *Organ specificity.* Patterns of movement occur which are specific to one region of the digestive tract but are not found in other regions. These patterns are appropriate to the state of ingesta at that site, and to the function of the adjacent epithelial surfaces (absorption, secretion).

Again, it must be emphasized that a comprehensive picture of these spatio-temporal patterns is still lacking. In general, regions which are more easily accessible to investigation (oesophagus, stomach) are better understood, but this is an imperfect generalization; efforts to define physiological patterns of activity in the rectosigmoid region have not, so far, led to generally agreed conclusions. Notwithstanding, it seems reasonable to assume that *motility disorders occur when a physiological pattern of motility is disrupted, or absent, or is replaced by an aberrant pattern.*

Physiological patterns of motor activity. The classification of patterns of motility is dictated by the fact that these patterns are time-specific as well as organ-specific. That regional variation occurs is self-evident; the effect of time less so. Within the digestive tract, there are two main time phases, *postprandial* and *interdigestive.* The postprandial phase comprises the assimilation of a meal, from ingestion to the completion of absorption. The interdigestive phase, originally assumed to be a phase of motor inertia, refers to the period when the digestive tract is void of exogenous nutrient, and contains only resting secretions, cellular debris, and indigestible food residues. Some motility disorders are clearly meal-related, while others are not; for these reasons, it is necessary to understand the different patterns which characterize the two phases.

Postprandial motor activity. *Pharynx and oesophagus.* The upper oesophageal sphincter, represented by the cricopharyngeus muscle, a voluntary muscle, is normally tonically contracted due to tonic discharge of the somatic nerves by which it is served. Swallowing is initiated voluntarily by the striated muscle of the oropharynx and pharynx, and also requires the stimulation of local sensory receptors. Impulses from the swallowing centre in the brain stem induce a series of co-ordinated movements which propel a bolus through the pharynx, and through the temporarily relaxed upper oesophageal sphincter. As the bolus progresses to the smooth muscle portion of the oesophagus, control is assumed by autonomic nerves, which are non-adrenergic inhibitory nerves. Normally, there is no tone in the oesophageal smooth muscles, but activation of the autonomic inhibitory nerves is followed by a rebound contraction; it is this contraction, progressing down the oesophagus, which forms a peristaltic wave. The progression of the contraction is neurally determined, but is modulated by a gradient of excitability within the smooth muscle itself. As the bolus, propelled by a peristaltic wave, reaches the lower oesophageal sphincter, this sphincter relaxes, and the bolus passes into the stomach.

The stomach. The major physiological function of the stomach is *not* the chemical digestion of ingesta by acid and pepsin (as witness the fact that individuals with complete gastric achlorhydria have no apparent functional deficit) but the mechanical breakdown of solid ingesta, and the regulation of the delivery of chyme (ingesta reduced to a liquid or fine particulate consistency) to the small intestine at a rate which will not overwhelm the digestive and absorptive capacity of the small intestine. These physiological functions are reflected in the clinical problems which sometimes occur as sequelae of gastric surgery.

In terms of function, the human stomach may be considered as two separate but linked organs, the *proximal stomach* (fundus and corpus) and the *distal stomach* (antrum and pylorus). The proximal stomach serves primarily as a reservoir, while both mechanical breakdown and emptying are accomplished by the distal stomach. Normal gastric function depends equally upon both these properties.

The passage of a bolus through the lower oesophageal sphincter is accompanied by *receptive relaxation*, or accommodation, of the proximal stomach. This is required not only to accommodate an increased volume, but also to ensure that the intragastric pressure is transiently lowered while the lower oesophageal sphincter remains open, and this relaxation is mediated through the vagus nerve. Beyond this function, the postprandial activity of the proximal stomach is not well understood.

Mixing and emptying are accomplished by contraction waves starting in the corpus and sweeping over the distal stomach to the pylorus. Following a meal, these contraction waves are of relatively low amplitude (in contrast with the contractions which occur during fasting) but persistent, occuring up to three times per minute (the maximal gastric contraction frequency). These contraction waves propel material through the distal stomach, towards the relaxed pyloric segment. As the contraction reaches the distal antrum, the leading portion of the bolus of chyme traverses the pylorus; but almost immediately, the contraction wave reaches the pylorus, which closes. Occlusion of the distal antrum combined with pyloric closure causes compression and retropulsion of chyme backwards towards the proximal stomach, ensuring both 'grinding' and mixing. Thus the bolus of chyme which traverses the pylorus is both small in volume, and predominantly fluid, since it is fluid which is propelled most rapidly by the contraction wave; larger particles are left behind, and propelled back to the proximal stomach. Not only do fluids empty more easily than particulate solids, but the lipid

phase (which is liquid at body temperature) empties more slowly than the aqueous phase from a mixed meal. That a pure aqueous load will be emptied more rapidly than a pure lipid load is partly a function of stimulation of duodenal receptors which have a negative feedback effect on gastric contractile activity, but the ability of the stomach to discharge lipid more slowly from a mixed meal probably reflects only the fact that the lipid forms a floating layer which, due to the J-shaped anatomy of the stomach, rarely forms the first part of the chyme to be propelled by the gastric contraction wave.

It must be emphasized most strongly that gastric emptying is not a function of gravity; the paralysed stomach does not empty.

Small intestine. The postprandial motor activity of the small intestine is complex and has not been precisely defined. There is general agreement that it is characterized by persistent contractile activity. Measured at any one point, this contractile activity appears to be irregular and lacking any regular periodicity or pattern, but radiology and manometric observations from adjacent sites suggest that there are ring contractions which are either stationary (segmenting) or moving (peristaltic) over short distances, serving both to mix and slowly propel chyme. There appears to be a degree of co-ordination between the antrum and the duodenal bulb; during an antral contraction, the duodenal bulb is relaxed so as to permit the influx of chyme through the pylorus.

Studies of transit of ingesta through the small intestine cannot be correlated with contractile activity, as imaging of precise locations along the convoluted small intestine is difficult, but such studies provide some idea of how a meal progresses along the bowel. After ingestion, the head of the meal appears to traverse the length of the small bowel within a short time (5 to 20 minutes), but only a small proportion travels at this speed. The bulk of the meal follows much more slowly, and the speed of the meal diminishes as it travels. It has been suggested that the duodenum and jejunum serve as a conduit, while the ileum is a reservoir. Although very little is known about the function of the ileocaecal valve, it is possible that it has a sphincteric action associated with the ileum functioning as a reservoir which is the final site of absorption.

The colon. The motor activity of the colon remains ill-defined to the point where it would be rash to regard any pattern of colonic motor activity as characteristically normal or abnormal; moreover, useful techniques for the clinical study of colonic motor activity are virtually non-existent. It is known that both longitudinal and ring contractions (*haustrations*) occur, and that colonic contents may be propelled in both directions. The transit time of ingesta through the colon in normal subjects varies between hours and days.

However, there is some evidence that colonic motor activity varies with feeding. *Mass movements* of faeces along the colon were described by Cannon, a pioneer of gastrointestinal radiology, and ingestion of a meal appears to activate the *gastrocolic reflex*. This reflex activity involves the mass movement of faeces from the descending and sigmoid colon into the rectum, initiating the signal for defaecation. Evidence of increased postprandial sigmoid motor activity has been obtained using intraluminal electromyography, although it has to be remembered that increased muscle activity is not conclusive proof of propulsion of faeces. But although the detailed mechanism may remain obscure, the postprandial call to stool is a reality, best observed in infants unrestrained by social inhibition.

Rectum and anus. Since defaecation is the major function of the rectum and anus, and since the desire to defaecate is commonly postprandial, it is logical to include a brief description of this specialized function in a review of postprandial motor activity.

In healthy subjects, continence is maintained by three mechanisms. It is now known that the muscles of the pelvic floor, although voluntary, are normally in a state of tonic contraction (cf. the upper oesophageal sphincter), elevating the anorectum, and producing an acute angle at the rectosigmoid junction. This maintains an empty rectum until there is active propulsion of faeces caudad from the sigmoid colon. In addition, the internal anal sphincter, composed of smooth muscle, is tonically contracted, closing the anal canal: the voluntary external anal sphincter may also be contracted, while the smooth muscle walls of the rectum itself are relaxed. Entry of faeces into the rectum stimulates mechanoreceptors, initiating a complex sequence of events constituting a defaecation reflex. First, the pelvic floor and the internal sphincter relax. Subsequently, the rectum is emptied by relaxation and opening of the external anal sphincter, and elevation of intra-abdominal pressure by voluntary muscle contraction, which may even involve a Valsalva manoeuvre. When the rectum is emptied, the sensory stimulus is abolished, and the tonic mechanisms of continence return.

Interdigestive motor activity. Although the greater part of the organized motor activity of the digestive tract is related to the correct disposal of a meal, activity also occurs during the interdigestive, or interprandial phase. Some of this activity occurs at the extreme ends of the digestive tract and is subject, although not invariably, to conscious regulation. Possibly of greater physiological and pathophysiological importance is the interdigestive activity of the stomach and small intestine.

Entry and exit. The sphincteric mechanisms which normally seal the digestive tract operate intermittently throughout the day and night.

At the proximal end, swallowing is required to dispose of saliva and nasal secretion; the latter is often augmented in the presence of respiratory infection by mucopurulent secretion from the upper respiratory tract or, through coughing, from the lower respiratory tract. 'Dry swallowing', or swallowing in the absence of food or drink, usually propels a bolus of air in the stomach; if by this means, the gastric air bubble becomes excessively large, belching, or *eructation*, results. It should be remembered that air-swallowing, or *aerophagy*, is to some extent a normal physiological function; it may become a clinical problem when it is excessive.

At the distal end of the digestive tract, excessive colonic gas is eliminated as *flatus*. This gas is a mixture of swallowed gas which has traversed the length of the digestive tract, and gas derived from the bacterial fermentation of residual ingesta in the colon; this moiety is predominantly methane and hydrogen sulphide. Some foods provide particularly favourable substrates for gas formations; beans of the type served as 'baked beans' are deservedly notorious in this respect.

The mechanism of elimination of flatus involves the propulsion of gas along the colon to the rectum. It is not always remembered that the sensory receptors of the rectum not only respond to distension, but can also discriminate between gaseous, liquid, and solid distension. Elimination of flatus is a simpler mechanism than defaecation, requiring only sphincteric relaxation and expulsion of gas, without a rise in intra-abdominal pressure. Although the passage of flatus is to some extent under voluntary control, this is clearly not always so. The ability of the rectum to distinguish between gaseous and liquid or solid distension means that flatus may be passed 'involuntarily' while, in the socially trained individual, faeces are not. Clinically, the cessation of the passage of flatus in the post-surgery patient is an important sign of an adynamic bowel.

Interdigestive migrating complex. That at the conclusion of digestion, the digestive tract should remain in a state of motor quiescence might seem to be a reasonable and logical deduction, and has been widely assumed to be the case since the early days of digestive physiology. At the beginning of the 20th century, W. N. Boldyreff, a physiologist working in Pavlov's laboratory in St Petersburg, noted that in fasted dogs, brief periods of high-amplitude gastric contractions coinciding with copious pancreatic secretion recurred at 90-minute intervals, and that this periodic activity was abolished for several hours by the ingestion of a meal. These observations excited some interest among his contemporaries: W. B. Cannon recorded similar 'hunger contractions' in a human subject. The phenomenon was neglected, and this work was largely forgotten until 1969, when J. H. Szurszewski, at the Mayo Clinic, demonstrated in dogs that periodic fasting motor activity migrated from the stomach along the entire length of the small bowel to the terminal ileum; moreover, feeding interrupted this activity at all levels, inducing the persistent but irregular contractile activity which has already been described. Since then, the phenomenon has been confirmed in a number of mammalian species, and has been conclusively demonstrated in man.

Because Szurszewski's observations were made using electromyography with electrodes implanted at multiple sites along the digestive tract, the phenomenon was originally termed the 'interdigestive migrating myoelectric complex'. Since it may be demonstrated using manometry to show contractile patterns as well as by electromyography, and since there is some doubt as to whether it only occurs in the absence of digestive activity, it is now best referred to as the 'migrating myoelectric complex' or 'migrating motor complex', dependig upon the mode of observation, or, most simply, by the common abbreviation *MMC*.

Recording of motor activity at a single point in the distal stomach or small intestine reveals a remarkably consistent pattern during fasting. A phase of *motor quiescence*, lasting about 50 minutes, is succeeded by a phase of *irregular motor activity* which may persist for about 30 minutes. The irregular phase culminates in a brief period of *regular motor activity*, sometimes known as the *activity front*, in which the smooth muscle contracts at its maximum frequency (three per minute in the human stomach, 11 per minute in the human proximal duodenum) for about five minutes. This phase terminates abruptly in a new period of motor quiescence. The whole complex starts virtually simultaneously in the lower oesophageal sphincter, antrum, and duodenal bulb, and migrates slowly down the small intestine, reaching the terminal small bowel after 100 minutes. The activity front constitutes a true peristaltic wave, sweeping down the entire small bowel, and propelling onwards any residual content.

In recent years, the MMC has been the subject of intense study, and a number of features can be regarded as established. First, in man, the periodicity appears to be variable; 85 minutes is the median interval between MMCs, but much longer (and shorter) intervals may occur in healthy subjects. Secondly, in dogs, MMCs are rapidly suppressed at the beginning of a meal, and do not return for some hours. Thirdly, the appearance of the MMC in the stomach and duodenum is accompanied by a burst of augmented gastric, pancreatic, and biliary secretion. Finally, the contractions which occur during the activity front (regular contractile activity) are easily recognizable because of their regularity and their high amplitude; there is some evidence to suggest that large pieces of ingested solids which have not been adequately broken down in the stomach are only emptied by the gastric activity front of the MMC because digestive, or post-prandial, antral contractions are of sufficient force.

The importance of the MMC in clinical practice remains uncertain. Various functions have been ascribed to it, and it has been described as an intestinal 'housekeeper' (C.F. Code). Absence of the MMC in some individuals seems to be associated with bacterial overgrowth of the small bowel, while chronic post-vagotomy diarrhoea has been associated with premature return of the MMC pattern following a meal. What is clear, and which was previously obscure, is that the pattern of motor activity in the stomach and small intestine is completely different following a meal from the pattern during fasting, and that the change from one pattern to another involves a complex sequence of receptor stimulation, neural activity, and the release of peptides. The importance of the MMC to the scientist is that it provides a consistent and reproducible phenomenon for study, and also clear evidence of integrated motor activity dependent on neural networks in the myenteric plexus. For the clinician, it provides a means of detecting whether the motor activity in the stomach and small bowel is appropriate to the physiological status of the patient; there is preliminary but accumulating evidence associating clinical disturbances with the failure of the proximal digestive tract to switch to the appropriate pattern.

The MMC does not traverse the colon and, at present, no distinctive pattern of activity resembling the MMC has been recorded in the colon.

Abnormal motility

The classification of motility disorders is, in the present state of knowledge, a problem. The pathological basis of some motility problems remains uncertain; further, it is even uncertain to what extent some syndromes, currently labelled as 'functional', are primarily disorders of motility. Moreover, disorders of motility become apparent not because of symptoms arising from local lesions of the neuromuscular apparatus of the digestive tract, but because of the abnormal propulsion—or lack of propulsion—of ingesta and/or secretions.

The classification of motility disorders on either a pathological basis (Table 1) or a functional basis (Table 2) represents an individual choice rather than a generally agreed taxonomy; the latter does not yet exist. The functional approach may prove more useful to the practitioner since, clinically, it is apparently disordered transit rather than specific muscle dysfunction which commonly requires investigation.

Investigation of abnormal motility. At the present time, the methods available for the investigation of motility disorders are largely directed at documenting disorders of transit. Techniques for the direct evaluation of the neuromuscular system of the digestive tract are, for the greater part, not yet developed to the point where they yield reliable and reproducible information, and they remain in the domain of the research worker. A scheme of possible investigations is presented in Table 3; the range of investigations available to the individual practitioner will depend upon available resources, and a measure of ingenuity is sometimes necessary to supplement conventional techniques. The aim of this section is to review available techniques and to stress the limitations of existing techniques. With few exceptions, standard 'motility tests' do not exist at present.

Radiology. Except in the oesophagus, where a barium swallow is often diagnostic of a motility disorder, conventional gastrointestinal radiology is often unhelpful, and a 'normal barium meal' or 'normal barium enema' by no means excludes a motility disorder. As has been pointed out, the motor activity of the digestive tract is markedly altered in the presence of food. Barium sulphate is not a nutrient substance, and the transit of barium through the digestive

Table 1   Primary disorders of motility: pathological classification

	Oesophagus	Stomach	Small bowel	Colon	Anus/rectum
1. Myopathic	abnormal contractions contraction rings	hypertrophic pyloric stenosis 'tachygastria'	chronic pseudo-obstruction		
2. Neuropathic	achalasia	post-vagotomy ileus .... diabetes mellitus		Hirschsprung .... 'cathartic colon'	
3. Inflammatory	stricture	pyloric stenosis	sub-acute obstruction .... (Crohn's, TB, etc.)		
4. Psychomotor	globus hystericus	vomiting aerophagy rumination	irritable colon syndrome .... constipation		incontinence
5. Invasive	Chagas' disease				

Table 2   Primary disorders of motility: disordered transit

	Oesophagus	Stomach	Small intestine	Colon	Anus/rectum
1. Delay	obstruction	post-vagotomy pyloric stenosis	chronic pseudo-obstruction subacute obstruction adynamic ileus		constipation Hirschsprung
2. Accelerated		post-surgery dumping syndrome	'irritable colon' 'intestinal hurry'	'irritable colon' purgative abuse	incontinence proctitis
3. Retrograde	hiatus hernia	biliary gastritis	bacterial overgrowth		

Table 3   Investigation of disordered transit (see Table 2)

	Oesophagus	Stomach	Small intestine	Colon	Rectum
1. Delay	barium swallow manometry	barium meal	barium meal and follow through	opaque markers	proctoscopy
2. Accelerated		barium meal barium mixed with food radionuclide with scan	breath hydrogen	opaque markers	
3. Retrograde	barium meal endoscopy and biopsy pH study	endoscopy and biopsy	breath hydrogen		

tract is dissimilar from the transit of food, except in the oesophagus. Barium radiology is effective in the observation of oesophageal motility because there is no difference in the oesophageal transit of a barium bolus from the transit of a nutrient bolus; the swallowing reflex activated in each case is identical. Distally, conventional barium radiology may yield some clues; a stomach which still contains significant residue after the normal period of fasting usually indicates delayed gastric emptying, and it is sometimes possible to suggest from the rate of transit of barium that the transit of food and secretions may be abnormal. Gastro-oesophageal reflux may be demonstrated radiologically, but failure to demonstrate reflux may reflect lack of skill on the part of the radiologist rather than the absence of reflux in the patient.

The admixture of contrast media with food, originally used by Cannon to study gastric emptying, is disliked by radiologists because the mucosal pattern is impaired, but this is the simplest relevant technique for the study of motility disorders. Barium sulphate can be incorporated into food during preparation, as a 'bariumburger', or more simply, the patient can be asked to take sips of barium sulphate between mouthfuls of food. Given close collaboration between physician and radiologist, the 'nutrient barium meal' can be established as a useful routine diagnostic procedure.

The investigation of the progress of the solid phase of a meal without conventional X-ray contrast media has been carried out by using *solid radio-opaque markers*; usually small pieces of plastic into which barium sulphate has been incorporated. These are most valuable for studying colonic transit. In the presence of normal gastric emptying and small intestinal transit, it is reasonable to assume that all the opaque markers eaten with a meal will have passed into the colon after six to eight hours. Subsequent radiological study of their distribution may give useful information about colonic stasis or accelerated transit. Essentially similar information which avoids exposing the patient to ionizing radiations can be obtained by X-raying all stool samples subsequent to marker ingestion until all the markers have been recovered.

The importance of radiology in the investigations of motility disorders resides in the fact that radiology services are widely available. While conventional examinations with contrast media may be unhelpful, particularly if the radiologist has not been clearly informed of the clinical problem, the intelligent use of radiology and the application of some ingenuity may yield a diagnosis as precise as that which can be obtained by more refined techniques.

Manometry. Manometric techniques remain largely within the domain of the research worker, but are likely to find an increasing place in clinical practice. In general, manometric techniques involve the sensing of pressure at the distal end of a tube introduced into the digestive tract, and the transmission of the pressure through a fluid or air column to the proximal end of the tube, where a transducer converts the physical change into a DC voltage for recording on a polygraph, or on magnetic tape. For pressure measurement in narrow regions (oesophagus, small bowel), pressure is sensed and transmitted through an open-tipped narrow bore tube slowly perfused with water or saline, whereas for large cavities (fundus, rectum) a closed balloon may be preferable. Artefacts and damping of the pressure change along perfused tubes can be minimized by the use of a pneumohydraulic pump to introduce the fluid; alternatively, a miniature strain-gauge transducer may be introduced at the site where pressure is to be measured. Some progress has been made with the use of ingested 'endoradiosondes'—pressure-sensitive capsules emitting a radio signal varying with pressure—for pressure movement; these capsules may be better tolerated for long periods of study than intubation systems. Pressure measurement at one point only gives no indication of the likely direction and velocity of propulsion of ingesta, but simultaneous observation of pressure at two or more sites separated by a short distance may be very helpful.

Oesophageal manometry using multiple perfused tubes is usually diagnostic of disordered oesophageal motility but is, in practice,

rarely required because radiology will also usually yield a diagnosis and is simpler and better tolerated by the patient. Manometry may be used to confirm the existence of a zone of increased pressure at the site of the lower oesophageal sphincter but the clinical value of this measurement is often dubious.

Gastric manometry as an isolated procedure is rarely helpful, but observation of motility in a selected region together with that in the adjacent viscus may be of clinical value. Gastro-oesophageal manometry will indicate whether the swallowing reflex in the oesophagus induces the appropriate receptive relaxation in the fundus. Gastroduodenal manometry will indicate the integrity of the antral contractile mechanism, and also the integrity of gastroduodenal co-ordination, whereby antral contraction should be closely associated with relaxation of the duodenal bulb.

Duodenojejunal manometry is becoming established as a reliable method for confirming the integrity of the migrating complex (MMC) and its abolition by food. Because of the prolonged observation required to observe several MMC cycles, radio-capsules have been employed to minimize patient discomfort. Absence of the MMC, or absence of the appropriate motor response to food may be indicative of enteric myopathy or neuropathy; it is to be expected that as this procedure is more widely adopted, it will increase in clinical importance.

Manometry of the colon is not, at the time of writing, either practical or useful as a routine clinical procedure, but anorectal manometry is helpful in the investigation of faecal incontinence in order to study the function of internal and external anal sphincters; it is also an essential component of biofeedback systems which have been employed in the treatment of faecal incontinence.

Clinical investigators should not be deterred from employing manometry by the technical refinements and complexities of interpretation which prevail among research workers. Research projects demand a degree of precision which is often in excess of that required to resolve a simple diagnostic point; absolute pressure values are not required in order to determine whether a normal pattern of motility such as swallowing or the MMC exists. Simple apparatus may be improvised, or borrowed from the cardiovascular or physiological laboratory, which may well serve to resolve a diagnostic problem.

Radionuclides. The problems of observing the transit of ingesta with radiology include the fact that X-ray contrast media do not resemble food, and also the radiation hazards of observation over long periods of time. Radionuclides, which can be incorporated in tracer quantities into palatable meals, offer an answer to the first problem, while imaging techniques using a gamma-camera scan allow detailed observation over prolonged periods of time. The current disadvantage of these techniques is the poor resolution of the image in comparison with radiology, and the difficulty of reconstructing continuous movements from serial scans.

Radionuclides offer the best available method of studying gastric emptying at the present time. Considerable ingenuity has been employed in developing methods of incorporating isotopes into food to ensure that the isotope remains with the solid phase of the meal. Two techniques have been widely employed: (*a*) technetium-sulphur colloid added, before cooking, to scrambled eggs; and (*b*) radio-labelled vitamin B_{12} administered to a chicken is incorporated into the liver: an hour later the chicken is killed, and its liver is used in the preparation of a meal. The nature of the method employed will depend upon the facilities available. Few isotope departments routinely offer such a diagnostic service, but co-operation if sought can usually be obtained.

Radionuclides have been used to study all levels of the digestive tract. The assessment of *gastric emptying*, particularly before and after gastric surgery, remains the principal application. The measurement of *oesophageal clearance* has recently become possible with the refinement of scanning and computer analysis techniques, although it remains to be seen whether the diagnostic yield is improved in comparison with contrast radiology and manometry. *Small bowel transit* can also be studied using isotopes, but the length and convolution of the small bowel do not allow anything less than major disturbances of transit to be studied; the same is true of the colon. The development, recently reported, of radio-labelled indigestible fibre may offer a new avenue for clinical study.

Breath tests. Breath tests have been introduced into various aspects of gastroenterological diagnosis, and the *hydrogen breath test* has proved to be useful in the assessment of small bowel transit time. It is based on the principle that bacterial fermentation of indigestible solids in the colon results in the formation of hydrogen, which is absorbed through the colonic mucosa and excreted in expired air. From this, it follows that the arrival of the residue of a meal in the colon will be signalled by a rise in breath hydrogen. Apparatus for the measurement of breath hydrogen down to a level of 10 parts per million is now commercially available, and the value of the test will be further increased when detectors with a sensitivity increased by one order of magnitude become generally available.

Endoscopy. The introduction of fibre-optic endoscopy, which has proved so fruitful in the accurate diagnosis of mucosal lesions in the digestive tract, has little to offer in the study of motility. This is hardly surprising, since the muscle and nerve of the digestive tract are out of sight, and beyond the reach of the biopsy forceps; moreover, the premedication required for endoscopy, and the need for a void viscus, mean that the movements observed through an endoscope do not represent any characteristic pattern. Endoscopy has a limited place in determining the degree of damage due to refluxed secretions, and endoscopic biopsy is a useful diagnostic adjunct in confirming the presence of oesophagitis due to refluxed gastric acid, and gastritis due to refluxed bile. Endoscopic visualization of bile reflux is not diagnostic, since a degree of bile reflux is physiological, but its appearance should prompt the endoscopist to biopsy the antral mucosa. Endoscopic diagnosis of hiatus hernia and pyloric stenosis is possible, but dynamic tests of function are required in order to determine whether the lesion that has been seen is of functional importance.

Electromyography. Gastrointestinal electromyography is widely used in motility research in animals, and should, in theory, offer a definitive means of investigation of motility disorders. This is not the case, because of the difficulty of placing sensors in relation to the smooth muscle, and because of the complexity of the recorded signal. In clinical practice, manometry offers a much simpler method of obtaining analogous information about muscle contraction. There are rare cases of gastrointestinal myopathy, in which electromyography might be regarded as definitive, and it is possible that the spectrum of such disorders will increase with advancing knowledge. Chronic pseudo-obstruction and tachygastria (atony associated with a gastric electrical slow wave of abnormally high frequency) are disorders of current research interest which require definitive electromyographic diagnosis, but they are thought to be uncommon problems. Electromyography of the sigmoid colon has been alleged to be of value in the diagnosis of the 'irritable colon syndrome', but the electromyographic abnormalities that have been reported are not always present in all cases with characteristic symptoms, and the putative abnormalities can only be detected by the application of sophisticated methods of computer analysis.

For the present, electromyography rests firmly in the domain of the specialist research worker who may, none the less, be able to offer useful assistance in the study of rare and baffling syndromes.

Plasma gut peptide assay. (See page 12.47.) Radio-immunoassay of a number of gut peptides ('gut hormones') in plasma samples is offered by a number of specialist centres. Such assays play no part *at present* in the diagnosis of motility disorders, but none the less deserve mention because of the likelihood that plasma profiles which are diagnostic of motility disorders will be described, since these peptides appear to be involved in the regulation of motility as humoral agents, or as neurotransmitters or neuromodulators.

Primary disorders of motility

Retrograde transit (reflux). *Reflux oesophagitis and hiatus hernia.* Reflux of gastric juice, containing hydrochloric acid and pepsin,

into the oesophagus causes pain and damage to the mucosal squamous epithelium. This is the commonest primary disorder of motility in Europe and North America. Gastro-oesophageal reflux commonly occurs in the presence of a *hiatus hernia*, or protrusion of the proximal stomach through the diaphragmatic hiatus into the chest (Fig. 2), but it may also occur without any apparent anatomical displacement. That a hiatus hernia should produce reflux is evidence that the sphincteric mechanism which normally prevents reflux is not only due to the intrinsic lower oesophageal sphincter, but also to the normal anatomical relationship of oesophagus, cardia, and proximal stomach.

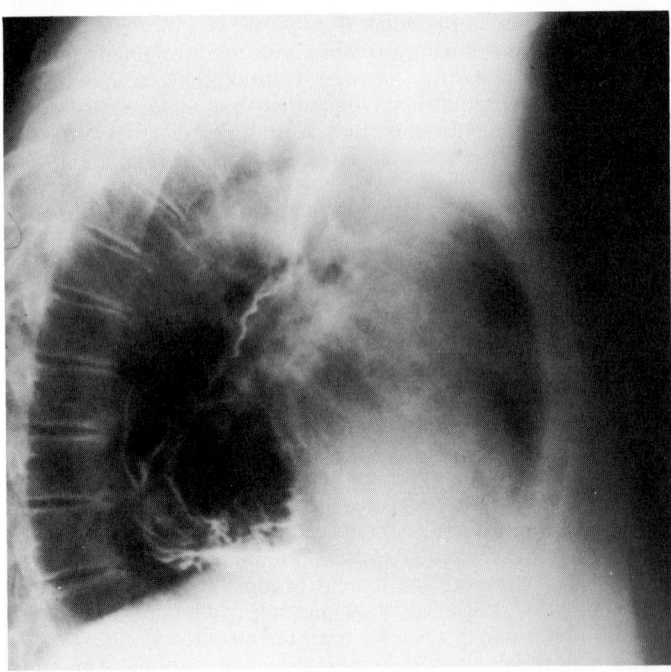

Fig. 2 Hiatus hernia, shown in this case by the presence of the gastric air bubble within the thoracic cavity. The anatomical distortion of the gastro-oesophageal junction impairs the resistance to reflux, which cannot be maintained by the intrinsic lower gastro-oesophageal sphincter.

Symptomatic reflux usually involves the association of two factors, hiatus hernia and obesity. It may occur in the absence of hiatus hernia, especially in the obese; conversely, a non-obese subject with a radiologically demonstrable hiatus hernia is often free of symptomatic reflux. Both duodenal ulcer and cholelithiasis are said to be associated with an increased degree of reflux, as is smoking.

The symptoms of reflux are, initially, retrosternal pain or burning associated with posture; symptoms occur on stooping, lying down, or even slumped in an armchair. Since the two latter postures may be adopted postprandially, postprandial symptoms are common. Patients may also experience 'water brash', as a bitter fluid, usually described as 'bile', welling up into the oropharynx, usually during the night, or on stooping. As reflux becomes established, so does oesophagitis, and this will lead to retrosternal pain during the consumption of food and drink, among which hot drinks and spicy foods are most troublesome. Apart from oesophagitis, complications of gastro-oesophageal reflux are few, but there is accumulating evidence that episodes of reflux may precipitate asthmatic attacks in susceptible subjects.

The diagnosis of reflux with or without hiatus hernia can usually be made on the basis of the history alone, but should be confirmed radiologically with a barium meal examination which includes screening in the Trendelenburg (head down and prone) position. Endoscopy will reveal oesophagitis which should be confirmed by biopsy, and an experienced endoscopist should be able to confirm the presence of a hiatus hernia. If there is doubt over the diagnosis, two further tests may be used. The *Bernstein test* involves the instillation of acid through an oesophageal tube; failure of this manoeuvre to provoke symptoms should cast doubt on the diagnosis. *Monitoring of oesophageal pH* with a pH probe may reveal repeated lowering of pH due to reflux, but there is little point in this test unless a range of values in subjects free from reflux has been established. It has to be remembered that episodes of reflux probably occur in all individuals from time to time.

The treatment of reflux has two aims; the alleviation of symptoms, and the treatment of underlying causes. Even in the presence of a hiatus hernia, treatment is initially medical, since it may result in the abolition of symptoms without further measures. The patient should be instructed to avoid lying flat at night, and when active, to squat rather than stoop; when, as is often the case, the patient is a housewife, she must be persuaded to delegate activities such as bedmaking to another member of the household. Lying flat at night is avoided by raising the head of the bed, either with blocks under the bed, or a large wedge-shaped piece of foam rubber or plastic under the pillows. The use of additional pillows is not helpful, because individuals accustomed to sleep with only one pillow will invariably push additional pillows to one side during the night. Medication with antacids is a helpful adjunct, but is usually inadequate as the only line of treatment. Antacids can be taken as required; there are a number of proprietary formulations intended for the treatment of reflux, but there is no convincing evidence that they are particularly effective. H_2-receptor antagonists (cimetidine, ranitidine) are as effective as antacids, but probably not more so, while being more expensive.

Obesity is the main cause of reflux, and there is typically a history of weight gain over the period during which symptoms developed. The treatment of obesity, when present (which is usual), is the main avenue of treatment, and a weight-reducing regimen should be prescribed (see Section 8). The patient can be motivated to follow a restricted calorie regimen by proper explanation of the problem; above all, the physician should not offer any expectation of effective treatment without the reduction of obesity. Gastro-oesophageal reflux in pregnancy is common, but the obesity is self-limiting.

The majority (about 90 per cent) of patients will lose their symptoms on regaining their normal body weight. This leaves a residue of patients who constitute a difficult problem, as they will require continued medication. If there is a significant hiatus hernia, they should be offered surgery, although only a proportion will be given complete relief by surgery. If there is no significant hiatus hernia, the diagnosis should be reviewed, and the presence of other lesions (such as peptic ulcer and gallstones) which might provoke similar symptoms should be rigorously excluded.

Many patients with reflux are referred to gastroenterologits, but specialist referral is not necessary; a careful history will establish the diagnosis, and logical treatment will relieve the condition.

Biliary gastritis. Experimentally, it has been shown that the gastric mucosa is damaged by bile acids, possibly due to their detergent action of the protective layer of mucus. It is also known that if the pylorus is a true sphincter, its major role is to prevent the reflux of duodenal contents into the antrum. It seems reasonable to assume that biliary gastritis may occur when the integrity of the pylorus is disturbed, or (at least, in theory) when there is loss of motor co-ordination between the antropyloric region and the duodenal bulb. Unfortunately, there are no histological features which, on light microscopy, distinguish the antrum damaged by bile from other forms of antral gastritis, although characteristic changes on scanning electron microscopy have been reported.

A diagnosis of biliary gastritis may reasonably be made when dyspeptic symptoms persist following vagotomy and pyloroplasty, provided that: (*a*) active ulcer disease is excluded; (*b*) antral gastritis is confirmed by biopsy; (*c*) biliary reflux is confirmed at endoscopy; and (*d*) gastric aspiration repeatedly confirms the presence of bile. To make the diagnosis without an antecedent history of gastric surgery is more contentious, and must lean heavily on the repeated demonstration of bile in the stomach.

Treatment of biliary gastritis is difficult; antacids are often inef-

fective, since the lesion is not acid-induced. Medical treatment is a matter of trial and error; some cases will respond to antacids, some to carbenoxolone, and some to metoclopramide, the latter being sometimes effective in improving gastric clearance and antro-duodenal motor co-ordination. Some cases do not respond to medical treatment, and if this is the case, and the persistence of antral damage is confirmed, surgery may be indicated. A Roux-en-Y gastrojejunostomy is the operation of choice, and has shown to be an effective, if drastic, treatment.

Delayed transit. Oesophageal spasm. Oesophageal spasm consists of uncoordinated, simultaneous, or spontaneous contraction of the oesophageal smooth muscle. Asymptomatic abnormal contractions are sometimes found by chance in elderly patients undergoing a barium meal; but, in other patients, oesophageal spasm presents with dysphagia, or pain, or both. The diagnosis can usually be made with a barium swallow, when the bolus of barium is seen to travel normally only as far as the smooth muscle segment of the oesophagus; thereafter it may be delayed, occluded, or compressed by a number of ring contractions ('corkscrew oesophagus') (Fig. 3).

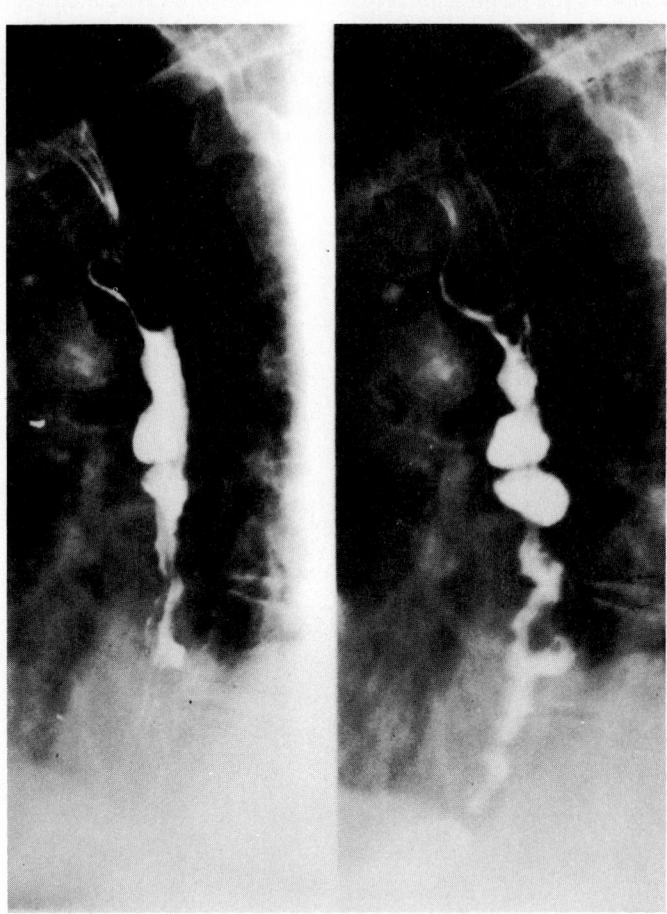

Fig. 3 Oesophageal spasm, shown here with the classic radiological appearance of 'corkscrew oesophagus'. Instead of proceeding as a smooth bolus, the barium column is indented by a series of ring contractions. (By courtesy of Dr Kreel.)

The appearances vary not only between patients, but also in the same individual on different occasions. Manometry provides confirmation, and occasionally, if the only abnormality is spontaneous contractions, may be required to make the diagnosis. Manometry may also be helpful in the detection of impaired lower sphincter relaxation, which sometimes occurs.

Angina pectoris is an important differential diagnosis; although the effect of exercise may be diagnostic, this is not always the case. Recently, it has been reported that diagnosis can be helped by the administration of ergometrine, which will provoke typical oesophageal spasm, but this should only be done after the possibility of cardiac ischaemia has been eliminated, and with both ECG control and the aid of oesophageal manometry to confirm the effect on the oesophagus.

The condition is largely unresponsive to treatment, and prognosis is variable. Some patients benefit from glyceryl trinitrate sublingually for the relief of pain arising from the spasm; others may benefit from anticholinergic drugs. In some patients, progression to the characteristic syndrome of achalasia has been documented.

Achalasia. Achalasia is chronic and progressive obstruction to the passage of contents through the lower oesophageal sphincter (LES). The cause is degeneration of the ganglion cells of the myenteric plexus, or vagal nuclei, and the pathophysiological consequence is failure of relaxation of the sphincter; although resting LES pressure may be mildly elevated, the previous term 'cardiospasm' is somewhat misleading. The condition occurs in middle or late adult life, and the aetiology is unknown except in Latin America where achalasia may be one manifestation of Chagas' disease (see Section 5).

The condition presents as dysphagia, sometimes associated with pain, occurring both with fluids and with solids. A barium swallow examination will reveal failure of the sphincter to relax, and, additionally, disordered peristalsis on swallowing in the distal oesophagus. The oesophagus becomes dilated and elongated, and acts as a reservoir of unassimilated nutrient (Fig. 4). Spillage from this reservoir into the airway may result in aspiration pneumonia, which is one (uncommon) presentation of achalasia.

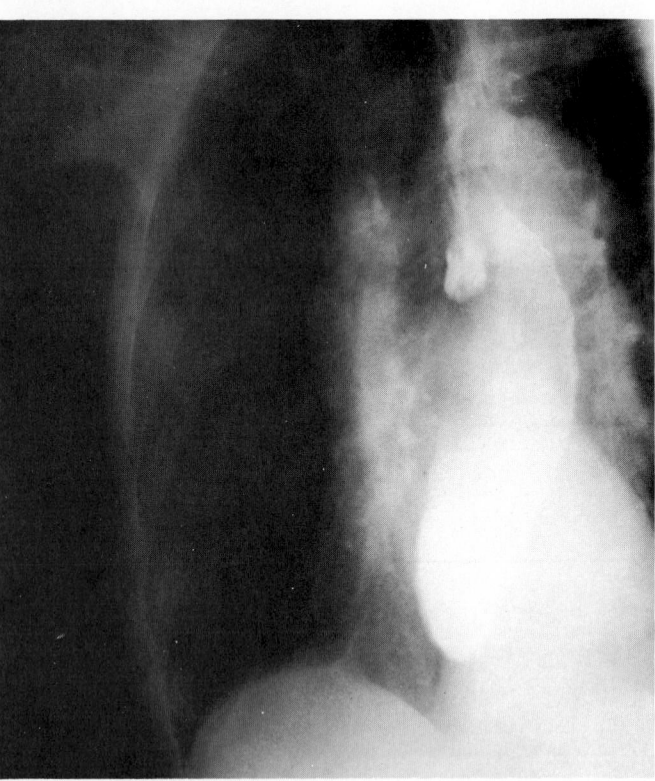

Fig. 4 Achalasia of the cardia, showing gross dilatation of the oesophagus, which is filled with food debris. (By courtesy of Dr Kreel.)

Oesophagoscopy will also reveal a dilated oesophagus, but the endoscope will traverse the LES, showing that the obstruction is not a true organic stenosis. Manometry is diagnostic, and will demonstrate the failure of relaxation. Because a tissue deprived of its autonomic nerve supply is unduly sensitive to the missing neurotransmitter, the diagnosis may be confirmed by the administration of small doses of methacholine (5–10 mg subcutaneously) during manometry, which will, in the achalasic patient, induce powerful,

prolonged, and sometimes painful, contractions of the oesophageal body.

The condition is progressive and the degenerative process is unresponsive to treatment. Therefore therapy must be directed to mechanical relief of the functional obstruction. The majority of patients will obtain lasting relief from forcible dilatation of the LES by bouginage, presumably because the procedure ruptures significant numbers of muscle fibres. The remainder of the patients will require surgery.

Heller's operation, in which a longitudinal myotomy with preservation of the mucosa is performed, is the most successful procedure; radical destruction of the sphincter is to be avoided because of the subsequent post-operative reflux and oesophagitis. After dilatation or surgery, patients should be given advice on posture similar to that offered to patients with established gastro-oesophageal reflux.

Apart from the pulmonary complications of achalasia, carcinoma of the distal oesophagus is a late, and rare, complication.

Gastric stasis. Gastric stasis may be non-obstructive, or due to distal outflow obstruction. Stasis due to obstruction is associated with pyloric stenosis, and usually presents with vomiting.

Congenital hypertrophic pyloric stenosis is a congenital thickening of the pyloric smooth muscle, and usually presents as projectile vomiting, with constipation and weight loss, 10 days to three months after birth. The condition occurs in about two per 1000 live births, and is four times as frequent in male infants. Physical signs may include visible gastric peristalsis, and a palpable mass; barium radiography will show an elongated and symmetrically-narrowed pylorus. The treatment is a surgical pyloromyotomy (Ramstedt's operation), after correction of nutritional and electrolyte deficiency.

Rare forms of congenital outflow of obstruction, such as duodenal bands or duodenal stenosis, may occur, and may not be diagnosed until early adult life, as the obstruction is usually less severe. These conditions are considered in more detail on page 12.142.

Adult pyloric stenosis occurs as a late complication of chronic duodenal ulcer disease. It is characterized by vomiting, usually of copious amounts of food some hours after a meal, in an individual with a long history of ulcer disease; occasionally a history of dyspepsia may not be volunteered, as the patient may have trained himself to disregard 'indigestion'. The stenosis may be due entirely to long-standing fibrosis of the pylorus and duodenal bulb; more commonly it presents during a period of active ulceration, in which case there is an inflammatory component which will respond to conservative treatment. Even if there is a rapid response to initial treatment, surgery is inevitable.

Non-obstructive gastric stasis is an acute sequel of section of the vagus nerve, and consequently occurs during the early post-operative period following a vagotomy. It rarely persists, as there is considerable functional adaptation following vagotomy. Adynamic ileus of the stomach also occurs as part of a generalized adynamic ileus (see below), and usually responds to a conservative 'drip and suck' regimen with correction of electrolyte imbalances. Chronic gastric stasis is a manifestation of autonomic denervation, typically as a complication of diabetes mellitus; radiology and manometry reveal a dilated hypotonic stomach with poor emptying. Stasis due to dysrhythmias of the gastric electrical slow wave has been reported, but the condition appears to be very uncommon; it has been termed *tachygastria*.

Gastric stasis may respond to treatment with metoclopramide, a procainamide analogue which is an *in vitro* dopamine antagonist. The mode of action of this drug *in vivo* is uncertain, as is the therapeutic benefit, but metoclopramide has been shown to be beneficial in some cases of diabetic gastroparesis.

Adynamic ileus. Adynamic ileus (or paralytic ileus) is a condition in which there is a functional motor paralysis of the digestive tract. It is the small intestine which is predominantly affected, but the colon and stomach may also be involved. It is a neurogenic condition, in which the normal electrical slow wave is present in the smooth muscle, but does not excite any action potentials. The mechanism is thought to be adrenergic inhibition, possibly involving dopamine release, but adrenoceptor blockade or dopamine inhibition have not been shown to be therapeutically effective. The motor inhibition is triggered by a variety of stimuli, the commonest being tactile stimulation during surgery and peritonitis; ileus is also sometimes associated with severe trauma outside the abdomen.

The signs of ileus are a cessation of any motor activity; bowel sounds are absent, flatus is not passed, and there is consequent gastric stasis which may lead to vomiting. The radiological appearances are diagnostic; a plain X-ray of the abdomen in the upright posture shows dilated loops of bowel with multiple fluid levels, indicating distension with fluid and air (Fig. 5).

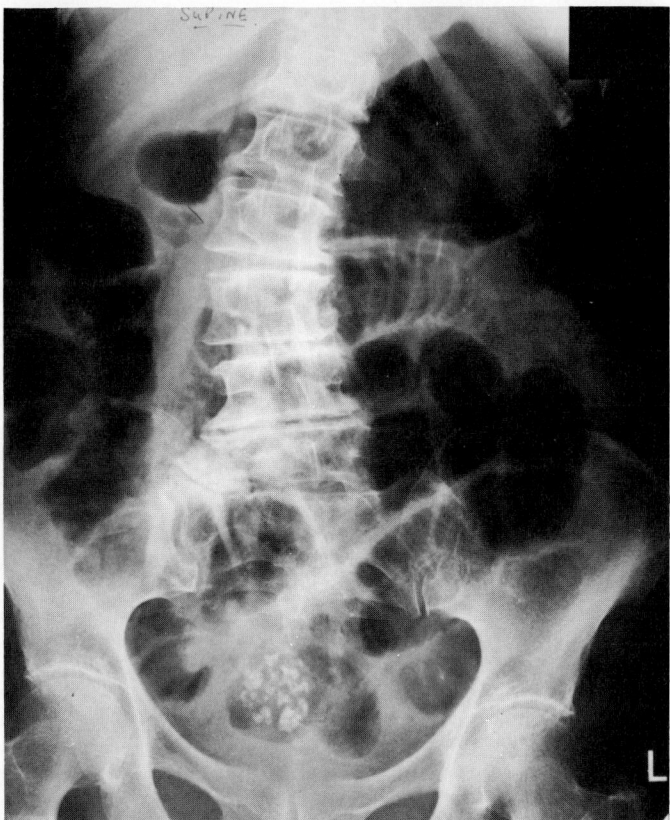

Fig. 5   Adynamic ileus of the small bowel, shown by dilated air-filled loops of bowel in this plain film taken in the supine posture. A few liquid levels were seen in an erect film taken at the same occasion. Severe degenerative changes in the spine and a calcified fibroid are also visible. (By courtesy of Dr Kreel.)

Treatment is conservative, as the condition is self-limiting. Recovery is hastened by the correction of any fluid or electrolyte imbalance, and by measures to 'defunction' the small bowel by aspirating gastric contents and administering fluid and nutrients by the parenteral route.

Sub-acute obstruction. Sub-acute intestinal obstruction occurs when there is any condition which creates a functional stenosis of the bowel which falls short of complete obstruction. The usual causes are intrinsic obstruction due to inflammatory disease of the bowel (Crohn's disease, tuberculosis) or extrinsic obstruction due to tumour or fibrous adhesions. The condition usually presents as episodes of colicky pain, sometimes associated with abdominal distension and vomiting. Localized tenderness may indicate the site of obstruction.

The diagnosis of subacute obstruction is not always simple. Any episode of abdominal pain in a patient at risk, such as a patient with known Crohn's disease, will give rise to the suspicion of subacute

obstruction, but many of these episodes are not obstructive. The diagnosis of subacute obstruction is important; in the absence of any known predisposing cause, explanatory laparotomy is indicated, but conversely, it is important to prevent unnecessary exploration of patients with known enteric disease.

It is probably true (although unproven) that sub-acute obstruction is always accompanied by abnormal transit proximal to the site of obstruction. Careful radiology may indicate abnormal transit of contrast medium. Recent evidence suggests that manometry will reveal a gross disturbance of the normal pattern of motility proximal to the site of obstruction, where repeated bursts of powerful contractions are seen at intervals of a few minutes; it is these bursts which are presumably projected into the sensorium as pain. This is an example of one condition in which the use of manometry for diagnostic purposes is likely to prove increasingly helpful.

Chronic pseudo-obstruction. (See page 12.100.) The label of chronic pseudo-obstruction includes a variety of rare disorders in which the patient presents, usually in childhood or early adult life, with the clinical features of subacute or acute intestinal obstruction, but in whom no actual obstruction can be found. The cause of pseudo-obstruction is an intrinsic disorder of function of the bowel, which is usually due to a myopathy. The disorder may be familial, and some varieties of pseudo-obstruction are associated with disorders of other smooth muscle, usually in the urinary tract. One of the commoner presentations of this uncommon clinical problem is that of *megaduodenum*, which appears to be due to a localized neuropathy of the duodenum; duodenojejunostomy is indicated. Chagas' disease may also result in chronic intestinal pseudo-obstruction (see Section 5).

The rarity of pseudo-obstruction is such that the physician will always be relatively unfamiliar with the condition, and the lack of consistent pathology means that there is no established routine of investigation. Ingenuity and perseverance is required from the physician, as well as understanding for a patient who has often previously been dismissed as a malingerer or neurotic and who faces a lifetime of likely disability.

Hirschsprung's disease. Hirschsprung's disease (see also page 12.146) is a congenital disorder, occurring about one in 2000 live births, in which there is an aganglionic segment in the distal colon. In the affected segment, ganglia are absent, and the muscle is persistently contracted; the colon proximal to the aganglionic segment is dilated, with normal or increased ganglia, and hypertrophied muscle. The condition usually presents in the neonate as an episode of intestinal obstruction, and repeated episodes occur thereafter with severe constipation and, occasionally, visible colonic peristalsis. Radiology will reveal, on plain X-ray, an ovoid faecal mass outlined by small irregular gas shadows. The presence of a narrowed segment is demonstrated by barium enema (Fig. 6). The treatment is surgical, although if the aganglionic segment is very short and close to the anus, a normal bowel habit can be maintained by the regular use of laxatives and enemas.

Simple constipation. By definition, constipation implies delayed transit of faeces. In the absence of neuropathy (as in Chagas' disease and Hirschsprung's disease), or systemic disorders such as myxoedema, there is no evidence that it is due to any local lesion in the colon, and it has, therefore, been considered as a functional or psychomotor disorder (see below).

Diverticular disease. The presence of colonic diverticula is not a motility disorder, nor do diverticula cause disordered motility. There is some evidence that they occur more readily in chronic constipation, possibly as a result of the attempt of colonic muscle to move inspissated faeces. In the absence of complications, such as inflammation or perforation, management should be along the lines suggested for simple constipation. It is fashionable nowadays to prescribe high residue diets for patients with diverticular disease, just as a few decades ago it was fashionable to prescribe low residue diets. The truth of the matter appears to be that, as in constipation, manipulation of the constituents of the diet may improve colonic evacuation. This condition is considered further on page 12.153.

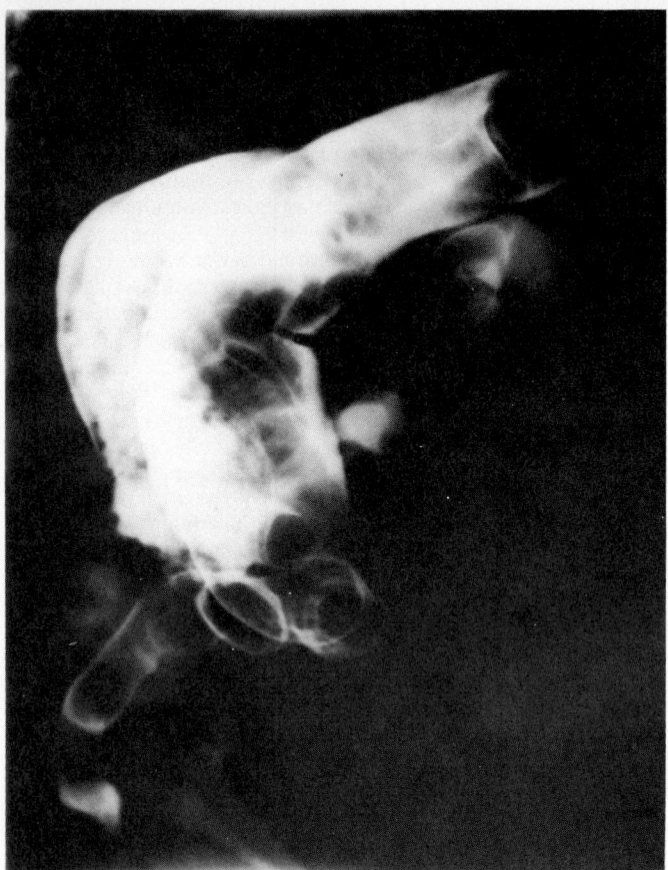

Fig. 6 Hirschprung's disease in an infant, shown by a film after the evacuation of barium. A narrowed distal aganglionic segment of the colon is visible together with gross dilation proximal to the narrowing. (By courtesy of Dr Kreel.)

Accelerated transit.   *Gastric incontinence.* Gastric incontinence, or excessively rapid gastric emptying is an uncommon sequel of gastric surgery which included a procedure to alter gastric drainage, usually pyloroplasty. The presence of gastric incontinence is indicated by manifestations of excessive input into the small bowel, of which the commonest is the *dumping syndrome.* The syndrome of dumping includes postprandial weakness, sweating, flushing, and cramping abdominal pain. The mechanism is thought to be due both to the rapid delivery of hypertonic contents to the small intestine resulting in osmotic diminution of blood volume, and to disturbances of carbohydrate metabolism leading to excessive insulin activity. The problem is entirely food-related and does not occur during fasting; consequently it is best managed by the regulation of food intake. Small frequent meals should be substituted for large infrequent meals and carbohydrate intake should be reduced as it is the carbohydrate moiety of a meal which makes the greatest osmotic contribution. Recently, it has been shown that the addition of colloids, such as guar or pectin, to carbohydrate is also helpful in reducing the rate of effective delivery of carbohydrate to the small intestine.

The presence of a dumping syndrome is diagnostic of gastric incontinence, but if there is an associated motility disorder of the small bowel, as may occur after truncal vagotomy, gastric incontinence may lead to diarrhoea. Under these circumstances, further investigation of gastric emptying by methods outlined previously may be required; above all, the physician should remember that the rate of emptying of barium sulphate from the stomach may be a very poor, or even misleading indicator of the rate of emptying of a meal.

Where the problem cannot be managed by the adoption of a different pattern of eating by the patient, or the use of food addi-

tives, some form of surgery may be indicated. Reversal of a segment of proximal intestine, in combination with a Roux-en-Y procedure may be helpful, and it is likely that the success rate of this type of palliative surgery will increase as diagnostic techniques become more refined.

Intestinal hurry. Intestinal hurry is another ill-defined disorder of motility, in which the transit of ingesta through the small intestine is excessively rapid, too rapid to permit the normal assimilation of water and solute. The result is the delivery to the colon of an excess fluid and nutrient load, the latter being then subject to bacterial fermentation which causes osmotic dilution; the outcome is diarrhoea.

The circumstances in which intestinal hurry occur are far from clear. Damage to the intrinsic innervation of the bowel as in diabetes, or to the extrinsic innervation as a sequel of vagotomy, are known factors. Another possibility is the persistence of powerful peristaltic activity, resembling the interdigestive migrating complex, in the postprandial phase.

The truth is that too little is yet known about this condition; at the present time, the physician will continue to encounter occasional cases of chronic 'motor diarrhoea', in which the only abnormality is excessively rapid transit of the intestine, or intestinal hurry. Until further light is shed on this condition, specific therapy does not exist, and the only form of management is conventional antidiarrhoeal medication. This condition is sometimes labelled as one form of the 'irritable colon syndrome', but even though there may be a psychogenic component, the label is probably a misnomer.

Rectal incontinence. Chronic faecal incontinence is a distressing disability, which may occur in the absence of anorectal disease. The primary disorder appears to be defective tonic contraction of the internal anal sphincter, with defective compensation by the external sphincter, as shown by anorectal manometry. A variety of surgical procedures have been attempted in this condition, but the results have been variable.

A new approach to this procedure, pioneered in the United States, is treatment by biofeedback, using 'operant conditioning'. With this technique, the pressure changes recorded on manometry are displayed to the patient on a visual display which also shows a normal manometric trace. The patient is encouraged to attempt to achieve a normal manometric pattern, and is able to compare his, or her, performance with the normal pattern. Where there is no associated organic disease or remediable anatomical defect, a high rate of success is claimed for this technique.

Proctitis. Proctitis, or inflammation of the rectal mucosa, deserves a brief mention for, although not a motility disorder, it results in disordered defaecation. The rectal mucosa appears to be unduly sensitive to the presence of any content, and this can result in frequent, and often unproductive, calls to stool which are often socially inconvenient. Treatment is directed towards the underlying cause.

Secondary disorders of motility
Metabolic.   *Diabetes mellitus.* Disordered motility is encountered in severe cases of diabetes mellitus as a consequence of autonomic neuropathy. The precise nature of the lesion has not been defined, but there are two types of disorder, which may coexist in the same patient. *Diabetic gastroparesis* is delayed gastric emptying due to gastric atony. The prolonged retention of food may be diagnosed by radiology, or endoscopy, and it may provoke vomiting in addition to abdominal distension and discomfort. Metoclopramide has been shown to be beneficial in some, but not all, cases. *Diabetic diarrhoea* is uncommon and is assumed to be due to autonomic denervation in the small bowel. It is characterized by intestinal atony, can be detected manometrically, and results in variable combinations of diarrhoea and steatorrhoea. It is refractory to treatment, but since bacterial overgrowth of the small intestine may occur, antibacterial therapy sometimes affords a degree of relief.

Thyroid dysfunction. Diarrhoea may be one presenting feature of hyperthyroidism, and, conversely, hypothyroidism is usually accompanied by constipation. It is assumed, on the basis of very little evidence, that these extremes are due to disordered motility, although altered smooth muscle activity in thyroid disease has been demonstrated. Treatment is that of the underlying metabolic disorder. Given the incidence of these symptoms in the normal population, it must not be assumed that these symptoms are always a consequence of the disease, or that their occurrence should always provoke investigations of thyroid status.

Adrenal insufficiency. Abdominal pain and vomiting form one presentation of adrenal insufficiency. Although it is not clear whether this is due to disordered motililty, the assumption seems to be at least reasonable. The symptoms disappear with appropriate adrenocortical supplementation.

Porphyria. Autonomic neuropathy may occur in porphyria, but there is no characteristic manifestation.

Neuropathic. *Oropharyngeal dyskinesia.* Under this heading may be grouped disorders of the voluntary muscles involved in swallowing. These include bulbar poliomyelitis, and vascular disease of the brain stem; both may lead to permanent impairment. *Myasthenia gravis* is an important cause of oropharyngeal dyskinesia, because of the risk of aspiration pneumonia.

Invasive. *Chagas' disease.* Chagas' disease (see Section 5) is caused by the protozoan *Trypanosoma cruzii*, the vector being a beetle. It is endemic in parts of South America, affecting poverty-stricken people in particular, as it is the barefoot and those who sleep on the ground who get bitten. Infection also occurs through transfusion with blood from an infected donor. It has been estimated that at present, there are 10 000 000 sufferers in Brazil alone. The parasite has a predilection for smooth muscle regions, but it is the digestive tract which is particularly affected. The result of infection is destruction of the autonomic nerves, and the disease is characterized by various manifestations of denervation: achalasia of the cardia, chronic pseudo-obstruction, and aganglionic colon may occur independently or in combination. Once denervation has occurred, treatment consists only of palliative surgery; current therapeutic efforts are directed towards the development of an effective prophylactic vaccine.

Autoimmune. *Scleroderma.* The digestive tract may be affected in scleroderma (progressive systemic sclerosis). The regions most commonly affected are the oesophagus and small intestine, where replacement of smooth muscle by collagen, and destruction of autonomic nerves may occur. These lesions result in failure of oesophageal peristalsis, leading to dysphagia, and an adynamic small intestine in which bacterial overgrowth may occur. Manometry of the small intestine has shown diminished or absent MMC activity in affected intestine.

Functional and psychomotor disturbances of motility. Functional disorders of the digestive tract constitute the most frequent disorders confronting physicians. Their classification as motility disorders is not, for the greater part, based on scientific grounds, but simply because the presenting symptoms suggest a disturbance of motility, or manifest themselves, as in vomiting, by an actual disorder of function.

The psychogenic nature of some of these complaints is also for the most part, an unverified assumption. Yet the assumption does not appear to be without justification, for of the major functions of the digestive tract—secretion, absorption, and motility—it is motility which is modulated from moment to moment in accordance with the function of the whole individual, and it is motility which appears to be under neural control. The 'brain–gut axis', although still largely unexplored, is not a scientific myth. The stressful effect of emotional and social life, as well as overt psychiatric illness, produce dysfunction in all systems of the body, as somatic pain, migraine, asthma, etc. The digestive tract is no exception, and it

appears to be motility which is the gastrointestinal function which is most susceptible to stress, psychiatric illness, and—most commonly—unhappiness.

These considerations mean that the physician who wishes to deal effectively with the majority of patients presenting with apparent dysfunction of the digestive tract must understand that many of these symptoms are manifestations of unsuccessful adaptation to the demands of life. Successful management of these patients includes some common principles.

1. *A careful history.* Gastrointestinal diagnosis depends little on physical signs of disease, but very largely on an accurate history, which should not only consist of an enumeration of symptoms, but also the chronology of the illness (periodicity, duration, association with environment, and activity) and also some consideration of the psychosocial aspects of the patient's life.

2. *A positive diagnosis.* Many patients with functional disorders fear that they are suffering from some serious disease, usually malignancy. It is important that the physician makes a positive diagnosis, and not a diagnosis by exclusion. The attitude of: 'Well, we've done all the tests that we can think of and we can't find anything wrong' is not reassuring to the patient who may well assume that the diagnostic routine omitted a crucial test. Once sure that the problem is indeed functional (and a long history of symptoms combined with manifest physical well-being is often a sure indicator), the physician should refrain from further investigations, and should explain to the patient that a positive diagnosis is now clear.

3. *A full explanation.* The physician who dismisses functional symptoms as of little importance is not likely to help a patient whose social and private life may be considerably impaired by discomfort. An explanation of the problem, and any possible association with provocative factors in the lifestyle of the patient must be offered. The limitations of effective therapy must be explained, and the patient must be firmly reassured that he is not suffering from the prodromal manifestations of serious organic disease. The prognosis of most functional complaints is that, by and large, there will be little change, and this should not be concealed from the patient. In fact, when the patient gains insight into the problem, symptoms often lessen or even disappear; alternatively, the provocative factors in the patient's life may be removed with the passage of time. Even so, this should be regarded as an unexpected bonus; the wisest attitude for the physician is that of 'no disease and no cure'. A sensible physician will also avoid attribution of symptoms to a specific occupational or conjugal situation, since not only are individuals rarely free to change these circumstances at will, but also the association of symptoms with such specific circumstances may be coincidental rather than causal.

Although functional symptoms may present in a bewildering variety of permutations, certain syndromes predominate, and are more easily recognized.

Globus hystericus. This curious condition presents as apparent dysphagia at the level of the upper oesophageal sphincter, which may be only related to swallowing, or also as a persistent feeling of 'a lump'. Investigation reveals no abnormality, but anxiety is a common feature of this condition. Since the syndrome is remarkably specific, it may well be that this is a sensory disorder of motility, in which abnormal tension of voluntary muscle plays a part. As the principal fear of the patient is usually of oesophageal malignancy, adequate investigation followed by strong reassurance is required.

Rumination. Rumination, or *merycism*, comprises the effortless regurgitation of a meal into the mouth. This condition is not now well recognized, although this was not the case at the beginning of the 20th century. Rumination is normal in infants, and is perpetuated through childhood in mentally retarded children. Children are taught not to regurgitate, and the presence of rumination in later childhood or early adult life should be regarded as a failure of early training. In rumination boluses of food are retropelled into the mouth at intervals during the first one or two postprandial hours, when the acidity of gastric contents is still insufficient to render them unpalatable. The retropulsion is due to a complex sequence of efforts which involve a rise in intra-abdominal pressure at the moment when the lower oesophageal sphincter opens during swallowing. Patients tend to be encouraged to seek medical attention by their relatives or spouses; halitosis is one of the side-effects of the habit. It is important not to confuse this syndrome with normal gastro-oesophageal reflux. There is no known method of treatment beyond persuasion, which is rarely successful.

Aerophagy. Aerophagy, or air-swallowing, is not a true disorder of motility. It is well recognized that repeated attempts at belching actually result in more air being swallowed than expelled, and the usual cause of aerophagy is attempts by an individual to 'bring up wind', usually a consequence of postprandial epigastric distension or 'bloating' which may be real or imagined. This type of discomfort often occurs in ulcer or gallstone disease, and the occurrence of excessive belching or flatulence should raise the suspicion of some associated organic disorder.

Many cases of aerophagy are not associated with any actual lesion, and whether or not the patient is aware of attempting to belch, they are almost invariably unaware that they are swallowing air. The problem should be explained to them, and this usually results in the habit being discontinued. Because air-swallowing is commonest in the early postprandial phase, and because air-swallowing can only be done with a closed mouth, it is often helpful to advise patients to keep an open mouth after meals. The traditional remedy of sitting with a cork gripped between the teeth is most effective but rarely socially acceptable.

Psychogenic vomiting. Unlike the retropulsion of rumination, which is often intrinsically satisfying to the patient, psychogenic vomiting which is self-induced is a conversion symptom; that is, a symptom designed to draw attention to the patient as an invalid. Patients are commonly adolescent girls, but not invariably so. There is usually a discrepancy between the alleged profuseness and frequency of vomiting, and an apparently adequate state of nutrition. Treatment of this condition requires the elimination of the existence of possible organic causes of vomiting, and attention to the underlying psychological disturbance. As with other functional complaints with a presumed psychogenic origin, admission to hospital for close observation often results in complete remission.

One cause of vomiting, which is not psychogenic and with which this should not be confused, is retching associated with spasms of coughing in bronchitis. This usually occurs on getting out of bed in the morning, and is usually found in heavy smokers.

Irritable colon syndrome. The irritable colon syndrome, also known as 'irritable bowel' and 'spastic colon', is a heading used to cover a variety of miscellaneous disorders characterized by various combinations of abdominal pain and altered bowel habit. There is no evidence that the 'irritable colon syndrome' is a single diagnostic entity, although attempts have been made to demonstrate an underlying disorder of colonic smooth muscle. An eminent contemporary has commented that such '. . . diagnostic terms are used to conceal ignorance rather than to clarify thinking' (J. Christensen), and this is undoubtedly true. Even so, patients continue to present with symptoms that require the attention of the physician, and some sort of definition must be attempted. It has been estimated that up to 50 per cent of all patients referred to gastroenterology clinics suffer from this type of disorder.

The common presentation of this syndrome is a history, usually longstanding, of altered bowel habit with alternating constipation and (so-called) diarrhoea. Remissions and relapses are common. Episodes of defaecation are often associated with cramping lower abdominal pain. Investigations are not helpful in making the diagnosis, except in a negative sense; occasionally, the barium enema may reveal an unusually contracted colon, or one with abnormal haustration, but this is not usually the case. The stools usually vary between hard, small, scybala ('rabbit's droppings') and loose, semi-formed stools sometimes accompanied by mucus. The important differential diagnoses are inflammatory disease of the bowel, or

malignancy of the large bowel, and these can usually be excluded simply on the basis of the length of history, the age of the patient, physical well-being, and the absence of blood in the stools. Diarrhoea is not present, although the term is often used by patients to distinguish between different types of bowel habit. In the sense that diarrhoea implies water malabsorption with an increased daily stool volume, it is absent in the irritable colon syndrome in which the daily stool weight is normal or less than normal.

If the history is short, increased attention must be paid to the differential diagnosis. Useful and relatively inexpensive screening investigations are a blood count and a sedimentation rate; if these are normal on two successive occasions, the presence of organic disease of the bowel is highly unlikely, especially in the young. The confidence and experience of the physician play a large part in making a correct diagnosis without undue investigation, but the experienced physician will also learn to review his patients from time to time to make sure that the symptoms do not represent the prodrome of organic disease. Some physicians assert that the diagnosis can only be made with confidence after barium radiology of the entire digestive tract, cholecystography, and sigmoidoscopy with rectal biopsy, but the diagnostic load implied by this routine in every such patient demand some discrimination in the use of these techniques. Review of the patient's symptoms, physical state, and haematological profile at regular intervals is often more helpful in detecting the insidious onset of organic disease than an extensive (and expensive) battery of investigations on one occasion.

Since the irritable colon syndrome is a disorder, or spectrum of disorders, in which the pathophysiology is unknown, it is to be expected that there is no effective specific therapy, and this is indeed the case. The general management follows the lines indicated at the beginning of this section. Some patients benefit from the consumption of bran, or of stool-bulking agents, while others find that a reduction in carbohydrate intake with elimination of white bread from the diet is helpful. Various medications have been formulated for treatment of this condition, but there is little convincing evidence that their effect is other than that of a placebo.

Constipation. Since the bowel habit of normal individuals is so varied, constipation defies precise definition. Empirically, it may be defined as occurring when defaecation is sufficiently infrequent to cause the sufferer discomfort or alarm, and to induce recourse to self-medication or medical attention. Some individuals are content to open their bowels once every two or three days, while others are not. The aim of the physician should be to increase the regularity of defaecation by the patient to a frequency which satisfies the patient, and also to persuade the patient to discontinue self-medication with potentially hazardous purgatives.

Constipation in children may be an expression of psychological disturbance, in which there is conscious forced retention of faeces, or *encopresis.* This may lead to spurious diarrhoea, in which there is leakage of liquid faeces around mass of hard, retained faeces. Expert paediatric management is required in these cases, as attempts to treat only the bowel disorder may aggravate the situation.

Constipation in the elderly, where a hypotonic colon and a lax abdominal musculature may be provocative factors may also present as spurious diarrhoea. In the elderly, anal problems such as haemorrhoids which render defaecation painful are often additional aggravating factors, and will require treatment. In the elderly, manual movement of a retained mass may be required before a normal bowel habit can be regained.

Apart from the special circumstances which may obtain in the very young and in the elderly, constipation in the majority of patients in the absence of any organic disease resolves around twin defects: the suppression of the defaecation reflex, and the absence of habit. In the normal individual, sensory stimulation of the rectum when it fills with faeces initiates the defaecation reflex. Since the rectum normally fills as a result of the postprandial gastrocolic reflex, which initiates a mass movement, the act of defaecation becomes a reflex which is perpetuated as a postprandial habit; one act of defaecation following the first meal of the day is sufficient for the majority of individuals. Constipation develops when the habit is disturbed. This may be because a change of job requires the individual to leave the house in a hurry, whereas previously there was time for adequate defaecation. Overcrowding may mean lack of access to a lavatory at the appropriate time. School children may dislike the lack of privacy and cleanliness which are too often the hallmark of communal school facilities. As the habit is abolished, so is rectal sensation suppressed from consciousness, and the patient becomes unaware of the call for stool. Once the reflex is disturbed, attempts at self-regulation of defaecation may be unsuccessful; with the loss of rectal sensation, the patient may be straining to void an empty rectum out of sense of social obligation. Suppression of defaecation leads to gradual colonic distension with inspissated faeces, causing a sensation of abdominal discomfort. In addition, patients may complain of a host of generalized somatic discomforts, such as headache, fatigue, and nausea; these do not arise from constipation, but more probably from the patient's need to convert an undignified inadequacy into an illness. One curious feature of simple constipation is that sufferers in early adult life are almost invariably female. There is no satisfactory explanation for this phenomenon, but the fact that constipation is sometimes eased during menstruation and during pregnancy suggests that endocrine factors may be responsible.

When a patient presents with constipation, the history should be directed into determining under what circumstances did an acceptable bowel habit lapse into constipation, in addition to simple enquiries about the frequency of bowel habit and the nature of the patient's diet. Physical examination will usually reveal a palpable firm descending colon, and often a rectum loaded with faeces; if the latter is the case, the patient will usually deny any sensation of rectal fullness or desire to defaecate.

Treatment should be directed towards restitution of a lost habit. Bran and hydrophilic colloids may provide faeces which give stronger stimulation to the colon. Laxatives are permissible initially, but should be prescribed so as to induce a physiological bowel habit. Anthracene purgatives (such as senna) should be avoided; osmotic laxatives (such as lactulose and magnesium sulphate) are better. The patient's diet is of less consequence than is generally imagined, since myriads of individuals live with a great variety of diet but an acceptable bowel habit, but emphasis on breakfast, preferably including a bran cereal is important, as it is following breakfast that attempts to establish a normal bowel habit are most likely to be successful. Reassurance and explanation to the patient are important, and the physician should explain the logic of the regimen he is advocating. Adjunctive therapy may include treatment of anal and peri-anal discomfort which sometimes causes the individual to strain at stool with a closed external anal sphincter. Self-medication should be firmly discouraged, and the dangers of anthracene purgatives which cause gradual autonomic denervation of the colon with prolonged use should be emphasized to the patient (see also page 12.14).

Purgative abuse. Given the degree of cultural concern over the alleged dangers of constipation (a concern which has been assiduously cultivated by the vendors of patent medicines since the invention of advertising), self-medication with purgatives is to be expected. Less expected is the fact that some individuals may surreptitiously take purgatives to the point where troublesome chronic diarrhoea prompts recourse to the physician. The psychopathology which leads such an individual to deny the use of purgatives is varied, and the causes are often obscure. Diarrhoea due to purgative abuse must be differentiated from other forms of chronic diarrhoea. Suggested features include hypokalaemia, finger clubbing, and persistence during abstention from food. If anthracene purgatives are being used, pigmentation of the colonic mucosa may be present (melanosis coli). Barium enema may reveal a colon lacking in haustrations, similar to the appearance of chronic ulcerative colitis, but the mucosal pattern is normal, and this may be confirmed by endoscopic examination and biopsy. Analysis of the urine may reveal traces of cathartics.

The condition is only treatable when the purgatives are found and the patient is confronted with the evidence; this usually requires hospital admission. Removal of the purgatives results in prompt remission; if the colonic innervation has been damaged by prolonged use of anthracene derivatives, such as senna, the diarrhoea may be replaced by troublesome constipation; this should be treated with osmotic purgatives. Psychiatric referral may be helpful in determining the cause of the habit.

References

Basic and clinical physiology

Code, C. F. (ed.) (1968). *Handbook of physiology, Section 6: Alimentary canal. Vol IV: Motility.* American Physiology Society, Washington, DC.
Davenport, H. W. (1977). *Physiology of the digestive tract*, 4th edn. Year Book Medical Publishers, Chicago.
Earlam, R. W. (1976). *Clinical tests of oesophageal function.* Crosby Lockwood Staples, London.
Johnson, L. R. (ed.) (1981). *Physiology of the gastrointestinal tracts*, vols. 1 and 2. Raven Press, New York.
Thomas, P. A. and Mann, C. V. (eds.) (1981). *Alimentary sphincters and their disorders.* Macmillan, London.

Disorders of motility

Fordtran, J. H. and Sleisenger, M. H. (eds.) (1973). *Gastrointestinal disease.* W. B. Saunders, Philadelphia.

Recent research

Christensen, J. (ed.) (1979). *Gastrointestinal motility.* Raven Press, New York.
Duthie, H. (ed.) (1978). *Gastrointestinal motility in health and disease.* MTP Press, Lancaster.
Wienbeck, M. (ed.) (1982). *Gastrointestinal motility.* Raven Press, New York.

Hormones and the gastrointestinal tract

R. G. Long, J. M. Polak, and S. R. Bloom

In 1902, Bayliss and Starling showed that acidification of denervated duodenum caused secretion of alkaline pancreatic juice. They also demonstrated that if extracts of duodenum were injected intravenously a similar pancreatic response was seen. In this way the first gut hormone, secretin, was discovered. Cholecystokinin and gastrin soon followed, but it has only been in the last 20 years that it has been possible to sequence and measure these peptide hormones.

In the last 10 years there has been an explosion of knowledge about gut hormones and other peptides in the gastrointestinal mucosa and muscle. Initially it was thought that they acted as hormones, being released into plasma after a physiological stimulus and acting on distant tissues. This is undoubtedly true for many of these peptides (Table 1). However, some of the peptides, for example cholecystokinin, gastrin, neurotensin, somatostatin, vasoactive intestinal polypeptide, substance P, bombesin, and the endorphins have been also demonstrated to occur in the brain, and the concept of neuracrine peptides with neurotransmitter roles has arisen. In the peripheral nervous system it is thought that these peptides mediate the postganglionic intrinsic nerves of the non-cholinergic non-adrenergic inhibitory pathways. Somatostatin was initially discovered as a hypothalamic peptide inhibiting growth hormone secretion but subsequently it has been found to have widespread inhibitory effects, and it is thought that it is released locally and then has effects on neighbouring cells, for example inhibiting insulin and gastric acid secretion. This has become known as a paracrine effect and is thought to be the main mode of action of somatostatin; many other peptides classified as hormones or neurotransmitters may also have such a role.

Table 1 Classification of gut regulatory peptides into probable main physiological mode of action

Hormonal (endocrine)	Local (paracrine)	Neurotransmitter (neuracrine)
Secretin	Somatostatin	Vasoactive intestinal polypeptide
Cholecystokinin		Bombesin
Gastrin		Substance P
Motilin		Endorphins
Gastric inhibitory polypeptide		
Pancreatic glucagon		
Pancreatic polypeptide		
Neurotensin		
Enteroglucagon		

Gut peptides have in general been found to have a biological effect and it has then been possible to isolate and determine their amino acid sequence. Measurement by specific radioimmunoassays has allowed very low concentrations to be demonstrated in plasma and tissue and has helped to elucidate the pathophysiology. Using immunocytochemistry and specific antibodies, it has been possible to find peptide containing cells and nerves in both the gut and brain (Fig. 1). Electron microscopy can finally be used to define specific peptide storage granules (Fig. 2). This section describes the basic biochemistry and physiology of gut peptides and outlines abnormalities in gastrointestinal disease and in functioning gut peptide tumour syndromes.

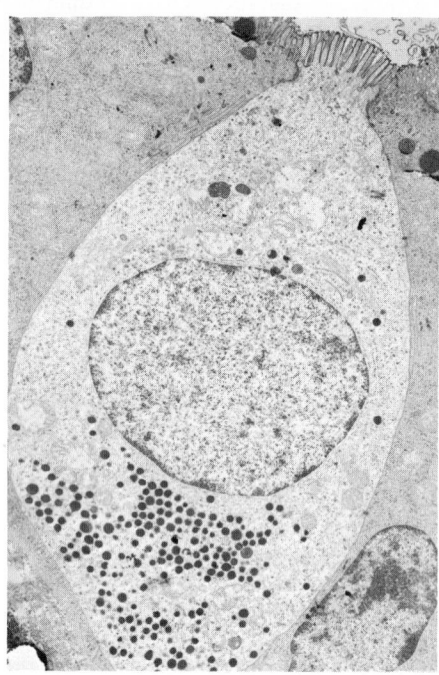

Fig. 2 Electronmicrograph of mucosal endocrine cell showing well-developed microville and secretory granules grouped at the basal membrane (×5500).

Hormones

Gastrin. Gastrin occurs in multiple molecular forms but all the biological activity is present in the C-terminal four amino acids (tetrin). The molecule originally described is composed of 17 amino acids (G17) and has a molecular weight of 2098 dalton. Other molecular forms include pentagastrin, G14, big gastrin (G34), and big big gastrin which may be artefactual and is of similar size to plasma proteins. In man gastrin is predominantly localized to the gastric antrum where G17 predominates but also occurs in the upper small intestine where G34 is the main form. Gastrin is localized to the G cell and on electron microscopy the granules are large and electronlucent.

Gastrin release is particularly stimulated by protein ingestion and gastric distension. Its main physiological action is the stimulation of gastric acid secretion, and it has been shown that infusion of gastric to mimic the postprandial plasma rise results in similar gastric acid secretion to that seen after a meal. Other important physiological roles are thought to be powerful trophic effects on the gastric mucosa, pancreas, small intestine, and colon, the stimulation of gastric motor activity, and contraction of the lower oesophageal sphincter.

Secretin. Secretin is a 27-amino-acid polypeptide with a molecular weight of 3056. It appears to occur in only one molecular form and the whole molecule is needed for full biological activity. Plasma concentrations are lower than those usually seen with gut hormones. It is localized to the S cell of the mucosa of the upper small intestine where it is stored in characteristic secretory granules.

Secretin release can be demonstrated if acid is instilled into the duodenum or if a subject drinks an acid drink. Secretin is probably also secreted after a meal but the timing and quantities of this secretion are uncertain. Pharmacological amounts of secretin cause profuse bicarbonate secretion by the exocrine pancreas, but how

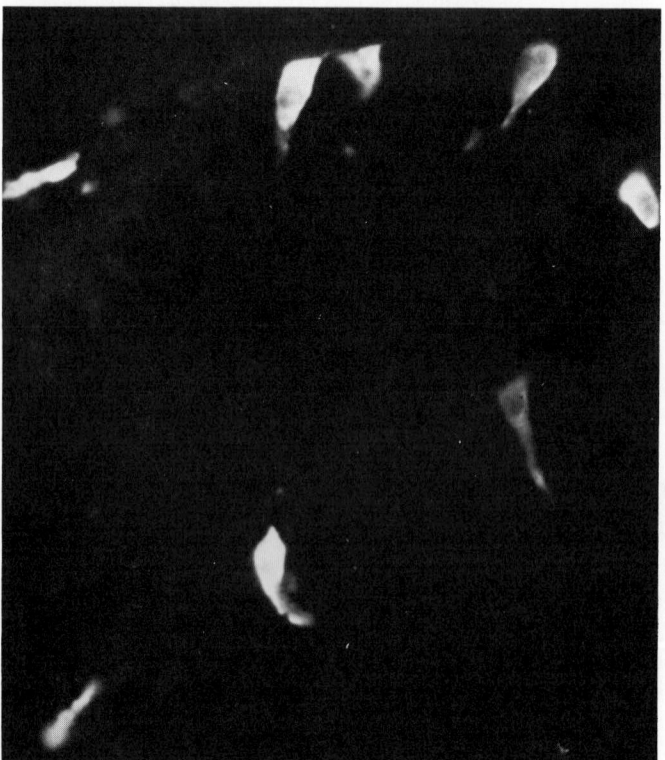

Fig. 1 Somatostatin cells, immunostained using the technique of indirect immunofluorescence, in the mucosa of human colon (×300).

physiologically important secretin is in stimulating postprandial pancreatic bicarbonate is uncertain.

Cholecystokinin (CCK). Cholecystokinin occurs in multiple molecular forms but its biological activity resides in the last eight C-terminal amino acids (molecular weight 1143). This octapeptide CCK is thought to circulate in plasma but other known forms include 33 and 39 amino-acid moieties which may also circulate. CCK is present in both the brain and gut and is therefore a neuropeptide, possibly with a neurotransmitter role, as well as a hormone. In the gut the highest tissue concentrations are in the upper small intestine but it can be detected in the ileum. CCK is present in both the mucosa and muscle of the intestine and in the mucosa it is present in the endocrine I cell.

The physiology of CCK is poorly understood because plasma measurement is difficult. It is thought that CCK is released into the plasma by the presence of fat or amino acids in the duodenum. CCK may stimulate the postprandial secretion of pancreatic enzymes and cause contraction of the gallbladder but this remains unproven and the postulated chymodenin may be important in these roles.

Gastric inhibitory polypeptide (GIP or glucose-dependent insulinotrophic polypeptide). This is a 43-amino-acid polypeptide with a molecular weight of 5105. Its N-terminal amino-acid sequence bears considerable similarities to those of secretin, glucagon, and vasoactive intestinal polypeptide. GIP is found in endocrine cells in the mucosa predominantly of the upper small intestine but can be demonstrated from the gastric antrum to the ileum. It is stored in large granules.

Plasma GIP concentrations rise rapidly after a meal and glucose, fat, and amino acids have all been shown to cause GIP release. Infusions of GIP in man have shown that it causes insulin secretion and it appears that it may be the gastrointestinal 'incretin' factor which causes a much greater release of insulin after oral compared to intravenous glucose administration. GIP also causes inhibition of gastric acid secretion and reduced gastric motor activity but it is not known if this role is physiologically important.

Motilin. This is a 22-amino-acid polypeptide with a molecular weight of 2700. It appears to be present in two major molecular forms but the amino-acid sequence of the second larger form has not been elucidated. Motilin is localized to endocrine cells in the upper small intestine. Fasting plasma motilin concentrations vary and rises are seen at the onset of duodenal myoelectric complex formation. It has therefore been suggested that motilin is the hormone which controls this reflex motor activity which in the fasting state starts at two hourly intervals in the duodenum and progresses to the terminal ileum, thus keeping the small intestine empty.

Plasma motilin concentrations rise after a meal and after drinking water. Motilin infusion with physiological plasma increments has been shown to stimulate the gastric emptying of liquids and solids, to hasten small intestinal transit time, and to cause motor activity in the colon. Motilin may therefore have physiological roles in accelerating gastric emptying, controlling small intestinal transit, and stimulating the gastrocolic reflex.

Pancreatic polypeptide (PP). This is a 36-amino-acid peptide with a molecular weight of 4226. It was first discovered as a contaminant of insulin and appears to be almost entirely localized to the PP cell of the pancreas. After pancreatectomy plasma PP levels are consequently indetectable. PP is present more in the head than the tail of the pancreas. PP cells occur around the islets of Langerhans and also between the acinar cells and in the duct walls. On electron microscopy the granules are small and electron dense.

PP rises dramatically after a meal, particularly if the food contains large amounts of protein. This rise is largely under cholinergic control as it can be much reduced by atropine. Infusion studies have shown that at physiological plasma concentrations it causes inhibi-

tion of pancreatic and biliary secretions and it has therefore been suggested that it is responsible for the inhibition of these secretions.

Neurotensin. Neurotensin is a 13-amino-acid polypeptide with a molecular weight of 1673. It was initially isolated in the bovine hypothalamus but subsequently shown to be present in large quantities in an identical molecular form in the mucosal endocrine NT cells of the ileum.

Plasma neurotensin concentrations rise after a meal, the rise being proportional to the size of the meal. Babies show much larger rises than adults. Intravenous infusions of physiological amounts of neurotensin have shown that it causes a delay in gastric emptying and reduces gastric acid secretion. As neurotensin seems to rise when food reaches the ileum, it may be the physiological feedback mechanism by which gastric emptying of nutrients is controlled.

Enteroglucagon. Enteroglucagon is the term used to describe the large molecular-weight peptide found in the intestine which cross-reacts with some pancreatic glucagon antisera. There are probably multiple molecular forms but one form (called glicentin) has been purified from the pig intestine and found to be approximately 100 amino acids in length. Enteroglucagon is found in high concentrations in the mucosa of the ileum, colon, and rectum and has been demonstrated to occur in the EG cell.

Large amounts of enteroglucagon are released by a mixed meal. Enteroglucagon, like gastrin, is believed to have a trophic effect on small intestinal mucosa and like neurotensin may have a feedback effect on gastric function. Its exact physiological roles can, however, only be elucidated when pure material becomes available for infusion studies.

Paracrine peptides

Paracrine substances are those which are secreted by cells and have effects only on neighbouring cells. It is possible that many of the gastrointestinal hormones and putative neurotransmitters have such roles but this is difficult to prove. Somatostatin, however, is thought to act primarily in this way in peripheral tissue but in the central nervous system it acts as a transmitter or neuro-modulator substance. It is also present in the circulation and may occasionally act as a hormone.

Somatostatin. This is a 14-amino-acid peptide with a molecular weight of 1640 but there is evidence for a 28-amino-acid molecular form which may be a precursor. Somatostatin was initially demonstrated in the hypothalamus where it was found to inhibit growth hormone secretion. Subsequently it has been demonstrated in the D cell in the pancreas and mucosa of the gastrointestinal tract from stomach to rectum. Somatostatin may be present in gastrointestinal nerves as well as being present in D cells.

Infusion studies have shown that somatostatin has many inhibitory actions (Table 2). It appears, however, to stimulate the formation of interdigestive myoelectric complexes and to hasten gastric emptying of solids and liquids. Studies with isolated perfused

Table 2 Inhibitory effects of somatostatin

Hormone release	Physiological function
Growth hormone	Lower oesophageal sphincter contraction
Thyroid-stimulating hormone	Gastric acid secretion
Insulin	Pepsin secretion
Glucagon	Pancreatic secretions
Pancreatic polypeptide	Biliary secretion
Gastrin	Nutriment absorption
Secretion	Coeliac blood flow
Gastric inhibitory polypeptide	
Motilin	
Neurotensin	
Enteroglucagon	

organs, for example the stomach and pancreas, have shown that small amounts of somatostatin are secreted into the plasma when some physiological stimuli are applied. As relatively small amounts of infused somatostatin have such widespread effects, it seems unlikely that it acts as a hormone but instead is physiologically a very important local mediator.

Peptide neurotransmitters

A number of gastrointestinal regulatory peptides have been demonstrated in the brain. These include gastrin, cholecystokinin, neurotensin, somatostatin, vasoactive intestinal polypeptide, substance P, bombesin, and the endorphins. The evidence suggests that they have a neurotransmitter role in the brain and studies have, for example, shown that cerebral substance P concentrations are reduced in the substantia nigra of patients with Huntington's chorea. All these peptides may also act as neurotransmitters in gastrointestinal tissue, but it is thought that this is the primary mode of action of vasoactive intestinal polypeptide, substance P, and bombesin.

Vasoactive intestinal polypeptide (VIP). This is a 28-amino-acid polypeptide with a molecular weight of 3326. Multiple molecular forms have been demonstrated both in the colon and in the plasma of patients with VIP-secreting tumours (vipomas). It is found in large quantities in the brain and in the mucosa and muscle of the gastrointestinal tract. In the gut it appears to be present in postganglionic intrinsic nerves (Fig. 3) although some may also be present in

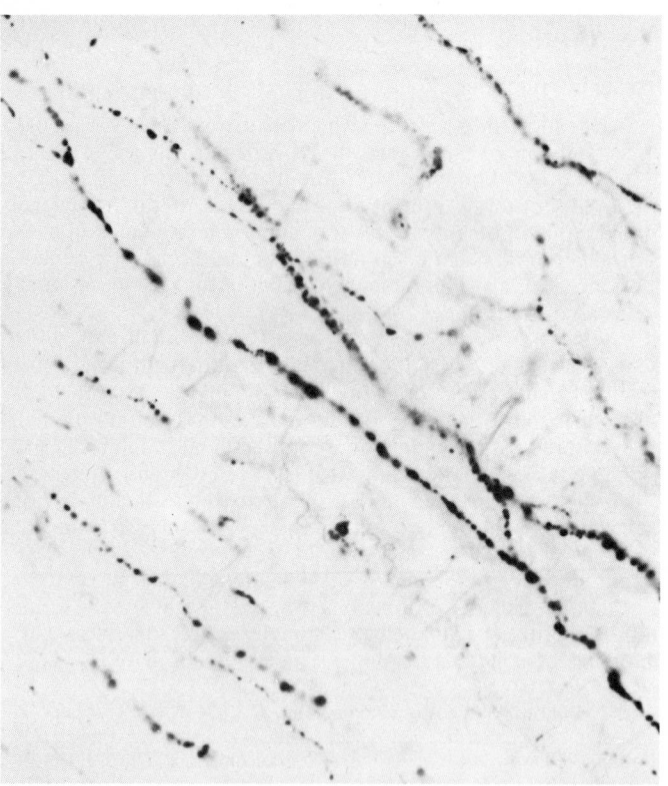

Fig. 3 Vasoactive intestinal polypeptide fibres, immunostained using the unlabelled antibody enzyme (PAP) method, in the submucosa of human colon (×500).

endocrine cells. VIP secretion has been demonstrated after direct neural stimulation. Infusions of VIP have shown it to have many biological effects including the stimulation of small intestinal and colonic secretion with a rise in gut mucosal cyclic AMP concentrations, the production of diarrhoea, hypercalcaemia, and glycogenolysis, the stimulation of pancreatic bicarbonate secretion, the inhibition of gastric acid output, and the lowering of systemic blood

pressure. No rise in plasma VIP concentrations is seen after a meal in normal subjects.

Bombesin. This is a 14-amino-acid polypeptide with a molecular weight of 1620. It is part of a family of peptides initially isolated in the amphibian *Bombina bombina*. Bombesin-like peptides are found in large quantities in the brain of mammals and can also be demonstrated in gastrointestinal nerves. In birds, however, it is found primarily in endocrine cells, particularly in the proventriculus, and may thus play a paracrine or endocrine role in certain species. Infusions of bombesin in man have shown it to have many effects including the stimulation of gastric acid and gastrin secretions, the stimulation of pancreatic secretions, and the stimulation of the release of numerous gut hormones. It is not yet known whether bombesin circulates in plasma in man.

Substance P. Is an 11-amino-acid polypeptide with a molecular weight of 1345. Its existence was first demonstrated in 1931 and its characteristics have consequently been widely studied. It is found in the human brain, particularly in the hypothalamus, in the spinal cord, and in nerves in the gastrointestinal tract. It is possible that it may also be present in enterochromaffin cells in the human gut. Infusions of substance P have shown that it is a potent vasodilator and has a spasmogenic effect on smooth muscle. It causes a reduction in plasma insulin and a rise in plasma glucagon concentrations and thus results in hyperglycaemia. It inhibits pancreatic bicarbonate and amylase secretion and bile flow and stimulates salivation. It acts on the kidney to cause a natriuretic diuresis. It is not yet known if substance P circulates in plasma in man or responds to different physiological stimuli.

Endorphins. The smallest of the endorphins are the two 5-amino-acid enkephalins which differ by one amino acid—methionine enkephalin and leucine enkephalin (respective molecular weights 574 and 556). These *endo*genous m*orphine*-like peptides are widely present in the brain, adrenal medulla, carotid body, and in cells and nerves of the gastrointestinal tract. They are thought to have major roles in determining pain threshold. A study of cerebrospinal fluid met-enkephalin levels during electro-acupuncture showed that this peptide rises and suggested that it may mediate acupuncture analgesia. Opiates are known to greatly inhibit bowel motility and endorphins may play a role in reducing diarrhoea. It seems likely that the primary physiological role of these peptides is as a neurotransmitter substance but endocrine and paracrine functions may also exist.

Gut hormones in gastrointestinal disease

Achlorhydria is associated with very high plasma gastrin concentrations due to a loss of the negative feedback of gastric acid. In patients with fasting hypergastrinaemia it is important to assess basal and pentagastrin-stimulated gastric acid secretion because it is possible to confuse hypergastrinaemia due to a gastrinoma and that due to hypochlorhydria or achlorhydria.

In *coeliac disease* there is loss of the villous pattern in the upper small intestine as a result of dietary gluten sensitivity. Groups of fasting patients with untreated and treated coeliac disease have been given a standard 530 calorie test breakfast and have been followed with regular blood samples for three hours. Greatly reduced concentrations of the hormones secretin and gastric inhibitory polypeptide which originate in the area of the affected bowel have been found in the untreated patients compared to the treated ones and a group of normal controls. This failure of secretin release explains the functional failure of pancreatic bicarbonate secretion which occurs in coeliac disease. In contrast the ileal hormones enteroglucagon and neurotensin were markedly raised in the untreated patients compared to the other two groups (Fig. 4). The raised neurotensin concentrations may be acting to delay gastric emptying and the raised enteroglucagon to delay gastrointestinal

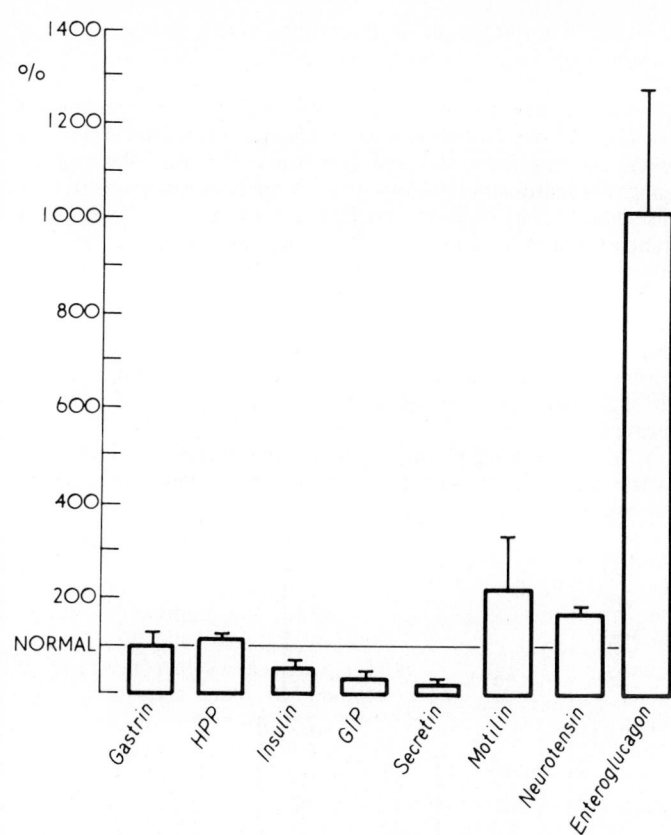

Fig. 4 The percentage incremental rise following a standard test breakfast in blood glucose and some gut hormones compared to normal controls in patients with coeliac disease.

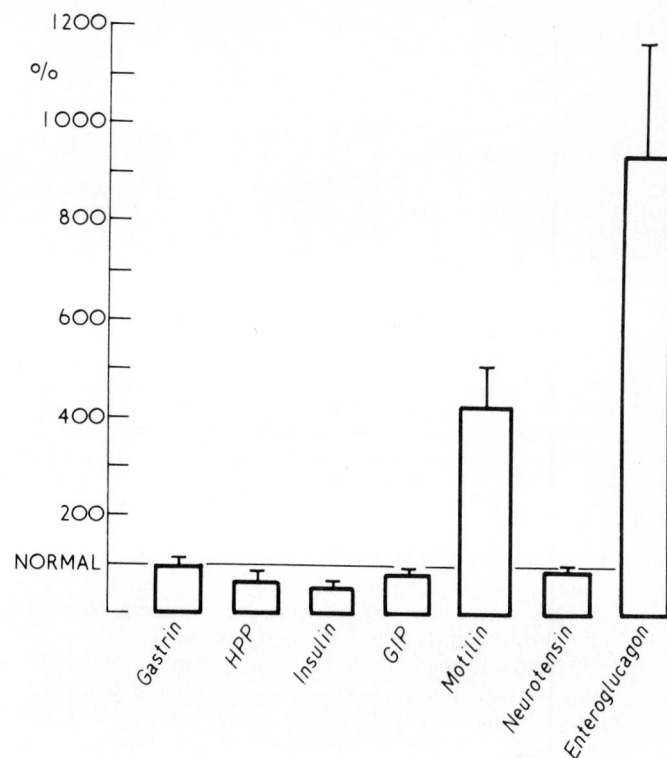

Fig. 5 The percentage incremental rise following a standard test breakfast in blood glucose and in some gut hormones compared to normal controls in patients with tropical sprue.

transit time and to have a trophic effect on the remaining small intestinal mucosal cells. The release of other hormones such as gastrin and pancreatic polypeptide was normal.

Tropical sprue affects the whole length of the small intestine and in these patients a different hormone profile is seen from untreated coeliac disease after a standard test breakfast (Fig. 5). Elevated basal motilin and enteroglucagon concentrations occur and these levels remain elevated for the three hours following the meal. Rises in plasma motilin are known to have stimulatory effects on gastric emptying and small intestinal mucosa. The other plasma gut hormones including neurotensin remain normal in tropical sprue patients.

Fasting and postprandial gut hormone profiles have been studied in massively obese patients before and after treatment by *jejuno-ileal bypass surgery*. Before operation the patients had increased plasma insulin and glucose responses compared to normal weight controls, but no other abnormal gut hormone results. When studied after jejuno-ileal bypass the plasma gastric inhibitory polypeptide response was almost totally lost and the consequent insulin response much reduced. Undigested nutrients were reaching the ileum and presumably for this reason there was a mean 16-fold increase in enteroglucagon responses and an 8-fold increase in the neurotensin response. It is known that the unbypassed bowel greatly hypertrophies following these operations and enteroglucagon is a major candidate for mediating this response.

Patients with *acute infective diarrhoea* have much raised plasma motilin concentrations but no significant changes in other gut hormones. This rise may mediate some of the gastrointestinal motility abnormalities which these patients have.

In patients with *partial ileal resections*, plasma enteroglucagon concentrations are raised, but if the colon is resected, the concentrations are subnormal. This suggests that enteroglucagon is released by the large bowel when the small intestine is diseased and

stimulates the small bowel to hypertrophy and thus absorb more nutrients.

Patients with *ulcerative colitis* have high basal and meal-stimulated plasma gastrin concentrations and this probably reflects reduced gastric acid secretion. Both patients with ulcerative colitis and Crohn's disease with diarrhoea have raised plasma motilin concentrations. The incremental enteroglucagon response to a meal is also raised in patients with Crohn's disease.

Partial postgastrectomy and postvagotomy patients with the dumping syndrome develop symptoms of hypotension and prostration after meals. After 75 g oral glucose tolerance test patients with dumping symptoms have raised plasma concentrations of the known hypotensive peptides neurotensin and VIP. These latter peptides must therefore be considered as candidates for mediating some of the symptoms of this syndrome. Physiologically neurotensin is presumably trying to feedback on the upper small intestine to delay gastric emptying and glucose transit time. Plasma enteroglucagon concentrations are normal in the fasting state but rise to a higher level that controls after the glucose.

The possibility that the *irritable bowel syndrome* might be mediated by gut peptides was intriguing. However, measurement of fasting and meal-stimulated gut hormones has shown no abnormality in groups of patients with pain and constipation and pain alone. Gut hormones cannot therefore be considered as the mediators of this syndrome.

Gut hormones in pancreatic disease

Patients with chronic pancreatitis commonly have insulin-dependent diabetes mellitus. Plasma basal and arginine-stimulated glucagon concentrations vary from high to low. Basal and meal-stimulated pancreatic polypeptide concentrations are usually low in patients with chronic pancreatitis and steatorrhoea but normal in chronic pancreatitis without steatorrhoea (Fig. 6). Patients with steatorrhoea have a reduced response to an intravenous injection of Boot's secretin. The mean response of pancreatic polypeptide to insulin hypoglycaemia is also subnormal in chronic pancreatitis. It

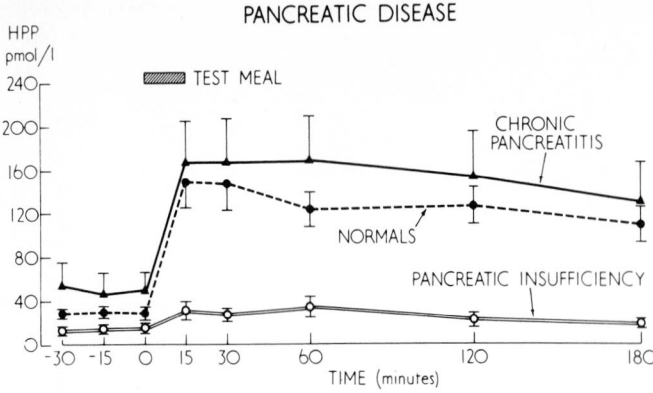

Fig. 6   The plasma human pancreatic polypeptide (HPP) response (pmol/l) following a mixed breakfast in normal controls and patients with chronic pancreatitis with and without steatorrhoea. A markedly reduced response was seen in patients with steatorrhoea.

thus appears that the order of destruction of hormone cells in chronic pancreatitis is pancreatic polypeptide, insulin, and glucagon. The early destruction of pancreatic polypeptide presumably reflects the position of its cells in the periphery of the islets in the pancreatic head and scattered in the acini and in the epithelium lining the pancreatic ducts. However, as occasional patients with very severe chronic pancreatitis may have normal plasma pancreatic polypeptide secretion, assessment of this peptide cannot be considered a reliable diagnostic test.

Patients with chronic pancreatitis have raised basal and stimulated enteroglucagon levels which presumably reflect malabsorption. Plasma motilin concentrations are commonly raised to a moderate degree. Raised plasma cholecystokinin concentrations are also reported.

Gut hormone responses have not been studied in acute pancreatitis but the pancreatic hormones have been assessed. It appears that insulin secretion is usually reduced and plasma glucagon concentrations during initial attacks are raised. Repeated attacks are associated with falling plasma glucagon concentrations. Other stress hormones producing hyperglycaemia such as cortisol and the catecholamines may also contribute to the glucose intolerance.

In children and young adults with cystic fibrosis, diabetes mellitus commonly develops. Fasting plasma pancreatic polypeptide concentrations are usually reduced and fail to respond to a milk drink stimulus. Plasma gastric inhibitory polypeptide concentrations fail to rise after a milk stimulus and this is associated with glucose intolerance; this result suggests that there is a failure in the entero-insular axis as well as the failure of insulin secretion caused by the reduced beta cell mass. Milk-stimulated enteroglucagon concentrations are also reduced in patients with cystic fibrosis.

There is good evidence that there are major neural components in the secretion of insulin, pancreatic glucagon, and pancreatic polypeptide. Study of patients with chronic autonomic failure (the Shy–Drager syndrome) has shown reduced pancreatic glucagon and pancreatic polypeptide release during insulin hypoglycaemia. Patients with gastrointestinal Chagas' disease have reduced insulin secretion to oral glucose and reduced pancreatic glucagon and pancreatic polypeptide during hypoglycaemia. These studies suggest that pancreatic endocrine cell denervation occurs in these two syndromes.

Deficiency of somatostatin—nesidioblastosis. Nesidioblastosis occurs in neonates and is a syndrome of hypoglycaemia associated with plasma insulin concentrations inappropriately high for the prevailing blood glucose levels. The possibility of this syndrome being due to somatostatin deficiency is strongly suggested by the findings of reduced pancreatic somatostatin D cells in affected children and of normalization of blood glucose concentrations by low dose somatostatin infusions. These results suggest that nesi-

dioblastosis is due to a deficiency of paracrine somatostatin allowing hyperinsulinaemia and hypoglycaemia.

Neuracrine peptides in gastrointestinal disease. Biochemical and immunohistochemical studies have been performed in two types of bowel denervation associated with loss of intrinsic nerve fibres, Chagas' disease, and Hirschsprung's disease. In patients with Chagas' disease and megaoesophagus or megacolon, VIP and substance P concentrations and nerve fibres are reduced in affected bowel and in rectal biopsy specimens. In patients with chronic autonomic failure (the Shy–Drager syndrome) who have loss of preganglionic extrinsic nerves, the rectal peptide nerves are normal (Fig. 7). These results support the concept of VIP and substance P nerves mediating intrinsic nerve transmission. Children with Hirschsprung's disease also have reduced VIP nerves in affected segments of colon.

Patients with Crohn's disease have a considerable increase in VIP in affected segments. The significance of this striking increase is not yet explained.

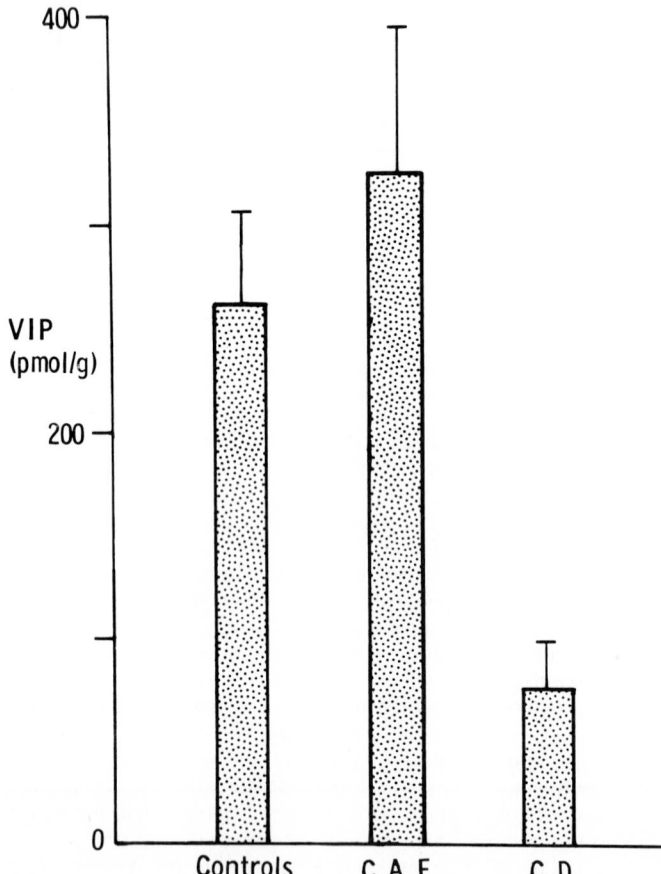

Fig. 7   Rectal vasoactive intestinal polypeptide concentrations (pmol/g wet tissue) in controls and patients with chronic autonomic failure (CAF) and Chagas' disease (CD) with gastrointestinal involvement. Reduced concentrations were seen in Chagas' specimens (reproduced from *Lancet* (1980), **i**, 559, by permission).

Pancreatic endocrine tumours

Pancreatic endocrine tumours have been described which secrete insulin (insulinomas, see Section 9), gastrin (gastrinomas, the Zollinger–Ellison syndrome), glucagon (glucagonomas), vasoactive intestinal polypeptide (vipomas), pancreatic polypeptide (PP-omas), and somatostatin (somatostatinomas). These tumours are derived from APUD cells which have the ability of *a*mine *p*roduction *u*ptake and *d*ecarboxylation and have thus become known as apudomas. On occasions pancreatic tumours may also secrete other hormones, for example adrenocorticotrophic hormone (ACTH) or parathyroid hormone. A major feature of all these tumours, except for PP-omas, is that they present, usually when still small, with the metabolic symptoms of the polypeptide which the tumour is synthesizing rather than with the local symptoms of invasion characteristic of pancreatic carcinomas.

Pancreatic endocrine tumours commonly occur in association with a parathyroid adenoma causing primary hyperparathyroidism and with functioning pituitary adenomas (for example, prolactinomas). This association should be sought in all patients by checking plasma calcium and phosphate concentrations and X-raying the pituitary fossa and is called *Wermer's syndrome* or multiple endocrine adenomatosis *Type 1 (MEA Type 1)*. Recent evidence has suggested that in some MEA Type 1 families, if one of the triad occurs in an individual, the other two tumours eventually also manifest themselves. *MEA Type 2 (Sipple's syndrome)* is the association between parathyroid adenomas, medullary carcinomas of the thyroid, and phaeochromocytomas. Pancreatic endocrine tumours were originally thought only to secrete one major peptide. Subsequently it was shown that large numbers of these tumours also secrete excessive amounts of pancreatic polypeptide, for example 77 per cent of vipomas and 50 per cent of glucagonomas. Some patients may start with the symptoms of a vipoma and then develop those of an insulinoma, and an insulinoma becoming a glucagonoma is also recorded. This indicates that these tumours often have the potential to synthesize multiple peptides and may sometimes be related to a disparity between immunoassayable and biologically active fragments. Plasma measurement by radioimmunoassay of the dominant peptide is diagnostic in these patients, but it is worth measuring the other peptides as these may be raised and become clinically important later in the patient's illness.

Diagnosis of pancreatic endocrine tumours can usually be made by radioimmunoassay of a single fasting plasma sample and by a small number of confirmatory tests. Localization of the tumours can be very difficult even with selective arteriography. This problem has led to the use of percutaneous trans-hepatic portal venous sampling and measurement of plasma from different veins draining the pancreas to try and demonstrate a peptide peak indicating the site of tumour drainage. When surgery is performed, it is useful to perform standard histology and to perform specific immunocytochemical and ultrastructural studies on the tumour tissue. Radioimmunoassay of tumour extracts provides absolute tumour concentrations and chromatography may be used to assess the prevalence of different molecular forms.

Treatment of pancreatic endocrine tumours is varied but, except with gastrinomas, an attempt should always be made to excise the primary tumour if there is no evidence of metastases. In the presence of metastases a number of symptomatic treatments may be used for the specific tumour symptoms. Somatostatin or long-acting subcutaneous analogues may be of considerable use in reducing tumour secretion in the future. Attempts may be made to reduce tumour mass by the nitrosourea cytotoxic drug streptozotocin and embolization of hepatic artery metastases via a catheter often greatly reduces plasma hormone concentrations and the associated symptoms.

Vipomas. Two types of VIP-secreting tumour exist: pancreatic endocrine tumours and, more rarely, ganglioneuroblastomas which originate from the sympathetic chain or adrenal medulla. Both types of tumour occur equally in both sexes but pancreatic tumours occur in adulthood while the majority of ganglioneuroblastomas occur in children. Most ganglioneuroblastomas are benign, but at the time of operation about 50 per cent of the pancreatic tumours have metastasized, usually to lymph nodes and the liver.

Major clinical and biochemical characteristics of vipomas are listed in Table 3. These characteristics accord well with the known biological effects of VIP (see above). The diarrhoea may undergo spasmodic remissions and steatorrhoea is usually minimal or absent. Diarrhoea in adults is always more than 1 litre per day and

may be greater than 10 litres daily. Loss of weight and varying degrees of dehydration occur. Colicky abdominal pain is a major symptom in more than half the patients. Spontaneous cutaneous flushing and flushing on tumour palpation, sometimes with a marked fall in systemic blood pressure, occur in some patients.

Table 3 Clinical and biochemical features of vipomas

Clinical	Biochemical
Secretory diarrhoea	Raised plasma VIP
Loss of weight	High tumour VIP
Dehydration	Raised plasma pancreatic polypeptide
Abdominal colic	Raised plasma urea
Cutaneous flushing	Hypokalaemic acidosis
	Achlorhydria
	Hypercalcaemia
	Diabetic glucose tolerance

Vipomas are associated with very high plasma VIP concentrations. Plasma concentrations in 62 vipomas (52 pancreatic and 10 ganglioneuroblastomas) ranged from 48 to 760 pmol/l whereas in 41 controls, the range was 1–21 pmol/l (Fig. 8). Plasma VIP estimation is thus of diagnostic use in these patients. Tumour VIP concentrations, as assessed by extraction and radioimmunoassay, are also usually very high. Immunocytochemistry shows VIP to be present in cells in the tumours and electron microscopy shows characteristic small secretory granules. The majority of pancreatic tumours secrete pancreatic polypeptide and some may secrete gastrin, calcitonin, glucagon, and insulin. Some ganglioneuroblastomas secrete

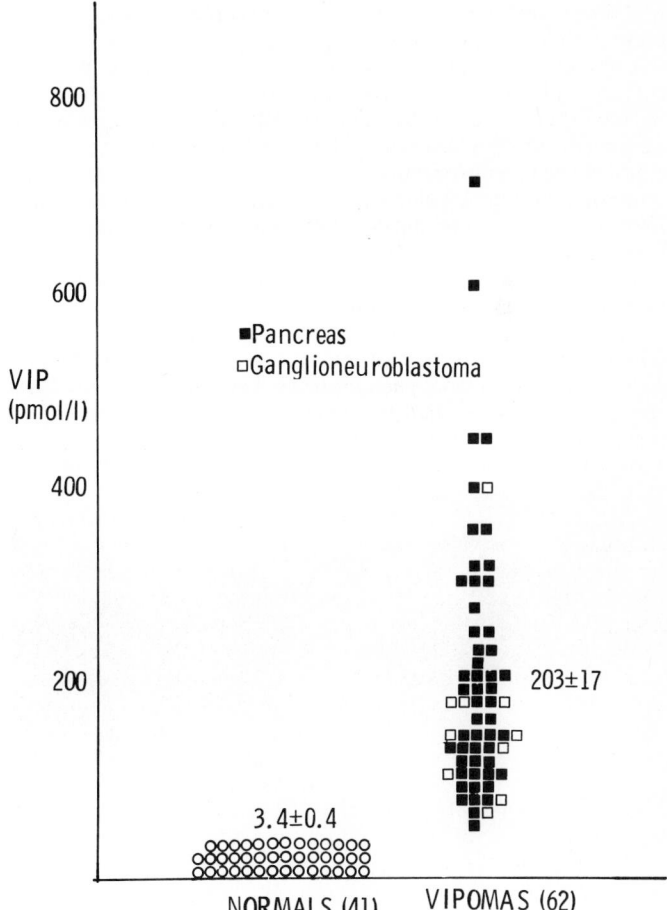

Fig. 8 Plasma vasoactive intestinal polypeptide (VIP) concentrations in normal controls (O) and VIP-secreting pancreatic (□), and ganglioneuroblastoma tumours (■).

adrenaline and noradrenaline and these patients may have raised 24-hour urinary vanillylmandelic acid (VMA) concentrations.

The plasma urea rises because of dehydration and possibly also because of increased catabolism. The faeces contain high concentrations of sodium, potassium, and bicarbonate, and patients consequently have a hypokalaemic acidosis. Achlorhydria or hypochlorhydria are common but not always present and therefore the eponym the *WDHA syndrome* (watery diarrhoea, hypokalaemia and achlorhydria) seems inappropriate. At operation the gallbladders are often dilated. Hypercalcaemia may occur with normal plasma parathyroid hormone and 25-hydroxy vitamin D concentrations, and although dehydration may play a part, a direct action of VIP is probably the main cause. Mild hyperglycaemia occurs in some patients but this rarely requires treatment.

The treatment of choice is surgical resection after correction of acute metabolic problems. The majority of ganglioneuroblastomas are resectable but in about half of the patients with pancreatic tumours unresectable metastases are present. In these latter patients streptozotocin may produce remissions lasting several years.

A number of drugs have produced a symptomatic improvement. Corticosteroids usually reduce stool volumes but the symptoms often relapse after a few weeks. Somatostatin may be helpful by reducing plasma VIP concentrations. It is possible that VIP may act through prostaglandins and indomethacin sometimes reduces the diarrhoea. Metoclopramide, by reducing absolute amounts of 28-amino-acid VIP, lithium carbonate, and opiates may also reduce the diarrhoea.

Glucagonomas. Glucagonomas are alpha cell tumours of the pancreas which synthesize pancreatic glucagon and similar peptides. They occur in adulthood, appear to be slightly more common in women, and the majority have metastasized at the time of presentation.

The patients usually have diabetes mellitus and present with a characteristic necrolytic migratory erythematous rash which particularly involves the perineum and if undiagnosed may persist for many years. Bullae occur with the rash, break down, and then gradually heal, only to recur in another site (Fig. 9). Other common symptoms include angular stomatitis, glossitis, weight loss, diarrhoea, crumbling nails, and those of venous thrombosis and pulmonary embolism.

The diagnosis can be confirmed by demonstrating raised fasting plasma glucagon concentrations by radioimmunoassay. The tumour tissue has large quantities of extractable glucagon present and immunocytochemistry shows this to be present in typical alpha cells. Electron microscopy demonstrates dense homogeneous secretory granules. About half the tumours also synthesize pancreatic polypeptide and some may produce gastrin and insulin.

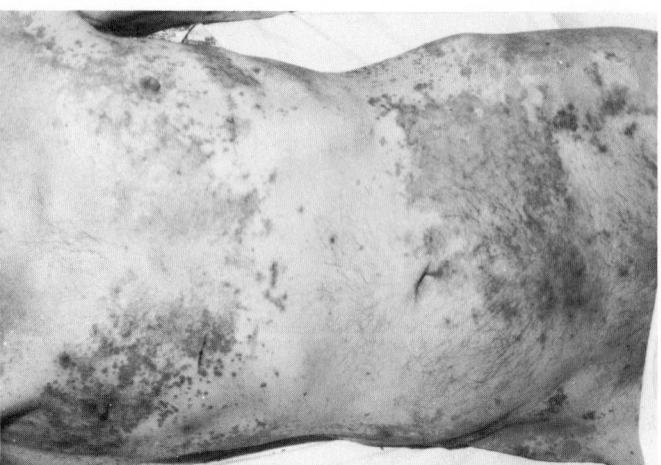

Fig. 9 Typical necrolytic migratory erythematous rash seen in a patient with a pancreatic glucagonoma.

The majority of glucagonomas are associated with diabetes mellitus, which is commonly insulin-dependent, but not associated with complications or ketoacidosis. Skin biopsy of early lesions shows necrolysis of the upper layers of the stratum Malpighi of the epidermis whilst late lesions show only a non-specific dermatitis. A normochromic normocytic anaemia is usually present and the serum iron may be low although marrow iron is normal. Iron supplements normalize the serum concentrations but do not appear to improve the haemoglobin or the cutaneous or oral lesions. Hypokalaemia may occur when diarrhoea is present. Barium studies show coarse jejunal and ilial folds but normal jejunal histology is seen. Steatorrhoea is absent or minimal and exocrine pancreatic function is normal unless a tumour is obstructing the pancreatic duct. Plasma amino acid and tissue zinc concentrations are greatly reduced.

Surgical excision of the pancreatic tumour is the treatment of choice for non-metastasized cases and produces resolution of all the problems including the rash and diabetes. In patients with unresectable primary tumours or metastases, streptozotocin often reduces tumour size and improves symptoms. Hepatic metastases may be treated with arterial embolization. The rash has some similarities to the childhood zinc deficiency syndrome acrodermatitis enteropathy and oral zinc supplements usually greatly improve the skin of glucagonomas. Anticoagulants may be helpful in preventing deep vein thrombosis and the pulmonary emboli of which these patients commonly die. On occasions oral tetracycline, corticosteroids, and azathioprine have also been shown to benefit the rash.

Gastrinomas. (see also page 12.60). Gastrinomas usually originate in the pancreas but raised plasma gastrin levels producing gastric hyperacidity may also occur with duodenal and antral tumours and antral G-cell hyperplasia. Tumours producing many problems may be only a few mm in diameter. They usually occur in adulthood and tend to follow a very slowly progressive malignant course.

Zollinger and Ellison in 1955 described the classic association of pancreatic non-beta islet cell tumours, severe duodenal ulcer disease, increased gastric acid secretion, and a poor response to ulcer therapy. The duodenal ulcers are usually severe and multiple and may be associated with perforation, bleeding, pyloric stenosis, oesophagitis, and oesophageal stricture. Diarrhoea and steatorrhoea are prominent features in some patients. About a third of the patients have associated functioning parathyroid adenomas or pituitary adenomas, and some patients also have multiple primary gastrinomas.

Investigations show a raised fasting plasma gastrin concentration associated with raised basal gastric acid secretion. The majority of gastrin is usually in the G17 rather than the G34 form. The duodenal ulcers, prominent gastric folds, and oesophageal abnormalities can be best demonstrated by upper gastrointestinal endoscopy. Further jejunal ulcers can sometimes be demonstrated by barium studies. Confirmation of gastrinoma-related hypergastrinaemia can be obtained by either the secretin or calcium tests. In the secretin test, the patients are fasted, pure secretin is injected intravenously, and in gastrinoma patients an inappropriate rise in plasma gastrin occurs. In the calcium test a greater than normal rise in plasma gastrin occurs. Localizing gastrinoma tumours is usually very difficult by standard pancreatic visualization techniques (including arteriography) but portal venous sampling and measurement of plasma gastrin concentrations may be helpful.

The treatment of gastrinomas used to be excision of the target organ, i.e. total gastrectomy. This treatment is effective but may be associated with the symptoms of a severe dumping syndrome and of various nutritional deficiencies. The development of cimetidine has resulted in many patients' symptoms being controlled on doses of 1–3 g daily. Radical surgery to remove primary tumours should probably only be performed if a single primary tumour can be localized pre-operatively and there is no evidence of metastases. In the presence of metastatic disease streptozotocin reduces tumour size and plasma gastrin concentrations markedly in some patients.

Somatostatinomas. Somatostatinomas have been described originating in the pancreas and gut and on occasions calcitonin may also be secreted. Calcitonin has not been demonstrated in pancreatic D cells but both calcitonin and somatostatin occur in thyroid C cells. The tumours have only been described in adults and the majority have hepatic metastases present at operation.

Major clinical problems are cholelithiasis, diabetes mellitus, steatorrhoea, hypochlorhydria, anaemia, and weight loss. The first four abnormalities can be respectively explained by the known inhibitory effects of somatostatin on biliary secretion, insulin secretion, intestinal absorption, and gastric acid secretion whilst the latter two problems presumably reflect widespread malignancy.

The diagnosis can be confirmed by demonstrating raised concentrations of plasma somatostatin by radioimmunoassay. Multiple molecular forms of somatostatin occur in the plasma and tumour extracts of these patients. Diabetes is usually mild and neither the plasma insulin nor glucagon responses are completely abolished. Other effects which have been demonstrated include reduced growth hormone secretion, reduced gastric inhibitory polypeptide secretion, increased numbers of myoelectric complexes, and reduced pancreatic exorcine bicarbonate and enzyme secretion.

Radical pancreatic surgery would be expected to be of help but three of the four reported patients so treated died after the procedure (the one surviving having non-metastatic disease). Streptozotocin or other cytotoxic drugs have not yet been assessed. No drugs have been demonstrated to improve symptoms.

PP-omas. Apudomas secreting only pancreatic polypeptide (PP-omas) are rare and usually present with the problems of local expansion, metastatic spread, or common bile duct obstruction rather than with any metabolic symptoms. The diagnosis, which usually follows finding characteristic apudoma histology, can be confirmed by demonstrating raised plasma fasting PP and tumour PP concentrations. Treatment is with surgery or, if impossible, with streptozotocin.

Secretion of PP is typical of pancreatic apudomas and raised fasting plasma PP concentrations and is seen in some 77 per cent of vipomas, 50 per cent of glucagonomas, and 25 per cent of gastrinomas and insulinomas. Plasma PP is not raised in ganglioneuroblastomas and consequently a raised plasma PP in a vipoma indicates a pancreatic primary site. Pancreatic adenocarcinomas are not associated with PP secretion. Plasma PP measurement is thus useful in the diagnosis and follow-up of pancreatic apudomas.

Enteroglucagonoma. Only one tumour secreting enteroglucagon has been described. The tumour originated in the right kidney. The patient had severe constipation, peripheral oedema, and a transient erythematous skin rash. Investigation revealed a very high plasma enteroglucagon concentration, hypoalbuminaemia, mild steatorrhoea, and a diabetic oral glucose tolerance test. A barium follow-through showed a dilated small intestine with coarse thickened mucosal folds and a slow transit time, and jejunal histology revealed gross villous hypertrophy. Resection of the renal tumour produced clinical and biochemical resolution.

Carcinoid syndrome

Primary gastrointestinal carcinoid tumours occur in the area of the embryological foregut (including thyroid, bronchus, stomach, common bile duct, and pancreas), midgut, or hindgut, and their behaviour is partly dependent on their origin. The most common primary gastrointestinal site for carcinoid tumours is the terminal ileum. Primary carcinoid tumours of the appendix are common but very rarely metastasize. Hindgut, usually rectal, carcinoids are commonly benign, may have multicentric origins, and, even when they metastasize, usually do not cause metabolic symptoms. Symptoms of the carcinoid syndrome do not develop when the tumour drainage is through an intact liver so that gut tumours have to have metastasized, usually to the liver, before any metabolic symptoms develop. Carcinoid tumours may on occasions originate in the bronchi, testes, or ovaries, and in these patients symptoms may develop before metastases have developed.

Clinical picture. The classic symptom of the carcinoid syndrome is the flush. The carcinoid flush predominantly involves the head and neck, and a tachycardia, fall in systolic blood pressure, and a rise in skin temperature occur. The patients have a sensation of intense heat, and some have associated wheezing. In severe cases the flush may spread to the trunk and limbs and be associated with lacrimation, facial oedema, and great distress. Precipitating factors include alcohol, ingestion of food, stress, and emotion. Ileal tumours with metastases cause generalized flushing which usually only lasts a few minutes but may become almost continuous as the disease progresses; these patients tend to have a chronically reddened and cyanotic facial hue with widespread telangiectasia. In contrast the gastric carcinoids often have raised localized wheal-like areas of flushing which are usually pruritic and may migrate. Bronchial carcinoids, like rectal carcinoids, are often metabolically inactive, but when they cause flushing the patients can have severe flushes which may last for hours or days and be associated with such severe falls in blood pressure that anuria results.

Secretory diarrhoea is the main symptom in some patients with carcinoid tumours. The diarrhoea is often profuse (more than 1 litre per day) and may be associated with abdominal pain, nausea, and vomiting. Intestinal obstruction due to tumour should be excluded but the primary intestinal tumours are usually small, being less than 1 per cent of total body tumour weight in the typical gastrointestinal carcinoid syndrome patient. Weight loss is common and may be due to a poor dietary intake, malabsorption, and increased catabolism. Pellagra with dermatitis of sun-exposed areas may occur. Right hypochondrial pain is commonly associated with hepatomegaly, and acute severe pain with peritonism commonly occurs when hepatic metastases become hypoxic. Peptic ulcer disease is also said to be more common in patients with the carcinoid syndrome.

Involvement of the tricuspid and pulmonary valves by a fibrotic process is common and may cause both tricuspid and pulmonary stenosis and regurgitation. Right-sided cardiac failure with oedema and breathlessness is the usual clinical problem and may cause death. Left-sided cardiac valvular lesions are rare but may occur with bronchial carcinoids and atrial septal defects with right to left shunts.

Occasionally carcinoid tumours synthesize ACTH and a relatively common cause of the ectopic ACTH syndrome is a primary carcinoid tumour in the pancreas not associated with the carcinoid syndrome. On occasions carcinoid tumours may be associated with functioning parathyroid adenomas and with gastrinomas.

Biochemistry. Metastatic carcinoid tumours take up the amino-acid tryptophan, form 5-hydroxy tryptophan, and then decarboxylate it to 5-hydroxy tryptamine (serotonin, 5-HT) (Fig. 10). The latter is the biologically active molecule of the metabolic pathway and appears to play a role in the pathogenesis of some carcinoid symptoms, particularly increased intestinal gastrointestinal motility, diarrhoea, and bronchoconstriction. 5-hydroxyindole acetic acid (5HIAA) is formed by the action of monoamine oxidase and aldehyde dehydrogenase enzymes and accounts for more than 95 per cent of urinary excretion.

Flushing can be provoked in patients by alcohol and intravenous noradrenaline and peptides such as pentagastrin but how the flushing is actually mediated is unknown. It has been shown that after stimulation of the tumour by noradrenaline, activation of tumour kallikrein occurs and bradykinin is consequently released into the plasma; the latter may contribute to the production of the flush. Gastric carcinoids tend to contain much histamine and this probably plays a major role in the aetiology of the wheals of geographical flushing. Other possible flushing mediators include vasoactive peptides and prostaglandins (but flushing is rarely prevented by prostaglandin inhibitors such as indomethacin).

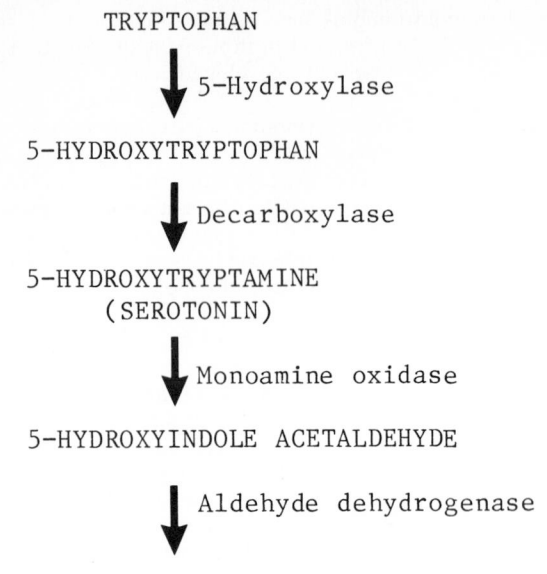

TRYPTOPHAN

↓ 5-Hydroxylase

5-HYDROXYTRYPTOPHAN

↓ Decarboxylase

5-HYDROXYTRYPTAMINE
(SEROTONIN)

↓ Monoamine oxidase

5-HYDROXYINDOLE ACETALDEHYDE

↓ Aldehyde dehydrogenase

5-HYDROXYINDOLE ACETIC ACID

Fig. 10 Biochemical pathway for the synthesis and degradation of serotonin (5-HT).

5-HT and histamine have been demonstrated in carcinoid tumours. There is also evidence for small quantities of pancreatic polypeptide, substance P, neurotensin, enteroglucagon, and motilin occurring in some carcinoid tumours but their roles are, as yet, unclear.

Investigations. Raised urinary 5-HIAA concentrations are used to confirm the diagnosis of the carcinoid syndrome and serial quantitative 24-hour urinary samples give an index of tumour progression. False positive results may be seen with food containing high concentrations of 5-HT, for example bananas, pineapples, and walnuts, and false negative results may occur in patients taking phenothiazines. Whole blood or platelet 5-HT concentrations may be measured but do not replace urinary 5-HIAA results. Plasma histamine concentrations are often raised in association with gastric carcinoids. Many patients have raised fasting plasma pancreatic polypeptide concentrations and this can be used as a tumour marker; plasma motilin concentrations are usually raised when diarrhoea occurs. Carcinoid tumours may also be associated with raised plasma concentrations of gastrin, glucagon, insulin, ACTH, parathyroid hormone, and calcitonin.

Other investigations to document tumour site are important and should include isotopic liver scans to demonstrate metastases and liver function tests, particularly serum albumin which may be reduced as a result of a poor diet, reduced liver function, and increased bowel loss. When the syndrome is present but no hepatic secondaries can be demonstrated, every effort should be made to define the tumour site as surgical cure may be impossible.

Histology is useful and can usually be obtained by percutaneous liver biopsy. The cells reduce silver salts and this argentaffin-positive characteristic can be demonstrated by numerous silver stains.

Treatment. Patients with the carcinoid syndrome need regular careful assessment and treatment of new problems. Careful attention should be paid to diet and any evidence for pellagra investigated and treated with nicotinamide. Drugs such as codeine phosphate, diphenoxylate (Lomotil), and loperamide may reduce diarrhoea, and, if terminal ileal resection has been performed, cholestyramine may reduce the associated bile acid-induced diarrhoea. Cardiac problems should be treated in the usual way and valve replacement may sometimes be indicated.

Cyproheptadine and methysergide are specific 5-HT antagonists which may be very helpful in controlling diarrhoea and flushing, but

the latter should be used guardedly in view of its potential for causing retroperitoneal fibrosis. The alpha-adrenergic blocking drug phenoxybenzamine and phenothiazines with alpha-adrenergic blocking activity, for example prochlorperazine, may be helpful in controlling flushing and probably act by preventing kallikrein release. Parachlorophenylalanine is an inhibitor of the rate-limiting enzyme tryptophan hydroxylase in 5-HT synthesis; it usually reduces diarrhoea but is rarely used because of the high incidence of allergic complications. The main product of gastric carcinoids is usually histamine and a combination of H_1 and H_2 receptor blockade may greatly help these patients. Continuous intravenous infusions of somatostatin have been shown to greatly reduce flushing and diarrhoea; this peptide may be useful prior to surgery but there is a danger of an exacerbation of symptoms when it is stopped. In so-called 'carcinoid crisis' when symptoms are severe and continuous, corticosteroids, plasma volume expansion, methoxamine (not catecholamine-derived drugs as these may worsen the situation), and antibiotics appear of use. Cytotoxic drugs, for example 5-fluorouracil, streptozotocin, cyclophosphamide, and cytosine arabinoside, have been used but the tumours are relatively insensitive to this approach. Such drug therapy should be monitored very carefully (see Section 19).

Surgery may be curative for the rare gonadal and pulmonary tumours. Excision of primary gut carcinoids is indicated when intestinal destruction occurs, but otherwise is unhelpful. Hepatic metastases can often be 'shelled out' at laparotomy and such surgical debulking may cause long remissions. An alternative technique not requiring laparotomy is to selectively embolize hepatic metastases via a hepatic artery catheter.

Prognosis. Many carcinoid tumours are slow growing and follow a prolonged course of up to 20 or more years from the development of the first carcinoid symptoms. Medical treatment can provide a good quality of life and, when symptoms worsen, treatment by surgical debulking or hepatic arterial embolization should create a further remission.

References

Allison, D. J., Modlin, I. M., and Jenkins, W. J. (1977). Treatment of carcinoid liver metastases by hepatic artery embolization. *Lancet* ii, 1323.
Besterman, H. S., Bloom, S. R., Sarson, D. L., Blackburn, A. M., Johnston, D. I., Patel, H. R., Stewart, J. S., Modigliani, R., Guerin, S., and Mallinson, C. N. (1978). Gut-hormone profile in coeliac disease. *Lancet* i, 785.
—, Cook, G. C., Sarson, D. L., Christofides, N. D., Bryant, M. G., Gregor, M., and Bloom, S. R. (1979). Gut hormones in tropical malabsorption. *Br. med. J.* i, 1252.
Bloom, S. R. (1972). An enteroglucagon tumour. *Gut* 13, 520.
— (ed.) (1978). *Gut hormones*. Churchill Livingstone, Edinburgh.
— and Polak, J. M. (1980). Glucagonomas, vipomas and somatostatinomas. *Clins Endocr. Metab.* 9, 285.
— and — (1980). Gut hormones. *Adv. clin. Chem.* 21, 177.
— and — (1980). Plasma hormone concentrations in gastrointestinal disease. *Clins Gastroent.* 9, 785.
Buchanan, K. D. (1980). Gut hormones and gut endocrine tumour syndromes. *Br. J. hosp. Med.* 24, 190.
Grahame-Smith, D. G. (1972). In *The carcinoid syndrome*. Heinemann, London.
Hirsch, H. J., Loo, S., Evans, N., Crigler, J. F., Filler, R. M., and Gabbay, K. H. (1977). Hypoglycaemia of infancy and nesidioblastosis—studies with somatostatin. *New Engl. J. Med.* 296, 1323.
Holst, J. J. (1979). Gut endocrine tumour syndromes. *Clins Endocr. Metab.* 8, 413.
Krejs, G. J., Orci, L., Conlon, J. M., Ravazzola, M., Davis, G. R., Raskin, P., Collins, S. M., McCarthy, D. M., Baetens, D., Rubenstein, A., Aldor, T. A. M., and Unger, R. H. (1979). Somatostatinoma syndrome: biochemical, morphologic and clinical features. *New Engl. J. Med.* 301, 285.
Long, R. G., Adrian, T. E., and Bloom, S. R. (1981). Gastrointestinal hormones in pancreatic disease. In *Pancreatic disease in clinical medicine* (eds. C. J. Mitchell and J. Kelleher). Pitman Medical, Tunbridge Wells.
—, Barnes, A. J., Adrian, T. E., Mallinson, C. N., Brown, M. R., Vale,

W., Rivier, J. E., Christofides, N. D., and Bloom, S. R. (1979). Suppression of pancreatic endocrine tumour secretion by long-acting somatostatin analogue. *Lancet* **ii**, 764.

—, Bishop, A. E., Barnes, A. J., Albuquerque, R. H., O'Shaugnessy, D. J., McGregor, G. P., Bannister, R., Polak, J. M., and Bloom, S. R. (1980). Neural and hormonal peptides in rectal biopsy specimens from patients with Chagas' disease and chronic autonomic failure. *Lancet* **i**, 559.

—, Bryant, M. G., Mitchell, S. J., Adrian, T. E., Polak, J. M., and Bloom, S. R. (1981). Clinopathological study of pancreatic and aganglioneuroblastoma tumours secreting vasoactive intestinal polypeptide (vipomas). *Br. med. J.* **282**, 1767.

—, Peters, J. R., Bloom, S. R., Brown, M. R., Vale, W., Rivier, J. E., and Grahame-Smith, D. G. (1981). Somatostatin, gastrointestinal peptides and the carcinoid syndrome. *Gut* **22**, 549.

Mallinson, C. N., Bloom, S. R., Warin, A. R., Salmon, P. R., and Cox, B. (1974). A glucagonoma syndrome. *Lancet* **ii**, 1.

Roberts, L. J., Marney, S. R., and Oates, J. A. (1979). Blockade of the flush associated with metastatic gastric carcinoid by combined H_1 and H_2 receptor antagonists. *New. Engl. J. Med.* **300**, 236.

Stadil, F. and Stage, J. G. (1980). The Zollinger–Ellison syndrome. *Clins Endocr. Metab.* **8**, 433.

Turner, R. C., Lee, E. C. G., Morris, P. J., Harris, E. A., and Dick, R. (1978). Localisation of insulinomas. *Lancet* **i**, 515.

Peptic ulcer

J. J. Misiewicz and R. E. Pounder

Introduction. Chronic duodenal ulcer (DU) and chronic benign gastric ulcer (GU) are often grouped together as peptic ulcers. Although the two diseases have many similarities, they differ in some important aspects such as epidemiology, natural history, outcome, and management. These differences are important clinically, and it is therefore sensible always to establish a precise diagnosis of either DU or GU and to manage them clinically as separate, although related, diseases.

Duodenal ulcer

Definition. Duodenal ulcer (DU) is a distinct break in the mucosa of the duodenum, almost invariably in the duodenal bulb. The ulcer may be superficial, or may penetrate to the serosa.

Aetiology. It is not known why certain patients develop duodenal ulceration, nor why the clinical course is characterized by episodes of intermittent ulcer relapses. Many aetiological factors may affect the incidence of DU; the relative importance of each of them in particular geographical areas or particular individuals is impossible to judge with certainty. Epidemiological evidence suggests that DU first became common in Western Europe around the turn of the twentieth century: similar observations cannot be made in other areas because of lack of reliable records. The clinical characteristics of DU appear to be changing quite rapidly with time, towards a less severe clinical form: why this should be so is not known.

Acid and pepsin. Although the presence of acid and pepsin is essential for the appearance of a DU it is probably only one of several aetiological factors operating in most patients. Ulceration is generally thought to be caused by an imbalance between the damaging effects of acid and pepsin attack and the body's mucosal defences. This simplistic hypothesis does fit the extremes of acid secretion: duodenal ulcers do not occur in anacidic patients, but are almost inevitable in the presence of gross hypersecretion of acid in the Zollinger–Ellison syndrome.

As a group DU patients secrete more acid than healthy people, but there is a considerable overlap between DU patients and healthy subjects (Fig. 1). Four factors may account for the tendency of DU patients to hypersecrete acid and pepsin: (*a*) increased parietal cell mass; (*b*) increased stimulation of acid secretion; (*c*) increased parietal cell sensitivity to stimulants; and (*d*) decreased inhibitory control of acid secretion. The evidence for these four factors is incomplete but, on average, DU patients do have more parietal cells than normal; their peak acid output increases as the years of disease continue (perhaps due to pyloric obstruction, antacid consumption, or bile/alkaline reflux into the antrum). DU patients have high basal and nocturnal unstimulated gastric acid outputs; they also have an exaggerated gastrin response to food and

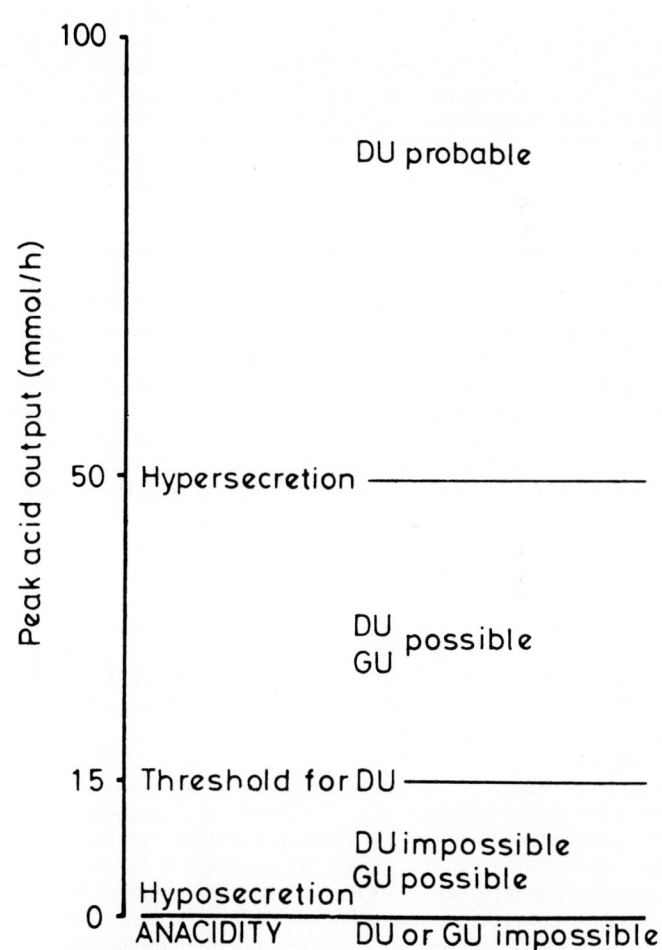

Fig. 1 Peak gastric acid secretion rates and possibility of development of DU or GU. (From Baron, H. (1972). *Chronic duodenal ulcer*, ed. C. Wastell, Butterworth, London, by permission.)

continue to secrete gastrin despite increasing acidification of the antrum. Finally, increased sensitivity to exogenous pentagastrin has been reported in DU patients, when compared with controls.

A great deal is known about the physiology of acid secretion, but the abnormalities of acid output and gastrin release described above are subtle, difficult to investigate, and based on evidence collected from intensive study of few patients: it is uncertain whether they apply to all the DU patients. Much less is known about the importance of pepsin secretion, while knowledge of factors affecting mucosal defence and integrity is fragmentary, especially in relation to the mucosa of the duodenal bulb. It is tempting to speculate that DU is a disease of multifactorial origin and that the importance of various factors differs. For example, excess acid output may be of greater importance in some cases with frank hypersecretion of acid (Fig. 1), while other reasons, such as faulty mucosal defence, may predominate in others.

Gastric emptying. The pH in the duodenal lumen is lower (more acid) more frequently and for longer periods in patients with duodenal ulceration than in controls. DU patients empty food from their stomachs faster so that after a meal there is less food available to buffer secreted acid as it passes into the duodenum. Acid is neutralized in the duodenum by bicarbonate secreted partly by the duodenal mucosa and partly by the exocrine pancreas. DU patients do not have a gross defect of pancreatic alkaline secretion, but little is known about the alkaline secretions of the duodenal mucosa.

Ulcerogenic drugs. Much has been written about the ulcerogenic potential of drugs, such as corticosteroids, aspirin, and other non-steroidal anti-inflammatory agents, but the evidence that they cause chronic DU (or GU) is not convincing. Patients with chronic diseases, such as rheumatoid arthritis, possibly have an increased incidence of peptic ulcer, but there are no strong indications that anti-inflammatory drugs with which they are treated have a decisive influence on the frequency, chronicity, or complication of these ulcers. Anti-inflammatory agents can damage the gastric mucosa and are frequently used to produce ulcer models in experimental animals for the testing of drugs. Extrapolation from these models to humans, however, should be viewed with a certain amount of scepticism.

Psychological factors. Stress of modern life is often invoked as an important cause of DU, but life has always appeared modern and stressful to people living in a given period of history. Chronic (as opposed to acute) stress is difficult to measure and reproduce experimentally. Stress is a non-specific stimulus and will aggravate practically any pre-existing chronic condition. The aetiological importance of stress in DU is difficult to determine, but it can be associated with exacerbation of pre-existing duodenal ulcer. Rapid urbanization in emergent countries is said to coincide with increased incidence of DU, but other diseases also change their pattern and the effects of stress, environment, dietary changes, and better diagnostic facilities are difficult to disentangle.

Epidemiological factors. Duodenal ulceration is very common and may affect 10–15 per cent of many populations. The prevalence of DU is subject to marked geographic variation; for example, DU is much more common in Scotland and northern England than in southern England; it is more common in the south of India than the north. Clinical attributes of DU are also affected by geographical location; for example the rate of perforation in Scotland is greater than in metropolitan London. The characteristics of the disease appear to change with time, as evidenced by the decreasing incidence of perforated DUs (Fig. 2). Duodenal ulceration is more common in men than women, although this difference is becoming less exaggerated, mainly because the incidence of DU in women appears to be increasing. DU is more frequent in women after the menopause, suggesting that sex hormones may be important in the aetiology of the disease. The condition probably reached its European peak in the 1950s, but is now declining. In India and Africa the prevalence of DU is higher in populations who eat a low residue diet; an American study suggested that coffee and soft drinks provoke ulceration. There are weak associations between duodenal ulceration and smoking, alcohol intake, and anti-inflammatory drugs. Although duodenal ulceration has been reported to have positive associations with other medical conditions (such as cirrhosis, chronic lung disease, and hyperparathyroidism), these correlations are probably artefactual and due to intensive investigation of patients who are liable to a second common disease. It is possible that there is a genetic predisposition to duodenal ulcers: it is more common in close family members, patients with blood group O, and non-secretors.

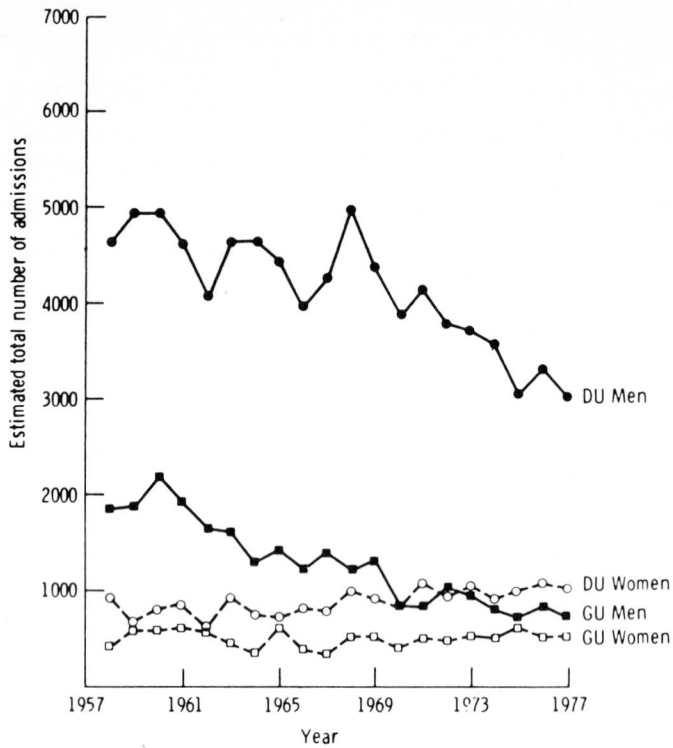

Fig. 2 Estimated admissions for perforated DU and GU in England and Wales, 1958–77. (From Coggon, D., Lambert, P. and Langmann, M. J. S. (1981). *Lancet* **ii**, 1302, by permission.)

Clinical picture and natural history. The major symptom of duodenal ulceration is pain. Although the pain is classically epigastric, related to food, and occurs during the night, it is clear that there can be great individual variation. Indeed, severe ulceration to the point of perforation or haemorrhage can be virtually symptomless. The exact cause of ulcer pain is not clear: it is not always directly related to intraduodenal acidity, but is rapidly and frequently relieved by antacids.

Nausea and vomiting are relatively unusual, unless there is severe pain or pyloric stenosis; vomiting quite often brings relief from pain. Posterior penetration of a duodenal ulcer into the pancreas may cause mid-back pain, or acute pancreatitis. Complication rates are difficult to assess, but major complications are rare—perhaps 1 per cent per year of patients under follow-up. Haemorrhage may cause haematemesis, melaena, or iron deficiency anaemia. Perforation can cause acute, severe pain, collapse, and peritonitis.

Duodenal ulceration is a condition of spontaneous relapses and remissions. The change in the clinical picture from relapse to remission is remarkable. The patient, made miserable by severe epigastric pain and loss of sleep due to night-time symptoms, may return a few days later, feeling perfectly well. It is therefore unwise to make decisions about surgery during a relapse of DU as the patient's reactions may be imbalanced by the symptoms. Recent trials suggest that within a year of ulcer healing, 60 per cent of patients receiving a placebo will have had a symptomatic relapse (Fig. 3), but in addition 27 per cent of asymptomatic DU patients have recurrent active ulceration when examined by endoscopy. The course of the illness is variable—some patients suffer only a single episode of ulceration, while in others the illness is progressive, with rare remissions and severe complications. Spontaneous DU healing may be delayed in patients who continue to smoke cigarettes.

The natural history of untreated duodenal ulceration is unclear. Although it appears that the disease may go into prolonged remission after 10–15 years of intermittent illness, this may be an artefact due to surgical treatment of patients with more aggressive ulcers.

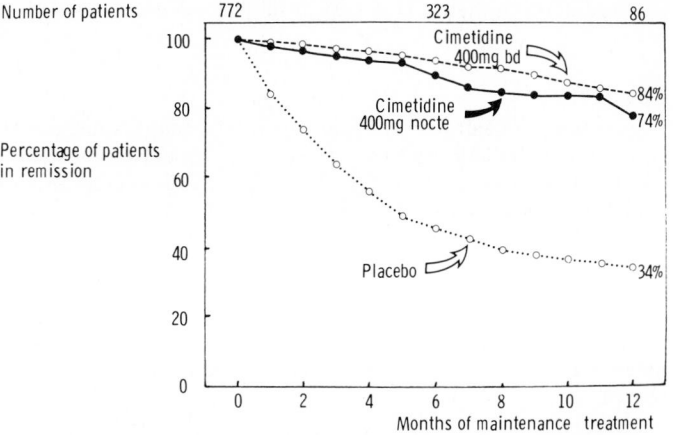

Number of patients

772   323   86

Cimetidine 400mg bd

Cimetidine 400mg nocte

84%

74%

Percentage of patients in remission

Placebo

34%

Months of maintenance treatment

Fig. 3 Maintenance treatment of DU with cimetidine: results of double-blind trials from 22 centres. (From Burland, W., Hawkins, B. W., and Beresford, J. (1980). *Post-grad. med. J.* **56**, 173, by permission.)

Diagnosis. Duodenal ulcer cannot be diagnosed by clinical history, because similar symptoms occur in other diseases, such as gastric ulcer, gastric cancer, or the irritable bowel syndrome. The patient often points to the epigastrium as site of the pain, but this is not reliable. Physical examination may show epigastric tenderness, but is otherwise unhelpful. In rare cases of severe pyloric stenosis, visible gastric peristalsis and a succussion splash are present.

The diagnosis of DU must be established by radiology or endoscopy. A barium meal, preferably air-contrast, will show deformity of the duodenal cap, but the differentiation between scarring, mucosal folds, and an active ulcer crater is less certain. Where available, fibre-optic endoscopy is the best method of diagnosis for DU. Even then, pyloric stenosis with retention of gastric contents, mucosal oedema, haemorrhage, or incomplete inspection of the base of duodenal cap with commonly used end-viewing instruments can all cause the DU crater to be missed. Diagnostic endoscopy in suspected DU should preferably be done at the time of a relapse. Previous therapy with ulcer-healing drugs may make the diagnosis of DU more difficult or impossible. Duodenal ulcers are usually single, circular areas of discrete ulceration resembling oral aphthous ulcers, usually with a creamy-yellow base. The surrounding duodenal mucosa may be normal, or may be erythematous with punctate haemorrhages due to duodenitis.

Gastric secretory tests have no place in the routine diagnosis or management of duodenal ulceration. The fasting plasma gastrin concentration should always be measured in patients with severe or ectopic ulceration, or in those with continuing ulceration after adequate surgery, to exclude the Zollinger–Ellison syndrome.

Chronic benign gastric ulcer

Definition. A benign gastric ulcer (GU) is usually a single circular or semi-circular discrete break in the gastric mucosa. Ulcers can occur anywhere in the stomach, but most develop on the lesser curvature at the junction between the acid-secreting mucosa and the mucosa of the antrum. Gastric ulcers may occur in the antrum: special care must be taken to exclude malignancy in antral ulcers. Pre-pyloric ulcers resemble DUs endoscopically and are probably best managed clinically on the lines indicated for duodenal ulcers. A benign gastric ulcer can vary in size from a few millimetres to several centimetres in diameter; it often penetrates deeply into the muscularis mucosae.

Aetiology
Acid secretion and duodenogastric reflux. The cause of benign GU is uncertain. The gastric mucosa is probably injured by the combination of acid secreted by the stomach and the reflux of duodenal contents into the stomach. The duodenal juice contains bile, lysolecithin, and pancreatic enzymes, all of which may damage the gastric mucosa. A number of studies have demonstrated that patients with gastric ulcer do tend to reflux their duodenal contents, a tendency that is aggravated by smoking cigarettes. Gastric emptying time in patients with GU tends to be prolonged and retention of contents predisposes to gastric ulceration.

Gastric ulcers do not develop unless there is a degree of intragastric acidity. Patients with severe gastritis due to free biliary reflux after antrectomy rarely develop benign gastric ulceration, presumably because they secrete a negligible amount of acid. Hitherto it had been considered that GU patients secrete a relatively low amount of gastric acid (Fig. 1). This hyposecretion may be due to a decrease in the parietal cell mass produced by chronic atrophic gastritis, or it may be an artefact due to neutralization of gastric acid by duodenogastric reflux of pancreatic bicarbonate. Another factor may be back-diffusion of acid through a gastric mucosa damaged by gastritis. As GU and gastritis are more prevalent in older patients, gastritis is likely to be aetiologically important in the aetiology of gastric ulcer. Gastritis is dealt with fully on page 12.70.

It is thought that one of the defences of the gastric mucosa is a small amount of bicarbonate secreted by the mucosa into the gastric mucus. This alkaline gradient may be an important factor for mucosal integrity and it may be deficient in patients with gastric ulceration.

Epidemiology. In the nineteenth century gastric ulceration was a disease of young women but it is now commoner in men, in older age groups, and in patients of low socio-economic class. It is less common than DU. Associations with other medical conditions are doubtful, but anti-inflammatory drugs may cause gastric ulceration.

Clinical picture and natural history. Benign gastric ulceration typically presents with epigastric pain which cannot be distinguished from pain due to other causes. Although exacerbations of discomfort after meals, unremitting pain, weight loss, and a long history are relatively common in this group of patients, a confident diagnosis cannot and must not be made on clinical evidence alone. Acute or occult gastrointestinal haemorrhage, or perforation, are the commonest complications.

Gastric ulceration is a recurrent chronic condition. The outcome seems to differ from that of DU with up to a half of the patients not developing recurrence of the ulcer.

Diagnosis. As in duodenal ulceration, neither clinical history nor physical examination provides evidence for a positive diagnosis. A barium meal examination, especially if double contrast, may detect even superficial ulceration (Fig. 4). However, the major advantage of upper gastrointestinal endoscopy is that it allows a tissue diagnosis to be made using both biopsy and brush cytology. As the important differential diagnosis is between early gastric cancer and a benign gastric ulcer, all patients with GU should be endoscoped, with multiple, targeted biopsies taken from the ulcer rim and base, followed by exfoliative brush cytology. The greater the number of biopsies, the greater the likelihood of picking up early intramucosal gastric carcinoma: the minimum number of biopsies is four, one from each quadrant of the crater. The importance of diagnosing early gastric cancer lies in its good prognosis after total gastrectomy.

Acute erosive ulceration

Multiple superficial ulcers may develop in the oesophagus, stomach, or duodenum of acutely stressed patients, particularly after major trauma, extensive burns, or during shock or hypoxia. In only one situation (*Cushing's ulceration* following head injury) is there a positive relationship between mucosal damage and high gastric acid secretion. Some acid secretion is apparently necessary for stress ulceration to develop, but the main damage appears to be due to hypoxia, or perhaps increased back-diffusion of gastric acid.

This type of ulceration, which must not be confused with chronic DU or GU, usually presents with haemorrhage some days after the initial insult. The patient is best investigated by endoscopy because

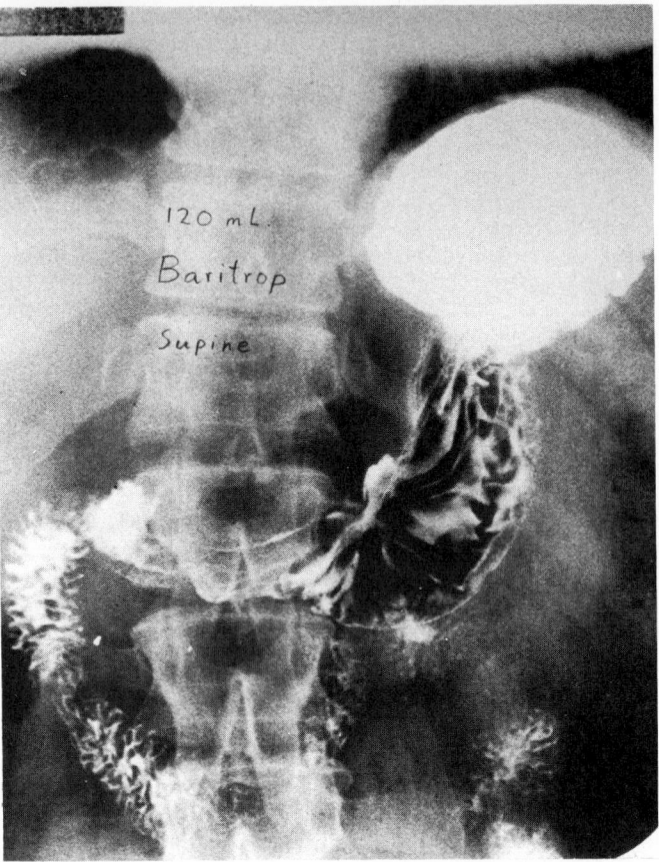

120 mL.
Baritrop
Supine

Fig. 4 Benign gastric ulcer demonstrated by air-contrast barium meal examination. Mucosal folds reach the rim of the ulcer crater.

the superficial ulceration is often not visible on conventional barium meal radiographs. The gastrointestinal haemorrhage may be aggravated by coagulopathies associated with the primary stressful event. Prophylactic high dose antacids given every hour, or H$_2$-receptor blockers can prevent this type of ulceration and haemorrhage. The available evidence has not established whether high doses of antacids (up to 200 ml per day) or histamine H$_2$-receptor antagonists are better in the prevention of haemorrhage from acute erosive ulceration of the upper alimentary tract. H$_2$-antagonists, such as cimetidine or ranitidine, are more convenient, and cimetidine should be given orally whenever feasible: the intravenous route should only be used when oral administration is definitely contra-indicated by other considerations. The dosage can be monitored by sampling the gastric secretions via an indwelling nasogastric tube: the pH of gastric juice should not be allowed to fall below 5.0. Treatment should begin at once, because it is the preventative effect of suppressing acid secretion that is important. In the presence of renal insufficiency the dose of cimetidine should be decreased, as the drug is mainly excreted by the kidney. Watch must be kept on the patient's mental state, because cimetidine occasionally causes coma in severely ill people.

Erosive ulcers can also develop in patients whose upper gastrointestinal mucosa is damaged by either non-steroidal anti-inflammatory drugs or alcohol. Indeed, these forms of stress ulceration are frequently used in experimental animal models and are usually prevented by pre-treatment with cimetidine, high dose antacid, or prostaglandin analogues.

The management of patients with established stress ulceration involves blood transfusion, correcting of clotting defects, and the use of cimetidine or antacids. Unfortunately the benefit from these drugs is smaller than when used for prophylactic treatment. Surgery is to be avoided if at all possible, because the diffuse nature of mucosal damage means that radical surgery would be needed to stop the bleeding.

Oesophagitis

Oesophagitis is dealt with fully on page 12.41, but it is mentioned here, because patients with peptic ulcer, and particularly those with duodenal ulcer, often complain of heartburn and regurgitation of acid. Inflammation of distal oesophageal mucosa is not infrequently seen at endoscopy. The presence of oesophagitis in a patient with duodenal ulceration does not generally call for any modification of the adopted plan of therapy. The oesophagitis may be expected to improve as the DU goes into remission, but advice regarding weight reduction, elevation of the head of the bed, and avoidance of large meals before going to bed may be needed, if oesophageal symptoms persist.

Non-ulcer dyspepsia

History of typical ulcer symptoms—epigastric pain, related to food and relieved by antacids—is not sufficient to make the diagnosis of GU or DU. Many patients have the typical symptoms, but no ulcer can be demonstrated radiologically or endoscopically, even if the investigations are done in the symptomatic phase. The duodenal cap may be completely normal to endoscopic inspection, or may show minor changes of duodenitis: biopsies will likewise be normal, or display mild inflammation.

The mechanism of pain in these patients is not clear. It is possible that the duodenal mucosa may be sensitive to acid or pepsin without frank ulceration, but this is speculative. In any case, short-term therapy with cimetidine has little effect on either symptoms or on endoscopic and biopsy appearances. Another explanation is that the pain originates not in the duodenum, but in the transverse colon reflexly contracting in response to meals, so that the condition is really a variant of the irritable colon syndrome. These hypotheses need to be further studied before any definite statements can be made. Meanwhile the treatment remains symptomatic and the physician may have to search empirically for a preparation that will relieve the patient's symptoms. It is not known how many patients with non-ulcer dyspepsia eventually develop frank duodenal ulceration.

Duodenitis

Duodenitis is an ill-defined condition, characterized at endoscopy by inflamed, haemorrhagic, and friable duodenal cap mucosa; duodenal biopsies show acute inflammatory changes. If erosions are present, the condition is called erosive duodenitis, although where erosions end and duodenal ulcers proper begin is somewhat difficult to define precisely. Erosive duodenitis may give rise to symptoms indistinguishable from those of duodenal ulcer and may be complicated by haemorrhage leading to haematemesis and/or melaena. Duodenitis is best regarded as forming one end of the spectrum of duodenal ulcer disease. Frank duodenal ulcers are often surrounded by areas of duodenitis and the latter may persist after the ulcer crater has healed.

There are few trials of treatment of duodenitis. Cimetidine 1 g daily in divided doses may relieve the symptoms and improve the endoscopic and histopathological appearances. Other patients may respond to antacids, or to carbenoxolone sodium. In some patients environmental factors, such as heavy drinking, can be identified and attention to those will lead to improvement of the duodenal inflammation.

The Zollinger–Ellison syndrome

Definition. In 1955 Zollinger and Ellison described a syndrome encompassing severe peptic ulceration, hypersecretion of gastric acid, and an islet cell tumour of the pancreas (see page 12.60).

Pathophysiology. The islet cell tumours in these patients have been shown to secrete gastrin. Gastrinomas are usually found in the body or tail of the pancreas; the tumours may be multiple and they can be both histologically and clinically malignant. The gastrin secreted by the tumours is usually the G17 form (little gastrin), but smaller and larger molecular species have also been reported. Prolonged high plasma gastrin concentrations cause an increase of the parietal cell mass with consequent high basal and maximal acid secretion. Occasionally a pancreatic gastrinoma is associated with hyperparathyroidism in Wermer's syndrome (multiple endocrine adenomatosis I) (see page 12.53).

The majority of patients (95 per cent) have aggressive peptic ulceration. But the second major symptom is diarrhoea, present in 40 per cent of the patients, although diarrhoea may be the only symptom. Peptic ulcers may occur in the duodenum, stomach, or oesophagus, but they tend to be larger, to penetrate deeper, and to be multiple. Ulceration often extends beyond the first part of the duodenum. Haemorrhage or perforation occurring soon after gastric surgery is characteristic of the Zollinger–Ellison syndrome.

The diarrhoea is not due to hypergastrinaemia itself, for diarrhoea does not occur in patients with pernicious anaemia who often have high plasma gastrin concentrations. The diarrhoea is probably due to low intestinal pH produced by sustained acid hypersecretion. The low pH denatures pancreatic enzymes causing steatorrhoea and precipitates bile salts, causing bile salt malabsorption which in turn provokes water secretion by the colon.

Diagnosis. The diagnosis of the Zollinger–Ellison syndrome initially depends on the detection of an elevated concentration of gastrin in fasting plasma in the presence of acid in the stomach. As gastrin is measured by radioimmunoassay using antibodies with varying affinity to the different molecular species of gastrin, there is variation between the normal ranges of different laboratories. Most laboratories would be suspicious of a fasting plasma gastrin level of more than 50–100 pmol/l.

Three conditions can cause hypergastrinaemia with increased acid output and aggressive peptic ulceration, but without the presence of a gastrinoma. Firstly, hyperplasia of the gastrin secreting cells of the antrum, called confusingly the Zollinger–Ellison syndrome type I (the classical condition is type II), which may represent the upper part of the normal range of gastrin and acid secretion. Secondly, a cuff of antral mucosa inadvertently retained at the end of the oversewn blind loop of a Polya partial gastrectomy results in the excluded antrum being bathed in alkaline duodenal and pancreatic secretion, thereby causing profound gastrin release. Thirdly, for a short time after massive small intestinal resection plasma gastrin levels rise markedly with consequent gastric hypersecretion: this is possibly due to transient deficiency of an inhibitory gastrointestinal polypeptide.

Excessive histamine release is found in rare patients with either systemic mastocytosis, or mast cell leukaemia (see Section 19. Thus continuous histamine stimulation of the stomach may cause profound gastric hypersecretion, with normal or low plasma gastrin concentrations. High plasma gastrin concentrations are usually found in patients with pernicious anaemia but they are anacidic.

A number of criteria can be used to define the hypersecretion of acid in the Zollinger–Ellison syndrome: (a) basal acid output of more than 15 mmol/hour or basal acidity greater than 100 mmol/l (pH less than 1.0); (b) basal acid secretion at the level of 60 per cent or more, of maximal or peak acid output. Measurements of acid output and pH of gastric juice are simple and within the capabilities of most hospitals, but unfortunately they cannot be relied on to establish the diagnosis of the syndrome.

The most reliable confirmatory investigation is the secretin test. Two units GIH secretin per kg are given by slow intravenous injection with the patient fasting. In normal individuals the plasma gastrin concentration drops, but in patients with the Zollinger–Ellison syndrome there is an immediate rise to more than 50 per cent above basal values. Patients with type I Zollinger–Ellison syndrome have a normal response to secretin, but those with an

excluded antrum may still be confused with type II Zollinger–Ellison syndrome. As the retained cuff of antrum will concentrate technetium in its gastric mucosa, it can sometimes be identified using a gamma camera, particularly if the patient has not received oral perchlorate before the scan.

The pancreatic tumour may be small and difficult to identify even at laparotomy. However, selective arteriography, ultrasound, or an abdominal CT scan may help to localize the tumour before surgery, but none of these techniques is completely reliable. Percutaneous trans-hepatic sampling of splenic vein gastrin concentration may also aid pre-operative tumour localization.

Treatment. The management of the classical Zollinger–Ellison syndrome is controversial. Until the mid-1970s the only possible treatment was a total gastrectomy, thus removing the target organ for gastrin. This some surgeons combined with exploration and perhaps resection of the pancreas. As many patients already had previous failed gastric operations, were malnourished and catabolic, the mortality and morbidity of surgery were high.

Two advances have altered the outlook for these patients: the availability of gastrin radioimmunoassay and the histamine H₂-receptor antagonists. The former has made early diagnosis possible, and the latter have allowed pharmacological blockade of the hypergastrinaemia.

As cimetidine and ranitidine are competitive H₂-antagonists, in the face of uncontrolled gastrin release large amounts (up to six times the normal dose) of the antagonist may be needed to control acid secretion. The optimal dose can be determined by measuring intragastric pH during the day after breakfast and lunch: successful treatment should keep the gastric contents between pH 2.0 and 7.0. If an H₂-antagonist alone is ineffective, the anticholinergic propantheline, 30 mg four times a day, can be added.

The role of surgery is now controversial. Some recommend a laparotomy to see whether the tumour is resectable; a highly selective vagotomy done at the same time may moderate later acid secretion without extra hazard to the patient. Post-surgery plasma gastrin concentrations provide a convenient marker for tumour activity. Others argue that pancreatic surgery is hazardous, that the outlook is good with maintenance cimetidine or ranitidine, and that surgery should be reserved for those in whom medical treatment fails. Inoperable and progressive malignancy may respond to streptozotocin.

Complications of peptic ulcer

Perforation. Perforation is a serious complication of peptic ulcer: it is more common in men and more frequent in duodenal than in gastric ulcers. A proportion of patients—estimated at approximately 10 per cent in various studies—perforate without any antecedent history of dyspepsia. The most common site of perforation is the anterior wall of the duodenal cap in DU or the lesser curve of the stomach in GU. Rarely, ulcers may perforate into the biliary tract, filling it with air.

The diagnosis is not difficult in most cases. The history is of a sudden onset of very severe abdominal pain. The abdomen is rigid, there is rebound tenderness, the abdominal respiratory movements and bowel sounds are absent, and the liver dullness to percussion is diminished. A plain abdominal radiograph may show free air between the upper border of the liver and the diaphragm, but absence of this sign does not exclude perforation. Leucocytosis usually appears promptly. The symptoms are so stereotyped that the condition is eminently suitable for accurate computer diagnosis. Difficulties in diagnosis arise in the elderly, or in the mentally ill, in patients hospitalized for chronic illness, or in those on high doses of steroids. In this group of patient 'silent' or painless perforations may occur; unexplained shock is the most common clinical finding.

Treatment of perforation is surgical, medical management being reserved only for moribund patients, or for those who are rendered inoperable by severe coexisting disease. Medical management consists of continuous nasogastric suction, treatment of shock, electrolyte and fluid replacement, and antibiotic therapy with ampicillin, gentamicin, and metronidazole. Failure of the perforated ulcer to heal leads to surgery.

Oversewing a perforated ulcer provides first-aid treatment, but no long-term cure. To avoid recurrent ulceration the patient may need either maintenance treatment with an H_2-antagonist or an elective, definitive re-operation.

Haemorrhage. Haemorrhage from the stomach and duodenum is the commonest life-threatening gastrointestinal emergency. The main causes of upper gastrointestinal haemorrhage are peptic ulceration or variceal bleeding secondary to chronic liver disease; both are conditions with a highly variable prevalence throughout the world. Thus variceal haemorrhage is a relatively rare cause of upper gastrointestinal haemorrhage in the United Kingdom, although the incidence is increasing. Duodenal ulcer, gastric ulcer, erosive gastritis, and the Mallory–Weiss syndrome are all more common, in descending order of frequency (see page 12.15).

Symptoms and signs. Most patients will have a history of dyspepsia, although haemorrhage may be the first evidence of peptic ulceration, particularly if the patient is physically stressed by trauma or illness.

The first symptom of upper gastrointestinal haemorrhage is often an episode of sudden collapse, with weakness, sweating, and palpitations. The patient may vomit blood or may notice active bowel sounds due to stimulation of gastrointestinal motility by the blood. This is often followed by lower abdominal colic, as in acute gastroenteritis, finally relieved by defaecation of normal stools and later melaena. The melaena is usually dark red or black, due to partial digestion of the blood, but fresh blood may be passed per rectum even if the haemorrhage is in the stomach or duodenum. The bleeding usually stops spontaneously and the patient gradually recovers to be left with symptoms of anaemia.

Management. Any patient with melaena or haematemesis within the preceding 48 hours should be admitted to hospital because of the risk of further haemorrhage. Repeated bleeding rarely occurs more than 48 hours after the first episode. There are three phases in the management of a patient with an acute upper gastrointestinal haemorrhage: resuscitation, exact diagnosis, and treatment.

Resuscitation. As soon as an upper gastrointestinal haemorrhage is diagnosed a cannula should be placed in a peripheral vein: even without evidence of further bleeding this cannula should be kept patent for 48 hours.

A patient should be transfused for one of two reasons: shock, or anaemia. Before cross-matched blood is available, the patient may need resuscitation with plasma or a colloid volume expander. The precision and safety of rapid blood transfusion can be much improved by the use of a central venous-pressure (CVP) line, particularly in elderly patients, or in those with cardiac or renal disease. Patients with life-threatening haemorrhages tend to arrive in hospital with a relatively normal haemoglobin concentration; this is because brisk haemorrhage causes urgent hospital admission before there is time for haemodilution of the depleted red cell mass. If the patient is anaemic, yet has a CVP of 0 cm or higher, a potent diuretic such as frusemide should be given intravenously to compensate for the volume of rapidly transfused packed red blood cells. It is advisable to treat anaemia by transfusion so that the patient's haemoglobin is at least 10 g/dl; this leaves the patient in a better condition should there be further bleeding. As a general rule, one pack of blood is needed to raise an adult's haemoglobin by 1 g/dl. It is sometimes wise to measure the patient's serum B_{12}, red cell folate, and ferritin prior to transfusion, in case there is an associated nutritional anaemia.

Two units of cross-matched blood should be kept available for 48 hours after the haemorrhage stops to ensure immediate treatment of rebleeding. The amount of blood cross-matched at the time of admission depends on availability, but ideal standards are set out in Table 1.

Table 1 Blood cross-matching requirements on admission for acute haemorrhage from peptic ulcer, based on clinical state and initial haemoglobin levels

Clinical condition	Admission haemoglobin	Blood requirements (500 ml packs)			
		For resuscitation	For anaemia	For rebleeding	Total
Not shocked	> 10.0 g/dl	0	0	+2	2
Shocked	> 10.0 g/dl	4	0	+2	6
Not shocked	* X g/dl	0	+ 10−X*	+2	10−X+2
Shocked	* Y g/dl	4	+ 10−Y*	+2	10−Y+6

* X and Y represent values of Hb < 10 g/dl

Diagnosis of the source of bleeding. Either endoscopy or a barium meal X-ray can be used to make an exact diagnosis of the origin of bleeding; both can be conveniently done approximately 12 to 24 hours after hospital admission. Emergency endoscopy is expensive in terms of hospital resources and possible damage to endoscopes by blockage of suction or biopsy channels with blood. In the presence of active haemorrhage it is difficult to establish the diagnosis anyway. Prospective studies have shown that emergency endoscopy does not influence the clinical outcome of haemorrhage from DU or GU. More urgent investigation is only needed if liver disease is suspected, particularly if there is splenomegaly thus making portal hypertension likely, or if the patient is exsanguinating. Urgent endoscopy in the operating theatre after endotracheal intubation may be useful, provided that it does not delay surgery. If a patient presents with melaena alone, introduction of a nasogastric tube at the time of admission may show blood in the stomach, thereby saving later unnecessary investigation of the lower bowel.

Endoscopy has two major advantages: firstly it provides the highest rate of correct diagnosis; secondly it can detect ongoing haemorrhage, or predict the likelihood of a rebleed. Rebleeding is much more likely if the endoscopist reports the presence of a protruding blood vessel, or a blood clot in the base of the ulcer. The disadvantages are that it needs an experienced endoscopist, that brisk bleeding may obscure the site of haemorrhage, and that being an invasive procedure there is a limited, but definite, morbidity and mortality.

A barium meal examination, particularly if the air-contrast technique is used, can identify lesions, but it can neither identify the site of active bleeding nor can it differentiate between active DU and old scars of the duodenum. However, it might be the best available test for the very young adult who will not swallow an endoscope, or for the patient with severe cardiovascular or respiratory disease, or because of limited resources.

Occasionally selective coeliac arteriography may be useful if results of endoscopy are inconclusive. A catheter is passed via the femoral artery and active bleeding can be identified as a pool of extravasated contrast medium. Unless there is an arteriovenous malformation, the technique is only useful when there is brisk active bleeding. It has been argued that a precise diagnosis makes little difference to the outcome of gastrointestinal haemorrhage in most patients, but this attitude is probably too negative.

Detection of rebleeding is easy if haematemesis or melaena recur. A drop in haemoglobin, sudden rise in the pulse rate, hypotension, peripheral vasoconstriction and sweating, a decrease in CVP, or the reappearance of fresh blood on aspiration through a nasogastric tube, all point to recurrence of haemorrhage.

Treatment. The major objective in the management of an upper gastrointestinal haemorrhage is to ensure the patient's survival. Figure 5 shows that survival has improved in recent years, but most studies still show that approximately 10 per cent of patients die. However, the average age of patients presenting with haemorrhage has gradually increased, so that in Europe approximately half are 60 years or older.

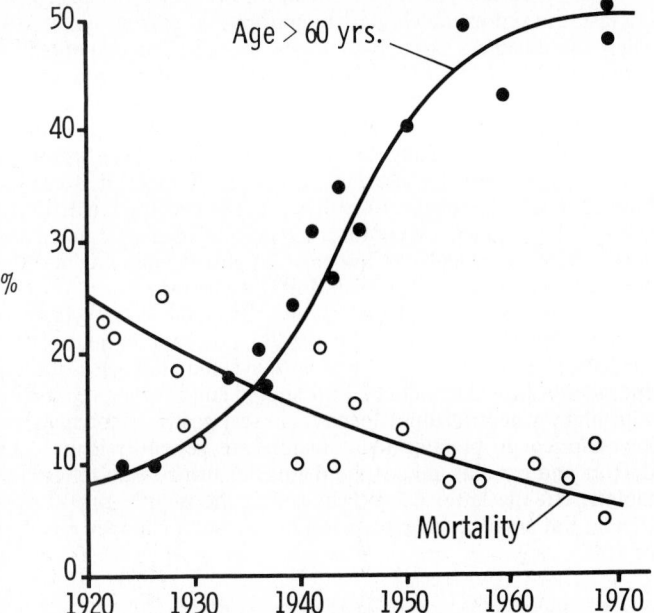

Fig. 5 Percentage of patients over 60 years and mortality rate from gastro-intestinal bleeding in major European studies 1920–70. (Modified from Allan, R. and Dykes, P. (1976). *Q. Jl Med.* **45**, 534, by permission.)

Analysis of causes of death suggests that, although occasional patients do die from exsanguination, the majority die from medical, rather than from surgical post-operative complications, or else the gastrointestinal haemorrhage has been a final insult in an inevitable decline of health.

The death rate from exsanguination should be minimized by appropriate resuscitation, but post-operative deaths pose more of a problem. Do the complications arise because the patients are in poor condition when presented for surgery, and would earlier surgery decrease these complications? Or would early surgery result in unnecessary operations, thereby exposing more patients to the hazards of post-operative recovery? Available data do not provide a clear answer to this problem.

The exact criteria for recommending emergency surgery are difficult to define. They include: (*a*) a suitably experienced surgeon; (*b*) continuing severe haemorrhage but the use of modern infusion techniques should mean that the majority of patients are fully resuscitated prior to surgery; and (*c*) a combination of the high risk factors that makes major rehaemorrhage likely. Elderly patients, those with gastric ulceration, and those who have suffered a brisk initial bleed, are all more liable to recurrent haemorrhage. Endo-scopy may further identify those who have high risk of rebleeding. These high risk patients need urgent and careful resuscitation with early medical and surgical co-operation. This co-operation might usefully be carried through to the post-operative period, allowing physicians rather than surgeons to manage the medical problems.

There are no medical treatments that decrease the incidence or severity of rebleeding. H₂-receptor antagonists do not help, indeed their use may encourage complacency. The underlying causes of haemorrhage should receive standard medical treatment, aiming to speed ulcer healing. Most patients will require oral iron supplements but should be warned that they will notice a grey discoloura-tion of their stools. Ferrous sulphate 200 mg three times daily is convenient and inexpensive.

Pyloric stenosis. Pyloric stenosis due to long-standing peptic ulcer disease must be differentiated from infantile and adult hyper-trophic pyloric stenosis. More than 80 per cent of cases are due to DU. The diagnosis is suggested by a long history of peptic ulcer pain, with a more recent onset of vomiting. The vomitus contains food and articles of diet consumed the previous day may sometimes be identified. Weight loss is present in most patients. Visible gastric peristalsis and a succussion splash are the physical signs, but they may be absent, especially if the patient is examined soon after vomiting. Dehydration, pre-renal uraemia, or metabolic alkalosis may complicate the picture.

The diagnosis can be made on the history and clinical examina-tion. A barium meal examination will show a dilated, often atonic stomach; food debris may be present in the lumen. Gastric empty-ing of barium will be grossly prolonged. Endoscopy is helpful, but the stomach must be first emptied and washed out.

Gastric outlet obstruction due to pyloric stenosis caused by chronic DU must be differentiated from malignant tumours, the commonest being antral carcinoma. Cancer of the head of the pancreas or lymphoma can also interfere with gastric emptying. Other causes are benign tumours (adenomatous polyp or annular pancreas), adult hypertrophic pyloric stenosis, and occasionally, a pyloric or duodenal diaphragm. The treatment is surgical, after correction of water, electrolyte, and metabolic abnormalities.

Gastric outlet obstruction can occur during exacerbations of DU and is probably due to oedema surrounding the duodenal or pyloric channel ulcers. The oedema and the obstruction are relieved by medical treatment and pyloric stenosis should not be diagnosed in these patients.

Medical treatment of DU and GU

General strategy. In common with many other alimentary disor-ders, many patients with DU and GU are ideally best managed jointly by a physician and a surgeon. Apart from emergencies such as haemorrhage or perforation, complications such as pyloric sten-osis or suspicion of malignancy, unusual circumstances such as patients residing in remote areas with established chronic peptic ulcer disease presenting for definitive treatment, all ulcer patients should be treated medically in the first instance. The exceptions are those in whom it is certain that previous adequate medical therapy (adequate in terms of time, drugs used, and dosage) has been given and failed.

Evaluation of the results of ulcer therapy. The aims of treatment in duodenal and gastric ulcer are the relief of symptoms, the healing of the ulcer crater, the prevention of recurrence, and the prevention of complications. Only the first two of these aims can be achieved with a substantial measure of success by medical therapy; preven-tion of recurrence is only partly successful and, as far as is known, depends on continuous treatment. It is not clear whether long-term therapy influences the incidence of ulcer complications.

Symptomatic relief, although of paramount importance to the patient, is very difficult to measure accurately because of the sub-jective nature of the symptoms: measurements of antacid consump-tion are also unreliable. It is now generally accepted that evaluation of ulcer-healing drugs must be monitored by fibreoptic endoscopy and that the end-point of treatment must be the complete healing of the ulcer crater. This is because changes of ulcer size are difficult, or impossible to measure accurately endoscopically and also because a partly healed ulcer is a doubtful therapeutic benefit. Relapses of gastric ulcer must also be endoscopically confirmed. The difficulties of accurately evaluating effects of treatment on ulcers are com-pounded by the observation that correlation between remissions and relapse of symptoms, and the healing or recurrence of the ulcer crater is poor, especially in gastric ulcer. In both duodenal and gastric ulceration typical symptoms may be present in the absence of the ulcer crater. On the other hand, close surveillance of patients with duodenal ulcer studied in maintenance trials of cimetidine has shown that approximately 30 per cent of recurrences are asymptomatic.

Additionally, the clinical attributes of both gastric and duodenal ulcer are subject to considerable variation by ill-defined factors such as race, geographical location, diet, and the tendency of the disease to alter, quite rapidly, with passage of time. It is therefore unwise to accept uncritically results from clinical trials, important as these results are for the scientific basis of ulcer therapy. Not only may data collected in one country be not applicable to another, but it must also be remembered that clinical trials are conducted on relatively small, highly selected populations of patients and the results may not apply to everyone. The results of trials are essential if effects of treatment are to be scientifically measured, but circumstances will often modify the management of individual patients.

Diet. Diet looms very large in the consciousness of most patients with peptic ulcer. Avoidance of fatty, fried, spicy, and rich meals is almost universal, and it is sometimes difficult to be certain how much of this is due to powerful folklore, and how much to some undefined pathophysiological mechanism. The factor that has been convincingly shown to relate directly to peptic ulcer pain is low intragastric or intraduodenal pH: neutralization of acid, or its removal by vomiting or nasogastric suction leads in most cases to rapid relief of ulcer dyspepsia. Studies exploring the possibility of other factors being involved in the production of peptic ulcer pain, e.g. gastroduodenal motility, have not been convincing. It is therefore not clear how certain foods trigger ulcer dyspepsia, and it is quite possible that in a proportion of patients the discomfort may originate from areas other than the ulcer crater, such as the colon.

Be this as it may, the patient with a peptic ulcer will have almost invariably excluded from the diet those foods that produce pain and distention. Although many elaborate dietary regimens have been advocated in the management of peptic ulcer disease in the past, there is no evidence that any of them affects the natural history of the disease. Detailed dietary advice is therefore unnecessary and can be summed up as: avoid what upsets you and eat little and often. There is some scientific backing for advising frequent, small meals, because food is a powerful buffer and it has been shown that intragastric pH rises after meals. Only highly obsessive individuals need detailed dietary guidance, and that for their own peace of mind, rather than for any good it does to their ulcers.

Smoking and alcohol. There is now such ample evidence of the deleterious effects of smoking on various body systems, that advice to give up should be given to everyone who smokes, regardless of the pathology. Having said that, there is little evidence to show that giving up smoking has an effect on the healing rate of duodenal ulcer, although faster healing rates of gastric ulcer have been reported in those patients who gave up smoking, compared with those who continued to smoke.

Similar considerations apply to alcohol consumption. Excessive drinking must be discouraged to avoid alcoholic disease, but total abstinence is not a condition required for ulcer healing.

Rest, sedation, and psychotrophic drugs. Rest and removal from stressful circumstances at home, or in the workplace will act as a non-specific adjuvant to the treatment of peptic ulcer. Admission to hospital, however, is indicated only in extreme cases and is hardly ever necessary: indeed, it is contra-indicated in the vast majority. Sedation has no part to play in the management of either gastric or duodenal ulcer. Indiscriminate prescribing of anxiolytics, such as diazepam, to patients with duodenal ulcer is not good practice. Discussion of the particular life circumstances and lifestyle with the patient can often be more helpful and more productive of introducing changes—often quite small adjustment is all that is needed—to achieve better symptom control. There is evidence from a small number of controlled trials that tricyclic antidepressants accelerate the healing of duodenal ulcers in the short-term, when compared with a placebo. At the time of writing there is insufficient evidence to recommend this class of drugs as an established therapy for duodenal ulcer: depression co-existing with peptic ulcer disease should be treated on its own merits. How tricyclic antidepressants act in peptic ulcer disease is unknown.

Antacids. Antacids are the backbone of symptomatic treatment for both gastric and duodenal ulcer and are very effective in providing fast, but unfortunately only temporary, relief from symptoms. Their effectiveness is testified to by the very large number of commercial antacid preparations available over the counter in chemist's shops. Rapid relief of pain from peptic ulcer by antacids suggests that the mechanism of action is due to neutralization of intraluminal acid, bringing the pH up to the level at which stimulation of pain-mediating afferent nerves in the ulcer area ceases. Unfortunately the relief is short-lived, partly because the action of antacids is curtailed by continued secretion of gastric acid, and partly because antacids are lost through gastric emptying into the jejunum, where they are useless for ulcer therapy.

The numerous antacid preparations available differ widely in physical properties, flavour, palatability, cost, and in neutralizing capacity (Fig. 6); they also tend to leave the stomach at different rates. Rational antacid therapy should employ the preparation with highest neutralizing capacity, slowest gastric emptying, and lowest price: in practice these factors are generally ignored by doctors and patients alike. Liquid antacids bring faster relief than tablets, but the latter can be chewed in the mouth, providing a steady, but small, trickle of base into the stomach over a period of time.

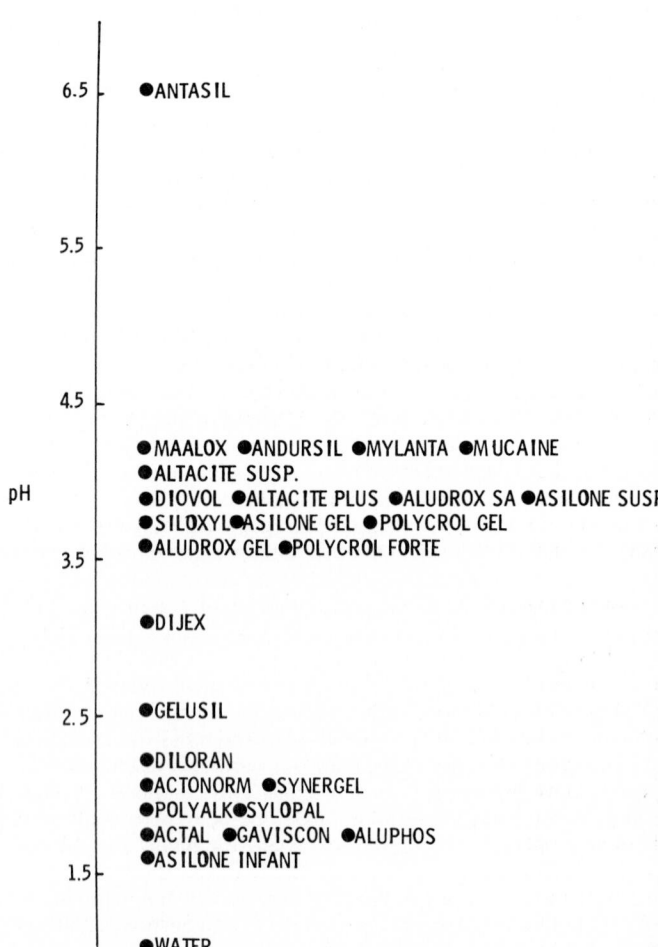

Fig. 6 *In vitro* acid neutralizing activity of some proprietary antacids available in 1980 in the United Kingdom showing final pH after adding 2.5 ml antacid to 50 ml 0.1 mmol HCl (90 min at 37 °C). (By permission of W. Brampton, and R. E. Pounder).

Antacids are used for mainly symptomatic relief of peptic ulcer symptoms. There is some evidence that very large doses (over 200 ml or 1000 mmol H^+ neutralizing capacity) will significantly accelerate the healing of duodenal ulcer in the short-term: there are no similar data concerning gastric ulcer and no evidence that prolonged medication with antacids affects the natural history of either type of peptic ulceration. High-dose antacids regimens are inconvenient for the patient, associated with diarrhoea or constipation, and in general have not found acceptance in the day-to-day management of peptic ulcer as healing therapy.

In general antacids are very safe to use. The commonest unwanted effect is diarrhoea produced by Mg-based antacids or constipation produced by Al-based antacids: this is best treated by reducing the dose, switching to another antacid, or giving a 'balanced' mixture of Al and Mg salts, although the balance is difficult to achieve. This aspect of unwanted action of antacids can be utilized to good effect, constipated patients with a peptic ulcer being given Mg-based preparations, and vice-versa.

$NaHCO_3$ is an efficient antacid, but watch has to be kept on its high sodium content: it is of course contra-indicated for patients with cardiac or renal insufficiency. All antacids, if consumed in large amounts, are theoretically capable of producing a clinically significant metabolic alkalosis, but in practice this is very rare. The *milk-alkali syndrome* is a condition produced by a high calcium and base intake and is characterized by hypercalcaemia, alkalosis, and renal failure. Although widely known, the syndrome is uncommon.

Sustained hypersecretion of acid—the so-called acid rebound—may be shown to be present after administration of calcium carbonate. It is uncertain whether acid rebound is clinically important in the treatment of peptic ulcer. Aluminium-containing antacids (but not aluminium phosphate) can theoretically lead to phosphate depletion by the formation of insoluble phosphate salts, but in practice this is very rare. Absorption of aluminium does occur from the gastrointestinal tract after giving aluminium hydroxide.

By the time the doctor is consulted, the patient will have usually used antacids bought over the counter. Advice is needed regarding the best kind of antacid to use and the frequency and timing of medication. There is no point in taking antacids during remissions of either gastric, or of duodenal ulcer, as they have not been shown to decrease the frequency of relapses. During exacerbations antacids should be used liberally, until the discomfort of the ulcer is relieved. Patients usually take antacids by swallowing 10 ml after meals. Both the dose and timing are wrong. The dose is too small, and on average 30 ml of a liquid antacid preparation will be needed to neutralize the gastric contents. After meals the intragastric pH rises as the acid is buffered by the food. The correct way is therefore to cover the period one to two hours after food and until the next meal with antacids, using additional doses every two hours if discomfort is not relieved. Up to seven 30 ml doses of a patent antacid (Fig. 6) may be needed in each 24 hours.

Anticholinergics. Gastric acid secretion is stimulated, at least in part, via a cholinergic pathway, mainly mediated by the efferent vagal fibres. Interruption of the vagal pathway by surgical vagotomy leads to healing of duodenal ulcer. In theory, anticholinergic drugs also block the cholinergic pathway and should have beneficial effects on the ulcer: in practice this class of compounds has been disappointing. The size of the dose is severely limited by the occurrence of unwanted effects involving other cholinergically mediated functions such as ocular accommodation, salivary secretion, and bladder emptying in men. Blurred vision, dry mouth, and difficulty in micturition generally prevent the administration of effective doses of anticholinergics. As patients vary greatly in their tolerance of anticholinergic therapy, the dose should be determined for each patient individually. Ideally, the dose should be gradually increased until intolerable side-effects occur and then decreased slightly, but this is a time-consuming procedure and few physicians, or for that matter patients, are prepared to do it.

There is no good evidence that anticholinergics are useful in the

short or long-term healing of either gastric or duodenal ulcer. Various workers have advocated administration of anticholinergics together with other drugs, such as antacids, where slowing of gastric emptying might increase the length of time during which the antacid is available for neutralization of acid, but systematic data are scanty. Similarly, administration of anticholinergics together with histamine H_2-receptor antagonists has been advocated by some workers, whilst others could not demonstrate the existence of any synergistic effect between them. Prolonged duration of action of some anticholinergic compounds might make them suitable for nocturnal dosage, when the side-effects should be masked by sleep, but again systematic data are not available. More recently, claims have been made for a new anticholinergic drug (pirenzepine) which, by virtue of its antimuscarinic activity, is said to be more selective in blocking cholinergic receptors on or near gastric parietal cells. Early results are encouraging but more evidence, unavailable at the time of writing, is needed before pirenzepine can be properly compared with anticholinergics such as propantheline bromide, poldine methylsulphate, atropine, or other ulcer-healing drugs.

In practice the place of anticholinergics in the management of peptic ulcer disease is uncertain. Anticholinergics may be given in addition to antacids, when the control of symptoms with the latter is incomplete, but they should not be regarded as a therapy producing ulcer healing. Anticholinergics are contra-indicated in patients with glaucoma. They also probably should not be used in patients with heartburn because, by lowering oesophageal sphincter pressure, they might make this condition worse.

Bismuth. Bismuth has been used for a long time to give relief from symptoms of peptic ulcer. Administration of bismuth salts carries an appreciable risk of neurotoxicity and they have no place in the treatment of peptic ulcer. Complexed bismuth however, such as tri-potassium di-citrato bismuthate, seems safe. This compound has been shown in a number of controlled short-term trials to accelerate significantly the healing of gastric or duodenal ulcer, when compared with placebo medication. The rate of healing over four to six weeks of outpatient therapy is approximately 80–90 per cent and comparable to the healing rates achieved with H_2-receptor blocking drugs (Tables 2 and 3). Results of long-term therapy with bismuth have not been explored: in its present form complexed bismuth is not suitable for maintenance therapy because of its strong ammoniacal odour. The way in which complexed bismuth speeds up healing of peptic ulcers is unclear. It is claimed that the drug forms a complex with exudative and mucus proteins in the base of the ulcer crater, providing protection from the actions of acid and pepsin, thus allowing the ulcer to heal. This idea needs further experimental evidence before it is accepted.

Table 2 Results of short-term double-blind trials in DU. Diagnosis and healing of ulcer confirmed endoscopically in all patients, who had unlimited access to antacids

Drug	Daily dosage	Duration of treatment in weeks	Number of patients (studies)	Percentage of ulcers healed on	
				Active treatment	Placebo
TDB*	5 ml × 4	4–6	251 (7)	82	29
Carbenoxolone†	1 capsule × 4	6–12	336 (6)	68	30
Cimetidine‡	0.8–2 g	4–6	924 (13)	76	36

* Tripotassium dicitrato bismuthate
† In the positioned-release capsule formulation containing 50 mg carbenoxolone solution
‡ In 7 out of 13 studies the dose was 1 g/day, one only used 2 g/day

Complexed bismuth has the great advantage of apparent safety and cheapness and deserves further evaluation in controlled trials,

Table 3   Results of short-term double-blind trials in GU. Conditions as in Table 2

Drug	Daily dosage	Duration of treatment in weeks	Number of patients (studies)	Percentage of ulcers healed		
				studied treatment	control treatment	
TDB*	5 ml × 4	4	49 (2)	90	25	placebo
Carbenoxolone†	300 mg for 1 week, then 150 mg	4–5	176 (3)	50	36	placebo
Carbenoxolone†		6	54 (1)‡	52	78	cimetidine
Cimetidine	0.8–1g	4–6	172 (4)	75	38	placebo

* Tripotassium dicitrato bismuthate
† In the 50 mg tablet formulation
‡ Results of one study show no significant difference from control treatment

so that its usefulness as a healing agent can be firmly assessed. It provides a useful and inexpensive alternative to other ulcer-healing drugs.

Carbenoxolone sodium. Carbenoxolone sodium is a synthetic derivative of glycyrrhizinic acid, which is a naturally occurring constituent of liquorice. Liquorice root has been traditionally used for the treatment of dyspepsia.

The mechanism of action of carbenoxolone sodium is unclear. The drug is apparently rapidly absorbed from the stomach and excreted by the liver after conjugation with glucuronic acid. There is some experimental evidence to suggest that carbenoxolone prolongs the life-span of gastric mucosal cells and that it can alter the chemical properties of mucus, but how these observations relate to ulcer healing is not certain. Nor is it certain whether the drug acts locally or systemically. Thus the two formulations of carbenoxolone sodium as tablets (Biogastrone), for the treatment of gastric ulcer, and as the so-called positioned-release capsules, that are claimed to release the drug directly into the duodenal cap (Duogastrone), are not based on sound experimental evidence.

Data collected from endoscopically controlled trials suggest that carbenoxolone sodium is useful in accelerating the healing rate of either gastric or duodenal ulcer. The effect in duodenal ulcer is probably comparable to cimetidine results, but the treatment has to be given for longer (12 weeks) and symptomatic relief is slower. Healing of chronic benign gastric ulcer is probably faster during carbenoxolone therapy than on placebo (Tables 2 and 3). There are no controlled data available relating to long-term therapy with carbenoxolone in either gastric, or duodenal ulcer.

The main limitation of carbenoxolone therapy are the unwanted effects of this drug, which has aldosterone-like activity. Sodium and water retention, hypertension, and hypokalaemia have all been reported and are potentially dangerous, especially in the elderly or in those with cardiorespiratory or renal insufficiency. These effects make the close supervision of patients treated with carbenoxolone sodium very important. Ideally, weekly measurement of weight and blood pressure should be done and plasma electrolytes should be checked every two weeks. Side-effects of carbenoxolone therapy can be treated by decreasing the dose of the drug, or by giving thiazide diuretics, but oral potassium supplements must also then be prescribed, as both drugs increase renal potassium excretion. Aldosterone antagonists such as spironolactone also prevent the appearance of unwanted effects of carbenoxolone, but the healing effect (on gastric ulcer) is concomitantly abolished.

Attempts have been made to get over toxicity of carbenoxolone sodium by synthesis of analogues and by producing a preparation of deglycyrrhizinated liquorice, i.e. liquorice from which the precursor of carbenoxolone, glycyrrhizinic acid, had been removed. None of these preparations have so far been shown to be therapeutically active.

At present, carbenoxolone sodium has a limited place in short-term therapy of peptic ulcer. Similarly to bismuth, it can be given to patients who cannot tolerate histamine H_2-receptor antagonists, or whose ulcers have not healed on the latter. How many will heal after thus changing the treatment is not clear, as no adequate controlled observations have been published so far.

Histamine H_2-receptor antagonists. Histamine, together with an enzyme system that controls its synthesis and degradation, is abundantly present in the human gastric mucosa and is a powerful stimulant of gastric acid and pepsin secretion. It is as yet unsettled whether histamine forms the final common pathway for acetylcholine (released by the efferent vagal nerve endings) and gastrin (released by the antral G cells) in the stimulation of acid output, or whether separate receptors for the three substances directly mediating acid output exist on, or near the parietal cell. Experimental observations indicate that there is a close inter-relationship between the three secretory stimulants, and that the inhibition of one will markedly decrease the effects of the others. Antagonism of the secretory effects of histamine powerfully inhibits gastric secretion produced by hormonal or neurogenic stimulation.

Histamine H_2-receptor antagonists are a new class of antihistaminic drugs, whose main pharmacological action in the body is the inhibition of gastric acid secretion. The effects of histamine on various body systems are apparently mediated through two populations of receptors, termed H_1 and H_2 histamine receptors. The effects of histamine on smooth muscle of the gut, the bronchial tree, and the arterial vasculature are mediated via the H_1-receptors and are blocked by the classical antihistaminic drugs such as chlorpheniramine maleate. H_1-receptor antagonists do not inhibit the powerful stimulatory effects of histamine on gastric acid and pepsin output. This observation was well known for many years, when histamine was used as a gastric stimulant for gastric secretory tests, the patient being protected from the systemic effects of histamine by pre-treatment with a conventional antihistaminic drug. It is only fairly recently, however, that the concept of H_1 and H_2-histamine receptors has been clearly formulated, and this then paved the way to the development of specific drugs to block the action of histamine at H_2-receptor sites.

The pharmacology of histamine H_2-receptor antagonists has been studied very extensively in laboratory animals and in man. The first drug to find widespread clinical application was cimetidine, ranitidine being another compound extensively researched. In man, histamine H_2-receptor blockade with either cimetidine or ranitidine results in inhibition of acid secretion evoked by all known agonists. Thus either cimetidine or ranitidine administered orally or intravenously will markedly decrease acid and pepsin output stimulated by histamine, gastrin, or its analogues, cholinergic drugs, the vagus, and most importantly, food. Basal and nocturnal acid secretion can be inhibited completely, whilst doses of cimetidine (200 mg thrice daily and 400 mg at night), or ranitidine (150 mg twice daily) will inhibit acid output by about 70 per cent and significantly decrease intragastric acidity (Fig. 7). This decrease in stimulated acid secretion is similar to that produced by vagotomy, which undoubtedly has a bearing on the ulcer-healing properties of H_2-receptor antagonists. The only other major acute phar-

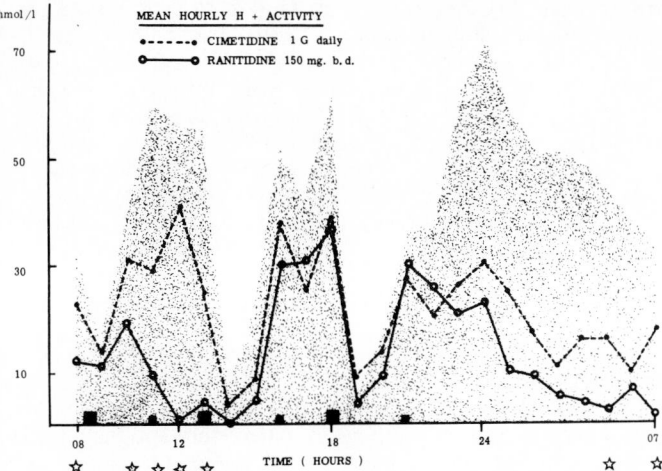

Fig. 7 Mean hourly H+ activity (i.e. intragastric acidity) during a 24 hour period in 10 patients with DU receiving placebo (hatched area), cimetidine 1 g daily (------), or ranitidine 150 mg twice daily (———). Dark squares on horizontal axis mark meals. * =significantly greater inhibition of acidity by ranitidine, than by cimetidine. (From Walt, R. P., Male, P.-J., Rawlings, J., Hunt, R. H., Milton-Thompson, G. J., and Misiewicz, J. J. 1981). *Gut* **22**, 49.)

nacological action of H₂-receptor blockade in the human is the abolition of that part of histamine-induced vasodilatation (histamine flush) that is not blocked by conventional antihistaminics. This is because peripheral blood vessels probably have both H₂ and H₁ receptors on or near their smooth muscle. This effect is of no clinical importance.

Histamine H₂-receptor antagonists are rapidly absorbed from the upper small intestine and excreted largely unchanged by the kidneys. The metabolites, which include sulphoxide derivatives, have not been shown to have any important pharmacological effects. Neither cimetidine nor ranitidine accumulates in the body.

Early histamine H₂-receptor antagonists were not evaluated clinically in large numbers of patients either because absorption was erratic (burimamide) or because of reversible granulocytopaenia occasionally produced by the drug (metiamide). Cimetidine was the drug first generally available for clinical use. Other H₂-antagonists with improved specificity, notably ranitidine, have now been developed and tested clinically. Ranitidine differs from cimetidine in being a substituted furan instead of an imidazole and in having a different side-chain. Although both drugs bind at H₂-receptors, cimetidine also binds at other sites in the body and some of these interactions may give rise to side-effects in some patients. Cimetidine binds at cytochrome P450 which forms part of the mixed oxygenase metabolizing system in the liver. Inhibition of this enzyme by cimetidine can potentiate the action of drugs such as warfarin or diazepam. Cimetidine may also bind at androgen receptors and at, as yet uncharacterized, binding sites in the brain. Ranitidine does not appear to bind at these additional sites and may therefore be less likely to cause side-effects of this type. Ranitidine is, on a molar basis, five to eight times more powerful than cimetidine. The two drugs have a similar half-life in the peripheral circulation (approximately 120 min) and it is likely that their duration of action is also similar.

Short-term treatment of DU and GU with H₂-receptor antagonists. The main bulk of evidence as to the efficacy and safety of H₂-receptor blockade in the treatment of peptic ulcer pertains to cimetidine, as this drug has been in widespread and intensive use for more than five years at the time of writing. Similar data are beginning to accumulate for ranitidine, but the number of patients treated is much smaller.

Short-term treatment usually means outpatient therapy over a period of four to eight weeks with oral cimetidine 0.8 to 2.0 g daily in divided doses, or oral ranitidine 150 mg twice daily. Tables 2 and

3 show that approximately 70 to 80 per cent of either gastric, or duodenal ulcers will heal under this regimen, the proportion of ulcers healed being significantly higher in patients receiving the drug compared with those receiving a placebo, both groups having unlimited access to antacids. The customary dose of cimetidine in the United Kingdom and European countries has been 1 g daily: 200 mg three times a day and 400 mg at night. In the USA a 300 mg tablet is used and the daily dose is usually 1.2 g daily. Recent evidence suggests that cimetidine 400 mg twice daily may be as effective as the higher dose, but the number of patients thus treated in trials is small at the time of writing. Controlled comparisons between cimetidine 1 g/day and ranitidine 150 mg twice daily suggest that the two H₂-receptor blockers are equipotent in terms of percentage of duodenal ulcers healed.

Whether H₂-receptor blockade should be continued for longer than eight weeks at full dose if the DU fails to heal is difficult to decide, as there are no systematic data on which to base the decision. Some of the ulcers will presumably heal because of spontaneous remission. In general, the likelihood of more prolonged treatment at full dose with H₂-receptor blockers being effective after eight weeks is low. Administration of H₂-antagonists is accompanied by rapid relief of dyspepsia, the symptoms usually subsiding completely within a week of starting treatment.

These findings are now generally accepted, but there are certain interesting discrepancies. Firstly, in a small number of controlled trials no significant advantage could be shown for cimetidine when compared with placebo. Secondly, the benefit conferred by cimetidine therapy as measured by the increase in the number of duodenal ulcers healed in the treated group compared with placebo, varies considerably in different trials (Fig. 8). The reasons for these differences are not clear, but must depend, at least in part, on dissimilarities in environment, selection of patients, and antacid consumption. It has been shown for example, that patients in the USA with gastric ulcer consume daily 10 or 20 times the amount of antacid taken by patients in England or France.

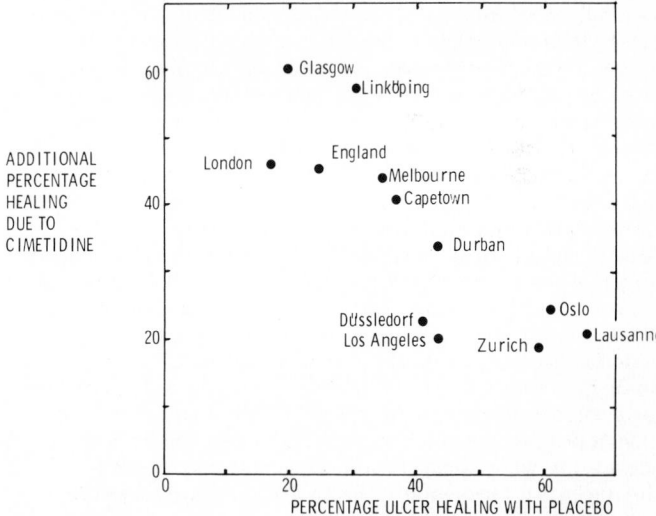

Fig. 8 Results of short-term trials of cimetidine in DU in different centres. Percentage of DUs healed on placebo compared with additional healing on cimetidine therapy. (From Blum, A. L., Siewert, J. R., and Halter, F. (1978). *Deutsche Medizinische Wochenschrift* **103**, 135).

Unwanted effects of H₂-receptor blockade. Hypergastrinaemia does occur during H₂-receptor blockade. The release of gastrin from the antral G cells is controlled by a negative feedback mechanism dependent on the pH in the antral lumen. Decreased intragastric acidity produced by cimetidine or ranitidine leads to excessive release of gastrin. As gastrin is a trophic hormone for the parietal cells, it is possible that prolonged hypergastrinaemia could lead to parietal cell hyperplasia, with consequent hypersecretion of acid once treatment is stopped, leading to severe re-ulceration. Parietal cell hyperplasia has been reported in rats receiving very high doses of cimetidine, but has never been detected in man, even after 12 months of treatment. Recurrence rate of DU is similar in patients who have had 12 months' maintenance treatment and in those who have not. At present, therefore, rebound hypersecretion after prolonged H_2-receptor blockade is not clinically demonstrable.

In experimental animals and in *in vitro* models cimetidine has been shown to have a weak anti-androgenic action. Sporadic instances of male erectile impotence have been reported, but this is not a serious problem in practice; ranitidine has no anti-androgenic properties. Prolactin levels increase after bolus intravenous cimetidine (but not after ranitidine), while oral cimetidine does not affect prolactin metabolism. Gynaecomastia in men and galactorrhoea in women has been occasionally reported: this rare unwanted effect is commonest in patients treated with cimetidine for the Zollinger—Ellison syndrome. Cimetidine (but not ranitidine) affects the blood levels of drugs metabolized by the hepatic microsomal enzymes. Blood concentrations of warfarin, labetolol, diazepam, and phenytoin are significantly higher in patients receiving cimetidine, so that smaller doses of these drugs may be necessary. Other interactions may emerge. Both cimetidine and ranitidine cross the blood–brain barrier in healthy subjects and are present in low concentrations in CSF obtained at lumbar puncture. This is probably of little significance in healthy people. However, instances of reversible mental confusion and coma have been reported in elderly or severely ill patients in intensive care units receiving cimetidine, and this unwanted effect has to be borne in mind.

Probably the commonest side-effect of cimetidine is mild sedation and tiredness, which disappears when the drug is withdrawn. It is rarely severe enough to interfere with treatment. Cimetidine may cause a minor, and unimportant rise in creatinine or hepatic transaminases; marrow-toxic effects are not a problem.

Concern has been expressed recently about possible carcinogenic effects of long-term treatment with cimetidine. Inhibition of acid secretion by cimetidine favours bacterial colonization of the stomach. Bacterial enzymes favour the conversion of dietary nitrates to nitrites, with consequent formation of carcinogenic nitrosamines. It is theoretically possible that cimetidine itself may be converted to nitrosocimetidine which could be carcinogenic. This derivative has never been recovered in *in vivo* human studies, but there are serious technical difficulties in detecting it reliably. Gastric anacidity in pernicious anaemia and gastric hypoacidity after partial gastrectomy are associated with increased incidence of gastric cancer. In both these conditions, however, additional factors, such as gastritis and severe bile reflux, are also present. The anecdotal reports of gastric carcinoma in patients on cimetidine can probably all be explained by the diagnosis of neoplasia having been missed initially. So far there have been no reports of cancer developing in animals receiving large doses of cimetidine for prolonged periods. However, another H_2 histamine receptor antagonists (tiotidine—not available for human use) produced histopathological abnormalities in antral mucosa of rats. At the time of writing there are no grounds for withholding cimetidine treatment because of possible carcinogenesis, but obviously this area needs further careful experimental and clinical research.

Short-term management of DU or GU. The management begins with the diagnosis and, as outlined above, this has to be established either radiologically or, perferably, endoscopically. The patient is given general common-sense advice regarding frequent small meals and is started on ulcer-healing drugs. Strict dietary schedules are unnecessary, except for the obsessive. Smoking should be discouraged on general medical grounds; the same applies to excessive consumption of alcohol. Admission to hospital is virtually never necessary.

The main difference between the short-term management of DU and GU lies in the need to exclude the presence of gastric carcinoma in patients with a gastric ulcer. It is therefore mandatory to endoscope every patient with gastric ulcer at the start of treatment. Multiple targeted biopsies from the rim and base of the ulcer crater and exfoliative cytology brushings must be taken. The endoscopist should take the minimum of four biopsies from the ulcer edge, spaced evenly apart, in addition to two or three from the base. Increasing the number of biopsies diminishes the chances of missing a carcinoma *in situ*. It is then mandatory to re-endoscope the patient after 6–10 weeks of medical therapy to check that the ulcer has healed: if not, then histopathological evaluation must be repeated. This is because the diagnosis of early intramucosal carcinoma can be difficult to establish, while results of resection of early gastric cancer are good and quite different from the gloomy prognosis of advanced neoplasm of the stomach. The failure of an even apparently benign gastric ulcer to heal also influences the management (see below).

By contrast, once the diagnosis of duodenal ulcer is established, repeated endoscopy or radiology is unnecessary and the management is based on symptomatic assessment of the patient. Re-investigation is only needed if the pattern of symptoms changes suggesting the need to revise the diagnosis, if complications occur, or prior to operation to provide the surgeon with up-to-date anatomical information.

Choice of short-term drugs for DU or GU. There is now available a range of drugs, all apparently active in accelerating the healing of gastric and duodenal ulcers. Results of clinical trials (Tables 2 and 3) indicate that there is apparently very little difference between results of any of these agents in the short-term treatment of peptic ulcer. This is highly surprising, because the drugs have such dissimilar pharmacological properties. Neither carbenoxolone sodium nor tripotassium dicitrato bismuthate affect acid secretion. Antacids neutralize acid in the gastric lumen, while H_2-receptor antagonists suppress acid and pepsin output to a variable extent. Despite these differences, all the drugs produce a 70–80 per cent healing rate after 4–12 weeks of outpatient treatment. Why the remaining 30 per cent of ulcers fail to heal is not clear, and analysis of variables such as age, sex, length of history, acid secretion, of consumption of tobacco and alcohol has failed to provide an answer: failure to take the tablets must play a part in some cases.

Taking the results of available therapeutic trials at their face value, therefore, the efficacy of treatment is not apparently of prime importance in deciding which drug to use in the short-term management of peptic ulcer, and the choice of therapeutic agent must depend on other factors, such as safety, convenience, and cost.

H_2-receptor antagonists are the most thoroughly researched drugs for the treatment of peptic ulcer and they are based on good pharmacological principles with well-defined, specific action on acid output. On present evidence H_2-blockers are very safe in short-term usage and are the first choice for drug therapy of peptic ulcer.

Their main disadvantage is high cost. Antacids serve as adjuvant therapy, used to control symptoms at the start of H_2-blockade treatment; they can be tailed off as soon as symptoms improve. It is important to encourage patients to take enough antacid to control peptic ulcer symptoms: the routine use of 10 ml thrice daily after meals is inadequate. It is also important to realize that not every patient with duodenal ulcer needs cimetidine therapy each time symptoms occur. The diagnosis of duodenal ulcer should not lead to automatic prescribing of cimetidine by physicians: minor relapses can be well managed with antacids. Tripotassium dicitrato bismuthate deserves further intensive evaluation, but it would appear to provide a cheap and safe alternative to cimetidine. Its main disadvantage is the ammoniacal smell making some patients reluctant to take the medication. The use of carbonoxolone sodium has declined with the introduction of other compounds, but it remains available for patients who, for some reason, are unable to take the other drugs. The need for close supervision with regular measurements of weight, blood pressure and serum K is a serious disadvantage; elderly patients, and those with compromised cardiorespiratory function need to be watched especially closely.

Anticholinergics, and especially pirenzepine, are also useful in some patients and can be used if H_2-receptor antagonists are ineffective, badly tolerated, or unavailable. There is no need for routine prescribing of psychotropic or anxiolytic drugs, unless there is a specific clinical reason.

Long-term management of DU or GU. Only H_2-receptor antagonists have been shown to affect the incidence of relapses of peptic ulcer.

The evidence is provided by data collected in maintenance trials, in which patients with ulcer healing confirmed at endoscopy were followed for six or 12 months, whilst receiving cimetidine 400 mg at night, or cimetidine 400 mg twice daily, or a placebo. Endoscopic examinations were done at predetermined intervals, or when symptoms recurred and show that long-term administration of cimetidine results in a highly significant decrease in the incidence of relapses of duodenal ulcer, there being little difference between the two doses of the drug (Fig. 3). Maintenance therapy of gastric ulcer with cimetidine gives similar results, but the evidence is less strong than for duodenal ulcer, as the number of patients studied in controlled trials is smaller. There are no data to predict the relapse rate of either type of ulcer on cimetidine maintenance therapy extending beyond twelve months, but there is no theoretical reason why the drug should not remain effective for long periods. As Fig. 3 shows, however, there is a definite, if slow, tendency of duodenal ulcers to recur despite maintenance treatment. The reasons for this are not clear, but failure to take the tablets probably plays a part: it is notoriously difficult to persuade well people to take any treatment regularly—with the possible exception of the contraceptive pill. Any consideration of very prolonged maintenance therapy with cimetidine, or any other agent must take into account the fact that a number of subjects will relapse despite medical treatment.

A choice of therapeutic strategies is available for the long-term medical management of duodenal ulcer with cimetidine: continuous therapy with 400 mg at night, or 400 mg twice daily with increase to 1 g daily if symptoms suggest a relapse, is one alternative. Another is to withhold continuous maintenance medication, but to treat individual relapses promptly with cimetidine 1 g daily for four to six weeks: each period on the full dose may be followed by a few weeks' treatment on the maintenance level. The best general guide to decide which regimen is best for the individual patient is the previous history of ulcer symptoms. The patient who has three or four well-defined relapses of DU each year, but who remains well otherwise, clearly does not need continuous maintenance medication. On the other hand the individual with continuous symptoms, or whose symptom-free periods are short will tend to do better on continuous therapy. Preliminary attempts have been made to compare the clinical efficacy of the two regimens, but at present it is not possible to come to a definite conclusion, nor is it easy to lay down firm rules as to how long to continue H_2-receptor antagonist maintenance therapy in duodenal ulcer patients. There is little or no evidence to suggest that long-term treatment affects the natural history of duodenal ulcer, so that once treatment is discontinued the ulcer recurrence rate reverts to pretreatment levels. Despite reports to the contrary, there is no convincing evidence to show that 'rebound' ulceration is a serious problem in the post-cimetidine period. Some physicians prefer to tail off maintenance cimetidine treatment rather than stopping the drug abruptly. There are no experimental data to support this, but it is probably good practice.

The safety of prolonged medication with cimetidine has been studied intensively in a small number of patients, and additional general clinical experience in practice involving very large numbers of patients suggests that the drug is safe within those limits. Administration of the drug for periods longer than 12 months is also probably safe, but more experience is needed in this area. In patients with persistent symptoms not satisfactorily controlled by

antacids and in whom the risk of elective surgery is unacceptable because of concurrent cardiorespiratory or other problems, H_2-receptor blockade is justified for prolonged periods. It can also be given to those who are judged psychologically unfit for surgical treatment, or who are unwilling to have it. In other patients, the situation is best reviewed after one year of maintenance therapy and the position discussed with the patient. An attempt to stop the treatment can be made, and if the DU recurs the advantages and disadvantages of surgery, or continued medical treatment can be discussed with the patient. The severity of the symptoms also enters into the decision-making process: severe symptoms would make surgical treatment more likely.

The general view is that recurrent gastric ulcers should be treated surgically and that one failure of medical maintenance chemotherapy should lead to a partial gastrectomy. We would not disagree with this. Exceptions to the rule are patients in whom the risk of operation is unacceptable, or younger patients in whom the long-term metabolic consequences and the slightly increased risk of carcinoma in the gastric remnant would make one persevere longer with medical treatment.

Surgical treatment of DU and GU

Indications for surgery. As no permanent medical cure exists for either type of ulcer and as both are chronic, relapsing conditions, it could be said that all patients with both DU and GU will ultimately come to operation. This is not so in practice, because of the mild course of the disease in some patients and unsuitability or unwillingness to undergo surgery of others.

In duodenal ulcer absolute indications for surgical intervention are continuing or life-threatening haemorrhage, perforation, or organic pyloric stenosis. In the uncomplicated case, frequent and severe recurrences that interfere with social or professional life, poor response to, or poor compliance with medication, residence in remote areas with limited access to medical facilities, and occupations where a sudden haematemesis or perforation may endanger the life of others all indicate the need for surgical intervention.

The general answer to the question of when is surgery indicated in the uncomplicated case of DU is when medical treatment has failed to control the symptoms adequately. This rule should not be applied indiscriminately, however. It is better not to push patients into accepting surgery if they are reluctant to have it. Some individuals need time to adjust to the idea of an operation and more than one consultation, with full discussion of what an operation entails is needed. It is very helpful for the surgeon to see the patient together with the physician. There is no need to wait for the patient to 'earn' his operation through years of discomfort: a two to three year history of duodenal ulcer is more than enough.

In gastric ulcer absolute indications for surgery are similar to those for duodenal ulcer, except that pyloric stenosis does not occur and that suspicion of carcinoma should lead to thorough re-evaluation: if a neoplasm cannot be confidently excluded, it is safer to proceed to operation. As already stated, most gastroenterologists advocate early, rather than late surgery for benign, uncomplicated gastric ulcers, although there are a few studies suggesting that the outcome of unoperated GU may not be as bad as generally believed.

Choice of operation for DU and GU. Uncomplicated duodenal ulcer is now almost invariably treated by some variant of vagotomy: either a truncal vagotomy with a drainage procedure (pyloroplasty or gastroenterostomy), or by selective, or highly selective vagotomy. The latter operation denervates only the parietal cell mass, leaving the innervation of the antral pump, and thus control of gastric emptying, undisturbed. Gastric ulcers are usually dealt with by a Billroth-type partial gastrectomy: surgical texts can be consulted for details.

Outcome of operations for DU and GU. Surgical treatment works well for properly selected patients with either type of ulcer. Highly selective vagotomy for DU is attractive, because it is a physiologically logical and least mutilating operation. The incidence of unwanted effects is very low; the main disadvantage is a relatively high recurrence rate, reported from various centres as 5–15 per cent. Other types of vagotomy have a lower recurrence rate, but the incidence of side-effects such as post-vagotomy diarrhoea, or dumping, is higher at about 5 per cent. Vagotomy and antrectomy carries the lowest recurrence rate, but mortality is slightly higher than after vagotomy and drainage, where it is less than 1 per cent in good centres.

Recurrence is rare after elective partial gastrectomy for chronic GU, but the mortality is at around 3 per cent, mainly because GU tends to be the disease of elderly patients from a low socio-economic group. Late or early dumping is an unwanted sequel of partial gastrectomy. Early dumping is due to hypovolaemia caused by copious secretion of fluid into the intestinal lumen provoked by the rapid emptying of a hyperosmolar load into the small gut. Late dumping is associated with hypoglycaemia: rapid absorption of a large carbohydrate load causes hypersecretion of insulin with consequent overswing of blood glucose levels to below normal. Symptoms of dumping can be controlled in most patients by decreasing the carbohydrate intake in the diet and by advising them not to take fluids with, or immediately after meals.

Late sequelae of partial gastrectomy include weight loss, iron-deficiency anaemia (see Section 19), mild steatorrhoea, and occasionally osteomalacia. There is also a slightly increased incidence of carcinoma in the gastric remnant. For these reasons it is important that all patients with partial gastrectomy should be seen yearly at a follow-up clinic. At each visit the haemoglobin and the serum Ca, P, and alkaline phosphatase should be measured and the patient's weight recorded. The anaemia usually responds to oral iron supplements. Abnormalities in Ca, P, and an elevated alkaline phosphatase level should lead to bone biopsy to confirm, or refute the presence of osteomalacia which, if present, can be treated by oral calcium and vitamin supplements. Recurrence of symptoms, anorexia, further sudden weight loss, or loss of well-being should alert to the possibility of a neoplasm and lead to a gastrectomy.

Post-surgical recurrent ulcers. Duodenal ulcer may recur after any type of vagotomy, but recurrence is most common after the highly selective (parietal cell) type. Re-ulceration becomes apparent by return of the previous ulcer symptoms usually within 12 or 18 months after the original operation. Haemorrhage from the recurrent ulcer may be the presenting symptom. Duodenal ulcers may recur at or near their original site in the duodenal cap. If the gastroenterostomy had been fashioned, ulcers may form just distal to the stoma in the jejunal mucosa. The vast majority of recurrences after vagotomy are due to the incomplete division of the vagal fibres by the surgeon: a few are previously undiagnosed cases of the Zollinger–Ellison syndrome.

A great deal of time and effort has been devoted to the development of a reliable test for completeness of vagotomy. Most of the work is based on measurements of gastric acid secretion produced by vagal stimulation through insulin-induced hypoglycaemia. Vari-ous criteria, based on the original work of Hollander have been proposed, but none have proved very satisfactory in practice and the predictive value of such tests is poor. There is no point in performing insulin stimulation tests routinely following vagotomy, as after several months a proportion of negative tests will become positive without recurrent ulceration.

The diagnosis of recurrent duodenal ulcer after vagotomy is best established by endoscopy. Treatment of recurrent DU is either by re-operation, at which undivided vagal trunks are identified and cut, or a highly selective vagotomy is converted to another type, or a partial gastrectomy is performed. Results of re-operation are good, but repeated surgical procedures carry a higher morbidity and mortality than the original operations. The alternative is medical treatment with H_2-receptor antagonists. The few controlled therapeutic trials available in this area have dealt with small numbers of patients, but in general results are favourable, a significant number of recurrent ulcers healing after a few weeks of therapy. It would be illogical however, to expect the recurrent ulcer to heal permanently after a short period of medical treatment and one is therefore committed to long-term administration of cimetidine or ranitidine. In the otherwise fit patient, re-operation is usually preferable, especially as stomal ulcers have a tendency to bleed.

References

Avery Jones, F., Hunt, T. C., and Reed, P. I. (eds.) (1980). Carbenoxolone symposium. *Scand J. Gastroent.* **15** suppl. 65.
Baron, J. H. (1978). Diagnostic value. In *Clinical tests of gastric secretion*, 79. Macmillan Press, London.
— (ed.) (1981). *Cimetidine in the 80s.* Churchill Livingstone, Edinburgh.
—, Langman, M. J. S., and Wastell, C. (1980). Stomach and duodenum. In *Recent advances in gastroenterology* (ed. I. A. D. Bouchier), 23. Churchill Livingstone, Edinburgh.
British Medical Journal (1981). After gastrectomy. *Br. med. J.* **282**, 1096.
— (1981). Does cimetidine cause gastric cancer? *Br. med. J.* **282**, 1178.
Brogden, R. N., Pinder, R. M., Sawyer, Phyllis R., Speight, T. M., and Avery, G. S. (1976) Tripotassium dicitrato bismuthate: a report of its pharmacological properties and therapeutic efficacy in peptic ulcer. *Drugs* **12**, 401.
Burland, W. L., Hawkins, B. W., and Beresford, J. (1980).Cimetidine treatment for the prevention of recurrence of duodenal ulcer: an international collaborative study. *Post-grad. med. J.* **56**, 173.
Carter, D. C. (1980). Aetiology of peptic ulcer. In *Scientific foundations of gastroenterology* (eds. W. Sircus and A. N. Smith), 344. Heinemann, London.
Chierichetti, S. M., Gaetani, M., and Petrin, G. (eds.) (1979). Pharmacokinetic and clinical studies on pirenzepine, a new antiulcer drug. *Scand. J. Gastroent.* **14**, suppl. 57.
Conn, H. O. (1981). To scope or not to scope. *New Engl. J. Med.* **304**, 967.
Langman, M. J. S. (1979). Peptic ulcer in *The epidemiology of chronic digestive disease*, 9. Arnold, London.
McGuigan, J. E. (1981). A consideration of the adverse effects of cimetidine. *Gastroenterology* **80**, 181.
Misiewicz, J. J. and Sewing, K-Fr. (eds.) (1981). First international symposium on ranitidine. *Scand. J. Gastroent.* **16**, suppl. 69.
Wastell, C., Ellis, E., and Tanner, N. C. (1972). Surgical treatment. In *Chronic duodenal ulcer* (ed. C. Wastell), 134. Butterworth, London.

Gastritis

K. B. Taylor

Before 1950 the term gastritis was almost exclusively a clinical one and largely synonymous with non-ulcer dyspepsia. Clinicians applied the term to epigastric discomfort or pain, nausea, and even heartburn, occurring in the absence of radiological findings of peptic ulcer.

The diagnosis and classification of gastric mucosal diseases depend largely on technical developments during the past 30 years. At the beginning of this century it had been emphasized how misleading was post-mortem gastric material for the study of mucosal pathology unless formalin was instilled into the stomach immediately after death to prevent autolysis. Surgical specimens were also shown to undergo significant change as a consequence of ischemia and trauma caused by manipulation at the time of operation. Wood in Australia obtained gastric biopsies free from significant artefact by suction, using a flexible instrument 'blind' or under fluoroscopic control. Studies by the Melbourne group using this technique paved the way for better understanding of the gastritic process and for achieving a more precise diagnosis. The recently introduced fibre-optic, biopsying gastroduodenoscope has made it possible to obtain mucosal tissue under direct vision from standardized locations in the stomach and duodenum. Current histological classification of gastritis is based on studies of such material.

During the same period significant advances have been made in measurements of gastric secretory functions. Hydrochloric acid secretion can be reproducibly estimated both under resting conditions and following stimulation of the parietal-cell mass by ingestion of food or injection of specific drugs and hormones. Radio-immune assays have been used to quantify the secretion of pepsinogens, intrinsic factor, and the hormone gastrin. Further, measurements of humoral and cell-mediated immune responses to gastric mucosal and other antigens have provided another tool for making distinctions between groups of subjects with gastric lesions.

The structural and functional abnormalities associated with peptic ulceration, mucosal erosion and varying degrees of mucosal inflammation, atrophy, and metaplasia can now be scrutinized with some precision and observed sequentially with the probes available. Understanding of the biological nature of gastric and duodenal mucosal lesions has, in consequence, expanded significantly in the past decade. However, the aetiological factors involved in the development of almost all gastric lesions have still to be identified and current classifications are based on structural, functional, and immune changes rather than differences in causation. It must be emphasized that correlation between these three is incomplete.

Gastric physiology. The important functions of the stomach are its roles as a reservoir or hopper for ingested foods and liquids, as a muscular mill to reduce ingested food to liquid chyme, and as a secretory organ. Its main secretions derive from the glands of the body of the stomach and include hydrochloric acid, pepsinogens, and intrinsic factor (IF), a glycoprotein which uniquely mediates the absorption of cobalamin (vitamin B_{12}) into the epithelial cell of the ileum. Acid and IF are secreted in man and many other mammals by the parietal or oxyntic cells, although in some other species, such as rodents, the IF is secreted by the chief or pepsinogen-secreting cells.

Gastric proteolytic enzymes are almost exclusively pepsins and are derived from pepsinogens by autocatalysis. There are seven pepsinogens, characterized by differences in antigenicity and electrophoretic mobility. They are secreted by the chief cells and mucous cells of the gastric mucosa. They are designated pepsinogens 1–5 (Group I) and pepsinogens 6–7 (Group II). The secretion of the Group I pepsinogens is restricted to the acid-secreting, body mucosa, whereas pepsinogens of Group II are secreted by body, antral, and duodenal mucosa.

The mucosa of the gastric antrum, also termed the pyloric glandular area, is very different from that of the body of the stomach (Fig. 1). It contains few parietal cells and chief cells, but present in the mucosa adjacent to the lumen are neuroendocrine cells termed G cells. These secrete the polypeptide gastrin in response to such stimulants as stretching of the antrum, a rise in pH of the contents of the antral lumen, and nerve impulses transmitted through vagal fibres.

The body-type of mucosa of the stomach occupies all of its internal surface except that comprising the first centimetre beyond the gastro-oesophageal junction proximally, which is termed the cardiac region, in which the mucosal glands are loosely packed, contain no parietal cells, and sometimes display cystic changes, and that comprising the antral or pyloric glandular region distally which, on the side of the greater curve, is restricted to the immedi-

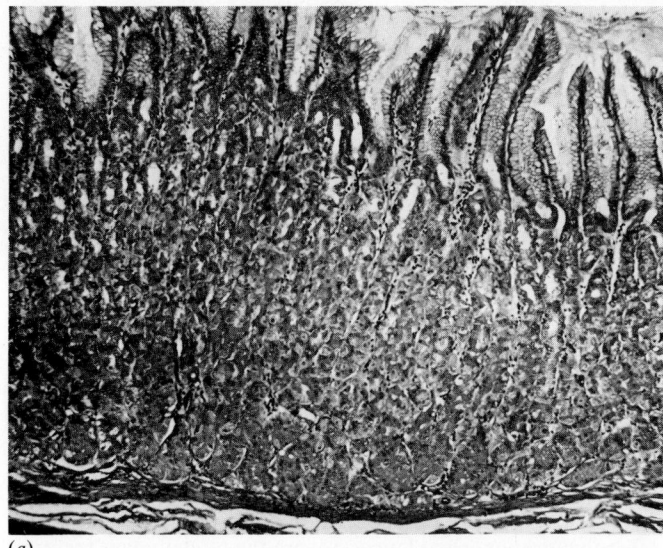

(a)

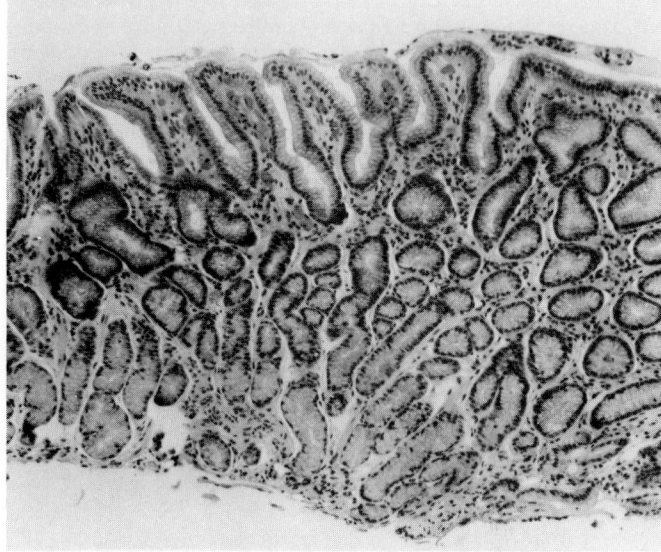

(b)

Fig. 1 Normal gastric mucosa: (a) body, (b) antrum. (Courtesy of Dr K. Lewin, Department of Pathology, University of California, Los Angeles).

ate prepyloric region, but on the lesser curve may extend to the angulus of the stomach or even more proximally, on occasions becoming continuous with the cardia. The boundaries between the different zones are not sharply demarcated; there are transitional bands of varying width.

Although inflammatory changes in the mucosa of the body and antrum are both termed gastritis and both regions may on occasions appear to be equally affected, there is persuasive evidence that these two parts of the stomach behave, both in health and diseased states, largely as separate though contiguous organs which influence each other through changes in content of their secretions into the gastric lumen and hormonal fluctuations. The difference between body and antrum is supported by structural, functional, and immunological studies and has provided an important concept in our understanding of how the stomach works in health and disease states.

Classification of gastritis

This has been attempted on the basis of studies of (a) histology, (b) secretory function, (c) endoscopic appearances, (d) association with other diseases, (e) immunological responses, and (f) clinical picture.

None of these can be considered wholly satisfactory. For example, histological findings do not show close concordance with disturbances of function, endoscopic appearances correlate well with histology in chronic atrophic gastritis but poorly in chronic superficial gastritis, and when symptoms are attributed to gastritis, functional and histological confirmation is commonly lacking. Conversely, most diffuse gastric mucosal lesions are not associated with a consistent pattern of symptoms.

Histological criteria. Currently these provide the basis of the classification most commonly used. The major division is into acute and chronic gastritis.

Acute gastritis. This may involve both the gastric body and antrum. The response of the gastric mucosa to trauma is similar to that in other tissues and due to release or disinhibition of an array of physiologically active substances. The causes may be ingestion of irritants such as aspirin, alcohol, ferrous sulphate, or phenylbutazone, uremia, or streptococcal septicaemia, but often no cause is found.

Erythema, oedema, and infiltration of the interglandular spaces with polymorphonuclear leucocytes are the predominant features. If the insult is more severe, the response may likewise be more florid and direct injury to tissues and indirect effects of anoxia due to interruption of the microcirculation may lead to necrosis. Necrosis of the mucosa results in erosions of variable depth (acute erosive gastritis), the superficial epithelium being shed at the level of the necks of the gastric glands. Damaged capillaries at this level may bleed profusely (acute haemorrhagic gastritis). The inflammatory

process may extend more deeply to involve sub-mucosal structures and the lesion is then, by definition, an acute ulcer. The mucosal involvement may be patchy or homogeneous.

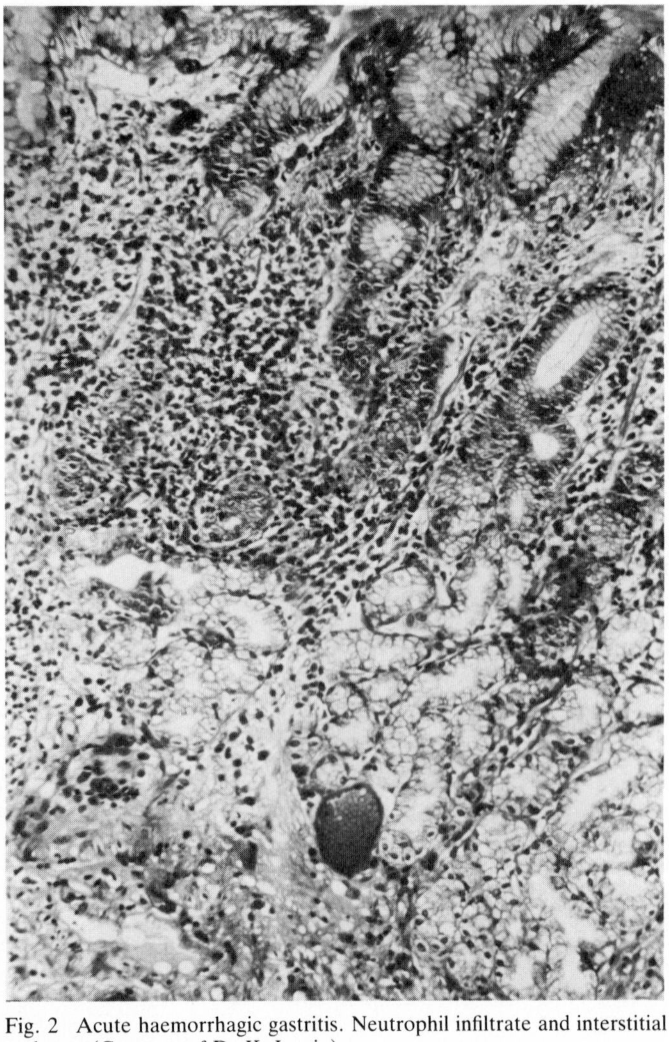

The cellular infiltrate, which consists predominantly of polymorphonuclear leucocytes, may contain in addition variable numbers of eosinophils and mononuclear cells. The latter may invade the epithelium and appear to be destroying it. The lamina propria is filled with neutrophils, the vascular tree is dilated, and there is variable interstitial oedema (Fig. 2).

The appearances are, therefore, those of acute inflammation. Mild acute inflammation usually terminates in resolution or, when necrosis has occurred, in regeneration and repair. Unlike most other tissues, gastric mucosa possesses, as does the pancreas, its own specialized secretory mechanisms capable of producing powerful proteolytic activity. Under certain conditions it is possible but not proven that these properties may contribute to local damage of the mucosa of the gastric body and prolong or perpetuate it.

Chronic gastritis. This may involve both gastric body and antrum but there may be differences between the two, which are discussed later. There is at present no generally agreed upon histological classification of chronic gastritis. The terms chronic superficial gastritis, chronic atrophic gastritis, gastric atrophy, and intestinal metaplasia are widely used. There is in the literature a lack of consistency in terminology well exemplified by such terms as superficial gastritis with minimal atrophy and mild atrophic gastritis, used by different authors to describe similar or identical appearances. The following section is based on systematic examination of gastric mucosal specimens obtained by biopsy under direct vision.

Chronic superficial gastritis. The inflammatory cellular infiltrate does not extend deeper than the gastric pits (Fig. 3). The changes

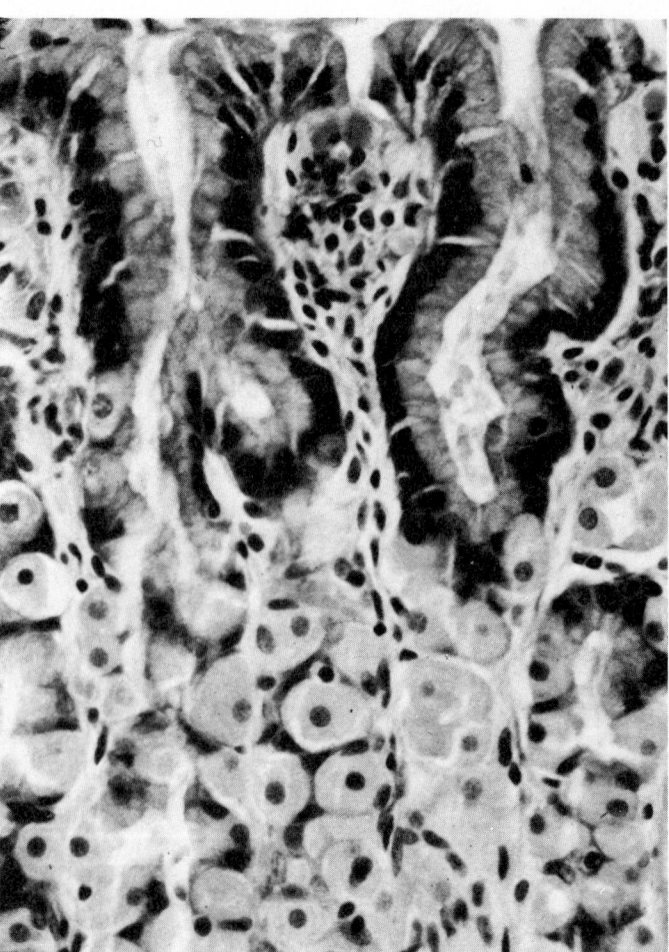

Fig. 2 Acute haemorrhagic gastritis. Neutrophil infiltrate and interstitial oedema. (Courtesy of Dr K. Lewin).

Fig. 3 Chronic superficial gastritis. Mononuclear cell infiltrate limited to zone superficial to gastric glands. (Courtesy of Dr K. Lewin).

may be confluent or patchy. No glandular atrophy occurs but the epithelial cells are more cuboidal than normal and have diminished cytoplasmic content.

Chronic atrophic gastritis. The infiltrate involves the mucosa down to the muscularis mucosae and there is a variable degree of glandular atrophy, classed as mild, moderate, or severe according to the numbers of persisting parietal and chief cells (Fig. 4). An extreme form is called *gastric atrophy* (Fig. 5). In this, the inflammatory infiltrate is usually slight, there is virtually complete loss of parietal cells and marked reduction in chief cells, and there are often pyloric or intestinal glands. The epithelium shows similar changes to those seen in chronic superficial gastritis except in areas of intestinal metaplasia.

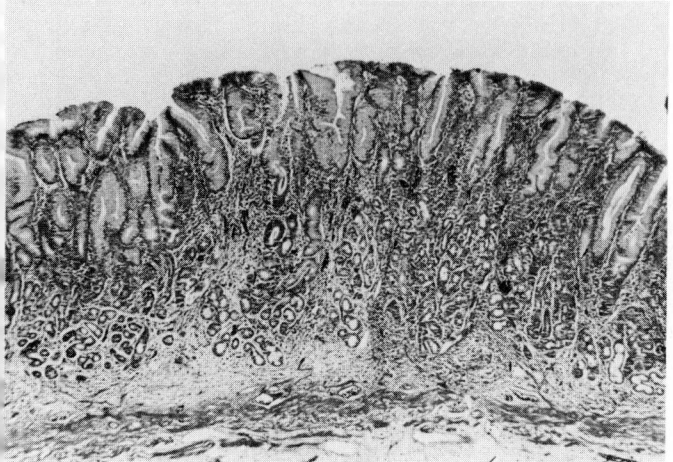

Fig. 4   Chronic atrophic gastritis (severe). (Courtesy of Dr K. Lewin).

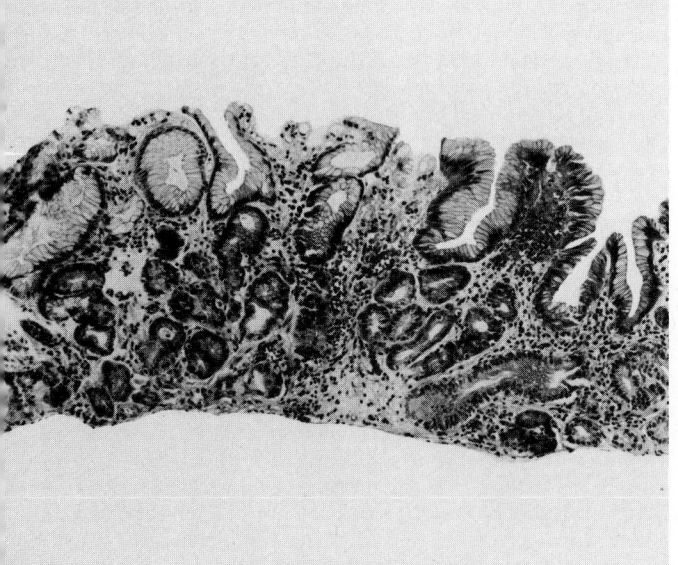

Fig. 5   Gastric atrophy. (Courtesy of Dr K. Lewin).

From currently available data it is not possible to conclude that one form may progress or revert to another. There are insufficient longitudinal studies of individuals and attempts to integrate cross-sectional biopsy studies of groups of different ages and degrees of chronic gastritis have not been convincing to date. Thus the proposed term 'chronic progressive atrophy of the gastric mucosa' seems to represent an over-interpretation of histological appearances.

The inflammatory infiltrate. Common to all forms of chronic gastritis is infiltration of the epithelium and lamina propria with greater than normal numbers of lymphocytes and plasma cells. Sometimes lymphoid follicles may be seen and such cases have been termed follicular gastritis but probably these do not represent a separate entity. In addition variable numbers of polymorphs and eosinophils are usually present. The principle zone of infiltration may be quite superficial or may involve the whole thickness down to the muscularis mucosae. The activity of the lesion is estimated by some observers by the proportion of polymorphs seen. This may vary markedly in different subjects with persisting, chronic disease. In the mucosa of the gastric body there is a considerable variation in the relationship between the intensity of the inflammatory response and the degree of glandular atrophy. A scanty, diffuse inflammatory infiltrate may be found in a mucosal biopsy in which there is little atrophy and differentiated glandular cell types are present in apparently normal numbers or in biopsies displaying complete loss of glandular tissue. Conversely, a heavy inflammatory infiltrate may occur with little loss of glandular mass or with marked atrophy.

Metaplasia. This occurs very frequently in chronic atrophic gastritis. The mucosa of the gastric body undergoes transformation either to one resembling that of small intestine or gastric pylorus. In the former the epithelium has the structural histo-chemical and functional characteristics of small intestinal mucosa. There are mucin-containing goblet cells, a prominent brush-border of microvilli, and Paneth cells are often present in large numbers. None of these is seen in normal gastric body mucosa. Occasionally the arrangement of villi and crypts is indistinguishable from normal small intestine, though villi are often not present (Fig. 6).

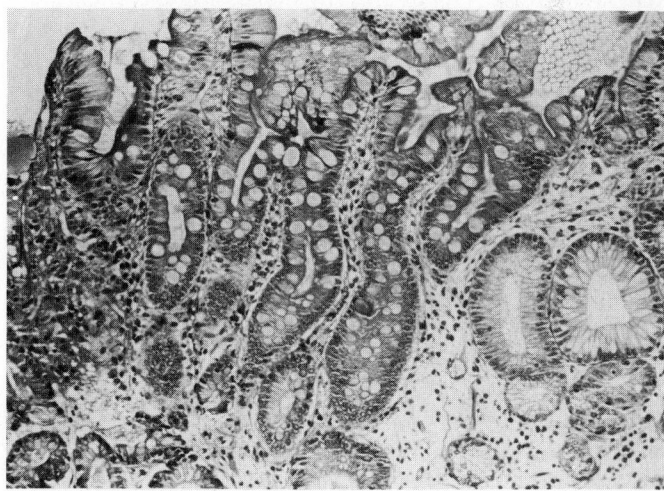

Fig. 6   Intestinal metaplasia of gastric body. (Courtesy of Dr K. Lewin).

Pyloric metaplasia (the term pseudo-pyloric metaplasia is redundant) occurs only in atrophic gastritis. The appearances are of absence of glands containing differentiated parietal and chief cells, the cells being of the pyloric type (Fig. 7). Since in the region of the lesser curve of the stomach the extent of the pyloric glandular mucosa is very variable in the normal stomach, biopsies from this area are difficult to interpret. It has been claimed that the presence of some parietal cells indicates normal pyloric glands whereas in metaplastic mucosa none is seen.

The presence of intestinal metaplasia at the margins of human gastric adenocarcinomas is interpreted by some experienced pathologists as evidence of its carcinomatous potential. This is supported by the presence of intestinal metaplasia in the stomachs of rats treated with *N*-methyl-*N*-nitro-*N*-nitrosoguanidine which produces gastric cancers. Others have claimed, however, that in a Japanese population gastric carcinoma may occur in the complete absence of intestinal metaplasia and that the site of maximal intestinal metaplasia correlates better with gastric ulcer than carcinoma.

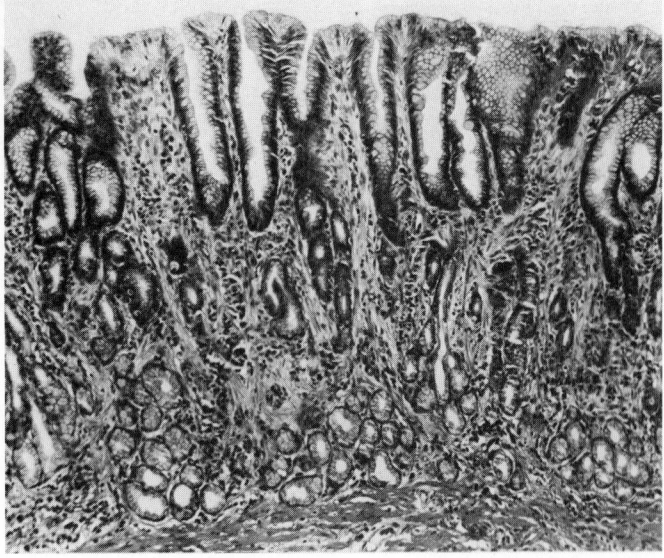

Fig. 7 Pyloric metaplasia of gastric body. (Courtesy of Dr K. Lewin).

Some uncommon histological types of chronic gastritis should be mentioned in this section. *Chronic cystic gastritis* describes a rare finding of dilatation of glands in the deeper zones of the lamina propria, which are lined with flattened epithelium. Another rarity is *giant hypertrophic gastritis* or *Menetrier's disease*. It is probably incorrect to apply the term gastritis to this condition. The gastric mucosal folds are much enlarged by marked hyperplasia of epithelial cells and consequently appear polypoid. The gastric glands are elongated, branched, and tortuous with dilated cystic spaces lined by epithelium and they penetrate deep to the muscularis mucosae. The changes may be generalized or there may be areas of normal gastric mucosa. In affected areas the mucosal surface may be infiltrated with red cells and erosions are common. Inflammatory infiltrates of the lamina propria occur in the region of erosions but a generalized inflammatory response is not a feature of the condition.

The limitations of the histological classification are that it provides inadequate information about gastric function and very little, if any, about aetiology and pathogenesis. Like most structures in the gastrointestinal tract the repertory of response of the gastric mucosa to injury is limited. By ordinary histological examination of biopsies a distinction cannot be made between chronic atrophic gastritis in which secretion of IF is adequate to mediate absorption of sufficient cobalamin and the lesion in established pernicious anaemia, for instance. Similarly, the biopsy appearances of the gastritis associated with gastric ulcer may be indistinguishable from those found in iron deficiency anaemia.

Secretory criteria

Acid secretion. The introduction of the standardized augmented histamine test of gastric acid secretion 30 years ago resulted in a decade or more of intense study of acid production by gastric mucosa in various stages of disease. Today pentagastrin is used (6.0 μg/kg) instead of a combination of histamine and H_1 blocking agent, or the response to ingestion of food can be measured, using an intragastric titration technique. The site, extent, and degree of gastritic involvement all play important roles in determining the degree of reduction of acid secretion and the volume of total secretion. In the predominantly antral or prepyloric gastritis associated with duodenal ulcer disease gastric acid secretory activity is usually in the high normal range and, in response to a meal, can be shown to be abnormally high. By contrast both superficial and atrophic gastritis of the body of the stomach may be associated with reduced or absent acid secretion. There is good correlation between the amount of acid secreted in the augmented histamine test and the histological appearance of the gastric body mucosa in atrophic gastritis and gastric atrophy, but in chronic superficial gastritis there is frequently an unexpectedly large reduction of acid output. Total volumes of gastric juice show the same trend (Table 1). The cause of this hypochlorhydria in superficial gastritis is not clear. The parietal cell mass appears not to be reduced and microscopically there is no evidence of structural change. It has been postulated that as a consequence of an inflammatory response there is a breakdown in the mechanism responsible for retaining hydrogen ions in the gastric lumen. Significant exchange of hydrogen with sodium ions occurs and measurements of acid in the gastric juice may underestimate parietal cell function. A similar underestimate is implicit in the widely accepted two-component theory of gastric secretion, which postulates that an alkaline secretion from the non-parietal mucosa in part or wholly neutralizes secreted acid. When small amounts of acid are secreted there may appear to be no acid secretion.

Table 1 Gastric histology, acid secretion, and volume of gastric juice

Histology	No.	Mean total acid (mol)	Mean volume (ml)
Normal	36	22.00	188
Superficial gastritis	25	10.00	116
Atrophic gastritis	22	3.54	61
Gastric atrophy	14	0.02	11

Derived from Bock, O. A. A., Richards, W. C. D., and Witts, L. J. (1963), *Gut* 4, 112.

Pepsinogen secretion. Estimations of gastric pepsinogen secretion, either directly in stimulated gastric secretions, or indirectly in plasma or urine were done by measuring proteolytic activity, a method now supplanted by radioimmunoassay techniques. A sensitive and specific screening test of good predictive value for chronic atrophic gastritis has been developed, which depends on estimation of serum pepsinogen I content.

IF secretion. The amount of IF secreted by the parietal cells of the healthy stomach is enormously in excess of what is required for the absorption of the daily requirement of cobalamin. In chronic gastritis reduction of the parietal cell mass results in a corresponding decrease in IF secretion. Even a 95 per cent loss of parietal cells is compatible with production of adequate IF, providing the residue of parietal cells is functional. In some patients virtual achlorhydria may be consonant with normal absorption of cobalamin. The number of IF-secreting parietal cells, the pH of gastric contents, and the presence of IF antibodies which may inhibit IF binding to cobalamin in the lumen or block binding of the IF-cobalamin complex at the ileal receptor site all affect cobalamin absorption. Very low or absent IF activity in gastric juice, histological evidence of marked atrophic gastritis or gastric atrophy, achlorhydria, and, in more than 80 per cent of subjects, the presence of IF antibodies in serum and gastric juice co-exist in established pernicious anaemia. Other subjects may meet the second and third of these criteria and yet not have the lesion of pernicious anaemia.

The clinically important issue is whether cobalamin is absorbed in sufficient amounts and this is best estimated by the urinary excretion test of Schilling, or by total body-counting after oral administration of small amounts of radio-cobalt labelled cobalamin, either alone or complexed with biologically active IF (see Section 19).

Gastrin secretion. Estimation of serum gastrin by radioimmunoassay provides another probe for the indirect assessment of gastric mucosal function. In 60–80 per cent of patients with pernicious anaemia serum gastrin levels in the fasting subject are abnormally high (normal is less than 100 pmol/l). This phenomenon has been interpreted as being the result of reduced or absent acid secretory activity of the mucosa of the body of the stomach with relative sparing of the antral mucosa, which contains the gastrin-secreting G cells. The activity of these cells is high, since the luminal pH is high. There is also evidence that the G-cell mass is greater than normal. The reason for this hyperplasia is not clear. In the absence of high acid secretion (which would suggest the presence of a gastrinoma, i.e. the Zollinger–Ellison syndrome) a high serum gastrin indicates atrophic gastritis or gastric atrophy. The predictive value of this for chronic gastritis, taken in conjunction with evidence of gastric auto-immune responses, is discussed in a later section.

In summary, none of these secretory tests alone or in conjunction provides a basis for more than a very crude classification of chronic gastritis, though some are sensitive and specific indicators of this condition. Tests of cobalamin absorption (providing other causes of its malabsorption, such as small intestinal or pancreatic disease have been excluded) discriminate between the chronic gastritis of pernicious anaemia and the rest, which even histological examination of the gastric mucosa by standard techniques cannot do.

Endoscopic appearances. Until publication of Wood's studies no histological data for comparison with endoscopic findings were available. It is now possible to state unequivocally that the endoscopic diagnosis of *chronic atrophic gastritis* and *gastric atrophy* agree well with the histology. The mucosa is grey, folds are absent or much reduced, and blood vessels, including their finer branches, are seen with abnormal clarity. Chronic superficial gastritis, conversely, is hard to recognize by endoscopy.

In both acute and chronic gastritis the mucosa of the body of the stomach may appear glossy with adherent mucus and show marked reddening and contact friability, especially along folds and ridges. The appearance of a multiple, erosive gastritis may be seen in both acute gastritis *de novo* and also when acute gastritis supervenes in chronic atrophic gastritis, the cause of which may be exposure to alcohol or drugs such as aspirin, but is often unknown.

Chronic hypertrophic gastritis is found occasionally in otherwise healthy subjects who complain of dyspepsia. The salient features are diffuse erythema of the mucosa and a prominence of the gastric folds which mimics polypoid change. Dilatation of the stomach with air may diminish but does not eradicate the abnormal appearance of the folds. The mucosa is friable to contact and acute erosions may occur, but ulcers are not associated with this condition. It is generally believed that the changes are those of an actively secreting gastric mucosa. In the Zollinger–Ellison syndrome the gastric mucosa appears identical. Estimation of resting serum gastrin should always be done in such cases.

In giant hypertrophic gastritis or Menetrier's disease the endoscopic appearances are similar to but usually more marked than those in chronic hypertrophic gastritis but the histological changes are quite different (see page 12.74). It must be emphasized that in none of these three conditions is inflammation a feature and the term gastritis is inappropriate.

Association with other diseases. Implicit in much written about gastric mucosal disease is a classification based on association with other diseases, such as pernicious anaemia, hypochromic anaemia, thyroid diseases, diabetes mellitus, hypoparathyroidism, vitiligo, and many others. This raises a number of objections. First, some of the so-called 'other diseases' may be caused by the primary gastric defect as in pernicious anaemia and possibly in iron-deficiency anaemia. Secondly, some of the claimed associations may not be true but apparent ones due to underestimates of the real prevalence or incidence of either condition and to bias inherent in the clinical sampling process. Chronic gastritis, in which studies have shown that the majority of those affected are asymptomatic, is particularly susceptible to such error and is compounded by the latency of much endocrine disease. Thirdly, some of the associated diseases may be expressions of the same underlying disturbance as the gastric

disease. The last is not a strong proscription and the greater knowledge of aetiopathogenesis may subsequently validate this type of classification.

Apparent predisposition to develop auto-antibodies of organ-specific type in diseases such as pernicious anaemia, thyrotoxicosis, and adrenalitis, and the overlap of humoral immune responses in patients with these diseases and in close relatives of affected probands, support the possibility of associations, but at present available evidence does not provide a firm basis for classification. Provided this is recognized, it is convenient to refer to the chronic gastritis of pernicious anaemia, of iron deficiency anaemia, of thyrotoxicosis, of diabetes mellitus, and so on.

There are sufficient studies of chronic gastritis in association with gastric and duodenal ulcer, gastric adenocarcinoma, and following gastric surgery to provide convincing evidence of true associations. In the case of ulcers of the body of the stomach it has been shown that there is usually a widespread zone of chronic gastritis around an ulcer, often involving most of the stomach, in which intestinal metaplasia is found in more than one-third of subjects studied. Treatment of the ulcer to complete healing either medically or by vagotomy and pyloroplasty is not accompanied by consistent reduction of the extent or activity of the gastritis. This and related phenomena are dealt with later in the section on aetiology. It is likely that the chronic gastritic change associated with gastric ulcer is not secondary to the ulcer but is the primary lesion.

Thus, ulcer-associated gastritis and post-surgical gastritis are useful descriptive terms for defining clinical categories.

Immunological classification

Humoral antibodies. Discovery of circulating gastric auto-antibodies in patients with pernicious anaemia provided the first non-invasive marker of chronic gastritis. The two auto-antigens implicated are Castle's intrinsic factor (Fig. 8) and a lipoprotein compo-

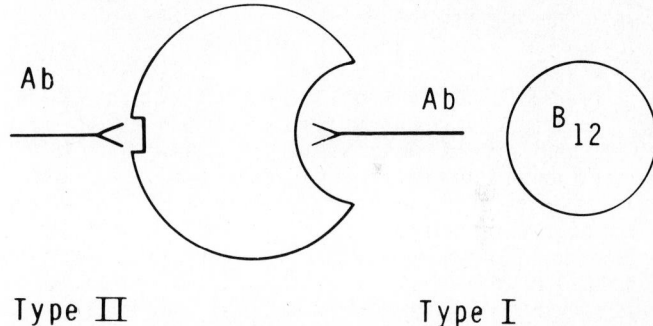

Type II   Type I

Fig. 8   Antibodies to intrinsic factor: blocking, or type I, inhibits IF–B$_{12}$ binding, while binding, or type II, reacts with IF or IF–B$_{12}$ complex.

nent of the microvilli of the parietal cell canaliculi (Fig. 9). Both are completely parietal-cell specific. Studies of sera from patients with acute gastritis have been negative for gastric antibodies except in a proportion of those patients in whom an acute gastritis supervenes on chronic atrophic gastritis. However, immunological techniques have provided a means of separating chronic gastritis into two major categories, namely those in which auto-allergic responses are detectable and those in which they are not. There is some evidence that the distribution of the gastric changes is significantly different in these categories, the antral mucosa being relatively spared in subjects in whom gastric antibodies are present. These have been classified as having type A gastritis and comprise mainly patients with pernicious anaemia and some close relatives. The rest have type B gastritis, whether associated with gastric ulcer, carcinoma, gastric surgery, or arising apparently spontaneously. In these there is no evidence of sparing of the antral mucosa, which may show histological disease of a severity similar to that in the body. The antral mucosa in type A gastritis may show a variable increase in the number of gastrin-producing cells (G cells) and elevated circulating

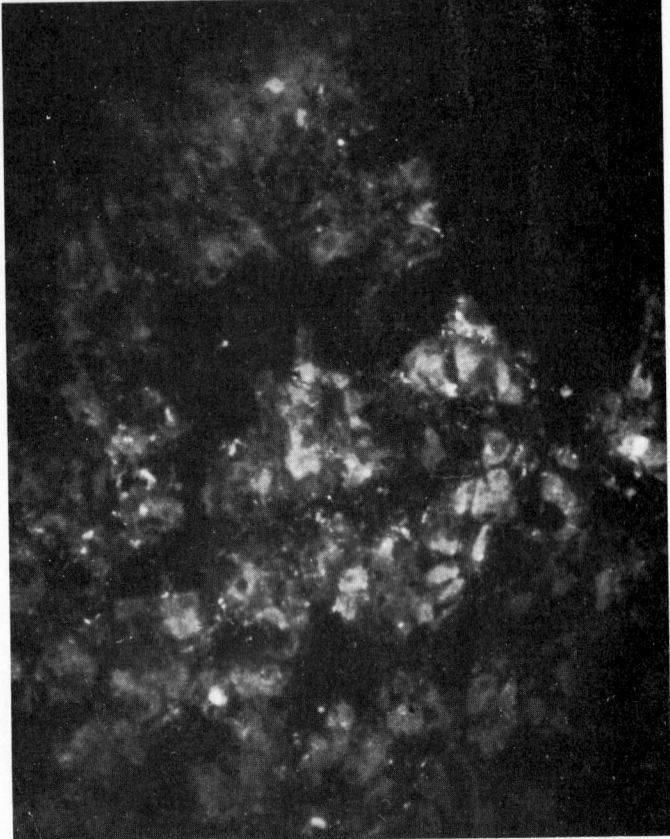

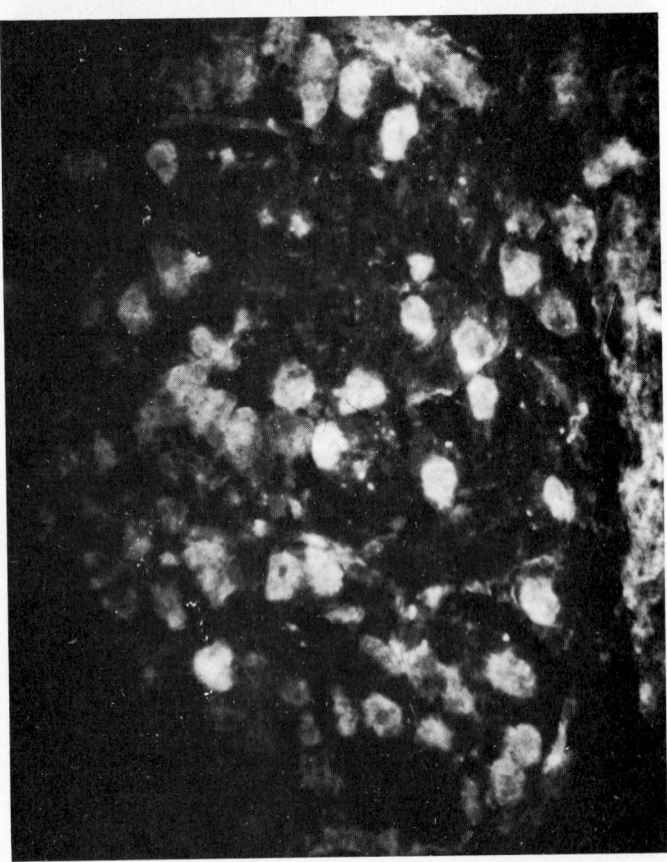

Fig. 9   Normal human gastric mucosa treated with (above) normal serum, (below) pernicious anaemia serum containing parietal canalicular antibody. Both subsequently treated with fluorescein-labelled antihuman gamma-globulin (indirect Coombs' technique).

gastrin-activity is found in some but not all patients with pernicious anaemia. However, though relative sparing of the antral mucosa is found in 60–80 per cent of patients with pernicious anaemia, this phenomenon has not been demonstrated in relatives of pernicious anaemia patients, subjects with iron deficiency anaemia, thyroid diseases, Addison's disease, or juvenile diabetes mellitus, in a proportion of whom parietal cell canalicular antibodies are found (Table 2). Unfortunately studies in which gastric mucosal histology

Table 2   Frequency of parietal cell canaliculi antibody in pernicious anaemia, first-order relatives of pernicious anaemia patients, and other diseases

Pernicious anaemia	
< 60 years	93%
> 60 years	76%
Pernicious anaemia relatives	40%
Iron-deficiency anaemia	30%
Thyroid disease	30%
Juvenile diabetes mellitus	20%
Adrenalitis	30%

has been correlated with humoral antibody findings in these various diseases have not been reported. As is shown in Table 3 gastric mucosal disease does not occur in all patients with chronic iron deficiency, but we do not know whether those patients with histologically proven chronic gastritis have circulating gastric antibodies and the others do not. However, good correlation has been shown in iron-deficient subjects between hypo- or achlorhydria and the presence of parietal canalicular antibodies in the serum.

Table 3   Gastric histology in iron deficiency anaemia

	Controls	Iron deficient
Normal	71	26
Superficial gastritis	6	31
Atrophic gastritis	10	33
Gastric atrophy	13	10

Derived from Davidson, W. M. B. and Markson, J. L. (1955), *Lancet* ii, 639.

It is of interest that in a small percentage of subjects with chronic antral gastritis circulating antibodies to a G cell, cytoplasmic antigen have been detected, the nature of which is not yet known. The frequency is clearly too low for this finding to provide a useful screening test, but it may later prove to have discriminatory power.

The weaknesses of the immunological classification are manifold. For example, humoral antibodies to gastric antigens are not detected in all subjects with proven pernicious anaemia; in other diseases such as adrenalitis, thyrotoxicosis, or juvenile diabetes mellitus, gastric antibodies are found in lower but significant frequency, as well as adrenal, thyroid, or β-islet cell antibodies. A number of these subjects, both with and without detectable gastric antibodies, have the functional lesion of pernicious anaemia, but the distribution of the gastritic process has not been evaluated, and many published reports of humoral gastric antibodies have not been correlated with corresponding studies of gastric histology.

In a number of studies of gastric histology it has been claimed that humoral antibodies to the gastric parietal cell may be detected in the absence of demonstrable gastritic change. These claims are based on methods of antibody detection which involve the use of rat gastric mucosa as the antigen-containing tissue. This is known to give a large percentage of false positive values with human sera. In our own experience and that of others humoral parietal canalicular antibodies have 100 per cent specificity. The sensitivity is of the order of 85 per cent for the gastric lesion of pernicious anaemia. In the chronic gastritis associated with gastric and duodenal ulcer disease tests for gastric antibodies are invariably negative.

Cell-mediated immunity. Studies by several groups using lymphocyte transformation or macrophage migration inhibition suggest that in almost 100 per cent of subjects with pernicious anaemia there is evidence of auto-allergic response to human or porcine intrinsic factor or various human gastric mucosal extracts, even in patients in whom tests for humoral antibodies are negative. The lymphocytes of some subjects with biopsy-proven chronic atrophic gastritis without the demonstrable lesion of pernicious anaemia may also give positive results. The subsequent course of these subjects is not known; they may develop pernicious anaemia later. The most consistent results with regard to cellular immunity have been obtained with intrinsic factor as antigen. There are reports that in some patients, who have pernicious anaemia and variable dysgammaglobulinaemia, tests of cell-mediated immunity are sometimes positive, though no humoral auto-antibodies are detected.

In chronic atrophic gastritis not associated with the lesion of pernicious anaemia there have been few studies of cellular immunity. It has been shown that cell-mediated immune responses do not occur in subjects with peptic ulcer disease, gastric or duodenal, either before or after various types of surgery.

Clinical classification of gastritis

Clinically, acute and chronic gastritis diagnosed by gastroscopic biopsy are both frequently asymptomatic and their clinical significance lies in various complications or sequelae such as haemorrhage from erosions, gastric ulceration, pernicious anaemia, and gastric carcinoma. The following clinical classification applies to gastritis associated with symptoms for which the patient seeks medical care.

Acute gastritis. Endoscopic studies have shown that acute gastritis following ingestion of drugs such as salicylates, phenylbutazone, or alcohol is often asymptomatic although there may be mild anorexia. Bleeding may produce the first clinical evidence of the gastritic process. In staphylococcal toxin or salmonella food poisoning the resulting acute gastritis is associated with anorexia, epigastric discomfort or pain, and nausea, suggesting that another factor than mucosal damage is responsible. Vomiting, followed by dry heaving or retching may prostrate the patient, who is initially pale and sweating and later dehydrated.

If haematemesis occurs, the sequence of events is important in making a diagnosis. If the vomitus is bloody from the start, haemorrhagic gastritis or bleeding peptic ulcer are the likely causes. It must be emphasized that acute haemorrhagic gastritis is an important cause of upper gastrointestinal bleeding, constituting in some series 30 per cent or more of all cases.

If haematemesis occurs after one or more bouts of vomiting, there is a strong possibility of a mucosal tear in the cardiac region or less commonly in the oesophagus (*Mallory–Weiss syndrome*).

For periods ranging from hours to one to two days after the onset, fluids and food may not be retained; intravenous fluid support is then necessary. During the attack there is reduction or absence of acid secretion, which is presumed to be due to breakdown in the mucosal barrier with back-diffusion of hydrogen ions into the blood but could in part be due to buffering of acid by serum proteins and blood. Recovery is the rule and occurs quite rapidly. Histologically the mucosa may be normal within one week or less from onset and sometimes in a matter of hours.

It is clear from systematic biopsy and endoscopic studies that acute gastritis may be asymptomatic. Beaumont's description in 1833 of the gastric mucosa of Alexis St Martin, who had a permanent gastric fistula as a consequence of a gunshot wound, following excessive intake of alcohol is not only the first recorded description of acute erosive gastritis, but is also notable for the absence of

symptoms associated with these changes. The introduction of aggressive gastric endoscopy in cases of haematemesis and melaena stressed the importance of haemorrhagic gastritis as a source of upper gastrointestinal bleeding. In some series almost 30 per cent of clinically significant upper gastrointestinal bleeding has been due to acute gastric mucosal lesions. Various types of blood loss have been described. Diffuse weeping is sometimes observed by the endoscopist or the surgeon at gastrectomy, when recognizable erosions or ulcers are not apparent. It occurs from any part of body or antrum. However, small multiple discrete erosions with bleeding or dark, clotted bases are the commoner lesion. Some observers arbitrarily classify erosions as less than 10 mm in diameter, larger lesions being described as acute ulcers, but others restrict the use of the term ulcer to lesions penetrating below the mucosa.

Acute infectious gastritis. Anorexia, nausea, and sometimes vomiting occur in febrile illnesses, and histological changes are seen in gastric mucosa similar to those observed in gastritis due to an exogenous agent. Frequently gastritis-producing medications have been ingested by such patients. However, there does seem to be a true association with the illness itself in addition to iatrogenic gastritis, and the extremest expression may be the acute, phlegmonous gastritis, now very rare, which has been described in children and occasionally in adults as a complication of septicaemia. In these patients invasion of the gastric mucosa and deeper structures with pyogenic organisms occurs and the clinical picture is one of an acute abdominal catastrophe involving threatened or actual perforation.

Acute corrosive gastritis. Corrosives, both strong acids and alkalis, and fixatives, such as phenol and formaldehyde, may produce severe damage to oesophagus and stomach when ingested by accident or in suicidal attempts. Severe burning substernal and epigastric pain ensue immediately following ingestion. Vomiting sometimes follows. Hypotensive shock and collapse are common. Perforation may occur if the full thickness of the stomach wall is involved.

Chronic gastritis. Uncomplicated chronic atrophic gastritis is usually asymptomatic. However, some patients who complain of chronic dyspepsia and in whom peptic ulcer disease has been excluded radiologically and endoscopically, are found on gastric endoscopy and biopsy to have chronic gastritis. The possible contribution of reflux oesophagitis to the patient's complaint is not always entertained and there is in consequence some persisting uncertainty about the symptomatology of chronic gastritis. In the past 25 years I have seen a few patients whose symptoms provide persuasive evidence that gastric inflammatory disease without ulcer can be symptomatic. They have had anorexia and persistent epigastric pain unrelieved by antacids, and have been found to be hypochlorhydric or achlorhydric in the face of maximal doses of histamine or pentagastrin, and they have biopsy-proven chronic atrophic gastritis of considerable severity in the absence of other demonstrable disease.

Chronic gastritis therefore usually presents clinically as a finding associated with an attack of acute erosive gastritis, with peptic ulcer disease, gastric carcinoma, pernicious anaemia, or hypochromic microcytic anaemia.

It must be clear from the foregoing that no useful clinical classification of gastritis is possible.

Prevalence of gastritis

Acute gastritis must be a frequent event that is usually undiagnosed. It is also an important cause of clinically significant upper gastrointestinal bleeding. For this reason emergency gastroduodenoscopy is recommended by many in patients presenting with haematemesis, since surgery in unequivocal acute erosive gastritis is rarely indicated. Emergency endoscopy has not been shown to reduce mortality but it makes it possible to manage such patients conservatively with greater confidence.

Acute gastric erosions are the cause of about 10–25 per cent of significant upper gastrointestinal bleeds depending on the patient population. In the majority there is a history of exposure to alcohol, aspirin, or other drugs but in approximately one-quarter of such patients no predisposing cause is found.

The prevalence of chronic gastritis in any population has yet to be determined, since non-invasive markers of gastric mucosal disease have only recently been developed and have still to be evaluated by correlation with mucosal biopsy findings. Circulating parietal canalicular antibodies are detectable in apparently healthy individuals without any history of gastrointestinal disease. These subjects, for reasons already given, almost certainly have chronic gastritis. The percentage of positive serological findings increases with age and is as high as 15–20 per cent over the age of 60. There have been no gastric biopsy studies of large numbers of healthy subjects selected randomly to determine what percentage of the gastric serologically negative individuals have chronic gastritis. Similar difficulties apply to other potentially useful markers such as serum pepsin and gastrin values. Gastric serology is negative in almost all subjects who have or have had peptic ulcer disease and in most patients with gastric carcinoma, except those with precedent pernicious anaemia. Our knowledge of the prevalence of chronic gastritis is restricted to special groups of patients with pernicious anaemia, iron deficiency anaemia, peptic ulcer, and some endocrine conditions.

Causes of gastritis

Acute gastritis. The factors involved in pathogenesis are not clearly understood in spite of the clear endoscopic and histological evidence that ingestion of certain drugs and bacterial toxins is associated with acute mucosal inflammation and erosions in man and in experimental animals. Also well documented as causes of acute gastritis are systemically administered cancer chemotherapeutic agents, thermal injury, ionizing radiation, and stressful events such as severe trauma, surgery outside the gastrointestinal tract, and Gram-negative septicaemic shock. Similar mucosal changes have been produced in experimental animals by a variety of means, including the stress of induced exhaustion. Two theories, not mutually exclusive, have been advanced. The first, which is supported by cell-turnover studies in animals, is that inhibition of epithelial regeneration, with consequent failure to maintain integrity of the surface of the mucosa, is an important factor. The second is that cell-protective mechanisms, which may involve prostaglandins E_1, E_2, and A are impaired, permeability of protective surfaces is increased, and damage is produced by a range of cytotoxic agents which includes hydrochloric acid and proteolytic enzymes.

To date the important issue, namely how to prevent acute gastritis consequent on necessary therapy, has not been resolved.

Chronic gastritis. Many factors have been proposed for the pathogenesis of chronic gastritis of the body of the stomach.

Some of the unresolved problems are: do repeated insults to the gastric mucosa, each causing an acute gastritis, ultimately produce chronic gastritis; do the majority of cases of less severe chronic gastritis tend to progress, as Faber believed, through chronic atrophic gastritis to gastric atrophy?

There is evidence that the habit of drinking very hot fluids results in chronic gastritis and regular ingestion of ethanol in amounts sufficient to produce repeated acute gastritis may have a similar effect, though this has been disputed. Follow-up studies of the effects of ionizing radiation on the gastric mucosa in man emphasize the remarkable ability of the mucosa to restore itself to normal after severe injury in all but a few subjects. The well-established increase of chronic gastritis and gastric atrophy with advancing age does not support specially any theory of causation (Fig. 10).

It is possible that genetic or other environmental factors mediate or modify the action of mechanical, physical, chemical, or other

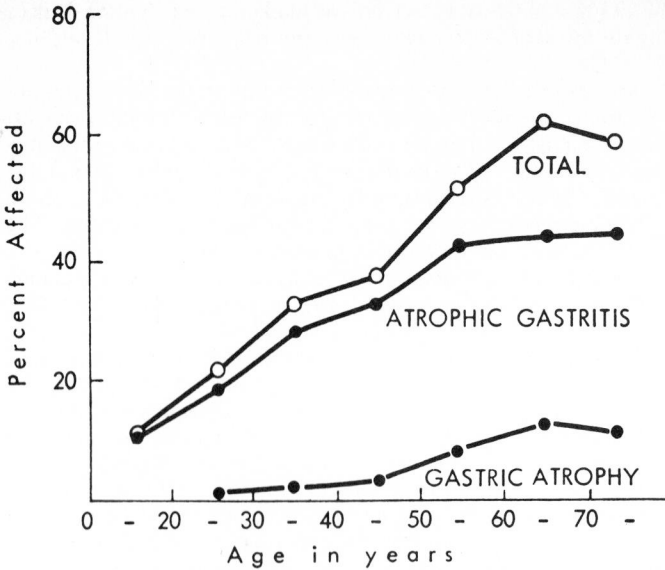

Fig. 10 Prevalence of chronic gastritis with age. (In Witts (1966), based on data of Joske, R. A., Finckh, E. S., and Wood, I. J. (1955). Gastric biopsy: study of 1000 consecutive successful biopsies. *Q. Jl Med.* **24**, 269).

trauma so that in some cases a self-perpetuating series of events occurs, the predominant features of which are: (*a*) chronic inflammatory response to the mucosa; (*b*) rapid turnover of stem cells in the neck region of the mucosal glands and of mucosal epithelial cells; (*c*) inhibition of normal differentiation into parietal and chief cells or possibly more rapid destruction of newly-formed cells of these types; and (*d*) metaplasia.

Infection, nutritional deficiencies, or endocrine disturbances have been proposed as causal or contributory factors but in none of these is there unequivocal evidence of aetiological involvement. There appears to be a true association between chronic gastritis and hypochromic anaemia due to iron deficiency. However, coexistence of the two is not invariable (Table 3) and similar changes are not seen in experimental iron deficiency. Other factors, such as other nutritional deficiencies or disturbed immune homeostasis, may have had an adjuvant effect in those subjects in whom the anaemia and chronic gastritis coexist. There is an excellent review of the debate as to whether the gastric lesion precedes the development of iron deficiency or vice versa by L. J. Witts in his monograph *The Stomach in Anaemia.* Currently both views are tenable and it is likely that in some subjects iron deficiency may be the primary event and in others the chronic gastritis.

In chronic gastritis associated with immunological responses, currently referred to as type A, there is much evidence to support the concept that these responses have pathogenic roles. The alternative hypothesis, that the immune phenomena are secondary to mucosal damage, is untenable in the light of clinical observation and experimental evidence. No gastric mucosal injury of any kind has been shown to be followed by humoral or cell-mediated immune reactions to gastric antigens. In type A gastritis there is, at least in the later stages, significantly greater pathological change in the gastric body than the antrum and the auto-allergic responses are directed against antigens in the parietal cells which are largely confined to the gastric body. Gastric antibodies are found not only in serum but in gastric juice and in immunoglobulin-containing plasma cells in the chronically inflamed body mucosa. Human parietal canalicular antibodies inhibit acid secretion of parietal cells *in vitro* and their repeated injection into animals results in reduction of the parietal cell mass with, however, little inflammatory response. In some species atrophic gastritis and reduced gastric acid secretion follow immunization with antigens from the gastric body.

IF antibodies are also found in the gastric juice, and gastric mucosal plasma cells of patients with pernicious anaemia. There is convincing evidence that their presence inhibits the biological activity of IF and in some patients may be the decisive event in the full expression of IF deficiency.

There is some evidence of sensitization to IF and other gastric antigens of lymphocytes from patients with pernicious anaemia and from some with atrophic gastritis without pernicious anaemia, although there are disparities which may in part be due to variations in antigen purity. But no direct cell-mediated cytotoxicity has yet been established.

What initiates the gastric immune responses in unknown. No evidence of exogenous antigens derived from micro-organisms and cross-reactive with IF or parietal canalicular antigen has been obtained. Genetic susceptibility has been explored, since pernicious anaemia occurs at least 20 times more frequently in first-order relatives of patients with the disease and parietal canalicular antibodies are found in up to 40 per cent of such relatives. However, studies of histocompatibility antigen haplotypes have not yet provided any support for such genetic susceptibility.

Other aetiological factors must be considered in the majority of cases of chronic gastritis. One is that the integrity of the mucosa depends in part on trophic factors, either hormonal or mediated by the vagus. Gastrin itself has a trophic effect on gastric body mucosa, but lack of circulating gastrin is not evident in most subjects with chronic atrophic gastritis. With regard to vagal influences observations of the consequences of truncal or highly selective vagotomy in the gastric mucosa are of interest. In subjects with duodenal ulcer disease there is almost invariably present some degree of chronic gastritis which tends, as in pre-pyloric ulcer disease, to be most severe in the antrum and lower lesser curve, with relative sparing of the fundus, body in the greater curve and high lesser curve. Following vagotomy improvement occurs in the chronic antral gastritis but deterioration is seen in the more proximal areas, including the fundus, in which atrophic areas occur. These studies suggest loss of some vagally mediated trophic influence. They also provide a positive answer to the question whether chronic mucosal lesions may regress or progress and, further, make it highly unlikely, at least in this situation, that biliary reflux is an important cause of chronic gastritis as has been suggested. Whether reflux of duodenal contents is a significant cause of gastritis has still to be demonstrated.

Further, these observed changes parallel those suggested by an integrated, cross-sectional analysis of gastric biopsy studies of a substantial Finnish population of first-order relatives of patients with pernicious anaemia. An apparent improvement in antral gastritis appears to occur as the body mucosa becomes increasingly atrophic and non-secretory.

Thus a possible sequence of events might be that the antral mucosa is sometimes chronically damaged by secretions of the body mucosa and that when the latter decrease as a consequence of vagal interruption or auto-allergic damage, the antrum undergoes partial recovery. The question whether a minor degree of atrophic gastritis usually or invariably progresses towards total atrophy remains unanswered. In some special cases in which evidence of auto-immunity is present, such progression has been documented. In the majority of subjects with chronic gastritis progression to the lesion of pernicious anaemia is clearly rare.

Management

Acute gastritis almost always responds to conservative treatment. Only antacids should be given by mouth and, since early recovery is the rule, total parenteral feeding is unnecessary and only water, glucose, and electrolytes are given intravenously. It is always advisable, if there is a background of alcoholism, to include B complex vitamins, especially thiamin.

If bleeding continues, there may be need for replacement with blood and intermittent suction is maintained through a nasogastric tube, which is kept in position to monitor loss and keep the gastric lumen empty. Frequent lavage with cold or iced water keeps the lumen of the tube patent, but probably does not affect bleeding.

The rate of loss of blood from extensive erosive gastritis may be surprisingly high to the inexperienced.

No medications have been shown to be effective. Secretion of gastric acid appears to be reduced or absent, because of buffering by blood in the lumen and possibly because of back diffusion of hydrogen ions. On this assumption, we routinely give 50–100 mmol liquid antacid every two hours after significant bleeding has ceased. Cimetidine, an H_2 inhibitor, is currently also much used. The value of either is unproven. The acute phase usually terminates within 72 hours and the patient should be given oral liquids and a soft but otherwise normal diet as soon as hunger returns.

Less than 5 per cent of patients with significant haemorrhagic gastritis require surgery. Unfortunately such patients are frequently those with complicating disease, especially alcoholic cirrhosis and present a poor surgical risk, complicated by coagulopathy associated with hepatic damage, malnutrition, and massive transfusion of blood. The surgical treatment of choice is not agreed upon. Vagotomy with pyloroplasty is widely done and seems to be successful in arresting haemorrhage in a majority of patients, for reasons which are not clear. In a few cases partial gastrectomy and, rarely, total gastrectomy are performed, usually when vagotomy with pyloroplasty has failed and as a last resort. The mortality is high. Physicians and surgeons should work together in the care of all patients with haemorrhagic gastritis, as in other cases of gastro-intestinal bleeding.

Following recovery the patient requires careful counselling, particularly about use of gastric irritants. Medications must be reviewed and substitutes found for any suspected of causing mucosal damage, if possible, or, if not, their mode of use changed.

There is no treatment of chronic gastritis as such, only of associated conditions, such as iron-deficiency or the sequelae, such as cobalamin deficiency.

Corticosteroids have been shown to improve transiently function of the gastric body mucosa but the doses required are relatively large and there is no place for these drugs in maintenance treatment. Opinions differ about aggressive screening for early detection of gastric carcinoma. This must involve serial endoscopy, gastric cytology or radiography, procedures poorly tolerated by the aged who constitute the population at risk. The value of examining the stool for occult blood as a means of improving outcome has not been established. My own practice is to recommend patients visit the outpatient clinic every six months and that gastroscopy be done annually if the patient wishes it.

Prognosis. The prognosis in acute gastritis must depend largely on whether patients change their habits and reliable figures are not available.

In chronic atrophic gastritis the two potential sequelae are pernicious anaemia and gastric adenocarcinoma. The latter may occur in the absence of the lesion of pernicious anaemia and on occasion in stomachs still capable of secreting detectable amounts of acid, or may complicate established pernicious anaemia. The estimated chances of the latter are approximately three times that in the general population and the risk of carcinoma of the stomach in subjects with simple atrophic gastritis may be twenty times greater than in the general population, though there are population or regional variations.

References

Faber, K. (1935). *Gastritis and its consequences.* Oxford University Press, London.
Ivey, K. J. (1971). Acute haemorrhagic gastritis: modern concepts based on pathogenesis. *Gut* **12**, 750.
Morson, B. C. and Dawson, I. M. P. (1979). *Gastrointestinal pathology*, 2nd edn. ch. 10. Blackwell Scientific Publications, Oxford.
Taylor, K. B. (1976). Immune aspects of pernicious anaemia and atrophic gastritis. *Clinics Haemat.* **5**, 497.
Whitehead, R., Truelove, S. C., and Gear, M. W. L. (1972). The histological diagnosis of chronic gastritis in fibroptic gastroscope biopsy specimens. *J. clin. Path.* **25**, 1.
Witts, L. J. (1966). *The stomach and anaemia.* Athlone Press, London.

Immune disorders

A. D. B. Webster

Introduction

Morphology of the gut associated lymphoid tissue (GALT). The gastro-intestinal tract contains numerous plasma cells which are mainly situated in the lamina propria of the bowel wall. The majority of these cells in normal subjects secrete the IgA isotype although IgG, IgM, and IgE secreting cells are also present. Experiments in mice indicate that these cells are derived from immunoblasts which were initially sensitized in the gut and which then migrated via the thoracic duct and the blood back to the gastrointestinal tract.

Lymphocytes are also found between the epithelial cells (intra-epithelial lymphocytes). Most of these are T lymphocytes. Their role is not known but it is likely that they are actively engaged in an immune reaction rather than just leaking out of the bowel.

Peyers' patches and appendix. These are specialized lymphoid organs which have been extensively studied in animals such as rabbits. Their precise role in man is not known.

Peyers' patches appear at 24 weeks' gestation and are most numerous at 12 years of age when they number up to 305. They are present throughout the intestinal tract but are most numerous in the distal ileum. They consist of a variable number of lymphoid nodules which have distinct regions (Fig. 1). The lymphoid nodules in the

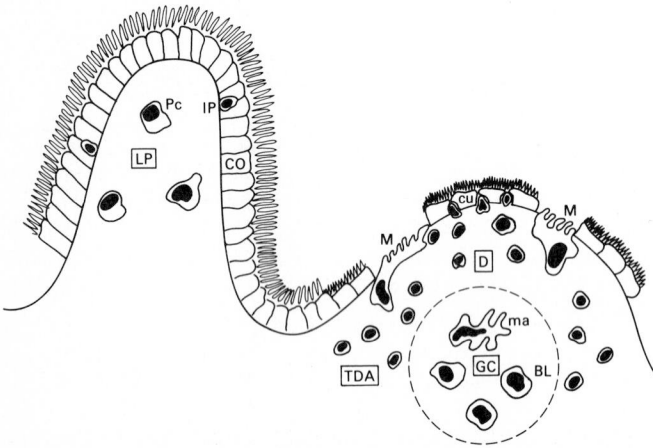

Fig. 1 Diagram showing the immune apparatus of the gastrointestinal tract. On the left, plasma cells (Pc) can be seen in the lamina propria (LP), together with intra-epithelial lymphocytes (IP) between the columna epithelial cells (CO). On the right, there is a Peyer's patch covered by cuboidal epithelium (CU) with occasional 'M' cells (M). The Peyer's patch consists of three areas: (*a*) the dome (D) where there are many intra-epithelial lymphocytes; (*b*) the thymus dependent area (TDA) containing small lymphocytes; and (*c*) the germinal centre (GC) containing macrophages (ma) and B lymphoblasts (BL).

appendix are similar but much larger. The mucosa overlying these nodules is different from that in the rest of the small bowel by being cuboidal instead of columna. The mucosa also contains specialized M cells, so-called because they have microfolds instead of villi. The germinal centres contain predominantly B lymphocytes and macrophages while the thymic-dependent areas consist of T lymphocytes. These cells enter the nodule via the circulation because there are no afferent lymphatics. However, there are efferent lymphatics through which cells can re-enter the circulation. It is thought that the specialized nature of the overlying epithelium of the nodules, particularly the presence of M cells, allows direct access of bacteria and other antigens which can stimulate a local immune response.

Secretory immunoglobulins. There are immunoglobulins in the saliva, and in the gastric and intestinal secretions. IgA predominates in saliva although in jejunal and colonic juice the concentration of IgA and IgG is similar. IgM is not normally present in saliva but is found in small bowel juice. The IgA secreted by plasma cells in the lamina propria passes through the epithelial cells where secretory piece is added to the J chain of the immunoglobulin molecule. IgA with secretory piece (SIgA) is then released into the bowel lumen where it tends to become concentrated in the mucous layer overlying the epithelial cells. The presence of secretory piece offers some protection against proteolytic enzymes and hence increases the life of the molecule in the bowel lumen. Secretory piece can also bind to IgM but not to IgG. The immunoglobulin concentration in the intestine of rats is enhanced by the selective excretion of monomeric plasma IgA into the bile. It is not yet certain whether this also occurs in man.

It is not known whether secretory immunoglobulins play a major role in protection against intestinal infection despite the fact that oral immunization with organisms such as polio virus leads to the production of specific IgA antibodies which will prevent disease. However, British patients with primary antibody deficiency do not usually suffer from significant gastrointestinal infection. Nevertheless, the situation may be very different in the tropics where gastrointestinal infections are common.

Secretory IgA may also form complexes with potential allergens in food and prevent their absorption. Against this view is the fact that most patients with selective IgA deficiency do not suffer from food allergy. It is well known that repeated oral feeding of antigens in animals can induce a state of specific tolerance to the antigen. The precise mechanism is unknown but this unresponsiveness can be transferred to other animals of the same strain by T 'suppressor' lymphocytes obtained from mesenteric lymph nodes. This may be a very important mechanism in preventing immune reactions to food proteins and commensal intestinal bacteria.

Immunodeficiency diseases

See also Section 4.

Selective IgA deficiency. *Definition.* It is useful to be precise about the terminology of selective IgA deficiency. A serum level of IgA below the level of detection by radial immunodiffusion (about 1 mg/100 ml) is referred to as 'IgA deficiency'. Levels between 1 and 10 mg/100 ml are referred to as 'low serum IgA'. By definition, the serum IgG and IgM are normal.

Aetiology. Primary IgA deficiency is an autosomal dominant or recessive disorder which occurs in about 1 in 700 of the population. It is also associated with defects in chromosome 18 and is common in the autosomal recessive syndrome of ataxia telangiectasia. Both IgA deficiency and low serum IgM may be due to drugs such as phenytoin or penicillamine, and to virus infections such as congenital rubella.

Auto-antibodies. Patients with selective IgA deficiency commonly have serum antibodies to food proteins. For instance, about 36 per cent of IgA deficient blood donors have serum antibodies to milk as compared to 0.3 per cent of healthy controls. IgA deficient subjects also tend to have auto-antibodies to antigens such as IgA itself and collagen. Although antibodies to IgA may cause reactions during blood transfusions, the other auto-antibodies are usually harmless.

Clinical features. *Infection*. There is good evidence for an association between low serum IgA and recurrent upper respiratory tract infections. Paradoxically, there is no convincing evidence of an increase in upper or lower respiratory tract infections in patients with complete IgA deficiency.

Gastrointestinal complications. Chronic diarrhoea and malabsorption is common in patients with IgA deficiency after truncal vagotomy and gastroenterostomy for duodenal ulcer. This is due to overgrowth of commensal bacteria in the upper intestinal tract, presumably because of a deficiency of local antibody and achlorhydria. Impairment of gastrointestinal motility is probably also important since vagotomy alone in IgA deficient patients does not predispose to diarrhoea.

There is about an eight-fold increase of IgA deficiency in patients with coeliac disease as compared to the general population. One possibility is that the IgA deficiency exacerbates the reaction to gluten in the intestine in genetically susceptible individuals, probably because IgG-gluten complexes form which activate complement.

It is a widely held view that secretory IgA helps prevent absorption of food antigens through the mucosal surface. This is supported by the relatively high serum antibody titres to milk protein in infants during the first three months of life when their serum IgA is very low. Furthermore, infants with a family history of atopy who have particularly low levels of serum IgA are prone to infantile eczema when they are fed on cows milk. Infants with weight loss, vomiting, and diarrhoea related to cows milk also tend to have a low serum IgA and a family history of allergy. It is not known whether the combination of low IgA and allergy to milk in infants predisposes to allergic eczema and asthma in later childhood. One important issue in interpreting IgA levels in infancy is that the normal ranges are very wide and some normal infants have extremely low levels. The failure to establish normal ranges in the majority of studies because of ethical considerations has cast some doubt on the significance of these findings.

General strategy and management. Patients undergoing truncal vagotomy with gastroenterostomy should be screened for IgA deficiency before operation. The necessity for operation should be reconsidered in those with IgA deficiency and gastroenterostomy avoided if possible. Current information suggests that it is reasonable to advise mothers to breast feed infants for at least the first three months of life when there is a family history of atopy. It is not known whether such children should continue to avoid potential allergens if their serum IgA remains low.

Hypogammaglobulinaemia. (See also Sections 4 and 19.)
Definition. Primary hypogammaglobulinaemia is a rare condition which is usually non-familial although there is an X-linked type which starts in early childhood. The disease can occur at any age and the lifetime prevalence of the syndrome for males is about 15 per million and for females, 4 per million of the population. Most patients have very low or unmeasurable levels of all serum immunoglobulin classes although there are some who retain the ability to make significant amounts of IgM. The association of hypogammaglobulinaemia and thymoma probably constitutes a distinct syndrome. The aetiology of these diseases is not known.

Secondary hypogammaglobulinaemia commonly occurs in chronic lymphatic leukaemia and myeloma. Hypogammaglobulinaemia also occurs in severe protein-losing enteropathy, the main effect being a lowering of the serum IgG which is usually not severe enough to cause symptoms.

Clinical features. Recurrent upper and lower respiratory tract infections are the main problem. However, clinically significant gastrointestinal complications also occur in about 10 per cent of patients in England.

Periodontal disease and caries. There is an impression that patients with hypogammaglobulinaemia have a low incidence of caries. This is surprising in view of the evidence that specific antibodies to *Streptococcus mutants*, a commensal cariogenic organism in the mouth, protect against caries in monkeys. However, further work is needed to clarify whether the frequent taking of antibiotics by hypogammaglobulinaemic patients protects them against caries.

The stomach. Achlorhydria occurs in about 30 per cent of patients with the adult onset type of primary hypogammaglobulinaemia. The incidence in the X-linked and childhood onset type is not known. A minority of patients also fail to secrete intrinsic factor and may present with pernicious anaemia (PA). Histological examination of the stomach shows inflammatory changes and mucosal atrophy which usually affects all areas of the stomach. These patients have normal serum gastrin levels in contrast to the high levels often found in patients with classical PA. These differences are probably explained by the severity of the inflammation around the antral gastrin secreting cells, patients with classical PA having relatively little antral involvement.

There is about a 50-fold increase in gastric carcinoma in patients with primary hypogammaglobulinaemia as compared to the general population. This is much higher than the five-fold increase in patients with classical PA. Both these groups of patients have considerable numbers of nitrate-reducing organisms in their stomachs and hypogammaglobulinaemic patients with achlorhydria have particularly high gastric juice nitrite levels. This could be the explanation for the high incidence of gastric carcinoma in hypogammaglobulinaemia since nitrites are readily converted to carcinogenic nitrosamines.

Nodular lymphoid hyperlasia (NLH). Multiple sub-mucosal lymphoid nodules commonly occur in the small bowel, and occasionally in the stomach and colon of patients with adult onset primary hypogammaglobulinaemia. Such patients usually retain some ability to produce IgM immunoglobulin. The ultrastructure of these nodules is similar to Peyers' patches and lymphoblasts containing IgM are found in the centres of the follicles. The condition probably represents hypertrophy of the gut associated lymphoid tissue in response to antigens in the gut lumen. It is not premalignant in patients with primary hypogammaglobulinaemia although it has been observed in other apparently immunocompetent patients who have intestinal lymphomas. NLH can occur transiently in normal children in the terminal ileum or colon where it may cause abdominal pain or rectal bleeding.

Gastrointestinal infection. *Giardiasis*. This is an important cause of malabsorption in patients with primary hypogammaglobulinaemia. To make the diagnosis, the stools should first be examined for parasite cysts. If none are found, then trophozoites should be looked for either in a sample of jejunal juice or in the mucous smeared onto a slide from a jejunal biopsy. The treatment is either a seven day course of metronidazole (2 g daily as a single dose) or mepacrin (100 mg three times daily for 10 days). Animal models of the disease have so far taught us very little about defence mechanisms against giardia parasites, although the high incidence of giardiasis in hypogammaglobulinaemia suggests that antibodies are important. Another factor in these patients may be the common occurrence of achlorhydria which may allow large numbers of organisms to reach the intestines.

Campylobacter enteritis. Patients with hypogammaglobulinaemia are particularly prone to Campylobacter infection which usually causes diarrhoea, sometimes with malabsorption, and may rarely cause an ascending chlolangitis and hepatitis. The organisms can usually be cultured from the stools. The treatment is a two-week course of erythromycin (500 mg four times daily) after which the stools should again be cultured to check that the treatment has been effective.

Other parasites. Cryptosporidium infection of the intestine has been reported in a few patients with either primary hypogammaglobulinaemia or with lymphomas being treated with cytotoxic drugs. This parasite belongs to the suborder Eimeria which also includes

Gastroenterology

toxoplasma and isospora, the latter being a documented cause of diarrhoea and malabsorption in immunosuppressed patients. Cryptosporidiosis seems to be a more serious condition than isosporiasis and most of the patients described have had intractable malabsorption with bouts of torrential watery diarrhoea requiring emergency electrolyte and water repletion. These cholera-like episodes are a useful clue to the diagnosis which can be confirmed by finding the parasites on the villous brush border of a jejunal biopsy by light microscopy. Electron microscopy is required to identify the organism formally. A negative finding on the first biopsy does not rule out the diagnosis and further biopsies may have to be taken if there is a high suspicion for the disease.

Some patients with isosporiasis have been cured by either stopping the immunosuppressive drugs or by giving co-trimoxazole. However, there is no known drug for cryptosporidiosis and most of the patients reported have eventually died of malnutrition.

Commensal gut bacteria. Most patients with primary hypogammaglobulinaemia in England and the USA only have a slightly raised number of bacteria in their jejunal juice (about 10^5 organisms/ml). This is well below the number of organisms found in the jejunal juice of patients with the blind loop syndrome ($\simeq 10^8$ organisms/ml). However, this is sometimes the only abnormal finding in patients with primary hypogammaglobulinaemia who complain of abdominal discomfort and steatorrhoea. At all events, it is common practice to treat these patients empirically with courses of tetracycline and metronidazole which sometimes improves their symptoms.

Miscellaneous syndromes. (See also Section 4). Intractable diarrhoea and malabsorption occurs in most infants with the syndrome of *severe combined immunodeficiency* where there is a defect of both humoral and cellular immunity. This is partly responsible for the characteristic wasting in this condition. The precise cause of the diarrhoea is usually not found but intestinal infection with *Candida albicans*, bacteria, or viruses has been described. Infants with selective T cell defects do not usually suffer from gastrointestinal complications.

Children with the *Wiskott–Aldrich syndrome* have a partial immunodeficiency together with thrombocytopenia and may develop bloody diarrhoea. This could possibly be due to food allergy as these children are frequently atopic with very high serum IgE levels.

Chronic mucocutaneous candidiasis is a disease of unknown aetiology which may be based on an immunological abnormality. Such patients may develop candidiasis of the intestinal tract with oesophageal strictures.

Patients with *chronic granulomatous disease* of childhood (see Section 19) have an autosomal or X-linked inherited defect which prevents their neutrophils and macrophages from killing certain bacteria. There may be hepatosplenomegaly due to granulomas and there is sometimes unexplained diarrhoea. Lactose intolerance with malabsorption also occurs. Jejunal biopsy is usually macroscopically normal although with special fixation procedures vacuolated histiocytes, similar to those seen in Whipple's disease, are often found in the lamina propria.

Acrodermatitis enteropathica. This autosomal recessive condition is due to zinc deficiency caused by inadequate zinc absorption. There is some evidence that the basic defect is a failure of the gut to secrete prostaglandins which facilitate zinc absorption. The clinical features appear shortly after weaning with diarrhoea, eczematous lesions on the extremities and around the mouth and anus, growth retardation, alopecia, and a mental state similar to autism. There may be a protein-losing enteropathy with secondary hypogammaglobulinaemia and there is often a marked depression of cellular immunity. A similar disease may occur in older children who are zinc deficient because of an inadequate diet. The condition responds completely to oral zinc supplements.

Immunodeficiency secondary to gut disease. Hypogammaglobulinaemia, particularly when IgG is mainly depressed, may be due to increased intestinal loss of gammaglobulin. A useful clue to this possibility is a low serum albumin, because there are no known conditions where gammaglobulin is selectively lost from the gut. The various conditions causing protein losing enteropathy are discussed on page 12.101.

Intestinal lymphangiectasia is one condition of particular immunological interest. The basic abnormality is an abnormal dilatation of the lymphatic vessels in the intestine which leads to leakage of protein and lymphocytes. There is a primary familial form in children who present with diarrhoea, malabsorption, and growth retardation. Such children may have abnormal lymphatics elsewhere in the body causing chylous ascites, pleural effusions, and localized areas of oedema. The condition may occur secondarily to lymphatic obstruction due to lymphomas in the intestine or constrictive pericarditis (see Fig. 3c, page 12.89).

The diagnosis is suspected when there is lymphopenia, hypoalbuminaemia, and hypogammaglobulinaemia. The diagnosis can be confirmed by finding dilated lymphatics in a jejunal biopsy. The primary form of the disease responds well to a low-fat diet with additional medium chain triglycerides. Steroids are useful when the condition is secondary to inflammatory bowel disease (see also pages 12.99 and 12.144).

Food hypersensitivity

Introduction. This is an area of medicine bedevilled by the generally unscientific manner in which it has been investigated. One reason for this has been the lack of knowledge of the basic mechanism of food hypersensitivity while another is the difficulty of carrying out controlled clinical studies in affected patients. Nevertheless, there are rare patients with convincing food hypersensitivity who develop anaphylactic type reactions, skin rashes, and even asthma when they eat foods such as nuts and fish. Whether food hypersensitivity is a common cause of eczema, asthma, and abdominal pain in children remains a controversial issue.

Definition. State of hypersensitivity to one or more food substances usually associated with the presence of specific IgE antibodies and positive immediate skin tests. The symptoms include anaphylaxis, eczema, asthma, and abdominal pain which cease after allergen avoidance, and recur after allergen challenge.

Aetiology. It used to be a commonly held view that potentially immunogenic food antigens could not cross the gut mucosa in significant amounts to induce an immune reaction; either because the molecules were too large or because they were complexed with IgA. However, experiments in the 1920s clearly demonstrated that food antigens can penetrate the gut to enter the circulation. This was initially shown by injecting serum from a patient with known sensitivity to cows' milk protein into the skin of a normal subject. A flare at the skin test site (positive Prausnitz–Kustner reaction) was then observed shortly after the normal subject ate the appropriate antigen, showing that this must have crossed the gut and triggered sensitized mast cells at the skin test site to release histamine. Further studies have shown that non-IgE antibodies to proteins in cows' milk and eggs do occur in infants, but only if a large amount of the relevant protein is ingested. However, these antibodies gradually disappear in the first few years of childhood. In contrast, relatively small amounts of protein are sufficient to induce antibodies, including those of the IgE type, in allergic children. Such infants tend to retain high levels of serum antibody throughout childhood. A similar situation occurs in allergic rhinitis due to pollen sensitivity where the difference between non-allergic and allergic subjects has been worked out in greater detail. In essence, allergic subjects have a genetically determined predisposition to make high levels of all classes of specific antibody when immunized with minute quantities of pollen.

Prevalence. There are no reliable estimates; probably about 0.5 per cent of infants are affected. This frequency declines with age, overt food hypersensitivity being extremely rare in adults.

Signs and symptoms. *Early or immediate reactions*. Table 1 shows the various symptoms which can occur within minutes up to two hours after exposure to allergens. IgE antibodies are predominantly involved in these reactions. Although a wide variety of food proteins might theoretically produce reactions, in practice only nuts, cows' milk, hens' eggs, and soya beans are documented examples.

Table 1 Symptoms and signs associated with early (less than 2 hours) and late (more than 2 hours) reactions to food allergens. These are listed with decreasing frequency. Those in italics are either rare or have not been substantiated adequately with a blind challenge test.

Early reactions	Late reactions
Asthma	Diarrhoea
Abdominal pain	Vomiting
Vomiting	*Asthma*
Urticaria	*Urticaria*
Anaphylaxis	*Dermatitis*
Diarrhoea	*Malabsorption*
Rhinitis	*Protein-losing enteropathy*
Angio-oedema	*Gastrointestinal bleeding with anaemia*
Dermatitis	*Alveolitis*
	Growth retardation

Late reactions. Table 1 also shows the symptoms which can occur several hours to days after allergen ingestion. Some of these reactions are probably mediated by IgE, although other classes of antibody may also be involved. The delay in the symptoms is attributable to the time taken for the target organ (e.g. the skin) to manifest an inflammatory reaction. It is not known what excites this reaction although there is some evidence that immune complexes may be involved. There is no evidence that the lesions are caused by a classical delayed hypersensitivity reaction.

Gastroenteropathy in infants. Severe diarrhoea and vomiting may develop 12–36 hours after ingestion of certain foods, particularly cows' milk. Jejunal biopsies taken during the acute phase show villous atrophy and lymphocyte infiltration similar to that seen in gluten enteropathy. It is likely that this disease has an immunological basis although this is still to be demonstrated. IgE antibodies do not seem to be involved and there is usually no family history of allergy. The treatment is to remove the offending food from the diet. However, the disease is usually only transient and such children can start taking a normal diet again at about two to three years of age.

There is a chronic form of gastroenteropathy in infants characterized by mild or intermittent diarrhoea, hypochromic anaemia, hypoproteinaemic oedema, and retarded growth. There is often an eosinophilia and jejunal biopsies show eosinophilic infiltration of the lamina propria without villous atrophy. Affected infants have high titres of precipitins to milk proteins in their serum. The treatment is to eliminate milk from the diet but the children can usually start taking milk again after about six months. The mechanism of this disease is not known.

Diagnosis. *Skin tests*. There is controversy over the usefulness of skin tests in the diagnosis of food hypersensitivity. This may be partly due to some patients having only small amounts of specific IgE fixed to skin mast cells together with a failure to confirm the diagnosis by double blind challenge. However, the general impression is that skin tests are useful in making a diagnosis.

Immediate hypersensitivity 'prick' tests are the most useful, a wheal and flare reaction occurring within minutes in allergic patients. This is mediated by reaginic IgE antibodies on mast cells which, when they combine with antigen, trigger the mast cell to release histamine. An IgG antibody to milk protein was found in some children with allergic symptoms developing about 24 hours after milk ingestion. It has been suggested that such an antibody may account for the transient positive prick tests which are sometimes seen in non-allergic children after first exposure to milk.

In vitro *tests*. There has been much recent enthusiasm for radio-alergosorbent (RAST) tests for identifying serum IgE antibodies to a variety of allergens. However, it is likely that such tests have no advantage over properly performed skin tests and may even be less sensitive. One problem is that IgE antibody may be rapidly fixed to tissue mast cells and consequently not be measurable in serum.

Challenge tests. The suspected foods should first be eliminated from the diet so that the patient is asymptomatic at the time of the test. When the offending food is not known, then the patient may need to take an elimination diet which consists essentially of rice, canned fruit, and vegetables until he is asymptomatic. The patient should be unaware of what is being offered to him during the challenge test. If possible, the foods to be tested should be in the dried form and placed in capsules. A suitable placebo should be used. Such tests are unnecessary and dangerous in patients who have had anaphylactic reactions.

Differential diagnosis. The diagnosis is obvious when patients have anaphylactic reactions following ingestion of certain foods. However, patients with chronic symptoms such as abdominal pain, diarrhoea, and vomiting must be investigated for other causes (e.g. infection or Crohn's disease). Disaccharide intolerance, which may be secondary to an allergic gastroenteropathy, should be suspected in patients with chronic diarrhoea, particularly if the stools have a pH below 6 and contain reducing substances. Gluten enteropathy must always be considered in patients with malabsorption and steatorrhoea. If the jejunal biopsy shows villous atrophy, then a trial of a gluten-free diet is indicated. Psychologically unstable adults who are chronic purgative 'addicts' are often very difficult to diagnose and may be thought to have a food hypersensitivity. The diarrhoea in such patients usually improves when they are in hospital under observation.

Treatment. The only effective treatment is to eliminate the offending food from the diet. Oral disodium cromoglycate is still under trial but there is no compelling evidence so far that this is effective. Corticosteroids are useful in severe gluten-sensitive enteropathy and eosinophilic gastroenteropathy as a method of reducing the intestinal inflammation rapidly in very ill patients. Although hyposensitization has been used extensively to treat patients with allergy to pollen and ragweed, there is inadequate information about its efficacy in food hypersensitivity.

Alpha-chain disease

See also page 12.98.

Definition. An immunoproliferative disease involving the small intestine, and sometimes the bronchi, which particularly affects patients living in countries around the Mediterranean. The lymphoproliferation involves plasma cells which secrete fragments of IgA immunoglobulin (alpha-chains).

Aetiology. Virtually all the patients reported have come from countries around the Mediterranean: particularly Greece, Israel, and Algeria. A few patients have been reported in South America, Pakistan, and Japan. The disease affects about 8 per 100 000 Arabs in Israel; it is not familial.

The geographical distribution suggests that environmental factors are important. One possibility is that the disease is initiated by a chronic infection in the gut which causes proliferation of IgA-producing cells, and eventually the emergence of a malignant clone. The fact that a few patients in the early stages of the disease have been cured with antibiotics supports this view.

Signs and symptoms. Most of the patients are young men in the third decade who present with chronic diarrhoea with malabsorption, abdominal pain, and wasting. Finger clubbing is common and tetany may occur due to calcium malabsorption. There may be a protein-losing enteropathy with hypoproteinaemia, hypogamma-globulinaemia, and oedema.

Investigations. There is usually malabsorption of fat, vitamin B_{12}, and lactose. The stools may contain parasites, particularly *Giardia lamblia* and hookworm. Barium follow-through shows a characteristic widening of the intestinal loops. The disease only seems to affect the small bowel, particularly the proximal jejunum. Jejunal biopsy shows a heavy infiltrate of plasma cells and lymphocytes. Various degrees of mucosal atrophy are seen and the crypts of the glands are characteristically sparse and very small.

Serum electrophoresis is abnormal in 50 per cent of cases, showing hypogammaglobulinaemia with an abnormal band representing the alpha-heavy chains. Further characterization of the abnormal protein can be carried out using zone electrophoresis and showing that the abnormal protein does not contain light chains. In doubtful cases, physicochemical analysis of the abnormal protein may be required.

Prognosis and treatment. The disease shows a spectrum of severity, which probably parallels the chonicity of the condition. Patients in the early stages have a good response to a combination of alkylating agents, tetracycline, and steroids and usually remain in good health for many years. A few patients have been completely cured but the majority have persistent lymphoproliferation in the bowel and retain alpha chains in the serum. Most patients eventually develop a malignant plasmacytoma or reticulum cell sarcoma of the bowel. It is hoped that earlier diagnosis and treatment will improve the prognosis.

References

Ament, M. E., Ochs, H. D., and Davis, S. D. (1973). Structure and function of the gastrointestinal tract in primary immunodeficiency disorders: a study of 39 patients. *Medicine, Baltimore* **52**, 227.

Asherson, G. L. and Webster, A. D. B. (1980). *The diagnosis and treatment of immunodeficiency diseases*. Blackwell Scientific Publications, Oxford.

Doe, W. F. (1978). Alpha chain disease. In *Immunology of the gastrointestinal tract* (ed. P. Asquith), 306. Churchill Livingstone, Edinburgh.

Ganguly, R. and Waldman, R. H. (1980). Local immunity and local immune responses. *Prog. Allergy* **27**, 1.

May, C. D. (1979). Food hypersensitivity. In *Cellular, molecular and clinical aspects of allergic disorders* (eds. S. Gupta and R. A. Good), 321. Plenum, New York.

Waksman, B. H. and Ozer, H. (1976). Specialized amplification elements in the immune system. *Prog. Allergy* **21**, 1.

Malabsorption

M. S. Losowsky

Functions of the small intestine

The functions of the small intestine are the digestion of food substances, the absorption of the products of digestion (and of substances, such as salt and water, which can be absorbed without prior digestion), the secretion of hormonal substances, and participation in the immune defensive system.

Digestion and absorption of carbohydrate. In the usual diet in the United Kingdom most of the carbohydrate is starch, most of the remainder is sucrose, and a small proportion of the total is lactose. Although there is a salivary amylase and digestion of starch can commence in the mouth and continue in the stomach, most of the digestion of starch is by pancreatic amylase to produce maltose (two glucose molecules joined together), maltotriose (three glucose molecules joined together in a straight chain), and alpha-limit dextrins (five or more glucose molecules joined in a branching pattern). This is the limit of carbohydrate digestion within the lumen of the upper part of the small intestine. Digestion of lactose and sucrose does not commence within the lumen. Further digestion of carbohydrate takes place at the microvilli which form the luminal surface of the mucosal cells. The disaccharidases and oligosaccharidases present within the microvilli split the carbohydrates present into their component monosaccharides, glucose, galactose, and fructose.

Transfer of the monosaccharides into the cell can occur against a concentration gradient and thus is by active transport. The active transport of glucose and galactose involves a specific carrier mechanism, dependent on simultaneous transfer of sodium and the availability of energy in a suitable form. Fructose is probably transported by a different carrier mechanism, independent of sodium. It is possible that there are other carrier mechanisms involving disaccharides and independent of sodium, which are of nutritional significance.

Disorders of the digestion and absorption of carbohydrate may be due to primary deficiencies of single enzymes or may be secondary to mucosal disease or nutritional disorders which usually cause deficiencies of multiple enzymes.

Digestion and absorption of protein. The protein to be digested and absorbed consists not only of dietary protein but also of endogenous protein, secreted in significant amounts.

Protein digestion commences with gastric pepsin but its contribution is minor.

The major digestion of protein is by the pancreatic proteolytic enzymes trypsin, chymotrypsin, and elastase acting on internal molecular bonds, and carboxypeptidase acting on terminal amino acids. All these pancreatic proteolytic enzymes are initially secreted as inactive pro-enzymes. The presence of food in the duodenum stimulates the release of the brush border enzyme enterokinase which activates trypsinogen to trypsin. Trypsin itself further activates trypsinogen and also activates the other pro-enzymes.

The activated pancreatic proteolytic enzymes act sequentially at their appropriate sites on the molecules and break down proteins and large polypeptides to oligopeptides and amino acids suitable for absorption. The oligopeptides are further digested by peptidases of the brush border, releasing their constituent amino acids. It is now clear, however, that some di- and tripeptides are absorbed directly into the cell by active transport, in quantities sufficient to be of nutritional significance, and here are hydrolysed by cytosol enzymes to their constituent amino acids.

Amino acids released in the lumen or in the brush border are absorbed into the cell by active transport and involve a multiplicity of carriers for different types of amino acid.

Digestion and absorption of fat (Fig. 1). Dietary fat is, of course, insoluble in water and consists largely of triglycerides of which the fatty acid portions are long chain, approximately 16–18 carbon atoms. Dietary fat also contains small amounts of cholesterol and fat-soluble vitamins.

The initial phase in the digestion of fat is the formation of a coarse emulsion in the stomach and this is emptied slowly through the pylorus into the duodenum. There the hydrolysis of triglyceride by pancreatic lipase is commenced, and for effective hydrolysis a pH greater than four is required. Two fatty acid molecules are removed from the triglyceride leaving beta-monoglyceride. In the lumen the fatty acid and monoglyceride, resulting from luminal digestion, meet bile salts coming down the bile duct either directly from the liver or in high concentration from contraction of the gall-bladder stimulated by a meal. These bile salts are present as water-soluble conjugates and when in sufficiently high concentration (the critical micellar concentration), they form into large structured molecular aggregates. These are called micelles and are water-soluble since the bile salt molecules are so arranged that their hydrophilic portions are to the outside. The hydrophobic portions, facing the inside of the micelle, provide a site where lipids can be carried. Thus in the centre of the micelle monoglyceride, fatty acid, fat-soluble vitamins, phospholipid, and cholesterol accumulate and the structure is then called a mixed micelle. These remain in the water phase.

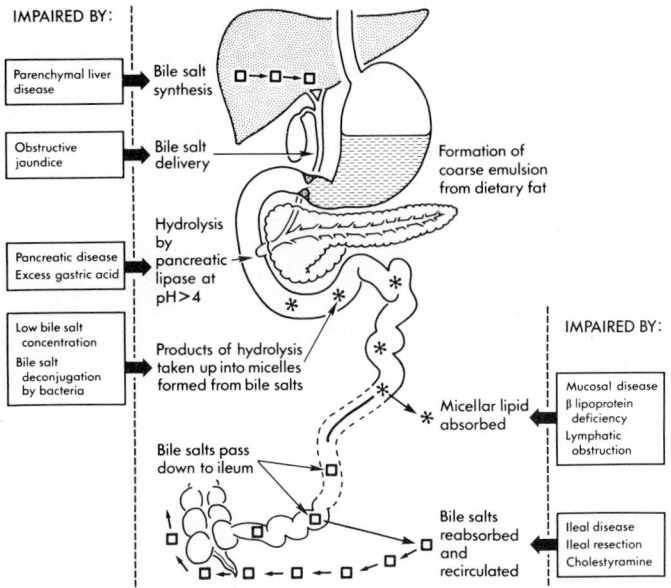

Fig. 1 Digestion and absorption of fat. Steatorrhoea may be caused by disease processes which impair different stages in the sequence of events.

The mixed micelles reach the brush border of the enterocytes, having crossed the unstirred water layer, and there the lipid contents of the micelles are absorbed into the cells by dissolving in the lipid of the cell membrane. The bile salts remain in the lumen and pass down the intestine to be absorbed by a very efficient specific absorptive mechanism in the terminal ileum. Only a few per cent of the bile salts reaching the terminal ileum escape absorption and enter the colon to be largely lost from the body. The absorbed bile salts return to the liver where they are recirculated to the duodenum. Such is the magnitude of this bile salt recirculation that the total body pool of bile salts may be circulated through the duodenum twice in a meal. Thus a relatively small increase in the proportion of bile salts lost at each circulation will impose a large requirement on the liver for additional bile salt synthesis, and the capacity of the liver to do this is limited.

Disorders which affect this part of the process of fat digestion (Fig. 1) include disorders affecting the actions of pancreatic enzymes and those affecting the actions of bile salts. Disorders affecting the actions of pancreatic enzymes are insufficiency of pancreatic lipase due to disease of the pancreas, and inactivation of pancreatic lipase by a gross excess of gastric acid. Disorders affecting actions of the bile salts attack all aspects of their metabolism. The bile salt concentration in the duodenum may be low, due to deficient synthesis as a result of severe parenchymal liver disease, or due to failure of delivery of bile salts into the duodenum consequent upon obstruction of the bile ducts either outside the liver or within the liver. Bile salts may be inactivated by deconjugation due to bacterial overgrowth within the lumen. Reduced concentrations of bile salts in the lumen may be consequent upon ileal disease, leading to excessive loss of bile salts from the body.

Most of the fat is absorbed in the upper jejunum in the normal subject but fat absorption can take place further down the small intestine. Thus mucosal disease of the upper small intestine needs to be extensive to produce a marked impairment of fat absorption.

Once within the enterocytes, long-chain fatty acids and monoglycerides are resynthesized intracellularly to triglycerides. Within the cell, aggregates of triglyceride are formed and coated with phospholipid and protein to form chylomicrons which also carry a certain amount of cholesterol and fat-soluble vitamins. These exit via the base of the enterocytes and enter the intestinal lymphatics, the lacteals, and hence the blood stream. it appears that beta-lipoprotein is necessary for the formation of chylomicrons since absence of betalipoprotein leads to deficient chylomicron formation. Interference with free flow through the lacteals, in the condition of intestinal lymphangiectasia, results in deficient fat absorption (Fig. 1).

Although the above complex mechanism is the most efficient means of absorption of most forms of dietary lipid, even if this is interfered with in some of the ways indicated a substantial proportion of fat absorption still occurs.

Triglycerides containing fatty acids of medium chain length, from six to 12 carbon atoms, are more easily digested and absorbed than those with long-chain fatty acids, being more readily hydrolysed and taken up in micelles. The importance of medium-chain triglycerides in treatment, however, lies in the fact that a significant proportion of dietary medium-chain triglyceride can be taken up by the enterocytes in unsplit form, hydrolysed by a mucosal lipase, and the medium-chain fatty acid formed can enter the portal vein directly without the necessity for re-esterification.

The causes of malabsorption

The main causes of malabsorption are summarized in Table 1, in which an attempt is made to relate defective absorption to the underlying disorder of structure or function of the small bowel.

Clinical presentation of malabsorption

There are symptoms and signs which occur in the malabsorption syndrome, whatever the cause:

1. *Diarrhoea with features to suggest steatorrhoea.* In the severe case the stools are typically loose, bulky, offensive, greasy, light coloured, and difficult to flush away. Although there may be only one bulky stool per day, stool frequency is usually increased, but not to the extent seen in colonic disease. The stools may, however, appear normal and even constipated although steatorrhoea is shown by faecal fat measurement. Steatorrhoea may be absent in any of the diseases of the small intestine.

2. *Abdominal symptoms* including discomfort, borborygmi, and distension. The discomfort may follow food and thus mimic peptic ulcer, or it may be to some extent relieved by bowel action thus mimicking the irritable colon syndrome.

3. *Nutritional deficiency.* A patient with malabsorption may present with an apparently isolated nutritional deficiency, for example anaemia due to iron, folate or vitamin B_{12} deficiency, bleeding due to increased prothrombin time secondary to vitamin K deficiency, or bone disease secondary to vitamin D deficiency. Such deficiencies may be reflected by a variety of symptoms and signs including glossitis, pallor, pigmentation of the skin, petechiae or bruising, muscle pain, neurological abnormalities, a positive Chvostek or Trousseau sign, and skeletal abnormalities.

4. *Features of general ill health.* These include anorexia, weight loss, lethargy, tiredness on little effort, dyspnoea, and general irritability. In contrast to the usual anorexia, some patients have hyperphagia and a very high food intake. Finger clubbing occurs in some cases. In the patient with severe or prolonged disease hypoalbuminaemia, oedema, electrolyte deficiencies, and dehydration may occur.

5. *Features related to the underlying cause.* There may be clinical

Table 1 The classification of causes of malabsorption

1 *Mucosal*—definitive investigation: intestinal
    biopsy
  Structure
    Food sensitivities:
      * Gluten-sensitive enteropathy
      Dermatitis herpetiformis
      Cows' milk sensitivity in infants
      Soya protein sensitivity
      * Tropical sprue
    Whipple's disease
    Intestinal lymphangiectasia
    Mast cell disease
  Function
    Alactasia
    Abetalipoproteinaemia

2 *Structural*—definitive investigation: usually
    small bowel radiology
  * Crohn's disease
  Intestinal resection
  * Gastric surgery (see below)
  Mesenteric arterial insufficiency
  Small intestine lymphoma or other malignancy
  Blind loops, fistulae, diverticula, strictures
  Idiopathic chronic ulcerative enteritis
  Amyloidosis
  Eosinophilic gastroenteropathy
  Mechanisms of malabsorption after gastric
    surgery
    Poor mixing   ⎫ not important
    Decreased gastric digestion ⎬
    Lack of stimulus to bile and pancreatic secre-
      tion
    Rapid gastric emptying
    Intestinal hurry
    Afferent loop pooling of bile and pancreatic
      secretions
    Afferent loop bacterial overgrowth
    Pancreatic atrophy
    Unmasking of other disease: gluten sensi-
      tivity, alactasia, jejunal diverticula
    Inadvertent gastro-ileostomy ⎫ rare
    Gastro-colic fistula   ⎬

3 *Infective*
  Acute enteritis
  * Travellers' diarrhoea
  Intestinal tuberculosis
  Parasitic disease of the intestine
  Whipple's disease
  Contaminated small bowel
    Anatomical: blind loops, fistulae, diver-
      ticula, strictures
    Motility disturbance: systemic sclerosis,
      intestinal pseudo-obstruction, diabetes
      mellitus, abdominal radiotherapy
  Achlorhydria
  Hypogammaglobulinaemia

4 *Defective luminal digestion*
  Pancreatic
    Chronic pancreatitis
    * Carcinoma of the pancreas
    * Cystic fibrosis
    Pancreatectomy
    Zollinger-Ellison syndrome
    Defective stimulation: intestinal
      disease, gastric surgery
    Malnutrition
  Bile salt mediated
    * Parenchymal liver disease
    * Biliary obstruction
    Bacterial degradation (see contaminated
      small bowel)
    * Terminal ileum disease
    * Terminal ileum resection
    Cholestyramine

5 *Drugs*
  Neomycin
  Cholestyramine
  Colchicine
  Para-amino salicylic acid
  Irritant purgative abuse
  Phenindione
  Metformin
  Methyldopa
  Methotrexate
  Liquid paraffin
  Ethyl alcohol
  Antacids

6 *Lymphatic obstruction*
  Congenital lymphangiectasia
  Acquired   lymphangiectasia: lymphoma,
    tuberculosis, cardiac disease
7 *Disease outside the gastrointestinal tract*
  Endocrine disorders: hyperthyroidism,
    hypothyroidism, Addison's disease,
    hyperparathyroidism, hypoparathyroidism,
    diabetes mellitus, carcinoid syndrome
  Collagen diseases
  Ulcerative colitis
  Widespread skin disease
  Malnutrition

8 *Specific deficiences of metabolic disorders*
  Pancreatic enzyme deficiencies, with normal
    structure
  Enterokinase deficiency
  Disaccharidase deficiency
  Cystinuria
  Hartnup disease
  Congenital chloridorrhoea
  Vitamin B_{12} malabsorption
  Folate malabsorption
  Acrodermatitis enteropathica

* Relatively common
  Some disorders cause malabsorption by more than one mechanism and are thus classified under more than one heading. This has the advantage of allowing consideration of different forms of treatment in the same patient.

features which give a clue to the underlying cause of the malabsorption syndrome. These include the finding of an abdominal mass in intestinal lymphoma or regional enteritis, the dermatological changes of scleroderma, facial flush and large liver suggestive of the carcinoid syndrome, signs of hypo- or hyperthyroidism, neurological impairment associated with abetalipoproteinaemia, occular or neurological changes suggestive of diabetes mellitus, lymph node enlargement, arthritis and lung disease characteristic of Whipple's disease, or the dermatological changes characteristic of systemic mast cell disease.

Although the above features may suggest the malabsorption syndrome, and other clinical features may suggest the correct diagnosis, definitive diagnosis requires special investigations. There is a bewildering variety of tests available for the patient suspected of malabsorption. These can, in general, be divided into two groups. Firstly, those which document a defect in the integrated processes of digestion and absorption and hence are useful in confirming a disorder of this type, in documenting its severity, and in monitoring the effects of treatment. Measurement of faecal fat is the important investigation in this group. Secondly, there are definitive investigations,

such as intestinal biopsy and radiology, appropriate to particular diseases, and these are required for making a precise diagnosis.

Investigation of the patient suspected of malabsorption

Documentation of defective absorption. For most substances defective absorption cannot be demonstrated simply by comparing intake in the diet with output in the stool because of the intervention of other processes such as endogenous secretion and bacterial breakdown. Direct demonstration of defective absorption by intestinal intubation and perfusion is not of practical clinical importance. Thus, with the exception of fat, the demonstration of defective absorption is indirect.

In the estimation of faecal fat an abnormal result does not distinguish between inadequate digestion and inadequate absorption. Indirect assessments of the malabsorption of other substances, by the use of plasma levels or by the demonstration of deficiencies, can clearly be affected by factors other than problems of digestion and absorption and the results need to be interpreted with due caution.

Faecal fat. Simple measurement of the quantity of fat put out in the stools in one day is unsatisfactory for a number of reasons. The reservoir function of the colon is variable from day to day so that the output of fat varies greatly. Thus faeces need to be collected for several days, preferably at least five, and the result expressed as average daily excretion. Even this may not be reliable in patients with irregular bowel habits. Faecal markers, intermittent or continuous, improve the accuracy. The use of continuous markers allows reduction in the period of collection of faeces.

The quantity of fat in the stool depends on the intake of fat in the diet. Although there is a small quantity of endogenous fat in the stool, of the order of 1–2 g per day, this does not increase to any significant extent in patients with steatorrhoea: in such patients the excess faecal fat is unabsorbed dietary fat. In ambulant patients being investigated for malabsorption, dietary fat intakes may differ by a factor of four or five. Thus for interpretation of the faecal fat the dietary intake of fat must be known. Expressing the faecal fat as a percentage of dietary fat gives a meaningful basis of comparison between patients on different fat intakes and from time to time in the same patient if the fat intake varies with the clinical state. Ninety-three per cent absorption is the approximate limit of normal.

Faecal fat determined in this way is useful in diseases associated with maldigestion or malabsorption since it gives an overall assessment of major physiological functions. Repeated estimations are of proven value in assessing the progress of certain diseases and the effects of treatment. However, most functions concerned in digestion and absorption have considerable reserve capacity and in the case of the small intestine adaptation may occur with compensatory increased function in non-diseased areas. Thus fat absorption may be normal with established disease in organs involved in digestion and absorption, for example the small intestine, the pancreas, and the liver.

To minimize collection and handling of faeces many indirect methods of estimation of fat absorption have been devised. These include the use of radioactive fats, macroscopic or microscopic examination of faeces, and fat tolerance tests. Most correlate moderately well with faecal fat measurements.

Carbohydrate absorption. The absorption of glucose cannot be directly assessed but the glucose tolerance test, which measures blood levels after a standard oral dose of glucose, tends to give a lower rise than normal with most causes of malabsorption but a higher rise than normal in patients with pancreatic disease. There are, however, so many other factors which affect the result of this test that it is of little value in the context of malabsorption.

The test which is usually used to assess carbohydrate absorption is the xylose absorption test. An oral dose of xylose is given and the excretion in the urine measured for the ensuing five hours. Excretion of greater than 22 per cent of a 5 g dose and greater than 17 per cent of a 25 g dose may be regarded as normal, although the limits of normal show some variation from one laboratory to another. This test rarely gives normal results in untreated coeliac disease or tropical sprue and abnormal results rarely occur in patients with pancreatic disease. Abnormal results occur, however, for reasons other than malabsorption. These include delayed gastric emptying, low urine flow, or poor renal function.

A lactose tolerance test may be performed in a similar way to the glucose tolerance test. In patients with low levels of lactase in the intestinal mucosa (alactasia), either primary or secondary to intestinal mucosal disease, oral lactose is followed by little rise in the blood glucose (see page 12.97). The unabsorbed lactose reaching the colon is converted by bacteria to volatile fatty acids which may cause inhibition of the absorption of salt and water by the colon and consequent abdominal discomfort and diarrhoea. These symptoms following oral lactose are presumptive evidence of alactasia. Direct measurement of lactase in mucosal biopsy specimens is a better test for alactasia than is the lactose tolerance test.

Protein absorption. Faecal nitrogen is a measure of protein malabsorption, especially when there is gross maldigestion as in severe pancreatic disease, and parallels faecal fat in some conditions. It is, however, rarely used in diagnosis since much of the faecal nitrogen derives from sources other than dietary protein, for example bacteria and mucus.

Excessive loss of protein (protein-losing enteropathy) is a feature of many disorders of the gastrointestinal tract and is commonly responsible for hypoproteinaemia. Faecal nitrogen does not reflect this process since most of the protein in the lumen is digested and reabsorbed. Protein-losing enteropathy is assessed by measuring faecal radioactivity after intravenous injection of radioactive protein or other substance of similar molecular weight (see page 12.101).

Vitamin B_{12} absorption. (See also Section 19.) In the absence of other reasons for it to be malabsorbed, the absorption of vitamin B_{12} may be used as a test of function of the terminal ileum. The Schilling test consists of an oral dose of radioactive vitamin B_{12} followed by an intramuscular large, 'flushing' dose of non-radio active vitamin B_{12} and measurement of urinary radioactivity, which reflects the amount absorbed. Confirmation that a low value is not due to pernicious anaemia or other gastric pathology can be obtained by repeating the test and giving intrinsic factor with the oral dose of vitamin B_{12}. If malabsorption is due to ileal disease, the result will remain abnormal. Vitamin B_{12} absorption can also be determined using a whole-body counter.

Small bowel biopsy. Small intestinal biopsy is now widely available, extremely safe, and is an invaluable aid to the diagnosis of small bowel disease.

Probably most widely used is the Crosby–Kugler capsule in which a spring-loaded blade is activated by suction through a fine tube. This has the disadvantages of producing only a single specimen and of requiring the capsule to be removed before recovery of the specimen. If, for any reason, a satisfactory specimen is not obtained, the patient must swallow the capsule again. An alternative is a hydraulic capsule in which the specimen is flushed to the surface with the capsule still in position in the small intestine. The blade is automatically reset so that multiple specimens can be obtained before removal.

There are remarkably few complications to these procedures. Bleeding may occur but this is exceedingly rare provided that neither prothrombin time nor platelet count is grossly abnormal. In our experience, on the rare occasions when bleeding has occurred it has terminated spontaneously and rarely needed transfusion. Perforation of the intestine is a theoretical possibility and has occasionally been described in severely malnourished subjects. The procedure is sufficiently free of complications for us to carry it out routinely with adult outpatients, provided the patients can be observed for a few hours after completion.

Processing. The specimen can be examined and orientated on a plastic mesh, using the dissecting microscope. This enables an immediate rough assessment of the likelihood of pathology, certain recognition of severe villous loss, and an indication for sections at multiple levels if a patchy lesion is seen. The mounting and orientation of the specimen are important to obtain the best information, even though severe lesions can be diagnosed with imperfect orientation.

Histological interpretation. The biopsy of the normal upper small bowel in temperate zones shows a mixture of finger-shaped and leaf-shaped villi (Fig. 2a). Histologically the epithelial cells are tall and columnar with basal, palisaded nuclei. There are a few lymphocytes between the epithelial cells. There is a scanty infiltrate of inflammatory cells in the lamina propria. The villi are several times as long as the depth of the crypts (Fig. 2b).

Duodenal samples with underlying Brunner's glands may show villi which are rather flattened and this may apply in areas of jejunal samples which overlie lymphoid nodules. In tropical areas a wider

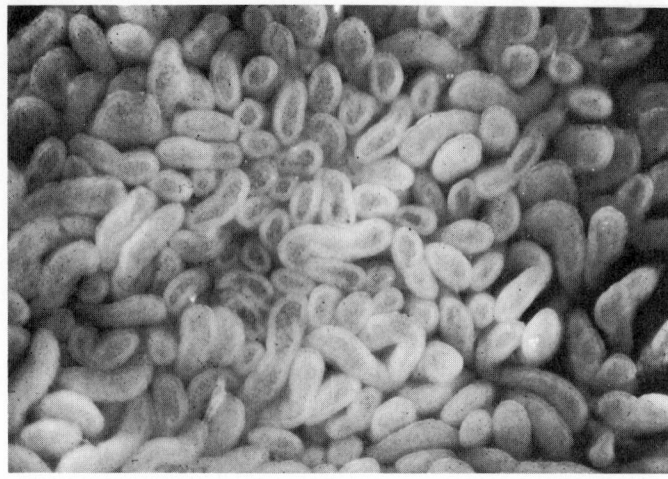

Fig. 2 (a) Dissecting microscope appearance of normal jejunal mucosa showing finger-shaped and leaf-shaped villi.

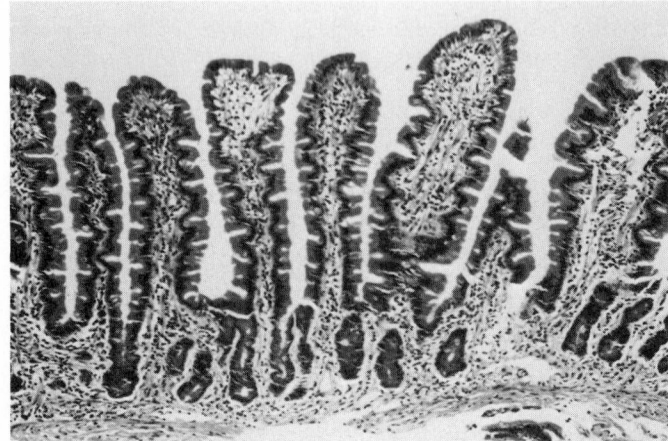

(b) Histological appearance of normal jejunal mucosa showing tall villi, several times as long as the crypts are deep. The epithelial cells are columnar with basal nuclei. There is a scattering of inflammatory cells deep to the epithelium.

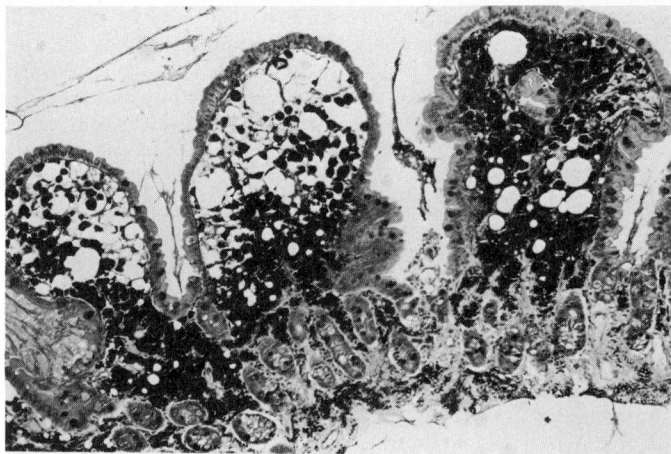

Fig. 3 Some examples of conditions which may be diagnosed or suspected from jejunal biopsy material.
(a) Whipple's disease. The villi are distended but the overlying epithelium is relatively normal. This PAS stain demonstrates macrophages stuffed with deposits of glycoprotein, and distended lymphatic spaces within the villi.

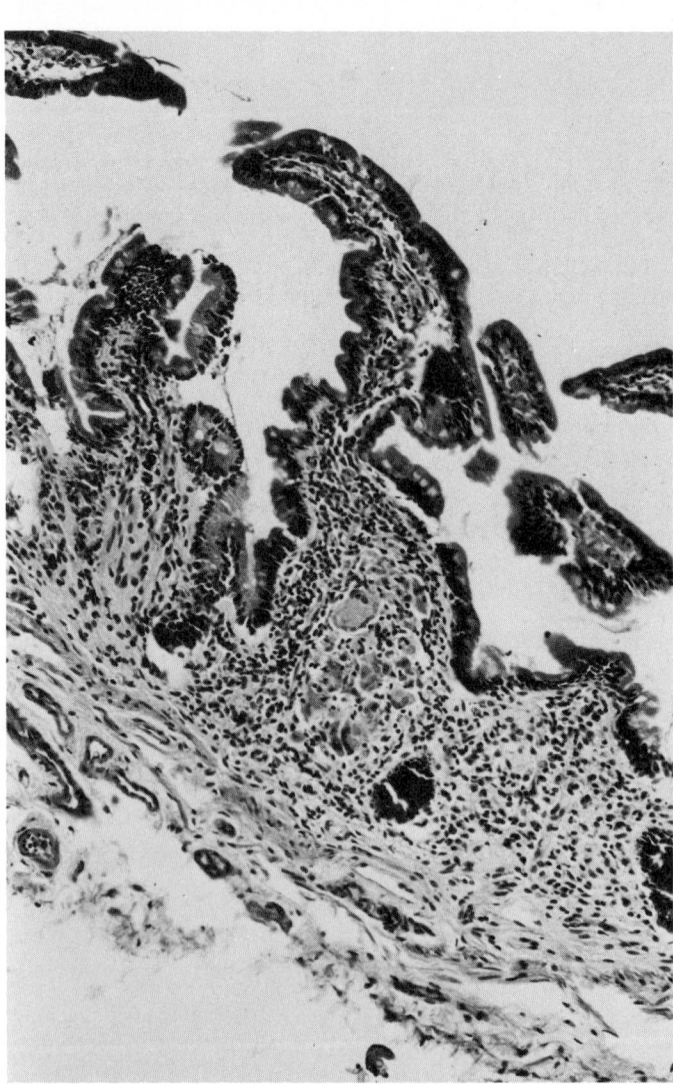

(b) Crohn's disease. At the base of a villus is a granuloma containing giant cells.

range of appearances may be found in subjects with no evidence of disease.

The small intestine responds in a similar way to many different diseases. Milder lesions, which consist of (*a*) broadening of the villi which may be branched or fused, (*b*) oedema and excess of inflammatory cells beneath the surface epithelium, and (*c*) reduction in the height of the epithelial cells and loss of their regular nuclear arrangement, are very non-specific. Causes include malignancy anywhere in the body, malnutrition, small bowel ischaemia, severe skin disease, bacterial overgrowth in the small intestine, excess secretion of gastric acid as in the Zollinger–Ellison syndrome, and numerous other conditions. A severe lesion with total loss of villi and crypt hypertrophy is highly suggestive of coeliac disease but a similar lesion may be seen occasionally in other pathologies, notably severe tropical sprue, cows' milk sensitivity in young children, and gastroenteritis in young children.

Diseases with specific features (Fig. 3) by which a confident diagnosis may be made from the intestinal biopsy include Whipple's disease (in which the villi are seen to be stuffed with macrophages containing PAS-positive material), abetalipoproteinaemia (in which the epithelial cells are distended with lipid), diffuse lymphoma, giardiasis and other infestations in which the parasites may be found, lymphangiectasia (in which distended lymphatics can be identified in some of the villi), and humoral immune deficiencies (in which all grades of villous abnormality may be seen together with a deficiency of plasma cells in the lamina propria).

There are certain other conditions in which a presumptive diagnosis may be made from the biopsy. Crohn's disease may show granulomas with giant cells (Fig. 3b). The small bowel lesion which

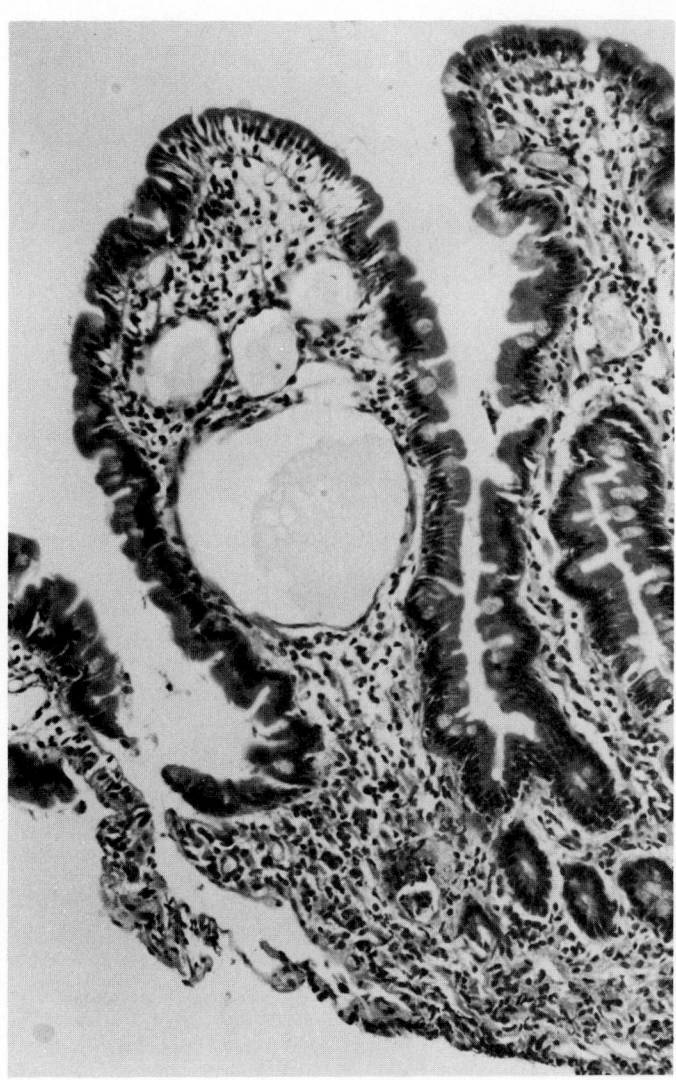

Fig. 3 *cont.* (c) Intestinal lymphangiectasia. A villus is shown with grossly distended lymphatics in its core.

follows abdominal radiotherapy may show villous loss without crypt hyperplasia (a similar lesion is sometimes seen in severe coeliac disease or tropical sprue). Specific stains may reveal amyloid infiltration.

Endoscopic biopsy. With the ready availability of upper gastrointestinal endoscopy, small biopsy samples from the duodenum are frequently available. Coeliac disease may be strongly suspected from the endoscopic appearances of the duodenum. Endoscopic biopsy may reliably refute coeliac disease, if normal villi are shown, or suggest coeliac disease if the characteristic lesion is seen. There are, however, a number of pitfalls in interpreting duodenal biopsies. Villous flattening over Brunner's glands is mentioned above. The proportion of leaf-shaped villi is higher in the duodenum and histologically this may appear as broadening of the villi. Duodenal mucosa from the vicinity of a peptic ulcer may show inflammatory changes. The relatively common condition of duodenitis must be appreciated to avoid misinterpretation. In occasional patients with coeliac disease the duodenal mucosa is much less severely affected than the jejunal mucosa.

Enzyme measurements. Determination of enzyme activity in biopsy tissue reveals multiple deficiencies associated with gross histological abnormalities. Isolated deficiency of lactase is diagnostic of primary alactasia.

Small bowel radiology. The purpose of small bowel radiology is to reveal anatomical lesions as the cause of malabsorption and as complications of other disorders, and to indicate gross defects of motility. A small bowel follow-through can be performed as a sequel to a barium meal when metoclopramide can be used to speed the progress of the contrast medium, but we prefer the technique of small bowel enema in which a fine tube is passed into the duodenum, and barium sulphate is followed by a propellant such as methycellulose suspension (Fig. 4).

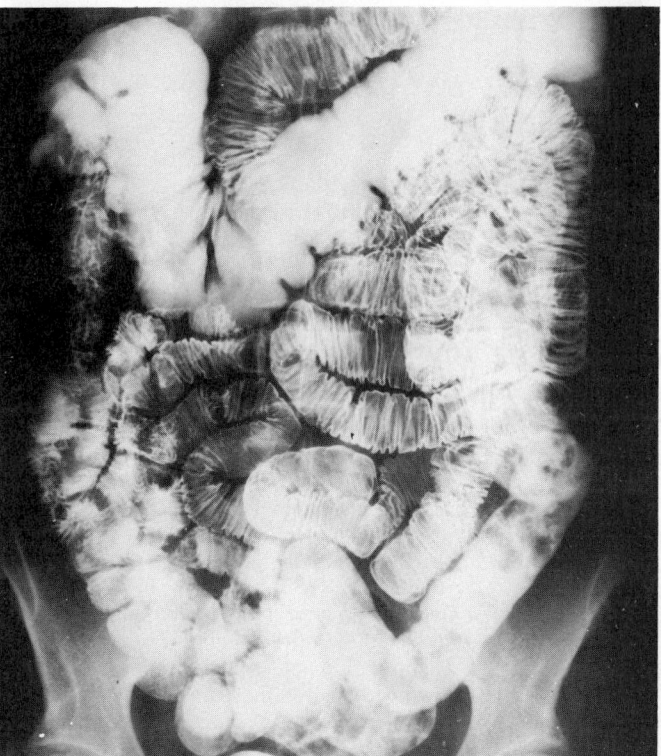

Fig. 4 Normal small intestine shown by the technique of small bowel enema. The loops of the small intestine and their transverse folds are well shown. The large intestine is also partially filled on this film.

Non-specific findings. Non-specific findings such as dilatation, thickened folds (suggesting oedema), and poor motility occur in many small bowel disorders which are accompanied by malabsorption. Flocculation of the contrast medium is minimized by the technique of small bowel enema and by the newer, relatively non-flocculating media, but when it does occur it is a non-specific indication of excessive secretion.

Specific findings. A definitive diagnosis of a cause for malabsorption may be obtained with diverticula, blind loops, strictures, or fistulae (Fig. 5).

In systemic sclerosis a severe motility disturbance may be accompanied by the diagnostic feature of dilatation of the small bowel, particularly affecting the duodenum, but with the folds remaining close together (the 'hidebound' bowel) in contrast to spreading of the folds seen in other causes of dilatation (Fig. 6).

A diagnosis of Crohn's disease may be made with considerable confidence if ulceration, narrowing of the lumen, and thickening of the wall are seen, particularly if present in the terminal ileum and more particularly if multiple short segments of small bowel are affected ('skip lesions'). Differential diagnosis of such appearances includes tuberculosis of the small intestine, lymphoma, Henoch–Schönlein lesions, and mesenteric venous thrombosis which sometimes occurs in young females taking the contraceptive pill.

Tumours of the small intestine, usually lymphomas, may appear as mass lesions or merely as rigidity or thickening of the wall.

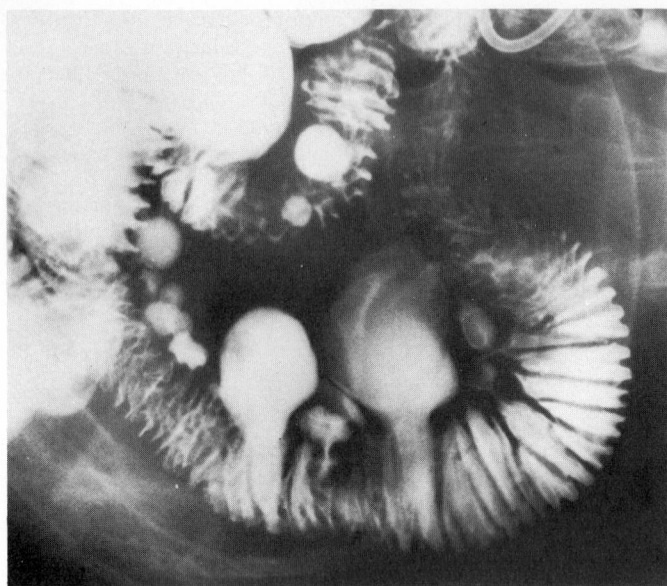

Fig. 5   Multiple diverticula of the small intestine shown by the technique of small bowel enema.

Lymphoma of the small intestine may, however, be present with entirely normal appearances by this technique.

Complications of other disorders. In coeliac disease strictures and ulcers may occur. A similar condition, which has been termed idiopathic chronic ulcerative enteritis, may occur in the absence of coeliac disease.

In conditions of defective humoral immunity multiple small lymphoid nodules may be found in the small intestine, (nodular lymphoid hyperplasia) and should not be mistaken for lymphoma.

After abdominal or pelvic radiation there may be defective motility of a region of small intestine and this may be accompanied by scarring, shown by tethering or rigidity of the wall, or by strictures.

Nutritional status. Deficiencies of the major nutrients, reflected in a general way by loss of body weight and low serum albumin, respond to treatment of the cause of the malabsorption. If the underlying condition cannot be corrected, nutritional support may be given in the form of medium-chain triglyceride, 'elemental' diets (perhaps better termed chemically defined diets), or intravenous nutrition.

Investigation for deficiencies of haematinic factors (iron, folic acid, and vitamin B_{12}) and fat-soluble vitamins (A, D, and K) must be undertaken and appropriate therapy given (see Sections 8, 17 and 19).

Deficiencies of water-soluble vitamins are uncommon and appropriate tests for most of these are not widely available. If there is any clinical indication of deficiency, supplements should be given orally or parenterally.

If diarrhoea is severe, water and electrolyte deficiencies need to be confirmed and managed in the usual way.

Magnesium deficiency may be suspected from low plasma and urine magnesium levels. Treatment is by oral magnesium chloride or sulphate which may exacerbate the diarrhoea, or by intramuscular or intravenous magnesium sulphate.

Hypocalcaemia may need emergency treatment by intravenous calcium if tetany or other acute problems occur. Magnesium deficiency may need to be treated concurrently.

Coeliac disease

For practical purposes coeliac disease may be defined as the condition in which there is a morphological abnormality of the mucosa of the small intestine brought on by contact with dietary gluten.

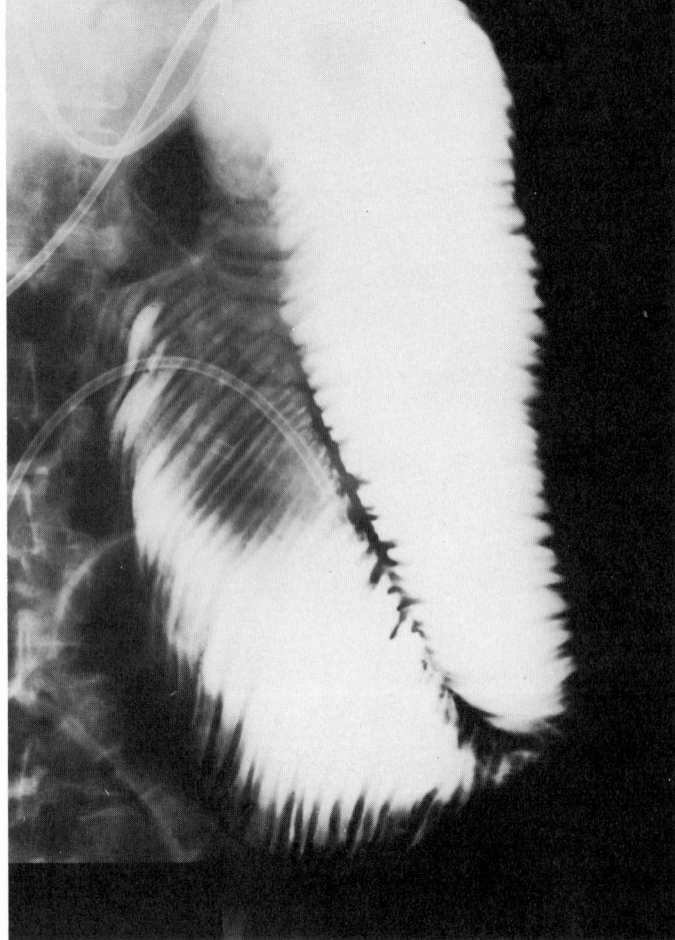

Fig. 6   Dilated small intestine with the transverse folds remaining very close together (the 'hidebound' bowel) diagnostic of systemic sclerosis of the small intestine.

Gluten is the term applied to a group of protein substances which occur in various forms of grain. The toxic material is present in wheat, barley, rye, and probably also in oats. The alternative name for the condition, gluten-sensitive enteropathy, encompasses these features. Other terms include non-tropical sprue, idiopathic steatorrhoea, and in the USA, coeliac sprue. The morphological abnormality of the intestinal mucosa is reversible by withdrawal of gluten from the diet and the sensitivity to gluten is permanent. In contrast, it is possible that there is a temporary sensitivity to dietary gluten associated with certain other conditions including cows' milk sensitivity in young children and tropical sprue.

The prevalence of coeliac disease in England is usually considered to be about 1 in 2–3000, but recent indications suggest that this may be an underestimate. In the west of Ireland the prevalence is probably of the order of 1 in several hundred.

Genetic aspects. Coeliac disease has a clearcut familial susceptibility. The evidence suggests that the familial predisposition has a genetic basis.

The histocompatibility antigen HLA-B8 is very much commoner in patients with coeliac disease than in controls. In most series some 80 per cent or more of patients have this antigen compared with about 20 per cent of controls. A much closer association is found with the DRW3 antigen and with certain B cell antigens. It seems likely that, when methods have been standardized to allow comparison of data in large numbers of patients, combinations of such antigens will show the closest correlation with the disease.

Pathogenesis. The mechanism by which gluten induces damage in the intestinal mucosa is not understood. The two main theories are (a) deficiency of a mucosal enzyme involved in the breakdown of either a toxic component of gluten or a toxic material formed during digestion, and (b) an immunological reaction, directed against gluten or one of its components, which incidentally and misguidedly causes damage to the intestinal mucosa. A third theory is that a constituent of gluten may be acting as a plant lectin and bind to the cell membrane of the intestinal epithelium because of some unusual configuration of that membrane in the coeliac subject.

Currently the immunological theory is most favoured and a variety of types of evidence may be quoted in its favour. There is an abundance of evidence of cell-mediated and humoral immune reactions to gluten in coeliac subjects. There is evidence suggesting immune reactions to gluten by intestinal mucosa from coeliac subjects, cultured *in vitro*. There is an association of coeliac disease with other disorders thought to be auto-immune in origin. Some patients with otherwise typical coeliac disease have selective deficiency of IgA. However, none of these factors establishes that an immune reaction is responsible for the damage. Current thinking is that histocompatibility antigens may be markers of immune response genes and thus a reflection of particular patterns of immune responsiveness which are necessary, but not sufficient, for the development of the disease. Other factors required for the disease to develop are not, at the moment, clear.

It is possible that combinations of mechanisms may be necessary for the disease to occur. Thus, for example, an abnormal membrane configuration of the intestinal mucosal cell might allow binding of one of the constituents of gluten in such a way that in an individual with a particular immune response gene, it initiated an immune response which subsequently led to the damage.

Pathology. Normally the mucosa of the jejunum shows finger- or leaf-shaped villi which are several times as long as they are thick (Fig. 2). In coeliac disease typically the villi are lost, the mucosal surface is flat, and the mouths of the crypts are seen as indentations (Fig. 7a). The lesion is less severe further down the small intestine, presumably in keeping with diminished exposure to the toxic material. In some patients with coeliac disease the abnormality is less severe and stunted, broad villi are seen.

Histology (Fig. 7b) confirms the absence of villi or that they are short and stunted. The depth of the crypts is increased. There is an increase in inflammatory cells beneath and within the epithelium. The epithelium itself is abnormal, the normal tall columnar epithelial cells with palisaded basal nuclei and a regular brush border seen on electron microscopy, are replaced by multi-layered, flattened

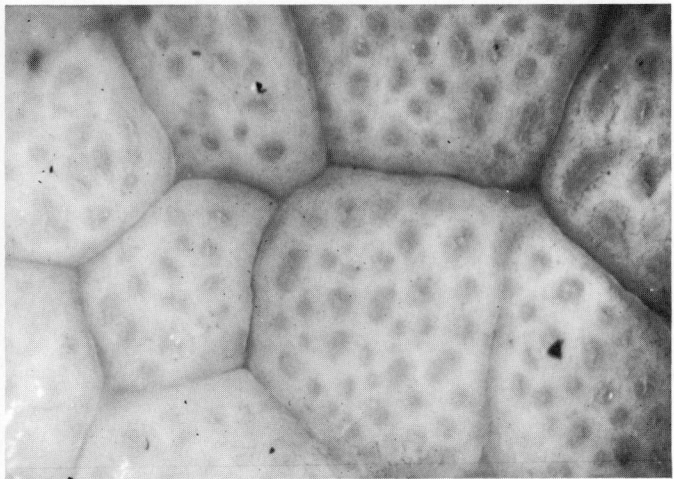

Fig. 7 (a) Dissecting microscope appearance of jejunal mucosa in untreated coeliac disease. There are no villi. The mucosa is flat, with a mosaic pattern. The mouths of the crypts are seen as indentations.

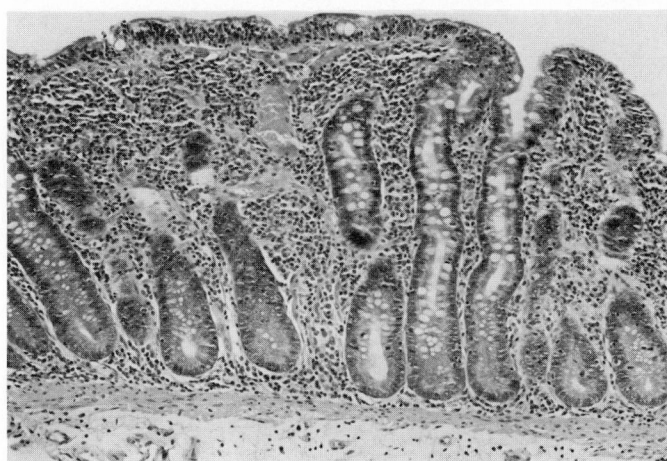

(b) Histology of jejunal mucosa in untreated coeliac disease. There are no villi. The crypts are deeper than normal so that the total thickness of mucosa is not reduced. There are abundant inflammatory cells between the crypts. The surface epithelium is multi-layered, the cells are flattened, and the nuclei arranged haphazardly.

epithelial cells with irregularly placed nuclei, and with a stunted and less regular brush border on electron microscopy. Occasional findings, suggested as predictors of poor response to a gluten-free diet, are a heavy subepithelial deposit of collagen and lack of hypertrophy of the crypts.

The severe mucosal lesion with absence of villi is highly suggestive of coeliac disease, but not diagnostic. Other rare causes of a complete loss of villi include infectious enteritis in children, lymphoma, Whipple's disease, hypogammaglobulinaemia especially if complicated by *Giardia lamblia* infestation, the condition of idiopathic chronic ulcerative enteritis, kwashiorkor, severe tropical sprue, and sensitivity to cows' milk or soya protein in children. The milder abnormalities, with short and broad villi, may occur in very many diseases including disorders not primarily involving the small intestine.

Clinical course. A common time of presentation is in the infant after weaning but presentation may be at any time of life.

The classical features of the condition, well described by Gee in 1888, are pale, bulky, loose, offensive stools associated with abdominal distension and discomfort, loss of weight, and the development of nutritional complications.

When the patient presents in this way, clinical features which are frequently present include oedema, glossitis, anaemia, and nocturia. Other features which may be present are finger clubbing, aphthous ulceration in the mouth, hypotension and, less frequently, polyneuritis, paraesthesiae and tetany, dryness of the skin, and generalized pigmentation. A rare neurological syndrome including cerebellar signs and extensor plantar responses, with autopsy changes in brain and spinal cord, does not appear to respond to withdrawal of dietary gluten.

It is increasingly recognized that many, and perhaps most, patients with coelic disease do not present in this classical fashion. Indeed some patients, discovered as a result of family surveys, or the chance finding of changes of hyposplenism on a bloodfilm, have complained of no symptoms. Some patients appear well-nourished at the time of diagnosis. Others present with pure nutritional deficiencies; the disorder may present at any time including old age with refractory iron deficiency anaemia, megaloblastic anaemia, or skeletal symptoms and signs secondary to vitamin D deficiency. Some children present with impaired growth and development (Fig. 8). Permanent short stature may result if diagnosis is delayed until adult life. A large group presents with only trivial or apparently unrelated symptoms. In many patients the symptoms are of very long duration before diagnosis.

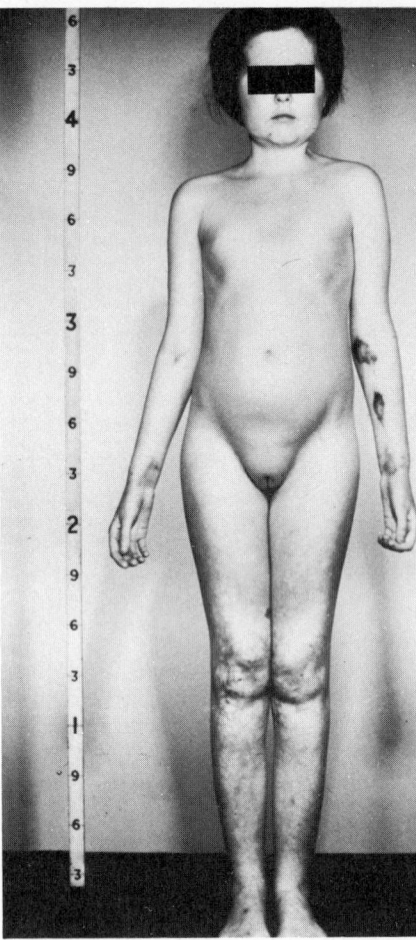

Fig. 8 Patient with untreated coeliac disease aged 19½ years at presentation. Superficially she does not appear malnourished but there is short stature and failure to attain puberty. Growth and development occurred rapidly after starting on a gluten-free diet.

In some patients there are long, apparently asymptomatic, intervals. There may be suggestive symptoms during infancy and then nothing further until middle life or even later.

Symptoms may be precipitated by other events, for example, pregnancy, gastric surgery, or infection. A small proportion of patients, otherwise apparently typical, fail to respond to all forms of treatment. The nature of this disorder is not understood.

Associated disorders. Thyroid disease and other auto-immune disorders are described in association with coeliac disease.

Pancreatic dysfunction occurs, perhaps secondary to malnutrition since it may recover on a gluten-free diet.

Diabetes mellitus and various forms of liver disease have been described in association with coeliac disease.

Investigation. Diagnosis demands at least two biopsies of the small intestinal mucosa. Abnormality must be shown, with improvement on a gluten-free diet. In young children a third biopsy, to demonstrate relapse on a gluten challenge, is usually recommended since cows' milk sensitivity and infectious enteritis are not uncommon causes of a similar mucosal lesion and morphological improvement may occur while on a gluten-free diet without being due to the diet.

Faecal fat estimation is not necessary but may be used as an indication of severity and of progress. Nutritional measurements such as serum iron, serum and red cell folate, and serum B_{12} should be performed since if abnormal appropriate supplements will cause rapid improvement in symptoms.

The gut hormones in coeliac disease are described on page 12.51.

Treatment. The cornerstone of treatment is the gluten-free diet. In general the younger the patient the more rapid the clinical response to the diet. In adults the diet may need to be continued for six months, or even a year, before symptomatic improvement occurs. Once a gluten-free diet is established continued nutritional supplements are unnecessary.

Achieving a strictly gluten-free diet poses considerable problems to the patient. Initially the burden is great but most patients adjust so that they can live full and normal lives.

Failure of clinical response to the diet should not be accepted in the adult until at least a year of strict adherence, particularly if there is histological improvement. If there is no histological response, the diagnosis should be re-assessed and a search made for complications of the disease. In the absence of complications pancreatic enzymes, a lactose-free diet, and corticosteroids should be tried sequentially, while continuing the gluten-free diet. If there is still no improvement, then serious consideration must be given to the possibility of intestinal ulceration or lymphoma. Laparotomy may be the only means of diagnosing these lesions.

In the occasional patient who is severely ill at presentation, steroids, intravenous fluid and electrolytes, and even parenteral nutrition, may be necessary initially.

The gluten-free diet should be continued for life.

Complications. Coeliac disease must be regarded as a pre-malignant condition since *lymphoma of the small intestine* may supervene, usually in middle age or beyond. Although usually reported as Hodgkin's disease or reticulum cell sarcoma, it has recently been suggested that these lymphomas should be classified as a malignant histiocytosis. Symptoms suggesting lymphoma include deterioration in health or recurrence of abdominal discomfort and diarrhoea despite keeping to the gluten-free diet, gastrointestinal bleeding, and skin rashes. Signs include fever, anaemia, lymphadenopathy, clubbing, abdominal distension, and hepatomegaly. Obstruction or perforation of the small intestine may occur. Unless superficial lymph nodes are involved, the diagnosis requires laparotomy; even at laparotomy the diagnosis may not be obvious. Prognosis is poor although occasional long survival is reported. In the management, local resection is recommended where possible: radiotherapy, corticosteroids, and cytotoxic drugs, alone or in combination, are used. There are no studies enabling rational choice of therapy.

In addition to lymphomas, there is an increased incidence of *carcinoma* in coeliac disease. The best-documented association is with carcinoma of the oesophagus but carcinoma of the jejunum and of other parts of the gastrointestinal tract and, indeed, elsewhere in the body are described.

Ulceration of the small intestine, usually in the jejunum, may be followed by stricture formation. The clinical presentation is as intestinal perforation, gastrointestinal bleeding, or subacute obstruction, but there may be merely general ill health raising the suspicion of lymphoma, which may coexist. Ulcers may not be seen radiologically but strictures are more easily identified. The diagnosis usually requires laparotomy. The condition has a bad prognosis and does not appear to respond to a gluten-free diet. Surgical excision is recommended although corticosteroids may be tried if the patient is not fit for surgery. The evidence for pre-existing coeliac disease has been good in some such patients, while others have been shown to have a histological lesion compatible with coeliac disease but have not had a demonstrated morphological response to a gluten-free diet. Yet others have had normal villous architecture. The term 'idiopathic, chronic, ulcerative enteritis' may be applied to this entire group of patients until their relationship to coeliac disease is clarified.

Atrophy of the spleen occurs in some adult patients with coeliac disease.

Dermatitis herpetiformis (See also Sections 19 and 20.) Most patients with the blistering skin condition dermatitis herpetiformis also have a small bowel enteropathy which responds to the withdrawal of gluten from the diet. Thus, by definition, they have coeliac disease. Dermatitis herpetiformis has the same association with histocompatability antigens as coeliac disease. The intestinal lesion in dermatitis herpetiformis is, however, usually mild and is thought to be more patchy than in coeliac disease. The clinical features suggesting malabsorption are also usually mild, often producing no symptoms or signs or obvious nutritional deficiencies. Splenic atrophy occurs commonly.

It is not clear why some patients with coeliac disease develop dermatitis herpetiformis and others do not.

The skin lesion usually improves with a gluten-free diet but, as in other forms of coeliac disease, lymphoma may develop.

Tropical sprue (See also page 12.137)

The term tropical malabsorption may be used to include both post-infective malabsorption and tropical sprue (see also page 12.137). Post-infective malabsorption is the term used when the onset is acute and the symptoms relatively short-lived, with return to normal in weeks or occasionally a few months. Malabsorption may, however, be demonstrated for a period after the symptoms have largely resolved. The term tropical sprue is reserved for the chronic condition.

Tropical sprue is defined as a chronic malabsorption syndrome, without definable cause, in a subject who lives or has lived in the tropics. The term is usually applied only to subjects in whom malabsorption of more than one substance can be demonstrated. The period in the tropics may have been brief and may have predated the symptoms by months or even years.

The problem of post-infective diarrhoea and its relationship to tropical sprue is considered on pages 12.133 and 12.137.

Epidemiology. Tropical sprue is endemic in the Middle East, the Far East, India, and the Caribbean. Within these areas the distribution is patchy. Small and large epidemics are recorded. The condition seems to be relatively uncommon in Africa.

Aetiology. In apparently healthy subjects, bowel habit, nutrition, and jejunal biopsy appearances differ in tropical areas from those in temperate zones. The findings in tropical sprue represent an exaggeration of these differences. The epidemiology suggests, however, that tropical sprue is a distinct entity and not merely the extreme end of a spectrum.

It seems likely that tropical sprue is due to infection of the gastrointestinal tract and the best evidence for this is the response to antibiotics. Delayed transit in the small intestine has been demonstrated and this may favour colonization with responsible organisms. No single type of organism has been incriminated and perhaps different organisms can produce similar effects. The condition is not the same as the stagnant bowel syndrome since the characteristic bacterial flora is not consistently found and there is not, apparently, deconjugation of bile salts in the upper small intestine.

Clinical features. Characteristic clinical features are diarrhoea of small bowel type, abdominal discomfort, abdominal distension, and anorexia. Weight loss may be as much due to anorexia as to diarrhoea. Glossitis and stomatitis are common and soreness of the mouth may be one of the main complaints. Pigmentation of the skin and oedema are also common.

Often the condition starts acutely and in the early stages there may be severe diarrhoea, fever, and blood and mucus in the stools raising the question of dysentery. The symptoms may be persistent or remittent. Nutritional deficiencies persist even when the symptoms remit. Remission commonly, but not necessarily, occurs on leaving the tropics. With increasing duration of disease the initial general lethargy passes on to more clearcut nutritional deficiency

syndromes. Eventually megaloblastic anaemia and even subacute combined degeneration of the spinal cord occur.

The frequencies of the various clinical manifestations and nutritional deficiencies differ in different descriptions and apparently from one geographical area to another. This may depend on the definition of the disorder used, the stage at which patients present, and the industry with which various manifestations are sought, but it remains possible that there are real differences in the disease in different parts of the world.

Investigation. If the onset is acute, and particularly if there are blood and mucus in the stools, amoebic and bacillary dysentery must be excluded. Those parasitic infestations which are found in the area concerned must be excluded. Giardiasis is the most important, being capable of producing all the features of tropical sprue and sometimes being accompanied by abnormal bacterial colonization of the upper small intestine. Infestations with strongyloides, capillaria, and isospora may produce a similar syndrome (see Section 5).

Malabsorption may be confirmed by finding steatorrhoea, or by demonstrating deficiencies of other nutrients such as folic acid, vitamin B_{12} or iron by the usual methods. Vitamin B_{12} deficiency and folate deficiency are common at all stages of the disorder. In contrast to coeliac disease, vitamin D deficiency is much less common in sprue.

Jejunal biopsy reveals changes similar to those found in coeliac disease but usually less severe. There is villous atrophy of variable severity, the epithelium is abnormal, and there is an excess of subepithelial inflammatory cells. Suggested differences from coeliac disease are minor and include a relatively greater number of eosinophils in the lamina propria and a greater tendency for the lesion to extend into the ileum. The relatively severe folate deficiency may produce megaloblastosis of the crypt cells and indeed folate deficiency may be responsible for some part of the villous blunting. Occasionally the biopsy findings are so severe as to resemble those usually seen in coeliac disease; on the other hand the abnormalities may be extremely mild. Thus the biopsy findings, while suggestive, are in no way diagnostic. Interpretation is made more difficult by the wide range of jejunal biopsy appearances in control subjects in the tropics.

An abnormal xylose test, an abnormal glucose tolerance test, secondary hypolactasia, and non-specific abnormalities on small bowel radiology confirm small bowel disease, but are not helpful in differential diagnosis. The gut hormones in sprue are described on page 12.51.

Treatment. Antibiotics are effective. The best documented is tetracycline. Folic acid alone produces some improvement but does not reverse all manifestations. If folic acid is given with the tetracycline, recovery is more rapid. In view of the frequency of deficiency of vitamin B_{12} this should be given too, at the start of the treatment. Clinical improvement is rapid, within days or weeks, and morphological improvement of the jejunal biopsy is also rapid.

Other deficiencies should be treated. In a severely ill patient fluid and electrolyte repletion may be necessary. Symptomatic treatment for the diarrhoea may be necessary.

Treatment must be continued for at least six months, probably longer if the disease has been severe or if the history is long. Complete normality may not be restored and relapses occur, particularly in those who continue to visit or live in the tropics. Thus follow-up should be prolonged.

The contaminated small bowel syndrome

An abnormal bacterial flora in the upper small intestine may lead to a malabsorption syndrome usually manifested particularly by defective absorption of fat and vitamin B_{12}. Malabsorption of carbohydrate, protein, and other nutrients also occurs.

The normal flora of the small intestine. The upper part of the small intestine has a transient and variable flora which is received from the stomach and is derived from the resident mouth organisms and from organisms ingested in the food. The normal gastric acid helps to minimize the load of bacteria transmitted to the small intestine. In residents of temperate zones in the fasting state the upper part of the small intestine is remarkably free of organisms and those few present are aerobes. The further down the small intestine, the more abundant the bacterial flora becomes and the greater the concentration of anaerobes. As the terminal ileum is approached, the spectrum of organisms comes to resemble that in the proximal colon but in much lower concentrations. The microflora in the lumen of the small intestine has beneficial nutritional effects, synthesizing vitamin K and sometimes folic acid, and also deleterious nutritional effects, consuming or binding vitamin B_{12} and deconjugating bile salts.

Causes of bacterial overgrowth. An increase in the bacteria entering the small intestine may be due to reduced gastric acid or to entry of organisms from elsewhere, for example from an infected bile duct. These circumstances rarely result in a clinically significant overgrowth. In contrast a fistula from the colon to the stomach or to the upper small intestine gives entry to a much greater load of bacteria and clinical consequences follow.

The second reason for an abnormally profuse overgrowth of organisms in the small intestine is interference with immune defence mechanisms. The hereditary or acquired agammaglobulinaemias and the much rarer deficiencies of cell-mediated immunity are examples. Impairment of immune mechanisms may be secondary to malnutrition which itself may be secondary to malabsorption. Occasional cases of specific deficiencies of gastrointestinal immune mechanisms have been described, without deficiency of immune mechanisms elsewhere.

Bacterial overgrowth follows stasis of luminal contents in the small bowel which may be due to congenital or acquired anatomical abnormalities including diverticula, strictures, fistulae, and surgically created blind loops. Resection of the ileocaecal valve, particularly if there is also resection of ileum, predisposes to backwash infection of the jejunum.

Stasis may be due to impaired motility. Causes include systemic sclerosis, autonomic neuropathy as occurs in diabetes mellitus, chronic intestinal pseudo-obstruction, and the after effects of radiotherapy to the abdomen. Perhaps the bacterial overgrowth found in the small intestine of otherwise healthy elderly people can be attributed to a combination of decreases in immune mechanisms together with decrease in gastric acid and impaired motility.

Pathogenesis of the malabsorption. When there is bacterial overgrowth in the small intestine the development of the clinical syndrome correlates well with the concentration of anaerobic bacteria. Anaerobes may eventually come to predominate.

The major factor in steatorrhoea is thought to be deconjugation of bile salts, so that the concentration of conjugated bile salts is insufficient for optimal fat absorption.

The overgrowth of bacteria may cause some degree of morphological abnormality in the jejunal mucosa but this is mild in comparison with, for example, coeliac disease and tends to be rather patchy. It seems unlikely that this makes a major contribution to the malabsorption.

Malabsorption of vitamin B_{12} is due to binding or utilization by the bacteria; the absorptive mechanism remains intact.

Diagnosis. Diagnosis of the presence of bacterial overgrowth in the small intestine requires quantitative bacteriology on jejunal aspirates, with particular attention to anaerobes.

The xylose tolerance test usually gives abnormal results in those patients with clinical effects of bacterial overgrowth in the small intestine.

Presumptive evidence of small bowel bacterial overgrowth may be obtained by the bile acid breath test (Fig. 9). A conjugated bile acid, with the amino acid portion labelled with ^{14}C, is given by mouth. If there are abnormal bacteria in the upper small intestine, the bile salt is deconjugated and the radioactively labelled amino acid is absorbed, transported to the liver, and rapidly metabolized to carbon dioxide. The radioactive carbon dioxide excreted in the breath is collected and the amount of radioactivity indicates the amount of deconjugation of the bile salt which occurred in the upper small intestine. In the normal subject very little deconjugation occurs and the conjugated bile salt passes down the small intestine, to be reabsorbed intact in the terminal ileum. In disease of the terminal ileum the conjugated bile salt is not absorbed and enters the colon where deconjugation is produced by colonic bacteria and radioactive carbon dioxide is excreted in the breath. This false positive result in ileal disease can be recognized by measuring the faecal excretion of radioactivity, which is high in ileal disease but not in bacterial overgrowth in the upper small intestine. The bile acid breath test may give false negative results which presumably depend on the particular type of bacteria inhabiting the upper small intestine.

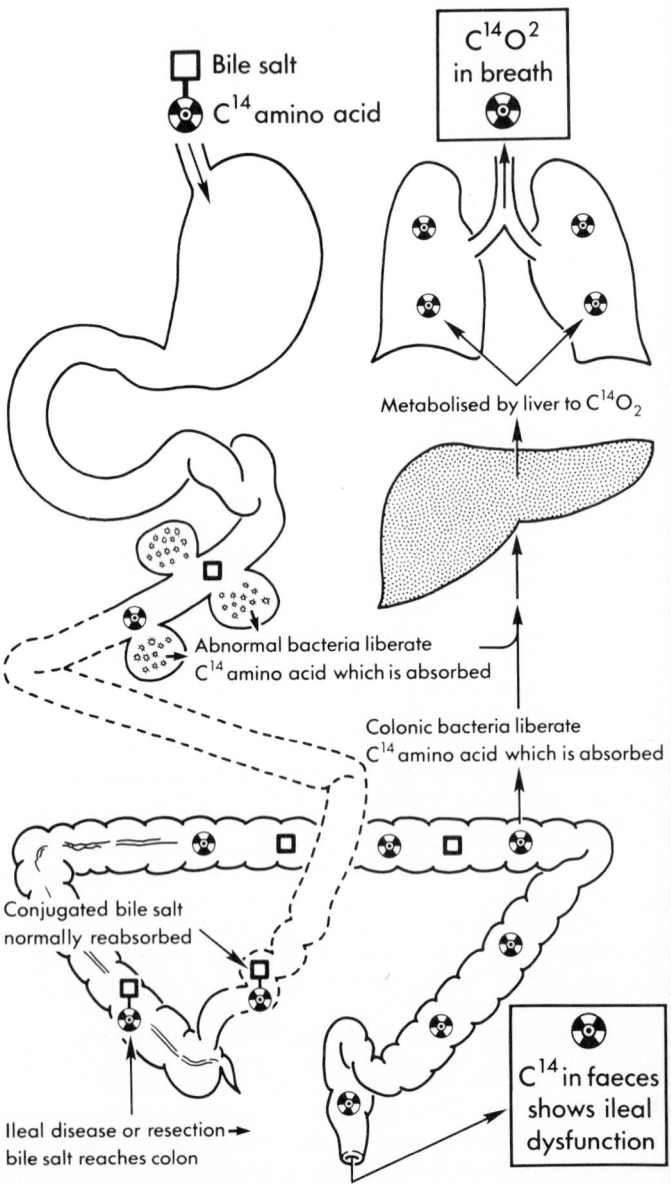

Fig. 9 The radioactive bile acid breath test for detection of bacterial overgrowth in the small intestine. A false positive result may be caused by ileal disease or resection but there is also excess radioactivity in the faeces (see text).

Having established the presence of bacterial overgrowth, investigation is directed at determining the cause. In many cases the cause will be obvious or can be presumed from the history, as for example surgical blind loops or radiotherapy. In some patients the cause may be presumed from other features, such as the skin lesions of scleroderma suggesting systemic sclerosis involving the bowel. If the cause is not clear then an early investigation should be radiological demonstration of the small intestine to seek an anatomical abnormality or disordered motility.

Treatment. An anatomical cause for the condition should be remedied if possible. For example, excision of strictures or of surgical blind loops may give dramatic improvement. If there is an anatomical lesion which cannot be cured then long term follow-up is mandatory.

In preparation for surgery, or if surgery is not possible, antibiotics should be given. The effect of antibiotics on the symptoms and on the absorption of fat and vitamin B_{12} is so reliable as to be useful confirmatory evidence of the diagnosis. Tetracycline is well documented as effective. Antibiotics which are particularly effective against anaerobes, for example metronidazole and lincomycin, are also useful. Neomycin is not consistently effective and, in view of its potential for causing malabsorption, is not recommended. In many patients a brief course of antibiotics for a few weeks gives an effect lasting many months. A further course of the same antibiotic may then be effective. In some patients antibiotics need to be rotated to maintain their effect. Some patients need continuous antibiotics.

Nutritional deficiencies, particularly of vitamin B_{12}, need to be sought and corrected. Provided the malabsorption is adequately treated, long-term nutritional supplements should not be necessary.

If the malabsorption cannot be controlled, which is rarely the case, reduction of long-chain fat in the diet and its substitution by medium-chain triglyceride may be used to maintain weight and nutrition.

The short bowel syndrome

The short bowel syndrome is a term used to describe effects which may follow resection of part of the small intestine. The small intestine has a large reserve for most functions so that it is only after major resection that serious problems are likely. The proximal half of the small intestine may be removed without expectation of serious effects.

The severity of effects depends on (a) the extent of resection (more correctly the length of residual small intestine); (b) the site of resection (adaptation is better in ileum than jejunum, preservation of terminal ileum is important in minimizing loss of bile salts); (c) whether the ileocaecal valve is also resected; (d) whether there is disease of the residual small bowel; (e) whether there is disease of the colon or resection of part of the colon; and (f) whether other organs involved in digestion, such as the liver and the pancreas, are functioning normally.

Crohn's disease is the commonest reason for resection of the small intestine. Other reasons are mesenteric vascular occlusion, volvulus, trauma, lesions due to the effects of abdominal radiotherapy, and rare lesions such as malignancy of the small intestine or multiple strictures or ulcers.

Modern techniques of parenteral nutrition enable long-term survival even with no effective functioning small intestine.

Pathophysiology (Fig. 10). Although the jejunum has a larger mucosal surface area per unit length than the ileum, paradoxically, resection of jejunum gives rise to less severe effects than resection of ileum. Reasons for this include relatively slow transit in the ileum allowing time for digestion and absorption, adaptation of ileal structure and function occurring with time, and retention of the specific ileal functions of absorption of vitamin B_{12} and bile salts which cannot be efficiently undertaken elsewhere in the intestine.

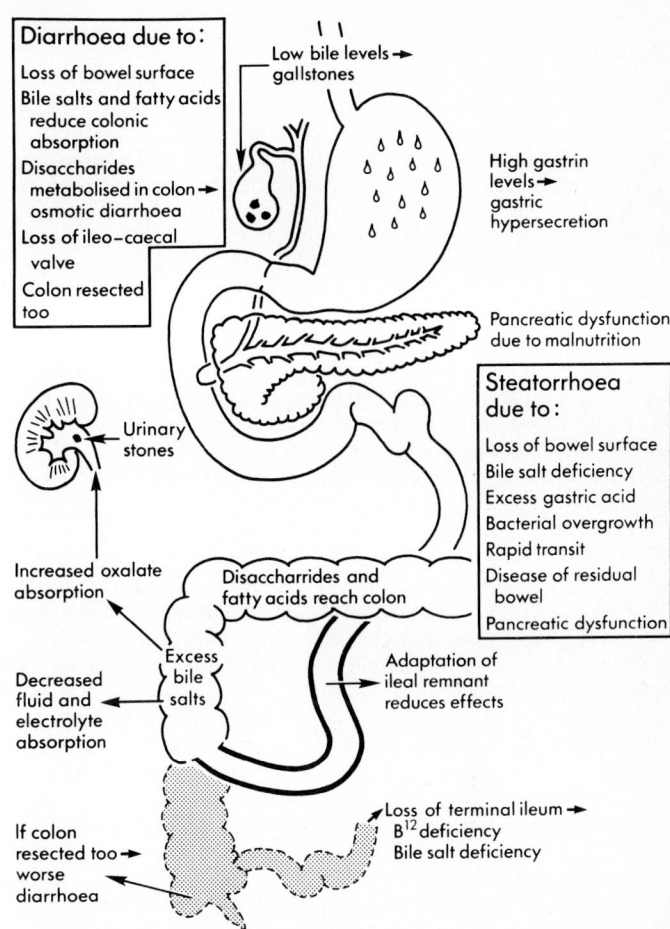

Fig. 10 Pathophysiology following resection of ileum (see text).

Problems which arise particularly after jejunal resection are folic acid deficiency, since folic acid is preferentially absorbed in the upper small intestine, and lactose intolerance, presumably because a large amount of lactase-bearing mucosa has been resected and also in some subjects because an underlying alactasia has been unmasked. Resection of duodenum and jejunum removes the site of cholecystokinin and secretin formation necessary for normal stimulation of the pancreas. Pancreatic exocrine impairment may also be secondary to severe malnutrition consequent on intestinal resection.

Following resection of the ileum vitamin B_{12} deficiency is likely, after an interval of months or years dependent on the magnitude of body stores. Although there is compensatory increase in bile salt synthesis by the liver, unabsorbed bile salts lost into the colon after resection of the terminal ileum may not be entirely replaced and this leads to diminution in the body pool of bile salts and a consequent defect in fat absorption. This is the most important reason for severe steatorrhoea after ileal resection. The unabsorbed bile salts reach the colon and cause excessive loss of water and electrolytes resulting in watery diarrhoea. The storage of bile salts synthesized overnight often results in the watery diarrhoea being more severe in the morning. Unabsorbed fatty acids contribute to the diarrhoea by their action on the colon, as do short-chain fatty acids formed by colonic bacteria acting on unabsorbed disaccharides.

Bile salts also affect colonic absorption of oxalate, paradoxically causing increased absorption. This, and other mechanisms, result in a high level of urinary oxalate and an increased risk of urinary oxalate stones.

There is an increased likelihood of gallstones after ileal resection and this may be related to diminished bile salt concentrations available for solubilization of cholesterol in the bile.

Gastric hypersecretion occurs after resection of the small intestine, more severe with jejunal than ileal resection and more severe in the early months after operation. The mechanism is not well understood but high serum gastrin levels are found and it may be that the small intestine normally inactivates gastrin or that it produces an inhibitor of gastric secretion (see page 12.51). The excessive acid secretion may exacerbate steatorrhoea by inactivating pancreatic lipase (as in the Zollinger–Ellison syndrome) and it may cause peptic ulceration. The excessive loss of chloride may even produce a hypochloraemic alkalosis. All of these clinical manifestations are, however, rare and gastric secretion need only be investigated if diarrhoea persists after the more usual forms of treatment, or if the other complications of hypersecretion of acid occur.

Resection of the ileocaecal valve along with ileal resection is associated with more severe diarrhoea. This is probably dependent on the functions of the ileocaecal valve in delaying transit and in preventing reflux of colonic bacteria. Bacterial colonization of the small intestine may then contribute to steatorrhoea.

Management

Fluid and electrolytes. In the early post-operative period severe watery diarrhoea with massive loss of fluid and electrolytes is common. Careful intravenous repletion is life-saving. An isotonic oral solution of saline and glucose, as has been found useful in cholera, may be helpful. Parenteral nutrition may be necessary if this stage is prolonged.

Bowel motility. Antiperistaltic drugs such as codeine, diphenoxylate (combined with atropine as Lomotil), and loperamide may be used. Particularly in the early stages, the absorption of these drugs may be impaired and they may need to be given parenterally.

Diet. After the early days or weeks, oral feeding should be introduced. Oral feeding tends initially to aggravate the diarrhoea and thus should be commenced gradually with easily digested foods such as sugars, small peptides, and medium-chain triglyceride, without lactose, and given as nearly isotonic as possible. 'Elemental' diets may be used, diluted, by slow drip, via a nasogastric tube.

With time a more normal diet may be introduced, initially given as small frequent feeds, with a low fat content. In the long term a relatively high calorie intake may be necessary to compensate for poor absorptive function. Frequent small meals should be encouraged. Fat restriction reduces calorie intake directly and also by making the diet less appetising. Thus fat intake should be allowed to the extent that it does not cause significant increase in the diarrhoea. Medium-chain triglyceride may be taken in addition to or, preferably, instead of long-chain fat. In the short term this is very useful but patients may not tolerate useful amounts of medium-chain triglyceride for long.

Nutritional supplements. Nutritional deficiencies of folic acid, vitamin B_{12}, and iron are easily tested for and corrected.

Methods of assessment of vitamin D status are now becoming available, enabling diagnosis prior to severe clinical manifestations of tetany and osteomalacia (see Section 17). Estimation of plasma levels of vitamin D metabolites is however, unfortunately not yet widely available. Bone biopsy has revealed sub-clinical osteomalacia to be more common than hitherto suspected, even without disturbance of serum calcium, phosphorus, alkaline phosphatase, or urinary calcium.

Assessment of deficiencies of other fat soluble vitamins and of minerals such as magnesium and possibly zinc should also be undertaken at intervals. Deficiencies of water-soluble vitamins, other than vitamin B_{12} and folic acid, rarely occur.

Because of these potential nutritional deficiencies, follow-up must be life-long.

Other measures. If the clinical state remains unsatisfactory or if complications arise, then other measures, deduced from the pathophysiology, may be helpful.

Watery diarrhoea, due to the effects of bile salts on the colon, may be helped by cholestyramine. This, however, tends to exacerbate the steatorrhoea, particularly after extensive ileal resection, by increasing the excretion of bile salts. Symptomatic benefit must be balanced against this. If there is severe gastric hypersecretion of acid, H_2 receptor antagonists may help to reduce steatorrhoea. Peptic ulcer should be treated by these drugs rather than surgery which would tend to exacerbate steatorrhoea and cause other problems. Secondary pancreatic exocrine dysfunction, which will contribute to steatorrhoea, may be treated by pancreatic supplements.

If gallstones are found, unless they are causing severe symptoms, cholecystectomy should be avoided so as to preserve the reservoir function of the gallbladder. If urinary oxalate stones occur, they should be treated on their merits, and it may be thought wise to avoid high oxalate foods and maintain a high urine volume.

If the ileocaecal valve has been removed, and if there is evidence of overgrowth of organisms in the small intestine, antibiotics such as tetracycline may be helpful.

Reversal of a short segment of the distal end of the remaining small intestine has been undertaken as a means of slowing intestinal transit. Other ingenious surgical manoeuvres have also been described. Although benefit has resulted in individual cases, such surgical manoeuvres are not generally recommended.

For the most severely affected patients, long term parenteral nutrition may be necessary.

Gastric surgery

A minor degree of steatorrhoea is common after all types of gastric surgery for peptic ulcer, with the probable exception of highly selective vagotomy (see also page 12.69). It causes no symptoms, requires no treatment, and is unrelated to the weight loss which is so common after gastric surgery. Symptomatic malabsorption occurs in a small proportion of patients, sometimes early but sometimes not until years after surgery, and should lead to a search for a complicating disorder. With time, deficiencies of iron and folic acid occur relatively commonly, and deficiency of B_{12} less commonly. Total gastrectomy is almost always followed by malabsorption and this combines with diminished intake to induce nutritional deficiencies, especially of vitamin B_{12}, which may be severe.

Mechanisms of malabsorption. Loss of the function of the pylorus, and thus of the reservoir action of the stomach, leads to rapid gastric emptying which, particularly with liquid meals, dilutes the bile and pancreatic juice. This is probably more important in limiting the early stages of digestion than loss of the normal mechanism of stimulation of bile and pancreatic juice which follows some types of gastric surgery. Poor mixing of the food with bile and pancreatic enzymes may play a part.

If there is a long afferent loop, malabsorption may be due to bacterial contamination of the small intestine; reduction of gastric acid output contributes to bacterial overgrowth. Pancreatic atrophy may be an early or delayed feature of gastric surgery and pancreatic exocrine deficiency contributes to steatorrhoea. The operation may unmask concomitant conditions which have hitherto been asymptomatic. These include gluten-sensitive enteropathy, alactasia, and jejunal diverticula.

Occasional anatomical abnormalities such as a gastrocolic fistula and an inadvertent gastro-ileostomy are important because they are correctable. It must be remembered that the small stomach remaining after some forms of gastric surgery may lead to malnutrition of dietary origin.

Management. Frequent small meals should be recommended. Nutritional deficiencies should be treated. Symptomatic management of diarrhoea may help.

Investigation for mechanisms of malabsorption, and concomitant conditions listed above, should be undertaken and will suggest appropriate therapy. Oral pancreatic supplements may allow weight gain even without clear evidence of pancreatic insufficiency.

If medical measures prove unsatisfactory, various types of revisional surgery are available depending on the nature of the problem and of the original operation.

Follow-up should be life-long.

Disaccharidase deficiency and malabsorption

The enzymes responsible for splitting disaccharides into monosaccharides are found in the brush border of the intestinal epithelial cells, the concentration of the enzymes being highest in the proximal small intestine. Deficiencies of these disaccharidases may occur either as an isolated deficiency of an enzyme (primary deficiency) or as a result of small intestinal disease (secondary deficiency).

Hypolactasia. This is a common condition. Congenital lactase deficiency, however, is rare. It presents in neonates and is thought to be inherited as an autosomal recessive. The majority of patients with primary hypolactasia develop symptoms later in life, and although a role for inheritance has been suspected, the pattern is not yet clear.

Distribution. In Europe and North America, primary hypolactasia is found in 3–20 per cent of the population—the figure for the United Kingdom is about 6 per cent. However, it occurs in about 75 per cent of the American Black population and approaches 100 per cent in certain African and Oriental races. To what degree the lactase deficiency is contributed to by villous abnormalities caused by infections and parasites in these populations is unknown.

Aetiology and pathogenesis. In many animals, including mammals, intestinal lactase activity declines within a few weeks of weaning. This pattern has now been observed in many human populations who have a high incidence of hypolactasia in the adult. The persistence of lactase activity in whites of European origin can therefore be regarded as abnormal. It has been suggested that this is related to the continuing ingestion of milk but the evidence for this hypothesis is not strong. Secondary hypolactasia can occur in association with any disease that damages the small intestinal villi, e.g. coeliac disease, tropical sprue, Crohn's disease, infestation with *Giardia lamblia*, bacterial overgrowth, rotavirus infections in children, and cholera.

The inability to split disaccharides results in defective absorption of these sugars and hence they pass into the colon. Diarrhoea is caused partly by the increased osmotic load and partly by the products of bacterial fermentation. This latter process is responsible for the gaseous distension, which is a common clinical feature, and for the high lactic acid content of the stools. In children, the pH of the stool can be a useful diagnostic clue for disaccharidase deficiency but it is seldom helpful in adults.

Clinical features. Lactase deficiency is associated with loose or watery diarrhoea, intermittent abdominal distension, audible borborygmi, and the passage of excess flatus. There is usually no systemic upset or weight loss. Many patients may be symptom-free while others have marked symptoms and this presumably relates to dietary lactose intake and the severity and extent of the hypolactasia. Some patients present with symptoms of an irritable colon syndrome but these usually persist despite treatment.

Diagnosis. The definitive diagnostic test is the measurement of lactase activity in a jejunal biopsy. Other tests that can be used are the lactose tolerance test and the measurement of breath hydrogen following an oral dose of lactose. The lactose tolerance test, in which blood glucose is measured following oral lactose, correlates poorly with lactase activity measured directly and is associated with a high false positive and false negative rate. The hydrogen breath

test, in contrast, correlates well with biochemical assays and is the test of choice since it is simple and non-invasive. The oral dose of lactose used in these tests (50 g) usually causes symptoms in hypolactasic patients.

Treatment. Lactose-free diets usually bring about a marked improvement in symptoms. Patients with secondary hypolactasia may also benefit from a temporary lactose-free diet while the underlying disorder is being treated. A common pitfall is to ignore the lactose content present in many pharmaceutical tablets, e.g. diazepam, nitrazepam, soluble aspirin, benzhexol, and a variety of iron and vitamin tablets. This source of lactose may be quite sufficient to cause symptoms in patients with a severe lactase deficiency.

Sucrase–isomaltase deficiency. As a secondary deficiency, this is always associated with hypolactasia and rarely causes symptoms in its own right. Congenital sucrase–isomaltase deficiency is rare and is probably inherited as a autosomal recessive. It usually presents with watery diarrhoea and failure to thrive at about four weeks of age when sugar is being introduced into the diet. Treatment is by eliminating sugar from the diet. As the child grows older, sugar tolerance usually increases.

Malabsorption due to drugs

Many drugs can be shown to cause malabsorption of individual nutrients, in a small proportion of patients. Common and clinically significant malabsorption is, however, restricted to a very few drugs, the commonest being neomycin and cholestyramine. Colchicine and para-aminosalicylic acid are also well documented causes of steatorrhoea. Ethyl alcohol, while not strictly a drug, may be considered here.

Malabsorption produced by drugs is reversible and dose-related. Multiple mechanisms are involved including structural damage to the mucosa, inhibition of mucosal or luminal enzymes, precipitation of bile acids and fatty acids, other physico-chemical alterations which affect absorption, and alteration of bowel flora.

Neomycin. This is the best documented example of drug-induced malabsorption. Neomycin is a poorly absorbed antibiotic, used long-term in the management of patients with hepatic encephalopathy. It produces a reversible malabsorption of nutrients including fat, nitrogen, carotene, iron, vitamin B_{12}, and glucose. Neomycin also causes malabsorption of other drugs. The effect is dose dependent and, while commoner with larger doses, may be seen at doses of 2–3 g per day which are commonly used. Similar effects have been described for other antibiotics of this group such as kanamycin.

The mechanism of the malabsorption is multifactorial. Histological changes in the villi have been demonstrated, binding and precipitation of fatty acids and bile acids occur in the lumen, and inhibition of cellular and luminal enzymes probably contributes.

Cholestyramine. Cholestyramine is a resin used for its property of binding bile salts in the bowel lumen. Common uses are in patients with itching due to obstructive jaundice and in patients with diarrhoea induced by bile salts escaping into the colon as a consequence of ileal resection or disease.

By virtue of its function of binding bile salts cholestyramine causes excessive loss of bile salts from the body. In the normal individual this can be largely compensated by increased synthesis, and marked steatorrhoea does not occur. When used in the context of obstructive jaundice or ileal disease, in both of which there is a diminished concentration of bile salts in the duodenal lumen, increased bile salt loss may give rise to marked steatorrhoea and consequent malabsorption of fat soluble vitamins. Cholestyramine also binds nutrients such as iron and vitamin B_{12} and also certain other drugs.

Colchicine. Colchicine is well documented as a cause of steatorrhoea, if given long term in doses of 2 g or more per day. Malabsorption of fat, carbohydrate, vitamin B_{12} and carotine has been demonstrated. The mechanism is probably direct injury to the mucosa.

Para-aminosalicylic acid. This is well documented as a cause of steatorrhoea. Malabsorption of carbohydrate, vitamin B_{12}, folate, and iron are also documented.

Ethyl alcohol. Ethyl alcohol produces a direct effect on the small intestine, probably causing damage to sub-cellular organelles. Other causes of malabsorption in alcoholic subjects include liver damage, pancreatic damage, the effect of folate deficiency on the small bowel mucosa, and the administration of neomycin to control encephalopathy. Malabsorption of fat, fat soluble vitamins, carbohydrate, vitamin B_1, folic acid, and vitamin B_{12} has been demonstrated.

Other drugs. The biguanides, used as oral antidiabetic drugs, have been shown to cause malabsorption of fat, amino acids, carbohydrates, and vitamin B_{12}. This is probably produced by direct mucosal damage.

Chronic abuse of irritant purgatives may give rise to malabsorption of fat and carbohydrate, and probably also other substances. Methotrexate, and other drugs used in the chemotherapy of malignant disease, cause damage to the epithelium of the small intestinal mucosa because of its rapid rate of turnover. Drugs causing either an increase or a decrease in intestinal motility may alter rates of absorption particularly of other drugs, the precise effect varying from substance to substance, presumably depending on the site, efficiency, and rapidity of absorption. Methyldopa has occasionally been reported to cause malabsorption, probably by damage to the mucosa.

It is possible that one of the causes of folic acid deficiency in patients taking anticonvulsants is malabsorption of folic acid (see Section 19).

Lymphoma of the small intestine

The small intestine may be involved in lymphoma which arises primarily elsewhere in the body. Malabsorption is not a major consideration.

Localized lymphoma may arise primarily in the small intestine and this may present with general features of malaise, fever, and anorexia, or with local features of perforation, obstruction, or a palpable mass. Malabsorption is rarely a problem except for those arising in association with coeliac disease.

There is a type of primary lymphoma which presents with generalized disease of the small intestine and mesenteric lymph nodes. Malabsorption is a prominent feature. This condition is closely related to alpha chain disease (see page 12.98). Although well under 200 cases have been reported worldwide, the condition may not be excessively rare in some Mediterranean areas such as North Africa (see page 12.98).

Generalized lymphoma of the small intestine. The early lesion consists of a diffuse infiltration, with plasma cells and lymphocytes, of the lamina propria of the whole length of the small intestine and also of mesenteric lymph nodes. In some, probably most, such patients excessive production of free polypeptide, which bears a close resemblance to the alpa chain portion of the IgA immunoglobulin molecule, can be demonstrated. If this material can be detected, in serum or in intestinal fluid or in cells, the term alpha chain disease is applied. Careful analysis shows that the material does not consist of entire normal alpha chains and there are probably subtle differences between the molecules produced in different patients. Rare cases of alpha chain disease primarily involve other organs which have a secretory immunoglobulin system, notably the respiratory tract and other parts of the gastrointestinal tract.

Pathogenesis. Several features of the disease have led to the suggestion that it may commence as a reaction to prolonged local antigenic stimulation. It occurs predominantly among underprivileged peoples with a high prevalence of intestinal infections and infestations, the infiltrate consists of plasma cells and lymphocytes, alpha chains are part of the IgA molecule which is the major intestinal secretory immunoglobulin, and there appears to be a premalignant phase with long remission following treatment with antibiotics.

In view of the possibility of a pre-malignant phase it has been suggested that the term *immunoproliferative small intestinal disease* (IPSID) is preferable to referring to all patients as having lymphoma.

Clinical features. Characteristically this is a condition of young people, usually not beyond the third decade. Early descriptions centred on the Mediterranean but cases have now been described in many parts of the world, mainly in underprivileged peoples.

The usual symptoms are abdominal pain, vomiting, and anorexia, often for some years. Diarrhoea and weight loss are almost invariable. Fever and finger clubbing are common. Peripheral lymphadenopathy occurs rarely. Severe malabsorption is nearly always present.

Investigation. The diagnosis is made by jejunal biopsy. There is generalized, massive infiltration of the lamina propria, predominantly with plasma cells but also with lymphocytes. In some patients there is no clear evidence of malignancy, the plasma cells appear benign and are confined to the lamina propria. The villi are flattened and the crypts separated out and not hypertrophied. The overlying epithelium is remarkably normal. The whole length of the small intestine is affected but the lesion varies in severity from place to place. The presence of cytological features of malignancy also differs from place to place.

Fat, xylose, and vitamin B_{12} absorption are diminished. Nutritional deficiencies are usual. A raised level of plasma alkaline phosphatase may be shown to be due to the intestinal iso-enzyme.

Radiology of the small intestine may, or may not, show strictures and filling defects and evidence of enlarged mesenteric lymph nodes.

In some patients excess alpha chains may be suspected from an abnormal band on electrophoresis of plasma proteins. Excess alpha chains may, however, be present without such a band. They may be demonstrable only in intestinal juice, or occasionally in cells. Sensitive and specific immunological methods are necessary to be certain of the presence of alpha chains. This question was discussed earlier on page 12.83.

At the moment it seems that not all patients with the generalized form of lymphoma of the small intestine have alpha chain disease.

Course and management. Untreated, the course of the disease is variable, some patients having partial remission. Nevertheless, in the present state of knowledge all patients should be treated.

If there is no overt malignancy, one approach is to undertake staging laparotomy at the outset, with biopsies of small intestine from several places and removal of several lymph nodes to try to detect malignancy. Alternatively, tetracycline may be given and intestinal biopsy and assays for alpha chains in blood and intestinal fluid repeated after several weeks. Even if there is apparent disappearance of the disease, follow up must be life-long since eventual malignancy is to be expected, even after intervals of many years. Lack of response to tetracycline would be an indication for staging laparotomy. Antilymphoma therapy (see Section 19) should probably be given to all patients who have not had improvement after some months on antibiotics and to those who have not achieved complete remission by 12 months.

If there is histological evidence of malignancy, chemotherapy is indicated, or radiotherapy or both. Antibiotics should also be given and perhaps steroids as well. Remission may follow.

It seems reasonable to stop treatment some six months after a complete remission has been obtained. Further experience is necessary for firm treatment guidelines.

Termination with disseminated malignancy has been described.

Recent developments. Initially the picture of 'Mediterranean' lymphoma and alpha chain disease was of a remarkably uniform condition. More recently the clinical and pathological spectrum has been extended. It is now clear that there may be no diarrhoea or malabsorption even though there is extensive infiltration of the small intestine. The condition may present with lymphoma in peripheral lymph nodes. Distant organs including liver, lung, and bone may be involved. There may be only segmental involvement in the gastro-intestinal tract, with sparing of the proximal small intestine. The distribution of alpha chain disease may be as lymphomatous polyps of the small intestine with normal mucosa between.

Whipple's disease

Whipple's disease (see also Section 19) is a very rare condition with the pathognomonic feature of massive periodic acid Schiff (PAS) positive deposits of glycoprotein within the macrophages in the lamina propria of the small intestine. Similar deposits occur in the abdominal lymph nodes and elsewhere but are not diagnostic in these situations. Electron microscopy suggests that the glycoprotein deposits are residues of bacteria. The response to antibiotics is further evidence of an infective cause. The organism involved, if indeed a single organism is responsible, has not been identified. A defective immune response by the host may well be a pre-requisite.

Clinical features. Most patients are middle-aged men of Caucasian stock. The disease has been recorded in siblings.

There is usually a long history prior to diagnosis. Weight loss and diarrhoea, with features suggesting steatorrhoea, are almost invariable. Most patients have episodes of migratory polyarthritis affecting large joints and receding without leaving deformity. Spondylitis may occur. The arthritis may precede other manifestations by a long period. Pyrexia is not uncommon and there may be a long history of undiagnosed episodes of pyrexia.

Other relatively common features are abdominal pain without specific diagnostic features, peripheral lymphadenopathy, pigmentation of the skin (but not the buccal mucosa), and clubbing of the fingers.

Symptoms and signs reflecting nutritional deficiencies, consequent upon the steatorrhoea, are common.

In a minority of patients other manifestations occur, including pleural effusion, pericardial effusion, endocarditis, and central nervous system involvement.

Investigation. The definitive investigation is jejunal biopsy (Fig. 3a, page 12.88). The villi are swollen, distorted and flattened because the lamina propria is stuffed with foamy macrophages which stain with PAS reagent. This is diagnostic. Distended lymphatic spaces may be seen within the villi. The overlying epithelium is not severely abnormal, a point of distinction from coeliac disease with which there might just be confusion if the villi are severely flattened. The lesion in the small intestine may be rather patchy.

Steatorrhoea and multiple nutritional deficiencies are almost invariable.

X-rays of the small bowel show only oedema of the folds and the bowel wall, but suggestive evidence of grossly enlarged lymph nodes may be obtained and may give a clue to the diagnosis.

Treatment. The response to antibiotics is dramatic and life-saving. Responses have been recorded to many different antibiotics. Prolonged therapy is necessary. A recommended regimen is intramuscular penicillin one to two million units per day and intramuscular streptomycin 1 g daily for two weeks, followed by tetracycline 1 g per day for a year. Other antibiotic regimens are probably equally effective.

Corticosteroids are not to be recommended except perhaps in a desperately ill patient while awaiting response to antibiotics.

Clinical response to antibiotics should occur within a week or two, but morphological response in the small intestine takes much longer.

Lymphangiectasia

Dilatation of lacteals within the villi may be secondary to obstruction of lymphatic vessels by abdominal malignancy or infection, or may be secondary to constrictive pericarditis and other conditions affecting the heart and pericardium (see also Section 13). A similar dilatation of lacteals within the villi occurs, as a very rare disorder, without obvious underlying disease, usually presenting in children but sometimes in young adults, and is presumed to represent congenital hypoplasia of lymphatic vessels (see pages 12.82 and 12.144).

Clinical features. Mild diarrhoea and steatorrhoea may occur, probably caused by failure of lipid transport in the lymphatics. Severe steatorrhoea occurs in a minority of patients. Hypoproteinaemia is thought to be due to rupture of the dilated lacteals into the lumen of the gut resulting in loss of protein as well as lipid. Oedema of the legs, which may be asymmetrical, is a manifestation of hypoproteinaemia and also frequently of associated abnormalities of lymphatic vessels from the legs. There may be chylous effusions into peritoneal or pleural cavities.

Investigation. Diagnosis is made by jejunal biopsy which shows distended lymphatics in the cores of a small proportion of the villi (Fig. 3c, page 12.88). Thus the abnormality is more likely to be seen if multiple biopsies are taken and if the entire biopsy is examined by the dissecting microscope or by sections for histology at many levels.

Radiology of the small bowel may show no abnormality, or coarse folds due to oedema, or non-specific features of malabsorption.

There is hypoproteinaemia and lymphocytopenia, the latter due to loss of lymphocytes into the gut lumen. Protein loss into the gut can be demonstrated by the appropriate tests. Abnormalities of lymphatic vessels in the legs may be shown by lymphangiography.

Treatment. A very low fat intake minimizes the loss of fat, protein, and lymphocytes from the bowel. This diet is, however, unpalatable and may not be tolerated. Medium-chain triglycerides may be tried. In some children the lymphatic abnormality is localized to a short length of intestine. This can be decided only at laparotomy and, if found, resection should be attempted and may give considerable benefit (see page 12.144). There is a report of amelioration by a lymphatic-venous anastomosis but this must rarely be an option.

Primary hypogammaglobulinaemia and the small intestine

Patients with defective immune mechanisms frequently have gastrointestinal symptoms. The syndrome of severe combined immune deficiency may have malabsorption as a feature. Chronic granulomatous disease may be associated with partial villous atrophy of the small intestine. However, primary hypogammaglobulinaemia (see page 12.81) is much the commonest primary immune deficiency and gastrointestinal features which may occur in this condition are described below.

Diarrhoea. In this condition there are several causes of diarrhoea. An important and common superimposed infection is giardiasis. There is dispute as to whether bacterial overgrowth explains symptoms in many of these patients. Bacterial overgrowth may be due more to achlorhydria, which is a feature of such patients, than to the deficiency of humoral immunity. Disaccharidase deficiency is common and may be partly due to bacterial overgrowth.

Malabsorption. Malabsorption occurs in a significant proportion of patients, perhaps one in four. The malabsorption is usually mild but is occasionally overt and leads to gross nutritional deficiencies. Malabsorption is rare in childhood.

Giardiasis is responsible for the malabsorption in many if not most of these patients. Giardia may be difficult to demonstrate and should be sought not only in the stools but also in the jejunal aspirate and by smearing the mucosal biopsy on to a microscope slide. Giardia is responsible for various degrees of villous atrophy, even severe villous atrophy, and the lesions may be patchy. It is justifiable to treat for giardiasis even if the organism is not found.

Even in the absence of giardiasis, a few patients have a mucosal lesion, which may be severe enough to suggest coeliac disease. The diagnostic feature histologically is absence, or extreme paucity, of plasma cells. In a very few such cases suggestive evidence of a response to a gluten-free diet has been reported. The evidence is not as clear cut as in some patients with selective deficiency of IgA, in whom coeliac disease is well documented. Rarely patients with selective IgA deficiency have a villous lesion which does not respond to gluten withdrawal.

There is conflicting evidence as to the importance of bacterial overgrowth in the small intestine in causing malabsorption in these patients. Broad spectrum antibiotics such as tetracycline may be tried. Injections of immune globulins may be added but there is little evidence to justify this.

Associated conditions. Nodular lymphoid hyperplasia, consisting of multiple, small (3–5 mm) nodules of lymphoid hyperplasia demonstrated on small bowel X-ray, is a feature of various immunoglobulin deficiency syndromes, perhaps particularly if there is giardia infection.

Exocrine pancreatic deficiency has been described in association, in a few patients.

A variety of liver disorders has been described in association, and presumably bile salt deficiency may contribute to malabsorption in these patients.

Idiopathic chronic ulcerative enteritis has been described as a complication: steroids and antibiotics have been used in treatment.

Abetalipoproteinaemia

This is a very rare, genetic disorder probably with autosomal recessive inheritance (see Section 9 for more detailed discussion). There is absence, or virtual absence, of betalipoproteins in the plasma probably dependent on a deficiency of the apoprotein. There is an inability to synthesize chylomicrons and other low density lipoproteins. Plasma cholesterol, triglyceride, and phospholipid are all low.

Clinical features. Early in life there is malabsorption, which is often mild, and coeliac disease may be erroneously diagnosed. The red cells are of abnormal shape with multiple spikes (acanthocytosis) (see Section 19). The full syndrome which develops by adolescence or adult life consists of a progressive neurological disorder (with cerebellar and posterior column signs and sometimes other features), atypical retinitis pigmentosa, steatorrhoea, and acanthocytosis (see also Section 9). Partial syndromes occur.

Diagnosis. A low serum cholesterol and a low ESR (the abnormal red cells do not aggregate) may suggest the diagnosis. Absent betalipoproteins, acanthocytes (best seen on wet blood films), and failure to form chylomicrons after a fatty meal are confirmatory. Jejunal biopsy shows normal villous morphology with pronounced cytoplasmic vacuolation of the enterocytes over the upper parts of the villi. Specific stains show the vacuoles to contain neutral fat. There is little fat in lacteals in the central portions of the villi.

Management. There is no effective treatment. A low fat diet and medium chain triglyceride are usually recommended. Vitamin A deficiency is common and should be treated. Deficiencies of the other fat-soluble vitamins and of essential fatty acids should be sought and treated. It is possible that treatment with large doses of vitamin E may have some effect in slowing the rate of deterioration.

Systemic sclerosis affecting the small intestine

It seems likely that visceral accompaniments, of this skin disorder are relatively common, but often asymptomatic (see also Section 16). Visceral lesions are described with minimal skin involvement and may precede the skin lesions. Very rarely similar visceral abnormalities occur without obvious skin lesions.

Clinical features. When symptoms due to intestinal involvement occur, they consist of abdominal distension and discomfort, nausea and vomiting, and loose stools. If the colon is involved, there may be constipation or even faecal impaction. Diarrhoea and constipation may alternate. Dysphagia and oesophageal reflux, with abnormal oesophageal motility, are features of the syndrome and help in diagnosis if there is doubt about the skin lesions.

Investigation. Radiology of the small intestine may show gross duodenal distension and, less commonly, distension of other parts of the small intestine. Motility of affected regions is poor. The distended small intestine shows folds which are crowded together, in contrast to the appearance in other forms of distension (Fig. 6, page 12.90).

Intestinal biopsy shows mild inflammatory changes in the villi in some patients. Full thickness biopsy is necessary to see the submucosal collagen and focal muscle atrophy which occur.

Steatorrhoea and bacterial overgrowth in the small intestine occur.

Management. Corticosteroids are probably of no benefit to the bowel lesion. Antibiotics may reduce the small bowel bacterial overgrowth and hence improve the steatorrhoea but the response is usually only temporary. Medium-chain triglyceride may be tried. Nutritional deficiencies should be repleted. Eventually parenteral feeding may be felt necessary and justified.

Intestinal pseudo-obstruction (See also page 12.43)

This may be defined as a clinical syndrome with features suggesting intestinal obstruction but without a mechanical cause. The syndrome is not identical to that of mechanical obstruction in that there is usually diarrhoea and not constipation, and flatus continues to be passed. Thus the clinical features are nausea and vomiting, colicky abdominal pain, and abdominal distention, usually with diarrhoea. Radiology shows disordered motility of the small intestine and, by definition, absence of mechanical obstruction.

There are three forms of intestinal pseudo-obstruction, acute, chronic, and idiopathic recurrent. All are rare. Acute intestinal pseudo-obstruction is a complicating feature in other illnesses, including pneumonia, pancreatitis, congestive heart failure, and many other acute and chronic conditions. The main effect is on the colon and malabsorption is not a feature. Chronic intestinal pseudo-obstruction affects many parts of the gastrointestinal tract and may be secondary to other disorders, gastrointestinal or not. Gastrointestinal disorders associated with this condition include jejunal diverticulosis, systemic sclerosis or other collagen disease affecting the gut, and amyloidosis affecting the gut. Non-gastrointestinal conditions include hypothyroidism, diabetes mellitus, chronic neurological disorders such as muscular dystrophy, Parkinson's disease, and Chagas' disease, and the effect of some drugs such as phenothiazines, tricyclic antidepressants, and some of the drugs used to treat Parkinson's disease. In coeliac disease pseudo-obstruction is a rare complication and tends to be episodic thus being more similar to the idiopathic recurrent variety.

Idiopathic recurrent intestinal pseudo-obstruction. This is a very rare condition, sometimes starting early in life. By the time the patient is seen there may be a long history and several previous laparotomies. Each episode lasts some days to a week or more: with time the symptoms tend to become more persistent. Characteristically there is diarrhoea but this may alternate with constipation. In a few instances members of the family have been similarly affected and family studies may reveal milder manifestations in other members, and in some there is also atony of the bladder.

Investigation discloses steatorrhoea during the attack and often in between attacks. Nutritional sequelae of steatorrhoea may be found. Radiology shows distended small bowel and very slow transit and there may be evidence of disordered motility. The distension may be limited to the duodenum and upper jejunum as in systemic sclerosis. Other parts of the gastrointestinal tract may be distended, particularly the colon.

Broad spectrum antibiotics may help the malabsorption, presumably because of bacterial overgrowth secondary to the stagnation. Such help is usually only transient. Unless the dilatation is localized, surgery should be avoided if mechanical obstruction is confidently excluded. Parenteral nutrition may be necessary.

Protein-losing enteropathy

Hypoalbuminaemia may occasionally result from excessive loss of serum proteins into the intestine. This is an important condition to recognize because the resulting oedema or ascites may overshadow the intestinal symptoms and hence the condition is easily missed.

Aetiology. This condition (Table 2) has been found in association with a wide variety of inflammatory or neoplastic disorders of the small bowel and abdominal lymphatic system. It has also been observed rarely in association with allergic disorders involving the small bowel (see page 12.83).

Table 2 Some causes of protein-losing enteropathy

1 Mucosal ulceration
Gastric or colonic tumours
Multiple gastric ulcers
Ulcerative colitis
Crohn's disease

2 Without ulceration
Coeliac disease
Sprue
Whipple's disease
Allergic enteritis
Post-infective
Giant rugae of stomach (Menetrier's disease)
Villous adenoma of colon
Fistulae

3 Lymphatic disorders
Lymphoma
Lymphangiectasia
Infestation (*Capillariasis philippinensis*)
?Constrictive pericarditis

Clinical features. The condition is characterized by marked peripheral oedema and occasionally by ascites and pleural effusions. There is marked hypoalbuminaemia in the absence of liver or renal disease. In many but not all cases there are associated symptoms relating to the underlying disorder.

Diagnosis. The diagnosis is made by determining the rate of loss of protein into the intestine using a radioactive label. The most suitable compound for this purpose is ^{51}Cr-labelled albumin. After intravenous injection the rate of excretion of the chromium label into the stool is measured. In normal individuals about 5–25 ml of plasma is cleared daily into the gastrointestinal tract; in patients with protein-losing enteropathy this level is very much elevated. ^{67}Cu-labelled ceruloplasmin may also be used for estimating the loss of protein into the bowel. The further diagnosis of the condition is directed towards determining the underlying cause as indicated in Table 2.

Treatment. The treatment is directed towards albumin replacement and correction of the underlying disorder. For example, cases associated with neoplasms of the stomach or colon should be treated by surgical resection. Those secondary to coeliac disease, sprue, Whipple's disease, or allergic gastroenteropathies should be treated accordingly (see appropriate entries in this section). If the underlying cause can be eradicated, the prognosis for this condition is extremely good.

Miscellaneous causes of malabsorption

Some of the malabsorption syndromes are described elsewhere in this book. These include allergic disorders of the stomach and small bowel (page 12.82), infections of the small bowel (page 12.137), amyloidosis (Section 19), and endocrine disorders including thyrotoxicosis, hypoparathyroidism, and diabetes (Section 10). Isolated disorders of vitamin B_{12} absorption are considered in Section 19. The primary immune disorders of the bowel are considered in further detail on page 12.80. The problem of post-infective malabsorption is considered in detail on page 12.138. The carcinoid syndrome is described on page 12.55 and systemic mastocytosis in Sections 19 and 20.

References

Alexander-Williams, J. and Hoare, A. M. (1979). Postsurgical syndromes: the stomach, part II. Partial gastric resection. *Clins Gastroent.* **8**, 321.

Alpers, D. H. and Seetharam, B. (1977). Pathophysiology of involving intestinal brush-border proteins. *New Engl. J. Med.* **296**, 1047.

Baer, A. N., Bayless, T. M., and Yardley, J. H. (1980). Intestinal ulceration and malabsorption syndromes. *Gastroent.* **79**, 754.

Borriello, P., Hudson, M., and Hill, M. (1978). Investigation of the gastrointestinal bacterial flora. *Clins Gastroent.* **7**, 329.

Cooper, B. T., Holmes, G. K. T., Ferguson, R., and Cooke, W. T. (1980). Celiac disease and malignancy. *Medicine, Baltimore* **59**, 249.

Donaldson, R. M. (1978). Carbohydrate intolerance. In *Gastrointestinal disease* (eds. M. H. Sleisenger and J. S. Fordtran), 1181. W. B. Saunders, Philadelphia.

Faulk, D. L., Anuras, S., and Christensen, J. (1978). Chronic intestinal pseudoobstruction. *Gastroent.* **74**, 922.

Freeman, H. J., Kim, Y. S., and Sleisenger, M. H. (1979). Protein digestion and absorption in man: normal mechanisms and protein-energy malnutrition. *Am. J. Med.* **67**, 1030.

Friedman, H. I. and Nylund, B. (1980). Intestinal fat digestion, absorption and transport. *Am. J. clin. Nut.* **33**, 1108.

Gray, G. M. (1975). Carbohydrate digestion and absorption—role of the small intestine. *New Engl. J. Med.* **292**, 1225.

— (1978). Intestinal disaccharidase deficiencies and glucose-galactose metabolism. In *The metabolic basis of inherited disease*, 2nd edn. (ed. J. B. Stanbury, J. B. Wyngaarden, and D. S. Fredrickson). 1526. McGraw-Hill, New York.

Herlinger, H. (1978). A modified technique for the double-contrast small bowel enema. *Gastrointest. Radiol.* **3**, 201.

Longstreth, G. F. and Newcomer, A. D. (1975). Drug-induced malabsorption. *Mayo Clinic Proc.* **50**, 284.

Losowsky, M. S., Walker, B. E., and Kelleher, J. (1974). *Malabsorption in clinical practice.* Churchill Livingstone, Edinburgh.

Marshak, R. H., Lindner, A. E., and Maklansky, D. (1979). Lymphoreticular disorders of the gastrointestinal tract: roentgenographic features. *Gastrointest. Radiol.* **4**, 103.

Perera, D. R., Weinstein, M. D., and Rubin, C. E. (1975). Small intestinal biopsy. *Human Pathol.* **6**, 157.

Sahi, T. (1978). Dietary lactose and the aetiology of human small-intestinal hypolactasia. *Gut* **19**, 1074.

Scott, B. B. and Losowsky, M. S. (1977). The definition and diagnosis of coeliac disease. *J. Roy. Col. Phycns.* **11**, 405.

Sleisenger, M. H. and Brandborg, L. L. (1977). *Malabsorption.* W. B. Saunders, Philadelphia.

Sturman, R. M. (1968). The Bassen–Kornzweig syndrome: 18 years in evolution. *J. Mt. Sinai Hosp.* **35**, 489.

Thaysen, E. H. (1977). Diagnostic value of the ^{14}C-cholylglycine breath test. *Clins Gastroent.* **6**, 227.

Weser, E. (1979). Nutrition aspects of malabsorption; (short gut adaptation). *Am. J. Med.* **67**, 1014.

Williamson, R. C. N. (1978). Intestinal adaptation—structural, functional, and cytokinetic changes. *New Engl. J. Med.* **298**, 1393.

— (1978). Intestinal adaptation—mechanisms of control. *New. Engl. J. Med.* **298**, 1444.

Crohn's disease

D. P. Jewell

Crohn's disease is a chronic inflammatory disease of the gastrointestinal tract, the cause of which remains unknown. It is characterized by a granulomatous inflammation affecting any part of the gastrointestinal tract, frequently in discontinuity, and by the tendency to form fistulae.

History. The first clear description of the disease affecting the terminal ileum (regional ileitis) was given by Crohn, Ginzburg, and Oppenheimer in 1932. However, the disease certainly existed long before then and many of the early descriptions of ulcerative colitis would now be regarded as Crohn's disease. Dalziel, in 1913, described an inflammatory process of the ileum and colon consisting of ulceration, submucosal oedema, fibrosis, and mesenteric lymphadenopathy. He reported the presence of granulomata on microscopy but could find no evidence of tuberculosis. Similar cases were described in the 1920s by Moschowitz and Willensky.

Following the description by Crohn and his colleagues, it was clearly recognized that the colon could also be involved and, on occasions, it could be the sole site of the disease. The disease therefore became known as regional enteritis or, preferably, Crohn's disease. Colonic disease is referred to as Crohn's disease of the colon, Crohn's colitis, or granulomatous colitis.

Epidemiology. Crohn's disease is well recognized in Europe, Scandinavia, North America, and Australasia but it is rarely seen in India, tropical Africa, and South America. This may be largely due to the difficulty of diagnosing Crohn's disease in areas where intestinal tuberculosis is common and to the problems of long-term follow-up. The disease is also said to be rare in Japan but its prevalence there appears to be increasing.

There has been a striking increase in the incidence and prevalence of Crohn's disease in Europe and Scandinavia since 1950 (Table 1). This is also shown by examining the Annual Discharge Rates in England and Wales. For Crohn's disease, the rate rose from 2.8 per 100 000 in 1958 to 7.2 per 100 000 of the population in 1971 whereas the rate for ulcerative colitis during the same period was unchanged at 10–12 per 100 000. Recent studies in Scotland and in Stockholm have suggested that the incidence has begun to decline.

Table 1   Incidence of Crohn's disease per 100 000 population

Aberdeen	1955–61	1.7	Uppsala	1956–61	1.7
	1964–66	3.3		1962–67	3.1
	1967–69	4.5		1968–73	5.0
	1970–72	4.3	Stockholm	1955–59	1.5
	1973–75	2.6		1960–64	2.2
Cardiff	1934–70	1.1		1965–69	3.6
	1971–77	4.6		1970–74	4.5
Malmö	1958–65	3.5		1975–79	4.1
	1966–73	6.0			

The reasons for the changing patterns of incidence are not clear. Much of the increased incidence is due to an increased frequency of colonic disease and it might be argued that this represents diagnostic transfer from ulcerative colitis to Crohn's disease. The Annual Discharge Rates for England and Wales, quoted above, make this explanation unlikely. Whether similar changes in frequency have occurred in North America is uncertain although the data available suggest that the incidence has probably not altered. It is possible that the changing incidence may result from an infective or environmental factor.

Crohn's disease occurs in all age groups but it is rare in early childhood and most commonly affects young adults. There is no marked sex difference, and no association with social class or occupation. In the USA, there may be an increased incidence amongst Jews.

Genetics. There is a definite familial incidence of the disease, reports varying from 6–15 per cent, and the affected members of a given family may have Crohn's disease or ulcerative colitis. However, there is no clear mode of inheritance and there is no established association with HLA types, apart from those patients who also have ankylosing spondylitis who usually have the HLA-B27 phenotype. Discordance for the disease in a pair of identical twins suggests that environmental factors may be operating but the extreme rarity of ulcerative colitis or Crohn's disease in both husband and wife makes it unlikely that environmental factors alone are responsible for the disease.

Aetiology. The aetiology is unknown but there is current interest in the role of diet, the presence of an infective agent, and the extent to which immunological mechanisms are involved in the pathogenesis of the disease.

Diet. Several workers have reported that patients with Crohn's disease have a higher intake of refined sugar than a control population or a matched group of patients with ulcerative colitis. Patients with Crohn's disease also have a reduced intake of fibre, especially that derived from fruit and vegetable. The significance of these changes, however, remains in doubt.

Infective agents. Conventional techniques have failed to isolate any specific bacterium, mycobacterium, or virus from tissue involved with Crohn's disease or from the faeces of affected patients. Recently extracts from Crohn's tissue have induced cytopathogenic effects in tissue culture cell lines but whether this represents the presence of a specific virus is far from established. The isolation of *Mycobacterium kansasii* from a mesenteric node of one patient with Crohn's disease was an interesting finding but further studies in a large group of patients were negative. Cell-wall deficient pseudomonads have also been isolated from Crohn's tissue but this observation has neither been confirmed nor refuted. There is, therefore, no substantial evidence of an infective agent and this is supported by the absence of case-clustering.

Immune mechanisms. Patients with Crohn's disease usually have normal serum concentrations of immunoglobulins and complement components, although raised concentrations may be found in association with active disease. Neutrophil and monocyte functions, *in vitro*, show no defect, although inhibitors of cell motility are often present in the serum of patients with active disease. There may be some reduction in the absolute numbers of circulating T lymphocytes and this may explain the depressed responses to non-specific mitogens and the relative anergy to delayed hypersensitivity skin testing that have been variously reported. The histological features suggest that a cell-mediated response may be involved but there is little immunological evidence for this. Lymphocytes from some patients appear to be sensitized to colonic epithelium or coliform antigens, and circulating lymphocytes may be cytotoxic to colonic epithelium. However, similar findings are present in many patients with ulcerative colitis and therefore they may be secondary to inflammation rather than primary effector mechanisms. Antigen–antibody reactions may be another important effector mechanism in the pathogenesis of the disease as suggested by increased consumption of complement and the presence of circulating small immune complexes. Impairment of suppressor cell activity during active disease has been found which might account for the increased circulating antibody titres to dietary and bacterial antigens but, so far, no basic defect in immuonregulatory control has been observed.

Pathology. Crohn's disease may occur anywhere in the gastro-intestinal tract although the commonest pattern is an ileocolitis. The disease is often discontinuous giving rise to the so-called skip lesions. Isolated involvement of the mouth, oesophagus, stomach, and anus is recognized but such cases are extremely rare. Macro-scopically the bowel is thickened and frequently stenosed. The serosal surface may be inflamed and the mesentery becomes oede-matous. The regional mesenteric nodes are usually enlarged. The earliest macroscopic lesion on the mucosal surface is an aphthoid ulcer—a small superficial lesion often surrounded by hyperaemia. In areas of more severe disease, deep fissuring ulcers occur in the oedematous and inflamed mucosa giving rise to a cobblestone pattern. Long, serpiginous ulcers are a further characteristic fea-ture. Strictures occur as a result of submucosal fibrosis and, because of serosal inflammation, the affected intestine may become adher-ent to adjacent loops of intestine or other structures (e.g. bladder or vaginal vault) with the subsequent formation of fistulae.

Histologically, the inflammation is transmural and consists prin-cipally of lymphocytes, histiocytes (tissue macrophages), and plasma cells. Granulomata are found in only 65 per cent of patients and they occur more commonly the more distal the disease; that is, they are present in most cases with rectal disease but are much less common in ileal disease. The mucosal architecture is well preserved despite heavy inflammation and, in the colon, goblet cells are usually present even though the glands are being infiltrated with inflammatory cells. Fissures penetrating into the submucosa and lined with histiocytic cells are frequently present.

Quantitative histology and enzyme studies have suggested that the whole of the gastrointestinal tract is abnormal in patients with Crohn's disease even though only one segment may be overtly involved at any one time.

Immunofluorescent and immunoperoxidase studies have shown a large increase in IgG- and IgM-containing cells with a smaller rise in IgA-containing cells. Even in quiescent disease, the IgG- and IgM-containing cells appear to be increased compared with the normal intestine.

Clinical features. The manifestations of Crohn's diseaee are pro-tean and are partly determined by the anatomical location of the disease. The majority of patients complain of diarrhoea (70–90 per cent), abdominal pain (45–66 per cent), and weight loss (65–75 per cent). Fever is also common (30–40 per cent). Colonic disease causes rectal bleeding more commonly than ileal disease but even so it is present in only about 50 per cent of patients with Crohn's colitis. Colonic disease is also associated with peri-anal disease (in about one-third of patients) and with the extra-intestinal manifesta-tions which are uncommonly seen when the disease is confined to the ileum. Symptoms of anaemia are common and usually occur as a result of iron deficiency from intestinal blood loss or, less fre-quently, from vitamin B_{12} or folate deficiency. Other features of malabsorption are infrequent but in patients with extensive small bowel disease, symptoms and signs of osteomalacia may occur and there may be a bleeding tendency secondary to vitamin K malabsorption. Nutritional deficiencies may also be present, e.g. deficiencies of magnesium, zinc, ascorbic acid, and the B vitamins, but these are rare and are usually due to inadequate intake.

A few patients present with the clinical features of acute appendi-citis but at operation they are found to have an acute terminal ileitis. Only a minority of these prove to be due to Crohn's disease. Diagnostic difficulties may also occur when the disease presents without gastrointestinal symptoms. These include patients present-ing with fever, weight loss, and anaemia without diarrhoea or abdominal pain and patients with ileocaecal disease presenting with urinary frequency and dysuria due to ureteric involvement.

Physical examination may be normal but many patients will show evidence of anaemia. Glossitis and aphthous ulcers in the mouth, beaking or frank clubbing of the nails, evidence of weight loss, and a tachycardia are common features. Abdominal examination often reveals tenderness over the affected bowel which can often be felt to be thickened. An abdominal mass is frequently palpable when small intestinal disease is present. Anal examination often shows the presence of fleshy skin tags which have a characteristic viol-aceous hue. Anal fissures, perianal fistulae, and abscesses are particularly associated with colonic disease.

The extra-intestinal manifestations of Crohn's disease are similar to those of ulcerative colitis. Table 2 lists those that are most frequently seen.

Table 2 Extra-intestinal manifestations of Crohn's disease

	Frequency (%)	Comment
Related to disease activity		
Apthous ulceration	20	
Erythema nodosum	5–10	
Pyoderma gangrenosum	0.5	
Acute arthropathy	6–12	large joints affected; transient, non-destructive
Eye complications:	3–10	
Conjunctivitis		
Episcleritis		
Uveitis		
Unrelated to disease activity		
Sacro-iliitis	15–18	usually asymptomatic; may be present in up to 50% using isotope scan-ning; unrelated to HLA-B27
Ankylosing spondylitis	2–6	75% patients possess HLA-B27 phenotype
Liver disease		
Pericholangitis	5–6	
Primary sclerosing cholangitis		very rare and poorly documented in Crohn's disease
Gallstones	very common	due to malabsorption of bile salts from ileum
Chronic active hepatitis	2–3	
Cirrhosis	2–3	
Fatty change	6	very common in ill patients requiring surgery
Amyloid	rare	
Granulomas		

Complications. Patients with Crohn's disease can develop an acute dilatation of the bowel (defined as a colonic diameter of 5 cm or more on a plain radiograph), perforation, or massive haemorrhage especially when the disease involves the colon. These complica-tions, however, occur less frequently than they do in ulcerative colitis. The more usual complications are intestinal obstruction due to strictures in the small or large intestine and fistulae. The latter may occur between other parts of the gastrointestinal tract (e.g. gastrocolic, enterocolic) or between the affected loop of intestine and the bladder or vagina. Pneumaturia, the passage of faeces in the urine or a faecal vaginal discharge are cardinal features of the latter forms of fistula formation. The gross malabsorption that occurs with a gastrocolic or ileocolic fistula is largely due to bac-terial overgrowth of the small intestine. External fistulae to the skin also occur but this is usually secondary to surgical intervention. Crohn's disease affecting the terminal ileum or the right side of the colon may involve the right ureter giving rise to frequency with a sterile pyuria, a frank urinary tract infection, or a ureteric stric-ture with subsequent hydronephrosis. Left-sided disease may oc-casionally involve the left ureter but this is very uncommon.

Hyperoxaluria and oxalate stones may be complications of ileal disease associated with steatorrhoea. The mechanism is currently thought to be due to binding of calcium to unabsorbed fat leaving the oxalate free to be absorbed from the colon.

Carcinoma of the colon may complicate Crohn's colitis. The incidence is about 3–5 per cent—a frequency similar to that of carcinoma associated with ulcerative colitis. However, the risk factors are not yet established although histological dysplasia has been noted in some cases of Crohn's colitis. Small bowel carcinomas have been reported in association with ileal Crohn's disease.

Amyloid is another complication of Crohn's disease which may occur within the bowel or systemically, e.g. liver, spleen, and kidney. If renal function is deteriorating, the affected bowel should be resected as the amyloid may then regress with concomitant improvement in renal function.

Radiological appearances. A plain X-ray of the abdomen should always be obtained together with decubitus films. These are often normal but may show evidence of intestinal obstruction or suggest an inflammatory mass in the right iliac fossa. In acute Crohn's colitis, evidence of mucosal oedema and ulceration may be clearly seen on the plain films. This appearance may obviate the need for barium studies which should, if possible, be avoided in the presence of severe, active disease. The plain film can also provide evidence of sacro-iliitis or ankylosing spondylitis.

Examination of the oesophagus, stomach, and duodenum is best done endoscopically because the radiological appearances are often non-specific and biopsies are required for histological confirmation. The small intestine may be examined with a standard barium meal and follow-through but much more information is obtained using the barium infusion technique (small bowel enema, enteroclysis). Following colonic preparation, a tube is passed until the tip lies just beyond the ligament of Treitz and a dilute barium suspension is infused (800–1200 ml). The earliest lesions are thickening of the valvulae coniventes and small, discrete aphthoid ulcers. In more severe disease, cobblestoning, fissure ulcers, and thickening of the wall occur (Fig. 1). Longitudinal ulcers may also occur but these are uncommon. Areas of stenosis and dilatation may be present and sinus tracts and fistulae may be demonstrated. Asymmetry of the bowel is often present, although this may be an unreliable sign. The abnormal segment of the intestine is usually well demarcated from the normal bowel.

Radiological examination of the colon is performed using a double-contrast barium enema following a thorough but gentle preparation. Characteristically there is rectal sparing but the appearances of Crohn's colitis are otherwise similar to those described for the small intestine (Fig. 2). Table 3 lists the main features which differentiate the radiological appearances of Crohn's colitis from ulcerative colitis. The barium enema is a good means of showing internal fistulae and fistulae to other organs.

If fistulae to the surface are present, sinograms should be performed to delineate the anatomy.

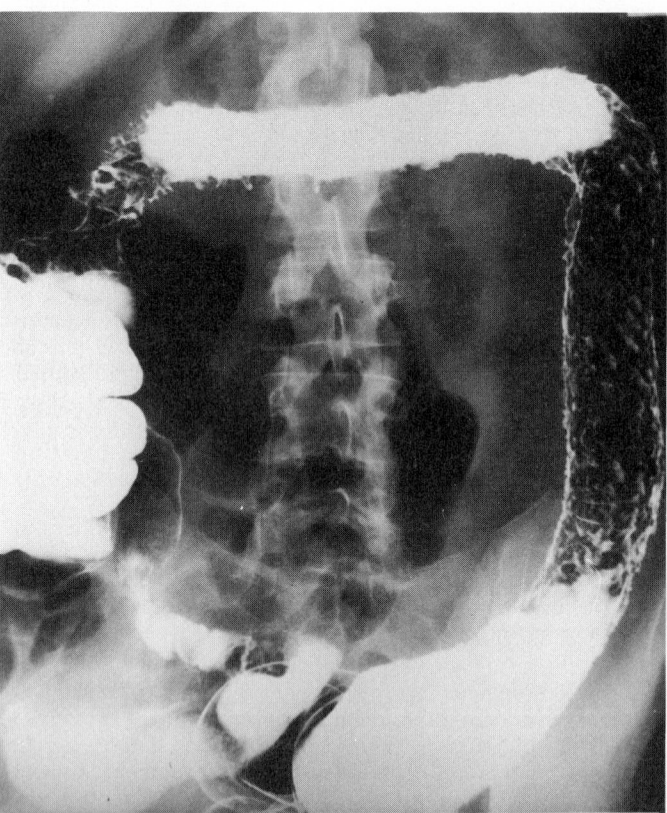

Fig. 2 Barium enema showing Crohn's disease of the colon and terminal ileum. Distal sigmoid, rectum, and a segment of ascending colon are normal. The diseased segments show loss of haustration, shortening, and fissure ulcers. (Courtesy of Dr D. J. Nolan.)

Endoscopy. Sigmoidoscopy and rectal biopsy should be performed in all patients. The rectal mucosa is frequently normal but may show a granular proctitis and occasionally the typical appearances of Crohn's disease.

The indications for colonoscopy are: (*a*) to examine the colon and obtain biopsies in suspected cases in whom the barium enema is normal or equivocal; (*b*) to obtain biopsies from strictures; (*c*) to

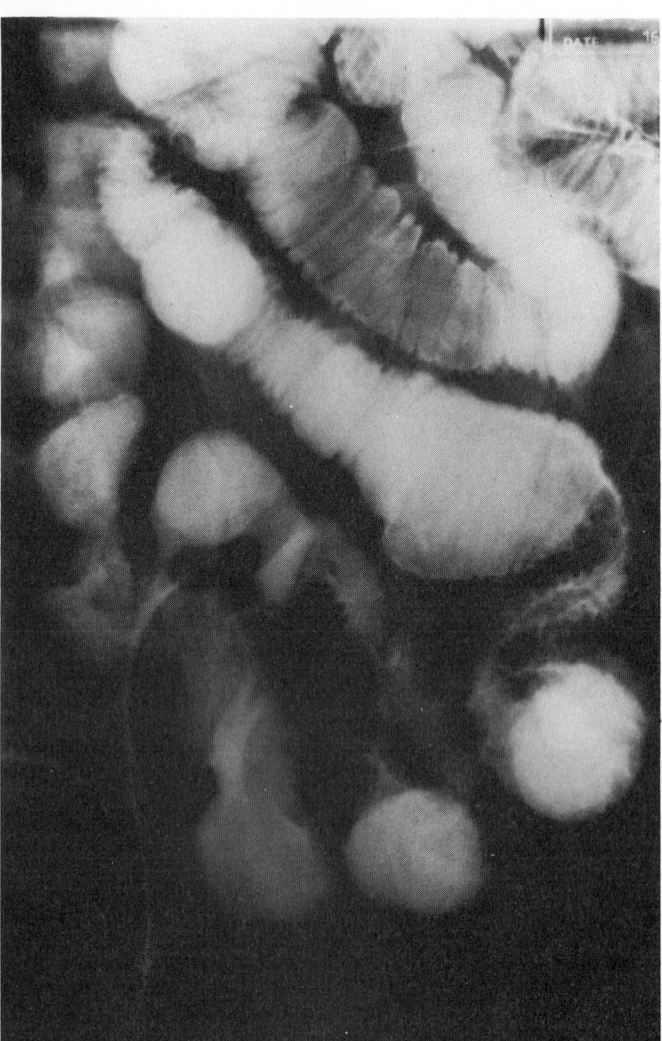

Fig. 1 Small bowel enema demonstrating Crohn's disease of the terminal ileum with fissure ulcers, ileocaecal fistulae, and partial obstruction. (Courtesy of Dr D. J. Nolan.)

Table 3 Differential diagnosis of Crohn's disease and ulcerative colitis

	Crohn's disease	Ulcerative colitis
Clinical features		
Bloody diarrhoea	less common	common
Abdominal mass	common	rare
Peri-anal disease	common	less common
Malabsorption	frequent (ileal disease)	never
Radiological features		
Rectal involvement	frequently spared	invariable
Distribution	segmental, discontinuous	continuous
Mucosa	cobblestones	fine ulceration
	fissure ulcers	'double-contour'
Strictures	common	rare
Fistulae	frequent	rare
Histological features		
Distribution	transmural	mucosal
Cellular infiltrate	lymphocytes, plasma cells, macrophages	polymorphs, plasma cells, eosinophils
Glands	gland preservation	mucus depletion gland destruction crypt abscesses
Special features	apthoid ulcers granulomata histiocyte-lined fissures	none

obtain biopsies when the differential diagnosis is in doubt; and (d) to assess activity and extent of disease in symptomatic patients when there is little clinical evidence of activity. A further advantage of colonoscopy is that biopsies can often be obtained from the terminal ileum.

Endoscopically the earliest lesion of colonic Crohn's disease is a small aphthoid ulcer surrounded by normal mucosa with a normal vascular pattern. This contrasts with the erythema and loss of vascular pattern seen in ulcerative colitis. In more severe disease the mucosa becomes oedematous and is penetrated by fissuring ulcers to give a cobblestone appearance. The ulcers are often linear and may eventually become confluent. A diffusely inflamed granular, friable, and dark red mucosa is typical of ulcerative colitis although discrete ulceration may occur in severe cases. Pseudopolyps and mucosal bridges occur in both diseases.

Multiple biopsies should be taken even from apparently normal areas of mucosa since granulomata may be present which allows a precise diagnosis to be made.

Upper gastrointestinal endoscopy is not routinely required in these patients and is only indicated in the presence of appropriate symptoms or if abnormalities are noted on a barium meal. Although Crohn's disease of the stomach or duodenum may occur as an isolated phenomenon, most cases are associated with disease elsewhere in the gastrointestinal tract. Deep longitudinal ulcers may occur in the stomach together with rugal hypertrophy and a cobblestone appearance. In the duodenum the major differential diagnosis is duodenal ulcer but there is usually a 'cobblestone' mucosa surrounding the frank ulceration. Biopsies are usually helpful although granulomata are found infrequently.

Laboratory data. Anaemia is common and is often due to mixed deficiencies. Iron deficiency from intestinal blood loss is the commonest cause but serum folate and vitamin B_{12} concentrations may also be low. The blood film and MCV may therefore show microcytosis or macrocytosis. Combined deficiences may result in a normochromic anaemia. Serum ferritin is the best indicator of iron stores in these patients with chronic disease. A neutrophil leucocytosis is usually, but not invariably, associated with active disease and there may also be a thrombocytosis. The total lymphocyte count and the absolute number of circulating T lymphocytes may be reduced.

Hypokalaemia is associated with severe diarrhoea and the

plasma urea concentration is often low, reflecting a poor dietary intake of nitrogen. Serum albumin is reduced in the presence of active disease and studies with ^{51}Cr-labelled albumin often demonstrate a protein-losing enteropathy. Serum immunoglobulins are normal or mildly elevated and there may be a rise in the alpha-2 globulins. A low serum calcium, when corrected for albumin, is unusual unless there is extensive small bowel disease and a low urinary calcium is more likely to reflect a poor diet rather than osteomalacia. Liver function tests are frequently abnormal, usually consisting of mild elevations of the aspartate transaminase (AST) and the alkaline phosphatase. Persistence of abnormal liver function tests suggests associated liver disease and should be investigated by liver biopsy and visualization of the biliary tree. Patients with extensive ileal disease or with ileal stricture may have increased faecal fat excretion. This is usually secondary to bacterial overgrowth rather than loss of absorptive surface, and is compounded by the low circulating pool and increased excretion of bile salts which is often present in patients with long-standing ileal disease. It is important not to miss magnesium and zinc deficiencies which are occasionally present.

Diagnosis. This may be delayed for several years. Intermittent abdominal symptoms and diarrhoea without systemic symptoms are often labelled as the irritable colon syndrome. Weight loss, fever, and anaemia without gastrointestinal symptoms are another source of misdiagnosis. The diagnosis of Crohn's disease in children may be considerably delayed when it presents as failure to thrive or delayed puberty but without gastrointestinal symptoms.

Even when the clinical diagnosis seems sound, all patients must have: (a) stool examination to exclude pathogens; (b) sigmoidoscopy and rectal biopsy: characteristic features (e.g. a granuloma) may often be present in the biopsy specimen even when the mucosa is macroscopically normal; (c) radiology of the small and large intestine to confirm the diagnosis and establish the extent of the disease; and (d) colonoscopy with multiple biopsies is indicated where the above investigations are equivocal or normal and there are strong clinical reasons for suspecting Crohn's disease. Colonoscopy should also be performed if the differential diagnosis is in doubt or if strictures are present.

Differential diagnosis. Few patients with an acute ileitis and a clinical picture of an acute appendicitis subsequently develop Crohn's disease. Serological examination helps to diagnose those cases caused by Yersinia; the aetiology of the remainder is unknown. The main differential diagnosis of ileal Crohn's disease is tuberculosis, especially when the disease occurs in patients from areas where intestinal tuberculosis is common. Laparoscopy may be helpful if serosal tubercles are present as they can be biopsied and cultured. Stool culture and circulating antibodies to mycobacteria are unhelpful. If genuine doubt exists, corticosteroid therapy for Crohn's disease must be covered with antituberculosis therapy. Other differential diagnoses include abdominal lymphoma, alpha chain disease, actinomycosis, amyloid, Behçet's disease, and carcinoma of the small bowel.

The major differential diagnosis of Crohn's colitis is ulcerative colitis (Table 3). Crohn's disease should also be considered in patients presenting with proctitis since 30 per cent of patients with ileal Crohn's disease may have a proctitis and may present in this way. When a segmental colitis occurs, ischaemia, tuberculosis, and lymphoma have to be excluded. Young adults may present with an acute segmental colitis which is self-limiting. The cause is unknown although, in women, oral contraceptives have been implicated. Crohn's disease can be overlooked on the barium enema when it occurs in association with severe diverticular disease.

As indicated above, Crohn's disease may have to be considered in the differential diagnosis of a fever with weight loss, malabsorption, and delayed development.

Assessment of activity. There is no satisfactory method of assessing activity of the disease and this poses a major clinical problem. Symptoms such as fever or continuing weight loss are obvious indicators but severe disease can be present in the absence of any major symptom. Laboratory evidence of activity includes reduced serum albumin levels and increased C-reactive protein concentration (a much more sensitive indicator than the ESR). Recently a number of elaborate indices have been developed—the American Crohn's disease activity index (CDAI) and the Dutch activity index (AI)—but they are not ideal for general use.

Management. The management of Crohn's disease involves medical therapy, surgical treatment, and nutritional support at various times during the course of the disease. Patients are therefore best managed by a physician and a surgeon working as a team.

The role of diet is controversial although it appears that many patients have diets deficient in vegetable and fruit fibre and rich in refined sugar. Whether a change to a high fibre, low sugar diet will alter the course of the disease is currently being evaluated. In general, patients should be advised to take a well-balanced diet. A low-residue diet is indicated for patients with strictures and a low-fat diet for those with steatorrhoea. Patients with hypolactasia may benefit from a lactose-free diet.

Medical treatment. Deficiencies of folic acid, vitamin B_{12}, and vitamins B, C, and D are treated with appropriate supplements. Similarly, electrolyte deficiencies are also corrected. Iron deficiency can be treated with oral supplements but patients with this disorder are often intolerant to oral iron and in such cases intravenous total dose infusion is the best form of treatment.

In general, Crohn's disease is only treated if it is causing symptoms; there is no indication for giving corticosteroids or other forms of therapy to asymptomatic patients. Corticosteroids are indicated, however, in symptomatic patients with evidence of active disease. In the presence of severe disease, an intravenous regimen of nutrients, fluids, electrolytes, and pednisolone 21-phosphate (60–80 mg daily) should be employed. Patients are allowed only water by mouth. A good clinical response usually occurs and at the end of five to seven days oral feeding can be resumed together with oral corticosteroid therapy. Patients with less severe disease can be treated with prednisolone 20–40 mg daily by mouth. There is no defined duration of corticosteroid therapy although most patients will have made a good symptomatic response after four to six weeks; the dose can then be reduced over a further four to six weeks and then stopped. Sulphasalazine (Salazopyrin, Azulfidine) has also been shown to have some effect on active colonic Crohn's disease although this has not been a universal experience. There is no evidence that long-term treatment with either corticosteroids or sulphasalazine is beneficial.

Azathioprine is ineffective in the treatment of active disease and its use as a maintenance agent is controversial. Certainly, some patients appear to derive benefit from it and it should probably be given to patients who are not responding to corticosteroids or who relapse as soon as the corticosteroid dose is reduced. Although azathioprine was originally described for the treatment of Crohn's fistulae, it is now thought to be of little value for the management of this complication.

Many other treatments have been tried (levamisole, dapsone, transfer factor, cromoglycate) but there is little evidence to support the use of any of them. Metronidazole may be useful if there is bacterial infection superimposed on active Crohn's disease, e.g. peri-anal sepsis, abscesses associated with fistulae, and small bowel overgrowth secondary to ileal stasis. However, metronidazole probably has no direct effect on the disease process. Elemental diets are currently in vogue and anecdotal experience is promising in those patients who can tolerate the diet for prolonged periods.

Surgery. The majority of patients (70–80 per cent) will require at least one operation during the course of their disease. Indications for surgery include: disease failing to respond to medical therapy and continuing to cause symptoms; strictures causing mechanical obstruction; fistulae; and other local complications such as abscess and perforation. Severe peri-anal disease is not necessarily an indication because it is frequently asymptomatic.

When surgery is required, the following principles apply. Resection should be limited to removing only the most severely affected bowel, and end-to-end anastomoses should be performed, even if there is inflammation in the tissue being anastomosed. Bypass procedures (e.g. ileotransverse colostomy for ileocolitis) should be avoided as they are associated with a high risk of recurrence. When fistulae are present, surgical management should be staged. For example, an ileostomy can be made above all the fistulae as a first procedure. This allows the active disease to settle and the patient to gain weight and restore his nutrition. A second operation can then be performed in order to resect the diseased bowel and the fistulae. Panproctocolectomy may be required for extensive Crohn's colitis and this operation is probably preferable to an ileorectal anatomosis which is associated with a high risk of recurrence. In Oxford, Crohn's colitis which has not responded to medical therapy is treated with a split ileostomy. Corticosteroids are then dripped daily into the isolated colon. After one to two years, the majority of patients have healed and anatomical continuity can be restored. This procedure is often followed by a prolonged remission although not all centres have this experience.

All surgical procedures should be covered with corticosteroids to minimize the risk of a major flare-up of the disease in the post-operative period.

Management during pregnancy. Crohn's disease should be treated in the pregnant woman along the lines outlined above. Overall, the outcome of the pregnancy is not influenced by the disease except in very severe cases where there may be an increased risk of abortion. Corticosteroids and sulphasalazine are safe to use and have not been associated with fetal abnormalities. Likewise, azathioprine has not been clearly demonstrated to be teratogenic and can be used if there is sufficient clinical indication.

Management in children. There is no essential difference in the principles of management from those described for adults, although dosages may need to be reduced. Alternate day steroids should be employed especially if long-term treatment seems likely. Excellent but uncontrolled results have been reported in adolescents using maintenance corticosteroids, as an alternate day regimen, which allowed puberty and growth to develop normally. One of the major effects of the disease in children is growth retardation. Corticosteroid therapy often promotes a growth spurt but great emphasis should be paid to the child's nutrition. Dietary intake should be assessed and supplemented to provide a high calorie, high nitrogen intake.

Course and prognosis. Patients are never cured of Crohn's disease and they are subject to relapses of their disease and to recurrence following surgical resection. The majority of patients (70–80 per cent) will receive surgical treatment at some point during the course of their illness. Following a resection, the disease recurs in about 30 per cent of patients during the subsequent five years and in 50 per cent of patients during the subsequent ten years; of these, half will require further surgery. Although there is still some controversy, the balance of evidence suggests that the risk of requiring second or third operations is no greater than the risk of requiring the initial operation. Patients with Crohn's colitis who have a panproctocolectomy appear to have a lower risk of recurrence than those who have an ileal or ileo-colic resection.

The overall mortality of Crohn's disease varies from 10–15 per cent in different studies. Some of these reports have suggested a worse prognosis for women than for men and for patients over the age of 50, although this was mainly associated with a higher operative mortality. Overall, age and sex probably have little influence on the outcome of the disease. The Oxford experience has suggested that mortality is not appreciably increased during the first five years of the disease but then becomes progressively greater during subsequent follow-up. In contrast, however, recent data from Birmingham suggests that the highest mortality occurs in young people during the early stages of the disease.

In general, the majority of patients with Crohn's disease will have a good prognosis with a mortality of only about twice that expected. Considerable morbidity can be expected but this will be intermittent and the overall quality of life should be good.

References

Pena, A. S., Weterman, I. T., Booth, C. C., and Strober, W. (1981). *Recent advances in Crohn's disease.* Martinus Nijhoff, The Hague, Boston, London.

Shorter, R. G. and Kirsner, J. B. (1980). *Inflammatory bowel disease,* 2nd edn. Lea and Febiger, New York.

Thomas, H. C. and Jewell, D. P. (1979). *Clinical gastrointestinal immunology.* Blackwell Scientific Publications, Oxford.

The National Cooperative Crohn's Disease Study (1979). *Gastroent.* **77**, 829.

Ulcerative colitis

S. C. Truelove

Ulcerative colitis is the term applied to a chronic disease of unknown aetiology in which a part or the whole of the mucosa of the large bowel becomes diffusely inflamed and may ulcerate. As a result, the patient suffers from diarrhoea which is usually bloody.

Pathology. The mucosa of the affected part of the large bowel is diffusely inflamed. Initially, there is hyperaemia and granularity of the mucosa without naked-eye ulceration. In more severe disease, multiple ragged ulceration of the mucosa can be seen. In the most severe instances, blood oozes spontaneously from the inflamed mucosa so that the underlying ulceration is obscured.

Microscopically, in mild disease, the mucosa shows a heavy infiltration of the lamina propria with plasma cells predominating, a diminution in the number of goblet cells in the epithelium of the crypts of Lieberkühn, flattening of the surface epithelium and loss of goblet cells, and dilatation of the small blood vessels within the lamina. In more active disease, the inflammatory infiltrate contains many polymorphs and some of the crypts are distended with these cells, a condition known as a crypt abscess. The crypt abscess may rupture on to the surface and create a microscopic ulcer.

The disease is primarily a mucosal inflammation which does not penetrate the muscularis mucosae. However, in severe disease, the inflammation spreads through the muscularis mucosae into the submucosa where abscesses are formed which rupture into the lumen and create gross ulceration. Occasionally, in severe disease, the proper muscle coat of the bowel is penetrated and this may lead to perforation of the colon.

This diffuse inflammatory process appears to begin in the rectum and then usually speads proximally to a variable extent around the colon. If it remains confined to the rectum, it is often known as haemorrhagic proctitis. If it involves the rectum, sigmoid, and descending colon, it is often described as distal ulcerative colitis. Involvement of the transverse colon in addition represents extensive colitis, and when the entire colon is affected, the term universal or total colitis is commonly applied.

Epidemiology. The prevalence of ulcerative colitis varies greatly from one part of the world to another. It occurs most frequently in Western society and is rare in many other societies. For example, formal epidemiological studies in England, Denmark, and USA show that approximately one in 1500 of these populations are affected. In the USA, whites are more liable to develop the disease than blacks, and Jews are more liable than non-Jews. In South Africa, the prevalence in whites appears to be much the same as in Europe but the disease is decidedly uncommon among the blacks, although it does occur. In New Zealand, the Maoris are reported as having only one-twentieth the incidence of ulcerative colitis as their compatriots of English stock. In Japan, ulcerative colitis was formerly rare, but it is now on the increase, although its incidence is still low by European standards.

Aetiology. This is still unknown but many theories have been advanced, the main ones being as follows.

Infective. Repeated attempts have been made to identify a specific infective agent in ulcerative colitis but so far without success. At various times, the disease has been considered to be due to dysentery bacilli, a diplostreptococcus, fungi, bacillus necrophorum, or a virus. At the present time, there is still interest in viruses and cell-wall deficient bacteria (L-forms), both of which have been cultured from homogenates of the inflamed mucosa. The difficulty is to know whether these organisms are a primary pathogenic factor or whether they merely invade and settle in a mucosa which is already inflamed.

While ordinary bacteria can probably be ruled out as a cause of the disease, it is likely that they are of great importance as secondary invaders of the inflamed mucosa in the more severe cases, especially in causing local complications and possibly by inducing allergic reactions.

Nutritional. As diarrhoeal states can occur in some deficiency diseases, such as pellagra and folic acid deficiency, the possibility that ulcerative colitis might be the consequence of a similar process has been entertained. It is sufficient to say that there is no convincing evidence to support this view.

Psychosomatic. Formerly, the notion that ulcerative colitis was a psychosomatic disease was widely held. This theory dates from 1930, when Murray investigated the psychological aspects of ulcerative colitis in 12 patients and found a 'well-marked relationship between the outbreak of an emotional disturbance and the onset of symptoms'. In another study, it was found that, in the majority of the patients, 'a clear-cut emotional trauma, serious enough to be regarded as a precipitating agent, immediately preceded the onset of the colitis'. Engel reviewed the psychosomatic hypothesis and found that four factors appeared to be of importance: (a) defects in personality preceding the colitis; (b) dependent relationships with other people; (c) psychological disturbances in the mothers; and (d) lack of full heterosexual development.

More recent psychological studies of patients with ulcerative colitis have failed to find such striking evidence of personality disorders. For example, Feldman and his colleagues in Los Angeles found that the majority of the patients they studied were psychologically normal and that only a small minority experienced an emotional disturbance shortly before the onset of the colitis. This more sceptical view of the importance of psychological factors in the induction of ulcerative colitis is in line with the general experience of gastroenterologists, most of whom do not regard ulcerative colitis as a psychosomatic disease.

Although it seems improbable that psychological factors are the primary cause, it must be noted that an emotional disturbance is not infrequently the apparent precipitant of a relapse in patients already suffering from the disease.

Immunological. Some of the clinical features of ulcerative colitis are compatible with its being an allergic disorder. Some studies have found an excess of known allergic diseases, such as hay fever and infantile eczema, in patients with ulcerative colitis and also in their close relatives.

The American physician, Andresen, advanced the view that ulcerative colitis was an example of food allergy in at least two-thirds of the patients. He based this opinion on the results he obtained with elimination diets. In his opinion, the food most likely to be responsible was cows' milk, but other foodstuffs included eggs, wheat, tomatoes, oranges, and potatoes. In the only formal controlled therapeutic trial of different diets yet published, it was found that the relapse rate on a gluten-free diet was identical to that on a normal diet, but that a milk-free diet was attended by a lower relapse rate. The results suggested that approximately one in five of the patients benefited from the milk-free diet. However, the issue has since become complicated by the discovery that temporary hypolactasia is quite common in sharp attacks of ulcerative colitis so that a milk-free diet may be beneficial because of the exclusion of lactose rather than the milk proteins. This issue is still undecided.

Another possibility is that the patients with ulcerative colitis have become sensitized to one or more of the various chemical additives present in the modern diet of Western society. Such additives are very diverse and are said to number 10 000 or so. It is plain that this possibility would furnish one possible explanation of why populations previously singularly free from ulcerative colitis, such as the Japanese, become increasingly prone to develop it as they adopt Western habits.

The discovery of auto-antibodies to human colonic epithelial cells raised the possibility of ulcerative colitis being an auto-immune disease. The antigen is a lipopolysaccharide contained in the epithelial cells and it cross-reacts with lipopolysaccharide antigens in certain colonic bacteria, such as varieties of *Escherichia coli*. In animals, antibodies to colonic apithelium have been induced by immunizing them with a variety of bacteria. However, the weight of evidence is against these auto-antibodies being responsible for the mucosal damage in ulcerative colitis. Their experimental production in animals is not attended by mucosal inflammation. In patients with ulcerative colitis, auto-antibodies are not universally found and, when demonstrated, they do not correlate with any particular clinical course. Human sera containing auto-antibodies have no damaging effect on human colonic cells growing in tissue cultures.

By contrast, the circulating lymphocytes of patients with ulcerative colitis kill human colonic epithelial cells growing in tissue culture. The lymphocytes of all patients with ulcerative colitis show this capacity to kill colonic epithelial cells and the reaction is specific to ulcerative colitis and Crohn's disease. The exact mechanism of action is unknown. It is interesting that the circulating lymphocytes of healthy subjects can be rendered cytotoxic to human colonic epithelial cells by incubating them with sera from patients with ulcerative colitis or with a lipopolysaccharide extract of *E. coli*.

There is also evidence that immune complexes containing IgG are present in the inflamed mucosa in ulcerative colitis. This suggests that an Arthus reaction (type III) may be wholly or partly responsible for the tissue damage. In addition, some patients with ulcerative colitis have been found to have small immune complexes containing IgG in their sera and this finding is positively correlated with clinical activity and with certain complications of the disease, such as uveitis, erythema nodosum and arthritis.

Clinical features. The disease may occur at any age, from early infancy to extreme old age, but in the majority the onset is during late adolescence or early adult life. The mode of onset is variable, being either gradual or sudden. In the gradual type of onset, the illness begins either with the passage of blood per rectum or with mild diarrhoea. In those patients who commence by passing blood as the sole symptom, this takes the form of small quantities of blood being passed at the time of defaecation, although blood and mucus may also be passed separately; if left untreated, diarrhoea super-venes after some weeks or months, and the blood is then intimately mixed with the unformed faeces. In those in whom the illness begins with simple diarrhoea, at some point in time this becomes bloody, indicating the presence of gross organic disease. Less commonly, the onset is acute, with diarrhoea which may be bloody from the start or which rapidly becomes so. The most acute type of onset is when the patient has a sudden severe haemorrhage from the bowel but this is rare.

Constitutional symptoms are common. When the disease is confined to the rectum (haemorrhagic proctitis) or to the rectum and sigmoid colon (proctosigmoiditis), the main effect is usually anaemia but few other symptoms. With more extensive disease, especially if the diarrhoea is severe, pronounced constitutional disturbances occur and the patient may become severely ill in the course of a few days or weeks. It is convenient to classify an attack in terms of severity, especially when considering treatment, and a simple classification is as follows.

Mild attack. Not more than four motions a day with only small amounts of macroscopic blood in them. No evidence of appreciable constitutional disturbance.

Moderate attack. Intermediate between mild and severe.

Severe attack. At least six loose motions a day with large amounts of blood in the faeces. Pronounced constitutional disturbance as manifested by severe general malaise, fever, tachycardia, a falling haemoglobin level, leucocytosis, much raised ESR, and rapid loss of weight.

In severe attacks the diarrhoea may be profuse, with twenty or more bowel actions a day. The stools are liquid and consist of a mixture of blood, mucopus, and faeces. Anorexia is common and nausea and vomiting may also occur. Electrolyte disturbances may be profound. Diffuse abdominal discomfort is common but frequently is notable by its absence.

Course of the disease. This is of three main types.

Chronic intermittent. The majority of patients suffer from recurrent attacks with intervals of complete freedom from symptoms between the attacks. The recurrent attacks occur at irregular intervals, which may be weeks, months, or years in length. Various factors may precipitate a relapse, such as psychological disturbances, upper respiratory infections, broad-spectrum antibiotics given by mouth for an unrelated condition, the gastrointestinal infections even of the sort causing only a brief diarrhoeal illness in otherwise healthy subjects. However, the majority of relapses occur without any apparent cause.

Chronic continuous. A much smaller number of patients never become free from colitic symptoms once the disease has become manifest, although these symptoms wax and wane in severity. This chronic continuous type has become relatively uncommon as a result of improvements in medical treatment and also because, if medical treatment is ineffective, such continuous symptoms are commonly regarded as an indication for treatment by radical surgery.

Single attack. A few patients suffer from an attack of bloody diarrhoea, diagnosed as ulcerative colitis, and never have another attack. It is possible that in many of these patients the original diagnosis was incorrect. For example, in recent years, infection with campylobacteria has been found to be responsible for out-breaks of diarrhoea, the cause of which was previously unknown as special methods are necessary for the culture of the organism. Although campylobacter infection normally causes a simple diarrhoea which clears up in a week or two even without treatment, in some instances it gives rise to bloody diarrhoea with sigmoidoscopic appearances closely resembling those of ulcerative colitis and with biopsy appearances which demand expert interpretation if they are to be distinguished from those of ulcerative colitis. In the past, such patients would almost certainly have been diagnosed as suffering from ulcerative colitis.

Ulcerative colitis beginning in childhood. Although ulcerative colitis is not common in childhood, when it does occur it often runs a severe course. In the past, the outlook for these patients was poor. For example, a large study at the Mayo Clinic found that 20 per cent of the subjects died each decade after the onset and that the risk of developing cancer of the large bowel was 20 per cent per decade after ulcerative colitis had been in progress for more than ten years. Modern medical treatment has improved the outlook but a considerable proportion of these patients need to be treated by radical surgery. Such radical surgery may be required as an emergency procedure in order to save the patient's life if an attack is severe. Some of the patients have repeated troublesome attacks in spite of medical treatment and in such circumstances radical surgery is required to restore general health and activity.

Ulcerative colitis and pregnancy. As ulcerative colitis frequently begins in early adult life, it often occurs in women during their reproductive years. It is therefore a matter of great consequence to know whether ulcerative colitis influences fertility and conversely whether pregnancy affects the course of the disease. All adequate studies of the problem have shown that fertility is normal in women with ulcerative colitis. In the past, pregnancy often appeared to have a deleterious effect upon the colitis, but modern medical treatment has changed the picture. The most recent large-scale study of women attending an ulcerative colitis clinic reached the following conclusions.

'Fertility was normal and the women as a whole had the same expectation of producing a healthy full-term baby as women in the general population. There was no maternal mortality in the series, which covered 119 women who had 216 pregnancies after the development of ulcerative colits.

'Women who were symptom-free at the time of conception had an excellent chance of remaining so throughout pregnancy and the puerperium. When relapse did occur, the symptoms were readily held in check by medical treatment.

'Women who had symptoms of colitis at the time of conception usually continued to have symptoms throughout pregnancy but in most instances medical treatment ensured that they were not unduly troublesome. A few of these women had severe symptoms, and in these the expectation of the pregnancy ending in a healthy full-term baby was considerably reduced.

'Women who developed their first attack of ulcerative colitis during pregnancy or the puerperium generally had mild attacks which responded well to medical treatment. In the past, ulcerative colitis beginning in this way often ran a severe course.

'Medical treatment with corticosteroids or sulphasalazine appeared to have no obvious deleterious effects on the fetus or new-born child.'

It is therefore recommended that, whenever feasible, a woman with ulcerative colitis should plan her family so that she conceives only when the colitis is quiescent. Active ulcerative colitis in pregnancy should be treated with corticosteroids and sulphasalazine in the same way as non-pregnant patients (see section on Medical treatment below).

Complications. The complications of ulcerative colitis are numerous and diverse. They can be divided into two main categories:

Local complications are those arising in and around the inflamed large bowel.

Remote complications, sometimes known as systemic or extraintestinal complications, are those occurring in distant organs.

Local complications. These may occur either during a clinical attack or as a consequence of chronic disease.

The dangerous local complications of an attack of ulcerative colitis are liable to occur when the attack is clinically severe. There are three major complications:

Perforation of the colon is an uncommon but highly dangerous complication which requires emergency colectomy if the patient is

to be saved. It is especially liable to occur in a first attack of the disease if this happens to be severe, but it can also occur in a severe relapse. It is often difficult to diagnose on clinical evidence as a patient who is already seriously ill may not show the classical symptoms and signs of perforation. It should always be suspected in any patient whose general condition deteriorates and plain abdominal X-rays, using a horizontal beam, should be obtained to see if free gas is present.

Acute dilatation of the colon, sometimes known as *toxic megacolon,* is liable to occur in any severe attack. The dilatation affects principally the transverse and ascending colon. Although the condition can be regarded as a paralytic ileus of the colon, it must be emphasized that the patient invariably continues to have liquid diarrhoea. The patient may show abdominal distension and it is sometimes possible, in a thin patient, to observe visually the localized distension of the transverse colon from the contours of the abdominal wall, and gentle palpation may also define the dilated colon, which is usually tender. There is almost invariably evidence of severe constitutional disturbance, such as general malaise, fever, and tachycardia. The crucial investigation is a plain abdominal X-ray with overhead tube. This will show the greatly dilated transverse colon filled with gas and with no haustra. In addition to the dilatation, polypoid mucosal swellings may be seen, either in profile at the borders of the colon or *en face* as rounded opacities outlined by the intraluminal gas. These appearances, which are known as 'mucosal islands', are a consequence of very severe and widespread ulceration of the colon so that most of the mucosa has been destroyed, while the remaining pockets of mucosa are swollen with inflammation to form the polypoid masses visible on X-ray. If a toxic megacolon shows these appearances, emergency colectomy is indicated. In their absence, intensive medical treatment can be tried and the decision to operate be deferred while the effect of medical treatment is observed. Various factors have been suggested as precipitants of a toxic megacolon. Antidiarrhoeal drugs, such as anticholinergics, loperamide, opium, and codeine have been incriminated, but it is difficult to be certain how large a part they play; however, it is certainly wise to stop any such medication in a patient with toxic megacolon and, in any event, they are not indicated in the treatment of ulcerative colitis. Superadded infection with pathogenic bacteria, such as dysentery bacilli, salmonellae, and *Clostridium difficile* has also been considered to be a precipitant in some patients and, if such an infection is identified, it should be treated appropriately in addition to giving the standard treatment for a severe attack of ulcerative colitis as set out later. Severe electrolyte abnormalities, especially potassium depletion, have been judged to be a cause of toxic megacolon, but such abnormalities are a common feature of any severe attack of ulcerative colitis; needless to say, they require correction by appropriate intravenous therapy. A metabolic acidosis has also been judged to be a relevant factor and it is claimed that correction of this by intravenous therapy will result in rapid improvement in the lesser grades of toxic megacolon. A toxic megacolon is frequently complicated by perforation of the colon, but it must be emphasized that perforation of the colon can occur in the absence of a dilated colon.

Massive haemorrhage from the bowel may occur but this is rare, unless there is some predisposing condition such as the patient suffering from haemophilia or other bleeding disease. Haemorrhage usually responds to blood transfusion and is only occasionally the sole reason for an emergency colectomy.

Various complications around the rectum may occur, either during an acute attack or as a consequence of chronic disease even if the bowel symptoms are mild at the time. The main ones are ischiorectal abscess, fistula-in-ano, and rectovaginal fistula. Abscesses require immediate surgical drainage, but surgery for the other pararectal complications should not be attempted if the ulcerative colitis is active but should be deferred until medical treatment has rendered the colitis quiescent. These pararectal complications are much less common in ulcerative colitis than they are in Crohn's disease (see page 12.105) and therefore, if they occur, the diagnosis should be reviewed.

Other local complications include pseudopolyposis of the colon, fibrous strictures of the colon, and cancer of the colon. Pseudopolyposis is the result of severe ulceration of the colon, with the formation of polypoid swellings of inflamed mucosa in between extensive areas of ulceration. They tend to persist, although they may diminish if the colitis is quiescent for a long time. Fibrous strictures of the colon may occur in the course of chronic disease but the discovery of a smooth stricture on barium enema should always raise the suspicion that the patient may be suffering from Crohn's disease or that the stricture is malignant. Cancer of the colon is an important late complication of ulcerative colitis and it is dealt with in a separate section (see page 12.123).

Remote complications. Skin complications are common and assume many forms, such as scarlatiniform, morbilliform, or purpuric rashes, urticaria, erythema multiforme, and erythema nodosum. Some of these eruptions are caused by *drug reactions* and this is the first possibility to be considered. Assuming that drugs do not appear to be responsible, the essential is to treat the ulcerative colitis with corticosteroids and the skin complications will usually disappear as the colitis comes under control. An important, although rare, skin complication is *pyoderma gangrenosum*, a condition which is almost specific for ulcerative colitis and Crohn's disease. It usually occurs as a complication of a severe attack of ulcerative colitis but may arise when the bowel symptoms are mild, although sigmoidoscopy and biopsy will then invariably show that the colitis is active. The early lesions consist of intra-epidermal bullae filled with clear fluid which is sterile. The fluid soon becomes milky and purulent. The bullae burst leaving ulcerated areas which frequently coalesce forming large denuded areas which become covered with scabs. Secondary infection supervenes and renders the patient very ill. Pyoderma gangrenosum was once a dangerous complication requiring protocolectomy for its cure but it usually responds rapidly to treatment with large doses of corticosteroids and is nowadays only occasionally an indication for proctocolectomy.

Eye complications are common. The usual clinical manifestation is angular conjunctivitis (episcleritis) which often affects only one eye. Treatment is with eye drops containing a water-soluble corticosteroid. There may also be iridocyclitis (uveitis) which is often not frankly symptomatic although slit-lamp examination shows that it occurs in at least 10 per cent of the patients.

Severe aphthous ulceration of the mouth may occur. Moniliasis of the mouth is also sometimes seen; it requires to be treated promptly because of the risk that it may extend into the oesophagus or the lungs.

Arthritis is another complication, typically affecting one or more of the large joints. Tests for rheumatoid factor are negative.

Patients with ulcerative colitis are unduly prone to suffer from ankylosing spondylitis. The two sexes are equally at risk, which contrasts sharply with the heavy male preponderance in the generality of subjects with ankylosing spondylitis. Patients who suffer from both ulcerative colitis and ankylosing spondylitis belong predominantly to HLA-B27 whereas ulcerative colitis patients as a whole do not differ from the general population. It appears that ulcerative colitis and ankylosing spondylitis are two separate diseases that are associated with one another for genetic reasons. The onset of the spondylitis may either precede or follow that of the ulcerative colitis and the two conditions appear to progress independently of each other. Proctocolectomy does not halt the progression of an associated ankylosing spondylitis.

Liver disease is not uncommon in patients with ulcerative colitis. During severe attacks of colitis, the liver shows marked fatty change but gradually reverts to normal after the colitis goes into remission. The commonest abnormality is pericholangitis (portal triaditis). It is possible that this may progress to cirrhosis but there is no general agreement on this point. A chronic hepatitis may occur and may lead on to cirrhosis. The combination of chronic liver disease and ulcerative colitis carries a bad prognosis. There is some evidence that proctocolectomy may arrest the progression of a chronic hepatitis but this possibility is not well established.

Primary sclerosing cholangitis is a rare condition which is especially liable to occur in patients with ulcerative colitis, although it also occurs in other subjects. The patient shows features of an obstructive jaundice. The diagnosis may be made by ERCP (endoscopic retrograde cholangio-pancreatography) which shows a characteristic diffuse irregular narrowing of the bile ducts. The changes extend into the intra-hepatic ducts and a liver biopsy may show a fibrotic thickening of the duct wall with a diffuse inflammatory infiltrate composed chiefly of lymphocytes. The condition progresses to a secondary biliary cirrhosis with portal hypertension.

Carcinoma of the bile duct is another rare complication of ulcerative colitis, especially when the entire colon is affected by the colitis.

Diagnosis. The symptoms immediately focus attention on the large bowel as the likely seat of disease and the diagnosis of a fresh case can usually be made with confidence on the basis of the following investigations.

Sigmoidoscopy. The sigmoidoscopic appearances vary according to the severity of the disease and can be classified as follows.
Mild. The mucosa shows diffuse hyperaemia and tiny petechiae. The normal vascular pattern of the mucosa is obscured. The mucosa is fragile as shown by the occurrence of bleeding when it is rubbed with a piece of gauze held in forceps introduced through the sigmoidoscope.
Moderate. Hyperaemia, granularity, and contact bleeding are much more pronounced. Haemorrhagic flares are seen, rather than small petechiae. Areas of purulent exudate may be present and discrete ulceration may be seen.
Severe. The mucosa is intensely inflamed and blood often oozes spontaneously from its surface. Purulent exudation and gross ulceration may be seen.
In the case of the inflammation being confined to the rectum (haemorrhagic proctitis) the sigmoidoscope will show normal mucosa proximal to it, usually with a fairly sharp line of demarcation.
Rectal biopsy. A rectal biopsy taken through the sigmoidoscope will show the microscopic features already mentioned in the section dealing with the pathology of the disease.
Barium enema. A double-contrast enema will almost invariably show abnormalities if performed by a skilled radiologist. In mild disease, there is an abnormal mucosal pattern. In more severe disease, evidence of multiple ulceration is seen. The chief value of the barium enema is in providing evidence of the extent and severity of the disease process. If the attack is clinically severe, the barium enema should not be carried out until plain radiographs have been taken. If these show evidence of dilatation of the colon (toxic megacolon), it may be decided to forego the barium enema; in any event, the barium enema should be carried out with caution in patients in a severe attack of ulcerative colitis and the contrast medium should be introduced under a low hydrostatic pressure.
Bacteriological examination of the faeces. This is essential to exclude an infective dysentery as the cause of the symptoms.
Other investigations may sometimes be necessary, especially in tropical countries, where diseases such as amoebic dysentery, schistosomiasis, and lymphogranuloma venereum need to be considered.

Management. As ulcerative colitis is a chronic disease which persists for the rest of the patient's life, it is best if he can remain under the long-term supervision of a physician with a special interest in the disease. The principles of management can be summarized as follows: (a) attacks should be treated promptly in the hope of obtaining rapid remission; (b) maintenance therapy should be used to reduce the relapse rate; and (c) certain patients need to be treated by radical surgery.

Treatment of an attack. General medical measures are of great importance in the treatment of a severe attack. They involve measures to overcome dehydration, electrolyte deficiencies, anaemia, and poor nutritional state. Although such measures will combat some of the harmful effects of the disease, they do nothing to cut short the attack. For this purpose, only two types of medical treatment have been shown by controlled therapeutic trials to have a major effect. They are the corticosteroids and sulphasalazine.

It has been shown that oral corticosteroids improve the chance of obtaining a rapid remission whatever the grade of severity of the attack. Corticosteroids can also be used topically as retention enemata or as a rectal drip, and it has been shown that the combination of oral and topical corticosteroid therapy is more effective than a single type of administration. Water-soluble corticosteroids can also be given intravenously and this is valuable when dealing with a severe attack. Such intravenous therapy has supplanted ACTH for the treatment of ulcerative colitis.

Sulphasalazine is also a useful treatment for an attack of ulcerative colitis although it does not result in a rapid remission as frequently as combined oral and topical corticosteroid therapy. However, it can be used in conjunction with corticosteroids and this combined therapy appears to be an advantage. Sulphasalazine has a number of side-effects. The common ones are dose-related and consist of anorexia, nausea, vomiting, headache, and general malaise. Such side-effects are not very common if the dose of sulphasalazine is limited to 2 g daily, but affect many patients if larger doses are employed. Sulphasalazine may also cause a rash, fever, and adenitis, but patients can be desensitized to this type of reaction by stopping the drug temporarily and then starting with a very low dose (1 mg daily) which is then gradually increased. Occasionally, a severe photosensitive eruption or an exfoliative dermatitis may occur; the drug should then be stopped for ever and the skin condition treated by corticosteroids. Sulphasalazine frequently causes oligospermia with impaired fertility in men but this is only an important factor if it is being used for a long time, as fertility is rapidly restored when the drug is stopped. The most serious complication of sulphasalazine is agranulocytosis; fortunately this is rare, but a number of fatal cases have been reported. A few cases of Heinz-body haemolytic anaemia have also been reported.

Treatment of a mild attack. Prompt and decisive treatment is necessary, but the patient can proceed with his normal life. A suitable regimen is as follows: (a) prednisolone by mouth 5 mg four times a day; (b) sulphasalazine 0.5 g four times a day; and (c) predsol retention enemas nightly on retiring to bed.

The great majority of patients become symptom-free in the course of a week or two. If so, the regimen should be continued for a total period of one month, after which the corticosteroids can be tailed off fairly rapidly, but the sulphasalazine should be continued, for reasons given below. In the event of no improvement occurring during the first two weeks, more vigorous treatment, as for a moderate attack, should be tried. Actual worsening of the symptoms may require the patient to be admitted to hospital for more intensive treatment.

Treatment of a moderate attack. The patient should be admitted to hospital and general medical measures instituted if they appear to be indicated. Suitable specific treatment is as follows: (a) prednisolone by mouth 10 mg four times a day; (b) sulphasalazine 0.5 g four times a day; and (c) topical corticosteroid treatment morning and evening.

As with a mild attack, a good response should mean that the corticosteroids should be continued for a total period of one month before being tailed off. Failure to respond, or actual deterioration, should be an indication for treating the patient as for a severe attack.

Treatment of a severe attack. Immediate admission to hospital and rapid institution of appropriate treatment. In Oxford it has become standard practice to commence treatment with five days of intensive intravenous therapy, usually applied through a central line. This enables dehydration to be overcome, electrolyte deficiencies to be made good, blood transfusion to be given if required, parenteral feeding to be employed where necessary, and for a water-soluble corticosteroid to be given intravenously, a suitable preparation being prednisolone 21-phosphate, 60 mg daily in divided doses. The question of whether an antibiotic should be included in this intravenous regimen remains uncertain. Many of the patients treated with this intravenous regimen remains uncertain. Many of the patients treated with this intravenous regimen respond swiftly and are then put back to normal feeding together with drug treatment similar to that for a moderate attack. Failure to respond after five days intravenous therapy should be taken as an indication for emergency colectomy. Any deterioration in the patient's general condition during the five-day course, and in particular the occurrence of perforation of the colon or severe toxic megacolon, should be taken as absolute indications for emergency colectomy. By using these indications for emergency colectomy, the deaths from these severe attacks can be kept to a very small number, whereas previously a severe attack frequently ended fatally.

Maintenance treatment to prevent relapse. No medical method has yet been found which will prevent relapses from occurring and the best that can be done is to lower the relapse rate. Most of the agents that have been subjected to controlled trial have proved to be disappointing. The corticosteroids, although of great value in the treatment of an attack, have proved to be totally ineffective when used in moderate doses as maintenance therapy to prevent recurrence. Furthermore, when used for a long time, corticosteroid therapy is liable to cause dangerous side-effects whereas it appears to be relatively harmless when used in short courses in the treatment of actual attacks of colitis. Immunosuppressive drugs, such as azothioprine, are of limited value in reducing the relapse rate. A milk-free diet has also been found to benefit a minority of patients. Disodium cromoglycate (Intal or Nalcrom) appeared at one stage to be of value, but subsequently large controlled trials have shown that it is virtually useless. At present, the only agent which has been shown to bring about a major reduction in the rate of recurrence is sulphasalazine. Maintenance therapy with this in a dose of 2 g a day results in the recurrence rate being reduced to a quarter of the rate experienced without treatment. This suppressive effect of sulphasalazine appears to persist indefinitely and therefore long-term maintenance therapy is advisable unless there are side-effects of therapy. Unfortunately, such side-effects are fairly common. As virtually all the side-effects are due to the sulphapyridine contained in the sulphasalazine molecule, while the therapeutic activity appears to depend on the 5-amino-salicylic acid which makes up the other part of the molecule, there is a strong possibility that sulphasalazine will soon be replaced by a safer and more effective drug.

Surgical treatment. The majority of the patients with ulcerative colitis can be managed satisfactorily throughout their lives by medical treatment but a substantial minority, of the order of one in every four or five, need to be treated surgically. The indications for surgery are as follows.

1. Emergency colectomy to save life in patients suffering from a severe attack because of (a) perforation of the colon, (b) severe toxic megacolon, or (c) general deterioration in spite of intensive medical therapy.

2. Elective colectomy to restore health in chronic disease in patients suffering from: (a) chronic continuous symptoms, (b) frequent troublesome attacks, (c) severe fistula-in-ano, rectovaginal fistula, or other pararectal complications, (d) cancer of the colon.

3. Preventive colectomy to eliminate the risk of cancer in high-risk subjects.

Some patients with ulcerative colitis have a greatly increased risk of developing cancer of the colon. It is a late complication of the disease, the risk being negligible during the first few years after the onset of the colitis but becoming appreciable after 10 years and being specially prone to occur round about 20 years after the onset. One of the aims of long-term management is to eliminate this risk which at present can only be done by protocolectomy. This, however, does not mean that all patients with ulcerative colitis should have their large bowel removed when the colitis has been present for ten years or more. The risk of cancer is not spread evenly among the sufferers from ulcerative colitis and certain bad risk factors can be identified. They are a severe first attack, universal involvement of the colon, chronic continuous symptoms, and onset of the colitis in childhood or early adult life.

One approach to the cancer risk is to recommend preventive colectomy to patients with two or more of these factors when the colitis has been present for more than 10 years. Another approach is to rely on regular colonoscopy with multiple biopsy and to recommend colectomy if there is severe epithelial dysplasia, which is considered to be a precancerous condition. Neither method is perfect and it is still too early to be certain that colonoscopic surveillance represents a big advance on the earlier method of relying on clinical criteria as the indications for preventive colectomy.

Types of surgical operation. The surgical procedure most commonly used is proctocolectomy with a permanent ileostomy. When the operation is performed electively, the operative fatality rate is low (about 2 per cent), but when done as an emergency the rate may be much higher, especially if there is much delay in resorting to surgery when a patient with a severe attack is failing to respond to medical treatment. After recovering from the operation, the patient is at some risk during the first year, chiefly because he may develop small-intestinal obstruction and perforation, requiring rapid surgical treatment. Thereafter, ileostomists have an expectation of life which is not very greatly worse than that of the general population. They can indulge in virtually all forms of physical activity and their general health is good. Some of them have psychological problems related to the ileostomy, including psychosexual difficulties. These difficulties appear to be less if, instead of a standard ileostomy emptying into a bag, the so-called continent ileostomy devised by the Swedish surgeon, Kock, is made. In this, the terminal small intestine is converted surgically into an internal pouch which opens onto the skin as an inconspicuous mucous fistula, merely requiring a small gauze pad over it. However, there are various complications with the pouch so it remains to be seen whether it will become the standard procedure when an ileostomy is necessary.

A minority of the patients requiring to be treated by major surgery do well with colectomy and ileorectal anastomosis. However, there is then the risk that the retained rectum may develop a cancer and, for this reason, some surgeons regard the operation as specially suitable as a temporary procedure for children and adolescents because it may enable them to reach full adulthood without an ileostomy even though it may be wise then to remove the rectum and eliminate the risk of cancer.

A further possibility is proctocolectomy with ileo-anal anastomosis and the formation of an internal pouch analogous to Kock's continent ileostomy pouch. However, this procedure is still in an experimental phase.

Prognosis. Ulcerative colitis was formerly a most serious disease with a high mortality and severe morbidity. This can be illustrated by considering the long-term fate of patients dealt with in their first attack at the Radcliffe Infirmary, Oxford during the period 1938–52. Patients presenting with a mild first attack did fairly well with a survival curve not greatly different from expected. In those presenting with a severe or moderately severe first attack the long-term course was persistently unfavourable, with 50 per cent dying during the next 20 years.

Modern medical and surgical treatment has transformed the prognosis for the better. However, a severe attack of ulcerative colitis remains a most dangerous illness, especially if complicated by perforation of the colon or toxic megacolon, and some fatalities still occur as a result.

Virtually all patients with ulcerative colitis are prone to recurrent attacks throughout the rest of their lives and there is no truly effective preventive measure other than proctocolectomy. However, the frequency of attacks can be greatly reduced by maintenance therapy with sulphasalazine.

Patients with ulcerative colitis have a greatly increased risk of developing cancer of the colon when the disease has been present for more than 10 years. The factors associated with this high risk are a severe first attack, involvement of the entire colon, chronic continuous symptoms, and onset of the colitis in childhood or early adult life. Patients with a combination of two or more such factors require preventive colectomy to eliminate the risk.

References

Azad Khan, A. K., Howes, D. T., Piris, J., and Truelove, S. C. (1980). Optimum dose of sulphasalazine for maintenance treatment in ulcerative colitis. *Gut* **21,** 232.
Edwards, F. C. and Truelove, S. C. (1963, 1964). The course and prognosis of ulcerative colitis. *Gut* **4,** 299, 309; **5,** 1, 15.
Goodman, M. J. and Sparberg, M. (1978). *Ulcerative colitis.* Wiley, New York.
Kirsner, J. B. and Shorter, R. G. (eds.) (1980). *Inflammatory bowel disease.* Lea and Febiger, Philadelphia.
Truelove, S. C. and Jewell, D. P. (1974). Intensive intravenous regimen for severe attacks of ulcerative colitis. *Lancet* **i,** 1067.
—, Willoughby, C. P., Lee, E. G., and Kettlewell, M. G. W. (1978). Further experience in the treatment of severe attacks of ulcerative colitis. *Lancet* **ii,** 1086.

Tumours of the gastrointestinal tract

M. L. Clark, A. B. Price, and C. B. Williams

Oesophageal tumours

Benign. Leiomyomas are the commonest benign tumours of the oesophagus. They are often discovered accidentally or at autopsy and only rarely, if ever, give any symptoms that can be related to the oesophagus. Barium swallow examination performed for vague oesophageal symptoms reveals an intramural lesion which must be distinguished from extrinsic compression. If a leiomyoma is found, surgical enucleation without resection is often possible and the prognosis is good.

Fibrovascular polyps, lipomas, and other benign tumours are found, but are all extremely rare.

Malignant. The majority of malignant tumours occur in the middle (50 per cent) and lower third (25 per cent) of the oesophagus. They are usually squamous carcinomas but adenocarcinomas occur in the lower third and at the cardia. It is often difficult to decide whether these adenocarcinomas arise primarily from the fundus of the stomach or whether they arise from a localized area of columnar epithelium which is sometimes found in the lower oesophagus and when ulcerated is known as a *Barrett's ulcer*. Other malignant tumours are rare and consist of malignant melanomas, secondary tumours, plasmacytomas, and leiomyo sarcomas.

Epidemiology and aetiological factors. In the United Kingdom the overall incidence of oesophageal carcinoma varies from five to ten cases per 100 000 people, or 2.5 per cent of all malignant disease. The incidence varies considerably throughout the world, being high in China, parts of Africa, and the Caspian region of Iran where the incidence is the highest observed for any type of cancer anywhere in the world. Because of this high incidence cytological screening studies have been introduced in asymptomatic subjects. The variation in incidence throughout the world is greater than for any other commonly occurring cancer and is unusual in that sharp differences occur between regions only a few hundred miles apart. There is no simple explanation for this geographic variability which is probably multifactorial. A relationship with soil type, diet, urban versus rural dwelling, and other environmental considerations has been investigated without a definite conclusion. In most areas the tumour is commoner in males (approximately 4:1) but there is considerable variation throughout the world. The median age for oesophageal cancer is 67.9 for males and 68.2 for females and the disease is virtually unknown in children.

There is an increased incidence of malignancy in patients with oesophageal strictures due to ingestion of corrosives as well as in patients treated with irradiation. An increased incidence also occurs in patients with achalasia, possibly due to stasis above the narrowed segment. There is, however, no clear relationship between carcinoma and reflux oesophagitis or a hiatus hernia. The Paterson–Kelly (Plummer–Vinson) syndrome, in which hypochromic anaemia and an associated post-cricoid web occurs, is associated with carcinoma of the oesophagus. In this syndrome women are affected 10 times more than men and carcinomas occur at the younger age of 40–50. This syndrome is decreasing in incidence as most patients with iron deficiency anaemia are treated early.

In all parts of the world there is strong association between carcinoma of the oesophagus and excess consumption of alcohol. This association is probably significant although it is difficult to separate drinking habits from smoking, which has also been associated with oesophageal carcinoma. In some areas of high incidence there seems to be an association with the use of opium. Repeated minor trauma (e.g. ingestion of hot liquids, dry bread, etc.) may result in increased individual susceptibility and the combination of trauma and other factors may be additive.

Tylosis, a rare skin disease inherited as an autosomal dominant trait, is characterized by hyperkeratosis of the palms and soles. Oesophageal carcinomas occur in up to 45 per cent of such patients.

Clinical features. The early symptoms of oesophageal carcinoma may be vague and unimpressive. Dysphagia is the commonest single symptom and is a complaint which should always be taken seriously and investigated in the hope of making earlier diagnosis of oesophageal cancers. The dysphagia of malignancy is progressive, initially only being present with solids but eventually dysphagia with liquids occurs. Benign strictures, in contrast, often produce intermittent dysphagia. Impact pain after eating occurs but more persistent pain in the front and back of the chest suggests infiltration and is a bad prognostic feature. Loss of appetite and weight loss often occur, partly because of the difficulty in swallowing but also because the patient may have advanced disease. Metastases, most commonly to regional lymph nodes, are found at diagnosis in approximately 50 per cent of cases, the earliest spread being through the mediastinal tissues around the oesophagus but subsequently downwards to the gastric glands and to the liver. Direct spread of the tumour involves neighbouring structures, especially the bronchi, lungs, and pleura, but also the aorta. Perforation and local sepsis may occur resulting in tracheo-oesophageal or other fistulas or mediastinitis. Involvement of the recurrent laryngeal nerve causes hoarseness. By the time that oesophageal obstruction is causing difficulty in swallowing saliva, cough and other features of aspiration are common and they result in terminal bronchopneumonia.

Diagnosis usually involves both radiology and endoscopy. A barium swallow, which is usually the first investigation performed, gives an accurate picture of the extent of any deformity (Fig. 1a) and also demonstrates fistulation. Oesophageal carcinoma characteristically shows itself as a narrowing with an abrupt shoulder and an irregular mucosa as opposed to the smooth narrowing of a benign stricture. Oesophagoscopy with fibre-optic instruments gives a more detailed view of the mucosal surface and biopsies can be taken. Cytology samples can also be obtained with a small rotatable brush and combining biopsies with brushings a diagnostic accuracy rate of over 95 per cent is achieved.

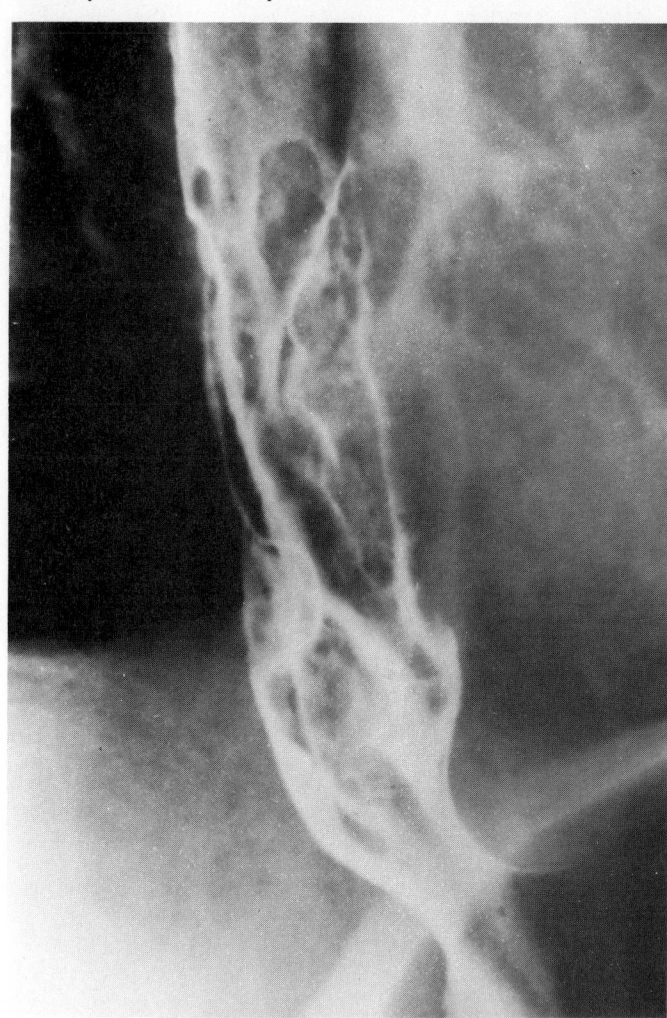

Fig. 1(a)   Oesophageal carcinoma on barium swallow.

On X-ray, endoscopy, and on the tissue samples it is important in tumours of the distal oesophagus to differentiate between squamous carcinoma of the oesophagus and adenocarcinoma of the cardia or fundus since these can only be treated surgically. The differential diagnosis is a 'peptic stricture' following reflux oesophagitis, which can sometimes produce extremely similar symptomatology and radiological appearances. At endoscopy some of the irregularity apparent on X-ray may prove to be due to food residue.

Treatment. The overall results of treatment of carcinoma of the oesophagus are poor and often only symptomatic palliation is possible and preferable to suffering major surgery on top of terminal illness. Symptomatic relief can be achieved by dilating the stricture over an endoscopically placed guide-wire and then placing an oeso-phageal tube (Fig. 1b) through the tumour. This technique is preferable to tube insertion using either a rigid endoscope or at surgery. A single successful intubation under sedation is frequently sufficient for the few months life-expectancy of patients for whom it is selected. Intubation is particularly indicated when there is a tracheo-oesophageal fistula, simultaneously blocking off the fistula and maintaining the oesophageal lumen. The tube allows passage of saliva and soft food but the patient is usually unable to eat a completely normal diet. Unblocking of the tube may be necessary with fizzy drinks or repeat endoscopy. Tube placement in the upper third of the oesophagus gives unpleasant sensations and is therefore only used for a short period during palliative radiotherapy.

Results of surgical treatment depend on the site of the tumour and more importantly on the histological type. Adenocarcinoma

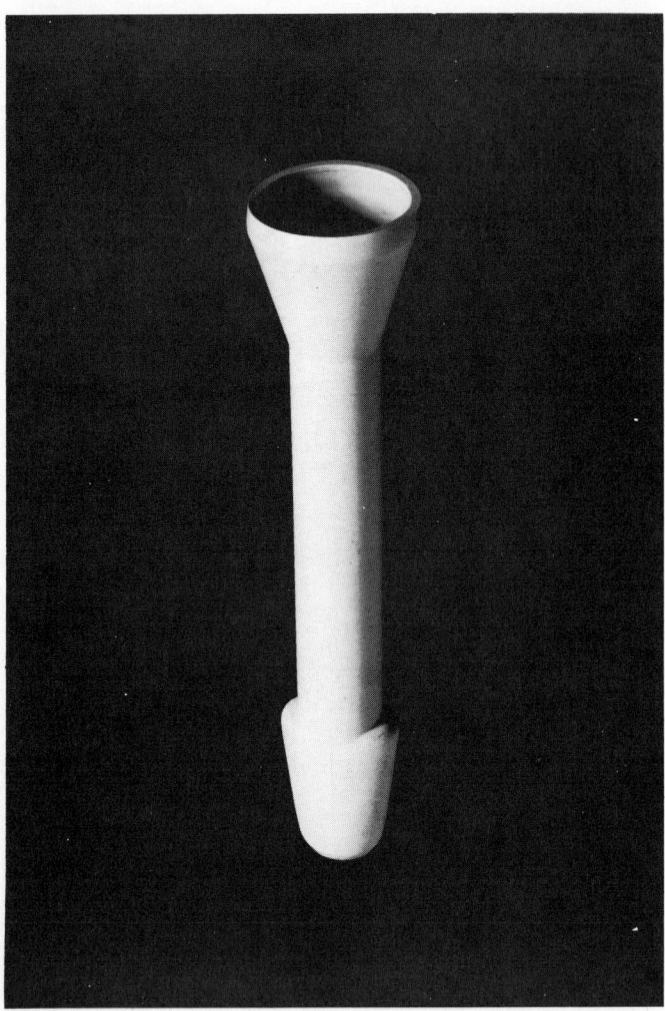

Fig. 1(b) Oesophageal tube suitable for endoscopic placement.

involving the lower oesophageal segment is accompanied by a relatively low operative mortality (10 per cent) and surgery is usually the treatment of choice although palliation is the most that can be expected as most tumours have already spread distally. Surgical palliation for squamous carcinoma at any level either by insertion of a tube or resection and re-anastomosis between the oesophagus and stomach is often performed but operative mortality is high (approximately 30 per cent) and the long-term results are also poor. 'Curative' surgery can only be performed in approximately 20 per cent of all cases of carcinoma of the oesophagus and heroic surgical procedures may be involved, such as a colonic-swing in which a segment of the colon is transposed to the chest. Selection of the few cases that can be so treated is difficult and can

often only be made at laparotomy or thoracotomy. In ideal circumstances high cure rates of around 50 per cent at five years have been claimed but the numbers in which cure is achieved is small and the overall five year survival for all cases is less than 5 per cent.

X-ray therapy for squamous carcinoma has a number of advocates and the use of megavoltage radiation has apparently produced extremely good results with reported 20 per cent survival at five years. This compares very favourably with the surgically treated group and the immediate mortality related to treatment is much lower. There seems to be no evidence at present that either combined therapy with irradiation and surgery or additional chemotherapy improves prognosis.

Stomach tumours

Benign tumours and polyps. The most common benign tumour of the stomach at autopsy is a leiomyoma. In life this tumour is usually found incidentally during investigation of other problems although occasionally it can ulcerate and result in haematemesis. Although a leiomyoma may appear to protrude into the stomach, endoscopic removal is not possible since the tumour is intramural, arising from the muscularis mucosa. Management is usually by surgical removal and the prognosis is good. Other benign gastric tumours include lipomas and angiomas and are rare.

Gastric polyps are relatively uncommon lesions usually found by chance in a patient being investigated for unrelated dyspepsia. The commonest gastric polyp is the regenerative or hyperplastic polyp and may be the end result of previous inflammation. It has no malignant potential. Adenomatous (tubular, villous, and borderline) polyps of the stomach occur but their classification and natural history is confused in the literature compared to the relatively clear cut situation of neoplastic colonic polyps and colonic cancer. It is difficult for the pathologist to distinguish these gastric polyps from certain patterns of early gastric cancer and it is important that if a polyp is biopsied and shown to be adenomatous the whole of it should be removed for microscopy, either by endoscopy or surgery. Although some gastric adenomas may contain carcinoma, there is no evidence to suggest that gastric cancers usually arise from pre-existing adenomas. In rare cases a large pedunculated polyp may ulcerate, bleed, or obstruct the pyloric outflow.

Carcinoma of the stomach

Epidemiology and aetiological factors. The occurrence of gastric carcinoma varies considerably throughout the world with a high incidence in Japan and Chile and low incidence in the United States of America. In the United Kingdom 45 per 100 000 males per year are affected. It is the third most fatal cancer in the United Kingdom and accounts for about 10 per cent of all deaths from malignant disease. At the present time there appears no obvious reason for the dramatic fall in the worldwide incidence of gastric carcinoma, including Japan. The incidence of gastric carcinoma increases with age, with a higher incidence in males at age of 60 by 2:1. It has been suggested that differences in incidence may be related to racial and ethnic factors but it is difficult to exclude environmental behavioural factors and social class differences. A genetic factor is suggested by the observed higher incidence of gastric cancer in individuals with blood group A compared with suitable controls but this is thought to play only a minor role compared with environmental factors. Migrants from countries such as Wales or Japan with a high incidence of carcinoma in their own country continue at high risk when they migrate to a low risk area such as America; a decreased incidence, however, occurs in succeeding generations, which suggests an environmental factor such as change in dietary habits. There is an increased incidence of carcinoma amongst the lower socio-economic groups which might relate either to environment or occupation. Dietary factors are of particular interest since they are preventable. Recent evidence has linked levels of dietary or water nitrate ingestion with high incidence areas for gastric carcinoma. Nitrates can be converted by bacteria to nitrosamines which are known to be carcinogenic in animals and are present in increased concentrations in achlorhydria or after gastric surgery where both bacterial colonization and increased cancer risk are recognized.

Precancerous conditions. The incidence of the development of cancer in a proven peptic ulcer, or unequivocal evidence of a previous peptic ulcer having occurred at the site of a proven carcinoma, is probably less than 1 per cent. Hence a benign gastric ulcer is rarely a premalignant condition. It can of course be very difficult to differentiate clinically, radiologically, and endoscopically between some benign and malignant ulcers, and some malignant ulcers have been known to heal on treatment. It is for these reasons that it was originally thought that gastric ulcers could become malignant.

There are a number of reports suggesting that patients with pernicious anaemia have a higher incidence of gastric carcinoma but much of this evidence does not stand up to critical review and reassessment of the association is necessary. Any association that may exist may well be explained on the precancerous nature of the gastric atrophy which is present in pernicious anaemia, particularly in the body and fundus of the stomach.

Many gastric cancers develop in areas of atrophic gastritis but the epithelial change which particularly predisposes to malignancy is intestinal metaplasia. Intestinal metaplasia occurs more frequently in stomachs that contain a carcinoma. In some early cases of carcinoma of the stomach there appears to be a transition between metaplastic mucosa and carcinoma.

Intestinal metaplasia and chronic gastritis are also found in the resected stomach and in many series there is an increased incidence of gastric cancer after gastrectomy (especially with a gastrojejunostomy). This is the case whether the gastric resection was for a gastric or duodenal ulcer. A prolonged contact of bile with the stomach remnant leading to gastritis is the suggested mechanism.

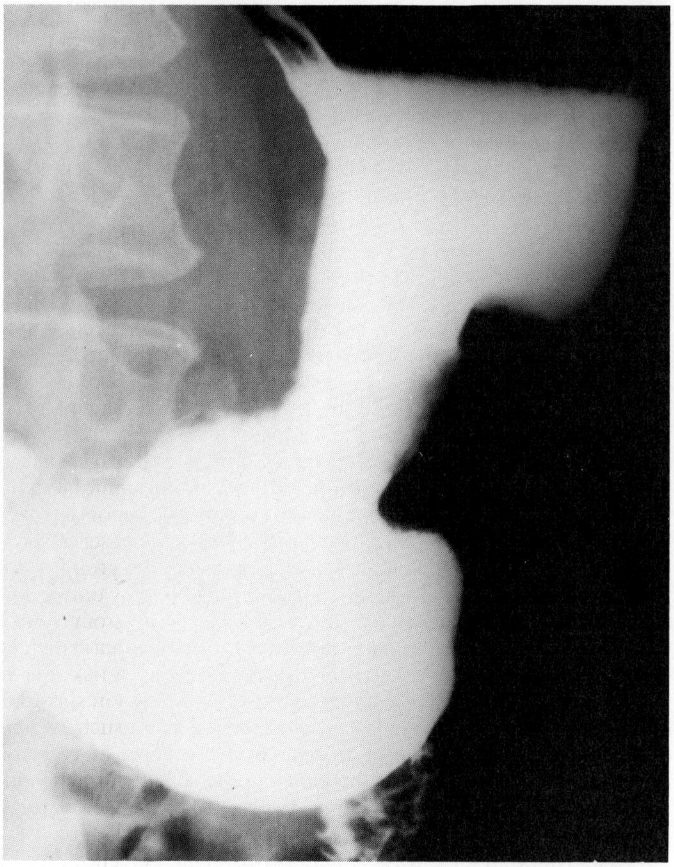

Clinical features. Outside Japan early gastric cancer is rarely diagnosed except by chance when it is found either in symptomless patients or in those with non-specific or unrelated symptoms. Large-scale screening programmes of asymptomatic volunteers in Japan yield one cancer per 1000 persons examined, half of which are early tumours. In the United Kingdom the overall incidence of gastric cancer is about a quarter of that of Japan and screening of asymptomatic individuals is not warranted, although when the stomach is examined for other reasons, more careful inspection using Japanese criteria reveals some early gastric cancers in European subjects, which would previously have been missed.

Most patients with carcinoma of the stomach have advanced disease at the time of diagnosis (Fig. 2), the common symptoms being anorexia, weight loss, and epigastric pain. The pain is often vague but may be indistinguishable from that of peptic ulcer and may also be relieved by food and alkalis. Vomiting occurs in approximately half the patients. Gross haematemesis is unusual but anaemia from occult blood loss is frequent. The presence of palpable epigastric mass has been reported in up to 50 per cent of patients. Carcinoma of the stomach is the cancer most frequently associated with dermatomyositis and acanthosis nigricans.

Pathology. Gastric cancer occurs most frequently in the antrum of the stomach. It is almost invariably an adenocarcinoma. The most widely accepted histological classification recognizes two patterns of carcinoma. The intestinal (or gastric) pattern occurs in high frequency areas, in elderly patients, and is usually polypoid; it is often associated with intestinal metaplasia in the surrounding mucosa. The diffuse pattern is composed of scattered solitary or small clusters of cells and occurs in low frequency areas and in younger people. It is associated with extensive submucosal spread which may result in the picture of 'linitis plastica', and has a worse prognosis than the intestinal type.

Early gastric cancer is defined as carcinoma limited to the mucosa or submucosa and not invading the muscle layer (Fig. 3). The complex Japanese classification of early gastric cancer is not used worldwide, differentiation often being made simply between tumours that are raised and those that are ulcerated. Early

Fig. 2 Carcinoma of the stomach demonstrated on barium meal.

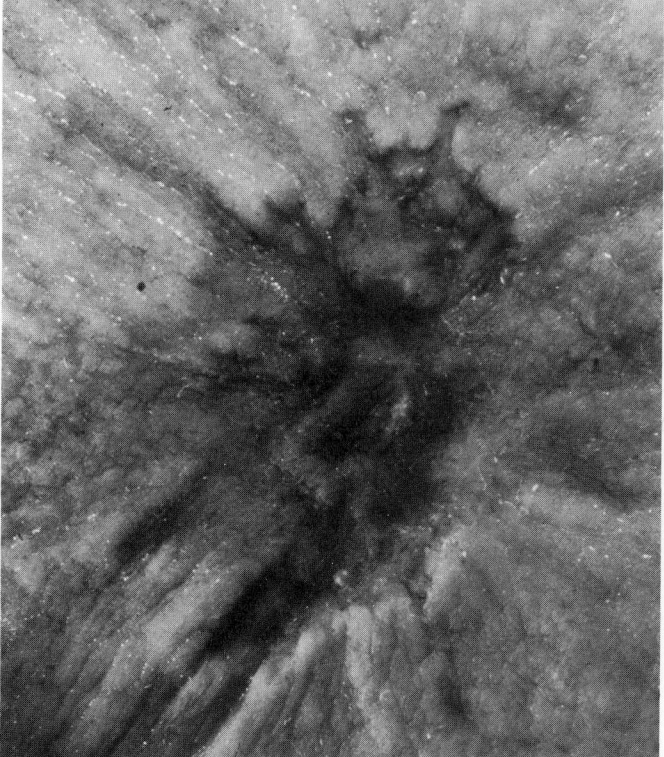

Fig. 3 Early gastric cancer (operation specimen, close-up view).

gastric cancers are not necessarily small and may spread superficially to cover a considerable area.

Diagnosis. Barium meal examination is the main technique used for diagnosis, and with good quality double-contrast radiology provides a correct diagnosis in a high percentage of cases. Japanese screening surveys rely on mobile units using double-contrast X-rays, endoscopy being used only on selected patients for visualization and biopsy of any abnormality found on X-ray study (see Fig. 2). Although gastroscopy with modern miniaturized fibre-optic instruments is a relatively easy technique, it is less acceptable to the patient. X-rays can be more difficult to interpret but they provide a permanent record and can be easily reviewed. A few centres feel that direct visualization and the ability to take biopsies justifies gastroscopy as the primary procedure in symptomatic patients. In practice the relative role of the two techniques is determined largely by the skills and experience of the personnel available.

Diagnosis of early gastric cancer requires fastidious technique since the lesions are often inconspicuous (see Fig. 3). Positive biopsies can be obtained in almost all cases of obvious carcinoma in spite of the small size of the biopsy that is obtained. However, one or more negative biopsies from the edge of an ulcer does not rule out malignancy and it is recommended that eight to 10 biopsies should be taken around the ulcer margin and from its base. Taking superficial brushing specimens for exfoliative cytology during the same procedure, in addition to the biopsies, will further improve the diagnostic rate.

Treatment. The five-year survival rate of resected early gastric cancer patients is 90 per cent but since less than 10 per cent of the at-risk population in Japan undergoes screening there has been no apparent decrease in the overall gastric cancer mortality, other than that attributable to the decline in the incidence of gastric cancer.

Surgery for more advanced gastric cancers gives only a 10 per cent five-year survival rate; this figure has not changed over the past 25 years. Total gastrectomy is now seldom performed since the operative morbidity is high and the five-year survival rate no better than sub-total or partial gastrectomy. Sixty-five per cent of tumours are found to be inoperable at the time of surgery but a palliative resection is sometimes performed to prevent obstruction and haemorrhage.

Treatment with chemotherapy has been attempted, 5-fluorouracil being the drug most widely used. This drug is now usually combined with other agents such as adriamycin and nitrosourea derivatives such as CCNU. The results of clinical trials are poor and although survival may be prolonged by a few months the serious toxicity of the drugs limits their use. At the present time chemotherapy should normally only be administered as part of a clinical trial and its indiscriminate use is not justified.

Other malignant tumours of the stomach. Primary lymphomas of the stomach make up about 10 per cent of all gastric malignancies and, in addition, systemic lymphoma may involve the stomach. The clinical features are indistinguishable from those of adenocarcinoma, except that nausea and vomiting seem to be more frequent. Treatment is surgical, usually combined with postoperative irradiation, and the prognosis is good with 50 per cent five-year survival.

Small bowel tumours

The small intestine is relatively resistant to the development of neoplasia and only 3–6 per cent of all gastrointestinal tumours and less than 1 per cent of all malignant lesions occur in the small bowel. This contrasts with its long length and the complexity of its different histological structures. The reason for the rarity of these tumours is not known; explanations include the fluidity and relative sterility of the small bowel contents and the rapid transit time which reduces the time of exposure to potential carcinogens. It may also be due to the unique role that the gut plays in immunological surveillance. It is possible that IgA, secreted mainly by the gut mucosa, may play an

important role in preventing malignancy, possibly by forming complexes with agents such as viruses or chemical carcinogens.

Malignant tumours, 90 per cent of which are symptomatic, are more common than benign tumours. The diagnosis is difficult to make pre-operatively, however, because the condition is so uncommon in clinical practice and because the symptoms are often vague and non-specific.

Benign. Adenomas, leiomas, and lipomas are the three commonest solitary benign tumours (excluding *Peutz–Jeghers syndrome* and other forms of polyposis discussed later). They are frequently asymptomatic and often found incidentally at operation or necropsy. If symptoms occur, pain is the most common, usually due to intussusception, but insidious loss of blood leading to anaemia is another frequent manifestation. Haemangiomas are rare but can occur as small polyps which are usually not seen on conventional barium meal studies of the small bowel or small intestine but may be found on angiography or by pre-operative fibre endoscopy of the small intestine. The length of history is extremely long in some of these cases, the diagnosis being unsuspected because of its rarity. Resection is curative.

Malignant. Malignant tumours of the jejunum and ileum account for only 1–5 per cent of alimentary tract malignancies and carcinoma in these regions is 40–60 times less common than colonic cancers. It is of interest that, despite this 'resistance' to malignancy, the small bowel is the commonest site in the gastrointestinal tract to find metastatic melanoma.

Adenocarcinoma is the commonest malignancy accounting for about 50 per cent of primary tumours. Carcinoid tumours form the next major group and lymphoma and smooth muscle tumours make up the remainder. Adenocarcinomas are found most often in the duodenum, peri-ampullary region, and jejunum, and lymphomas and carcinoid tumours most often in the ileum.

Epidemiology and predisposing factors. There appears to be no geographic or population cluster in small bowel malignancies and thus genetic and environmental factors seem to be unimportant. However, several chronic bowel diseases predispose to malignancies.

Gluten enteropathy. In coeliac disease and dermatitis herpetiformis there is an increased incidence of both lymphoma and adenocarcinoma of the small bowel. There is, in addition, an increased incidence of all malignancies throughout the body. In both conditions the upper intestinal mucosa is abnormal (sub-total villous atrophy) due to sensitivity to the gluten fraction of wheat (see page 12.90). The reason for the development of malignancy is unknown but it may be related to the mucosal lymphoid cell hyperplasia and abnormal mitotic activity. There is an altered immune status, both cellular and humoral, and an increased incidence of HLA-B8 associated with this disorder. It is now accepted that coeliac disease is a premalignant condition. There is no identifiable risk factor predisposing to malignancy in coeliac disease and no association with poor response to a gluten-free diet or chronicity of symptoms. The duration of symptoms of previous disease seems to be the same for both lymphoma and carcinoma, and there is no evidence that treatment of the coeliac disease with a gluten-free diet protects against the development of malignancy. The histology of the lymphoma associated with coeliac disease shows an overwhelming number of histiocytic cells and as the tumour has other features of malignant histiocytosis.

Crohn's disease. Crohn's disease of long duration results in increased incidence of adenocarcinoma of the small bowel but this is rare and does not influence management of the disease. The association with epithelial dysplasia in some cases suggests that the chronic inflammatory process is responsible (see Cancer in ulcerative colitis below).

Alpha chain disease. Alpha chain disease (see also pages 12.83 and 12.98) occurs mainly in countries surrounding the Mediterranean, and in South America and the Far East, and may progress to lymphoma of the bowel. It seems to be related to poor hygiene and intestinal infestation. There is proliferation of plasma cells in the lamina propria of the small bowel, predominantly in the duodenum and jejunum, producing IgA 'heavy chains' which can be detected in the gut mucosa by immunofluorescence, in the serum, and also in small quantities in the urine.

Clinical features. Malignant tumours, in contrast to benign tumours, are invariably symptomatic. They present with abdominal pain, diarrhoea, anorexia, weight loss, or anaemia. A palpable mass may be present. Most lesions can be detected on small bowel X-ray examination but it is sometimes necessary to use an intubation technique with air insufflation as the lesion can be extremely small.

Jejunal biopsies sometimes show an associated flat biopsy and may also yield histological evidence of malignancy.

Most patients, however, require a laparotomy in order for the diagnosis to be made and resection is usually performed at this time if possible. Over 50 per cent of patients with small intestinal adenocarcinoma already have involvment of the regional lymph nodes, and radiation therapy and chemotherapy are usually necessary.

Primary gastrointestinal lymphomas are of the non-Hodgkin's type and they must be differentiated from generalized lymphomas involving the gut secondarily, which are more common. The criteria for acceptance of a primary tumour involves freedom from disease elsewhere; at laparotomy the liver and spleen should be free of tumour and the bowel lesion should predominate with only closely related lymph nodes being involved. The treatment of non-Hodgkin's lymphoma depends partly on the staging of the disease at laparotomy and partly on the precise histological grading. Both are complex and not universally accepted. Chemotherapy as well as radiation is almost invariably used and the two-year survival rate varies from 60 to 80 per cent depending on the histological grade (see also section 18).

Carcinoid tumours. The carcinoid syndrome is described on page 12.55.

Colon polyps and polyposis syndromes

A polyp is an elevation above the mucosal surface, the word deriving from the Greek *polypos* for an octopus, which a stalked polyp broadly resembles. The majority of colorectal polyps prove to be adenomas with malignant potential (whereas they are the minority in the stomach) and thus their detection and removal is important.

Polyps range in appearance from tiny translucent and almost invisible bumps only 1–2 mm in diameter to those having a head of 1–3 cm in diameter on a vascular stalk or peduncle of normal tissue. A small number are sessile, little raised, and 1–10 cm in diameter. Polyps may be single, may occur together in small numbers, or in hundreds, or carpet the colon in thousands as part of the rarer polyposis syndromes. Histology is essential because it is usually impossible to be sure of the type of polyp by direct macroscopic or radiological inspection; the pathologist prefers to examine representative whole polyps rather than small biopsies in order to assess malignancy. Table 1 gives a general classification of large bowel polyps, most individual types occasionally occurring as polyposis.

Non-neoplastic polyps. The non-neoplastic polyps most commonly seen by a clinician on proctosigmoidoscopy are metaplastic (hyperplastic) polyps which are seen as 2–5 mm pale nodules in the rectum, where they are a normal finding. They have characteristic histology with 'saw-toothing' of the elongated mucosal crypts but have normal-looking nuclei. This makes microscopic distinction from the dysplastic crypts of adenomas easy. Metaplastic polyps or metaplastic polyposis have no clinical consequence although the occasional larger ones may need removal for reassurance that they are not adenomas.

Table 1 Classification of colorectal polyps

	Solitary	Multiple (polyposis syndromes)
Neoplastic	adenomas tubular tubulo-villous villous carcinoid	familial adenomatous polyposis malignant lymphoid polyposis
Non-neoplastic Hamartomas	Peutz–Jeghers juvenile (mucus retention)	Peutz–Jeghers syndrome juvenile polyposis
Inflammatory	lymphoid inflammatory	benign lymphoid polyposis inflammatory polyps ulcerative colitis, Crohn's disease, schistosomiasis, etc.
Miscellaneous	metaplastic (hyperplastic) connective tissue polyps: fibroma, leiomyoma, lipoma, neurofibroma	metaplastic polyposis Cronkhite–Canada syndrome

Inflammatory polyps may be equally numerous and extremely variable in size and shape although classically filiform (thread-like). Inflammatory polyps are seen in the healed phase after one or more severe attacks of colitis (ulcerative, Crohn's, schistosomal, etc.) and, while sometimes dramatic-looking on endoscopy or X-ray, are usually unimportant and, on histology, appear to be little more than tags covered by normal or slightly deranged epithelium. Larger inflammatory polyps may be composed of granulation tissue and may be sufficiently inflamed to cause bleeding or protein loss; they may also require removal for biopsy for distinction from adenomas.

Hamartomatous polyps, principally juvenile or Peutz–Jeghers in type, are developmental malformations containing a disorganized mixture of normal intestinal tissues and having practically no malignant potential. They are commonly large and stalked, the histology of juvenile polyps showing mucus retention cysts and inflammation (Fig. 4), whereas Peutz–Jeghers polyps have characteristic fibromuscular fronds radiating between the disorganized mucosal crypts. Juvenile polyps are a cause of bleeding in childhood, which may be acute if the head twists and auto-amputates; they may intussuscept and present at the anus; they also may be an incidental finding in middle-age. Juvenile polyposis, defined as more than 10 colonic polyps (the small intestine is not involved) may require colectomy and ileorectal anastomosis since these patients seem to have a considerably increased risk of colon cancer. There is no evidence that sporadic juvenile polyps have neoplastic potential. Histologically similar polyps occur throughout the intestine in the rare *Cronkhite–Canada syndrome*, resulting in diarrhoea and steatorrhoea. The full syndrome includes ectodermal abnormalities such as alopecia, nail dystrophy and skin hyperpigmentation.

Peutz–Jeghers syndrome of mucocutaneous pigmentation (circumoral, hands and feet) the gastrointestinal polyposis is, like adenomatous polyposis, inherited as a Mendelian dominant. Peutz–Jeghers polyps may occur anywhere in the intestine but definite association with malignancy is rare and mainly affects the duodenal region where carcinomas may arise. Lip and mouth pigmentation (Fig. 5) is a very useful clinical marker, indicating that it may be necessary to resect small intestinal polyps prophylactically or at least to operate early if symptoms of intussusception occur, since there is a risk of infarction and a resultant short-bowel syndrome. Gastroduodenal and colonic polyps may cause anaemia and are easily removed by endoscopic snare polypectomy.

Other non-neoplastic polyps are less common. Lipomas are found usually in the right colon and, as in the skin, do not require removal. Fatty enlargement of the ileocaecal valve may produce worrying radiographic appearances but is equally unimportant. Endometriosis involving the bowel is usually on the serosal aspect

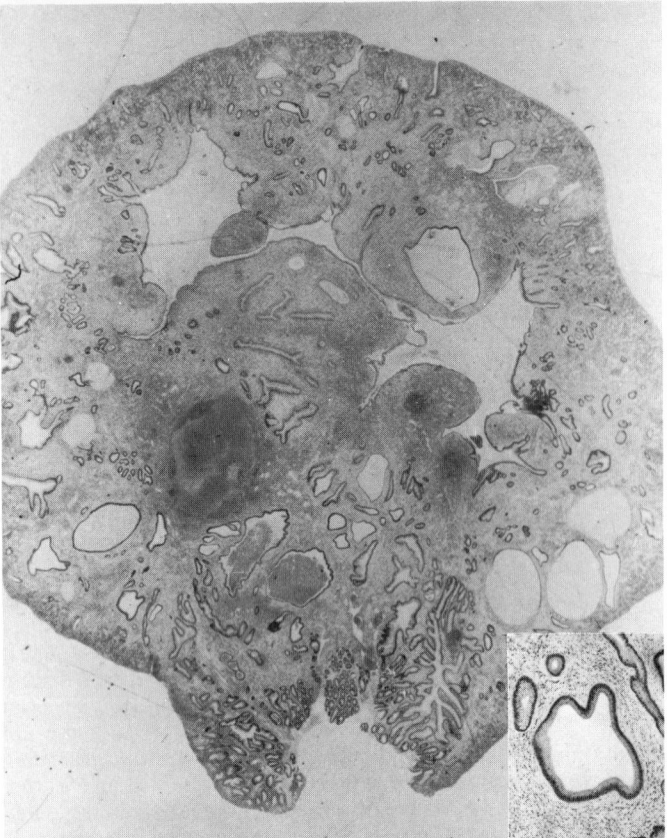

Fig. 4 Photomicrograph of juvenile (hamartomatous) polyp showing mucus retention cysts but normal covering epithelium. The glands are not dysplastic (inset).

or in the muscle layers of the distal colon, causing deformity but no symptoms; rarely it may result in a submucosal polypoid mass which bleeds and needs differentiation from carcinoma (see page 12.120). As might be expected, benign tumours can also arise from other tissue elements of the wall of small or large intestine and include neurofibromas, leiomyomas, and polypoid haemangiomas. Lymphoid tissue is present in the colon as tiny follicles dotted across the mucosa. They are normally only visible in childhood at which time nodular lymphoid hyperplasia may cause radiological appearances which in the colon resemble polyposis and in the terminal ileum mimic Crohn's disease. Pneumocystic disease (pneumatosis cystoides) causes multiple raised colonic mucosal blebs, sometimes haemorrhagic, which can be punctured and collapsed (see page 12.154).

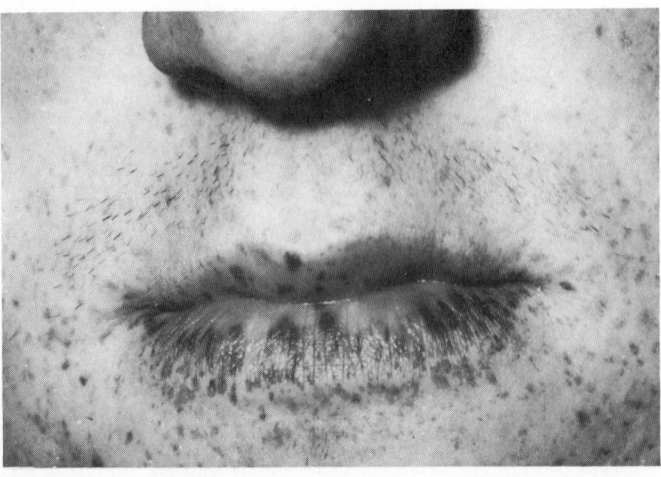

Fig. 5 Peutz–Jeghers patient with characteristic lip pigmentation.

Neoplastic polyps. The majority of neoplastic polyps in the colorectum are adenomas, a generic name covering the spectrum of benign epithelial growths with malignant potential. They range from the most frequent, tubular adenomas, to those with mixed or intermediate tubulovillous characteristics and to the rarer, larger, and often sessile villous adenomas (villous papilloma) which have the greatest tendency to malignancy (Fig. 6). The differing use of histological terms in the literature can be confusing. The nomenclature used here is that recommended by the World Health Organization.

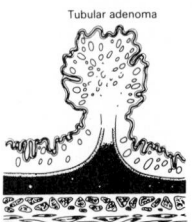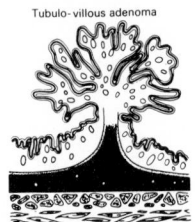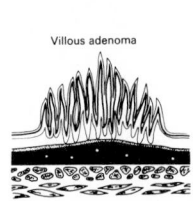

Fig. 6 Diagrammatic representation of the histology of the three histological patterns of adenomatous polyps.

Aetiological factors and pathology. Adenomas occur, usually asymptomatically, in at least 10 per cent of the Western populations but more rarely in Africa, Asia, and South America. They are uncommon in Japanese unless they adopt a Western diet, whether at home or after emigration, and the factors affecting adenoma development are probably the same as those relating to carcinoma. All observations suggest the influence of environmental or ecological factors, probably diets which may result in changed bacterial flora and the production of chemical carcinogens by bacterial action. Additionally there is evidence of genetic influences, of which the most obvious is the dominant inheritance of familial adenomatous polyposis, which seems to occur with approximately equal incidence throughout the world. The concept which emerges from these studies is of a change in the normal processes of epithelial cell maturation resulting in an unstable epithelium with abnormally large and hyperchromatic nuclei (Fig. 7) and disordered crypt architecture. Contrary to common belief this neoplastic epithelium has a normal rate of cell turnover. Available clinical evidence also suggests that adenomas are extremely slow growing, in most cases taking several years to reach 1 cm in size and often causing no sequelae in the lifespan of the patient.

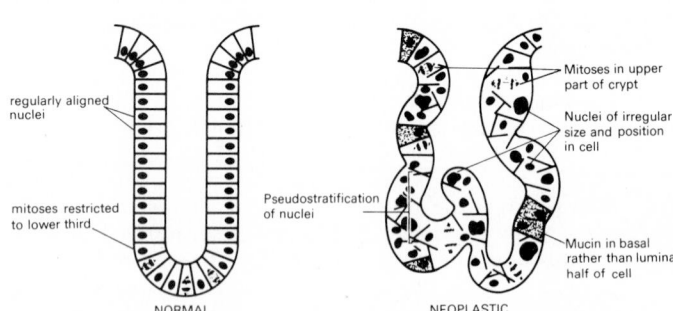

Fig. 7 The histological difference between normal and neoplastic (dysplastic) colonic epithelium.

All forms of adenoma have similar abnormal or 'dysplastic' epithelium, analogous to pre-neoplastic changes in bronchial epithelium or cervix uteri. The severity of the changes may be graded as mild, moderate, or severe, and reflect the malignant potential of the polyp. There is a junction clearly visible between the darker red neoplastic epithelium and pale shiny normal mucosa which makes local excision easy. Only histological examination can determine if dysplastic epithelium has invaded across the muscularis mucosae into the submucosa of the head of the polyp (Fig. 8). This is the only acceptable proof that carcinomatous change has occurred.

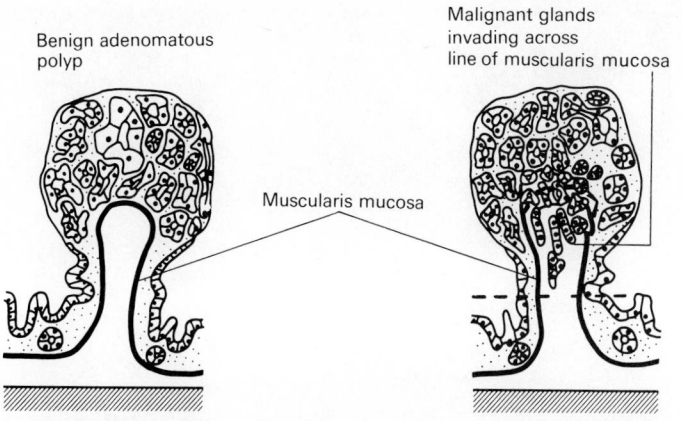

Benign adenomatous polyp

Malignant glands invading across line of muscularis mucosa

Muscularis mucosa

Fig. 8 Diagrammatic representation of the histology of carcinoma invading the head of an adenomatous polyp (dotted line indicates extent of section/electrocoagulation after snare polypectomy).

Although localized foci of severe dysplasia may occur on the surface of the adenoma and are sometimes described as 'carcinoma *in situ*', this term is best avoided, since, without invasion across the muscularis mucosae, there is no contact with lymphatics and therefore no possibility of metastases. The frequency with which invasive carcinoma arises in adenomas increases with the size of polyp and degree of dysplasia (Table 2). It is greater in villous adenomas because they are often large and severely dysplastic. Data from surgical series suggest an average incidence of carcinoma in adenomas of 10 per cent whereas large endoscopic series find it to be around 5 per cent, including some polypoid carcinomas. The difference between these results is probably due to case selection since the surgical figures are biased by the inclusion of polyps found during cancer resection.

Table 2 Frequency of invasive carcinoma in different types and sizes of adenomas in an endoscopic series

	Type as % of all adenomas	% of type with carcinoma			
		<1 cm	1–2 cm	>2 cm	Total
Tubular	75	1	3	10	2
Tubulo-villous	20		4	11	6
Villous	5		5	38	18

The adenoma–adenocarcinoma sequence. There is considerable circumstantial evidence that most if not all colon carcinomas originate from an adenoma. No one disputes that some adenomas progress to invasive carcinoma; the average latent interval for a medium-size adenoma to develop malignancy is thought to be about five to seven years. Many small carcinomas contain areas of benign adenomatous change but these are less often found in more advanced cancers. It is presumed that the carcinoma has engulfed and destroyed the benign tissue. Very small or intramucosal carcinomas are rarely found except in association with the unique flat pattern of dysplasia of chronic long-standing ulcerative colitis. Patients with adenomas have a higher risk of coexisting (synchronous) colon carcinomas or of developing one subsequently, the risk of cancer increasing with the numbers of adenomas found up to the 100 per cent risk in familial adenomatous polyposis. The distribution of colorectal carcinomas and adenomas is similar with increasing incidence distally towards the rectum; the small increased incidence of caecal carcinomas may parallel a similar increased tendency to villous adenoma formation in the caecum. Epidemiological patterns for colorectal cancer also mirror those for adenomas, for instance Japanese emigrating to Hawaii acquire a raised incidence of both adenomas and cancer. Systematically destroying adenomas in the rectum of asymptomatic subjects or familial adenomatosis patients is found to decrease markedly the expected local incidence of carcinoma formation.

The rare occurrence of a carcinoma of 1 cm or so in diameter can be explained by the existence of 'microadenomas' in which only one or more individual epithelial crypts show neoplastic changes; such a tiny initial focus would be undetectable after development of carcinoma. Although small foci of adenoma presumably carry a lower statistical chance of malignant change than large masses, their existence means that even the most careful surgery or follow-up regimens are unlikely completely to remove the risk of carcinoma formation.

Clinical features in management of colonic polyps. Most colonic polyps are symptomless and diagnosed on X-ray (Fig. 9) or endoscopy. Larger ones may bleed intermittently and can cause mild anaemia. Obvious mucus production, altered bowel habit, or abdominal pain are exceedingly rare and only result from very large polyps. The largest are the sessile villous adenomas of the rectum which can rarely present with profuse mucoid diarrhoea and electrolyte depletion, especially hypokalaemia. Even small colonic polyps definitely identified on X-ray are probably worth destroying because they are usually adenomatous and because, when the colon is known to be polyp-free, the patient can be spared frequent follow-up examinations which is the alternative if the polyp is left. If the radiologist reports a 'ring shadow', this usually means that he is in doubt whether the small abnormality shown is a polyp, an air-bubble, or a blob of faeces; careful review of the films will often decide the matter.

Once found on X-ray or endoscopy, a polyp should usually be removed completely for histological assessment. The introduction of fibre-optic endoscopes makes any polyp accessible and almost

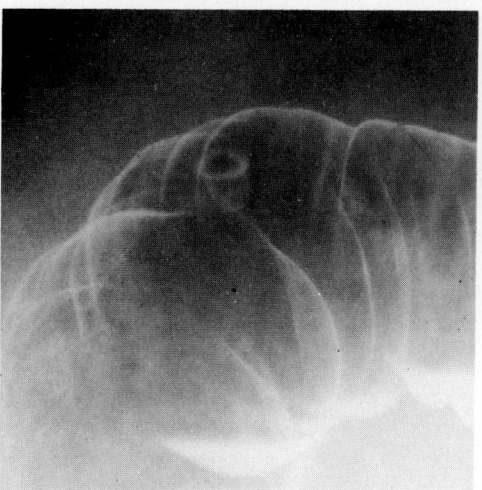
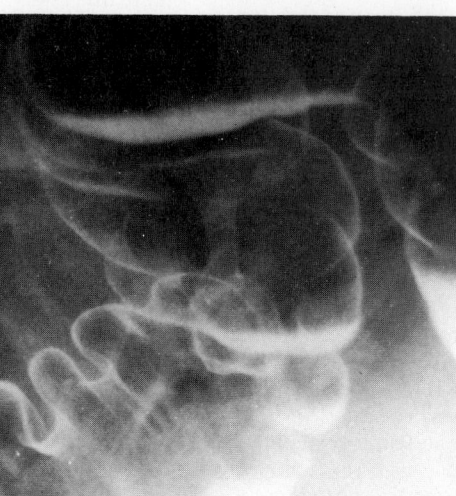

Fig. 9 Air-contrast radiographs of (left) a 5 mm colonic polyp (note the characteristic double ring-shadow or 'hat sign') and (right) a 1.5 cm stalked polyp.

always completely removable by snare polypectomy or local elec- trocoagulation. The mucosal surface of the colon is without pain sensation so that the action of snaring and electrocoagulating the polyp stalk to prevent bleeding is not felt by the patient and can be performed on an out-patient basis with or without sedation. Ninety per cent of patients with polyps have only one or two, and the same percentage are under 2 cm in diameter, thin-stalked, and easy to snare. Bigger polyps have larger feeding vessels with a greater tendency to bleed after polypectomy; patients with these lesions should be admitted overnight after polypectomy for observation. Very large or sessile polyps may have to be removed 'piecemeal' in multiple portions but few are so large as to need surgical resection. Within 5 cm of the anus the likelihood of pain sensation makes general anaesthesia advisable for polypectomy. Skilled manage- ment by a colorectal surgeon is needed for local removal of large sessile villous adenomas in the rectum.

When carcinoma is identified in a resected adenoma the decision for or against further surgical resection of the bowel is a matter of balancing the very small chance of finding resectable metastatic carcinoma in the draining lymph nodes against the risks of operation, as the subject is often elderly. If the pathologist finds the carcinoma to be limited to the head, well-differentiated, and not apparently invading lymphatics or veins, operation is usually not advised.

Follow-up. Once a patient has had one or more polyps removed and shown to be adenomas, some form of follow-up surveillance is recommended for life because over the ensuing years adenomas are found in at least 30 per cent of patients and carcinomas in 2–4 per cent. Existing data on follow-up regimens based on rigid procto- sigmoidoscopy and barium enema examination is inexact and few carefully controlled studies are available using fibre-endoscopy. Which follow-up technique is adopted depends on the relative availability of colonoscopy and good quality double-contrast bari- um enema. The standard or single contrast barium enema is shown to be highly inaccurate for demonstrating any but the largest polyps and should not be employed. The high concentration of adenomas in the rectum and sigmoid colon suggests the combination of fibre- sigmoidoscopy to check the distal colon and barium enema to demonstrate the proximal colon. The interval between follow-up examinations is debatable; patients at high-risk for development of further lesions, including those with multiple adenomas, malig- nancy or a family history of adenomas or cancer, are often recom- mended one to two yearly examinations until no adenomas are found, whereas three-yearly checks are thought to be adequate for low-risk patients with one or two adenomas. Villous adenomas are associated with high incidence of invasive carcinomas and a remarkable tendency to recure locally, thus requiring frequently repeated examination after attempted removal.

Familial adenomatous polyposis. Familial adenomatous polypo- sis (adenomatosis) is now known to affect the whole gastrointesti- nal tract, and since the duodenal region and small intestine are usually involved, the term 'polyposis coli' is best avoided, even though the colon is the area of main involvement and clinical interest. At least a hundred and often thousands of polyps are present throughout the colon (Fig. 10). The qualification 'adeno- matous' is included to ensure distinction from other non-neoplastic forms of polyposis. The condition is inherited as a Mendelian dominant with equal incidence in males and females and probably in all races. It can also occur without a preceding family history, presumably via a spontaneous mutation. The prime reason for concern is the inevitable occurrence of colorectal carcinoma in all polyposis patients followed for long enough; cases of carcinoma of the duodenum, ampulla, and bile ducts have also been reported. *Gardner's syndrome*, in which adenomatosis coexists with meso- dermal tumours (dermoid tumours of the abdomen, osteomas of the mandible and skull, sebaceous cysts, and soft-tissue tumours of the skin) and the even rarer *Turcot's syndrome* in which there are

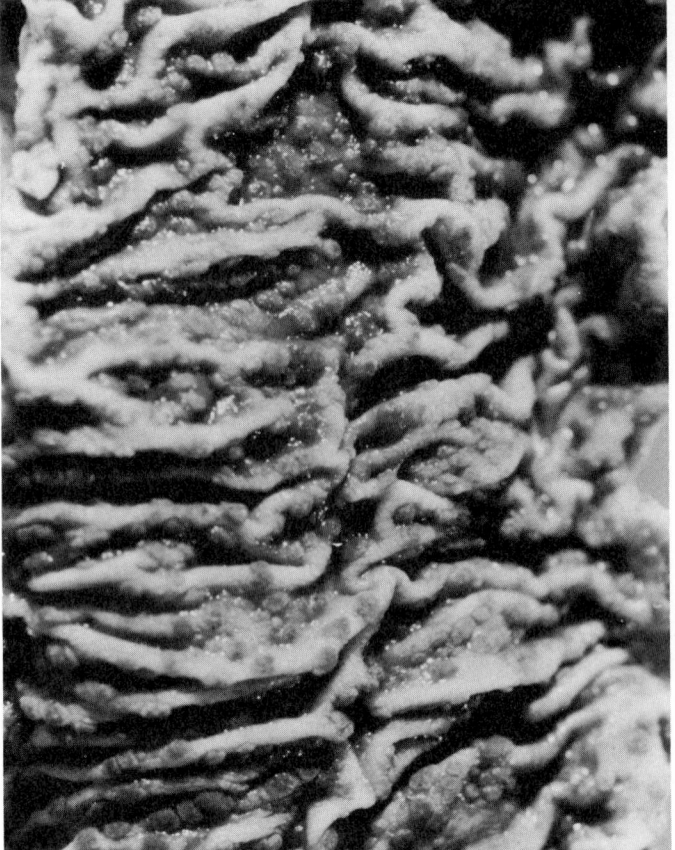

Fig. 10 Familial adenomatous polyposis: part of operation specimen showing carpeting of the colon by hundreds of adenomas.

brain tumours and adenomatosis, are both variants within the broad spectrum of clinical presentation of familial adenomatous polyposis.

It is rare for the adenomas to develop before adolescence, and if screening examinations are not performed, symptoms usually only occur when a carcinoma has developed. The mean age of sympto- matic presentation in the St Mark's polyposis registry is 36 years whereas the diagnosis can be made much earlier and before the development of cancer if all members of known 'polyposis families' are called to attend a screening clinic aged 12–14 years. Fibre- sigmoidoscopy in such patients is a more accurate examination than rigid proctosigmoidoscopy. If no polyps are seen distally there is no need for further procedures other than re-examination every two to three years until the age of 30 and possibly at infrequent intervals thereafter. Any polyps seen, however small, must be biopsied to differentiate between adenomatous and non-neoplastic forms of polyposis. Procto-colectomy with ileo-anal anastomosis or ileos- tomy is usually performed at the age of 17–18 years for social convenience since there is no significant risk of carcinoma before this. Careful long-term follow-up is needed if rectal mucosa is left, with repeated electrocoagulation of any new polyps seen. Ten per cent of the St Mark's familial polyposis patients with ileo-rectal anastomosis developed rectal stump cancer over a 30-year period.

A cancer screening programme is necessary for all blood relatives including cousins, nephews, and nieces of the relevant age, in addition to constructing a careful family tree and keeping a register of affected families. By such precautions, familial adenomatous polyposis has become the classic example of practical cancer pre- vention.

Colorectal cancer

Adenocarcinomas of the colon and rectum present a major chal- lenge to medical practice, being common, potentially curable, and possibly preventable. The other malignancies of the region, lymphoma, sarcoma, and carcinoid are very rare.

Epidemiology and aetiological factors. Colorectal carcinoma is the commonest malignancy in the United Kingdom after lung cancer and in the United States after skin cancer. In the United Kingdom 16 000 deaths are reported annually, separated into 10 000 from colon carcinoma and 6000 from rectal carcinoma. Exact statistics are uncertain since anatomical distinction between rectum and colon is sometimes arbitrary. At least another 6000 colorectal cancers a year are successfully resected and do not enter these statistics. There is evidence from the United States that the percentage of colon cancers is steadily increasing compared to rectal cancers. There are differing reports on sex incidence but men appear to be slightly more at risk for rectal cancer and women for colon cancer. The incidence of both cancers increases with age, the average age at diagnosis being around 60–65 years.

The epidemiology of colorectal cancer suggests that environmental (probably dietary) and genetic factors are both important. The incidence of colorectal cancer is higher in Northern Europe and North America than in Southern Europe and South America or in Africa and Asia. Japan is a low-risk area for carcinoma of the colon compared to carcinoma of the rectum, but Japanese of higher socio-economic status who adopt a 'Westernized' diet or who emigrate to America change to 'high-risk' for colon cancer. Sporadic examples of colorectal cancer occur even in low-risk countries, unfortunately often in young people who develop an anaplastic carcinoma with poor prognosis. Heavy meat-eating groups in otherwise low-risk areas show a high incidence of colon cancer and conversely vegetarians in high-risk areas have a lower incidence. There is some evidence that carcinogens or co-carcinogens may be produced by bacterial metabolism of bile salts or other sterols derived from animal fat. The higher incidence of colorectal cancer in populations eating a low-fibre diet may be explained by slow colonic transit which gives more time for carcinogen production, concentration, and contact with the mucosa. Besides the extreme example of familial polyposis, the importance of genetic factors is suggested by an increased incidence of cancer within families. Fifteen per cent of siblings and 10 per cent of children of colorectal cancer patients develop the disease and other 'colon cancer families' have been described with a very high incidence in first degree relatives, without evidence of adenomatous polyposis. Other factors must be invoked to explain the raised incidence in association with breast, ovarian, or prostatic cancer and with chronic extensive ulcerative colitis. Surgical implantation of the ureters into the sigmoid colon results after 10–20 years in a high incidence of colonic adenoma or carcinoma adjacent to the ureteric stoma, possibly due to carcinogen formation from bacterial action on substances excreted in the urine.

Putting the various theories and factors together the suggested hypothesis for the aetiology of colorectal cancer is that predisposition to adenomas occurs if a recessive gene is inherited from each parent; that dietary factors result in altered bacterial flora and carcinogen production promoting first adenoma formation and then eventual malignant transformation. The redeeming factor from the clinical point of view is that the sequence of events is slow-moving, giving a chance to find and remove the lesion at its precancerous stage; additionally, most colorectal cancers are well or moderately well differentiated and usually present without metastases. Furthermore, colorectal neoplasms, whether precancerous or invasive, tend to grow into the lumen of the bowel which makes them easier to diagnose and resect.

Pathology. The majority of bowel carcinomas occur distally in the rectosigmoid. A convenient rule, acceptably accurate considering the difficulties of definition and measurement of site, is that 30 per cent occur in the rectum, 30 per cent in the sigmoid colon and 30 per cent proximal to that.

The typical carcinoma is a polypoid mass with central ulceration

and irregular easily-bleeding edges, which may spread to become a stricture (Fig. 11); infiltrating scirrhous colon carcinomas are rare. Colorectal carcinoma initially spreads by local invasion rather than by venous or lymphatic routes, which accounts for its good prognosis when confined to the bowel wall. It invades through the submucosa and muscle coats of the bowel to penetrate the extramural tissues and may involve adjacent organs such as the bladder giving rise to secondary complications such as fistula formation. Involvement of veins, particularly thick-walled veins, results in early spread to the liver and poor prognosis, although occasionally liver metastases may be single and resectable. If lymphatics are invaded, the spread is to nodes nearest to the growth before those lying more centrally in the mesentery. This gradual progression through mainly free-slung and easily resected tissues improves the chances of complete surgical removal of large bowel cancer.

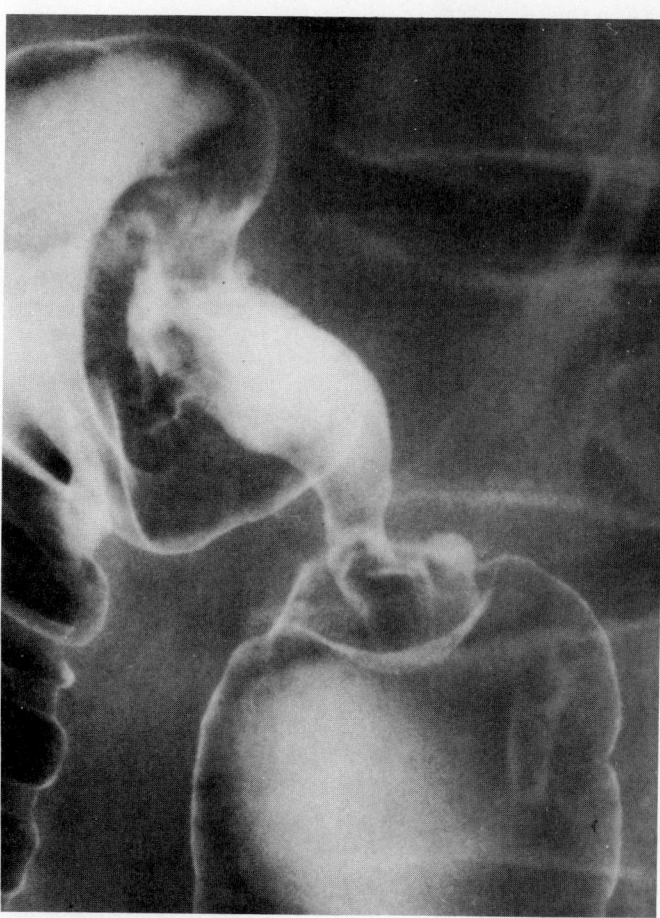

Fig. 11 Air-contrast radiograph of characteristic 'apple-core' stricture caused by colonic carcinoma.

In 1932 Dukes described a staging classification for resected carcinoma of the rectum, subsequently applied to colonic carcinomas as well, in which the extent of local spread and presence or absence of lymph node metastases was related to five-year survival (Fig. 12). Classification is also possible by histological grade (well differentiated, moderately-well differentiated, poorly differentiated) but is less accurate than the Dukes' classification in predicting survival. The poorly differentiated carcinomas are usually the most extensive and have a poorer prognosis, disproportionately worse if larger veins are involved. The most frequent sites of metastases are liver (over 60 per cent), lung (over 50 per cent), peritoneum or skeleton (each 15 per cent).

Clinical features. Once a colorectal carcinoma has reached moderate size, it is likely to produce symptoms, which will depend on its site in the colon. Rectal and sigmoid colon cancers usually bleed

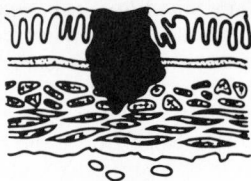

DUKES A
Tumour limited
to bowel wall

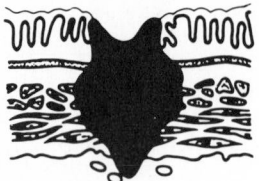

DUKES B
Tumour has
penetrated through
the bowel wall
but lymph nodes are
not involved

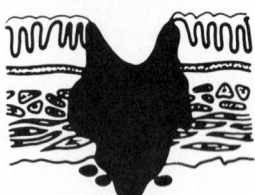

DUKES C
The lymph nodes
are now involved

Fig. 12 Dukes' classification of colorectal carcinoma.

because the friable tumour surface is buffetted by solid stool, the blood being mixed in with the stool (in contrast to the bright red and separated blood of haemorrhoids). Alteration in previously regular habit, whether bowel frequency or constipation, is more likely when the tumour obstructs the passage of solid stool in the narrow left colon, whereas the flow of liquid contents through the capacious caecum or ascending colon is unaffected even by large tumours. For this reason the caecum is known as a 'silent area' in which large symptomless carcinomas may occur, eventually presenting with iron-deficiency anaemia. This is a consequence of the long-continued minor blood loss, altered by bacterial action and therefore unnoticed in the stools. The problem of diagnosis in the caecum is further compounded by the difficulty of cleansing it completely and of obtaining good X-rays of the area. Pain, suggesting obstruction or invasion, and weight-loss are late symptoms which are most common in advanced cancers in the right colon. Even at this stage the slow-moving nature of colon cancer means that it may be resectable. The presence of a palpable mass does not invariably mean a bad prognosis, for the carcinoma may be small with considerable faecal hold-up or most of the mass be due to surrounding inflammatory change or abscess formation.

The problem in clinical diagnosis of colorectal cancer is that the symptom patterns are very variable and non-specific. The commonest causes of anorectal bleeding are trivial haemorrhoids or fissures and the patients most troubled by colonic pain, altered bowel habit, or mucus loss are those with an irritable or spastic colon, who often also have an obsessive and cancerphobic personality. Nonetheless the importance of early diagnosis of colon cancer is such that any new colonic symptoms should be taken seriously, particularly bleeding and especially in patients over 45 years of age. Every patient should be clinically examined with initial digital examination of the rectum and rigid proctosigmoidoscopy; if a trivial cause is diagnosed he should be frequently reviewed so that if symptoms persist or recur expert opinion is sought and further investigations performed.

Diagnosis. The fibre-sigmoidoscope will probably in future replace or supplement proctosigmoidoscopy in any patient with bleeding or particular cancer risk. Fibre-sigmoidoscopy requires a single enema as preparation, needs no sedation, and takes only two to three minutes longer to perform than the rigid examination but

examines three to four times the extent of colon with proportionately increased reassurance and pathological yield. Its range over the distal colon (sometimes to the splenic flexure) covers both the highest risk area for adenomas and carcinoma and the region where most radiological misses occur. Examination of the proximal colon is also most accurate with the fibre-optic colonoscope but the technique is difficult and traumatic in about 30 per cent of patients so that some sedation is normally required. The air- or double-contrast barium enema (DCBE) gives comparable accuracy for large lesions such as cancers and is considerably easier and quicker to perform, with films available for expert review. If preceded by fibre-sigmoidoscopy and an efficient bowel cleansing regimen and followed with colonoscopy in those cases where doubt remains, the DCBE should retain its initial diagnostic role in most centres. Patients with unexplained and persistent rectal bleeding must nonetheless have fibre-endoscopy even if the barium enema appears normal, and 20 to 30 per cent of those referred are found to have radiologically missed polyps or cancer. Conversely, patients with strictures of the colon can have malignancy excluded more certainly by the passage of a small calibre fibrescope than by diagnostic laparotomy, because of the mucosal view and biopsy capability of the endoscope. Even those patients with the diagnostic 'apple core' appearance of stricturing colon carcinoma (see Fig. 11) on X-ray need high-quality examination of the rest of the colon, either radiologically or by endoscopy, because of the 20 per cent incidence of coexisting benign or malignant neoplasms.

Differential diagnosis must be made from other benign lesions such as localized ischaemic areas, solitary ulcer of the rectum, granulation tissue masses, endometriosis or inflammatory lesions such as amoebomas, all of which can exactly mimic carcinoma on X-ray and endoscopy. Palpable masses with radiological features stimulating carcinoma can be caused in the caecal area by an appendix abscess, tuberculosis, actinomycosis, Crohn's disease or an amoeboma, and in the sigmoid colon by diverticular disease with pericolic abscess formation. Strictures which cause suspicious X-ray appearances but prove to be benign on endoscopic biopsy or cytology occur in Crohn's disease, ulcerative colitis, or after severe ischaemic colitis. Whenever practicable, a forceps biopsy should be taken before operating on a carcinoma.

Other indirect diagnostic approaches such as haemoglobin estimation or sedimentation rate make limited contribution to diagnosis. The lack of specificity of serological tests such as the carcino-embryonic antigen (CEA) has so far been a disappointment; they are now used routinely only in a few institutions and then mainly postoperatively in the hope that early diagnosis and management of recurrent tumour will improve prognosis. Screening studies have been attempted on large asymptomatic populations over the age of 40 using commercially available occult blood test packs. Those cancers that are found by such screening (about 1 per 1000 persons tested) are usually at an earlier stage, with improved prognosis. However, the costs of screening are enormous, especially the further investigations by endoscopy or X-ray of the 30 to 40 subjects per 1000 tested who show positive results, most of whom then have no significant pathology found. Most workers conclude that to extend such screening programmes to the general population is unrealistically demanding on resources; however, annual occult blood testing has been made available free of charge to those over 45 in Germany and the long-term results will be awaited with interest.

Treatment and results. The best treatment for colorectal carcinoma is excision, usually by surgical resection except for polyps which have been snared and show invasion limited to the head, or small and circumscribed rectal cancers suitable for local excision. There have been enthusiastic reports on radiotherapy for rectal carcinoma, but this method is usually reserved for unfit patients with inoperable tumours, especially for pain relief. Chemotherapy with 5-fluorouracil alone or in combination with other agents has not shown any improvement in survival time whether used in advanced disease or as adjuvant therapy in patients undergoing curative surgery. The hope of the surgeon is to be able to perform a radical operation, removing the growth with an adequate margin of normal tissue and the entire draining lymphatic field. Even in the 20 per cent of patients in whom the presence of metastases or extensive infiltration makes radical surgery impossible, the resection of the primary tumour is desirable as palliative treatment in order to avoid obstruction and the unpleasantness of bloody discharge.

Pre-operatively as part of the general examination the surgeon attempts to assess by palpation the resectability of any tumour accessible to digital examination. Urography is usually performed to check for ureteric involvement. The bowel is prepared for surgery by cleansing with oral lavage or a purgative regimen with enemas and an antibiotic combination to reduce the risk of postoperative sepsis. Obstructing carcinomas make effective cleansing impossible, spillage more likely, and the hazards of surgery greater.

The choice of operation is usually straightforward since the object is to remove a wide area of the supplying vasculature and the associated lymphatic field. Substantial resections are therefore performed such as a right hemicolectomy for proximal lesions, transverse colectomy, left hemicolectomy, or sigmoid colectomy distally, the feeding artery or arteries to the region being tied off and dissected close to their origin from the aorta. Improved surgical suturing techniques or the use of the stapling gun have made it possible to resect and re-anastomose rectal carcinomas down to less than 10 cm above the anus. The exact limit depends on circumstances including the apparent extent of tumour spread, since a 3–5 cm margin of excision is desirable. 'Low' anterior resections are now commonplace and the results of restorative surgery or local excision is so good that rectal excision is often avoidable. When the tumour involves the region of the anal sphincter, there is no alternative to rectal excision and a permanent colostomy. A temporary colostomy is sometimes performed when the likelihood of postoperative anastomotic leakage or sepsis is high, for instance after low anterior resections, technically difficult operations or when there is obstruction and imperfect preparation. The operative mortality of colorectal resections is around 5 per cent.

The long-term results of surgery for colorectal cancer depend on the centre reporting as well as on stage and grade of tumour. Specialist centres quote over 90 per cent of cases as being suitable for radical or curative surgery with corrected five-year survival of 50–60 per cent overall and 100 per cent for Dukes' A cases (Table 3). District general hospitals find only 50 per cent to be suitable for radical surgery and even so have only 30 per cent corrected five-year survival. The overall figures reflect the problems of less experienced surgeons in general hospitals, elderly patients with a more advanced stage of disease due to later referral or inadequate diagnostic methods, and emergency operations (obstruction, perforation) performed under unfavourable conditions. Even so the results for colorectal cancer are cheerful in comparison to those for gastric or pancreatic cancer, reflecting the difference in pathology rather than medical skill. Surgical technique and advances in anaesthesia, post-operative care, and antibiotic cover have in the past improved the results considerably but they have not changed in the past 30 years. Further improvement in survival figures must rest on public attitude towards early reporting of bleeding or bowel symptoms and early referral for investigation with modern diagnostic techniques.

Table 3 Prognosis and Dukes' classification for colorectal cancer

Dukes' classification	Cases resected %	5-year survival (corrected for other causes of mortality) %
A	15	95–100
B	40	65–75
C_1	35	30–40
C_2	10	10–20

Carcinoma in ulcerative colitis. Patients who have ulcerative colitis (see also page 12.110) for more than 10 years affecting the whole colon are at increased risk to develop colon cancer. A similar tendency may also exist in the few patients with long-standing extensive Crohn's colitis. The risk remains even when the ulcerative colitis is inactive and the patient symptom-free, but is probably greater when the colitis has been persistently active or started in childhood. After 20 years from the onset of symptoms of extensive ulcerative colitis 5–10 per cent of patients are likely to have developed carcinoma. Unlike other colon cancers, these are more likely to be multifocal, intramucosal, and histologically of mucinous or signet-ring type, although any variety may occur. Though this risk is a matter for concern in the individual patient, the numbers involved are small and account for less than 0.5 per cent of all colon cancers. There appears to be no significant risk in patients with a short history or in those with only left-sided colitis.

A number of centres report success in screening long-standing extensive colitis patients with periodic rectal and colonoscopic biopsies, looking for precancerous or severely dysplastic changes analagous to those in adenomas or in the cervix uteri. The rectum of patients with previous ileorectal anastomosis is similarly at risk and requires surveillance. Symptomless patients with persistent severe dysplasia on biopsy may be recommended to have surgery for this alone. This dysplasia surveillance policy is still under evaluation but appears to offer a reasonable alternative to the blunderbuss approach of performing total colectomy on all patients with chronic extensive colitis.

Other colonic and anal tumours

Carcinoid tumours of the large bowel occur mainly as yellowish rectal nodules which are usually benign, do not produce the carcinoid syndrome, and can be locally resected. Primary lymphoma of the colon is rare but polyposis-like involvement occurs as part of generalized lymphoma with multiple umbilicated nodules present in the distribution of the lymphoid follicles in the colon and elsewhere in the gastrointestinal tract; diagnosis is made on forceps biopsy, the polyps disappearing on chemotherapy. Localized lymphoma may be treated by resection or irradiation, depending on its site.

In the anal region a number of tumours may occur relating to the different structures and embryology of the area. They include (cloacogenic) anal gland tumours, condylomas, and malignant melanomas. Rarely the anal region may be the site of precancerous skin conditions such as leucoplakia, Paget's disease, or Bowen's disease.

References

Bussey, H. J. R. (1970). Gastrointestinal polyposis (progress report). *Gut.* **11**, 970.

Butt, J. H., Lennard-Jones, J. E., and Ritchie, J. K. (1980). A practical approach to the risk of cancer in inflammatory bowel disease. *Med. Clins N. Am.* **64**, 1203.

Correa, P. and Haenszel, W. (1978). The epidemiology of large bowel cancer. *Adv. Cancer Res.* **26**, 1.

Earlham, R. and Cunha-Melo, J. R. (1980). Oesophageal squamous cell carcinoma. I. Review of surgery. II. Review of radiotherapy. **67**, 381, 457–61.

Kawai, K. (1978). Screening for gastric cancer in Japan. *Clins Gastroent.* **7**, 605.

Lipkin, M. and Good, R. A. (1978). *Gastrointestinal tract cancer.* Plenum, New York.

Moertel, C. G. (1976). Chemotherapy of gastrointestinal cancers. *Clins Gastroent.* **5**, 743.

Morson, B. C. and Dawson, I. M. P. (1979). *Gastrointestinal pathology.* Blackwell Scientific Publications, Oxford.

Panish, J. (1979). Management of patients with polypoid lesions of the colon—current concepts and controversies. *Am. J. Gastroent.* **71**, 315.

Schein, P. S. and Woolley, P. V. (1976). Colon carcinoma. *Semin. Oncol.* **3**, 329.

Seidman, H., Scherberg, E., and Holleb, A. I. (1976). Cancer statistics 1976. *Cancer* **26**, 14.

Sherlock, P., Lipkin, M., and Winawer, S. J. (1980). The prevention of colon cancer. *Am. J. Med.* **68**, 917.

Terz, J. J., and Beatty, J. D. (1979). Chemotherapy and cancer of the gastrointestinal tract. *Surg. Ann.* **11**, 149.

Winawer, S. J., Sherlock, P., Schottenfeld, D., and Miller, D. G. (1976). Screening for colon cancer. *Am. J. Gastroent.* **70**, 783.

Wright, R. (1980). *Recent advances in gastrointestinal pathology.* W. B. Saunders, Philadelphia.

Vascular and collagen disorders

G. Neale

Clinical disorders of the gastrointestinal tract caused by vascular and collagen diseases are rare in general medical practice. In this group of disorders the major syndromes are caused by intestinal ischaemia sufficient to cause cell death. This in turn gives rise to three major pathological pictures: (*a*) transient tissue damage with ulceration of the mucosa and an inflammatory response which resolves completely leaving structure and function unimpaired; (*b*) more severe damage causing structural changes in the submucosal tissues as well as to the mucosal cells followed by the development of strictures; and (*c*) necrosis of all layers of the wall of the intestine leading to perforation of the gut.

Gastroenterologists have become increasingly aware of the clinical correlates of these pathological processes but have made slow progress in developing methods for assessing the adequacy of blood flow to the intestine in human subjects. Thus the medical management of many of the conditions described in this section remains unsatisfactory; all too often a potentially life-threatening acute episode is the first indication of gastrointestinal involvement.

Ischaemic disease of the gut

Aetiology and pathogenesis. Ischaemic lesions may occur in the small or large intestine with or without evidence of gross vascular occlusion. The stomach is rarely affected. A list of causes is shown in Table 1.

Table 1   Causes of ischaemic disease of the gut

Atheromatous occlusion of arteries
Thrombosis of major vessels
Systemic emboli
Inflammation of blood vessels with secondary thrombosis
Miscellaneous lesions damaging or compressing the arterial tree
Diffuse microthrombosis
Non-occlusive intestinal infarction
Occlusion of large veins

Atheromatous occlusion of the major arteries is the commonest cause of mesenteric vascular insufficiency but the majority of cases remain undiagnosed in life probably because the slowness of the pathological process allows for the development of a compensatory collateral circulation. Intestinal infarction secondary to atheromatous occlusion of one major vessel is uncommon. Indeed, all three vessels may be occluded without visceral damage.

Thrombosis often develops on an ulcerated atheromatous plaque but may also occur as a result of such disorders as polycythaemia, sickle cell disease, cryoglobulinaemia, thrombotic thrombocytopenic purpura, and amyloidosis.

Systemic arterial embolism has accounted for up to one-third of cases of mesenteric vascular occlusion in some series. Emboli arise from the heart especially in patients with mitral stenosis and atrial fibrillation, with myocardial infarction and endocardial thrombosis, and with bacterial endocarditis. Paradoxical embolism through a patent foramen ovale and embolism from aortic mural thrombi are uncommon causes.

Systemic vasculitis associated with a number of conditions, particularly the 'collagen' disorders, may involve the stomach, small intestine, and colon. It may cause oedema, mucosal haemorrhages, focal ulceration, and focal necrosis with perforation. Occasionally the healing process leads to the development of intestinal strictures.

Primary gastrointestinal angiitis without systemic lesions has been described but in such cases one must take care to exclude conditions which may cause secondary inflammation of vessels such as inflammatory bowel disease, potassium-induced ulceration, and eosinophilic granuloma.

Granulomatous diseases, including Wegener's disease and lethal midline granuloma, may also cause angiitis of the gastrointestinal tract.

Irradiation of the abdomen leads to vascular necrosis and thrombosis which in turn may cause ischaemic ulceration and on healing leaves a fibrosed intima and a poorly perfused segment of intestine. This will be at special risk if mesenteric vascular disease subsequently develops.

Miscellaneous lesions. Many other conditions occasionally cause frank intestinal ischaemia. For example, blood vessels may be compressed, by retroperitoneal haematomata from leaking aneurysms and following trauma; by neoplastic infiltration; and rarely by proliferating fibrous tissue such as occurs in retroperitoneal fibrosis and very rarely around carcinoid tumours.

The walls of mesenteric arteries may be involved in fibro-elastic hyperplasia and in Takayasu's disease. In malignant hypertension intimal hyperplasia and fibrinoid necrosis of arteriolar walls may lead to patchy ischaemia of the intestine.

Damage to the arterial wall in the splanchnic circulation may also occur a few days after surgical correction of co-arctation of the aorta. There is necrotizing arteritis with fibrinoid necrosis most marked at arterial bifurcations, and similar changes may be seen in the small vessels of the liver, kidney, and spleen. These changes, which appear to be related to the sudden sustained increase in blood pressure, in most cases probably resolve spontaneously but may occasionally lead to intestinal infarction requiring operative intervention.

Diffuse microthrombosis may occur as a result of disseminated intravascular coagulation (as in the Shwartzman reaction) although this usually gives rise to the haemolytic-uraemic syndrome and only rarely causes intestinal damage.

Non-occlusive intestinal infarction. Sporadic and epidemic cases of necrotizing enteritis presumably due to ischaemia have been described from many parts of the world and in all age groups, from premature neonates to the very elderly.

The mechanisms remain poorly defined and in most cases microvascular occlusion cannot be demonstrated in the affected segment of gut although disseminated intravascular coagulation may occur as a result of bacterial endotoxins and the release of tissue thromboplastins from necrotic intestine.

In the Western world infarction of the gastrointestinal tract without vascular occlusion is seen mainly in the elderly with severe low-output cardiac failure and occasionally in the severely shocked. In tropical and subtropical areas the condition occurs at any age and may be related to environmental factors including diet, infection, and infestation.

Irrespective of the cause, necrosis of the intestinal mucosa is initiated by factors such as underperfusion, bacterial cytotoxins, and local hypersensitivity reactions which may be precipitated by intraluminal antigens such as migrating parasitic larvae. Invading bacteria may cause the necrotic areas to extend sometimes to the level of rapidly progressive gangrene. The β-toxin of *Clostridium welchii* type C is most frequently implicated in this process.

Venous occlusion. In experimental studies mesenteric venous occlusion has to be very extensive before there is obvious intestinal damage. In such cases there is haemorrhagic infarction with gross oedema and often it is impossible to decide whether the original lesion was on the arterial or venous side of the circulation. The colon appears to be at most risk.

Clinical syndromes. The clinical effects of mesenteric vascular insufficiency are becoming more clearly recognized. Four major syndromes have emerged in medical literature (unfortunately under a variety of titles): (*a*) acute intestinal ischaemia (affecting much of the intestine); (*b*) chronic intestinal ischaemia; (*c*) focal ischaemia of the small intestine; and (*d*) ischaemic colitis.

Acute intestinal ischaemia. Acute intestinal ischaemia is primarily a condition of older people, with degenerative cardiovascular disease. Occasionally it may cause an acute abdomen in the newborn infant. It correlates with necrosis, threatened or complete, of that part of the gut supplied by the superior mesenteric artery.

Clinical features. The onset of the condition is usually abrupt but may be insidious. Often the patient is already under treatment in hospital for an associated condition. Abdominal pain is the key symptom and at the onset is generally colicky in nature and poorly localized. As the condition progresses the pain becomes constant and unremitting. Initially it is felt in the right iliac fossa and then spreads over the entire abdomen. Diarrhoea is usual and frequently the motions contain blood. Vomiting occurs in some cases but haematemesis is rare.

In the early stages of illness the distress of the patient is out of all proportion to the physical signs. There may be slight tenderness in the right iliac fossa and some exaggeration of bowel sounds. As the condition develops over the course of hours (or at the most a day or two) the abdomen becomes distended and silent with increasing tenderness and a positive rebound sign. At the same time there are usually signs of peripheral circulatory failure. The patient is pale, anxious, sweating, and tachypnoeic. Later the blood pressure falls, the patient becomes cyanosed and anuric. At this stage intestinal necrosis has almost certainly gone beyond the point of recovery.

The diagnosis may be suspected on the basis of clinical correlations but is often difficult and delayed. It may depend on the efficiency with which other causes of abdominal catastrophe can be excluded. Needling the peritoneal cavity usually produces blood-stained fluid.

Straight X-rays of the abdomen may show non-specific dilatation of loops of intestine with multiple fluid levels. The presence of gas bubbles in the portal vein is diagnostic of intestinal necrosis at a stage when the patient is beyond recovery. The place of aortography is not yet clearly defined.

Management. In the management of this condition the clinician has to combat the effects of: (*a*) loss of water, electrolytes and protein leading to hypovolaemia and impaired tissue perfusion; (*b*) bacterial invasion; and (*c*) disseminated intravascular coagulation. The value of pharmacological agents such as phenoxybenzamine, glucagon, or dopamine to improve the mesenteric circulation remains uncertain. Similarly there is not clear evidence regarding the potential beneficial effect of large doses of corticosteroids.

As soon as the patient is sufficiently fit laparotomy must be performed. If a large vessel is occluded, the surgeon may be able to undertake embolectomy or reconstruct an occluded artery. In both occlusive and non-occlusive vascular disease it is necessary to decide how much intestine to resect. If there is doubt regarding the viability of the residual intestine, the abdomen may be closed and 24 hours later, re-explored. Infiltrating the coeliac and mesenteric plexuses with local anaesthetic may help relieve vascular spasm.

The mortality of patients with acute intestinal ischaemia causing necrosis is high. Those who do recover may present major problems in the management of their nutrition.

Chronic intestinal ischaemia. All too often warning symptoms of impending mesenteric vascular occlusion go unnoticed or undiagnosed. The prodromal period is usually short but the history of a quite characteristic abdominal pain occurring shortly after eating may raise the possibility of chronic intestinal ischaemia. Unfortunately in the absence of any test to show functionally significant intestinal ischaemia the diagnosis often remains uncertain. Atheroma of the visceral arteries commonly involves the coeliac axis and superior mesenteric artery. The inferior mesenteric artery is affected to a much lesser extent. Stenotic lesions occur at the aortic origins of the vessels. Diffuse severe atheroma throughout the intestinal arterial tree is uncommon and therefore arterial reconstruction may be very rewarding.

Clinical features. Classically the patient suffers cramping abdominal pain 20–60 minutes after eating. This may be relieved by simple analgesics or by vasodilator drugs. As the condition progresses the patient becomes afraid to eat and loses weight.

The finding of a loud systolic bruit on auscultation of the abdomen is a doubtfully valid physical sign. Bruits may be detected in normal subjects, young as well as old, and may be absent in patients with severe visceral arterial disease.

In practice the diagnosis is made by excluding the conditions which cause obscure abdominal pain and weight loss. It depends on the correlation of clinical symptoms with angiographic findings. Standard tests of intestinal function are usually normal and are not helpful in assessing intestinal blood flow.

The descriptions of methods for the correction of arterial abnormalities leave one more impressed by the degree of surgical enthusiasm and ingenuity than by the standard of care in evaluating the results. The subject is well reviewed by Marston (1977).

Coeliac axis compression. In occasional patients with chronic abdominal pain and an abdominal bruit (which may be exacerbated by inspiration) aortography shows apparent constriction of the coeliac axis by the median arcuate ligament. It has been claimed that the arteries in the territory of the coeliac axis 'steal' blood from that of the superior mesenteric artery thereby causing intestinal angina which may be relieved by dividing the median arcuate ligament and possibly by reconstructing the coeliac axis.

Unfortunately, symptomless coeliac axis compression has been demonstrated frequently and some symptomatic patients are not helped by operation. Although patients claim to have been cured by coeliac axis surgery the validity of the syndrome remains uncertain.

Focal ischaemia of the small intestine. Ischaemia of a segment of small intestine may cause local ulceration which on healing leads to stenosis. This may occur as a result of any of the vascular disorders already described as causing diffuse, acute intestinal ischaemia whether these be thrombotic, embolic, or non-occlusive.

More specific entities include ischaemic damage caused by a *strangulated hernia*, by an episode of *blunt trauma to the abdomen*, by irradiation, and rarely by localized vasculitis secondary to infective disease (e.g. typhoid or leprosy) or collagen-vascular disorders (e.g. polyarteritis).

Drug-induced ulceration is an important entity, of which that associated with the ingestion of potassium salts is the most clearly defined. It has been shown that a high concentration of potassium in the lumen of the intestine causes venous spasm and subsequently local arterial thrombosis. This may lead to ulceration and fibrosis of a segment of intestine especially if there is preexisting large vessel disease.

Clinical features. The patient presents with features of subacute obstruction of the small intestine. Colicky abdominal pain occurs two to three hours after meals associated with nausea, abdominal distension, and occasional vomiting. The stricture is located by radiological examination of the small intestine and the obstruction needs to be relieved by operation.

Ischaemic colitis. The colon has distinctive features which makes it more prone to ischaemic damage than the small intestine. The transverse and descending segments of the colon are supplied by marginal branches of the middle colic (superior mesenteric artery) and left colic (inferior mesenteric artery) arteries. An arterial and lymphatic watershed exists close to the splenic flexure which is supported to a variable extent by an additional vascular arcade. A deficient marginal artery or an absent anastomotic arcade may imperil the blood supply of the splenic flexure in occlusive disease of either mesenteric artery.

If the blood supply fails, damage to the large intestine may be more rapid and more severe than that occurring in the small intestine because of the effects of the high concentration of bacteria in the faecal stream.

Again blood flow to the colon may be impaired by any of the mechanisms described previously. In addition, colonic obstruction may reduce blood flow by increasing the intraluminal pressure. Thus the pathological changes of ischaemic colitis may occur in the segment of intestine immediately proximal to an obstructing carcinoma (stercoral ulceration) or in association with prolapse or volvulus of the colon.

Venous occlusion is also a possible cause of ischaemic colitis. Inevitably the contraceptive pill has been incriminated as a cause but the condition has been described in young men as well as in young women. The evidence regarding the pill remains suggestive rather than conclusive.

Clinical features. In the acute phase of ischaemic colitis the clinician has to differentiate between mild disease which responds quickly and effectively to supportive measures and treatment with appropriate antibiotics; and severe disease in which gangrene may develop. Most patients are between the ages of 50 and 70 years and often have a background history of atheromatous arterial disease, collagen disorder, or local colon pathology. Typically the affected person complains of pain in the left iliac fossa, nausea, and vomiting followed by the passage of a loose motion containing dark blood.

Marked tenderness in the left iliac fossa is the most constant physical sign. At colonoscopy the mucosa may be blue and swollen with contact bleeding. The rectum is invariably spared. Straight X-ray of the abdomen may show an abnormal segment of large intestine outlined with gas. Angiography may be helpful in showing occlusive arterial disease. More often than not it is unhelpful.

Contrast enema examination of the colon is a most useful way of demonstrating ischaemic damage. In the early phase 'thumb-printing' is the characteristic sign which may persist for several days (Fig. 1). Subsequently the mucosal appearances may return to normal or progress to the next phase of mucosal ulceration giving an appearance which may be indistinguishable from segmental ulcerative colitis or Crohn's disease although the haustral pattern is usually not seriously disrupted and the ulcers are patchy and do not penetrate deeply.

Again these changes may resolve spontaneously or progress to tubular narrowing of the intestine with or without sacculation on the anti-mesenteric border.

Ischaemic colitis may be confused with dysenteric conditions, acute diverticular disease of the colon, acute inflammatory bowel disease, perforation of a hollow viscus, or left-sided peritonitis secondary to pancreatitis. The most important distinguishing features are the characteristic age range, the association with degenerative cardiovascular disease, and the distinctive radiological and colonoscopic appearances.

Management. On establishing the diagnosis of ischaemic colitis the treatment is initially expectant. The patient is observed in hospital, given intravenous fluid as necessary together with systemic broad-spectrum antibiotics (on the basis of experimental rather than clinical evidence).

Well over 90 per cent of recognized cases resolve spontaneously.

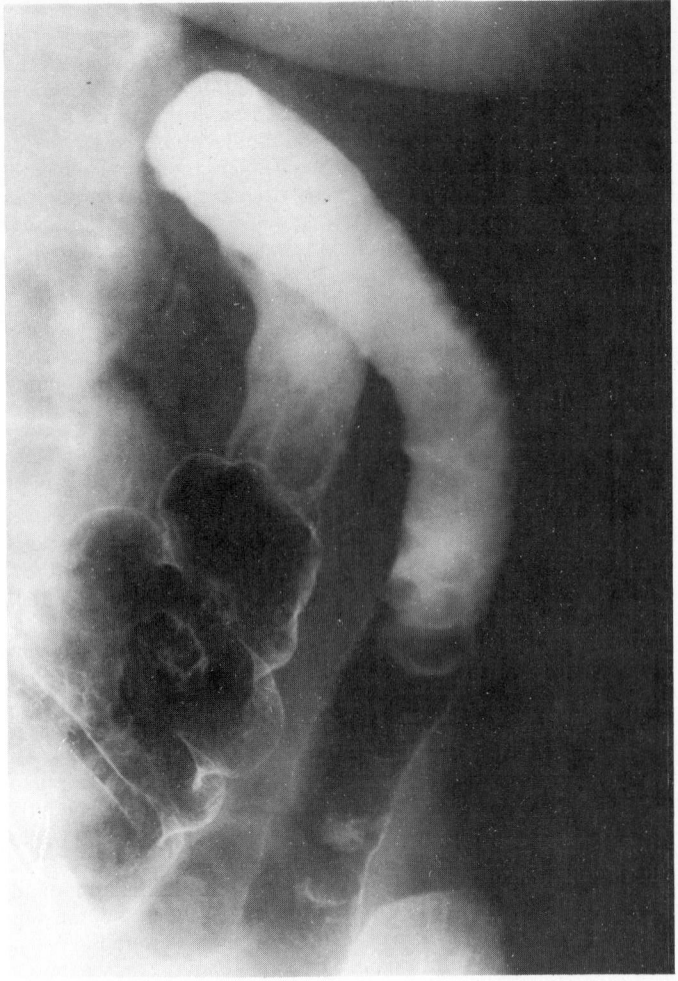

Fig. 1 Ischaemic colitis: barium enema showing thumb-printing at the splenic flexure. (Courtesy of Dr A. Freeman, Addenbrooke's Hospital).

A stricture may develop in up to a third of patients but this is usually asymptomatic and only rarely needs to be resected.

Surgery is indicated if there is evidence of peritonitis (gangrene of the colon), persistent bleeding, or evidence of an underlying colonic disorder (such as carcinoma).

Vascular malformations in the gut

Haemangiomata. Haemangiomata are uncommon lesions of the gut which may cause painless bleeding especially from the jejunum.

Intestinal telangiectasia. These lesions occur most commonly with Osler–Weber–Rendu disease (see Sections 19 and 20) and may lead to microscopic bleeding with anaemia especially in adult life.

Vascular dysplasia. This is a more recently recognized and not uncommon disorder causing occult bleeding from the gut in older subjects. The lesions occur as small arteriovenous malformations or as foci of ectatic capillaries or veins with little supporting stroma predominantly in the caecum and ascending colon. There may be an association with aortic stenosis but none with cutaneous telangiectases and no family aggregations are yet described.

Patients give a history of recurrent anaemia or episodes of bleeding from the gut; usually have been investigated repeatedly without getting a firm diagnosis; and sometimes have had one or more operations, including resection of a segment of the gastrointestinal tract, without relief of symptoms. The diagnosis of vascular dysplasia should be considered in all cases of obscure gastrointestinal haemorrhage and may be made by direct visualization of the colonic mucosa (Fig. 2) or by selective mesenteric arteriography (Fig. 3). The lesions may be multiple in which case resection of the affected segment of gut may be necessary. Most cases however can be treated successfully by fulguration of the lesion through a colonoscope.

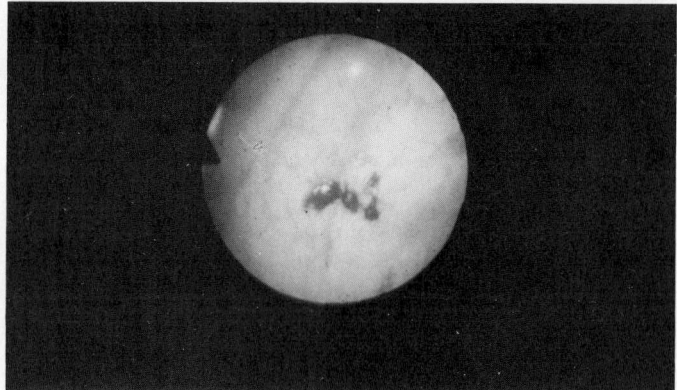

Fig. 2   Angiodysplastic lesion in the caecum, photographed through a colonoscope. (Courtesy of Dr R. Hunt, R. N. Hospital, Haslar).

Superior mesenteric artery syndrome. A syndrome of postprandial epigastric pain, distention and vomiting may occur in asthenic young people especially those who have lost weight or who are fixed in a position of hyperextension after spinal injury.

Barium studies show a distended proximal duodenum with a sharp cut off at the line where the superior mesenteric artery crosses the duodenum. Symptoms may be relieved if the patient adopts the prone position after meals and may disappear as the patient gains weight. Occasionally surgery is necessary.

The condition must be distinguished from duodenal ileus caused by bands associated with partial malrotation of the mid-gut.

Collagen disorders

The gut is frequently involved in the systemic collagen disorders. Vasculitis is a major feature in all such conditions. This may lead to focal ischaemic damage of the intestine and any of the syndromes described previously. In addition the visceral muscle may be involved and this may cause dysphagia, delayed gastric emptying, small intestinal stasis with bacterial overgrowth, and colonic inertia. Gas may infiltrate the tissues giving rise to pneumatosis intestinalis.

The specific pathological diagnosis is usually based on the systemic features of the illness and the laboratory findings rather than on the mostly non-specific abdominal complications. But the inquisitive physician may also recognize curious associations in patients with multi-system disorders. Thus intestinal malabsorption and protein-losing enteropathy have been described in association with systemic lupus erythematosus and rheumatoid arthritis, pancreatic insufficiency with systemic sclerosis, acute pancreatitis during the course of Behçet's disease, and apparently classical inflammatory bowel disease with systemic lupus erythematosus.

Thus it is difficult to provide clear cut clinical descriptions of typical disorders of the gut in this group of conditions.

Systemic sclerosis

Pathology. In primary systemic sclerosis (see Section 16) fibrous connective tissue proliferates. In the gastrointestinal tract it may replace smooth muscle, especially in the oesophagus (involved in 80 per cent of cases), to a lesser extent, in the small intestine (although duodenal involvement is quite common), and rather rarely in the colon.

Overt vasculitis is a less common feature but occasionally causes intestinal infarction. Pneumatosis cystoides intestinalis is also described especially in association with intestinal pseudo-obstruction or pneumoperitoneum.

Symptoms. Difficulty in eating may be caused by induration of the gums, by restriction of the size of the oral cavity as a result of subcutaneous fibrosis, and in advanced cases by impaired sensation because of atrophy of the buccal mucosa and taste buds.

Progressive dysphagia is the most frequent gastrointestinal symptom in systemic sclerosis. Initially there is a decrease in the incidence and amplitude of contractions of the lower oesophagus and incomplete relaxation of the lower oesophageal sphincter. In addition, the resting tone of the sphincter is reduced allowing reflux of gastric juices, oesophagitis, shortening of the oesophagus, and occasionally stricture formation. Associated hiatal herniation is common.

Malnutrition due to difficulty in eating and swallowing is not uncommon in patients with systemic sclerosis.

Rarely the stomach is also involved causing delayed emptying which on occasion is exacerbated by associated stenosis of the pyloric canal. Changes lower down the gastrointestinal tract are readily found when looked for. Characteristically the duodenum is dilated, the valvulae of the small intestine are thickened, and pseudodiverticulae may form. These changes may give rise to ab-

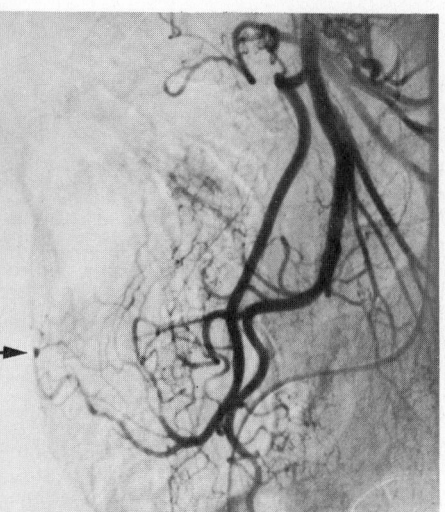 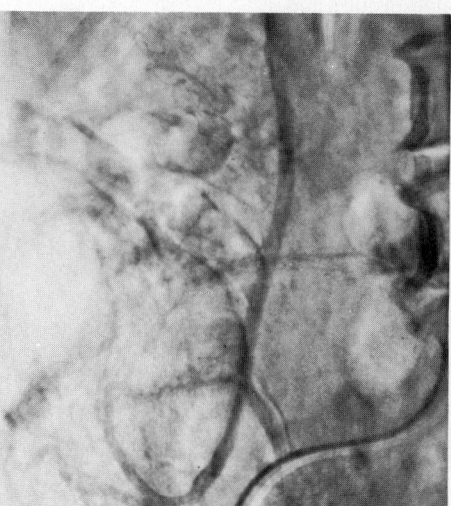 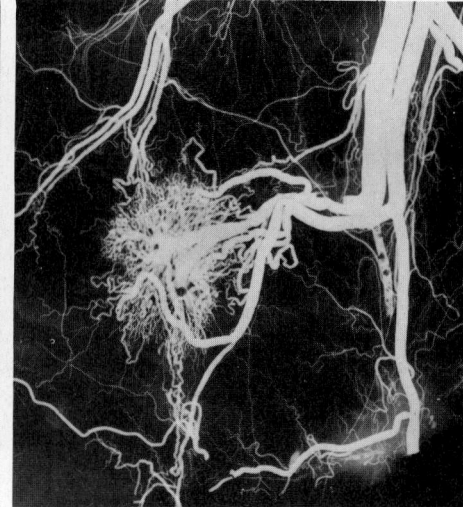

Fig. 3   Angiodysplastic lesion in the caecum: Superior mesenteric angiogram in a 53 year old man with anaemia for 20 years (no lesion found at two previous operations). (a) Vascular lake in caecum (arrowed). (b) Capillary phase, showing early-filling vein arising from lesion. (c) Injected specimen (magnified ×30). (Courtesy of Dr D. J. Allison, Royal Postgraduate Medical School and reprinted with permission of the Editor of the *British Journal of Hospital Medicine*).

dominal discomfort, distention, and borborygmi, especially after the taking of meals. The impaired motility of the small intestine leads to stasis of its contents and bacterial overgrowth causing malabsorption, especially of fat and vitamin B_{12} (see pages 12.89 and 12.100). Occasionally this is sufficiently severe to cause acute or chronic pseudo-obstruction with persistent abdominal distention and vomiting.

Colonic involvement is rare. Clinically, there is progressive constipation sometimes going on to large bowel obstruction secondary to impaction of faeces. Radiologically there is a loss of the normal haustral pattern, the development of wide-necked pseudodiverticuli on the antimesenteric border of the transverse and descending colon and generalized dilatation of the lumen. On examination with a colonoscope one sees a rigid large intestine with a pale mucosa but this examination should not be undertaken lightly because of the danger of precipitating pneumatosis.

If the internal sphincter (smooth muscle) of the rectum is involved, it will not relax normally with rectal distention. This will exacerbate the already troublesome constipation. A significant reduction of intestinal secretions (gastric, biliary, and pancreatic) appears to occur in perhaps one-third of patients with primary systemic sclerosis but rarely, if ever, is this severe enough to cause malabsorption.

Management. There is no specific treatment for primary systemic sclerosis. Lesions in the gastrointestinal tract need management on their merits. It is important to recognize early the patient with gastro-oesophageal reflux. Antacids should be used to try to prevent the ravages of acid-peptic digestion of the oesophageal mucosa, and cimetidine given to reduce the secretion of acid. The patient may need dietary advice regarding the make-up of meals which can be taken with minimal discomfort and yet will maintain a good nutritional state. Repeated oesophagoscopy is the best way of documenting the progress of disease, and when strictures occur these should be dilated by bouginage. If a stricture becomes fixed and unyielding, surgical intervention may be necessary. It is important to remember that cardiopulmonary complications significantly increase the operative risks and prolonged postoperative ileus is not unusual following abdominal surgery on a patient with systemic sclerosis affecting the intestine.

The bile salt breath test (see page 12.94) is a useful screening test for delayed passage of contents and bacterial proliferation in the small intestine. To obtain a valid result it may be necessary to instil the bile salt solution directly into the duodenum to overcome the problem of concomitant gastric stasis. Patients with a positive breath test should be assessed for evidence of malabsorption and, if this is found, intermittent therapy with antibiotics for an indefinite period may be of clinical value.

Patients with severe colonic disease are often difficult to manage. Efforts should be made to avoid the development of severe constipation. A combination of a high roughage diet and aperients as necessary are usually sufficient but occasionally it may be necessary to resort to the repeated use of enemas.

Systemic lupus erythematosus. Systemic lupus erythematosus (SLE) (see Section 16) frequently causes abdominal symptoms which may arise from any part of the gastrointestinal tract. Anorexia, weight loss, nausea, vomiting, and diarrhoea are relatively common. Dysphagia, abdominal pain, distention due to ascites, and gastrointestinal bleeding are less frequent symptoms. Occasionally, a patient with SLE develops an acute abdomen which may be due to localized or widespread lupus vasculitis causing ischaemic damage to the gut or its related organs including the gall bladder and pancreas.

Diagnosis. The diagnosis of SLE is usually made from the general pattern of disease with associated laboratory evidence. Presentation with abdominal symptomatology is rare and in such cases diagnosis is usually delayed. Radiological examination of the intestine may show mucosal ulceration and thickening of the folds. If arteriography is performed to identify an obscure cause of gastrointestinal bleeding, one may see diffuse irregularities of the branches of the mesenteric vessels.

Treatment. Treatment with oral corticosteroids usually relieves minor abdominal symptoms and will lead to rapid resolution of simple ascites. In the acute stage of the disease, however, surgery may be necessary to deal with infarcted intestine, serious bleeding or intestinal obstruction.

Rheumatoid arthritis. Vasculitis secondary to rheumatoid arthritis is associated with long-standing disease, seropositivity, and florid subcutaneous nodule formation. It may affect small arteries, arterioles, capillaries, and venules, and often causes little in the way of symptoms. Occasionally, a severe diffuse and necrotizing angiitis causes infarction in the gall bladder, pancreas, or intestine.

Symptoms vary from vague abdominal pain with or without diarrhoea to the development of an acute abdomen. Malnutrition is present in many such patients and for the most part is due to a decreased intake of nutrients rather than malabsorption although this has been described in association with rheumatoid arthritis.

Treatment will depend on the severity of the lesion and is discussed in Section 16.

Dermatomyositis. This inflammatory disease (Section 16) of muscle and skin only rarely causes damage to the viscera. Thrombosis of small vessels occasionally causes gastrointestinal ulceration.

Behçet's syndrome. The trial of relapsing iritis, painful ulcers of the mouth and genital ulceration is only a segment of the manifestations of this multi-system disorder (see page 12.33 and Section 20). Again vasculitis appears to be the underlying histopathological lesion. In the gastrointestinal tract this may lead to ulceration of colon, malabsorption (sometimes with lymphangiectasia), and pancreatitis.

Primary vasculitis

Henoch–Schönlein or anaphylactoid purpura. This is a self-limited disorder of unknown cause causing small-vessel vasculitis (see Section 19). Gastrointestinal involvement occurs in at least two-thirds of cases and is manifest as abdominal pain or gastrointestinal bleeding. Intramural haematomata are common and rarely may be complicated by intussusception, gross infarction, or perforation.

Polyarteritis nodosa. Abdominal pain and other gastro-intestinal symptoms are common in patients with polyarteritis nodosa (see Section 16). The underlying cause is usually recognised by evidence of systemic disease such as skin lesions, renal involvement, hypertension, and eosinophilia. Mesenteric angiography is useful as a diagnostic tool because up to two-thirds of cases have recognizable micro-aneurysms of mesenteric and renal vessels. A small proportion of patients with polyarteritis have acute abdominal episodes including ulceration, haemorrhage, perforation, and segmental necrosis of intestine; cholecystitis, pancreatitis, and hepatic infarction. *Kohlmeier–Degos* syndrome is a variant of polyarteritis characterized by a papular skin eruption and occlusive lesions of small arteries.

References

Arseculeratna, S. N., Panabokke, R. G., and Navaratnam, C. (1980). Pathogenesis of necrotizing arteritis with special reference to intestinal hypersensitivity reactions. *Gut* **21**, 265.

Lancrault, G. and Jacobson, E. D. (1976). The gastrointestinal circulation. *Gastroent.* **71**, 851.

Marston, A. (1977). *Intestinal ischaemia*. Arnold, London.

Tarin, D., Allison, D. J., Modlin, I. M., and Neale, G. (1978). Diagnosis and management of obscure gastrointestinal bleeding. *Br. med. J.* **iii**, 751.

Infections of the gastrointestinal tract

A. M. Tomkins

Introduction. Diarrhoea is still a major public health and clinical problem especially in developing countries where it frequently causes death and precipitates malnutrition. It has been estimated that there are 500 million episodes in children each year in Africa, Asia, and Latin America resulting in 5–18 million deaths. Diarrhoea also kills adults, but in millions more the chronic ill health from dysentery, intestinal parasites, and malabsorption syndromes is considerable.

Infective diarrhoea of adults in the United Kingdom is usually the problem of the international traveller, whether businessman or holidaymaker, and in most cases the disease is mild. However, an important number of patients are very ill and some even die. Tragically, a significant proportion of these are undiagnosed because the various pathogens are not sufficently considered. The continuing mortality from amoebiasis in the United Kingdom is just one example.

In the last decade there have been considerable advances in knowledge of the physiology of different diarrhoea syndromes. This has been particularly helpful in explaining the mechanisms of fluid and electrolyte secretion in watery diarrhoea due to enterotoxins such as those produced by *Escherichia coli*. Several treatment regimens have been developed which simply and successfully restore fluid and electrolyte balance even in severe diarrhoea. In previous years many cases of diarrhoea were diagnosed as nonspecific, meaning that classical pathogens such as shigella, salmonella, or certain serotypes of *E. coli* could not be isolated. Several techniques have been developed by microbiologists in recent years which make it possible to identify more of the great variety of enteropathogens that are responsible for diarrhoea.

It is also recognized that many diarrhoeas are self-limiting (i.e. caused by enteropathogens that colonize the intestine for short periods only). Several practical features arise from drug trials in infective diarrhoea. Firstly, that in many cases of diarrhoea those who receive antibiotics do not recover faster than those taking placebo. Secondly, that excretion of the pathogen may actually be prolonged by the administration of antibiotics. Thirdly, there is a disturbing national and international trend for the emergence of enteropathogens with multiple antibiotic resistance patterns. The net effect is that contempory treatment regimens for diarrhoeal disease contain fewer antibiotics than those that were written in previous years. However, there are still clear indications for antibiotics in many specific diarrhoeal syndromes.

This chapter will describe the pathophysiology and clinical features of different infective diarrhoea syndromes and examine the way in which the clinician may suggest appropriate clinical and microbiological investigations for accurate diagnosis. We shall then discuss appropriate treatment regimens. The microbiology of the various organisms discussed here will be found in the appropriate parts of Section 5.

Factors favouring colonization by enteropathogens

Although some of these factors have been referred to in Section 5, there are specific features which are important in diarrhoea. These are either (*a*) host factors or (*b*) enteropathogen factors.

Host factors. The intestinal microflora which is established during infancy and early childhood remains relatively stable during adulthood. This stability is controlled by several complex interdependent protective mechanisms, breakdown of which facilitates colonization.

Gastric juice. Most intestinal bacteria are inhibited by H^+ ions, and conversely, patients with hypochlorhydria are more susceptible to salmonellosis. The administration of sodium bicarbonate to volunteers receiving doses of *E. coli* lowers the critical number of organisms required to produce diarrhoea. Those American volunteer workers in Bangladesh who regularly consumed marijuana, which is known to decrease gastric acidity, had an increased incidence of diarrhoea. There is gastric atrophy and impaired acid secretion in protein energy malnutrition in children and in chronic tropical sprue in Indian adults. Hypochlorhydia may be an important factor in the bacterial colonization which is characteristic of both these syndromes. It is of interest that the bacterial colonization of the upper intestine in hypogammaglobulinaemic adults in the United Kingdom may be due to the associated hypochlorhydria rather than the immunological defect.

Motility. Alterations in peristalsis as a result of various drugs (e.g. ganglion blockers) is associated with increased bacterial numbers in the upper intestine. This is dangerously true for lomotil which may encourage the incubation of large numbers of toxin-producing enteropathogens within the intestine.

Resident microflora. Soon after birth the intestine becomes colonized by a variety of organisms. The pattern of the microflora is markedly influenced by the type of feeding; that of bottle-fed babies is quite different from that in breast-fed babies. The latter are characteristically colonized by large numbers of *Bifidobacteria* with low numbers of *E. coli* and tend to have a lower faecal pH than bottle-fed babies. *In vitro* studies on the bacteriostatic activity of faeces from babies shows it to be particularly active at low pH. It is likely that the low pH of the gut in the breast-fed baby also facilitates production of metabolites that are toxic to certain enteropathogens. Volatile fatty acids, excreted in greater quantities by breast-fed than bottle-fed babies are inhibitors of *Shigella* spp. for example. Bile acids also have potent *in vitro* activity against *Shigella* spp. They are excreted in greater concentrations by adults who eat a western diet which is high in protein and animal fat compared with adults in developing countries who typically eat less protein and animal fat. However, in view of the extreme differences in environment it is not clear whether the bile acid concentrations in the colon are protective against dysentery in real life.

Immunity. There is a highly developed series of humoral and cell-mediated reactions in the intestine. In general these contribute to: (*a*) the resistance to colonization by enteropathogens; (*b*) the clearance of pathogens; and may (*c*) be involved in the processes whereby mucosal damage occurs. An example of (*a*) is the resistance to colonization by polio virus which is determined by IgA antibody secreted into the intestine. An example of (*b*) is the delayed clearance of intestinal nematodes after experimental infection in immunologically deprived animals. An example of (*c*) is the failure of such animals to produce an inflammatory infiltration in response to the intestinal nematode, the inference being that the mucosal lesions during intestinal parasitism may be, in part, the result of toxic products of T cells which are active against the nematode.

A proportion of asymptomatic residents in the contaminated environments common in developing countries excrete pathogens such as *Campylobacter*, enterotoxin-producing *E. coli*, *Shigella* spp., and *Giardia Lamblia*, but when visitors from cleaner environments become colonized, they usually develop diarrhoea. The immune mechanisms involved in the carrier state are largely undefined although circulating antibodies to heat labile (LT) enterotoxin have been demonstrated in American visitors to Kenya who developed acute watery diarrhoea. Circulating antibodies to giardia cyst antigen and enterobacteria are demonstrable in patients with severe giardiasis (associated malabsorption) but are not usually found in mild giardiasis (mild mucosal lesions without malabsorption). Agglutinating antibody is present in the duodenal fluid and serum of some infants with enteropathogenic *E. coli* gastroenteritis. Early in the infection the antibodies are mainly of the IgM class; later they are predominantly IgA. Increased quantities of IgM are detected in the intestinal mucosa from infants with acute diarrhoea and in adults with post-infective malabsorption. Although these and other antibodies cross react with a wide range of enterobacteria, it is not clear whether this is sufficient to protect against subsequent infection by similar organisms.

Infection with intestinal viruses is associated with development of circulating antibodies but subsequent rotavirus infections in the same individual are common. It is now recognized that there are several different antigenic types or rotavirus; exposure to one may not confer immunity against others. Host variability appears to be important in Norwalk agent diarrhoea. Some of the adult volunteers infected with Norwalk agent developed long-term immunity for repeated experimental infection while others had only brief protection. A further, interesting group of volunteers who failed to develop any demonstrable immunity on laboratory testing also failed to develop the disease after repeated inoculation. Absence of appropriate virus receptor sites on the enterocytes has been suggested.

Perhaps the greatest disappointment in bacterial immunology has been the failure to develop efficient vaccines against diarrhoeal disease. The failure of currently available cholera vaccine to protect against the development of cholera in several epidemiological studies despite the development of circulating antibody emphasizes that it is gut immunity rather than systemic immunity that matters. However, new methods are under development and efficient vaccines against rotavirus and LT and heat stable (ST) producing *E. coli* may become available in the future.

Breast milk. Many constituents of breast milk have potent antibacterial activity. Significant quantities of IgA are secreted in breast milk and the levels are highest in the colostrum from women in developing countries, suggesting that colostral IgA may be primed by maternal infection. Iron binding proteins including lactoferrin and transferrin, normally in the unsaturated state, are found in human milk. A combination of these and antibodies have powerful bacteriostatic activity towards *E. coli in vitro*. It is interesting that in both the United Kingdom and developing communities there is considerable variation in *in vitro* bacteriostatic activity of breast milk between mothers in the same community. A heat labile antiviral factor has been demonstrated recently; it appears to be different from interferon.

Enteropathogen factors. The concept that 'stickiness' of an enteropathogen is an important part in the development of diarrhoea has been introduced in recent years following the demonstration of specific adhesion factors on the *E. coli* that cause porcine diarrhoea. In these the adhesion (K-88) antigen, which is plasmid-mediated and can therefore be removed, must be present for the organism to colonize and produce diarrhoea by secretion of a potent enterotoxin. Inoculation of enterotoxin positive *E. coli* which were K-88 negative did not result in diarrhoea.

A comparable phenomenon was observed in adults with diarrhoea due to enterotoxin producing *E. coli* in Bangladesh and Mexico; *in vitro* tests showed adhesion to rabbit intestine. Some strains of *E. coli* isolated from diarrhoea in children in the United Kingdom adhere to fetal human intestine *in vitro*. The plasmid which possessed this adhesion property has been identified. However, several other studies have failed to show consistent colonization factors in *E. coli* that cause diarrhoea. Nevertheless, in acute diarrhoea and in infective malabsorption syndromes in adults, there are considerable numbers of organisms that lie in the mucus adjacent to the enterocytes. Their ability to stay appears to be an

important, but unexplained, determinant of their ability to multiply and induce fluid and electrolyte secretion and damage the structure of the intestinal mucosa.

A further unexplained variable is the number of infective organisms that are required to produce diarrhoea, 10^8–10^{10} *E. coli* are usually given to produce watery diarrhoea in volunteers; any less does not produce disease. By contrast an inoculum of only 10–200 shigella bacteria will produce severe dysentery.

Pathogenesis of acute infective diarrhoea

In health there is a remarkably efficient absorption of the 6–8 litres of fluid which enter the intestine every day so that only 100–200 ml is excreted in the faeces of a subject on a western diet and perhaps 500 ml in adults on a high-fibre diet. Similarly, of the 1000 mmol of sodium and the 100 mmol of potassium that enter the intestine every day, only 5 mmol and 10 mmol respectively leave it. Most of the absorption occurs in the small intestine. Each villus is covered by enterocytes which originate as cuboidal cells in the crypts (Fig. 1). These immature cells have not yet developed microvilli and therefore possess virtually no brush border enzymes. As they migrate up the villus, taking 48–72 hours to reach the villus tip, they become columnar and acquire microvilli and brush border enzymes. In general the crypt cells are secretory cells and the villus tip cells are absorptive cells. In the intact villus the absorptive cells predominate and there is net absorption of fluid and electrolytes. Although most of the absorption of fluid and electrolytes takes place in the jejunum and ileum, the colonic mucosa also has an important role. Figure 1 shows the various ways in which enteropathogens may disturb the normal physiology to produce diarrhoea.

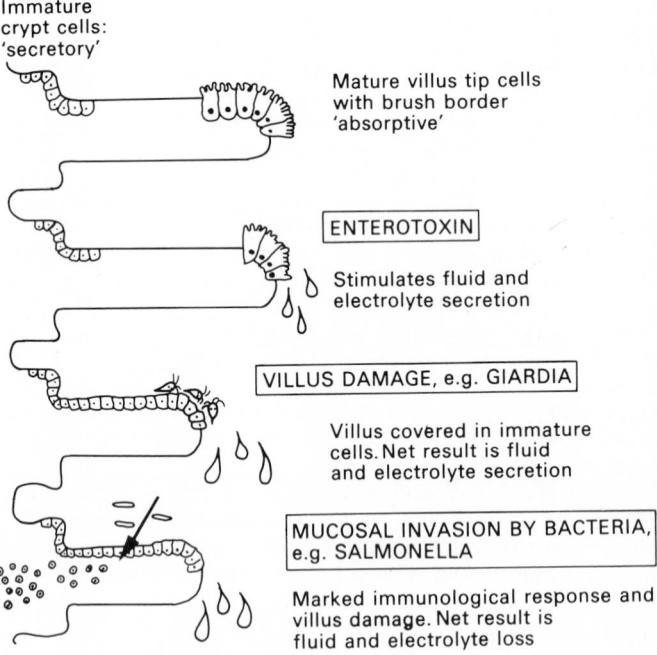

Fig. 1   Pathogenesis of acute infective diarrhoea.

Enterotoxin production. Several species of bacteria produce toxins which stimulate secretion from the enterocytes. The most classic example is cholera toxin produced by *Vibrio cholerae* but certain strains of *E. coli* and *Shigella dysenteriae* type 1 also produce potent enterotoxins. They act in a stepwise manner: (*a*) they bind to the cell membrane of the enterocyte; (*b*) they penetrate the cell and increase the intracellular concentration of adenylate cyclase; and (*c*) this in turn increases the concentration of the cyclic nucleotides, (either cGMP or cAMP) which control the flux of fluid and electrolytes across the enterocyte membrane. This is achieved by chemical means alone; jejunal biopsy appearances in patients with these infections are usually normal.

The original studies showed that when *V. cholerae* organisms were introduced into isolated loops of rabbit ileum there was marked fluid secretion and distension of the gut. Later, bacteria-free supernatents of cultures of *V. cholerae* were shown to produce the same effect. This has also been demonstrated for strains of *E. coli* that cause watery diarrhoea by the production of an entero-toxin. *E. coli* may produce two enterotoxins; one is heat stable (ST) and the other is heat labile (LT). Because of the large numbers of animals required for the rabbit ileal loop assay, alternative methods for detection of enterotoxin have been developed.

Tissue culture. When certain cell lines such as VERO, CHO, and YI adrenal cells are inoculated with bacteria-free filtrates of organisms that produce enterotoxin, these cells develop characteristic cytopathic changes. LT enterotoxin from *E. coli* may be detected in this way. ST has no effect.

Immunological methods. The enterotoxin of *V. cholerae* and the LT enterotoxin of *E. coli* are large molecular weight (100 000) proteins and may be detected using antisea. It is now possible to use the ELISA technique for this assay.

Weanling mouse assay. The ST enterotoxin of *E. coli* is of low molecular weight (5000) and immunological methods for detection are not yet satisfactory. It may be detected by measuring the weight of intestine plus fluid secretion/weight of carcass, after injection of a bacteria-free filtrate. Several other groups of bacteria produce enterotoxins but knowledge of their structure and function is less developed. The important food poisoning group includes *Staphylococcus aureus*, *Clostridium perfringens*, *Vibrio parahaemolyticus*, and *Bacillus cereus*. In some cases the enterotoxin is swallowed in food; in others it may develop within the intestine. This explains why the severe watery diarrhoea in some food poisoning may develop at various times after eating bad food.

Although *Shigella* spp. is classically a causal pathogen of bacillary dysentery, it is now recognized that some strains also produce an enterotoxin with potent activity on the mucosa of the small intestine. Enterotoxin-producing strains of *Sh. dysenteriae* type 1, *Sh. flexneri*, and *Sh. sonnei* must first penetrate the mucosa of the large intestine; the enterotoxin then circulates in the blood to the entero-cytes of the small intestine. This explains why some attacks of dysentery (blood and mucus) are complicated by a stage of severe watery diarrhoea.

The diarrhoea of *Salmonella* spp. is classically caused by mucosal invasion and infiltration of the lymphoid tissue in the ileum but certain strains (*S. typhimurium* and *S. enteritidis*) also produce enterotoxins which are active stimulators of secretion in the upper intestine.

Finally there is a group of bacteria which have been isolated from the upper intestine of children with protracted diarrhoea, many of whom are malnourished, and from the upper intestine of adults with a variety of infective malabsorption syndromes. They include species such as *Klebsiella*, *Enterobacter*, *Proteus*, and *Serratia* which are not regarded as classical pathogens. However, when bacteria-free filtrates of these organisms are introduced into certain test systems for enterotoxins, they frequently produce positive responses.

Production of mucosal lesion of small intestine. The organisms which have been isolated from cases of diarrhoea with lesions of the small intestine are listed in Table 1, but in the majority of cases it is not clear how the enteropathogen causes the damage. Nevertheless there are some clear examples. Rotavirus has been identified in the damaged villi of children with acute diarrhoea. Volunteers who receive Norwalk agent have villus atrophy when jejunal biopsy samples are examined 48 hours later. Electron micrographs of villi in acute giardiasis show severe lesions at the interface between trophozoites and microvilli.

It is not so certain whether bacteria can produce mucosal damage. There are considerable numbers of bacteria in the upper

Table 1 Enteropathogens which may cause malabsorption

Parasites	Bacteria
Giardia	Klebsiella
Strongyloides	E. coli
Capillaria	Enterobacter
Coccidia	V. cholerae
Ascaris	Staphylococcus
Hookworm	Shigella
Fish tapeworm	Salmonella
Viruses	Fungus
Rotavirus	Candida
Norwalk agent	

intestine of patients with the blind loop syndrome and yet mucosal changes are minimal. However, in acute tropical sprue the presence of enterobacteria is associated with mucosal atrophy. Bacteria-free filtrates of these organisms produce damage to villi when perfused along rat intestine. When bacteria-free filtrates of various organisms isolated from the upper intestine of children with protracted diarrhoea and malnutrition are perfused into rat intestine, many reduce the lactase activity of the mucosa indicating microvillus damage. Mucosal lesions of the jejunum and ileum occur in *Campylobacter* infection. Pig-bel, a severe necrotic and haemorrhagic disease of the jejunum and ileum develops in response to *Cl. perfringens* enterotoxin. It is a particular danger for those who eat contaminated pig, as in some parts of Papua New Guinea and Uganda.

The overall effect of any mucosal lesion is twofold. Firstly, there is a decrease in surface area, and malabsorption often occurs during the acute and/or recovery phase. Secondly, there are more immature enterocytes on the villus than normal. The effect of these secretory cells is that net absorption can be turned into net secretion even without the presence of an enterotoxin. The acute dehydrating diarrhoea of rotavirus infection is probably caused by a severe villus atrophy in which mature absorptive cells have been lost. Diarrhoea will continue until the villi regenerate. This takes two to three days in healthy children but the impaired ability to regenerate enterocytes in protein energy malnutrition and folate deficiency may explain why malnourished children tend to have rather protracted episodes of diarrhoea.

Enteropathogenic mechanisms. There is a large body of epidemiological evidence which suggests that certain strains of *E. coli* are associated with outbreaks of diarrhoea. Classically, in the United Kingdom these organisms have been associated with outbreaks of 'summer diarrhoea' which had devastating effects on children in the 1920s and 1930s. Since then it has largely declined in significance but is still responsible for some outbreaks of diarrhoea. These organisms produce a watery diarrhoea but the mechanism by which they produce their disease is largely unknown. They do not produce typical LT or ST responses in tissue culture or weanling mouse assay respectively. Two possible mechanisms are suggested at present. Firstly, using a perfused rat intestine system, bacteria-free filtrates of these enteropathogenic *E. coli* (EPEC) stimulate water secretion. Secondly, the filtrates produce an effect on VERO cells which is distinct from that produced by LT toxin.

Production of mucosal lesion of large intestine. Damage to the mucosa of the large intestine characteristically causes blood loss and increased secretion of mucus—the dysentery syndrome. Although considerable fluxes of fluid and electrolytes occur across the membranes of the epithelial cells of the colon and rectum, there is no recognized way in which enteropathogens produce their effects by altering these fluxes. Many histological studies have shown that invasion of the colonic mucosa is the major event.

Certain strains of *E. coli* (the entero-invasive *E. coli*, EIEC) can produce a dysentery illness. *Campylobacter* and *Yersinia* also produce a severe mucosal lesion.

Pathogenesis of protracted infective diarrhoea

In the majority of cases of acute infective diarrhoea there is rapid improvement as the enteropathogen is cleared from the intestine and/or the mucosal lesion recovers. However, in a proportion of cases protracted diarrhoea may occur for a variety of reasons (Fig. 2).

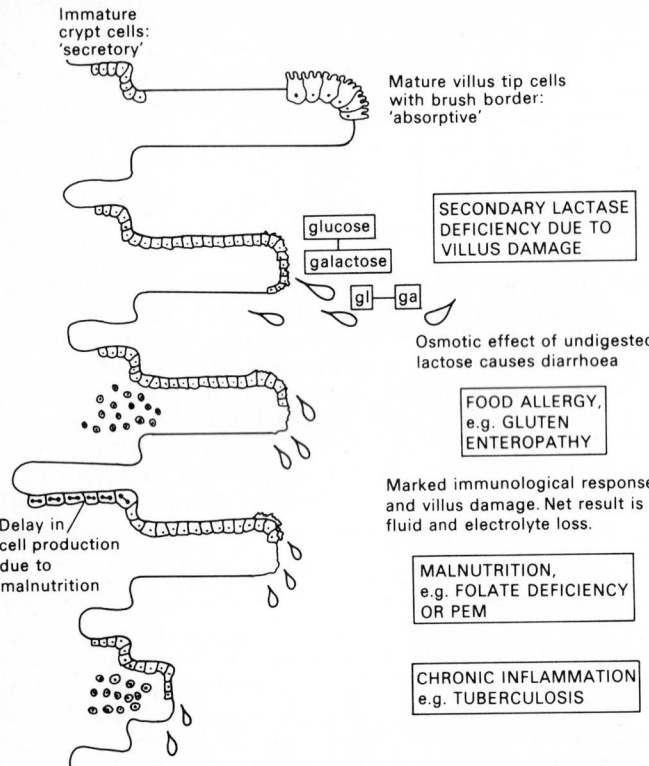

Immature crypt cells: 'secretory'

Mature villus tip cells with brush border: 'absorptive'

glucose
galactose
gl ga

SECONDARY LACTASE DEFICIENCY DUE TO VILLUS DAMAGE

Osmotic effect of undigested lactose causes diarrhoea

FOOD ALLERGY, e.g. GLUTEN ENTEROPATHY

Marked immunological response and villus damage. Net result is fluid and electrolyte loss.

Delay in cell production due to malnutrition

MALNUTRITION, e.g. FOLATE DEFICIENCY OR PEM

CHRONIC INFLAMMATION e.g. TUBERCULOSIS

Fig. 2 Pathogenesis of protracted diarrhoea. (PEM = protein energy malnutrition.)

Persistent mucosal lesion of the small intestine. This may be due to (*a*) continued infection with an agent such as *Giardia lamblia* which damages the villi as long as it is present, or (*b*) inadequate regeneration of enterocytes because of malnutrition. It is possible that (*a*) and (*b*) may co-exist and the combination of an infective agent (e.g. enterobacteria) and folate deficiency (limiting the regeneration of enterocytes) is the likely cause of the mucosal lesion of tropical sprue.

Lactose intolerance. Persistent lactose intolerance (see page 12.97) sometimes occurs for months after an acute diarrhoea. It is probably due to a delay in complete recovery of the normal villus architecture and lactase concentrations in jejunal biopsy specimens are often low. The severity of lactose intolerance in infective diarrhoea syndromes (where jejunal lesions are mild) contrasts with the minimal problem of lactose intolerance in gluten enteropathy (where jejunal lesions are severe). The probable explanation is that in gluten enteropathy the ileum is usually normal with sufficient lactase to digest lactose entering the ileum from the damaged jejunum, whereas in infective diarrhoea syndromes there is often an ileal lesion as well as jejunal atrophy thereby decreasing the total lactase concentration of the small intestine such that lactose enters the colon. Once in the colon, bacterial fermentation reactions produce gases (hydrogen especially) to produce abdominal distension. The watery diarrhoea is the result of a high osmotic load drawing water into the intestine.

Food allergies (including gluten enteropathy). This category was too loosely defined previously but a number of dietary antigens are now recognized to stimulate an immunological reaction in the mucosa

and villus atrophy results. Among children who develop protracted infective diarrhoea, cows' milk protein intolerance is an important syndrome to diagnose. Diarrhoea will only cease if they are placed on soya protein 'milks' or chicken-based formulae. In a proportion of children and adults with continued villus atrophy after infective diarrhoea, gluten withdrawal is followed by marked improvement. Conversely, when challenged with gluten after temporary recovery there is a rapid relapse, i.e. the characteristic features of gluten enteropathy. It is not clear why intestinal infection should precipitate transient or even long-term gluten enteropathy but studies on the interaction of lectins (of which gluten is an example) with enterocyte membranes shows that lectins are particularly avid binders to immature crypt cells. It is therefore likely that during the mucosal atrophy of acute infection the greater numbers of crypt cells that cover the villi present a particularly good opportunity for gluten-induced enteropathy to occur in susceptible individuals.

Intestinal parasites which do not cause mucosal atrophy. Persistent diarrhoea, usually accompanied by abdominal pain is a characteristic feature of some cases of infection with *Ascaris lumbricoides*. There is little evidence of villus atrophy, most of the diarrhoea appears to be due to increased peristalsis as a result of the bulky nature of the parasite. Although malnutrition is described in severe cases, it is not clear how much is due to the anorexia that severe ascariasis can produce. Hookworm (either *Ancylostoma duodenale* or *Necator americanus*) disease may present with diarrhoea but there is little evidence of generalized villus atrophy. Its main effect is to cause significant blood loss from the intestine and this is discussed elsewhere (see Section 5).

Chronic inflammatory conditions. Several infective agents elicit inflammatory cell responses and mucosal damage is characteristic. These conditions of which tuberculosis is a classic example will be discussed later.

Irritable colon. A considerable proportion of patients who experience acute infective diarrhoea affecting the colon (by dysentery organisms such as *Shigella* or EIEC, for example) continue to have pain, intestinal hurry, and abdominal distension after the acute attack. Many of these patients have been investigated and in very few is there any evidence of persisting mucosal abnormality. It seems likely, but unproven, that transient mucosal invasion triggers off the irritable colon syndrome but the physiological explanation for this symptom complex is far from clear.

Clinical syndromes of infective diarrhoea

A careful clinical history and examination will often enable the clinician to diagnose the category of infective diarrhoea and sometimes enable him to make a reasonable suggestion about the identity of the infective agent. An epidemiological history is essential. The onset of acute watery diarrhoea during or soon after return from a holiday in India suggests enterotoxin producing *E. coli* (ETEC), whereas a more protracted diarrhoea with malabsorption symptoms developing during a visit to Leningrad or Aspen, Colorado has, until recently when the contaminated water supply was repaired, been very suggestive of giardiasis. Chronic diarrhoea with abdominal pain and intermittent passage of blood and mucus per rectum after travel in Central or South America might suggest amoebiasis, whereas an acute dysentery syndrome in United Kingdom schoolchildren might suggest a source of *Shigella* spp. The clinician should be informed about the changing nature of epidemiological patterns of diarrhoeal pathogens and will find that regular valuable reports are published by the Public Health Laboratory Service in the United Kingdom.

It is unusual to discuss treatment regimens before diagnosis but this is done to emphasize that mortality and patient comfort from many diarrhoeas can be remarkably improved by early, enthusiastic attention to restoration of hydration and electrolyte balance

The development of oral rehydration schemes (see below) has been a major advance in the last decade. While clinical presentations, differential diagnosis, and microbiological techniques are discussed below, it should be emphasized that rehydration should be commenced as soon as the patient is seen. The decision to use antibiotics or antidiarrhoeal agents can usually wait for a microbiological diagnosis.

In general infective diarrhoeal syndromes are of four types: (*a*) acute watery diarrhoea; (*b*) acute dysentery; (*c*) protracted diarrhoea with malabsorptions syndromes; and (*d*) chronic diarrhoea.

Acute watery diarrhoea

Acute traveller's diarrhoea (turista). The commonest infective diarrhoea syndrome among British citizens is acute traveller's diarrhoea or *turista* which has rather more descriptive names according to the source of infection (Hong Kong dog, Delhi belly, Aztec two step, Rangoon runs, Gypi tummy, Basrah belly, etc.). It is also experienced by indigenous subjects in these areas. In adults the commonest enteropathogen appears to be enterotoxigenic *E. coli*, of whom about 15 per cent produce ST, 10 per cent produce LT, and about 8 per cent produce both depending on the geographical region. There is frequently a single source of infection, a classic example being an epidemic of diarrhoea among British soldiers visiting the Middle East in whom a single serotype (O148:H28) of *E. coli* was found in faecal samples from most of those with diarrhoea. Subsequent studies on this strain, which produced diarrhoea in a laboratory worker, demonstrated enterotoxin production.

Clinical features and diagnosis. The incubation period varies but is usually from one to five days and is followed by sudden onset of severe diarrhoea, sometimes 10–20 times per day, accompanied by nausea, fever, and mild abdominal pain. The stool is fluid and usually does not contain mucus or blood. In the majority there is marked improvement in diarrhoea within a few days whatever treatment is given but up to 20 per cent may still have diarrhoea by 10 days later. A minority, for reasons that are largely unexplained, may go on to develop a malabsorption syndrome which is discussed later.

Stool microscopy during the acute stage shows no pus cells or erythrocytes. If reference laboratory facilities are available, the *E. coli* isolated from the faeces may be tested for enterotoxin production. Recent studies show that ETEC are usually in a restricted range of serogroups and serotypes, so it may be possible to use serotyping in the future. However, all these identification tests are time-consuming and investigation in most health facilities should aim at excluding other causes of diarrhoea such as *V. cholerae* (if epidemiologically indicated), *Shigella* spp., *Salmonella* spp., and *Campylobacter* (henceforth described as classical pathogens).

Treatment. The fluid loss in this syndrome may be severe, especially in children, and rehydration is important. Bed rest and avoidance of any solid foods is usually sufficient treatment but symptomatic relief may be achieved by Lomotil (diphenoxylate 2.5 mg and atropine sulphate 0.025 mg) which may be given in a dose of two tablets every four to six hours. This should only be given to adults. If cramping abdominal pain is severe, codeine phosphate given as 30 mg four times daily may be given. Although a standard mixture of kaolin and morphine is frequently taken, its action is limited to bulking of the stool and reduction of urgency of defaecation rather than reduction of the volume of diarrhoea. Many antibiotics have been used including tetracycline, neomycin, guanamycin, and sulphonamides. When these have been objectively evaluated, none has improved diarrhoea faster than a placebo.

Prophylaxis. Despite firmly held beliefs in the efficacy of medicines for preventing diarrhoea, there are few convincing studies of their value. There was a reduction in the incidence of traveller's diarrhoea (from 17 per cent in the control group compared with 13 per cent in the treatment group) in those taking Streptotriad (streptomycin 65 mg, sulphadimidine 100 mg, sulphadiazine 100 mg, and sulphathiazole 100 mg) when taken as one tablet twice daily for two weeks and then once daily for one week. Doxycycline, a tetracycline, protected all except one of eighteen Peace Corps volunteers during their first three weeks after arrival in Kenya compared with a control group of 21 individuals nine of which developed diarrhoea. Clioquinol (sold as Enterovioform) has been widely used by travellers but in view of the serious neurotoxic side-effects, especially in some populations, it cannot be recommended. The disturbance of the intestinal microflora that prophylactics induce might account for the greater incidence of salmonella infection among Swedish travellers who took prophylactic oxyquinolone. The potential development of antibiotic resistance is of even greater concern. In practice it is best to advise travellers to take extreme care about what they eat and drink and to take a supply of Lomotil or codeine phosphate with them. If they absolutely insist on a prophylactic, suggest they take Streptotriad. They should be warned against the overenthusiastic practitioners who may wish to prescribe a variety of dangerous and useless antibiotics if acute diarrhoea develops.

Virus infection. Virus infection can now be reliably diagnosed and is recognized to be an important cause of acute watery diarrhoea. In children, rotavirus may be responsible for 20–30 per cent of cases of acute diarrhoea especially during winter in the United Kingdom and during the cool dry season of the tropics. Although children from three months to three years are especially susceptible, adults are also infected. Other viruses such as Norwalk agent, coronavirus, and parvovirus are likely causes of acute diarrhoea. In the case of rotavirus, diagnosis is readily made by the electron microscopic features of infected faeces or by immunological methods such as ELISA which may be performed on faecal or serum samples. Diagnosis of the other viral agents is less satisfactory at present.

Clinical features. There is a sudden onset of watery diarrhoea, usually without abdominal pain but there may be associated upper respiratory tract signs and fever. Stool microscopy shows no pus cells or erythrocytes. The incubation period is two to three days and generally the disease lasts only for two to three days.

Treatment. Intensive rehydration should be instituted. There is little indication for anti-diarrhoeal drugs in adults and no indication for them in children.

Prophylaxis. The best prevention for infants is breast feeding because antirotavirus antibodies are secreted in the maternal milk.

Cholera. Cholera is a life-threatening watery diarrhoea which differs from acute traveller's diarrhoea by virtue of its greater severity. The mechanisms by which it produces diarrhoea and its bacteriology are described in Section 5.

Clinical features. The incubation period is from a few hours to five days. There is a sudden onset of profuse diarrhoea sometimes accompanied by vomiting. The volume of diarrhoea may be enormous, in tens of litres daily, and the stools are characteristically odourless and consist predominantly of water with flecks of mucus and epithelial cell debris—hence the term 'rice water' because it looks like the water that is drained off after boiling rice. If the patient is untreated, there is a high mortality from dehydration and electrolyte loss. If inadequately treated, circulatory failure may cause renal failure which may become irreversible.

Diagnosis is by dark ground illumination of freshly passed faeces and by culture on selective media (discussed in Section 5). Stool microscopy shows no pus cells or erythrocytes. Again, there are characteristic epidemiological features which should alert the clinician to the possibility of cholera. It is now endemic in parts of India but one of the mysteries of tropical gastroenterology is why it does not occur more widely in Africa except in epidemic form.

Treatment. If adequate hydration techniques are used, the mortality can be reduced almost to zero. The difficulty in measuring fluid and electrolyte balance can be improved by the use of a cholera bed whereby the watery faecal losses pass effortlessy into a bucket with measuring device. The faecal losses average 140 mmol of sodium, 10 mmol of potassium, 110 mmol of chloride, and 140 mmol of bicarbonate per litre and the resultant metabolic acidosis should be treated at the same time as replacing sodium, potassium, and water. This may be achieved by oral or intravenous fluid replacement or both. Tetracycline has been used in doses of 250 mg four times daily, its claimed advantage being to shorten the duration of diarrhoea (which it probably does in the case of El Tor vibrios) and to prevent the spread of infection in the community. Currently many cases are infected by *V. cholerae* which are resistant to tetracycline and not surprisingly the duration of excretion does not appear to be influenced by the tetracycline. As the acute diarrhoea is usually improved after 48 hours and the patient is clinically improved if rehydration has been successful, there are few advocates for antibiotics in cholera.

The management of cholera is discussed in detail in Section 5.

Food poisoning bacteria. Several organisms produce a severe watery diarrhoea by the production of toxins. The species and some clinical features are shown in Table 2.

Staphylococcal gastroenteritis is due to consumption of an enterotoxin already produced in food which has been inadequately heated or refrigerated after cooking. Salads and dairy products such as cream may also contain enterotoxin. After a four to eight hour incubation there is onset of severe nausea and vomiting accompanied by watery diarrhoea. The dehydration may be severe in children. Stool microscopy shows no pus cells or erythrocytes. Treatment is by rehydration therapy as described below.

Vibrio parahaemolyticus is an important cause of food poisoning especially from shellfish. The enterotoxin is eaten and after two to 48 hours there is a sudden onset of diarrhoea which lasts for two to three days. The diarrhoea is usually watery but may in addition contain blood. Fever may be present. Stool microscopy may show some pus cells or erythrocytes indicating mucosal invasion. Treatment consists of rehydration; tetracycline 250 mg four times daily is claimed to decrease the duration of excretion of the organism.

Salmonella. Certain species, notably typhimurium and enteritidis, produce watery diarrhoea by enterotoxins which are similar to those produced by *E. coli*. A watery diarrhoea develops six to 48 hours after ingestion of the contaminated food. There may be chronic abdominal pain and some dysenteric symptoms suggesting that the organisms also invade the mucosa. Stool microscopy may show pus cells and erythrocytes. Treatment consists of rehydration therapy; antobiotics should not be used.

Pig bel disease. This disease, which has been described in Papua New Guinea and Uganda, is due to a toxin produced by *Cl. perfringens*. Colonization of the intestine characteristically occurs after eating pork prepared under unhygienic conditions. The toxin produces extensive haemorrhagic lesions in the small intestine. Initially there is severe watery diarrhoea and this is followed by severe blood loss, peritonitis and intestinal perforation. In some series, over half the patients died. Treatment consists of public health education; there is a vaccine which has been used with good protective effect in Papua New Guinea. In the established cases,

intravenous fluids including blood transfusions and laparotomy may be necessary. Penicillin and type C gas gangrene antisera are also useful.

Diseases affecting the colon predominantly. Several infections which are described in the next sections are primarily diseases of the colon but may be present with watery diarrhoea. This is true of *Shigella dysenteriae* type 1, *Yersinia enterocolitica*, *Campylobacter*, and also entero-invasive *E. coli*.

Rehydration regimens

The most dramatic reductions in mortality from infective diarrhoea have been achieved during the last decade since the introduction of simple, successful rehydration regimens. This has been most striking in areas of the developing world which are endemic for cholera; efficient village health centre based regimens of oral rehydration have reduced the mortality from 50 per cent to almost zero. Similarly, oral rehydration is effective in watery diarrhoeas due to ETEC and rotavirus among adults and children in developing and more developed country alike.

The emphasis on oral rehydration came as a result of the demonstration that sodium and water transport from the lumen across the enterocyte membrane and into the mucosa could be stimulated by the presence of intraluminal glucose, even when the enterocyte was being stimulated to secrete fluid into the lumen by cholera toxin. Subsequently it has been shown that iso-osmolar sucrose can stimulate electrolyte and water absorption just as well. There has been considerable debate about the most advisable concentration of sodium in oral rehydration solutions (ORS). This largely arose because of the concern by many paediatricians that cases of hypernatraemic dehydration would be made worse by solutions containing large amounts of sodium. At the time when ORS was being introduced (the late 1960s) up to 20 per cent of children admitted to some hospitals in developing countries had hypernatraemia before the administration of the ORS. Much of this may be attributed to the high sodium concentrations of formula milks that were taken by bottle-fed babies who subsequently developed diarrhoea and were admitted with dehydration. The proportion with hypernatraemia seems to have fallen over the years; this is probably the result of change in composition of commercial milk formula. Where breast feeding is the main food supply for the infant hypernatraemia is very rare. The WHO now recommend a single formula for ORS which is suitable for all ages (Table 3), although there are also commercially available packets which provide only 30 mmol of sodium per litre (i.e. a third of the sodium in the WHO formula).

The doses of ORS to be used are included in Table 3. In many cases the volumes to be administered can be given by mouth provided careful, patient nursing or maternal encouragement is given. If this fails, the fluid may be given via a nasogastric tube. Some patients vomit to begin with. This is not an indication to abandon the attempt but the volumes should be decreased and given more

Table 2 Differential diagnosis of acute watery diarrhoea

Organism	Abdominal pain	Fever	Dysentery	Faecal pus cells	Mucosal lesion of small intestine	Mucosal lesion of large intestine	Enterotoxin production
V. cholerae	∓	−	−	−	−	−	+
E. coli (ETEC)	∓	+	−	−	−	−	+
E. coli (EPEC)	∓	+	−	−	−	−	?(probably+)
Giardia	∓	∓	−	−	+	−	−
Rotavirus	∓	+	−	−	+	−	−
Shigella (certain species)	+ +	+ +	+ +	+	−	+ +	+
Salmonella (certain species)	+	+	+	+	−	+	+
Food poisoning group*	+	+	−	−	−	−	+ †

* Food poisoning group includes *Staph. aureus*, *Cl. perfringens*, *V. parahaemolyticus*, and *Bacillus cereus*
† Many, but not all cause diarrhoea by production of enterotoxin

Table 3 Rehydration regimens

(a) Oral glucose electrolyte solution (WHO formula)

Concentration (mmol/l)	Can be provided (in 1 litre) by	
Sodium 90	Sodium chloride	3.5 g
Potassium 20	Sodium bicarbonate	2.5 g
Chloride 80	Potassium chloride	1.5 g
Bicarbonate 30	Glucose*	20.0 g
Glucose 110		

* Sucrose may be substituted for glucose. It should be given as 40.0 g/l., i.e. 220 mmol/l

(b) Volumes to be given (WHO recommendations for children)

Hydration status	Immediate replacement	Further replacement
Normal	100 ml/kg body weight in 24 hours	100 ml/kg body weight in 24 hours
Moderate (fluid loss up to 50 ml/kg body weight)	100 ml/kg body weight in 6 hours. (In practice give 30 ml every 15 min. for 1 hour, 60 ml every 15 min. for 2 hours, then give remainder)	200 ml/kg body weight
Severe (fluid loss up to 100 ml/kg body weight)	Intravenous*: 100 ml/kg in 6 hours (give half in first hour) *plus* oral: 100 ml/kg body weight in 6 hours	200 ml/kg body weight in 24 hours

* If a good drip cannot be established give the fluid intraperitoneally 50 ml/kg body weight

frequently. Attention to signs of fluid overload such as peri-orbital oedema, cough, or slight dyspnoea, etc. are just as important in oral as in intravenous rehydration.

Some patients are too ill to drink or their state of dehydration is so severe that the fluid replacement they require must, initially at least, be given by intravenous route. Such patients usually have severe metabolic acidosis and the ideal solution, developed in Bangladesh, consists of the following in 1 litre of water: 8 g glucose, 4 g sodium chloride, 6.5 g sodium acetate (or 5.4 g sodium lactate), and 1 g of potassium chloride. Other suitable solutions in decreasing order of value are Hartmann's solution, half strength Darrows solution, and normal saline. Dextrose 5 per cent has no value because of its lack of electrolytes. These solutions should be given intravenously using a peripheral vein (a scalp vein in a child). However, if it is impossible to establish a good intravenous line, 50 ml/kg of the fluid may be given intraperitoneally in children.

Using 'village technology' approaches, many programmes advise the use of sugar and salt regimens (1 level 5 ml teaspoon of salt and 8 level teaspoons of sugar per litre of water gives virtually the same concentration as the WHO formula) made up at home. While this may be the best available, it suffers from the absence of potassium. This can be provided by orange juice or mashed bananas. Limes, though commonly recommended, contain little potassium.

Acute dysentery syndromes
Definition. Diarrhoea in which there is increased passage of mucus and blood.

The prognosis is more serious than watery diarrhoea and, particularly in the elderly, the very young, and the malnourished, if diagnosis and treatment are delayed the illness may be fatal. In the treatment of dysentery it is important to rehydrate and even give blood transfusions as soon as the patient presents. Antibiotics have an important role to play but in selected cases only. Table 4 gives a differential diagnosis for dysentery syndromes.

Shigella. There is a spectrum of illness from mild diarrhoea to fulminating dysentery with severe systemic features. In general the milder cases are caused by *Sh. sonnei* and more severe illness is caused by *Sh. flexneri* and *Sh. boydi*. The most serious illness is caused by *Sh. dysenteriae* type 1 (Shiga's bacillus). In recent years Shiga dysentery has caused serious epidemics with high mortality in Central America (where it was estimated that 120 000 cases occurred with a 10 per cent mortality in Guatemala during one year alone) and in Bangladesh. In these areas a disturbing antibiotic resistance pattern emerged. Initially sulphonamides were used. When organisms became resistant to them tetracycline was introduced. When organisms became resistant to tetracycline, ampicillin was introduced; resistance to ampicillin is now present in 50 to 90 per cent of Shigella strains isolated in some areas. In the United Kingdom the most frequently isolated Shigella is *Sh. sonnei* and fortunately shigellosis is rarely fatal.

Clinical features. After an incubation period of one to five days there is onset of diarrhoea. Sometimes this is sudden and voluminous from the start. In other cases it gradually worsens over several days as the bacilli invade the mucosa. Stool microscopy shows the presence of pus cells and erythrocytes. Proctoscopy or sigmoidoscopy shows hyperaemia of the mucosa with excess mucus in the early stages and later becomes frankly haemorrhagic with micro-ulcers. The appearances are very similar to those of ulcerative colitis.

There may be severe systemic features including fever, leucocytosis, and meningism (especially in infants and young children) in all the Shigella syndromes but especially with *Sh. dysenteriae* type 1. The leucocytosis may be severe and a haemolytic/uraemic syndrome may develop. Other features include pneumonia, myocardial involvement, ocular lesions, arthropathy, and peripheral neuropathy. Bacteraemia seldom occurs and it is thought that these systemic clinical features are the result of hypersensitivity reaction to toxin.

Treatment. Rehydration is essential. In severe cases with fever,

Table 4 Differential diagnosis of acute dysentery

Organism	Sudden onset	Rapid dehydration	Brief illness	Onset gradual and relapsing	Fever	Voluminous watery stools	Stool microscopy			Trophozoites
							Pus cells	Red cells	Mononuclear cells	
Shigella	++	+	+	−	+	++	++	++	−	−
E. coli (EIEC)	++	+	+	−	+	+	++	++	−	−
Inflammatory bowel disease	∓	−	−	++	+	−	+	++	−	−
Salmonella	+	∓	+	∓	+	+	∓	++	++	−
Campylobacter	+	∓	+	−	+	−	++	++	−	−
Amoeba	−	−	−	++	+	+	++	++	−	++
Antibiotic-associated colitis	∓		−	+	+	+	++	++	−	−

aspirin and tepid sponging should be used to reduce the pyrexia. If convulsions occur, intravenous diazepam should be used. Abdominal pain may be severe and codeine phosphate 60 mg four times daily may be used. In mild cases, the majority of patients stop excreting the organism and improve clinically after one week. There is no indication for antibiotics in healthy adults but in infants or young children, the elderly or where host resistance is low, or in malnourished patients, antibiotics should be given. Severe cases with systemic manifestations and frequent passage of mucus and blood should all be given antibiotics. Ampicillin 500 mg should be given four times daily for five days, or tetracycline 500 mg four times daily for five days. Recently a single bolus of tetracycline 2.5 g has been shown to be very effective in adults. The management of Shigella infections is likely to become beset with problems in the future as more antibiotic resistance emerges. Various regimens have been suggested for the treatment of asymptomatic carriers. The administration of lactobacilli or lactulose has been tried in order to reduce faecal pH and increase fatty acid concentrations both of which are inhibitors to Shigella. However, neither of these have any constant effect on Shigella excretion. The pressures to treat are greatest with those whose job makes it dangerous to be a carrier (e.g. a food handler or a nurse in a children's ward). At present the best management seems to be to perform regular faecal microbiology until the organism clears spontaneously. If the Shigellae are still excreted by four weeks after the first consultation a course of ampicillin may be prescribed but there has never been a systematic study to evaluate whether this really does expedite clearance.

Salmonella. In general, acute watery diarrhoea and dysentery are caused by *S. typhimurium*, *S. enteritidis*, and *S. heidelberg* whereas enteric fever, in which diarrhoea may be a prominent feature, is caused by *S. typhi*, *S. paratyphi* A, and *S. paratyphi* B. Diarrhoea develops as the bacteria invade the mucosa and become taken up by the lymphoid tissue. In some cases the bacteria pass through and invade the blood stream. This is especially likely to occur in conditions with abnormalities of the reticulo-endothelial system due to blockade (e.g. malaria and sickle cell disease) or as part of a decreased host response to infection (e.g. protein energy malnutrition).

Clinical features. After an incubation period of one to five days diarrhoea with blood and mucus develops. Stool microscopy shows the presence of pus cells and erythrocytes although this is less marked than in shigellosis. Proctoscopy and sigmoidoscopy show a haemorrhagic mucosa which is very similar to that produced by *Shigella* spp. or ulcerative colitis. In some patients watery diarrhoea predominates and in others a typhoid fever syndrome develops. The diagnosis and management of which are dealt with in more detail elsewhere (see Section 5).

Treatment. Rehydration is essential. In mild cases antibiotics should not be used because the disease improves spontaneously, and excretion of organisms is often prolonged by antibiotics. In more severe cases, chloramphenicol should be used at a dose of 250 mg every eight hours for seven days. If there is failure to improve or if drug resistance is demonstrated *in vitro*, other drugs which may be used are amoxicillin 250 mg four times daily for 10 days or trimethoprim and sulphamethoxazole tablets which should be taken as two tablets three times daily for 10 days.

Campylobacter. (see also Section 5). Considerable advances have been made in the diagnosis of this genus in the last decade, mainly as a result of the design of appropriate media and incubation conditions. Mucosal lesions are described in the jejunum and ileum but the main damage appears to be in the colon. *In vitro* tests of organisms isolated from patients with diarrhoea show tissue invasion of chicken embryo cells, and in the weanling mouse assay (the standard test for ST enterotoxin from *E. coli*) a small proportion of the campylobacters produce a positive response.

Clinical features. After an incubation period of three to five days, there is often a prominent systemic illness (pyrexia, headache, and myalgia) before the onset of diarrhoea. Initially stools are watery and later become blood-stained and contain mucus. In most patients the symptoms improve spontaneously after a week even though organisms are excreted for much longer. In some patients there is severe abdominal pain, and in children an incorrect diagnosis of appendicitis has sometimes been followed by a laparotomy which has shown diffuse hyperaemia of the ileum and colon. Stool microscopy shows pus cells and erythrocytes, and if a fresh specimen is examined using dark ground or phase contrast microscopy, the campylobacters can be recognized by their characteristic motility.

Treatment. In mildly symptomatic patients no antibiotics are needed but if symptoms are more severe or prolonged, erythromycin 500 mg may be given eight hourly for seven days. In those with severe dysentery or systemic infection gentamycin or chloramphenicol should be used. As there have been no controlled clinical trials it is not possible to recommend one rather than the other.

Entero-invasive E. coli (EIEC). Certain strains of *E. coli* can invade mucosal cells of the colon to produce acute dysentery. Outbreaks of this disease, which have often been associated with a common contaminated food source, have been described in all age groups and from many countries. These strains of *E. coli* are often atypical and may be non-lactose fermenting; therefore they are sometimes reported as *Shigella* spp. However several fermentation characteristics and motility appearances are easily recognized differentiating features. Rabbit ileal loop and guinea pig eye (Sereny) test are positive.

Clinical features. A one to three day incubation period is followed by abrupt onset of watery diarrhoea which rapidly becomes dysenteric with severe abdominal pain. Stool microscopy shows pus cells and erythrocytes. Sigmoidoscopy shows a haemorrhagic mucosa. The disease usually improves spontaneously after five days.

Treatment is the same as for ETEC-producing watery diarrhoea.

Amoebiasis. The epidemiology, life-cycle and biological features of amoebiasis are described in Section 5. It is an important cause of bloody diarrhoea in developing countries and is, unnecessarily, an important cause of death in some more developed countries largely as a result of inadequate awareness of its presence. Two features are important to physicians in developed countries. Firstly, that the disease may present many years after return from overseas (a gap of over 37 years has been recorded), and secondly that the disease may occur in some individuals without ever leaving the United Kingdom. The reasons for this are unknown.

Clinical features. Several syndromes occur. A gradual onset of watery diarrhoea associated with cramping central and lower abdominal pain may be followed by passage of mucus and blood. Stool microscopy shows pus cells and erythrocytes. Symptoms may improve spontaneously and then relapse quite suddenly. In those with protracted symptoms for several weeks there may be marked weight loss; blood loss may lead on to anaemia and hypoproteinaemia. Sigmoidoscopy shows ulcers in some but not all cases; the most common appearance is of an easily bleeding mucosa with necrotic areas surrounded by relatively healthy looking mucosa on which there is excessive mucus. The problem is that these are just the appearances in some cases of ulcerative colitis in which corticosteroid therapy and intestinal surgery are indicated, with fatal consequences if the patient has amoebiasis. It is essential to look for cysts or trophozoites of *Entamoeba histolytica* in all cases of chronic diarrhoea and in all cases of inflammatory bowel disease before they are subjected to corticosteroid therapy or surgery. The faecal specimen must be examined fresh, within half an hour of being passed, if trophozoites are to be diagnosed. The onus is on the physician to examine the mucus obtained at sigmoidoscopy himself using the microscope which should be on every ward. Cysts of *Entamoeba histolytica* are more hardy and will maintain morphology for many hours but two problems exist. Firstly, they may be intermittently excreted and a minimum of three samples should be examined, preferably after a formol ether concentration method prior to microscopy. Secondly, as a result of lack of experience and training in parasitological diagnosis by laboratory workers in some developed countries, there is a real risk of the parasite being missed. It is almost impossible to identify *Entamoeba histolytica* for two weeks after a barium study. Rectal biopsies should be taken in any suspected case of amoebiasis if faecal microscopy is negative; they should preferably be examined using immunofluorescent methods as well as by light microscopy. Serology is helpful, particularly the indirect fluorescent antibody test which is positive in about 85 per cent of cases of acute invasive intestinal amoebiasis. The indirect haemagglutination test is also positive in nearly all cases of acute amoebiasis. The tests remain positive for months after clinical improvement as discussed elsewhere.

Some patients may develop a fulminent amoebic colitis from the onset. The disorder resembles the toxic megacolon of ulcerative colitis, dangerously so because the management is entirely different. Early warning signs of this problem are increasing abdominal tenderness and distension, together with the passage of sloughs of mucosa. The patient becomes very toxic with pyrexia, dehydration, and tachycardia. If untreated, perforation and peritonitis occur which are nearly always fatal.

Treatment. This is directed towards the patient and the parasite. The *patient* may require rapid rehydration, and blood loss should, if severe, be treated with blood transfusion. For the *parasite*, the drug of first choice is metronidazole which should be given at a dose of 800 mg three times daily for 10 days. The majority of patients will be able to take it by mouth but if there are severe side-effects, or for severely ill patients, parenteral forms are now available. Some patients fail to respond to metronidazole and the more old-fashioned emetine hydrochloride may be used. Several field studies indicate that tinadazole is effective but so far it has only been evaluated in mild, chronic cases. A common problem is what to do with the chronic cyst carrier. As millions of people excrete cysts throughout the world without developing invasive amoebiasis, it is difficult to know how far to go. In the United Kingdom, cyst carriage is infrequent and should probably be treated. Diloxanide furoate 500 mg three times daily for 10 days should be given; metronidazole is not as effective against cysts.

Antibiotic-associated colitis (pseudomembranous colitis). This syndrome is included here because it is an important differential diagnosis in a patient with infective diarrhoea, many of whom will have received antibiotics before being referred to a specialist clinic. The pathogenesis is discussed elsewhere (see Section 5). In a high proportion toxins produced by *Cl. difficile* are demonstrable.

Clinical features. The diarrhoea is usually watery or mucoid but in a proportion there is blood as well. Stool microscopy often shows pus cells.

Treatment. Emphasis should be placed on rehydration and electrolyte replacement and withdrawal of the antibiotic which has produced the condition. Several regimens have been used. Vancomycin, to which nearly all strains of *Cl. difficile* are susceptible, may be given in doses of 125 mg four times daily for at least one week. Metronidazole has *in vitro* activity against *Cl. difficile* but is less successful than vancomycin. Cholestyramine, which binds the cytotoxin produced by *Cl. difficile*, produces a decrease in diarrhoea as long as the patient can take it because of its unpleasant taste, but does not improve the morphological lesion.

Yersinia enterocolitica. This organism, which is transmitted by animals, although certain commercial foods may also be implicated, produces a cellular infiltration of the lower ileum and colon. In the acute phase there is frank ulceration with acute bloody diarrhoea. The disease may be persistent. Differential diagnosis is from appendicitis, tuberculosis, or Crohn's disease. The histology of resected specimens suggests a Shwartzman type of reaction to the bacteria. Sometimes severe systemic features are dominant with

pyrexia and weight loss. Diagnosis is by serology in most cases but the organism can be identified in the stools. Treatment is with tetracycline or chloramphenicol 250 mg four times daily for two weeks.

Balantidiasis. The disease, caused by the protozoan *Balantidum coli*, is commonest in areas where pigs are kept close to humans. The life history and clinical features are similar to those of *Entamoeba histolytica*. The mucosal lesion is frequently severe with large ulcers throughout the large intestine. Fortunately metronidazole used in the same doses as for amoebiasis seems to be effective.

Protracted diarrhoea with malabsorption syndromes. A proportion of patients who present with acute diarrhoea fail to improve rapidly. Some of them have conditions, such as lactose intolerance, food allergies including gluten enteropathy, and irritable colon, already discussed on page 12.86.

This section will deal with infective malabsorption syndromes. As Table 1 shows, there are many enteropathogens which cause a mucosal lesion and malabsorption. In practical terms, when patients present with persistent malabsorption, it is most important to diagnose parasitic infection because these are relatively easily treated. This leaves an important group of patients without parasites in whom there is malabsorption. Figure 3 gives a working classification for diagnosis and management. Although these syndromes are often called tropical malabsorption because of their widespread presence in many tropical countries, they may occur in patients with post-infective malabsorption who have never left the United Kingdom. The term 'infective malabsorption' is therefore preferred.

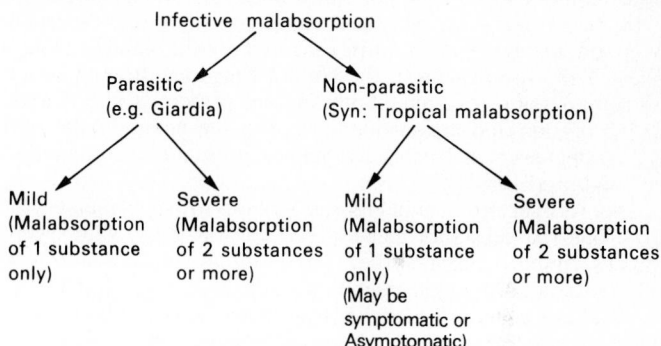

Fig. 3 A classification of infective malabsorption syndromes.

There is clearly a spectrum of severity. At one end there is mild malabsorption (of one test substance only) which may occur without intestinal symptoms. At the other end are cases of severe malabsorption (of two or more test substances) most of whom have severe diarrhoea and various nutritional deficiencies (often called tropical sprue). The aetiology of these various degrees of malabsorption is complex and almost certainly due to different pathogens in different regions.

Infective malabsorption in residents in developing countries. The small bowels of babies throughout the world have similar, characteristic 'finger-like' villi. These remain the same throughout life in Western subjects and are regarded as the normal pattern for adults. However, during the first year of life in an unhygienic environment, as for instance in many developing countries, the villi of most infants become blunted such that 'leaf' or even 'ridge-shaped' appearances become the normal pattern. These appearances remain throughout adult life unless the subject emigrates to a 'cleaner' environment, in which case his villi become more 'Western'. These morphological changes are accompanied by changes in absorption of glucose, xylose, amino acids, and dipeptides. It seems likely that the villi are damaged by repeated infection, whether clinical or subclinical.

Against this background of villus damage, often called tropical enteropathy, there are some who have more severe malabsorption which may occur in endemic or epidemic form. The term 'tropical sprue' is conventionally used to describe patients with malabsorption of two test substances or more in the absence or parasitic or 'non-tropical' cause for the malabsorption (see page 12.93). It is still not certain whether tropical sprue is really separate from tropical enteropathy but epidemiological features suggest that they are different. Whereas tropical enteropathy is common among adults throughout the developing world including Africa, the Far East, some parts of the Middle East, and India, it is very rare to find tropical sprue in Africa although cases have been reported in Zimbabwe and South Africa. Epidemics of tropical sprue have been described in southern India, an area where tropical enteropathy is common.

Tropical sprue has been most extensively studied in the Caribbean and southern India. In the former area there is a characteristic colonization of the upper intestine by enterobacteria but in southern India a much wider range of organisms has been isolated.

The tropical sprue of expatriates and that in indigenous subjects are similar in terms of objective tests of malabsorption; the different clinical picture may be largely due to variability in the underlying nutritional status and access to medical treatment at any early stage.

Infective malabsorption in expatriates. The early classic accounts concentrated on the severe cases which were frequent in the days before haematinics or antibiotics were used. Indeed, among cases of tropical sprue in expatriates who were brought back to the United Kingdom largely from India and China in the 1920s there was a 20 per cent mortality. Patients died from malnutrition which was a consequence of the prolonged uncontrolled diarrhoea.

In recent years the increased popularity of travel, especially overland, to developing countries has changed the pattern of infective malabsorption seen in the United Kingdom. Instead of the missionaries and government officials who presented with chronic malabsorption and malnutrition, we now see young adults with similar degrees of malabsorption but who present earlier than their colonial predecessors.

There is a spectrum, as in Fig. 3, from cases with mild malabsorption (one test substance malabsorbed only) to those with severe malabsorption (tropical sprue). There are no clinical features to differentiate between the conditions though, in general, if weight loss is severe or there is megaloblastic anaemia due to folate deficiency, the patient will nearly always have tropical sprue. Investigations should aim at diagnosing easily treatable parasitic conditions causing malabsorption (the majority of young adults returning to the United Kingdom with infective malabsorption after overseas travel have giardiasis). Patients should also receive formal investigation of the small intestine including xylose and vitamin B_{12} absorption tests together with measurement of fat excretion while on a constant fat intake. A jejunal biopsy should be performed to exclude gluten enteropathy (a small but important proportion of patients with 'latent' gluten enteropathy appear to be precipitated into clinical malabsorption after an acute intestinal infection), and also giardiasis (by providing portions of mucus and tissue for microscopy for the trophozoites of Giardia lamblia) (see Section 5).

Many studies indicate that enterobacteria are important in the aetiology of infective malabsorption. In healthy western adults the upper intestine is colonized by lactobacilli or streptococci predominantly. Enterobacteria are normally absent. However, intubation studies of the luminal fluid and mucosa from the upper intestine of patients with mild malabsorption and tropical sprue show that colonization by enterobacteria, especially E. coli, Klebsiella pneumoniae, and Enterobacter cloacae, is a frequent finding. Tests on bacteria-free filtrates of these organisms show that they can produce fluid secretion in perfused rat intestine and can also induce morphological lesions. When strains of these organisms which have been isolated from the upper intestine of patients with blind loop syndrome are tested in the perfused rat intestine, they have no enterotoxin effect. An indirect indication that bacterial colonization

is significant in infective malabsorption is the rapid response in vitamin B_{12} absorption following antibiotic therapy. Other infective agents have been suggested, such as coronavirus, but these are also widely present in the faeces of children and adults without tropical sprue in India and Africa.

Treatment of mild cases (xylose malabsorption alone and minimal changes on jejunal biopsy) is by dietary advise to restrict fat, avoid alcohol (patients with infective malabsorption seem particularly susceptible to the intestinal toxic effects of alcohol), and restrict lactose, and the administration of folic acid 5 mg daily. The majority will improve over the next few months. Treatment of more severe cases is the same, together with a course of tetracycline, 250 mg six-hourly for four weeks. If diarrhoea continues, sulphadimidine 0.5 g four times daily for four weeks should be given. The majority of cases improve provided they remain in the United Kingdom but a proportion relapse when they return to a developing country. Such attacks should be treated with further courses of antibiotics and folic acid. In previous decades the risk of developing chronic tropical sprue was considered so great that many expatriates were strongly advised against return to the tropics (especially those areas which are endemic for tropical sprue such as India). It seems that patients with acute tropical sprue who receive early energetic treatment are not likely to be at such risk for chronic sprue, and foreign travel is not absolutely contra-indicated. If expatriates who regularly work in developing countries suffer repeated diarrhoea every time they return to their overseas post, conditions other than infective malabsorption such as inflammatory bowel disease and irritable colon should be considered.

Chronic diarrhoeas

Tuberculosis. The infection may be caused by Mycobacterium tuberculosis or Mycobacterium bovis. Several possible modes of infection are possible including swallowing of acid-alcohol-fast bacilli (AAFB), by haematogenous spread, and by invasion from locally infected organs such as lymph glands. The mucosa is usually ulcerated and there is variable fibrosis. In some cases the former predominates; in others stricture formation is the dominant feature. The characteristic pathology of tuberculosis is present, i.e. granulomas with epithelioid cells and giant cells with central caseating necrosis. In most cases of intestinal tuberculosis bacteriological diagnosis is made by culture of the mesenteric glands and special staining of histological sections to detect the AAFB. Search for AAFB in the stools is usually unrewarding. Several clinical syndromes may occur.

Ileocaecal tuberculosis. This often causes symptoms of weight loss, fever, abdominal pain, and diarrhoea. Barium follow-through studies shows strictures. There is usually a normal chest X-ray and no signs of tuberculosis elsewhere in the body. Differential diagnosis should include lymphoma, Crohn's disease, and yersinia enterocolitis. In the United Kingdom many of the patients with ileocaecal tuberculosis are immigrants from Asia. In most cases, antituberculous chemotherapy will have to be started without microbiological proof. If there is no improvement after three months, laparotomy should be considered to enable a tissue diagnosis to be made.

Tuberculous peritonitis (see also page 12.150). The patient presents rapid onset of ascites, sometimes with abdominal pain or diarrhoea. There is frequently a large number of granulomatous lesions on the serosa which cause the intestine to stick together, thereby giving a characteristic 'dough' feeling on palpating the abdomen. The ascitic fluid protein level is usually high and it may contain large numbers of lymphocytes. If sufficient ascitic fluid is present a peritoneal biopsy can be performed using an Abrams needle. This sample, together with staining of a centrifuged deposit of ascitic fluid, enables a diagnosis to be made in the majority of cases. Differential diagnosis is from carcinomatosis, hepatoma with secondaries, and constrictive pericarditis. There is an increased incidence of tuberculous peritonitis in cirrhotic patients and tuberculosis should be considered whenever a patient with cirrhosis deteriorates. Treatment is by antituberculous therapy and improvement should occur within two months.

Glandular tuberculosis. Although this rarely presents with diarrhoea, tuberculous infection of the mesenteric glands is so common that it must be mentioned. It is usually as part of a generalized adenopathy involving cervical, aortic, mediastinal, and peritoneal glands. The main symptoms are fever and abdominal pain. Children may be incorrectly diagnosed as having acute appendicitis. In some the fever may continue and if cervical glands appear, microbiological diagnosis may be made by biopsy, and if fever persists, antituberculous therapy should be started. In many there is spontaneous resolution of the glands and in later life calcific shadows are visible on plain X-ray of the abdomen. Differential diagnosis is from other causes of glandular enlargement such as lymphoma and infective mononucleosis.

Schistosomiasis. The life cycle and pathology of this infection are dealt with in greater detail in Section 5. The symptoms are those of the systemic invasion (e.g. the local swimmer's itch followed by a more generalized reaction including fever, muscle pain, and urticaria) and the local tissue reaction. There may be mild diarrhoea or severe dysentery in some cases, while in others severe fibrosis of the intestine can occur without symptoms. The intestinal mucosa may become granular and hyperaemic. In some cases there is polyp formation which may cause sudden profuse haemorrhage. It is essential to perform microscopy on rectal scrapes and histology on biopsies of abnormal mucosa, as excretion of the ova is very intermittent and even with concentration techniques results are often negative. Occasionally, liver biopsy may demonstrate the parasite. Serological diagnosis and treatment is discussed elsewhere.

Chagas' disease (South American trypanosomiasis). There is destruction of the nerve plexus of Auerbach so that motility alters, causing dilation of the colon which presents with alternating constipation and diarrhoea. An epidemiological history is important because this condition is limited to the lower socio-economic groups in South America in whose environment the reduvid bug is able to transmit *Trypanosoma cruzi* (see Section 5). Complement fixation tests are useful but the most definitive test is xenodiagnosis in which uninfected reduvid bugs are put on the skin and subsequently examined for the presence of trypanosomes. There is, unfortunately, no satisfactory treatment for established disease.

Lymphogranuloma venereum (Tropical bubo). This is primarily a venereal disease caused by chlamydia in which a shallow ulcer develops transiently and is followed by the development of painful swollen lymph glands in the groin which, if untreated, discharge pus and even develop fistulae (see Section 5). In later stages there is infiltration of the colon and anal region, with stricture formation which is characteristically felt on rectal examination. Diarrhoea and incontinence occur. Differential diagnosis is from rectal carcinoma. Mucosal ulceration may resemble that in ulcerative colitis. Treatment for established intestinal disease is the same as for the primary venereal disease, i.e. tetracycline or chloramphenicol 250 mg four times daily or sulphamethoxazole/trimethoprim two tablets twice daily. Treatment is usually continued for two months or more before the intestinal lesions improve which may happen quite dramatically. In severe cases, surgery is necessary but results are often unsatisfactory.

Granuloma inguinale (Chancroid). This is also primarily a venereal disease caused by *Haemophilus ducreyi* (see Section 5). It produces a diffuse ulcerating lesion over the perineum which may spread to the anus. A fibrotic reaction around the anus may cause abnormal function of the anal sphincter in advanced cases. Treatment is by tetracycline, chloramphenicol, or sulphamethoxazole/trimethoprim in the same doses as for lymphogranuloma venereum.

Intestinal parasites. Several parasites, discussed in more detail elsewhere (see Section 5), may cause diarrhoea. Trichuris may induce diarrhoea and rectal prolapse especially in malnourished children. Strongyloides and ascaris may cause diarrhoea and abdominal pain.

References

Dean, A. G., Ching, Y. C., Williams, R. G., and Harden, L. B. (1972). Test for *Escherichia coli* entertoxin using infant mice: application in a study of diarrhoea in children in Honolulu. *J. infect. Dis.* **125**, 407.

Dolby, J. M., Honour, P., and Rowland, M. G. M. (1980). Bacteriostasis of *Escherichia coli* by milk. V. The bacteriostatic properties of milk of West African mothers in the Gambia: *in vitro* studies. *J. Hyg.*, *Camb.* **85**, 347.

Dupont, H. L. (1981). Modern views on travellers' diarrhoea (emporiatric enteritis). *Trans. R. Soc. trop. Med. Hyg.* **75**, 137.

Frost, J. A., Rowe, B., Vandepitte, J., and Threlfall, E. J. (1981). Plasmid characterization in the investigation of an epidemic caused by multiple resistant *Shigella dysenteriae* type 1 in Central Africa. *Lancet* ii, 1074.

Harrison, M. and Walker-Smith, J. A. (1977). Reinvestigation of lactose intolerant children: lack of correlation between continuing lactose intolerance and small intestinal morphology, disaccharidase activity, and lactose tolerance tests. *Gut* **18**, 48.

Kapikian, A. Z., Wyatt, R. G., Greenberg, H. B., Kalica, A. R., Kim, H. W., Brandt, C. D., Rodriguez, W. J., Parrott, R. H., and Chanock, R. M. (1980). *Rev. infect. Dis.* **2**, 459.

Keusch, G. T. (1979). Shigella infections. *Clins Gastroent.* **8**, 645.

McNeish, A. S., Turner, P., Fleming, J., and Evans, N. (1975). Mucosal adherence of human enteropathogenic *Escherichia coli*. *Lancet* ii, 946.

Pickering, L. K., Dupont, H. L., and Olarte, J. (1978). Single dose tetracycline therapy for shigellosis in adults. *J. Am. Med. Ass.* **239**, 853.

Rahaman, M. M., Aziz, K. M. S., Patwari, Y., and Munshi, M. H. (1979). Diarrhoeal mortality in two Bangladesh villages with and without community based oral rehydration therapy. *Lancet* ii, 809.

Ridley, M. J. and Ridley, D. S. (1976). Serum antibodies and jejunal histology in giardiasis associated with malabsorption. *J. clin. Path.* **29**, 30.

Rohde, J. E. and Northrup, R. S. (1976). Taking science where the diarrhoea is. In *Acute diarrhoea in childhood*, 339. Ciba Foundation Symposium 42 (new series). North Holland, Amsterdam.

Sack, D. A., Kaminsky, D. C., Sack, B. R., Itotia, J. N., Arthur, R. R., Kapikian, A. Z., Ørskov, F., and Ørskov, I. (1978). Prophylactic doxycycline for travellers' diarrhoea. *New Engl. J. Med.* **298**, 758.

—, —, —, Wamola, I. A., Ørskov, F., Ørskov, I., Slack, R. C. B., Arthur, R. R., and Kapikian, A. Z. (1977). Enterotoxigenic *Escherichia coli* diarrhoea of travellers: a prospective study of American Peace Corps volunteers. *Johns Hopkins Med. J.* **141**, 63.

Smith, H. W. and Linggood, M. A. (1971). Observations on the pathogenic properties of the K88, Hly and ENt plasmids of *Escherichia coli* with particular reference to porcine diarrhoea. *J. med. Microbiol.* **4**, 467.

Spiers, J. I., Stavric, S., and Konowalchuk, J. (1977). Assay of *Escherichia coli* heat labile enterotoxin with Vero cells. *Infect. Immun.* **16**, 617.

Tomkins, A. M. (1979). Folate malnutrition in tropical diarrhoeas. *Trans. R. Soc. trop. Med. Hyg.* **73**, 498.

— (1981). Tropical malabsorption: recent concepts in pathogenesis and additional significance. *Clin. Sci.* **60**, 131.

—, Bradley, A. K., Oswald, S., and Drasar, B. S. (1981). Diet and the faecal microflora of infants, children and adults in rural Nigeria and urban UK. *J. Hyg.*, *Camb.* **86**, 285.

—, Drasar, B. S., and James, W. P. T. (1975). Bacterial colonizaton of jejunal mucosa in acute tropical sprue. *Lancet* i, 59.

—, James, W. P. T., Cole, A. C. E., and Walters, J. H. (1974). Malabsorption in overland travellers to India. *Br. med. J.* iii, 380.

—, Smith, T., and Wright, S. G. (1978). Assessment of early and delayed responses in vitamin B_{12} absorption during antibiotic therapy in tropical malabsorption. *Clin. Sci.* **55**, 533.

Wellcome Trust Collaborative Study (1971). *Tropical sprue and megaloblastic anaemia*. Churchill Livingstone, Edinburgh.

World Health Organization Scientific Working Group (1980). Cholera and other Vibrio-associated diarrhoeas. *Bull. Wld Hlth Org.* **58**, 353.

Wright, S. G., Tomkins, A. M., and Ridley, D. S. (1977). Giardiasis: clinical and therapeutic aspects. *Gut* **18**, 343.

Yadar, M. and Iyngkaran, N. (1981). Immunological studies in cows' milk protein-sensitive enteropathy. *Archs Dis. Childh.* **56**, 24.

Yolken, R. H., Wyatt, R. G., Zissis, G., Brandt, C. D., Rodriguez, W. J., Kim, H. W., Parrott, R. H., Urrutia, J. J., Mata, L. J., Greenberg, H. B., Kapikian, A. Z., and Chanock, R. M. (1979). Epidemiology of human rotavirus types 1 and 2 as studied by enzyme-linked immunosorbent assay. *New Engl. J. Med.* **299**, 1156.

Congenital abnormalities of the gastrointestinal tract

J. A. Walker-Smith and V. Wright

Introduction. Congenital disorders of the gastrointestinal tract may present shortly after birth, but presentation may be delayed for months or even for years, on occasion. For example, duodenal atresia presents in the first few days of life whereas a duodenal diaphragm may not present for many years, sometimes not until adult life. A general classification of these conditions is shown in Table 1.

In this chapter the embryology of congenital abnormalities of the gastrointestinal tract will be briefly reviewed and then the most important syndromes will be discussed commencing with disorders of the oesophagus and concluding with imperforate anus.

Table 1   Congenital disorders of the gastrointestinal tract

1 Developmental failures
  Atresia and stenosis
  Duplication
  Failure of innervation
  Failure of development of abdominal wall
2 Errors of rotation
3 Persistence of vestigial structures
4 Miscellaneous, e.g. meconium ileus

Embryology of the congenital abnormalities of the gastrointestinal tract. The primitive gut is initially a simple tube of endoderm, the muscular and connective tissue developing from the splanchno-pleuric mesoderm. Cranially, the gut terminates at the bucco-pharyngeal membrane and caudally at the cloacal membrane. Both membranes disappear, failure of the cloacal membrane to do so resulting in one of the rarer forms of imperforate anus. The primitive foregut diverticulum gives rise to the respiratory system, oeso-phagus, stomach, duodenum to the level of the ampulla of Vater, liver, and pancreas. The primitive oesophagus lengthens rapidly, becomes narrow, and frequently the lumen is transiently obliter-ated. A longitudinal ventral diverticulum of the foregut forms the trachea with ridges on either side which fuse, initially caudally with progression cranially until the primitive respiratory system is sepa-rated from the oesophagus. Failure of this complex process results in the various forms of oesophageal atresia and tracheo-oesopha-geal fistula. Dilatation of the foregut distal to the oesophagus produces the stomach, initially slung from the dorsal body wall by the dorsal mesentery and from the septum transversum by the ventral mesentery. Rapid differential growth results in the stomach rotating through 90 degrees on its long axis, the dorsal border becoming the greater curvature, and the ventral border the lesser curvature. The dorsal mesentery forms the greater omentum. The ventral mesentery, into which the liver bud grows, forms the falci-form ligament and coronary ligaments attaching the liver to the diaphragm, and the lesser omentum. Congenital abnormalities of the stomach are excessively rare. The liver arises as a shallow groove on the ventral aspect of the duodenum. The groove becomes tubular and invades the septum transversum and the ventral mesentery. Bile is secreted from the fifth month, and gives meconium its characteristic dark green appearance. The mesoderm of the septum transversum forms the fibrous tissue of the liver.

The pancreas develops as two outgrowths of the duodenum. One comes from the dorsal aspect, the other from the ventral aspect. The dorsal bud grows into the dorsal mesentery and the ventral bud is swept around dorsally into the mesentery when the duodenum rotates to the right. These two primordia fuse, the ducts fuse, and the main pancreatic duct joins the bile duct to enter the duodenum at the ampulla of Vater.

If the ducts do not fuse, an accessory pancreatic duct persists. Annular pancreas is a congenital anomaly where the pancreas surrounds the duodenum which may be atretic or intrinsically sten-osed. Annular pancreas is not the primary cause of the duodenal obstruction in these cases.

The duodenum is derived partly from foregut and partly from the midgut. The loop of primitive duodenum is fixed at the pyloric end, and by the ligament of Treitz at the duodeno-jejunal flexure to the left of the first lumbar vertebra. By rotating to the right, the entire duodenum comes to lie retroperitoneally in a curve around the head of the pancreas. Failure of the duodenum to fix in this position is a fundamental reason for the gut failing to rotate correctly. During rapid growth the duodenal lumen is obliterated and partial or total failure of recanalization will result in the anomalies of duodenal atresia or stenosis. The small intestine and colon, sus-pended on the dorsal mesentery, rapidly lengthen and outgrow the primitive peritoneal cavity, and herniation occurs into the umbilical sac during the fifth week of development. Growth in length contin-ues, the loop of bowel rotating through 180° anticlockwise, the cranial limb lengthening more than the caudal limb. About the tenth week the loops of bowel return to the peritoneal cavity. The small intestine goes first, the large intestine subsequently. Thus the large intestine lies in front of the small. The caecum is initially subhepatic, but then descends to the right iliac fossa. The caecum, ascending colon, and descending colon become fixed to the poster-ior abdominal wall, thus the small bowel is suspended from a mesentery which runs from the left side of the first lumbar vertebra to the right iliac fossa. Failure of the duodenum to rotate and fix, coupled with a failure of normal rotation of the bowel with conse-quent lack of normal fixation, gives rise to malrotation of the intestine. Abnormal bands run from the caecum which lies to the left of the midline, to the region of the gallbladder and may com-press the duodenum. The narrow mesentery of the small intestine predisposes to a volvulus of the entire midgut.

At the apex of the midgut loop, the primitive gut is in continuity with the extra-embryonic yolk sac via the vitello-intestinal duct which runs in the umbilical cord. Obliteration and disappearance of this duct occurs and allows the bowel to return from the umbilical sac to the enlarged peritoneal cavity. Failure of the duct to dis-appear may result in a Meckel's diverticulum, a band connecting the ileum to the umbilicus, a communication between the lumen of the ileum and the umbilicus, or failure of the gut to return comp-letely to the peritoneal cavity, resulting in a small umbilical hernia.

Persistence of the umbilical sac will result in an exomphalos with the sac containing a variable amount of gut and much of the liver. The embryology of gastroschisis is disputed. It may be due to early rupture of the umbilical sac allowing the primitive gut to extrude into the extra-embryonic coelom, or failure of fusion of the lateral body folds producing a defect in the anterior abdominal wall adja-cent to the umbilicus.

The midgut comprises the duodenum distal to the ampulla of Vater, jejunum, ileum, caecum, and colon as far as the left trans-verse colon. Atresia affecting the midgut may occur at a single site or multiple sites. The aetiology is probably intra-uterine interfer-ence with the blood supply to that part of the gut which is affected, with consequent resorption of the ischaemic bowel.

The hindgut gives origin to the left third of the transverse colon, the descending colon, sigmoid, rectum, and upper part of the anal canal and a considerable part of the urogenital system. The hindgut terminates in the primitive cloaca which is separated from the proctodaeum (a shallow ectodermal depression) by the cloacal membrane. The primitive cloaca communicates with the hindgut and the allantois. Early in development the cloaca is joined by the pronephric ducts. A coronal septum (the urorectal septum) arises in the angle between the allantois and hindgut, grows caudally, fuses with the cloacal membrane, and divides the cloaca into a dorsal primitive rectum and a ventral primitive urogenital sinus. The cloacal membrane breaks down, establishing continuity between the endodermal hindgut and the ectodermal part of the anal canal. There are many varieties of imperforate anus. Absence of a variable length of rectum and anal canal, known as the 'high' anomaly, is frequently associated with the bowel terminating via a recto-urethral or rectovaginal fistula. Ten per cent of babies with an imperforate anus will have oesophageal atresia with or without a fistula, suggesting that the division of trachea and oesophagus and urogenital system and rectum must be occurring at a similar time in gestation, with possibly a similar mechanism producing the division. Anomalies of the urogenital system occur in a very high proportion of affected infants. Abnormalities of the ectodermal component of the anal canal result in 'low' imperforate anus.

The ganglion cells of the gut lie in the submucosa and intermyenteric plane. Ectodermal in origin, they migrate caudally along the length of the gut. Failure of migration down to the internal sphincter of the anal canal results in an aganglionic segment extending for a variable distance proximally, and is the underlying abnormality in Hirschsprung's disease.

Mucosal differentiation occurs in the early months. The inner circular muscle differentiates earlier than the outer longitudinal. Thus the fetal intestinal tract is prepared for digestion, absorption, and propulsion at a comparatively early stage in development.

Oesophageal atresia and tracheo-oesophageal fistula. The incidence of this condition is approximately 1 in 3500 live births.

The upper oesophagus ends in a blind pouch. In the majority of cases the lower oesophagus communicates at its upper end with the trachea, i.e. there is a tracheo-oesophageal fistula. Although much less common, there are a number of well-recognized anatomical variations illustrated in Fig. 1.

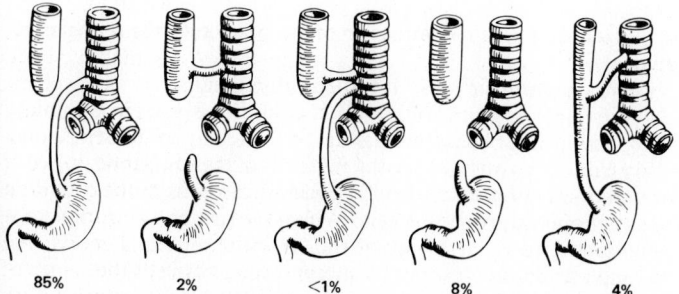

| 85% | 2% | <1% | 8% | 4% |

Fig. 1 Anatomical variations of oesophageal atresia and tracheo-oesophageal fistula, indicating the relative frequency.

Clinical features. Frequently the infant is premature or small for gestational age. In 50 per cent there is history of polyhydramnios. Shortly after birth, because swallowing is impossible, copious amounts of frothy saliva dribbles from the mouth associated with choking, dyspnoea, and cyanotic episodes. Frequent suction is required to keep the airway clear.

Over 50 per cent of infants will have significant associated anomalies. Of particular importance are cardiac, anorectal, urogenital, and skeletal anomalies. The premature or small for gestational age infant is more likely to have multiple anomalies than is the full-term infant.

The infant with isolated tracheo-oesophageal fistula coughs, chokes, and becomes cyanosed during feeds. Because air escapes through the fistula into oesophagus, marked gaseous distension of the abdomen is frequently present. Aspiration of feed into the airway results in pulmonary collapse/consolidation initially involving the right upper lobe but becoming rapidly more extensive. The infant who is small, has associated major congenital abnormalities or pre-operative pneumonia, may require pre-operative respiratory support and more than one operative procedure. Where a primary anastomosis of the oesphagus cannot be achieved initially, because the distance between the two ends of the oesophagus is too great, a gastrostomy is performed for feeding purposes. A decision on whether to attempt an oesphageal anastomosis after a delay of four to six weeks, having left the upper oesophageal pouch intact and kept empty of saliva by continuous suction, or to perform a cervical oesophagostomy with the intention after some months of establishing continuity between mouth and stomach, using a length of colon, or a tube fashioned from the greater curve of the stomach, will depend on the clinical situation and the surgeon's preference.

Survival of infants with oesophageal atresia depends on birth weight and associated abnormalities. All infants with a birth weight greater than 1.8 kg and no associated abnormalities or pneumonia should survive, this is also being true of the larger infant with a moderately severe associated abnormality or pneumonia. The mortality for the small infant or one with multiple severe congenital abnormalities remains in the region of 20–30 per cent.

Diagnosis. When oesopheal atresia is suspected a size 10 or 12 FG catheter is passed through the mouth and into the oesophagus. If the oesophagus is obstructed, the catheter characteristically meets a resistance 9–11 cm from the gum margin. A smaller catheter may curl up in the upper pouch and the diagnosis be missed. Contrast studies of the oesophagus are rarely necessary. A chest and abdominal X-ray will show the position of a radio-opaque tube in the upper oesophagus, and the presence of gas in the distal bowel, if a tracheo-oesophageal fistula (TOF) is present. Complete absence of gas in the abdomen is diagnostic of an oesophageal atresia without a distal TOF. The X-ray will also reveal any rib or vertebral abnormalities, signs of pneumonia, and may provide evidence of an associated cardiac abnormality.

In isolated tracheo-oesophageal fistula very careful contrast studies of the oesophagus are required to demonstrate the fistula.

Management. In the full-term infant with no significant associated anomalies, a right thoracotomy is performed. The tracheo-oesophageal fistula is divided and the upper and lower oesophagus anastomosed. Post-operatively respiratory problems may require tracheal intubation and ventilation but usually the full-term infant with no pre-operative pulmonary complications only needs careful suction of the nasopharynx to maintain a clear airway. A gastrostomy or a nasogastric transanastomotic tube is used to enable the infant to be fed within 48 hours of the operation.

Anterior abdominal wall defects. The incidence of *exomphalos* and *gastroschisis* is approximately 1 in 3000 births. An exomphalos occurs because the intra-abdominal contents herniate through the umbilical ring into the base of the umbilical cord and are covered by a translucent membrane composed of peritoneum and amnion. Exomphalos major indicates that the diameter of the defect is greater than 5 cm, exomphalos minor that the defect is less than 5 cm. The contents of the exomphalos almost always includes liver and a variable amount of bowel. On occasions a very small amount of bowel alone herniates into the base of the cord. Of the babies born with exomphalos, almost half are stillborn or die shortly after birth. Exomphalos is particularly associated with anencephaly, autosomal trisomies, major cardiac anomalies, and the Beckwith-Wiedemann syndrome. In gastroschisis there is a full thickness defect in the anterior abdominal wall usually to the right of the umbilical cord. The defect is small but most of the gastrointestinal tract may be extruded through it, and appears grossly thickened, very short and covered with a densely adherent gelatinous membrane. In contrast to exomphalos, other intra-abdominal organs are rarely eviscerated and abnormalities outside the gastrointestinal are unusual.

Exomphalos. *Clinical features.* The lesion will be obvious at birth. Occasionally the membrane will rupture during, or shortly after delivery. Careful examination for associated defects is essential.

Management. A nasogastric tube is passed to keep the bowel decompressed and prevent unnecessary enlargement of the exomphalos by air-filled bowel. The sac can be very satisfactorily covered and supported by wrapping clingfilm around the exomphalos and the baby's trunk. Plain X-rays of chest and abdomen are taken pre-operatively in order to study the cardiac contour, the intestinal gas pattern, and to look for evidence of an associated diaphragmatic hernia. If the contents of the sac can be reduced into the peritoneal cavity, the abdominal wall can be closed in layers. If closure of all layers of the abdominal wall is impossible, skin closure alone may be used, with or without excision of the membrane, or a synthetic material such as Silastic sheeting or Teflon mesh is used to enclose the sac after suturing it to the margins of the defect. Gradual reduction, over a number of days, of the contents into the peritoneal cavity is then possible with delayed closure of the abdominal wall. An alternative is to paint the sac with an antiseptic solution such as 70 per cent alcohol, or one of the iodine-based preparations. This results in the formation, after a few days, of a dry eschar which separates, after some weeks, leaving a granulating surface which gradually epithilializes. Any method which does not achieve muscle closure will leave a ventral hernia which requires surgery at a later date.

Post-operatively, ventilatory support may be necessary. Antibiotics commenced pre-operatively are continued post-operatively, particularly if an artificial material is used. Parenteral nutrition will be necessary if oral feeds cannot be given. Survival is related to the size of the lesion and the presence of severe associated abnormalities.

Gastroschisis. *Clinical features.* Babies with this abnormality are frequently small form gestational age. Heat loss from the exposed bowel rapidly causes hypothermia. Hypoproteinaemia is very common. The small size of the defect in the anterior abdominal wall and the often narrow pedicle from which the bowel is suspended, may impair the blood supply and result in infaction of much of the extruded intestine. Atresia may have occurred because of intra-uterine impairment of the blood supply.

Management. A nasogastric tube is passed and the bowel decompressed. The bowel can be enclosed in clingfilm wrapped around the baby's trunk, or the baby can be placed in a large polythene bag taped around the chest. This keeps the bowel moist and prevents excessive heat loss. Antibiotics are commenced pre-operatively and plasma is given to counteract the existing hypoproteinaemia. At operation the anterior abdominal wall is stretched and the bowel contents washed out to reduce bulk. Reduction of the extruded bowel is attempted and abdominal wall closure achieved where possible.

In a high proportion of cases Silastic sheeting is used to form an artifical sac over the intestine. The sheeting is sutured to the margins of the defect and the size of the sac gradually reduced over some days, squeezing the bowel back into the peritoneal cavity until closure of the abdominal wall becomes feasible—usually after 10–14 days. Ventilatory support post-operatively is often necessary. Parenteral nutrition is essential and may need to be continued for many weeks until gastrointestinal motility and absorption become adequate. Sepsis is a considerable hazard. The mortality is now 10–20 per cent compared with 80 per cent 10 years ago. Improved post-operative management is largely responsible for this.

Pyloric stenosis. The incidence is 2 per 1000 live births. The aetiology is unknown. Theories include primary muscle hypertro-

phy, abnormalities of the maturation of ganglion cells, absence of a certain type of ganglion cell, or a response to abnormally high levels of circulating gastrin. Genetic and environmental factors play an important role. There is a greatly increased incidence of pyloric stenosis in siblings of an affected child and in the offspring of a women who has had the condition. Environmental factors include social class, type of feeding, and a seasonal variation with an increase in the winter months. In any large series the male to female ratio is 3 or 4 to 1 and half the cases will be first born.

Clinical features. The onset of symptoms is usually between three and six weeks of age, but may present shortly after birth. Vomiting of increasing severity is the cardinal symptom eventually occurring after most feeds and becoming projectile. The vomitus is milk and mucus and may contain altered blood suggesting an oesophagitis or gastritis; bile is never present. The baby stops gaining weight and becomes constipated. Characteristically the baby is alert, anxious, and hungry.

Examination reveals evidence of weight loss and in advanced cases signs of dehydration will be evident. When the stomach is full, waves of peristalsis travelling from left to right in the epigastrium will be seen (visible peristalsis).

The thickened pylorus is felt as an olive-sized tumour lying deep to the edge of the right rectus and is often most easily felt when the stomach is empty. The diagnosis of pyloric stenosis is made on clinical grounds in the majority of cases. A plain X-ray of the abdomen may be very helpful in revealing a large stomach with a paucity of distal gas. A barium meal is diagnostic when the 'string' sign of the elongated pylorus is demonstrated, the barium study may also reveal marked gastro-oesophageal reflux which is commonly associated with pyloric stenosis.

Management. In the child presenting early, electrolyte disturbance and dehydration are minimal. In the later case, dehydration with hypochloraemic alkalosis and marked potassium depletion occurs. Pre-operative correction of water and electrolyte deficits is essential. The operation of pyloromytomy, described by Ramstedt in 1912, splits the hypertrophied muscle longitudinally allowing the mucosa to bulge through the defect thus enlarging the pyloric canal. Post-operatively, various feeding regimes are advocated; all aim to have the baby on a normal feeding regime 48–72 hours post-operatively. The prognosis is excellent.

Congenital intrinsic obstruction of the small intestine (atresia and stenosis)

Definition. Intrinsic small intestinal obstruction may produce either complete or partial obliteration of the bowel lumen. Complete obliteration may be due to a diaphragm occluding the lumen. It may also be due to a gap between the two ends of the small intestine with or without a connecting band between these ends. Such complete obstruction is known as atresia. When obstruction is incomplete it may be due to a narrowing of the lumen known as stenosis. An incomplete diaphragm may also occur, especially in the duodenum, partially occluding the bowel lumen and producing a clinical picture identical to that found in children who have stenosis. Small intestinal atresia is a more common finding than is stenosis.

In an analysis of 42 consecutive admissions to the Royal Alexandra Hospital for Children, Sydney, atresia occurred most often and was found in 30 children. Stenosis occurred in the remaining 12.

The duodenum is most often involved, followed by the jejunum and then the ileum. These disorders are often associated with other abnormalities of the gastrointestinal tract as study of these 42 children revealed. (Table 2). Duodenal lesions are particularly associated with lesions outside the gastrointestinal tract (Table 3).

Clinical features. Intrinsic obstruction of the small intestine of congenital origin presents most often in the neonatal period but when the obstruction is partial it may first present much later, in infancy and childhood.

Table 2 Associated abnormalities of the gastrointestinal tract at Royal Alexandra Hospital for Children

	Duodenum	Jejuno-ileum
Number of children	24	18
Malrotation of midgut loop	10	3
Meckel's diverticulum	1	3
Oesophageal atresia	4	–
Imperforate anus	2	–
Volvulus	–	4
Meconium peritonitis	1	2
Meconium ileus	–	2
Perforation	2	–
Annular pancreas	2	–
Atresia of the bile ducts	3	–

Table 3 Associated abnormalities outside the gastro-intestinal tract at Royal Alexandra Hospital for Children

	Duodenum	Jejunum	Ileum
Number of children	24	11	7
Urogenital	7	–	–
Musculoskeletal	4	2	–
Down's syndrome	11	–	–
Cardiovascular	6	–	–

Congenital intrinsic duodenal obstruction. When duodenal obstruction is complete, vomiting usually occurs within a few hours of birth and is characteristically bile-stained except when the obstruction is proximal to the ampulla of Vater. Vomiting does not occur when there is an accompanying oesophageal atresia, a well-recognized association of this disorder. Meconium at first may be passed normally and there may be no obvious epigastric distension. In view of the frequent association with other abnormalities outside the gastrointestinal tract these should be sought for carefully, once the diagnosis has been established. In particular the infant should be examined carefully for evidence of Down's syndrome. This is an important association of this syndrome and occurs in 20–30 per cent of cases.

When obstruction is incomplete the symptoms may be intermittent and the diagnosis delayed.

Congenital intrinsic duodenal obstruction may be accompanied by an annular pancreas. This is a congenital disorder in which the pancreas grow around the second part of the duodenum and rarely occurs in isolation. Indeed it is a sign of failure of duodenal development rather than an obstructive lesion *per se*. It may accompany intrinsic duodenal atresia, a duodenal diaphragm, or sometimes malrotation with Ladd's bands. In children with duodenal atresia at operation it often looks as if there is an annular pancreas because there is inter-position of the pancreas between the two ends of the duodenal atresia.

Congenital intrinsic duodenal obstruction is not in general associated with multiple atresias in the remainder of the small intestine.

Jejuno-ileal obstruction. Symptoms, typically vomiting and abdominal distension, usually occur within the first two days of life. When obstruction is complete, once the initial meconium has been passed, there is no further stool.

In some infants no meconium is passed at all. When obstruction is incomplete the diagnosis may again be long delayed and the child may present with intermittent vomiting, abdominal distension, and even with features of malabsorption, and a clinical picture that may resemble coeliac disease.

Diagnosis. Plain X-ray of the abdomen is usually diagnostic in infants who present acutely. In duodenal atresia there is the characteristic 'double bubble' (Fig. 2). When duodenal obstruction is incomplete there may be small amounts of air in the lower bowel. A barium meal may be useful to demonstrate associated malrotation which could suggest additional extrinsic pressure causing obstruction due to Ladd's bands.

When there is complete jejuno-ileal obstruction, there are usually dilated loops of small intestine apparent on plain X-ray of the abdomen and there is no colonic gas. A barium enema may reveal an unused microcolon. When obstruction is incomplete a barium follow-through may be needed to establish the diagnosis. Laparotomy may be the final court of appeal in these circumstances.

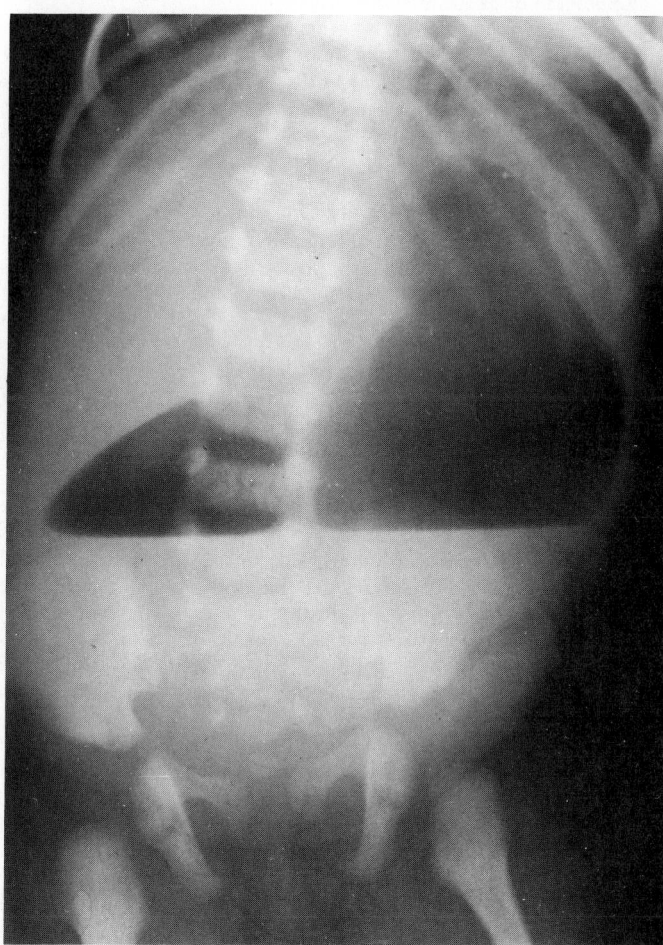

Fig. 2 Plain X-ray of the abdomen of an infant with duodenal atresia showing characteristic 'double bubble'.

Management. Delay in diagnosis leads to poor surgical results. Unfortunately, such delay sometimes occurs because of the lack of appreciation of the significance of bile-stained vomiting in the first 24 hours of life and, therefore, failure to ask for a surgical opinion.

Correction of fluid and electrolyte disturbances, if present, should precede surgery. At laparotomy, care should be taken to exclude any accompanying gastrointestinal abnormality. In duodenal obstruction, the operation of choice is duodeno-duodenostomy or duodeno-jejunostomy. Some surgeons use a feeding enterostomy during the immediate post-operative period. A gastrostomy is used to drain the stomach. In jejuno-ileal lesions, resection is obviously indicated but there should be adequate resection of the proximal dilated gut as, post-operatively, gut immediately proximal to an atresia may remain flabby and dilated with in effective peristalsis.

It is recommended that 10–15 cm of the proximal blind end of jejuno-ileal atresias and 2–3 cm of the distal end should be resected. This reduces the great discrepancy is size between the two blind ends and so facilitates end-to-end anastomosis, although an oblique-to-end anastomosis is still sometimes necessary.

Despite these manoeuvres, post-operative diarrhoea may occur and this may be related to the stagnant loop syndrome producing sugar malabsorption acutely in the post-operative period or steatorrhoea months or even years later. Sometimes further surgery is necessary to correct this complication by resecting the area of proximally dilated bowel where there is stasis of gut contents above the previous anastomosis. So unfortunately surgical treatment of this disorder may often result in considerable shortening of the bowel, especially when multiple atresias are present.

Duplication of gastrointestinal tract

Definition. Duplications are cystic or tubular structures whose lumen is linked by a mucous membrane, usually supported by smooth muscle. They occur most often within the dorsal mesentery of the gut. They are also sometimes described as enteric cysts, neurenteric cysts, and reduplications, but the term duplications seems the most suitable, taking into account their alimentary tract but they are found most often in relation to the small intestine, particularly the ileum. Only occasionally do they communicate directly with the gastrointestinal tract. Duplications may be found in association with intestinal atresias. Sometimes those in association with small intestine may be lined by gastric mucosa and peptic ulceration and bleeding may occur. Those associated with the colon never have ectopic gastric mucosa.

Clinical features. These are congenital malformations that present most often in early infancy. They may present later in childhood but far less often, but may even occasionally present in adult life. Duplications may present in infancy as small intestinal obstruction, sometimes by the production of an intussusception. A palpable abdominal mass in infancy as well as rectal bleeding and volvulus may also be modes of presentation of this disorder. The clinical diagnosis is often difficult and the diagnosis may sometimes be made only on laparotomy. A technetium scan may be helpful diagnostically by demonstrating ectopic gastric mucosa. Some cases may present as a posterior thoracic space occupying lesion and frequently may go through the diaphragm and may be related to an extensive upper small intestinal duplication as well.

Small intestinal malrotation with or without volvulus. Malrotation of the small intestine is due to disordered movement of the intestine around the superior mesenteric artery during the course of embryological development.

Two main abnormalities that produce clinical syndromes may occur. First, there is a gross narrowing of the fixation of the mesentery which may allow the midgut to twist around and cause a volvulus. This may occur acutely, causing complete obstruction, or it may occur intermittently producing bouts of partial or complete obstruction which may at times release themselves spontaneously. Secondly, there may be partial duodenal obstruction from extrinsic compression of the small intestine by peritoneal bands (Ladd's bands) which extend from the caecum or hepatic flexure.

Malrotation may also be associated with duodenal atresia or stenosis. It may also be found in association with diaphragmatic hernia, omphalocele, and gastroschisis. However, malrotation may not produce symptoms and may sometimes be discovered only as an incidental finding on a barium study. The majority of children who develop symptoms related to malrotation do so within the neonatal period, presenting with features of intestinal obstruction, complete or incomplete. When there is volvulus there may also be obstruction to the blood supply to the bowel which, if complete, will lead to extensive gangrene of the small bowel with perforation and peritonitis. The passage of melaena stools may be an early sign of their complication.

Those children with malrotation who present later in childhood may do so with features of intermittent obstruction such as episodes of vomiting, often bile-stained, and abdominal pain, but sometimes they may manifest with features of malabsorption and many clinical features suggestive of coeliac disease. This is due to intestinal stasis with bacterial overgrowth in the lumen of the small intestine. Such steatorrhoea may be accompanied at times by protein-losing enteropathy due to obstructing of the mesenteric lymphatics and sometimes chylous ascites may also be found.

Diagnosis. The diagnosis needs to be considered in the differential diagnosis of small intestinal obstruction in infancy.

Plain X-ray of the abdomen may be very useful, typically revealing some distension of the stomach and duodenum, but unlike duodenal atresia this is accompanied by some gas scattered through the lower part of the abdomen. However, volvulus of the midgut may not be accompanied by any abnormality on plain X-ray of the abdomen and a barium meal and follow-through study may then be necessary to reveal the presence of malrotation. A barium enema may be useful to demonstrate the presence of malrotation of the colon by the position of the caecum and thus suggest accompanying malrotation of the small intestine, but a barium follow-through is often more useful, although in chronic cases repeated barium study may be necessary to make the diagnosis.

Management. Surgical intervention is indicated when symptoms occur and resection of the gut may be necessary when there is strangulation. Ladd's operation is usually the procedure of choice. This involves, in general, the placement of the caecum on the left and the small intestine on the right, having divided any bands and adhesions between the duodenum and large bowel and by dissection broadened the base of the mesentery as much as possible.

Small intestinal lymphangiectasia (See also pages 12.89 and 12.99.) The syndrome of idiopathic hypoproteinaemia without proteinuria and with normal hepatic function has been shown to result from excessive loss of plasma proteins into the alimentary tract. Dilation of the small intestinal lymphatics, usually known as lymphangiectasia, has been a frequent finding in many infants with this syndrome.

Small intestinal lymphangiectasia has been described as a primary or congenital abnormality or as a secondary manifestation of some other disease process such as constrictive pericarditis. The primary abnormality may be accompanied by generalized lymphatic abnormalites outside the alimentary tract, including lymphoedema, chylous ascites, and hypoplasia, or aplasia of the peripheral lymphatic system but the lymphatic abnormality may be confined to the small bowel and its mesentery. It is usually, but not invariably, accompanied by hypoproteinaemic oedema. Radioisotope studies in these patients have demonstrated that the hypoproteinaemia is due to abnormal protein loss into the gut. The pathogenesis of the hypoproteinaemia in such patients has been attributed to the rupture of dilated lymphatic channels or to protein exudation from intestinal capillaries via an intact epithelium, where there is obstruction of lymphatic flow.

Clinical features. It is a rare condition which may present throughout life, but most often in the first two years of life with diarrhoea and failure to thrive and, later, generalized oedema with hypoproteinaemia. The clinical picture may closely resemble coeliac disease.

Characteristically, these patients are found on investigation to have lymphopenia in the presence of a normal bone marrow and extreme reduction of serum albumin and serum immunoglobulins, in particular serum IgG, and carrier proteins such as protein-bound iodine. Owing to the lymphopenia and immunoglobulin deficiency, there is increased susceptibility to infection. The severe protein loss may be accompanied by enteric calcium loss leading to hypocalcaemia. Steatorrhoea is also found in this disorder (page 12.99).

Diagnosis. The diagnosis is established definitively by demonstrating the characteristic lymphatic abnormality on small intestinal biopsy, i.e. dilated lacteals. However, the lesion is patchy and one negative biopsy does not exclude the diagnosis. The radioisotope demonstration of abnormal enteric protein loss using a technique such as intravenous $^{51}CrCl_3$ is helpful in diagnosis but is not specific.

Barium studies in most cases show coarse mucosal folds without dilation of the small intestine.

Pathology. Post-mortem studies reveal a considerable variation in the distribution of the lymphatic abnormality along the length of the small intestine. Indeed dilated lacteals may occur irregularly along the entire length of the small bowel and there may be large globular structures which are made up of grossly dilated lymphatics projecting into the lumen.

Lymphatic proliferation and dilatation may also occur within the mesentery, as well as the serous, muscular, and submucosal layers of the small intestinal wall. This overgrowth of lymph vessels may also extend into the lymph nodes and occupy part of the nodal tissue.

Treatment. This is usually dietetic, since the lymphangiectasia is rarely localized enough to allow surgical excision of the involved gut in order to effect a permanent cure. The basis of dietetic management is to limit the amount of long-chain fat in the diet which is normally absorbed via the intestinal lymphatics. This leads to a reduction in the volume of intestinal lymph and to the pressure within the dilated lymphatics. It is best done by placing the child on a low fat diet (5–10 g/day) and adding medium-chain triglycerides, instead of the usual long-chain dietary fats, in unrestricted amounts. A milk containing medium-chain triglyceride such as Pregestimil may be used with medium-chain triglyceride oil for cooking. A diet based on medium-chain triglycerides usually leads to a clinical remission, but some children may be resistant to this dietetic therapy when the abnormality is very extensive and, on occasion, death may result despite therapy. Albumin infusions are of little value in management as their benefit is so transitory. Corticosteroids have been advocated for severe cases but there is little evidence to justify their use in these circumstances.

A follow-up study of children has shown that, although there was a continuing chyle leak, as evidenced by persistent lymphopenia and hypoalbuminaemia, a rapid and sustained improvement in dependent oedema following the use of the diet recommended above, although asymmetrical oedema from peripheral lymphatic abnormalities was unaffected. Their growth rate improved on the diet. Clinical relapse occurred quickly when the diet was relaxed. Continued adherence to a strict diet, at least through puberty is, therefore, recommended. Indeed it seems probable that this is a life-long disorder and that dietetic managment may usually need to be permanent.

Surgical resection can offer some hope when the lesions are localized to one part of the small intestine, but this may be difficult to determine even at laparotomy, and localization seems to be an unusual event in this disorder.

Meckel's diverticulum. This diverticulum is the vestigial remnant of the vitello-intestinal duct. Although most people who have such a diverticulum are asymptomatic, complications may arise which may present in a variety of ways. In children these complications chiefly arise in association with the presence of ectopic gastric mucosa in the diverticulum. Other ectopic tissue, for example, pancreatic tissue and coloric mucosa, may be found in some causes.

The diverticulum is located in the distal ileum within 100 cm of the ileocaecal valve. It is always antimesenteric in position.

Clinical features. Rectal bleeding is the main symptom. This is usually the passage of bright blood rather than tarry melaena stools. Typically the stool is at first dark in colour but later bright red. Bleeding may be acute with shock requiring urgent blood transfusion or it may be chronic. From a practical viewpoint any child who has a massive painless rectal bleed should be regarded as having Meckel's diverticulum until proved otherwise. Most often bleeding

from a Meckel's diverticulum is associated with ulceration of ectopic gastric mucosa but this is not always the case as such bleeding on occasion may occur in the absence of ectopic gastric mucosa.

Small intestinal obstruction may also be a mode of presentation. This may be as a volvulus, intussusception with diverticulum as the leading part, or as acute diverticulitis which may produce a picture indistinguishable from acute appendicitis.

Diagnosis and management. This depends upon the mode of presentation. When rectal bleeding occurs other causes such as anal fissure, volvulus, intussusception, peptic ulcer, and colonic polyps must be considered. Investigation may include colonoscopy to exclude colonic causes and upper endoscopy to exclude peptic ulceration, etc.

Barium follow-through is usually an unrewarding investigation but introduction of barium via a duodenal tube may be more successful. Angiography to exclude a haemangiomatous malformation may sometimes be done but a technetium scan is usually the most important investigation. The radionuclide $^{99}Tc^m$ concentrates in the gastric mucosa. When it is given intravenously, ectopic gastric mucosa appears as an abnormal localization on abdominal imaging with a gamma-ray camera. In this way a Meckel's diverticulum with ectopic gastric mucosa or indeed a duplication with such ectopic tissue may be diagnosed. However, although the use of this technique should lead to an earlier and more accurate diagnosis of Meckel's diverticulum, a negative result in a child with severe bleeding should not deter a surgeon from proceeding with a diagnostic laparotomy which even now remains the final diagnostic test.

Indeed, when considering the other modes of presentation of Meckel's diverticulum, it is often only at laparotomy that the role of a Meckel's diverticulum in the child's intestinal obstruction is appreciated.

Meconium ileus (see page 12.166.) This is a manifestation of cystic fibrosis. Meconium ileus is the earliest mode of presentation of this disorder during the neonatal period. A similar syndrome in older children and young adults who have cystic fibrosis may occur. It is usually known as the *meconium ileus equivalent*. The abnormally viscid consistency of the meconium is usually believed to account for this syndrome. It may result from several factors, including the lack of pancreatic enzymes during fetal life, which may, in turn, account for its high protein content, a characteristic of the meconium from these children. There is also evidence of reduced secretion of water and electrolytes in such infants which may further render the meconium more viscid. The meconium, because of its high viscosity, cannot be propelled along the bowel and so small intestinal obstruction results. This occurs most often in the distal ileum.

Clinical features. The neonate with this disorder usually develops signs of intestinal obstruction within the first 24–48 hours of life and with the classical signs of bile-stained vomiting, progressive abdominal distension, and scant or absent meconium. In simple meconium ileus the meconium is the sole source of the obstruction but meconium ileus may be complicated by perforation of the gut, and when this occurs *in utero*, small calcified areas in the peritoneum may be observed on plain X-ray of the abdomen, providing evidence of complications former meconium peritonitis. Such perforation may also occur in the neonatal period. Volvulus and atresia may also complicate meconium ileus.

Sudden acute abdominal distension, especially when accompanied by signs of tympany or ascites, strongly suggests this diagnosis. Plain X-ray of the abdomen may show a dilated bowel but unaccompanied by many fluid levels. Sometimes there is a homogenous shadow in the region of the lower ileum with a stippled appearance. If a Gastrografin enema is done, a microcolon, a consequence of disuse, may be demonstrated. The finding of such an X-ray appearance in the presence of a family history of cystic fibrosis makes the diagnosis of meconium ileus highly probable but the situation may be confused when there is an associated ileal astresia.

Management. When meconium ileus is complicated by atresia or perforation, gangrene, peritonitis, or associated volvulus, surgical intervention is essential. In these circumstances resection of the affected segments with an end-to-side anastomosis is usually the treatment of choice, the distal end being brought to the surface as an ileostomy (Bishop Koop). Various irrigations through the ileostomy have been advocated, including pancreatic enzymes, mucolytic agents such as acetyl cysteine, and the industrial detergent 'Tween 80'. Non-operative treatment of uncomplicated meconium ileus, using enemata containing such agents, has been advocated for some time but only relatively recently has such non-operative management been widely employed with success. Noblett in Melbourne, in 1969, advocated the use of Gastrografin enemata to relieve intraluminal obstruction. Gastrografin is a radio-opaque hypertonic solution that is effective because of its tonicity. This technique should not be used until: (a) plain X-ray of the abdomen has failed to demonstrate any calcification, free gas, or fluid in the peritoneal cavity; (b) a barium enema has excluded Hirschsprung's disease and demonstrated a microcolon extending to the proximal colon; and (c) the retrograde passage of contrast medium through the ileocaecal valve has demonstrated an obstructing meconium mass with a proximal dilated ileum, thus excluding ileal atresia.

Although there may be no signs clinically or radiologically of pulmonary complications at this stage, immediate, cautious physiotherapy of the chest and inhalation therapy should be started together with vigorous treatment of chest infections with antibiotics when they occur (as for older children with cystic fibrosis). A pancreatic enzyme preparation should also be started, at first in small dosage when milk feedings have begun. The child's ultimate prognosis depends upon the prognosis of his cystic fibrosis. This diagnosis should be confirmed by sweat electolyte estimations, which is the corner stone for diagnosis of cystic fibrosis. Concentrations of sweat sodium above 60 mmol/l are definitely abnormal (see p.12.166).

Congenital short intestine. There is a syndrome of congenital short intestine in association with malrotation with clinical features like those following massive intestinal resection. There is also another syndrome of congenital short intestine in association with pyloric hypertrophy and malrotation. This latter syndrome is due to an absence or diminution of argyrophil ganglion cells in the small intestinal wall. These cells normally organize peristalsis and ensure that the bolus move forward at the correct speed. In the absence of such innervation, smooth muscle of the small intestinal wall contracts spontaneously and rhythmically, but segmentation is not co-ordinated and the food bolus does not move forward, and there is work hypertrophy of smooth muscle.

Both syndromes are rare and often are only diagnosed at laparotomy.

Colonic atresia. Atresia of the large intestine is rare. In any series of cases of intestinal atresias, less than 10 per cent will have isolated colonic atresia.

Clinical features. The baby presents in the first 24–48 hours with marked abdominal distension, vomiting, and failure to pass meconium.

Diagnosis. Abdominal X-rays reveal multiple dilated loops of bowel with fluid levels, the position of the loops may suggest a large bowel obstruction. Confirmation of the level of the atresia is obtained by barium enema.

Management. Nasogastric suction and intravenous fluids are commenced pre-operatively. At laparotomy the lesion may be an isolated atresia or associated with multiple atresias of small and large

bowel. If the atresia is solitary, it may be possible to perform an anastomosis after resection of the atresia and a length of the grossly dilated proximal bowel. Frequently a colostomy is performed to allow the dilated proximal bowel to contract before performing an end-to-end anastomosis some weeks later.

Hirschsprung's disease. In this condition ganglion cells are absent in the bowel wall. The distal rectum is always aganglionic and the aganglionosis extends proximally for a variable distance.

In 70 per cent the rectosigmoid is involved, in 20 per cent the colon is involved proximal to the sigmoid, and in 10 per cent the aganglionosis extends proximally into the small intestine. The aganglionic bowel is incapable of co-ordinated peristalsis and passively constricts resulting in a mechanical obstruction. The incidence is approximately 1 in 5000 births.

Clinical features. Hirschsprung's disease is not associated with a high incidence of prematurity, and the majority of the babies have a birth weight appropriate for gestational age. This contrasts sharply with most of the other congenital alimentary tract obstructions. Associated abnormalities are rare. The most important association is with Down's syndrome.

Symptoms of Hirschsprung's disease are present in the first few days of life in almost all cases. Exceptionally a baby will have no symptoms during the early neonatal period. The major symptoms are failure to pass meconium within 36 hours of birth, abdominal distension, vomiting, and poor feeding. These may occur simply or in combination. Frequently a rectal examination will relieve the obstruction by passively dilating the aganglionic segment. The significance of these early symptoms is often not appreciated and 20–50 per cent of patients with Hirschsprung's disease are not diagnosed in the early weeks of life. Later presentation is with constipation which dates back to the neonatal period. It is not accompanied by soiling and is frequently associated with failure to thrive. Presentation may be delayed for months or years. Hirschsprung's enterocolitis may be the mode of presentation in the infant of a few weeks of age. This condition, the precise aetiology of which is unknown, presents with abdominal distension, profuse diarrhoea and circulatory collapse. The infant is gravely ill and the mortality is 20 per cent. The child with this complication successfully treated initially may have absorptive problems for some time, suffer recurrent episodes of enterocolitis despite successful surgery and the surgery is attended by a higher rate of complications. The incidence of enterocolitis can be greatly reduced if the diagnosis of Hirschsprung's disease is made in the first week of life.

Diagnosis. In the neonatal period a plain abdominal X-ray will reveal distension of small and large bowel. A barium enema may show the narrow aganglionic bowel with dilated proximal bowel but a normal barium enema does not exclude Hirschsprung's disease (Fig. 3). A 24-hour film showing retained barium in the colon is often more helpful than the actual enema in confirming the clinical suspicion of Hirschsprung's disease. The definitive diagnostic procedure is a rectal biopsy. Suction biopsy enables the pathologist to look for ganglion cells in the submucosal plexus, a full thickness biopsy providing the intermyenteric plexus as well but this is usually unnecessary. In Hirschsprung's disease ganglion cells are absent, hypertrophied nerve trunks are present, and if a histochemical stain for acetylcholinesterase is used, this reveals excessive amounts of this enzyme in the bowel wall. Anorectal manometry in Hirschsprung's disease typically shows failure of relaxation of the internal sphincter in response to rectal distension but this reflex is frequently absent in normal-term babies until after the second week of life. This method of diagnosis is therefore unreliable in the neonatal period, requires considerable expertise to obtain reliable results, and cannot be regarded as suitable for the routine diagnosis of Hirschsprung's disease.

Management. Having established the diagnosis, the initial pro-

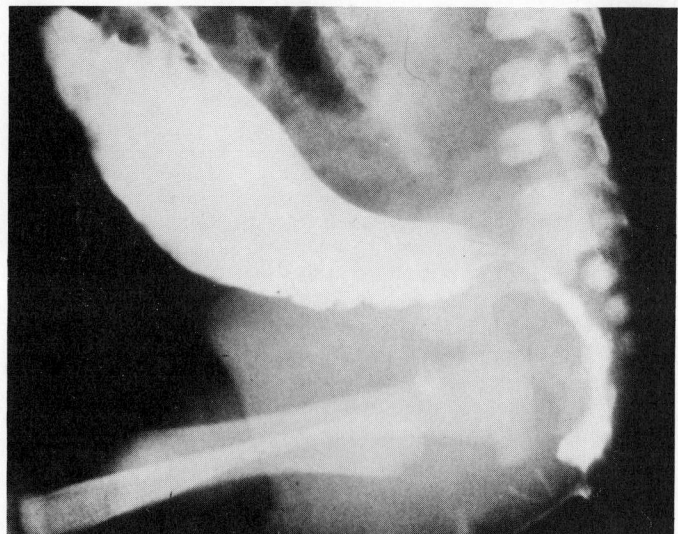

Fig. 3   Barium enema in Hirschsprung's disease illustrating a narrow aganglionic rectum with dilatation proximally.

cedure in the majority of patients is a colostomy performed in ganglionic bowel to relieve the obstruction and allow the dilated hypertrophied proximal bowel to return to normal. If the diagnosis is made in the neonatal period, the colostomy is left for four to 12 months to allow the child to reach a reasonable size. Definitive surgery consists of excision of aganglionic bowel with a 'pull through' procedure enabling an anastomosis to be performed between the anus and ganglionic colon. The three operations most often performed are those described by Swenson, Duhamel, and Soave. Providing the surgery is uncomplicated, the long-term complications, which include faecal and urinary incontinence and impotence, should be minimal. Bowel control is likely to be imperfect for a number of years with soiling as a major problem but good bowel control will be achieved in the majority of patients treated by experienced surgeons.

Imperforate anus. The exact incidence of these abnormalities is not known but the usual incidence quoted is 1 in 5000 births. The basic classification differentiates between the high anomalies, where the bowel terminates above the pelvic floor, the bowel narrowing down to communicate with the urethra in the male—a recto-urethral fistula—and the vagina in the female—a rectovaginal fistula—in the majority of cases. In the low anomalies, the bowel passes through the pelvic floor and either terminates in an abnormal perineal position, or just beneath the perineal skin-covered anus. The high anomaly is more likely to occur in boys, the low anomaly in girls. Overall, more boys than girls present with an imperforate anus. Associated anomalies of the urogenital tract, oesophagus, heart, and skeletal system are common.

Clinical features. Early examination of the perineum will establish the presence of an anorectal anomaly. In the male the presence of meconium on the perineum indicates a low anomaly. In the female careful inspection is necessary to differentiate meconium being passed per vaginum, indicating a high anomaly, from meconium emerging from a perineal site suggesting a low anomaly. Careful probing of any opening will enable the direction in which the bowel is running to be established. In the female doubt about the precise anatomy of the anomaly may be resolved by contrast studies. In the male differentiating a completely covered anus from a high anomaly may be difficult in the early hours after birth. Examination of the urine microscopically may reveal the presence of squamous cells or debris, suggesting a fistula between bowel and urethra. Occasionally meconium is passed per urethra.

A film of the inverted baby's pelvis with the blind-ending bowel outlined with air may indicate the level (Fig. 4) but this film cannot

be reliably interpreted in the first few hours after birth because air may not have reached the distal bowel. A micturating cysto-urethrogram will demonstrate a recto-urethral fistula in a high proportion of cases, but is rarely necessary in the neonate. Having defined the nature of the anorectal anomaly, evidence of any associated abnormality should be sought by careful clinical examination and X-rays of chest, abdomen and the vertebral column.

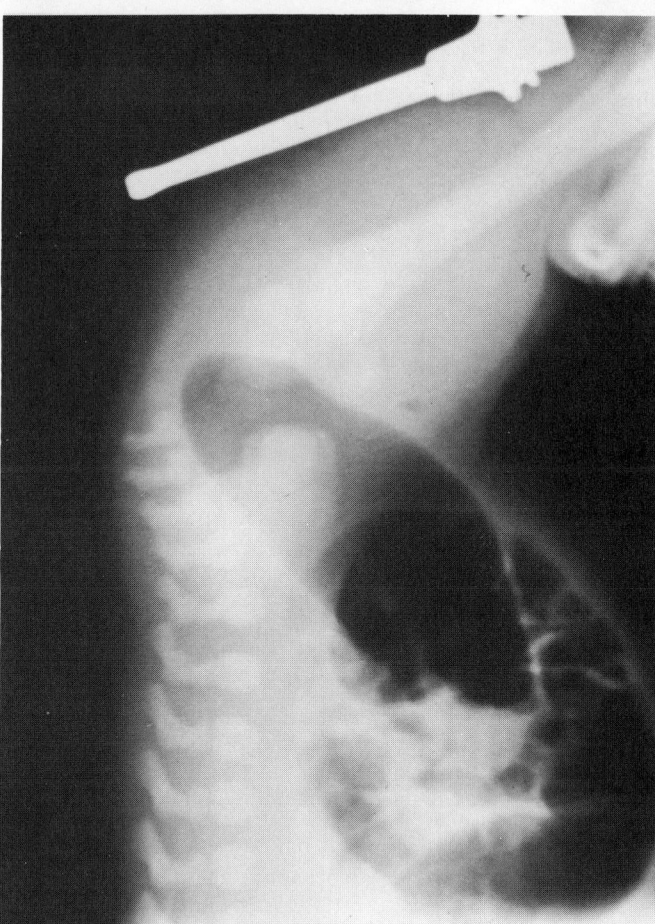

Fig. 4   Inverted X-ray with a marker on the anus and air outlining the dilated colon terminating above the pelvic floor—a 'high' anomaly.

Management. A low anomaly usually requires a perineal procedure to enlarge the opening. Dilatation alone may suffice but in the majority of cases a simple anoplasty produces a more satisfactory result. In the long term the functional results for the low anomalies should be very good. A high anomaly necessitates a defunctioning colostomy in the neonatal period. The fistula is divided and the bowel pulled through the puborectalis sling to the perineum when the infant is six to 12 months old. Delay in achieving bowel control is common and a number of secondary operations designed to improve control have been advocated. However, if the initial surgery is meticulous and the importance of the puborectalis sling is recognized, acceptable continence should be achieved in over 80 per cent of children within the first 10 years. A permanent colostomy should rarely be necessary. The high incidence of associated genito-urinary abnormalities makes it mandatory to investigate carefully the urinary tract at an early stage. The mortality for anorectal anomalies is largely dictated by the presence of other serious abnormalities.

Reference

Rickham, P. P., Lister, J., and Irving, I. M. (1978). *Neonatal surgery*. Butterworth, London.

The appendix, the peritoneum, and omentum

E. G. Lee

This section deals with parts of the body in which diseases are usually thought to be diagnosed and treated almost exclusively by surgeons. However, it is often the general practitioner who is faced with the initial diagnosis of many of the common diseases of the region. A prime example is acute appendicitis, the diagnosis of which may be very difficult. In addition many chronic lesions which require surgical treatment may first be seen by a general physician or gastroenterologist.

The appendix

It has been estimated that up to 12 per cent of the population of western countries will suffer an acute attack of appendicitis at some time during their lives (Ashley 1967).

In a recent survey carried out by the OMGE (*Organization Mondiale de Gastroenterologica*) it was concluded from reports of acute appendicitis in 10 different countries that the disease presents in roughly the same fashion throughout the world and that the mortality is still significant. There were 27 deaths in the 6097 patients studied (0.5 per cent) (De Dombal 1979). In the United Kingdom more than 80 000 people are admitted to hospital each year with appendicitis.

Development and structure. The appendix develops as a blind out-pouching of the fetal caecum, and it occasionally grows with it. More commonly the antimesenteric and anterior sides of the caecum grow more rapidly, causing the organ to remain as a vestigal structure and to lie in its typical posteromedial position. Numerous variations of size, shape, and position can occur. It may even lie on the right side of the abdomen when malrotation or total intestinal transposition occurs.

Because of the asymetrical growth of the caecum opposite the ileocaecal valve, the base of the appendix usually lies retrocaecally, but its tip can be found in a variety of positions. Wakeley (1933) recorded the frequency of different positions in 10 000 specimens. In the adult the commonest sites are retrocaecal or pelvic, but rarely the organ can lie in front or behind the ileum or it may point straight downwards into the abdominal cavity. Quite apart from the obvious importance to the surgeon during an appendicectomy operation, these anatomical positions have a clinical significance, since the symptoms and mode of presentation of acute appendicitis may differ as a result of the site of the organ.

The structure of its wall is not different from the caecum apart from the narrowness of its lumen, the particular richness of its lymphoid follicles, and the fact that lymphatic channels in the submucosa tend to run in a longitudinal direction. The organ probably has little function but some authors have suggested that the numerous follicles may indicate that it has important immunological activity in the gut, at least during the first three decades of life when the lymphoid tissue is such a prominent feature.

Acute appendicitis
Aetiology. There is still considerable discussion about the reasons why the appendix should so commonly become infected. The fact that its lumen is open to the faeces and pathogenic organisms of the colon must play an important role, but the main factor that has been implicated is blockage of the lumen by faecolith, by hypertrophy of lymphoid follicles, or by fibrous stricture. This is made more likely by its narrow lumen. Abnormalities of its shape or position (such as occurs for example when a short appendicular artery holds the organ up retro-ileally) may predispose to infection because of kinking causing obstruction.

Diet appears to be an important factor in the aetiology of infection. Evidence is accumulating that acute appendicitis is much lower in communities on a high residue diet such as was the rule in Africa. The relationship of diet and race to the incidence of appendicitis has been the subject of discussion for a considerable time. As long ago as 1896 Matas reported that 'iliac phlegmons' were less common in the southern states of America than in the north, and that blacks in northern states had a lower incidence of the disease than did whites. This does not appear to be due to a genetic factor because when American blacks began moving to the north of the USA in large numbers, an increasing incidence of appendicitis occurred (Burkitt 1971). Burkitt has also described an increase of the disease in Africa associated with the adoption of a Western diet. Walker et al. (1973) reported the prevalence of appendicitis in South African students from different racial backgrounds, and ascribed the higher incidence to a lower intake of diet fibre. They also found a marked difference in different social groups. In one study they reported an annual rate of appendicitis of 7.8 cases per 1000 population of privileged white students eating a typical Western diet, but only 1.8 cases per 1000 in an underprivileged group of white students on a high fibre diet. These findings are comparable with those recorded in 1946 by Short in this country in his monograph on the causation of appendicitis when he compared the incidence of appendicitis in children from a public school with that of children in a local orphanage. It has also been shown that increasing the dietary fibre in a modern western society can reduce the incidence of appendicitis.

Age and sex. Acute appendicitis can occur at any age but it is rare in infants. The incidence rises rapidly in children above the age of five years and reaches a peak during the second and third decades. The disease is not uncommon in the elderly and can occur in extreme old age. Some authors have reported a sex difference in the younger age group (15–25 years) where it may be twice as common amongst males.

Diagnosis. The disease continues to produce a classical syndrome in the majority of patients and it can usually be diagnosed with little difficulty from the history and findings on physical examination. Nevertheless it is frequently misdiagnosed. This leads on the one hand to a large number of unnecessary operations, and on the other to a high morbidity and a significant mortality especially if operation is delayed until the appendix has perforated.

It is most commonly misdiagnosed at the extremes of life. Graham et al. (1980) reviewed more than 1000 children with appendicitis who were admitted to hospital during a 22-year period. During the last two years of their study there was a marked fall in the post-operative mortality, but a significant morbidity still occurred if the appendix was found at operation to be perforated. The over-all perforation rate was high (63 per cent), and had not fallen over the years. An interesting point was that nearly half of the children had been treated medically for some condition other than appendicitis which the community physicians failed to diagnose. Of the patients so treated, 83 per cent were found at operation to have a perforation.

The diagnostic accuracy may be even worse in the elderly. A high proportion, 40 per cent, of older patients may present with atypical symptoms and signs, and the majority of these may have a perforation of the appendix when operated upon. Women who develop acute appendicitis during the last trimester of pregnancy often present the clinician with a difficult diagnostic problem because the enlarging uterus progressively displaces the caecum so that the pain and tenderness may eventually become localized in the flank where they can easily be mistaken as the signs of an infection of the urinary tract.

Variations of the anatomical position may produce symptoms and signs which are quite different from the classical syndrome which usually occurs if the organ is lying in the retrocaecal, paracaecal, or pelvic positions. Infection in a high retrocolic organ may simulate an infection of the urinary tract because the pain and tenderness may radiate to the back and be associated with psoas spasm. Not infrequently erythrocytes and leucocytes can be found in the urine in quite large numbers. Patients with retro-ileal appendicitis often have little localized pain and tenderness in the abdomen since the parietal peritoneum is protected from irritation by the overlying small bowel which localizes inflammation even if an abscess develops. On the other hand, marked irritation of the ileum may occur and lead to severe diarrhoea and vomiting. The patient may therefore complain of minimal pain but may have symptoms which are strongly suggestive of gastroenteritis. Elderly patients with peritonitis may present as a subacute intestinal obstruction because of intestinal ileus, or with reflex urinary retention due to pelvic peritonitis. Long-standing herniae are sometimes thought to become strangulated if appendicitis develops, because abdominal distention occurs which makes the hernia difficult or impossible to reduce, and it may be associated with marked local pain and tenderness. The latter symptom is the result of peritonitis in the hernial sac.

Natural history of untreated appendicitis. Although making a wrong diagnosis often leads to a perforation, spontaneous resolution of acute appendicitis is possible. In other cases delay may lead to a generalized peritonitis or the development of an abscess in the region where the appendix lies. Bradley and Isaacs (1978) found that 2 per cent of 2621 cases had established abscesses when admitted to hospital. They reported a mortality of 3 per cent in cases with an abscess. Recurrent appendicitis has been reported to occur not infrequently at a later stage, a finding which supports the case for interval appendicectomy when the primary treatment has been by simple drainage of the abscess.

Rarely a delayed diagnosis may result in acute appendicitis progressing to an 'appendix mass'. This term should not simply be used to denote the presence of a lump palpable in the right iliac fossa, but should be restricted to the clinical syndrome in which early symptoms and signs gradually improve as the pain becomes localized in the iliac fossa where a well defined tender mass can be felt, but in which there are no signs of generalized peritonitis or ileus. The pathological lesion consists of a haemorrhagic oedematous mass in the ileo-caecal region and appendix, to which is attached a mass of inflamed matted omentum. This type of lesion is the typical phlegmon of the older literature. Most surgeons consider that surgery is contra-indicated at this stage, because the inflammatory mass may bleed severely if a dissection of the appendix is attempted. The condition is best treated conservatively. Usually the mass diminishes rapidly within four to five days. Whether a short course of antibiotics should be used is a point of great controversy. Foran *et al.* (1978) reported that of 30 patients treated conservatively only four required operation during the hospital admissions because an abscess developed. Jordan *et al.* (1981) have reported appendicectomies being carried out safely in a small number of patients with masses. However, some of the patients they describe appear not to have a lesion which could be classified as an abdominal phlegmon. Small appendicular masses can often be palpated on rectal examination, or bimanual examination or in the abdomen when the patient has been anaesthetized. These mobile masses are not a contra-indication to early appendicectomy.

Most surgeons consider that an interval appendicectomy should be carried out some months later, but recently it has been suggested that since recurrence of appendicitis is less common than previously described and that re-operation is associated with a significant incidence of post-operative complications, most patients should not be treated by operation unless they develop further trouble.

A point of major importance is that a number of other pathological lesions such as caecal carcinoma, Crohn's disease, ileocaecal tuberculosis, and schistosomiasis may produce a lesion which can simulate an appendix mass. Patients with a mass which does not diminish within a short time should be submitted to full intestinal investigations.

Differential diagnosis. So many conditions may simulate an acute appendicitis that it would serve no purpose to set out a full list. In children, mesenteric adenitis, gastroenteritis, Meckel's diverticulitis, intersusception, Henoch–Schönlein purpura, and primary peritonitis are the lesions most commonly misdiagnosed as acute appendicitis.

Non-specific mesenteric adenitis occurs most commonly in adolescence and appears to affect boys more frequently than girls. The cause is still not finally agreed upon but there have been recent reports of specific organisms such as adenovirus being implicated. It may be impossible to differentiate between lymphadenitis and early appendicitis but in the former case the pain is often colicky and enlarged lymph nodes may be palpated in other parts of the body. Occasionally a septic adenitis may occur in the nodes lying along the external iliac vein, due to infection spreading from a focus in the lower limb or some other site of lymphatic drainage. An abscess may develop, which, although retroperitoneal, is easily mistaken for appendicitis because of tenderness becoming localized in the right iliac fossa and because general signs of an infected process develop.

Primary peritonitis occurs most commonly in premenarchecal girls. It is usually due to infection with a pneumococcal organism which has gained access to the peritoneal cavity through the sex passages. After the menarche an increase of acidity in the vagina acts as a barrier to organisms and the condition is then very rare. During recent years there has been a change in the pattern of the disease. An increasing number of cases have been recorded in infants in whom the infection is more common in males.

In adults a host of other conditions may cause diagnostic difficulty. In young women, gynaecological lesions such as ruptured ectopic pregnancy, ovarian cysts undergoing torsion or haemorrhage, *mittelschmerz*, or infection of the Fallopian tubes are commonly misdiagnosed as appendicitis. Urinary tract infections are also found with great frequency. A higher proportion of young men than young women operated on with a history and physical examination suggestive of appendicitis have the disease.

As the age of patients increases, the number of other pathological conditions which can be mistakenly diagnosed as appendicitis increases. The most important of these are: perforated peptic ulcers, infection or perforation of the diverticular disease, and carcinoma of the colon. Rare conditions such as an acute inflammation of a solitary caecal diverticulum and acute and benign ulceration of the caecum are occasionally seen. The latter consists of an acute inflammatory thickening in the caecal wall or opposite the ileocaecal valve, in the centre of which a deep ulcer can be palpated at operation. The aetiology of the condition is obscure but it is known to resolve spontaneously. Surgical treatment should be conservative if it can be diagnosed pre-operatively. If found at operation, it is usually safe to leave this lesion. A hemicolectomy should not be undertaken as it is unnecessary and may well leave unpleasant sequelae such as diarrhoea. Caecal carcinoma or Crohn's disease occasionally perforate and may be mistaken for an acute appendicitis or an appendicular mass.

A problem which is encountered not infrequently is the finding of an acutely inflamed segment of ileum. Some cases of acute ileitis may become typical chronic Crohn's disease but during the last few years it has become recognized that infection with the pseudotuberbulous organism *Yersinia enterocolitica* can cause the inflammation. The diagnosis can be made by finding the organism in stool culture and by complement fixation tests on the serum. Treatment should be conservative because the infection usually resolves without sequelae.

An important problem is that a large number of patients, (particularly young women) who are diagnosed as having acute appendicitis are found at laparotomy to have normal appendices. It has been reported that nearly two-thirds of appendix specimens removed from young women are histologically normal. Many of the cases are probably suffering from the irritable colon syndrome. It is probable that these were the patients who in the past were said to have a grumbling appendix.

Treatment. Appendicectomy at the earliest possible time after onset of the symptoms is the treatment of choice unless the patient presents with an abdominal mass. This usually does not develop before seven to 10 days after the onset of the disease, by which time (if generalized peritonitis has not developed) the inflammation has become so well localized that conservative management is safer than operative treatment. Drainage of an abscess may be required if the infection breaks down into pus, but in many patients a phlegmonous mass resolves spontaneously.

The results of the surgical treatment of appendicitis have improved dramatically during the last few years because of the introduction of more effective antibiotics if peritonitis develops. Recently considerable attention has been directed to the prophylactic use of antibiotics. Foster and his colleagues (1981) halved the incidence of wound infection using a short course of metronidazole and pointed out that a reduction of this magnitude has important clinical and economic consequences for the health services as well as for the patient.

Tumours of the appendix. Benign neoplasms of the appendix are rare. Leiomyoma, fibroma, neuroma, neurofibroma, and ganglioneuroma have been recorded quite frequently but the most common tumour is the carcinoid. Whatever histological variant is found, metastases are rare and the development of a carcinoid syndrome is very uncommon. Other malignant tumours are very uncommon but adenocarcinomas, malignant mucocoele, and a variety of sarcoma have been described.

Tumours usually present as an acute appendicitis or as a mucocoele of the appendix caused by obstruction. Less commonly the tumour may present as an abdominal mass causing pain or obstruction. Occasionally a tumour may be found unexpectedly during a laparotomy for some other condition.

Diseases of the peritoneal cavity

The peritoneal cavity is a mesothelial-lined closed sac which is invaginated from behind by most of the intra-abdominal organs which also have a peritoneal lining on at least two or three surfaces as well as on each side of the vascular pedicles. In the gut these pedicles perform a line of attachment to the back of the bowel known as the mesentery. The sac contains small amounts of fluid which allow the organs to move freely without friction. Under normal circumstances the sac is completely empty in the male except for lubricating fluid, but in women the ovum shed at ovulation passes across the cavity to the tubes.

Peritonitis. Most cases of infective peritonitis are secondary to diseases of intra-abdominal organs. Most commonly, enteric organisms gain entry into the sac by passing through the wall of a diseased organ or by perforation of a hollow viscus. Among the commoner underlying disorders are: necrosis of bowel due to obstruction, infarction, or a neoplasm; inflammatory disease such as appendicitis, diverticulitis, or fulminant ulcerative colitis; and perforation of a peptic ulcer. Less commonly, peritonitis may occur in the absence of an intra-abdominal lesion. For example, patients with cirrhosis or the nephrotic syndrome and ascites are prone to peritonitis; the commonest infecting organism is *E. coli* but the pneumococcus or streptococcus may be implicated.

Bacterial contamination of the peritoneal cavity leads to the production of an exudate, paralytic ileus, and reflex spasm of the abdominal wall muscles. If the condition is not treated early it leads to volume depletion, shock, oliguria, and, occasionally, acute tubular necrosis. Many patients show the characteristic clinical picture of abdominal pain, guarding with rebound tenderness, vomiting, absent bowel sounds, tachycardia, hypotension, and pyrexia. It should be emphasized, however, that these clinical findings are not always present, particularly in the elderly in whom the abdominal findings may be minimal, and a rising pulse rate or falling blood pressure may be the only clues to the diagnosis. Similarly, patients who have been receiving corticosteroids may show very few of the classical signs of peritonitis. Because the peritoneum is often able to 'wall off' an inflammatory process, peritonitis may be restricted to one area of the abdomen over the inflamed or ruptured viscus.

The diagnosis of peritonitis is usually made on the clinical findings together with the history of a preceding abdominal inflammatory disorder. A plain X-ray of the abdomen may show air in the peritoneal cavity. Peritonitis is a major surgical emergency. The patient's general condition should be restored as rapidly as possible using intravenous fluid replacement, and if there is severe volume depletion fresh frozen plasma or fresh blood may be required. A naso-gastric tube should be passed and a broad-spectrum antibiotic regimen using gentamycin and metronidazole should be started. Adequate analgesia is necessary although should be used with care in the early stages of the disease because of the danger of masking the diagnosis. As soon as the patient is fit, surgical exploration should be carried out with appropriate drainage.

Tuberculous peritonitis. The diagnosis and management of this condition is described in Section 5. Unlike acute bacterial peritonitis, the symptoms are usually insidious and consist of fever, anorexia, malaise, and weight loss. In about 70 per cent of cases there is abdominal distension due to ascites; sometimes a mass can be palpated when the fluid has been removed. The diagnosis is made by examination of the peritoneal fluid for its cellular content (see below), biopsy of the peritoneum, or by culture of ascitic fluid or biopsy material.

Fungal and parasitic peritonitis. These rare forms of peritonitis present a similar clinical picture to tuberculous peritonitis. Fungal peritonitis usually occurs in patients who are immunosuppressed, particularly those on corticosteroids. For example, Boyer *et al.* (1976) described 31 cases of peritonitis due to *Candida albicans*; the infection was successfully treated with amphotericin B or 5-fluorocytosine given intraperitoneally or intravenously. Cryptococcal infections have also been reported in immunosuppressed patients. Peritoneal schistosomiasis has been observed occasionally, often stimulating a malignant disease.

Pseudomyxoma peritonei. In this rare condition the peritoneal cavity becomes distended with a semitranslucent mucinous material. It is usually associated with an ovarian tumour, most often a mucinous cystadenoma or cystadenocarcinoma. A few cases secondary to ovarian teratoma or fibromata have been recorded. Clinically, the condition presents with enlargement of the abdomen which is found to contain the characteristic fluid.

Starch-granulomatous peritonitis. Until the early 1950s talc powder, used to reduce stickiness of surgical rubber gloves after sterilization, caused a granulomatous peritonitis which sometimes resulted in adhesions, delayed healing, infection, and the formation of faecal fistulae. More recently a combination of starch and magnesium oxide has been used for treating surgical gloves but even this mixture can occasionally cause a chronic granulomatous peritonitis. The condition is characterized by postoperative fever, pain, and intestinal obstruction which may persist for a considerable time. At laparotomy there may be extensive adhesions with loculate fluid cavities, and the peritoneal lining is studded with granulomata.

Familial paroxysmal peritonitis. This condition, which occurs mainly in ethnic groups from the Mediterranean area, is part of the syndrome of familial polyserositis or familial Mediterranean fever. It is described in Section 23.

Subphrenic abscess. This condition usually arises secondary to a source of infection in the abdomen, especially a perforated appendix or diverticulum, cholecystitis, perforated peptic ulcer, pancreatitis, or as an extension of a hepatic abscess. Occasionally, a subphrenic abscess may occur without an obvious source of inveciton in the abdominal cavity.

The clinical picture is usually characterized by malaise, fever, pain either in the region of the abscess or referred to the shoulder tip, and a polymorphonulcear leucocytosis. In most cases there are minimal physical signs although there may be localized abdominal tenderness and a small pleural effusion on the affected side. Plain X-ray of the abdomen may show gas under the diaphragm and on screening there may be impaired movement of the diaphragm. The diagnosis may be facilitated by ultrasound examination, CT scanning or, occasionally, by gallium-67 scanning. Treatment is by surgical drainage together with appropriate antibiotic therapy.

Ascites. Several mechanisms may lead to accumulation of fluid in the peritoneal cavity. First, there may be an increase in the permeability of the peritoneal capillaries due to inflammatory or neoplastic disease of the peritoneum or of the organs which it covers. Secondly, there may be diminished plasma osmotic colloid pressure due to hypoalbuminaemia such as occurs with the nephrotic syndrome, protein-losing enteropathy, liver disease, or malnutrition. Thirdly, ascites may develop if there is an elevation of the hydrostatic pressure in the hepatic sinusoids. This occurs in patients with cirrhosis, hepatic congestion due to heart failure or constrictive pericarditis, or with inferior vena caval or hepatic vein obstruction. It may also result from portal vein occlusion. In patients with cirrhosis, or in other conditions in which there is an alteration in plasma volume or renal perfusion, ascites may be further aggravated by retention of sodium and water. Finally, ascites may occur in patients with myxoedema or benign ovarian tumours (Meigs' syndrome); the mechanism is unknown. The mechanism of the production of ascites in cirrhosis of the liver and related disorders is considered in detail on page 12.184.

Ascitic fluid is usually classified as either being an 'exudate' i.e. with a protein composition of 2.5 g/dl or more, or as a 'transudate' with a lower protein content. In fact, this is not always useful. Occasionally, 'transudative conditions' such as cirrhosis and congestive cardiac failure are associated with relatively high protein levels. Similarly, malignant ascites may sometimes have a low amount of protein.

Ascites is characterized by an increase in abdominal girth associated with shifting dullness and a fluid thrill. A plain abdominal X-ray may show an opaque appearance. The diagnosis is confirmed by paracentesis. The protein concentration and cellular composition of the fluid should be analysed. A blood-stained fluid usually indicates neoplastic disease; often this can be confirmed by cytological examination. A high polymorphonuclear leucocyte count usually reflects an underlying inflammatory disease although it is found occasionally in malignant disease. A high lymphocyte count is suggestive of tuberculous peritonitis. The fluid should always be cultured for routine organisms, and, when appropriate, for acidfast bacillae. An elevated amylase level is indicative of pancreatic disease. A reduced sugar level (less than 60 mg/100 ml) occurs quite commonly in neoplastic disease.

The management of ascites associated with liver disease is considered on page 12.188. Malignant effusions may be controlled temporarily by the use of intraperitoneal antitumour agents.

Ascites from other causes is managed by treating the underlying disease.

Chylous ascites. This condition is due to the presence of lymph lipoproteins and chylomicrons in the peritoneal cavity. It is diagnosed by finding ascites characterized by a white, turbid fluid on aspiration. Since not all turbid fluid is chylous the diagnosis must be confirmed by analysis of the fluid for neutral fat. It must be distinguished from *pseudochylous ascites* in which there is a turbid fluid due to the presence of cell debris; this is usually associated with neoplasia. In adults, chylous ascites is usually caused by lymphatic obstruction due to lymphoma. An acute form has been described after trauma or rupture of a chylous cyst. In children, the condition may be associated with intestinal lymphangiectasia (page 11.144).

Recurrent chylous ascites together with chylous pleural effusions occur in *lymphoangioleiomyomatosis*, a rare condition affecting young females. The condition is diagnosed by exclusion of other causes of chylous effusions and by characteristic biopsy and lymphangiogram appearances. There are anecdotal reports suggesting that this condition may respond to oophorectomy or to the administration of tamoxifen (Nolvadex).

'Urine ascites'. Urine may accumulate in the peritoneal cavity after trauma or in infants with congenital obstructive lesions of the urinary tract.

Tumours of the peritoneum. The vast majority of tumours in the peritoneal cavity are due to secondary metastases from carcinomas arising in the breast, the lung, the colon, the stomach, the pancreas, the uterus, the ovary, and the liver. Rarely a primary malignant tumour may occur. The commonest of these is a primary mesothelioma. It is an interesting tumour which may occur in the pleura or peritoneal cavity and is associated with exposure to asbestosis. Most males have been found to work in the textile industry, as brake-liners in the motor car industry or as insulators in the building trade, and occasionally on board ship where an asbestos was, at least in the past, widely used.

A number of interesting points have been described about this tumour. If the patient has been exposed to the asbestos for a considerable length of time, in 60–80 per cent of the cases there is evidence on underlying pulmonary asbestosis. Seventeen per cent of the patients have the tumour in the pleura and only 30 per cent develop primary peritoneal mesotheliomata.

Retroperitoneal fibrosis. Since the report of Ormond (1948), a host of reports have appeared describing various aspects of this interesting condition which consists of a marked fibrosis in the tissue of the retroperitoneal space which follows an initial nonsuppurative inflammation characterized by infiltration of lymphocytes, mononuclear cells, and plasma cells (see also section 23). Later, collagen is deposited in association with a marked vascular change. In the end the fibrosis becomes massive, with dense vascular collagen deposition.

Considerable fibrosis may be associated with radiotherapy, tumours (particularly carcinoids), chronic infection, leakage of intestinal contents, urine or blood, chronic lymphangitis, and trauma but the most interesting relationship is with the administration of drugs. The most important of these are methysergide and, more recently, beta-adrenoreceptor antagonists (Committee of Safety of Medicine 1981).

Clinical presentation. The disease can occur at any age although it is most commonly seen during middle age. Pain occurs commonly in the early stages followed by anorexia, fatigue, malaise, loss of weight, and, occasionally, oedema. In the late stages the symptoms result from obstruction to the urinary tract. Less commonly gastrointestinal symptoms may dominate the clinical picture due to obstruction. Fibrosis may involve the duodenum, small intestine, or colon. More frequently, gastrointestinal symptoms are caused by uraemia. Hypertension may be severe.

Diagnosis. The possibility of the disease should be kept in mind when abdominal symptoms and weight loss is associated with a raised ESR. Confirmation is usually made after investigation of the renal tract radiologically or at operation when biopsies should be taken to exclude malignant fibrosis. Treatment is surgical and is aimed at relieving the obstruction to the renal vessels, urinary tract, intestines, or peripheral arteries which rarely can be involved. Corticosteroids are often used post-operatively after ureterolysis in an attempt to prevent further fibrosis.

Diseases of the omentum

Lesions arising primarily in the omentum are rare although the organ is frequently involved with inflammatory or neoplastic disease in the abdominal cavity. Tumours and cysts may occasionally be the cause of abdominal masses.

A rare but interesting lesion is idiopathic segmental infarction of the omentum which may be more common than the 115 cases which have been reported in the English literature since the initial description. The condition may occur in children who develop a progressive peritoneal irritation usually misdiagnosed as acute appendicitis, but it has been reported at any age. Characteristic laparotomy findings are of a wedge-shaped infarction along the right inferior border of the greater omentum. The cause remains obscure but the condition may be associated with torsion of the omentum.

References

Ashley, D. J. B. (1967). Observations on the epidemiology of appendicitis. *Gut* 8, 533.

Bates, B. (1965). Granulomatous peritonitis secondary to corn starch. *Ann. intern. Med.* 62, 335.

Boyer, A. S., Blumenkrantz, J. S., Montgomerie, J. S., Gralpin, J. E., Cobur, J. W., and Guze, L. B. (1976). Candida peritonitis: a report of 22 cases and review of the English literature. *Am. J. Med.* 61, 832.

Bradley, E. L., and Isaacs, J. (1978). Appendiceal abscesses revisited. *Archs Surg.* 113, 130.

Burkitt, D. P. (1971). The aetiology of appendicitis. *Br. J. Surg.* 58, 675.

Carrington, D., Cugeii, D. W., and Gaensler, E. A. (1977). Lymphangioleiomyomatosis. *Am. Rev. Respir. Dis.* 116, 977.

Coder, D. M., and Olander, G. A. (1972). Granulomatous peritonitis caused by starch glove powder. *Archs. Surg.* 105, 83.

Committee of Safety of Medicine (1981). *Current problems*, no.6, July.

Creed, F. (1981). Life events and appendicetomy. *Lancet* i, 1381.

de Dombal F. T. (1979). Acute abdominal pain—an OMGE survey. *Scand. J. Gastroent.* 14, 56, 29.

—, Leaper, D. J., Staniland, J. R., McCann, A. P., and Horrocks, J. C. (1972). Computer aided diagnosis of acute abdominal pain. *Br. med. J.* ii, 9.

Donhauser, J. L. (1957). Primary acute mesenteric lymphadenitis. *Archs. Surg.* 74, 528.

Eisman, B., Sielig, M. G., and Womack, N. A. (1947). Talcum powder granulomata. A frequent and serious post-operative complication. *Ann. Surg.* 126, 820.

Foran, B., Berne, T. V., and Rosoff, L. (1978). Appendiceal abscesses revisited. *Archs Surg.* 113, 130.

Foster, G. E., Burke, J. B., Bolwell, J., Doran, J., Balfour, T. W., Holliday, A., Hardcastle, J. D., and Marshall, D. J. (1981). Clinical and economic consequences of would sepsis after appendicectomy and their modification by metronidazole or providine iodine. *Lancet* i, 769.

Gilmore, O. J. A., Brodribb, A. J. M., and Browett, J. P. (1975). Appendicitis and mimicing conditions. *Lancet* ii, 421.

Graham, J. M. Pokorny, W. J., and Harberg, F. J. (1980). Acute appendicitis in pre-school age children. *Am. J. Surg.* 139, 247.

Jess, P., Bjerregaard, B., Brynitz, S., Holst-Christensen, J., Kalaja, E., and Lund-Kristensen, J. (1981). Acute appendicitis. Prospective trial concerning diagnostic accuracy and complications. *Am. J. Surg.* 141, 232.

Jordan, J. S., Kovalcik, P. J., and Schwab, C. W. (1981). Appendicitis with a palpable mass. *Ann. Surg.* 193, 227.

McDougal, W. S., Izant, R. J., and Zollinger, R. M. (1975). Primary peritonitis in infants and childhood. *Ann. Surg.* 181, 310.

Matas, R. (1896). Iliac phlegmons. *Trans. Ann. Surg. Ass.* 14, 483.

Mosegaard, A., and Nielsen, O. S. (1979). Interval appendicectomy: a retrospective study. *Acta chir. scand.* 145, 109.

Nase, H. W., Kovalcik, P. J., and Cross, G. H. (1980). The diagnosis of appendicitis. *Am. Surg.* 46, 504.

Ormond, J. K. (1948). Bilateral ureteral obstruction due to envelopment and compression by an inflammatory retroperitoneal process. *J. Urol* 59, 1072.

Parsons, J., Gray, J., and Thorbarnson, B. (1970). Pseudomyxoma peritonei. *Archs. Surg.* 101. 545.

Prince, R. L. (1979). Evidence for an aetiological role for adenovirus type 7 in the mesenteric adenitis syndrome. *Med. J. Aust.* 2, 56.

Singh, M., Bhargava, A., and Jain K. (1969). Tuberculous peritonitis. *New Engl. Med. J.* 281, 1091.

Sohar, E., Prass, M., Heller, J., and Heller, H. (1961). Genetics of familial Mediterranean fever (FMF). A disorder with recessive inheritance in non-Ashkenazi Jews and Armenians. *Archs intern. Med.* 107, 529.

—, Gafni, J., Prass, M., and Heller, H. (1967). Familial Mediterranean fever. A survey of 470 cases and review of the literature. *Am. J. Med.* 43, 227.

Tomasian, A., Greenberg, M. S., and Rumeran, H. (1982). Tamoxifen, for lymphangioleiomyomatosis. *N. Eng. J. Med.* 306, 745.

Wakeley, C. P. G. (1933). The position of the vermiform appendix as ascertained by an analysis of 10 000 cases. *J. Anat.* 67, 277.

Walker, A. R. P., Walker B. F., Richardson, B. D., and Woolford, A. (1973). Appendicitis, fibre intake and bowel behaviour in ethnic groups in South Africa. *Post-grad. med. J.* 49, 243.

Watson, N., and Johnson, A. (1973). Cryptococcal peritonitis. *South med. J.* 66, 387.

Miscellaneous disorders of the gastrointestinal tract

D. J. Weatherall and D. P. Jewell

This section reviews some of the conditions which do not fall naturally into any of the other major sections which deal with disorders of the gastrointestinal tract.

Diverticula of the gastrointestinal tract

A diverticulum is a saccular pouch derived from one or more layers of the walls of the gut. With the exception of Meckel's diverticulum which is described on page 12.145, all diverticula seem to be acquired herniations of the mucosa through defects in the muscular wall of the gut. They frequently occur at weak points where vessels penetrate the serosal and muscular layers and hence tend to present later in life and probably result from long-term exposure to high intraluminal pressures.

Oesophagus. Oesophageal diverticula occur at the upper end, the middle, or the lower end of the oesophagus.

The commonest oesophageal diverticulum is the hypopharyngeal or Zenker's diverticulum. This lesion, which is seen in approximately 0.1 per cent of upper gastrointestinal X-rays, affects males over the age of 60 and is thought to represent a pulsion herniation between the fibres of the cricopharyngeal muscle. As it increases in size, it produces a swelling in the lateral part of the neck. If large enough, it may produce dysphagia and there may be spillage of the contents of the diverticulum into the pharynx and larynx leading to aspiration pneumonia and lung abscess formation. The diagnosis is made by barium swallow X-ray. If symptomatic, these lesions should be removed surgically.

The rarer mid-oesophageal or lower oesophageal (epiphrenic) diverticula are usually found by chance on barium swallow investigation and rarely require treatment. The lower oesophageal diverticula are sometimes associated with achalasia (see page 12.42).

Stomach. Gastric diverticula are rare. The most common site is high on the posterior wall of the stomach although occasionally they are found in the prepyloric region and, in this situation, they may result from pyloric stenosis. Gastric diverticula rarely require treatment.

Duodenum. Duodenal diverticula are usually found by chance on barium meal examination. Sometimes they are multiple and they may be associated with colonic diverticulosis. Rarely these diverticula may be associated with post-prandial pain and fullness in the epigastrium and occasionally they cause symptoms due to bleeding or even perforation. Occasionally they may present with obstructive jaundice or acute pancreatitis.

Small bowel. Most small bowel diverticula are asymptomatic. Occasionally they cause surgical complications such as obstruction, volvulus, intussusception, or bleeding. If they are large, small bowel diverticula may result in bacterial overgrowth with the production of a 'blind loop' syndrome (see page 12.94).

Colon. *Diverticulosis coli* is a common condition. Its frequency is strikingly correlated with age, and over the age of 60 approximately a third of the population will have a varying number of colonic diverticula. It is also a condition which has become more frequent during the 20th century and the prevalence in autopsy studies has risen from 5 per cent in 1910 to 50 per cent today. The condition is encountered 40 times more frequently in Western societies than in the developing countries. This difference has been attributed to the high fibre content of the diet in developing countries and it is noteworthy that the incidence of diverticulosis in native Africans or Japanese increases with time if they settle in the Western world.

Diverticular disease is a general term which encompasses diverticulosis, i.e. the presence of diverticula, and diverticulitis which implies frank inflammation or perforation of a diverticulum. The diverticula consist of herniations of mucosa and submucosa through the muscle wall at the points of weakness where blood vessels penetrate from serosa to submucosa. Ninety-five per cent of patients have diverticula of the sigmoid colon. Occasionally they are confined to the right side of the colon but this is uncommon. Solitary diverticula of the caecum or sigmoid may occur.

Pathogenesis. The pathogenesis of diverticulosis is not known. The role of dietary fibre appears to be important since, in epidemiological studies, the prevalence of diverticulosis is inversely correlated with the fibre content of the diet. However, this correlation has not always been found and there is no evidence to suggest that the natural history of diverticular disease is altered by a high fibre diet. Motility studies have shown that patients with diverticular disease show exaggerated sigmoid contractions with the development of areas of high pressure in response to food or cholinergic stimuli. More recent studies have shown that these disturbances in motility correlate with symptoms (i.e. pain) and that patients with asymptomatic diverticulosis have normal motility patterns. Thickening of the circular and longitudinal muscles is frequently associated with diverticula but the relationship between motility and muscle mass is unclear. Indeed, muscle thickening can occur in the absence of diverticula (so-called 'prediverticular' disease) and diverticula can be present in the absence of muscle thickening. Another possible factor in the development of diverticula is collagen. Since the type of collagen in some tissues is known to alter with age, it is conceivable that a similar process occurs in the colon.

Clinical features. The majority of patients with diverticulosis coli are asymptomatic. A few patients develop symptoms which are identical to those of the irritable colon syndrome, namely, abdominal pain associated with alteration of bowel habit—diarrhoea and/or constipation (see page 12.46); some patients have painless diarrhoea. These symptoms are due to motility disturbances and there is no good evidence that they are due to inflammation.

Acute diverticulitis occurs in less than 10 per cent of patients with diverticulosis. It probably occurs as a result of a faecolith becoming impacted in a diverticulum and causing either obstruction to the blood supply or ulceration. The sigmoid colon is almost always the site affected, possibly because the faeces become solid in the sigmoid whereas they are more liquid higher up in the colon. Symptoms may resemble a 'left-sided appendicitis'. There is usually a sudden onset of lower abdominal pain and tenderness associated with fever and constipation. On examination, there is acute tenderness and guarding in the left iliac fossa and an inflammatory mass may be palpable. Rectal examination usually elicits pain. A blood count shows a neutrophil leucocytosis and the sedimentation rate becomes elevated. The major complications that occur in a small proportion of patients who develop acute diverticulitis are: pericolic abscess, vesicocolic fistula, perforation of the colon with a generalized peritonitis, and rarely, a portal pyaemia.

Diverticulosis is the commonest cause of massive haemorrhage from the colon in middle-aged or elderly subjects. It is more liable to occur in patients with large numbers of diverticula affecting most of the colon and it is said that diverticula on the right side of the colon bleed more frequently than those on the left. The bleeding is usually self-limiting but may be recurrent. Diagnosis is based on the barium enema findings and the exclusion of other lesions, such as angiodysplasia, by colonoscopy and angiography.

The differential diagnosis of diverticular disease includes carcinoma of the colon, polyps, Crohn's disease, and ischaemic colitis. Since diverticulosis is so common, it is not unusual for it to be present in association with one of these other conditions. If the diverticulosis of the sigmoid is severe with considerable muscle thickening, then the radiologist may not be able to detect a coexistent carcinoma, polyp, or Crohn's disease.

Treatment. Diverticulosis presenting with symptoms of an irritable colon syndrome should be treated accordingly (see page 12.46). A combined regimen of a sedative, antispasmodic, and a bulking agent (e.g. Fybogel) should be used together with a high fibre diet. There is no place for antibiotics. Surgical resection should also be avoided because medical therapy is usually effective and the symptoms may recur following resection. In patients with intractable symptoms, a sigmoid myotomy can be performed although the symptomatic relief obtained is usually only temporary.

Patients with acute diverticulitis should be put to bed, usually in hospital. They should be given nothing by mouth except sips of water and should be given intravenous antibiotics to cover anaerobic as well as aerobic Gram-negative organisms, e.g. a combination of metronidazole with gentamicin or ampicillin. Antibiotics should be continued for at least seven days. Blood cultures should be taken before antibiotics are administered. Abdominal pain should be treated with pethidine—opiate derivatives should be avoided as they cause exaggerated rises in intraluminal pressure. The majority of patients settle well and should then probably be treated with a low residue diet for a few weeks; patients who have recurrent episodes of acute diverticulitis should be advised to take a low-residue diet long-term.

Indications for surgery in patients with acute diverticulitis include failure to respond to medical therapy and the development of one of the complications such as an abscess or a fistula. Elective surgery may be required for patients with recurrent attacks of acute diverticulitis, for obstruction due to stricture formation, and for those in whom a carcinoma cannot be excluded radiologically or by colonoscopy.

Giant sigmoid diverticula. These are rare and may result from dilatation of a small diverticulum as it is often associated with diverticulosis. They occur in the elderly and their size ranges from 6 to 27 cm. Patients may complain of intermittent lower abdominal pain and discomfort or they may develop an acute diverticulitis. A giant diverticulum may bleed or perforate and may initiate volvulus. Surgical resection is recommended even in the absence of complications.

Diaphragmatic hernia

Diaphragmatic hernias may be congenital or acquired. In *congenital partial thoracic stomach*, the descent of the developing stomach into the abdominal cavity fails to occur before the diaphragm is formed from the septum transversum. A variable amount of stomach is therefore trapped above the diaphragm and is associated with a short oesophagus. Most cases are asymptomatic but post-prandial discomfort, colicy pain, and vomiting may occur. Treatment is surgical. *Herniation* may occur through the foramina of Morgagni and Bochdalek. The foramina of Morgagni are situated anteriorly and the hernia, which usually contains the colon, is situated substernally. The foramina of Bochdalek are the posterior points of weakness of the diaphragm and the hernia may contain stomach or colon. If symptoms occur, treatment is surgical. Rarely, herniation may follow traumatic injury to the diaphragm. Traumatic hernia occurs more frequently on the left than the right. Eventration of the diaphragm is a congenital disorder in which there is absence of muscle from the central area of either the left or right part of the diaphragm. It is usually asymptomatic but may cause epigastric discomfort, flatulence, and even gastric outlet obstruction in middle-aged subjects. The condition responds well to surgical repair.

Hiatus hernia. A hiatus hernia is the protrusion of a portion of the stomach through a diaphragmatic hiatus into the chest. These hernias are usually divided into sliding, in which the gastro-oesophageal junction is displaced upwards into the chest, and rolling, in which the gastro-oesophageal junction remains in its normal position and a portion of the stomach herniates into the chest by rolling up and alongside the oesophagus. The vast majority of these hernias are asymptomatic and are found by chance on barium studies. Three-quarters of them are of the sliding type, the remaining being rolling or mixed rolling/sliding hernias. Herniation is much more common on the left side than the right. Rolling hernias are much more frequent in women than in men and are found with increasing frequency in the elderly.

Most hiatus hernias are asymptomatic and when symptoms are present they are usually related to reflux oesophagitis and include heartburn, acid reflux, flatulence, and dyspepsia. However, as mentioned elsewhere (see page 12.40) the two are not always related and the oesophageal reflux can occur without the hiatus hernia. Similarly, the presence of a hiatus hernia does not necessarily indicate that there is associated reflux. The subject of reflux oesophagitis with or without hiatus hernia is discussed in detail on page 12.40.

Chronic iron deficiency anaemia is a common complication of hiatus hernia since this condition can lead to blood loss of up to 500 ml per month. The bleeding results from either gastritis or from an ulcer within the hernia.

The herniated pouch itself may produce mechanical symptoms. These are usually associated with the rolling form of the condition. Symptoms include vague retrosternal discomfort, and although a variety of other symptoms have been ascribed to hiatus hernia, it is difficult to be certain about the relationship. Occasionally a rolling hiatus hernia may become incarcerated, leading to some substernal pain and symptoms of a high gastrointestinal obstruction.

The management of hiatus hernia with reflux is discussed in detail on page 12.40. Symptomatic rolling hernias are not amenable to medical treatment and require surgery. Emergency surgery is required for incarceration, strangulation, or perforation.

Cystic disorders of the bowel

There are a variety of disorders of the small and large bowel associated with cyst formation. All of them are rare and present major diagnostic and therapeutic problems.

Colitis cystica There are several varieties of benign cystic lesions involving the colonic mucosa. *Colitis cystica superficialis* occurs in patients with pellagra and has also been reported in adult coeliac disease. The presenting feature is usually diarrhoea and the condition is characterized by the presence of small mucus-filled cysts which lie superficial to the muscular layer of the colon. The disease seems to respond to therapy for pellagra. In *colitis cystica profunda* the cysts occur below the muscular layer of the colon. The pathogenesis and aetiology of this condition are unknown. It is usually characterized by cramping lower abdominal pain, tenesmus, and diarrhoea associated with blood and mucus in the stools. The diagnosis is made by sigmoidoscopy, rectal biopsy, and barium enema examinations. Treatment consists of local surgical excision.

Pneumatosis cystoides intestinalis This disorder is characterized by the presence of multiple gas-filled cysts in the submucosa of the large bowel and, less frequently, the small intestine. The condition usually occurs in middle-aged patients. It may be associated with chronic obstructive airways disease or peptic ulceration with some degree of pyloric obstruction. It has also been found in association with a variety of other conditions including mesenteric vascular disease, lymphosarcoma of the small bowel, Whipple's disease, or in patients who have had small bowel surgery. The aetiology and pathogenesis of the condition are completely unknown.

Pneumatosis cystoides usually is an incidental finding during radiological examination of the abdomen or intestinal tract. Occasionally it is associated with lower abdominal pain, recurrent diarrhoea, rectal bleeding, and tenesmus or partial intestinal obstruction. It is diagnosed by barium examination of the small bowel and colon.

Asymptomatic forms of the condition require no therapy. However, if there is severe pain, tenesmus, or diarrhoea, treatment is required. Initially this should be medical. Since the predominant gas in the cyst is nitrogen, prolonged breathing of oxygen reduces the partial pressure of other gases in the blood and therefore promotes diffusion of gas from the cystic spaces. Oxygen should be administered continuously through nasal catheters or a face mask. In some cases complete resolution of the cystic lesions will occur within a week of commencement of therapy. There is a tendency for the condition to recur but it may again respond to a further course of oxygen therapy. Antibiotics such as metronidazole and treatment with an elemental diet have also been used with favourable results. Extensive surgical resection of the small or large bowel may be required in severe cases but this should be avoided if possible since the cysts may recur in the remaining bowel.

Miscellaneous vascular disorders of the bowel

Intramural bleeding The commonest cause of bleeding into the wall of the bowel is anticoagulant therapy. Occasionally, intramural haematomata form in patients with congenital coagulation defects such as haemophilia or in conditions such as vasculitis. The usual presentation is with abdominal pain and symptoms of intestinal obstruction and bleeding. The diagnosis is made by barium follow-through or enema examination and the condition can usually be treated conservatively with blood replacement and, if necessary, nasogastric suction.

Aortic aneurysm. Aneurysmal dilatation of the aorta is relatively common in elderly patients, the usual site being the segment distal to the origin of the renal arteries. Aneurysms larger than 6–7 cm in size or those which show increasing enlargement are probably best resected. Rarely a spontaneous fistula into the duodenum may develop with catastrophic gastrointestinal haemorrhage.

In patients who have had prostheses inserted into the abdominal aorta or into other retroperitoneal arteries the complication of paraprosthetic-enteric fistula may occur. This is characterized by the abrupt onset of abdominal pain and shock. Treatment is surgical and the prognosis is extremely poor.

Vascular malformations The vascular ectasias of the colon are described on page 12.126. Haemangiomas of the small intestine are rare. They usually present as recurrent anaemia due to gastrointestinal bleeding. They are best diagnosed by angiography. Telangiectasia may also occur throughout the stomach and bowel as part of the Osler–Rendu–Weber syndrome.

Endometriosis

The term endometriosis describes the presence of extra-uterine endometrial tissue and its clinical manifestations. The disorder occurs most frequently between the ages of 30 and 40 years and is rare below the age of 20. Intestinal involvement is most common in those parts of the bowel adjacent to the uterus and Fallopian tubes, particularly the rectosigmoid colon. It is not certain how heterotopic endometrial tissue reaches the bowel, and spread may be direct, via the blood stream or via the lymphatics. The mucosa of the bowel is seldom penetrated by ectopic endometrial tissue and therefore gastrointestinal bleeding is an unusual accompaniment of endometriosis of the bowel.

The usual symptoms of endometriosis include dysmenorrhoea, menorrhagia, sterility, and intermenstrual pelvic pain and backache. If the rectosigmoid region is involved, there may be cyclic pains in the rectum and, occasionally, mild diarrhoea and tenesmus. Implants in the small intestine may produce symptoms of obstruction or volvulus.

The diagnosis of endometriosis requires a thorough pelvic examination to demonstrate tender nodules in the rectosigmoid region or in the rectovaginal area. The diagnosis may be suggested by radiological evidence of the presence of lesions in the rectosigmoid region, but ultimately depends on biopsy of these lesions. Laparoscopy is often helpful in making the diagnosis. The differentiation from carcinoma may be extremely difficult and when in doubt surgical exploration should be carried out.

The management of this condition requires expert gynaecological help. Mildly symptomatic cases are probably best managed by analgesics and sedation. More severe cases may require hormonal therapy with either progesterone or the more recently introduced anti-gonadotrophic agent, Danazol.

Malakoplakia

This is a rare granulomatous disease involving the urinary tract and occasionally the colon or stomach. Histologically the condition is characterized by the presence of histiocytes containing dark inclusions which are PAS positive and seem to contain both calcium and iron. There appears to be an acquired abnormality of macrophage function associated with defective digestion of phagocytozed bacteria.

Colonic malakoplakia is usually found as an incidental finding in elderly debilitated individuals, quite often in association with a malignant disease of the colon. Occasionally it presents as a systemic illness characterized by fever, diarrhoea, and other gastrointestinal symptoms. It can only be diagnosed by histological examination of the bowel. There is no effective treatment although there has been a recent report of improvement in otherwise unresponsive cases by the use of cholinergic drugs.

Isolated ulceration of the large bowel

Single ulcers may occur in the colon or rectum. Lesions in the colon may present with lower abdominal pain, fever, and leucocytosis whereas rectal ulcers usually present with tenesmus or bleeding. These non-specific ulcers must be differentiated from inflammatory disease of the bowel, tuberculosis, or neoplasms. Those which occur in the colon or caecum tend to heal but, in contrast, nonspecific ulcers of the rectum may remain static for many years. They are best treated symptomatically by maintaining a soft stool and only if they produce severe and incapacitating symptoms is surgical excision required.

Non-specific solitary ulcers of the colon and rectum must also be differentiated from stercoral ulcers which result from pressure necrosis following faecal impaction. The latter diagnosis is easily made on rectal examination. The treatment is as for faecal impaction i.e. manual removal of larger pieces of impacted faeces followed by gentle warm water or saline enemas together with oral agents such as lactulose or sodium picosulphate. Perforation of a stercoral ulcer usually follows vigorous attempts to treat high faecal impaction.

Melanosis coli and related disorders

The term melanosis coli is used to describe black or brown discoloration of the mucosa of the colon. It results from the presence of dark pigment in large mononuclear cells or macrophages in the lamina propria of the mucosa. The coloration is usually most intense just inside the anal sphincter and is less dark higher up in the sigmoid colon. Similar pigment has been found in the appendix and mesenteric nodes. The condition is thought to result from faecal stasis and the use of anthracene cathartics such as cascara. There may be an association between melanosis coli and carcinoma of the colon, and if this condition is found and there is no history of the use of anthracene laxatives or of chronic constipation, a radiological examination of the large bowel should be carried out.

Chronic cathartic abuse may also cause radiological changes of the colon which go under the general heading of cathartic colon. The changes are characterized by loss of haustral markings and appearances resembling multiple strictures although in fact these areas are capable of distention. These changes may involve all parts of the colon and the terminal ileum and have to be distinguished from those of ulcerative colitis, Crohn's disease, and other inflammatory bowel diseases.

References

Dockerty, M. B. (1972). Primary malakoplakia of the colon. *Mayo Clin. Proc.* **47**, 114.

Fleischner, F. G. (1971). Diverticular disease of the colon. New observations and revised concepts. *Gastroenterology* **60**, 316.

Folley, J. H. (1970). Ulcerative proctitis. Course and prognosis. *New Engl. J. Med.* **282**, 1362.

Ranney, B. (1975). The prevention, inhibition, palliation and treatment of endometriosis. *Am. J. Obstet. Gynec.* **123**, 778.

Skinner, D. B., Belsey, R. H. R., Hendrix, T. R., and Zuidema, G. P. (1972). *Gastro-esophageal reflux and hiatal hernia.* Little, Brown, Boston.

Sleisenger, M. H., and Fortram, J. S. (1978). *Gastrointestinal disease*, 2nd edn. W. B. Saunders, Philadelphia.

Steer, H. D., and Colin-Jones, D. G. (1975). Melanosis coli. Studies of toxic effects of irritant purgatives. *J. Pathol.* **115**, 119.

Diseases of the pancreas

K. G. Wormsley

Pancreatic disease in adults

Pancreatic disease in adults manifests as sudden, acute parenchymal destruction or as slowly progressive exocrine (acinar) failure, often also accompanied by destruction of the endocrine (islet) tissue. The acute sudden cellular necrosis of the pancreas may affect a previously healthy gland or a gland which is already the site of ongoing chronic inflammatory or neoplastic disease. The causes of these acute and chronic pathological processes are not known but many diseases of other systems or organs, or their attempted therapy, have been shown to precede, or be associated with, the pancreatic diseases.

Acute pancreatitis. When acute pancreatic parenchymal necrosis affects an otherwise apparently healthy gland, the disease is called acute pancreatitis. Successive episodes of such necrosis are termed recurrent acute pancreatitis. It seems quite extraordinary that we do not know what determines the precise point at which most, or all, of the pancreatic acinar cells (and often the islet cells also) die and, therefore, which patient is at risk. It is easy to visualize why massive parenchymal destruction occurs during the course of infections, or as a result of adverse reactions to drugs, or following occlusion of the arterial blood supply, but we do not understand why alcoholic patients develop acute pancreatic cellular death 36 to 48 hours after an alcoholic debauch, nor why some patients with gallstones sometimes actually die from pancreatic necrosis while the majority never develop this type of pancreatic disease.

Incidence. It is not possible to provide meaningful, precise values for the incidence of acute pancreatitis in any specified population because it is not yet possible to diagnose the disease accurately. Despite recent improvements in diagnostic techniques, the only means by which the occurrence of acute pancreatitis can be definitively established are laparotomy or autopsy. All other diagnostic criteria lack both sensitivity and specificity. We do not know how often acute pancreatitis occurs without the 'cardinal' diagnostic features of abdominal pain associated with raised circulating levels of amylase, while conversely, these 'diagnostic features' often occur in patients suffering from non-pancreatic diseases. In this connection it has been reported that up to 80 per cent of patients with confirmed acute pancreatitis may not be diagnosed clinically until laparotomy or autopsy, while an incorrrect diagnosis of acute pancreatitis is made in as many as 40 per cent of patients.

However, despite these diagnostic problems, it seems that the incidence of acute pancreatitis is increasing in most Western countries and sometimes reaches epidemic proportions, as in South African Black workers who have migrated to the big shanty towns from the kraals. In most countries acute pancreatitis affects especially males in the fourth and fifth decades and females a decade or so later.

Predisposing conditions. A number of clinical conditions are associated with acute pancreatitis more than expected on the basis of chance and are therefore thought to 'cause' the pancreatitis.

In Britain, much of Europe, and Israel acute pancreatitis occurs most frequently in patients who suffer from diseases of the biliary tract (such as cholecystitis, gallstones, and abnormalities of the bile ducts). Clinically obvious gallstones, mainly in the gall-bladder and less frequently in the bile duct or ampulla, are present six times more commonly in patients with acute pancreatitis than in control populations. It seems that acute pancreatitis is related especially to the combination of small stones and wide cystic ducts and, indeed, in one recent study, 85 per cent of patients with acute pancreatitis related to biliary disease had gallstones in their stool. It is important to recognize the association of acute pancreatitis with disease of the biliary tract because this type of acute pancreatitis, which occurs especially in females older than 60 years, tends to be severe and has a high mortality. Occurrence, and recurrence, of the acute pancreatitis associated with biliary disease can be prevented by elective surgical treatment of the diseased biliary tract.

In the USA, Australia, and South Africa 'acute pancreatitis' is most often associated with intake of large amounts of alcohol. In Europe and South America there is also a high, and increasing, incidence of alcohol-associated acute pancreatitis. The first attacks of this type of pancreatitis tend to be the most severe and may even be fatal. Subsequent episodes tend to be milder in British patients, although in other geographical areas (like the USA) any attack of alcohol-associated pancreatitis may be severe. Deterioration of exocrine function tends to occur if abstinence from alcohol is not virtually complete. Repeated episodes of acute pancreatitis associated with drinking of beer (in Northern Europe and South America) result ultimately in chronic non-calcific pancreatitis, while the acute episodes of the pancreatic disease associated with the drinking of wine or spirits in the USA, southern Europe, and South Africa are an aspect of, or develop into, chronic calcific pancreatitis.

Acute pancreatitis may follow abdominal surgery, particularly involving the biliary tract, pancreas, or stomach. This type of acute pancreatitis usually occurs within one to two days of the operation and often presents as shock, or ileus, so that the clinical diagnosis may be difficult. Acute pancreatitis has been described following transplantation and cardiac bypass surgery, with an incidence of about 2 per cent and mortality of nearly half. Acute pancreatitis may result from direct pancreatic trauma, such as blunt abdominal injury, seat-belt injury, or stab wounds, or following invasive clinical procedures such as endoscopic retrograde pancreatography and translumbar aortography.

Acute pancreatitis also occurs during the course of specific metabolic disorders. Thus, acute pancreatitis has been noted to occur during the course of hyperparathyroidism (in 5 to 20 per cent of cases), as well as in association with other hypercalcaemic states such as hypervitaminosis D and metastatic bone disease, and even following an intravenous infusion of calcium. Numerically more important is the association between acute pancreatitis and hyperlipidaemia. The hyperlipidaemia may be hereditary (Fredericksen's types I, IV, and V, see Section 9), alcohol-induced, or, more important, the consequence of taking oestrogen-containing contraceptive pills.

Attacks of acute pancreatitis have been noted in patients taking drugs for the treatment of many non-pancreatic diseases. For example, acute pancreatitis occurs within two weeks to 15 months after the start of therapy with diuretics such as thiazides and frusemide.

In addition, treatment with azathioprine (used for immunosuppression or in the therapy of Crohn's disease) or phenformin (particularly following the development of lactic acidosis) may result in the development of acute pancreatitis. Patients who have taken an overdose of paracetamol, or who are being treated with high doses of steroids, have also developed acute pancreatitis.

Acute pancreatitis may occur during the course of infections, including mumps, enteroviral infections such as Coxsackie group B viruses and echoviruses, and also during infections with *Myco-*

plasma pneumoniae. Acute pancreatitis has also been reported to occur following sting by a scorpion (*Tityus trinitatis*) in Trinidad.

Other disorders occasionally found in association with acute pancreatitis include anatomical abnormalities of the pancreatic duct, ranging from congenital disorders such as pancreas divisum to ampullary cancer, as well as duodenal anatomic anomalies, such as congenital diverticulae or the partial obstruction (afferent loop syndrome) which sometimes follows partial gastrectomy. Acute pancreatitis has been recorded quite commonly in patients suffering from hypothermia and also occasionally in individuals overfed after prolonged fasting. Up to 20 per cent of patients with malignant hypertension may develop acute pancreatitis.

Clinical manifestations. The clinical presentation and features of acute pancreatitis reflect the severity of the pancreatic necrosis. If the pancreatic inflammation is mild, the patient complains of abdominal pain and tenderness, plus vomiting and transient intestinal ileus. Ambulation is possible within a day or two of the start of the attack. With more severe pancreatic inflammation, the patient may develop some degree of hypovolaemic shock and more prolonged ileus. In a variable proportion of cases, depending in part on the associated condition and the age of the patient, the attack of pancreatitis results in an overwhelmingly severe disease, associated with pulmonary, renal, and hepatic failure and encephalopathy, often with fatal outcome.

The principal manifestation of acute pancreatitis is pain, which is most commonly sited in the epigastrium but may be localized to either subcostal region, to the lower abdomen, or which may be generalized. The pain is usually constant in intensity and ranges from catastrophically severe to quite mild, radiating to the back between the scapulae in about half the patients. The pain characteristically lasts from one to two days or longer and may be very difficult to relieve. Associated symptoms depend on the disturbed function of other organs or processes, or on defective repair of the necrotic pancreas.

The onset of the pain may be related to the associated, or predisposing, condition. Thus, alcohol-associated pancreatitis characteristically occurs following a latent period of 24 to 48 hours after the intake of alcohol. In patients with disease of the biliary system, the pain of acute pancreatitis may develop a few hours after a heavy meal. A similar interval has been recorded between an infusion of calcium and the onset of the pain of acute pancreatitis.

It is not known how often pain is absent in acute pancreatitis, since the only reliable information is available from autopsy data, which show that up to 20 per cent of fatal acute pancreatitis may be 'painless'.

Nausea and vomiting are associated with pain in up to 90 per cent of cases. Vomiting may dominate the clinical picture and may be associated with haematemesis.

The other clinical manifestations of acute pancreatitis are attributable to the local and systemic complications of the disease. Some of the complications, especially those affecting the pancreas itself and other parts of the alimentary system, are independent of the severity of the attack and may occur during or after even mild attacks of pancreatitis. On the other hand, the systemic complications often reflect severe disease, with fatal outcome.

Pancreatic complications. *Pseudocyst.* Pseudocysts, comprising collections of fluid within the pancreas or in the lesser sac, occur in more than half of the patients who suffer from acute pancreatitis. The pseudocyst gives rise to a palpable mass in about half the patients and is so large, or sited so close to the bile duct, that jaundice develops in about 10 per cent of affected individuals. In 25–50 per cent of patients, the pseudocyst resolves spontaneously. The remainder may develop complications such as hyperamylasaemia; infection; erosion of adjacent vessels with haemorrhage into alimentary tract or peritoneum; or leakage into serosal cavities, especially the peritoneum, resulting in ascites.

Abscess. Pancreatic abscesses occur in up to 5 per cent of patients

with acute pancreatitis. Development of the abscess may be delayed for as long as six months after an attack of acute pancreatitis, but usually occurs within the first two months. Fistulae, haemorrhage, and septicaemia are the most serious complications and mortality rates as high as 50 per cent have been reported.

Persistent pancreatitis. Occasionally, the inflammatory process persists for some weeks after the attack of acute pancreatitis, perhaps because pancreatic ductal obstruction has developed. Although the clinical manifestation of epigastric mass may be indistinguishable from pseudocyst or abscess, the treatment is different since pancreatic resection is usually necessary if there is ductal obstruction.

Alimentary complications. *Intestinal obstruction.* Paralytic ileus is common during attacks of acute pancreatitis and may be generalized when peritonitis is present, or localized giving rise to the characteristic radiological 'sentinel loop' obstruction of a short segment of jejunum, or the 'cut-off' sign of obstruction of the transverse colon. Alternatively, intestinal obstruction may be mechanical, when colonic, duodenal, or small intestinal stenosis may result from occlusion of mesenteric arteries and infarction of the affected segment of intestine.

Haemorrhage. Severe bleeding from the alimentary tract has been reported in as many as 10 per cent of patients with acute pancreatitis and is often lethal. The most severe haemorrhage results from the erosion of major arteries, such as splanchnic or colonic, or from bleeding varices secondary to obstruction of splenic or portal veins. Bleeding is also caused by acute erosive gastritis and duodenitis and may be aggravated by a haemorrhagic diasthesis.

Perforations. Perforation of the colon into the peritoneal cavity has been reported after acute pancreatitis. More commonly, pseudocysts rupture into the stomach or intestine or manifest as fistulae, with the development of serosal effusions, especially ascites, although pleural and pericardial effusions may also occur. The serosal effusions characteristically contain high concentrations of pancreatic enzymes.

Hepatobiliary complications. *Obstructive jaundice.* As many as 40 per cent of patients develop jaundice during an attack of acute pancreatitis. The jaundice is often obstructive and reflects either the underlying calculous disease of the biliary tract or pancreatic oedema or a pseudocyst in the head of the pancreas. It is always necessary to exclude ampullary carcinoma in patients who develop acute pancreatitis and obstructive jaundice.

Hepatocellular jaundice. Hepatocellular disease has been recorded in up to 70 per cent of patients with acute pancreatitis. Alcoholic patients tend to develop acute fatty liver (in as many as two-thirds of the individuals). When severe, the acute fatty change can cause hepatocellular failure and death. Liver cell necrosis may also occur, especially in patients suffering from shock or septicaemia.

Metabolic complications. *Hypocalcaemia.* Abnormally low serum calcium values occur in up to 30 per cent of patients with acute pancreatitis and signify a severe attack, with poor prognosis. The cause of the hypocalcaemia has not yet been satisfactorily defined but hypoalbuminaemia or abnormalities in the concentration of circulating parathyroid hormone have been reported.

Hyperglycaemia. Abnormalities in the secretion of insulin or glucagon are common during an attack of acute pancreatitis. The secretion of the pancreatic islet hormones may be partially, or wholly, impaired, so that the abnormalities of glucose homeostasis range from mild glucose intolerance to severe acute keto-acidosis. Hyperglycaemia occurs in 30 to 70 per cent of cases, with glycosuria in about 25 per cent. Transient diabetes mellitus, requiring treatment with insulin, occurs in about 5 per cent of patients during the episode of acute pancreatitis, but permanent diabetes is rare and occurs in less than 2 per cent of patients. Hypoglycaemia develops occasionally, presumably because there is dysfunction of the alpha cells of the islets.

Hyperlipidaemia. Abnormalities of circulating lipoproteins may precede and cause the pancreatitis, or may occur as a result of the pancreatitis, or both acute pancreatitis and hyperlipaemia may be manifestations of a common underlying cause, such as alcohol abuse. It has been estimated that about 2 per cent of patients with acute pancreatitis develop transient hyperlipidaemia during the course of an attack. In some patients, a circulating inhibitor of plasma lipoprotein lipase has been recorded, while in others it seems that levels of lipoprotein lipase are abnormally low. Alternatively, acute deficiency of insulin may result in a type I hyperlipoproteinaemia.

Haematological complications. Disorders of coagulation are occasionally an important aspect of the clinical picture of acute pancreatitis. Both excessive and impaired coagulability have been recorded. Disseminated intravascular coagulation results in widespread fibrin thrombi which, in turn, contribute to the hepatocellular, respiratory, and renal failure in severe acute pancreatitis.

Renal complications. The renal complications of acute pancreatitis range from mild reversible tubular defects (responsible for the increased clearance of amylase) to severe renal failure which is fatal in more than half the affected individuals. The degree of renal failure is related to the severity of the pancreatitis. Acute renal failure has been recorded in 2–20 per cent of patients and results from shock; from occlusion of the renal arteries in the pancreatitic process; or from the disseminated fibrin thrombi caused by diffuse intravascular coagulation.

Neurological complications. Neuropsychiatric changes are common during attacks of acute pancreatitis and range from mild confusion to acute delirium or coma, usually starting between the second and fifth day of the attack. The encephalopathy has been attributed, in part, to foci or diffuse areas of demyelination throughout the central nervous system, perhaps caused by circulating pancreatic lipolytic enzymes.

This type of organic delirium must be differentiated from delirium tremens which may accompany an attack of acute pancreatitis in an alcoholic patient.

Cardiovascular complications. *Circulatory failure.* Some degree of shock occurs in up to 60 per cent of patients with acute pancreatitis. Circulating plasma volume is reduced, with vasconstriction and sequestration of fluid. The changes have been attributed to diffuse vascular damage, caused by circulating proteases and kinins, as well as to accumulation of extracellular fluid in the serosal cavities, and to losses of blood as a result of alimentary haemorrhage.

Hypertension. Transient hypertension has been reported in as many as one-third of patients with acute pancreatitis and is considered to have a bad prognostic significance, since the hypertension is often followed by the development of complications such as shock and renal failure.

ECG changes. Acute pancreatitis can mimic cardiac infarction, since typical ischaemic ECG changes, as well as arrhythmias, may develop during an attack.

Pulmonary complications. Many of the patients with severe acute pancreatitis develop pleuro-pulmonary complications. About 5 per cent of patients develop acute respiratory failure with increasingly more severe hypoxaemia and death within 24 to 48 hours. The clinical respiratory distress is associated with an increase in pulmonary extravascular water and abnormal patterns of gas distribution. Clinically, anxiety and tachypnoea are associated with progressive arterial hypoxia and radiological development of diffuse bilateral pulmonary infiltrates.

About one-third of patients who die suffer from pulmonary failure, while the respiratory insufficiency contributes to death in another third.

Left basal effusions may occur in the absence of more extensive pulmonary involvement.

Cutaneous changes. Blood from a necrotic pancreas may track into the left flank to produce ecchymotic discoloration (Grey–Turner's sign). Less common peri-umbilical bruising is called Cullen's sign.

Fat necrosis. Occasionally, acute pancreatitis may present with disseminated necrosis of fat, or panniculitis occurs during the course of an episode of acute pancreatitis. Cutaneous panniculitis presents as fluctuant subcutaneous nodules which sometimes ulcerate and discharge necrotic tissue. The lesions resemble other types of panniculitis (like those of the Weber–Christian syndrome); or the nodules of erythema nodosum or cutaneous vasculitis. Necrosis of fat in synovial membranes presents as arthralgia and joint effusions, while necrosis of fat in the bone marrow produces necrosis of long bones. Necrosis of mesenteric and retroperitoneal fat is one of the causes of abdominal pain in this disease. There is often associated eosinophilia

Diagnosis. The clinical manifestations of acute pancreatitis are mainly so non-specific that the disease is often not recognized or, conversely, is incorrectly diagnosed. Investigational procedures are not yet sufficiently specific to improve diagnostic efficacy. Serum amylase levels are increased in about 80 per cent of patients with acute pancreatitis but absence of a diagnostic increase is common and attributed to 'mildness' of the attack or to associated hyperlipidaemia (which masks the increase in serum amylase), or to the passage of too long a period of time since the acute pancreatic necrosis. Unfortunately, it is not yet possible to estimate the 'diagnostic sensitivity' of elevated serum amylase levels in the detection of acute pancreatitis since the underlying problem—whether acute pancreatitis is or is not present—has never been resolved by an independent and more sensitive and specific diagnostic technique. The converse information is perhaps more valuable, since it has been shown that from 60 to 90 per cent of patients with elevated serum amylase levels do not have acute pancreatitis. Measurement of amylase in urine instead of blood, or expressing urinary excretion of amylase in terms of clearance ratios, has not improved diagnostic sensitivity or specificity. It seems possible that newer techniques, such as measuring the levels of the specific *p*-isoamylase and of immunoreactive trypsin in the circulation; or, alternatively, morphological investigations involving ultrasonographic examination or computerized abdominal tomography, may provide better means to distinguish between the normal and acutely inflamed pancreas, but sufficient information is not yet available to provide definitive guidelines for routine clinical use.

It must be emphasized that if there is any doubt about the diagnosis, exploratory laparotomy must be undertaken to exclude potentially fatal non-pancreatic causes of abdominal pain.

Differential diagnosis. Acute pancreatitis must be considered when patients have an acute episode of upper abdominal pain, especially if complicated by the development of shock, jaundice, an upper abdominal mass or ascites, hypocalcaemia or diabetes mellitus, or by abdominal cutaneous ecchymoses or an acute arthropathy.

The majority of patients with acute pancreatitis present with an 'acute abdomen'. When a patient has had previous episodes of acute pancreatitis, the recurrences are usually easily recognizable. Problems arise especially during the first attack. Acute pancreatitis can be distinguished from a perforated viscus by the board-like rigidity of the abdomen which characterizes the latter and the presence of free air under the diaphragms in many of the patients who perforate their intestine. About one-third of the misdiagnoses of acute pancreatitis have perforated peptic ulcers. Acute pancreatitis with ileus may be difficult to distinguish from mesenteric vascular occlusion and laparotomy is essential if there is any doubt about the diagnosis, particularly in patients suffering from atrial fibrillation. When accompanied by jaundice, acute pancreatitis must be differentiated from disease of the biliary system and from acute alcoholic hepatitis. High fever and rigors, with typical colicky pain, occur with gallstones and are unusual in patients with acute pancreatitis. Primary alcoholic involvement of the liver may be impossible to distinguish clinically from the secondary hepatobiliary involvement in acute pancreatitis, so the alternative pathologies must be kept in mind. Acute cholecystitis may also be difficult to distinguish clinically from acute pancreatitis and indeed, many patients diagnosed as acute pancreatitis are found to have acute cholecystitis at laparotomy.

If the abdominal pain is accompnied by development of an abdominal mass, acute pancreatitis must be distinguished from dissecting aneurysm of the aorta. The intra-abdominal haemorrhage which characterizes acute haemorrhagic pancreatitis may be mimicked by splenic rupture of an ectopic pregnancy. The former is usually the result of blunt trauma to the abdomen, or occasionally of an acute infection involving the spleen, while abnormalitis of menstruation point to an ectopic pregnancy. Occasionally, acute abdominal pain with some of the manifestations of acute pancreatitis (jaundice, encephalopathy) occurs during an acute episode of porphyria, with resulting diagnostic confusion especially because acute pancreatitis has been described in association with the latter disease. The occurrence, in acute pancreatitis, of acute abdominal pain with hypertension or, more commonly, with severe hypotension simulates myocardial infarction, the more so since arrhythmias and ischaemic electrocardiographic changes occur during attacks of acute pancreatitis.

Course and prognosis. The course of acute pancreatitis reflects the presence or absence of complications of the disease. In uncomplicated acute pancreatitis, patients suffer pain for two to three days, with transient ileus. The patient can be discharged within a week or so of admission to hospital. Such clinically benign course does not preclude the development of 'late' complications, such as pseudocyst.

During the initial few hours of a severe attack of acute pancreatitis, the principal manifestations are pain, fever, vomiting, meteorism, and paralytic ileus in 50–80 per cent of individuals. There is abdominal tenderness, without guarding, in about 90 per cent. Some patients present with transient hypertension (10–15 per cent), although more commonly shock dominates the clinical picture. Up to 40 per cent of plasma volume may become sequestrated. Shock is the principal cause of death early during the course of the disease. At this time, also, arrhythmias may develop, so that in the presence of ischaemic electrocardiographic changes, the clinical picture may resemble myocardial infarction.

During the first two to three days, the most serious complication is the development of hypoxaemia, with the nadir of blood oxygen tension occurring during the second to fourth day after the onset of pain. Coincident pulmonary oedema is maximal three to five days after the start of the disease. At this time, also, the affected patient is most likely to develop a toxic psychosis. Blood concentrations of glucose rise during this period, while the concentration of calcium falls. The haematocrit, which has risen as a result of fluid sequestration, may fall if the patient starts to bleed. The platelet count may fall, with rise in concentration of fibrinogen and fibrinogen degradation products. The concentration of blood urea rises as a result of acute renal failure, which manifests at this time.

During the first few days, the patient may develop Grey–Turner's sign and serous effusions, especially in peritoneal and pleural cavities.

The late complications of acute pancreatitis, which tend to develop two to four weeks after the onset of an attack, include especially the development of a pseudocyst or an abscess. The appearance of these complications has usually been preceded by subsidence of the symptoms of acute attack. These complications are heralded by recurrence of fever or rigors, with abdominal tenderness and the appearance of an upper abdominal mass. Other problems which occur at this time include thrombosis of the splenic vein; the development of duodenal or colonic stenosis or fistulae; the appearance of fatty changes in the liver; and secondary haemorrhage from erosion of visceral vessels, portal hypertension, or ulcers. Haemorrhage is one of the causes of late shock, the others being rupture of an abscess or pseudocyst.

Acute pancreatitis tends to be severe particularly during first attacks. In different studies, from 20 to 50 per cent of attacks have been considered severe. The average mortality is about 10 per cent, with about half the fatalities occurring during the first week of the disease. The causes of death include intractable circulatory collapse, septicaemia, alimentary haemorrhage, and respiratory, renal, or hepatic failure. Indeed, it has been noted that the clinical diagnoses of 'shock' and 'respiratory distress' are associated with death in more than 70 per cent of affected individuals. Of those who die, about 20 per cent die on the day of admission and 60 per cent within six days. Pulmonary pathology dominates the picture in those dying before the end of the first week of an attack. Patients dying late in the disease do so especially from infections such as septicaemia, abscesses, or peritonitis.

In view of the obviously lethal significance of some of the local and systemic complications of acute pancreatitis, prognostic inferences have been based on evidence of pulmonary involvement (such as tachypnoea and progressive arterial hypoxia), cardiovascular impairment with sequestration of blood and shock, bleeding, with associated progressive decrease in haematocrit, hepatic insufficiency, as shown by impaired output of urine and increasing blood levels of urea nitrogen, and metabolic complications, signalled by hypocalcaemia and diabetic ketoacidosis.

Emergency investigations therefore include blood levels of amylase, calcium, glucose, bilirubin, and liver enzymes, urea, PCV, white cell count, and blood gases. While the course of the disease is often unpredictable, the prognosis is considered to be bad if the patient is older than 55 years; has prolonged hypotension with systolic blood pressure less than 90 mmHg; has a white blood count of more than 15×10^9/l; a temperature higher than 39 °C; blood glucose greater than 10 mmol/l; an arterial Po_2 less than 60 mmHg (7.5 kPa); a GOT more than 100 IU./l and LDH more than 600 IU./l; plasma urea more than 15 mmol/l; a serum calcium less than 2 mmol/l; a fall in haematocrit more than 10 per cent and especially with combinations of these values. The presence of circulating methaemalbumin is also considered to denote the presence of haemorrhagic pancreatitis, with bad prognosis. Similarly, the aspiration by paracentesis of brown or blood-stained fluid from the peritoneal cavity denotes the more serious haemorrhagic pancreatitis.

Twenty-four hours after admission, it is worth carrying out an ultrasonic or isotopic scan of the gall-bladder, using diethyl acentanilido-imino diacetic acid. If the gall-bladder does not fill, the patient is probably suffering from gallstone-associated pancreatitis and it is necessary to operate to decompress the biliary system.

After one week (and thereafter at weekly intervals) the patient should be subjected to upper abdominal ultrasonographic scans to monitor the development of pseudocysts.

About half the patients have recurrences of acute pancreatitis, irrespective of whether the associated condition is alcoholism or disease of the biliary tract, unless the associated disease can be treated.

Treatment. *Medical therapy*. The treatment of acute pancreatitis remains unsatisfactory since therapy is symptomatic and devoted to correcting the systemic complications of the disease. Many of the measures are self-evident and supportive. All patients have a large-bore infusion set up on admission, are catheterized, and have blood gases monitored.

Relief of pain is often a problem, since pethidine and opiates cause contraction of the sphincter of Oddi and of the duodenal musculature. In practice, there is no evidence that these analgesics adversely affect the clinical course of acute pancreatitis, but it is perhaps worth attempting to control the pain with a drug such as buprenorphine which has a longer duration of action and therefore does not have to be given so frequently.

The treatment of shock involves the administration of blood if the haematocrit falls. Alternatively, and especially if there is no overt loss of blood, plasma can be used or, if available, fresh frozen plasma. Large volumes of electrolyte solutions may be necessary to keep urinary flow greater than 30 ml per hour and the haematocrit from rising above 40. In view of the renal shut-down which may accompany acute pancreatitis, and the circulation of proteases which increase capillary permeability, the potential occurrence of fluid overload must be monitored carefully, to prevent pulmonary oedema.

Patients are catheterized to permit accurate monitoring of urinary flow rate. Renal failure is serious and usually indicates a fatal outcome, but dialysis should be undertaken if urinary output remains persistently at less than 30 ml/hour.

The pulmonary failure requires frequent monitoring of blood gases and treatment with humidified oxygen. Since most patients with acute pancreatitis suffer from hypoxaemia, all should be given additional oxygen by mask or nasal catheters. With severe pulmonary failure (Po_2 less than 50 mmHg) it may become necessary to undertake intermittent or continuous positive end-expiratory pressure ventilation. Pulmonary atelectasis should be prevented by early physiotherapy to prevent the effects of diaphragmatic splinting. Pleural effusions must be aspirated and pulmonary infections treated with appropriate antibiotics.

The disturbed glucose homeostasis, presenting with hyperglycaemia, diabetic ketoacidosis, or non-ketotic hyperosmolar syndrome, requires treatment with insulin and electrolyte infusion.

Prophylactic antibiotics should not be used routinely. Antibiotics and biliary decompression are required for suppurative cholangitis. If a pancreatic abscess develops, the abscess must be drained and appropriate antibiotics administered.

Parenteral nutrition is not necessary unless there is prolonged ileus or some other complication of the disease which precludes oral therapy.

A number of unvalidated measures have been advocated in theoretically unfounded attempts to 'rest' the pancreas and to counteract the supposed 'autodigestion'. Thus, it has been reported that ingestion of food increases the mortality during acute attacks of pancreatitis and it has therefore been recommended that food must not be taken until clinical manifestations and serum levels of amylase have returned to normal. It seems reasonable to provide intravenous alimentation while the patients are seriously ill, have ileus, anorexia, and are vomiting, but there does not appear to be any evidence that food intake is disadvantageous once recovery has started. For the same reason (to rest the pancreas) nasogastric suction has been advocated, in order to prevent gastric contents from passing into the duodenum and stimulating pancreatic secretion. While there is no evidence that nasogastric suction beneficially influences the course of acute pancreatitis, nasogastric intubation is desirable during the early stages of an episode because vomiting is very painful. Antacids and gastric secretory inhibitors (such as anticholinergics and cimetidine) have also been recommended but no evidence is available to show that gastric inhibition is beneficial during attacks of acute pancreatitis and, indeed, serum amylase levels have been reported to be higher during treatment with cimetidine than without, while the incidence of tachycardia, ileus, and hypotension may be increased if anticholinergic drugs are used in the treatment of acute pancreatitis.

A number of alleged pancreatic secretory inhibitors have been recommended in order to decrease the effects of release of pancreatic enzymes from damaged pancreatic cells. These inhibitors include the peptides glucagon, calcitonin, and somatostatin but the evidence that these peptides beneficially affect the clinical course of acute pancreatitis has not yet been satisfactorily established and all have additional effects (e.g. glucagon increases blood sugar and decreases calcium; calcitonin further lowers blood calcium; somatostatin inhibits pancreatic islet cell function as well as many other

endocrine functions) which render management of the acute pancreatitis more difficult.

Intravenous administration of antiproteases, especially aprotinin (Trasylol) has been used in an attempt to counteract the pancreatic proteolytic enzymes released into the necrotic gland and into the circulation. The current consensus is that aprotinin does not influence the clinical course of acute pancreatitis. Recently, fresh frozen plasma has been used at a rate of 1 unit per 12 hours for five days, in view of its high content of powerful antiproteolytic activity. Peritoneal lavage with isotonic dialysate (36 to 48 litres) starting not later than 48 hours after admission has been used in an attempt to remove 'toxic factors' from the peritoneal cavity, since peritoneal fluid from patients with acute pancreatitis has been shown experimentally to produce hypotension and increase vascular permeability. It has been stated that the overall survival is not influenced by peritoneal dialysis, although the incidence of systemic complications may be reduced. However, the respiratory distress accompanying acute pancreatitis may be aggravated, as may the diabetic tendency. In addition, peripancreatic abscess is a complication of peritoneal lavage.

Surgical therapy. Surgical exploration is always required if the diagnosis is not certain or if the pancreatitis is traumatic or the result of afferent loop obstruction. Surgical treatment may also become necessary for some of the complications of the acute pancreatitis. Thus, drainage of pseudocysts or pancreatic abscesses is often necessary, as is surgical intervention to stop overt alimentary haemorrhage or mechanical obstruction of the intestine. Decompression of the biliary system is required in as many as 75 per cent of patients with gallstone-associated pancreatitis, in order to prevent or treat cholangitis and Gram-negative septicaemia, since these complications tend to be lethal. The role of definitive surgery, to remove impacted gallstones in acute pancreatitis, is under study at present, since contradictory reports have appeared about the hazard of this type of procedure during the acute episode. However biliary surgery should be undertaken before a patient is discharged from hospital after an attack of gallstone-associated pancreatitis, in view of the high incidence of recurrence of the acute pancreatitis (33 to 67 per cent) if the gallstones are not removed.

Surgery may also be required if a patient experiences recurrences of acute pancreatitis. Sometimes removal of the gall-bladder prevents further attacks even if the gall-bladder is radiologically and ultrasonographically normal, because the patient is suffering from biliary microlisthiasis. If endoscopic retrograde pancreatography shows ductal or papillary strictures, attempts may be made to remove or bypass the strictures, or pancreatectomy may become necessary.

There is still a lot of controversy about the desirability and effects of resection of necrotic pancreatic tissue early during acute attacks of pancreatitis. The indications have been taken to be the failure to prevent deterioration of the patient's general condition during the first 48 hours after the onset of pain. Surgical resection of the pancreas has been advocated, especially if there is a combination of respiratory failure requiring intubation with shock and hypocalcaemia, in view of the high mortality when these complications are treated medically. However, early surgery is often lethal, with increased pulmonary complications and severe intra-abdominal fat necrosis, unless the pancreatectomy is total.

Chronic pancreatitis
Definition. Chronic pancreatitis is the clinical manifestation of pathological processes which result in inflammation and progressive fibrotic destruction of the acinar and ductal tissues of the pancreas, often with parenchymal calcification or intraductal listhiasis. Occasionally, non-sclerotic atrophy, with replacement of the pancreatic acinar tissue by fat, is found in patients who present clinically with features of chronic pancreatitis.

Incidence. The incidence of chronic pancreatitis varies greatly in different parts of the world and in different population groups within individual countries. In the United Kingdom and Western countries, the mean age of onset of chronic pancreatitis is about 35 years (which is a decade or two younger than the mean age of patients with acute pancreatitis). In some Asian countries, malnutrition-associated chronic pancreatitis occurs earlier in life, with a mean age of onset less than 15 years and, in some areas, attains an overall incidence of more than 5 per cent in autopsy studies. Unlike the alcohol-associated type of chronic pancreatitis which is more common in men, the calcific chronic pancreatitis associated with malnutrition is equally common in males and females.

Chronic pancreatitis is also sometimes associated with other diseases, particularly hyperparathyroidism or hyperlipidaemia. The metabolic disease of these patients has often not been recognized before presentation of the pancreatic disease. Chronic pancreatitis rarely occurs in families and may then present in childhood. Rarely, chronic pancreatitis is the consequence of congenital abnormalities of the duodenum or biliary system, or of a slow-growing ampullary carcinoma.

Aetiology. It is not yet known whether 'chronic pancreatitis' represents the end result of one or of a number of different disease processes which cause the progressive destruction of the gland. Thus, pancreatic calcification is most frequently encountered in patients with chronic alcoholism, but has also been recorded in young people who suffer from malnutrition, as well as in 5–10 per cent of patients with hyperparathyroidism and in individuals with hereditary pancreatitis, or with the 'chronic pancreatitis' of old age. In all these situations, severe pancreatic destruction with clinical chronic pancreatitis may also occur without pancreatic calcification, so that the pancreatic calcification is a useful diagnostic criterion, but not an indication of the cause or of the severity of the pancreatic disease.

Attempts have been made to define nutritional causes of chronic pancreatitis. International surveys demonstrate that patients with chronic pancreatitis in Europe, North America, and South Africa tend to have a high intake of alcohol and also a high intake of fat and protein. The risk of developing chronic pancreatitis is stated to be logarithmically related to the quantity of alcohol consumed, with no lower limit. The amounts of alcohol required to produce chronic pancreatitis and the duration of consumption is less in women than in men. In southern Europe, chronic calcific pancreatitis is associated with high intake of carbohydrate, protein, and fat, together with alcohol in the form of wine, while in northern Europe, the chronic pancreatitis tends to be non-calcific and to be associated with high intake of protein and fat, with alcohol in the form of beer. In Asian and African countries, chronic calcific pancreatitis tends to be associated with protein-deficient diets, in the absence of alcoholism.

In alcoholic chronic pancreatitis, the mean duration of alcohol intake before clinical presentation of the disease ranges from five to 20 years in males and less in women (compared with the finding that alcohol intake precedes manifestation of cirrhosis of the liver by about 30 years).

In the United Kingdom, the cause of the chronic pancreatitis is not found in about half the patients and the condition is then labelled 'idiopathic'. In a small proportion of patients, acute pancreatitis is followed by chronic pancreatitis, especially if the acute attack has resulted in an irreversible complication such as pancreatic ductal stenosis or pseudocyst. Less than 5 per cent of patients with chronic pancreatitis are found to have gallstones, which are the 'cause' of the pancreatitis in some of these individuals and the consequence of the pancreatic disease in others.

Clinical manifestations. The clinical manifestations of chronic pancreatitis reflect the pathological processes involving the pancreas and the pathophysiological consequences of the exocrine and endocrine insufficiency.

The fibrotic process which characterizes chronic pancreatitis often results in pancreatic ductal strictures, so that recurrent episodes of pain afflict 90 per cent of affected individuals. The pain is usually indistinguishable from acute pancreatitis, but is often less severe and of shorter duration, so that in most individuals the pain lasts less than a day. Often, the severity of the attacks becomes less, and the frequency of attacks decreases, as the disease progresses. Occasionally, the converse is found, with increasingly severe and frequent attacks of pain, which may ultimately become continuous. A different type of pain has also been recorded in chronic pancreatitis. The pain occurs within 30 minutes or so after meals and lasts an hour or two, like the pain of intestinal ischaemia, although the occurrence of this type of pancreatic pain is not as regular as ischaemic pain. The frequency and severity of the attacks of pain are directly responsible for the high incidence of psychiatric problems, ranging from opiate addiction to depression and suicide. Pain in chronic pancreatitis is also sometimes caused by duodenal ulceration, which occurs in 10–20 per cent of affected patients.

Pancreatic fibrosis, with superadded oedema during acute episodes of pancreatitis, is also responsible for the cholestatic jaundice which affects about 10 per cent of the patients and may occur independently of pain. When jaundice accompanies the pain of an acute relapse of pancreatitis, the clinical picture may simulate biliary listhiasis, but high fever and rigors are rare in chronic pancreatitis with jaundice. The jaundice is usually transient and, when prolonged, indicates the development of ampullary stenosis or of a pseudocyst. Occasionally the jaundice is caused by gallstones, which have been reported in as many as 10 per cent of patients with chronic pancreatitis (because the bile salt pool is abnormally small as a consequence of abnormal faecal losses of bile salts in pancreatic steatorrhoea).

Fatty degeneration of the liver is also common and a variable proportion (ranging from 0 to 50 per cent with an average of about 10 per cent) of individuals have hepatic cirrhosis, which tends to be clinically quiescent. The cirrhosis is usually alcoholic, but biliary cirrhosis may develop as a result of biliary ductal stenosis. In some areas (like the USA and South Africa), chronic pancreatitis may be associated with excessive absorption of iron, so that the clinical picture resembles haemochromatosis. The tropical form of chronic pancreatitis, resulting from malnutrition, has an incidence of associated cirrhosis of about 15 per cent, so that the combination of chronic pancreatitis and cirrhosis is not specific for alcoholism.

Other results of the local fibrotic process include obstruction of adjacent beings, particularly the splenic vein, with resultant segmental portal hypertension, splenomegaly, varices and variceal bleeding, or splenic rupture. Partial obstruction of the abdominal lymphatics occurs in up to 10 per cent of patients and may be involved in the ascites which occurs in some patients with chronic pancreatitis.

The most important complication of chronic pancreatitis is the exocrine secretory insufficiency which characterizes this disease. The degree of abnormality of the processes involved in the assimilation of food is very variable, but at least one-third of the patients with chronic pancreatitis develop features of severe malassimilation, often late in the clinical course of the disease after many episodes of abdominal pain. However, in 5 to 10 per cent of patients steatorrhoea is the presenting feature of chronic pancreatitis, the disease having previously been 'painless'.

The most important pathophysiological abnormality in chronic pancreatitis is the impaired capacity to secrete digestive enzymes. Clinically, the maldigestion manifests as steatorrhoea, with creatorrhoea less common unless the exocrine secretory capacity is very severely impaired. If there are no aggravating factors, pancreatic secretory capacity has to be reduced to less than 10 per cent before maldigestion occurs. However, aggravating factors are common and may be functionally (and therefore therapeutically) more important than the impaired secretory capacity. For example, food intake may be markedly altered in chronic pancreatitis. Food intake may be reduced, especially if repeated episodes of pain, requiring analgesics, induce anorexia and depression. More commonly, the overall malassimilation of food alters the feelings of postcibal satiety so that patients with chronic pancreatitis tend to eat more than normal amounts of food and may, indeed, become severely hyperphagic.

In addition, patients with chronic pancreatitis often have abnormal gastric secretory and motor function. While some patients suffer from gastric hyposecretion, perhaps as a result of severe alcoholic gastritis, many patients have gastric hypersecretion as severe as in patients with duodenal ulcer. Patients with chronic pancreatitis also suffer from abnormally rapid emptying of gastric contents. Both gastric hypersecretion and abnormally rapid gastric emptying are attributable to impaired inhibition of the gastric secretory and motor functions as a consequence of lack of the breakdown products of fat in the duodenum. The net result of the abnormally rapid gastric emptying is that large amounts of food, ingested as a result of the hyperphagia, are emptied excessively rapidly into the upper small intestine together with abnormally large amounts of gastric juice. Not only does the influx of unprocessed food swamp the impaired digestive capacity of the pancreas, but the acidity of the duodenal contents rapidly and irreversibly denaturates those pancreatic enzymes which are still secreted by the damaged gland. As a consequence of all these functional disturbances, pancreatic steatorrhoea tends to be quantitatively the most severe form of malassimilation.

In addition to maldigestion, patients with chronic pancreatitis also suffer from malabsorption of fat because dietary lecithin (which is not hydrolysed to lysolecithin since insufficient phospholipase is secreted by the diseased pancreas) blocks the transfer of fatty acids from micelles to villous absorptive cells. There is also impaired absorption of fat-soluble vitamins, but clinical manifestations such as osteomalacia are uncommon. Defective absorption of vitamin B_{12} can be found in nearly half the patients with chronic pancreatitis, who lack a pancreatic protease-related factor necessary for the absorption of the vitamin. On the other hand, absorption of iron may be excessive in patients with alcoholic chronic pancreatitis.

Destruction or dysfunction of the islet cells in chronic pancreatitis can be clinically silent or can result in disturbances of glucose homeostasis, ranging from spontaneous or reactive hypoglycaemia (attributable to defective secretion of glucagon aggravated by defective assimilation of food) to diabetes mellitus responsive to diet, hypoglycaemic drugs, or requiring insulin. Overt diabetes occurs in more than 10 per cent of patients and impaired glucose tolerance is found in at least half the patients during the first 10 years of the disease. Diabetes may be the presenting feature of 'painless' chronic pancreatitis. It seems that the 'degenerative complications', involving retina, peripheral nerves, and kidneys, are less common than in the 'idiopathic' form of diabetes.

Occasionally, chronic pancreatitis manifests clinically with some of the features of acute pancreatitis. For example, during acute exacerbations of the chronic pancreatitis, patients may develop subcutaneous fat necrosis or acute arthralgia. Chronic pancreatitis may also present with serous effusions, especially in peritoneal or pleural cavities. The ascites is often massive, without any associated pancreatic pain, and is occasionally haemorrhagic or chylous. Complications such as the development of pseudocysts can also occur during the course of chronic pancreatitis but, unlike the lesions in acute pancreatitis, the pseudocysts do not resolve spontaneously.

Diagnosis. The diagnosis of chronic pancreatitis is confirmed by demonstrating pancreatic exocrine hypofunction following stimulation with the small intestinal hormones secretin and cholecystokinin. Impaired secretion of bicarbonate is present in at least 95 per cent of patients with chronic pancreatitis.

Chronic pancreatitis can be confirmed radiologically by the characteristic appearances of the parenchymal calcification or ductal listhiasis across the upper posterior abdomen at the level of the first lumbar vertebra. Endoscopic retrograde pancreatography also shows characteristic ductal abnormalities in about 80 per cent of patients with chronic pancreatitis, since the main and branch ducts become dilated, tortuous and develop areas of stenosis. Ultrasonography and CT scanning also demonstrate the dilated duct, as well as enlargement, with irregular consistency and outline of the gland.

When the diagnosis of chronic pancreatitis has been established, attempts must be made to ascertain the cause, from family and social history, measurement of blood levels of calcium and lipids, and endoscopic studies.

Differential diagnosis. The principal clinical pictures which arouse suspicion of chronic pancreatitis include recurrent episodes of upper abdominal pain, steatorrhoea, obstructive jaundice, or sudden onset of diabetes mellitus, especially when combined with one or more of the other clinical manifestations.

The differential diagnosis of the attacks of pain in patients with chronic pancreatitis includes recurrent attacks of acute pancreatitis, since the characteristics of the pain in the two conditions are identical. Differentiation between acute and chronic pancreatitis is necessary clinically, since removal of the cause of acute pancreatitis prevents relapses. Acute pancreatitis tends to affect older individuals, especially females, and to be associated with gallstones. Chronic pancreatitis occurs earlier in life and affects especially males. In acute pancreatitis, pancreatic function is normal between attacks, while patients with chronic pancreatitis have pancreatic exocrine hypofunction.

In pancreatic cancer, the pain tends to be continuous rather than intermittent. There is a greater tendency to lose weight than in chronic pancreatitis. Jaundice usually occurs early during the course of pancreatic cancer and is persistent and progressive. The presence of pancreatic calcification makes the diagnosis of chronic pancreatitis more likely.

Chronic pancreatitis with steatorrhoea and recurrent episodes of abdominal pain must be distinguished from intrinsic disease of the biliary tract causing intermittent obstruction, and from intestinal disorders such as Crohn's disease. Impairment of exocrine pancreatic function usually distinguishes pancreatic from other causes of steatorrhoea, but difficulties may arise when patients develop pain after gastrectomy, because it may be difficult or impossible to test pancreatic function under these circumstances. Laparotomy with biopsy of the pancreas may therefore be necessary to establish the diagnosis of chronic pancreatitis in patients who have had previous gastric operations.

The combination of steatorrhoea with diabetes mellitus is characteristic, but not diagnostic, of pancreatic steatorrhoea. Patients with coeliac disease have a greater than expected incidence of diabetes mellitus and may also suffer from pancreatic insufficiency. The presence of coeliac disease must be established by small intestinal biopsy, but the demonstration of villous atrophy does not preclude coincident chronic pancreatitis. The steatorrhoea which occurs in patients with diabetic autonomic neuropathy is distinguishable from the steatorrhoea of chronic pancreatitis with diabetes by the history of preceding diabetes for many years and by the presence of diabetic neuropathy, retinopathy, and nephropathy. Although pancreatic exocrine function may be impaired in long-standing diabetes mellitus, the degree of impairment is not as great as the virtual or total pancreatic achylia of patients with chronic pancreatitis complicated by diabetes.

Sudden onset of insulin-requiring diabetes mellitus or obstructive jaundice may be attributable to pancreatic disease, and although these presentations may signify the presence of chronic pancreatitis, it is always essential to exclude the presence of pancreatic cancer (see below).

Course and prognosis. The course of chronic pancreatitis usually involves slowly progressive deterioration of pancreatic exocrine function following episodes of abdominal pain of variable frequency and duration. Occasionally, the acute relapses become severe and may end fatally. Alternatively, the acute relapses may be painless and manifest as obstructive jaundice, arthropathy, or panniculitis.

In due course, as a result of the inexorable progression of the disease, the patient develops steatorrhoea and, some years later, diabetes mellitus. Destruction of the pancreas is then usually so severe that the attacks of pain become less frequent and ultimately disappear altogether. Occasionally the disease becomes clinically obvious only at this stage, having previously been 'pain free'.

At any time during the course of the disease, patients may present with severe psychiatric disturbances attributable to drug addiction and depression.

More than 50 per cent of the patients die within 20 years of diagnosis. Death results from complications such as haemorrhagic necrosis during an acute relapse or the subsequent development of a pseudocyst or an abscess. Patients die as a result of addiction to narcotics, or from suicide. Diabetic complications, especially ketotic or hypoglycaemic coma may also be fatal.

The prognosis is worst in patients who continue to drink alcohol. It has been estimated that if alcohol intake stops, 80 per cent of the affected individuals live for more than 10 years, while continuation of drinking reduces the 10-year survival rate to between 20 and 60 per cent.

Treatment. *Medical therapy*. The medical treatment of chronic pancreatitis involves counselling the patient to abstain from alcohol. Psychiatric treatment for addiction to alcohol and analgesics, as well as for depression, may be required. However, relapses of pain should be treated with adequate analgesics.

The steatorrhoea is controlled or abolished by reducing the intake of dietary fat and by replacing the pancreatic enzymes. In order to provide satisfactory replacement therapy it is necessary to use potent pancreatic extract, which should be administered in powder form and mixed with the food, although the appalling taste of most of the available extracts makes compliance impossible for some patients. Alternatively, pancreatic extract can be given in the form of granules or capsules, which are coated and therefore hide the taste. These forms of the extracts are unfortunately often not effective, since the enzymic activities are not released, or rapidly destroyed, in the upper small intestine.

Pancreatic extracts are irreversibly destroyed in the stomach if the patient secretes gastric juice. Such patients should receive ranitidine 150 mg 30 to 45 minutes before each meal in order to inhibit the gastric secretory response to the meal. It is usually also necessary to provide an antacid with the meal.

Supplements of fat-soluble vitamins are not usually required but if there is clinical evidence of osteomalacia, supplements of vitamin D must be given by injection.

The control of diabetes depends on the control of the maldigestion, so that stable control of the blood sugar is much more easily attained if the steatorrhoea has been corrected. The patients are liable to develop hypoglycaemic reactions because digestion is impaired and glucagon secretion is defective. The control of the hypoglycaemic attacks requires glucose or sucrose and must not be dependant on food which needs digestion. Each patient should also have a supply of glucagon for injection.

It has recently been suggested that pancreatic listhiasis can be improved by administration of citrate in the form of citric acid (2.6 g), potassium dihydrogen citrate (4 g), and sodium dihydrogen citrate (4 g) three times daily with meals.

Surgical treatment may be needed to relieve the complications of chronic pancreatitis.

By far the most important reason for operative treatment of chronic pancreatitis is the relief of pain. Quite early during the clinical course, the physician may have to make a decision whether the quality and duration of a patient's life will be better as a narcotic addict or after removal of the pancreas. This decision is difficult, because no satisfactory epidemiological information is available about the relative survival of potential or actual narcotic addicts with chronic pancreatitis compared with individuals who have undergone pancreatectomy.

Several types of operation have been used for the relief of pancreatic pain, but most achieve only transient success, or the relief of pain is attributable to progression of the disease, especially if accompanied by abstinence from alcohol. Thus, about 50 per cent of patients achieve temporary relief after drainage of the pancreatic ductal system, especially if the duct is dilated. Similarly, as many as 80 per cent of patients gain temporary relief of pain after partial pancreatectomy, but the operation is accompanied by a high incidence of infection (such as sub-phrenic abscess) and fistula formation, as well as long-term morbidity from steatorrhoea and diabetes.

The operation which gives most chance of success involves resection of 80 to 90 per cent of the pancreas. This operation has a high long-term morbidity, since the operated patients often develop diabetes mellitus and steatorrhoea. Patients also tend to develop stomal ulceration and may therefore require treatment with a gastric inhibitory drug like ranitidine. However, it seems to me that patients are much happier and healthier after near-total pancreatectomy than when treated with repeated or continuous courses of analgesic drugs—but that is merely a personal opinion. Recent claims that injection into the pancreatic duct of quickly setting solutions of amino acids destroys the residual acinar tissues of the pancreas and relieves pain without other adverse reactions will, perhaps, preclude the necessity for surgical intervention for the relief of pain in chronic pancreatitis.

Surgical treatment is also required for some of the other complications of chronic pancreatitis. Thus, obstruction of the bile duct necessitates some form of by-pass operation, taking care to exclude the presence of an ampullary carcinoma or cancer of the head of the pancreas. The development of portal hypertension is usually the result of thrombosis of the splenic vein and is cured by splenectomy. Pseudocysts and pancreatic abscesses require surgical drainage, either internally or externally. Pancreatectomy may have to be carried out to control pancreatic ascites, since the underlying fistulae are untreatable by medical means. Rarely recurrent episodes of fat necrosis may also cause sufficient disability to warrant pancreatectomy.

Pancreatic cancer

Pathology. Pancreatic cancer is usually an adenocarcinoma which arises in the head of the gland in about two-thirds of cases. However, the cancer is often multifocal, a finding which precludes partial resection as operative treatment of the condition.

The adenocarcinoma is generally stated to originate from pancreatic ductal tissue, on the grounds that histologically many of the cancers have 'ductal' morphology and some experimental pancreatic cancers (in hamsters) originate in the ductal system. However, other experimental cancers (in rats) arise in acinar tissue and precursor lesions, similar to those which precede carcinoma in rats, are found in about 50 per cent of human individuals, especially heavy smokers.

The cancer tends to spread locally, occluding the pancreatic duct so that acute or chronic pancreatitis develops distal to the occlusion, and also obstructing the bile duct, causing jaundice. The tumour invades especially by perineural spread, but also by veins, arteries, and lymphatics. Metastases are present in more than 75 per cent of cases at the time of diagnosis, with involvement particularly of regional lymph nodes and liver. Peritoneal spread is also quite common especially from tumours sited in the body or tail of the gland. The marked tendency of pancreatic cancer to spread and to metastasize determines the very low operability and short survival of affected patients.

Incidence. There has been a marked increase in the incidence of pancreatic cancer throughout the world during the past decade, so that deaths from the disease have almost doubled. It has been estimated that pancreatic cancer is present in approximately 2 per cent of the autopsies in France and Japan. However, the highest incidence of pancreatic cancer has been found in Polynesians such as the Maoris of New Zealand and in native Hawaiians. An unduly high incidence has also been recorded in Black males in the USA.

Pancreatic cancer affects individuals of all ages, but the incidence increases rapidly in patients older than 50 years. Males tend to be affected twice as frequently as females.

The development of pancreatic cancer has been related to smoking. The median age of smokers is about 15 years less than non-smokers at the time of development of the disease. It has also been stated that the risk of development of pancreatic cancer is directly proportional to the number of cigarettes smoked, especially by males. There also appears to be an increased risk in coffee drinkers.

The incidence of pancreatic cancer appears to be increased in some patients suffering from other diseases. For example, there appears to be a two-fold increase in the incidence of pancreatic cancer in patients with diabetes mellitus. Up to 20 per cent of individuals who are heterozygous for ataxia telangiectasia develop pancreatic cancer. A similar proportion of subjects with hereditary pancreatitis die from pancreatic cancer. However, whether or not there is an increased incidence of pancreatic cancer in patients with acquired chronic pancreatitis is still controversial. There is a geographical correlation of pancreatic cancer with areas of high incidence of alcohol-associated chronic calcific pancreatitis and it has been calculated that there is an increased incidence (up to 5 per cent) of pancreatic cancer in patients with chronic calcific pancreatitis and pancreatic listhiasis. It seems that there may also be a relationship between cholecystectomy and pancreatic cancer, which accounts in part for an unusually high incidence of pancreatic cancer in American Indian females, who undergo cholecystectomy because they suffer from a very high incidence of gallstones.

Aetiology. It has been noted that there is an unusually high incidence of pancreatic cancer in industrial chemists in the USA, from which it has been concluded that industrial carcinogens are involved in the pathogenesis of the disease. It has also been shown that the incidence of pancreatic cancer is directly related to the content of fat in the diet of different populations. As a result, environmental and dietary factors responsible for the development of pancreatic cancer are being sought.

The responsible industrial carcinogens have not yet been identified, but it has been shown in experimental animals that specific nitrosamine derivatives can selectively produce pancreatic cancer in hamsters and rats. Carcinogens from natural sources have also been shown to produce a high incidence of pancreatic cancer in experimental animals. For example, azaserine, an aminoacid analogue derived from a soil streptomyces, is selectively carcinogenic for the pancreas of rats.

The direct relationship between dietary content of fat and incidence of pancreatic cancer in different populations has been interpreted as indicating that the fat somehow increases the indidence of pancreatic cancer. In this connection, it has been shown that a diet rich in unsaturated fatty acids increases the incidence of pancreatic cancer produced by azaserine in rats.

Clinical manifestations. The mean age of onset of symptoms of pancreatic cancer is about 55 years. The duration of symptoms at the time of presentation is less than 6 months in more than 50 per cent of the patients, but despite the quite short prodrome, more than half the tumours are not resectable at the time of presentation.

The principal symptoms of pancreatic cancer are early and progressive loss of weight, abdominal pain, and jaundice. However, the sequence of presenting features depends on the location of the carcinoma within the pancreas. Carcinoma of the head of the pancreas presents as abdominal pain or painless jaundice, each in approximately one-third of the affected patients. Pain is the presenting feature in about 75 per cent of patients with cancer of the tail of the pancreas, while jaundice is the initial manifestation in two-thirds of the patients with ampullary cancer. Pain is present at some time in the great majority (up to 90 per cent) of patients with pancreatic cancer and jaundice occurs in most patients with cancer of the head of the pancreas and in ampullar cancer. Jaundice may be painless throughout the disease in half the cases of ampullary cancer and about 25 per cent of the cancers of the head of the

pancreas. Pain precedes jaundice by about three months when both symptoms are present. The jaundice usually becomes progressively more severe but occasionally fluctuates in intensity, perhaps because necrotic tumour material has sloughed and relieved the obstruction of the bile duct.

Pain, which is often the predominant symptom, is very variable in site, duration, and severity. Typically, the pain is upper abdominal, often epigastric, and penetrates to the back or is maximal there. The pain may be intermittent and can be precipitated by food and relieved by change in posture. The pain is sometimes attributable to invasion and dysfunction of adjacent organs and may mimic duodenal ulceration or small intestinal or colonic obstruction. In about 10 per cent of patients, there may be associated attacks of acute pancreatitis, which can antedate other manifestations of the cancer by up to two years.

Often the symptoms of pancreatic cancer are non-specific and include anorexia, lassitude, and loss of weight. The weight loss, which is often a presenting feature, is partly attributable to anorexia secondary to nausea and pain, and partly to maldigestion and malassimilation of food. Loss of weight does not have any serious prognostic implications and is not a contra-indication to surgical treatment.

Psychiatric abnormalities are common in patients with pancreatic cancer. Depression, which affects 75 per cent of the patients, is often a presenting feature.

Pancreatic cancer may also present as endocrine or metabolic disease. At least 20 per cent pf patients with pancreatic cancer develop some degree of diabetes mellitus and the acute onset of diabetes in elderly subjects, or failure of control in a previously mild and well-controlled individual is one of the ways in which pancreatic cancer presents. Rarely, pancreatic cancer may manifest as hypoglycaemia, for reasons which are not known. Pancreatic cancer can also produce peptide hormones or amines, so that the patients can present with Cushing's syndrome, hypercalcaemia, or the carcinoid syndrome.

Some patients with pancreatic cancer develop metastatic fat necrosis involving skin, joints, retroperitoneal tissue, and bone marrow. The clinical presentation of fat necrosis is fluctuant, tender subcutaneous nodules resembling erythema nodosum, or a polyarthritis affecting especially the large joints.

Patients with pancreatic cancer sometimes develop rather specific symptoms attributable to an abnormal thrombotic tendency which may be resistant to anticoagulants. Thus the cancer may present with thrombophlebitis migrans, or as non-bacterial verucous endocardiopathy, which can embolize throughout the systemic circulation.

Occasionally pancreatic cancer presents as a result of invasion of adjacent viscera or distant metastases. Thus, thrombosis of the splenic vein can cause portal hypertension and bleeding varices, while obstruction of the renal veins results in a nephrotic syndrome. Ascites is produced by peritoneal seeding, or by involvement of the portal vein in the neoplastic process.

The physical signs of pancreatic cancer are mainly non-specific. Hepatic enlargement is common and present in more than half of the patients. Usually the hepatomegaly reflects either obstruction of the bile ducts or hepatic metastases. Dilatation of the gall bladder is a more specific sign of ampullary or pancreatic cancer and the gall bladder is stated to be clinically palpable in half the ampullary cancers and one-third of the carcinomas of the head of the pancreas. However, this sign does not manifest until late in the course of the disease. When the pancreatic cancer is clinically palpable, as an upper abdominal mass, there is invariably involvement of lymph nodes and the cancer is no longer resectable. Splenomegaly, attributable to thrombosis of the splenic vein, has been reported in 15 per cent of patients with carcinoma of the tail of the pancreas. Ascites and dependent oedema are late manifestations of cancer of body or tail of the pancreas.

Diagnosis. At present the diagnosis of cancer involving the head of the pancreas is best confirmed by demonstrating morphological abnormalities (such as localized or generalized enlargement, different densities of parts of the gland, irregularity of the outline, invasion of surrounding structures, or ductal dilatation) by ultrasonographic examination of the pancreas. Ultrasonography is not as satisfactory in detecting cancers of the body or tail of the pancreas, which are perhaps better studied with CT scans. Endoscopic retrograde pancreatography satisfactorily demonstrates ductal abnormalities (such as papillary carcinoma, ductal occlusion, stricture, or necrotic tumour cavity) in the majority of cases of pancreatic cancer. However, the results of these procedures are often not sufficiently specific to differentiate pancreatic cancer from chronic pancreatitis. The definitive diagnosis of cancer necessitates histological confirmation of malignancy, by cytological examination of pancreatic juice or brushings obtained during retrograde pancreatography, or of duodenal juice obtained during test of function. Alternatively, tissue for histological examination may be obtained by pancreatic biopsy during laparoscopy, or by percutaneous needle biopsy during ultrasonic or CT examination. While a positive histological diagnosis confirms the presence of pancreatic malignancy, negative results even at laparotomy do not exclude the diagnosis of cancer (see also page 12.174).

Information about staging, or determination of resectability, is perhaps best obtained laparoscopically or by angiography. The latter technique identifies cancers which are not resectable because there is invasion of major blood vessels by the cancer, or because the cancer has metastasized.

Differential diagnosis. The pain of pancreatic cancer is not sufficiently specific in nature to permit differentiation from the many other causes of upper abdominal pain. However, it is worth emphasizing that persistent pain in the upper abdomen, especially if associated with loss of weight, raised ESR, and psychiatric changes, requires investigation with ultrasonography, endoscopic retrograde pancreatography, or laparoscopy.

The differential diagnosis of extrahepatic obstructive jaundice requires, in the first place, differentiation between pancreatic cancer and gallstones. Clinically, it has been repeatedly emphasized that a palpably enlarged gall bladder indicates neoplastic obstruction of the bile duct, since cholelisthiasis is usually associated with chronic cholecystitis and failure of the obstructed gall bladder to distend. The differential diagnosis is best made by percutaneous or laparoscopic cholangiography. If the jaundice is caused by obstruction at the lower end of the bile duct, the differential diagnosis is best established by endoscopy and, if necessary, retrograde pancreatography since this procedure differentiates between ampullary and other cancers, pancreatic cancer, and chronic pancreatitis as cause of the obstruction. The differentiation of pancreatic cancer from cancers of the ampulla, lower bile duct, or duodenum is of considerable prognostic importance since these neoplasms have progressively better resectability. For example, the five-year survival after resection of duodenal carcinoma is greater than 40 per cent.

In patients who present with recent onset of either steatorrhoea or of diabetes mellitus and who are found by function tests to suffer from exocrine hypofunction of the pancreas, the differential diagnosis lies between chronic pancreatitis and pancreatic cancer. The diagnosis is made by cytological examination of pancreatic juice or duodenal contents after stimulating the pancreas, or by biopsy under ultrasonographic or laparoscopic control. This type of investigation is desirable even in the presence of the pancreatic calcification in view of the occasional development of pancreatic cancer in the latter patients. Very rarely, the differential diagnosis is settled in favour of cancer because the calcification 'disappears' as the cancer progresses.

Course and prognosis. Carcinoma of the pancreas has one of the lowest survival rates, with only 1 per cent of patients surviving for longer than five years. The survival rate has not changed during the past two decades. The average interval between onset of symptoms and death has ranged from four to 10 months, with an 80 per cent mortality within one year of diagnosis.

The prognosis of pancreatic cancer depends largely on its location within the gland. Since jaundice tends to be an early symptom of cancer in the head of the pancreas, about one-third of the cancers presenting with jaundice are resectable and approximately one-third of the resected cancers have not spread locally or metastasized at the time of operation. Thus, only about 10 per cent of patients with cancer of the head of the pancreas have any chance of successful surgical treatment. On the other hand, the occurrence of symptoms in patients with cancer sited in the body or tail of the gland almost invariably indicates that the pancreatic cancer is no longer resectable and the prognosis of cancer in these sites is therefore very bad, with survival less than one year. Other prognostically bad features include the early onset of severe pain, symptomatic history longer than three months, angiographic involvement of major arteries, hepatic metastases, and obstruction of the bile duct within 4 cm of the bifurcation into hepatic ducts on percutaneous cholangiography.

The causes of death include cachexia in more than 50 per cent of patients, with cholangitis, hepatic coma, and pulmonary emboli each in a further 10 per cent.

Treatment. *Surgical.* Dissemination of the pancreatic cancer makes resection impossible. Under these circumstances, bypass procedures should be carried out to decompress the biliary tract (and relieve jaundice and pruritus) and to establish a gastrojejunostomy, since duodenal obstruction by the pancreatic cancer necessitates reoperation in more than 25 per cent of patients in whom a duodenal bypass has not been performed. The average duration of survival after biliary and duodenal bypass procedures ranges from four to eight months, so that this type of palliative surgical treatment does not alter the prognosis of pancreatic cancer.

The only chance of curing the disease is adequate resection. Three types of operation have been carried out. Whipple's procedure involves duodenectomy and partial pancreatectomy. The mortality of this operation is low in specialist units but ranges up to 40 per cent in general hospitals. The morbidity is high, with early formation of pancreatic fistulae and a high incidence of pancreatic insufficiency and diabetes mellitus. Anastomotic ulceration is a late complication. As an alternative, total pancreatectomy has been advocated because pancreatic cancer is often, if not always, multifocal. In addition, jejuno-pancreatic anastomosis is avoided, so that there is no possibility of fistula formation and no post-operative pancreatitis. The removal of lymph nodes is more complete than with a Whipple operation. Total pancreatectomy is nowadays therefore preferred to partial pancreatectomy as operative treatment for pancreatic cancer, with an average survival of 10 to 20 months. The operation of regional pancreatectomy is more radical than total pancreatectomy and involves removal of major vessels as well as lymph nodes and viscera in the upper abdomen. The operation has a high mortality and the results are not as good as after total pancreatectomy.

After total pancreatectomy, patients require pancreatic replacement therapy. Insulin requirements are small, since the patients are sensitive to insulin and only rarely develop ketoacidosis. Hypoglycaemic attacks may occur frequently and affect 20–50 per cent of patients. After pancreatectomy, patients should therefore be provided with standby glucagon.

Chemotherapy. A number of single drugs have been used in the treatment of pancreatic cancer, but none have proved to have any value. Combinations of cytotoxic drugs have also been studied and have increased life expectancy by six to 12 months. A number of multicentre trials of combinations of drugs is in progress, especially in the USA, but no definitive information is available at present.

Radiotherapy. At laparotomy, the tumour mass is outlined with clips so that radiation can be applied, either at operation or subsequently. The benefit of radiation is dose-related and there are occasional long-term survivors. Better results have been claimed in response to treatment with a combination of radiotherapy and 5-fluorouracil. However, the mean survival is not much longer than six months, so that further studies of combined treatments are in progress.

Pancreatic disease in childhood

Hereditary disease

Cystic fibrosis. Cystic fibrosis is a hereditary disease affecting exocrine glands and characterized by abnormal composition of the exocrine secretions. The disease is the commonest cause of pancreatic insufficiency in childhood.

Incidence. Cystic fibrosis affects mainly individuals of European ancestry, occurring in about 1 in 2000 live births on the basis of autosomal recessive inheritance. The frequency of the gene has been estimated to be 2–5 per cent of the general Caucasian population. In the USA, less than 2 per cent of patients are black. The sex incidence is approximately equal.

Aetiology. The defect underlying the abnormal exocrine secretions has not yet been defined. Characteristically, the secretions contain too little water relative to the content of proteins or electrolytes, causing 'mucoviscidosis' and giving rise to the diagnostically high concentrations of sodium and chloride in the sweat of affected individuals.

Clinical manifestations. The clinical expression of cystic fibrosis ranges in severity from apparently 'normal' to markedly impaired health and even death in the first year of life.

The most important clinical abnormalities result from disease of the respiratory tract. The symptoms of pancreatic involvement may be quite insignificant or, alternatively, can antedate the respiratory complications by many years. The affected children often present with diarrhoea and failure to thrive, despite marked hyperphagia. 20 per cent of infants have developed rather characteristic rectal prolapse by the age of two years. Alternatively, meconium ileus may be the earliest presentation and affects 15 per cent of infants with cystic fibrosis. The infants or children present less commonly with hypoalbuminaemic oedema, portal hypertension or heat exhaustion. In about 20 per cent, the diagnosis of cystic fibrosis is not made until the patient is in the late teens, and then usually as a consequence of chronic respiratory disease.

The initial pancreatic changes, which are often present at birth, consist of ducts blocked by inspissated secretions. Dilatation of the ducts follows, with inflammatory changes in the gland and subsequent disappearance of acinar tissue which is replaced by fat and fibrous tissue. Clinical pancreatic exocrine insufficiency may already present in the neonatal period and result in steatorrhoea, creatorrhoea and diarrhoea, with hyperphagia. Undernutrition is common in affected infants, but less usual in older children and adolescents, whose stature may be normal. Symptoms attributable to malabsorption of fat-soluble vitamins are rare, but deficiency of vitamin A or K has been recorded and minor abnormalities of calcium metabolism are common. In other children, pancreatic function is normal early in life but eventually deteriorates, following attacks of abdominal pain suggestive of recurrent pancreatitis. Older children may present with diabetes mellitus although ketoacidosis is rare compared with the usual form of 'juvenile diabetes'.

Hepatic changes (see page 12.226) result from blockage of the bile ductules by inspissated secretions. Pericholangitis and periportal fibrosis, followed by biliary cirrhosis, affect less than 5 per cent and the hepatic disease is symptomatic in less than 2 per cent of children with cystic fibrosis. Surgical treatment may be necessary for hypersplenism or, more frequently, for protal hypertension which has resulted in variceal bleeding. Children with cystic fibrosis also have an increased incidence of gallstones, which occur in about 10 per cent of older individuals.

The intestinal changes in cystic fibrosis depend on the secretion of excessive amounts of abnormally viscid mucus. Clinically the abnormal mucus secretion causes 'meconium ileus', which presents as intestinal obstruction in 10–20 per cent of affected neonates (see page 12.145). There may be associated volvulus or intestinal atresia. The infants do not pass meconium after birth and X-rays show no colonic gas, while the dilated small intestine contains no fluid levels. Older children and adults may suffer from recurrent attacks of abdominal pain with palpable masses of faeces, intussusception, and subacute or acute intestinal obstruction. The 'meconium ileus equivalent' may be precipitated by withdrawal of pancreatic supplement therapy.

The most important pathological abnormalities in cystic fibrosis are found in the lungs. Although the respiratory system appears normal at birth, inspissated mucus causes bronchiolar obstruction with resultant atelectases and infection, leading to progressive destruction of alveolar tissues, bronchiectasis, and emphysema and ultimately pulmonary insufficiency and cor pulmonale. In the upper respiratory tract, sinusitis and nasal polyposis is common.

Abnormalities of the reproductive system in males, such as atresia or absence of seminal vesicles, vas deferens, and epididimis, are a consequence of maldevelopment of mesonephric derivatives. Spermatogenesis is often defective or absent.

Diagnosis. The diagnosis of cystic fibrosis in infants is confirmed by the finding that concentrations of sodium in sweat are greater than 60 mmol/l. Sweating is best elicited by pilocarpine iontophoresis in duplicate tests on different days. Sweat samples must be greater than 100 mg.

Increased concentrations of albumin in meconium have also been used for diagnostic purposes.

Pancreatic involvement in the disease is confimed by the demonstration of pancreatic hyposecretion or achylia. About 25 per cent of children without steatorrhoea secrete low volumes of pancreatic juice with very high concentrations of enzymes, indicating that primarily there is selective impairment of pancreatic water and electrolyte secretion.

Differential diagnosis. The steatorrhoea of cystic fibrosis in infancy and childhood must be distinguished from other causes of steatorrhoea and, specifically, from other causes of pancreatic insufficiency.

Villous atrophy usually easily differentiates the steatorrhoea of coeliac disease from cystic fibrosis but it is necessary to keep in mind that cystic fibrosis and coeliac disease may segregate in the same sibship and that infants with cystic fibrosis may therefore develop coeliac disease when weaned. Conversely, pancreatic exocrine insufficiency sometimes occurs as a complication of coeliac disease.

The pancreatic insufficiency of cystic fibrosis must be distinguished from congenital hypoplasia. Children with the latter condition have hypoplasia of the bone marrow and metaphyseal dysostosis and normal concentrations of sweat sodium.

It may be difficult to establish the diagnosis of cystic fibrosis in adolescents and adults since the concentration of sodium in sweat may be more than 60 mmol/l in normal individuals. It seems that values greater than 100 or 110 mmol/l are more likely to be diagnostic of cystic fibrosis, although it has been reported that up to one-third of patients with calcific chronic pancreatitis have concentrations of sweat sodium above 90 mmol/l and 14 per cent have concentrations above 120 mmol/l. These very high values of sweat sodium concentration have led to the suggestion that some patients with chronic calcific pancreatitis are suffering from a 'forme fruste' of cystic fibrosis.

Course and prognosis. Both pancreatic and pulmonary disease are progressive and tend to become more severe as the child grows older. Children who retain some pancreatic function suffer from attacks resembling acute pancreatitis. About 50 per cent of adolescents develop glucose intolerance.

With satisfactory treatment, more than 80 per cent of individuals suffering from cystic fibrosis attain the third decade. As a result, cystic fibrosis is the most common cause of chronic obstructive pulmonary disease and of pancreatic insufficiency in the first three decades of life in Western countries. The pulmonary disease is the main cause of morbidity and mortality in adolescents and adults with cystic fibrosis. The steatorrhoea persists, but is clinically less obtrusive than in childhood.

Treatment. The treatment of cystic fibrosis is not satisfactory, since the aetiology has not been defined and no means are available for modifying the defective exocrine secretions. Therapeutic measures are therefore confined to replacing the essential components of the defective secretions (such as pancreatic enzymes) and treating the consequences of the blockages of tubes and ducts (particularly, therefore, pulmonary infections and intestinal obstruction).

The pancreatic exocrine insufficiency is not satisfactorily treated with pancreatic extract alone, since the steatorrhoea persists with this simple form of treatment. In part, the unsatisfactory nature of replacement therapy results from poor compliance, because most pancreatic extracts taste so revolting. The extract therefore tends to be administered in enteric-coated form but the digestive efficacy of these preparations is low. In addition, some children with cystic fibrosis have gastric hypersecretion and pancreatic extract is therefore destroyed during gastric transit or, in the case of the enteric-coated preparations, in the upper small intestine since the latter is flooded with acid. Treatment of the steatorrhoea of cystic fibrosis is improved if ranitidine is administered 30–45 minutes before each meal in order to suppress the gastric secretion stimulated by food. In addition, it seems probable that the steatorrhoea is partly attributable to lack of bile salts, because in children with cystic fibrosis there may be failure of secretion, and there is often interruption of the normal enterohepatic recirculation of bile salts with excessive faecal losses. Satisfactory replacement of bile salts has not yet been achieved, but adequate pancreatic replacement therapy decreases faecal losses of bile salts sufficiently to diminish the formation of gallstones in these patients. Fat-soluble vitamins should be given regularly, by injection.

The intestinal obstruction may require surgical relief. Treatment with oral or colonically-administered acetyl cysteine, or gastrigrafin enemas has also been advocated.

The main impediment to survival of affected individuals is the development of recurrent pulmonary infections, with consequent destruction of the lungs. The principal therapeutic efforts must therefore be devoted to relieving bronchiolar obstruction by regular postural drainage and to administration of appropriate antibiotics when pulmonary infections occur. Whether antibiotic therapy should be continuous or intermittent is still controversial, but in the first year of life, continuous therapy is probably indicated.

Pancreatic hypoplasia. Pancreatic hypoplasia (Shwachman–Diamond syndrome) is a familial disorder which involves not only the pancreas but also the haemopoietic and skeletal system of affected individuals. The condition, which is present in the newborn, appears to be worldwide in distribution and is the second most common cause of pancreatic exocrine insufficiency in infants (after cystic fibrosis).

The disease is characterized by total, or almost complete, absence of the pancreatic exocrine tissue, with fatty replacement. The islet tissue is apparently normal. The pancreatic insufficiency is often clinically manifest as severe steatorrhoea in neonates or early infancy, but diarrhoea may be slight or absent. Birth weight may be low, there is often failure to thrive, and growth retardation or dwarfism are present in about half the children.

The children also suffer from repeated infections, especially of lungs and middle ears, because of the persistent or cyclic neutropenia, which reflects the hypoplasia of the bone marrow, characteristic of the syndrome (see also Section 19). There may also be mild or severe associated deficiency of IgA.

The skeletal abnormalities present first as flaring of the anterior ends of the ribs during infancy. When the children are older than about two years, metaphyseal growth abnormalities affect especially knees and hips.

The normal concentrations of sodium and chloride in sweat, as well as the associated haematological and skeletal clinical features, differentiate the disease from cystic fibrosis. The overall prognosis is reasonably good, provided infections are correctly treated.

The steatorrhoea seems to be fairly easily managed with supplements of oral pancreatic extract. However, the skeletal abnormalities cannot be treated and residual dwarfism is often severe.

Pancreatic hypoplasia has been recorded in association with situs inversus.

Deficient secretion of single pancreatic enzymes. A few reports have described children with 'isolated enzyme deficiency'. The absence of lipase from pancreatic juice has resulted in severe steatorrhoea, often with persistent anal seepage of oil. The general nutrition of the children is satisfactory because 50–80 per cent of the dietary fat is absorbed (for reasons which have not yet been satisfactorily explained). The diagnosis is based on the absence of lipase from the duodenal contents after pancreatic stimulation, despite secretion of normal amounts of the other enzymes and bicarbonate.

Defective secretion of trypsinogen has been recorded in a few children presenting with failure to thrive, diarrhoea, vomiting, and especially oedema attributable to hypoalbuminaemia. Some of the children probably suffered from the somewhat more common deficiency of small intestinal enterokinase. The latter enzyme is required to convert secreted trypsinogen, which is enzymically inactive, to active trypsin in the duodenal lumen, so that the clinical presentation of enterokinase deficiency is similar to failure of secretion of the proteolytic enzymes. The two conditions can be diagnosed from the absence of proteolytic enzymic activity in the duodenal contents after pancreatic stimulation, while lipolytic activity and bicarbonate secretion are normal. Incubation of the duodenal aspirate with exogenous enterokinase differentiates defective secretion of trypsinogen from deficiency of enterokinase. In children with enterokinase deficiency, normal proteolytic activity of duodenal aspirate can be demonstrated after activation, while added exogenous enterokinase does not uncover proteolytic activity in children who do not secrete trypsinogen. Both trypsinogen deficiency and enterokinase deficiency may initially require treatment with protein digests, but subsequently therapeutic oral pancreatic extract is usually adequate to maintain normal nutrition.

Hereditary pancreatitis. Chronic pancreatitis may occur with either autosomal recessive or autosomal dominant types of inheritance in several generations.

The affected children complain of recurrent attacks of abdominal pain, lasting for one to two days, for which no cause is usually found. After some years, steatorrhoea and pancreatic calcification make the diagnosis obvious. Thrombosis of portal and splenic veins is common. As many as 20 per cent of individuals develop pancreatic cancer.

The diagnosis is made on the basis of increased values of serum amylase or lipase during the attacks of pain and by the demonstration of steatorrhoea with pancreatic calcification and hypofunction. Some families show aminoaciduria, with cystine and lysine predominant.

The differential diagnosis includes cystic fibrosis, hereditary hyperparathyroidism, and hereditary hyperlipoproteinaemias (types I and V, see Section 9), all of which may also present with acute episodes of pancreatitis and result in chronic pancreatitis. The calcific pancreatitis associated with malnutrition usually presents with steatorrhoea rather than recurrent abdominal pain, and does not have the characteristics of hereditary transmission. Occasionally, exposure to alcohol during childhood has resulted in chronic alcoholic pancreatitis at this age.

Developmental abnormalities

Annular pancreas. When the embryological elements of the pancreas do not migrate normally during developmental rotation of the duodenum, the result may be partial or complete encirclement of the duodenum by pancreatic tissue. This type of abnormality is associated with other developmental abnormalities in as many as 70 per cent of children and 15 per cent of adults. The annular pancreas comprises the whole pancreas, or may join the body and tail normally. Symptoms can occur in infancy, as the result of the development of high small intestinal obstruction and obstructive jaundice. Radiologically, the 'double bubble' of air in stomach and duodenal bulb is characteristic of annular pancreas.

Later in life, fibrosis may give rise to duodenal obstruction, after repeated attacks of pancreatitis have resulted in chronic pancreatitis, sometimes together with peptic ulceration. Treatment involves surgical bypass of the duodenum since direct attack on the stricture generally results in multiple complications.

Pancreas divisum. Incomplete fusion of ventral and dorsal elements of the embryonic pancreas results in partial or complete division of the organ into two parts. As a result, much or most of the pancreas drains into the duodenum through the accessory duct. It has been suggested that drainage through the accessory duct and papilla may be inadequate, with obstruction to the flow of pancreatic juice from the dominant dorsal segment of the pancreas causing recurrent attacks of pancreatitis.

Acquired diseases. Acute pancreatitis in children is uncommon and has the same clinical features as the adult disease. However, in view of the rarity of the condition, the diagnosis is often not suspected when children complain of acute abdominal pain, so that about one quarter of affected individuals are only diagnosed at autopsy. The principal associated conditions differ from those encountered in adults. Thus, abdominal trauma accounts for as many as 30 per cent of cases, often as a result of child battering. Intake of drugs (especially high doses of corticosteroids) accounts for about one quarter of cases, while viral infection (such as mumps and mycoplasma pneumoniae) or infestation with ascaris are also relatively common causes of acute pancreatitis. When acute pancreatitis is associated with biliary disease, there are usually underlying congenital abnormalities of the biliary tract.

Chronic pancreatitis, with exocrine insufficiency, diabetes mellitus, and radiologically visible disseminated calcification has been reported from Africa and South Asia in large numbers of adolescents. The disease has been attributed to malnutrition, perhaps associated with intake of (undefined) dietary toxins.

References

Banks, P. A. (1979). *Pancreatitis*. Plenum, New York.
Cohn, I. (1979). Pancreatic cancer. *Semin. Oncol.* **6**, no. 3.
Cushieri, A. and Wormsley, K. G. (1980). The pancreas. In *Recent advances in gastroenterology*, vol. 4 (ed. I. A. D. Bouchier), 223. Churchill Livingstone, Edinburgh.
Di Sant'Agnese, P. A. and Davis, P. B. (1979). Cystic fibrosis in adults. *Am. J. Med.* **66**, 121.
Forell, M. M. (1976). Pankreas. In *Handbuch der inneren medizin*. Band 3, *Verdauungsorgane*, teil 6. Springer Verlag, Berlin.
Howat, H. T. (1972). The exocrine pancreas. *Clin. Gastroent.* **1**, no. 1.
— and Sarles, H. (1979). *The exocrine pancreas*. W. B. Saunders, London.
Lebenthal, E. and Shwachman, H. (1977). The pancreas—development, adaptation and malfunction in infancy and childhood. *Clin. Gastroent.* **6**, 397.
Levison, D. A. (1979). Carcinoma of the pancreas. *J. Path.* **129**, 203.
Mallory, A. and Kern, F. (1980). Drug-induced pancreatitis: A critical review. *Gastroent.* **78**, 813.
Wood, R. E., Boat, T. F., and Doershuk, C. F. (1976). Cystic fibrosis. *Am. Rev. resp. Dis.* **113**, 833.

Diseases of the gall bladder and biliary tree

J. A. Summerfield

Anatomy. The biliary system comprises the collection of ducts extending from the biliary canaliculus of each hepatocyte to the ampulla of Vater opening into the duodenum. The biliary canaliculi drain into interlobular and then septal bile ducts. These further ramify to form the intrahepatic bile ducts which are visible on cholangiography (Fig. 1). They eventually form the right and left hepatic ducts draining bile from the right and left lobes of the liver respectively. The junction of the hepatic ducts at the porta hepatis forms the common hepatic duct. The cystic duct, linking the gall bladder to the bile duct, arises from the lower end of the common hepatic duct. The gall bladder rests in a fossa under the right lobe of the liver. Anatomical variations in the size and position of the gall bladder and the insertion of the cystic duct into the bile duct are of major surgical importance. The common hepatic duct becomes the common bile duct below the insertion of the cystic duct. The common bile duct passes through the head of the pancreas and the sphincter of Oddi to drain into the duodenum via the ampulla of Vater. The bile duct usually exits through a common channel with the pancreatic duct in the ampulla of Vater, although anatomical variations are frequent.

The investigation of biliary disease

Objectives. The clinical and laboratory features of biliary disease may also be caused by hepatic disorders. Consequently, the primary objective of the investigation is to establish that the cause is due to biliary and not hepatic disease. The secondary objective is to define the anatomy of the lesion to permit a rational choice of the many surgical and non-surgical therapeutic options which are now available. To achieve these objectives requires not only a careful history and physical examination, but also the use of various imaging techniques and sometimes aspiration liver biopsy.

Symptoms and signs. Disorders of the biliary system usually give rise to the symptoms and signs of biliary obstruction (cholestasis). The repertoire is rather limited; pain, jaundice, itching, nausea and vomiting, fevers, and rigors. The pain can range between abdominal discomfort described as 'dyspepsia' to severe right hypochondrial colic caused by a sudden rise in biliary pressure. Jaundice, dark urine, and pale stools indicate obstruction of the bile duct. Itching is another important sign of biliary obstruction. Nausea and vomiting may be prominent in sudden obstruction of the bile duct, usually by a gallstone. The milder symptoms of flatulence and intolerance of fatty food are more common. Fever and rigors indicate bacterial infection of the biliary tract which frequently accompanies partial obstruction. In jaundiced patients weight loss is usual and results from fat malabsorption due to the lack of bile acids reaching the gut; it may also indicate a malignant tumour. Prolonged biliary obstruction leads to skin changes; increased pigmentation (due to melanin) and cholesterol deposits (xanthelasma and xanthoma). Finally, biliary cirrhosis may develop causing the signs of portal venous hypertension and liver-cell failure.

Laboratory investigations. In general, disorders of the biliary system give rise to the biochemical picture of *biliary obstruction* (*cholestasis*). A notable exception is gallstones in the gall bladder (cholelithiasis) where the liver function tests are usually normal. In cholestasis, the serum bilirubin concentration may be normal or raised and most of the bilirubin is esterified (conjugated). Bilirubinuria is

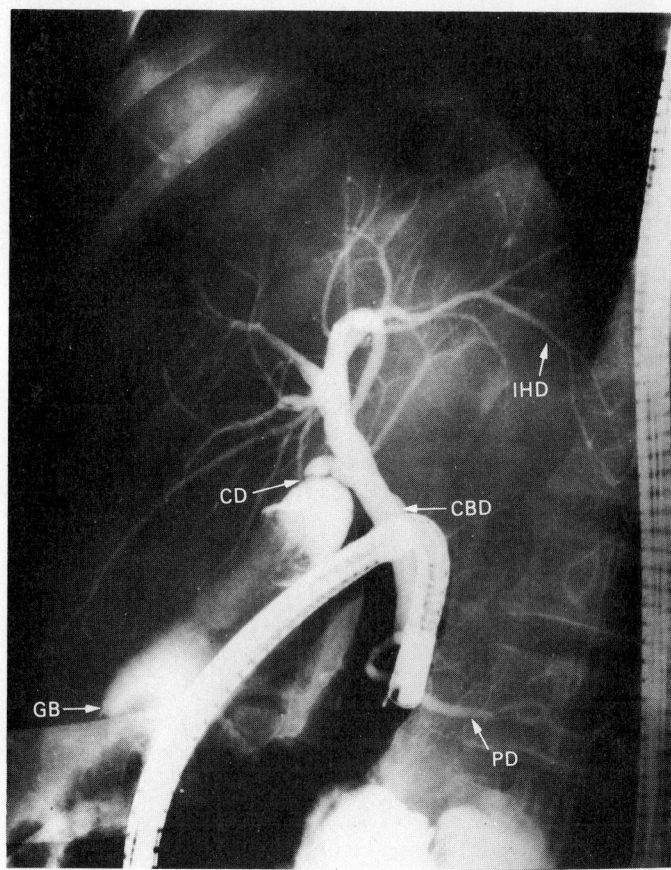

Fig. 1   The normal biliary tree. The intrahepatic bile ducts (IHD) taper smoothly and extend deep into the liver. The gall bladder (GB) drains via the cystic duct (CD) into the common bile duct (CBD). The pancreatic duct (PD) has also been opacified in this endoscopic retrograde cholangiogram (ERCP).

present. The disappearance of urobilinogen from the urine indicates complete biliary obstruction. Elevation of the serum alkaline phosphatase is an important, but not invariable, sign of biliary obstruction; the rise is usually greater than three times normal. Other biliary canalicular enzymes accumulate in the blood, including 5′-nucleotidase and γ-glutamyl transpeptidase. 5′-nucleotidase (which is only found in the liver) is estimated if there is doubt as to whether the alkaline phosphatase is of bony or hepatic origin. This may be required in children and patients with malignancy. Serum transaminases, such as aspartate aminotransferase, show only modest elevations in contrast to the rises which occur in hepatitis. The serum cholesterol concentration rises and may cause abnormalities of red cell shape (target cells) (see Section 19). A raised serum bile acid concentration is a sensitive index of biliary disease. Hypoprothrombinaemia reflects intestinal malabsorption of fat-soluble vitamin K due to a lack of bile acids. Vitamin A and D deficiency may also develop. The serum albumin and gamma globulin levels are normal until biliary cirrhosis develops. A polymorphonuclear leucocytosis accompanies bacterial infections of the biliary system.

Imaging techniques. A plain X-ray of the abdomen is mandatory; it may reveal an enlarged liver, calcified gallstones, or air in the biliary tree. This should be followed by a non-invasive technique such as grey scale ultrasonography (ultrasound) or computerized tomography (CT scan) (see page 12.9). These reveal dilated bile ducts and may also indicate the position of the obstruction in the biliary tree and dense structures such as gallstones. Hepatic scintiscanning with 99Tcm-labelled HIDA (dimethyl acetanilide iminodiacetic acid) (see page 12.8) is an alternative and is of value in the

diagnosis of acute cholecystitis. However, these investigations often provide insufficient anatomical detail for diagnosis or planning of treatment. In the non-jaundiced patient the next step should be an oral cholecystogram, and if this is unsatisfactory, an intravenous cholangiogram. In the jaundiced patient and those with poor liver function an invasive cholangiographic technique such as percutaneous transhepatic cholangiography (PTC) and endoscopic retrograde cholangiopancreatography (ERCP) are performed. If the non-invasive technique shows that the intrahepatic bile ducts are dilated, PTC is most likely to succeed. However, in patients with non-dilated ducts or blood clotting disorders ERCP is the preferred approach. Both these techniques carry risks including haemorrhage, biliary peritonitis and cholangitis (PTC), and bowel perforation and cholangitis (ERCP). Should cholangiography reveal a normal biliary system in a jaundiced patient, a liver biopsy is indicated.

This diagnostic approach is ideal but expensive both in terms of human and material resources. The apparatus required is costly and procedures such as ERCP require considerable expertise. Obviously local factors will determine the diagnostic pathway that is adopted. Nevertheless, these techniques have revolutionized the management of the patient with biliary disease. It is now a routine matter to rapidly achieve a precise diagnosis. In addition, a series of non-operative therapeutic options ranging from the introduction of endoprostheses for the management of benign and malignant biliary structures to endoscopic sphincterotomy for the removal of the biliary calculi are direct consequences of these new diagnostic approaches.

Bile composition and gallstone formation

Bile composition. Bile is secreted by the hepatocytes and its water and electrolyte composition is altered during its passage down the biliary system. Between meals much of the bile is diverted to the gall bladder where it is concentrated by the removal of sodium, chloride, bicarbonate, and water. In response to food, the gall bladder contracts, emptying bile into the duodenum. Apart from water (97 per cent) the major components of bile are bile acids, phospholipids, and cholesterol. Bile is also the major excretory route of other compounds including bilirubin and certain drugs and their metabolites. Cholesterol is insoluble in water but is held in solution by the detergent action of bile acids with the aid of phospholipids.

Cholesterol is synthesized primarily in the liver and small intestine. The rate-limiting enzyme for cholesterol production is hydroxymethylglutaryl-CoA reductase which catalyses the first step, the conversion of acetate to mevalonate. Subsequently, non-esterified (free) cholesterol is secreted into bile. Dietary cholesterol also contributes to biliary cholesterol secretion. The control of cholesterol metabolism is complex. It is not yet clear what proportion of biliary cholesterol is derived from circulating lipoproteins and what proportion is newly synthesized by the liver.

The primary bile acids, cholic and chenodeoxycholic acid, are synthesized in the liver from cholesterol. The economy of the bile acid pool is preserved by efficient reabsorption, principally in the terminal ileum. About 95 per cent of the bile acids are reabsorbed and pass back to the liver in the portal venous system (enterohepatic circulation). The remainder enters the colon where bacteria form the secondary bile acids, deoxycholic and lithocholic acid, from cholic acid and chenodeoxycholic acid respectively. Some of the secondary bile acids are absorbed from the colon but most are excreted in the faeces. The normal bile acid pool is about 3–5 g and circulates 6 to 10 times each day. Synthesis is controlled by the negative feedback of bile acids returning in the portal venous blood which act on the rate limiting hepatic enzyme, cholesterol-7α-hydroxylase. The principal phospholipid in bile is lecithin. It is produced in the liver and secreted into the bile. In the intestine lecithin is hydrolysed to lysolecithin by pancreatic phospholipase and is subsequently reabsorbed.

Above a certain level (the critical micellar concentration) bile acids coalesce to form micelles that have a hydrophilic external surface and hydrophobic internal surface. Cholesterol is incorporated into the hydrophobic interior. Phospholipids are inserted into the micellar wall so that the micelles are enlarged; these 'mixed micelles' are thus able to hold more cholesterol.

Consequently, the solubility of cholesterol in bile depends on the concentrations of bile acid and phospholipid. In the presence of a relative excess of bile acid and phospholipid (on a molar basis) the cholesterol holding capacity of bile is increased and it is said to be unsaturated. However, if there are insufficient micelles of bile acid and phospholipid to hold the cholesterol, the solution is referred to as saturated and the excess cholesterol tends to precipitate. With a knowledge of the molar concentrations of cholesterol, phospholipid, and bile acid, the cholesterol saturation of bile can be predicted using triangular co-ordinate diagrams.

Gallstone formation. Gallstone disease is common and afflicts between 10 and 20 per cent of the world's population. Gallstones are classified according to their composition into two main groups: *cholesterol stones* and *bile pigment stones*. Cholesterol stones are composed mainly of cholesterol (more than 70 per cent) and can be sub-divided into pure cholesterol stones, usually solitary, and cholesterol–pigment–calcium stones ('mixed stones') composed of a mixture of cholesterol, bile pigment, and calcium (Figs. 2 and 3). They are usually multiple and faceted. Bile pigment stones can also be divided into two main groups. Bile-pigment–calcium stones which are brown, soft, and pliable, and pure pigment stones ('black stones') which are black, hard, and brittle. Gallstones are rare before the age of 10. The incidence increases progressively with age. Cholesterol gallstones account for about 75 per cent of the gallstones in Europe and the USA.

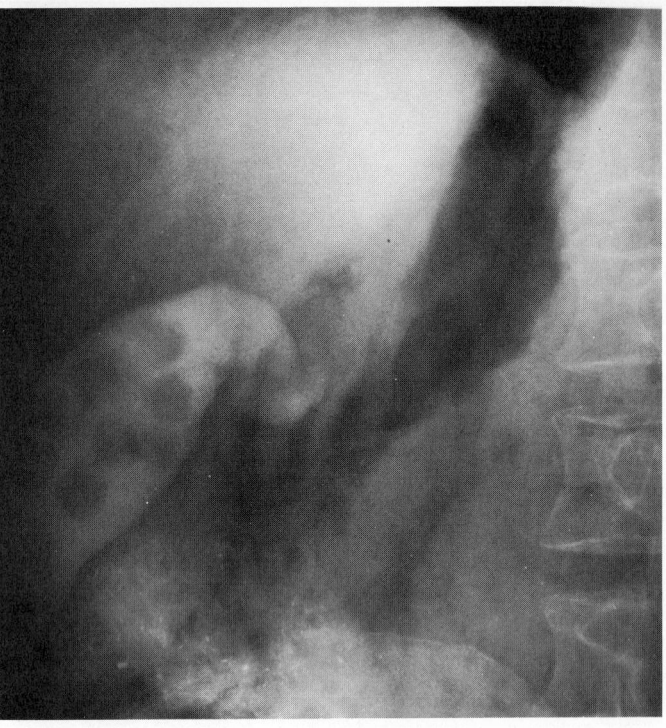

Fig. 3 Cholesterol gallstones. An intravenous cholangiogram has opacified the gall bladder showing multiple faceted radiolucent gallstones. These are typical features of cholesterol stones.

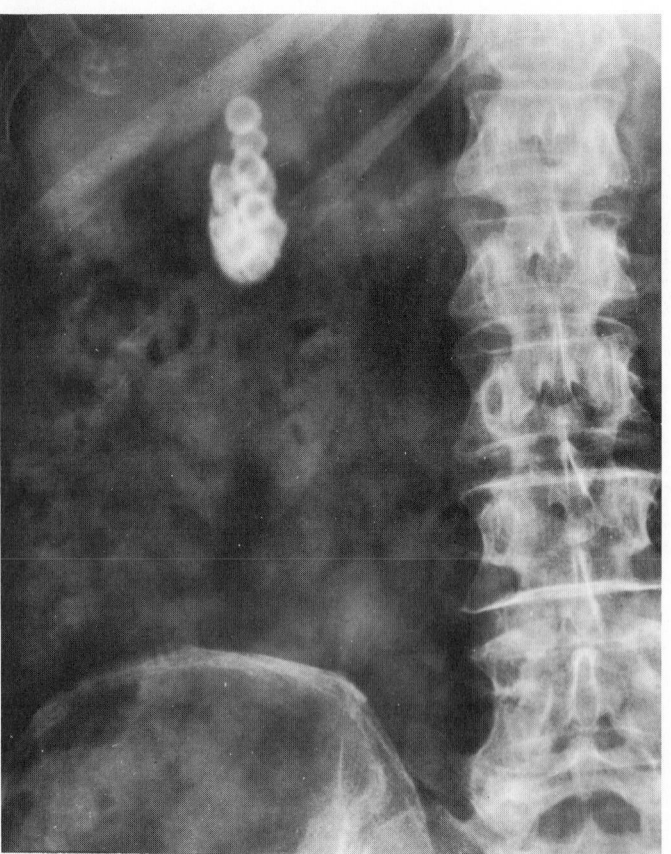

Fig. 2 Calcified gallstones. Gallstones contain sufficient calcium to be visible on a plain abdominal X-ray in about 10 per cent of patients. The gall bladder stones are surrounded by a ring of calcium salts. (From Sherlock, S., and Summerfield, J. A. (1979). *A colour atlas of liver disease*, Wolfe Medical Publications, London, with permission.)

Cholesterol gallstones. Cholesterol gallstones result from the secretion of cholesterol saturated bile by the liver. The cause of this saturation is unclear. Gallstone patients usually have a smaller bile acid pool than controls and it circulates more frequently. The rapid recycling of bile acids may be responsible for the smaller bile acid pool by excessive inhibition of the enzyme which controls bile acid synthesis, cholesterol-7α-hydroxylase. However, diminished bile acid synthesis is probably not the most important factor in the production of saturated bile. This appears to be an elevated biliary cholesterol secretion rate, due either to increased hepatic cholesterol synthesis or increased transfer of plasma lipoprotein cholesterol into bile. Nevertheless, saturated bile may be encountered in normal subjects, especially during fasting. It is therefore likely that other factors such as the condition of the gall bladder, the mechanism of seeding (nucleation) of gallstones and the control of gallstone growth are important. Furthermore, racial differences, advancing age, female sex, obesity, diet, drugs (such as the contraceptive pill and clofibrate), and gastrointestinal disease (such as Crohn's disease) are known to have a significant influence on the development of gallstones.

Bile pigment gallstones. In contrast to cholesterol stones, little is known of the aetiology of bile pigment stones. The soft, brown, pliable *bile-pigment–calcium* stones are expecially common in the Far East and are associated with *E. coli*, bacteroides, and clostridium infections of the biliary tract. It is probable that these bacteria contribute to stone formation by producing β-glucuronidase which deconjugates bilirubin diglucuronide to form free unconjugated bilirubin. This combines with calcium to form sparingly soluble calcium bilirubinate which precipitates.

The black, hard and brittle *pure pigment* stones are the type commonly encountered in the West. The incidence of pure pigment stones increases with age and they are found in patients with cirrhosis, chronic bile duct obstruction (e.g. biliary strictures), chronic haemolytic anaemias including prosthetic heart valve induced haemolysis, and malaria. Pure pigment stones affect both sexes equally. The mechanism of stone production is unclear, but does not appear to be due to cholesterol saturation of hepatic or gall-bladder bile. About 50 per cent of all pigment stones are radio-opaque, and they account for about 70 per cent of all opaque stones.

Natural history of gallstones. The majority of gallstones remain in the gall-bladder (cholelithiasis) and may give rise to no symptoms ('silent' gallstones) being discovered incidentally during investigation or at autopsy. Impaction of gallstone in the neck of the gall bladder results in gall-bladder inflammation and the symptoms and signs of acute or chronic cholecystitis. Acute cholecystitis will subside if the stone spontaneously disempacts or may progress to gangrene and perforation of the gall bladder or empyema of the gall bladder. Gallstones may pass through the cystic duct into the bile duct (choledocholithiasis) resulting in biliary obstruction and jaundice. Bacterial infection (cholangitis) commonly accompanies choledocholithiasis and can lead to a liver abscess. Gallstones may perforate through the inflamed gall-bladder wall to form an internal fistula, usually to the small intestine or colon. A large gallstone passing into the small intestine may impact in the ileum resulting in intestinal obstruction (gallstone ileus). Finally, surgical treatment for gallstones, while usually curative, may result in a post-cholecystectomy syndrome or a benign stricture of the bile duct.

Treatment. The mainstay of treatment for gallstones remains cholecystectomy although medical dissolution may now be employed in selected patients (see below). Treatment is obviously indicated for symptomatic gallstones and for their complications. However, in patients in whom 'silent' gallstones are discovered incidentally, and in patients with minimal symptoms, it is by no means clear that treatment is always the best solution. The problem revolves around the probability of serious complications in the future and on this point the information is inadequate. At present, it is appropriate to offer treatment to young patients (who, with many years ahead of them, will have a greater likelihood of developing the complications of gallstones) and to advise against treatment in the elderly with other major medical problems. However, in fit middle-aged patients with no or minimal symptoms it is reasonable to tell the patient of the finding and to withhold surgery until it is warranted by symptoms or complications.

Gallstone dissolution. Cholesterol gallstones can be dissolved in a proportion of patients with chenodeoxycholic acid. Oral chenodeoxycholic acid, a normal constituent of bile, reduces the cholesterol saturation of bile and results in the leaching of cholesterol from gallstones. It appears to act by reducing the hepatic synthesis and biliary excretion of cholesterol.

Patient selection and dosage. Chenodeoxycholic acid treatment is only suitable for patients with cholesterol gallstones in a functioning gall bladder (as judged by an oral cholecystogram). It will dissolve gallstones in about 60 per cent of patients fulfilling these criteria. Radiolucent gallstones are usually, but not always, composed of cholesterol. Calcified gallstones do not dissolve. The treatment is protracted and although it appears safe, this has not been established. At present, chenodeoxycholic acid should be reserved for patients with mild or no symptoms in whom the risk of cholecystectomy is high, including those with pre-existing disease, the elderly, and the very obese. It is also of value in patients who refuse surgery. Drugs which increase the cholesterol saturation of bile should be avoided; these include oestrogens, the oral contraceptive pill, and clofibrate. Chenodeoxycholic acid should not be taken during pregnancy. The dosage of chenodeoxycholic acid that consistently produces an unsaturated bile is 13–15 mg/kg body weight. Obese patients (more than 125 per cent ideal body weight) require a larger dose (18–20 mg/kg body weight). Gallstone dissolution usually requires 6–24 months of therapy, depending on stone size. Oral cholecystograms are performed every six months to assess progress.

Side-effects and toxicity. The most frequent symptom is diarrhoea. It is dose-related and usually mild and transient. It can be minimized by slowly increasing the dose to the required level. Transient elevations of serum transaminase activity are also common; liver function tests should be monitored. Gallstone recurrence remains a major problem with chenodeoxycholic acid therapy. One year after gallstone dissolution about 30 per cent of patients will have had a recurrence. The prevention of recurrences by low dosage or intermittent maintenance therapy with chenodeoxycholic acid or a high fibre diet is being evaluated.

Ursodeoxycholic acid. This agent is a promising agent for dissolving gallstones. Structurally, it is closely related to chenodeoxycholic acid. Ursodeoxycholic acid appears to have several advantages over chenodeoxycholic acid; smaller doses are required, it dissolves gallstones more rapidly, and it does not cause diarrhoea or elevations of the serum transaminases. At present it is more expensive than chenodeoxycholic acid.

Acute cholecystitis
Aetiology. Acute cholecystitis is associated with gallstones in over 90 per cent of patients. It follows the impaction of a gallstone in the cystic duct. Continued secretion by the gall bladder leads to a rise in pressure. Inflammation of the gall-bladder wall results from the toxic effects of the retained bile and bacterial infection. The gall-bladder bile is usually turbid but may become frank pus (empyema of the gall bladder). Intestinal organisms, especially anaerobes, are commonly cultured from the gall bladder. Ischaemia in the distended gall-bladder wall may lead to infarction and perforation. Generalized peritonitis may follow but the leak is usually localized to form a chronic abscess cavity. Some patients have repeated attacks of acute cholecystitis which are probably exacerbations of chronic cholecystitis.

Symptoms and signs. The typical patient is an obese, middle-aged female, and the acute attack is often precipitated by a large or fatty meal. However, there are many exceptions to this pattern. The principal symptom is pain, of fairly sudden onset, which is severe, continuous or minimally fluctuating, and localized to the epigastrium or right hypochondrium. The pain often radiates to the back. The constancy of the pain is in contrast to the repeated short bouts of biliary colic. In uncomplicated cases the pain gradually subsides over 12–18 hours. Flatulence and nausea are common but persistent vomiting suggests the presence of a stone in the common bile duct. Examination reveals an ill, sweating patient with shallow, jerky respirations. Fever indicates a complicating bacterial cholangitis. Jaundice may accompany acute cholecystitis but is usually a sign of a stone in the bile duct. The abdomen moves poorly with respiration. Right hypochondrial tenderness is present and is exacerbated by inspiration (Murphy's sign). Muscle guarding and rebound tenderness are common. The gall bladder is usually impalpable but occasionally a tender mass of omentum and gall bladder may be felt under the liver.

Laboratory investigations. The white cell count is usually moderately elevated ($12-15 \times 10^3$) due to a polymorphonuclear leucocytosis. Serum bilirubin concentrations between 17–68 μmol/l (1–4 mg/dl) may be seen in uncomplicated acute cholecystitis but should raise the suspicion of a stone in the bile duct. Modest rises in the serum alkaline phosphatase, aspartate transaminase, and amylase may also be seen. An abdominal X-ray will show gallstones in about 10 per cent of patients. Intravenous cholangiography is helpful; opacification of the gall bladder usually rules out the diagnosis and opacification of the bile duct without the gall bladder is evidence of blockage of the cystic duct. Scintiscanning with ^{99}Tc^{m}-labelled HIDA provides similar information. If these techniques fail, intravenous cholangiography with large doses of contrast medium may be employed. It is important to establish the correct diagnosis before surgery is performed.

Differential diagnosis. Acute cholecystitis may be confused with other abdominal emergencies including perforated peptic ulcer, acute pancreatitis, retrocaecal appendicitis, perforated carcinoma, or diverticulum of the hepatic flexure of the colon and liver abscess. Cardiac infarction and pneumonia with right-sided pleurisy should also be considered.

Complications. *Gangrene of the gall bladder.* Pain, tenderness, and fever progressively increasing or persisting for longer than 24–48 hours are indications of gangrene of the gall bladder. The prognosis is poor if necrosis and perforation occur. In the elderly and obese perforation of the gall bladder can occur without definite signs. Perforation into an adjacent viscus may produce a cholecystenteric fistula and may lead to gallstone ileus.

Cholangitis. Intermittent high temperatures sometimes accompanied by rigors indicate bacterial infection of the bile duct and usually follow the passage of a stone into the bile duct.

Treatment. In most patients acute cholecystitis subsides in a few days with conservative treatment. Cholecystectomy is performed either a few days after the symptoms have settled or two to three months later. In the latter event, if the symptoms recur during the interval, cholecystectomy is performed without delay. Surgery is mandatory if signs of gangrene or perforation develop.

Conservative treatment. Oral feeding is stopped. Intravenous fluids, and analgesia with pentazocine or pethidine (demerol) and atropine are administered. Antibiotics are given to all but the most mild cases; tetracycline, ampicillin, or a cephalosporin are satisfactory for general use. The patient should be observed frequently with abdominal examination and sequential leucocyte counts to detect signs of gangrene of the gall bladder or cholangitis.

Surgical treatment. Cholecystectomy is the operation of choice. Operative cholangiography should be performed at the time of surgery to determine whether bile-duct stones are present. About 10 per cent of patients with acute cholecystitis will also have stones in the common bile duct. In poor-risk patients and when technical difficulties are encountered a cholecystotomy may be performed.

Chronic cholecystitis. This is the most common form of gall-bladder disease that results from gallstones. Pathologically it is characterized by chronic inflammation and thickening of the gall-bladder wall. In addition to stones the gall-bladder may contain a brown sediment ('biliary mud'). A proportion of these patients have cholesterolosis of the gall-bladder ('strawberry gall-bladder'). This describes the deposition of yellow specks of cholesterol in the pink gall-bladder wall and is a consequence of cholesterol-saturated bile. Cholesterolosis of the gall bladder is asymptomatic but about half the patients develop gallstones. Chronic cholecystitis usually develops insidiously but may follow an attack of acute cholecystitis.

Symptoms and signs. Some patients complain of bouts of constant right hypochondrial or epigastric pain. If it is intermittent, i.e. biliary colic, the height of the pain is separated by 15–60 minute intervals. The pain may last several hours or be as brief as 15–20 minutes. It may radiate to the right shoulder or the back. More commonly the symptoms are vague and ill-defined and include abdominal discomfort and distension, nausea, flatulence, and intolerance of fatty foods. Unfortunately, many patients who do not have chronic cholecystitis complain of these symptoms. Examination of the abdomen may reveal tenderness over the gall bladder and a positive Murphy's sign. Laboratory investigations are usually unhelpful.

Imaging techniques. A plain X-ray of the abdomen may reveal calcified stones or opacification of the gall bladder caused by high concentrations of calcium carbonate ('limey bile'). An ultrasound examination is a useful initial investigation to detect gallstones. An oral cholecystogram should be performed next. This may show the

stones or may fail to opacify the gall bladder. In the latter event an intravenous cholangiogram is employed, which will usually opacify the bile duct and gall bladder (unless a stone obstructs the cystic duct). If these tests fail, PTC or ERCP should be performed in order to establish the diagnosis before surgery is performed.

Differential diagnosis. Dyspepsia and fat intolerance are common symptoms that may be caused by many conditions including peptic ulcers, hiatus hernia, irritable bowel syndrome, chronic relapsing pancreatitis, and tumours of the stomach, pancreas, colon, or gall bladder. Other functional disorders may also mimic chronic cholecystitis.

Complications. The complications of chronic cholecystitis include acute exacerbations (acute cholecystitis), passage of stones into the bile duct (choledocholithiasis or Mirizzi's syndrome), pancreatitis, cholecystenteric fistula formation, and gallstone ileus, and rarely carcinoma of the gall-bladder. Occasionally the accumulation of mucus and gallstones produces hydrops of the gall bladder which is characterized by a tender mass without the occurrence of acute cholecystitis.

Treatment. In established cases of chronic cholecystitis the treatment of choice is cholecystectomy. When the diagnosis is in doubt, especially when vague symptoms are associated with a well-functioning gall bladder containing stones, a conservative approach is worth trying. This includes weight reduction and a low fat diet especially if fatty food is associated with the symptoms. Treatment with chenodeoxycholic acid may also be considered.

Prognosis. Chronic cholecystitis carries a good prognosis. Cholecystectomy is curative and should have a mortality below 1 per cent. However, if cholecystectomy is performed indiscriminately on patients with 'dyspeptic' symptoms who happen to have incidental gallstones the results will be unpredictable and often unsatisfactory.

Choledocholithiasis. Most stones in the common bile duct originate in the gall bladder. About 15 per cent of patients with cholelithiasis have common duct stones. This proportion rises with age so that in the elderly nearly 50 per cent of patients with cholelithiasis may have common duct stones. Stones may develop in the bile duct in diseases causing chronic biliary obstruction such as benign bile duct strictures and sclerosing cholangitis.

Clinical features. The classical triad of symptoms is right upper abdominal pain, jaundice, and fever. The abdominal pain is typically colicky, severe, and persists for hours. It is often associated with vomiting. Fever and rigors indicate cholangitis which commonly accompanies bile duct stones. Jaundice is variable; it may be mild or deep and is often intermittent. The urine is dark due to conjugated bilirubin and the faeces pale. Frequently, the amount of pigment in the faeces varies. Itching may be prominent. However, common bile duct stones may also be silent, especially in the elderly. Alternatively, only one of the triad of symptoms may be present; the patient presenting with jaundice, abdominal pain, or cholangitis. The liver is moderately enlarged and there may be tenderness in the right upper quadrant. Prolonged biliary obstruction lasting months or years eventually leads to a biliary cirrhosis with portal venous hypertension and liver cell failure.

Laboratory investigations. Liver function tests show a cholestatic (biliary obstructive) pattern. The prothrombin time may be prolonged due to inadequate absorption of vitamin K. A polymorphonuclear leucocytosis is common and indicates biliary infection. Blood cultures should be performed repeatedly during the fevers to isolate the organism and determine sensitivities.

Imaging techniques. A plain X-ray of the abdomen may show gallstones. Ultrasonography is useful for demonstrating the dilated biliary tree that results from obstruction and may reveal the biliary gallstones. Intravenous cholangiography will succeed if the serum bilirubin is below 51 μmol/l (3 mg/dl). In deep jaundice cholangiography will require the use of ERCP or PTC (Fig. 4).

Differential diagnosis. Common duct gallstones are the most common cause of cholestatic (biliary obstructive) jaundice. Next in frequency are carcinomas of the head of the pancreas, ampulla of Vater, and bile duct (see Table 1). Certain intrahepatic diseases may also cause a cholestatic jaundice and must be considered. These include viral and alcoholic hepatitis, jaundice due to drugs, and the jaundice of pregnancy.

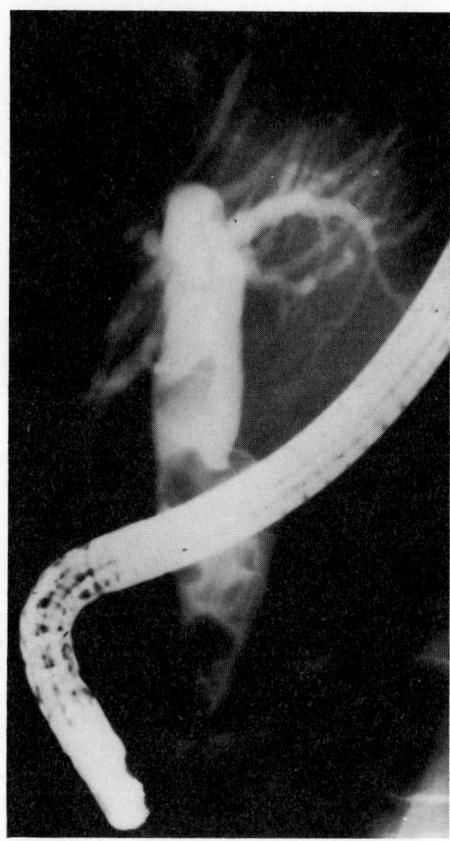

Fig. 4 Choledocholithiasis. An endoscopic retrograde cholangiogram shows multiple faceted radiolucent stones in a dilated bile duct. The gall bladder has not been opacified.

Table 1 Causes of bile duct obstruction

Intrinsic causes
  Common bile duct gallstones
  Cholangitis
  Carcinoma of the bile duct
  Carcinoma of the gall bladder
  Benign post-traumatic stricture
  Sclerosing cholangitis (primary and secondary)
  Haemobilia
Extrinsic causes
  Carcinoma of the pancreas
  Carcinoma of the ampulla of Vater
  Metastatic carcinoma
  Reticulosis
  Pancreatitis (acute and chronic)
  Pancreatic cysts
Congenital causes
  Biliary atresia
  Choledochal cyst
  Congenital intrahepatic biliary dilatation (Caroli's disease)

Treatment. The treatment of common bile duct stones is cholecystectomy and exploration of the common bile duct. Pre-operative preparation includes appropriate antibiotics for cholangitis, the correction of fluid and electrolyte balance, nutrition, and anaemia, and if the prothrombin time is prolonged, parenteral vitamin K. Pre-operative percutaneous biliary drainage for several days may be performed to reduce the jaundice or to drain infected bile before surgery. Endoscopic sphincterotomy is employed for the removal of common duct gallstones in patients unfit for surgery. Stones overlooked at surgery (residual calculi) are best treated by non-operative procedures. If a T-tube is in place, the stones may be removed by a steerable basket-catheter manipulated down the T-tube track; otherwise endoscopic sphincterotomy is performed.

Post-cholecystectomy syndromes. After cholecystectomy a proportion of patients continue to complain of symptoms such as right-upper quadrant pain, flatulence, and fatty food intolerance. However, the vast majority of patients with gallstones are improved by surgery. The persistence of symptoms in many is probably a consequence of the wrong diagnosis being made before surgery and other diseases such as oesophagitis, pancreatitis or functional bowel disease should be sought. In others technical problems during surgery may have resulted in a benign post-traumatic biliary stricture or residual calculi. However, there remains a group of patients where the cause appears to be due to some less common biliary disorder such as a long, dilated cystic duct remnant, amputation neuroma of the cystic duct, and spasm or stenosis of the sphincter of Oddi. The biliary tract must always be carefully investigated in these patients especially if colicky pain, fever, jaundice, or cholestatic liver function tests persist. Biliary tract manometry may be of value when spasm or stenosis of the sphincter of Oddi is suspected.

Biliary infections

Bacterial cholangitis (suppurative cholangitis). This is usually associated with common bile duct calculi and benign biliary strictures. Malignant strictures produce complete obstruction and the bile remains sterile. Other conditions associated with cholangitis are biliary enteric fistulas, both spontaneous and surgical, sclerosing cholangitis, and congenital intrahepatic biliary dilatation (Caroli's disease). Organisms of the gut flora are usually cultured in these infections including aerobes, such as *E. coli, Str. faecalis, Pr. vulgaris*, and staphylococci, and anaerobes such as bacteroides, aerobacter, and anaerobic streptococci.

Clinical features and treatment. The onset of malaise, fever and rigors is followed by pain, vomiting, jaundice, and itching. The urine turns dark and the faeces pale. The biliary obstructive features are probably due to oedema of the bile duct wall. Recurrent attacks are common. Hepatic abscesses may result. Repeated blood cultures are performed during the fever to isolate the organisms. Culture of a liver biopsy fragment may also yield the organism. The main element of treatment is surgical drainage of the biliary tract. Additionally, appropriate antibiotics such as gentamicin and metronidazole are given. For recurrent attacks of cholangitis, tetracycline, ampicillin, or a cephalosporin are usually effective.

Infestations. Infestations (see Section 5) with the round worm *Ascaris lumbricoides* and the liver fluke *Clonorchis sinensis* are particular problems of the Far East. Both lead to cholangitis. *C. sinensis* infestation predisposes to bile duct carcinoma and primary liver cancer. The common sheep fluke *Fasciola hepatica* may be encountered as a cause of cholangitis in Europe during wet summers.

Benign biliary strictures. In about 95 per cent of patients these are a consequence of biliary tract surgery. The remainder are caused by gallstones eroding the bile duct and rarely, blunt injury to the abdomen. Signs of biliary stricture may be detected in the immediate post-operative period but are often delayed. Disasters such as ligation or section of the bile duct present early with jaundice, and drainage of bile from the wound drains. With lesser damage to the duct the patient presents after an interval with cholangitis and jaundice. Liver function tests reveal a cholestatic pattern and blood cultures may yield an organism. The precise delineation of the stricture requires PTC or ERCP. Biliary stricture is not a benign condition; untreated it will often progress to biliary cirrhosis with portal venous hypertension and liver-cell failure. Treatment is surgical and should be performed by a surgeon skilled in this difficult repair.

Malignant biliary stricture. This is most commonly due to adenocarcinoma of the head of the pancreas but may also be caused by adenocarcinoma of the bile ducts, carcinoma of the ampulla of Vater, and rarely gall-bladder carcinoma. Occasionally the cause is lymph node enlargement at the porta hepatis due to malignant metastases or reticulosis (see also page 12.163).

Symptoms and signs. Cancers of the pancreas and biliary tree (Figs. 5 and 6) usually affect the middle aged and elderly. The onset is insidious with deepening jaundice, itching, and weight loss. A dull nagging upper abdominal pain, which radiates to the back, is common. In contrast to choledocholithiasis and benign strictures, cholangitis is unusual. Examination reveals a deeply jaundiced patient often excoriated from scratching. The liver is enlarged but not tender. If the malignant obstruction is below the level of the cystic duct, the gall bladder is distended and may be palpable (Courvoisier's law). The urine is dark and the stools pale. In cancer of the ampulla of Vater a film of blood on the pale stool gives it a silvery colour ('silver stools').

Laboratory investigations. The standard liver function tests reveal a cholestatic pattern. The serum bilirubin may be very high (600 μmol/l; 35 mg/dl). A microcytic hypochromic anaemia indicates blood loss from the tumour.

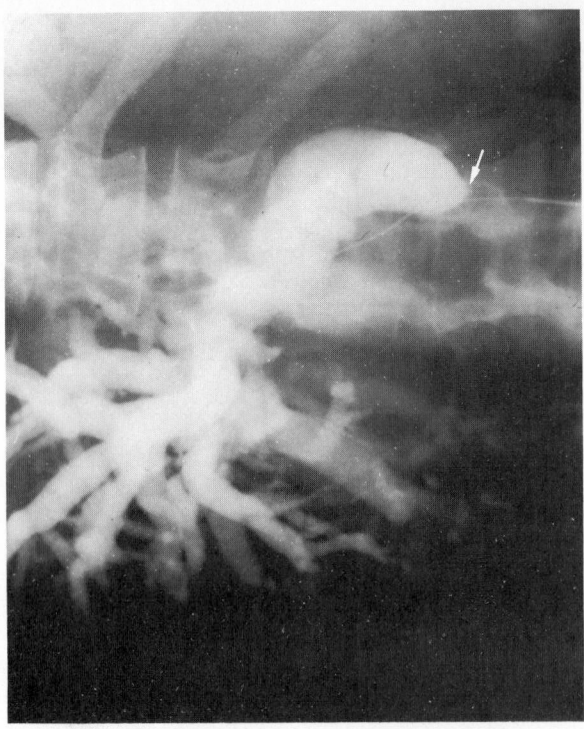

Fig. 6 Carcinoma of the pancreas. The percutaneous transhepatic cholangiogram (PTC) shows a very dilated biliary tree which terminates in a blunt 'nipple-like' obstruction (arrow) at the lower end of the common bile duct. This is the usual finding in cancers of the head of the pancreas which obstruct the biliary system.

Imaging techniques. An abdominal X-ray shows an enlarged liver. An ultrasound or CT scan examination will reveal dilatation of the biliary tree and may demonstrate the level of the obstruction. Ultrasound guided percutaneous needle biopsy may be employed to provide a histological diagnosis. In deeply jaundiced patients oral and intravenous cholangiography will not succeed. Bile duct carcinoma frequently causes obstruction at the porta hepatis and consequently at laparotomy the biliary tract appears non-dilated. Even if operative cholangiography is performed, the contrast medium frequently fails to pass the obstruction and fill the dilated intrahepatic biliary tree. However, it is important to pursue the diagnosis before surgery is performed because of the therapeutic options that are available. Consequently patients who have dilated intrahepatic ducts determined by ultrasound should then be submitted to a PTC to delineate the lesion precisely.

Treatment. Small tumours confined to the head of the pancreas and ampulla of Vater may be treated curatively by a Whipple's operation. Usually, however, carcinoma of the pancreas can only be treated palliatively with a bypass procedure such as a cholecystojejunostomy. The prognosis for these patients is poor. An alternative non-operative treatment, the percutaneous transhepatic introduction of endoprostheses through the stricture may be more suitable for patients with advanced tumours. In contrast, carcinoma of the bile duct tends to be a scirrhous slow-growing tumour which forms metastases late. Although excision of the tumour is not often possible, an endoprosthesis placed through the stricture may give several years of jaundice free life.

Other causes of bile duct obstruction. Pancreatitis may obstruct the common bile duct during its passage through the head of the pancreas. Transient jaundice is common in acute pancreatitis, due to compression by pancreatic oedema. In chronic pancreatitis, especially alcoholic, persistent jaundice can develop requiring a surgical bypass procedure such as a cholecystojejunostomy. This biliary obstruction is probably a consequence of pancreatic fibrosis.

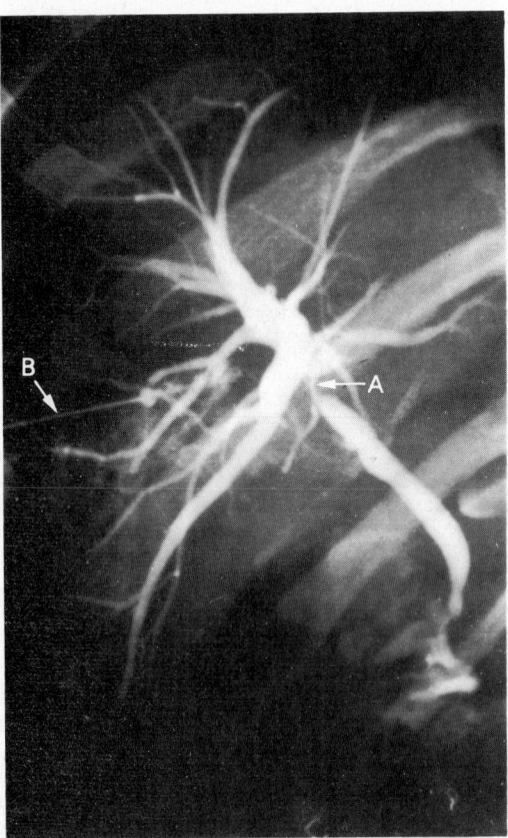

Fig. 5 Carcinoma of the bile duct. A percutaneous transhepatic cholangiogram (PTC) shows a stricture (A) high in the bile duct at the porta hepatis. The intrahepatic bile ducts are moderately dilated. The transhepatic track of the 'skinny' needle used for the PTC is also visible (B).

Pancreatic cysts may rarely cause extrinsic compression of the bile duct. Haemobilia or haemorrhage into the biliary tract is uncommon but may follow trauma, liver biopsy, biliary tumours, and gallstones. In addition to jaundice, the blood clots cause biliary pain. Massive gastrointestinal haemorrhage may occur. The diagnosis of these conditions relies on adequate cholangiography.

Sclerosing cholangitis. Sclerosing cholangitis is the description applied to multiple strictures and bead-like dilatations of the intrahepatic and extrahepatic biliary tree. Secondary sclerosing cholangitis is a consequence of recurrent bacterial cholangitis due to gallstones or benign biliary strictures.

Primary sclerosing cholangitis (Fig. 7). This should only be diagnosed if the following criteria are satisfied; (*a*) absence of gall-stones; (*b*) absence of previous biliary surgery; and (*c*) sufficiently long follow-up to exclude carcinoma of the bile duct. Primary sclerosing cholangitis affects males more than females (2:1) and about 70 per cent of patients have ulcerative colitis. The usual clinical presentation is cholestatic jaundice and cholangitis. However, a significant proportion of patients are asymptomatic or present with cirrhosis and portal venous hypertension. There is associated retroperitoneal fibrosis or Riedel's thyroiditis in some cases. Serum biochemistry shows cholestatic liver function tests. A raised serum alkaline phosphatase is almost invariable. Consequently the diagnosis should be considered in cirrhotic patients whose liver function tests show cholestatic features. The IgM concentration is commonly elevated. Liver biopsy may be helpful and usually indicates large bile duct obstruction. The diagnosis is established by cholangiography with ERCP or PTC. Laparotomy should not be performed routinely to establish the diagnosis but should be reserved for the small number of patients with complete obstruction of the main ducts or to remove stones or sludge. Primary sclerosing cholangitis is being recognized more frequently as a result of the widespread use of ERCP and PTC. It may be confused with primary biliary cirrhosis, but the serum mitochondrial antibody is always negative in primary sclerosing cholangitis. Treatment is unsatisfactory, neither corticosteroids nor azothiaprine are of proven value. Pruritus may be helped by cholestyramine. The prognosis is variable. Bile-duct adenocarcinoma is a late complication.

Congenital disorders of the gall bladder and biliary tract. This subject is discussed on page 12.227.

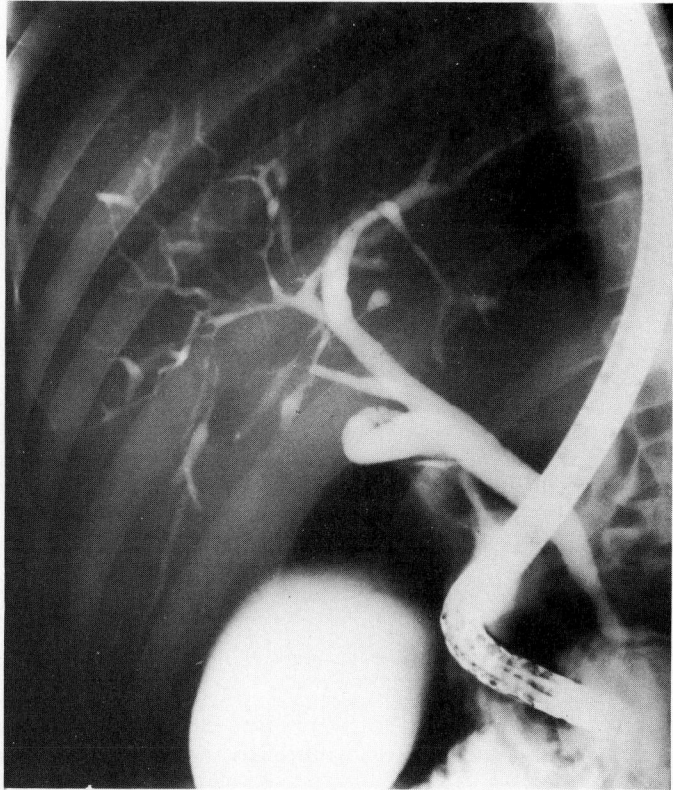

Fig. 7 Primary sclerosing cholangitis. The intrahepatic bile ducts show alternate strictures and dilatations ('beading'). The common bile duct, cystic duct, and gall bladder appear normal in this study but may also be involved.

References

Bouchier, I. A. D. (1980). Medical treatment of gallstones. *Ann. Rev. Med.* **31**, 59.

Chapman, R. W. G., Arborgh, B. A. M., Rhodes, J. M., Summerfield, J. A., Dick, R., Scheuer, P. J., and Sherlock, S. (1980). Primary sclerosing cholangitis: a review of its clinical features, cholangiography and hepatic histology. *Gut* **21**, 870.

Classen, M. and Ossenberg, F. W. (1977). Non-surgical removal of common bile duct stones. *Gut* **18**, 760.

Elias, E. (1976). Cholangiography in the jaundiced patient. *Gut* **17**, 801.

Schiff, L. (1975). *Diseases of the liver*, 4th edn. Lippincott, Philadelphia.

Sherlock, S. (1981). *Diseases of the liver and biliary system*, 6th edn. Blackwell Scientific Publications, Oxford.

— and Summerfield, J. A. (1979). *A colour atlas of liver disease*. Wolfe Medical Publications, London.

Soloway, R. D., Trotman, B. W., and Ostrow, J. D. (1977). Pigment gallstones. *Gastroent.* **72**, 167.

Weissmann, H. S., Badia, J., Sugarman, L. A., Kluger, L., Rosenblatt, R., and Freeman, L. M. (1981). Spectrum of 99 m-Tc-IDA cholescintigraphic patterns in acute cholecystitis. *Am. J. Radiol.* **138**, 167.

Jaundice

E. Elias

Jaundice is the yellow discolouration of sclerae, mucous membranes, and skin caused by accumulation of bilirubin. Involvement of the sclerae helps distinguish jaundice from other causes of pigmentation such as melanosis, hypercarotenaemia, and mepacrine therapy. Bilirubin is the major bile pigment in man and is formed as an end-product of the catabolism of haem-containing proteins. Jaundice results from either excessive production or defective elimination. There may be detectable differences in the tint produced by haemolytic (lemon-yellow), hepatocellular (orange-yellow), and cholestatic (greenish-yellow) causes of jaundice but no diagnostic reliance should be based on such impressions alone. In medicine *icterus*, from the Greek ἴκτερος, is used synonymously with jaundice, though it can also refer to a disease of plants in which the leaves turn yellow, or to a certain yellowish-green bird.

Metabolism of bilirubin

Production. Bilirubin is a tetrapyrrole compound formed when the ring structure of haem is broken open by microsomal haem oxygenase, liberating a bridge carbon as carbon monoxide (Fig. 1). Biliverdin and carbon monoxide are formed in equimolar amounts but because haem oxygenase and biliverdin reductase are present in man in all tissues where senescent red cells are destroyed, bilirubin is formed instantaneously so there is virtually no biliverdin detectable in plasma. Haem oxygenase exhibits maximal activity for free haem, intermediate activity for haemoproteins such as haemoglobin, cytochrome P450, and catalase (in all of which the haem and apoprotein are linked solely through the iron and therefore freely dissociable), and lesser activity for compounds such as carboxyhaemoglobin in which the haem is tightly bound to its apoprotein.

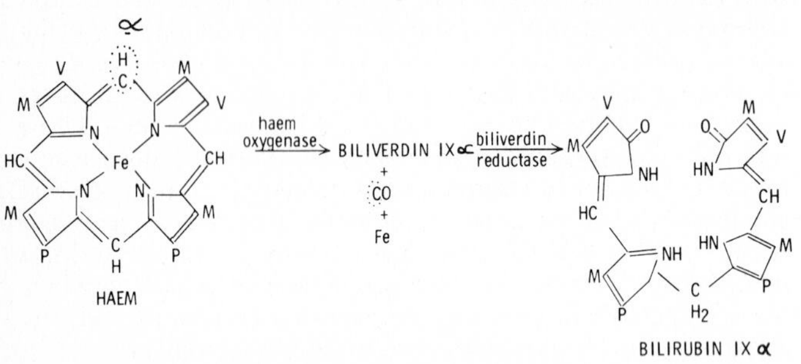

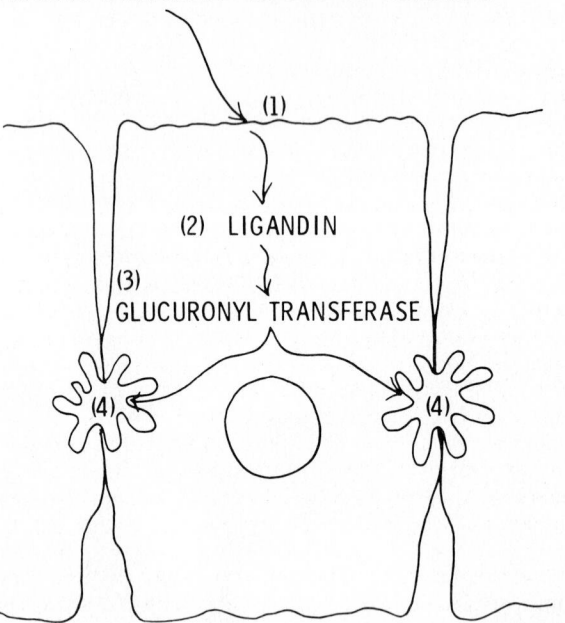

Fig. 1   Production of bilirubin from haem. $M = CH_3$; $V = CH=CH_2$; $P = CH_2-CH_2-COOH$. Of the four bridge carbon atoms ($\alpha, \beta, \gamma, \delta$), the ring is usually opened at α.

The major source of bilirubin in man is from breakdown of red cells. Since all four nitrogen atoms are derived from glycine, it is possible to investigate haem metabolism after administration of ^{15}N-glycine. As would be expected, peak production of ^{15}N-bilirubin and its derivatives occurs between 90 and 120 days later and coincides with the disappearance of ^{15}N-labelled erythrocytes from the circulation. However, a significant peak of ^{15}N-bilirubin production is seen within two weeks and does not appear to be due to destruction of circulating erythrocytes. This has been termed 'early labelled bilirubin' and is thought to result from ineffective erythropoieses and catabolism of non-haemoglobin haemoproteins such as hepatic cytochromes, catalase, or myoglobin. An increase of the early labelled bilirubin peak occurs in pernicious anaemia, erythropoietic porphyria, the thalassaemia syndromes, shunt hyperbilirubinaemia, refractory sideroblastic anaemia, and lead poisoning. In these conditions it may be due to defective synthesis of haemoglobin, but destruction of erythrocytes in the bone marrow before they have entered the circulation will also enhance production of early labelled bilirubin (see Section 19). A third component of ^{15}N-bilirubin production of uncertain origin spans the interval between the early labelled peak and senescent erythrocyte removal.

Although bilirubin may be regarded as a waste product of haem catabolism, the constituent amino acids of its apoproteins (e.g. globin in haemoglobin) and iron are conserved and re-utilized. Other minor degradation pathways for haemoglobin have been described in which biliverdin and bilirubin may not be intermediates and in one such pathway the denatured haemoglobin of Heinz bodies is converted to water-soluble compounds which are not detected by the van den Bergh reaction.

Transport in plasma. Bilirubin is transported from its site of production to the liver bound to albumin. The molecular configuration of bilirubin secludes potentially polar groups and renders it non-polar and lipophilic. Even physiological concentrations of plasma bilirubin vastly exceed its solubility in water and are only possible because of protein binding. Each albumin molecule has one binding site for bilirubin which is of such high affinity that when molar ratios of bilirubin:albumin do not exceed 1:1 there is virtually no free bilirubin in solution. Each albumin molecule has two additional binding sites of moderately high affinity and a third group of low affinity binding sites. However, when bilirubin:albumin ratios exceed 1:1 binding affinities are such that there is a disproportionate increase of the unbound, freely diffusable fraction of bilirubin in plasma, and in newborn infants brain damage leading to kernicterus may occur. A molar ratio of 1:1 exists between albumin 40 g/l and bilirubin 578 µmol/dl, but in newborn infants there is danger of saturation with relatively less bilirubin. The situation is exacerbated by agents which compete with bilirubin and displace it from the binding sites on albumin (e.g. salicylates, sulphonamides, diazepam, and fat-soluble vitamin K analogues). Drugs which are not protein bound may be used safely. The brain is not susceptible to kernicterus in later life though in deep jaundice all tissues other than the brain may become pigmented. Rarely bilirubin in the eye will produce yellow vision (xanthopsia).

Hepatic uptake (Fig. 2). Uptake of bilirubin by the liver is very rapid and occurs independently of albumin uptake. It is assumed that a

PLASMA BILIRUBIN (BOUND TO ALBUMIN)

STEPS IN HEPATIC TRANSPORT AND METABOLISM OF BILIRUBIN

1.   UPTAKE BY SINUSOIDAL PLASMA MEMBRANE AND INTERNALISATION
2.   INTRACELLULAR BINDING BY LIGANDIN AND Z PROTEIN
3.   CONJUGATION   (mainly to glucuronides)
4.   CANALICULAR SECRETION OF CONJUGATE

Fig. 2   The hepatic transport metabolism of bilirubin.

transport receptor exists on the hepatocyte's sinusoidal plasma membrane. Within the cell bilirubin is bound by ligandin (formerly known as Y protein) and Z protein (also known as fatty acid binding protein). Other organic anions including bromsulphthalein (BSP), and indocyanine green (ICG) and cholecystographic agents compete with bilirubin for hepatocyte uptake and for binding to ligandin and Z protein. Clearance of these agents is enhanced by phenobarbitone, which increases ligandin synthesis, and reduced by fasting or oestrogen therapy which diminish hepatic levels of ligandin and Z protein.

Conjugation. Within the liver-cell free bilirubin is rendered water soluble by conjugation with glucuronic acid. This reaction is catalysed by the microsomal enzyme glucuronyl transferase or UDPGT (bilirubin uridine diphosphate glucuronate glucuronyl transferase). The major conjugate in human bile is bilirubin diglucuronide with lesser quantities of monoglucuronide and other conjugates, e.g. glucosides and xylosides. There is controversy as to whether bilirubin diglucuronide is formed as a direct consequence of glucuronyl transferase activity or whether monoglucuronides are formed which subsequently condense to form bilirubin diglucuronide under the influence of a transesterase enzyme within the bile canalicular plasma membrane. The unconjugated bilirubin in this scheme returns to the microsomes (Fig. 3).

(a) Bilirubin + 2UDPGA $\xrightarrow{\text{microsomal UDPGT}}$ Bilirubin diglucuronide + 2UDP

(b) Bilirubin + UDPGA $\xrightarrow{\text{microsomal UDPGT}}$ Bilirubin monoglucuronide + UDP
2 Bilirubin monoglucuronide $\xrightarrow{\text{canalicular transesterase}}$ Bilirubin diglucuronide + bilirubin

Fig. 3 Two proposed pathways for bilirubin diglucuronide formation.

Biliary excretion. The concentration of bilirubin in bile greatly exceeds that in the liver but the nature of the concentrative step is unknown. It has been proposed that bile acids, by incorporating bilirubin into mixed micelles effectively decrease its concentration in the aqueous phase of bile and thus alter the concentration gradient to favour a net transport from hepatocyte to canaliculus. When bilirubin or BSP are administered by intravenous infusion, their plasma concentration and biliary excretion rise until a plateau level of biliary excretion is reached. Further infusion produces a progressive rise of plasma concentration without an increment of biliary excretion. Reflux of increasing amounts of conjugated bilirubin into plasma then occurs, suggesting that canalicular excretion rather than conjugation is the rate limiting step. Transport of bile acids and bilirubin into the canaliculus appear to be mediated by separate transport processes. Thus, in the Dubin–Johnson syndrome transport kinetics for bile acids are usually normal though there is a marked excretory defect for the organic anions bilirubin, BSP, and indocyanine green.

Urobilinogen. Metabolism of bilirubin by intestinal bacteria produces a number of breakdown products which include the readily-absorbable, water-soluble urobilinogen. Most of the absorbed urobilinogen is immediately extracted by the liver and excreted in bile, thus undergoing an enterohepatic circulation. The small fraction of urobilinogen which passes through the liver to enter the systemic circulation is available for urinary excretion. An increased urinary urobilinogen output may be caused by a diminished hepatic fractional extraction rate, when its detection is a very sensitive index of early liver disease. Alternatively, increased urinary urobilinogen may occur in the face of a normal hepatic fractional extraction rate when it has been produced and absorbed in proportion to excessive bilirubin production, e.g. in haemolysis. If there is complete biliary obstruction, absence of bile from the gut will be reflected by absence of urobilinogen from the urine.

Clinical chemistry. Plasma bilirubin may be measured by the van den Bergh reaction. Conjugated bilirubin forms a violet colour immediately on addition of sulphanilic acid (direct reacting bilirubin); the colour is intensified by unconjugated bilirubin following addition of alcohol (indirect reacting bilirubin). Urobilinogen in the urine may be detected by addition of Ehrlich's reagent (2 per cent *p*-dimethylaminobenzaldehyde in 50 per cent HCl) which produces a red colour. Both urobilinogen and porphobilinogen produce a red colour, but only that due to urobilinogen may be extracted by chloroform.

Additional liver function tests. The measured levels of various substances in blood, including bilirubin, have traditionally been described as liver function tests though, as can be seen from the preceding discussion, the concentration of serum bilirubin depends on many factors of which liver function is only one. The term is equally inappropriate for the measurements of hepatocellular enzymes in serum since these more precisely reflect the degree and extent of damage to hepatocytes; thus the highest levels are found in massive hepatic necrosis. Liver function is more truly reflected by levels of circulatory proteins which are exclusively synthesized by the liver (e.g. albumin and some clotting factors: II, V, VII, IX, X) and by the liver's ability to clear certain substances (e.g. bile acids and bromsulphthalein) from the blood, though for each of these too there are important determinants other than the health of hepatocytes and patency of the biliary tree.

Hepatocellular damage is reflected by a rise in the activity of serum aspartate aminotransferase (AsT) or glutamic oxalacetic transaminase (GOT), and alanine aminotransferase (AlT) or glutamic pyruvic transaminase (GPT). Some laboratories prefer isocitrate dehydrogenase (ICD). Because the enzymes are not specific for the liver, elevated serum levels of, say, AsT and lactate dehydrogenase (LDH), could reflect either muscle or hepatic damage. Even when the tissue of origin is known with certainty, the diagnostic significance of individual values must be interpreted with caution; nevertheless, in liver disease when serum AsT or AlT activity reaches levels which exceed normal by more than 30-fold, jaundice is almost certainly due to a hepatitis, whether of viral, drug, or toxic origin.

High levels of serum alkaline phosphatase (SAP) activity are characteristic of cholestasis of both intra- and extrahepatic origin. Electrophoresis permits discrimination between isoenzymes of alkaline phosphatase which are characteristic of liver, bone, kidney, placenta, and intestinal mucosa. Total SAP levels which exceed two-and-a-half times normal due to an increase of the hepatic isoenzyme are rare in jaundice due to hepatocellular disease but common in biliary disorders. Serum 5'-nucelotidase is more specific to liver than alkaline phosphatase and its estimation can be substituted for isoenzyme analysis in order to discriminate between hepatic and bony origins of raised SAP activity. Measure of the serum bile acid concentration has a high level of both sensitivity and specificity for detection of minor degrees of hepatic dysfunction. The sensitivity is enhanced by performing estimations on blood taken two hours after a fatty meal, when hepatic clearance has been stressed by the bile acid load returning in the portal blood as part of their enterohepatic circulation.

Bromsulphthalein (BSP) is a compound which, when injected into the circulation of normal subjects, is rapidly extracted by the liver and excreted in bile as its glutathione-conjugate; in normal subjects less than 5 per cent of the injected dose (5 mg/kg body weight) remains in the circulation after 45 minutes but this retained fraction is increased in most forms of liver disease. Though, in a clinical setting, the test is rarely necessary it still provides a sensitive index of liver dysfunction. Rarely, anaphylactoid reactions occur and therefore intravenous hydrocortisone should always be at hand when BSP is being administered.

Causes and pathophysiology of jaundice. Hyperbilirubinaemia with jaundice may result from excessive bilirubin production, reduced hepatic uptake of bilirubin, reduced hepatic conjugation of bilirubin, or reduced excretion of conjugated bilirubin (Fig. 4).

Excessive production of bilirubin. Excessive production of bilirubin occurs in the haemolytic anaemias. It also may occur in patients with a marked degree of ineffective erythropoiesis and intramedullary destruction of red cell precursors, as occurs, for example, in thalassaemia and pernicious anaemia. These conditions are considered in detail in Section 19.

Reduced uptake of bilirubin. A defect in the transfer of bilirubin to the hepatocyte may explain the unconjugated hyperbilirubinaemia associated with Gilbert's syndrome, severe congestive heart failure, portocaval shunts, and the action of certain drugs.

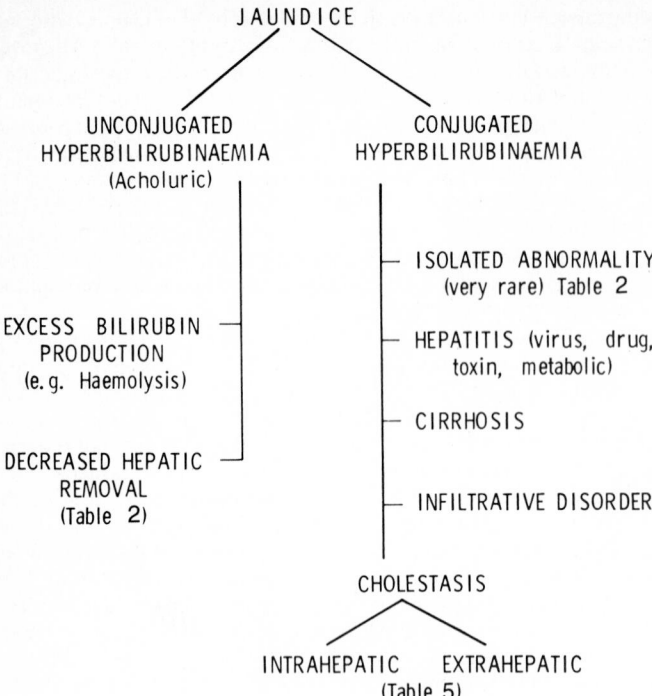

Fig. 4   Classification of jaundice.

Reduced hepatic conjugation of bilirubin. Reduced hepatic conjugation of bilirubin is probably the cause of neonatal jaundice and occurs in the Crigler–Najjar syndrome where it results from a specific deficiency of glucuronyl transferase. Inhibition of the activity of the latter by steroids excreted in maternal milk is a rare cause of neonatal jaundice.

Reduced excretion of conjugated bilirubin. This may occur either due to congenital defects in hepatic excretion as occur in the Dubin–Johnson and Rotor syndromes, hepatocellular injury, as in virus hepatitis, or the abnormalities of liver cell metabolism, due to the action of a variety of different drugs. It may also be due to inflammatory, granulomatous, or neoplastic infiltration of the liver, or to extra-hepatic bile duct obstruction by gallstones, strictures, or carcinoma and other malignant disorders.

Clinical approach to the jaundiced patient. Urine testing differentiates between unconjugated and conjugated hyperbilirubinaemia (Table 1). If bilirubin is *absent* from the urine, the detection of excess urinary urobilinogen, splenomegaly, anaemia, reticulocytosis, and a family history of anaemia suggest a haemolytic cause for jaundice. If there is no haemolysis or ineffective erythropoiesis,

and other liver function tests are normal, the patient may be fasted for 48 hours to differentiate between benign hepatic hyperbilirubinaemia (see below) and liver disease such as inactive cirrhosis. In newborn babies action may be required to prevent brain damage.

If bilirubin is *present* in the urine, the common causes are hepatitis and obstruction of the biliary system. Inquiry should be made regarding family history, travel, exposure to toxins, viral hepatitis, drugs, or a recent anaesthetic. In viral hepatitis, jaundice is usually preceded by a prodromal phase involving anorexia, nausea, and aversion to smoking, sometimes with an influenza-like illness; the liver is characteristically enlarged and tender at the onset, and serum transaminase levels (AlT, AsT) are markedly elevated. When the typical features of hepatitis are absent, jaundice with bilirubinuria, especially if accompanied by pale stools and pruritus, prompts the question of whether cholestasis is due to intrahepatic causes or biliary obstruction. In certain cholestatic conditions (e.g. primary biliary cirrhosis or sclerosing cholangitis) jaundice may be a very late sign, preceded by raised serum alkaline phosphatase levels, pruritus, and xanthelasma for several years. Severe abdominal pain of abrupt onset preceding jaundice by a couple of days suggests gallstone obstruction. A rigor in association with dark urine due to bilirubinuria is extremely strong evidence that mechanical biliary obstruction is causing cholangitis. Painless cholestatic jaundice when accompanied by the absence of urinary urobilinogen and a palpable gall bladder usually indicates a neoplastic cause (Courvoisier's law). Ultrasonography is used to determine the diameter of the bile ducts, and when the ducts are not dilated may be followed by liver biopsy or endoscopic retrograde cholangiography (ERCP), and when the ducts are dilated, percutaneous transhepatic cholangiography (PTC) may be the preferred method for clarifying the diagnosis.

When jaundice and bilirubinuria are accompanied by none of the features mentioned above, and liver function tests are otherwise normal, one of the rare familial causes of conjugated hyperbilirubinaemia is probable. During examination of the jaundiced patient other features which may indicate that liver disease is chronic or due to alcoholism should be sought, including spider naevi, bruises, parotid enlargement, gynaecomastia, testicular atrophy and loss of body hair, leuconychia, palmar erythema, and Dupuytren's contracture. Fetor hepaticus, mental impairment, and asterixis may accompany hepatic encephalopathy. In addition, portal hypertension may be suspected because of dilated veins on the abdominal wall, splenomegaly, and ascites. In cirrhosis the liver may be enlarged or very small. Absence of any signs of chronic liver disease in a jaundiced patient with an enlarged, irregular hard liver suggests the presence of an infiltrative disorder, possibly a secondary neoplasm.

Unconjugated hyperbilirubinaemia. The main causes of unconjugated hyperbilirubinaemia are summarized in Table 2.

Table 1   Scheme for differentiation of types of jaundice by testing of urine and observation of stool colour

	Gilbert's Crigler–Najjar	Haemolysis	Hepatitis	Bile duct obstruction
Blood				
Unconjugated hyperbilirubinaemia	↑	↑	↑	–
Conjugated hyperbilirubinaemia	–	–	↑	↑
Urine				
Bilirubin	–	–	↑	↑
Urobilinogen	N	↑	↑ early may be ↓ late	↓/O
Stool				
Faecal urobilin	N	↑	↓	↓

Table 2   Hyperbilirubinaemia in the absence of overt liver or biliary tract disease or haemolysis

Unconjugated	Conjugated
Gilbert's syndrome	Dubin–Johnson syndrome
Crigler–Najjar type I	Rotor syndrome
Crigler–Najjar type II	
Physiological jaundice of the newborn	
Transient familial neonatal hyperbilirubinaemia	
Breast-milk jaundice	

Gilbert's syndrome. In 1901, Gilbert noticed the familial occurrence of hyperbilirubinaemia in the absence of apparent liver disease. He subdivided subjects according to whether or not there was splenomegaly, the former group later being shown to be due to haemolysis. Gilbert's syndrome now refers to mild unconjugated hyperbilirubinaemia in the absence of liver disease or overt haemolysis, although, if red cell survival studies are performed, up to half the cases are shown to have slightly diminished values. Estimates of its frequency vary from 0.5–8 per cent, giving a mean incidence of 1–2 per cent of the population.

It is even argued whether Gilbert's syndrome exists as a distinct population or merely represents the upper end of a normal distribution curve for plasma bilirubin. Plasma concentration of bilirubin depends on the rate of bilirubin production and the hepatic capacity for bilirubin clearance. It may be that both these determinants follow a normal distribution, and yet because their effects are multiplied, inheritance of a high normal rate of production combined with low normal rates of hepatic clearance will produce a skewed distribution for plasma bilirubin levels. Thus, doubling the rate of bilirubin production and halving the rate of its hepatic clearance quadruples the plasma bilirubin concentration.

Some patients with Gilbert's syndrome complain of abdominal pain, weakness, and malaise, but these symptoms are non-specific and may represent a coincidental occurrence rather than true association. Plasma bilirubin levels fluctuate markedly, and are usually not sufficiently high to produce jaundice. Most patients are discovered incidentally, many as a result of scleral icterus brought on by reduced caloric intake during an illness which causes anorexia.

Though a strong familial tendency exists, the precise mode of inheritance is unclear. An autosomal dominant defect has been suggested, but it is likely that Gilbert's syndrome embraces a heterogeneous group of biochemical defects including abnormalities of hepatic uptake, intracellular binding, and conjugation. In most cases hepatic UDPGT acivity is diminished, suggesting a primary defect in glucuronidation. However, this is a highly inducible enzyme, and decreased levels may be due to decreased hepatic uptake. Furthermore, in some, clearance of indocyanine green (ICG) is defective though this organic anion is excreted unconjugated, and in another subgroup abnormal BSP clearance also suggests a defect in hepatic uptake. Conventional liver function tests are normal. Liver histology is grossly normal, though an increase of lipofuscin may be seen especially in centrolobular hepatocytes. Electron microscopy suggests heterogeneity between patients with evidence of mitochondrial changes and proliferation of the smooth endoplasmic reticulum in some. The diagnosis is based on clinical and laboratory findings. Demonstration of unconjugated hyperbilirubinaemia with otherwise normal liver function tests and no overt haemolysis may suffice. Plasma bilirubin levels approximately double in both normal individuals and those with Gilbert's syndrome when dietary intake is reduced to 1680J (400 cal) daily for 48 to 72 hours. The percentage increase is similar in normals and Gilbert's subjects; however, the increment and final value are much higher in Gilbert's, which may be diagnostically useful since such increases are not seen in patients with hyperbilirubinaemia due to hepatocellular disease or cirrhosis. Liver biopsy is required when there is reasonable doubt about the diagnosis but is not essential.

The prognosis is excellent, and there is no substantive evidence for the association of Gilbert's syndrome with other more serious disorders. Plasma bilirubin levels are reduced when phenobarbitone is administered to patients with Gilbert's syndrome but there is no theoretical benefit to justify its use, and most patients need no more than reassurance derived from an understanding of the commonness of their condition and its totally benign nature.

Crigler–Najjar syndrome. The Crigler–Najjar syndrome results in severe unconjugated hyperbilirubinaemia in the absence of other evidence of hepatic dysfunction or haemolysis. Where they have been studied, hepatic clearance of BSP and ICG, red cell survival, and 'early labelled bilirubin' peak are all normal. The underlying defect appears to be a deficiency of UDPGT activity. There are two genetically distinct groups, types I and II.

In Type I Crigler–Najjar there appears to be complete absence of UDPGT activity, and no bilirubin glucuronide is formed though other compounds may be glucuronidated by the liver. Severe unconjugated hyperbilirubinaemia occurs in the neonatal period leading to kernicterus and early death in most infants. A minority survive without apparent brain damage but they may succumb in later childhood.

The diagnosis is based on clinical and laboratory findings. There is no rhesus, ABO, or other blood group incompatibility and no haemolysis. Other liver function tests are normal and there is no bilirubin in the urine. Bilirubin conjugates are not present in bile which may be colourless. Nevertheless, the colour of faeces has been normal, and urobilin is present though quantitatively diminished in the faeces. The explanation for this is unclear, but is thought to result from diffusion of a small amount of unconjugated bilirubin into the bowel lumen across the intestinal mucosa and biliary tract. Consanguinity is common in the parents of affected offspring, suggesting an autosomal recessive mode of inheritance. Heterozygotes are usually not jaundiced.

Type II Crigler–Najjar is associated with only partial deficiency of UDGPT activity, and is a less well-defined entity than type I embracing those unconjugated hyperbilirubinaemias of hepatic origin which are intermediate between Gilbert's syndrome and type I Crigler–Najjar. Jaundice is usually of less acute onset and less severe than in type I and occasionally may not be apparent in early childhood. Kernicterus is rare. Bile contains bilirubin glucuronides and therefore is deeply pigmented. Familial occurrence is common. Gilbert's syndrome is frequently found in relatives, and in some families Crigler–Najjar type II syndrome appears to represent the homozygous state for a variant of Gilbert's syndrome present in both parents, but the incidence of Crigler–Najjar is much lower than it would be if this was true for all cases.

Treatment. In Crigler–Najjar type II syndrome the time-course of the response to phenobarbitone therapy suggests that an enzyme with a relatively long half-life is being induced. The lack of any such responsiveness to phenobarbitone in type I suggests complete absence of the enzyme, and constitutes the most useful method for clinically differentiating the two types. In type II, phenobarbitone treatment reduces plasma bilirubin levels which patients may welcome for its cosmetic effect.

Phototherapy is effective in alleviating hyperbilirubinaemia in infants. Bilirubin has an intense absorption band in the visible spectrum between 425 and 475 nm, and exposure of the skin to light of this wavelength reduces the plasma bilirubin concentration. A series of highly polar water-soluble derivatives of bilirubin result from its photodegradation, and these pass readily into urine, bile, or across the intestinal wall. This treatment has become established as a means of preventing kernicterus in neonatal units. However, it is probably impractical as a lifelong measure, even in patients with Crigler–Najjar type I syndrome, and its freedom from undesirable side effects in the long term is unproven. Photodegradation may be enhanced by riboflavin.

Diagnosis of unconjugated hyperbilirubinaemia. The main points of difference between Gilbert's and Crigler–Najjar syndromes are summarized in Table 3.

Physiological jaundice of the newborn. A rise in plasma bilirubin concentration occurs very commonly in the first few days of life, but infants born prematurely with low birth weights are most likely to become jaundiced. *In utero* bilirubin is transported across the placenta and removed by the maternal liver. After birth the fetal liver may be incapable of maintaining low plasma bilirubin levels, its immaturity being shown by low levels of ligandin, glucuronyl transferase activity, and capacity for excretion of conjugated bilirubin into bile. This susceptibility to hyperbilirubinaemia in the neonate may be compounded by a shortened red cell life-span, a reduced calorie intake, or shunting past the liver through a patent ductus venosus.

Plasma bilirubin levels must be monitored in jaundiced infants since a risk of kernicterus exists. Although levels in excess of 340 μmol/l have, traditionally, been thought to be dangerous,

Table 3   Points which differentiate the familial unconjugated hyperbilirubinaemias   s.e.r. = smooth endoplasmic reticulum

	Gilbert's syndrome	Crigler–Najjar syndrome	
		Type I	Type II
Defect in bilirubin metabolism	decreased hepatic uptake decreased UDPGT activity	absent UDPGT activity	markedly decreased UDPGT activity
Jaundice	mild, occasional	severe	moderately severe
Kernicterus	never	usual	seldom
Haemolysis	mild haemolysis may be detected by red-cell survival studies in about half of patients	no	no
BSP clearance	may be decreased in some	normal	normal
Liver biopsy	may contain excess lipofuscin and hyperplasia of the s.e.r.	normal	normal
Response to phenobarbitone	yes	no	yes
Animal model	previously regarded as Southdown sheep but they have defective bild acid transport not seen in Gilbert's	homozygous Gunn rat	heterozygous Gunn rat

recent work suggests that plasma levels half as high may be associated with some impairment of subsequent psychomotor development. This problem can be averted by reduction of plasma bilirubin concentrations with phototherapy or exchange transfusions. In addition reabsorption of unconjugated bilirubin formed in the intestine by the action of β-glucuronidase may be prevented by the oral administration of a non-absorbable agar which binds the bilirubin. Drugs which displace bilirubin from albumin should be avoided.

Transient familial neonatal hyperbilirubinaemia. Occasionally, there is a familial tendency to develop neonatal hyperbilirubinaemia, and affected infants are at risk of developing kernicterus even following full-term gestation. There is no haemolysis, and the onset of jaundice occurs earlier than is seen with breast-milk jaundice. The management is the same as for physiological jaundice. Jaundice is transient and the long-term prognosis excellent. Neonatal jaundice associated with glucose 6-phosphate dehydrogenase deficiency is considered in Section 19.

Breast-milk jaundice. A small number of infants has been reported in whom jaundice due to unconjugated hyperbilirubinaemia occurred, apparently as a result of breast feeding. Kernicterus was not a complication. There appears to be an icterogenic factor in breast milk which is not detectable in maternal serum. Siblings of affected individuals are also liable to jaundice if breast fed. High levels of the steroid 3(α),20(β)-pregnanediol, an inhibitor of glucuronyl transferase, in the milk of these mothers, has been implicated. However, whether this is the true icterogenic factor remains to be confirmed.

Conjugated hyperbilirubinaemia. Conjugated hyperbilirubinaemia results from reflux in plasma of bilirubin which has previously been taken up and conjugated by the liver. In most instances it is found in association with retention of other biliary constituents such as bile acids, but typical families have been described in which defective excretion of conjugated bilirubin occurs as an isolated defect.

The Dubin–Johnson syndrome. Although many patients with the Dubin–Johnson syndrome complain of vague symptoms of anorexia, malaise, easy fatiguability, right hypochondrial pain, and occasional diarrhoea, most are asymptomatic until jaundice is dis-

covered. This may be brought on by pregnancy or oral contraceptives, or the diagnosis may only be made during family studies. There is a high incidence of consanguinity in reported families suggesting an autosomal recessive mode of inheritance.

The level of plasma bilirubin varies widely and fluctuates in the individual patient. Bilirubin and excess urobilinogen are found in the urine in the absence of haemolysis or abnormalities of liver function tests. In addition to bilirubin and urobilinogen, other organic anions are affected, and non-visualization of the gall bladder with cholecystographic media is the rule. The pattern of BSP clearance is also helpful diagnostically. Early plasma disappearance of BSP appears normal and retention at 45 minutes may not be markedly deranged. However, plasma levels subsequently rise so that levels at 90 minutes exceed those at 45 minutes, due to reflux of glutathione-conjugated BSP. The diagnosis may be confirmed by measurement of urinary coproporphyrin excretion. In the homozygous state for the Dubin–Johnson syndrome the ratio of urinary coproporphyrin I to coproporphyrin III is at least 4:1 compared to a ratio of approximately 1:3 in normal subjects. The intermediate ratios found in heterozygous carriers support an autosomal recessive mode of inheritance. Similarly increased ratios occur in erythropoietic porphyria but the markedly increased overall excretion of coproporphyrins seen in that situation are not a feature of the Dubin–Johnson syndrome.

The liver is deeply pigmented, and the diagnosis may be suspected if a liver biopsy specimen appears black to the naked eye. Histologically, liver cells contain much granular pigment which is not bilirubin and which has been variously ascribed to lipofuscin and melanin.

There is no recognized treatment for the condition, which is benign, and the patient can be reassured accordingly. Very rarely there has been a co-existent dyserythropoietic anaemia or defect in blood coagulability.

Rotor syndrome. Rotor described the familial occurrence of conjugated hyperbilirubinaemia in natives of the Philippines. Originally considered a variant of the Dubin–Johnson syndrome, it is now thought to have a different pathology with demonstrable uptake and storage defects similar to those found in Southdown sheep and Indigo snake. There is no apparent abnormality of bile acid transport and other liver function tests are normal. Plasma concentrations of bilirubin fluctuate widely as in the Dubin–Johnson syndrome but formal testing distinguishes between the two conditions.

The main differences between the Dubin–Johnson and the Rotor syndromes are summarized in Table 4.

Table 4 Differential features of the two commoner types of familial conjugated hyperbilirubinaemia

	Dubin–Johnson syndrome	Rotor syndrome
Cholecystography	usually unsuccessful	usually successful
Liver biopsy	pigment loaded	no excess pigment
BSP clearance	normal initial phase late rise of BSP–GSH	slow initial clearance no late rise of BSP–GSH
Urinary coproporphyrin		
Total excretion	normal	raised
Ratio I:III	raised	raised

Intrahepatic cholestasis. Cholestasis describes a constellation of clinical, biochemical, and histological findings in which the predominant abnormality is failure of bile secretion. The earliest detectable abnormality may be elevation of serum bile acid levels, but accumulation of other biliary constituents including cholesterol and conjugated bilirubin often follows. Derangement of liver function test characteristically produces an elevation of alkaline phosphatase and 5'-nucelotidase as the more striking features. Liver histology may show accumulation of bile pigment in hepatocytes and Kupffer cells, and bile plugs within the canaliculi, especially in centrolobular zones. Absence or diminution of intestinal bile acids may lead to steatorrhoea, and if cholestasis is prolonged, deficiency states affecting the fat soluble vitamins A, D, E, and K may be anticipated. The classical triad of symptoms in cholestatic disorders is dark urine, pale stools, and pruritus. When biliary obstruction is incomplete pruritus is often first to appear and may be the sole feature for an extended period of time.

Cholestasis may result from obstruction of the extrahepatic biliary system (see page 12.174), and from obstruction of intrahepatic interlobular bile ducts, e.g. in primary biliary cirrhosis (see page 12.190) sclerosing cholangitis (see page 12.175) or parasites (see page 12.220) (Table 5). However, intrahepatic cholestasis may be due to secretory failure at the level of the hepatocellular canaliculus in the absence of any obstruction to flow within the bile ductules or ducts (Table 4). This is seen with drug-induced cholestasis (see page 12.213) and occasionally when liver disease is due to alcohol (see page 12.209) or viral hepatitis (see page 12.195). Only those intralobular cholestatic conditions which do not fit into any of the above categories will be dealt with here.

Table 5 Classification of cholestatic disorders

Intrahepatic
  Without structural liver disease
    Pregnancy
    Hormones, e.g. contraceptive steroids; methyltestosterone
    Benign recurrent intrahepatic cholestasis
    Hodgkin's disease
    Total parenteral nutrition
    (Benign) post-operative cholestasis
  With structural liver disease
    Drugs, e.g. chlorpromazine
    Viral hepatitis
    Alcoholic hepatitis
    Biliary hypoplasia: arteriohepatic dysplasia; Byler's syndrome; alpha-1 antitrypsin deficiency
    Primary biliary cirrhosis
    Sclerosing cholangitis
Extrahepatic
  (obstruction of the major biliary tree including the major divisions of the biliary tree within the liver, i.e. the term extrahepatic is used loosely to denote the causes of mechanical biliary obstruction which it may be possible to relieve by mechanical methods)

Benign recurrent intrahepatic cholestasis. This is a relatively rare condition, affecting males more than females, characterized by recurrent attacks of cholestasis in the absence of any mechanical biliary obstruction and with restoration of completely normal hepatic structure and function between attacks. The first attack usually occurs during childhood or adolescence; attacks last several weeks or months and are separated by intervals of normality lasting many months or years. Pruritus usually precedes jaundice and may sometimes subside without occurrence of jaundice. Patients tend to recognize a pattern common to all of their attacks, though the features vary between individuals. There may be vague right hypochondrial pain and malaise preceding pruritus but fever and chills are not a feature.

Serum bile acids and alkaline phosphatase levels are characteristically raised during attacks. Jaundice is due to conjugated hyperbilirubinaemia, bilirubin is present in the urine, and urinary urobilinogen is extremely low. Disappearance from plasma of unconjugated bilirubin is always normal, but during episodes of jaundice, there is a subsequent rise of conjugated bilirubin. Cholestasis may also cause steatorrhoea and significant hypoprothrombinaemia with bruising. If the diagnosis is not established, retrograde cholangiography may be performed to rule out mechanical obstruction. Histological examination of the liver reveals centrolobular cholestasis. The appearances on electron microscopy show changes which are common to many forms of cholestasis, namely canalicular dilation with loss of canalicular microvilli, widening of the pericanalicular ectoplasm, enlargement of the Golgi, and proliferation of the smooth endoplasmic reticulum.

Benign recurrent intrahepatic cholestasis has a familial incidence but no hereditary pattern is apparent. One family has been reported in which there were several members with benign recurrent intrahepatic cholestasis, cholestasis of pregnancy, or contraceptive steroid-induced cholestasis, which suggests a related mechanism in these conditions. Several possible explanations have been advanced but none is substantiated. Because of the early changes in bile acid metabolism in each attack, it has been postulated that the bile acids have a primary pathogenic role. Another possible explanation is that progressively larger bile constituent molecules diffuse from bile to plasma across abnormally leaky tight junctions; these 'tight junctions' normally restrict passage to bile acids, bilirubin, etc. from the bile canaliculus to the plasma via the intercellular space.

Patients can be reassured of the benign, non-progressive nature of their disease. Corticosteroids appear to hasten the resolution of attacks in some but not all patients, and cholestyramine may relieve pruritus.

Cholestasis of pregnancy. Intrahepatic cholestasis which clinically resembles that described under benign recurrent intrahepatic cholestasis is seen in some women during pregnancy, usually in the third trimester. Pruritus is usually the first symptom and cholestasis may progress to give jaundice with conjugated hyperbilirubinaemia, bilirubinuria, and low urinary urobilinogen levels. Hypochondrial pain is uncommon and fever is not a feature. Liver function tests characteristically reveal elevations of bile acids, alkaline phosphatase, and 5'-nucleotidase, but transaminases are not markedly raised. Steatorrhoea may be produced with hypoprombinaemia which corrects rapidly following parenteral administration of vitamin K. Pruritus is much commoner than jaundice in cholestasis of pregnancy but should probably be regarded as a mild form of the same condition. Cholestasis characteristically resolves rapidly following parturition, and normality is usually restored within two to three weeks. Incomplete resolution of the cholestasis following delivery may indicate underlying liver disease such as primary biliary cirrhosis which has been unmasked by pregnancy. The differential diagnosis includes cholelithiasis which has an increased incidence during pregnancy; even so cholangiography can usually be avoided in cholestasis of pregnancy if the course is typical. Also viral hepatitis is a more common cause of jaundice during pregnancy than either intrahepatic cholestasis of pregnancy or choledocholithiasis. The viral illness is usually less cholestatic and proportionately higher serum transaminase levels reflect the hepatitic nature of the illness.

There is a strong tendency for cholestasis to recur in subsequent pregnancies, and these women also are predisposed to develop cholestasis if given oral contraceptive steroids. There is a relatively strong familial tendency, though the precise mode of inheritance is unclear. Particularly high incidences of recurrent intrahepatic cholestasis of pregnancy have been observed in certain countries, notably in Scandinavia and Chile. The outcome is usually benign, but there may be an increased risk of fetal distress and premature labour. No long-term ill effects on infant or mother have been described.

Histological examination of the liver reveals a purely cholestatic disorder without hepatocellular necrosis. The features for both light and electron microscopy are the same as those described for benign recurrent intrahepatic cholestasis above.

The concurrence of cholestasis with the third trimester of pregnancy when oestrogen levels are at their highest, and the predisposition of the same subjects to develop cholestasis when given contraceptive steroids points to a pathogenetic role for oestrogens. The importance of progestogens is less certain. At present it appears that cholestasis occurs in women who have an unusual susceptibility to respond in this way to normal oestrogens, rather than from formation of an abnormal compound with cholestatic properties.

Contraceptive-steroid induced cholestasis. Pruritus progressing to jaundice occurs in some women taking oral contraceptive steroids (see Section 11). Symptoms usually appear during the first three monthly cycles, and recede spontaneously when 'the pill' is discontinued. Those who have experienced cholestasis on the 'contraceptive pill' have a high likelihood of developing cholestasis of pregnancy and vice versa. If possible, oral contraceptive steroids should be avoided in women with a prior history of cholestasis of pregnancy or benign recurrent intrahepatic cholestasis. Rarely, progressive biliary disorders such as primary biliary cirrhosis or sclerosing cholangitis may first become symptomatic due to the unmasking effect of contraceptive steroids and also constitute contra-indications to their use. There is no evidence to suggest an increased risk of oral contraceptive-induced cholestasis during convalescence from viral hepatitis.

References

Bondy, P. K. and Rosenberg, L. E. (1980). *Metabolic control and disease*, 8th edn. W. B. Saunders, Philadelphia and London.
Popper, H. and Schaffner, F. (1979). *Progress in liver diseases*, vol. 6. Grune and Stratton, New York.
Schiff, L. (1975). *Diseases of the liver*. 4th edn. Lippincott, Philadelphia.
Sherlock, S. (1981). *Diseases of the liver and biliary system*. 6th edn. Blackwell Scientific Publications, Oxford.

Cirrhosis of the liver

S. Sherlock

Definition. Cirrhosis is defined anatomically as a chronic diffuse process with fibrosis and nodule formation. It has followed hepatocellular necrosis. Although the causes are many, the end result is the same. The liver architecture is irreversibly destroyed so that complete recovery is impossible. Cirrhosis results in two major events, failure of liver-cell function and portal hypertension. Prognosis and treatment depend on the magnitude of these two factors. In clinical terms, the types are either latent and well-compensated or active and decompensated.

Mechanisms. The responses of the liver to necrosis are strictly limited; the most important are collapse of hepatic lobules, formation of diffuse fibrous septa, and nodular regrowth of liver cells. Thus, irrespective of the aetiology, the ultimate histological picture of the liver is similar.

When the liver cells become necrotic, the reticulin framework collapses with approximation of portal and central zones (bridging). Some cells regrow to form nodules of various sizes. The nodules distort the hepatic vascular tree so that portal blood flow is impeded and protal hypertension results.

Sinusoids persist at the periphery of the regenerating nodules at the site of the portal-central bridges. Portal blood is diverted past functioning liver tissue leading to vascular insufficiency at the centre of the nodules. Basement membranes form in the Dissë (perisinusoidal) space, so impeding metabolic exchange between blood in the sinusoids and the liver cells.

Aetiology. This depends on the geographical location. In the Western world, alcohol (see page 12.209) and hepatitis B (see page 12.197) account for the majority. A large number are termed cryptogenic and the aetiology of this heterogeneous group is unknown. The incidence of the latter varies in different parts of the world; in the United Kingdom it is about 30 per cent, whereas in other areas, such as France or in urban parts of the USA, where alcoholism is prevalent, the level drops. As specific diagnostic criteria appear, so the percentage of cryptogenic cirrhosis falls. The advent of serum markers for hepatitis B transferred many previously designated cryptogenic cirrhotics to the post-hepatic group. Estimations of serum smooth muscle and mitochondrial antibodies and better interpretation of liver histology separated others into the chronic active hepatitis–primary biliary cirrhosis category. Some of the remainder may be in alcoholics who deny alcoholism. Some are due to non-A, non-B hepatitis.

The metabolic group includes iron overload states, Wilson's disease, alpha-1 antitrypsin deficiency, type IV glycogenosis, galactosaemia, and congenital tyrosinosis (see page 12.221).

Prolonged cholestasis, whether due to intrahepatic causes, such as primary biliary cirrhosis (see page 12.190), or extrahepatic lesions such as biliary stricture or sclerosing cholangitis lead to biliary cirrhosis.

Hepatic venous outflow obstruction, due to such causes as veno-occlusive disease, Budd–Chiari syndrome or constrictive pericarditis, leads to cardiac cirrhosis. Disturbed immunity leads to an auto-immune type chronic active hepatitis followed by cirrhosis (see page 12.204). Cirrhosis can follow adverse reactions to certain drugs including methotrexate, isoniazid, and methyldopa. Rare causes of cirrhosis include intestinal bypass for obesity, and Indian childhood cirrhosis (see page 12.222).

The terminal stages of the various types may be identical and differences must not be stressed. The aetiological distinction, however, is important both for prognosis and for specific treatment such as alcohol withdrawal, venesection in haemochromatosis or corticosteroids in the auto-immune type of chronic active hepatitis. Finally, comparison of cirrhosis in different parts of the world must allow for different aetiologies, although the basic pattern of liver-cell failure and portal hypertension may be similar. Results for the treatment of one type cannot be compared with those for another.

Clinically latent cirrhosis

The disease may be discovered at a routine examination or bio-chemical screen, or at operation undertaken for some other condition. Cirrhosis may be suspected if the patient has mild pyrexia, vascular spiders, palmar erythema, or unexplained epistaxis or oedema of the ankles. Firm enlargement of the liver and splenomegaly are helpful diagnostic signs. Vague morning indigestion and flatulent dyspepsia may be early features in the alcoholic cirrhotic. Confirmation should be sought by biochemical tests and, if necessary, by needle liver biopsy.

Biochemical tests may be quite normal in this group. The most frequent changes are a slight increase in the serum transaminase or gammaglutamyl transpeptidase levels and a constant excess of uro-bilinogen in the urine.

These patients may remain compensated until they die from another cause. Some proceed, in a period from months to years, to the stage of hepatocellular failure. In others, the problems of portal hypertension with oesophageal bleeding arise. The course in the individual patient is very difficult to predict.

Table 1 Investigation of the patient with cirrhosis

General information
  Age, sex, occupation, birthplace
Clinical history
  Fatigue and weight loss
  Abdominal pain
  Jaundice, colour of urine and faeces
  Swelling of legs or abdomen
  Haemorrhage—nose, gums, skin
  Gastrointestinal bleeding: number, dates, transfusions, symptoms,
    treatment
Past
  Jaundice, hepatitis, drugs ingested
  Previous biochemical tests
Social
  Family history of liver disease
  Alcohol consumption
Examination
  Nutrition (weight), fever, fetor hepaticus, jaundice,
    pigmentation, purpura and bruising, clubbing, white nails,
    vascular spiders, liver palms, gynaecomastia, testicular
    atrophy, body hair, parotid enlargement, Dupuytren's contracture,
    blood pressure
  Abdomen: ascites, veins, liver, spleen
  Peripheral oedema.
  Neurological changes: mental functions, stupor, tremor
Special investigations
  Serum biochemical: bilirubin, alkaline phosphatase, albumin
    and globulin, transaminase
  If ascites present: sodium, potassium, bicarbonate, chloride
    and urea
  Serum immunological: quantitative immunoglobulin, smooth
    muscle, mitochondrial, and nuclear antibodies. Hepatitis B
    surface antigen, and (if positive), 'e' antigen, alpha-1 fetoprotein
  Haematology: haemoglobin, absolute values, WBCs and
    platelets, prothrombin time
  Plain X-ray, abdomen and chest
  Barium swallow and meal
  Endoscopy
  Needle liver biopsy if blood coagulation permits
Additional investigations
  Hepatic scan or ultrasound
  EEG if neuropsychiatric changes
  Transplenic portal venography
  Intrasplenic pressure
  Hepatic vein catheterization
  Selective splanchnic arteriography

Decompensated cirrhosis

The patient usually seeks medical advice because of ascites and/or jaundice. General health fails with weakness, muscle wasting, and weight loss. Continuous mild fever (37.5–38 °C) is often due to Gram-negative bacteriaemia, to continuing hepatocellular necrosis, or to a complicating liver-cell carcinoma. Fetor hepaticus may be present. Cirrhosis is the commonest cause of hepatic encephalopathy.

Jaundice. Jaundice is largely due to failure of the liver-cells to metabolize bilirubin, so it is some guide to the severity of liver-cell failure. In the patient with cirrhosis, jaundice may be absent or mild. This is due to the balance achieved between hepatic necrosis and regeneration. When present, it represents active hepatocellular disease and a bad prognosis. Diminished erythrocyte survival adds a haemolytic component to the jaundice.

Hyperkinetic circulation. In advanced cases the circulation is hyperdynamic shown by flushed extremities, bounding pulses, and capillary pulsations. The blood pressure tends to be low in all forms of cirrhosis, whatever the stage.

Vasomotor tone is decreased and the circulation resembles that found in association with systemic arteriovenous fistulae. It seems possible that large numbers of normally present but functionally inactive arteriovenous anastomoses have opened under the influence of a vasodilator substance. The diseased liver might produce such a vasodilator or fail to metabolize one formed elsewhere. False neuromuscular transmitters of gut origin, which are not metabolized by the diseased liver, have been invoked as the cause; this has not been proven.

Pulmonary changes and cyanosis. About one-third of patients with decompensated cirrhosis have reduced arterial oxygen saturation and are sometimes cyanosed. This is probably due to intrapulmonary shunting through microscopic arteriovenous fistulae. Reduction of diffusing capacity is likely to be due to dilatation of small pulmonary blood vessels. Reduction in transfer factor is perhaps related to thickening of alveolar walls and small veins and capillaries by a layer of collagen.

Skin changes. Vascular spiders are found in the vascular territory of the superior vena cava, and very rarely below a line joining the nipples. Common sites are the necklace area, the face, forearms, and dorsum of the hand.

The arterial vascular spider consists of a central arteriole radiating from which are numerous small vessels resembling a spiders' legs. If sufficiently large it can be seen, or felt, to pulsate. Pressure on the central prominence with a pin head causes blanching of the whole lesion, as would be expected from an arterial condition.

The selective distribution of vascular spiders is not understood. The number does not correlate with the hyperdynamic circulation. The vascular spiders have been traditionally attributed to oestrogen excess. They are also seen in pregnancy when circulating oestrogens are increased. Oestrogen certainly enlarges and dilates the spiral arterials of the endometrium. The liver inactivates oestrogens. Higher plasma oestradiol levels are found in patients with vascular spiders than in those without. However, vascular spiders appear and disappear irrespective of changes in plasma oestradiol. Palmar erythema (liver palms) is characterized by a bright red colouration, especially on the hypothenar and thenar eminences and pulps of the fingers. The hands are warm. The soles of the feet may be similarly affected. Like vascular spiders the mechanism of production is unknown.

Vascular spiders and palmar erythema are most frequent with cirrhosis, especially of the alcoholic. They may appear transiently in virus hepatitis. Rarely they are found in normal persons, especially children. During normal pregnancy vascular spiders appear between the second and fifth months, disappearing within two months of delivery. A few spiders should not be sufficient to diagnose liver disease, but many new ones, with increasing size of old ones, arouse suspicion.

White nails are due to opacity of the nail bed and are very frequent in patients with cirrhosis. A pink zone is seen at the tip of the nail, and in a severe example, the lunula cannot be distinguished.

Endocrine changes. These are most common in cirrhosis of the alcoholic, and if the patient is in the active, reproductive phase of life. In the male, the changes are towards feminization, and in the female, towards masculinization or gonadal atrophy.

Diminished libido and potency are frequent in men with active cirrhosis, and many are sterile. The testes are soft and small. Secondary sexual hair is lost, and men shave less often. Patients with well-compensated disease may have large families.

In the female gonadal changes are not conspicuous, for the patients are usually post-menopausal and any breast or uterine atrophy is of little significance. In younger patients, libido is lowered and the patient is usually infertile. Menstruation is diminished or absent but rarely excessive. The breasts and uterus usually atrophy.

Gynaecomastia occasionally complicates cirrhosis, usually in alcoholics but also in young men with chronic active hepatitis. The breasts may be tender. Spironolactone therapy is the commonest cause of gynaecomastia in cirrhotic patients. The changes of feminization are particularly common in alcoholics.

Despite improved biochemical techniques for measuring sex hormones in blood, the mechanism of the endocrine changes remains unclear.

Ascites. There are two important factors in the formation of ascites, the plasma colloid osmotic pressure exerted by the plasma proteins which retains fluid in the vascular compartment, and the portal venous pressure which forces fluid into the tissue spaces.

In cirrhosis albumin synthesis is decreased and plasma albumin and colloid osmotic pressure are reduced. Portal hypertension is also present. Regenerating nodules compress hepatic veins causing a hepatic outflow block. This results in hepatic lymph over-production and this extravasates into the peritoneal cavity. More fluid enters the peritoneal cavity than leaves it and ascites develops. This results in depletion of the effective intravascular volume which causes the renal tubules to retain sodium and water. The effect on the distal tubules is presumably through aldosterone; the mechanism of the proximal tubular urinary sodium retention is uncertain.

By these various methods sodium and water are retained, body fluids are again replete, more ascites is formed, and the whole cycle starts again.

Clinical features. Ascites may appear suddenly or develop insidiously over the course of months. Sudden onset may be associated with reduction of hepatic function, for instance by haemorrhage, infection, or an alcoholic debauch. The insidious onset carries a worse prognosis because it is not associated with any rectifiable factor. The increasing abdominal distension results in dyspnoea.

Examination. The patient is dehydrated and sweating is diminished. Muscle wasting is obvious. The thin limbs contrast with the protuberant belly (Fig. 1).

The abdomen is distended, not only with fluid but also by air in the dilated intestines. The fullness is particularly conspicuous in the flanks and the umbilicus is everted. The increased intra-abdominal pressure favours the protrusion of hernias in the umbilical, femoral, or inguinal regions, or through old abdominal incisions. Scrotal oedema is frequent. Distended abdominal veins radiating from the umbilicus represent portal-systemic collaterals. Inferior vena-caval collaterals result from pressure on the cava from the peritoneal fluid. They are seen in the flanks. Abdominal striae may develop. Dullness on percussion in the flanks is the earliest sign. With tense ascites it is difficult to palpate the abdominal viscera, but with moderate amounts of fluid the liver or spleen may be ballotted.

A fluid thrill means much free fluid; it is a very late sign of fluid under tension. A pleural effusion is found in about 6 per cent of cirrhotics and in 67 per cent of these it is right-sided. It is due to defects in the diaphragm allowing ascitic fluid to pass into the

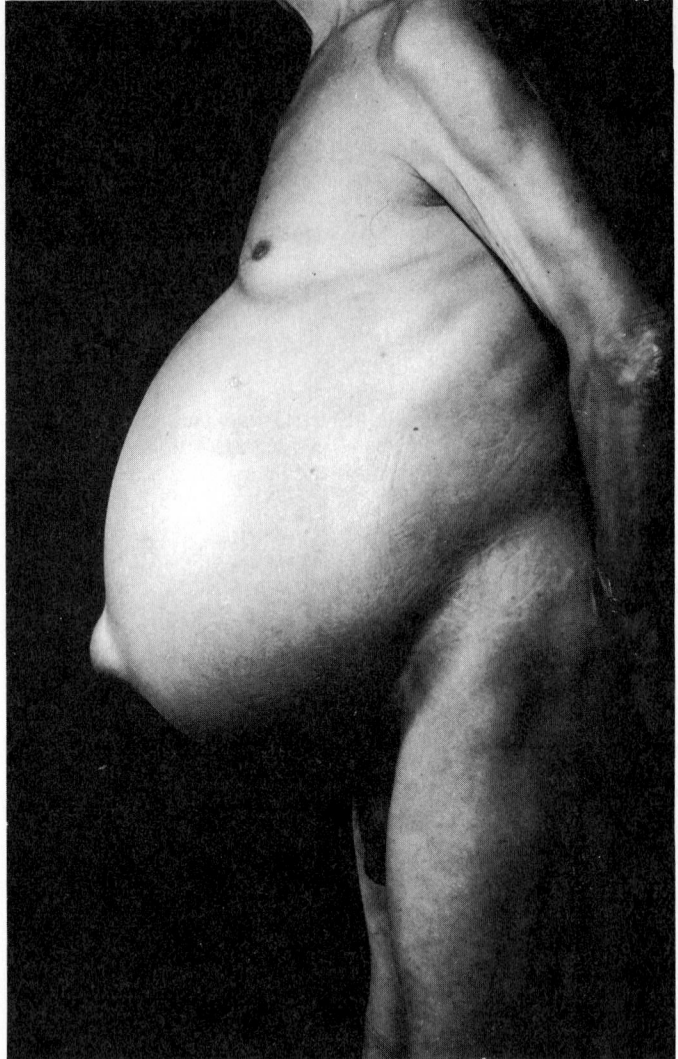

Fig. 1 Patient with cirrhosis and gross ascites. Note also umbilical hernia and marked muscle wasting.

pleural cavity. Oedema usually follows ascites and is related to hypoproteinaemia.

Ascitic fluid and paracentesis abdomenis. Diagnostic paracentesis (of about 50 ml) is always performed. Theurapeutic paracentesis is very rarely necessary unless the patient is in severe discomfort.

Protein concentration rarely exceeds 10–20 g/l. Higher values suggest infection, obstruction to the hepatic veins, malignant peritonitis, or pancreatic ascites. The fluid appears clear, green, straw coloured, or bile-stained. The volume is variable and up to 70 litres have been recorded. A blood-stained fluid indicates malignant disease or a recent paracentesis or an invasive investigation such as splenic venography or liver biopsy.

Infection of the ascitic fluid is very common. This develops spontaneously in about 8 per cent of cirrhotic patients with ascites. The cirrhosis is usually severely decompensated. The infection is usually part of a septicaemia. Infection may also follow a previous paracentesis. Spontaneous bacterial peritonitis should be suspected if the patient with known cirrhosis undergoes sudden deterioration particularly with encephalopathy. Pyrexia, local abdominal pain and tenderness, and systemic leucocytosis may be noted. These features are by no means constant, however, and a diagnosis is made on the index of suspicion with examination of the ascitic fluid. This shows a leucocyte count exceeding 500 per mm^3 with 75 to 100 per cent polymorphs. Although the values are not conclusive evidence of bacterial peritonitis, they are sufficiently alarming to merit antibiotic therapy. The infecting organisms are usually Gram-negative coliforms or streptococci. The infection may be mixed. Centrifuged deposits of ascitic fluid must be stained by Gram's method and the fluid cultured. Tuberculous peritonitis should be suspected, particularly in the severely malnourished alcoholic. The cells in the ascitic fluid are usually mononuclear. The deposit must always be stained for tubucle bacilli and suitable cultures set up. Cytology of ascitic fluid is of little value. The normal peritoneal endothelial cells resemble malignant ones, so leading to an over-diagnosis of cancer.

Urine. The urine volume is diminished and it is deeply pigmented and of high osmolarity. The daily output of sodium is greatly reduced, usually less than 5 mmol and in the severe case less than 1 mEq.

Radiological features. Plain X-ray of the abdomen shows a diffuse, ground-glass appearance. Distended loops of bowel may simulate intestinal obstruction. Ultrasound shows an echo-free space around the liver and can be used to demonstrate quite small amounts of fluid.

Hepatic encephalopathy

Aetiology. Patients with hepatic cirrhosis of all types suffer from a variable, fluctuant organic mental reaction with an associated neurological disturbance. There are various factors in the aetiology (Table 2). The most important is the failure of the liver cell to detoxicate nitrogenous compounds, usually with an alimentary portal of entry, or produced elsewhere in the body. The intestinal toxic substance is produced by bacterial action on protein in the colon. The failure of the liver cell may be enhanced by such precipitating factors as haemorrhage, usually gastrointestinal, infection, acute alcoholic excess, or electrolyte imbalance provoked by diuretics.

Table 2 Aetiological factors precipitating hepatic encephalopathy in cirrhotic patients

	Survival	Precipitant
No precipitant	50%	
Precipitant	70–80%	diuresis, haemorrhage, diarrhoea and vomiting, paracentesis, surgery, sedatives, alcohol excess, infections
Chronic	100%	dietary protein, constipation, sedatives

Every patient presenting the features of hepatic encephalopathy has a circulatory pathway through which portal blood may enter the systemic veins and reach the brain without being metabolized by the liver. In patients with poor hepatocellular function the shunt is through the liver itself. The damaged cells are unable to metabolize the contents of the portal venous blood completely, so that they pass unaltered into the hepatic veins. In addition, in patients with cirrhosis, the portal blood bypasses the liver cells through large natural portal systemic collaterals. The portal hepatic vein anastomoses developing around the nodules in a cirrhotic liver may also act as internal shunts. The picture is a common complication of porta-caval shunt operations.

The brain of the patient with liver disease seems unduly sensitive to insults that would be without effect in the normal individual. A small dose of morphine for instance, can initiate pre-comatous changes in a patient with cirrhosis. A similar sensitivity is shown to electrolyte imbalance. Indeed, whether cause or effect, cerebral metabolism is undoubtedly abnormal in liver disease. Ammonia has been the most widely postulated toxic substance. The syndrome may be reproduced in some patients by ammonium salts and arterial ammonium levels may be high. Ammonia can be derived from the nitrogenous contents of the intestine by bacterial action. It is present in high concentration in portal blood and is metabolized

by the liver to urea. However, there is no clear evidence associating the amounts of ammonia in the brain and the mental state. The raised blood ammonia level in hepatic coma may well be more a non-specific indicator of disturbed brain metabolism than the causative factor.

Estimations of blood ammonia levels are time-consuming and do not always correlate with severity or prognosis. The estimation is not necessary for routine use.

Other pharmacologically active amines can be formed by intestinal bacteria acting on protein and are present in portal blood. They are difficult to determine in biological fluids and their place in inducing hepatic encephalopathy remains uncertain.

Intestinal bacterial decarboxylation results in the production not only of ammonia but also of amines such as octopamine which is formed from tyramine. These bacterial products could act as false neurochemical transmitters competing with the true transmitters, noradrenaline and dopamine. A Parkinsonian-like syndrome with akinesia, rigidity, tremor, and mask-like facies could thus be induced. High levels of serum and urinary octopamine are found in hepatic encephalopathy. However, intraventricular infusion of enormous quantities of octopamine with resulting depression of brain dopamine and noradrenaline failed to cause coma in normal rats. Neurotransmitter synthesis is controlled by the brain concentration of the precursor amino-acids. The aromatic amino acids, tyrosine, phenylalanine, and tryptophan, are increased in liver disease, perhaps due to failure of hepatic deamination. The branched chain amino acids, valine, leucine, and isoleucine, are decreased, perhaps due to increased catabolism by skeletal muscle and the kidneys secondary to the hyperinsulinism of chronic liver disease. The reduced ratio between the branched chain and the aromatic amino acids has been related to the development of hepatic encephalopathy. However, in a large group of cirrhotic patients the ratio was reduced both in those with and without encephalopathy.

Other metabolic abnormalities include hypoxia, hypokalaemia, and an increase in serum short-chain fatty acids. All of these abnormalities could disturb cerebral metabolism.

Hypoglycaemia may complicate fulminant hepatitis but is rare with chronic hepatic encephalopathy.

Finally such factors as *infection, hypotension,* or *anoxia* act both on the liver and the brain. Multiple factors may operate in the individual patient.

Clinical associations. The neuropsychiatric picture is complex and affects all parts of the brain. Disturbed consciousness is usual. This is progressive from confusion with altered mood and behaviour to deep coma with no response to painful stimuli. A rough clinical grading should be used and made frequently (Table 3).

Table 3 Grades of hepatic encephalopathy

1 Confused. Altered mood or behaviour; psychometric tests defective
2 Drowsy. Inappropriate behaviour
3 Stuporose, but speaking and obeying single commands. Inarticulate speech. Marked confusion
4 Coma

Personality changes are conspicuous with advanced liver disease. These include childishness, irritability, and loss of concern for family. Intellectual deterioration varies in severity. The disturbances in visual, spatial gnosis lead to constructional apraxia, shown by inability to reproduce designs with matches. Psychometric tests confirm intellectual impairment. Speech is slow and slurred.

The most characteristic neurological abnormality is the 'flapping' tremor (*asterixis*). It is demonstrated with the patient's arms outstretched and fingers separated, or by hyperextending the wrists with the forearm fixed. It can occasionally be appreciated by gentle elevation of a limb or by the patient gripping the physician's hand.

A flapping tremor is not specific for hepatic encephalopathy. It can also be observed in uraemia, in respiratory failure, and in severe heart failure. Deep tendon reflexes are usually exaggerated, although in deep coma the patient becomes flaccid and loses his reflexes.

The clinical course is very fluctuant and frequent observation of the patient is necessary.

The cerebrospinal fluid is usually clear and under normal pressure. Patients in hepatic coma may show an increased CSF protein concentration but the cell count is normal. Glutamic acid and also glutamine may be increased.

The electro-encephalogram shows slowing of the frequency from the normal alpha range of 8–13 Hz right down to the delta range of below 4 Hz. The changes should be graded using frequency analysis. The EEG is useful for diagnosis and to assess the results of treatment. Similar EEG changes are seen with uraemia, carbon dioxide retention, Vitamin B_{12} deficiency, and hypoglycaemia. These changes however in a conscious patient with liver disease are virtually diagnostic.

Clinical types. There are two main types. In the acute form, the syndrome may appear spontaneously or following a precipitating event. In the chronic form the major factor is a large portal-systemic collateral circulation.

Acute type. The syndrome may appear spontaneously without a precipitant, usually in a deeply jaundiced patient with ascites and in the terminal stages. Precipitating factors act by depressing liver cell or cerebral function, increasing nitrogenous material in the intestine, or increasing the portal collateral flow.

The commonest precipitant is a brisk response to a potent diuretic. Paracentesis may also precipitate coma; the mechanism is uncertain. Electrolyte imbalance following removal of large quantities of electrolytes and water, changes in hepatic circulation, and hypotension may contribute. Other causes of fluid and electrolyte depletion such as diarrhoea or vomiting may be precipitants. Gastrointestinal haemorrhage, usually from oesophageal varices, is another common precipitant.

Surgical procedures are tolerated extremely poorly in the cirrhotic patient. Hepatic function is depressed by the blood loss, anaesthesia and 'shock', and coma may follow.

Acute alcoholism precipitates coma both by depressing cerebral function and by the associated acute alcoholic hepatitis. Morphia and barbiturates depress cerebral function and have a prolonged action when hepatic detoxication is delayed.

Infections, especially with bacteraemia and including 'spontaneous' bacterial peritonitis may be the precipitant.

Coma may occasionally be initiated by a large protein meal or by severe constipation.

Chronic type. Portal-systemic collateral circulation is particularly extensive. This may consist simply of small anastomotic vessels or, more often, one major collateral channel such as the umbilical vein or inferior mesenteric vein, predominates. The construction of a surgical portal-systemic shunt is often followed by chronic neuropsychiatric symptoms.

Fluctuations are related to dietary protein and diagnosis can be confirmed by noting the effect clinically and on the EEG of a precipitant such as a high protein diet, or by demonstrating improvement by dietary protein withdrawal. Clinical and biochemical evidence of liver disease may by equivocal or absent, and the neuropsychiatric disorder may dominate the picture.

The disturbance may continue for many years and the diagnosis is very liable to fall between the various specialist's interests, including psychiatrists, neurologists, and hepatologists. The patient may be seen for the first time in coma or in remission, adding to the diagnostic difficulty.

Acute psychiatric changes may be paranoid, schizophrenic, or manic. Rarely paraplegia may develop insidiously. Chronic cerebellar and Parkinsonian syndromes may occasionally develop after years of chronic hepatic encephalopathy.

Portal hypertension

Pathogenesis. All forms of cirrhosis lead to intrahepatic portal hypertension. The mechanism is complex. The portal vascular bed is distorted and diminished and the portal blood flow is mechanically obstructed. The hepatic venous radicles and sinusoids are also rigidly compressed by the nobules. The obstruction to portal venous flow is at all levels from portal zones through the sinusoids to the hepatic venous outflow.

Some of the portal venous blood is diverted into major collateral venous channels and some bypasses the liver cells and is shunted directly into the hepatic venous radicles in the fibrous septa. These portal-hepatic anastomoses develop from pre-existing sinusoids enclosed in the septa. The hepatic vein is displaced further and further outwards until it lies in the septum linked with the portal venous radical by the original sinusoid. The regenerating nodules become divorced from their portal blood supply and are nourished by the hepatic artery. About one-third of the total blood flow perfusing the cirrhotic liver may bypass sinusoids, and hence functioning liver tissue, through these channels.

Clinical associations. Haematemesis, usually from ruptured oesophageal varices is the commonest presentation. Portal-systemic collaterals in ileostomies, colonic mucosa, or rectum may also bleed sometimes. The number and severity of previous haemorrhages should be noted, together with their immediate effects, whether there was associated confusion or coma and whether blood transfusion was required.

A number of prominent collateral veins radiating from the umbilicus is termed *caput Medusae*. This is rare, and usually one or two veins, frequently epigastric, are seen. The blood flow is away from the umbilicus, whereas in inferior vena-caval obstruction the collateral venous channels carry blood upwards to reach the superior vena-caval system. In portal hypertension the blood comes from the left branch of the portal vein which is diverted via para-umbilical veins to the umbilical region and hence to reach veins of the caval system.

A venous hum may be heard, usually in the region of the xiphoid or umbilicus, occasionally radiating to the sternum or over the liver. A thrill, detectable by light pressure, may sometimes be felt at the site of maximum intensity. The sound may be accentuated during systole, in inspiration, or in the erect or sitting positions. It is due to blood rushing through a large umbilical or para-umbilical channel in the falciform ligament from the left branch of the portal vein to the veins of the anterior abdominal wall.

The spleen enlarges progressively. The edge is firm. Size bears little relation to the portal pressure. It is larger in young people and in macronodular rather than micronodular cirrhosis. An enlarged spleen is the single most important diagnostic sign of portal hypertension. If the spleen cannot be felt or is not enlarged radiologically, the diagnosis of portal hypertension is questionable.

Diagnosis
Endoscopy. This is a reliable method of demonstrating oesophageal varices. They show as blue, rounded projections under the mucosa. Gastric and duodenal varices may also be visualized.

Radiology. Oesophageal varices are shown as filling defects in the regular contour of the oesophagus (Fig. 2). They are most often seen in the lower third but may spread upwards so that the entire oesophagus is involved. Widening and gross dilatation are helpful signs. Care must be taken that the oesophagus is not overfilled with contrast material as the varices may be masked.

Visualizing the portal venous system. *Scanning.* The least invasive techniques are CT scanning and ultrasound which visualize the portal vein at the hilum of the liver. A normal portal vein is easily seen. In portal hypertension the main vein is dilated. If re-canalization is in progress, the vein is irregular and reduced in diameter. A

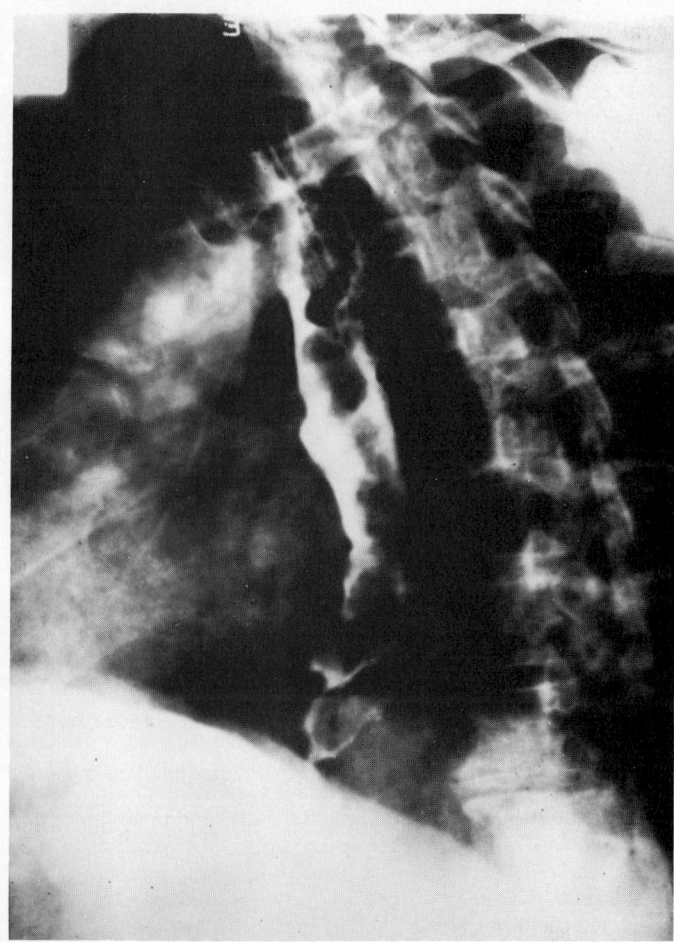

and portal veins. In adults, local anaesthesia is used, but children require a general anaesthetic. This technique gives excellent visualization of the splenic and portal veins and any collateral circulation. The intrasplenic pressure is measured at the same time and gives a good indication of the portal venous pressure. Deep jaundice, impaired clotting, thrombocytopenia, and tense ascites are contraindications. In cirrhosis the intrasplenic pressure is usually raised. The splenic and portal veins are patent, and collaterals, usually gastro-oesophageal, are visualized. The intrahepatic vascular pattern is usually distorted ('tree in winter appearance'). Occlusion of the main portal vein usually implies a complicating primary liver cancer. However, a non-filled vein may sometimes reflect only a very large extrahepatic portal-systemic collateral circulation.

Selective visceral angiography. The coeliac axis or superior mesenteric artery is catheterized via the femoral artery with a pre-formed opaque catheter and contrast material is injected. This returns to the splenic and superior mesenteric veins to produce a splenic and portal venogram of variable quality. Collateral channels tend not to be very clearly defined. The portal venous pressure cannot be measured. The procedure has the advantage that in the cirrhotic patients the presence of an intrahepatic tumour circulation may allow a previously unrecognized primary liver cancer to be diagnosed. Knowledge of splenic and hepatic arterial anatomy may be useful if surgery is contemplated. The procedure may be done with defects in blood coagulation that would contra-indicate splenic venography.

Trans-hepatic portography. This technique gives excellent visualization of the portal and splenic veins and the portal systemic collateral circulation. Portal pressure is measured. It is, however, technically difficult and carries a greater risk than the other procedures. It is usually performed as a preliminary to transhepatic obliteration of varices.

Measuring portal pressure. This can be done by the splenic or transhepatic routes. Alternatively, a catheter may be introduced into a hepatic venous radical until it goes no further and the wedged hepatic venous pressure measured. This reflects intrasinusoidal venous pressure. The standard of reference is the pressure in the inferior vena cava measured before or after entering the liver. The technique is relatively easy, safe, and can be performed in patients with a bleeding tendency. In cirrhosis the wedged pressure is increased. Repeated measurements may be used to assess progress.

Laboratory investigations in cirrhosis

Biochemical. In the well compensated cirrhotic patient, biochemical tests may be quite normal. The most frequent changes are a slight increase in the serum transaminase or γ-glutamyl transaminase level and a constant excess of urobilinogen in the urine.

In the decompensated cirrhotic patient, the urine shows urobilinogen excess. Bilirubin may be present. The urinary sodium is diminished in the presence of ascites. Serum shows a variably raised serum bilirubin level, depression of albumin and a raised gamma-globulin. The serum alkaline phosphatase is usually raised to about twice normal; very high readings are occasionally found. Serum transaminase values are variably increased.

Haematological. There is usually a mild normochromic, normocytic anaemia; it is occasionally macrocytic, especially in the alcoholic patient. Gastrointestinal bleeding leads to hypochromic anaemia. The leucocyte and platelet counts are reduced (hypersplenism). The prothrombin time is prolonged and does not return to normal with vitamin K therapy. The haematological changes in liver disease are considered further in Section 19.

Needle biopsy diagnosis. If there are no contra-indications, such as ascites or a coagulation defect, this should always be done. It may give a clue to aetiology and to activity.

Diagnosis may be difficult as the soft parenchyma is readily aspirated leaving fibrous tissue behind. Large nodules provide a

Fig. 2 Barium swallow X-ray shows a dilated oesophagus. The margin is irregular. There are multiple filling defects representing oesophageal varices.

thrombosed vein is not detected. The collateral circulation is not well seen.

Trans-splenic portal venography (Fig. 3). Contrast material, injected percutaneously into the pulp of the spleen, is absorbed into the portal blood stream with sufficient rapidity to outline the splenic

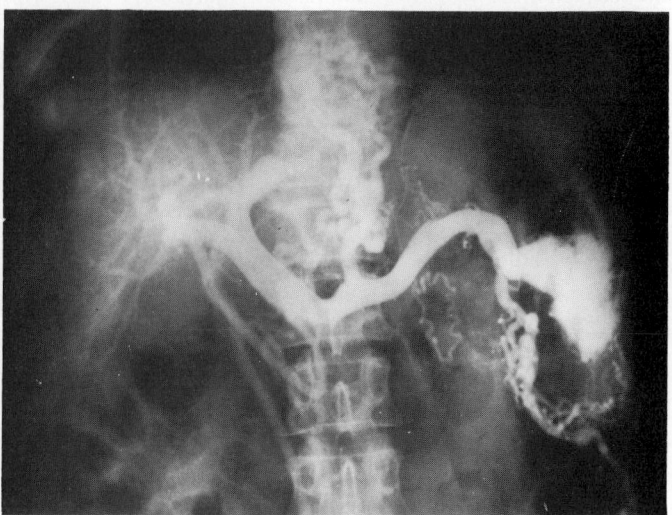

Fig. 3 Splenic venogram from a patient with cirrhosis of the liver. The splenic pulp is shown. The portal vein is patent. A collateral circulation can be seen running to the oesophagus. The umbilical vein can be seen running downwards from the left branch of the portal vein. The intrahepatic portal vascular tree is distorted ('tree in winter' appearance).

special difficulty in interpretation. Reticulin and collagen stains are essential. Helpful diagnostic points include fragmentation of the specimen, fibrous tissue at the margins, absence of portal tracts, abnormal vascular arrangements, nodules with fibrous septa, variable cell size and appearance, and thickened liver-cell plates.

Radioisotope scanning. $^{99}Tc^m$, which is taken up by reticulo-endothelial cells, is the usual isotope employed. Cirrhosis is suggested by a generalized decrease in uptake, an irregular pattern, and by uptake of technetium by the spleen and bone marrow. This picture may be useful diagnostically when a bleeding tendency contraindicates liver biopsy. Widespread hepatic metastases may produce a somewhat similar pattern but without splenic uptake.

In the presence of severe hepatocellular disease, for instance advanced cirrhosis, the isotope is hardly taken up by the liver as the blood shunts past the reticulo-endothelial cells.

Ultrasound and CT scanning. These methods are of limited value in the investigation of cirrhosis. False negative and false positive results are frequent, especially if the cirrhotic nodules are large. Fatty liver may be shown as a lower radiodensity than normal, whereas in haemochromatosis the density is greater. Ascites can be demonstrated, but this is usually possible by less sophisticated methods.

Treatment

Results are at the same time depressing and encouraging. The cirrhotic liver will never regain normal structure, but the liver cells retain such an enormous regenerative capacity that functional compensation may be attained.

General measures. The patient with well-compensated cirrhosis requires no specific treatment.

A high protein diet may be of particular value in the alcoholic, but usually 80–100 g protein and 10.5 kj (2.5 kcal) daily suffice. Additional choline or methionine or various 'hepatoprotectives' are unnecessary. The avoidance of butter and other fats, eggs, coffee, or chocolate is not of therapeutic value. The development of ascites or hepatic encephalopathy demands a stricter diet and this will be considered later. Alcohol should in general be avoided. However, if the cirrhosis is definitely not of an alcoholic aetiology, one glass of wine or a beer daily will not be harmful.

Sedatives should be avoided as most of them are metabolized by the liver and have prolonged actions in cirrhotic patients. Nitrazepam for night sedation is usually safe and oxazepam, which is not metabolized by the liver, is also a useful drug.

Specific measures. Where the aetiology is known, specific measures may be possible. These include corticosteroids and antiviral therapy in some forms of chronic active hepatitis with cirrhosis, penicillamine for Wilson's disease, and venesections and iron chelation therapy for haemochromatosis. Alcohol abstinence and adequate nutrition are clearly of vital importance in the alcoholic. These specific measures are described on page 12.212.

Treatment of major complications. Three major complications may require treatment. Ascites, hepatic encephalopathy, and portal hypertension.

Treatment of ascites (Table 4). The mere presence of ascites does not merit active treatment. Over-vigorous measures may precipitate hepatic encephalopathy or induce renal failure (*hepatorenal syndrome*). Indications must always be clear cut and caution the working rule. Indications include uncertain diagnosis, to allow better palpation, abdominal pain and dyspnoea, and threatening rupture of an umbilical hernia.

The patient is admitted to hospital. For initial control the patient is confined to bed. He is weighed at the same time daily. Urine volume is measured. Urinary electrolyte determinations are helpful

Table 4   Treatment of ascites

1 Bed rest, 0.5 g (22 mmol) Na diet
   Restrict fluids to 1 litre daily
   Check serum (if possible urinary) electrolytes
   Weigh daily
   Measure urinary volume
   Add KCl 7.5 g (100 mmol) daily
2 After four days, if weight loss less than 1 kg, start amiloride 10 mg daily or spironolactone 100 mg daily. Reduce KCl to 3.75 g (50 mmol) daily
3 After one more day check serum electrolytes. Add frusemide 80 mg or bumetamide 1 mg daily as required
4 After four more days check serum electrolytes. If weight is less than 2 kg amiloride 10 mg twice daily or spironolactone 200 mg daily
5 If necessary raise frusemide to 120 mg daily. Stop diuretics if pre-coma ('flap'), hypokalaemia, azotaemia, or alkalosis, or weight loss more than 0.5 kg daily

but are costly and not essential. Urine volume and body weight provide a satisfactory guide to progress. Abdominal girth is unreliable because gaseous distension is common. Serum electrolytes and urea are measured twice weekly while in hospital. Diagnostic abdominal paracentesis is performed (see above).

The patient who is accumulating ascites excretes very little sodium in the urine. For control of the fluid retention dietary sodium must be severely restricted to less than 0.5 g (22 mmol) daily. Fluid intake is restricted to 1 litre daily. Food is cooked without salt. Salt substitutes may be used at table. Bread and butter are salt free. Anything containing baking powder is omitted—this includes cakes, biscuits, and ordinary bread. Obviously salty foods such as ham, sausages, kippers, cheese, and ice cream are omitted. Meat, poultry, and fish are confined to 100 g daily, and in addition, one egg is allowed. Only a quarter litre of milk is permitted daily. The patient can take as much as he likes of fresh fruit and vegetables, boiled rice, and salt-free bread and butter. Flavourings such as garlic, lemon juice, pepper, herbs, and salt-free ketchup and mayonnaise add palatability to the diet. Protein intake is maintained by low sodium supplements such as casilan. Very low sodium foods are now available commercially. The patient should be virtually a vegetarian. Failure to adhere to a low sodium diet is the usual reason for ascites to become 'resistant'. In a severe case, even combinations of the newer diuretics in high doses will not compensate for a high dietary sodium intake.

Diuretics should be given only if the weight loss is less than 1 kg after four days on the dietetic and fluid restriction regime. The dose and frequency must be calculated for each individual patient. Too rapid diuresis must be followed by stopping the diuretic; too slow by increasing the dose or frequency. A start is made with a diuretic which conserves potassium at the same time as being natriuretic. This can be amiloride 10 mg or spironolactone 100 mg. If ineffective alone, either frusemide 80 mg or bumetamide 5 mg daily are added. Potassium chloride supplements will probably be required. If the serum potassium is low, it is advisable to add 7.5 g (100 mmol) potassium chloride daily from admission to hospital. Long-acting diuretics such as thiazides or ethacrynic acid have the disadvantage that the action may continue when electrolyte disturbances have already developed.

Using a combination of diuretics and a salt-free diet satisfactory control of ascites is usual and failures are in those with poor hepatocellular function who are usually dead within six months of starting therapy.

Complications include encephalopathy which follows any profound diuresis, or electrolyte disturbance particularly hypokalaemia, hyponatraemia, and hypochloraemic alkalosis. The most dreaded complication is azotaemia (*hepatorenal syndrome*). This reflects altered renal cortical perfusion rather than any lesion of the renal parenchyma. It is diagnosed when the plasma creatinine level exceeds 1.5 mg/dl while tubular function is good as shown by a urine to plasma osmolarity ratio exceeding 1, urine to plasma creatinine ratio exceeding 30, and urine sodium concentration less than 0.23 g/dl. It is often initiated by reduction in the intravascular volume due to over-vigorous diuretic therapy, paracentesis, vomiting, or diarrhoea. It may develop without a precipitant. The classical features of uraemia are usually absent. The syndrome is particularly common in the end-stage cirrhosis of the alcoholic.

Treatment of the hepatorenal syndrome is very unsatisfactory. The problem is the failure of the liver rather than that of the kidney. Conservative measures include restriction of fluid intake, sodium, potassium, and protein, and withdrawal of potentially nephrotoxic drugs, such as neomycin or gentamicin. Blood cultures should be taken and any septicaemia treated appropriately. The ascitic fluid should be further sampled to detect spontaneous bacterial peritonitis. Mannitol and high doses of frusemide are unavailing. Renal dialysis does not improve survival. The renal-cortical circulatory failure has been related to the action of false neurotransmitter amines of intestinal origin. This has lead to the administration of such drugs as l-dopa; they have not been successful.

Failure to respond to the dietetic and diuretic regime indicates either failure to comply or advanced liver failure. In some patients, however, ascites is gross and diuretics have to be pushed to extreme doses. In such refractory patients there is particular danger of depletion of the intravascular compartment and the development of the hepatorenal syndrome. In such patients ascites reinfusion techniques must be considered. The rhodiascit automated ultrafiltration apparatus removes ascitic fluid via a peritoneal dialysis catheter and passes it over an ultra-filter. The concentrate, which contains two to four times as much protein as the ascitic fluid, is returned to the patient intravenously. Up to 13 litres of ascites can be removed in 24 hours.

The Le Veen peritoneal venous shunt system gives more continuous treatment over many months. The peritoneal cavity is drained by a long plastic tube which connects with a special pressure sensitive valve lying extraperitoneally and deep to the abdominal muscles. This connects in turn with a silicone rubber tube which passes subcutaneously from the abdominal wound towards the neck and so into the internal jugular vein. The end of the tube is left in position in the superior vena cava. Complications include fever, leakage of peritoneal fluid, blocked shunt, infections, both subcutaneous and systemic, and bacterial endocarditis. Disseminated intravascular coagulation always occurs to a variable extent and may be severe and fatal. Complications are numerous and severe in those who have advanced hepatocellular failure. The patient with well-compensated cirrhosis who has ascites as a major problem may do exceedingly well with improved nutrition, rise in serum albumin levels, increased urinary flow, and continued control of ascites.

With modern diuretic and dietetic regimens, such measures as the concentration reinfusion technique and the Le Veen shunt are really necessary. They may be useful in those who cannot co-operate with diet and diuretics, the alcoholic who insists on imbibing, and those coming from countries where medical services are insufficient to manage the diet and diuretic regime.

Treatment of hepatic encephalopathy. Hepatic coma is of multiple causation, and the factors acting in the particular patient must be defined and treated (Table 5). The major ones are toxic nitrogenous substances formed in the colon by bacterial action on proteins.

All dietary protein is stopped. At least 6.7 kJ (1.6 kcal) are supplied daily as glucose drinks or as 20 per cent glucose through a gastric drip. During recovery protein is added in 20 g increments on alternate days. The protein is divided between four meals. In patients with an acute episode, a normal protein intake is soon achieved. In the chronic group, permanent protein restriction is needed to control mental symptoms; the limits of tolerance are usually 40–60 g per day. Protein derived from vegetables may be tolerated better than animal protein.

Neomycin, given orally, is very effective in decreasing gastrointestinal ammonia formation. Little is absorbed, although blood levels have been detected and impaired hearing may follow its long-

Table 5 Treatment of hepatic encephalopathy

Acute
1 Identify precipitating factor, e.g., haemorrhage, infection, bacterial peritonitis, alcoholism, electrolyte imbalance, sedatives, constipation, large protein meal
2 Empty lower bowel—enema and magnesium sulphate purge
3 Withdraw dietary protein
4 Neomycin 1 g, four times daily by mouth for seven days
5 Maintain calorie, fluid, and electrolyte balance
6 Stop diuretics

Chronic
1 Dietary protein, largely vegetarian, at limit of tolerance (about 50 g daily)
2 Ensure two semi-solid motions daily using 10–30 ml lactulose, three times a day
3 If symptoms worsen, adopt regimen for acute encephalopathy
4 Consider trial of bromocriptine

term use. It remains the most satisfactory antibiotic for the treatment of acute short-term coma; 4–6 g are given daily in divided doses. The EEG improves, blood ammonium levels fall, and fetor hepaticus diminishes.

Lactulose is a synthetic disaccharide not split by intestinal lactases. When given by mouth, the bulk reaches the caecum where it is broken down by bacteria to lactic acid and small amounts of acetic acid, and the faecal pH falls. Neuropsychiatric symptoms are relieved and blood ammonia levels fall. The mechanism of the beneficial action in chronic hepatic encephalopathy is uncertain. Improvement precedes changes in bacterial flora and the drug works in those taking neomycin who have no lacto-bacilli in the faeces. The antibiotic might act by reducing de-amidization of ammonium to ammonia and so increasing faecal ammonia, but this is not so. It may simply provide a carbohydrate source to facilitate ammonia utilization by gut bacteria.

The aim is to produce acid stools without diarrhoea. The dose is 10–30 ml three times a day and is adjusted to produce two semisolid stools daily. Lactulose is non-toxic and should be used in the chronic case. It should not be given in acute hepatic coma where nitrogenous intoxication is best controlled by neomycin.

If hepatic encephalopathy is related to a defect in dopaminergic neurotransmission, then replenishment of cerebral dopamines should be beneficial. Levodopa can cause temporary arousal in acute hepatic encephalopathy and is sometimes of benefit in the chronic case although in only a few patients Nausea and psychiatric disturbances are side-effects. Bromocriptine is a specific dopamine receptor agonist with a prolonged action. In a dose of up to 15 mg daily it causes improvement in patients with portal systemic encephalopathy. It should be considered in the rare patient with chronic encephalopathy resistant to dietary protein restriction and lactulose.

Infusions high in branch chain and low in aromatic amino acids are said to be beneficial, but the results have been uncontrolled.

Portal hypertension. Prophylactic treatment of gastro-oesophageal varices is not indicated. It is impossible to predict on the basis of size or height of portal pressure which patient will suffer from bleeding varices, or when. The enlarged spleen results in mild anaemia, thrombocytopenia, and leucopenia. This is symptomless and splenectomy should not be performed.

Bleeding gastro-oesophageal varices. This may present as a slow ooze, as sudden haematemesis, or as melaena. The bleeding is liable to continue for days. Hepatocellular failure may be precipitated.

The patient should be hospitalized. He should be managed by an intensive care team, with participation of both physicians and surgeons. Endoscopy will usually visualize the site of bleeding if performed within eight hours. Blood transfusion is a first priority and large quantities (at least 4 units) should be available. Saline infusions are avoided. Clotting is liable to be defective and fresh blood, fresh packed red cells, fresh frozen plasma and platelets may be necessary. Vitamin K, intramuscularly is given routinely. Cimetidine is given in full dosage. This may be helpful in preventing stress-induced acute mucosal ulcers. Hepatic encephalopathy is anticipated and treatment for it instituted. Sedation is avoided. Chlorodiazepoxide or heminevrin may be used if delirium tremens is expected in the alcoholic. If the haemorrhage stops, the patient is either treated conservatively or considered for surgery. If bleeding continues, the patient is given intravenous vasopressin 20 units in 100 ml 5 per cent dextrose in 10 minutes. This results in facial pallor, intestinal colic, and defaecation. If these features are absent, the vasopressin is probably inactive.

Vasopressin acts as a vasoconstrictor reducing splanchnic (and hepatic) blood flow, and so portal venous pressure. It also constricts coronary arteries and must not be given to those with a history of myocardial ischaemia or where there is an abnormal ECG. the advantage is in its simplicity of administration. The short duration of action is obviously unsatisfactory.

Vasopressin may be repeated in four hours if bleeding recurs, but efficacy drops with continued use. At this stage some method or variceal sclerosis or emergency surgery has to be considered. Either procedure is preceded by use of oesophageal tamponade using the Sengstaken–Blakemore tube. This compression tube is very successful in controlling the bleeding from oesophageal varices. There are, however, many complications, particularly discomfort to the patient and oesophageal ulceration. The oesophageal balloon should not be kept inflated for longer than 24 hours. Recurrence of bleeding after intravenous vasopressin or removal of the Sengstaken–Blakemore tube reflects defective hepatic function and blood clotting rather than portal hypertension *per se*. The decision as to whether to introduce the Sengstaken tube repeatedly, or to keep it in position for days, or to give many injections of vasopressin with diminishing effect, is hard to make. Emergency surgery is to be avoided if at all possible. Trans-hepatic variceal sclerosis can be performed under local anaesthesia. The main collateral venous supply of the gastro-oesophageal varices is visualized by transhepatic portal venography. A catheter is introduced into the portal vein and the dangerous variceal supply veins selectively catheterized and injected with human thrombin and gel foam, so obliterating them. The hole in the liver is plugged with gel foam as the catheter is withdrawn. This is an excellent method of stopping variceal bleeding, particularly in those with severe liver failure. The duration of occlusion, however, is uncertain.

Direct injection sclerotherapy using an oesophagoscope and ethanolamine oleate is done under local anaesthesia. Injection is difficult if the patient is actually bleeding, and control of haemorrhage must be achieved before injection by such methods as the Sengstaken tube. Fundal varices are not obliterated. Complications include bleeding, oesophageal stenosis, mediastinitis, and pneumonia. Recanalization is a long-term problem. Injection sclerotherapy has also been used long-term, the veins being injected about every two months.

Surgical procedures. Surgical oesophageal transection is a 'last ditch' procedure in patients with intractable variceal bleeding. Mortality is very high.

Surgical portal-systemic shunts such as the end-to-side portacaval shunt, the mesocaval, and the splenorenal are being performed less often because of the high incidence of complicating encephalopathy and the reduction of liver function post-operatively. They are not performed as emergency procedures. The most popular is the selective distal splenorenal shunt (Warren shunt). This aims to divide veins feeding the dangerous oesophago-gastric collaterals while allowing drainage or portal blood through short gastric and splenic veins through a splenorenal shunt to the inferior vena cava. Portal blood flow is maintained. The technique is difficult and time consuming. Encephalopathy, however, is reduced. It does not always achieve its object of long-term preservation of portal blood flow.

Prognosis. In an individual patient, many factors are concerned in determining the prognosis. If there is a known aetiological factor which can be treated, such as alcoholism or haemochromatosis, the outlook is better. If a known correctable precipitating factor such as haemorrhage or infection can be identified the prognosis is better than if decompensation is spontaneous.

Initial response to therapy is important; failure to improve within one month of entering hospital is a bad sign. Persisting jaundice, a serum albumin level less than 2.5 g/dl, hypoprothrombinaemia, serum sodium values less than 12.0 mmol/l (off diuretics) are also grave signs.

Hepatic histology may be a useful indication of the outlook.

Necrosis and marked inflammation are bad signs, but a fatty liver responds well to treatment. The prognosis is always grave after ascites has developed and especially if it is resistant to treatment or if large doses of diuretics are required for control. Hepatic encephalopathy unrelated to extensive portal systemic shunting is also a bad sign.

The prognosis of bleeding oesophageal varices depends on adequate treatment, and in particular on the extent of underlying hepatocellular failure. The combination of deep jaundice, ascites, and coma with bleeding is usually fatal.

Primary liver cancer (see page 12.215) is a frequent complication of all forms of cirrhosis except the biliary and cardiac types. It should be suspected if a patient with cirrhosis shows deterioration of general health, weight loss, right upper quadrant pain, refractory ascites, or develops a local mass in the liver. It is confirmed by scanning, selective hepatic arteriography, and serum alpha-feto-protein determination.

Primary biliary cirrhosis

This is a condition of progressive destruction of intrahepatic bile ducts. It is termed primary biliary cirrhosis although in the early stages the nodular hepatocellular regeneration of cirrhosis is inconspicuous and this is not in fact a cirrhosis. The term 'chronic non-suppurative destructive cholangitis' is a better one although too cumbersome to replace the popular 'primary biliary cirrhosis' (PBC).

Aetiology. The aetiology remains unknown but immunological mechanisms have been invoked in the initiation of the bile duct injury.

There is an association with diseases believed to have an immunological basis, particularly the collagen diseases. Granulomas, the hallmark of disturbed cell-based immunity, are found near damaged bile ducts (Fig. 4) and also in lymph nodes at the porta-hepatis and elsewhere. There is skin test anergy. These disturbances seem

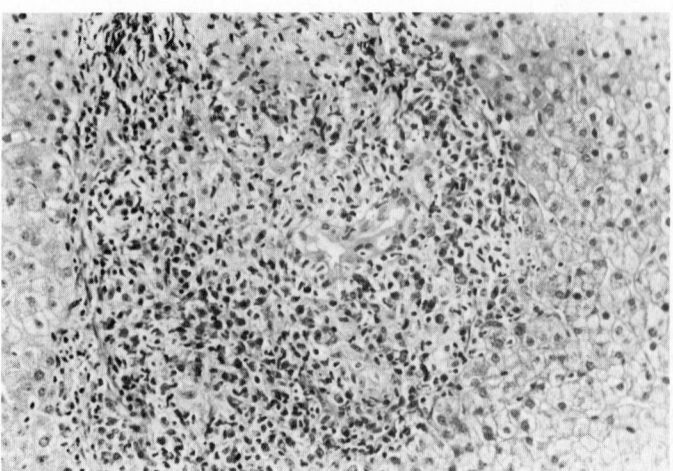

Fig. 4 Primary biliary cirrhosis. A portal zone shows a damaged bile duct surrounded by a granulomatous inflammation. Stained with haematoxylin and eosin (× 165).

to bear little relation to the severity and may be effects of the disease rather than aetiological.

The serum of patients with primary biliary cirrhosis show circulating large immune complexes and these might mediate bile duct damage. They may be produced in the walls of bile ductules or surrounding tissue—a reaction in many ways analogous to Arthus' reaction. An antigen absorbed from the bile may combine with antibody derived from the portal circulation and result in complex formation in the bile ductule wall and portal tracts. A spillover of complexes into the systemic circulation may explain the association of primary biliary cirrhosis with extrahepatic conditions such as arthritis, vasculitis, and glomerulonephritis. Such immune complexes might also contribute to the state of anergy. Although this hypothesis describes the possible mechanism of bile duct damage and granuloma formation in primary biliary cirrhosis, the antigen involved and the way in which it enters the tissues of the portal zones of the liver are unknown.

Many of the ductular and extraductular features of primary biliary cirrhosis, including immune complex formation and macroglobulinaemia, are seen in chronic graft-versus-host disease following bone marrow transplantation. In graft-versus-host reaction the immune response is to the histocompatibility complex antigens which are present in high density on biliary ductular epithelial cells. A similar mechanism may be operative in primary biliary cirrhosis, either because of altered antigenicity of epithelial cell histocompatibility antigens or because of failure of the HLA dependent T cell self-recognition system.

Genetic factors. There seems to be familial clustering, and primary biliary cirrhosis has been reported in sisters, twins, and in mothers and daughters.

There is a significant increase in the incidence of serological antibodies, including the mitochondrial antibody in healthy relatives with primary biliary cirrhosis. This raises the question of genetic and environmental factors or indeed interaction between the two. The disease is not associated with any particular pattern of histocompatibility antigens.

Clinical features
Presentation. Ninety per cent of patients are females usually between the ages of 40 and 59. The disease starts insidiously, usually with pruritus. Jaundice may never develop but in the majority appears within six months to two years of the onset of pruritus. In about a quarter jaundice and pruritus start simultaneously. Pruritus can start during pregnancy.

Examination shows a well-nourished pigmented woman. Jaundice is slight or absent. The liver is usually enlarged and firm and the spleen palpable.

The patient may also be diagnosed when asymptomatic. This may follow detection of hepatomegaly or raised serum alkaline phosphatase or positive auto-antibody tests at the time of examination for routine screening or for a related condition such as rheumatoid arthritis. Such patients tend to be diagnosed younger; it can be recognized as early as 23 years old.

Course. Earlier diagnosis has made the duration seem much longer. The rate of progress is very variable. Patients can remain asymptomatic for longer than 10 years. The development of symptoms cannot be predicted by biochemical tests or hepatic histology.

The course of those diagnosed with symptoms is six to seven years (range four to 14 years).

Serum bilirubin levels remain stable for a variable period (about four years) and then rise rapidly until death some two years later. Diarrhoea may be due to steatorrhoea. Weight loss is slow. The patient feels surprisingly well and has a good appetite. The course is afebrile and abdominal pain is unusual.

Skin xanthomas develop frequently but not in all patients. Terminally xanthomas may disappear. The skin may be thickened and tough over fingers, ankles, and legs.

The bone changes complicating chronic cholestasis are particularly profound in the deeply jaundiced. The patient complains of backache and pains over the ribs, sometimes with pathological fractures. These bone changes are enhanced by prolonged corticosteroid therapy. Duodenal ulceration and haemorrhage are common.

Bleeding oesophageal varices may be a presenting feature, even before nodules have developed in the liver. Haemorrhage from varices also accompanies the late cirrhotic stage.

Hepatocellular carcinoma is a very rare termination.

Associated diseases. Extrahepatic disorders are found in 69 per cent of patients. Associated collagen diseases include rheumatoid arthritis and dermatomyositis. The CRST syndrome of calcinosis, Raynaud's phenomena, sclerodactyly, and telangiectasia may be present in whole or in part.

The 'sicca complex' of dry eyes and mouth occurs in about 70 per cent of patients. Auto-immune thyroiditis is another association. Finger clubbing is common and occasionally hypertrophic osteoarthropathy.

Renal complications include IgM associated membranous glomerulonephritis and renal tubular acidosis. Weight loss may sometimes be explained by the steatorrhoea of coeliac disease. Gallstones, usually of pigment type, have been seen by endoscopy in about a third of patients.

Diagnosis
Biochemical findings. The serum reflects prolonged cholestasis with a serum bilirubin level usually between 17 and 85 IU (1–5 mg/100 ml). The serum bilirubin may fluctuate and may be within normal limits for some months. The alkaline phosphatase is usually increased to about three times the upper limit of normal. The serum IgM may be very high.

Serum mitochondrial antibody test. A non-organ specific antibody against mitochondria is present in over 96 per cent of patients. It is usually absent in patients with mechanical bile duct obstruction or with the cholestasis associated with inflammatory bowel disease. In a patient with cholestasis, a negative result means that primary biliary cirrhosis is not the correct diagnosis. A positive result in an icteric patient throws considerable doubt on whether the jaundice is due to a mechanical block to bile ducts.

Liver biopsy. Four stages of the disease are recognized.
Stage 1: The florid duct lesion. This is diagnostic. The larger intra-hepatic bile ducts are damaged and surrounded by lymphocytes, plasma cells, and a few eosinophils (Fig. 4). Lymphoid aggregates may be found. Granulomas are often seen, usually near a damaged duct in the portal tract. Cholestasis is rarely severe.
Stage 2: Ductular proliferation. There is fibrosis, acute and chronic inflammatory infiltration, and ductular proliferation. Ducts are reduced and their place taken by ill-defined lymphoid aggregates which, with the fibrosis and inflammation, give a rather characteristic appearance.
Stage 3: Scarring. The inflammation has subsided and a cellular septa extends from the portal tracts into and around the lobules. Lymphoid aggregates may still be seen. Periportal cholestasis may be severe. These appearances are not pathognomonic but may be interpreted as compatible with the diagnosis.
Stage 4: Cirrhosis. Regenerating nodules are seen and the picture is of end-stage liver disease. The diagnosis may still be suggested by paucity of bile ducts or by accumulation of lymphocytes.

There is much overlap between the stages. Although diagnosis is more confident with large, laparotomy liver biopsies, diagnosis nowadays is usually made on needle biopsy specimens.

Treatment. The symptomatic treatment is that of chronic cholestasis with intramuscular fat-soluble vitamins and calcium supplements particularly important. Pruritus is controlled, usually with cholestyramine.

Corticosteroids increase bone thinning and are contra-indicated. Azathioprine has been proved ineffective in controlled trials.

D-penicillamine therapy is useful. It is effective in reducing liver copper which, because of failure of biliary excretion, is very high in all forms of chronic cholestasis including primary biliary cirrhosis. It also reduces serum immune complex levels. Liver function tests improve. It is not indicated in the early pre-symptomatic stages but survival is increased when the drug is given in the later stages shown as grade 3 and 4 on liver biopsy. The initial dose is 150 mg daily. This is built up to a maintenance of 600 mg daily over nine weeks. Unfortunately the side-effects are numerous. Nausea, vomiting, and transient loss of taste are frequent. Skin rashes may necessitate withdrawal. Proteinuria and blood dyscrasias are more serious and necessitate stopping the drug. Urine tests and blood counts should be performed weekly for the first month and then monthly during therapy.

Portal systemic shunts should be considered for bleeding oesophageal varices in those without hepatocellular failure. Such operations are tolerated well and the incidence of encephalopathy is low.

Gallstones should be left *in situ* unless present in the common bile duct. Cholecystectomy is rarely indicated.

Prognosis. The prognosis of the asymptomatic patient is unpredictable but is usually compatible with a virtually normal life expectancy. Once jaundice develops, the prognosis is much worse. There seems to be no correlation between the severity of the liver lesions and the duration of symptoms. Bleeding from oesophageal varices in the deeply jaundiced is particularly ominous.

The terminal stages are marked by rapid deepening of jaundice with disappearance of both xanthomas and pruritus. Serum albumin and total cholesterol levels fall. Oedema and ascites develop. The final events include hepatic encephalopathy, uncontrollable bleeding, and septicaemia, often Gram negative.

References

Deering, T. B., Dickson, E. R., Fleming, C. R., Geall, M. G., McCall, J. T., and Baggenstoss, A. H. (1977). Effect of D-penicillamine on copper retention in patients with primary biliary cirrhosis. *Gastoent.* **72**, 1208.

Epstein, O., Jain, S., Lee, R. G., Cook, D. G., Boss, A. M., Scheuer, P. J., and Sherlock, S. (1981). D-penicillamine treatment improves survival in primary biliary cirrhosis. *Lancet*, **i**, 1275.

—, Thomas, H. C., and Sherlock, S. (1980). Primary biliary cirrhosis is a dry gland syndrome with features of chronic graft-versus-host disease. *Lancet* i, 1166.

Long, R. G., Scheuer, P. J., and Sherlock, S. (1977). Presentation and course of asymptomatic primary biliary cirrhosis. *Gastroent.* **72**, 1204.

Millward-Sadler, G. H. and Wright, R. (1979). Cirrhosis: and appraisal. In *Liver and biliary disease* (eds. R. Wright, K. E. M. M. Alberti, S. Karran, and G. H. Millward-Sadler), 688. W. B. Saunders, London.

Scheuer, P. J. (1980). *Liver biopsy interpretation*, 3rd edn., 117. Bailliere Tindall, London.

Schiff, L. and Schiff, E. (eds.) (1982). *Diseases of the liver*, 5th edn. Lippincott, Philadelphia.

Sherlock, S. (1978). Portal circulation and portal hypertension. *Gut* **19**, 70.

— (1981). *Diseases of the liver and biliary system*, 6th edn., 227, 322. Blackwell Scientific Publications, Oxford.

— and Summerfield, J. A. (1979). *Colour atlas of liver disease*, 65. Wolfe Medical Publications, London.

Disorders of the hepatic veins and arteries

D. J. Weatherall

The important vascular disorders of the liver include underperfusion in conditions of shock, and the wide variety of diseases which give rise to portal hypertension. Although cirrhosis of the liver is the commonest cause of portal hypertension, there are other conditions which can produce this clinical picture. A simple classification is shown in Table 1. They can be divided broadly into pre-, intra-, and post-hepatic. The main prehepatic causes are obstruction to flow in the portal veins, or increased flow due to massive splenomegaly (see Section 19). The intrahepatic causes of portal hypertension include cirrhosis, veno-occlusive disease, and obstruction to the portal tracts by a variety of conditions including parasitic infestations, myeloproliferative diseases, lymphomas, sarcoidosis, and congenital hepatic fibrosis. Blockage of the hepatic venous outflow results from disorders which cause obstruction or thrombosis of the hepatic veins.

Acute cardiac failure and shock. Reduced hepatic blood flow may lead to centrilobular necrosis. This occurs frequently in acute congestive heart failure or in severe hypotension from any cause.

In acute congestive cardiac failure, the liver may be enlarged and tender if the central venous pressure is elevated. There may be biochemical features of liver cell damage or intrahepatic cholestasis. Liver function may be interfered with sufficiently to cause a reduction of prothrombin synthesis and hence increased sensitivity to anticoagulant drugs.

In patients with severe hypovolaemic shock there may be marked biochemical changes of deranged liver function, and, in severe cases, jaundice. These changes are transient and revert rapidly to normal following restoration of a normal blood pressure and perfusion.

Chronic venous congestion and cardiac cirrhosis. A persistently elevated central venous pressure due to right-sided heart failure or constrictive pericarditis results in hepatic venous congestion and hepatomegaly. The associated histological changes are characterized by centrilobular congestion with surrounding fatty change (the typical 'nutmeg liver'). If the disorder is of long standing, there may

Table 1 Some disorders of hepatic blood supply

Reduced perfusion	Shock
	Hepatic artery disease
Portal hypertension	
Prehepatic	Portal vein thrombosis
	Splenomegaly (for causes, see Section 19)
	Developmental abnormalities
Intrahepatic	Cirrhosis from any cause
	Veno-occlusive disease
	Portal tract obstruction
	Parasites
	Lymphoma
	Myeloproliferative disorders
	Sarcoidosis
	Hepatitis
	Felty's syndrome
Post-hepatic	Budd–Chiari syndrome
Acute and chronic venous congestion	Cardiac failure
	Constrictive pericarditis

be progressive fibrosis extending peripherally from centrilobular to portal areas, although regenerative nodules are not prominent.

Apart from the underlying cardiac lesion, this disorder is characterized by hepatic enlargement and signs of congestive cardiac failure. The serum bilirubin level is usually increased and there may be a slight elevation in the serum alkaline phosphatase level and in the transaminases.

It should be emphasized that although the changes outlined above are relatively common in patients with long-standing heart failure, true cirrhosis of the liver with regenerative nodules is very rare, as is the clinical picture of portal hypertension which accompanies other forms of cirrhosis of the liver; it is very unusual to find oesophageal varices in patients with cardiac cirrhosis.

Hepatic artery occlusion. This is a rare condition. It usually follows surgical trauma but has been found in association with arteritis and bacterial endocarditis.

The condition is characterized by an acute onset of pain in the upper abdomen, tenderness over the liver, and progressive shock and liver failure. Most cases have a fatal outcome.

Hepatic artery aneurysm. This condition is recognized by the triad of upper abdominal pain, jaundice, and haematemesis following rupture of the aneurysm into the stomach or duodenum. The diagnosis is made by hepatic angiography. Treatment is by surgical resection.

Budd–Chiari syndrome

Definition. The Budd–Chiari syndrome is the clinical disorder which results from an obstruction to the hepatic venous outflow.

Aetiology. In his early descriptions of this disease, Budd described pseudomembranes of the hepatic veins, fibrous tissue in the portal veins, and extensive adhesions involving the liver, spleen, heart, and lungs. Chiari considered that his cases were due to primary phlebitis with secondary thrombosis of the hepatic vein.

It is now apparent that there are many different conditions which can cause blockage of outflow of the hepatic venous system. These fall into two main groups: tumour infiltration, and thrombosis of the hepatic veins. Of the former, hepatoma, carcinoma of the right kidney, retroperitoneal sarcoma invading the hepatic veins, and metastatic tumours are the commonest.

There are many well-documented causes of thrombosis of the hepatic veins. In the larger series, blood dyscrasias such as polycythaemia vera, other myeloproliferative conditions and paroxysmal nocturnal haemoglobinuria are the commonest disorders. Other causes include the use of oral contraceptives, pregnancy, liver abscess, alcoholic liver disease, antileukaemic agents, and hydatid disease or fungal infections. Interestingly, about one-third to one-half of reported cases have been associated with no obvious underlying aetiology. The contribution of such factors as congenital webs and bands remains uncertain, although there is some evidence that there may be a form of the disorder associated with membranous obstruction of the inferior vena cava and of the hepatic veins caused by endothelial folds.

Pathology. The liver is usually enlarged and congested and shows a prominent 'nutmeg' pattern with centrilobular haemorrhages and a surrounding yellow appearance in the rest of the hepatic lobules. Histologically, there is marked centrilobular congestion, while the rest of the liver shows either fatty or other degenerative changes.

Clinical features. This syndrome is usually associated with a fairly dramatic clinical onset characterized by hepatic enlargement with pain and tenderness, and rapidly developing ascites. These symptoms are usually associated with systemic symptoms including nausea and vomiting, fever and, sometimes, profound shock. A less acute form, with progressive liver failure and ascites, may occur.

Diagnosis. This condition should always be considered in a patient who develops an acute illness characterized by hepatomegaly and rapidly developing ascites. This is particularly the case in those with myeloproliferative disorders or paroxysmal nocturnal haemoglobinuria. There is usually biochemical evidence of liver cell dysfunction although this does not fall into any specific pattern. Liver biopsy is not particularly helpful in making a diagnosis, and if there is an underlying haematological disorder, may be dangerous.

Colloid liver scanning shows hepatic and splenic enlargement with patchy uptake, and, particularly, unequal distribution of the colloid between the lobes of the liver with a considerable uptake by the bone marrow. Although these findings occur in other liver diseases, the most striking feature in the Budd–Chiari syndrome is that there is often a region of increased uptake located centrally between the right and left lobes. (Recent studies have cast some doubt on the reliability of this finding.) This corresponds to the caudate lobe which may remain relatively uninvolved, possibly because it drains by small veins directly into the vena cava. It may be possible to demonstrate the occlusion of the hepatic veins directly by ultrasound examination.

Other useful investigations include an intravenous pyelogram which will help to exclude a renal or retroperitoneal tumour. An inferior venacavagram may demonstrate thrombus in the hepatic veins, and hepatic venography may define the obstruction directly.

It should be remembered that patients with the Budd–Chiari syndrome are often extremely ill and prolonged investigation with repeated intravenous injections of radio-opaque material should be avoided as they may lead to further dehydration and may activate complement, possibly due to endotoxin contamination. For this reason it is best to proceed directly to a liver scan and ultrasound examination, and only if there are skilled personnel available to carry out a hepatic venogram. If none of these aids are at hand, it should be remembered that the ascitic fluid has an extremely high protein content in this condition, which may give some clue as to the diagnosis.

Management. Although much has been written about the management of the Budd–Chiari syndrome, very little is known about the value of any particular therapeutic approach. It has been suggested recently that early heparinization may be of some value, particularly if there is an underlying haematological disorder such as polycythaemia vera or paroxysmal nocturnal haemoglobinuria. In the former condition this should be combined with venesection to lower the packed cell volume to a safe level (see Section 19). It may be necessary to continue intravenous heparin therapy at a full therapeutic dose (see Section 19) for weeks or even longer. Experience with other anticoagulants, aspirin, and fibrinolytic agents has been disappointing. The same goes for corticosteroid therapy and various surgical approaches. The management of the ascites follows the same lines as that described for the management of the ascites of hepatic cirrhosis (see page 12.188).

Recent studies have stressed the importance of making a rapid diagnosis followed by early heparinization and hydration. It is too early to say whether this approach will have a genuine effect on the outcome of this illness but certainly none of the other therapeutic regimens appear to be of any value.

Prognosis. This depends to some extent on the underlying cause. In many patients there is progression to acute or chronic liver damage with cirrhosis and death from hepatic failure. However, there is no doubt that a small proportion of patients recannalize the hepatic veins and the condition may regress completely. This outcome has been well documented in patients with underlying haematological disorders.

Hepatic veno-occlusive disease. A condition with some features resembling the Budd–Chiari syndrome occurs in response to the ingestion of various toxic alkaloids and other agents (see also Section 6).

Aetiology and pathogenesis. Hepatic veno-occlusive disease affects mainly children in the Caribbean area, Israel, and India and is believed to be caused by the ingestion of alkaloids derived from various types of 'bush tea', probably brewed from *Senecia* (ragwort) or *Crotalaria*. Similar findings have been observed occasionally in patients with the hypereosinophil syndrome or after bone marrow transplantation.

Histologically, the condition is characterized by occlusion of sublobular and central hepatic veins by swelling and proliferation of the intima. In the later stages of the illness there may be centrilobular cirrhosis and portal hypertension.

Clinical features. Typically, the condition affects young children in the first five years of life. They are often undernourished and in some cases show clinical evidence of protein energy malnutrition.

In acute stage of the illness, which often follows an intercurrent disorder such as pneumonia, there is loss of weight and rapidly developing hepatomegaly and ascites. In the second phase, there may be a symptomatic hepatomegaly, and finally the condition culminates in the typical clinical picture of chronic cirrhosis with portal hypertension. At this stage the children are wasted and have massive, protruberant bellies due to a combination of hepatic enlargement and ascites.

Treatment is symptomatic (see Section 6).

Portal venous obstruction. Obstruction to the portal vein causes the syndrome of extrahepatic portal hypertension.

Aetiology. Thrombosis of the portal vein results from a variety of causes. It may follow an ascending infection along the umbilical vein at birth secondary to umbilical sepsis. It may also result from any form of sepsis arising in the abdominal cavity at any time in life. This leads to septic endophlebitis of the mesenteric and portal venous system. There is increasing evidence that procedures for the trans-hepatic injection of oesophageal varices are accompanied by a significant risk of causing portal vein thrombosis. The incidence of this complication has ranged from 25 to 40 per cent in several recent series. Rarer causes include occlusion of the portal vein by a pancreatic neoplasm, an underlying haematological disorder such as polycythaemia vera, or the use of the contraceptive pill. It has also been reported to occur spontaneously in the post-partum period.

Clinical features. When this condition presents early in life, there may be a history of umbilical sepsis or of an exchange transfusion for rhesus incompatibility. Cases which present later may give a history of intra-abdominal sepsis such as appendicitis. On the other hand, some patients present with no preceding history of such an event and the clinical picture may develop without any evidence of an underlying disease. In this case, presentation may be either with a complication of portal hypertension such as haematemesis or melaena, or the finding of splenomegaly on routine clinical examination. The other features of portal hypertension such as ascites and liver failure are rarely seen in this condition.

Diagnosis. Certainly in the early stages of the illness, liver function tests are normal and there may be no abnormalities on liver biopsy. However, as the disease progresses, there may be evidence of developing derangement of liver function with elevation of the serum alkaline phosphatase and bilirubin levels. Oesophageal varices may be present on barium swallow. The condition is diagnosed by the finding of occlusion of either the splenic or portal veins and the appearance of many collateral channels on a splenic venogram.

Complications. Bleeding from oesophageal varices is the most important complication. There may be progressive splenomegaly and the clinical picture of hypersplenism may complicate the picture and lead to a bleeding tendency due to a low platelet count, or to repeated infections (see Section 19).

Management. With blood replacement, patients with this condition usually stop bleeding from their varices and there is much less risk of them developing hepatic failure than is the case in patients with portal hypertension due to hepatic cirrhosis. However, bleeding may be severe and tends to recur, and if possible surgical correction should be attempted. If the portal venogram shows that there is a high portal vein obstruction leaving a suitable length of portal vein for anastomosis, a porta-caval shunt should be carried out. If this is impossible, it is sometimes feasible to carry out a superior mesenteric-caval anastomosis. If neither of these procedures are possible, it may be necessary to attack the oesophageal varices directly (see page 12.190).

Complications of porta-caval shunt operations. Some of the problems of porta-caval shunt surgery were mentioned briefly in the previous chapter. Since this operation is carried out for several of the conditions mentioned above, its complications will be briefly summarized here.

The most common and incapacitating complication of any form of porta-caval shunt surgery is the development of neuropsychiatric change due to hepatic encephalopathy. Although this may only be transient in the post-operative period, long-term changes occur in a varying proportion of patients. Its development depends, to a large degree, on the state of liver function and the indications for the shunt operation. For example, in patients with well-maintained liver function associated with prehepatic portal hypertension, the results may be good and encephalopathy is relatively uncommon, whereas if the operation is carried out in patients with advanced hepatic cirrhosis with poor liver function, there is almost invariably progressive encephalopathy. The symptoms of this condition are described elsewhere (see page 12.185). Apart from this clinical picture, there may be a gradual deterioration of personality which seems to occur in about one-third of all patients who undergo shunt surgery. These complications are managed by scrupulous attention to the treatment of intercurrent illness or bleeding episodes and by careful regulation of the amount of protein in the diet.

The other complications of porta-caval shunt surgery are less common. They include the development of jaundice after the operation, refractory dependent oedema, myelopathy with paraplegia, and a mild form of iron loading due to increased intestinal absorption.

Septic venous thrombosis of the portal system. This condition results from infection anywhere in the abdominal cavity leading to pylephlebitis of the portal venous system. It may occasionally result from a systemic septicaemia or from inflammatory disorders of the bowel, such as ulcerative colitis.

The acute phase of the disorder is usually characterized by features related to the underlying abdominal sepsis. This is followed by an episode of high fever, worsening abdominal pain, and rigors. There may be obvious evidence of septic embolization to the liver. This may lead to abdominal pain and hepatic tenderness with mild jaundice. All the systemic features of a severe infection develop and there is usually a polymorphonuclear leucocytosis and abnormal liver function tests. Occasionally, multiple large intrahepatic abscesses may develop (see page 12.219).

The condition should be suspected in any patient with abdominal sepsis who develops an acute systemic illness with abdominal pain and deranged liver function. Management consists of intensive antibiotic treatment directed particularly towards Gram-negative organisms. The management of liver abscess is considered on page 12.220. In some patients the clinical picture associated with portal venous thrombosis may develop after the acute phase has settled.

References

Bolt, R. J. (1976). Diseases of the hepatic blood vessels. In *Gastroenterology*, 3rd edn. (ed. H. L. Backus), 471. W. B. Saunders, Philadelphia.
Bras, G., Brooks, S. E. M., and Walter, D. C. (1961). Cirrhosis of the liver in Jamaica. *J. Path. Biochem.* **82**, 503.

Brooks, S. E. M., Miller, C. G., McKenzie, K., Audretsch, J. J., and Bras, G. (1970). Acute veno-occlusive disease of the liver: fine structure in Jamaican children. *Arch. Path.* **89**, 507.

Gibson, J. B., Johnston, G. W., Fulton, T. T., and Rodgers, M. W. (1965). Extra-hepatic portal-venous obstruction. *Br. J. Surg.* **52**, 129.

Leibowitz, A. I. and Hartmann, R. C. (1981). The Budd–Chiari syndrome and paroxysmal nocturnal haemoglobinuria. *Br. J. Haemat.* **48**, 1.

Sherlock, S. (1981). *Diseases of the liver and biliary system* 6th edn. Blackwell Scientific Publications, Oxford.

Acute hepatitis and fulminant hepatic failure

A. L. W. F. Eddleston

Acute hepatitis

A self-limiting episode of liver-cell damage can be caused by various virus infections, drugs, chemicals, and toxins (Table 1). Although some of these agents produce specific histological changes, the basic lesions are often similar irrespective of the aetiology. Although commonly asymptomatic, the presentation and course in those patients who do develop a clinical illness frequently conforms to a recognizable pattern which can be operationally defined as an acute hepatitis.

Table 1 Causes of acute liver damage

Causative agents	Particular clinical features
Viruses	
Hepatitis viruses	
A	Predominantly liver damage with prominent prodromal 'flu-like' illness
B	
Non-A, non-B	
Epstein–Barr (infectious mononucleosis)	Subclinical liver disease very common; mild clinical hepatitis in 15 per cent
Cytomegalovirus	Rare but sometimes severe in immunosuppressed or immunodeficient patients
Herpes simplex	
Herpes zoster	
Coxsackie A	
Coxsackie B	Liver disease uncommon even with widespread organ involvement
Echoviruses	
Measles	
Lassa fever	Imported from Africa; severe generalized organ damage including liver
Marburg virus	
Ebola virus	
Rickettsial, mycoplasma and systemic fungal infections	Liver damage as part of generalized organ involvement
Septicaemia	Liver abscesses and intrahepatic cholestasis
Drugs	
Almost unlimited number	See page 12.213
Chemicals	
Alcohol	Hyaline inclusions and fatty change; sometimes marked cholestasis
Carbon tetrachloride	Marked fatty change; renal failure may be fatal
Trichlorethylene	Centrilobular hepatic necrosis in glue sniffers
Iron	Periportal necrosis in children after 'mummy's sweeties' overdose
Copper sulphate	Cholestasis and centrilobular necrosis
Phosphorus	Marked fatty change, often fatal
Mycotoxins	
Amanita phalloides (toadstool poisoning)	Severe vomiting, abdominal pain and diarrhoea; frequently coma and death
Aflatoxins (aspergillus contamination of stored foods)	Acute liver damage and carcinogenic (primary hepatoma) in animals, but not proven in man
Heart failure	Intrahepatic cholestasis and centrilobular congestion in right heart failure; hepatocellular necrosis in acute left ventricular failure

Clinical features. Many patients describe an initial 'flu-like' illness which may be followed from a few days to two weeks later by the appearance of jaundice. Malaise, myalgia, anorexia, nausea, and fever are common. These prodromal symptoms are not restricted to those with hepatitis virus infection but can also occur in drug-associated liver injury and acute alcoholic hepatitis. Up to 25 per cent of patients with hepatitis B virus infection may have arthralgia and skin rashes, ascribed to circulating immune complexes, and in occasional cases a more florid, serum sickness-like syndrome with arthritis, urticaria, and angioneurotic oedema has been described. The history of a prodromal illness is very useful clinically in suggesting acute hepatocellular injury and should be sought carefully by direct questioning in any patient with an acute onset of jaundice. Another symptom of considerable importance in the differential diagnosis is itching, which often precedes or parallels the jaundice in patients in whom there is biliary obstruction, but is usually absent or delayed in patients with acute hepatitis, only becoming of major clinical importance in those who have an unusually cholestatic course. Important exceptions to this general rule are acute alcoholic hepatitis, where cholestasis may sometimes be a dominant early feature, and hepatitis associated with some drugs and chemicals in which the whole emphasis is on disturbance of biliary secretion rather than hepatocellular damage. While patients commonly notice dark urine and pale stools, this is of no help in distinguishing acute hepatitis from other causes of jaundice.

In contrast to the history, which may point strongly to the diagnosis, the physical examination is often unremarkable in patients with acute hepatitis. Cutaneous stigmata of liver disease such as spider naevi, liver palms, leuckonychia, and Dupuytren's contracture are important clues against the diagnosis of simple acute hepatitis suggesting that this apparently acute episode may instead be a manifestation of chronic liver disease (see page 12.183). The most common finding in acute hepatitis is tender hepatomegaly with minor splenomegaly being present in a small proportion of those with virus infection. Lymphadenopathy is usually insignificant. Again, acute alcoholic hepatitis is an exception to these general rules. Signs of chronic liver disease including splenomegaly, ascites, and cutaneous stigmata may be found in cases with no histopathological features of cirrhosis or chronic liver disease, and most of these patients can make a complete clinical and histological recovery if they remain abstinent.

Once jaundice has appeared there is often rapid symptomatic improvement although in the rare clinical syndrome of fulminant hepatic failure, deterioration continues and proceeds within one to eight weeks to the development of coma (see later). At the other extreme there may be incomplete recovery from an otherwise unremarkable acute illness and progression to one of a number of forms of chronic hepatitis (see page 12.203). The frequency of this complication depends upon the aetiology of the acute hepatitis. Type A viral hepatitis always appears to be a self-limiting acute disease, while type B and non-A, non-B progress to chronic liver disease in from 10 to 40 per cent of cases. The vast majority of drug-induced cases will make a complete recovery provided the responsible agent is identified and withdrawn (see page 12.209). About

10 per cent of cases of acute alcoholic hepatitis progress to cirrhosis in spite of continued abstinence.

Liver function tests. Although the biochemical tests routinely used as indices of liver damage are usually referred to as liver function tests, most are not true tests of function but rather reflect hepatocellular damage or cholestasis. The pattern of biochemical changes found in acute hepatitis is variable and must be interpreted in the light of clinical findings and the results of other investigative procedures. In most cases aspartate and alanine aminotransferases (AST and ALT), enzymes found within hepatocytes, are released from damaged liver cells and levels in the serum are characteristically elevated during the prodrome and early icteric phase (Fig. 1).

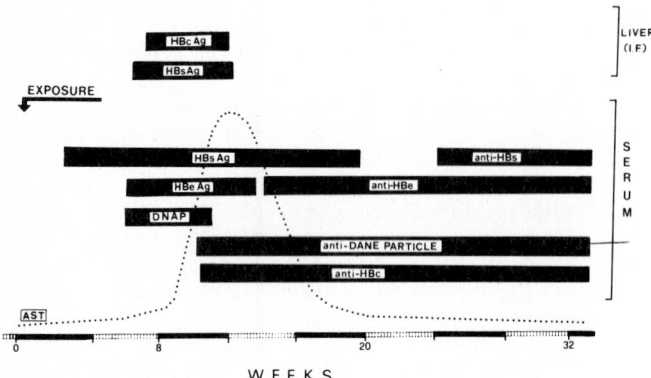

Fig. 1 Virological events in acute hepatitis B in relation to serum aminotransferase (AST) peak.

Peak enzyme levels are commonly seen at the time of presentation, about seven to 10 days before the maximum bilirubin levels. The aminotransferase levels then fall slowly during the recovery phase, and in patients who have an uncomplicated course, the values should have returned to normal within three months from presentation. Persistently elevated levels after this time may indicate progression to chronic liver disease, although delayed recovery is still possible. In most cases of acute hepatitis there is only a small increase in levels of alkaline phosphatase in serum, but if cholestasis becomes a prominent feature, levels may rise to those found in extrahepatic biliary obstruction. The liver variety of this enzyme is found predominantly at the microvilli of the bile canaliculi and serum levels rise in both extra and intrahepatic cholestasis. As mentioned earlier, cholestasis may be particularly pronounced in alcohol- and drug-induced hepatitis, and here there may be real difficulty in distinguishing these from cases of extrahepatic biliary obstruction. Very high levels of another liver enzyme, γ-glutamyl transferase, may be an important pointer to alcoholism (see page 12.212). When intrahepatic cholestasis complicates an acute hepatitis, the clinical course is often prolonged, but eventual complete recovery is still the rule.

Synthetic liver function is almost always normal in acute viral or drug-induced hepatitis with serum albumin levels being well preserved in all but the most severe cases. Likewise, the prothrombin time is usually normal except in those cases with unusually severe cholestasis or where there is a serious risk of progression to fulminant hepatic failure. An exception is alcoholic hepatitis where synthetic liver function may be markedly impaired, with low albumin and prolonged prothrombin time reminiscent of cirrhosis. If the prothrombin time is prolonged, administration of vitamin K parenterally is an excellent test of liver function. Failure to correct the prothrombin time is a very reliable indicator of severe hepatocellular damage. Total globulin and individual immunoglobulin levels (particularly IgG) are often slightly raised in acute hepatitis but these changes are of little diagnostic assistance.

Other investigative procedures. In many cases of acute hepatitis the characteristic clinical history and liver function tests will

strongly suggest the correct diagnosis and further investigations will concentrate on a specific aetiological diagnosis. However, in a few cases—those with an exaggerated cholestatic component and those with some features of chronic liver disease—further tests are indicated to establish a broad diagnostic grouping. Extrahepatic biliary obstruction is best excluded by showing no dilated intrahepatic bile ducts on ultrasound examination of the liver by an experienced observer, and if doubt still exists by visualizing the biliary tree via endoscopic retrograde choledochopancreatography (ERCP) (see page 12.8). Chronic liver disease is best excluded by liver biopsy, and if the clinical course is prolonged, it may be of considerable value in management. It is not indicated in uncomplicated acute hepatitis unless the diagnosis cannot be established by less invasive tests.

Histopathology. Essentially there is liver-cell death and degeneration, replacement regeneration, and a mesenchymal reaction. Specific features due to different aetiological factors may be superimposed on this general pattern of 'lobular disarray'. Cell damage is most obvious in the centrilobular area irrespective of aetiology. Damaged hepatocytes show ballooning degeneration and acidophil degeneration (Fig. 2). In the former, hepatocytes are swollen to

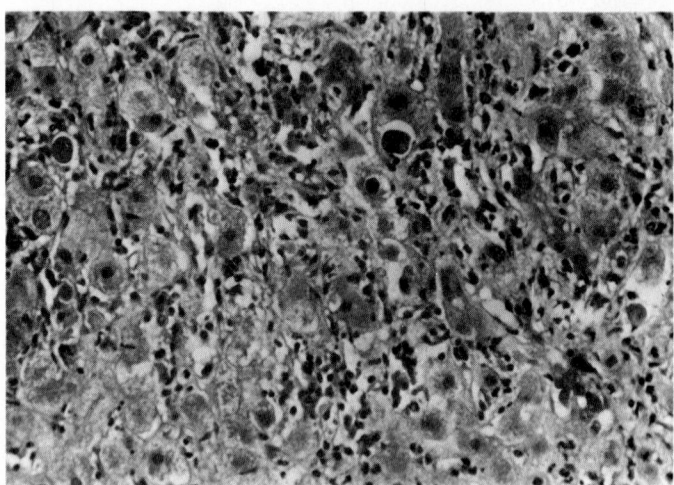

Fig. 2 Prominent acidophil bodies with associated acute inflammatory infiltrate in acute viral hepatitis.

about twice their normal size. There is a granular cuff of cytoplasm surrounding a central nucleus which is usually normal in appearance. Fine strands of cytoplasm radiate from the perinuclear cuff to the plasma membrane but the bulk of the periphery of the cell is not stained, giving an overall impression of peripheral pallor. While ballooning degeneration may affect many cells and seems to be reversible, acidophil degeneration is less frequent and represents cell death. Affected cells are small with uniformly acidophilic, deeply staining cytoplasm and pyknotic nuclei. Fatty change in hepatocytes is rarely seen in acute viral hepatitis but may be a more common feature of non-A, non-B viral hepatitis. It is usually a prominent feature in alcoholic hepatitis where the presence of hyaline inclusions also point to the correct diagnosis (see page 12.209). Reticulin stains show the passive collapse of the normal framework consequent on loss of hepatocytes. Occasionally this may link portal tracts with central veins when it has been called bridging hepatic necrosis. In retrospective studies this was thought to carry a poor prognosis with frequent progression to cirrhosis but a recent prospective evaluation has not supported this concept. Bile duct damage can occasionally be seen and may be another feature of non-A, non-B viral hepatitis.

The mesenchymal reaction is widespread in the lobules but also affects the portal tracts. A mixed mononuclear and polymorphonuclear infiltrate is found throughout the parenchyma but is also focal, particularly around hepatocytes showing acidophilic degeneration (Fig. 2). There is diffuse Kupffer cell hyperplasia and these phagocytes often contain lipofuscin, ceroid, and haemoglobin presumably from ingestion of hepatocyte debris. The inflammatory infiltrate in the portal tracts is predominantly lymphocytic but includes some macrophages, plasma cells, and neutrophil leucocytes. An excessive number of eosinophils may be one of the features suggestive of drug-associated hepatitis (see page 12.213). Although the portal mononuclear infiltrate is largely confined to the tracts, there may be some 'spill over' into the periportal region producing changes akin to the 'piecemeal necrosis' found in chronic active hepatitis (page 12.204). The proper interpretation of these periportal changes depends upon a careful assessment of the clinical features and results of virological, immunological, and biochemical tests as discussed in detail in the following contribution.

Although mitoses are not commonly seen, there are several signs of regeneration, including binucleate hepatocytes, pleomorphism, and double cell plates (seen best on reticulin stains).

Virological studies. Full details of the viruses which can damage the liver and the test systems available for the detection of their associated antigens and antibodies can be found elsewhere (see Section 5). Their use in patients with acute hepatitis is to confirm a clinical diagnosis and also to identify the specific aetiological agent. This may assist in determining prognosis; hepatitis A virus infection does not lead to chronic liver disease while B and non-A, non-B may do so in a proportion of cases. In the case of hepatitis B virus infection serial studies of the viral markers in serum can be particularly useful in identifying those at risk of such progressive disease. The absence of the usual steady fall in serum HBsAg levels and persistence of e antigen (or virion-associated DNA polymerase) in those centres where the test is available all point to persistence of viral replication and the need for careful follow-up (Fig. 3).

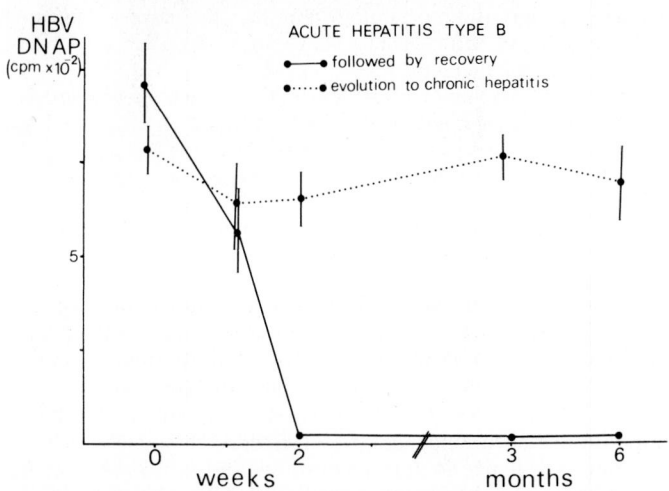

Fig. 3 Persistence of virus-associated DNA polymerase in serum is an early indicator of persistent hepatitis B virus infection.

Immunological studies. There has been considerable interest in the last 10 years in the role of cellular and humoral immunity to viral and hepatocyte antigens in the production of liver-cell damage in acute type B hepatitis and in determining the progression to chronic hepatitis in some cases. The basic mechanisms involved in drug-induced hepatitis may be similar.

Pathogenesis of acute hepatitis B. The existence of healthy carriers of the hepatitis B virus, some of whom have a histologically normal liver biopsy in the face of active virus replication strongly suggests that the hepatitis B virus is not cytopathic to the hepatocytes in which it replicates. The liver cell damage in acute type B hepatitis must then be associated with some other mechanism triggered by the virus infection. In experimental studies in animals

infected with other non-cytopathic viruses such as lymphocytic choriomeningitis virus, cell damage is thought to be mediated by cytotoxic T lymphocytes recognizing viral determinants on the surface of infected cells. In the early stages of acute type B hepatitis, HBsAg has been detected on the surface of infected liver cells, and cytotoxic T lymphocytes recognizing this antigen have been demonstrated in the peripheral blood of patients with acute and chronic hepatitis B virus infection. Although these ingredients could be an important part of the pathogenesis of acute hepatitis B, translation of these *in vitro* observations to the *in vivo* situation is hazardous and much further work is needed before the complex host–virus interactions can be fully appreciated. Thus, recent studies have emphasized the role of antibodies on the surface of infected liver cells in suppressing virus replication rather than mediating cell death, and the importance of a specific antivirion antibody in neutralizing virus particles released from damaged hepatocytes and preventing progression to chronic liver disease (Fig. 4).

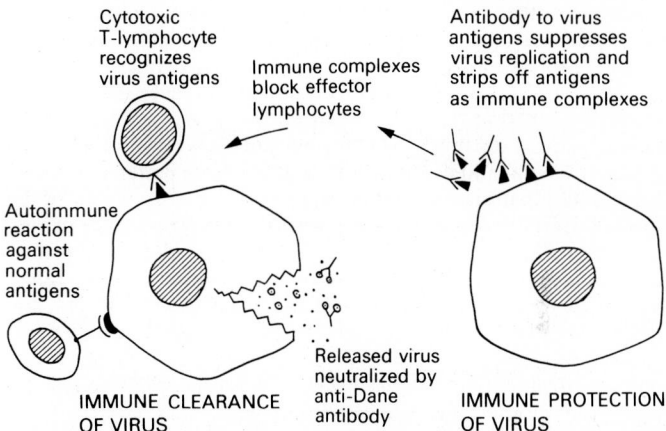

Fig. 4 The left-hand-side illustrates immune mechanisms acting to kill virus infected cells and eliminate the infection. The right-hand-side illustrates other immune reactions which may interfere with the processes depicted on the left.

Other immunological changes. In addition to immune responses to virus or drug-altered antigens on liver cells, transient auto-immune responses also develop in many patients with acute hepatitis. Of the conventional non-organ specific auto-antibodies usually sought in standard tests, anti-smooth muscle antibodies are most frequently positive, but in low titre. Antibodies reacting with a liver membrane lipoprotein complex (anti-LSP antibodies) are found using a radioimmunoassay in 60–100 per cent of cases of acute viral hepatitis and in some types of drug-associated hepatitis. Interest here has focused on the links these observations provide between acute and chronic hepatitis, where auto-immune reactions may contribute to the progressive liver damage and cirrhosis.

Treatment. The vast majority of cases of acute viral hepatitis will proceed to complete recovery without any therapeutic intervention. Treatment of the very occasional patient who develops fulminant hepatic failure will be described later. Early identification of those patients with type B or non-A, non-B infection who are most at risk of chronic sequelae would be of great value if specific non-toxic antiviral therapy were available. However, drugs that are currently available are still in the experimental stage and are only successful in exerting a permanent effect on viral replication in a small proportion of cases. Corticosteroids are of little value in most cases of chronic viral hepatitis and there is no evidence that they offer any therapeutic benefit in acute hepatitis except for rare cases in which there is prolonged cholestasis. In this situation corticosteroids usually produce a prompt fall in plasma bilirubin levels and relieve itching. Relapse may occur when the dose is reduced.

Bed rest, a favourite supportive therapy for many years, probably does nothing to speed resolution as judged by early controlled trials. On the other hand, anecdotal evidence suggests that vigorous exercise in the prodrome may increase the severity of the illness. Conventionally, a low fat diet is often recommended and some patients do feel less nauseous on such a regimen. However, instructions to 'eat what you fancy' are probably just as beneficial.

Essential therapy in drug-induced and alcoholic hepatitis is to withdraw the causative agent. The major problem here is of awareness in order to make the right diagnosis. Drug-induced hepatitis can mimic hepatitis virus infection and a full drug history must be obtained, particularly if the serological tests do not allow a specific virological diagnosis to be made.

Fulminant hepatic failure

This is a rare, but very serious, complication of almost any of the conditions listed in Table 1, but with the majority of cases being due to virus or drug-induced hepatitis. One of the best definitions of the syndrome is that used in the Fulminant Hepatic Failure Surveillance Study set up in Boston, USA, in which it was defined as a clinical syndrome developing as a result of massive necrosis of liver cells or following any other cause of sudden and severe impairment of hepatic function. It is characterized by progressive and severe mental changes starting with confusion and often rapidly advancing to stupor, coma, and death (Table 2). Only those patients in whom signs of fulminant hepatic failure appear within eight weeks of the onset of the illness, and in whom there has been no evidence of liver disease previously are included within this definition. Other features seen within the pattern of the clinical syndrome include renal, electrolyte and acid–base disturbances, coagulation disorders, and hypoglycaemia.

Table 2 Grades of cerebral function in acute hepatic failure

Grade	Mental state
1	Euphoria; occasionally depression; fluctuant mild confusion; slowness of mentation and affect; untidy; slurred speech; disorder in sleep rhythm
2	Accentuation of (1); drowsy; inappropriate behaviour
3	Sleeps most of time but is rousable; incoherent speech; marked confusion
4	Unrousable; may or may not respond to noxious stimuli

Mortality is high, and even with full intensive care facilities, has been more than 80 per cent in several large series. Of those who survive, few develop cirrhosis probably because of the remarkable regenerative capacity of the liver, and in recent years considerable effort has been directed towards improving supportive care, better management of complications, and the development of liver support systems, to give more time for regeneration to overtake cell destruction.

Aetiology. Although almost all the agents listed in Table 1 can cause fulminant hepatic failure, the majority of cases are related to hepatitis virus infection or drug reactions. Thus in England hepatitis virus infection is the aetiological factor in about 40 per cent of patients with severe liver damage while an equal proportion are due to direct hepatotoxicity from paracetamol overdose. The remaining 20 per cent are secondary to 'halothane hepatitis' and other drug reactions.

Viruses. The term 'fulminant viral hepatitis', generally refers to the primary hepatotrophic viruses: A (HAV), B (HBV), and non-A, non-B (see Section 5). The recent development of a sensitive radio-immunoassay to detect IgM antibodies to hepatitis A virus together with the well-established tests for hepatitis B surface antigen have provided a clearer picture of the aetiology of fulminant viral hepatitis and emphasized the importance of non-A, non-B infection. For example, in a serological study from Copenhagen

the aetiological agent was sought in 21 patients with fulminant viral hepatitis. Seven (33 per cent) had no serological evidence of either HAV or HBV infection and by exclusion of other identifiable viruses were characterized as having non-A, non-B fulminant hepatitis. In another study six patients with underlying liver disease developed non-A, non-B hepatitis after receiving factor IX concentrates and this proved fatal in three. The current non-A, non-B exposure risk is estimated at 1 per 100 units of blood transfused with a very small percentage developing fulminant hepatic failure. With this in mind, it is to be hoped that specific serological tests for the diagnosis of non-A, non-B hepatitis similar to those so successfully developed for the detection of hepatitis A and B will soon be available so that treatment with blood or blood products can be made even safer.

Drugs. While paracetamol overdose continues to be the most important drug-associated cause of fulminant hepatic failure, severe halothane-associated liver damage has been the subject of considerable interest and controversy. It seems clear that two kinds of clinical picture may follow multiple halothane anaesthetics. Minor asymptomatic liver damage, detected by monitoring AST levels is relatively common but clinically unimportant while fulminant hepatic failure is a very rare but often fatal complication. Rifampicin–isoniazid therapy and monoxamine oxidase inhibitors are other rare causes.

Other conditions. Two additional rare causes of fulminant hepatic failure worthy of special mention are pregnancy and Weil's disease.
Acute fatty liver of pregnancy is a rare but very serious complication of the last trimester, in which there is accumulation of fine deposits of fat in hepatocytes and a clinical picture of fulminant hepatic failure. Fetal death *in utero* is common and early delivery is essential as the mother often shows a rapid clinical improvement afterwards. Toxaemia may also be associated with severe liver damage but here the morphology is of hepatic infarcts associated with evidence of intravascular coagulation. Heparin may be of value in the management.
Weil's disease is due to infection with the spirochaete, *Leptospira icterohaemorrhagica*. Although the deep jaundice and altered level of consciousness focuses attention on the liver, the associated renal failure, haemorrhage, and haemolysis are most important in determining mortality. Histological changes in the liver are very variable and even in fatal cases the liver can be normal (see also Section 5).

Pathogenesis

Fulminant viral hepatitis. The reasons why viral hepatitis may follow, albeit rarely, a fulminant course are not known. In the case of the HBV, however, the identification of its specific antigenic markers has provided striking evidence of the variability of clinical and serological outcomes of HBV infection. This variation in clinical response has been emphasized by retrospective analysis of early experimental hapatitis transmission studies in volunteers. Although HBsAg-positive sera were infectious to almost all recipients, less than half had evidence of clinical disease. Furthermore, the range of clinical disease seen, including the development of a chronic carrier state in some and fulminant hepatitis in others, suggested that the outcome of HBV infection may be influenced by host factors rather than by the dose, virulence, and strain of the virus. Similarly, in the transmission of non-A, non-B hepatitis to chimpanzees, the volume of innoculum did not seem to influence the severity of the ensuing disease. There is also evidence that the HBV itself is not directly cytopathic and that liver damage is the result of immune-mediated mechanisms. In fulminant hepatitis B the humoral antibody response may be enhanced. There is a significantly faster rate of clearance of HBs antigen in patients with fulminant hepatitis than in those with severe uncomplicated acute hepatitis. In one study, the mean duration of antigenaemia was 10.7 days in patients with fulminant hepatitis compared to 44.1 days in patients with a non-fulminating course. On admission, anti-HBs as well as HBsAg has been found in about 40 per cent of patients with fulminant hepatitis whereas anti-HBs is very rarely detected at this time in patients with uncomplicated hepatitis.

Other, indirect evidence supports the hypothesis that host-immune factors determine the fulminant clinical course in HBV infection. HBV specific DNA polymerase levels are no different in patients with fulminant hepatitis than in those with uncomplicated acute hepatitis. As DNA polymerase is a known marker of active replication of the complete virus, this finding suggests that the severity of liver damage is not directly related to the degree of virus replication. In special circumstances, however, massive hepatocellular necrosis may follow a 'superinfection' in the hepatocytes. For example, fulminant hepatic failure has been observed after the withdrawal of immunosuppressive therapy in patients with malignant disease, who had acquired HBV infection after treatment commenced (Fig. 5). A possible explanation for this finding is that immunosuppressed HBsAg carriers, when compared to the normal healthy HBsAg carriers, have serological and tissue evidence of continuing viral replication which may result in a more widespread infection of hepatocytes than usual. Hence in these patients it may have been the return of cell-mediated immunity following the withdrawal of therapy which led to the destruction of a large number of infected hepatocytes and massive liver cell necrosis.

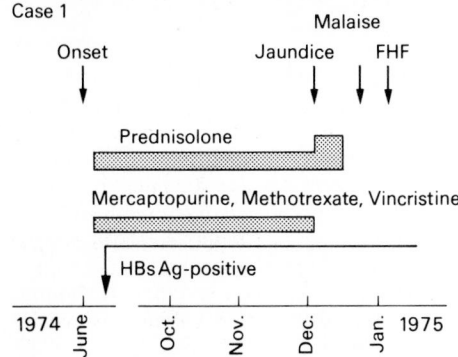

Fig. 5 Development of fulminant hepatitis B following the withdrawal of cytotoxic drug therapy in a man with chronic myeloid leukaemia. (From Galbraith (1975). *Lancet* ii, 528, by permission).

Halothane hepatitis. In fulminant hepatic failure following repeated halothane anaesthesia a heightened specific antibody response may also be implicated. In a recent study, we have shown that serum from patients with fulminant hepatic failure, following repeated exposure to halothane, contained antibodies reacting with a halothane-altered liver-cell membrane antigen. This antibody has not been found in any of several control groups, including those exposed to halothane but not developing severe liver damage and those with fulminant hepatic failure not related to halothane anaesthesia. Further *in vitro* experiments have shown that the antigen on the surface of hepatocytes with which the antibody reacts is associated with the oxidative metabolism of halothane and presumably represents a normal membrane constituent which has been altered by the metabolite. Although it seems unlikely that this very interesting immune reaction is of no relevance to pathogenesis, formal proof has not yet been provided that it is responsible for the severe liver damage.

Paracetamol liver damage. In marked contrast to those cases associated with halothane anaesthesia, there is no evidence that immune reactions to normal or drug-altered liver components play any part in the pathogenesis of the liver damage which follows paracetamol overdose. Hepatocyte necrosis is almost certainly due to the formation of reactive intermediary products of paracetamol metabolism which bind to vital intracellular proteins, interfering directly with cellular metabolism. Early administration of compounds like methionine which can inactivate these reactive metabolites can prevent or modify liver cell damage after a paracetamol overdose.

Pathophysiology. Knowledge of the pathogenesis of acute hepatic coma is derived from studies in patients with this disorder and from animal models of experimentally induced hepatic coma. Both approaches have limitations; studies in humans cannot yield details about the intracerebral metabolic abnormalities which occur in fulminant hepatic failure and animal models usually involve coma which is very rapidly and irreversibly induced by extirpation or devascularization of the liver. However, much has been learned in recent years about the multifactorial origin of acute hepatic coma, particularly in relation to coma-producing or toxic substances. These can be divided into two main groups, those which act directly on cellular systems and those which indirectly lead to metabolic derangement. High levels of ammonia have long been implicated in the pathogenesis of hepatic coma although it is clear from clinical and experimental studies that hepatic coma cannot be caused solely by an excess of ammonia. Additional toxins include free fatty acids, mercaptans, phenols, bilirubin, and bile acids. Studies in rats suggest that the first three compounds act synergistically in the brain to produce coma. For example, the dose of ammonium chloride required to produce coma in normal rats was reduced by the co-administration of (sub-coma) doses of the free fatty acid octanoate or the mercaptan methaneiol.

Gross elevations of all amino acids, except the branch chain amino acids valine, leucine, and isoleucine, are also seen in fulminant hepatic failure, and may contribute to the encephalopathy. Experimental studies have shown that the aromatic amino acids phenylalanine, tyrosine, and also tryptophan compete with the branch chain compounds for uptake into the central nervous system and it has been suggested that increased entry of the aromatic amino acids into the brain leads to the formation of inhibitory 'false neurotransmitter substances' such as octopamine and phenylethanolamine. Indeed, in animal models of acute liver failure the accumulation of these false neurotransmitters has been shown to correlate with the onset of encephalopathy. Similar studies in patients do not show such a striking relationship and again the impression is that the false neurotransmitter hypothesis is only one of several mechanisms leading to coma in fulminant hepatic failure.

Additional information about the pathogenesis of hepatic encephalopathy has been derived from recent animal studies which have suggested that middle molecular weight substances (1500–5000) might alter the permeability of the blood–brain barrier, allowing the entry of toxic metabolites into the brain and thus contribute to the development of cerebral oedema which is so often a feature of the terminal case. In fact, cerebral oedema is a major cause of death and in one post mortem study was found in 32 per cent of patients who died of fulminant hepatic failure. The exact stage at which cerebral oedema develops is difficult to determine. Papilloedema is seldom present and bradycardia with pyrexia and hypotension are common. All too often the first clinical sign of cerebral oedema is a sudden respiratory arrest followed by the development of fixed dilated pupils and absent brainstem reflexes indicating tentorial herniation. In pigs with surgically induced hepatocellular necrosis and implanted subdural pressure transducers progressive rises in intracranial pressure were observed (Fig. 6) and post mortem examination of the brains revealed gross oedema with flattened gyri and evidence of tonsillar herniation.

Clinical features. The occurrence of encephalopathy is of central importance in the syndrome of fulminant hepatic failure. The first signs often relate to the encephalopathy with the appearance of mild confusion, irrational behaviour, or even euphoria and psychosis. Characteristically the encephalopathy is associated with a widely fluctuating but progressive deterioration in mental condition. If coma rapidly ensues, then clinical jaundice is often not apparent and whilst encephalopathy usually appears within a few days of the onset, the whole illness from the first symptoms to death may be less than a week.

Important signs at examination include fetor hepaticus, a flapping tremor of the outstretched hand (asterixis), slurred speech, and

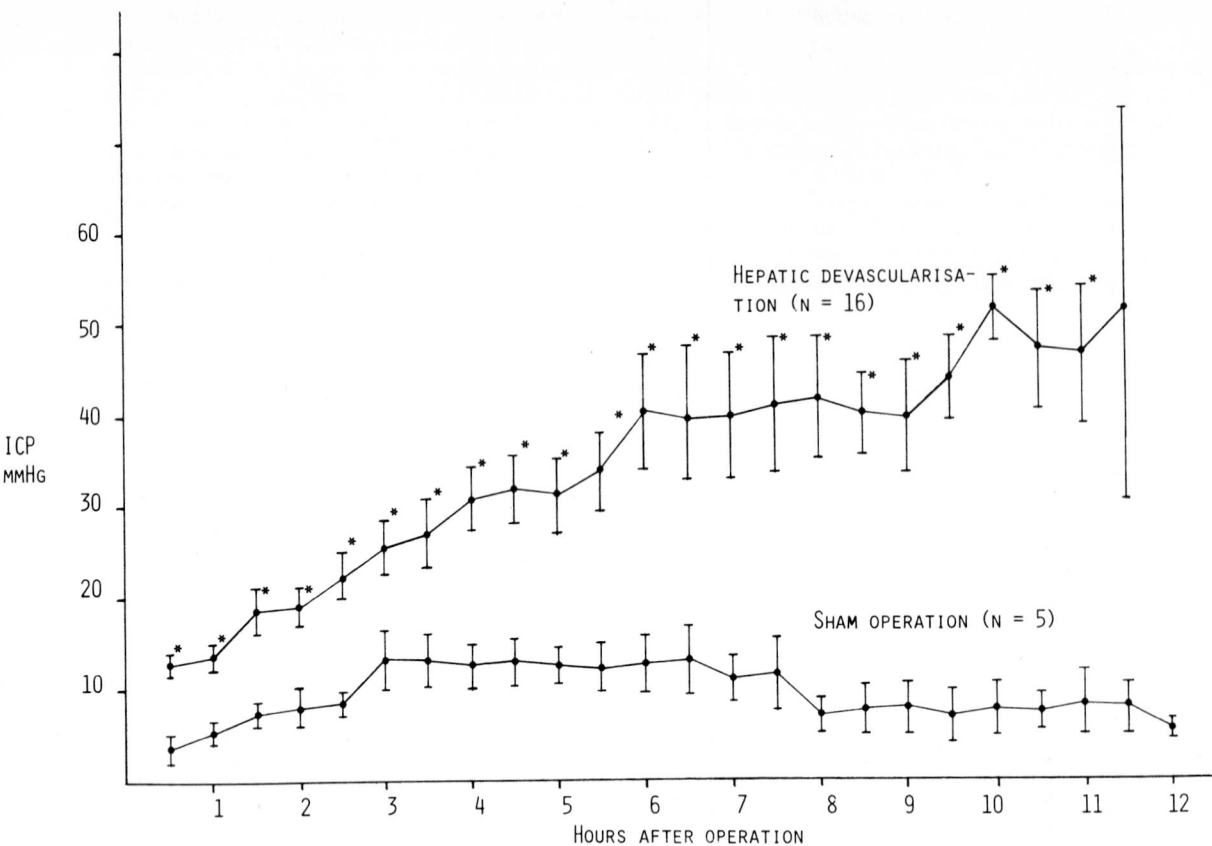

Fig. 6 A comparison of the sequential intracranial pressure levels (ICP mmHg) in control sham operated animals (lower trace) and animals following hepatic devascularization (upper trace).

difficulty in writing and copying simple diagrams (constructional apraxia). Jaundice deepens and at a later stage is associated with reduced liver size on percussion. Whilst cutaneous stigmata of chronic liver disease are absent, spider naevi are occasionally evident in the protracted but fulminant course. By this stage serum transaminase levels are raised often by 40-fold or more and the prothrombin time is considerably prolonged.

Whilst not necessary for diagnosis, an electroencephalogram at the onset of encephalopathy shows a slowing of the alpha rhythm and, with increasing drowsiness, this is replaced by lower frequency theta activity. When coma deepens, high amplitude delta waves become prominent and the characteristic triphasic waves appear. Preterminally the amplitude of these waves decreases and finally the electroencephalogram becomes isoelectric (Fig 7).

Once in grade IV coma (see Table 2, page 12.198), hyperventilation is common and the pupils are dilated and react sluggishly to light. Hypertonia and grasp reflexes are readily elicited, and in deep coma, decerebrate or decorticate postures are seen. Loss of the oculovestibular reflex invariably precedes a fatal outcome but other brainstem reflexes, including the occulocephalic reflex, may disappear transiently in patients who ultimately survive. Hypotension, cardiac arrhythmias and respiratory arrest may also occur and preterminally hypothermia and areflexea are commonly witnessed.

Renal and electrolyte abnormalities. Complex alterations in fluid and electrolyte balance occur in severe fulminant hepatic failure, and these are often aggravated by renal failure. In one study 43 per cent of 100 patients developed renal failure during the course of their fulminant disease. In about half of the patients the renal failure is associated with evidence of intact renal tubules and is termed 'functional renal failure'. It is characterized by low urine sodium concentration (less than 12 mmol/l), a hyperosmolar urine (urine/plasma osmolality ratio greater than 1:10), and normal renal histology. In other patients acute tubular necrosis occurs and is associated with high urine sodium concentration (greater than 20 mmol/l), isosmolar urine, and histological evidence of tubular

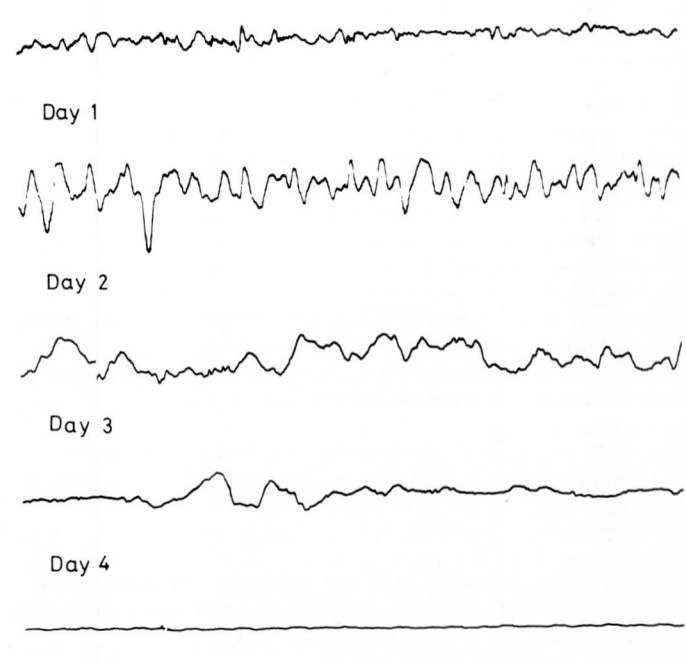

Day 1

Day 2

Day 3

Day 4

Day 5

Fig. 7 An EEG illustration of the steady decrease in amplitude and frequency associated with a terminal course in fulminant hepatic failure.

necrosis. The cause of renal failure in patients with fulminant hepatic failure is not known. It appears to be unrelated to the severity of the liver disease but has a particularly poor prognosis. Some evidence suggests that endotoxin (lipopolysaccharide components of the cell wall of Gram-negative bacteria) may be involved. Such bacteria are of course, normal commensals in the gut and small amounts of endotoxin are normally absorbed into the portal venous blood and filtered by the Kupffer cells of the liver. In severe hepatocellular necrosis with Kupffer cell dysfunction there may be a 'spill-over' of endotoxins into the systemic circulation in the absence of true Gram-negative infection (Fig. 8).

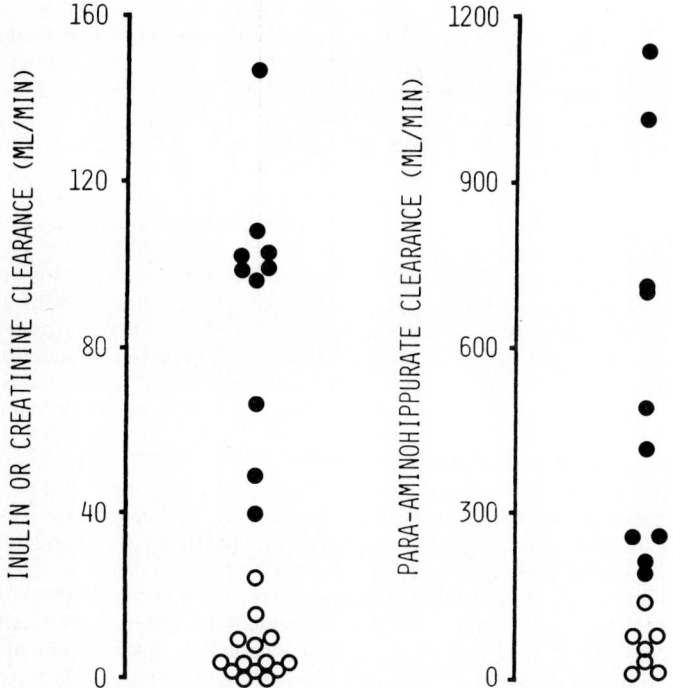

Fig. 8   Relationship of renal function to endotoxaemia in fulminant hepatic failure: ● = endotoxin not detected; ○ = endotoxaemia. (From Wilkinson (1974). *Lancet* **i**, 521, by permission.)

Acid–base disturbance. Alkalosis is a common finding in fulminant hepatic failure and is usually of respiratory origin. Hyperventilation leading to respiratory alkalosis is frequently seen in the early stages of coma. Respiratory alkalosis is associated with impaired oxygen dissociation from haemoglobin, reduced cerebral and peripheral perfusion, and diminished cerebral oxygen consumption. It may in addition result in neurological and electroencephalopathic changes similar in some respects to those of experimental ammonia toxicity and will be potentiated by a coexistent metabolic alkalosis. Metabolic alkalosis occurring early in the illness may be due to hypokalaemia or to a failure to alkalinize the urine—and continuous gastric aspiration may potentiate this abnormality at a later stage. Other potential causes of metabolic alkalosis include accumulation of basic compounds in the circulation and movement of hydrogen ions into the intracellular space.

Patients with fulminant hepatic failure, particularly those with a rapidly progressive downhill course associated with peripheral circulatory failure, often develop lactic acidosis. This complication, particularly in association with hypoglycaemia, suggest that lactic acidosis may be due to both failure of hepatic gluconeogenesis and increased anaerobic metabolism.

Abnormalities of haemostasis and coagulation. There may be widespread abnormalities of the haemostatic mechanism including thrombocytopenia, multiple clotting factor deficiencies, and disseminated intravascular coagulation. These changes are further considered in Section 19.

Proneness to infection. There is a marked increase in proneness to bacterial infection, particularly Gram-negative organisms derived from the gastrointestinal tract.

Cardiovascular system. The cardiac output is commonly raised and transient, often unexplained, hypotension is frequently seen. Inappropriate vasodilation may be responsible in some cases, perhaps secondary to central vasomotor depression. Cardiac arrhythmias in one series of patients included multiple ventricular ectopics (20 per cent), heart block and bradycardia (18 per cent). The arrhythmias probably arose as a result of alterations in myocardial oxygenation, plasma potassium, or intracranial pressure.

Management. Management of patients with fulminant hepatitis must be based on an understanding of the way in which the different signs and symptoms making up the clinical syndrome develop during the course of the illness. Basic supportive therapy is essential whatever other measures are used, and intensive monitoring is the only way to detect complications at an early stage when they are potentially reversible. The patient should be nursed in an intensive care ward or, better still, in a separate liver failure unit.

Coma. The same general supportive measures apply in fulminant hepatic failure as in coma complicating cirrhosis (see page 12.184). As soon as signs of hepatic decompensation appear dietary protein is withdrawn. A magnesium sulphate enema (80 ml of a 50 per cent solution w/v) is administered to empty the bowel. Lactulose is given orally, the dose adjusted to produce two soft motions daily; diarrhoea must be avoided as this aggravates any abnormality in fluid and electrolyte balance. Neomycin (1 g orally six-hourly) may also be given if renal function is normal.

Nutritional support. Infusions of dextrose are the mainstay of nutritional support in these patients. Blood glucose levels must be monitored regularly, however, as they can fluctuate widely. In addition, unsuspected hypoglycaemia can exacerbate hepatic encephalopathy. Insulin resistance occurs in severe acute hepatitis and as a result carbohydrate tolerance is impaired and plasma levels of tricarboxylic acid intermediates are high.

Generally, up to 3 litres of 10 per cent dextrose daily can safely be administered and in consequence the calorie intake is limited to 4.2–5 kJ (1–1.2 kcal) per day. Intravenous lipid preparations are contraindicated because they are poorly utilized and also will exacerbate an increase in plasma levels of free fatty acids caused by the disease itself.

Abnormalities in sodium and potassium are common and require particular attention. Hypokalaemia often occurs in the early stages of a fulminant illness and can be life threatening. The hyponatraemia so frequently seen in patients with acute liver failure is often associated with an inappropriately high renal retention of sodium and water, hence administration of sodium is contra-indicated. Gastric aspiration and purgation, however, can lead to true sodium depletion if the intake is inadequate, and this state may be impossible to distinguish from dilutional hyponatraemia, since in both states urinary sodium content is low.

Gastrointestinal haemorrhage. More than 50 per cent of patients with fulminant hepatic failure develop severe gastrointestinal haemorrhage from acute erosions in the stomach and oesophagus. Coagulation disorders are likely to increase any tendency the patient may have to bleed. Although many factors may promote the development of gastric erosions, acid appears to be one important basic ingredient in their pathophysiology. Maintenance of intragastric pH above 5 by the use of antacids has lowered the incidence of bleeding in patients with fulminant hepatic failure. H_2 receptor antagonists are more efficient than antacids for maintaining a consistently raised intragastric pH over long periods of time and in a controlled trial proved to be very effective in reducing the incidence of gastrointestinal bleeding in fulminant hepatic failure.

Bleeding into the lungs, retroperitoneal haemorrhage, epistaxis, and haemorrhage from peptic ulceration may also occur. The value of fresh frozen plasma in replacing the clotting deficiencies seen in fulminant hepatic failure is not proven. Only in those patients with unequivocal haematological evidence of disseminated intravascular coagulation should heparin therapy be given and then the levels should be monitored (see Section 19).

Respiratory problems. As in all comatose patients, a major problem is protection of the patient's airway from the risk of aspiration of blood or stomach contents. Early intubation is desirable and is performed as soon as the patient's gag reflex becomes depressed. Respiratory arrest may occur at any time and facilities for rapid intubation and ventilation must be available. Respiratory infection is common and must be treated with appropriate antibiotics with careful monitoring of their plasma levels.

Cerebral oedema. Continuous recordings from sub-dural pressure transducers in patients with fulminant hepatic failure have shown fluctuations in intracranial pressure in all cases with marked elevations in patients who eventually died. Mannitol infusions often lead to quite marked reversal of pressure increases (Fig. 9), and should be given as soon as a sustained pressure rise is detected.

Other approaches to management

Corticosteroids. The role of corticosteroids in the management of fulminant hepatic failure remains uncertain. Several years ago, the use of corticosteroids in the treatment of acute hepatic encephalopathy was advocated but controlled trials failed to show any definite improvement in survival. Indeed in one study of patients with severe viral hepatitis it was suggested that corticosteroids may be deleterious. We have shown, in an animal model of fulminant hepatic failure, that methyl prednisolone administered prior to hepatic devascularization can prevent the rise in intracranial pressure so often seen in this syndrome, perhaps by reducing the increased permeability of the plasma membranes of brain capillary endothelial cells. However, if the prednisolone was given after raised intracranial pressure was established, it had no beneficial effects suggesting that irreversible damage to the blood-brain barrier had already occurred.

Artificial liver support. The specific purpose of artificial liver support systems is to aid the removal of toxic metabolites which accumulate in fulminant hepatic failure and hence to keep patients alive long enough for liver regeneration to provide enough functioning liver tissue to allow recovery to occur.

Early attempts at liver support were based on techniques such as extracorporeal animal liver perfusion, human cross circulation, and exchange transfusion. These led to improvements of conscious level in some cases, although in most the improvement could not be maintained with repeated use of the systems and few patients survived to leave hospital. It soon became apparent that an artificial system with reproducable function was essential. Such is the complexity of the metabolic abnormalities that occur in fulminant hepatic failure, however, that at present it is not possible to separate those of primary importance from those that are only of secondary importance in the pathogenesis of the clinical syndrome. An additional factor which further complicates the management of these patients is the likelihood that both water-soluble and protein-bound compounds contribute to the range of toxic metabolites which accumulate in acute hepatic failure.

Water-soluble substances can be removed during perfusion of blood through activated charcoal, and using this technique it has been possible to show prolongation of survival in animal models of liver failure. In an initial study of 37 patients with fulminant hepatic failure treated at the Liver Unit, King's College Hospital, 14 (38 per cent) survived, a figure which compared favourably with the 16 per cent survival in a previous series of 25 patients treated with a conservative but vigorous medical regimen. However, as the number of patients treated increased, the survival figures fell, with many developing severe unresponsive hypotension during haemoperfusion. The close temporal relationship between these episodes and the formation of cellular aggregates in the blood suggested that problems of biocompatibility were being encountered. Later work has shown that platelet aggregates were formed as the blood was passed over charcoal and it is possible that the hypotension was caused by the release of vasoactive amines from the platelets. Meanwhile Opolon, using the Rhône-Poulenc haemodialysis system, which has a highly permeable polyacrylonitrile membrane to remove middle molecular weight substances (up to 5000), had reported a significant improvement in conscious level in patients with stage IV coma. Although final percentage survival figures were not appreciably better than those achieved by conservative therapy alone, the prolonged periods of survival obtained in some patients were encouraging. This haemodialysis system was used at King's College Hospital from 1976 to 1979 and of 108 patients treated, 31 survived (29 per cent). Recently the King's group have again returned to the use of charcoal haemoperfusion but have added prostacyclin, a potent inhibitor of platelet aggregation, to the perfusion

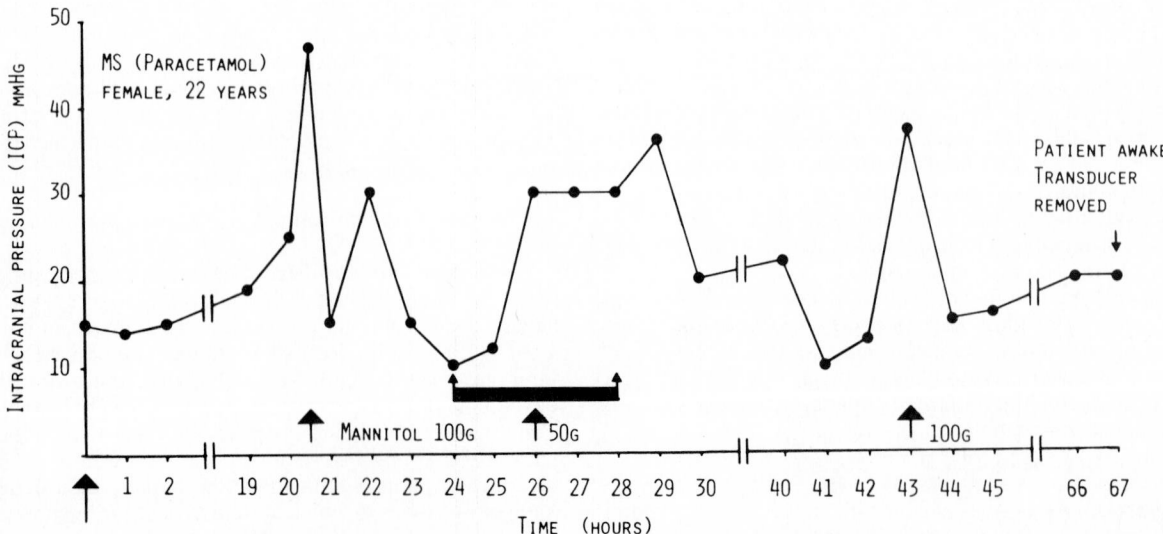

Fig. 9   Serial intracranial pressure measurements in a patient with fulminant hepatic failure. The shaded area was a four-hour period of polyacrylonitrile membrane haemodialysis.

system. The problems of platelet clumping and hypotension during perfusion seem to have been overcome and initial clinical results are encouraging. In addition to the removal of water-soluble toxins, the ideal artificial liver support system would probably also need to remove protein-bound toxins. The resins of the Amberlite series are most effective in absorbing protein-bound toxins, but during preliminary experiments in an animal model of acute liver failure prohibitive platelet losses were observed. Recent studies, however, have shown that it is possible to bind human serum albumin tightly to Amberlite XAD-7 resin and this system has substantially improved the biocompatibility of the resin with respect to platelet losses. Hence, it should now be possible to assess the effect of treatment with combined extracorporeal support systems.

Lastly, and most importantly, it has now become evident that no form of liver support therapy will be effective if it is continually instituted at a preterminal stage in the illness. Once the oculovestibular reflex has been lost, no form of therapy is likely to affect the outcome. A retrospective analysis of 92 cases admitted to the King's Liver Unit has shown that 90 per cent of those admitted in grade III coma ultimately progressed to grade IV coma, and it seems logical to begin supportive therapy at this earlier stage before irreversible metabolic events have already prejudiced survival.

References

Alberti, A. and Eddleston, A. L. W. F. (1981). Determinants of chronicity in hepatitis B virus infection. In *Clinical immunology update*, vol. 3 (eds. R. H. Buckley, D. Doniach, J. L. Fahey, C. W. Parker, W. F. Rosse, and E. C. Franklin). Elsevier North-Holland, New York.

Chalmers, T. C., Eckhardt, R. D., Reynolds, W. E., Cigarroe, J. G., Deane, N., Reifenstein, R. W., Smith, C. W., and Davidson, C. S. (1955). The treatment of acute infectious hepatitis. Controlled studies of the effects of diet, rest and physical reconditioning on the acute course of the disease and on the incidence of relapses and residual abnormalities. *J. Clin. Invest.* **34**, 1163.

Desmet, V. J. and De Groote, J. (1974). Histological diagnosis of viral hepatitis. *Clins Gastroent.* **3**, 337.

Gocke, D. J. (1975). Extrahepatic manifestations of viral hepatitis. *Am. J. med. Sci.* **270**, 49.

Gregory, P. B., Knaver, C. M., Kempson, R. L., and Miller, R. (1976). Steroid therapy in severe viral hepatitis. A double blind, randomized trial of methyl-prednisolone versus placebo. *New Engl. J. Med.* **294**, 681.

Jenkins, P. and Williams, R. (1980). Fulminant viral hepatitis. *Clins Gastroent.* **9**, 171.

Redecker, A. G. (1975). Viral hepatitis: clinical aspects. *Am. J. med. Sci.* **270**, 9.

Shaldon, S. and Sherlock, S. (1957). Virus hepatitis with features of prolonged bile retention. *Br. med. J.* **ii**, 734.

Chronic hepatitis

H. C. Thomas

Chronic hepatitis is defined as hepatic inflammation continuing without improvement for longer than six months. Inflammation of the intrahepatic biliary tree is usually excluded from this group of diseases. The diagnosis is made by liver biopsy. When there is historical evidence of an attack of acute hepatitis, then the biopsy should not be undertaken earlier than six months after that acute episode. Premature biopsy usually gives an equivocal result: chronic persistent hepatitis cannot usually be differentiated from the changes of resolving acute hepatitis. Early biopsy may be indicated when there is no historical evidence of an acute hepatitis and the duration of the symptoms and signs and the liver biochemistry are consistent with a chronic disease process which has already progressed to a severe stage. A prolonged period of lethargy, jaundice, fluid retention, or gastrointestinal bleeding from oesophageal varices would suggest advanced disease. Laboratory data such as a low serum albumin, high gamma globulin, and a markedly prolonged prothrombin time would support this diagnosis. In these cases, liver biopsy must be undertaken to establish the type and severity of the disease process. In some cases, fresh frozen plasma may be needed to correct the coagulopathy before percutaneous biopsy can be safely undertaken. If this therapy is ineffective, transjugular hepatic biopsy may be tried.

Several aetiological factors may initiate chronic hepatitis. These are listed in Table 1 and include a primary defect in the regulation of the immune response (auto-immune), persistent viral infection (type B and the non-A, non-B hepatitis viruses), prolonged administration of drugs (oxyphenisatin, methyldopa, isoniazid, and nitrofurantoin), and alcohol, Wilson's disease, and a substantial group where no aetiological agent can be identified.

The distribution of the inflammatory infiltrate in the portal tracts and hepatic lobules, established by hepatic biopsy, allows a further classification (Fig. 1) which is justifiable on prognostic grounds. These lesions may be seen with any of the aetiological factors.

Chronic persistent hepatitis

Definition. This diagnosis can only be made by liver biopsy. The histological picture is of a mononuclear cell infiltrate of the portal tracts with no spillover into the periportal area (Fig. 1). There may, however, be areas of focal liver cell necrosis in the lobule, and in these cases the histological picture should be described as chronic persistent hepatitis with a lobular component.

Table 1 Aetiological classification of chronic hepatitis

1 Primary auto-immune: characterized by the presence of high titre antibodies to nuclear, smooth muscle, liver/kidney microsomal, and mitochondrial antigens
2 Hepatitis B virus (HBV)-related: usually characterized by the presence of HBs antigenaemia
3 Non-A, non-B hepatitis virus-related: characterized by the absence of auto-antibodies and markers of HBV infection; no positive serological markers identified
4 Drug-related: oxyphenisatin, methyldopa, nitrofurantoin, and isoniazid
5 Alcohol-related: (histological features of alcohol-induced liver injury, i.e. Mallory's hyalin, pericellular centrilobular fibrosis, and fat, are usually present)
6 Wilson's disease: characterized and diagnosed by identification of the metabolic abnormalities of this disease

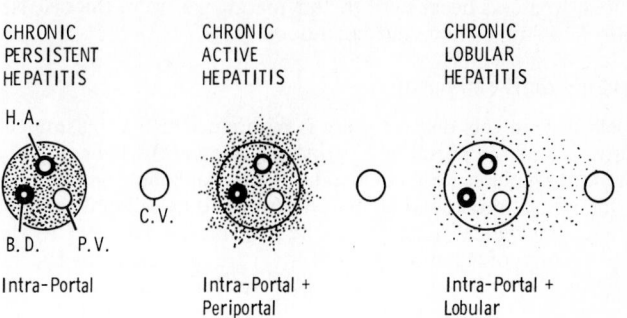

H.A. = Hepatic Artery, B.D. = Bile Duct, P.V. = Portal Vein, C.V. = Central Vein, ◯ = Limiting plate of portal tract, ⋰ = Inflammatory cells

Fig. 1 Histological classification of chronic hepatitis dependent on distribution of inflammatory infiltrate.

Clinical features. These patients are asymptomatic with no physical signs of chronic liver disease. The liver and spleen are not enlarged. The aspartate and alanine aminotransferase levels are increased approximately 2–5 times the upper limit of the normal range. The bilirubin, alkaline phosphatase, serum albumin, globulin, and prothrombin time are normal.

Many cases present because abnormal aminotransferases are found six or more months after an episode of acute hepatitis. Others come to clinical attention during auto-analyser biochemical screening, and presumably have followed asymptomatic acute hepatitis. In the majority of cases no aetiological agent can be identified. Only a few cases are attributable to hepatitis B virus infection and the magnitude of the role of the non-A, non-B viruses cannot be determined until satisfactory serological markers have been defined.

Prognosis and treatment. The disease has a good prognosis. The majority of cases do not progress to chronic active hepatitis and cirrhosis. Hepatitis B surface antigen-positive patients who have evidence of active viral replication (HBe antigen positivity) may progress slowly to active hepatitis and cirrhosis over many years. These patients may need anti-viral therapy (see below), but in HBs antigen-negative cases no therapy is required.

Chronic lobular hepatitis

Definition. The histological picture is virtually identical to acute lobular hepatitis, chronicity being recognized by careful biochemical follow-up. The hepatic lobule is infiltrated from portal to central areas with chronic inflammatory cells and there are scattered areas of necrosis of hepatocytes (focal necrosis) (Fig. 1).

Clinical features. These patients are usually icteric with symptoms of general malaise. The course is often fluctuating. A viral aetiology is usual (type B or non-A, non-B), but in some cases high titre smooth muscle and nuclear antibodies suggest an auto-immune aetiology.

The biochemical picture is similar to that seen in acute hepatitis. The aspartate and alanine aminotransferase and bilirubin are markedly elevated. A low serum albumin and prolonged prothrombin time indicate severe disease.

Prognosis and treatment. Hepatitis-B virus-induced chronic lobular hepatitis has a variable prognosis. A benign course has been described but others progress rapidly to cirrhosis. Chronic lobular hepatitis due to non-A, non-B virus infection may have a more benign course. Patients with high titre auto-antibodies also have a benign prognosis.

The administration of antiviral therapy would be a logical approach in some of these patients. Clinical experience with such therapy, however, is not yet available. In patients with auto-antibodies, immunosuppressant therapy has been tried. Its value is difficult to assess because of the fluctuating course of the disease: controlled studies have not been done.

Chronic active hepatitis

Definition. In this disease there is mononuclear and plasma cell infiltration of the portal and periportal areas of the liver (Fig. 1). The limiting plate, which delineates the portal zone from the periportal area of the hepatic lobule, is breached by the infiltrate and there is 'piecemeal' necrosis of the hepatocytes adjacent to this plate. Groups of hepatocytes ('rosettes') are surrounded by chronic inflammatory cells. When liver cells are destroyed, the reticulin framework may collapse. This may be followed by collagen accumulation and regeneration of hepatocytes, resulting in disorganization of the lobular architecture and the development of a coarse macronodular cirrhosis. The picture of chronic active hepatitis may be accompanied by varying degrees of chronic lobular hepatitis and occasionally by cholangitic features. When the degree of piecemeal

necrosis is severe, bands of necrotic tissue may extend from one portal tract to another or to the central vein (bridging hepatic necrosis). This histological picture is usually seen in patients with subacute hepatic necrosis, a term used to describe patients who develop fluid retention and encephalopathy between one and two months after the onset of acute hepatitis.

The histological entity of chronic active hepatitis may be the result of a variety of pathogenic processes (see Table 1) which will be dealt with under separate headings.

Auto-immune chronic active hepatitis (CAH). In normal subjects the regulatory cells of the immune system (suppressor cells) permit responses to foreign antigens (protective immunity) but suppress or control those directed to 'self components' (auto-immunity). In spite of this system, a transient auto-aggressive response does occur in normal subjects when subjected to tissue damage (Fig. 2a), and only when this response is prolonged does it represent a pathological state. Chronic auto-immunization may thus occur secondary to prolonged liver damage resulting from exposure to a toxin or infection with a virus in the presence of a normal immunoregulatory system (Fig. 2b), or as a primary event due to failure of this system (Fig. 2c). Auto-immune CAH is probably an example of a primary auto-immune disease in which the defective immunoregulatory system permits a prolonged and exaggerated response to a liver membrane antigen. This defect has been poorly defined because of the limitation of techniques available for measuring the function of the suppressor cells which fulfill regulatory function. Thus, at the moment, a diagnosis of primary auto-immune CAH can often only be made when the disease continues after all identifiable inciting factors have been removed. Additional clues may stem from the specificity of the auto-antibody. Current information would suggest that lupoid (primary auto-immune) CAH is characterized by the presence of a liver membrane antibody (LMA) which is mainly found in this disease and is distinct from the auto-antibody associated with virus and toxin-induced CAH (antibody to liver-specific protein). In the latter, the auto-immune response is presumably secondary to the denaturation of liver antigens during toxic or viral exposure. Further features, including high titre nuclear (dsDNA) and smooth muscle (actin) antibodies, high serum immunoglobulin—particularly IgG—concentrations, and an association with other auto-immune disease states (Hashimoto's thyroiditis, haemolytic anaemia, and thrombocytopenia), suggest a primary disorder of the immune system as the major precipitating or permissive factor in these patients. That this defect may be genetically determined is suggested by the finding of an increased incidence of auto-antibodies and raised globulin in the relatives of these patients and an association of the disease with the human leucocyte antigen (HLA) B8. The latter suggests that the inheritance of a gene or genes close to the locus of the major histocompatibility complex on chromosome 6 predisposes to the development of the disease either spontaneously or in response to some environmental trigger factor.

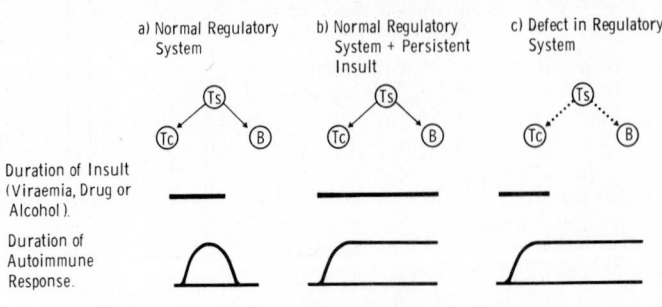

a) Normal Regulatory System　　b) Normal Regulatory System + Persistent Insult　　c) Defect in Regulatory System

Ts = suppressor T-lymphocyte;　Tc = cytotoxic T-lymphocyte;　B = B-lymphocyte

Fig. 2 Acute and chronic auto-immunization. Note the transient auto-immune response after acute liver injury (a). When the insult continues (b) the auto-immune response is protracted in spite of a normal regulatory system. When the immunoregulatory system is abnormal (c), the auto-immune reaction continues after removal of the insult.

Clinical features. Most patients (70 per cent) have established cirrhosis at the time of the first liver biopsy. Three-quarters of the patients are female, and although all ages may be affected, peak incidence is seen between 10–25 and 50–65 years. The disease has an insidious onset in the majority of cases, but occasionally may present abruptly with features suggestive of acute viral hepatitis. In these cases the disease is probably brought to light by an intercurrent viral hepatitis (type A, B, or non-A, non-B) rather than being initiated by these viruses. In others, the condition is diagnosed during surgery or by routine biochemical screening during medical investigations for coincidental problems. The patients usually complain of general malaise for several months before jaundice is noted.

The clinical signs include mild to moderate icterus and the stigmata of chronic hepatocellular liver disease including spider naevi and palmar erythema. The liver is usually normal or small in size and there is clinically detectable splenomegaly. Additional features are abdominal striae, acne, gynaecomastia, and amenorrhoea. Approximately half of the patients have other 'immunological' disorders including arthralgia or arthritis, vasculitis, ulcerative colitis, glomerulonephritis, fibrosing alveolitis, Hashimoto's thyroiditis, auto-antibody positive haemolytic anaemia, leucopenia and thrombocytopenia, and diabetes mellitus.

The biochemical picture is of chronic hepatocellular disease (aminotransferases 2–30 times normal, and normal alkaline phosphatase) with a variable degree of impairment of hepatic synthetic function (normal or low serum albumin and 2–8 second (15–70 per cent) prolongation of prothrombin time). There is often haematological evidence of hypersplenism secondary to portal hypertension (leucopenia and thrombocytopenia). The serum immunoglobulin G is usually elevated with smaller changes in M and A levels. Antinuclear factor (ANF), antibodies to double-stranded (ds) DNA and to smooth muscle (actin) are present in high titre (usually greater than 1:40 by immunofluorescence tests). The term lupoid CAH should be restricted to ANF-positive patients but the term is also used for those with only smooth muscle antibodies. More recently additional auto-antibodies have been described (liver/kidneys microsomal and 'non-PBC' mitochondrial) and the 'auto-immune' group of patients has been subdivided according to the specificity of these auto-antibodies (Table 2). It remains to be determined whether these divisions are useful clinically.

Table 2 Auto-immune chronic active hepatitis; auto-antibody specificities

Nuclear (dsDNA, ribonucleoprotein, and others)
Smooth muscle (actin)
Liver/kidney microsomal
Mitochondrial
Liver membrane (LMA and LSP)

The differential diagnosis involves exclusion of the other causes of chronic active hepatitis (Table 1). Additional problems may lie in differentiating the disease from: (a) primary biliary cirrhosis: approximately 20 per cent also have mild periportal piecemeal necrosis. These patients have cholestatic features and are mitochondrial antibody-positive; (b) primary sclerosing cholangitis: the majority have piecemeal necrosis. Cholangiography usually establishes the cholangitic component and makes the diagnosis. These patients are usually clinically and biochemically cholestatic.

Management. Until we are able to correct the specific defect in the immune system of these patients, immunosuppression represents the mainstay of therapy. Corticosteroids (prednisolone or prednisone) are usually started at a dosage of 20–30 mg per day, continued for one month, and then reduced by 5 mg every month until a maintenance dose of 10–15 mg is established. The patients respond symptomatically within a few days and biochemical improvement is clearly evident by two weeks. The dosage should be adjusted to maintain the aminotransferases within the normal or near-normal range. This is usually achieved in three to six months and is accompanied by an improvement in hepatic synthetic function (increase in albumin and reduction in prothrombin time). In some cases, poor coagulation may prohibit liver biopsy and steroid therapy is started on the basis of a clinical, biochemical, and serological diagnosis. In these cases, sufficient improvement may be evident within one month so that confirmatory liver biopsy can be undertaken.

When adequate control can only be obtained at the expense of corticosteroid side-effects, azathioprine may be added at a dosage of 1–2 mg/kg body weight. Corticosteroid therapy should always be continued, albeit at reduced dosage, because azathioprine has been shown to be ineffective by itself.

Prognosis. The cumulative mortality rate is much reduced by this programme of management. In a recent follow-up study of the Royal Free Hospital trial, the survival rate at 10 years in the treated group was 63 per cent compared to 27 per cent in the control group. The duration of therapy varied considerably, and at the moment there are no firm criteria which allow one to predict whether therapy can be safely withdrawn. However, in the control group of the above trial, the mortality rate was high in the first two years after diagnosis and thereafter disease activity was low and the majority of patients had a well-compensated inactive macronodular cirrhosis. It seems probable that prednisone therapy should be continued for at least two years. At this stage the patient should be rebiopsied and if the level of inflammatory activity is minimal, a gradual withdrawal of therapy may be attempted. Relapse, indicated by a significant increase in aminotransferase, occurs in 60–70 per cent of cases, particularly those that are still auto-antibody (SMA and ANF)-positive. In these cases therapy should be restarted and a further attempt at withdrawal made after another year.

Hepatitis-B virus (HBV)-induced chronic active hepatitis. There are probably 150–200 million people in the world who are chronically infected with the hepatitis B virus, the highest prevalence being in tropical Africa, Central and South America, China, and Indonesia. The virus may produce chronic persistent, lobular or active hepatitis and some progress to develop cirrhosis and primary hepatocellular carcinoma. In others there is no significant inflammatory or malignant liver disease (Fig. 3). In occasional patients, usually those with mild inflammatory liver disease (chronic persistent hepatitis or inactive cirrhosis), extrahepatic pathology—polyarteritis nodosa or membranoproliferative glomerulonephritis—may be evident.

The factors which determine whether an individual suffers an

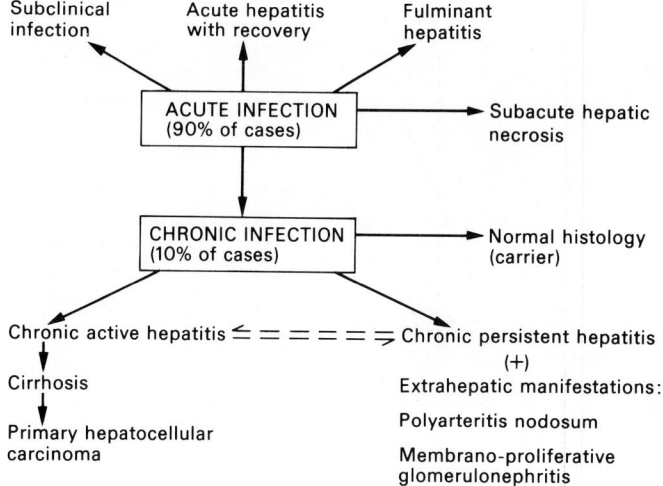

Fig. 3 Clinical syndromes associated with acute and chronic HBV infection.

acute or chronic infection are unknown. Various immune defects, genetically determined or acquired, have been described but none of these is of proven pathogenic significance. At some stage the viral genome integrates with the hepatocyte DNA but the relationship of this event to the development of persistent infection and to malignant transformation is unknown. The virus is not directly cytopathic and the variety of pathology exhibited in chronically infected people is related to variation in the ability of the host's immune system to respond to the virus. An analogy may be usefully drawn to the tuberculoid and lepromatoid reactions to *Mycobacterium leprae* infection. Patients with chronic active hepatitis mount a vigorous cell-mediated immune response ('tuberculoid reaction') to the virus, while those with extrahepatic disease mount a predominantly humoral response ('lepromatoid reaction'). Those who are carriers with no inflammatory liver disease are tolerant to the surface antigens of the virus.

The mechanism of liver damage is not fully established. There is certainly a cell-mediated immune response to some viral antigens (HBs) and in addition a response to native liver membrane antigens such as liver-specific protein (LSP). The relative importance of these cellular responses to viral and hepatocyte membrane antigens in mediating liver cell damage is unknown. Humoral responses to these antigens are also present and may play a role in virus neutralization or in hepatocyte necrosis. Immune complexes containing viral antigens have been demonstrated in the serum and tissues of patients with polyarteritis and glomerulonephritis.

Clinical features. The majority of patients are asymptomatic, coming to medical attention as a result of testing for HBs antigenaemia during blood donation or routine screening during hospital admission for non-hepatic problems. These patients usually have chronic persistent hepatitis or are carriers with normal hepatic histology, and more rarely have chronic active hepatitis or cirrhosis. They rarely give a history of acute hepatitis, and presumably have suffered either a subclinical attack or have been infected at birth. Infection during the neonatal period or in early childhood is common in the Tropics and Far East, but probably of lesser importance in Western Europe and North America, where infection probably occurs in the second and third decades of life as a result of sexual contact or drug abuse.

Some cases follow acute hepatitis. Between 90 and 95 per cent of patients will have cleared the virus and its antigens (HBs) from the blood within three months of the clinical onset of the hepatitis (Fig. 4). Additional patients will clear the virus up to one year after infection but thereafter the spontaneous recovery from infection is rare. The majority of persistently infected patients will develop chronic active hepatitis. During the first years of the chronic infection the virus replicates at a high rate and virus particles can be demonstrated in both the liver and blood. At this stage the patient is

HBe antigen-positive and is highly infectious. At a later stage the level of replication is lower and the virus cannot be detected in the blood in spite of the continued presence of HBs antigen. These patients are HBe antibody-positive and are of much lower infectivity. In some cases, many years after the onset of infection, the HBs antigen may be undetectable in the blood but can be found in the liver. These patients usually produce antibodies to HBc but not to HBs antigen.

Some cases present relatively late in the course of the infection, usually with the complications of cirrhosis, including ascites, oesophageal variceal bleeding, and hepatic failure.

The importance of HBV infection as a cause of chronic active liver disease (CAH with or without cirrhosis) varies considerably in different countries, and in general parallels the incidence of HBV carriage. In the United Kingdom, Western Europe, and North America it accounts for less than 5 per cent of the clinically overt cases. In Tropical Africa, India, Japan, and China it is probably the most common cause. It is more common in men.

Management. The initial assessment will require the determination of: (*a*) the level of viral replication; (*b*) the severity and type of inflammatory liver disease; (*c*) the degree of fibrosis or cirrhosis.

The level of replication will determine the infectivity of the patient's blood. In general, blood from HBe antigen-positive patients is highly infectious, less than 0.01 ml being sufficient to transmit the disease. These patients may infect their sexual partners by oral or genital contact. Of epidemiological importance is the fact that HBe antigen-positive mothers have a 95 per cent probability of infecting their infants and approximately half of these children develop chronic infections. HBs antigen-positive patients who are HBe antibody-positive are of much lower infectivity. Larger volumes of their blood is required to transmit the infection and therefore sexual transmission is uncommon. The infants of HBs antigen-positive HBe antibody-positive mothers have a less than 5 per cent chance of being infected at birth.

The level of inflammatory activity will influence the prognosis of the patient. Those with severe CAH or active cirrhosis have progressive disease and should be offered appropriate therapy (see below). Those with CPH and inactive cirrhosis have quiescent disease and should only be treated if they have evidence of active viral replication (HBe antigen-positivity) and therefore a high level of potential infectivity.

An assessment of the degree of fibrosis or cirrhosis is an indication of the amount of damage already accrued. It is of prognostic value only.

Treatment of HBe antigen-positive patients. *Interferons* have been shown to cause transient inhibition of viral replication and in some cases treatment for several months has produced permanent inhibition with conversion from HBe antigen to antibody. No controlled studies of the effectiveness of long-term therapy have been published and the usefulness of these natural antiviral compounds remains to be determined when they are available in clinically useful quantities. The recent cloning, in bacteria, of the gene for interferon production may permit larger scale production of the material for clinical studies. However, because of the current limited availability of interferon, various synthetic antiviral compounds have been evaluated.

Vidarabine (adenine arabinoside) has been subjected to controlled trial and was shown to be effective in producing an increased rate of conversion from HBe antigen to antibody, a reduction in HBs antigen concentration, and improvement in liver biochemical tests. More recently, adenine arabinoside 5′-monophosphate, a water-soluble derivation of the parent compound, has been shown to be effective when given twice daily by intramuscular injection for three to four weeks. In a small study, the majority of cases showed permanent inhibition of viral replication (Fig. 5) and long-term follow-up is in progress.

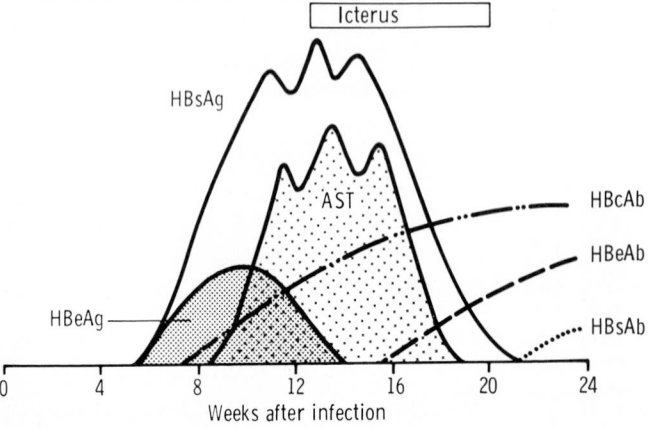

NB During phase of HBe Antigenaemia HBV particles are present in blood

Fig. 4   Acute type B hepatitis—viral antigens (HBs and HBe).

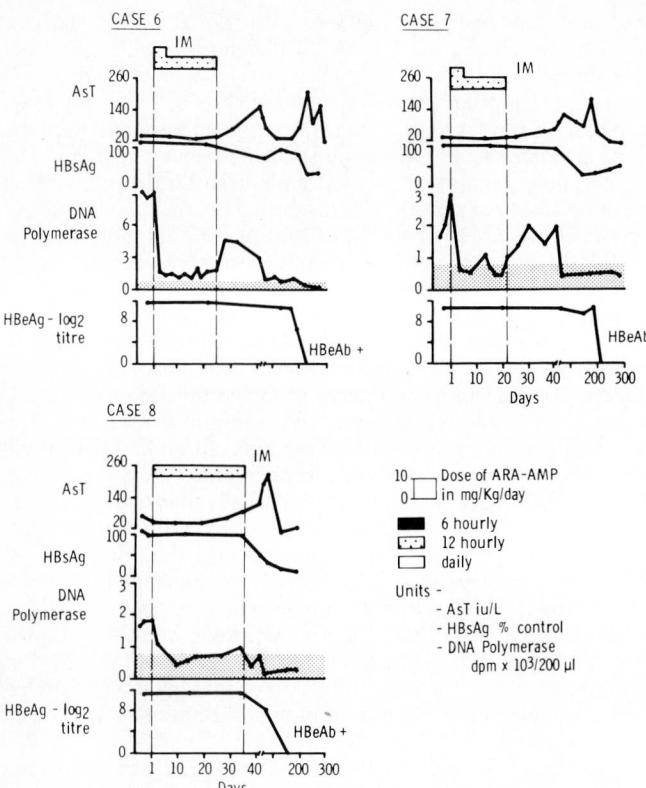

Fig. 5 Vidarabine monophosphate (Ara-A-AMP) in the treatment of chronic HBV infection (HBeAg positive). Note that three consecutive patients lost HBe antigen and developed HBe antibody after treatment. This change is associated with a reduction in infectivity and in the level of hepatic inflammatory activity. (From Weller, I. V. D. *et al.* (1982). *Gut*, in press.)

Immunostimulation has been proposed as an alternative approach. Synthetic (levamisole) and bacterial (BCG) adjuvants have been studied. No beneficial effect has yet been established and they should still be considered as experimental procedures. The aim in such therapy is to stimulate the host's immune system to facilitate clearance of the virus. Their use may be in combination with the synthetic antiviral agents.

Immunosuppression has been shown to result in increased replication of the virus with no improvement in the level of inflammatory activity in the liver. It is contra-indicated in patients with active viral replication.

Treatment of HBe antibody-positive patients. *Antiviral therapy* with adenine arabinoside has been shown to have no effect on HBs antigen concentrations or on liver function tests.

Immunostimulation has not been evaluated.

Immunosuppression may have some value in this group of patients but has not been evaluated in controlled trials. Moderate dosage (10–15 mg) of prednisone or prednisolone does not cause an increased level or replication: they do not revert to HBe antigenaemia.

Prognosis. The natural history of HBV-induced chronic active hepatitis is variable. In a few cases the disease may progress rapidly to cirrhosis but in most the evolution is slow. In general, progression is fastest during the early stage of infection when the level of viral replication is high and the patient is HBe antigen-positive. When the patient converts to a lower level of replication associated with the presence of HBe antibody, the inflammatory activity subsides. Thus CAH may become CPH and active cirrhosis changes to inactive cirrhosis. The rate of conversion from HBe antigenaemia to HBe antibody-positivity varies from 5–10 per cent per annum in different populations.

Non-A, non-B (NANB)-hepatitis virus-induced chronic active hepatitis. There are at least two parenterally transmitted NANB hepatitis viruses which can be distinguished by differing incubation periods (two to four and seven to 10 weeks) but have not yet been morphologically or serologically characterized (see Section 5). More recently, enterically transmitted epidermic and sporadic forms of NANB hepatitis have also been described.

In the United Kingdom 10–15 per cent of sporadic acute hepatitis and an unknown but significant proportion of post-transfusion hepatitis is attributable to these viruses. Between 20 and 50 per cent of these patients develop chronic infection and it seems probable that the NANB agents are a major cause of chronic liver disease. The proportion of the crytogenic cases of CAH and cirrhosis which are the result of this infection must await the development of adequate diagnostic serological tests. Epidermic and sporadic NANB hepatitis do not result in chronic hepatitis.

Clinical features. Several clinical pictures have been described, but whether each type is related to a specific virus cannot be established.

Several groups have reported NANB hepatitis as a relatively mild illness which is usually asymptomatic. The transaminases fluctuate rapidly during the early course of the illness, the peak values becoming gradually lower (Fig. 6). This pattern has been prominent in haemophiliac patients infected by a virus (or viruses) transmitted by factor VIII concentrates. About 80 per cent of these patients develop chronic hepatitis, the lesions ranging from chronic persistent to active hepatitis and cirrhosis, and being characterized by the presence of an intense lobular infiltrate of mononuclear cells. These patients exhibit a predominantly short (two to four weeks) incubation period.

Other groups have reported chronic hepatitis developing after blood transfusion or plasma donation (plasmapheresis). In the majority of these patients the incubation period was seven to 10 weeks and the hepatic biopsies showed predominantly chronic persistent hepatitis with a low incidence of periportal piecemeal necrosis and lobular hepatitis. It seems possible that this milder lesion, occurring after a longer incubation period, is the result of infection with a different agent. Alternatively, these differences

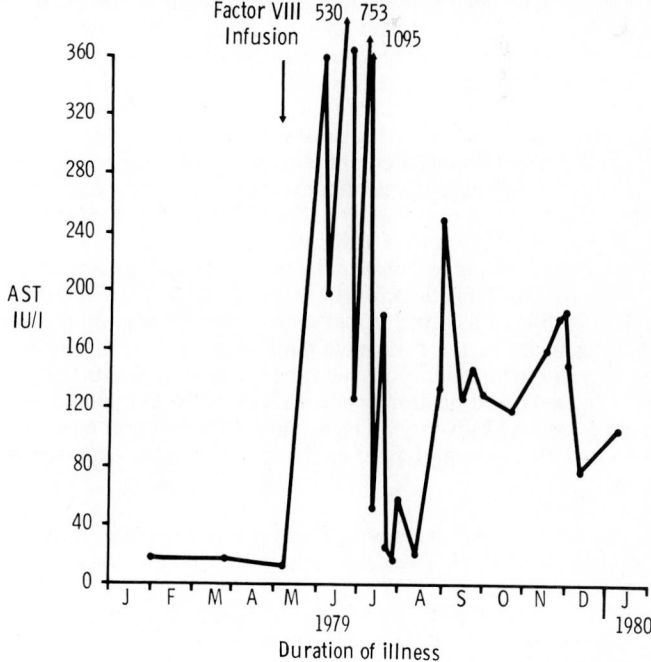

Fig. 6 Non-A, non-B hepatitis in a haemophiliac following infusion of factor VIII concentrate (prepared from a pool of about 500 donors). Note the rapid onset (two to four week incubation period) and fluctuating pattern of aminotransferase activity. Biopsy showed chronic active hepatitis with lobular component.

may be the result of variation in the size of the innoculum of a single agent.

The immunological features of this form of chronic hepatitis are more similar to HBV-induced disease than to the auto-immune type. Serum immunoglobulins are normal until the stage of advanced cirrhosis when IgG levels increase. Smooth muscle and nuclear antibodies may be found in patients with chronic active hepatitis or cirrhosis, but the titres are much lower than those found in auto-immune CAH and cirrhosis.

Management and prognosis. The rate of progression of the disease is variable. In some cases cirrhosis may develop in five to 10 years but in the majority the prognosis is good. In some series there has been a tendency for the inflammatory process to subside over a period of several years, and in others progression is very slow. Once again this variation may reflect the involvement of different viruses and a more precise study of the natural history of this disease must await the availability of serological methods for identification of the causative viruses.

At the moment the indications for and approaches to treatment are unknown. Corticosteroids have been used in patients with symptomatic chronic active liver disease and clinical and biochemical improvement has been noted. Controlled trials are currently in progress.

Drug-induced chronic active hepatitis. (See also page 12.213.) An increasing number of widely used and generally well-tolerated drugs can cause hepatic injury. This may range from a transient elevation of serum aminotransferase concentrations, or, after prolonged exposure, to the development of chronic liver disease. Both the acute and chronic lesions are often clinically, biochemically, and histologically indistinguishable from virus-induced or auto-immune forms of liver injury, and thus a causative role for a drug cannot always be established. For this reason the list of drugs which are suspected of inducing liver injury is much larger than that of drugs of proven involvement.

Drug-induced liver injury may be the result of either direct toxicity or an idiosyncratic reaction.

Direct toxicity occurs within a few hours in all patients exposed, is dose-dependent and does not cause chronic hepatitis. Paracetamol may cause hepatic necrosis and when taken for a prolonged period at high dosage has been suggested as a possible cause of chronic liver disease. Chronic liver necrosis would be expected to result in fibrosis and possibly cirrhosis, but chronic inflammation and piecemeal necrosis are not expected or observed during this process.

Idiosyncratic reactions occur infrequently in an exposed population, occur at varying intervals after exposure, are not dose related, and are usually characterized by the presence of an inflammatory reaction (hepatitis). Such a response implies either an unusual metabolic or immune response to the drug or its metabolites in the patient afflicted. Genetic or environmental factors may influence the metabolism of the drug so that varying degrees of alteration of the antigenicity of the liver membrane might occur. The host's immune and inflammatory response to the altered membrane, as well as genetic and environmental influences, would then determine the type and severity of liver injury. In some cases an initial episode of toxic necrosis is followed by an idiosyncratic hypersensitivity response.

Clinical features and management. Several drugs have been reported to cause chronic hepatitis by an idiosyncratic hypersensitivity reaction.

Oxyphenisatin was the first to be described. The onset of the disease is often delayed for several months after starting therapy. The biopsy appearance in the acute stage is similar to viral hepatitis and progression to chronic active hepatitis has been described. The patients often exhibit serological features similar to those seen in auto-immune chronic hepatitis (high titre ANF and smooth muscle antibodies). On withdrawal of the drug, inflammatory activity sub-

sides, and immunosuppressant therapy is not required. Patients may be left with inactive cirrhosis. The diagnosis may be confirmed by careful re-exposure.

Isoniazid is another important cause of chronic active hepatitis. The picture is similar to that seen with oxyphenisatin but often the lesions are more severe including subacute hepatic necrosis. The drug is mildly hepatotoxic, raised aminotransferase levels being seen in up to 20 per cent of patients during the first two months of therapy. However, in about 1 per cent of exposed individuals, a hypersensitivity reaction to a metabolite occurs, resulting in a more severe hepatic lesion occurring usually during the third and fourth months of therapy. Biopsy at this stage will reveal an acute hepatitis indistinguishable from viral hepatitis. The most severe reactions are seen in fast acetylators and in patients taking enzyme inducers. Rifampicin is an inducer of mixed function microsomal oxidase activity and when given with isoniazid causes more frequent and possibly more severe reactions. In all cases isoniazid must be stopped and alternative antituberculous therapy initiated. Clinical and biochemical improvement usually then occurs over the ensuing weeks. Subacute hepatic necrosis and chronic active hepatitis are seen in patients who continue to take the drug. In these patients there is a significant mortality. Once the diagnosis is made and the drug is withdrawn, inflammatory activity always subsides. The patient may be left with inactive cirrhosis. Steroid therapy is not usually required. Diagnostic rechallenge is not justified in symptomatic cases, but re-introduction of therapy may be undertaken cautiously in cases of asymptomatic transient elevation of aminotransferases.

Alpha methyldopa may result in a similar sequence of clinical and histological events. Acute hepatitis, subacute hepatic necrosis, and chronic active hepatitis have all been described often in association with auto-antibodies (ANF and smooth muscle), elevated immunoglobulins, and other auto-immune manifestations (Coombs' positive haemolytic anaemia). Inflammatory activity will subside on withdrawal of the drug but restoration of hepatic function may take several weeks, particularly in the middle-aged and older patients.

Nitrofurantoin may cause a hypersensitivity reaction resulting in fever, a macular rash, and a mixed hepatitic/cholestatic liver lesion. Eosinophilia has been described. Following prolonged administration, chronic active hepatitis may develop. Management involves withdrawal of the offending drug and monitoring of liver biochemistry to ensure that improvement does occur.

Wilson's disease. Between five and 10 per cent of patients with Wilson's disease (see also page 12.221 and Section 9) present with symptoms of chronic active liver disease. These patients are homozygotes for the recessive gene; heterozygotes are not afflicted.

Clinical features. Patients present with symptoms of liver disease including general malaise, jaundice, ascites, and variceal bleeding, in the first and second decades of life. Coexistent neurological dysfunction (spastic gait, ataxia, and dysarthria) is evident in only a minority of cases (less than 15 per cent) and these are usually slightly older (15–25 years). Hepatosplenomegaly is present in the majority of patients. A few patients exhibit evidence of liver failure. Kayser–Fleischer rings may be found by slit lamp examination in approximately 50 per cent of cases: these are usually the older patients.

The liver test abnormalities are similar to those seen in other types of CAH. The majority of patients have an elevated bilirubin and an aspartate aminotransferase 5–10 times the upper limit of the normal range. Albumin concentrations are often low and prothrombin times increased, changes indicative of severe hepatocellular liver disease. Immunoglobulin G levels are elevated. Auto-antibodies (smooth muscle and nuclear) are absent or present in low titre (less than 1:20 by indirect immunofluorescence). Haemolytic anaemia may be present particularly in the most severe cases.

Liver biopsy shows portal and periportal mononuclear cell infiltration and piecemeal necrosis. The majority of patients have established cirrhosis at diagnosis. Diagnostic features are not present but fine droplet fat and nuclear vacuolation are almost always present. The diagnosis is made by measurement of the liver copper. In normal subjects this is usually less than 250 μg/g of dry liver and in hepatic Wilson's disease is more than 300 μg/g dry liver. Histochemical stains for copper are not useful. Serum copper and caeruloplasmin levels are usually low but during periods of active liver cell necrosis and hepatic inflammation, the caeruloplasmin concentration may rise to the lower end of the normal range. Urinary copper is elevated in the majority of cases and increases further when D-penicillamine is administered. The uptake of radiocopper by the liver is reduced in Wilson's disease but this test is prohibitively expensive.

Management. Wilson's disease must be excluded in all cases of CAH. Whereas the auto-immune form of the disease responds to steroids, Wilson's CAH must be treated by copper chelation. D-penicillamine should be given at a dosage of 1–1.5 g/day for the rest of the patient's life. When the drug is not tolerated, other copper chelating compounds may be tried at specialist centres. During treatment the urine copper will rise and the liver copper falls. The dosage may be reduced when the urinary copper starts to fall. In patients with severe liver failure steroid therapy may be added to D-penicillamine.

All siblings of the patient should be screened by measuring serum copper and caeruloplasmin, urinary copper, and liver copper. Asymptomatic cases must be treated (see also Section 9).

Prognosis. Most cases present late. The overall mortality is 50 per cent in the first two years after diagnosis. The greatest mortality is in those with severe hepatic necrosis and haemolysis. Long-term survival on D-penicillamine is possible.

References

Chadwick, R. G., Galizzi, J., Heathcote, J., Lyssiotes, T., Cohen, B. J., Scheuer, P. J., and Sherlock S. (1979). Chronic persistent hepatitis: hepatitis B virus markers and histological follow-up. *Gut* **20**, 372.

Popper, H. and Schaffner, F. (1971). The vocabulary of chronic hepatitis. *New Engl. J. Med.* **284**, 1154.

Thomas, H. C. and Bamber, M. (1981). Clinical aspects of non-A, non-B hepatitis. In *Advances in medicine*. Medical London.

—, Bassendine, M. F., and Weller, I. V. D. (1981). Treatment of chronic hepatitis B virus infection. In *Developments in antiviral therapy* (eds. L. H. Collier and J. Oxford). Academic Press, London.

— and Jewell, D. P. (1979). Acute and chronic viral hepatitis; Autoimmune chronic active hepatitis. In *Clinical gastrointestinal immunology*. Blackwell Scientific Publications, Oxford.

Wilkinson, S. P., Portmann, B., Cochrane, A. M. G., Tee, D. E. H., and Williams, R. (1978). Clinical course of chronic lobular hepatitis. *Q. J. Med.* **47**, 421.

Alcohol and the liver

P. W. Brunt

Alcohol is a major cause of liver disease. It vies with hepatitis viruses for pride of place in both acute and chronic morbidity and mortality. In worldwide terms the scale of the problem is enormous. In the USA between 1950–74, while cardiovascular deaths actually fell slightly (by 2 per cent), deaths from cirrhosis, mostly alcoholic, rose by 72 per cent making it now the fourth commonest cause of death in white, male adults. The socio-economic toll of alcohol abuse in the USA, in terms of medical care, crime, accidents, and industrial losses, is now said to top $70 000 million yearly. In the United Kingdom the figure is much less but still considerable, and the annual cost of alcohol-related traffic accidents alone exceeds £100 million.

There is a consistent relationship between alcohol consumption in a community and deaths from cirrhosis; countries with the highest consumption like France and Portugal having the highest recorded death rates. However, the use of this relationship to estimate alcoholism prevalence (the 'Jellinek formula') is unreliable since mortality statistics are known to give a serious underestimate of the true prevalence of alcoholic cirrhosis. About two in every three cases of cirrhosis in Britain are alcohol-induced and the proportion is even higher in France and USA. In most tropical countries and communities where alcohol is proscribed (e.g. some Islamic societies) the ratio is very much smaller.

Of great interest in alcohol-induced liver disease is the protean spectrum of its presentation ranging from fatty liver to hepatitis, cirrhosis, and carcinoma. It remains uncertain whether these are distinctive responses, or steps in an inevitable progressive process, albeit very slow in some individuals. At least half of all clinically significant disease is non-cirrhotic.

Definitions. The terms 'alcoholism' and 'alcoholic' are difficult to define with universal acceptance and are best avoided in the context of alcohol-related liver disease. Physical addiction or dependance, an essential component for many definitions of 'alcoholism', is not a prerequisite for liver damage. This has important implications for treatment since curtailment rather than abstinence may be applicable in many patients with milder forms of alcoholic liver disease.

Since there is no evidence that small amounts of alcohol are damaging, a definition or a diagnosis of 'alcohol-related disease' implies excessive intake and in many individuals this can be difficult to prove. It is easy to beg the question when preconceived ideas about clinical or histological features suggest the diagnosis in an individual who denies excessive intake. Problems arise in those conditions which can mimic alcoholic disease (certain drugs for example) and in those rare patients with abnormalities not usually recognized as alcoholic (e.g. chronic aggressive hepatitis) whose alcohol intake is excessive.

Pathology

Clinico-pathological considerations. In both acute and chronic alcoholic injury the liver is almost invariably enlarged. Only in advanced macronodular cirrhosis is the liver contracted and small. It is unlikely that a patient with a small liver is drinking excessively.

In the non-cirrhotic liver hepatomegaly is due to accumulation of fat and retention of intracellular protein. When cirrhosis has developed, and drinking continues, the liver is large, fibrous, finely nodular, and noticeably fatty; the 'hob-nail liver' described by Laennec. In both fatty liver and micronodular cirrhosis the liver is smoothly and regularly enlarged. Irregular or nodular enlargement suggests tumour.

Some degree of inflammation is common and accounts for pain and tenderness. Persisting or severe pain in alcoholic cirrhosis, however, suggests the development of primary liver cancer, which supervenes in about one in five alcoholic cirrhotics.

Histopathology. *Minimal change disease.* Following moderate alcohol ingestion histological changes are primarily sub-cellular. The mitochondria become swollen and disorganized with abnormal borders and irregular cristae. The smooth endoplasmic reticulum may be increased. Diminished export of cellular protein and accumulation of water and salts leads to hydropic changes and ballooning of cells.

Fatty liver. Fat deposition is highly characteristic of alcohol excess but is not pathognomonic and occurs in diabetes, obesity, malnutrition, and severe wasting. While the presence of fat is not a diagnostic essential, its absence from a liver biopsy should question an alcoholic basis. However, fat may disappear quite rapidly from the liver (within possibly two to three weeks) with abstinence. Fat droplets may be small, or large and coalescent, and occur most characteristically in the centrizonal cells.

Two additional histological features in the fatty liver (steatosis) presage future trouble. Firstly, small inflammatory foci may be seen with swollen fat-laden and necrotic cells surrounded by a ring of chronic inflammatory cells ('jackal lesion'). As this feature develops, it merges into alcoholic hepatitis. Secondly, perivenular sclerosis may be seen in up to 40 per cent of fatty livers. Collagen fibrils laid down around the central (terminal hepatic) veins lead to stellate scarring and incomplete septum formation. If observations in alcohol-fed baboons can be extrapolated to man, this lesion can be the first step in a cirrhotic process, apparently without the development of frank hepatitis.

Hepatitis. Alcoholic hepatitis is a distinctive pathological entity characterized by widespread necrosis, inflammatory reaction, usually fat, and sometimes hyaline (Fig. 1). Alcoholic hyaline, described by Mallory in 1905, is a fine fibrillary mesh of new protein material appearing predominantly in centrilobular hepatocytes as eosinophilic bodies. While characteristic of alcohol injury, especially if centrizonal, it is not exclusively alcoholic and may be seen in drug-induced hepatitis (e.g. perhexilene), chronic cholestasis, Wilson's disease, and Indian childhood cirrhosis.

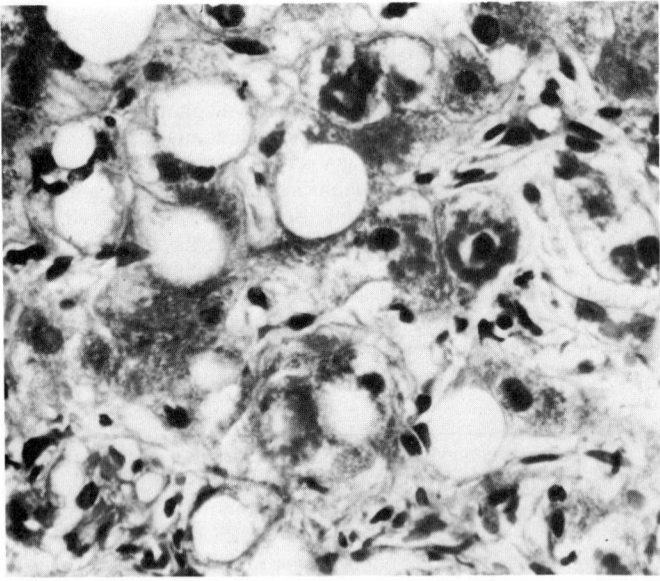

Fig. 1 Alcoholic hepatitis with fatty change, cell necrosis, and inflammation.

It is a curious fact that the apparent histological severity of the hepatitis may not be reflected in the clinical picture; a similar histological change may be seen both in patients with florid clinical hepatitis and in asymptomatic or minimally disturbed patients. This reflects in part the inability to differentiate acute from chronic hepatitis on histological grounds alone.

Increased collagen synthesis is invariable in hepatitis, and laying down of fibrous tissue around central veins ('central sclerosing hyaline necrosis') may be associated with the acute development of reversible portal hypertension. Changes of chronic aggressive hepatitis with little or no fat or hyaline have been described in alcohol abusers and in the absence of other recognized causes of chronic hepatitis.

Cirrhosis. With the development of fibrous septa and bridging between central veins and portal zones, cirrhosis gradually supervenes. Distortion of the architecture and formation of short-circuiting vascular channels are early changes of cirrhosis. The picture is completed in active cirrhosis by regenerative nodules, which are mainly small (less than 3 mm), i.e. micronodular cirrhosis. These nodules, though containing functioning hepatocytes, are poor performers because of vascular shunting.

Fat is commonly present in a micronodular cirrhosis but if drinking lessens or ceases it may disappear, and a more coarsely irregular, inactive, macronodular cirrhosis develops. Hepatoma is more likely to develop in this setting than in active micronodular cirrhosis. Mild iron deposition is common especially in wine drinkers.

Pathogenesis. There are three fundamental problems which remain unresolved: (a) the toxic role of alcohol and the importance of nutrition; (b) the significance of dose, duration, and type of alcoholic beverage; and (c) the reason why a significant proportion (85 per cent) of long-standing heavy drinkers escape irreversible disease.

Nutrition. Malnutrition as a cause of 'alcoholic' disease held sway for many years until the last decade. It is plausible enough as an explanation; alcoholics tend to eat poorly and alcohol interferes with small bowel absorptive function. Furthermore, alcohol displaces energy foods as a fuel, and yet provides only 'empty' calories (see below).

Animal studies in rats, for example, have shown little or no alcoholic injury where dietary intake has been well maintained. Unfortunately, extrapolation from rat data to humans is questionable. Moreover, while deficiency of certain nutrients such as choline in rats seems to cause cirrhosis, there is no convincing evidence that such deficiency or indeed malnutrition *per se* causes cirrhosis in humans. Experience in following patients with kwashiorkor lends support to this.

Some alcoholics eat good diets and still develop cirrhosis. Carefully controlled studies in normal volunteers, in alcoholics, and in baboons in which protein/vitamin intake has been more than adequate have shown alcohol to be hepatotoxic. In the case of baboons, progression to cirrhosis over about five to six years has been observed. Alcohol certainly can impair digestion and absorption but, while protein and nutrient deficiency may increase susceptibility to cellular injury, it also impairs fibrogenesis. It seems reasonable to conclude that malnutrition may play some role in alcoholic liver disease but certainly not an essential one.

Alcohol toxicity. The metabolic consequences of alcohol ingestion are far-reaching, reflecting the nature of the molecule and its degradation. It is small and freely miscible in water and lipid, and therefore rapidly distributes through tissues. Metabolism is obligatory; there is no excretion pathway (apart from small amounts in urine and breath) and no feedback control. Degradation occurs mainly in hepatocytes and at the expense of other cellular processes. As a fuel alcohol provides 29.5 kJ/g (7 kcal/g) but the process is oxygen-dependent and results in an embarrassing generation of unwanted hydrogen ions. During breakdown of alcohol to acetaldehyde, and acetaldehyde to acetate, nicotine adenine dinucleotide (NAD) acts as hydrogen acceptor and the $NADH^+$ produced alters the redox state of the cell with many potential metabolic effects. Increased lactate/pyruvate ratios with lactacidaemia and acidosis decreases urate excretion and may precipitate gout. Both gluconeogenesis and urea formation are impaired. Excess $NADH^+$ production drives the mitochondria to effect 'shuttle' removal of hydrogen ions with consequent depression of the citric acid cycle. Complex effects on lipid metabolism result in accumulation of triglycerides, depressed oxidation, and removal of lipids and the deposition of fat in cells.

Some of the effects of alcohol on the hepatocyte on protein metabolism, for example, depend partly on dose-size and on whether it is acute or chronic ingestion. Furthermore, acutely, occupation of the microsomal enzyme systems impairs metabolism of some drugs whereas, chronically, induction of the systems leads to enhanced clearance of both alcohol and some drugs. However, most alcohol degradation is catalysed by alcohol dehydrogenase, a non-microsomal enzyme, and normally only a small fraction is controlled by the microsomal enzyme oxidizing system.

There is growing evidence that the major biochemical lesion is the accumulation of acetaldehyde. This molecule produces a vicious circle by impairing the mitochondrial shuttles essential for disposal of reducing equivalents. It probably increases lipid membrane peroxidation and depletes glutathione and these may be crucial factors in producing cellular injury. Furthermore, acetaldehyde seems to bind to tubulin, thereby inhibiting polymerization with a decrease in the microtubular structures of the cell.

Thus, there is an ample basis for alcohol, and acetaldehyde derived from it, having a primary toxic role in liver injury.

Dose response in injury. There is plentiful evidence from Germany, France, the United Kingdom, and elsewhere that the 'risk' of developing steatosis, hepatitis, and cirrhosis can be related to daily intake and duration. Most patients with cirrhosis drink regularly in excess of 80–120 g alcohol daily (equivalent to ⅓–½ a bottle of spirits). It probably takes 8–10 years of such drinking to produce cirrhosis. Women seem more susceptible than men and cirrhosis develops more rapidly. There is some evidence to suggest that steady ('inability to abstain') drinkers are more susceptible than binge ('loss of control') drinkers. Racial variability may account, in part, for the curious geographical inhomogeneity of alcohol liver disease (for example, the greater frequency of florid alcoholic hepatitis in the USA as compared with the United Kingdom).

There is no convincing evidence that the type of alcoholic drink is important, the small amounts of toxic congeners in beverages contributing little to the damage.

Individual susceptibility. The crux of the problem lies in individual response. Most, if not all, individuals exposed to moderate amounts of alcohol will show some abnormality, notable fatty change. This rapidly regresses with abstinence and there is no good evidence that, of itself, it is of any permanent significance. Heavy alcohol ingestion will, if the dose is large enough, probably produce a hepatitis in most people. It is puzzling why florid alcoholic hepatitis is such a rare clinical event considering the vast alcohol consumption, and indeed why irreversible disease is not universal among heavy drinkers.

A variety of both humoral and cell-mediated immunological phenomena are associated with alcoholic injury (Table 1) but their significance remains questionable. The consistency of these findings, especially in patients with hepatitis (and active cirrhosis) as compared with steatosis, certainly marks out hepatitis as an important 'immunological event'. The fact that cirrhosis may supervene

upon hepatitis, not simply when drinking continues, but also apparently in the setting of abstinence, suggests a self-perpetuation mechanism. It has been suggested that Mallory's hyaline may act as a neo-antigen and it does seem to be related in some way to the microtubule system. More evidence is required before it can be firmly concluded that these findings are pathogenetic rather than epiphenomena.

Fibrogenesis is a crucial factor in the development of cirrhosis. The Ito cells—potential fibroblasts—lurking in the sinusoids are important. Laying down of collagen along the spaces of Disse has the effect of converting the sinusoid from an open to a closed system thereby jepordizing the hepatocytes' nutritional supply. Pericellular fibrosis, death of cells with collapse of the stroma and formation of septa signal the development of cirrhosis. The mechanisms for initiation of collagen deposition and release of 'collagen-stimulating factors' are imperfectly understood. They may well be enhanced by some metabolic changes, notably lactacidaemia.

Great individual variation has led to the obvious speculation that genetic factors are responsible, either for susceptibility to toxic damage or to perpetuation, or both. There is no evidence that genetic variations in rates of alcohol metabolism are of significance. A search for association with known genetic markers such as blood groups has been unfruitful, but recently several workers have shown an association between irreversible liver damage and HLA status, mainly HLA-B8.

Further aetiological considerations. It remains entirely possible that alcoholic cirrhosis is multifactorial and that its development is associated with an independant factor, pre-existing or co-existing. This factor could be an environmental pollutant, food additive, virus, etc. The obvious candidate is hepatitis B virus which of itself produces cirrhosis in a small proportion of individuals. Recent work tends to confirm an earlier observation that serological evidence of previous hepatitis B infection is significantly commoner in patients with alcoholic hepatitis and cirrhosis than in alcohol abusers with normal or fatty livers.

Conclusions. It seems reasonable to conclude that alcohol is a predictable liver poison, regardless of nutritional state, which in some individuals leads to permanent damage. Irreversibility is, in part, an expression of individual endogenous response, probably mediated immunologically, and possibly of coexistent factors such as hepatitis B. Risk of cirrhosis is directly correlated with dose and duration of drinking.

Clinical features. Approximately one-third of heavy drinkers have no clinically significant liver disease. A further third have fatty liver, commonly symptomless and detected at routine examination. Of the remainder with hepatitis and cirrhosis, some will be detected incidentally but many present with the features of hepatocellular failure and portal hypertension.

Non-specific alimentary symptoms are the commonest forms of presentation. Mild or moderate right upper quadrant pain (and liver tenderness) is surprisingly common. Anorexia, early morning nausea, and diarrhoea reflect gastric and small bowel irritation.

Fluid retention is the presenting feature in about one in eight with cirrhosis. Oedema reflects the lowered plasma albumin but ascites also indicates portal hypertension and lymphatic obstruction. Sudden development of ascites suggests portal vein thrombosis which raises the spectre of hepatoma.

Jaundice has many facets. If mild, it suggests a well-compensated cirrhosis and occasionally occurs in simple fatty liver. Deep cholestasis is a major problem. In the established cirrhotic it is almost invariably a poor prognostic sign. In *acute alcoholic hepatitis* cholestasis may be combined with pain, fever, leucocytosis (sometimes of leukaemoid proportions), ascites, and variceal bleeding. It is easily mistaken for viral hepatitis or worse still for biliary obstruction when an unnecessary laparotomy can be fatal.

Cholestasis may also be due to gallstones (which occur at an

Table 1   Altered immune mechanisms in alcohol-induced liver disease

Increased susceptibility to infection
Humoral mechanisms
   Increase in IgA
   Bacterial antibodies
   Tissue antibodies—smooth muscle
   Hyaline antibodies
Cell-mediated mechanisms
   Loss of delayed hypersensitivity
   Inhibition of PHA lymphocyte transformation
   Decreased T-rosette formation
   Decreased circulating T cells
   Altered cell-mediated immunity to liver antigens
   Lymphocyte cytotoxicity

increased frequency in cirrhosis) and, occasionally, alcoholic pancreatitis. Rarely alcohol may cause intrahepatic cholestasis without evidence of hepatitis.

Hepatocellular necrosis contributes to the jaundice of hepatitis and very rarely submassive necrosis may be a cause of rapid death.

Haemolysis is occasionally seen in association with hyperlipaemia (Zieve's syndrome) (see Section 19).

Haematemesis is common. In a proportion, varying from 20 to 60 per cent according to different series, it is due to varices. Peptic ulcer, erosions, and Mallory–Weiss tears are common sources and endoscopy is usually required in management. Haemorrhagic diathesis due to liver damage and hypersplenism is common and epistaxis may be confused with gastric haemorrhage.

Encephalopathy carries a better prognosis in alcoholic compared with other forms of cirrhosis. Distinction from subdural haematoma and alcoholic dementia is important and CT scanning and EEG are valuable diagnostic tools.

Management. Successful treatment involves three steps: (*a*) recognition and diagnosis; (*b*) treatment; and (*c*) rehabilitation.

Recognition and diagnosis. *Recognition of liver disease.* Usually the liver is enlarged and palpable and may be tender. Signs of decompensation such as spider naevi, palmar erythema, telangiectasia, gynaecomastia, and testicular atrophy reflect hepatitis or cirrhosis. Occasionally a cirrhotic liver may be undetectable clinically and be associated with normal or near-normal liver chemistry. Liver biopsy is the surest diagnostic procedure and deserves wider employment. However, radionuclide and ultrasonic scanning are reasonably reliable indicators of parenchymal damage and ultrasound may distinguish fat from fibrosis.

Recognition of alcohol abuse. A high degree of awareness is required and many alcohol abusers go undetected even by their family practitioners. High risk groups include occupations with high stress levels, 'drinking culture', or exposure to alcohol (such as business executives, entertainers, seamen, lawyers, doctors, and those in the licensed trade) and divorcees, the middle-aged single male, and the socially deprived or misfit. Poor work performance, frequent job changes, broken homes, repeated accidents, and violent behaviour should all suggest alcohol abuse. Features of dependance should be sought for; these include amnesic attacks, fits, tremulousness, unexplained tachycardia and night sweats, loss of libido, and abnormal drinking patterns.

Other physical manifestations of alcohol abuse, such as macrocytic anaemia, cardiomyopathy, pseudo-Cushing's disease, peripheral neuropathy, and Wernicke–Korsakoff syndromes, are helpful pointers.

Laboratory screening tests are useful. Raised mean corpuscular volume and macrocytosis are very frequent and sensitive and may persist long after drinking ceases. Raised γ-glutamyl transpeptidase is sensitive but more transient. Uric acid may be raised. Aminotransferases are less reliable indicants.

Treatment. *General measures.* Malnutrition results from penury, anorexia, vomiting, and malabsorption (due to pancreatic and small bowel damage). Folate and thiamine deficiencies are common. In the advanced cirrhotic wasting may be extreme. A high protein intake, provided encephalopathy is watched for, is advisable and the B group vitamins should be given parenterally.

Hypoglycaemia is an important complication especially following a binge. Hypomagnesaemia and hypokalaemia (even in the absence of diuretics) may occur and should be treated appropriately.

Opportunistic infections, such as Gram-negative septicaemia and infected ascites, are common and should be routinely sought. A chest X-ray to exclude tuberculosis is also important.

Major features of withdrawal such as fits and delirium tremens should be managed as described in Section 24. Chlormethiazole is the drug of choice, given either by titratable slow intravenous infusion or orally: 2–6 g day, to be reduced over two to three weeks. Chlordiazepoxide is the best alternative. Precipitating factors should be sought for and causes of confusion or coma other than withdrawal rigorously excluded; these include subdural haemorrhage, hepatic encephalopathy, and Wernicke's syndrome (Table 2).

Table 2 Hepatic encephalopathy and other alcohol-associated conditions

Feature	Hepatic encephalopathy	Withdrawal syndrome	Wernicke's syndrome	Subdural haemorrhage
Conscious level	lowered	heightened	variable	fluctuating
Anxiety	−	+	−	−
Hallucinations	−	+	+	−
Speech	slurred	rapid	slurred	normal
Pulse	normal	very rapid	rapid	slow

Specific therapy. Generally this has proved disappointing. The high mortality of hepatitis has prompted trials of corticosteroids with equivocal results in the dozen studies reported. They may be of value in severe hepatitis with encephalopathy, especially in females. It seems logical to use them in those patients with a chronic active hepatitis picture. Prevention of progression by penicillamine or colchicine is currently under trial (Table 3).

Table 3 Treatment of patients with alcoholic liver disease

Nutrition	
Usually poor; beware saline infusions (e.g. during surgery)	High protein diet, except where signs of encephalopathy Limited salt intake: in cirrhosis 'no added salt'; in the presence of ascites, dietician-supervised 20 mmol sodium diet Vitamin replacement: 5 days high potency polyvitamin injection (i.m. or i.v.) Oral folic acid 15 mg/day Vitamin K 10 mg i.m. × 3 doses Long-term oral vitamin B group replacement
Withdrawal	
Watch for from 1–9 days after removal of alcohol	Severe cases: i.v. chlormethiazole 1–2 mg/min through Y-connection Mild cases: oral chlormethiazole days 1–3: 1.5 g 3 times daily days 4–6: 1.0 g 3 times daily days 7–9: 0.5 g 3 times daily *or* chlordiazepoxide 5–10 mg 3 times daily
Fits	
Check electrolytes, CT brain scan where appropriate, and CSF	i.v. diazepam (with respiratory support available), occasionally phenytoin
Opportunistic infections	
Culture urine, blood, ascitic fluid, and, if appropriate, CSF	Broad spectrum antibiotics of low toxity, e.g. ampicillin
Specific therapy (alcoholic hepatitis)	
Especially in women with encephalopathy and prolonged prothrombin time	Prednisolone 40 mg/day for 2–6 weeks; then gradually withdraw

Rehabilitation. Crucial to the management of many patients is the maintenance of abstinence, although in those with less severe damage who are not addicted there is a case for controlled drinking. A few patients require formal psychiatric care; many will benefit from long-term support from family practitioners and agencies such as Alcoholics Anonymous, Councils on Alcoholism, and social work services (see Section 24).

Prognosis. For the many patients with mild or moderate disease (fatty liver) the prognosis is good if they can stop drinking. Frank hepatitis has a significant mortality and survival in this group is affected by abstinence (being in one series at seven years 80 per cent in abstainers and only 50 per cent in continuing drinkers). Similarly, with established cirrhosis medium-term survival is doubled by abstinence. However, some features, notably haemorrhage and deep jaundice, imply a very poor prognosis regardless of abstinence. In a recent British survey of deaths under 50 years, one-quarter of the patients with non-traumatic alcohol-related deaths had died within a month of first recognition.

Prevention of alcohol related disease depends primarily on sensible drinking habits, development of healthy social and cultural attitudes in communities, and upon careful application of fiscal and legal constraints on consumption.

References

Lieber, C. S. (ed.) (1977). *Metabolic aspects of alcoholism*. MTP Press, Lancaster.

Marks, V. and Wright, J. (eds.) (1978). Metabolic effects of alcohol. *Clin. Endocr. Metab.* **17**, no. 2.

Mowat, N. A. G. and Brunt, P. (1976). Alcohol and the gastrointestinal tract. In *Recent advances in gastroenterology* (ed. I. A. D. Bouchier), 150. Churchill Livingstone, Edinburgh.

Nicholson, G. (1980). Alcoholic liver disease. In *Medical consequences of alcohol abuse* (eds. P. M. S. Clarke and L. J. Kricka), 51. Ellis Horwood, Chichester.

Drugs and liver damage

J. M. Trowell

The liver is a major site of drug metabolism and many drugs or their metabolites are excreted in the bile. In addition, many drugs affect the metabolism of liver cells. The alteration in metabolic patterns induced by a drug may not cause irreversible cell damage and the changes may revert when the drug is stopped. On the other hand such chaos may be induced within the mitochondria and endoplasmic reticulum that irreversible structural damage and cell necrosis follows. The clinical manifestations of drug-induced liver damage can mimic many forms of liver disease, although particular patterns of clinical and pathological changes are recognized and associated with certain drugs or groups of drugs (Table 1). Drugs which cause forms of chronic hepatitis are considered on page 12.208; those which cause acute hepatic failure are described on page 12.198.

Table 1 Patterns of liver damage caused by different drugs

Clinical pathological changes	Drugs
Hepatic necrosis	paracetamol methotrexate

Hepatitis
  acute
  chronic
  proceeding to cirrhosis
	halothane
	methyldopa
	oxyphenisatin
	antituberculosis drugs

Cholestasis	chlorpromazine methyltestosterone oral contraceptives
Granulomatous hepatitis	phenylbutazone allopurinol
Thrombosis/obstruction of hepatic and portal veins	oral contraceptives busulphan
Hepatic fibrosis/sclerosis of portal venules	arsenic

The effect of liver failure on drug metabolism. Liver disease may alter drug metabolism in several ways which include changes in plasma binding by reducing serum protein levels, reducing the rate of clearance by decreasing hepatic blood flow or causing cholestasis, or by direct cell damage leading to a decreased ability to metabolize the drug. These effects are unpredictable and do not correlate well with the degree of liver damage as assessed by

biochemical tests of liver function. However, in any patient with liver disease it is important to bear in mind the possibility that toxic levels of drugs or their metabolites may occur at dosages which would be perfectly safe in a patient with normal liver function (see Section 7, page 7.12, Table 11).

Mechanisms of liver damage. Some drugs are predictably hepatotoxic. They produce damage to the liver in all patients who receive a high enough dose, although there may be considerable variation in the dose which is required to produce a toxic effect in an individual patient. Such liver damage is also produced in many animals and the mechanism of the damage can be defined. The toxic agent may be a metabolite and it is only when particular conditions exist, such as a dose adequate to saturate the normal metabolic pathways, that the toxic metabolite appears and damage occurs. This explains why higher doses may produce liver damage while 'therapeutic doses' do not. Paracetamol (acetaminophen or *N*-acetyl *p*-aminophenol) produces hepatic necrosis only in high doses when toxic metabolites are formed. The severity of liver damage following the ingestion of a large dose of paracetamol can be reduced by infusions of cysteamine, acetylcysteine, or methiamine which alter the relative amounts of the drug metabolized by different routes and thus reduce the amount of toxic metabolites produced.

Not all drugs behave as predictably as this. Liver damage may occur after small doses of a drug in some patients, and not at all after prolonged high dose in others. These drugs and their toxic effects can rarely be studied in animal models and the mechanism of this type of toxicity is poorly understood. However, the pattern of illness and the hepatic histology in those patients who are affected are often sufficiently characteristic for a particular drug or group of drugs for the association to be recognized. These unpredictable side-effects are sometimes called 'sensitivity' reactions and some markers of hypersensitivity, such as elevated blood eosinophil counts or an increase in eosinophils in the liver, may be found in some instances, but often a typical hypersensitivity reaction cannot be recognized and the term is best avoided. The individual variability in toxic reactions to these drugs may be related to some extent to genetic variations in metabolic pathways of drug metabolism within the liver but, since a family history is a poor predictor of hepatic drug toxicity, other factors must be involved. Previous exposure to enzyme-inducing agents may play a significant part and may influence the levels of toxic metabolites produced, as may, for example, renal disease which may prevent the renal excretion of a drug and cause its accumulation in liver cells.

Interactions of drugs. Many drugs produce enzyme induction in the liver cells and while this is not strictly a toxic effect, as there is no structural damage to the cell, it can have significant clinical implications by altering the metabolism and therefore the effects of other drugs administered at the same time (see Section 7). This is most frequently seen in patients who have regularly drunk significant quantities of alcohol and who then become resistant to the sedative effects of other drugs, but it may also occur in patients on regular medication with barbiturates and many other agents.

The importance of correct diagnosis. The detection of liver damage and its attribution to a particular drug, are both important as damage may become chronic and irreversible if the drug is continued indefinitely, but the changes will often remit with complete regeneration of the liver if the drug is discontinued. Re-exposure to a toxic drug may also produce more serious, or fatal, illness while an initial exposure had produced only a brief, trivial illness. If a drug is not suspected as the cause of liver damage, and an incorrect diagnosis made, especially in patients with pronounced cholestasis, an inappropriate laparotomy can precipitate liver failure.

The recognition of drug-related liver damage. Whatever the mechanism of the damage to the liver, the diagnosis is only made by a clinician who suspects that a drug may be responsible for liver damage and elicits a full and accurate drug history. The patient may be poorly informed about his medication, or may have forgotten drugs which have been taken in the recent past but not at the time of interview. The patient may be too ill to provide a full history and the responsibility for the patient's care may have changed to different doctors with the presentation of a liver problem. The time over which the drug history should be checked must vary with the chronicity of the process involved; in acute damage any drug started during the month before the onset of the symptoms is suspect, while in some cases a drug may have been taken for years before liver toxicity is manifest.

The pattern of liver injury may be well recognized and characteristic of a particular drug or group of drugs and exposure to these can be specifically sought. But in a patient who is receiving drugs, new drugs, or those less often used are more likely to have unrecognized side-effects and to be the cause of the liver damage. However, the incrimination of a particular drug is often difficult and all non-essential drug therapy should be discontinued to allow recovery and regeneration to occur. In most patients alternative drugs can be given without difficulty but in a few with the need for recurrent or long-term exposure to a particular drug, a direct challenge may be justified.

In other circumstances it may be difficult to show that a drug is hepatotoxic. This may be related to long-term administration of the drug and the chronicity and insidious onset of the symptoms. In these patients an awareness of the drug therapy and exclusion of any other cause may suggest the association but this is often difficult to prove. The fact that a patient improves when a drug is discontinued may be entirely fortuitous but continuation of the drug is rarely justified once the association is suspected. Systems of reporting of drug-associated reactions may accumulate case reports and strengthen the suspicion that a drug is toxic to the liver. A drug which is frequently prescribed may produce severe toxicity only rarely and this may therefore not be recognized as related to the drug exposure. Further confusion occurs if many therapeutic agents are given within a few days as at the time of a surgical operation with a general anaesthetic. The prolonged controversy as to whether the anaesthetic halothane was hepatotoxic is an example of the difficulties in showing the toxicity of a particular drug. The toxic reaction attributed to halothane mimicked viral hepatitis, and only prospective randomized control trials could show that the liver damage occurred more often after halothane used repeatedly than after other commonly used anaesthetics.

Clinical diagnosis of liver damage due to drugs. A patient whose liver has been damaged by drugs may become jaundiced or, if the damage is more acute, may present with features of hepatic encephalopathy and fulminating liver failure. Those with a more chronic illness or an obstruction to the portal or hepatic circulation may develop abdominal distension with hepatosplenomegaly and ascites and other complications of portal hypertension such as bleeding from oesophageal varices.

Now patients are monitored with frequent automated laboratory tests, elevation of the bilirubin, alkaline phosphatase, and serum transaminases may be detected without the patient being aware of any alteration in his symptoms. These biochemical changes frequently indicate early liver damage and in a patient who is being treated with potentially hepatotoxic drugs, it is unreasonable to continue the drugs to await more serious effects. However, if the underlying disease may also affect the liver function test, more precise diagnosis may be required. The pattern and timing of the abnormalities may be characteristic, but X-ray, isotope, and ultrasound scanning, and liver histology obtained by needle biopsy, may be required. Although the liver histology in drug-induced liver damage is never unique to a particular drug, the patterns associated with various forms of liver damage are sufficiently different for the different types of drugs for this to be diagnostically valuable. It can also be valuable to obtain liver histology where there is doubt as to whether the abnormalities are drug-induced or related to some other underlying pathology for which the drug was prescribed. If there is damage to the liver due to drugs, the risk of delaying diagnosis or of introducing other inappropriate therapy more than justifies pursuing the diagnosis by invasive techniques when the diagnosis would otherwise be obscure or delayed.

Some specific examples of agents which cause liver damage. Poisoning due to agents such as carbon tetrachloride and phenacetin are described in Section 7, and injury to the liver due to the effects of alcohol is discussed on page 12.209. Although many drugs can cause liver damage, there are some which are worthy of special mention because of the frequency of the reaction or the severity of their effects (Table 1).

Androgens. Methyl testosterone and related C-17 alkyl substituted corticosteroids frequently cause intrahepatic cholestasis with jaundice. This is rapidly reversible after withdrawing the drug.

Oral contraceptives. The possible association between the use of oral contraceptives and the Budd–Chiari syndrome was mentioned earlier (see page 12.193). These agents occasionally cause a cholestatic jaundice. There may be an association between the occurrence of benign adenomas of the liver, primary hepatocellular carcinoma, and oral contraceptives.

Antituberculosis drugs. Although some evidence of biochemical liver damage occurs in about one-fifth of patients receiving antituberculosis drugs, symptomatic illness is seen in less than 1 per cent of patients receiving these drugs.

Reactions occur in patients receiving rifampicin, para-aminosalicylic acid, and isoniazid.

Chlorpromazine. A small proportion of patients who receive chlorpromazine develop an obstructive jaundice. The condition usually regresses after stopping the drug, although a disorder resembling primary biliary cirrhosis has been described as a sequel to this complication.

Halothane anaesthesia. Although there has been considerable debate about the hepatic toxicity of halothane, it is now accepted that hepatitis can follow exposure to this agent. It occurs more commonly if several anaesthetics follow at close intervals, and in those patients liver failure may occur. Recovery is usually complete and the course resembles that of a viral hepatitis.

Methyldopa. Hepatitis occurs occasionally in patients receiving methyldopa. Although full recovery usually occurs after stopping the drug, there have been several well-documented cases of progressive liver failure and the development of cirrhosis.

Other hepatic disorders related to drug therapy are summarized on pages 12.198 and 12.208.

References

Sherlock, S. (1972). Liver disease due to drugs. In *Drug induced disease* (ed. L. Meyler and H. M. Peck). Excerpta Medica Foundation, Amsterdam.

— (1981). *Diseases of the liver and biliary system*, 6th edn. Blackwell Scientific Publications, Oxford.

Zimmerman, M. J. (1978). The adverse effects of drugs and other chemicals on the liver. In *Hepatotoxicity*, 357. Appleton-Century-Crofts, New York.

Liver tumours

I. M. Murray-Lyon

Benign and malignant tumours may arise in the liver from the hepatocytes, bile duct epithelium, or supporting mesenchymal tissue. With the exception of hepatocellular carcinoma all the primary malignant tumours are rare but the liver is frequently the site of secondary (metastatic) deposits of malignant tumours elsewhere in the body.

Hepatocellular carcinoma. This occurs either as a single mass or as scattered nodules of tumour and in around 80 per cent patients there is pre-existing cirrhosis. The tumour tends to invade the portal and hepatic veins and spread occurs to the abdominal lymph nodes, lungs, and bones. Histologically the tumour is typically composed of cells resembling hepatocytes which are arranged in cords but a number of other distinct histological subtypes are now recognized.

Epidemiology. Although this is a comparatively rare tumour in Western Europe and North America where the annual incidence is around 1–2 per 100 000 population, it seems to be becoming more common, and in Africa and Southeast Asia the incidence is 20–30 times higher. The highest annual incidence is recorded in Mozambique (98 per 100 000 males). In patients with underlying cirrhosis males greatly outnumber females but in non-cirrhotic cases this sex difference is less striking. In areas of high incidence the peak age is in the third and fourth decades but in Europe and North America most cases occur in the fifth and sixth decades.

Aetiology. In all countries of the world cirrhosis, particularly the macronodular form, is present in about 80 per cent cases and in Western Europe and USA this is due usually to chronic alcoholism or chronic active hepatitis and at least 10–15 per cent such patients will develop a hepatocellular carcinoma. In Africa and Asia the chronic liver disease is usually associated with hepatitis B virus infection and the percentage of these patients who develop this tumour is probably higher than in other types of cirrhosis. Rare cases may follow prolonged use of the oral contraceptive pill or prior investigations using the radioactive contrast agent Thorotrast. In parts of Africa and the Far East there is circumstantial evidence implicating aflatoxin. This is a potent carcinogen derived from the mould *Aspergillus flavus* which often contaminates food, and a number of field surveys have shown a correlation between aflatoxin levels in food and the incidence of hepatocellular carcinoma.

The hepatitis B virus (HBV) is now strongly suspected to have an important role in the development of hepatocellular carcinoma especially in areas of high incidence. Evidence comes from several lines including the similar geographic distribution of areas of high prevalence of the HBV and hepatocellular carcinoma, and viral markers of HBV infection are found in a substantially higher proportion of patients with the tumour than in matched controls. Recent long-term follow-up studies of large numbers of HBV carriers have confirmed that the risk of developing hepatocellular carcinoma is much higher than in matched uninfected controls. The HBV can be identified in tumour as well as the surrounding liver and integration of viral DNA in the genome of hepatocellular carcinoma has recently been shown.

Clinical features. In Africa and other high incidence areas the patients usually present with a short history of right upper abdominal pain, often associated with fever and weight loss. There may be considerable abdominal swelling due to liver enlargement with or without ascites. Sometimes catastrophic intraperitoneal bleeding occurs due to tumour rupture. In low incidence areas the disease is often more insidious and presents as a general deterioration in health of a patient already known to have cirrhosis. There is usually hepatomegaly and a bruit may be heard over the liver. A number of non-metastatic systemic manifestations may also rarely occur such as hypoglycaemia, hypercalcaemia, and prophyria cutanea tarda.

Investigations. The haematological and biochemical changes apart from alpha-fetoprotein are non-specific and reflect the space occupying lesion as well as the underlying cirrhosis present in about 80 per cent of cases.

Alpha-fetoprotein is a glycoprotein synthesized by fetal liver and plasma levels reach their maximum at the end of the first trimester (3–4 mg/ml) and then decline. After birth concentrations fall rapidly to adult levels (1–10 ng/ml). Raised levels are found in about 80 per cent of patients with hepatocellular carcinoma and tend to be higher in those in Africa and Far East than in the low incidence areas. Levels above 1000 ng/ml in a patient with liver disease are highly suggestive of hepatocellular carcinoma but in interpreting alpha fetoprotein values it should be remembered that high plasma levels are found in some patients with germinal cell tumours of the testis and ovary as well as occasional patients with carcinoma of the stomach or pancreas, usually with hepatic metastases. Below 1000 ng/ml there is a diagnostic 'grey zone', for such levels may be found in patients with severe viral hepatitis and active cirrhosis, but in these conditions subsequent readings tend to fall towards normal whereas in patients with hepatocellular carcinoma the levels rise exponentially. Sequential readings are therefore of great diagnostic value.

Other tumour markers for hepatocellular carcinoma have been described in the serum including an abnormal vitamin B_{12} binding protein, and tumour specific alkaline phosphatase and ferritin.

Liver imaging

Radioisotope scintiscanning. The liver image using $^{99}Tc^{m}$-sulphur colloid is abnormal in 80–90 per cent patients but in many it is difficult to know whether or not a hepatocellular carcinoma is superimposed on the uneven pattern of colloid uptake due to cirrhosis. Subsequent scanning with ^{75}Se-selenomethionine may be useful (Fig. 1). For technical reasons tumours of less than 2 cm in diameter cannot be detected by scintiscanning.

Grey scale ultrasound of the liver is a useful adjunct to scintiscanning and picks up hepatocellar carcinoma in 80–90 per cent cases. It will not detect small tumours in a cirrhotic liver and visualization of the left lobe is often difficult.

Abdominal CT scanning. This technique is probably no more accurate in detecting hepatocellular carcinoma than scintiscanning and ultrasound and should be reserved for cases in which doubt persists.

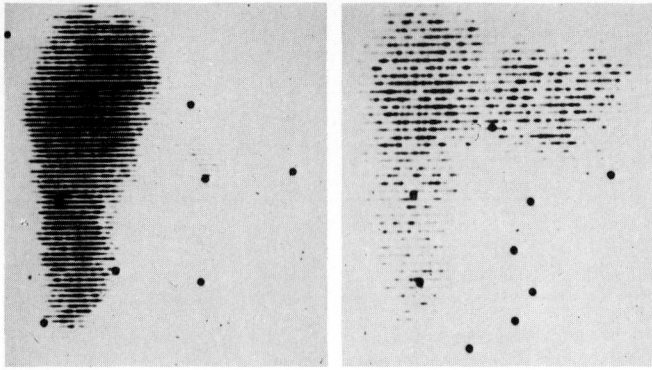

Fig. 1   Liver scan on left using technetium ($^{99}Tc^m$) sulphur colloid shows a filling defect in the left lobe. The scan on the right on the same patient after ^{75}Se-selenomethionine shows uptake into the liver and the area of the filling defect. The presence of hepatocellular carcinoma in the left lobe was confirmed on biopsy.

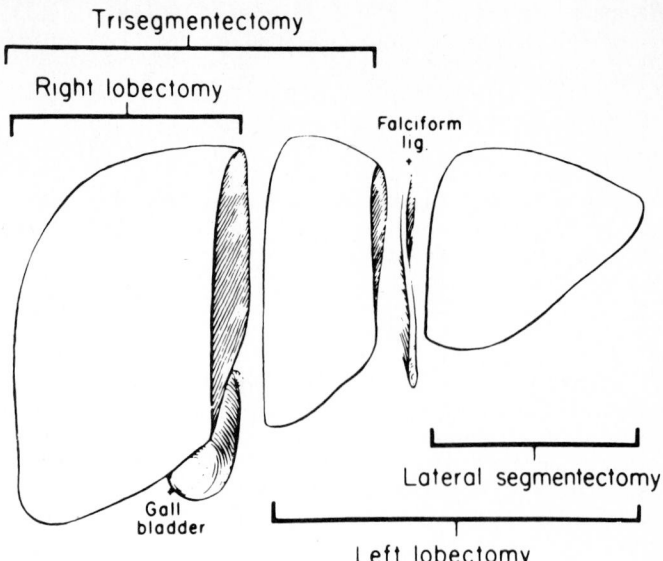

Fig. 2   Diagram to illustrate the main types of hepatic resection.

Hepatic arteriography. Excellent visualization of the hepatic artery can usually be obtained by selective catheterization using the Seldinger technique. As the major vascular supply to hepatocellular carcinoma is usually arterial, diagnostic changes are seen in a high proportion of cases. Information gained on the anatomical distribution of the tumour and the vascular anatomy is essential if surgical resection is being contemplated, and consideration can also be given at the time of arteriography to intra-arterial chemotherapy and hepatic artery embolization.

Liver biopsy. For definitive diagnosis liver biopsy is essential, although this is not always possible because of prolongation of the prothrombin time. The diagnosis can be considered highly likely without liver biopsy proof if the alpha fetoprotein level is greater than 1000 ng/ml and the hepatic arteriogram shows a tumour circulation. Biopsy may be conveniently performed at the time of laparoscopy and suspicious areas can be sampled under direct vision.

Prognosis. This is usually a highly malignant tumour and the mean survival in most series is around four months. In Africa the disease tends to run a more malignant course. Patients with encapsulated tumours and those with a special histological pattern (fibrolamellar) have a better prognosis.

Treatment. *Curative.* Only complete resection and orthotopic transplantation hold out any chance of cure and these procedures should be considered in every case. Resection is possible, however, in only about 10 per cent of cases because of underlying cirrhosis or spread to both lobes. In the presence of cirrhosis a limited resection only is possible as liver regeneration is defective but this procedure may be curative if the tumour is small. Usually a more major resection is needed and the anatomical possibilities are illustrated (Fig. 2). Many prolonged survivals are recorded following surgery. There are also some long-term survivors after transplantation but all too often micrometastases are present at the time of operation and tumour recurrence later occurs.

Palliation. X-irradiation alone has not produced consistent improvement and results are no better when used in combination with the cytotoxic drugs so far available.

Adriamycin (doxorubicin) is the only cytotoxic drug tried so far which has produced worthwhile regression but only 20–30 per cent of cases respond. It is given intravenously as a bolus every three weeks in a dose of 60 mg/m². The total dose is usually limited to 540 mg/m² because of cardiotoxicity, and the only other significant side-effects are hair loss and marrow depression. In patients with raised plasma alpha fetoprotein levels the response can be gauged after one or two courses by the change in alpha fetoprotein levels. These fall in patients with responsive tumours and there is no point in continuing adriamycin treatment in patients in whom the levels

are unchanged or rise and an alternative drug such as 5-fluorouracil may be tried.

Intra-arterial cytotoxic therapy may be given via an indwelling catheter in the hepatic artery. This approach has the advantage of delivering high concentrations of the drug into the tumour and, as adriamycin and other cytotoxic drugs are metabolized by the liver, systemic toxicity may be less. Side-effects such as catheter displacement, occlusion of the hepatic artery, and sopticaemia are troublesome, however, and this method of treatment has not yet been shown to improve the survival statistics.

Embolization of the hepatic artery with foreign material such as gelatin foam can be achieved at the time of hepatic arteriography and may result in substantial tumour necrosis particularly in highly vascular tumours which derive the bulk of their blood supply from the hepatic artery. In patients with cirrhosis and those with portal vein occlusion the procedure is more hazardous and embolization should be limited to the branches of the hepatic artery supplying the tumour. Total occlusion of the hepatic arterial vasculature should be avoided. Broad spectrum antibiotics are given for some days because of the risk of anaerobic infection in the ischaemic liver. Tumour necrosis is never complete and embolization of the tumour should be followed by chemotherapy.

Cholangiocarcinoma. Carcinoma may arise in the biliary tree in any part from the small intrahepatic bile ducts down to the lower end of the common bile duct. Two clinical varieties occur in the liver—a peripheral form which consists of multiple nodules often scattered throughout both lobes, and a hilar form usually situated at the confluence of the right and left hepatic ducts. This invades locally and causes obstruction of the biliary tree. Microscopically it is an adenocarcinoma with a simple ductular arrangement of columnar or cuboidal cells usually with a prominent fibrous stroma and the histological appearances are identical whatever the site of origin.

Epidemiology. This tumour is much less common than hepatocellular carcinoma and accounts for about 7–10 per cent of primary malignant tumours, except in the Far East where it makes up about 20 per cent. The peak age is in the sixth and seventh decades and is older than for hepatocellular carcinoma. The sex incidence shows only a slight male predominance.

Aetiology. Thorium dioxide (Thorotrast) is a well-recognized but rare cause of the intrahepatic variety of tumour. In the Far East infestation with one of a variety of distomes (*Clonorchis sinensis; Opisthorchis viverrini*) is probably commonly related for patients with intrahepatic cholangiocarcinoma are parasitized more frequently than matched controls and the tumours are usually found close to the heavily parasitized second order bile ducts close to the hilum. Patients with long-standing ulcerative colitis occasionally develop carcinoma in the biliary tract and the risk is about 10 times greater than for the general population. Patients with total involvement of the colon of more than 10 years duration are the ones usually affected and the tumour may develop some years after panproctocolectomy. Either the intra- or extrahepatic biliary tree may be affected. Various types of cystic disease of the biliary tree such as congenital hepatic fibrosis, polycystic disease of the liver, and Caroli's disease may all be complicated by the development of malignant change. The role of gallstones has been emphasized in the aetiology of extrahepatic cholangiocarcinoma but the association does not necessarily indicate causation. Unlike hepatocellular carcinoma neither long-standing hepatitis B virus infection nor cirrhosis seem to predispose to cholangiocarcinoma but secondary biliary cirrhosis may develop due to prolonged biliary obstruction.

Symptoms and signs. In the peripheral intrahepatic type patients present with upper abdominal pain, anorexia, malaise, and weight loss. With hilar tumours jaundice is an early feature. Hepatomegaly is usual and splenomegaly may be found if secondary biliary cirrhosis develops.

Diagnosis. The liver function tests show cholestatic features with elevation of bilirubin and alkaline phosphatase. Alpha-fetoprotein levels are usually normal or only slightly raised and tests for hepatitis BB virus infection are negative.

Radioisotope scintiscanning may show hilar or intrahepatic filling defects and these do not take up ^{75}Se-selenomethionine. Ultrasonography and CT scanning may demonstrate the tumour mass and with hilar tumours show dilatation of the intrahepatic biliary tree. On hepatic angiography the tumour tends to be avascular but encasement and occlusion of vessels occurs. Biliary tree obstruction in the hilum may be demonstrated by percutaneous transhepatic cholangiography using the skinny (Chiba) needle or by endoscopic retrograde cholangiography (ERCP).

Prognosis. Most patients deteriorate progressively with average survival from diagnosis around four to six months. If biliary drainage can be achieved in patients with hilar tumours, the prognosis is considerably better, for these tumours are often slow growing.

Treatment. For the peripheral tumours the principles of treatment are the same as for hepatocellular carcinoma (see above) but the response to chemotherapy with adriamycin is disappointing. A variety of different drug combination with or without radiotherapy are being tried but none can currently be recommended.

Hilar tumours may sometimes be resectable with re-anastomosis of the biliary tree or anastomosis of a Roux loop of jejunum to the biliary tree in the hilum. If curative excision is not possible, the aim must be to establish biliary drainage. A polythene tube can be placed through the growth at laparotomy, or more recently, via the percutaneous trans-hepatic route, thus avoiding surgery. Conventional radiotherapy may also produce useful symptomatic relief, and recently high dose local irradiation has been given within the biliary tree by means of iridium-192 wire. Excellent palliation can be achieved by these procedures and survival for one to two years is not unusual.

Angiosarcoma. (*Kupffer cell sarcoma; malignant haemangioendothelioma*). This is a rare tumour consisting of malignant endothelial cells supported on a reticulin framework. It is often multifocal and may arise in a cirrhotic liver.

Considerable progress has been made in identifying aetiological agents. Like hepatocellular carcinoma and cholangiocarcinoma, it

occurs in patients who were exposed to Thorotrast 15–25 years earlier, and chronic exposure to arsenic has also been implicated. More recently the tumour has been found in workers in the vinyl chloride industry, particularly those exposed to high concentrations of vinyl chloride monomer while cleaning the autoclaves. Since this discovery strict safety regulations have been introduced but because of the long latent period new cases continue to present. A few cases have occurred in long-term androgen takers but in the majority of patients no aetiologic factor has yet been identified.

As with other liver tumours patients present with abdominal pain and hepatic enlargement and blood-stained ascites is common.

This is a highly malignant tumour and curative resection is rarely possible. No form of palliative treatment has so far proved effective.

Other primary malignant tumours. These are extremely rare and include fibrosarcoma, leiomyosarcoma, and lymphoma. Children develop both hepatoblastoma and hepatocellular carcinoma. The former usually occurs in the first two years of life and the latter after the age of five. Both are frequently associated with raised alpha-fetoprotein levels. Resection may be curative.

Hepatic metastases. The liver is a favoured site for metastatic spread and about 50 per cent of malignant tumours in the portal venous drainage area eventually give rise to hepatic metastases.

Diagnosis. The diagnosis is easy when physical examination reveals a large nodular liver but detection of small or solitary deposits is difficult. Liver function tests may be normal, but as the tumour mass enlarges, the alkaline phosphatase usually rises. Liver scintiscanning should pick up tumours greater than 2 cm in diameter but false positive and negative scans are common. Accuracy is greatest when the metastases are large and numerous. In one large autopsy study metastatic deposits were all less than 2 cm in diameter in one-third of the cases. The diagnostic accuracy of ultrasonagraphy is similar to scintiscanning. 'Blind' liver biopsy is positive in only about 50 per cent of cases but accuracy can be greatly increased by target biopsy at the time of laparoscopy.

Prognosis. The prognosis is obviously worse when there is extensive liver replacement by tumour with severe disturbance in liver function tests or ascites. The site of the primary growth is also relevant and deposits from colorectal cancer have a better prognosis (untreated mean survival 9–12 months) than most other tumours, especially if the deposits first appear some years after resection of the primary.

Treatment. The range of possible treatments is the same as has been discussed for hepatocellular carcinoma. Partial hepatectomy to remove a solitary deposit may occasionally lead to prolonged survival or cure and the results are best in patients with colorectal cancer. The number of cases, however, with solitary deposits suitable for resection is small. A special situation exists with respect to hepatic metastases from the carcinoid tumour (see page 12.55). This is often a slowly growing neoplasm and the main problem is the distress caused by flushing and diarrhoea. Resection of tumour bulk without any attempt at total removal often gives symptomatic relief for some years.

Chemotherapy. The choice of drugs will be determined by the origin of the primary tumour and this will not be discussed in detail here. The most common drug used for deposits from gastrointestinal cancer is 5-fluorouracil but responses are infrequent (10–15 per cent) and short lasting. There is some indication that the results are better when 5-fluorouracil is combined with methyl CCNU, with or without vincristine.

As with hepatocellular carcinoma the poor results with systemic chemotherapy led to trials with intra-arterial perfusion. While objective tumour regression may occur, there is as yet no certain evidence that survival is prolonged and the technique cannot be recommended for general application.

Ligation of the hepatic artery at laparotomy or embolization at the time of hepatic arteriography by the Seldinger technique is best reserved for patients with severe pain due to their metastases. It may produce tumour shrinkage and give pain relief for a time.

X-irradiation may also give good palliation in some cases and should be considered when pain is troublesome. It can be combined with cytotoxic drugs.

Benign tumours

Haemangioma. This is the commonest benign tumour and is usually asymptomatic being found incidentally at laparotomy or autopsy. Occasionally it may cause abdominal pain or shock due to rupture. Rarely it may be associated with thrombocytopenia, hypofibrinogenaemia, or micro-angiopathic haemolytic anaemia.

A similar tumour also occurs in infants and usually presents before the age of six months with cardiac failure secondary to the arteriovenous shunt. Many of these tumours regress as the child develops but if symptoms are troublesome, involution may be speeded by corticosteroids or X-irradiation. Ligation of the hepatic artery which feeds the angioma may be needed as a life saving measure.

Hepatic adenoma. The incidence of this tumour seems to have increased markedly since the introduction of the oral contraceptive pill and most reported cases have occurred in females who have been on the pill for five years or more. It should be emphasized, however, that the risk for the individual woman is infinitessimal. Patients are often asymptomatic and a mass is discovered on physical examination but some complain of upper abdominal pain and others present acutely with shock due to intraperitoneal bleeding. The tumour is usually solitary but may be multiple and it consists of cords or acini of hepatocytes without bile ducts or portal tracts and fibrous tissue septa are sparse. It may be encapsulated. There is little or no disturbance in liver function and alpha fetoprotein levels are normal. A filling defect is seen on the isotope scan and hepatic arteriography demonstrates a highly vascular mass. In some cases the tumour has regressed after withdrawal of the pill but surgical resection is usually recommended because of the risk of intraperitoneal bleeding and the occasional development of malignant change.

Focal nodular hyperplasia. This is a benign condition of uncertain pathogenesis which is frequently confused with the hepatic adenoma. It is much more frequent in women than men but no relationship to the contraceptive pill has been established. The liver mass is usually solitary and is divided into nodules by bile duct containing fibrous tissue septa which radiate out from a central focus. It is usually asymptomatic but rupture with intraperitoneal bleeding occasionally occurs. The findings on investigation are closely similar to those for a hepatic adenoma. The prognosis is excellent and malignant change is not recorded. Surgical excision is usually recommended, however, for diagnostic certainty.

Other benign tumours. These are very much rarer and include fibroma, lipoma, leiomyoma, and cystadenoma.

References

Cameron, H. M., Linsell, C. A., and Warwick, G. P. (eds.) (1976). *Liver cell cancer*. Elsevier, Amsterdam.
Foster, J. H. and Berman, M. M. (1977). *Solid liver tumours*. W. B. Saunders, Philadelphia.
Klatskin, G. (1977). Hepatic tumors: Possible relationship to use of oral contraceptives. *Gastroent.* **73**, 386.
Lee, Y.-T. N. (1978). Nonsystemic treatment of metastatic tumors of the liver—a review. *Med. pediat. Oncol.* **4**, 185.
Murray-Lyon, I. M. (1981). Primary and secondary cancer of the Liver. In *Carcinoma of the liver, biliary tract and pancreas* (ed. J. C. Gazet). Arnold, London.
Okuda, K. and Peters, R. K. (eds.) (1976). *Hepatocellular carcinoma*. Wiley, New York.

Infections of the Liver

S. G. Wright

The specific infections which involve the liver are described in detail under the heading of each individual organism in Section 5. In the brief account which follows the clinical aspects of the different forms of infection of the liver are summarized so that the clinician is able to gain some insight into the range of different clinical presentations of liver infection and of the types of organisms which are associated with particular clinical pictures. This section should be read in conjunction with the description of the specific infectious diseases in Section 5.

Infections causing fever and hepatitis. The *hepatitis viruses, A, B, and non-A, non-B* are the organisms which infect the liver most frequently (see also page 12.195). When patients present in the prodomal phase of the illness with fever, anorexia, and sweats, viral hepatitis is only one of a considerable range of causes. Defervescence occurs when the patient becomes jaundiced and the diagnosis is usually obvious. In contrast there are a number of viral infections which may involve the liver and cause hepatomegaly with abnormal liver function tests and persisting fever. Jaundice is not a usual feature. Infections with the *Epstein–Barr virus* and the *cytomegalovirus* are two examples. Other physical signs are usually present to suggest the diagnosis clinically and serological tests confirm which agent is involved. Typical intranuclear inclusions are found within macrophages in cytomegalovirus infection and these may be seen in liver biopsies. Cytomegalovirus is important as a cause of fever in patients who are immunosuppressed by diseases or treatment and in patients who have received multiple blood transfusions, for example with cardiac surgery.

Yellow fever has long been recognized as a cause of fever and jaundice in the tropics. The disease is endemic in Africa and South America, and there have been outbreaks in Central America and Trinidad. High fever, severe myalgia, jaundice, and a bleeding tendency are typical features but there is a considerable range in the severity of the disease. Travellers to endemic areas should be protected by yellow fever vaccination. Two French tourists who were not vaccinated developed the disease and died on their return to France from a short stay in Senegal. The liver may be affected in disseminated *herpes simplex infection* which is particularly likely to occur in immunosuppressed patients. Hepatomegaly with fever and abnormal liver function tests occurs in *secondary syphilis*. Lymphadenopathy and mucocutaneous lesions may also be present. Liver function tests are mildly abnormal and liver biopsies show evidence of liver cell damage. Serological tests for syphilis are strongly positive. The liver is occasionally involved in *toxoplasmosis* with a mild biochemical hepatitis. The clinical diagnosis is supported by finding lymphadenopathy, and a strongly positive toxoplasma dye test with IgM antibodies indicates active infection. *Leptospirosis* is relatively common in some parts of the world with jaundice and hepatomegaly occurring in up to 18 per cent of cases. Despite the jaundice and high bilirubin levels plasma transaminases are only mildly abnormal. The diagnosis is confirmed by serological tests or by culturing the organism. *Malaria* must be considered in the differential diagnosis of a patient with fever, jaundice, and hepatosplenomegaly if he is or has recently returned from an endemic area. These features are usually associated with heavy infections and parasites are found in stained blood films.

Infections causing granulomatous hepatitis. Infectious diseases are prominent among the causes of granulomatous hepatitis. In general jaundice is not a common finding and there may be only mild abnormalities of plasma transaminases but plasma alkaline phosphatase levels are often considerably raised. The patient is usually febrile and fever may have been present for a considerable time. Hepatosplenomegaly is a common finding in these conditions. *Q fever*, *typhoid*, *secondary syphilis*, *brucellosis*, *tuberculosis*, and *leprosy* may involve the liver in this way. Liver biopsy may give proof of the diagnosis in miliary tuberculosis with the demonstration of granulomas containing acid-fast bacilli. Liver biopsy may also give the diagnosis in those patients with tuberculosis who have a prolonged fever but no evidence clinically of which organ is involved. Most of the *fungi* that cause the deep mycoses may spread to the liver. Granulomas are found around fungal elements but the cellular constituents of the granulomas vary with the different species and there is a tendency for microabscesses to form. Special stains may be needed to show fungi in liver biopsy specimens and serological tests may also be of help. *Visceral leishmaniasis* is an important cause of prolonged fever associated with hepatosplenomegaly, leucopenia, anaemia, and hyperglobulinaemia. This diagnosis is readily considered in the endemic areas but it should be remembered that these areas include many countries of the Mediterranean littoral. Liver biopsies show granulomas containing macrophages stuffed with Leishman–Donovan bodies.

Although *hepatic granulomas* are commonly due to infections, they also occur in patients with sarcoidosis, Hodgkin's disease, and in various forms of poisoning, notably with beryllium. Furthermore, patients are quite frequently encountered in whom there may be hepatomegaly and evidence of deranged liver function tests, and in whom a needle biopsy of the liver establishes the diagnosis of granulomatous disease. Despite extensive investigation, a cause for the granulomatous disorder of the liver cannot be established. Although some of the cases may represent unusual forms of sarcoidosis, quite frequently there is no other evidence for this condition. Some patients of this type undergo a spontaneous remission with restoration of the liver histology to normal, while others go on to develop Hodgkin's disease or other lymphomas.

Infections causing space occupying lesions in the liver. Amoebic liver abscess is one of the commonest causes of this abnormality. *Entamoeba histolytica* reaches the liver via the portal vein from sites where trophozoites have penetrated the colonic epithelium and the vessels of the submucosa. Necrosis and lysis of liver cells are the main features, and one or more cavities which may or may not intercommunicate form in the liver. The cavity contains a thick liquid which is referred to as amoebic pus. This term is something of a misnomer as it does not contain many inflammatory cells and is sterile on culture for bacteria. Typically the pus is described as anchovy sauce coloured, a pinkish-brown colour, but this appearance is not invariable and the pus may be yellowish in colour. The clinical presentations of patients with amoebic liver abscesses depend on the site and the size of the abscess. When the abscess is small, fever, night sweats, and anorexia may be the only symptoms and minimal hepatic tenderness on springing the lower rib cage may be the only sign to indicate a hepatic abnormality. Larger abscesses cause localizing symptoms and signs in addition to systemic upset with pain as the most usual symptom. Pain may be felt in the right hypochondrium, in the epigastrium, or in the right shoulder. The pain may also be felt over the lower chest and may be pleuritic. If

the abscess is in the lower part of the liver, tender hepatomegaly is found. In some cases a tender swelling is found on the surface of the liver. Where the abscess is in the upper part of the right lobe of the liver there may be no signs in the abdomen but considerable elevation of the hemidiaphragm with loss of diaphragmatic excursion with respiration. A range of abnormal signs can be found at the lung base overlying the abscess. Dullness to percussion with absent breath sounds indicates a pleural effusion while there may be a pleural friction rub or signs of collapse or consolidation. Inspection of the chest wall occasionally reveals a swelling in an intercostal space and on palpation this area is very tender. In all patients the intercostal spaces should be carefully palpated for point tenderness. The right lobe of the liver is most commonly affected. With left lobe abscesses a tender mass may be found in the epigastrium or left hypochondrium or the left hemidiaphragm may be elevated with signs at the left lung base. Occasionally, left lobe abscesses may rupture into the pericardium with signs of a pericardial tamponade.

Laboratory tests show a normochromic, normocytic anaemia with a leucocytosis. The sedimentation rate is raised. Serum albumin levels decrease while globulin levels are increased. Plasma transaminase levels are often slightly increased by jaundice is not commonly seen. Plasma alkaline phosphatase levels are often raised. These changes are entirely non-specific.

The diagnosis of amoebic liver abscess is usually made on the history of residence in the tropics together with the symptoms and signs discussed above and a positive serological test for amoebiasis, most commonly in indirect fluorescent antibody test. This test is positive in over 90 per cent of patients with this condition. Only about 50 per cent of patients have a history of amoebic dysentery and less than half the patients have cysts or trophozoites of the parasite in their stools. A chest radiograph shows abnormalities at the lung base overlying the abscess. As well as elevation of the diaphragm, a localized bulge may be seen on the contour of the diaphragm. Recent developments in scanning techniques have allowed much more accurate localization of liver abscesses. Technetium scans show the abscess as a 'cold' area. Ultrasound scans provide more accurate localization of the abscess and also can give an accurate assessment of the size of the lesion. This type of scan will indicate the depth of the abscess beneath the skin and can show the point on the skin that is closest to the cavity.

Metronidazole is currently the drug of first choice in the treatment of this condition (see Section 5). Symptoms and signs improve within 48 hours of starting treatment. Tinidazole, another nitroimidazole compound, is also effective. The need for aspiration must be considered in every patient with an amoebic abscess. Aspiration should be performed at the outset when the abscess is very large, causing considerable hepatomegaly or considerable elevation of the diaphragm. It should also be performed when there is a risk that the abscess will rupture. In many parts of the world aspiration of typical amoebic pus is the only way to confirm the diagnosis because serological tests are not available. Percutaneous aspiration of the abscess through the point of maximal tenderness can be performed safely under local anaesthesia using a wide-bore aspirating needle. There is a very low incidence of complications. The mortality from amoebic abscess rises considerably when rupture occurs and so it is imperative that this complication be prevented. Aspiration on more than one occasion may be needed in the treatment of large abscesses. Drug treatment alone is sufficient for smaller abscesses but if symptoms and signs do not improve aspiration may be needed. There is no evidence to suggest that aspiration hastens resolution of the pathological changes in the liver at the site of the abscess. These changes may take up to a year to resolve. Diloxanide furoate should be given for ten days to eradicate any amoebae which remain in the intestinal lumen.

Pyogenic liver abscess is a relatively uncommon condition but is one that should be considered in the differential diagnosis of patients with fever of undetermined origin. Pyogenic abscess causes symptoms and signs that are similar to those of an amoebic abscess but there are some differences. The patient with a pyogenic abscess usually has a shorter duration of symptoms, is more ill, and often has a history of co-existing or pre-existing diseases which predispose to development of this condition. These diseases include diverticulitis, appendicitis, pancreatitis, cholelithiasis and ascending cholangitis, alcoholic liver disease, perihepatic sepsis, and penetrating abdominal wounds. Previous bowel or biliary tract surgery may also be complicated by pyogenic liver abscess. A number of cases occur in patients who have no predisposing condition. High fever, rigors, anorexia, and malaise are usual systemic symptoms with pain in the upper abdomen or lower chest in relation to the site of the abscess. Diaphragmatic irritation may cause referred pain in the shoulder, as may occur in amoebic abscess. The physical signs are similar to those discussed above for amoebic abscess.

Investigations show a raised white cell count with a neutrophil leucocytosis. Other changes in the blood are non-specific and are similar to those found with amoebic abscess. Blood cultures are positive in 50 per cent of patients and so must be set up. Serological test for amoebiasis must be performed because the two conditions cannot be distinguished clinically. These are negative in pyogenic abscess. Technetium and ultrasound scans localize the lesions in the liver but amoebic abscesses cannot be distinguished from pyogenic abscesses unless the ultrasound scan shows numerous small cavities through the liver, in which case bacterial infection is the likely cause. Gallium scanning shows increased uptake in pyogenic abscesses while amoebic abscesses do not take up this isotope.

Treatment comprises surgical drainage of the abscess and antibiotic therapy. At operation a large volume of pus, 20–30 ml, should be obtained for bacteriological examination. Enterobacteria were thought to be the organisms which caused this condition, but the importance of anaerobic bacteria from the colonic microflora and *Streptococcus milleri* have been recognized recently. Gas in the abscess cavity, foul smelling pus, the morphology of the organisms on Gram staining, and the lack of growth in aerobic culture are features which suggest the presence of anaerobic infection. The choice of antibiotics depends on the sensitivities of the organisms grown, but if there is an urgent need to start treatment before culture results are available, parenteral penicillin, metronidazole, and gentamicin should be given. This regimen should be changed as necessary when sensitivities are known. The duration of treatment depends on the response of the patient but four to six weeks of treatment with antibiotics are usually needed. Where there are numerous small abscesses throughout the liver, surgical drainage cannot be effectively carried out and intensive antibiotic treatment should be given.

Pseudomonas pseudomallei occasionally causes liver infections in man. Geographically these are limited to the countries of Southeast Asia. It may cause intrahepatic abscesses.

Hydatid cysts of the liver are common in many parts of the world often causing symptomless hepatomegaly. Liver function is normal and these patients often have no eosinophilia in the peripheral blood, and serological tests for hydatid are often negative or only weakly positive. Liver biopsy should not be performed in any patient who may have a hydatid cyst in the liver without first excluding the presence of a cyst by isotope or ultrasound scanning. Daughter cysts may be spilled from the main cyst when it is punctured by a biopsy needle and these may seed into the peritoneal cavity. This can also occur as a result of blunt abdominal trauma. Local pain and allergic manifestations, which range from urticaria to anaphylaxis, may accompany leakage of cyst contents.

Elective removal of hepatic hydatid cysts that are causing no symptoms should be avoided. Where the cyst is growing progressively larger and causing symptoms or likely to rupture, surgical removal of the cyst is indicated. Ultrasound scanning of the liver is a useful technique for assessing changes in cysts. Computerized axial tomography can also be used but has no advantage over ultrasound scans. When hydatid cysts become infected, the clinician is faced with a difficult problem of diagnosis and management. This complication of hydatid disease must be distinguished from amoebic abscess and amoebic serology is helpful. Blood cultures may be positive in patients with infected hydatid cysts and those with pyogenic liver abscess. Ultrasound scans may be of help because the cavities of pyogenic and amoebic abscesses are irregular while the hydatid cyst is regular and well-demarcated from surrounding liver tissue. There may be some increase in echoes around an infected hydatid cyst which may make this distinguishing feature less sure. Treatment comprises antibiotics and surgical drainage. Adequate drainage for the infected cyst contents must be provided and yet peritoneal contamination by possibly viable daughter cysts must be avoided.

Helminthic infections and the liver. *Schistosomiasis* causes liver damage because of granulomas that form around eggs that have embolized to the liver and impacted in the presinusoidal branches of the portal vein. The granuloma resolves with residual, irreversible fibrosis occluding the small vessel. When this process goes on over many years in a patient with a heavy infection, schistosomal hepatofibrosis results and the patient develops portal hypertension with gastric and oesophageal varices and congestive splenomegaly. Despite the hepatofibrosis, liver function is well-preserved, so that if the patient bleeds from oesophageal varices, he will not develop portosystemic encephalopathy unless he has some co-existing hepatic parenchymal disease such as cirrhosis. If blood volume can be restored by transfusion and further losses prevented by measures such as pitressin infusion and as balloon tamponade, the patient with hepatofibrosis alone has a fairly good prognosis. Ascites may also occur and the congestive splenomegaly may cause a dragging pain in the left hypochondrium and haematological changes such as anaemia and pancytopaenia. Splenic infarcts may also occur. The newer antischistosomal drugs, oxamniquine and praziquantel (Section 5), can be used in the presence of schistosomal and other liver diseases but niridazole is contra-indicated.

The hermaphroditic flukes, *Clonorchis sinensis* and *Opisthorcis viverrini*, infect the biliary tree and cause similar symptoms, signs, and pathological changes. Those patients who have few worms have no symptoms. Those with moderate numbers of worms may develop upper abdominal pain and diarrhoea while those with heavy infections have upper abdominal pain and hepatomegaly, and they may develop obstructive jaundice, ascending cholangitis, septicaemia, cholelithiasis, and eventually cholangiocarcinoma. Pancreatitis may be caused by flukes obstructing the pancreatic ducts. The diagnosis is confirmed by finding eggs of the parasite in stools or in fluid aspirated from the duodenum. Praziquantel is effective in the treatment of both infections.

Fasciola hepatica, a hermaphroditic fluke also parasitizes the biliary tree. Patients may present early in the course of this infection with fever, upper abdominal pain, tender hepatomegaly and eosinophilia. This occurs when the larvae have burrowed through the wall of the duodenum to reach the liver through which they migrate until they enter a bile duct. At this stage the diagnosis can only be established by a positive serological test for fascioliasis. Eggs are not produced by the immature worm. Patients with established infections often have upper abdominal pain and hepatomegaly. Those with heavy infections may develop obstructive jaundice and cholangitis. Rarely very heavy infections are found and these may cause severe bleeding from the biliary tree. Long-standing infections are not complicated by cancer of the biliary tree. The parasitological diagnosis is made by finding eggs in stools or duodenal fluid. Bithionol is an effective treatment.

Toxocara canis may cause fever, hepatosplenomegaly, and eosinophilia in the syndrome of visceral larva migrans. Granulomas may be found in liver biopsies but the diagnosis is confirmed by serological tests. Diethylcarbamazine kills any living larvae and the infection resolves. Infective filarifom larvae of *Strongyloides stercoralis* invade the liver when massive auto-infection occurs. Granulomas are found around degenerating worms.

References

References to each specific infection mentioned in this chapter will be found in Section 5.

Barbour, G. L. and Juniper, K., Jr. (1972). A clinical comparison of amebic and pyogenic abscess of the liver. *Am. J. Med.* **53**, 323.

Danis, M., Brucker, G., Gentilini, M., Richard-Lenoble, D., and Smith, M. (1977). Treatment of hepatic hydatid disease. *Brit. medical J.* **ii**, 1356.

Moore-Gillon, J. C., Eykyn, S., and Phillips, I. (1981). Microbiology of progressive liver abscess. *Br. med. J.* **283**, 819.

Sabbaj, J., Sutter, V. L., and Finegold, S. M. (1972). Anaerobic pyogenic liver abscess. *Ann. Intern. Med.* **77**, 629.

Schiff, L. (1975). *Diseases of the liver*, 4th edn. Lippincott, Philadelphia.

Sherlock, S. (1981). *Diseases of the liver*, 6th edn. Blackwell Scientific Publications, Oxford.

Metabolic, genetic, and congenital disorders of the liver and biliary tract

A. P. Mowat

Introduction. This section will concentrate on metabolic, genetic, and congenital disorders in which the most prominent clinical manifestations are deranged hepatic metabolism or structure. The conditions which will be stressed are those for which effective treatment is available and early diagnosis is essential. Accurate diagnosis of other disorders for which no treatment is as yet available is also important as a guide to prognosis and particularly for accurate genetic counselling. An ever-increasing number of such genetic disorders can be diagnosed by amniocentesis early in pregnancy. The advice of a specialized centre should always be sought when considering antenatal diagnosis so that the family may have the benefit of the most up-to-date information available.

Many of the conditions described below are considered in greater detail elsewhere in this book and the sections which follow deal mainly with their hepatic aspects.

Abnormalities of metal metabolism

Wilson's disease

Definition. Wilson's disease (see also Section 9) is an inherited error of metabolism associated with the accumulation of toxic amounts of copper in the liver, brain, kidneys, and cornea. The basic genetic defect is unknown. There is diminished biliary excretion of copper, and in over 90 per cent of cases impaired production of caeruloplasmin, a copper-containing glycoprotein found in serum.

Liver pathology. In the initial stages the liver is enlarged with fatty infiltration and focal necrosis but as the disorder progresses the features may mimic chronic aggressive hepatitis, and ultimately cirrhosis and its complications develop. It may be difficult to demonstrate copper in the liver by standard stains; it is usually distributed periportally associated with lipofuscin deposits.

Clinical features of the hepatic forms. The classical form of this disease, progressive lenticular degeneration with tremor, increasing muscular rigidity, asymptomatic cirrhosis, Kayser–Fleischer rings in the cornea, and disturbances of renal function, commonly has its onset in the second decade of life. In childhood the principal presentation is a hepatic disorder. This may mimic all forms of liver disease ranging from asymptomatic hepatomegaly, hepatosplenomegaly with vague gastrointestinal symptoms, jaundice with oedema and ascites, subacute or fulminant hepatitis, chronic aggressive hepatitis, asymptomatic cirrhosis, or gastrointestinal haemorrhage from portal hypertension.

Abnormalities such as clumsiness, slurring of the speech, difficulties with fine movements, deteriorating school performance, or changes in personality are common neurological presentations. Haemolytic anaemia, vitamin D resistant rickets, renal rickets, or the Fanconi syndrome may also be the first indication of disease.

Diagnosis. The diagnosis must be considered in any patient with liver disease whatever their age, or in any patient who develops a neurological abnormality in late childhood or early adult life.

Kayser–Fleischer rings, brown or greenish-brown deposits of copper just within the limbus, are pathognomonic of Wilson's disease unless there has been chronic cholestasis. Identification by slit-lamp examination is essential in every suspected case. They are not, however, present in every case. The caeruloplasmin is less than 20 mg/dl in over 90 per cent of cases, but similar low values may be found in fulminant hepatitis, chronic active hepatitis, and tyrosinosis, as well as protein-losing enteropathy, severe malabsorption, or the nephrotic syndrome. In addition, heterozygotes for Wilson's disease may have low caeruloplasmin levels. The urinary copper excretion is frequently in the range of 100–1000 μg/day as compared with the normal upper limit of 40 μg/day. With penicillamine in a dose of 0.5 g twice a day, urinary copper values of greater than 1000 are found in Wilson's disease. The liver copper is elevated to between one and a half to 25 times the upper limit of normal, except in the presence of advanced cirrhosis when it may fall within the normal range.

The uptake of copper into caeruloplasmin may be shown to be defective using radioactive copper.

Treatment. Untreated, Wilson's disease is invariably fatal. D-penicillamine in a dose of 500 mg twice daily in adults (up to 20 mg/kg daily in children), increasing to 1 g twice daily will gradually deplete the liver copper stores, prevent further progression of the liver disease, and may cause some improvement in liver function. Treatment given when fulminant hepatic failure or decompensated cirrhosis is established is rarely successful. If there are side-effects from penicillamine, tetraethylene tetraamine hydrochloride may be used. A diet low in copper should also be given. Further details are given in Section 9.

Haemochromatosis. Iron loading of the liver cells leads to hepatocellular damage and fibrosis. The pathology is similar whether the iron accumulation results from idiopathic haemochromatosis or from secondary iron overloading states. The severity of liver damage is proportional to its iron content and is most marked in the periportal regions where iron is concentrated. The mechanism of liver damage by iron is uncertain. There is some evidence that iron loading of lysosomes results in their increased fragility, possibly leading to an inappropriate release of hydrolases and other enzymes. It has been suggested that lysosomal instability and lipid peroxidation of their membranes, and defective release of lysosomal collagenases, may all play a role in producing hepatic damage and fibrosis although there is limited experimental data to support this hypothesis. Iron loading may occur either in idiopathic haemochromatosis or it may be secondary to the increased iron absorption which occurs in various iron loading anaemias or as the result of transfusion.

Idiopathic haemochromatosis and the iron loading anaemias are considered in Section 19. Only those aspects which relate particularly to the liver are discussed briefly below.

Hepatic aspects of idiopathic haemochromatosis. This disorder is characterized by a marked increase in iron absorption of unknown aetiology. It presents in middle age with pigmentation, hepatomegaly, diminished sexual activity, and diabetes. The liver is usually large and firm. Abdominal pain and hepatic tenderness are common features. However, signs of hepatocellular failure are unusual, as is ascites. Similarly, oesophageal varices and portal hypertension occur rarely. Primary liver cancers develop in about 14 per cent of cases and may be the mode of presentation. Interestingly, these tumours may develop even after intensive iron-removal therapy.

Idiopathic haemochromatosis is best diagnosed by liver biopsy. The findings include a marked increase in iron deposition and pigmentary cirrhosis. On the whole, the amount of iron in the biopsy correlates well with the total body iron load. If the liver iron is less than 1.5 per cent dry weight, the diagnosis is unlikely to be idiopathic haemochromatosis. It is possible to monitor therapy with repeated biopsies.

Early iron loading of the liver is one of the most useful indicators of the existence of haemochromatosis before the disease is clinically apparent. Hence it may be used, together with HLA typing, for screening relatives of patients for the disease. The serum iron and percentage iron saturation are also useful for this purpose although serum ferritin levels may be normal in the presence of quite severe parenchymal iron loading of the liver. This is because parenchymal loading occurs early, and reticulo-endothelial loading, which seems to be required to elevate the plasma ferritin level, occurs late. It is becoming increasingly apparent that the liver iron content is the most sensitive marker of the disease.

The management of primary idiopathic haemochromatosis is described in Section 19.

Secondary iron loading. The causes of secondary iron loading are described in Section 19. Transfusion siderosis has been most intensively studied in transfusion-dependent β-thalassaemia. The iron is deposited first in the reticulo-enothelial cells and later in the parenchymal cells. Despite massive iron loading of the liver in this condition, liver failure and cirrhosis are relatively rare causes of death. Where this has occurred, there is evidence that there may have been previous liver damage resulting from B virus hepatitis following transfusion therapy.

Liver damage which occurs secondary to iron loading anaemias such as sideroblastic anaemia has a similar pattern to that which occurs in thalassaemia.

Iron loading of the liver is also seen commonly in alcoholic cirrhosis. The mechanism is not understood. There is some increase in gastrointestinal iron absorption in many patients with cirrhosis irrespective of the cause. Many alcoholic beverages are rich in iron and the association of chronic pancreatitis may increase duodenal iron absorption. The hepatic histology shows the features of alcoholic liver damage (see page 12.209) and iron deposition in liver cells but not so marked in reticulo-endothelial cells. There may be rapid accumulation of iron in the liver after a porta-caval shunt. Again the mechanism is uncertain. The iron deposition in the liver which occurs in the South African Bantu is the result of preparing foods, particularly porridge, in iron pots at an acid pH.

The management of secondary iron overload is described in Section 19.

Indian childhood cirrhosis. There has been great interest recently in a form of cirrhosis which occurs in certain areas of India and which may result from both genetic and environmental factors.

The liver pathology in this condition is characterized by the presence of a fine, micronodular cirrhosis associated with typical hyaline bodies (Mallory's bodies) identical to those which are seen in alcoholic hepatitis. The hepatic copper level is markedly increased but its distribution is not the same as that of Wilson's disease.

It is still not clear whether this condition has a major genetic component and whether copper metabolism is abnormal in these children, or whether the copper loading of the liver results from increased dietary intake. Furthermore, there is insufficient evidence to determine whether removal of copper has any effect on the progression of the liver damage. Since this condition is extremely common in some areas of India, and since it is invariably fatal, its pathogenesis requires urgent study.

Hepatic porphyrias

The hepatic porphyrias (see Section 9) are inherited disorders of the haem synthesis pathway. The three which are best defined are acute intermittent porphyria, hereditary coproporphyria, and variegate porphyria. Each of these conditions is inherited as an autosomal dominant. Although the liver seems to be the main site in which the inborn error of haem synthesis is expressed, the genetic lesions are not limited to the liver cells and can be demonstrated in other tissues such as erythrocytes, fibroblasts, and amniotic fluid cells.

The three genetically determined hepatic porphyrias have a number of clinical features in common. The acute phrase of each of the disorders is characterized by neuropsychiatric manifestations and increased production and urinary excretion of delta amino laevulinic acid (ALA) and porphobilinogen. The three conditions are associated with exacerbations precipitated by a variety of drugs, most of which are lipid-soluble inducers of hepatic cytochrome P450 and of hepatic ALA synthetase. Despite the fact that the liver is the main site of the production of abnormal porphyrins in these conditions, they are rarely associated with liver damage. Their clinical and biochemical manifestations are described further in Section 9.

The other form of porphyria, porphyria cutanea tarda, may be associated with severe liver disease. This condition is described in detail in Section 9 and this discussion is restricted to the hepatic manifestations.

Porphyria cutanea tarda (PCT). There has been considerable controversy over the years about the aetiology of this disorder and of the relative importance of genetic as compared with environmental factors in its pathogenesis. It is now thought that it results from a genetic deficiency of the enzyme uroporphyrinogen decarboxylase (UD). However, the full clinical syndrome probably requires the interaction of acquired factors including alcohol, iron overload, or steroid hormones to become fully manifest. Interestingly, sensitivity to drugs such as barbiturates does not occur in this condition. There is considerable experimental evidence that the synthesis of UD can be inhibited by excess iron, alcohol, or various phenols.

The pathological changes in the liver in PCT include subacute hepatitis, iron loading, and frank cirrhosis. Uroporphyrin can be demonstrated by its red fluorescence in ultraviolet light.

The clinical picture is characterized by skin photosensitivity, blistering, and scarring pigmentation with hypertricosis. Acute attacks similar to those which occur in the other forms of hepatic porphyria are not characteristic of PCT. There is usually chemical evidence of liver dysfunction and in some cases there may be all the clinical findings of advanced cirrhosis.

The management of PCT is difficult because its pathogenesis is still not fully understood. For example, it is not clear whether the iron loading which is so common occurs as part of the primary metabolic defect or whether it is secondary to alcoholic cirrhosis. However, iron chelation therapy with desferrioxamine (see Section 19) or iron removal by repeated venesection may lead to a clinical remission; many months treatment may be required.

Hepatomas have been found in a significant percentage of patients with PCT. Although these may have been related to the cirrhosis and iron loading rather than to the porphyria, it is interesting to note that tumours have been observed in the livers of patients with this disorder who had no evidence of cirrhosis. Interestingly, in several of these reports it was noted that the tumours, but not the surrounding liver tissues, showed porphyrin fluorescence. There has been at least one report of the remission of PCT after removal of an apparently benign porphyrin-laden hepatic adenoma. These observations suggest that PCT may occasionally arise from defective porphyrin metabolism in a hepatic tumour.

Erythopoietic protoporphyria. This rare condition results from a genetic deficiency in haem synthetase and it affects the red cell precursors and the erythrocytes predominantly. It is described in detail in Section 9. There have been a few reports of deaths from liver failure in this disorder although the cause is unknown.

Secondary coproporphyrias. An increased excretion of coproporphyrin in the urine occurs in a variety of conditions including lead poisoning, several liver diseases, the Dubin–Johnson syndrome (see page 12.180), and after drug therapy. It has also been described in a patient with a hepatic adenoma who developed a light sensitivity with skin blistering. Removal of the adenoma was associated with a complete remission.

Disorders of carbohydrate metabolism

Disorders of carbohydrate metabolism are considered in detail elsewhere in this book (see Section 9 for accounts of diabetes mellitus and the genetic disorders of carbohydrate metabolism). In this section we will review briefly the hepatic aspects of some of these conditions.

Diabetes mellitus. Hepatic complications of diabetes mellitus are relatively uncommon and form a small part of the clinical spectrum of the disorder. In the juvenile, insulin-sensitive type of diabetes some hepatic enlargement may occur, particularly during episodes of ketosis. For example, in one series liver enlargement was noted in about 10 per cent of well-controlled diabetics but in 60 per cent of poorly controlled cases and in all patients with ketoacidosis. The hepatomegaly regresses when the diabetes is controlled and is thought to be due to increased amounts of glycogen in the liver cells. Sometimes the liver is enlarged in maturity-onset diabetes, in this case due to the deposition of fat in the liver cells.

Hepatomegaly is seen more commonly in childhood diabetes. Again it appears to be due to a combination of fatty infiltration and increased amounts of glycogen. In the *Mauriac syndrome* there is massive hepatomegaly associated with growth retardation, obesity, and hypercholesterolaemia. However, portal hypertension and its accompaniments are not usually observed.

Whether there is a genuine association between cirrhosis and diabetes is still unresolved.

Glycogen storage disease. The heterogeneous series of genetic disorders of glycogen metabolism which are grouped under the general term glycogenoses are described in detail in Section 9. The majority of them appear to be inherited as autosomal recessives except for subtype VI which is sex-linked. All these conditions are associated with inefficient glycogen utilization which leads to hypoglycaemia and glycogen deposition in various tissues.

Hepatic enlargement occurs in association with glycogenoses III, V, VI, VIII, IX, and X, but although some degree of hepatic fibrosis may develop, severe cirrhosis is not a feature of these conditions.

In *type I glycogenosis* there is marked glycogen deposition in the liver but cirrhosis does not occur. Occasionally, however, hepatocellular adenomas and even carcinomas occur late in the course of the illness. The condition presents in early infancy with hypoglycaemia, convulsions, coma, acidosis, hepatomegaly, and slow growth. Less severely affected infants usually present in the first or second year with massive hepatomegaly without splenomegaly.

In *type IV glycogenosis* a curious variety of cirrhosis may develop associated with many giant cells in the liver. Liver biopsies also show the presence of deposits of abnormal glycogen which shows characteristic staining patterns with iodine and PAS. Affected children develop marked hepatosplenomegaly and signs of portal hypertension and liver failure.

The diagnosis and management of these disorders is considered in Section 9.

Galactosaemia (See also Section 9)
Definition. Galactosaemia is a rare recessive disorder in which there is deficiency of the enzyme galactose-l-phosphate uridyl transferase which metabolizes galactose-l-phosphate to allow its participation in carbohydrate metabolism. In galactosaemia galactose, galactose-1-phosphate, and galactitol accumulate in all body tissues.

Hepatic pathology. Early hepatic changes include fatty infiltration and hepatic necrosis proceeding to pseudoglandular transformation of hepatocytes, hepatic fibrosis, and cirrhosis in patients who survive. The pathogenesis of these lesions and of the brain damage is not clear. Galactitol is thought to cause the cataracts.

Clinical features. Symptoms may start following the first lactose-containing feed with vomiting, jaundice, spontaneous bleeding and, in severe cases, early death from septicaemia. Some patients have a more indolent course presenting with features of cirrhosis at the age of two to six months by which time mental retardation and cataracts may be apparent. Rarely, patients present even later in life with cataracts, mental retardation, and latent hepatic involvement.

Diagnosis. The diagnosis may be suspected by the finding of galactosuria demonstrable for one to two hours after a lactose-containing feed. The urine gives a positive result for reducing substances, e.g. with Clinitest tablets, but there is a negative reaction with glucose oxidase tests. Galactosuria is not present in every case and the diagnosis must be excluded in patients with the above features by demonstrating normal enzyme activity in red blood cells.

Treatment. A galactose-free diet will prevent progression of the neurological changes, allow some improvement in hepatic function unless cirrhosis is already established, and may cause reabsorption of the cataracts. Even if such a diet is instituted at birth, some patients will have mental retardation suggesting possible intrauterine brain damage. It has been suggested that this may be prevented by a galactose-free diet during pregnancy.

Fructosaemia (See also Section 9)
Definition. Dietary fructose is converted to glucose in the liver by the action of the enzyme fructose-1-phosphate aldolase. This enzyme is deficient in fructosaemia causing an accumulation of fructose and fructose-1-phospate in serum, fructosuria, and hypoglycaemia.

Liver pathology and clinical manifestations. Steatosis and necrosis of hepatocytes in the early stages progress to intralobular fibrosis and ultimately cirrhosis and its complications. Symptoms start when fructose is introduced to the diet. Vomiting and hepatomegaly are almost always present as is failure to thrive. In the first two months of life jaundice and a bleeding diathesis with deranged coagulation is found. There may be features of hypoglycaemia. A distaste for sweet foods may be apparant before one year of age.

Diagnosis. The diagnosis may be confirmed by the regression of symptoms when fructose is withdrawn from the diet and the demonstration of low activity of fructose-1-phosphate aldolase in liver or intestinal mucosa.

Treatment. In the acute stages treatment for liver failure may be required. If the patient survives, and fructose and sucrose are excluded from the diet, progress is excellent with regression of the liver damage. Vitamin C supplements are required.

Amino acid disorders

Hereditary tyrosinaemia. This disorder (see Section 9) is characterized by the accumulation in serum and urine of tyrosine and its metabolites. This is associated with severe liver damage, initially in the form of fatty infiltration but proceeding to cirrhosis, and a renal tubular defect causing glycosuria, hyperamino-aciduria, and phosphaturia. Rickets and hypoglycaemia are frequent complications. The exact biochemical basis of this condition is unknown.

In its acute form the disease presents in the first six months of life with vomiting, diarrhoea, hepatosplenomegaly, ascites, a bleeding diathesis, and severe failure to thrive. A chronic form characterized by cirrhosis, renal tubular defects, and rickets may continue from this acute presentation or develop as the initial manifestation later in childhood.

The diagnosis is suspected on the basis of clinical features, the abnormal amino acid content of the serum and urine, grossly abnormal liver function tests, and raised serum alpha-fetoprotein levels. Galactosaemia and fructosaemia are the main differential diagnosis.

Urea-cycle disorders. (See Section 9.) Genetically determined deficiency has been identified for five separate enzymes in the liver involved in the conversion of ammonia to urea. These disorders are characterized by a high blood ammonia, an accumulation of ornithine, citrulline, arginosuccinic acid, or arginine depending on the site of the metabolic block. The principal pathological change is brain damage but the liver usually shows an increase in fat and glycogen. The clinical features include a dislike of protein-containing food, and vomiting, irritability or lethargy following ingestion of such foods. Failure to thrive, mental retardation, and hepatomegaly occur. The diagnosis is suspected by the finding of a high blood ammonia, but is established by the demonstration of deficiency of the particular enzyme involved.

The management of amino acid disorders are considered in Section 9.

Glycoprotein disorders

Hepatic aspects of alpha-1 antitrypsin deficiency.

Aetiology. Over 30 alleles of alpha-1 antitrypsin can now be distinguished by acid starch gel electrophoresis or isoelectric focusing. These are inherited in an autosomal co-dominant fashion. The normal allele is designated Pi^M (Pi =protease inhibitor). The normal phenotype is written MM, therefore. There is a variant which is called Z. Individuals who are heterozygous for this gene, with the phenotype MZ, have approximately 60 per cent of the normal concentration of the enzyme inhibitor in their blood. Liver disease occurs in individuals who are homozygous for this variant, i.e. the phenotype ZZ (incidence 1:3400 in the United Kingdom), or who have no glycoprotein in the serum, with the Pi Null phenotype. In a large survey in Norway the gene frequency for Pi^z was 0.026 and that for Pi^0 (null) was 0.001. Individuals with the MZ phenotype may have an increased incidence of chronic obstructive airways disease. Despite much speculation it is still not clear why enzyme-deficient individuals develop lung or liver disease.

Hepatic pathology. Histological examination of the liver in PiZZ individuals shows characteristic diastase-resistant periodic-acid-Schiff positive magenta coloured granules which by histochemical, immunochemical, and electromicroscopic techniques are shown to be accumulations of abnormal alpha-1 antitrypsin in the cisternae of the endoplasmic reticulum. Current evidence indicates that the alpha-1 antitrypsin gene modifies the protein core of the glycoprotein causing secondary changes in its carbohydrate content. Such abnormalities are present whether or not the liver shows any functional or structural abnormality.

Clinico-pathological features. Liver disease is usually first detected in infancy by the appearance of a conjugated hyperbilirubinemia with pale stools, dark urine, hepatomegaly, splenomegaly, and failure to thrive. Liver function tests are deranged. There may be a bleeding diathesis. Histological examination of liver biopsy tissue shows a wide variety of structural change ranging from a mild hepatitis to marked portal tract widening by fibrous tissue with prominent bile duct reduplication and even cirrhosis. If the patient survives the acute phase, the jaundice gradually fades after weeks or months but liver function tests remain abnormal. Approximately

25 per cent of such jaundiced infants die of cirrhosis in early childhood, while 40–50 per cent have chronic persisting liver disease with features of a compensated cirrhosis. Some of these develop features of decompensation in late childhood or early adolescence and thereafter death occurs rapidly. A few children survive a period of jaundice without hepatosplenomegaly and in these the liver function tests may gradually revert to normal if the initial histological changes in the liver have been mild. Rarely, children, adolescents, or adults are found to have cirrhosis without prior history of jaundice in infancy. Hepatoma may occur as a complication of the cirrhosis. At present no treatment has been shown to modify liver disease associated with alpha-1 antitrypsin deficiency.

Genetic counselling. Genetic counselling poses particular difficulties. The deficiency state is inherited in an autosomal recessive fashion. Antenatal diagnosis is possible by fetal blood sampling at 17-weeks gestation at which time termination of the pregnancy is possible. The problem comes in knowing what the prognosis for the ZZ fetus might be, given that not all will develop liver or lung disease. Our evidence from families in which the proband has liver disease, is that subsequent ZZ siblings commonly follow a course similar to the proband.

Genetic 'storage' disorders

An increasing number of conditions are being recognized in which deficiency of an enzyme causes the accumulation within tissues of its substrate and related metabolites. This causes enlargement of organs such as liver and spleen, together with infiltration and interference in function and structure of the brain, bones, skin, gums, gastrointestinal system, and lungs. These disorders are rare but with the advent of antenatal diagnosis by amniocentesis and fibroblast culture, are of great importance in that genetic counselling is available for affected families. The precise diagnosis is therefore essential. They are considered in detail in Section 9. Some of the principal enzyme defects together with clinical and diagnostic features of those who present with marked hepatomegaly are given in Tables 1 and 2.

Reye's syndrome

The association of acute encephalopathy with fatty change of the liver and other viscera was reported by Reye and his colleagues in 1963. The neurological aspects and management of this disorder are described in Section 21.

This condition is of unknown aetiology although much has been learnt in the last few years about the underlying biochemical abnormalities. It appears to occur in children who are recovering from a mild viral illness, small clusters of cases being associated with epidemics of viral infection, particularly influenza A and influenza B. An additional causative factor may be an environmental toxin, e.g. insecticides or salicylates. Certainly, it is not clear why some children suffering from a particular viral infection should develop this clinical picture. There are striking metabolic changes which appear to be related to a temporarily reduced activity of mitochondrial enzymes, particularly in the liver, but also in muscles and brain.

The condition is characterized by vomiting, which is persistent and profuse, and neurological deterioration coming on during the recovery period following a viral illness. There is commonly no clinical evidence of liver involvement. Histological and electron microscopic examination of the liver shows glycogen depletion, panlobular micro-vesicular lipid accumulation and distortion and swelling to the mitochondria. There is usually no hepatic necrosis. These histological abnormalities are associated with elevated serum transaminases and creatine-phosphokinase and, in the majority of cases, by a raised blood ammonia and a prolonged prothrombin time. The serum bilirubin is usually normal. Hypoglycaemia may occur, particularly in young children.

Table 1 Complex carbohydrate storage disorders in which hepatomegaly is a major feature

Disorder	Material abnormally stored	Enzyme deficient	Clinical features	Diagnostic investigation Specific enzyme activity (SEA) Preferred investigation
Mucopolysaccharidosis				
Hurler syndrome	heparin and dermatan sulphates	α-L-iduronidase	cloudy cornea bone/joint deformity mental retardation	SEA in leucocytes or fibroblast excess heparin sulphate (HS) and dermatan sulphate (DS) in urine
Scheie syndrome	heparin and dermatan sulphates	α-L-iduronidase	late onset slow progression no mental retardation	SEA in leucocytes or fibroblast excess HS and DS in urine
Hunter syndrome (X-linked inheritance)				
Sanfilippo syndrome type A	heparin sulphate	heparin sulphoglucosamine sulphatase	mental regression from 6 years of age with bony abnormalities	SEA in leucocytes and fibroblasts. Excess heparin sulphate in the urine
Sanfilippo syndrome type B	heparin sulphate	N-acetyl glucosaminidase	mental regression from 6 years of age with bony abnormalities	SEA in leucocytes and fibroblasts. Excess heparin sulphate in the urine
Maroteaux–Lamy syndrome	dermatan sulphate	aryl-sulphatase	like Hurler's syndrome, but no mental retardation	SEA in leucocytes or fibroblasts and dermatan sulphate excess in urine
Lipoprotein storage diseases				
Mannosidosis	mannose rich oligosaccharides	acid α-mannosidase	mental retardation, coarse facies, skeletal abnormalities, lens opacities, vacuolated lymphocytes, hypogammaglobulinemia	SEA in leucocytes or fibroblasts
Fucosidosis	fucose rich glycoproteins and glycolipids	α-fucosidase	dementia, cardiomegaly, thick skin, excessive sweat with high sodium content	SEA in leucocytes or fibroblasts
Mucolipidoses				
Sialidosis	complex lipoglycoproteins appearing in fome cells in bone marrow	acid neuraminidase	like Hurler's syndrome but with cherry red spot at the macula	SEA in fibroblasts and increased sialic acid in fibroblasts
I cell disease	sialic acid-rich material	unknown	severe features of Hurler's syndrome but with minimal corneal clouding and marked gingival hypertrophy	abnormal fibroblasts elevated serum lysosomal enzymatic activity no mucopolysaccharides in urine

Table 2 Lipid storage disorders in which hepatomegaly is a major feature

Disorder	Material abnormally stored	Enzyme deficient	Clinical features	Diagnostic investigation Specific enzymatic activity (SEA) Preferred investigation
Sandoff's disease	ganglioside GM2	hexosaminidase A & B	dementia with a cherry red spot at the macula bone and joint abnormal	SEA in serum and fibroblasts
Generalized gangliosidosis GM1	ganglioside GM1	β galactosidase	dementia, hyperacusis, flexion deformities	SEA in leucocytes and fibroblasts
GM3	ganglioside GM3	sialidase	as above	SEA in serum and leucocytes
Gaucher's disease	glucosyl-ceramide	glucosyl ceramide β glycosidase	infantile form; dementia and spasticity. Childhood form: hypersplenism, bone skin and lung infiltration	SEA in fibroblasts or liver biopsy
Sphingomyelin storage diseases				
Neimann–Pick disease	spingomyelin	sphingomyelinase	dementia; pulmonary infiltration	SEA in leucocytes or fibroblasts
Sphingomyelin disease with supranuclear ophthalmoplegia	unidentified sphingomyelin	unknown	progressive dementia starting with supranuclear ophthalmoplegia; abnormal liver architecture	bone marrow and liver biopsy with special staining for lipids and 'sea-blue' histiocytes
Wolman's disease	cholesterol esters and triglycerides	acid esterase	vomiting and diarrhoea starting in infancy; developmental delay, calcified adrenals	SEA in leucocytes, fibroblasts and liver biopsy
Cholesterol ester storage disease	as above	as above	malabsorption, splenomegaly	SEA in leucocytes and fibroblasts
Familial hyperlipoproteinemia				
Type 1	fat	lipoprotein, lipase	xanthoma, abdominal pain, lipaemia retinalis	chylomicronaemia
Type IV	fat	unknown	xanthoma, premature atherosclerosis	marked increase of very low density lipoproteins
Type V	fat	unknown	xanthoma with severe abdominal pain	marked increase in chylomicrons and very low density lipoproteins

The diagnosis is suspected on the basis of the clinical history and the above abnormalities in liver function tests and confirmed by the percutaneous liver biopsy findings. The conditions to be considered in the differential diagnosis include genetic deficiency of ornithine transcarbamylase and systemic carnitine deficiency.

Hepatic aspects of cystic fibrosis

Cystic fibrosis is a genetically determined disorder of exocrine secretory glands which causes them to produce tenacious viscoid secretions. The abnormal mucus stagnates in small ducts causing destruction of cells draining into or associated with them, a process aggravated by infection. The respiratory system and pancreas are principally involved, but other organs with mucus-producing glands in their duct systems, such as the biliary system are also affected. The condition is considered in detail on page 12.166 and only its hepatic manifestations are summarized briefly here.

Pathology of liver disease in cystic fibrosis. The main cause of chronic liver disease is thought to be inspisated biliary secretions causing focal biliary obstruction and fibrosis which is present to a minor degree in all patients. In 20 per cent of cases the gall bladder is pathologically small and a further 20 per cent are unable to concentrate cholecystographic agents, while 8 per cent have gallstones. Hepatocytes frequently contain excessive accumulations of fat suggesting the action of a nutritional or toxic effect, the exact nature of which still remains unidentified. Drugs, infection, and abnormal immune mechanisms have all been implicated in causing chronic liver damage. A biliary type of cirrhosis may appear in the first year of life, but more often cirrhosis becomes evident in late childhood or early adolescence. It is estimated that approximately 15 per cent may be so affected.

Clinical features. Obstructive jaundice, starting in the newborn period as a neonatal hepatitis and persisting for up to one year of age, is a rare presentation. Only a small minority of patients die of liver disease in the first few years of life, however. Equally uncommon is the massive hepatomegaly which may occur in the newborn period due to excessive fat accumulation in the liver.

Cirrhosis is found in approximately 10–15 per cent of adolescents with cystic fibrosis. It is usually found by chance with the detection of a large, hard liver and splenomegaly on clinical examination. On the other hand it may present with complications due to portal hypertension with alimentary bleeding from varices, splenic pain, or hypersplenism. Liver function tests are mildly deranged with elevation of the aspartase transaminase, alkaline phosphatase, and γ-glutamyl transpeptidase, but usually the serum albumin is normal. Decompensated cirrhosis with ascites is rare, except when cor pulmonale develops.

Management of hepatic complications. No treatment which influences the underlying process is available. Since alimentary bleeding commonly follows aspirin ingestion, this must be forbidden. Surgical obliteration of the varices by portacaval anastomosis is possible but it is a formidable undertaking causing acute chest problems and having an uncertain effect on subsequent hepatic function. Sclerosing the varices by endoscopically injecting ethanolamine oleate on five or six occasions under a general anaesthetic may prove to be a better option. Rarely, the pain from splenic infarction may be so severe as to require splenectomy which is usually combined with a splenorenal shunt.

Fibropolycystic disease

The term fibropolycystic disease covers a heterogeneous group of genetically determined disorders of the liver and intrahepatic biliary system. The conditions range from those in which the main lesions are cystic, such as adult and infantile fibropolycystic disease, to those in which fibrosis predominates, in particular congenital hepatic cirrhosis. An additional disorder, focal intra-hepatic biliary dilatation (Caroli's disease) is usually considered as part of this group. The latter condition differs from the other syndromes in that

the kidneys are not usually involved. Brunt has grouped all these conditions together as a family of genetic disorders of the hepatobiliary system under the general heading of fibropolycystic disease of the liver and biliary tract.

Adult fibropolycystic disease. This condition, which is inherited in an autosomal dominant fashion, is characterized by the occurrence of multiple cysts in the liver, often associated with polycystic disease of the kidney.

Pathology. Cysts may be distributed diffusely through the liver or restricted to one area, usually the left lobe. They vary in size but are rarely greater than 10 cm in diameter. The lobular architecture of the liver is preserved and the cystic areas appear to be related to bile ducts in the portal areas. They are surrounded by a dense fibrous tissue which is lined with columnar epithelium. Very frequently there is cystic disease of the kidneys, spleen, pancreas, ovary, and lungs. There may be associated congenital anomalies such as spina bifida.

Clinical features. The condition may present incidentally in a patient who is being investigated for another disorder or with polycystic kidneys. Otherwise it presents in the fourth or fifth decades, usually with gradual swelling of the abdomen. On examination the liver may be impalpable or may be massively enlarged and sometimes the cystic swellings can be palpated. Liver function is usually normal and portal hypertension is rare.

The condition can usually be diagnosed by ultrasound or liver scan and the diagnosis confirmed by hepatic arteriography.

Treatment is rarely required but unusually large cysts may be excised if they are causing symptoms.

Infantile fibropolycystic disease of the kidney and liver. This autosomal recessive disorder is characterized by the development of cysts and fibrous tissue in both organs with the loss of functioning tissue. It may present *in utero*, in infancy, or in late childhood. The earlier the onset, the more marked the renal features and it is only in infancy and later that hepatic problems arise. Each variety appears to be a distinct genetic entity. Only the hepatic aspects of the problem will be considered here.

Pathology. The liver is enlarged and smooth. In the portal tracts there is increased fibrous tissue and an abundance of dilated bile ductules lined by cuboidal epithelium. The hepatic lobular architecture is maintained and the liver cells are normal. The portal vein branches become distorted. Portal hypertension with oesophageal and gastric varices, splenomegaly, and hypersplenism are common findings.

Clinical features. In infancy the predominant features are renal failure, growth retardation and incidental, asymptomatic hepatosplenomegaly.

Cases presenting in later childhood show features of portal hypertension with alimentary bleeding and hypersplenism. Liver function tests are frequently normal although the alkaline phosphatase level may be elevated. There may be evidence of impaired renal function but in some cases it is only the intravenous pyelogram which shows abnormalities such as bluntened, shortened, indistinct calyxes, a persistent nephrogram, or alternating dense and radiolucent streaks on the nephrogram. There may be renal cysts demonstrated by ultrasonography.

An intermediate form with both portal hypertension and renal failure developing at eight to 12 years of age has also been described.

Treatment is limited to dietary measures to combat the renal failure. Aspirin should be avoided, since it may provoke alimentary bleeding. Surgical relief of portal hypertension should be considered in patients who have bled from varices; portasystemic shunting appears to be well tolerated by these individuals.

Congenital hepatic fibrosis. Congenital hepatic fibrosis is not a single distinct entity but may be found in association with a range of congenital syndromes also affecting the kidneys. These include infantile polycystic disease of the liver and kidneys, Ivemark's familial dysplasia, Meckel's syndrome, adult-type polycystic disease, nephronophthisis, medullary sponge kidney, and cortical or medullary renal cysts. Rarely, it may occur without renal disease.

Pathology. The unique pathological feature of this condition is the presence throughout the liver of bands of fibrous tissue clearly demarcated from the hepatic parenchyma and containing elongated or circular spaces lined by bile duct cells. Portal vein branches are small and sparse. The liver is large and hard. Portal hypertension occurs.

Clinical features. The clinical features are the result of portal hypertension or associated complications such as abdominal pain and fever due to cholangitis. There may be abdominal distension due to hepatosplenomegaly. Haematemesis may be the presenting symptom at any age from eight to 60 years. The outcome is dependent on the nature of the renal involvement. The natural history of cases without renal involvement is uncertain.

Diagnosis. The diagnosis is established by the typical histological appearances in a trucut liver biopsy. Renal assessment with intravenous pyelography and ultrasonic scanning is essential.

In general, porta-systemic shunting is better tolerated than in patients with cirrhosis, but hepatic decompensation can occur after such operations. They should therefore be reserved for patients in whom bleeding has occurred unprovoked by aspirin and in whom varices cannot be obliterated by direct injection. Cholangitis must be treated by appropriate antibiotics.

Focal intrahepatic biliary dilatation (Caroli's disease). This condition is characterized by non-obstructive sacular dilatation of the intrahepatic bile ducts. The dilated ducts are liable to become infected and gallstone formation is common. The liver may show the features of congenital hepatic fibrosis. There is no evidence that the condition is genetically determined, and the renal lesions which are associated with the disorders described in previous sections are not found in this condition.

Clinical features. The disorder usually presents in childhood or early adult life, often with abdominal pain and fever, and sometimes with septicaemia. Jaundice is not usually present except during acute episodes of cholangitis. The condition is often associated with a malabsorption syndrome. Portal hypertension rarely develops.

The diagnosis depends on ultrasound appearances, and percutaneous endoscopic operative cholangiography confirms the saculated and dilated appearance of the intrahepatic ducts.

The condition is managed with antibiotic therapy to control the attacks of cholangitis and removal of calculi as required.

Biliary atresia

The various syndromes of biliary atresia are of considerable importance in paediatric practice because if treatment is to be successful they must be recognized early. Both extra- and intrahepatic forms occur.

Extrahepatic biliary atresia. In this disorder there is an inability to secrete bile due to an obstruction of the bile duct anywhere between the duodenum and the first or second order branches of the hepatic ducts. The obstruction may be associated with obliteration or absence of the bile ducts and is extremely variable in site and extent. These changes are associated with intrahepatic periductular fibrosis and marked proliferation of the ducts leading to the development of a biliary cirrhosis. The rate at which this occurs varies considerable but without surgical treatment the mean age of death is about 21 months.

Aetiology. This is unknown although recent studies suggest that extrahepatic biliary atresia results from a progressive obstructive cholangiopathy. Intra-uterine infection has been suggested as a possible basis for this process, but it has not been possible to incriminate any particular pathogen.

Clinical features. Usually, affected infants are born following a normal pregnancy and have no perinatal problems. Jaundice usually dates from birth although its onset may be as late as six weeks. Features of cirrhosis become apparent by about eight months but can appear at any time between the second and sixteenth month.

Diagnosis. This disorder should be considered in any infant who develops features of hepatitis and acholic stools. The diagnosis is confirmed by exclusion of known metabolic causes of hepatitis in this age group and hepatitis B infections, and by finding typical appearances on liver biopsy together with the faecal excretion of less than 10 per cent of an injected dose of ^{141}I RoseBengal in 72 hours. The diagnosis must be confirmed by laparotomy.

Management. Treatment, where feasible, is surgical although this must be carried out before cirrhosis is established.

Intrahepatic biliary hypoplasia. The syndrome of intrahepatic biliary hypoplasia is characterized by the absence or diminution in size and number of intralobular, intrahepatic bile ducts. The term is usually applied to patients with patent extrahepatic ducts. It may occur with other genetic abnormalities such as alpha-1 antitrypsin deficiency and there may be associated cardiac abnormalities or other congenital defects.

Some cases present in infancy with features of hepatitis complicated by pruritis. In some of these infants the jaundice fades after several months but pruritis, biochemical features of hepatocellular necrosis, hypercholesterolaemia and xanthelasma, often develop around the age of six to eighteen months. Other patients present in the second or third year of life with pruritis, hepatomegaly, deranged liver function tests, and, ultimately, cholestasis. The majority of these infants go on to develop chronic liver disease. Some develop cirrhosis and its complications by the age of two years, while others progress to liver failure only towards the end of childhood.

There is no specific treatment for this disorder. Cholestyramine may be helpful in controlling the pruritis. Fat soluble vitamin supplements should be administered, as is the case in other forms of cholestasis.

Choledochal cysts. Choledochal cysts are localized dilatations of the common bile duct which may arise as a result of congenital weakness. They vary in size; some of them reach enormous dimensions with a capacity of up to 8 litres. In adult life they may be associated with recurrent pancreatitis, gallstone formation and malignant neoplasms in the cyst itself or in the biliary tract.

Choledochal cysts usually present in the early years of life with intermittent jaundice or abdominal pain, and or a palpable mass in the abdomen. In infancy they may cause obstructive jaundice. They may be associated with congenital hepatic fibrosis or Caroli's disease. They are diagnosed by ultrasound, CT scanning, or percutaneous or retrograde cholangiography. Untreated, they cause biliary cirrhosis.

Treatment is by excision of the cysts with restoration of the biliary tract by choledochojejunostomy.

Other hepatic cysts. Cysts of the liver, other than those caused by parasites, are rare. Solitary cysts are occasionally found, usually as an incidental observation, and occasionally small cysts arise from the intra- or extrahepatic biliary system. These may contain mucus, blood, or even lymph if they arise from obstruction or congenital dilatation of the hepatic lymphatic system.

Congenital abnormalities of the biliary tract

Numerous congenital abnormalities of the biliary tract have been recorded which can be related to defects in the original budding from the primitive foregut or from failure of vacuolization of the solid gall bladder and bile diverticulum. They are frequently associated with other congenital abnormalities and many of them are of little clinical importance except where they result in bile stasis and the production of gallstones.

There are several forms of congenital absence of the gall bladder which result either from failure of the outgrowth from the hepatic diverticulum of the foregut or defective vacuolization of the gall bladder. The latter condition is usually associated with atresia of the extrahepatic ducts and presents at birth with deepening jaundice. A more common defect is failure of vacuolation of the solid biliary bud. Occasionally this involves only the cystic duct, and the gall bladder then becomes enlarged and cystic and contains mucus. However, if the common bile duct or hepatic duct are involved the syndrome of biliary atresia occurs (see above).

There are a variety of other congenital abnormalities of the gall bladder and bile ducts, most of which are of little clinical significance. Congenital deformities of the gall bladder include a variety of forms of double gall bladder, bi-lobed gall bladders, kinking between the body and the infundibulum giving the so-called 'hour-glass' gall bladder, a variety of different forms of diverticulae of the gall bladder, and abnormal siting of the organ which may be under the left lobe of the liver, or in its normal relation to the liver on the left side of the abdomen in cases of total situs inversus. The gall bladder may be buried in hepatic tissue; this condition is associated with a high incidence of infection and gallstone formation. Occasionally the gall bladder is contained at the end of a long mesentery and may hang 2–3 cm below the liver. Such floating gall bladders tend to twist with impairment of their blood supply and the organ may become infarcted in this way.

Congenital abnormalities of the bile duct are rare. Accessory ducts may join the common hepatic duct between the junction of the right and left hepatic ducts and the entry of the cystic duct, or may join the cystic duct, the gall bladder or the common bile duct. Occasionally, cholecystohepatic ducts occur following persistence of connections between the gall bladder and the liver parenchyma with failure of recanalization of the hepatic ducts. Continuity of drainage may be maintained if the cystic duct enters a common hepatic duct or the duodenum. These abnormalities have no significance except that they may be damaged during biliary surgery.

Finally, abnormalities of the cystic duct are relatively common. In about 20 per cent of individuals it runs parallel to the hepatic duct for some distance before joining it. Occasionally the cystic artery arises from the left hepatic artery or accessory cystic arteries may also arise from this vessel.

References

Further references to prophyria, diabetes mellitus, storage disease, and the amino acid disorders are given in Section 9. References to haemochromatosis are given in Section 19.

Wilson's disease

Sass-Kortsak, A. (1975). Wilson's disease—A treatable liver disease in children. *Pediat. Clins N. Am.* **22**, 963.
Sternlieb, I. and Scheinberg, I. H. (1979). Wilson's disease. In *Liver and biliary disease* (eds. R. Wright, K. G. M. Alberti, S. Karran, and G. H. Millward-Sadler), 774. W. B. Saunders, London.

Porphyria

Bissell, D. M. (1979). Haem metabolism and porphyrias. In *Liver and biliary disease* (eds. R. Wright, *et al.*), 324. W. B. Saunders, London.
Bloomer, J. R. (1976). Hepatic porphyrias: pathogenesis, manifestations and management. *Gastroent.* **71**, 689.
Lamon, J. M., Frykholm, B. C., Hess, R. A., and Tschudy, D. P. (1979). Haematin therapy in acute porphyria. *Medicine, Baltimore* **58**, 252.

Glycogen storage disease

Greene, H. L., Slonim, A. E., Burr, I. M., and Moron, J. R. (1980). Type I glycogen storage disease: five years of management with nocturnal intra gastric feeding. *J. Pediat.* **96**, 590.

Howell, R. R. (1978). The glycogen storage diseases. In: *The metabolic basis of inherited diseases*. 4th edn. (eds. J. B. Stanbury, J. B. Wyngaar den, and D. S. Fredrickson). McGraw-Hill, New York.
Igarashi, Y., Otomo, H., Narisawa, K., and Tada, K. (1979). A new variant of glycogen storage disease type I: probably due to a defect in glucose 6-phosphate transport system. *J. inher. metab. Dis.* **2**, 45.
Leonard, J. V., Francis, D. E. M., and Dongar, D. B. (1979). The dietary management of hepatic glycogen storage disease. *Proc. Nutr. Soc.* **38**, 321.

Galactosaemia

Monk, A. M., Mitchell, A. G. H., Milligan, D. W. A., and Holton, J. B. (1977). The Diagnosis of classical galactosaemia. *Arch. Dis. Child.* **52**, 943

Fructosaemia

Baerlscher, K., Giltzelman, R., Steinmann, B., and Giltzelman-Cumara samy, N. (1978). Hereditary fructose intolerance in early childhood. *Helv. paediat. Act.* **33**, 465.
Odievre, M., Gontil, C., Gautier, M., and Alagille, D. (1978). Hereditary fructose intolerance in childhood; Diagnosis, management and course in 52 infants. *Am. J. Dis. Child.* **132**, 605.

Amino acid disorders

Grenier, A., Belanger, L., and Laberge, C. (1976). Alpha-1 fetoprotein measurement in hereditary tyrosinaemia. *Clin. Chem.* **22**, 1001.
Hill, A., Nordin, P. M., and Zaleski, W. A. (1970). Dietary treatment of tyrosinosis *J. Am. diet. Ass.* **56**, 308.
Skiver, C. R. and Rosenberg, L. E. (1973). Tyrosine in aminoacid metabo lism and its disorders. In *Major problems in clinical paediatrics*, vol. 10, 338.
Weinberg, A. G., Mize, C. E., and Worthen, H. G. (1976). The occurrence of hepatoma in a chronic form of hereditary tyrosinemia. *J. Pediat.* **88**, 434.

Urea cycle disorders

Palmer, T., Oberholtzer, B. G., Burgess, E. A., Butler, L. J., and Levin, B. (1974). Hyperammonaemia in 20 families. *Arch. Dis. Child.* **49**, 443.

Alpha-1 antitrypsin deficiency

Aagenaes, Ø. and Sveger, T. (1976). Clinical aspects of liver disease in children with alpha-1 antitrypsin deficiency. In *Liver disease in infancy and childhood* (ed. S. R. Berenberg). Martinhus Nijhoff, The Hague.
Bearn, A. G. and Litwin, S. D. (1978). Deficiencies of circulating enzymes and plasma proteins. In *The metabolic basis of inherited disease*, 4th edn. (eds. J. W. Stanbury, J. B. Wyngaarden, and D. S. Fredrickson). McGraw-Hill, New York.
Psacharopoulos, H. T., Mowat, A. P., Portmann, B. T., and Williams, R. (1980). The prognosis in childhood of liver disease associated with alpha-1 antitrypsin deficiency. In *Cholestasis in infancy* (ed. Japanese Medical Research Council), 133. University of Tokyo Press. Tokyo.
Sveger, T. (1978). Alpha-1 antitrypsin deficiency in early childhood. *Pe diat., Springfield* **62**, 22.
Trigger, D. R. and Millward-Sadler, G. (1979). In *Liver and biliary disease* (ed. R. Wright, K. G. M. Alberti, S. Karran, and G. H. Millward-Sadler), 805. W. B. Saunders, London.

Genetic storage disorders

Ishak, K. G. and Sharp, H. L. (1979). Metabolic errors and liver disease. In *Pathology of the liver* (eds. R. N. M. MacSween, P. Anthony and P. J. Scheur), 88.
Mowat, A. P. (1979). Inborn errors of metabolism causing hepatomegaly or disordered liver function. In *Liver disorders in childhood*, 162. But ter worth, London.

Reye's syndrome

Pollack, J. D. (ed.) (1975). *Reye's syndrome*. Grune and Stratton, New York.

Cystic fibrosis

Isenberg, J. M., L'Heurex, P., Warwick, J. W., and Sharp, H. L. (1976). Clinical observations on the biliary system in cystic fibrosis. *Am. J. Gastroent.* **65**, 134.

Mowat, A. P. (1979). Hepato-biliary disease in cystic fibrosis. In *Liver disorders in childhood*, 269. Butterworth, London.

Infantile polycystic disease of the kidneys and liver, and congenital hepatic fibrosis

Lake, D. N. W., Smith, P. M., and Wheeler, H. (1977). Congenital hepatic fibrosis and choledochal cyst. *Br. med. J.* **ii**, 1259.

Mowat, A. P. (1979). Familial and genetic structural abnormalities in the liver and biliry system. In *Liver disorders in childhood*, 202. Butterworth, London.

Murray-Lyon, I. M., Ockenden, B. G. and Williams, R. (1973). Congenital hepatic fibrosis—is it a single clinical entity? *Gastroent.* **44**, 653.

NOTES

NOTES

NOTES

NOTES

NOTES

NOTES

NOTES

NOTES

NOTES

NOTES

NOTES

NOTES

NOTES

NOTES

NOTES

NOTES

NOTES

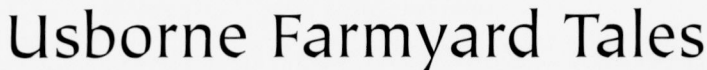

Usborne Farmyard Tales

The Complete Book of
Farmyard Tales

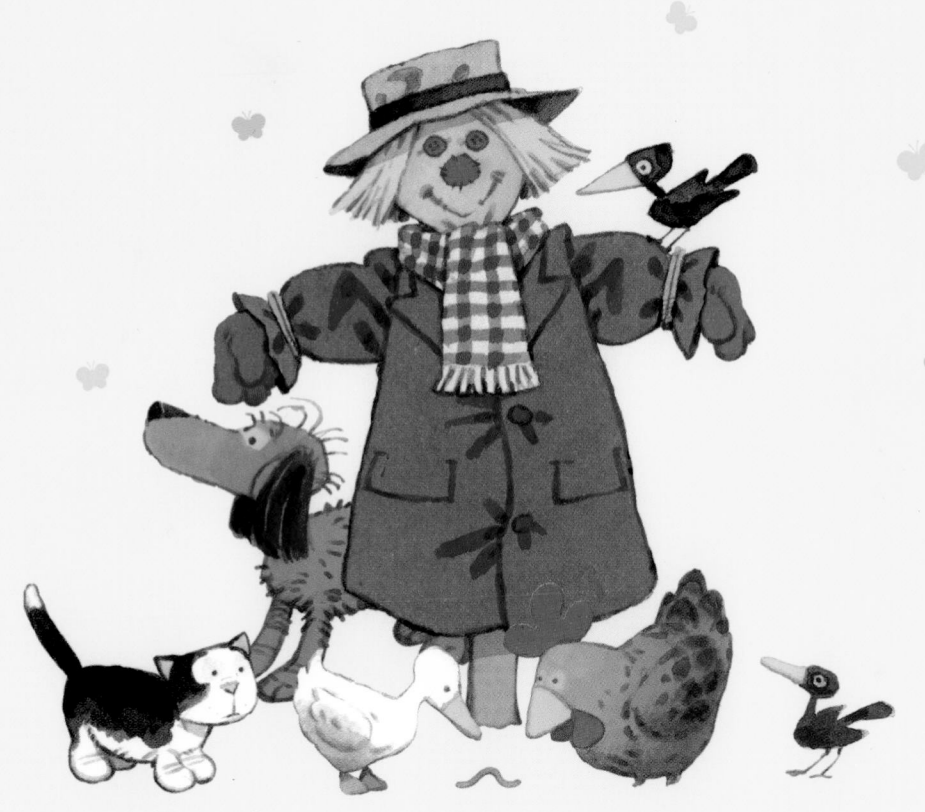

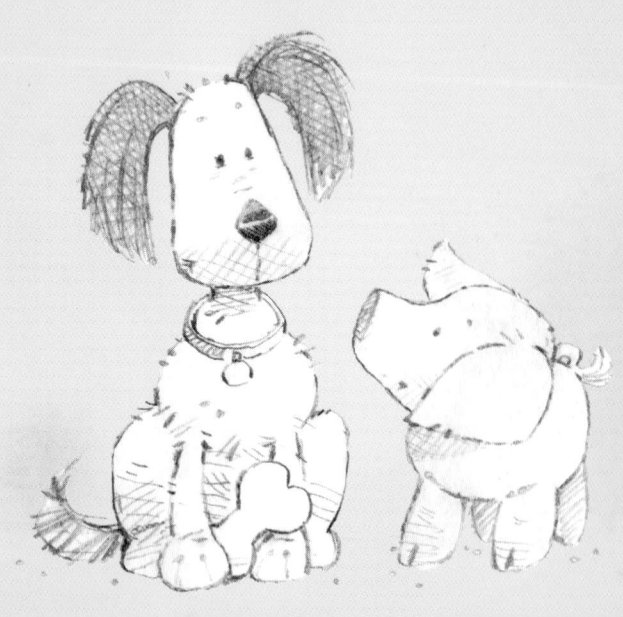

Cover design by Hannah Ahmed
Digital manipulation by Sarah Cronin, Natacha Goransky and Nelupa Hussain.

First published in 2004 by Usborne Publishing Ltd. 83-85 Saffron Hill, London EC1N 8RT, England. www.usborne.com
Copyright © 2004, 1999, 1996, 1995, 1994, 1992, 1990, 1989 Usborne Publishing Ltd.
The name Usborne and the devices ♀ ♔ are Trade Marks of Usborne Publishing Ltd. All rights reserved. No part of this publication may be reproduced, stored in a retrieval system, or transmitted in any form or by any means, electronic, mechanical, photocopying, recording or otherwise, without prior permission of the publisher. UE. First published in America in 2004. Printed in China.

Usborne Farmyard Tales

The Complete Book of
Farmyard Tales

Heather Amery

Illustrated by Stephen Cartwright

Language consultant: Betty Root
Series editor: Jenny Tyler

There's a little yellow duck to find in every picture.
Can you find it?

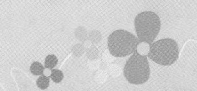

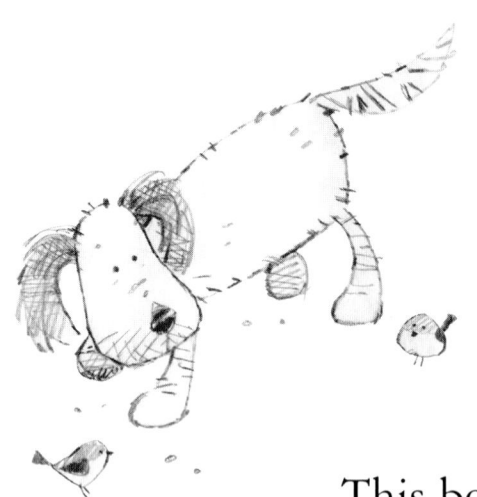

This book is dedicated
to the memory of
Stephen Cartwright
1948 - 2004

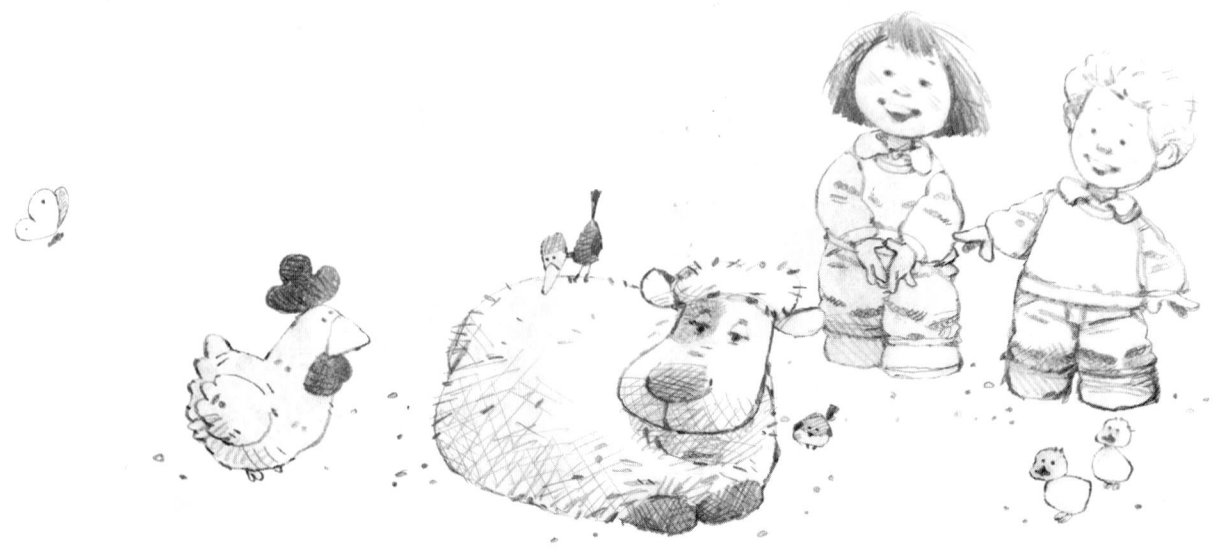

These are some of Stephen Cartwright's original
pencil drawings for the characters of Farmyard Tales.

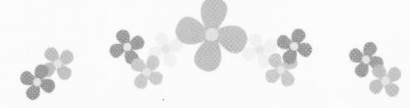

Contents

Pig Gets Stuck   1

The Naughty Sheep   17

Barn on Fire   33

The Runaway Tractor   49

Pig Gets Lost   65

The Hungry Donkey   81

Scarecrow's Secret   97

Tractor in Trouble   113

The Silly Sheepdog   129

Kitten's Day Out   145

The New Pony   161

The Grumpy Goat   177

The Snow Storm   193

Surprise Visitors   209

Market Day   225

Camping Out   241

The Old Steam Train   257

Dolly and the Train   273

Rusty's Train Ride   289

Woolly Stops the Train   305

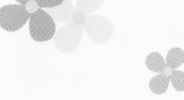

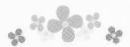

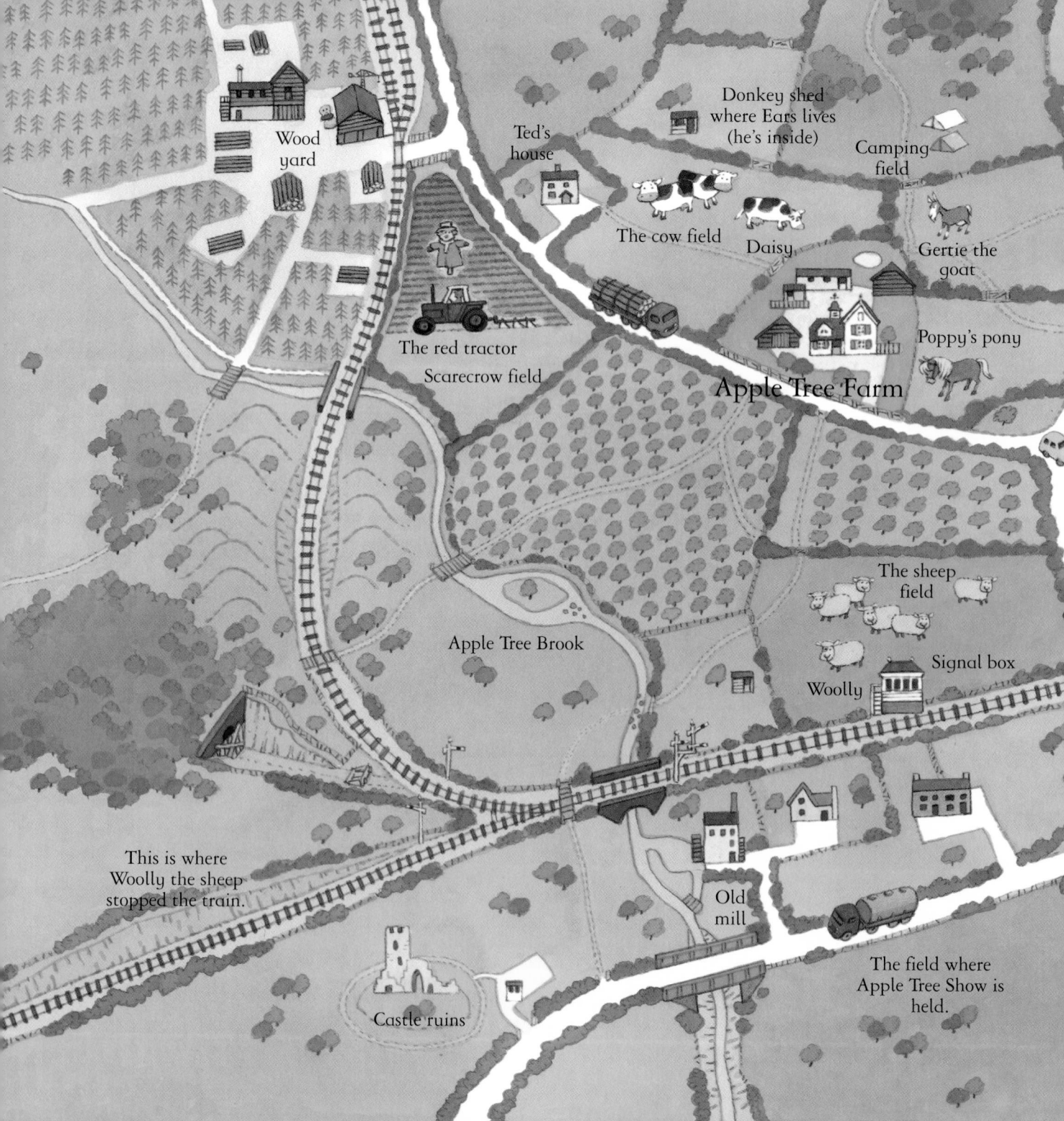

Wood yard

Ted's house

Donkey shed where Ears lives (he's inside)

Camping field

The cow field

Daisy

Gertie the goat

The red tractor
Scarecrow field

Poppy's pony

Apple Tree Farm

The sheep field

Signal box

Apple Tree Brook

Woolly

This is where Woolly the sheep stopped the train.

Old mill

The field where Apple Tree Show is held.

Castle ruins

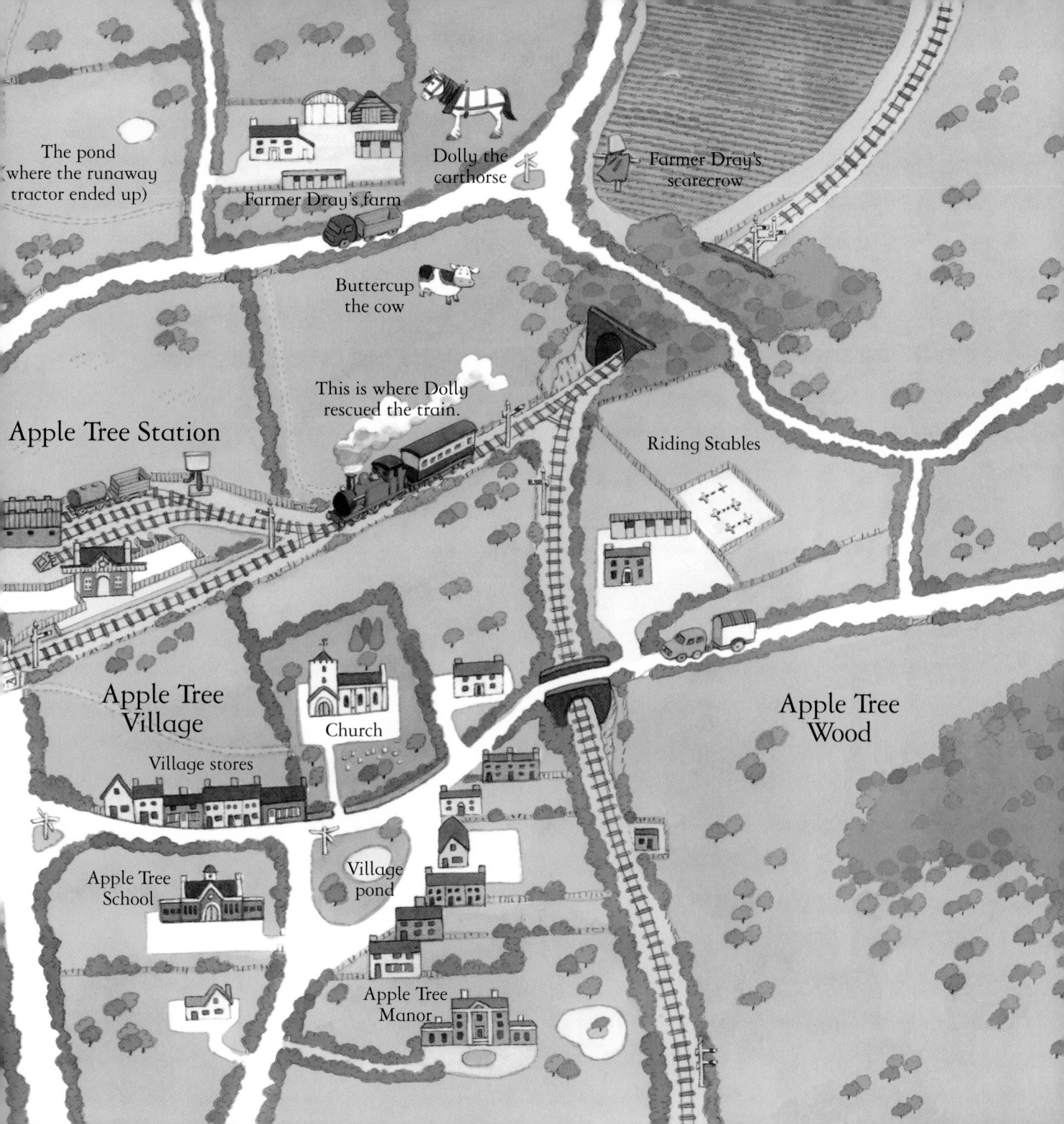

The pond
(where the runaway
tractor ended up)

Farmer Dray's farm

Dolly the
carthorse

Farmer Dray's
scarecrow

Buttercup
the cow

This is where Dolly
rescued the train.

Apple Tree Station

Riding Stables

Apple Tree
Village

Apple Tree
Wood

Church

Village stores

Apple Tree
School

Village
pond

Apple Tree
Manor

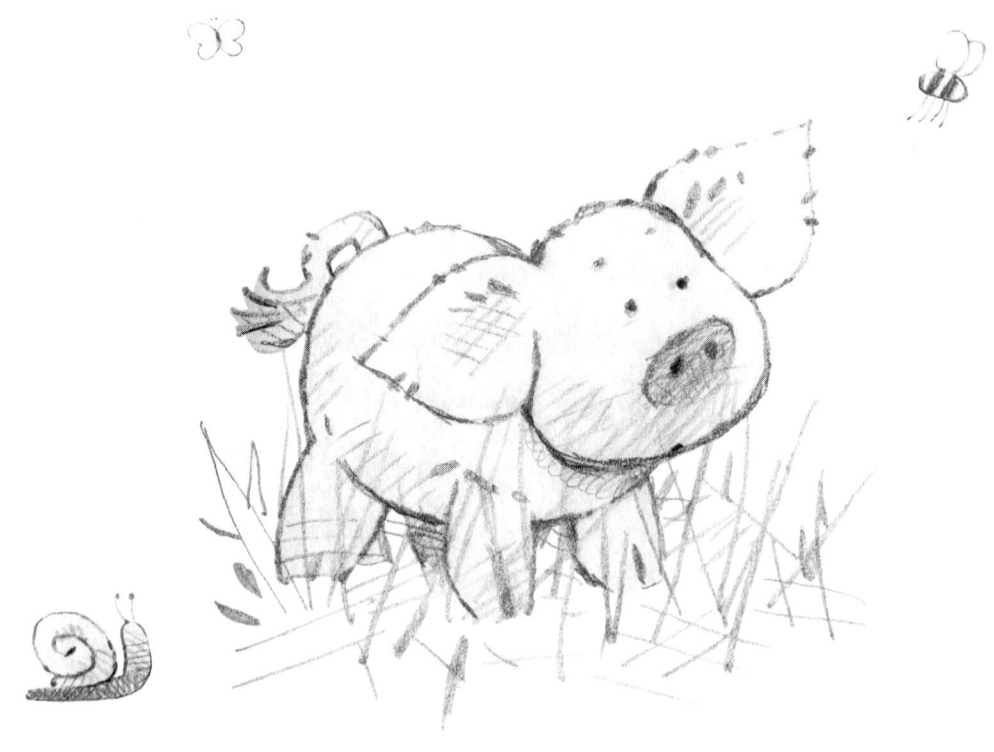

Curly the pig

Pig Gets Stuck

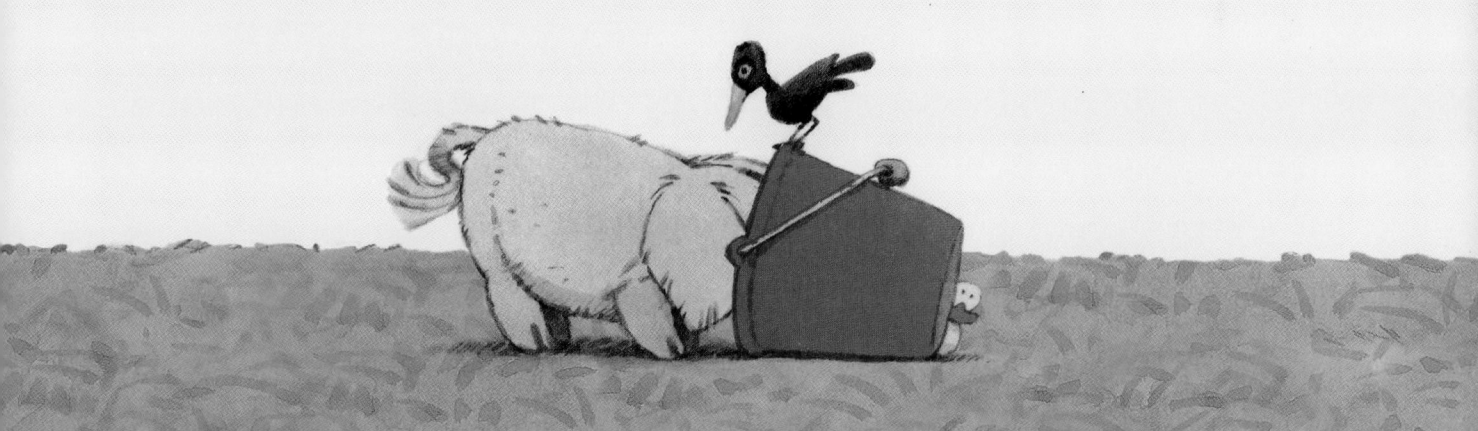

This is Apple Tree Farm.

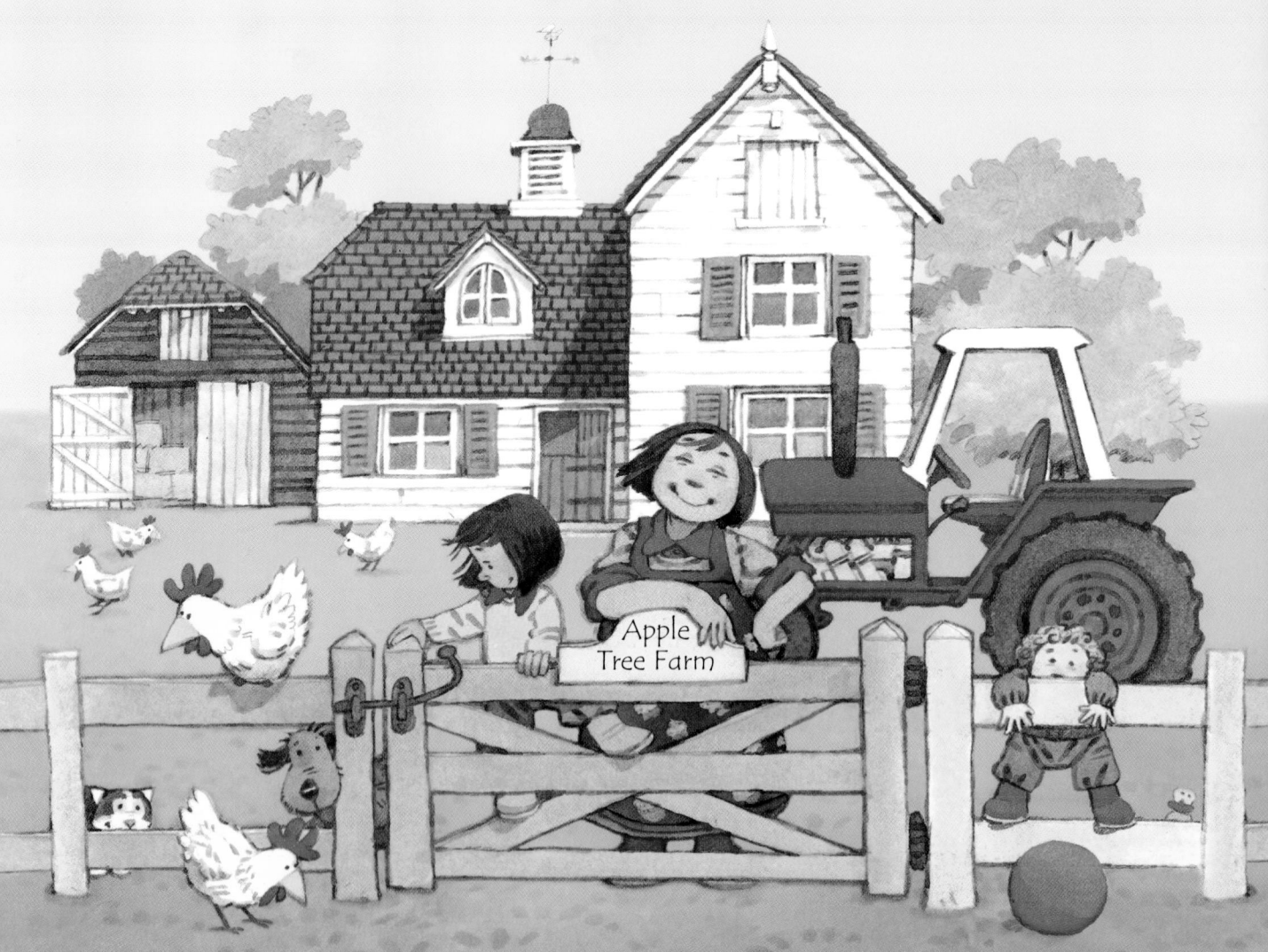

This is Mrs. Boot, the farmer. She has two children, called Poppy and Sam, and a dog called Rusty.

2

On the farm there are six pigs.

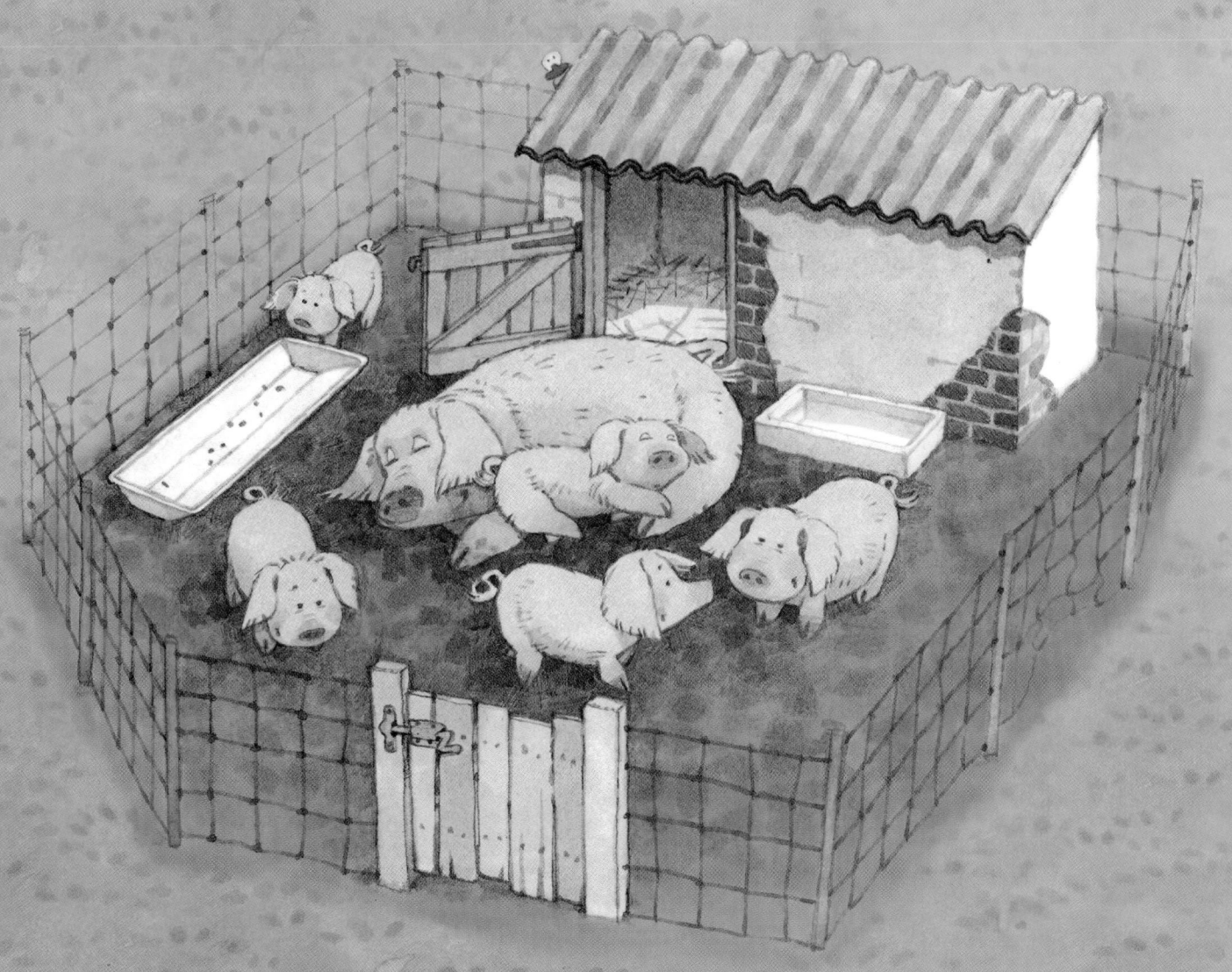

The pigs live in a pen with a little house.
The smallest pig is called Curly.

It is time for breakfast.

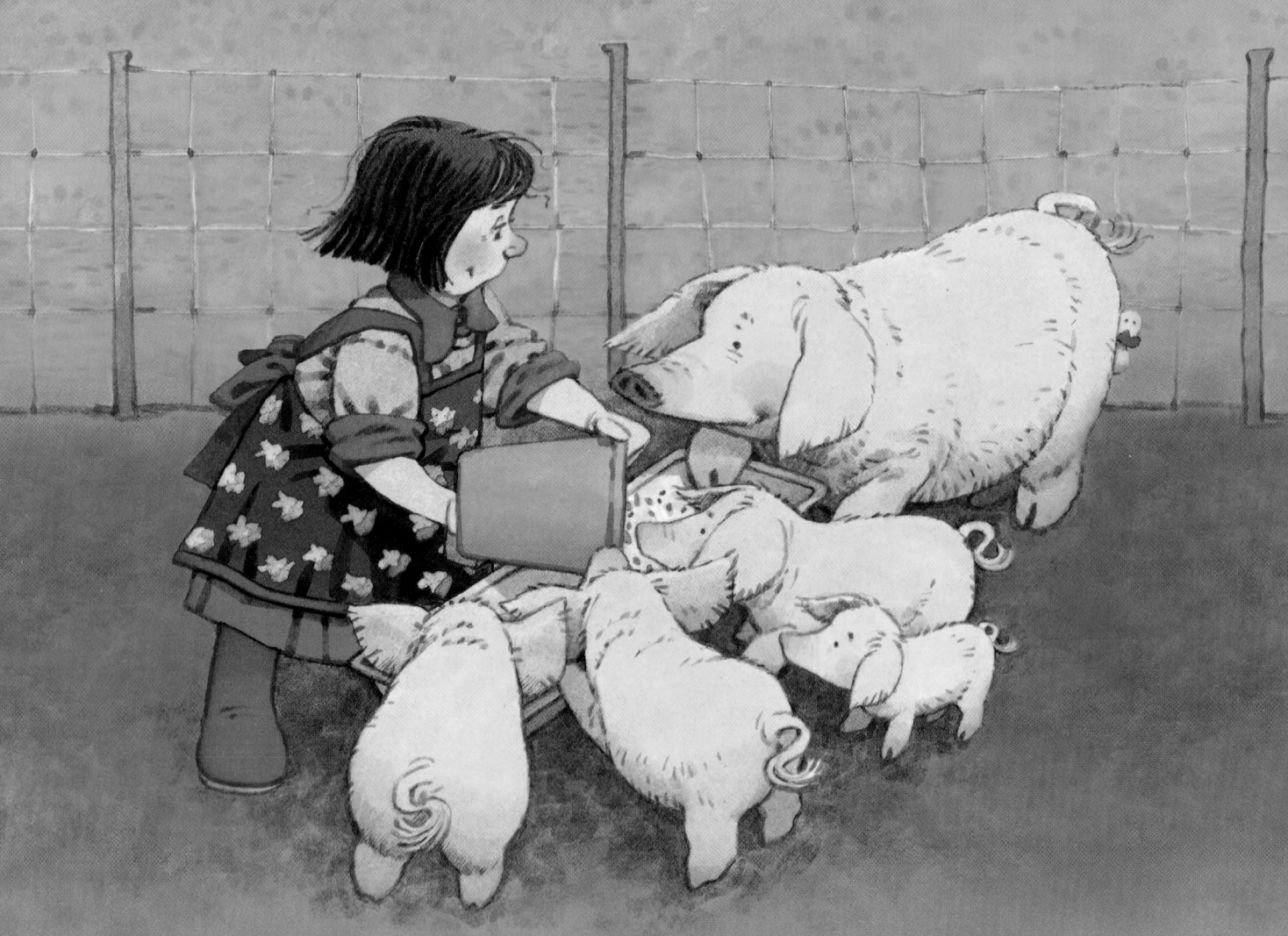

Mrs. Boot gives the pigs their breakfast.
But Curly is so small, he does not get any.

Curly is hungry.

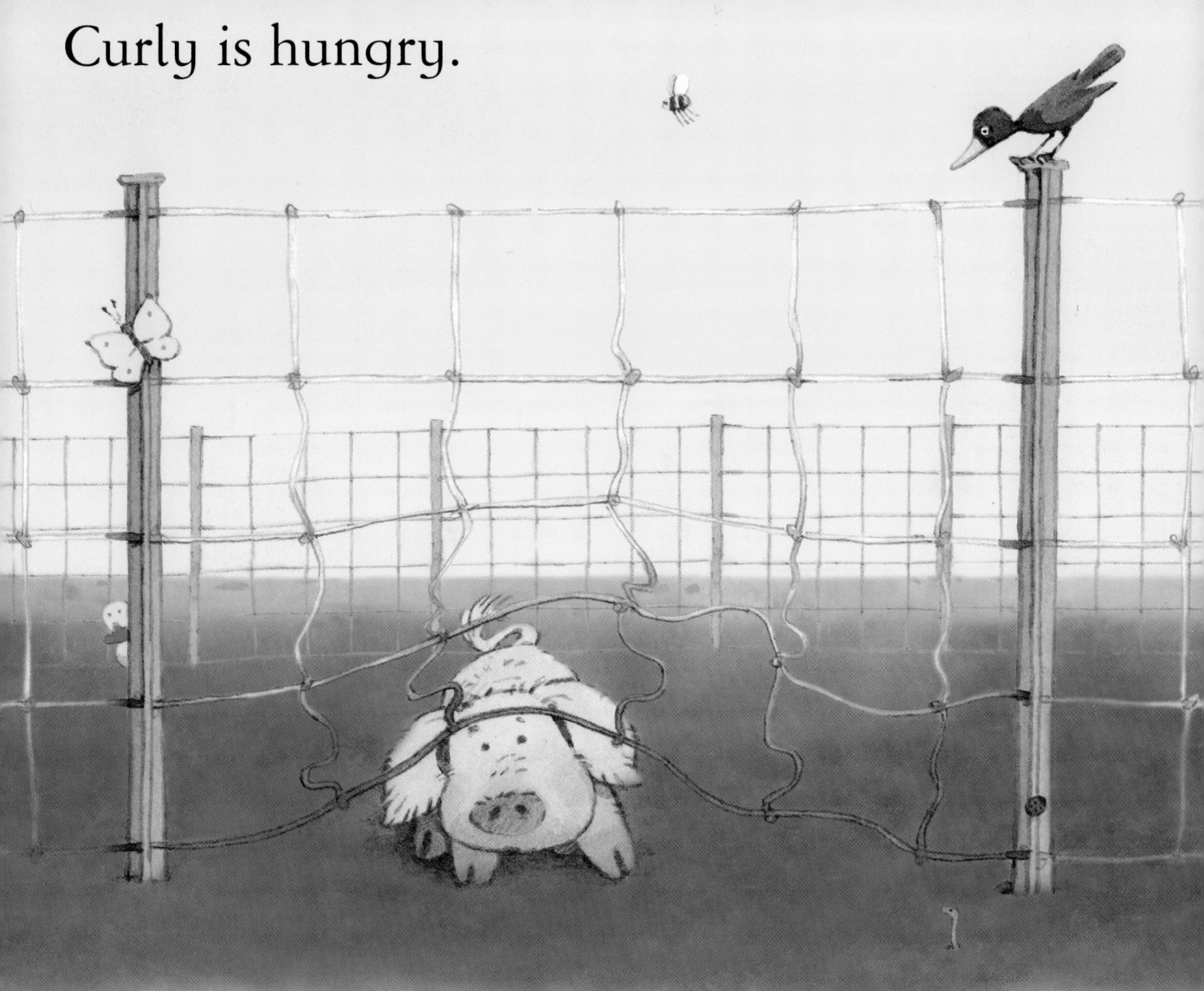

He looks for something else to eat in the pen.
Then he finds a little gap under the wire.

Curly is out.

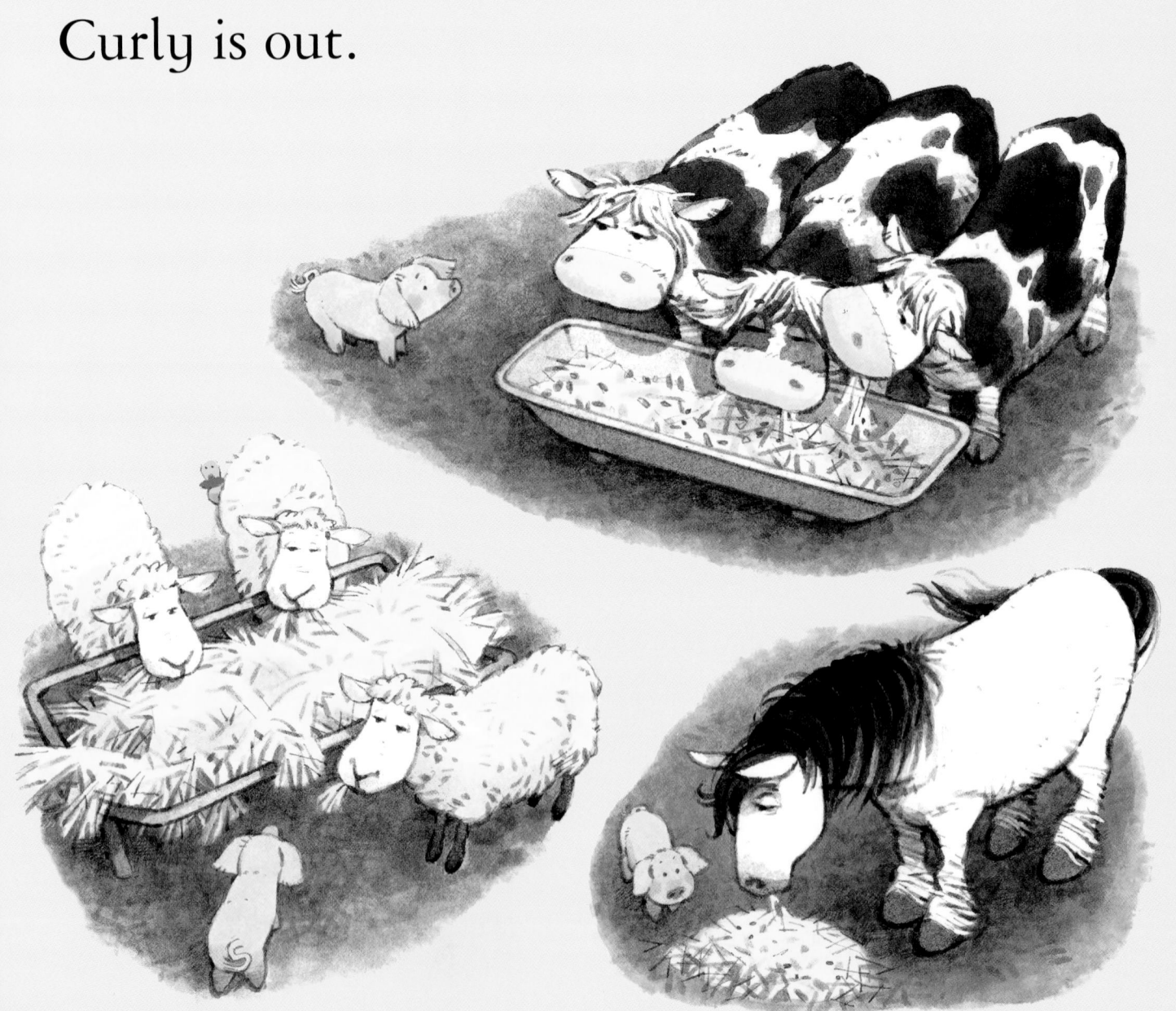

He squeezes through the gap under the wire.
He is out in the farmyard.

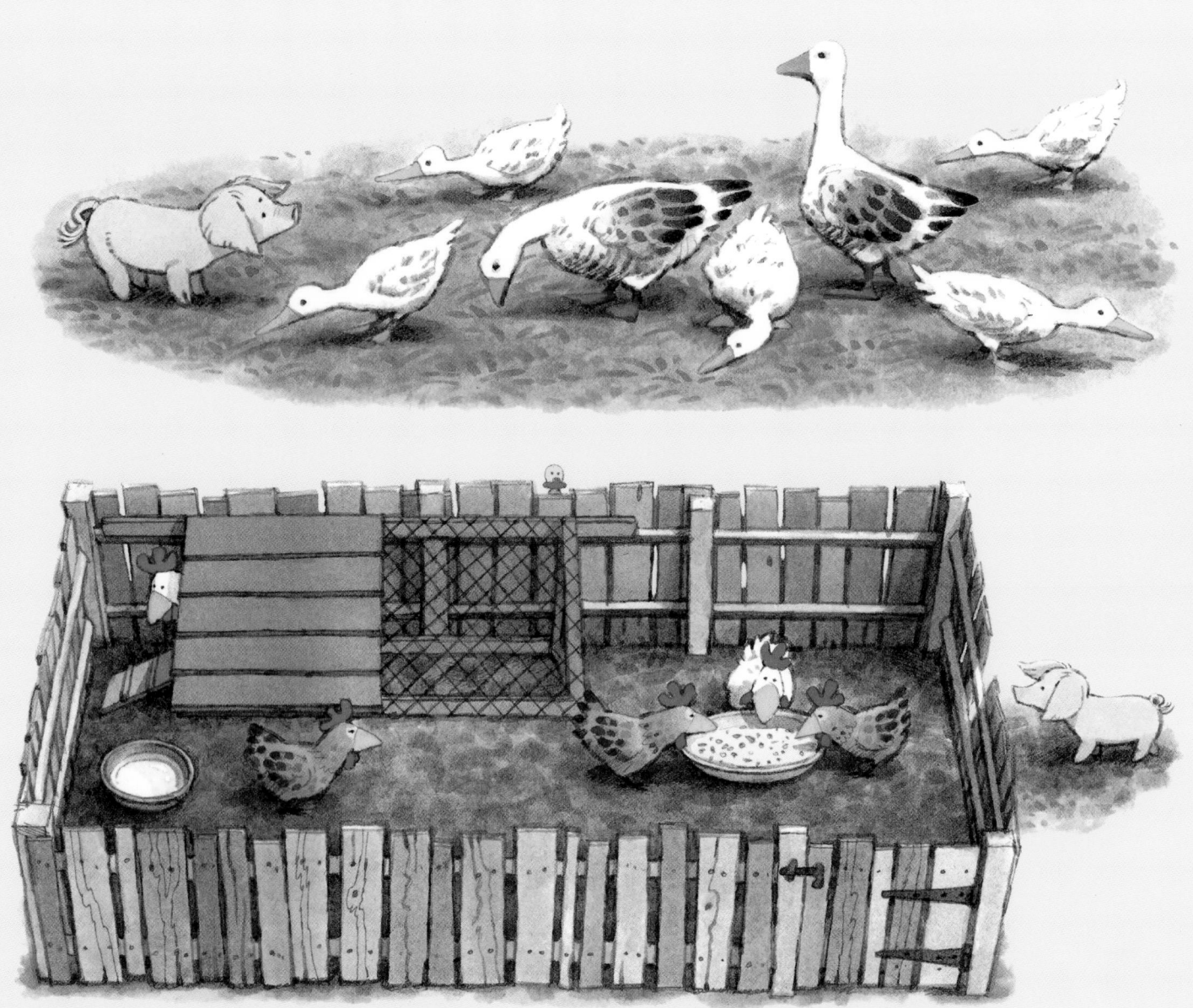

He meets lots of other animals in the farmyard.
Which breakfast would he like to eat?

Curly wants the hens' breakfast.

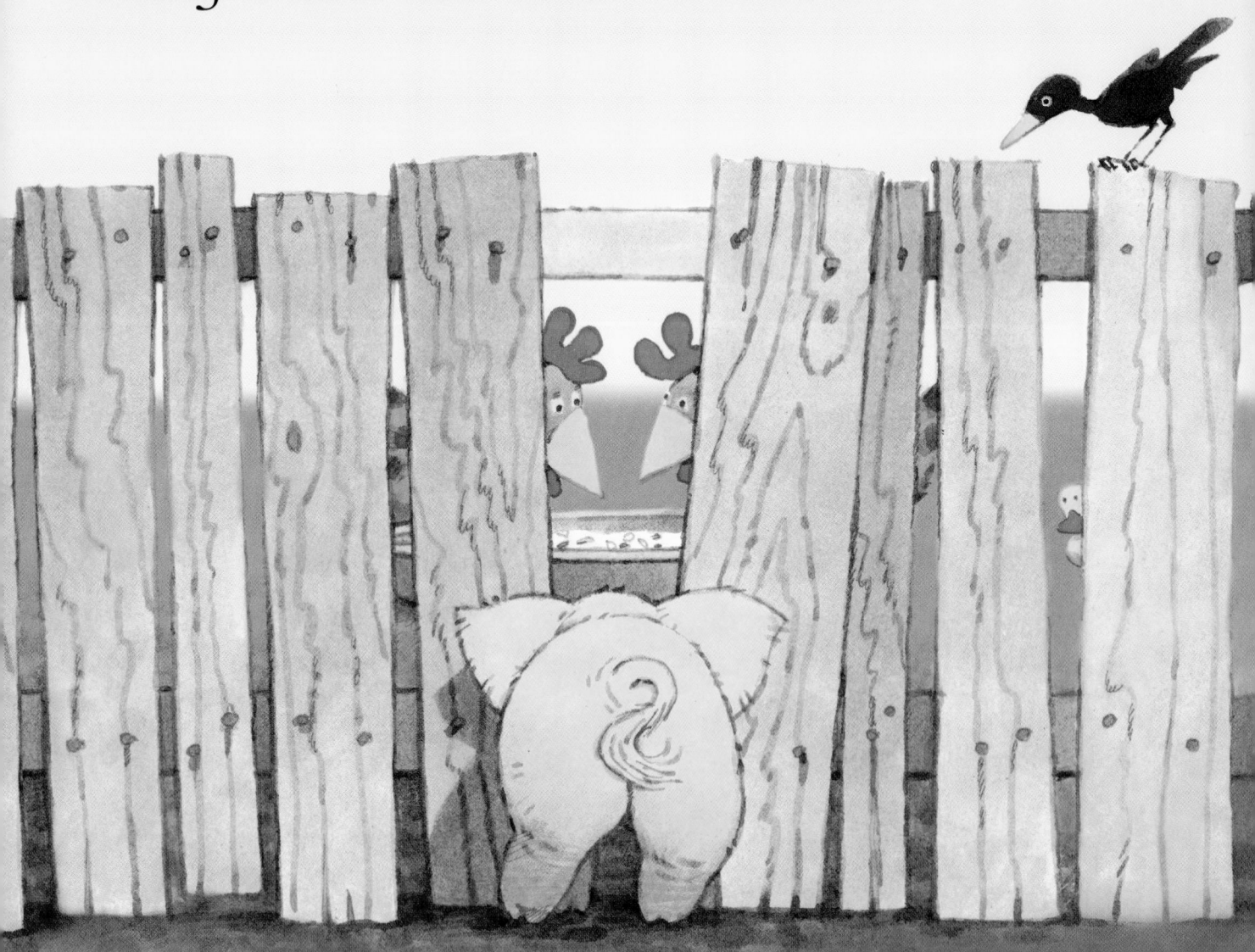

He thinks the hens' breakfast looks good.
He squeezes through the gap in the fence.

8

Curly tries it.

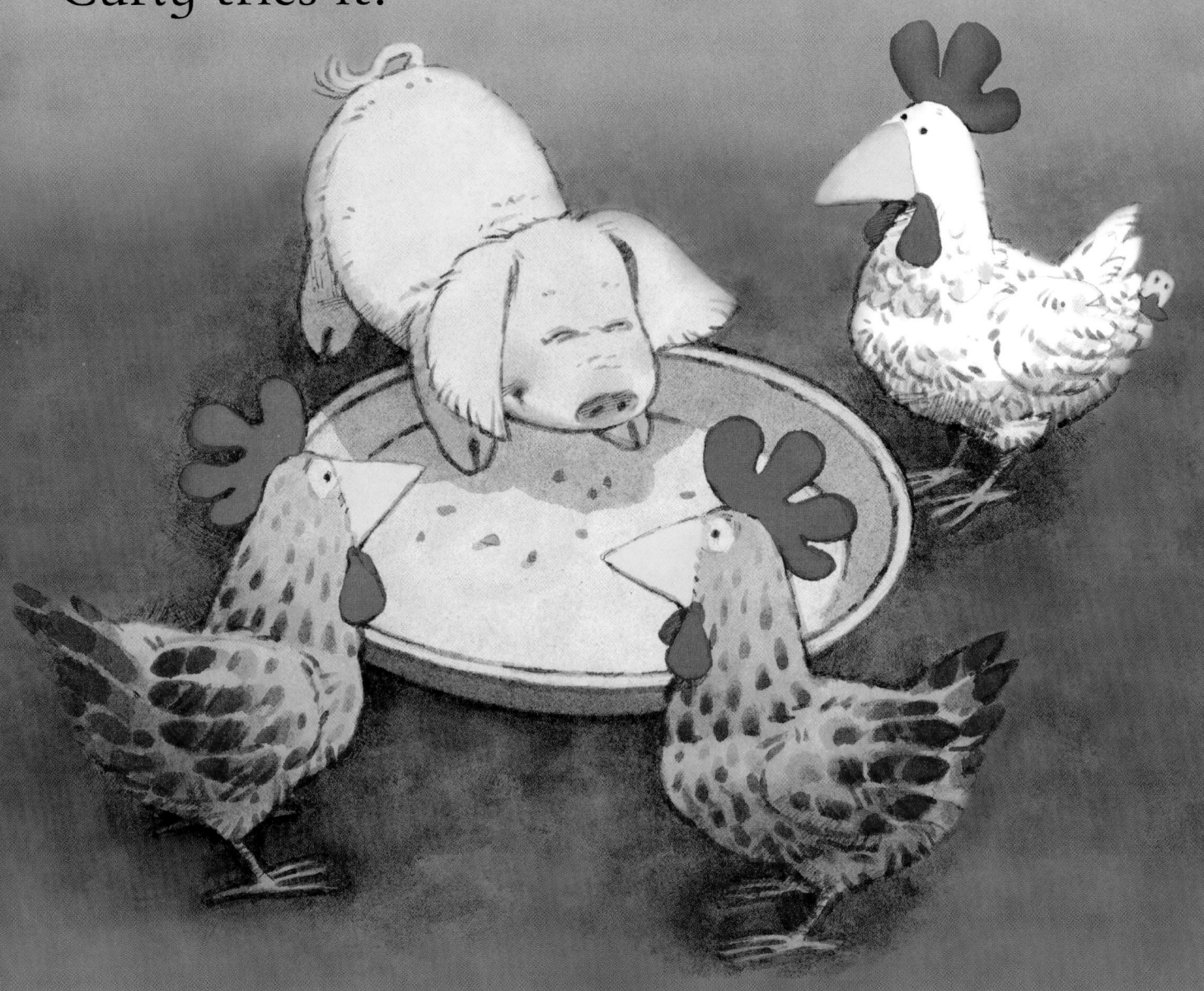

The hens' food is so good, he gobbles it all up.
The hens are not pleased.

Mrs. Boot sees Curly.

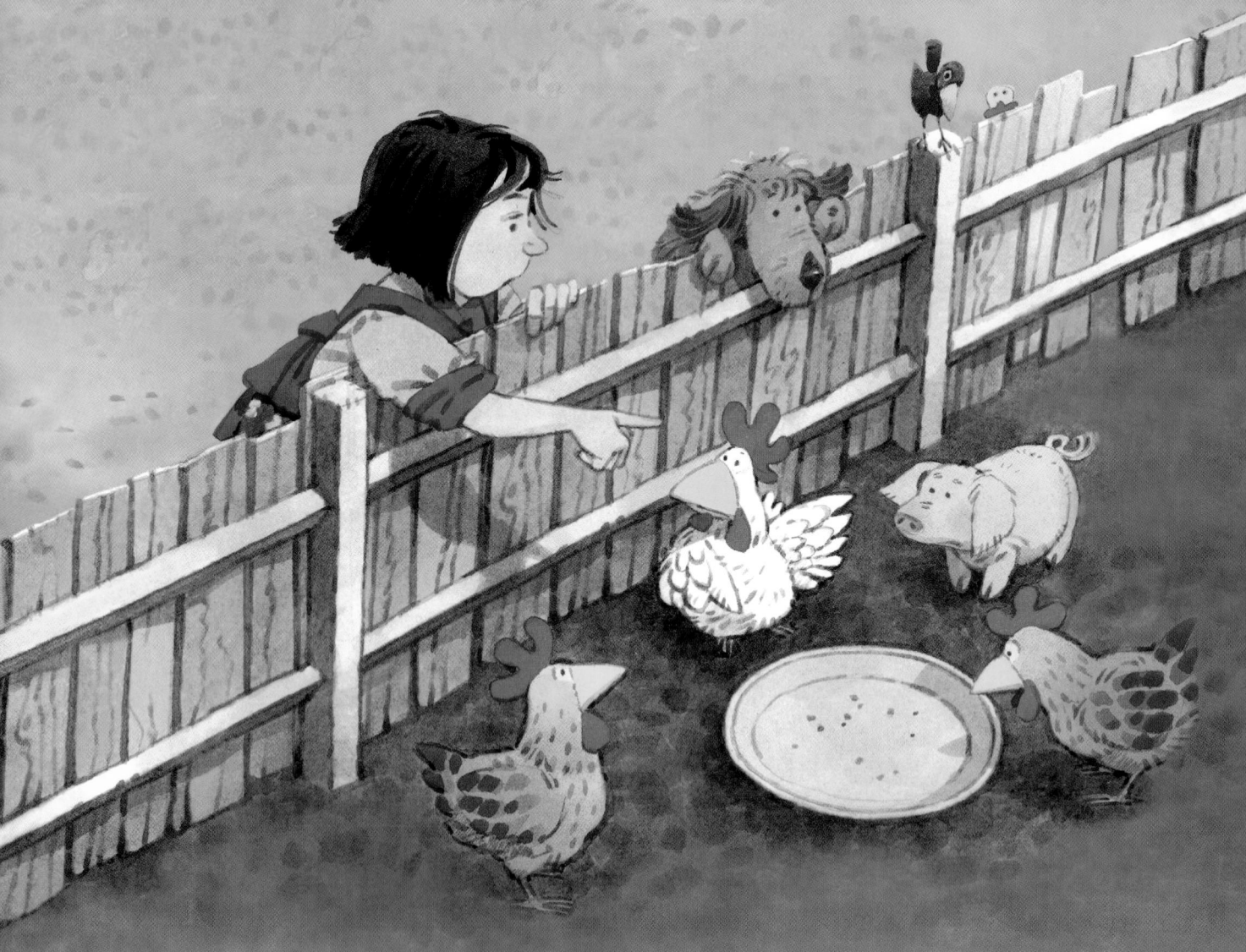

Curly hears Mrs. Boot shouting at him.
"What are you doing in the hen run, Curly?"

10

He runs to the fence.

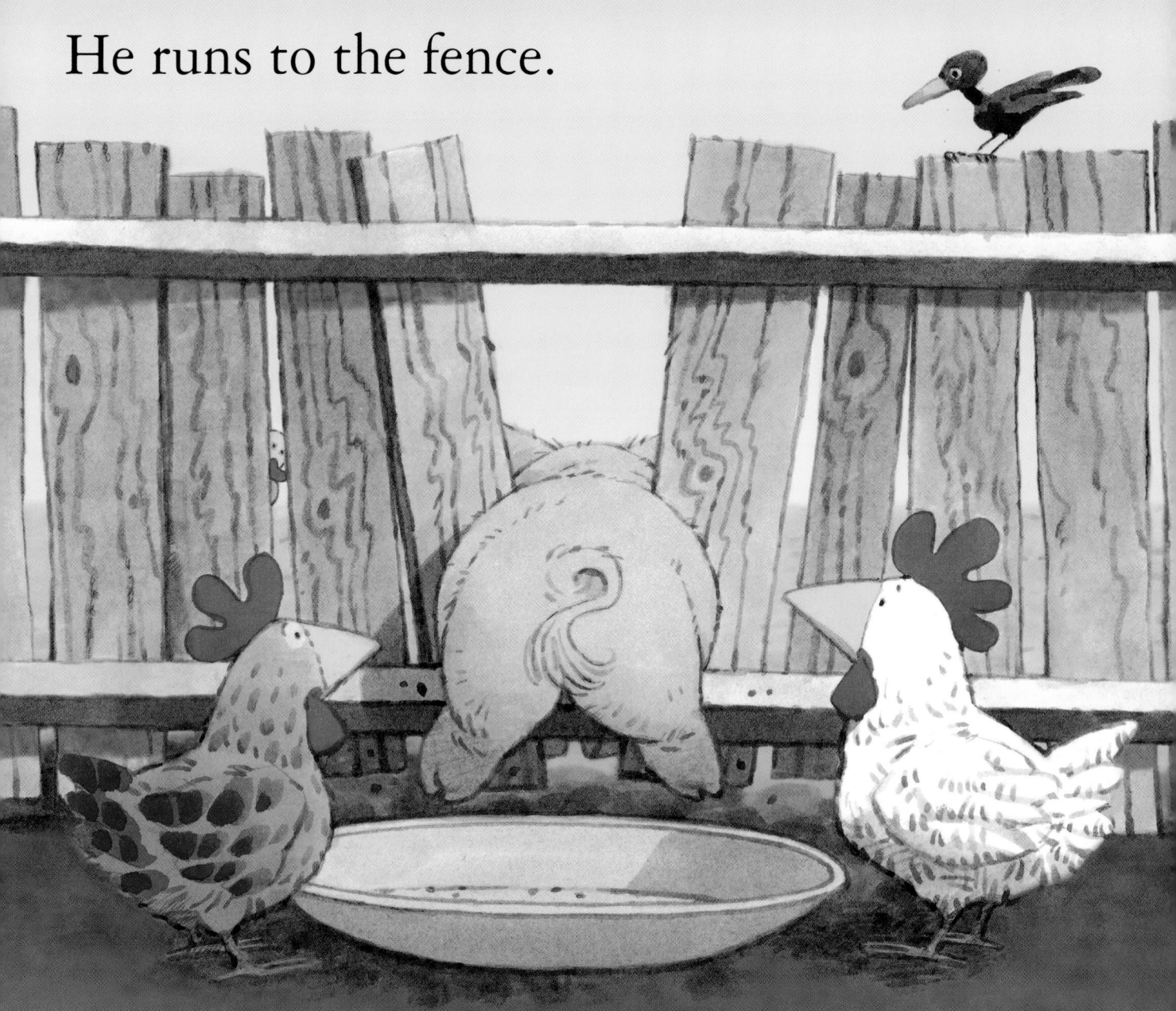

He tries to squeeze through the gap. But he has eaten so much breakfast, he is too fat.

11

Curly is stuck.

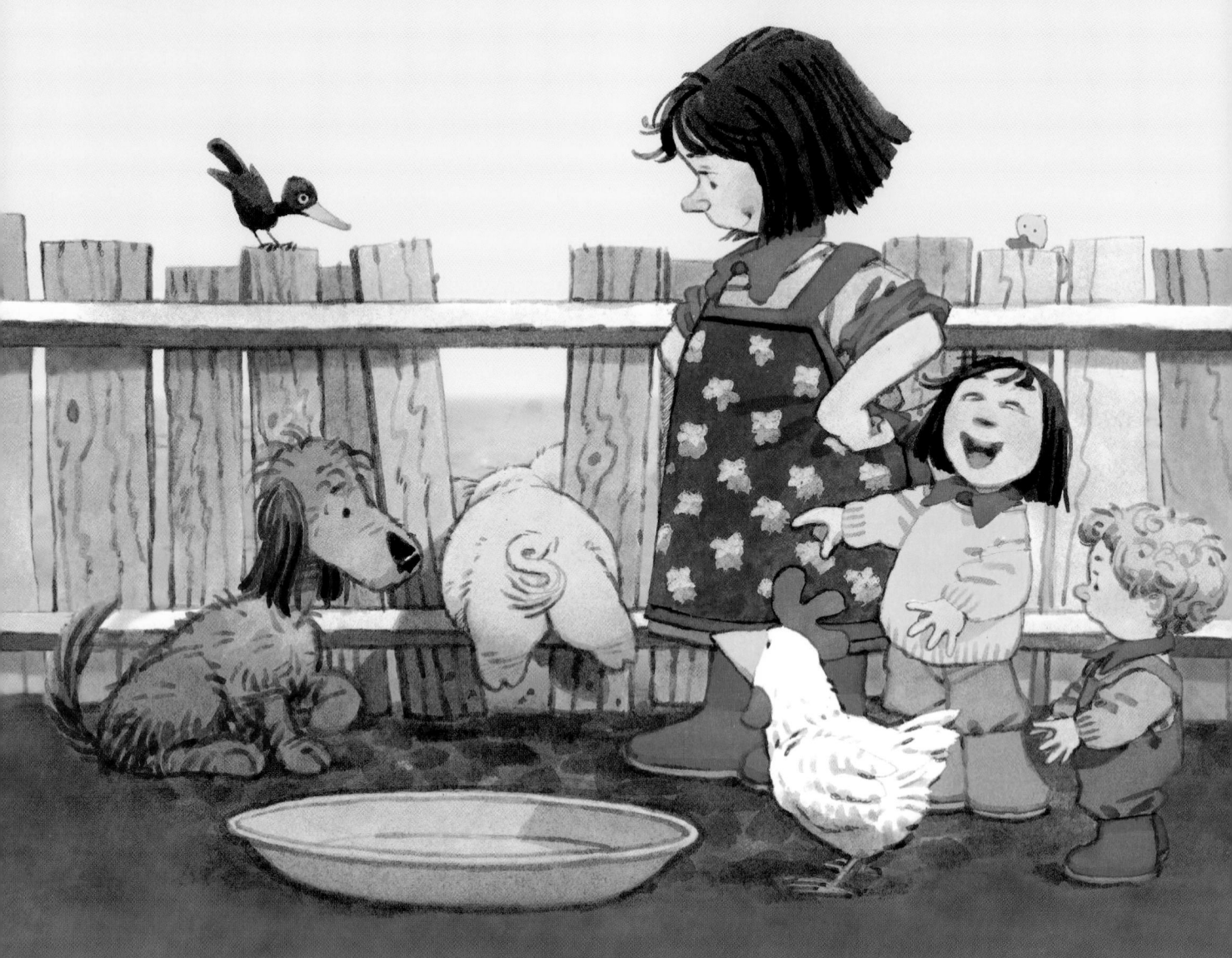

Curly pushes and pushes but he can't move.
He is stuck in the fence.

They all push.

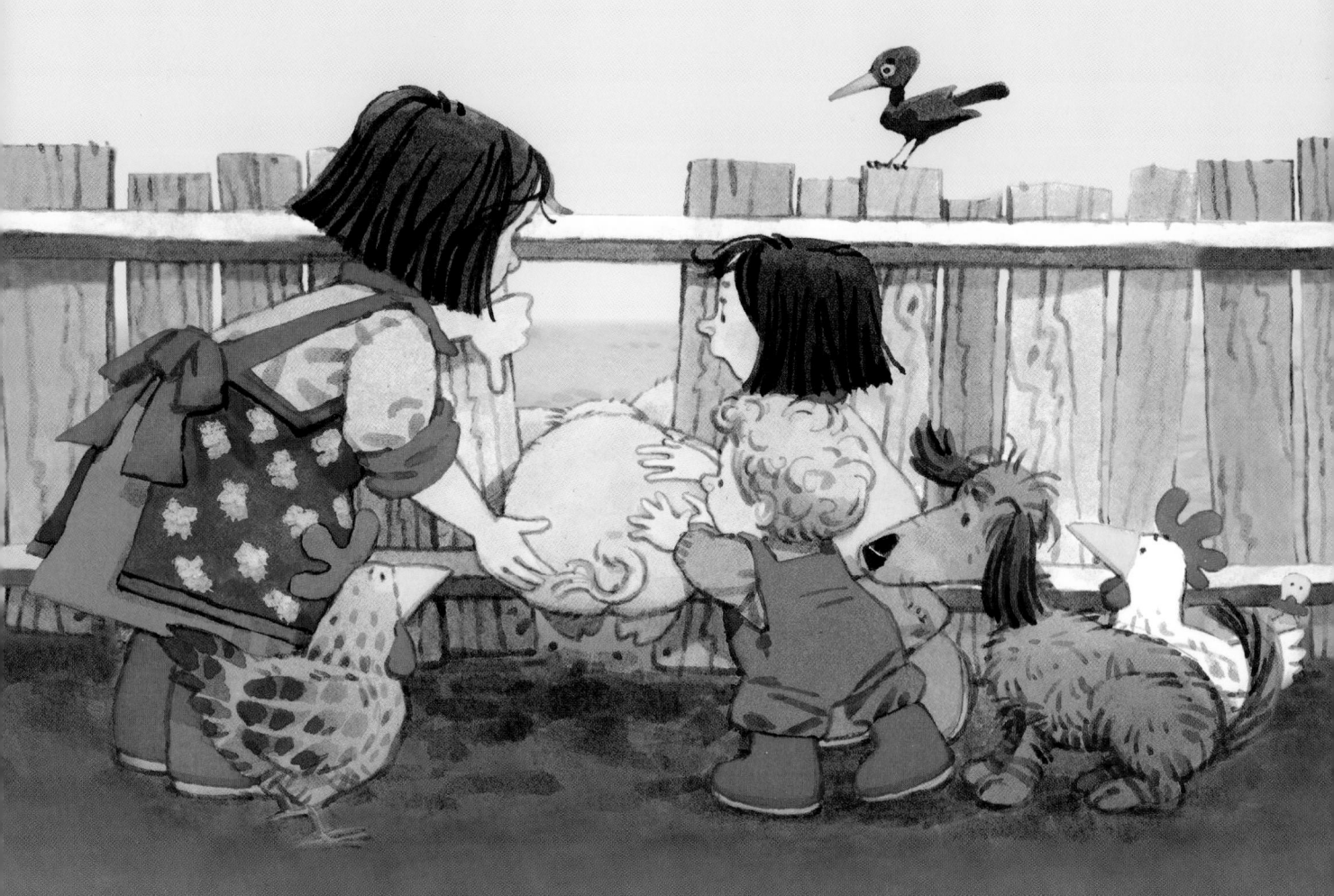

Mrs. Boot, Poppy and Sam all push Curly.
He squeals and squeals. His sides hurt.

Curly is out.

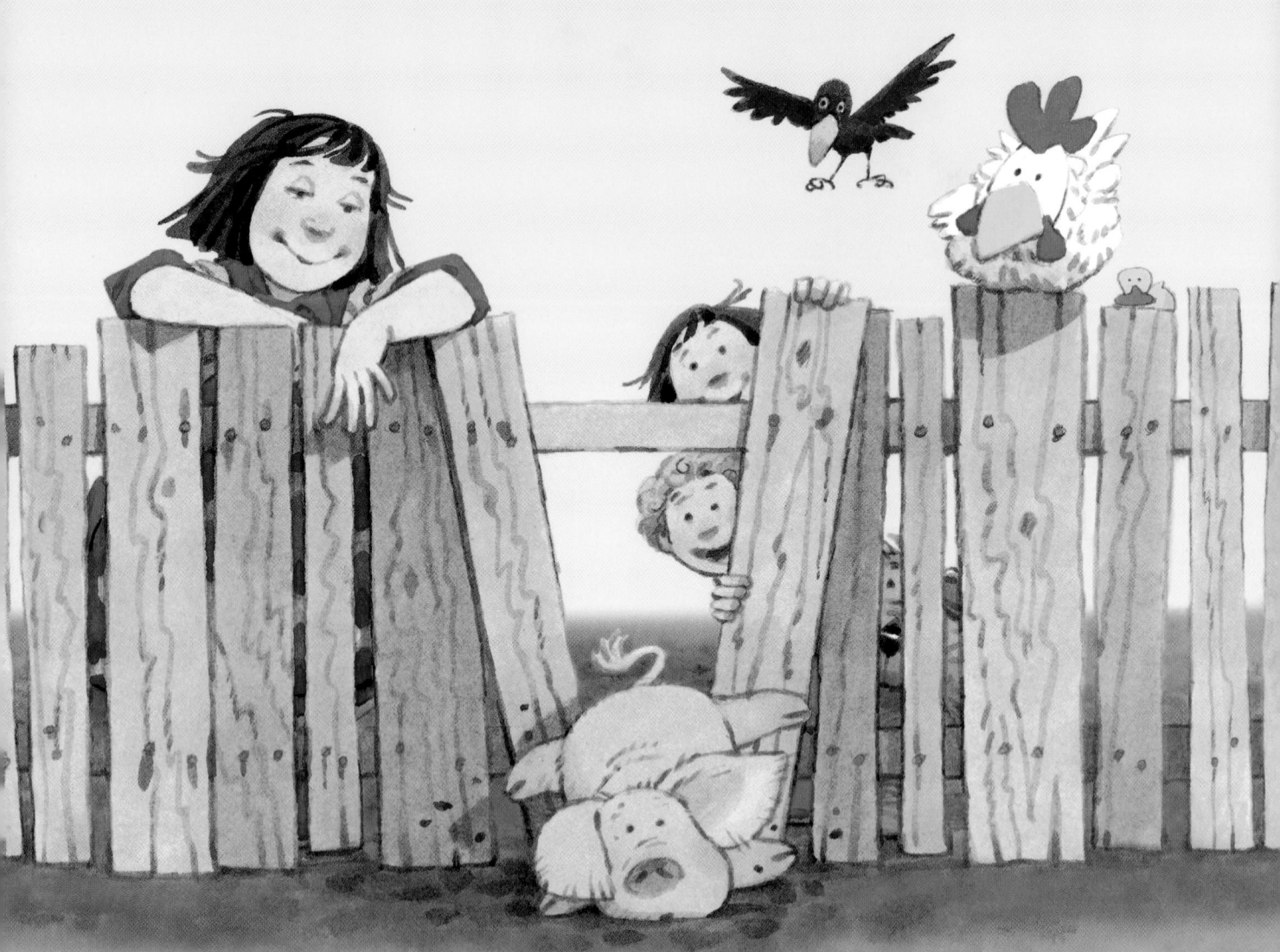

Then with a grunt, Curly pops through the fence.
"He's out, he's out," shouts Sam.

14

He is safe now.

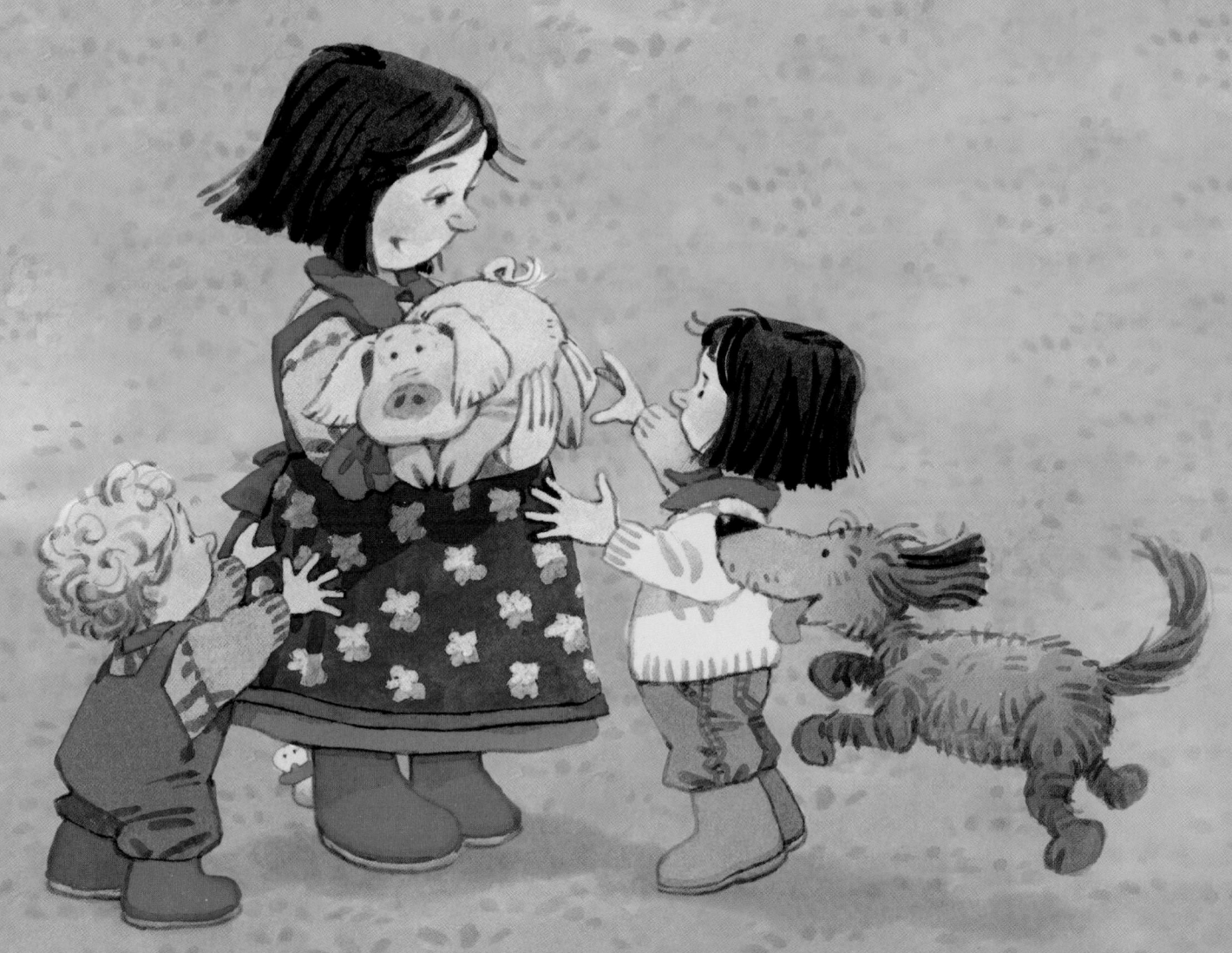

Mrs. Boot picks up Curly. "Poor little pig," she says. And she carries him back to the pig pen.

Curly is happy.

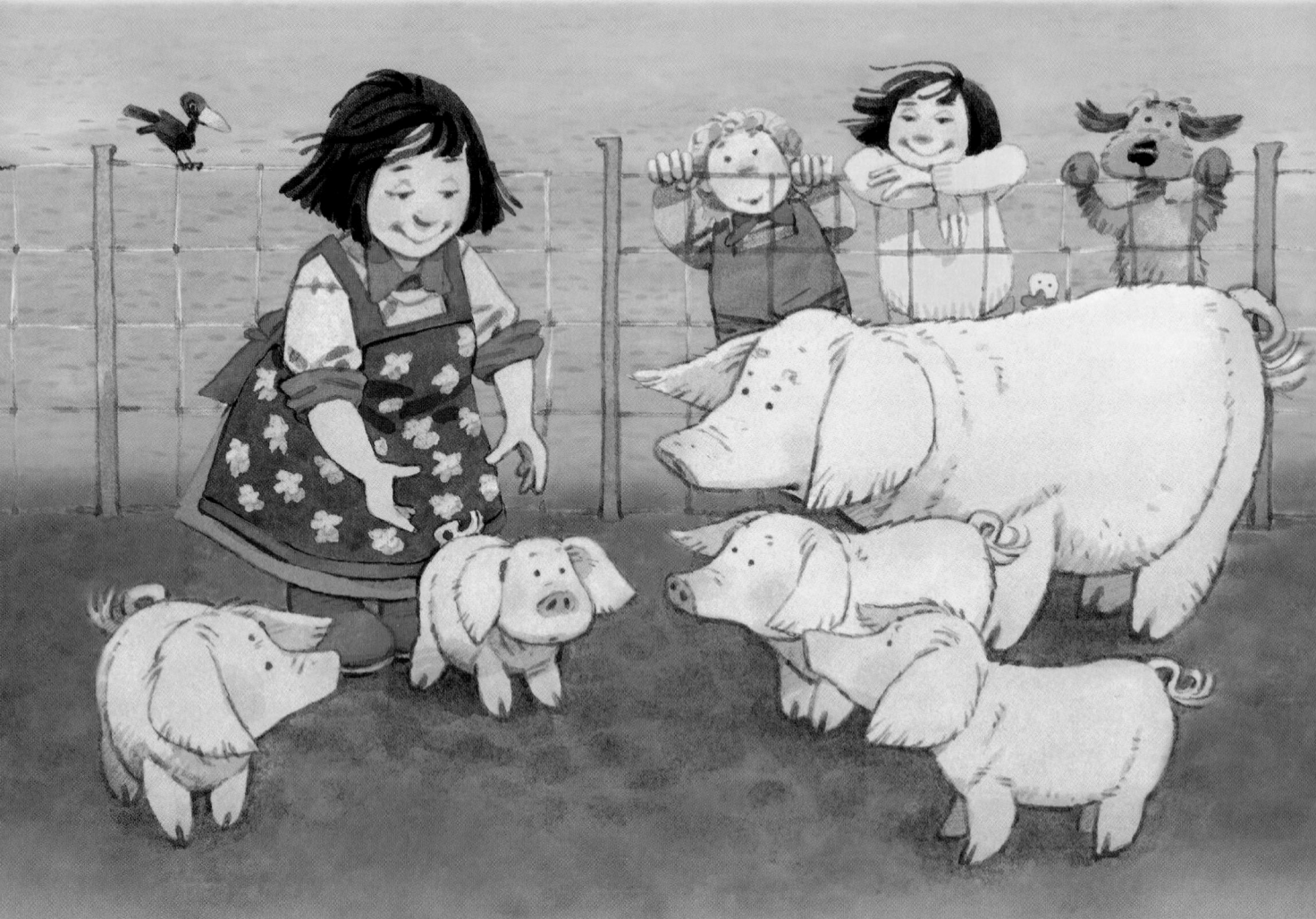

"Tomorrow you shall have lots of breakfast," she says. And Curly was never, ever hungry again.

The
Naughty Sheep

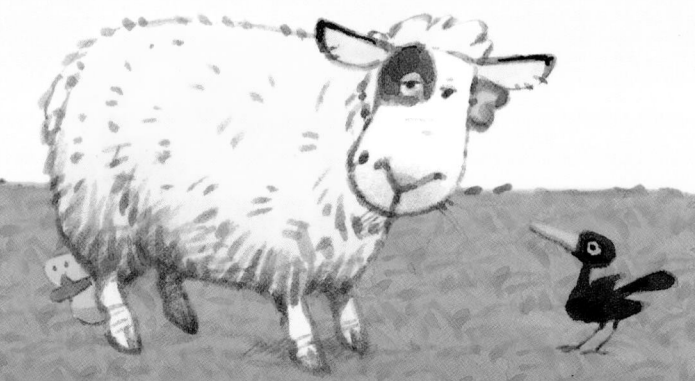

This is Apple Tree Farm.

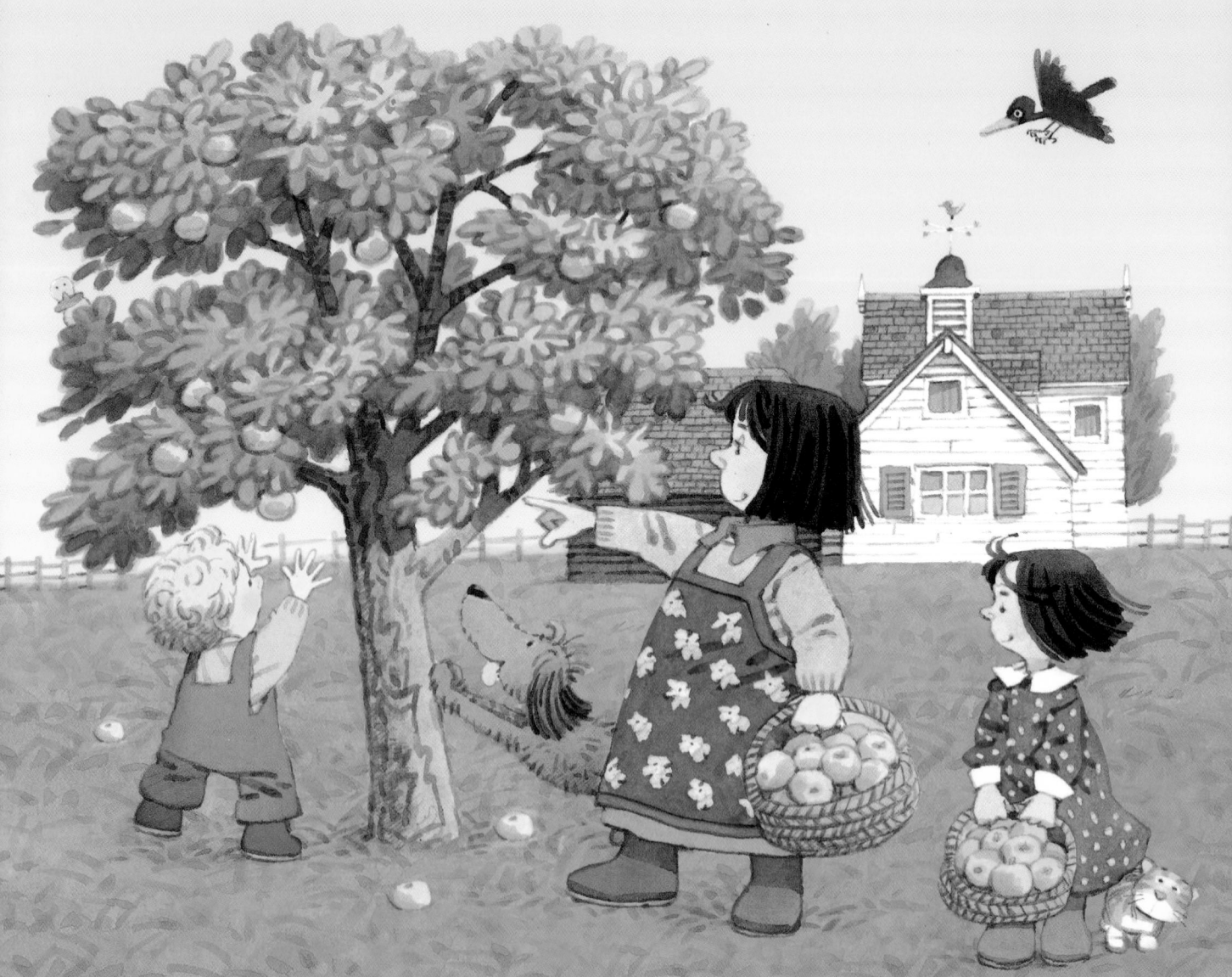

This is Mrs. Boot, the farmer. She has two children, called Poppy and Sam, and a dog called Rusty.

On the farm there are seven sheep.

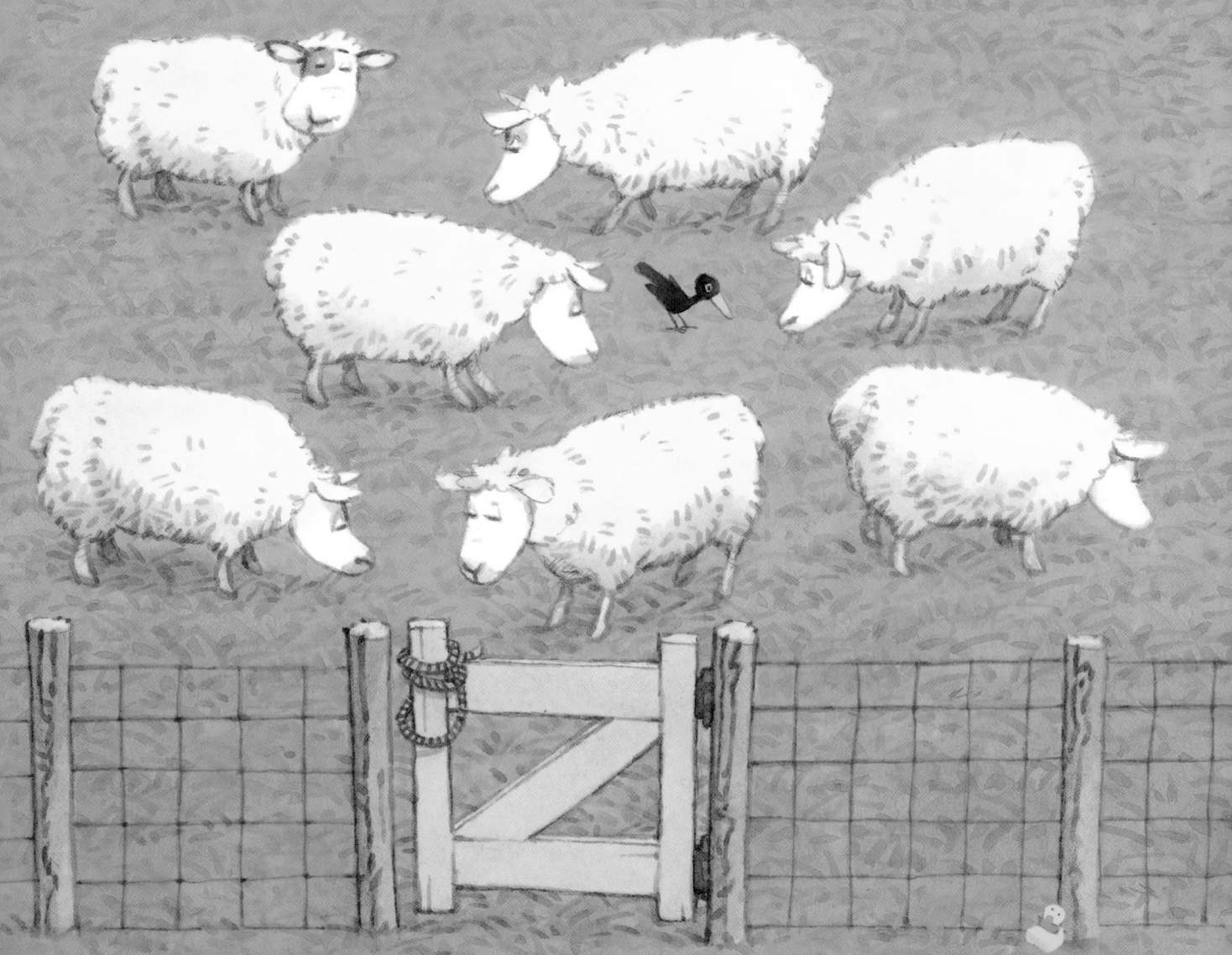

The sheep live in a big field with a fence around it.
One sheep has a black eye. She is called Woolly.

Woolly is bored.

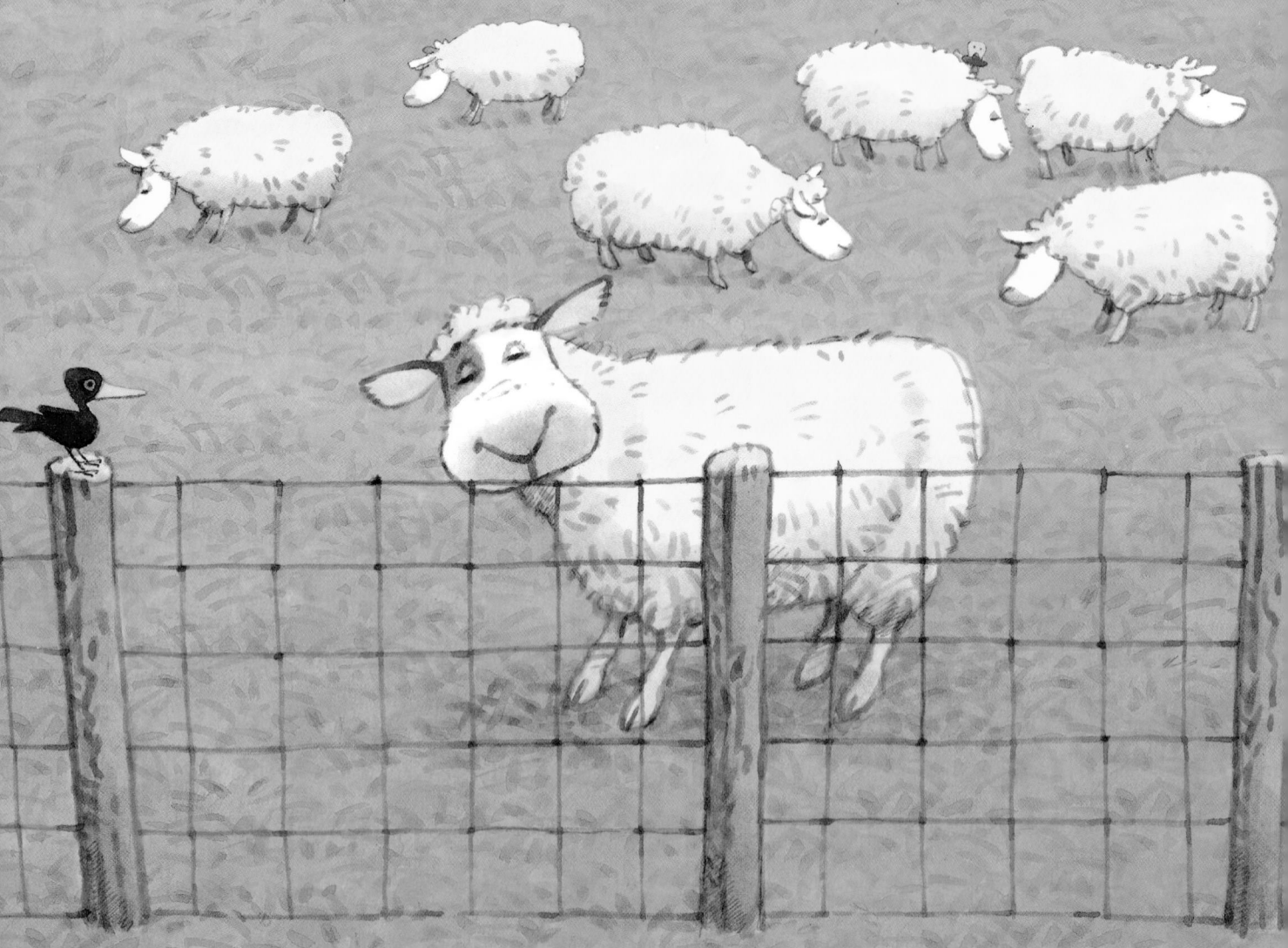

Woolly stops eating and looks over the fence.
"Grass," she says, "nothing but grass. Boring."

Woolly runs out of the gate.

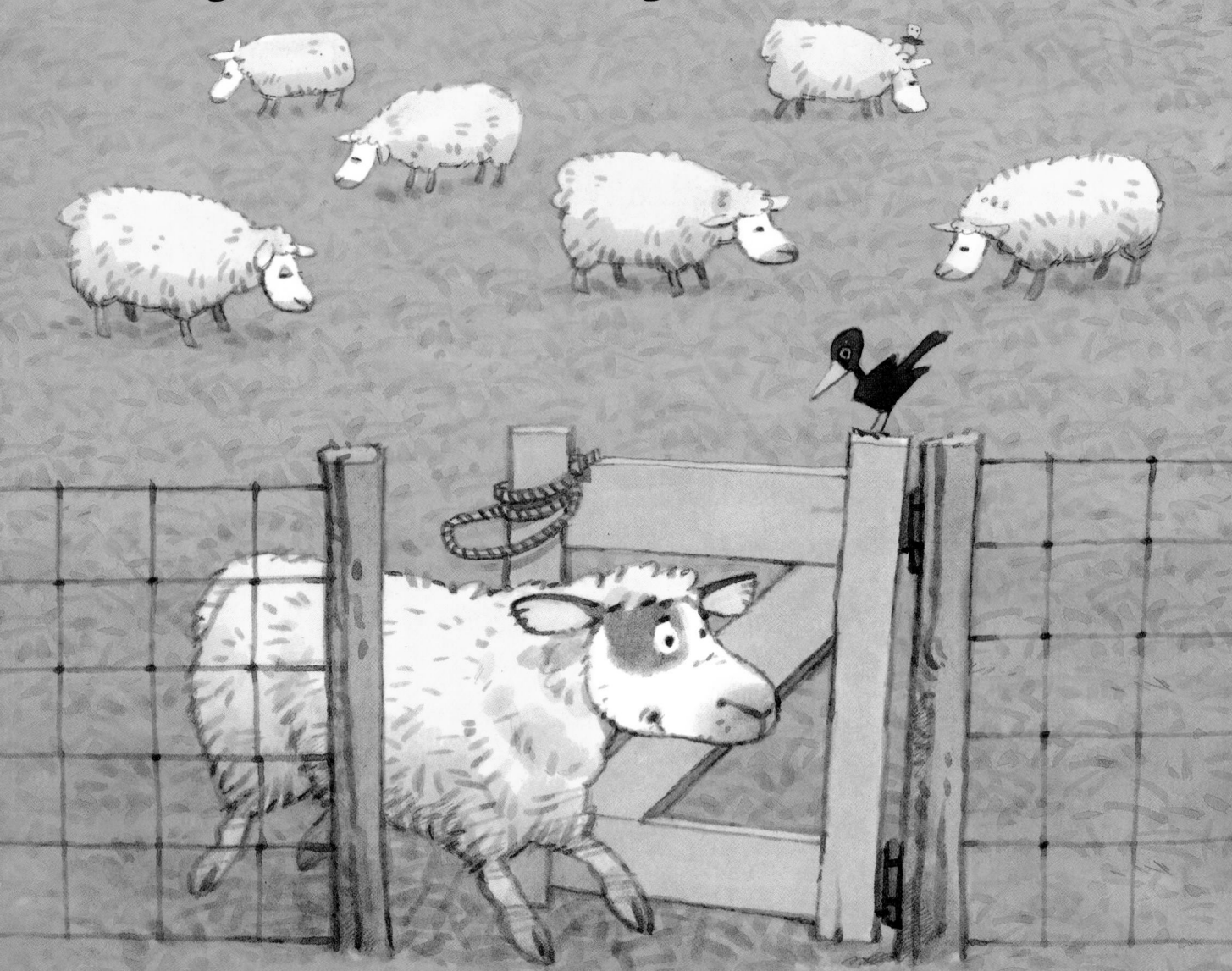

She runs out of the field into the farmyard. Then she runs through another gate into a garden.

Woolly sees lots to eat in the garden.

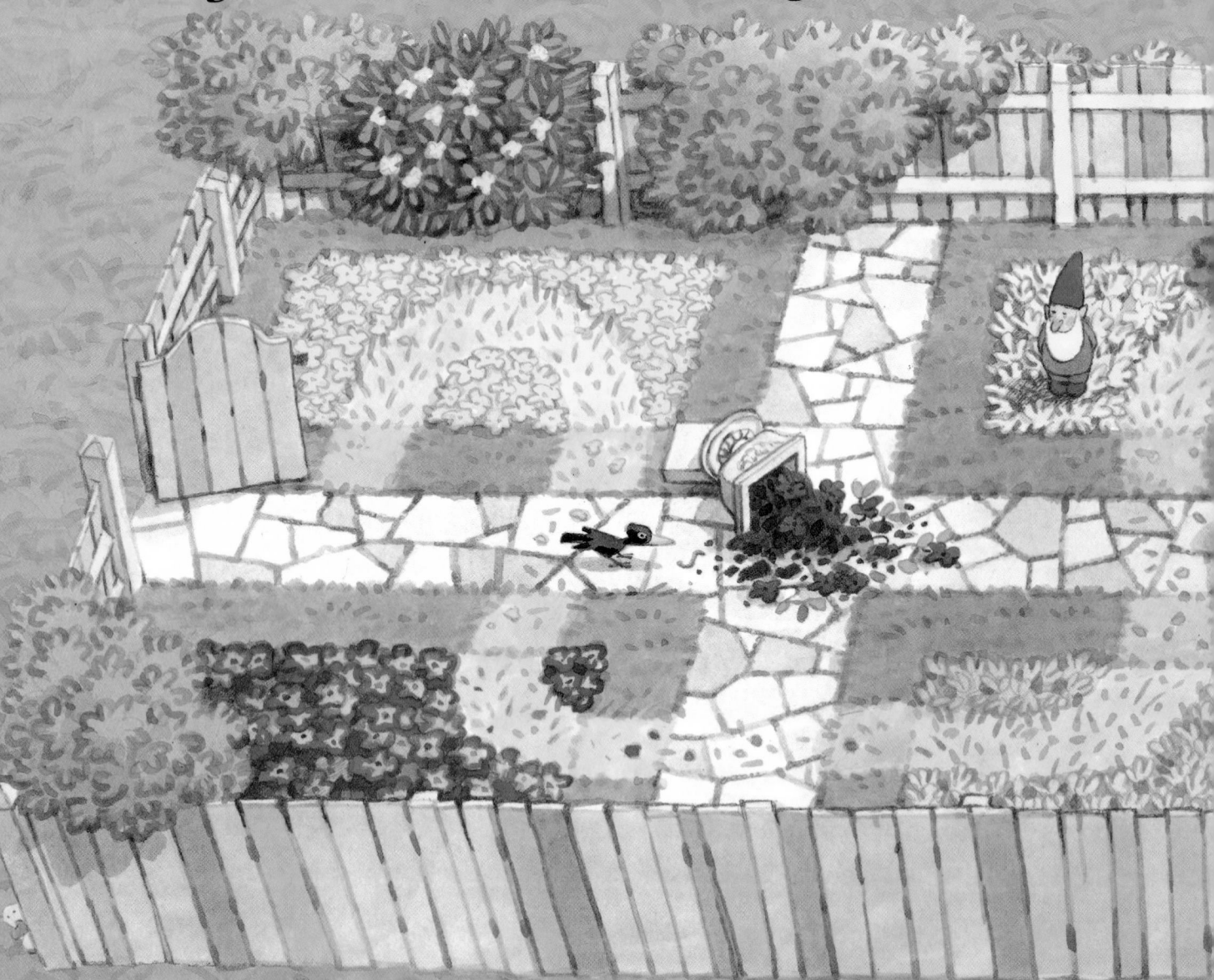

She tastes some of the flowers. "Very good,"
she says, "and much prettier than grass."

Can you see where Woolly walked?

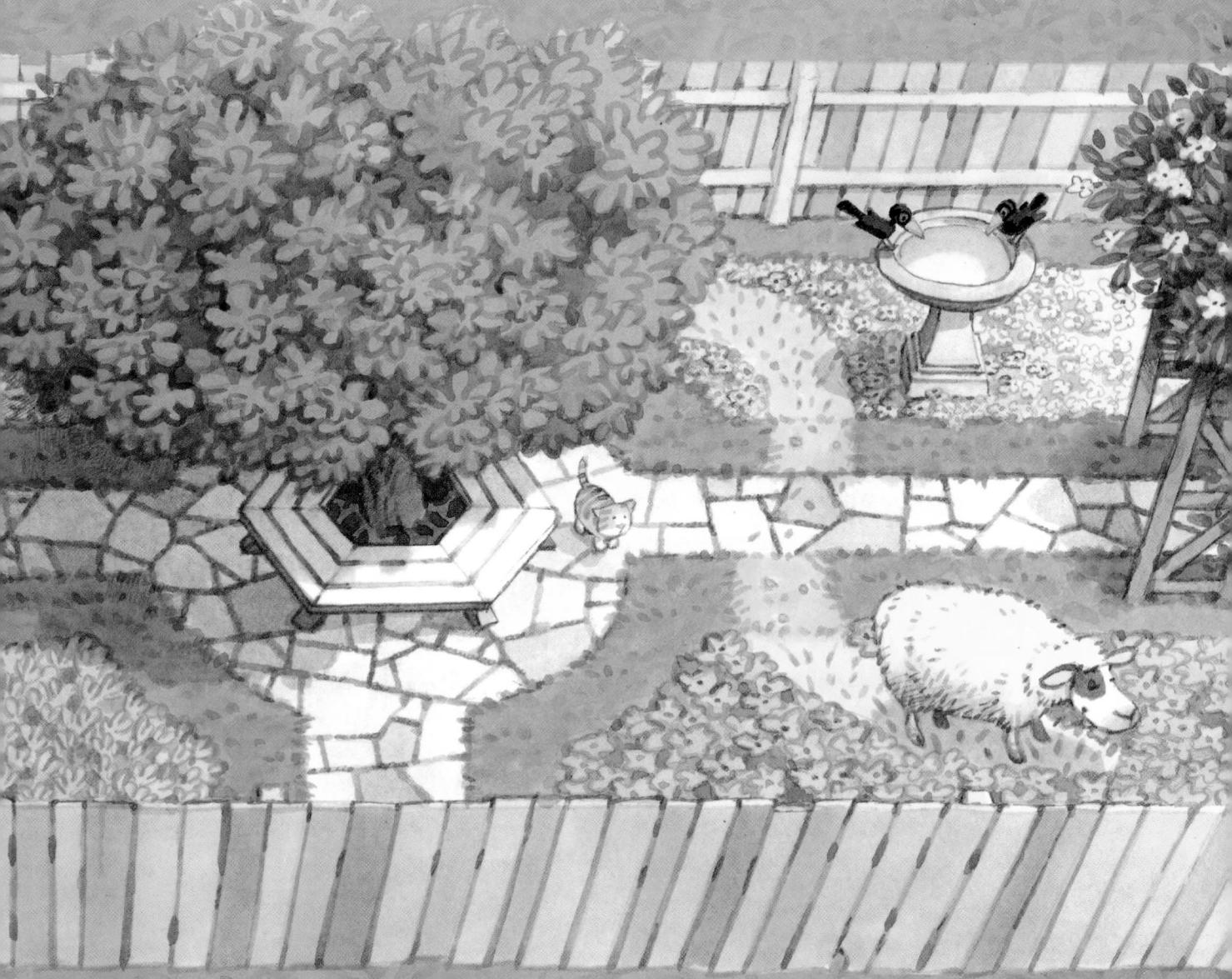

She walks around the garden, eating lots of the
flowers. "I like flowers," she says.

Mrs. Boot sees Woolly in the garden.

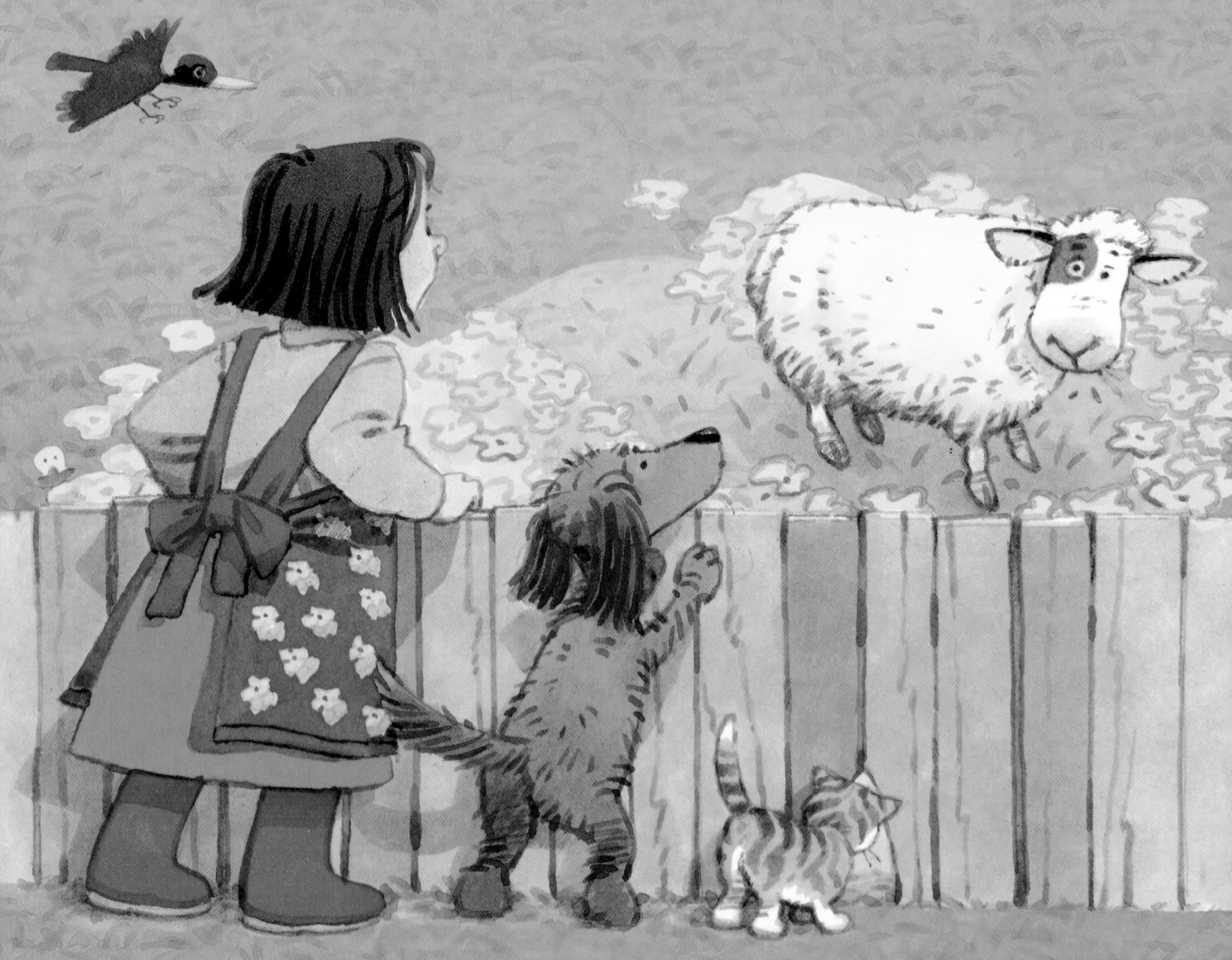

"What are you doing in my garden?" she shouts.
"You've eaten my flowers, you naughty sheep."

24

Mrs. Boot is very cross.

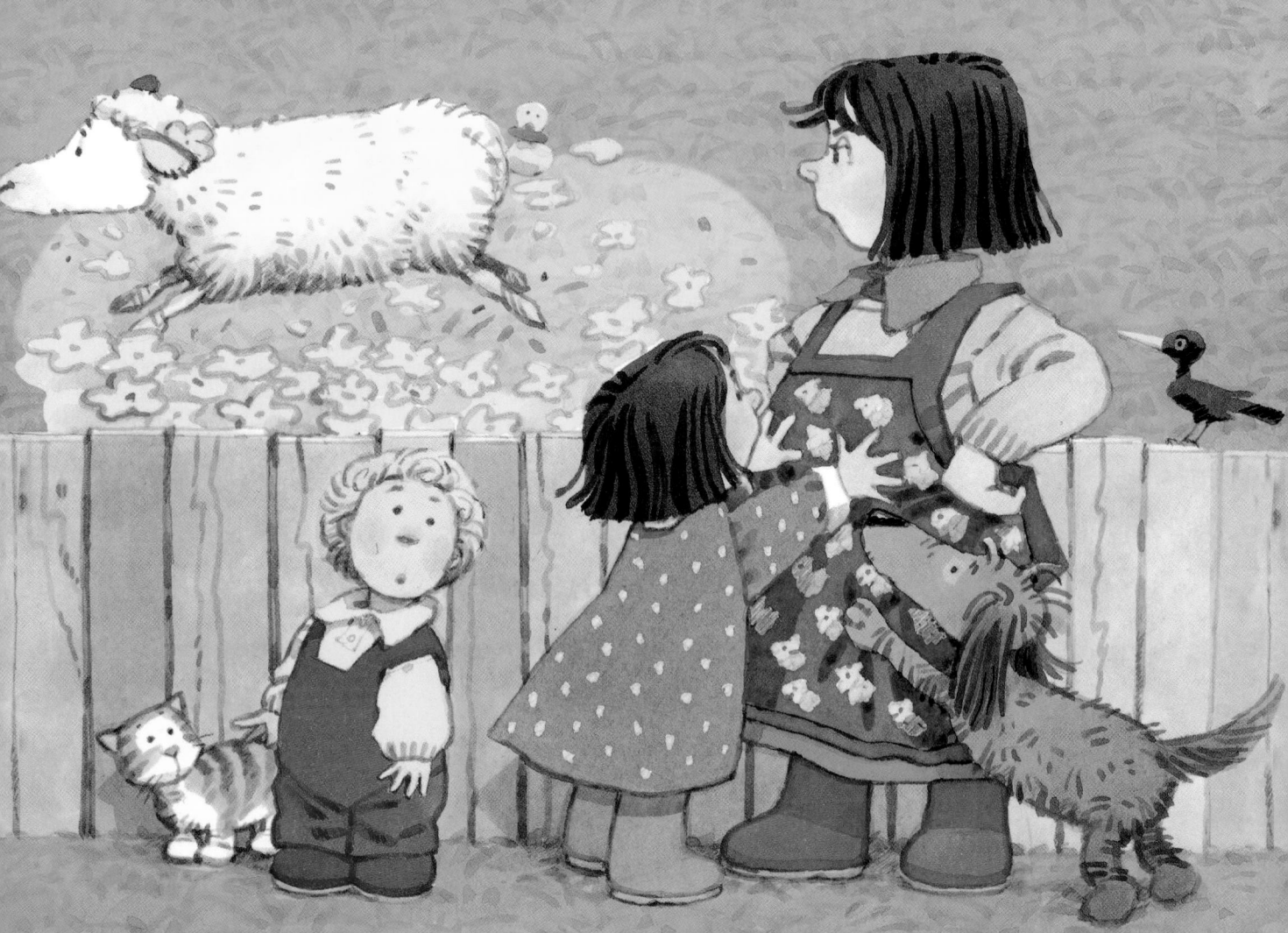

"It's the Show today," she says. "I was going to pick my best flowers for it. Just look at them."

25

It is time for the Show.

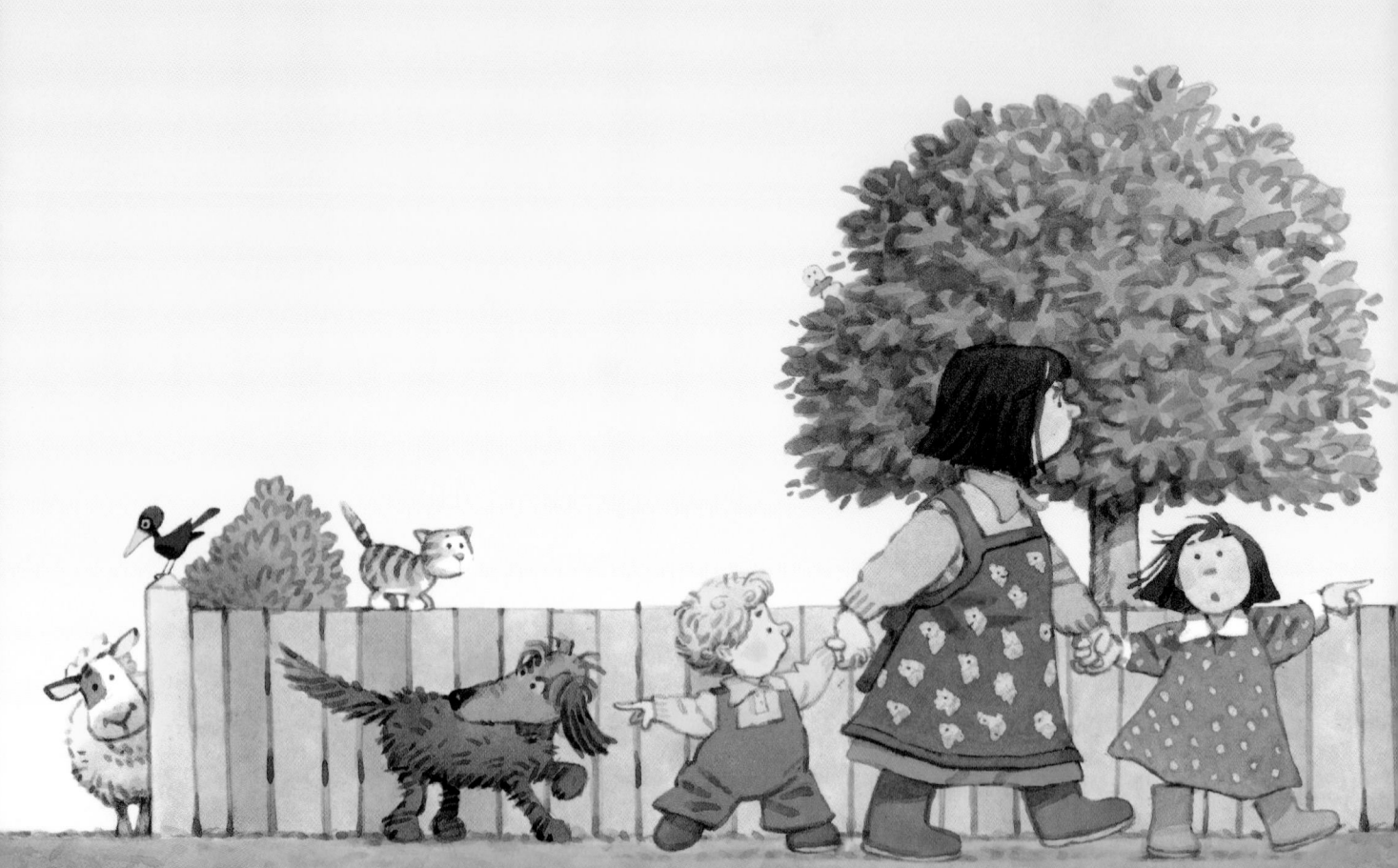

"Come on," says Poppy. "We must go now. The Show starts soon. It's only just down the road."

They all walk down the road.

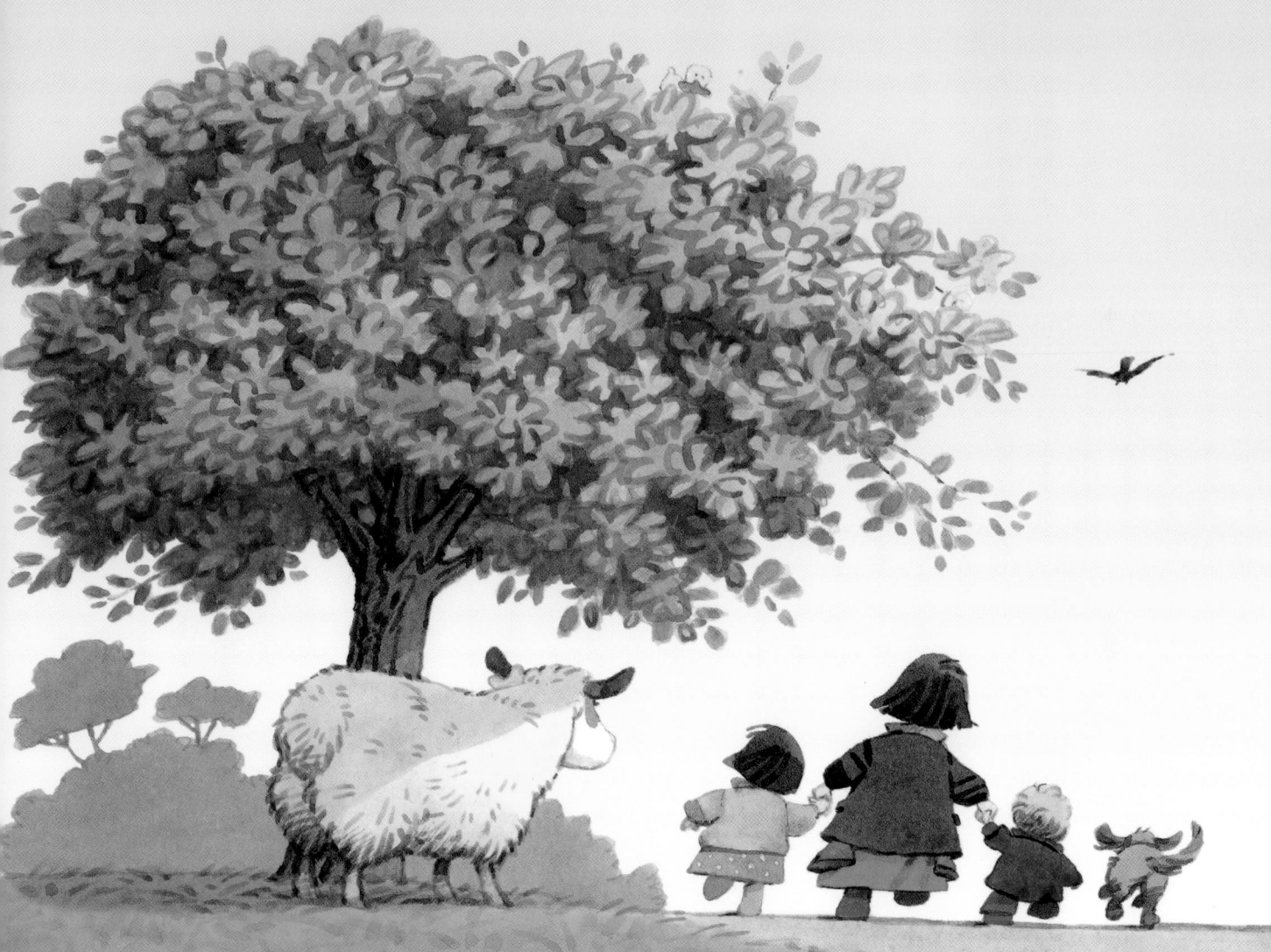

Woolly watches them go. She chews her
flower and thinks, "I'd like to go to the Show."

27

Woolly goes to the Show.

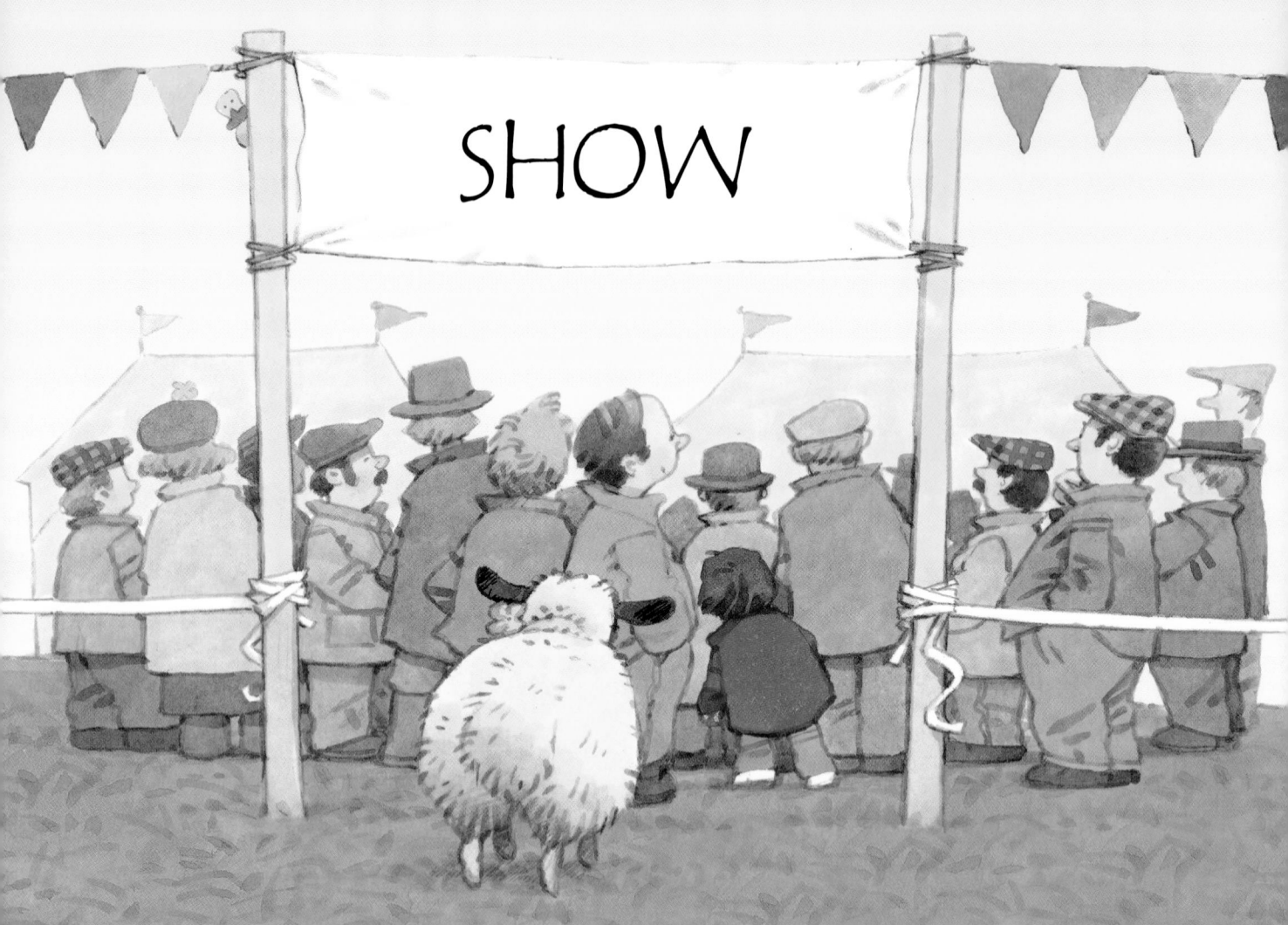

Woolly runs down the road. Soon she comes to
a big field with lots of people in it.

Woolly goes into the ring.

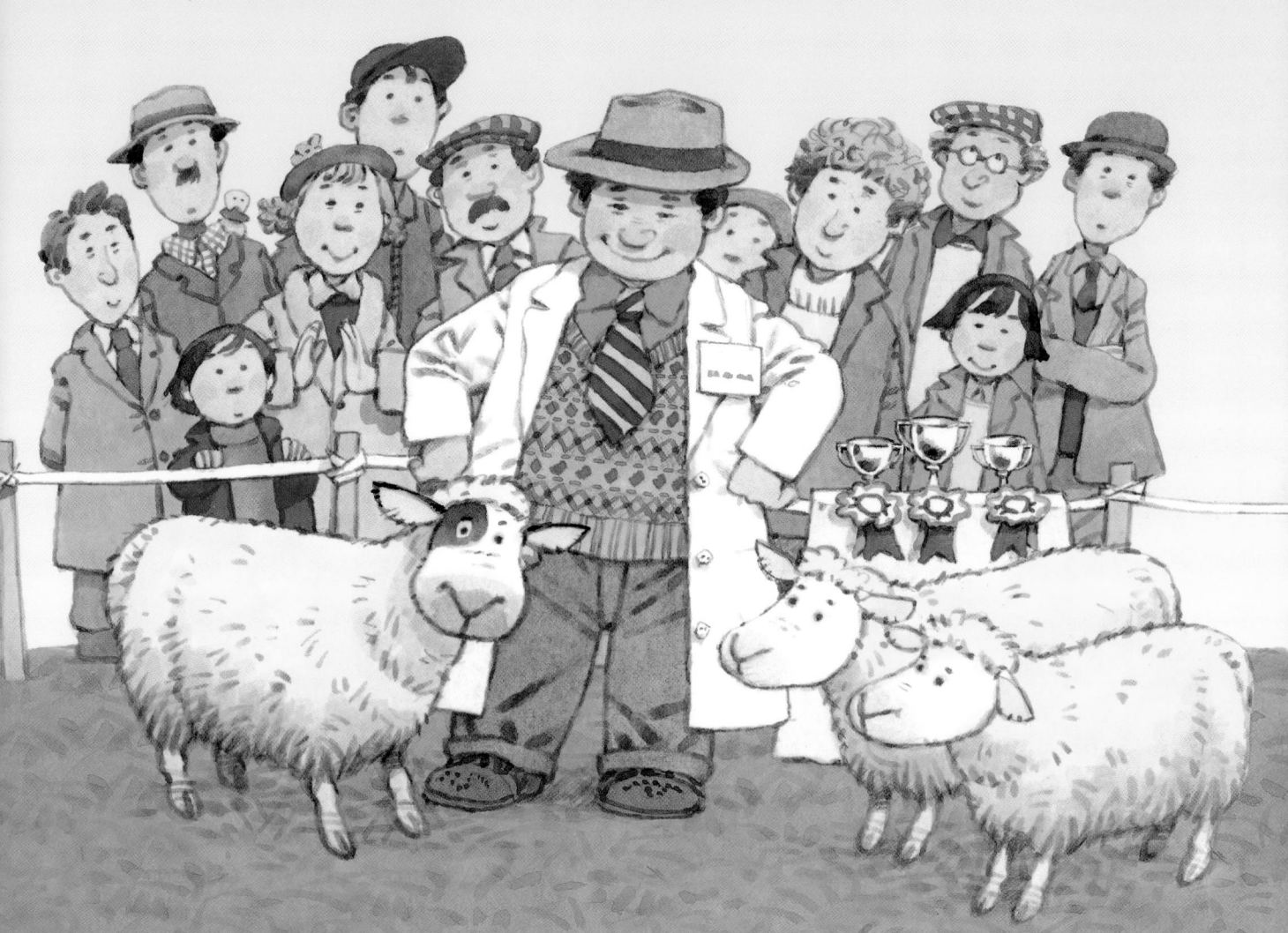

She pushes past the people and into the field.
She stops by a man in a white coat.

Mrs. Boot finds her.

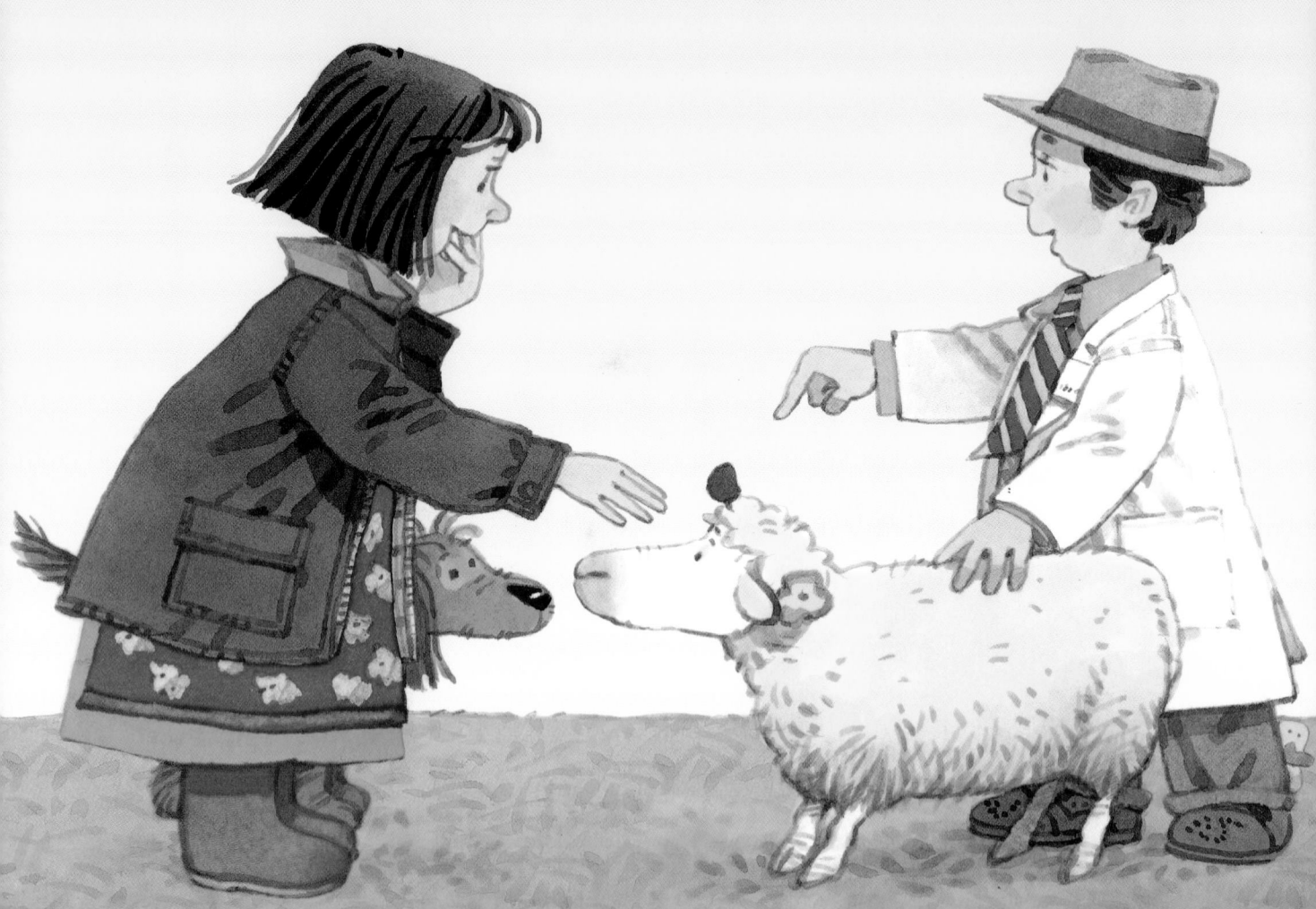

"What are you doing here, Woolly?" says Mrs. Boot.
"She has just won a prize," says the man.

Woolly is the winner.

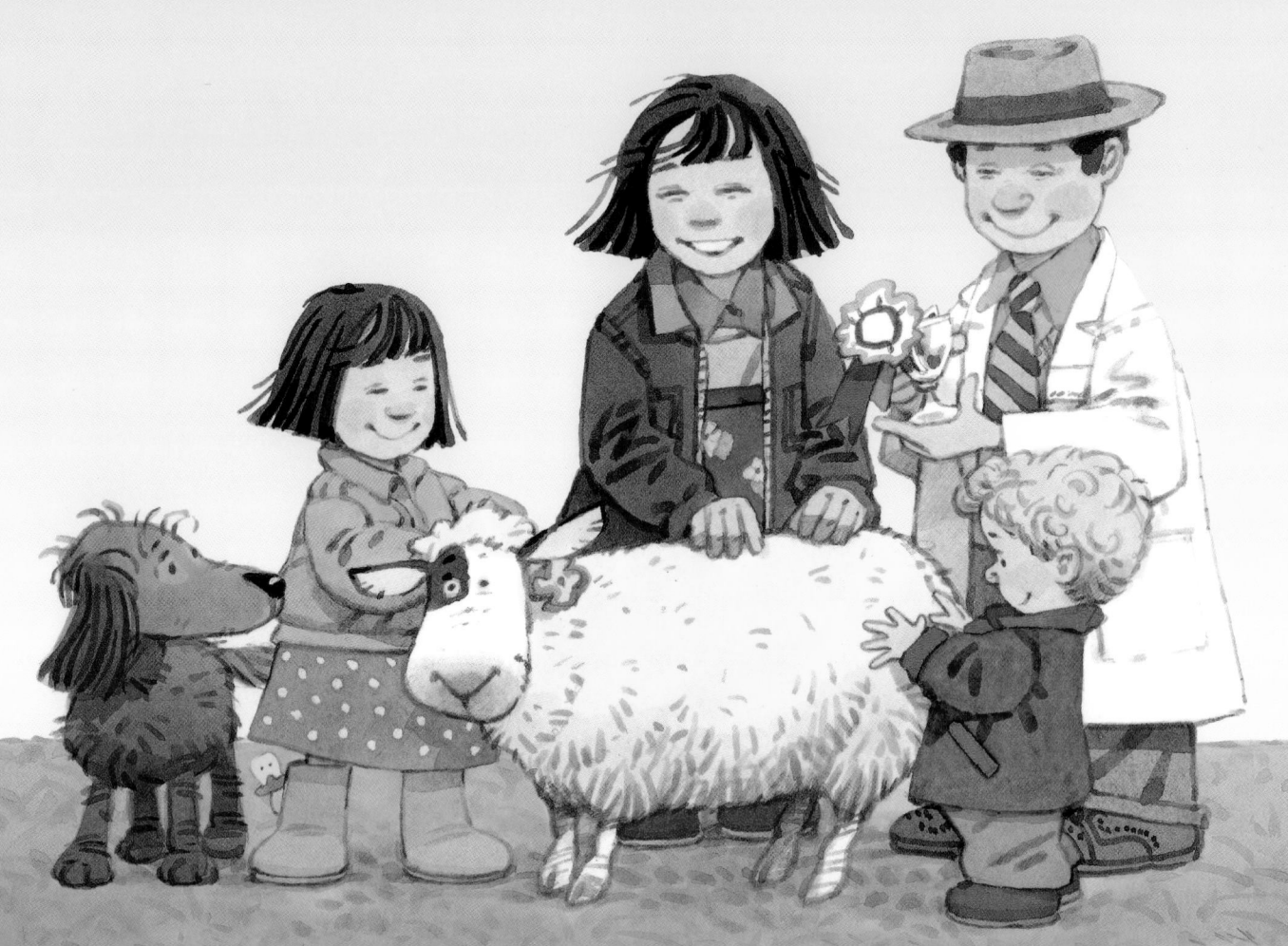

"This cup is for the best sheep," says the man.
"Oh, that's lovely. Thank you," says Mrs. Boot.

It is time to go home.

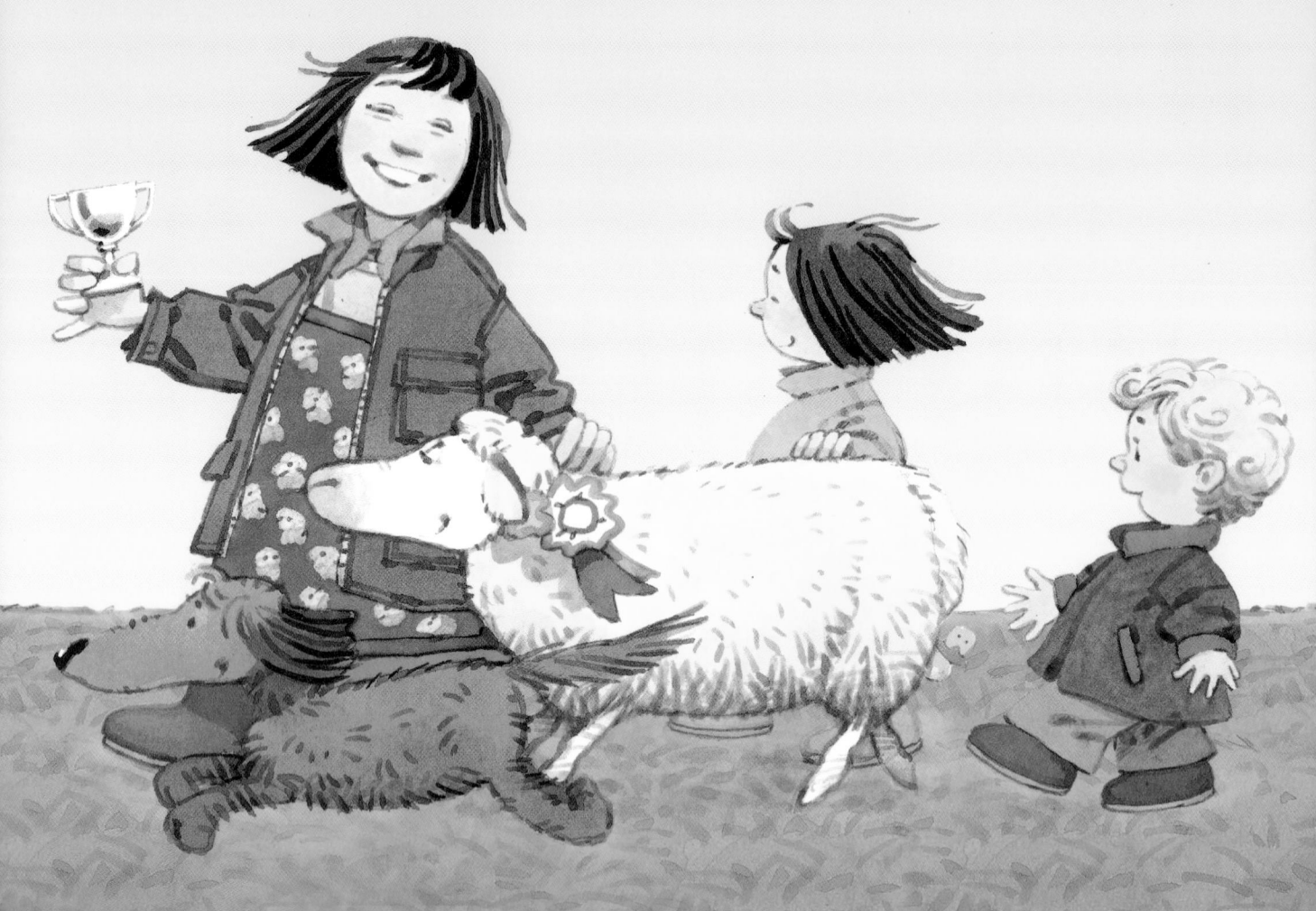

"Come on, Woolly," says Mrs. Boot. "We'll take you back to your field, you naughty, clever sheep."

Barn on Fire

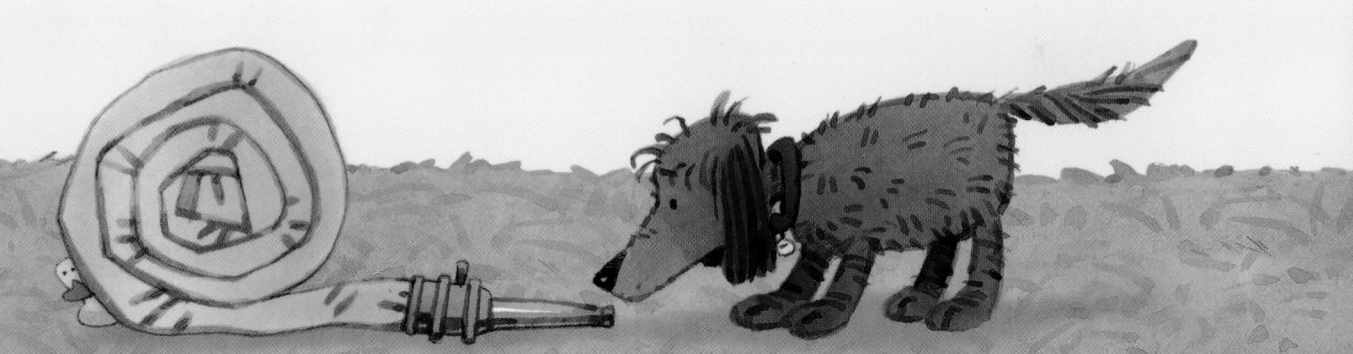

This is Apple Tree Farm.

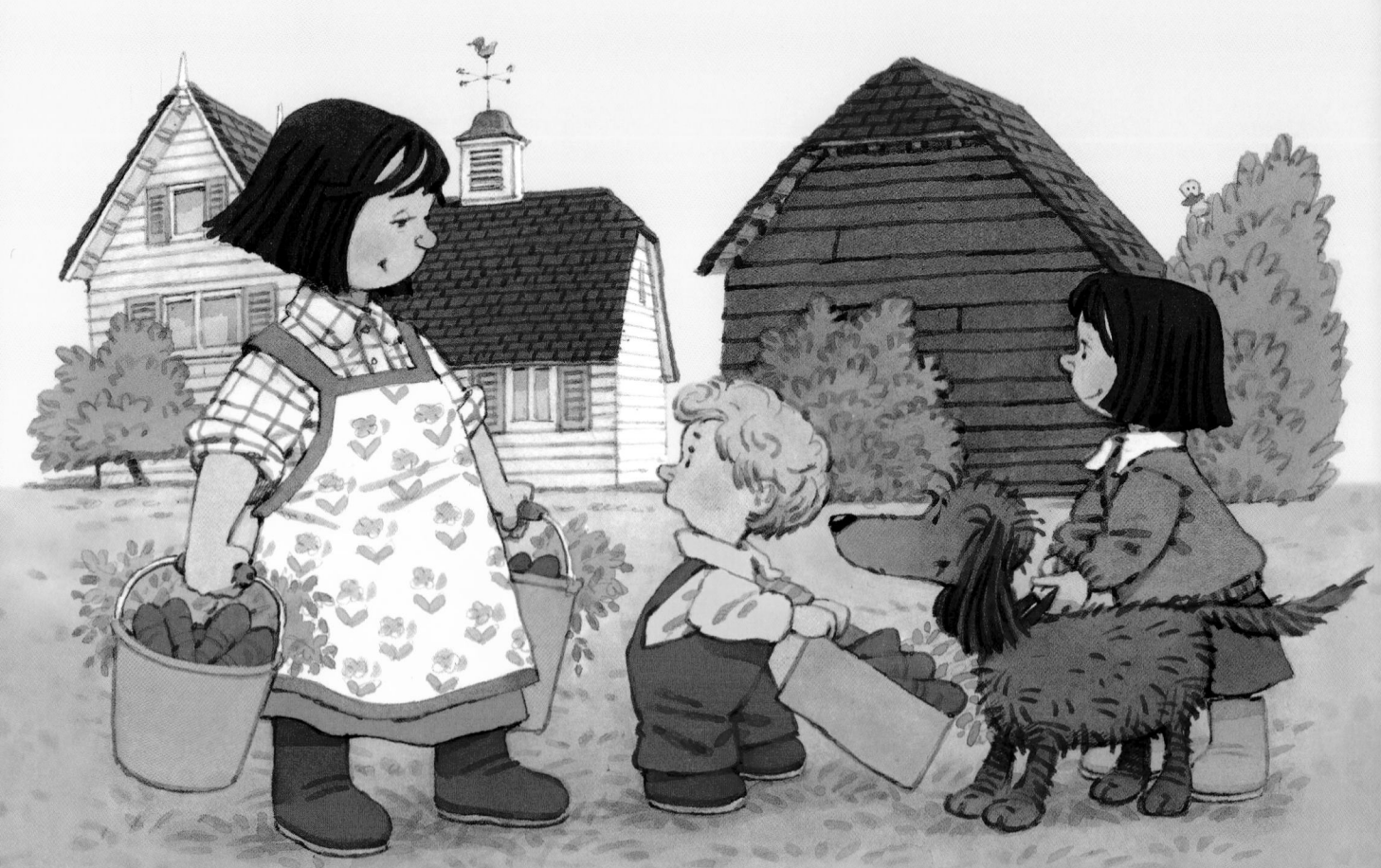

This is Mrs. Boot, the farmer. She has two children, called Poppy and Sam, and a dog called Rusty.

This is Ted.

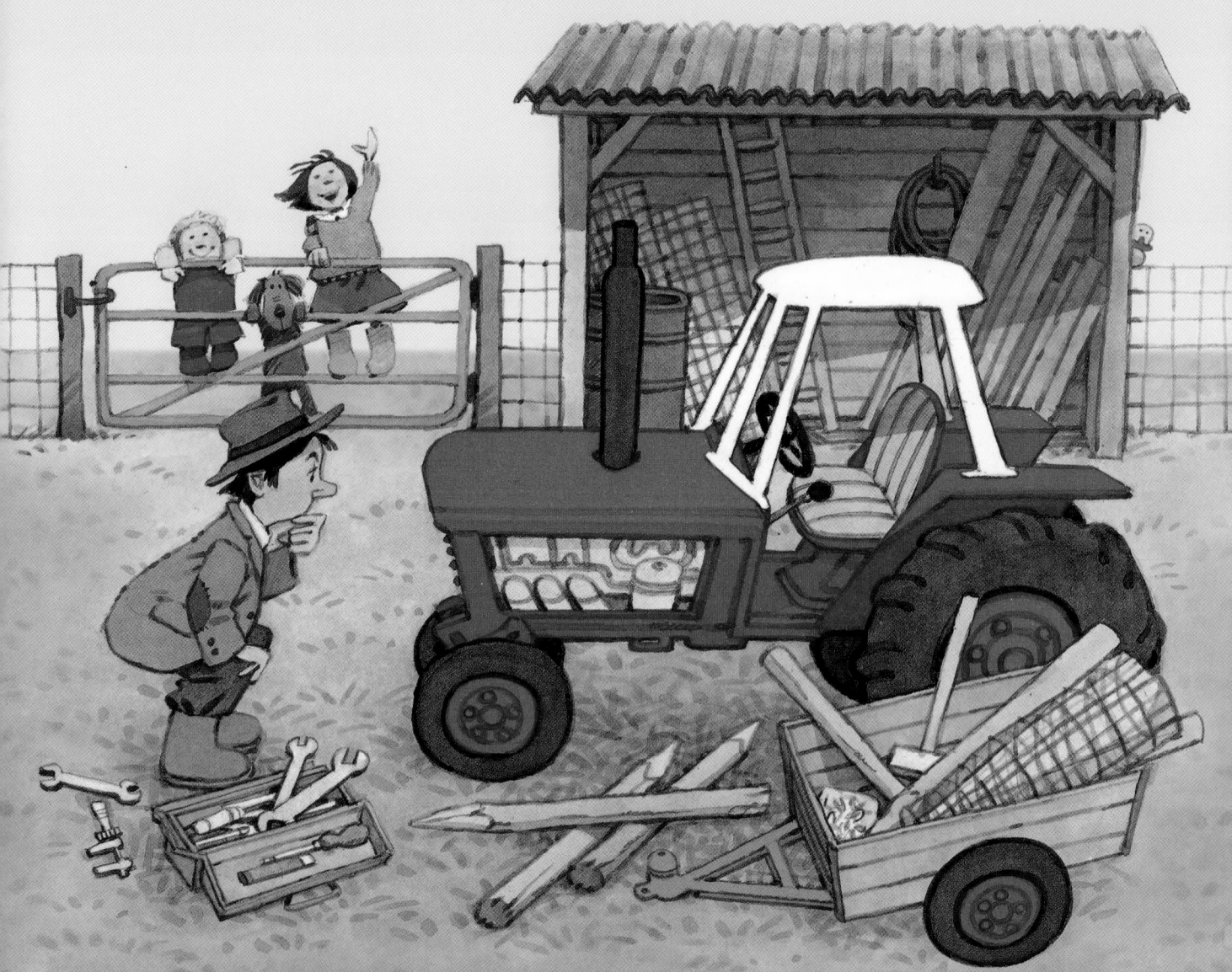

Ted works at Apple Tree Farm. He looks after the tractor and all the other farm machines.

Poppy and Sam help Ted.

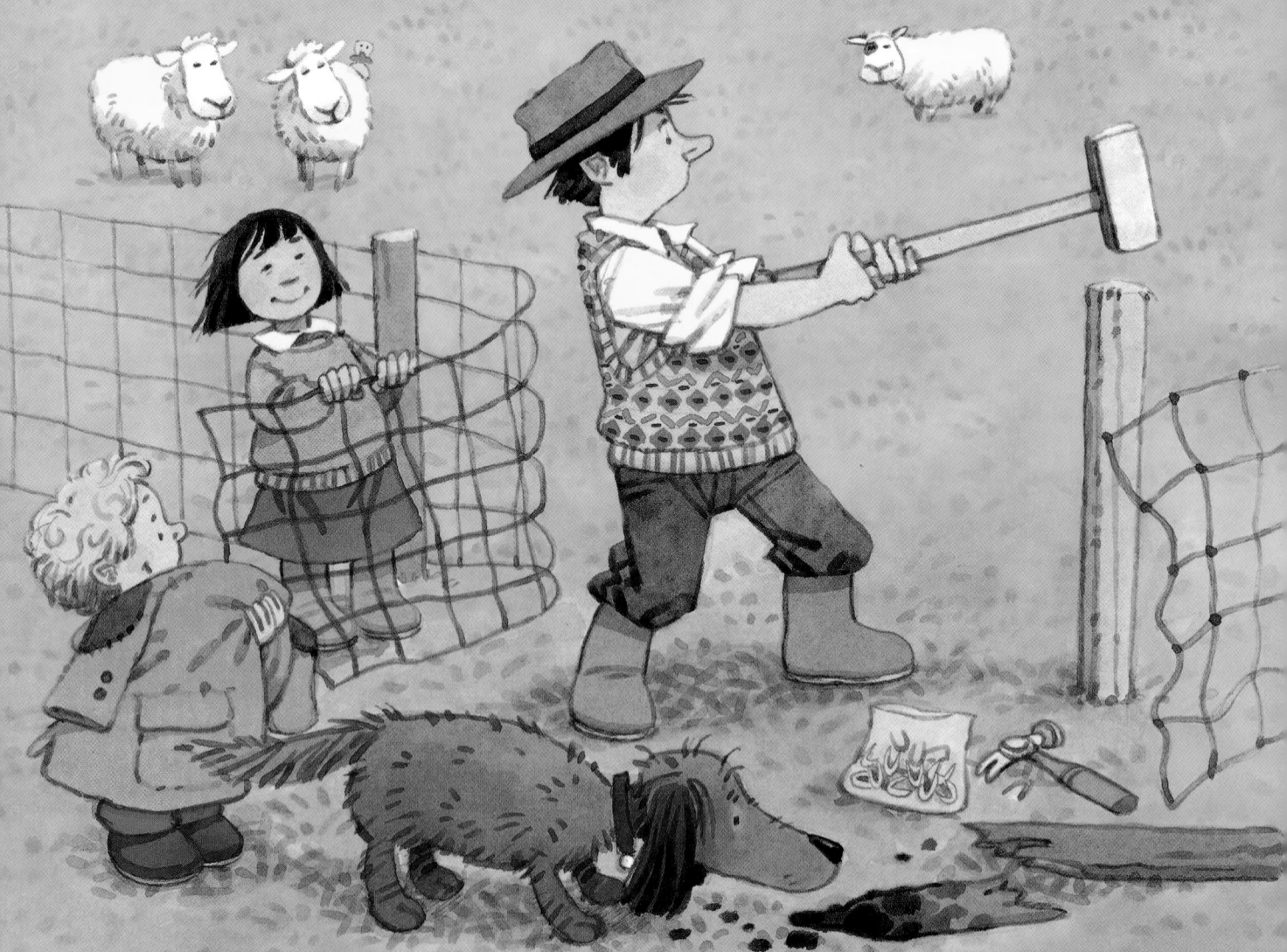

They like helping Ted with jobs on the farm. Today he is fixing the fence around the sheep field.

Sam smells smoke.

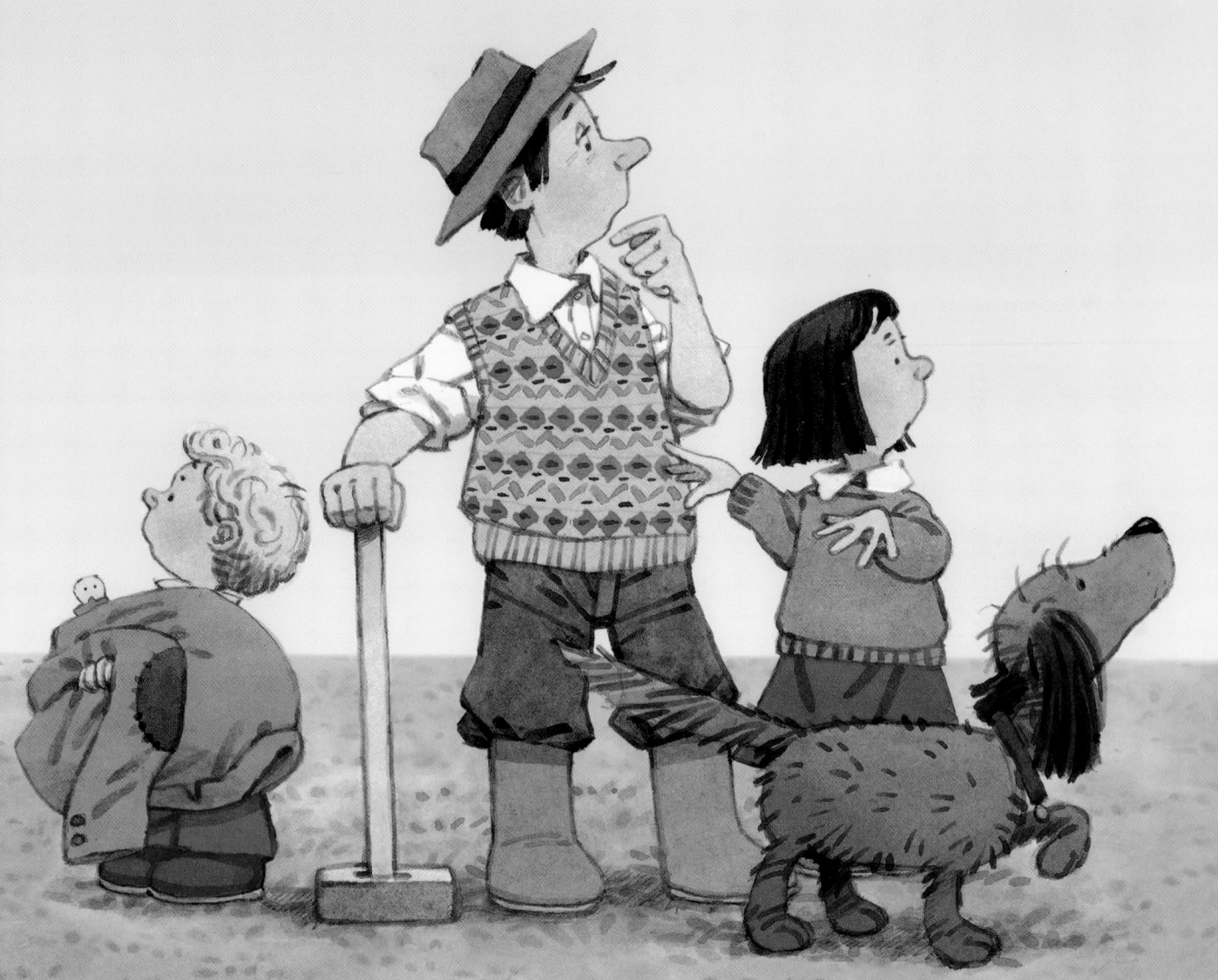

"Ted," says Sam, "I think something's burning."
Ted stops working and they all sniff hard.

The barn is on fire.

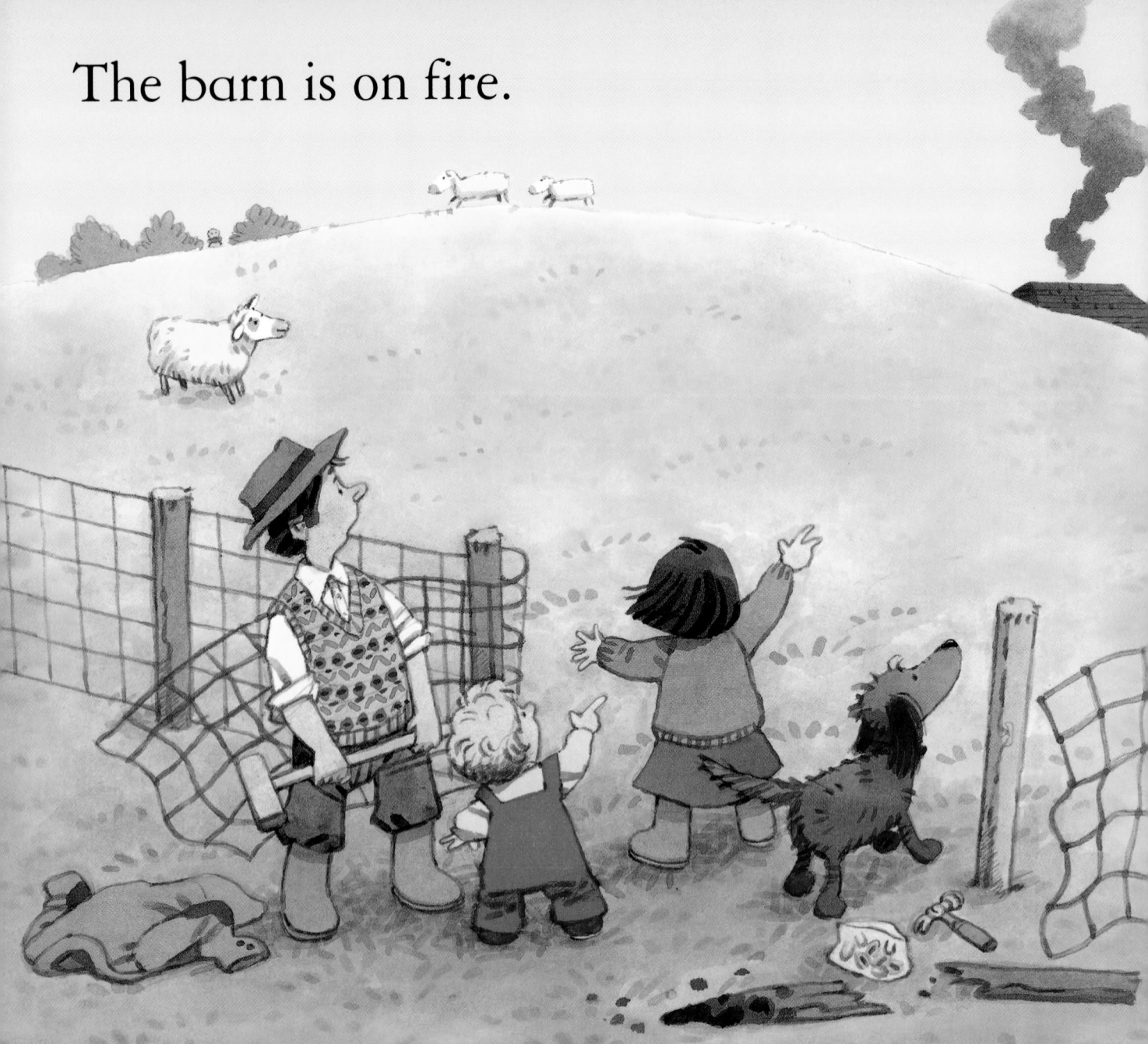

"Look," says Poppy, "there's smoke coming from the hay barn. It must be on fire. What shall we do?"

"Call a fire engine."

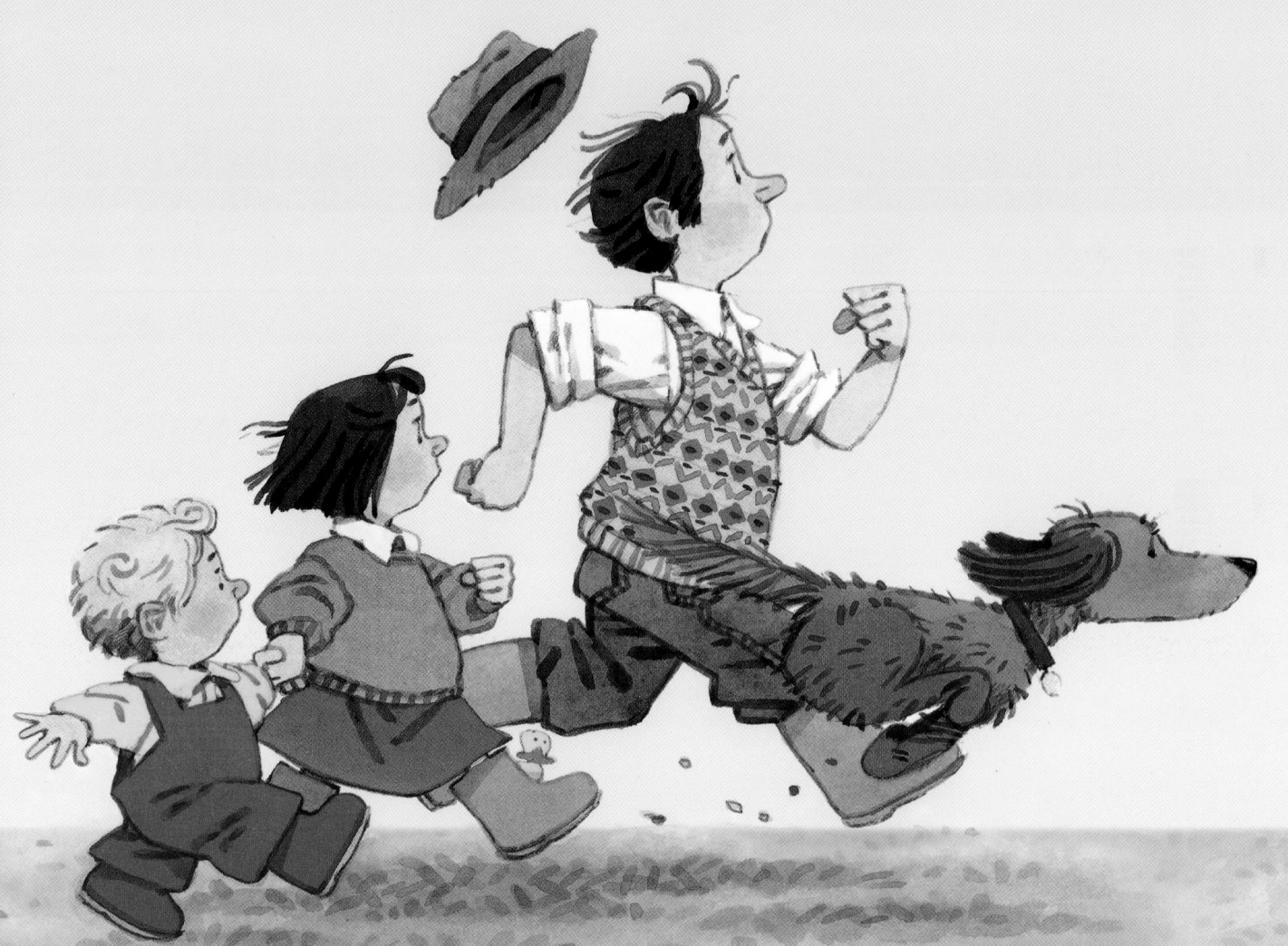

"Come on," says Ted. "Run to the house. We must call a fire engine. Run as fast as you can."

Poppy and Sam run to the house.

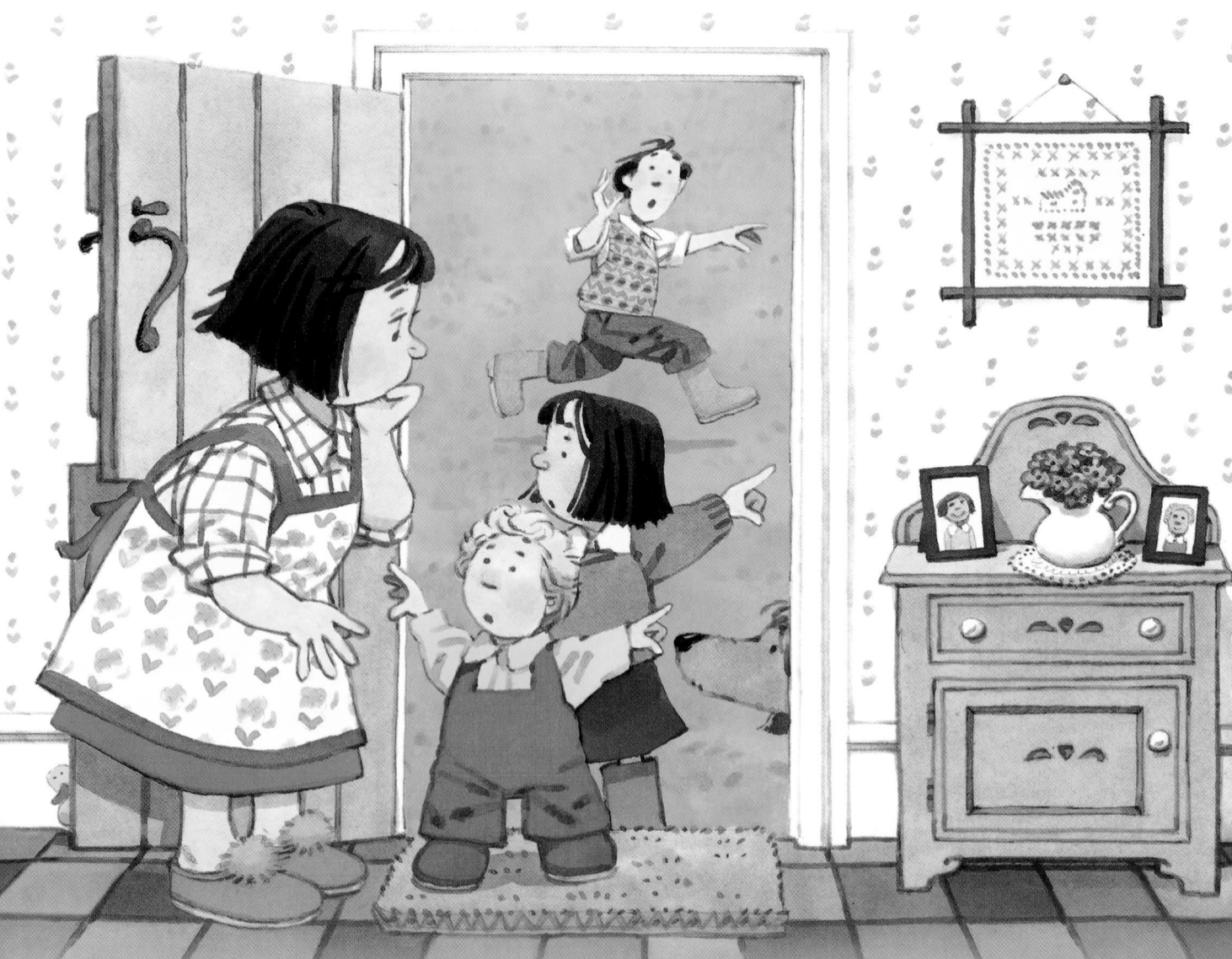

"Help!" shouts Poppy. "Call a fire engine.
Quickly! The hay barn is on fire."

Mrs. Boot dials the number.

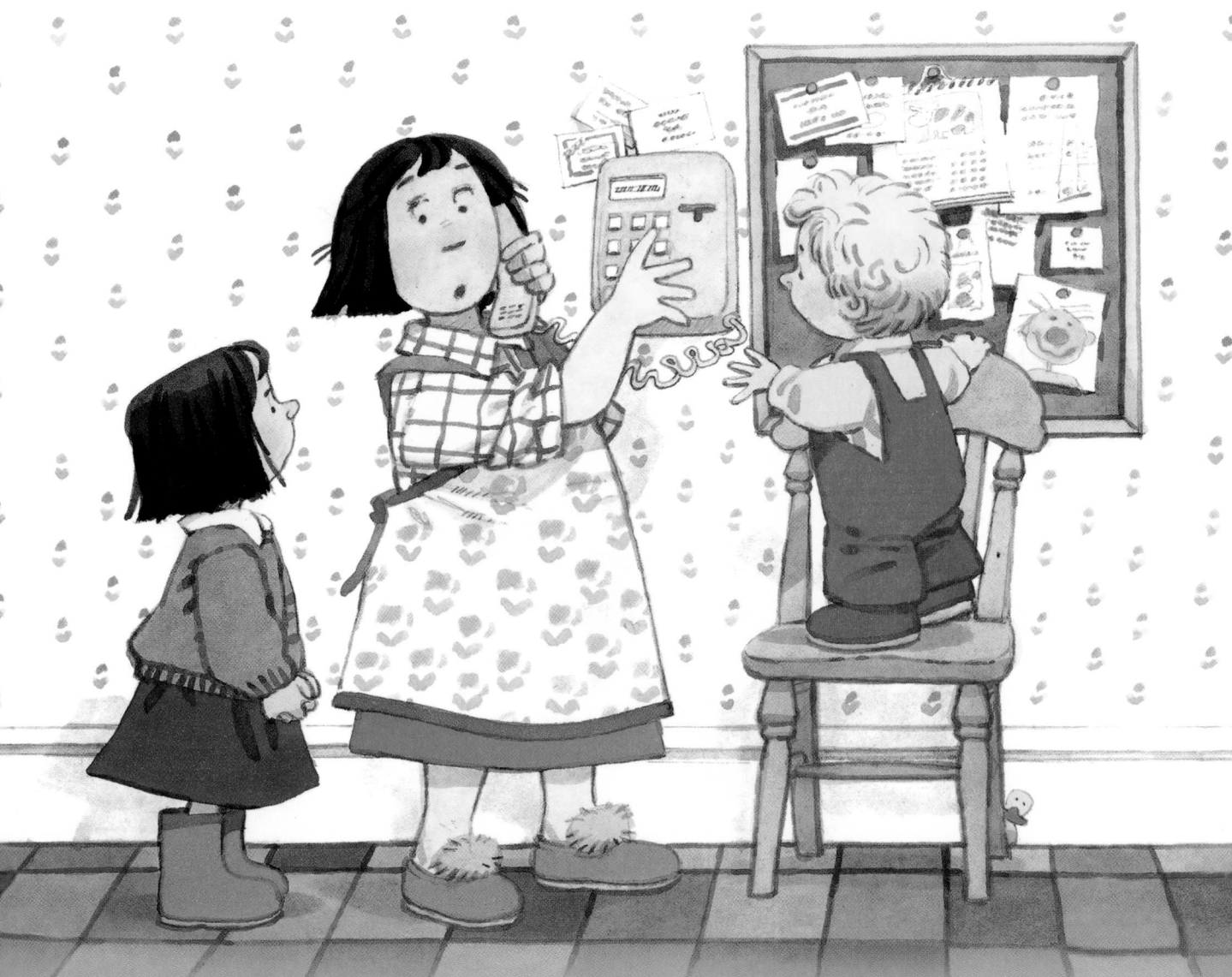

"It's Apple Tree Farm," she says. "A fire engine please, as fast as you can. Thank you very much."

"You must stay here."

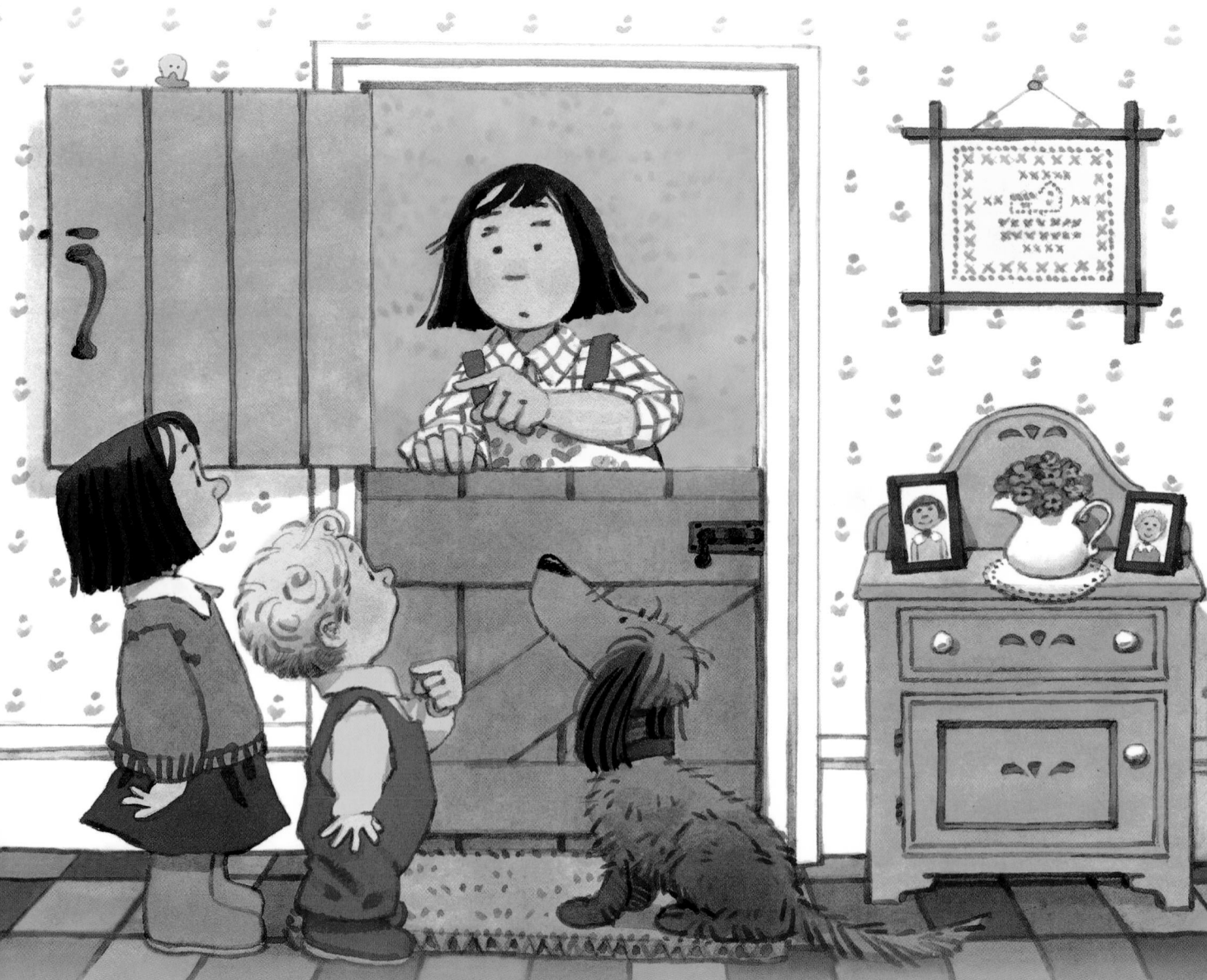

"Now, Poppy," says Mrs. Boot. "I want you and Sam to stay indoors. And don't let Rusty out."

Poppy and Sam watch from the door.

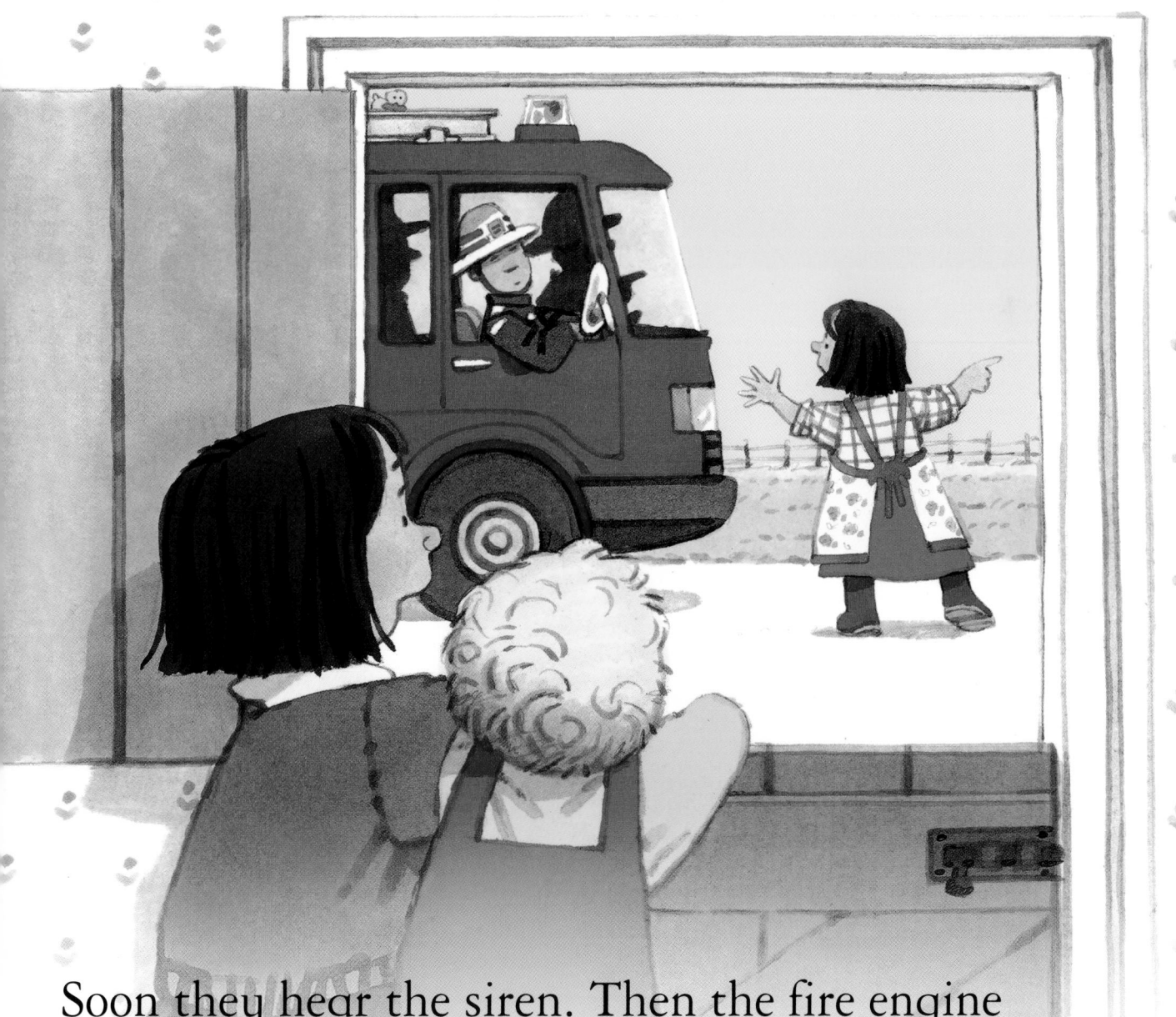

Soon they hear the siren. Then the fire engine
roars up the road and into the farmyard.

"The firemen are here."

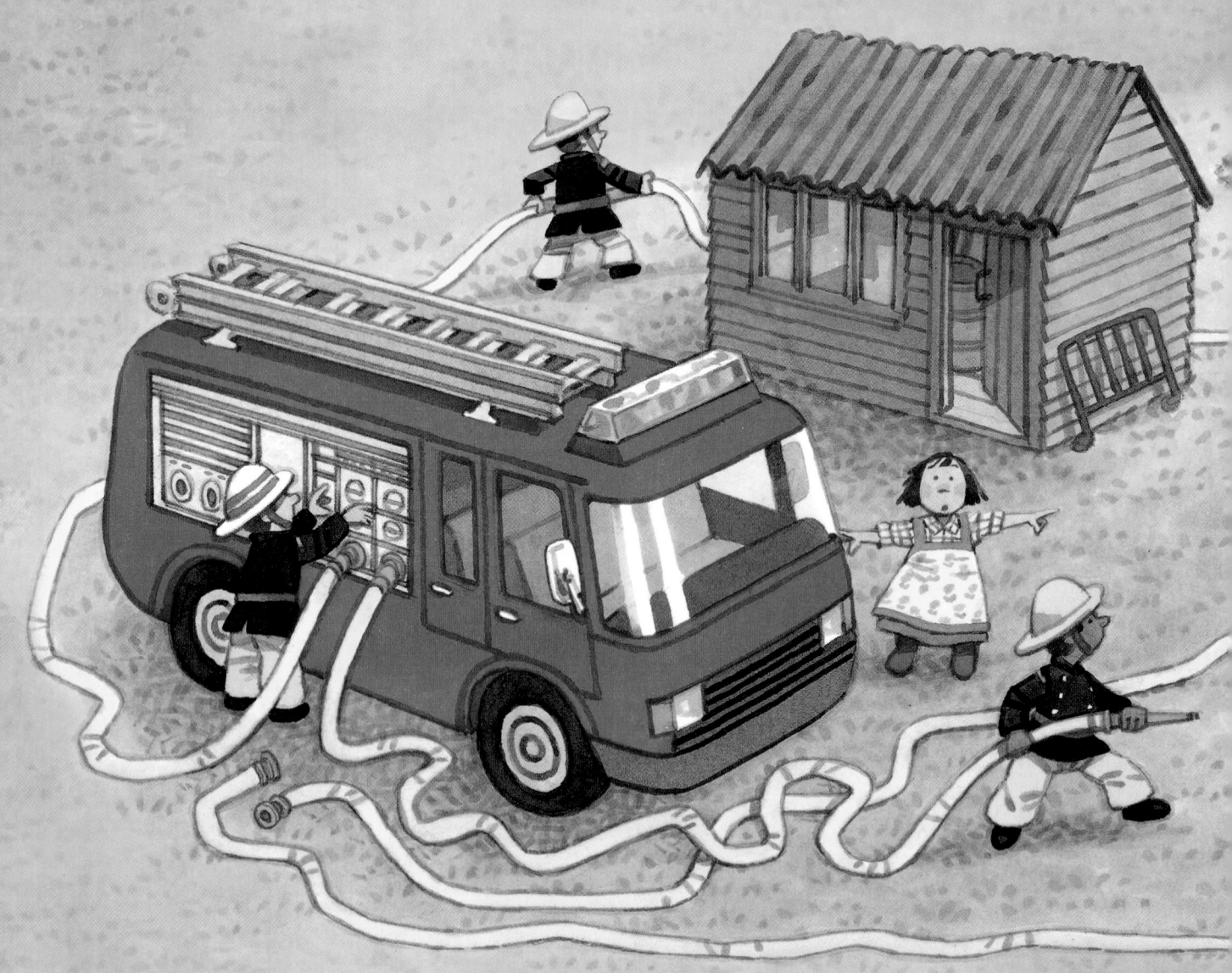

The firemen jump down from the engine.
They lift down lots of hoses and unroll them.

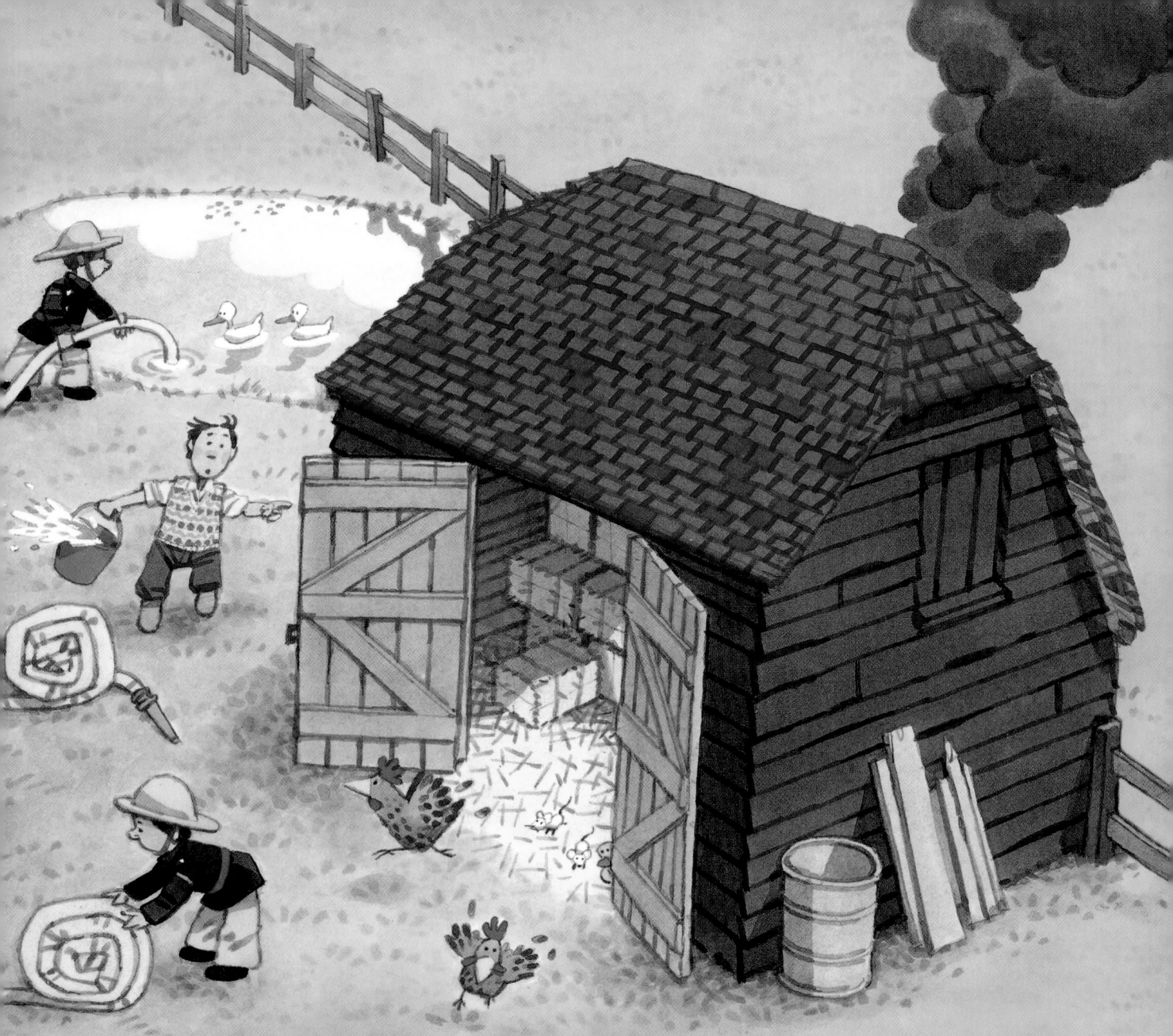

The firemen run over to the barn with the hoses.
Can you see where they get the water from?

The firemen squirt water onto the barn.

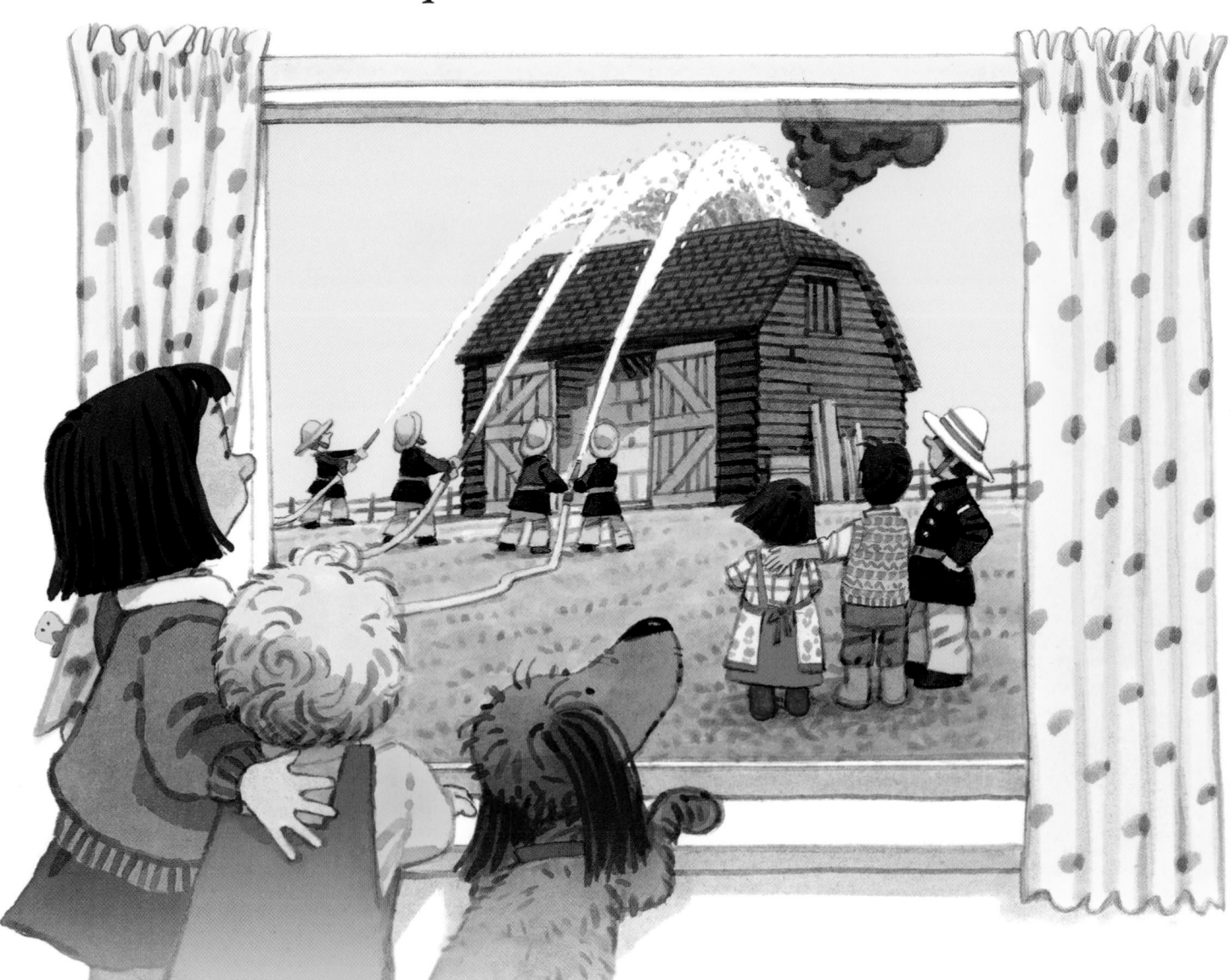

Poppy and Sam watch them from the window.
"It's still burning on the other side," says Poppy.

"There's the fire."

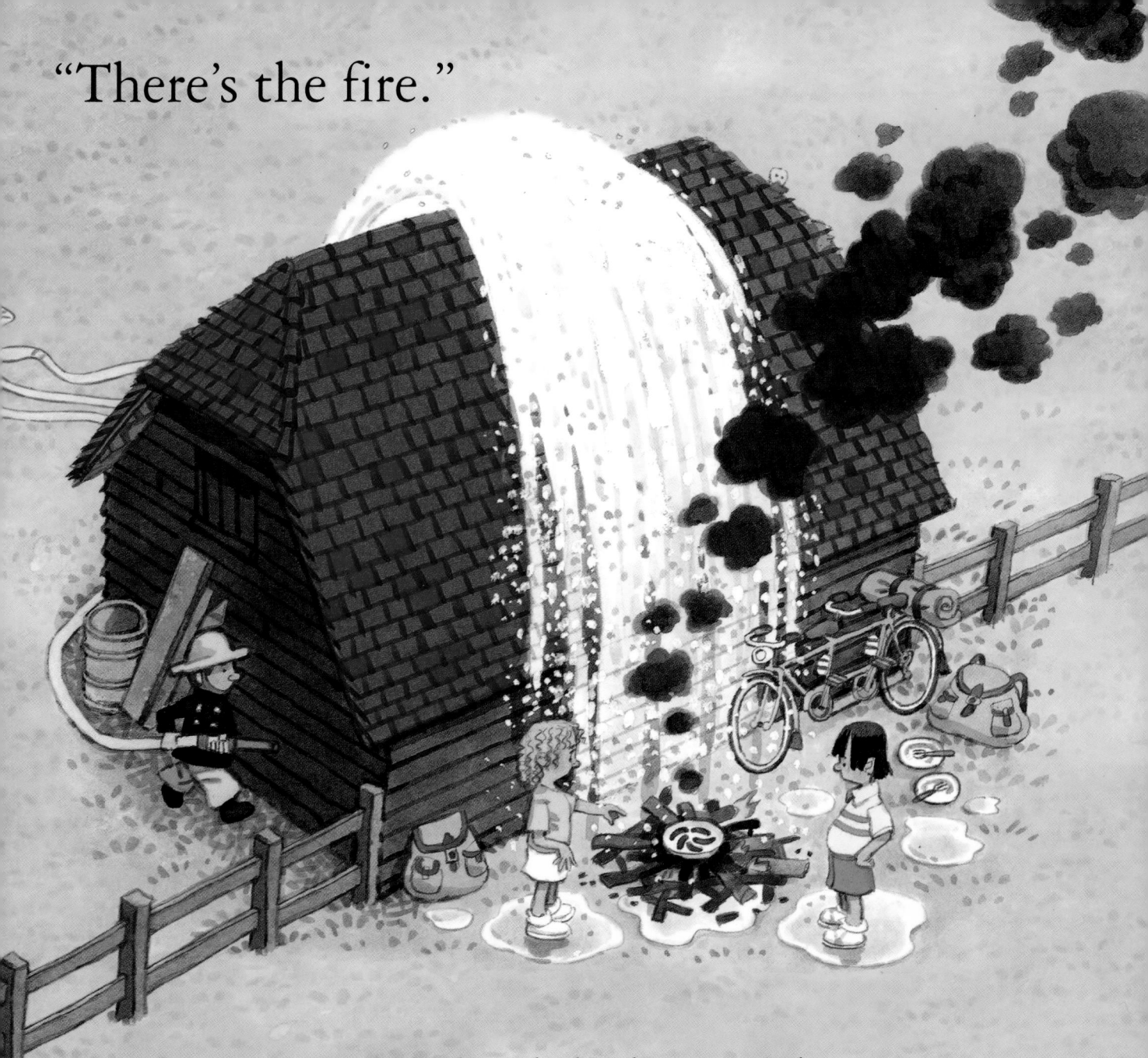

One fireman runs behind the barn. What a surprise!
Two campers are cooking on a big wood fire.

The fire is out.

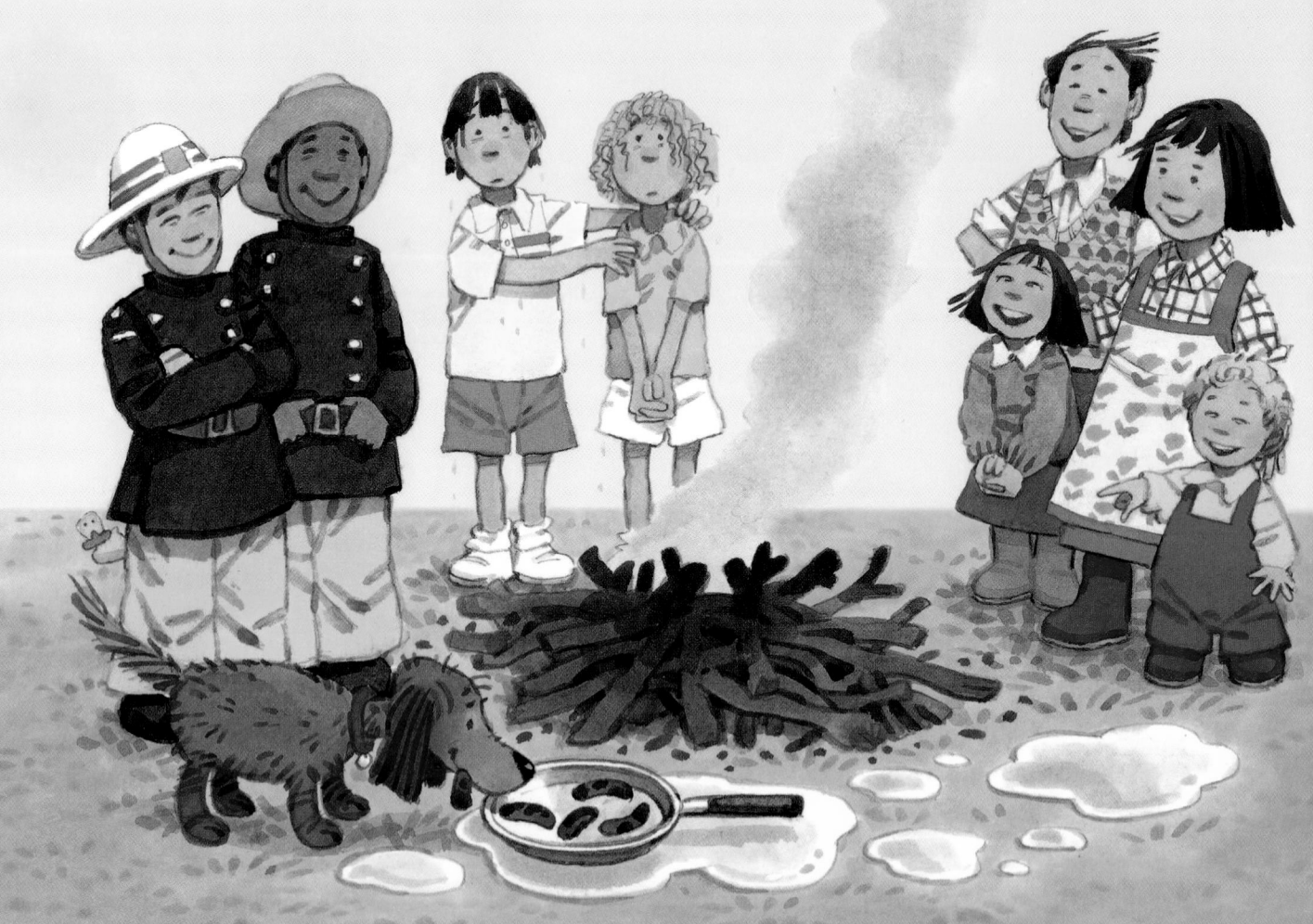

"We're sorry," say the campers. "It was exciting," says Sam, "but I'm glad the barn is all right."

The
Runaway Tractor

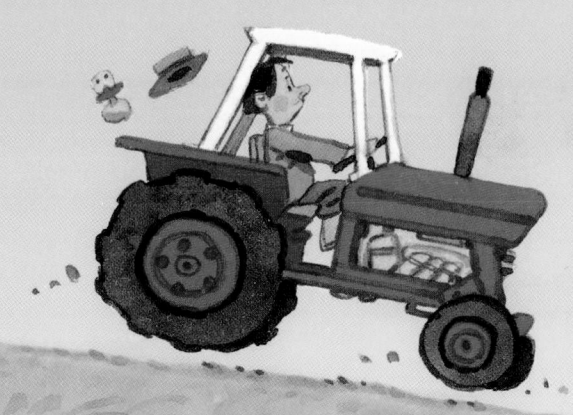

This is Apple Tree Farm.

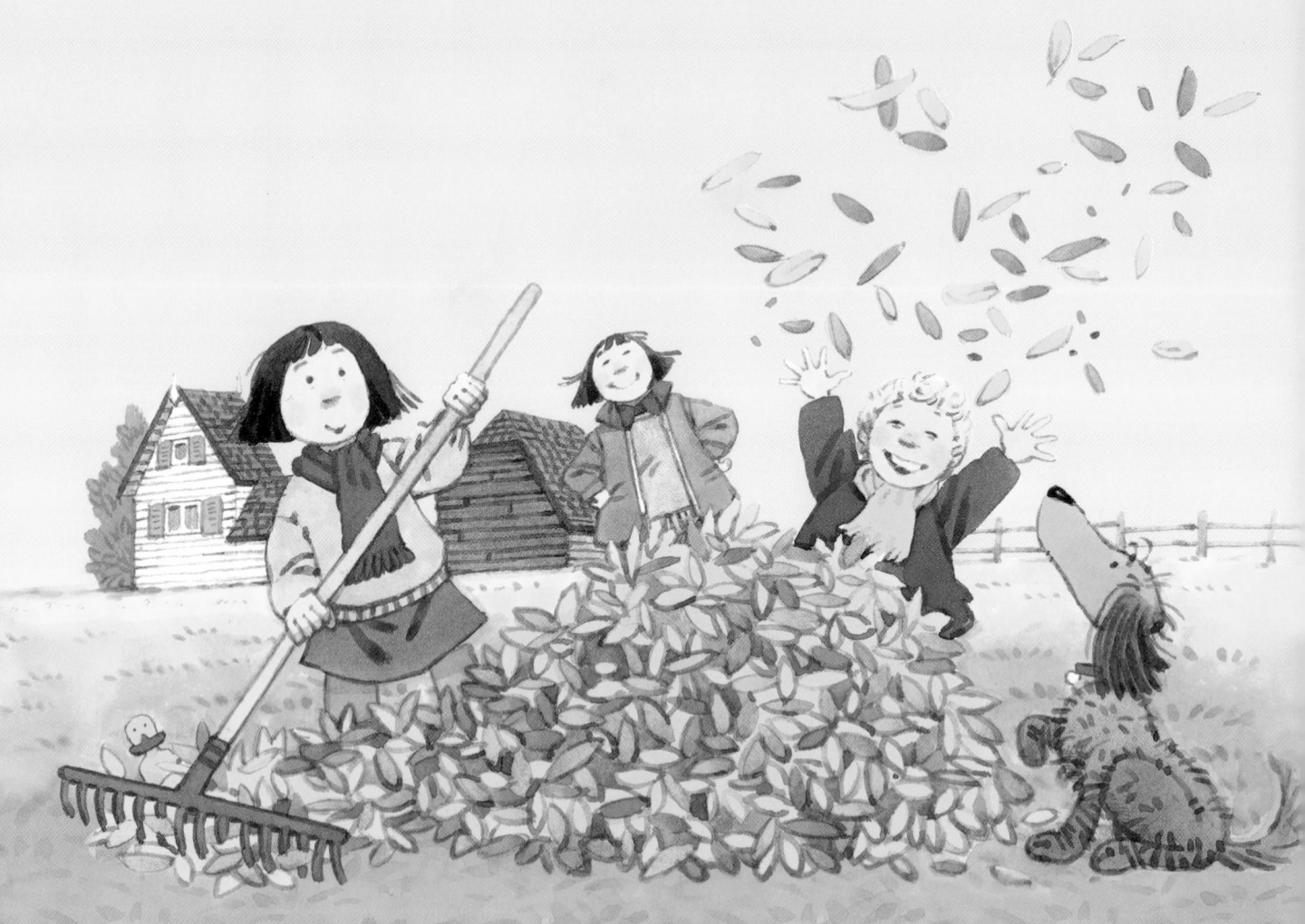

This is Mrs. Boot, the farmer. She has two children, called Poppy and Sam, and a dog called Rusty.

Ted is the tractor driver.

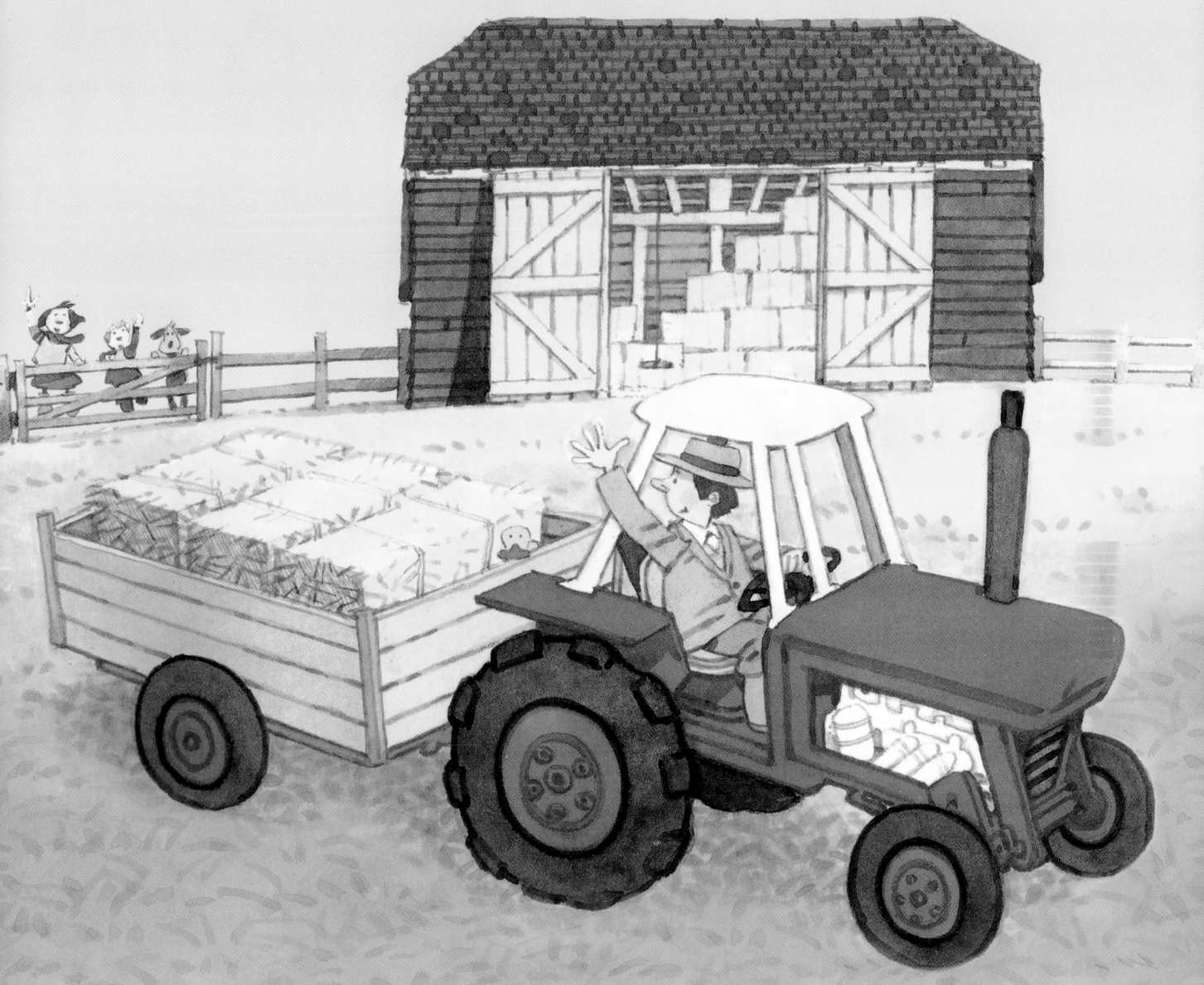

He has filled the trailer with hay. He is taking
it to the fields to feed the sheep.

Poppy and Sam hear a funny noise.

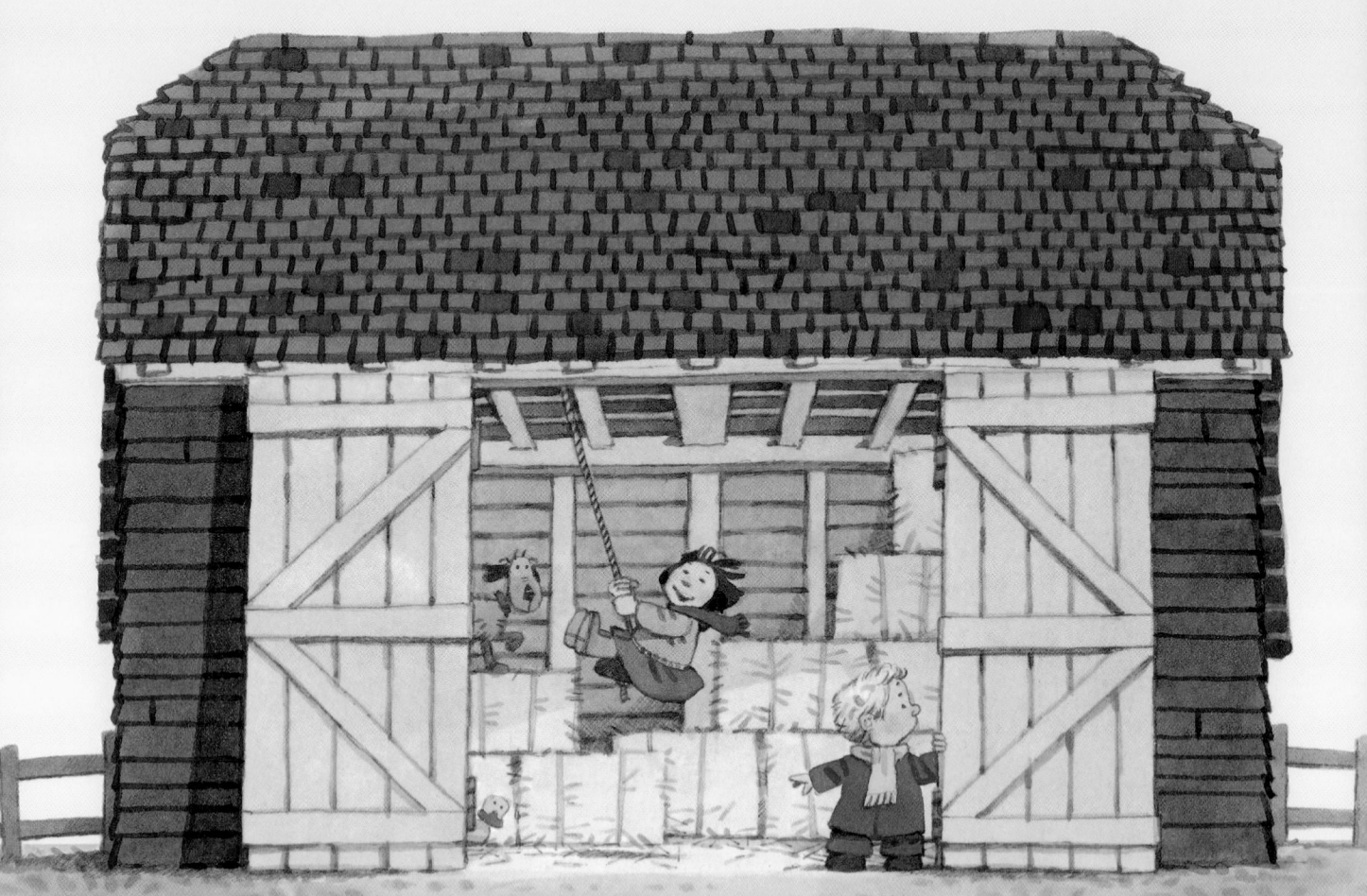

"Listen," says Sam. "Ted is shouting and the tractor is making a funny noise. Let's go and look."

They run to the top of the hill.

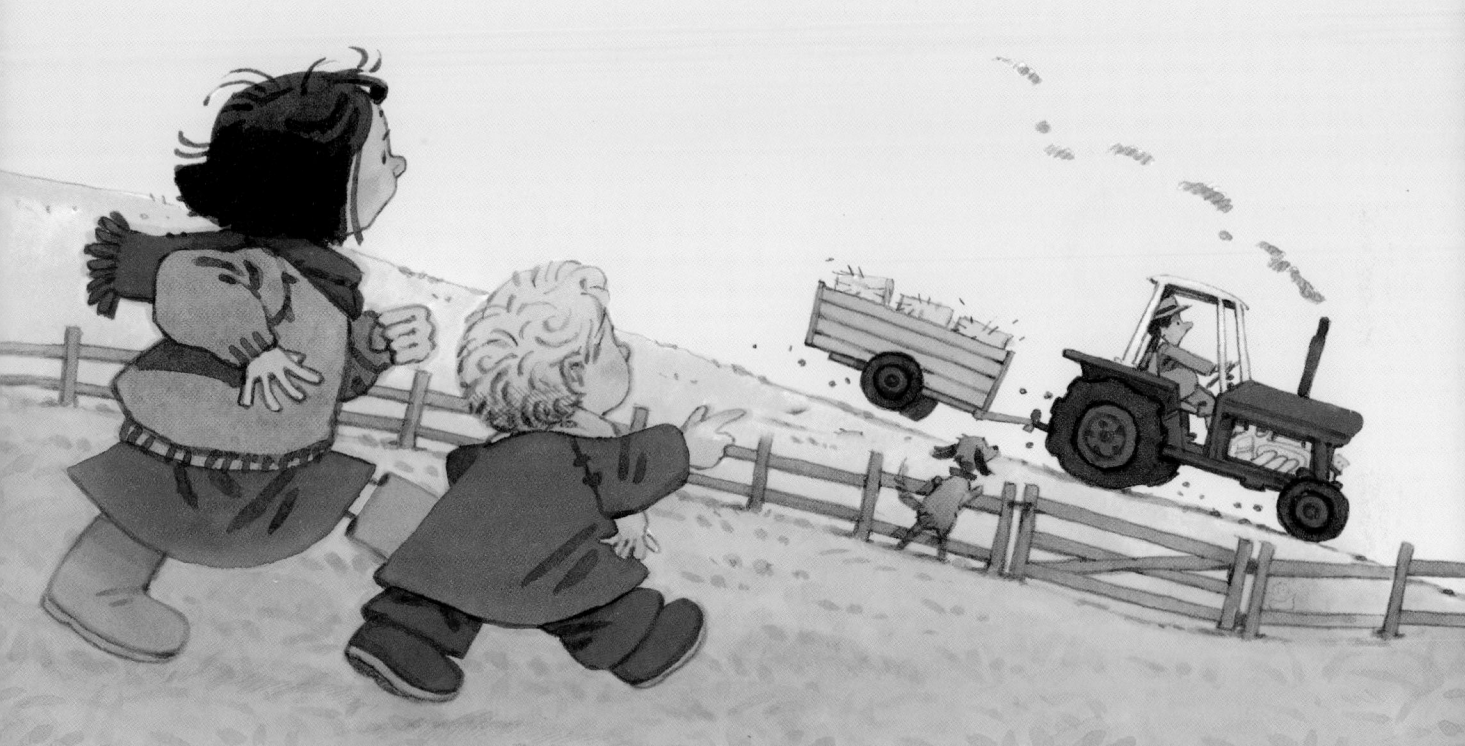

The tractor is racing down the hill, going faster
and faster. "It won't stop," shouts Ted.

The trailer comes off.

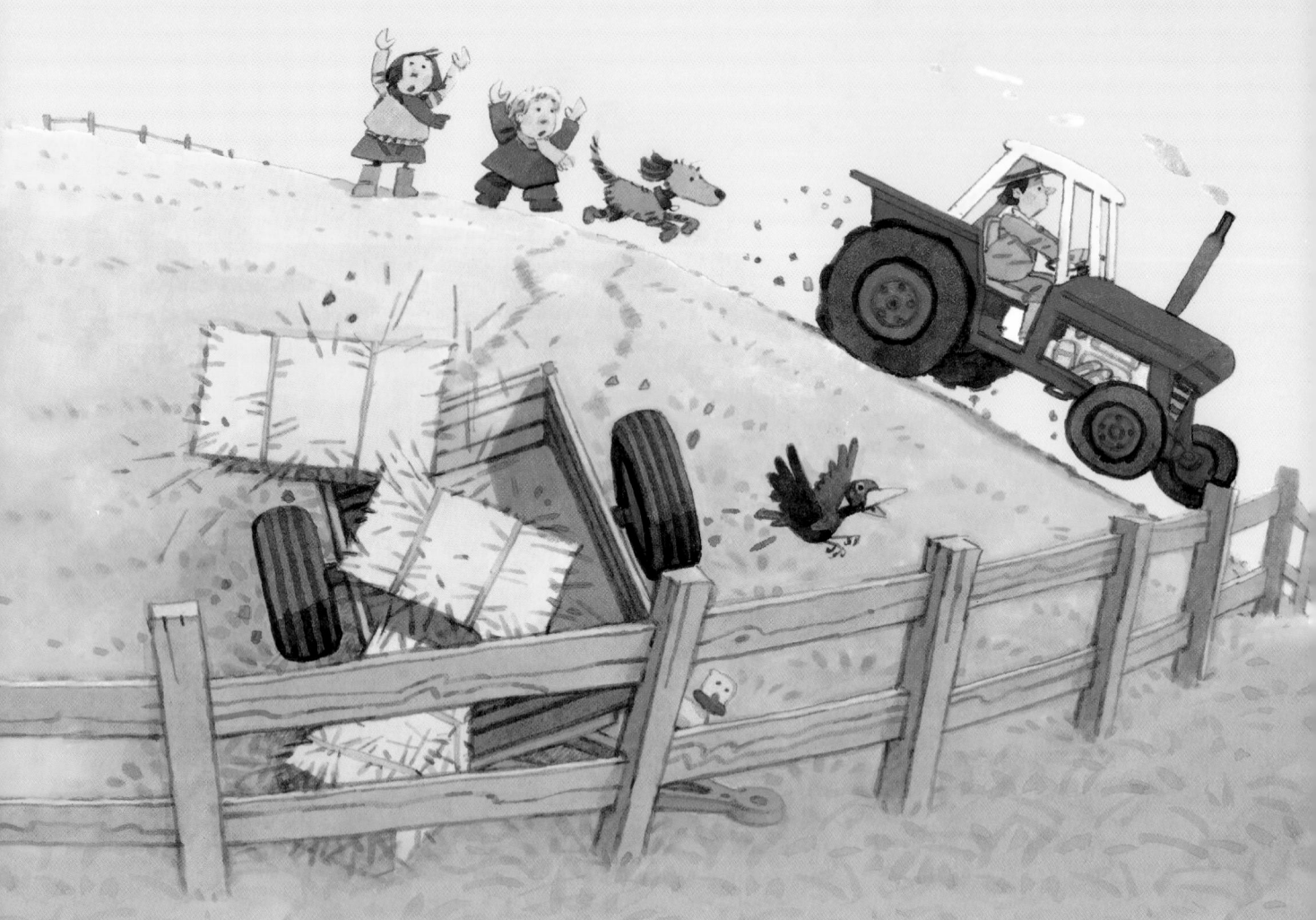

The trailer runs down the hill and crashes into a fence. It tips up and all the hay falls out.

The tractor runs into the pond.

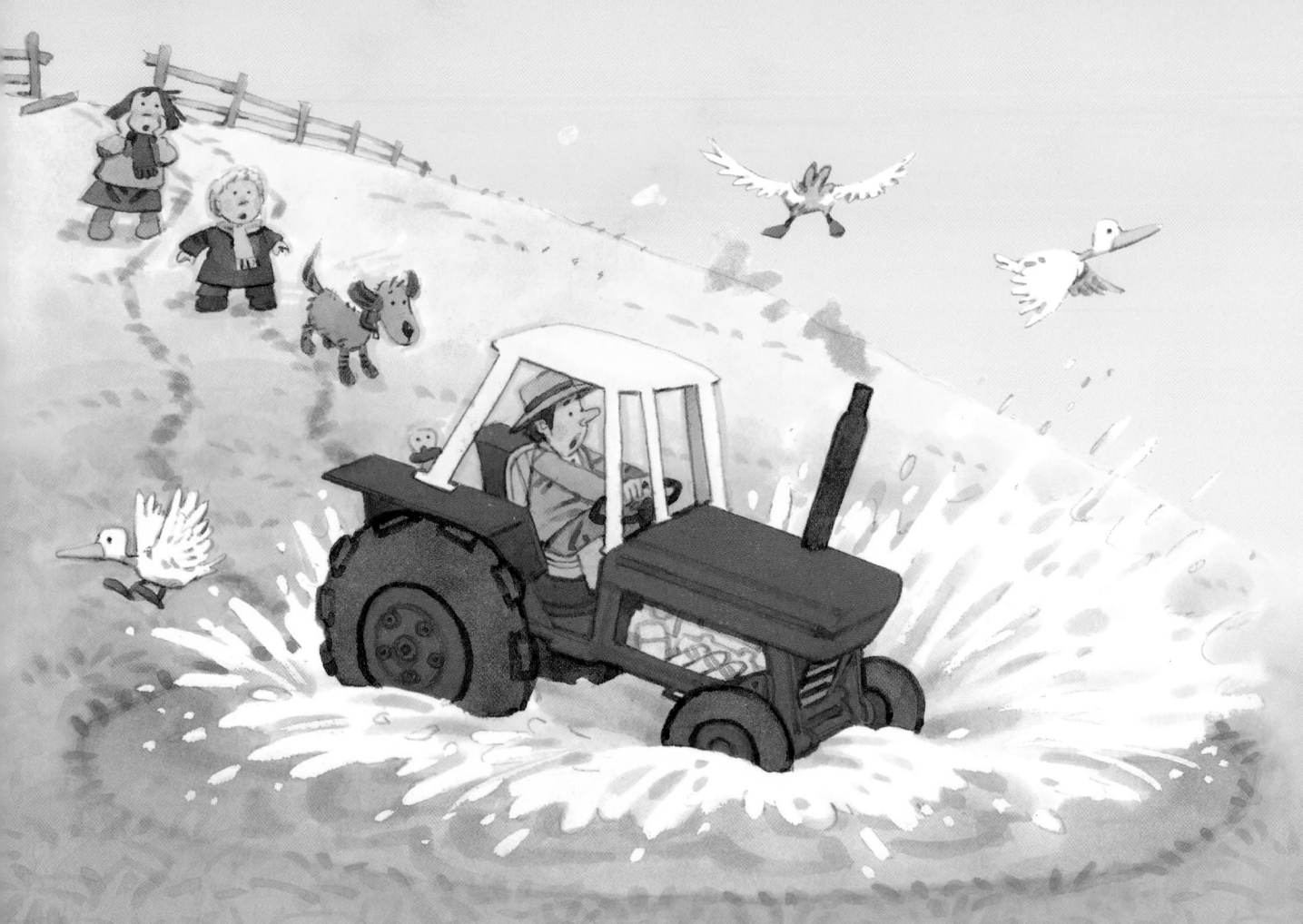

The tractor hits the water with a great splash. The
engine makes a loud noise, then it stops with a hiss.

Ted climbs down from the tractor.

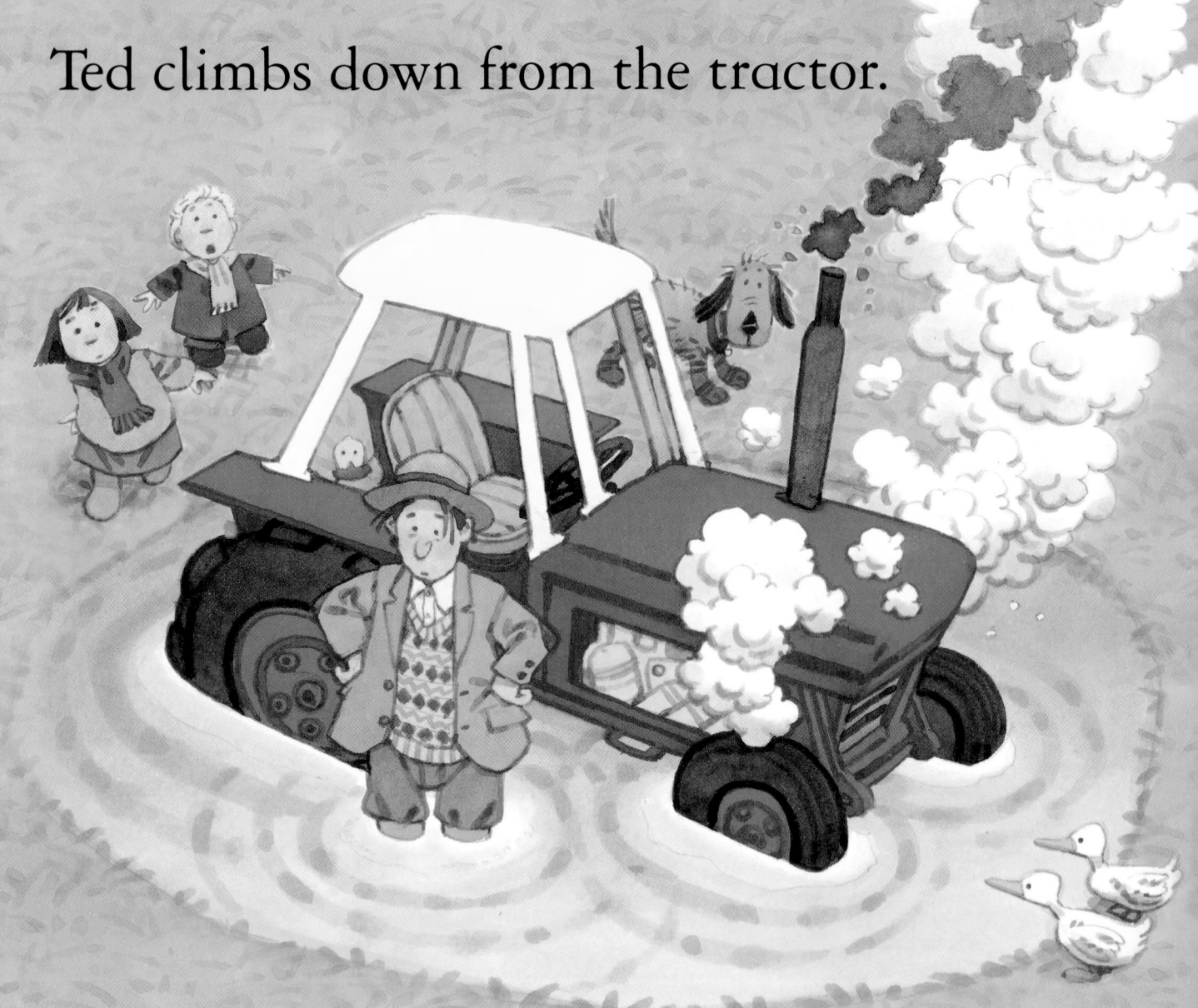

Ted paddles through the water and out of the
pond. Poppy and Sam run down the hill.

Ted is very wet.

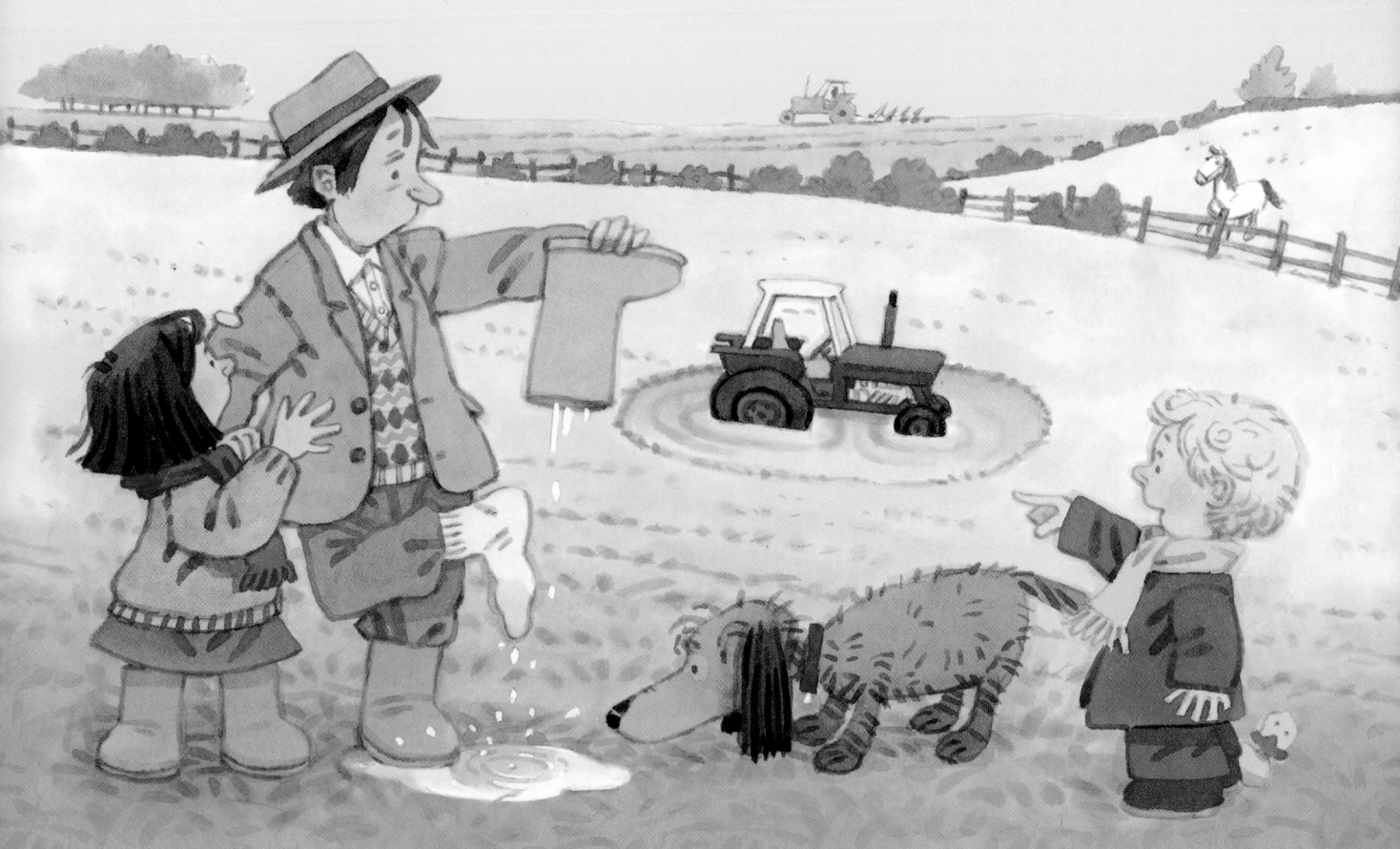

Ted takes off his boots and tips out the water.
How can he get the tractor out of the pond?

"Go and ask Farmer Dray to help."

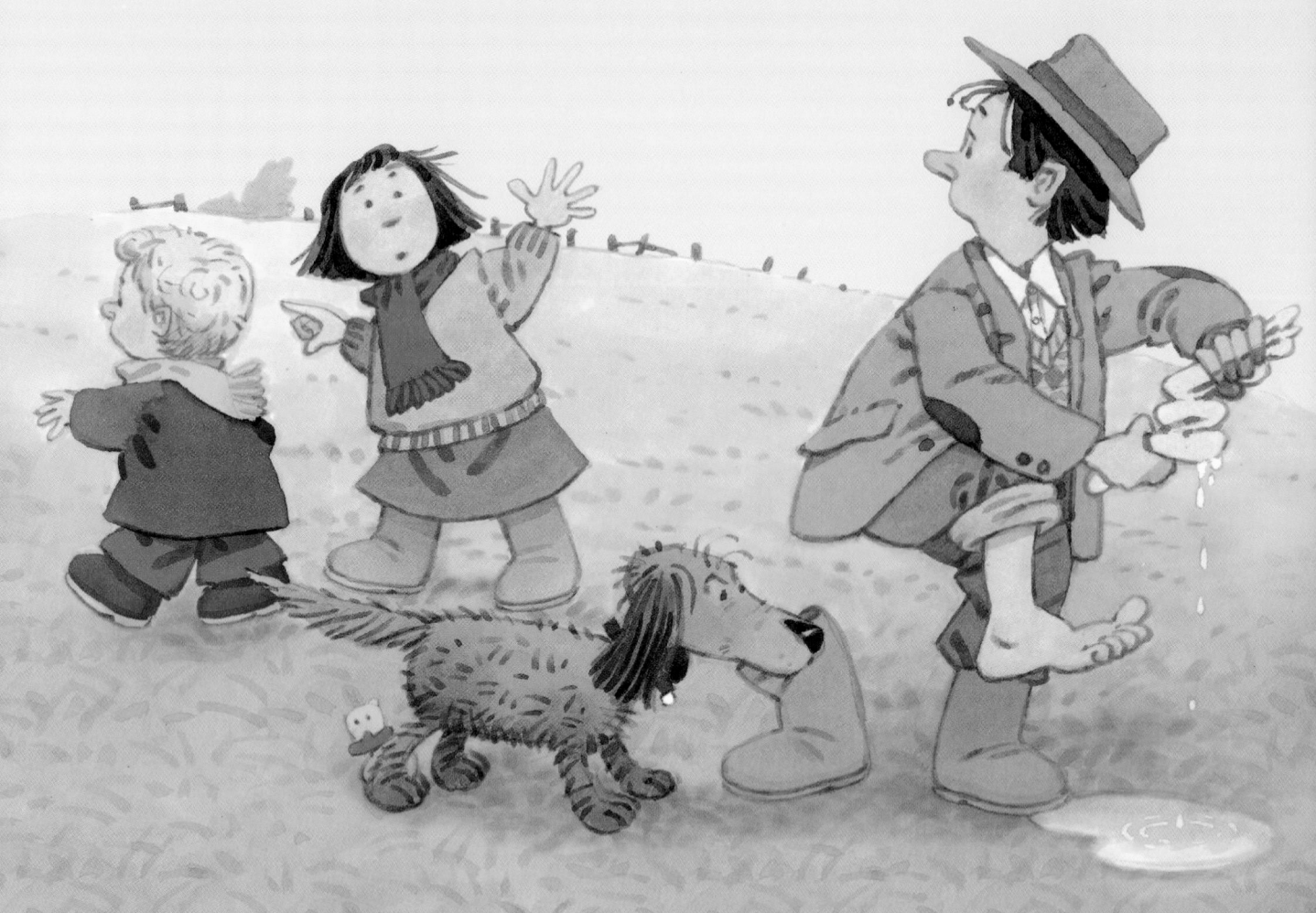

"Ask someone to telephone Farmer Dray," says Ted.
Poppy and Sam run off to the house.

Farmer Dray has a big horse.

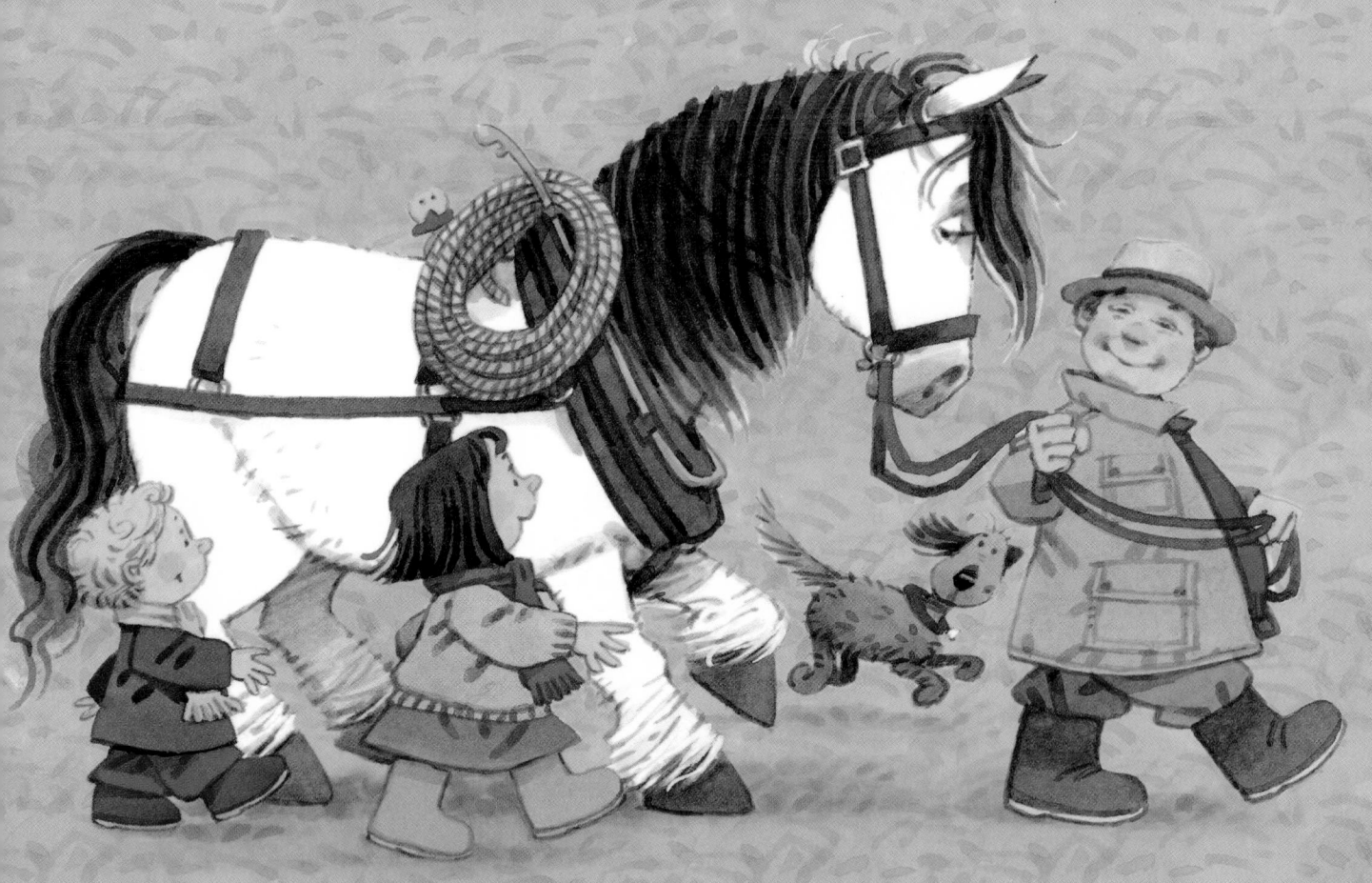

Soon he walks down the hill with his horse.
It is a huge carthorse, called Dolly.

Ted helps with the ropes.

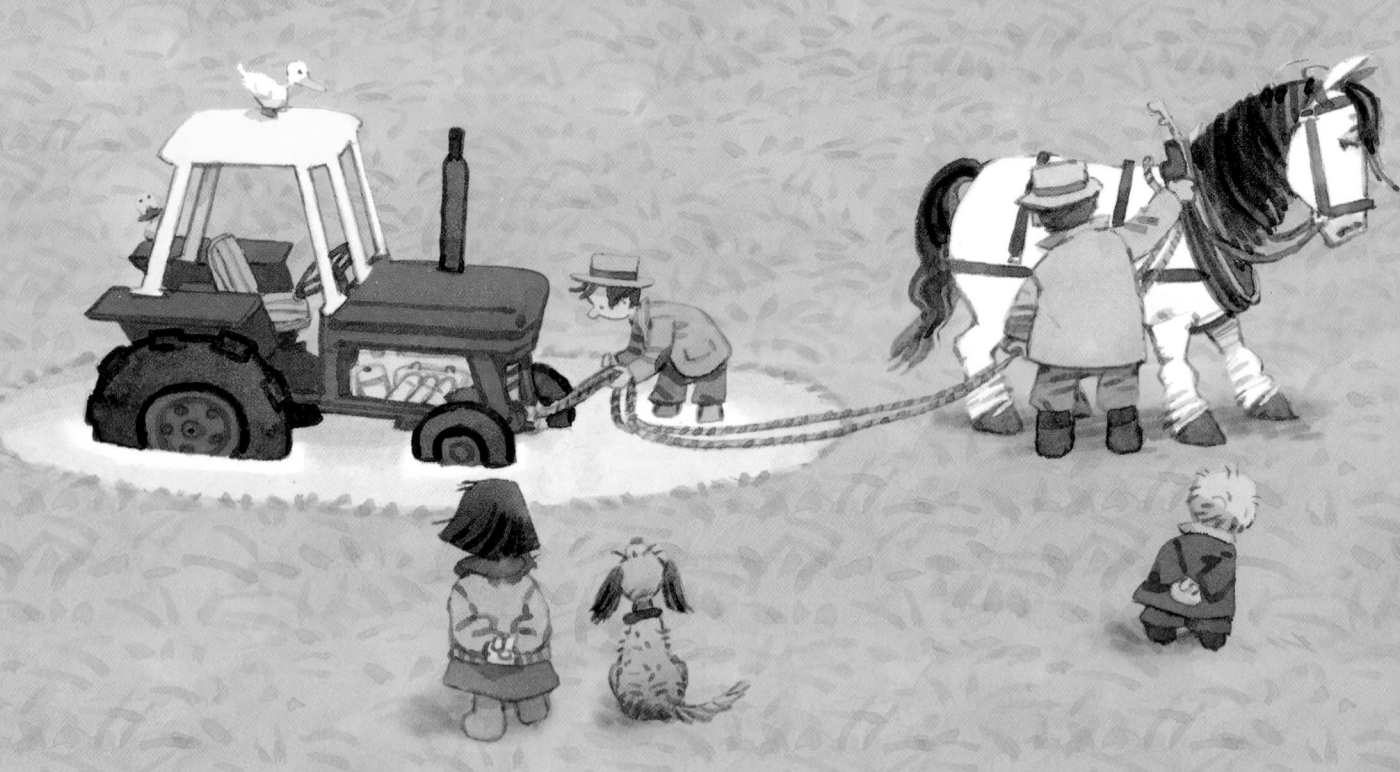

Farmer Dray ties the ropes to the horse. Ted ties
the other ends to the tractor.

Dolly pulls and pulls.

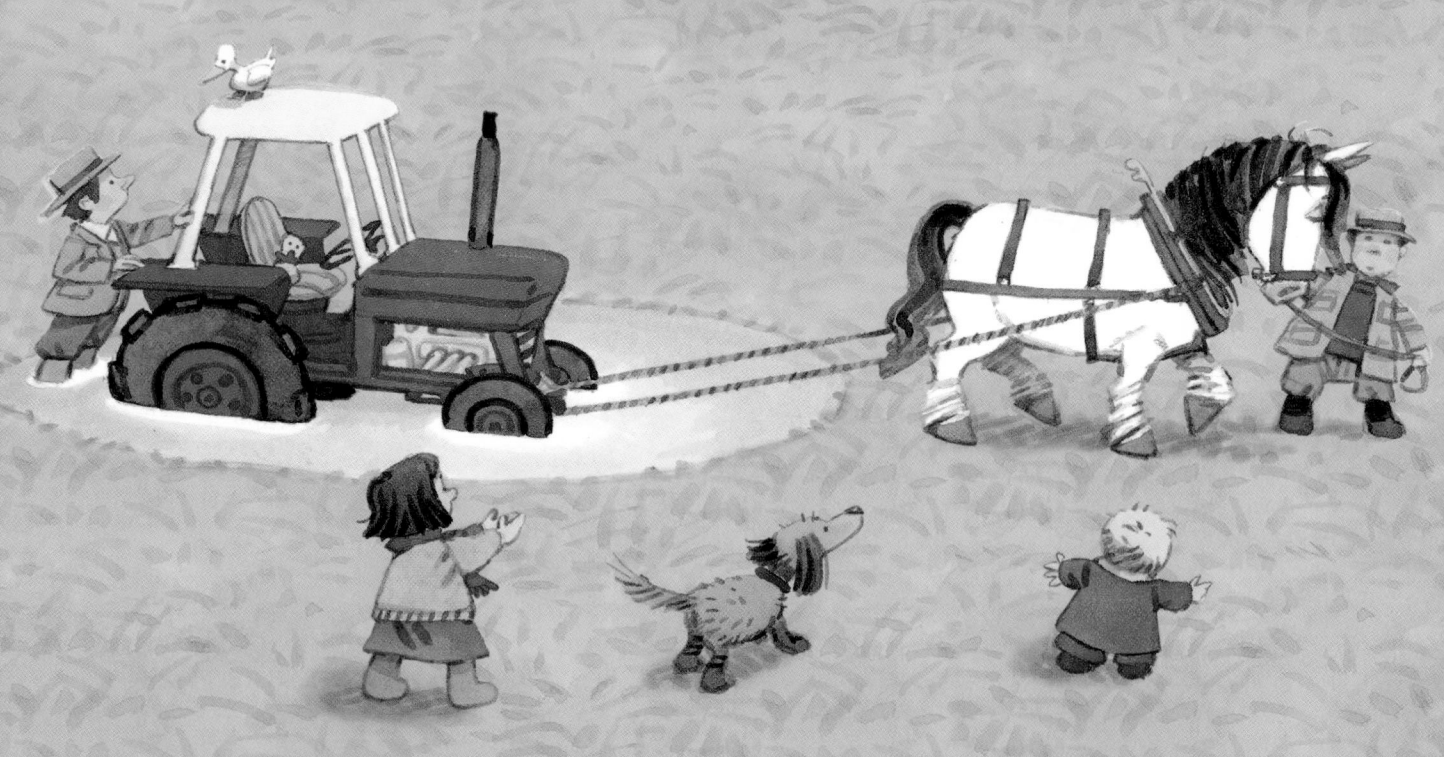

Very slowly the tractor starts to move. Ted pushes as hard as he can and Dolly pulls.

Ted falls over.

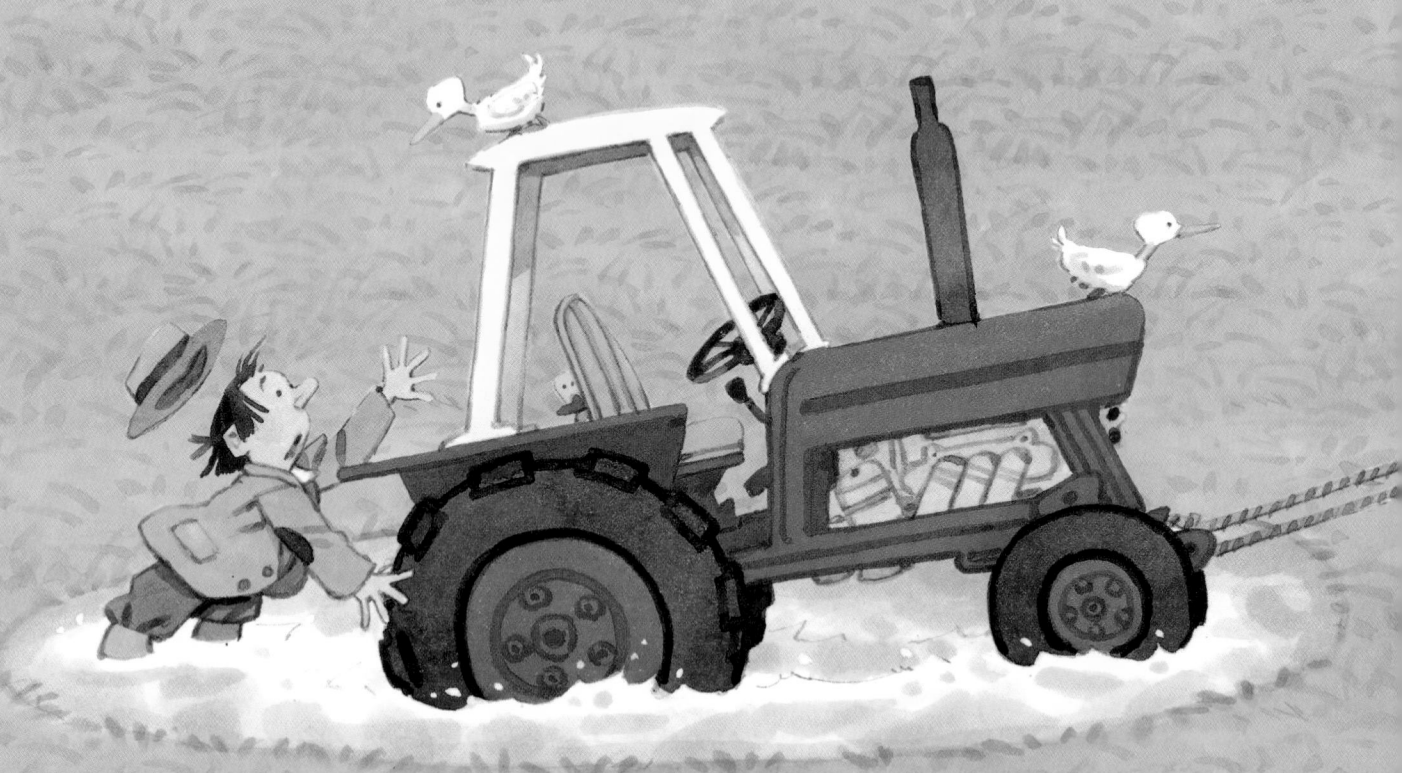

The tractor jerks forward and Ted falls in the water. Now he is wet and muddy all over.

The tractor is out of the pond.

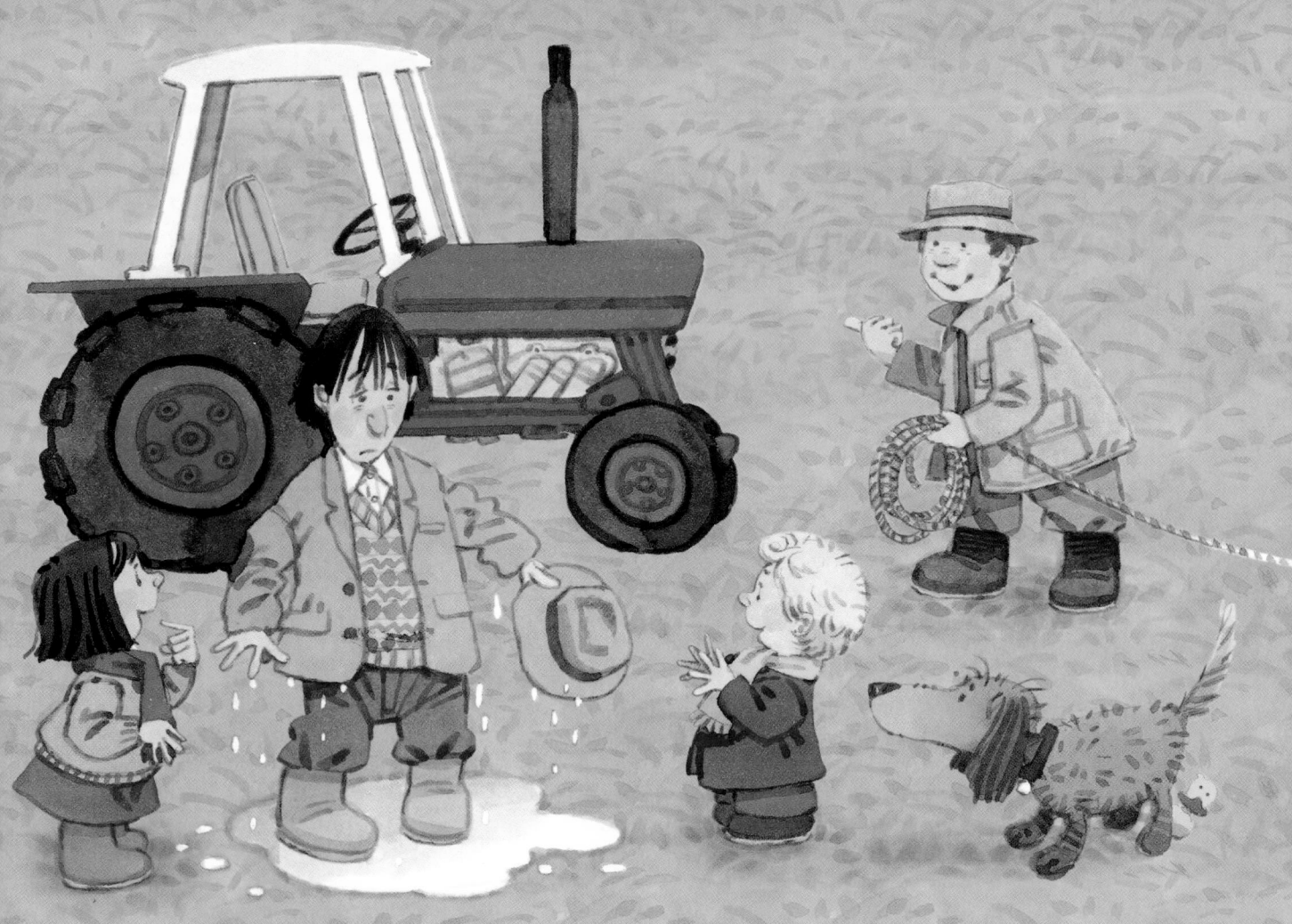

"Better leave the tractor to dry," says Farmer
Dray. "Then you can get the engine going again."

Poppy and Sam ride home.

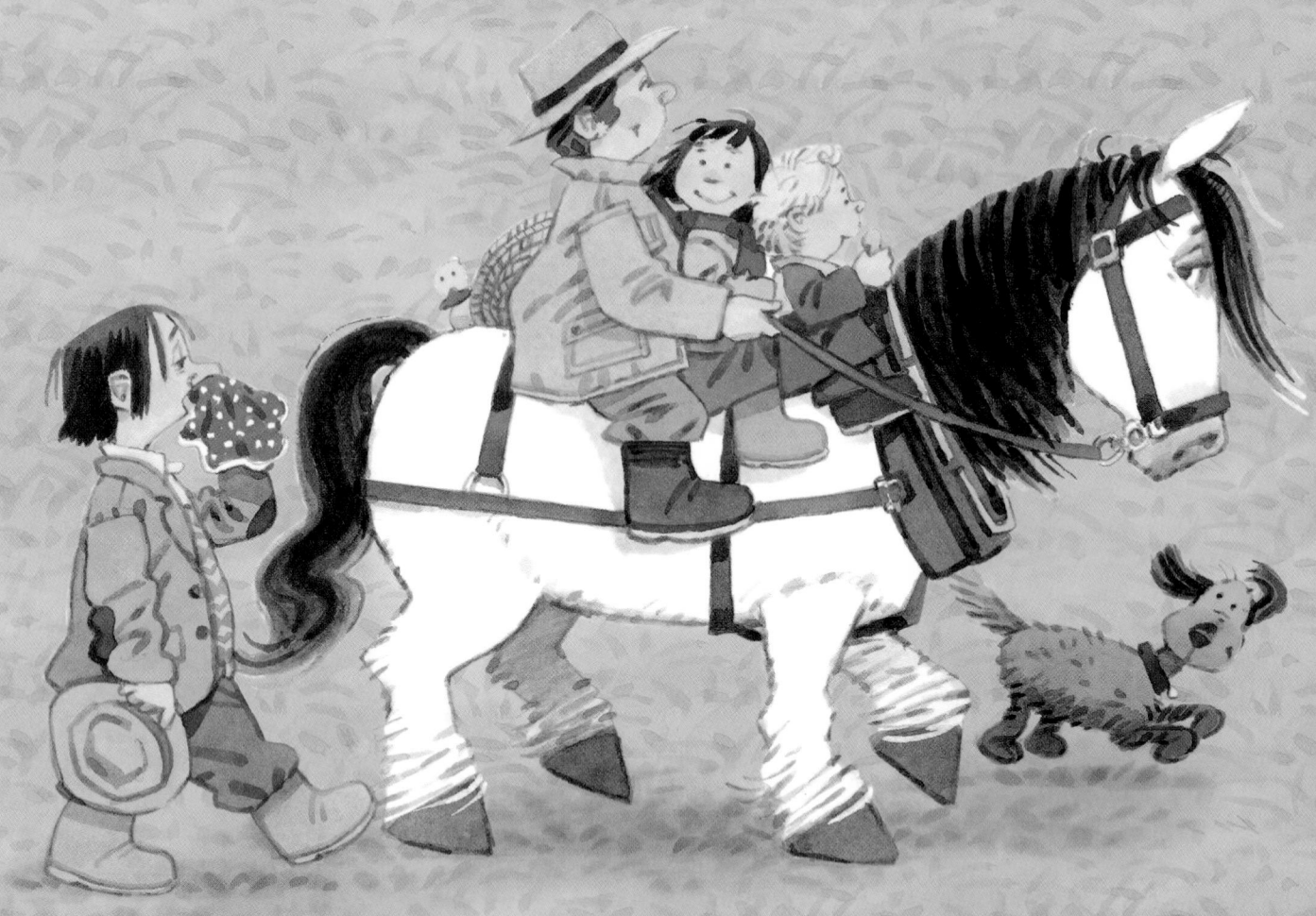

Farmer Dray lifts them onto Dolly's back.
But Ted is so muddy, he has to walk.

Pig Gets Lost

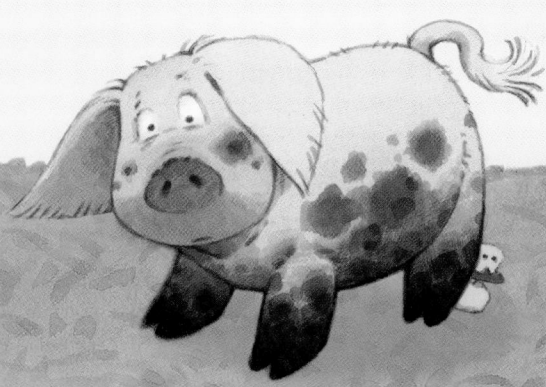

This is Apple Tree Farm.

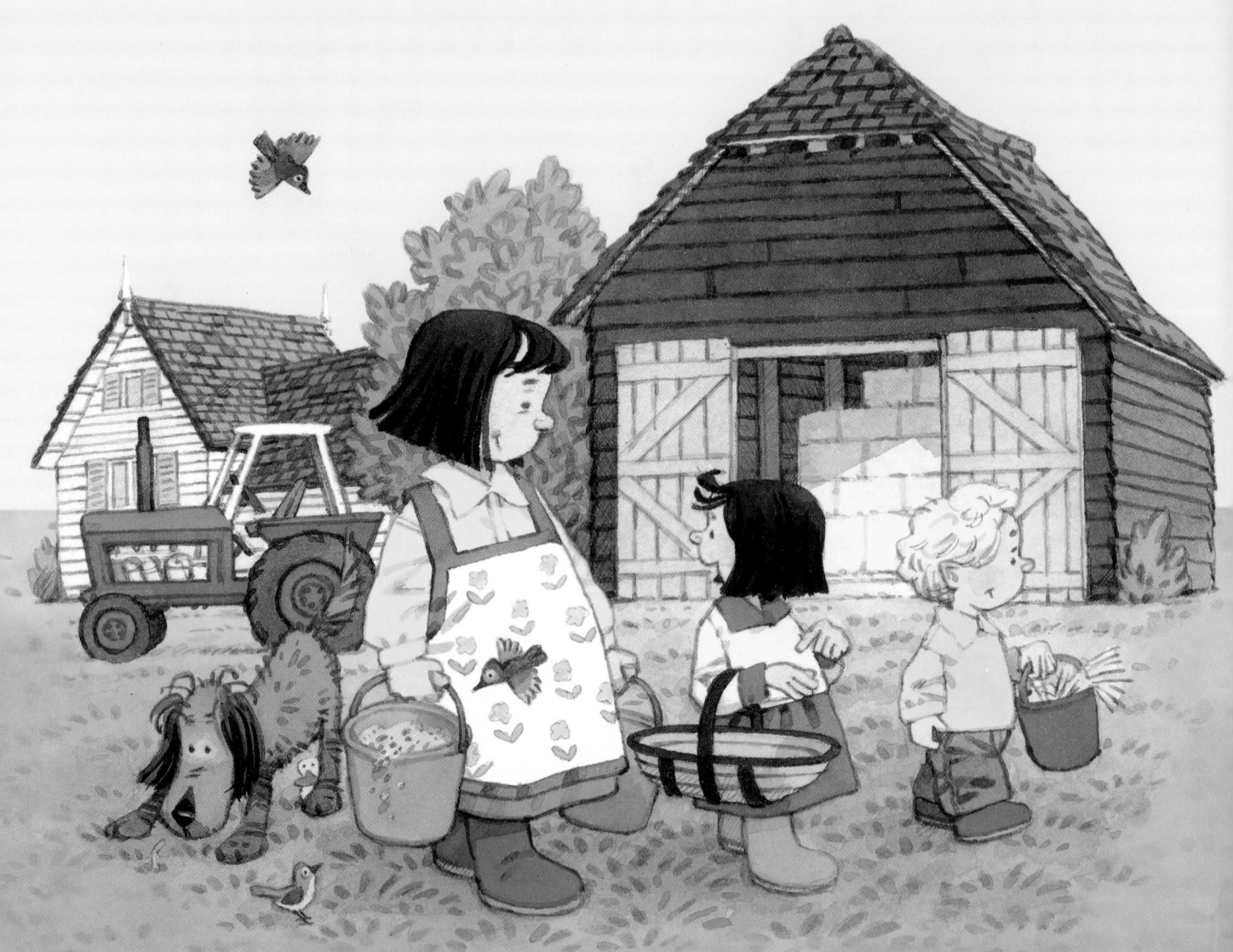

This is Mrs. Boot, the farmer. She has two children, called Poppy and Sam, and a dog called Rusty.

Mrs. Boot has six pigs.

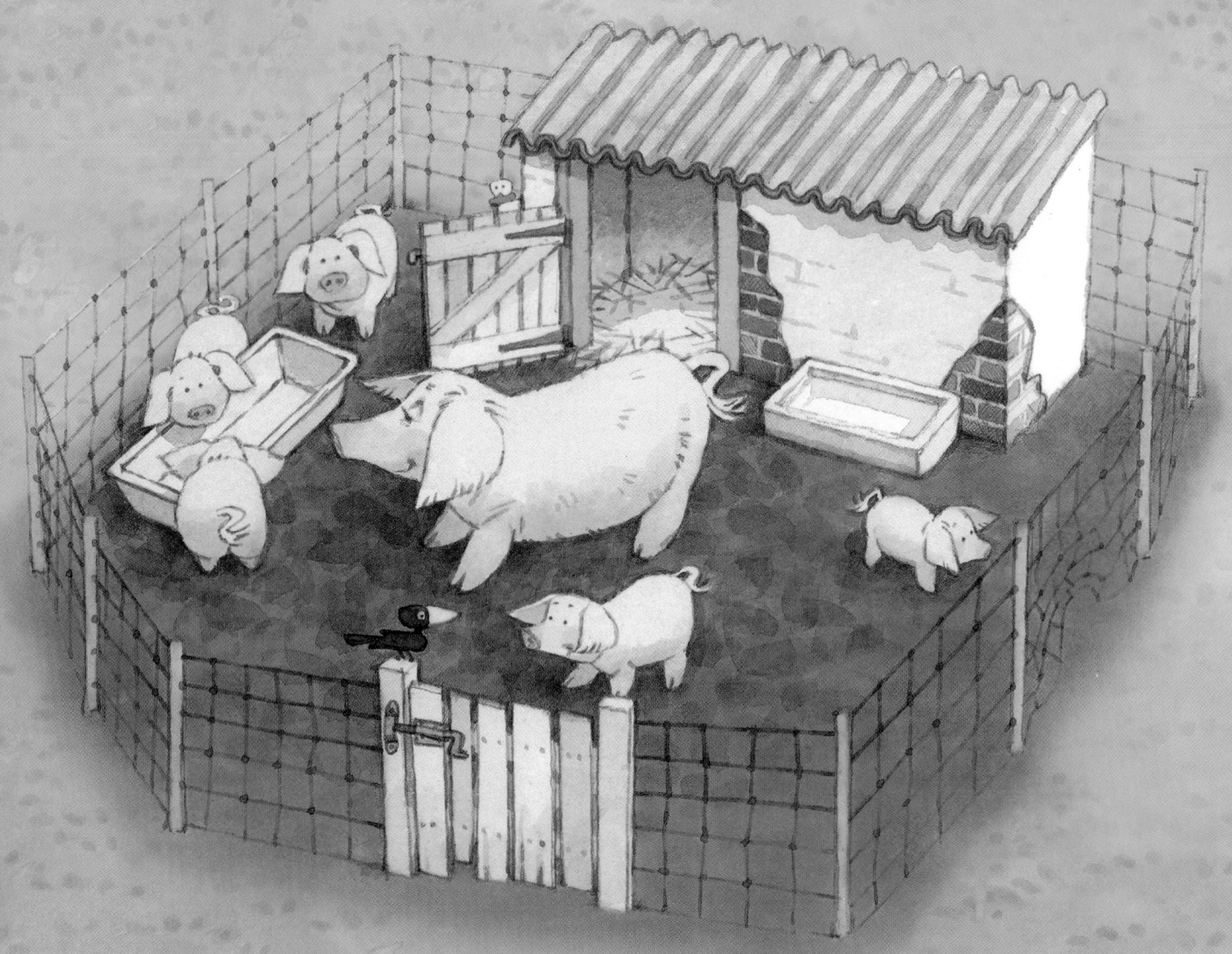

There is a mother pig and five baby pigs.
The smallest pig is called Curly. They live in a pen.

Mrs. Boot feeds the pigs every morning.

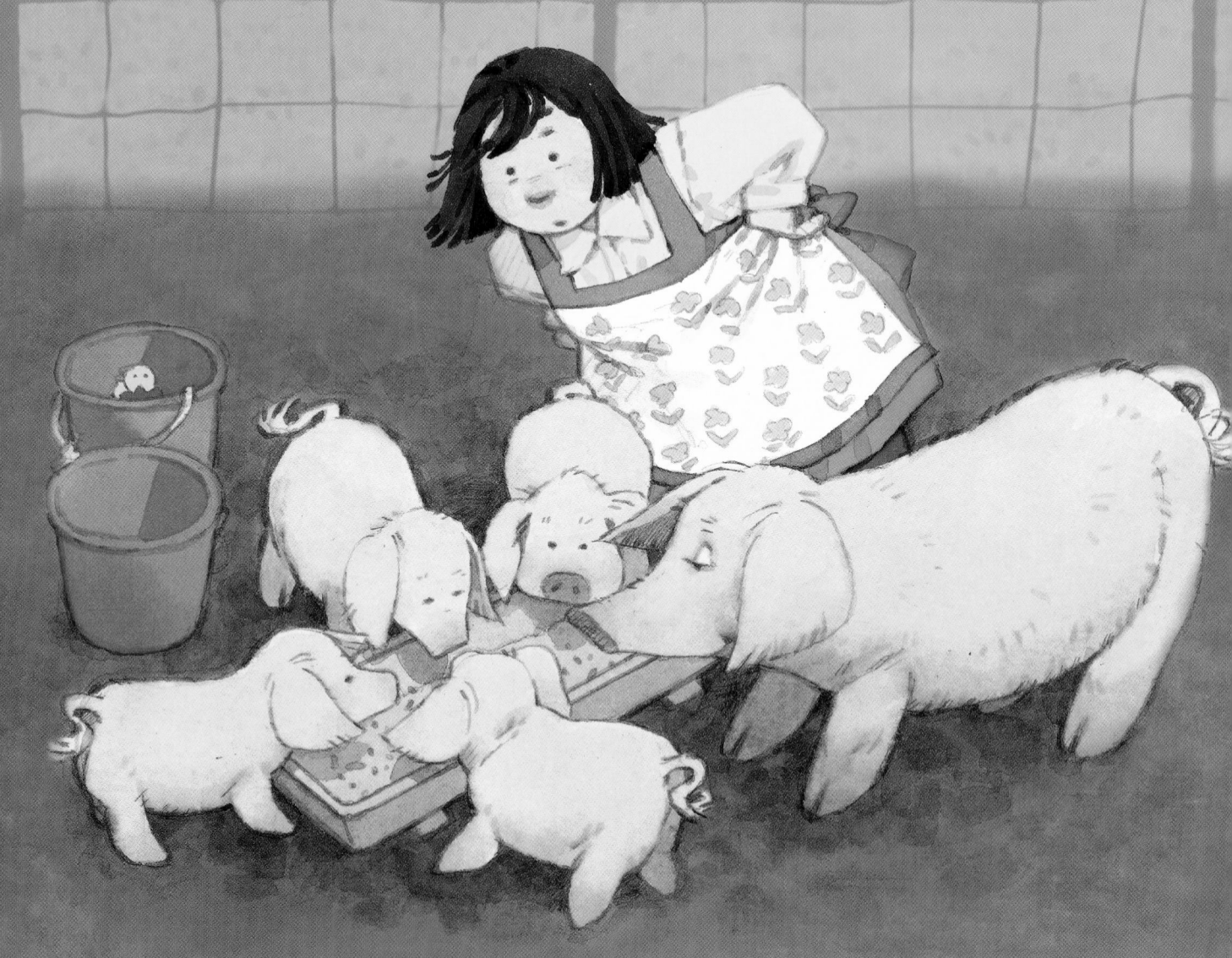

She takes them two big buckets of food.
But where is Curly? He is not in the pen.

She calls Poppy and Sam.

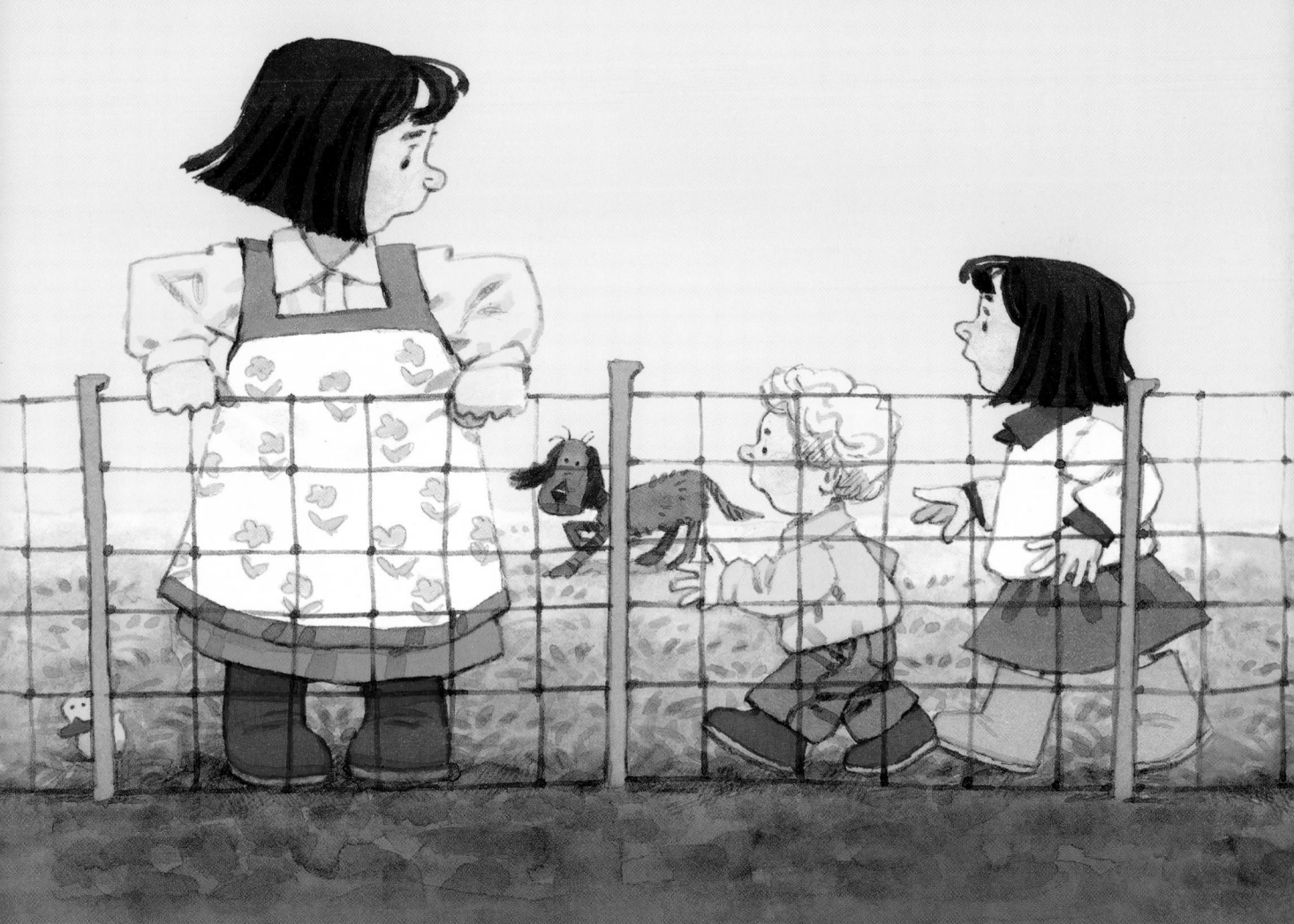

"Curly's gone," she says. "I need your help to find him."

"Where are you, Curly?"

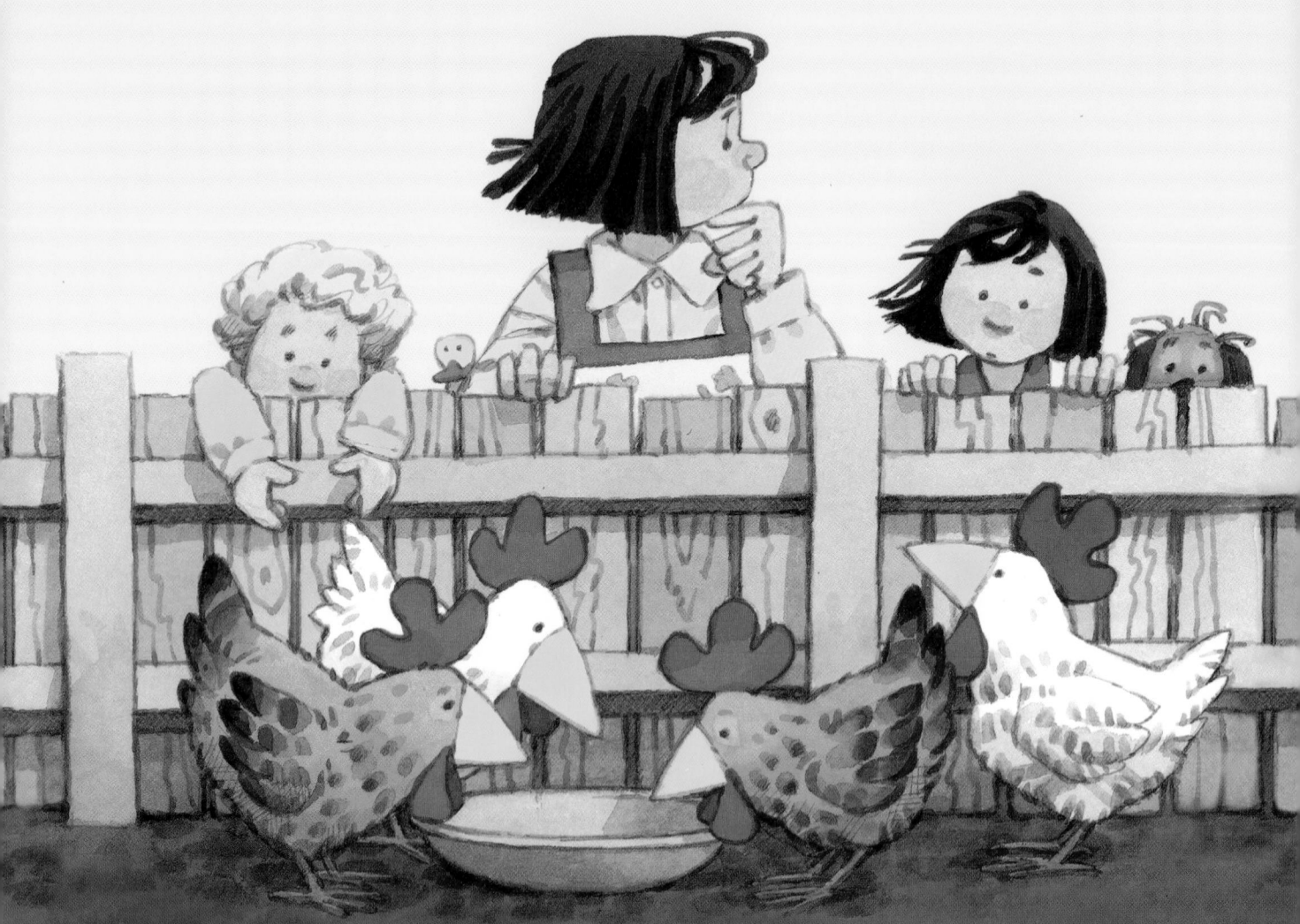

Poppy and Sam call to Curly. "Let's look in the hen run," says Mrs. Boot. But Curly is not there.

"There he is, in the barn."

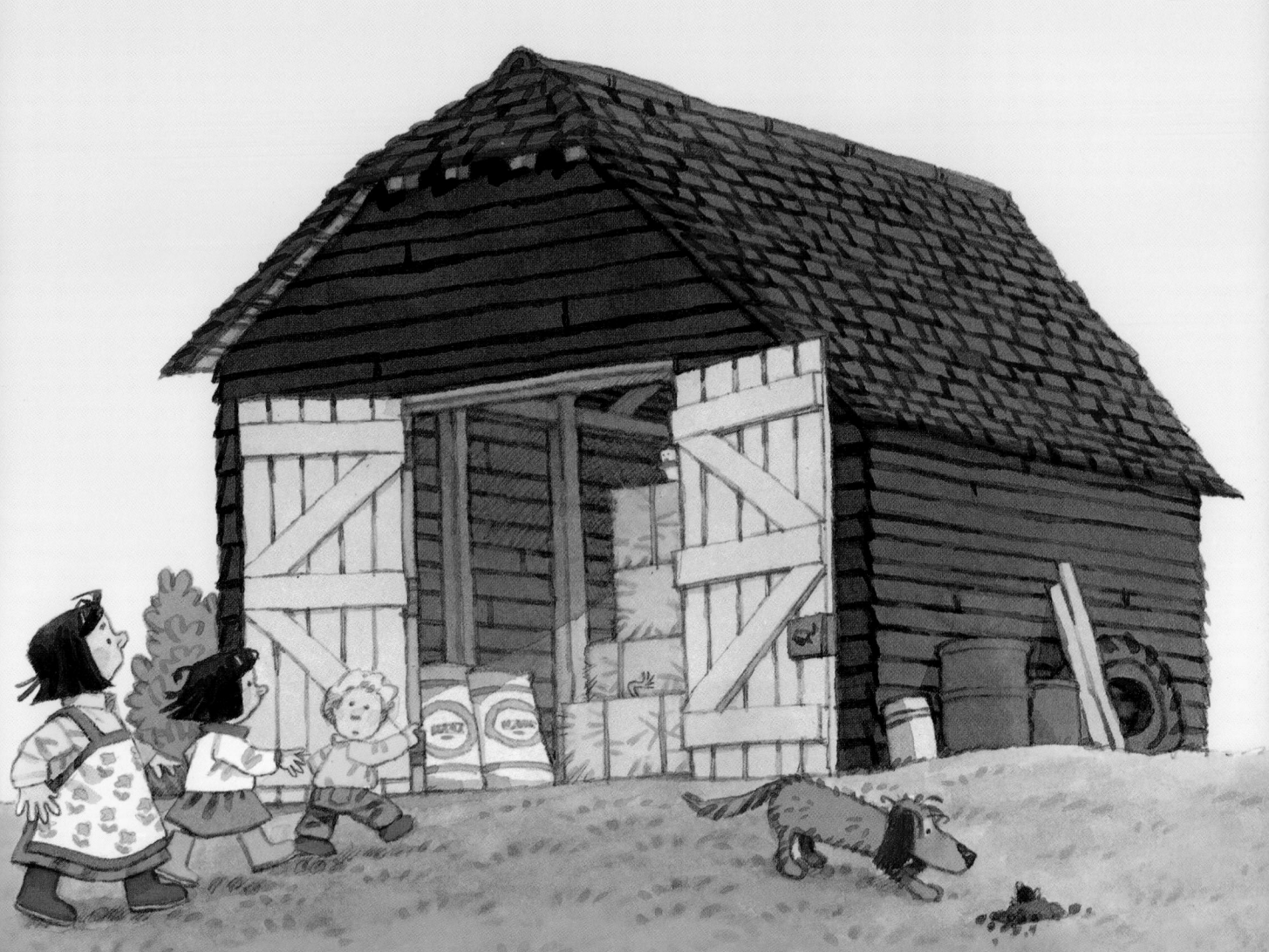

"He's in the barn," says Sam. "I can just see his tail." They all run into the barn to catch Curly.

"That's not Curly."

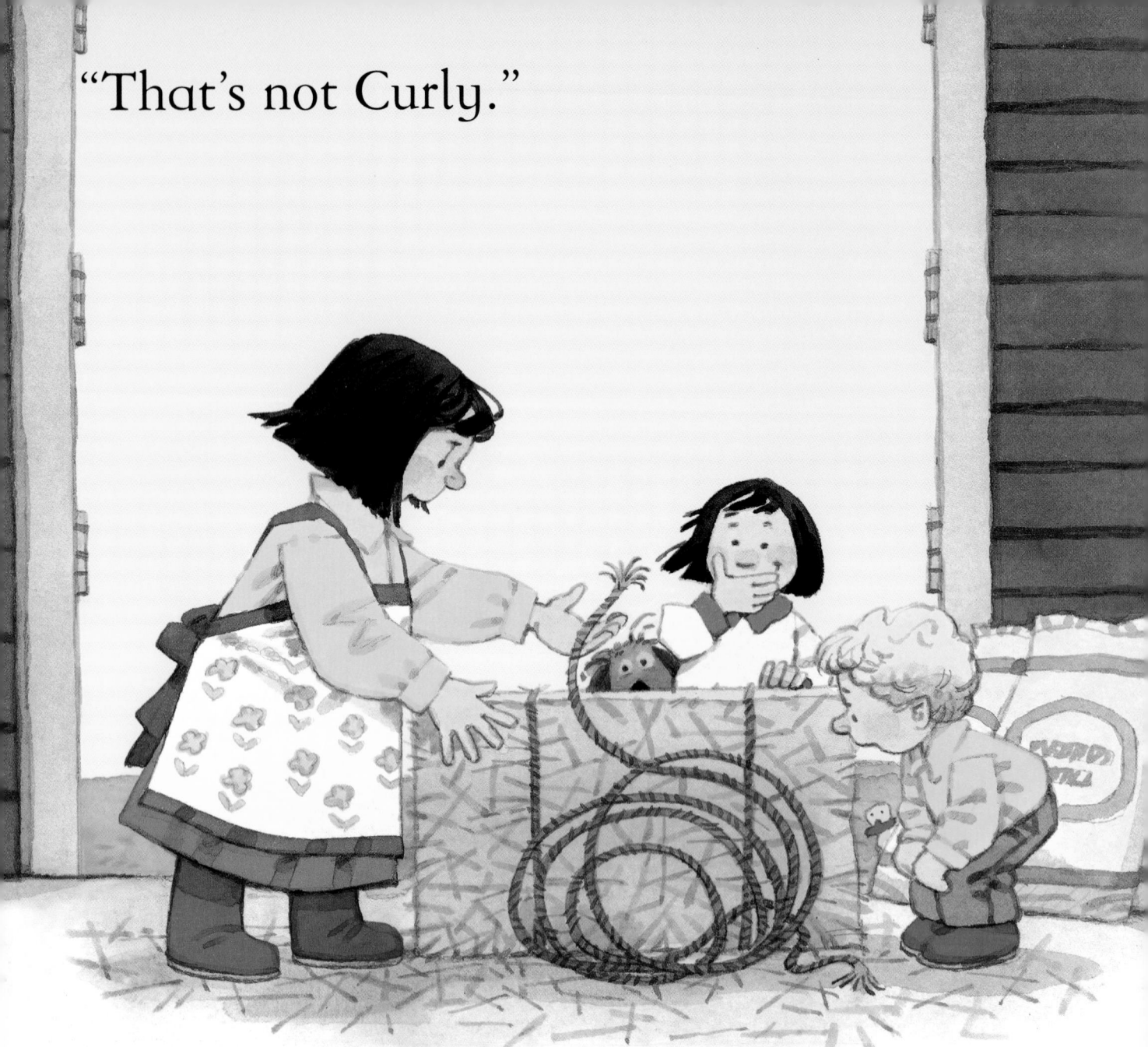

"It's only a piece of rope," says Mrs. Boot. "Not Curly's tail." "Where can he be?" says Poppy.

"Maybe he's eating the cows' food."

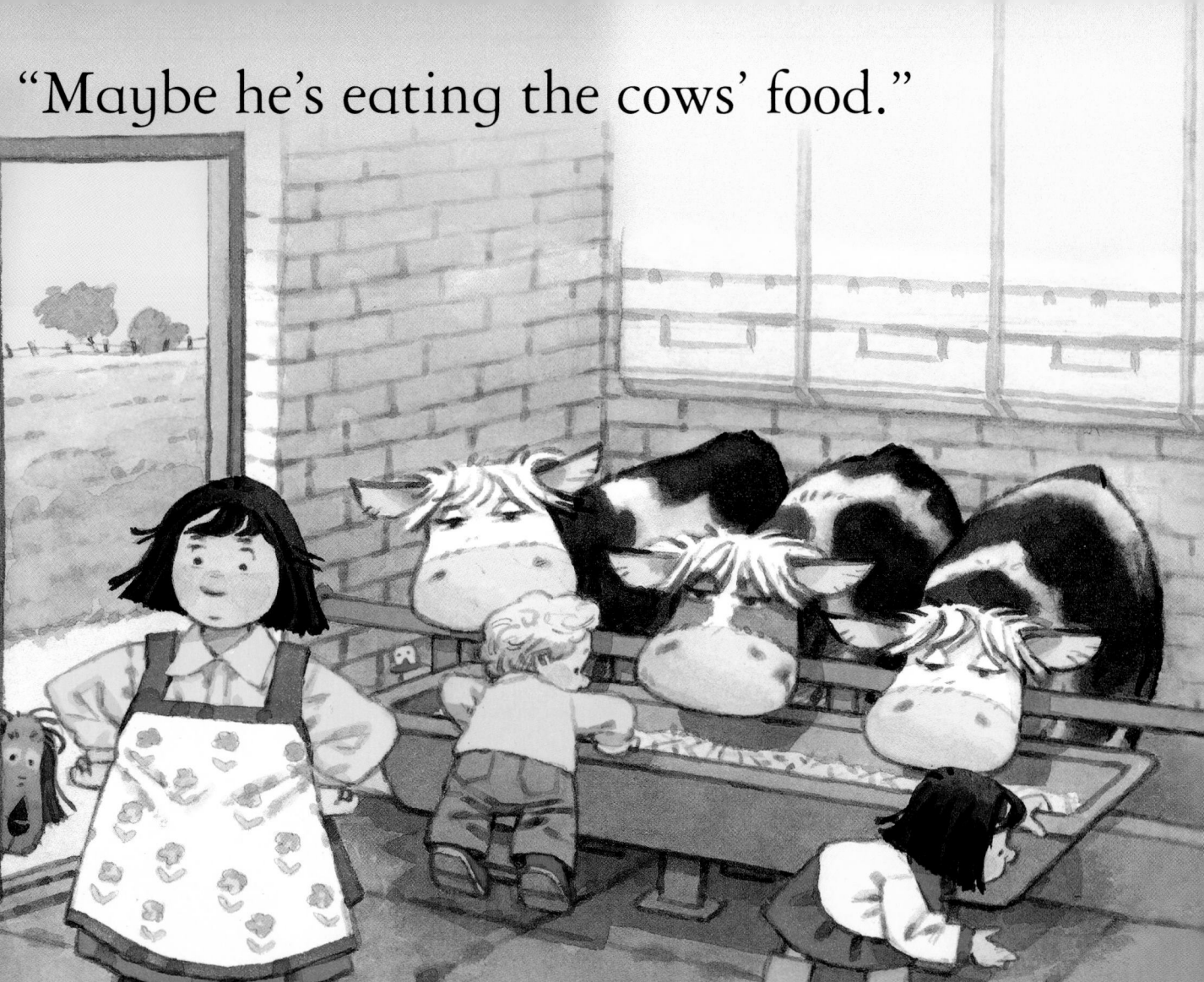

But Curly is not with the cows. "Don't worry,"
says Mrs. Boot. "We'll soon find him."

"Perhaps he's in the garden."

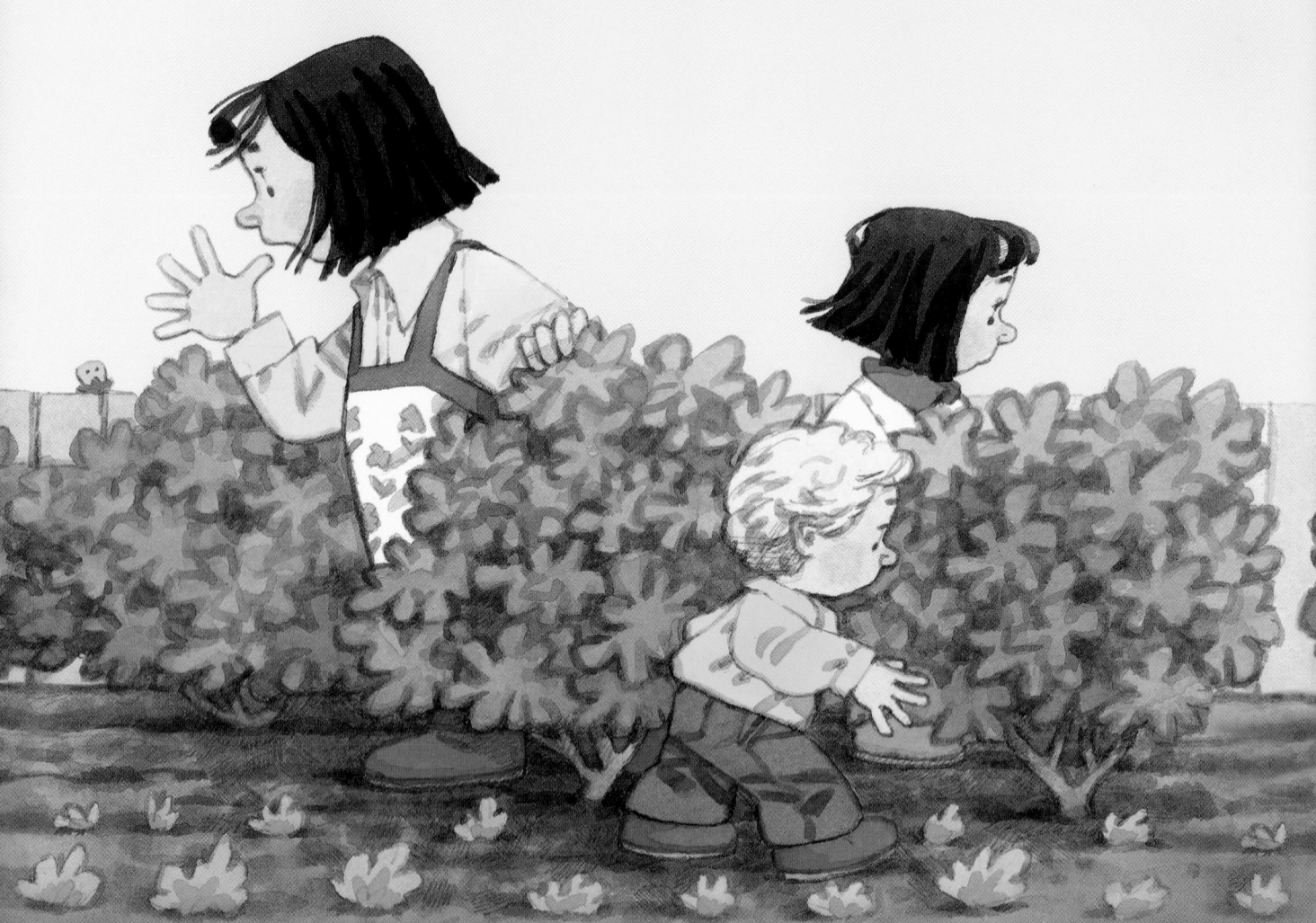

They look for Curly in the garden, but he is not there. "We'll never find him," says Sam.

"Why is Rusty barking?"

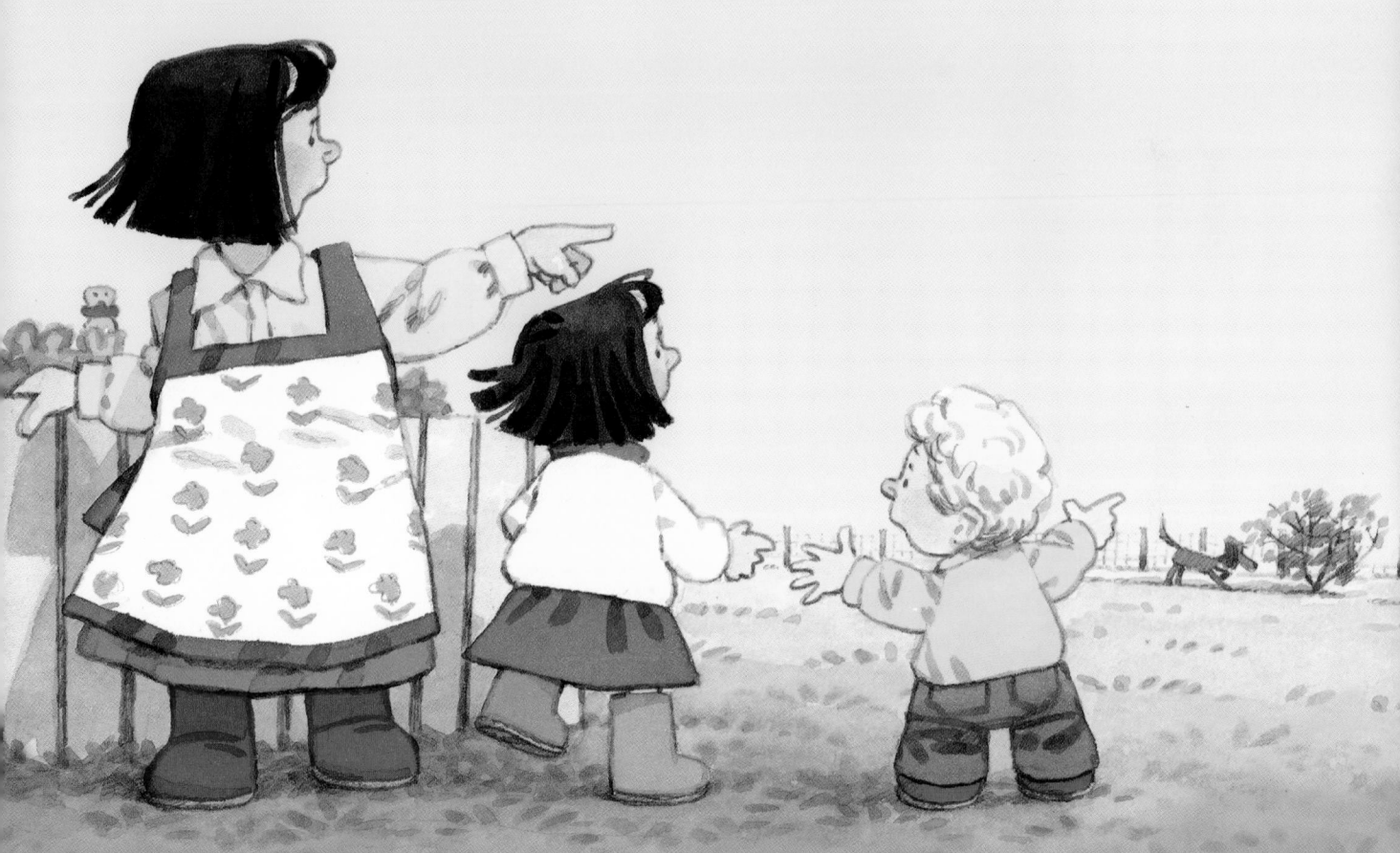

Rusty is standing by a ditch. He barks and barks.
"He's trying to tell us something," says Poppy.

"Rusty has found Curly."

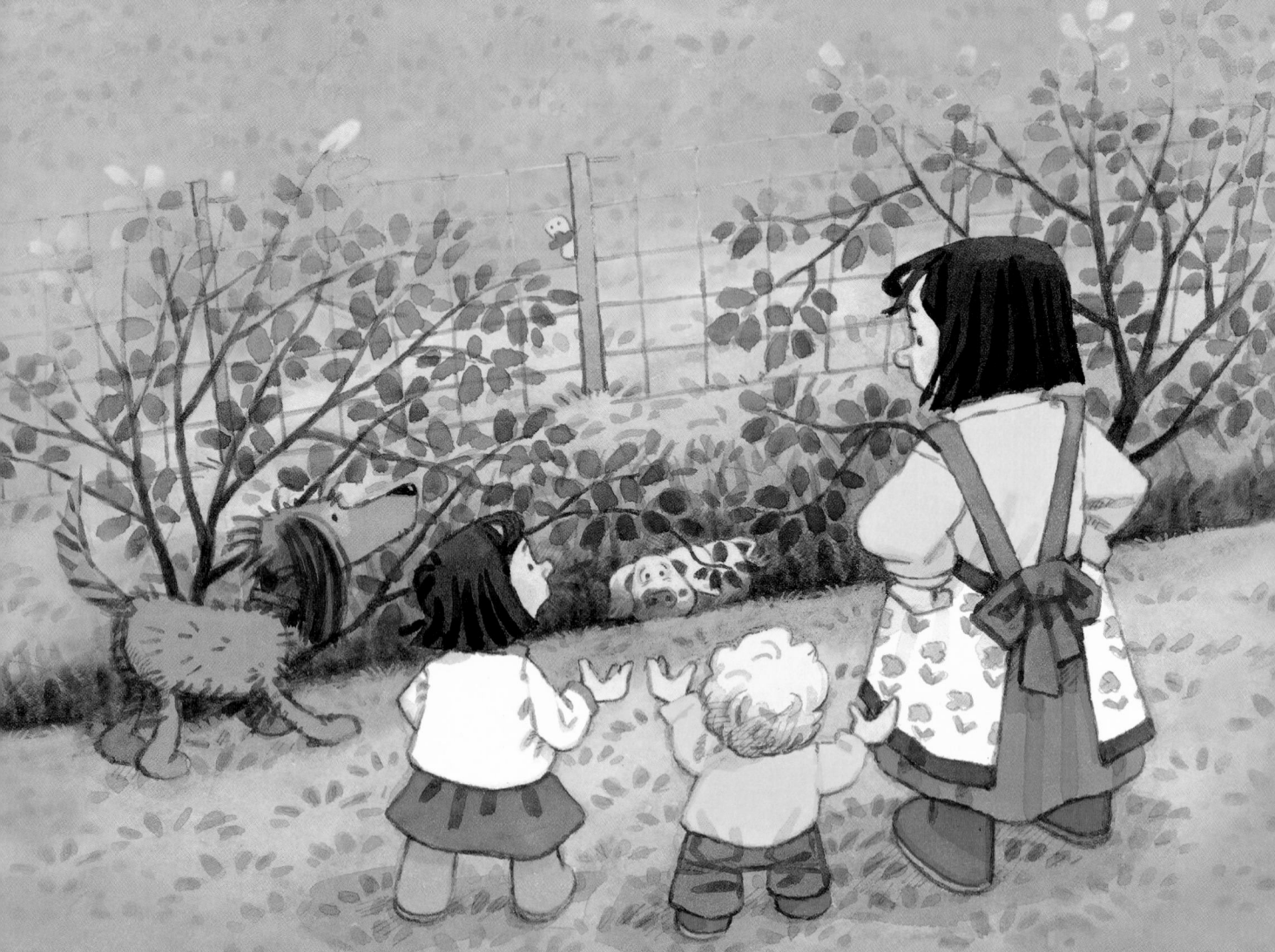

They all look in the ditch. Curly has slipped down into the mud and can't climb out.

"We'll have to lift him out."

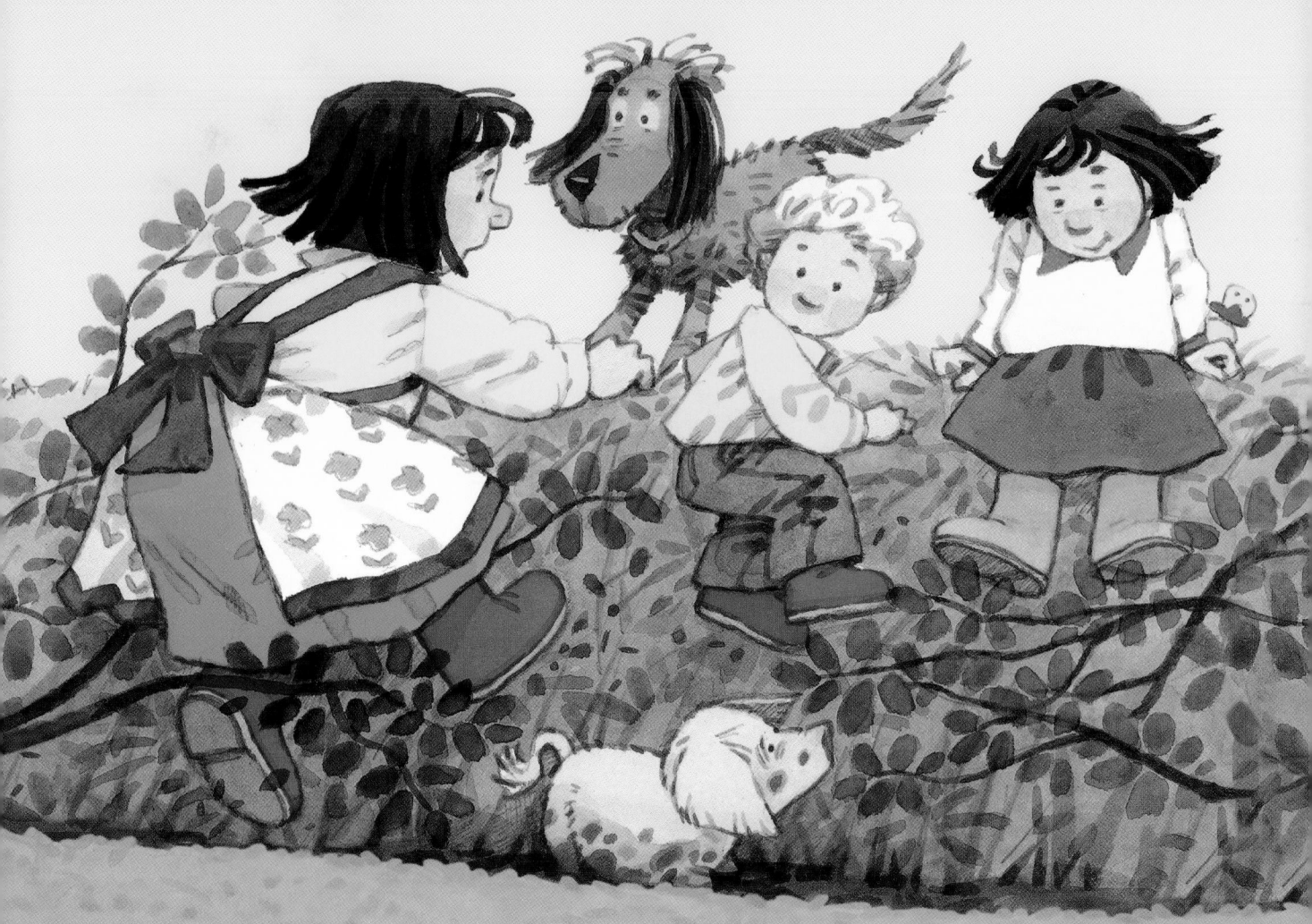

"I'll get into the ditch," says Mrs. Boot. "I'm coming too," says Poppy. "And me," says Sam.

Curly is very muddy.

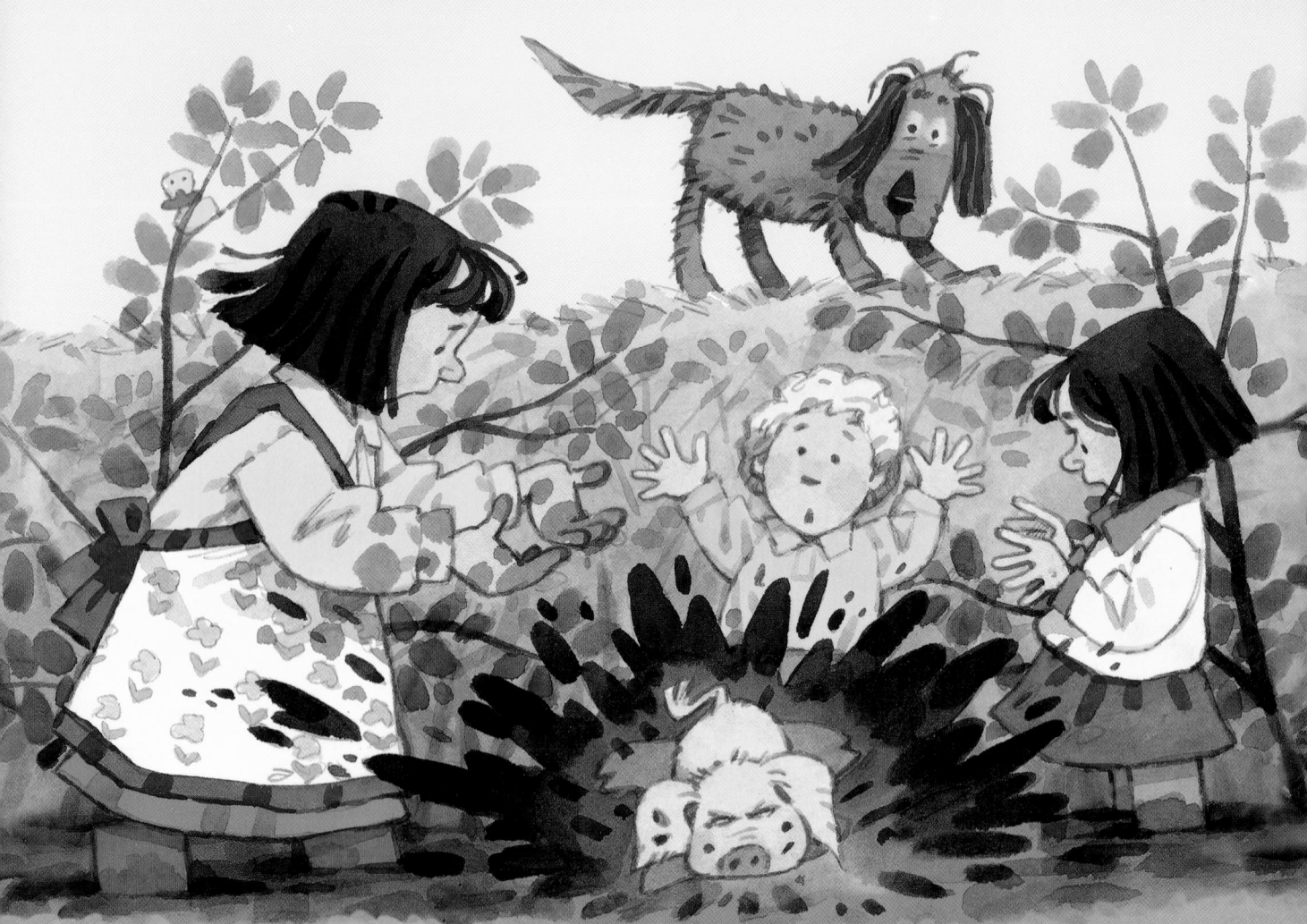

Mrs. Boot picks Curly up but he struggles. Then he slips back into the mud with a splash.

Now everyone is very muddy.

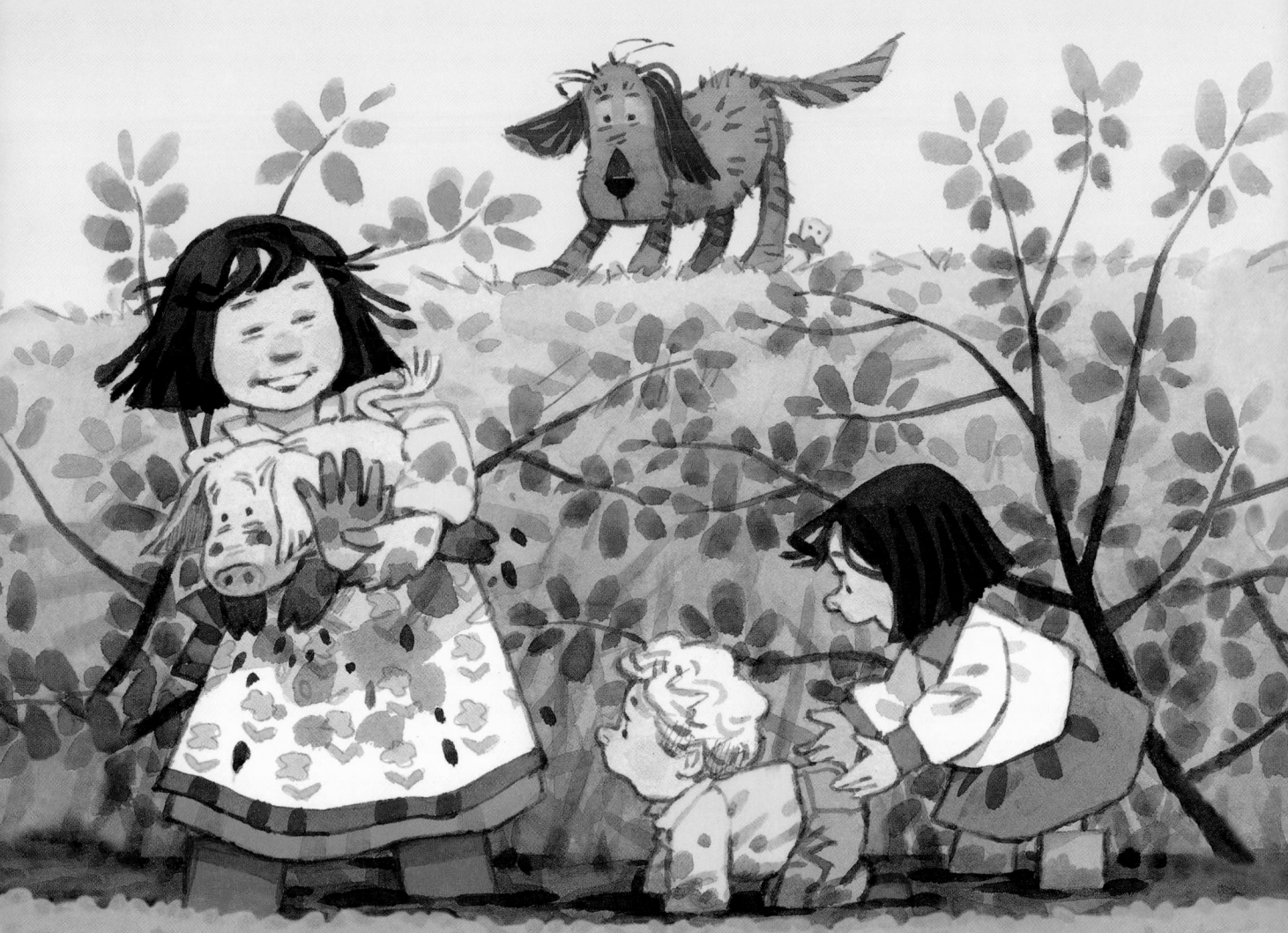

Sam tries to catch Curly but he falls into the mud.
Mrs. Boot grabs Curly and climbs out of the ditch.

They all climb out of the ditch.

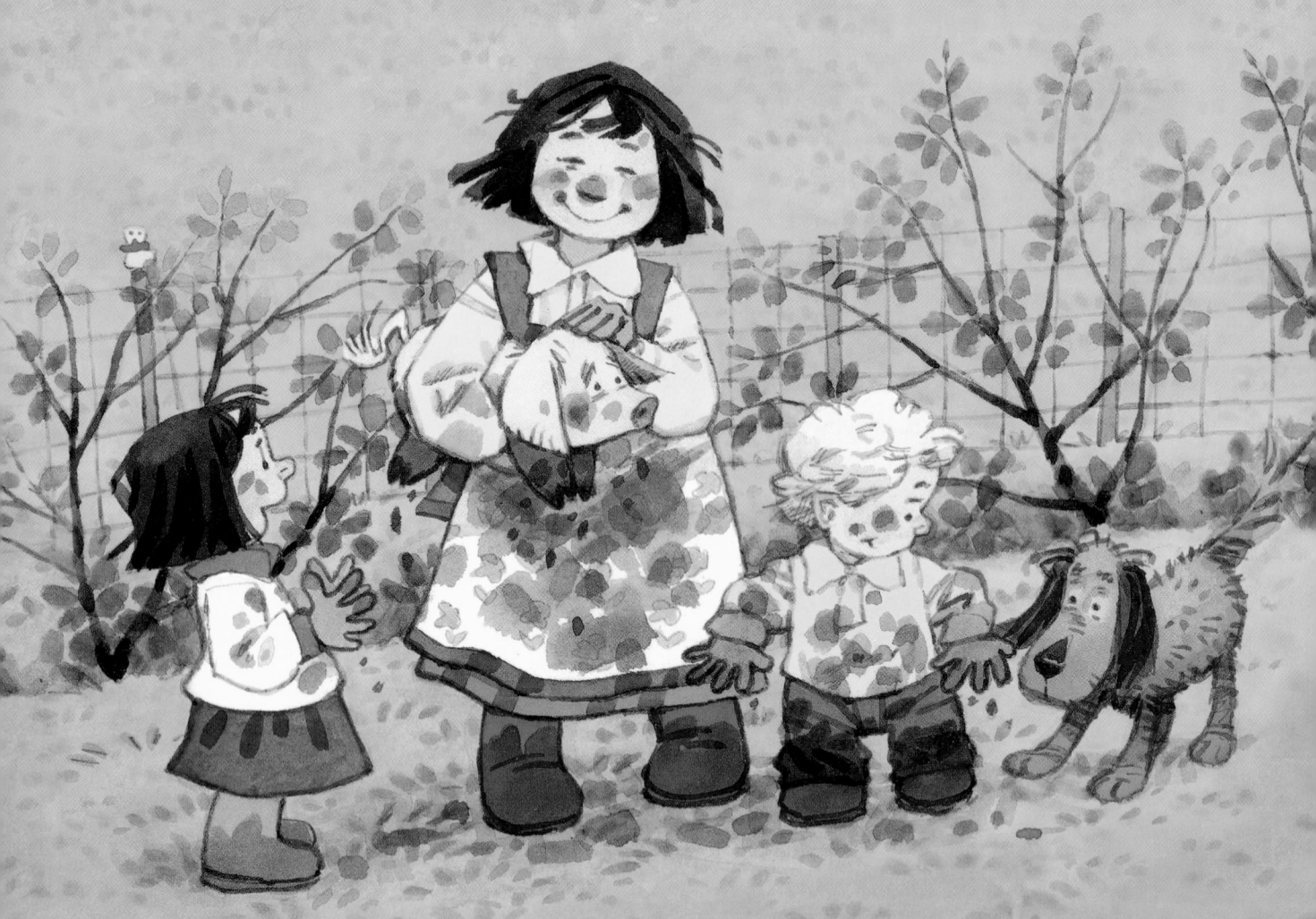

"We all need a good bath," says Mrs. Boot.
"Rusty found Curly. Clever dog," says Sam.

The
Hungry Donkey

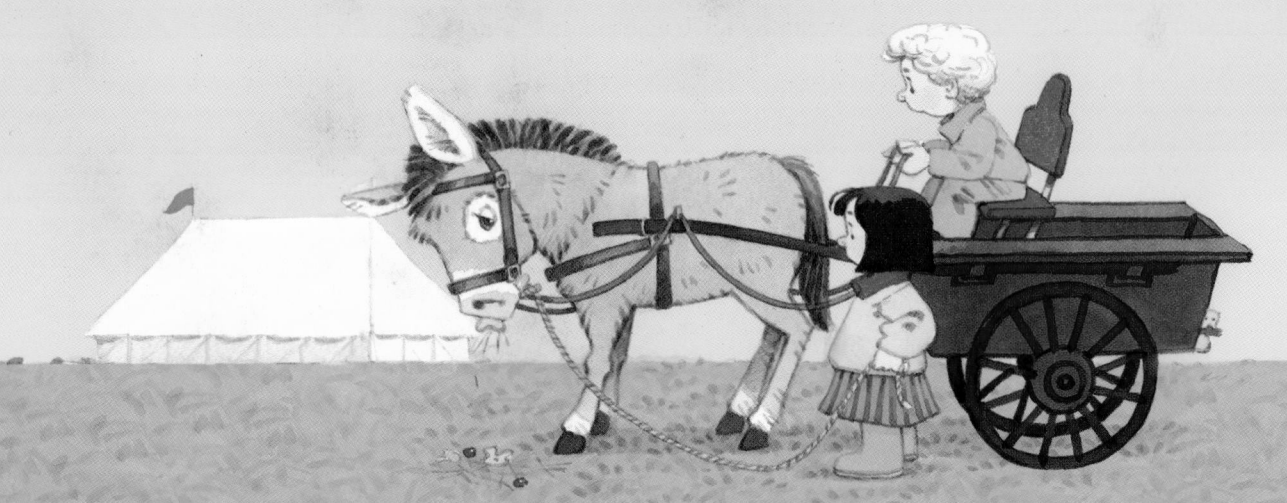

This is Apple Tree Farm.

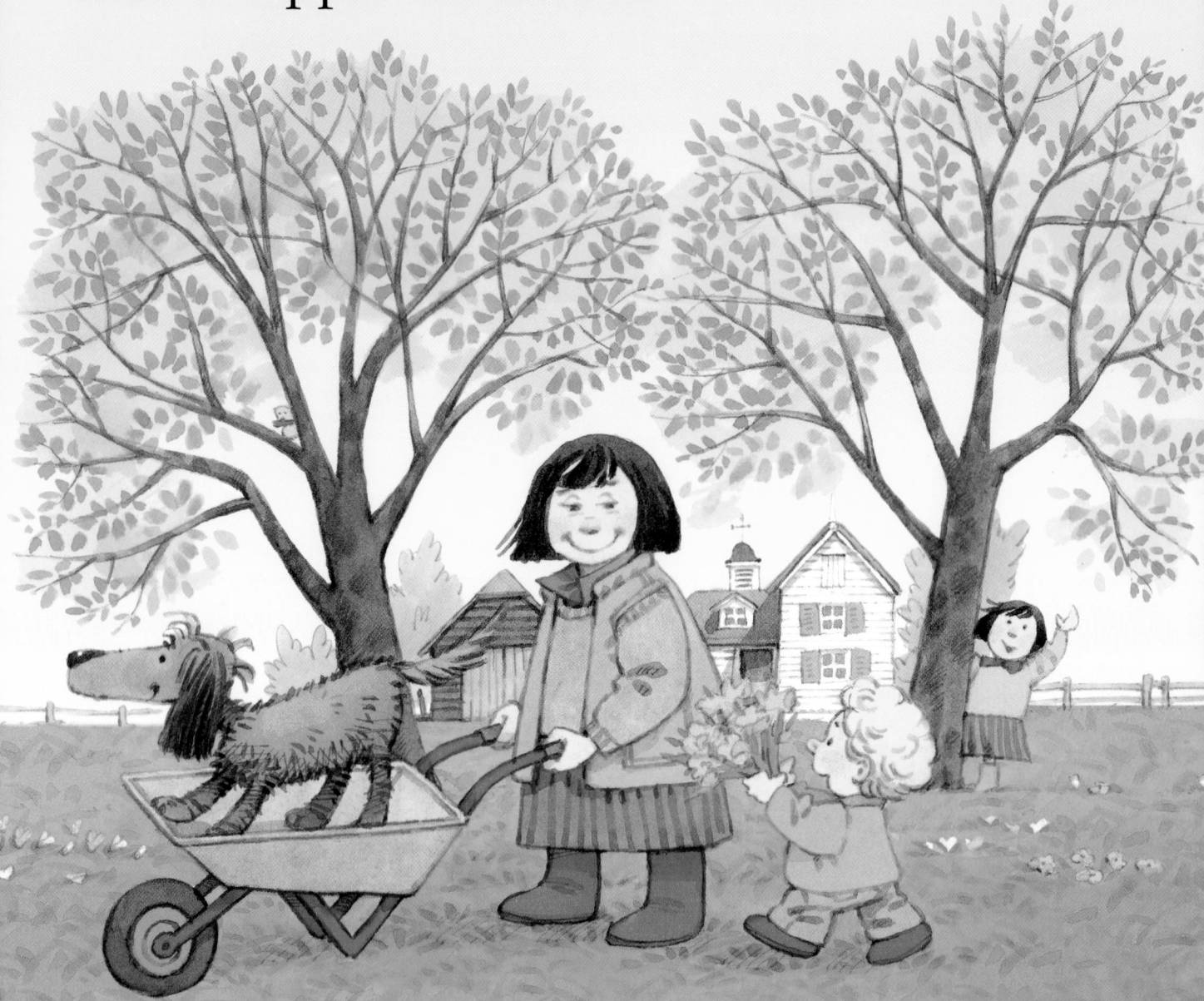

This is Mrs. Boot, the farmer. She has two children, called Poppy and Sam, and a dog called Rusty.

There is a donkey on the farm.

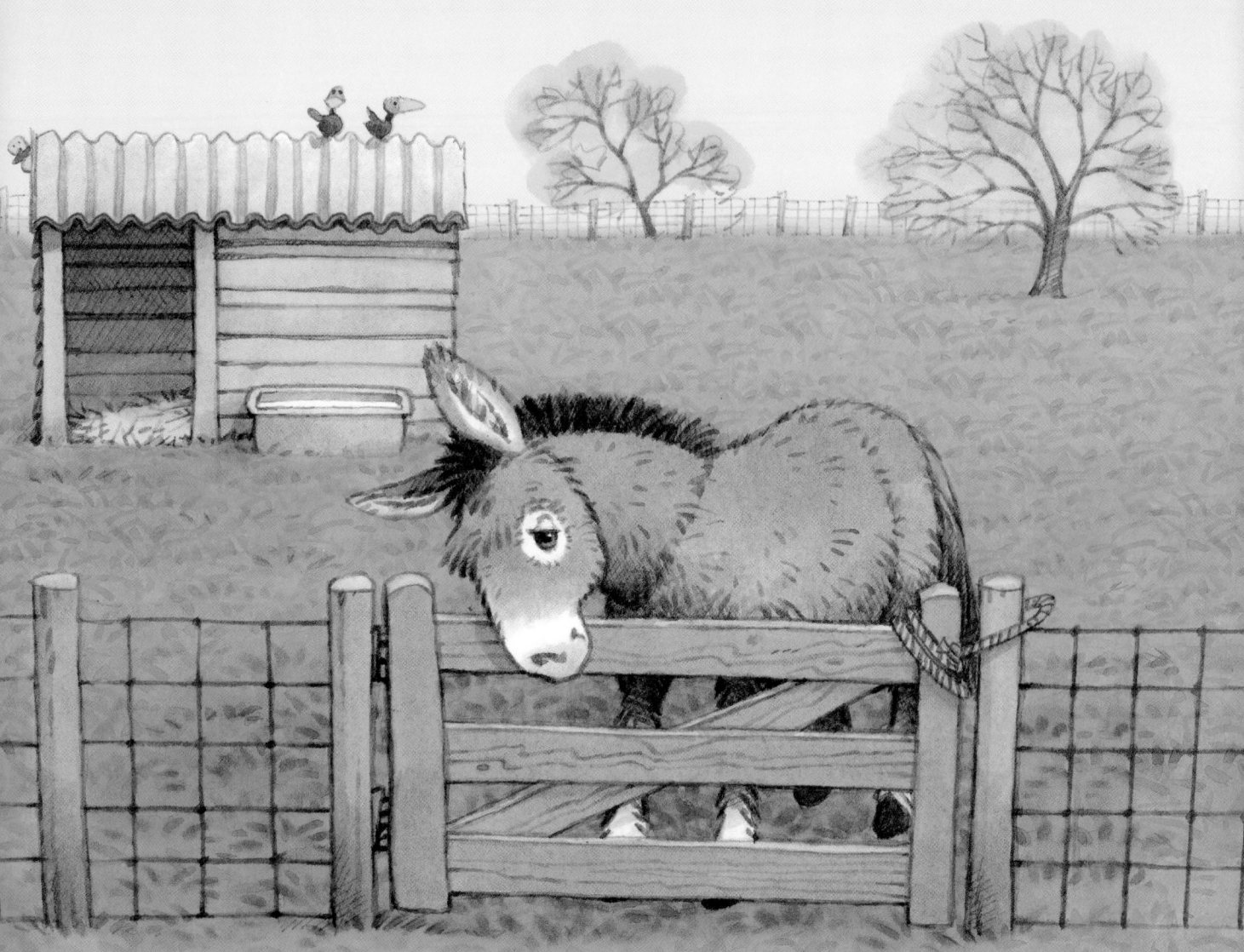

The donkey is called Ears. She lives in a field
with lots of grass, but she is always hungry.

Ears, the donkey, is going out.

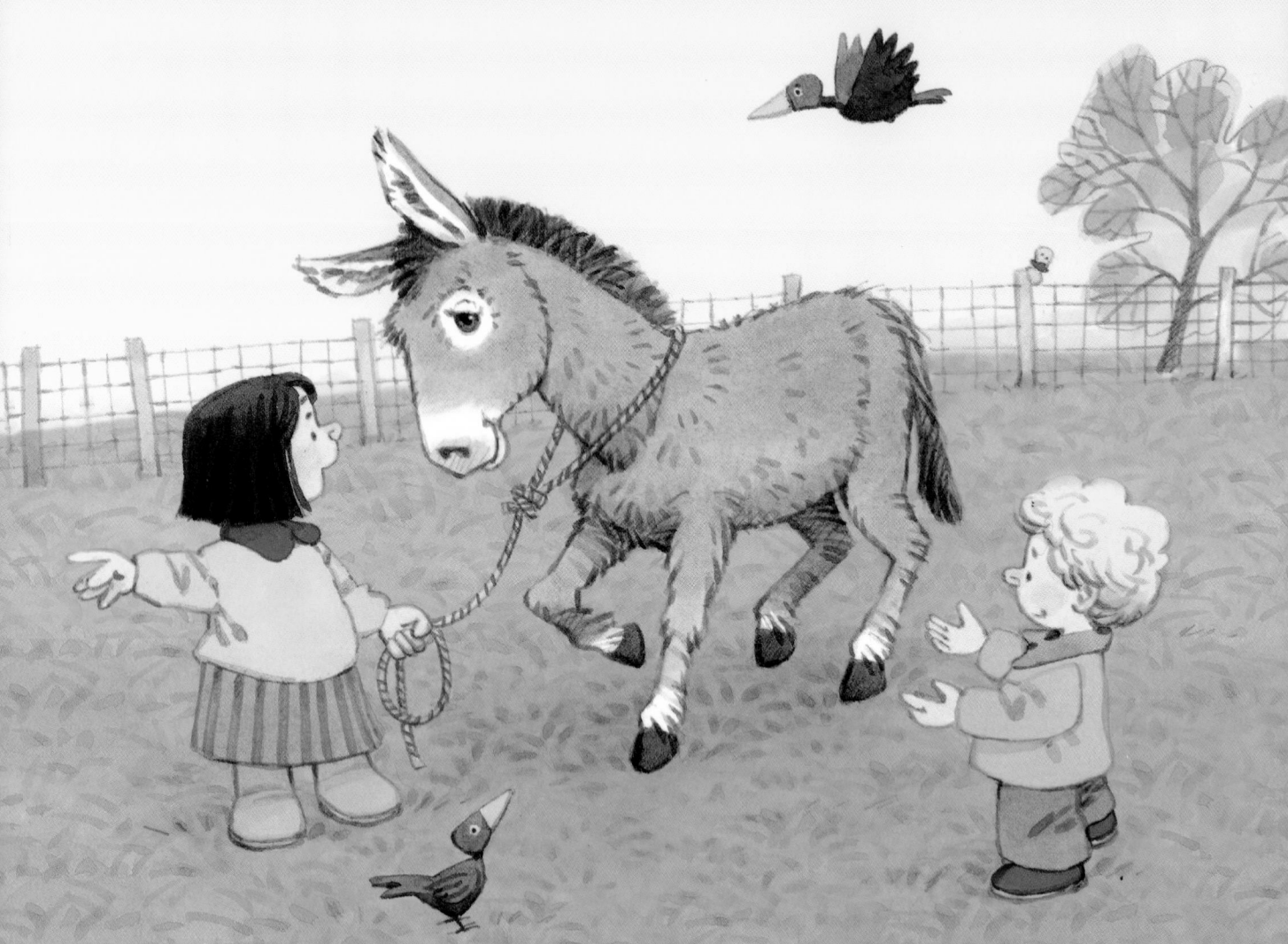

Poppy and Sam catch Ears and take her to the farmyard. Today is the day of the Show.

Ears has a little cart.

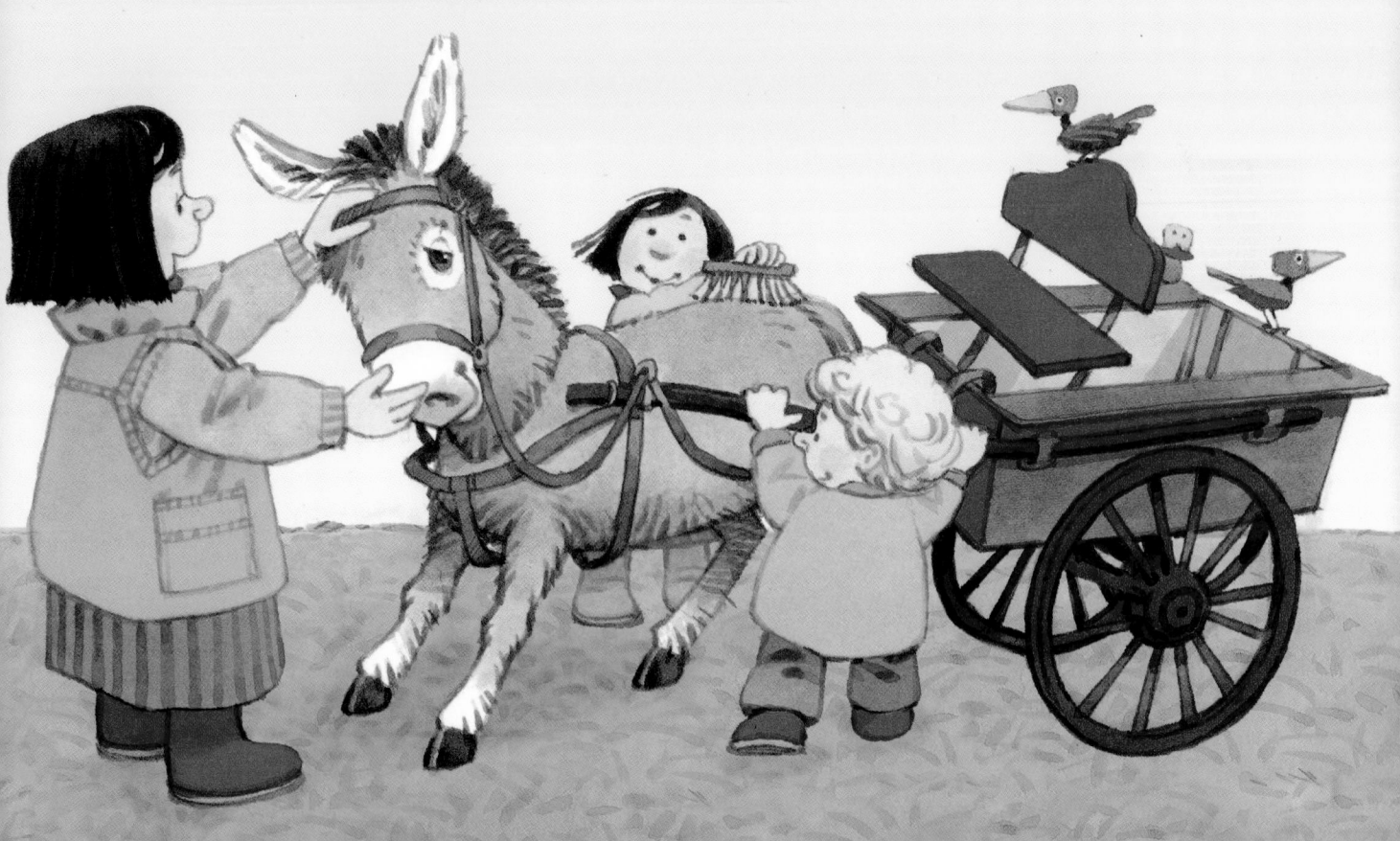

They brush her coat, comb her tail and clean
her feet. Mrs. Boot puts her into her little cart.

Off they go to the Show.

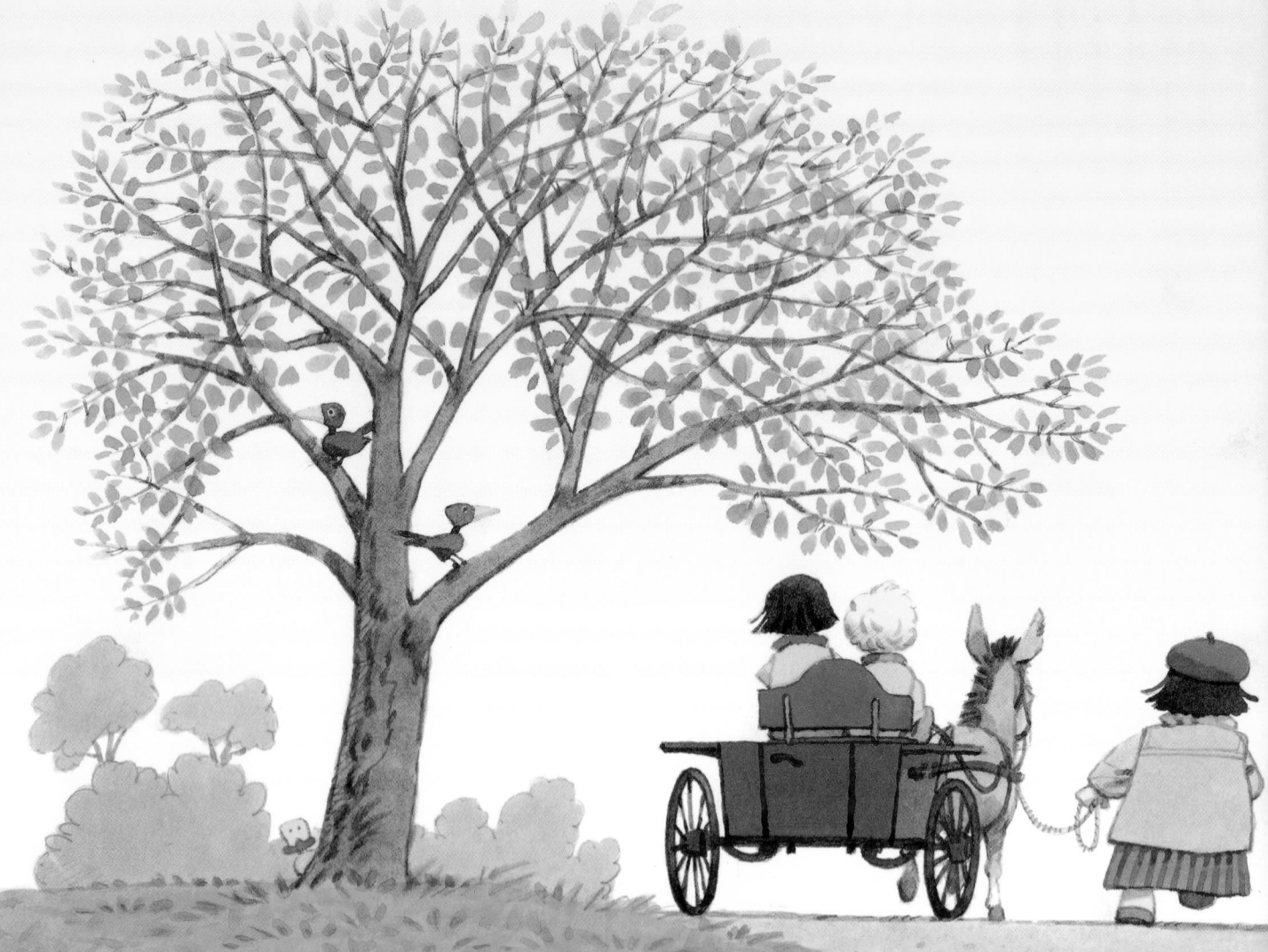

Poppy and Sam climb up into the cart. They all go down the lane to the show ground.

"You stay here, Ears."

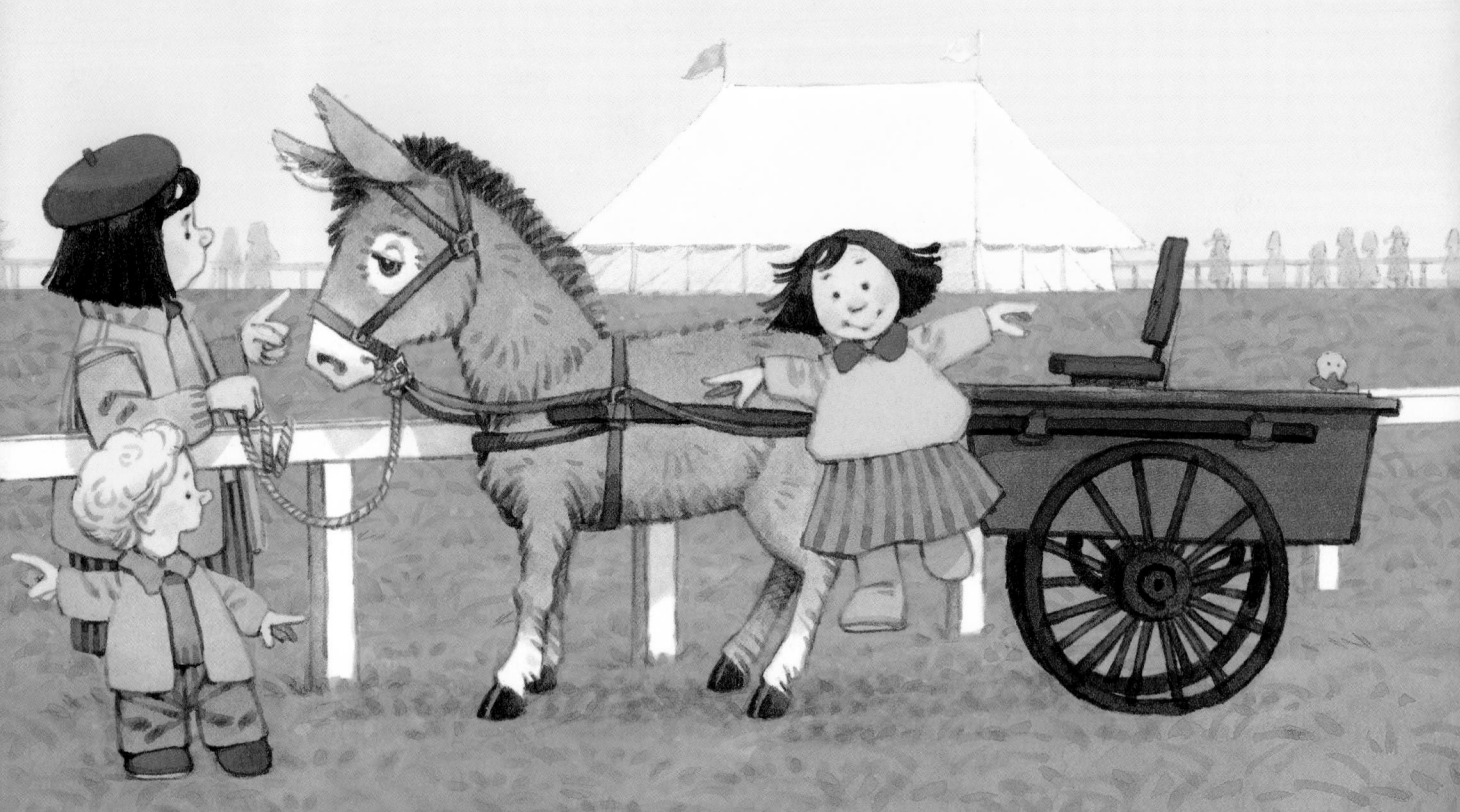

At the show ground, Mrs. Boot ties Ears to a fence. "Stay here. We'll be back soon," she says.

Ears gets free.

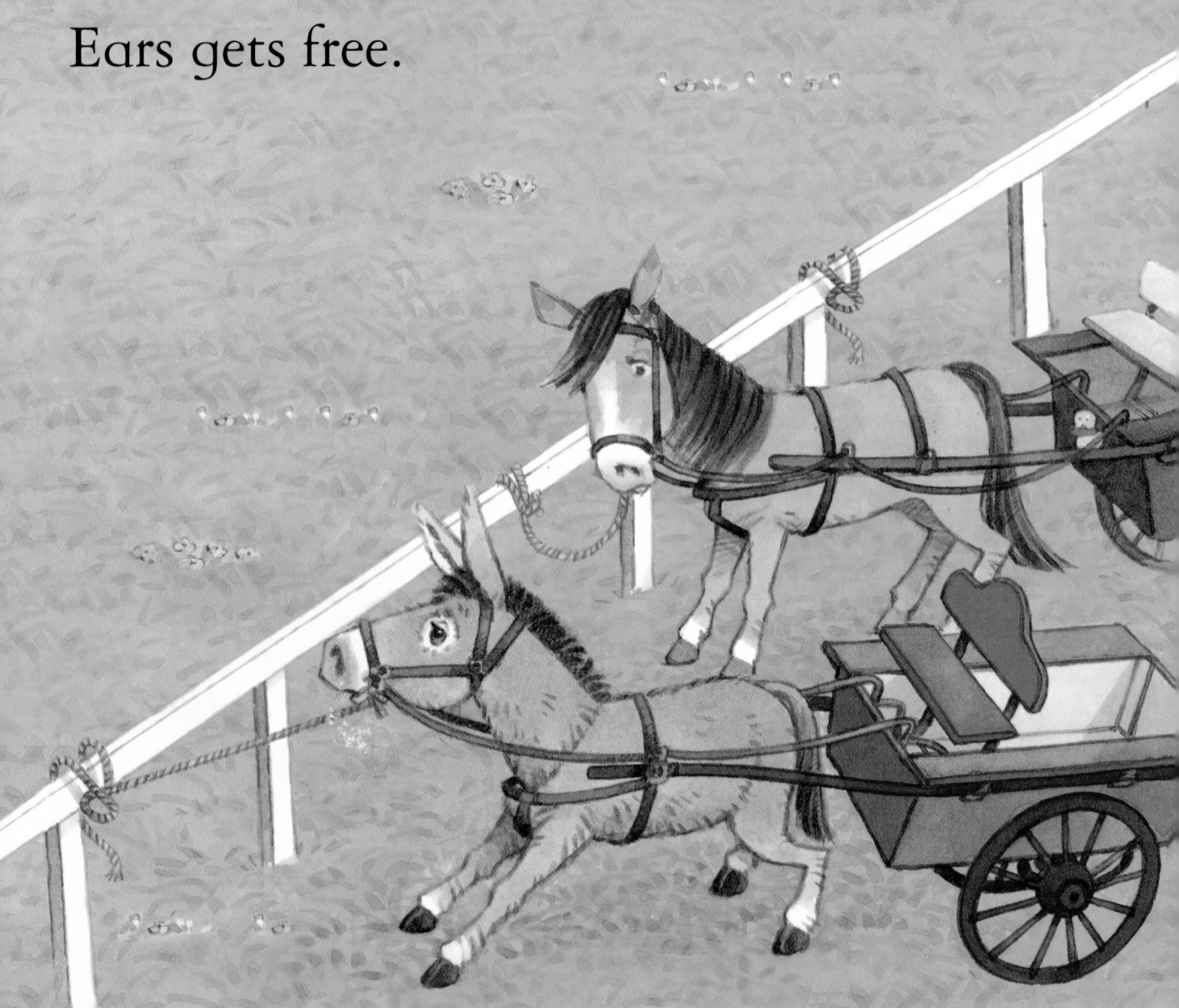

Ears is hungry and bored with nothing to do.
She pulls and pulls on the rope until she is free.

Ears looks for food.

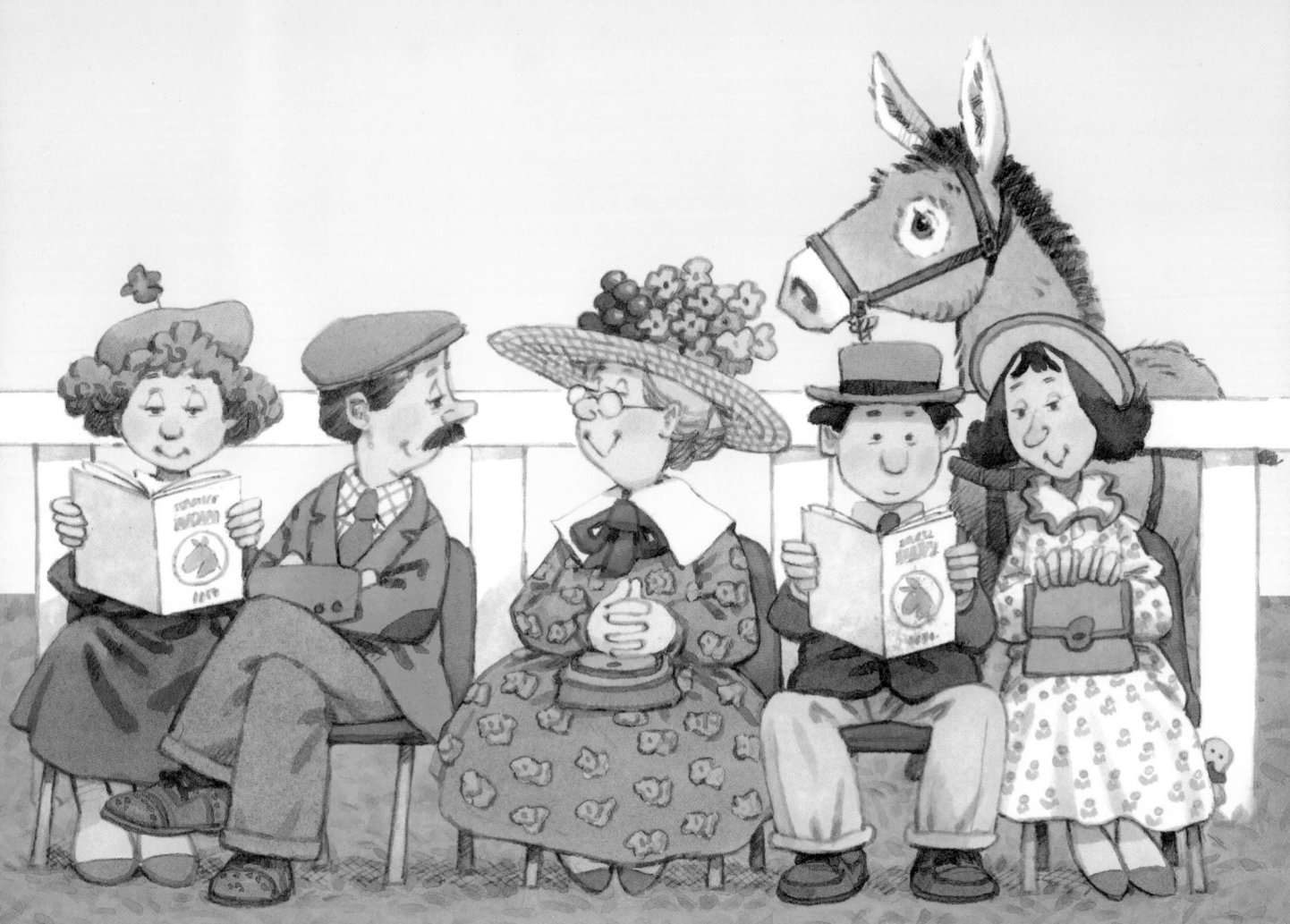

Ears trots across the field to the show ring.
She sees a bunch of flowers and some fruit.

"That looks good to eat."

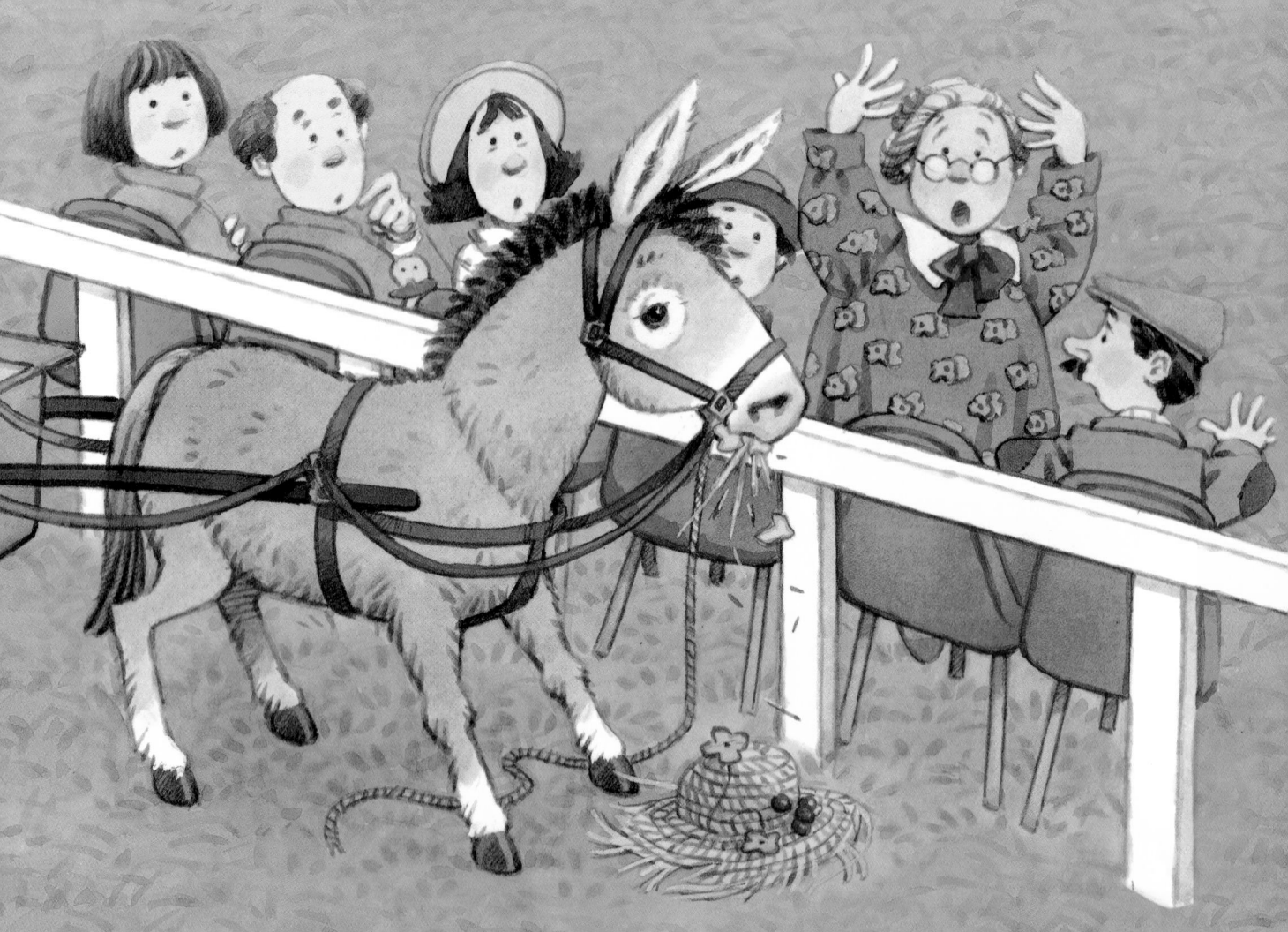

She takes a big bite, but the flowers do not taste very nice. A lady screams and Ears is frightened.

Ears runs away.

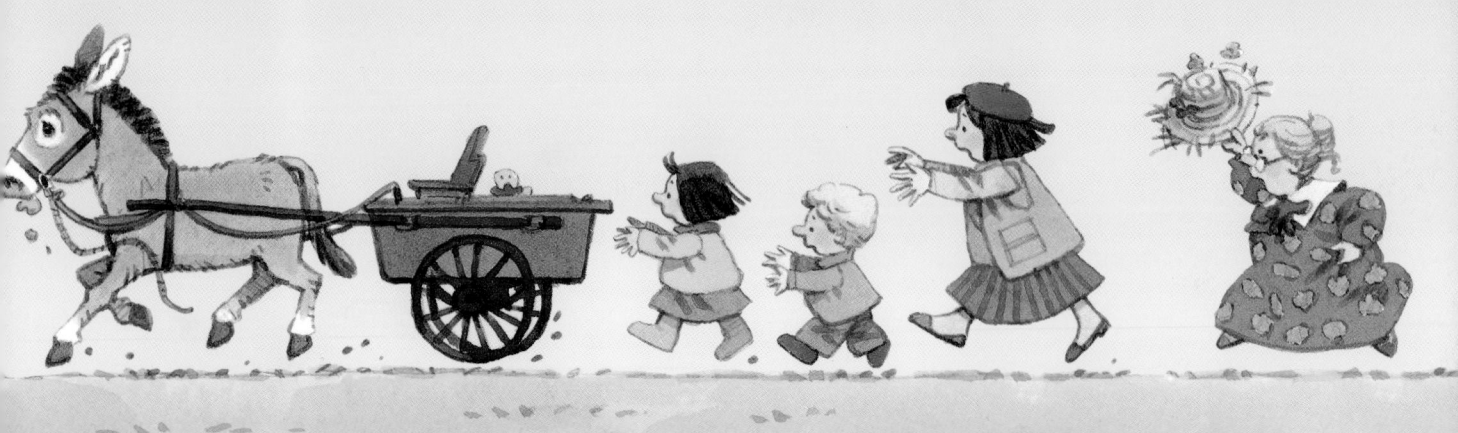

Mrs. Boot, Poppy and Sam and the lady run
after her and catch her.

"Naughty donkey," says Sam.

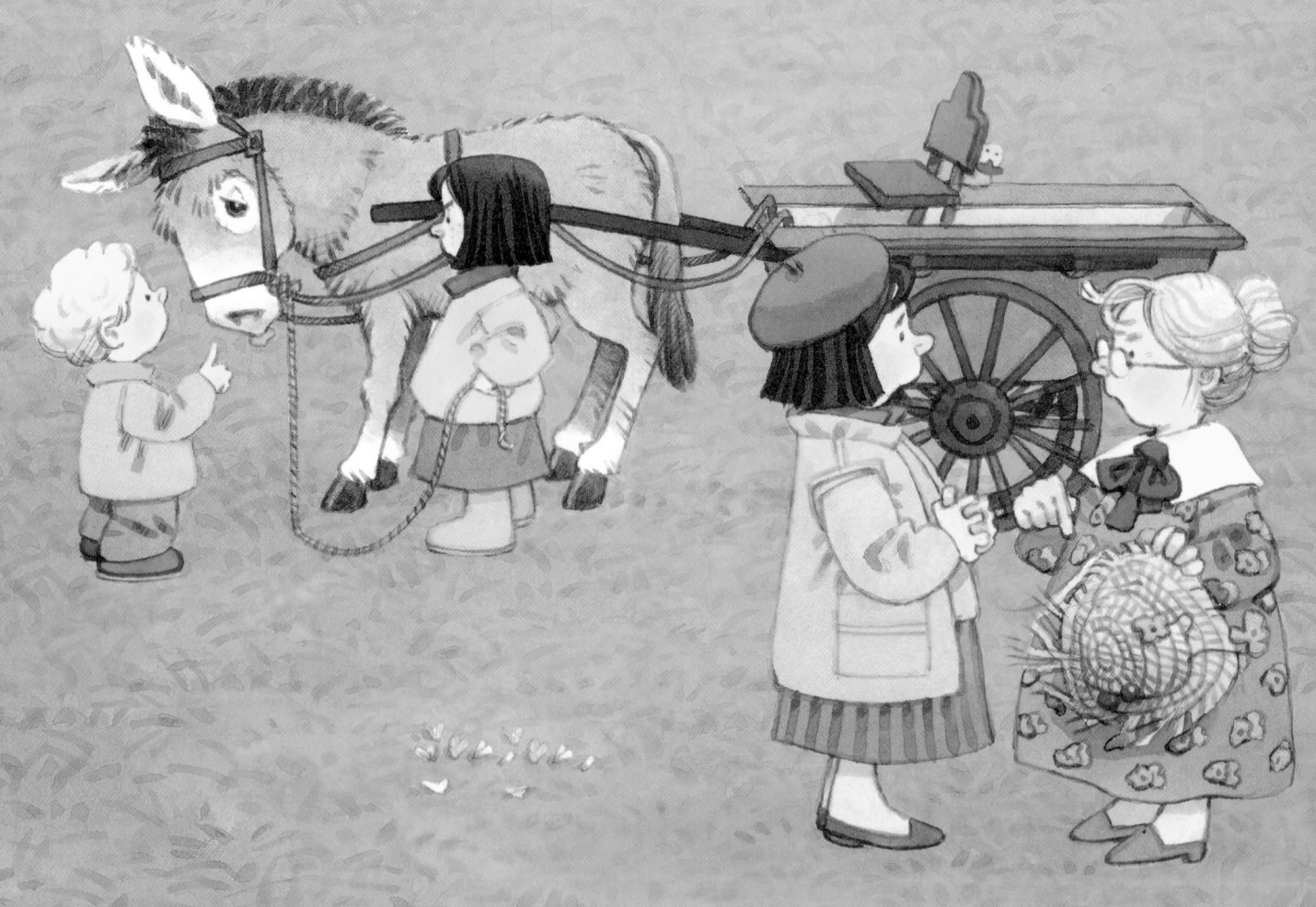

"I'm sorry," Mrs. Boot says to the lady. "Would you like to take Ears to the best donkey competition?"

Ears is very good now.

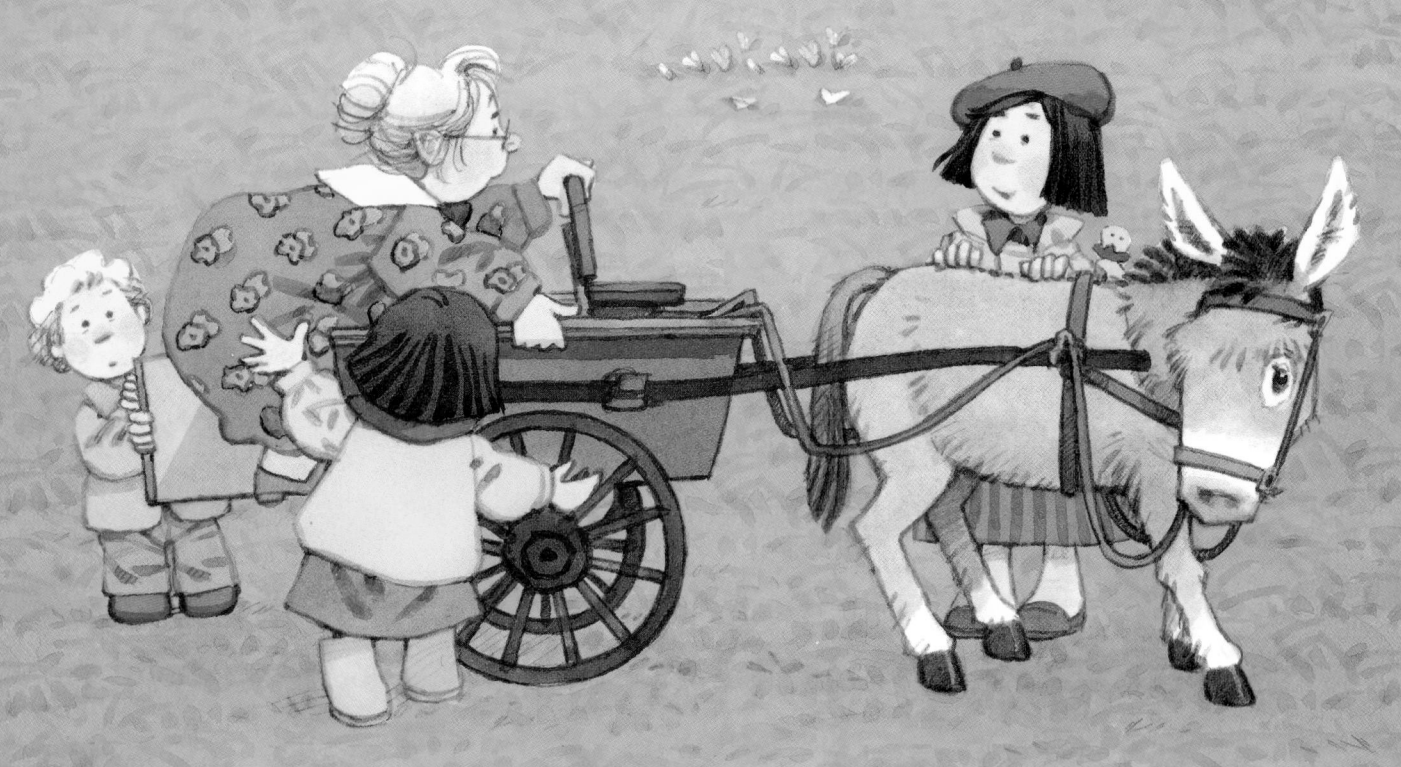

The lady is called Mrs. Rose. She climbs into the
cart. "Come on," she says, and shakes the reins.

Ears pulls the cart into the show ring.

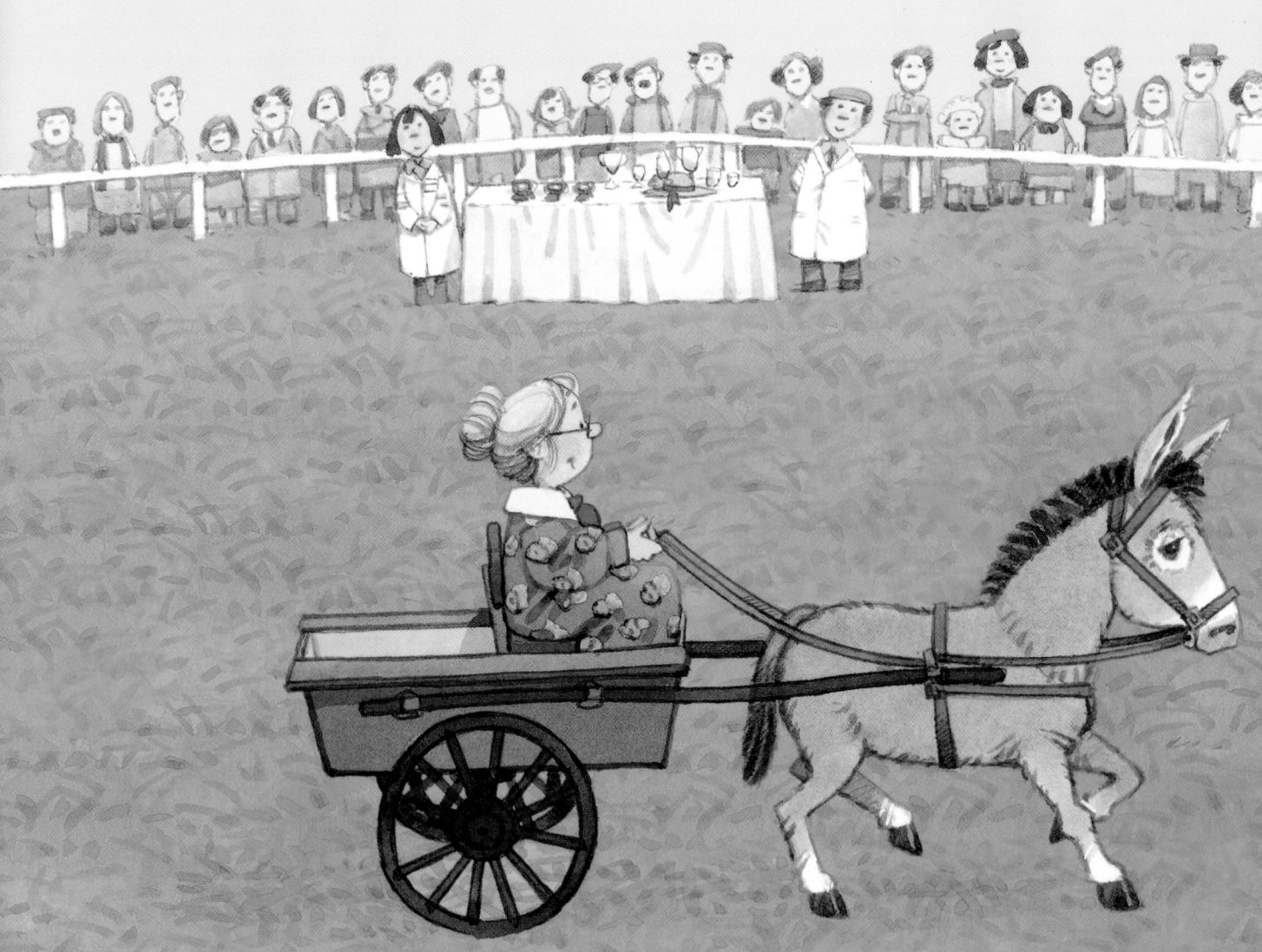

She trots in front of the judges. She stops and goes when Mrs. Rose tells her.

Ears wins a prize.

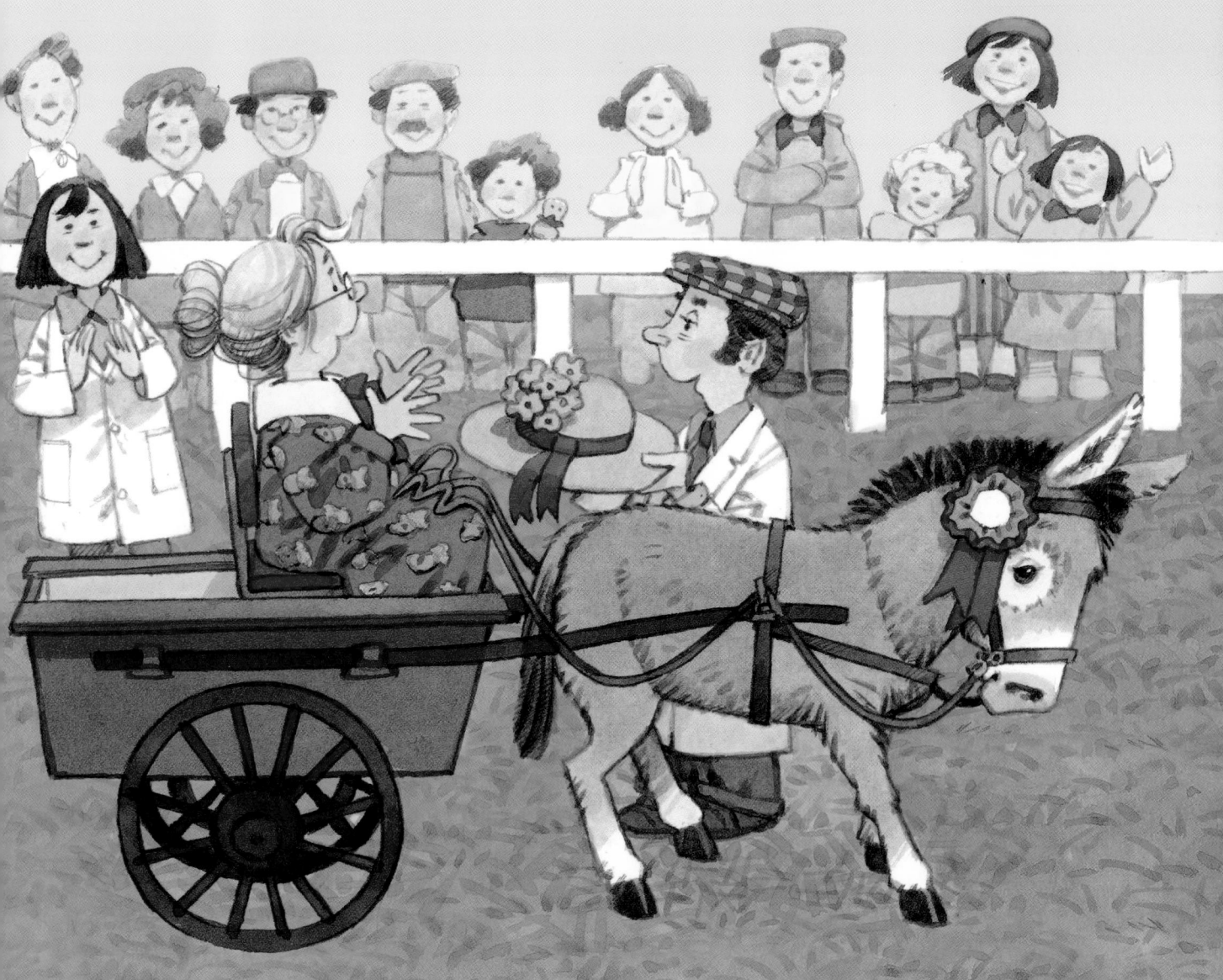

"Well done," says the judge, giving her a rosette.
He gives Mrs. Rose a prize too. It is a hat.

It is time to go home.

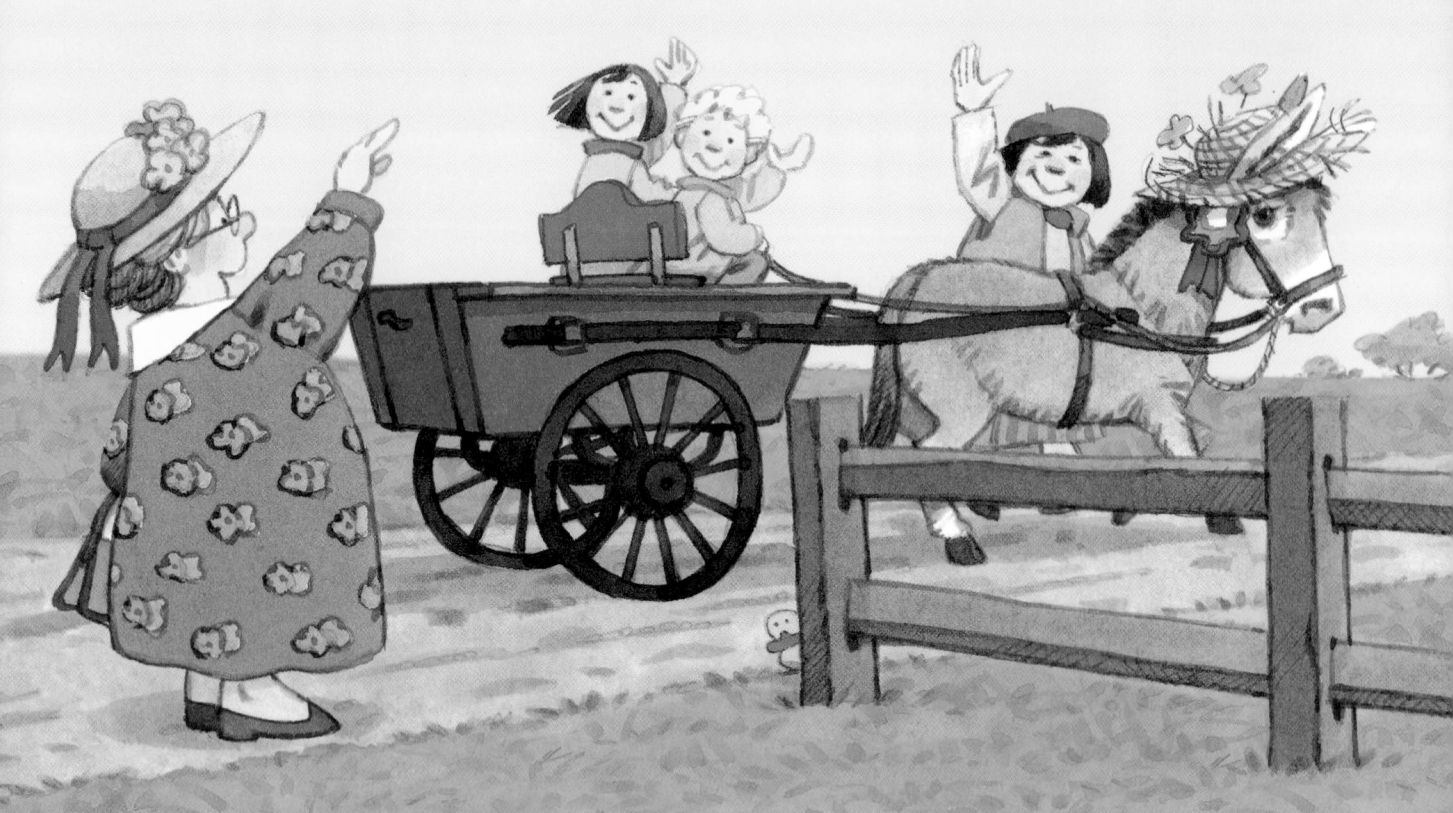

Mrs. Rose waves goodbye. "That was such fun," she says. Ears trots home. She has a new hat too.

Scarecrow's Secret

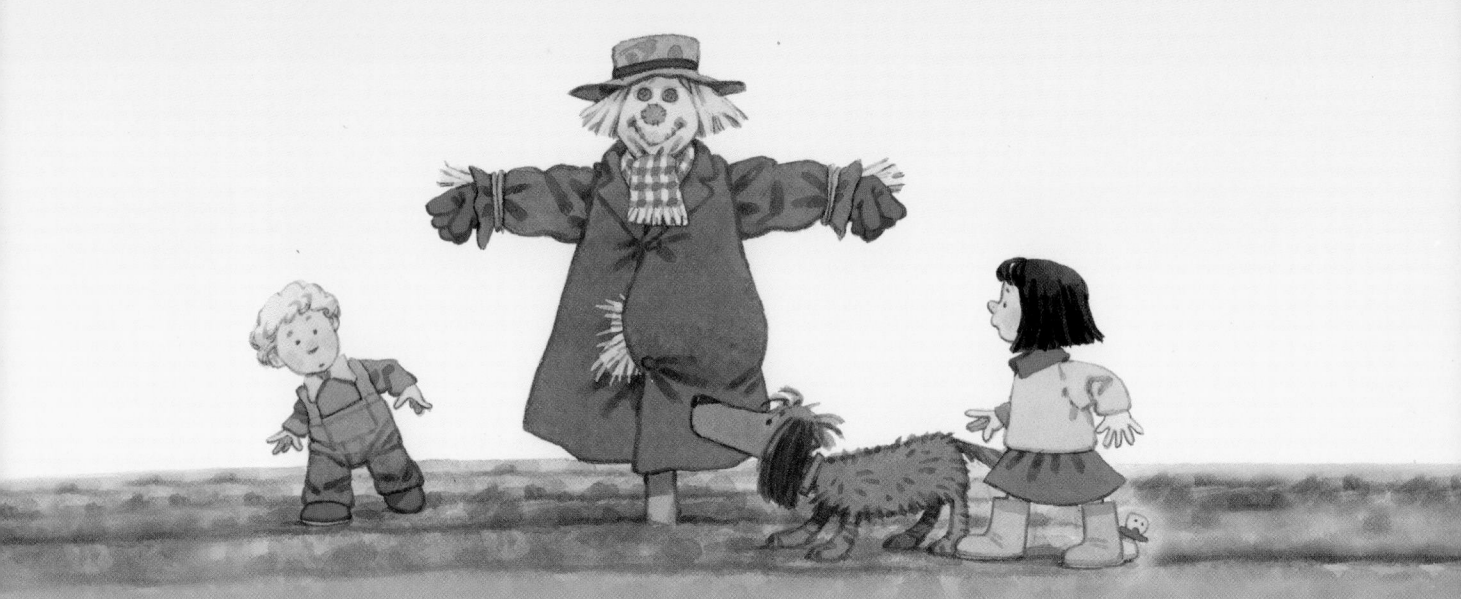

This is Apple Tree Farm.

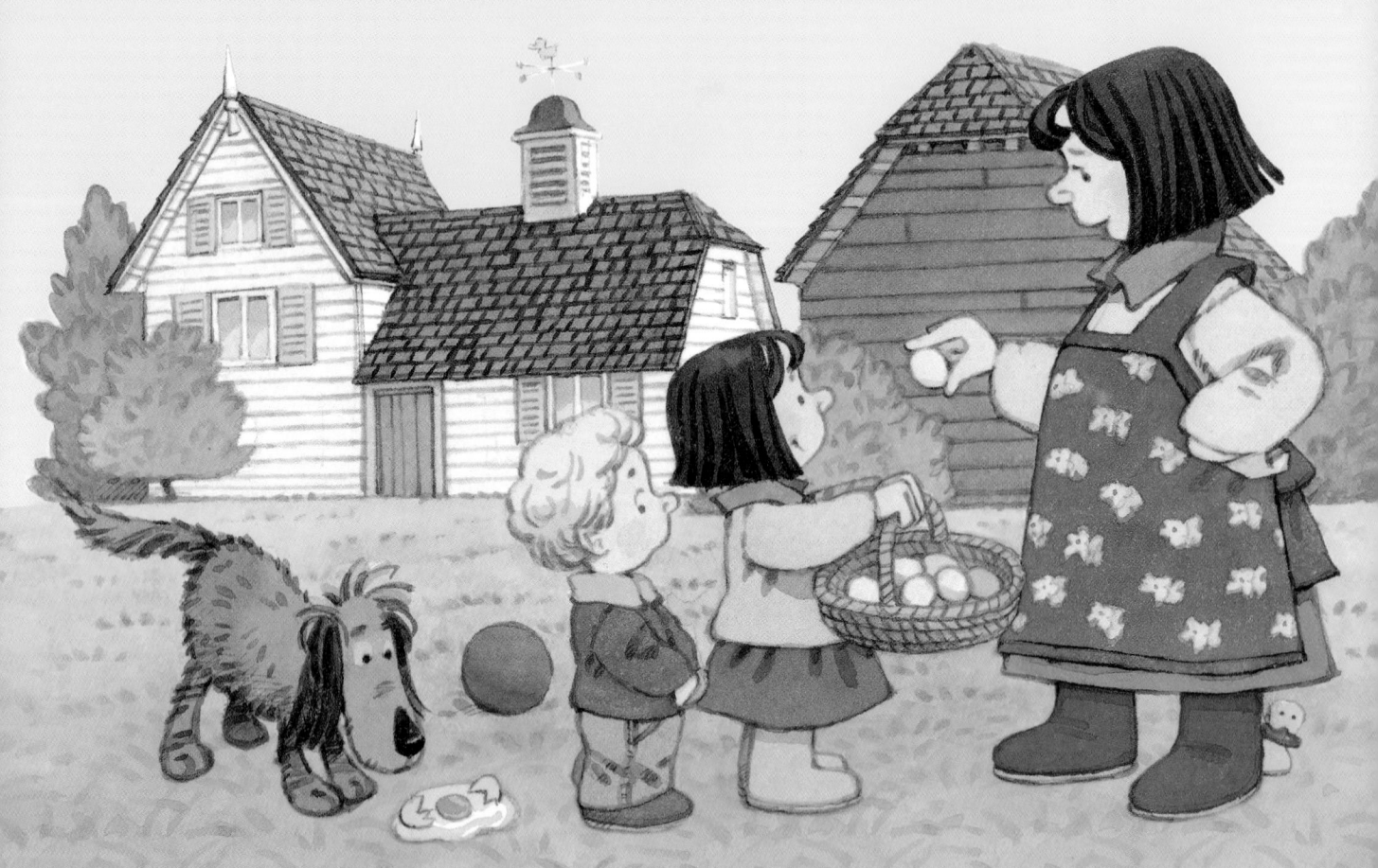

This is Mrs. Boot, the farmer. She has two children, called Poppy and Sam, and a dog called Rusty.

Mr. Boot is working in the barn.

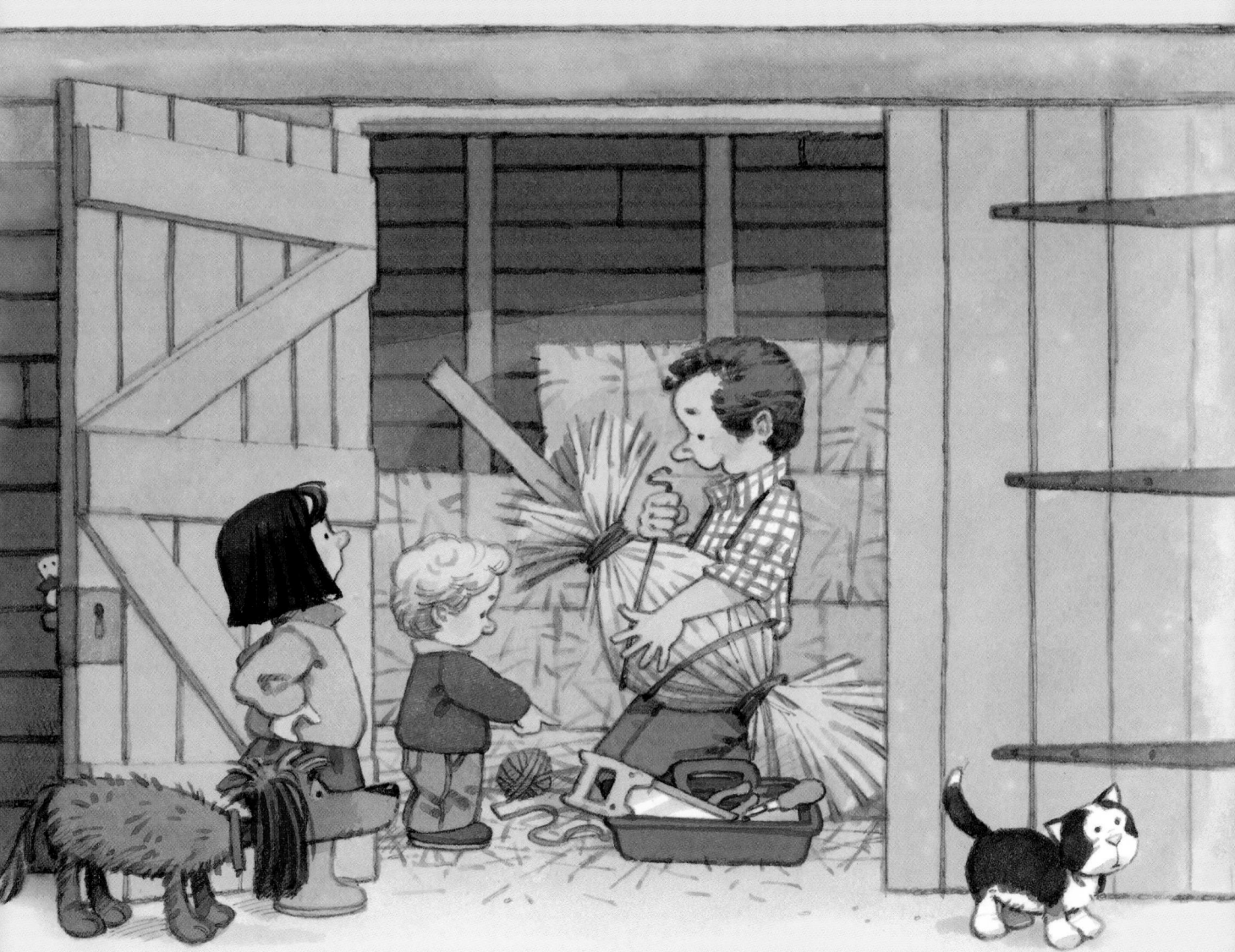

"What are you doing, Dad?" asks Sam. "I'm tying lots of straw on these poles," says Mr Boot.

"What is it?"

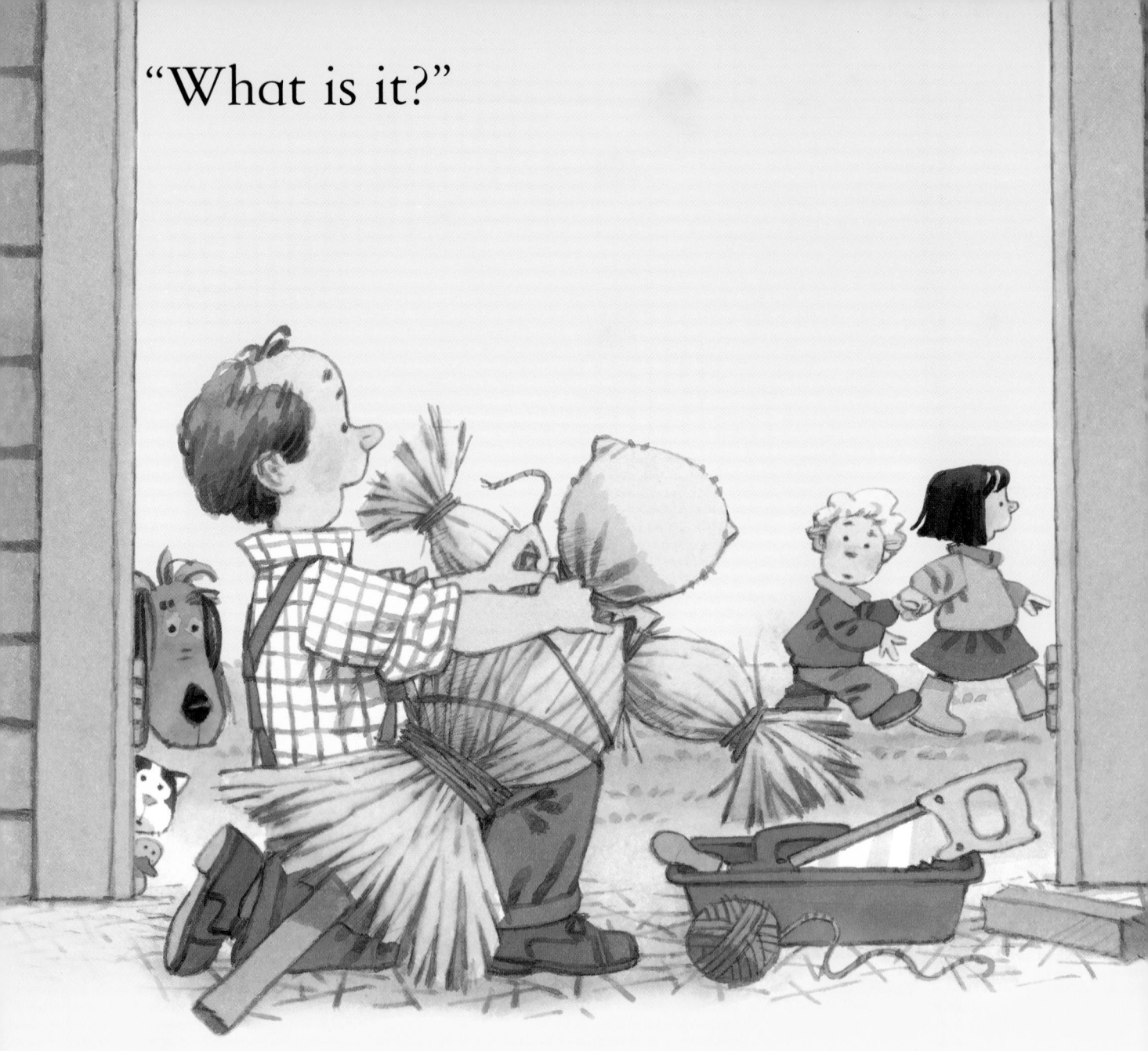

"You'll soon see," says Mr. Boot. "Go and get my old coat from the shed, please. Bring my old hat too."

"It's going to be a scarecrow."

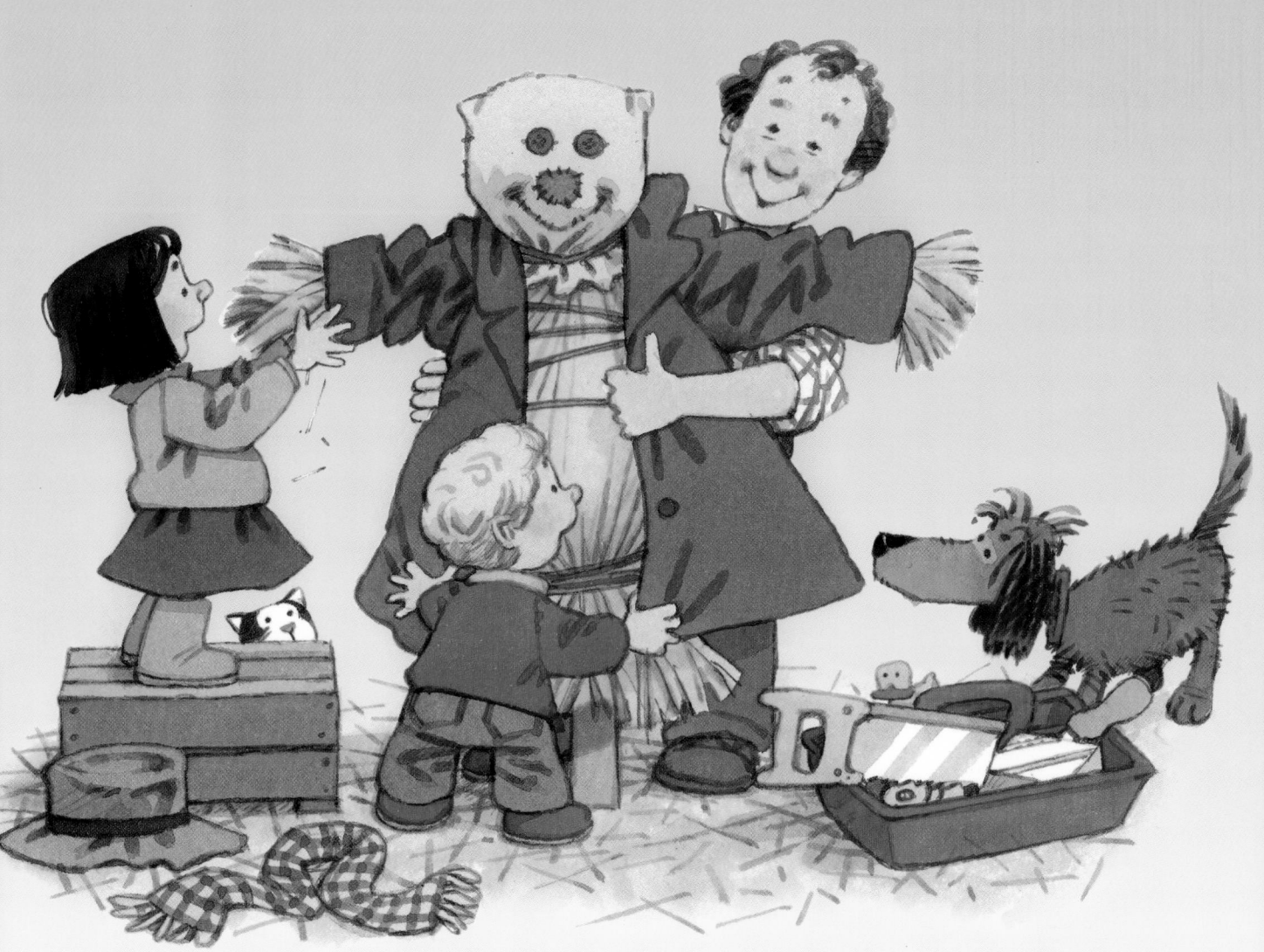

Poppy and Sam come back with the coat and hat.
Then they help Mr. Boot put them on the scarecrow.

"He's just like a nice old man."

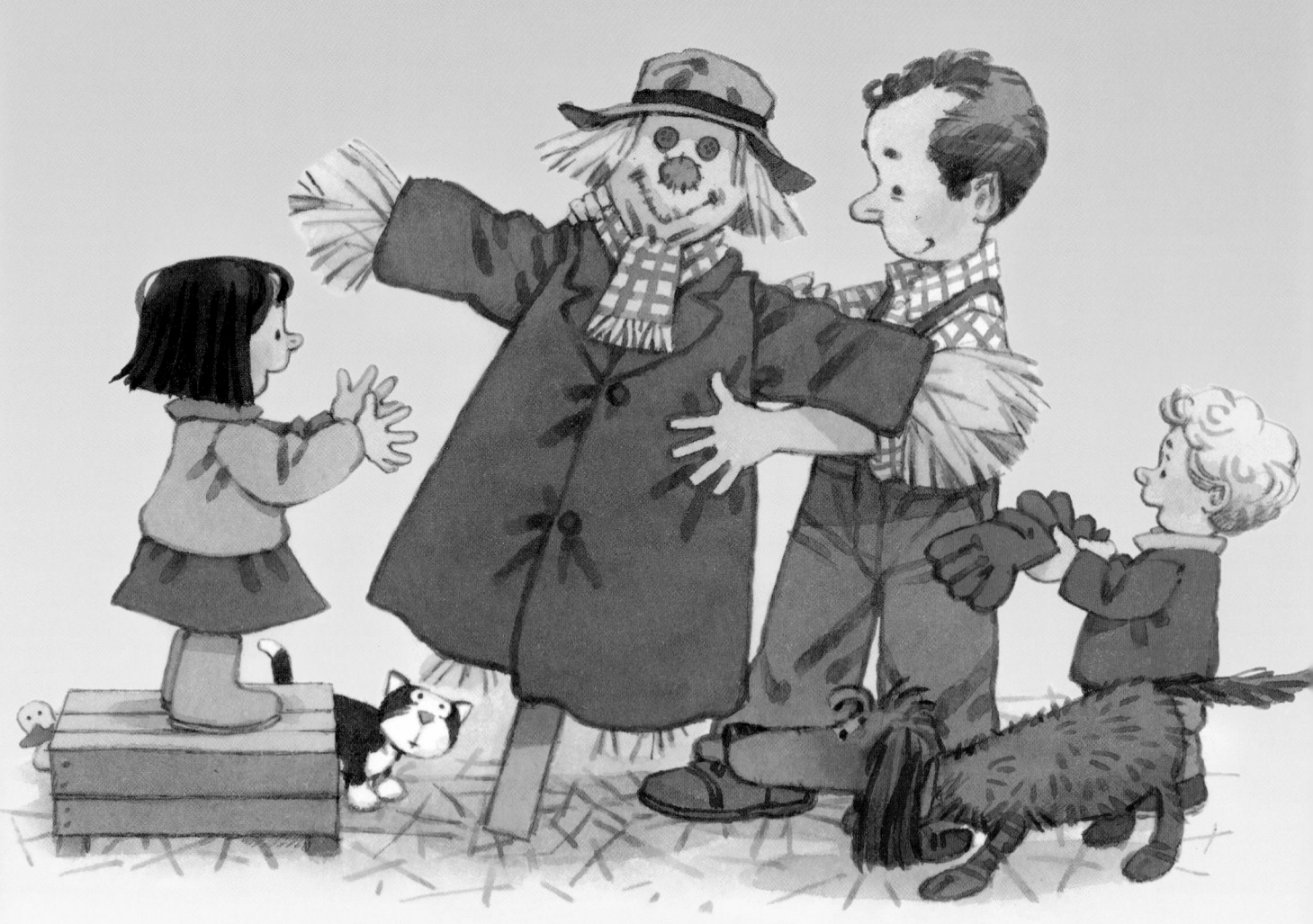

"I've got some old gloves for him," says Sam.
"Let's call him Mr. Straw," says Poppy.

"He's finished now."

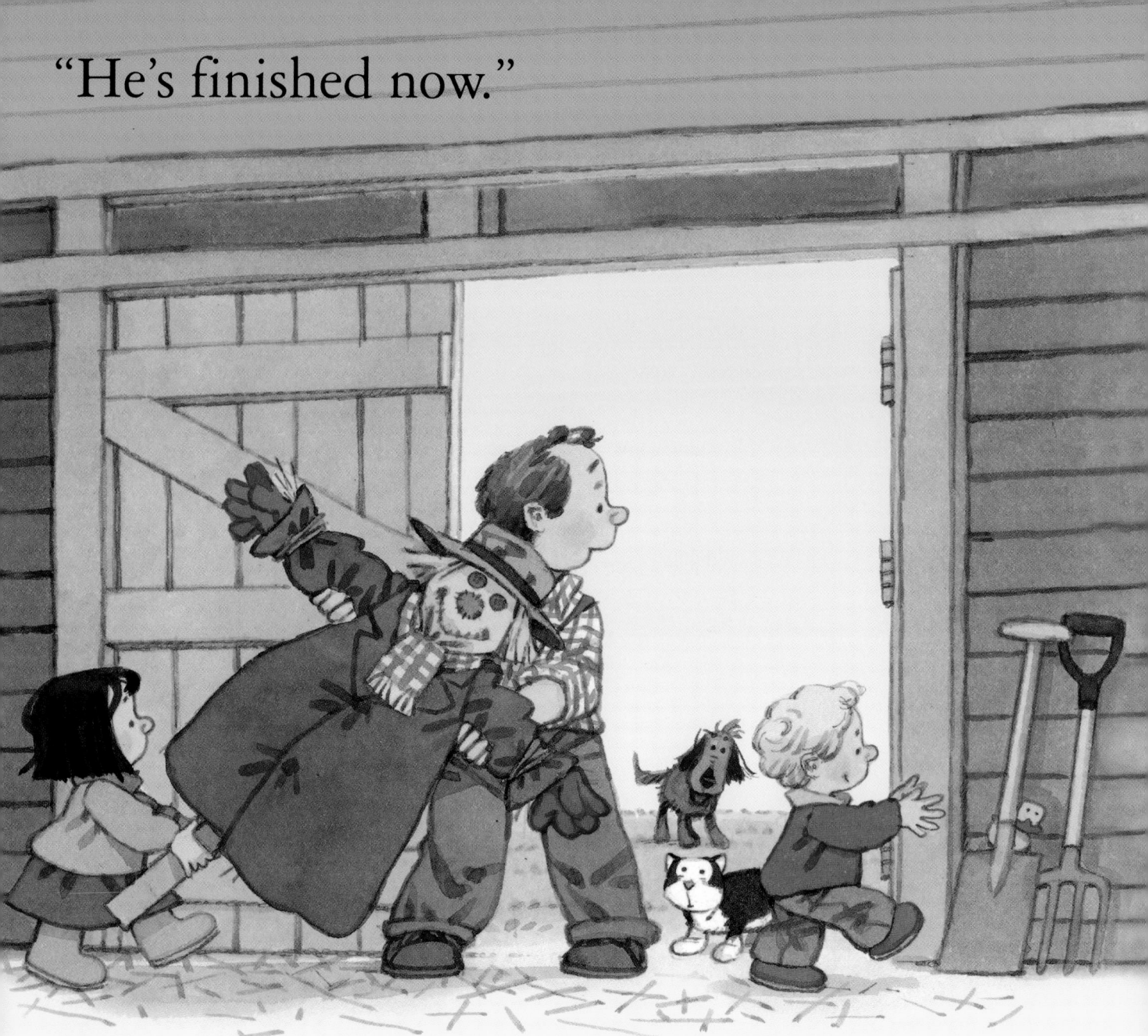

"Help me carry him, please, Poppy," says
Mr. Boot. "You bring the spade, Sam."

They all go to the cornfield.

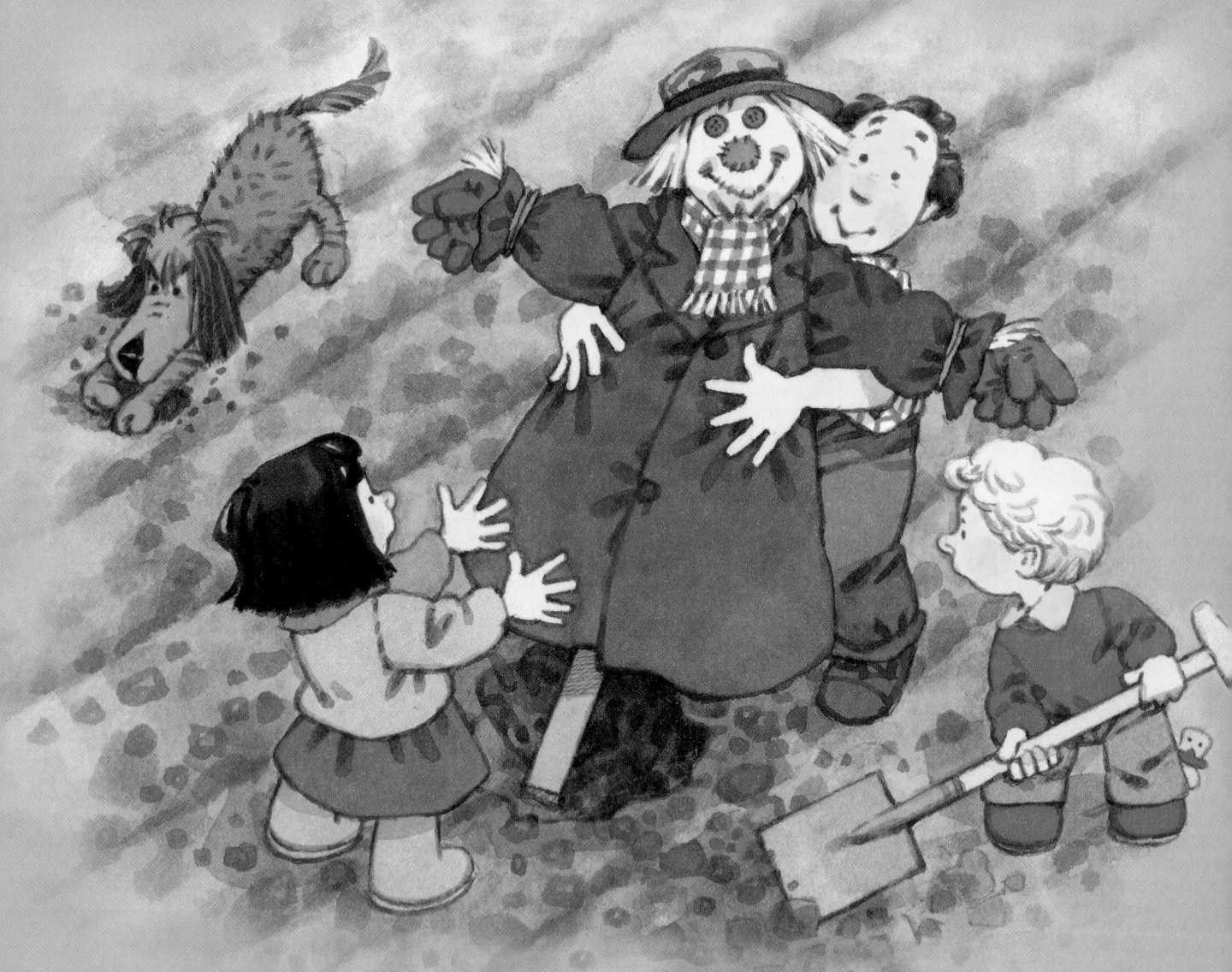

Mr. Boot digs a hole in the field. Then he pushes
in the pole so that Mr. Straw stands up.

"He does look real."

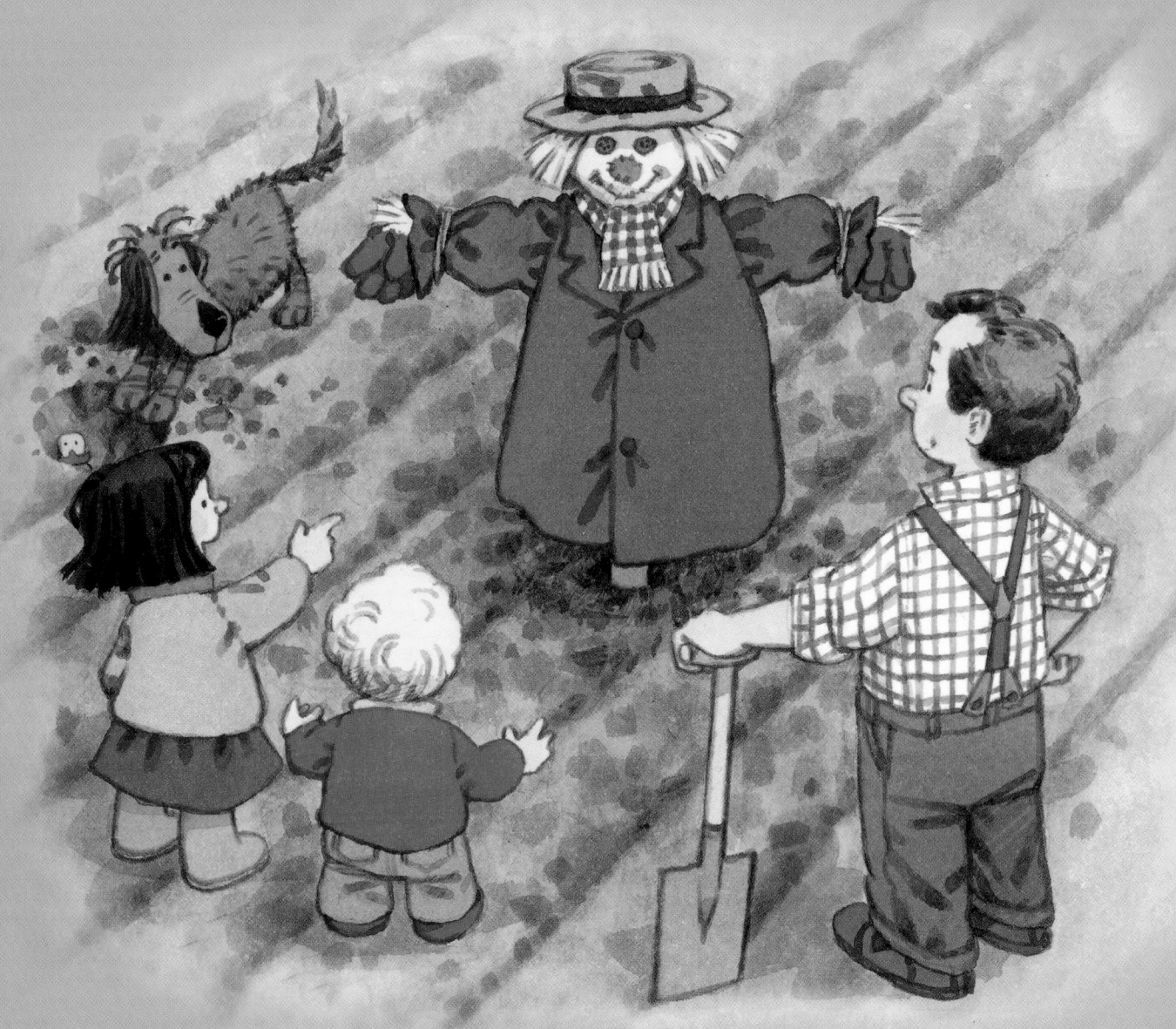

"I'm sure Mr. Straw will scare off all the birds,"
says Sam. "Especially the crows," says Poppy.

Mr. Straw is doing a good job.

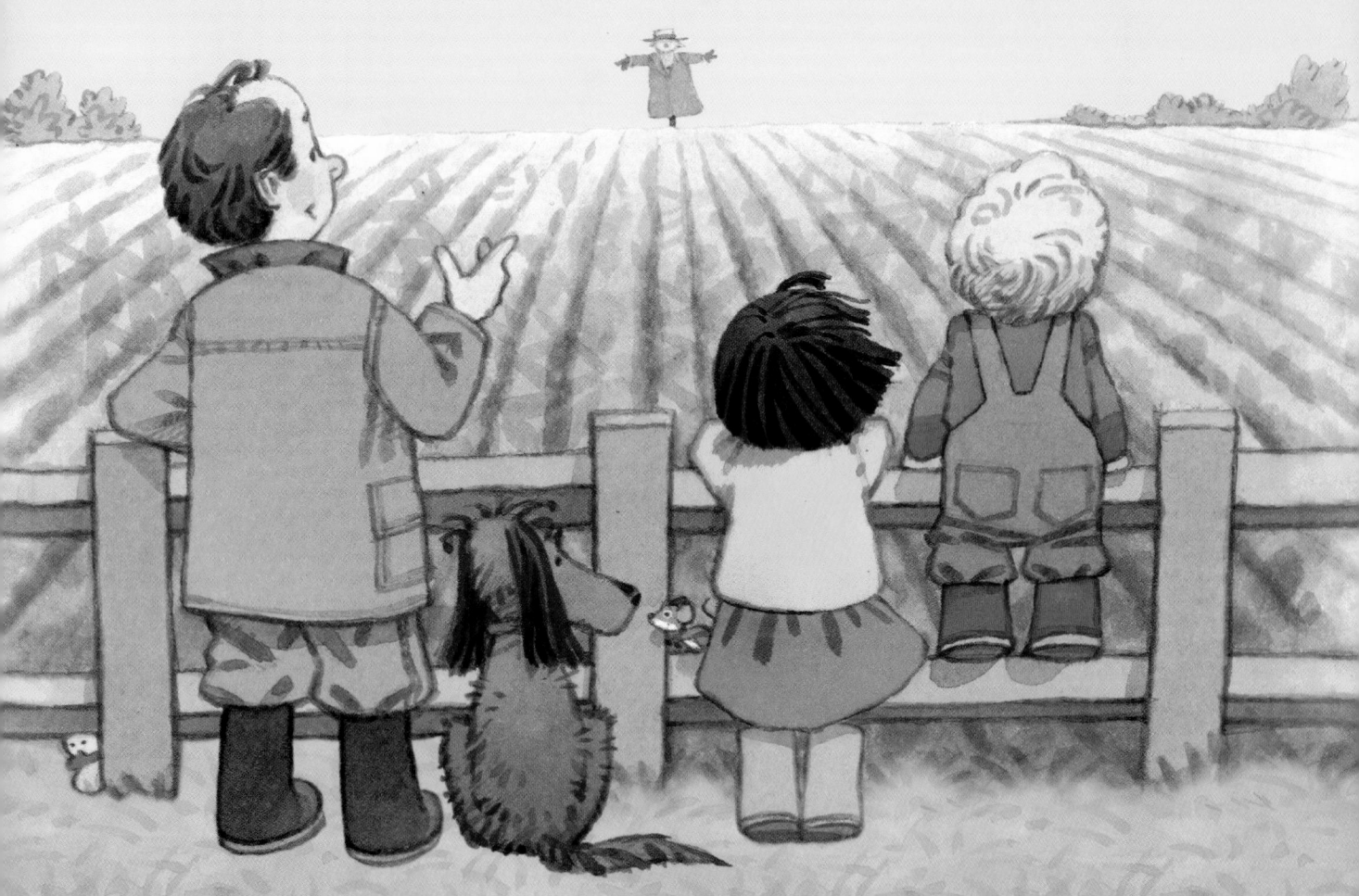

Every day Mr. Boot, Poppy and Sam look at
Mr. Straw. There are no birds in the cornfield.

"There's Farmer Dray's scarecrow."

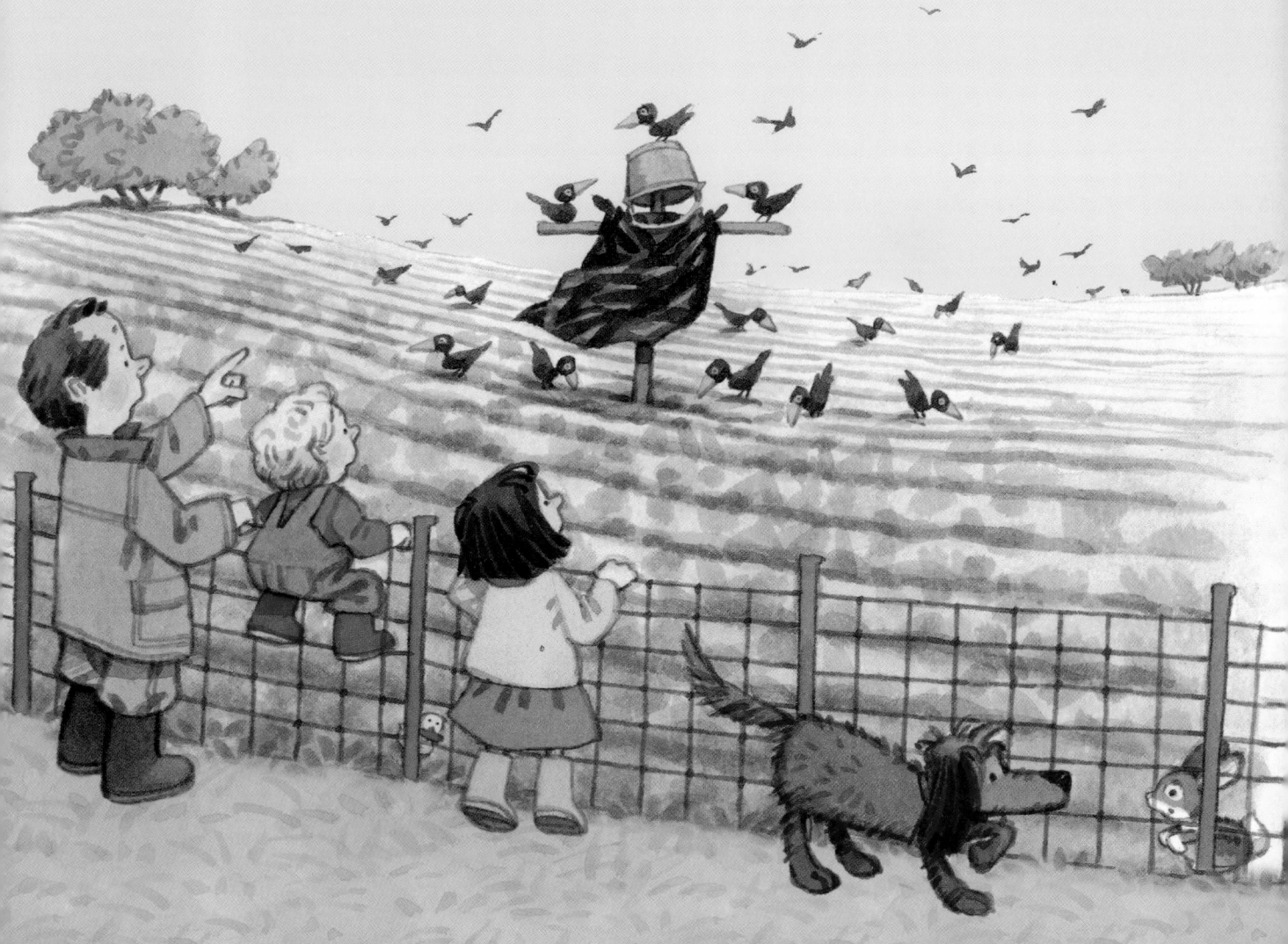

"He's no good at all," says Sam. "The birds are eating all the corn and standing on the scarecrow."

107

"Why is Mr. Straw so good?"

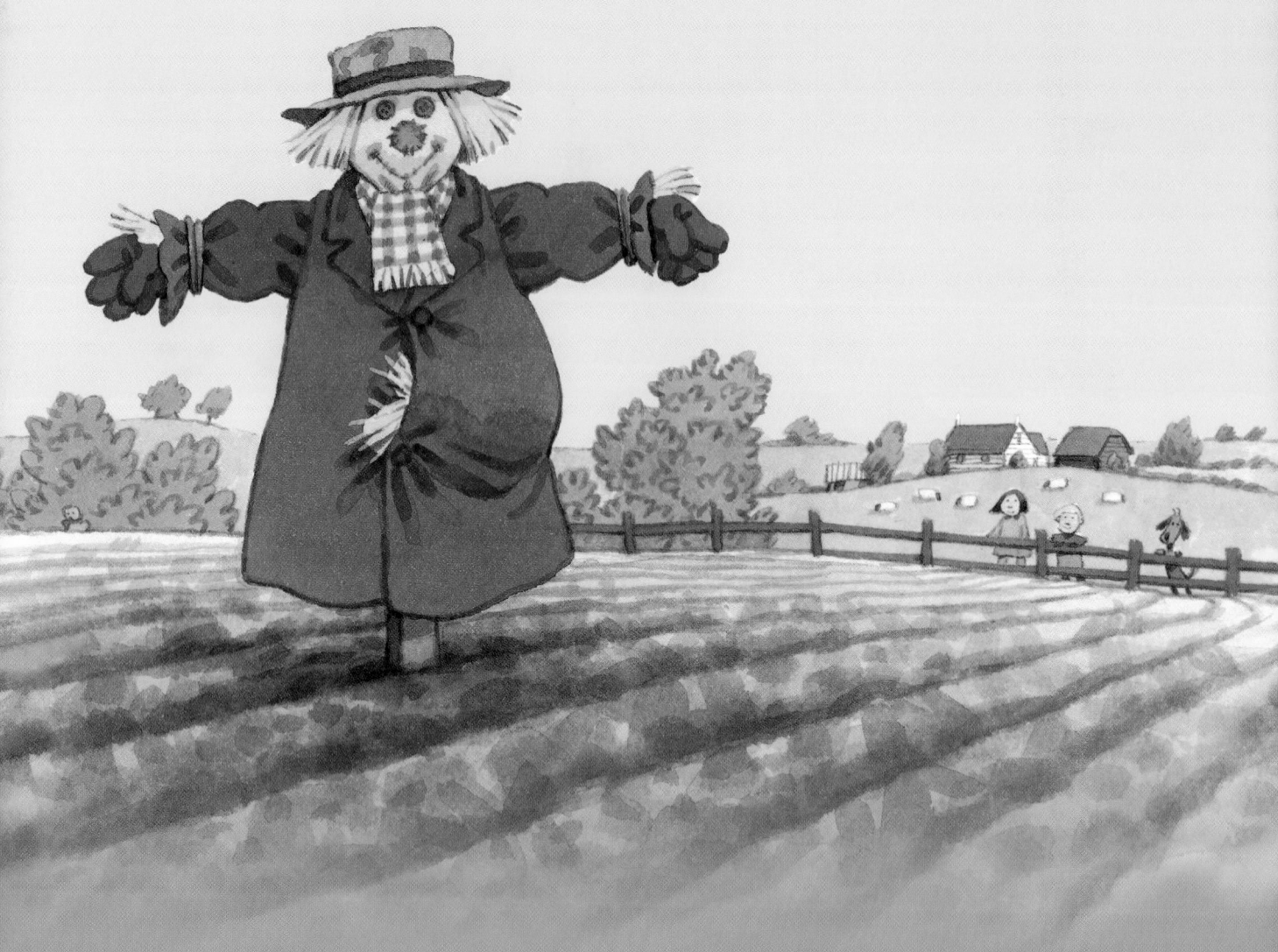

"Sometimes he looks as if he is moving," says
Poppy. "His coat goes up and down. It's very odd."

"Let's go and look."

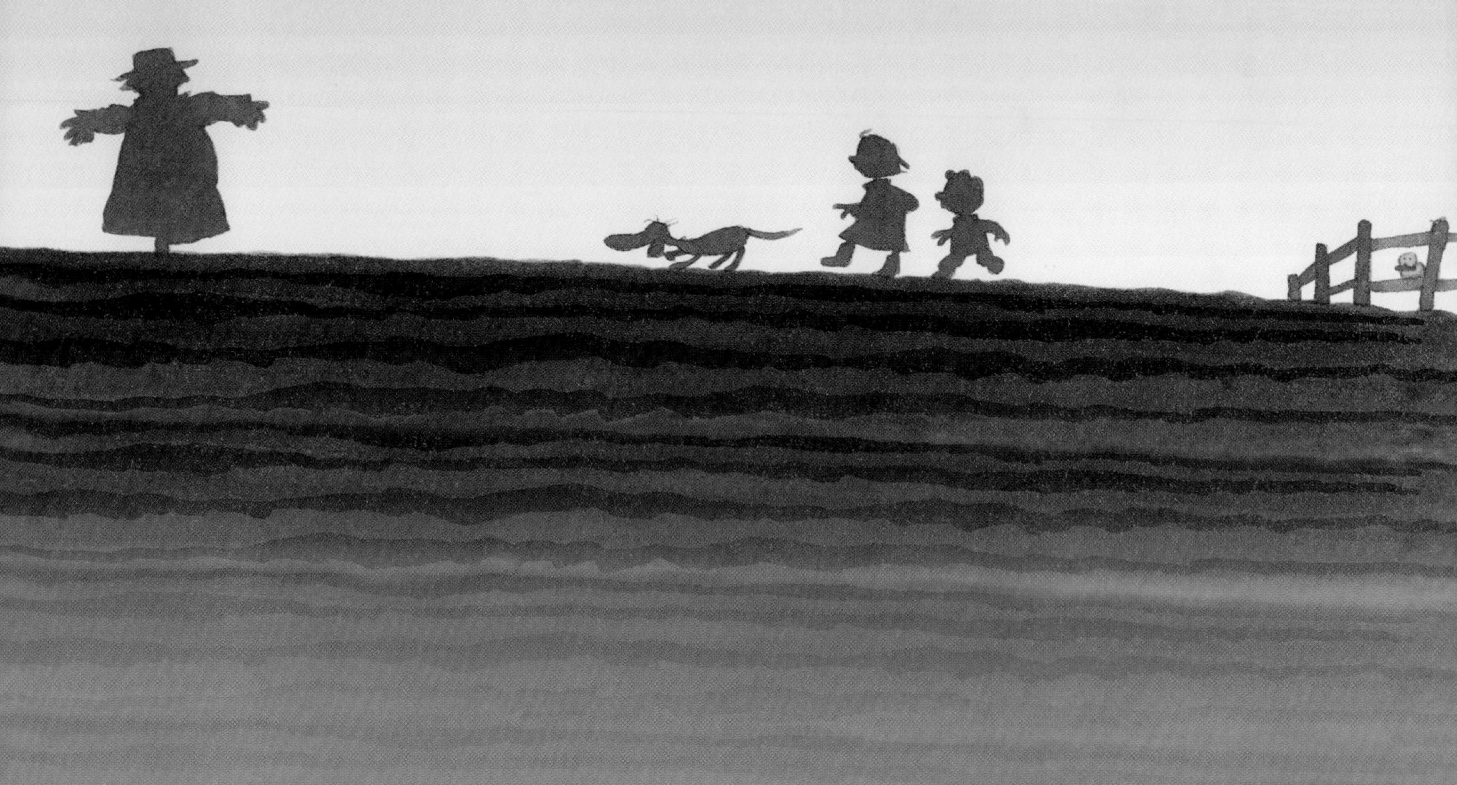

"Let's creep up very quietly," says Sam. And they tiptoe across the cornfield to look at Mr. Straw.

"There's something inside his coat."

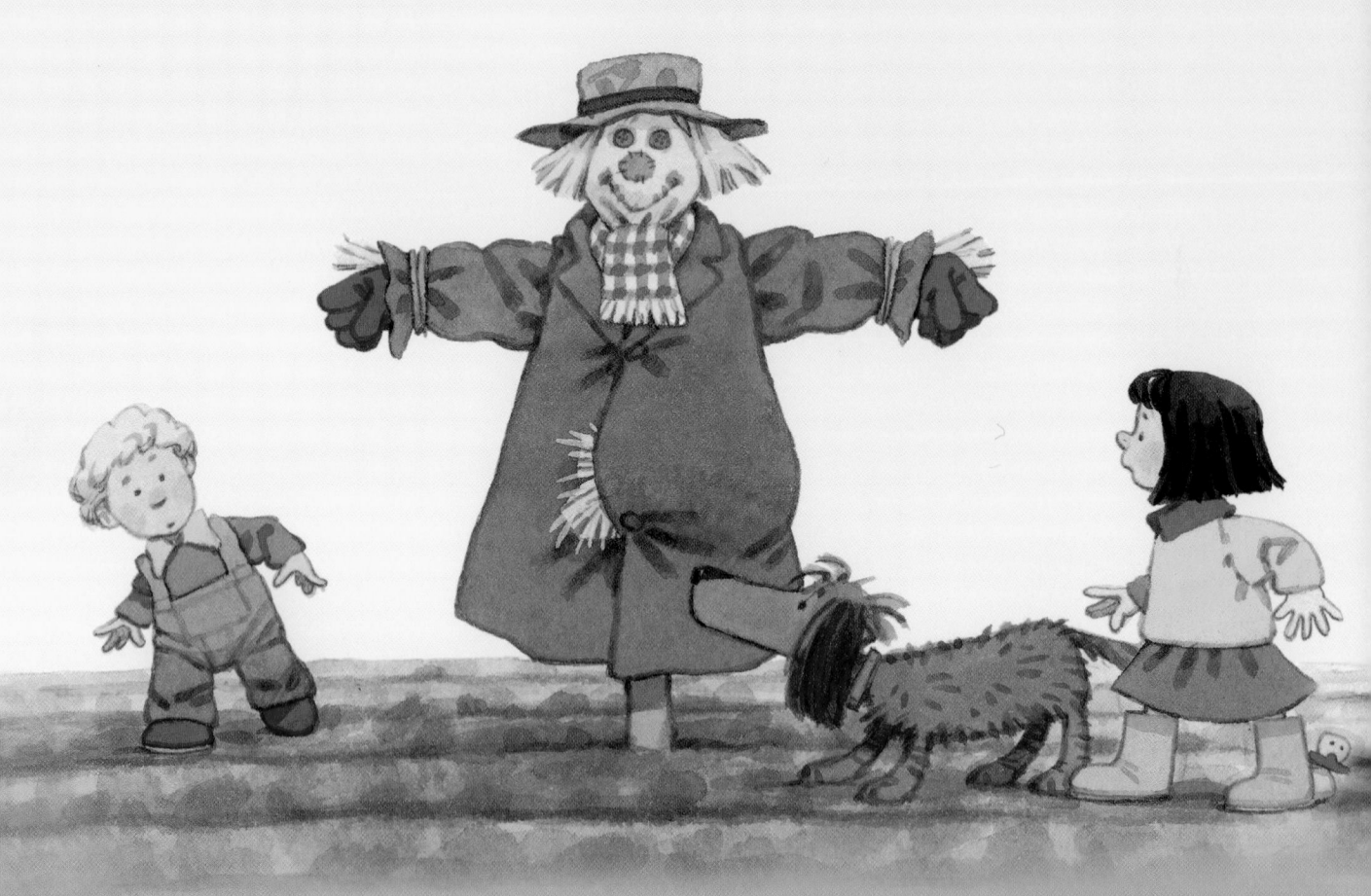

"It's moving," says Poppy. "And it's making a funny noise. What is it?" says Sam.

"It's our cat and her kittens."

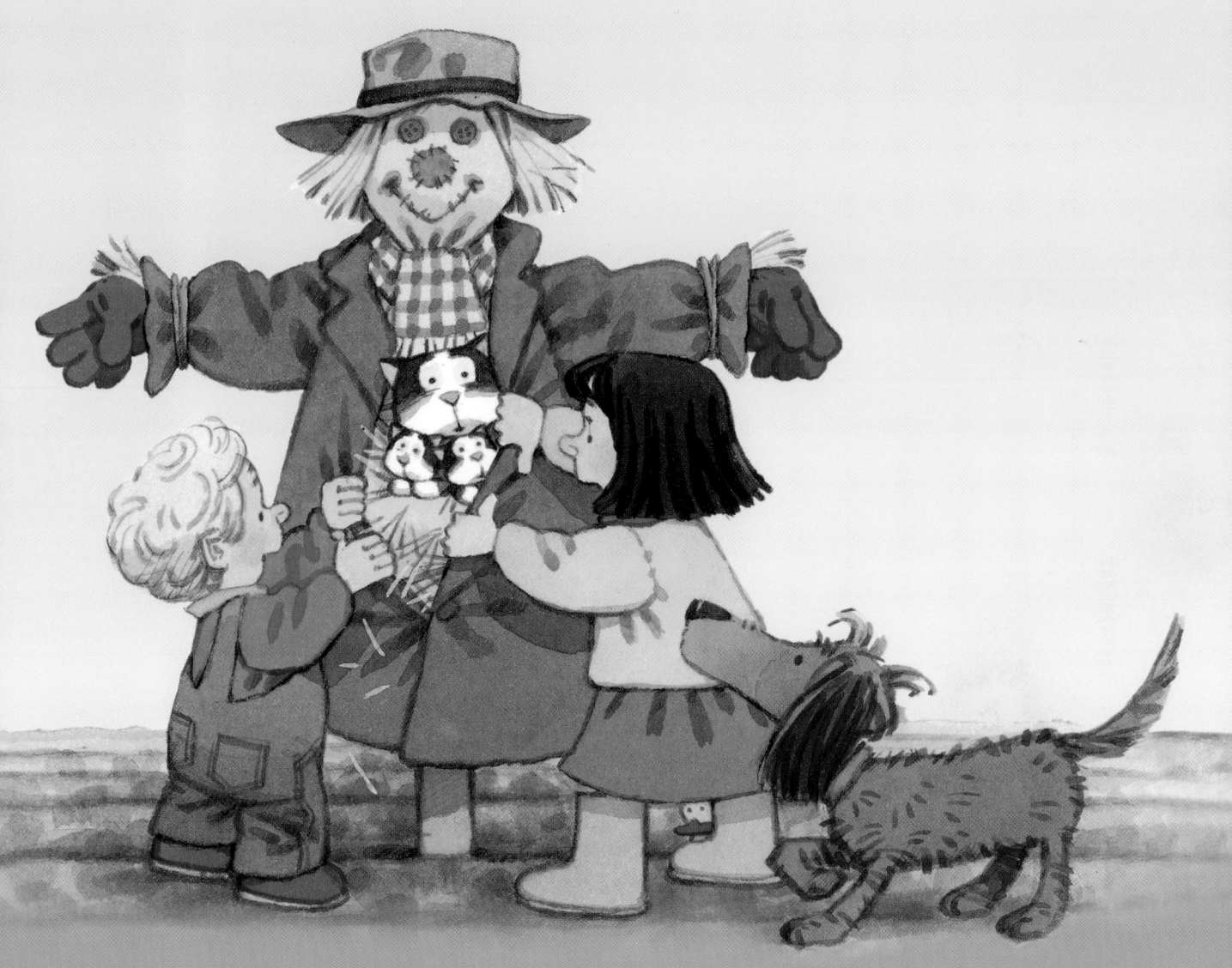

Carefully they open the coat. There is Whiskers,
the cat, and two baby kittens hiding in the straw.

"So that's the scarecrow's secret."

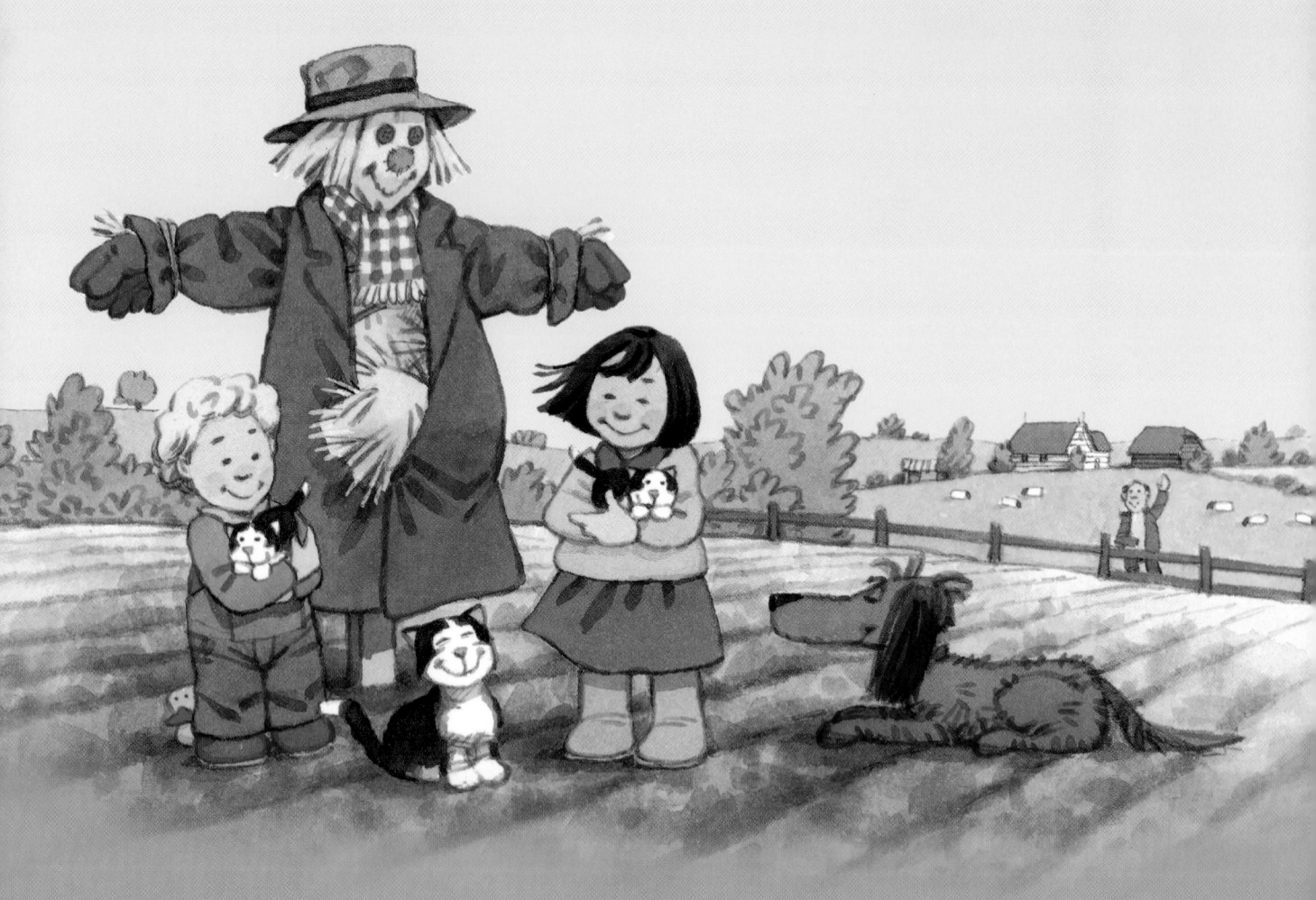

"Whiskers is helping Mr. Straw to frighten off the birds," says Poppy. "Clever Mr. Straw," says Sam.

Tractor in Trouble

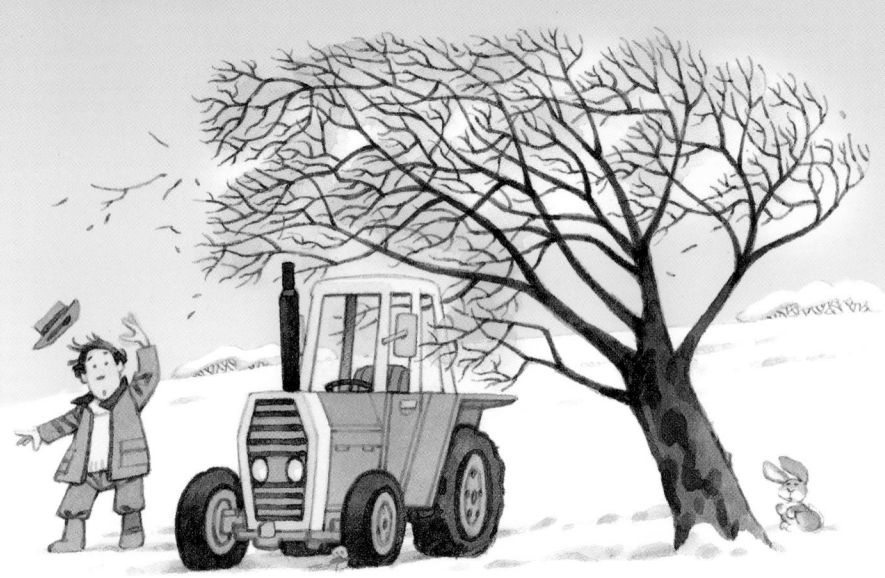

This is Apple Tree Farm.

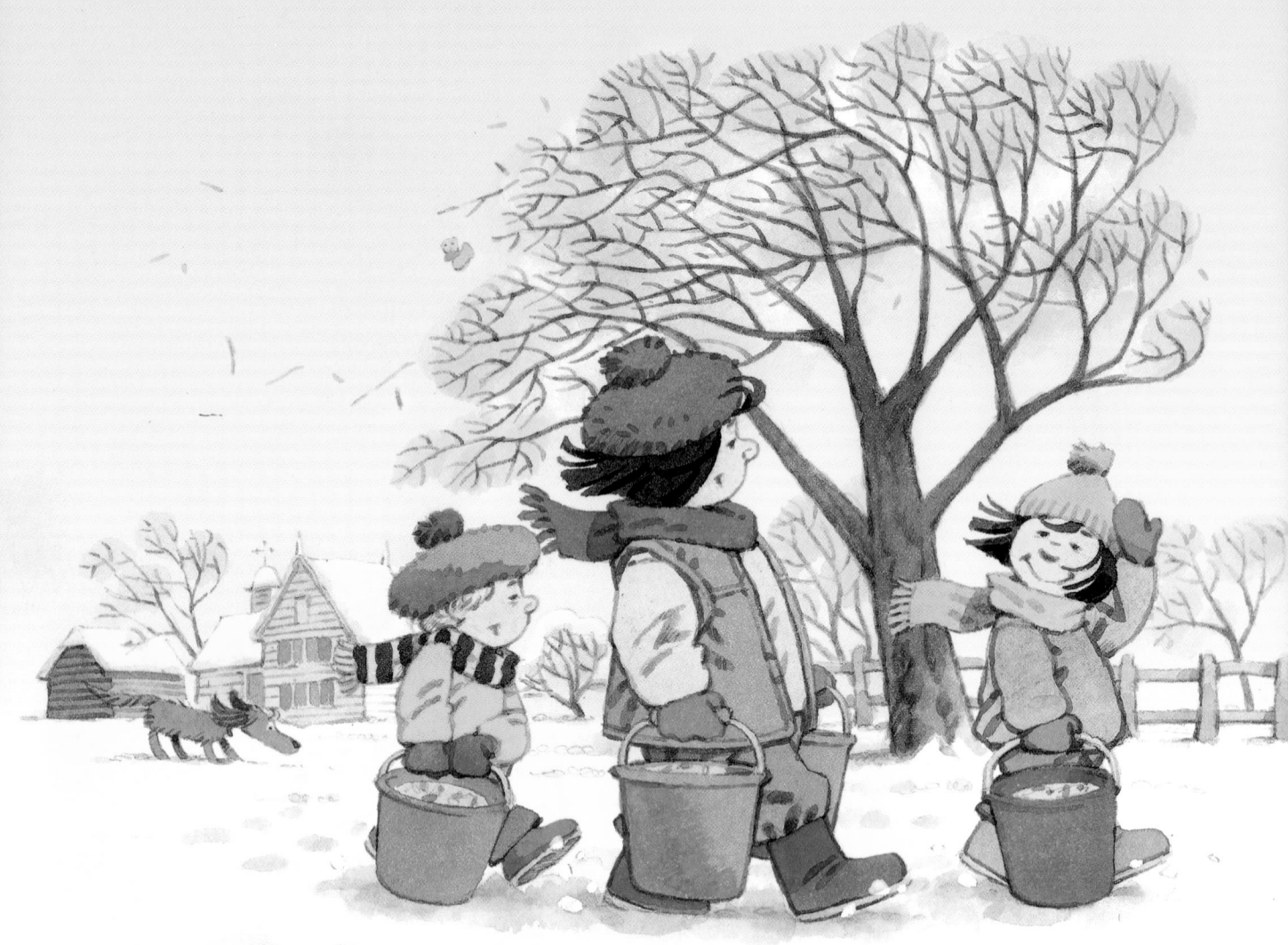

This is Mrs. Boot, the farmer. She has two children, called Poppy and Sam, and a dog called Rusty.

Ted works on the farm.

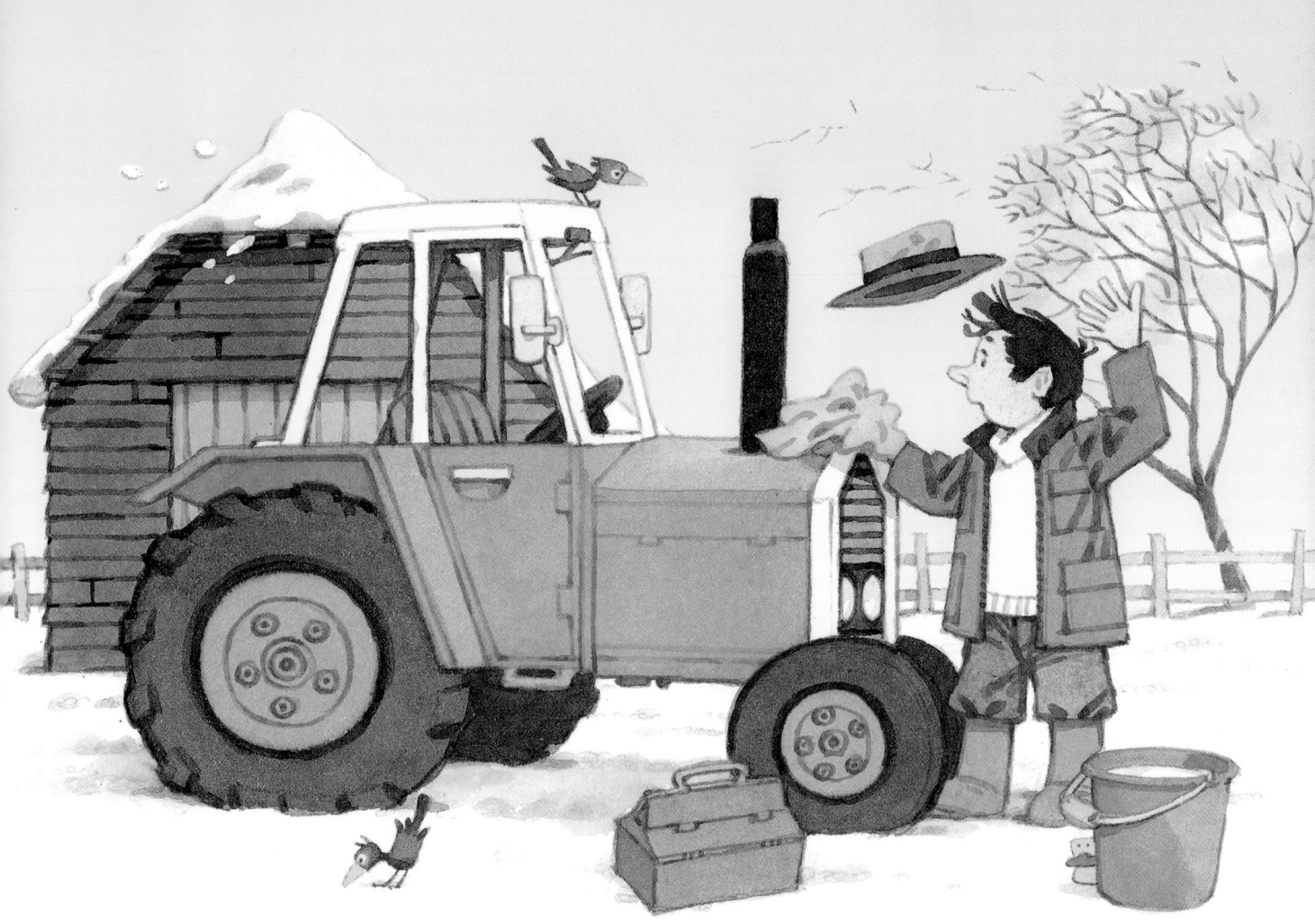

He helps Mrs. Boot. Ted looks after the tractor and
all the farm machines.

Today it is very windy.

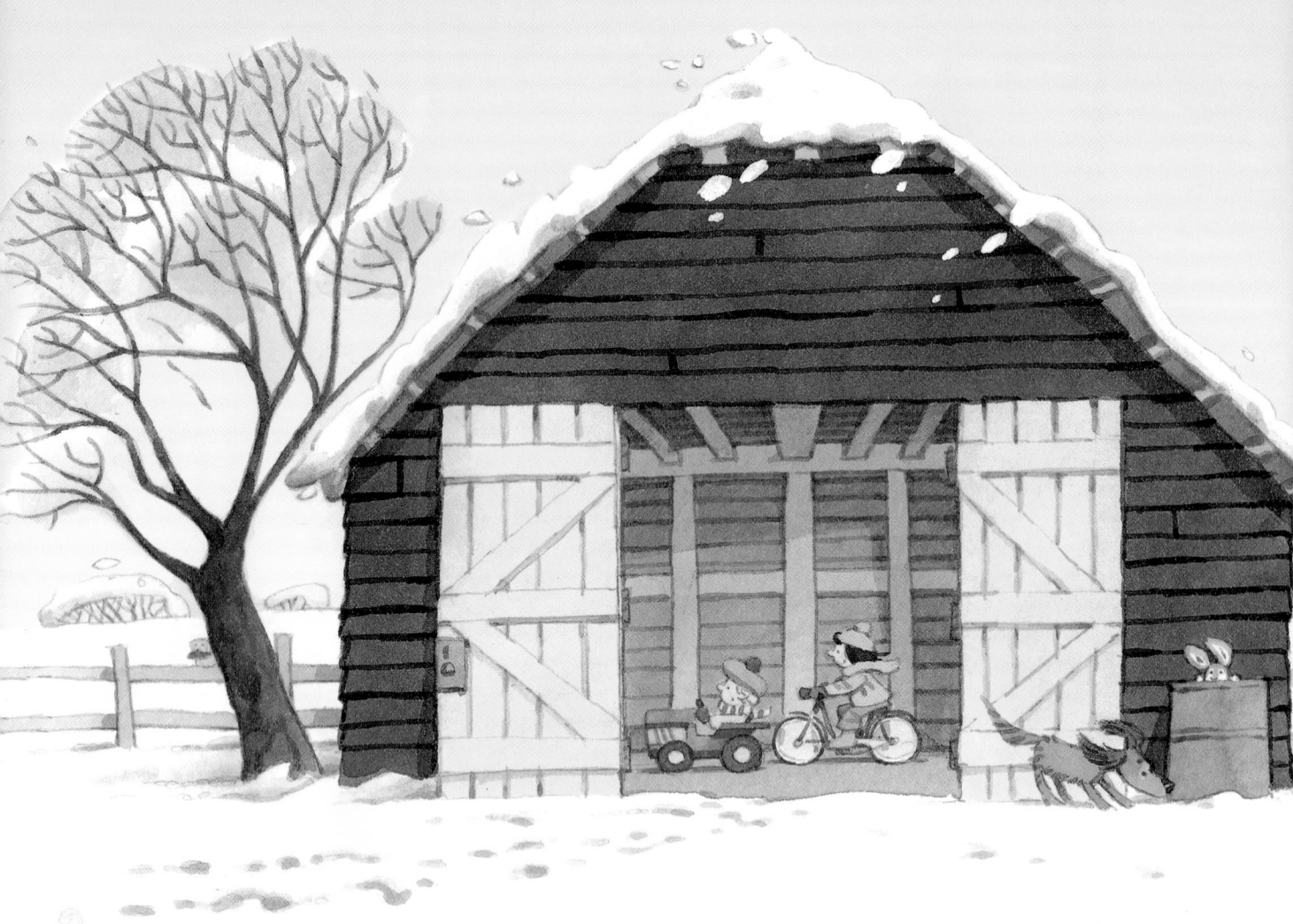

The wind is blowing the trees and it is very cold.
Poppy and Sam play in the barn.

"Where are you going, Ted?"

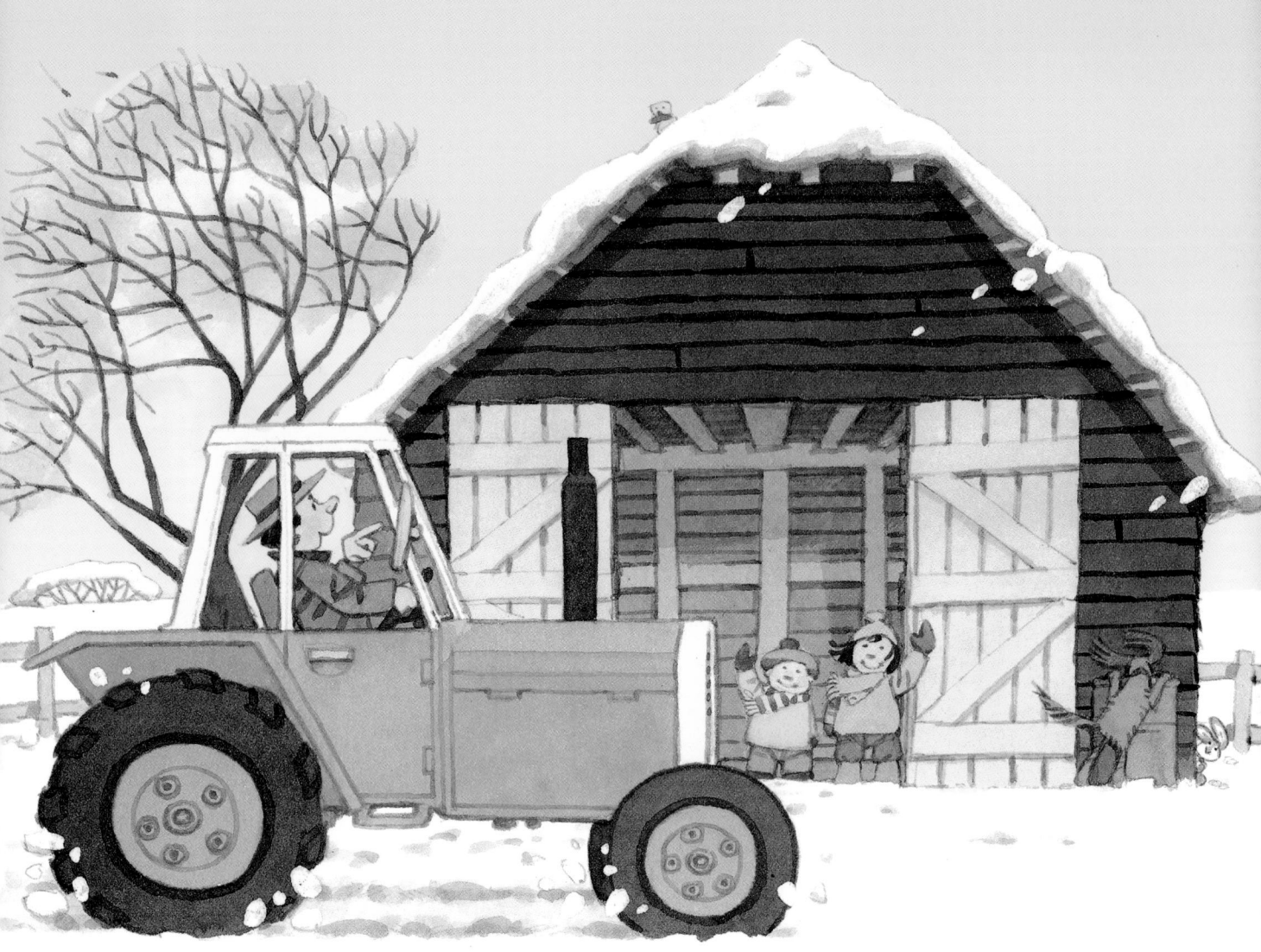

Ted is driving the tractor out of the yard. "I'm just going to see if the sheep are all right," he says.

Ted stops the tractor by the gate.

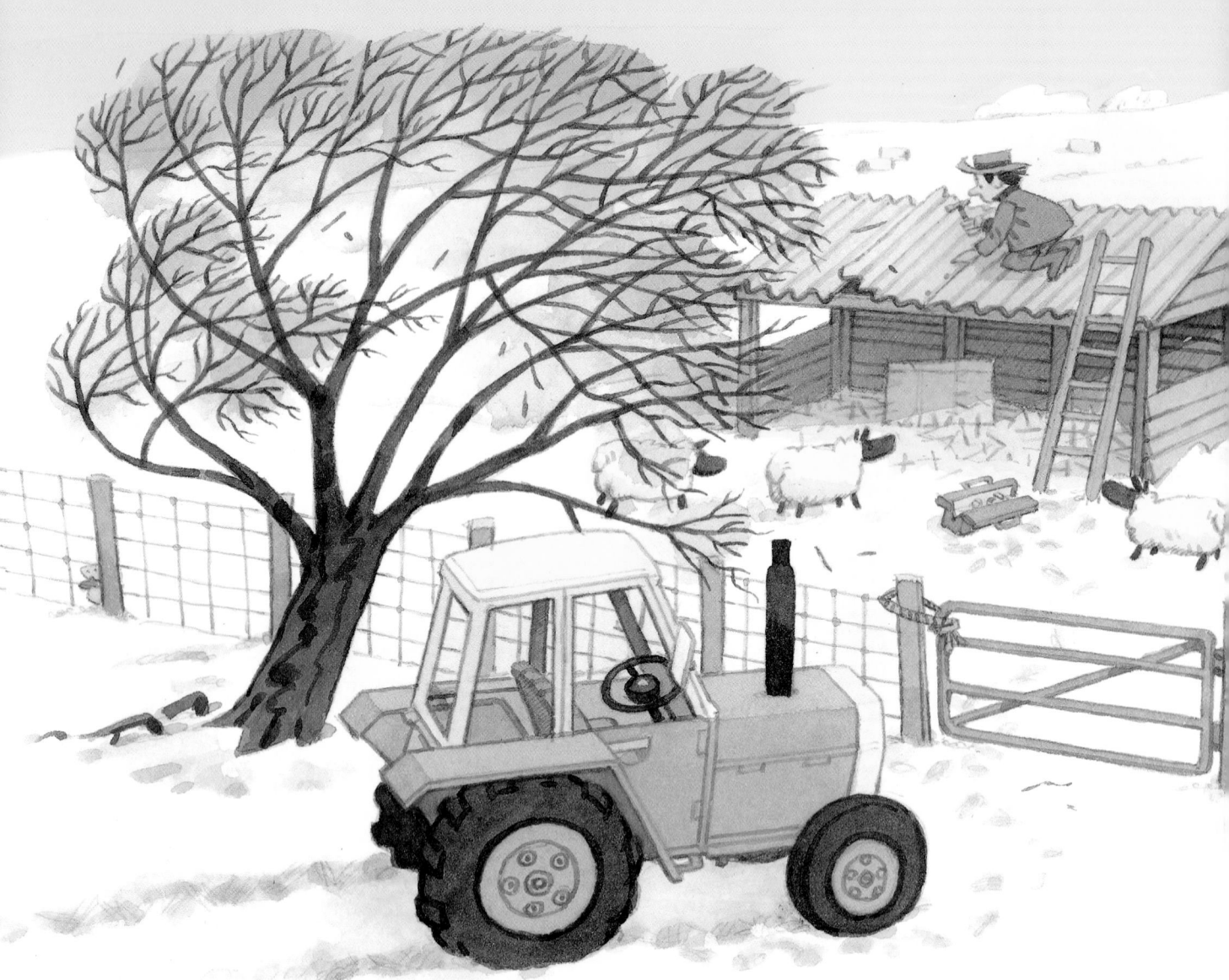

He goes into the sheep field. He nails down
the roof of the sheep shed to make it safe.

Poppy and Sam hear a terrible crash.

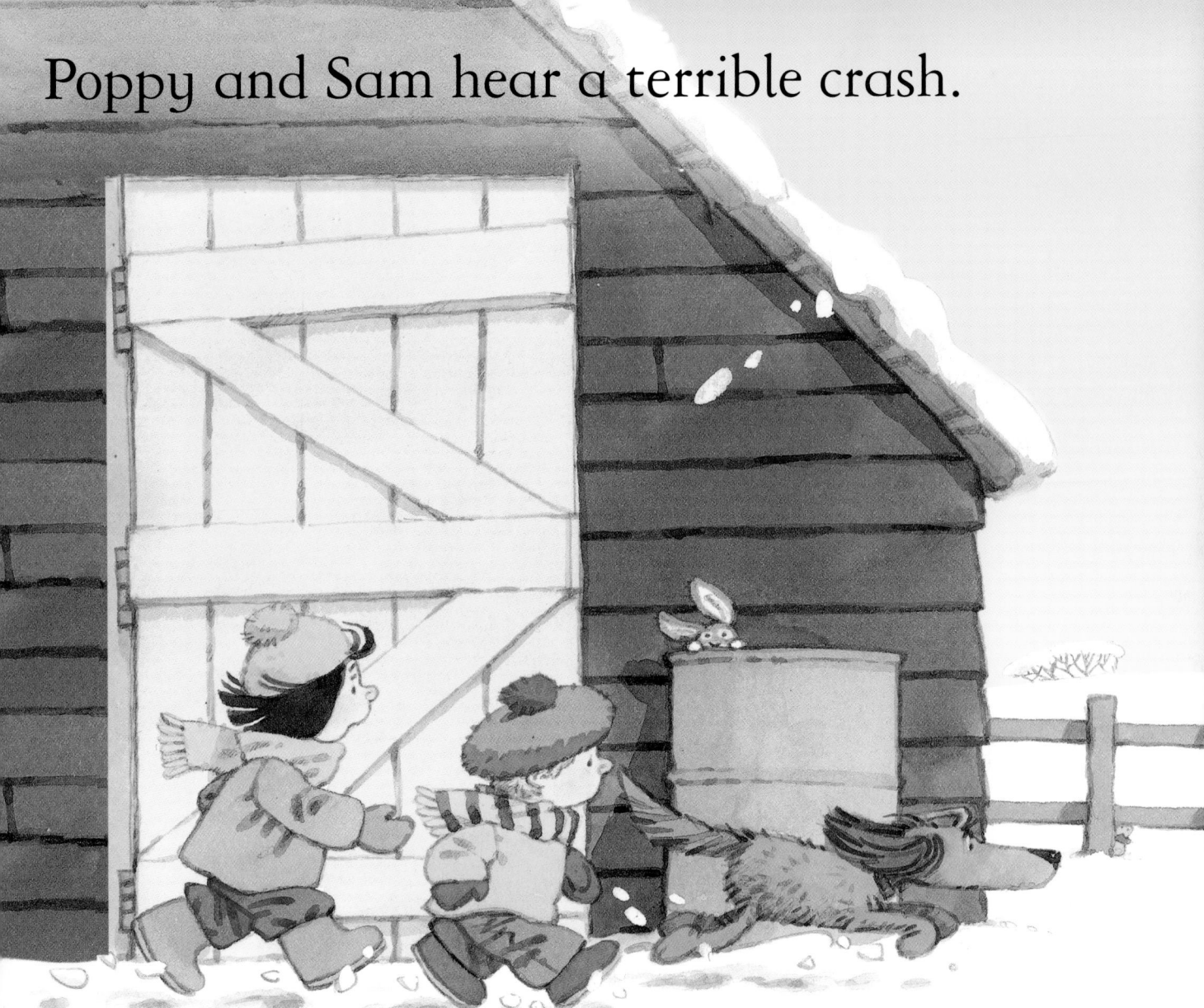

"What's that?" says Sam. "I don't know. Let's go
and look," says Poppy. They run down the field.

"A tree has blown down."

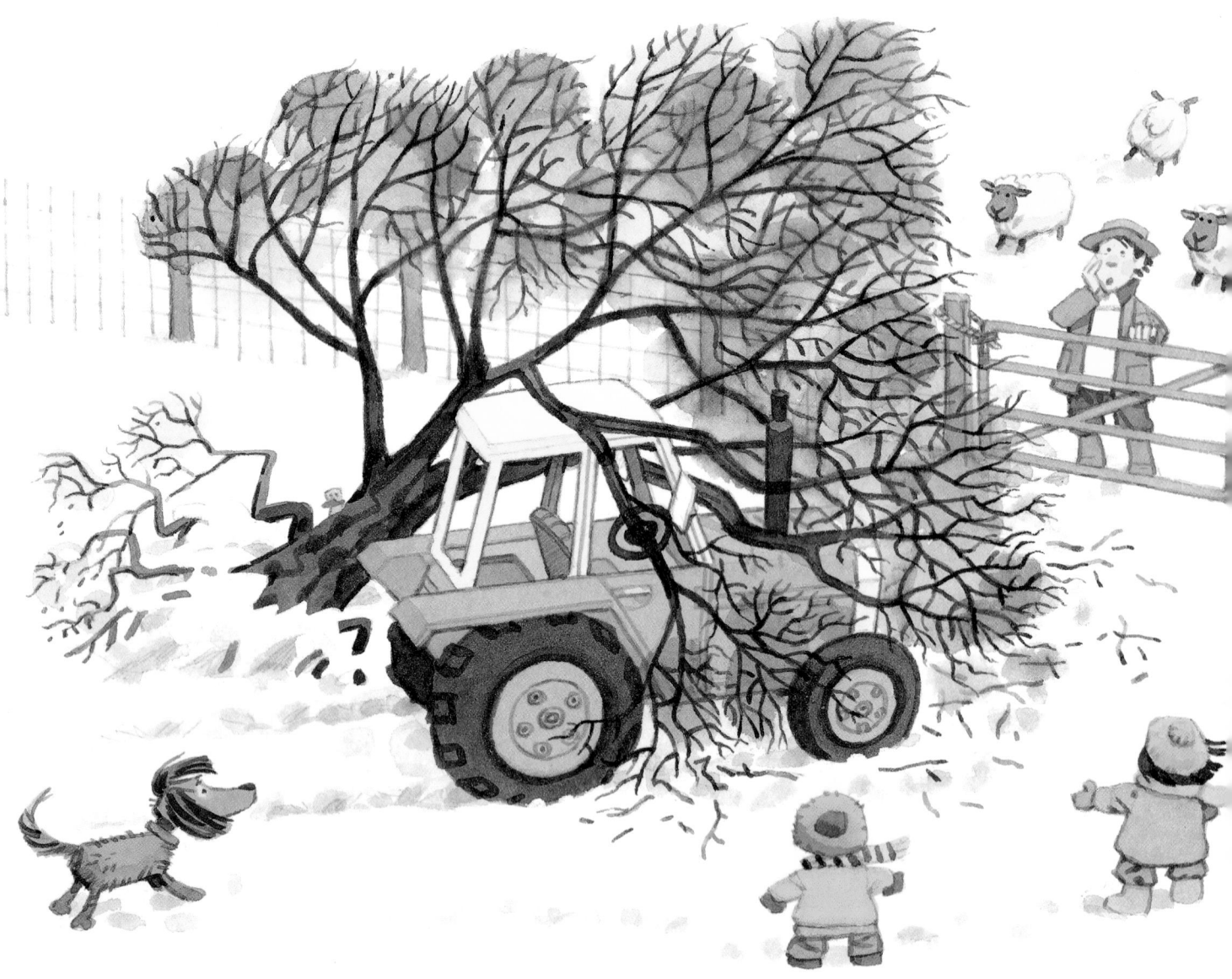

"It's coming down on Ted's tractor," says Poppy.
"Come on. We must help him," says Sam.

"What are you going to do, Ted?"

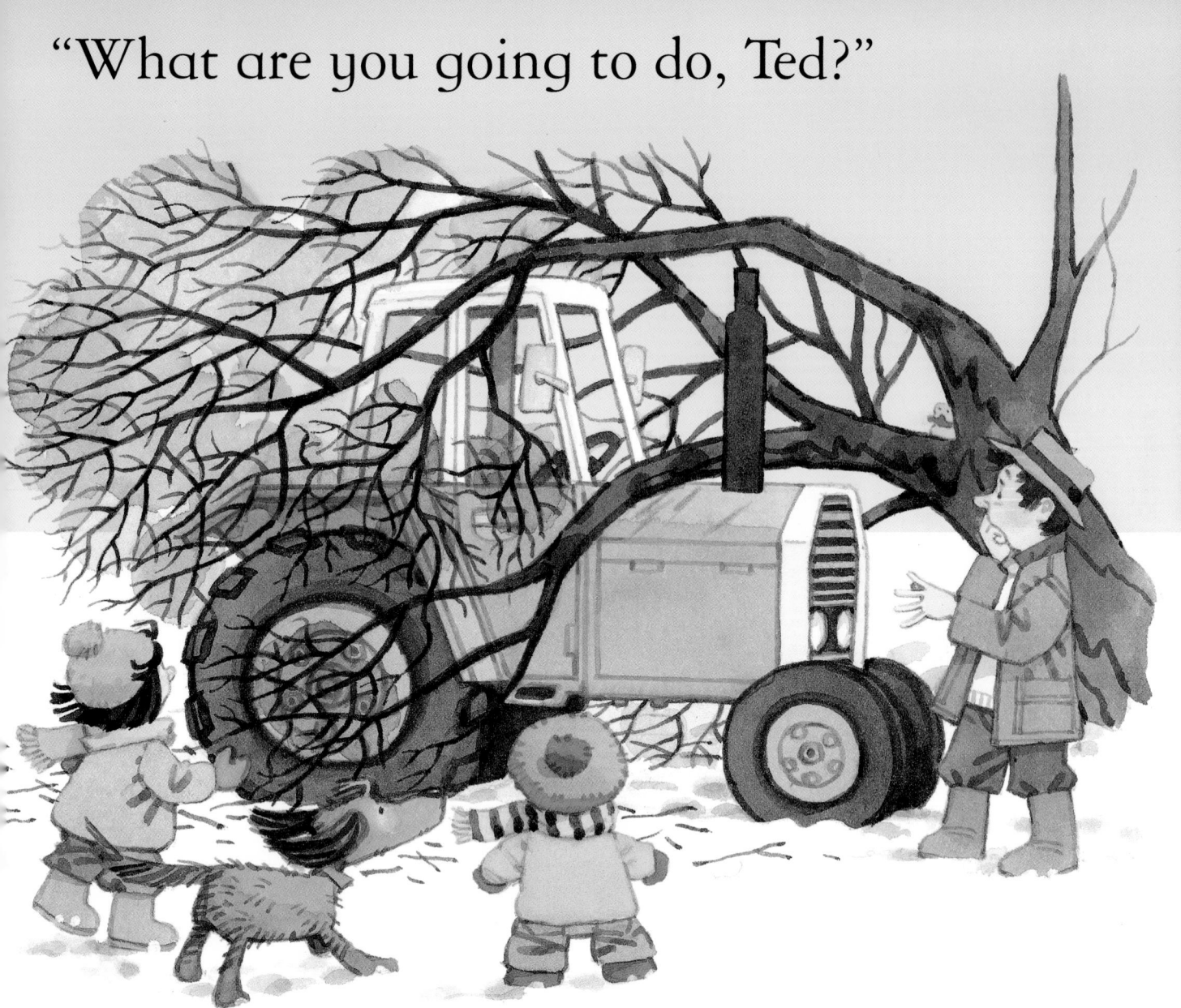

Poor Ted is very upset. The tree has scratched his new tractor. He can't even get into the cab.

"Ask Farmer Dray to help."

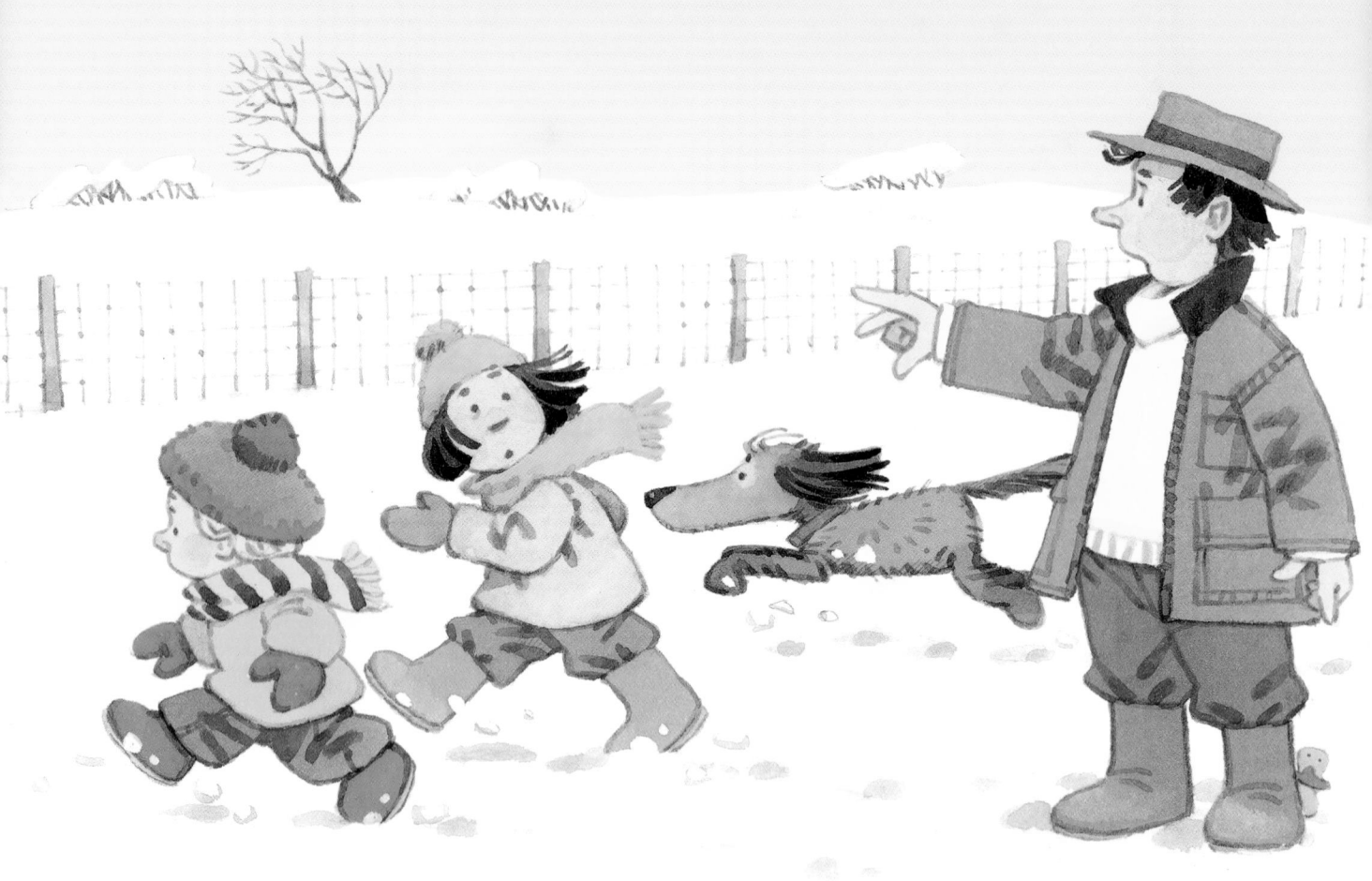

"I think I can see him on the hill," says Ted.
Poppy and Sam run to ask him.

Soon Farmer Dray comes with his horse.

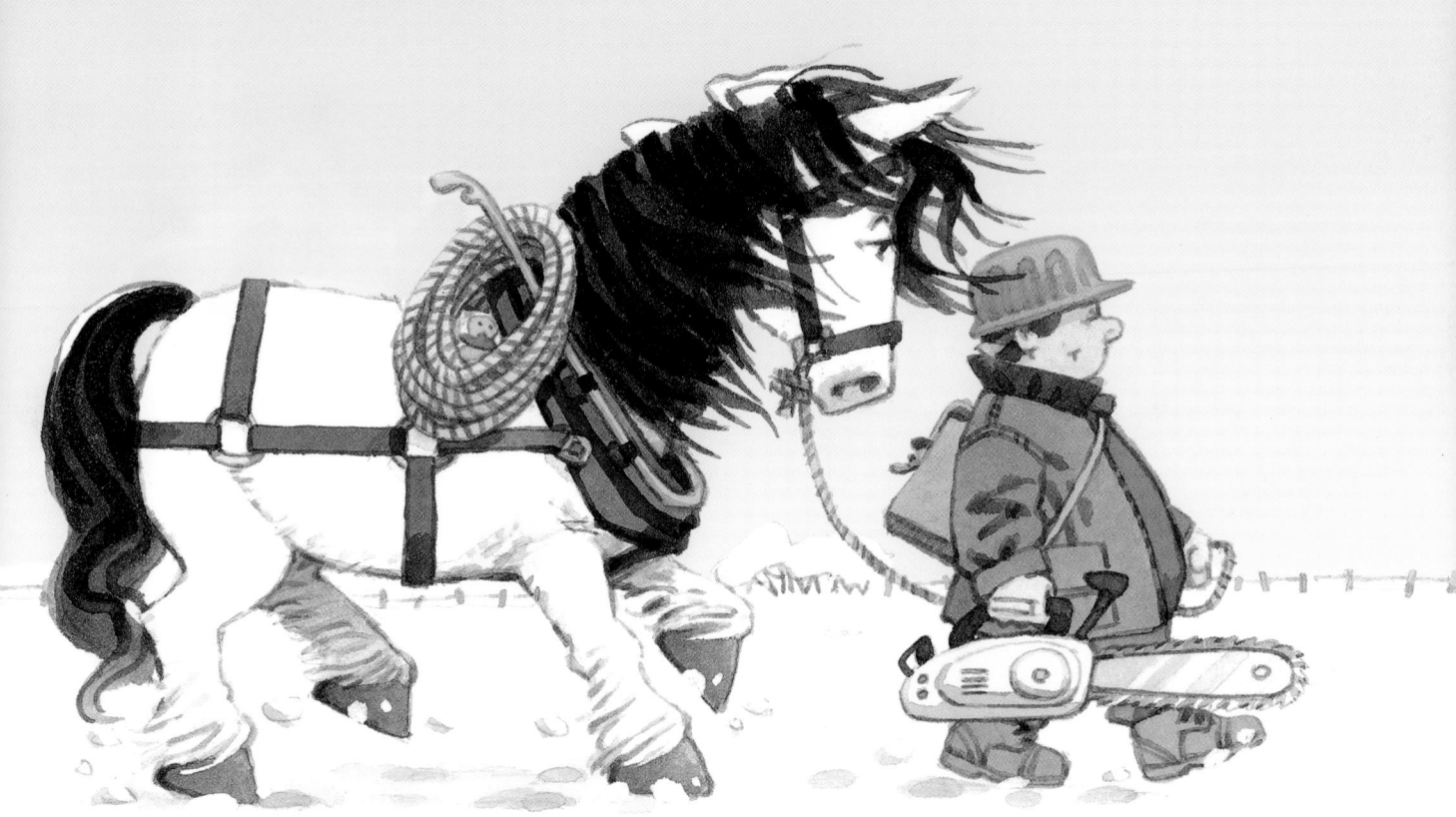

Farmer Dray has a big, gentle carthorse, called
Dolly. They have come to help Ted.

123

"I'll cut up the tree first."

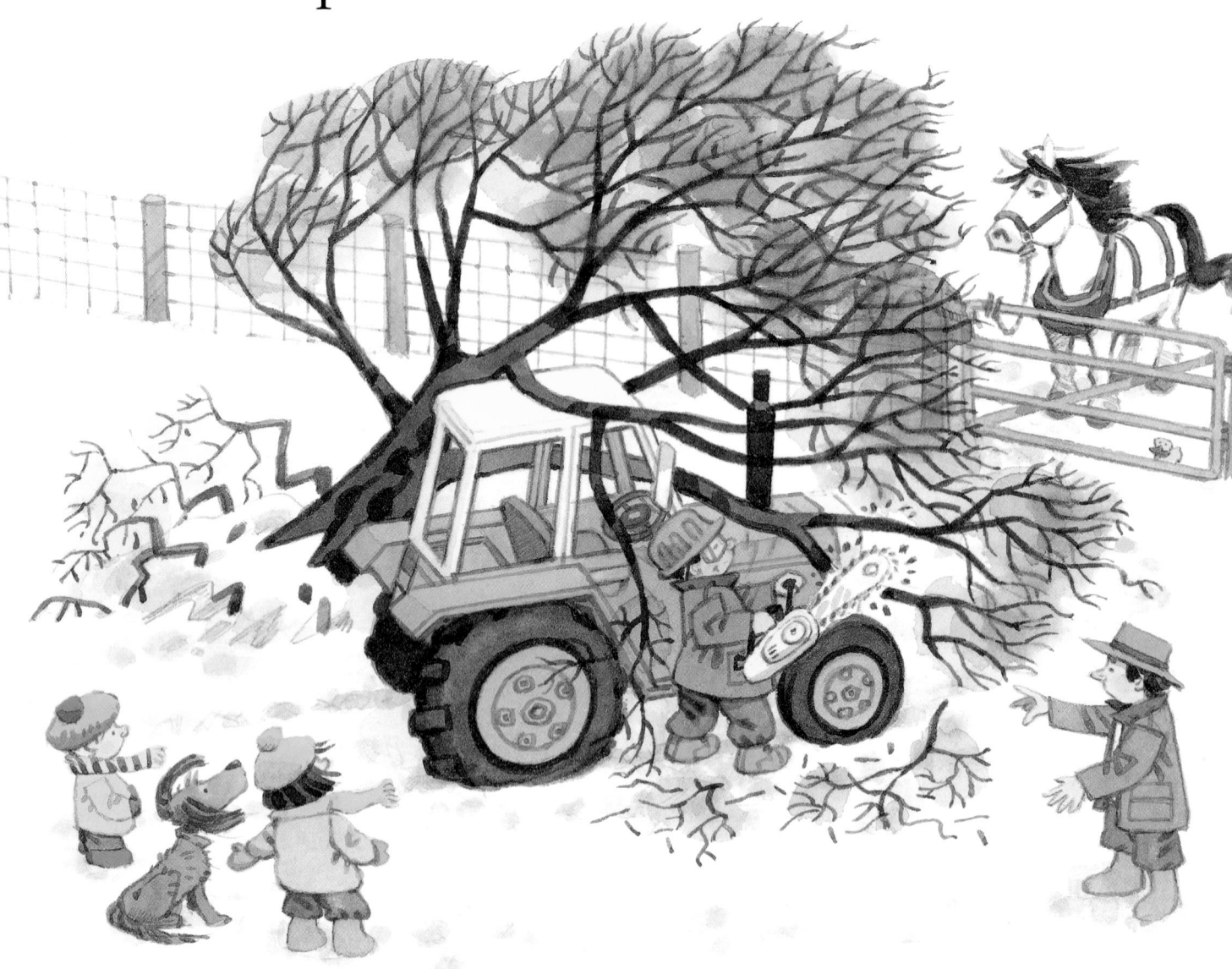

Farmer Dray starts up his chain saw. Then he cuts
off the branches which have fallen on the tractor.

Dolly starts to work.

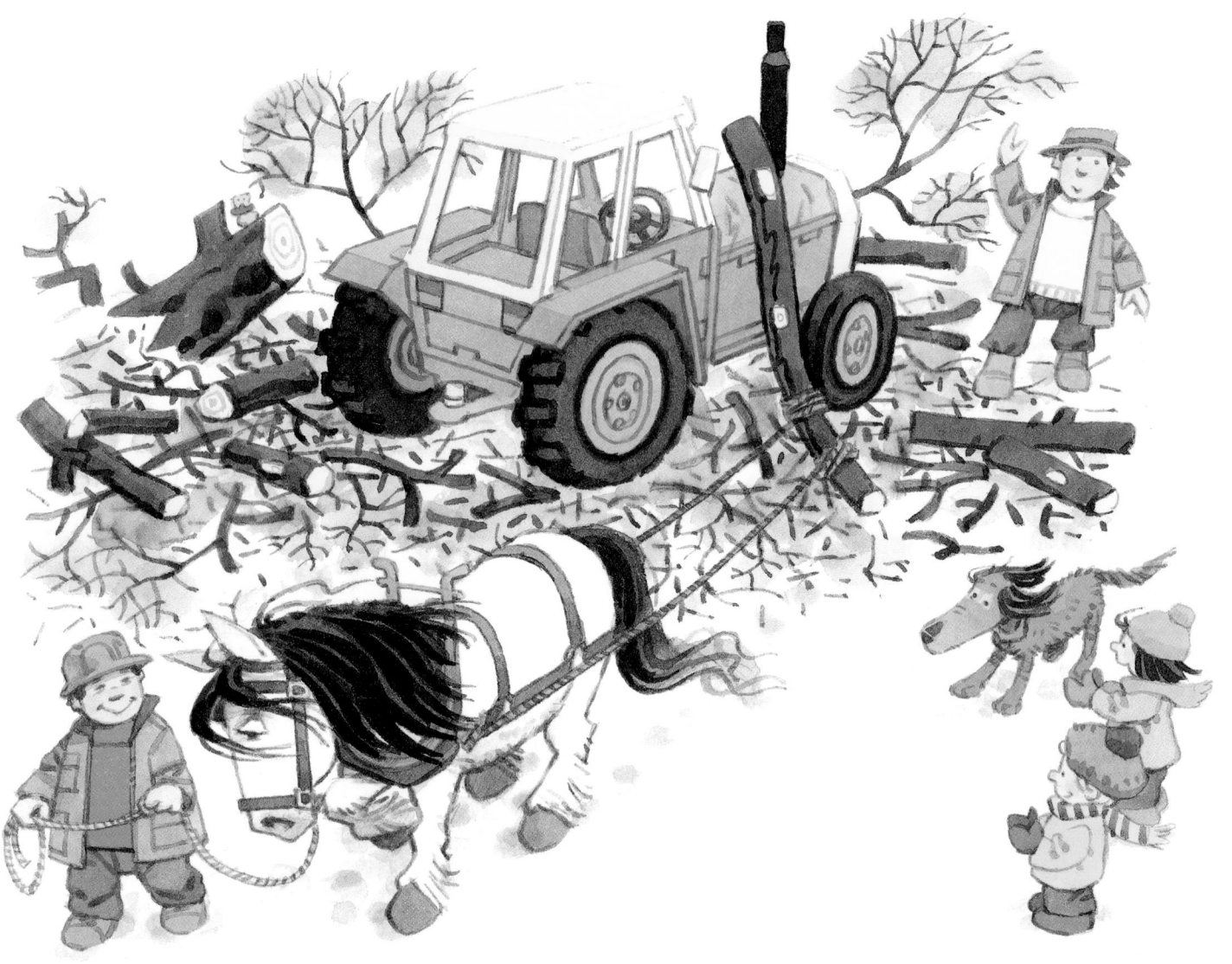

Farmer Dray ties two ropes to Dolly's harness.
Ted ties the other ends to the big branches.

Dolly pulls and pulls.

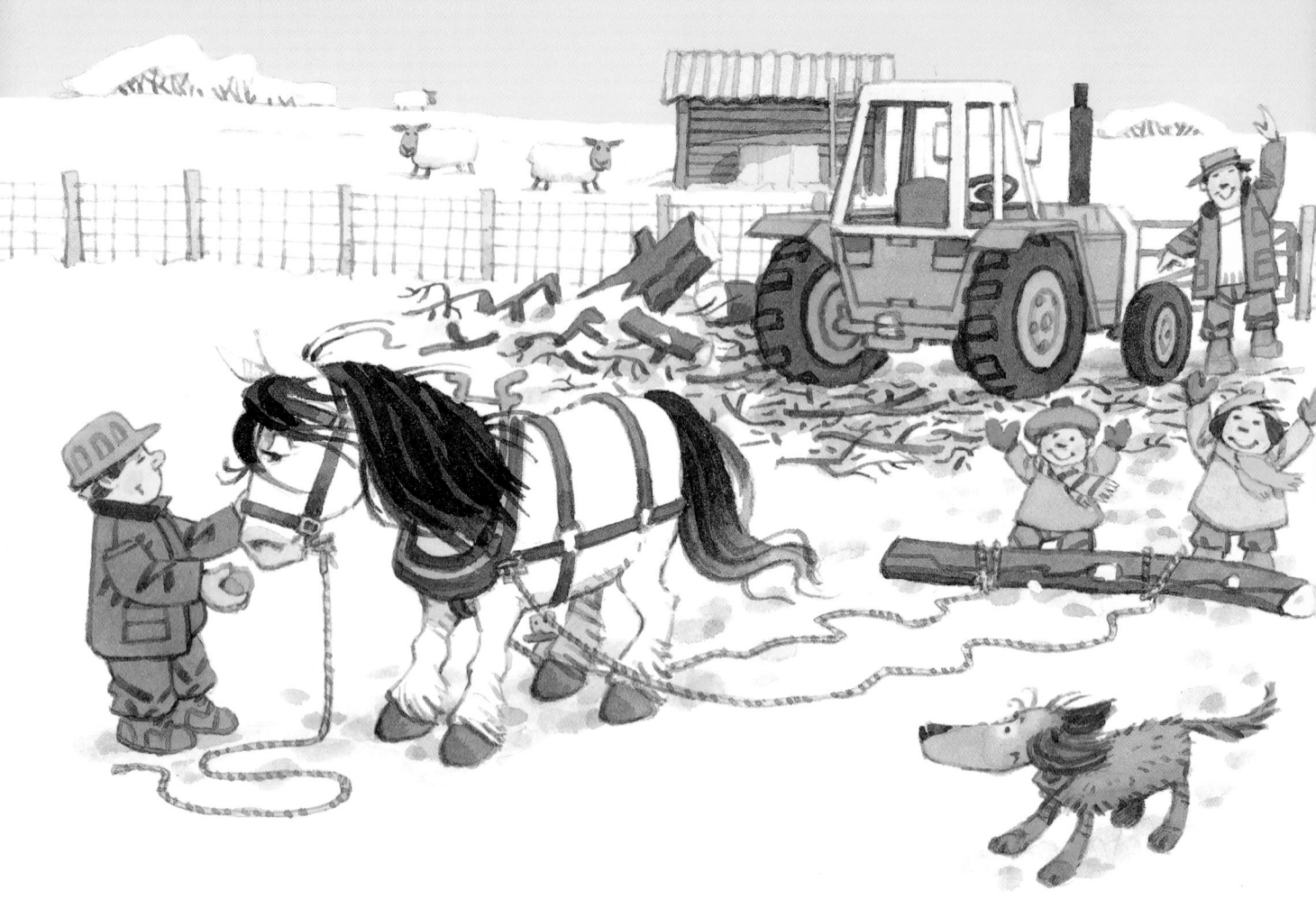

She works hard until all the branches are off the tractor. "Well done, Dolly," says Farmer Dray.

Ted climbs up into the cab.

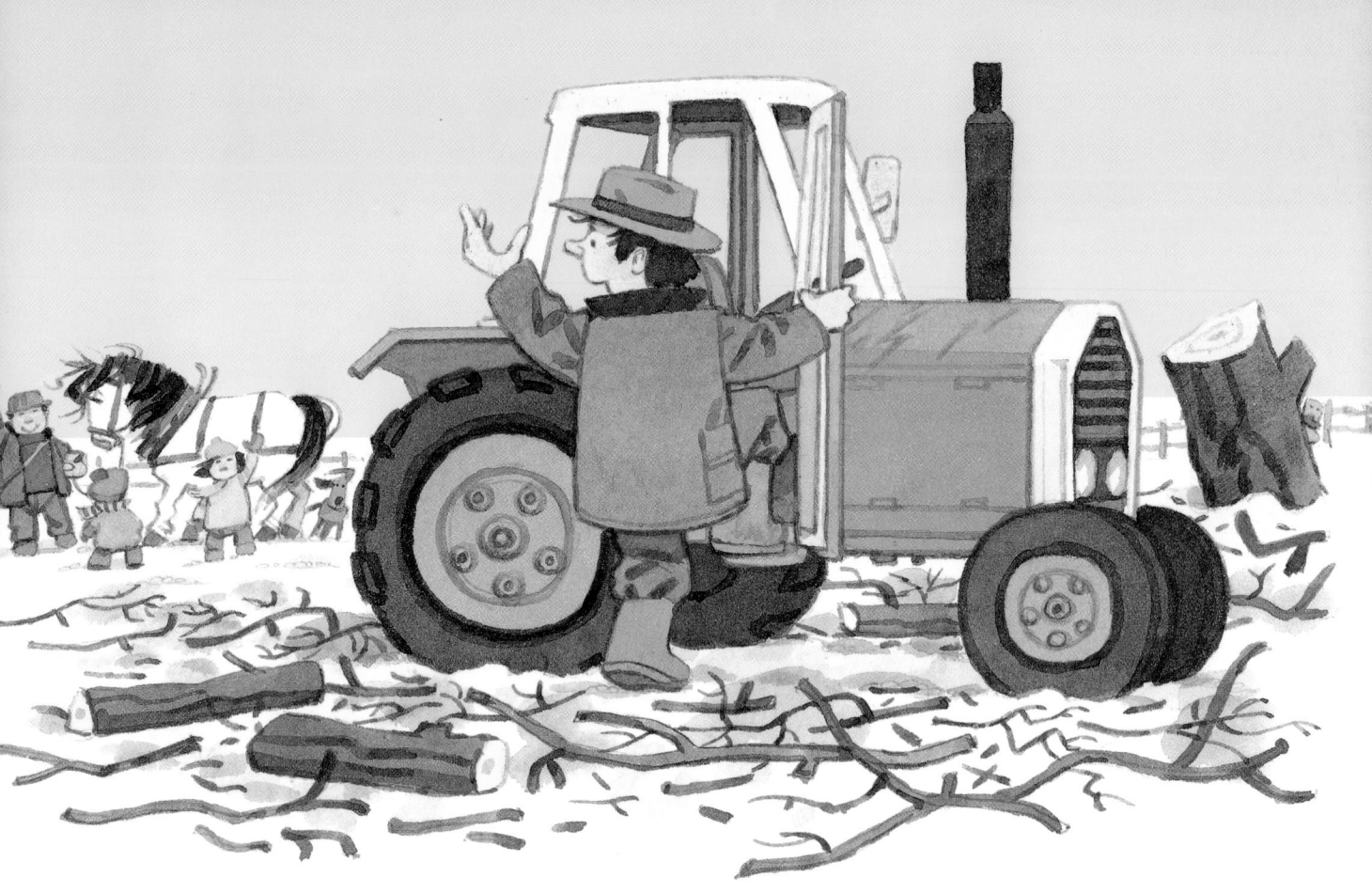

"Thank you very much, Farmer Dray and Dolly,"
he says. And they all go back to the farmyard.

The tractor looks a little messy.

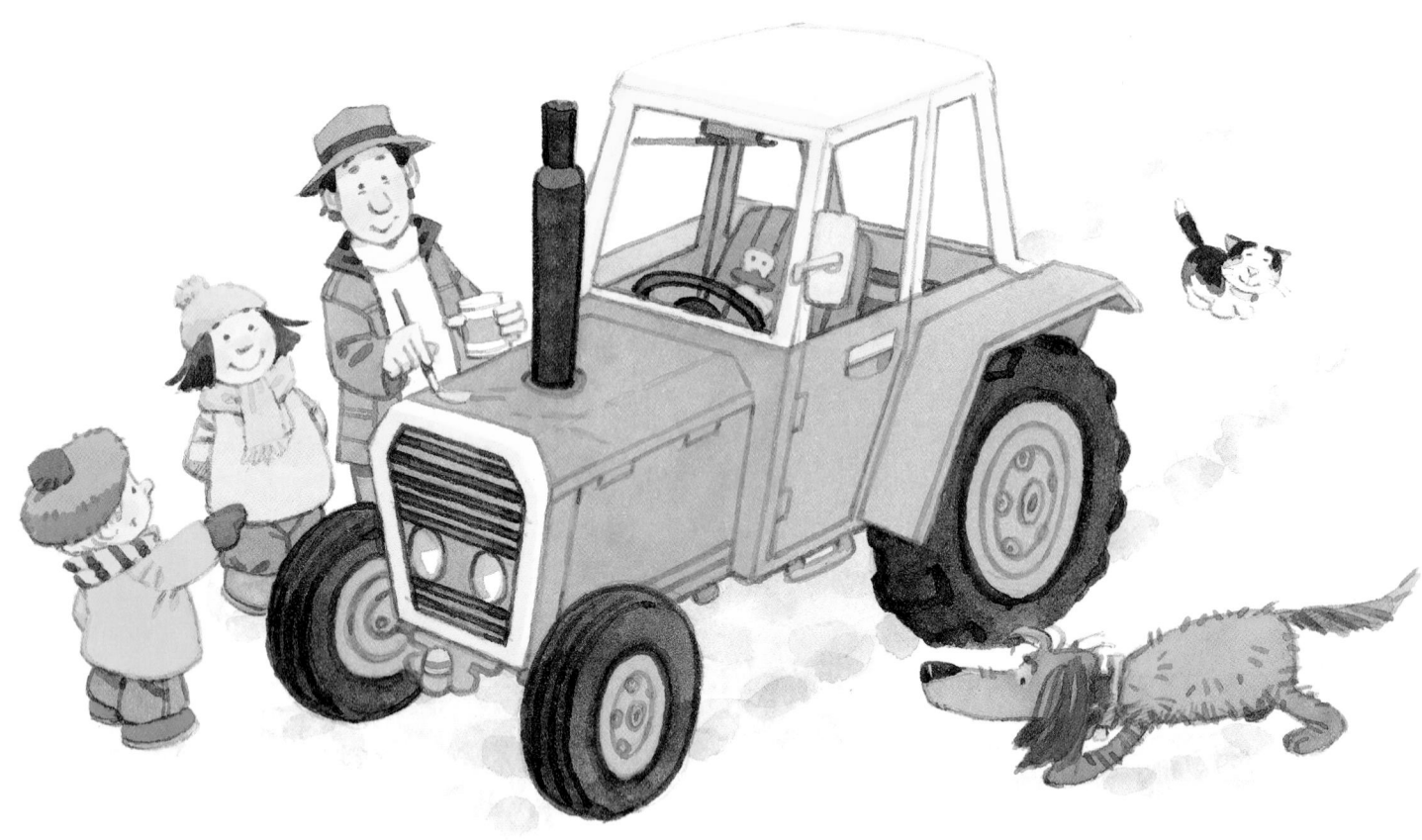

Ted finds a brush and paints over all the scratches.
"It will soon be as good as new," he says.

The
Silly Sheepdog

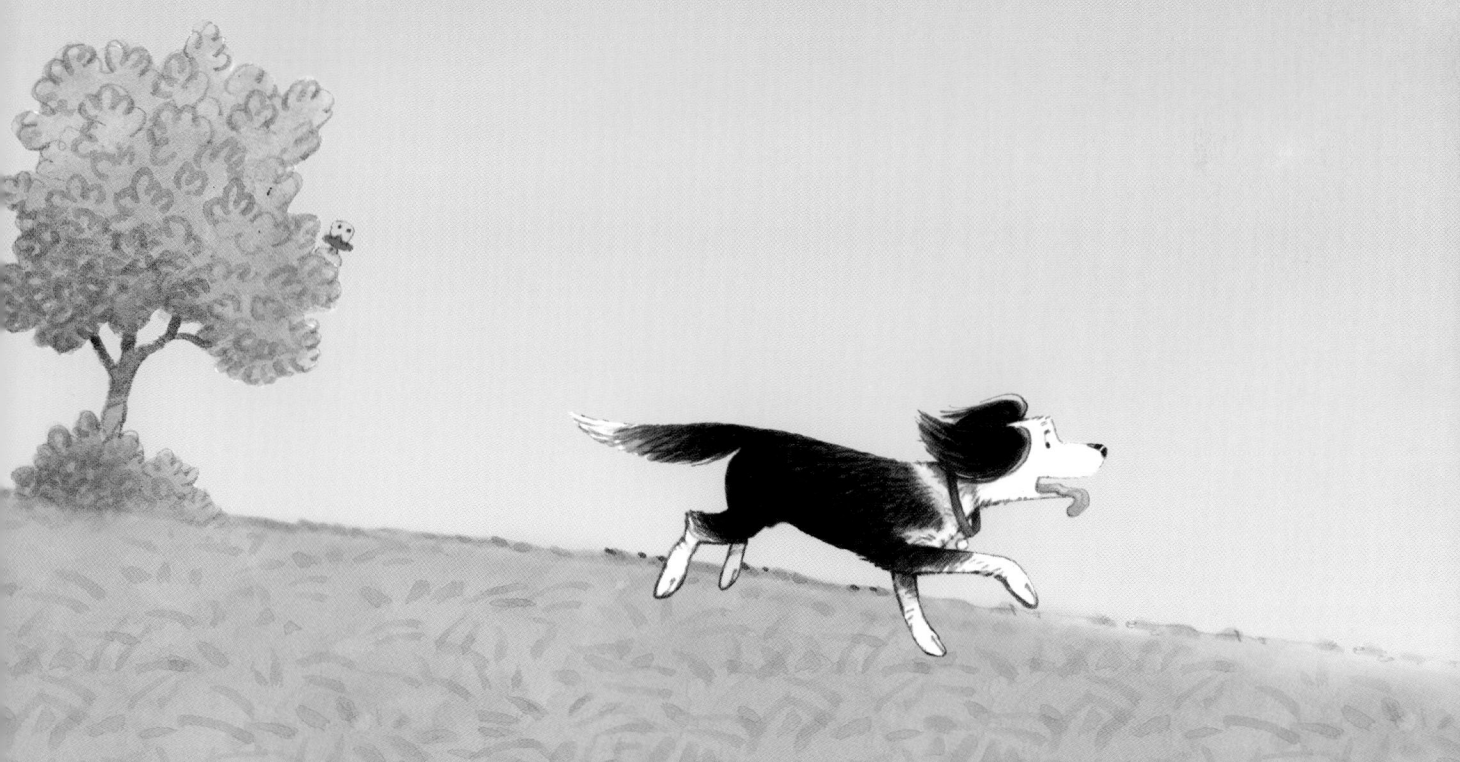

This is Apple Tree Farm.

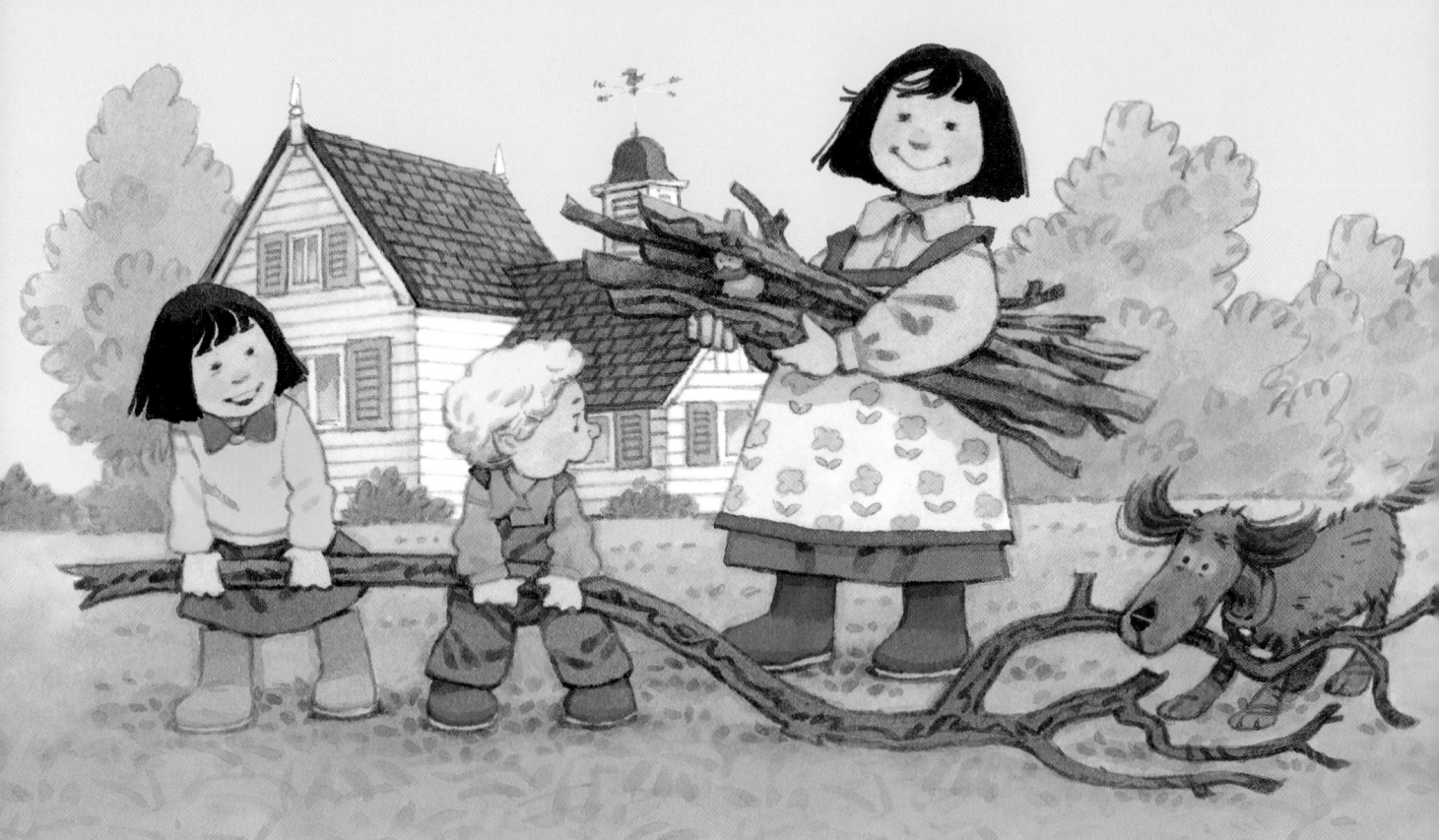

This is Mrs. Boot, the farmer. She has two children, called Poppy and Sam, and a dog called Rusty.

Ted works on Apple Tree Farm.

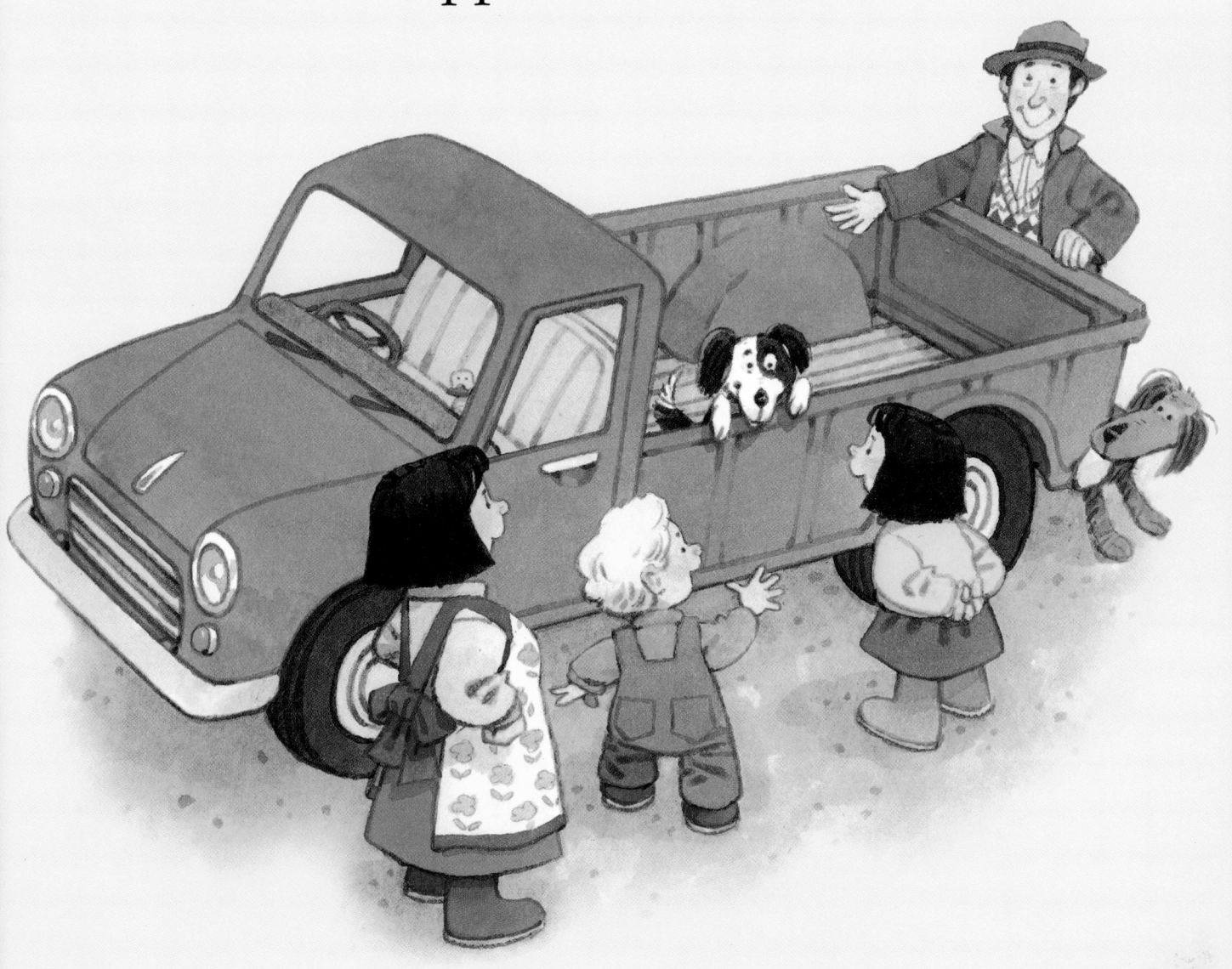

He has just bought a sheepdog to help him with the sheep. The sheepdog is called Patch.

Poppy, Sam and Rusty say hello to Patch.

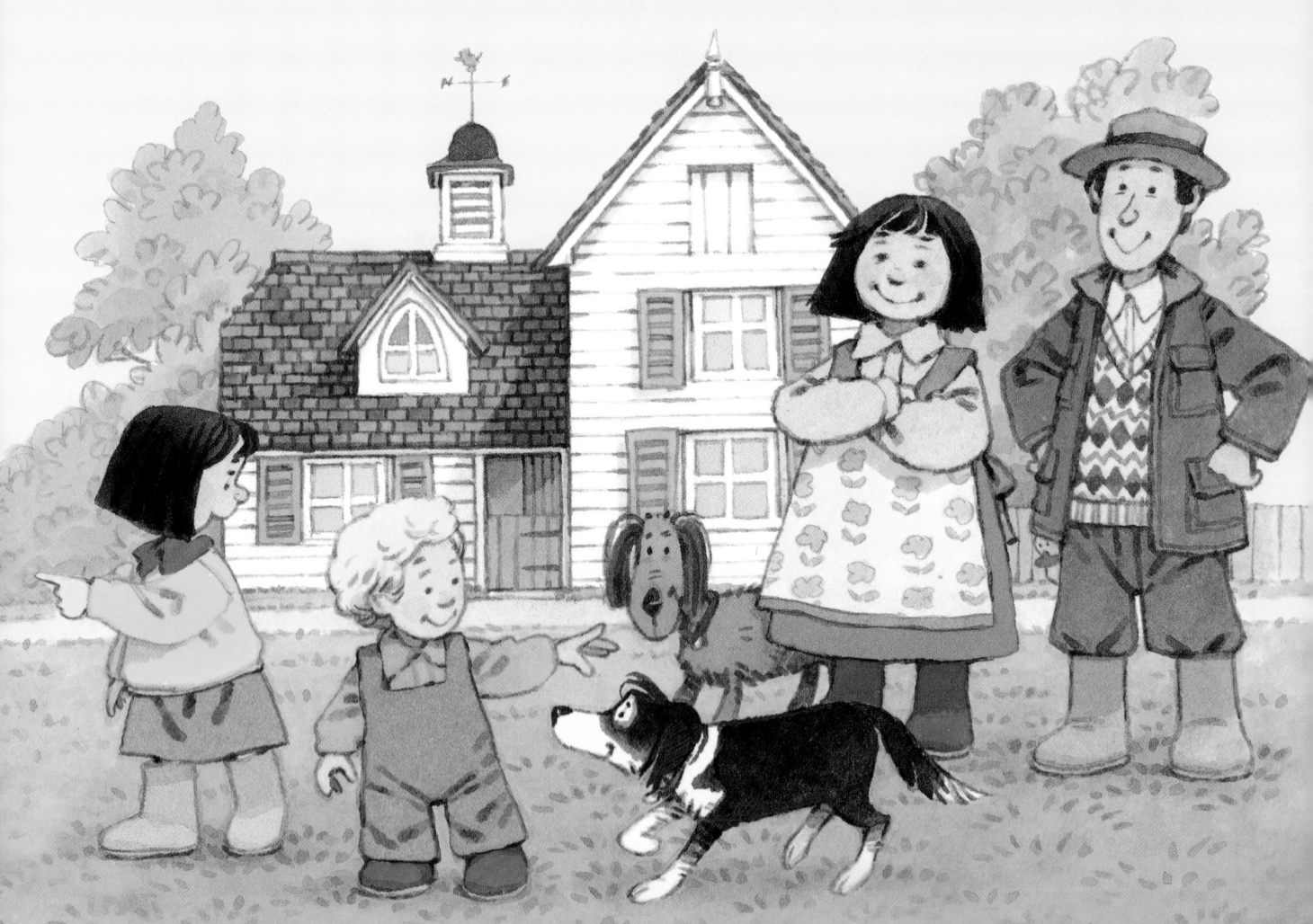

"Come on, Patch," says Sam. "We'll show you all the animals on our farm."

First they look at the hens.

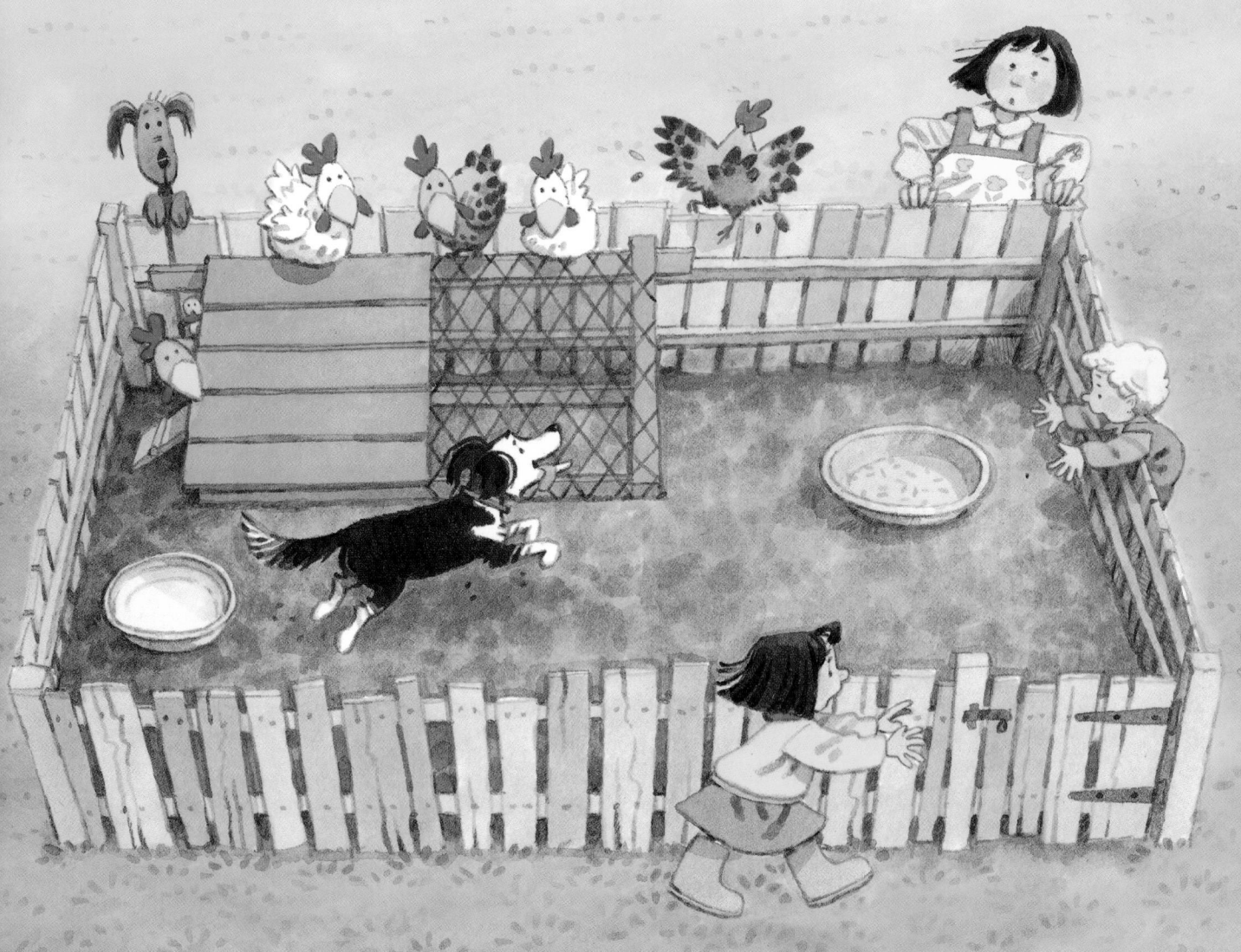

Patch jumps into the hen run and chases the hens.
They are frightened and fly up onto their house.

"Now we'll go and see the cows."

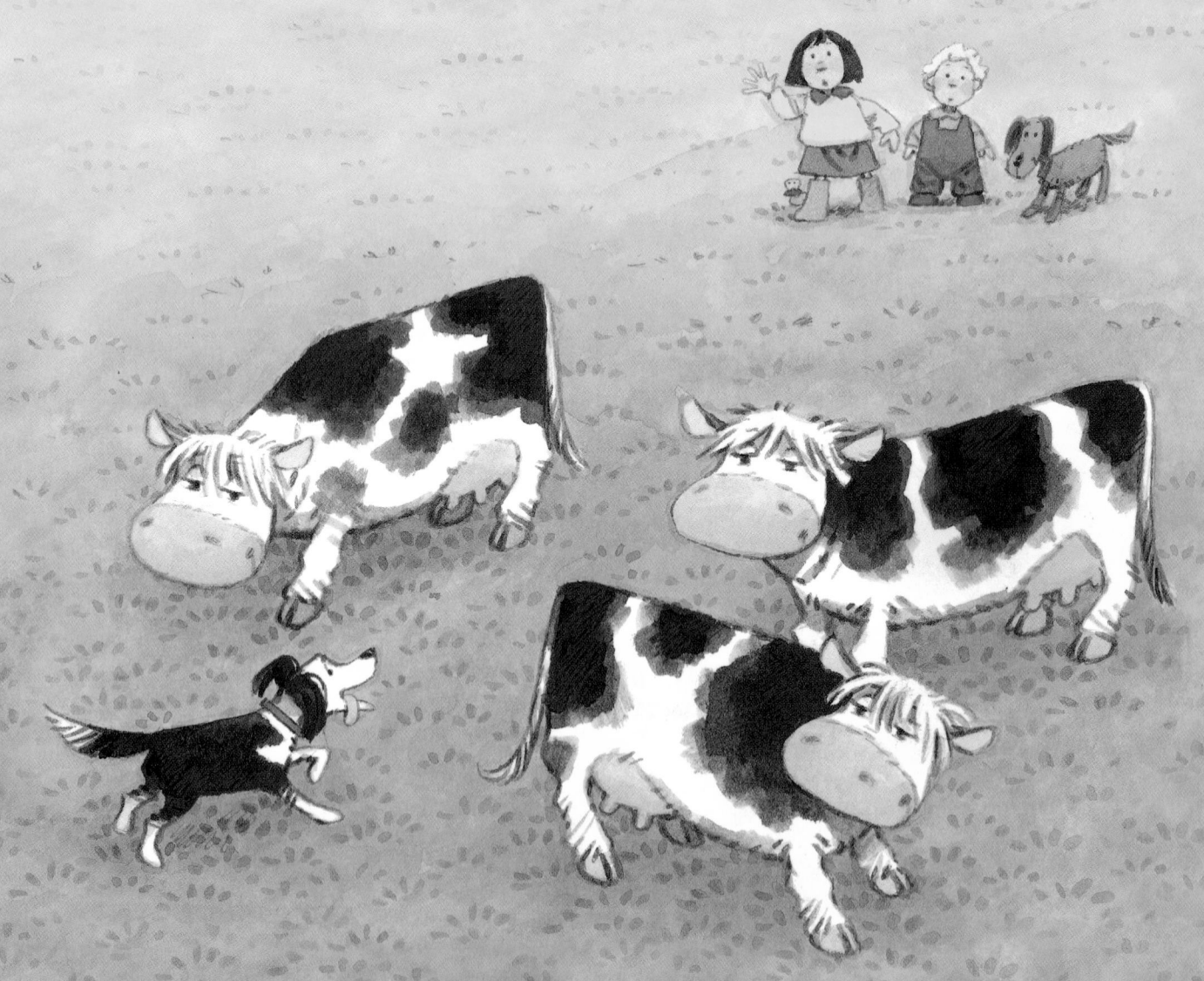

Patch runs into the field and barks at the cows.
But they just stand and stare at him.

Then they look at the pigs.

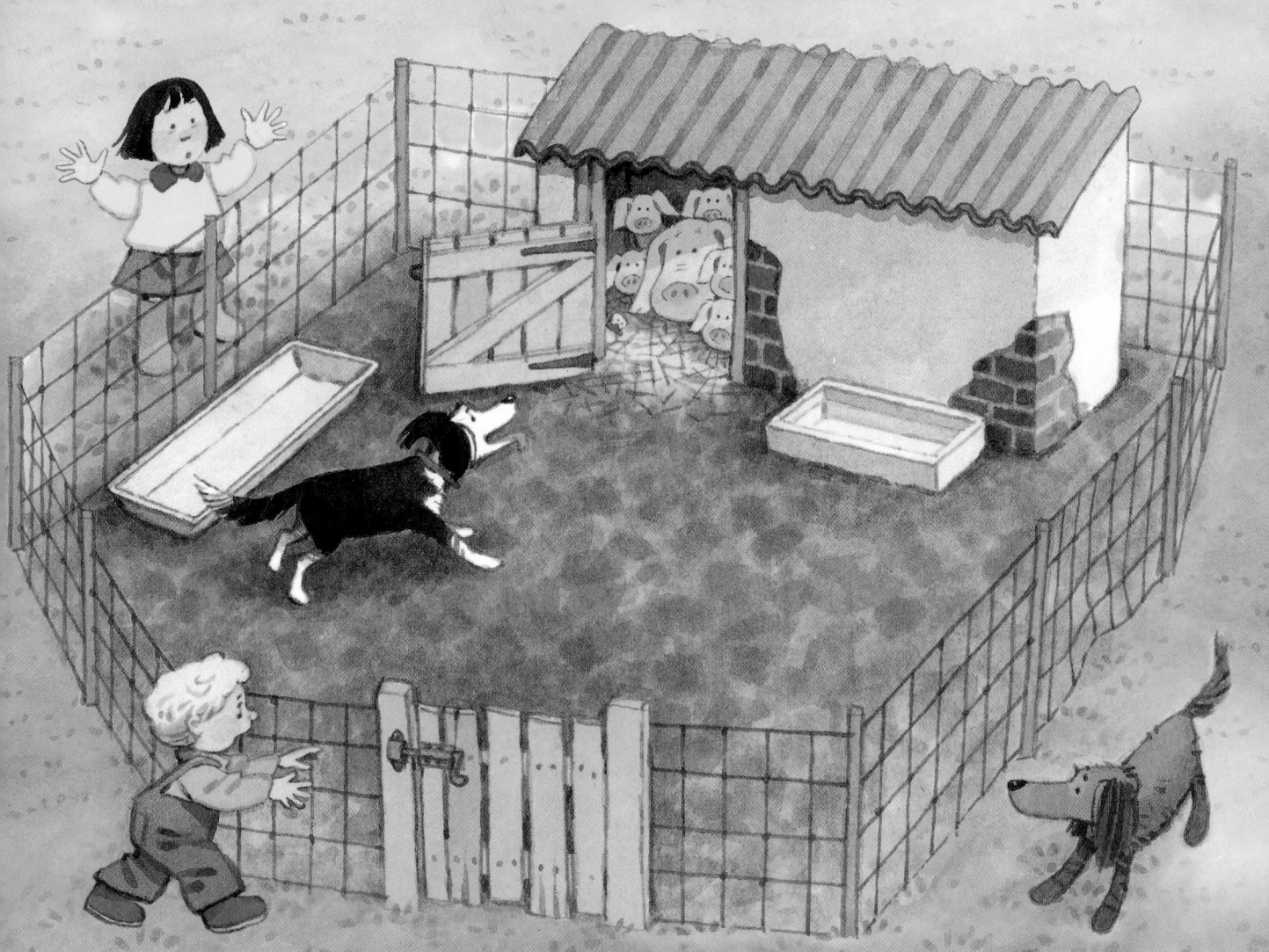

Patch jumps into the pig pen and chases all the pigs
into their little house.

Sam shouts at Patch.

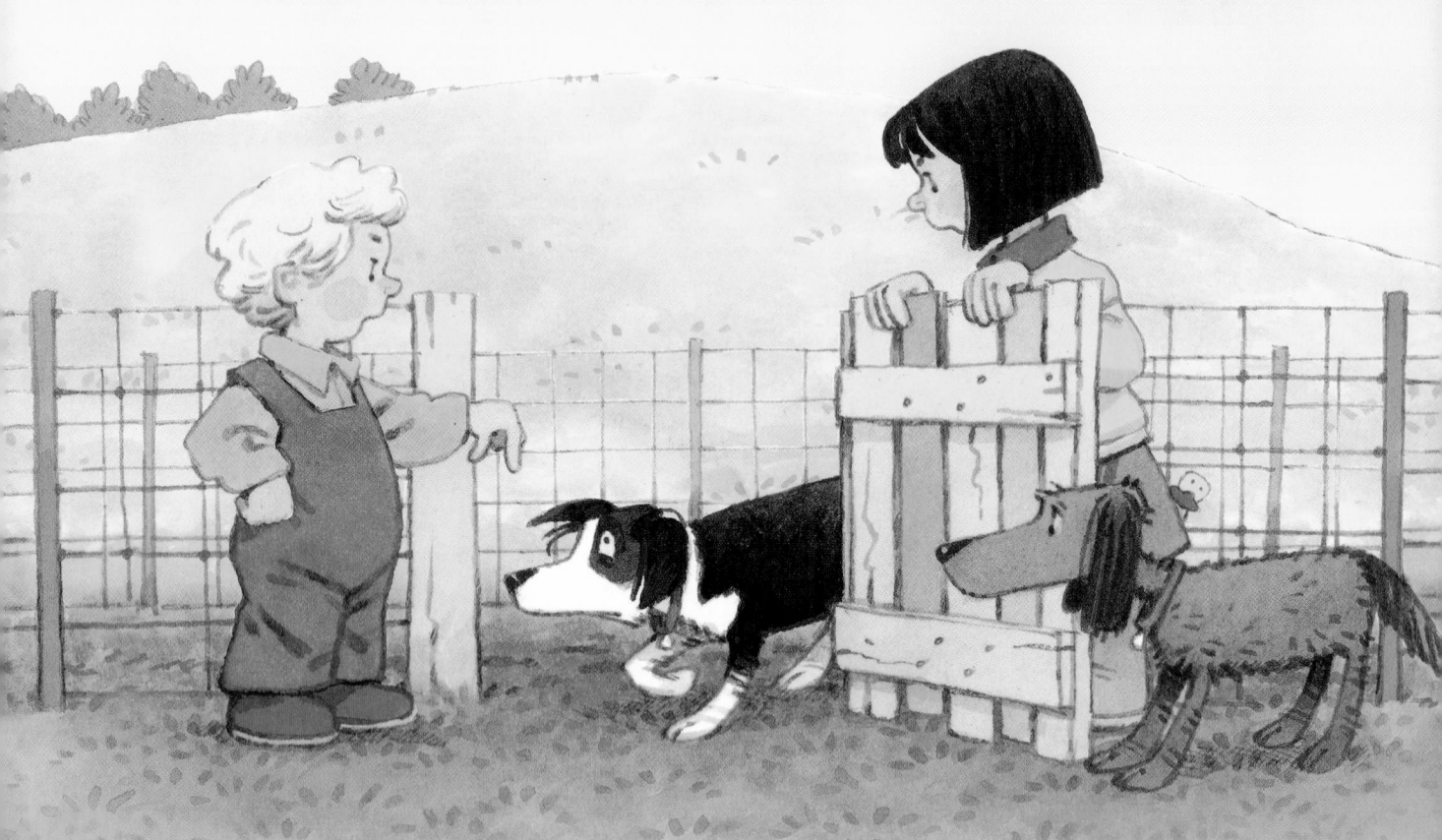

"Come here, you silly thing. You're meant to be
a sheepdog. Ted will have to send you back."

They go to the sheep field.

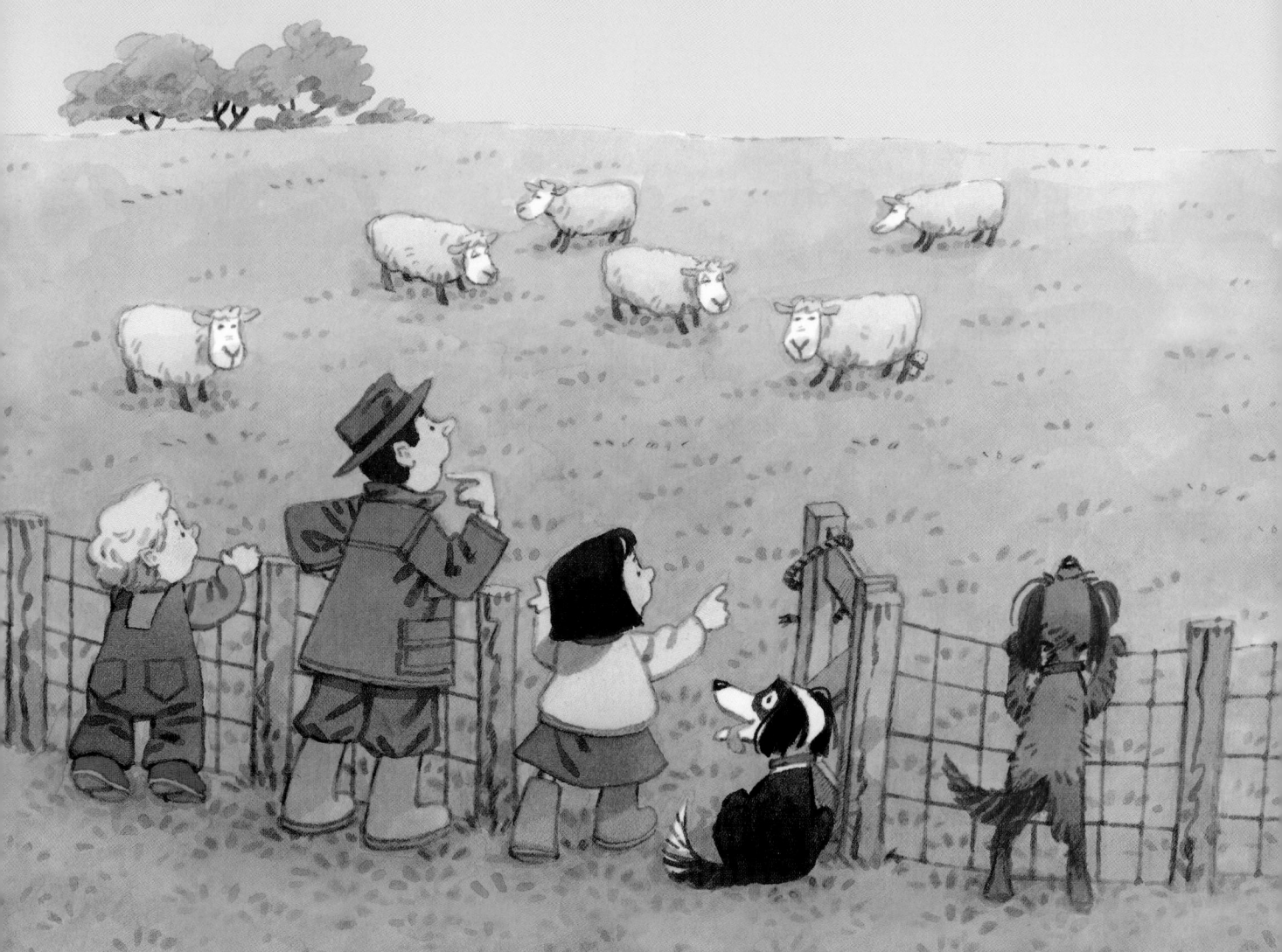

"Look," says Sam. "One sheep is missing." "Yes, it's
that naughty Woolly again," says Ted.

"Where's Patch going?" says Sam.

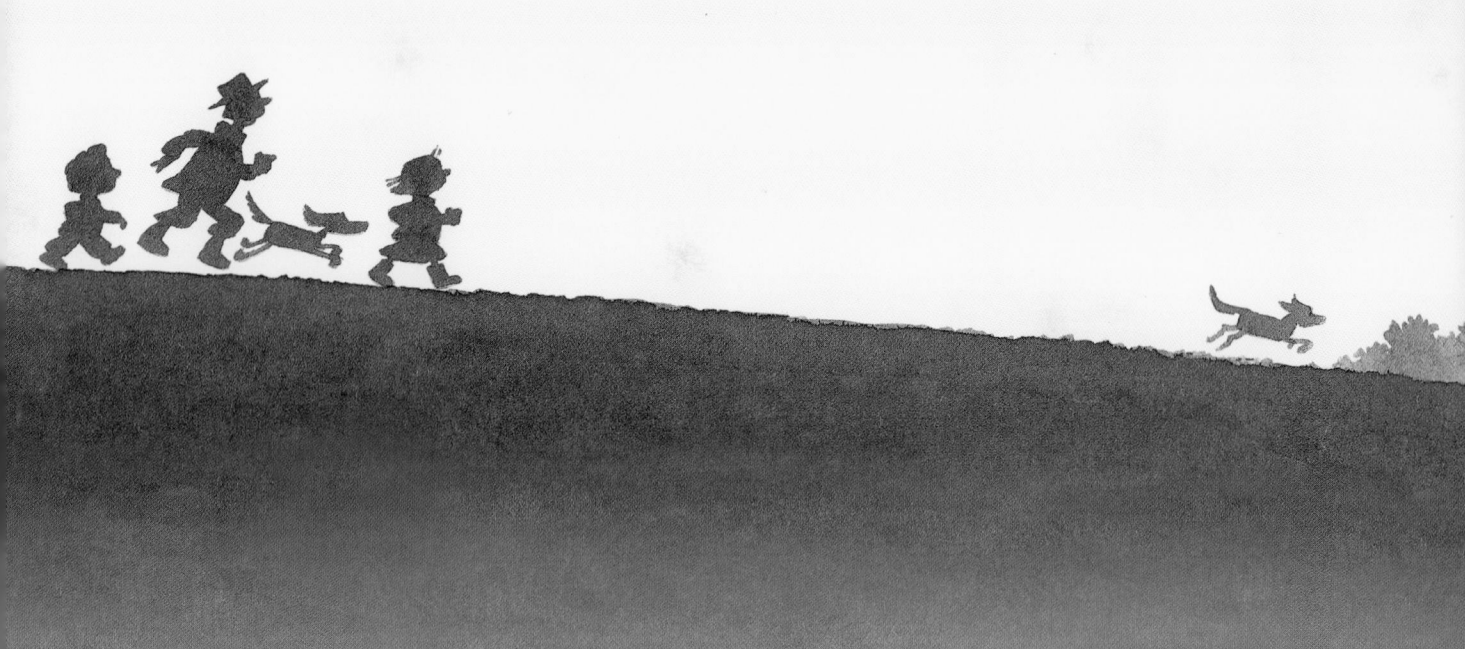

Patch runs away across the field. Ted, Sam, Poppy
and Rusty run after him.

Patch dives through the hedge.

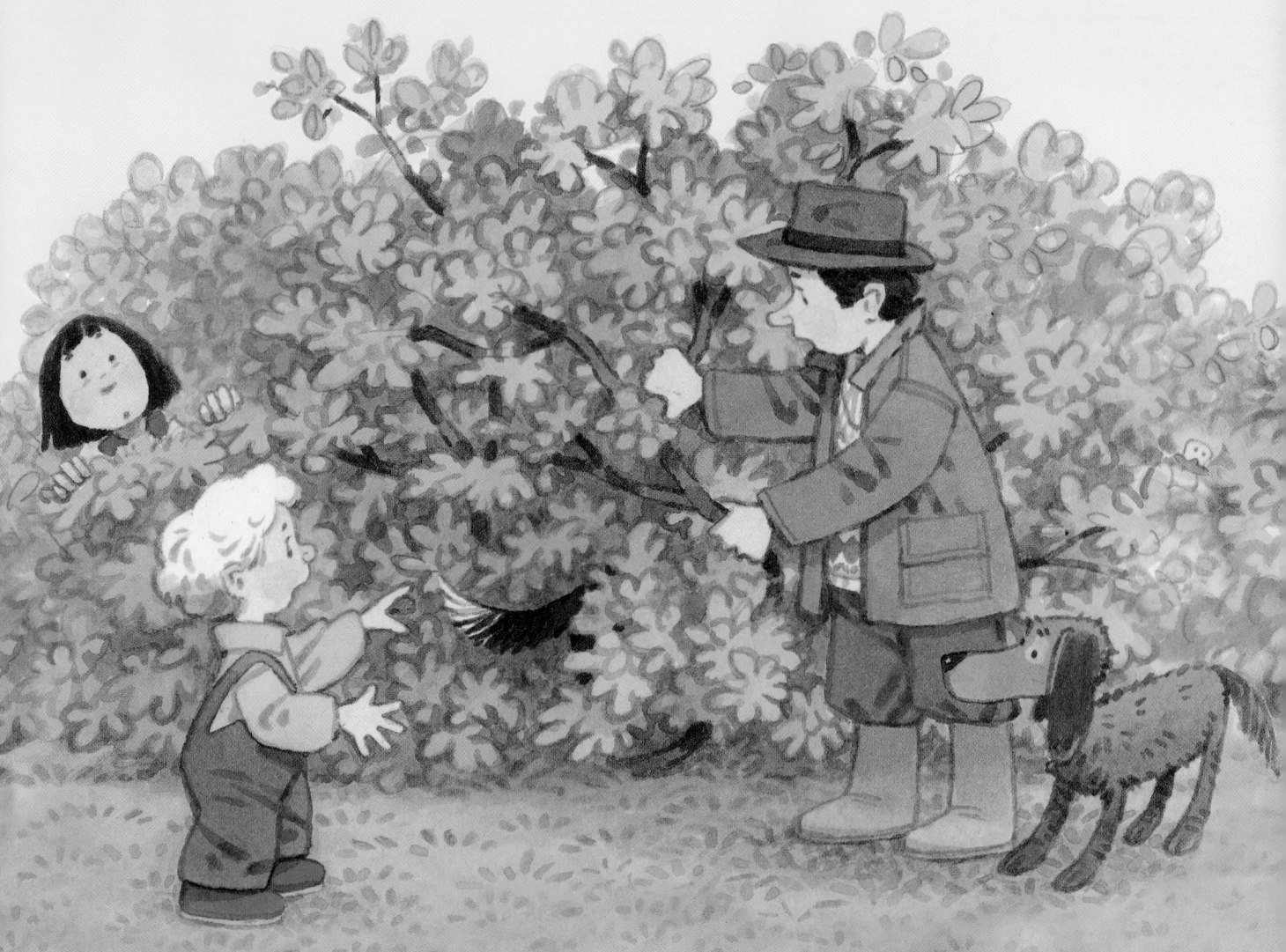

Patch barks and barks. "What has he found?"
says Sam. They all go to look.

Patch has found a boy.

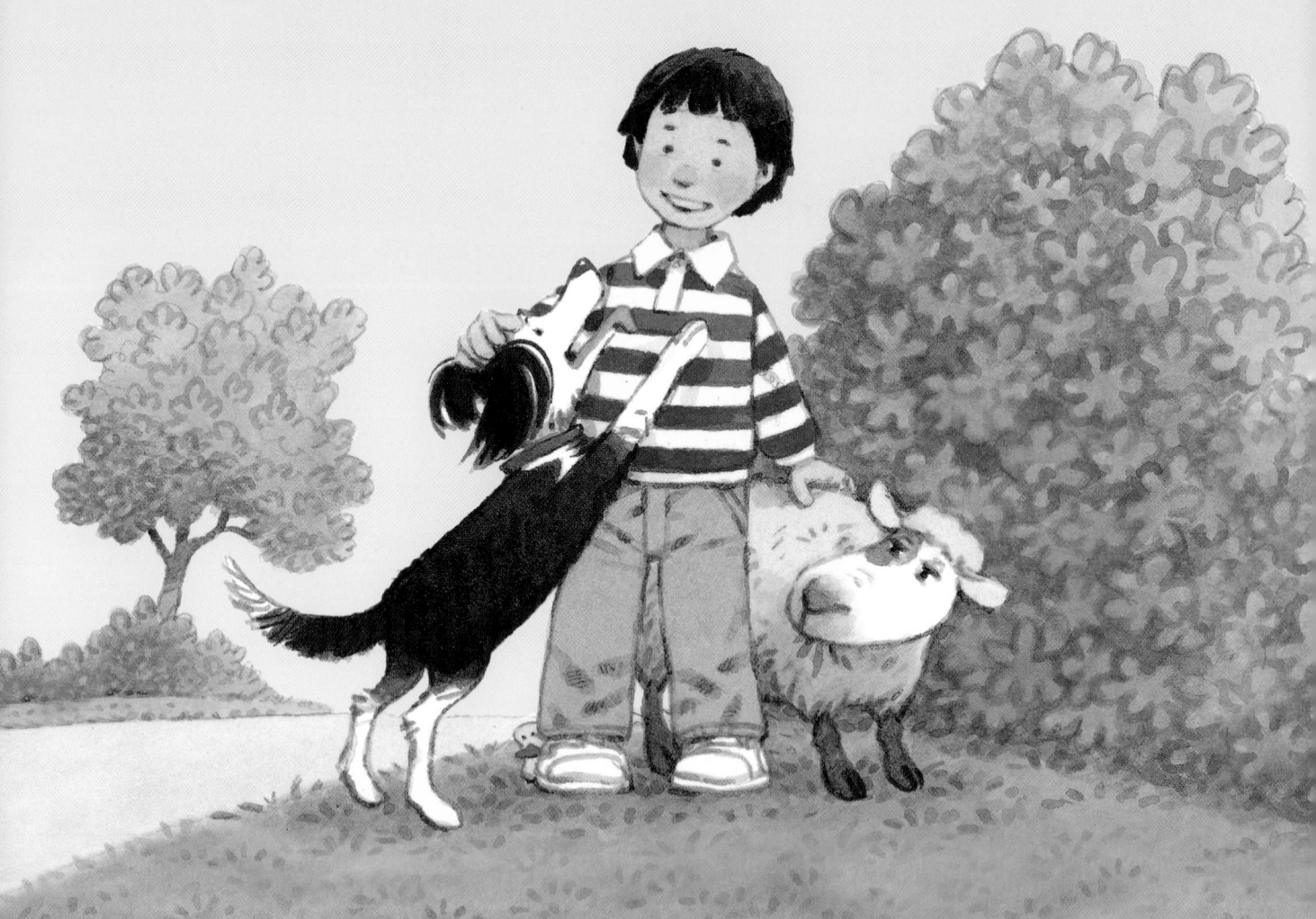

The boy pats Patch. "Hello," he says. "I wondered who bought you when my dad sold his farm."

The boy has found a sheep.

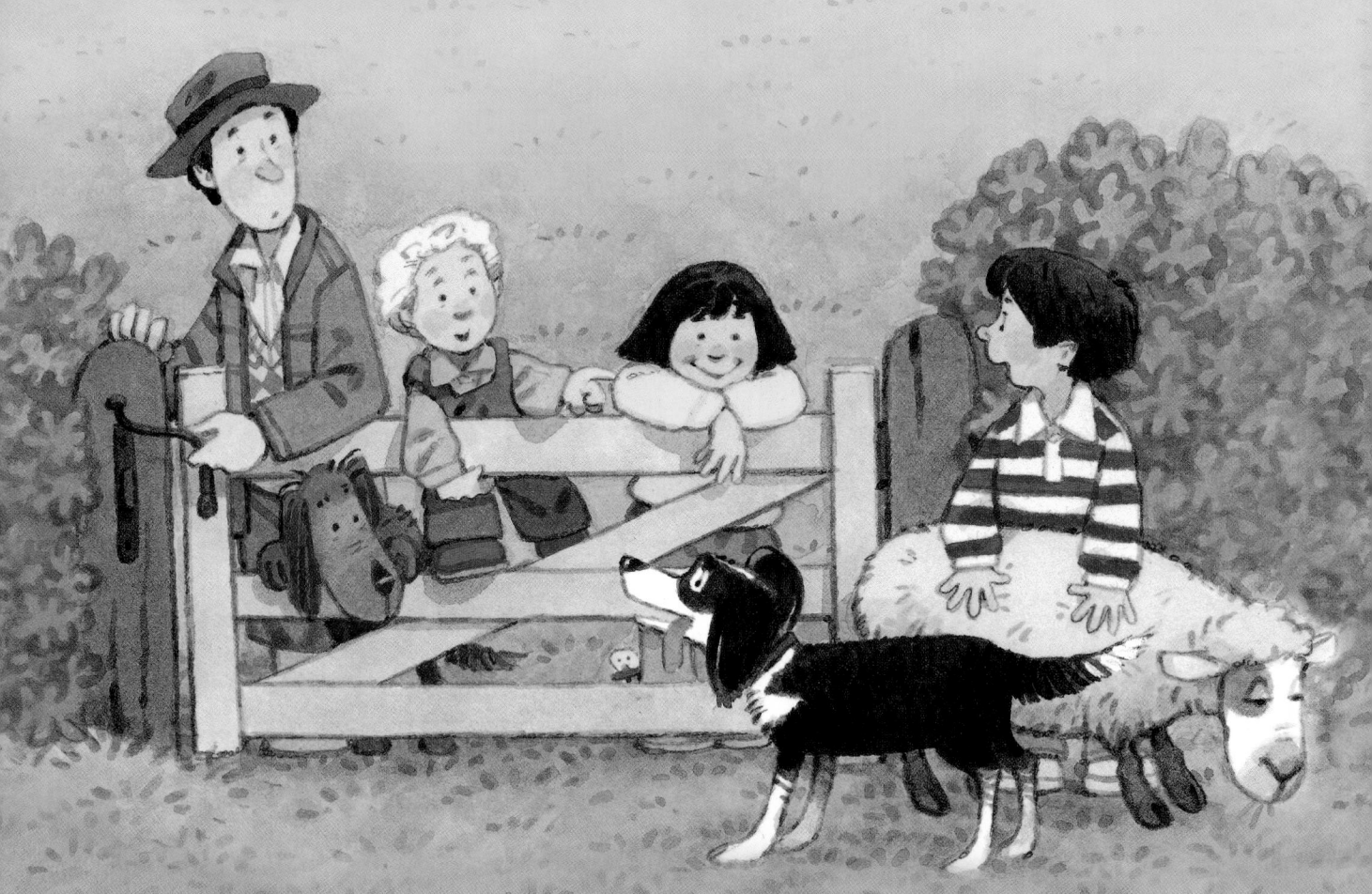

"There's Woolly," says Sam. "I found her on the
road," says the boy. "I was bringing her back."

The boy whistles to Patch.

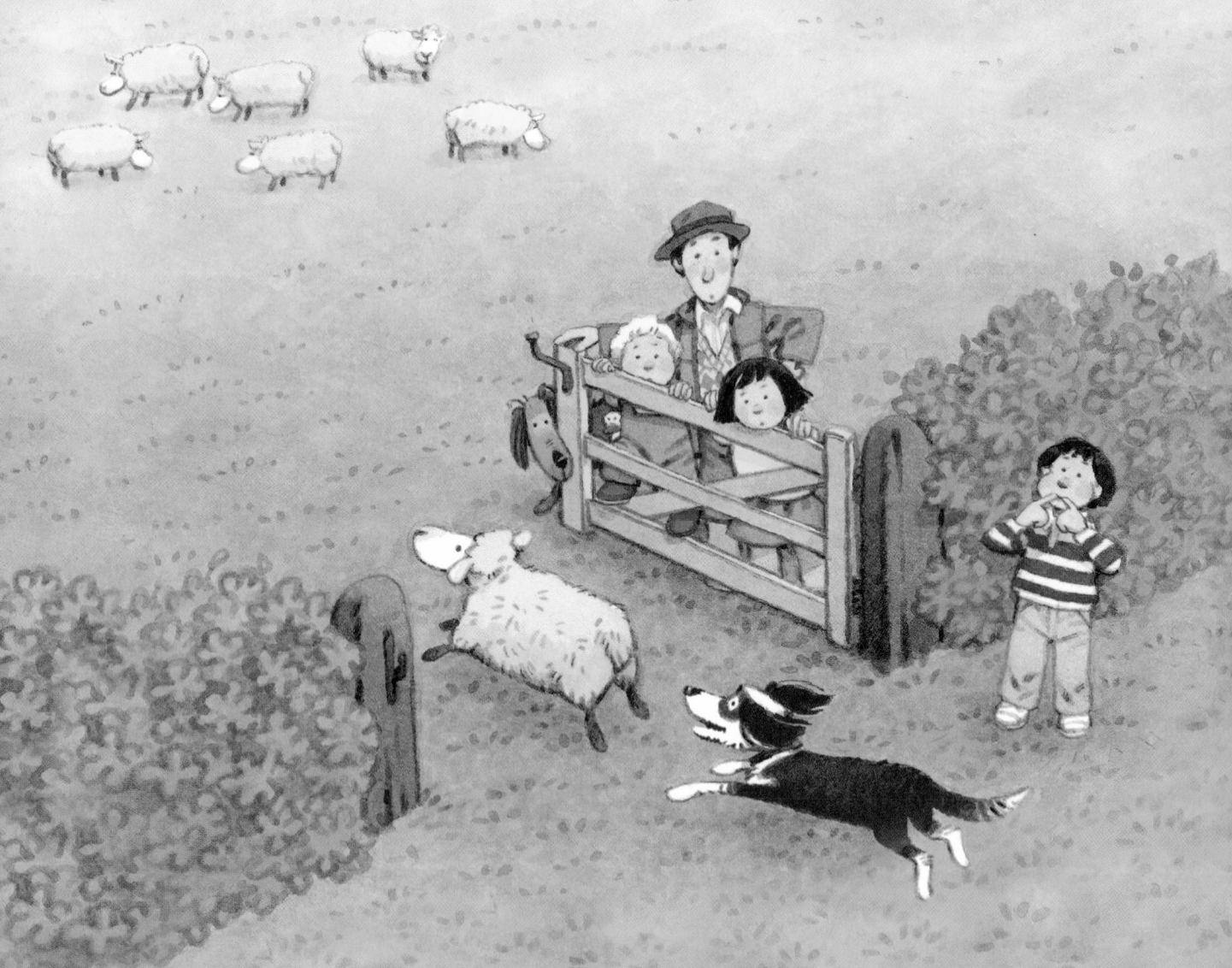

Patch chases Woolly back through the gate.
She runs into the field with the other sheep.

Ted stares in surprise.

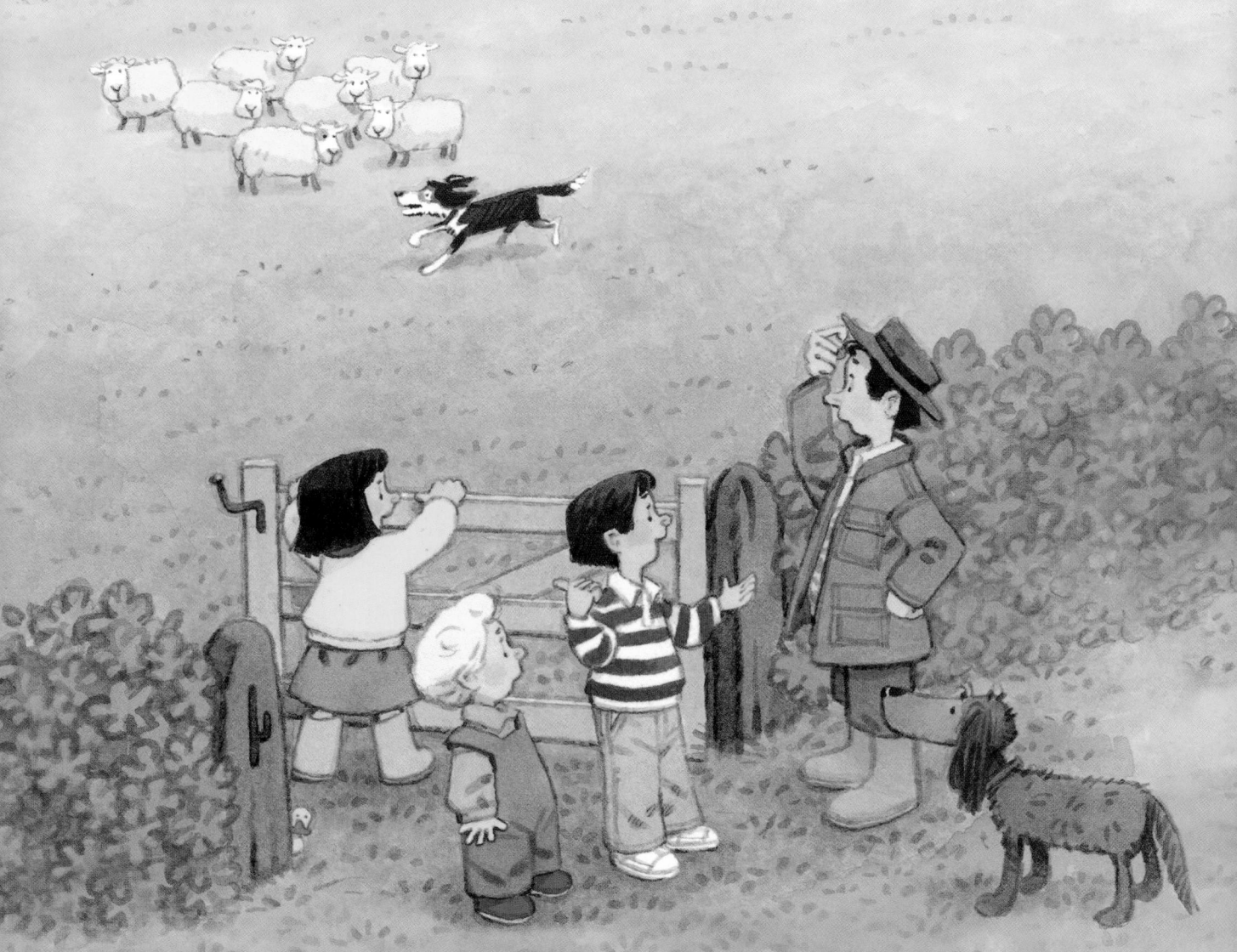

"Patch doesn't do anything I tell him," says Ted.
"You don't know how to whistle," says the boy.

Patch runs back to them.

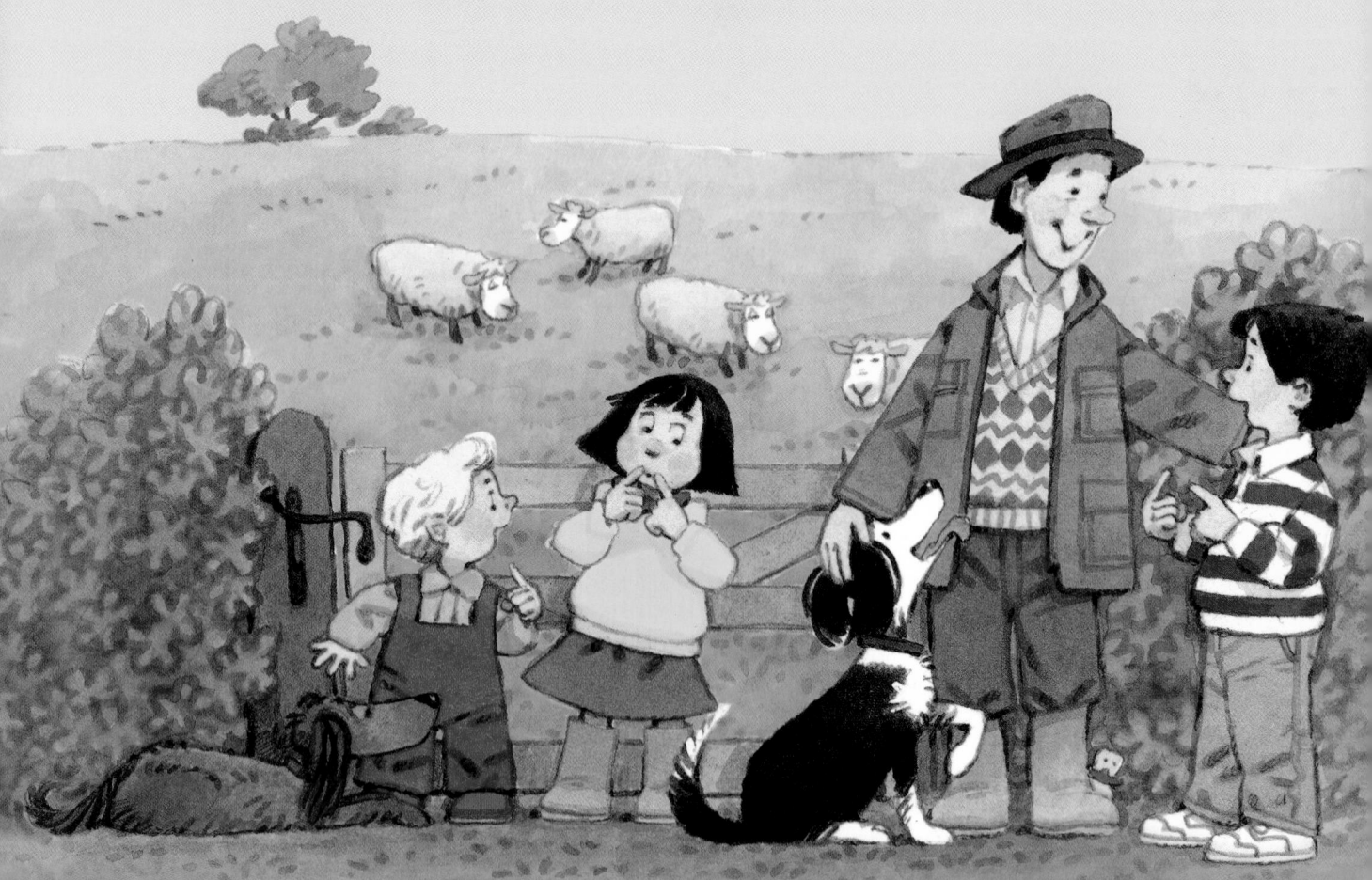

"You must teach me how to whistle to Patch,"
says Ted. "He's not a silly dog after all," says Sam.

Kitten's Day Out

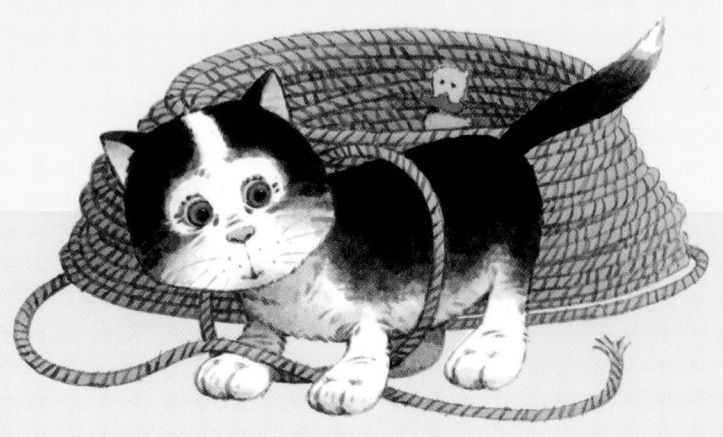

This is Apple Tree Farm.

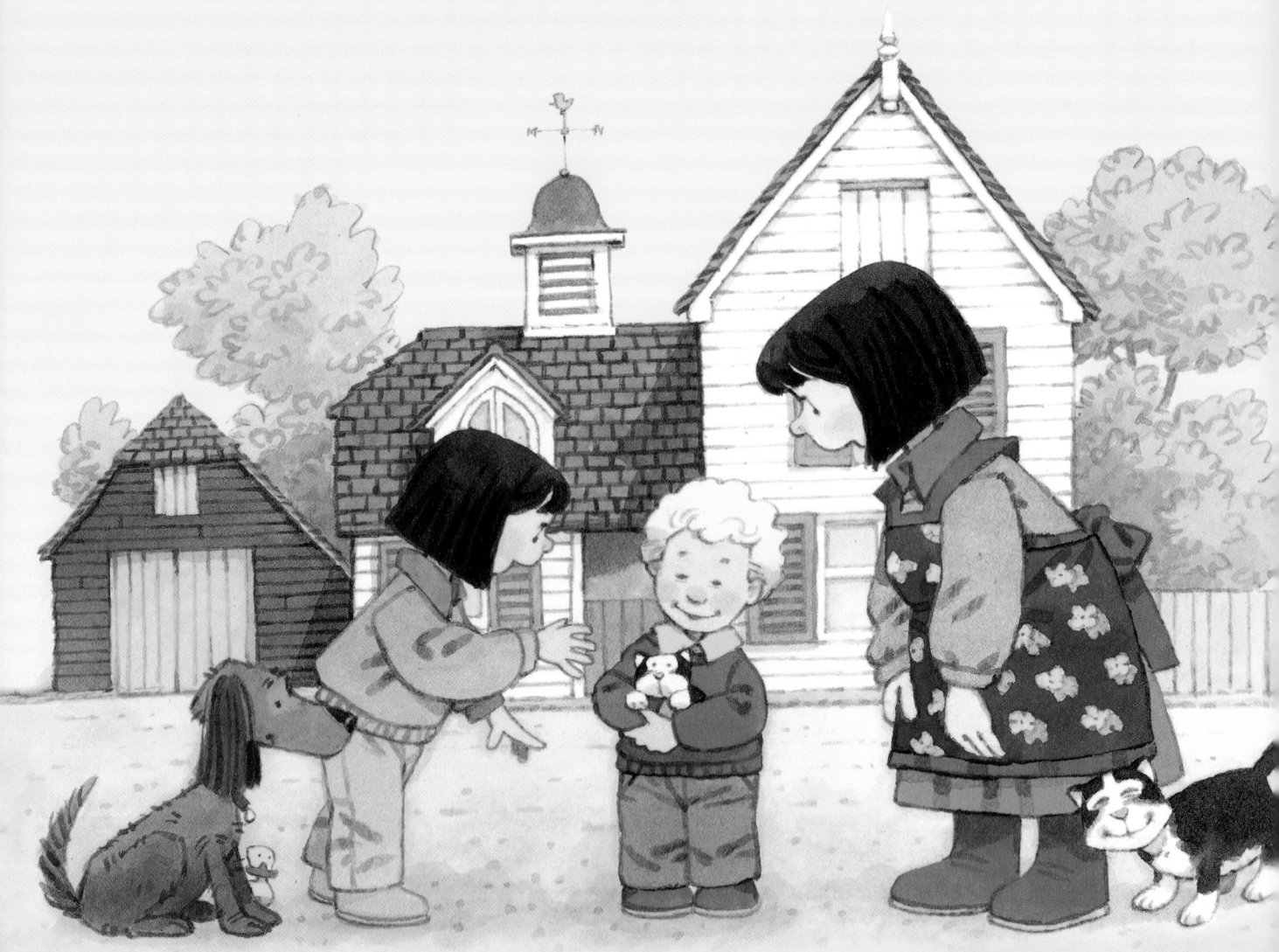

This is Mrs. Boot, the farmer. She has two children, called Poppy and Sam, and a dog called Rusty.

Ted works on the farm.

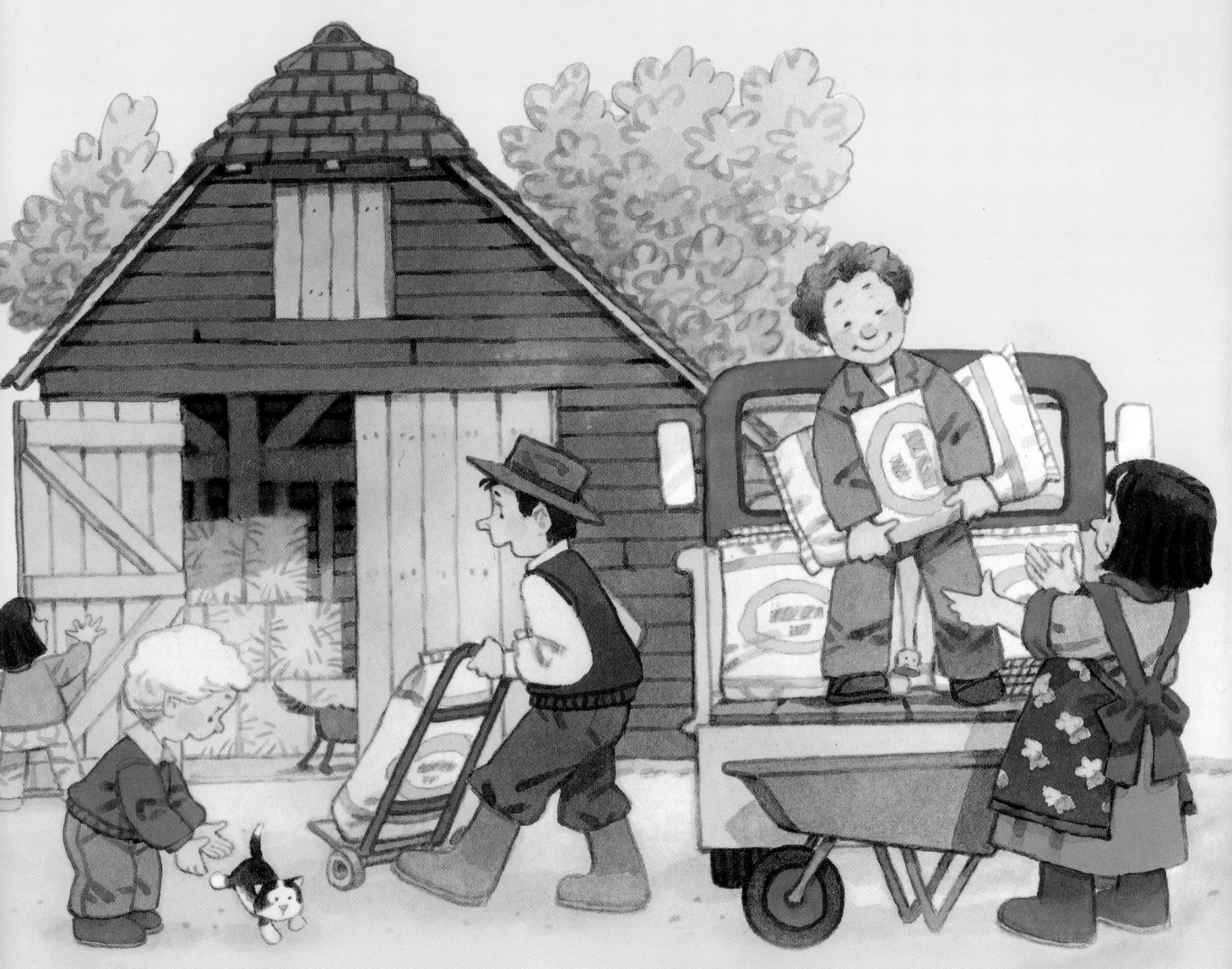

He is helping Mr. Bran, the truck driver. Mr. Bran
has brought some sacks of food for the cows.

They say goodbye to Mr. Bran.

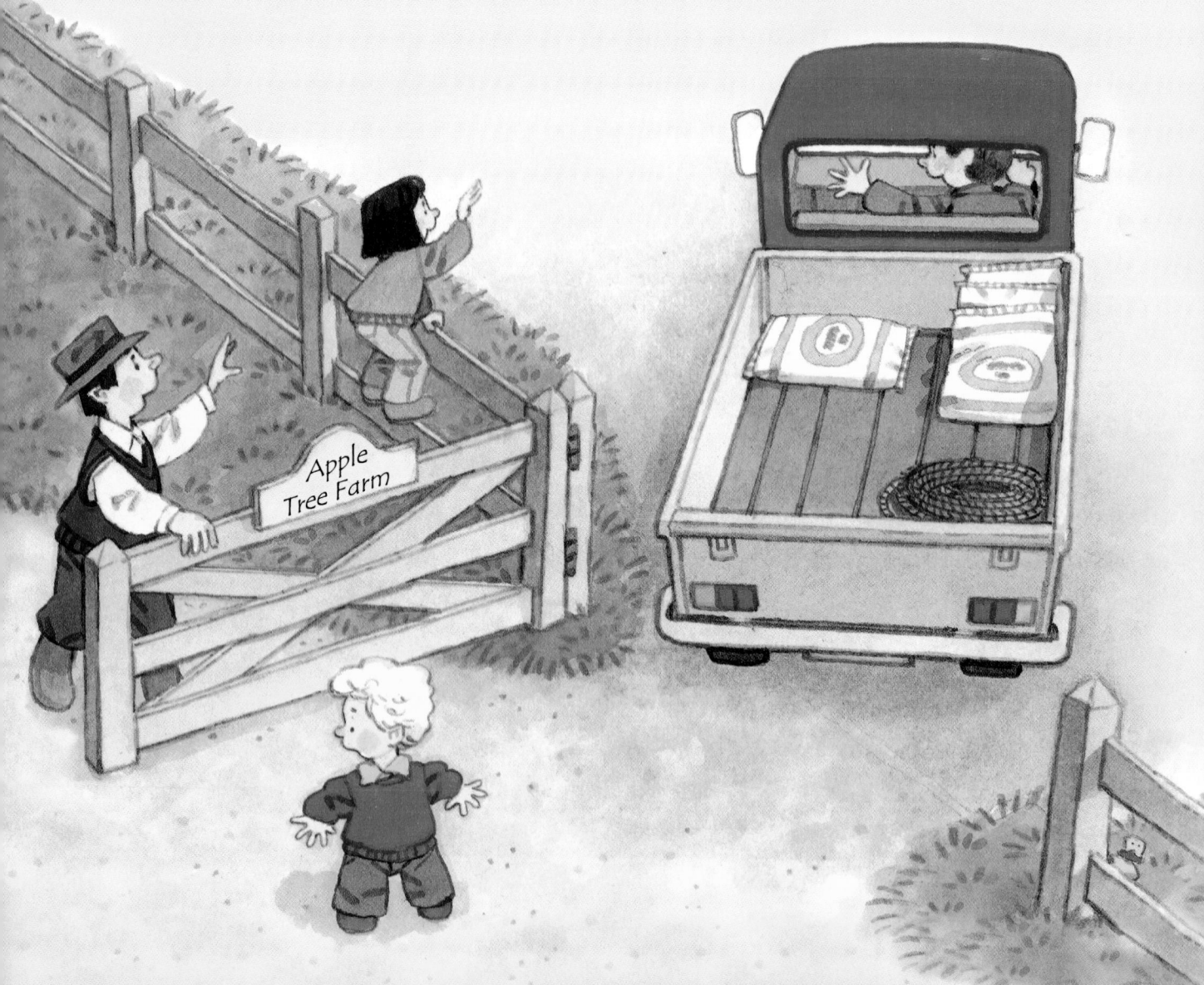

Mr. Bran waves as he drives his truck out
of the farmyard. Ted and Poppy wave back.

148

"Where's my kitten?"

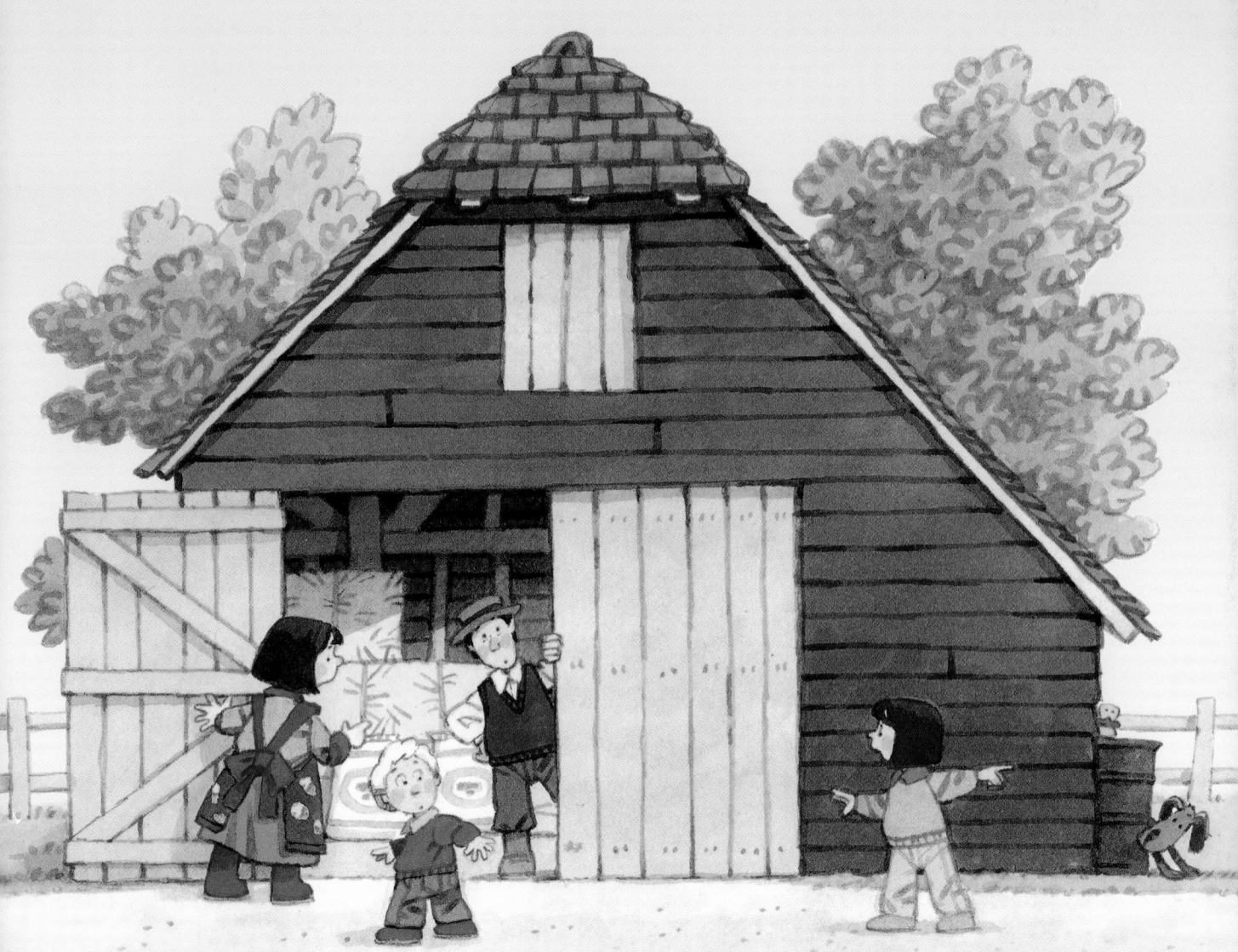

"Where's Fluff?" says Sam. They all look everywhere for Fluff. But they can't find her.

"Perhaps she jumped on the truck."

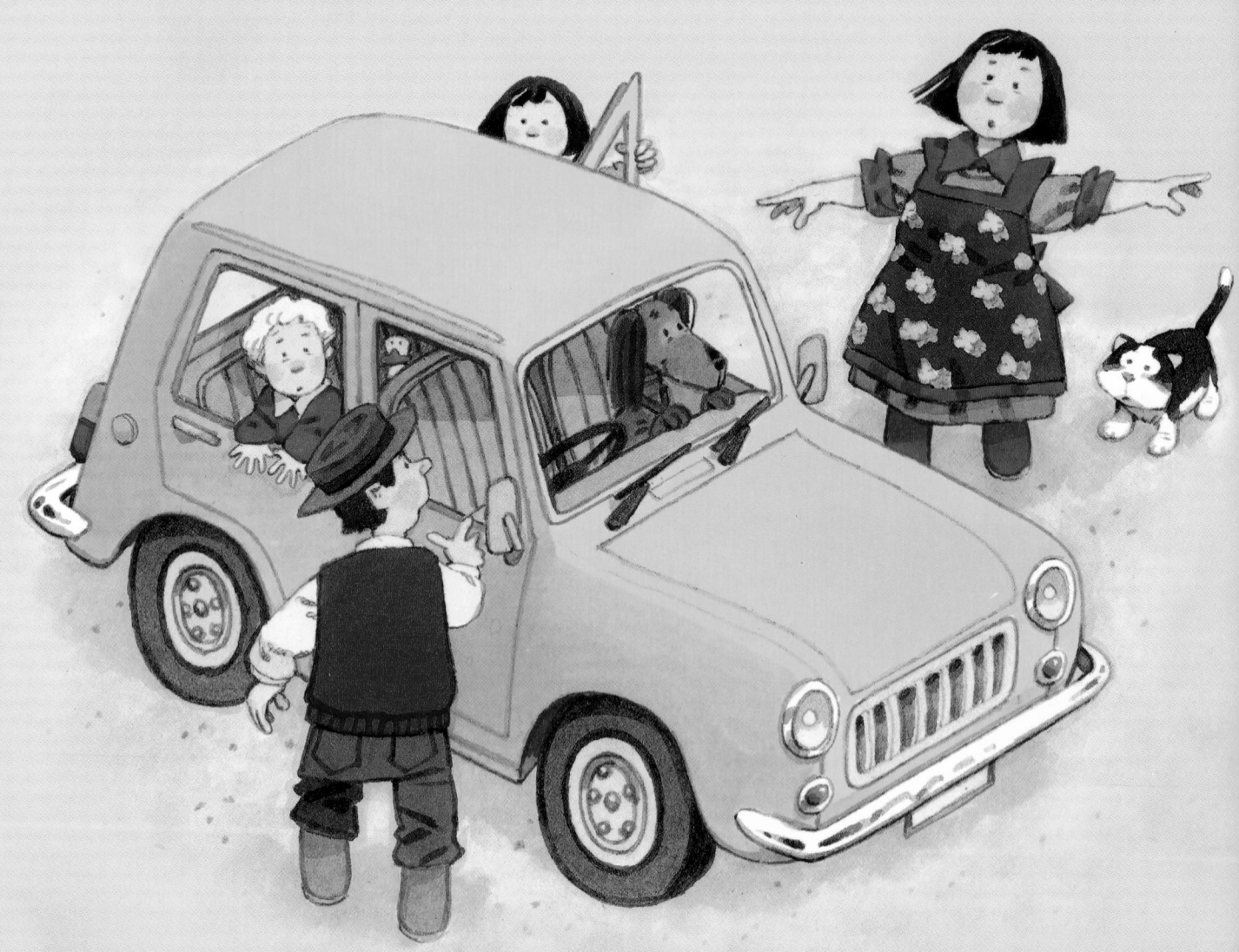

"Take my car and go after the truck, Ted," says Mrs. Boot. They jump in the car and drive off.

Ted stops the car at the crossroads.

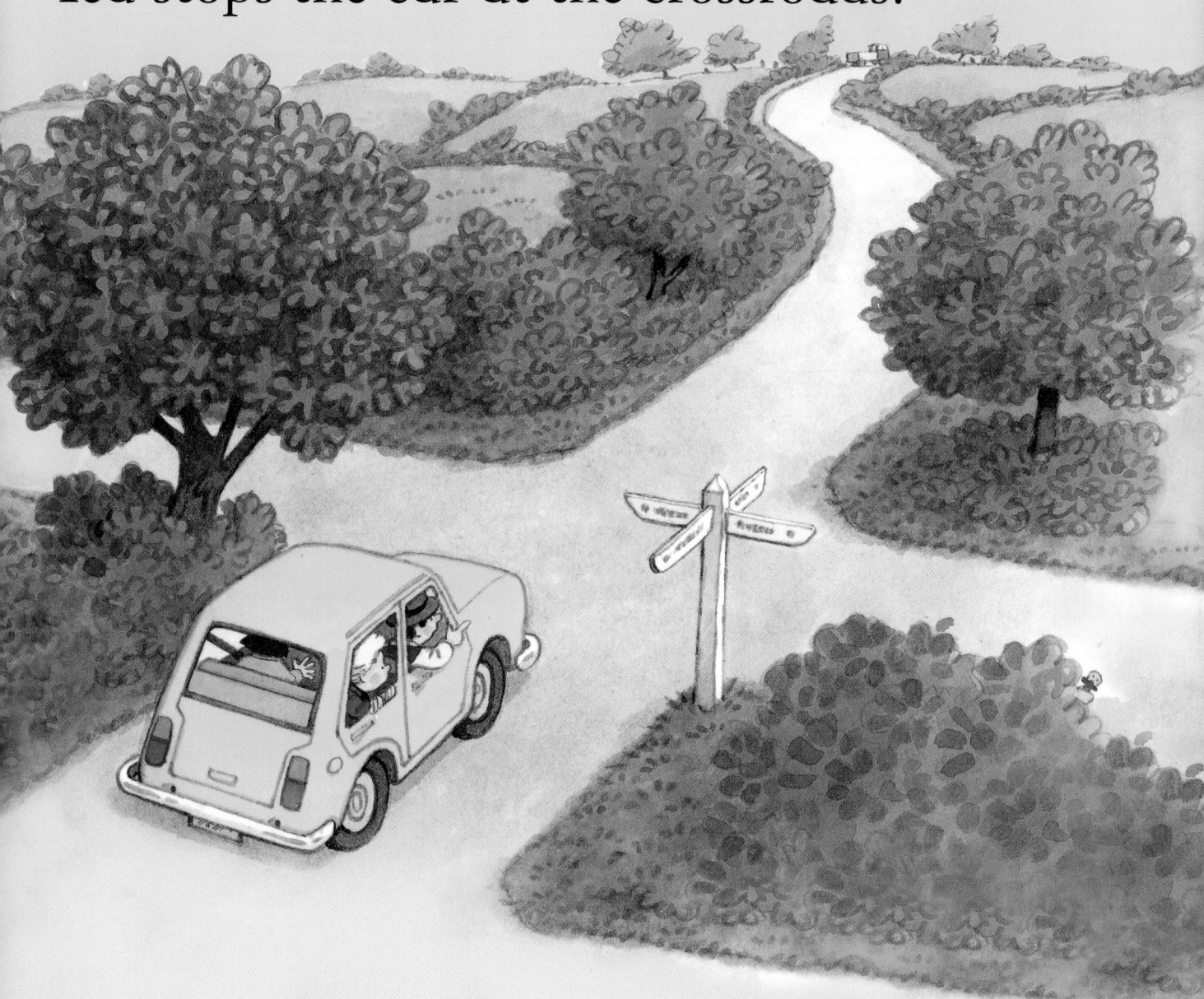

"Which way did Mr. Bran go?" says Ted. "There's a truck," says Sam. "It's just going around the bend."

Ted drives down a steep hill.

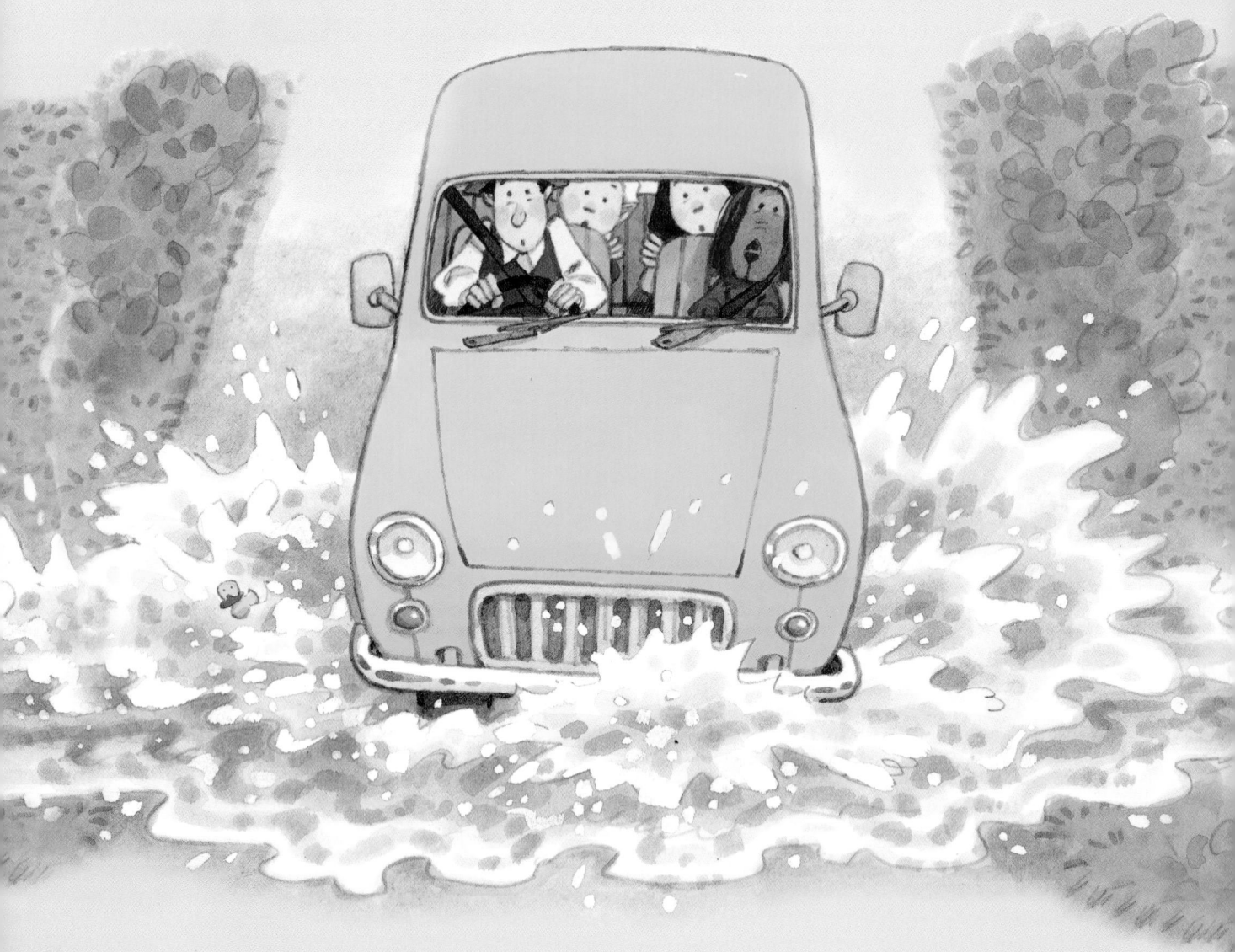

"Look out Ted," says Poppy. There's a stream at the bottom. The car splashes into the water.

The car stops in the stream.

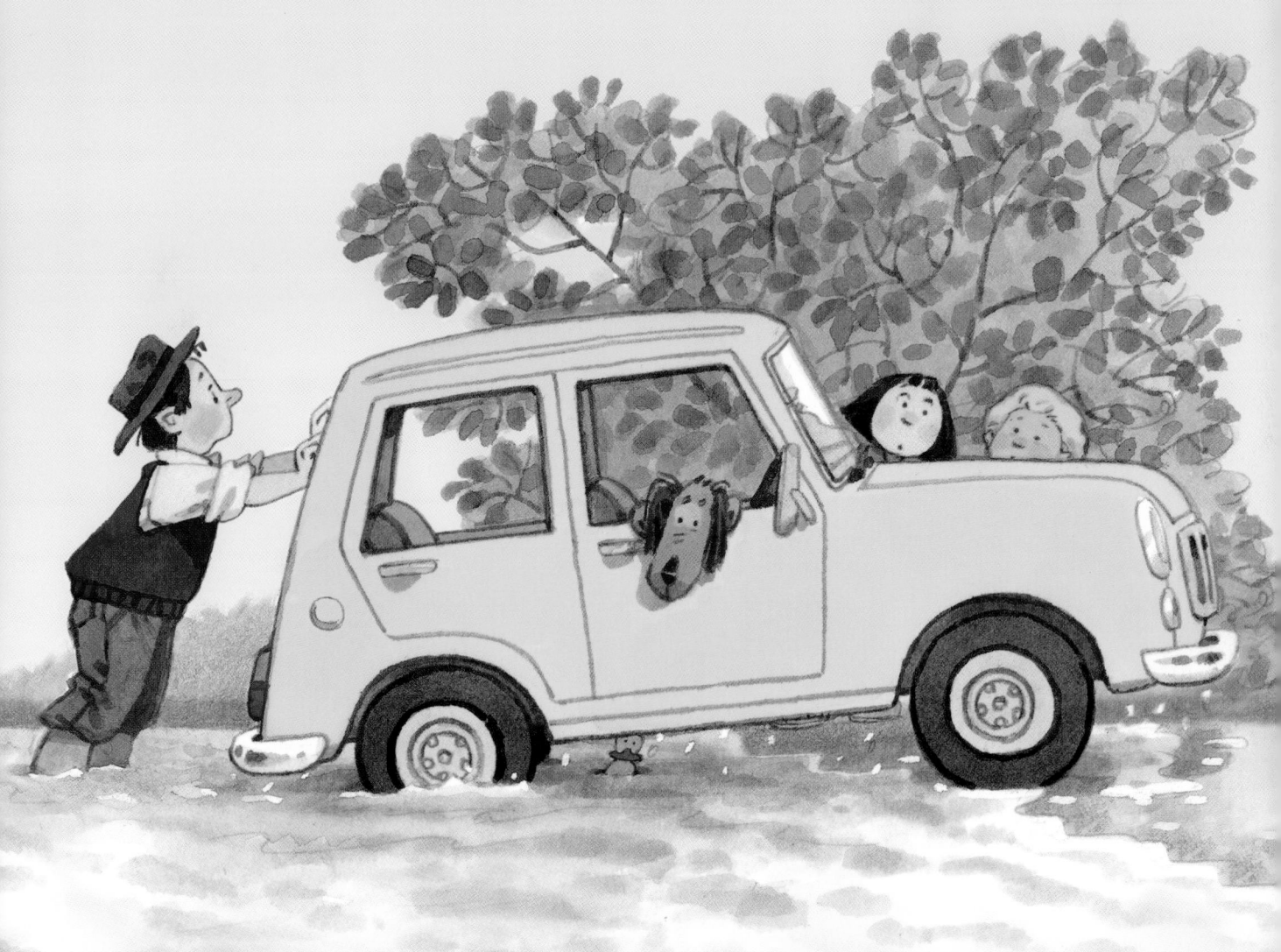

"Water in the engine," says Ted. "I'll have to push."
"We'll never find the truck now," says Sam.

Ted looks inside the car.

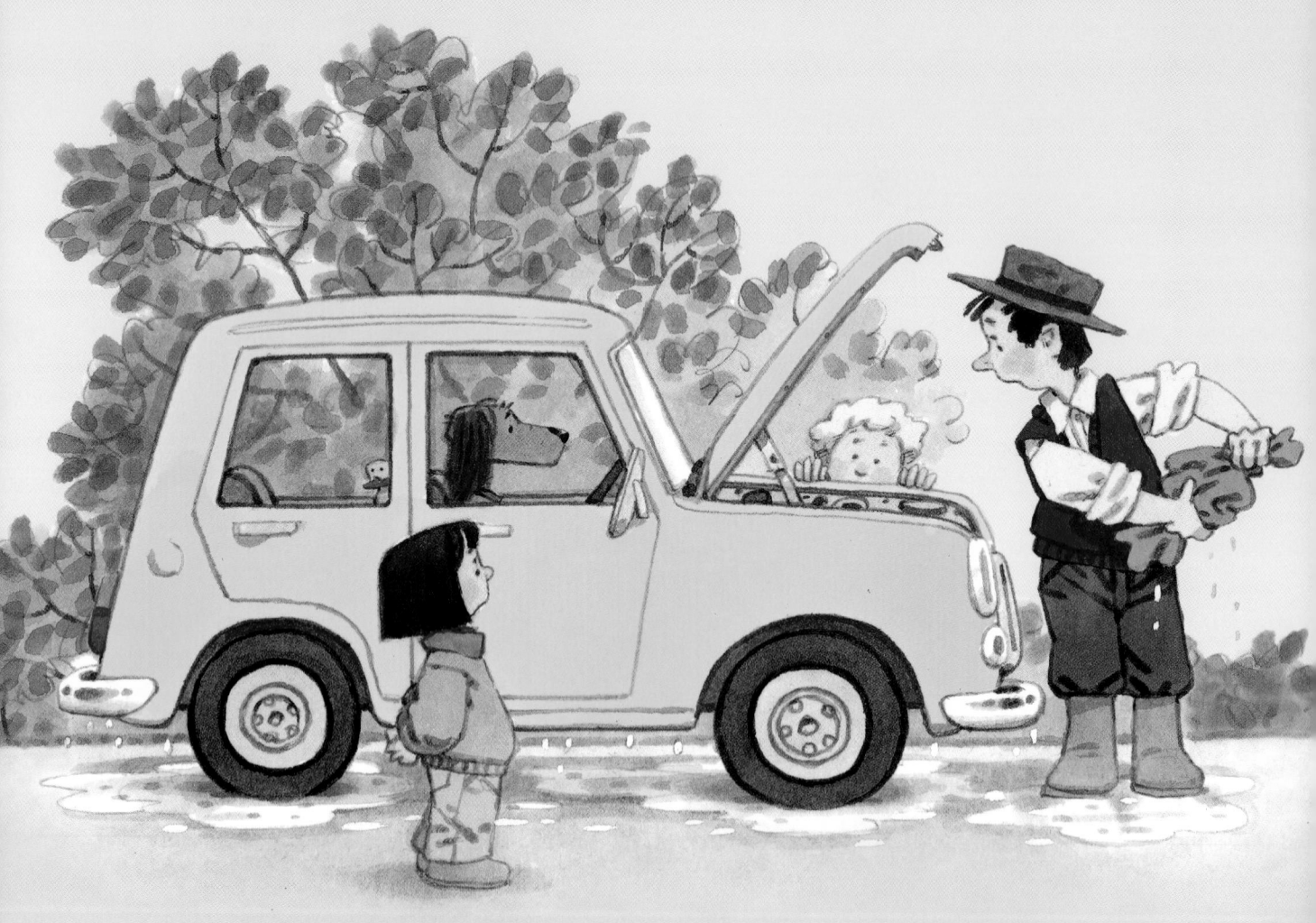

He mops up all the water. Soon he gets the car
to start again. They drive on to look for the truck.

There are lots of sheep on the road.

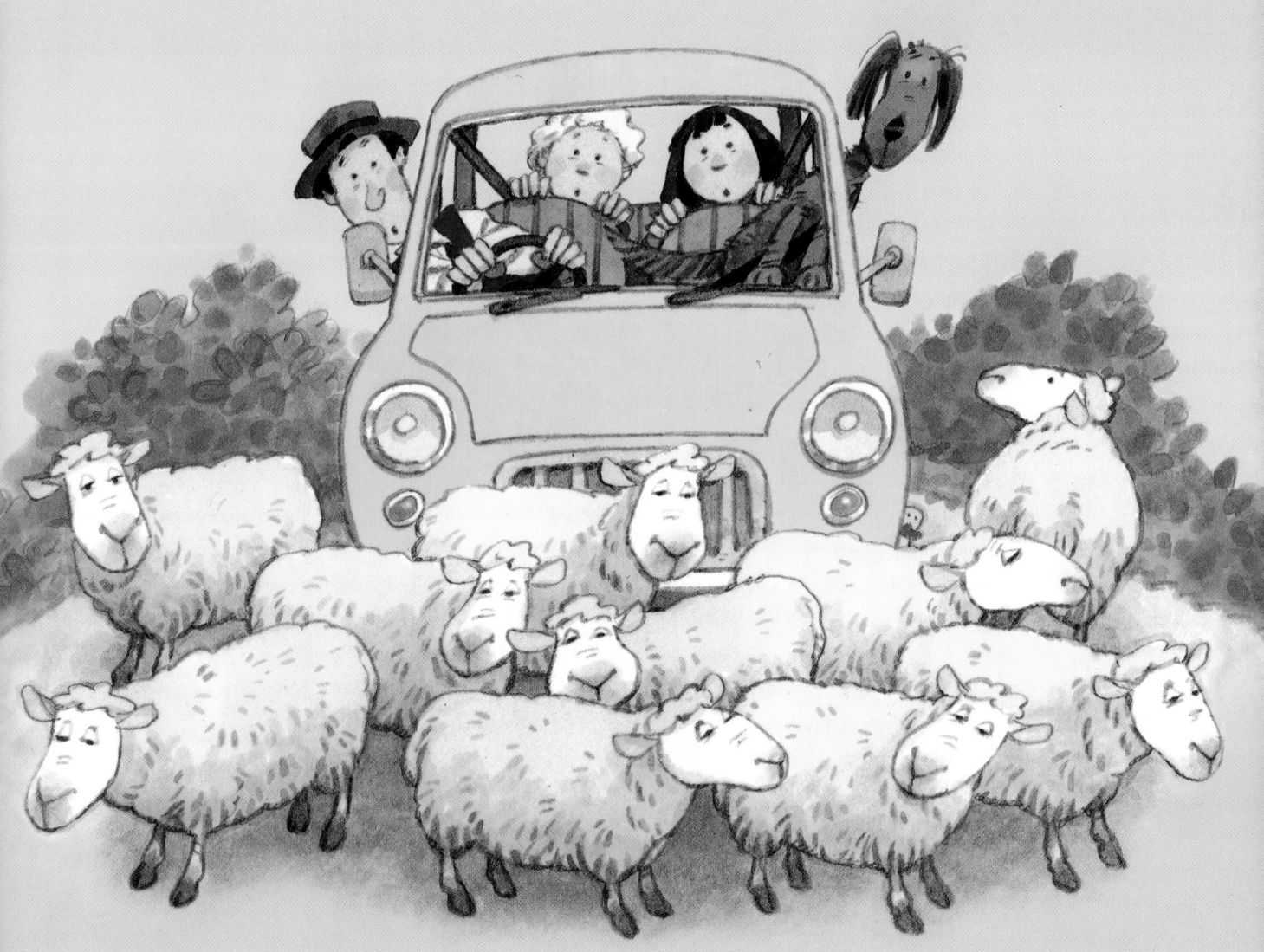

"The sheep came out of the field. Someone left the gate open," says Ted. "We must get them back."

Ted, Poppy and Sam round up the sheep.

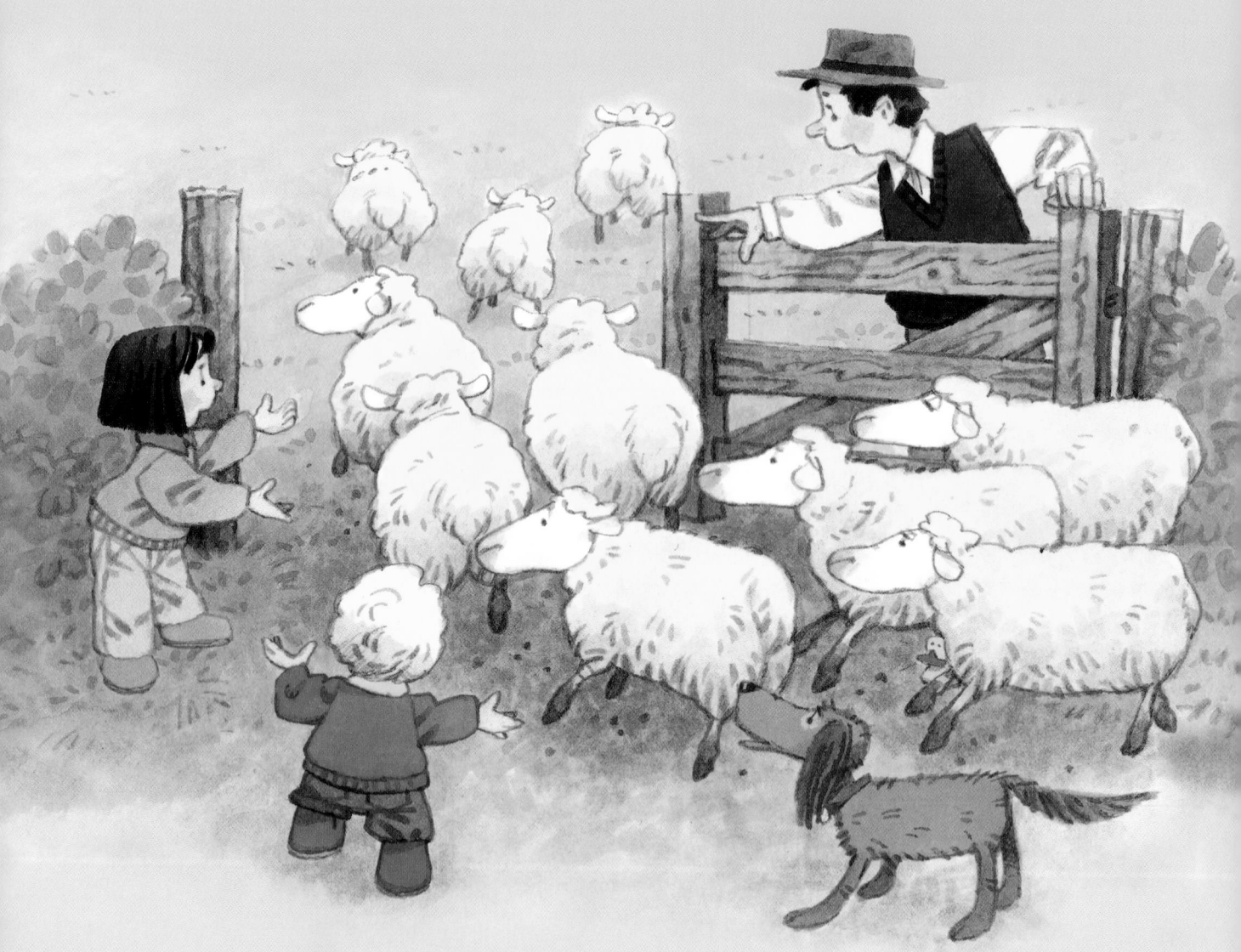

They drive them back into the field. Ted shuts the gate. "Come on, we must hurry," says Sam.

"Stop, Ted, there's a truck."

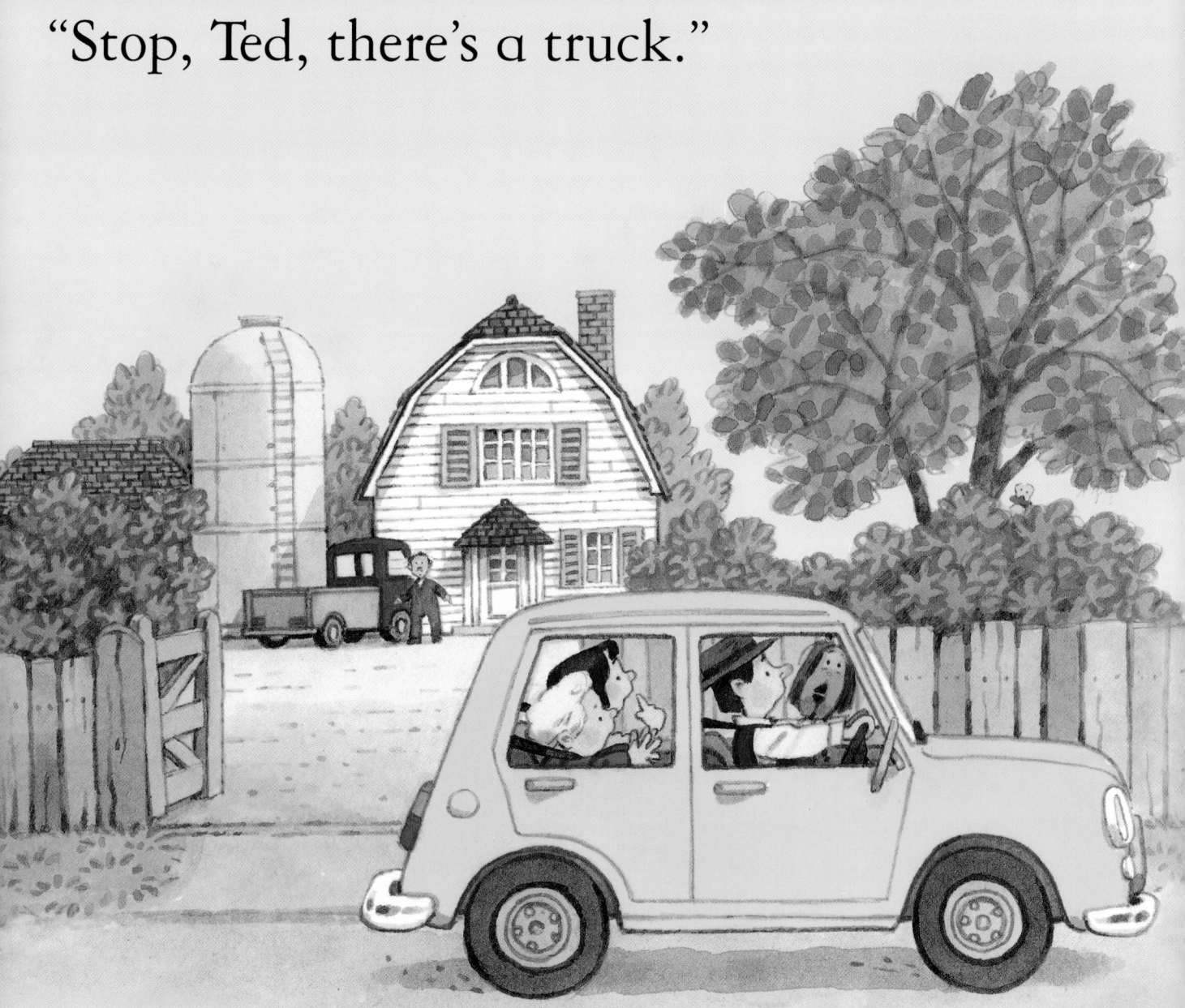

"I'm sure that's Mr. Bran's truck in that farmyard," says Sam. Ted drives in to see.

157

"It's the wrong truck."

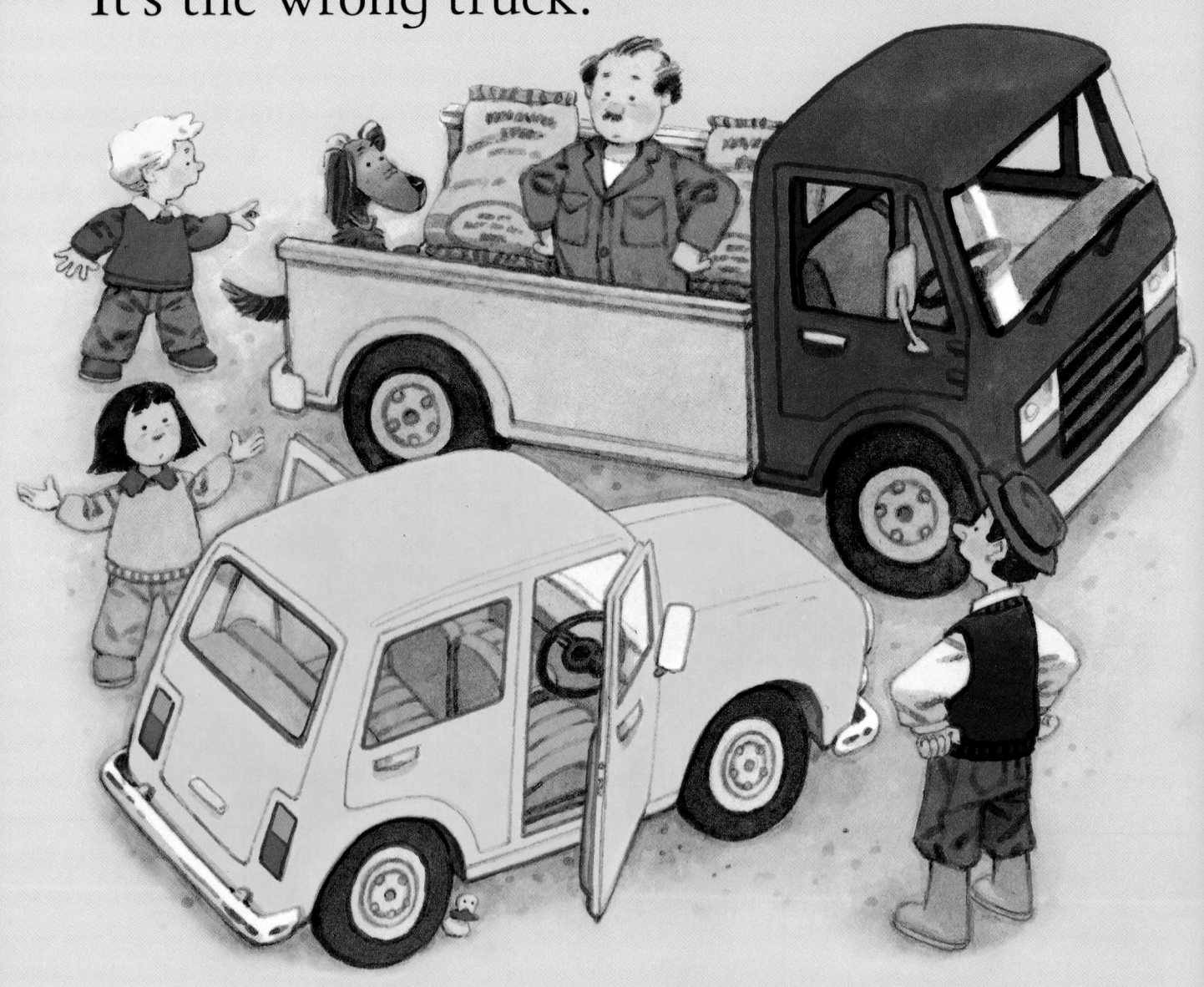

"Oh dear," says Poppy. "It's not Mr. Bran, and that's not Mr. Bran's truck."

Ted drives them home.

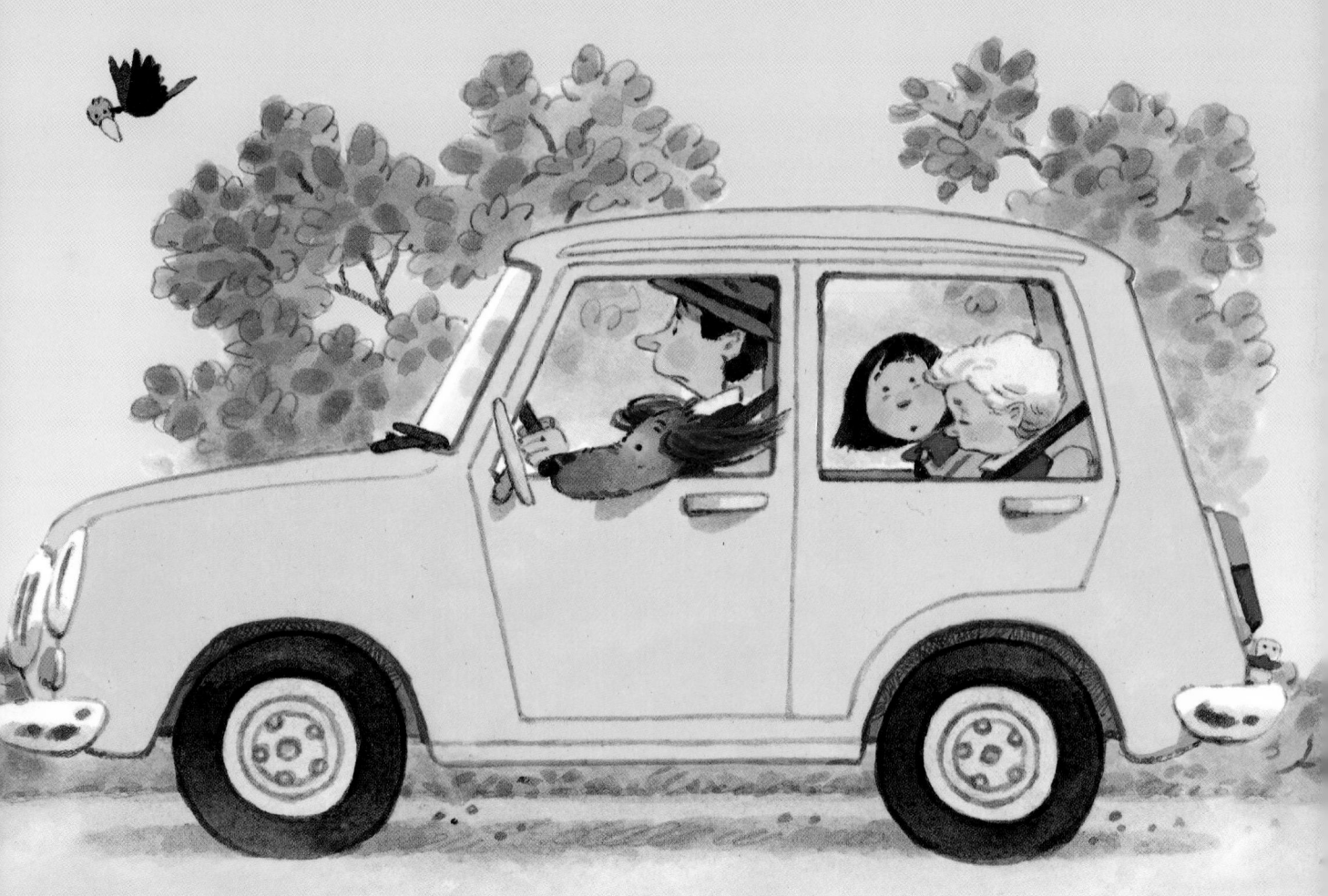

"We'll never find my kitten now," says Sam.
"I'm sure she'll turn up," says Poppy.

There's a surprise at Apple Tree Farm.

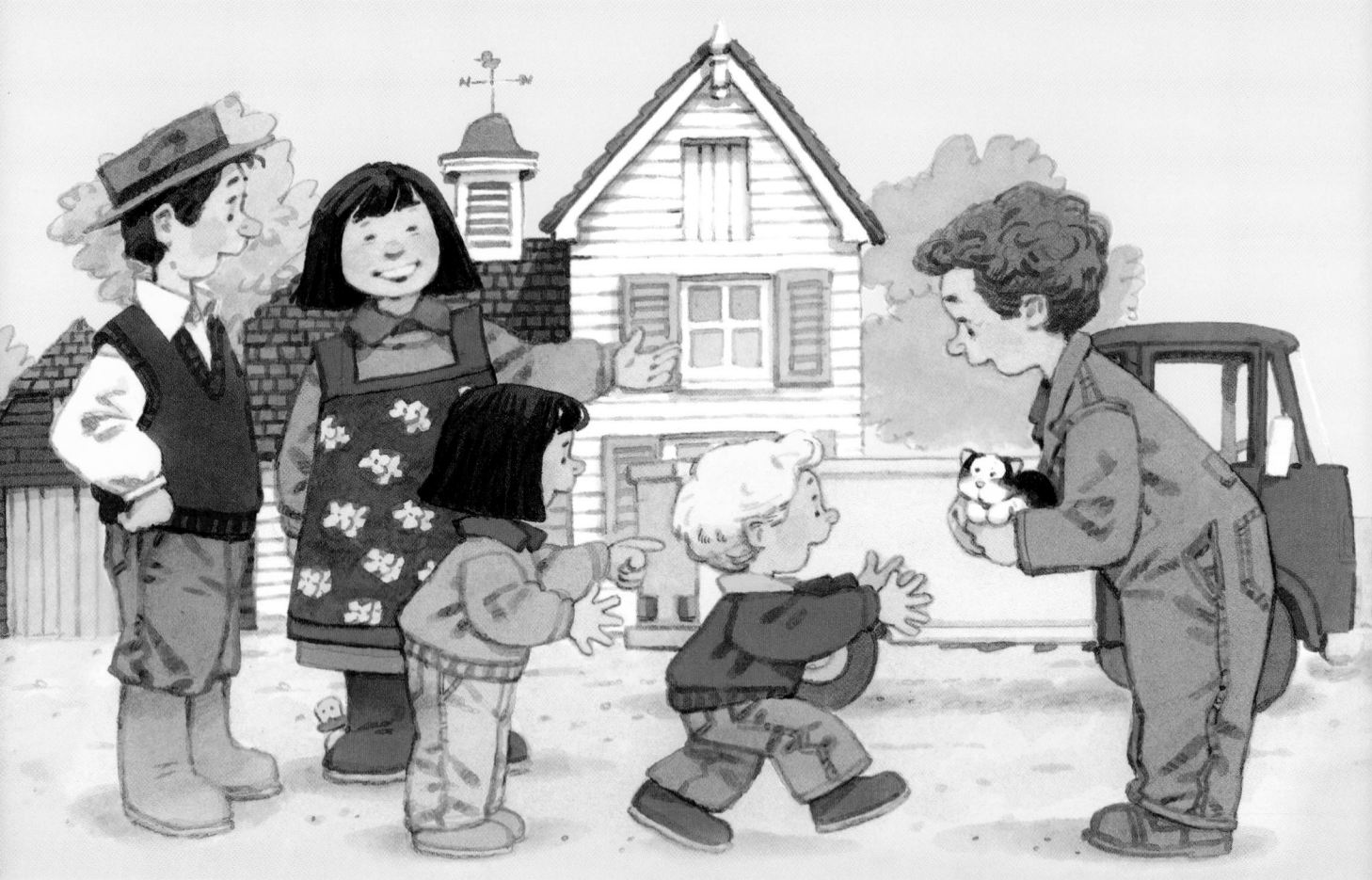

"Here's your kitten," says Mr. Bran. "She's been in my truck all day and now I've brought her home."

The New Pony

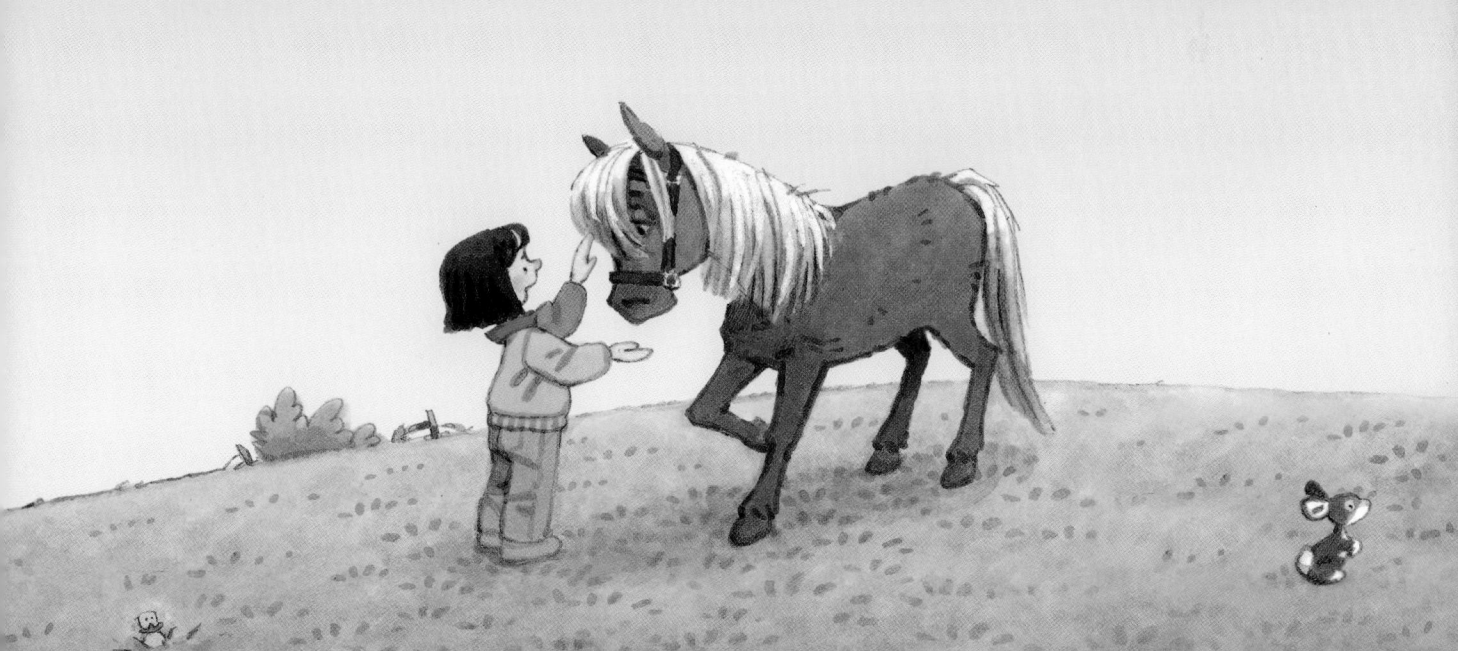

This is Apple Tree Farm.

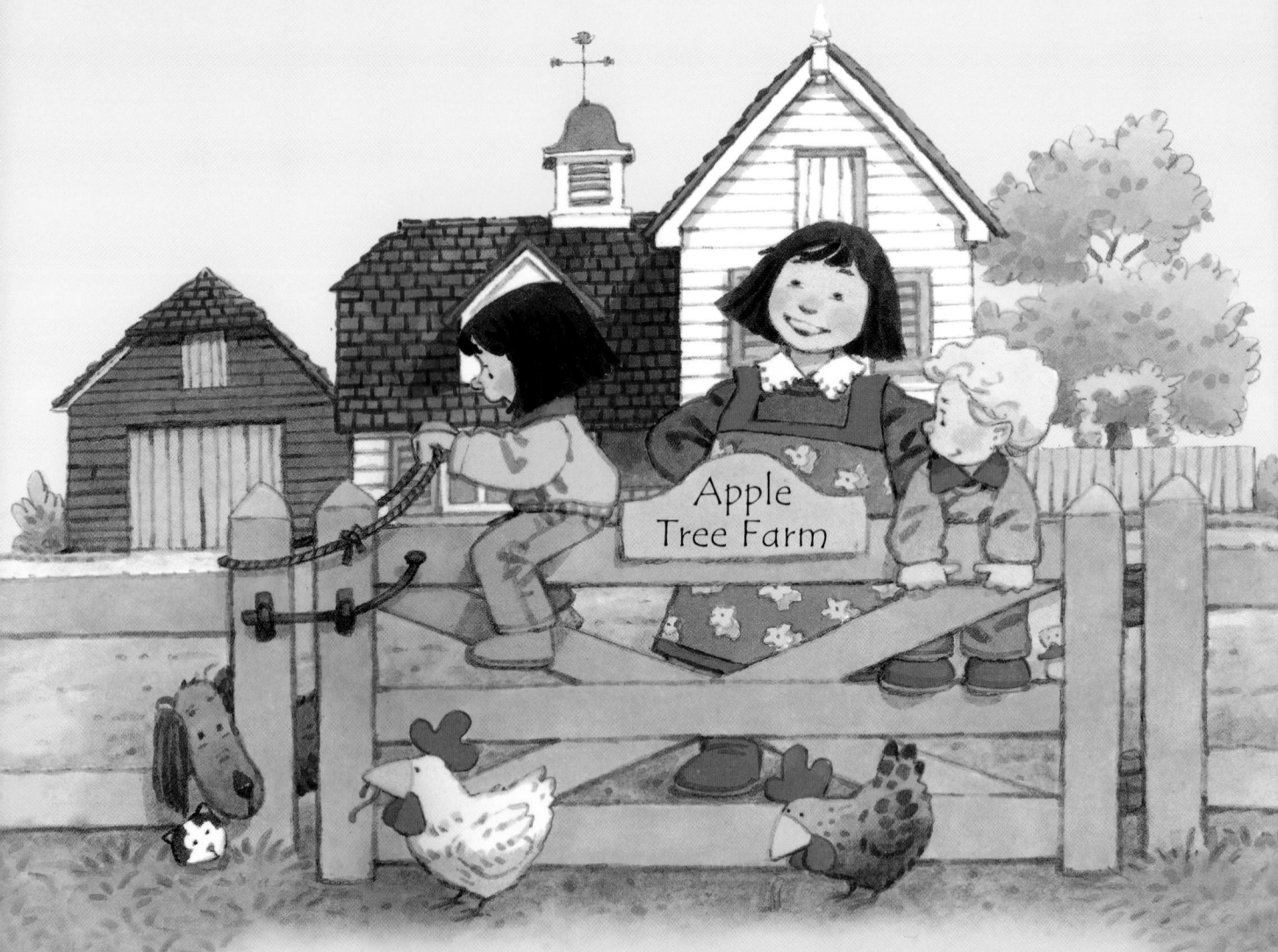

This is Mrs. Boot, the farmer. She has two children, called Poppy and Sam, and a dog called Rusty.

Mr. Boot, Poppy and Sam go for a walk.

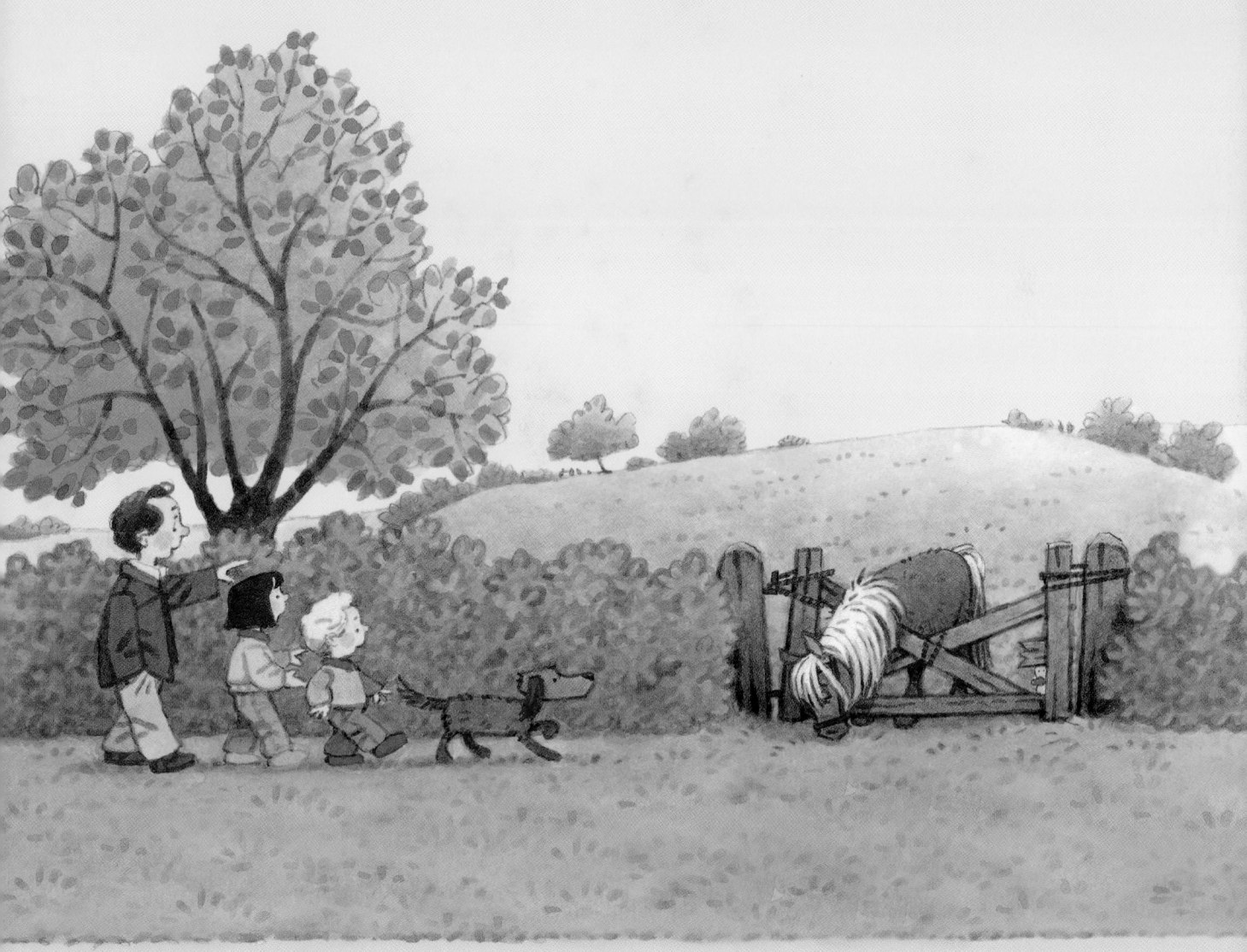

They see a new pony. "She belongs to Mr. Stone, who's just bought Old Gate Farm," says Mr. Boot.

The pony looks sad.

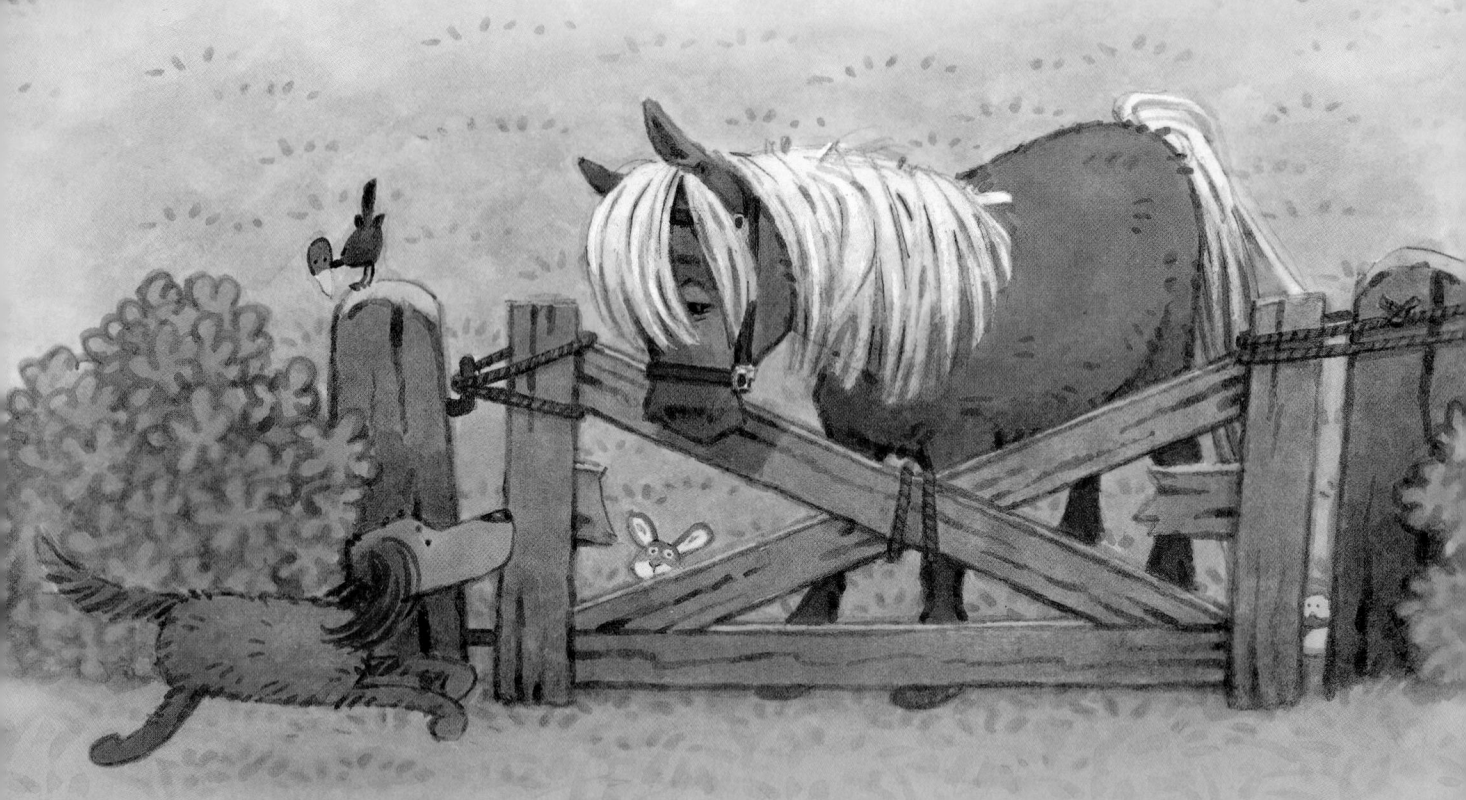

Her coat is rough and dirty. She looks hungry.
It looks as though no one takes care of her.

Poppy tries to stroke the pony.

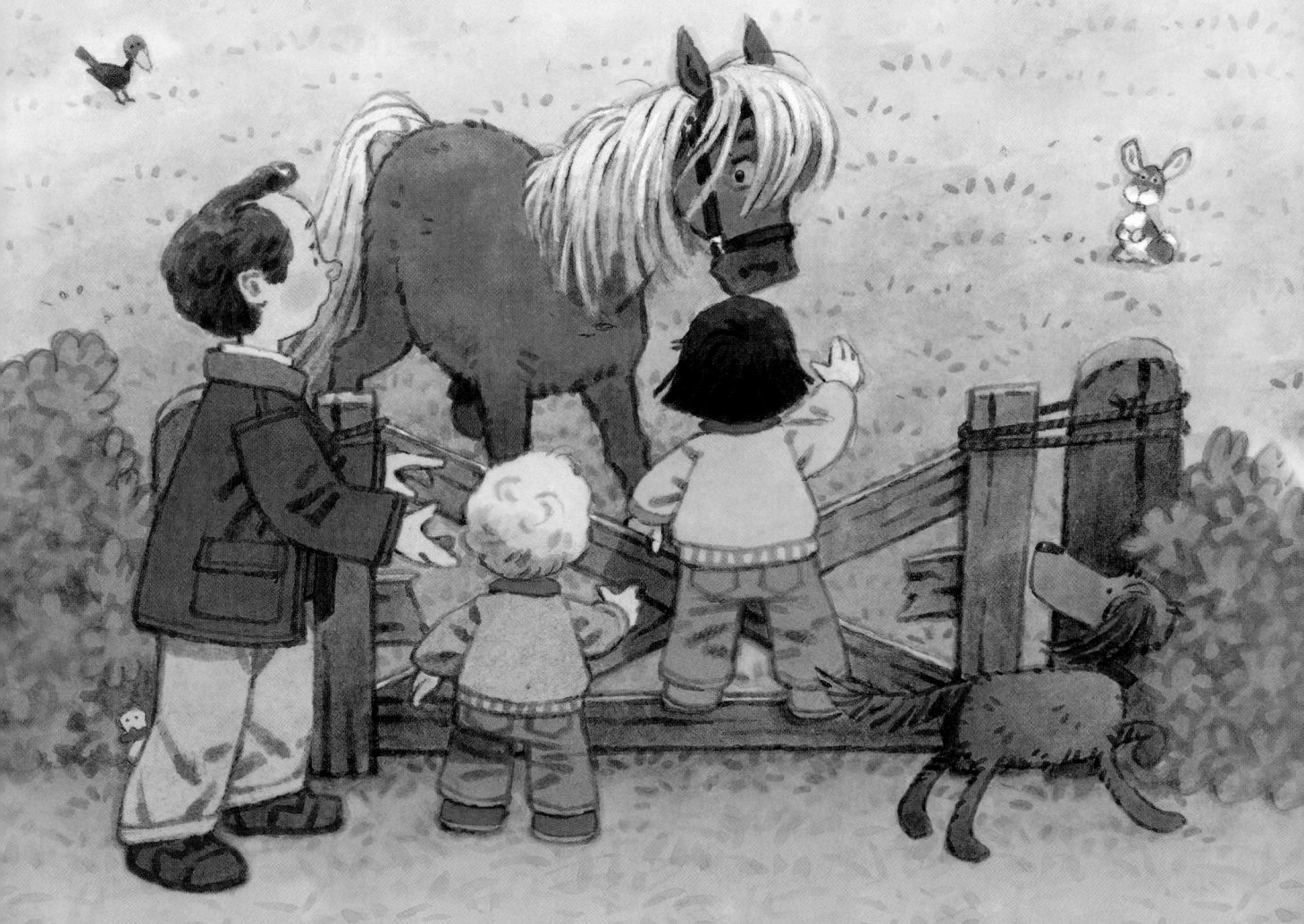

"She's not very friendly," says Sam. "Mr. Stone says she's bad tempered," says Mr. Boot.

Poppy feeds the pony.

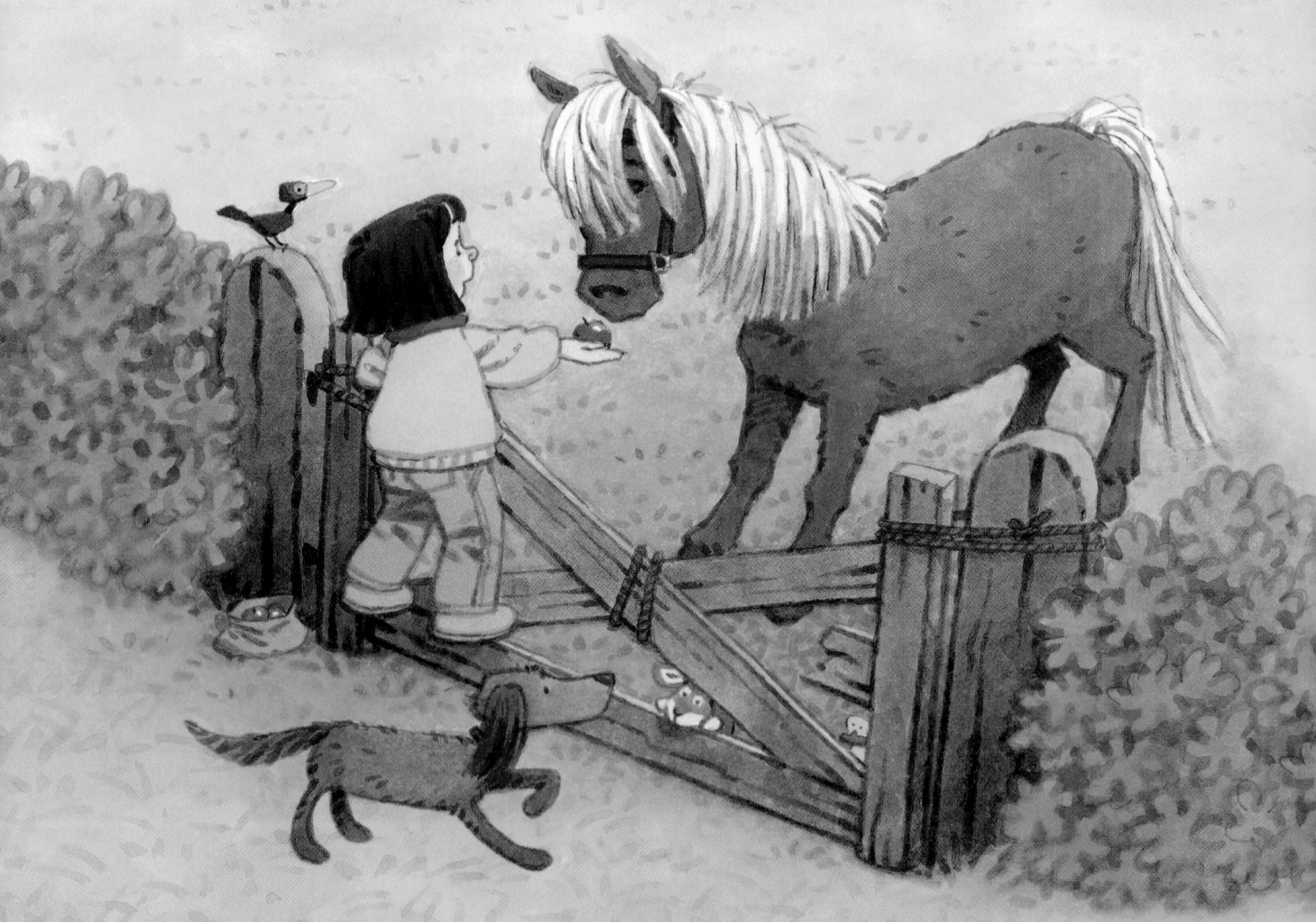

Every day, Poppy takes her apples and carrots.
But she always stays on the other side of the gate.

166

One day, Poppy takes Sam with her.

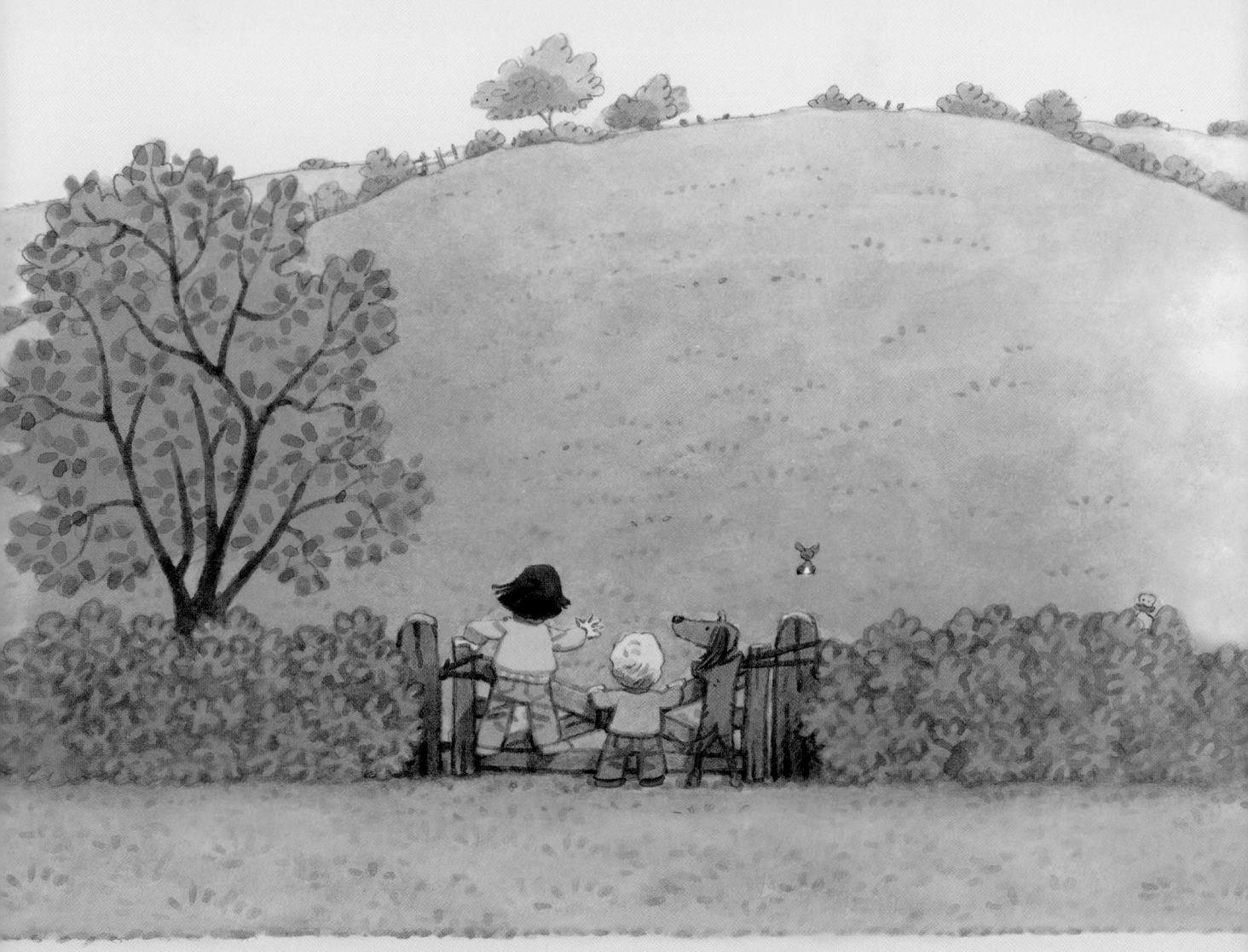

They cannot see the pony anywhere. The field looks empty. "Where is she?" says Sam.

Poppy and Sam open the gate.

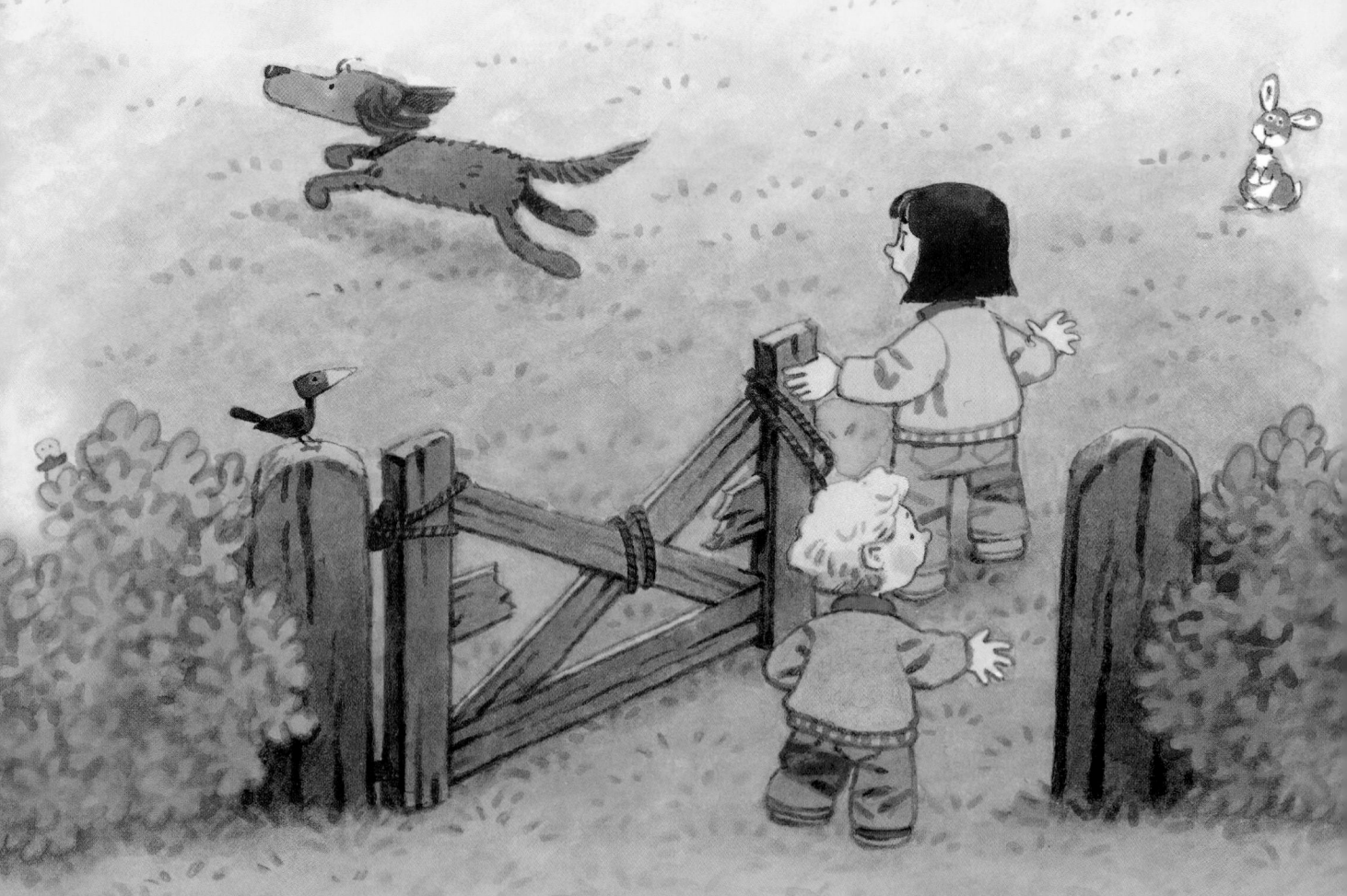

Rusty runs into the field. Poppy and Sam are a
bit scared. "We must find the pony," says Poppy.

"There she is," says Sam.

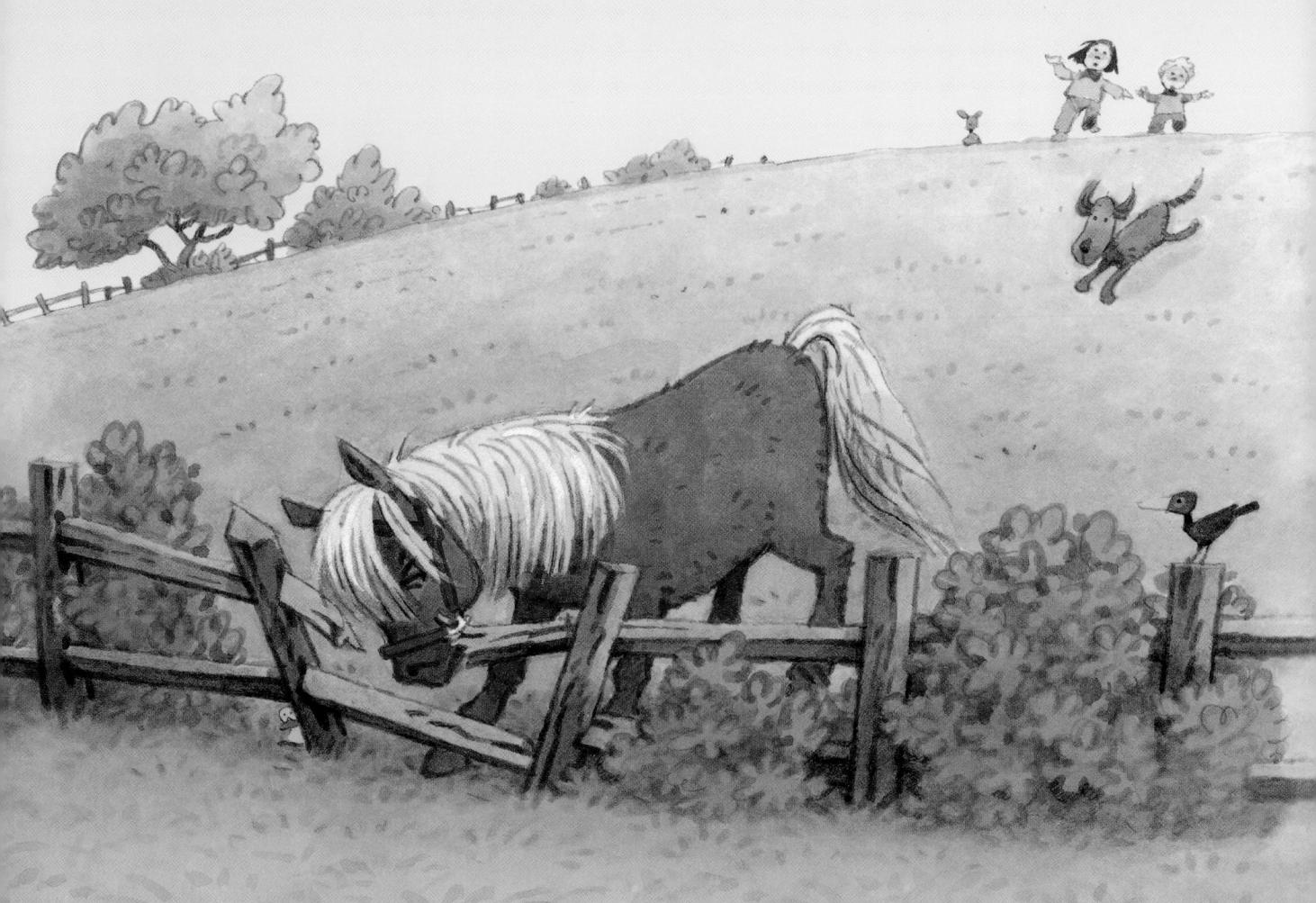

The pony has caught her head collar in the fence.
She has been eating the grass on the other side.

Poppy and Sam run home to Mr. Boot.

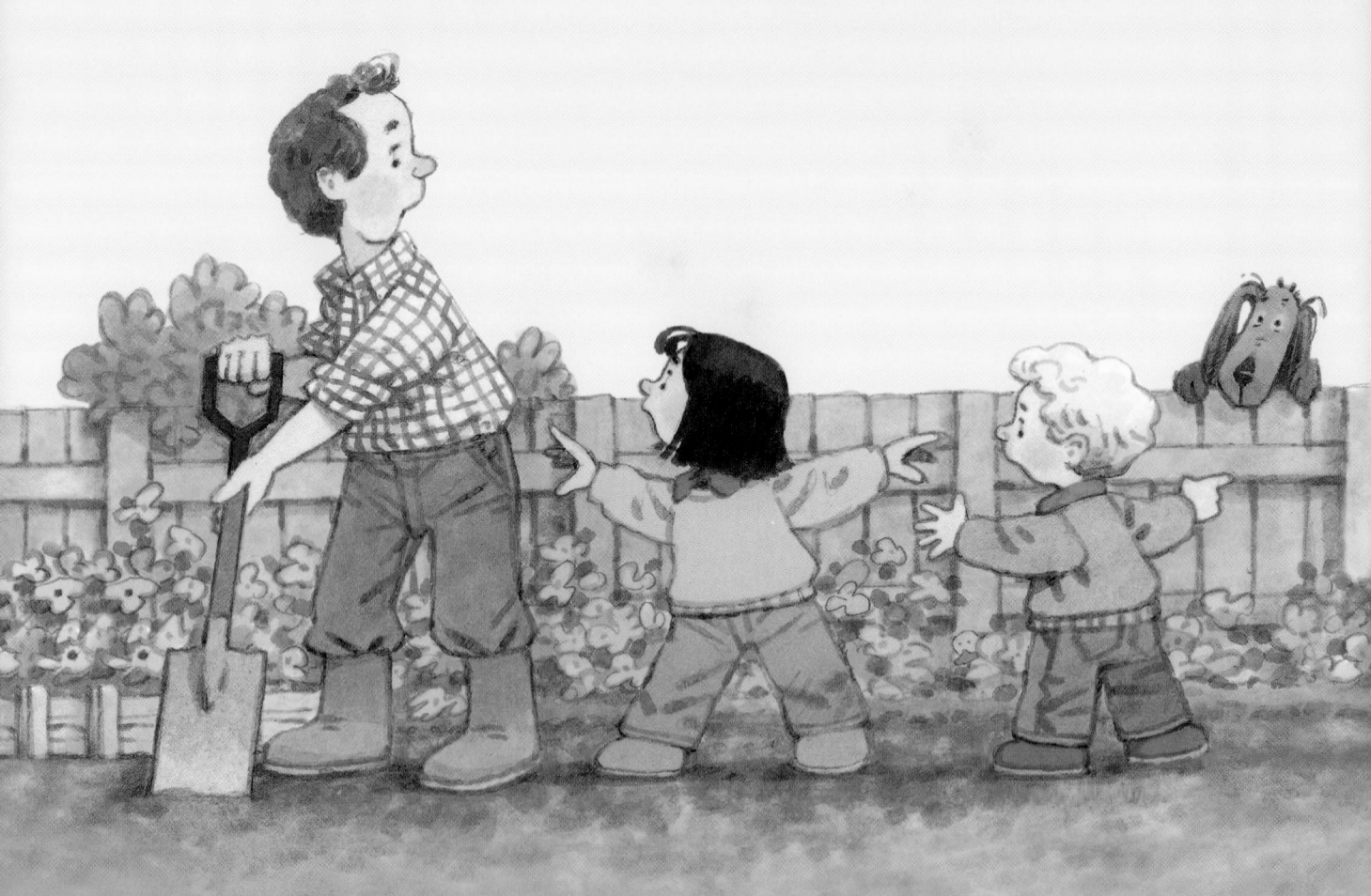

"Please come and help us, Dad," says Poppy. "The pony is caught in the fence. She will hurt herself."

Mr. Boot walks up to the pony.

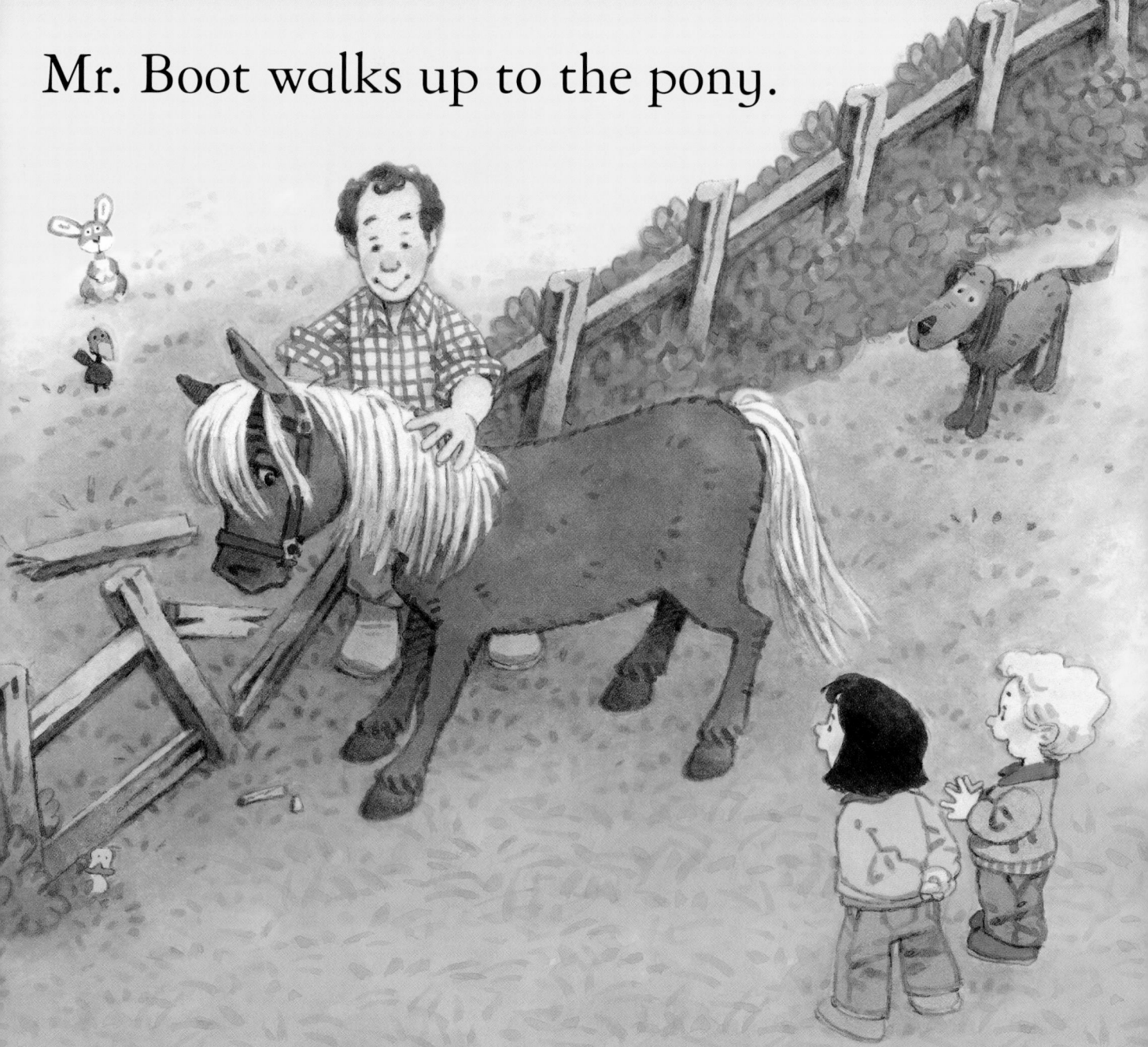

He unhooks the pony's head collar from the fence.
"She's not hurt," says Mr. Boot.

"The pony's chasing us."

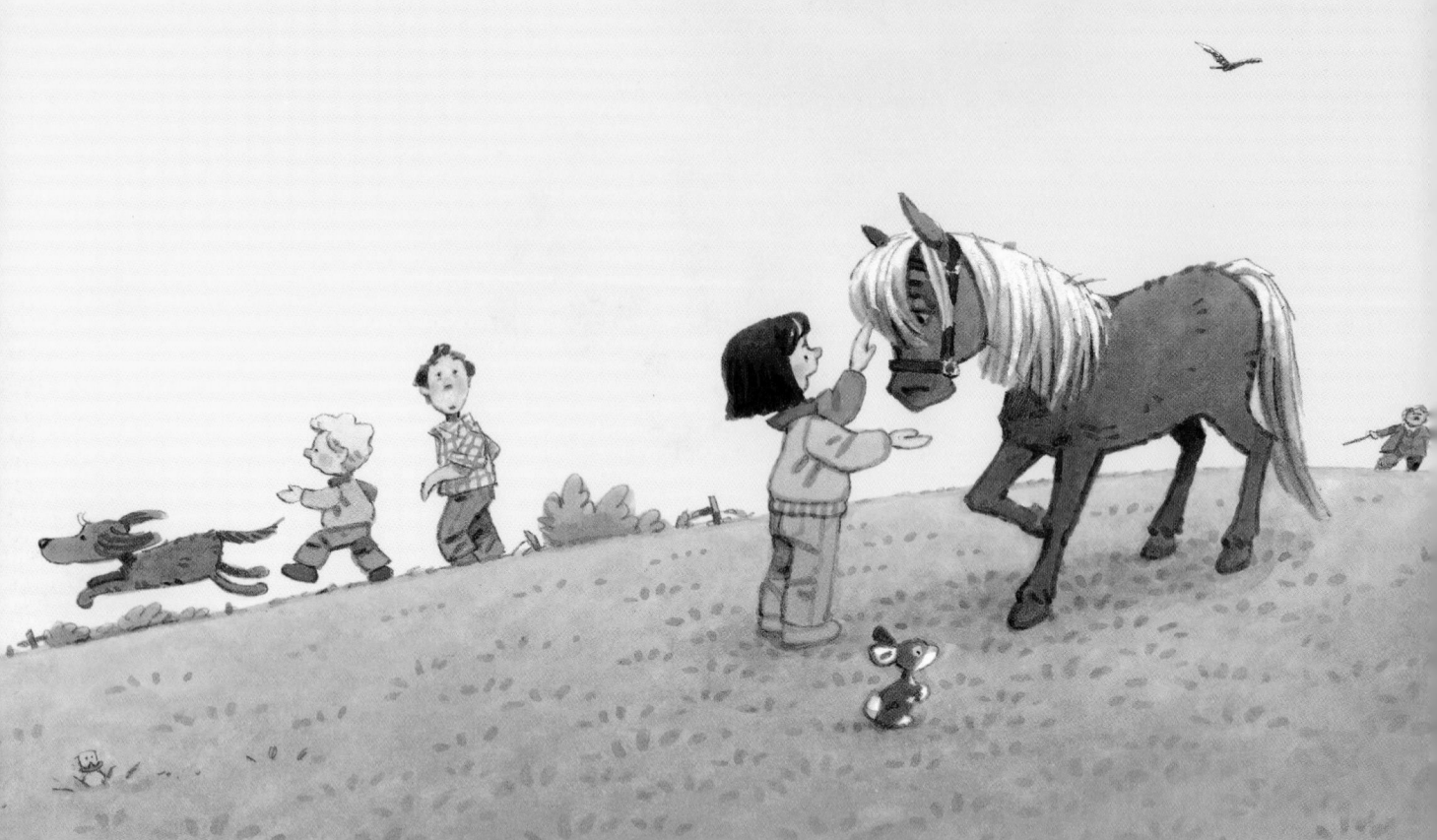

"Quick, run," says Sam. "It's all right," says Poppy,
patting the pony. "She just wants to be friends."

They see an angry man. It is Mr. Stone.

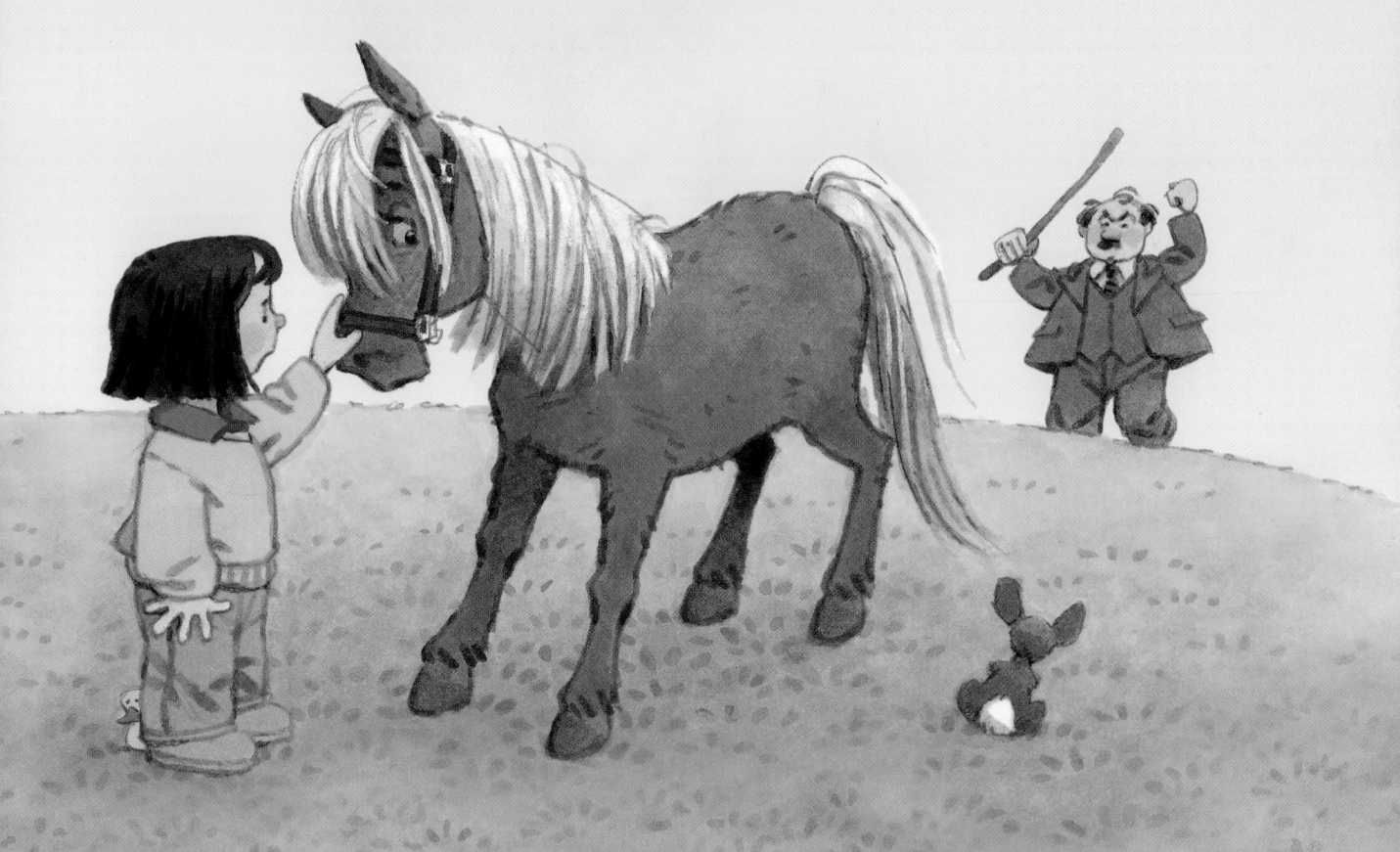

"Leave my pony alone," says Mr. Stone. "And get out of my field." He waves his stick at Poppy.

The pony is afraid of Mr. Stone.

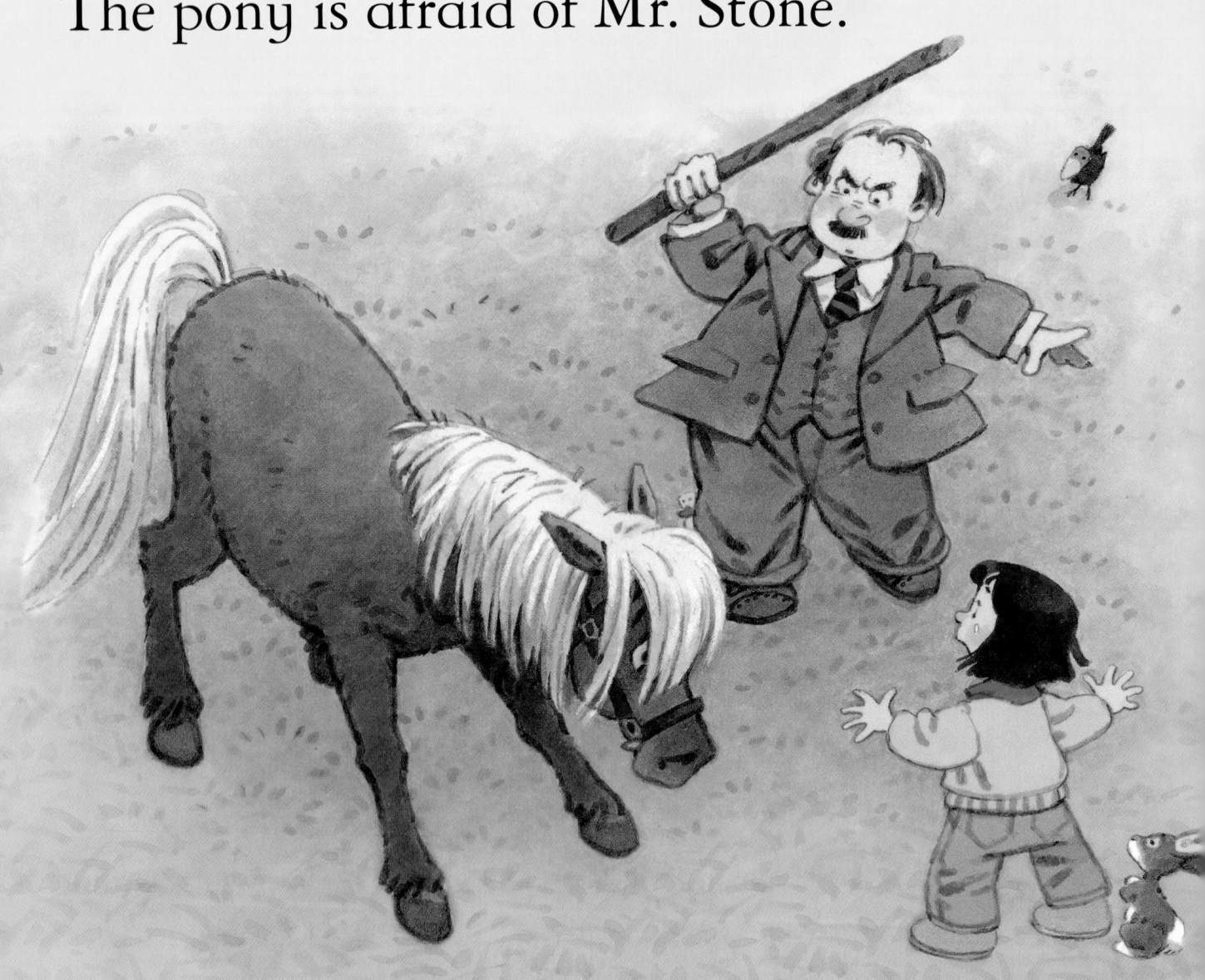

Mr. Stone tries to hit the pony with his stick. "I'm going to get rid of that nasty animal," he says.

Poppy grabs his arm.

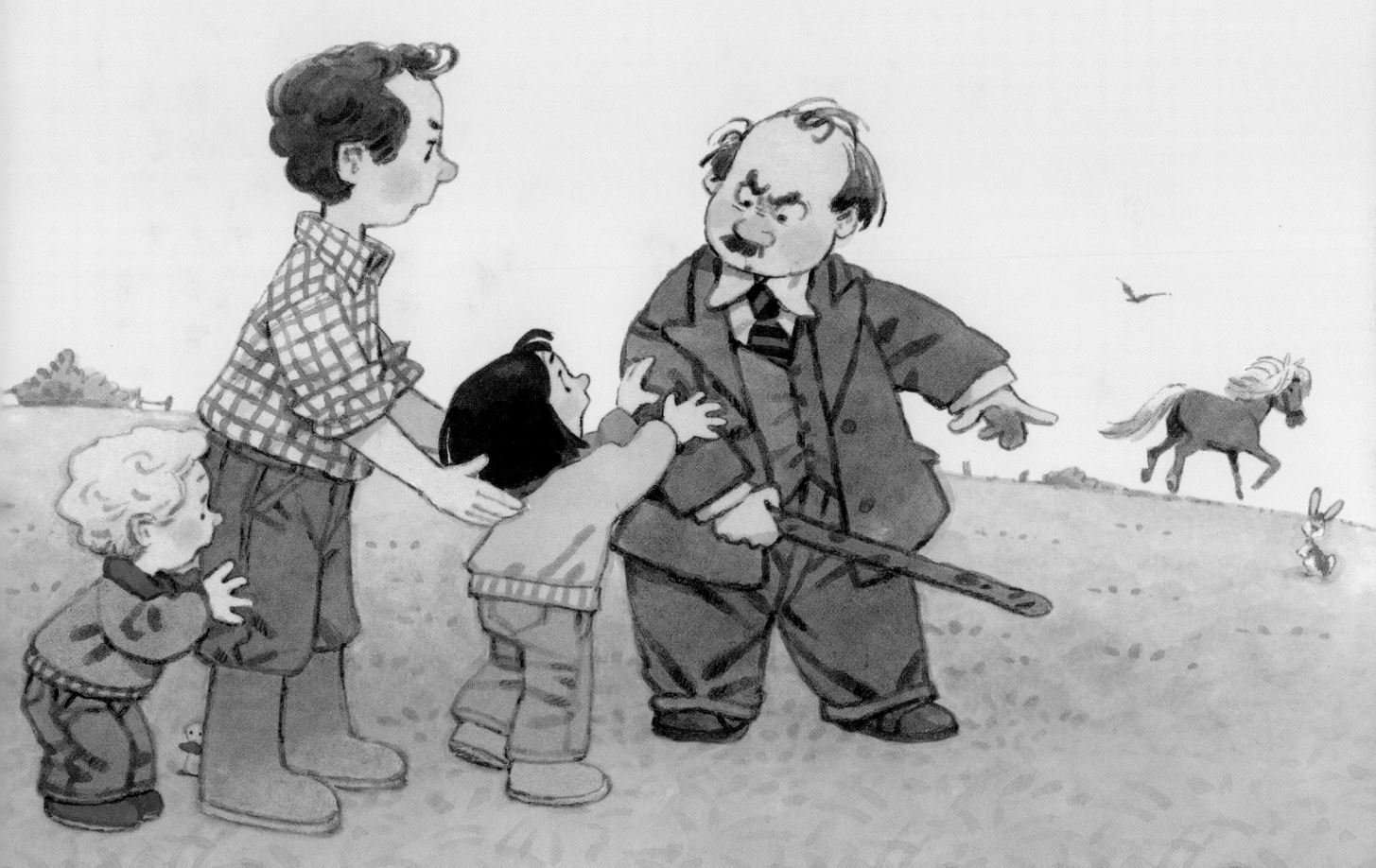

"You mustn't hit the pony," she cries. "Come on
Poppy," says Mr. Boot. "Let's go home."

Next day, there's a surprise for Poppy.

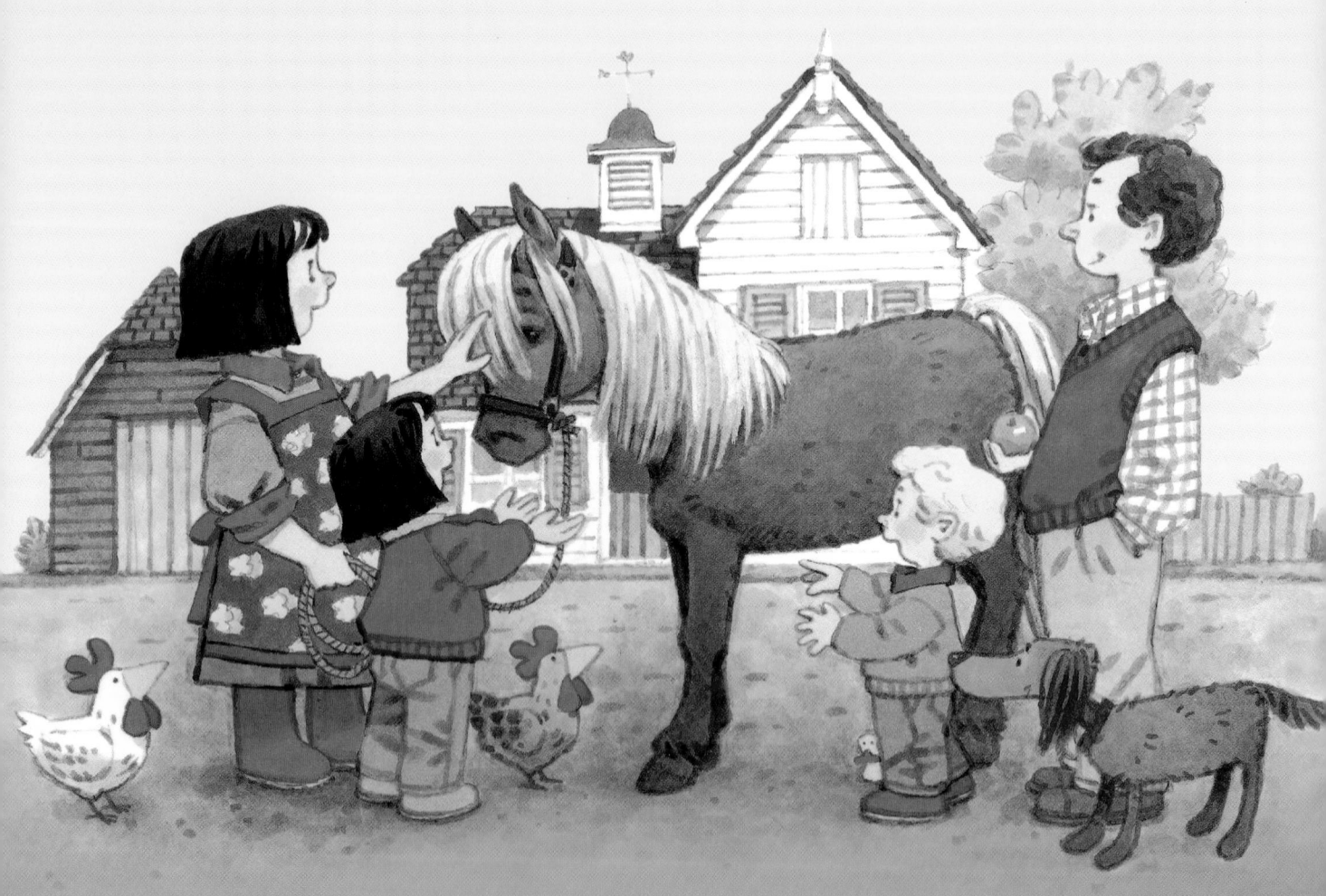

The pony is at Apple Tree Farm. "We've bought her for you," says Mrs. Boot. "Thank you," says Poppy.

The
Grumpy Goat

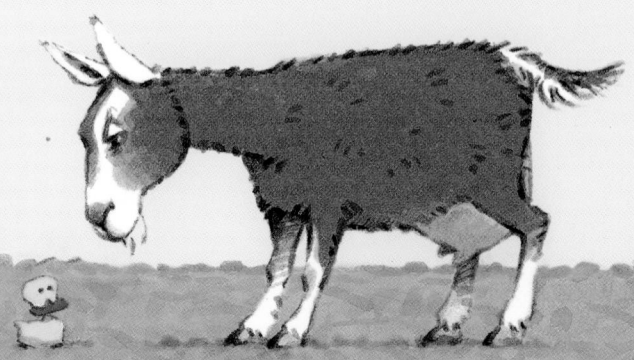

This is Apple Tree Farm.

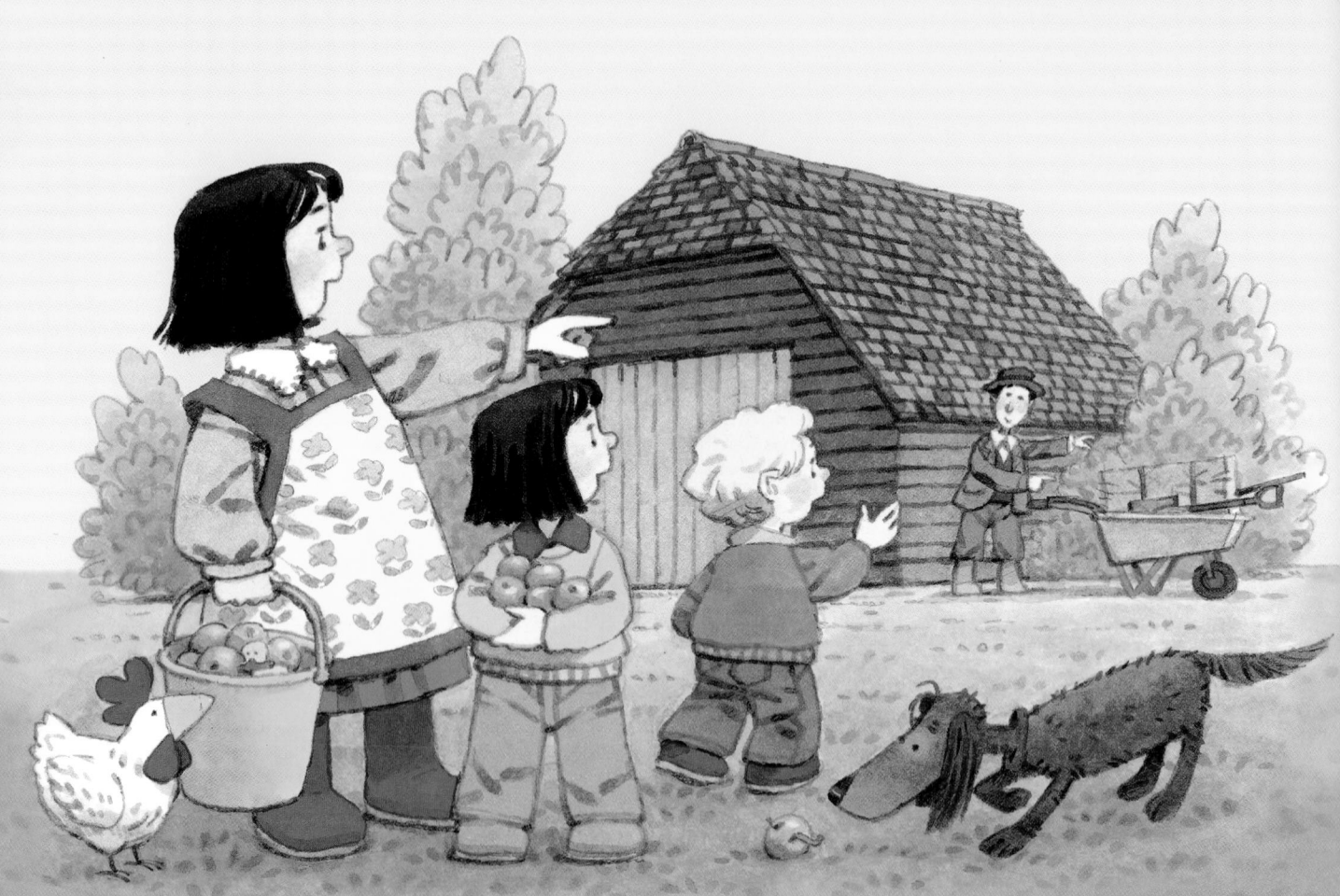

This is Mrs. Boot, the farmer. She has two children, called Poppy and Sam, and a dog called Rusty.

Ted works on the farm.

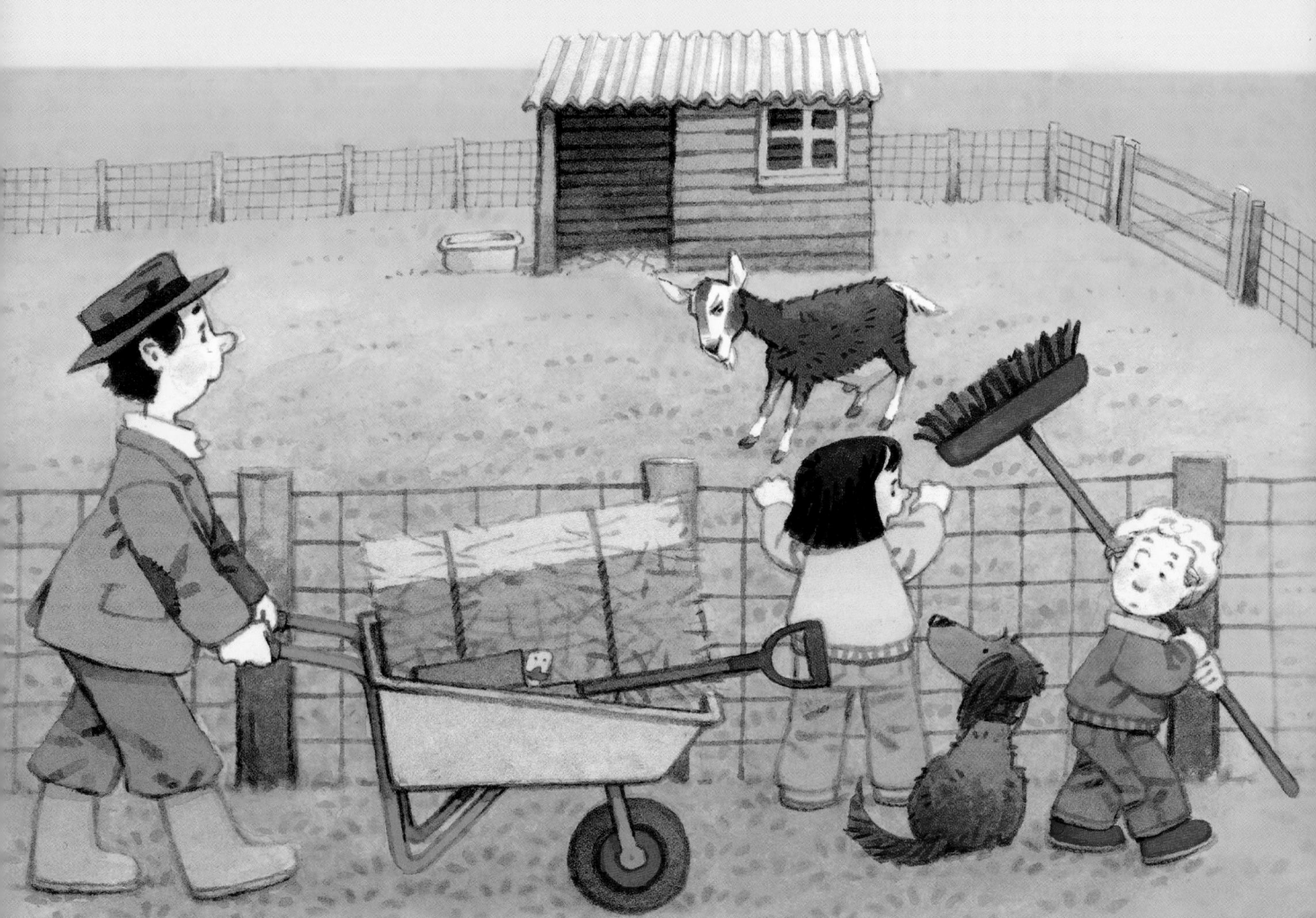

He tells Poppy and Sam to clean the goat's shed.
"Will she let us?" asks Sam. "She's so grumpy now."

Gertie the goat chases Sam.

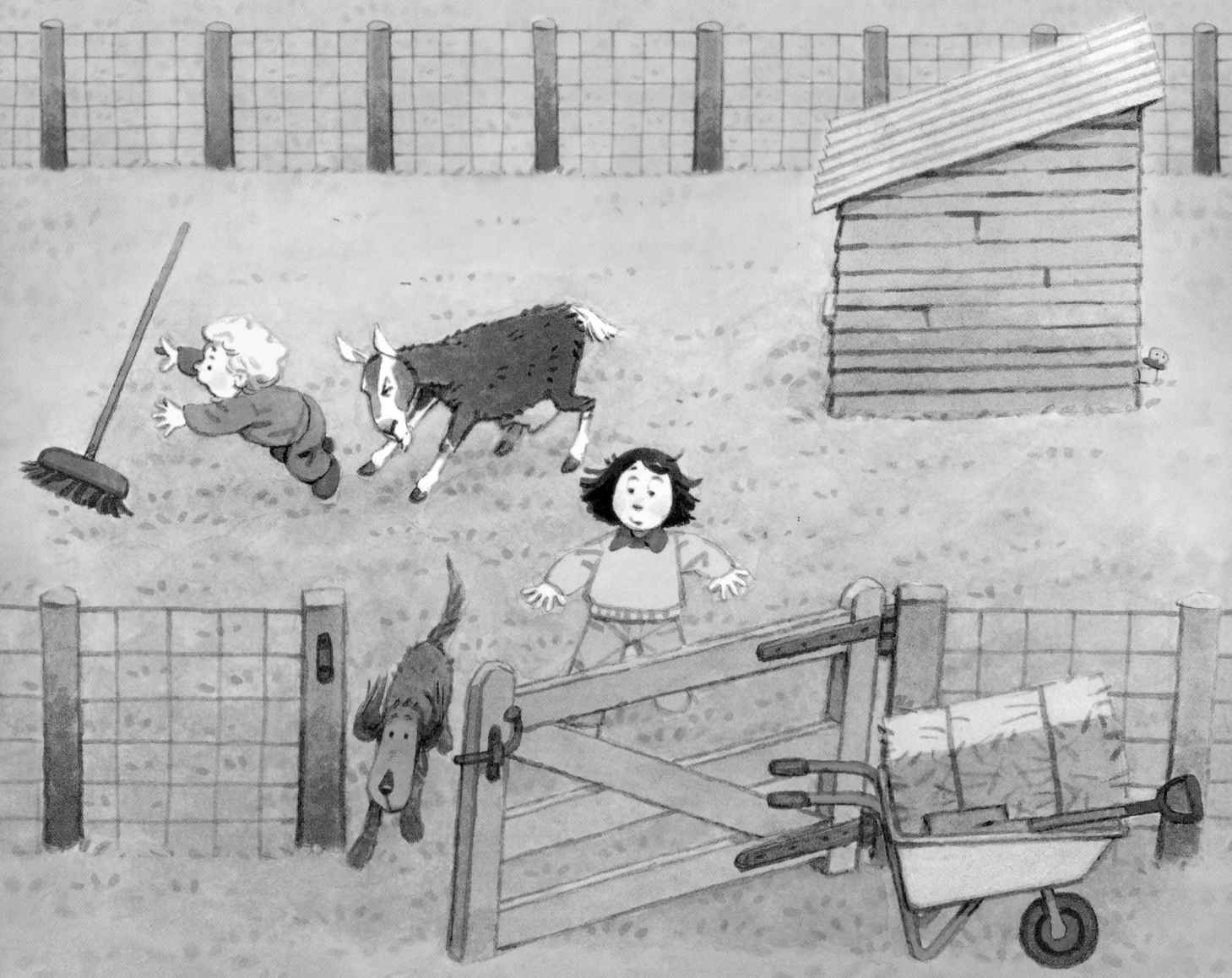

She butts him with her head. He nearly falls over.
Sam, Poppy and Rusty run out through the gate.

Poppy shuts the gate.

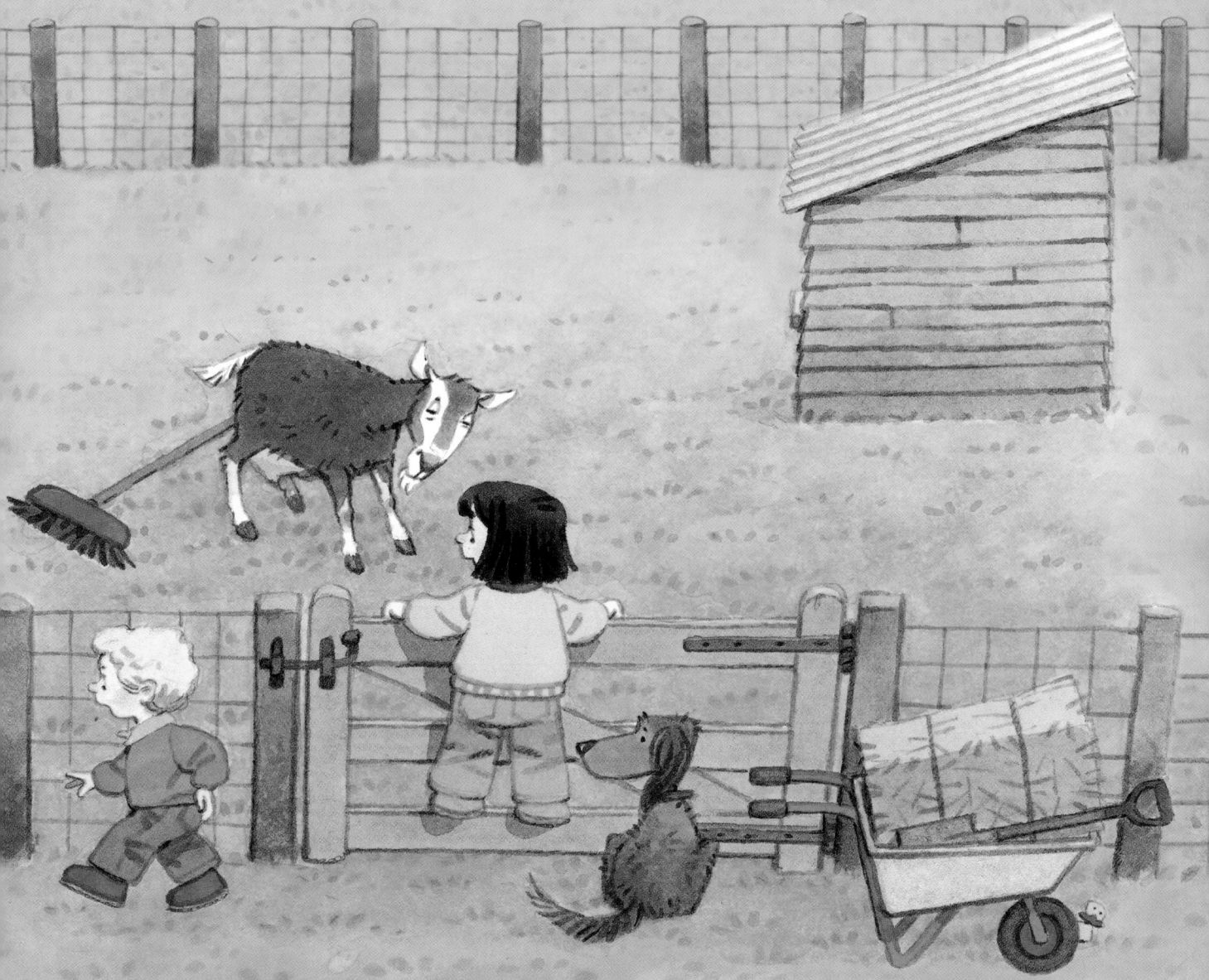

They must get Gertie out of her pen so they can get to her shed. "I have an idea," says Sam.

Sam gets a bag of bread.

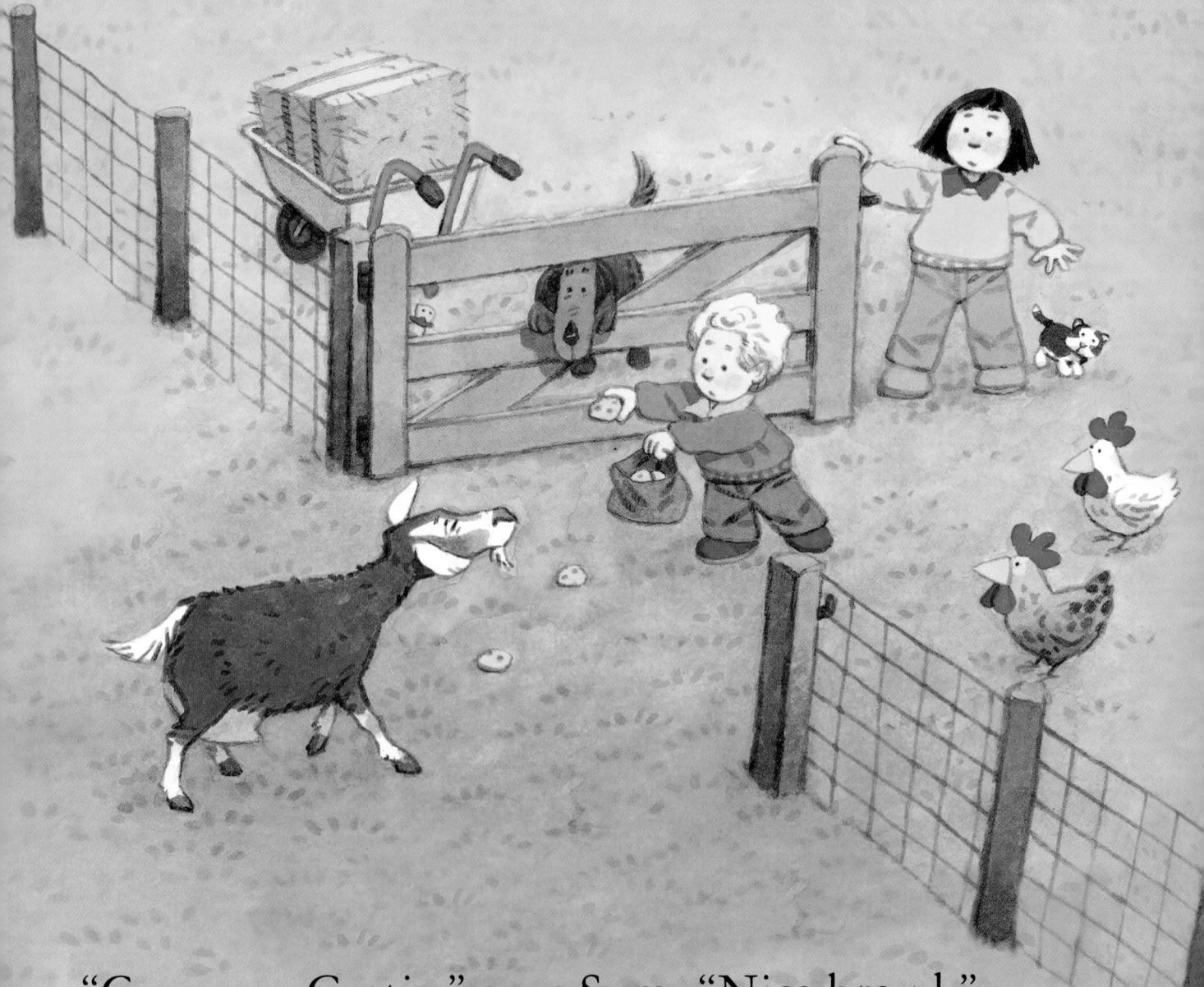

"Come on, Gertie," says Sam. "Nice bread."
Gertie eats it and the bag, but stays in her pen.

"Let's try some fresh grass," says Poppy.

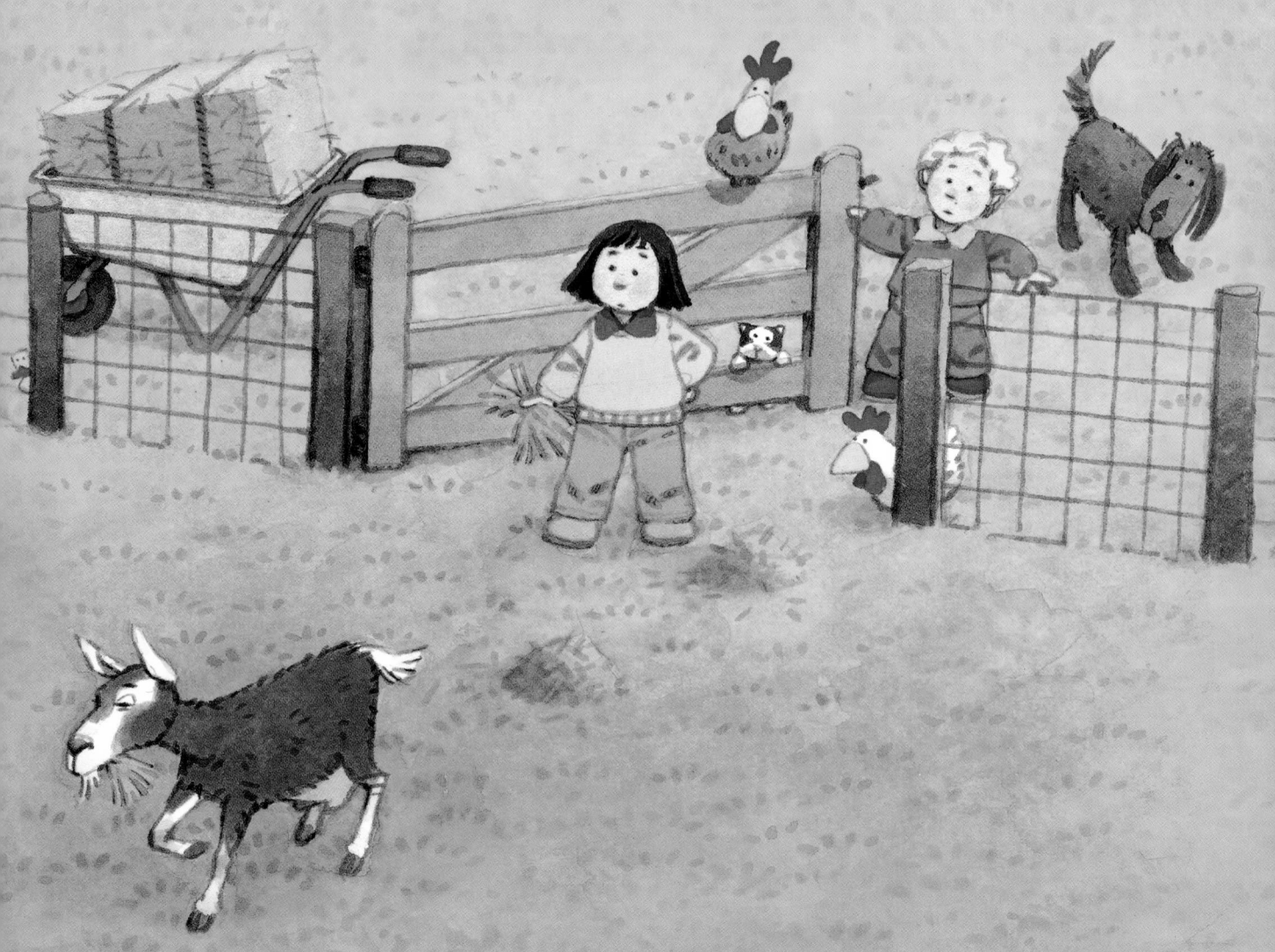

Poppy pulls up some grass and drops it by the gate.
Gertie eats it but trots back into her pen.

"I have another idea," says Sam.

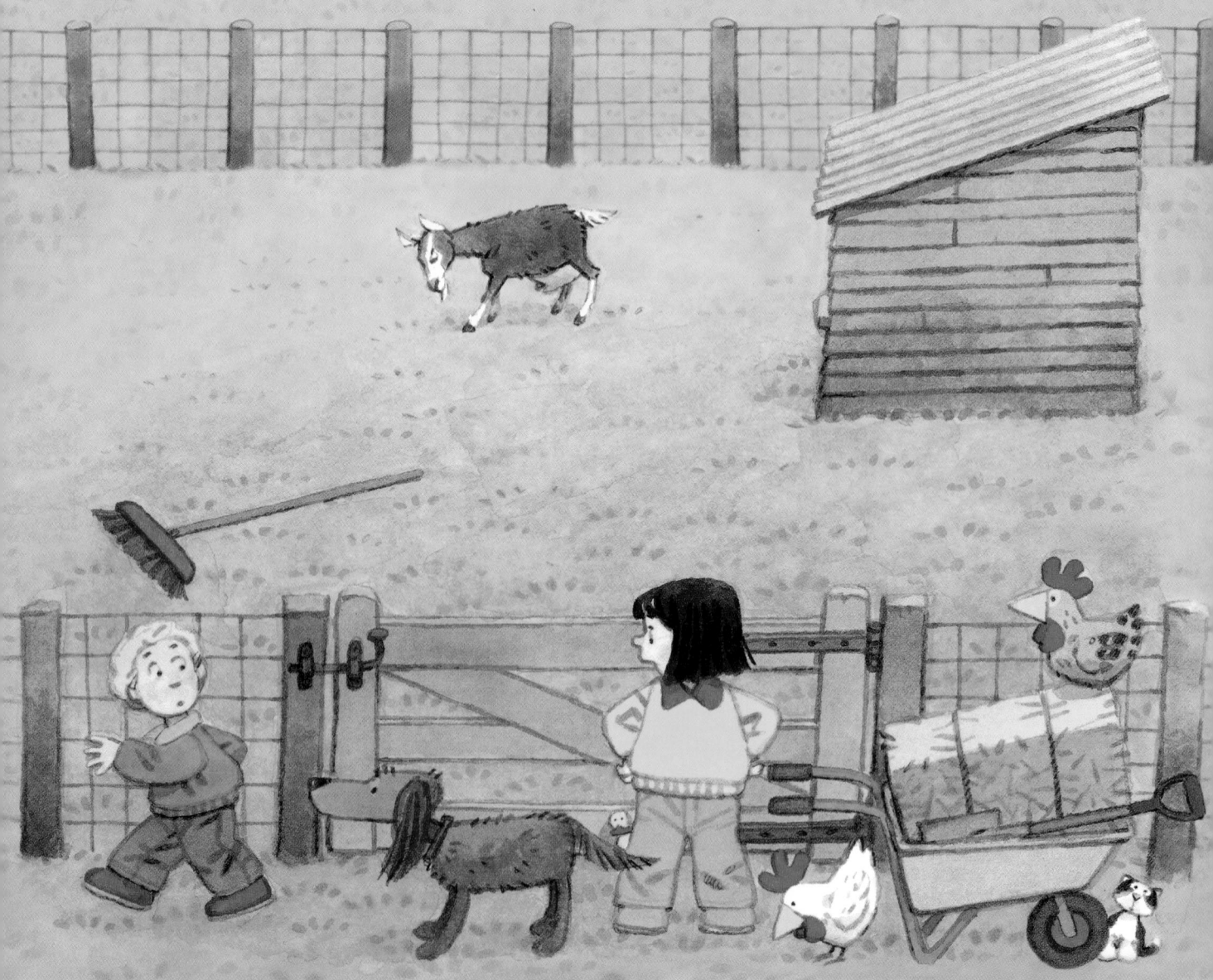

"Gertie doesn't butt Ted. She wouldn't butt me if
I looked like Ted," says Sam. He runs off again.

184

Sam comes back wearing Ted's clothes.

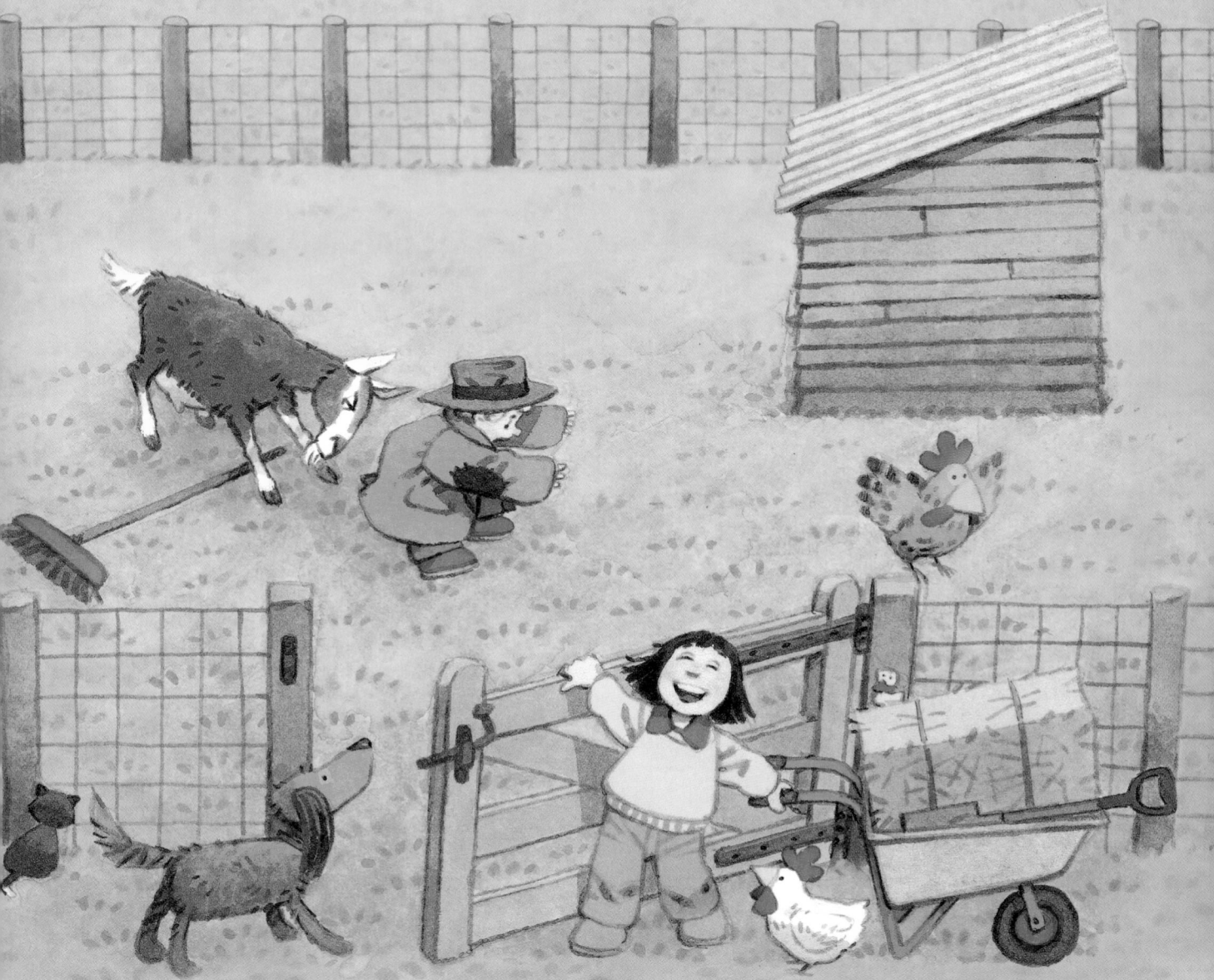

He has found Ted's old coat and hat. Sam goes
into the pen but Gertie still butts him.

"I'll get a rope," says Poppy.

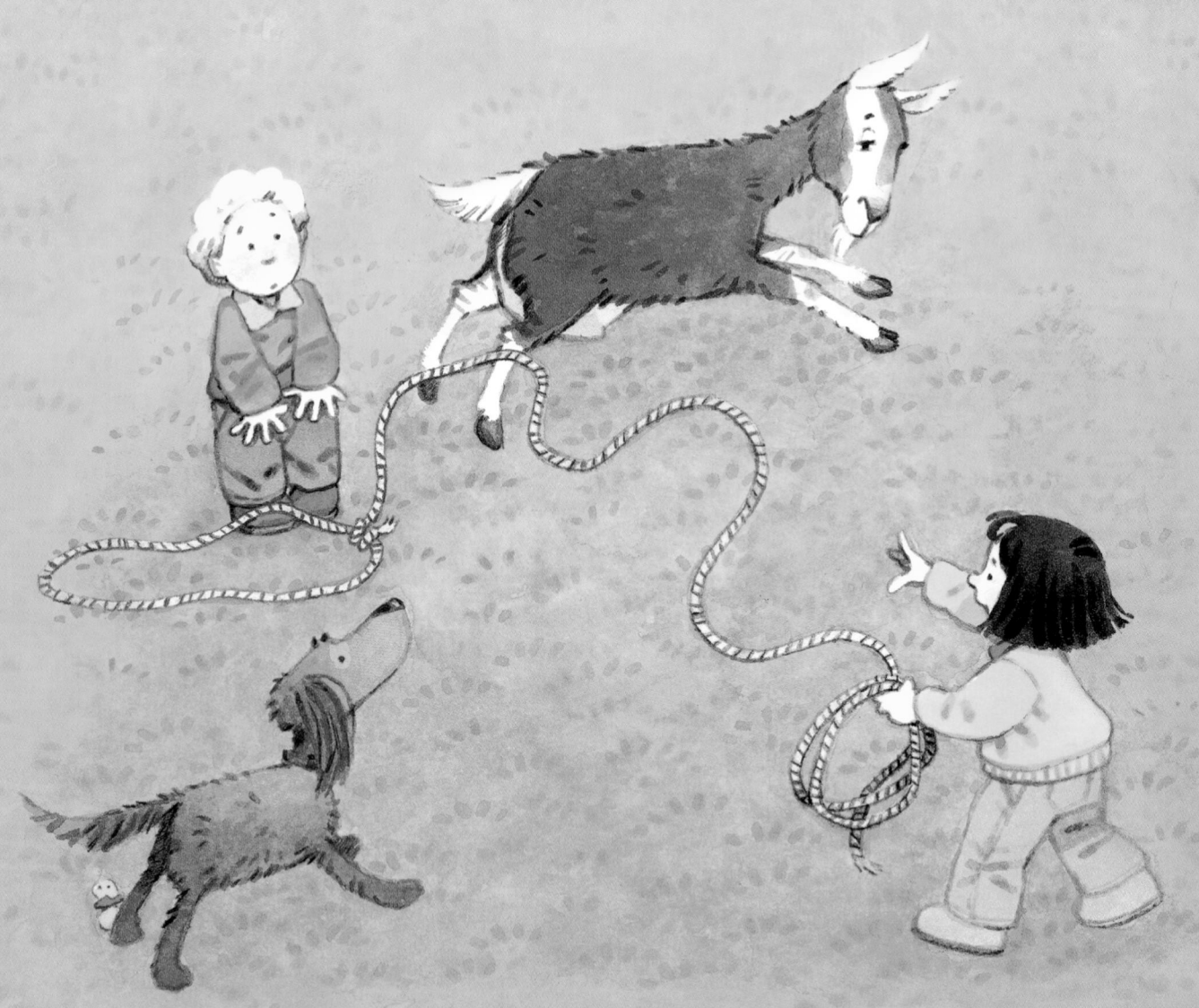

They go into the pen. Poppy tries to throw the rope over Gertie's head. She misses.

Gertie chases them all.

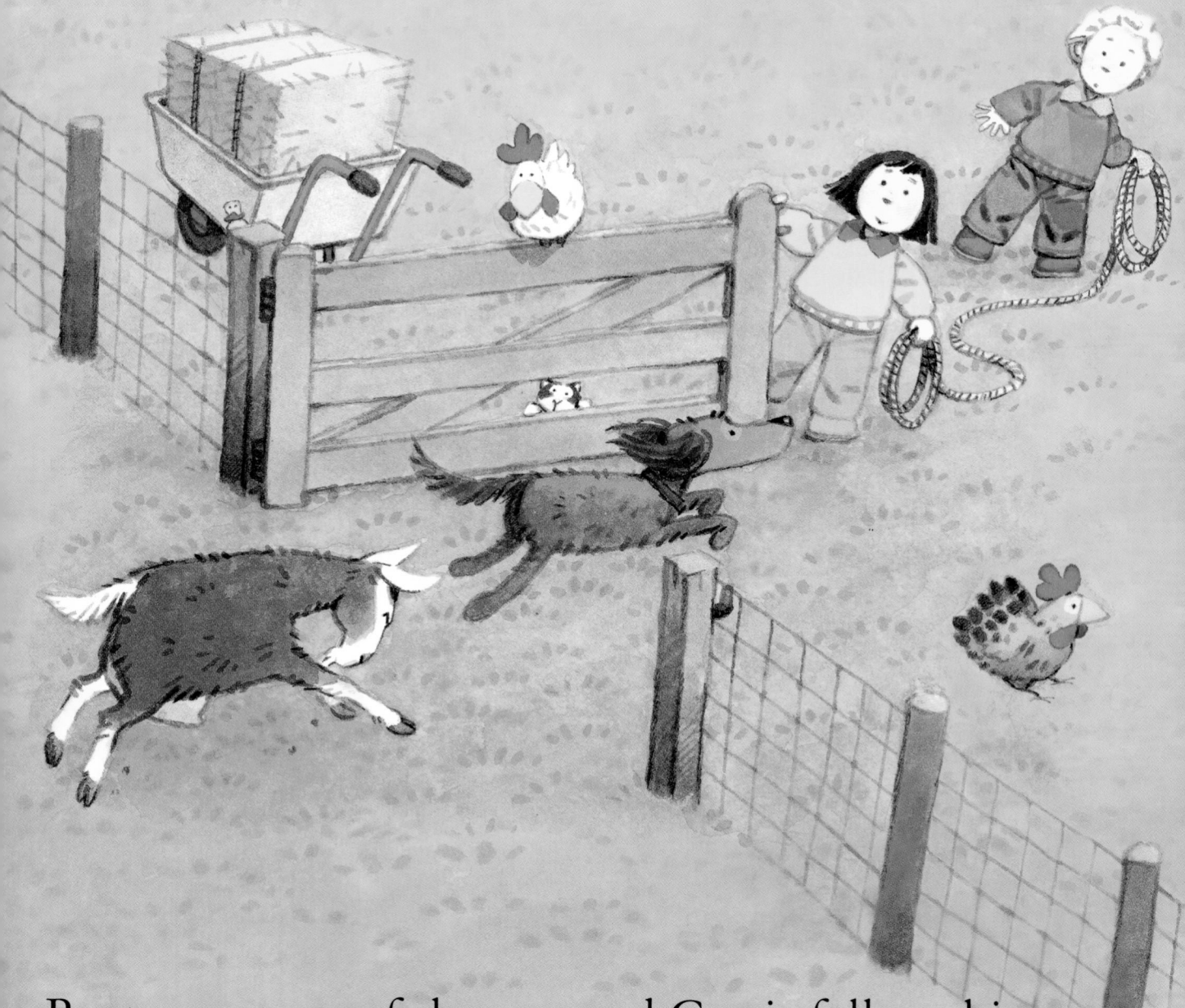

Rusty runs out of the pen and Gertie follows him.
"She's out!" shouts Sam. "Quick, shut the gate."

Sam and Poppy clean out Gertie's shed.

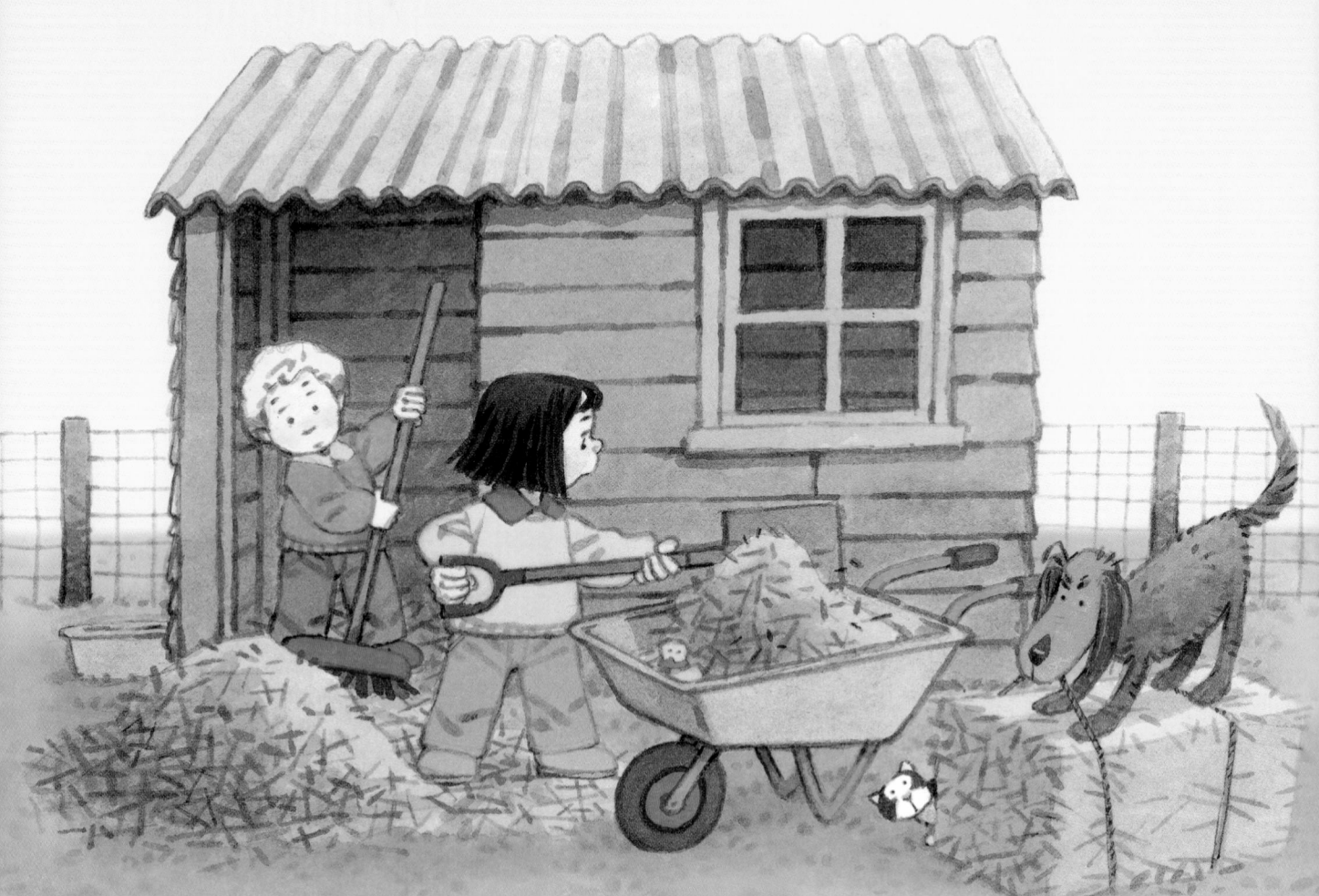

They sweep up the old straw and put it in the wheelbarrow. They spread out fresh straw.

Poppy opens the gate.

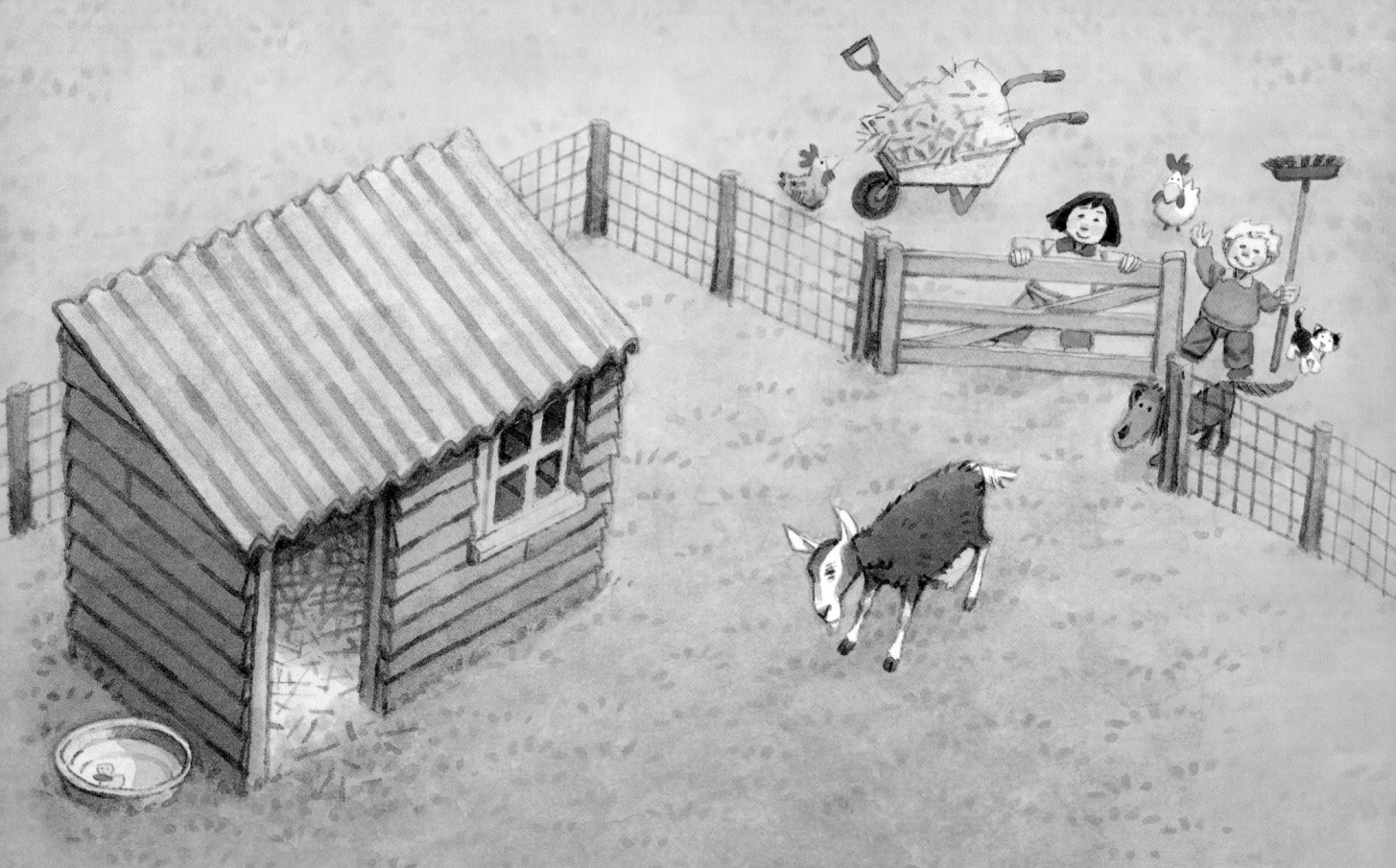

"Come on, Gertie. You can go back now," says Sam.
Gertie trots back into her pen.

"You are a grumpy old goat," says Poppy.

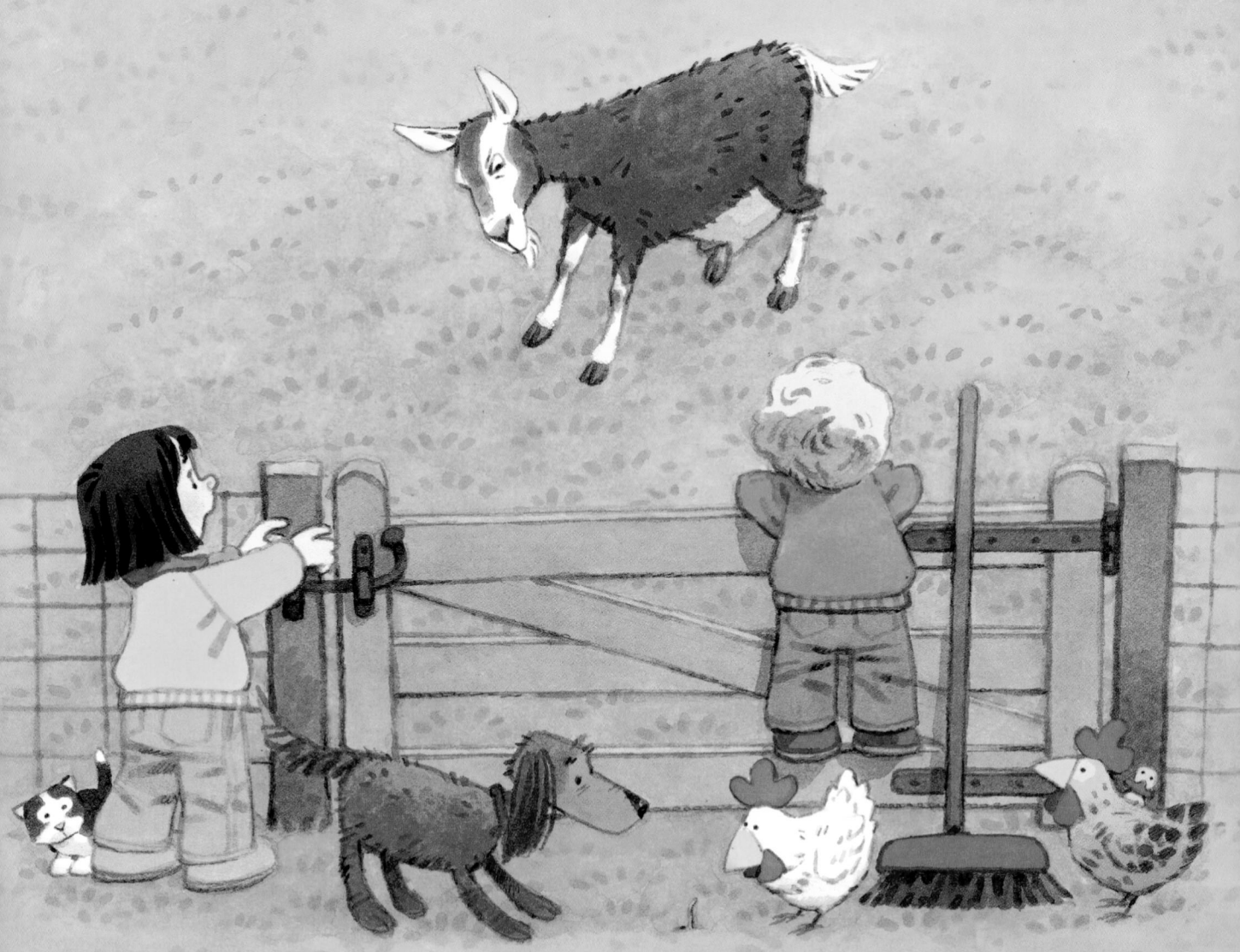

"We've cleaned out your shed and you're still grumpy," says Sam. "Grumpy Gertie."

Next morning, they meet Ted.

"Come and look at Gertie now," says Ted. They all
go to the goat pen.

Gertie has a little kid.

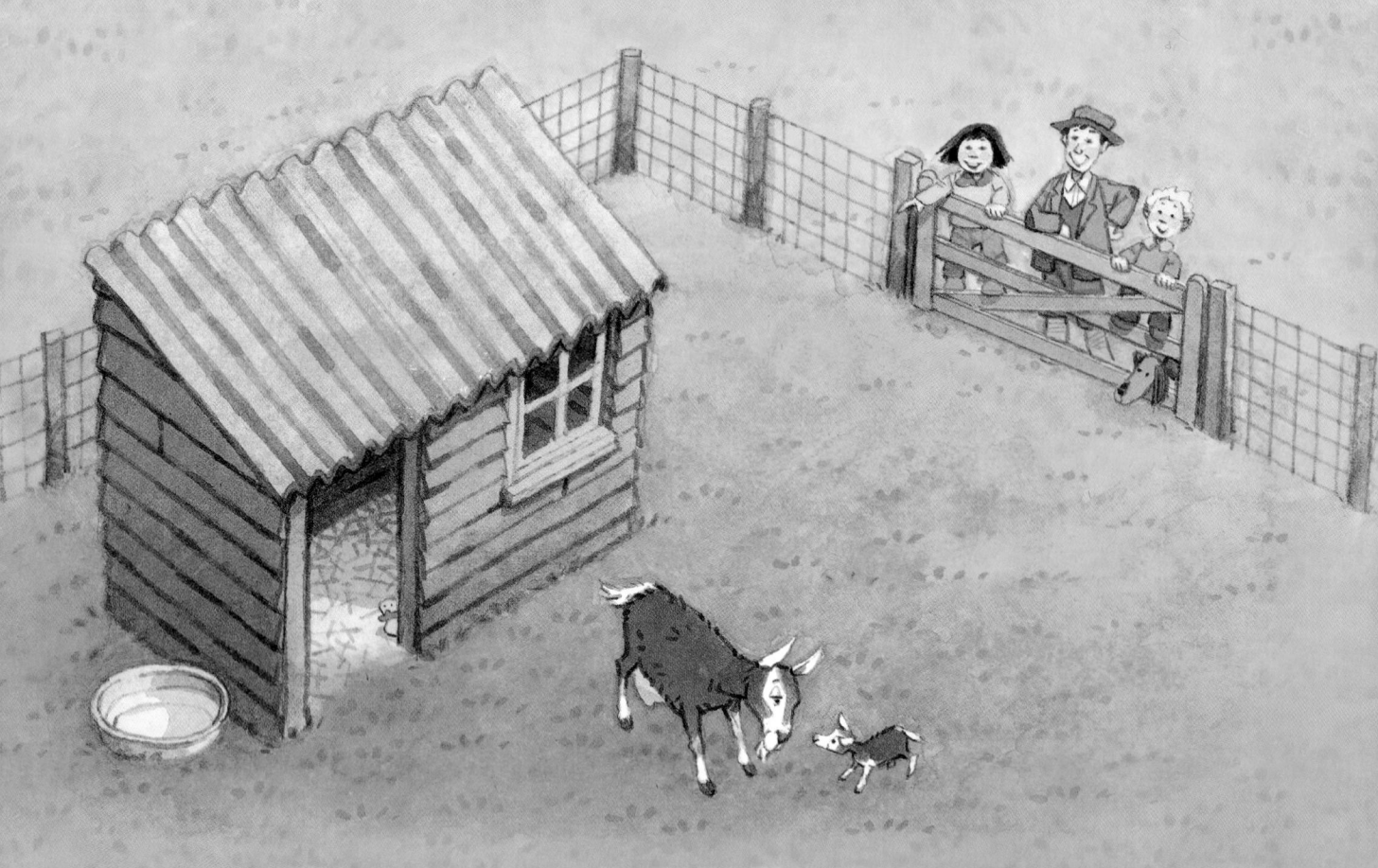

"Oh, isn't it sweet," says Poppy. "Gertie doesn't look grumpy now," says Sam.

The Snow Storm

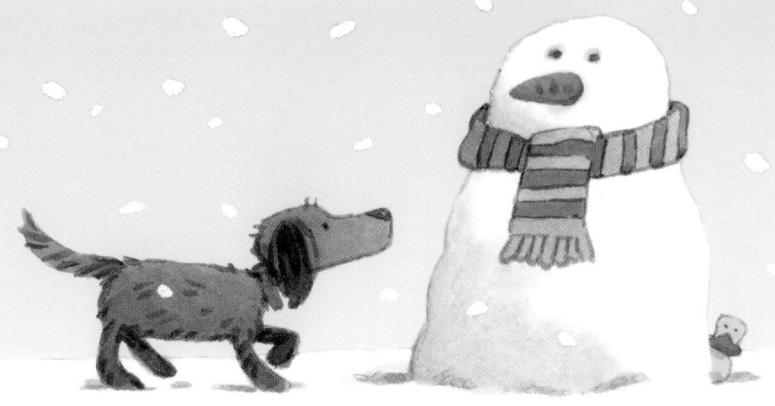

This is Apple Tree Farm.

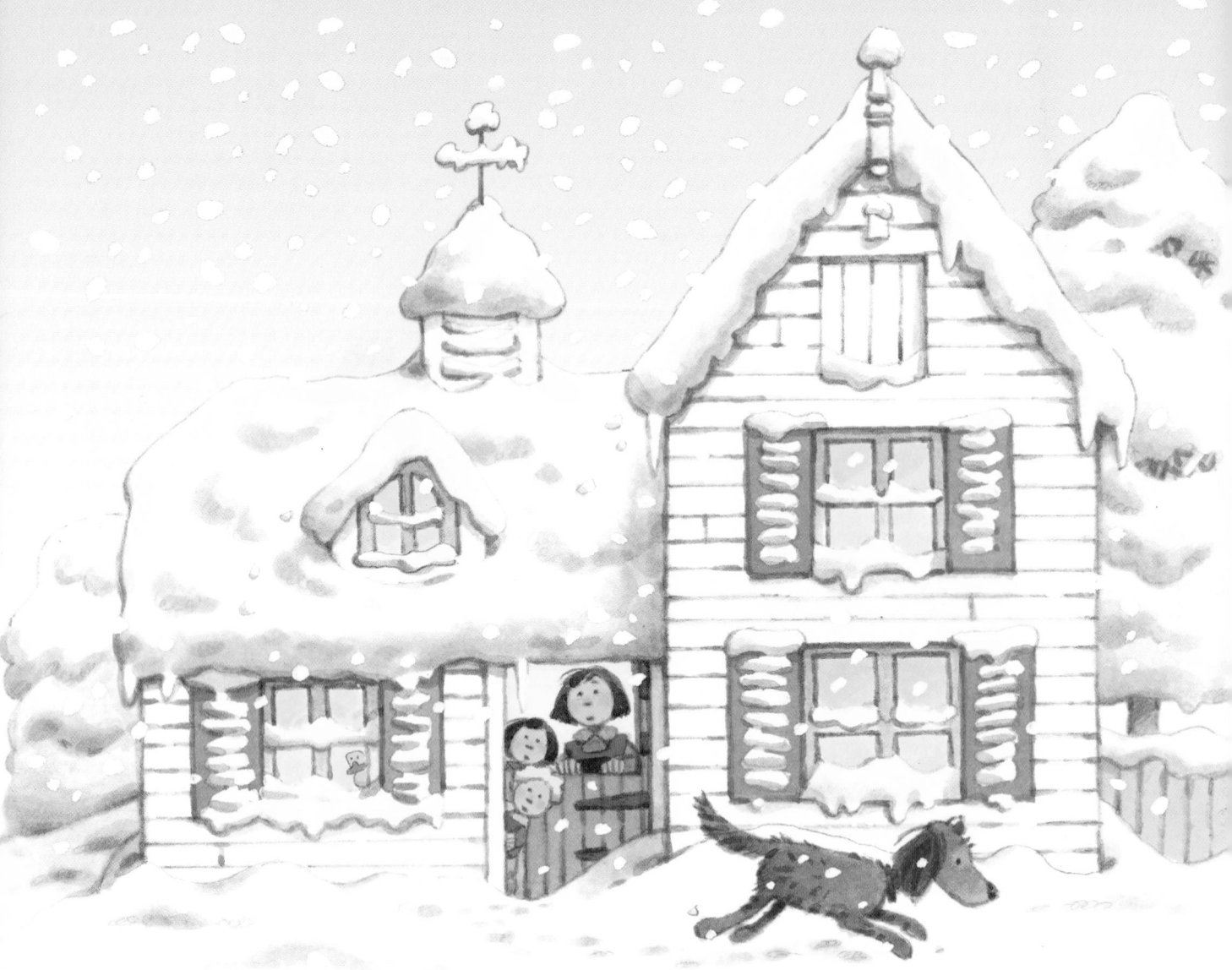

This is Mrs. Boot, the farmer. She has two children, called Poppy and Sam, and a dog called Rusty.

In the night there was a big snow storm.

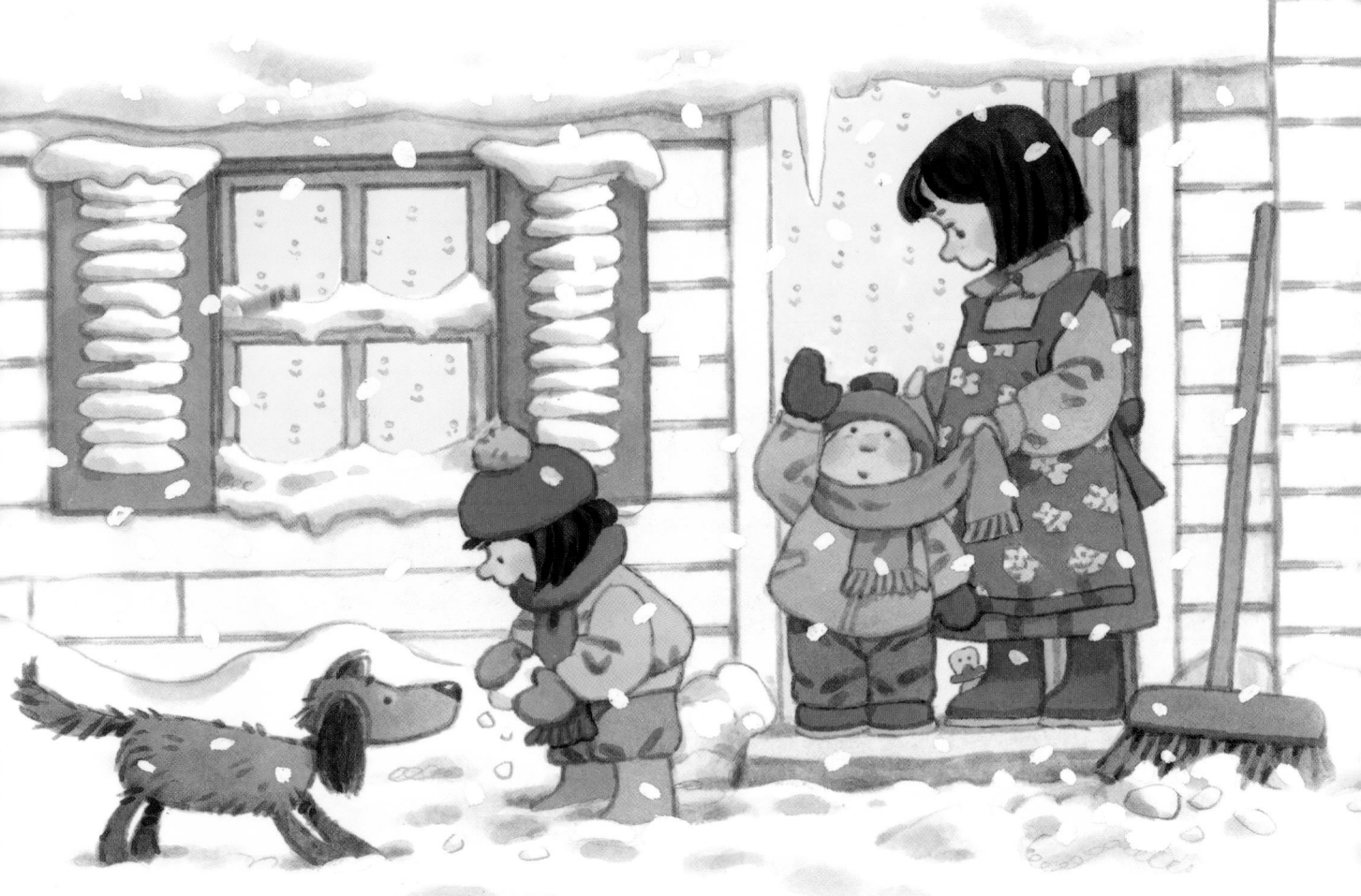

In the morning, it is still snowing. "You must wrap up warm," says Mrs. Boot to Poppy and Sam.

195

Ted works on the farm.

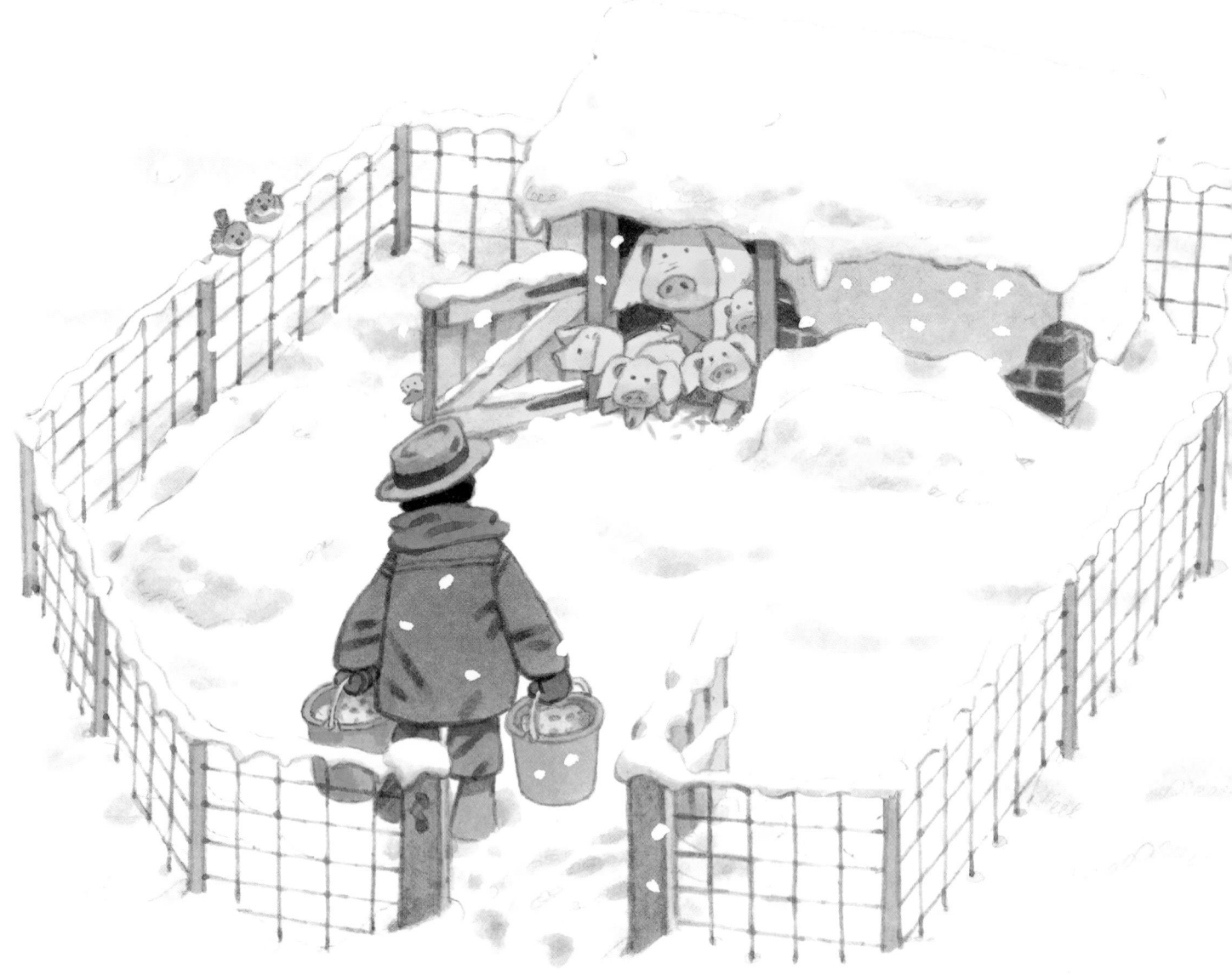

He helps Mrs. Boot look after the animals.
He gives them food and water every day.

"Come and help me," calls Ted.

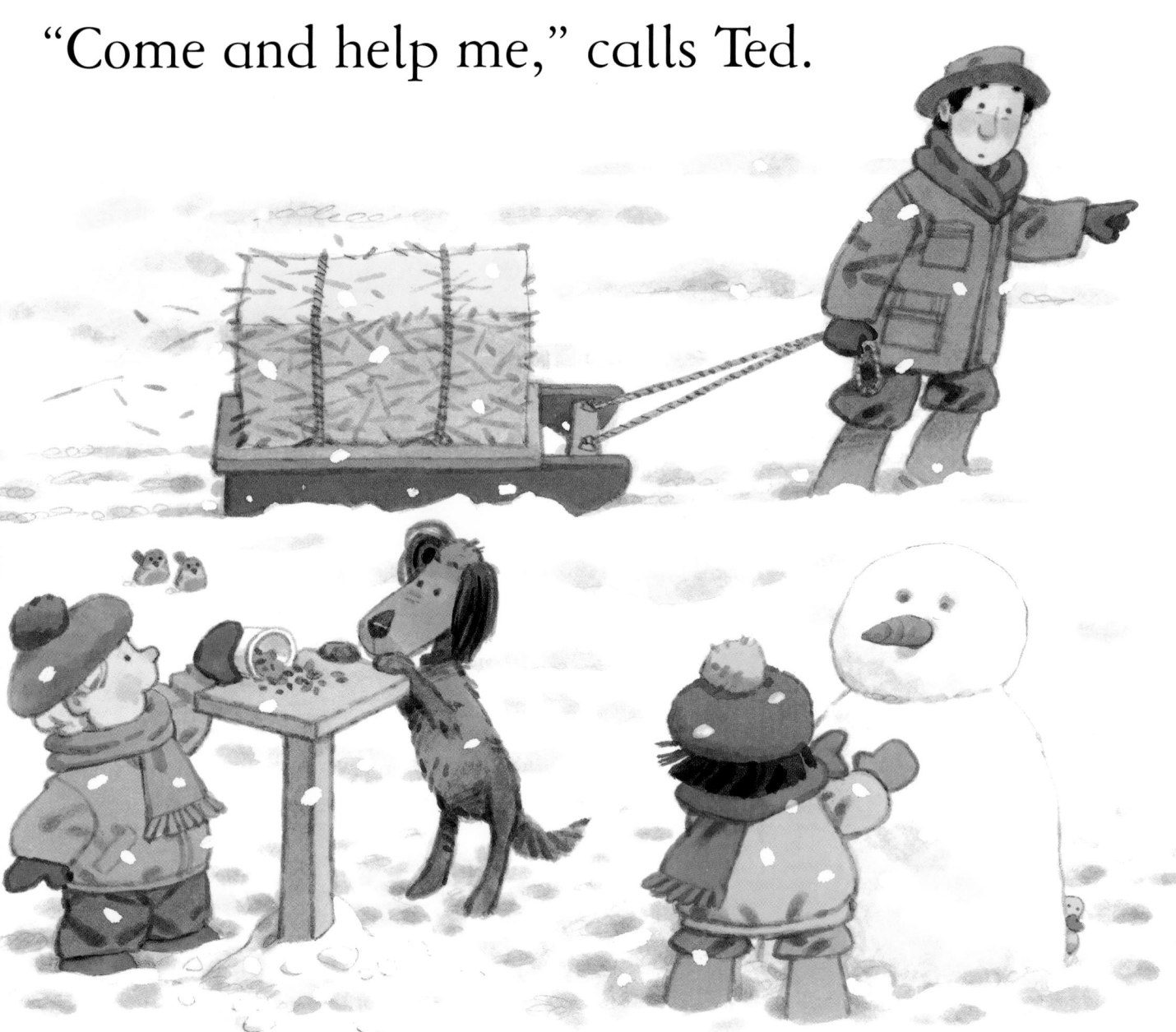

"Where are you going?" says Poppy. "I'm taking this hay to the sheep," says Ted.

Poppy and Sam pull the hay.

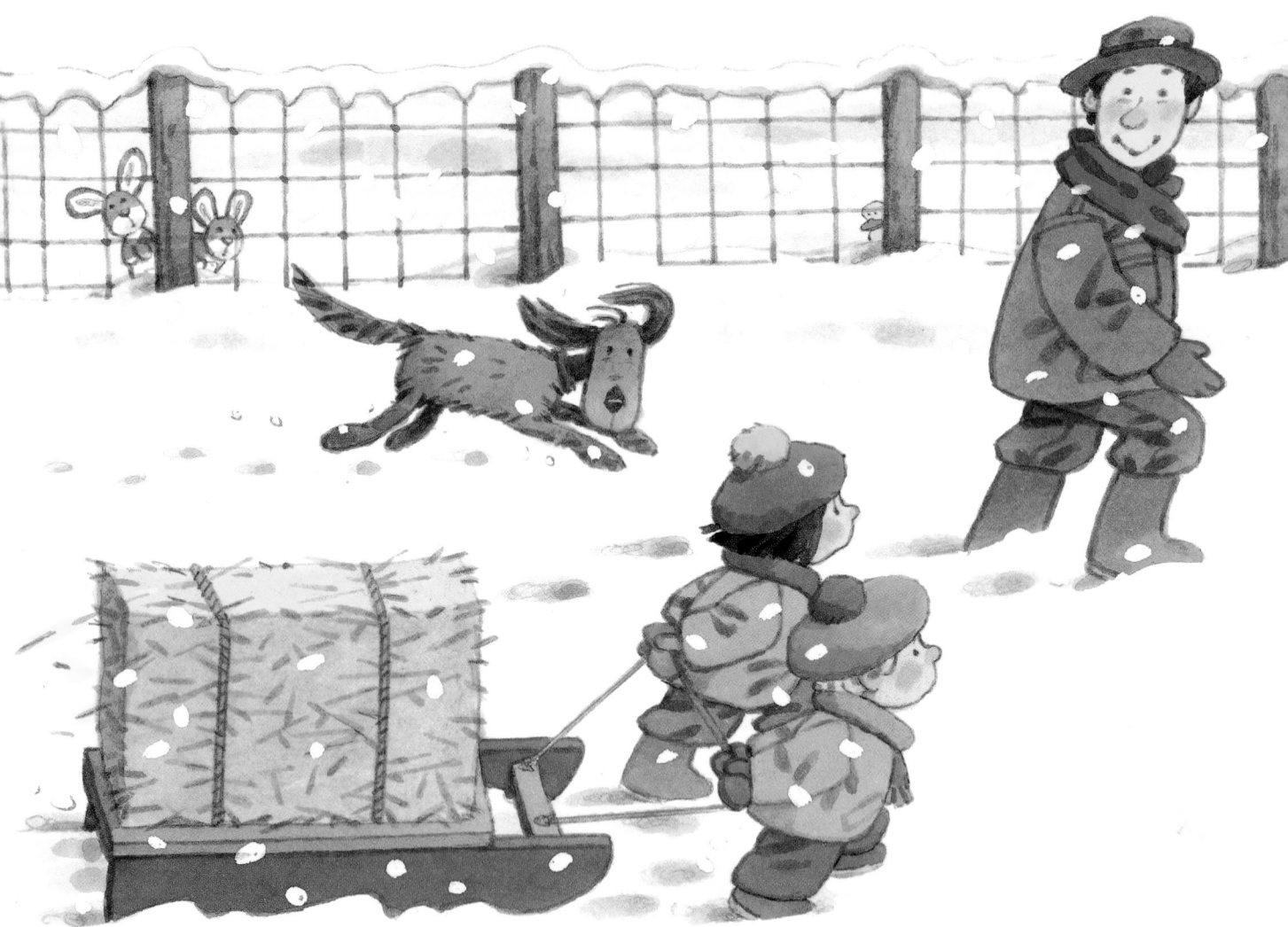

They go out of the farmyard with Ted. They walk
to the gate of the sheep field.

"Where are the sheep?" says Sam.

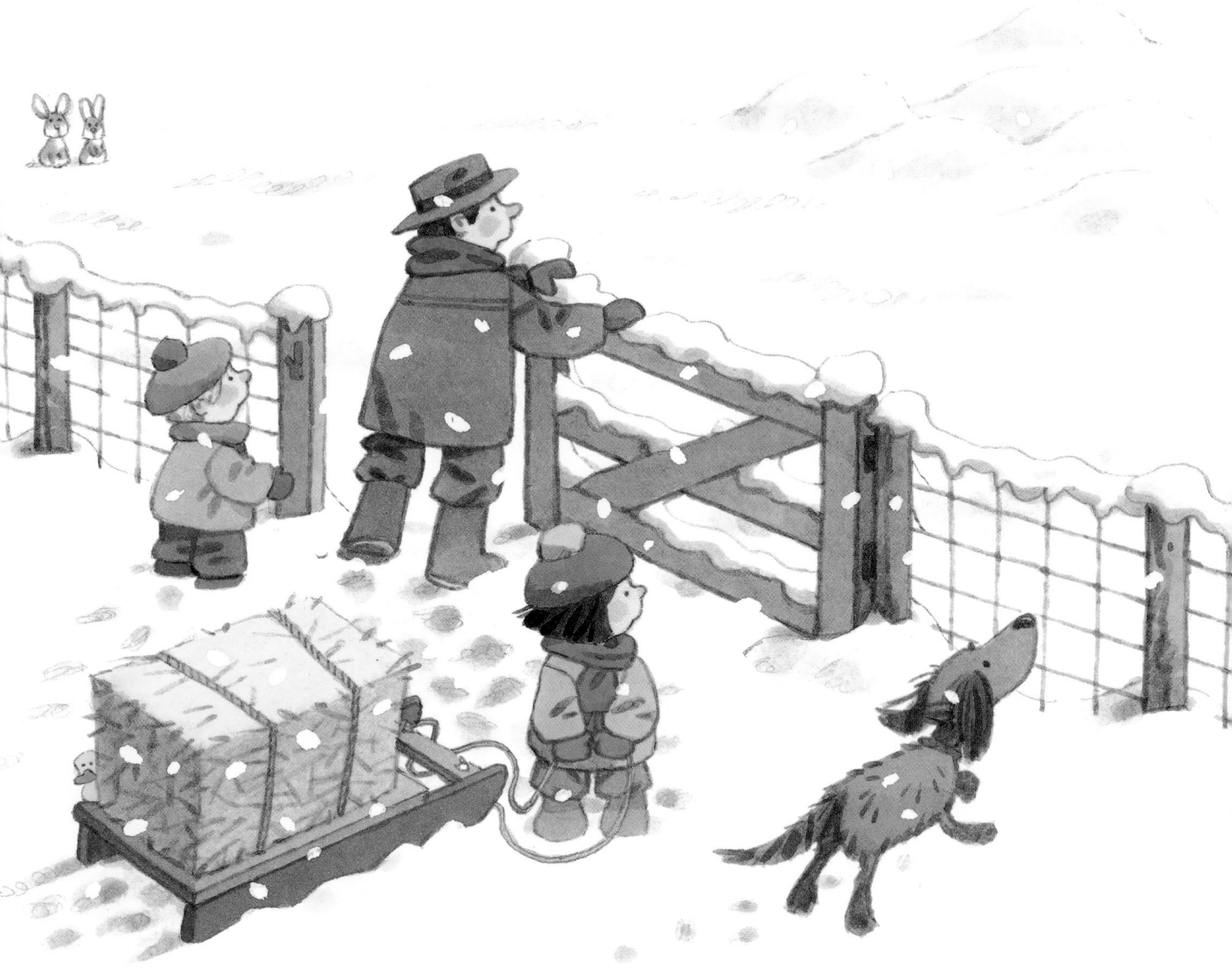

"They are all covered with snow," says Ted.
"We'll have to find them," says Poppy.

They brush the snow off the sheep.

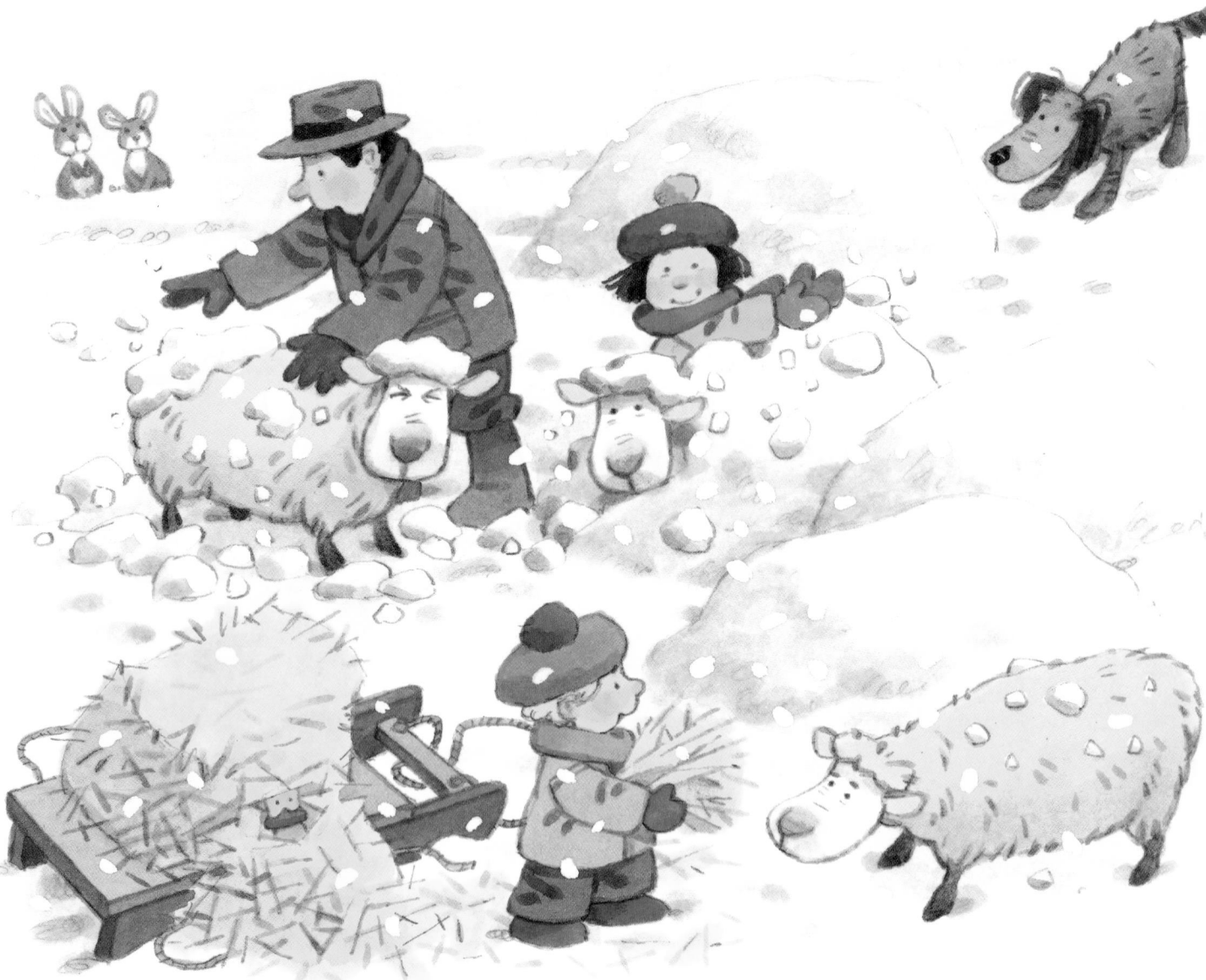

Ted, Poppy and Sam give each sheep lots of hay.
"They've got nice warm coats," says Sam.

Poppy counts the sheep.

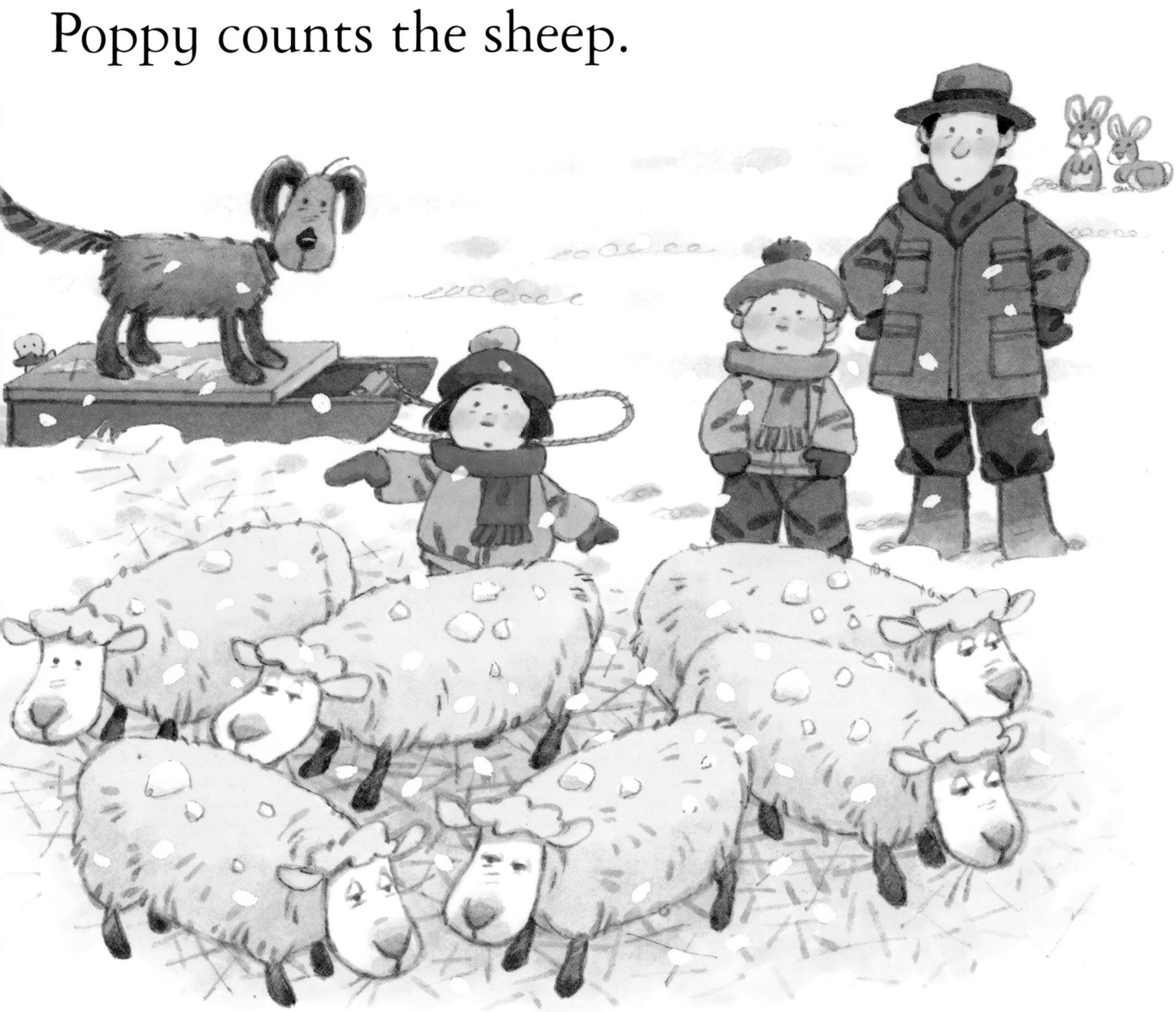

"There are only six sheep. One is missing," says
Poppy. "It's that naughty Woolly," says Ted.

They look for Woolly.

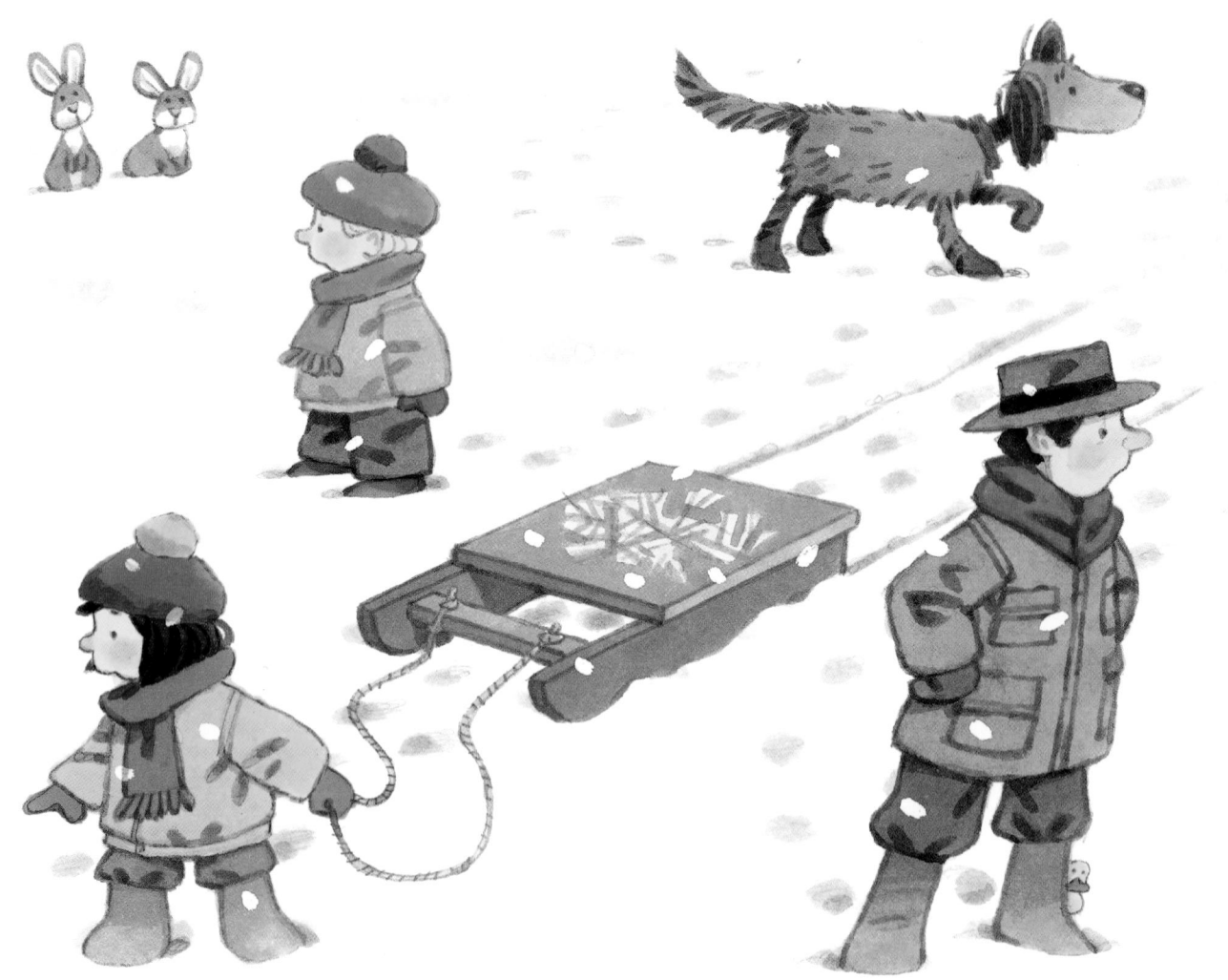

They walk around the snowy field. "Rusty, good
dog, find Woolly," calls Sam.

Rusty runs across the field.

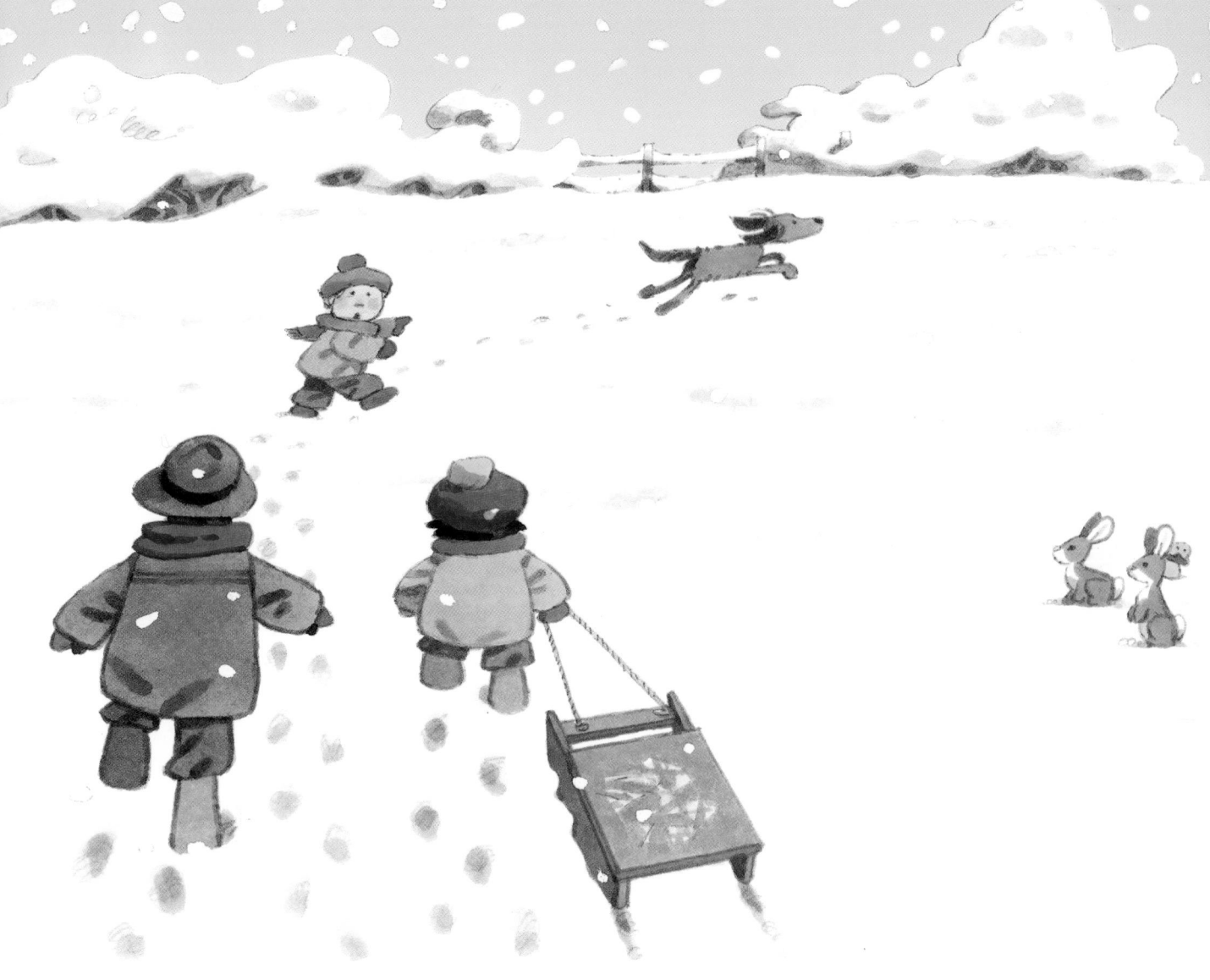

Ted, Poppy and Sam run after him. Rusty barks
at the thick hedge.

Ted looks under the hedge.

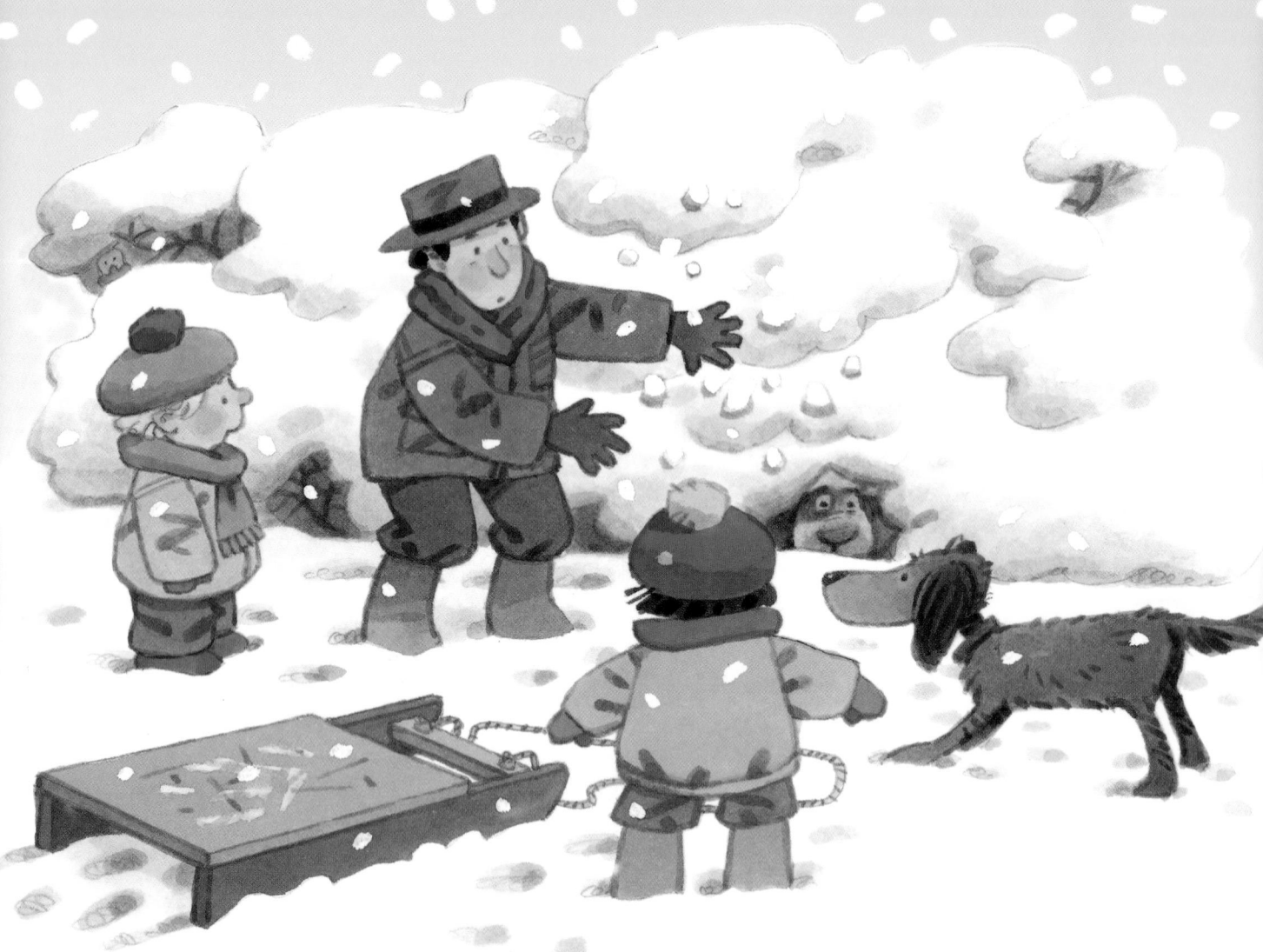

"Can you see anything?" says Sam. "Yes, Woolly is hiding in there. Clever Rusty," says Ted.

"Come on, Woolly."

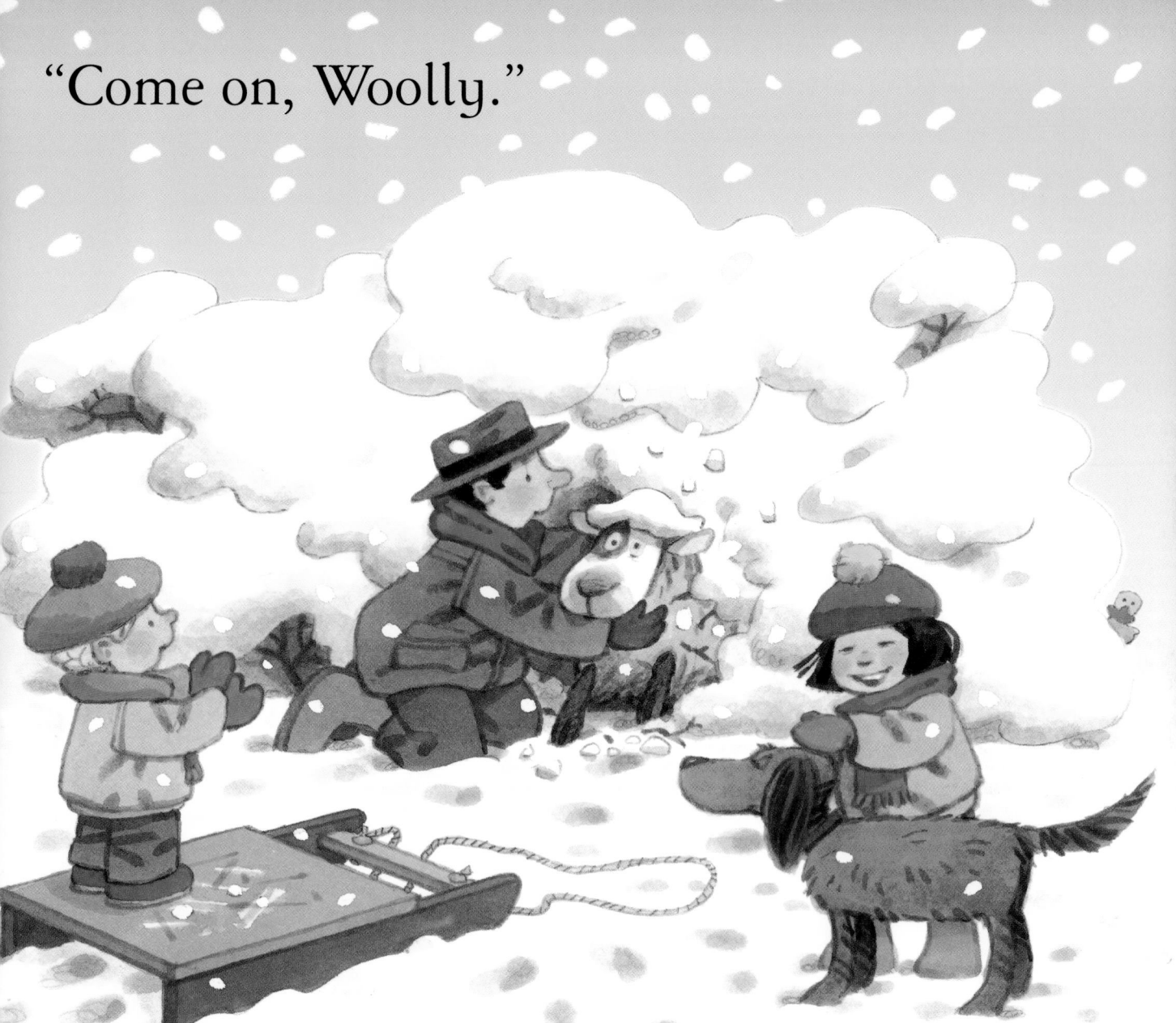

"Let me help you out, old girl," says Ted.
Carefully he pulls Woolly out of the hedge.

"There's something else!"

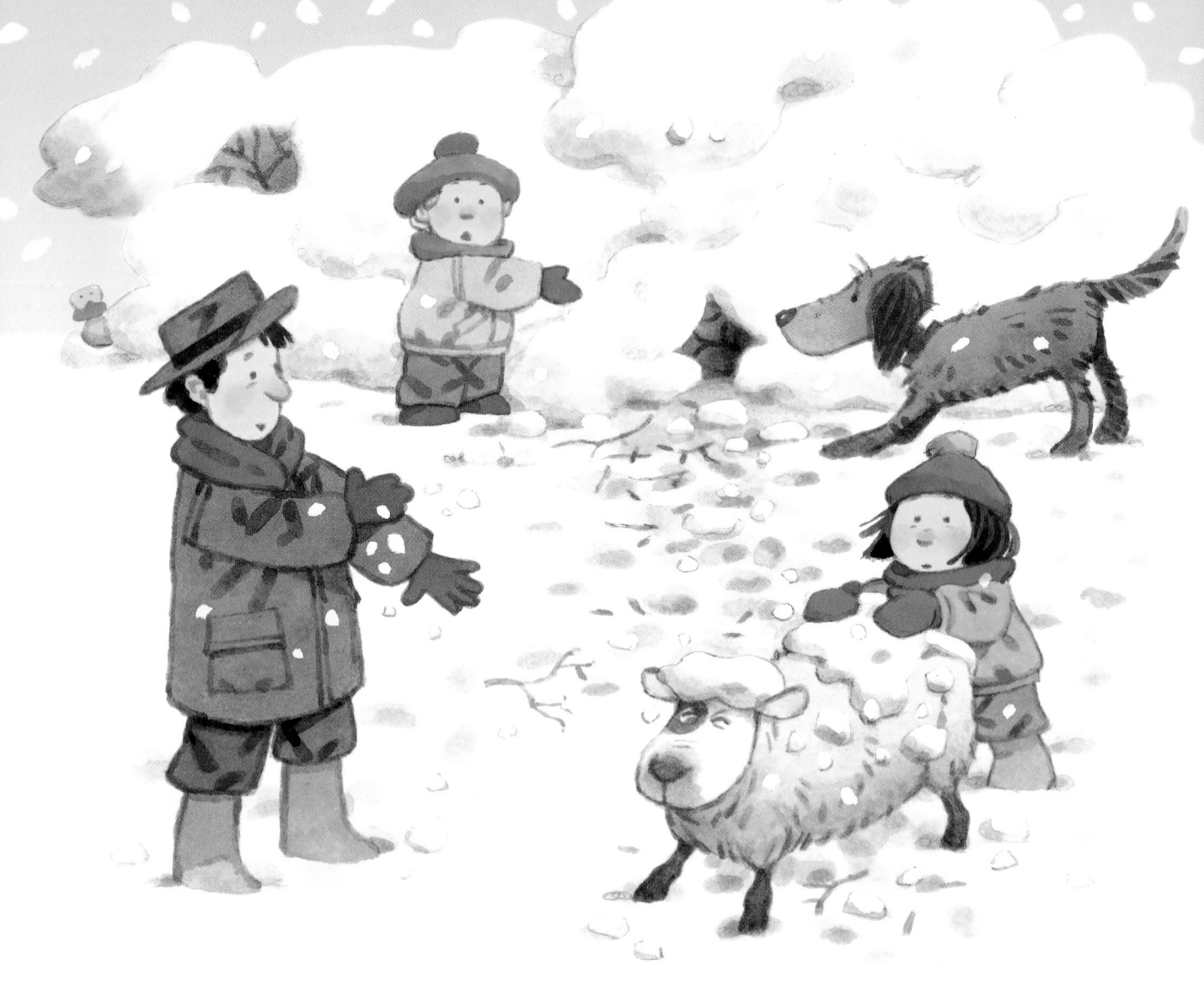

"Look, I can see something moving," says Sam.
"What is it, Ted?" says Poppy.

Ted lifts out a tiny lamb.

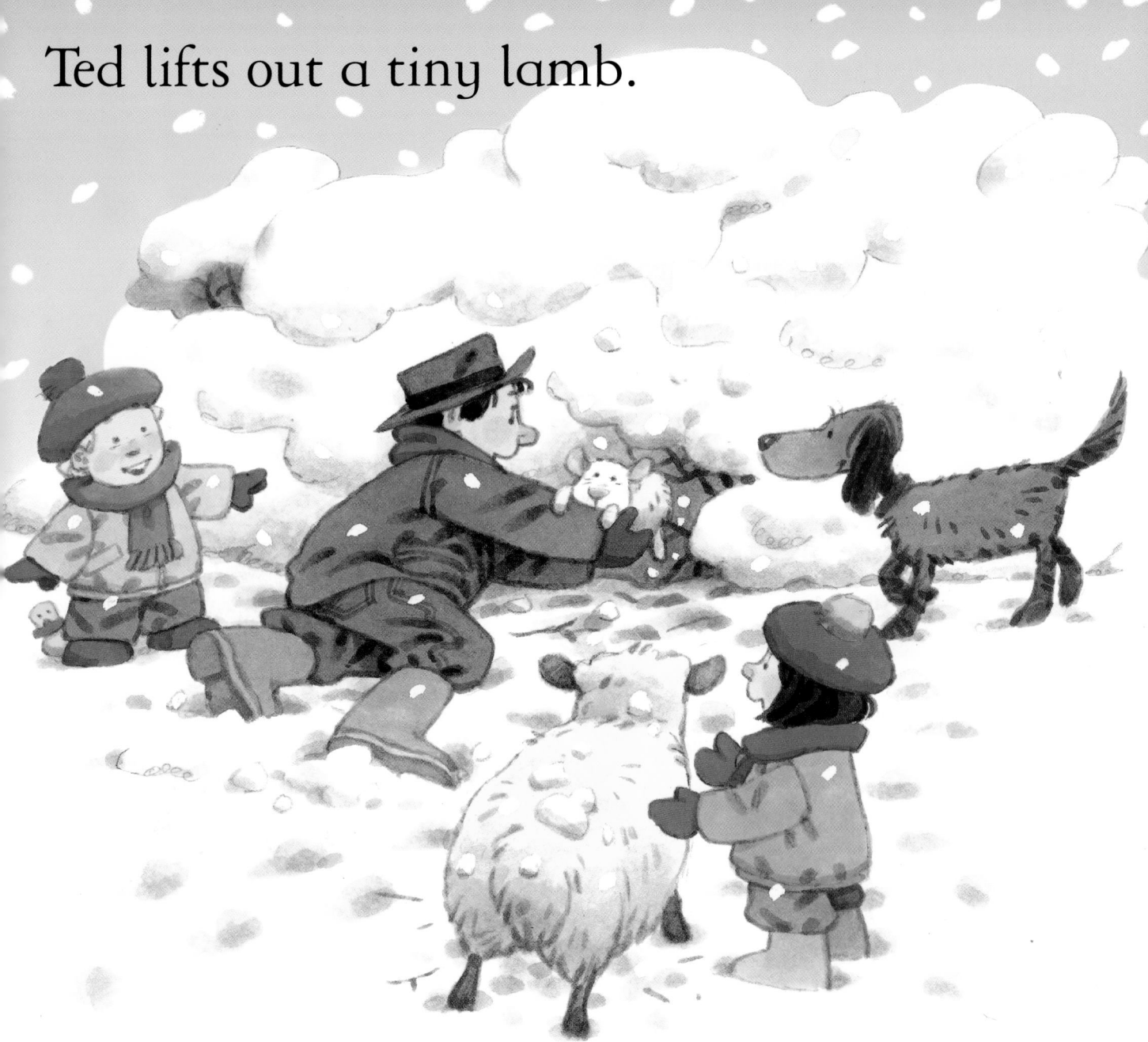

"Woolly has had a lamb," he says. "We'll take it and Woolly to the barn. They'll be warm there."

Poppy rides home.

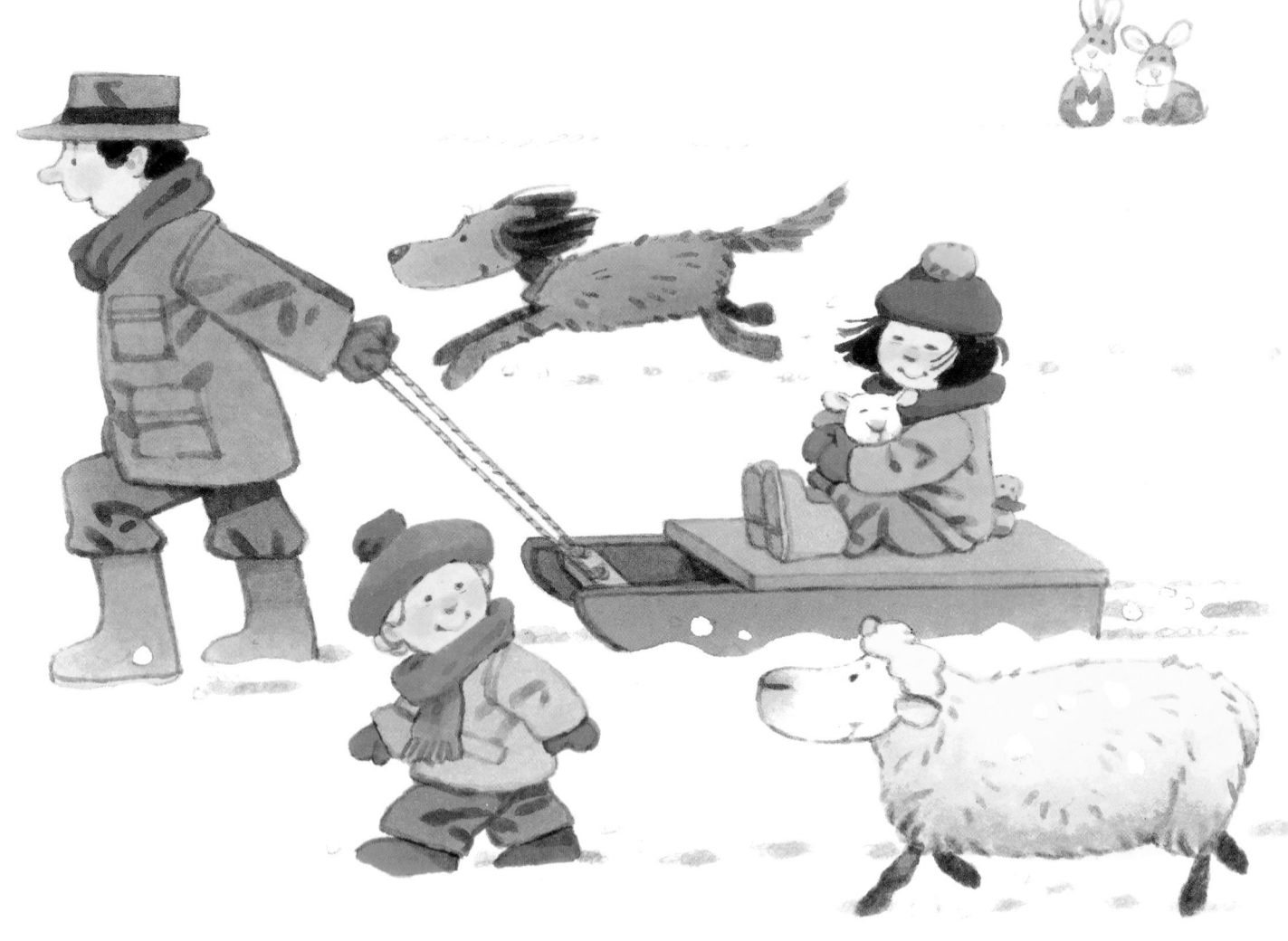

She holds the lamb. "What a surprise!" she says.
"Good old Woolly."

Surprise Visitors

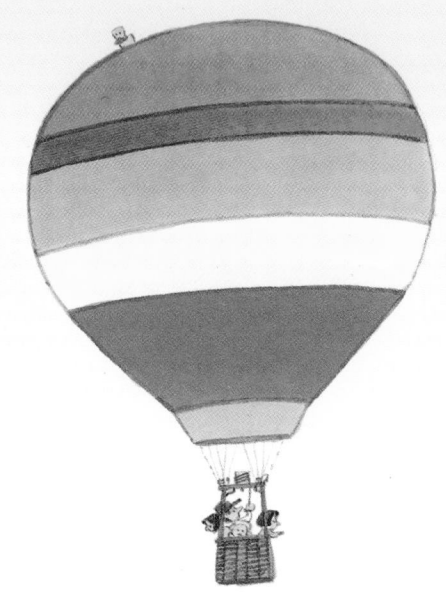

This is Apple Tree Farm.

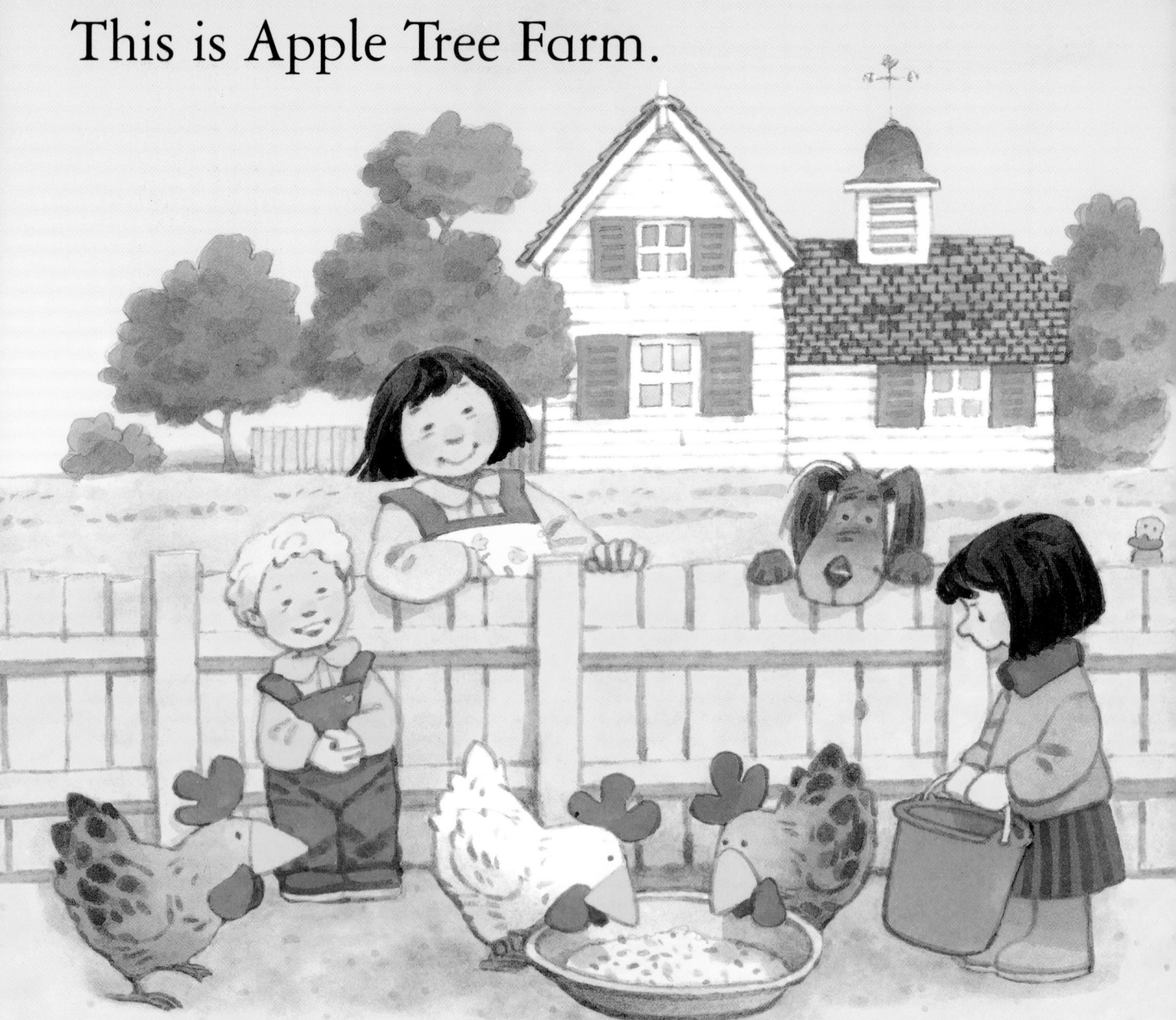

This is Mrs. Boot, the farmer. She has two children, called Poppy and Sam, and a dog called Rusty.

Today is Saturday.

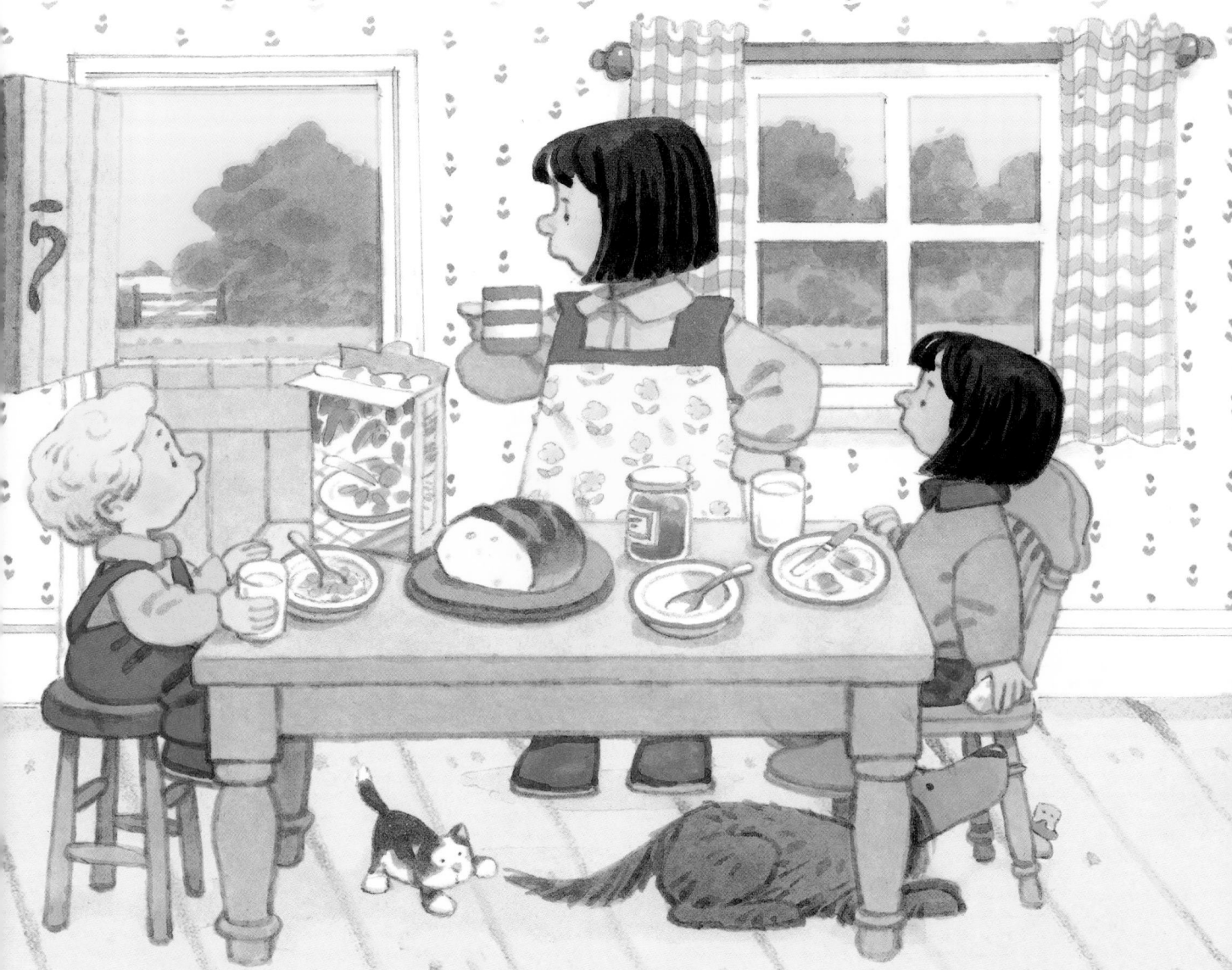

Mrs. Boot, Poppy and Sam are having breakfast.
"Why are the cows so noisy?" asks Sam.

They all run out to the field.

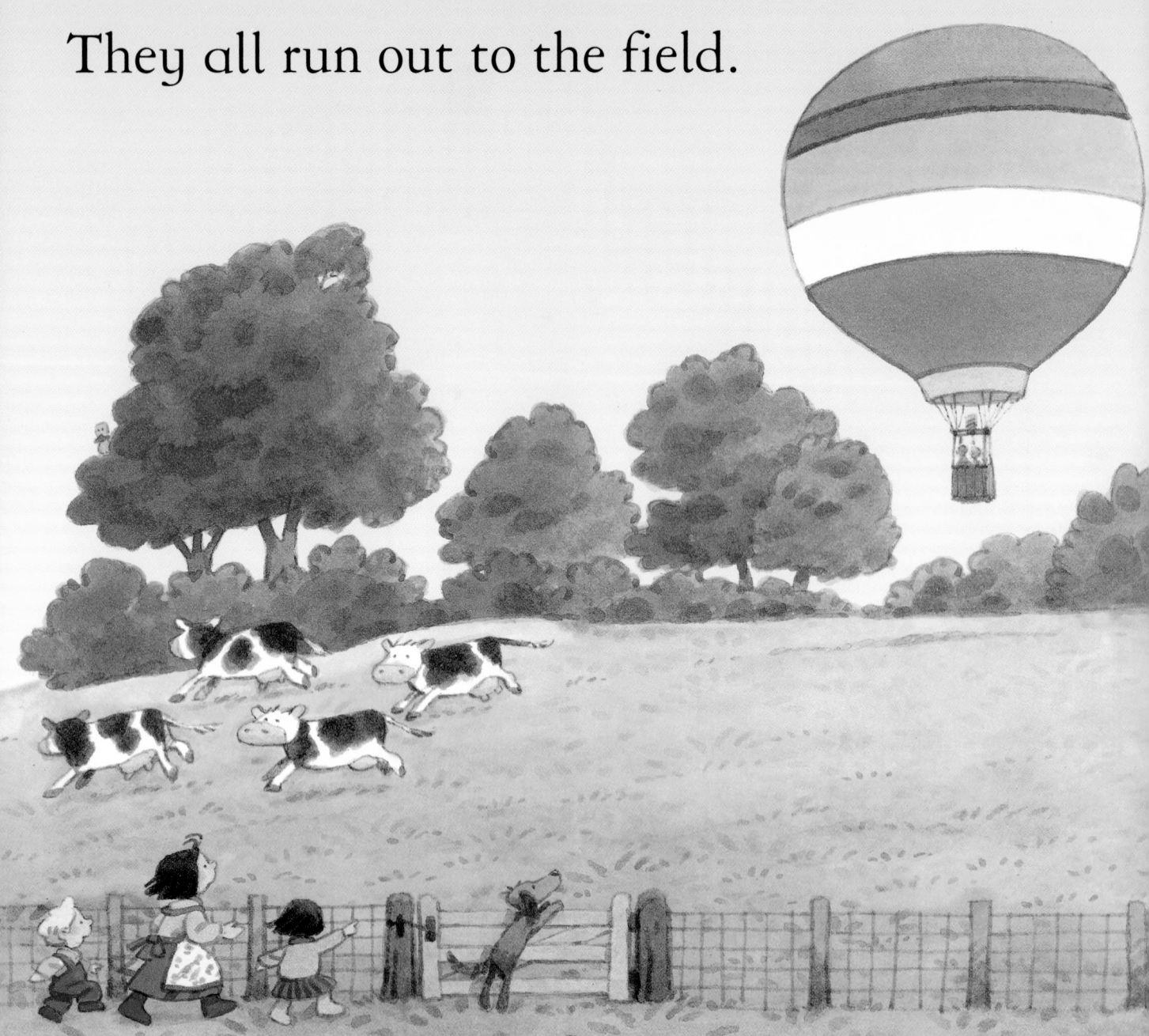

The cows are running around the field. They are scared. A big balloon is floating over the trees.

"It's a hot air balloon."

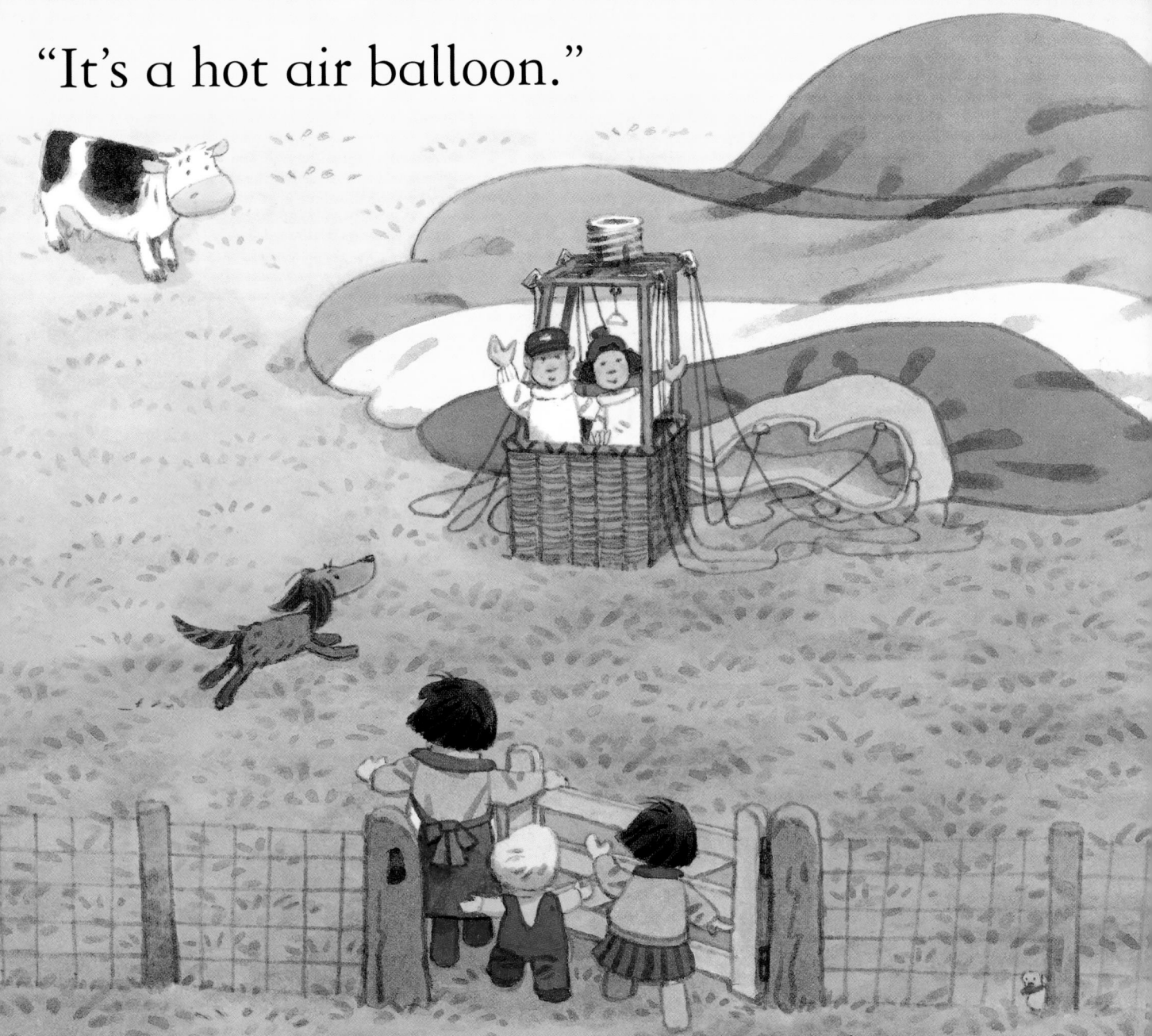

"It's coming down," says Mrs. Boot. "It's going to land in our field." The balloon hits the ground.

213

There are two people in it.

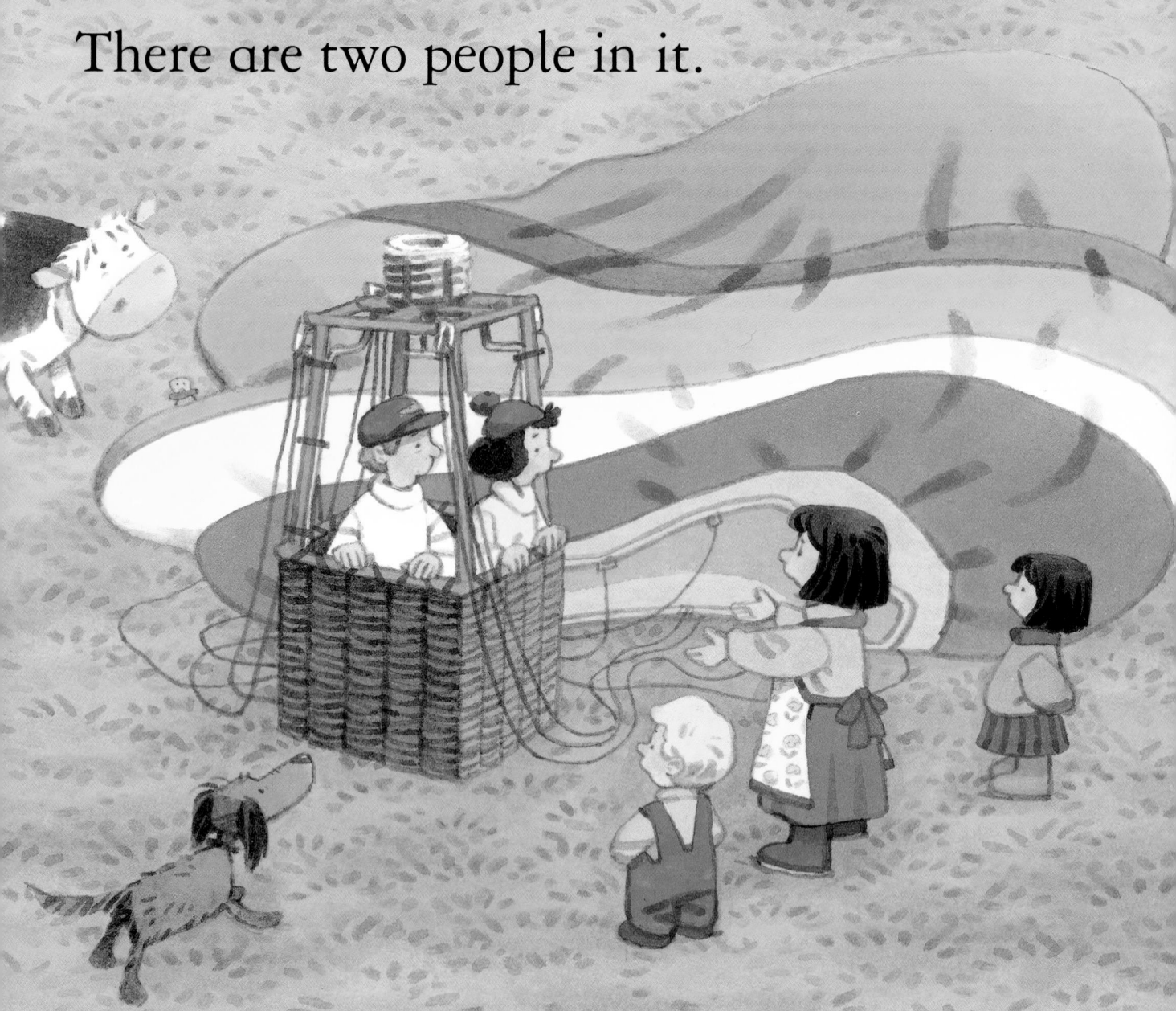

"Where are we?" asks the man. "This is Apple Tree Farm. You frightened our cows," says Mrs. Boot.

The man climbs out.

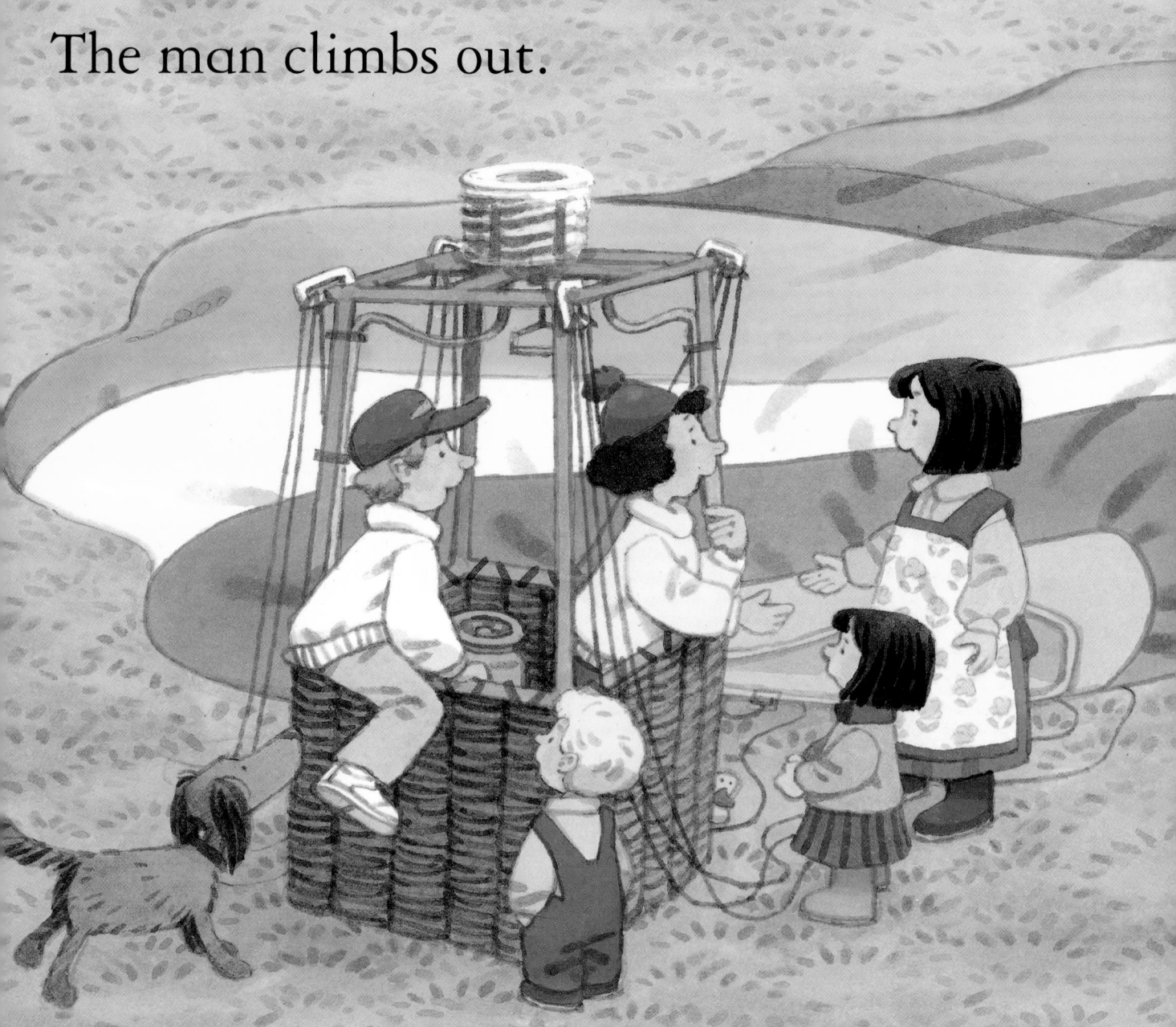

"I'm Alice and this is Tim," says the woman.
"We ran out of gas. Sorry about your cows."

"A truck is following us."

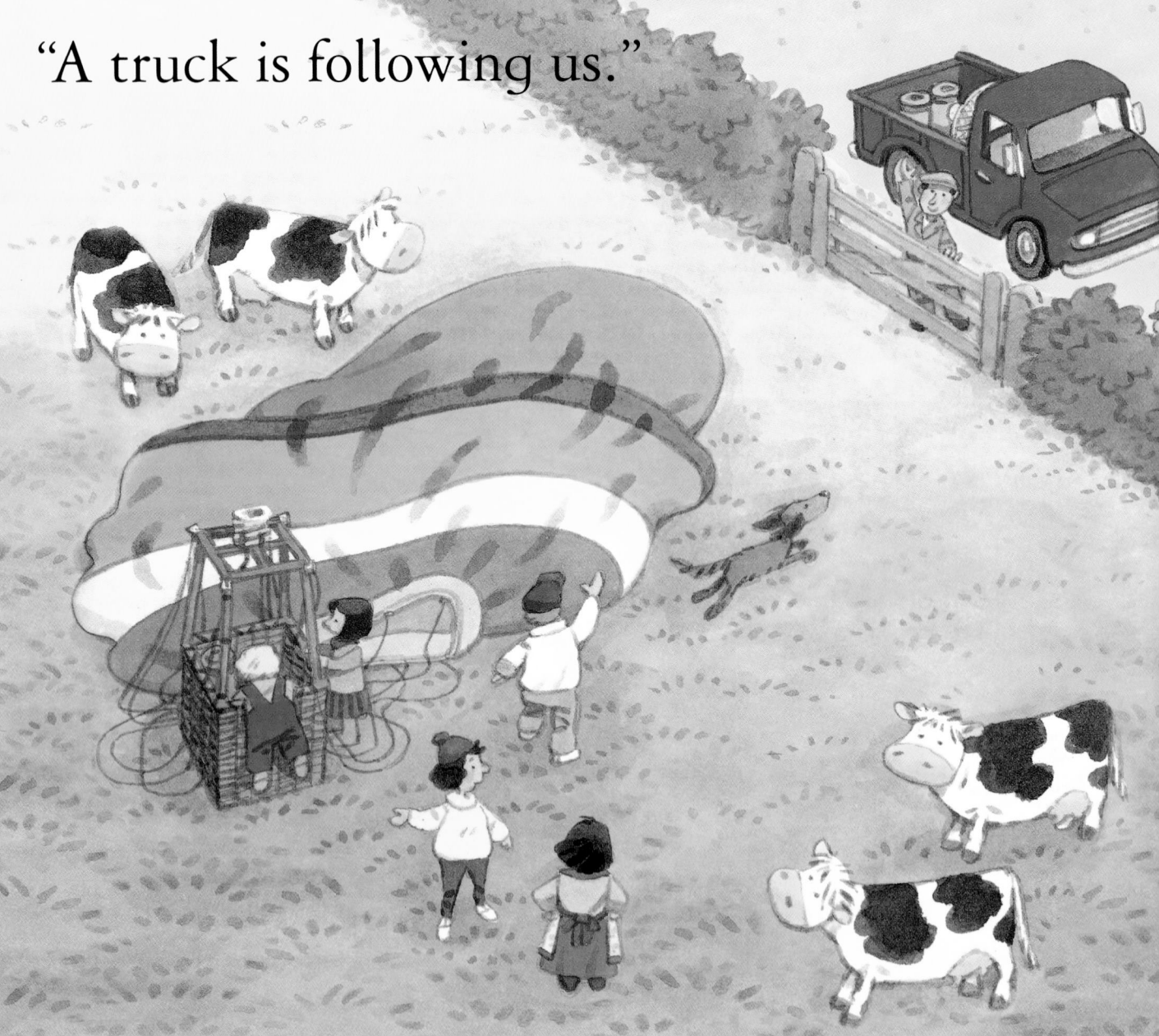

"There it is now," says Alice. "Our friend is bringing more cylinders of gas for the balloon."

216

Alice helps to unload the truck.

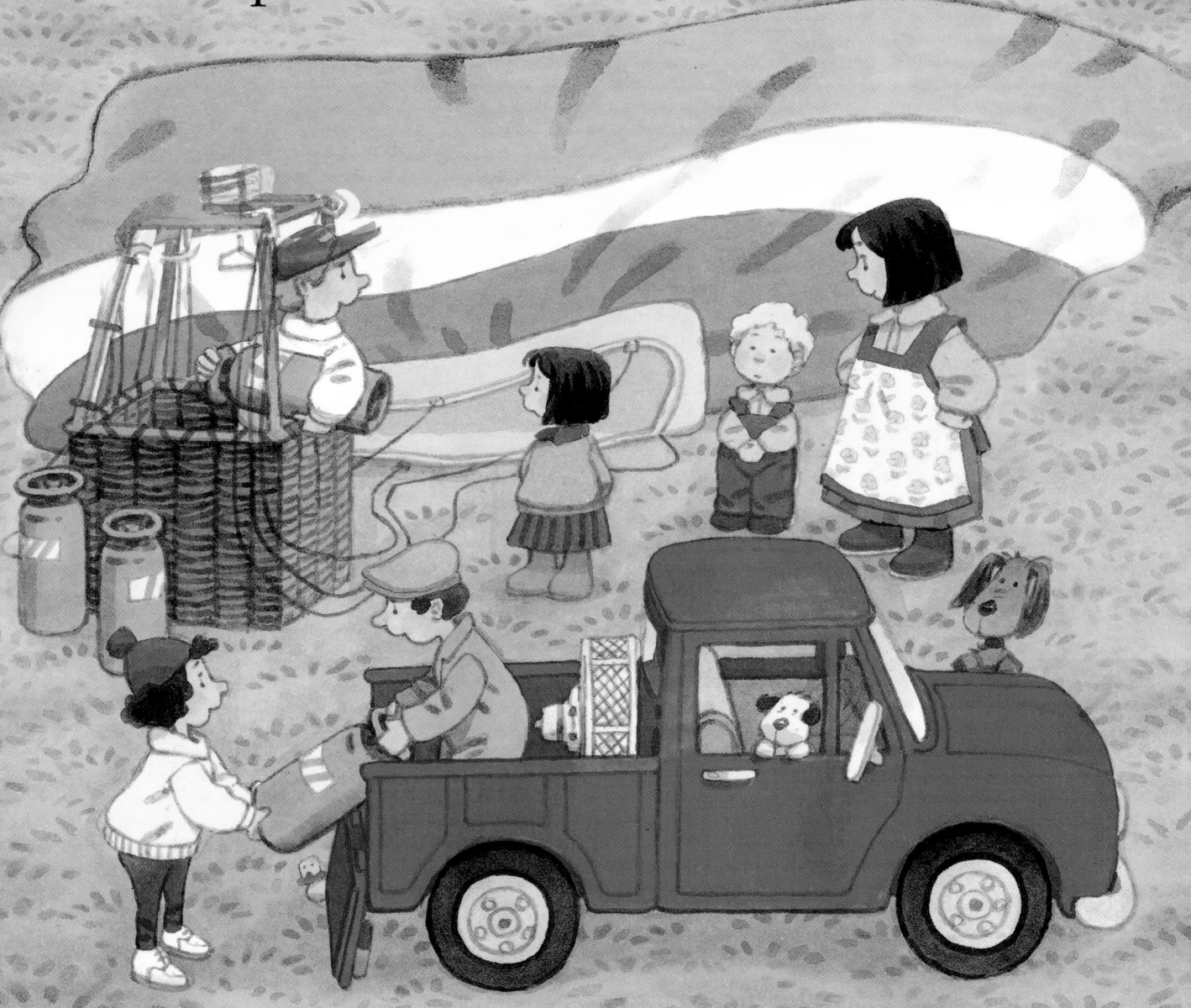

Tim unloads the empty cylinders. Then he puts the
new ones into the balloon's basket.

They blow up the balloon.

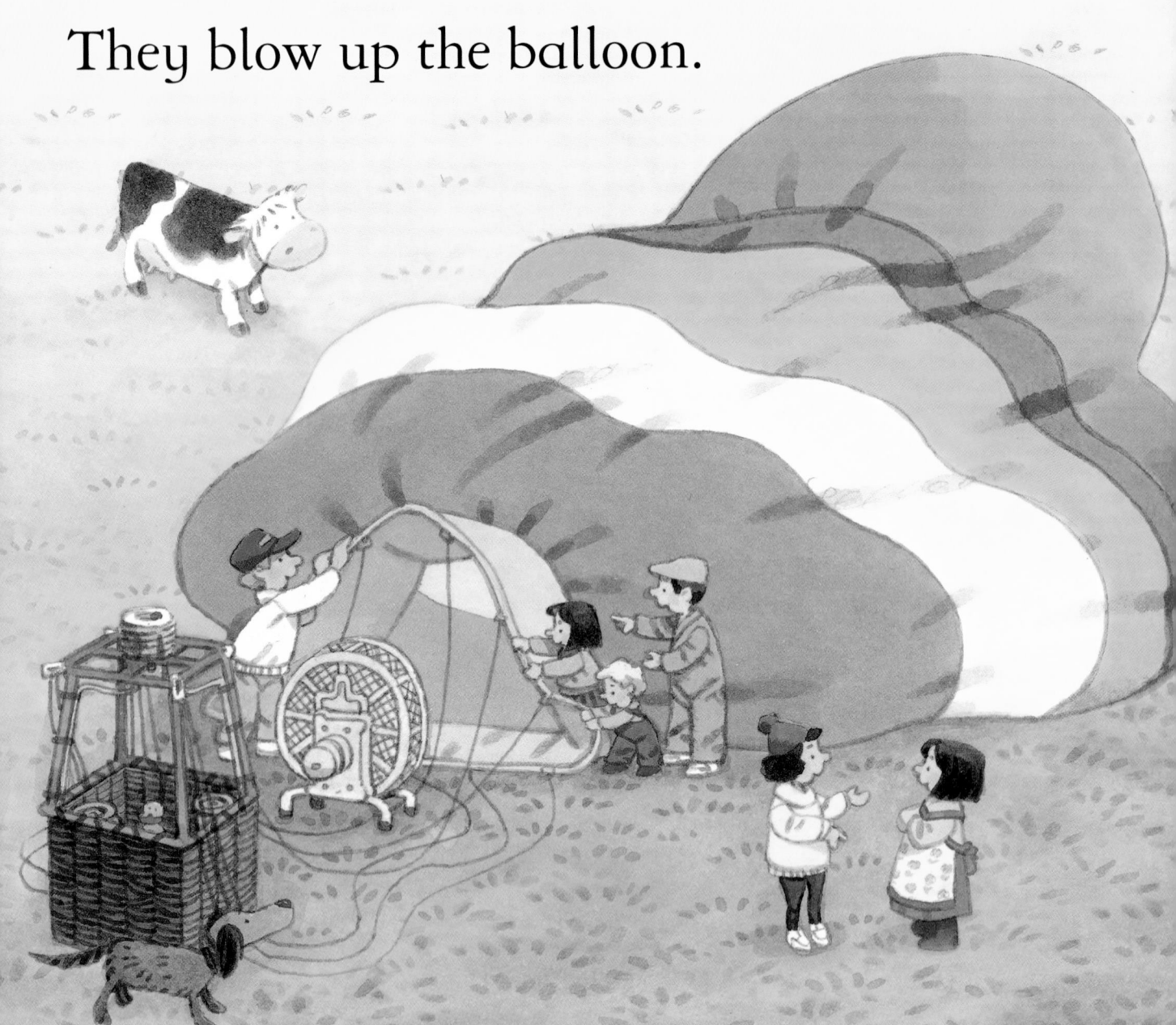

Poppy and Sam help Tim hold open the balloon.
A fan blows hot air into it. It gets bigger and bigger.

"Would you like a ride?"

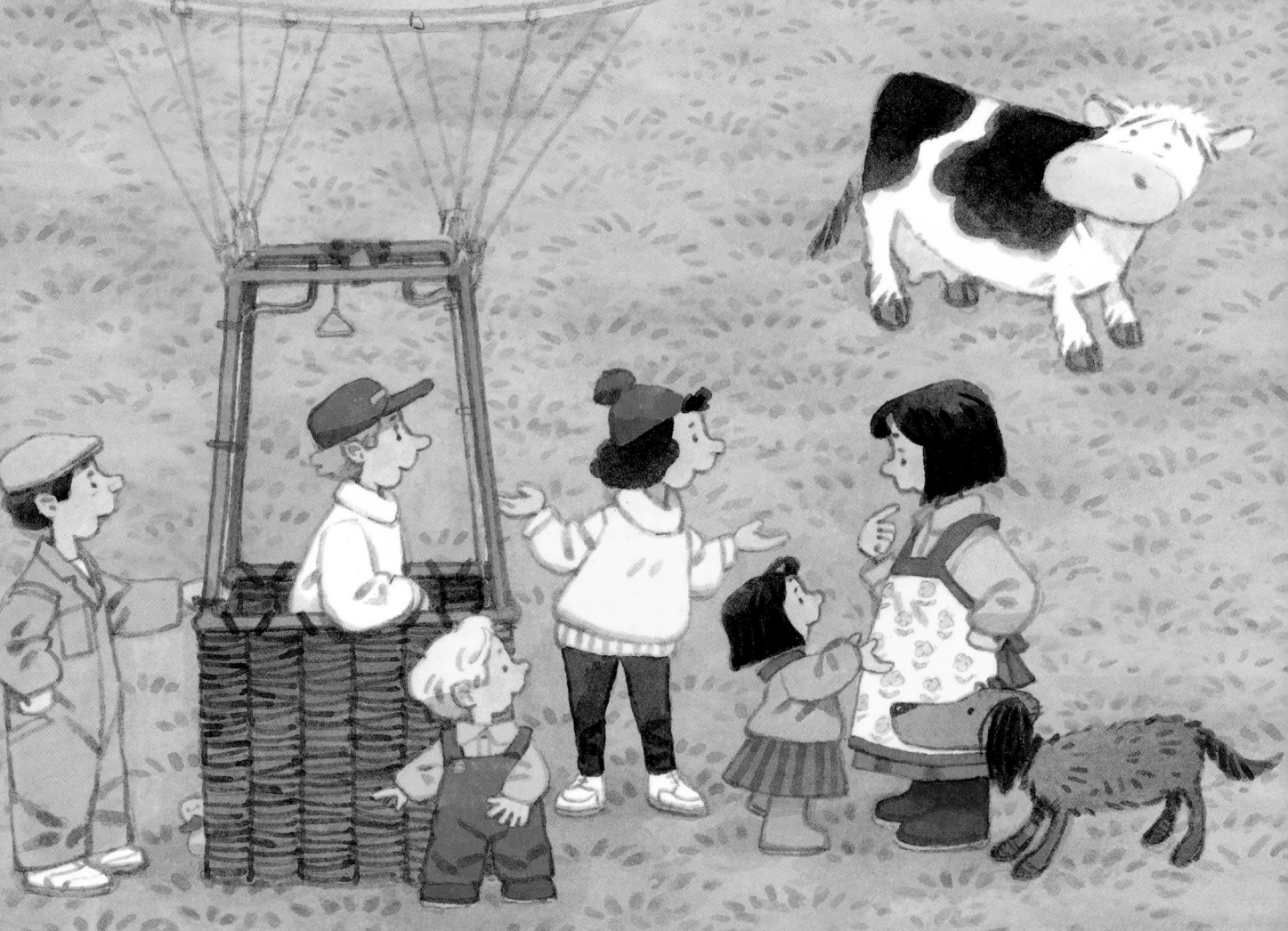

"Oh, yes please," says Poppy. "Just a little one,"
says Tim. "The truck will bring you back."

Mrs. Boot, Poppy and Sam climb in.

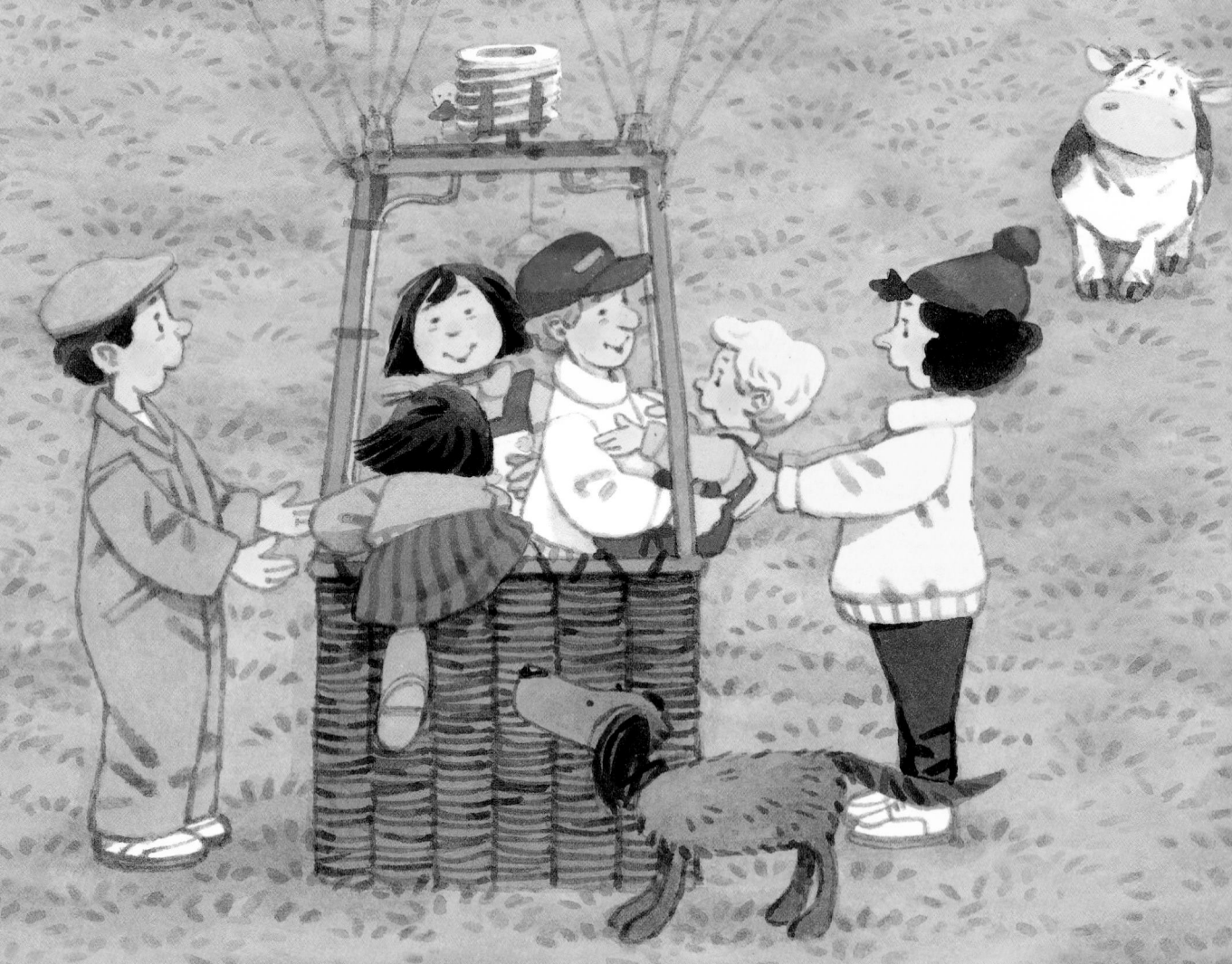

Tim lights the gas burner. The big flames make
a loud noise. "Hold on tight," says Alice.

The balloon goes up.

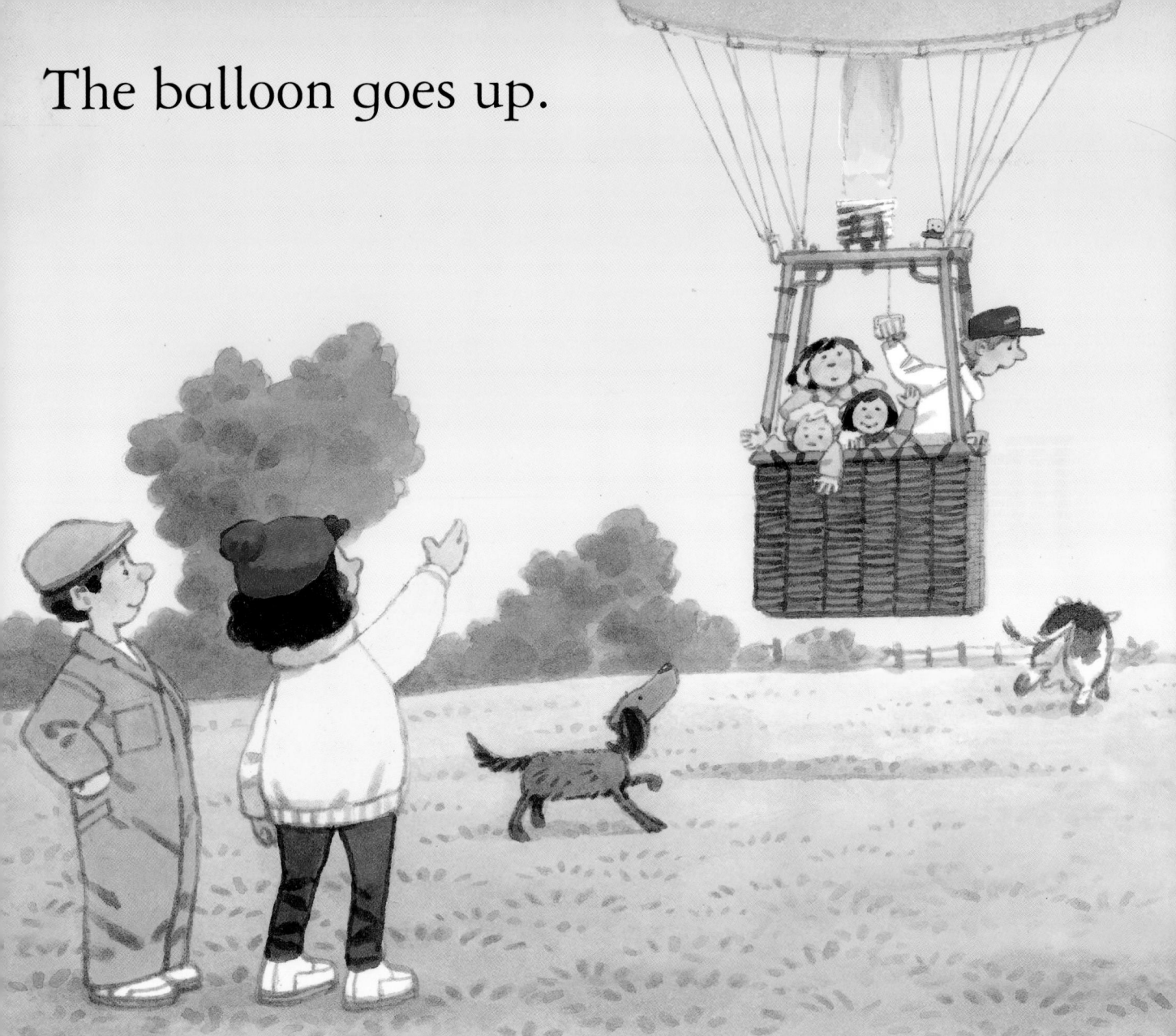

Slowly it leaves the ground. Tim turns off the burner. "The wind is blowing us along," he says.

The balloon floats along.

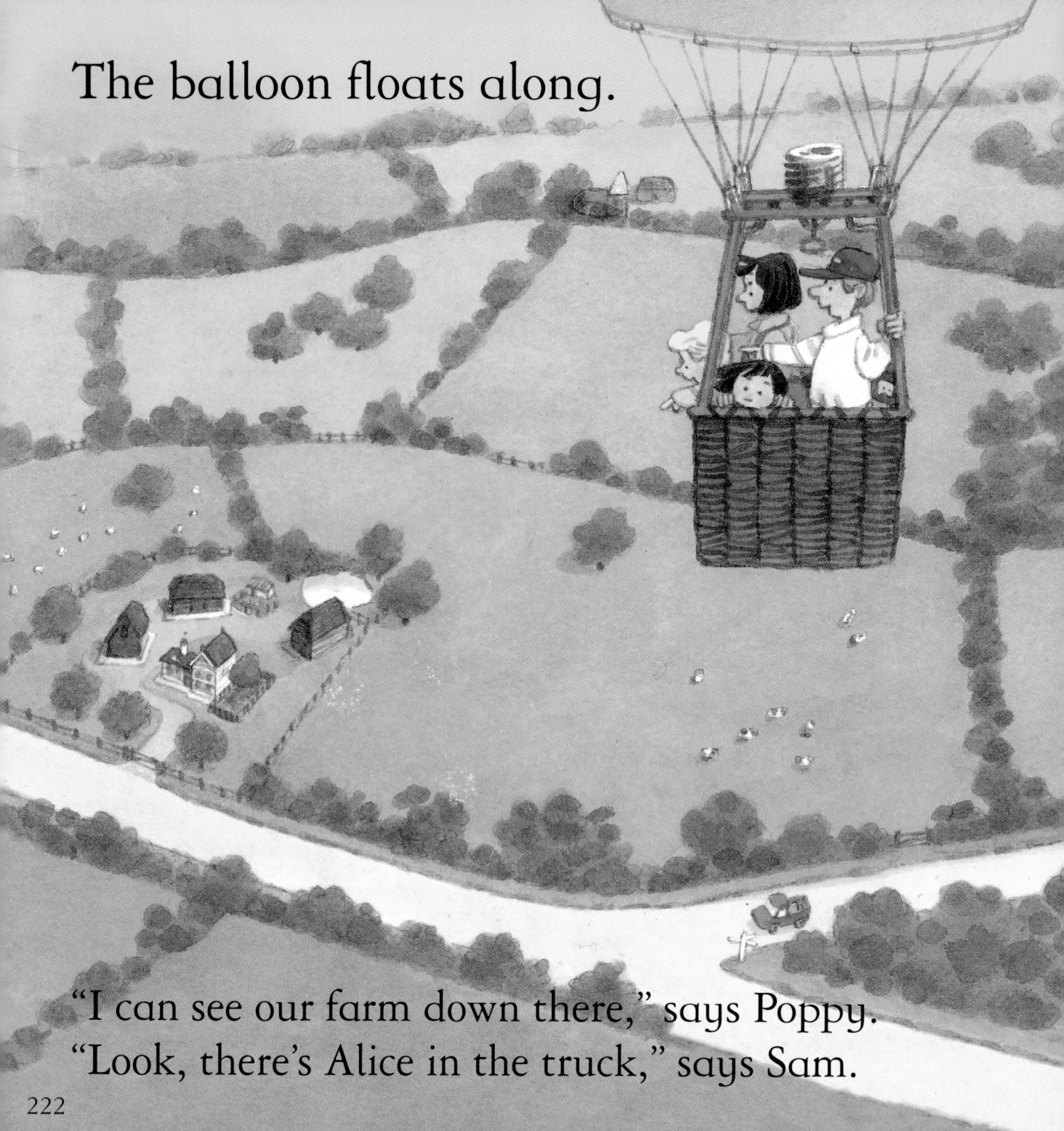

"I can see our farm down there," says Poppy.
"Look, there's Alice in the truck," says Sam.

"We're going down now," says Tim.

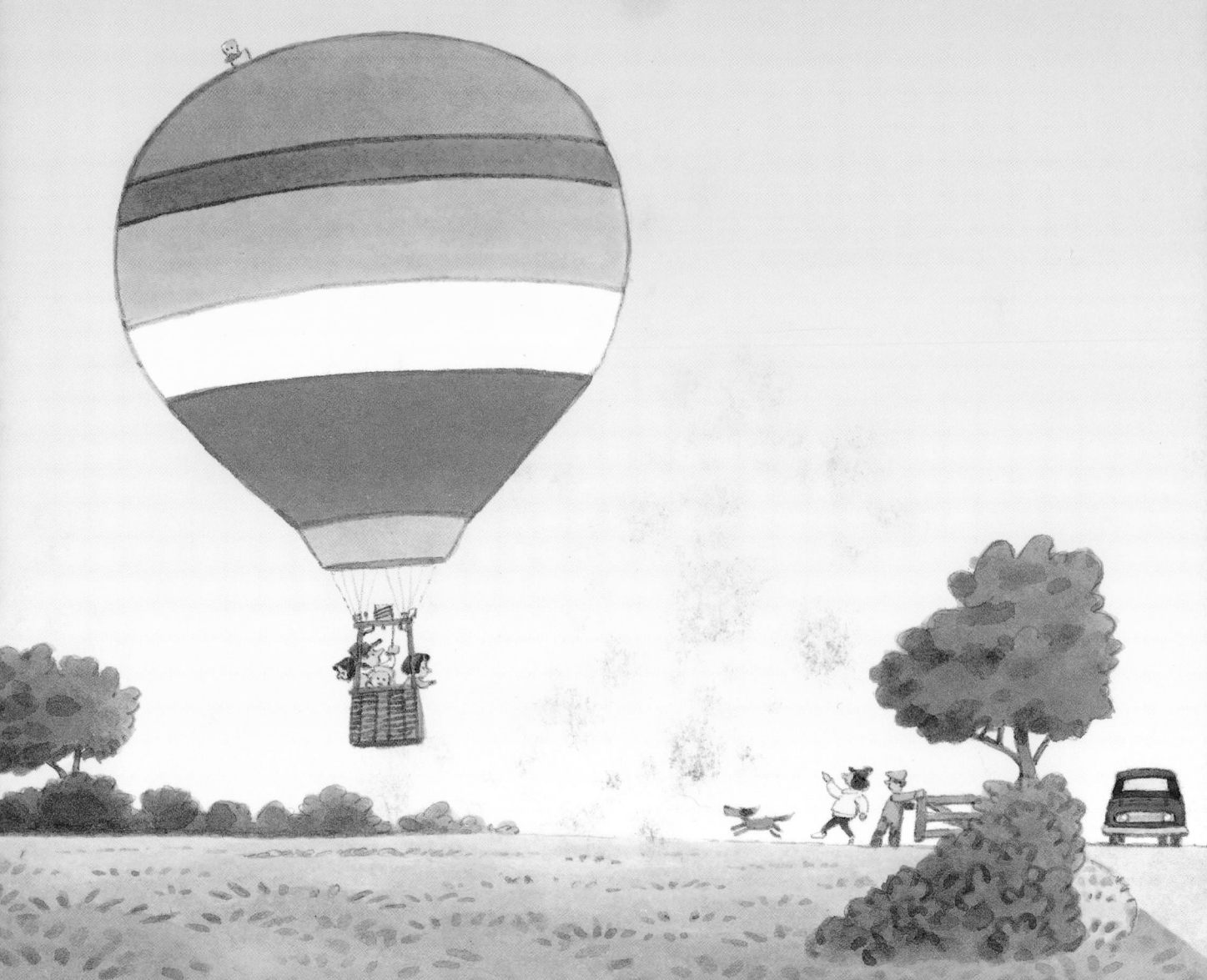

The balloon floats down and the basket lands in a field. Mrs. Boot helps Poppy and Sam out.

"Thank you very much."

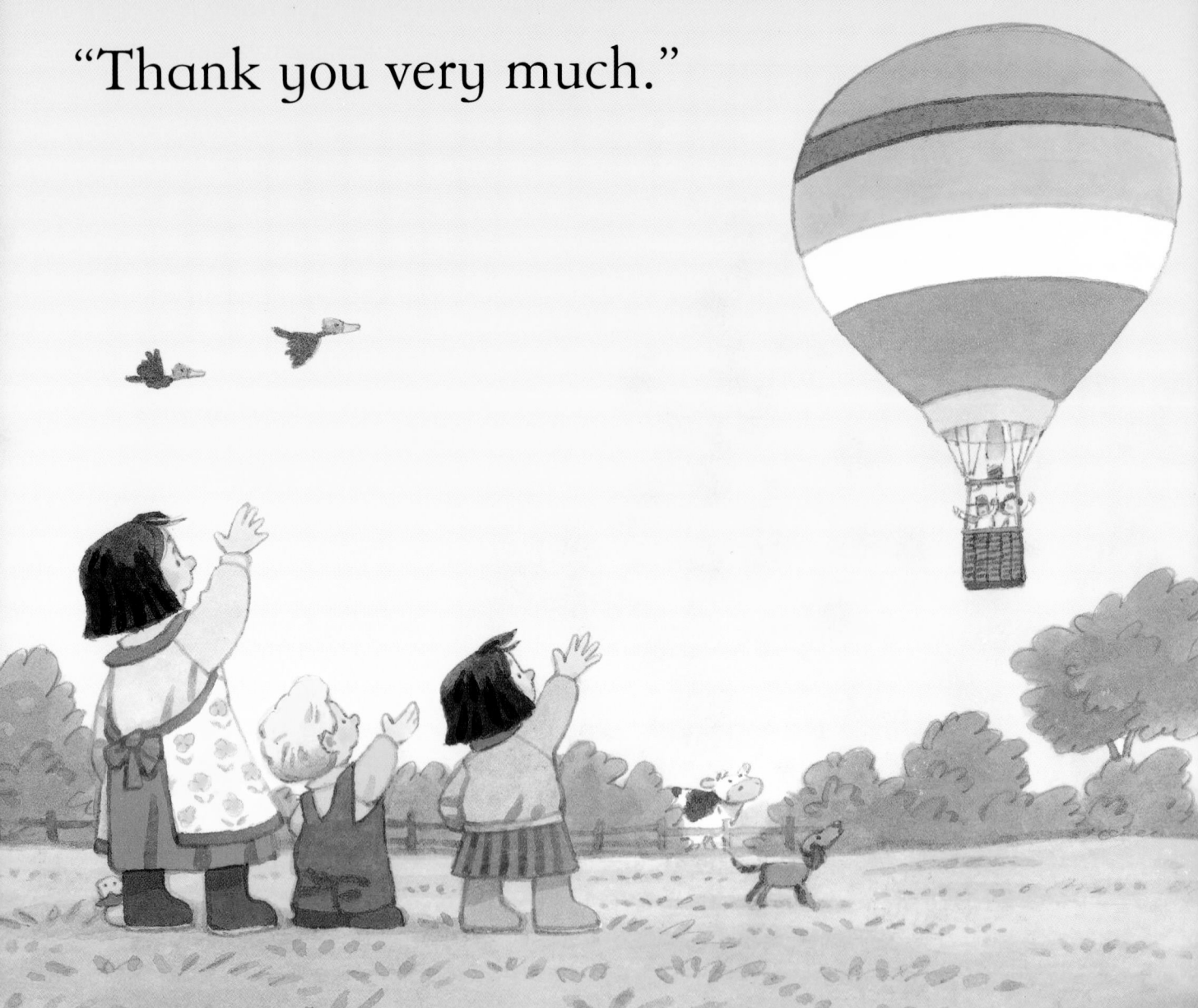

They wave as the balloon takes off again.
"We were flying," says Sam.

Market Day

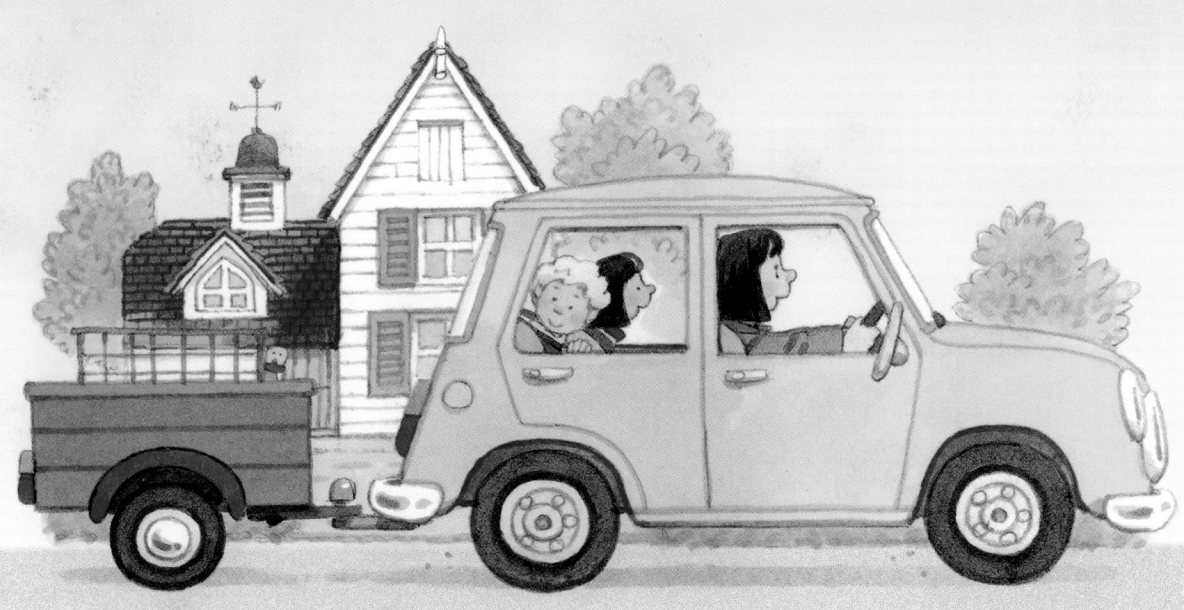

This is Apple Tree Farm.

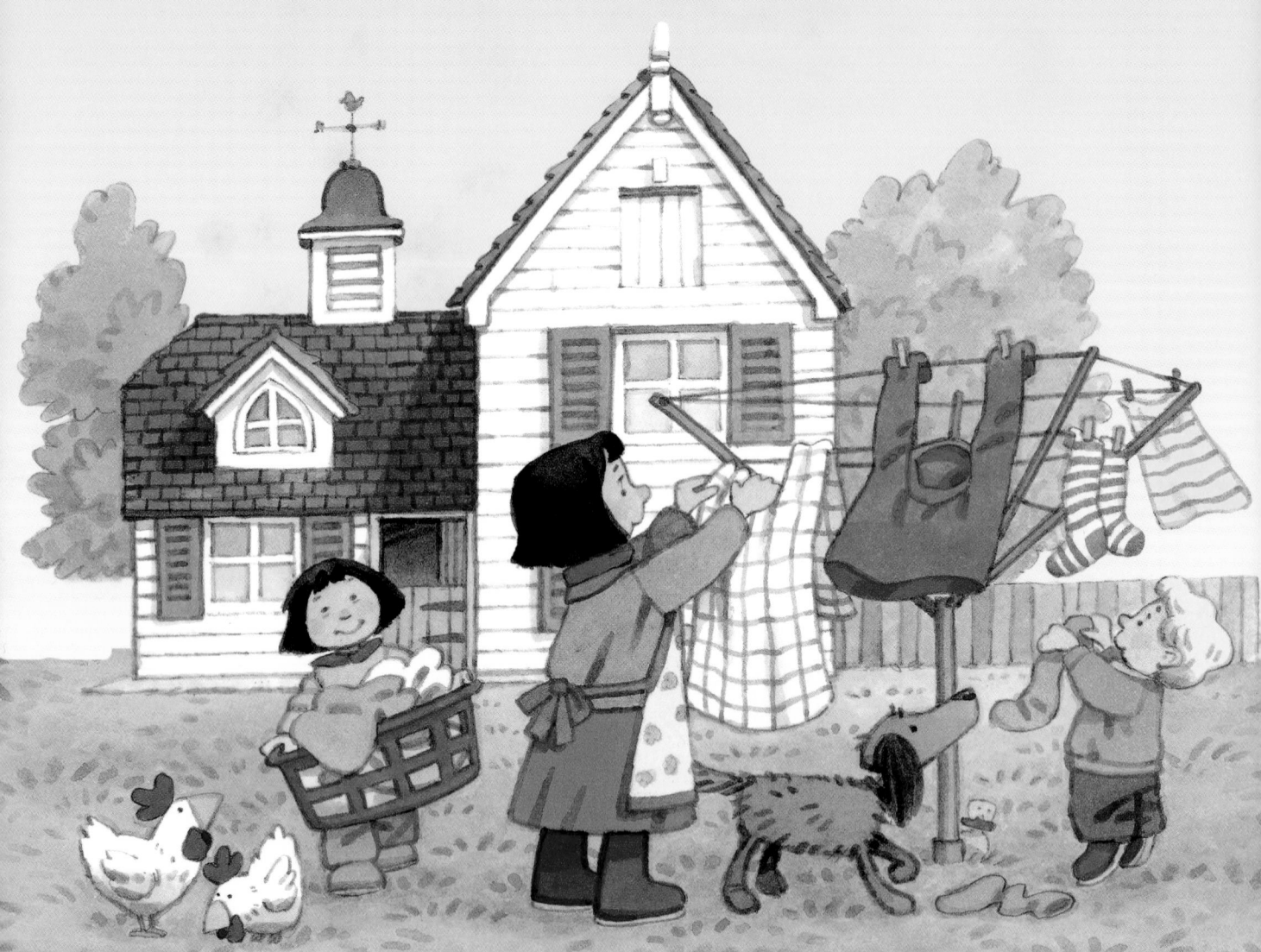

This is Mrs. Boot, the farmer. She has two children, called Poppy and Sam, and a dog called Rusty.

Today is market day.

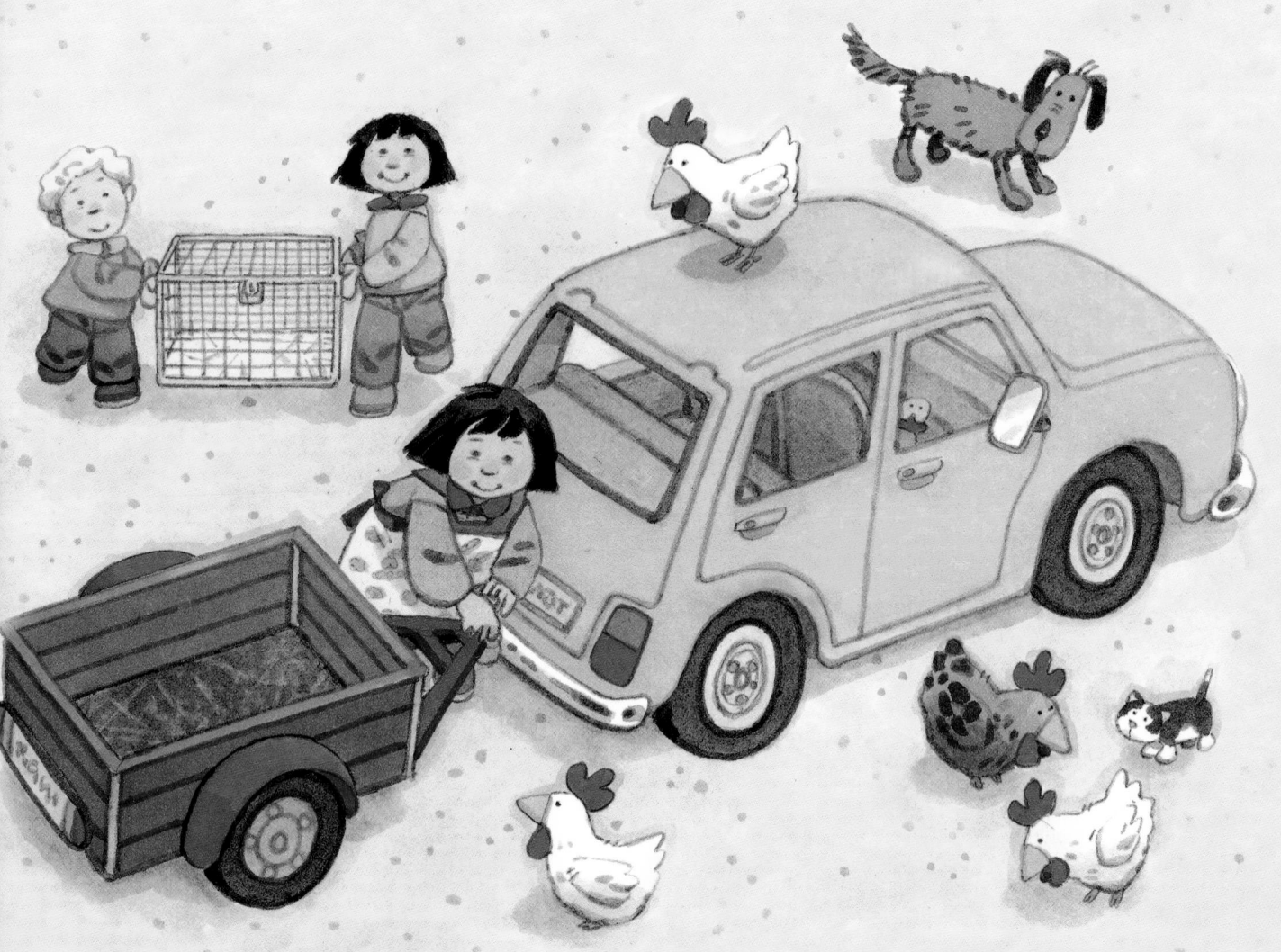

Mrs. Boot puts the trailer on the car. Poppy and
Sam put a wire crate in the trailer.

They drive to the market.

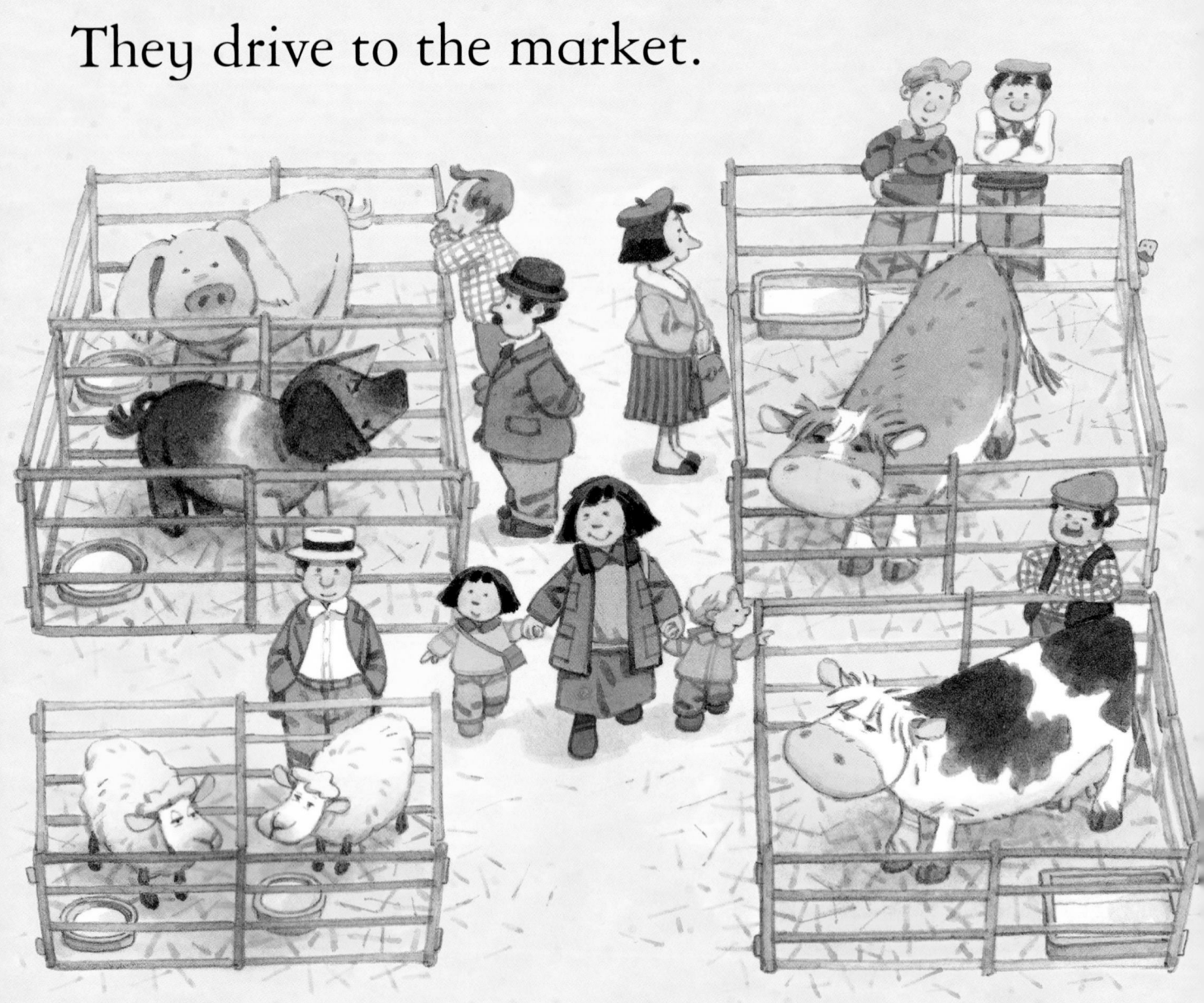

Mrs. Boot, Poppy and Sam walk past cows, sheep and pigs. They go to the shed which has cages of birds.

There are different kinds of geese.

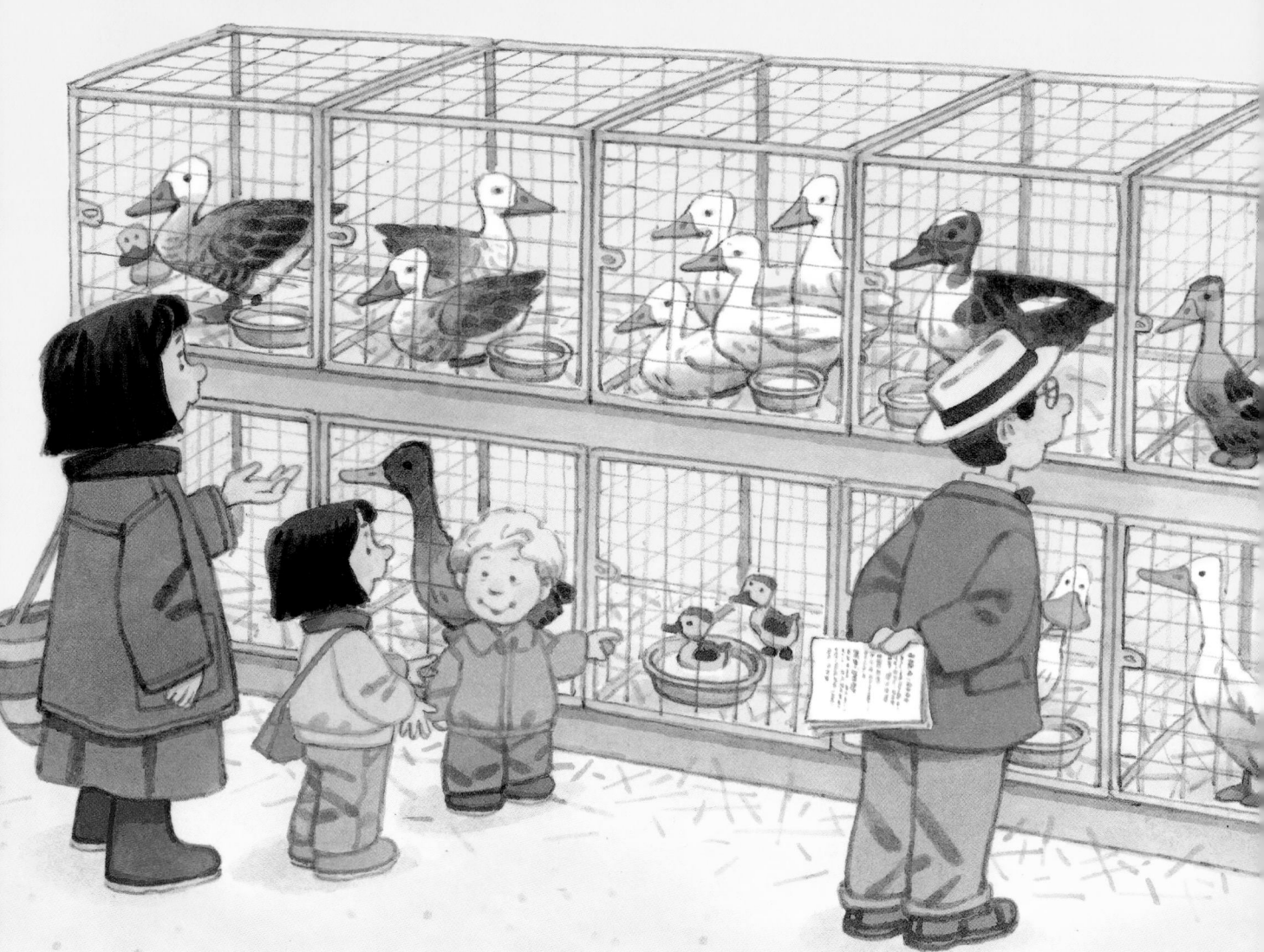

"Let's look in all the cages," says Mrs. Boot.
"I want four nice young geese."

"There are four nice white ones."

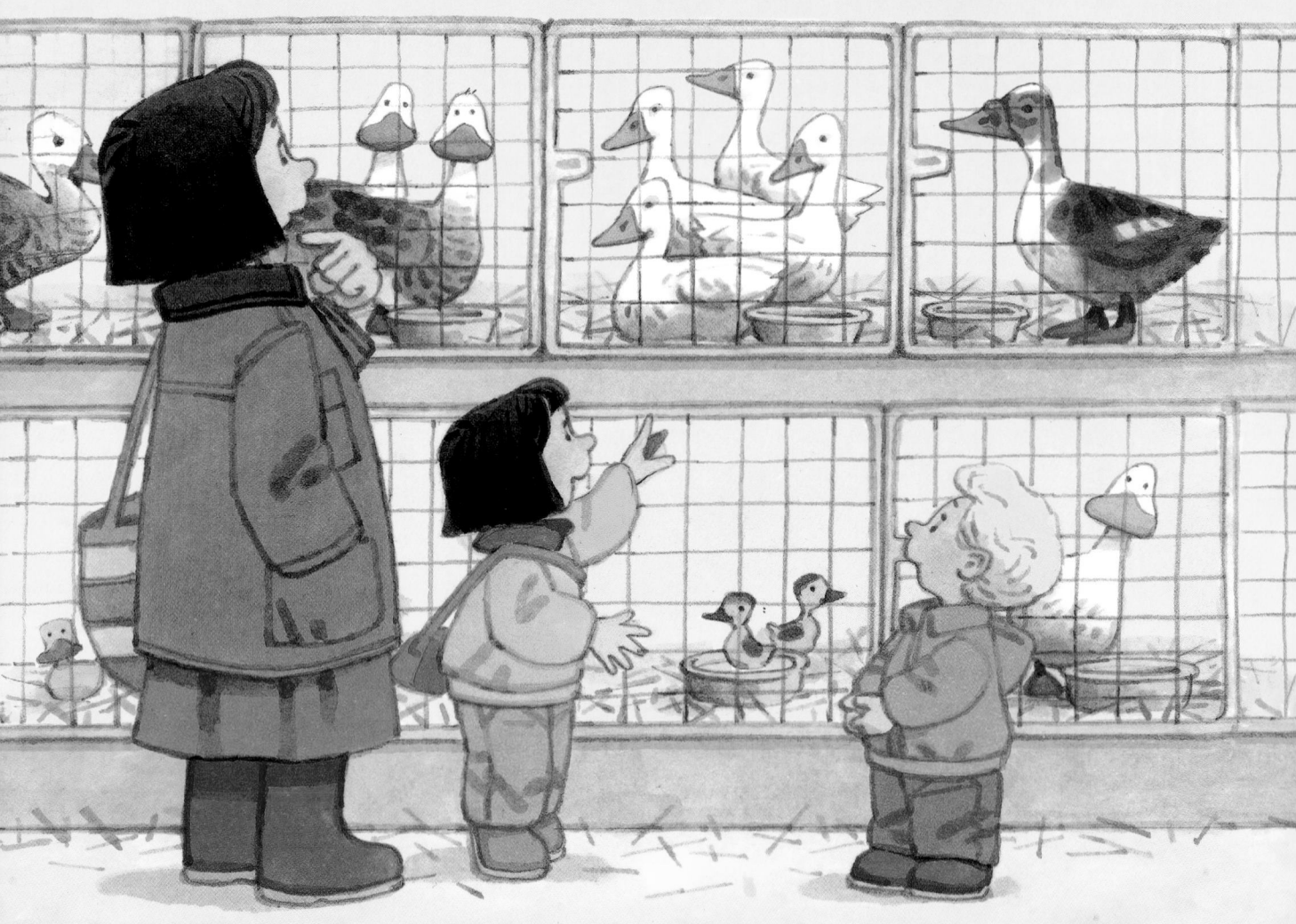

"They look nice and friendly," says Poppy.
"Yes, they are just what I want," says Mrs. Boot.

A woman is selling the geese.

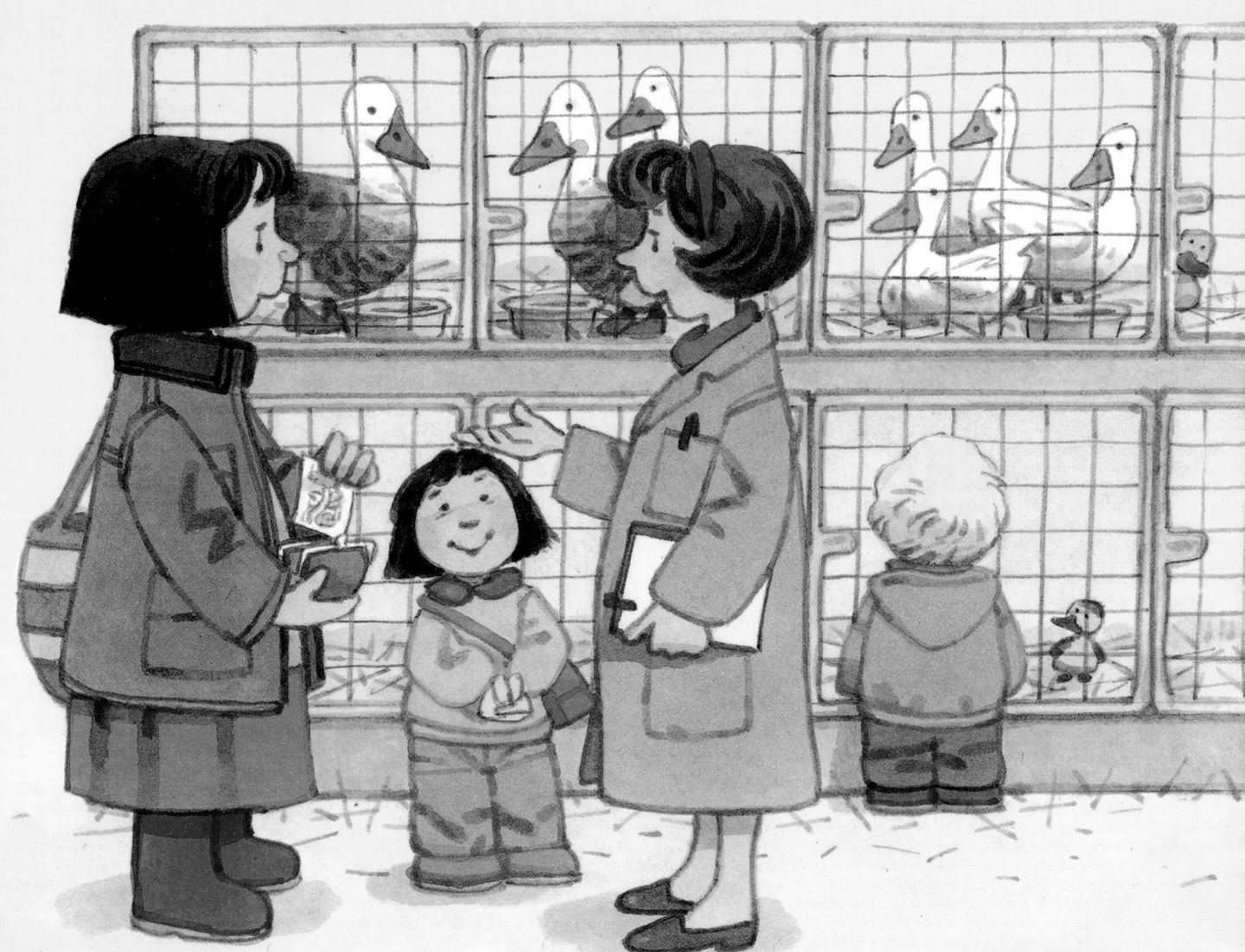

"How much are the four white ones?" asks Mrs. Boot. "I'll buy them, please." She pays for them.

"We'll come back later."

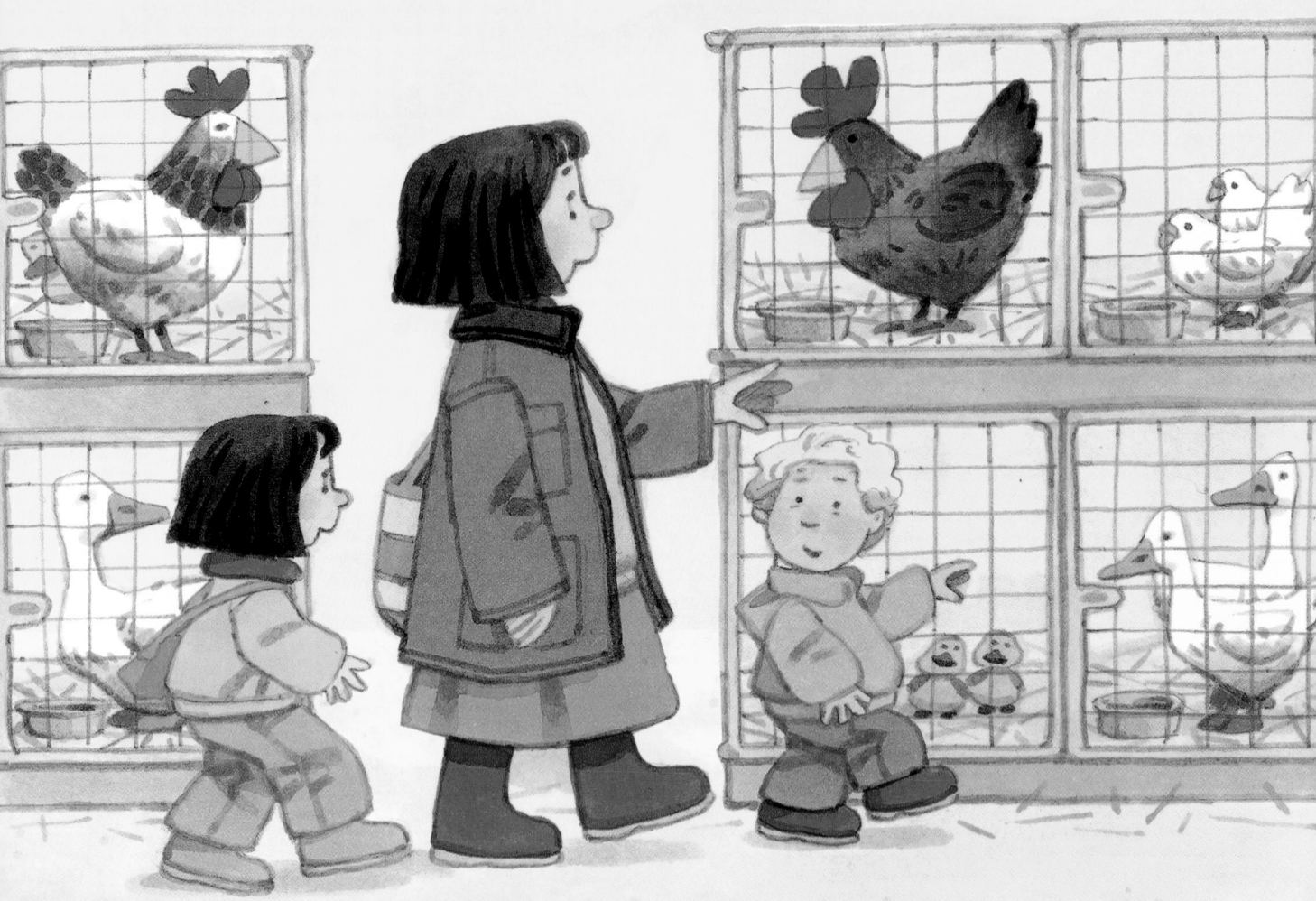

"Let's look at the other birds," says Sam. There are cages with hens, chicks, ducks and pigeons.

"Look at the poor little duck."

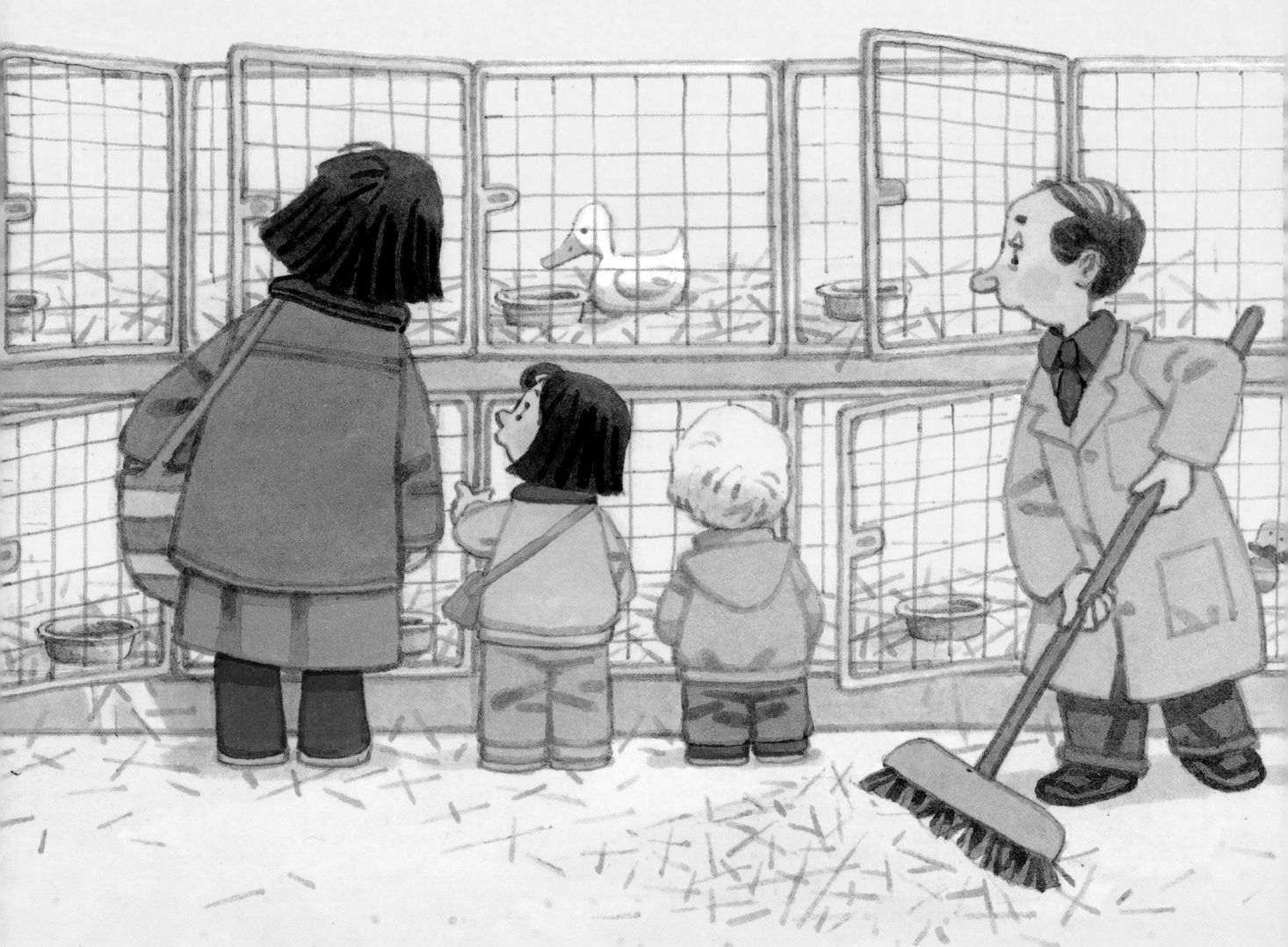

"It's lonely," says Poppy. "Please may I buy it?
I can pay for it with my own money."

"Yes, you can buy it."

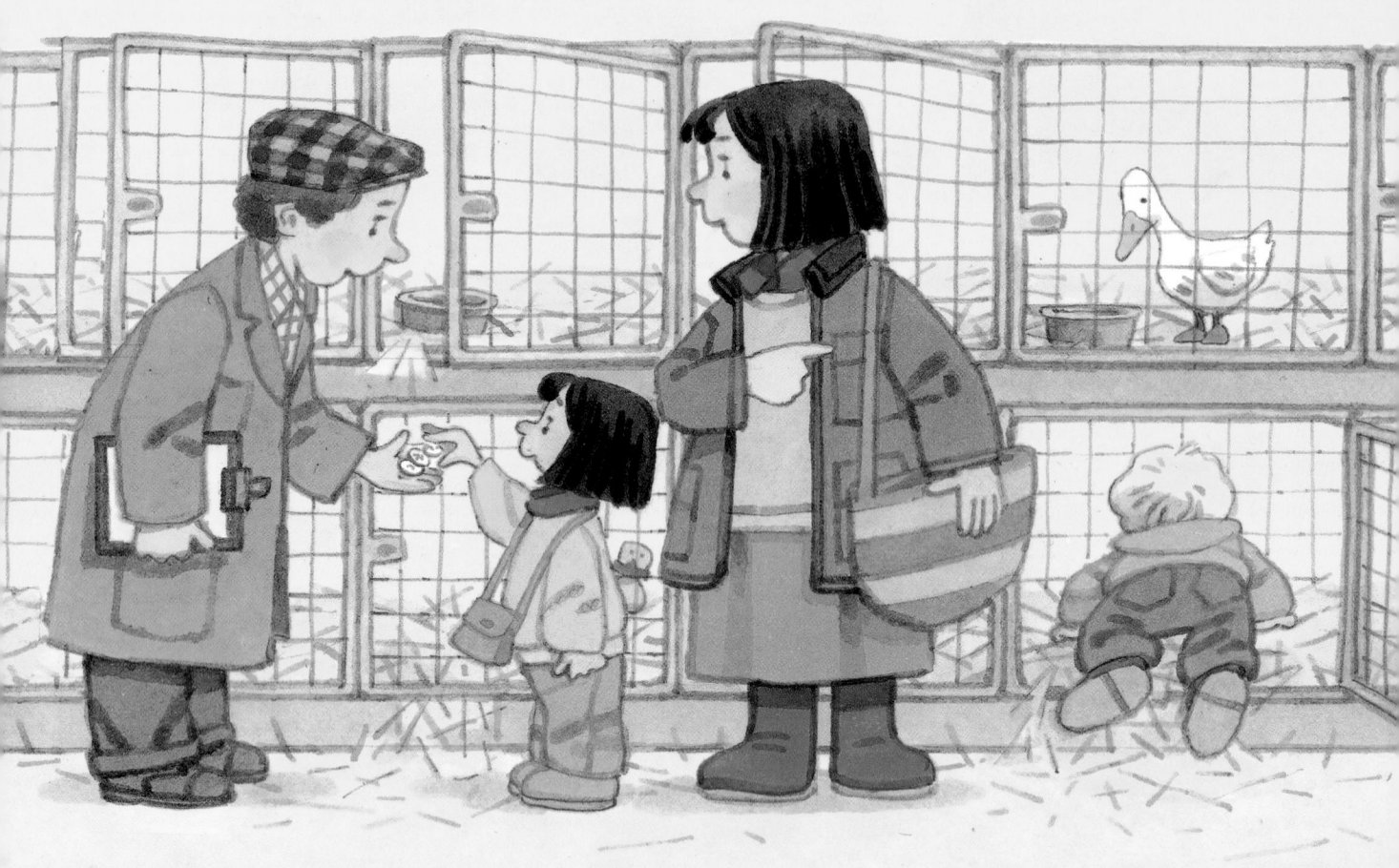

"We'll get it when we come back for the geese,"
says Mrs. Boot. Poppy pays the man for the duck.

Mrs. Boot brings the crate.

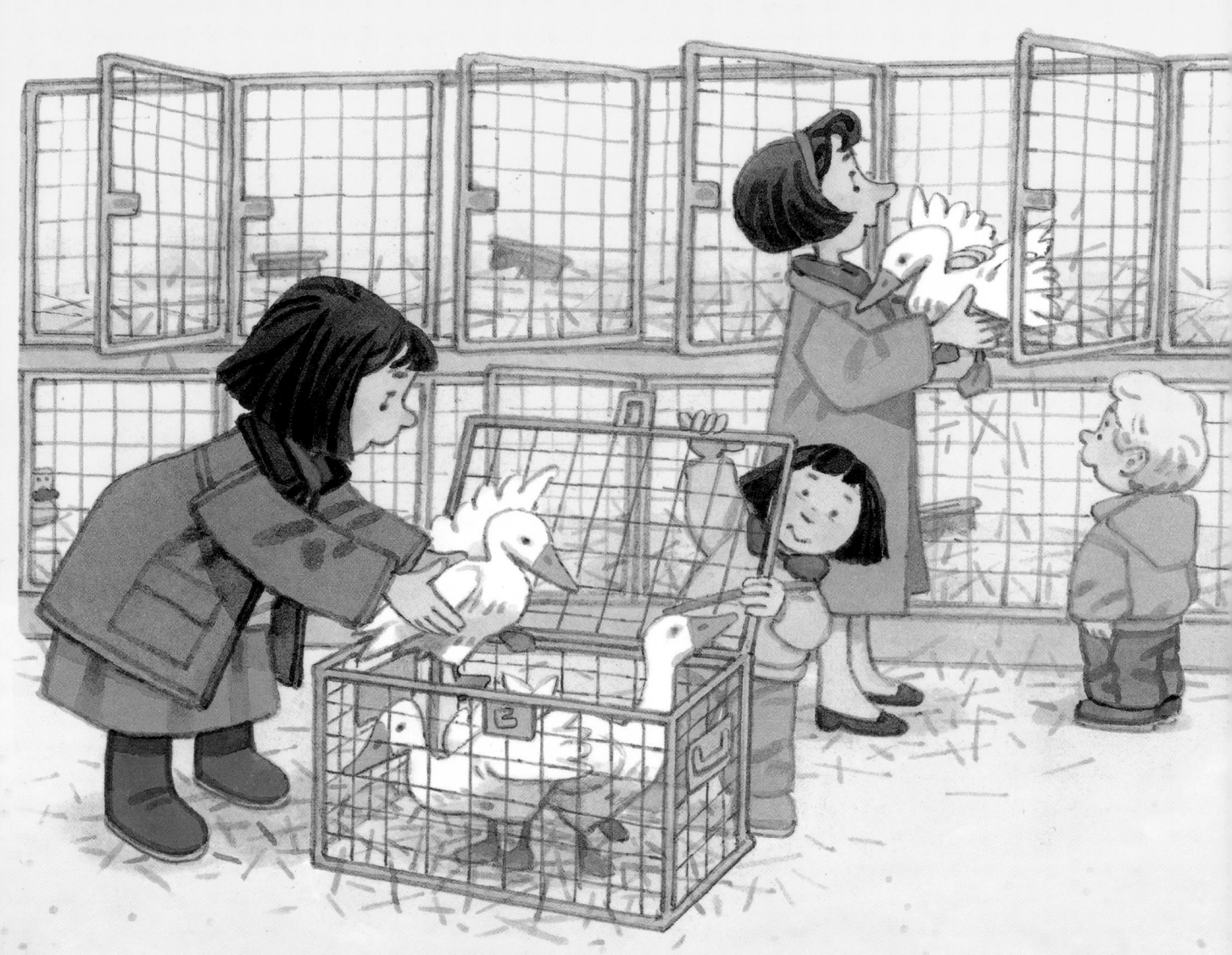

Poppy opens the lid. The woman passes the
geese to Mrs. Boot. She puts them in the crate.

One of the geese runs away.

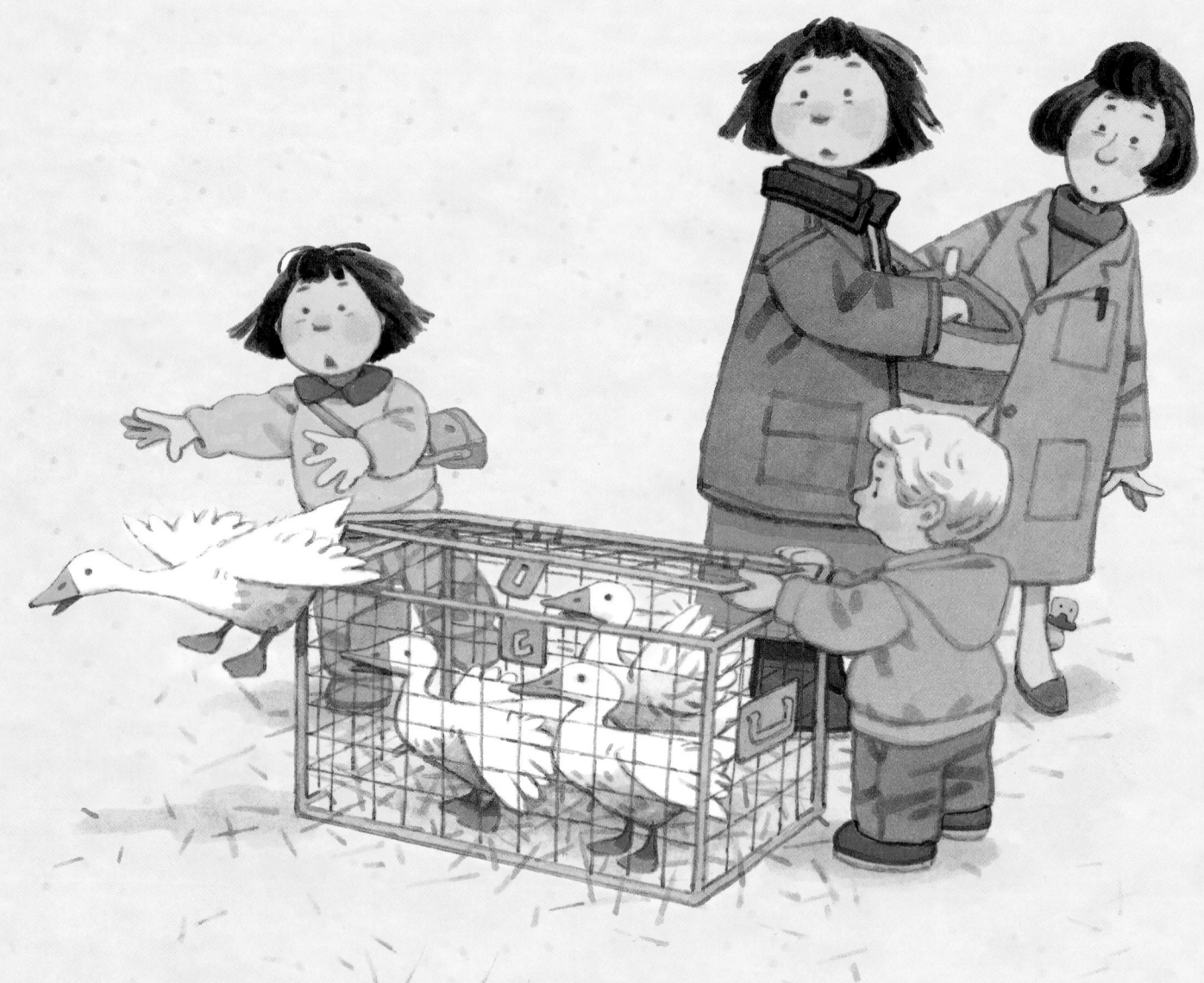

A goose jumps out of the crate just before Sam
shuts the door. It runs very fast out of the shed.

"Catch that goose."

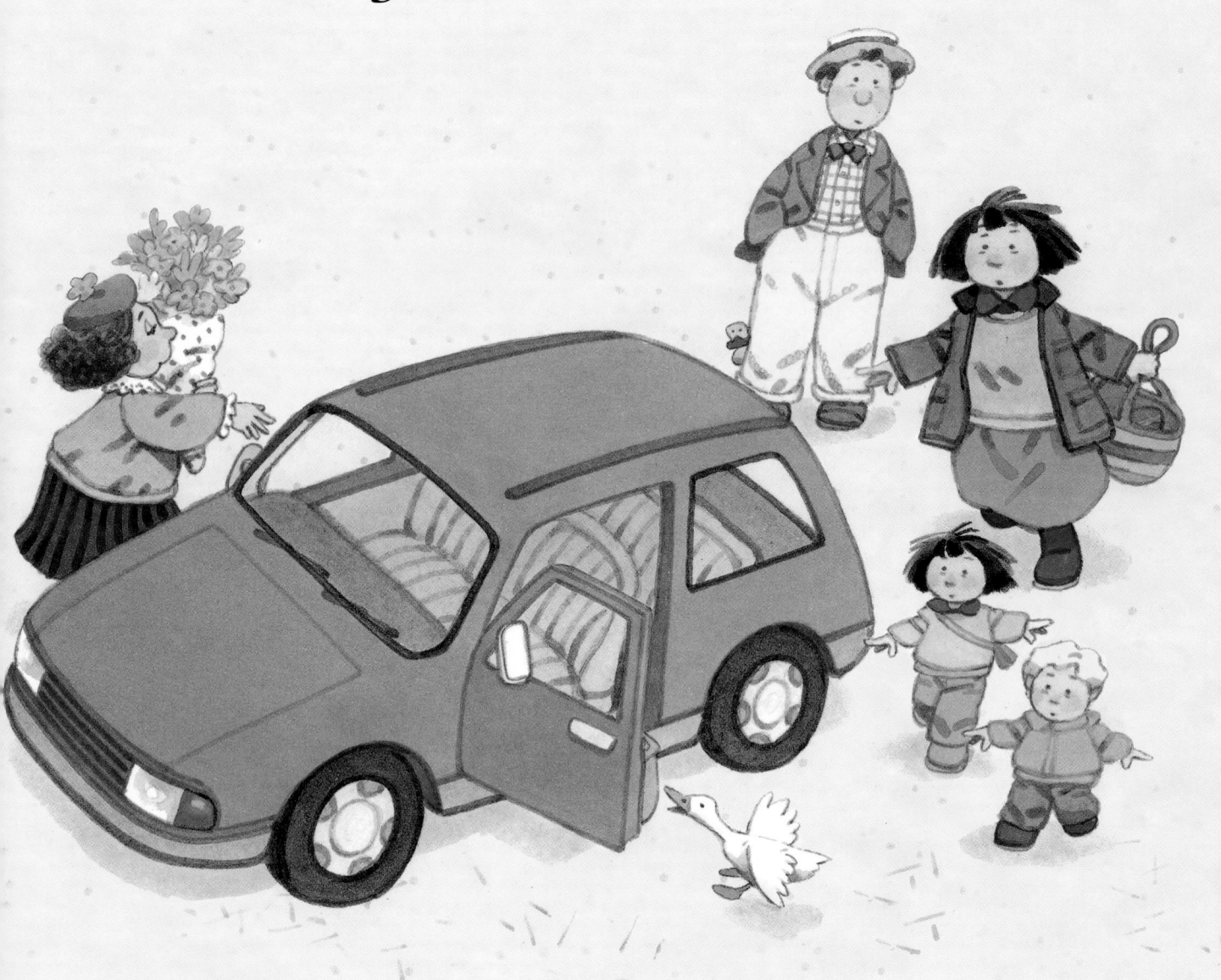

Mrs. Boot, Poppy and Sam run after the goose.
The goose jumps through an open car door.

"Now we've got it," says Sam.

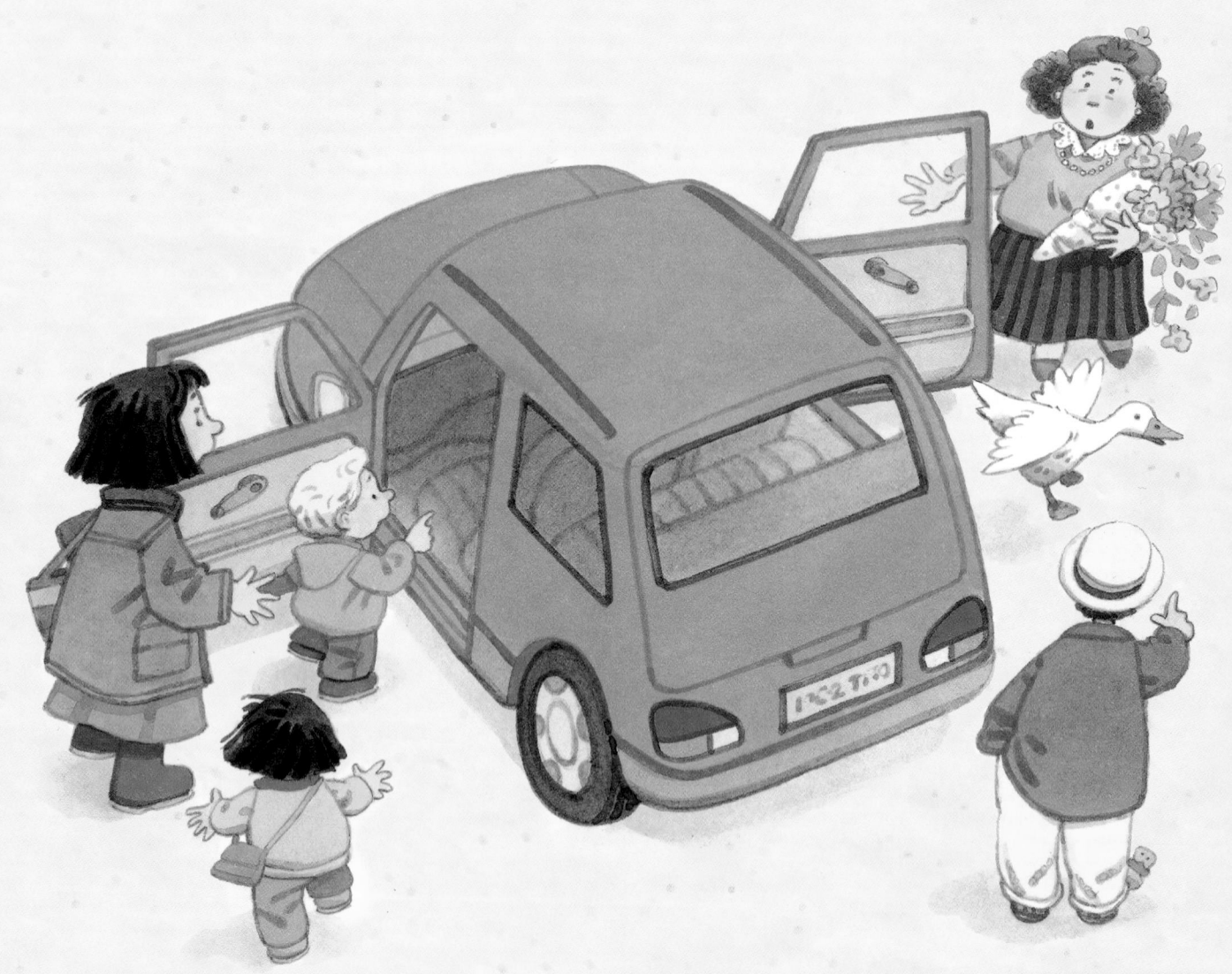

But a woman opens a door on the other side.
The goose jumps out of the car and runs away.

"Run after it," says Mrs. Boot.

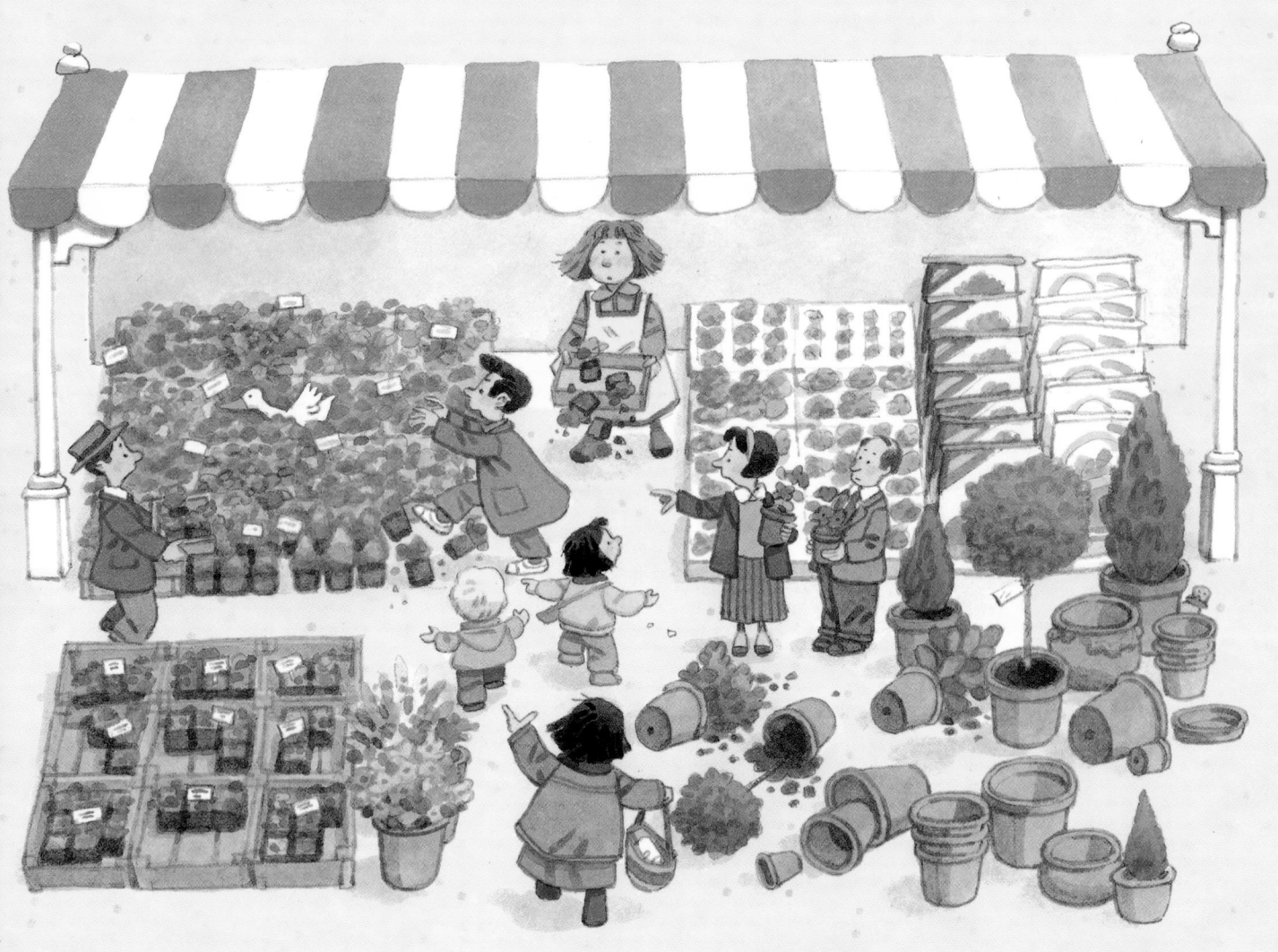

The goose runs into the plant tent.
"There it is," says Sam, and picks it up.

"Let's go home," says Mrs. Boot.

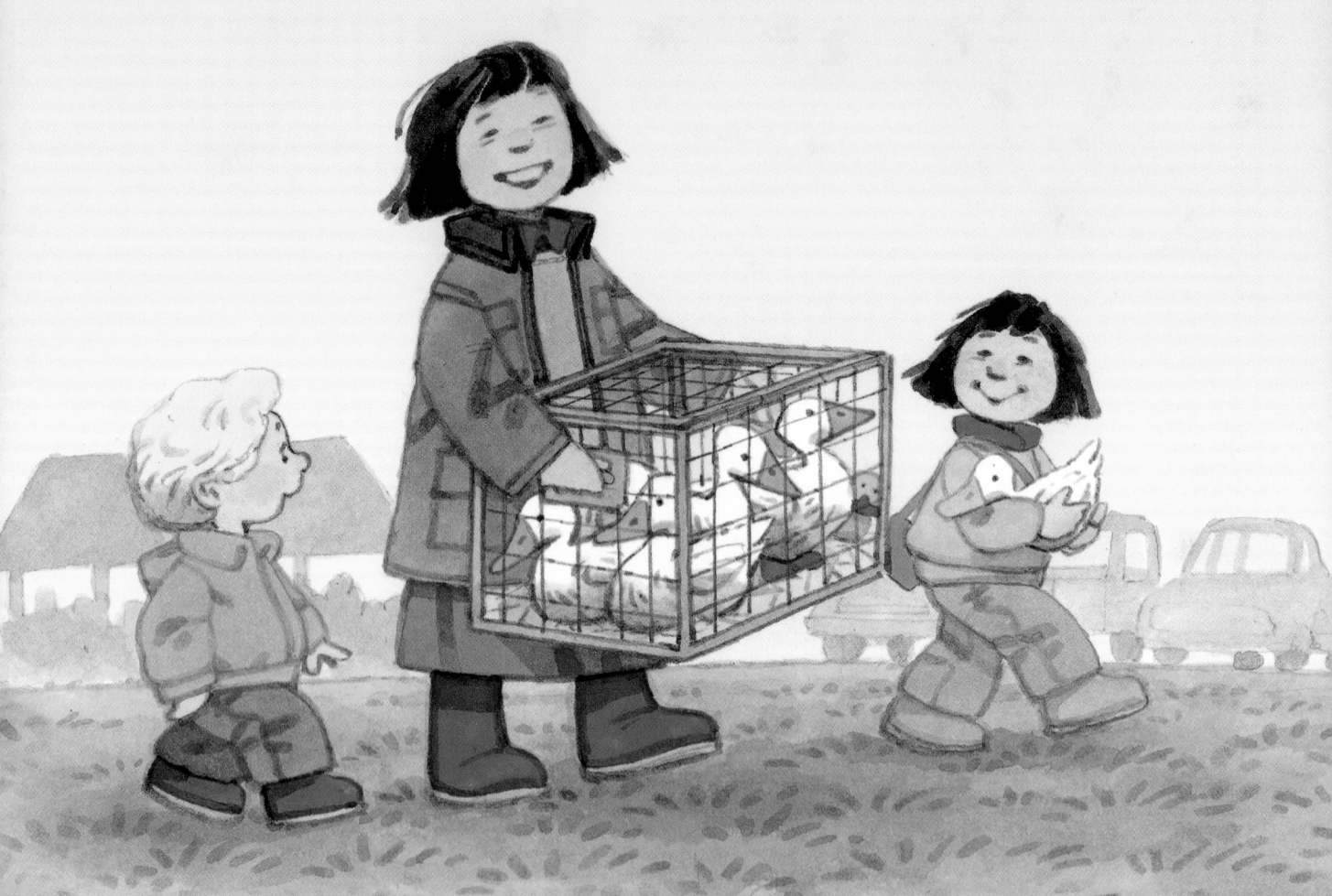

"I've got my geese now." "And I've got my duck," says Poppy. "Markets are fun," says Sam.

Camping Out

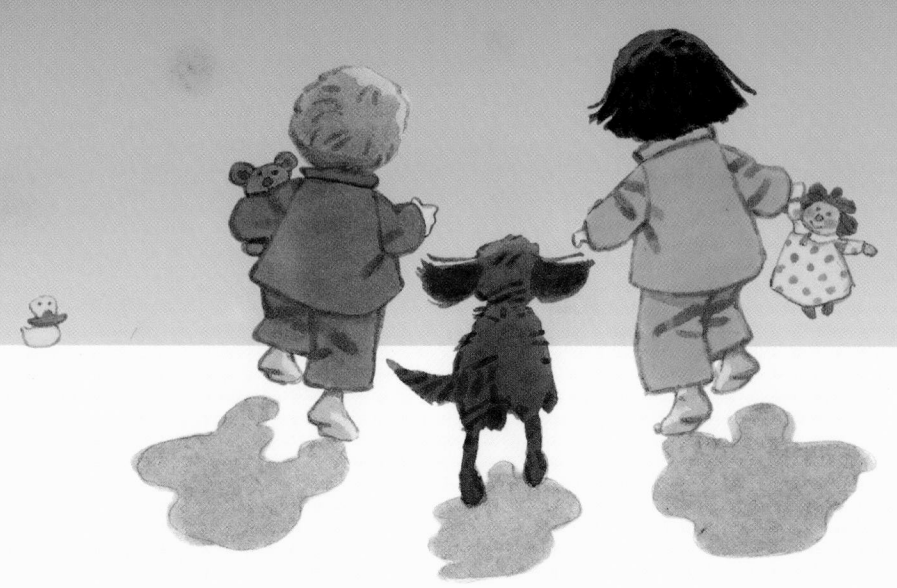

This is Apple Tree Farm.

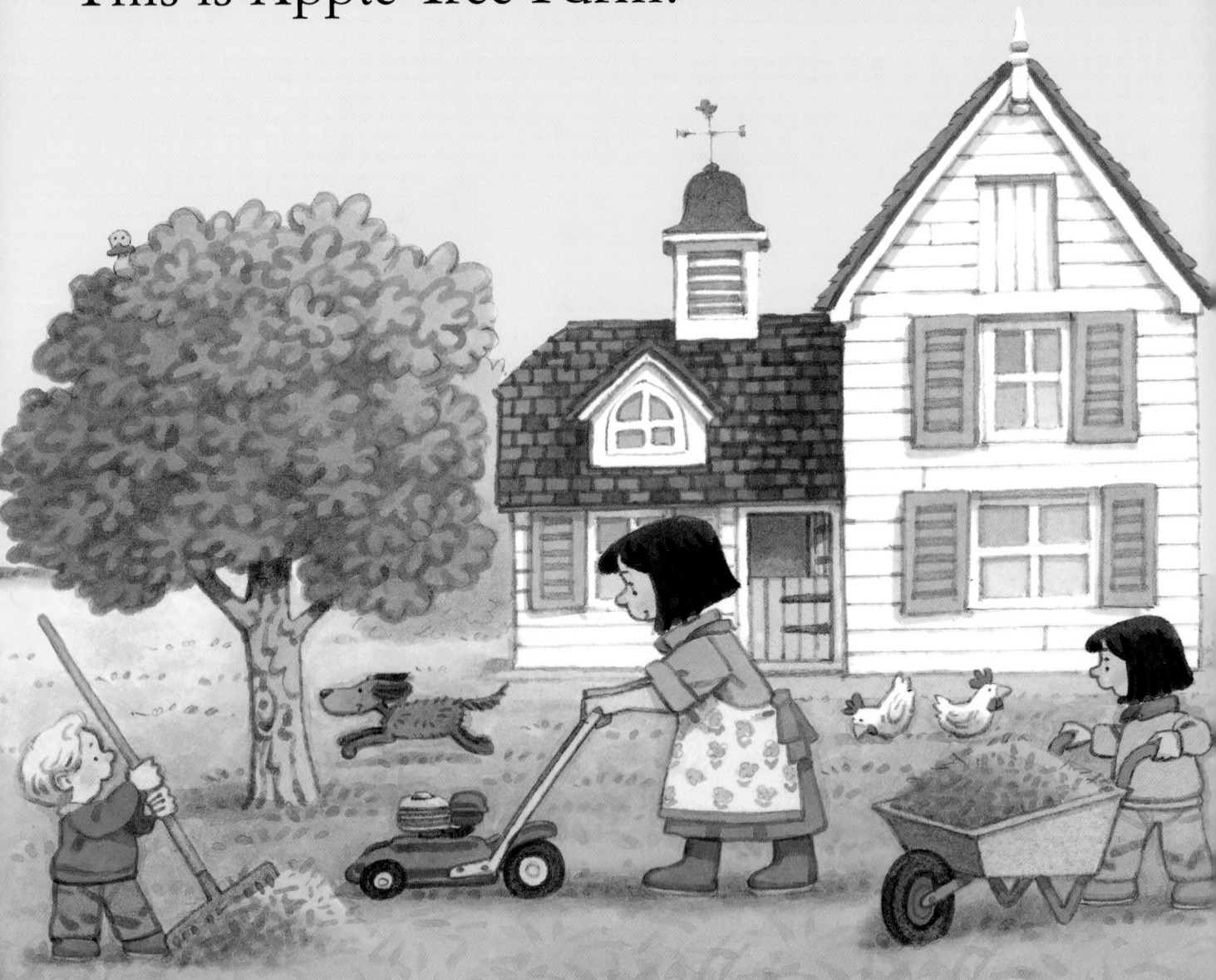

This is Mrs. Boot, the farmer. She has two children, called Poppy and Sam, and a dog called Rusty.

A car stops at the gate.

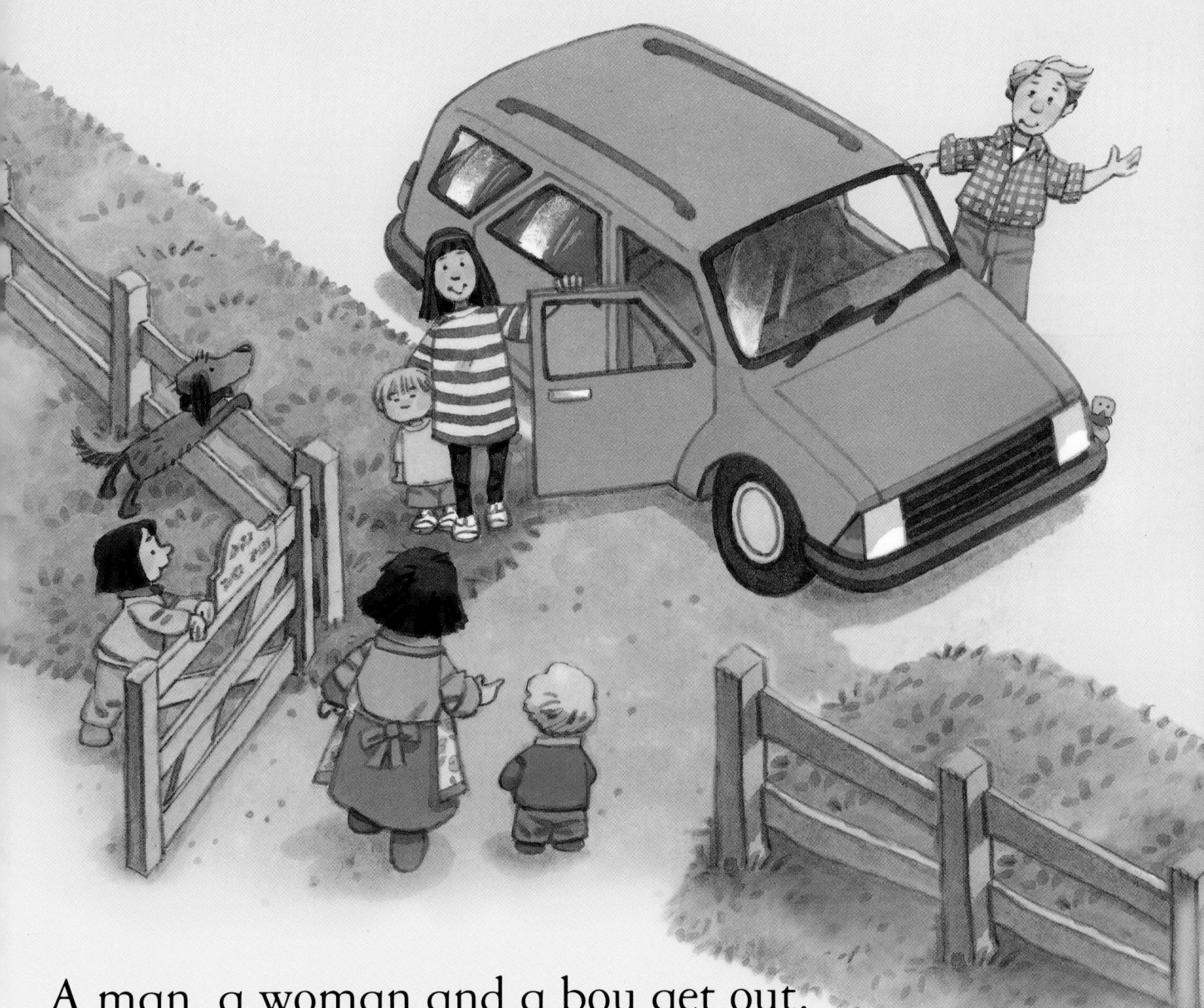

A man, a woman and a boy get out.
"Hello," says the man. "May we camp on your farm?"

"Yes, you can camp over there."

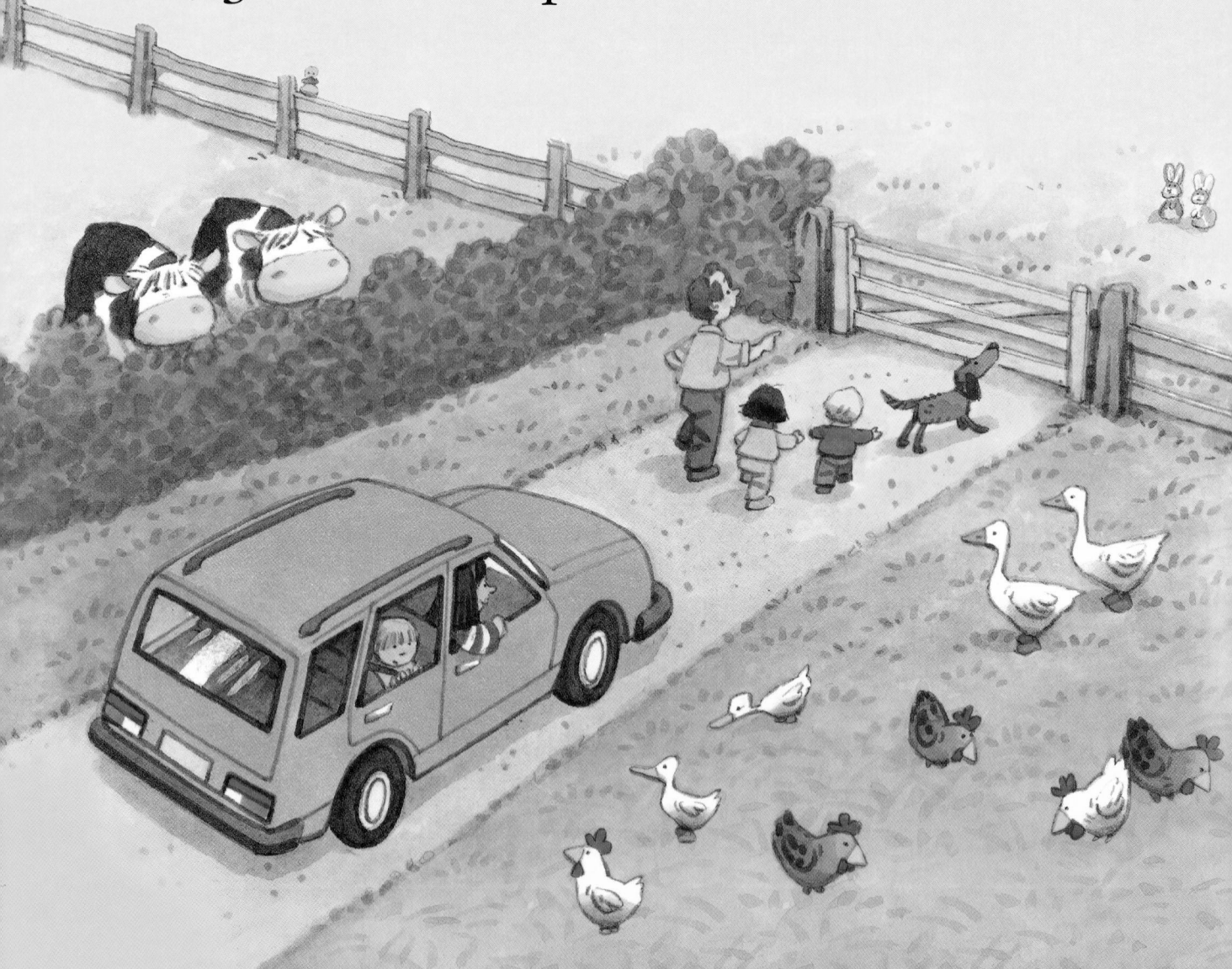

"We'll show you the way," says Mr. Boot.
The campers follow in the car.

244

The campers put up their tent.

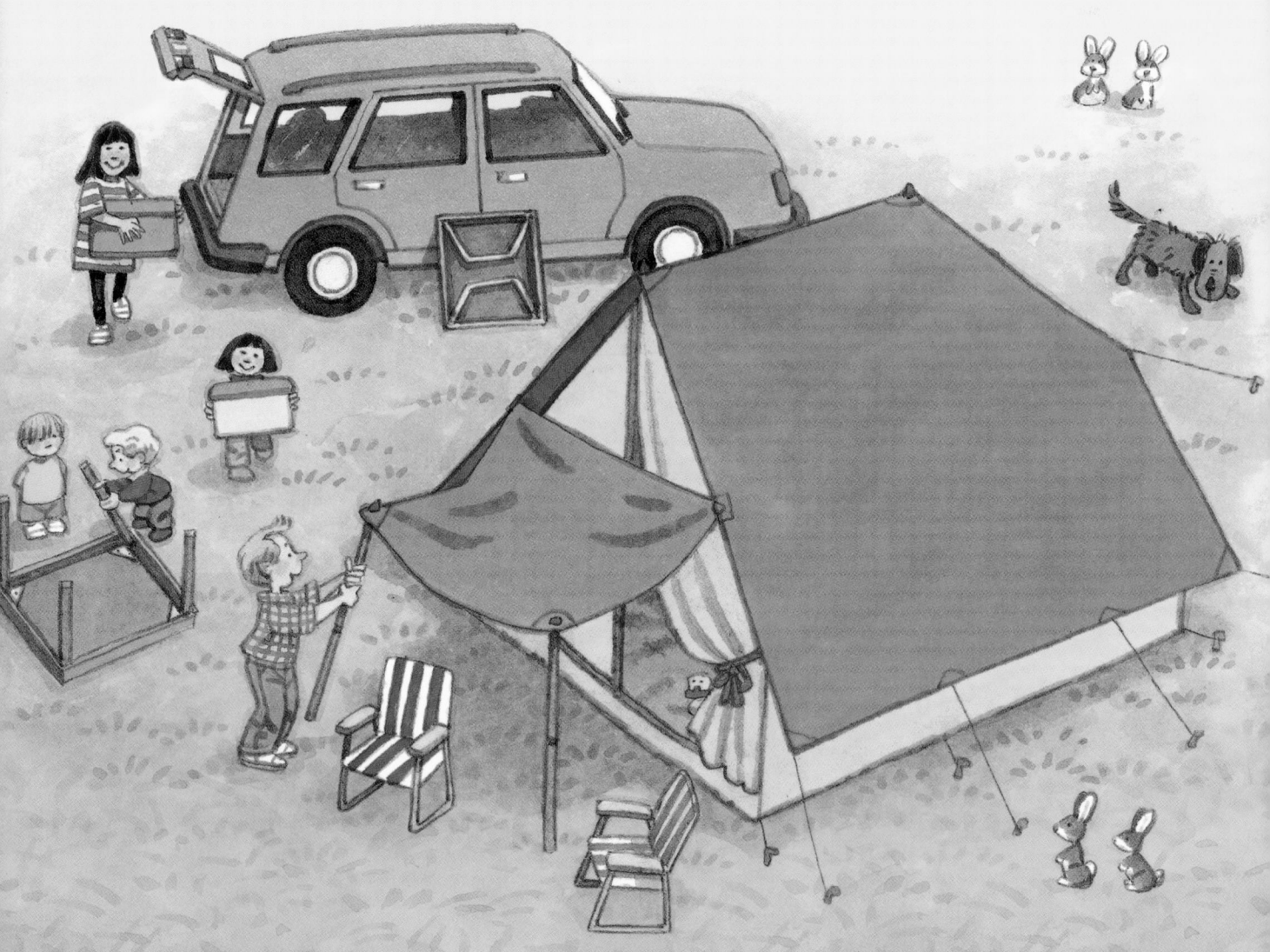

Poppy and Sam help them. They take chairs,
a table, a cooking stove and food out of the car.

Then they all go to the farmhouse.

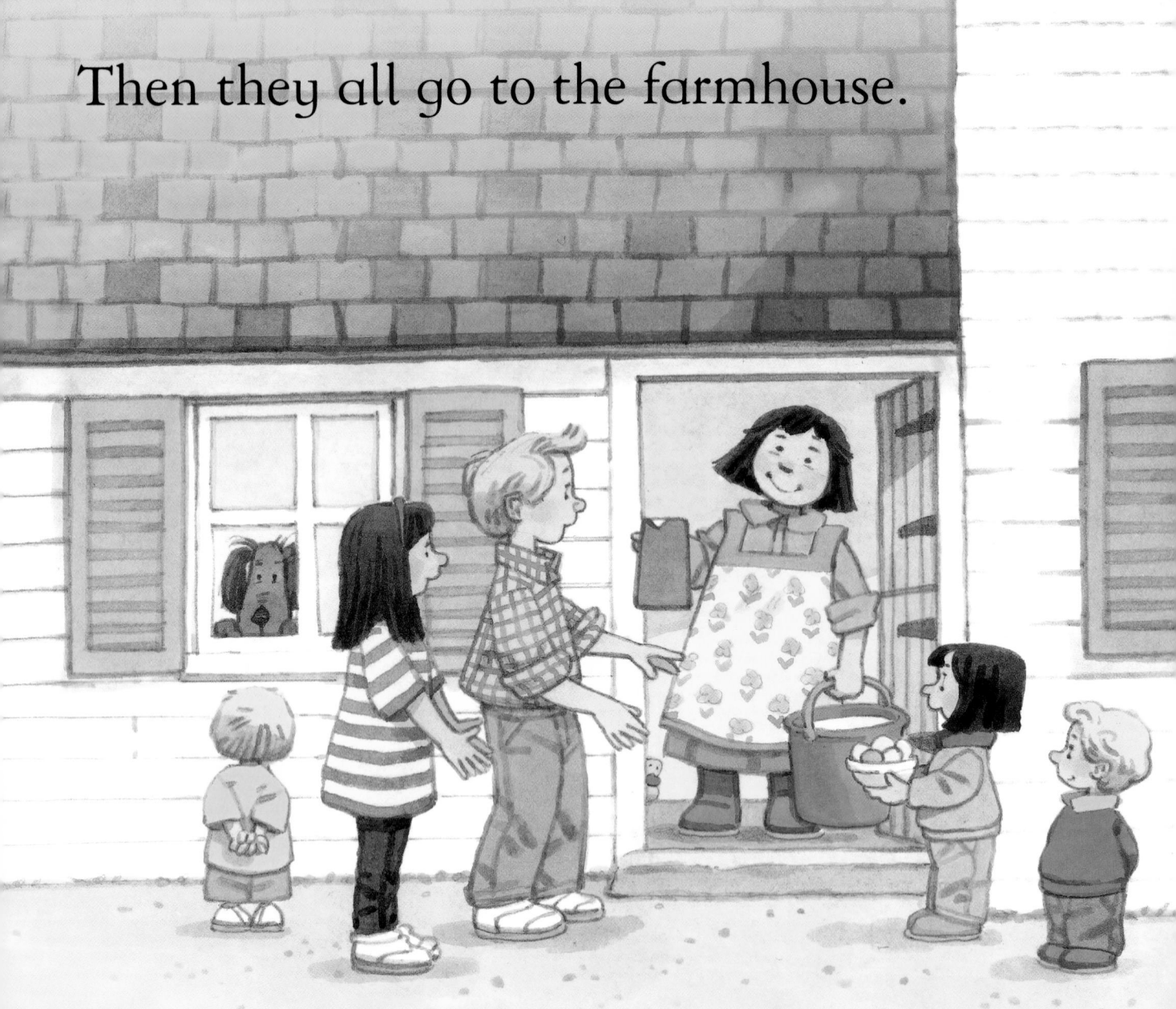

Mrs. Boot gives the campers a bucket of water
and some milk. Poppy and Sam bring some eggs.

"Can we go camping?"

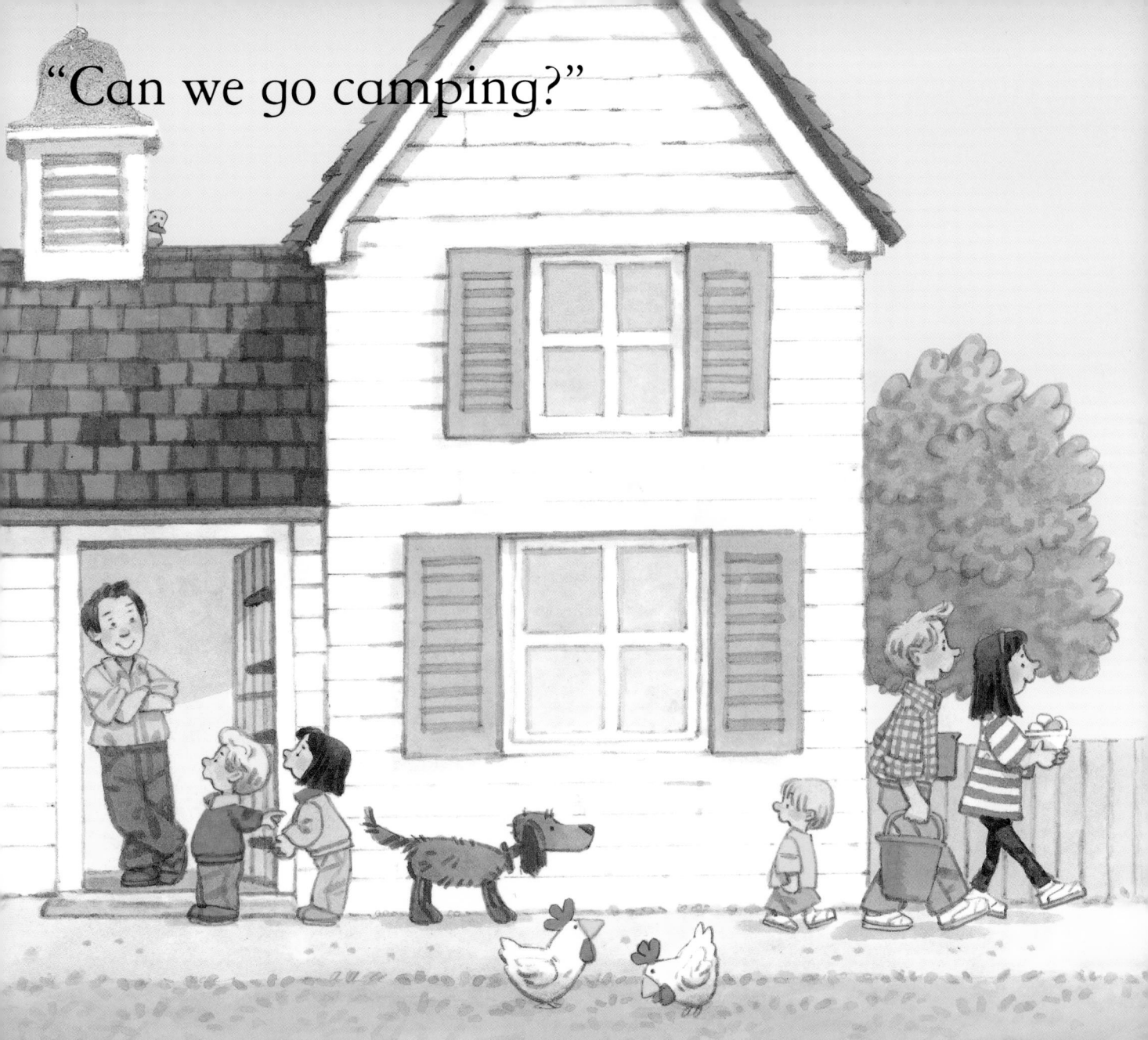

"Please Dad, can we put up our tent too?"
says Poppy. "Oh yes, please Dad," says Sam.

247

Mr. Boot gets out the tent.

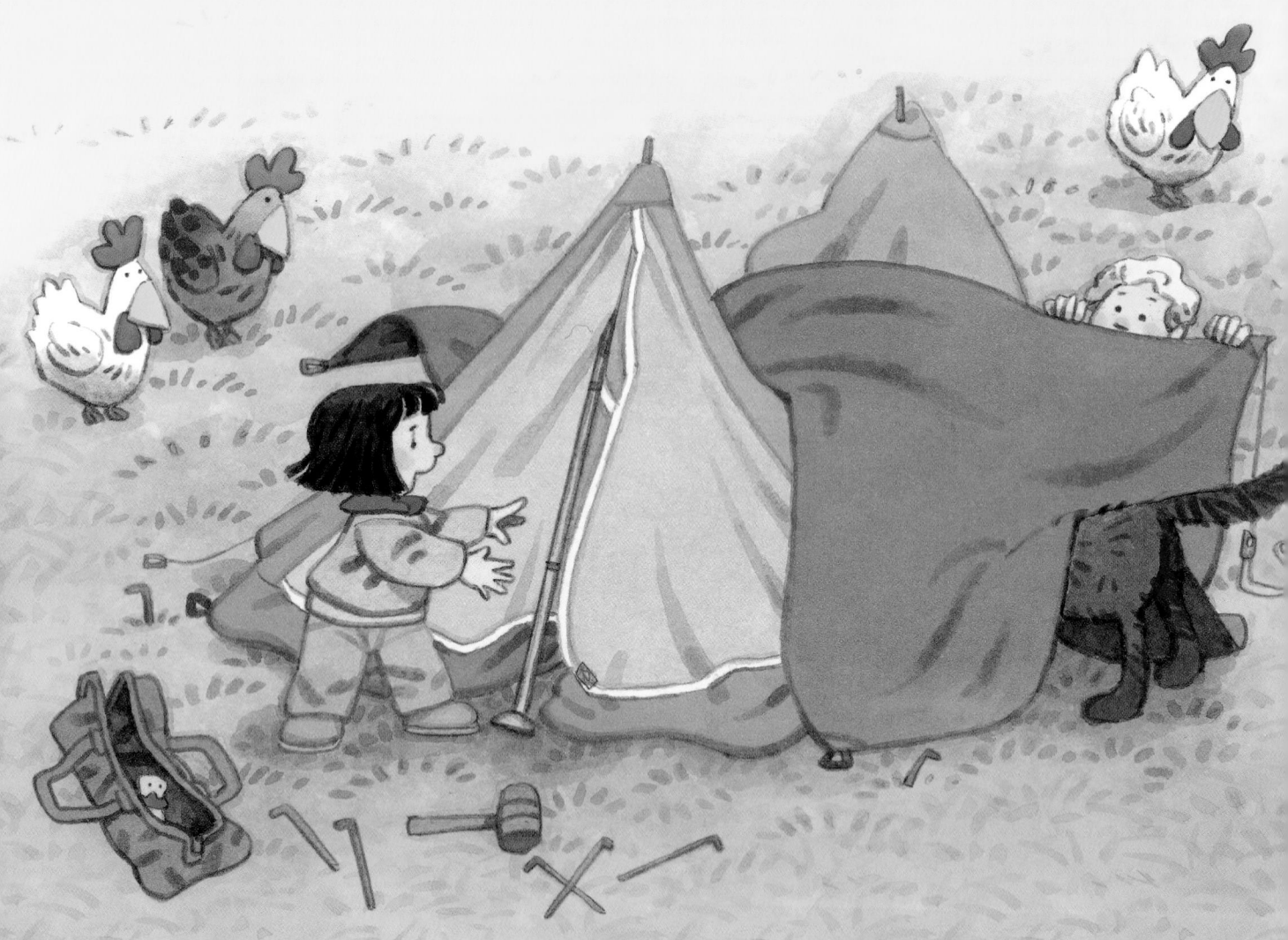

Poppy and Sam try to put up the little blue tent
but it keeps falling down. At last it is ready.

"Come and have supper."

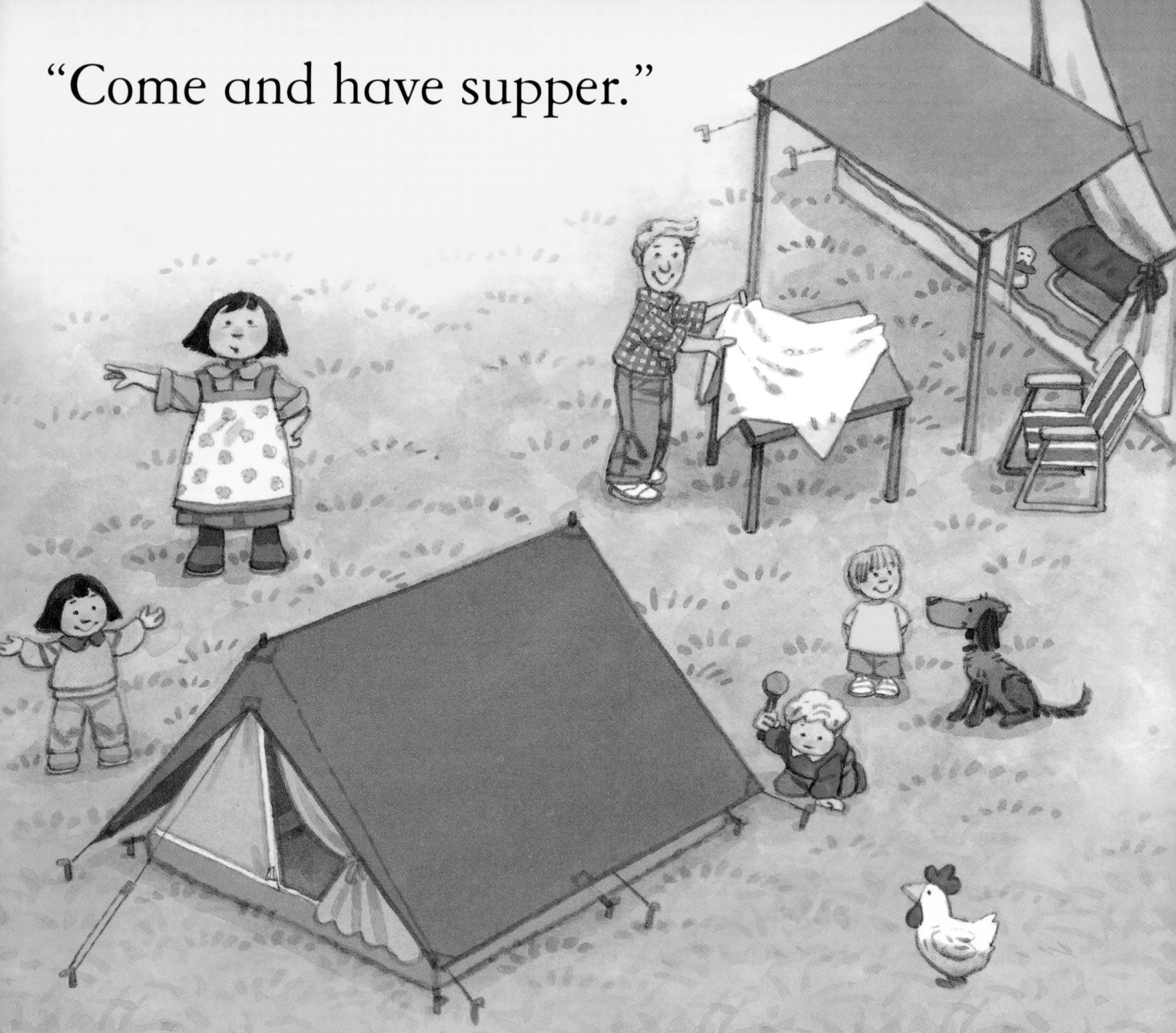

"Then you can go to the tent," says Mrs. Boot.
"But you must wash and brush your teeth first."

249

Poppy and Sam go to the tent.

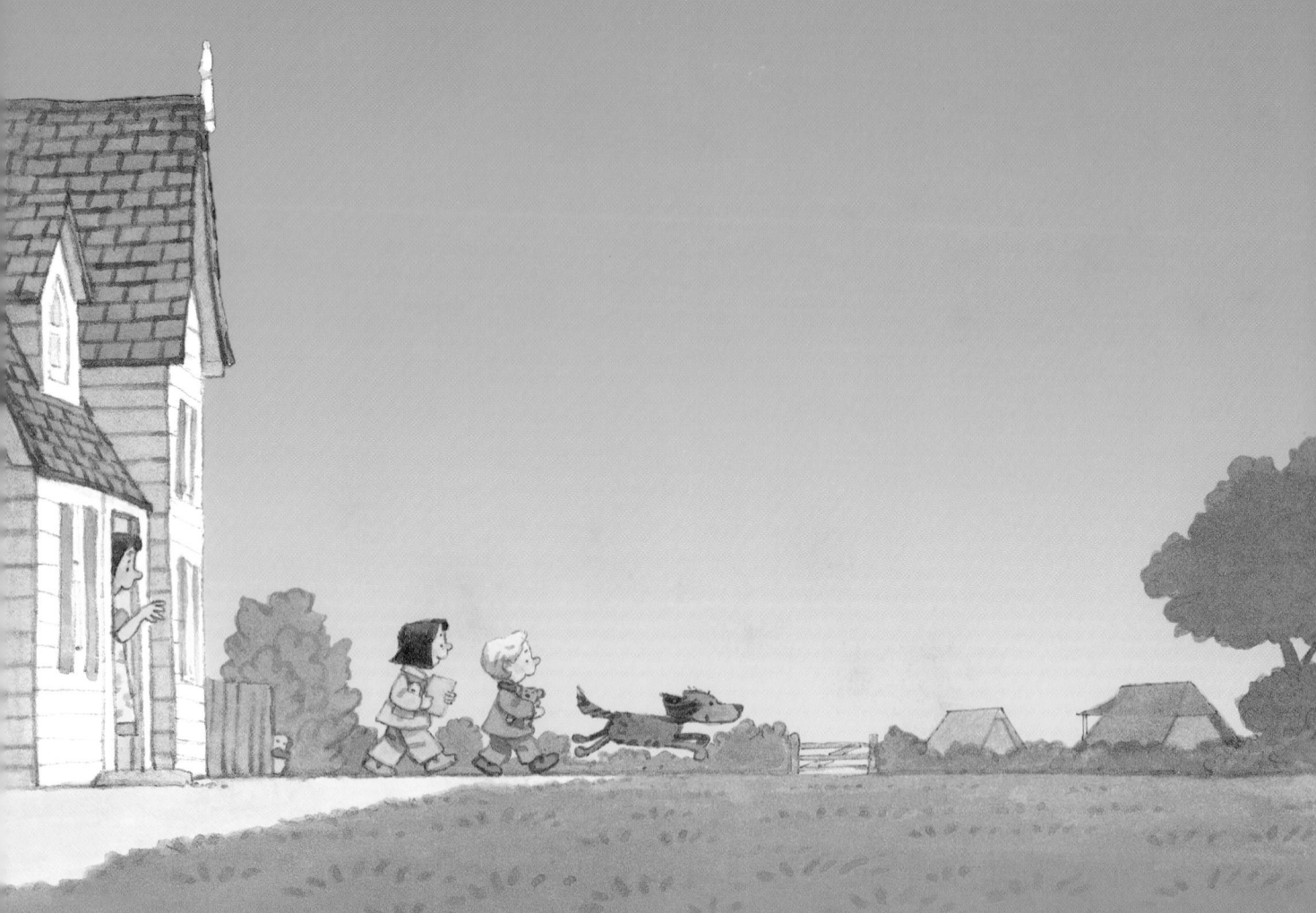

"It's not dark yet," says Sam. "Come on, Rusty.
You can come camping with us," says Poppy.

Poppy and Sam go to bed.

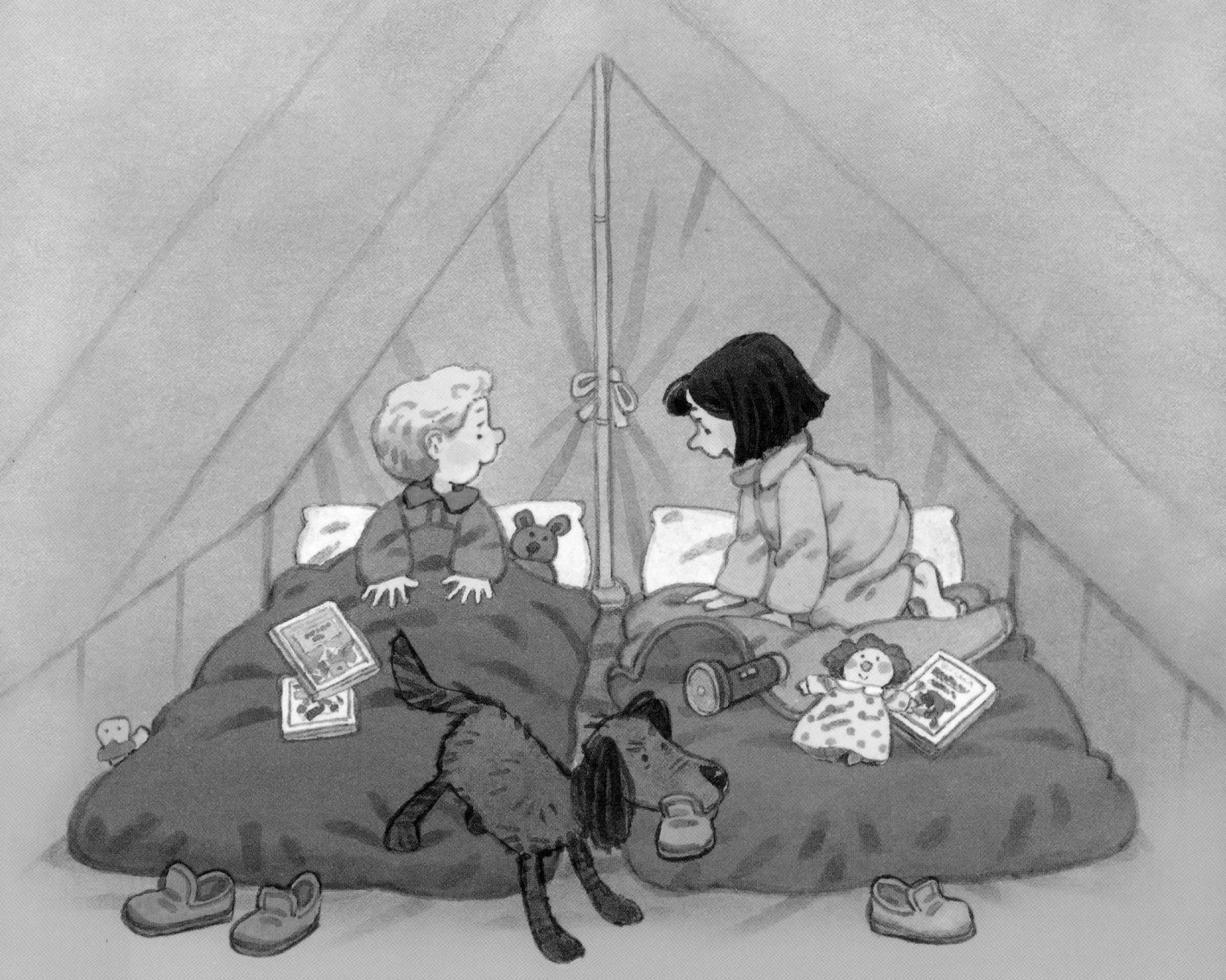

They crawl into the tent and tie up the door.
Then they wriggle into their sleeping bags.

"What's that noise?"

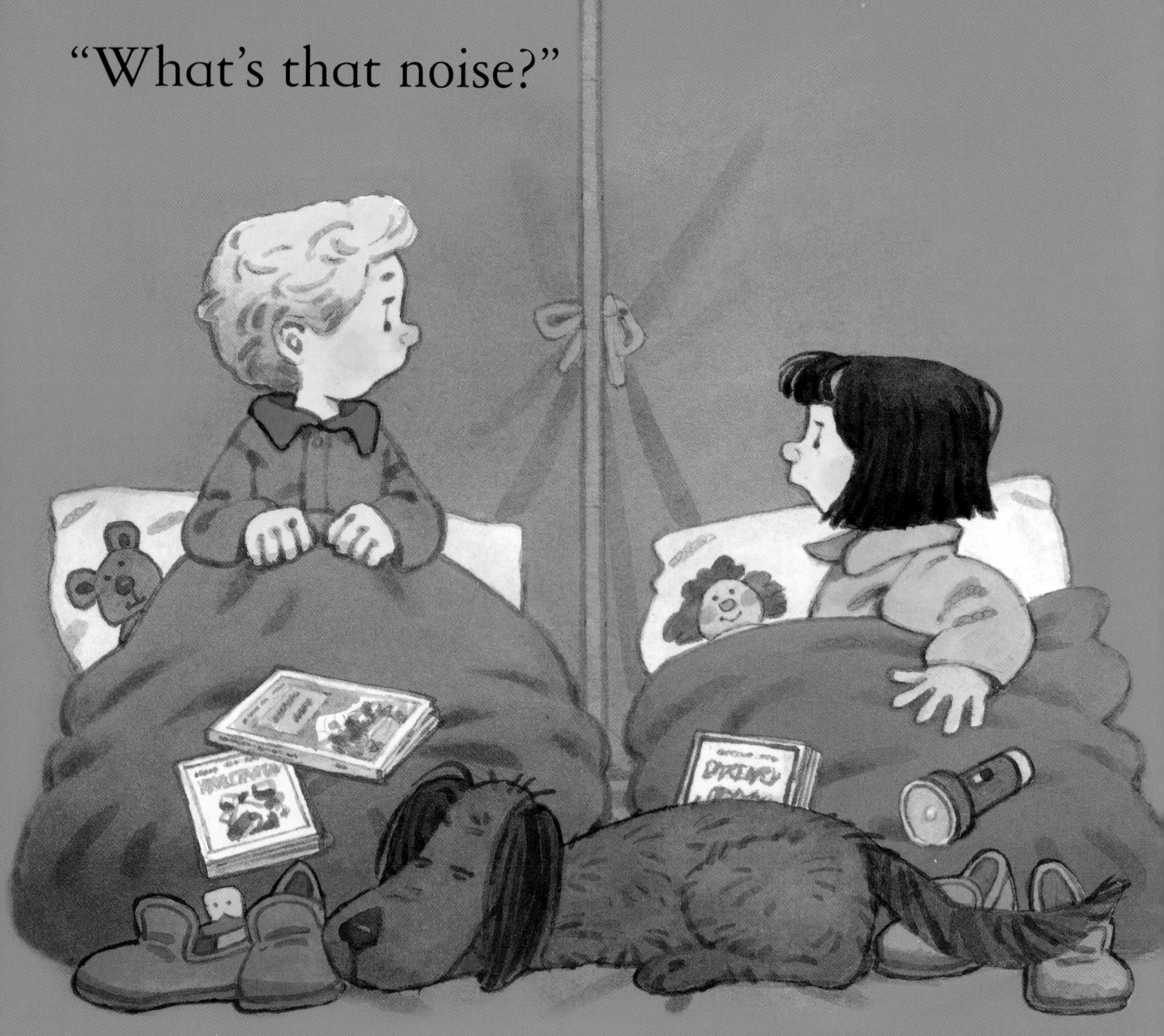

Sam sits up. "There's something walking around outside the tent," says Sam. "What is it?"

Poppy looks out of the tent.

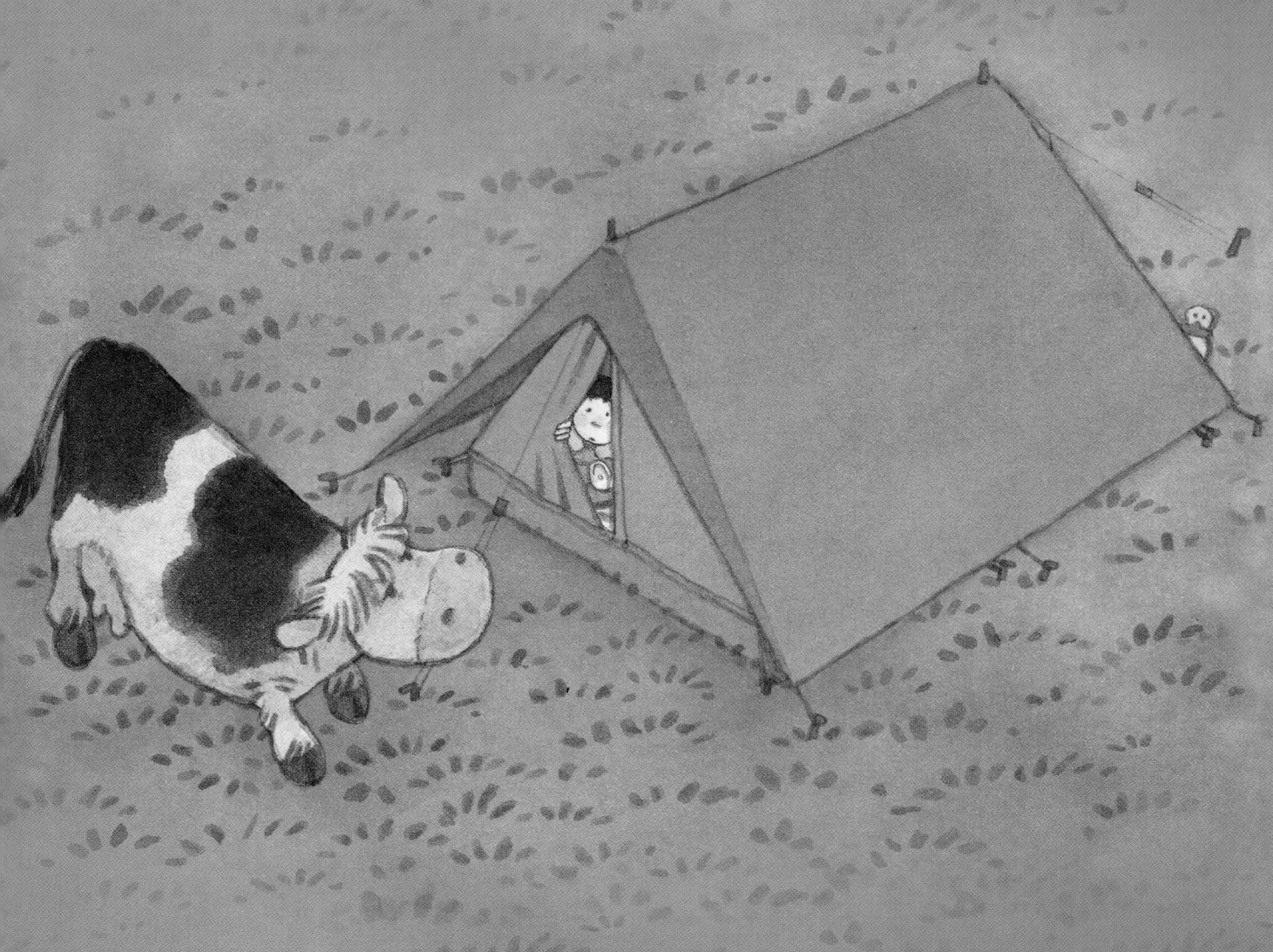

"It's only Daisy, the cow," she says. "She must have strayed into this field. She's so nosy."

Daisy looks into the tent.

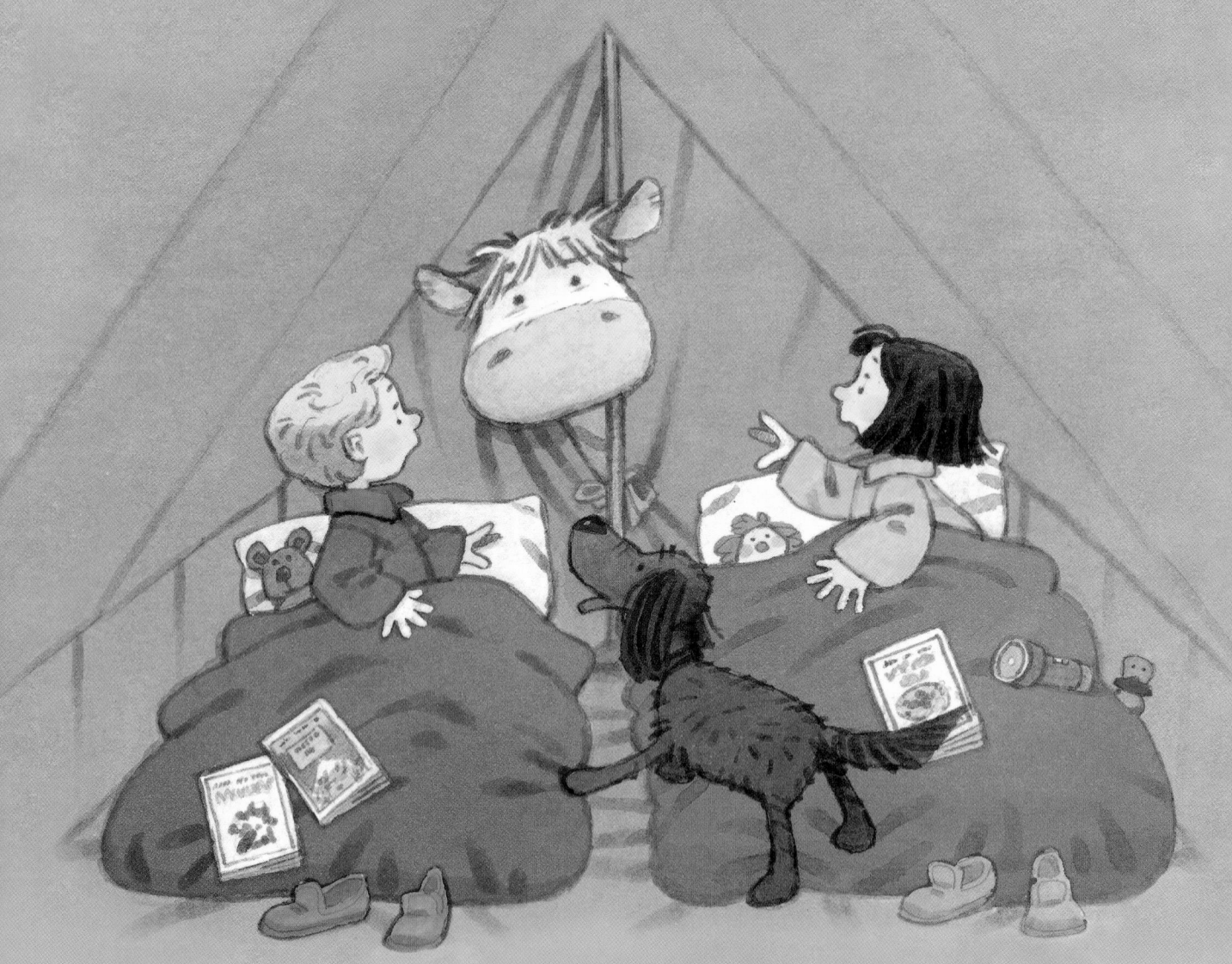

Rusty barks at her. Daisy is scared. She tries to back away but the tent catches on her head.

Daisy pulls at the tent.

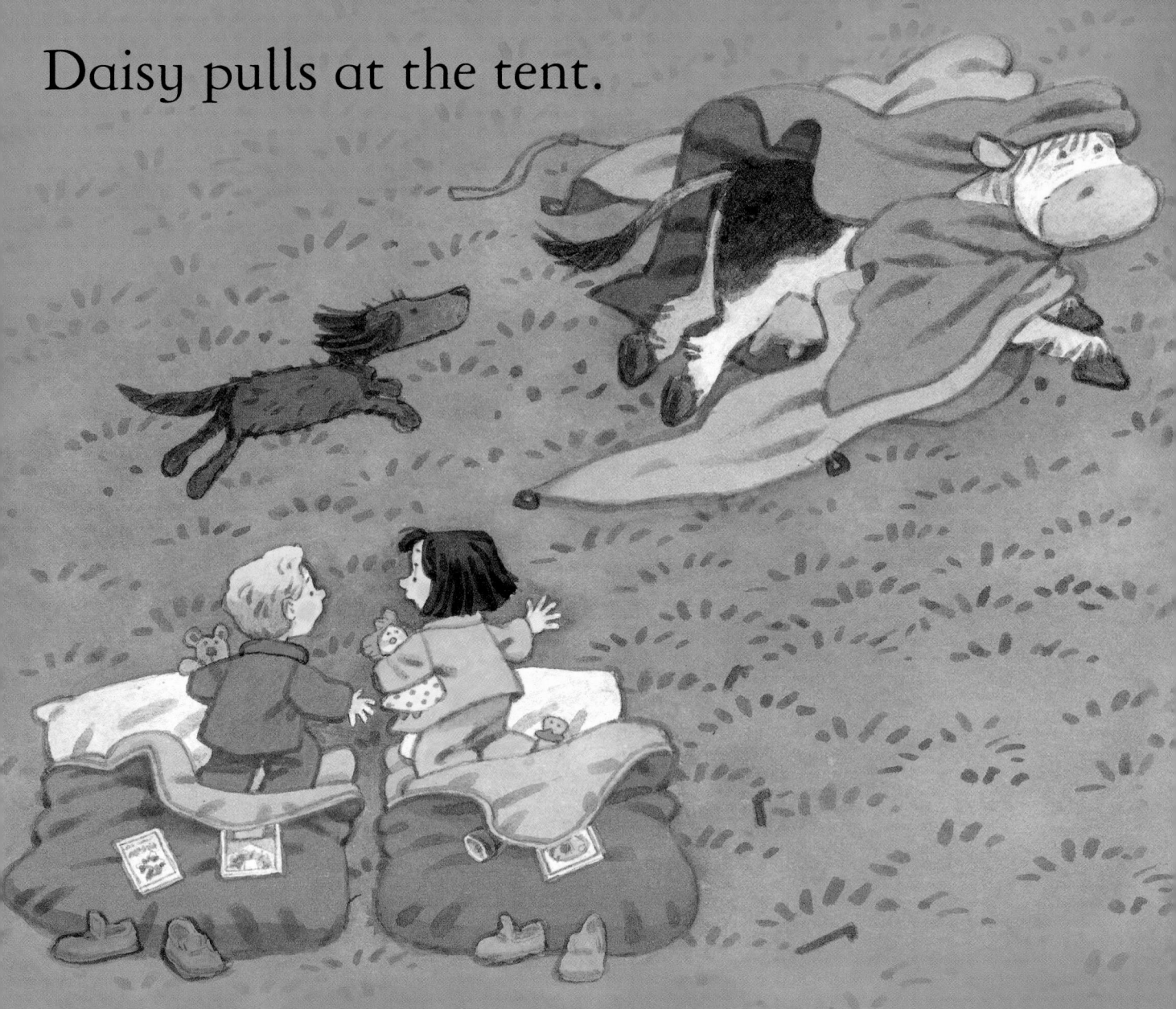

She pulls it down and runs off with it. Rusty chases
her. Poppy and Sam run back to the house.

Mr. Boot opens the door.

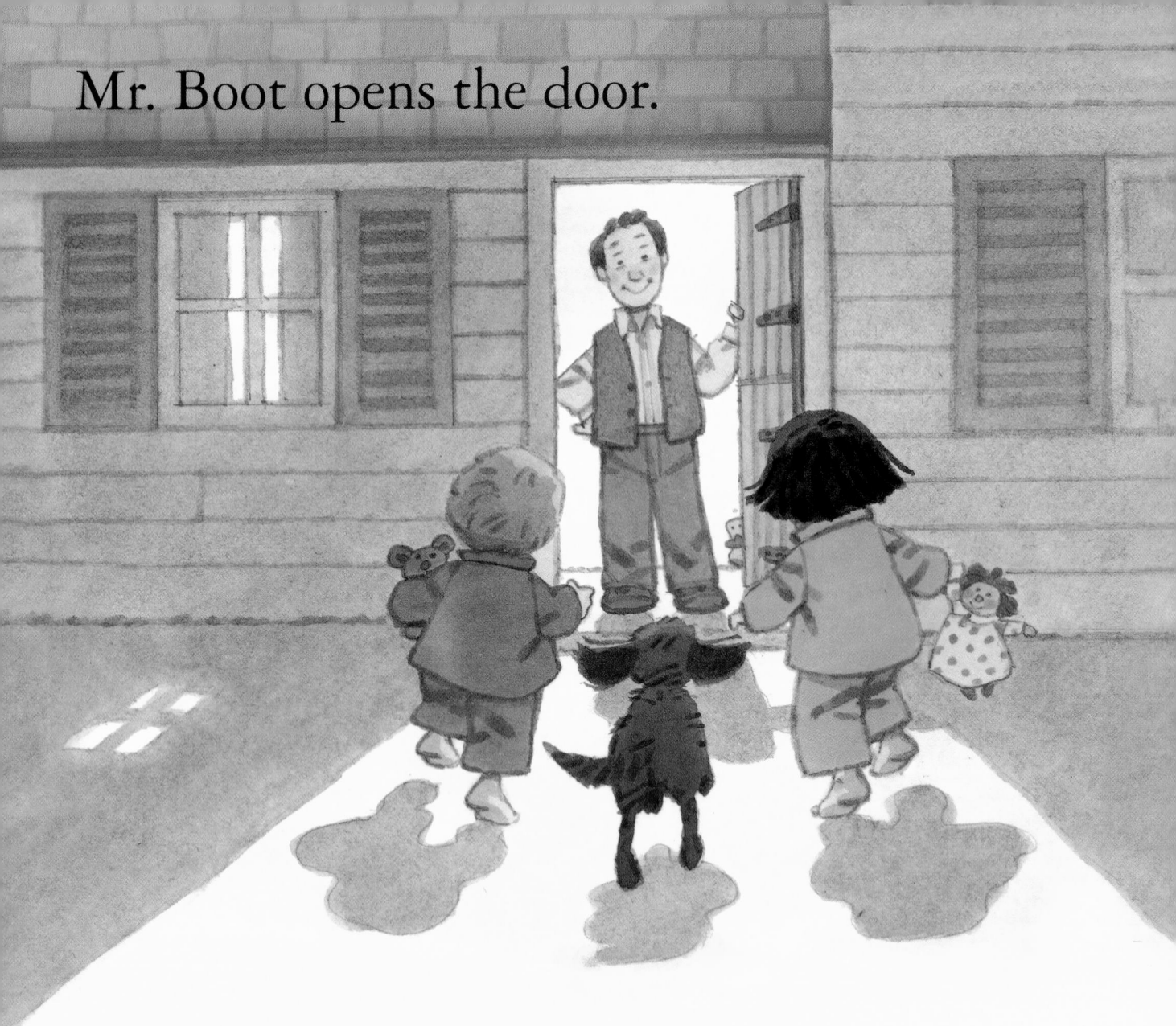

"Hello, Dad," says Sam. "Daisy's got our tent."
"I think camping is fun," says Poppy.

The
Old Steam Train

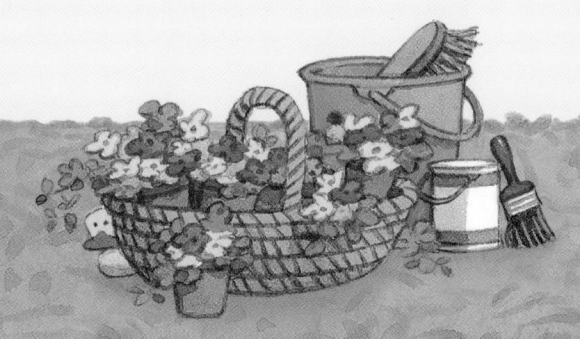

This is Apple Tree Farm.

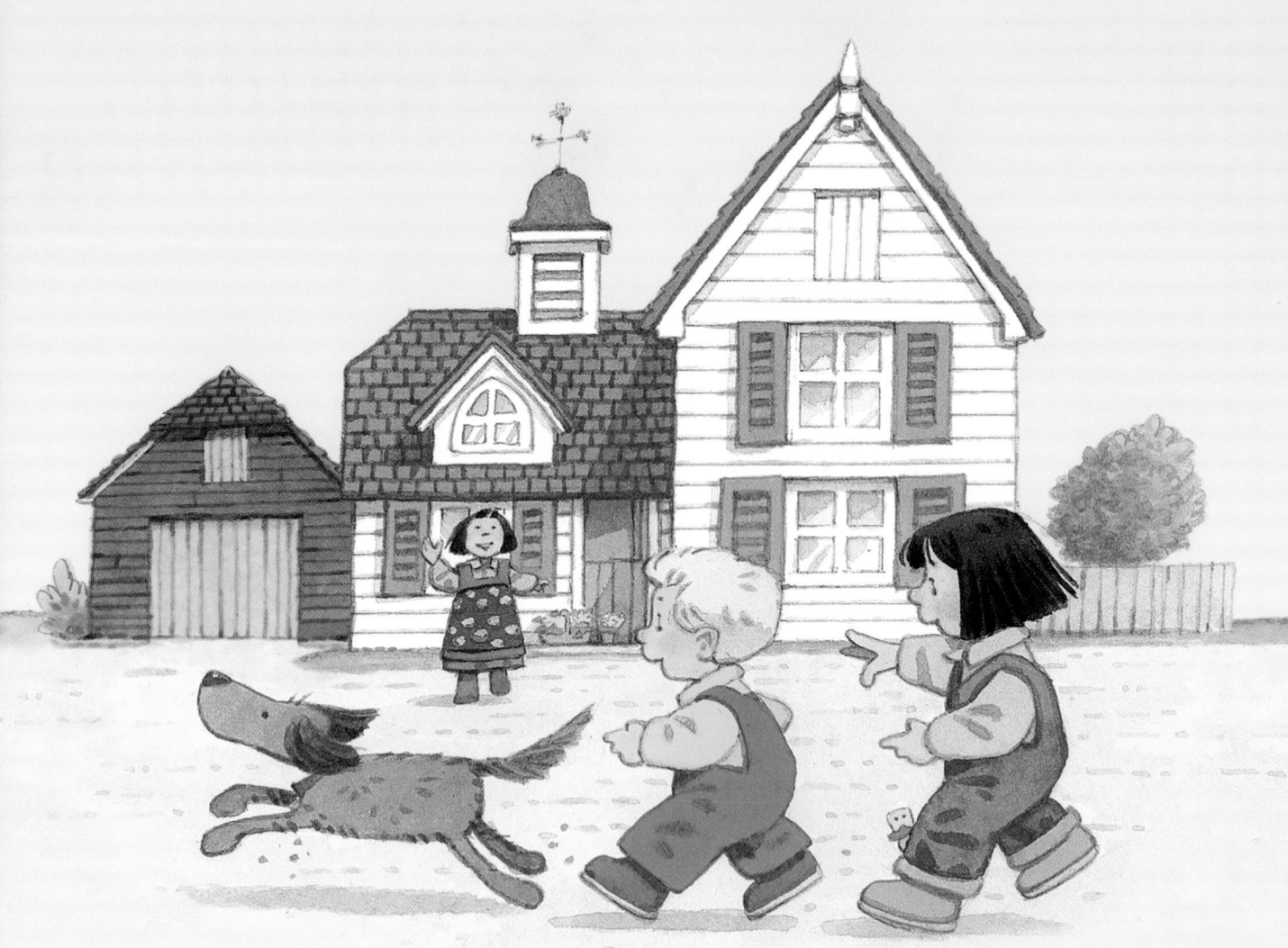

This is Mrs. Boot, the farmer. She has two children, called Poppy and Sam, and a dog called Rusty.

"Hurry up," says Mrs. Boot.

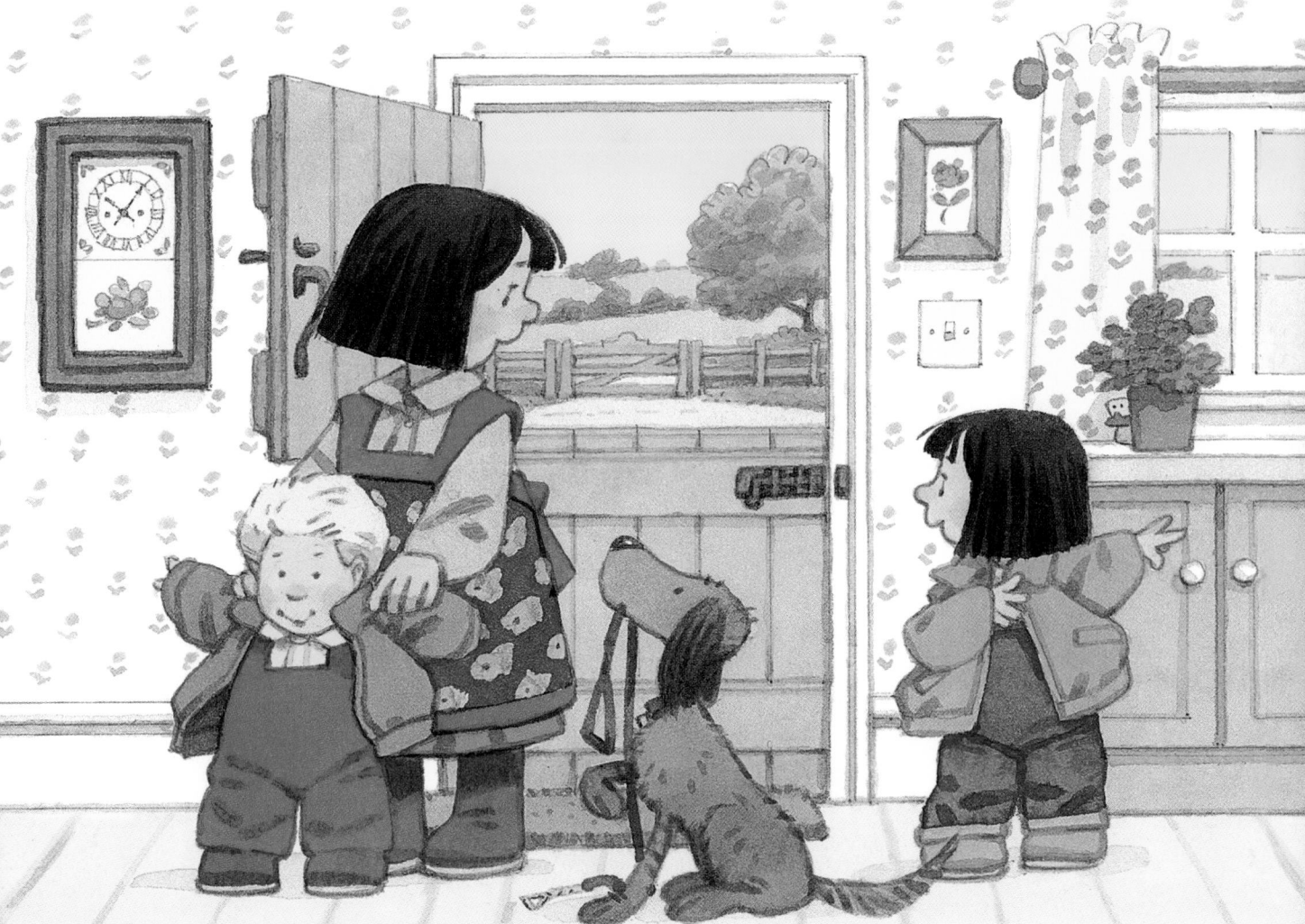

"Where are we going today?" asks Poppy.
"To the old station," says Mrs. Boot.

259

They walk down the lane.

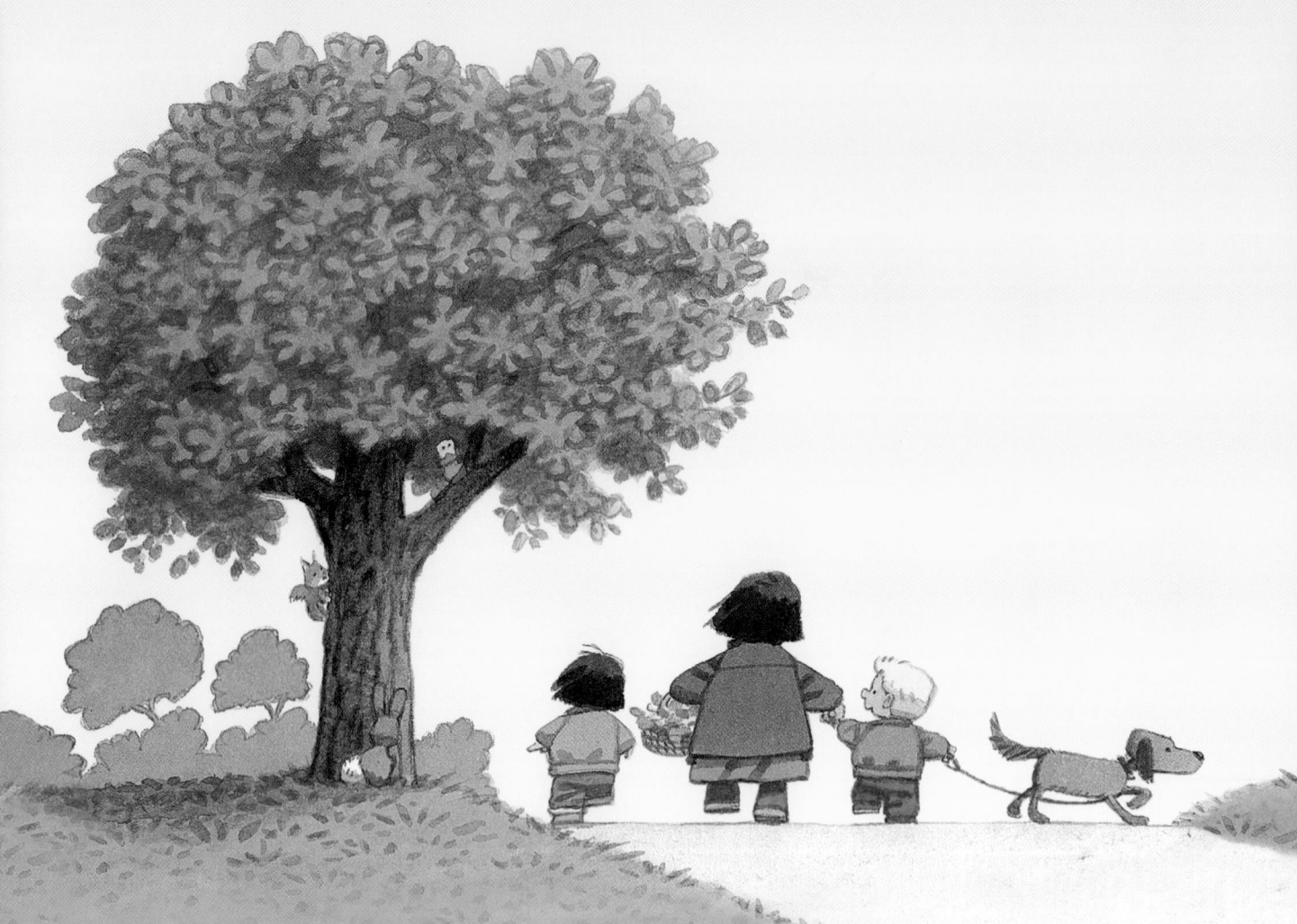

"Why are we going? There aren't any trains," says Sam. "Just you wait and see," says Mrs. Boot.

"What's everyone doing?" asks Poppy.

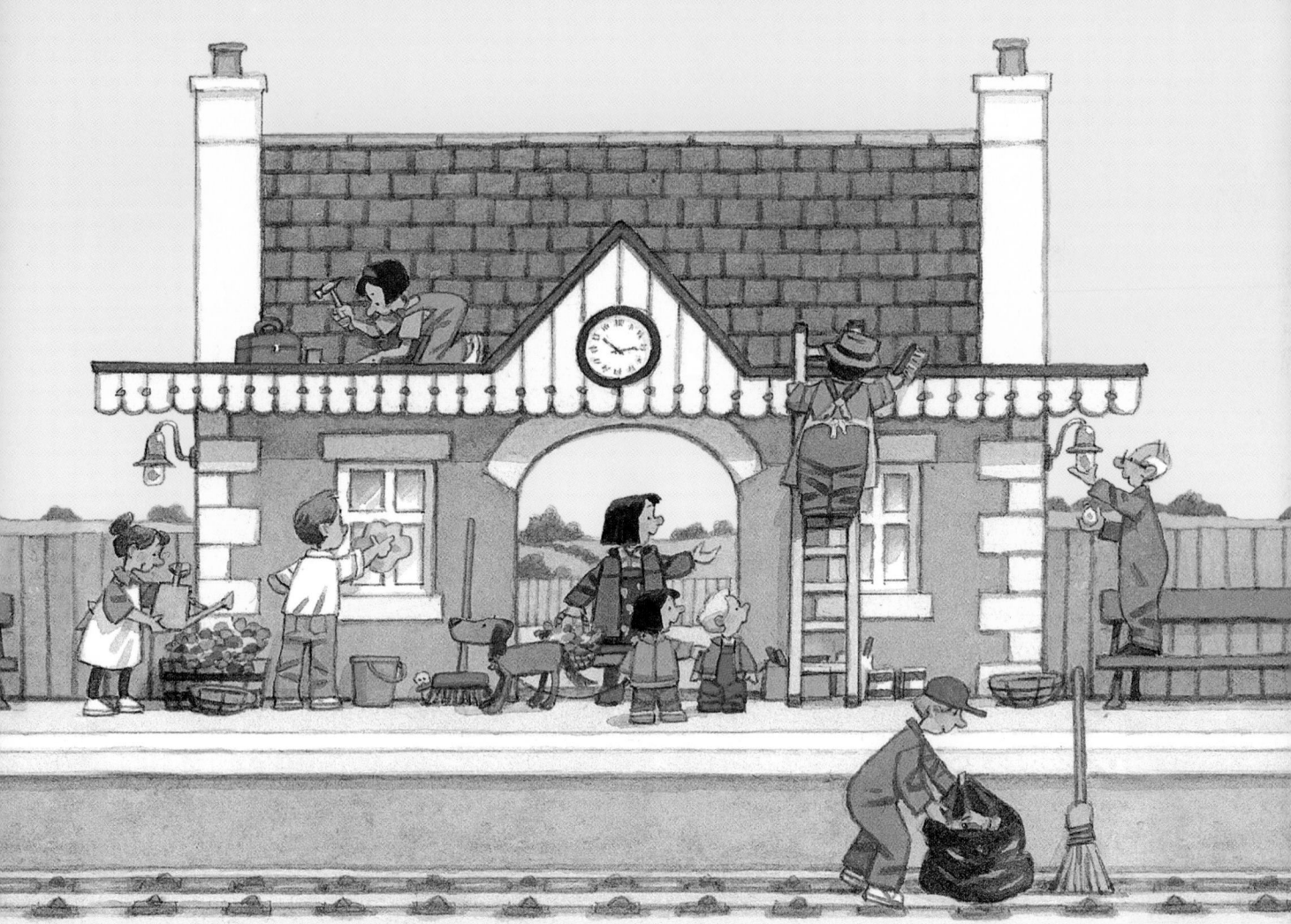

"They're cleaning up the old station," says
Mrs. Boot. "Everyone's helping today."

261

"There's lots to do."

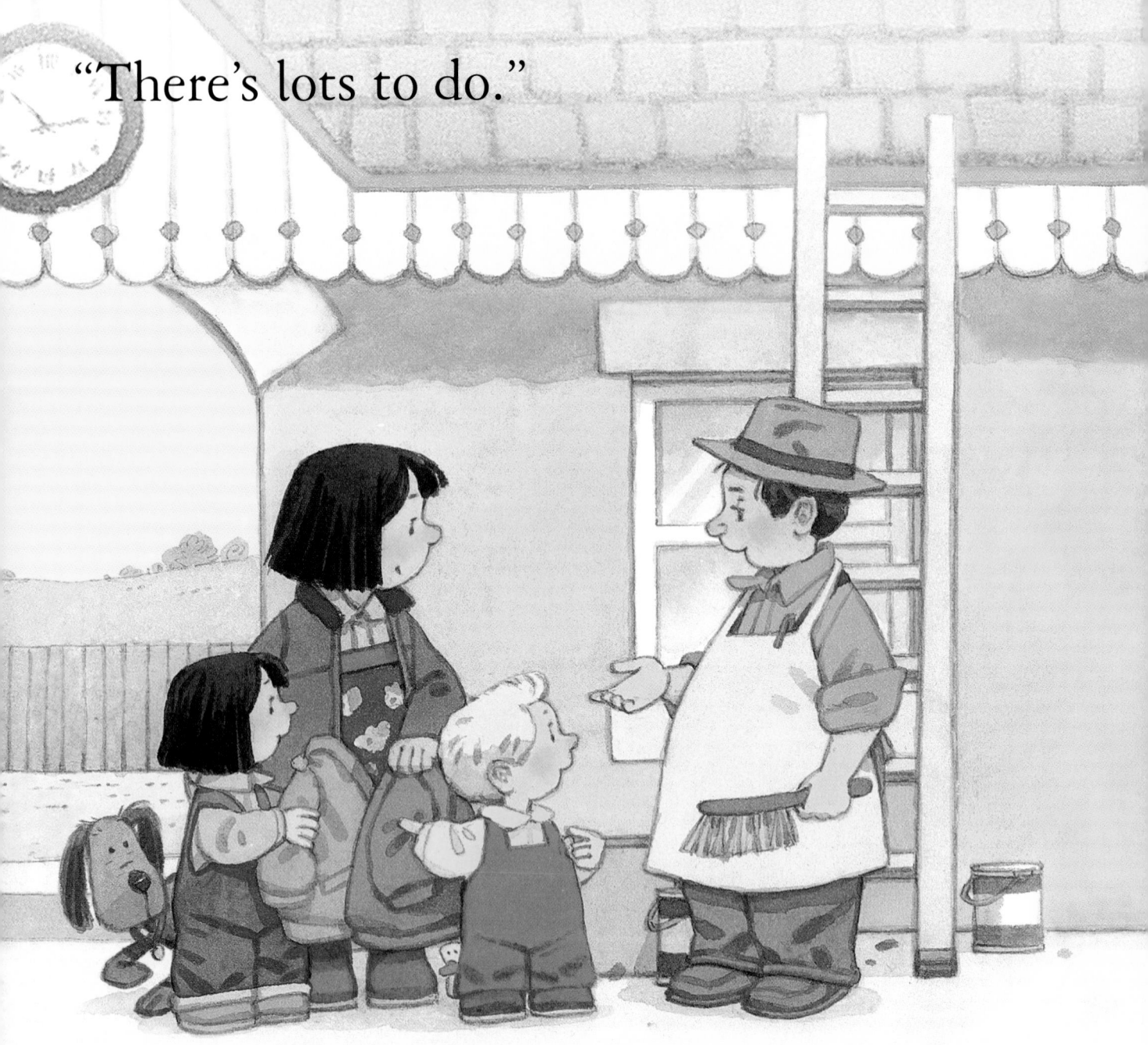

"Poppy and Sam can help me," says the painter.
"Coats off and down to work," says Mrs. Boot.

Poppy and Sam work hard.

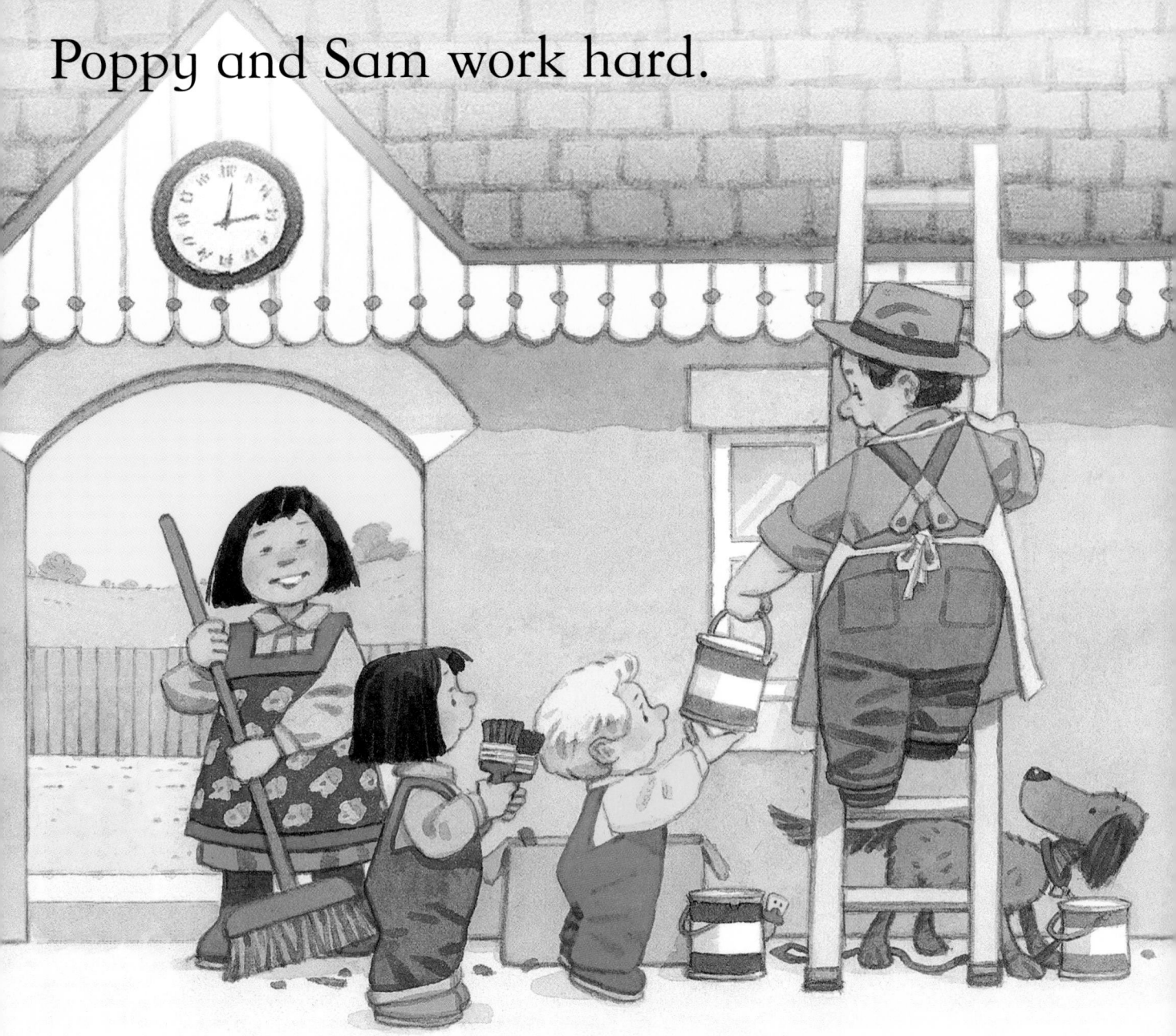

Sam brings pots of paint and Poppy brings the brushes. Mrs. Boot sweeps the platform.

"What's that noise?"

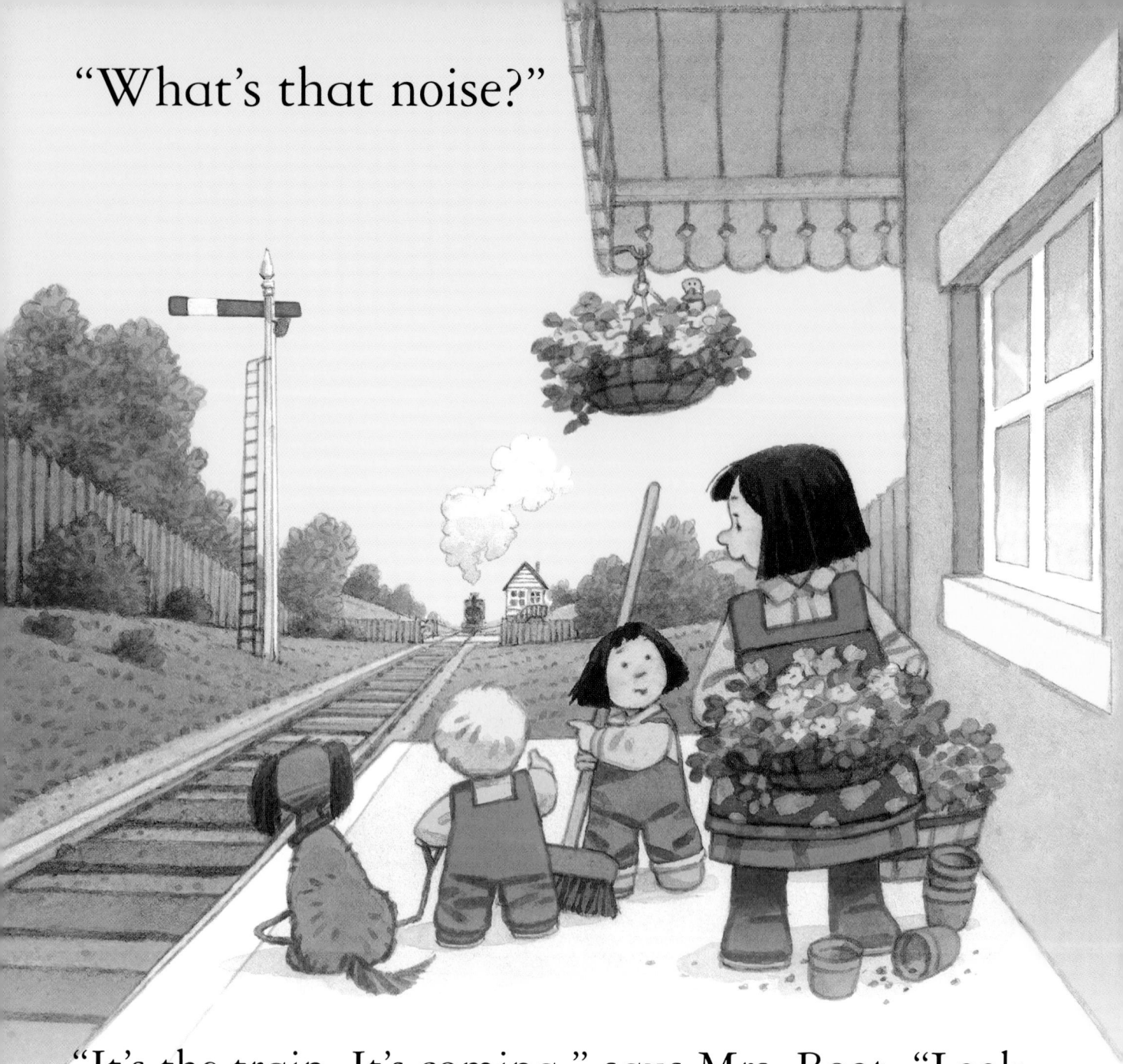

"It's the train. It's coming," says Mrs. Boot. "Look,
it's a steam train," says Poppy. "How exciting."

The train puffs down the track.

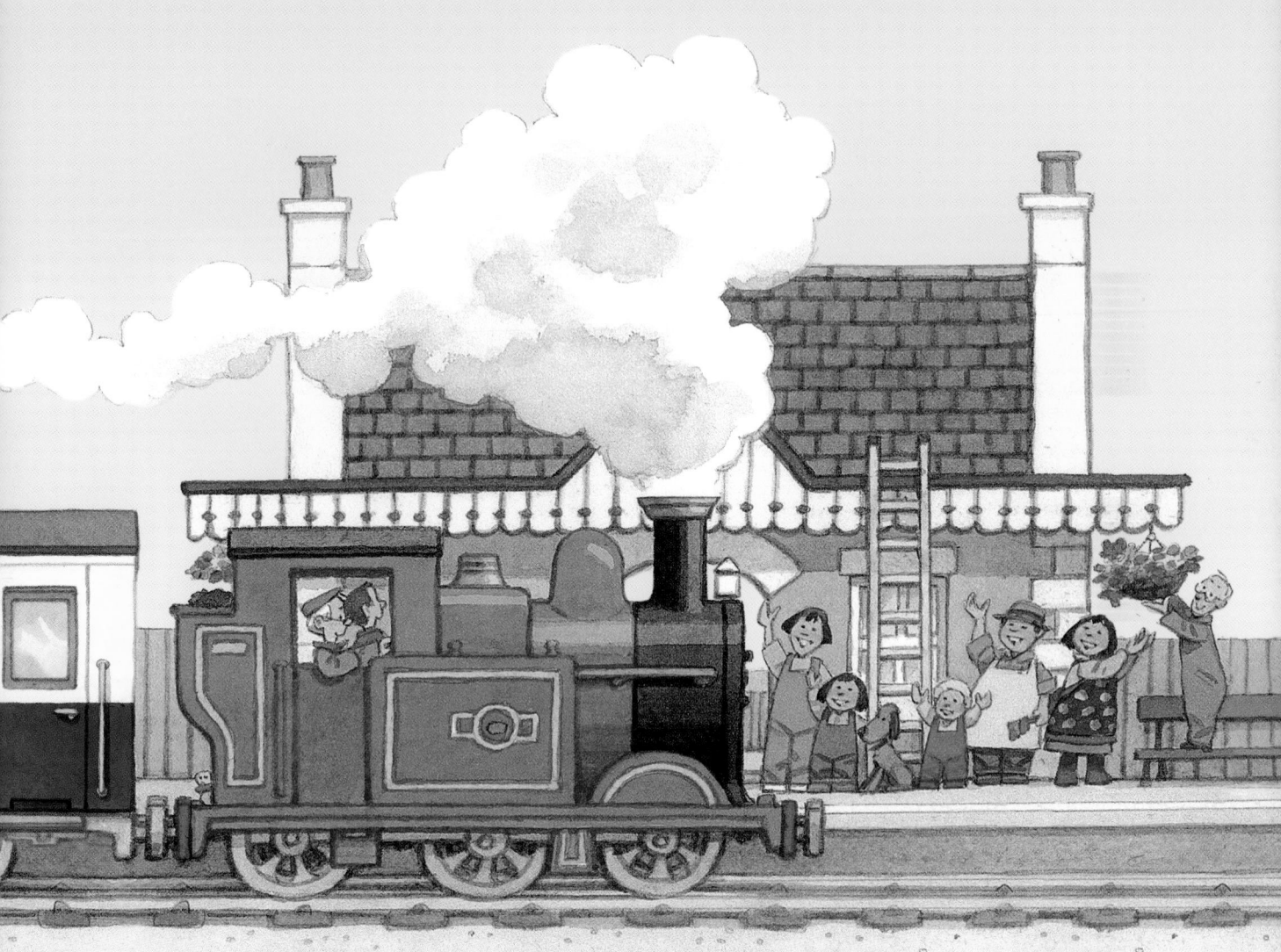

It stops at the platform. The engine gives a long whistle. Everyone cheers and waves.

"Look, there's Dad," says Sam.

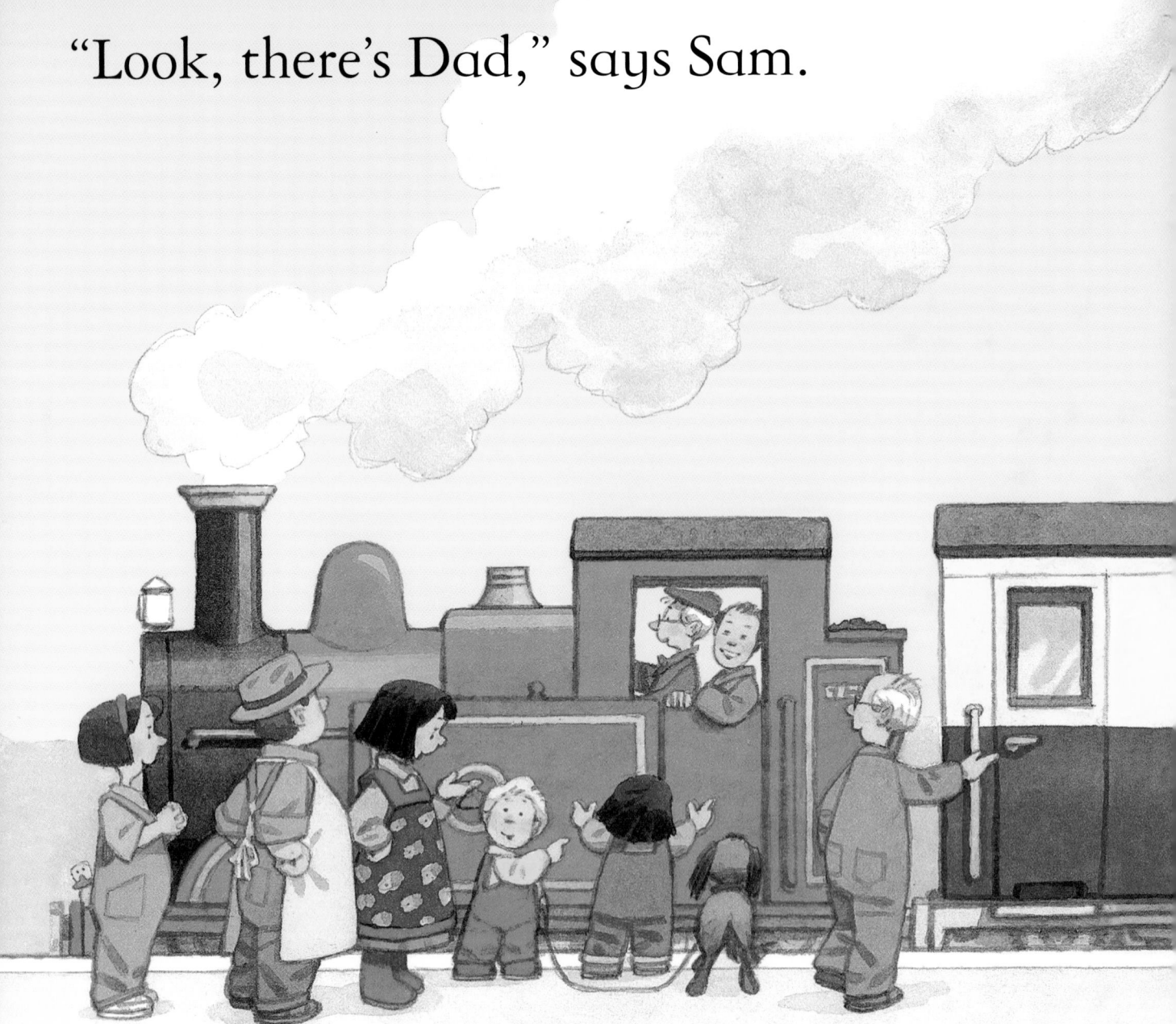

"He's helping the driver, just for today," says
Mrs. Boot. "Isn't he lucky?" says Poppy.

"All aboard," says Mrs. Boot.

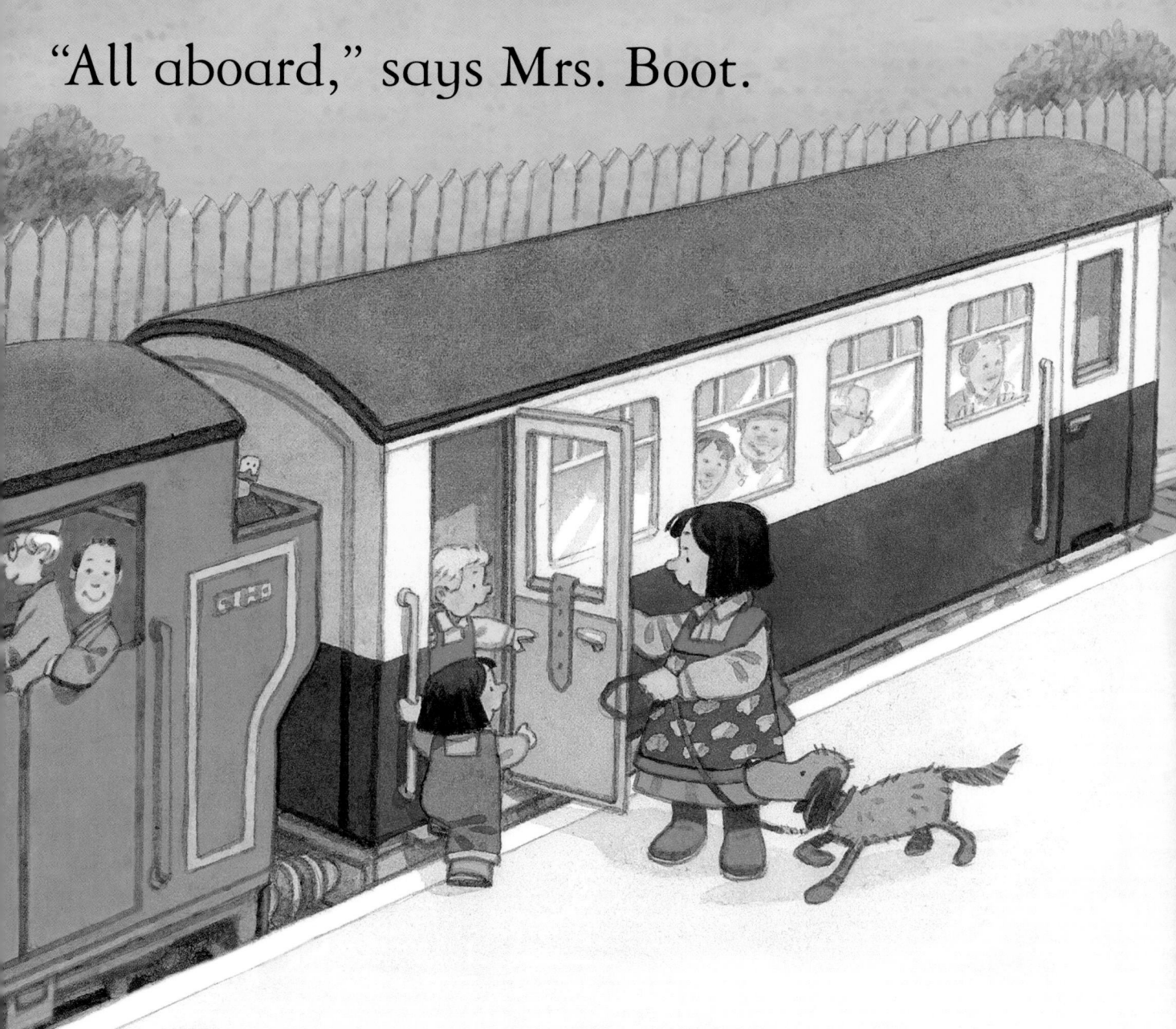

"I'll get on here," says Poppy. "Come on, Rusty," says Sam. "I'll shut the door," says Mrs. Boot.

"Where are you going?"

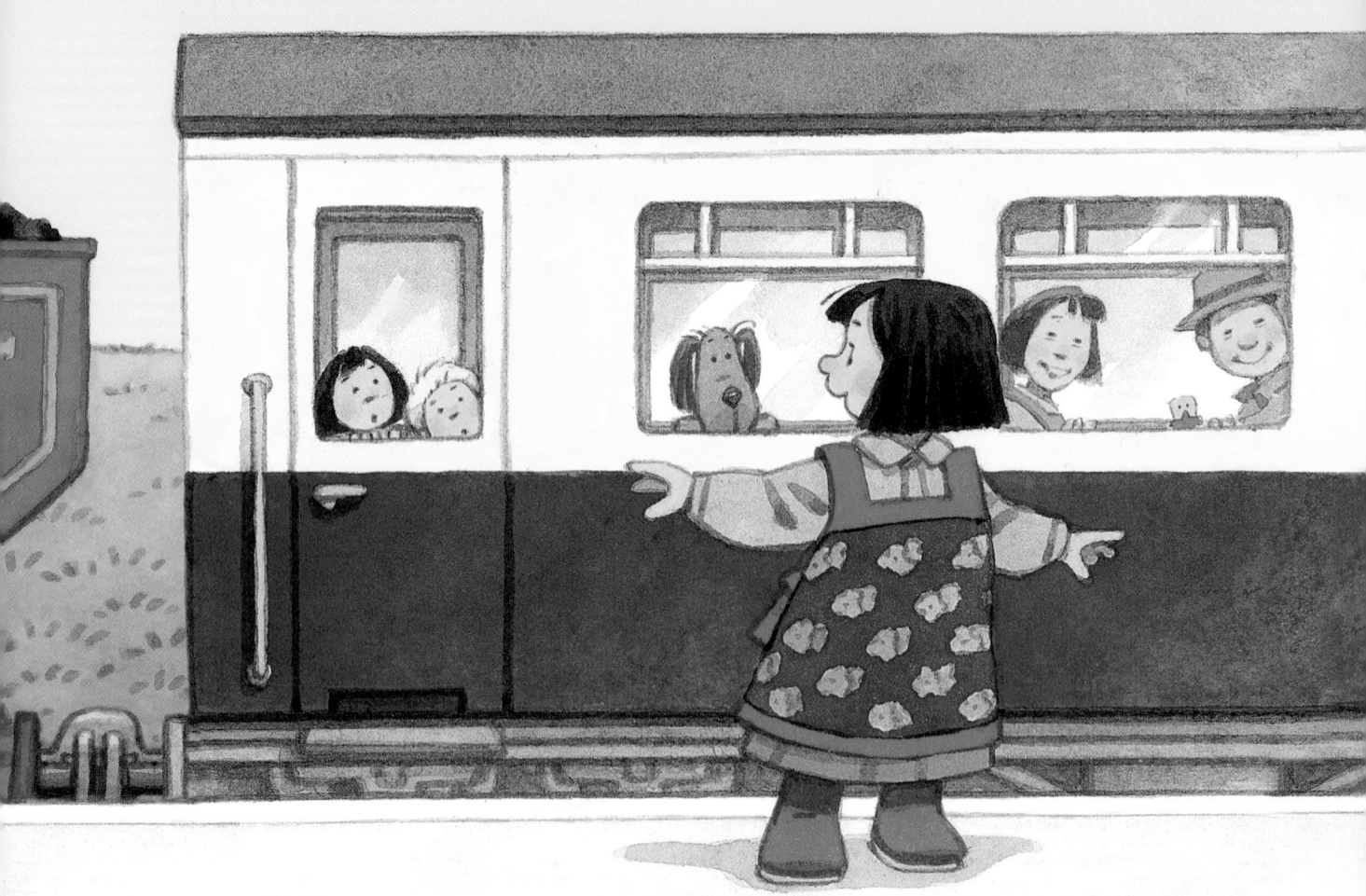

"Aren't you coming with us?" asks Sam. "You stay on the train," says Mrs. Boot. "I'll be back soon."

"Look, there she is."

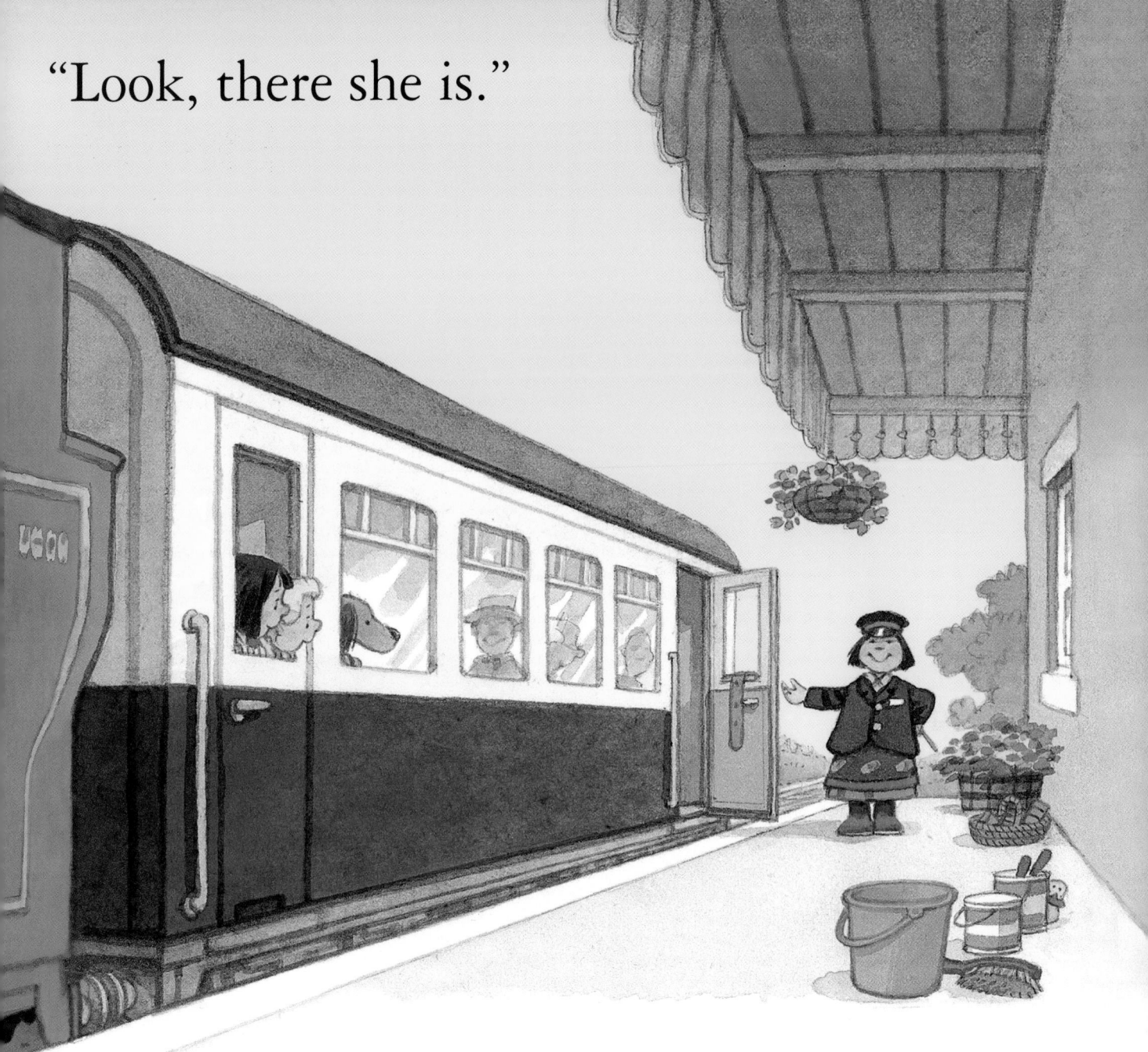

"She's wearing a cap," says Poppy. "Yes, I'm the guard, just for today," says Mrs. Boot.

Mrs. Boot waves a flag.

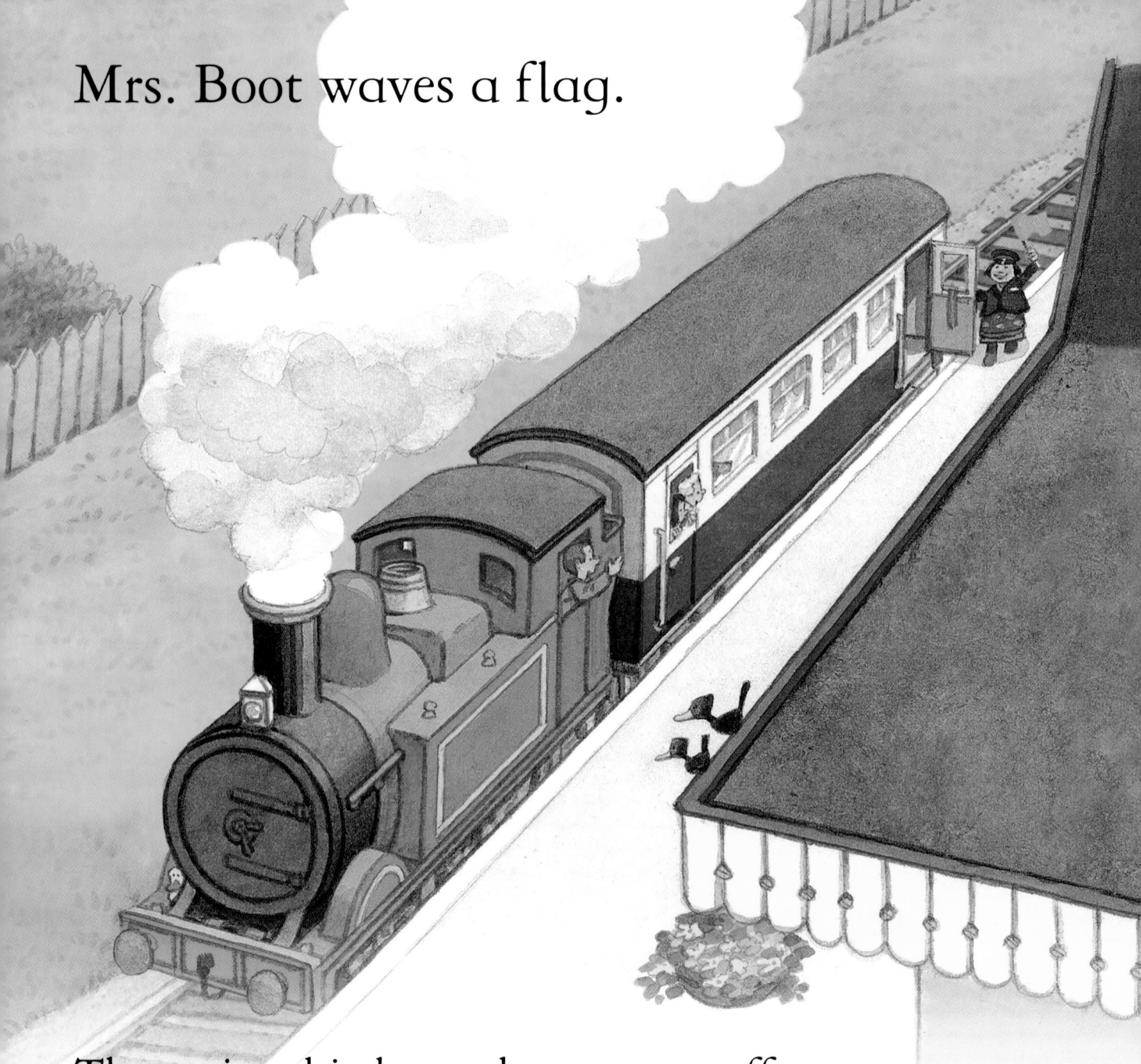

The train whistles and starts to puff away.
Mrs. Boot jumps on the train and shuts the door.

"We're off," says Sam.

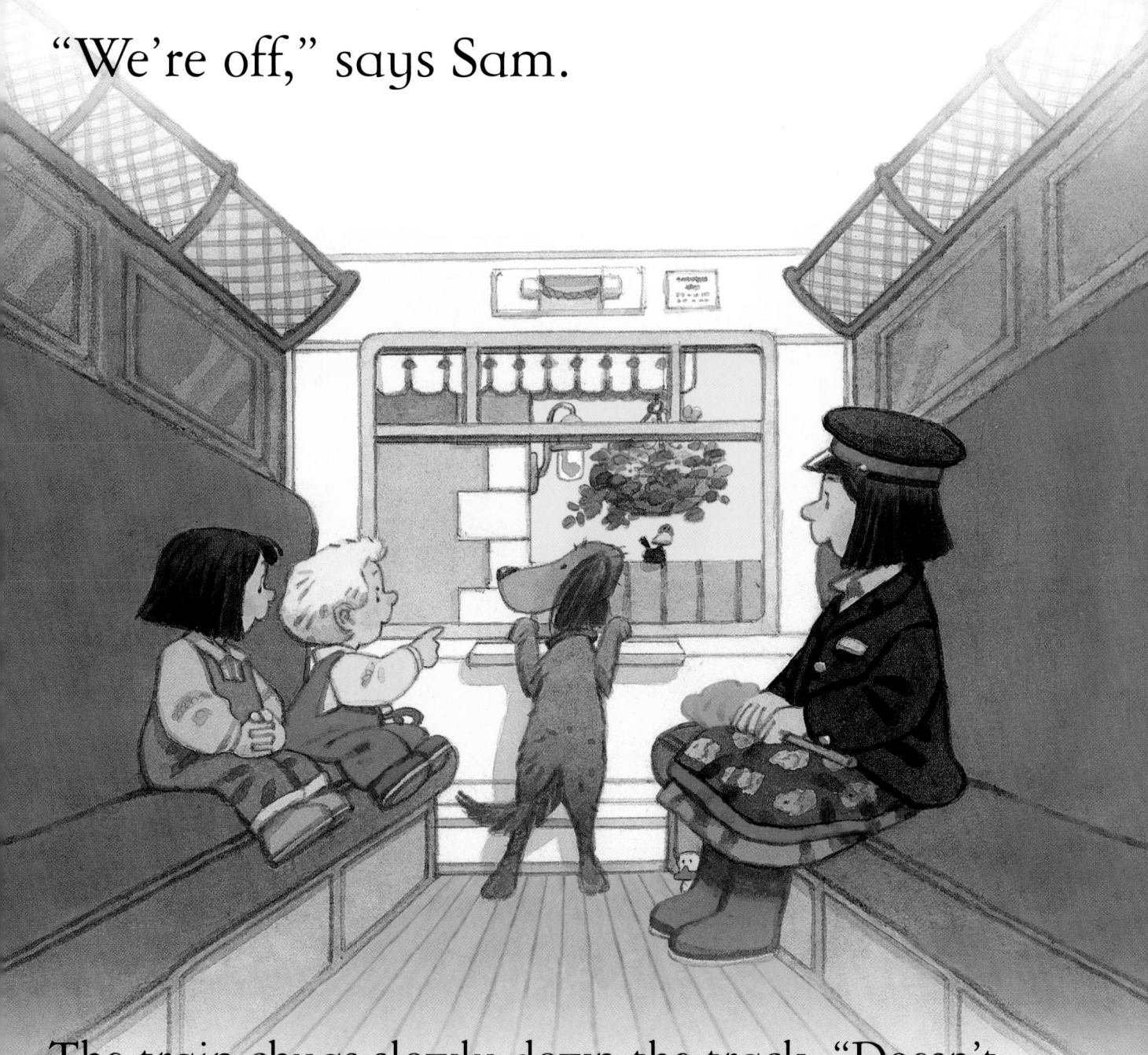

The train chugs slowly down the track. "Doesn't the old station look good now?" says Poppy.

"I like steam trains," says Sam.

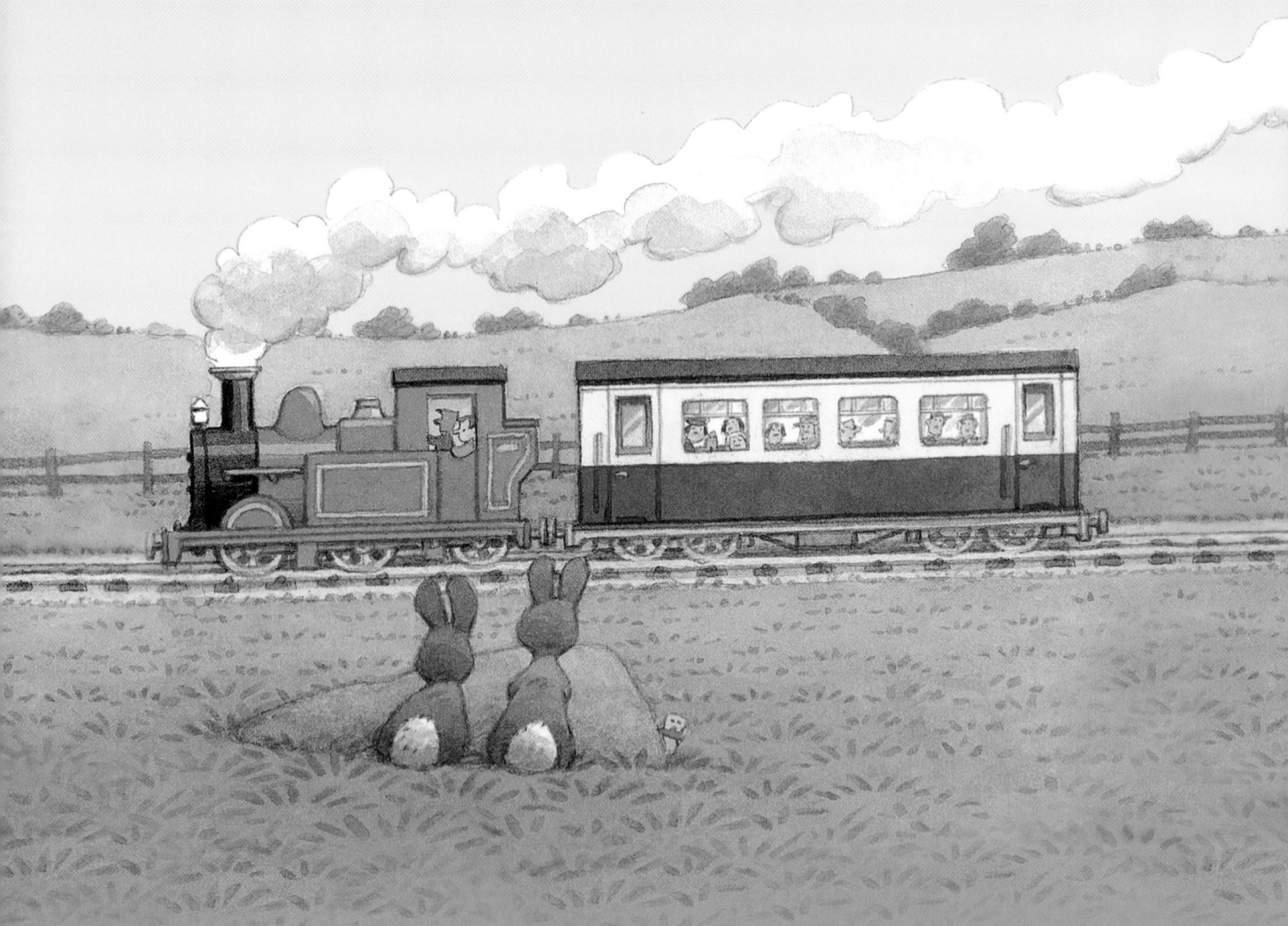

"The station is open again," says Mrs. Boot. "And we can ride on the steam train every weekend."

Dolly and
the Train

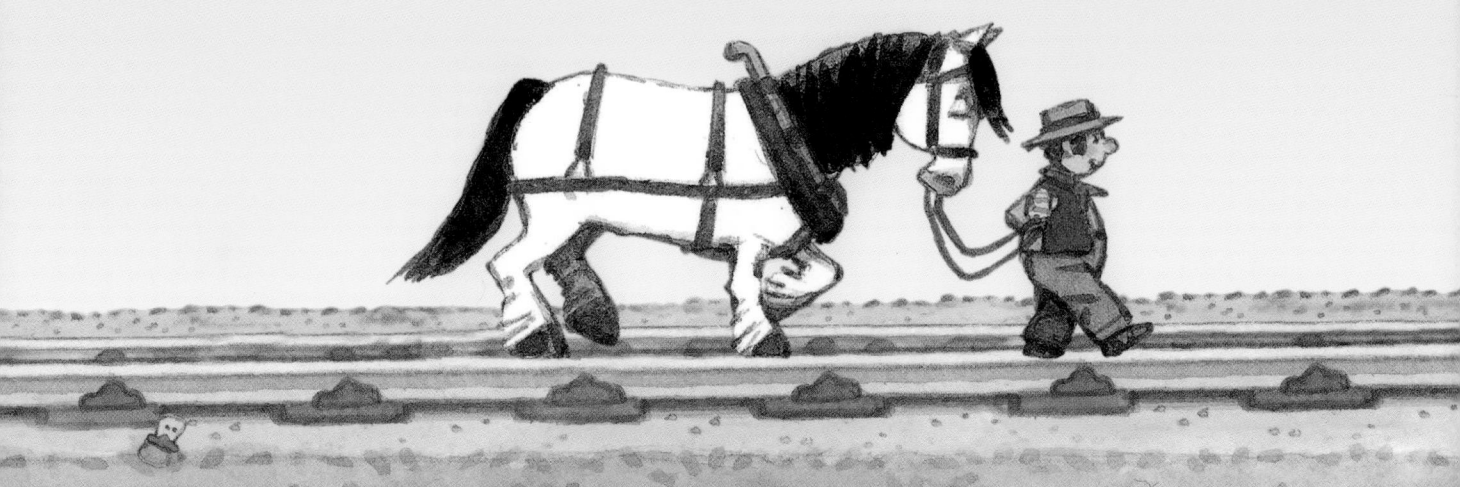

This is Apple Tree Farm.

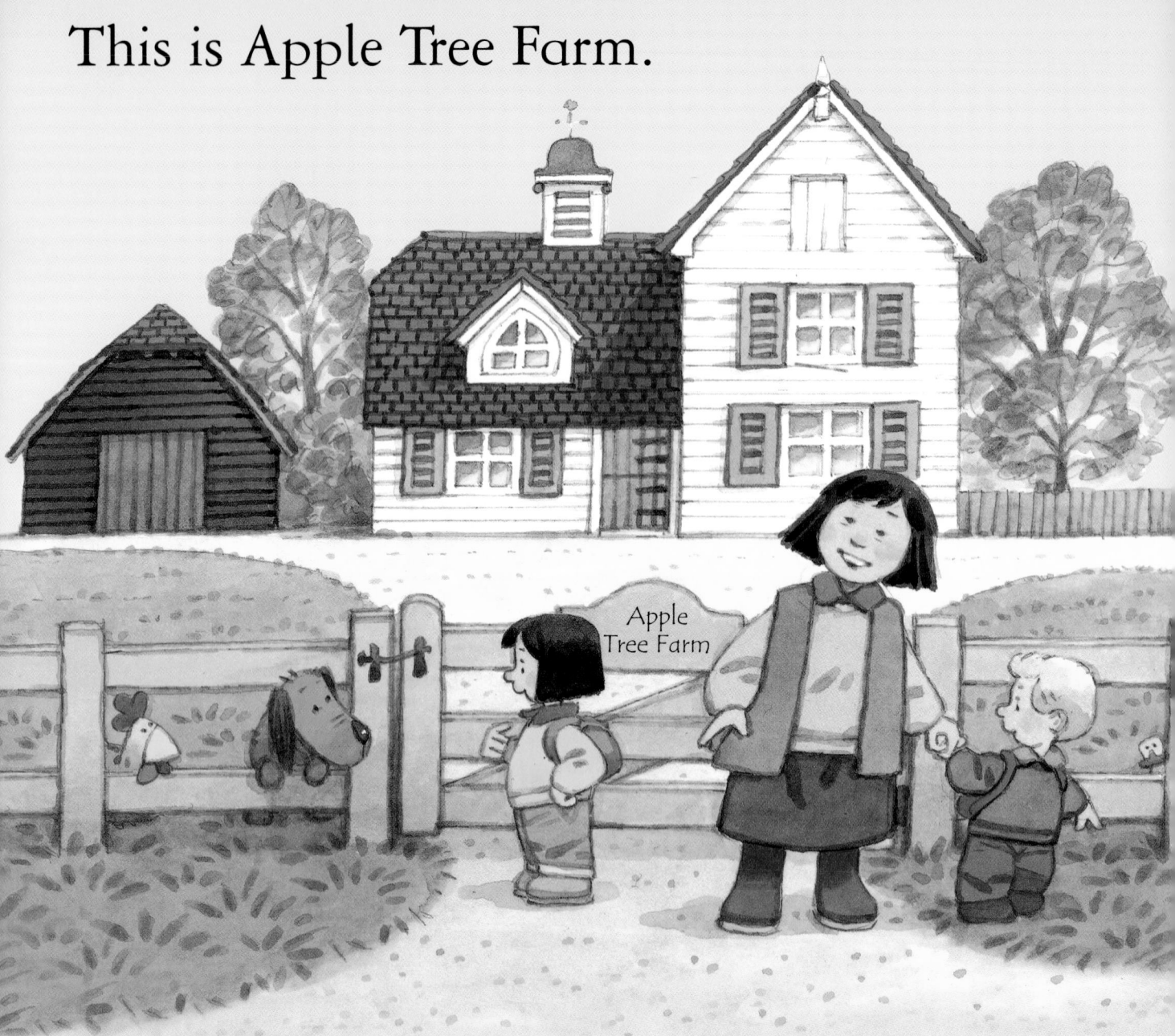

Apple Tree Farm

This is Mrs. Boot, the farmer. She has two children, called Poppy and Sam, and a dog called Rusty.

Today there is a school outing.

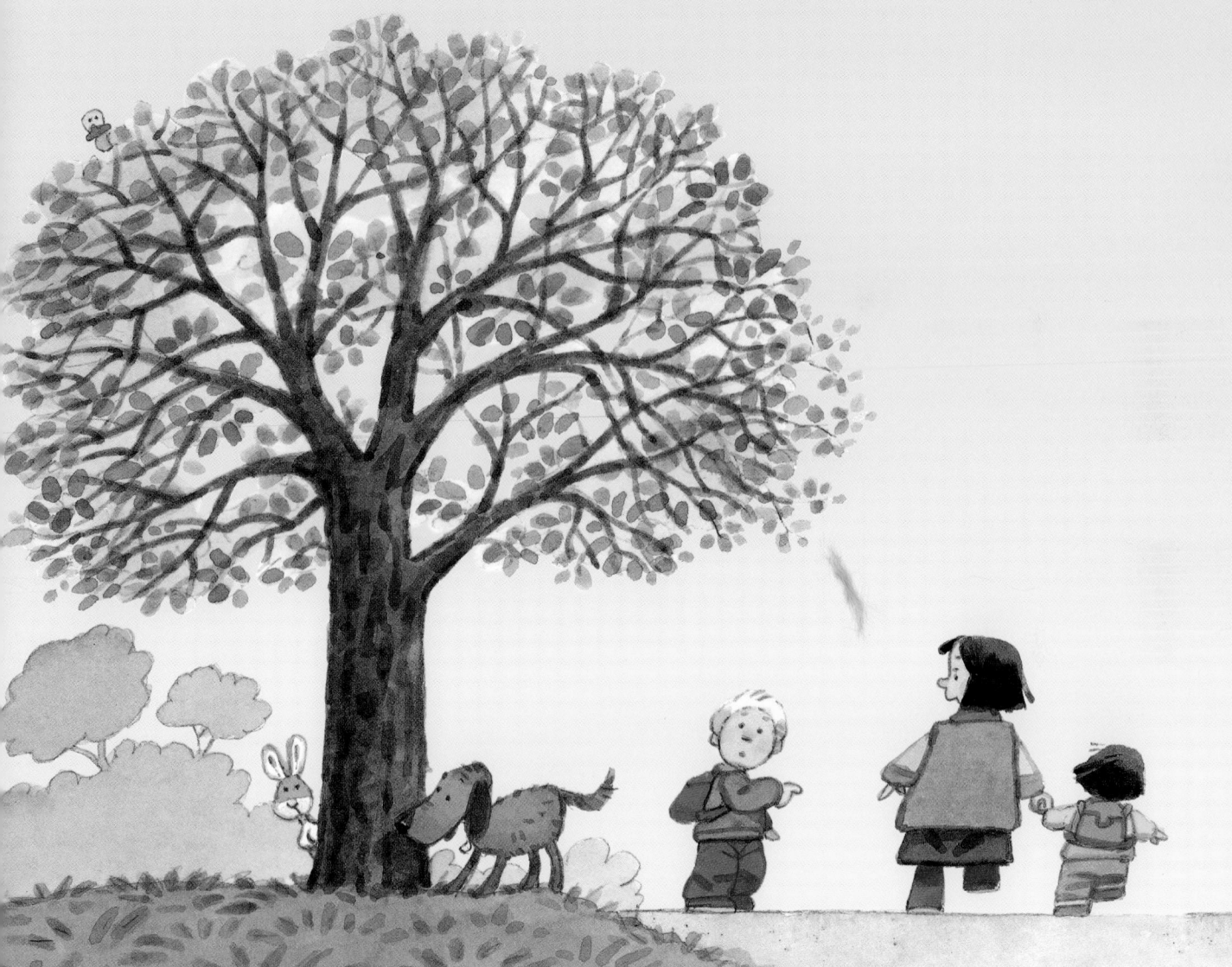

Mrs. Boot, Poppy and Sam walk down the road to the old station. "Come on, Rusty," says Sam.

"There's your teacher," says Mrs. Boot.

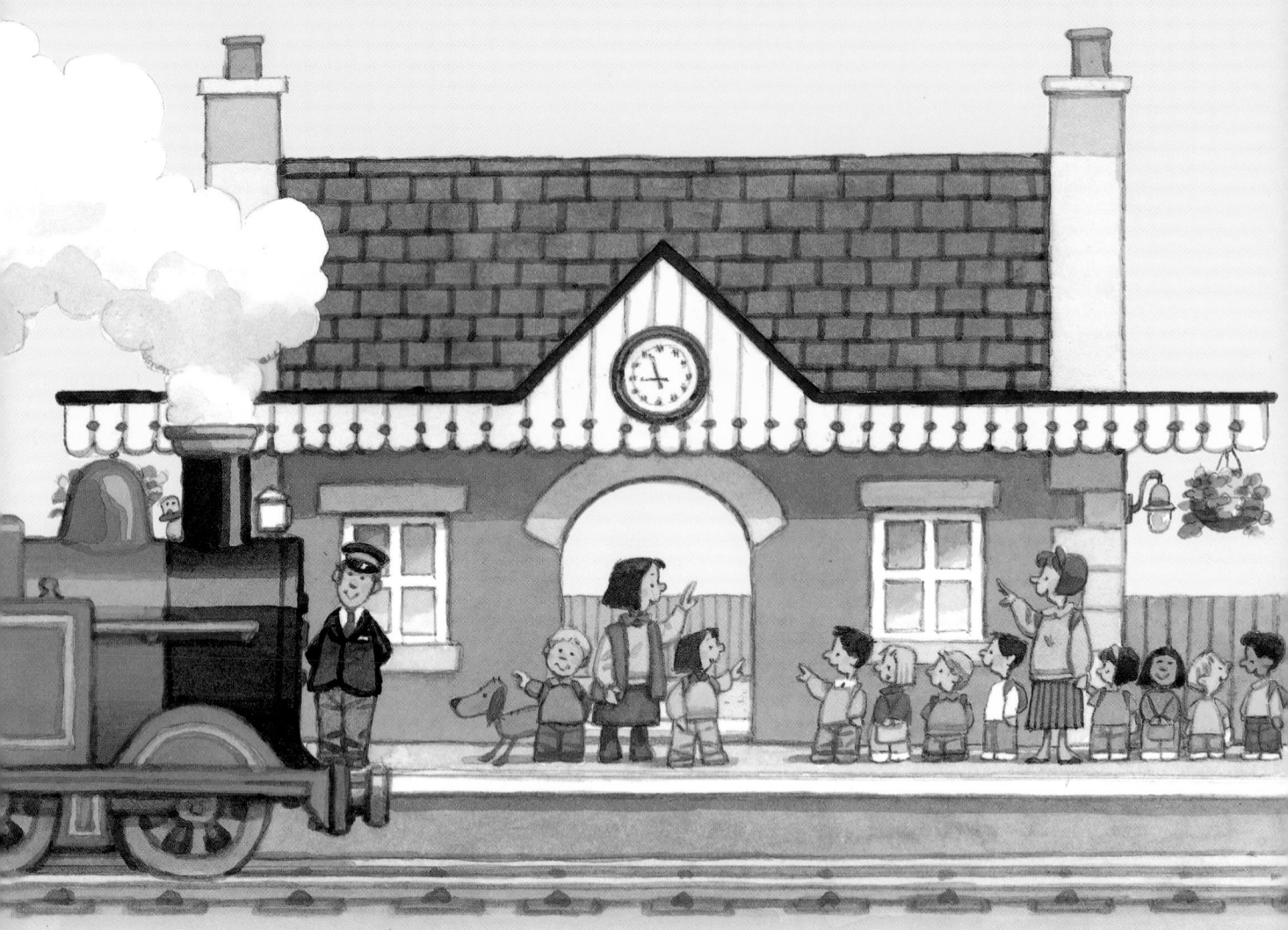

"And there's the old steam train, all ready for our outing," says Poppy.

"All aboard," says the driver.

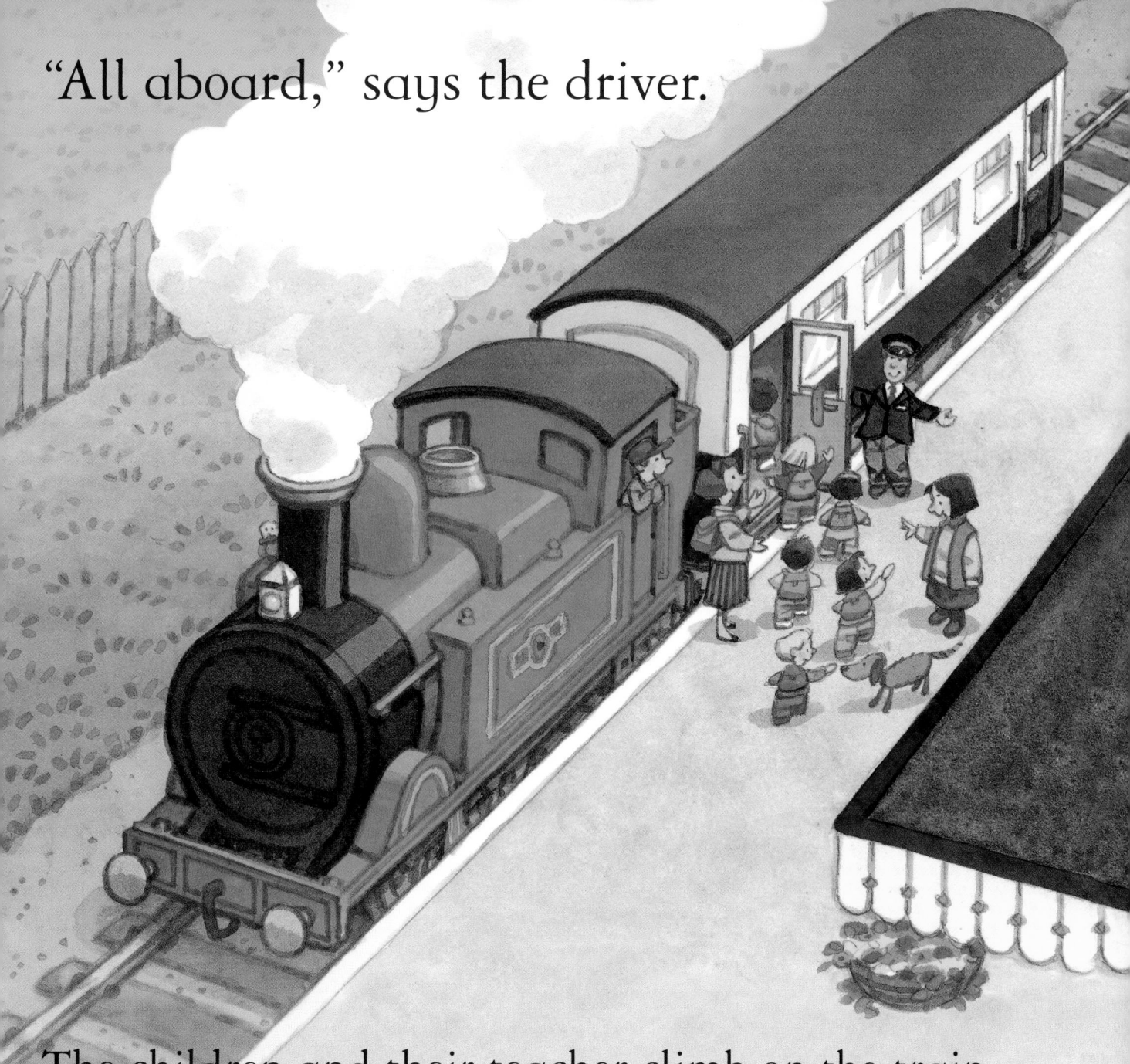

The children and their teacher climb on the train.
The guard closes the door and blows his whistle.

Mrs. Boot waves goodbye.

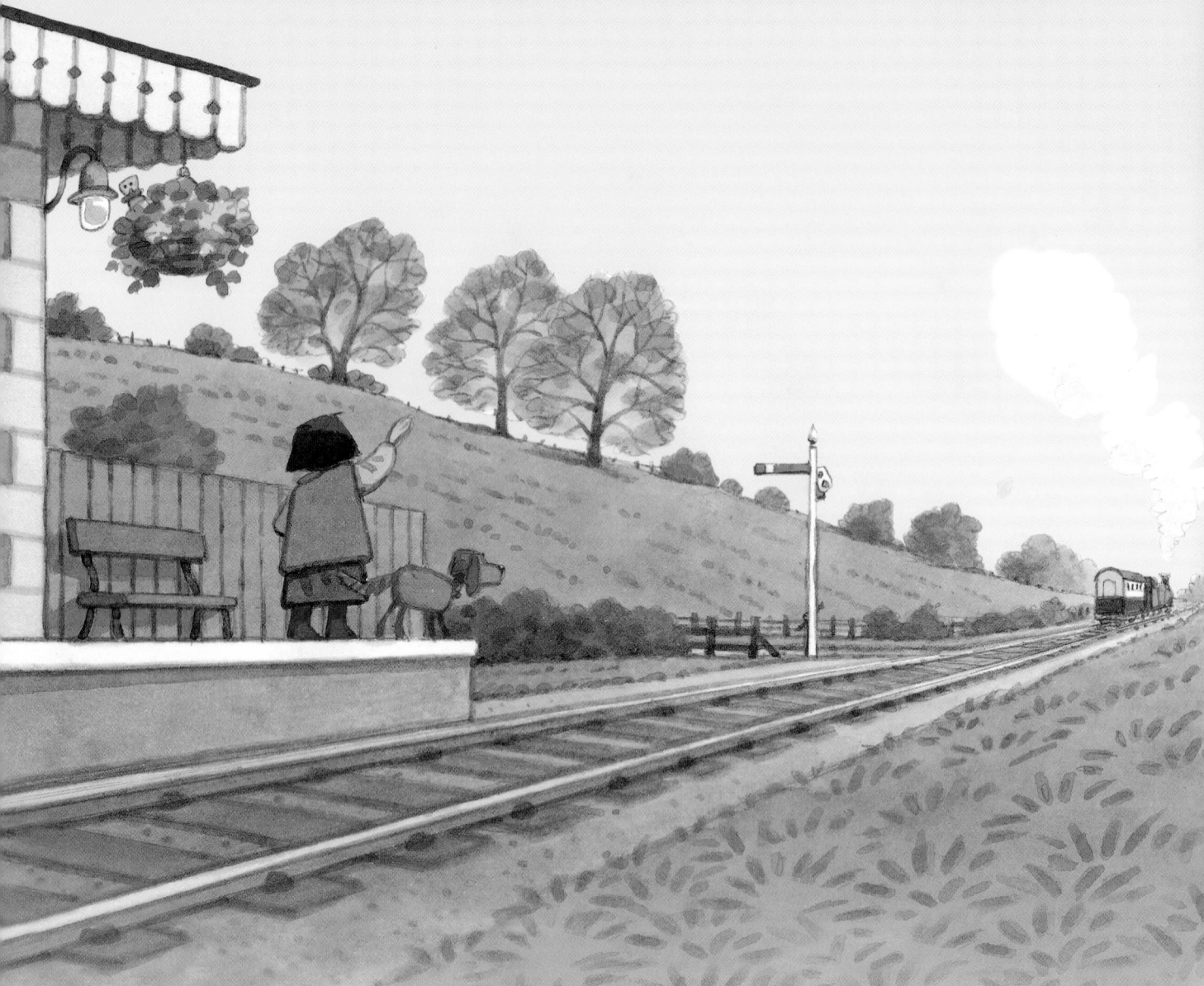

The train puffs slowly down the track. Rusty barks at it. He wants to go on the outing too.

The children look out of the window.

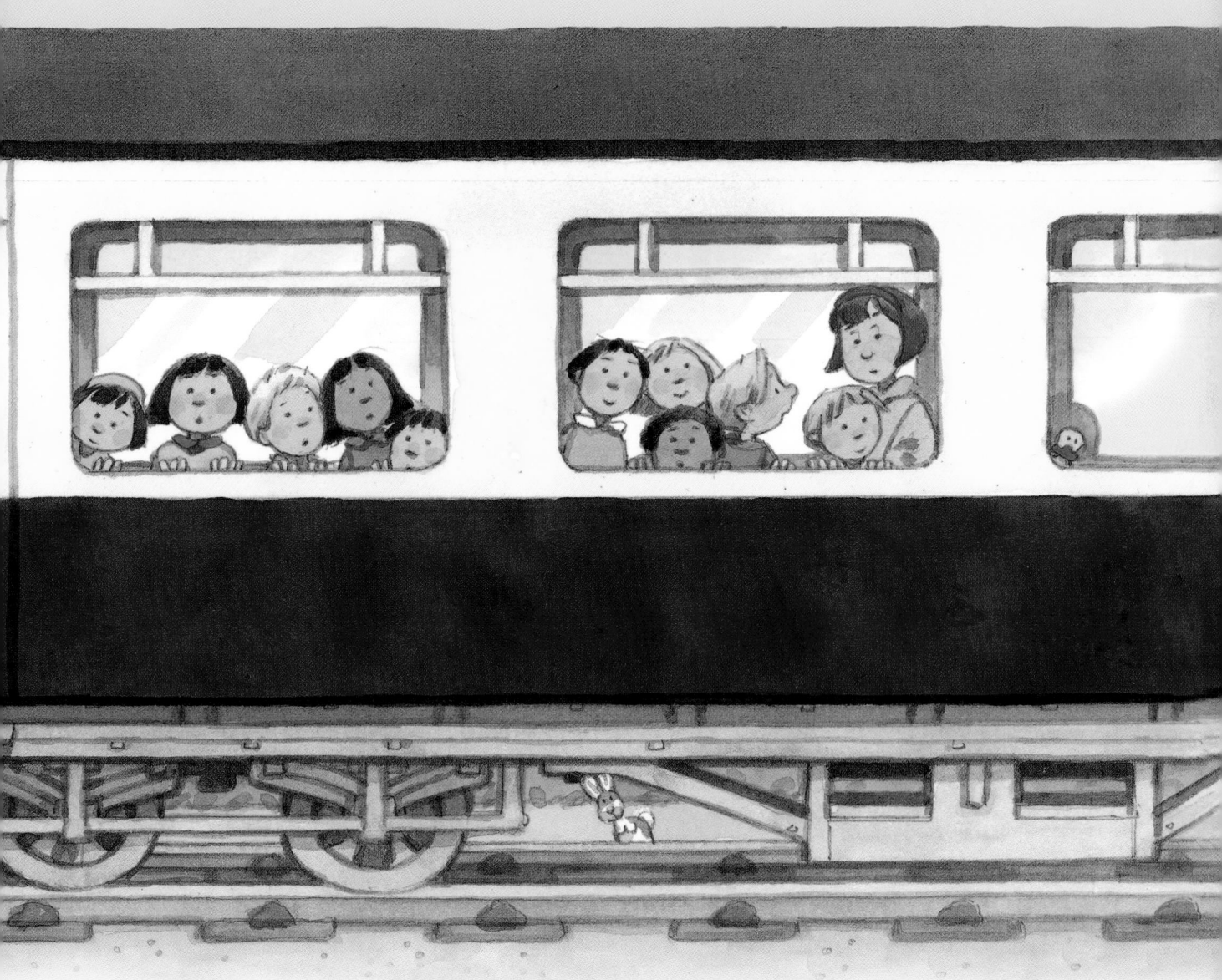

"I can see Farmer Dray's farm," says Sam.
"Why has the train stopped?" asks Poppy.

"The engine has broken down."

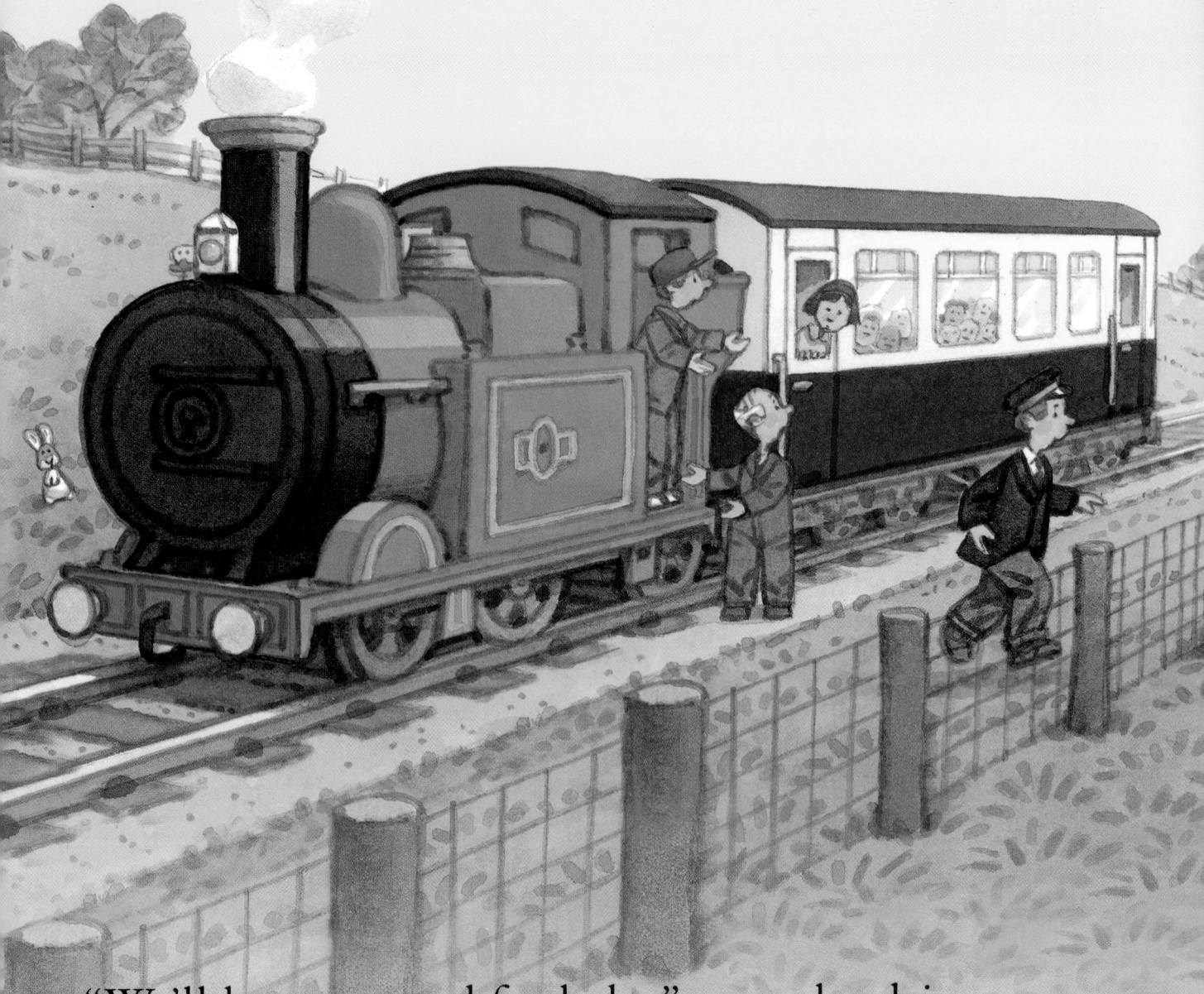

"We'll have to send for help," says the driver.
"It won't be long." The guard runs across the fields.

"Here's a ladder."

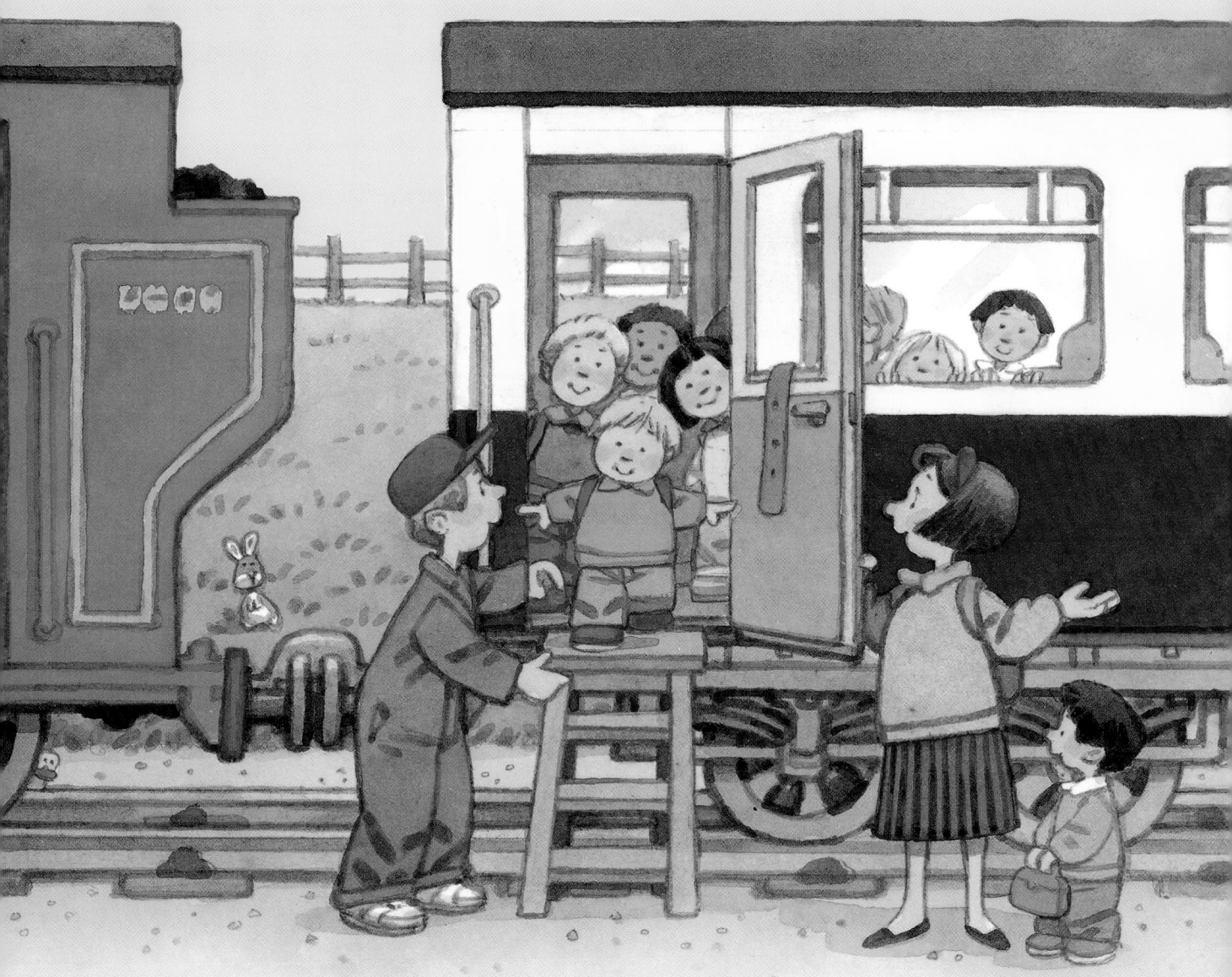

"You can all get off now," says the driver. "We can have our picnic here," says the teacher.

"Let's go into the field," says Sam.

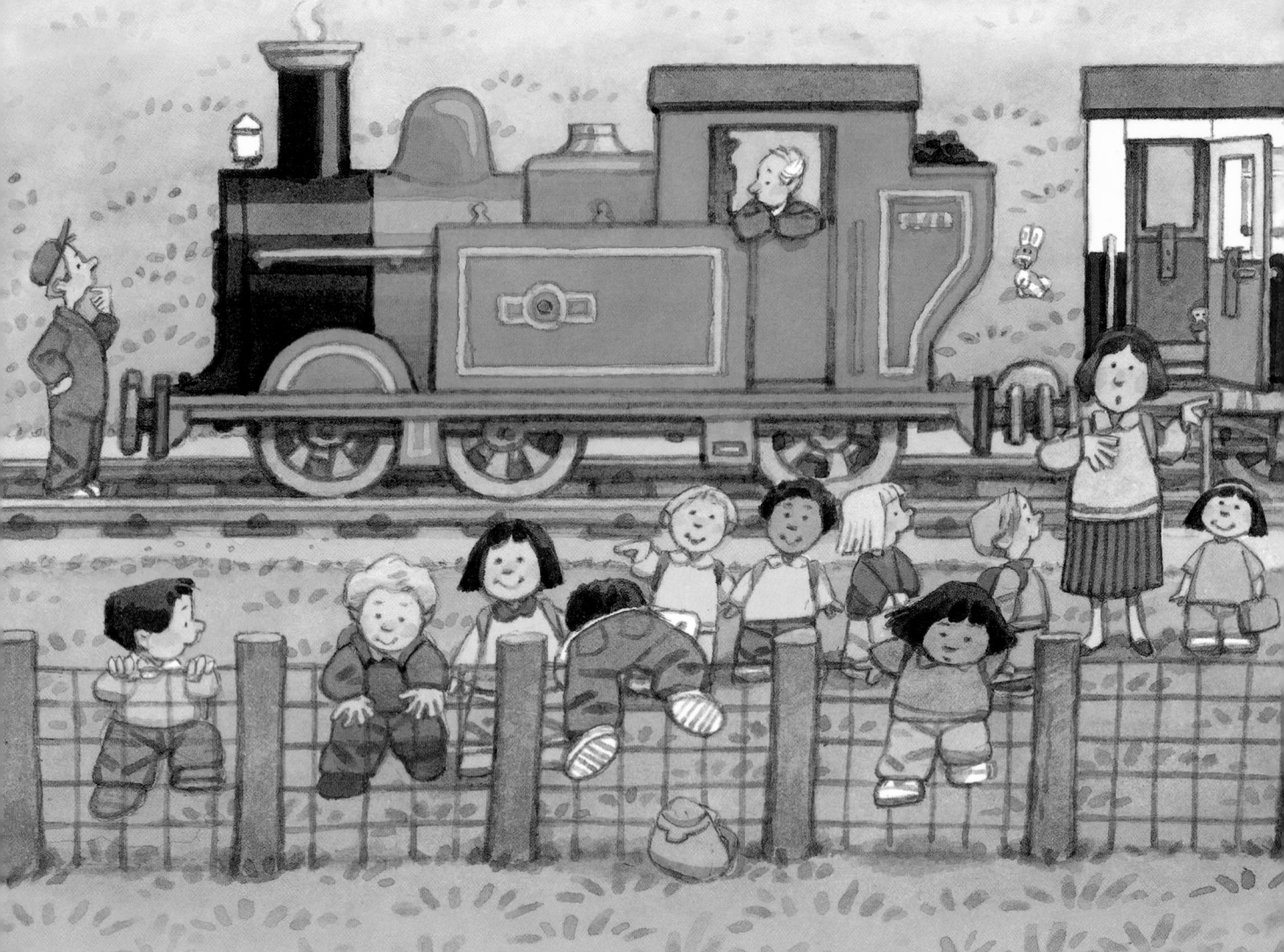

The children climb over the fence. "Stop! Come back, children," says the teacher. "There's a bull."

"It's only Buttercup."

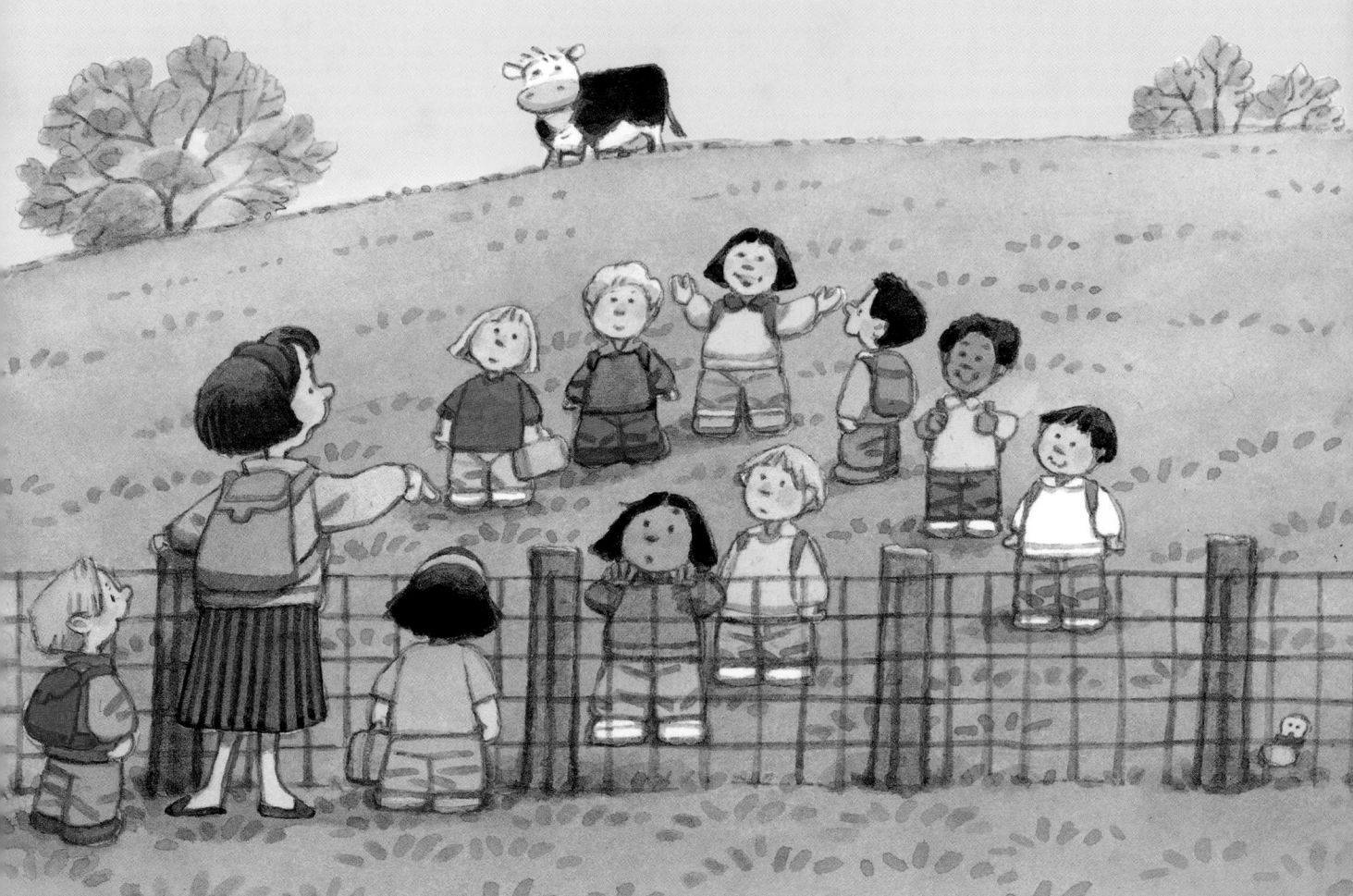

"She's not a bull. She's a very nice cow," says Poppy.
"Well, come back here," says the teacher.

"Look, there's Farmer Dray."

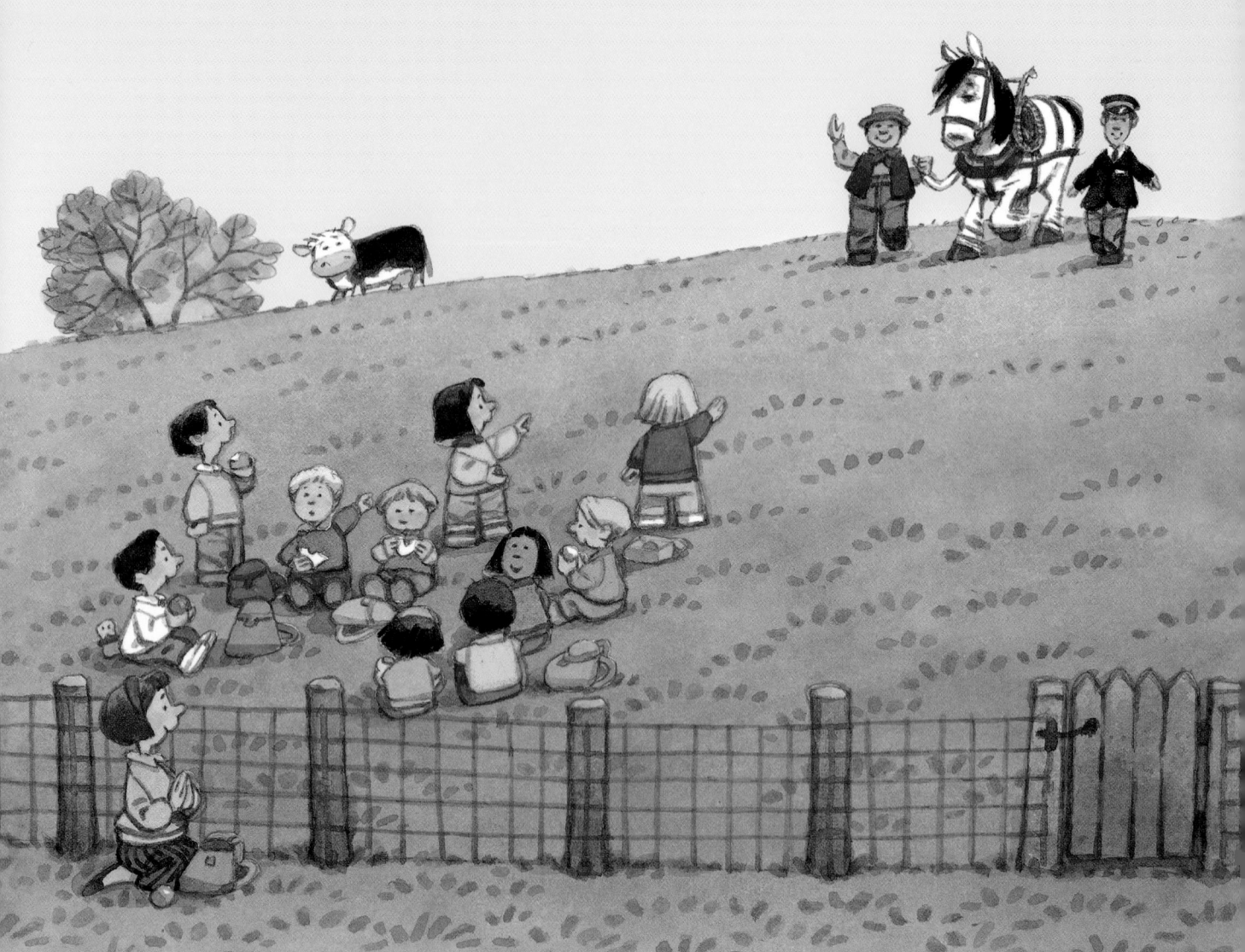

"He's brought Dolly with him," says Sam. "A horse is no good. We need an engine," says the teacher.

The children watch.

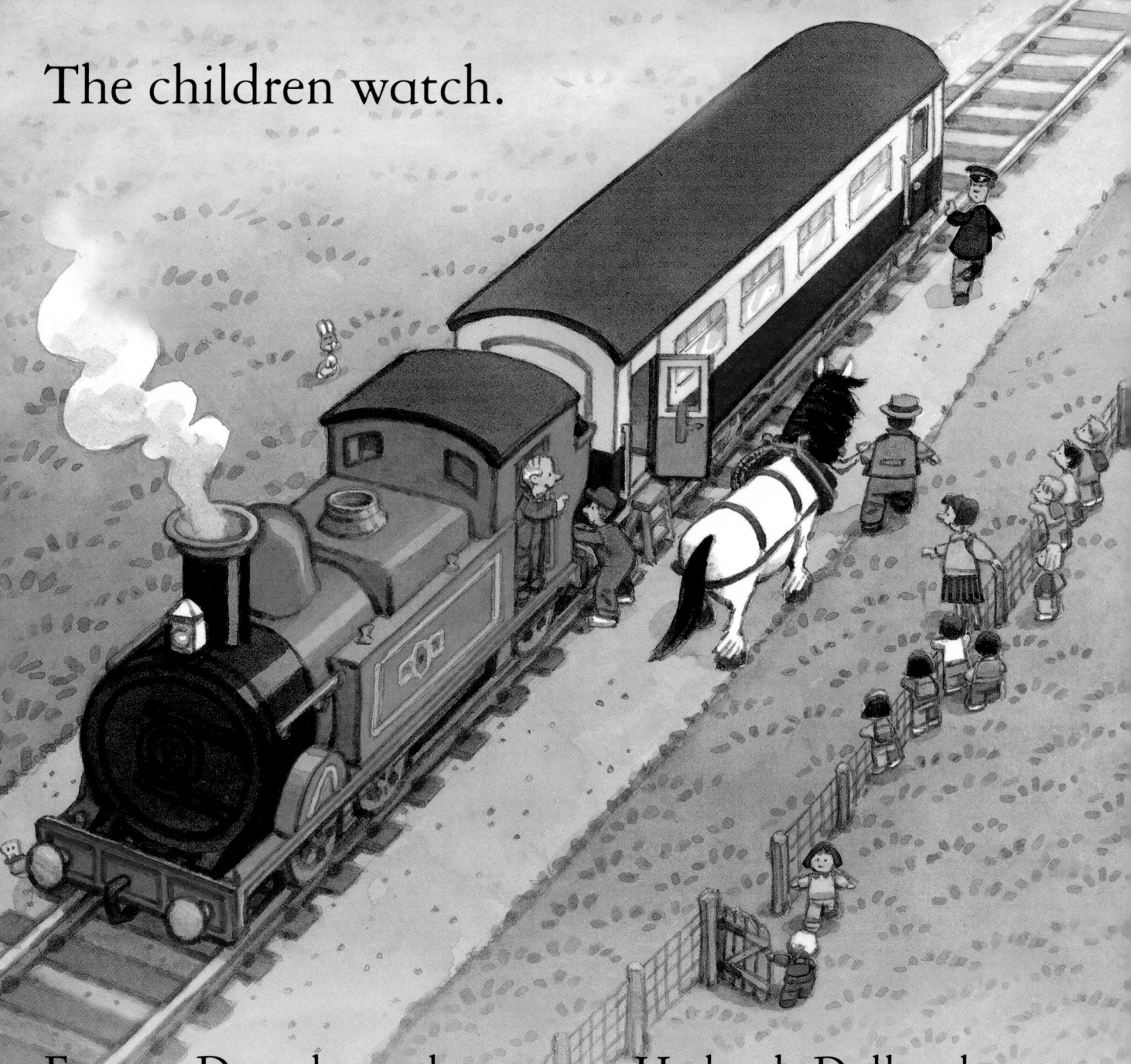

Farmer Dray has a long rope. He leads Dolly along the train. The driver unhitches the engine.

The children climb back on the train.

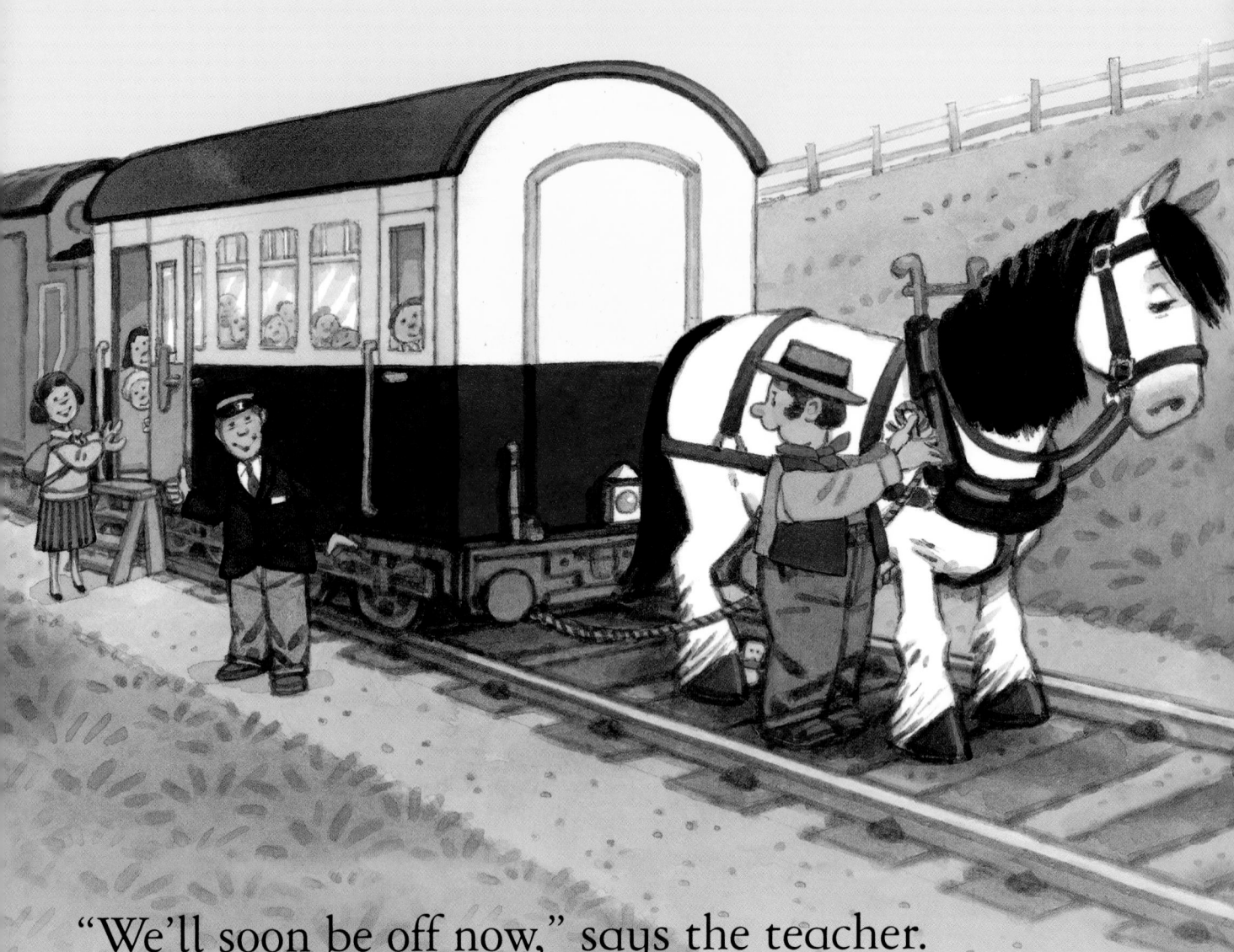

"We'll soon be off now," says the teacher.
"Dolly's ready," says Farmer Dray.

"Pull away, Dolly."

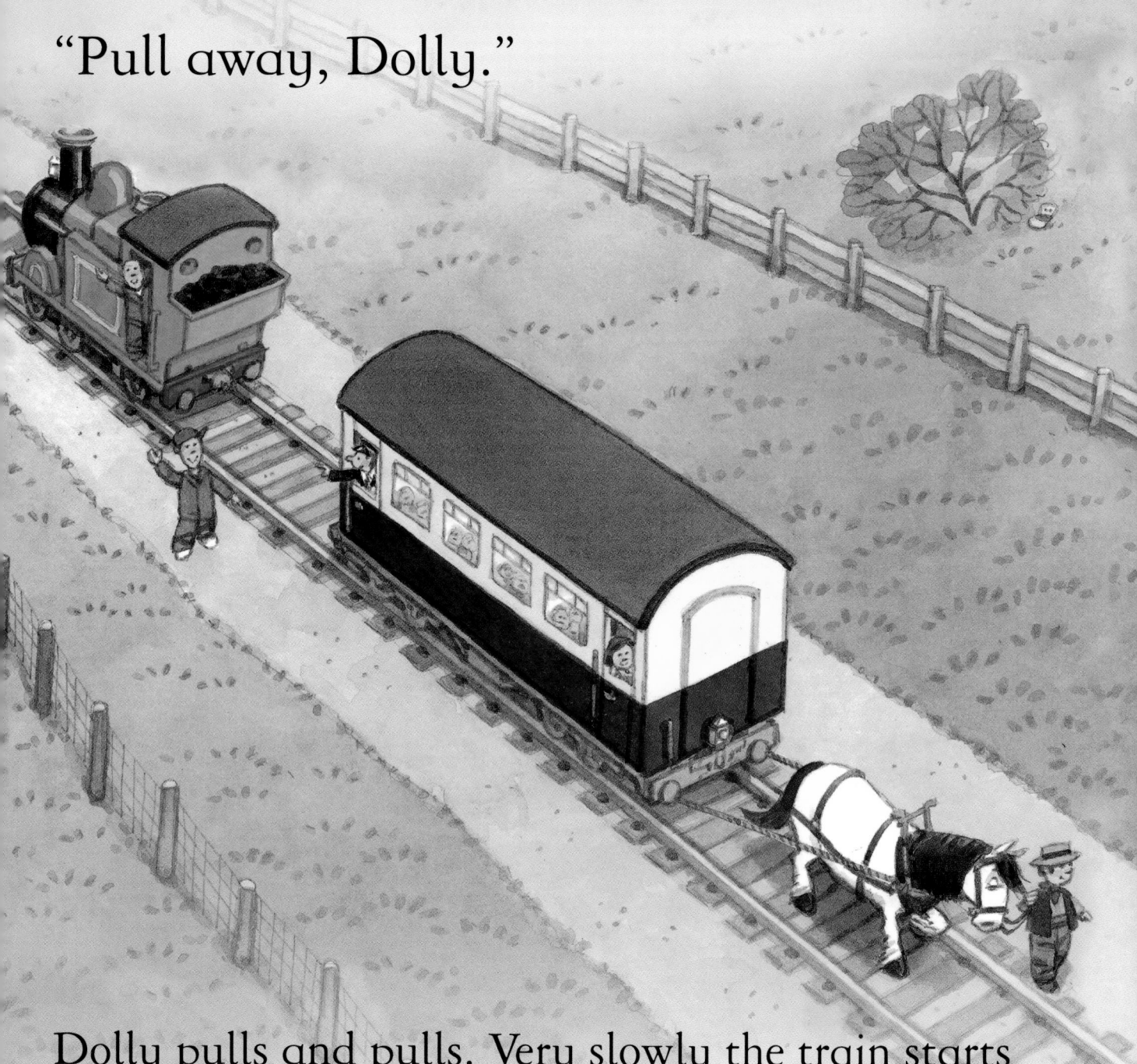

Dolly pulls and pulls. Very slowly the train starts to move. Farmer Dray walks along with Dolly.

They reach the station.

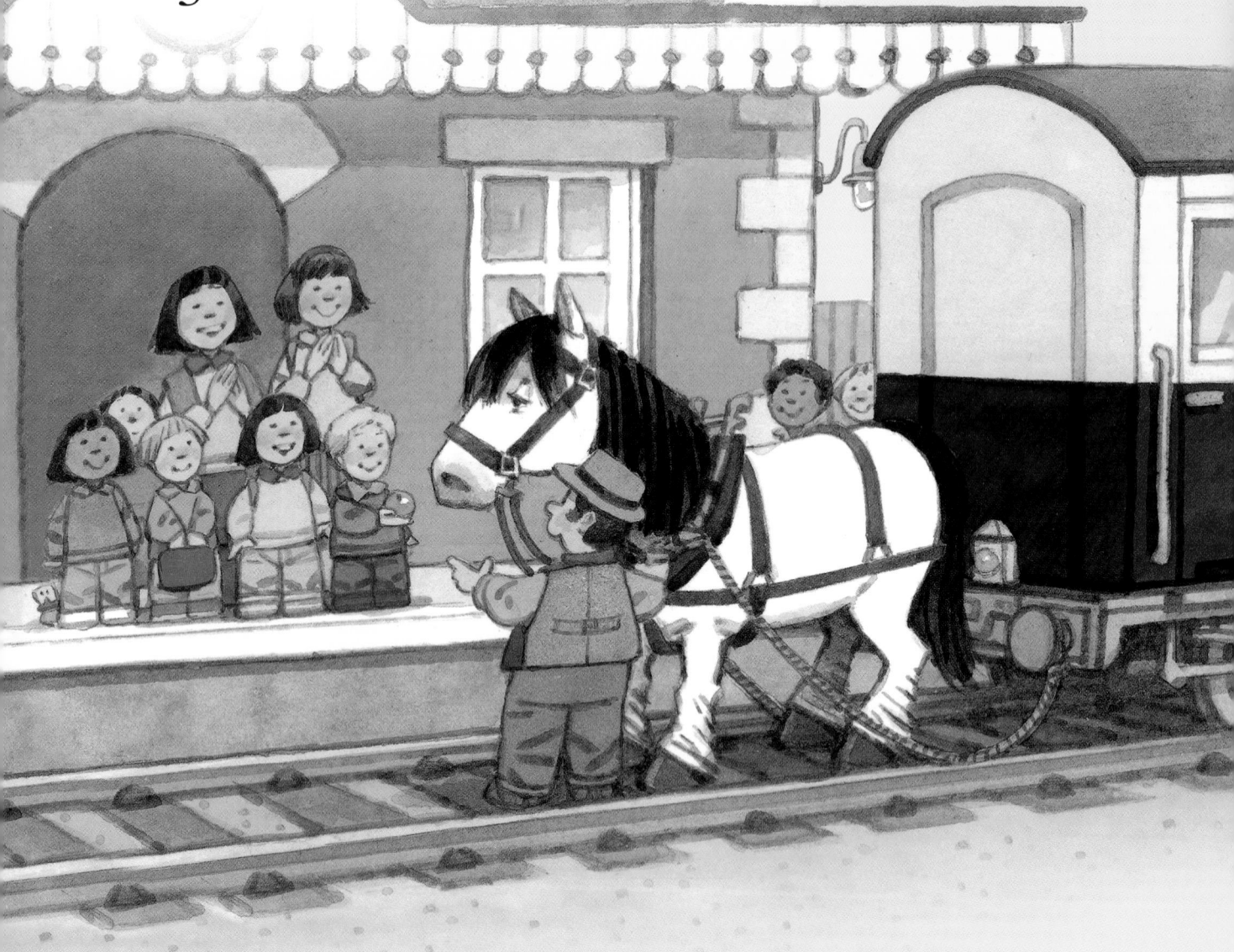

"Out by engine, back by horse," says Farmer Dray.
"That was a good outing," says Sam.

Rusty's Train Ride

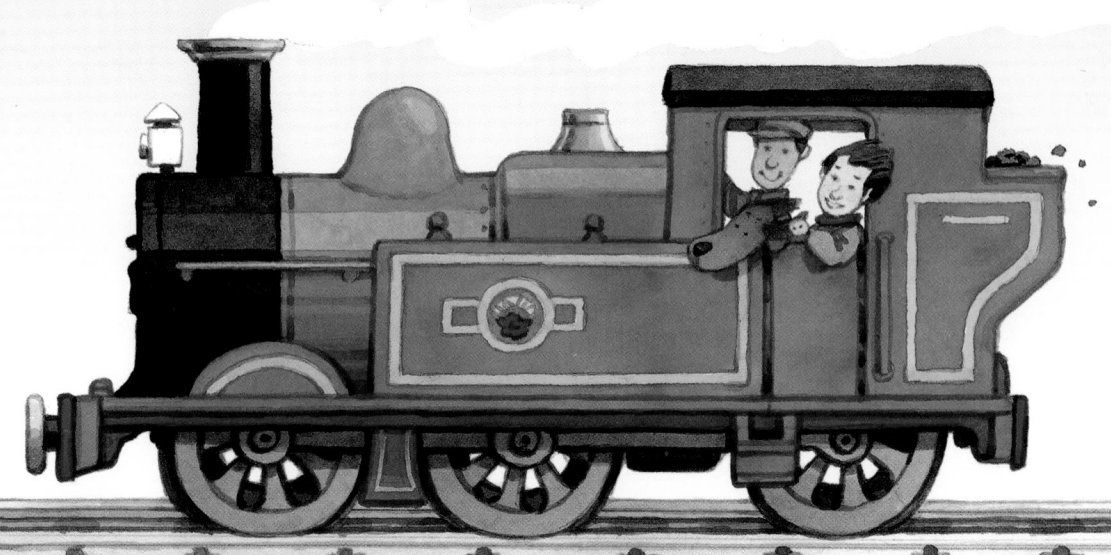

This is Apple Tree Farm.

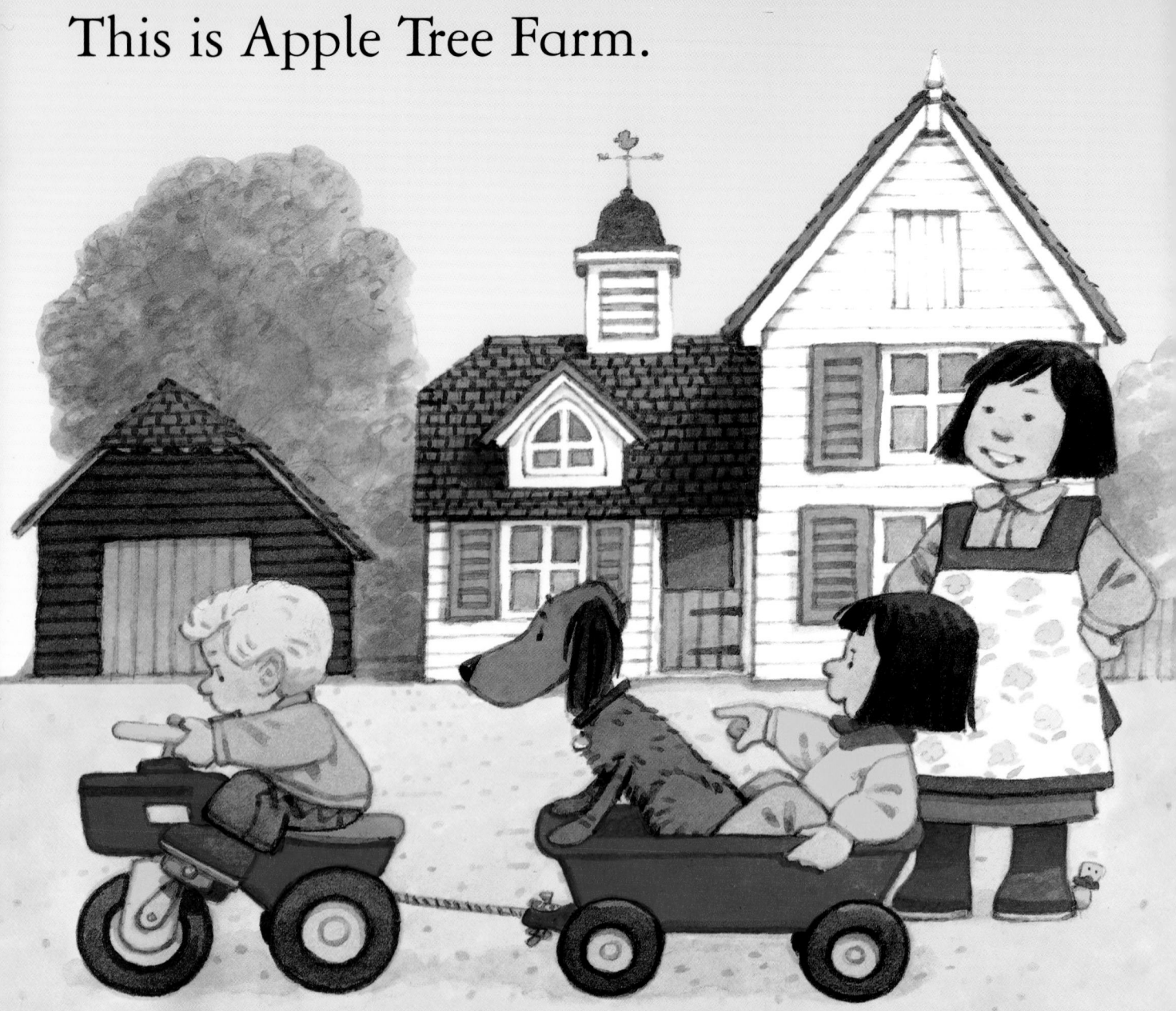

This is Mrs. Boot, the farmer. She has two children, called Poppy and Sam, and a dog called Rusty.

They are having breakfast.

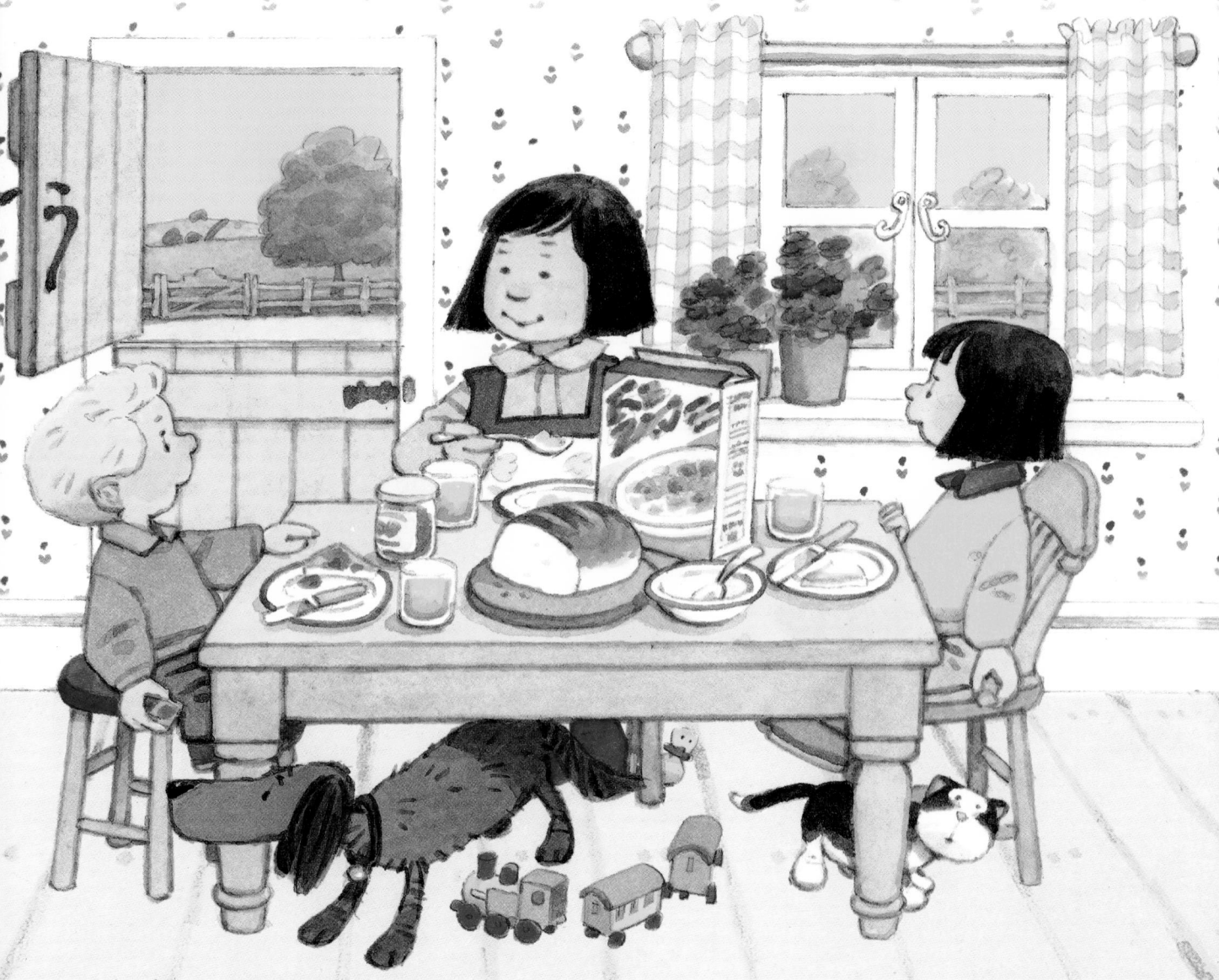

"What are we doing today?" says Sam. "Let's go and see the old steam train," says Mrs. Boot.

"Come on, Rusty," says Sam.

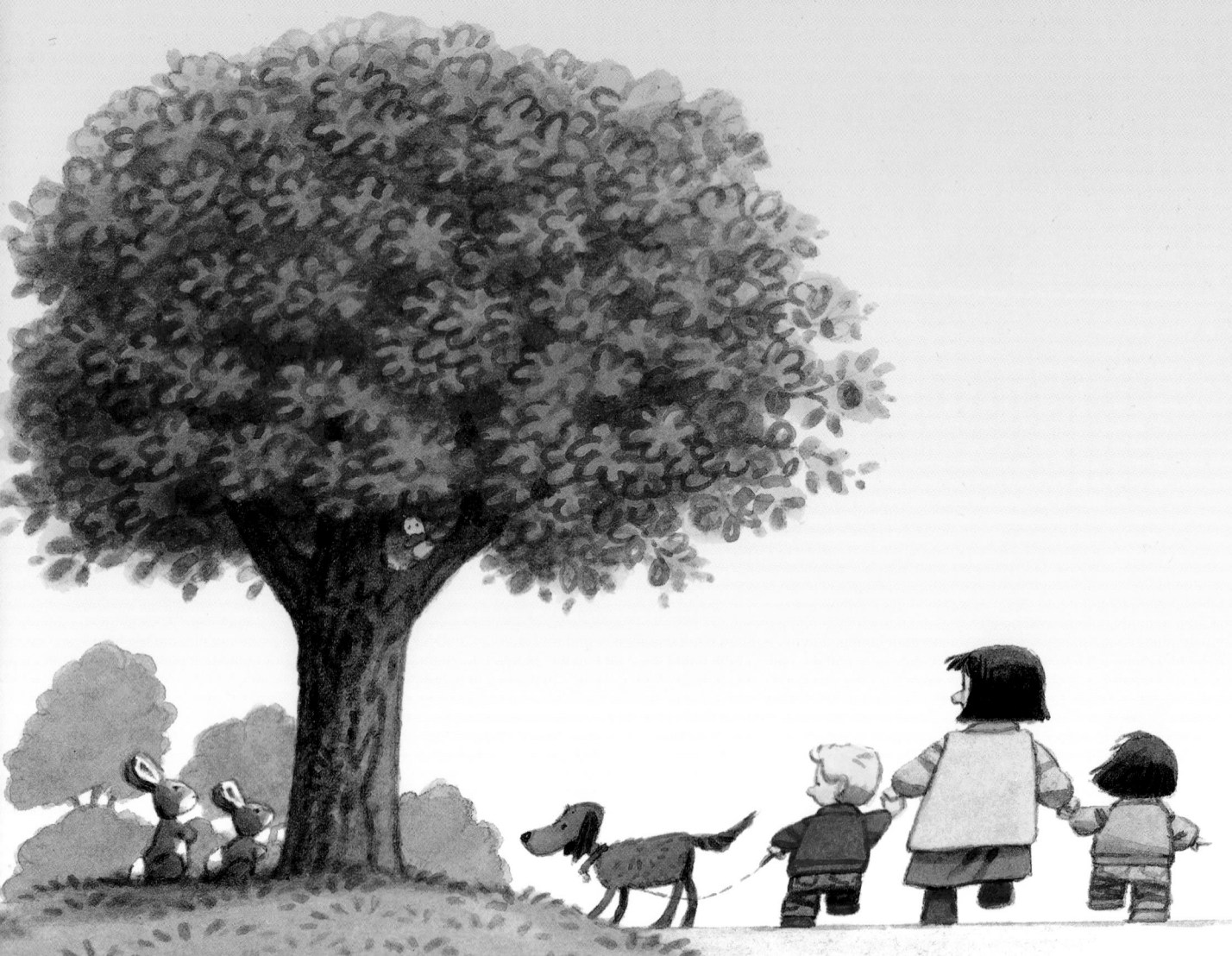

They walk down the road to the station. "Don't let
Rusty go. Hold him tight," says Mrs. Boot.

They wait on the platform.

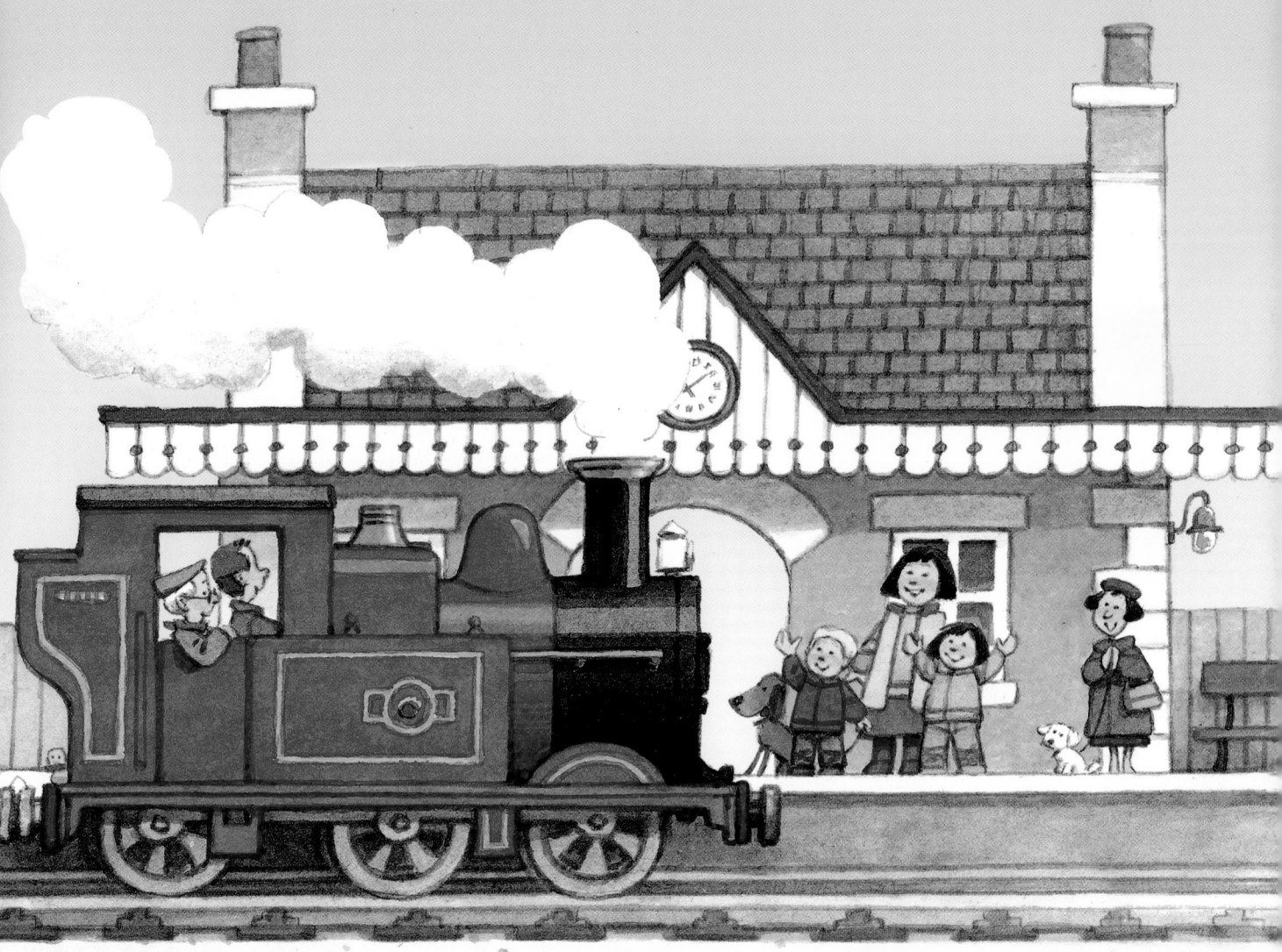

Mrs. Boot, Poppy and Sam watch the train come in.
Mrs. Hill and her puppy watch with them.

The train is ready to go.

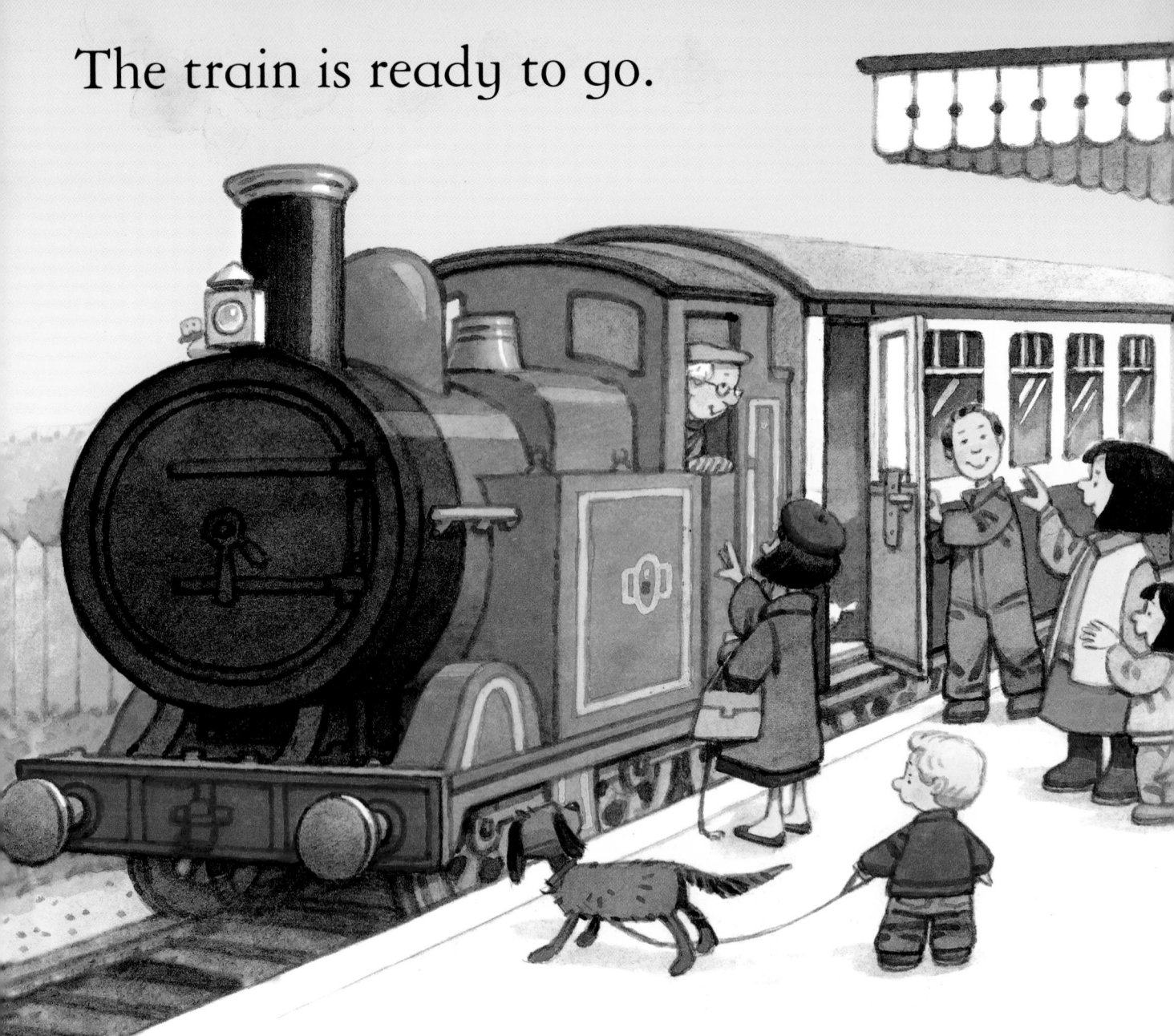

Everyone talks to the train driver. The fireman shuts
the doors. He climbs on the train.

"Where's my puppy?"

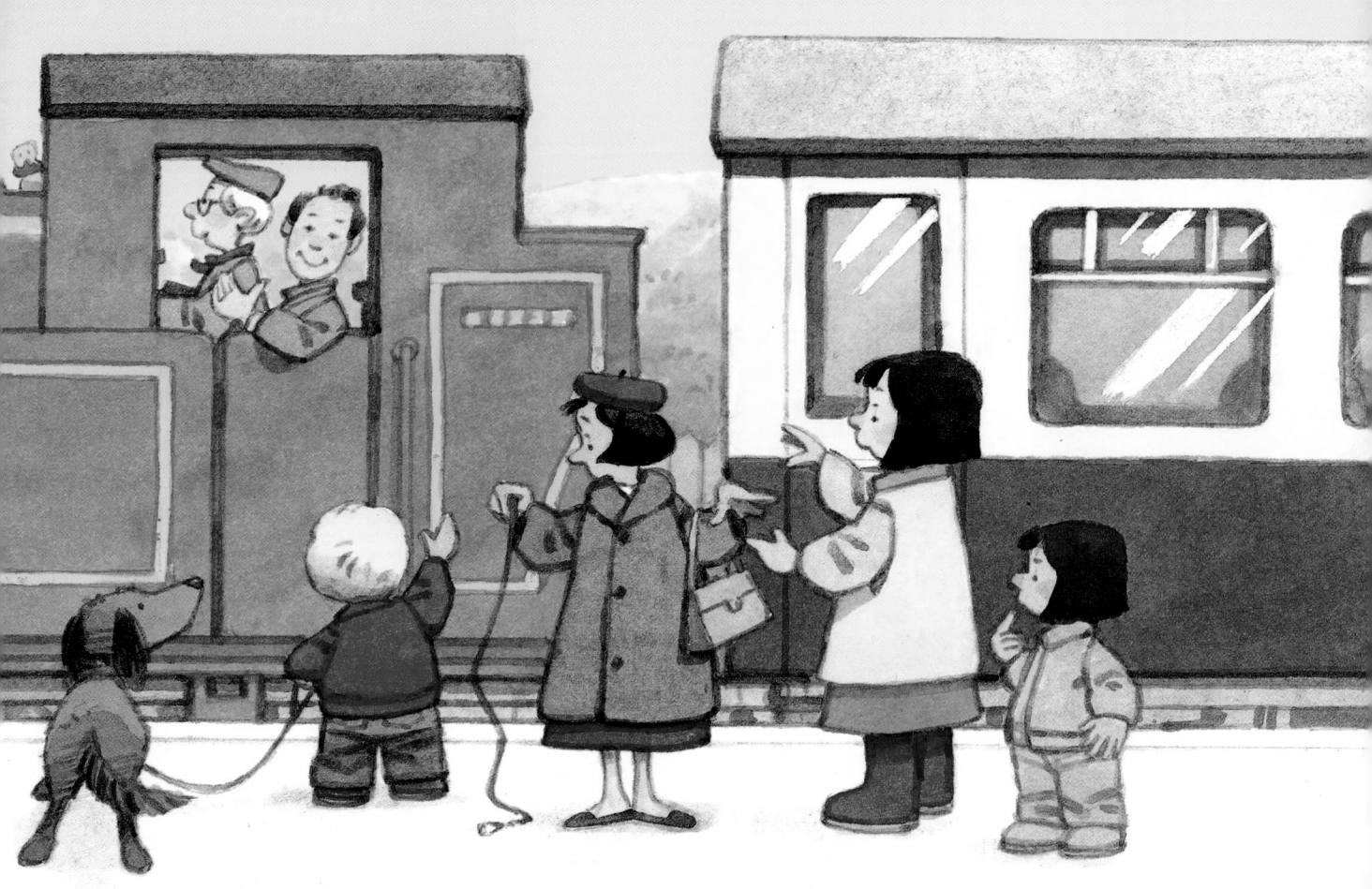

"Mopp was with me on the platform," says Mrs. Hill.
"Now he's gone." The train starts to move.

Rusty watches it go.

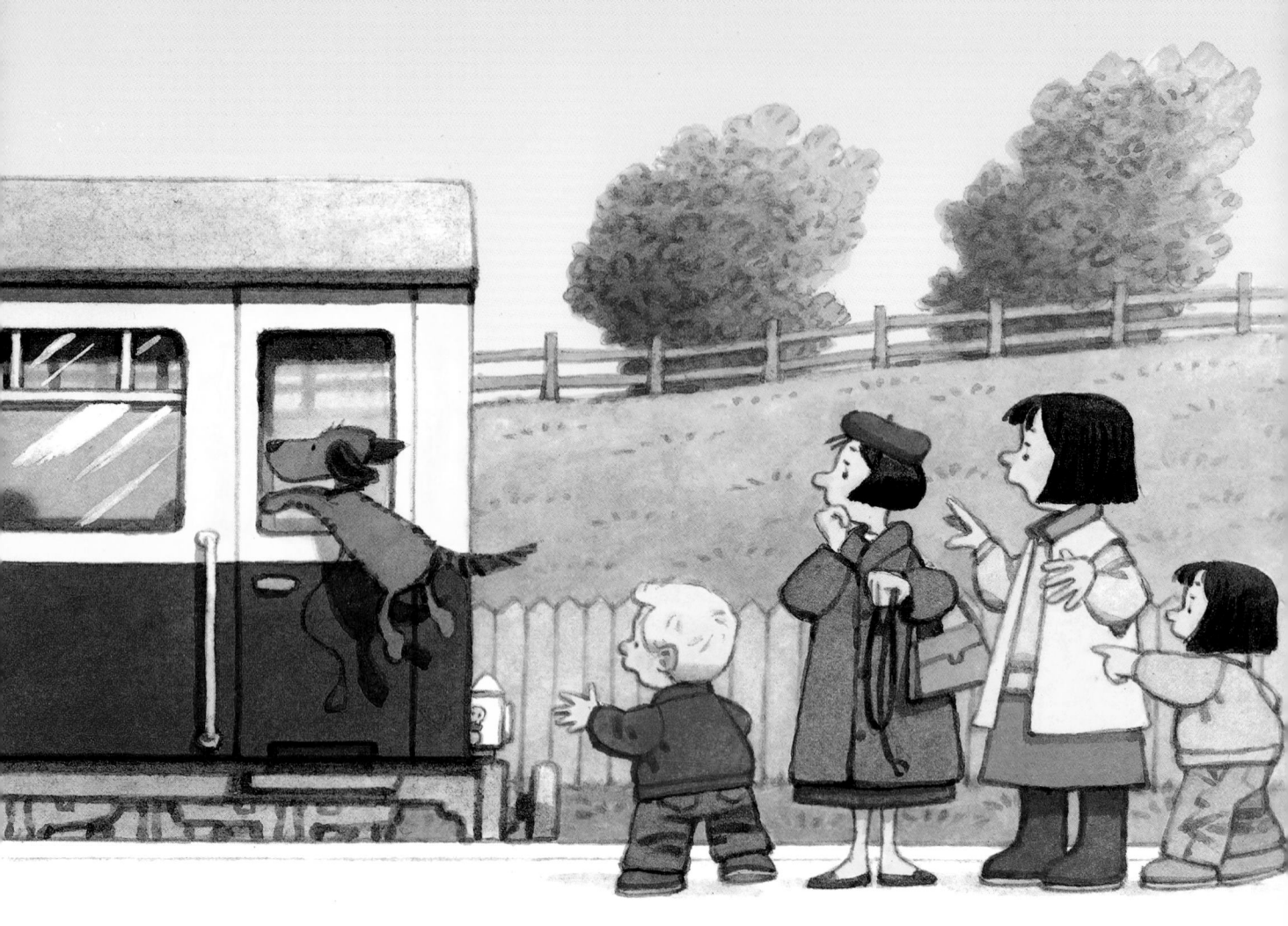

He pulls and pulls and runs away. Then he jumps through an open carriage window.

"Come back, Rusty," shouts Sam.

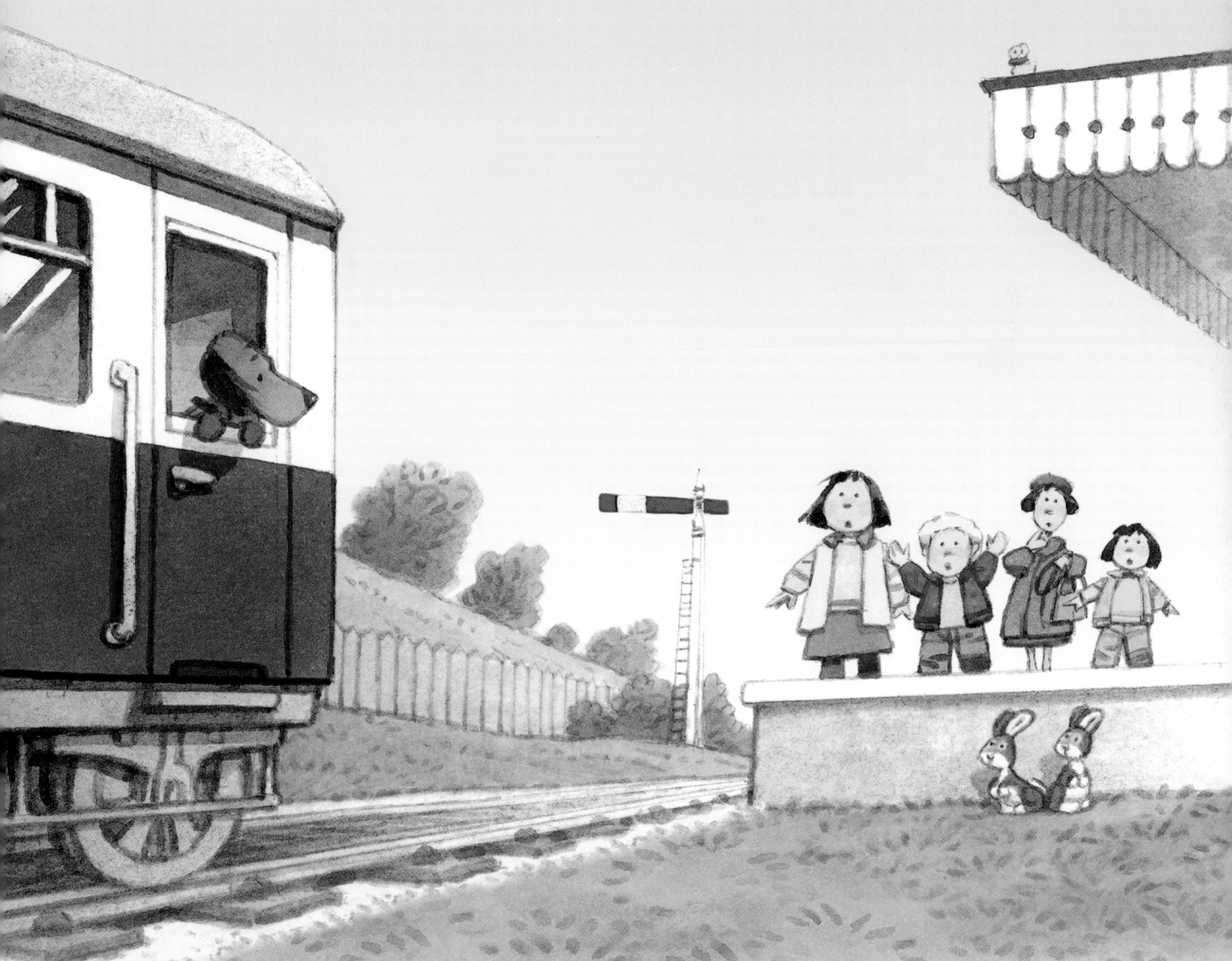

Rusty looks out of the window. "There he is," says
Poppy. "He's going for a train ride on his own."

"Stop, stop the train," shouts Sam.

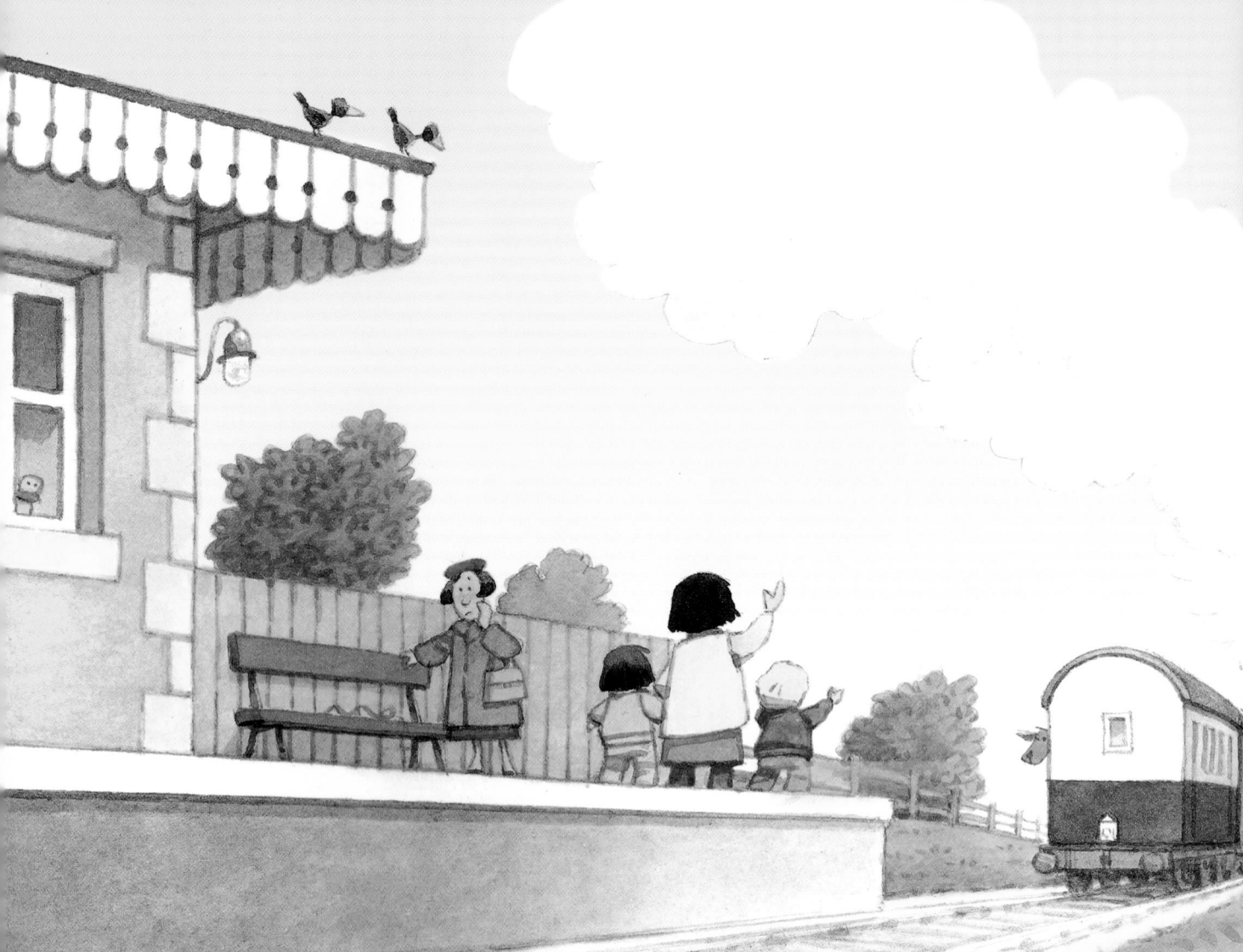

Mrs. Boot, Poppy and Sam shout and wave.
But the train puffs away down the track.

"What shall we do?"

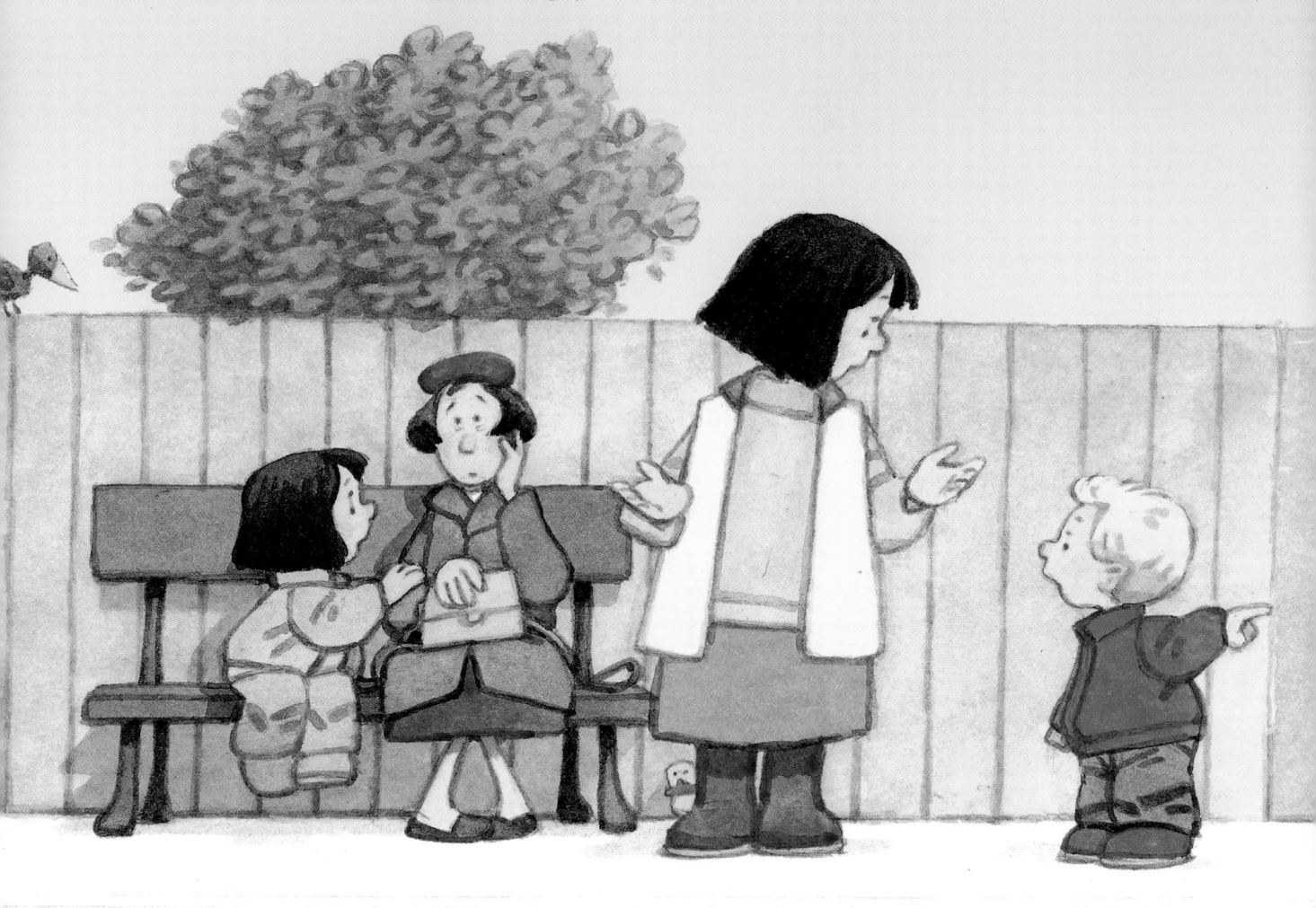

"Both dogs have gone," says Sam. "We'll have to wait for the train to come back," says Mrs. Boot.

At last, the train comes back.

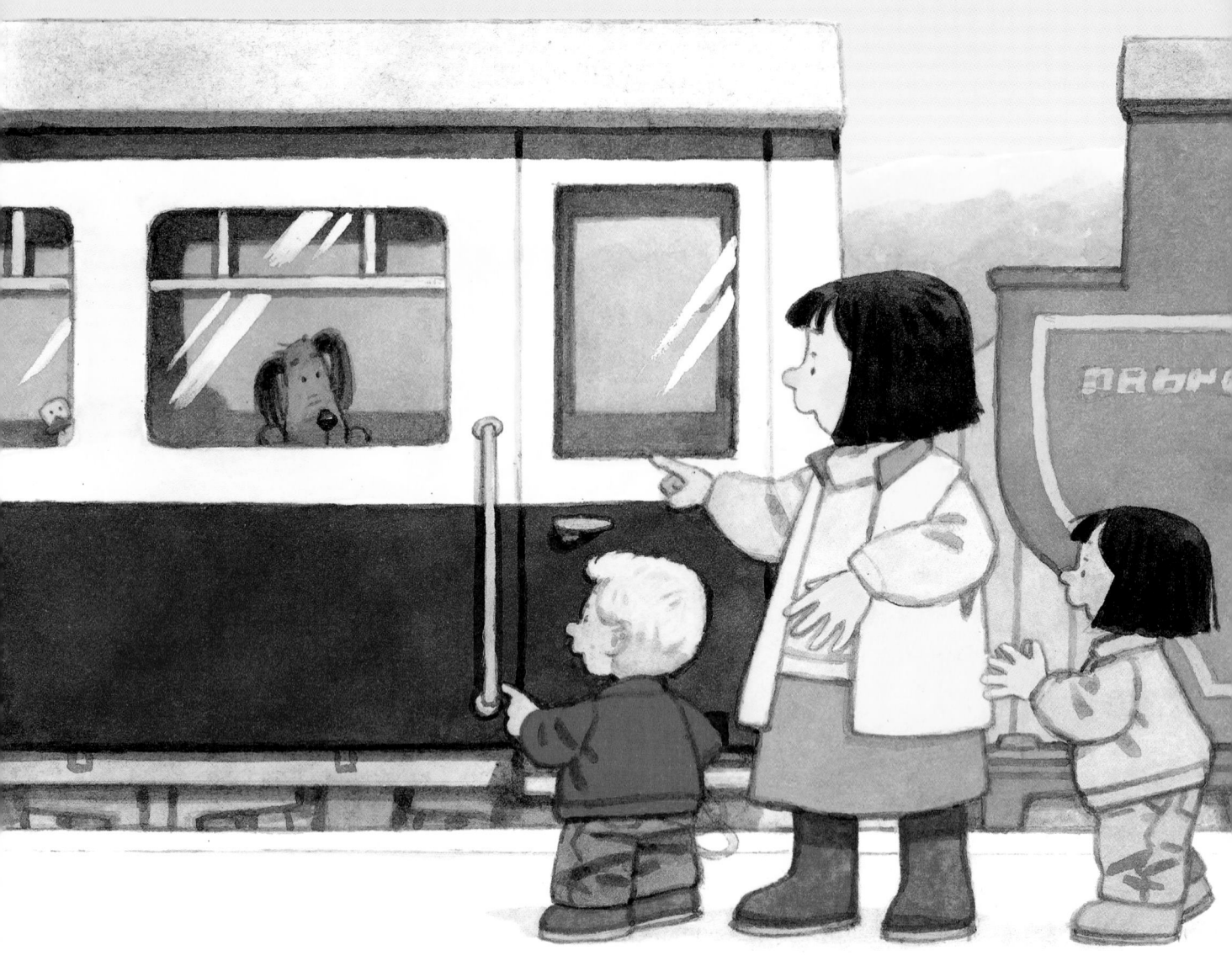

"Look, there's Rusty," says Sam. "You naughty dog, where have you been?" says Poppy.

The train stops at the station.

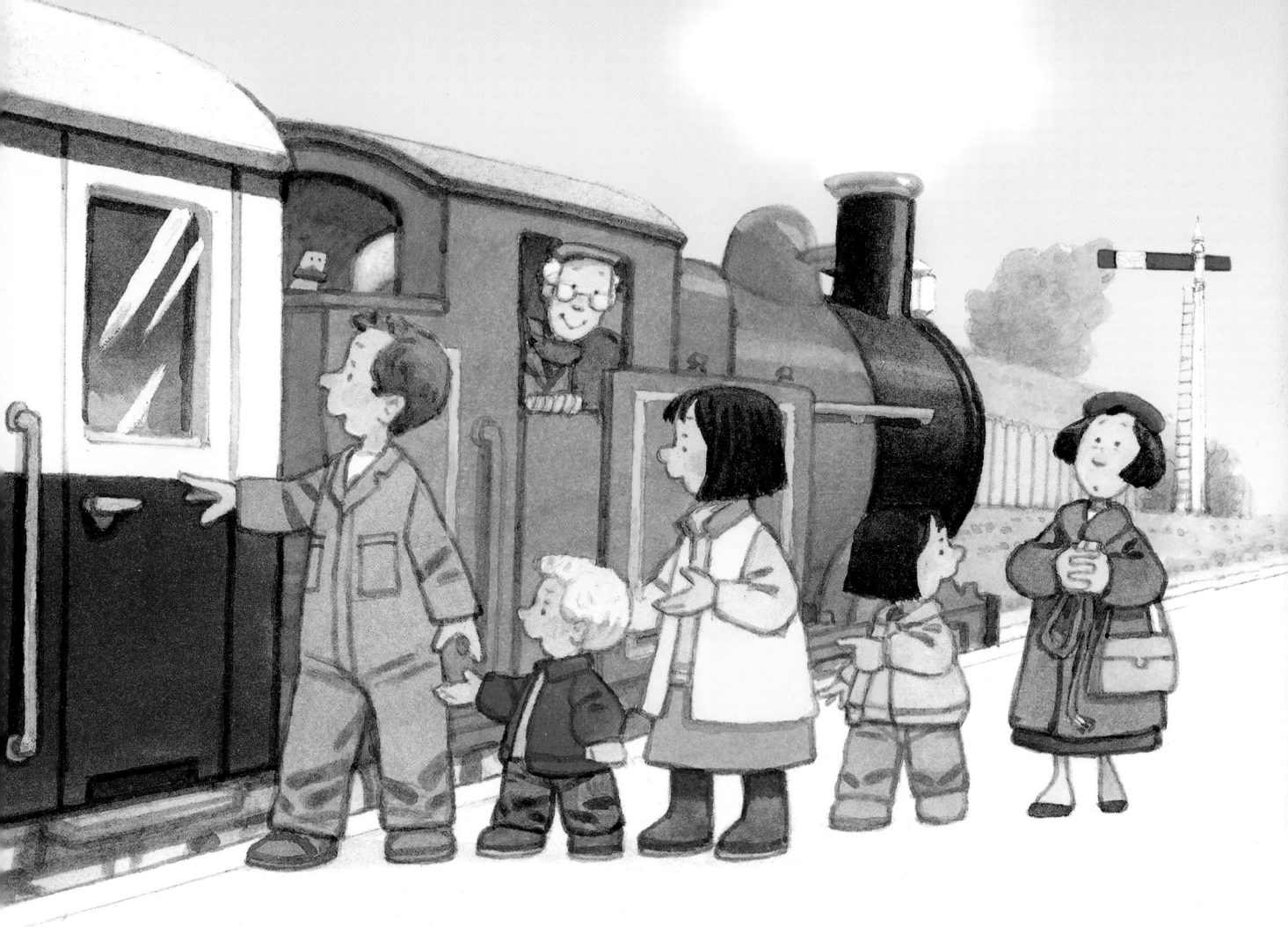

The fireman climbs down from the engine. He opens the carriage door.

"Come on, Rusty."

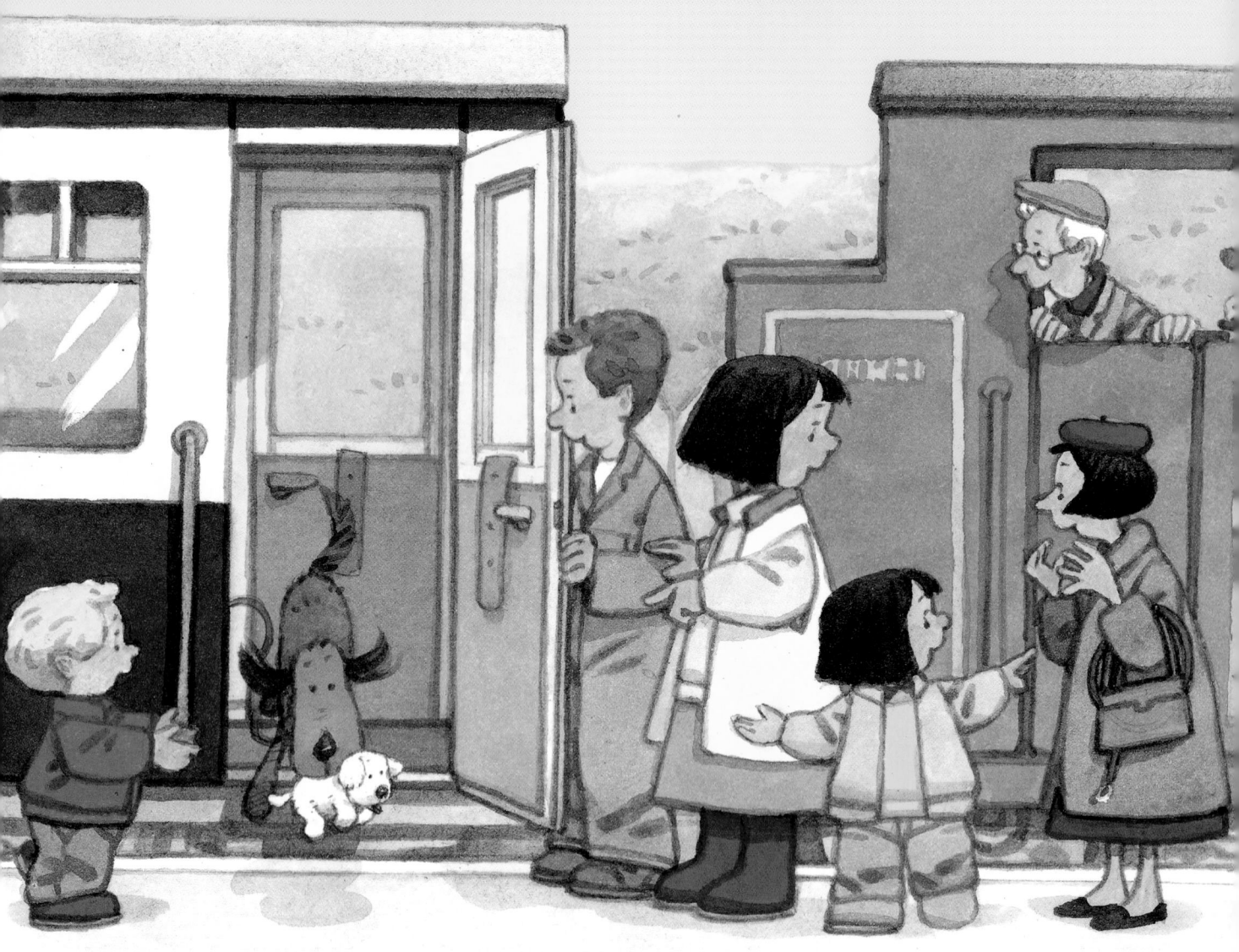

"Your ride on the train is over," says Mrs. Boot.
Rusty jumps down. "What's he got?" says Sam.

"It's my little Mopp."

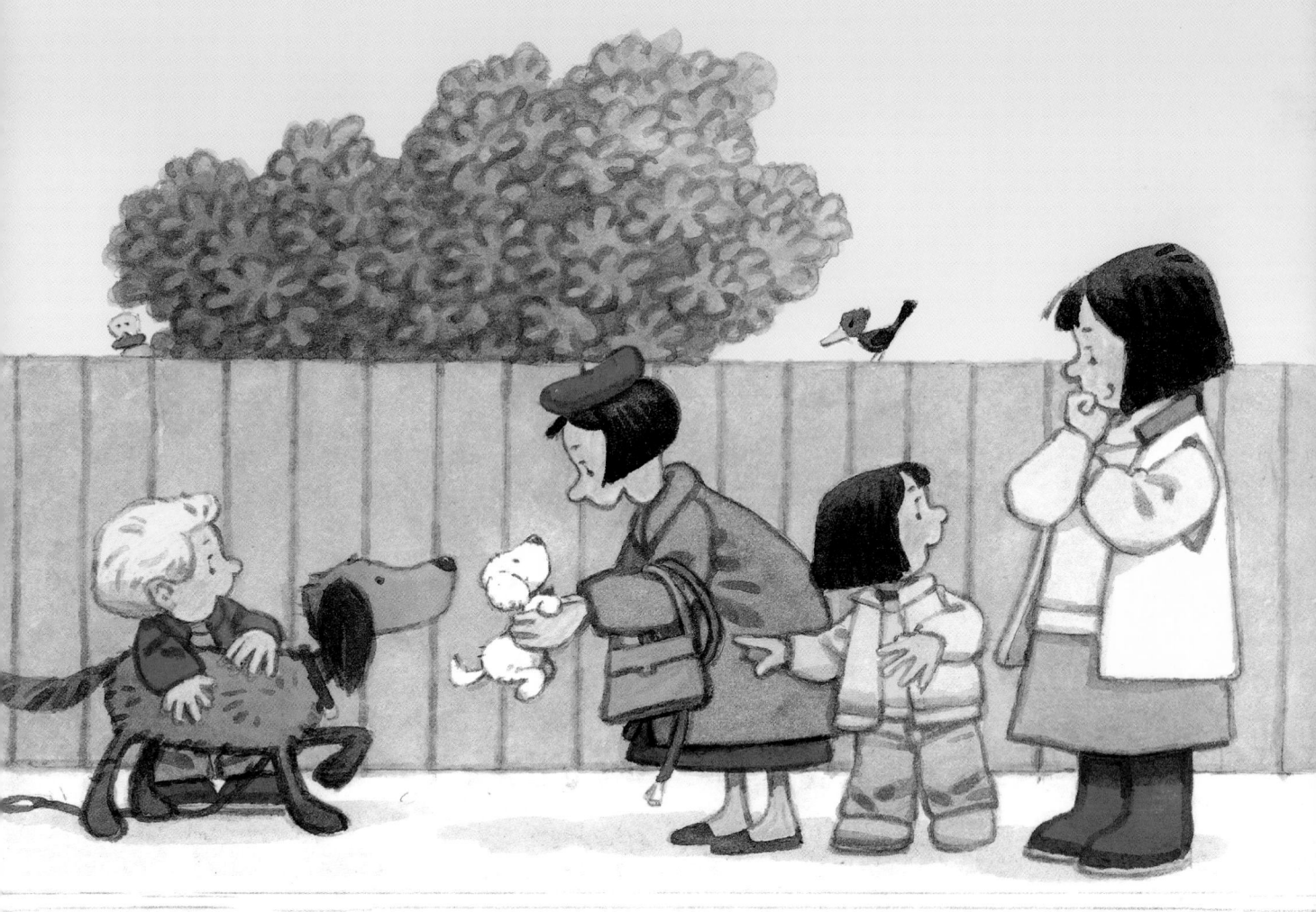

Mrs. Hill picks up her puppy. "Poor little thing.
Did you go on the train all by yourself?"

"Rusty went with him," says Sam.

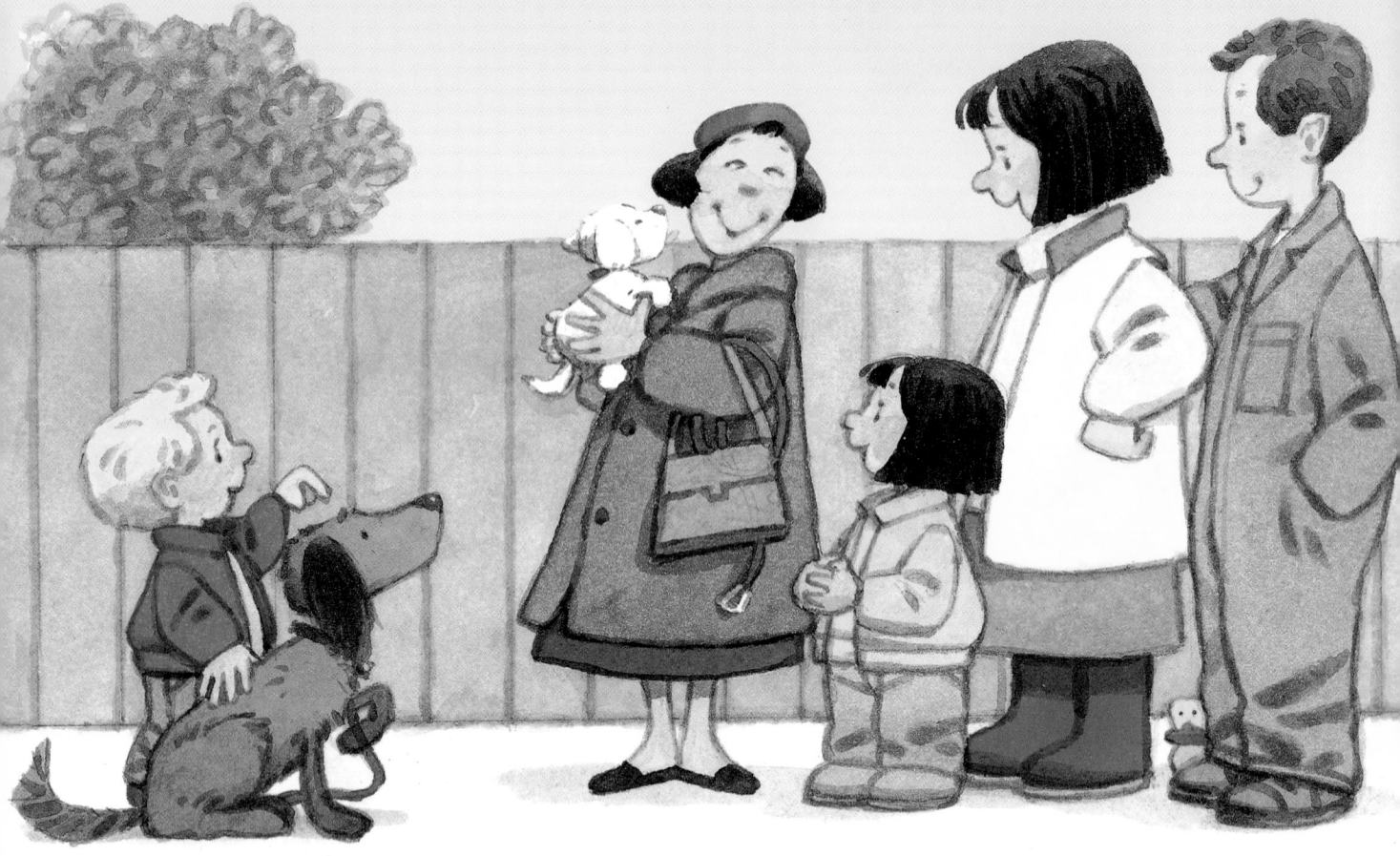

"That's why he jumped on the train," says Poppy.
"Clever Rusty," says Sam.

Woolly Stops
the Train

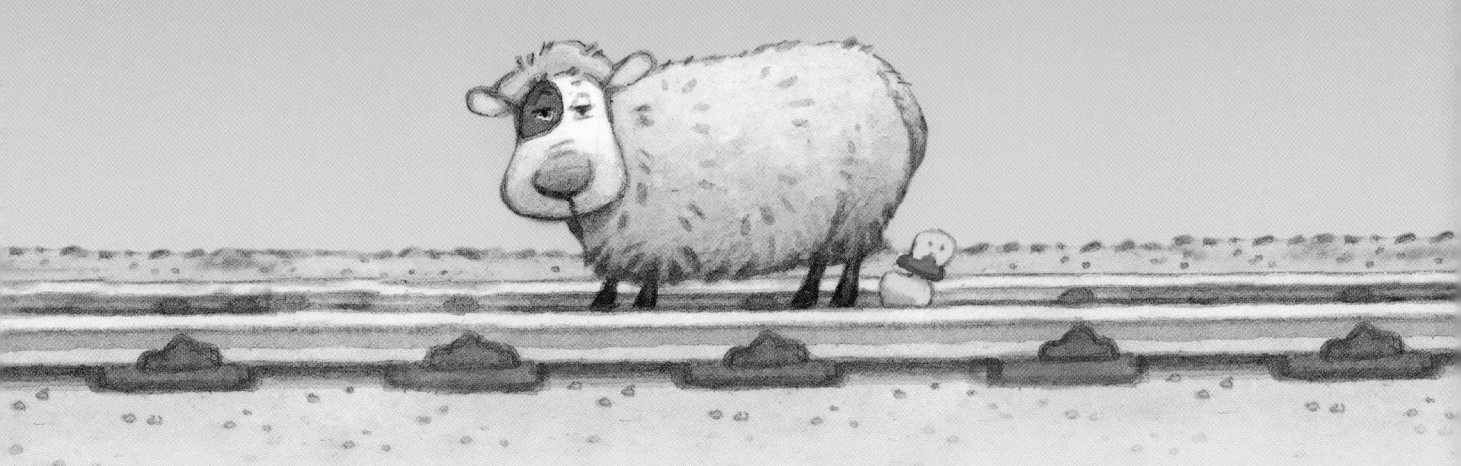

This is Apple Tree Farm.

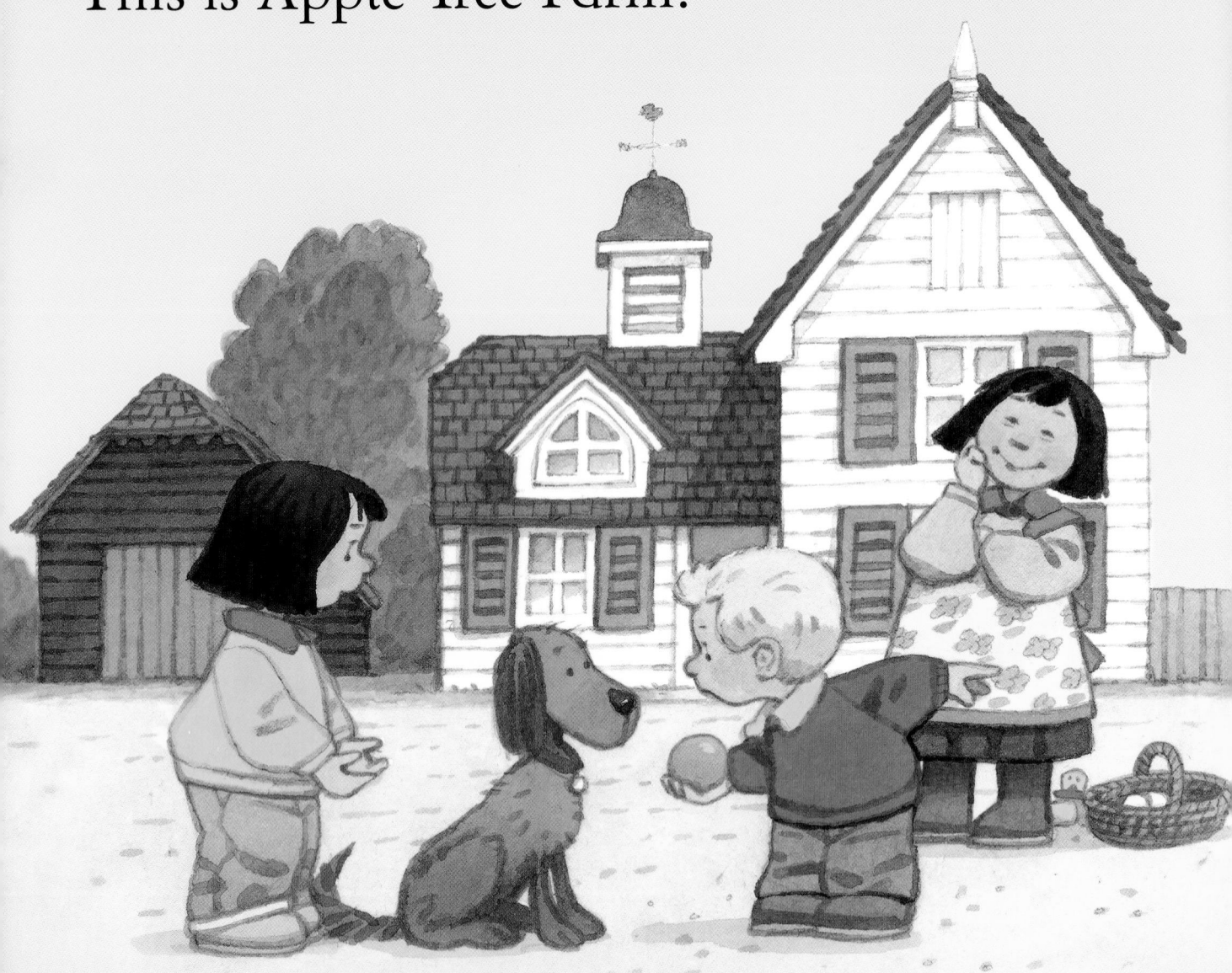

This is Mrs. Boot, the farmer. She has two children, called Poppy and Sam, and a dog called Rusty.

This is Ted.

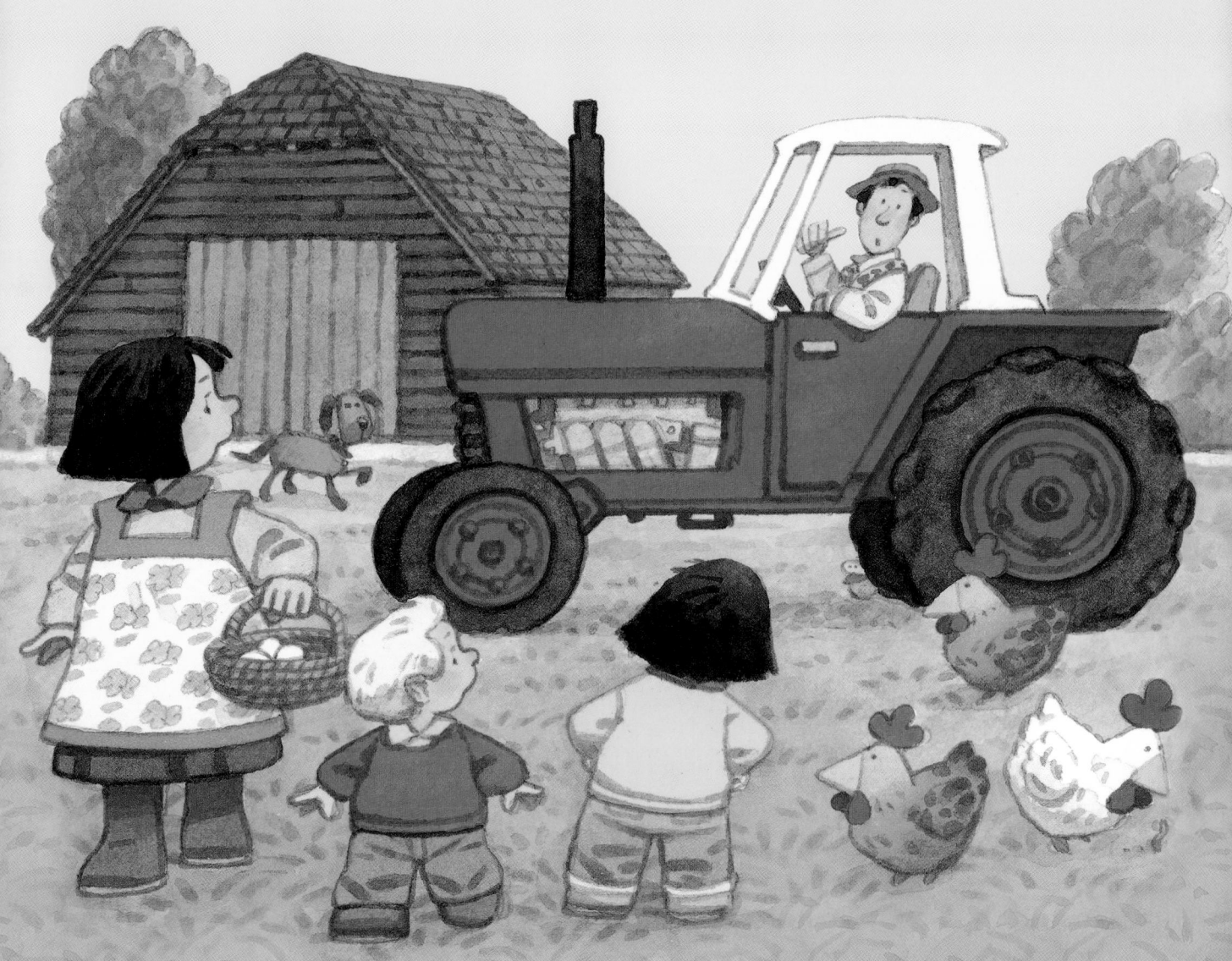

He drives the tractor and helps Mrs. Boot on the
farm. He waves and shouts to Mrs. Boot.

"What's the matter, Ted?" asks Mrs. Boot.

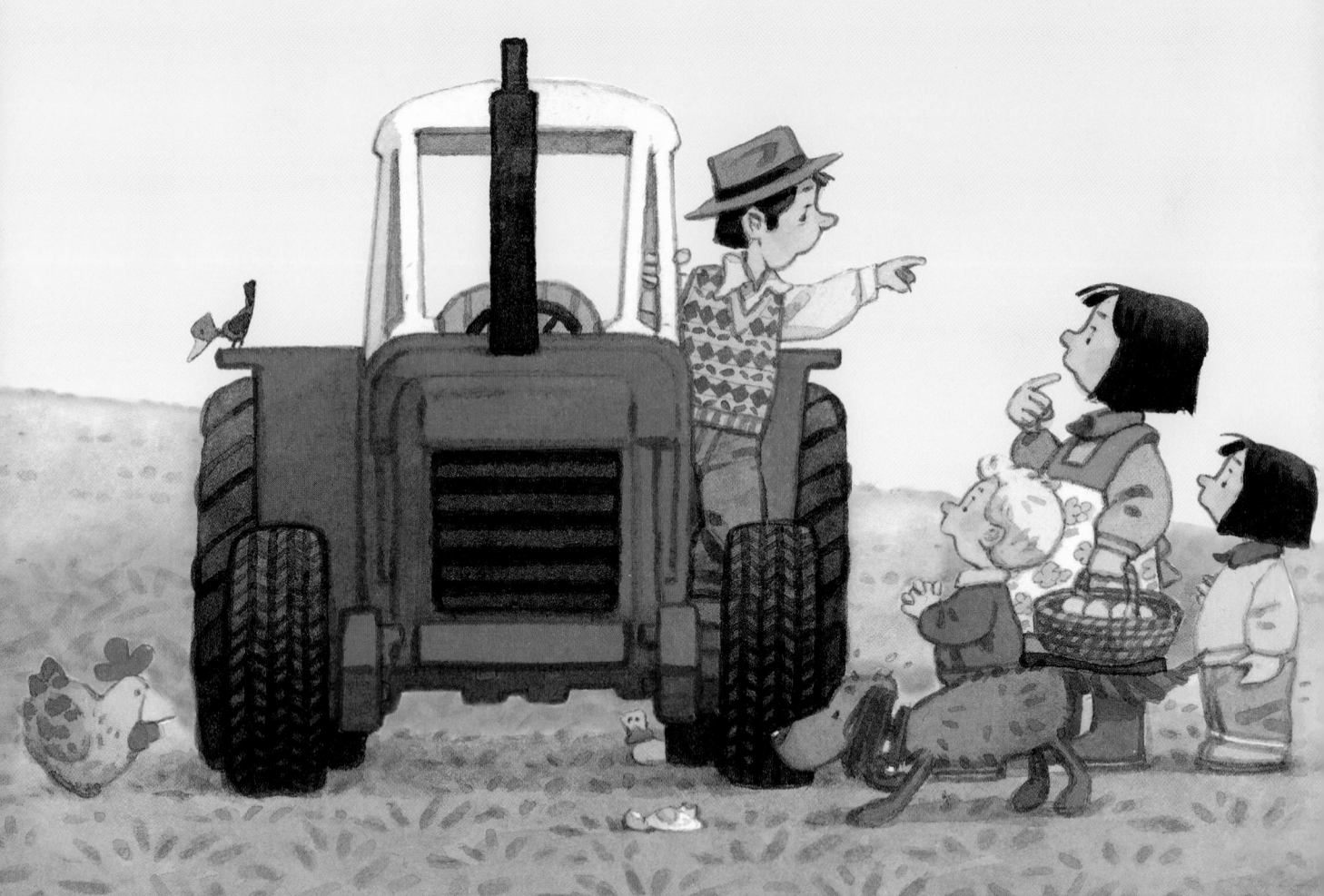

"The train is in trouble. I think it's stuck. I can hear it whistling and whistling," says Ted.

"We'll go and look."

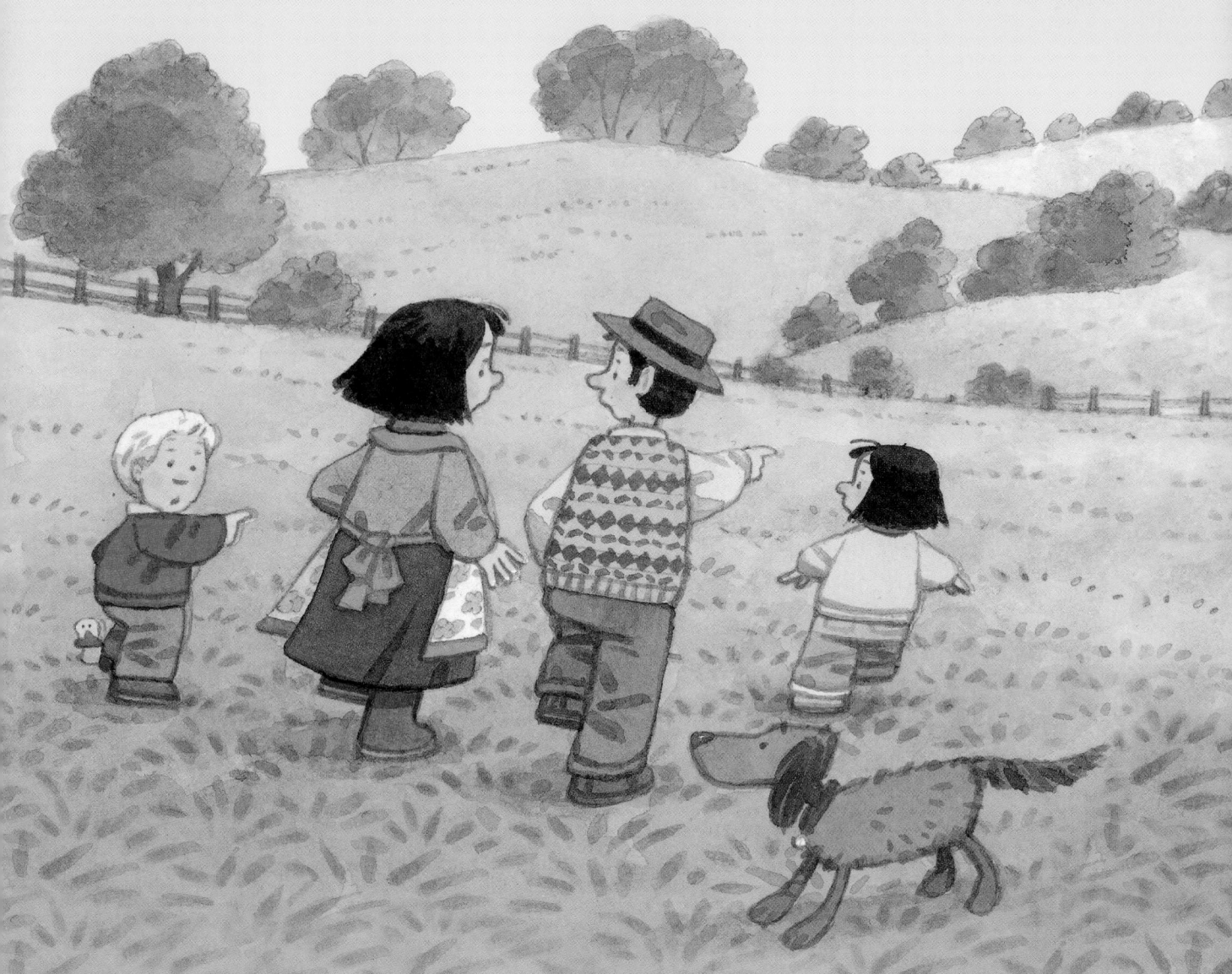

"Poppy and Sam can come too," says Mrs. Boot.
"And Rusty," says Sam. They walk across the fields.

Soon they come to the train track.

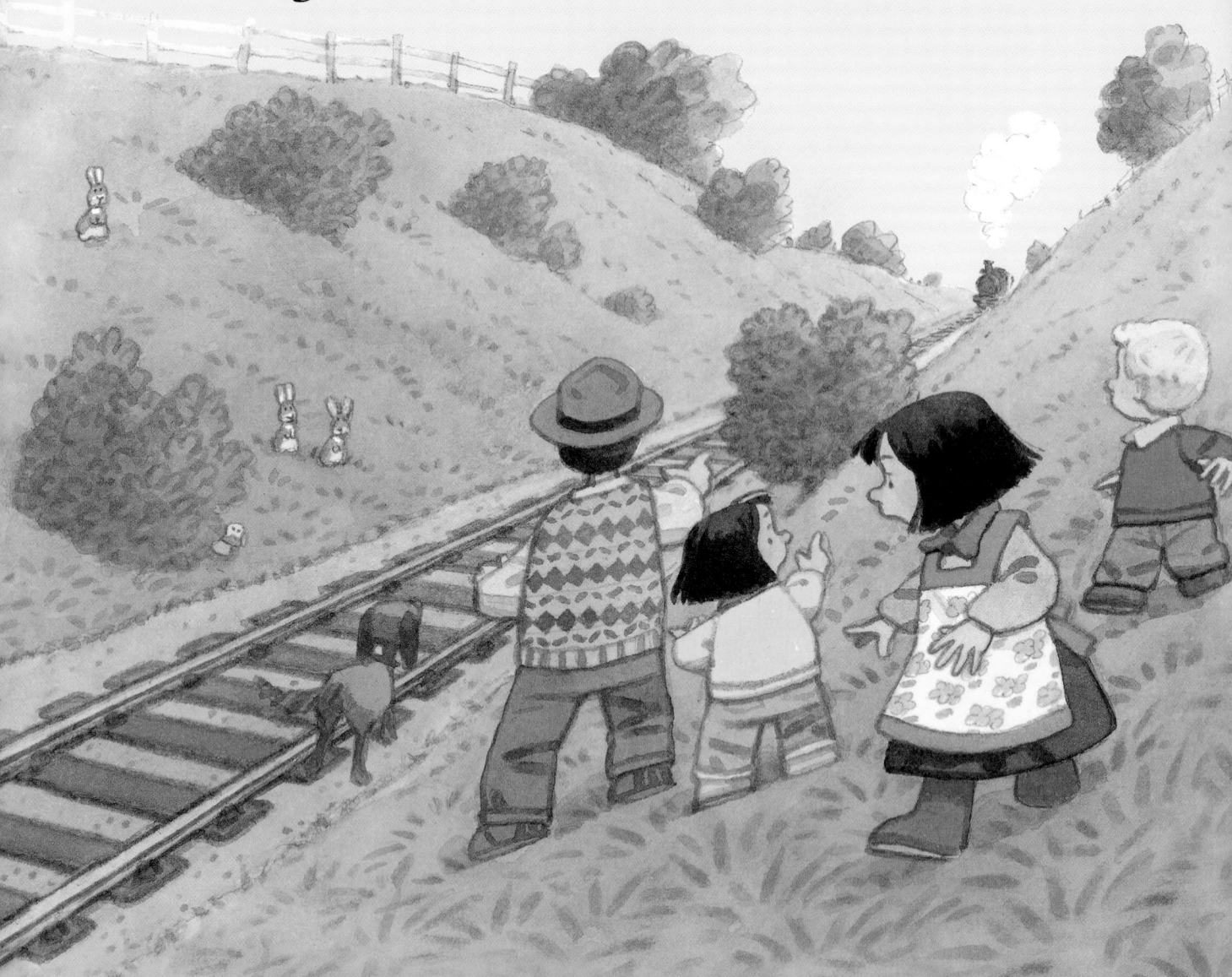

They can just see the old steam train. It has stopped but is still puffing and whistling.

"Look at those sheep."

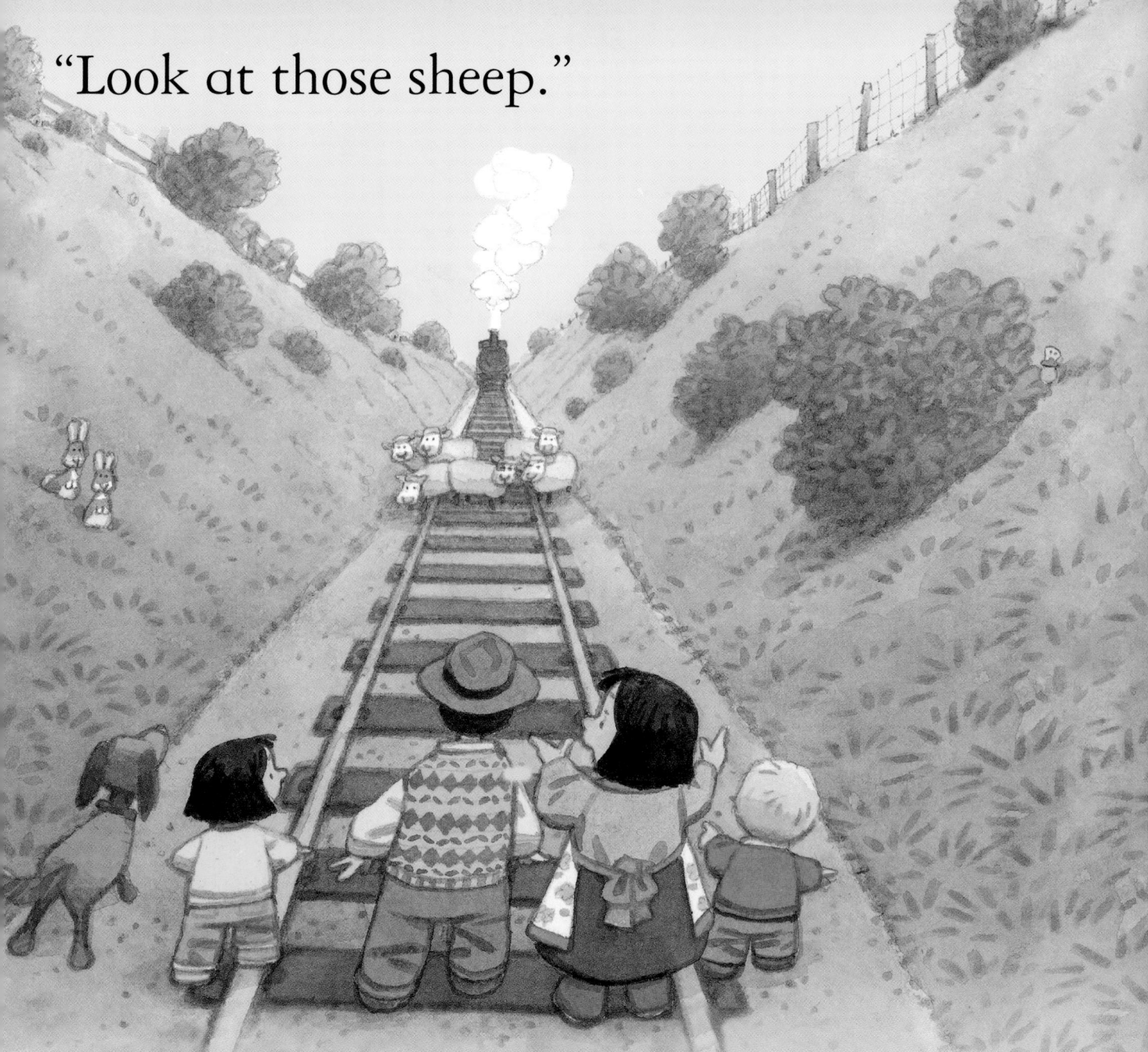

"They are on the track," says Poppy. "That's why the train has stopped." "Silly sheep," says Sam.

"It's that naughty Woolly."

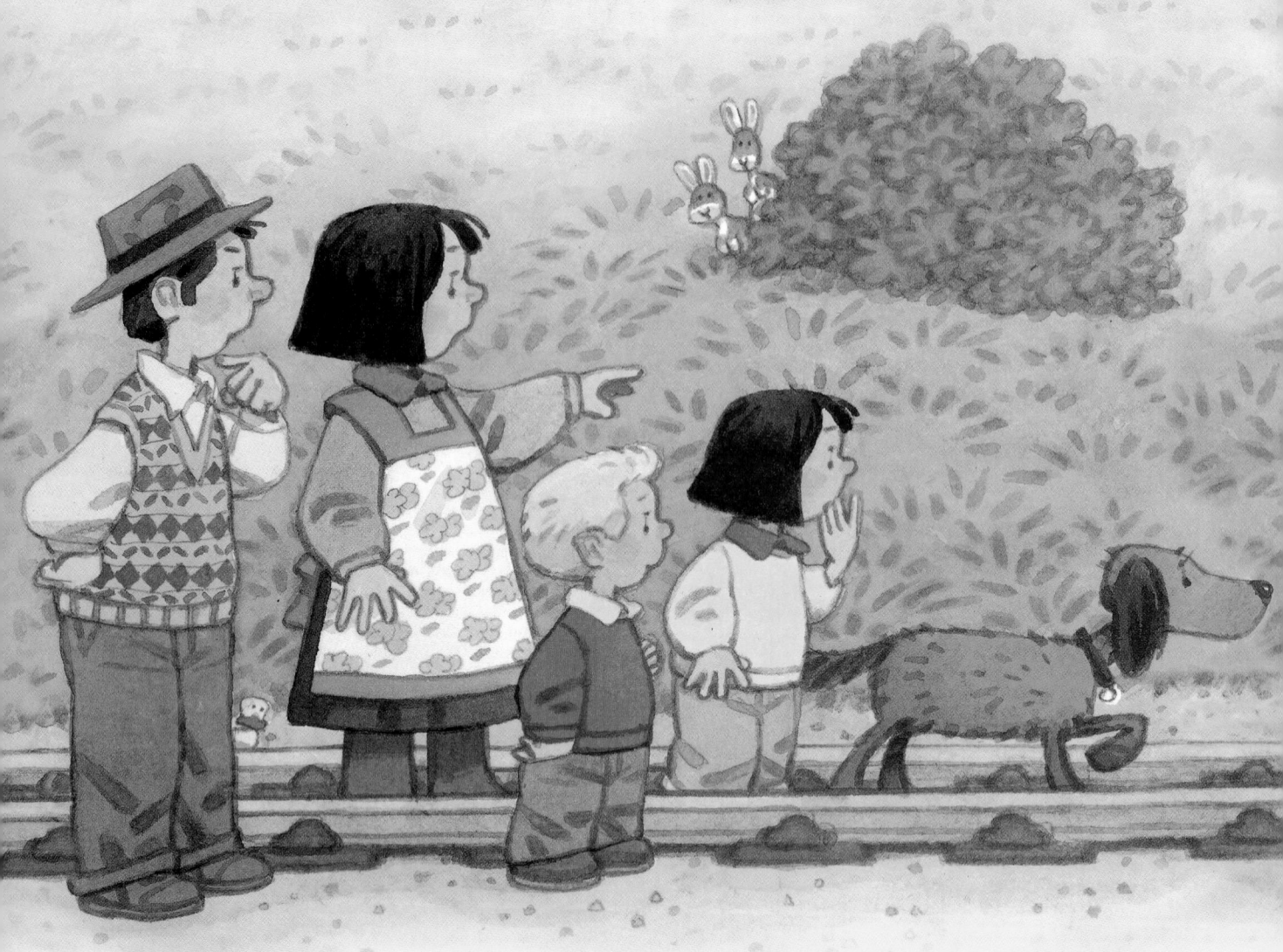

"She's escaped from her field again," says Poppy.
"She wanted to see the steam train," says Sam.

"We must move them."

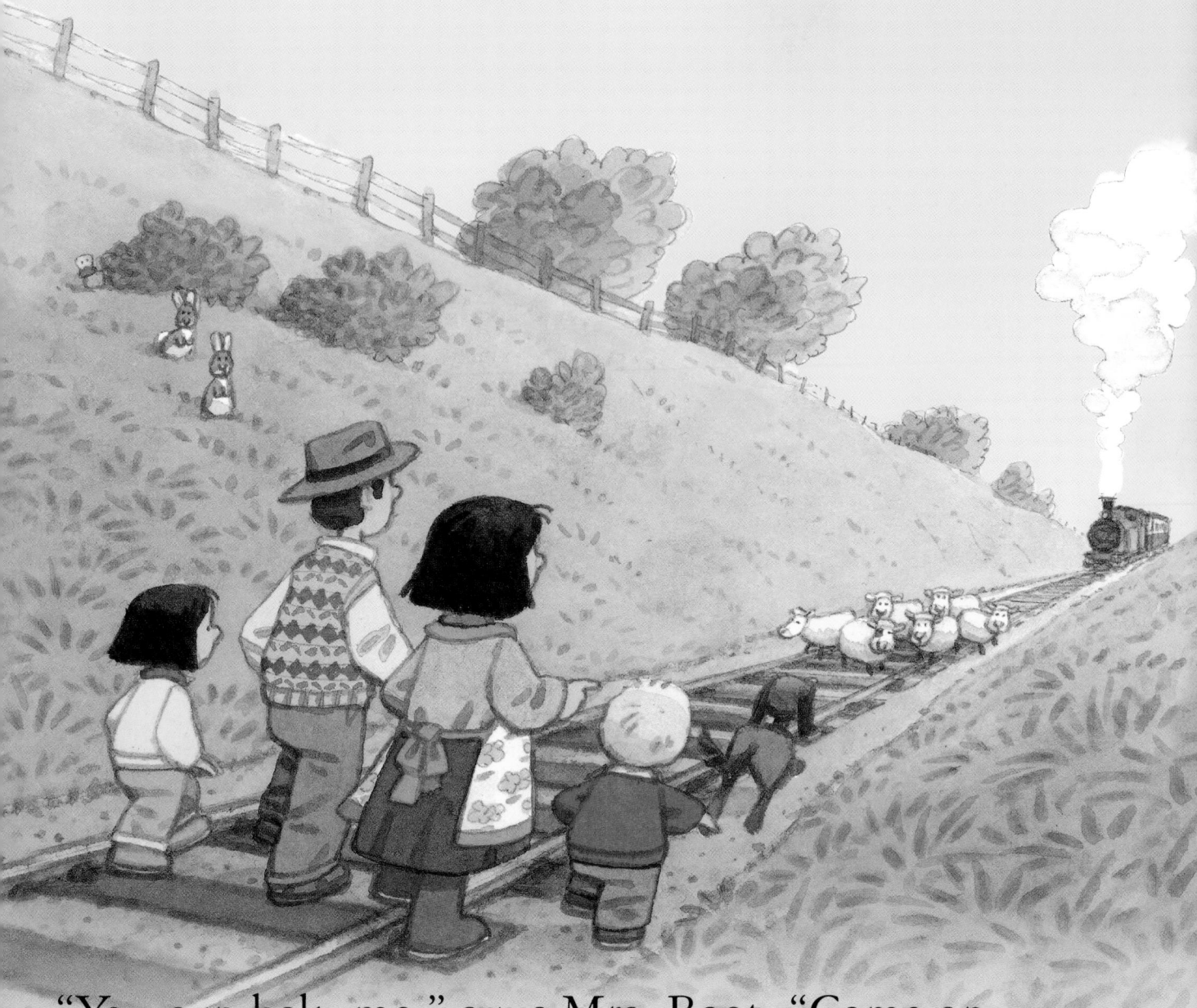

"You can help me," says Mrs. Boot. "Come on,
Rusty," says Sam. They walk up to the sheep.

"How can we get them home?"

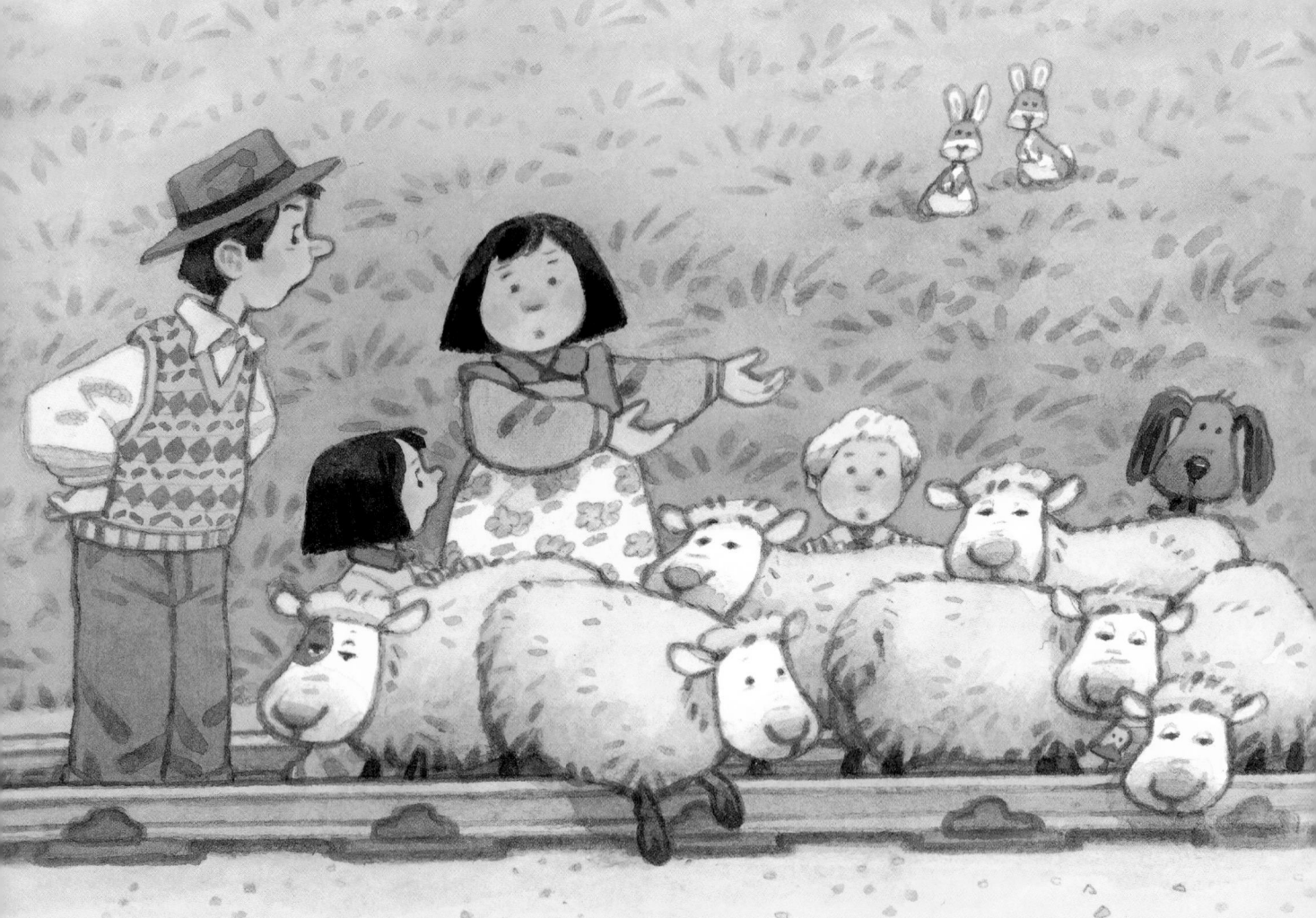

"We can't get them up the bank," says Ted.
"We'll put them on the train," says Mrs. Boot.

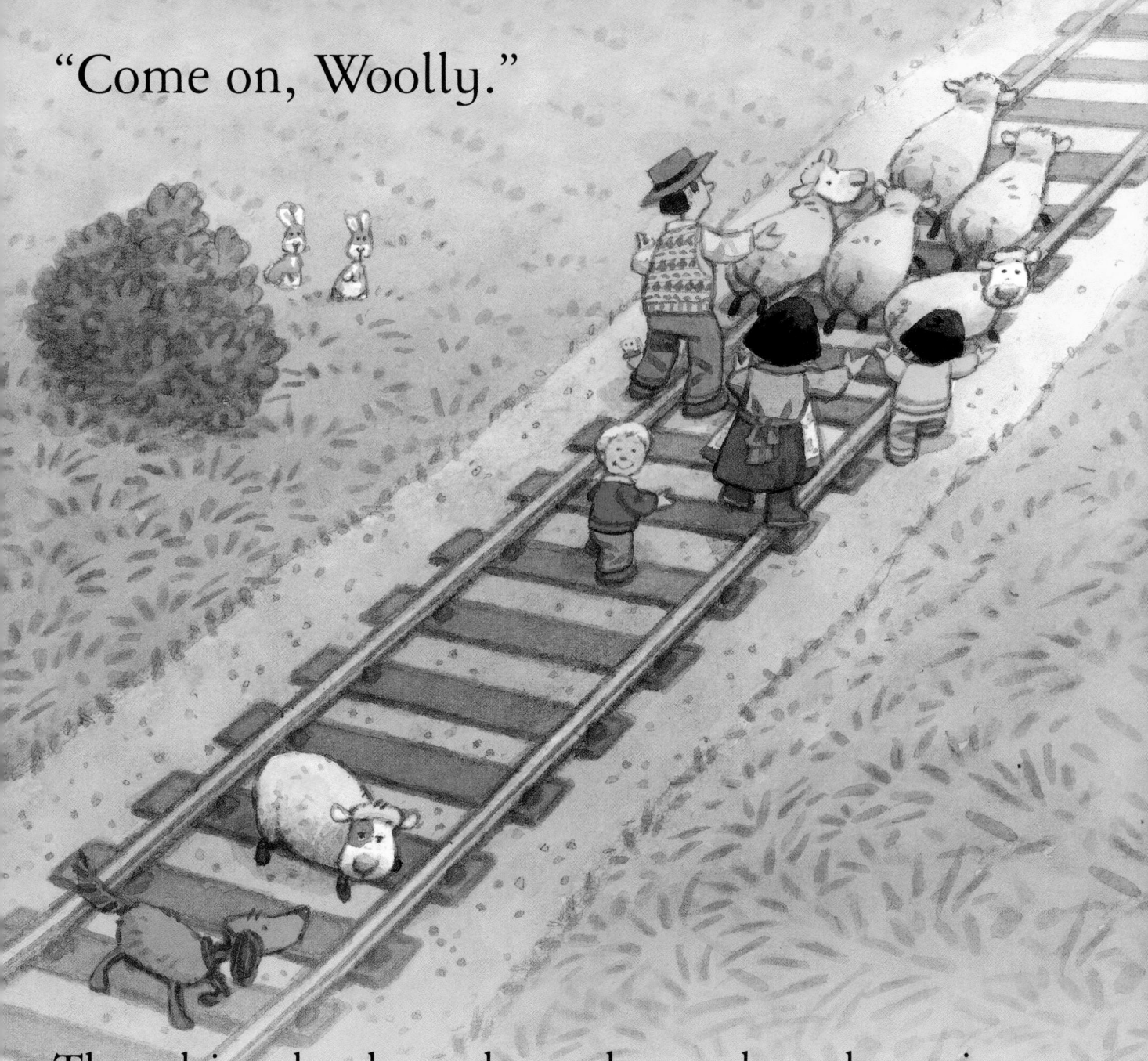

"Come on, Woolly."

They drive the sheep down the track to the train.
Woolly runs away but Rusty chases her back.

315

"We'll lift them up."

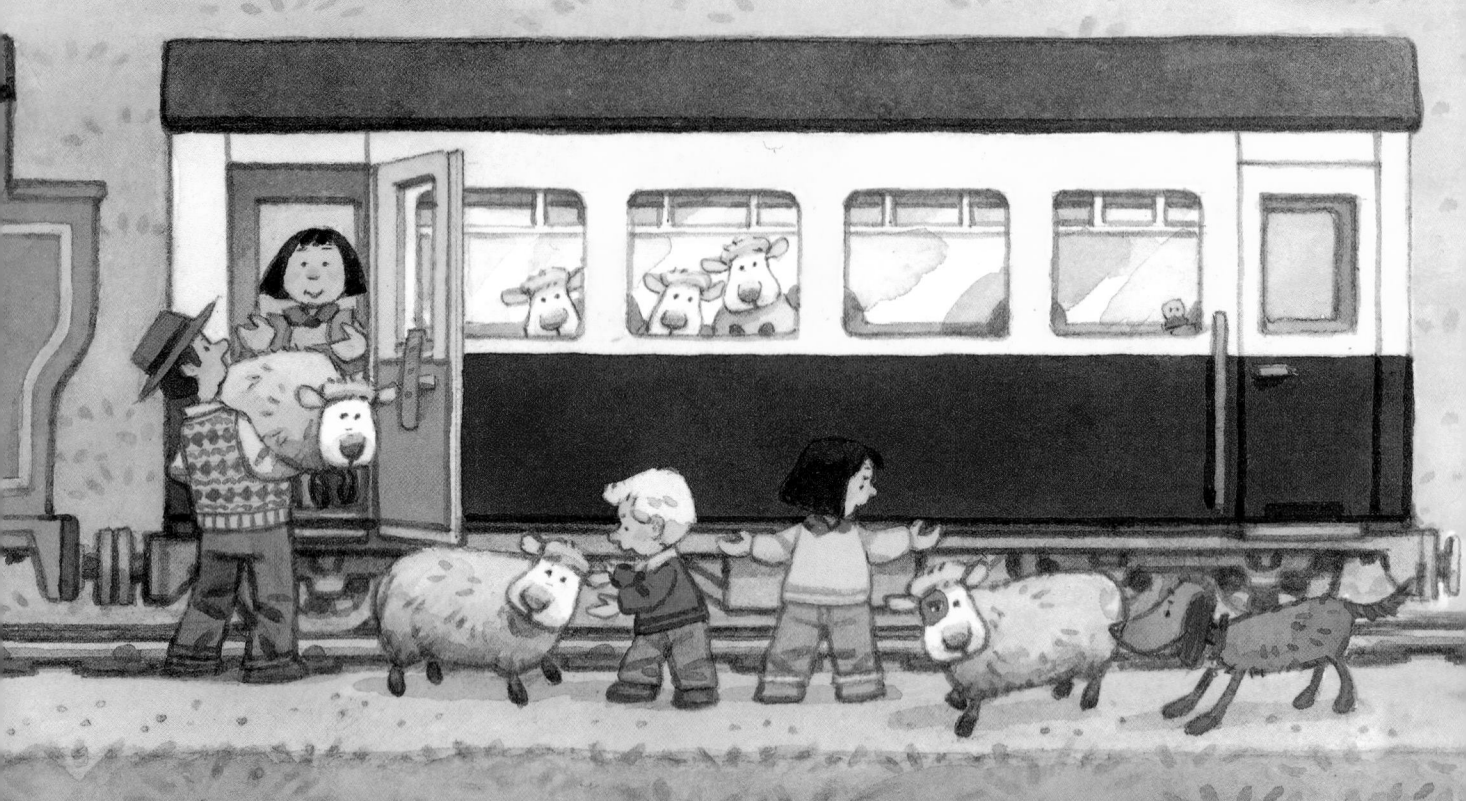

"Please help me, Ted," says Mrs. Boot. Ted and Mrs. Boot lift the sheep up into the carriage.

"All aboard!"

Poppy, Sam, Mrs. Boot, Ted and Rusty climb up
into the carriage. Mrs. Boot waves to the driver.

The train puffs along.

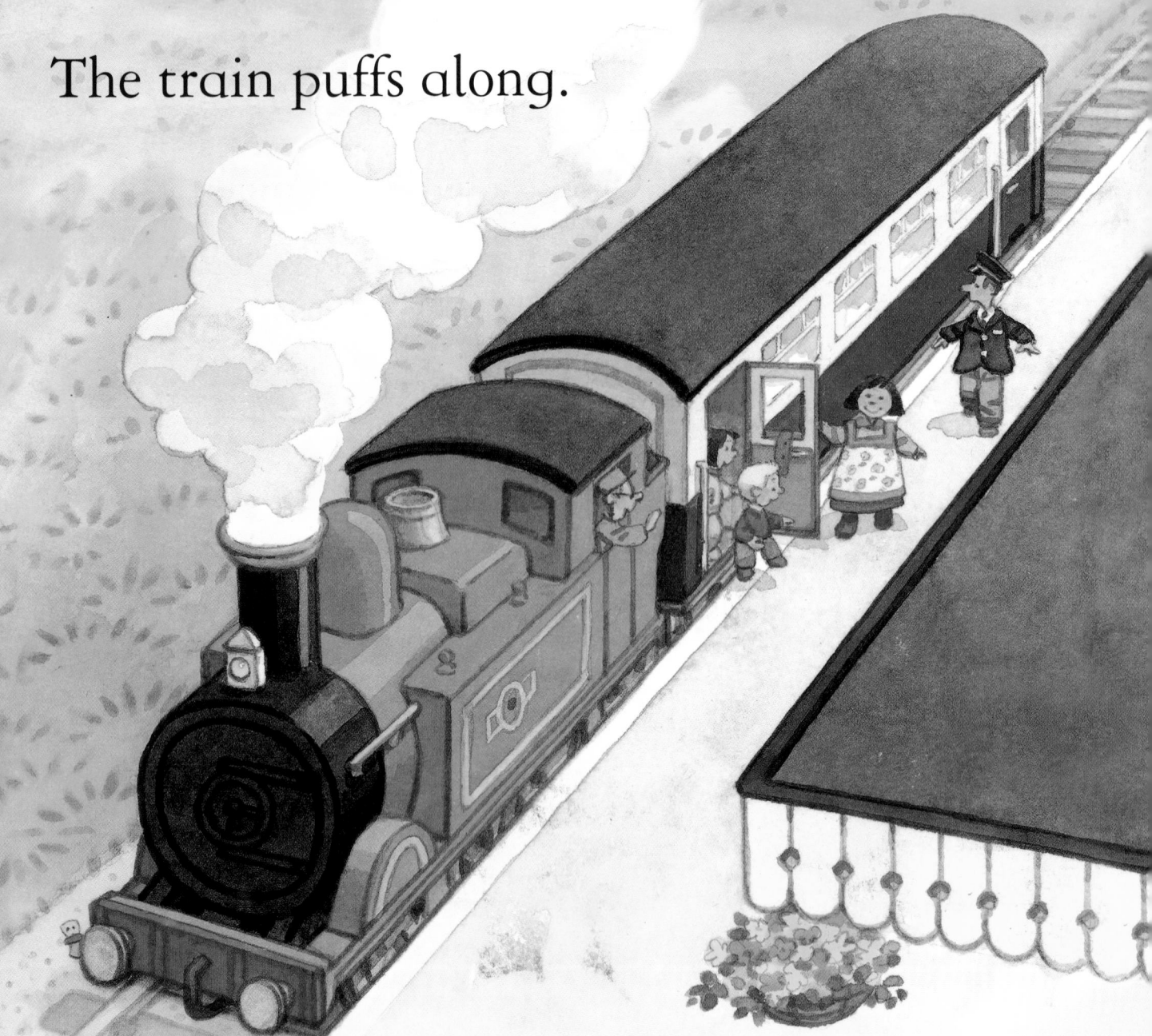

It stops at the station. Mrs. Boot opens the door.
Poppy and Sam jump down onto the platform.

"How many passengers?" says the guard.

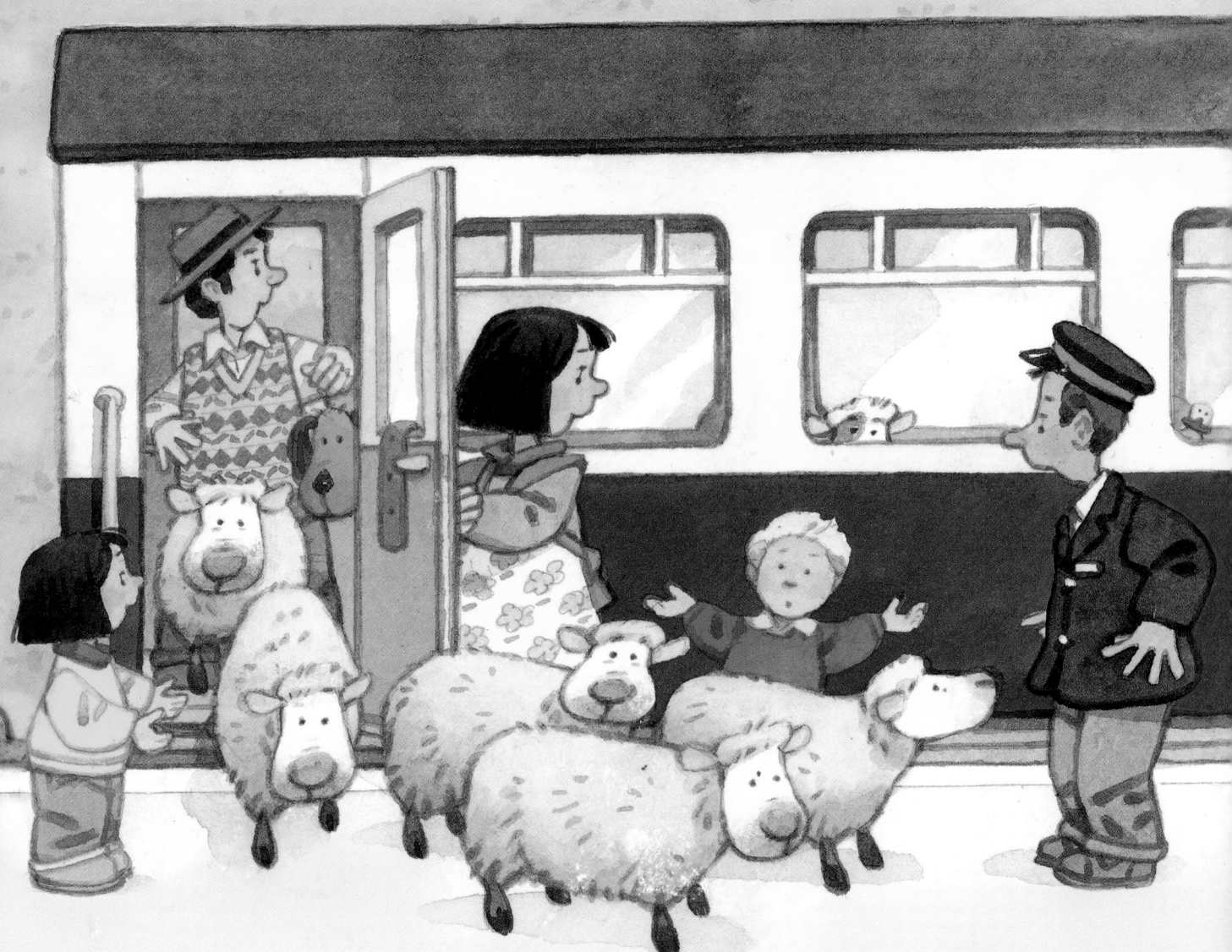

"Six sheep, one dog and four people," says Mrs. Boot.
"That's all."

"Let's all go home now," says Mrs. Boot.

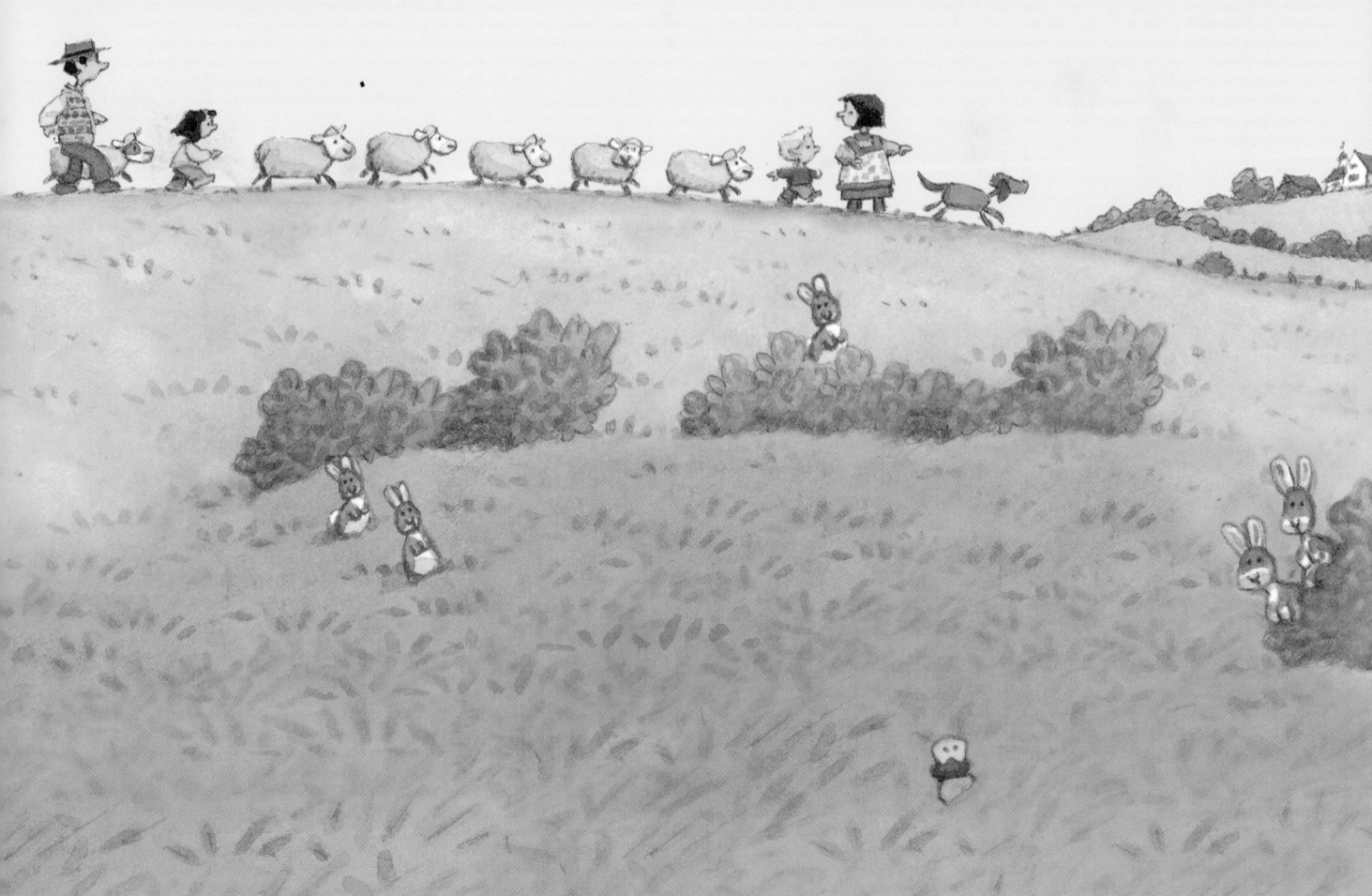

They take the sheep back to the farm. "I think Woolly just wanted a ride on the train," says Sam.